# DISEASES/CONDITIONS AND ICD-9-CM CODES

| | |
|---|---|
| Abruptio placentae | 641.2** |
| Acne vulgaris | 706.1 |
| Acromegaly | 253.0 |
| Actinic keratosis | 702.0 |
| Acute bronchitis | 466.0 |
| Acute and chronic viral hepatitis | 070.9 |
| Acute diarrhea (NOS) | 787.91 |
| Acute leukemia (plain leukemia) | 208.0** |
| Acute myocardial infarction | 410.9** |
| Acute otitis media | 382.9 |
| Acute pancreatitis | 577.0 |
| Acute peripheral facial paralysis (Bell's palsy) | 351.0 |
| Acute renal failure | 584.9 |
| Acute respiratory failure | 518.81 |
| Acute stress disorder | 308.9 |
| Adrenocortical insufficiency | 255.4 |
| Adverse reactions to blood transfusions | 999 |
| Alcoholism | 303.9** |
| Allergic reactions to drugs | 995.2 |
| Allergic reactions to insect stings | 989.5 |
| Allergic rhinitis | 477.8 |
| Alopecia areata | 704.01 |
| Alzheimer's disease | 331.0 |
| Amebiasis | 006.9 |
| Amenorrhea | 626.0 |
| Anal fissure, | 565.0 |
| Anaphylaxis, NOS | 995.0 |
| Angina pectoris | 413.9 |
| Angioedema | 995.1 |
| Ankle fracture | 824.8 |
| Ankylosing spondylitis | 720.0 |
| Anorectal abscess | 566. |
| Anorexia nervosa | 307.1 |
| Aortic aneurysm and dissection | 441.00 |
| Aplastic anemia | 284.9 |
| Asthma | 493.9** |
| Atelectasis | 518.0 |
| Atopic dermatitis | 691.8 |
| Atopic fibrillation | 427.31 |
| Attention deficit/hyperactivity disorder | 314.01 |
| Autoimmune hemolytic anemia | 283.0 |
| Bacterial meningitis | 320 |
| Bacterial pneumonia | 482.9 |
| Bacterial vaginitis | 616.1 |
| Benign prostatic hyperplasia | 600 |
| Blastomycosis | 116.0 |
| Bleeding esophageal varices | 456.0 |
| Brain abscess | 324. |
| Brain tumors | 239.6 |
| Breast cancer | 174 |
| Brucellosis | 023 |
| Bulimia nervosa | 307.51 |
| Bullous diseases | 694 |
| Burns | 940-949 |
| Bursitis | 726-727 |
| Cancer of the endometrium | 182.0 |
| Cancer of the skin | 172-173 |
| Cancer of the uterine cervix | 180 |
| Cardiac arrest, sudden cardiac death | 427.5 |
| Care after myocardial infarction | 414.8 |
| Cellulitis | 682. |
| Chancroid | 099.3 |
| Chlamydia trachomatis infection | 079.88 |
| Cholelithiasis and cholecystitis | 574.1-574.9 |
| Cholera | 001 |
| Chronic fatigue syndrome | 780.71 |
| Chronic leukemia | 208.1** |
| Chronic obstructive pulmonary disease | 491.2** |
| Chronic pancreatitis | 577.1 |
| Chronic renal failure | 585 |
| Chronic serous otitis media | 381.1** |
| Coccidioidomycosis | 114* |
| Colorectal cancer | 153 |
| Concussion | 850 |
| Congenital heart disease | 745-747 |
| Congenital rubella | 771.0 |
| Congestive heart failure | 428.0 |
| Conjunctivitis, acute | 372.0** |
| Connective tissue disease | 710* |
| Constipation | 564.0 |
| Contact dermatitis | 692 |
| Cough | 786.2 |
| Cushing's syndrome | 255.0 |
| Delirium | 780.0 |
| Dementia, multi-infarct, uncomplicated | 294.8 |
| Depression psychosis | 298.0 |
| Depression with anxiety | 300.4 |
| Diabetes insipidus | 253.5 |
| Diabetes mellitus, I | 250.01 |
| Diabetes mellitus, II | 250.02 |
| Diabetic ketoacidosis | 276.2** |
| Diphtheria | 032* |
| Diseases of the mouth | 528* |
| Disseminated intravascular coagulation | 286.6 |
| Diverticulitis | 562.11 |
| Drug abuse (nondependent) | 305.9** |
| Dysfunctional uterine bleeding | 626.6 |
| Dysmenorrhea | 635.5 |
| Dysphagia and esophageal obstruction | 530.3 |
| Ectopic pregnancy | 633* |
| Elbow dislocation | 832.0** |
| Encephalitis | 323* |
| Endometriosis | 617* |
| Enuresis | 786.30 |
| Epididymitis | 604** |
| Episodic vertigo | 386.11 |
| Erythema multiforme | 695.1 |
| Fetal lung immaturity | 770.4 |
| Fever | 780.6 |
| Fibrocystic diseases of the breast | 610.1 |
| Fibromyositis | 729.1 |
| Fifth disease | 057.0 |
| Finger dislocation, closed | 834.0** |
| Finger fracture | 816.0** |
| Fistula (anal) | 565.1 |
| Fitting of diaphragm | V25.02 |
| Folliculitis | 704.8 |
| Food allergy | 693.1 |
| Food poisoning | 005* |
| Foot fracture | 825.2** |
| Frostbite | 991* |
| Gangrene | 785.4 |
| Gastritis | 535** |
| Gastroesophageal reflux disease (GERD) | 530.81 |
| Generalized anxiety disorder | 300.02 |
| Generalized epilepsy | 345.1** |
| Genital warts (condylomata acuminata) | 078.11 |
| Giant cell arteritis | 446.5 |
| Giardiasis | 7.1 |
| Gilles de la Tourette syndrome | 307.23 |
| Glaucoma | 365** |
| Gonorrhea | 098.0 |
| Gout | 274.9 |
| Granuloma inguinale (donovanosis) | 099.2 |
| Guillain-Barré syndrome | 357.0 |
| Headache | 784.0 |
| Heart block | 426.1** |
| Heat exhaustion | 992.3 |
| Heat stroke | 992.0 |
| Hemochromatosis | 285.0 |
| Hemolytic disease of the fetus and newborn | 773.2 |
| Hemophilia and related conditions | 286.0 |
| Hemorrhoids | 455.6 |
| Herpes gestationis | 646.8** |
| Herpes simplex | 054* |
| Herpes zoster | 053* |
| Hiccups | 786.8 |
| High-altitude sickness | 993.2 |
| Histoplasmosis | 115** |
| HIV-associated infections | 042.0 |
| HIV infection, asymptomatic | V08 |
| HIV infection, early symptomatic | 042 |
| HIV infection, late symptomatic | 042 |
| Hyperlipoproteinemias | 272* |
| Hyperparathyroidism | 252.0 |
| Hyperprolactinemia | 253.1 |
| Hypersensitivity pneumonitis | 495 |
| Hypertension (essential) | 401* |
| Hyperthyroidism | 242** |
| Hypertrophic cardiomyopathy | 425.4 |
| Hypoparathyroidism | 252.1 |
| Hypothyroidism | 244* |
| Immunization practices | V03, VO4, VO5, VO6** |
| Impetigo | 684 |
| Impotence | 302.72 |
| Indigestion | 536.8 |
| Infectious diarrhea | 009.2 |
| Infectious mononucleosis | 075 |
| Infective endocarditis | 424.9** |
| Influenza | 487.2 |
| Ingrowing nail | 703.0 |
| Insect and spider bite | 989.5 |
| Insertion of intrauterine device | V25.1 |
| Insomnia (NOS) | 780.52 |

# DISEASES/CONDITIONS AND ICD-9-CM CODES (Continued)

| | |
|---|---|
| Intracerebral hemorrhage | 431 |
| Iron deficiency anemia | 280.0-280.9 |
| Irritable bowel syndrome | 564.1 |
| Jellyfish sting | 989.5 |
| Juvenile rheumatoid arthritis | 714.3** |
| Keloids | 701.4 |
| Laryngitis | 464.00 |
| Lead poisoning | 984* |
| Legionnaires' disease | 482.84 |
| Leishmaniasis | 085* |
| Leprosy | 030* |
| Lichen planus | 697.0 |
| Low back pain | 724.2 |
| Lyme disease | 088.81 |
| Lymphogranuloma venereum | 099.1 |
| Malabsorption | 579* |
| Malaria | 084.6 |
| Measles (rubeola) | 055.9 |
| Meconium aspiration | 770.1 |
| Melanoma, malignant | 172* |
| Ménière's disease | 386.0** |
| Meningitis | 320-322 |
| Menopausal | 627.2 |
| Migraine headache | 346** |
| Mitral valve prolapse | 424.0 |
| Monilial vulvovaginitis | 121.1 |
| Multiple myeloma | 203.0** |
| Multiple sclerosis | 340 |
| Mumps | 072.9 |
| Myasthenia gravis | 358.0** |
| Mycoplasmal pneumonias | 483.0 |
| Mycosis fungoides | 202.1** |
| Nausea and vomiting | 787.01 |
| Neoplasm of the vulva | 239.5 |
| Neutropenia | 288.0 |
| Nevi | 216* |
| Newborn physiologic jaundice | 774.6 |
| Nongonococcal urethritis | 099.4** |
| Non-Hodgkin's lymphomas | 202.8** |
| Non-autoimmune hemolytic anemia | 283.1** |
| Normal delivery | 650 |
| Obesity | 278.0** |
| Obsessive-compulsive disorders | 300.3 |
| Onychomycosis | 110.1 |
| Optic neuritis | 377.3** |
| Osteoarthritis | 715** |
| Osteomyelitis | 730** |
| Osteoporosis | 733.00 |
| Otitis externa | 380.10 |
| Paget's disease of bone | 731.0 |
| Panic disorder | 300.01 |
| Pap smear | V72.3 |
| Parkinsonism | 332.0 |
| Paronychia | 681.0** |
| Partial epilepsy | 345.4** |
| Patent ductus arteriosus | 747.0 |
| Pediculosis | 132* |
| Pelvic inflammatory disease | 614* |
| Peptic ulcer disease | 533* |
| Pericarditis | 432.9 |
| Peripheral arterial disease | 443.9 |
| Peripheral neuropathies | 356* |
| Pernicious anemia | 281.0 |
| Personality disorder | 301** |
| Pheochromocytoma | 227.0 |
| Phobia | 300.2** |
| Pigmentary disorders—vitiligo | 709.01 |
| Pinworms | 127.4 |
| Pityriasis rosea | 696.3 |
| Placenta previa | 641** |
| Plague | 020* |
| Platelet-mediated bleeding disorders | 287.1 |
| Pleural effusion | 511.9 |
| Polycythemia vera | 238.4 |
| Polymyalgia rheumatica | 725 |
| Porphyria | 277.1 |
| Postpartum hemorrhage | 666.1** |
| Post-traumatic stress disorder | 309.81 |
| Pregnancy | V22.2 |
| Pregnancy-induced hypertension | 642** |
| Premature beats | 427.6** |
| Premenstrual tension syndrome (PMS) | 625.4 |
| Prescribed oral contraceptive | V25.01 |
| Pressure ulcers | 707.0 |
| Preterm labor | 644.2** |
| Primary glomerular disease | 581-583 |
| Primary lung abscess | 513.0 |
| Primary lung cancer | 162.9 |
| Prostate cancer | 185 |
| Prostatitis | 601* |
| Pruritus | 698.9 |
| Pruritus ani | 698.0 |
| Pruritus vulvae | 698.1 |
| Psittacosis (ornithosis) | 073* |
| Psoriasis | 696.1 |
| Pulmonary embolism | 415.1 |
| Pyelonephritis | 590** |
| Q fever | 083.0 |
| Rabies | 071 |
| Rat-bite fever | 026* |
| Relapsing fever | 087* |
| Renal calculi | 592 |
| Reye syndrome | 331.81 |
| Rheumatic fever | 390 |
| Rheumatoid arthritis | 714.0 |
| Rib fracture | 807.0** |
| Rocky Mountain spotted fever | 082.0 |
| Rosacea | 695.3 |
| Roseola | 057.8 |
| Rubella | 056* |
| Salmonellosis | 003.0 |
| Sarcoidosis | 135 |
| Scabies | 133.0 |
| Schizophrenia | 295** |
| Seborrheic dermatitis | 690.1** |
| Septicemia | 038* |
| Sézary's syndrome | 202.2** |
| Shoulder dislocation | 831.0** |
| Sickle cell anemia | 282.6** |
| Silicosis | 502 |
| Sinusitis, chronic | 473* |
| Skull fracture | 800, 801, 803 |
| Sleep apnea | 780.57 |
| Sleep disorders | 780.50 |
| Snakebite | 989.5 |
| Stasis ulcers | 454.0 |
| Status epilepticus | 345.3 |
| Stomach cancer | 151* |
| Streptococcal pharyngitis | 034.0 |
| Stroke | 436 |
| *Strongyloides* infection | 127.2 |
| Subdural or subarachnoid hemorrhage | 852** |
| Sunburn | 692.71 |
| Syphilis | 090-097 |
| Tachycardias | 785.0 |
| Tapeworm infections | 123* |
| Telogen effluvium | 704.02 |
| Temporomandibular joint syndrome | 524.6** |
| Tendonitis | 726.90 |
| Tetanus | 037 |
| Thalassemia | 282.4** |
| Therapeutic use of blood components | V59.0** |
| Thrombotic thrombocytopenic purpura | 446.6 |
| Thyroid cancer | 193 |
| Thyroiditis | 245* |
| Tinea capitis | 110.0 |
| Tinnitus | 388.3** |
| Toe fracture | 826.0 |
| Toxic shock syndrome | 040.82 |
| Toxoplasmosis | 130* |
| Transient cerebral ischemia | 435* |
| Trauma to the genitourinary tract | 958,959 |
| Trichinellosis | 124 |
| Trichomonal vaginitis | 131.01 |
| Trigeminal neuralgia | 350.1 |
| Tuberculosis, pulmonary | 011** |
| Tularemia | 021* |
| Typhoid fever | 002.0 |
| Typhus fevers | 080, 081 |
| Ulcerative colitis | 556* |
| Urethral stricture | 598* |
| Urinary incontinence | 788.30 |
| Urticaria | 708* |
| Uterine inertia | 661.0** |
| Uterine leiomyoma | 218* |
| Varicella | 052* |
| Venous thrombosis | 453.8 |
| Viral pneumonia | 480.9 |
| Viral respiratory infections | 465.9 |
| Vitamin deficiency | 264-269 |
| Vitamin K deficiency | 269.0 |
| Warts (verrucae) | 078.10 |
| Wegener's granulomatosis | 446.4 |
| Whooping cough (pertussis) | 033* |
| Wrist fracture | 814.0** |

*4th digit needed
**5th (or 4th and 5th) digit needed

# CONN'S
# Current Therapy 2008

# CONN'S
# Current
# Therapy
## 2008

**Robert E. Rakel, MD**
Professor, Department of Family and
    Community Medicine
Baylor College of Medicine
Houston, Texas

**Edward T. Bope, MD**
Director, Riverside Family Practice Residency Program
Clinical Professor, Department of Family Medicine
The Ohio State University College of Medicine
Columbus, Ohio

LATEST APPROVED METHODS
OF TREATMENT FOR
THE PRACTICING PHYSICIAN

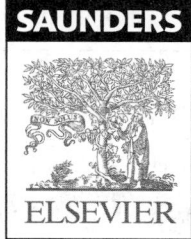

SAUNDERS

ELSEVIER

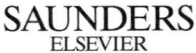

1600 John F. Kennedy Blvd.
Ste 1800
Philadelphia, PA 19103-2899

CONN'S CURRENT THERAPY 2008        ISBN: 978-1-4160-4435-2

---

**Notice**

Knowledge and best practice in this field are constantly changing. As new research and experience broaden our knowledge, changes in practice, treatment, and drug therapy may become necessary or appropriate. Readers are advised to check the most current information provided (i) on procedures featured or (ii) by the manufacturer of each product to be administered, to verify the recommended dose or formula, the method and duration of administration, and contraindications. It is the responsibility of the practitioner, relying on his or her experience and knowledge of the patient, to make diagnoses, to determine dosages and the best treatment for each individual patient, and to take all appropriate safety precautions. To the fullest extent of the law, neither the Publisher nor the Editors assume any liability for any injury and/or damage to persons or property arising out of or related to any use of the material contained in this book.

The Publisher

---

**Library of Congress Cataloging-in-Publication Data**
Current therapy; latest approved methods of treatment for the practicing physician.
Editors: H. F. Conn and others
   v. 28 cm. annual
     ISBN 978-1-4160-4435-2
   1. Therapeutics.    2. Therapeutics, Surgical.    3. Medicine—Practice.
   I. Conn, Howard Franklin, 1908–1982 ed.

   RM101.C87 616.058 49–8328 rev*

*Acquisitions Editor:* Druanne Martin
*Developmental Editor:* Lucia Gunzel
*Publishing Services Manager:* Frank Polizzano
*Project Manager:* Jeff Gunning
*Design Direction:* Steve Stave

Printed in the United States of America

Last digit is the print number:  9  8  7  6  5  4  3  2  1

# Contributors

**Charles S. Abrams, MD**
Associate Professor of Medicine, University of Pennsylvania School of Medicine; Staff Physician, Division of Hematology-Oncology, Hospital of the University of Pennsylvania, Philadelphia, Pennsylvania
*Platelet-Mediated Bleeding Disorders*

**Mark J. Abzug, MD**
Professor of Pediatrics (Infectious Diseases), University of Colorado School of Medicine; Staff Pediatrician, The Children's Hospital, Denver, Colorado
*Viral Meningitis and Encephalitis*

**Suraj Achar, MD**
Assistant Clinical Professor, Department of Family and Preventive Medicine, and Associate Director, Sports Medicine Fellowship, University of California, San Diego, School of Medicine, La Jolla; Staff Physician, UCSD Thornton Hospital, La Jolla, and UCSD Medical Center, Hillcrest, California
*Common Sports Injuries*

**Sujeet S. Acharya, MD**
Resident Physician, The University of Chicago Medical Center, Chicago, Illinois
*Renal Calculi*

**Tod C. Aeby, MD**
Residency Program Director, Department of Obstetrics, Gynecology, and Women's Health, University of Hawaii John A. Burns School of Medicine, Honolulu, Hawaii
*Uterine Leiomyomas*

**Carl M. Allen, DDS, MSD**
Professor, Department of Oral Pathology, The Ohio State University College of Dentistry; Director, Oral & Maxillofacial Surgery and Pathology, University Hospital; Professor, Department of Pathology, The Ohio State University College of Medicine and Public Health, Columbus, Ohio
*Diseases of the Mouth*

**Antonio Almeida, MD**
Assistant Professor, Universidade Nova de Lisboa School of Medicine; Consultant Hematologist, Instituto Portugês de Oncologia, Lisbon, Portugal
*Sickle Cell Disease*

**Tina S. Alster, MD**
Clinical Professor of Dermatology, Georgetown University School of Medicine; Director, Washington Institute of Dermatologic Laser Surgery, Washington, DC
*Keloids*

**Navin M. Amin, MD**
Professor of Family Medicine, University of California, Irvine, School of Medicine, Irvine; Associate Professor of Medicine, David Geffen School of Medicine at UCLA, Los Angeles; and Associate Professor of Medicine, Stanford University School of Medicine, Stanford, California
*Infective Endocarditis*

**Girish Anand, MD**
Fellow in Gastroenterology, Albert Einstein Medical Center, Philadelphia, Pennsylvania
*Dysphagia and Esophageal Obstruction*

**Deverick J. Anderson, MD**
Clinical Associate, Duke University Medical Center, Durham, North Carolina
*Rickettsial and Ehrlichial Infections*

**Vinicius C. S. Antao, MD, MSc, PhD**
Adjunct Assistant Professor, Community Medicine Department, West Virginia University College of Medicine, Morgantown, West Virginia
*Silicosis and Asbestosis*

**Karim Aoun, MD**
Associate Professor, University of Tunis Faculty of Medicine; Attending Physician, Pasteur Institute of Tunis, Tunisia, Tunisia
*Leishmaniasis*

**Baha M. Arafah, MD**
Professor of Medicine, Case Western Reserve University School of Medicine; Attending Physician, Division of Endocrinology, University Hospitals/Case Medical Center, Cleveland, Ohio
*Hyperprolactinemia*

**Paul M. Arguin, MD**
Captain, U.S. Public Health Service; Chief, Domestic Malaria Unit, Centers for Disease Control and Prevention, Atlanta, Georgia
*Malaria*

**Aydin Arici, MD**
Professor of Obstetrics and Gynecology, Yale University School of Medicine, New Haven, Connecticut
*Dysfunctional Uterine Bleeding*

**Isao Arita, MD**
Chairman, Agency for Cooperation in International Health, Kumamoto, Kumamoto City, Japan
*Smallpox*

**Noel A. Armenakas, MD**
Clinical Associate Professor, Department of Urology, Cornell Weill Medical School; Attending Surgeon, Lenox Hill Hospital and New York–Presbyterian Hospital, New York, New York
*Trauma to the Genitourinary Tract*

**Ramesh Ayyala, MD**
Associate Professor; Director, Residency Program in Ophthalmology; and Director, Glaucoma Service, Department of Ophthalmology, Tulane University School of Medicine, New Orleans, Louisiana
*Conjunctivitis*

**Claus Bachert, MD, PhD**
Professor, University of Ghent Faculty of Medicine; Chief of Clinics, Ear-Nose-Throat Department, University Hospital of Ghent, Ghent, Belgium
*Nonallergic Perennial Rhinitis*

**Gopal H. Badlani, MD**
Vice Chairman, Department of Urology, Long Island Jewish Medical Center, New Hyde Park, New York
*Benign Prostatic Hyperplasia*

**Adrianne Williams Bagley, MD**
Clinical Associate Professor, Johns Hopkins University School of Medicine; Associate Staff, Johns Hopkins Hospital, Baltimore, Maryland
*Pelvic Inflammatory Disease*

**David A. Baker, MD**
Professor, Department of Obstetrics, Gynecology, and Reproductive Medicine, State University of New York at Stony Brook Health Sciences Center School of Medicine, Stony Brook, New York
*Vulvovaginitis*

**David M. Bamberger, MD**
Professor of Medicine and Vice-Chair of Educational Affairs, Department of Medicine, University of Missouri–Kansas City School of Medicine; Chief, Infectious Diseases Section, Truman Medical Center, Kansas City, Missouri
*Gonorrhea*

**Raymond L. Barnhill, MD**
Clinical Professor of Dermatology and Pathology, University of Miami Miller School of Medicine, Miami; Staff Pathologist, University of Miami Medical Group and Sylvester Comprehensive Cancer Center, Coral Gables, Florida
*Nevi*

**James C. Barton, MD**
Clinical Professor, Department of Medicine, University of Alabama at Birmingham School of Medicine; Medical Director, Southern Iron Disorders Center, Birmingham, Alabama
*Iron Deficiency*

**Nurcan Baykam, MD**
Associate Professor of Infectious Diseases, University of Ankara Faculty of Medicine; Staff, Infectious Diseases and Clinical Microbiology Clinic, Ankara Numune Education and Research Hospital, Ankara, Turkey
*Brucellosis*

**Carolyn E. Beck, MD, MSc**
Assistant Professor, University of Toronto Faculty of Medicine; Staff Paediatrician, Division of Paediatric Medicine, The Hospital for Sick Children, Toronto, Ontario, Canada
*Parenteral Fluid Therapy for Infants and Children*

**Meg Begany, RD, CSP, LDN**
Clinical Neonatal Dietitian, The Children's Hospital of Philadelphia, Philadelphia, Pennsylvania
*Normal Infant Feeding*

**Jerome Belinson, MD**
Staff, Department of Obstetrics and Gynecology, Taussig Cancer Institute; Director, Gynecologic Oncology Fellowship Program, Cleveland Clinic, Cleveland, Ohio
*Ovarian Cancer*

**Nicholas P. Bell, MD**
Clinical Assistant Professor, Department of Ophthalmology and Visual Science, University of Texas Medical School at Houston, Houston, Texas
*Glaucoma*

**Pelayo C. Besa, MD**
Radiation Oncology Head, Santiago, Chile
*Hodgkin's Disease: Radiation Therapy*

**Karl R. Beutner, MD, PhD**
Associate Clinical Professor of Dermatology, University of California, San Francisco, School of Medicine, San Francisco, California
*Condyloma Acuminatum (Genital Warts)*

**Zulfiqar A. Bhutta, MB, BS, PhD**
Husein Lalji Dewraj Professor of Pediatrics, Aga Khan University and Medical Center, Karachi, Pakistan
*Typhoid Fever*

**Joseph Biederman, MD**
Professor of Psychiatry, Harvard Medical School; Chief of Clinical and Research in Pediatric Psychopharmacology, Massachusetts General Hospital, Boston, Massachusetts
*Attention Deficit Hyperactivity Disorder*

**John P. Bilezikian, MD**
Professor of Medicine and Pharmacology, Columbia University College of Physicians and Surgeons; Attending Physician, NewYork–Presbyterian Hospital, New York, New York
*Primary Hyperparathyroidism and Hypoparathyroidism*

**Warren P. Bishop, MD**
Professor of Pediatrics, University of Iowa Carver College of Medicine; Director, Division of Gastroenterology, University of Iowa Children's Hospital, Iowa City, Iowa
*Constipation*

**Soenke Boettger, MD**
Fellow, Memorial Sloan-Kettering Cancer Center, New York, New York
*Delirium*

**Jonathan Bond, MB, MRCPI**
Specialist Registrar in Hematology, The Adelaide and Meath Hospital, Dublin, Ireland
*Chronic Leukemias*

**Herbert L. Bonkovsky, MD**
Professor, University of Connecticut School of Medicine, Farmington, Connecticut; Professor, University of North Carolina College of Medicine; Vice President for Research, Carolinas Health Care System, Charlotte, North Carolina
*Porphyria*

**Patrick Borgen, MD**
Chief, Breast Service, Department of Surgery, Memorial Sloan-Kettering Cancer Center, New York, New York
*Diseases of the Breast*

**Harisios Boudoulas, MD, PhD**
Professor of Medicine and Pharmacy Emeritus, The Ohio State University College of Medicine and Public Health, Columbus, Ohio; Director, Center of Clinical Research, Academy of Athens, Athens, Greece
*Mitral Valve Prolapse: The Floppy Mitral Valve, Mitral Valve Prolapse, and Mitral Valvular Regurgitation*

**Aida Bouratbine, MD**
Professor, University of Tunis Faculty of Medicine; Head, Laboratory of Parasitology, Pasteur Institute of Tunis, Tunis, Tunisia
*Leishmaniasis*

**Krystene I. Boyle, MD**
Clinical Instructor, Department of Obstetrics and Gynecology, University of Cincinnati College of Medicine; Clinical Fellow, Department of OB/GYN, Division of Reproductive Endocrinology, University of Cincinnati Medical Center, Cincinnati, Ohio
*Menopause*

**Robert Bradsher, MD**
Richard V. Ebert Professor of Medicine, University of Arkansas College of Medicine; Program Director, Internal Medicine Residency and Infectious Diseases Fellowship Training Program; Vice-Chairman, Department of Internal Medicine; Director, Division of Infectious Diseases, University of Arkansas for Medical Sciences, Little Rock, Arkansas
*Blastomycosis*

**Daniel M. Brailita, MD**
Fellow in Gastroenterology, University of Texas Southwestern Medical Center, Dallas, Texas
*Acute and Chrunic Hepatitis*

**Marc Brand, MD**
Assistant Professor of Surgery, Rush Medical College; Attending Surgeon, Rush University Medical Center, Chicago, Illinois
*Tumors of the Rectum and Colon*

**Chad M. Braun, MD**
Assistant Professor, Department of Family Medicine, University of Illinois at Chicago College of Medicine, Chicago, Illinois
*Nausea and Vomiting*

**Mark E. Brecher, MD**
Professor and Vice Chair, Department of Pathology and Laboratory Medicine, University of North Carolina at Chapel Hill School of Medicine; Director, McLendon Clinical Laboratories, Chapel Hill, North Carolina
*Therapeutic Use of Blood Components*

**Patricia D. Brown, MD**
Associate Professor of Medicine, Division of Infectious Diseases, Wayne State University School of Medicine; Chief of Medicine, Detroit Receiving Hospital, Detroit, Michigan
*Pyelonephritis*

**J. James Bruno II, MD**
Lenox Hill Hospital, New York, New York
*Trauma to the Genitourinary Tract*

**John Brusch, MD**
Assistant Professor of Medicine, Harvard Medical School, Boston; Associate Chief of Medicine, Cambridge Health Alliance, Cambridge, Massachusetts
*Streptococcal Pharyngitis*

**Peter Buckley, MD**
Professor of Psychiatry, Medical College of Georgia; Staff Psychiatrist, MCG Medical Center, Augusta, Georgia
*Schizophrenia*

**Cathy L. Budman, MD**
Associate Professor of Psychiatry, New York University School of Medicine, New York; Director, Movement Disorders Program in Psychiatry, North Shore–Long Island Jewish Health System, Manhasset, New York
*Gilles de la Tourette Syndrome*

**Irina Burd, MD, PhD**
Instructor, Department of Obstetrics and Gynecology, University of Pennsylvania School of Medicine; Staff, Hospital of the University of Pennsylvania, Philadelphia, Pennsylvania
*Menopause*

**Kevin A. Bybee, MD**
Assistant Professor of Medicine, University of Missouri–Kansas City School of Medicine; Consulting Cardiologist, Mid-America Heart Institute, Cardiovascular Consultants, PA, Kansas City, Missouri
*Acute Myocardial Infarction*

**John Byrne, MCh**
Assistant Professor of Surgery, Albany Medical College; Member, The Vascular Group, Albany Medical Center, Albany, New York
*Acquired Diseases of the Aorta*

**Alexander Bystritsky, MD, PhD**
Professor, Department of Psychiatry and Biobehavioral Sciences, David Geffen School of Medicine at UCLA; Director, Anxiety Disorder Program, The Semel Institute for Neuroscience and Human Behavior, Los Angeles, California
*Panic Disorder*

**Diego Cadavid, MD**
Associate Professor, Department of Neurology and Neuroscience, UMDNJ–New Jersey Medical School, Newark, New Jersey
*Relapsing Fever*

**Grant R. Caddy, MD**
Consultant Physician and Gastroenterologist, Ulster Hospital, Belfast, Northern Ireland
*Cholelithiasis and Cholecystitis*

**Thomas R. Caraccio, PharmD**
Associate Professor of Emergency Medicine, State University of New York at Stony Brook Health Sciences Center School of Medicine, Stony Brook; Assistant Professor of Pharmacology and Toxicology, New York College of Osteopathic Medicine, Old Westbury, New York
*Medical Toxicology: Ingestions, Inhalations, and Dermal and Ocular Absorptions*

**Enrique V. Carbajal, MD**
Associate Clinical Professor of Medicine, University of California, San Francisco, School of Medicine, San Francisco; Staff Physician–Cardiology, VA Central California Health Care System, Fresno, California
*Premature Beats*

**Stephen D. Cassivi, MD, MSc, FRCSC, FACS**
Associate Professor of Surgery, Mayo Clinic College of Medicine; Director of Lung Transplantation, Division of General Thoracic Surgery, Mayo Clinic, Rochester, Minnesota
*Pleural Effusion and Empyema Thoracis*

**Serguei A. Castaneda, MD**
Research Associate, Cancer Research Center, Boston University School of Medicine, Boston, Massachusetts
*Thalassemia*

**Frank R. Cerniglia, Jr., MD**
Director of Pediatric Urology, Urologic Institute of New Orleans, New Orleans, Louisiana
*Childhood Enuresis*

**Joumana T. Chaiban, MD**
Fellow in Endocrinology, Case Western Reserve University School of Medicine and University Hospitals/Case Medical Center, Cleveland, Ohio
*Hyperprolactinemia*

**Sarah L. Chamlin, MD**
Assistant Professor of Pediatrics and Dermatology, Northwestern University Feinberg School of Medicine; Staff Physician, Children's Memorial Hospital, Chicago, Illinois
*Atopic Dermatitis*

**Miriam M. Chan, RPh, PharmD**
Clinical Assistant Professor of Family Medicine, College of Medicine, and Clinical Assistant Professor of Pharmacy, College of Pharmacy, The Ohio State University; Director of Pharmacy Education, Riverside Family Medicine Residency Education, Riverside Methodist Hospital, Columbus, Ohio
*Popular Herbs and Nutritional Supplements; New Drugs*

**Sam S. Chang, MD**
Associate Professor of Urologic Surgery, Vanderbilt University School of Medicine, Nashville, Tennessee
*Malignant Tumors of the Urogenital Tract*

**Gary C. Chen, MD**
Resident Physician, Internal Medicine, Cedars-Sinai Medical Center, Los Angeles, California
*Bleeding Esophageal Varices*

**Stella T. Chou, MD**
Instructor in Pediatrics, University of Pennsylvania School of Medicine; Attending Physician, The Children's Hospital of Philadelphia, Philadelphia, Pennsylvania
*Nonimmune Hemolytic Anemia*

**Bart L. Clarke, MD**
Assistant Professor of Medicine, Mayo Clinic College of Medicine; Consultant, Mayo Clinic, Rochester, Minnesota
*Osteoporosis*

**Claus-Frenz Claussen, MD**
Professor Extraordinarius in Neuro-otology, Julius-Maximilaus University Faculty of Medicine, Wuerzburg, Germany; Acting Director, Neuro-otological Research Institute of 4GF, Bad Kissingen, Germany
*Tinnitus*

**Harris R. Clearfield, MD**
Professor of Medicine, Drexel University College of Medicine; Section Chief, Gastroenterology, Hahnemann University Hospital, Philadelphia, Pennsylvania
*Diverticula of the Alimentary Tract*

**Donald Clemons, MD**
Clinical Assistant Professor, Department of Family Practice, Quillen School of Medicine, Johnson City, Tennessee
*Premalignant Lesions*

**Melanie W. Conway, MD**
Attending Psychiatrist, Texarkana Living Hope, Texarkana; Dardanelle Hospital, Dardanelle; Levi Hospital, Hot Springs; and White River Medical Center, Batesville, Arkansas
*Mood Disorders*

**Michael S. Cookson, MD**
Associate Professor of Urologic Surgery, Vanderbilt University School of Medicine, Nashville, Tennessee
*Malignant Tumors of the Urogenital Tract*

**John F. Coyle II, MD**
Clinical Professor, Department of Medicine, University of Oklahoma College of Medicine–Tulsa, Tulsa, Oklahoma
*Disturbances Caused by Heat*

**Lester M. Crawford, PhD**
Former Research Professor, Georgetown University School of Medicine, Washington, DC; Former Head, Department of Physiology, University of Georgia College of Medicine, Athens, Georgia
*Foodborne Illness*

**Burke A. Cunha, MD**
Professor of Medicine, State University of New York at Stony Brook Health Sciences Center School of Medicine, Stony Brook; Chief, Infectious Disease Division, Winthrop-University Hospital, Mineola, New York
*Viral and Mycoplasmal Pneumonias; Urinary Tract Infections in Women*

**Stella Dantas, MD**
Physician, Department of Obstetrics and Gynecology, Beaverton Medical Office, Northwest Permanente PC Physicians and Surgeons, Beaverton, Oregon
*Uterine Leiomyomas*

**R. Clement Darling III, MD**
Professor of Surgery, Albany Medical College; Chief, Division of Vascular Surgery, Albany Medical Center Hospital, The Vascular Group, PLLC, Albany, New York
*Acquired Diseases of the Aorta*

**Andre Dascal, MD, FRCPC**
Associate Professor of Medicine, Microbiology and Immunology, McGill University Faculty of Medicine; Senior Infectious Disease Physician, Sir Mortimer B. Davis Jewish General Hospital, Montreal, Quebec, Canada
*Acute Infectious Diarrhea; Toxic Shock Syndrome*

**Susan Davids, MD, MPH**
Assistant Professor of Medicine, Medical College of Wisconsin; Associate Program Director, Internal Medicine Residency, Clement J. Zablocki Veterans Affairs Medical Center, Milwaukee, Wisconsin
*Acute Bronchitis*

**Susan A. Davidson, MD**
Associate Professor, University of Colorado School of Medicine; Chief, Gynecologic Oncology, University of Colorado Hospital, Denver, Colorado
*Neoplasms of the Vulva*

**Prakash C. Deedwania, MD**
Professor of Medicine, University of California, San Francisco, School of Medicine, San Francisco; Chief, Cardiology Section, VA Central California Health Care System, Fresno, California
*Premature Beats*

**Albert A. Del Negro, MD**
Clinical Assistant Professor of Medicine, Georgetown University School of Medicine, Washington, DC; Medical Director, Cardiac Pacemaker Clinic, and Cardiac Electrophysiologist, Inova Fairfax Hospital, Fairfax, Virginia
*Heart Block*

**Marie-France Demierre, MD**
Associate Professor of Dermatology and Medicine, Boston University School of Medicine; Director, Skin Oncology, and Director, Photopheresis Program, Boston Medical Center, Boston, Massachusetts
*Cutaneous T Cell Lymphoma*

**Stephen R. Deputy, MD**
Assistant Professor of Neurology, Louisiana State University School of Medicine; Staff Neurologists, Children's Hospital, New Orleans, Louisiana
*Traumatic Brain Injury in Children*

**Sarah E. Dick, MD**
Senior Dermatology Resident, Hospital of the University of
Pennsylvania, Philadelphia, Pennsylvania
*Bullous Diseases*

**Ram Dickman, MD**
Research Fellow, Southern Arizona VA Health Care System, Neuro-
Enteric Clinical Research Group, Tucson, Arizona
*Gaseousness and Indigestion*

**Alice N. Do, DO**
Research Fellow, Solano Clinical Research, Division Dow
Pharmaceutical Sciences, Vallejo, California
*Condyloma Acuminatum (Genital Warts)*

**Sunil Dogra, MD, DNB, MNAMS**
Assistant Professor, Department of Dermatology, Venereology and
Leprology, Postgraduate Institute of Medical Education and Research,
Chandigarh, India
*Leprosy*

**Basak Dokuzoguz, MD**
Chief, Infectious Diseases and Clinical Microbiology Clinic, Ankara
Numune Education and Research Hospital, Ankara, Turkey
*Brucellosis*

**Douglas A. Drevets, MD, DTM&H**
Associate Professor of Medicine, University of Oklahoma School of
Medicine; Staff Physician, Oklahoma City VA Medical Center,
Oklahoma City, Oklahoma
*Plague*

**Jean Dudler, MD**
Associate Professor of Medicine, Division of Rheumatology, Centre
Hospitalier Universitaire Vaudois and University of Lausanne,
Lausanne, Switzerland
*Rat-Bite Fever*

**Kamryn T. Eddy, PhD**
Clinical Fellow, Massachusetts General Hospital, and Research Fellow,
Harvard Medical School, Boston, Massachusetts
*Bulimia Nervosa*

**Libby Edwards, MD**
Associate Clinical Professor of Dermatology, University of North
Carolina at Chapel Hill School of Medicine, Chapel Hill; Chief,
Division of Dermatology, Carolinas Medical Center and Southeast
Vulvar Clinic, Charlotte, North Carolina
*Pruritus Ani and Vulvae*

**George E. Ehrlich, MD**
Adjunct Professor, Department of Medicine, University of
Pennsylvania School of Medicine, Philadelphia, Pennsylvania; Adjunct
Professor of Clinical Medicine, New York University School of
Medicine, New York, New York
*Osteoarthritis*

**Kimberly May Eickhorst, MD**
Chief Resident, St. Luke's–Roosevelt Hospital Center, New York, New York
*Diseases of the Hair*

**Brandon D. Einstein, BA**
Medical Student, University of Pennsylvania School of Medicine,
Philadelphia, Pennsylvania
*Nevi*

**Julian Elliott, MB, BS, FRACP**
Conjoint Senior Lecturer, National Centre in HIV Epidemiology and
Clinical Research, University of New South Wales, Sydney; Infectious
Diseases Physician, Alfred Hospital, Melbourne; HIV Clinical Advisor,
International Health Research Group, Macfarlane Burnet Institute for
Medical Research and Public Health, Melbourne, Australia
*Psittacosis*

**John M. Embil, MD, FRCP(C), FACP**
Associate Professor, Department of Medicine and Medical
Microbiology, Section of Infectious Diseases, University of Manitoba
Faculty of Medicine; Director, Infection Prevention and Control Unit,
Health Science Centre, Winnipeg, Manitoba, Canada
*Necrotizing Skin and Soft Tissue Infections*

**Elizabeth D. Ennis, MD**
Clinical Assistant Professor, Department of Surgery, Division of
Neurosurgery, University of Alabama at Birmingham School of
Medicine; Vice President of Medical Education and Research, Baptist
Health System–Birmingham; Director, Internal Residency Program,
Baptist Health System, Birmingham, Alabama
*Diabetic Ketoacidosis and Hyperglycemic Hyperosmolar Syndrome*

**Helen Enright, MD**
Department of Haematology, Adelaide and Meath Hospitals, Tallaght,
Dublin, Ireland
*Chronic Leukemias*

**Alexander Espinoza, MD**
University of California, Los Angeles School of Medicine, Los Angeles,
California
*Common Sports Injuries*

**Chukwuemeka N. Etufugh, MD**
Resident, Department of Pathology, Baylor University Medical Center,
Dallas, Texas
*Venous Stasis Ulcers*

**Amanda Nickles Fader, MD**
Clinical Fellow in Gynecologic Oncology, Cleveland Clinic, Cleveland,
Ohio
*Ovarian Cancer*

**Ruth Falik, MD**
Associate Professor of Medicine, Baylor College of Medicine;
Attending Physician, Ben Taub General Hospital, Houston, Texas
*Pain; Atrial Fibrillation*

**Ronnie Fass, MD**
Professor of Medicine, University of Arizona School of Medicine;
Director, GI Motility Laboratories, University of Arizona Health
Sciences Center and Southern Arizona VA Health Care System,
Tucson, Arizona
*Gaseousness and Indigestion*

**Fred G. Fedok, MD, FACS**
Professor, Department of Surgery, Chief, Division of
Otolaryngology—Head and Neck Surgery, Penn State Hershey
Medical Center, Hershey, Pennsylvania
*Bell's Palsy (Idiopathic Acute Peripheral Facial Paralysis)*

**Seth I. Felder, BA**
Medical Student, University of South Florida College of Medicine,
Tampa, Florida
*Nevi*

**Steven R. Feldman, MD, PhD**
Professor of Dermatology, Wake Forest University School of
Medicine, Winston-Salem, North Carolina
*Acne Vulgaris and Rosacea*

**Eve S. Ferdman, BA**
Managing Editor, *Brachytherapy*, Memorial Sloan-Kettering Cancer Center, New York, New York
*Brain Tumors*

**L. Jaime Fitten, MDS**
Professor of Psychiatry and Biobehavioral Sciences, David Geffen School of Medicine at UCLA; Director, Geriatric Psychiatry, Greater Los Angeles Veterans Administration, Sepulveda Campus, Los Angeles, California
*Alzheimer's Disease*

**Alan B. Fleischer, Jr., MD**
Professor and Chair, Department of Dermatology, Wake Forest University School of Medicine, Winston-Salem, North Carolina
*Acne Vulgaris and Rosacea*

**Adriana Foster, MD**
Assistant Professor, Department of Psychiatry and Health Behavior, Medical College of Georgia; Staff Psychiatrist, MCG Medical Center, Augusta, Georgia
*Schizophrenia*

**Melvin H. Freedman, MD**
Professor Emeritus, Department of Pediatrics, University of Toronto Faculty of Medicine; Honorary Consultant, Hematology-Oncology; Senior Scientist Emeritus, Research Institute; and Chair, Research Ethics Board (IRB), The Hospital for Sick Children, Toronto, Ontario, Canada
*Neutropenia*

**Ellen W. Freeman, PhD**
Research Professor, Department of Obstetrics/Gynecology and Department of Psychiatry, University of Pennsylvania School of Medicine, Philadelphia, Pennsylvania
*Premenstrual Syndrome*

**Eugene P. Frenkel, MD**
Professor of Internal Medicine and Radiology, University of Texas Southwestern Medical School at Dallas; Patsy R. & Raymond D. Nasher Distinguished Chair in Cancer Research; Elaine Dewey Sammons Distinguished Chair in Cancer Research in honor of Eugene P. Frenkel, M.D.; and A. Kenneth Pye Professorship in Cancer Research, Harold C. Simmons Comprehensive Cancer Center, Southwestern Medical Center, Dallas, Texas
*Pernicious Anemia and Other Megaloblastic Anemias*

**Jermy N. Friedman, MB, ChB**
Associate Professor, Department of Paediatrics, University of Toronto Faculty of Medicine; Head, Division of Paediatric Medicine, The Hospital for Sick Children, Toronto, Ontario, Canada
*Parenteral Fluid Therapy for Infants and Children*

**Neil J. Friedman, MD**
Adjunct Clinical Associate Professor, Department of Ophthalmology, Stanford University School of Medicine, Stanford; Private Practice, Mid-Peninsula Ophthalmology, Palo Alto, California
*Vision Correction Procedures*

**Deborah K. Froh, MD**
Associate Professor of Pediatrics, University of Virginia School of Medicine, Charlottesville, Virginia
*Cystic Fibrosis*

**Maisie M. Fung, MD**
Staff Physician, Camino Medical Group, Mountain View, California
*Peripheral Arterial Disease*

**Joseph M. Furman, MD, PhD**
Professor, Departments of Otolaryngology and Neurology, University of Pittsburgh School of Medicine, Pittsburgh, Pennsylvania
*Episodic Vertigo*

**Steven L. Galetta, MD**
Ruth Wagner Van Meter and Ray Van Meter Professor of Neurology, University of Pennsylvania School of Medicine, Philadelphia, Pennsylvania
*Optic Neuritis*

**R. Michael Gallagher, DO**
Director, Headache Center of Central Florida, Melbourne, Florida
*Headache*

**Andrea Gallina, MD**
Vita-Salute University; Resident in Training, San Raffaele Hospital, Milan, Italy
*Prostatitis*

**Juan Armando Garcia, MD**
Staff-Intensivist, Cardiovascular ICU, The Methodist Hospital, Houston, Texas
*Management of Chronic Obstructive Pulmonary Disease*

**Christopher S. George, MD**
Attending Physician, Department of Hematology and Medical Oncology, Riverside Methodist Hospital, Columbus, Ohio
*Primary Lung Cancer*

**James N. George, MD**
George Lynn Cross Professor of Medicine, University of Oklahoma College of Medicine; Hematology-Oncology Section, Department of Medicine, University of Oklahoma Health Sciences Center, Oklahoma City, Oklahoma
*Thrombotic Thrombocytopenic Purpura*

**Teresa M. George, MD**
Assistant Program Director, Internal Medicine Residency Program, Riverside Methodist Hospital, Columbus, Ohio
*Primary Lung Cancer*

**Glenn S. Gerber, MD**
Associate Professor of Surgery/Urology, Director of Endourology, and Director of Residency Program and Student Clerkship, University of Chicago Pritzker School of Medicine, Chicago, Illinois
*Renal Calculi*

**Paul L. F. Giangrande, MD**
Senior Lecturer in Haematology, University of Oxford; Consultant Haematologist, Oxford Haemophilia Centre and Thrombosis Unit, Churchill Hospital, Oxford, United Kingdom
*Venous Thrombosis*

**David B. K. Golden, MD**
Associate Professor of Medicine, Johns Hopkins University School of Medicine; Director, Allergy-Immunology, Sinai Hospital, Baltimore, Maryland
*Allergic Reactions to Insect Stings*

**Monica Peterson Gordon, MD**
Geriatric Psychiatry Fellow, David Geffen School of Medicine at UCLA, Los Angeles, California
*Alzheimer's Disease*

**E. Ann Gormley, MD**
Professor of Surgery (Urology), Dartmouth Medical School;
Staff Urologist, Dartmouth-Hitchcock Medical Center, Lebanon,
New Hampshire
*Urinary Incontinence*

**Eduardo Gotuzzo, MD**
Principal Professor of Medicine, Universidad Peruana Cayetano
Heredia; Chief, Department of Infectious, Tropical, and Dermatologic
Diseases, Hospital National Cayetano Heredia, Lima, Peru
*Cholera*

**John E. Gough, MD, FACEP**
Professor, Department of Emergency Medicine, Brody School of
Medicine at East Carolina University; Attending Physician, Emergency
Department, Pitt County Memorial Hospital, Greenville, North
Carolina
*Marine Trauma, Envenomations, and Intoxications*

**Mark A. Granner, MD**
Associate Professor of Neurology, University of Iowa Carver College
of Medicine; Director, Iowa Comprehensive Epilepsy Program,
University of Iowa Hospitals and Clinics, Iowa City, Iowa
*Seizures and Epilepsy in Adolescents and Adults*

**Charles S. Greene, DDS**
Clinical Professor and Director of Orofacial Pain Studies, University
of Illinois College of Dentistry; Orofacial Pain Consultant, Illinois
Masonic Hospital, Chicago, Illinois
*Temporomandibular Disorders*

**Joseph Greensher, MD**
Professor of Pediatrics, State University of New York at Stony Brook
Health Sciences Center School of Medicine, Stony Brook; Medical
Director and Associate Chair, Department of Pediatrics, Long Island
Regional Poison and Drug Information Center, Winthrop-University
Hospital, Mineola, New York
*Medical Toxicology: Ingestions, Inhalations, and Dermal and Ocular
Absorptions*

**Charles Grose, MD**
Professor of Pediatrics, University of Iowa Carver College of
Medicine; Director of Infectious Diseases Division, Children's
Hospital of Iowa, Iowa City, Iowa
*Varicella (Chickenpox)*

**Marlon A. Guerrero, MD**
Chief Surgical Resident, St. Luke's Episcopal Health System, Houston,
Texas
*Thyroid Cancer*

**Abdo Haddad, MD**
Fellow, Hematology and Medical Oncology, Cleveland Clinic
Foundation, Cleveland, Ohio
*Aplastic Anemia*

**Frank G. Haluska, MD, PhD**
Tufts University School of Medicine; Deputy Director and Clinical
Director, Cancer Center, Tufts-New England Medical Center, Boston,
Massachusetts
*Melanoma*

**Rashidul Haque, MB, PhD**
Scientist, Laboratory Sciences Division, International Centre for
Diarrhoeal Disease Research, Bangladesh (ICDDR, B), Dhaka,
Bangladesh
*Amebiasis*

**Rachel Haroz, MD**
Assistant Professor of Emergency Medicine, UMDNJ–Robert Wood
Johnson Medical School at Camden; Attending Physician,
Department of Emergency Medicine, Cooper University Hospital
Camden, New Jersey
*Spider Bites and Scorpion Stings*

**E. John Harris, Jr., MD**
Professor of Surgery, Division of Vascular Surgery, Stanford University
School of Medicine, Stanford, California
*Peripheral Arterial Disease*

**Umur Hatipoğlu, MD**
Clinical Assistant Professor of Medicine, University of Illinois at
Chicago College of Medicine; Section Chief, Pulmonary and
Critical Care Medicine, Mercy Hospital and Medical Center, Chicago,
Illinois
*Bacterial Pneumonia*

**Dana M. Hayden, MD, MPH**
General Surgery Resident, Rush University Medical Center, Chicago,
Illinois
*Tumurs of the Rectum and Colon*

**Emil R. Heinze, MD**
Assistant Clinical Professor of Medicine, David Geffen School of
Medicine at UCLA, Los Angeles; Senior Rheumatology Fellow, UCLA
San Fernando Valley Program, Olive View–UCLA Medical Center,
Sylmar, California
*Bursitis, Tendinitis, Myofascial Pain, and Fibromyalgia*

**J. Claude Hemphill III, MD, MAS**
Associate Professor of Clinical Neurology and Neurological Surgery,
University of California, San Francisco, School of Medicine; Director,
Neurocritical Care, San Francisco General Hospital, San Francisco,
California
*Intracerebral Hemorrhage*

**William Henderson, MD**
Clinical Assistant Professor, University of British Columbia Faculty of
Medicine, Vancouver; Attending Physician, Royal Columbia Hospital,
New Westminister, British Columbia, Canada
*Acute Respiratory Failure*

**David B. Herzog, MD**
Professor of Psychiatry (Pediatrics), Harvard Medical School,
Cambridge; Director, Eating Disorders Unit—Child Psychiatry
Service, and Director, Harris Center for Education and Advocacy in
Eating Disorders, Massachusetts General Hospital, Boston,
Massachusetts
*Bulimia Nervosa*

**Camile Hexsel, MD**
Research Fellow, Department of Dermatology, Henry Ford Hospital,
Detroit, Michigan
*Sunburn*

**David G. Hill, MD**
Waterbury Pulmonary Associates, Waterbury; Yale University School
of Medicine, New Haven, Connecticut
*Cough*

**Christopher D. Hillyer, MD**
Transfusion Medicine Program, Department of Pathology and
Laboratory Medicine, Emory University School of Medicine, Atlanta,
Georgia
*Adverse Effects of Blood Transfusion*

**Darryl T. Hiyama, MD**
Professor of Clinical Surgery, David Geffen School of Medicine at UCLA; Staff Surgeon, UCLA Center for Health Sciences, Los Angeles, California
*Parenteral Nutrition in Adults*

**Brian D. Hoit, MD**
Professor of Medicine, Physiology and Biophysics, Case School of Medicine; Director, Echocardiography, University Hospitals of Cleveland, Cleveland, Ohio
*Pericarditis*

**M. Ekramul Hoque, MBBS, MPH (Hons), PhD**
Research Fellow, School of Population Health, University of Auckland, Auckland, New Zealand
*Giardiasis*

**Duane R. Hospenthal, MD, PhD**
Associate Professor of Medicine, Uniformed Services University of the Health Sciences, F. Edward Hébert School of Medicine, Bethesda, Maryland; Clinical Professor of Medicine, University of Texas Medical School at San Antonio, San Antonio; Chief, Infectious Disease Service, Brooke Army Medical Center, Fort Sam Houston, Texas
*Coccidioidomycosis*

**Tamara Salam Housman, MD**
Procedural Dermatology/Mohs Micrographic Surgery Fellow, Dermatologic Surgery, University of Washington Medical Center, Seattle, Washington
*Warts (Verrucae)*

**Samuel S. Hsu, MD**
Assistant Professor, University of Maryland School of Medicine, Baltimore, Maryland
*Tetanus*

**Katherine Hughes, MB, ChB**
Specialist Registrar in Endocrinology and Diabetes, Endocrinology Unit, Centre for Cardiovascular Science, Queen's Medical Research Institute, Edinburgh, United Kingdom
*Thyroiditis*

**Scott A. Hundahl, MD**
Professor of Clinical Surgery, University of California, Davis, School of Medicine; Chief of Surgery, VA Northern California Health Care System, Sacramento VA Medical Center, Sacramento, California
*Tumors of the Stomach*

**Nader Husseinzadeh, MD**
Professor, University of Cincinnati School of Medicine, Cincinnati, Ohio
*Cancer of the Uterine Cervix*

**Neil H. Hyman, MD**
Samuel B. and Michlle D. Labow Professor of Surgery, University of Vermont College of Medicine; Chief, Division of General Surgery, Fletcher Allen Health Care, Burlington, Vermont
*Hemorrhoids, Anal Fissure, and Anorectal Abscess and Fistula*

**Robert D. Inman, MD**
Professor of Medicine and Immunology, University of Toronto Faculty of Medicine; Director, Arthritis Center of Excellence, University Health Network, Toronto, Ontario, Canada
*Ankylosing Spondylitis*

**Matilde Iorizzo, MD**
Department of Dermatology, University of Bologna, Bologna, Italy
*Diseases of the Nails*

**Jon E. Isaacson, MD**
Division of Otolaryngology, Head and Neck Surgery, Department of Surgery, Penn State University College of Medicine, Hershey, Pennsylvania
*Bell's Palsy (Idiopathic Acute Peripheral Facial Paralysis)*

**Alan C. Jackson, MD, FRCPC**
Professor of Medicine (Neurology) and Medical Microbiology, University of Manitoba Faculty of Medicine; Head, Section of Neurology, Winnipeg Regional Health Authority, Winnipeg, Manitoba, Canada
*Rabies*

**Aleda A. Jacobs, MD**
Mohs Fellow, Procedural Dermatology, Baylor College of Medicine/Baylor Clinic, Houston, Texas
*Cancers of The Skin*

**Robert M. Jacobson, MD**
Professor of Pediatrics, Mayo Clinic College of Medicine; Chair, Department of Pediatric and Adolescent Medicine, and Consultant in Pediatric and Adolescent Medicine, Mayo Clinic, Rochester, Minnesota
*Office-Based Immunization Practices*

**Mamta K. Jain, MD, MPH**
Assistant Professor, University of Texas Southwestern Medical School at Dallas, Dallas, Texas
*Acute and Chronic Hepatitis*

**James J. James, MD, DrPH, MHA**
Director, Center for Disaster Preparedness and Emergency Response, American Medical Association, Chicago, Illinois
*Toxic Chemical Agents Reference Chart: Symptoms and Treatment; Biologic Agents Reference Chart—Symptoms, Tests, and Treatment*

**Stephen G. Jenkinson, MD**
Chief, Pulmonary Diseases Section, Audie Murphy VA Medical Center, San Antonio, Texas
*Management of Chronic Obstructive Pulmonary Disease*

**Gordon L. Jensen, MD, PhD**
Professor and Head, Department of Nutritional Sciences, and Professor of Medicine, Pennsylvania State University, Hershey, Pennsylvania
*Obesity*

**Jeffrey Jim, MD, MS**
Resident Physician, Department of Surgery, UCLA Medical Center Los Angeles, California
*Parenteral Nutrition in Adults*

**Michael Johns, MD**
Assistant Professor of Otolaryngology, Emory University School of Medicine, Atlanta, Georgia
*Hoarseness and Laryngitis*

**Candice E. Johnson, MD, PhD**
Clinical Professor of Pediatrics, University of Colorado Health Sciences Center School of Medicine; Volunteer Faculty, The Children's Hospital, Denver, Colorado
*Bacterial Infections of the Urinary Tract in Girls*

**James F. Jones, MD**
Research Medical Officer, Chronic Viral Diseases Branch, National Center for Zoonotic, Vector-Borne, and Enteric Diseases, Centers for Disease Control and Prevention, Atlanta, Georgia
*Chronic Fatigue Syndrome*

**Michael P. Jones, MD**
Associate Professor of Medicine, Division of Gastroenterology, Northwestern University Feinberg School of Medicine; Attending Physician, Northwestern Memorial Hospital, Chicago, Illinois
*Irritable Bowel Syndrome*

**Joseph L. Jorizzo, MD**
Professor, Founding and Former Chair, Department of Dermatology, Wake Forest University School of Medicine, Winston-Salem, North Carolina
*Cutaneous Vasculitis*

**Rome Jutabha, MD**
Associate Professor of Medicine, David Geffen School of Medicine at UCLA; Director, UCLA Center for Small Bowel Diseases, UCLA Medical Center, Los Angeles, California
*Bleeding Esophageal Varices*

**S. Patrick Kachur, MD**
Commander, U.S. Public Health Service; Chief, Malaria Strategic Applied Science Unit, Centers for Disease Control and Prevention, Atlanta, Georgia
*Malaria*

**Tamilarasu Kadhiravan, MD**
Senior Resident, Department of Medicine, All India Institute of Medical Sciences, New Delhi, India
*Management of the Patient with HIV Disease*

**Pierre I. Karakiewicz, MD**
Associate Professor, Department of Urology, University of Montreal Faculty of Medicine; Urologic Oncologist and Director, Cancer Prognostics and Health Outcomes Unit, University of Montreal Health Center, Montreal, Quebec, Canada
*Prostatitis*

**Matthew E. Karlovsky, MD**
Staff Urologist (Voiding Dysfunction/Female Urology), Private Practice, Center for Urological Services, PC, Phoenix, Arizona
*Benign Prostatic Hyperplasia*

**Andreas Katsambas, MD, PhD**
Professor and Chairman, 1st Department of Dermatology, University of Athens School of Medicine; Attending Physician, "Andreas Sygros" Hospital for Skin and Venereal Diseases, Athens, Greece
*Parasitic Diseases of the Skin*

**Philip O. Katz, MD**
Clinical Professor of Medicine, Jefferson Medical College of Thomas Jefferson University; Chairman, Division of Gastroenterology, Albert Einstein Medical Center, Philadelphia, Pennsylvania
*Dysphagia and Esophageal Obstruction*

**Andrew M. Kaunitz, MD**
Professor, Department of Obstetrics and Gynecology, University of Florida College of Medicine, Jacksonville, Florida
*Contraceptive Methods*

**Sean Keenan, MD**
Clinical Assistant Professor of Medicine, University of British Columbia Faculty of Medicine, Vancouver; Head, Department of Critical Care Medicine, Royal Columbia Hospital, New Westminister, British Columbia, Canada
*Acute Respiratory Failure*

**Jennifer Kelly, DO**
Assistant Professor of Medicine, Division of Endocrinology, SUNY Upstate Medical University, Syracuse, New York
*Diabetes Insipidus*

**Rebecca Lewis Kelso, MD**
Assistant Professor, Department of Dermatology, University of Texas Medical Branch School of Medicine, Galveston, Texas
*Fungal Diseases of the Skin*

**Stephen F. Kemp, MD**
Associate Professor of Medicine and Assistant Professor of Pediatrics, University of Mississippi School of Medicine; Director, Allergy and Immunology Fellowship Program, University of Mississippi Medical Center, Jackson, Mississippi
*Anaphylaxis and Serum Sickness*

**James W. Kendig, MD**
Professor of Pediatrics, Pennsylvania State University School of Medicine; Staff Pediatrician, Division of Newborn Medicine, Penn State Children's Hospital, Hershey, Pennsylvania
*Hemolytic Disease of the Newborn*

**Sripathi R. Kethu, MD**
Assistant Professor of Medicine, Brown University School of Medicine, Providence, Rhode Island
*Gastric and Peptic Ulcer Disease*

**Sundeep Khosla, MD**
Professor of Medicine, Mayo Clinic College of Medicine; Consultant, Mayo Clinic, Rochester, Minnesota
*Osteoporosis*

**Craig S. Kitchens, MD**
Professor of Medicine, University of Florida College of Medicine; Associate Chief of Staff for Education, Malcolm Randall VA Medical Center, Gainesville, Florida
*Snakebite*

**Joel D. Klein, MD, FAAP**
Professor of Pediatrics, Jefferson Medical College of Thomas Jefferson University, Philadelphia, Pennsylvania; Chief, Division of Pediatric Infectious Diseases, Alfred I. duPont Hospital for Children, Wilmington, Delaware
*Mumps*

**Jonathan Kolitz, MD**
Associate Professor of Medicine, New York University School of Medicine, New York; Director, Leukemia Service, Monter Cancer Center, North Shore University Hospital, Lake Success, New York
*Acute Leukemias in Adults*

**Luciano Kolodny, MD**
Endocrinologist, HealthPartners Medical Group, Woodbury, Minnesota
*Erectile Dysfunction*

**Gerald B. Kolski, MD, PhD, FAAAAI, FAAP**
Clinical Professor of Pediatrics, Temple University School of Medicine; Adjunct Clinical Professor of Pediatrics, Drexel University School of Medicine, Philadelphia; Chairman, Department of Pediatrics, Crozer Chester Medical Center, Upland, Pennsylvania
*Asthma in Children*

**John Koo, MD**
Professor and Vice Chairman, Department of Dermatology, University of California, San Francisco, School of Medicine; Director, UCSF Psoriasis Treatment Center, Phototheraphy Unit and Clinical Research Unit, University of California San Francisco Medical Center, San Francisco, California
*Papulosquamous Disorders*

**Stephen L. Kopecky, MD**
Professor of Medicine, Mayo Clinic College of Medicine, Rochester, Minnesota
*Acute Myocardial Infarction*

**Frederick K. Korley, MD**
Robert E. Meyerhoff Assistant Professor of Emergency Medicine,
Johns Hopkins University School of Medicine; Staff, Johns Hopkins
Medical Institutions, Baltimore, Maryland
*Disturbances Due To Cold*

**Milind J. Kothari, DO**
Professor of Neurology and Vice Chair of Education and Training,
Pennsylvania State College of Medicine, Hershey, Pennsylvania
*Myasthenia Gravis and Related Disorders*

**Jeffrey A. Kraut, MD**
Chief of Dialysis, Veterans Affairs Greater Los Angeles Healthcare
System; Professor of Medicine, David Geffen School of Medicine at
UCLA, Los Angeles, California
*Chronic Renal Failure*

**Robert A. Kreisberg, MD**
Distinguished Professor Emeritus, University of South Alabama,
Mobile; Clinical Professor of Medicine, University of Alabama at
Birmingham School of Medicine, Birmingham; Teaching Faculty,
Baptist Health System, Birmingham, Alabama
*Diabetic Ketoacidosis and Hyperglycemic Hyperosmolar Syndrome*

**Jacques Kremer, PhD**
Post-Doctoral Program, Institute of Immunology, National
Laboratory of Health, Luxembourg, Luxembourg
*Measles (Rubeola)*

**John N. Krieger, MD**
Professor of Urology, University of Washington School of Medicine
and Public Health; Attending Surgeon, University of Washington
Medical Center and Hanborview Medical Center; Chief of Urology,
VA Puget Sound, Seattle, Washington
*Epididymitis; Nungonococcal Urethritis*

**Leonard R. Krilov, MD**
Professor of Pediatrics, State University of New York at Stony Brook
Health Sciences Center School of Medicine, Stony Brook; Chief,
Pediatric Infectious Disease, and Vice-Chairman of Pediatrics,
Winthrop-University Hospital, Mineola, New York
*Infectious Mononucleosis*

**Michael Kroll, MD**
Associate Professor of Medicine, Baylor College of Medicine; Staff
Hematologist-Oncologist, Michael E. DeBakey VA Medical Center,
Houston, Texas
*Polycythemia Vera*

**Bhushan Kumar, MD, MNAMS**
Former Professor and Head, Department of Dermatology,
Post-Graduate Institute of Medical Education and Research,
Chandigarh, India
*Leprosy*

**Paul Y. Kwo, MD**
Associate Professor of Medicine, Division of
Gastroenterology/Hepatology, Indiana University School of Medicine,
Indianapolis, Indiana
*Cirrhosis*

**Norman J. Lacayo, MD**
Assistant Professor, Department of Pediatrics, Division of
Hematology-Oncology, Stanford University School of Medicine,
Stanford; Attending Physician, Lucile Packard Children's Hospital,
Palo Alto, California
*Acute Leukemia in Children*

**Lori M. B. Laffel, MD, MPH**
Associate Professor of Pediatrics, Harvard Medical School; Chief,
Pediatric, Adolescent, and Young Adult Section, and Investigator,
Section on Genetics and Epidemiology, Joslin Diabetes Center,
Boston, Massachusetts
*Diabetes Mellitus in Children and Adolescents*

**Gabriella Lakos, MD, PhD**
Visiting Assistant Professor of Medicine, Northwestern University
Feinberg School of Medicine, Chicago, Illinois
*Connective Tissue Disorders*

**Paul R. Lambert, MD**
Professor and Chairman, Department of Otolaryngology, Medical
University of South Carolina, Charleston, South Carolina
*Ménière's Disease*

**Barbara A. Latenser, MD**
Clara L. Smith Professor of Burn Treatment and Clinical Professor of
Surgery, University of Iowa Carver College of Medicine; Medical
Director, Burn Treatment Center, University of Iowa Hospitals and
Clinics, Iowa City, Iowa
*Burn Treatment Guidelines*

**Yung R. Lau, MD**
Associate Professor of Pediatric Cardiology, University of Alabama of
Birmingham School of Medicine, Bimingham, Alabama
*Congenital Heart Disease*

**Mark Layton, MD**
Reader, Imperial College; Consultant, Hammersmith Hospital,
London, United Kingdom
*Sickle Cell Disease*

**Luca Lazzarini, MD**
Department of Infectious Diseases and Tropical Medicine, San
Bortolo Hospital, Vicenza, Italy
*Osteomyelitis*

**Andrew G. Lee, MD**
Professor of Opthalmology, Neurology, and Neurosurgery, University
of Iowa Carver College of Medicine, Iowa City, Iowa
*Optic Neuritis*

**Chai Sue Lee, MD**
Assistant Professor, Department of Dermatology, University of
California, Davis, School of Medicine, Davis; Director, Psoriasis and
Phototherapy Treatment Center, UC Davis Medical Center,
Sacramento, California
*Papulosquamous Disorders*

**Jason T. Lee, MD**
Assistant Professor of Surgery, Division of Vascular Surgery, Stanford
University School of Medicine, Stanford, California
*Peripheral Arterial Disease*

**Julie Leegwater-Kim, MD, PhD**
Fellow in Movement Disorders, Department of Neurology, Columbia
University Medical Center, New York, New York
*Parkinsonism*

**Jerrold B. Leikin, MD**
Professor of Emergency Medicine, Northwestern University Feinberg
School of Medicine; Professor of Medicine, Rush Medical College,
Chicago; Director of Medical Toxicology, Evanston Northwestern
Healthcare–Omega, Glenbrook Hospital, Glenview, Illinois
*Disturbance Due to Cold*

**Marcel Levi, MD**
Professor of Medicine, University of Amsterdam Faculty of Medicine;
Chairman, Department of Medicine, Academic Medical Center,
Amsterdam, The Netherlands
*Disseminated Intravascular Coagulation*

**Moshe Levi, MD**
Professor of Medicine, University of Colorado School of Medicine;
Nephrology Fellow, University of Colorado Hospital, Aurora,
Colorado
*Hyponatremia*

**Eyal Levit, MD**
Assistant Clinical Professor of Dermatology, Columbia University
College of Physicians and Surgeons; Director of Dermatologic and
Cosmetic Surgery, St. Luke's Hospital; Director, Procedural
Dermatology Fellowship, New York–Presbyterian Hospital and
St. Luke's–Roosevelt Hospital, New York, New York
*Diseases of the Hair*

**Henry W. Lim, MD**
Chairman and C.S. Livingood Chair, Department of Dermatology,
Henry Ford Hospital, Detroit, Michigan
*Sunburn*

**Gary H. Lipscomb, MD**
Professor and Vice Chairman, University of Tennessee College of
Medicine; Director, Division of Gynecologic Specialties, University of
Tennessee Health Science Center, Memphis, Tennessee
*Ectopic Pregnancy*

**James A. Litch, MD, DTMH**
Clinical Assistant Professor, University of Washington School of
Medicine and School of Public Health, Seattle, Washington
*High-Altitude Illness*

**Virginia Litle, MD**
Assistant Professor of Surgery, Mount Sinai School of Medicine;
Assistant Attending, Department of CT Surgery, Mount Sinai Medical
Center, New York, New York
*Primary Lung Abscess*

**Jonathan S. Lopresti, MD, PhD**
Associate Professor of Clinical Medicine, Keck School of Medicine at
USC; Attending Physician, LAC/USC Medical Center, Los Angeles,
California
*Hypothyroidism*

**Jacqueline M. Losi-Sasaki, MD**
Private Practice, The Dermatology Clinic, PLLC, Gulfport, Mississippi
*Viral Diseases of the Skin*

**James M. Lyznicki, MS, MPH**
Senior Scientist, Center for Disaster Preparedness and Emergency
Response, American Medical Association, Chicago, Illinois
*Toxic Chemical Agents Reference Chart: Symptoms and Treatment;
Biologic Agents Reference Chart—Symptoms, Tests, and Treatment*

**Jaroslaw P. Maciejewski, MD, PhD**
Staff, Hematologic Oncology and Blood Disorders; Section Head,
Experimental Hematology and Hematopoiesis; and Associate Professor,
Cleveland Clinic Lerner College of Medicine, Cleveland, Ohio
*Aplastic Anemia*

**Douglas W. MacPherson, MD, MSc (CTM)**
Professor, Department of Pathology and Molecular Medicine, Faculty
of Health Sciences, McMaster University, Hamilton; President,
Migration Health Consultants Inc., Cheltenham, Ontario, Canada
*Intestinal Parasites*

**Carl D. Malchoff, MD, PhD**
Professor of Internal Medicine, University of Connecticut School of
Medicine, Farmington, Connecticut
*Adrenocortical Insufficiency*

**Brian F. Mandell, MD, PhD**
Professor of Medicine, Cleveland Clinic Lerner College of Medicine at
Case Western Reserve University; Vice Chairman of Medicine,
Department of Rheumatic and Immunologic Disease, Cleveland
Clinic, Cleveland, Ohio
*Hyperuricemia and Gout*

**Susan Manzi, MD, MPH**
Associate Professor of Medicine and Epidemiology and Co-Director,
Lupus Center of Excellence, University of Pittsburgh School of
Medicine; Attending, UPMC Magee and UPMC Presbyterian,
Pittsburgh, Pennsylvania
*Connective Tissue Disorders*

**Ali J. Marian, MD**
Center for Cardiovascular Genetic Research and The Brown
Foundation Institute of Molecular Medicine, The University of Texas
Health Science Center; Staff Physician, The Methodist Hospital;
Professional Staff, St. Luke's Episcopal Hospital/Texas Heart Institute,
Houston, Texas
*Hypertropic Cardiomyopathy*

**Vickie Martin, MD**
Resident, Department of Obstetrics and Gynecology, Kingston
General Hospital, Kingston, Ontario, Canada
*Amenorrhea*

**Maria Mascarenhas, MBBS**
Associate Professor of Pediatrics, University of Pennsylvania School of
Medicine; Section Chief, Nutrition Division of Gastroenterology and
Nutrition; Director, Nutrition Support Service, The Children's
Hospital of Philadelphia, Philadelphia, Pennsylvania
*Normal Infant Feeding*

**Wissam E. Mattar, MD**
Indiana University School of Medicine, Indianapolis, Indiana
*Cirrhosis*

**Eric L. Matteson, MD, MPH**
Professor of Medicine, Mayo Clinic College of Medicine; Consultant
in Rheumatology, Mayo Clinic, Rochester, Minnesota
*Rheumatuid Arthritis*

**Martin J. McCaffrey, MD**
Associate Professor of Pediatrics, Division of Neonatal and Perinatal
Medicine, University of North Carolina at Chapel Hill School of
Medicine; North Carolina Children's Hospital, Chapel Hill, North
Carolina
*Resuscitation of the Newborn*

**Anthony L. McCall, MD, PhD**
James M. Moss Professor of Diabetes, University of Virginia School of
Medicine; Endocrinologist, University of Virginia Health Care System,
Charlottesville, Virginia
*Diabetes Mellitus in Adults*

**Michael T. McCann, MD**
Clinical Assistant Professor, Baylor College of Medicine, Houston,
Texas
*Spine Pain*

**Laura J. McCloskey, PhD**
Assistant Professor of Pathology, Anatomy, and Cell Biology, Jefferson Medical College of Thomas Jefferson University; Associate Director, Clinical Laboratories, and Director, Jefferson Hospital for Neurosciences Laboratory, Thomas Jefferson University Hospital, Philadelphia, Pennsylvania
*Reference Intervals for the Interpretation of Laboratory Tests*

**Jacqueline Carinhas McGregor, MD**
Director, Baylor Child Psychiatry Clinic; Associate Professor, Menninger Department of Psychiatry and Behavioral Sciences, Baylor College of Medicine, Houston, Texas
*Anxiety Disorders*

**Michael McGuigan, MD**
Medical Director, Long Island Regional Poison and Drug Information Center, Winthrop-University Hospital, Mineola, New York
*Medical Toxicology: Ingestions, Inhalations, and Dermal and Ocular Absorptions*

**Stephen H. McKellar, MD**
Chief Resident, Cardiothoracic Surgery, Department of Surgery, Mayo Clinic, Rochester, Minnesota
*Pleural Effusion and Empyema Thoracis*

**Dilcia McLenan, MD**
Assistant Professor of Pediatrics, Baylor College of Medicine, Pearland, Texas
*Care of the High-Risk Neonate*

**D. Scott McMeekin, MD**
Presbyterian Foundation Presidential Professor, University of Oklahoma College of Medicine; Section Chief, Gynecologic Oncology, University of Oklahoma Health Sciences Center, Oklahoma City, Oklahoma
*Cancer of the Endometrium*

**J. Scott McMurray, MD**
Associate Professor of Pediatric Otolaryngology, Department of Surgery, University of Wisconsin School of Medicine and Public Health, Madison, Wisconsin
*Otitis Media*

**Donald McNeil, MD**
Associate Professor of Clinical Medicine, Department of Immunology, The Ohio State University College of Medicine and Public Health, Columbus, Ohio
*Allergic Reactions to Drugs*

**Anupama Menon, MD, MPH**
Assistant Professor of Medicine, Division of Infectious Diseases, University of Arkansas for Medical Sciences; Staff Physician, Central Arkansas Veterans Healthcare System, Little Rock, Arkansas
*Blastomycosis*

**Ted A. Meyer, MD, PhD**
Assistant Professor, Department of Otolaryngology, Medical University of South Carolina, Charleston, South Carolina
*Ménière's Disease*

**Merry N. Miller, MD**
Professor and Chair, Department of Psychiatry and Behavioral Sciences, Quillen College of Medicine, East Tennessee State University; Attending Psychiatrist, Woodridge Psychiatric Hospital, Johnson City, Tennessee
*Mood Disorders*

**Paul D. Miller, MD**
Distinguished Clinical Professor of Medicine, University of Colorado School of Medicine; Medical Director, Colorado Center for Bone Research, Lakewood, Colorado
*Paget's Disease of Bone*

**Peter A. Millward, MD**
Assistant Professor of Pathology, Pennsylvania State College of Medicine; Medical Director, Blood Bank and Apheresis Service, Milton S. Hershey Medical Center, Hershey, Pennsylvania
*Therapeutic Use of Blood Components*

**Howard C. Mofenson, MD**
Professor of Pediatrics and Emergency Medicine, State University of New York at Stony Brook Health Sciences Center School of Medicine, Stony Brook; Professor of Pharmacology and Toxicology, New York College of Osteopathic Medicine, Old Westbury, New York
*Medical Toxicology: Ingestions, Inhalations, and Dermal and Ocular Absorptions*

**Alladi Mohan, MD**
Adjunct Professor, Department of Medicine, Sri Venkateswara Institute of Medical Sciences, Andhra Pradesh, India
*Sarcoidosis; Tuberculosis and Other Mycobacterial Diseases*

**Robert M. Moldwin, MD**
Assistant Professor of Urology, Albert Einstein College of Medicine of Yeshiva University, Bronx; Director, Interstitial Cystitis Center, North Shore–Long Island Jewish Health Care System, New Hyde Park, New York
*Bacterial Infections of the Urinary Tract in Males*

**Eugene W. Monroe, MD**
Assistant Clinical Professor of Dermatology, Medical College of Wisconsin; Staff, Advanced Healthcare, Milwaukee, Wisconsin
*Urticaria and Angioedema*

**Angela Yen Moore, MD**
Arlington Center for Dermatology, Arlington, Texas
*Viral Diseases of the Skin*

**Terry L. Moore, MD**
Professor of Internal Medicine, Pediatrics, and Molecular Microbiology and Immunology, Saint Louis University School of Medicine; Director, Division of Pediatric Rheumatology and Adult Rheumatology, Saint Louis University Medical Center, St. Louis, Missouri
*Juvenile Idiopathic Arthritis*

**Enrique Morales, MD**
Attending Nephrologist, Hospital 12 de Octubre, Madrid, Spain
*Primary Glomerular Diseases*

**John F. Moran, MD**
Professor of Medicine, Loyola University Stritch School of Medicine, Maywood, Illinois
*Angina Pectoris*

**Arnold M. Moses, MD**
Professor of Medicine, State University of New York Upstate Medical University College of Medicine; Attending Physician, University Hospital, Syracuse, New York
*Diabetes Insipidus*

**Scott Moses, MD**
Medical Staff, Fairview Lakes Regional Medical Center, Wyoming, Minnesota
*Pruritus*

**Alan C. Moss, MD**
Instructor, Harvard Medical School; Fellow in Gastroentrology, Beth Israel Deaconess Medical Center, Boston, Massachusetts
*Inflammatory Bowel Disease*

**Steven F. Moss, MD**
Associate Professor of Medicine, The Warren Alpert Medical School of Brown University; Director, Gastroenterology Fellowship Training Program, Rhode Island Hospital, Providence, Rhode Island
*Gastric and Peptic Ulcer Disease*

**Claude P. Muller, MD**
Immunology, University of Trier Faculty of Medicine; Experimental Medicine, University of Horburg, Germany; HOD Institute of Immunology, National Laboratory of Health, Luxembourg, Luxembourg
*Measles (Rubeola)*

**Tashanna K.N. Myers, MD**
Fellow in Gynecologic Oncology, University of Oklahoma Health Sciences Center, Oklahoma City, Oklahoma
*Cancer of the Endometrium*

**Ashwatha Narayana, MD**
Associate Professor, Department of Radiology, New York University School of Medicine; Residency Program Director and Associate Chair of Clinical Research, Department of Radiation Oncology, New York University Medical Center, New York, New York
*Brain Tumors*

**Lisa R. Nash, DO**
Assistant Professor, Department of Family Medicine, University of Texas Medical Branch School of Medicine, Galveston, Texas
*Postpartum Care*

**Laeth S. Nasir, MBBS**
Professor, Department of Family Medicine, University of Nebraska College of Medicine; Staff Physician, University of Nebraska Medical Center, Omaha, Nebraska
*Dysmenorrhea*

**Gideon Nesher, MD**
Start Clinical Associate Professor of Medicine, The Hebrew University Medical School; Head, Department of Internal Medicine A, Share-Zedek Medical Center, Jerusalem, Israel
*Polymyalgia Rheumatica and Giant-Cell Arteritis*

**David N. Neubauer, MD**
Assistant Professor, Johns Hopkins University School of Medicine; Associate Director, Johns Hopkins Sleep Disorders Center, Baltimore, Maryland
*Sleep Disorders*

**Ronald Lee Nichols, MD**
William Henderson Professor of Surgery–Emeritus and Professor of Microbiology and Immunology, Tulane University School of Medicine, New Orleans, Louisiana
*Bacterial Diseases of the Skin*

**Electra Nicolaidou, MD, PhD**
Lecturer in Dermatology, 1st Department of Dermatology, University of Athens School of Medicine; Lecturer in Dermatology, "Andreas Sygros" Hospital for Skin and Venereal Diseases, Athens, Greece
*Parasitic Diseases of the Skin*

**John T. Nicoloff, MD**
Professor of Medicine and Senior Associate Chair for Research, Department of Medicine, Keck School of Medicine at USC; Attending Physician, LAC/USC Medical Center, Los Angeles, California
*Hypothyroidism*

**Maureen M. O'Brien, MD**
Instructor, Division of Pediatric Hematology/Oncology, Stanford University School of Medicine, Stanford; Staff, Lucile Packard Children's Hospital, Palo Alto, California
*Acute Leukemia in Children*

**David L. Olive, MD**
Professor of Obstetrics and Gynecology, University of Wisconsin School of Medicine and Public Health, Madison, Wisconsin
*Endometriosis*

**Brian Olshansky, MD**
Professor of Medicine, University of Iowa Carver College of Medicine; Cardiologist, University of Iowa Hospitals and Clinics, Iowa City, Iowa
*Tachycardias*

**Steven M. Opal, MD**
Professor of Medicine, The Warren Alpert Medical School of Brown University, Providence; Director, Infectious Disease Service, Memorial Hospital of Rhode Island, Pawtucket, Rhode Island
*Severe Sepsis and Septic Shock*

**Ida F. Orengo, MD**
Professor of Dermatology, Baylor College of Medicine; Chief of Mohs Surgery, Baylor Clinic and VA Medical Center, Houston, Texas
*Cancers of the Skin*

**Richard R. Orlandi, MD**
Associate Professor, Division of Otolaryngology–Head and Neck Surgery, University of Utah School of Medicine; Associate Director, Center for Therapeutic Biomaterials, University of Utah Health Sciences Center, Salt Lake City, Utah
*Sinusitis*

**Finbar D. O'Shea, MB, MRCPI**
Spondylitis Fellow, Arthritis Center of Excellence, Toronto Western Hospital, Toronto, Ontario, Canada
*Ankylosing Spondylitis*

**Matthew T. Oughton, MD, FRCPC**
Post-Doctoral Research Fellow, Department of Medicine, McGill University Faculty of Medicine, Montreal, Quebec, Canada
*Acute Infectious Diarrhea*

**Gary D. Overturf, MD**
Professor of Pediatrics and Pathology University of New Mexico College of Medicine; Medical Director, Infectious Diseases, TriCore Reference Laboratories, Albuquerque, New Mexico
*Bacterial Meningitis*

**Paul M. Palevsky, MD**
Professor of Medicine, University of Pititsburgh School of Medicine; Chief, Renal Section, VA Pittsburgh Healthcare System, Pittsburgh, Pennsylvania
*Acute Renal Failure*

**Charles J. Parker, MD**
Professor of Medicine, University of Utah School of Medicine, Salt Lake City, Utah
*Autoimmune Hemolytic Anemia*

**John E. Parker, MD**
Professor of Medicine, West Virginia University of College of Medicine; Section Chief, Pulmonary and Clinical Care Medicine, WVU Health Sciences Center, Morgantown, West Virginia
*Silicosis and Asbestosis*

**Manisha J. Patel, MD**
Clinical Instructor, Johns Hopkins University School of Medicine, Baltimore, Maryland
*Cutaneous Vasculitis*

**Eleni Patrozou, MD**
Teaching Fellow in Medicine Infectious Diseases, The Warren Alpert Medical School of Brown University, Providence; Infectious Disease Fellow, Memorial Hospital of Rhode Island, Pawtucket, Rhode Island
*Severe Sepsis and Septic Shock*

**Ian M. Paul, MD, MSc**
Associate Professor of Pediatrics and Health Evaluation Sciences, Pennsylvania State College of Medicine, Hershey, Pennsylvania
*Fever*

**Mark A. Peppercorn, MD**
Professor of Medicine, Harvard Medical School; Senior Consultant, Center of Inflammatory Bowel Disease, Beth Israel Deaconess Medical Center, Boston, Massachusetts
*Inflammatory Bowel Disease*

**Nancy D. Perrier, MD**
Associate Professor, University of Texas M.D. Anderson Cancer Center, Houston, Texas
*Thyroid Cancer*

**Andrew C. Peterson, MD**
Assistant Professor of Surgery, Uniformed Services University of the Health Sciences F. Edward Hébert School of Medicine, Bethesda, Maryland; Urology Residency Program Director, Madigan Army Medical Center, Tacoma, Washington
*Management of Urethral Stricture Disease*

**William A. Petri, MD, PhD**
Chief, Division of Infectious Disease and International Health, University of Virginia Medical Center, Charlottesville, Virginia
*Amebiasis; Travel Medicine*

**Tania J. Phillips, MD**
Professor of Dermatology, Boston University School of Medicine; Consulting Dermatologist, Boston Medical Center, Boston, Massachusetts
*Venous Stasis Ulcers*

**Michael E. Pichichero, MD**
Professor of Microbiology and Immunology, Pediatrics, and Medicine, Department of Microbiology and Immunology, University of Rochester School of Medicine and Dentistry, Rochester, New York
*Pertussis*

**Bianca Maria Piraccini, MD, PhD**
Department of Dermatology, University of Bologna, Bologna, Italy
*Diseases of the Nails*

**Pierre-François Plouin, MD**
Professor of Cardiovascular Medicine, Université Paris-Descartes; Head, Hypertension Unit, Hôpital Emopeen G. Pompladh, Paris, France
*Pheochromocytomas*

**Michael J. Pollack, MD**
Gastroentrology Fellow, University Hospitals of Cleveland, Cleveland, Ohio
*Hiccups*

**Susan P. Perrine, MD**
Professor of Pediatrics, Medicine, and Pharmacology and Experimental Therapeutics, Boston University School of Medicine; Hematologist, Boston Medical Center, Boston, Massachusetts
*Thalassemia*

**Uday Popat, MD**
Associate Professor of Medicine, University of Texas M.D. Anderson Cancer Center, Houston, Texas
*Non-Hodgkin's Lymphoma*

**Lawrie W. Powell, MD, PhD**
Professor Emeritus, School of Medicine, The University of Queensland Faculty of Health Sciences; Director of Research, Teaching and Research Unit, Royal Brisbane and Women's Hospitals, Brisbane, Queensland, Australia
*Hemochromatosis*

**Manuel Praga, MD**
Associate Professor of Medicine, Universidad Complutense; Head, Nephrology Department, Hospital 12 de Octubre, Madrid, Spain
*Primary Glomerular Diseases*

**Richard A. Prinz, MD**
Professor of Surgery, Rush Medical College; Chief, General Surgery, Rush University Medical Center, Chicago, Illinois
*Acute and Chronic Pancreatitis*

**L. Michael Prisant, MD**
Professor of Medicine, Medical College of Georgia; Director of Hypertension and Clinical Pharmacology, MCG Medical Center, Augusta, Georgia
*Hypertension*

**Gregory Proctor, MD**
Nephrology Fellow, University of Colorado School of Medicine/University of Colorado Hospital, Aurora, Colorado
*Hyponatremia*

**Beth W. Rackow, MD**
Assistant Professor, Department of Obstetrics and Gynecology, Yale University School of Medicine, New Haven, Connecticut
*Dysfunctional Uterine Bleeding*

**Sharow S. Raimer, MD**
Professor and Chair, Department of Dermatology, University of Texas Medical Branch School of Medicine, Galveston, Texas
*Fungal Diseases of the Skin*

**Kirk D. Ramin, MD**
Associate Professor and Director, Maternal-Fetal Medicine Fellowship Program, Department of Obstetrics and Gynecology, University of Minnesota Medical School, Minneapolis, Minnesota
*Antepartum Care*

**Julio A. Ramirez, MD**
Professor of Medicine, University of Louisville School of Medicine; Chief, Division of Infectious Diseases, Department of Veterans Affairs Medical Center, Louisville, Kentucky
*Legionellosis*

**Didier Raoult, PhD**
Faculty of Medicine, Rickettsial Unit, Université de la Mediterranée, Marseille, France
*Q Fever*

**Susan E. Reef, MD**
Centers for Disease Control and Prevention, Atlanta, Georgia
*Rubella and Congenital Rubella Syndrome*

**Adam Reich, MD, PhD**
Assistant Professor, Department of Dermatology, Venereology and Allergology, Wroclaw Medical University, Wroclaw, Poland
*Pigmentary Disorders*

**Robert L. Reid, MD**
Professor, Department of Obstetrics and Gynecology, Queen's University Faculty of Medicine; Chair, Division of Reproductive Endocrinology and Infertility, Kingston General Hospital, Kingston, Ontario, Canada
*Amenorrhea*

**Martin Reite, MD**
Professor of Psychiatry, University of Colorado School of Medicine; Medical Staff, University Hospital, Denver, Colorado
*Treatment of Insomnia*

**Robert W. Rho, MD**
Assistant Professor of Medicine, Division of Cardiology, University of Washington School of Medicine, Seattle, Washington
*Cardiac Arrest: Sudden Cardiac Death*

**Lawrence Rice, MD**
Professor of Medicine and Professor of Thrombosis Research, Baylor College of Medicine; Staff Physician, The Methodist Hospital, Houston, Texas
*Non-Hodgkin's Lymphoma*

**James R. Roberts, MD**
Professor of Emergency Medicine and Senior Consultant of Medical Toxicology, Drexel University College of Medicine; Chairman of Emergency Medicine and Director, Division of Toxicology, Mercy Hospital of Philadelphia, Philadelphia, Pennsylvania
*Spider Bites and Scorpion Stings*

**Jenice Robinson, MD**
Assistant Professor of Neurology, Pennsylvania State College of Medicine, Hershey, Pennsylvania
*Myasthenia Gravis and Related Disorders*

**Robb L. Romp, MD**
Assistant Professor of Pediatric Cardiology, University of Alabama at Birmingham School of Medicine, Birmingham, Alabama
*Congenital Heart Disease*

**Leon Rosenthal, MD**
Sleep Medicine Associates of Texas, Dallas, Texas
*Sleep Apnea*

**Richard N. Rosenthal, MD**
Professor of Clinical Psychiatry, Columbia University College of Physicians and Surgeons; Chairman, Department of Psychiatry, St. Luke's–Roosevelt Hospital Center, New York, New York
*Alcoholism*

**Michael B. Rothberg, MD, MPH**
Assistant Professor of Medicine, Tufts University School of Medicine, Boston; Director of Scholarly Activities, Internal Medicine Residency Program, Baystate Medical Center, Springfield, Massachusetts
*Influenza*

**Israel Rubinstein, MD**
Professor of Medicine and Biopharmaceutical Sciences, University of Illinois at Chicago College of Medicine, Chicago, Illinois
*Bacterial Pneumonia*

**Chirag Sandesara, MD**
Electrophysiology Fellow, University of Iowa Hospitals and Clinics, Iowa City, Iowa
*Tachycardias*

**Karl J. Sandin, MD, MPH**
Adjunct Professor of Sociology, Westmont College, Santa Barbara, California
*Rehabilitation of the Stroke Patient*

**J. Terry Saunders, PhD**
Assistant Professor of Medical Education in Internal Medicine, University of Virginia School of Medicine, Charlottesville, Virginia
*Diabetes Mellitus in Adults*

**Peter C. Schalock, MD**
Instructor in Dermatology, Harvard Medical School; Assistant in Dermatology, Massachusetts General Hospital, Boston, Massachusetts
*Contact Dermatitis*

**Ralph M. Schapira, MD**
Professor and Vice Chair, Department of Medicine, Medical College of Wisconsin; Staff Physician, Milwaukee Veterans Affairs Medical Center, Milwaukee, Wisconsin
*Histoplasmosis; Acute Bronchitis*

**Randall T. Schapiro, MD**
Clinical Professor of Neurology, University of Minnesota Medical School, Minneapolis; Director, The Schapiro Center for Multiple Sclerosis at The Minneapolis Clinic of Neurology, Golden Valley, Minnesota
*Multiple Sclerosis*

**Michael Schatz, MD, MS**
Clinical Professor, Department of Medicine, University of California, San Diego, School of Medicine; Chief, Department of Allergy, Kaiser Permanente, San Diego, California
*Asthma in Adolescents and Adults*

**Stacey A. Scheib, MD**
Resident Physician, Department of Obstetrics and Gynecology, Thomas Jefferson University Hospital, Philadelphia, Pennsylvania
*Menopause*

**Lawrence R. Schiller, MD**
Clinical Professor of Internal Medicine, University of Texas Southwestern College of Medicine at Dallas; Attending Physician, Digestive Health Associates of Texas; Program Director, Gastroenterology Fellowship, Baylor University Medical Center, Dallas, Texas
*Malabsorption*

**Kerrie Schoffer, MD, FRCPC**
Assistant Professor in Neurology, Dalhousie University Faculty of Medicine; Neurologist, QEII Health Sciences Centre, Halifax, Nova Scotia
*Peripheral Neuropathies*

**Craig Michael Schramm, MD**
Associate Professor, Department of Pediatrics, University of Connecticut School of Medicine, Farmington; Chief, Pediatric Pulmonary Division, Connecticut Children's Medical Center, Hartford, Connecticut
*Atelectasis*

**Kathryn G. Schuff, MD**
Associate Professor of Endocrinology and Clinical Research Compliance Manager, General Clinical Research Center, Oregon Health and Science University School of Medicine, Portland, Oregon
*Cushing's Syndrome*

**W. Cooper Scurry, Jr., MD**
Fellow, McCollough Plastic Surgery Clinic, Gulf Shores, Alabama
*Bell's Palsy (Idiopathic Acute Peripheral Facial Paralysis)*

**Carlos Seas, MD**
Associate Professor of Medicine, Universidad Peruana Cayetano Heredia; Chief, Inservice Department, Hospital National Cayetano Heredia, Lima, Peru
*Cholera*

**Daniel J. Sexton, MD**
Professor, Duke University School of Medicine, Durham, North
Carolina
*Rickettsial and Ehrlichial Infections*

**Mrunal Shah, MD**
Clinical Assistant Professor of Family Medicine, The Ohio State
University College of Medicine; Assistant Program Director, Riverside
Family Practice Residency Program, Riverside Methodist Hospital,
Columbus, Ohio
*Syphilis*

**Rupali Shah, MD**
Resident Physician, UNC Hospitals, Chapel Hill, North Carolina
*Hoarseness and Laryngitis*

**Prateek Sharma, MD**
Professor of Medicine and Fellowship Program Director, University of
Kansas School of Medicine/Medical Center, Kansas City Missouri
*Gastroesophageal Reflux Disease*

**Surendra K. Sharma, MD, PhD**
Chief, Division of Pulmonary and Critical Care Medicine, All India
Institute of Medical Sciences, New Delhi, India
*Management of the Patient with HIV Disease; Sarcoidosis;
Tuberculosis and Other Mycobacterial Diseases*

**Chelsea A. Sheppard, MD**
Transfusion Medicine Program, Department of Pathology and
Laboratory Medicine, Emory University School of Medicine, Atlanta,
Georgia
*Adverse Effects of Blood Transfusion*

**Raj D. Sheth, MD**
Director, Comprehensive Epilepsy Program; Professor, University of
Wisconsin–Madison School of Medicine, Madison, Wisconsin
*Epilepsy in Infancy and Childhood*

**Marc A. Silver, MD**
Clinical Professor of Medicine, University of Illinois at Chicago
College of Medicine, Chicago; Adjunct Professor, Department of
Biomedical Engineering, Illinois Institute of Technology, Chicago;
Chairman, Department of Medicine, and Director, Heart Failure
Institute, Advocate Christ Medical Center, Oak Lawn, Illinois
*Heart Failure*

**Peter A. Singer, MD**
Professor of Clinical Medicine, Keck School of Medicine of USC;
Chief, Clinical Endocrinology, Department of Medicine, LAC–USC
Medical Center, Los Angeles, California
*Hyperthyroidism*

**Arti Sinha, MB, BS**
Guy's, King's and St. Thomas' School of Medicine; Foundation Year 2
Physician, St. Thomas' Hospital; London, United Kingdom
*Conjunctivitis*

**Michael J. Smith, MD**
Instructor, Department of Pediatrics, University of Pennsylvania
School of Medicine; Fellow, Division of Infectious Diseases, The
Children's Hospital of Philadelphia, Pennsylvania
*Cat-Scratch Disease*

**Cynthia B. Snider, MD, MPH**
Department of Medicine, University of Virginia School of Medicine,
Charlottesville, Virginia
*Travel Medicine*

**Carmen C. Solorzano, MD**
Assistant Professor of Surgery, University of Miami Miller School of
Medicine; Chief, Endocrine Surgery, University of Miami/Sylvester
Cancer Center, Miami, Florida
*Acute and Chronic Pancreatitis*

**Suman Sood, MD**
Instructor in Medicine, Hematology-Oncology, University of
Pennsylvania School of Medicine; Staff, Hospital of the University of
Pennsylvania, Philadelphia, Pennsylvania
*Platelet-Mediated Bleeding Disorders*

**Thomas Spencer, MD**
Associate Professor of Psychiatry, Harvard Medical School; Assistant
Director of Clinical and Research Program in Pediatric
Psychopharmacology and Director of Depression and Tourette's
Clinic, Massachusetts General Hospital, Boston, Massachusetts
*Attention Deficit Hyperactivity Disorder*

**Stanley M. Spinola, MD**
David H. Jacobs Professor and Director, Division of Infectious
Diseases, Indiana University School of Medicine, Indianapolis,
Indiana
*Chancroid*

**Richard K. Sterling, MD**
Professor of Medicine, Medical College of Virginia–Virginia
Commonwealth University School of Medicine, Richmond, Virginia
*Cirrhosis*

**Catherine Stevens-Simon, MD**
Associate Professor of Pediatrics, Division of Adolescent Medicine,
University of Colorado School of Medicine; Staff Physician, Children's
Hospital, Denver, Colorado
*Chlamydia trachomatis*

**A. Keith Stewart, MB, ChB**
Senior Associate Consultant, Mayo Clinic Arizona, Scottsdale, Arizona
*Multiple Myeloma*

**Christopher D. Still, DO**
Medical Director, Center for Nutrition and Weight Management,
Department of Gastroenterology and Nutrition, Geisinger Health
Care System, Danville, Pennsylvania
*Obesity*

**Erik K. St. Louis, MD**
Assistant Professor of Neurology, University of Iowa Carver College of
Medicine; Co-Director, Iowa Comprehensive Epilepsy Program,
University of Iowa Hospitals and Clinics, Iowa City, Iowa
*Seizures and Epilepsy in Adolescents and Adults*

**Mark W. J. Strachan, MD**
Consultant Endocrinologist, Metabolic Unit, Western General
Hospital, Edinburgh, United Kingdom
*Thyroiditis*

**David J. Straus, MD**
Professor of Clinical Medicine, Weill Cornell Medical College;
Attending Physician, Memorial Sloan-Kettering Cancer Center, New
York, New York
*Hoogkin's Disease: Chemotherapy*

**Paniti Sukumvanich, MD**
Fellow, Breast Service, Department of Surgery, Memorial Sloan-
Kettering Cancer Center, New York, New York
*Diseases of the Breast*

**Scott Swanson, MD**
Professor of Surgery, Mount Sinai School of Medicine; Attending
Surgeon, Mount Sinai Medical Center, New York, New York
*Primary Lung Abscess*

**Jessica P. Swartout, MD**
Fellow in Maternal-Fetal Medicine, Department of Obstetrics and
Gynecology, University of Minnesota Medical School, Minneapolis,
Minnesota
*Antepartum Care*

**Misha F. Syed, MD**
Assistant Professor, Department of Ophthalmology and Visual Sciences,
University of Texas Medical Branch School of Medicine, Galveston, Texas
*Glaucoma*

**Jacek C. Szepietowski, MD, PhD**
Professor and Vice Chair, Department of Dermatology, Venereology
and Allergology, Wroclaw Medical University; Director, Institute of
Immunology and Experimental Therapy, Polish Academy of Sciences,
Wroclaw, Poland
*Pigmentary Disorders*

**Mahsa Tehrani, MA**
Medical Student, George Washington University School of Medicine
and Health Sciences, Washington, DC
*Keloids*

**Marty S. Teltscher, MD, CM**
Infections Diseases and Medical Microbiology Fellow, McGill
University Faculty of Medicine/SMED–Jewish General Hospital,
Montreal, Quebec, Canada
*Toxic Shock Syndrome*

**Victor J. Test, MD, FCCP**
Assistant Professor of Clinical Medicine, Division of Pulmonary
Medicine and Critical Care, University of California, San Diego,
School of Medicine, La Jolla, California
*Pulmonary Embolism*

**Manish Thapar, MD**
Instructor, University of Missouri College of Medicine; Attending
Physician, University Hospital, Columbia, Missouri
*Porphyria*

**David R. Thomas, MD**
Professor of Medicine, Saint Louis University School of Medicine;
Attending Physician, Saint Louis University Hospital, St. Louis,
Missouri
*Pressure Ulcers*

**Rodger E. Tiedemann, MB, ChB, PhD**
Clinical Senior Lecturer in Medicine, University of Auckland Faculty
of Medicine, School of Medicine, Auckland, New Zealand; Research
Associate, Mayo Clinic Arizona, Scottsdale, Arizona
*Multiple Myeloma*

**Joyce A. Tinsley, MD**
Associate Professor, Department of Psychiatry; Director of Psychiatric
Residency Training and Director of Addiction Psychiatry Training,
University of Connecticut School of Medicine, Farmington,
Connecticut
*Drug Abuse*

**Lama L. Tolaymat, MD, MPH**
Assistant Professor, Department of Obstetrics and Gynecology,
University of Florida College of Medicine; Director of Ultrasound and
Prenatal Diagnosis, UF Health Science Center Jacksonville,
Jacksonville, Florida
*Contraceptive Methods*

**Linus H. Santo Tomas, MD, MS**
Assistant Professor of Pulmonary Critical Care Medicine, Medical
College of Wisconsin, Milwaukee, Wisconsin
*Histoplasmosis*

**Marcia G. Tonnesen, MD**
Associate Professor of Dermatology and Medicine, State University of
New York at Stony Brook Health Sciences Center School of Medicine,
Stony Brook; Chief of Dermatology, Veterans Affairs Medical Center,
Northport, New York
*Erythema Multiforme, Stevens-Johnson Syndrome, and Toxic Epidermal
Necrolysis*

**Peter P. Toth, MD, PhD**
Chief of Medicine, CGH Medical Center; Visiting Clinical Associate
Professor, University of Illinois at Chicago College of Medicine,
Chicago; Director of Preventive Cardiology, Sterling Rock Falls Clinic,
Sterling, Illinois
*Dyslipoproteinemias*

**Maria Trent, MD, MPH**
Assistant Professor of Pediatrics, Johns Hopkins University School of
Medicine; Active Staff, Johns Hopkins Hospital Children's Center,
Baltimore, Maryland
*Pelvic Inflammatory Disease*

**Arvid E. Underman, MD, FACP, DTMH**
Clinical Professor of Medicine and Microbiology, Keck School of
Medicine of USC, Los Angeles; Director of Graduate Medical
Education, Huntington Hospital, Pasadena,
California
*Salmonellosis*

**Nicholas Van Bruaene, MD**
ENT in Training, Department of Oto-Rhino-Laryngology, University
Hospital Ghent, Ghent, Belgium
*Nonallergic Perennial Rhinitis*

**Mary Lee Vance, MD**
Professor of Medicine and Neurosurgery, University of Virginia
School of Medicine; Attending Physician, University of Virginia
Hospital, Charlottesville, Virginia
*Acromegaly; Hypopituitarism*

**Brian A. VanderBrink, MD**
Chief Resident, North Shore–Long Island Jewish Health Care System,
New Hyde Park, New York
*Bacterial Infections of the Urinary Tract in Males*

**John Varga, MD**
Gallagher Professor of Medicine, Northwestern University Feinberg
School of Medicine, Chicago, Illinois
*Connective Tissue Disorders*

**Donald C. Vinh, MD, FRCP(C), Dip(ABIM)**
Division of Infectious Diseases, Department of Medicine, and
Department of Medical Microbiology, McGill University Health
Center, Montreal General Hospital, Montreal, Quebec,
Canada
*Necrotizing Skin and Soft Tissue Infections*

**Todd W. Vitaz, MD**
Assistant Professor, Department of Neurological Surgery, University
of Louisville School of Medicine; Director of Neurosurgical
Oncology; Co-Director, Neurosciences ICU, Norton Hospital,
Louisville, Kentucky
*Management of Head Injuries*

**Jeffery T. Vrabec, MD**
Associate Professor, Department of Otolaryngology–Head and Neck Surgery, Baylor College of Medicine; Clinical Associate Professor, Department of Head and Neck Surgery, M.D. Anderson Cancer Center; Active Staff, Otolaryngology–Head and Neck Surgery, The Methodist Hospital; Courtesy Staff, Otolaryngology Service, Texas Children's Hospital, and Head and Neck Surgery, M.D. Anderson Cancer Center, Houston, Texas; Chair, Facial Nerve Disorders Committee, and Member, SIPac Committee, American Academy of Otolaryngology–Head and Neck Surgery; Chair, ByLaws Committee, American Neurotology Society Membership Committee
*Otitis Externa*

**Sachin Wani, MD**
Gastroenterology and Hepatology Fellow, University of Kansas School of Medicine/VA Medical Center, Kansas City, Missouri
*Gastroesophageal Reflux Disease*

**Shobha Wani, MD**
Fellow, Section of Rheumatology, Washington Hospital Center, Washington, DC
*Lyme Disease*

**Thomas T. Ward, MD**
Associate Professor of Medicine, Oregon Health and Science University School of Medicine; Chief, Infectious Diseases, Portland Veterans Affairs Medical Center, Portland, Oregon
*Toxoplasmosis*

**Cheryl Waters, MD**
Albert and Judith Glickman Professor, Department of Neurology, Columbia University College of Physicians and Surgeons, New York, New York
*Parkinsonism*

**Richard W. Weber, MD**
Professor of Medicine, University of Colorado School of Medicine and National Jewish Medical and Research Center, Denver, Colorado
*Allergic Rhinitis Caused by Inhalant Factors*

**Arthur Weinstein, MD, FACP, FACR**
Professor of Medicine, Georgetown University School of Medicine; Associate Chairman, Department of Medicine, and Director, Section of Rheumatology, Washington Hospital Center, Washington, DC
*Lyme Disease*

**Steven D. Weisbord, MD, MSc**
Assistant Professor of Medicine, University of Pittsburgh School of Medicine; Staff Physician, Renal Section, and Core Faculty Member, Center for Health Equity Research and Promotion, VA Pittsburgh Healthcare System, Pittsburgh, Pennsylvania
*Acute Renal Failure*

**David G. Weismiller, MD**
Associate Professor and Vice Chair for Academic Affairs, Department of Family Medicine, Brody School of Medicine at East Carolina University, Greenville, North Carolina
*Hypertensive Disorders of Pregnancy*

**Mitchell J. Weiss, MD, PhD**
Associate Professor of Pediatrics, University of Pennsylvania School of Medicine; The Children's Hospital of Philadelphia, Philadelphia, Pennsylvania
*Nonimmune Hemolytic Anemia*

**Robert C. Welliver, Sr., MD**
Professor, University at Buffalo State University of New York School of Medicine; Co-Director, Division of Infectious Diseases, Women and Children's Hospital of Buffalo, Buffalo, New York
*Viral Respiratory Infections*

**Victoria Werth, MD**
Professor, Department of Dermatology, University of Pennsylvania School of Medicine; Chief, Dermatology, Philadelphia VA Medical Center, Philadelphia, Pennsylvania
*Bullous Diseases*

**Derek S. Wheeler, MD**
Assistant Professor of Clinical Pediatrics, University of Cincinnati College of Medicine; Associate Medical Director, Division of Critical Care Medicine, Cincinnati Children's Hospital Medical Center, Cincinnati, Ohio
*Resuscitation of the Newborn*

**Timothy Wilens, MD**
Associate Professor of Psychiatry, Harvard Medical School; Director of Substance Abuse Services, Clinical and Research Pediatric Psychopharmacology, Massachusetts General Hospital, Boston, Massachusetts
*Attention Deficit Hyperactivity Disorder*

**Kira Williams, MD**
Chief Resident in Psychiatry, Anxiety Disorders Clinic, Department of Psychiatry and Biobehavioral Sciences, Neuropsychiatric Institute and Hospital, Los Angeles, California
*Panic Disorder*

**Steven R. Williams, MD**
Clinical Assistant Professor, Department of Obstetrics and Gynecology, The Ohio State University College of Medicine and Public Health, Columbus, Ohio
*Infertility*

**Phillip M. Williford, MD**
Associate Professor of Dermatology and Director of Mohs Micrographic Surgery, Department of Dermatology, Wake Forest University School of Medicine, Winston-Salem, North Carolina
*Warts (Verrucae)*

**Elzbieta Wirkowski, MD**
Associate Professor of Clinical Neurology, SUNY at Stony Brook, Long Island; Director of Cerebrovascular Disorders and Co-Director of Neurological Intensive Care Unit, Withrop University Hospital, Mineola, New York
*Ischemic Cerebrovascular Disease*

**Andrew L. Wong, MD**
Professor of Clinical Medicine, David Geffen School of Medicine at UCLA, Los Angeles; Chief of Rheumatology, Olive View–UCLA Medical Center, Sylmar, California
*Bursitis, Tendinitis, Myofascial Pain, and Fibromyalgia*

**Wing-Yen Wong, MD**
Associate Professor of Pediatrics, Keck School of Medicine at USC; Voluntary Faculty/Attending Staff Physician, Children's Hospital Los Angeles, Los Angeles; Medical Director, Clinical Research and Development, Baxter BioScience, Baxter Health Care Corp., Westlake Village, California
*Hemophilia and Related Disorders*

**Jamie R. S. Wood, MD**
Instructor in Pediatrics, Harvard Medical School; Research Associate, Sections on Genetics and Epidemiology and Vascular Cell Biology, and Staff Physician, Pediatric, Adolescent, and Young Adult Section, Joslin Diabetes Center, Boston, Massachusetts
*Diabetes Mellitus in Children and Adolescents*

**Jon B. Woods, MD**
Associate Professor of Pediatrics, Uniformed Services University of the Health Sciences F. Edward Hébert School of Medicine, Bethesda, Maryland; Pediatric Infectious Diseases, Wilford Hall Medical Center, Lackland Air Force Base, San Antonio, Texas
*Anthrax*

**Charles F. Wooley, MD**
Professor of Medicine Emeritus, Division of Cardiology, Heart and Lung Research Institute/The Ohio State University School of Medicine and Public Health, Columbus, Ohio
*Mitral Valve Prolapse: The Floppy Mitral Valve, Mitral Valve Prolapse, and Mitral Valvular Regurgitation*

**Jennifer Wright, MD**
Fellow in Hematology/Oncology, Baylor College of Medicine, Houston, Texas
*Polycythemia Vera*

**Ronald F. Young, MD**
Director of Neurosurgery, California Neuroscience Institute, St. John's Regional Medical Center, Oxnard, California
*Trigeminal Neuralgia*

**William F. Young, Jr., MD, MSc**
Professor of Medicine, Mayo Clinic College of Medicine; Consultant, Division of Endocrinology, Diabetes, Metabolism, and Nutrition, Mayo Clinic, Rochester, Minnesota
*Primary Aldosteronism*

**Michael C. Zacharisen, MD**
Associate Professor of Pediatrics and Medicine (Allergy/Immunology), Medical College of Wisconsin; Staff Physician, Children's Hospital of Wisconsin, Milwaukee, Wisconsin
*Hypersensitivity Pneumonitis*

**Jami Star Zeltzer, MD**
Associate Professor, Department of Obstetrics and Gynecology, Division of Maternal-Fetal Medicine, University of Massachusetts Medical School, Worcester, Massachusetts
*Vaginal Bleeding in Late Pregnancy*

**Kathryn A. Zug, MD**
Associate Professor of Medicine(Dermatology), Dartmouth Medical School, Hanover; Staff Physician, Dartmouth Hitchcock Medical Center, Lebanon, New Hampshire
*Contact Dermatitis*

Starting in 1949, *Conn's Current Therapy* has provided a yearly update on the practical treatment of nearly 400 diseases and disorders. Howard Conn was the initial developer and author, who set out to provide a concise and up-to-date reference on the most recent advances in therapy for conditions most commonly encountered in practice. Some less common conditions also are included, because certain disorders can have serious consequences if not diagnosed early and managed appropriately. Well-known scholar and clinician Robert Rakel, MD, took over editorship in 1984 after Dr. Conn's death and remains today as the editor. Edward Bope, MD, joined him in 2001 to share the editor responsibilities.

Each year, new experts are chosen to write on the topics. They are selected on the basis of recommendations from other authorities, or scholarly activity and/or research. Changing authors with each edition keeps the book crisp in coverage, fresh in tone, and brimming with the latest in practical advice. The authors give references for their discussions but also tell you how they manage the problem in their own clinical practice. Such practical wisdom is of immense value to today's physician, who typically is inundated with sometimes conflicting information from multiple sources. New topics are included every year, so the book remains current with the problems likely to be encountered in practice.

Now with the purchase of *Conn's Current Therapy 2008* you also can have your favorite or commonly referenced topics available on your computer or handheld device. In fact, you will have access to the 2006, 2007, and 2008 editions for downloading your favorite articles from the book. Readers are encouraged to compare the treatments presented in these editions to see how different experts manage the same problem.

*Conn's Current Therapy* is indeed an international book. Contributing authors from around the world offer advice about the diagnosis and management of conditions not common to the United States. The contribution of these international experts adds greatly to the comprehensive nature of the book, and given the amount of international travel, it is quite possible to see unusual disorders far from the homeland of their origin.

Each chapter includes Key Diagnostic and Key Therapeutic boxes for quick reference. As always, tables, graphs, and figures are used when possible to present in-depth data in a convenient format. References for further reading provide some options for additional information if needed. In keeping with today's emphasis on evidence-based medicine, the clinician is pointed toward good evidence, when available, for treatment success. Careful attention is given to ensuring that the information included is correct and up to date. All of the material is reviewed by a pharmacist, Dr. Rakel or Dr. Bope, and multiple copy editors for accuracy and readability. Trade names are included alongside the generic drug names to help the clinician identify the medicines by whatever name is most familiar. The treatments recommended are those found to work best in the experience of the author. When a drug is not FDA approved for that use, this is indicated by a footnote; such notations may merely reflect that approval for that indication was never requested.

We greatly appreciate the assistance of the very capable editorial staff at Elsevier and particularly the contribution of our pharmacist reviewers, Miriam Chan, RPH, PharmD, and Grace Kuo, PharmD.

*Robert E. Rakel, MD*

*Edward T. Bope, MD*

xxv

# Contents

## SECTION 3
# Diseases of the Head and Neck

## SECTION 4
# The Respiratory System

# SECTION 7
# The Digestive System

# SECTION 8
# Metabolic Disorders

SECTION 9
# The Endocrine System

SECTION 10
# The Urogenital Tract

SECTION 11
# The Sexually Transmitted Diseases

## SECTION 17
# Psychiatric Disorders

## SECTION 18
# Physical and Chemical Injuries

## SECTION 19
# Appendices and Index

# Symptomatic Care Pending Diagnosis

## Pain

Method of
*Ruth Falik, MD*

Pain is one of the most common patient complaints. According to population-based surveys, it has been estimated that 75 million American adults experience chronic pain. Of these, one third report a significant impact on their quality of life. The annual cost in direct medical expenditures, informal costs, and lost productivity has been estimated at greater than $100 billion. Chronic pain is the most common cause of long-term disability—more than 5 million American workers receive disability compensation for chronic pain.

Pain is subjective. The physician depends on the patient's description to determine intensity, quality, location, and duration of pain. The patient's perception of pain is the best available tool for evaluation. Intellectual, emotional, and cultural variables affect the patient's experience and description of pain. Pain is commonly underappreciated by the physician and hence undertreated. Whether pain is acute or chronic, inadequate treatment can slow recovery, impair patient functioning, and adversely affect the quality of life.

## Definitions

Pain can be considered a successful adaptive response to a hostile environment. The experience of pain provides protective information that contributes to survival either by preventing injury or by promoting attention to healing when injury has occurred. Pain becomes maladaptive when it is divorced from noxious stimuli and instead represents a pathologic process of the nervous system.

Several distinct types of pain have been described. *Nociceptive* pain is defined as transient pain in response to a noxious stimulus; it is protective and confers a survival benefit. *Inflammatory pain* is defined as spontaneous pain and hypersensitivity to pain in response to inflammation and the resulting damage to tissue. *Neuropathic pain* is the result of damage to the nervous system itself, such as lesions to the peripheral nervous system seen in patients with diabetic or AIDS neuropathy. *Functional pain* is the result of abnormal central processing of normal input; no neurologic deficit or peripheral abnormality can be identified. Functional pain is maladaptive; it is a dysfunctional amplification in the responsiveness of the nervous system.

Inflammatory, neuropathic, and functional pain share some characteristics. Pain can arise spontaneously in the absence of any apparent peripheral stimulus *(allodynia)* or it can arise in response to normally innocuous stimuli *(hyperalgesia),* such as light touch. Spontaneous pain and changes in sensitivity to stimuli are basic to the disease entity of chronic pain. Current research tries to define the underlying neuro-biological mechanisms so that therapy can be targeted to the particular mechanism. The aim is to move from mere symptom control to mechanism-specific modalities that can eradicate or even abort the development of pain.

## Epidemiology

There are at least 600 identifiable pain syndromes, ranging from fibromyalgia to low back pain. Risk factors for developing chronic pain include trauma, surgery, a prior history of back or breast surgery, cholecystectomy, thoracotomy, and advanced age.

Among the noninstitutionalized elderly, 25% to 65% report chronic pain. For those in long-term care facilities, more than 80% have chronic pain. Sensitivity to pain changes with aging. The elderly

### CURRENT DIAGNOSIS

- Pain is subjective. The physician is dependent on the patient's description to determine intensity, quality, location, and duration of pain.
- Intellectual, emotional, and cultural variables affect the patient's experience and description of pain.
- Nociceptive pain is transient pain in response to a noxious stimulus; it is protective and confers a survival benefit.
- Inflammatory, neuropathic, and functional pain can arise spontaneously in the absence of apparent noxious stimulus (allodynia) or in response to normally innocuous stimuli (hyperalgesia).
- Chronic pain persists despite attempts to alleviate it. The duration of pain is not the criterion by which chronic pain is distinguished from acute pain; it is the inability to restore the pain-free state. Chronic pain is not merely a symptom but is itself a disease.
- Addiction is rare in patients who first use opioids for pain relief. Tolerance and dependency are likely with long-term use. Close follow-up is mandatory.

might not manifest the classic symptoms of such painful syndromes as myocardial infarction or appendicitis. Although the response to acute pain can diminish with age (possibly due to deterioration of peripheral C-fibers), the elderly have an increased incidence of chronic pain, possibly due to age-related reduction in the functioning of the antinociceptive pathways and reduced levels of endorphins and enkephalins.

Perception of pain may be gender specific. Women seek treatment for chronic pain more often than do men. Many clinical entities with chronic pain as a major component (fibromyalgia, temporomandibular disorder, interstitial cystitis) are far more prevalent in women. For the most part, the published literature shows that women a have a lower pain threshold and a lower tolerance of painful stimuli. Researchers have postulated that differences in women's experience of pain are linked to primitive survival strategies. Cultural, emotional, and behavioral influences also affect gender differences in the experience of pain. Recent studies have shown that there are gender differences in the opioid receptor system; this might someday provide the basis for gender-based therapy.

## Treatment

### PHARMACOLOGIC TREATMENT

#### Nonopioid Analgesics

The goal of treatment for any pain is to remove the cause. Correct diagnosis is essential.

Acute pain, typically caused by tissue injury or infection, requires only temporary therapy. Treating the underlying condition might not immediately ameliorate the pain for some conditions (e.g., burns, trauma, and sickle cell crisis). Analgesic medications are then the first line of therapy.

In treating acute mild pain, aspirin, acetaminophen, and nonsteroidal anti-inflammatory agents (NSAIDs) are the drugs of choice. Currently, more than 20 NSAIDs are available. Aspirin and NSAIDS inhibit cyclooxygenase (COX), thereby preventing the subsequent formation of prostaglandins responsible for inflammation. Aspirin and NSAIDs are also antipyretic and analgesic. Acetaminophen has antipyretic and analgesic actions, but it does not

### CURRENT THERAPY

- Aspirin, acetaminophen, and nonsteroidal anti-inflammatory drugs (NSAIDs) are first-line choices in the treatment of mild to moderate pain.
- If pain persists despite optimal dosing, then opioid drugs should be given. Administer orally whenever possible.
- Although opioid effects are dose-related, there is great variability among patients. Optimal pain relief with minimal side effects requires titration of both dose and interval.
- Side effects can be anticipated and should be treated proactively.
- Adjuvant drugs may be used in addition to traditional analgesic medication. Adjuvant drugs can enhance the analgesic effect of opioid and nonopioid medications, allowing a lower dose of the opioid or nonopioid drug and a lower incidence of side effects.
- Nonpharmacologic modalities, such as exercise and cognitive behavior therapy, can improve functioning and the quality of life.
- Address the *four As* of pain management outcomes (analgesia, activities of daily living, adverse side effects, and aberrant drug-taking behavior) at each encounter.

have anti-inflammatory properties. These over-the-counter medications alleviate common types of pain, such as headache and musculoskeletal pain. Gastrointestinal absorption is excellent, and side effects are minimal with occasional use.

NSAIDS and aspirin, by inhibiting COX-1, undermine gastric mucosal integrity and can lead to bleeding. Aspirin also irreversibly acetylates platelets, impairing their aggregative function. NSAIDs, when used chronically, can impair renal function and, in some persons, increase blood pressure. Acetaminophen does not impair platelet function or cause gastric irritation. Acetaminophen is hepatotoxic at large doses (>4 g/day), and at not-so-large doses (>2.5 g/day) in patients with impaired liver function.

*Ketorolac tromethamine* (Toradol), a parenteral NSAID, extends the usefulness of this class of compounds in managing acute severe pain, for example, postoperatively. Because it is more nephrotoxic than orally administered NSAIDs, it is recommended for short-term use only. A lower dose should be given to patients who weigh less than 50 kg or who are older than 65 years.

COX-2 inhibitors have been marketed as more selective NSAIDs. These drugs act primarily on COX-2, which is an inducible form of COX and an important mediator of inflammation and pain. They were thought to have little or no effect on platelets or gastric mucosa, but because of an increased incidence of cardiovascular events noted in patients taking some COX-2 inhibitors, rofecoxib (Vioxx) and valdecoxib (Bextra) were withdrawn from the market. Celecoxib (Celebrex) is still available, as is meloxicam (Mobic), a less selective COX-2 inhibitor.

#### Opioid Analgesics

Opioids are the most powerful analgesic medications available. They are pharmacologically similar to opium or morphine and are the drugs of choice when aspirin, NSAIDS, and acetaminophen fail. They have the broadest range of efficacy. They are rapid acting and reliable. For the most part, side effects are mild and well tolerated. Respiratory depression, the most serious side effect, can be readily reversed with the narcotic antagonist naloxone (Narcan).

Oral opioids typically prescribed in the ambulatory care setting include codeine, oxycodone (OxyContin, Roxicodone), and hydrocodone (typically in combination with acetaminophen [e.g., Vicodin]). The choice and dose of opioid medication vary depending on the route of administration, severity of pain, known side effects, and cost. These drugs are often given in combination with aspirin or acetaminophen for additive analgesia, but doses of these combination medications are limited by the nonopioid component. When this occurs, the opioid and nonopioid medications should be given separately to allow further upward titration of the opioid.

Oral dosing is preferred but might not be feasible in the setting of nausea, vomiting, dysphagia, or abnormal gastrointestinal absorption. Rapid pain relief requires parenteral administration. Intravenous administration is preferred; intramuscular injection should be avoided if possible. Acute side effects include nausea, vomiting, and sedation; the most serious side effect is respiratory depression. Patients receiving parenteral opioids should be closely monitored, preferably with an oxygen saturation monitor, and naloxone should be readily available.

Opioid effects are dose related, but there is great variability among patients. Optimal pain relief with minimal side effects requires titration of both dose and interval. Side effects can be anticipated and should be treated proactively. It is imperative that pain relief and side effects be assessed frequently and the dose adjusted accordingly.

Morphine remains the standard against which all other opioids are measured. Constant pain requires continual (around-the-clock) analgesic medication, preferably with a longer-acting drug, as well as a supplementary, shorter-acting medication for breakthrough pain. If frequent supplementation is required, then the maintenance dose of the long-acting analgesic should be increased or the dosing interval decreased. If adequate pain relief cannot be achieved at the maximum recommended dose of one narcotic preparation (or if side effects become intolerable), the patient should be switched to another opioid medication starting at the equivalent dosage (Table 1).

Codeine is usually given in combination with aspirin or acetaminophen. It provides excellent analgesia for mild to moderate pain as well

**TABLE 1 Equianalgesic Doses of Selected Opioids**

| Drug | Route | | Duration |
| --- | --- | --- | --- |
| | Parenteral | Oral | |
| Morphine* | 10 mg | 60 mg* | 3-6 h |
| Extended release morphine (MS Contin, Kadian) | NA | 15 mg | 8-12 h |
| Codeine | 60 mg | 120 mg | 4-6 h |
| Oxycodone (OxyContin, Roxicodone) | NA | 20 mg | 4-6 h |
| Methadone | 10 mg | 15 mg | 6-8 h |
| Fentanyl injectable (Sublimaze) | 100 μg | NA | 1-2 h |
| Fentanyl patch (Duragesic Transdermal) | 25 μg/h | | 1 patch/72 h |
| Hydromorphone (Dilaudid) | 1.5 mg | 7.5 mg | 2-4 h |
| Meperidine (Demerol) | 75 mg | 300 mg | 2-4 h |
| Hydrocodone† (Vicodin, Lortab) | NA | 30 mg | 3-4 h |

*For single or intermittent dosing. For chronic or scheduled dosing, 30 mg.
†Combined with acetaminophen at varying doses of component drugs.
*Abbreviation:* NA = not applicable.

as excellent cough suppression (particularly useful for pleuritic pain management). Oxycodone and propoxyphene (Darvon) are given for moderate to severe pain. Immediate-release and sustained-release morphine sulfate preparations (MS Contin, Kadian) are available as pills or liquid.

Methadone (Dolophine) is very effective when taken orally and suppresses the symptoms of withdrawal from other opioids because of its extended half-life (8-59 hours) and slow release from liver and other tissues. Its analgesic duration (6-8 hours) is much shorter. Tramadol (Ultram) is not an opioid but has similar analgesic properties and is thought to be less addictive. It comes in pill form only.

Hydromorphone (Dilaudid) is a morphine derivative that can be given orally, intramuscularly, subcutaneously, or, with caution, intravenously. It also comes in a rectal suppository formulation. Fentanyl (Sublimaze, Duragesic) can be given parenterally as well as transdermally (Duragesic patch) and transmucosally (Actiq) using a lollipop for drug delivery.

Meperidine (Demerol) is contraindicated in patients with impaired renal function or those taking MAO inhibitors. Meperidine should not be used for more than 48 hours or at doses greater than 600 mg/24 hours because accumulation of the toxic metabolite, normeperidine, can result in seizures.

Patient-controlled analgesia (PCA) has been successfully used in postoperative and terminally ill patients. PCA typically delivers drug via a continuous infusion of an opioid. An agent with a short half-life should be used. Additional doses can be given when the patient pushes a button. The system is set up to limit the total hourly dose that can be delivered to prevent overdosing. PCA can also be provided subcutaneously, intrathecally, or epidurally. It requires an alert, oriented patient who can understand the dosing principle and who can physically push the button. Early studies have shown better pain relief than with conventional analgesic therapy without an increase in the total amount of drug used.

### Adjuvant Analgesics

Successful relief of pain can require more than opioid and nonopioid drugs. In addition to traditional analgesic medications, adjuvant drugs may be used. Antidepressants, anticonvulsants, systemically administered local anesthetics, corticosteroids, neuroleptics, N-methyl-D-aspartate (NMDA) antagonists, and bisphosphonates are often used to enhance pain relief. The choice of adjuvant drug should be directed at the specific type of pain. Adjuvant analgesics are standard therapy for treating diabetic neuropathy, postherpetic neuralgia, and trigeminal neuralgia.

Antidepressant drugs are commonly used to treat neuropathic pain. Tricyclic antidepressants have been widely used for diabetic neuropathy. Low-dose amitriptyline (Elavil) can provide significant relief for some patients. At higher doses, serious side effects including cardiac dysrhythmias can occur, limiting the usefulness of this group of drugs. Currently, the FDA has approved medications for only two neuropathic pain syndromes: gabapentin (Neurontin) and 5% lidocaine patch (Lidoderm) for postherpetic neuralgia and carbamazepine (Tegretol) for trigeminal neuralgia (Table 2).

Bisphosphonates are used for bone pain in cancer patients: pamidronate (Aredia) and zoledronic acid (Zometa) are parenteral formulations that are also useful for treating hypercalcemia. Corticosteroids are also used in cancer patients who have bone, visceral, or neuropathic pain. Additional benefits of corticosteroids include an antiemetic effect, mood elevation, and appetite stimulation. Adjuvant pharmacologic therapy can boost the analgesic effect of opioid and nonopioid medication. This allows a lower dose of the opioid or nonopioid and a lower incidence of their side effects.

## NONPHARMACOLOGIC TREATMENT

### Physical Therapy

Although medications can diminish pain and its concomitant symptoms (fatigue, depression), nonpharmacologic therapies can improve the dysfunction induced by chronic pain. The two most studied nonpharmacologic modalities studied are exercise and cognitive behavior therapy. For musculoskeletal pain, massage, guided mobilization and manipulation, stretching, strengthening, thermotherapy, and neurostimulatory modalities are of value in alleviating pain and maintaining function. Biofeedback, individual counseling, group therapy, and relaxation techniques can provide support and improve the patient's sense of well-being. The challenge is to improve long-term adherence and compliance. The role of

**TABLE 2 Adjuvant Drug-Dosing Regimens**

| Medication | Starting Dose | Maximum Dose | Comments |
| --- | --- | --- | --- |
| Gabapentin (Neurontin) | 300 mg hs | 3600 mg/day (1200 mg q8h) | Can increase by 100-300 mg/d every 7 days. Adjust dose amount and frequency when renal function is impaired |
| 5% Lidocaine (Lidoderm) | 1 patch daily for 12 h | 3 patches daily for 12 h | Do not apply to broken or inflamed skin; caution in patients with impaired liver function |
| Amitriptyline (Elavil) | 10-25 mg hs | 150 mg/day | Start at lowest dose in elderly given anticholinergic side effects; monitor QRS duration |
| Carbamazepine (Tegretol) | 100 mg bid | 600 mg bid | Take with food; therapeutic levels 4-12 μg/mL |

complementary and alternative medicine in managing chronic pain is an area of ongoing research; the original funding in 1992 for the National Institutes of Health Office of Alternative Medicine was $2 million; currently it is more than $115 million.

## Issues in Chronic Pain Management

Chronic pain is seen with chronic disease (e.g., arthritis, AIDS). It can also be seen with one-time injury to the central or peripheral nervous system (e.g., stroke, varicella zoster infection).

Chronic pain persists despite attempts to alleviate it. The duration of pain is not the criterion by which chronic pain is distinguished from acute pain; the criterion is the inability to restore the pain-free state. Chronic pain is not merely a symptom but is itself a disease. The original tissue injury heals, but either central or peripheral sensitization occurs, and there is persistent pain in the absence of apparent damage. The International Association for the Study of Pain defines chronic pain as "an unpleasant sensory and emotional experience associated with actual or potential tissue damage"; the pain experienced might not correlate well with tissue damage.

Some patients experience both acute and chronic pain; cancer patients, for example, can have chemotherapy-induced neuropathy along with acute pain caused by procedures or metastatic spread of disease. Patients with chronic pain can undergo surgery or experience significant trauma, and the acute pain superimposed on chronic pain is challenging to manage.

The long-term use of opioids to treat pain caused by malignant disease is accepted, but there is still resistance to such therapy for pain of nonmalignant origin. Addiction is rare in patients who first use opioids for pain relief. Tolerance and physical dependency are likely with long-term use. Close follow-up is mandatory.

Patients with pain can have concomitant aberrant drug-taking behavior. Addiction manifests as out-of-control behavior, with compulsive and harmful drug use. This needs to be distinguished from pseudoaddiction, which occurs when pain is inadequately treated, driving the patient to unilateral dose increases or use of alcohol or street drugs. Patients with comorbid conditions can benefit from a multidisciplinary approach that includes physical and occupational therapy, social service support, and psychological counseling.

The *four As* of pain management outcomes are *a*nalgesia (pain relief), *a*ctivities of daily living (psychosocial functioning), *a*dverse side effects, and *a*berrant drug-taking behavior (addiction-related activities). These domains should be explicitly assessed, discussed, and documented at each encounter.

### REFERENCES

American Academy of Pain Medicine: Home page. Available at http://www.painmed.org (accessed July 12, 2007).

Furlan AD, Sandoval J, Mailis-Gagnon A, Tunks E: Opioids for chronic noncancer pain: A meta-analysis of effectiveness and side effects. CMAJ 2006;174(11):1589-1594.

Gilron I, Watson CPN, Cahill CM, Moulin DE: Neuropathic pain: A practical guide for the clinician. CMAJ 2006;175(3):265-275.

Loeser JD, Medzack R: Pain: An overview. Lancet 1999;353(9164): 1607-1609.

MedlinePlus: Pain. Available at http://www.nlm.nih.gov/medlineplus/pain.html (accessed July 12, 2007).

Olorunto WA, Galankiuk S: Managing the spectrum of surgical pain: Acute management of the chronic pain patient. J Am Coll Surg 2006;202(1): 169-175.

Passik SD, Weinreb HJ: Managing chronic nonmalignant pain: Overcoming obstacles to the use of opioids. Adv Ther 2000;17(2):70-83.

Schnitzer TJ: Non-NSAID pharmacologic treatment options for the management of chronic pain. Am J Med 1998;105(1B):45S-52S.

Wilson JF: The pain divide between men and women. Ann Intern Med 2006;144(6):461-464.

Woolf CJ: Pain: Moving from symptom control toward mechanism-specific pharmacologic management. Ann Intern Med 2004;140(6):441-451.

# Nausea and Vomiting

Method of
*Chad M. Braun, MD*

Nausea and vomiting are protective reflexes caused by a wide range of etiologies spanning from benign conditions to emergent disorders. Nausea and vomiting can occur independently but most often are associated. Usually nausea precedes vomiting and is often accompanied by skin pallor, increased sweating, and feeling flushed. It is also described as the urge to vomit. Vomiting (emesis) is the forceful oral expulsion of the contents of the stomach. Retching is the repetitive contraction of the muscles of the diaphragm and abdominal wall that often precede or accompany vomiting. Nausea and vomiting are mediated by efferent stimuli from the vomiting center in the brain to the musculature in the abdomen and chest. The neurotransmitters commonly associated with nausea and vomiting are acetylcholine, histamine, serotonin, and dopamine. These neurotransmitters are important in the treatment of persistent or severe nausea and vomiting. Most episodes of nausea and vomiting are acute, self-limited, and easily diagnosed based on the clinical picture. Chronic nausea and vomiting (1 month or more) is a diagnostic and therapeutic challenge for the clinician.

## Differential Diagnosis

Causes of nausea and vomiting are numerous and varied (Table 1). Of these causes, one of the most common is an adverse reaction to a medication. Nonsteroidal anti-inflammatories, chemotherapeutic agents, antidepressants, narcotics, antibiotics, and oral contraceptives are all commonly associated with nausea and vomiting. It is important to note, however, that almost any medication can cause nausea. An accurate medication history thus is very important.

Viral and bacterial infections are another common cause of nausea and vomiting. This manifestation is often as an acute syndrome with fever and diarrhea. Common viral agents are rotavirus, enterovirus, and adenovirus. Bacterial causes such as *Salmonella, Campylobacter,* and *Shigella* are usually seen with the consumption of tainted food or water and can be associated with bloody diarrhea.

Disorders of the gastrointestinal tract can cause nausea and vomiting. Common examples of this are peptic ulcer disease, gastroparesis, dyspepsia, and irritable bowel disease. In addition, gastrointestinal emergencies such as acute appendicitis, acute cholecystitis, mesenteric ischemia, and intestinal obstruction can be associated with nausea and vomiting.

Nausea and vomiting are also exhibited during pregnancy. This is usually most frequent in the first trimester and manifested as "morning sickness." It is most common in the first pregnancy and is usually self-limited. Rarely seen is hyperemesis gravidarum, a condition characterized by intractable vomiting and weight loss that is often accompanied by fluid and electrolyte abnormalities.

 **CURRENT DIAGNOSIS**

- Acute and chronic nausea and vomiting must be differentiated.
- Nausea and vomiting have a wide range of possible causes.
- Control patient symptoms and then look for an underlying etiology.
- Few evidence-based therapy guidelines exist outside of postchemotherapy and postoperative nausea and vomiting.

## TABLE 1 Differential Diagnosis of Nausea and Vomiting

**Medications**

Analgesics—acetaminophen, aspirin, nonsteroidal anti-inflammatory drugs (NSAIDs), rheumatologic and antigout drugs, opioids (codeine, morphine, oxycodone [Roxicodone])

Anesthetic agents—halothane, fentanyl (Sublimaze)

Antiasthmatics—theophylline

Anticonvulsants—phenobarbital, phenytoin (Dilantin)

Antidepressants—selective serotonin reuptake inhibitors (SSRIs)

Antimicrobials—acyclovir (Zovirax), erythromycin, itraconazole (Sporanox), metronidazole (Flagyl), sulfonamides, tetracycline

Antiparkinsonian drugs—levodopa (Dopar), carbidopa (Lodosyn)

Cancer chemotherapy—cisplatin (Platinol-AQ), cyclophosphamide (Cytoxan), dacarbazine (DTIC-Dome), nitrogen mustard

Cardiovascular agents—antiarrhythmics, antihypertensives, β-blockers, calcium channel antagonists, digoxin, diuretics

Corticosteroids—prednisone

Diabetic drugs—sulfonylureas, metformin (Glucophage)

Ergot alkaloids—dihydroergotamine (Migranal), ergotamine (Ergomar), methysergide (Sansert)

Gastrointestinal agents—azathioprine (Imuran), sulfasalazine (Azulfidine)

Hormonal agents—estrogen, progesterone, oral contraceptives

Iron replacement—ferrous sulfate

Substance abuse—alcohol, nicotine

**Infectious Causes**

Gastroenteritis—viral, bacterial, parasitic

Other—otitis media, systemic sepsis

**Gastrointestinal Disorders**

Functional disorders—chronic intestinal pseudo-obstruction, gastroparesis, irritable bowel syndrome, nonulcer dyspepsia

Mechanical obstruction—gastric outlet obstruction, small bowel obstruction

Organic gastrointestinal disorders

Appendicitis

Hepatobiliary disease—biliary colic, cholecystitis, hepatitis, neoplasia

Inflammatory bowel disease—Crohn's disease

Mesenteric ischemia

Peptic diseases—esophagitis, *Helicobacter pylori*, nonulcer dyspepsia, peptic ulcer disease

Pancreatic disease—pancreatitis, pancreatic adenocarcinoma

Paralytic ileus

Peritoneal irritation—peritonitis, metastases

Postoperative gastric surgery

Retroperitoneal fibrosis

**Central Nervous System (CNS) Disorders**

Increased intracranial pressure—abscess, hemorrhage, hydrocephalus, infarction, malignancy, meningitis, pseudotumor cerebri

Demyelinating disorders

Labyrinthine disorders—labyrinthitis, Méniére's disease, motion sickness

Migraine headaches

Parkinsonian disorders

Seizures—complex partial

**Psychologic/Psychiatric Disorders**

Anxiety

Depression

Eating disorders—anorexia nervosa, bulimia nervosa

Pain

Psychogenic vomiting

**Medical Conditions**

Cardiac—acute myocardial infarction, congestive heart failure

Genitourinary—acute nephritis, nephrolithiasis, ovarian torsion, pyelonephritis, testicular torsion

Endocrinologic and metabolic conditions—acute intermittent porphyria, Addison's disease, diabetic ketoacidosis, hypercalcemia, hyperparathyroidism, hyperthyroidism, hypoparathyroidism, uremia

Pregnancy—hyperemesis gravidarum, morning sickness

**Postoperative Nausea and Vomiting**

**Radiation Therapy**

**Idiopathic Conditions**

Cyclic vomiting syndrome

Gastric dysrhythmias

---

Psychological disorders are also associated with nausea and vomiting. These can be seen in anxiety, depression, eating disorders such as anorexia and bulimia, and in psychogenic vomiting. Note that patients with psychogenic vomiting usually maintain a normal level of nutrition because they vomit only a small amount of the ingested food.

Other causes of nausea and vomiting not to be overlooked include central nervous system (CNS) disorders such as acute labyrinthitis, Méniére's disease, and motion sickness. In addition, any condition that causes increased intracranial pressure can cause nausea and vomiting. Further, approximately three fourths of all surgical procedures are complicated by postoperative nausea and vomiting. Most of this is thought to be anesthesia related.

## Clinical Assessment

To narrow the wide differential associated with nausea and vomiting, it is important for the clinician to use a thoughtful approach to determine the underlying cause. Assessment begins with the differentiation of these symptoms from regurgitation (passive retrograde flow of gastric or esophageal contents into the mouth) and rumination (an effortless regurgitation of recently digested food into the mouth followed by spitting or reswallowing). With a thorough history and physical examination, the clinician can determine whether the patient can be effectively treated as an outpatient or requires hospitalization for treatment and further evaluation. To do this, the clinician must effectively characterize the patient's symptoms with special attention to the onset, duration, frequency, and severity of the symptoms. Some sample questions and scenarios follow.

When did the symptoms begin? How long have they been present? Acute causes of nausea and vomiting such as gastroenteritis or an adverse reaction to a medication has a much different course than chronic causes such as gastroparesis or irritable bowel syndrome. When does the vomiting occur? Is it in the morning or after meals? The temporal course is important. Early morning vomiting is often associated with pregnancy and uremia, whereas nausea and vomiting after meals can be seen with a motility disorder or an obstruction. It is also important to explore the character of the vomitus, specifically if it contains food, bile, or blood. In addition, the clinician should query the patient about any exacerbating or alleviating factors and whether or not the patient has experienced any weight loss or recently traveled.

After completing the history, the clinician should perform a focused physical examination. Here the key is to search for any consequences or complications of vomiting and to identify any signs that may point to the cause of the symptoms. Areas to be highlighted would be as follows. Vital signs, mucous membranes, and skin turgor should be examined for signs of dehydration. Bowel sounds should be quantified as normal, hyperactive, or hypoactive. The abdomen should be evaluated for distention and tenderness because specific sites of discomfort can give a clue to a diagnosis. Any visible hernias, surgical scars, or peristalsis should be noted. A neurologic exam should also be performed, including an assessment of the patient's optic fundus and gait. The teeth should be inspected for signs of enamel breakdown. A brief screening for any signs of psychological disease such as anxiety or depression should also be undertaken.

## Diagnostic Testing

The history and physical examination guides the clinician to any further diagnostic testing that is required. Many cases of nausea and vomiting do not require any further testing. If necessary, screening laboratory testing should include serum chemistries, which may detect electrolyte abnormalities, dehydration or uremia, and a complete blood count, which may detect signs of infection. Depending on the clinical picture, an erythrocyte sedimentation rate (ESR), thyroid-stimulating hormone, and liver and pancreatic function testing can be considered. All women of childbearing age should have a pregnancy test. Stool studies can also be considered (e.g., giardiasis). Serum drug levels for toxicity should be considered in appropriate patients.

Further diagnostic testing is dictated by the patient presentation. If any obstruction or perforation is suspected, flat and upright abdominal radiographs can be obtained. Note that these can be normal in early or intermittent obstruction. Further studies such as an upper gastrointestinal barium study or a small bowel followthrough can be helpful if obstruction is considered. Esophagogastroduodenoscopy (EGD) is used to evaluate the mucosa of the esophagus, stomach, and duodenum for signs of inflammation. Additional testing that may be helpful depending on symptomatology includes an abdominal ultrasound, abdominal computed tomography (CT) scan, enteroclysis, and electrogastrography. For hypothesized gastric motility disorders, a gastric emptying study and antroduodenal manometry can be pursued.

If nausea and vomiting are persistent or severe and a gastrointestinal cause is not found, other etiologies such as systemic disease, CNS disorders, and psychological causes must be considered. CNS causes are best evaluated by head CT or magnetic resonance imaging (MRI). MRI provides better visibility of a posterior fossa lesion if that is of concern. Patients with chronic unexplained nausea and vomiting should also be screened for psychiatric disorders. If the clinician has pursued this diagnostic evaluation and is still unsure of the cause of persistent symptoms, consultation with a specialist should be obtained. Most often this would begin with a gastroenterologist but would depend on the symptom picture.

## Treatment

Effective treatment of nausea and vomiting depends on identification and correction of the underlying cause. Most cases of nausea and vomiting require no specific treatment. However, patients may require evaluation for fluid and electrolyte disorders associated with nausea and vomiting. Symptomatic therapy should be based on symptom severity and the clinical presentation. Except in the case of pregnancy or drug overdose, antiemetic agents are often used empirically for relief. Oral rehydration, or intravenous if necessary, can then be pursued. If abdominal pain is also present, surgical consultation may be warranted.

With mild nausea and vomiting, dietary changes may be sufficient. Patients should be counseled to try small amounts (1–4 ounces/serving) of cool, clear liquids and advance as tolerated. A goal of 1 to 2 liters of fluid a day is a good one. If the patient successfully tolerates clear liquids, addition of small portions of easily digested foods such as bananas, rice, bouillon, and toast are in order. Dietary fat content should be reduced. Dairy products should be avoided. The diet can gradually be advanced with easily tolerated foods such as plain chicken

## CURRENT THERAPY

- Most cases of nausea and vomiting do not require any therapy except dietary change.
- Hydration status must be monitored.
- Depending on symptom severity, antiemetics can be given by a variety of routes: oral, intravenous, and rectal.
- Use of medications is often limited by adverse effects.

or turkey and vegetables, bland soups, and fruit. Food should be consumed deliberately, and the patient should take care not to overeat. Increased physical activity around times of eating should be avoided. Note that nausea and vomiting associated with pregnancy can very often be treated with dietary changes alone.

With persistent or severe nausea and vomiting, antiemetic agents may be warranted. Most of these agents are centrally acting and can be divided into nine families (Table 2). By using medications from different families as needed or in combination, the likelihood of adverse drug reactions can be lessened. Because these agents work in the CNS, most adverse effects are also central, such as sedation, lethargy, and extrapyramidal effects. Outside of postoperative and postchemotherapy nausea and vomiting, there are few trials that identify an antiemetic of choice. Commonly used antiemetics are prochlorperazine (Compazine), promethazine (Phenergan), metoclopramide (Reglan), and trimethobenzamide (Tigan).

## Antiemetic Drugs

### SEROTONIN ANTAGONISTS

Ondansetron (Zofran), granisetron (Kytril), and dolasetron (Anzemet), especially when introduced prior to treatment, are effective in the prevention of chemotherapy- and radiation-associated emesis. They are also effective in postoperative nausea and vomiting, but less expensive options (e.g., droperidol [Inapsine] and dexamethasone [Decadron][1]) are equally effective. The serotonin antagonists are usually well tolerated.

### DOPAMINE ANTAGONISTS

The phenothiazines, butyrophenones, and substituted benzamides are all examples of antiemetics that work through dopaminergic blockade. Phenothiazines are often not effective for severe vomiting and have a high incidence of side effects including sedation, hypotension, and extrapyramidal effects. Metoclopramide (Reglan) is more effective for severe nausea and vomiting but again has a high incidence of adverse effects. This agent has been especially effective in treating gastroparesis. It should be noted that droperidol (Inapsine) has been associated with QT prolongation and electrocardiogram (EKG) monitoring is recommended with administration.

### ANTIHISTAMINES AND ANTICHOLINERGICS

Antihistamines and anticholinergics are of value in the prevention of nausea and vomiting associated with inner ear disturbances, motion sickness, vertigo, and migraines. They often cause drowsiness.

### BENZODIAZEPINES

These medications can be helpful in psychogenic and anticipatory vomiting.

[1]Not FDA approved for this indication.

## TABLE 2 Commonly Used Medications for Nausea and Vomiting

| Class/Medication | Usual Dosage | Route(s) | Adverse Effects |
|---|---|---|---|
| **Anticholinergic** | | | |
| Scopolamine (Transderm Scop) | 1 patch every 3 d | Transdermal | Dry mouth, drowsiness, impaired eye accommodation; rare: disorientation, memory disturbance, dizziness, hallucinations |
| **Antihistamines** | | | |
| Diphenhydramine (Benadryl) | 25-50 mg q4-6h | IM, IV, PO | Sedation, dry mouth, constipation, confusion, blurred vision, urinary retention |
| Hydroxyzine (Atarax, Vistaril) | 25-100 mg q6h | IM, PO | |
| Meclizine (Antivert) | 25-50 mg q6h | PO | |
| Promethazine (Phenergan) | 12.5-25 mg q4-6h | IM, IV, PO, PR | |
| **Benzamides** | | | |
| Metoclopramide (Reglan) | 5-15 mg q6h | IM, IV, PO | Sedation, restlessness, diarrhea, agitation, central nervous depression, extrapyramidal effects, hypotension, neuroleptic syndrome, supraventricular tachycardia |
| Trimethobenzamide (Tigan) | 250 mg q6-8h | IM, PO, PR | |
| **Benzodiazepines** | | | |
| Lorazepam (Ativan)[1] | 0.5-2.5 mg q8-12h | IM, IV, PO | Sedation, amnesia, respiratory depression, ataxia, blurred vision, hallucinations, emotional reactions |
| **Butyrophenones** | | | |
| Droperidol (Inapsine) | 0.625-1.25 mg q3-4h[3] | IM, IV | Sedation, hypotension, tachycardia, extrapyramidal effects, dizziness, blood pressure increase, hallucinations, chills, QT prolongation, torsade de pointes |
| Haloperidol (Haldol)[1] | 05.-5 mg q8h | IM, IV, PO | |
| **Cannabinoids** | | | |
| Dronabinol (Marinol) | 2.5-5 mg q8h | PO | Drowsiness, euphoria, vision difficulties, somnolence, vasodilation, abnormal thinking, dysphoria, diarrhea, flushing, tremor, myalgias |
| **Corticosteroids** | | | |
| Dexamethasone (Decadron)[1] | 4 mg q6h | IM, IV, PO | Gastrointestinal upset, anxiety, insomnia, hyperglycemia, facial flushing, euphoria, peritoneal itching |
| **Phenothiazines** | | | |
| Chlorpromazine (Thorazine) | 10-25 mg q4-6h | IM, PO, PR | Sedation, lethargy, skin irritation, cardiovascular effects, extrapyramidal effects, cholestatic jaundice, hyperprolactinemia, neuroleptic malignant syndrome, blood abnormalities |
| Prochlorperazine (Compazine) | 5-10 (25PR) mg q6h | IM, IV, PO, PR | |
| Thiethylperazine (Torecan) | 10-20 mg q6h[3] | IM, IV, PO | |
| **5-HT3 Serotonin Antagonists** | | | |
| Ondansetron (Zofran) | 8 mg q8h | IV, PO | Headache, constipation, fever, asthenia, arrhythmias, diarrhea, dizziness, ataxia, tremor, somnolence, thirst, nervousness, elevated hepatic transaminases |
| Granisetron (Kytril) | 2 mg per 24 h | IV, PO | |
| Dolasetron (Anzemet) | 100 mg per 24 h | IV, PO | |

[1]Not FDA approved for this indication.
[3]Exceeds dosage recommended by manufacturer.
*Abbreviations:* IM = intramuscular; IV = intravenous; PO = orally; PR = per rectum.

## CORTICOSTEROIDS

Dexamethasone (Decadron)[1] is commonly used in combination with other antiemetics. Use of steroids and serotonin antagonists is effective in chemotherapy-associated nausea and vomiting, and steroids and low-dose droperidol (Inapsine) is useful in postoperative nausea and vomiting.

## CANNABINOIDS

Marijuana is used as an antiemetic and an appetite stimulant. Its efficacy is increased when combined with prochlorperazine (Compazine).

[1]Not FDA approved for this indication.

Dronabinol (Marinol) is a synthetic cannabinoid available by prescription. CNS side effects are very common with these drugs.

## NONPHARMACOLOGIC OPTIONS

Note that both ginger and acupressure are effective in the treatment of nausea and vomiting.

# Special Circumstances

## CHEMOTHERAPY INDUCED

Attempt to treat patients prophylactically to avoid nausea and vomiting. Use combination therapy. Try to avoid using medications from the same family to decrease the chance of adverse reactions. Note that chemotherapy-induced emesis may begin as long as 24 hours post treatment and may require therapy for 4 to 7 days.

## DIABETES

Use promotility agents such as metoclopramide (Reglan) for gastroparesis-associated nausea and vomiting.

## PREGNANCY

Morning sickness is common in the first trimester of pregnancy but usually resolves by the second. Reassurance, frequent small meals, and dietary changes are usually sufficient. For some patients, pyridoxine (vitamin $B_6$)[1] is helpful. In most cases, antiemetics are avoided in pregnancy. In severe cases involving protracted symptoms and fluid and electrolyte abnormalities (hyperemesis gravidarum), hospitalization and intravenous hydration may be required. No antiemetics are approved for use in pregnancy. Selection of any medication to be used in pregnancy should be with careful consideration of the severity of symptoms and potential risk to the fetus. Meclizine (Antivert) and promethazine (Phenergan) are used in pregnancy but neither is FDA-approved for this indication.

## MOTION SICKNESS

Anticholinergics and antihistamines are effective here. Transdermal scopolamine patches (Transderm Scop) are convenient for those exposed to motion for long periods (cruise ships).

## POSTOPERATIVE

Approximately 80% of patients who undergo anesthesia experience nausea and vomiting in the perioperative or postoperative period. Serotonin antagonists or combination therapy with dexamethasone (Decadron)[1] and droperidol (Inapsine) are effective here.

## REFERENCES

American Gastroenterological Association: Medical position statement: Nausea and vomiting. Gastroenterology 2001;120(1):261-262.
Anthony L: Nausea and vomiting. *Conn's Current Therapy*, 2004.
Hasler WL, Chung O: Approach to the patient with gastrointestinal disease. *Harrison's Principles of Internal Medicine*, 16th ed. 2005.
McQuaid KR: Nausea and vomiting. *Current Medical Diagnosis and Treatment*. 2006.
Miser WF: Nausea and vomiting. *Conn's Current Therapy*. 2005.
Pasricha PJ: Treatment of disorders of bowel motility and water flux; antiemetics; agents used in biliary and pancreatic disease. *Goodman and Gilman's The Pharmacological Basis of Therapeutics*, 11th ed. 2005.

# Gaseousness and Indigestion

Method of
*Ram Dickman, MD, and Ronnie Fass, MD*

## Gaseousness

Gaseousness includes bloating, belching, and flatulence, which are among the most common gastrointestinal symptoms reported by patients who seek their physician's advice and especially by those with functional bowel disorders. Despite the clinical importance of gaseousness, the pathophysiology of this disorder is not fully understood. Bloating and flatulence are frequently attributed to excess gas within the gut lumen; however, gas transit studies in patients with bloating have not demonstrated an increased amount of gas within the gut. The current mainstays of treatment of gaseousness include lifestyle and diet modifications.

## BLOATING

*Abdominal bloating* is a sensation of a swollen or distended abdomen. The term is sometimes used to describe a sensation of excess gas or a full belly.

Abdominal bloating may affect between 10% and 30% of the general population. Bloating is a very common complaint, especially in patients with functional bowel disorders, such as irritable bowel syndrome (IBS) and functional dyspepsia (FD).

### Objective Evidence

The gastrointestinal lumen of a normal subject contains less than 200 mL of gas, which is a combination of swallowed air ($N_2$, $O_2$) and gases that are produced during acid neutralization ($CO_2$) and bacterial fermentation ($H_2$, methane, $CO_2$). Measurement of a patient's abdominal girth using abdominal impedance plethysmography allows objective assessment of reports of bloating.

Studies in IBS patients show a greater 24-hour fluctuation in abdominal girth as compared to healthy controls. Abdominal distention (objective parameter) peaks 4 to 6 hours before bedtime and was correlated with bloating (subjective parameter) only in the subgroup of patients with constipation-predominant IBS. However, in other subgroups of IBS patients, there was no association between symptoms and changes in abdominal girth.

Interestingly, studies that assessed intestinal gas dynamics found that IBS patients have delayed transit of gas along the gut and a significant increase in gas retention as compared to controls. Specifically, gas retention within the jejunum seems to be the main cause for the patients' symptoms. However, other studies found that the total amount of gas within the gut in symptomatic patients (mainly IBS) who complained of bloating was the same as in asymptomatic controls. In one study, for example, during gas infusion into the gut, patients

---

 **CURRENT DIAGNOSIS**

**Gaseousness**

- History: drugs (narcotics, calcium channel blockers, anticholinergics), surgery (vagotomy, adhesions, Nissan fundoplication), diabetes, celiac sprue, intestinal myopathies, diet (consumption of starch, lactose, fructose, sorbitol, beans, cabbage, cauliflower, Brussels sprouts)
- Alarm symptoms: weight loss, anemia, anorexia, fever, and gastrointestinal bleeding
- Blood tests: complete blood count, glucose and electrolytes, thyroid-stimulating hormone
- Upper or lower endoscopy and/or 24-hour pH monitoring
- Breath testing for lactose and fructose intolerance

**Indigestion**

- Upper endoscopy with biopsies for *Helicobacter pylori*
- 24-hour pH monitoring
- Gastric emptying rate measurement
- Water-load test
- Psychological evaluation

---

[1]Not FDA approved for this indication.

with IBS and bloating complained of greater discomfort and gaseousness than did controls. Thus, it appears that the key mechanism for bloating in patients with functional bowel disorders is an abnormal perception of intestinal gas.

## BELCHING

Belching is the expulsion of gas from the stomach while retaining solid and fluid material. Occasional belching is a normal physiologic process aimed to remove air from the stomach, typically during or after meals. The air is commonly swallowed during meals or introduced into the stomach through carbonated beverages and other food products. Repetitive belching not related to meals is secondary to esophageal air aspiration. Excessive belching is almost always associated with functional gastrointestinal disorders (functional dyspepsia and aerophagia) and with gastroesophageal reflux disease (GERD). Patients may also complain of an inability to belch. Common causes of the latter include esophageal achalasia and post-Nissan fundoplication ("gas-bloat syndrome"). In one large study, 17% of 8351 healthy subjects reported having excessive belching with a similar frequency in men and women.

### Patient Evaluation

Evaluation of patients with excessive belching is appropriate only if an underlying organic cause is suspected and should include an upper endoscopy, esophageal pH monitoring, and esophageal manometry (the latter to rule out achalasia). Radiographic studies of the esophagus and stomach may also be helpful in patients with co-morbid factors.

## FLATULENCE

Studies of healthy subjects found that the frequency of flatus passed per day ranges from 10 to 14 times. Flatus volume is difficult to measure in clinical practice. Thus, clinicians should rely on their patient's reported average frequency of flatus episodes per day over a predetermined period of time (1 to 2 weeks).

Increased flatus production (more than 22 times per day) may be caused by malabsorption of carbohydrates in patients with celiac sprue, pancreatic insufficiency, and short bowel syndrome. Additionally, in susceptible patients, malabsorption of lactose, fructose, sorbitol, and starch can result in excessive flatus production because of colonic bacterial fermentation of these unabsorbable carbohydrates.

### CLINICAL ASSESSMENT

The clinical assessment of gaseousness is aimed to rule out more serious conditions that have clinical manifestations similar to benign functional bowel disorders.

### TREATMENT

Treatment of gaseousness includes recommendations to reduce ingestion of gas-forming food products and drugs that facilitate intestinal passage. Patients need to reduce air swallowing (aerophagia) by avoidance of carbonated beverages, gum chewing, and smoking and by drinking from a straw. Dietary modifications include avoidance of dietary fibers, caffeine, cabbage, Brussels sprouts, beans, broccoli, and cauliflower. Loperamide (Imodium) may increase intestinal fluid absorption in patients with rapid transit. Tegaserod (Zelnorm) may improve bloating in constipation-predominant IBS patients. Antibiotics may be beneficial in the case of bloating caused by bacterial overgrowth.

# Indigestion (Dyspepsia)

Dyspepsia is a persistent or recurrent pain or discomfort in the epigastrium associated with a feeling of fullness, early satiety, bloating, belching, and nausea. It is estimated that up to 40% of the adults in the United States experience dyspeptic symptoms at least once a year.

## CURRENT THERAPY

**Gaseousness**
- Bloating and flatulence
  - Reduce air swallowing (avoidance of carbonated beverages, gum chewing, smoking; drinking from a straw)
  - Dietary modifications (avoidance of dietary fibers, caffeine, beans, cabbage, broccoli, cauliflower)
  - Loperamide (Imodium), 2 mg PO 1–2/d, for malabsorption because of rapid transit
  - Tegaserod (Zelnorm), 6 mg PO 2/d, for constipation-predominant irritable bowel syndrome
  - Short courses of antibiotics for bacterial overgrowth
  - Simethicone (Mylicon)
- Belching
  - Reduce air swallowing

**Indigestion**

**DYSPEPSIA**
- Prokinetics
  - Metoclopramide (Reglan),[1] 10 mg PO 1–3/d
  - Tegaserod (Zelnorm),[1] 6 mg PO 3/d
  - Domperidone (Motilium),* 40 mg PO 3/d
- Proton pump inhibitors (PPIs)
  - Omeprazole (Prilosec),[1] 20 mg PO 1–2/d
  - Rabeprazole (AcipHex),[1] 20 mg PO 1–2/d
  - Pantoprazole (Protonix),[1] 40 mg PO 1–2/d
  - Lansoprazole (Prevacid),[1] 30 mg PO 1–2/d
  - Esomeprazole (Nexium),[1] 40 mg PO 1–2/d
- Combination PO therapy for *H. pylori* infection: 10–14 d: PPI 2/d + 1 g amoxicillin 2/d + 500 mg clarithromycin 2/d

**FUNCTIONAL DYSPEPSIA**
- Antidepressants
  - Nortriptyline (Aventyl/Pamelor),[1] amitriptyline (Elavil/Endep),[1] Doxepin (Sinequan), 50 mg PO qhs
  - Trazodone (Desyrel), 100–150 mg PO 1/d
- Hypnotherapy
- Psychological treatments

---

[1]Not FDA approved for this indication.
*Investigational drug in the United States.
*Abbreviation:* PO = orally.

## ETIOLOGY

In most of the patients with dyspepsia (60%), no significant organic finding underlies patients' symptoms. These patients are defined as having functional dyspepsia. Other causes include peptic ulcer disease (15% to 25%), *Helicobacter pylori* infection (30% to 60%), GERD, gastric cancer, and nonsteroidal anti-inflammatory drug (NSAID) use. The underlying mechanisms for functional dyspepsia include antral hypomotility, impaired gastric accommodation, disordered gastric electrical activity, and visceral hypersensitivity. Additionally, studies found that psychological co-morbidity (anxiety, neuroses, and depression) are more common in FD than in controls.

## CLINICAL ASSESSMENT

Because of the many symptoms included in the category of dyspepsia, the clinical evaluation of dyspeptic patients implies that many other conditions are included in the differential diagnosis such as gastroesophageal reflux disease, *H. pylori* infection, and gastric cancer.

Consequently, an appropriate workup for patients with dyspepsia may include upper endoscopy, 24-hour esophageal pH monitoring, *H. pylori* assessment, gastric emptying studies, and the water-load test. In patients with functional dyspepsia, psychological consultation is an important part of the patient's evaluation.

## TREATMENT

Physicians should tailor their treatment approach to dyspepsia according to the severity and frequency of the patient's symptoms. Evaluation for psychosocial abnormalities may be essential in a significant subset of dyspeptic patients. Although not systematically validated, therapeutic recommendations include dietary and lifestyle modifications such as eating smaller and frequent meals and avoiding foods with high fat and fiber content. Antisecretory medications, promotility drugs, and pain modulators should be considered in the proper clinical scenario. Hypnotherapy is more effective in FD patients as compared to medical therapy. Psychological intervention is an essential therapeutic modality in patients with psychological disturbances.

## REFERENCES

Kellow J, Lee OY, Chang FY, et al: An Asia-Pacific, double blind, placebo controlled randomised study to evaluate the efficacy, safety, and tolerability of Tegaserod in patients with irritable bowel syndrome. Gut 2003;52:671-676.

Mertz H, Fass R, Krodner A, et al: Effect of amitriptyline on symptoms, sleep, and visceral perception in patients with functional dyspepsia. Am J Gastroenterol 1998;93:160-165.

Moayyedi P, Forman D, Braunholtz D, et al: The proportion of upper gastrointestinal symptoms in the community associated with *Helicobacter pylori*, lifestyle factors, and nonsteroidal anti-inflammatory drugs. Leeds HELP Study Group. Am J Gastroenterol 2000;95:1448-1455.

Salvioli B, Serra J, Azpiroz F, et al: Origin of gas retention and symptoms in patients with bloating. Gastroenterology 2005;128:574-579.

Serra J, Azpiroz F, Malagelada JR, et al: Impaired transit and tolerance of intestinal gas in the irritable bowel syndrome. Gut 2001;48:14-19.

Talley NJ, Vakil NB, Moayyedi P: American Gastroenterological Association technical review on the evaluation of dyspepsia. Gastroenterology 2005;129:1756-1780.

# Hiccups

Method of
*Michael J. Pollack, MD*

Hiccups are a common and usually benign phenomenon that affects nearly everyone at some time. It is more accurately termed *singultus*, derived from the Latin word *singult*, which means the act of catching one's breath while sobbing. Hiccups are caused by synchronous contractions of the diaphragmatic and intercostal muscles followed by the immediate and sudden closure of the glottis. The forcefully inspired air meeting the closed glottis creates the hiccup sound. Most episodes are transient and resolve without medical therapy. Rarely, hiccups are the only symptom of a serious systemic illness. The role of the practitioner is to know when to initiate the appropriate workup and how to treat the hiccups until the underlying problem, if identified, is resolved.

## Classification

Hiccups can be classified as transient, persistent, or chronic. An episode of hiccups that lasts less than 1 day is transient. This type of episode is usually a benign, often physiologic phenomenon. An episode lasting up to 1 month is deemed persistent. Beyond this time it is considered chronic. Practically speaking, hiccups should be viewed as either transient or chronic. Most people experience some

form of hiccups throughout their lives. The majority of these episodes are a transient nuisance. Chronic hiccups are quite rare with an estimated prevalence of approximately 1 in 100,000 people but can lead to significant adverse effects including malnutrition, weight loss, fatigue, and generalized debilitation. Those patients who present to their practitioner with hiccups most often experience them chronically. Hiccups can occur in utero, but they have no known physiologic function. Chronic hiccups occur more often in males, but transient hiccups affect both males and females equally.

## Mechanism

The precise mechanism of hiccups is unknown. Three neural pathways are described in the hiccup reflex: afferent (phrenic and vagus nerves); a poorly characterized hiccup center in the brainstem; and efferent (phrenic, vagus, cervical, and thoracic nerves). The hiccup center is thought to involve a complex interaction among the brainstem, respiratory centers, phrenic nerve nuclei, the reticular activating center, and the hypothalamus. Theoretically, pathology in or around any of these areas can trigger hiccups. The frequency of hiccups is known to increase with a decline in arterial $PCO_2$ and to decrease as $PCO_2$ rises. This is the physiologic basis for the home remedy of breathing into a paper bag to stop hiccups.

## Etiology

Transient hiccups are usually caused by overdistention of the stomach by air (such as during endoscopy), overeating, eating too fast, or alcohol or tobacco use; these typically resolve without medical therapy. Other benign causes include sudden changes in ambient or gastrointestinal temperature, sudden excitement, or emotional stress. Chronic hiccups may be caused by many underlying processes (Table 1). Processes affecting either the vagus or the phrenic nerve are the most common cause. Examples of precipitating irritants include foreign bodies in contact with the tympanic membrane (auricular branch of the vagus), pharyngitis, laryngitis or neck tumors (recurrent laryngeal nerve of the vagus), mediastinal masses, subdiaphragmatic abscesses, and gastroesophageal reflux (phrenic nerve).

Central nervous system (CNS) disorders, toxic-metabolic disorders, and psychogenic factors are also implicated, to some extent, in the etiology of hiccups. CNS disorders include structural, vascular, and infectious processes. Toxic-metabolic disorders include uremia, alcoholic intoxication, and general anesthetic agents. Psychogenic factors associated with both transient and persistent hiccups include stress, anxiety, and even malingering.

## Medical Evaluation

The approach to the patient with an attack of hiccups depends on its duration. Transient hiccups are both common and benign and do not require investigation. However, chronic hiccups may be the only symptom of an underlying medical condition, and they require a thorough evaluation. The initial approach to identify the cause of chronic hiccups is a complete patient history and comprehensive physical

### CURRENT DIAGNOSIS

- Hiccups are usually transient and benign.
- The hiccup reflex arc, which consists of afferent/efferent phrenic and vagus nerves as well as a poorly characterized hiccup center in the brainstem, is key in understanding the underlying cause.
- Chronic hiccups may be a symptom of a serious underlying condition and warrant a thorough medical evaluation.

## TABLE 1  Selected Causes of Persistent Hiccups

| Phrenic/Vagus Nerve Irritation | CNS Disorders | Toxic-Metabolic Disorders | Postoperative Factors | Drugs | Psychogenic Factors |
|---|---|---|---|---|---|
| Pharyngitis | Meningitis | Alcohol | General anesthesia | Barbiturates | Stress |
| Laryngitis | Encephalitis | Uremia | Tracheal intubation | Steroids | Excitement |
| Pneumonia | Cerebrovascular | Hypoglycemia | Neck extension | Benzodiazepine | Malingering |
| Esophagitis | accident | Hyponatremia | Gastric distention | Methyldopa | Conversion |
| Aortic aneurysm | Arteriovenous | Hypocalcemia | Organ manipulation | | |
| Mediastinal | malformation | Septicemia | | | |
| tumors | Brain abscess | | | | |
| Pancreatitis | Neoplasms | | | | |
| Peptic ulcer | Trauma | | | | |
| disease | Temporal arteritis | | | | |
| Subphrenic | Multiple sclerosis | | | | |
| abscess | Hydrocephalus | | | | |
| Myocardial | Ventriculoperitoneal | | | | |
| infarction | shunts | | | | |
| Gallbladder | | | | | |
| disease | | | | | |
| Gastric | | | | | |
| distention | | | | | |

*Abbreviation:* CNS = central nervous system.

examination, with a focus on the duration, frequency, alleviating factors, and aggravating factors.

Laboratory tests should start with a complete blood count and renal function with full electrolyte panel. A chest radiograph is important to aid in the detection of possible anatomic irritants to the phrenic or vagus nerves. An electrocardiogram helps detect pericardial disease or even pacemaker dysfunction. If the radiograph and electrocardiogram are unrevealing, second-level testing should be pursued guided by the relevant history and clinical findings, including a computed tomography of the head, chest, and abdomen; lumbar puncture; upper endoscopy; or bronchoscopy. Further testing, if required, would include magnetic resonance imaging of the head, an electroencephalogram, pulmonary function tests, and esophageal manometry.

## Treatment

Because chronic hiccups are usually a sign of an underlying systemic disease, priority should be given to treating the condition. For example, proton pump inhibitors can be used if gastroesophageal reflux is implicated, or systemic chemotherapy can be administered if a neoplasm is detected.

When a cause cannot be determined and hiccups persist, empirical therapy is warranted. It can be used to palliate chronic, transient, or persistent hiccups while treatment of the underlying condition is ongoing.

No single modality or agent is universally accepted as the treatment of choice.

Interventions can be divided into pharmacologic (Table 2) and nonpharmacologic therapies (Table 3). Examples of nonpharmacologic treatments include the age-old and well-known home remedies that include breath holding, breathing into a paper bag, swallowing a teaspoon of sugar, the Valsalva maneuver, and gargling with ice water. Some of these maneuvers have a physiologic basis because they are based on an attempt to interrupt the vagally mediated afferent limb of the hiccup reflex arc.

Several drugs are successful anecdotally in the treatment of hiccups. The most widely used agent is chlorpromazine (Thorazine), a phenothiazine antipsychotic. It is the only agent that has achieved U.S. Food and Drug Administration (FDA) approval for treatment of hiccups.

## CURRENT THERAPY

- Most transient hiccups resolve spontaneously.
- Numerous nonpharmacologic and pharmacologic therapies are proposed for treating chronic hiccups.
- Although symptom control is important, a search for an underlying etiology is essential.

## TABLE 2  Pharmacotherapy for Persistent Hiccups

| Antipsychotics | Anticonvulsants | Muscle Relaxants | Dopamine Antagonists | Antidepressants |
|---|---|---|---|---|
| Chlorpromazine (Thorazine) | Phenytoin (Dilantin)[1] | Baclofen (Kemstro)[1] | Metoclopramide (Reglan)[1] | Amitriptyline (Elavil)[1] |
| Haloperidol (Haldol)[1] | Carbamazepine (Tegretol)[1] | Cyclobenzaprine (Flexeril)[1] | | |
| | Valproic acid (Depakene)[1] | | | |
| | Gabapentin (Neurontin)[1] | | | |

[1]Not FDA approved for this indication.

## TABLE 3  Home Remedies to Treat Hiccups

Breath holding
Forcible traction on the tongue
Direct pharyngeal stimulation
Biting on a lemon
Valsalva maneuver
Ice-water gargles
Swallowing granulated sugar
Fright
Breathing into a bag
Rubbing back of neck (C5 dermatome)

Chlorpromazine is a centrally acting agent whose precise mechanism in terminating hiccups is unknown. Intravenous administration is considered to be most effective and frequently used in an emergency department setting. Its side effects include hypotension, dystonic reactions, and excessive drowsiness. These are usually rare occurrences and avoidable if the drug is administered slowly. Oral formulations in doses of 25 to 50 mg three to four times daily as needed can be used up to 7 to 10 days. Metoclopramide (Reglan),[1] a dopamine antagonist and promotility agent, is often used when chlorpromazine does not alleviate the hiccups. It has a more favorable side-effect profile but is not as effective as chlorpromazine. The usual dose is 10 mg three to four times a day. Baclofen (Kemstro),[1] an analogue of γ-aminobutyric acid, has shown some success in limited case series, and it has fewer side effects than the other agents used to treat hiccups. The usual dosage is 10 mg three times a day. Various anticonvulsants, antidepressants, and CNS agents are all reported to terminate intractable hiccups. When the therapies just cited fail, both nonconventional and invasive modalities may be successful. Both hypnosis and acupuncture have been tried, and case reports laud their success. Phrenic nerve blocking and crushing are successful as well. Diaphragmatic pacing ameliorates those afflicted with chronic hiccups.

In summary, hiccups are a common annoyance that most people experience at some point in their lives. Their self-limiting nature usually obviates the need for medical intervention. Hiccups rarely are chronic and can be the sole symptom of a serious underlying condition. The approach to the management of patients with symptomatic hiccups is the search for and treatment of the underlying problem as well as the implementation of the numerous methods known to resolve hiccups.

### REFERENCES

Friedman NL: Hiccups: A treatment review. Pharmacotherapy 1996;16:986-995.
Kolodzik PW, Eilers MA: Hiccups: Review and approach to management. Ann Emerg Med 1991;20:565-573.
Lewis JH: Hiccups: Causes and cures. J Clin Gastroenterol 1985;7:539-552.
Rousseau P: Hiccups. South Med J 1195;88:175-181.
Souadjian J, Cain J. Intractable hiccups: Etiological factors in 220 cases. Postgrad Med 1968;43:72-77.

# Acute Infectious Diarrhea

Method of
*Matthew T. Oughton, MD, FRCPC, and Andre Dascal, MD, FRCPC*

Diarrhea is defined as production of at least 200 g of stool per day. However, accurate measurement of stool mass is impractical and is most often used only in clinical trials. A more functional definition of diarrhea is an increase in stool frequency and liquidity compared to the patient's usual bowel habit. Diarrhea is generally classified as acute if it lasts no more than 14 days, persistent if longer than 14 days, and chronic if longer than 30 days.

Clinically, there are two major types of diarrhea. Secretory diarrhea is watery, is usually produced in large volumes, and contains little or no blood or leukocytes. Inflammatory diarrhea is bloody, usually has leukocytes, and is produced in smaller volumes. Recognizing the class of diarrhea can be useful in suggesting etiologies and in managing the diarrhea.

The precise cause of a case of diarrhea is usually difficult to ascertain, because diarrhea is a nonspecific reaction by the intestine to numerous insults, including infections, toxins, and autoimmune disorders. Acute infectious diarrhea, by definition, is caused by a microbial pathogen. Although infections are the leading cause of diarrhea, many different pathogens cause acute infectious diarrhea, and the likelihood of any particular agent depends on the patient's age, symptoms, and epidemiologic risk factors (Boxes 1 and 2).

In immunocompetent adults in the developed world, acute infectious diarrhea is most often a minor and self-resolving ailment. Recent data for the United States estimate an annual burden of between 211 million and 375 million cases, with more than 900,000 hospitalizations and 6000 deaths. However, acute infectious diarrhea can cause severe illness in infants, immunocompromised patients, and malnourished patients; it remains a major cause of global morbidity and mortality. The World Health Organization (WHO) estimates that more than 4 billion cases of acute infectious diarrhea occur each year

## BOX 1  Clinical History for Acute Infectious Diarrhea

- Description of diarrhea
  - Duration
  - Frequency
  - Presence of blood, pus, "grease" in stool
  - Symptoms of fever, tenesmus, dehydration
  - Weight loss
- Other GI symptoms
  - Anorexia
  - Cramping
  - Emesis
  - Nausea
- Previous episodes with similar symptoms
- Ill contacts with similar symptoms
- Recent antibiotic exposure
- Other medication exposure
  - Anticholinergics
  - Antimotility agents
  - Aspirin (ASA)
  - Proton pump inhibitors (PPIs)
- Recent dietary history
  - Shellfish
  - Undercooked meat (chicken)
  - Unsanitary water
- Animal contacts
  - Turtles
  - Other reptiles
- Travel history
  - Travel to endemic or epidemic areas
- Sexual history
- Vaccination history
- Contact with institutions, e.g., hospitals, nursing homes, daycare facilities
- Employment history
- Immune status
  - Presence of HIV
  - Presence of other congenital or acquired immunodeficiencies

___
[1]Not FDA approved for this indication.

## BOX 2  Physical Examination for Acute Infectious Diarrhea

- Vital signs
  - Blood pressure (look for postural changes)
  - Heart rate (look for postural changes)
  - Respiratory rate
  - Temperature
  - Weight (particularly useful to assess effects of rehydration)
- Cardiovascular examination
  - Volume status (jugular venous pressure)
- Respiratory examination
- Rule out hyperventilation (compensatory respiratory alkalosis for metabolic acidosis due to dehydration and loss of bicarbonate)
- Abdominal examination
  - Focal tenderness
  - Guarding
  - Hepatosplenomegaly
  - Consider rectal examination (look for bloody stool)
- Integument examination
  - Lymphadenopathy
  - Rashes (rose spots)

## BOX 3  Etiologic Agents of Predominantly Secretory Diarrhea

**Bacterial**
- Enteroaggregative *Escherichia coli* (EAEC)
- Enterotoxigenic *E. coli* (ETEC)
- *Vibrio cholerae*

**Viral**
- Adenovirus (types 40 and 41)
- Astrovirus
- Caliciviruses (Norwalk, Sapporo)
- Rotavirus

**Protozoal**
- *Cryptosporidium*
- *Cyclospora*
- *Dientamoeba fragilis*
- *Giardia lamblia*
- *Isospora belli*
- Microspora species (especially *Enterocytozoon bieneusi*)

worldwide and attributes 2 million deaths (5% of all deaths) to diarrheal diseases annually. Most of these deaths are in children who are younger than 5 years and live in developing countries.

Thorough investigation of a patient with acute diarrhea should include a detailed history, physical examination, and laboratory tests (see Boxes 1 and 2). In general, clinical investigation of an individual case of acute infectious diarrhea is more useful in identifying sequelae of diarrhea, such as dehydration, than it is in revealing the exact etiologic agent. However, identification of the causative organism can sometimes reveal the existence of a common-source outbreak. One well-known example occurred in 1994, when the state public health laboratory in Minnesota noted an increase in *Salmonella* serotype enteritidis detected in submitted samples; this ultimately led to the recognition of a multistate *Salmonella* outbreak related to improperly cleaned ice cream trucks.

## Etiology

It is uncommon to identify the exact etiologic agent in a case of acute infectious diarrhea. However, in some clinical situations, exact identification is important for determining optimal management or possible sequelae. The treatment of inflammatory diarrhea varies depending on the causative organism, and some diseases require alterations in therapy (e.g., suspected *Campylobacter* resistance to fluoroquinolones) or even avoidance of antibiotic therapy (e.g., enterohemorrhagic *Escherichia coli*, in which antibiotic therapy has been associated with more frequent adverse outcomes) (Boxes 3 and 4).

### BACTERIA

#### *Escherichia coli*

*E. coli* is a versatile pathogen that causes a wide spectrum of disease affecting numerous organ systems. This is illustrated by the wide variety of diarrheagenic *E. coli*, including enterotoxigenic (ETEC), enteroaggregative (EAEC), enterohemorrhagic (EHEC), enteropathogenic (EPEC), and enteroinvasive (EIEC) strains. In general, people are exposed to diarrheagenic *E. coli* by consuming contaminated food and water.

ETEC is a major cause of infantile diarrhea and traveler's diarrhea. Infantile diarrhea affects infants usually in developing countries, particularly during warm and wet conditions, and traveler's diarrhea

affects the immunologically naive tourist under similar conditions. In both cases, a large inoculum is required to cause disease. Major virulence factors of ETEC strains include species-specific fimbriae for enterocyte adherence, as well as heat-stable and heat-labile plasmid-encoded enterotoxins. After a relatively brief incubation period of 1 to 2 days, the infected patient develops a secretory diarrhea that lasts up to 5 days. The cornerstones of management are prevention (through dietary hygiene) and adequate rehydration. Antibiotics use is controversial and usually reserved for moderate to severe disease.

EAEC is recognized as a major cause of children's and traveler's diarrhea. Since the initial identification of EAEC in 1985, studies have identified numerous putative virulence factors, including specific aggregative adherence fimbriae. However, no one factor has been identified in all EAEC strains. This suggests that apart from their aggregative adherence to enterocytes, EAEC strains are probably a heterogeneous collection. However, the clinical disease caused by EAEC is relatively consistent and includes persistent secretory diarrhea with low-grade fever. Management of disease from EAEC requires adequate rehydration; the role of antibiotics remains controversial.

The notorious virulence of EHEC (also known as Shiga-like toxin–producing *E. coli*) has led to frequent media reports of "hamburger disease." *E. coli* O157:H7 is the most common strain of EHEC, although several others have been documented. Unlike most other categories of diarrheagenic *E. coli*, EHEC can cause disease with

## BOX 4  Etiologic Agents of Predominantly Inflammatory Diarrhea

**Bacterial**
- *Aeromonas* sp.
- *Bacteroides fragilis* (enterotoxigenic strains)
- *Campylobacter* sp. (particularly FQ-resistant strains)
- *Clostridium difficile* (toxigenic strains)
- *Escherichia coli* (enterohemorrhagic, enteroinvasive)
- *Pleisomonas* sp.
- *Shigella* sp.
- *Salmonella enterica* serotypes *typhi* and *paratyphi*
- Nontyphoid *Salmonella* species
- Noncholera *Vibrio* species
- *Yersinia*

**Protozoal**
- *Entamoeba histolytica*

an infectious dose as low as 10 to 100 organisms. Sequelae of EHEC infection include hemorrhagic diarrhea, hemolytic-uremic syndrome, and thrombotic thrombocytopenic purpura. The primary virulence factor is Shiga-like toxin, which damages ribosomes. The gene for Shiga-like toxin is transmitted between EHEC strains by a bacteriophage vector. A separate virulence plasmid has been identified in certain strains of EHEC, but its significance is uncertain. Management of EHEC disease is supportive, because some evidence suggests that antibiotics can enhance the release of Shiga-like toxin and increase the risk of developing hemolytic-uremic syndrome.

EPEC has been associated most strongly with pediatric diarrhea in both epidemic and sporadic forms. EPEC adheres to enterocytes, causing the pathognomic attaching and effacing lesion seen on pathologic section. It then secretes proteins that initiate signal transduction within the enterocyte, ultimately resulting in secretory diarrhea. Because EPEC causes persistent diarrhea that can lead to significant dehydration, rehydration and antibiotic therapy are usually indicated.

As its name implies, EIEC invades enterocytes, where it then replicates and spreads to adjacent cells. The resulting diarrhea may be secretory or inflammatory and lasts up to 7 days. EIEC is closely related to *Shigella* genetically and in the clinical disease that they both cause. As with *Shigella*, antibiotic treatment reduces duration of symptomatic illness.

### *Shigella* Species

The genus *Shigella* consists of four serovars pathogenic to humans: *Shigella sonnei* (Group A), *Shigella flexneri* (Group B), *Shigella boydii* (Group C), and *Shigella dysenteriae* (Group D). *S. sonnei*, the most commonly isolated species, typically causes secretory diarrhea, and the remaining *Shigella* species cause bacillary dysentery with fever, bloody diarrhea, cramping, and tenesmus. As with the typhoid group of *Salmonella*, humans are the sole host for *Shigella* species; however, the low infectious dose required by *Shigella* species to cause disease is more similar to the nontyphoid *Salmonella* species.

### *Salmonella* Species

For clinical purposes, the genus *Salmonella* can be divided into two broad groups: typhoid and nontyphoid.

The typhoid group, consisting of *Salmonella enterica* serotypes *typhi* and *paratyphi*, causes typhoid (enteric) fever. These organisms exclusively infect human hosts and are transmitted via contaminated food or water. A large inoculum of typhoid group bacteria is required to experimentally produce infection. Some infected persons become chronic carriers who can transmit infection to others, such as the infamous Typhoid Mary. Typhoid fever is endemic in the developing world. The classic presentation of typhoid fever evolves over 3 weeks: a stepwise fever with temperature-pulse dissociation in the first week, abdominal pain and rose spots on the trunk in the second week, and hepatosplenomegaly with intestinal bleeding in the third week. Because these species are only transmitted between human hosts, identification of one case of typhoid fever becomes a public health issue that mandates contact tracing. Possible complications include bacteremia, gastrointestinal bleeding or perforation, cholangitis, pneumonia, and osteomyelitis.

The nontyphoid group consists of all *Salmonella* species except *S. enterica* serotypes *typhi* and *paratyphi*. These species generally incubate in animals and are transmitted to humans through consumption of contaminated food or water; direct human-to-human transmission is exceedingly rare. In contrast to the typhoid group, nontyphoid *Salmonella* species can cause disease with inocula as low as 10 to 100 colony-forming units (CFU). The disease that results is most often a gastroenteritis with fever, emesis, and diarrhea that can be secretory or inflammatory, lasting up to 7 days. Possible complications include bacteremia, endovascular infection from seeding of atherosclerotic plaques or prosthetic grafts, and Reiter's syndrome

### *Campylobacter* Species

*Campylobacter* species are common bacterial causes of acute infectious diarrhea; *Campylobacter jejuni* is the major species that causes human disease. Infection is contracted through consumption of contaminated poultry, milk, or water. After an incubation period of 2 to 7 days, the patient develops bloody diarrhea. *Campylobacter* diarrhea is also notable for its manifold extraintestinal complications, including autoimmune phenomena such as reactive arthritis and Guillain-Barré syndrome. Antibiotic therapy is usually reserved for severe disease or immunocompromised patients, in whom recurrent disease is more frequent.

### *Vibrio cholerae*

*Vibrio cholerae* is the prototype of an enterotoxic bacterium that causes secretory diarrhea. It is almost exclusively a disease of developing countries with poor sanitation. There have been several pandemics in the last century, with the most recent affecting South America and Central America as well the more typical regions in Africa and Asia. The only two serotypes to cause human disease are O1 and O139; serotype O1 is divided into biotypes *cholerae* and *eltor*. Cholera toxin affects enterocytes to produce a secretory diarrhea described as *rice-water stools*. Disease severity ranges from mild to severe with profound dehydration. Rehydration is the cornerstone of treatment, via oral or intravenous routes as dictated by clinical severity.

### *Clostridium difficile*

*Clostridium difficile* has been recognized as one cause of antibiotic-associated diarrhea and the leading cause of pseudomembranous colitis since the late 1970s. *C. difficile*–associated diarrhea was conventionally thought to only be a health issue for institutionalized patients who have had recent exposure to antibiotics or chemotherapy. In the last 3 years, however, significant expansions in *C. difficile*–associated diarrhea disease severity and host range have been described by researchers in North America and Europe. Disease severity ranges broadly from asymptomatic colonization to mild diarrhea to fulminant pseudomembranous colitis.

### Other Bacteria

Several other bacteria are less-common causes of acute infectious diarrhea. They merit some discussion because of their specific clinical presentations or potential for causing severe disease.

### *Vibrio parahemolyticus*

*Vibrio parahemolyticus* causes gastrointestinal illness associated with consumption of raw or undercooked oysters and other seafood. The spectrum of illness varies widely. Immunocompetent patients usually develop self-limited secretory diarrhea or gastroenteritis with fever lasting from 1 to 3 days, and immunocompromised patients present with severe diarrhea, septicemia, and a profound hemolytic anemia.

### *Staphylococcus aureus*

*Staphylococcus aureus* causes a variety of gastrointestinal illnesses. It is a common cause of enterotoxin-mediated foodborne illness, manifesting with emesis, watery diarrhea, and cramping after a brief incubation period of 1 to 6 hours. *S. aureus*, particularly methicillin-resistant *S. aureus* (MRSA), is also an uncommon but recognized cause of pseudomembranous colitis.

### *Bacteroides fragilis*

Although *Bacteroides fragilis* is recognized as part of the normal flora of the large intestine, certain strains produce a metalloprotease that has been associated with diarrhea in several studies of human and animal populations. Some studies have suggested that these enterotoxigenic *B. fragilis* strains may be more likely than nontoxigenic strains to cause blood infections.

### Clostridium perfringens

*Clostridium perfringens* is a ubiquitous pathogen that is a common cause of enterotoxin-mediated secretory diarrhea. Its specific enterotoxin (CPE) has been found in all five toxinotypes of *C. perfringens*. Gastrointestinal disease can result from ingestion of preformed toxin, with a short incubation period before clinical disease, or ingestion of a large bacterial inoculum, requiring a longer incubation before disease. Treatment is usually supportive.

## PROTOZOA

### Giardia lamblia

*Giardia lamblia* is a protozoan pathogen that causes diarrhea that can be chronic and refractory to treatment. The infectious cyst form is ingested in contaminated food or water, and the trophozoite then attaches to the intestinal wall. *Giardia* has expanded its environmental niche in recent years from the beaver fever endemic to isolated rivers and lakes, becoming a global pathogen.

### Entamoeba histolytica

*Entamoeba histolytica* can cause amoebic dysentery, which can manifest as acute, subacute, or chronic diarrhea. Diagnosis of *E. histolytica* is complicated by the highly similar but nonpathogenic *Entamoeba dispar*. Other than the rare situation where microscopy of stool detects ingested erythrocytes (pathognomic of *E. histolytica*), the two species are morphologically identical and can only be distinguished by methodologies such as serology, antigen detection, or nucleic acid testing.

## VIRUSES

### Rotavirus

Rotavirus primarily affects infants and children from 3 to 36 months of age, resulting in a spectrum of disease from asymptomatic shedding to severe gastroenteritis with dehydration. Globally, it is the leading viral cause of severe gastroenteritis. Other groups affected include travelers, the immunocompromised, and patients in hospitals or other institutions.

### Calicivirus

Norwalk virus is the most well-known member of the calicivirus family. Outbreaks of Norwalk often occur in long-term care facilities, cruise ships, and hospitals. It is highly contagious, with attack rates often greater than 10%. The clinical syndrome of Norwalk infection usually features rapid onset of severe nausea and emesis along with varying degrees of diarrhea.

## Differential Diagnosis

### OTHER INFECTIONS

Infections that cause diarrhea are not necessarily primarily gastrointestinal (Box 5). Systemic infections that result in diarrhea are probably underrecognized as a distinct etiology; however, the astute clinician should usually be able to recognize a systemic infection after a proper history, physical examination, and appropriate laboratory tests. Bacterial infections such as Group A streptococcosis, legionellosis, leptospirosis, and some tick-borne infections (including borreliosis, ehrlichiosis, tularemia, and Rocky Mountain spotted fever) can manifest with diarrhea as an initial symptom. Septicemia, caused by a variety of pathogens such as gram-negative enteric organisms, can also cause diarrhea and other gastrointestinal symptoms. Viremia is another cause of diarrhea; the most common cause is probably influenza, but other viruses including severe acute respiratory syndrome–associated coronavirus (SARS-CoV), hantaviruses, dengue

---

> **BOX 5   Diseases That Can Mimic Acute Infectious Diarrhea**
>
> **Infectious Etiologies**
> - Dengue fever
> - *Francisella* sp.
> - Hantavirus
> - *Legionella* sp.
> - Leptospirosis
> - Lyme borreliosis
> - Malaria
> - SARS
>
> **Noninfectious Etiologies**
> - Antibiotic-associated diarrhea
> - Bacterial overgrowth
> - Brainerd diarrhea (infectious etiology suspected but unproved)
> - Endocrinopathies (e.g., VIPoma)
> - Inflammatory bowel disease
> - Irritable bowel syndrome
> - Other medications
>
> *Abbreviations:* SARS = severe acute respiratory syndrome; VIP = vasoactive intestinal peptide.

virus (*Flavivirus* sp.), and hemorrhagic fever viruses should be considered in the presence of correlating exposures. *Plasmodium falciparum* malaria can result in diarrhea severe enough to mimic bacillary dysentery, and severe diarrhea has been associated with poor outcome.

### OTHER NONINFECTIOUS ETIOLOGIES

A variety of noninfectious causes can result in acute diarrhea (see Box 5). For instance, diarrhea is a common adverse effect of antimicrobial agents and other medications. The mechanism varies by antibiotic, but common reasons include direct stimulation of gut motility, increased gut osmolality, and disruption of the normal gut flora.

Although not strictly an infection, diarrhea is one of the most common symptoms of bacterial overgrowth. This disease occurs after disruption of host mechanisms that normally regulate bacterial intestinal colonization, such as pancreatitis or intestinal dysmotility. Definitive treatment should address the underlying condition, but broad-spectrum antibiotics can result in a long-lasting cure.

Brainerd diarrhea was initially described after an outbreak in Brainerd, Minnesota, in 1983. It manifests as an acute secretory diarrhea that can last for several months. Its etiology remains unknown, but several outbreaks have demonstrated epidemiologic links to consumption of unpasteurized milk and undertreated water.

Some endocrinopathies, such as VIPoma, can cause profuse diarrhea. Inflammatory bowel diseases (e.g., Crohn's disease, ulcerative colitis) can manifest with an inflammatory diarrhea and constitutional symptoms. Irritable bowel syndrome can result in periods of diarrhea; however, there are alternating periods of constipation and a lack of constitutional symptoms.

## Special Cases

### TRAVELER'S DIARRHEA

According to the Centers for Disease Control and Prevention (CDC), 20% to 50% of international travelers develop diarrhea related to their travels. The etiologic agents vary by exposure, geographic region, and local outbreaks. Bacteria are the most commonly implicated pathogens, with ETEC being the most commonly identified cause. Other etiologic agents include the other common bacterial, viral, and protozoal enteric pathogens described earlier. Diarrhea is usually mild to moderate and self-limited; 90% of patients report resolution of symptoms after 1 week, and 98% after 4 weeks. Although it is usually a nuisance rather than a severe threat to health, diarrhea can significantly limit the traveler's activities.

Because traveler's diarrhea is self-limited, investigations of the cause are usually reserved for diarrhea that is prolonged or manifests with higher-risk features such as fever or bloody stool. Stool should be examined for ova and parasites (O&P) if the travel history is supportive.

The focus for management should be supportive care. People seen for travel medicine advice should be counseled to avoid consuming water or food not known to be safe. The safest diet for travelers consists of freshly prepared foods served thoroughly heated, fruits and vegetables that are peeled or are washed with safe water, and beverages that are bottled or boiled before consumption. Ice and tap water should be considered contaminated. Patients for whom diarrhea could be catastrophic should be advised to avoid traveling unless it is strictly necessary.

After the traveler has developed diarrhea, a variety of medications are available for treatment. See the discussion of management of acute infectious diarrhea later in this chapter.

## IMMUNOCOMPROMISED STATES

Gastrointestinal illness is a common problem in immunocompromised patients. Apart from the infectious etiologies of diarrhea described earlier, other causes found in immunocompromised patients include the agent causing the immunocompromised state (such as HIV or chemotherapeutic agents), opportunistic organisms, adverse effects of medications, dysfunction of intestinal absorption, and idiopathic enteropathies.

Opportunistic organisms that can cause diarrhea include parasites (e.g., *Cryptosporidium parvum*, *Cyclospora cayetanensis*, *Isospora belli*, microsporidia), fungi (e.g., disseminated fungal infections from *Histoplasma capsulatum* and *Cryptococcus neoformans*), bacteria (e.g., *Mycobacterium avium-intracellulare* complex), and viruses (e.g., cytomegalovirus, herpes simplex virus). In general, treatment requires prolonged courses of antimicrobial agents and can be complicated by concomitant medications or diseases; consultation with an appropriate specialist is suggested.

## Prevention

Methods of prevention are listed in Box 6.

### AVOIDANCE

An effective method for preventing acute infectious diarrhea is to eliminate exposures that put one at risk. This applies particularly to patients who would be at high risk for contracting acute infectious diarrhea or having adverse outcomes, for example, patients who are immunocompromised or physically debilitated. Exposure avoidance is

usually situational and patient-specific, such as suggesting that travel be postponed to a region currently undergoing a cholera epidemic or cautioning against consumption of raw seafood.

### HYGIENE

Proper handwashing by health care workers caring for patients with acute diarrhea is essential to prevent institutional transmission, and its importance cannot be overstated. Barrier precautions are also commonly implemented, particularly if the patient is incontinent of stool. Other precautions, such as tailoring environmental cleaning practices to specific pathogens during outbreaks, are also proven effective.

### PROPHYLACTIC ANTIBIOTICS

There is a limited role for antibiotics in preventing acute infectious diarrhea, particularly traveler's diarrhea. The normally mild severity and self-limited nature of the disease, along with the risk of adverse effects from antibiotics, means that prophylactic antibiotics are most often reserved for brief durations in patients at high risk for contracting acute infectious diarrhea or for experiencing adverse outcomes.

### PROBIOTICS

There has been a surge of publications concerning the role of probiotics in preventing diarrhea of varying etiologies. Although individual studies have produced varied results for diarrhea caused by *C. difficile*–associated diarrhea and traveler's diarrhea, a recent meta-analysis of 34 studies supported a role for probiotics in preventing diarrhea, with an overall risk reduction of at least 21%. Stratification by type of diarrhea found a much larger reduction in antibiotic-associated (52%) than traveler's (8%) diarrhea. Protective effects seemed relatively conserved despite different probiotic organisms being used, which might imply a common protective mechanism shared between organisms or a common host response. The variety of probiotic organisms and dosing regimens described in the literature has not yet led to a standardized formulation.

---

 **CURRENT DIAGNOSIS**

**History**

- Duration and frequency of diarrhea
- Other gastrointestinal symptoms (emesis, tenesmus, abdominal pain)
- Presence of bloody stool, fever
- Medication use, including recent antibiotic use
- Recent contact with ill persons, travel, and animal contact
- Consumption of raw or undercooked poultry or seafood
- Immunocompromised state (rule out)

**Physical Examination**

- Hydration status
- Gastrointestinal examination
- Other systems as indicated by symptoms

**Laboratory Tests**

- For limited secretory diarrhea: usually none
- For bloody diarrhea: complete blood count (CBC), stool for culture (rule out O157:H7); consider ova and parasites test (O&P)
- For chronic diarrhea: consider *C. difficile* assay, O&P
- For traveler's diarrhea: CBC, stool for culture and O&P
- For immunocompromised patients: CBC, stool for culture and O&P

---

| **BOX 6**   **Prevention of Acute Infectious Diarrhea** |
|---|

- Avoidance
- Hygiene
- Prophylactic antibiotics
- Probiotics
- Vaccines
  - Cholera/ETEC (Dukoral)[2]
  - Rotavirus (RotaTeq)
  - *Salmonella typhi* (Vivotif Berna, Typhim Vi)

---

[2]Not available in the United States.
*Abbreviation:* ETEC = enterotoxigenic *Escherichia coli*.

## VACCINES

### Rotavirus

A live human-bovine reassortant rotavirus oral vaccine (RotaTeq) has been licensed since February 2006 in the United States for infants 6 to 32 weeks of age. The vaccine appears efficacious in preventing rotaviral gastroenteritis, and consequently it reduces the need for outpatient and inpatient assessment. A large phase III trial demonstrated no increased risk over placebo of intussusception, an adverse effect that led to the withdrawal of a previous rotavirus vaccine.

### *Vibrio Cholerae* and ETEC

An oral inactivated cholera vaccine (Dukoral), available in Canada but not in the United States, has demonstrated some efficacy in preventing traveler's diarrhea. The B subunit of *V. cholerae* toxin used in this vaccine has sufficient structural homology with ETEC heat-labile toxin to provide moderate short-term protection against this common cause of traveler's diarrhea, lasting up to 3 months. This vaccine is limited to patients with high-risk medical conditions, such as immunodeficiencies.

### *Salmonella typhi*

Enteral and parenteral vaccines are available to prevent typhoid. The enteral form (Vivotif Berna) is a live attenuated strain of *S. typhi*, which is taken as four capsules over 7 days and confers immunity for approximately 5 years. The parenteral form (Typhim Vi) is purified capsular polysaccharide that is given as a single intramuscular injection. This is the preferred route for patients with contraindications to live attenuated vaccines, such as immunocompromised status. Neither vaccine is completely protective, and neither provides protection against *S. paratyphi*.

## Treatment

Management of acute infectious diarrhea is listed in Box 7.

### REHYDRATION

Maintaining adequate hydration is usually the cornerstone of management for acute diarrhea. The route of administration depends on the patient's hydration status and disease severity; enteral hydration is preferred to parenteral, if possible.

---

### CURRENT THERAPY

- Supportive care
- Rehydration (always replace previous losses and provide maintenance)
    - Enteral
    - Parenteral (intravenous, intraosseus, enteroclytic)
- Antidiarrheal medications (only if patient is afebrile and stools are not bloody)
    - Morphine derivatives
    - Bismuth subsalicylate (Pepto-Bismol)
- Antibiotics (only if necessary as indicated by symptoms, severity, and risk factors)
    - Empiric therapy
        - Adults
            - Ciprofloxacin (Cipro) 500 mg PO bid for 3-5 d
            - Levofloxacin (Levaquin)[1] 500 mg PO qd for 3-5 d
        - Children
            - Azithromycin (Zithromax)[1] 5-10 mg/kg PO qd for 3-5 d
            - Trimethoprim-sulfamethoxazole (Septra) 5-25 mg/kg/d PO in two equally divided doses for 3-5 d *plus*
            - Erythromycin 10 mg/kg/d PO qid for 5 d
    - Specific therapy as directed by pathogen identification and susceptibilities
- Probiotics

---

In 2003 the WHO reformulated their well-known oral rehydration solution (ORS). The new lower-osmolarity formula has been found to reduce stool volume, emesis, and the need for switching to intravenous therapy in children with diarrhea. This new formulation has 75 mmol/L sodium, 75 mmol/L glucose, and a total osmolarity 245 mOsm/L, which can be achieved with a recipe of 2.6 g sodium chloride, 13.5 g anhydrous glucose, 1.5 g potassium chloride, 2.5 g sodium bicarbonate and 1.5 g trisodium citrate dihydrate per liter of water.

A homemade solution can be prepared with 40 mL sugar and 5 mL table salt per liter of clean water; however, this preparation lacks potassium. Furthermore, commercially prepared rehydration solutions should be preferred to homemade in order to minimize the chance of errors in preparing the solution. Most sports drinks are not equivalent to actual rehydration solutions, because sports drinks often have higher carbohydrate and lower electrolyte loads.

Parenteral rehydration is usually intravenous, although intraosseus administration can be used for infants in whom intravenous access cannot be obtained and enteroclysis can be used in adult patients with difficult vascular access who do not require large volumes of replacement fluid. Sufficient volumes of fluid should be given to replace preexisting fluid deficits as well as ongoing losses and maintenance requirements.

### ANTIDIARRHEAL MEDICATIONS

Some medications reduce intestinal motility by affecting the myenteric motor plexus to inhibit peristalsis. Opioid derivatives, such as loperamide (Imodium), are the class of medications most commonly used for this purpose. Although licensed for use with acute, chronic, and traveler's diarrhea, loperamide is contraindicated in the presence of fever or bloody stool or in situations where inhibition of peristalsis is otherwise undesirable or potentially harmful.

Other medications are classified as antidiarrheal but have different mechanisms of action. Bismuth subsalicylate (Pepto-Bismol) appears

---

### BOX 7   Management of Acute Infectious Diarrhea

**Rehydration**
- Enteral
    - World Health Organization formulation
    - Commercially available rehydration solutions
    - Home remedies
- Parenteral
    - Intravenous
    - Intraosseus
    - Enteroclysis

**Medications**
- Antidiarrheals
    - Bismuth subsalicylate
    - Morphine derivatives
- Antibiotics
- Probiotics

**TABLE 1** Empiric Therapy of Diarrheal Disease

| Clinical Syndrome | Adult Patients | Pediatric Patients |
|---|---|---|
| Febrile dysenteric diarrhea in industrialized regions, or moderate to severe traveler's diarrhea | Ciprofloxacin (Cipro) 500 mg PO bid *or* levofloxacin (Levaquin)[1] 500 mg PO qd for 3-5 d | Azithromycin (Zithromax)[1] 5-10 mg/kg PO qd for 3-5 d *or* trimethoprim-sulfamethoxazole (Septra) 5-25 mg/kg/d PO in two divided doses for 3-5 d *plus* erythromycin[1] 10 mg/kg PO qid for 5 d |
| Persistent diarrhea (≥14 d in duration) in industrialized countries | Consider anti-*Giardia* therapy: metronidazole (Flagyl)[1] 250 mg PO tid for 7 d | Consider anti-*Giardia* therapy: metronidazole (Flagyl)[1] 20 mg/kg/d PO in three divided doses for 7 d |

Adapted from Montes M, DuPont HL: Enteritis, enterocolitis and infectious diarrhea syndromes. In Cohen J, Powderly WD: Infectious Diseases, 2nd ed. St Louis: Mosby, 2004, pp 477-489.

to function by multiple mechanisms including intestinal secretion reduction, intestinal reabsorption of fluids and electrolytes, toxin binding, and direct antimicrobial effects. It has proven efficacy in the management of traveler's diarrhea, although its dosing frequency may be difficult for some patients. Racecadotril (or acetorphan)[2] is a new synthetic enkephalinase inhibitor that acts by the same mechanism as the opioid derivatives and has been studied for its antidiarrheal effect in pediatric patients.

## ANTIBIOTICS

Antibiotics should be used cautiously in the treatment of acute infectious diarrhea. Most clinical cases adequately resolve without antibiotic therapy. Furthermore, their use can sometimes cause diarrhea

[2]Not available in the United States.

(such as antibiotic-associated diarrhea or *C. difficile*–associated diarrhea), and indiscriminate use can contribute to selective pressures that favor development of antibiotic-resistant organisms. Recommendations in the empiric and pathogen-specific treatment of acute infectious diarrhea are given in Tables 1 and 2.

## PROBIOTICS

As with the prevention of diarrhea, a growing body of evidence supports the use of probiotics for treating acute infectious diarrhea. One of the major limitations to using probiotics is the variation in species and doses used in different clinical trials. However, there seems to be a class effect that is most likely a combination of competition for intestinal binding sites or nutritional resources, elaboration of antibacterial compounds, and immune stimulation. Another recognized limitation is the rare but serious case of blood infection from the probiotic organism; documented cases have occurred not only in recipients but also in other patients being cared for in close proximity to the recipient.

**TABLE 2** Pathogen-Specific Therapy of Diarrheal Disease

| Pathogen | Adult Patients | Pediatric Patients |
|---|---|---|
| *Campylobacter jejuni* | Azithromycin (Zithromax)[1] 500 mg PO qd for 3 d | Erythromycin stearate[1] 40 mg/kg/d in four divided doses for 5 d *or* azithromycin[1] 10 mg/kg/d |
| *Clostridium difficile* | Initial disease: metronidazole (Flagyl) 250 mg PO qid for 10-14 d or vancomycin (Vancocin) 125-500 mg PO qid for 10-14 d | Initial disease: metronidazole 20 mg/kg/d in three divided doses for 10-14 d or vancomycin 125-500 mg PO qid for 10-14 d |
| EAEC, EIEC, EPEC, ETEC | Same as empiric therapy for febrile dysentery and traveler's diarrhea (see Table 1) | Azithromycin[1] 10 mg/kg/d. If resistance is suspected, use ceftriaxone (Rocephin),[1] cefixime (Suprax),[1] or cefotaxime (Claforan)[1] |
| EHEC* | No antimicrobial therapy (increased risk of increasing toxin release and hemolytic-uremic syndrome) | No antimicrobial therapy (increased risk of increasing toxin release and hemolytic-uremic syndrome) |
| *Entamoeba histolytica* | Metronidazole 500 mg PO tid for 10 d or tinidazole (Tindamax) 1 g PO bid for 3 d. Follow with paromomycin (Humatin) 500 mg PO tid for 7 d | Metronidazole 50 mg/kg/d IV in three divided doses plus diiodohydroxyquin (Yodoxin) 40 mg/kg/d in three divided doses for 20 d |
| *Giardia lamblia* | Metronidazole[1] 250 mg PO tid for 7 d *or* albendazole (Albenza)[1] 400 mg PO qd for 5 d *or* tinidazole 2 g PO in one dose | Metronidazole[1] 20 mg/kg/d in three divided doses for 7 d or furazolidone (Furoxone) 6 mg/kg/d divided in four doses for 7 d |
| *Shigella* sp. | Ciprofloxacin (Cipro) 500 mg PO bid for 3-5 d *or* levofloxacin (Levaquin)[1] 500 mg PO qd for 3-5 d | Azithromycin[1] 10 mg/kg/d. If resistance is suspected, use ceftriaxone,[1] cefixime,[1] or cefotaxime[1] |
| *Salmonella* sp. non-typhoid group | Asymptomatic or mild: no antimicrobial therapy. At risk for complications: ciprofloxacin[1] 500 mg PO bid or levofloxacin[1] 500 mg PO qd for 5-7 d. Alternatives: azithromycin[1] or erythromycin stearate (Erythrocin stearate)[1] 500 mg PO bid for 5 d | ≤6 mo old: ceftriaxone[1] 50 mg/kg IV qd. >6 mo old and healthy, and asymptomatic or with mild illness: no antimicrobial therapy. At risk for complications: ceftriaxone[1] 50 mg/kg IV qd (not to exceed 2 g/d) |
| typhoid group | Ciprofloxacin (Cipro) 500 mg PO bid for 7-10 d or levofloxacin (Levaquin)[1] 500 mg PO OD for 7-10 d or ceftriaxone 2 g IV q 24h for 14 d | Ceftriaxone 75-100 mg/kg IV q24h for 14 d (not to exceed 4 g/d) or azithromycin 20 mg/kg PO OD for 5-7 d (not to exceed 1 g/d) |

**TABLE 2  Pathogen-Specific Therapy of Diarrheal Disease—cont'd**

| Pathogen | Adult Patients | Pediatric Patients |
|---|---|---|
| *Vibrio cholerae* | Doxycycline 300 mg PO for one dose or ciprofloxacin[1] 1 g PO for one dose Recurrent disease can require prolonged courses of antibiotics or adjunctive therapy (e.g., IVIG,[1] resins[1]) | TMP-SMX (Septra)[1] 1 DS tab PO bid for 3 d or azithromycin[1] 20 mg/kg PO for one dose (not to exceed 1 g) |

Adapted from Montes M, DuPont HL: Enteritis, enterocolitis and infectious diarrhea syndromes. In Cohen J, Powderly WD: Infectious Diseases, 2nd ed. St Louis: Mosby, 2004, pp 477-489.
[1]Not FDA approved for this indication.
[2]Not available in the United States.
*Shiga toxin and Shiga-like toxin–producing *E. coli*.
*Abbreviations:* DS = double strength; EAEC = enteroaggregative *E. coli*; EHEC = enterohemorrhagic *E. coli*; EIEC = enteroinvasive *E. coli*.
    EPEC = enteropathogenic *E. coli*; ETEC = enterotoxigenic *E. coli*; IVIG = intravenous immunoglobulin; TMP-SMX = trimethoprim-sulfamethoxazole.

## REFERENCES

Aranda-Michel J, Giannella RA: Acute diarrhea: A practical review. Am J Med 1999;106:670-676.

DuPont HL: What's new in enteric infectious diseases at home and abroad. Curr Opin Infect Dis 2005;18:407-412.

Dupont HL, and the Practice Parameters Committee of the American College of Gastroenterology: Guidelines on acute infectious diarrhea in adults. Am J Gastroenterol 1997;92(11):1962-1975.

Guerrant RL, Van Gilder T, Stiner TS, et al: Practice guidelines for the management of infectious diarrhea. Clin Infect Dis 2001;32:331-350.

Hahn S, Kim Y, Garner P: Reduced osmolarity oral rehydration solution for treating dehydration due to diarrhea in children: Systematic review. Br Med J 2001;323:81-85.

Helton T, Rolson DD: Which adults with acute diarrhea should be evaluated? What is the best diagnostic approach? Cleve Clin J Med 2004; 71(10):778-785.

Musher DM, Musher BL: Contagious acute gastrointestinal infections. N Engl J Med 2004;351(23):2417-2427.

Reisinger EC, Fritzsche C, Krause R, Krejs GJ: Diarrhea caused by primarily non-gastrointestinal infections. Nat Clin Practice Gastroenterol Hepatol 2005;2(5):216-222.

Sazawal S, Hiremath G, Dhingra U, et al: Efficacy of probiotics in prevention of acute diarrhoea: A meta-analysis of masked, randomised, placebo-controlled trials. Lancet Infect Dis 2006;6:374-382.

Thielman NM, Guerrant RL: Acute infectious diarrhea. N Engl J Med 2004; 350:38-47.

World Health Organization: Oral rehydration salts: Production of the new ORS. 2006. PDF available at http://www.who.int/child-adolescent-health/New_Publications/CHILD_HEALTH/WHO_FCH_CAH_06.1.pdf (accessed April 5, 2007).

# Constipation

Method of
*Warren P. Bishop, MD*

Constipation is not as easily defined as one might imagine. Patients may report being constipated in response to several different symptoms. Decreased defecation frequency is perhaps the most common symptom.

What is normal bowel frequency? This varies throughout life. In infants who are exclusively breast-fed, initial bowel frequency can be more than 10 stools per day. After several weeks of age, breast-fed infants can produce less than one stool per week without any evident distress or distention. In bottle-fed infants and throughout childhood, one or two stools per day is typical. Stool frequency remains stable throughout most of adult life, varying between one stool every 3 days and three stools per day.

Fewer than three stools per week is considered to be abnormal in adults, as defined by the Rome II Committee on Functional Gastrointestinal Disorders in 1999. Other criteria for constipation defined by this committee are listed in Box 1. At least two of the listed criteria must be met to make the diagnosis.

## Etiology and Physiology

The major physiologic causes of constipation include slow colonic transit and blocked defecation. The first requirement for normal defecation is normal colonic motility, or transit. *Slow colonic transit* can be caused by many factors, such as neuromuscular disorders, hypothyroidism, diabetes mellitus, conditions obstructing the colon, and medications (Box 2). The act of defecation itself is a complex process requiring normal rectal sensation, reflex relaxation of the internal anal sphincter, voluntary relaxation of the external sphincter, and contraction of pelvic floor muscles. Interference with this sequence of events leads to *obstructed defecation*. Many interacting factors can contribute, including poor-quality diet, physical inactivity, low calorie intake, poor social situation, cultural taboos, fear of painful stools (especially in young children), sexual abuse, medications, and physical ailments that reduce muscle strength, reduce CNS control, or block the anal canal.

Blocked defecation in children is most commonly the result of voluntarily withholding stool. This usually occurs during toilet training, and the resultant large, hard stools cause pain and continued fecal withholding. Congenital anorectal anomalies typically result in blocked defecation in infants. In older persons, cancers, sigmoid and rectal intussusception, solitary rectal ulcer syndrome, poor pelvic floor function, and pregnancy may be responsible (Box 3).

---

**BOX 1  Diagnostic Criteria for Constipation**

At least 12 wk, which need not be consecutive, in the preceding 12 mo of two or more of:
- Straining in >1 of 4 defecations
- Lumpy or hard stools in >1 of 4 defecations
- Sensation of incomplete evacuation in >1 of 4 defecations
- Sensation of anorectal obstruction or blockage in >1 of 4 defecations
- Manual maneuvers to facilitate >1 of 4 defecations (e.g., digital evacuation, support of the pelvic floor)
*plus*
- Fewer than three defecations per wk
- Loose stools are not present, and there are insufficient criteria for diagnosis of irritable bowel syndrome

## BOX 2 Causes of Slow Colonic Transit

**Functional**
- Irritable bowel syndrome

**Endocrine or Metabolic**
- Anticholinergics
- Antipsychotics
- Diabetes mellitus
- Hypercalcemia
- Hypokalemia, hypomagesemia
- Hypothyroidism
- Renal failure

**Medications**
- Aluminum antacids
- Antidiarrheal agents
- Antiparkinson drugs
- Calcium channel blockers
- Cholestyramine (Questran)
- Diuretics
- Opiates
- Tricyclic antidepressants

**Neuromuscular**
- Amyloidosis
- Botulism
- Chagas' disease
- Dysautonomia
- Hirschsprung's disease
- Pseudo-obstruction
- Sarcoidosis

**Obstructive**
- Colon cancer
- External compression
- Strictures

## BOX 3 Causes of Blocked Defecation

**Congenital (Infants)**
- Anal stenosis
- Anteriorly displaced anus
- Hirschsprung's disease
- Imperforate anus
- Spinal cord dysraphism

**Acquired Structural Conditions**
- Pregnancy
- Rectocele
- Sigmoid or rectal intussusception
- Solitary rectal ulcer syndrome
- Strictures

**Functional**
- Anal fissure or painful defecation
- Pelvic floor dysfunction
- Voluntary stool withholding (functional fecal retention)

## Evaluation

After a careful history of the onset, characteristics, and associated symptoms of constipation (see Box 1), the physical examination must include careful evaluation of the abdomen. Care should be taken not to mistake abdominal or pelvic tumors for fecal masses. Rectal examination must be performed in all cases. The rectal evaluation should include documenting perianal lesions, tenderness, anal stenosis, pelvic mass lesions, perineal descent when bearing down, strength of external sphincter and perineal ascent during voluntary clenching, the force of expulsion when asked to expel the examiner's finger, evidence of fecal soiling, and the presence or absence of rectal dilation.

History of difficult defecation with excessive straining, sensation of incomplete emptying, or use of manual assistance will serve to differentiate blocked defecation from slow colonic transit. Patients with these symptoms can benefit from further evaluation by a gastroenterologist, who might consider further diagnostic testing such as anorectal manometry, colonic motility studies, or defecography. Patients with suspected slow transit constipation can be further evaluated by selective use of colonic transit studies (using radiopaque markers or scintiscan) or barium enema, or both. Most patients with constipation do not require specialized studies and can be treated empirically as outlined next.

## Treatment

### EDUCATION

Patients need to understand the physiology of defecation, including the importance of using the toilet in response to the urge to defecate and toilet-sitting immediately on awakening and after meals, times when propulsive colonic activity is most likely. The mechanism of action, safety, and precautions of all prescribed drugs should be discussed. Patients are often unduly afraid that even nonabsorbable osmotics like polyethylene glycol (e.g., MiraLax) may be habit-forming, and thus deny themselves adequate therapy.

### CURRENT DIAGNOSIS

- Constipation can be defined in several ways. Stools that are hard, infrequent, or pebbly are common symptoms. Other criteria include excessive straining, need for manual assistance during defecation, or a sensation of incomplete emptying.
- History must include the symptoms listed above, painful defecation, rectal bleeding, fecal soiling, and a detailed history of laxatives used. The presence of abdominal pain relieved by defecation suggests irritable bowel syndrome.
- Rectal examination must always be performed to evaluate for obstruction, inflammation, and function of pelvic floor and sphincter muscles.
- Etiologic categories include blocked defecation (physical obstruction, voluntary retention due to pain or fear of defecation, anismus), slow-transit constipation, and irritable bowel syndrome with constipation.

### CURRENT THERAPY

- Increased fiber should be taken orally, generally given as a twice-daily fiber supplement.
- A saline or osmotic laxative, such as milk of magnesia or polyethylene glycol (MiraLax or GlycoLax), should be used if fiber alone is not sufficient.
- Saline laxatives containing phosphate carry a risk of electrolyte disturbance and should be used with caution.
- Fermentable osmotic agents, such as sorbitol and lactulose, can cause cramping, flatulence, and perianal skin irritation.
- Stimulant laxatives such as bisacodyl and senna derivatives are of questionable safety for long-term use, but they are reasonable for acute relief.

**TABLE 1** Fiber Therapy Products

| Fiber Type | Brand Name | Fiber Content |
|---|---|---|
| Bran | All Bran | 10.4 g per ½ cup |
| Psyllium | Metamucil | 3.4 g/Tbs |
|  | Konsyl | 6 g/tsp |
| Methycellulose | Citrucel | 2 g/Tbs |
| Calcium polycarbophil | FiberCon | 1 g/ 2 tabs |
| Guar gum | Benefiber | 3 g/Tbs |

*Abbreviations:* tabs = tablets; Tbs = tablespoon (5 mL); tsp = teaspoon (15 mL).

**TABLE 2** Medical Treatment of Constipation

| Type | Example | Usual Dose |
|---|---|---|
| Fermentable osmotic agents | Lactulose, sorbitol | 15-30 mL bid |
| Fiber supplements | See Table 1 | Start 2-3 g bid, increase for effect |
| Lubricant | Mineral oil | Usual dose: 15-45 mL qd-bid |
| Nonfermentable osmotic agent | PEG 3350 (MiraLax) | Adult 17-68 g/d* Child 0.5-1.5 g/d* |
| Saline laxatives | Milk of magnesia | Adult: 15-30 mL bid Child: 2-4 mL/kg/d |
| Stimulants | Bisacodyl (Dulcolax) | One 10-mg suppository up to 3 × per wk |
| Surfactant stool softener | Docusate sodium (Colace) | 100 mg bid |

*Start with lower dose and adjust for effect.
*Abbreviation:* PEG = polyethylene glycol.

## MEDICAL THERAPY

If a fecal impaction is present on rectal examination, it should be evacuated immediately before beginning maintenance therapy. Enemas should be used only when absolutely necessary and with caution; complications have occurred, especially with repeated administration or poor expulsion of the solution. Potential complications include intestinal perforation, hyperphosphatemia, hypocalcemia, hypovolemic shock, and sepsis. Oral polyethylene glycol solutions (MiraLax, GlycoLax, GoLYTELY[1], CoLyte[1]), taken over several days, are gentle and effective disimpaction agents.

After disimpaction for adult patients, most authorities recommend beginning maintenance therapy with fiber supplements, some of which are listed in Table 1. Often, fiber alone is simply not adequate. Milk of magnesia is a relatively inexpensive next step and works well for most adult patients, but palatability limits its use in children. Electrolyte-free polyethylene glycol with an average molecular weight of 3350 (e.g., MiraLax, GlycoLax) is now the standard laxative therapy in many centers, especially for children, due to its excellent efficacy, safety, and palatability. The average effective pediatric dose is around 0.8 g/kg/day. It is generally mixed at a hypotonic strength of around 2 g/30 mL, which allows some water absorption while also increasing fecal water content. Adult dosing has been variously reported between 17 and 68 g/day.

For all patients, response to the chosen initial dose should be evaluated and then adjustments made as appropriate. Phosphate-based laxatives and nonabsorbable disaccharides are less desirable because of potential side effects and poor palatability. Stimulants such as bisacodyl (Dulcolax) or senna (Senokot) can be very effective for occasional use to treat exacerbations or as part of a disimpaction regimen. Chronic use of these agents should be limited to patients unresponsive to adequate doses of osmotic laxatives such as polyethylene glycol. Medical therapies for constipation are summarized in Table 2.

## SURGICAL THERAPY

Very few cases of constipation merit consideration of surgery. Obvious candidates are patients with congenital anorectal malformations, strictures, or cancer. Cecostomy for antegrade enemas is helpful in spinal cord injury and meningomyelocele patients, who cannot provide the voluntary muscle contractions required for efficient defecation. Colectomy is reserved for the most severe cases of colonic inertia unresponsive to maximum medical management. Placement of a stoma is a reversible action that can benefit some patients with distal colonic dysmotility.

## REFERENCES

DiPalma JA, DeRidder PH, Orlando RC, et al: A randomized, placebo-controlled, multicenter study of the safety and efficacy of a new polyethylene glycol laxative. Am J Gastroenterol 2000;95:446-450.

Heaton KW, Radvan J, Cripps H, et al: Defecation frequency and timing, and stool form in the general population: A prospective study. Gut 1992;33:818-824.

Mollen RM, Claassen At, Kuijpers JH: The evaluation and treatment of functional constipation. Scand J Gastroenterol 1997;223:8-17.

Pashankar DS, Bishop WP: Efficacy and optimal dose of daily polyethylene glycol 3350 for treatment of constipation and encopresis in children. J Pediatr 2001;139:428-432.

Sandler RS, Jordan MC, Shelton BJ: Demographic and dietary determinants of constipation in the U.S. population. Am J Pub Health 1990;80:185-189.

Smith B. Pathologic changes in the colon produced by anthraquinone laxatives. Dis Colon Rectum 1973;16:455-458.

Thompson WG, Longstreth GF, Drossman DA, et al: Functional bowel disorders and functional abdominal pain. Gut 1999;45(suppl 2):II43-II47.

# Fever

Method of
*Ian M. Paul, MD, MSc*

Fever is both sign and symptom of an underlying disease process that often produces anxiety for patients, parents, and health care providers. This so-called fever phobia can cause inappropriate management of the illness and fever. Fever is typically a transient phenomenon that only requires treatment when it is accompanied by discomfort or otherwise compromises a patient's health.

## Definitions

Fever is characterized by an elevated core body temperature that occurs as a protective response to a pathogen. Observations by Wunderlich in 1868 defined normal body temperature at 37°C (98.6°F) and febrile temperature at 38°C (100°F) or higher. Studies also show diurnal variation and differences in temperature based on temperature site (mouth, rectum, ear, or temporal artery),

---

[1]Not FDA approved for this indication.

## CURRENT DIAGNOSIS

- Temperatures taken by oral, rectal, tympanic, or temporal artery thermometers of 38.0°C (100.4°F) or more are consistent with fever.
- Fever is a normal physiologic response but can cause dehydration and increase metabolic rate. Benign febrile seizures can occur in young children with fevers.
- The other symptoms accompanying a fever help determine the severity of the febrile illness.
- Fever in infants younger than 3 months or in neutropenic patients is considered a medical emergency until proved otherwise.
- Fevers lasting 8 or more days without a clear cause are considered a fever of unknown origin (FUO). They may warrant more extensive evaluation.

but most clinicians classify a temperature of 38°C (100.4°F) or greater as fever.

Many clinicians, patients, and parents also use the term *high fever*, although this is not based on consistent objective criteria. Nonetheless, a temperature of 40°C (104°F) or greater is considered by many to be a high fever because nearly universally, patients are uncomfortable when experiencing a body temperature of this magnitude. Some worry that without treatment body temperature continues to rise during fever. This fear is unjustified, however, because only rarely do temperatures exceed 41.1°C (106°F), the temperature considered to be the physiologic limit of the febrile response. If a temperature recorded is greater than 41.1°C (106°F), superimposed hyperthermia is probable. Hyperthermia is distinguished from fever and characterized by a temperature above the hypothalamic set point. This is related to a hypothalamic insult or a disruption in normal homeostatic mechanisms that balance heat production and dissipation.

Two other definitions related to fever are fever without a source and fever of unknown origin (FUO). Both terms are used when no cause is determined for the fever and/or its associated illness. The majority of cases in both have infectious etiologies; the difference relates to duration of the fever. Fever without a source is used in the first week of an illness, whereas FUO is used for a fever lasting 8 or more days or occurring at intervals over weeks or months.

## Physiology and Pathophysiology

Fever begins with an inciting stimulus that triggers an inflammatory response. Most often this stimulus is infectious and causes leukocytes to release cytokines including interleukin-1β, tumor necrosis factor-α, interleukin-6, and interferon-γ. These and other cytokines interact with the temperature regulatory tissues in the anterior hypothalamus and release prostaglandin $E_2$ ($PGE_2$). $PGE_2$ then alters the firing rate of neurons in the preoptic area of the anterior hypothalamus, increasing the thermoregulatory set point.

Other systems respond to increase body temperature as this set point rises. Examples of these responses include shivering to increase heat production and peripheral vasoconstriction to reduce heat loss. Behavioral responses such as wearing warm clothes or covering up with a blanket may also occur.

The febrile response to an antigenic challenge is a beneficial one. Numerous studies show improved outcomes in those who manifest proper febrile responses and that many components of the immune system function better at higher temperatures (e.g., enhanced neutrophil migration, increased T-cell proliferation, and production of interferon). Clinical studies supporting this concept show treatment with acetaminophen prolonged the duration of active varicella in children, and aspirin therapy prolonged the shedding of rhinovirus in adults.

## Fever Phobia and the Complications of Fever

*Fever phobia*, the fear surrounding fever, termed by Dr. Barton Schmitt, has been recognized for several decades. Schmitt found some startling results when questioning parents about fever. His study shows that 56% of parents gave antipyretics for temperatures less than 37.8°C (100°F), and 58% thought temperatures less than 38.9°C (102°F) constituted a "high fever." Further, 62% thought fever caused permanent harm, with "brain damage" a common concern. In 2001, a similar study found equally troubling results. These authors found that 85% of parents woke their child to give antipyretics, 52% checked their child's temperature every hour or less, and most worrisome, 58% gave antipyretics too often.

Fever is the normal physiologic process previously described. Complications are rare and usually well tolerated. Common adverse events are dehydration and, in children 6 months to 6 years of age, benign febrile seizures, which are a common occurrence in young children without subsequent focal findings. The belief that seizures are caused by a rapid rise in temperature has been contradicted. In addition, no evidence suggests that aggressive use of antipyretics prevents a febrile seizure.

Fever is generally a protective physiologic response, but under some circumstances, it is harmful. For example, the metabolic rate steadily increases as body temperature rises. Further, myocardial depression, orthostatic dysfunction, and increases in oxygen consumption, respiratory minute volume, and respiratory quotient may not be tolerated by patients, especially those with chronic conditions. Severe complications such as death or so-called brain damage occurring during febrile illness are related to the underlying disease process, not fever.

## Treatment of Fever

It is important to overcome the desire to focus on a thermometer's reading when treating a fever by evaluating and treating the underlying illness and treating the discomfort associated with the febrile illness. The underlying condition may be age or disease specific. For example, infants younger than 3 months and neutropenic patients with fever are considered medical emergencies and require aggressive evaluation. Fever in the absence of a condition like one of these requires treatment only when accompanied by discomfort or other morbidity.

## CURRENT THERAPY

- Treat the underlying illness and the discomfort associated with the febrile illness, not the number on the thermometer.
- If antipyretic/analgesic medications are used, appropriate choices for *children* are:
  - Acetaminophen (Tylenol) 15 mg/kg every 4 to 6 h up to five times per d as needed for children older than 3 mo.
  - Ibuprofen (Motrin, Advil) 10 mg/kg every 6 h as needed for children older than 6 mo.
- If antipyretic/analgesic medications are used, appropriate choices for *adolescents and adults* are:
  - Acetaminophen (Tylenol), 650 to 1000 mg every 4 to 6 h as needed (maximum 4000 mg per d).
  - Ibuprofen (Motrin, Advil), 200 to 400 mg every 6 h as needed.
  - Aspirin, 325 to 650 mg every 6 h as needed.
- Sponge bathing, if chosen, should use tepid water with an antipyretic medication and no alcohol.

## ACETAMINOPHEN

Acetaminophen (Tylenol) is the most commonly used medication to treat fever. This drug is well absorbed from oral and rectal routes and widely available in liquid and tablet preparations around the world. Acetaminophen produces its antipyretic effect by inhibiting the release of $PGE_2$ yet does not possess the anti-inflammatory properties of nonsteroidal anti-inflammatory agents. Children at least 3 months or older may be given acetaminophen at a dose of 15 mg/kg every 4 to 6 hours up to a maximum of 75 mg/kg per day. Remember that children less than 3 months of age require evaluation when presenting with fever, and acetaminophen should be used with caution so as not to miss a serious bacterial infection. Doses of 650 to 1000 mg every 4 to 6 hours with a maximum daily dose of 4000 mg may be given to adolescents and adults. An extended-release preparation of 1300 mg maximum every 8 hours is also available for adolescents and adults.

## IBUPROFEN

Ibuprofen (Motrin, Advil) is a nonsteroidal anti-inflammatory drug (NSAID) that has analgesic and anti-inflammatory properties in addition to its antipyretic effects. This drug is highly effective and generally well tolerated with short-term administration when given orally. Ibuprofen's antipyretic mechanism of action blocks prostaglandin synthesis through inhibition of cyclooxygenase. This converts arachidonic acid to cyclic endoperoxides. Ibuprofen may be given to febrile children 6 months or older at a dose of 10 mg/kg every 6 to 8 hours. This dose has similar efficacy to that of acetaminophen. Adolescents and adults may take doses of 200 to 400 mg every 6 hours as needed.

## ASPIRIN

Aspirin (acetylsalicylic acid) is used less than it was in recent years. This drug was the standard treatment of fever for many years but is no longer used with children because of an association with Reye's syndrome. It has anti-inflammatory, analgesic, and antipyretic properties similar to ibuprofen and remains an effective treatment for adults. Adults may be given doses of 325 to 650 mg every 4 to 6 hours as needed. Bleeding commonly occurs with aspirin therapy because of its antiplatelet effect (e.g., in the gastrointestinal tract).

## MEDICATION COMBINATIONS

Combinations or alternating regimens of antipyretics should be used with caution, although studies show that aspirin and acetaminophen combinations are more effective. The American Academy of Pediatrics (AAP) cautions against using multiple antipyretics because of an increase in the likelihood of dosing errors. The AAP also cites a lack of evidence to support the joint use of acetaminophen with ibuprofen.

## NONPHARMACOLOGIC TREATMENT

External cooling, most commonly sponge bathing, is used to reduce fever. Some have advised against its use because it can cause discomfort. Discomfort is less likely to occur during sponging when using tepid water and antipyretic administration, but the efficacy of this treatment is questioned. Alcohol should not be a component of the bath because it may cause dehydration and hypoglycemia.

## REFERENCES

Acetaminophen toxicity in children. Pediatrics 2001;108(4):1020-1024.
Aronoff DM, Neilson EG: Antipyretics: Mechanisms of action and clinical use in fever suppression. Am J Med 2001;111(4):304-315.
Bouchama A, Knochel JP: Heat stroke. N Engl J Med 2002;346(25):1978-1988.
Crocetti M, Moghbeli N, Serwint J: Fever phobia revisited: Have parental misconceptions about fever changed in 20 years? Pediatrics 2001;107(6):1241-1246.
Doran TF, De Angelis C, Baumgardner RA, Mellits ED: Acetaminophen: More harm than good for chickenpox? J Pediatr 1989;114(6):1045-1048.
Kluger MJ: Fever: Role of pyrogens and cryogens. Physiol Rev 1991;71(1):93-127.
Kluger MJ: Fever revisited. Pediatrics 1992;90(6):846-850.
Mackowiak PA, Worden G: Carl Reinhold August Wunderlich and the evolution of clinical thermometry. Clin Infect Dis 1994;18(3):458-467.
Schmitt BD: Fever phobia: Misconceptions of parents about fevers. Am J Dis Child 1980;134(2):176-181.
Sharber J: The efficacy of tepid sponge bathing to reduce fever in young children. Am J Emerg Med 1997;15(2):188-192.
Simons SHP, Anderson BJ, Tibboel D: Analgesic agents. In Yaffe SJ, Aranda JV (eds): Neonatal and Pediatric Pharmacology: Therapeutic Principles in Practice, 3rd ed. Philadelphia, Lippincott Williams & Wilkins, 2005, pp 638-662.
Stanley ED, Jackson GG, Panusarn C, et al: Increased virus shedding with aspirin treatment of rhinovirus infection. JAMA 1975;231(12):1248-1251.

# Cough

Method of
*David G. Hill, MD*

Cough is among the most common presenting complaints of outpatients in the United States. It serves as a protective reflex against foreign material and as a method to clear secretions from the airway. The cough center is located in the medulla, and the cough reflex is mediated by way of multiple nervous system pathways including the trigeminal, glossopharyngeal, vagus, and phrenic nerves. Cough is mediated by separate neural pathways from bronchoconstriction. When cough occurs there is a synchronized activation of muscles, the glottis opens, and the lungs expand. At the peak of inspiration the glottis closes and expiratory muscles contract. This results in increased intrathoracic pressure; when the glottis opens airflow can reach 500 miles per hour. The cough reflex varies in different patient populations. Women have a more sensitive cough reflex than men. Smokers' cough reflexes are depressed despite the increased frequency of cough in this population. Patients who have a decreased cough sensitivity following cerebral vascular accidents have an increased incidence of pneumonia. Angiotensin-converting enzyme (ACE) inhibitors increase cough reflex sensitivity and have been shown to decrease the risk of pneumonia in patients with cerebrovascular accidents. The evaluation of cough as a patient complaint may best be pursued by examining the duration of the symptoms. Cough can be subcategorized into acute and chronic cough. Cough that occurs following an acute respiratory infection may narrow the differential diagnosis and is addressed separately.

## Acute Cough

Acute cough may be defined as cough that has been present for less than 8 weeks. Because all causes of chronic coughs initially cause acute symptoms, patients with acute cough may actually have cough caused by one of the etiologies discussed later in this section; however, acute cough more commonly is the result of a less indolent process (Box 1).

---

**BOX 1  Causes of Acute Cough**

- Viral upper respiratory infections (the common cold)
- Acute sinusitis (usually viral, occasionally bacterial)
- Exacerbation of chronic obstructive pulmonary disease
- Allergic rhinitis
- *Bordetella pertussis* infection

Infectious etiologies are a frequent cause of acute cough. Most acute cough is the result of viral infections, specifically the common cold. Most cough resulting from the common cold is self-limited and lasts less than 3 weeks. Most episodes of sinusitis are of viral etiology; however, bacterial sinusitis can also result in acute cough. The presence of a significant smoking history raises the possibility of an acute exacerbation of chronic obstructive pulmonary disease (COPD) as the cause of acute cough, especially in patients with previously documented COPD. *Bordetella pertussis* infection may also be the etiology of an acute episode of cough. Noninfectious processes that lead to acute cough include allergic rhinitis, congestive heart failure, asthma, and aspiration. The clinical history, physical examination, and diagnostic testing are of particular importance in differentiating these disease states and often point to the diagnosis.

## Postinfectious Cough

Postinfectious cough begins with an acute upper respiratory tract infection but persists following the resolution of the other acute symptoms (Box 2). Postnasal drip syndrome may present following the common cold or sinusitis. Bronchospasm may lead to postinfectious cough either as a result of a single episode of postinfectious wheezing or an exacerbation of underlying asthma. Postinfectious cough may be the initial presentation of asthma. Recurrent episodes of airflow obstruction are required to confirm the diagnosis of this chronic illness. Because *B. pertussis* can present with an indolent course, this infection can be confused with a postinfectious cough. Similarly, bacterial sinusitis can be confused with postinfectious cough. Both of these etiologies of cough are the result of ongoing infection rather than true postinfectious cough. *Mycoplasma pneumoniae* and *Chlamydia pneumoniae* infections may also result in postinfectious cough likely because of persistent airway inflammation and increases in cough reflex sensitivity.

## Chronic Cough

Chronic cough presents the most difficult diagnostic dilemma for the health care practitioner. Cough of greater than 8 weeks' duration can be considered chronic. Lesser duration of symptoms may still be indicative of one of the etiologies discussed in this section, but such cough is more likely the result of one of the infectious or postinfectious etiologies described previously. In patients who have never smoked, chronic cough is most likely the result of asthma, postnasal drip syndrome, or gastroesophageal reflux. These three etiologies are the most common cause of chronic cough regardless of patient age. In nonsmokers with a normal chest radiograph who are not taking an ACE inhibitor, these three etiologies alone or in combination are the cause of more than 85% of chronic cough (Box 3). Postnasal drip syndrome is the most common of these etiologies. Cough may be the sole presenting symptom of any of these conditions; they are not mutually exclusive and may coexist, particularly in the patient with troublesome, persistent symptoms. Most patients with problematic, persistent cough have multiple etiologies contributing to their symptoms. COPD must be considered in current smokers and in those patients with a significant smoking history. Smokers can have a cough of any etiology, however, and it should not be assumed that their cough is the result of smoking or COPD. Although smokers frequently

---

### BOX 2 Causes of Postinfectious Cough

- Postnasal drip syndrome
- Bronchospasm
- *Bordetella pertussis* infection
- Bacterial sinusitis
- *Mycoplasma pneumoniae/Chlamydia pneumoniae* infection

---

### BOX 3 Causes of Chronic Cough

- Postnasal drip syndrome
- Asthma
- Gastroesophageal reflux disease (GERD)
- Eosinophilic bronchitis
- Angiotensin-converting enzyme inhibitors

---

admit to cough when a history is taken, they infrequently seek medical attention for this symptom. Cough resulting from the use of ACE inhibitors must be considered in all patients being treated with these medications. Less common, yet frequent causes of cough include chronic bronchitis from irritants other than tobacco smoke and eosinophilic bronchitis. Occasionally, chronic cough may be the result of:

- Bronchogenic carcinoma
- Metastatic carcinoma
- Bronchiectasis
- Sarcoidosis
- Pulmonary fibrosis
- Pneumoconiosis
- Hypersensitivity pneumonitis
- Congestive heart failure
- Chronic infection, such as tuberculosis or *Mycobacterium avium* complex
- Recurrent aspiration because of pharyngeal or esophageal abnormalities

## Key Diagnostic Points

The evaluation of acute cough should focus on the history and physical examination. Most acute cough will be the result of self-limited viral upper respiratory infections. More thorough evaluation is necessary in the workup of cough of longer duration particularly if the cough has been present for more than 2 months. The history of onset of the cough and whether it was associated with an acute infectious episode should be elicited. Exposure to sick contacts particularly to a known case of *B. pertussis* are important historic considerations. The timing and nature of the cough and any associated sputum must be described. Factors that mitigate or worsen the cough should be examined, and prior history of episodic cough, allergies, wheezing, asthma, and gastroesophageal reflux should be questioned. A thorough medication history particularly regarding use of ACE inhibitors must be obtained. Environmental factors both at home and in the work place should be reviewed. Although smoking history is important, it is again noted that smoking-related cough is an infrequent reason for a patient to seek medical attention. The physical examination should focus most on the head, neck, and thorax with a thorough examination of the upper respiratory tract including the auditory canal, nose, and oropharynx. The cardiopulmonary examination should also be thorough to elicit signs of less common illnesses.

Acute cough associated with an acute respiratory illness and prominent upper airway symptoms can be assumed to be secondary to the common cold. Diagnostic testing is not indicated in such patients; a chest radiograph would be normal and is thus not recommended. Patients who have abnormal sinus transillumination, purulent nasal secretions, sinus pain or tenderness, or maxillary toothache could possibly have bacterial sinusitis. Again, a viral etiology of sinusitis is more likely than bacterial sinusitis, and antibiotic therapy should be initiated only in patients with persistent symptoms despite symptomatic therapy. Patients with documented COPD who present with acute cough, purulent sputum, dyspnea, and wheezing have an exacerbation of their underlying COPD and should be treated appropriately. Allergic rhinitis usually presents with a clear clinical history of episodic nasal and other allergy symptoms, and allergen avoidance can be initiated. It is important to note that allergic rhinitis can present with perennial symptoms.

Postinfectious cough should be evaluated with thorough history and physical examinations followed by limited diagnostic evaluation and empiric therapies. Patients should be treated for postnasal drip syndrome, particularly in the setting of described rhinitis, postnasal drip, or frequent throat clearing. The presence of nasal inflammation and congestion, cobblestoning of the pharyngeal mucosa, or mucus in the oropharynx should also lead to empiric therapy for postnasal drip syndrome. If cough persists in the patients with suspected postnasal drip syndrome, evaluation of the sinuses with imaging and treatment of those patients with evidence of bacterial sinusitis should be pursued. Computed tomography (CT) imaging of the sinuses is the gold standard for diagnosing bacterial sinusitis. Patients with postinfectious cough and an abnormal respiratory examination should have a chest radiograph. Patients with a normal radiograph and evidence of bronchospasm can be empirically treated for airway hyperreactivity. Again, the diagnosis of asthma requires recurrent airflow obstruction and cannot be made on the basis of a single episode of postinfectious wheezing or airway hyperreactivity. In subjects with cough and vomiting, known exposure to a case of B. pertussis, or in the presence of a B. pertussis epidemic in the community, empiric therapy for this illness should be pursued.

Before the vaccine era, B. pertussis was an endemic disease, which occurred in cyclic epidemics. It has been documented that B. pertussis continues to circulate in the adult population despite control of the disease in the pediatric population by vaccination. Immunity to B. pertussis, whether as a result of primary infection or immunization, is shortlived. The longer the elapsed interval since prior infection or immunization and repeat infection, the more likely repeat infection will be symptomatic. Perhaps repeat adolescent and adult booster immunization programs should be implemented to effectively control or eliminate this infection.

History and physical examinations remain paramount in the patient presenting with chronic cough. The majority of patients should have a chest radiograph obtained as part of their evaluation. If the history and physical examination suggest that postnasal drip, asthma, or gastroesophageal reflux is the etiology of a patient's symptoms, empiric therapy for these conditions should be initiated. Cough triggered by environmental factors or changes may be secondary to rhinitis and postnasal drip or airway hyperreactivity and asthma. Substernal burning or a sour taste in the mouth, particularly when triggered by supine positioning or bending, should increase the suspicion of gastroesophageal reflux.

If asthma is suspected, spirometry should be performed to document whether airflow obstruction is present. Response to inhaled bronchodilator with normal spirometry is indicative of airway hyperreactivity. Improvement in symptoms and spirometry with empiric asthma therapy even in the setting of normal baseline flow rates also confirms an asthmatic etiology. A methacholine challenge can be performed to confirm airway hyperreactivity. If cough in the setting of a positive methacholine challenge shows absolutely no response to empiric asthma therapy with inhaled corticosteroids and bronchodilators, consider a trial of systemic steroids. If the cough does not respond to aggressive asthma therapy, the methacholine challenge test results were probably false positive; asthma therapy can be discontinued and diagnostic efforts focused elsewhere.

Cough patients being treated with ACE inhibitors should cease these medications. Up to 30% of patients treated with ACE inhibitors will develop a persistent cough, more commonly in women, nonsmokers, and patients of Chinese ancestry. It may take 4 weeks or more for cough caused by ACE inhibitors to resolve following cessation of these medications. In the presence of ACE inhibitor use, further evaluation of dry cough should not be pursued until the patient has been withdrawn from these medications for 1 month.

An abnormal chest radiograph can direct further diagnostic studies and therapies, whereas a normal chest radiograph makes less common etiologies of chronic cough such as carcinoma, congestive heart failure, sarcoidosis, or interstitial lung disease unlikely. Evidence of basilar infiltrates or fibrosis may suggest interstitial lung disease or chronic aspiration. Severe gastroesophageal reflux must be considered in those patients with radiographic evidence of chronic aspiration.

Chronic cough without a definitive etiology can be troubling to both patient and health care provider. A systematic approach can simplify both diagnosis and treatment (Figure 1). It is again stressed

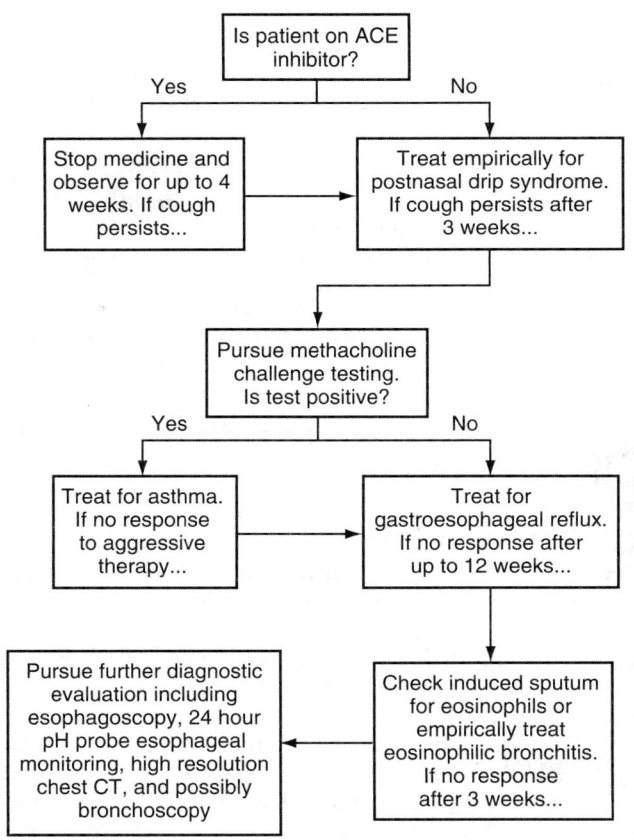

**FIGURE 1.** Approach to chronic cough of uncertain origin. ACE = angiotensin-converting enzyme; CT = computed tomography

Cough

25

## CURRENT DIAGNOSIS

### All Patients Presenting With Cough

- Perform thorough history and physical examination.
- Review timing and nature of cough along with exacerbating or mitigating factors.
- Review prior history of cough, allergies, asthma, or gastroesophageal reflux.
- Take medication history, particularly use of ACE inhibitors.
- Focus physical examination on head, neck, and thorax.

### Patients With Postinfectious or Chronic Cough

- Obtain chest radiograph, particularly in patients with an abnormal respiratory examination.
- Evaluate airflow obstruction with spirometry.
- Stop ACE inhibitors and assess for improvement.
- Administer empiric therapy for postnasal drip, asthma, or gastroesophageal reflux.
- Consider methacholine challenge testing to evaluate for airway hyperreactivity.
- Induce sputum for eosinophils or empiric trial of corticosteroids for eosinophilic bronchitis.
- If cough persists, consider esophagoscopy, 24-hour pH probe monitoring, high-resolution chest CT, or bronchoscopy.

*Abbreviations:* ACE = angiotensin-converting enzyme; CT = computed tomography.

that such a cough may be the result of multiple etiologic factors. In the absence of specific factors that help to point to an etiology of chronic cough, empiric treatment for postnasal drip syndrome should be pursued. Methacholine challenge testing will rule out asthma if it is negative and should also be performed early in the evaluation of chronic cough. Cough may be the sole manifestation of asthma in nearly 60% of patients presenting with chronic cough. A positive methacholine challenge does not have 100% predictive value but should lead to empiric asthma therapy.

Empiric therapy for silent gastroesophageal reflux should be initiated in those who do not respond to treatment for postnasal drip syndrome and do not have evidence of or respond to treatment for asthma. Cough may be the only manifestation of gastroesophageal reflux up to 30% of the time. Definitive diagnosis of gastroesophageal reflux requires invasive testing and may require more than one testing modality. Therefore it is recommended that empiric therapy for reflux be pursued before diagnostic testing. Reflux therapy should include conservative approaches such as dietary and lifestyle changes, bed positioning, and pharmacologic treatment. Gastroesophageal reflux–related cough can be particularly troublesome and persistent and may take weeks or months to respond to appropriate and intensive antireflux therapy. This may include higher-than-normal doses of proton pump inhibitors and promotility agents. Surgical treatment of reflux may be necessary to effectively treat reflux related cough in some patients. In patients with persistent cough, the common etiologies of cough often coexist and exacerbate one another. Therapy should often be additive, for instance treating both asthma and reflux, rather than mutually exclusive. Persistent cough should result in further diagnostic

 **CURRENT THERAPY**

### Treatment of Acute Cough

- Common cold: Supportive care with dexbrompheniramine, 6 mg, and pseudoephedrine, 120 mg (Drixoral Cold and Allergy Tablets); or ipratropium nasal spray (Atrovent, 0.06%), two 42-mcg sprays in each nostril 3 times daily for 4 to 7 d depending on duration of symptoms.
- Acute sinusitis: Treat as a common cold. Add oxymetazoline (Afrin), two sprays twice daily for three days. If symptoms persist, consider antibiotic therapy directed against *Haemophilus influenzae* and *Streptococcus pneumoniae* such as azithromycin (Zithromax), 500 mg daily for 3 d.
- Exacerbation of chronic obstructive pulmonary disease: Antibiotics directed against *H. influenzae* and *S. pneumoniae* for 3 to 7 d such as clarithromycin (Biaxin), 500 mg twice daily for 7 d; systemic corticosteroids such as prednisone (Deltasone), 40 mg tapered over 10 d; inhaled anticholinergics such as tiotropium (Spiriva), one inhalation daily; and short-acting β-agonists such as albuterol (Proventil), two inhalations every 4 h as needed; smoking cessation.
- Allergic rhinitis: Nasal corticosteroids such as mometasone (Nasonex), two sprays in each nostril daily; nonsedating antihistamines such as fexofenadine (Allegra), 180 mg daily; allergen avoidance if possible.
- *Bordetella pertussis*: Erythromycin 500 mg four times daily for 14 d or trimethoprim 160 mg/sulfamethoxazole (Bactrim DS),[1] 800 mg twice daily for 14 d. Other macrolide antibiotics such as azithromycin (Zithromax)[1] or clarithromycin (Biaxin)[1] are likely effective and may be better tolerated.

### Treatment of Postinfectious Cough

- Postnasal drip syndrome: Dexbrompheniramine, 6 mg, and pseudoephedrine (Drixoral Cold and Allergy Tablets), 120 mg for up to 3 wk; ipratropium (Atrovent), 0.06% nasal spray for up to 3 wk; azelastine (Astelin) nasal spray (137 mcg), two sprays each nostril twice daily for up to 3 wk.
- Bronchospasm: Inhaled corticosteroid such as budesonide (Pulmicort),[1] two inhalations daily with or without inhaled long-acting β-agonist such as formoterol (Foradil), two inhalations twice daily; short-acting β-agonist such as albuterol (Ventolin), two puffs every 4 h as needed. Oral steroids such as prednisone (Deltasone), 40 mg tapered over 10 d.
- *Bordetella pertussis*: Erythromycin, 500 mg four times daily for 14 d, or trimethoprim 160 mg/sulfamethoxazole, 800 mg (Bactrim DS)[1] twice daily for 14 d. Other macrolide antibiotics such as azithromycin (Zithromax)[1] or clarithromycin (Biaxin)[1] are likely effective and may be better tolerated.
- Bacterial sinusitis: Dexbrompheniramine, 6 mg, and pseudoephedrine (Drixoral Cold and Allergy Tablets), 120 mg for up to 3 wk; oxymetazoline (Afrin), two sprays twice daily for 3 d; azithromycin (Zithromax), 500 mg daily for 3 d.
- Chlamydia/mycoplasma: Clarithromycin (Biaxin), 500 mg twice daily for 14 d.

### Treatment of Chronic Cough

- Postnasal drip syndrome
  Nonallergic: Dexbrompheniramine, 6 mg, and pseudoephedrine (Drixoral Cold and Allergy Tablets), 120 mg for up to 3 wk; ipratropium (Atrovent), 0.06% nasal spray for up to 3 wk; azelastine (Astelin) nasal spray (137 mcg), two sprays each nostril twice daily for up to 3 wk.
  Allergic: Fluticasone (Flonase) (50 mcg), two sprays each nostril daily; fexofenadine (Allegra), 180 mg daily; allergen avoidance.
- Asthma: Albuterol (Proventil), two puffs every 4 hours as needed; inhaled corticosteroid such as budesonide (Pulmicort), two inhalations daily with or without inhaled long-acting β-agonist such as formoterol (Foradil), two inhalations twice daily; combination of long-acting β-agonist and inhaled steroid such as fluticasone/salmeterol (Advair) (100/50 mcg), inhaled twice daily; montelukast (Singulair), 10 mg daily; prednisone (Deltasone), 40 mg daily with tapering dose over 10 d.
- Gastroesophageal reflux: Dietary and lifestyle modifications, lansoprazole (Prevacid), 30 mg daily for up to 3 mo; metoclopramide (Reglan), 10 mg before meals and sleep.
- Eosinophilic bronchitis: Fluticasone (Flovent)[1] (110 mcg), two inhalations twice daily; prednisone (Deltasone), 30 mg daily for 3 wk.
- ACE inhibitor: Discontinue medication.

[1]Not FDA approved for this indication.

evaluation including sputum studies, esophagoscopy, 24-hour pH probe esophageal monitoring, high-resolution chest CT, and possibly bronchoscopy. In the presence of normal chest imaging, bronchoscopy is unlikely to yield beneficial diagnostic information in the patient with chronic cough.

Eosinophilic bronchitis in the absence of asthma is also a frequent cause (up to 13% of cases) of chronic cough. Patients with eosinophilic bronchitis will have normal spirometry and a negative methacholine challenge. The disease may be diagnosed by appropriate induced sputum analysis showing at least 3% eosinophils. Alternatively it can be empirically treated with a course of inhaled corticosteroids. Most patients appear to respond to inhaled corticosteroids within 3 weeks. Systemic corticosteroids may be required to improve the symptoms in some cases. There may be an association of gastroesophageal reflux with eosinophilic bronchitis. Patients with gastroesophageal reflux have been found to have increased sputum eosinophilia.

Bronchiectasis may infrequently result in chronic cough. Bronchiectasis is characterized by the abnormal dilatation of one or more branches of the bronchial tree. It can effectively be diagnosed by high resolution CT scan of the thorax. Bronchiectasis may occur following a severe infection, distal to an area of airway obstruction, congenitally, from chronic inflammatory processes, and as a result of chronic parenchymal scarring and traction. Patients with bronchiectasis may present with productive or nonproductive coughs. They may have recurrent episodes of infection resulting from persistent colonization of the abnormal bronchial segment. Infectious agents may include routine bacterial organisms and typical or atypical mycobacterium. Bronchiectasis may be seen in a variety of chronic illnesses. The presence of bronchiectasis in a patient without a known predisposing cause should prompt the clinician to look for appropriate clinical states, such as:

- Primary or acquired immunodeficiencies
- Abnormalities of ciliary function, such as ciliary dyskinesia or cystic fibrosis
- Postinfectious inflammatory processes, such as allergic bronchopulmonary aspergillosis
- Collagen vascular diseases
- Inflammatory bowel disease
- Sarcoidosis
- Yellow nail syndrome

The presence of localized bronchiectasis may be an indication to pursue flexible fiberoptic bronchoscopy to rule out an obstructing lesion and to obtain appropriate culture specimens. Treatment of bronchiectasis is aimed at the underlying disease state if one can be identified. Infections should be treated with appropriate antibiotics. Clearance of bronchial secretions can be aided with mucolytics and chest physiotherapy including use of percussive devices. In some cases surgical therapy to remove the bronchiectatic segment can be considered.

## Treatment

The key treatments for cough are best described based on the suspected etiology. Acute cough therapy should focus on supportive treatment of the underlying suspected etiology, which will likely be a viral upper respiratory infection. Therapy for exacerbation of chronic obstructive pulmonary disease, allergic rhinitis, bacterial sinusitis, or *B. pertussis* infection is more specific. Postinfectious cough should focus on therapy for postnasal drip syndrome or airways reactivity if suspected. In chronic cough of uncertain etiology (see Figure 1), cough therapy should begin with empiric treatment of postnasal drip syndrome, evaluation and treatment of asthma, empiric treatment of gastroesophageal reflux syndrome, and finally evaluation or empiric therapy for eosinophilic bronchitis.

Cough is a frequent and troublesome symptom for both patient and health care provider. Acute cough although at times troubling is usually self-limiting. Postinfectious cough and chronic cough are more problematic, but can effectively be evaluated and treated by performing a thorough history and physical examination and pursuing a systematic approach to diagnostic evaluation and both empiric and guided therapies. The resolution of chronic troubling cough is a therapeutic relief for the patient and a gratifying experience for the caregiver.

## REFERENCES

Barnes TW, Afessa B, Swanson KL, Lim KG: The clinical utility of flexible bronchoscopy in the evaluation of chronic cough. Chest 2004;126:268-272.
Breitling CE, Ward R, Goh KL: Eosinophilic bronchitis is an important cause of chronic cough. Am J Respir Crit Care Med 1999;160:406-410.
Cherry JD: Epidemiological, clinical, and laboratory aspects of pertussis in adults. Clin Infect Dis 1999;28(suppl2):S112-S117.
Cohen M, Sahn SA: Bronchiectasis in systemic diseases. Chest 1999;116:1063-1074.
Irwin RS, Madison JM: Symptom research on chronic cough: A historical perspective. Ann Intern Med 2001;134:809-814.
Irwin RS, Madison JM: The diagnosis and treatment of cough. N Engl J Med 2000;343:1715-1721.
Irwin RS, Madison JM: The persistently troublesome cough. Am J Respir Crit Care Med 2002;165:1469-1474.
Kiljander TO: The role of proton pump inhibitors in the management of gastroesophageal reflux disease-related asthma and chronic cough. Am J Med 2003;115(3A):S65-S71.

# Treatment of Insomnia

Method of
*Martin Reite, MD*

Three things should be remembered when considering treatment of an insomnia complaint. First, insomnia is more often a symptom, than a specific disorder. Second, it is important to perform a systematic differential diagnosis, keeping in mind the possibility that there will be very likely more than one cause of an insomnia complaint. Finally, the cause of the complaint usually can be determined, and most patients complaining of insomnia can be helped. Also, insomnia must not be trivialized.

Insomnia is among the most frequent complaints in the population; untreated insomnia is associated with increases in new-onset anxiety and depression, increased daytime sleepiness, and increased health-related concerns.

Insomnia can include difficulty in getting to sleep (sleep-onset insomnia), difficulty staying asleep (sleep-maintenance insomnia), or early morning awakening (terminal insomnia). Because such subtypes are not stable over time, this method of subtyping may have little clinical usefulness. As a rule, insomnia complaints are more frequent in women, elderly persons, and patients of lower socioeconomic status.

## Screening for Sleep Complaints

Three routine questions, illustrated in Box 1, will detect most significant sleep problems. A positive answer to any of these questions merits consideration of a more detailed sleep history to determine whether in fact a sleep disorder is present. Box 2 outlines the items to be covered in a sleep history.

Sources of diagnostic information should include the bed partner whenever possible because many sleep-related symptoms are apparent only to the bed partner. A several-week daily sleep diary also can be

---

**BOX 1  Detection of Specific Sleep Disorders**

Are you content with your sleep? (identifies most insomnia complaints)
Are you excessively sleepy during the day? (identifies most disorders of excessive sleepiness)
Does your bed partner complain about your sleep? (identifies most parasomnia disorders)

## BOX 2 Sleep History Questionnaire

When did the symptoms start, and what was going on at
the time?

What has been the symptom pattern across time?

Are symptoms stress or situationally related?

What is your typical daily schedule, hour by hour?

What medications and treatments have been and are
currently being used to date?

Is there a presence of familial sleep-related symptoms?

## BOX 4 Medications Often Associated with Insomnia

| | |
|---|---|
| Anticholinergics | Corticosteroids |
| Antidepressants | Decongestants |
| Antihypertensives | Diuretics |
| Antineoplastic agents | Histamine-2 (H2) |
| Bronchodilators | blockers |
| CNS stimulants | Smoking cessation aids |

useful at this stage of the evaluation because it can provide a detailed
daily description of sleep/wake activity patterns.

# Transient and Short-Term Insomnia

Transient (1 to several days) and short-term (up to 3 weeks) insomnias
are typically stress related, and respond well to pharmacologic (short-
term hypnotic) intervention. They should be considered for active treatment, because untreated short-term insomnia can lead to a state of
"conditioned arousal" resulting in a chronic insomnia.

# Differential Diagnosis of the Chronic Insomnia Complaint

The differential diagnosis of a chronic insomnia complaint can represent a more challenging task and requires a thorough differential diagnostic evaluation, which includes systematically considering the
conditions or combinations of conditions that are most likely to result
in insomnia complaints. General practice parameters for the
evaluation of chronic insomnia complaints can be found at:
http://www.aasmnet.org/ PDF/ChronicParameter.pdf. Box 3 lists the
common causes of insomnia (not necessarily listed in order of
frequency). Each cause is briefly discussed.

## MEDICAL CONDITIONS AND TREATMENT

Medical conditions, and in susceptible patients, many pharmacologic
treatments of medical conditions, can result in insomnia complaints.
The endocrinopathies are notorious for being associated with sleep-
related complaints, as are conditions associated with chronic pain,
breathing difficulties, cardiac arrhythmias, arthritis, renal failure, and
central nervous system (CNS) disorders. Box 4 lists the more
commonly used medications that can result in insomnia complaints.

The treatment of insomnia associated with medical conditions is
first to isolate and appropriately treat the medical condition and the
symptoms (e.g., pain) causing the insomnia. If the insomnia complaint
persists, evaluate the possibility of an additional cause for the sleep

## BOX 3 Common Causes of Insomnia

Medical conditions and/or pharmacologic treatment of
medical conditions

Psychiatric disorders (especially depression, anxiety, and
post-traumatic stress disorder [PTSD])

Substance abuse disorders

Circadian rhythm disorders presenting as insomnia

Periodic limb movements in sleep (PLMS)

Central sleep apnea

The primary insomnia, conditioned insomnia, and
sleep-state misperception group

complaint. Supplementary use of a short half-life hypnotic agent [e.g.,
zolpidem (Ambien), 5-10 mg at bedtime] may be helpful. Insomnia
associated with fibromyalgia and chronic fatigue syndrome is
frequently resistant to treatment, although small doses of amitriptyline
(Elavil)[1] (10-50 mg at bedtime) or cyclobenzaprine (Flexeril)[1] (10 mg
three times a day) have been reported to be helpful; occasionally,
zolpidem (5-10 mg) will help with the associated insomnia complaints.

Dementing illnesses are often associated with severe insomnia
complaints that are quite disruptive to patients and families and often
are the factors precipitating institutional care. Sleep is often disturbed
in such disorders on the basis of disease-associated CNS lesions, and
different specific pathophysiologies (not yet well understood) may
respond to different treatments. Until such specific treatments can be
based on specific pathophysiology, we should adhere to optimal environmental circadian principles (quiet, dark nocturnal environment;
bright, socially stimulating daytime environment). Appropriate use of
hypnotics may be helpful, although responses may be variable.

## PSYCHIATRIC DISORDERS

Psychiatric disorders, especially those associated with anxiety or
depression, frequently include insomnia (delayed sleep onset, frequent
awakening, or early morning awakening) as an associated symptom.
Effective treatment of the psychiatric condition will often relieve the
insomnia complaint, although a supplemental hypnotic might be indicated early in treatment. Different antidepressant agents have quite
different effects on sleep as illustrated in Table 1, and the initial choice
of an antidepressant might profitably take such effects into account.

If, for a patient already complaining of insomnia, an antidepressant
with a known high incidence of insomnia side effects is chosen, it may be
useful to augment it with a hypnotic agent early in the course of treatment.

## SUBSTANCE USE SLEEP DISORDERS

Alcohol abuse remains a significant problem in the etiology of sleep
complaints, as do stimulants and other drugs of abuse. Treatment
includes withdrawal of the offending substance, with long-term abstinence as the goal. Treatment of substance abuse-related insomnia should
emphasize behavioral treatment strategies to the fullest extent possible,
because psychoactive agents have already proved to be a problem.

## CIRCADIAN RHYTHM DISORDERS

Disturbances in the regulation of the circadian system frequently present as sleep-related complaints, although the source of the problem lies
in the circadian system rather than sleep pathology. Sleep per se may be
adequate, but it occurs at the wrong time. Delayed sleep-phase
syndrome (DSPS) is the most common, and is likely a genetically based
disorder with frequent onset in adolescence or early adulthood. These
individuals cannot get to sleep (because of phase delay in the body
temperature rhythm) until 3 to 4 a.m., and if allowed to sleep, 8 to
9 hours may do well. If they have to arise at 7 a.m. for school or work,
they will be sleep deprived and complain of insomnia.

---

[1]Not FDA approved for this indication.

**TABLE 1** Effect of Antidepressants on Sleep Scale*

| Effects on EEG Sleep Drug | Trade Name | Continuity | SWS | REM | Sedation Effects |
|---|---|---|---|---|---|
| **TCAs** | | | | | |
| Amitriptyline | Elavil | I (3) | I (1) | D (3) | 4 |
| Doxepin | Sinequan | I (3) | I (2) | D (2) | 4 |
| Imipramine | Tofranil | I (0-1) | I (1) | D (2) | 2 |
| Nortriptyline | Pamelor | I (1) | I (1) | D (2) | 2 |
| Desipramine | Norpramin | (0) | I (1) | D (2) | 1 |
| Clomipramine | Anafranil | I (0-1) | I (1) | D (4) | 0 |
| **MAOIs** | | | | | |
| Phenelzine | Nardil | D (1) | (0) | D (4) | 0 |
| Tranylcypromine | Parnate | D (2) | (0) | D (4) | 0 |
| **SSRIs** | | | | | |
| Fluoxetine | Prozac | D (1) | D (0-1) | D (0-1) | 0 |
| Paroxetine | Paxil | D (1) | D (0-1) | D (2) | 0 |
| Sertraline | Zoloft | (0) | (0) | D (2) | 0 |
| Citalopram | Celexa | D (1) | (0) | D (1) | ND |
| Fluvoxamine | Luvox | D (1) | (0) | D (1) | ND |
| Escitalopram | Lexapro | (0) | (0) | D (2) | 0 |
| **Other** | | | | | |
| Bupropion | Wellbutrin | D (0-1) | (0) | I (1) | 0 |
| Venlafaxine | Effexor | D (1) | D (1) | D (3) | 2 |
| Trazodone | Desyrel | I (3) | I (0-1) | D (1) | 4 |
| Mirtazapine | Remeron | I (3) | I (2) | (0) | 3 |
| Nefazodone | Serzone | I (1) | (0) | I (1) | 1 |

*Abbreviations:* EEG = electroencephalogram; MAOIs = monoamine oxidase inhibitors; REM = rapid eye movement; SSRIs = selective serotonin reuptake inhibitors; SWS = slow-wave sleep; TCAs = tricyclic antidepressants.
*Scale 0-4: 0 = no significant effect; I = increase and D = decrease.

Early morning bright-light exposure, with restriction of light exposure in the evening, has been found to be effective for phase-advancing the circadian system in DSPS. Evening bright-light treatment is effective in treating advanced sleep-phase syndrome. Low-dose (1-3 mg) melatonin[1,*] at bedtime may help regulate circadian rhythms in some individuals.

Jet lag and shift-work–related sleep problems also fall in the category of circadian rhythm problems. A detailed discussion of these problem areas is beyond the scope of this article, but recently emerging data suggest that properly timed bright-light exposure, supplemented with melatonin[1,*] administration and appropriate hypnotic use, can significantly reduce associated symptoms.

## PERIODIC LIMB MOVEMENTS OF SLEEP AND RESTLESS LEGS SYNDROME

Both restless legs syndrome (RLS) and periodic limb movements of sleep (PLMS) are associated with a variety of medical conditions, including iron deficiency, but they may occur in otherwise healthy individuals (especially the elderly). A polysomnogram (PSG) is usually required for accurate diagnosis of a PLMS disorder, quantifying both the number of events and their association with awakenings or arousals. Table 2 lists the drugs currently used in the treatment of PLMS and RLS.

## CENTRAL SLEEP APNEA

Central sleep apnea with frequent arousals is a relatively rare cause of chronic insomnia except at higher altitudes, and may require a PSG for accurate diagnosis. Both oxygen and continuous positive airway pressure (CPAP) can be used in the treatment of central apnea in patients with medical disorders. The efficacy of pharmacologic agents in the treatment of central sleep apnea has yet to be clearly established in well-controlled studies. Acetazolamide (Diamox)[1] (250 mg twice a day) may be effective for the prevention of high altitude-induced central apnea.

## THE PRIMARY INSOMNIA, CONDITIONED INSOMNIA, AND SLEEP-STATE MISPERCEPTION SYNDROME GROUP

Although there are several more rare causes of a chronic insomnia complaint, most often it is generally safe to assume that once the aforementioned specific causes have been systematically excluded or appropriately treated (and the insomnia complaints remain), we are in all probability left with either a primary insomnia disorder (DSM-IV 307.42), a conditioned insomnia, a sleep-state misperception syndrome (SSMS), or some combination thereof.

A treatment approach that combines both behavioral and pharmacologic approaches is generally recommended. Such a combined treatment approach offers the advantage of a pharmacologic agent that can produce rapid relief of the sleep complaint, along with behavioral strategies, which take longer to become effective but provide long-term results that are under a patient's control. Active and continued involvement of the patient is important for any chronic insomnia treatment.

## Sleep Laboratory Studies

All night PSGs, which monitor multiple physiologic variables during sleep, are rarely needed in the evaluation of insomnia complaints, except for symptoms associated with PLMS or for a sleep-related breathing disorder, where a PSG is usually required for accurate diagnosis. A recent review of the use of PSGs in the insomnia complaints can be found at: http://www.aasmnet.org/PDF/260616.pdf.

[1]Not FDA approved for this indication.
*Available as a dietary supplement.

[1]Not FDA approved for this indication.

**TABLE 2  Beginning Dose Schedules for PMLS and RLS**

| Drug | Dose (mg) | Administration |
|---|---|---|
| **Dopa Agonists** | | |
| Carbidopa/Levodopa | 25/100-50/200 | Bedtime/(Sinemet)[1] symptom onset |
| Controlled-release | 25/100-50/200 | Bedtime/Carbidopa/Levodopa symptom onset (Sinemet CR)[1] |
| Bromocriptine (Parlodel)[1] | 2.5-5 | Bedtime |
| Baclofen (Lioresal)[1] | 20-40 | Bedtime |
| Pergolide (Permax)[1] | 0.05 | Bedtime/symptom onset |
| Pramipexole (Mirapex)[1] | 0.125 | Bedtime |
| Ropinirole (Requip)[1] | 0.25 | Bedtime |
| **Other Agents** | | |
| Oxycodone (Roxicodone)[1] | 5-15 | Bedtime |
| Codeine[1] | 10-60 | Bedtime |
| Triazolam (Halcion)[1] | 0.125-0.25 | Bedtime |
| Temazepam (Restoril)[1] | 15-30 | Bedtime |
| Clonazepam (Klonopin)[1] | 0.5-1.5 | Bedtime |
| Gabapentin (Neurontin)[1] | 100-300 | Bedtime |

[1]Not FDA approved for this indication.

The 24-hour recording of activity (Actigraphy) can also be useful in the diagnosis of circadian rhythm-based sleepcomplaints (e.g., see: http://www.aasmnet.org/PDF/260315.pdf ).

# Treatment

After completing the evaluation of a chronic insomnia complaint and arriving at a diagnostic formulation, a treatment plan should be developed addressing all likely contributing causes. The treatment plan will likely include both behavioral and pharmacologic components, and should be discussed in detail with the patient. Patients might be encouraged to visit the web pages of the American Sleep Disorders Association (www.asda.org) and the National Sleep Foundation (www.nsf.org) to learn more about factors influencing sleep. Patient education facilitates effective treatment.

## BEHAVIORAL TREATMENTS

Behavioral treatment strategies are aimed at (a) breaking bad sleep habits and replacing them with sleep-promoting habits; (b) directly decreasing physiologic arousal levels using cognitively based or learned strategies; and (c) providing the patient with several types of cognitive strategies to deal with sleep difficulties, thus promoting a sense of competence and diminishing anxiety about sleep. First and foremost among the behavioral strategies is good sleep hygiene—the behaviors and habits that foster good sleep. Box 5 highlights the principles of good sleep hygiene. It is helpful to prepare a handout for patients summarizing good sleep hygiene practices that they can take with them. Box 6 lists additional behavioral strategies.

## PHARMACOLOGIC TREATMENTS

Benzodiazepine (BZ) compounds and newer nonbenzodiazepine agents active at the level of the BZ receptor are the most commonly used hypnotic agents. Older hypnotic agents (chloral hydrate, paraldehyde [Paral], barbiturates) may have limited usefulness for very short-term use in specific patients, but they cannot be recommended for the treatment of chronic insomnia.

BZ agents activate all BZ receptors (hypnotic, anxiolytic, muscle relaxant, anticonvulsant), and different agents demonstrate relatively little receptor specificity.

The BZ compounds differ substantially in terms of half-life and are illustrated in Table 3. The clinician can choose the agent with a half-life most appropriate for the clinical situation.

Long half-life BZ agents may be associated with residual daytime sedation and impairments in psychomotor performance. All BZ agents interfere with memory consolidation, the more potent agents (e.g., triazolam [Halcion]) most prominently. All BZ agents are prone to the development of tolerance, dependence, and rebound insomnia in response to rapid withdrawal. BZ agents also tend to decrease stages 3 to 4 sleep, and increase fast activity in the waking and sleeping electroencephalogram (EEG). These results may continue after drug discontinuation. Clearly useful for the treatment of insomnia associated with anxiety, the use of long-term BZ treatment of primary

---

**BOX 5  Good Sleep Hygiene**

Establish a regular sleep schedule that does not vary by more than 1 hour.

Maintain a state of good aerobic fitness with regular exercise (but not within 3 hours of sleep onset).

Do not use caffeine or alcohol to excess.

Ensure a quiet, dark, cool bedroom.

Provide a time to wind down in the evening before sleeping.

Consider a high-tryptophan snack (milk, cookies, banana) before bed.

Use the bedroom for sleep and sex but not for reviewing or thinking about the affairs of the day.

Minimize exposure to late evening bright light to avoid phase-delaying the circadian system.

---

**BOX 6  Other Behavioral Strategies for the Treatment of Insomnia**

Biofeedback (EMG and EEG): teaches subjects to decrease autonomic arousal

Progressive relaxation: training in systematic total body relaxation

Sleep restriction: good for subjects spending excessive time in bed with poorly consolidated sleep

Yoga, transcendental meditation (TM): self-control strategies

Cognitive behavioral therapy (several types): improved self-confidence and self-control

## TABLE 3 Benzodiazepines

| Name | | Dose (mg) | | | |
|---|---|---|---|---|---|
| Generic | Trade Name | Adult | Elderly | Onset | Half-Life (Hours) |
| Triazolam | Halcion | 0.125-0.25 | 0.125-0.25 | Rapid | 1.5-5.5 |
| Estazolam | ProSom | 1-2 | 0.5-1 | Rapid | 20-30 |
| Temazepam | Restoril | 15-30 | 7.5-15 | Intermediate | 8-20 |
| Quazepam | Doral | 7.5-15 | 7.5 | Intermediate | 15-120 |
| Flurazepam | Dalmane | 15-30 | 7.5 | Intermediate | 36-250 |

insomnia is problematic, especially in light of the research and development of new, apparently safe and effective nonbenzodiazepine agents designed to be selectively more active on the hypnotic receptor.

Newer non-BZ agents selectively active at the omega$_1$ BZ receptor include zolpidem and zolpidem-MR (Ambien and Ambien-CR), zaleplon (Sonata), and eszopiclone (Lunesta). These agents do not appear to alter sleep architecture, and appear less prone to induce significant tolerance, dependence, or withdrawal compared to conventional benzodiazepines. All have relatively rapid onset of action, but differ in half life and duration of action. Approximate half lives are zaleplon ~1 hr, zolpidem ~1-3 hr, zolpidem MR ~2-4 hr, and eszopiclone ~6 hr. Neither zolpidem-MR or eszopiclone have restrictions on duration of use.

The melatonin receptor agonist ramelteon (Rozerem) has also been recently released for the treatment of insomnia (possibly most effective in circadian regulation problems), and has no duration of use restriction.

Antidepressant agents, especially sedative tricyclics, are frequently used at low doses to manage chronic insomnia despite the relative lack of well-controlled double-blind studies demonstrating efficacy. These agents are clearly indicated in insomnia that accompanies depressive disorders, where their effectiveness is clear. These agents are normally taken about one hour before bedtime so their sedative effects have time to emerge. This effectively teaches the patient to take a pill to sleep, which is counterproductive for treating insomnia. The new non-BZ hypnotics with their rapid onset of action can be placed at the bedside and are taken if the patient has not fallen asleep within 30 minutes.

Several agents more directly involved in modulating γ-aminobutyric acid (GABA) activity, such as tiagabine (Gabitril)[1] and sodium oxybate (Xyrem),[1] have been used in limited studies to promote slow-wave sleep, but there are insufficient published data to make specific recommendations as to their potential usefulness in insomnia at this time.

### LONG-TERM USE OF HYPNOTIC AGENTS

Current thinking suggests we might best conceptualize primary insomnia as a chronic disorder that will likely require long-term treatment. Considering the known adverse effects of chronic sleep loss, in the context of the present availability of relatively safe and effective hypnotic agents, there would appear to be no reason to withhold or severely limit pharmacologic treatment in those responsible patients for whom a comprehensive and thorough diagnostic evaluation has established the presence of a primary insomnia disorder. It should go without saying, however, that behavioral treatment also should be actively implemented in those patients who are being considered for long-term pharmacologic management.

---

[1]Not FDA approved for this indication.

# Pruritus

Method of
*Scott Moses, MD*

Because pruritus is the most common symptom in dermatology, clinicians are often asked to reduce its distressing effect on comfort and sleep. Left untreated, itch and its associated persistent scratching increases risk of chronic skin changes and secondary infection. Although pruritus is most often caused by a dermatologic condition, it can also be a symptom of underlying systemic disease.

The sensation of itch starts in the skin's free nerve endings, travels via unmyelinated C-fibers to the spine, and finally travels via the spinothalamic tract to the brain. Histamine, commonly associated with allergic rhinitis and urticaria, is only one of several chemical mediators of pruritus. Serotonin is integral to the pruritus of uremia, cholestasis, polycythemia vera, lymphoma, and morphine-associated pruritus. In atopic dermatitis, proinflammatory mediators (e.g., cytokines) are released in an immune-mediated response. Pruritus has been attributed to neuropathy in a wide variety of conditions including herpes zoster, brachioradial pruritus, notalgia paresthetica, spinal tumors, and multiple sclerosis.

## Diagnosis

History is the key to identifying the cause of pruritus. Most causes are evident from the associated dermatitis (Box 1), distribution (Figure 1), or exogenous exposure history (Box 2). Clinicians should focus on the timing of pruritus and associated rash development, food and medication exposures, possible allergen and irritant exposures, pet exposure, and travel history.

In children, pruritus rarely has a systemic cause. However, clinicians should be alert for children who demonstrate red flag symptoms

---

 **CURRENT DIAGNOSIS**

- Reassuring findings that suggest a nonorganic cause include recent onset, localized itch, pruritus limited to exposed skin, household members also with pruritus, and recent travel history.
- Underlying systemic disease is responsible for up to 50% of pruritus in older adults and is uncommon in children.
- Laboratory testing to consider in atypical cases includes a complete blood count, ferritin, thyroid-stimulating hormone, serum bilirubin, alkaline phosphatase, serum creatinine, blood urea nitrogen, HIV test, and skin scrapings, biopsy, and culture.

## BOX 1 Dermatitis-Associated Causes of Pruritus

**Allergic Contact Dermatitis**
- Sharply demarcated erythematous lesion with overlying vesicles
- Reaction within 2-7 d of exposure (see Box 4)

**Atopic Dermatitis**
- Atopic patients (allergic rhinitis, asthma) with the itch that rashes
- Affects flexor wrists and ankles, antecubital and popliteal fossa

**Bullous Pemphigoid**
- Initially pruritic urticarial lesions, often in intertriginous areas
- Tense blisters form after urticaria

**Cutaneous T-Cell Lymphoma (Mycosis Fungoides)**
- Oval eczematous patch on non–sun-exposed skin (e.g., buttocks)
- Can also manifest as erythroderma (exfoliative dermatitis)
- Can also manifest as a new eczematous disorder in older adults

**Dermatitis Herpetiformis**
- Rare vesicular dermatitis affects lumbosacral spine, elbows, knees

**Folliculitis**
- Pruritus out of proportion to appearance of dermatitis
- Papules and pustules at follicular sites on chest, back, or thighs

**Lichen Planus**
- Lesions often on the flexor wrists
- 6 Ps: pruritus, polygonal, planar, purple papules and plaques

**Lichen Simplex Chronicus**
- Complication of chronic scratching (e.g., atopic dermatitis)

- Thickened plaques over lower legs, posterior neck, and groin

**Parasitic Skin Infections**
*Insects*
- Chigger bites (harvest mite): Southeastern United States
- Cutaneous myiasis (bot fly): Central and South America, Africa
- Leishmaniasis (sand fly): Central and South America, Africa, Asia

*Pediculosis (lice)*
- Occiput of school-aged child
- Genitalia affected in adults (STD)

*Scabies*
- Burrows at hand web spaces, axillae, and genitalia
- Hyperkeratotic plaques, pruritic papules or scale present
- Face and scalp affected in children but not adults

**Prurigo nodularis**
- Complication of chronic scratching (variant of lichen simplex)
- 1-2 cm nodules on extensor arms and legs

**Psoriasis**
- Plaques on extensor extremities, low back, palms, soles, and scalp

**Sunburn**
- Consider photosensitizing causes (e.g., NSAIDs, cosmetics)

**Xerotic Eczema**
- Intense itching during winter in northern climates
- Involves back, flanks, abdomen, waist, and distal extremities

*Abbreviations:* NSAIDs = nonsteroidal anti-inflammatory drugs; STD = sexually transmitted disease.

such as growth failure, anorexia, fatigue, associated bowel or bladder changes, and nighttime awakenings due to pruritus.

Underlying systemic disease is responsible for up to 50% of pruritus in older adults and should be considered in refractory cases and where skin findings are absent. Reassuring findings that suggest a non-systemic cause include recent onset, localized itch, pruritus limited to exposed skin, household members also with pruritus, and recent travel history.

Dermatitis distribution and appearance often indicate the cause. The examination can also reveal the chronicity of pruritus. Excoriations and impetigo are seen acutely, and postinflammatory pigment changes and lichenification are seen with chronic scratching. Clinicians should be alert for findings consistent with thyroid disease, renal disease, liver disease, anemia, and hematologic malignancy. Examination should include careful palpation of the lymph nodes, liver, and spleen. Systemic causes of pruritus are listed in Box 3. Pruritic conditions specific to pregnancy are summarized in Box 4.

In cases refractory to 2 weeks of symptomatic therapy or in which an underlying systemic cause is considered, a limited laboratory evaluation is indicated and is summarized in Table 1. When itch persists or is refractory to general measures, remember that up to one half of older adults have pruritus caused by an underlying systemic problem.

# Treatment

Pruritus is usually self-limited and responds well to nonspecific measures such as liberal use of skin lubricants and avoidance of provocative factors (Box 5). Oral antihistamines are not uniformly effective in all

---

**CURRENT THERAPY**

- Pruritus is usually self-limited and responds well to nonspecific measures such as liberal use of skin lubricants and avoidance of provocative factors.
- Antihistamines are not uniformly effective in reducing itch.
- Left untreated, itch and its associated persistent scratching increases risk of impetigo and cellulitis in the short term and lichen simplex chronicus and prurigo nodularis in chronic cases.

## CAUSES OF PRURITUS

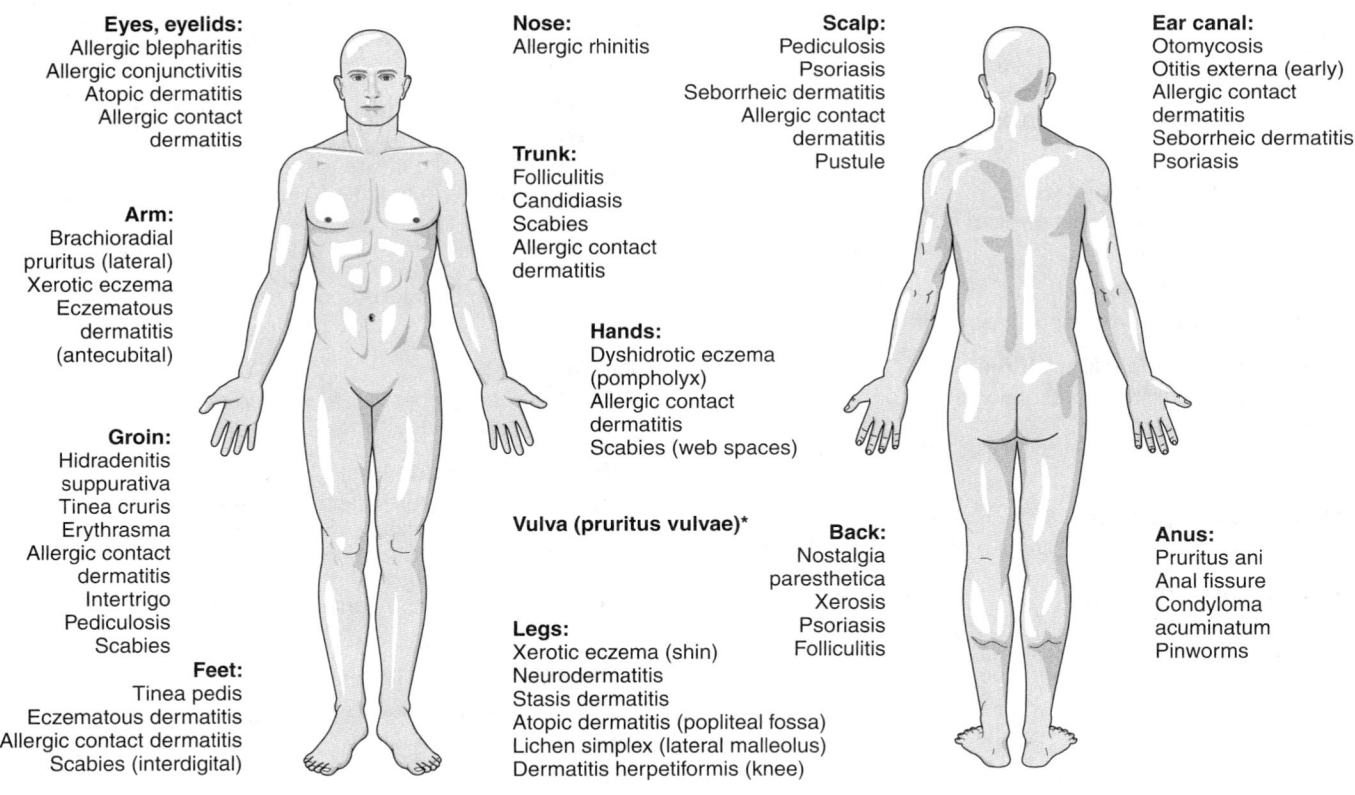

**Eyes, eyelids:**
Allergic blepharitis
Allergic conjunctivitis
Atopic dermatitis
Allergic contact
dermatitis

**Arm:**
Brachioradial
pruritus (lateral)
Xerotic eczema
Eczematous
dermatitis
(antecubital)

**Groin:**
Hidradenitis
suppurativa
Tinea cruris
Erythrasma
Allergic contact
dermatitis
Intertrigo
Pediculosis
Scabies

**Feet:**
Tinea pedis
Eczematous dermatitis
Allergic contact dermatitis
Scabies (interdigital)

**Nose:**
Allergic rhinitis

**Trunk:**
Folliculitis
Candidiasis
Scabies
Allergic contact
dermatitis

**Hands:**
Dyshidrotic eczema
(pompholyx)
Allergic contact
dermatitis
Scabies (web spaces)

**Vulva (pruritus vulvae)***

**Legs:**
Xerotic eczema (shin)
Neurodermatitis
Stasis dermatitis
Atopic dermatitis (popliteal fossa)
Lichen simplex (lateral malleolus)
Dermatitis herpetiformis (knee)

**Scalp:**
Pediculosis
Psoriasis
Seborrheic dermatitis
Allergic contact
dermatitis
Pustule

**Back:**
Nostalgia
paresthetica
Xerosis
Psoriasis
Folliculitis

**Ear canal:**
Otomycosis
Otitis externa (early)
Allergic contact
dermatitis
Seborrheic dermatitis
Psoriasis

**Anus:**
Pruritus ani
Anal fissure
Condyloma
acuminatum
Pinworms

*—Causes of pruritus vulvae: prepubertal girls—poor hygiene, streptococcal infection, Escherichia coli infection, pinworms, scabies, allergic contact dermatitis; young women—vaginitis, allergic contact dermatitis, hidradenitis suppurativa, lichen simplex chronicus; postmenopausal women—atrophic vaginitus, lichen sclerosus, vulvar cancer, Paget's disease; females with diabetes mellitus—candidiasis, other dermatophyte infections.

**FIGURE 1.** Causes of pruritus (by distribution). Adapted from Moses S: Pruritus. Am Fam Physician 2003;68:1135-1146.

---

**BOX 2  Exposure-Related Pruritus**

**Allergic Contact Dermatitis**
- Topical medications: Neomycin, benzocaine (Americaine)
- Nickel, latex, cosmetics, black hair dye
- Laundry detergents or fabric softeners
- Paint-on tattoos (paraphenylenediamine)
- Tattoo dye: cadmium yellow, mercuric sulfide (red)
- Ointments highly concentrated in inert oil

**Heat Exposure**
- Miliaria rubra (prickly heat)
- Cholinergic urticaria (response to hot bath, fever, exercise)

**Occupational Exposure**
- Dyes (e.g., glyceryl monothioglycolate)
- Potassium dichromate in cements and dyes
- Rosins or epoxy resins in adhesives
- Rubber, methyl methacrylate, fiberglass

**Systemic Medications**
- Drug hypersensitivity (rifampin [Rifadin], vancomycin [Vancocin])
- Itraconazole (Sporanox), fluconazole, ketoconazole (Nizoral)
- Niacinamide (niacin), B vitamins, aspirin, quinidine (Quinidex)
- Nitrates (food preservatives)
- Spinal narcotics (pruritus affects face, neck, and upper chest)

**Water Exposure**
- Aquagenic pruritus (associated with polycythemia vera)
- Cholinergic urticaria (response to warm water)
- Itching within 15 min of any water contact
- Polycythemia vera
- Swimmer's itch (7-d eruption after freshwater swimming)

## BOX 3  Systemic Causes of Pruritus

**Cholestasis**
- Intense itching, worse at night
- Affects hands, feet, and pressure sites
- Reactive hyperpigmentation spares midback (butterfly appearance)

**Chronic Renal Failure**
- Severe paroxysms of generalized itching
- Worse in summer

**Delusions of parasitosis**
- Focal erosions on exposed areas of arms and legs

**Human Immunodeficiency Virus**
- Pruritus is a common presenting symptom due to secondary causes
- Causes: Eczema, drug reaction, eosinophilic folliculitis, seborrhea

**Hodgkin's Lymphoma**
- Prolonged generalized pruritus often precedes diagnosis

**Hyperthyroidism**
- Skin is warm and moist
- Pretibial edema may be present
- Onycholysis, hyperpigmentation, and vitiligo have been associated

**Iron-Deficiency Anemia**
- Other dermatologic signs include glossitis and angular cheilitis

**Malignant Carcinoid**
- Intermittent head and neck flushing
- Explosive diarrhea

**Multiple Myeloma**
- Affects elderly with bone pain, headache, cachexia, anemia, and renal failure

**Neurodermatitis or Neurotic Excoriations**
- Bouts of intense itching that can awaken the patient from a sound sleep

- Affects scalp, neck, wrist, extensor elbow, outer leg, ankle, perineum

**Parasitic Infection (usually in returning travelers or immigrants)**
- Filariasis: Tropical parasite responsible for lymphedema
- Onchocerciasis: Transmitted by black fly in Africa, Latin America
- Schistosomiasis: Fresh water exposure in Africa, Mediterranean, South America
- Trichinosis: Undercooked pork, bear, wild boar, or walrus meat

**Parvovirus B19**
- Slapped cheek appearance in children
- Arthritis in some adults

**Peripheral Neuropathy**
- Brachioradial pruritus: Affects lateral arms of white patients in the tropics
- Notalgia paresthetica: Midback pruritus with hyperpigmented patch
- Herpes zoster: Accompanies painful prodrome 2 d before rash

**Polycythemia Rubra Vera**
- Pricking-type itch persists for hours after hot shower or bath

**Scleroderma**
- Nonpitting extremity edema, erythema, and intense pruritus
- Edema phase with pruritus precedes fibrosis of the skin

**Urticaria**
- Response to allergen, cold, heat, exercise, sunlight, or direct pressure

**Weight Loss (Rapid) in Eating Disorders**
- Other signs include hair loss or fine lanugo hair on back and cheeks
- Also yellow skin discoloration and petechiae

## BOX 4  Causes of Pruritus in Pregnancy

**Pruritic Urticarial Papules and Plaques of Pregnancy**
- Common in the third trimester
- Intense pruritus involves abdomen
- Spreads to thighs, buttocks, breasts, and arms

**Prurigo of Pregnancy**
- Common in second half of pregnancy
- Extensor arms and abdomen with excoriated papules and nodules
- Associated with atopic dermatitis

**Herpes Gestationis or Pemphigoid Gestationis**
- Uncommon
- Autoimmune condition associated with Graves' disease
- Vesicles and bullae on abdomen and extremities in second half of pregnancy
- Responds to prednisone[1] 0.5 mg/kg (Level A)

**Intrahepatic Cholestasis of Pregnancy**
- Uncommon
- Trunk and extremity itching without rash in late pregnancy
- Jaundice not present in the mild form (prurigo gravidarum)
- Responds to cholestyramine (Questran) and Vitamin $K_1$ (Aquamephyton)[1] (Level B)

**Pruritic Folliculitis of Pregnancy**
- Uncommon, occurs in second half of pregnancy
- Erythematous follicular papules over trunk, with spread to extremities
- May be a variant of prurigo of pregnancy

**Other Common Pruritic Conditions Exacerbated in Pregnancy**
- Atopic dermatitis
- Contact dermatitis

---

[1]Not FDA approved for this indication.
Levels of evidence: Level A: Evidence from high-quality randomized controlled clinical trials or meta-analyses; Level B: Evidence from nonrandomized clinical studies or nonquantitative systematic reviews.

**TABLE 1  Diagnostic Evaluation of Pruritus for Atypical, Persistent, or Refractory Cases**

| Tests | Findings |
|---|---|
| Complete blood count,* serum ferritin* | Iron deficiency anemia, polycythemia rubra vera, Hodgkin's lymphoma, multiple myeloma, parasitic infection |
| Serum bilirubin, alkaline phosphatase* | Cholestasis (e.g., cirrhosis) |
| Serum creatinine, blood urea nitrogen* | Uremia (e.g., chronic renal failure) |
| Thyroid stimulating hormone* | Hyperthyroidism |
| Microscopy of skin scrapings, skin culture, skin biopsy | Dermatophytes, scabies; skin bacterial, fungal or viral infection; mastocytosis, mycosis fungoides, bullous pemphigoid |
| HIV test | HIV infection |
| Chest radiograph | Hodgkin's lymphoma, multiple myeloma |
| Stool tests | Parasites, *Helicobacter pylori* |
| | Children: pinworms, perianal streptococcus |

*Denotes a first-line test. Unmarked tests are performed if history indicates.

causes of pruritus. Specific management of dermatitis, as with atopic dermatitis, scabies, and contact dermatitis, can relieve symptoms.

In the atypical case, where these measures fail, a systemic condition may be uncovered. In these patients, the itch should be alleviated by treating the underlying condition, as with thyroid replacement in hypothyroidism or iron supplementation in iron deficiency anemia. Uremia and cholestasis-related pruritus have established effective therapies beyond treating the causative chronic renal or hepatic insufficiency (Box 6).

## Complications

Itch and the scratch it induces are not benign. When scratching is left unchecked, fingernails introduce bacteria into abraded skin, and impetigo or cellulitis can ensue. Lichen simplex chronicus and prurigo nodularis are chronic skin changes seen with long-term scratching and in particular with atopic dermatitis.

Medications to treat pruritus are also not without adverse effects. Antihistamines can affect alertness and learning if used during the day, and with chronic use, the associated dry mouth can predispose to tooth decay.

## Follow-Up

General measures to treat pruritus should be reviewed at each visit. Consistent practice of these simple home strategies can prevent sleepless nights, frequent evaluations, unnecessary medications, and the complications of scratching.

---

**BOX 5  Nonspecific Management of Pruritus**

- Use skin lubricants liberally
  - Petrolatum or skin lubricant cream at bedtime
  - Apply alcohol-free, hypoallergenic lotions frequently during day
- Avoid excessive bathing
  - Briefly pat dry after bath and immediately apply skin lubricants
  - Decrease bathing frequency
  - Limit bathing to brief exposure to tepid water
- Limit soap use
  - Use mild, unscented, hypoallergenic soap 2 or 3 times per wk
  - Daily use of soap only in groin and axillae; spare legs, arms, and torso
- Minimize dryness
  - Humidify dry indoor environment (especially in winter)
- Choose clothing that does not irritate the skin
  - Doubly rinsed cotton clothes and silk are best
  - Add bath oil (e.g., Alpha Keri) to rinse cycle when washing sheets
  - Avoid heat-retaining fabrics (synthetics)
  - Avoid wool and smooth-textured cotton clothes
- Avoid vasodilators
  - Avoid caffeine, alcohol, spices, hot water, and excessive sweating
- Avoid provocative topical medications
  - Avoid prolonged topical corticosteroids (risk of skin atrophy)

- Avoid topical anesthetics and antihistamines
  - May sensitize exposed skin and risk contact dermatitis
- Standard antipruritic topical agents
  - Menthol and camphor (e.g., Sarna Lotion)
  - Oatmeal baths (e.g., Aveeno)
  - Pramoxine[1] (e.g., PrameGel [pramoxine + menthol], Pramosone [pramoxine + hydrocortisone])
  - Calamine lotion (Use on weeping lesions only, not on dry skin)
- Antipruritic topical agents for refractory cases (used in severe atopic dermatitis)
  - Doxepin 5% cream (Zonalon)
  - Burow's solution (wet dressings with aluminum acetate 5% in water)
  - Unna's boot[1] (zinc oxide paste bandages)
  - Coal tar emulsion[1] (Zetar)
- Systemic antipruritic agents (used in allergic and urticarial disease)
  - Doxepin (Sinequan)[1] 1 mg/kg up to 25 mg at bedtime (Level A)
  - Hydroxyzine (Atarax) 0.5 mg/kg up to 25-50 mg at bedtime
  - Nonsedating antihistamines (e.g., Fexofenadine [Allegra], Level A)
- Prevent complications of scratching
  - Keep fingernails short and clean
  - Rub skin with palms if urge to scratch is irresistible

[1]Not FDA approved for this indication.
Level A: Evidence from high-quality randomized controlled clinical trials or meta-analyses.

---

**BOX 6  Specific Management of Pruritic Conditions**

**Cholestasis**

- Cholestyramine (Questran) (Level B)
  - Adult: 4 g 30 min before meals
  - Child: 240 mg/kg/d divided tid (up to 6 g/d)
- Ursodiol (Actigall)[1] 15 mg/kg/d divided before meals
- Ondansetron (Zofran)[1] 4-8 mg IV, then 4 mg PO q8h (Level B)
- Opioid receptor antagonist (Level A)
  - Naloxone (Narcan)[1] 0.002 mcg/kg/h IV, titrate to max 0.25 mcg/kg/h
  - Naltrexone (Revia)[1] 12.5 mg PO qd (advance to 50 mg PO qd)
- Rifampin (Rifadin)[1] 10 mg/kg/d divided bid (max: 300 mg bid) (Level B)
- Bile duct stenting from extrahepatic cholestasis (Level A)
- Lidocaine (Xylocaine)[1] IV has been used
- Bright light therapy (Level B)
- Plasmapheresis

**Neurotic Excoriation**

- Pimozide (Orap)[1] for delusions of parasitosis
- Selective serotonin reuptake inhibitor (SSRI)

**Notalgia Paresthetica**

- Topical capsaicin (Zostrix)[1] applied 4-6 times per d for several wk (Level B)

**Polycythemia Vera**

- Aspirin[1] 500 mg PO q8-24h (Level B)
- Paroxetine (Paxil)[1] 10-20 mg PO qd (Level B)
- Interferon-α (Intron A)[1] 3-35 million IU/wk (Level B)

**Spinal Opioid–Induced Pruritus**

- Ondansetron (Zofran)[1] 8 mg IV concurrent with opioid (Level A)
- Nalbuphine (Nubain)[1] 5 mg IV concurrent with opioid (Level B)

**Uremia**

- UV B phototherapy twice weekly for 1 mo (Level A)
- Activated charcoal[1] 6 g/d (Level A)
- Topical capsaicin[1] 0.025% cream to localized areas (Level A)
- Ondansetron and naltrexone are not efficacious in uremia (Level A)

---

[1]Not FDA approved for this indication.
Levels of evidence: Level A: Evidence from high-quality randomized controlled clinical trials or meta-analyses; Level B: Evidence from nonrandomized clinical studies or nonquantitative systematic reviews.

## REFERENCES

Belsito DV: The diagnostic evaluation, treatment and prevention of allergic contact dermatitis in the new millennium. J Allergy Clin Immunol 2000;105:409-420.

Bender BG: Sedation and performance impairment of diphenhydramine and second-generation antihistamines: A meta-analysis. J Allergy Clin Immunol 2003;111:770-776.

Bergasa NV: An approach to the management of the pruritus of cholestasis. Clin Liver Dis 2004;8:55-66.

Berger R, Gilchrest BA. Skin disorders. In Duthie EH, Katz PR (eds): Practice of Geriatrics, 3rd ed. Philadelphia: WB Saunders, 1998, pp 467-472.

Boiko S, Zeiger R: Diagnosis and treatment of atopic dermatitis, urticaria, and angioedema during pregnancy. Immunol Allergy Clin North Am 2000;20:839.

Callen JP, Bernardi DM, Clark RAF, Weber DA: Adult-onset recalcitrant eczema: A marker of noncutaneous lymphoma or leukemia. J Am Acad Dermatol 2000;43:207-210.

Correale CE, Walker C, Lydia M, Craig TJ: Atopic dermatitis: A review of diagnosis and treatment. Am Fam Physician 1999;60:1191-1210.

Cyr PR, Dreher GK: Neurotic excoriations. Am Fam Physician 2001;64:1981-1984.

Diehn F, Tefferi A: Pruritus in polycythaemia vera: Prevalence, laboratory correlates and management. 2001;115:619-621.

Fagan EA: Intrahepatic cholestasis of pregnancy. Clin Liver Dis 1999;3:603-632.

Finn AF, Kaplan AP, Fretwell R, et al: A double-blind, placebo-controlled trial of fexofenadine HCl in the treatment of chronic idiopathic urticaria. J Allergy Clin Immunol 1999;103:1071-1078.

Fisher AA: Aquagenic pruritus. Cutis 1993;51:146-147.

Gelfand JM, Rudikoff D: Evaluation and treatment of itching in HIV-infected patients. Mt Sinai J Med 2001;68:298-308.

Ghent CN: The pruritus of cholestasis. Hepatology 1999;29:1003-1006.

Gupta MA, Gupta AK, Voorhees JJ: Starvation-associated pruritus: A clinical feature of eating disorders. J Am Acad Dermatol 1992;27:118-120.

Habif TP. Clinical Dermatology, 3rd ed. Chicago: Mosby–Year Book, 1996.

Harrigan E, Rabinowitz LG: Atopic dermatitis. Immunol Allergy Clin North Am 1999;19:383-396.

Heymann WR: Chronic urticaria and angioedema associated with thyroid autoimmunity: Review and therapeutic implications. J Am Acad Dermatol 1999;40:229-242.

Koblenzer CS: Itching and atopic skin. J Allergy Clin Immunol 1999;104:S109-S113.

Krajnik M, Zylicz Z: Understanding pruritus in systemic disease. J Pain Symptom Manage 2001;21:151-168.

Kroumpouzos G, Cohen LM: Dermatoses of pregnancy. J Am Acad Dermatol 2001;45:1-19.

Leung AKC: Pruritus in children, J Roy Soc Health 1998;118:280-286.

Lidofsky S, Scharschmidt BF: Jaundice. In Feldman M, Scharschmidt BF, Sleisenger MH, Fordtran JS (eds): Sleisenger and Fordtran's Gastrointestinal and Liver Disease, 6th ed. Philadelphia: WB Saunders, 1998, pp 230-231.

Moses S: Pruritus, Am Fam Physician 2003;68:1135-1146.

Parker F. Structure and function of skin. In Goldman L, Bennett JC (eds): Cecil Textbook of Medicine, 21st ed. Philadelphia: WB Saunders, 2000, pp 2266.

Paus R, Schmeiz M, Biró T, Steinhoff M: Frontiers in pruritus research: Scratching the brain for more effective itch therapy. J Clin Invest 2006;116:1174-1185.

Robinson-Bostom L, DiGiovanna JJ: Cutaneous manifestations of end-stage renal disease. J Am Acad Dermatol 2000;43:975-986.

Shellow WVR: Evaluation of pruritus. In Goroll AH, Mulley AG (eds): Primary Care Medicine, 4th ed. Philadelphia: Lippincott Williams & Wilkins, 2000, pp 1001-1004.

Stambuk R, Colvin R: Dermatologic disorders. In Gabbe SG, Niebyl JR, Simpson JL (eds): Obstetrics: Normal and Problem Pregnancies, 4th ed. New York: Churchill Livingstone, 2002, pp 1283-1290.

Tennyson H: Neurotropic and psychotropic drugs in dermatology. Dermatol Clin 2001;19:179-197.

Tormey WP, Chambers JPM: Pruritus as the presenting symptom in hyperthyroidism. Br J Clin Pract 1994;48:224.

Valsecchi R, Cainelli T: Generalized pruritus: A manifestation of iron deficiency. Arch Dermatol 1983;119:630.

Veien NK, Hattel T, Laurberg G. Spaun E: Brachioradial pruritus. J Am Acad Dermatol 2001;44:704-705.

Villamil AG, Bandi JC, Galdame OA, et al: Efficacy of lidocaine in the treatment of pruritus in patients with chronic cholestatic liver disease. Am J Med 2005;118:1160-1163.

Waxler B, Dadabhoy Z, Stojiljkovic L, Rabito SF: Primer of postoperative pruritus for anesthesiologists. Anesthesiology 2005;103:168-178.

Zirwas MJ, Seraly MP: Pruritus of unknown origin: A retrospective study. J Am Acad Dermatol 2001;45:892-896.

# Tinnitus

Method of
*Claus-Frenz Claussen, MD*

Tinnitus is noise(s) in the ear, which is usually subjective and can be extremely disturbing and frustrating to those affected. According to studies of the American Tinnitus Association, approximately 36 million Americans older than 40 years suffer from tinnitus.

Tinnitus has been regarded as a disease entity for many centuries. During the second half of the 20th century, physicians were able to discriminate among several different kinds of tinnitus including bruits, maskable tinnitus, and nonmaskable tinnitus. Under the influence of Shulman and his team, the term *tinnitology* was coined.

The present interest of researchers in the field of tinnitology is split into two fields of action: suggestions for improvement of objective and quantitative differential diagnostics in tinnitus and research and development to improve various types of treatment for different kinds of tinnitus.

## General Phenomena of Tinnitus

A noise without any human information function, a tinnitus, can be a normal as well as a pathologic function of human hearing. On the one hand, tinnitus can be regarded as a problem of acoustic resolution of the inner ear microphone, that is, the cochlear noise-to-signal ratio. In a well-dampened soundproof chamber, most normal-hearing persons experience a sizzling sound in their ears because of their perception of molecular vibrations from inner ear fluids (as known from thermodynamics). Yet this underlying percept is masked in everyday life by normal environmental noise.

On the other hand, tinnitus patients regularly tell their physicians about subjective ear noises that they describe, for example, as pulsating, humming, roaring, whistling, hissing, fullness of the ear, and pressure and/or pain in the ear.

Table 1 presents the subjective sensational qualities of tinnitus in 823 tinnitus patients (77.52% male and 22.48% female with a mean age of 50.87 years ± 8.68 years) from Bad Kissingen, Germany, who underwent clinical inpatient rehabilitation therapy for several weeks for severe disabling tinnitus.

In these same patients, we looked for descriptions of different time/intensity patterns of their tinnitus (Table 2), and the subjective background of discomfort was investigated as shown in Table 3. Additionally, the patients named the most irritating factors related to their tinnitus (Table 4).

Sleep disturbance is a common and frequent complaint. Scientific studies report decreased tolerance and increased discomfort when insomnia and depression are associated with tinnitus.

In 1991, a sample of 338 New Zealanders regularly experiencing tinnitus completed and returned questionnaires to associations for people with tinnitus or hearing impairment. Nearly half the sample was sometimes depressed because of tinnitus. Those reporting depression and those reporting more severe problems as a consequence of the tinnitus saw more health care professionals and used more coping

## CURRENT DIAGNOSIS

Irritating subjective or objective perception of irritating acoustic noise or sound in the ear, head, or body that may be described, for example, as:
- Pulsating
- Humming
- Roaring
- Whistling
- Hissing

strategies. Most respondents did not remember exactly when they first noticed the tinnitus.

A questionnaire investigation comprising 1091 patients from Bispebjerg Hospital, Copenhagen (1993), concerning "tinnitus-incidence and handicap," was conducted at a hearing center. A majority of patients, 59%, claimed that they were troubled by tinnitus. Neither a greater degree of hearing loss nor a longer duration of tinnitus was associated with more severe tinnitus. Among patients with both subjective hearing loss and tinnitus, 23% stated that tinnitus was the greater problem, and 38% said that tinnitus and hearing loss were equally troublesome. The corresponding figures for patients with hearing impairment of such a degree that a hearing aid was deemed necessary were 9% and 41%, respectively. Stress symptoms such as headache, tension of facial muscles, and sleep disturbances were correlated to tinnitus. Of patients with tinnitus, 83% were interested in obtaining treatment for it.

The so-called Copenhagen Male Study reported on the results from a 10-year follow-up examination concerning hearing and factors known to cause hearing problems. The original sample comprised 5050 subjects, and at the present examination, 3387 (67%) men at a median of 63 years of age (range, 53 to 75 years) participated. An increasing prevalence of 30% to 40% of hearing problems was demonstrated with increasing age. A prevalence of 17% of tinnitus of more than 5 minutes' duration was found; 3% indicated that tinnitus was so annoying that it interfered with sleep, reading, and/or concentration. The prevalence of tinnitus increased up to 70 years of age and seemed to remain constant thereafter.

In Norway, 15% of the adult population has experienced shorter or longer periods of tinnitus. Three percent of these, in total approximately 7000 to 10,000 persons, suffer from continuous tinnitus followed by symptoms that represent a handicap or occupational disability. Similar observations were reported from many other countries.

## Clinical Types

Tinnitus is no longer considered to be a syndrome or a single disease. Because of improvements in neuro-otometry, several different types of tinnitus can be differentiated.

By means of modern audiometry, the framework for normal hearing can be described objectively and quantitatively. Therefore, in any tinnitus case, a thorough analysis of the hearing function and pathways needs to be performed including threshold audiometry, audiometric

**TABLE 1 Subjective Classification of Ear Noises in 823 (= 100%) Tinnitus Patients**

| Complaints | Right Ear (%) | Left Ear (%) |
| --- | --- | --- |
| Pulsating | 1.94 | 1.94 |
| Humming | 7.41 | 6.93 |
| Roaring | 14.10 | 14.22 |
| Whistling | 50.67 | 51.76 |
| Hissing | 9.96 | 10.81 |
| Pressure in the ear | 6.32 | 5.83 |
| Pain in the ear | 14.10 | 14.22 |

**TABLE 2 Subjective Classification of Different Time/Intensity Patterns of Tinnitus in 823 (= 100%) Patients**

| Time/Intensity Patterns | % |
| --- | --- |
| Permanent | 59.17 |
| Intermittent | 19.97 |
| Swelling up and going down | 43.26 |

**TABLE 3 Subjective Classification of Subjective Background of Discomfort in 823 (= 100%) Patients**

| Subjective Complaints About Factors of Discomfort | % |
| --- | --- |
| Headache | 69.02 |
| Migraine | 4.13 |
| Exhaustion | 59.99 |
| Lacking in drive | 42.16 |
| Feeling of weakness | 55.29 |
| Forgetfulness | 68.41 |
| Disorientation | 0.49 |
| Daze | 44.84 |
| Tiredness | 63.91 |
| Insomnia | 69.50 |

tinnitus masking (if possible), acoustic dynamics between the measurable thresholds of hearing and acoustic discomfort, speech audiometry, otoacoustic emissions, acoustic brainstem-evoked potentials, and acoustic late-evoked potentials. Thereby signs of pathology within the hearing pathways between the ear and the human brain cortex can be measured.

Thus, we know from thorough neuro-otologic studies that approximately 24% of cases of disabling tinnitus have their source within the otoacoustic periphery (i.e., inner ear and the eighth cranial nerve). Approximately 35% originate from the acoustic pathways within the brainstem. Approximately 41% have their cause within supratentorial structures and/or functions. These pathologies also should serve as basic information for planning systematic pharmacotherapy directed to the central nervous system (CNS) focus of dysfunction.

At least four different kinds of tinnitus (Figure 1) can be discriminated, which can be determined by the physician using a simple question-and-answer procedure as follows.

## BRUITS

Q: Has someone informed you that he or she could hear a noise coming from your head?
A: Yes. Their description of what they heard listening from outside my head is similar to what I perceive.

By means of auscultation through a stethoscope or a microphone, a real sound can be objectively heard emanating from the patient's skull. Patients frequently report, for example, a bubbling, hissing, or pulsating sound.

The cause can be vascular in origin, that is, abnormal curling of blood caused by atheromas, vascular dissections, scars, compressions, or high blood pressure amplitudes, for example.

Bruits also can originate from the middle ear and its connections toward the epipharynx: middle ear inflammations with bubbling sounds

**TABLE 4 Subjective Classification of Most Irritating Factors Related to Their Tinnitus in 823 (= 100%) Patients**

| Most Irritating Factors Related to Tinnitus | % |
| --- | --- |
| All patients with specific additional statements | 25.76 |
| Difficulties in going to sleep | 10.69 |
| Difficulties in sleeping through the night | 11.06 |
| Depression | 0.24 |
| Abnormal sounds (also hallucinations) | 2.67 |
| Acute hearing loss | 8.38 |

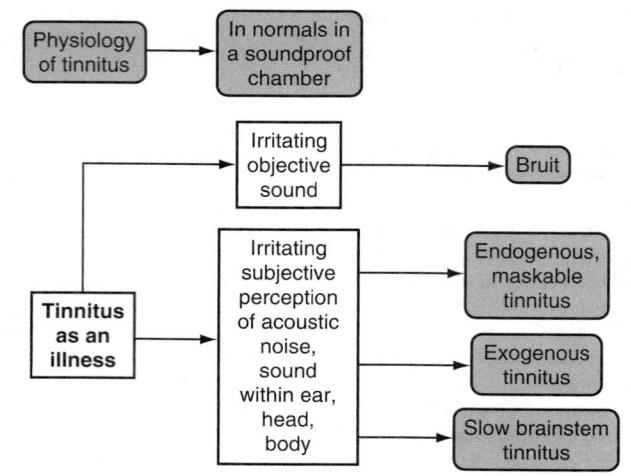

**FIGURE 1.** Categories of physiologic and clinical types of tinnitus.

of gas from within the effusions, whizzing middle ear muscles, or an open eustachian tube.

Cracking sounds, which are misinterpreted as tinnitus, are reported from arthritic and other mandibular joint disorders. Also, sounds can be transferred from the cervical spine and its joints as well as its vessels into the cranial structures so that they become misinterpreted as tinnitus.

## ENDOGENOUS TINNITUS

Q: Where is your feeling of well-being better, in a busy and noisy environment or in cavelike silence?
A: I much prefer a busy and noisy environment.

The patient with a maskable or endogenous tinnitus prefers covering it with external sounds. When using masking procedures, easily three zones of tinnitus can be discriminated within the hearing field:

1. Low-tone tinnitus (at and below 750 Hz)
2. Middle-frequency tinnitus (1 to 2 kHz)
3. High-frequency tinnitus (above 2 kHz until 10 kHz or even 12 kHz)

Low-tone tinnitus is more frequently found in Ménière's disease and some other cochlear-apical disorders, and middle-tone tinnitus is more frequently found in diseases such as otosclerosis. Most frequently tinnitus is matched in the high-tone range and is related, for example, to noise trauma, whiplash, head and skull trauma, cardiovascular failure, stress, acoustic neuromas, and toxic events including those associated with pharmaceutical, nicotine, or drug abuse. Also, several masking points may exist simultaneously.

Dysfunctions of the inner ear contribute to the development of tinnitus. But tinnitus by itself depends on a cortical process of the human brain. A sleeping patient does not suffer from any kind of tinnitus.

Since approximately 1985, the Würzburg neuro-otology group of Claussen et al. has been able to detect by means of vestibular evoked potentials (VestEP) and brain electrical activity mapping (BEAM) groups of patients suffering from a maskable or endogenous tinnitus that respond cortically in a typical, reproducible, and measurable manner:

1. Location of the site of the potentials around the upper gyrus of the temporal lobe (Brodmann's area 41)
2. Typical shortening of the latencies of evoked quantitative electroencephalograms (QEEGs) (i.e., VestEP waves I, II, III)
3. Enlarged DC shift of the evoked QEEGs (i.e., difference between VestEP waves III and IV)
4. Typical cortical electrical burst expansion in three phases on the brain surface

Since approximately 1990, the New York group of Shulman, Strashun, and Goldstein has followed a neuroradiologic path for deciphering the cortical modalities in tinnitus patients by using single-photon emission computer tomography (SPECT). They discovered remarkably elevated metabolic processes in the temporal lobes of patients suffering from a maskable tinnitus.

Thereafter we were able to prove in therapeutic trials with pharmacotherapy (e.g., extractum ginkgo biloba [EGB 761]*), as well as with physiotherapy (competitive kinesthetic interaction therapy [KKIT]), that the subjective reduction or abolition of tinnitus goes together with an electrophysiologic measurable normalization of the VestEP with BEAM or QEEG. So the endogenous tinnitus could be proven to be a CNS network phenomenon.

## EXOGENOUS TINNITUS

Q: Where is your feeling of well-being better, in a busy and noisy environment or in cavelike silence?

A: I much prefer a cavelike silence because noise and/or a group of people speaking at the same time are most confusing. It provokes ringing and shrieking sounds within my ears.

Unlike endogenous tinnitus, patients suffering from exogenous tinnitus cannot benefit from masking noises from their surroundings. Some physicians wrongly call this condition *hyperacusis*, but these patients do not hear better as this term suggests. Seemingly better is the named syndrome of the hypersensitive ear.

In exogenous tinnitus, pure-tone audiometry may be normal or exhibit regular deficits of the hearing threshold, but there is no maskable tinnitus. However, when measuring the acoustic dynamics by adding the audiometrically recorded discomfort threshold, the discomfort level, which is usually between 1 and 8 kHz below 95 dB, rises below this level to values of 90 to 60 dB or even 50 dB. The person being exposed to sound exceeding the level of his low discomfort threshold experiences a loss of understanding together with subjective pain and noise in the ears accompanied by possible vegetative reactions.

Hearing aids can adjust the incoming sounds by filtering, peak clipping, and cleaning of the sound signals so they fit optimally into the remaining acoustic dynamics of the individually existing hearing field. Thus, hearing aids are the first choice for treating exogenous tinnitus. Some other methods for treating this type of tinnitus are physiotherapy, psychotherapy, stress reduction, and supportive pharmacotherapy.

## TINNITUS IN SLOW BRAINSTEM SYNDROME (CLAUSSEN)

Q: How would you best describe your tinnitus?

A: I am becoming increasingly more in a daze and more disoriented and hear ringing and other sounds, which I cannot really localize in my ears or my head. The noise disturbs me as much as my mental instability.

We regularly see older patients who complain about a hazy tinnitus in combination with vertigo, giddiness, and dizziness and also report a reduced state of alertness. These patients have a connected statoacoustic problem. Objectively, affected patients exhibit an increase in the latencies of the experimentally provoked vestibular nystagmus as well as of the acoustically evoked brainstem potentials.

Especially in this group, we have noted by evaluating our therapeutic responses that a combination of cocculus† (picrotoxin), conium† (coneine), amber and petrol oil (Vertigoheel†) has a so-called tuning-up effect on the brainstem. Then the typical symptoms also disappear.

---

*Available as dietary supplement.
†Available as homeopathic remedy.

## COMBINED ENDOGENOUS AND EXOGENOUS TINNITUS

A combination of both types of subjective tinnitus, endogenous and exogenous, is also found in tinnitus patients. Affected patients report that the noise they hear is present during both the day and night; however, the noise fluctuates. Especially the intensity of the noise can be very increased, for example when the patient is in a noisy environment or busy place or in a conversation with several participants.

Even though patients with combined endogenous and exogenous tinnitus have maskable tinnitus, they report that therapeutic acoustic maskers do not reduce their symptoms. They need a thorough audiometric and neuro-otologic workup.

# Contemporary and Practical Treatment

Modern therapy of tinnitus appears to be complex and sometimes incomprehensible. But when talking about therapy of disabling tinnitus, we emphasize a main therapeutic approach in the sense that we have to break and inhibit the psychosomatic cycle of deterioration from tinnitus to stress, to insomnia, to panic. Some aspects of this reactional behavior are similar to pain.

The steps for individual tinnitus therapy must be chosen according to the kind of tinnitus diagnosed. Tinnitus is frequently associated with conditions such as stress, hearing loss, noise trauma, otorhinolaryngologic disorders (e.g., Ménière's disease, otosclerosis, perilymphatic fistula, acoustic neuroma), high blood pressure, metabolic disorders, allergy, intoxications, whiplash and other head and neck traumas, functional disorders of the neck, burnout syndrome, mandibular joint problems, and extracranial and intracranial vascular problems.

The Current Therapy box lists different therapeutic approaches to tinnitus. These ten therapies must be individually interrelated with the different types of tinnitus (see Figure 1). Besides the severe disabling types of tinnitus, minor forms of tinnitus also occasionally occur that may be event related or may be time limited.

## NOISE AVOIDANCE AND BASICS OF THERAPY

Avoidance can help in noise-related tinnitus by the prevention of noise exposure or at least by wearing ear protection. The use of ototoxic drugs must be controlled and limited. Inflammatory ear disease needs specific treatment of the external and the middle ear with antibiotics and anti-inflammatory drugs. Control and maintenance of a satisfactory degree of aeration of the middle ear is necessary. Acoustic neuroma calls for surgical removal of the tumor. Surgery is also necessary in otosclerosis and perilymphatic fistula. Specific gnatholic therapy by a dentist is recommended in a temporomandibular joint syndrome.

## INSTRUMENTATIONS FOR THERAPY

Instrumentations currently available and frequently used according to the type and the chronicity of tinnitus are as follows:

1. Tinnitus maskers/tinnitus instruments, tapes/CDs for masking and relaxation
2. Acoustic ultra-high-frequency stimulation
3. Hearing aids
4. External electrical stimulations
5. External magnetic stimulation

## PHARMACOTHERAPY

Pharmacotherapy, that is, treatment with pharmaceutical agents, is important in the management of tinnitus. It may be the main therapy or may play only a supportive, palliative, or intermittent role. The four lines of therapeutic agents used in the treatment of tinnitus may overlap and may be combined.

### First-Line Agents

First-line therapeutic agents can relieve tinnitus either slowly or quickly. Lidocaine (Xylocaine),[1] a local anesthetic drug, only has a temporary effect in suppressing tinnitus. It is an aminoethylamide, which is well soluble in water.

A daily intravenous dose of lidocaine of 1 mg per kg of body weight can temporarily alleviate the phenomenon of endogenous tinnitus. The duration, however, depends on the blood level. As soon as the level of lidocaine in the blood is lowered below a threshold, tinnitus returns.

In tinnitus, lidocaine is best applied by iontophoresis through an electrical field with an active electrode in the external ear and a passive electrode at an arm, after instillation of a solution of lidocaine (1:100,000) into the external meatus.

This therapy temporarily relieves the disturbing tinnitus, so that the patients at least get some hours of rest and sleep. However, the untoward side effects of lidocaine also have to be taken into consideration.

Some forms of tinnitus also have an acoustic hallucinatory component, as in epilepsia. Therefore, carbamazepine (Tegretol),[1] which is an important antiepileptic agent used for bipolar affective disorders, is also used in tinnitus with a supratentorial focus. We have seen beneficial effects in very specific cases of endogenous tinnitus. Chemically, carbamazepine belongs to the tricyclic antidepressants. In adults, we give a daily dose of 200 mg. However, renal, hepatic, and hematologic parameters have to be monitored thoroughly.

### Second-Line Agents

This group of drugs is especially used to treat the emotional effects seen in endogenous tinnitus, exogenous tinnitus, and combined endogenous and exogenous tinnitus, which can lead via sleeplessness

---

[1]Not FDA approved for this indication.

**40**

## CURRENT THERAPY

- Avoidance of noise, ototoxic drugs, allergens
- Treatment of bruits by medical or surgical measures
- Instrumental therapy
- Tinnitus maskers
- Hearing aids
- Electrostimulation
- Specific pharmacotherapy
  - Lidocaine (Xylocaine)[1]
  - Carbamazepine (Tegretol)[1]
- Calming pharmacotherapy
  - Diazepam (Valium)[1]
  - Amitriptyline (Elavil)[1]
- Nontropic pharmacotherapy
  - Gingko*
  - Flunarizine[2]
- Neurotransmitter-directed pharmacotherapy
  - Betahistine*
  - Gabapentin (Neurontin)
- Psychotherapy
  - Retraining therapy (TRT)
- Physiotherapy
  - Competitive kinesthetic interaction therapy (KKIT)
- Other therapies
  - Hypnotherapy
  - Counseling
  - Acupuncture

---

[1]Not FDA approved for this indication.
[2]Not available in the United States.
*Available as dietary supplement.

to anxiety and panic. Here we see an indication for alprazolam (Xanax)[1] and similar substances. Alprazolam is administered to tinnitus patients in a daily dosage of 0.75 to 1.5 mg. Also chlordiazepoxide (Librium)[1] can alternatively be applied in a daily dosage of 15 to 30 mg. Even diazepam (Valium)[1] is used in a daily dosage of 4 to 30 mg.

The mood changes associated with tinnitus can lead to psychosis and insomnia. Here a tricyclic antidepressant such as amitriptyline (Elavil)[1] in a daily dosage of 75 to 150 mg can be helpful.

Additionally, this agent has a desired sedative component. Other sedatives and psychotropic drugs are also used to treat the psychologic effects associated with tinnitus, but they must be applied very carefully.

### Third-Line Agents

Third-line therapeutic agents comprise the so-called nootropic drugs. These are pharmacologic agents that activate brain function through improved metabolism, leading to a better adaptation and interconnection. They were originally developed to treat senile dementia. Within this group, in Germany, we use piracetam (Nootrop, Normabraïn) in a daily dosage of 800 to 1200 mg.

We have seen very beneficial effects from extract of ginkgo biloba (EGB 761*) (Tebonin, Rökan), which is administered in a daily dosage of 120 mg.

We also use calcium channel antagonists, among which flunarizine (Sibelium),[2] in a daily dosage of 15 to 30 mg, is effective in tinnitus with irritative foci, especially in mesencephalic and diencephalic areas. Cinnarizin[2] was the predecessor. This holds especially for the endogenous tinnitus group.

### Fourth-Line Agents

The fourth line of therapy involves neurotransmitter-directed pharmacotherapy. According to the chemical structures of the neurotransmitters, we mainly use one system of the amines (i.e., the histamine mechanism) and one system of amino acids (i.e., $\gamma$-aminobutyric acid [GABA]).

Because it is known that inner ear functions are regulated at the neurotransmission level of the histaminergic $H_1$, $H_2$, and $H_3$ receptors, betahistine (Serc)[2] plays an important role in inner ear receptor-targeted therapy. The daily dosage that we administer in peripheral cochlear tinnitus is 16 to 48 mg.

The inhibitory neurotransmitter GABA is extremely potent in its ability to alter neuronal discharges because of failures in the supratentorial CNS neurotransmission. According to recent findings, endogenous tinnitus with a supratentorial dysregulation can be influenced by gabapentin (Neurontin).[1] It is used in dosages starting with 300 mg daily and can be increased to 900 mg daily. Originally gabapentin was used as an additional therapy in partial epilepsia without secondary generalized seizures. Like with other antiepileptic drugs, the parameters from kidney, liver, and blood have to be supervised.

### ADAPTED PSYCHOTHERAPY

Nowadays so-called tinnitus retraining therapy (TRT) is widely applied. It includes a therapeutic wide-band low-level noise generator. It is based on habituation, which is defined as a reduced response to a stimulus after repeated exposure. It is a state in which the tinnitus signal no longer elicits any response. Resetting or reprogramming neuronal networks involved in subcortical signal detection brings about habituation.

Also, in cases with a known interrelation of stress and tinnitus, a stress–diathesis model for tinnitus was proposed by Shulman et al. Stress management techniques require a counselor and the close

---

[1]Not FDA approved for this indication.
*Available as dietary supplement.
[2]Not available in the United States.

cooperation of the patient, physician, biofeedback therapist, and psychologist.

A cognitive therapy that provides significant support to the patient with severe disabling tinnitus, particularly for control of the effect, is strongly recommended and encouraged.

## ADAPTED PHYSIOTHERAPY

A specific program of physiotherapy successfully applied in endogenous tinnitus is KKIT. This therapy uses expressive movements of body language. In a special rehabilitation program, different groups of muscles in the hand, arm, leg, foot, and body, rising from the feet up to the face, are activated, which guides the tinnitus patient into a situation of peaceful resting, reduction of tension, and finally into relaxation. This scheme was adapted from a program of treating pain. KKIT points toward mechanisms of interference of expressive gestural movements with facilitating tinnitus from around the basal ganglia of the brain.

## OTHER METHODS OF THERAPY

Other methods of tinnitus therapy recommended in the literature include acupuncture, counseling, group therapy, and hypnotherapy.

## REFERENCES

Alster J, Shemesh Z, Ornan M, Attias J: Sleep disturbance associated with chronic tinnitus. Biol Psychiatry 1993;34:84-90.

Arnesen AR, Engdahl B: Tinnitus—etiology, diagnosis and treatment. Tidsskr Nor Laegeforen 1996;116:2009-2012.

Bergmann JM, Bertora GO: Cortical and brainstem topodiagnostic testing in tinnitus patients—a preliminary report. Int Tinnitus J 1996;2:151-158.

Bertora GO, Bergmann JM: Tinnitus: Supratentorial areas study through brain electric tomography (LORETA). ASN 2004;2:2, ISSN 1612-3352. Available at http://www.neurootology.org

Claussen CF: Treatment of the slow brainstem syndrome with Vertigoheel. Biol Med 1985;3:447-470, 4:510-514.

Claussen CF: Medical classification of tinnitus between bruits: Exogenous and endogenous tinnitus and other types of tinnitus. ASN 2004;2, ISSN 1612-3352. Available at http://www.neurootology.org

Claussen CF, Kolchev C, Schneider D, Hahn A: Neurootological brain electrical activity mapping in tinnitus patients. Proceedings of the 4th International Tinnitus Seminar, Bordeaux, 1991;1092:351-355.

Claussen CF, Schneider D, Koltchev C: On the functional state of central vestibular structures in monaural symptomatic tinnitus patients. Int Tinnitus J 1995:1:5-12.

George RN, Kemp S: A survey of New Zealanders with tinnitus. Br J Audiol 1991;25:331-336.

Jastreboff PJ, Hazell JWP: A neurophysiological approach to tinnitus: Clinical implications. Br J Audiol 1993;27:1-11.

Parving A, Hein HO, Suadicani P, et al: Epidemiology of hearing disorders. Some factors affecting hearing. The Copenhagen Male Study. Scand Audiol 1993;22:101-107.

Quaranta A, Assennato G, Sallustio V: Epidemiology of hearing problems among adults in Italy. Scand Audiol Suppl 1996;42:9-13.

Shulman A: A final common pathway for tinnitus—the medial temporal lobe system. Tinnitus J 1996;2:115-126.

Shulman A, Aran JM, Feldmann H, et al: Tinnitus diagnosis/treatment. Philadelphia, Lea & Febiger, 1991.

Shulman A, Strashun AM, Afriyie M, et al: SPECT imaging of brain and tinnitus—neurotologic/neurologic implications. Int Tinnitus J 1995:1:13-29.

## ACKNOWLEDGMENT

Sponsored by grant Projekt D. 1417, durch die LVA Baden-Württemberg, Stuttgart, Germany.

# Spine Pain

Method of
*Michael T. McCann, MD*

Back pain is one of the most common musculoskeletal complaints seen in primary care practices; empirical treatment is frequently based on conjecture. Our understanding of the pathophysiology of spine and radicular pain has increased dramatically over the last decade as a result of new technology and more advanced diagnostic testing. Early and accurate diagnosis is imperative if we are to provide specific lesion-based treatment to optimize patient outcomes and health care spending.

Although patients are satisfied with their care for most major illnesses, 20% to 25% of surveyed patients were dissatisfied with their care for back pain. Only headache treatment also received such poor scores. The top reason patients listed for dissatisfaction with their physician's care was inadequate explanation of why they hurt.

Although muscle strain is the most common reason given to patients as the cause of their back pain, it is actually highly unlikely to be the etiology for back pain severe enough for a patient to seek medical care or for pain that lasts more than 2 weeks. An underlying spinal disorder is usually present, leading to overlying myofascial tenderness and tightness. Isolated back pain is not a neurologic problem. Rather, it is an orthopedic problem, as will be evident from the following discussion.

## Epidemiology

Eighty percent of the U.S. population develops back pain, limiting day-to-day activities, at some time in their lives. The peak incidence of such pain is between 35 and 65 years of age, declining thereafter. Based on radiographic degeneration alone, we would expect the incidence to increase linearly with age. In 80% of patients, episodes are self-limited, but in 15% to 20%, the pain chronically restricts function. Direct and indirect economical costs are estimated to be between $80 and $100 billion per year in the United States and, from an insurer's standpoint, costs may exceed expenditures on pediatric and obstetrical care combined. The majority of treatment expenditures are on the 20% of patients whose pain does not resolve spontaneously: recurrent or chronic back pain sufferers. To limit expenditures and optimize patient outcomes, it is vital that we prevent progression to a chronic state. Such prevention can best be achieved by early and accurate diagnosis and treatment.

## Pathophysiology

Somatic (nociceptive) pain is caused by noxious stimulation of nerve endings in the vertebrae, joints, ligaments and disks, whereas radicular (neuropathic) pain is produced by evoked ectopic impulses in the dorsal root ganglia (Figure 1).

## Somatic Pain

In primary somatic back pain, we try diagnostically to separate the pain generators into two anatomic categories based on their relation to the spinal canal. Treatment is significantly different based on the site of the lesions. Note that primary spinal nerve or cord pathology does not in and of itself produce axial back pain.

Pain generators in the anterior column are the disks and vertebral bodies. Only the outer third of a disk's annulus is innervated. Tears of these outer annular fibers produce exquisite pain and back spasm even without complete disruption of the disk. This is a frequent missed cause of nonspecific back pain because these internal disk disruptions are rarely visualized on routine spine magnetic resonance imaging (MRI) or computer tomography (CT) scans. If noted on MRI,

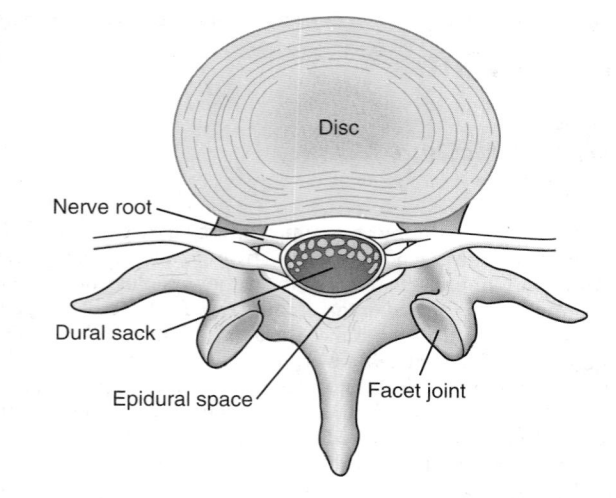

**FIGURE 1.** Spine cross section.

a high-intensity zone (HIZ) finding in a disk is highly suggestive of a painful internal annular tear. Definitive diagnosis is established with manometric provocative CT diskography. Diskitis, although rare, is also suggested by MRI findings, although aspiration may be necessary to establish an inflammatory or infectious etiology definitively.

Vertebral compression fractures, whether osteoporotic, traumatic, or pathologic, also contribute to anterior column primary axial pain. CT scanning or plain radiographs generally confirm the diagnosis; however, bone scanning may be necessary to confirm acuteness of a finding and to help rule out metastatic foci. Osteomyelitis should also be considered in any fracture with associated fever or a recent septic source.

The posterior column sources of back pain include the facet joints from the atlanto-occipital articulation caudad to the sacroiliac joints. All are true diarthrodial joints. The surfaces are capped with articular cartilage and lined with a synovial membrane. These paired innervated structures are subject to degeneration and painful traumatic injuries. In double-blind placebo controlled studies, the cervical facets appear to be the source of pain in 59% of patients with postwhiplash cervicalgia. Estimates regarding the lumbar spine place the incidence of facet-based low back pain between 15% and 40%, and the incidence increases significantly after 65 years of age.

Spondylolisthesis refers to a shift in the alignment between two vertebrae. With associated stress fractures of the pars interarticularis (spondylolysis), it is another posterior column source of pain. In chronic cases, instability leads to associated fibrosis under the pars fractures that produce radicular compression and neuropathic extremity pain. The slippage may also lead to central and foraminal stenosis with neurogenic claudication.

## Neuropathic Pain

The most common cause of lumbar radicular pain in young patients is disk herniation (98%). Nerve compression alone, however, does not offer a satisfactory explanation for the pain produced. In human studies, root compression alone produces distal extremity paresthesias and numbness but no pain. Isolated lumbar radiculopathy does not cause significant back pain, and disk herniation size does not correlate with severity of pain on straight leg raise testing. Nucleus pulposus placed within the epidural space produces extreme inflammation with a 100,000-fold increase in phospholipase-$A_2$ immunoreactivity that can be directly correlated with mechanical hyperalgesia. In the complete absence of root compression, nucleus pulposus stimulates sustained discharges of A$\delta$ and A$\beta$ pain fibers in the dorsal root ganglia and causes a conduction delay in the roots. Intravenous methylprednisolone

(Solu-Medrol)[1] prevents this conduction delay. Radicular pain appears to be caused by a combination of mechanical irritation in an otherwise chemically sensitized root.

Other sources of radicular pain include central spinal and lateral recess stenosis caused by facet arthropathies, ligamentous hypertrophy, and spondylolisthesis. Even more etiologies include neuromeningeal anomalies, neoplasms, infections, and vascular malformations. Peripheral neuropathies, including thoracic outlet, cubital and carpal tunnel syndromes, piriformis syndrome, tarsal tunnel, and other primary mononeuropathies, may also mimic or exist in conjunction with radiculopathies.

## Assessment

The goal of the initial assessment is to screen for emergent causes of back or radicular pain including aneurysms, infections, segmental instability, fractures, tumors, and myelopathy. A careful history and examination should help delineate referred cardiac, pulmonary, gastrointestinal, urologic, gynecologic, and vascular sources.

## History

For all patients presenting with back or radicular pain, the screening history should include weight loss, recent fevers or infections, and significant change in bowel or bladder function, including incontinence. For patients with cervicothoracic or upper extremity radicular pain, a cardiac history should be added. Abdominal symptoms, hematuria, dysuria, or vaginal discharge should be included for lumbar pain.

Radicular pain is lancinating with superficial and deep components that extend in distinct, but not necessarily dermatomal, distributions. Pain may extend partially or entirely in the distribution of the affected spinal nerve. Somatic referred pain is deep, aching, and diffuse. It can overlap with radicular symptoms in the proximal extremities. Proximal extremity pain can be radicular, whereas distal extremity pain is not necessarily always radicular.

Diffuse distal symptoms with dysesthesia, complaints of bowel or bladder urgency or incontinence, and a history of balance difficulties are red flags for myelopathy. Most patients also give a history of cervicothoracic or associated radicular pain. If accompanied by severe low back pain and complaints of saddle numbness, consider cauda equina syndrome, a surgical emergency.

Claudication symptoms are suggestive of spinal stenosis and usually there is little pain at rest. Differentiation from vascular claudication is sometimes difficult, but pain with neurogenic claudication is usually not worsened with supine positioning and leg elevation.

## Examination

Although clinical exam may establish the presence of a radiculopathy or localize the segmental pain level, etiology must be established by other means. Tumors, cysts, stenosis spondylolisthesis, and disk herniations may all cause very similar clinical signs.

Muscle pain and spasm should not be considered the primary source of the patient's back pain unless all other potential sources are ruled out and an objective rheumatologic etiology is identified pointing to a myositis. An antalgic gait from distal degenerative joint disease may cause lumbar muscular aching, but rarely is the back the site of greatest pain. This is not to say that muscles cannot be painful, but rather that in the majority of primary back pain cases, the muscles are simply reacting to an underlying derangement in the spine itself.

More specifically, examination should note hyperreflexia and clonus and test for Babinski's and Hoffmann's signs to note upper motor

---

[1]Not FDA approved for this indication.

## CURRENT DIAGNOSIS

**Emergent or Urgent Conditions Associated with Back Pain (Red Flags)**

| ASSOCIATED SYMPTOMS | CONDITION |
| --- | --- |
| ■ New onset bowel or bladder incontinence | Myelopathy |
| ■ Balance difficulties | Myelopathy |
| ■ Diffuse distal weakness or immobility | Myelopathy |
| ■ Recent weight loss | Tumor |
| ■ Severe chest or abdominal pain | Aortic aneurysm |

| HISTORY | CONDITION |
| --- | --- |
| ■ Osteoporosis | Fracture |
| ■ Recent trauma | Fracture |
| ■ Intravenous drug use | Infection |
| ■ Recent infection | Infection |
| ■ Immunosuppressed state | Infection |

| AGE | CONDITION |
| --- | --- |
| ■ <15 y or >60 y | Tumor suspicion |
| ■ Male >55 y (M:F 4:1) | Aortic aneurysm |

| ASSOCIATED SIGNS | CONDITION |
| --- | --- |
| ■ Tender abdomen | Aortic aneurysm |
| ■ Saddle sensory loss | Cauda equina syndrome |
| ■ Hyperreflexia with positive clonus, Babinski's sign, and Hoffmann's sign | Myelopathy |

neuron irritability. Screening cardiovascular and abdominal examination helps rule out other sources of back pain.

## Natural Course of the Disease

For lumbar radicular pain in patients treated conservatively, 50% of patients can expect to have resolution of radicular symptoms after 4 weeks. At 12 months, in 49% of males and 33% of females, radicular pain remains improved. Unfortunately, 60% to 70% of these patients developed back pain by 4 weeks that persisted at 12 months regardless of the radicular pain improvement.

For patients treated surgically versus conservatively, at 10 years there appears to be little statistically significant difference in outcome for radicular pain, with both groups achieving approximately 60% good results and poor results in 7% to 8%. This only holds true if surgery is not applied randomly, but as a last resort for patients who fail to respond to conservative care.

For cervical radiculopathic symptoms, 70% can be expected to improve with time and 20% become asymptomatic. In patients for whom surgery was an option, 90% are improved or only mildly incapacitated at long-term follow-up. Isolated recurrences are seen in 32% of cases, whereas 10% have moderate to severe persistent disability.

Although studies exist detailing favorable outcomes overall for radicular symptoms, the same does not necessarily hold true for mechanical back pain. Although 80% of patients appear to have resolution of initial symptoms independent of their course of care, 20% develop progressive or unrelenting pain. It appears that approximately 35% of persons have intermittent recurrences that limit their activities.

## Management

Take an algorithmic approach to the patient presenting with back and/or radicular symptoms of new onset. If initial history and examination suggest an emergent cause for these symptoms, appropriate additional diagnostic testing and referral should be made. Indications for urgent surgical interventions are few but include progressive motor deficit and cauda equina syndrome—progressive neurologic deterioration with loss of bowel and bladder function.

Once an emergent source of pain is ruled out, studies show that primary care physicians who prescribe the least amount of analgesics and place the fewest restrictions on activities have the best patient outcomes. In many cases, a more aggressive approach may reinforce illness behavior and foster a fear of future debilitation.

## Radicular Pain Predominating

If radicular pain predominates in a minimally distressed patient, simple reassurance and an explanation of the natural course of recovery may suffice. Avoiding bed rest and activity modification to prevent axial loading should be discussed (no lifting in a forward flexed position and no repetitive flexion activities). A 2-week reassessment allows any insidious red flag conditions to be picked up, provides reassurance, and allows adjustment of treatment.

For more significantly distressed patients with acute radicular pain, additional analgesics and more frequent follow-up may be required. Although no analgesic regimen alters the natural course of recovery, based on the inflammatory pathogenesis of radicular pain a pulse dose of prednisone or methylprednisolone with a taper can be considered over a week. However, in randomized controlled trials, the nonsteroidal anti-inflammatory drugs (NSAIDs) piroxicam (Feldene) and indomethacin (Indocin) did not offer any greater analgesia or enhance recovery more than placebo. A limited course of muscle relaxants and opioid analgesics may be prescribed but often provide little relief in cases of true neuropathic pain. The limited duration of these prescriptions should be explained to the patient at the outset. Despite ongoing pain, the goal is to avoid dependency and reliance on these medications for activities that may be detrimental to the natural course of the disorder.

Currently, greater success may be found with early initiation and titration of gabapentin (Neurontin)[1] for radicular pain. With low toxicity and few side effects, tolerance is usually good. Initiate dosing at night with 100 to 300 mg (lower dosing in patients >65 years old), escalating every 1 to 3 days as tolerated up to 1200 mg three times daily. If improvement is not obtained by 600 mg three times daily, further escalation is unlikely to be efficacious.

For distressed patients, duloxetine (Cymbalta)[1] may be efficacious while providing additional anxiolysis and antidepressive effects. Because nausea is a frequent side effect for the first few days upon initiation of dosing, we start with 30 mg every morning and advance to 60 mg every morning after 1 week. If sedation occurs, change to every-evening dosing. Symptomatic improvement is often seen by 7 to 10 days.

If at follow-up significant progress is not made and reassessment still lacks red flags, physical therapy with instructions for a McKenzie assessment and therapy over 2 weeks is indicated, with a home program to follow. Again, no scientific studies validate any particular regimen of therapy. However, from a spinal education standpoint, and as an impetus to maintaining function, an empirical recommendation can be made. Follow-up should be scheduled and if progress is partial, another 2 weeks of therapy could be considered.

Failure to improve or deterioration of function at any point would be an indication for additional imaging studies. An MRI provides the most comprehensive survey of causes for radicular symptoms. It does not, however, guarantee that anatomic changes are definitively the source for a patient's symptoms. In asymptomatic patients younger than 40 years, 30% had abnormal spine MRIs, whereas 60% to 70% of patients older than 40 years had abnormal MRIs. The prevalence of

---

[1]Not FDA approved for this indication.

**CURRENT THERAPY**

**Acute Presentation without Red Flags: Treatment Ladders (Frequent Reassessment as Indicated)**

BACK OR NECK PAIN PREDOMINATING

- Education, activity modification, and reassurance
- Limited course of analgesics dependent on stress
    - NSAIDs
    - Opioids
    - Muscle relaxants
    - Consider steroid taper regimen
- Physical therapy with spinal stabilization regimen
- Screening radiographs with flexion and extension views (rule out gross instability)
- Referral for spinal diagnostic assessment or orthopedic spine evaluation
- Fusion or disk replacement as indicated

RADICULAR PAIN PREDOMINATING

- Education, activity modification, and reassurance
- Early treatment of inflammation with steroid taper regimen
- Limited course of analgesics and muscle relaxants
- Early initiation of neuropathic pain medications
    - Gabapentin (Neurontin)[1]
    - Duloxetine (Cymbalta)[1]
    - Pregabalin (Lyrica)[1]
- Physical therapy guided by McKenzie assessment
- MRI (with gadolinium contrast for cancer, spinal cord pathology, and postoperative spine cases)
- Selective transforaminal steroid injection
- Surgical assessment for decompression

[1]Not FDA approved for this indication.
*Abbreviations:* NSAIDs = nonsteroidal anti-inflammatory drugs.

---

asymptomatic disk herniations alone ranged between 20% and 40% in patients between 40 and 60 years of age.

Evidence-based review of the literature currently does not support the use of electromyogram and nerve conduction velocity (EMG/NCV) studies) for diagnosis in cases of radiculopathic pain. Pain is mediated through $A\delta$ and C fibers, and an EMG tests activity in $A\alpha$ motor fibers. H and F reflexes similarly lack specificity in clinical trials with radiculopathy, despite proposed theoretical foundations. EMG/NCV testing would be indicated in cases where peripheral neuropathy or nerve entrapment is suspected and when objective muscle strength testing is suspect or primary myopathy may be present.

Recent prospective randomized blinded studies support selective nerve root injection (i.e., fluoroscopically guided transforaminal epidural steroid or epiradicular injections) as the next line of treatment. This highly selective procedure may reduce the need for surgical intervention in up to 59% of radicular cases and should be considered in cases where lack of improvement is noted as soon as 2 weeks. Serial MRI studies in humans show statistically significant improvement in the rate of disk reabsorption and symptoms in patients treated with transforaminal injections as compared to controls. The older regimen of translaminar epidural steroid injections is not nearly as efficacious and in some studies appears no more effective than placebo. Partial improvement at 10- to 14-day follow-up would be an indication for repeat injection. An automatic series of three injections is no longer considered standard of care, and response to a single transforaminal injection should guide additional treatment.

Lack of improvement or further functional decline would lead to surgical assessment.

Long-term management of a patient with radicular pain either unrelieved with surgery or in the patient for whom surgical options do not exist falls into the realm of neuropathic pain control. Narcotic regimens should be avoided because long-term efficacy has never been demonstrated. Medications options are limited, but gabapentin (Neurontin)[1] and duloxetine (Cymbalta)[1] are efficacious in reducing pain for a large number of patients with both radicular and other sources of neuropathic pain. The newest drug with indications for neuropathic pain is pregabalin (Lyrica)[1]. Efficacy for radicular pain is as yet undetermined but is expected to approximate gabapentin with fewer dose-related side effects. Other drugs to be considered include mexiletine (Mexitil)[1], tricyclic antidepressants,[1] and some of the newer anticonvulsants including levetiracetam (Keppra),[1] oxcarbazepine (Trileptal),[1] zonisamide (Zonegran),[1] and tiagabine (Gabitril).[1] All modify neuropathic pain in the presence and absence of associated depression.

For patients in whom neuropathic extremity pain far exceeds any mechanical back pain, despite optimization of all conservative treatment and surgical options, spinal cord stimulation may be considered. This modality is efficacious in between 60% and 70% of patients with neuropathic extremity pain predominating. It is not indicated for mechanical back pain. For permanently implanted patients, 70% continue to have approximately 50% improvement in neuropathic pain at 5-year follow-up.

## Axial Pain Predominating

For patients with nonurgent acute back or neck pain, again the level of distress helps guide care. Studies regarding early treatment and analgesic regimens for nociceptive back pain lack validity and specificity because early diagnosis is not usually sought because of the high incidence of spontaneous improvement. Early treatment thus remains empirical.

In a minimally distressed patient, supportive education and activity modification support the natural course of recovery. For an initial episode, physical therapy with spinal stabilization exercises, followed by a home program, is recommended to provide back education and to help reduce recurrences.

For the more distressed patient, oral analgesics may be indicated. Because the source of axial pain is nociceptive, NSAIDs should be considered as a first-line analgesic, with opioids reserved for very severe pain and again only for a limited duration. Failure to improve is not an indication for continued daily use of opioids. For moderate to severe pain where a significant inflammatory component is suspected, a bolus/taper dose of steroids over 1 week is often efficacious, and risks are low with this regimen. Muscle spasms are best managed with gradual stretching and paced activities. In severe cases, however, muscle relaxants may be beneficial, and even a limited course of benzodiazepines can be considered.

If at 2-week reassessment progress is not seen, physical therapy over 1 month (usually 3 to 4 times per week) for range of motion and stabilization exercise should be considered. Partial improvement would be an indication for another month of therapy or, in the motivated patient, another month of a home exercise program.

The goal of therapy is to maintain range of motion, strengthen supportive musculature, and maintain activities of daily living without additional injury. To this end, almost all exercise regimens claim efficacy, although no valid studies as yet show that any specific therapy actually alters the natural history.

Should a patient with primary back or neck pain fail to improve with therapy, screening radiographs may be indicated. Plain radiographs for mechanical back pain should always be obtained with flexion and extension views to rule out gross instability as well as other mechanical derangements, including spondylolisthesis, spondylolysis, and compression fractures.

Unfortunately, although all radiographic studies of the spine demonstrate anatomic abnormalities, they cannot show whether these

---

[1]Not FDA approved for this indication.

abnormalities are painful. With physical examination also notoriously unreliable for making a definitive diagnosis, referral for more advanced spinal diagnostic assessment may often be indicated in patients who fail to improve or who have frequent recurrences.

For the 20% of patients whose function remains limited by back pain despite maximized conservative care, identification of the exact pain source is imperative to improving outcomes. These patients are prone to seek numerous opinions, undergo fruitless operations, and pay for unproven modality-based treatments. Physicians tend toward making diagnoses based on response to treatment as opposed to the other way around. An early definitive diagnosis allows realistic treatment options and prognosis to be given. Patients can thus adjust their lifestyle to function within the limits imposed by their spinal condition.

Significant advances are being made in the field of diagnosing back pain. Select spinal injection techniques are refined to isolate the exact source of a patient's pain in the majority of cases. Validity testing can also determine if a patient's complaint has an anatomic basis or if symptom magnification is present.

CT-provocative diskography is the only test available to document internal disk anatomy precisely and to determine if a disk is the source of a patient's back pain. Studies show that compared with surgical findings, its anatomic accuracy exceeds MRI and CT myelography. With the use of manometry, intradiskal symptomatic pressures help determine the proper surgical technique to optimize patient outcomes. Diagnostic facet injections can also identify a symptomatic joint precisely, further helping determine options for treatment.

New nonsurgical or minimally invasive treatments are now validated, including radiofrequency thermocoagulation (RFTC) lesioning for desensitization of painful facet joint arthropathies, intradiskal electrothermal therapy (IDET) for treatment of painful disk lesions, and percutaneous disk decompression by both mechanical and laser techniques. For vertebral compression fracture, vertebroplasty and kyphoplasty may offer remarkable and rapid relief of associated fracture pain but do carry a risk of severe neurologic injury and embolism. Treatment outcomes for all of these procedures rely heavily on obtaining an exact diagnosis using the preceding tests.

Surgical assessment for nonemergent back pain should be reserved for those patients who fail conservative management and are not candidates for minimally invasive treatment or who have identifiable gross segmental spinal instability. Unlike radicular pain, decompression alone does not improve primary back pain. For mechanical back pain from segmental instability, the only surgical option is fusion. Poor pain relief is seen most frequently in patients who undergo fusion procedures for back pain based on radiographic findings alone. Provocative testing to isolate the actual pain generators and to determine the integrity of surrounding support structures maximizes the chances for success. For patients with isolated diskogenic pain, validated with manometric CT diskography, newer disk replacement techniques hold promise. Fusions cause a load shift to adjacent spinal motion segments causing degeneration. This leads to a 30% reoperation rate for fusion patients within 10 years. The hope is that disk replacements will prevent this transitional zone degeneration and lower the reoperation rate.

Not all patients are candidates for surgical reconstruction. In many cases, surgical intervention may only serve to worsen a patient's state. Tolerance of symptoms with acceptance of functional limitations is the preferred course.

To conclude, patients presenting with pain of spinal origin should be divided into those with predominantly radicular symptoms and those with primarily mechanical back or neck pain. In the vast majority of

**TABLE 1  Clinical Pearls**

Muscle strain is a very unusual cause of back pain severe enough to seek medical attention.
For back pain, think facets, disks, and vertebrae.
Referred back and neck pain can extend into the extremities and mimic radicular patterns.
Radicular pain does not always extend into the distal extremities (L5 radiculopathy can mimic hip trochanteric bursitis).
Magnetic resonance imaging (MRI) cannot tell you what hurts, only what might be causing pain.
MRI does not rule out all spinal pathology that can cause pain.
Order MRI with gadolinium contrast only if:
    You suspect cancer.
    You suspect a primary spinal cord lesion.
    Spine surgery was performed in the suspect region.
Laminectomy alone should not be used to treat predominant back pain (only radicular pain).
Fusions and disk replacements are for predominant back pain.
Only spinal diagnostic testing (selective computer tomography [CT] diskography, facet blocks, and transforaminal injections) can isolate the source of pain in refractory cases.
Electromyogram and nerve conduction velocity (EMG/NCV) studies should be used only if you:
    Suspect an underlying peripheral neuropathic process (double crush).
    Suspect lack of effort on motor testing.
    Suspect a primary myopathy.
Early referral for accurate diagnostic testing is the key to optimizing care: the more accurate the diagnosis, the more accurate the care.

cases, back and neck pain originates from derangements of the facets, disks, or vertebrae, not the muscles. Radicular pain is most likely secondary to a compressive lesion with associated underlying inflammation.

Proper diagnosis is paramount to optimizing patient treatment (both conservative and surgical) and to prevention of progress to a chronic dysfunctional state. MRIs have limitations in what they are able to visualize and do not guarantee that anatomic derangements are actually the source of the patient's pain. For an accurate diagnosis in a patient who fails to respond to initial conservative care, more specialized interventional spinal diagnostic testing is indicated (Table 1).

Identification and isolation of specific spinal pain generators has allowed for the development of specific lesion-based minimally invasive treatments. These include transforaminal injections for radiculopathy, RFTC desensitization for facet-based pain, and percutaneous decompression for disk displacement pain. Decompressive surgery is very effective at relieving severe radicular pain unresponsive to conservative care and injections, but it is complicated by post-laminectomy spinal instability. Spinal fusion surgery for well-diagnosed painful segmental instability remains the definitive treatment for this disorder; newer disk replacement surgery may offer an alternative to fusion for primary diskogenic back or neck pain.

# The Infectious Diseases

## Management of the Patient with HIV Disease

Method of
*Surendra K. Sharma, MD, PhD, and*
*Tamilarasu Kadhiravan, MD*

AIDS was described initially in the United States in 1981 among several case clusters of previously healthy young men who had sex with men, presenting with unusual infections such as *Pneumocystis jiroveci* pneumonia (PCP), mucosal candidiasis, disseminated cytomegalovirus (CMV) disease, and Kaposi's sarcoma. The cause of AIDS remained elusive then, leading to several speculations. A few years later, amid much controversy, the causative agent was established as HIV, which has a predilection to infect and destroy the immune effector cells, primarily the CD4+ T lymphocytes. The discovery of HIV led to the development of definitive diagnostic tests that unearthed, to everyone's dismay, a widespread, hitherto invisible, smoldering pandemic in evolution.

## Epidemiology

Since the beginning of the epidemic, approximately 25 million people have died of AIDS worldwide, making it one of the most devastating epidemics of all times. An estimated 40 million people are living with HIV/AIDS globally, including 17.5 million women and 2.3 million children younger than 15 years. In 2005 alone, an estimated 5 million people got newly infected, and approximately 3 million people died because of AIDS. More than half of the burden of HIV/AIDS is borne by sub-Saharan Africa, particularly the southern African nations. In countries such as Botswana, South Africa, Zimbabwe, Swaziland, and Namibia, the prevalence of HIV infection among expectant mothers is consistently in excess of 20%.

North America accounts for approximately 1.2 million people living with HIV/AIDS, most of them in the United States. Every year, more than 35,000 new cases are reported in the United States. Blacks and Hispanics are disproportionately represented among them, and pediatric AIDS accounts for approximately 1% of the cases. With the widespread implementation of preventive measures, a marginal but significant fall in HIV infection rates was observed for the first time among non-Hispanic blacks and injection drug users.

## The Causative Agent

HIV is an enveloped single-stranded RNA virus (family: Retroviridae; subfamily: Lentivirinae). Embedded in its envelope are glycoprotein spikes (gp120, gp41) that are crucial for binding with the host cell surface receptors such as CD4, CCR5, and CXCR4 and subsequent entry into the host cell. HIV is a retrovirus that elaborates the enzyme reverse transcriptase. It enables transcription of genomic RNA to proviral DNA for integration into the host cell DNA. Host cells that bear CD4+ (helper T cells, macrophages, etc.) are the main targets of HIV infection. There are two human immunodeficiency viruses, HIV-1 and HIV-2. Compelling genetic evidence suggests that they originated from the simian immunodeficiency viruses, of the chimpanzee (SIVcpz) and the sooty mangabey monkeys (SIVsm), respectively, in Africa several decades back. HIV-1 is global in distribution, whereas HIV-2 is confined mainly to western Africa. HIV-2 infection is less effectively transmitted and results in lower levels of viremia and slower disease progression compared to HIV-1.

Isolates of HIV-1 across the globe exhibit marked genetic heterogeneity and are classified into three groups (M, O, and N) and several clades. Clade C is the most common form worldwide. In North America and Europe, clade B is the predominant subtype. Genetic recombination among co-circulating clades often occurs, and such a recombinant subtype AE is the most prevalent form in Southeast Asia. Clade AE viruses are transmitted more effectively by the heterosexual route than the clade B virus. The genetic heterogeneity of HIV has to be taken into consideration in the development and evaluation of HIV vaccines.

## Modes of Transmission

Transmission of HIV occurs through contact with the body fluids of a HIV-infected person. The routes of transmission are sexual, both male to male as well as heterosexual contact; mother to child; transfusion of HIV-tainted blood and blood products; injection drug use; and occupational exposure in health care and laboratory workers. No evidence suggests that HIV is transmitted by casual contact and insect bites. Heterosexual transmission is the most prevalent route of HIV transmission worldwide, especially in developing countries. In the United States, male-to-male sexual contact is the most common route of transmission; however, the proportion of cases caused by heterosexual transmission is steadily increasing.

The average risk of HIV transmission per coital act in sero-discordant heterosexual couples is approximately 0.1%. Several factors, such as the presence of other sexually transmitted infections (ulcerative as well as nonulcerative) and higher viral load, increase the risk of transmission; condom use and male circumcision considerably reduce the risk. Female-to-male transmission is less effective than male-to-female transmission. Commercial sex is associated with a higher risk of transmission of approximately 5% to 10%. Receptive anal intercourse is associated with a higher risk of transmission as compared to vaginal intercourse. Even though the risk of transmission by oral sex is very low, it should not be considered completely safe.

Mother-to-child transmission of infection can occur during pregnancy, during delivery, or by breast-feeding. More than half of the transmissions occur intrapartum, mediated by direct contact of infant mucosa with HIV-laden maternal blood, amniotic fluid, and cervical/vaginal secretions. Placental microtransfusion also plays a role. High maternal plasma viremia, prolonged rupture of membranes, and chorioamnionitis increase the risk of mother-to-child transmission, whereas cesarean delivery and use of peripartum antiretroviral prophylaxis decrease the risk markedly.

With the implementation of mandatory testing practices, transmission through infected blood and blood products is almost eliminated in the developed world. However, despite using the highly sensitive nucleic acid-based tests, given the enormous number of transfusions in clinical practice, the risk of transfusion-transmitted HIV infection cannot be overlooked. It is estimated that each year 16 infectious donations are available for transfusion in the United States.

Although injection drug use is responsible for approximately 20% of HIV transmission in the United States, it is the driving force behind the HIV epidemic in Southeast Asian countries and China. Apart from direct transmission through sharing of contaminated needles and other paraphernalia, injection drug use also promotes risk-taking behavior and unsafe sexual practices. In developing countries, unsafe injections administered at health care facilities are a potential, but underappreciated, route of HIV transmission. Occupational transmission occurs through percutaneous needle stick injuries and after mucous membrane or nonintact skin exposure to infected body fluids. The risk of HIV infection following a contaminated needle stick injury is approximately 0.3% and is approximately 0.09% following mucous membrane exposure.

## Pathogenesis and Natural History of HIV Infection

Following infection, HIV localizes to the lymphoid organs of the body where it productively infects the CD4+ helper T lymphocytes in the milieu provided by the dendritic cells and subsequently spills over into the circulation. In the absence of an immune response, this results in intense viremia in the early weeks following primary infection. During this phase, extensive dissemination of the virus occurs throughout the body. In approximately 50% to 70% of individuals, this might become clinically manifest as a self-limited, mononucleosis-like illness known as "acute HIV syndrome" (Table 1). Soon, with the elaboration of HIV-specific cell-mediated as well as humoral immune responses, viremia is brought under control albeit incompletely. A balance thus is struck between the opposing influences of viremia and the host immune response, establishing the viral load around a relatively low, stable level known as the virologic setpoint. The virologic setpoint is one of the important determinants of the pace of subsequent disease progression. Even if the viremia gets suppressed to below-detectable limits, despite the disease being clinically silent, active viral replication occurs throughout the course of HIV disease.

Some aspects of viral dynamics in vivo are important from a therapeutic point of view. An enormously large amount of virions ($10^{10}$ to $10^{11}$) are produced and cleared every day. Thus, the chances of a drug-resistant strain emerging under the selection pressure exerted by antiretroviral therapy are very high. Even in patients who achieve undetectable viral loads for prolonged periods of time following treatment, ongoing active viral replication occurs. If therapy is stopped in these patients, viral load promptly bounces back. Further, antiretroviral therapy does not eliminate the large reservoir of latently infected cells that

### TABLE 1   Acute HIV Syndrome*

| Clinical Features | Differential Diagnosis |
| --- | --- |
| **Common (> 50%)** | |
| Fever | Infectious mononucleosis |
| Malaise | Acute cytomegalovirus |
| Lymphadenopathy | infection |
| Pharyngitis | Secondary syphilis |
| Rash—erythematous, | Acute toxoplasmosis |
| maculopapular; urticarial; | Rickettsial infections |
| mucocutaneous ulcers | Rubella |
| Myalgia and arthralgia | Systemic lupus |
| | erythematosus |
| | Still's disease |
| **Frequent (10%–50%)** | |
| Diarrhea | |
| Headache | |
| Nausea and vomiting | |
| Hepatosplenomegaly | |
| Oral thrush | |
| Anorexia and weight loss | |
| **Occasional (<10%)** | |
| Aseptic meningitis | |
| Acute meningoencephalitis | |
| Guillain-Barré syndrome | |
| Myelopathy | |
| Brachial neuritis | |
| Facial palsy | |
| Peripheral neuropathy | |
| Opportunistic infections | |

*Occurs approximately 3–6 wk following primary infection; symptoms last for 1 to several weeks, followed by gradual, spontaneous resolution; in a small proportion (approximately 10%), despite resolution of initial symptoms, rapid immunologic deterioration follows.

are capable of giving rise to replication-competent virus. Theoretically, it would take several decades of uninterrupted viral suppression for this reservoir to get depleted on its own.

During the phase of clinical latency, continuous viral replication leads to progressive depletion of CD4+ helper T cells, resulting from direct cytopathicity as well as by diverse indirect mechanisms. When the CD4+ cell count falls below 200 cells/mL, the risk of opportunistic infections (OIs) increases greatly, culminating in AIDS. The CD4+ cell count, as an index of immunosuppression because of HIV infection, predicts strongly the risk of OIs and thereby the risk of progression to AIDS and subsequent death (Table 2). However, when the CD4+ counts are above 350 cells/mL, their usefulness in predicting the risk of disease progression is limited. Conversely, the plasma viral load is a more robust predictor of the risk of AIDS, independent of the CD4+ count at all levels (Table 2). The rate of decline in CD4+ count is highly variable among individuals. Some progress very rapidly, whereas a few others maintain normal levels of CD4+ counts and immunocompetence for prolonged periods without treatment. In Western populations, the median time to development of AIDS is approximately 10 years, and approximately 10% of patients remain asymptomatic beyond 20 years. The latter are known as long-term nonprogressors.

Apart from the viral load, several host-related factors also influence the rate of disease progression. It is well known that people who are homozygous for the deletion mutation CCR5-Δ 32, which codes for a nonfunctional CCR5, are highly resistant to HIV infection despite repeated exposure. HIV-infected individuals who are heterozygous for this allele have comparatively lower plasma viral loads and slower rate of progression to AIDS. Likewise, homo/heterozygosity for the mutant allele CCR2 64I, the product of which dimerizes with and decreases the expression of CXCR4 on the cell surface, results in slower disease

**TABLE 2** Predicted 6-Month Risk of AIDS in the CASCADE Project, Based on Age, Current CD4+ Count, and Plasma Viral Load

| Viral Load (copies/mL) | Predicted Risk at Current CD4+ Cell Count (cells/μL) | | | | | | | | | |
|---|---|---|---|---|---|---|---|---|---|---|
| | 50 | 100 | 150 | 200 | 250 | 300 | 350 | 400 | 450 | 500 |
| **Age 25 y** | | | | | | | | | | |
| 3,000 | 6.8 | 3.7 | 2.3 | 1.6 | 1.1 | 0.8 | 0.6 | 0.5 | 0.4 | 0.3 |
| 10,000 | 9.6 | 5.3 | 3.4 | 2.3 | 1.6 | 1.2 | 0.9 | 0.7 | 0.5 | 0.4 |
| 30,000 | 13.3 | 7.4 | 4.7 | 3.2 | 2.2 | 1.6 | 1.2 | 0.9 | 0.7 | 0.6 |
| 100,000 | 18.6 | 10.6 | 6.7 | 4.6 | 3.2 | 2.4 | 1.8 | 1.4 | 1.1 | 0.8 |
| 300,000 | 25.1 | 14.5 | 9.3 | 6.3 | 4.5 | 3.3 | 2.5 | 1.9 | 1.5 | 1.2 |
| **Age 35 y** | | | | | | | | | | |
| 3,000 | 8.5 | 4.7 | 3.0 | 2.0 | 1.4 | 1.0 | 0.8 | 0.6 | 0.5 | 0.4 |
| 10,000 | 12.1 | 6.7 | 4.3 | 2.9 | 2.0 | 1.5 | 1.1 | 0.9 | 0.7 | 0.5 |
| 30,000 | 16.6 | 9.3 | 5.9 | 4.0 | 2.8 | 2.1 | 1.6 | 1.2 | 0.9 | 0.7 |
| 100,000 | 23.1 | 13.2 | 8.5 | 5.8 | 4.1 | 3.0 | 2.3 | 1.7 | 1.3 | 1.1 |
| 300,000 | 30.8 | 18.0 | 11.7 | 8.0 | 5.7 | 4.2 | 3.1 | 2.4 | 1.9 | 1.5 |
| **Age 45 y** | | | | | | | | | | |
| 3,000 | 10.7 | 5.9 | 3.7 | 2.5 | 1.8 | 1.3 | 1.0 | 0.7 | 0.6 | 0.5 |
| 10,000 | 15.1 | 8.5 | 5.4 | 3.6 | 2.6 | 1.9 | 1.4 | 1.1 | 0.8 | 0.7 |
| 30,000 | 20.6 | 11.7 | 7.5 | 5.1 | 3.6 | 2.6 | 2.0 | 1.5 | 1.2 | 0.9 |
| 100,000 | 28.4 | 16.5 | 10.6 | 7.3 | 5.2 | 3.8 | 2.9 | 2.2 | 1.7 | 1.3 |
| 300,000 | 37.4 | 22.4 | 14.6 | 10.1 | 7.2 | 5.3 | 4.0 | 3.1 | 2.4 | 1.9 |
| **Age 55 y** | | | | | | | | | | |
| 3,000 | 13.4 | 7.5 | 4.7 | 3.2 | 2.3 | 1.7 | 1.2 | 0.9 | 0.7 | 0.6 |
| 10,000 | 18.8 | 10.7 | 6.8 | 4.6 | 3.3 | 2.4 | 1.8 | 1.4 | 1.1 | 0.8 |
| 30,000 | 25.4 | 14.6 | 9.4 | 6.4 | 4.6 | 3.3 | 2.5 | 1.9 | 1.5 | 1.2 |
| 100,000 | 34.6 | 20.5 | 13.3 | 9.2 | 6.5 | 4.8 | 3.6 | 2.8 | 2.2 | 1.7 |
| 300,000 | 44.8 | 27.5 | 18.2 | 12.6 | 9.1 | 6.7 | 5.0 | 3.9 | 3.0 | 2.4 |

*Abbreviation:* CASCADE = Concerted Action on Seroconversion to AIDS and Death in Europe.
Reproduced with permission from Phillips A; CASCADE collaboration: Short-term risk of AIDS according to current CD4 cell count and viral load in antiretroviral drug-naïve individuals and those treated in the monotherapy era. AIDS 2004;18(1):51-58.

progression. HLA alleles B*5701 and B*2705 also are strongly associated with long-term nonprogressor status. Conversely, individuals having the single nucleotide polymorphism at the promoter site of the inhibitory cytokine IL-10 (IL-10-5'-592A) are at a higher risk for HIV infection upon exposure, and they progress to AIDS more rapidly once infected. Certain exogenous factors might also influence the course of HIV infection. The orphan virus GB virus C slows down disease progression and is associated with better survival in patients dually infected with HIV and GB virus C. CMV co-infection possibly augments the rate of HIV disease progression. Incident OIs, especially tuberculosis and deficiency of micronutrients, also accelerate disease progression.

## Changing Face of HIV/AIDS

Highly active antiretroviral therapy (HAART) has dramatically changed the long-term outcome of patients with HIV/AIDS, which once was a rapidly fatal illness. HAART not only improves the CD4+ counts but also decreases the risk of OIs and reduces the mortality substantially. The benefit of HAART is evident even in those patients with advanced immunosuppression. From a public health perspective, HAART is a cost-effective intervention, in the developed world and the developing nations alike. In fact, HAART is comparatively more cost-effective than some of the widely accepted therapies for certain non-HIV diseases.

Since the introduction of HAART in 1995, AIDS-related mortality has declined considerably in the United States. With improved survival of patients with AIDS, noninfectious complications of AIDS such as AIDS-related malignancies and chronic renal failure are increasingly seen. Similarly, some novel problems of long-term antiretroviral therapy, such as lipodystrophy, insulin resistance syndrome, increased risk of cardiovascular events, and osteoporosis, are also being recognized.

However, the changing face of AIDS is not a global phenomenon; paradoxically, the populations that need it the most are the ones with poor access to HAART.

## Whom to Test for HIV Infection

HIV testing should be offered to all persons reporting any of the known risk factors for HIV acquisition and those requesting a HIV test on their own, irrespective of their risk behavior. Patients presenting with OIs and noninfectious illnesses possibly related to HIV, such as lymphoma, cervical cancer, and anal cancer, should also be tested for HIV infection. Subtle clinical clues of immunocompromise, such as oral thrush, herpes zoster in a young person, or failure to thrive in children, should alert the physician to the possibility of HIV infection. In developing nations, it is not uncommon for a young child to be the index case of a HIV-infected family. All women who are receiving antenatal care and, in underdeveloped nations, antenatal cases coming into contact with the health care system for the first time while in labor should be screened for HIV infection. In addition, patients seen in certain high-risk settings in which the prevalence of HIV infection is known to be high, such as sexually transmitted disease clinics, tuberculosis clinics, detoxification clinics, and correctional facilities, should also be offered HIV testing. HIV infection should be systematically excluded by testing while evaluating patients presenting with fever of unknown origin, autoimmune disorders such as Sjögren's syndrome, systemic lupus erythematosus, Reiter's syndrome, and polymyositis, and neurologic illnesses such as young-onset dementia and unexplained peripheral neuropathy. To say there are no contraindications for offering HIV testing to a patient is no overstatement.

It is estimated that every fourth HIV-infected person in the United States is not aware of his or her serostatus. This not only jeopardizes their own care but also places others at risk of potential transmission, which could be prevented if they are detected early. In recent times, the current trend of "HIV exceptionalism" has come under considerable criticism. This calls for a public health approach, based on standard principles of epidemic control, which encompasses a nonselective HIV testing strategy instead of the targeted-testing practices in vogue. Recent evidence suggests that nonselective HIV testing, in health care settings and possibly in the general population also, could be cost effective.

## Diagnosis of HIV Infection

All persons who are offered HIV testing should receive appropriate pretest counseling, and their explicit consent must be obtained. Notification of the result must be confidential and has to be accompanied by post-test counseling. Post-test counseling should focus on behavior modification for persons who test negative and for persons who test positive as well.

Laboratory diagnosis of HIV infection is based on a sequential testing strategy for the detection of antibodies to HIV-specific antigens. The first test is a highly sensitive enzyme immunoassay (EIA) that contains antigens of both HIV-1 and HIV-2. If the test is negative, further testing is not warranted, unless the exposure was within the past 3 months, in which case it has to be repeated in 3 months. If the first test returns positive or indeterminate, the test is repeated in duplicate. If the repeat EIA tests are positive or indeterminate, the HIV-1 Western blot assay is needed for confirmation. A Western blot demonstrating antibodies to products of all three major genes of HIV (gag, pol, and env) is conclusive evidence of HIV infection (rare false-positives can occur with the conventional Centers for Disease Control and Prevention criterion that does not require reactivity to products of pol); a negative assay shows no bands. Patterns that fall in between are considered indeterminate and must be repeated after an interval of 1 month. Alternatively, one may proceed to a specific test such as the p24 antigen capture assay or HIV-1 RNA assay. If the HIV-1 Western blot result is discordant with that of EIA, the possibility of HIV-2 infection should be considered, and HIV-2-specific testing is warranted.

Four rapid tests—OraQuick Advance, Uni-Gold Recombigen, Reveal G2, and Multispot HIV-1/HIV-2—are approved by the U.S. Food and Drug Administration for point-of-care testing in acute care settings and for on-site testing at outreach testing sites. A positive result by any of these tests should be considered only as "preliminary positive," and further confirmatory testing is essential.

## Management of the HIV-Infected Patient

Similar to any other disease, there seems to be a learning curve in the case of HIV care as well. It is well known that the outcome of patients with HIV/AIDS receiving treatment, at least to a certain extent, depends on the expertise of the care provider. However, this does not mean that all HIV-infected patients should be treated only by a specialist, which is not a feasible proposition. The sheer magnitude of the

### CURRENT DIAGNOSIS

- Threshold to offer HIV testing to a patient should be low; nonselective HIV testing in health care settings could be cost effective.
- A repeatedly reactive enzyme immunoassay, rapid test, or nucleic acid-based test for HIV infection needs confirmation with a Western blot assay.
- Estimation of CD4+ count and plasma viral load should be performed to assess the need for antiretroviral therapy and the risk of opportunistic infections.

problem calls for greater participation on the part of the primary care physician. The U.S. Department of Health and Human Services panel recommends care by a physician with at least 20, preferably 50, HIV-infected patients. It is essential for a primary care physician to be familiar with the initial care of patients with HIV/AIDS. Primary care physicians who have not cared for a considerable number of patients with HIV/AIDS should liaise with a specialist in the field. Referral to a specialist is warranted in cases of treatment-failure and for the management of complications. Care of HIV-infected patients is multifaceted, and it needs a multidisciplinary approach. Such a comprehensive care is delivered better by the primary care physician.

### INITIAL EVALUATION

Evaluation of the HIV-infected patient is carried out in several stages: assessment of the stage of disease and the need for antiretroviral therapy; symptom-oriented evaluation for opportunistic conditions; screening to assess the risk of opportunistic infections (OIs) in the future; screening for diseases that are co-transmitted, such as sexually transmitted infections and viral hepatitis; and prevention of further transmission of HIV infection.

History should be elicited with reference to the route and time of HIV acquisition. Time of exposure and earlier negative HIV tests are useful to assess reasonably the latter but may not be available in every case. More often than not, patients have multiple risk factors, and some patients may not report any of the known risk factors. A nonjudgmental approach is important while taking a sexual history. In addition, questions should focus on symptoms of other sexually transmitted infections such as urethral/vaginal discharge, genital ulcers, dysuria, dyspareunia in females, and perianal/oral ulcers and sore throat in those who report anal/oral sex. It is also important to elicit how the patient is coping with the diagnosis of HIV infection and the social and family support available to the patient. All patients have to be screened for depression and the presence of suicidal ideations, and they should be encouraged to inform their spouse/sexual partner of their HIV status. The physician has to be aware of the legal obligations regarding partner notification because they vary from place to place.

History should focus also on symptoms such as unexplained weight loss, prolonged fever, chronic diarrhea, recurrent oral ulcers, dysphagia, shortness of breath, cognitive decline, and new-onset seizures pointing toward the presence of opportunistic conditions that need further diagnostic evaluation. In treatment-experienced patients, details of previous antiretroviral treatment and the response to it should be meticulously looked into and properly recorded. This can be invaluable while changing the therapy in cases of treatment failure. Medication history should include details of allergic reaction to drugs such as cotrimoxazole (Bactrim), nevirapine (Viramune), and abacavir (Ziagen), and details of other drug-related adverse effects, such as pancreatitis, peripheral neuropathy, and hepatitis too. Details of past illnesses like tuberculosis and viral hepatitis, contact with cases of tuberculosis, and travel to areas endemic for certain infections such as histoplasmosis (Ohio and Mississippi river valleys), coccidioidomycosis (southwestern United States, northern Mexico), penicilliosis (Southeast Asia), and leishmaniasis (tropics, subtropics, and southern Europe) should be elicited.

A complete physical examination has to be performed at the time of initial evaluation and at subsequent visits. Attention should be paid to the presence of lymphadenopathy, hepatomegaly/splenomegaly, serosal effusions, and features of wasting or lipodystrophy. Examination of the nervous system should focus on possible peripheral neuropathy, proximal myopathy, focal neurologic signs, meningism, and cognitive impairment. If the latter is suspected, further neuropsychological testing is required. In patients presenting with OIs, skin lesions often hold the clue. Funduscopic examination should be done, and in patients with CD4+ less than 50 cells/mL, detailed examination by an ophthalmologist is needed to screen for cytomegalovirus (CMV) retinitis and other ocular manifestations of HIV. One should look for thrush, hairy leukoplakia, mucosal lesions of Kaposi's sarcoma, and aphthous ulcerations while examining the oral cavity. Diligent examination of the anogenital area for urethral discharge, genital/perianal ulcerations, condylomata, and adnexal tenderness in females is needed. Table 3 describes the laboratory evaluation of HIV-infected patients.

## ANTIRETROVIRAL THERAPY

Antiretroviral drugs fall into four classes: nucleoside/nucleotide reverse transcriptase inhibitors (NRTIs), non-nucleoside reverse transcriptase inhibitors (NNRTIs), protease inhibitors (PIs), and fusion inhibitors (Table 4). HAART is a combination of at least three potent antiretroviral drugs, typically a combination of two NRTIs as the backbone, along with either a PI or an NNRTI. Antiretroviral drugs act by inhibiting the enzyme reverse transcriptase either competitively (NRTIs) or noncompetitively (NNRTIs) or by inhibiting the viral protease that is essential for virion assembly (PIs), or by causing functional inhibition of gp41 that is important for entry into the host cell (fusion inhibitors). NNRTIs are specific for the HIV-1 reverse transcriptase and have no activity against HIV-2. HIV-2 carries, constitutively, many of the mutations associated with PI resistance that might limit the activity of PIs against HIV-2.

The goal of treatment is to achieve maximal and sustained suppression of plasma viremia to undetectable levels (less than 50 to 80 copies/mL for currently available tests). In this regard, HAART is far superior to dual and monotherapies and is the standard of care.

## CURRENT THERAPY

- History of any AIDS-defining illness, CD4+ count <200 cells/µL, and symptomatic HIV disease warrant initiation of highly active antiretroviral therapy (HAART).
- HAART should be offered also to patients with CD4+ counts 200–350 cells/µL, irrespective of viral load and symptoms.
- HAART can be deferred if CD4+ count is >350 cells/µL with plasma viral load below 100,000 copies/mL.
- Once initiated, HAART has to be continued lifelong without interruption.
- Adherence is a very important determinant of virologic outcome.
- Regular monitoring of viral load should be done to diagnose treatment failure early.
- At least two fully active drugs, based on treatment history and resistance testing, should be included in the salvage regimen.

## TABLE 3 Initial and Subsequent Laboratory Evaluation of the HIV-Infected Patient

| Baseline Testing | Follow-up Testing[a] |
|---|---|
| CD4+ count[b] | Once in 3–6 mo |
| Plasma HIV RNA load[c] | Once in 3–4 mo if not on treatment; at 2–8 wk after initiating/changing treatment, then q3–4mo |
| Viral resistance testing[d] | Recommended in virologic failure |
| Complete blood count | q3mo, especially in patients taking zidovudine (Retrovir) |
| Blood urea, creatinine, electrolytes | q3–6mo, especially in patients taking indinavir (Crixivan) or other nephrotoxic drugs |
| Transaminases, alkaline phosphatase, bilirubin, albumin | q2wk in first month, monthly for next 3 mo, then once in 3 mo |
| Fasting blood glucose | If on PIs, at 1–3 mo after initiation, then q3–6mo |
| Fasting serum lipids | If on PIs, at 3–6 mo, then annually |
| Urinalysis—proteinuria, sediments | q3–6mo, especially in patients taking indinavir (Crixivan) |
| Chest radiograph | As clinically indicated |
| Electrocardiogram | As clinically indicated |
| **Serologic Screening** | |
| Antitoxoplasma IgG[e] | If seronegative, when CD4+ <100/µL and unable to take cotrimoxazole (Bactrim) |
| Syphilis serology (VDRL or RPR) | Annually, if sexually active[f] |
| Anticytomegalovirus IgG[g] | As clinically indicated |
| HBsAg, HBsAb, HCV-Ab, HAV-Ab[h] | As clinically indicated |
| Antivaricella IgG[i] | Not indicated |
| Tuberculin skin test[j] | Not indicated |
| Urine-based (first-void) NAAT for *Chlamydia* species, *Neisseria gonorrhoeae*[k] | Annually, if sexually active[f] |
| **In Women** | |
| Cervical Papanicolaou smear | Annually, if sexually active[f] |
| Vaginal secretions for *Trichomonas* species | Annually, if sexually active[f] |
| Cervical specimen for NAAT for *Chlamydia* species (if sexually active) | Annually, if sexually active[f] |

[a]May be repeated more frequently if clinically indicated.
[b]Preferably 2 baseline values measured 1–4 wk apart; if discordant, repeat third time.
[c]Preferably 2 baseline values measured 1–4 wk apart.
[d]Optional in acute HIV infection and before starting treatment in chronic HIV infection.
[e]Seronegative patients should be counseled regarding proper preparation of meat and appropriate handling of cat feces.
[f]q3–6mo in asymptomatic persons at higher risk.
[g]Seronegative patients should be transfused CMV-negative or leukocyte-depleted blood products only.
[h]Vaccination recommended for hepatitis B and hepatitis A, if found susceptible; testing for antibody to hepatitis B core antigen is optional.
[i]May be tested if no history of chickenpox or shingles; if seronegative, postexposure prophylaxis with varicella zoster immune globulin is indicated.
[j]Unless a history of tuberculosis or positive test earlier.
[k]In men and women reporting receptive anal sex, culture rectal sample for *Chlamydia* species, and *N. gonorrhoeae*, and in those reporting receptive oral sex, culture pharyngeal sample for *N. gonorrhoeae*.
*Abbreviations:* HAV-Ab = hepatitis A antibody; HBsAb = hepatitis B surface antibody; HBsAg = hepatitis B surface antigen; HCV-Ab = hepatitis C antibody; NAAT = nucleic acid amplification test; PI = protease inhibitor; RPR = rapid plasma reagin test; VDRL = venereal diseases research laboratory test.

## TABLE 4 Currently Approved Antiretroviral Drugs

| Drug | Dosage | Food/Fasting Requirement |
|------|--------|--------------------------|
| **Nucleoside/Nucleotide Reverse Transcriptase Inhibitors (NRTIs)** | | |
| Abacavir (Ziagen) | 300 mg bid or 600 mg qd | No effect of meals |
| Didanosine (Videx) | 400 mg qd or 200 mg bid (≥60 kg); 250 mg qd or 125 mg bid (<60 kg) | ½ hr before or 2 hr after meals |
| Emtricitabine (Emtriva) | 200 mg qd | No effect of meals |
| Lamivudine (Epivir) | 150 mg bid or 300 mg qd | No effect of meals |
| Stavudine (Zerit) | 40 mg bid (≥60 kg); 30 mg bid (<60 kg) | No effect of meals |
| Tenofovir (Viread) | 300 mg qd | No effect of meals |
| Zalcitabine (Hivid) | 0.75 mg tid | No effect of meals |
| Zidovudine (Retrovir) | 300 mg bid or 200 mg tid | No effect of meals |
| **Non-Nucleoside Reverse Transcriptase Inhibitors (NNRTIs)** | | |
| Delavirdine (Rescriptor) | 400 mg tid | No effect of meals |
| Efavirenz (Sustiva) | 600 mg qd | At or before bedtime; empty stomach |
| Nevirapine (Viramune) | 200 mg qd for 14 d; then 200 mg bid | No effect of meals |
| **Protease Inhibitors (PIs)** | | |
| Amprenavir (Agenerase) | 1400 mg bid | No effect of meals; avoid high-fat meals[a] |
| Atazanavir (Reyataz) | 400 mg qd | With meal[b] |
| Fosamprenavir (Lexiva) | 1400 mg bid; 1400/rtv 200 mg qd[c] | No effect of meals |
| Indinavir (Crixivan)/rtv | 800/100–200 mg q12h[d] | No effect of meals; if given unboosted, 1 hr before or 2 hr after meals |
| Lopinavir/rtv (Kaletra) | 400/100 mg bid or 800/200 mg qd[e] | With meals |
| Nelfinavir (Viracept) | 1250 mg bid or 750 mg tid[f] | With meal or snack |
| Ritonavir (Norvir) | 100–400 mg/d[g] | With meals |
| Saquinavir hard gel (Invirase)/rtv | 1000/100 mg bid | Within 2 hr of meals |
| Saquinavir soft gel (Fortovase)/rtv | 1000/100 mg bid | With or up to 2 hr after meals |
| Tipranavir (Aptivus)/rtv | 500/200 mg bid | With meals |
| **Fusion Inhibitor** | | |
| Enfuvirtide (Fuzeon) | 90 mg SC bid | Injectable only |

Note: Fixed-dose combinations of various NRTIs with or without an NNRTI are also commercially available.
[a]Ritonavir, if given for boosting, should not be administered simultaneously.
[b]Not to be taken with antacids.
[c]Should be given only as 2 equally divided doses in PI-experienced patients.
[d]800 mg q8h if given unboosted.
[e]533/133 mg bid in patients taking nevirapine or efavirenz.
[f]In pregnant patients, 750 mg tid should not be used.
[g]Doses given for pharmacokinetic boosting.
*Abbreviations:* rtv = ritonavir-boosted; SC = subcutaneous.

Table 5 presents the regimens recommended currently for use in treatment-naïve HIV-1-infected patients. Selection among these regimens is made individually, taking into consideration factors such as pill burden, co-morbidities, potential drug interactions, and pregnancy. Triple NRTI regimens are inferior to PI- and NNRTI-based regimens in achieving durable viral suppression, and hence triple NRTI regimens are to be used only when PI/NNRTI-based regimens cannot be given. NNRTI-based regimens containing nevirapine (Viramune) should be avoided in females with CD4+ more than 250 cells/mL and in males with CD4+ more than 400 cells/mL because of the high risk of serious hepatotoxicity. Efavirenz (Sustiva) is the preferred NNRTI in such situations. Efavirenz-based regimens are equivalent to PI-based regimens in terms of efficacy and durability and have the advantage of low pill burden and limited long-term toxicity. Once initiated, for reasons mentioned earlier, HAART has to be continued lifelong. Structured treatment interruptions, aimed at preventing drug resistance, place the patient unduly at risk of disease progression and death during the period of interruption and are not recommended. Similarly, the strategy of withholding HAART once CD4+ counts improve following treatment (CD4+-guided therapy) is also inferior to uninterrupted treatment.

## WHEN TO INITIATE HAART?

The decision to start HAART is a fine balance between the potential benefits of delaying the treatment and the risk of progression to AIDS and death. The patient has to be fully apprised of the benefits as well as the risks involved, and he or she has to play an active role in decision making. Initiation of HAART is warranted in patients with history of any of the AIDS-defining illnesses (irrespective of CD4+ count and viral load) and in those with advanced immunosuppression (CD4+ less than 200 cells/μL, irrespective of viral load and symptoms). Conversely, initiation of HAART can be delayed safely in patients with CD4+ counts more than 350 cells/μL and plasma viral load less than 100,000 copies/mL. Data from randomized, controlled trials are lacking regarding the optimal time of initiating HAART in patients with CD4+ counts of 200 to 350 cells/μL. Observational data suggest that it is desirable to initiate HAART in these patients before their CD4+ counts drop below 200 cells/μL. Current consensus is that these patients should be offered treatment, especially if the viral load is more than 50,000 to 100,000 copies/mL or the decline in CD4+ count is rapid (more than 100 cells/μL per year). Treatment of patients having CD4+ more than 350 cells/μL with high viral loads

**TABLE 5** First-Line Antiretroviral Regimens for Treatment-Naïve HIV-1-Infected Patients

| Recommendation/Regimen Class | Antiretroviral Regimen |
| --- | --- |
| *Preferred* | |
| NNRTI-based | Efavirenz (Sustiva)* + (lamivudine [Epivir] or emtricitabine [Emtriva]) + (zidovudine [Retrovir] or tenofovir [Viread]) |
| | I-based (Lopinavir + rtv [Kaletra]) + (lamivudine [Epivir] or emtricitabine [Emtriva]) + zidovudine (Retrovir) |
| *Alternative* | |
| NNRTI-based | Efavirenz (Sustiva)* + (lamivudine [Epivir] or emtricitabine [Emtriva]) + (abacavir [Ziagen] or didanosine [Videx] or stavudine [Zerit]) |
| | Nevirapine (Viramune)[†] + (lamivudine [Epivir] or emtricitabine [Emtriva]) + (zidovudine [Retrovir] or stavudine [Zerit] or didanosine [Videx] or abacavir [Ziagen] or tenofovir [Viread]) |
| PI-based | Atazanavir (Reyataz) + (lamivudine [Epivir] or emtricitabine [Emtriva]) + (zidovudine [Retrovir] or stavudine [Zerit] or didanosine [Videx] or abacavir [Ziagen] or tenofovir [Viread] + rtv])[‡] |
| | (Fosamprenavir [Lexiva] ± rtv) + (lamivudine [Epivir] or emtricitabine [Emtriva]) + (zidovudine [Retrovir] or stavudine [Zerit] or didanosine [Videx] or abacavir [Ziagen] or tenofovir [Viread]) |
| | (Indinavir [Crixivan] + rtv or lopinavir + rtv [Kaletra] or saquinavir [Invirase/Fortovase]+ rtv) + (lamivudine [Epivir] or emtricitabine [Emtriva]) + (zidovudine [Retrovir] or stavudine [Zerit] or didanosine [Videx] or abacavir [Ziagen] or tenofovir [Viread]) |
| | Nelfinavir (Viracept) + (lamivudine [Epivir] or emtricitabine [Emtriva]) + (zidovudine [Retrovir] or stavudine [Zerit] or didanosine [Videx] or abacavir [Ziagen] or tenofovir [Viread]) |
| Triple NRTI[§] | Abacavir (Ziagen) + zidovudine (Retrovir) + lamivudine (Epivir) |

Note: Once-daily regimens can be tailored by selecting the appropriate drug among the interchangeable choices presented here.
*Contraindicated in women who are pregnant, plan to conceive, or are not using effective contraception.
[†]Avoid in women with CD4+ >250/μL and men with CD4+ > 400/μL (see text).
[‡]If combined with tenofovir (Viread), atazanavir (Reyataz) should be boosted with rtv.
[§]Should be used only if NNRTI-based and PI-based regimens should not or cannot be given (see text).
*Abbreviations:* NNRTI = non-nucleoside reverse transcriptase inhibitor; NRTI = nucleoside reverse transcriptase inhibitor; PI = protease inhibitor; rtv = low-dose ritonavir (Norvir), 100–400 mg/d for pharmacokinetic boosting; not considered as fourth drug in the regimen; ritonavir (Norvir) alone should not be used as the sole PI.
Based on Guidelines for the use of antiretroviral agents in HIV-1-infected adults and adolescents, U.S. Department of Health and Human Services, October 2005.

(more than 100,000 copies/mL) is considered optional, and if treatment is deferred, CD4+ count and viral load should be monitored closely (every 3 months). Likewise, in the absence of supporting evidence, treatment of patients with acute HIV infection and those in whom seroconversion occurred within the past 6 months is considered optional.

## MONITORING RESPONSE TO ANTIRETROVIRAL THERAPY

In a patient on treatment, CD4+ counts have to be monitored every 3 to 6 months and the viral load every 3 to 4 months. A reproducible change in absolute CD4+ count of at least 30% and/or 3 percentage point change in the CD4+ percentage are considered significant. Similarly, for viral load, a threefold or $0.5 \log_{10}$ copies/mL change is deemed significant. It is important that these estimations are not performed during an episode of intercurrent infection or vaccination because transient fluctuations in viremia and CD4+ counts can occur during such episodes. Because of large variations in absolute CD4+ count estimations and interassay differences in estimating viral load, serial evaluations should be obtained from the same laboratory using the same assay. Before making any treatment change based on the laboratory results, they should be repeated and reconfirmed.

Following the initiation of effective antiretroviral therapy, CD4+ counts rapidly improve within a few weeks, largely as a result of redistribution of cells, and they subsequently improve at the rate of approximately 100 cells/μL per year over the subsequent years until a plateau is reached. Plasma viral load rapidly falls in the initial weeks and becomes undetectable in approximately 4 to 6 months. The rate of initial decline in viral load depends on the potency of the HAART regimen, and it predicts the durability of viral suppression. Determination of viral load at 2 to 8 weeks after the initiation or change in treatment thus is also recommended. An adequate response is defined as a decrease of at least $1.0 \log_{10}$ copies/mL at 2 to 8 weeks after starting treatment; plasma viral load should become undetectable by 16 to 24 weeks.

## DRUG RESISTANCE AND RESISTANCE TESTING

A patient may be infected with a drug-resistant virus to begin with (primary resistance) or else resistance can emerge as a result of treatment (secondary). The latter is more common. With widespread use of antiretrovirals, primary resistance is increasing. Most NNRTI-associated resistance mutations confer cross-resistance to all other NNRTIs as well. Among NRTIs, cross-resistance is common but varies by drug. Paradoxically, lamivudine(Epivir) resistance related to the M184V mutation enhances the susceptibility to zidovudine (Retrovir). With PIs, initial mutations might confer limited resistance only; however, accumulation of sequential mutations leads to broad cross-resistance. Tipranavir (Aptivus)/ritonavir (Norvir) is active against such strains of HIV-1 resistant to multiple PIs.

Drug-resistance testing is done by either genotypic or phenotypic assays. Overall, the resistance tests have a limited sensitivity. Resistance may not be detected if viremia is less than 1000 copies/mL or the frequency of resistant quasispecies is less than 10% to 20%. These tests are to be performed while the patient is still taking the failing regimen or within 4 weeks after discontinuation to avoid overgrowth of the resistant quasispecies by the wild strain. The exact role of resistance testing in clinical practice is not yet clear. In patients receiving tailored regimens based on resistance testing, benefit in terms of improved virologic outcome is modest only. However, testing for drug resistance is indicated in patients failing treatment, those having suboptimal virologic response, and in those treated for acute HIV infection. Routine resistance testing in drug-naïve patients with chronic HIV infection may also be considered, especially if the prevalence of primary resistance is more than 4%. Failure to identify any resistance in a patient failing treatment points toward poor adherence.

## TREATMENT FAILURE

Failure of treatment can be classified into virologic failure, immunologic failure, and clinical progression. Virologic failure is evidenced by repeated detection of viremia more than 400 copies/mL after 24 weeks or more than 50 copies/mL after 48 weeks of treatment in a drug-naïve patient or by persistent viremia after achieving complete suppression (virologic rebound). Inadequate CD4+ response (improvement of fewer than 25 to 50 cells/μL in the first year) or a fall below the pretreatment CD4+ level constitutes immunologic failure. Occurrence or recurrence of HIV-related events after the third month of HAART, in the absence of an alternative explanation, is considered indicative of clinical progression. Usually virologic failure is the first to occur, to be

followed months to years later by immunologic failure, and finally by clinical progression. Sometimes discordant responses (i.e., immunologic failure and clinical progression despite suppressed viremia) may occur. Provided that viremia is well suppressed, changing the regimen may not be warranted in such settings.

In a patient with virologic failure, although drug resistance is the proximate cause of failure, one must carefully look for factors that contributed to the emergence of drug resistance in that particular patient and try to address them. Otherwise, the new regimen is also bound to fail. Such factors include inadequate regimen potency, high baseline viral load, poor adherence, drug intolerance, preexisting resistance, and suboptimal pharmacokinetics because of malabsorption, noncompliance with food/fasting requirements, and drug interactions. Past-treatment experience of the patient should also be evaluated to inform them about further treatment choices (Table 6). In general, the new regimen should include at least two, preferably three, fully active drugs. A fully active drug is one that is likely to be effective based on both the treatment history and susceptibility on resistance testing. Addition of a single drug may be justified if substitution is being made to manage toxicity in a patient with otherwise good response or in a patient failing treatment where no resistance is identified, after ruling

---

**TABLE 6  Salvage Therapy in Patients with Treatment Failure (Virologic Failure)**

| Initial Regimen | First Virologic Failure | | Subsequent Virologic Failures |
| --- | --- | --- | --- |
| | **Resistance Identified** | **No Resistance Identified** | |
| NNRTI-based (2 NRTIs + NNRTI) | 2 NRTIs (based on resistance testing) + PI (unboosted or rtv-boosted) | Check adherence to treatment; if poor, address compliance. Was the resistance testing properly timed? (see text); if not properly timed, continue same regimen; repeat genotypic testing in 2–4 wk or start a new regimen; repeat genotypic testing in 2–4 wk. | Include at least 2, preferably 3, fully active drugs (see text); add a drug from new class, if available. If 3-class virologic failure, start > 1 NRTI (based on resistance testing) + a new boosted-PI (based on resistance testing) ± enfuvirtide (Fuzeon). If only 1 fully active agent available, add to failing regimen only if CD4+ <100/μL; otherwise, continue failing regimen. If no fully active agent available, continue failing regimen; do not interrupt. |
| PI-based (2 NRTIs + PI [unboosted or rtv-boosted]) | 2 NRTIs (based on resistance testing) + NNRTI or 2 NRTIs (based on resistance testing) + a new boosted PI (based on resistance testing) or 1 or more NRTI(s) (based on resistance testing) + NNRTI + a new boosted PI (based on resistance testing) | If adherence and timing of testing are acceptable, start a new regimen; repeat genotypic testing in 2–4 wk or intensify by adding 1 NRTI (tenofovir [Viread]) or boost the PI with rtv. | |
| Triple NRTI (3 NRTIs) | 2 NRTIs (based on resistance testing) + NNRTI or PI (unboosted or rtv-boosted) or 1 or more NRTI(s) (based on resistance testing) + NNRTI + PI (unboosted or rtv-boosted) or NNRTI + PI (unboosted or rtv-boosted) | | |

Based on Guidelines for the use of antiretroviral agents in HIV-1-infected adults and adolescents, U.S. Department of Health and Human Services, October 2005.
*Abbreviations:* NNRTI = non-nucleoside reverse transcriptase inhibitor; NRTI = nucleoside reverse transcriptase inhibitor; PI = protease inhibitor; rtv = ritonavir (Norvir).

out poor adherence and improperly timed resistance testing. Although the goal of treatment remains complete suppression of viremia below detectable limits, in treatment-experienced patients with resistance to multiple drugs, this may not always be feasible. In such patients with limited options, even a 0.5 to 1.0 log10 reduction in viral load may be acceptable. In patients failing treatment with extensive prior treatment, if no fully active drug is available, continuing with the failing regimen might decrease the risk of clinical progression.

## ADHERENCE TO TREATMENT

Adherence to prescribed treatment is a complex issue but of utmost importance. Antiretroviral treatment is very exacting in terms of adherence when compared to other chronic diseases; missing as little as 5% to 10% of doses is known to affect virologic outcome adversely. The natural tendency is to miss a few doses, and physician estimates of adherence are known to be unreliable. It is thus important to suspect noncompliance in every patient. Before initiating treatment, the patient must be counseled regarding medication requirements, and readiness to take the treatment has to be ensured. It has to be impressed on the patient that the first regimen has the best chance for long-term success. Adherence counseling and assessment of adherence should be done at each clinical encounter. Adherence is conventionally assessed by patient self-reports, pill counting, and a patient-recorded medication diary. Microelectronic monitoring systems like Medication Event Monitoring System (MEMS Track Cap) and therapeutic drug monitoring could provide more objective assessment of adherence. However, all these methods have their limitations, and it is preferable to use more than one method simultaneously.

Noncompliance with treatment has many causes. Patient-related factors, such as substance abuse, depression, lack of social support, and age; medication-related factors, such as dosing frequency, pill burden, food/fasting requirements, and adverse effects; and health care system–related factors, such as attitude of staff, communication, and accessibility, all operate in tandem to influence the adherence. Adherence can be improved by simplifying the dosage schedules, providing pillboxes, tailoring to suit the lifestyle, entrusting medication intake to a family member, using reminder calls and alarms and community-based case managers, alerting to adverse effects, providing patient education materials, making the clinic appointments convenient, and making the health system encounter pleasant. In patients found nonadherent, enough time should be spent to identify the responsible factors and to find acceptable solutions while involving the patient actively in the process.

## ADVERSE DRUG REACTIONS AND DRUG INTERACTIONS

Adverse drug reactions (ADRs) are common with antiretroviral therapy and an important cause of nonadherence. They also contribute to a significant proportion of clinic visits and mortality. ADRs can be idiosyncratic, dose related, time related (delayed), or dose and time related (cumulative). A particular ADR may be common to all drugs of the same class (e.g., lactic acidosis and fatty liver because of NRTIs, lipodystrophy because of PIs), or it might be drug specific (e.g., hypersensitivity to abacavir [Ziagen], nephrolithiasis because of indinavir [Crixivan]). The patient often is on other drugs as well, with overlapping ADR profiles, apart from antiretrovirals. A symptom-based approach is useful from a practical point of view (Table 7). Although many of the ADRs can be managed conservatively, some, such as symptomatic lactic acidosis, systemic hypersensitivity reactions, Stevens-Johnson syndrome, acute pancreatitis, and severe hepatotoxicity, are potentially life threatening. Serious ADRs necessitate withdrawal of the offending drug, and rechallenge of the drug should not be attempted in these situations.

**TABLE 7** Approach to Adverse Drug Reactions in the HIV-Infected Patient[a]

| Adverse Effect | Manifestations | Causative Drug(s) | | Stepwise Action |
| | | Antiretroviral(s) | Other Drugs | |
| --- | --- | --- | --- | --- |
| Stevens-Johnson syndrome/toxic epidermal necrolysis[b] | Rash, mucosal ulcerations, fever, hepatic dysfunction | NNRTIs most commonly NVP; rarely APV, LPV/r, ATV, ABC, ZDV, ddI | Cotrimoxazole, sulfadiazine, dapsone, atovaquone, voriconazole | Discontinue all ARVs and any other possible drug; manage like severe burns; do not rechallenge offending drug. |
| Hypersensitivity reaction[c] | Fever, diffuse rash, malaise, arthralgia, respiratory and GI symptoms, circulatory collapse | ABC, enfuvirtide (Fuzeon) | Cotrimoxazole, sulfadiazine, dapsone | Discontinue all ARVs and any other possible drug; rule out other causes; do not rechallenge ABC/enfuvirtide. |
| Skin rash | Maculopapular rash only; no blisters, skin tenderness, mucosal ulceration, or fever | DLV > EFV > APV, fAPV = ATV > NVP > ABC, TPV[d] | Cotrimoxazole, sulfadiazine, dapsone, atovaquone, voriconazole | Antihistamines; continue offending drug; watch for progression of rash; if so, discontinue. |

[a]Only common and serious side effects are dealt with; side effects such as osteoporosis, avascular osteonecrosis (PIs), unconjugated hyperbilirubinemia, retinoid-like effects (IDV) and cranial malformations (EFV) are also known to occur.
[b]Approximately 0.3%-1% with NVP; a low dose, lead-in period for NVP (see Table 4) may decrease the risk; less common (0.1%) with DLV and EFV; occurs in the initial weeks after initiation; safety of replacing NVP with another NNRTI is unknown.
[c]Approximately 5% with ABC; once daily dosing possibly increases the risk; If ABC-related, symptoms resolve within 48 hrs after discontinuation of ABC.
[d]APV, fAPV, and TPV are sulfonamide derivatives; potential cross-hypersensitivity with sulfonamides.

*Continued*

**TABLE 7  Approach to Adverse Drug Reactions in the HIV-Infected Patient—cont'd**

| Adverse Effect | Manifestations | Causative Drug(s) Antiretroviral(s) | Other Drugs | Stepwise Action |
|---|---|---|---|---|
| GI intolerance[e] | Anorexia, nausea, vomiting, epigastric pain | PIs, ddl, ZDV | Isoniazid, rifamycins, pyrazinamide | Administer with food (not for ddl, unboosted IDV); antiemetics; switch to less emetogenic ARV. |
| | Diarrhea | PIs, especially NFV, LPV/r, and buffered ddl formulations | Clindamycin, atovaquone | Rule out OIs; antimotility agents, calcium salts, bulk forming agents; rehydration, if needed. |
| Hepatotoxicity[f] | Jaundice, fever, vomiting, hepatic necrosis, encephalopathy | NVP | Isoniazid, rifamycins, pyrazinamide | Discontinue all ARVs and any other possible drug; rule out viral hepatitis; supportive management; do not rechallenge NVP. |
| | Symptomatic or subclinical hepatic enzyme elevations | NNRTIs, d4T, ddl, ZDV, PIs, especially TPV | Isoniazid, rifamycins, pyrazinamide, azithromycin, clarithromycin, all azole antifungals | If symptomatic, discontinue all ARVs and switch to nonhepatotoxic ARVs after normalization; if asymptomatic, monitor closely. |
| Lactic acidosis, fatty liver[g] | Nonspecific GI symptoms, tachypnea, tachycardia, hepatomegaly, hyperlactatemia, multiorgan failure | NRTIs especially d4T, ddl, ZDV | Metformin | Discontinue all ARVs; hydration; supportive treatment; IV thiamine/riboflavin; switch to ABC/3TC/TDF or NRTI-sparing regimens. |
| Pancreatitis[g] | Epigastric pain-postprandial, vomiting, fever, elevated amylase, lipase | ddl, d4T, ddC, RTV; 3TC (in children) | Alcohol, cotrimoxazole, pentamidine | Discontinue offending drugs; manage like acute pancreatitis related to any other cause; do not rechallenge. |
| Peripheral neuropathy[g] | Numbness, paresthesia—often painful; recovery possibly incomplete | ddl, d4T, ddC | Isoniazid | Switch to ABC/3TC/TDF; gabapentin, tricyclic antidepressants, narcotic analgesics. |
| Myopathy[g] | Myalgia, muscle tenderness, proximal weakness, elevated creatine kinase | ZDV | Statins, fibrates, steroids | Switch to another NRTI; improves in 3–4 wk after discontinuation; coenzyme-Q, L-carnitine (unproven). |
| Nephrolithiasis, crystalluria[h] | Flank pain, nondescript abdominal pain, dysuria, hematuria, renal dysfunction | IDV | Cotrimoxazole, sulfadiazine, acyclovir | Discontinue IDV; hydration and analgesics; IDV can be resumed with plenty of oral fluids; if recurs, consider switching. |
| Nephrotoxicity | Renal dysfunction; nephrogenic diabetes insipidus; Fanconi syndrome | IDV, TDF | Acyclovir, amphotericin B, cotrimoxazole, pentamidine | Discontinue offending drug; hydration; generally reversible. |
| Hematologic | Anemia, neutropenia[i] | ZDV | Cotrimoxazole, dapsone, | Discontinue concomitant marrow suppressant, if |

[e]Symptoms begin with first doses; might abate with time.

[f]Low-dose, lead-in period for NVP might reduce the risk; monitoring: see Table 3; onset within the first few weeks with NNRTIs, after weeks to months with PIs, and after months to years with NRTIs; discontinuation of 3TC, FTC, or TDF in HBV co-infected patients might cause acute flare-up of hepatitis; safety of replacing NVP with another NNRTI is unknown.

[g]Class-specific adverse effect of NRTIs, because of mitochondrial toxicity; do not combine ddl/d4T/ddC; ABC, 3TC, and TDF are less prone; all 4 syndromes can occur in variable combinations; symptomatic lactic acidosis is rare but is associated with high mortality.

[h]Approximately 10% of patients taking IDV experience at least 1 episode of colic; monitoring: see Table 3; recurrence is seen in only 50%, if fluid intake is improved (at least 1.5–2 L of noncaffeinated fluid; water preferably).

[i]Almost all ZDV-treated patients have isolated macrocytosis; anemia and neutropenia occur in approximately 1%-4% and 2%-8% respectively; monitoring: see Table 3.

**TABLE 7** Approach to Adverse Drug Reactions in the HIV-Infected Patient—cont'd

| Adverse Effect | Manifestations | Causative Drug(s) Antiretroviral(s) | Other Drugs | Stepwise Action |
|---|---|---|---|---|
| | | | sulfadiazine, pyrimethamine, flucytosine, trimetrexate, amphotericin B, ganciclovir, valganciclovir, rifabutin | any; exclude marrow involvement by OIs/malignancy; erythropoietin or filgrastim; switch to another NRTI. |
| | Bleeding tendency in hemophiliacs | PIs | | Factor VIII infusion; consider NNRTI-based regimens. |
| | Eosinophilia | Enfuvirtide (Fuzeon) | Cotrimoxazole, dapsone, sulfadiazine | Exclude disseminated strongyloidiasis, malignancy; watch for hypersensitivity. |
| CNS symptoms[j] | Drowsiness, insomnia, vivid dreams, nightmares, hallucination, worsening of psychiatric disorders, suicidal ideation | EFV | Isoniazid, dapsone, steroids | Usually resolve in 2–4 wk; consider discontinuation, if persistent or exacerbates psychiatric illness. |
| Lipodystrophy | Loss of subcutaneous fat, buffalo hump, double chin, dyslipidemia, insulin resistance, diabetes mellitus | PIs (except ATV); NRTIs, especially d4T | Steroids | Assess cardiac risk factors; lifestyle modification; metformin, glitazones, statins, fibrates[k]; consider early switching to ATV- or NNRTI-based regimens. |

[j]Occurs during initial weeks of treatment; patients are to be warned to restrict risky activities.
[k]Only atorvastatin (Lipitor) and pravastatin (Pravachol) among statins, and gemfibrozil (Lopid) and fenofibrate (Triglide) among fibrates, can be co-administered with PIs.
*Abbreviations:* 3TC = lamivudine (Epivir); ABC = abacavir (Ziagen); APV = amprenavir (Agenerase); ATV = atazanavir (Reyataz); CNS = central nervous system; d4T = stavudine (Zerit); ddC = zalcitabine (Hivid); ddI = didanosine (Videx); DLV = delavirdine (Rescriptor); EFV = efavirenz (Sustiva); fAPV = fosamprenavir (Lexiva); FTC = emtricitabine (Emtriva); GI = gastrointestinal; IDV = indinavir (Crixivan); LPV/r = lopinavir/ritonavir (Kaletra); NFV = nelfinavir (Viracept); NNRTI = non-nucleoside reverse transcriptase inhibitor; NRTI = nucleoside reverse transcriptase inhibitor; NVP = nevirapine (Viramune), OI = opportunistic infection; PI = protease inhibitor; RTV = ritonavir (Norvir); TDF = tenofovir (Viread); TPV = tipranavir (Aptivus); ZDV = zidovudine (Retrovir).
Based on Guidelines for the use of antiretroviral agents in HIV-1-infected adults and adolescents, U.S. Department of Health and Human Services, October 2005.

Drug interactions are often the underlying cause of ADRs. PIs are metabolized by the hepatic cytochrome P450 (CYP) enzymes. At the same time, PIs are potent inhibitors of CYP. Conversely, NNRTIs, especially efavirenz (Sustiva), are a potent inducer of CYP. When antiretrovirals are co-administered with other drugs metabolized by or affecting CYP (antihistamines, prokinetics, lipid-lowering agents, antifungals, antitubercular drugs, anticonvulsants, etc.), complex pharmacokinetic interactions occur; this can lead to potentially toxic or subtherapeutic drug levels. In a patient on HAART, unnecessary prescriptions are to be avoided, and it is prudent always to check the compatibility and the dose modifications needed before prescribing.

## Management of Opportunistic Conditions

### GENERAL CONSIDERATIONS

OIs are the most common cause of disability and death in HIV-infected patients who are not receiving treatment. Hence, it is important that OIs are promptly recognized and treated. Different pathogens may cause similar disease patterns, and multiple OIs may occur concurrently. Although it is important to make a definitive diagnosis in these patients, diagnostic workup should not delay unduly the initiation of appropriate treatment. Empirical treatment based on clinical suspicion may be justified in acutely ill patients. In a patient

with a severe OI as the initial manifestation of HIV disease, management of the OI takes precedence over immediate initiation of HAART. This avoids potential drug interactions and possibly decreases the occurrence of immune reconstitution inflammatory syndrome (IRIS). However, in patients with OIs for which no effective treatment is available (cryptosporidiosis, microsporidiosis, progressive multifocal leukoencephalopathy, and Kaposi's sarcoma), HAART itself can result in improvement and hence should be initiated as soon as possible.

IRIS manifests as the occurrence of a new OI or worsening of a preexisting OI following initiation of HAART, usually in the first 3 months. Symptoms include fever, lymphadenopathy, serosal effusions, worsening or fresh pulmonary infiltrates, vitreitis, uveitis, and intracranial lesions. Occasionally life-threatening complications like acute respiratory distress syndrome (ARDS) and acute renal failure develop. Most instances of IRIS respond well to nonsteroidal antiinflammatory drugs. HAART and OI-specific treatment need to be continued without interruption. Steroids may be useful in patients with life-threatening complications.

OIs can be prevented by timely initiation of primary chemoprophylaxis (Table 8). It has to be stressed that OIs listed in the table can also occur, albeit less often, in patients with CD4+ counts above the cutoffs for initiation of prophylaxis. Following treatment for an episode of OI, lifelong secondary prophylaxis is needed to prevent relapse. However, if a sustained improvement in CD4+ count is achieved following HAART, secondary prophylaxis for most of the OIs and primary prophylaxis can be withdrawn safely. Table 9 presents the

**TABLE 8** Primary Chemoprophylaxis for Opportunistic Infections in the HIV-Infected Patient*,†

| Opportunistic Pathogen | Criteria for Initiation | Preferred Regimen | Alternative Regimens | Criteria for Discontinuation‡ |
|---|---|---|---|---|
| *Pneumocystis jiroveci* | CD4+ <200/μL; oropharyngeal candidiasis | TMP-SMX (Bactrim), 960 mg qd or 480 mg qd | TMP-SMX (Bactrim), 960 mg tiw, or dapsone, 100 mg qd, or aerosolized pentamidine (NebuPent), 300 mg monthly, or atovaquone (Mepron), 1500 mg qd | CD4+ >200/μL for ≥3 mo |
| *Toxoplasma gondii* | CD4+ ≤100/μL in IgG toxoplasma antibody-positive patients | TMP-SMX (Bactrim), 960 mg qd | TMP-SMX (Bactrim), 480 mg qd, or dapsone, 50 mg qd, + pyrimethamine, 50 mg qw, + leucovorin, 25 mg qw, or atovaquone (Mepron), 1500 mg qd | CD4+ > 200/μL for ≥3 mo |
| *Mycobacterium avium-intracellulare* | CD4+ <50/μL | Azithromycin (Zithromax), 1200 mg qw, or clarithromycin (Biaxin), 500 mg bid | Rifabutin (Mycobutin), 300 mg qd | CD4+ >100/μL for ≥3 mo |
| *Mycobacterium tuberculosis*§ | TST ≥5 mm; positive TST in past without treatment; contact with active case, irrespective of TST | Isoniazid (Laniazid) + pyridoxine, 300 + 50 mg qd or 900 + 100 mg biw, for 9 mo | Rifampicin (Rifadin), 600 mg qd for 4 mo | Not applicable |

*Apart from chemoprophylaxis, annual influenza immunization in all, pneumococcal vaccination in those with CD4+ ≥200/μL, and hepatitis A and hepatitis B vaccinations in susceptible patients are recommended.
†Primary chemoprophylaxis not recommended for cytomegalovirus, *Cryptococcus neoformans*, *Histoplasma capsulatum*, *Coccidioides immitis*, *Salmonella* species, herpes simplex, and *Candida* species
‡Primary prophylaxis to be restarted if CD4+ falls again below levels recommended for initiation.
§Not prophylaxis in strict sense. For isoniazid-susceptible *M. tuberculosis* only; if probability of exposure to isoniazid-resistant *M. tuberculosis* is high, rifampicin (Rifadin), 600 mg qd, or rifabutin (Mycobutin), 300 mg qd, for 4 mo.
*Abbreviations:* biw = twice weekly; TMP-SMX = cotrimoxazole (Bactrim); TST = tuberculin skin test; qw = once a week; tiw = 3 times a week.
Based on USPHS/IDSA guidelines for the prevention of opportunistic infections in persons infected with HIV, 2001.

possible etiology of opportunistic conditions. Management of common potentially life-threatening OIs is presented next.

### *PNEUMOCYSTIS JIROVECI* PNEUMONIA (PCP)

PCP is the most common OI in HIV-infected patients. Approximately 90% of cases occur among patients with CD4+ less than 200 cells/μL. Although the overall mortality is approximately 10% to 20%, it exceeds 50% in those requiring mechanical ventilation for respiratory failure. PCP manifests as a subacute febrile illness accompanied by nonproductive cough and progressive exertional dyspnea. In patients with mild disease, physical findings are often scanty, barring tachypnea and scattered so-called cellophane crackles. Hypoxemia is useful to assess the severity of disease, and moderate to severe hypoxemia ($PaO_2$ less than 70 mm Hg or [A-a]$DO_2$ more than 35 mm Hg while breathing ambient air) indicates severe disease. Chest radiograph demonstrates diffuse, bilateral, interstitial infiltrates in a perihilar distribution. Atypical radiographic appearances like upper lobe predominance (in patients on inhaled pentamidine [NebuPent] prophylaxis), nodular infiltrates, cysts, and pneumothorax are also seen. An apparently normal-looking radiograph in a patient with compatible clinical presentation does not rule out a diagnosis of PCP. Diagnosis is established by the demonstration of cysts and trophozoites of *Pneumocystis* in induced sputum (sensitivity, 50% to 90%), bronchoalveolar lavage (90% to 99%), and transbronchial lung biopsy (95% to 100%) specimens by Gomori methenamine silver, Giemsa, or calcofluor staining. Immunofluorescent staining has better sensitivity and specificity than the tinctorial stains. rRNA-PCR techniques are currently being evaluated and can be used on oral washings.

Cotrimoxazole (TMP-SMX, Bactrim) is the drug of choice. Mild to moderately severe cases can be managed with oral TMP-SMX (two double-strength tablets [Bactrim DS] three times daily for 21 days) on an ambulatory basis. Patients developing PCP despite TMP-SMX (Bactrim) prophylaxis can also be effectively treated with standard doses of TMP-SMX. Intravenous therapy (15–20 [TMP]/75–100 [SMX] mg/kg/day every 6 to 8 hours for 21 days) is indicated for patients with severe hypoxemia. In addition, steroids (prednisone,[1] 40 mg orally twice daily for days 1 to 5, 40 mg every day for days 6 to 10, and 20 mg every day for days 11 to 21) improve the mortality and reduce the need for mechanical ventilation in severe cases and should be started within 72 hours of starting anti-PCP treatment. Lack of clinical improvement or worsening hypoxemia after at least 4 to 8 days of anti-PCP treatment indicates failure and warrants changing of treatment. Serious ADRs related to TMP-SMX (Bactrim) also often necessitate a treatment change. The preferred alternative treatments are pentamidine (Pentam, 4 mg/kg intravenously [IV] every day) or clindamycin (Cleocin, 600 to 900 mg IV every 6 to 8 hours) plus primaquine[1] (15 to 30 mg [base] orally every day). Dapsone (100 mg orally every day) plus trimethoprim (Trimpex,[1] 15 mg/kg/day orally thrice daily), atovaquone (Mepron, 750 mg orally twice daily), or

---

[1]Not FDA approved for this indication.

**TABLE 9  Etiology of Opportunistic Conditions in the HIV-Infected Patient**

| System Affected | Etiology (Infectious as well as Noninfectious) | | |
| --- | --- | --- | --- |
| | *Very common* | *Somewhat common* | *Rare* |
| Pulmonary | PCP<br>*Streptococcus*<br>  *pneumoniae*<br>*Haemophilus*<br>  *influenzae*<br>*Myobacterium*<br>  *tuberculosis*[a] | *Pseudomonas aeruginosa*<br>*Staphylococcus aureus*<br>Enteric GNB<br>*Histoplasma* species<br>*Cryptococcus* species<br>Cytomegalovirus<br>Kaposi's sarcoma<br>*Aspergillus* species<br>Pulmonary lymphoma<br>Heart failure | *Nocardia* species<br>*Legionella* species<br>*Myobacterium avium* complex<br>*Toxoplasma gondii*<br>*Cryptosporidium*<br>*Rhodococcus equi*<br>*Strongyloides*<br>Primary pulmonary hypertension<br>DILS |
| Central nervous system (CNS) | *Cryptococcus*<br>  species<br>*Toxoplasmosis*<br>ADRs<br>Psychiatric illness<br>HIV dementia<br>PMLE<br>CNS lymphoma | *M. tuberculosis*[a]<br>Cytomegalovirus<br>Bacterial brain abscess | *Nocardia* species<br>*Histoplasma* species<br>*Coccidioides immitis*<br>*Aspergillus* species<br>*Listeria monocytogenes*<br>Varicella-zoster virus<br>Herpes simplex virus<br>*Treponema pallidum*<br>*Acanthamoeba* species<br>*Trypanosoma cruzi*<br>DILS |
| Gastrointestinal (GI) | Cytomegalovirus<br>*Clostridium difficile*<br>*Salmonella* species<br>*M. avium* complex<br>*Giardia lamblia*<br>ADRs | *Shigella* species<br>*Campylobacter* species<br>*Microsporum*<br>*Cryptosporidium Isospora*<br>*Cyclospora*<br>*Cryptococcus* species<br>*Histoplasma* species | Amebiasis<br>*Strongyloides*<br>GI lymphoma<br>Kaposi's sarcoma<br>Enteroaggregative<br>  *Escherichia coli*<br>DILS |
| Undifferentiated fever | *M. avium* complex<br>*M. tuberculosis*<br>Cytomegalovirus<br>ADRs<br>Sinusitis<br>Catheter-related<br>Early PCP<br>Acute HIV syndrome | Endocarditis<br>Lymphoma | Extrapulmonary<br>  *Pneumocystis*<br>*Bartonella henselae*<br>*Coccidioides immitis*<br>*Mycobacterium kansasii*<br>*Penicillium marneffei*<br>*Leishmania* species<br>*Toxoplasma gondii* |

*Incidence of tuberculosis varies greatly depending on the local prevalence.
*Abbreviations:* ADR = adverse drug reaction; DILS = diffuse infiltrative lymphocytosis syndrome; GNB = gram-negative bacilli; PCP = *Pneumocystis jiroveci*
  pneumonia; PMLE = progressive multifocal leukoencephalopathy.
Adapted from Sax PE: Opportunistic infections in HIV disease: Down but not out. Infect Dis Clin North Am 2001;15:433-455.

trimetrexate (Neutrexin, 1.2 mg/kg IV every day with leucovorin, 0.5 mg/kg IV every 6 hours) can be used also as alternatives in mild to moderately severe PCP. Following treatment, patients should be administered secondary prophylaxis, which has to be discontinued if the CD4+ counts improve to more than 200 cells/μL for 3 months after initiating HAART. However, in those who develop PCP while their CD4+ counts were more than 200 cells/μL, it is prudent to continue the secondary prophylaxis lifelong.

## CRYPTOCOCCOSIS

Cryptococcosis occurs mostly among patients with CD4+ less than 50 cells/μL. Although the route of infection is via the lungs, most often the disease manifests as meningitis. Disseminated infection is common in HIV-infected patients, and in fact approximately 60% of patients with AIDS-associated cryptococcal meningitis have fungemia. Pulmonary involvement occurs either as a part of disseminated disease or as primary pneumonia. Molluscoid skin lesions with central hemorrhagic crust may be seen. Patients typically present with subacute onset of fever, prominent headache, and vomiting. The classical signs of meningeal inflammation are often absent. Occasionally, cognitive decline and personality changes might be the only presenting symptoms. Cryptococcomas may present as a focal neurologic deficit.

Diagnosis is readily established by the demonstration of yeast cells by India ink staining of cerebrospinal fluid (CSF). Fungal culture and latex agglutination for cryptococcal antigen have better sensitivity than the India ink stain. The antigen can also be detected in the blood in most patients with meningitis. Untreated disease is uniformly fatal. Amphotericin B deoxycholate (Fungizone, 0.7 mg/kg IV every day for 2 weeks) is the preferred treatment. Infusion-related ADRs such as chills, rigors, and fever are common and can be reduced by premedicating with acetaminophen (Tylenol). Liposomal preparations of amphotericin B (AmBisome, 4 mg/kg/day) can be used also to reduce nephrotoxicity. Addition of flucytosine (Ancobon, 25 mg/kg orally four times a day for 2 weeks) sterilizes the CSF faster and reduces the rate of relapse but not mortality. Amphotericin B is to be followed by fluconazole (Diflucan, 400 mg orally every day) for at least 8 weeks or until the CSF cultures become sterile and then lifelong (200 mg every day) for secondary prophylaxis. In patients with immune recovery following HAART, secondary prophylaxis can be discontinued if the CD4+ count is more than 100 to 200 cells/μL for 6 months. Raised intracranial pressure is very common and associated with early deaths. If symptomatic, daily lumbar punctures to reduce the pressure are needed, and in refractory cases, CSF shunting should be performed.

## DISSEMINATED *MYCOBACTERIUM AVIUM* INFECTION

Like cryptococcosis and CMV disease, disseminated atypical mycobacterial infections occur more commonly in patients with CD4+ less than

50 cells/µL. Most infections are caused by *Mycobacterium avium-intracellulare*. Infections by *Mycobacterium kansasii* and *Mycobacterium haemophilum* are also known to occur. Symptoms are nonspecific and include fever, weight loss, diarrhea, and abdominal pain. Peripheral and axial lymphadenopathy, hepatosplenomegaly, anemia, elevated alkaline phosphatase, and bone marrow infiltration are common features. Localized manifestations occur commonly as a manifestation of IRIS. Pulmonary lesions in the form of miliary nodules and air-space infiltrates may be seen. Diagnosis is established by demonstrating mycobacteremia or by isolating the organism from involved tissue specimens.

Treatment should include at least two effective drugs, usually clarithromycin (Biaxin, 500 mg orally twice daily) and ethambutol (Myambutol,[1] 15 mg/kg orally every day). Addition of a third drug should be considered, especially when CD4+ is less than 50 cells/µL, effective HAART is unavailable, or the mycobacterial load is high (more than 2.0 log$_{10}$ colony-forming units/mL of blood). Rifabutin (Mycobutin,[1] 300 mg orally every day) is the preferred third drug. Fluoroquinolones and amikacin (Amikin)[1] can be used as alternative agents. Generally, if possible, HAART should be initiated within 1 to 2 weeks after initiating antimycobacterial therapy. Lack of clinical improvement accompanied by persisting mycobacteremia after 4 to 8 weeks of treatment indicates failure, and further selection of drugs should be guided by susceptibility testing. Treatment has to be continued lifelong for secondary prophylaxis. However, if the CD4+ count improves to more than 100 cells/µL for 6 months, it can be discontinued, provided the patient is asymptomatic and treatment has been given for at least 12 months.

## CYTOMEGALOVIRUS DISEASE

Retinitis is the most common manifestation of CMV disease. It presents as progressive painless loss of vision, and patients often experience floaters. Funduscopy reveals focal necrotizing retinitis, characterized by perivascular fluffy infiltrates with hemorrhages. Lesions spread centrifugally from the periphery, and those adjacent to the macula are sight threatening. Visual loss, if it occurs, is irreversible. Other manifestations include colitis, esophagitis, meningoencephalitis, and pneumonitis. Colitis causes persistent diarrhea and may result in extensive hemorrhage, perforation, and bacterial sepsis. CNS disease presents as dementia, ventriculoencephalitis, or ascending polyradiculomyelopathy. Viremia in the absence of end-organ disease may be seen but does not warrant immediate therapy.

Sight-threatening retinitis is treated with an intraocular ganciclovir implant (Vitrasert) along with valganciclovir (Valcyte, 900 mg orally every day) lifelong. For peripheral lesions, valganciclovir (Valcyte), 900 mg orally twice daily for 2 to 3 weeks is to be followed by 900 mg every day for life. Ganciclovir (Cytovene, 5 mg/kg IV every 12 hours), foscarnet (Foscavir, 60 mg/kg IV every 8 hours), or cidofovir (Vistide, 5 mg/kg IV every day) for 2 to 3 weeks can be used as alternatives. Colitis and esophagitis are treated with ganciclovir (Cytovene) or foscarnet (Foscavir) for at least 3 to 4 weeks or until symptoms resolve. A combination of ganciclovir (Cytovene) and foscarnet (Foscavir) until symptoms resolve is required for the treatment of neurologic disease. Secondary prophylaxis can be discontinued if CD4+ is more than 100 to 150 cells/µL for 6 months. However, regular ophthalmologic monitoring should be done to detect relapse early. IRIS occurs in most of the patients with CMV retinitis following initiation of HAART, resulting in vitreitis or uveitis. Periocular steroids or short courses of oral steroids often control the symptoms.

## TUBERCULOSIS IN HIV-INFECTED PATIENTS

Tuberculosis is the most common OI in HIV-infected patients from developing countries. In contrast to other OIs, tuberculosis can occur at any level of CD4+ count. Extrapulmonary and disseminated forms become more common as the immunosuppression worsens. Meningeal and miliary dissemination often occurs. In advanced immunosuppression, typical cavitary and sputum-smear-positive pulmonary disease are seldom seen. Diagnostic and therapeutic approaches to tuberculosis remain the same as in a HIV-negative patient, except that once-weekly rifapentine (Priftin) and if CD4+ counts are less than 100 cells/mL, twice-weekly rifabutin (Mycobutin)[1] should not be used. Standard four-drug short-course regimens (see chapter on tuberculosis) are equally effective in HIV-infected patients with drug-susceptible tuberculosis. All patients should receive directly observed treatment, and thrice-weekly intermittent regimens can be used. Extensive interactions occur between rifamycins, PIs, and NNRTIs. If the patient is already on HAART, rifabutin (Mycobutin) is the preferred rifamycin, and HAART has to be continued with appropriate changes (Table 10). If the patient is not on HAART, it is better started after the completion of the intensive phase in those with CD4+ more than 200 cells/mL. In those with CD4+ less than 200 cells/mL, it is preferable to initiate HAART early, after approximately 2 weeks of intensive-phase treatment.

# Management of the Pregnant HIV-Infected Woman

Apart from the usual indications for initiating HAART, in a pregnant HIV-infected woman, an additional aim is to prevent perinatal transmission. This is most effectively achieved by suppressing viremia to undetectable levels with HAART. From this perspective, all pregnant HIV-infected women should be initiated on HAART, irrespective of the viral load, CD4+ count, and symptoms. Efavirenz (Sustiva), a combination of didanosine (Videx) and stavudine (Zerit), nevirapine (Viramune) in those with CD4+ more than 250 cells/µL, and oral liquid formulations of amprenavir (Agenerase) should be avoided. Although NRTIs and nevirapine (Viramune) can be administered in the usual adult doses, nelfinavir (Viracept) has to be given only twice daily (Table 4). Initiation is better timed at the second trimester, to improve the tolerability and to avoid early fetal exposure to antiretrovirals. A detailed second-trimester fetal survey is indicated.

The goal of treatment, follow-up assessment, and indications for resistance testing all remain the same as in a nonpregnant patient. HAART has to be continued without interruption through delivery. Intrapartum, zidovudine (Retrovir) has to be administered IV until the umbilical cord is clamped and other drugs can be continued by oral route. The option of elective cesarean delivery should be offered to patients with viral loads higher than 1000 copies/mL despite HAART. If opted for, elective cesarean delivery is performed at 38 weeks' gestation, avoiding an amniocentesis to document fetal lung maturity. Following delivery, the infant should receive zidovudine (Retrovir) for 6 weeks. To avoid transmission through breast milk, nursing the infant should be avoided completely, if resources permit. Where the sole indication for initiating HAART was the prevention of perinatal transmission, HAART may be discontinued (in a staggered fashion, if nevirapine [Viramune] was included) after delivery. All infants exposed to antiretrovirals in utero should be followed up for possible adverse effects, regardless of the HIV status. Combined together, these interventions, namely HAART, cesarean delivery, and avoidance of breast-feeding, have brought down the risk of mother-to-child HIV transmission from approximately 25% to 1% to 2% in developed countries. In resource-limited settings and for HIV-infected women without prior HAART presenting in labor, peripartum prophylaxis with zidovudine (Retrovir), zidovudine with lamivudine (Combivir), nevirapine (Viramune), or zidovudine with nevirapine are acceptable alternatives.

# Postexposure Prophylaxis of HIV Infection

The importance of adhering to universal precautions in preventing occupational transmission of HIV cannot be overstated. Administration of postexposure prophylaxis (PEP) can substantially

[1]Not FDA approved for this indication.

[1]Not FDA approved for this indication.

**TABLE 10 Pharmacokinetic Interactions between Antiretrovirals and Rifamycins**

| Antiretroviral Drug | Compatibility with Rifampicin (Rifadin) | | Compatibility with Rifabutin (Mycobutin) | |
| --- | --- | --- | --- | --- |
| | Antiretroviral dose change | Rifampicin (Rifadin) dose change | Antiretroviral dose change | Rifabutin (Mycobutin) dose change |
| Saquinavir (Invirase, Fortovase) | Should not be used together | | Should not be used together | |
| Saquinavir/ritonavir (Invirase Fortovase/Norvir) | (↓ 400/↑ 400) mg bid | None | None | ↓ 150 mg qod* |
| Indinavir (Crixivan) | Should not be used together | | ↑ 1000 mg tid | ↓ 150 mg qd† |
| Nelfinavir (Viracept) | Should not be used together | | ↑ 1000 mg tid | ↓ 150 mg qd† |
| Amprenavir (Agenerase) | Should not be used together | | None | ↓ 150 mg qd† |
| Atazanavir (Reyataz) | Should not be used together | None | ↓ 150 mg qod* | |
| Lopinavir/ritonavir (Kaletra) | (400/↑ 400) mg bid | None | None | ↓ 150 mg qod* |
| Efavirenz (Sustiva) | ↑ 800 mg qd | None | None | ↑ 450 mg qd‡ |
| Nevirapine (Viramune) | None | None | None | None |
| Delavirdine (Rescriptor) | Should not be used together | | Should not be used together | |

Note: Increase or decrease in the doses are indicated with appropriately directed arrows.
*Can be administered as 150 mg tiw.
†Can be administered as 300 mg tiw.
‡Can be administered as 600 mg tiw.
Based on Centers for Disease Control and Prevention: Updated guidelines for the use of rifamycins for the treatment of tuberculosis among HIV-infected patients, 2004.

reduce the risk of HIV transmission following accidental occupational exposure in the health care setting. However, PEP is associated with significant morbidity and potentially serious side effects. HIV testing of the health care personnel should be done at the time of exposure, at 6 weeks, 12 weeks, and 6 months after exposure. Generally, all grades of percutaneous, mucous membrane, and nonintact skin exposure to a known HIV-infected source warrant administration of PEP. In the case of mucosal or nonintact skin exposure to a small volume (a few drops) of body fluid from a known HIV-infected source, the decision to initiate PEP should be made on a case-to-case basis, after discussing with the exposed person the benefits as well as the risks of PEP.

PEP should be initiated as soon as possible, preferably within hours following the exposure. The basic prophylaxis is with a two-drug regimen, usually a combination of two NRTIs (zidovudine + lamivudine [Combivir] or emtricitabine + tenofovir [Truvada]). If the exposure is more severe, three-drug regimens containing a PI are recommended. PEP is to be given for 4 weeks. If the source serostatus is unknown, administration of basic prophylaxis should be considered if the source is likely to be HIV infected and the exposure was percutaneous or involved a large volume of potentially infectious body fluid. The recommendations for PEP were extended recently to include nonoccupational exposures also (e.g., those reporting within 72 hours following an unanticipated sexual or injection drug use exposure to a known HIV-infected source).

## REFERENCES

Aberg JA, Gallant JE, Anderson J, et al: Primary care guidelines for the management of persons infected with human immunodeficiency virus: Recommendations of the HIV Medicine Association of the Infectious Diseases Society of America. Clin Infect Dis 2004;39:609-629.

Carr A, Cooper DA: Adverse effects of antiretroviral therapy. Lancet 2000;356:1423-1430.

Centers for Disease Control and Prevention: Treating opportunistic infections among HIV-infected adults and adolescents: Recommendations from CDC, the National Institutes of Health, and the HIV Medicine Association/Infectious Diseases Society of America. MMWR Morb Mortal Wkly Rep 2004;53(No. RR-15):1-112.

Centers for Disease Control and Prevention: Antiretroviral postexposure prophylaxis after sexual, injection-drug use, or other nonoccupational exposures to HIV in the United States: Recommendations from the U.S. Department of Health and Human Services. MMWR Morb Mortal Wkly Rep 2005;54(No. RR-2):1-19.

Centers for Disease Control and Prevention: Updated U.S. Public Health Service guidelines for the management of occupational exposures to HIV and recommendations for postexposure prophylaxis. MMWR Morb Mortal Wkly Rep 2005;54(No. RR-9):1-17.

Chesney MA: Factors affecting adherence to antiretroviral therapy. Clin Infect Dis 2000;30(Suppl 2):S171-S176.

Grinspoon S, Carr A: Cardiovascular risk and body fat abnormalities in HIV-infected adults. N Engl J Med 2005;352:48-62.

Hammer SM: Management of newly diagnosed HIV infection. N Engl J Med 2005;353:1702-1710.

Panel on clinical practices for the treatment of HIV infection, U.S. Department of Health and Human Services: Guidelines for the use of antiretroviral agents in HIV-1-infected adults and adolescents. October 6, 2005. Available at http://AIDSinfo.nih.gov (accessed February 1, 2006).

Sax PE: Opportunistic infections in HIV disease: Down but not out. Infect Dis Clin North Am 2001;15:433-455.

Yeni PG, Hammer SM, Hirsch MS, et al: Treatment of adult HIV infection. 2004 recommendations of the International AIDS Society—USA panel. JAMA 2004;292:251-265.

# Amebiasis

Method of
*Rashidul Haque, MB, PhD, and
William A. Petri, Jr., MD, PhD*

Amebiasis, a disease caused by the protozoan parasite *Entamoeba histolytica*, is estimated to be the third leading parasitic cause of deaths worldwide in humans. There are noninvasive species of ameba including *Entamoeba dispar* and *Entamoeba moshkovskii* that are morphologically indistinguishable from *E. histolytica* by traditional light microscopy. Amebiasis is distributed worldwide, but the majority of cases are found in developing countries. The World Health Organization estimates that approximately 50 million people suffer from invasive amebiasis each year, resulting in 40,000 to 100,000 deaths annually. For example, a prospective study of preschool children in an urban slum of Dhaka, Bangladesh, demonstrated a 39% incidence of *E. histolytica* infection during the first year of observation.

Human beings are the only known host of the parasite *E. histolytica*. Individuals become infected with *E. histolytica* when they ingest cysts in fecally contaminated food or water. When these cysts reach the intestine, they swell and release the motile, symptom-inducing form of *E. histolytica*, called the trophozoite. Trophozoites can remain in the intestine and even form new cysts without causing disease symptoms. They colonize the large intestine by adhering to colonic mucins via a galactose and *N*-acetyl-D-galactosamine (Gal/GalNAc)–specific lectin. Reproduction of trophozoites is without a recognized sexual cycle, and the overall population structure of *E. histolytica* appears to be clonal. Aggregation of amebae in the mucin layer likely signals encystation via the Gal/GalNAc lectin. Cysts excreted in stool perpetuate the life cycle by further fecal–oral spread. Invasive disease results when the trophozoite penetrates the intestinal mucus layer, which acts as barrier to invasion by inhibiting amebic adherence to the underlying epithelium and by slowing trophozoite motility. In addition, trophozoites can be carried through the blood to other organs, most commonly the liver, where they form life-threatening abscesses.

## Intestinal Amebiasis

There are several clinical classifications of amebiasis based on the invasiveness and site of infection with different treatments. Intestinal amebiasis is a term that encompasses the entire spectrum of clinical intestinal disease, including amebic colitis. Patients with amebic colitis typically present with a several week history of cramping abdominal pain, weight loss, and watery or, less commonly, bloody diarrhea. The insidious onset and variable signs and symptoms make diagnosis difficult, with fever and grossly bloody stool absent in most cases. Differential diagnosis of a diarrheal illness with occult or grossly bloody stools should include *Shigella*, *Salmonella*, *Campylobacter*, and enteroinvasive and enterohemorrhagic *Escherichia coli*. Noninfectious causes include inflammatory bowel disease, ischemic colitis, diverticulitis, and arteriovenous malformation.

Unusual manifestations of amebic colitis include acute necrotizing colitis, toxic megacolon, ameboma, and perianal ulceration with potential fistula formation. Acute necrotizing colitis is rare (<0.5% of cases) and is associated with a greater than 40% mortality. Patients with acute necrotizing colitis are typically very ill-appearing with fever, bloody mucoid diarrhea, abdominal pain with rebound tenderness, and peritoneal signs of irritation. Surgical intervention is indicated if there is bowel perforation or if the patient fails to improve on antiamebic therapy. Toxic megacolon is rare (approximately 0.5% of cases) and typically is associated with corticosteroid use.

## Amebic Liver Abscess

Amebic liver abscess is 10 times more common in men than women and is a rare disease in children. Approximately 80% of patients with amebic liver abscess present with symptoms that develop relatively acutely (typically <2 to 4 weeks in duration) with fever, cough, and a constant, dull, aching abdominal pain in the right upper quadrant or epigastrium. Involvement of the diaphragmatic surface of the liver may lead to right pleural pain or referred shoulder pain. Associated gastrointestinal symptoms occur in up to 10% to 35% of cases and include nausea, vomiting, abdominal cramping, abdominal distention, diarrhea, or constipation. Hepatomegaly with point tenderness over the liver, below the ribs, or in the intercostal spaces is a typical finding. Complications from amebic liver abscess may arise from rupture of the abscess with extension into the peritoneum, pleural cavity, or pericardium. Extrahepatic amebic abscesses have occasionally been described in the lung, brain, and skin, and presumably reach these sites hematogenously.

## Diagnosis

Historically, diagnosis of amebiasis was complicated and often unreliable for various reasons. The signs and symptoms of amebiasis can provide means to obtain clinical diagnosis. However, the confirmation of an amebic infection rests with laboratory identification. Over the last 25 years, various molecular diagnostic tests have been developed to diagnose *E. histolytica*. The diagnosis of intestinal amebiasis must be based on tests that distinguish *E. histolytica* from *E. dispar*. *E. histolytica*-specific antigen detection test and polymerase chain reaction (PCR) tests are now available for specific diagnosis of *E. histolytica* (Table 1). Enzyme-linked immunoabsorbent assay–based antigen detection kits are now commercially available. Field studies that directly compared PCR to stool culture or antigen-detection tests for the diagnosis of *E. histolytica* infection suggest that these three different methods perform equally well. An important aid to antigen detection and PCR-based tests is the detection of serum antibodies to amebae, which are present in 70% to 90% of patients with symptomatic *E. histolytica* infection. A drawback of current serologic tests is that patients remain positive for years after infection, making it difficult to distinguish new from past infection in regions of the world where amebiasis is endemic. Colonic mucosal biopsies and exudates can reveal a range in histopathologic appearance and severity of intestinal lesions associated with amebic colitis.

Amebic liver abscess patients may reveal a mild to moderate leukocytosis and anemia. Patients with an acute presentation of amebic liver abscess tend to have a normal alkaline phosphatase and elevated aspartate transaminase with the opposite true for patients with a chronic presentation. Ultrasound, abdominal computed tomography scan, and magnetic resonance imaging of the liver are all excellent imaging modalities for detecting liver lesions (most commonly single and in the right lobe) but are not specific for amebic liver abscess. The differential diagnosis of a liver mass should include pyogenic liver abscess, necrotic hepatoma, and echinococcal cyst (usually an incidental finding that would not be the cause of fever and abdominal pain). Patients with amebic abscess are more likely than patients with pyogenic liver abscesses to be male and younger than age 50 years; have immigrated from or traveled to an endemic country; and lack jaundice, biliary disease, or diabetes mellitus. Fewer than half of patients with amebic liver abscess have parasites detected in their stool by antigen detection. Helpful clues to the diagnosis include the presence of epidemiologic risk factors for amebiasis and the presence of serum antiamebic antibodies (present in 70% to 80% of patients at the time of presentation; see Table 1). Occasionally, aspiration of the abscess is required to rule out a pyogenic abscess. Amebae are visualized in the abscess pus in a minority of patients with amebic liver abscess. Traditional PCR and real-time PCR tests can be used for the detection of *E. histolytica* DNA in the stool and liver abscess pus samples and have been found to be sensitive and specific (see Table 1).

## Therapy

Therapy differs for invasive versus noninvasive infections (Table 2). Noninvasive infections can be treated with lumen active agents such as paromomycin (Humatin) to eradicate cysts and lumen-dwelling trophozoites. Nitroimidazoles, particularly metronidazole (Flagyl), are the mainstay of therapy for invasive amebiasis (see Table 2). Nitroimidazoles with longer half-lives (namely tinidazole [Tindamax], secnidazole,[2] and ornidazole[2]) are better tolerated and allow shorter duration of treatment; they are recently available in the United States. Approximately 90% of patients presenting with mild to moderate amebic colitis or dysentery respond to nitroimidazole treatment. In the rare case of fulminant amebic colitis, it is prudent to add broad-spectrum antibiotics to treat intestinal bacteria that may spill into the peritoneum, with patients occasionally requiring surgical intervention

---

[2]Not available in the United States.

## TABLE 1 Sensitivity of Laboratory Tests for the Diagnosis of Amebiasis

| Laboratory Tests | Amebic Colitis | Amebic Liver Abscess |
|---|---|---|
| Microscopy (stool)* | 25%–60% | 8%–44% |
| Microscopy (abscess fluid) | N/A | <20% |
| Stool antigen detection[†] | >90% | 40% |
| Serum antigen detection[†] | <65% | >90% (before therapy) |
| PCR/real-time PCR (stool) | >90% | >40% |
| PCR/real-time PCR (abscess fluid) | N/A | 90%–100% (before therapy) |
| Serology | | |
| Acute | 50%–70% | 70%–90% |
| Convalescent | >90% | >90% |

*Does not distinguish *Entamoeba histolytica* from the commensal parasites *Entamoeba dispar* and *Entamoeba moshkovskii*.
[†]TechLab *E. histolytica* II antigen detection test.
*Abbreviation*: PCR = polymerase chain reaction.

for acute abdomen, gastrointestinal bleeding, or toxic megacolon. Parasites persist in the intestine in as many as 40% to 60% of metronidazole (Flagyl)-treated patients. Therefore, metronidazole (Flagyl) treatment should be followed with paromomycin (Humatin) or the second-line agent diloxanide furoate (Furamide)2 to cure luminal infection (see Table 2). Do not treat with metronidazole (Flagyl) and paromomycin (Humatin) at the same time because the diarrhea, a common side effect of paromomycin, (Humatin) may make it difficult to assess response to therapy.

Therapeutic aspiration of an amebic liver abscess is occasionally required as adjunctive treatment to antiparasitic therapy. Abscess drainage should be considered in patients who fail to clinically respond to drug therapy within 5 to 7 days or those with high risk of abscess rupture as defined by cavity size greater than 5 cm or location in the left lobe. Bacterial coinfection of amebic liver abscess has been occasionally observed (both prior to and as a complication of drainage), and it is reasonable to add antibiotics or drainage, or both, to the treatment regimen if a prompt response to nitroimidazole therapy is not observed. Imaging-guided percutaneous treatment (needle aspiration or catheter drainage) has replaced surgical intervention over more recent years as the procedure of choice for therapeutically reducing abscess size.

## REFERENCES

Diamond LS, Clark CG: A redescription of *Entamoeba histolytica* Schaudin 1903 (amended Walker 1911) separating it from *Entamoeba dispar* (Brumpt 1925). J Eukaryot Microbiol 1993;40:340–344.

Haque R, Mollah NU, Ali IKM, et al: Diagnosis of amebic liver abscess and intestinal infection with the TechLab *Entamoeba histolytica* II antigen detection and antibody tests. J Clin Microbiol 2000;38:3235–3239.

Haque R, Ali IKM, Akther S, Petri WA Jr: Comparison of PCR, isoenzyme analysis, and antigen detection for diagnosis of *Entamoeba histolytica* infection. J Clin Microbio1998;36:449–452.

Haque R, Ali IKM, Sack RB, et al: Amebiasis and mucosal IgA antibody against the *Entamoeba histolytica* adherence lectin in Bangladeshi children. J Infect Dis 2001;183:1787–1793.

Haque R, Huston CD, Hughes M, et al: Current concepts: Amebiasis. N Engl J Med 2003;348:1565–1573.

Petri WA Jr, Haque R, Lyerly D, Vine RR: Estimating the impact of amebiasis on health. Parasitol Today 2000;16:320–321.

Petri, WA Jr, Singh U: State of the art: Diagnosis and management of amebiasis. Clin Infect Dis 1999;29:1117–1125.

Stanley SL Jr: Amoebiasis. Lancet 2003;22;361(9362):1025–1034.

Tanyuksel M, Petri WA Jr: Laboratory diagnosis of amebiasis. Clin Microbiol Rev 2003;16:713–729.

World Health Organization: Amoebiasis. Wkly Epidemiol Rec 1997;72:97–100.

## TABLE 2 Drug Therapy for the Treatment of Amebiasis*

| Type of Infection | Drug | Adult Dosage | Pediatric Dosage |
|---|---|---|---|
| Asymptomatic intestinal colonization | Paromomycin (Humatin) or | 25–35 mg/kg/d in 3 doses × 7 d | 25–35 mg/kg/d in 3 doses × 7 d |
| | Diloxanide furoate (Furamide)* | 500 mg tid × 10 d | 20 mg/kg/d in 3 doses × 10 d |
| Amebic liver abscess[†] | Metronidazole (Flagyl) or | 750 mg tid × 7–10 d in 3 doses × 7–10 d | 35–50 mg/kg/d |
| | Tinidazole (Tindamax) *followed by luminal agent* | 800 mg tid × 5 d[3] in 3 doses × 5 d | 60 mg/kg/d[3] |
| | Paromomycin (Humatin) or | 25–35 mg/kg/d in 3 doses × 7 d | 25–35 mg/kg/d in 3 doses × 7 d |
| | Diloxanide furoate (Furamide)[5] | 500 mg tid × 10 d in 3 doses × 10 d | 20 mg/kg/d |
| Amebic colitis[†] | Metronidazole (Flagyl) *followed by luminal agent (similar to amebic liver abscess)* | 500–750 mg tid × 7–10 d in 3 doses × 7–10 d | 35–50 mg/kg/d |

*The information is updated annually by the Medical Letter on Drugs and Therapeutics at http://www.medletter.com/htmlprm.htm#Parasitic.
[†] Treatment of amebic liver abscess and amebic colitis should be followed by a treatment with a luminal agent.
[3]Exceeds dosage recommended by the manufacturer.
[5]Investigational drug in the United States.

# Giardiasis

Method of
*M. Ekramul Hoque, MBBS, MPH (Hons), PhD*

## Background

Giardiasis is a parasitic infection of the upper small intestine caused by a flagellated protozoan, *Giardia lamblia* (also called *Giardia intestinalis* and *Giardia duodenalis*). This ubiquitous parasite is a major cause of intestinal infection among adults and children in developing and developed countries. The existence of this parasite was reported in the prehistoric era across the continents. However, pathogenicity of the organism among humans was known only in the latter part of the last century.

## Organism

*Giardia* is a microscopic organism that exists in two life forms. The trophozoite, which is environmentally unstable, causes clinical illness, and the resistant cysts are responsible for the transmission of infection. Trophozoites are binucleated, flagellated, and pear shaped, measuring 12 to 15 μm long and 6 to 8 μm wide. They have a pair of claw-shaped median bodies and a concave ventral disk used for nourishment and attachment on the wall of the small intestine of vertebrate hosts. Cysts are smaller and oval, usually 8 to 12 μm long and 7 to 10 μm wide, and contain four nuclei.

## Epidemiology

Giardiasis is one of the most common intestinal infections in the world. More than 200 million people are reported to have symptoms of giardiasis, and some 500,000 new cases are reported annually. Some estimates suggest the worldwide prevalence of giardiasis is 20% to 60%. Others report from 2% to 7% in industrialized countries and 20% to 30% in developing countries. In 2002, there were 21,300 giardiasis cases reported from 46 states of the United States, with an incidence rate of 7.6 cases per 100,000 population. The incidence varied by state from less than 0.1 to 23.5 cases per 100,000 population; rates were higher in northern states than southern states. *Giardia* infection is probably underreported by a factor of 10, and therefore the true burden of giardiasis in the United States is probably underestimated. Annually, 5,000 people are hospitalized in the United States due to severe giardiasis. New Zealand reports more than 30 cases of giardiasis per 100,000 population every year, which is one of the highest among the industrialized countries. *Giardia* infection is reported to be more prevalent in urban areas than in rural populations.

Humans are the primary reservoir of the parasite. Other possible hosts are farm, wild, and domestic animals. Polymerase chain reaction (PCR) testing of samples of human feces from different geographic locations has so far associated *G. intestinalis* genotypes (assemblages) A and B with human infections. The role of animals in transmitting *G. intestinalis* to humans and the most likely routes of infection remain unclear.

Transmission of the *Giardia* infection is through the fecal-oral route following direct or indirect contact with cysts of *Giardia*. Cysts are infectious immediately after being excreted in feces. An infected person can excrete a maximum of $10^9$ cysts per day for several months. Cysts may be killed by simple drying and heat, but they can survive for several weeks in cool and wet environments. Infectious dose is low; ingestion of as few as 10 cysts can cause infection. Commonly, the organism spreads by water or food or directly through person-to-person contact. Outbreaks of waterborne giardiasis have been reported year round, suggesting frequent contamination of water sources and longer survival of cysts in water.

Giardiasis shows a bimodal pattern of age distribution, peaking in children younger than 5 years and in adults 25 to 44 years (Figure 1). Incidence of infection varies by season, peaking in late summer and early autumn and dropping in winter. Persons at increased risk for infection include (among others) children of diaper age, children attending daycare centers, daycare workers, immunocompromised persons, pregnant women, institutionalized persons, travelers to endemic regions, people drinking contaminated water during outdoor activities, sewage and irrigation workers, and men who have sex with men.

It is not clear whether giardiasis causes malnutrition or malnutrition predisposes to *Giardia* infection. However, nutritional insufficiency can contribute to chronicity of the disease. Repeated exposure to the parasite can elicit an immune response, which might explain asymptomatic giardiasis cases. Breast-fed infants of immune mothers might acquire temporary protection against giardiasis, but this is not conclusive.

## Pathogenesis

Clinical illness results from the interaction of *Giardia* organisms with the human host and the host's subsequent response to the parasite. *Giardia* isolates can vary in virulence, which might further explain the intensity of the symptoms.

After a person ingests *Giarda* cysts, excystation begins in the duodenum in the presence of gastric acid, pancreatic enzymes, and parasite-derived cysteine protease. Two tropozoites are formed from each cyst by binary fission (miotic division). The motility of parasites and the inflammatory cytokine response to parasitic attachment on the mucosal brush borders results in secretion of fluid and electrolytes, hence diarrhea and malabsorption. Trophozoites frequently slough off villi, which are swept into the fecal stream and replaced by new sets. After 4 to 15 days of colonization, some trophozoites encyst in the jejunum under an alkaline environment of bile secretion. Immotile cysts undergo a single cell division to form four nuclei, which are then passed intermittently in the feces.

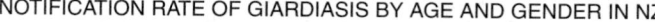

NOTIFICATION RATE OF GIARDIASIS BY AGE AND GENDER IN NZ

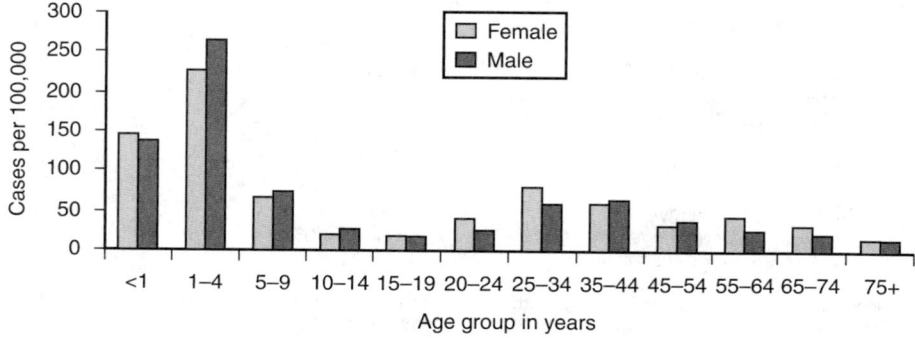

**FIGURE 1.** Notification rate of giardiasis in New Zealand by age and gender.

*Giardia* trophozoites remain adherent to the intestinal mucosa but are not invasive. This close association might directly affect the brush border and its enzyme system. Hospital-based investigation observed partial villous atrophy in up to 25% of patients. Malabsorption of vitamin $B_{12}$ occurs in 20% to 40% cases. Parasites are also found in extraintestinal sites such as the gallbladder and the urinary tract.

## Clinical Features

Clinical manifestations of giardiasis vary from asymptomatic infection to severe diarrhea. The incubation period for *Giardia* infection varies from 1 week to several weeks. However, a period of 5 to 25 days is average.

Freshly exposed persons in an endemic area can present with acute symptoms that usually begin about 15 days (range, 1-46 days) following exposure. The symptoms include nausea, anorexia, upper abdominal discomfort, malaise, low-grade fever, and chills followed by the sudden onset of explosive, watery, foul-smelling diarrhea associated with foul flatulence and abdominal distention. Generally, the acute stage resolves spontaneously within 2 to 4 weeks. Some patients become asymptomatic passers of cysts for a period. Others have periodic brief recurrences of acute symptoms.

About 30% to 50% of infected patients go on to a subacute or chronic stage. Overseas travelers to *Giardia*-endemic areas often do not recognize or remember the infection during their travel and subsequently present periodically with persistent or recurrent mild to moderate symptoms. Features of subacute to chronic *Giardia* infection include flatulence, mushy foul stools, upper abdominal cramps, abdominal distention, steatorrhea, marked weight loss, and fatigue. Uncommon manifestations are cholecystitis, pancreatitis, immunologic reactions (including arthritis, retinal arteritis, and iridocyclitis), and occasionally rash and urticaria, mostly in adults. In rare cases, symptoms persist for years, but most cases resolve spontaneously after a variable period of weeks or months.

Generally, 10% to 30% of infected people remain symptom free, but the true percentage may be as high as 60%. The prevalence of asymptomatic infection is higher among children than among adults, especially among those in daycare. The duration of the asymptomatic cyst-passing state is not determined.

## Diagnosis

Clinical signs and symptoms along with the history of risk behavior and exposure to *Giardia* risk factors can lead to a preliminary diagnosis of the disease. Laboratory diagnostic procedures are then applied to confirm the infection (Figure 2)

Traditionally, diagnosis is based on microscopic detection of *Giardia* cysts or trophozoites in the fecal specimens. At least three

 **CURRENT DIAGNOSIS**

- Giardiasis is a common parasitic infection of the small intestine.
- Children, caregivers, travelers, and persons exposed to contaminated water are at greater risk for infection.
- Clinical manifestations vary widely.
- A large fraction of infected persons remain asymptomatic.
- Infective cysts pass intermittently with patients' feces.
- Diagnosis is by detection of *Giardia* parasites in feces by repeated microscopy or by immunologic assays.
- Assays can give false positives in recently cured persons.
- Infection can resolve spontaneously or can go into a chronic stage lasting for months with marked weight loss.

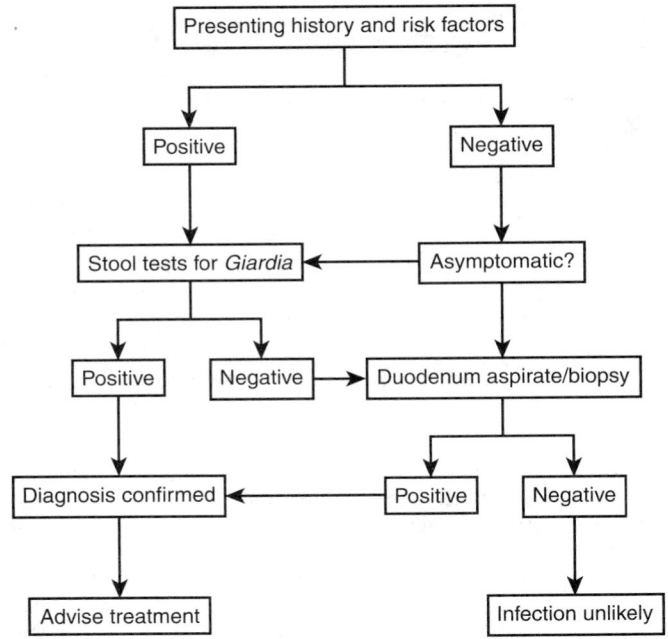

**FIGURE 2.** Diagnostic algorithm for giardiasis.

specimens of feces collected on consecutive days may be required to recover the parasite. The sensitivity of parasite detection is 50% to 70% in one specimen and 90% in three specimens.

Immunologic methods for detecting *Giardia* have superior sensitivity and specificity compared with other conventional methods of diagnosis. Widely used methods are enzyme immunoassay (EIA) detecting soluble antigens, direct fluorescent antibody (DFA) detecting intact organisms, and immunochromatographic lateral-flow immunoassays or rapid assay. Sensitivity of immunoassay varies between 94% and 97%, and specificity varies between 99% and 100%. EIA and rapid assay can pick up antigens of recently cured cases; DFA detects *Giardia* cysts. Immunoassay tests are quick and costs are reasonable.

Serologic tests do not have great diagnostic value in clinical practice because immunoglobulin G (IgG) persists even after infection; IgM, however, can indicate active infection. Negative serology does not exclude infection.

Duodenal aspirates or string test and duodenal mucosal biopsy are costly and invasive. They should be reserved for situations when giardiasis is strongly suspected despite persistent negative feces tests. PCR is used mostly in epidemiologic studies.

## Treatment

Giardiasis, if diagnosed, should be treated. There are unresolved debates on the significance of treatment of asymptomatic cases. However, asymptomatic cases can remain a potential source of infection and can turn symptomatic at any moment.

### PHARMACOLOGIC THERAPY

A number of effective antigiardial drugs are available (Table 1).

Metronidazole (Flagyl)[1] is preferred and widely used because of its broad-spectrum coverage. It is not approved by the FDA for routine treatment of giardiasis in the United States. Metronidazole is effective and well tolerated and has a cure rate of 80% to 95%. The common side effects are gastrointestinal upset, headache, nausea, leukopenia, and metallic taste in the mouth. It is contraindicated in the first

---

[1]Not FDA approved for this indication.

**TABLE 1  Therapeutic Doses of Antigiardial Drugs**

| Drugs | Adult Dose[h] | Pediatric Dose[h] |
|---|---|---|
| Metronidazole (Flagyl)[a] | 250 mg tid × 5-7 days | 5 mg/kg tid × 5-7 days |
| Tinidazole (Fasigyn)[b] | 2 g single dose | 50 mg/kg single dose (max, 2 g) |
| Ornidazole (Tiberal)[c] | 2 g single dose | 40-50 mg/kg single dose (max, 2 g) |
| Quinacrine (Atabrine)[c] | 100 mg tid × 5-7 days[f] | 2 mg/kg tid × 5-7 days (max 300 mg/d)[f] |
| Furazolidone[b,d] | 100 mg qid × 7-10 days | 1.25-2 mg/kg qid × 10 days |
| Paromomycin[a] | 7-10 mg/kg tid × 5-10 days[g] | 8-10 mg/kg tid × 5-10 days[g] |
| Paromomycin[a,e] | 7-30 mg/kg tid × 5-10 days[g] | |
| Albendazole[a] | 400 mg qd × 5 days | 15 mg/kg/day × 5-7 days (max 400 mg/d) |

[a]Not a U.S. FDA approved indication; [b]Not available in the U.S.; [c]No longer produced in the U.S.;
[d]Available in liquid formulation; [e]In pregnancy; [f] After meal; [g]With meal
[h]qd, once a day; bid, twice a day; tid, three times a day; qid, four times a day

trimester of pregnancy due to its suspected carcinogenic, teratogenic, and mutagenic effects. Other minor side effects are peripheral neuropathy, seizures, depression, irritability, restlessness, and insomnia. Drug resistance is not yet widespread.

Furazolidone (Furoxone)[2] is the primary drug choice in the United States. It is available in liquid form and is widely used to treat children. Cure rates are between 80% and 89%. It is not recommended in pregnancy. Side effects include gastrointestinal disturbances, hemolytic anemia, disulfiram-like reactions with alcohol, hypersensitivity reactions, brown discoloration of the urine, orthostatic hypotension, and hypoglycemia.

Albendazole (Albenza)[1] is an anthelminthic whose efficacy is equal to that of metronidazole and with cure rates of 62% to 95%. Absence of anorexia in using this drug is an advantage for treating children. Notable side effects are gastrointestinal upset, abdominal pain, nausea, vomiting, diarrhea, dizziness, vertigo, fever, increased intracranial pressure, alopecia, and (reversible) increase in serum transaminases after prolonged use. Albendazole is contraindicated in pregnancy due to teratogenicity. Paromomycin (Humatin)[1] is a poorly absorbed aminoglycoside that is excreted in the feces without being metabolized. Its efficacy rate is between 60% and 70%. It is recommended for giardial infection in pregnant patients. Common side effects are nausea, increased gastrointestinal motility, abdominal pain, and diarrhea. 5-Nitroimidazole compounds, tinidazole (Tindamax) and ornidazole (Tiberal),[1,2] are effective as first-line agents and have a cure rate of 90%.

They are effective in single doses. Common side effects are gastrointestinal upset, vertigo, and bitter taste. Quinacrine[2] was one of the most effective drugs against giardial infection, with a cure rate of 92% to 95%. This drug is no longer produced in the United States and elsewhere in the world due a number of pharmacokinetic issues and adverse effects. Other potential drugs include benzimidazole derivatives such as mebendazole (Vermox)[1] and a 5-nitrothiazole derivative (Nitazoxanide), which are not used widely. Nitazoxanide (Alinia) has been used successfully in France in resistant giardiasis patients infected with HIV.

## OTHER MEASURES

Diet modification can reduce acute symptoms, improve host defense mechanisms, and inhibit growth and replication of *Giardia* trophozoites in the lumen of the intestine. General advice is to consume a diet of whole foods that is high in fiber, low in simple carbohydrates, and low in fat.

# Follow-up

Follow-up stool tests are advised to ensure resolution of infection. Hygiene practices should be enhanced during outbreaks. Symptomatic persons should be kept away from public contact.

# Prognosis

Giardiasis is usually a self-limited intestinal infection. Effective antigiardial agents shorten the infection period. If untreated, giardiasis often resolves spontaneously in a few weeks. Prognosis is, therefore, generally excellent.

# Prevention

Eradication of giardiasis is not possible because the disease is endemic in the human population, animal population, and environment. Prevention and control methods are the way forward. Health departments in all countries, including the Centers for Disease Control and Prevention in the United States, publish recommendations for prevention and control of giardiasis. These include decontamination of water supplies and sanitary and hygiene practices. Potentially contaminated water may be treated by boiling for more than 1 minute or filtering through a pore size of 1 μm or smaller. Chlorination and iodination are unreliable. Laws and regulations to protect provisions of safe water should be enforced and monitored. Regular surveillance and reviews of sanitation can ensure quality.

[1]Not FDA approved for this indication.
[2]Not available in the United States.

## CURRENT THERAPY

- Metronidazole (Flagyl)[1] is widely used because of its broad-spectrum coverage, but it is contraindicated in the first trimester of pregnancy.
- Furazolidone (Furoxone)[2] is available in liquid form to treat children.
- Absence of anorexia with albendazole (Albenza)[1] is an advantage for treating children.
- Paromomycin (Humatin)[1] is recommended in pregnancy due to its poor absorption rate.
- Tinidazole (Tindamax) and ornidazole (Tiberal)[2] are effective in single doses.
- Nitazoxanide (Alinia) is used in drug-resistant giardiasis.
- Some diet modifications can reduce acute symptoms, improve host defense, and inhibit trophozoite replications.

[1]Not FDA approved for this indication.
[2]Not available in the United States.

People involved in recreational water activities and persons traveling overseas must be informed about the possibility of exposure to the parasite. Persons with symptomatic cases should not swim in a pool until 2 weeks after the treatment. Other occupational groups (e.g., daycare workers, medical personnel, irrigation and sewage workers) need to be cautioned. In daycare centers, hand washing with soap after changing diapers and a separate diaper-changing area should be implemented. All symptomatic family members, daycare center teachers, and children in daycare should be treated for giardiasis. Treatment of asymptomatic cases should be considered if the infected person is suspected to be a potential source of transmission of the disease.

## REFERENCES

Cacciò SM, Thompson RCA, McLauchlin J, Smith HV: Unravelling *Cryptosporidium* and *Giardia* epidemiology. Trends Parasitol 2005;21(9):430-437.

Centers for Disease Control and Prevention: Parasitic disease information: Giardiasis fact sheet. Available at http://www.cdc.gov/ncidod/dpd/parasites/giardiasis/factsht_giardia.htm (accessed April 5, 2007).

Gardner TB, Hill DR: Treatment of giardiasis. Clin Microbiol Rev 2001;14(1):114-128.

Hanson KL, Cartwright CP: Use of an enzyme immunoassay does not eliminate the need to analyze multiple stool specimens for sensitive detection of *Giardia lamblia*. J Clin Microbiol 2001;39(2):474-477.

Hetsko ML, McCaffery JM, Svard SG, et al: Cellular and transcriptional changes during excystation of *Giardia lamblia* in vitro. Exp Parasitol 1998;88(3):172-183.

Hlavsa MC, Watson JC, Beach MJ: Giardiasis surveillance—United States, 1998-2002. MMWR Surveill Summ 2005;54(SS01):9-16.

Hoque ME, Hope VT, Scragg R: *Giardia* infection in Auckland and New Zealand: Trends and international comparison. The N Z Med J 2002;115(1150):121-123.

Islam A, Stoll BJ, Ljungstrom I, et al: Giardia lamblia infections in a cohort of Bangladeshi mothers and infants followed for one year. J Pediatr 1983;103(6):996-1000.

Kulda J, Nohynkova E: Flagellates of the human intestine and of intestines of other species. In Kreier JP (ed). Protozoa of Veterinary and Medical Interest. Vol. II. New York: Academic Press, 1978, pp 69-104.

Lebwohl B, Deckelbaum RJ, Green PHR: Giardiasis. Gastrointest Endosc 2003;57(7):906-913.

Mineno T, Avery MA: Giardiasis: Recent progress in chemotherapy and drug development. Curr Pharm Des 2003;9:841-855.

New Zealand Ministry of Health: Communicable disease control manual. Wellington: New Zealand Ministry of Health, 1998.

# Severe Sepsis and Septic Shock

Method of
*Eleni Patrozou, MD, and Steven M. Opal, MD*

*Sepsis* is defined as a deleterious systemic inflammatory response to an infection. The precise incidence of sepsis is unknown, owing to the lack of a readily available and consistently applied definition, but a variety of epidemiologic studies indicate that it is increasing in incidence. The Centers for Disease Control and Prevention (CDC) has reported a threefold increase in the incidence of sepsis since the 1990s. Using hospital discharge coding data, it is estimated that there are between 660,000 and 750,000 episodes of severe sepsis each year in the United States. Severe sepsis accounts for 1 of every 10 intensive care unit (ICU) admissions and represents 2% to 3% of all hospital admissions.

Incidence of sepsis in the United States is projected to rise at a rate of 1.5% per year. The rising incidence of sepsis is primarily related to the aging of the population in developed countries, but the increased number of immunocompromised patients, the increased use of implantable devices in patient care, and the growing problem of antibiotic-resistant microorganisms probably contribute as well. Male patients are consistently and significantly more likely to develop sepsis than female patients.

Since the late 1980s, gram-positive organisms have surpassed gram-negative bacterial pathogens as the predominant causative organisms that lead to sepsis. There has also been a remarkable increase in the number of episodes of fungal sepsis. This is an unfavorable trend because fungal sepsis is associated with a worse outcome than bacterial sepsis.

Sepsis is now reported to be the tenth most common cause of death in the United States and is one of the most common causes of death in the noncoronary ICU.

## Systemic Inflammatory Response Syndrome and Sepsis

A major clinical issue in the recognition and early management of sepsis is the imprecise definitions and vague terminology used to describe the septic process. There is no single clinical or laboratory test that verifies the diagnosis of sepsis, severe sepsis, and septic shock. A constellation of physiologic and laboratory studies are employed in concert to make a diagnosis of sepsis (see the Current Diagnosis box).

The term *systemic inflammatory response syndrome* (SIRS) implies early evidence of an acute physiologic insult that may be induced by an infection. SIRS can result from a diverse group of insults such as trauma, severe drug reactions, burns, and pancreatitis. The term *sepsis* is used to define the SIRS response to a documented infection and generally implies a deleterious state in which the septic patient is at risk from both the infecting organism and the systemic host response itself. The lack of specificity in the clinical presentation of SIRS is problematic because the initial manifestations of sepsis mimic many other inflammatory states.

SIRS is operationally defined as the presence of two or more of the following:

- Temperature >38°C (100.4°F) or <36°C (96.8°F)
- Heart rate >90 beats per minute
- Respiratory rate >20 breaths per minute or $Paco_2$ <32 mm Hg
- White blood cell count (WBC) >12,000 cells/mm³, <4000 cells/mm³, or >10% immature band forms

Sepsis is the systemic inflammatory response to a documented infection. The diagnosis of sepsis requires the presence of at least two of the SIRS criteria as a response to an invasive infection in a normally sterile space (e.g., blood, lung parenchyma, renal interstitial space, cerebrospinal fluid). Uncomplicated sepsis can progress in a continuum of disease severity to severe sepsis and septic shock. *Severe sepsis* is defined as the presence of organ dysfunction or tissue hypoperfusion from the septic response. Perfusion abnormalities can include lactic acidosis, oliguria, or an acute alteration in mental status.

Sepsis-induced hypotension occurs when the systolic blood pressure falls to less than 90 mm Hg or falls more than 40 mm Hg from baseline systolic blood pressure. Septic shock is a subset of severe sepsis with hypotension despite adequate fluid resuscitation, along with the presence of perfusion abnormalities. Patients who require vasopressor agents to maintain blood pressure yet continue to present with hypoperfusion abnormalities or organ dysfunction are still considered to be in septic shock.

Multiple organ dysfunction syndrome (MODS) is sepsis-induced alteration of organ function. A gradation of organ dysfunction from mild biochemical abnormalities to complete organ failure necessitating interventional support exists in sepsis-related MODS.

In 2001, the International Sepsis Definitions Conference reaffirmed the basic usefulness of these clinical definitions originally proposed in 1991 by the American College of Chest Physicians and Society of Critical Care Medicine. The consensus conference generated a series of common signs and symptoms of sepsis (see the Current Diagnosis box).

---

**BOX 1  PIRO Staging of Sepsis**

*Predisposition*

Premorbid conditions that influence likelihood of infection, sepsis, morbidity, survival (age, gender, hormonal state, genetic polymorphisms for immune response and coagulation proteins)

*Infection*

Organism associated with the sepsis response (type of organism, virulence potential, toxins, community or nosocomial acquisition)

*Response*

Clinical and immunologic manifestations of the septic response (either hyperinflammation or hypoinflammation) (e.g., procalcitonin, IL-6, HLA-DR, TNF, PAF)

*Organ Dysfunction*

Type and number of dysfunctional organs (reversible versus irreversible dysfunction), severity of dysfunction

---

*Abbreviations:* HLA-DR = human leukocyte antigen-D related; IL = interleukin; PAF = platelet activating factor; TNF = tumor necrosis factor.
From Levy MM, Fink MP, Marshall JE et al: 2001 SCCM/ESICM/ACCP/ATS/SIS International Sepsis Definitions Conference. Crit Care Med 2003;31:1250-1256.

---

The conference participants also proposed a new classification scheme called the *PIRO system* (Box 1) to stratify septic patients on the basis of *p*redisposing factors, the nature of the *i*nfection, the host *r*esponse, and the pattern of *o*rgan dysfunction. The validity and practical usefulness of this proposed staging system to further the understanding of sepsis remain to be demonstrated.

## Pathogenesis

Sepsis often begins as a physiologic host response as the microbial clearance mechanisms of the innate immune system are called into play to eliminate a microbial invader. Sepsis becomes evident as the host response becomes excessive or dysfunctional, culminating in diffuse endothelial injury, MODS, and septic shock. The molecular pathogenesis of sepsis begins when the host response becomes a disadvantageous process in which host-derived mediators and coagulation factors induce damage to tissues remote from the site of the initiating infectious process. Generalized release of a network of proinflammatory and anti-inflammatory molecules and mediators produce a maladaptive state leading to dysfunctional cellular, tissue, and organ system injury. A complex and dynamic web of interacting inhibitors and activators of cell signaling events ensues, and these can deteriorate over time to refractory organ failure and shock unless appropriate interventions are instituted.

As the process unfolds, anti-inflammatory events dominate and an immune refractory state evolves. This immunodepressed state is now well recognized in the later stages of sepsis, and it is characterized by excess anti-inflammatory mediators and cytokine inhibitors, cellular apoptosis of CD4+ lymphocytes, follicular dendritic cells, and tissue refractoriness to endotoxin or other inflammatory signals. This paradoxically renders the patient susceptible to a variety of secondary infections by intrinsically less virulent pathogens such as fungal organisms, enterococcal pathogens, and a variety of antibiotic-resistant nosocomial pathogens.

Host factors responsible for the important first line of defense against the infectious insult include epithelial barriers, antimicrobial peptides, mucociliary flow, pH of body fluids, urine volume, and secretory immunoglobulins. Once the integument and mucosal barriers are

---

 **CURRENT DIAGNOSIS**

- Infection (documented or suspected) plus some of the following.

**General Variables**

- Fever (core temperature >38.3°C [101°F])
- Hypothermia (core temperature <36°C [96.8°F])
- Heart rate >90 bpm or >2 SD above the normal value for age
- Tachypnea
- Altered mental status
- Significant edema or positive fluid balance (>20 mL/kg for longer than 24 h)
- Hyperglycemia (plasma glucose >120 mg/dL or 7.7 mmol/L in absence of diabetes)

**Inflammatory Variables**

- Leukocytosis (WBC count >12,000/μL)
- Leukopenia (WBC count <4000/μL)
- Normal WBC count with 10% immature forms (bands)
- Plasma C-reactive protein >2 SD above the normal value
- Plasma procalcitonin >2 SD above the normal value

**Hemodynamic Variables**

- Arterial hypotension (systolic BP <90 mm Hg, MAP <70 mm Hg, or a systolic BP decrease >40 mm Hg in adults or <2 SD below normal for age)
- $SvO_2$ >70%
- Cardiac index >3.5 L/min/m²
- Organ dysfunction variables
- Arterial hypoxemia ($PaO_2/FiO_2$ < 300)
- Acute oliguria (urine output <0.5 mL/kg/h or <45 mmol/L for at least 2 h
- Creatinine increase >0.5 mg/dL
- Coagulation abnormalities (INR >1.5 or aPTT >60 sec)
- Ileus (absent bowel sounds)
- Thrombocytopenia (platelet count <100,000/μL)
- Hyperbilirubinemia (plasma total bilirubin >4 mg/dL or >70 mmol/L)

**Tissue Perfusion Variables**

- Hyperlactatemia (>1 mmol/L)
- Decreased capillary refill or mottling

---

*Abbreviations:* aPTT = activated partial thromboplastin time; bpm = beats per minute; INR = international normalized ratio; MAP = mean arterial pressure; SD = standard deviation; WBC = white blood cell.
From Levy MM, Fink MP, Marshall JC, et al: 2001 SCCM/ESICM/ACCP/ATS/SIS International Sepsis Definitions Conference. Crit Care Med 2003;31:1250-1256.

---

breached, the innate immune system of the host (neutrophils, monocytes, macrophages, dendritic cells, natural killer [NK] cells, alternate complement, and mannose-binding lectin pathways) provide key defenses against infectious insults. The adaptive arm of host immunity, composed of highly specific and clonal B cells and T cells, plays primarily a support role in sepsis. This adaptive response becomes more relevant to host defenses in repeated infection from the same or similar pathogens or as the septic process persists over days to weeks.

The innate immune system recognizes highly conserved, essential, and unique structures found only in microbial pathogens. These PAMPs (pathogen-associated molecular patterns) are detected by cognate pattern-recognition receptors. These receptors include CD14, complement receptors for C3b, and a remarkable group of 10 human transmembrane receptors known as the *Toll-like receptors* (TLR). TLR4 is the recognition receptor of bacterial endotoxin from gram-negative bacteria. TLR2 partners with TLR1 or TLR6 to recognize a variety of microbial structures including bacterial lipopeptides, peptidoglycans, outer membrane proteins, and mycobacterial antigens. TLR5 detects bacterial flagella, and TLR9, TLR8, and TLR3 recognize prokaryotic DNA sequences, single-stranded RNA, and double-stranded RNA, respectively. Engagement of the TLRs initiates a series of intracellular phosphorylation events that terminate as transcriptional activators for a large number of genetic programs for inflammation, coagulation, and other acute-phase responses.

Gram-positive organisms produce an array of potent exotoxins, some of which function as superantigens. Superantigens induce massive activation of mononuclear cells, macrophages, and T cells, leading to overproduction of inflammatory cytokines. The prototypic superantigenic disease entity is staphylococcal toxic shock syndrome caused by release of TSST-1 (toxic shock syndrome toxin-1). Streptococcal toxic shock from invasive group A streptococcal infections has now supplanted *Staphylococcus aureus* as the predominant superantigen-mediated form of toxic shock today.

Some of the more commonly recognized primary pro- and anti-inflammatory molecules and mediators are listed in Box 2. Included in the list of proinflammatory cytokines are tumor necrosis factor (TNF)-α, interleukin (IL)-1, IL-6, and interferon-γ (IFN-γ).

An overwhelming systemic inflammatory response results when the host is unable to contain the proinflammatory response locally at the site of microbial invasion. The massive, uncontrolled production of inflammatory signals induces diffuse endothelial dysfunction and systemic activation of the coagulation system. The result is microvascular thrombi and up-regulation of endothelial adhesion molecules, causing increased microvascular permeability, vasodilation, organ dysfunction, and shock.

# Treatment

In 2003, critical care and infectious disease experts representing 11 international organizations developed management guidelines for severe sepsis and septic shock based on the best available published evidence. These guidelines, produced by the Surviving Sepsis Campaign, were published in 2004 and updated in 2006 as new clinical trials data became available.

Management of sepsis and septic shock begins with prompt recognition of the process. Along with determination of the probable site of infection and causative microorganism, the initial management begins with an assessment of physiologic derangements. The general management strategy involves source control, restoration and maintenance of normal hemodynamic function, adequate oxygenation, ventilation, tissue oxygen delivery, and prevention of complications. The Current Therapy box outlines the general management principles.

## SOURCE CONTROL

Prompt and effective management of the source of the infection is the cornerstone of sepsis management. Necessary specimens should be sent for culture and susceptibility testing as early as possible and before antimicrobial therapy is initiated. This information will guide subsequent antimicrobial therapy to eradicate the causative pathogen(s). Recommendations for the initial antimicrobial regimen based on the source and likely pathogen are given in Table 1.

Intravenous antibiotic therapy should be started within an hour of recognizing severe sepsis. Effective antimicrobial administration within the first hour of documented hypotension has been associated with increased survival to hospital discharge in adult patients with septic shock. For every additional hour to effective antimicrobial initiation in the first 6 hours after onset of hypotension, survival drops an average 7.6%.

After the likely pathogen is identified, antibiotic selection should be guided by the susceptibility patterns of causative microorganisms. The antimicrobial therapy should then be appropriately tailored with the aim of using a narrow-spectrum antibiotic to prevent the development

**BOX 2  Potential Molecules Involved in the Pathogenesis of Severe Sepsis and Septic Shock**

**Proinflammatory Molecules**
- Arachidonic acid metabolites: Prostaglandins, prostacyclin, thromboxane, leukotrienes
- CD14, MD2
- Clotting factors, PAI-1
- Complement and activation of the complement cascade
- Cytokines and chemokines (ILs-1, -2, -6, -8, -12, TNF, IFN-γ, G-CSF, MCP-1)
- Elastase and lysosomal enzymes
- Endorphins
- Endotoxin and other microbial toxins and mediators
- High mobility group box 1 (HMGB1)
- Histamine and serotonin
- Kinases: Protein kinases, tyrosine kinases, serine/theonine kinases
- Kinins (e.g., bradykinin)
- Mannose-binding lectin
- Monocyte migration inhibitory factor (MIF)
- Neopterin
- NF-κB
- PAF, oxidized phospholipids
- Proteolytic enzymes
- Reactive nitrogen intermediates: Nitric oxide, peroxynitrite
- Soluble adhesion molecules
- Toll-like receptors (1-10)
- Toxic oxygen metabolites: Superoxide, hydroxyl radical, hydrogen peroxide
- Vasoactive neuropeptides

**Potential Anti-inflammatory Molecules**
- BPI
- Epinephrine
- Glucocorticoids and glucocorticoid receptors
- IL-1ra
- IL-1 receptor type II
- IL-4, IL-10, IL-13
- IκB
- Leukotriene B$_4$ receptor antagonist
- Soluble CD14
- sTNFr type 1 and type 2
- TGF-β

*Abbreviations:* BPI = bactericidal/permeability increasing protein; G-CSF = granulocyte colony-stimulating factor; IFN-γ = interferon-γ; IκB = inhibitor of NFκB; IL = interleukin; IL-ra = interleukin-1 receptor antagonist; MCP = monocyte chemoattractant protein; NFκB = nuclear factor κB; PAF = platelet-activating factor; PAI-1 = plasminogen activator inhibitor-1; sTNFr = soluble TNF receptor; TGF-β = transforming growth factor-β; TNF = tumor necrosis factor.

of resistance, reduce toxicity, and reduce costs. Once a causative agent is identified, there is no evidence that combination therapy is more effective than monotherapy. However, most experts recommend combination therapy for patients with *Pseudomonas* infections and for neutropenic patients with severe sepsis or septic shock. The duration of therapy should typically be 7 to 10 days and guided by clinical response.

All patients with severe sepsis should be evaluated for the presence of a focus of infection amenable to source-control measures, specifically drainage of an abscess or local focus of infection, débridement of

## CURRENT THERAPY

### Identify the Cause and Source of Infection

- Obtain suitable material for cultures, Gram stains, serologies, antigenic assays, and other diagnostic studies.
- Implement percutaneous or surgical drainage where appropriate.

### Initiate Appropriate Antibiotic Therapy

- Initial therapy is empiric, but tailored therapy should begin as soon as microbiological data are available.
- Survival is improved when the initial antibiotic therapy is effective against the isolated organism(s) and started early.

### Restore and Maintain Hemodynamic Function

- Implement an early goal-directed therapeutic approach.
- Fluids are the initial choice for volume resuscitation and may include crystalloids, colloids, volume expanders, or blood products.
- If hypotension and poor perfusion persist, then vasoactive agents should be used as necessary to ensure adequate hemodynamic function.
- Hemodynamic monitoring is often used to ensure the adequacy and effectiveness of therapy (arterial line, CVP, PA catheter).
- Physiologic dose corticosteroid replacement therapy may be beneficial for vasopressor-dependent patients who have an inadequate cortisol response.

### Provide Antithrombotic, Profibrinolytic, Anti-inflammatory Therapy

- Use drotrecogin alfa (activated) (Xigris) per package insert recommendations.

### Provide Metabolic Support

- Maintain early nutritional support.
- Maintain intestinal mucosa barrier function by the enteral route, the preferred method.
- Maintain tight glycemic control to decrease infectious complications; patient might need IV insulin therapy.

### Prevent Complications of Critical Illness

- Provide DVT prophylaxis.
- Prevent stress-related gastrointestinal bleeding.
- Prevent organ system dysfunction.
- Prevent nosocomial and secondary infections.
- Recognize critical illness polyneuropathy and myopathy.
- Anticipate anemia of critical illness.

*Abbreviations:* CVP = central venous pressure; DVT = deep vein thrombosis; PA = pulmonary artery.

**TABLE 1   Suggested Empiric Antibiotic Choices in Severe Sepsis**

| Likely Source of Infection | Antimicrobial Choice |
| --- | --- |
| Community-acquired pneumonia | Third-generation cephalosporin with a macrolide<br>Alternative: fluoroquinolones |
| Hospital-acquired pneumonia | Third- or fourth-generation cephalosporins, extended-spectrum penicillins ± an aminoglycoside<br>Alternatives: fluoroquinolones, carbapenems, β-lactam–β-lactamase inhibitors |
| Urinary tract infections | Extended-spectrum β-lactam agent ± an aminoglycoside<br>Add vancomycin (Vancocin) if MRSA is suspected<br>Add linezolid (Zylox) if VRE is suspected |
| Intraabdominal infections | Third- or fourth-generation cephalosporins with metronidazole (Flagyl) or clindamycin (Cleocin) *or*<br>Extended-spectrum penicillins or β-lactam–β-lactamase inhibitor ± an aminoglycoside or fluoroquinolones and metronidazole |
| Biliary tract infections | Extended-spectrum penicillin ± an aminoglycoside or fluoroquinolones |
| Neutropenic patients | Extended-spectrum β-lactam agent<br>Add vancomycin if MRSA is suspected<br>Add aminoglycoside or fluoroquinolone if *Pseudomonas aeruginosa* is suspected<br>Add a triazole antifungal or a β-glucan inhibitor if candidemia is suspected |

*Abbreviations:* MRSA = methicillin-resistant *Staphylococcus aureus*; VRE = vancomycin-resistant enterococci.

necrotic tissue, removal of a potentially infected device, or definite control of a source of ongoing microbial contamination. The source-control objective should be accomplished with the least invasive method; for example, percutaneous rather than surgical drainage should be used for abscess drainage, if possible.

## HEMODYNAMIC MANAGEMENT

Sepsis is characterized by vasodilative or distributive shock, and there is an increase in vascular capacitance along with the decrease in the systemic vascular resistance. Septic patients are functionally volume depleted in the intravascular space from increased permeability as a result of endothelial cell injury. Early recognition of significant hemodynamic derangements and restoration of normal tissue perfusion are vital to prevent organ dysfunction and failure. The goal of hemodynamic resuscitation should be to raise the mean arterial pressure above 65 mm Hg. The resuscitative efforts and the adequacy of tissue perfusion can be assessed at the bedside by monitoring heart rate, BP, orthostatic BP changes, mental status, hourly urine output, and skin perfusion.

The initial hemodynamic resuscitation should take the form of fluid for volume replacement. Debate continues regarding the appropriateness of colloid versus crystalloid fluids. Because the volume of distribution is much larger for crystalloids than for colloids, resuscitation with crystalloids requires about three times more fluid to achieve the same endpoints, and it results in more edema. The recent SAFE (Saline versus Albumin Fluid Evaluation) study indicated that albumin administration was indeed safe and as effective as crystalloid fluids. There was a nonsignificant decrease in mortality rates in a subset analysis of septic patients ($P = 0.09$). Previous meta-analyses of small studies of ICU patients had demonstrated no difference between crystalloid and colloid resuscitation. The lack of clear evidence of the benefit of colloid agents (albumin, dextran, and plasma expanders) and their high cost have generally resulted in the use of saline solutions for volume expansion.

**TABLE 2** Vasoactive Agents Commonly Used in Managing Severe Sepsis[1]

| Vasoactive Agent/ Receptor Activity | $\alpha_1$ | $\alpha_2$ | $\beta_1$ | $\beta_2$ | $V_1$ | $V_2$ | | | |
|---|---|---|---|---|---|---|---|---|---|
| Dopamine (Intropin) | 3+ | 3+ | 3+ | 2+ | | | <5 µg/kg/min | Vasodilation | Dopaminergic effects predominate Dilation of renal and mesenteric arteries Increased GFR and sodium excretion |
| | | | | | | | 5-10 µg/kg/min | ↑ Inotropy and chronotropy | β-Adrenergic effects predominate Increased CI, increased stroke volume |
| | | | | | | | >10 µg/kg/min | Vasoconstriction | α-Adrenergic effects predominate |
| Dobutamine (Dobutrex) | 1+ | | 3+ | 2+ | | 1+ | 2-20 µg/kg/min | ↑ Inotropy and chronotropy | 25% increase in CI decreases PAOP |
| Epinephrine | 3+ | 3+ | 3+ | 2+ | | 1+ | 0.1-0.5 µg/kg/min | ↑ Stroke volume and CI | Decrease splanchnic blood flow Increase oxygen consumption |
| Norepinephrine (Levophed) | 3+ | 2+ | 2+ | | | | 0.03-1.5 µg/kg/min | Vasoconstriction | Minimal change in heart rate or CI Can decrease lactate |
| Phenylephrine (Neo-Synephrine) | 3+ | | | | | | 0.5-8 µg/kg/min | Vasoconstriction | Increases MAP CI can decrease |
| Vasopressin (Pitressin)[1] | | | | | 1+ | | 0.01-0.04 U/min | Vasoconstriction | Vasoconstrictor effect on the up-regulated $V_1$, splanchnic vasoconstriction |

[1]Not FDA approved for this indication.
*Abbreviations:* CI = cardiac index; GFR = glomerular filtration rate; MAP. = mean aortic pressure; PAOP = pulmonary artery occluded pressure.

A delicate balance is required between maintaining tissue perfusion and preventing fluid overload, with its attendant risk of lung injury. Bolus infusions are typically administered using the clinical response or measurements of central venous pressure (CVP) or pulmonary capillary wedge pressure (PCWP) as a guide. A CVP of 8 to 12 mm Hg or a PCWP of 12 mm Hg is generally considered a reasonable resuscitation target.

Optimal fluid management in patients with acute lung injury is unknown. A recent large prospective, randomized study was performed to determine whether a liberal or a conservative strategy of fluid management was more effective in patients with established lung injury. Although there was no difference in 60-day mortality between the two treatment groups, patients in the group treated according to a conservative strategy of fluid management had significantly improved lung function and central nervous system function and a decreased need for sedation, mechanical ventilation, and intensive care.

Invasive vascular monitoring may be used to aid in determining adequate hemodynamic resuscitation. If a central venous catheter is present, the CVP can be measured to assess the adequacy of the intravascular volume status. In select patients with hemodynamic insufficiency, insertion of pulmonary artery catheters to measure the left-sided and right-sided filling pressures and the various hemodynamic parameters may be beneficial. The use of pulmonary artery catheters has declined because multiple randomized trials now indicate that pulmonary artery catheters are not useful for routine hemodynamic monitoring in critically ill patients and are associated with more complications than the CVC.

In shock states, estimation of blood pressure using a sphygmomanometer is commonly inaccurate. Insertion of an arterial line may be required, especially if the patient is unresponsive to initial volume resuscitation and requires the addition of vasopressor therapy for hemodynamic resuscitation.

## VASOPRESSOR MANAGEMENT

If adequate fluid resuscitation is insufficient to restore adequate hemodynamic function, then vasopressor or inotropic therapy, or both, will be necessary. There are a wide variety of vasoactive medications that are useful in the hemodynamic resuscitation of septic shock. Table 2 highlights the differences and advantages of some of the more commonly used agents. Despite a wide range of possible agents, dopamine (Intropin) and norepinephrine (Levophed) are typically used in most clinical units. Some centers prefer to use phenylephrine (Neo-Synephrine) in patients with tachycardia or a history of arrhythmias because this pure α-adrenergic agent causes less tachycardia and arrhythmia.

Unfortunately, there is a lack of large, prospective, randomized, protocol-controlled clinical trials that have compared dopamine and norepinephrine for managing patients who have septic shock. Dopamine has been the preferred agent in many units, in part because of its ease of use, the concept that it improves splanchnic and renal perfusion, and its safety record. Recent clinical trial results have revealed that there is no specific beneficial effect of renal dose dopamine in preventing the development of renal failure. A recent European observational study suggested that dopamine administration might actually be associated with increased mortality rates. Norepinephrine is a potent vasoconstrictor that also has some increased inotropic and chronotropic effects on the heart. A large observational study of French septic shock patients who required high doses of vasopressor therapy demonstrated a significant improvement in survival with the use of norepinephrine as compared with high doses of dopamine with or without the addition of epinephrine.

There has been renewed interest in the use of vasopressin (Pitressin)[1] in patients with vasodilative shock. The initial release of stored vasopressin from the posterior pituitary during hypotension depletes the body's store of the hormone. Unlike dopamine and epinephrine, vasopressin is a direct vasoconstrictor without inotropic or chronotropic effects. Vasopressin can lead to decreased cardiac output and hepatosplenic flow. Most published reports exclude patients from vasopressin treatment if the cardiac index is less than 2 to 2.5 L/min/m². Vasopressin should be used with caution in patients with cardiac dysfunction.

[1]Not FDA approved for this indication.

Some patients with severe sepsis and septic shock have a reversible biventricular myocardial dysfunction, which has been attributed to circulating TNF-α, IL-1, or nitric oxide that are elaborated as part of the SIRS response. Ventricular dilation and a reduced ejection fraction are the components of this myocardial depression. Inotropic agents such as dobutamine (Dobutrex) or epinephrine can improve the myocardial contractility and hemodynamic function in these patients. By increasing stroke volume and heart rate, dobutamine increases the cardiac index. Although epinephrine can also increase the cardiac index, its use should be limited in the septic patient because it can impair splanchnic blood flow and increase systemic and regional lactate concentrations.

## SUPPORT OXYGENATION AND VENTILATION

Abnormalities of the respiratory system are some of the most common evidence of organ system involvement in sepsis. Septic patients should be assessed for adequacy of oxygenation, oxygen delivery, ventilation, and the ability to protect the airway. Septic patients commonly have abnormalities of oxygenation and increased work of breathing. Patients who are hypoxemic should be given supplemental oxygen with a goal of achieving arterial oxygen saturation of at least 90%.

Another decision to make in caring for the septic patient is the need and timing for endotracheal intubation and ventilatory support. Acute lung injury (ALI) and acute respiratory distress syndrome (ARDS) are relatively common manifestations of pulmonary dysfunction in the patient with severe sepsis and septic shock. Up to 35% of septic patients present with ARDS. The goal of mechanical ventilation is to maintain the $PaO_2$ in the 55 to 70 mm Hg range while keeping the inspired oxygen concentration ($FiO_2$) below 60%. The traditional approach to mechanically ventilating patients who have ALI and ARDS has been to employ tidal volumes in the 10 to 15 mL/kg range. The Acute Respiratory Distress Syndrome Network (ARDSNet) trial used low tidal volume ventilation of 6 mL/kg ideal body weight, coupled with maintaining an end-inspiratory plateau pressure up to 30 cm $H_2O$ and a nomogram for positive end-expiratory pressure (PEEP) titration based on $FiO_2$ and oxygenation goals. This combination demonstrated an overall decrease in hospital mortality along with an increase in ventilator-free and organ failure–free days.

The risk of infection and ventilator-associated complications increases with the duration of ventilatory support. Patients should be removed from the ventilator as soon as they no longer need mechanical ventilatory support. The use of weaning protocols implemented by trained ICU support staff have been shown to speed the weaning process and improve the overall process of extubating the critically ill patient. It is also important to use sedation and analgesia appropriately in this critically ill population. Excessive sedation and analgesia have been linked to prolonged stays on mechanical ventilatory support and increased complications.

In a large multicenter controlled trial conducted in critically ill patients without ischemic cardiac disease or acute blood loss, the restrictive practice of packed red blood cell (RBC) transfusions in the management of anemia and low hemoglobin levels (7.0-9.0 g/dL) was shown to provide adequate oxygen delivery to the tissues. In a subgroup of younger patients and less ill patients, it was found to be associated with a lower mortality rate compared with a more liberal transfusion policy with hemoglobin levels maintained between 10.0 and 12.0 g/dL. Banked, stored RBCs are less deformable, are less efficient at releasing oxygen from their 2,3-diphosphoglycerate–depleted hemoglobin stores, and might have immunosuppressive effects. Aggressive use of packed RBC transfusions in an effort to achieve supernormal oxygen delivery states should be discouraged. The use of weekly recombinant erythropoietin (Epogen)[1] reduces the need for transfusions in critically ill patients but with no effect on clinical outcome, and therefore erythropoietin is not recommended as a standard treatment for anemia associated with severe sepsis.

## SUPPORTIVE CARE FOR THE CRITICALLY ILL PATIENT

Patients with severe sepsis and septic shock are critically ill and susceptible to the multiple complications common in the critically ill population. These complications include deep venous thrombosis (DVT) and pulmonary emboli, stress-related gastrointestinal bleeding, nosocomial infections, MODS, and critical illness polyneuropathy and myopathy.

Patients in the ICU who have sepsis or septic shock should receive prophylaxis for DVT with unfractionated heparin or low-molecular-weight heparin, unless they have contraindications to their use. Pneumatic compression devices may be used in patients who have a coagulopathy or increased risk of bleeding. In patients at high risk, such as those with severe sepsis and a history of DVT, trauma, or orthopedic surgery, a combination of pharmacologic and mechanical therapies is recommended unless contraindicated.

Prophylaxis for stress-related GI bleeding may be accomplished with $H_2$-receptor blockers,[1] proton pump inhibitors,[1] sucralfate (Carafate),[1] or early enteral feeding. Proper nutrition is important for maintaining the necessary immune function during the septic metabolic process. Enteral administration of nutrition can prevent stress-related GI bleeding and might prevent the translocation of bowel organisms or endotoxin by maintaining the integrity of the GI tract's mucosal barrier function.

Adequate nutrition is responsible for improved wound healing, decreased susceptibility of critically ill patients to infection, and optimized immune function. The following nutritional guidelines have been recommended for patients with sepsis:

- Daily caloric intake: 25 to 30 kcal/kg of usual body weight per day
- Protein: 1.3 to 2.0 g/kg per day
- Glucose: 30% to 70% of total nonprotein calories to maintain serum glucose lower than 150 mg/dL
- Lipids: 15% to 30% of total nonprotein calories
- Omega-6 polyunsaturated fatty acids: Reduce in septic patients, maintaining a level that prevents deficiency of essential fatty acids (7% of total calories)—generally 1 g/kg/day

Metabolic management also includes correction of electrolyte abnormalities as well as tight control of blood sugar, which might require constant insulin infusion. In medical and surgical ICU patients, tight glucose control aimed at keeping the blood sugar between 80 and 110 mg/dL was associated with a significant improvement in ICU and hospital survival. Tight glucose control should be the goal in critically ill patients if careful monitoring for prevention of hypoglycemia can be maintained.

## INNOVATIVE THERAPIES

### Corticosteroid Therapy

Experimental studies in animal models of sepsis and septic shock have demonstrated improved survival using pretreatment or early treatment with high doses of corticosteroids. As a result of multiple failed trials of high-dose steroids in patients with severe sepsis, this treatment practice has largely been abandoned.

Recently, the observation that basal cortisol levels and the cortisol response to the administration of adrenocorticotropic hormone (ACTH)[1] could predict survival in patients with severe sepsis and septic shock has renewed interest in steroid therapy. In a French study, patients who had septic shock and an intact pituitary-adrenal axis had a 74% survival rate. In comparison, patients who had impaired adrenal function, had a basal cortisol level of more than 34 μg/dL, and were unable to increase their cortisol level by at least 9 μg/dL had an 18% survival rate. Researchers hypothesized that patients with septic shock have a state of relative adrenal insufficiency and would benefit from the use of more physiologic corticosteroid replacement therapy.

---

[1]Not FDA approved for this indication.

[1]Not FDA approved for this indication.

A recent multicenter prospective randomized, controlled trial of 300 patients with vasopressor-dependent septic shock demonstrated an improved survival rate in patients with impaired adrenal function who were given physiologic corticosteroid replacement therapy. Subjects were given a stress dose of 50 mg of hydrocortisone (Solu-Cortef)[1] intravenously every 6 hours for 7 days combined with a once-daily oral dose of 50 μg of fludrocortisone (Florinef).

More recently, a randomized, double-blind clinical trial of patients with persistent ARDS found no beneficial effect of corticosteroids on survival in the hospital. Furthermore, the initiation of methylprednisolone (Solu-Medrol)[1] 2 or more weeks after the onset of ARDS was associated with an increased mortality rate as compared with that in the placebo group. Patients in the methylprednisolone group were able to breathe without assistance earlier than were patients in the placebo group, but they were also more likely to resume assisted ventilation. Possible explanations for this effect include complications of corticosteroid therapy, such as neuropathy; complications related to the withdrawal of steroids, including shock; and pulmonary parenchymal causes of hypoxemic respiratory failure, such as recrudescence of fibroproliferation as a result of corticosteroid withdrawal.

### High-Volume Continuous Venovenous Hemofiltration Therapy

The use of high-volume, continuous hemofiltration (either continuous arteriovenous or venovenous) benefits the hemodynamic course and outcome in patients with intractable circulatory failure resulting from septic shock. This form of management is expensive, requires defined expertise, and may be associated with metabolic and coagulation abnormalities. Further studies are needed to determine if this mode of therapy improves outcome in septic patients. Its use should probably be limited to patients with renal indications for hemofiltration.

### Antithrombotic Therapy

New therapies have been directed toward inhibitors of the coagulation system as a potential therapeutic strategy for patients with severe sepsis and septic shock. Among the therapies currently in use or under investigation are antithrombin tissue factor pathway inhibitor and recombinant human activated protein C.

The protein C system is one of the endogenous antithrombotic agents. Drotrecogin alfa (activated) (Xigris) is the recombinant form of human activated protein C. Two international multicenter controlled trials of drotrecogin alfa, the Recombinant Human Activated Protein C Worldwide Evaluation of Severe Sepsis (PROWESS) and Administration of Drotrecogin alfa (activated) in Early Stage Severe Sepsis (ADDRESS) trials, have produced inconsistent results. Drotrecogin alfa was approved on the basis of the favorable results of the PROWESS study, a phase III trial that demonstrated a significant survival benefit in 1690 patients with severe sepsis and septic shock. Treatment with a 96-hour infusion of drotrecogin alfa produced a 6.1% absolute risk reduction and a 19.4% relative risk reduction in the 28-day all-cause mortality in patients with severe sepsis ($P = 0.005$). The drotrecogin alfa–treated population experienced more serious bleeding complications (3.5%) compared with the placebo group (2.0%). The number needed to treat to save an additional life was 16.

The U.S. Food and Drug Administration (FDA) and 19 other regulatory bodies in other countries (including the European Union) have approved drotrecogin alfa to treat severe sepsis in adult patients with a high risk of mortality. The FDA gives the example of using the Acute Physiology and Chronic Health Evaluation (APACHE) II to estimate the risk of death (APACHE II score 25), and other regulatory agencies use sepsis-induced multiorgan failure as an indication for its use. Drotrecogin alfa is contraindicated in patients with known sensitivity to drotrecogin alfa and in patients with a high risk of death from or significant morbidity associated with bleeding.

However, the recently published ADDRESS trial demonstrated no evidence of benefit of drotrecogin alfa in patients with severe sepsis and at low risk of death. The results of the ADDRESS trial also failed to confirm the observation made in the PROWESS trial of a large reduction in mortality among patients with APACHE II scores of 25 or higher, although the number of patients (324) in this group was too small for a meaningful statistic comparison. Further trials of drotrecogin alfa in prospectively defined high-risk patients are required to clarify its optimal role in management of severe sepsis.

## Intensive Care of Patients with HIV Infection

Antiretroviral therapy has increased the life expectancy of patients who are infected with HIV and has reduced the incidence of illnesses associated with AIDS. However, the incidence of pulmonary, cardiac, gastrointestinal, and renal diseases that are often not directly related to underlying HIV disease has increased. Although the guiding principles of management in the ICU pertain to critically ill patients with HIV infection, antiretroviral therapy and unresolved questions regarding its use in the ICU add an additional level of complexity to already complicated cases.

Patients who are receiving antiretroviral therapy with evidence of virologic suppression (plasma HIV RNA below the limit of detection) before admission to the ICU should continue their antiretroviral regimen, if possible. Patients who continue to receive treatment should have no contraindications to continuation of treatment, such as major interactions between drugs used in the ICU and antiretroviral therapy. Drug interactions are particularly common and can be severe with hepatically metabolized agents via cytochrome P-450 3A (CYP 3A). In contrast, the benefits of continued antiretroviral therapy in the ICU are less clear for patients with detectable plasma HIV RNA. For these patients, practitioners should consult with an HIV expert.

Patients who did not receive antiretroviral therapy before ICU admission are the largest subgroup of patients with HIV infection admitted to the ICU. Initiation of antiretroviral therapy should be deferred in patients admitted to the ICU who have a condition that is not associated with AIDS. In these patients, the immediate prognosis is generally better than in those who have an AIDS-associated diagnosis, and the short-term outcome is most likely related to successful treatment of the underlying non-AIDS condition. However, antiretroviral therapy should be considered in patients whose CD4 cell count is less than 200 cells/mm[3] and whose stay in the ICU is prolonged. The risk of opportunistic infection is increased in patients whose CD4 count is less than 200 cells/mm[3]. For such patients, prophylaxis against opportunistic infections should also be prescribed (e.g., trimethoprim-sulfamethoxazole for *Pneumocystis* pneumonia), as recommended in current guidelines.

In contrast, antiretroviral therapy should be considered for patients who are admitted to the ICU with an AIDS-associated diagnosis. This recommendation especially applies to patients whose physiologic condition is worsening despite optimal ICU management and treatment for the AIDS-associated condition. Patients who receive antiretroviral therapy should be followed for development of the immune reconstitution syndrome.

## Prognosis

Despite the tremendous advances in the care of septic patients, the mortality rate for patients with severe sepsis and septic shock remains high. Mortality rates attributable to severe sepsis and septic shock remain in the 20% to 50% range. Factors associated with adverse outcome include advanced age, comorbid conditions, respiratory site of infection, virulent organisms, severity of illness, the number of organ system failures, and specific organ systems failing. In addition, a patient's genetic makeup or gender can have a dramatic impact on whether the patient develops sepsis as well as on the severity, clinical manifestations, and outcome of the sepsis. Survivors of sepsis have increased 6- and 12-month mortality rates compared with critically ill

---

[1]Not FDA approved for this indication.

patients who do not have sepsis. Patients who have survived an episode of sepsis have a reduced quality of life and more health-related issues. These observations underscore the importance of early aggressive management of the septic patient and suggest that our future focus should also be directed toward prevention of sepsis.

## REFERENCES

Dellinger RP, Carlet JM, Masur H, et al: Surviving Sepsis campaign guidelines for management of severe sepsis and septic shock. Crit Care Med 2004;32(3):858-873. Guidelines are also available at http://www.surviv-ingsepsis.org/node/156 (accessed April 18, 2007).

Friedrich JO, Adhikari NK, Meade MO: Drotrecogin alfa (activated): Does current evidence support treatment for any patients with severe sepsis? Crit Care 2006;10(3):145.

Huang L, Quartin A, Jones D, Havlir DV: Intensive care of patients with HIV infection. N Engl J Med 2006;355(2):173-181.

Kumar A, Roberts D, Wood KE, et al: Duration of hypotension before initiation of effective antimicrobial therapy is the critical determinant of survival in human septic shock. Crit Care Med 2006;34(6):1589-1596.

Martin GS, Mannino DM, Eaton S, et al: The epidemiology of sepsis in the United States from 1979 through 2000. N Engl J Med 2003;348:1546-1554.

Sakr Y, Reinhart K, Vincent JL, et al: Does dopamine administration in shock influence outcome? Results of the Sepsis Occurrence in Acutely Ill Patients (SOAP) Study. Crit Care Med 2006;34(3):589-597.

Steinberg KP, Hudson LD, Goodman RB, et al: Efficacy and safety of corticosteroids for persistent acute respiratory distress syndrome. N Engl J Med 2006;354(16):1671-1684.

Van den Burghe G, Wilmer A, Hermans G, et al: Intensive insulin therapy in the medical ICU. N Engl J Med 2006;354:449-461.

Wheeler AP, Bernard GR, Thompson BT, et al. Pulmonary-artery versus central venous catheter to guide treatment of acute lung injury. N Engl J Med 2006;354(21):2213-2224.

Wiedemann HP, Wheeler AP, Bernard GR, et al: Comparison of two fluid-management strategies in acute lung injury. N Engl J Med 2006;354(24):2564-2575.

# Brucellosis

Method of
*Basak Dokuzoguz, MD, and Nurcan Baykam, MD*

Brucellosis is a common bacterial zoonotic disease. It has become more significant in recent years as a bioterrorism agent. Brucellosis is known as a historic disease, and the sequencing of the *Brucella melitensis* genome was completed in 2002.

## Etiology

The disease is caused by bacteria of the genus *Brucella*, which are nonmotile, gram-negative, aerobic, unencapsulated cocci or short rods. *Brucella* species are divided into six subtypes based on the main host animals (Table 1). Of these, *B. abortus*, *B. melitensis*, *B. suis*, and *B. canis* are known human pathogens. Two new species, provisionally called *B. pinnipediae* and *B. cetaceae*, have been shown to cause human diseases.

## Epidemiology

Brucellosis is one of the major zoonotic diseases and occurs all over the world. Some countries in Europe and North America have achieved control and prevention of the disease based on vaccination programs. However, brucellosis remains endemic in other parts of the world, especially in the Mediterranean, the Middle East, Central Asia, Africa, and Latin America. The real incidence of the disease is not

**TABLE 1   Subtypes and Hosts of *Brucella* Species**

| Species | Host Animal | Human |
|---|---|---|
| *B. abortus* | Cows, camels, yaks, buffalo | + |
| *B. melitensis* | Goats, sheep, camels | + |
| *B. suis* | Pigs, wild hares, caribou, reindeer, wild rodents | + |
| *B. canis* | Canines | + |
| *B. neotomae* | Rodents | – |
| *B. ovis* | Sheep | – |
| *B. pinnipediae* | Minke whales, dolphins | + |
| *B. cetaceae* | Seals | + |

known because underreporting of the disease is believed to be common.

The most common causes of human brucellosis are reported as *B. melitensis* followed by *B. abortus*. The biotypes of *Brucella* species vary by geographic region.

The disease is transmitted to humans by direct contact with infected animals, by ingestion of raw or unpasteurized milk and milk products, through cuts and abrasions, or by inhalation of aerosols. It is an occupational disease of farmers, veterinarians, slaughterhouse workers, and health care workers, especially laboratory staff. Some individual cases occur as a result of ingesting contaminated dairy products, handling infected animal tissue or body fluids, or handling aborted animal fetuses and placentas. However, the transmission route for outbreaks is usually inhalation of aerosols. Human-to-human transmission of brucellosis is very rare, but there are a few case reports of humans infected through sexual contact, transplacental transmission, or transplantation.

## Pathogenesis

The *Brucella* species are pathogenic for humans and animals. *Brucella* species prefer to survive and multiply within phagocytic cells of the host. Unlike other pathogenic bacteria, they do not have classic virulence factors such as exotoxins, cytolysins, capsules, fimbria, plasmids, and endotoxic lipopolysaccharides. Instead of these factors, the bacteria have molecular determinants that are necessary for cell invasion and survival in the cellular compartment. The major one of these molecular determinants is S lipopolysaccharide (S LPS).

The bacteria are phagocytosed by M cells, macrophages, and neutrophils after invasion of mucosa. Fc receptors, complement, lectin, and fibronectin receptors mediate the bacteria for internalization. Most intracellular *Brucella* species are eliminated in phagolysosomes, but some of them reproduce in the acidic compartment. The intracellular mechanism of the organism is not completely described, but intracellular replication of bacteria does not destroy the cell or the cell's function.

After they are taken up by local tissue lymphocytes, the bacteria disseminate into the circulation, and with tropism to the reticuloendothelial system, they become localized within bone marrow, liver, spleen, and lymph nodes. The characteristic feature of the disease is the formation of granulomas in these tissues.

As a host humoral immune response to the disease, the titers of IgM antibodies increase within the first week of infection, and IgG synthesis follows after the second week. Cell-mediated immunity is probably the main mechanism for recovery from the infection.

## Clinical Features

Human brucellosis is a multisystem disease that can manifest with a broad spectrum of clinical features. The musculoskeletal, genital, cardiac, respiratory, and nervous systems are involved. The definition and the classification of cases recommended by the World Health Organization (WHO) is presented in Box 1. Some authors classify the disease course as acute, subacute, or chronic, but such a classification has no clinical significance.

## BOX 1 Recommended Case Definitions and Classifications by the World Health Organization

### Clinical Description

An illness characterized by acute or insidious onset, with continued, intermittent, or irregular fever of variable duration; profuse sweating, particularly at night; fatigue; anorexia; weight loss; headache; arthralgia and generalized aching. Local infection of various organs can occur.

### Laboratory Criteria for Diagnosis

- Isolation of *Brucella* spp. from clinical specimen *or*
- Brucella agglutination titer (e.g., standard tube agglutination tests: STA >160) in one or more serum specimens obtained after onset of symptoms *or*
- ELISA (IgA, IgG, IgM), 2-mercaptoethanol test, complement fixation test, Coombs' test, fluorescent antibody test (FAB), radioimmunoassay for detecting antilipopolysaccharide antibodies, counterimmunoelectrophoresis (CIE)

### Case Classification

#### Suspected

A case that is compatible with the clinical description and is epidemiologically linked to suspected or confirmed animal cases or contaminated animal products.

#### Probable

A suspected case that has a positive rose bengal test.

#### Confirmed

A suspected or probable case that is laboratory confirmed.

*Abbreviations:* ELISA = enzyme-linked immunosorbent assay; Ig = immunoglobulin.

## TABLE 2 Clinical Presentation and Laboratory Findings of Human Brucellosis

| Feature | Percentage |
|---|---|
| **Signs and Symptoms** | |
| Fever | 72-91 |
| Constitutive symptoms (e.g., malaise, arthralgias) | 26-90 |
| Hepatic involvement | 17-31 |
| Splenomegaly | 14-16 |
| Osteoarticular involvement | 9-22 |
| CNS disorder | 3-13 |
| Lymphadenopathy | 2-7 |
| Genitourinary involvement | 1-5.7 |
| Respiratory disorders | 0.2-6 |
| Cardiovascular disorders | 0.4-1.8 |
| Skin rashes | 0.4-3 |
| **Laboratory Findings** | |
| *Hematologic* | |
| Relative lymphocytosis | 40 |
| Anemia | 31 |
| Leukopenia | 2-27 |
| Thrombocytopenia | 5-15 |
| Pancytopenia | 2 |
| *Biochemistry* | |
| Elevated transaminase | 24-31 |

*Abbreviation:* CNS, central nervous system.
Data derived from Aygen B, Doganay M, Sümerkan B, et al: Clinical manifestations, complications and treatment of brucellosis: An evaluation of 480 patients. Med Mal Infect 2002;32:485-493; Dokuzoguz B, Ergonul O, Baykam N, et al: Characteristics of *B. melitensis* versus *B. abortus* bacteremias. J Infect 2005;50(1):1-5; Pappas G, Akritidis N, Bosilkovski M, Tsianos E: Brucellosis. N Engl J Med 2005;352:2325-2336.

The onset of symptoms can be insidious or acute after the incubation period, which is 2 to 8 weeks. A broad spectrum of symptoms such as fever, headache, back pain, weakness, profuse sweating, chills, depression, and joint pain can be observed. These symptoms can also mimic various infectious and noninfectious diseases. Usually an undulant fever pattern is accompanied by so much sweating that the patient needs to change clothes frequently. On the other hand, the physical examination might not reveal any specific finding (Table 2). In children, the range of clinical signs and symptoms may be different than in adults, because children have fewer constitutional symptoms but more hepatic and splenic involvement.

Hepatomegaly, elevated transaminase levels, and granulomatous lesions are the presentations of hepatic involvement in brucellosis. The most common complication of brucellosis is osteoarticular disease, which occurs as peripheral arthritis, sacroiliitis, and spondylitis. This complication is reported in 10% to 80% of cases, and this range may be related to the age and genetic predisposition (HLA-B39) of patients and the infecting *Brucella* species. Genitourinary system involvements exist in 2% to 20% of patients with brucellosis. Prostatitis, epididymoorchitis, cystitis, pyelonephritis, interstitial nephritis, exudative glomerulonephritis, and renal abscess are the clinical manifestations of this complication. Neurobrucellosis can develop at any stage of disease and can have widely variable manifestations, including encephalitis, meningoencephalitis, radiculitis, myelitis, peripheral and cranial neuropathies, subarachnoid hemorrhage, and psychiatric manifestations. Brucellosis can cause a variety of ocular lesions and different types of skin rash that are nonspecific and reported rarely. Another rare (<2%) but severe complication of brucellosis is endocarditis, which most often involves the aortic valve and requires surgery. Mortality from brucellosis is rare and is usually related to endocarditis.

## Diagnosis

The absolute diagnosis of brucellosis is based on identification of bacteria from blood, bone marrow, and materials from affected organs such as cerebrospinal fluid, liver, lymph nodes, synovial fluid, or prostatic fluid by culture. The rate of bacteria isolation from the blood is between 15% and 70%. Lysis centrifugation technique and automated systems improve the range of culture positivity.

Compatible clinical findings with a serum agglutinin titer of at least 1/160 in the standard tube agglutination test (STA) have diagnostic value. In endemic areas, the titer of at least 1/320 is recommended in the

 **CURRENT DIAGNOSIS**

- The common symptoms of brucellosis, which can also mimic various infectious and noninfectious diseases, are fever, headache, back pain, weakness, profuse sweating, chills, depression, and joint pain.
- The absolute diagnosis of brucellosis is based on identification of bacteria from blood, bone marrow, and materials of affected organs such as cerebrospinal fluid, liver, lymph nodes, synovial fluid, and prostatic fluid by culture.
- Compatible clinical findings with a serum agglutinin titer of ≥1/160 in the standard tube agglutination test (STA) have diagnostic value.

diagnosis. False-negative results of STA may be attributed to blocking antibodies; results can be improved by testing with 2-mercaptoethanol or antihuman immunoglobulin. Negative results in the early phase of the disease can be overcome by repeating the test after 2 weeks. Diagnosis of *B. canis* infection is unavailable with routine STA. False-positive results may be related to cross-reactions of some gram-negative bacterial infections.

Enzyme-linked immunosorbent assay (ELISA) is another serologic test that has higher specificity and sensitivity compared with STA. Although it is not used in current clinical practice because of standardization problems, polymerase chain reaction (PCR) is a promising diagnostic tool in brucellosis. Duration of diagnosis can be shortened by automated culture systems and PCR techniques. Rose bengal and a new dipstick test are also rapid tests useful for early diagnosis, but positive results should be confirmed by STA.

# Treatment

Because the *Brucella* species are intracellular pathogens, treatment requires not only combined regimens for their synergistic effect but also agents with good penetration into the macrophages. For success of the therapy, adequate duration of drug therapy is another important factor. At least 6 weeks of drug therapy is recommended by the WHO. This duration may be extended to 6 months, depending on such complications of the disease as neurobrucellosis, spondylodiskitis, and abscesses.

The drug combinations listed in Table 3 are widely used in brucellosis. Rifampin (Rifadin)[1] plus doxycycline (Vibramycin) treatment for human brucellosis was recommended by WHO two decades ago; it is still a favorable regimen and was found to be the most synergistic one. Rifampin may be replaced by streptomycin or gentamycin (Garamycin)[1] as first-line therapy choices. Combinations with trimethoprim-sulfamethoxazole (TMP-SMX, Bactrim)[1] is usually recommended in second-line treatment regimens. Combination rifampin plus a quinolone[1] is not preferred in the initial therapeutic regimen because of the reported decreased activity in pH 5 and lack of synergism between quinolones and other antibiotics that are used in brucellosis. Quinolones are alternative drugs for patients who have relapses or who have side effects from first-line drugs.

Rifampin[1] in combination with TMP-SMX[1] or an aminoglycoside are the main regimens for children younger than 8 years. The rifampin and TMP-SMX combination may be prescribed for pregnant patients.

Although the use of ceftriaxone (Rocephin)[1] is controversial in brucellosis, it may be preferred for treating central nervous system involvement. Because their activity is decreased in an acidic environment, macrolides are not used in brucellosis treatment.

Because there are no significantly important resistance problems for antibiotics targeted to *Brucella* species, susceptibility tests are not recommended routinely except in epidemiologic studies and for some

---

[1]Not FDA approved for this indication.

## TABLE 3 Drug Combinations Used to Treat Brucellosis

| Generic Name (Trade Name) | Adult Dose | Pediatric Dose | Dose Adjustment Renal Failure | Dose Adjustment Hepatic Insuffiency | Adverse Effects |
|---|---|---|---|---|---|
| Ciprofloxacin[1] (Cipro) | 500-750 mg PO q12h *or* 400 mg IVq8-12h | Not suggested | Necessary | No change | Drug fever, rash, seizures, Achilles tendon rupture or tendinitis |
| Doxycycline (Vibramycin, Vibra-tabs) | 100 mg PO q12h | 2.2-4.4 mg/kg[3] PO div. q12h (≥8 y) | No change | No change | Nausea, vomiting, eosinophilia, photosensitivity |
| Gentamicin[1] (Garamycin) | 2 mg/kg IM/IV q8h *or* 5 mg/kg IM /IV q24h[1] *or* 240 mg q24h | 2.5 mg/kg q8-12h IM/IV | Necessary | No change; blockade (rapid infusion) | Ototoxicity, nephrotoxicity, neuromuscular |
| Ofloxacin[1] (Floxin, Oflox) | 400 mg PO bid | Not suggested | Necessary | Moderate: no change Severe: necessary | Drug fever, rash, mild neuroexcitatory symptoms |
| Rifampin[1] (Rifadin, Rimactane) | 600-900 mg PO qd | 20 mg/kg PO qd Do not exceed 600 mg qd | No change | Moderate: caution Severe: avoid | Red/orange discoloration of body secretions, flu-like symptoms, elevated AST/ALT, drug fever, rash, thrombocytopenia |
| Streptomycin | 15 mg/kg IM q24h *or* 1 g IM qd for 2-3 wk | 20-40 mg/kg IM qd Do not exceed 1g qd | Necessary | No change | Ototoxic, nephrotoxic |
| TMP-SMX[1] (Bactrim, Septra) | 1 DS tab PO q12h (160 mg TMP/ 800 mg SMX) | 8-12 mg/kg TMP PO q12h | Necessary; avoid use | No change | Folate deficiency, hyperkalemia, leukopenia, thrombocytopenia, hemolytic anemia ± G6PD, aplastic anemia, elevated AST/ALT, hypersensitivity reactions (Stevens-Johnson syndrome, erythema multiforme) |

[1]Not FDA approved for this indication.
[3]Exceeds dosage recommended by the manufacturer.
*Abbreviations:* ALT = alanine aminotransferase; AST = aspartate aminotransferase; DS = double strength; G6PD = glucose-6-phosphate dehydrogenase; TMP-SMX = trimethoprim-sulfamethoxazole.

## CURRENT THERAPY

- The treatment requires combined regimens for their synergistic effect plus agents with good penetration capacity into the macrophages.
- At least 6 weeks of therapy may be extended to 6 months, according to the complications of the disease.
- Rifampin (Rifadin)[1] plus doxycycline (Vibramycin) treatment is a favorable regimen and the most synergistic one.
- Rifampin may be replaced by streptomycin or gentamycin (Garamycin)[1] as the first-line therapy choice.
- Combinations with trimethoprim-sulfamethoxazole (TMP-SMX; Bactrim)[1] is usually recommended in the second-line treatment regimens.
- Quinolones[1] are alternative drugs in cases with side effects due to first-line drugs and relapses.
- Rifampin in a combination with TMP-SMX[1] or an aminoglycoside are the main regimens for children younger than 8 years.
- Rifampin and TMP-SMX[1] combination is preferred in pregnancy
- Although the use of ceftriaxone (Rocephin)[1] is controversial in brucellosis, it could be preferred in the treatment of central nervous system involvement.
- Rifampin[1] (600-900 mg qd) plus doxycycline (100 mg bid) regimen for 2-3 weeks is recommended as postexposure prophylaxis.

[1]Not FDA approved for this indication.

## REFERENCES

Aygen B, Doganay M, Sümerkan B, et al: Clinical manifestations, complications and treatment of brucellosis: An evaluation of 480 patients. Med Mal Infect 2002;32:485-493.
Baykam N, Esener H, Ergonul O, et al: In vitro antimicrobial susceptibility of *Brucella* species. Int J Antimicrob Agents 2004;23(4):405-407.
Bossi P, Tegnell A, Baka A, et al: Bichat guidelines for the clinical management of brucellosis and bioterrorism-related brucellosis. Euro Surveill 2004;9(12):E15-E16.
Dokuzoguz B, Ergonul O, Baykam N, et al: Characteristics of *B. melitensis* versus *B. abortus* bacteremias. J Infect 2005;50(1):1-5.
Eren S, Bayam G, Ergonul O, et al: Cognitive and emotional changes in neurobrucellosis. J Infect. 2006;53:184-189.
Ergonul O, Celikbas A, Tezeren D, et al: Analysis of risk factors for laboratory-acquired *Brucella* infections. J Hosp Infect 2004;56:223-227
Falagas ME. Bliziotis IA: Quinolones for treatment of human brucellosis: Critical review of the evidence from microbiological and clinical studies. Antimicrob Agents Chemother 2006;50(1):22-33.
Giannacopoulos I, Nikolakopoulou NM, Eliopoulou M, et al: Presentation of childhood brucellosis in Western Greece. Jpn J Infect Dis 2006;59:160-163.
Joint Food and Agriculture Organization/World Health Organization: FAO-WHO Expert Committee on Brucellosis (sixth report). WHO Technical Report Series No. 740. Geneva: World Health Organization, 1986, pp 56-57.
Pan American Health Organization: Case definition: Brucellosis. Epidemiol Bull 2000;21(3):13. PDF available at http://www.paho.org/english/dd/ais/EB_v21n3.pdf (Accessed April 27, 2007).
Pappas G, Akritidis N, Bosilkovski M, Tsianos E: Brucellosis. N Engl J Med 2005;352:2325-2336.
Young EJ. *Brucella* species In Mandel GL, Bennett JE, Dolin R (eds): Mandell, Douglas and Bennett's Principles and Practice of Infectious Diseases, 6th ed. Philadelphia: Churchill Livingstone, 2005, pp 2669-2672.

rare recurrent cases. Most of the recurrences are related to noncompliance or to short duration of therapy. In tuberculosis-endemic populations, community-acquired rifampin resistance should be taken into consideration in treating brucellosis.

Supportive therapy might be useful depending on the clinical situation. The cognitive and emotional disturbances in neurobrucellosis can be improved by antibiotics without any antidepressant or antipsychotic therapy.

In the management of *Brucella* endocarditis, medical treatment alone is often effective in patients with early diagnosis and no cardiac failure. However, in most cases, surgery is required in addition to medical treatment.

## Prevention

Various vaccines have been applied to humans in some countries in the 20th century, but an acceptable vaccine has not yet been developed for humans. Although investigations of the *B. melitensis* outer membrane protein 25 and cytoplasmic protein BP26 are promising for future vaccine development, prevention of the disease in humans is related to controlling and eliminating animal brucellosis. In this respect, vaccination and slaughter programs of animals, pasteurization of milk and milk products, and education programs about contact precautions for persons at risk must be emphasized.

Because *Brucella* bacteria can be transmitted via the inhalational route, laboratory workers should be warned about the risk, and biosafety level 2 prevention measures should be applied.

Because of laboratory accidents and biological warfare, rifampin[1] (600-900 mg qd) plus doxycycline (100 mg bid) for 2 to 3 weeks is recommended as postexposure prophylaxis.

[1]Not FDA approved for this indication.

# Varicella (Chickenpox)

Method of
*Charles Grose, MD*

Chickenpox is caused by varicella zoster virus (VZV). After chickenpox occurs, VZV enters the sensory nerve and establishes latency in the dorsal root ganglia along the spinal cord. When VZV reactivates in late adulthood, the virus causes the disease known as shingles (herpes zoster).

## Pathogenesis of Chickenpox

Chickenpox is an airborne infection. The virus first infects the mucosa tissues of the nose and subsequently establishes an infection in the tonsils or lymph nodes around the neck. After 4 to 6 cycles of replication, the primary viremia occurs (Figure 1). The virus then disperses to

## CURRENT DIAGNOSIS

- Diagnosis of chickenpox is usually made by observation or rash.
- Diagnosis is confirmed by a rapid viral diagnosis kit performed on a vesicle smear.
- Diagnosis of past varicella infection is made by serology.
- Commercial antibody kits may not be sensitive enough to detect serum antibody after varicella vaccination.

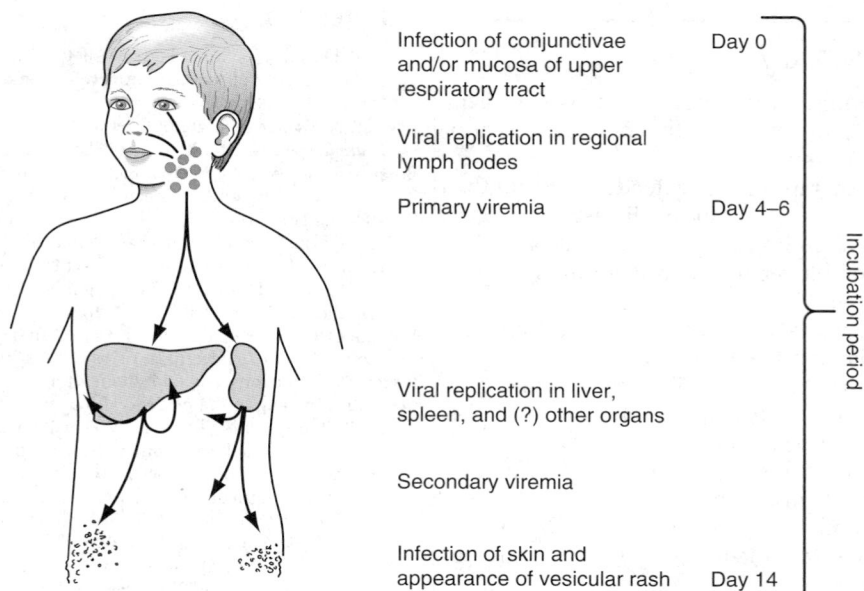

**FIGURE 1.** Diagrammatic representation of the pathogenesis of acute varicella infection. There are two viremias during the 14-day incubation period. The first viremia occurs after local replication at the site of infection. The typical chickenpox rash appears at the end of the second viremia. See Grose (2005) for a more detailed description.

multiple organs in the body. After a second period of replication, the second viremia occurs. The virus is carried within lymphocytes in the bloodstream. The vesicular lesions occur after the virus exits the capillaries and enters the epidermis.

# Epidemiology after Approval of the Vaccine

The varicella vaccine was approved for administration to children in the United States in 1995, and the vast majority of states have approved the administration of varicella vaccine to all young children. Approximately 4 million cases of chickenpox occurred annually in the United States prior to 1995. There were also approximately 100 deaths annually, the vast majority in otherwise healthy children, and more than 14,000 hospitalizations per year.

More than 10 years later, the effect of universal varicella immunization in the United States is dramatic. The number of hospitalizations and deaths was reduced by 75%. Similarly, the total number of cases of chickenpox in the United States has also decreased dramatically. Nevertheless, more than one half million cases of chickenpox will probably continue to occur annually. These cases will include many immunocompromised children who remain unimmunized.

## ADMINISTRATION OF VARICELLA VACCINE

Varicella vaccine is a live attenuated virus. Each dose of vaccine (0.5 mL) is administered subcutaneously. The virus must replicate in the infected child for an immune response to occur (Figure 2). The initial virus replication can cause a few vesicles near the site of infection. The replication can also lead to a viremia with a short-lived rash anywhere on the body. The vaccine virus can, in very few cases, replicate to a sufficient extent that the infection transfers to another person who will subsequently develop a mild case of vaccine-related chickenpox. In 1995, a single dose of varicella vaccine was originally recommended. As of 2007, two doses of varicella vaccine are recommended for every child. The first dose is given between 12 and 15 months. The second dose is routinely recommended between 4 and 6 years. Instead of single-dose vials of vaccine (Varivax), the vaccine can also be administered as a component of the 4-in-1 vials of measles-mumps-rubella-varicella vaccine (Pro Quad). This approach reduces the number of injections

given to a child. Children 13 years and above, who have never received varicella vaccine, should be given 2 doses of vaccine (Varivax), separated by a 4-week interval.

## RISK FACTORS FOR BREAKTHROUGH CHICKENPOX

Breakthrough chickenpox refers to a wild-type chickenpox that is usually a mild illness with less than 50 vesicles that occurs in children

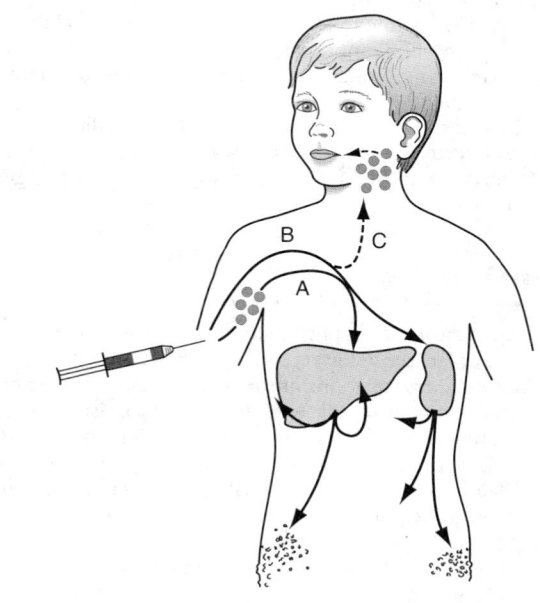

**FIGURE 2.** Pathways of infection following administration of varicella vaccine. Pathway A shows a rash that sometimes appears at the site of injection after local replication of the virus. Pathway B shows a viremia with appearance of a few small papulovesicular lesions on the skin distant from the site of injection. Pathway C shows the virus as it travels to the respiratory tract where infection can be spread on rare occasions to other individuals. See Grose (2005) for a more detailed description.

given varicella vaccine at least 42 days previously. Thus, breakthrough chickenpox is a form of vaccine failure. Breakthrough chickenpox was believed to be relatively uncommon during the prelicensure clinical studies. However, by 2000 it was apparent that breakthrough chickenpox was not a rare event. Several reports documented large outbreaks of wild-type chickenpox in immunized children who were attending large daycare facilities or grade schools.

A major risk factor is believed to be immunization with one dose of vaccine. The 2-dose regimen of varicella vaccine should eliminate most cases of breakthrough chickenpox.

## Treatment

### TREATMENT OF SEVERE CHICKENPOX IN HEALTHY CHILDREN

Chickenpox is considered a more severe disease in children younger than 1 year and in postpubertal adolescents. VZV is highly susceptible to acyclovir and two second-generation antiviral agents: famciclovir (Famvir) and valacyclovir (Valtrex). Acyclovir is now a generic drug and very economic. Every case of chickenpox in a child younger than 1 year should be treated with acyclovir. The oral dosage is 20 mg/kg four times a day for 5 to 7 days. Chickenpox in children older than 1 year can also be treated with acyclovir to reduce the severity and duration of disease. The maximum dosage is 800 mg four times a day. Acyclovir is available in a liquid suspension and tablets containing 200, 400, or 800 mg. The 800-mg tablet is very large and may be difficult for some children to swallow.

Famciclovir (Famvir) or valacyclovir (Valtrex) are the preferred antiviral agents for adolescents because these are better adsorbed than acyclovir. However, they are much more expensive. The dosage of famciclovir (Famvir) is 500 mg orally three times a day. The dosage of valacyclovir (Valtrex) is 1 g three times a day. For most adolescents, a 5-day regimen should be sufficient treatment.

### TREATMENT OF CHICKENPOX IN CHILDREN WITH AN UNDERLYING IMMUNODEFICIENCY

Children with HIV infection who contract chickenpox can usually be managed with oral acyclovir treatment as long as their HIV is under control. The majority of children diagnosed with acute chickenpox who have cancer or have undergone organ transplantation should be considered for admission to the hospital and begin immediate treatment with intravenous (IV) acyclovir. The dosage of IV acyclovir is 10 mg/kg every 8 hours. The dosage can be raised to 15 mg/kg every 8 hours in patients presenting varicella pneumonia or varicella encephalitis. The serum creatinine level should be monitored daily and the acyclovir dosage adjusted downward if the serum creatinine reaches 1 mg/dL.

The efficacy of oral famciclovir or valacyclovir is better than oral acyclovir, allowing older children with chickenpox and an immunosuppressive condition to be discharged more quickly from the hospital.

Discharge is generally considered after no new vesicle formation is noted for 24 hours. Antiviral therapy (combined IV and oral) for 10 to 14 days is usually suggested, although each case must be assessed individually. Children who have varicella encephalitis or varicella pneumonia may require more than 2 weeks of antiviral therapy.

### TREATMENT OF CHICKENPOX IN CHILDREN RECEIVING CORTICOSTEROIDS

Children receiving high-dose oral corticosteroid treatment for conditions such as acute asthma are also at high risk of severe chickenpox. These children should be treated with antivirals just as aggressively as those with cancer. Children receiving only intermittent inhaled corticosteroids do not appear to be at high risk of severe chickenpox.

### TREATMENT OF ZOSTER IN CHILDREN

Zoster in otherwise healthy children is usually a benign illness. The disease is normally improving by the time the diagnosis is made. However, zoster in immunocompromised children may persist for 2 weeks or longer, requiring immediate treatment with one of the oral antiviral drugs recommended. The dosage is the same as for severe chickenpox.

### ALTERNATIVES TO VARICELLA-ZOSTER IMMUNE GLOBULIN

Varicella-zoster immune globulin (VZIG) has been given in the past to infants and children with cancer who were exposed to chickenpox. VZIG has been discontinued after 2005. Physicians can consider the administration of IV gammaglobulin as a single infusion of 500 mg/kg for infants who are exposed to varicella shortly after birth. An alternative regimen is oral acyclovir suspension at 40 mg/kg per day divided every 6 hours. Acyclovir should be initiated on the day of exposure and continued for 10 days.

Prophylaxis with oral acyclovir also can be considered for VZV-nonimmune children with cancer after an exposure to chickenpox. The recommended dosage is one half of the therapeutic dosage, meaning oral acyclovir can be given at 40 mg/kg per day. The daily dosage for children who can swallow tablets can be divided three times a day rather than four times a day during the 10-day therapy period. Children who develop chickenpox despite oral acyclovir treatment should be admitted to the hospital for treatment with IV acyclovir at 10 mg/kg every 8 hours. There are extremely few examples of true acyclovir-resistant VZV; most failures are caused by inadequate absorption of the oral formulation.

### REFERENCES

Davis MM, Patel MS, Gebremariam A: Decline in varicella-related hospitalizations and expenditures for children and adults after introduction of varicella vaccine in the United States. Pediatrics 2004;114:786-792.

Grose C: Varicella vaccination of children in the United States: Assessment after the first decade, 1995-2005. J Clin Virol 2005;33:89-95.

Grose C, Widerman J: Generic acyclovir vs. famciclovir and valacyclovir. Pediatr Infect Dis J 1997;16:838-841.

Hay M, Kimura H, Oshiro M, et al: Varicella exposure in a neonatal medical center: Successful prophylaxis with oral acyclovir. J Hosp Infect 2003;54:212-215.

Nguyen HQ, Jumaan AO, Seward JF: Decline in mortality due to varicella after implementation of varicella vaccination in the United States. N Engl J Med 2005;352:450-458.

Takahashi M: Effectiveness of live varicella vaccine. Expert Opin Biol Ther 2004;4:199-216.

**CURRENT THERAPY**

- Severe chickenpox in infants and immunosuppressed children is treated with intravenous acyclovir (30 mg/kg/d).
- Severe chickenpox in healthy children is treated with oral acyclovir (80 mg/kg/d).
- Severe chickenpox in adolescents is treated with either famciclovir (Famvir) (500 mg tid) or valacyclovir (Valtrex) (1 g tid).
- Prophylaxis following exposure to chickenpox can be managed with a course of oral acyclovir (40 mg/kg/d).

# Cholera

Method of
*Carlos Seas, MD, and Eduardo Gotuzzo, MD*

Cholera is an ancient scourge recognized since the time of Hippocrates. More accurate descriptions of the disease began approximately in 1817. Since then, cholera has caused seven pandemics, affecting all continents, and it remains endemic in almost all affected areas. Recent examples of severe epidemics are the Latin American extension of the seventh pandemic in Peru in 1991, explosive epidemics among refugees in Africa, and unexpected epidemics of cholera due to a new serogroup in Asia since 1992. We can conclude from these epidemics that it is very difficult to predict when a new epidemic will start, that appropriate treatment reduces the mortality to values less than 1%, and that the pathogen continues to evolve in the environment despite interventions to control its spread.

## Etiology

Cholera is caused by a curved gram-negative bacillus that belongs to the family Vibrionaceae. Two serogroups, O1 and O139, are associated with clinical cholera, and both cause the same clinical entity. These serogroups have shown both regional and pandemic potential. *Vibrio cholerae* is a natural inhabitant of certain aquatic environments, where it lives attached to copepods, algae, and crustacean shells in a symbiotic association. If conditions are not favorable for growth, *V. cholerae* adopts a dormant state. In this state it remains metabolically inactive for long periods. The switch to a metabolically active state occurs when conditions become suitable for division. Humans get the infection by consuming contaminated water, beverages, or food. During epidemics, a single source can be identified, but usually multiple routes of transmission play a role simultaneously. Epidemics tend to occur during the warmest months of the year, and association with climate variability and El Niño southern oscillation has been recently documented.

*V. cholerae* O1 and O139 secrete a number of potent exotoxins that induce the characteristic isotonic dehydration of cholera. The better studied toxin is the cholera toxin, which has two subunits, A and B. The B subunit allows the toxin to attach to a specific receptor present along the small intestine of humans, and the A subunit activates the adenylate cyclase enzyme. The chain of events that follows this enzymatic activation is mediated by cyclic adenosine monophosphate (cAMP) and includes blockage of the absorption of sodium and chloride by the microvillus and promotion of secretion of chloride and water by crypt cells. The result of these events is the massive

## CURRENT DIAGNOSIS

- History of travel to an endemic area.
- Acute voluminous watery diarrhea with rice-water appearance, leading to severe dehydration in a matter of hours.
- Muscle cramps, vomiting, and signs of severe dehydration such as loss of skin elasticity (slow skin-pinch retraction), hoarse voice, sunken eyes, and wrinkled hands and feet (washerwoman hands).
- Fever is absent in most patients.
- Milder forms of dehydration cannot be distinguished from other common causes of acute diarrhea.
- Stool culture using proper media is positive for *V. cholerae* O1 or O139. Dark field microscopy of a fresh stool sample can detect the presence of vibrio; specific antisera confirm the serogroup.

liberation of water and electrolytes into the intestinal lumen, as shown in Table 1.

## Treatment

The objectives of therapy are to replace the fluid and electrolyte losses caused by diarrhea and vomiting, to maintain hydration, and to reduce the volume of diarrhea and excretion of vibrios to the environment. The treatment is divided into two phases: the rehydration phase and the maintenance phase.

### REHYDRATION PHASE

The objective of the rehydration phase is to replace the losses that occurred before the patient was admitted. This phase begins with a thorough evaluation of the degree of dehydration. Table 2 shows the clinical signs according to the degree of dehydration.

Patients with severe dehydration present with a constellation of signs that reflect a deficit of at least 10% of body weight. The pulse is feeble and very rapid, the blood pressure is not measurable, the skin elasticity is lost, the eyes are sunken, and the voice is inaudible or hoarse. The intravenous route is recommended for rehydrating all patients with severe dehydration. The rate and speed of the infusion is recommended at 50 to 100 mL/kg/hour for the first 2 to 4 hours. After this time, the patient must be fully rehydrated to begin the maintenance phase. The preferred intravenous solution is Ringer's lactate

## TABLE 1 Electrolyte Concentrations (mmol/L)

| Substance | Sodium | Chloride | Potassium | Bicarbonate | Osmolality |
|---|---|---|---|---|---|
| **Cholera Stool** | | | | | |
| Adults | | 130 | 100 | 20 | 44 |
| Children | | 100 | 90 | 33 | 30 |
| **Rehydration Solution** | | | | | |
| Ringer's lactate* | 130 | 109 | 4 | 28* | 271 |
| Normal saline | 154 | 154 | 0 | 0 | 308 |
| Rice-based ORS | 75 | 65 | 20 | 10 | 180 |
| WHO ORS‡ | 75 | 65 | 20 | 10† | 245 |

*Ringer's lactate contains lactate instead of bicarbonate.
†Bicarbonate is replaced with trisodium citrate, which stays fresh longer than bicarbonate in sachets.
‡Reduced osmolality formula.
*Abbreviations:* ORS = oral rehydration solution; WHO = World Health Organization.

## TABLE 2 Clinical Findings by Degree of Dehydration

| Clinical Finding | Degree of Dehydration | |
| --- | --- | --- |
| | Some | Severe |
| Loss of fluid (% of body weight) | 5%-10% | >10% |
| Mentation | Restless | Drowsy or comatose |
| Radial pulse rate | Rapid | Very rapid |
| Radial pulse intensity | Weak | Feeble or impalpable |
| Respiration | Normal or deep | Deep and rapid |
| Systolic blood pressure | Low | Very low or undetectable |
| Skin elasticity | Retracts slowly | Retracts very slowly |
| Eyes | Sunken | Very sunken |
| Voice | Hoarse | Not audible |
| Urine production | Scant | Oliguria |

solution. If this solution is not available, normal saline may be used, but the recovery from metabolic acidosis is less efficient. Oral rehydration solutions (ORS) should be started as soon a possible in these patients.

Milder forms of dehydration due to cholera cannot be clinically distinguished from other common causes of acute diarrhea. Symptoms due to some degree of dehydration are seen when water deficit is greater than 5% of body weight. The intravenous route may be used in these patients if the stool output is high

## CURRENT THERAPY

- Identify the degree of dehydration on admission.
- Register the intake and output regularly in predesigned charts.
- Rehydrate the patient in two phases. The rehydration phase lasts 2-4 hours. The maintenance phase lasts until diarrhea abates.
- Use the intravenous route for patients who have severe dehydration during the rehydration phase, those who purge more than 10-20 mL/kg/h, and those who do not tolerate the oral route during the maintenance phase. The amount and speed of the intravenous infusion vary between 50 and 100 mL/kg/h.
- The preferred intravenous solution is Ringer's lactate solution. Normal saline may be used, but the acidosis resolves less efficiently.
- Use the oral rehydration solution advised by the World Health Organization during the maintenance phase for severely dehydrated patients and for milder forms of dehydration in the rehydration phase. The amount of oral fluids advised is 500-1000 mL/h.
- Start antibiotics once the patient can tolerate the oral route. Doxycycline (Vibramycin) in a single dose of 300 mg, is the preferred regimen, given with a light meal.
- Start a normal diet as soon as the patient tolerates anything by mouth.
- Discharge patients when all the following criteria are fulfilled: oral tolerance <600-800 mL/h, stool output >400 mL/h, urine output <30-40 mL/h.

(<10-20 mL/kg/hour) or if the patient does not tolerate the oral route. The great majority of patients with milder forms of dehydration can be rehydrated by the oral route.

Laboratory abnormalities in patients with severe cholera reflect hemoconcentration and include a high hematocrit, increase in white blood cell count, azotemia, and elevation of specific gravity and total proteins. These laboratory parameters are good indicators of the degree of dehydration on admission, but they are not useful for following the rehydration status. Metabolic acidosis with a high anion gap is typically seen in patients with severe cholera. Hypokalemia or normal values (due to acidosis) and normal or low serum sodium and chloride are also observed in these patients. Hyperglycemia results from high levels of epinephrine, glucagon, and cortisol stimulated by hypovolemia. Hypoglycemia is rare but carries a poor prognosis, particularly in children.

### MAINTENANCE PHASE

The maintenance phase begins when the patient has been fully rehydrated. A good indicator of the recovery of the normal hydration status is not only the absence of clinical signs of dehydration but also the volume of urine output. Urine outputs greater than 0.5 mL/kg/hour are expected in fully hydrated patients. The maintenance phase has the objective of preserving the normal hydration status, and it lasts until the diarrhea abates.

The oral route is advised for the maintenance phase, and the ORS recommended by the World Health Organization (WHO) is the preferred oral solution. Recently, WHO has promoted the use of ORS with lower osmolality (75 mmol/L of sodium and total osmolality of 245 mOsm/L vs. the former solution containing 90 mmol/L of sodium and total osmolality of 311 mOsm/L) to treat all kinds of acute diarrheal diseases. Adults should be observed for hyponatremia when using this reduced-osmolality ORS. ORS uses the principle of common transportation of solutes, electrolytes, and water not affected by cholera in the intestine. ORS containing rice instead of glucose is also preferred, because the purging rate is lower with solutions containing rice than with glucose-based solutions. If ORS in packets is not available, a solution can be made with 2.6 g sodium chloride, 2.9 g sodium citrate, 1.5 g potassium chloride, and 13.5 g glucose or 50 g rice powder to 1 L of boiled water.

The amount of oral fluids should match the ongoing losses to prevent dehydration during this phase. Periodic review of the patient's chart is advised for this purpose. Predesigned forms to register intake and output and vital signs should be available to monitor the hydration status regularly. Cholera cots or cholera chairs facilitate the collection and measurement of stools and urine during treatment.

Discharging patients from the hospital is a critical issue, particularly when health centers are overloaded with patients with varying degrees of dehydration. Patients can be safely discharged if all the following criteria are met: oral intake between 600 and 800 mL/hour, urine output between 30 and 40 mL/hour, and stool output lower than 400 mL/hour. Case fatality rates in centers with experience in the treatment of cholera are extremely low, about 0.14%.

### PHARMACOLOGIC THERAPY

An oral antibiotic is advised to reduce the volume of diarrhea, the requirement for intravenous fluids, and the hospital stay. Antibiotics are not lifesaving and should not be offered if the patient cannot tolerate the oral route. A reduction in almost 50% of the volume and duration of diarrhea and a reduction in the excretion of vibrios to 1 to 2 days have been documented with the use of effective antimicrobials. Single-dose regimens are preferred over multiple-dose regimens. A single dose of doxycycline (Vibramycin) 300 mg, given with a light meal, is the preferred regimen. Alternative regimens are listed in Table 3.

The quinolones are the group of antimicrobials more extensively studied to date, and excellent results in both clinical and bacteriologic parameters have been reported in clinical trials. Quinolones should not be used in children or pregnant women. Resistance to the quinolones has emerged in endemic areas of India and Bangladesh.

**TABLE 3** Antimicrobial Regimens for the Treatment of Cholera

| Drug | Antimicrobial Regimen | |
| | Adult | Children |
| --- | --- | --- |
| **Preferred Regimen** | | |
| Doxycycline (Vibramycin) | 300 mg with food | |
| **Alternative Regimens** | | |
| Azithromycin (Zithromax)[1] | 1 g as a single dose | 20 mg/kg as a single dose |
| Ciprofloxacin (Cipro)[1] | 1g single-dose or 250 mg qd for 3 d or 500 mg bid for 3 d | Not recommended |
| Cotrimoxazole (Bactrim)[1] | TMP 160 mg and SMX 800 mg bid for 3 d | TMP 8 mg/kg and SMX 40 mg/kg divided in 2 doses for 3 d |
| Doxycycline (Vibramycin) | 300 mg as a single dose | Not evaluated |
| Erythromycin[1] | 250 mg qid for 3 d | 12.5 mg/kg q6h for 3 d |
| Furazolidone (Furoxone) | 100 mg qid for 3 d | 5 mg/kg qid for 3 d or 7 mg/kg as a single dose |
| Norfloxacin (Noroxin)[1] | 400 mg bid for 3 d | Not recommended |
| Tetracycline | 500 mg qid for 3 d | 50 mg/kg body weight qid for 3 d* |

[1]Not FDA approved for this indication.
*Only for children older than 8 years.
*Abbreviations:* SMX = sulfamethoxazole; TMP = trimethoprim.

Oral azithromycin (Zithromax)[1] (1g in a single dose) is an alternative to treat infections by quinolone-resistant strains in both children and adults. Chemoprophylaxis with antimicrobials to prevent transmission of cholera is not recommended.

## Complications and Prognosis

The most severe complication of cholera is acute renal failure. A careful evaluation of the medical charts of these patients disclosed improper replacement of fluids during the rehydration or maintenance phases. The nonoliguric form predominates. All age groups are affected, and the mortality rate is very high.

The presentation of cholera in children is similar to that in adults. Certain features are distinctive in children, however, such as fever, seizures, mental alteration, and hypoglycemia.

Cholera in the elderly carries a bad prognosis. The common presence of comorbidities, the difficulties in properly evaluating the hydration status, and the higher incidences of acute renal failure and pulmonary edema account for the higher mortality observed in this population.

Cholera in pregnant women is associated with more severe illness and with fetal losses.

---

[1]Not FDA approved for this indication.

## REFERENCES

Griffith DC, Kelly-Hope LA, Miller MA: Review of reported cholera outbreaks worldwide, 1995-2005. Am J Trop Med Hyg 2006;75:973-977.
Khan WA, Bennish ML, Seas C, et al: Randomized controlled comparison of single-dose ciprofloxacin and doxycycline for cholera caused by *Vibrio cholerae* O1 or O139. Lancet 1996;348:296-300.
Khan WA, Saha D, Rahman A, et al: Comparison of single-dose azithromycin and 12-dose, 3-day erythromycin for childhood cholera: A randomized, double-blind trial. Lancet 2002;360(9347):1722-1727.
Nalin DR, Hirschhorn N, Greenough W III, et al: Clinical concerns about reduced-osmolarity oral rehydration solution. JAMA 2004;291:2632-2635.
Sack DA, Sack RB, Nair GB, Siddique AK: Cholera. Lancet 2004;363:223-233.
Saha D, Karim MM, Khan WA, et al: Single-dose azithromycin for the treatment of cholera in adults. N Engl J Med 2006;354:2452-2462.
Seas C, Gotuzzo E: Cholera. In Mandell GL, Bennett JE, Dolin R (eds): Principles and Practice of Infectious Diseases. Philadelphia: Churchill-Livingstone, 2005, pp 2536-2544.

# Foodborne Illness

Method of
*Lester M. Crawford, PhD*

## History

In the 1920 edition of *Principles and Practice of Medicine*, Sir William Osler devoted three of the 1168 pages to food poisoning. He got virtually everything right, even by today's standards. He just had very little to report on a disease complex that was vitally important in his time. Today, the Centers for Disease Control and Prevention (CDC) estimates approximately 76 million illnesses, 325,000 hospitalizations, and 5000 deaths from foodborne disease each year in the United States. Viruses account for 67% of these infections, bacteria for 30%, and parasites for 2%.

Therapy of foodborne disease has passed through a variety of stages. In Osler's time, treatment primarily consisted of stomach lavage and enemas. After World War II, antibiotics were freely used. By the 1980s, competitive exclusion by antibiotic-resistant bacteria had dictated a more conservative approach that relied on supportive therapy including fluids. In severe cases, selective use of specific targeted antibacterials remained necessary. The remarkable success rate of oral rehydration therapy under primitive conditions in developing countries underscored the critical importance of maintaining fluid balance. Today, fluid therapy has become the cornerstone of the treatment of foodborne disease.

## Etiology, Diagnosis, and Treatment

There are 30 principal foodborne diseases. Waterborne diseases are classified as foodborne diseases. Six of the 30 diseases are dealt with in other chapters. These are hepatitis, salmonellosis, typhoid, cholera, giardiasis, and toxoplasmosis. This chapter deals with the remaining major causes of this group of diseases.

### *AEROMONAS* SPECIES

Although the role of *Aeromonas* in foodborne disease was elucidated in the 1890s, it has only recently been appreciated as the ubiquitous pathogenic organism that it is. These are, in fact, aquatic organisms, but *Aeromonas* has been isolated from a variety of plants, animals, and foodstuffs. *Aeromonas* has also been found in stool cultures, skin, and sputum samples from healthy persons. Gastrointestinal infections caused by this organism are characterized by mucoid, bloody stools, watery diarrhea typical of dysentery, and low-grade fever. This syndrome can progress to pneumonia, arthritis, osteomyelitis, endocarditis, and urinary tract infections, particularly in children, the elderly, and immunocompromised patients. *Aeromonas* can affect virtually any organ system and can cause hemolytic uremic syndrome.

The organism is amenable to antibiotic therapy and may be successfully treated with trimethoprim-sulfamethoxazole (Bactrim),[1] aminoglycosides, tetracyclines, cephalosporins, and the quinolones. Antibiotic resistance has now become a problem; it has been demonstrated that *Aeromonas* spp. can produce β-lactamases and transferable tetracycline R-plasmids. Therefore, it may be preferable to initiate therapy with trimethoprim-sulfamethoxazole or one of the fluoroquinolones when *Aeromonas* is isolated.

### BACILLUS CEREUS

*Bacillus cereus* was not recognized as a significant foodborne pathogen until the 1950s, and the first major outbreak was not until 1971 in England. This organism is ubiquitous in the environment but is not pathogenic until conditions favor its growth. Pathogenesis is accomplished through a wide variety of extracellular toxins and enzymes. There is a diarrheagenic toxin and an emetic toxin.

Foods become toxic when the levels of *B. cereus* approach millions of organisms per gram. The usual syndrome involves nausea (but not vomiting), watery diarrhea, rectal straining, and abdominal pain. There is an incubation period of 8 to 19 hours; the duration of illness is usually 12 to 24 hours. In some cases, an emetic syndrome occurs that is more severe and acute than the diarrheal syndrome. The emetic syndrome is characterized by an incubation period of approximately 3 hours and is typified by severe vomiting. Diarrhea is generally not present in the emetic syndrome. The emetic syndrome closely mirrors staphylococcal food poisoning.

The diarrheal syndrome generally requires minimal therapeutic intervention other than monitoring of fluid and food intake. The emetic syndrome, although brief, can require intravenous fluids and medication such as phenobarbital[1] to moderate the frequency of vomiting.

### CALICIVIRUSES

Caliciviruses cause the majority of foodborne illness in the United States and, most likely, the rest of the world. Indeed, without the cases caused by norovirus, cases of foodborne disease would be reduced by approximately two thirds according to some estimates, and there would likely be little need for or interest in this chapter.

Norwalk, Ohio, was the site of the first reported outbreak (1968) of this disease complex. The virus was therefore named *Norwalk virus*. The name was later changed to *Norwalk-like virus* (NLV), and the current name is *norovirus*.

There are three genotypes of enteric caliciviruses. In addition to norovirus, the calicivirus family includes Desert Shield virus, Hawaii virus, Mexico virus, Snow Mountain virus, and others.

### Etiology

Fecal-oral transmission is the most common route of infection, but vomitus can also transmit infectious doses of the agent. Although swimming pools and uncooked or partially cooked food can transmit the infection, the primary source is drinking water. The recent spate of cruise ship infections has generally been traced to drinking water. Properly chlorinated water is generally safe, but nonchlorinated water is problematic. Inadequately chlorinated or brominated water can transmit norovirus, as can chlorinated water that comes from an overwhelmingly contaminated source. Leakage of sewage into treated water can result in individual cases or outbreaks.

### Diagnosis

The disease entity is characterized by epidemic diarrhea. Symptoms include gastroenteritis, vomiting, diarrhea, headache, and 2 to 3 days of low-grade fever. People of all ages are affected. In the United States, older children and adults are more likely to be infected, and in the Third World, young children are more often involved. Diagnosis may be by isolation of the virus from feces and confirmation by radioimmunoassay (RIA) or enzyme-linked immunosorbent assay (ELISA), or both.

### Treatment

There is no specific treatment for norovirus infection. Supportive therapy, especially including fluids, is generally adequate for most patients. For patients in developing countries, oral rehydration therapy is generally the treatment of choice.

A specific vaccine for norovirus is being developed. The virus has been isolated, cloned, and sequenced, and an experimental vaccine is in clinical trials.

### CAMPYLOBACTER SPECIES

*Campylobacter* has gone from not being recognized as a human pathogen to being the leading cause of bacterial diarrhea in just over 25 years. The agent is estimated to cause about 2.5 million illnesses, which is 12% of all foodborne disease in the United States. Moreover, serious sequelae such as Guillain-Barré syndrome (1:1000 cases) and Reiter's syndrome (1:100 cases) infrequently supervene.

### Diagnosis

Difficulty in culturing *Campylobacter* prevented isolation and characterization of the organism until the early 1970s. *Campylobacter jejuni* is the species most associated with foodborne illness. Campylobacteriosis is characterized by abdominal pain, diarrhea, and fever lasting 2 to 5 days. Longer durations of illness and relapses are not uncommon. Diagnosis is confirmed by direct microscopic examination of the stool or through the use of selective media.

### Treatment

Seriously ill patients should be treated with antibiotics, as should infants, older people, and the immunosuppressed. Seriously ill patients are defined as those with persistent high fever or refractory or bloody diarrhea. Clarithromycin (Biaxin)[1] is generally accepted as the antibiotic of choice, and fluoroquinolones such as ciprofloxacin (Cipro)[1] are the first alternative. The tetracyclines are also useful. Campylobacteriosis is resistant to the cephalosporins, vancomycin (Vancocin), and rifampin (Rifadin). Supportive therapy aimed at electrolyte replacement and hydration is also important.

### CLOSTRIDIUM BOTULINUM

*Clostridium botulinum* elaborates one of the most potent substances in nature. One nanogram per kilogram of body weight is sufficient to paralyze an otherwise healthy person. When the toxin is ingested in food in sufficient quantities to cause illness, near total paralysis occurs in humans, often requiring artificial ventilation for extended periods. Mild botulism can consist of nothing more than double vision or a few days of dysphagia.

The mechanism of action of botulism is to block release of acetylcholine at the neuromuscular junction by attaching to specific receptors on the nerve terminal side of the junction. Nerve conduction restores activity at the neuromuscular junction.

Any food can contain botulinum toxin, but the most common vehicles in the United States are fruits and vegetables. Infant botulism is usually associated with consumption of honey.

### Diagnosis

Diagnosis is confirmed by isolation of botulinum toxin either from the suspect food or from the patient's blood serum or feces. Resorting to

---

[1]Not FDA approved for this indication.

[1]Not FDA approved for this indication.

symptomatic diagnosis can lead to confusing botulism with Guillain-Barré syndrome or even stroke.

## Treatment

Therapy must center around the management of respiratory impairment. This requires accessibility to an intensive care unit. The Centers for Disease Control and Prevention (CDC) can provide polyvalent vaccines[5, 10] that are effective against the six botulism toxins (A, B, C, D, E, F). The toxin can persist in the patient's serum for as much as a month after ingestion, and relapses and exacerbations are possible. The toxicity to the neuromuscular junctions can continue for months and, in rare cases, for as long as a year. Careful management and diagnostic advances have reduced mortality to well under 10%.

## *CLOSTRIDIUM PERFRINGENS*

McClane has written, "*Clostridium perfringens* is ideally suited for its role as a major foodborne pathogen." He was referring to its ubiquity in soil and in human and animal feces; moreover, the organism has a doubling time of less than 10 minutes once established in foods. Finally, *C. perfringens* is heat resistant and it elaborates two toxins that can induce specific pathology in the human intestinal tract. Indeed, *C. perfringens* is the third leading cause of foodborne illness in the United States, after norovirus and *B. cereus*.

## Diagnosis

The two forms of human disease caused by this organism are *C. perfringens* type A food poisoning and *C. perfringens* type C food poisoning, better known as necrotic enteritis. The type A syndrome is much more common but type C is a more serious disease.

Abdominal cramps and diarrhea typify the type A disease. These symptoms develop 8 to 16 hours after ingestion of contaminated food and persist for 12 to 24 hours, with a complete recovery in most patients. However, severe illness and even death can supervene in older or debilitated patients.

The necrotic enteritis form of the disease is characterized by vomiting, intense abdominal pain, bloody diarrhea, and severe gastroenteritis. The incubation period is 1 to 5 days after exposure. The more advanced cases can progress to jejunal necrosis and death if not managed well.

## Treatment

Treatment for the type A disease is supportive therapy. Necrotic enteritis can require surgical repair of the small intestine, including removal of the affected area. *C. perfringens* is quite susceptible to penicillin, and some authorities report that the antibiotic may be useful in the management of severe cases of type C.

## *ENTEROBACTER SAKAZAKII*

*Enterobacter sakazakii* causes meningitis or necrotizing enterocolitis in neonates, which results in a mortality rate of 40% to 80%. Surviving patients sometimes develop hydrocephalus, paralysis, or neurologic deficits. *E. sakazakii* has been isolated from dry infant formulas. The natural source of the organism is not well known.

Enterobacters are generally resistant to the cephalosporins but are responsive to medium-spectrum penicillins, such as carbenicillin (Geocillin),[1] piperacillin (Pipracil),[1] and ticarcillin (Ticar).[1] The aminoglycosides and the fluoroquinolones are also indicated.

## *ESCHERICHIA COLI* O157:H7

This variant of *Escherichia coli* burst on the scene in North America in the late 1970s, and now it can be found in practically every country in the world. The reservoir for the disease is believed to be cattle, but wildlife of various kinds can likewise harbor the organism. In cattle, the disease is silent, causing no overt signs.

In humans, the verocytotoxin, a Shiga-like toxin that has been genetically incorporated into the organism, can cause hemorrhagic colitis and hemolytic-uremic syndrome, which leads, in some cases, to disseminated intravascular coagulation (DIC). DIC can result in a layer of fibrin forming in the glomerular capillary bed and acute renal failure. These sequelae are most likely to occur in children and older persons and in pregnant women. The young patients generally fully recover but sometimes require dialysis.

The number of cases is low and the fatality rate is small, but the severity and permanence of some of the sequelae have given great prominence to the disease. Major outbreaks such as the Jack-in-the-Box event of 1993 and the 2006 spinach outbreak have focused public attention on *E. coli* O157:H7. Control of this organism depends on proper cooking and handling of food, assiduous hand washing, and effective water-treatment programs. There is much interest in a vaccine for cattle or humans for *E. coli* O157:H7.

## Diagnosis

Diagnosis is made by serotyping for specific antibodies to *E. coli* O157:H7. Transmission of the organism generally occurs from ingesting contaminated food but can occur from direct contact. The incubation period is 12 to 60 hours.

## Treatment

Therapy consists of fluid replacement. Antibiotics are of no use because the lesional insult is caused by a combination of toxins that continue to be pathogenic for a period of time after the elaborating organism is no longer active. In fact, the U.S. Food and Drug Administration (FDA) has issued (January 2007) a warning against the use of antibiotics in enterohemorrhagic *E. coli* cases because such therapy could adversely affect the outcome. Dialysis is indicated in cases that progress to kidney failure. In the more severe cases of intestinal hemorrhage, blood transfusion may be necessary.

## *LISTERIA MONOCYTOGENES*

Although *Listeria monocytogenes* infects a relatively small number of patients, listeriosis results in a 25% to 40% fatality rate, and severe aftereffects are relatively common in affected patients. It is extremely difficult to identify the specific food responsible because of the highly variable incubation period, which ranges from 3 to 70 days.

There are three modes of transmission: contaminated food, direct contact with the organism or with contaminated soil, and inhalation of the organism. Initial symptoms include fever, headache, and vomiting, but these may be followed by endocarditis, meningoencephalitis, and septicemia. These later symptoms can lead to hemorrhagic shock, disorientation, and coma. Listeriosis is a leading cause of stillbirth and miscarriage and must be handled aggressively in pregnant women. Neonatal cases likewise must be managed with care. Almost one half of all listeriosis cases are in neonates.

Confirmation of the diagnosis is accomplished by isolation of the organism from blood or cerebrospinal fluid. Virtually all β-lactam antibiotics are effective against *L. monocytogenes* including potassium penicillin G (Pfizerpen). Erythromycin (Ery-Tab),[1] tobramycin (Nebcin),[1] and other antibiotics in the macrolide and aminoglycoside families also are effective against *L. monocytogenes*.

## *STAPHYLOCOCCUS AUREUS*

Whereas most food borne illnesses have incubation periods of days and even weeks, *Staphylococcus aureus* infections usually trigger symptoms in 2 to 6 hours. The organism elaborates a complex system of

---

[1]Not FDA approved for this indication.
[5]Investigational drug in the United States.
[10]Available in the United States from the Centers for Disease Control.

---

[1]Not FDA approved for this indication.

toxins in food under certain conditions that results in nausea, vomiting, retching, and abdominal cramping. Severe cases result in muscle cramping, vacillations in blood pressure and heart rate, and severe headaches. The disease usually runs its course in 2 days, but some cases last longer. Death can occur in the young, the elderly, and the debilitated.

Incriminated foods in *Staphylococcal* outbreaks are generally those that require a great deal of human handling such as salads and various meats, although canned foods have caused clusters of infection. The usual inciting factor is not keeping the prepared foods hot enough or cold enough to prevent the proliferation of organisms and the formation of the causative toxins. Stored foods should be maintained at temperatures of 45°F (7.2°C) or kept warm at 140°F (60°C). Foods should be brought to these temperatures as rapidly as technologically possible.

Supportive therapy is indicated. Antibiotic therapy is not useful because the causative agent, the toxin, is not affected by antibiotics. Persistent vomiting or dehydration can indicate fluid therapy, such as 5% dextrose, together with electrolyte replacement, particularly potassium.

## REFERENCES

Allos BM, Blaster MJ: *Campylobacter jejuni* and the expanding spectrum of related infections. Clin Infect Dis 1995;20:1092-1101.

Ball JM, Graham DY, Opekum AR, et al: Recombinant Norwalk-like particles given orally to volunteers: Phase I study. Gastroenterology 1999;117: 40-48.

Bennett RW: *Bacillus cereus*. In Labbé RG, García S (eds): Guide to Foodborne Pathogens. New York: John Wiley and Sons, 2001, pp 51-60.

Gill DM: Bacterial toxins: A table of lethal amounts. Microbiol Rev 1982;46: 86-94.

Greatorex JS, Thorne GM: Humoral immune response to Shiga-like toxins and *Escherichia coli* O157:H7 lipopolysaccharide in hemolytic-uremic syndrome patients and healthy subjects. J Clin Microbiol 1994;32:1172-1178.

Lawrence GW: The pathogenesis of enteritis necroticans. In Rood JA, McClane, Songer JG, et al (eds). The Clostridia: Molecular Genetics and Pathogenesis. London: Academic Press, 1997, pp 198-207.

Lederberg J, Shope RE, Oaks SC (eds): Emerging Infections: Microbial Threats to Health in the United States. Washington, DC: National Academies Press, 1992.

Miliotis MD, Bier JW (eds): International Handbook of Foodborne Pathogens. New York: Marcel Dekker, 2003.

Olsen SJ, MacKinnon LC, Goulding JS, et al: Surveillance for foodborne-disease outbreaks—United States, 1993-1997. MMWR CDC Surveill Summ 2000;49(1):1-62.

Schlech WF: Foodborne listeriosis. Clin Infec Dis 2000;31:770-775.

# Necrotizing Skin and Soft Tissue Infections

Method of
*John M. Embil, MD, FRCP(C), FACP, and*
*Donald C. Vinh, MD, FRCP(C), Dip(ABIM)*

Necrotizing skin and soft tissue infections (SSTIs) are a heterogeneous group of infections that progress unimpeded across anatomic boundaries, producing destruction of the subcutaneous, fascial, or muscle layers of the integument, resulting in gangrenous cellulitis, necrotizing fasciitis, or myonecrosis, respectively. These infections have an acute onset, usually the patient appears toxic, and the infection is potentially limb- or life-threatening. Although necrotizing SSTIs are relatively uncommon, early recognition and appropriate interventions are crucial for optimal outcome. Thus, clinicians assessing a patient presenting with an SSTI should always consider the possibility of an underlying necrotizing process that would require consultation with a surgeon and infectious disease specialist.

## Etiology

Necrotizing SSTIs are most often bacterial in origin and can be either monomicrobial (type II) or polymicrobial (type I). Much less often, fungal pathogens cause such infections.

Polymicrobial necrotizing SSTIs are, by far, most common. These infections are caused by the synergistic interaction between mixed facultative anaerobic and obligate anaerobic gram-positive and gram-negative bacteria, such as *Escherichia coli*, *Klebsiella spp*, *Proteus spp*, the staphylococci, the streptococci, and *Bacteroides spp*. On average, 4 or 5 different organisms are involved. The polymicrobial nature can be suggested by the location of the infected site; most commonly, they occur in the head and neck area (especially if odontogenic), the abdominal area (e.g., postsurgical sites), the pelvic, genital, and perineal areas (e.g., Fournier's gangrene, infections following gynecologic procedures, and infections originating from sacral decubitus ulcers), and extremities with neglected care (especially diabetic foot infections). Culture and susceptibility testing (C&S) should be performed on any discharge or deep tissue to guide therapy.

Monomicrobial necrotizing SSTIs occur less often (Table 1). These pathogens should be especially considered among patients with certain risk factors (see Table 1) who present with community-acquired infections. By far the most common isolate responsible for this condition is group A streptococcus (*Streptococcus pyogenes*), which might or might not cause concomitant streptococcal toxic shock syndrome and which can have devastating consequences. Because no clinical features are absolutely diagnostic for a specific pathogen, cultures should be obtained.

Fungal pathogens are emerging as an important cause of acute necrotizing SSTIs. Most commonly, these are due to saprophytic septated molds (e.g., *Aspergillus spp*, *Fusarium spp*, *Paecilomyces spp*) and to the aseptated zygomycetes producing mucormycosis. Major risk factors

**TABLE 1  Causes and Risk Factors for Monomicrobial Acute Necrotizing Skin and Soft Tissue Infections**

| Pathogen | Risk Factors |
| --- | --- |
| *Aeromonas hydrophila* | Wounds contaminated by freshwater (e.g., lakes, rivers, streams) |
| *Clostridium perfringens* (gas gangrene) | Contamination of traumatic wounds (e.g., by soil) |
| | Deterioration in a postsurgical wound (e.g., dehiscence, duskiness, bullae) |
| *Clostridium septicum* | Malignancy (e.g., colon cancer, hematologic malignancy) |
| Community-acquired methicillin-resistant *Staphylococcus aureus* | No established regular risk factors |
| | Close contacts who have a recent history of furuncles or difficult-to-treat skin abscesses may be suggestive |
| Group A streptococci (*S. pyogenes*) | Breaks in integrity of skin |
| | Impaired lymphatic or venous circulation |
| | Diabetes mellitus |
| | Superinfection of chickenpox |
| *Pseudomonas aeruginosa* | Ecthyma gangrenosum: Immunocompromise (hematologic malignancy, neutropenia) |
| | Malignant otitis externa: Diabetes mellitus |
| *Vibrio vulnificus* | Wounds contaminated by saltwater (e.g., Atlantic Gulf Coast) |
| | Wounds exposed to saltwater crustaceans and other seafood |
| | Chronic liver disease or cirrhosis |
| | Chronic renal failure or dialysis |

**CURRENT DIAGNOSIS**

- Appropriate diagnosis and management of a necrotizing skin and soft tissue infection (SSTI) require early clinical suspicion and a prompt comprehensive examination. Focus on the following:
  - Systemic evaluation: Presence of certain risk factors, hemodynamic instability, respiratory distress, toxic appearance, delirium
  - Local features: Rapidly progressive erythema or pain, pain out of proportion to appearance of infection, dermal necrosis, bullae, crepitus, undermining of the skin, and tissue planes that separate when a blunt probe is passed through openings in the skin
  - Key laboratory investigations: Hematologic derangement, organ failure, gas in the soft tissues
- Diagnosis is best established by prompt surgical assessment of the involved soft tissue for gross and microscopic evaluation. Tissue specimens should be sent for immediate Gram stain, culture, and susceptibility testing.

include diabetic ketoacidosis, iron overload states and deferoxamine (Desferal) therapy, immunocompromised states (prolonged neutropenia, hematologic malignancy, corticosteroid therapy, solid organ or stem cell transplant), and soft tissue trauma (e.g., burns, contaminated wounds).

## Clinical Features

The distinction between necrotizing SSTIs and uncomplicated SSTIs (e.g., cellulitis) may be difficult. Both usually manifest with erythema, edema, and tenderness of a localized area of skin. A systematic approach for clinical features favoring the presence of a necrotizing SSTI should be undertaken, including a systemic evaluation of the patient, a focused assessment of the involved region, and laboratory investigations (Table 2).

## Diagnosis

A key component in diagnosing a necrotizing SSTI is to clinically suspect it. Imaging modalities (e.g., plain radiographs, computed tomographic [CT] scans, magnetic resonance image [MRI] scans) may be useful to delineate the depth and extent of infection. However, the time required to obtain such investigations can lead to inappropriate delays in diagnostic and life-saving interventions. The most important diagnostic procedure in suspected cases is surgical exploration to determine the gross and microscopic appearance of the subcutaneous, fascial, and muscle layers. Hence, early surgical consultation is necessary. Specimens of the tissue itself (rather than a swab) should be sent for Gram stain and microbiological culture and susceptibility testing; these results will help in guiding management.

## Treatment

Effective management of all forms of necrotizing SSTIs requires a combined surgical and medical approach. Early and aggressive débridement of gangrenous tissue is crucial. Repeated exploration and débridements are commonly necessary. Amputation is required in some cases.

Medical therapy consists of early initiation of appropriate antimicrobial therapy and supportive care (usually in an intensive care unit) (Table 3). In the case of STSIs, adjunctive therapy with intravenous immunoglobulin (IVIG, Baygam)[1] may be used. Because these infections may be difficult to treat, consultation with an infectious disease specialist is encouraged.

Because most necrotizing SSTIs are polymicrobial, it is usually most prudent to initiate broad-spectrum empiric antimicrobial therapy that covers the typical mixed aerobic and anaerobic flora of such infections. No single regimen is superior to others. Given the usual toxicity of such patients, intravenous therapy should be used, at least initially. In patients with a history of penicillin allergy, alternative regimens must be created that cover the same spectrum of pathogens

---

[1]Not FDA approved for this indication.

---

**TABLE 2   Clinical Clues to the Presence of Acute Necrotizing Skin and Soft Tissue Infections**

| Systemic Features | Local Features | Laboratory Investigations |
|---|---|---|
| Altered mental status (e.g., delirious, stuporous, obtunded) | Anesthesia of the affected area | Myonecrosis (e.g., increased creatine kinase, increased myoglobin) |
| | Crepitus | Radiography: Gas in the soft tissues |
| Hypotension (systolic BP <90 mm Hg or <5th percentile by age for children <16 years | Rapidly progressive spread of erythema or pain | WBC ≥12,000 cells/µL or ≤4000 cells/µL or >10% immature granulocytes |
| | Focal areas of dermal necrosis | |
| Hypothermia or fever (temperature ≤36°C or ≥38°C) | Foul smell | Acidosis |
| Hypoxia | Purulent discharge, particularly if grayish or blackish or with gas bubbles | Electrolyte derangements (e.g., hyponatremia, hypocalcemia) |
| Tachycardia (heart rate ≥90 bpm) | Dusky, violaceous, or brownish discoloration | Anemia |
| | Bullae (serum filled or blood filled) | |
| Tachypnea (respiratory rate ≥20 breaths/min) | Generalized erythematous macular rash with or without desquamation | Thrombocytopenia with or without DIC |
| Toxic appearance | Exquisite tenderness out of proportion to the appearance of the affected area | Organ dysfunction (e.g., increased serum creatinine, increased hepatic transaminase) |

*Note:* A patient who has a necrotizing soft tissue infection might also have limited clinical findings, and thus the history and clinical acumen will be of great value in helping to guide therapeutic interventions.
*Abbreviations:* DIC = disseminated intravascular coagulation; WBC = white blood cell count.

## CURRENT THERAPY

- Expeditious and aggressive surgical débridement is mandatory; second look surgeries with repeated débridements are usually required.
- Broad-spectrum antimicrobial therapy covering aerobic and anaerobic gram-positive and gram-negative organisms should be initiated empirically. Once culture results are available, the antimicrobial regimen can be tailored.

(gram-positive, gram-negative, and anaerobic bacteria). Examples of recommended regimens are provided in the Current Therapy box.

Monomicrobial necrotizing SSTIs do not, in theory, require empiric broad-spectrum therapy. However, because it may be difficult to confidently predict either the monomicrobial nature of the infection on initial presentation or the specific single pathogen involved, it may be most prudent to administer broad-spectrum antibiotic coverage empirically. Once results of cultures and susceptibilities become available, the regimen can be focused on the isolated pathogen.

Fungal necrotizing SSTIs should be empirically treated with amphotericin B (either deoxycholate [Fungizone] or lipid-based formulation [Abelcet, AmBisome]), because this is currently the only

**TABLE 3 Empiric Antimicrobial Therapy for Necrotizing Skin and Soft Tissue Infections**

| Pathogen(s) | Empiric Antimicrobial Therapy* | |
| --- | --- | --- |
| | **First Line** | **Alternative†** |
| **Polymicrobial** | | |
| Aerobic or anaerobic gram-negative or gram-positive bacteria | Ticarcillin-clavulanate (Timentin) 3.1 g IV q6h *or* Piperacillin/tazobactam (Tazocin, Zosyn) 3.375 g IV q6h *or* Meropenem (Merrem) 1 g IV q8h *or* Imipenem-cilastatin (Primaxin) 500 mg IV q6h | Vancomycin (Vancocin) 1 g IV q12h *plus* a fluoroquinolone *plus* metronidazole (Flagyl) 500 mg IV q8h *or* Vancomycin 1 g IV q12h *plus* aztreonam (Azactam) 1 g IV q8h *plus* metronidazole 500 mg IV q8h *or* Ceftriaxone (Rocephin) 1 g IV q24h *plus* clindamycin (Dalacin, Cleocin) 600 mg q8h |
| **Monomicrobial** | | |
| Group A streptococcus (*S. pyogenes*) | Penicillin G 4 million units IV q4h *plus* clindamycin 600-900 q4h *plus* mg IV q8h | Clindamycin 600-900 mg IV q8h |
| *Clostridium perfringens, Clostridium septicum* | Penicillin G 4 million units IV q4h plus clindamycin 600-900 mg IV q8h | Clindamycin 600-900 mg IV q8h or Metronidazole 500 mg PO or IV q8h |
| *Aeromonas hydrophila* | Ciprofloxacin (Cipro) 400 mg IV q12h or levofloxacin (Levaquin) 750 mg IV q24h | Trimethoprim-sulfamethoxazole (TMP/SMX, Septra, Bactrim)[1] 10 mg/kg/d (based on TMP) IV divided q6h or Ceftriaxone[1] 1 g IV q12h or Cefotaxime (Claforan)[1] 1 g IV q8h |
| *Vibrio vulnificus* | Minocycline (Minocin, Dynacin)[1] 100 mg IV q12h plus either ceftriaxone[1] 1 g IV q12h or cefotaxime[1] 1 g IV q8h | Ciprofloxacin (Cipro)[1] 400 mg IV q12h |
| *Pseudomonas aeruginosa* | Ciprofloxacin 400 mg IV q12h or Ceftazidime (Fortaz, Tazicef) 1 g IV q8h or Piperacillin-tazobactam 4.5 g IV q8h or Meropenem 1 g IV q8h | |
| Community-acquired methicillin-resistant *Staphylococcus aureus* | Vancomycin 1 g IV q12h | TMP/SMX[1] 10 mg/kg/d (based on TMP) IV divided q6h *or* Linezolid (Zyvox) 600 mg PO/IV q12h *or* Daptomycin (Cubicin) 4 mg/kg IV qd‡ |
| **Fungal** | | |
| Septated molds (e.g., *Aspergillus spp, Fusarium spp, Scedosporium spp*) | Amphotericin B deoxycholate (Fungizone) 1-1.5 mg/kg/d *or* Amphotericin B lipid-based formulations: Amphotericin B lipid complex (ABLC, Abelcet)[1] 5 mg/kg IV qd or Liposomal amphotericin B (L-AmB, AmBisome)[1] 5 mg/kg IV qd | Voriconazole (Vfend) 6 mg/kg IV q12h × 1 d, then 4 mg/kg IV q12h‡ |
| Zygomycetes or mucormycosis | Amphotericin B deoxycholate 1-1.5 mg/kg/d *or* Amphotericin B lipid-based formulations: Amphotericin B lipid complex[1] 5 mg/kg IV qd *or* Liposomal amphotericin B[1] 5 mg/kg IV qd | Posaconazole (Noxafil) 200 mg PO qid[1,‡,§] |

[1]Not FDA approved for this indication.

*The dosages of antimicrobial agents provided are based on normal renal function in adults weighing ≥70 kg and may need to be modified in patients with renal insufficiency. Drug serum levels should be monitored where appropriate.

†Alternative recommended regimens may be used in patients with a history of type 1 hypersensitivity reaction (anaphylaxis) to penicillin or other β-lactams. Other regimens with equivalent coverage are also appropriate.

‡Currently, there is a paucity of published clinical experience with these agents for necrotizing SSTIs.

§Posaconazole is available only orally.

antifungal agent with generally reliable coverage against septated molds and zygomycetes (although exceptions do occur). In addition, the underlying immunocompromised state, if possible, should be reversed (e.g., discontinue or decrease steroids and other immunosuppressive therapies).

Once the results of cultures and susceptibilities are available, the antimicrobial regimen can be tailored. The duration of antimicrobial therapy should be individualized.

## REFERENCES

Bisno AL, Stevens DL: Streptococcal infections of skin and soft tissues. N Engl J Med 1996;334:240-245.

DiNubile MJ, Lipsky BA: Complicated infections of skin and skin structures: When the infection is more than skin deep. J Antimicrob Chemother 2004;53:37-50.

Ellis MW, Lewis JS 2nd: Treatment approaches for community-acquired methicillin-resistant *Staphylococcus aureus* infections. Curr Opin Infect Dis 2005;18:496-501.

Eron LJ, Lipsky BA, Low DE, et al: Managing skin and soft tissue infections: Expert panel recommendations on key decision points. J Antimicrob Chemother 2003;52:3-17.

Nichols RL, Florman S: Clinical presentations of soft-tissue infections and surgical site infections. Clin Infect Dis 2001;33(suppl 2):S84-S93.

Lipsky BA, Berendt AR, Deery HG, et al, for the Infectious Disease Society of America: Diagnosis and treatment of diabetic foot infections. Clin Infect Dis 2004;39: 885-910.

Stevens DL, Bisno AL, Chambers HF, et al, for the Infectious Disease Society of America: Practice guidelines for the diagnosis and management of skin and soft-tissue infections. Clin Infect Dis 2005;41:1373-1406.

Vinh DC, Embil JM: Rapidly progressive soft tissue infections. Lancet Infect Dis 2005;5:501-513.

Vinh DC, Embil JM: Rapidly progressive soft tissue infections—Authors' reply. Lancet Infect Dis 2006;6:66-67.

# Toxic Shock Syndrome

Method of
*Marty S. Teltscher, MD, CM, and
Andre Dascal, MD, FRCPC*

Initially reported as early as 1927 as *staphylococcal scarlet fever*, toxic shock syndrome (TSS) was defined by Todd and colleagues in 1978, and it was brought to the forefront of public concern in the early 1980s when healthy young women were contracting severe systemic illness associated with use of highly absorbent tampons. Reports of a similar syndrome involving invasive streptococcal disease soon followed in the late 1980s.

TSS is a rapidly progressive, potentially lethal toxin-mediated syndrome characterized by hyperpyrexia, erythrodermic rash, and multiorgan dysfunction. Original descriptions were attributed to toxin-producing strains of *Staphylococcus aureus* (SA-TSS) and the invasive group A β-hemolytic streptococcus *Streptococcus pyogenes* (GAS-TSS). There have been case reports of TSS associated with infection by groups B, C, and G β-hemolytic streptococci and with *Clostridium sordellii*.

## Epidemiology

SA-TSS is categorized as either menstrual or nonmenstrual. Menstrual cases are defined as TSS occurring 2 days before menses or 2 days after menstruation. The vast majority of cases of menstrual SA-TSS were associated with tampon use, but it can occur during menses without tampon use. These cases demonstrate how noninvasive colonization by toxin-producing *S. aureus* can produce toxin-mediated disease. Nonmenstrual SA-TSS is associated with wound infections (surgical and nonsurgical), recalcitrant erythematous desquamating syndrome

(mainly in the HIV/AIDS population), presence of foreign bodies (including intrauterine devices, diaphragms, tampons, nasal packing), burns, osteomyelitis, septic arthritis, postinfluenza superinfection, and, increasingly, community-acquired methicillin-resistant *S. aureus* (CA-MRSA) infection.

Both forms of SA-TSS occur overwhelmingly in young women. Between 1979 and 1980, menstrual SA-TSS accounted for 91% of all TSS cases; surveillance through 1987 to 1996 noted a decline to 58% of cases. By the end of the 1980s, with change of tampon materials, removal of certain products from the market, and changes in patterns of tampon use, the incidence of SA-TSS diminished from 10 cases per 100,000 women of menstrual age to 1 case per 100,000 women.

In 2004, Schlievert and colleagues published data suggesting a reemergence of both menstrual and nonmenstrual cases of TSS, having observed the rate of 1 per 100,000 (in 2000) jump to nearly 4 per 100,000 by 2003. There was a concomitant 18% increase of all TSS reported by the Centers for Disease Control and Prevention (CDC). The reemergence of TSS is hypothesized to be associated with increased prevalence of CA-MRSA infection, earlier menarche, and a larger population of nonimmune menstruating women.

The case-fatality rate overall for SA-TSS was 3% between 1979 and 1980 and 5% between 1987 and 1996. Over the same time periods there was a marked decrease between case-fatality rates of menstrual cases from 5.5% to 1.8%; nonmenstrual rates remained relatively constant, diminishing only from 8.6% to 6%.

GAS-TSS most commonly occurs with GAS soft tissue infections such as cellulitis, necrotizing fasciitis, and myonecrosis. In up to 50% of cases, there is no identifiable portal of entry for GAS infection. Patients who develop GAS-TSS in the absence of invasive disease often develop an invasive infection over time. Because of the increasing frequency of invasive GAS infections, there are increased reports of GAS-TSS. GAS-TSS is estimated to have a prevalence of 1 to 5 cases per 100,000 persons. Risk factors include disruption of skin or mucosal barriers, diabetes, alcoholism, varicella infection, pregnancy, use of nonsteroidal anti-inflammatory medications (NSAIDs), immunocompromised state, recent surgery, and nonsurgical trauma. The morbidity and mortality rates for GAS-TSS are estimated at 30% to 80%.

## Pathogenesis

Toxic shock syndrome is the culmination of an exaggerated inflammatory immune response by bacterial endotoxins and exotoxins belonging to the superantigen (SAG) superfamily. Biochemical and genetic analyses demonstrate that SAG proteins likely have common ancestry and are homologous in structure and function. SAGs complex with the class II major histocompatibility molecule on antigen-presenting cells and facilitate the cross-linking with the variable β region on the T cell αβ receptor without normal antigen processing and outside of the standard antigen-presenting groove. A normal T-cell response recruits 1 in 10,000 T lymphocytes, but a SAG can activate up to 20% of all T lymphocytes. The end result is a rapid cytokine storm from T lymphocytes, macrophages, and other immune cells involving release of tumor necrosis factor α (TNF-α), interleukin-1 (IL-1), IL-2, and interferon-γ (INF-γ). Clinical manifestations of this immunologic process include hyperpyrexia, capillary leak syndrome, vasodilation, myocardial suppression, hypotension, erythroderma, coagulopathy, acute renal failure, and ultimately multisystem organ failure and death.

The host's immune system and ability to respond to the infectious agent are also implicated in disease severity. Immunocompromised patients and persons with low antibody titers to the offending toxin are likely to develop more severe disease. Superantigens contribute to further immune dysfunction by disrupting the reticuloendothelial system; increasing host susceptibility to endotoxin, causing shock; deleting T-lymphocyte populations mediating humoral immunity; and disrupting cellular immunity through T-cell anergy and accelerated apoptosis.

SA-TSS was initially associated with toxic shock syndrome toxin-1 (TSST-1). Ninety percent of strains isolated from menstrual cases produce TSST-1. Highly absorbent tampons facilitated toxin production by optimizing conditions for *S. aureus* toxin production, namely

**CURRENT DIAGNOSIS**

**Common Clinical Features**

- Fever, hypotension, and shock
- Multiorgan system dysfunction
- Diffuse macular erythroderma including the soles and palms
- Desquamation of soles and palms can occur in convalescent stages

**Type-Specific Clinical Features**

STAPHYLOCOCCAL TOXIC SHOCK SYNDROME

- History of current or recent menstruation
- Influenza-like prodrome
- Bacteremia in 5% of cases
- Microbiology: *Staphylococcus aureus* is isolated from the patient in 80% to 90% of cases but is not mandatory for diagnosis
- Serology: Lack of antibody to toxin at onset of illness is associated with severe illness
- Case fatality rate is 5%

STREPTOCOCCAL TOXIC SHOCK SYNDROME

- Presence of surgical or nonsurgical wound or foreign body
- Soft tissue infection, often invasive, including cellulitis, necrotizing fasciitis, or myonecrosis
- Dusky or gangrenous tissue carries a poor prognosis
- Bacteremia in 30%-60% cases
- Microbiology: Isolation of group A β-hemolytic streptococci
- Serology: Presence of antibody to toxin in convalescent stage confirmatory if initially absent
- Presence of anti-DNase B antibody and antistreptolysin O antibody are supportive
- Case fatality rate is 30%-80%

---

elevated $P_{O_2}$, elevated $P_{CO_2}$, neutral pH, and elevated protein levels. TSST-1 easily crosses mucosal barriers. In nonmenstrual SA-TSS, TSST-1 is only implicated in 50% of cases; the culprit toxins in the other half of these cases are staphylococcal enterotoxins (SEs), most commonly SEB and SEC.

GAS-TSS is mediated by streptococcal pyrogenic exotoxins (SPEs) and streptococcal mitogenic exotoxin Z. In addition, the cell surface M protein, a filamentous protein conveying antiphagocytic properties, is a contributing virulence factor. M serotypes 1 and 3 are associated with invasive streptococcal disease; these, in addition to serotypes 12 and 28, are associated with GAS-TSS.

## Diagnosis

Cases of TSS should be suspected in otherwise healthy persons presenting with rapidly progressing symptoms featuring fever, erythroderma, hypotension, and multiorgan dysfunction. Case definitions for SA-TSS and GAS-TSS are presented in Boxes 1 and 2, respectively.

Onset of SA-TSS occurs 2 to 3 days after surgery or onset of menses. Early manifestations include a diffuse red, macular rash that does not spare soles or palms. The rash might involve the mucosa. In some severe cases petechiae, ulcerations, vesicles, and bullae occur. During the convalescent phase of the illness, 1 to 2 weeks after onset of symptoms, a nonspecific maculopapular rash with desquamation of the palms and soles can occur.

---

**BOX 1  Case Definitions for *Staphylococcus aureus* Toxic Shock Syndrome**

**Standard Definition**

A definite case is an illness that meets 6 out of 6 original criteria. A probable case is an illness that meets 5 out of 6 criteria.

- Fever: Temperature >38.9°C
- Hypotension
  - Systolic blood pressure >90 mm Hg
  - Orthostatic drop in diastolic blood pressure >15 mm Hg
  - Orthostatic syncope or dizziness
- Rash: Diffuse macular erythroderma, often involving palms and soles
- Desquamation 1-2 wk after onset, particularly on the palms and soles
- Multisystem organ involvement (≥3)
  - CNS: Disorientation or altered level of consciousness without focal neurologic signs when fever and hypotension are absent
  - GI: Vomiting or diarrhea at onset of illness
  - Hematologic: Platelet count <100,000/mm³)
  - Hepatic: Total bilirubin, ALT, or AST >twice the upper limit of normal
  - Mucous membranes: Vaginal, oropharyngeal, or conjunctival hyperemia
  - Muscular: Severe myalgia or CK >twice the upper limit of normal
  - Renal: BUN or creatinine >twice the upper limit of normal or pyuria in the absence of UTI
- Negative results of
  - Blood, throat, or CSF cultures (blood cultures may be positive for *S. aureus*)
  - Serologic tests for Rocky Mountain spotted fever, leptospirosis, or measles

**Revised Definition**

A revised definition seeks to incorporate laboratory findings confirming presence of an agent and susceptibility of the host.
- Any of the following laboratory findings†
  - Isolation of *S. aureus* from a mucosal or normally sterile site
  - Production of TSS-associated SAG by isolate
  - Lack of antibody to the implicated toxin at the time of acute illness
  - Development of antibody to the toxin during convalescence

---

Standard definition adapted from Reingold AL, Hargrett NT, Shands KN, et al: Toxic shock syndrome surveillance in the United States, 1980 to 1981. Ann Intern Med 1982;96:875-880. Revised definition from Parsonnet J: Case definition of staphylococcal TSS: A proposed revision incorporating laboratory findings. In Arbuthnott J, Furman B (eds). European Conference on Toxic Shock Syndrome. International Congress and Symposium Series 229. London: Royal Society of Medicine Press, 1997.
*Abbreviations*: ALT = alanine aminotransferase; AST = aspartate aminotransferase; BUN = blood urea nitrogen; CK = creatine phosphokinase; CNS = central nervous system; CSF = cerebrospinal fluid; GI = gastrointestinal; SAG = superantigen; TSS = toxic shock syndrome; UTI = urinary tract infection.

A major review on the subject of TSS and superantigens in 2001 by McCormick and colleagues urges revision and modernization of the case definition by incorporating specific laboratory findings. The isolation of *S. aureus* from a mucosal or normally sterile site, production of TSS-associated SAG by isolated strains, lack of antibody to the implicated toxin at the time of acute illness, and development of antibody to the toxin during convalescence should contribute to the diagnosis of a likely case of SA-TSS. Although isolation of *S. aureus* from wounds and mucosal sites occurs in up to 90% of cases of SA-TSS, it is not required for the diagnosis. Bacteremia is present in only about 5% of cases.

In GAS-TSS, infection can begin within 1 to 3 days after a minor local trauma. Suspicions should be raised in cases with rapidly progressive localized or diffuse pain that might indicate invasive streptococcal soft tissue infection. Soft tissue disease is present in 80% of cases. Invasive disease is present in 50% of cases. Repeated meticulous physical examination is necessary to detect the manifestation of initially unidentified invasive soft tissue disease. An influenza-like prodrome occurs before toxic presentation in 20% of cases. Bacteremia is present in 60% of patients with GAS-TSS. Titers of antibody to DNase B and antistreptolysin O can be measured to confirm exposure to GAS.

The differential diagnosis of TSS includes septic shock, meningococcemia, Rocky Mountain spotted fever, scarlet fever, leptospirosis, ehrlichiosis, Kawasaki's disease, lupus erythematosus, measles, dengue fever, other viral exanthema, and adverse cutaneous drug eruption.

## Treatment

Management of TSS requires early and definitive treatment. Critical care expertise early in the presentation of these patients is desirable. Treatment focuses on stabilizing the patient, eradicating the culprit organism, minimizing the toxin-mediated effects, and modulating the inflammatory immune response. Initial therapy includes large volumes of crystalloid intravenous fluids and vasopressor support to minimize hypotension-induced end-organ damage. Blood products may be required to reverse coagulopathies and anemia. Surgical intervention in both GAS-TSS and SA-TSS should not be overlooked because it may be critical for exploration of affected tissues, débridement

## CURRENT THERAPY

**Initial Management**

- Volume and crystalloid resuscitation
- Vasopressors and inotropic agents to support blood pressure as needed
- Correction of coagulopathy and anemia (frozen plasma, cryoprecipitate, and packed red blood cells)
- Initiation of appropriate antibiotic therapy
- Surgical consultation should be considered early in manifestation
- Critical care and infectious disease consultation

**Staphylococcal Toxic Shock Syndrome**

- Antibiotics
- One penicillinase-resistant penicillin:
  - Oxacillin (Bactocill) 2 g IV q4h
  - Nafcillin (Unipen) 2 g IV q4h
  - Cloxacillin (Cloxapen) 2 g IV q4h*

*plus*

- Clindamycin (Cleocin) 900 mg IV q8h

*plus*

- Vancomycin (Vancocin) 2 g IV q12h†
- Adjust dose of penicillins and vancomycin for degree of renal dysfunction

**Streptococcal Toxic Shock Syndrome**

ANTIBIOTICS

- Penicillin 4 million U IV q4h

*with or without*

- Ceftriaxone (Rocephin) 2 g IV q12h

*plus*

- Clindamycin (Cleocin) 900 mg IV q8h
- Adjust dose of penicillins and vancomycin for degree of renal dysfunction

INTRAVENOUS IMMUNOGLOBULIN[1] (IVIG)

- 1.0 g/kg d 1, 0.5 g/kg d 2 and 3 of treatment
- Data are not sufficient to recommend IVIG in all cases
- May be beneficial in streptococcal toxic shock
- Reasonable in some severe cases of staphylococcal toxic shock
- Staphylococcal toxic shock may require higher doses

---

*Intravenous cloxacillin formulation is available only in Canada.
†The addition of vancomycin should be based on prevalence of community-acquired methicillin-resistant *S. aureus* in the patient's population. Discontinue if appropriate when sensitivities are known.

---

of necrotic tissues, and removal of foreign bodies. Antibiotics contribute to the management by reducing the number of toxin-producing organisms (β-lactams and vancomycin [Vancocin]), as well as reducing production of toxin (clindamycin [Cleocin]) and possibly by modulating immune response (clindamycin).

## ANTIBIOTICS

Antibiotics must be selected empirically, initially, and thereafter tailored to the specific resistance patterns of the organism. Penicillins and vancomycin should be appropriately adjusted for the degree of renal insufficiency. Patients who have allergies to β-lactams and therefore cannot take penicillins and cephalosporins should be treated with vancomycin. Macrolides are not recommended due to resistance patterns, despite their superiority to penicillin in vitro and in animal studies. Minimal data are available about the use of fluoroquinolones, quinpristin-dalfopristin (Synercid), and linezolide (Zyvox) in TSS.

Current recommendations for the treatment of SA-TSS include combination of a penicillinase-resistant penicillin such as oxacillin (Bactocill), nafcillin (Unipen), or cloxacillin (Cloxapen) (2 g IV q4h) and high-dose clindamycin (900 mg IV q8h). Due to increasing rates of toxin-producing CA-MRSA, the addition of vancomycin (2 g/day IV in divided doses) is advised until sensitivity to penicillinase-resistant penicillins is confirmed.

Current recommendations for the treatment of GAS-TSS include a combination of penicillin (4 million U q4h) and clindamycin (900 mg IV q8h). In severe GAS infections, ceftriaxone (Rocephin) (2g IV q12h) should be considered. Although GAS is susceptible to penicillin, in large numbers of organisms the efficacy is reduced, likely due to reduction in the penicillin-targeted penicillin-binding proteins (PBPs) when GAS enters the stationary phase of growth. Ceftriaxone may have preferred activity, likely due to the increased expression of PBPs that it targets. Clindamycin affects protein synthesis rather than structural cell wall building factors, and the number of organisms has no bearing on efficacy.

## ADJUNCTIVE THERAPY

### Immunomodulatory Therapy

Adjunctive therapies include intravenous immunoglobulin (IVIg)[1] and other immunomodulators of the exaggerated inflammatory reaction initiated by toxic superantigens.

Although there are minimal clinical trial data available on the use of IVIg in TSS, there is anecdotal and in vitro evidence supporting its early administration. It has been shown that polyclonal commercially available IVIg binds and inactivates toxins that mediate TSS; however, there is variability in efficacy from brand to brand, as well as between batches within brands. In vitro studies have demonstrated increased potency of IVIg against GAS toxins as compared with *S. aureus* toxins, raising doubt about appropriate protective doses of IVIg. In a 2003 survey of infectious disease and critical care specialists across Canada, 76% of respondents reported that they would use IVIg in GAS-TSS, but only 26% would add it to therapy for SA-TSS.

In a recent clinical trial, a trend toward a protective effect of IVIg (Endobulin) (1.0 g/kg on day 1, 0.5 g/kg on days 2 and 3) was elucidated. However, this trial was underpowered and halted prior to completion due to lack of enrollment. It is theorized that IVIg is particularly useful early in disease manifestation to minimize the inflammatory reaction until definitive antibiotic therapy is initiated.

The use of IVIg is not without risk. There have been case reports of acute tubular necrosis, aseptic meningitis syndrome, central retinal vein obstruction, myocardial infarction, and thromboembolic diseases associated with IVIG use. Furthermore, patients with immunoglobulin A (IgA) deficiency can have severe anaphylactic reactions to IVIg infusion.

In summary, due to lack of unequivocal objective data, IVIg therapy remains controversial, but it may be reasonable for treating TSS, especially GAS-TSS. Further research and well-formulated large-scale clinical trials are necessary.

Immunomodulatory therapy focuses on inhibiting the signaling cascades induced by superantigens as well as the cytokines that are ultimately expressed. A combination of in vivo and in vitro data has been reported using a variety of agents demonstrating the effectiveness of suppressing SEB-mediated effects of TSS. Pentoxifylline (Trental)[1] is a TNF-α inhibitor that has been shown to dampen the inflammatory reaction, as has the corticosteroid dexamethasone (Decadron).[1] Other synthetic compounds and antibiotics have also been proposed. These therapies have not yet been approved for use in TSS, and inadequate data are available to recommend their use at this time.

## Chemoprophylaxis

Chemoprophylaxis remains a controversial issue. The rate of secondary cases among close contacts of patients with invasive GAS disease is 200 times that of the general population. *Close contact* has been defined as persons spending more than 4 hours a day or 20 hours a week together, sharing sleeping arrangements, or having direct mucous membrane contact within 7 days of illness of the index patient.

In 1998, The CDC did not recommend antibiotic prophylaxis for all close contacts but rather individualization of prophylaxis for those exposed to patients with invasive GAS infection. The matter was revisited in a review in 2005 with a similar conclusion, stating that chemoprophylaxis was not warranted and that close contacts should be notified and urged to present for examination at the first signs of suspicious symptoms. Some public health authorities in Canada agree that close contacts should receive chemoprophylaxis with penicillin, first-generation cephalosporins, clindamycin, or erythromycin for 10 days. The official recommendations vary from province to province and depend on the type of invasive streptococcal disease.

The theoretical risks of empiric antibiotic use in the select few exposed to patients with this rare disease are probably negligible in the face of potentially new invasive GAS infections. Possible risks include antibiotic-associated diarrhea and *C. difficile* colitis.

## REFERENCES

Darenberg J, Ihendyane N, Sjolin J, et al; and the StreptIg Study Group: Intravenous immunoglobulin G therapy in streptococcal toxic shock syndrome: A European randomized, double-blind, placebo-controlled trial. Clin Infect Dis 2003;37:333-340.

Davies DH: Flesh-eating disease: A note on necrotizing fasciitis. Can J Infect Dis 2001;12:136-140.

Durand G, Bes M, Meugnier H, et al: Detection of new methicillin-resistant *Staphylococcus aureus* clones containing the toxic shock syndrome toxin 1 gene responsible for hospital- and community-acquired infections in France. J Clin Mircobiol 2006;44:847-853.

Gosbell IB: Epidemiology, clinical features and management of infections due to community methicillin-resistant *Staphylococcus aureus* (cMRSA). Intern Med J 2005;35:S120-S135.

Krakauer T: Chemotherapeutics targeting immune activation by staphylococcal superantigens. Med Sci Monit 2005;11(9):RA290-RA295.

Llewelyn M, Cohen J: Superantigens: Microbial agents that corrupt immunity. Lancet Infect Dis 2002;2:156-162.

McCormick JK, Yarwood JM, Schlievert PM: Toxic shock syndrome and bacterial superantigens: An update. Annu Rev Microbiol 2001;55:77-104.

Reingold AL, Hargrett NT, Shands KN, et al: Toxic shock syndrome surveillance in the United States, 1980 to 1981. Ann Intern Med 1982;96:875-880.

Schlievert PM: Use of intravenous immunoglobulin in the treatment of staphylococcal and streptococcal toxic shock syndromes and related illnesses. J Allergy Clin Immunol 2001;108:S107-S110.

Schlievert PM, Tripp TJ, Peterson ML: Reemergence of staphylococcal toxic shock syndrome in Minneapolis–St. Paul, Minnesota, during 2000-2003 surveillance period. J Clin Microbiol 2004;42:2875-2876. Correspondence and reply: Tierno PM: Reemergence of staphylococcal toxic shock syndrome in the United States since 2000. J Clin Microbiol 2005;43: 2032-2033.

Smith A, Lamagni TL, Olivier I, et al. Invasive group A streptococcal disease: Should close contacts routinely receive antibiotic prophylaxis? Lancet Infect Dis 2005;5:494-500.

Stevens DL. The flesh-eating bacterium: What's next? J Infect Dis 1999;179: S366-S374.

Todd J, Fishaut M, Kapral F, Welch T: Toxic-shock syndrome associated with phage-group-I Staphylococci. Lancet 1978;2(8100):1116-1118.

---

[1]Not FDA approved for this indication.

# Influenza

Method of
*Michael B. Rothberg, MD, MPH*

Influenza is a viral respiratory infection that occurs in winter epidemics, affecting one tenth of the world's population each year. Among children and persons living in closed environments such as nursing homes or military bases, infection rates are as high as 40%. In the United States alone, influenza is estimated to cause 35,000 deaths and 200,000 hospitalizations each year, mostly among the elderly and those with serious comorbid illnesses. Direct medical costs exceed $3 billion, and indirect costs stemming from lost productivity total $15 billion yearly in the United States.

Influenza types A and B cause illness in humans. Influenza A viruses are divided into subtypes based on the hemagglutinin (H) and neuraminidase (N) glycoproteins expressed on their surfaces. Currently circulating viruses include H3N2 and H1N1 subtypes. Minor variations in these glycoproteins (antigenic drift) occur almost yearly, resulting in new strains that cause localized outbreaks. Major variation (antigenic shift) occurs when two subtypes combine to create a new subtype, resulting in a global pandemic. Although infrequent, pandemics can have devastating consequences due to lack of immunity in the population. The H5N1 virus, or avian flu, has a mortality rate of 59%, but it cannot be considered a pandemic strain because it is not transmitted efficiently between humans.

Because treatment is only modestly effective, influenza control efforts have focused on vaccination and prophylaxis, especially of high-risk groups. More recently, vaccination programs have expanded to include lower-risk adults and preschool children. National surveillance networks can now identify local outbreaks quickly and communicate the information efficiently via the Internet to individual providers, allowing timely diagnosis and treatment with antiviral therapy. As the use of antiviral drugs has increased, so has resistance, creating a challenge to find newer, more effective therapies, as we stand on the brink of a global pandemic.

## Clinical Features

Influenza is spread via the respiratory route. Following an incubation period of 1 to 4 days, the virus typically causes abrupt onset of fever and dry cough, often accompanied by nasal congestion, headache, and myalgias. Fever can last for 3 to 5 days, during which time the patient is highly infectious. Recovery can last up to 2 weeks. Although the acute infection can cause a viral pneumonia, secondary bacterial infections—sinusitis, otitis media, bronchitis, and pneumonia—are more common. Elderly persons, infants, and those with comorbid conditions such as heart or lung disease are most susceptible to complications, accounting for the overwhelming majority of hospital admissions. Among community-dwelling elderly persons, there is considerable variability in the risk of hospitalization or death from influenza or pneumonia, ranging from 0.2% to 15% depending on age and comorbidities.

## Diagnosis

The signs and symptoms of influenza illness are nonspecific and cannot be reliably distinguished from those of other viral upper respiratory infections. One meta-analysis of diagnostic studies found that only fever (odds ratio [OR], 1.8) increased the likelihood of influenza, whereas absence of fever (OR, 0.40), cough (OR, 0.42), or headache (OR, 0.75) and lack of nasal congestion (OR, 0.49) all decreased it. Other symptoms typically associated with influenza, such as myalgia, malaise, and chills, had positive predictive value only for patients older than 60 years. Given the low odds ratios associated with clinical

## CURRENT DIAGNOSIS

- Influenza remains a clinical diagnosis based on the presence of fever, nasal congestion, and cough in the setting of local influenza activity.
- Rapid diagnostic testing can aid in diagnosis and surveillance early in the influenza season. Once influenza is detected, however, rapid testing gives too many false-negative results to be useful.

findings, signs and symptoms must be considered in the context of the local incidence of influenza at the time of presentation.

Rapid testing of nasal specimens is available. Two of these (Quickvue and ZStatFlu) can be conducted in the office in less than 30 minutes, allowing physicians to act on the diagnostic information. Others are restricted to laboratory use. Rapid tests have low sensitivity (65%-86%), especially among adults, but high specificity (>90%). Thus, a positive test confirms the diagnosis, but a negative test does not exclude it, especially when influenza is circulating locally.

Decision analyses and cost-effectiveness analyses have demonstrated that rapid testing is reasonable when clinical suspicion is low. In such cases, testing is superior to either empiric antiviral therapy or symptomatic therapy. When clinical suspicion is high, testing is not recommended, because the high false-negative rate can lead to patients with true influenza going untreated.

Until recently, clinicians rarely knew the local prevalence of influenza. Reports from state health departments and the Centers for Disease Control and Prevention (CDC) often lagged by several weeks and were not easily obtainable. Now, however, a number of Internet resources provide real-time surveillance. FluWatch.com and Flustar.com offer free twice-weekly reports of local influenza prevalence by zip code.

## Prevention and Treatment

Vaccination and antiviral medication are the two methods of prophylaxis. Antiviral medications are also used for treatment.

### VACCINE

Influenza vaccination is the mainstay of prevention. Annual vaccination prevents influenza illness, complications, hospitalizations, and death in high-risk patients, and it is cost saving in elderly patients. Annual vaccination is required because immunity wanes and because antigenic drift results in new viruses each year. Patients receiving vaccine 2 or more years in a row have heightened immunity.

Current influenza vaccines contain two strains of influenza A, an H3N2 and an H1N1, and a single strain of influenza B. The strains for

## CURRENT THERAPY

- Antiviral therapy is an adjunct to, not a replacement for, influenza vaccination.
- Antiviral therapy is most beneficial for high-risk patients and must be started within 48 hours of onset of symptoms to be effective. Earlier treatment is more effective.
- Due to current resistance patterns, only neuraminidase inhibitors should be used for treatment or prophylaxis.
- Choice of therapy depends on side effect profile, cost, and availability.

the coming season are chosen each spring by independent experts to allow time for vaccine production.

## Efficacy

Vaccine efficacy depends on the degree of similarity between the vaccine strains and those in circulation and on the age and immunocompetence of the vaccine recipient. For healthy adults younger than 65 years, a well-matched vaccine prevents 70% to 90% of influenza illness. The efficacy declines to 58% in community-dwelling elderly and 30% to 40% among nursing home patients. However, efficacy in preventing complications, including hospitalization and death, is much higher in elderly persons and nursing home patients, with vaccination preventing 80% of deaths, even among debilitated patients.

## Administration

The Centers for Disease Control and Prevention (CDC) recommends intramuscular administration of inactivated influenza vaccine for the following groups:

- Persons at high risk for influenza-related complications and severe disease
  - Children ages 6 to 59 months
  - Pregnant women
  - Persons older than 50 years
  - Persons of any age with certain chronic medical conditions
- Persons who live with or who care for persons at high risk
  - Household contacts who have frequent contact with persons at high risk and who can transmit influenza to persons at high risk
  - Health care workers.

Healthy persons wishing to decrease their risk of influenza may also be vaccinated, although such vaccination might not be cost-effective.

For the past several years, there has been a shortage of influenza vaccine in the United States. In an effort to improve the quantity and reliability of available vaccine, the FDA in 2006 approved 5 different vaccine formulations, each with a different indication (Table 1). The live attenuated influenza vaccine (LAIV) (FluMist), administered via the nasal passages, causes a localized influenza infection of the nasopharyngeal epithelium and is not approved for use in high-risk patients. It can be given to healthy children and adults ages 5 to 49 years,

although it is more expensive than the inactivated vaccine. After receiving LAIV, vaccinees might shed virus and should avoid contact with immunosuppressed patients for 7 days. Efficacy of LAIV in healthy adults is comparable with that of inactivated vaccine.

The optimal time for influenza vaccination is October or November, but clinicians should continue to offer vaccination throughout the influenza season. High-risk patients in the community may be offered vaccination in September. Nursing home patients should not be vaccinated before October to avoid declining antibody levels during the influenza season. Strategies demonstrated to improve vaccination adherence include reminder or recall systems and standing orders in hospitals. Annual influenza vaccination is now a measure of health care quality used by Medicare and others.

## Adverse Effects

Fear of side effects, including catching the flu from the vaccine, is the leading reason that elderly patients decline annual vaccination. Apart from local pain at the injection site, however, placebo-controlled trials in adults and the elderly show no difference in systemic symptoms following active and placebo injections. Moreover, inactivated vaccines contain killed virus and cannot cause influenza illness. LAIV does increase the rate of rhinorrhea and sore throat relative to placebo, but symptoms are mild and self-limited.

Any person could develop an anaphylactic reaction to one of the vaccine components. Because all current vaccines are grown in eggs, patients with severe hypersensitivity reactions (e.g., anaphylaxis) to eggs should not receive any vaccine formulation. However, desensitization can be considered for high-risk patients with egg allergies.

Guillain-Barré syndrome (GBS) was linked to the 1976 swine flu vaccine, occurring at a rate of less than 10 per million vaccinees. Subsequent vaccines have not been causally linked to GBS, although a weak association is hard to exclude, given that GBS has an annual incidence of only 10 per million. If there is a risk to vaccination, it does not exceed 1 per million, much less than the risk of more severe influenza complications, especially among high-risk patients.

## ANTIVIRAL MEDICATIONS

Two classes of antiviral medications are available for the treatment and prophylaxis of influenza: adamantanes (amantadine [Symmetrel] and rimantadine [Flumadine]) and neuraminidase inhibitors (oseltamivir [Tamiflu] and zanamivir [Relenza]). The adamantanes are not

**TABLE 1** Approved Influenza Vaccines for Different Age Groups—United States, 2007-2008 Season

| Trade Name | Manufacturer | Dose/Presentation | Thimerosal Mercury Content (µg Hg/0.5 mL Dose) | Age Group | No. of Doses | Route |
|---|---|---|---|---|---|---|
| **Inactivated (TIV)** | | | | | | |
| Fluzone | Sanofi Pasteur | 0.25-mL pre-filled syringe | 0 | 6-35 mo | 1 or 2* | IM† |
| | | 0.5-mL pre-filled syringe | 0 | ≥36 mo | 1 or 2* | IM† |
| | | 0.5-mL vial | 0 | ≥36 mo | 1 or 2* | IM† |
| | | 5.0-mL multidose vial | 25 | ≥6 mo | 1 or 2* | IM† |
| Fluvirin | Novartis Vaccine‡ | 0.5 mL pre-filled syringe | <1.0 | ≥4 yr | 1 or 2* | IM† |
| | | 5.0 mL multidose vial | 24.5 | ≥4 y | 1 or 2* | IM† |
| Fluarix | GlaxoSmithKline | 0.5-mL pre-filled syringe | <1.25 | ≥18 y | 1 | IM† |
| FluLaval | GlaxoSmithKline | 5.0-mL multidose vial | 25 | ≥18 y | 1 | IM† |
| **Live Attenuated (LAIV)** | | | | | | |
| FluMist | Medimmune | 0.2-mL sprayer | 0 | 5-49 y | 1 or 2§ | Intranasal |

*Two doses administered at least 1 month apart are recommended for children ages 6 months to <9 years who are receiving influenza vaccine for the first time.
†For adults and older children, the recommended site of vaccinations is the deltoid muscle. The preferred site for infants is the anterolateral aspect of the thigh.
‡Formerly Chiron Corporation.
§Two doses administered at least 6 weeks apart are recommended for children 5 years to <9 years who are receiving influenza vaccine for the first time.
*Abbreviations:* LAIV = live attenuated influenza vaccine; TIV = trivalent inactivated influenza vaccine.

**TABLE 2** Recommended Daily Dosages of Influenza Antiviral Medications for Treatment and Chemoprophylaxis—United States

| Age Group (y) | Zanamivir (Relenza) | | Oseltamivir (Tamiflu) | |
| | Treatment | Prophylaxis | Treatment* | Prophylaxis |
| --- | --- | --- | --- | --- |
| 1-12 | 10 mg bid[†] | 10 mg qd[‡] | ≤15 kg, 30 mg bid<br>15-23 kg, 45 mg bid<br>23-40 kg, 60 mg bid<br>>40 kg, 75 mg bid | ≤15 kg, 30 mg qd<br>15-23 kg, 45 mg qd<br>23-40 kg, 60 mg qd<br>>40 kg, 75 mg qd |
| 13-64 | 10 mg bid | 10 mg qd | 75 mg bid | 75 mg qd |
| ≥65 | 10 mg bid | 10 mg qd | 75 mg bid | 75 mg qd |

*A reduction in the dose of oseltamivir is recommended for persons with creatinine clearance <30 mL/min.
[†]Not approved for children ages 1-6 years.
[‡]Not approved for children ages 1-4 years.

effective against influenza B, and in the 2005 to 2006 season, more than 90% of influenza A viruses were resistant to adamantanes. The CDC now recommends that adamantanes not be used until circulating strains of influenza A demonstrate greater susceptibility.

Neuraminidase inhibitors (Table 2) are effective against both influenza A and B. To date, little resistance has been demonstrated. When administered within 48 hours of symptom onset, antiviral drugs shorten the duration of symptoms by approximately 1 day. In patients with fever and severe symptoms, symptoms can be shortened by up to 3 days, and in patients receiving therapy within 24 hours, symptoms can be shortened by almost 2 days. Both zanamivir and oseltamivir decrease the frequency of secondary bacterial infections, and pooled trials of oseltamivir suggest that it also reduces the risk of hospitalization by 59%.

Antiviral therapy offers a useful adjunct to vaccination, especially in high-risk patients who could not or would not be vaccinated and in years when the vaccine is not well matched to the prevailing strains. In contrast to vaccination, antiviral therapy is effective regardless of the severity of the epidemic or the circulating influenza strains. However, antiviral therapy should not be considered in place of vaccination. The decision about whether to prescribe antiviral therapy depends on the probability of influenza and the patient's risk of complications from the disease. High-risk patients and unvaccinated intermediate-risk patients with at least a 10% probability of influenza should receive empiric antiviral therapy with oseltamivir (Tamiflu) or zanamivir (Relenza). Intermediate-risk patients who are vaccinated should receive empiric therapy during local epidemics; when influenza prevalence is low, rapid testing should precede treatment. Cost-effectiveness studies also support treatment for healthy patients with high probability of influenza infection, but in cases of medication shortage, high-risk patients should be given priority.

There are no studies comparing oseltamivir and zanamivir, but they appear to have similar efficacy. Therefore, the choice of drug must be based on side-effect profile, cost, and availability. Zanamivir is inhaled and should not be used by patients with asthma or chronic obstructive pulmonary disease (COPD) due to risk of bronchospasm. In addition, some patients find the Diskhaler difficult to use. Zanamivir is otherwise well tolerated, with side effects similar to placebo. Oseltamivir causes nausea and vomiting in approximately 10% of patients; taking the medication with food can ameliorate this effect. The cost for a single course of treatment is approximately $60 for zanamivir and $80 for oseltamivir. Because of international stockpiling of neuraminidase inhibitors against a potential pandemic of avian flu, local shortages can develop. Both medications are recommended to be taken twice daily for 5 days, though a 3-day course is probably sufficient for most patients.

Chemoprophylaxis with oseltamivir should be given during institutional outbreaks of influenza to all residents regardless of vaccination status and to staff only during the first 2 weeks after vaccination. The prophylaxis dose is 75 mg daily and should continue throughout the period of the outbreak. High-risk patients in the community should also receive prophylaxis for 7 days if they are exposed to a known case of influenza (e.g., household contacts). Prophylaxis for the entire period that influenza is circulating (6-8 weeks) can be considered for high-risk patients and health care workers unable to be vaccinated and for immunosuppressed patients. Although neither medication is licensed for prophylaxis in young children, both have demonstrated efficacy in preventing household transmission to children. When used with inactivated vaccine, chemoprophylaxis should be continued for 2 weeks. Chemoprophylaxis should not be given with LAIV, because it can interfere with the viral reproduction necessary to stimulate an immune response.

## REFERENCES

Centers for Disease Control and Prevention: Prevention and control of influenza: Recommendations of the Advisory Committee on Immunization Practices (ACIP). MMWR Recomm Rep 2006;55(RR10);1-42.
Cooper NJ, Sutton AJ, Abrams KR, et al: Effectiveness of neuraminidase inhibitors in treatment and prevention of influenza A and B: Systematic review and meta-analyses of randomised controlled trials. BMJ 2003;326:1235-1243.
Demicheli V, Rivetti D, Deeks JJ, Jefferson TO: Vaccines for preventing influenza in healthy adults. Cochrane Database Syst Rev 2004;(3):CD001269
Kaiser L, Wat C, Mills T, et al: Impact of oseltamivir treatment on influenza-related lower respiratory tract complications and hospitalizations. Arch Intern Med 2003;163:1667-1672.
Nichol KL, Nordin J, Mullooly J, et al: Influenza vaccination and reduction in hospitalizations for cardiac disease and stroke among the elderly. N Engl J Med 2003;348:1322-1332.
Rothberg MB, Bellantonio S, Rose DN: Management of influenza in adults older than 65 years of age: Cost-effectiveness of rapid testing and antiviral therapy. Ann Intern Med 2003;139:321-329.
Smith KJ, Roberts MS: Cost-effectiveness of newer treatment strategies for influenza. Am J Med 2002;113:300-307.
Turner D, Wailoo A, Nicholson K, et al: Systematic review and economic decision modelling for the prevention and treatment of influenza A and B. Health Technol Assess 2003;7:iii-iv, xi-xiii, 1-170.
Uyeki TM: Influenza diagnosis and treatment in children: A review of studies on clinically useful tests and antiviral treatment for influenza. Pediatr Infect Dis J 2003;22:164-177.

# Leishmaniasis

Method of
*Karim Aoun, MD, and Aida Bouratbine, MD*

Leishmaniasis is a worldwide vector-borne disease caused by protozoan flagellates of the genus *Leishmania*. Metacyclic infective stages of these parasites are transmitted to humans and other mammalian hosts through the bites of sand flies belonging to the genus *Phlebotomus* in the Old World and *Lutzomyia* in the New World. Around 20 *Leishmania* species are anthropophilic and responsible for pathologic disorders ranging from localized cutaneous lesions to disseminated visceral leishmaniasis. The species is identified by parasite isoenzyme analysis or polymerase chain reaction (PCR) amplification of *Leishmania* DNA. Because no vaccine is available, many treatments are suggested for leishmaniasis without any definitive evidence. Treatment methods depend mainly on the clinical features, the involved species, the patient's immune status, the availability of effective drugs, and patients' access to health care.

## Pathogenesis

After a person is inoculated by sand fly bites, metacyclic promastigotes enter dermal mononuclear phagocytes and change into intracellular amastigotes. According to their tropism and their interaction with the host immune response, species can disseminate to different organs and determine the clinical expression of the infection. In cases of localized cutaneous lesions, parasites remain restricted to the initial injection sites by a strong cell-mediated inflammatory reaction.

Diffuse cutaneous leishmaniasis results from a large dissemination from the initial lesion to other skin sites because of the motility of the infected dermal macrophages. The parasite's spread is related to an insufficient cell-mediated immune response that is observed with *L. aethiopica*, *L. mexicana*, and *L. amazonensis* and in immunocompromised patients.

Visceral leishmaniasis is caused by *L. donovani* and *L. infantum*, which can induce spread of the parasites following the mononuclear phagocyte system route. All viscera are invaded, but spread is mainly to the spleen, the bone marrow, and the lymph nodes.

Mucocutaneous leishmaniasis is the result of an oronasal mucosa metastasis of some New World species, mainly *L. braziliensis*. The secondary local lesions can be delayed for a long time after the primary cutaneous ones, even if these original lesions are cured. The factors enabling that dissemination are not yet well understood.

## Epidemiology

Leishmaniasis is observed in tropical and temperate-climate regions where the weather is optimal for the life cycle of sand flies. More than 350 million people are exposed in endemic areas. Because of their high incidence and large geographic distribution, visceral leishmaniasis and localized cutaneous lesions are the most relevant forms. The estimated incidence of all forms of leishmaniasis is 2 million new cases per year, of which about 0.5 million are visceral leishmaniasis and about 1.5 million are localized cutaneous. Mucocutaneous and diffuse cutaneous leishmaniasis are more rarely observed.

### VISCERAL LEISHMANIASIS

Visceral leishmaniasis, also called *kala-azar*, is endemic in the Indian subcontinent, East Africa, the Mediterranean basin, the Middle East, and South America. Ninety percent of new cases are identified in just five countries: India, Bangladesh, Nepal, Sudan, and Brazil. India harbors the highest burden of leishmaniasis in the world, and around 90% of reported cases occur in Bihar.

In the Indian subcontinent and East Africa, visceral leishmaniasis is caused by *L. donovani*. The predominant mode of transmission is anthroponotic, and the major reservoir for ongoing transmission is constituted by humans with kala-azar or post–kala-azar dermal leishmanoid. In these areas, poverty, poor health care, military conflicts, and population movements contribute to irregular and incomplete treatment courses of visceral leishmaniasis, leading to rapid development of drug-resistant parasites.

In the Mediterranean, the Middle East, and Brazil, the disease caused by *L. infantum* is zoonotic. The domestic dog is the reservoir host, and human cases occur mostly in children or immunocompromised adults.

### CUTANEOUS LEISHMANIASIS

Based on its geographic distribution, cutaneous leishmaniasis can be divided into Old World (including southern Europe, the Middle East, parts of southwest Asia, and Africa) and New World (Central and South America) leishmaniasis. Afghanistan, Algeria, Brazil, Iran, Peru, Saudi Arabia, and Sudan account for 90% of cutaneous leishmaniasis cases.

Cutaneous leishmaniasis is caused by various *Leishmania* species and involves a broad spectrum of reservoir hosts. In the Old World, *L. tropica* and *L. major* are the most common species.

Mucocutaneous leishmaniasis is restricted to South America. It is sporadic and is subject to variation according to the region. Mucocutaneous leishmaniasis is mainly attributed to *L. braziliensis*, but cases caused by *L. panamensis*, *L. guyanensis*, and *L. amazonensis* have been described.

Most of the exceptional cases of diffuse cutaneous leishmaniasis are observed in East Africa and Central and South America, where *L. aethiopica*, *L. mexicana*, and *L. amazonensis* are endemic. Diffuse cutaneous leishmaniasis occurs elsewhere with other dermotropic species in immunocompromised patients.

## Clinical Features

Clinical symptoms of leishmaniasis appear following an incubation period varying from weeks to months after the infective sand fly bite. The common symptoms of visceral leishmaniasis, either in children or in adults, are fever, hepatosplenic enlargement, anemia, weight loss, and blood cytopenia. Unusual involvement of the lung or the digestive tract is reported in immunocompromised patients. If diagnosis is not established early and appropriate treatment is not given, the infection is uniformly fatal. The mortality number for visceral leishmaniasis is about 60,000 each year.

The typical localized cutaneous lesion starts as an erythematous papule of few millimeters in diameter that gradually expands and ulcerates. The lesions are single or multiple and affect uncovered parts of the body. Both wet and dry types are observed. Regression of localized cutaneous lesions is spontaneous within months to years, leaving depressed and usually disfiguring scars.

Old World species mostly cause benign and often self-limited cutaneous disease, but New World species cause a broad spectrum of conditions from benign to severe manifestations, including mucosal involvement. Tissues of the nose and the mouth are the most invaded during mucocutaneous leishmaniasis. Lesions consist of a long-lasting infiltration and erosion of mucosa that are not self-healing. Bacterial superinfection or obstruction of the airways or the digestive tract can complicate the course and cause death. Lesions of diffuse cutaneous leishmaniasis are disseminated and remain for a long time. They are nodular and nonulcerative, resembling those in lepromatous leprosy.

## Treatment

### PHARMACOLOGIC THERAPY

#### Pentavalent Antimonials

Pentavalent antimonials (Sb) meglumine antimoniate (Glucantime, Prostib)[2] for IM administration and sodium stibogluconate (Pentostam, Solustibosan, Stibanate)[10] for IV or IM administration have been the first-line drugs for treating all forms of leishmaniasis since 1940. Their respective Sb contents are 85 mg/mL and 100 mg/mL. Recently, studies comparing efficiency of generics with branded products established the worth of generics in terms of efficacy and safety in visceral leishmaniasis and cutaneous leishmaniasis.

---

[2]Not available in the United States.
[10]Available in the United States from the Centers for Disease Control and Prevention.

## CURRENT THERAPY

### Visceral Leishmaniasis

- Pentavalent antimonials (Glucantime,[2] Pentostam[10]): 20 mg Sb/kg/d for 28 d
- Amphotericin B (Fungizone): 0.75-1 mg/kg/d IV for 15-20 d
- Liposomal amphotericin B (AmBisome): Total dose of 18-20 mg ($2 \times 10$mg/kg/d or 3 mg $\times$ 6 (d 1 to 5 and d 10)
- Immunocompromised (HIV) patients: Secondary prophylaxis every 2-4 wk after cure

### Mucocutaneous Leishmaniasis

- Pentavalent antimonials: 20 mg Sb/kg/d for 28 d
- Amphotericin B: 0.75-1 mg/kg/d IV for 15-20 d

### Cutaneous Leishmaniasis

#### NEW WORLD

- Pentavalent antimonials: 20 mg Sb/kg/d IM for 20 d
- Pentamidine (Pentacarinat):[1] 3 mg/d IM for four injections (infection from French Guyana)

#### OLD WORLD

- 15% Paromomycin ointment (Humatin):[1,5-6] twice daily for 2-4 wk
- Pentavalent antimonials: 2 to 10 local infiltrations or 20 mg Sb/kg/d IM for 20 d
- Therapeutic abstention

#### OTHER

- Ketoconazole (Nizoral):[1] 600 mg/d for 28 d (*L. mexicana*)
- Fluconazole (Diflucan):[1] 200 mg/d for 6 wk (*L. major*)

---

[1]Not FDA approved for this indication.
[2]Not available in the United States.
[5]Investigational drug in the United States.
[6]May be compounded by pharmacists.
[10]Available in the United States from the Centers for Disease Control and Prevention.

The main target for Sb is the alteration of the bioenergetics mechanisms of the parasites. Pentavalent antimonials have many side effects, which include intolerance (fever, myalgias, arthralgias, abdominal pain) and toxic disorders that could be cardiac, renal, hematologic, or pancreatic.

The dose of Sb recommended by the World Health Organization (WHO) is 20 mg/kg/day for 28 days in fresh cases of visceral leishmaniasis, double duration (40-60 days) in relapse cases, and 20 mg/kg/day for 20 days for cutaneous leishmaniasis.

Resistance is still observed, mainly in Bihar, where leishmaniasis is hyperendemic; in Bihar, 40% to 60% of visceral leishmaniasis cases are unresponsive to Sb. In vitro studies conducted there have shown that *L. donovani* strains from nonresponder patients required five times the concentration of Sb as responders required to kill parasites.

The optimal duration of treatment with the dose of 20 mg/kg/day in cutaneous leishmaniasis is still debated. Some authors consider a 10-day course of treatment sufficient, but some studies indicate a clear positive correlation between treatment duration and efficacy.

Intralesional treatment of cutaneous leishmaniasis with Sb produces the maximum concentration in the lesions and has fewer side effects, but it does not reach metastatic localizations caused by New World species. The basic aim is to fill the infected part of the dermis. This requires carefully infiltrating the area around the lesion, including the base of the lesion, until the surface has blanched. Treatment should be given every 5 to 7 days for a total of two to ten treatments.

### Amphotericin B

Amphotericin B (AmpB) was originally developed as a systemic antifungal. Amphotericin B deoxycholate (Fungizone) has proven antileishmanial activity. Its activity was attributed to its selective affinity for ergosterol-like sterols, which are abundant in the membranes of *Leishmania* species. To address the increasing Sb unresponsiveness of visceral leishmaniasis in India, AmpB has been used successfully at a dosage of 0.75 to 1 mg/kg for 15 to 20 infusions administrated either daily or on alternate days. However, the major limiting factors include an almost universal occurrence of infusion-based reactions including high fever with rigor and chills, thrombophlebitis, and occasional serious toxicities such as myocarditis, severe hypokalemia, renal dysfunction, and death.

#### Lipid Formulations of Amphotericin B

Toxic effects of AmpB deoxycholate have been largely reduced with the advent of lipid formulations. In these compounds, deoxycholate has been replaced by lipids that mask AmpB from susceptible tissues, targeting its delivery to parasitized cells. This minimizes toxicity and emphasizes activity.

Three formulations are commercially available: liposomal AmpB (AmBisome); AmpB lipid complex (Abelcet), and AmpB colloidal dispersion (Amphocil, Amphotec).[1] Liposomal AmpB was the first one evaluated and is licensed in several European countries and the United States for treating visceral leishmaniasis. A total dose of 20 mg/kg is adequate to treat immunocompetent children and adults. The exact dosage schedule can be flexible and divided into doses of 10 mg/kg on two consecutive days or in smaller doses (3 mg/kg from the first to the fifth days then 3 mg/kg on the 10th day). However, liposomal AmpB pharmacokinetics suggests that an initial dose of at least 5 mg/kg will provide a better tissue level. The high cost of liposomal AmpB is the principal dose-limiting factor. Thus, the main purpose of recent clinical trials in India was to determine its lowest total dose with acceptable efficacy for Indian visceral leishmaniasis.

In patients with severe immunosuppression, relapse rates after treatment with Sb or liposomal AmpB are extremely high. However, because liposomal AmpB is less toxic, most clinicians consider it the antileishmanial drug of choice in patients coinfected with visceral leishmaniasis and HIV. Lipid AmpB has also been used successfully to treat cutaneous leishmaniasis in immunocompromised patients and children. However, because cutaneous leishmaniasis is usually a self-limited infection, the treatment cost appears to be disproportionate.

### Miltefosine

Miltefosine (Miltex, Impavido),[5] a phospholipid-derived hexadecylphosphocholine, was initially developed as an anticancer drug and is the first effective oral treatment for visceral leishmaniasis. Miltefosine induces modulation of cell surface receptors, inositol metabolism, phospholipase activation, and protein kinase C and other mitogenic pathways, culminating in apoptosis.

Its use is limited by gastrointestinal disturbances and renal toxicity, which are fortunately reversible. It is also teratogenic, so it is contraindicated in pregnancy.

Its prolonged half-life (6-7 days) might allow the emergence of resistance and relapses when it is used as monotherapy. In vitro studies have shown that miltefosine-resistant lines of *L. donovani* promastigotes can be selected.

---

[1]Not FDA approved for this indication.
[5]Investigational drug in the United States.

In many trials, miltefosine firmly established itself as a clinically effective antileishmanial compound in India. The recommended dose in India is 2.5 mg/kg/day for 28 days for patients 2 years and older. Concerning cutaneous leishmaniasis, the results of an uncontrolled trial in Colombia (phase I/II) are promising. However, further controlled studies with various species are needed before miltefosine can be proposed as a routine treatment for cutaneous leishmaniasis.

## Paromomycin (Humatin)

Paromomycin (identical to aminosidine) is an aminoglycoside that possesses antibacterial and antiprotozoal activity. It remained neglected until the 1980s, when topical formulations[6] were found to be effective in cutaneous leishmaniasis and a parenteral formulation[5] for visceral leishmaniasis was developed.

Action of paromomycin has been linked to the inhibition of cytochrome C reduction. However, mechanisms specific to *Leishmania* require further elucidation.

A resistance to paromomycin has been induced experimentally in vitro in *L. donovani* promastigotes. Development of the parenteral formulation of paromomycin for visceral leishmaniasis was slow, but phase III trials are currently under way in India. Preliminary analysis suggested an efficacy equal to that of other licensed drugs and an excellent tolerability.

As an ointment for topical use,[6] paromomycin has been tested in different formulations. The combination of paromomycin with methylbenzethonium appears to be more effective, but it causes local inflammatory reactions. A 15% paromomycin–methylbenzethonium chloride ointment[6] was applied with success in New World cutaneous leishmaniasis caused by *L. mexicana* and *L. panamensis* and Old World cutaneous leishmaniasis caused by *L. major*. A lack of efficacy is related to a variability of the response depending on the species involved (*L. tropica* in the Old World) and the type of lesion being treated (lesions with epithelial thickness). Topical formulations offer significant advantages over systemic therapy, such as easier drug use, fewer adverse effects, and lower cost.

## Azoles

Azoles, including ketoconazole (Nizoral),[1] fluconazole (Diflucan),[1] and itraconazole (Sporanox),[1] are essentially sterol biosynthesis inhibitors. They specifically block ergosterol synthesis, a membrane component of fungi and *Leishmania* species. They have the advantage of oral administration and few adverse effects, but they are only effective against some species. Most trials were conducted on cutaneous leishmaniasis.

Ketoconazole 600 mg daily for 28 days is effective against *L. mexicana* leishmaniasis. Fluconazole 200 mg daily for 6 weeks shows promising results in *L. major* leishmaniasis.

## Pentamidine (Pentacarinat)

Pentamidine is an aromatic diamidine. Its leishmanicidal activity has not been yet assessed. It might act on polyamine biosynthesis and mitochondrial potential.

Pentamidine was extensively used as a second-line drug for Sb-unresponsive visceral leishmaniasis in Bihar from the 1970s until 2003. Because of its declining efficacy and its unacceptable toxicity, including irreversible insulin-dependent diabetes mellitus, its use has been abandoned.

The isothionate salt of pentamidine (Pentacarinat) is the only formulation available for cutaneous leishmaniasis. It is used as the first-line treatment for cutaneous leishmaniasis in French Guyana, where *L. guyanensis* is responsible for more than 90% of the cases. Pentamidine is recommended as a short-course, low-dose regimen of

four injections containing 3 mg/kg/day every other day. At this dosage, no cases of new diabetes mellitus were observed.

## Sitamaquine (WR 6026)

Another oral drug that might be effective against visceral leishmaniasis is the 8-aminoquinoline derivative sitamaquine, which is currently in development. The common adverse events observed were vomiting, dyspepsia, cyanosis, and nephrotoxicity. Further clinical trials need to be done to assess its safety before it can be used in combination therapy with other antileishmanial agents.

## Imiquimod (Aldara)

Imiquimod is an antiviral compound used extensively for the topical treatment of genital warts caused by human papillomavirus. Imiqimod induces the production of cytokines and nitric oxide in infected macrophages. It has been used successfully in conjunction with standard antimonial chemotherapy to treat patients with cutaneous leishmaniasis whose lesions did not respond to antimonial therapy alone.

## PHYSICAL TREATMENTS

Cutaneous leishmaniasis has been treated in patients of all ages with a wide range of physical methods including cauterization, surgical excision, cryotherapy, local heat, and $CO_2$ laser. Cryotherapy is the most promising method. It is performed by repeated topical applications of liquid nitrogen with a cotton-tipped applicator or a cotton swab with moderate pressure to the lesion. The freezing time per application is 15 to 20 seconds. The procedure is repeated two or three times at short intervals.

## COMBINATION THERAPY

To solve the problems of resistance and relapse and to reduce the length of monotherapy regimens, combination of at least two antileishmanial drugs is the preferred option in visceral leishmaniasis. Miltefosine and paromomycin, which are potent antileishmanial drugs, must be reserved for combined therapy to prevent the emergence of resistance. Liposomal AmpB plus miltefosine or paromomycin should be tested.

Sb in a standard dose has already been combined with allopurinol (Zyloprim), which is an analogue of hypoxanthine. In visceral leishmaniasis patients, the association was found superior to Sb as monotherapy. In a prospective trial, Sb plus paromomycin for 21 days at 12 to 18 mg/kg/day was significantly more effective than Sb alone. However, an expert committee convened by WHO in 2005 recommended a combination regimen that does not include Sb when unresponsiveness to antimonial drugs exceeds a threshold of 10% to 20%.

Combination therapy has also been tested in cutaneous leishmaniasis. Cryotherapy plus Sb has shown better results than cryotherapy or Sb alone. Sb with allopurinol was more effective in *L. panamensis* infection than Sb alone. However, the addition of allopurinol to Sb provided no clinical benefit in mucocutaneous leishmaniasis cases.

## SPECIFIC RECOMMENDATIONS

### Anthroponotic Visceral Leishmaniasis (South Asia and East Africa)

Sb remains the treatment of choice in areas with a low rate of Sb resistance. When unresponsiveness to Sb exceeds a threshold of 10% to 20%, the WHO expert committee recommends that policymakers should strongly consider a shift to an alternative first-line regimen. AmpB deoxycholate has demonstrated a cure rate of nearly 100% in Sb-resistant areas. However, its use at peripheral health posts was prevented by frequent adverse events, the need for prolonged hospitalization, and close monitoring.

A possible alternative regimen is liposomal AmpB. However, its current price tends to be prohibitively expensive for poor countries.

---

[1]Not FDA approved for this indication.
[5]Investigational drug in the United States.
[6]May be compounded by pharmacists

Funding sources and the public health community should work in concert with governments and drug companies to provide it at the lowest possible price.

Despite its proven efficacy, no consensus has been reached about the use of oral miltefosine as a first-line drug.

### Zoonotic Visceral Leishmaniasis

In the Mediterranean basin, the Middle East, and Brazil, visceral leishmaniasis burdens are lower than in Asia and East Africa, and access to treatment is generally much better. Liposomal AmpB is the first-line drug in Europe. Elsewhere, because of cost constraints, Sb compounds are still used in WHO guidelines. However, in patients coinfected with visceral leishmaniasis and HIV, liposomal AmpB is considered the antileishmanial drug of choice. Secondary prophylaxis with doses of liposomal AmpB[1] every 2 to 4 weeks after initial clinical cure of visceral leishmaniasis is now the standard of care in Europe. However, data are insufficient to recommend a specific regimen.

### Cutaneous Leishmaniasis

To manage cutaneous leishmaniasis cases, three options involving systemic treatment, local treatment, or therapeutic abstention may be adopted.

Because of the risk of developing mucosal disease, systemic treatment is obvious for all New World species, except for *L. mexicana* infection, for which there is no risk. In fact, there is evidence that early and complete systemic treatment can prevent mucosal metastasis.

Parenteral Sb is still considered the gold standard treatment. A 20-day course of Sb 20 mg/kg is the most common schedule. Because the cure rate of Sb is low in patients infected with *L. guyanensis*, a short-course regimen of pentamidine[1] is recommended. Ketoconazole[1] may be used as the first choice for uncomplicated lesions caused by *L. panamensis*.

Local treatment should be used in self-limited cutaneous leishmaniasis caused by Old World species and *L. mexicana*. Treatment involves intralesional injections of Sb, application of paromomycin ointments,[6] or cryotherapy. The choice depends on the physician's experience and the availability of the method.

Based on expert opinion, systemic treatment is used in patients with multiple lesions (>5), large lesions (>5 cm) and para-articular or periorificial lesions. Systemic treatment is also recommended in patients with metastatic spread and in lesions not responsive to local treatment. If systemic treatment is indicated, ketoconazole[1] is an option for *L. mexicana*. Ketoconazole[1] and fluconazole[1] may be used for *L. major*. A recent study, using PCR for species-specific diagnosis, showed recurrent failure of local paromomycin and intralesional Sb treatment against *L. tropica*. Otherwise, it demonstrated a good response to a 10-day Sb systemic regimen. *L. tropica* appeared also to be less responsive to ketoconazole[1] than *L. major* is. However, local treatment is essential in patients with contraindications to systemic treatment, such as pregnant women or cardiac patients.

### Mucocutaneous Leishmaniasis

Sb given IM for 28 days is the first-line drug for mucosal infection. In cases of poor response or large tissue destruction, AmpB deoxycholate could be prescribed; 3 g of the product is sometimes necessary to achieve a total cure. To reduce side effects and the duration of treatment, liposomal AmpB is recommended when it is available. Pentamidine[1] at a tolerable dose of 2 mg/kg for seven injections every other day does not seem sufficiently effective against *L. brazilensis*. Surgery is sometimes necessary to repair deep mutilations.

### Diffuse Cutaneous Leishmaniasis

Diffuse cutaneous leishmaniasis is characterized by a lower sensitivity to classic drugs that are used in localized cutaneous lesions. Sb, pentamidine,[1] or AmpB should be used at the higher recommended doses, with close observation for side effects. To help therapeutic decision-making, clinical trials, which are constrained by the low number and the broad dispersion of cases, must be conducted with new and old drugs.

### REFERENCES

Alvar J, Croft S, Olliaro P: Chemotherapy in the treatment and control of leishmaniasis. Adv Parasitol 2006;61:223-274.
Bern C, Adler-Moore J, Berenguer J, et al: Liposomal amphotericin B for the treatment of visceral leishmaniasis. Clin Infect Dis 2006;43:917-924.
Blum J, Desjeux P, Schwartz E, et al: Treatment of cutaneous leishmaniasis among travellers. J Antimicrob Chemother 2004;53:158-166.
Croft SL, Seifert K, Yardley V: Current scenario of drug development for leishmaniasis. Indian J Med Res 2006;123:399-410.
Desjeux P: Therapeutic options for visceral leishmaniasis. Med Mal Infect 2005;35:S74-S76.
Jha TK: Drug unresponsiveness and combination therapy for kala-azar. Indian J Med Res 2006;123:389-398.
Sundar S, Chatterjee M. Visceral leishmaniasis: Current therapeutic modalities. Indian J Med Res 2006;123:345-352.

# Leprosy

Method of
### Bhushan Kumar, MD, MNAMS, and Sunil Dogra, MD, DNB, MNAMS

Leprosy is a chronic, very mildly infectious disease of the skin and peripheral nerves caused by *Mycobacterium leprae*. The first historical descriptions of leprosy came from India in about 600 BC when it was called *kushta*. Leprosy is also known as *Hansen's disease* after the demonstration of *M. leprae* by Gerhard Armauer Hansen in 1873. The damage to peripheral nerves results in sensory and motor impairment with the characteristic hideous deformities and disabilities so deeply associated with the disease. Leprosy was once widely distributed in Europe and Asia but now occurs mainly in resource-poor countries in tropical and warm temperate regions. Stigma remains a major obstacle to leprosy control, despite advances in bacteriology, chemotherapy, and epidemiology.

## Epidemiology

As of August 2006, leprosy remained a public health problem in six countries: Brazil, Congo, Madagascar, Mozambique, Nepal, and Tanzania. Global registered prevalence of leprosy at the beginning of 2006 was 219,826 cases. The number of new cases reported during 2005 was 296,499. The global detection of new cases continues to show a sharp decline; the number of new cases reported fell by more than 110,000 cases (27%) during 2005 compared with the number of new cases reported during 2004. India, which has the highest number of leprosy cases in the world, achieved national-level elimination of leprosy in December 2005. *Elimination* is defined as less than one case per 10,000 population, and the prevalence in India was 0.84 per 10,000 population as of the end of March 2006.

After the successful implementation of and subsequently very encouraging results reported with multidrug therapy (MDT), a highly effective treatment regimen, in 1991 the World Health Assembly developed the global strategy for eliminating leprosy as a public health problem by 2000. The goal to reduce the prevalence of leprosy to less

---

[1]Not FDA approved for this indication.
[6]May be compounded by pharmacists

---

[1]Not FDA approved for this indication.

than one case per 10,000 population at the global level by 2000 was achieved; however, several countries had not done so at the national level. Therefore, the deadline for achieving the goal for these countries was extended to the end of 2005.

Major achievements of the leprosy elimination strategy have included achieving elimination in more than 120 countries (including cure of more than 18 million patients), free supply of MDT drugs, increased coverage of leprosy services, and integration of the leprosy elimination strategy within general health services.

However, reaching a prevalence level of less than one per 10,000 population is not the end of leprosy or leprosy work. The new challenge is to build on the success of the leprosy campaign and deliver sustainable care for leprosy patients who have been treated successfully or who are likely to trickle in because of the long incubation of the disease.

## Etiopathogenesis

Modern-day leprosy dates from 1873 following the discovery of *M. leprae* (the first bacillus to be associated with a human disease). *M. leprae* is an acid- and alcohol-fast, gram-positive, obligate intracellular, noncultivable bacterium, which has been successfully inoculated and has multiplied in the nine-banded armadillo and nude mouse.

The principal means of transmission of *M. leprae* is probably through nasal or respiratory mucosa and skin-to-skin transmission in contacts of heavily infected multibacillary (MB) patients. The incubation period varies widely from months to 30 years, and the average time is usually 5 to 7 years. Apart from humans, nine-banded armadillos and, very rarely, sooty mangabey monkeys are the only known reservoir of infection.

More than 95% of adults are resistant to the infection. Subclinical infections occur more commonly in endemic areas, but clinical disease manifests in only a small fraction having specific impairment of cell-mediated immunity (CMI) to *M. leprae*.

The disease presents a broad spectrum of clinical and histopathologic manifestations ranging from bacteriologically scanty tuberculoid to highly bacilliferous lepromatous leprosy. The clinicopathologic bipolarity stems from the immunologic status, which guides the dual response of monocytes and macrophages to *M. leprae*. In cases located at the tuberculoid pole, these cells can destroy and eliminate all the bacilli; in cases near the lepromatous pole, the bacilli proliferate and persist in these cells and can be also partially killed simultaneously.

## Clinical Features

The clinical features of leprosy reflect the pathology, which in turn depends on the balance between bacillary multiplication and the host cell–mediated immune response (Table 1). Leprosy affects skin and nerves and produces systemic involvement in lepromatous disease. Patients commonly present with skin lesions, weakness or numbness caused by involvement of a peripheral nerve trunk, deformities, resorption of fingers and toes, or a burn or ulcer in an anesthetic hand or foot. Sometimes patients present with nerve pain, sudden palsy, new skin lesions, painful red eye, or a systemic febrile illness.

Inspection of the whole body in good light is important because otherwise lesions with faint erythema or slight hypopigmentation (more often on covered areas in borderline disease) might be missed. Skin lesions should be examined for hypoesthesia to light touch and temperature and for anhidrosis.

### TYPES OF LEPROSY

#### Indeterminate Leprosy

The classic skin lesion of indeterminate leprosy is most commonly found on the face, the extensors of the limbs, the buttocks, or the trunk. There may be one or more slightly hypopigmented or erythematous macules, a few centimeters in diameter, with poorly defined margins (Figure 1). Hair growth and nerve function are usually not affected. A biopsy might show perineurovascular infiltrate; however, acid-fast bacilli (AFB) are mostly not demonstrable. Many patients do not notice such lesions and present only with characteristic determinant lesions at some point. Perhaps three out of four indeterminate lesions heal spontaneously and the rest become determinate and enter the clinical spectrum.

#### Tuberculoid Leprosy

Tuberculoid leprosy (TT) often has one or few skin lesions, and lesions seldom measure more than 10 cm in diameter. The typical lesion is a well-defined erythematous plaque with a raised and clear-cut edge sloping toward a rather flattened and usually hypopigmented center, acquiring an annular configuration. Erythema might not be apparent on dark skin. The surface is dry, hairless, anesthetic, and sometimes scaly. Sensory impairment may be difficult to demonstrate on the face because of the generous supply of sensory nerve endings. Less commonly, the lesion is a dry, anesthetic macule with sparse hair; the lesion appears erythematous on light skin and hypopigmented (never depigmented) on dark skin. Usually, a solitary peripheral nerve trunk is thickened in the vicinity of a TT lesion—for example, a thickened ulnar nerve if the lesion is on the arm.

## TABLE 1  Characteristics of the Ridley-Jopling Classification*

| Observation | TT | BT | BB | BL | LL |
|---|---|---|---|---|---|
| Number of lesions | Usually 1 (up to 3) | Single, few (up to 10) | Several (10-30) | Many, asymmetric (>30) | Multiple, symmetric |
| Size of lesions | Variable, usually large | Variable, some are large | Variable | Variable, not very large† | Small |
| Surface | Very dry, scaly, lesions look turgid | Dry | Dull, slightly shiny | Shiny | Shiny |
| Sensations in lesions | Absent | Markedly diminished | Moderately diminished | Slightly diminished | Minimally diminished or not affected |
| Hair growth in lesions | Absent | Markedly diminished | Moderately diminished | Slightly diminished | Not affected |
| AFB in lesions | Nil | Nil or scanty | Moderate number | Many | Very many (globi) |
| Lepromin | Strongly positive (++++) | Weakly positive (+ or ++) | Negative | Negative | Negative |

*Compartmentalization of the features is not very stringent. All these features occur in various combinations as the disease progresses.
†Presence of large lesions indicates downgrading of the disease from a higher spectrum.
*Abbreviations:* AFB = acid fast bacilli; BB = borderline borderline leprosy; BL = borderline lepromatous leprosy; BT = borderline tuberculoid leprosy; LL = lepromatous leprosy; TT = tuberculoid leprosy.

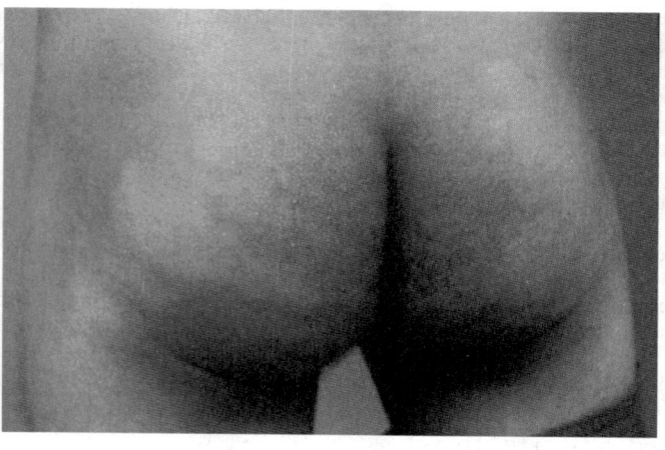

**FIGURE 1.** Indeterminate leprosy.

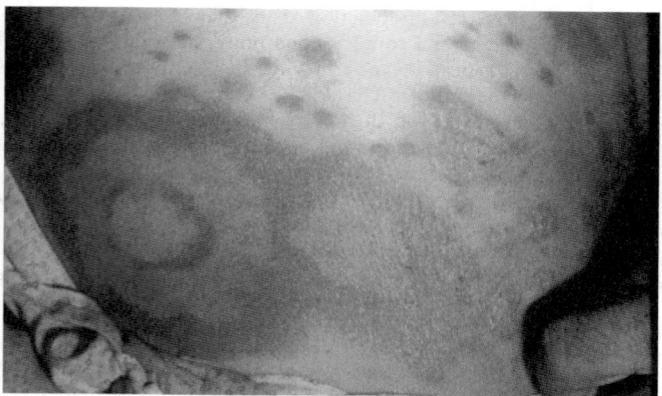

**FIGURE 3.** Borderline borderline leprosy.

## Borderline Tuberculoid Leprosy

The skin lesions of borderline tuberculoid (BT) leprosy resemble those of tuberculoid leprosy, but there is evidence that the disease is not contained. Individual lesions do not show the well-defined margins, and the edge in part might fade imperceptibly into normal skin (Figure 2). There may be satellite lesions. The number of lesions can vary from three to ten and show variation in size and contour. Loss of sensation is less intense than in the lesions of tuberculoid leprosy. Xerosis, scaling, and erythema or hypopigmentation are also less conspicuous than in the TL form.

Several of the peripheral nerves are likely to be enlarged irregularly and in an asymmetric pattern. Nerve damage is an important characteristic of BT leprosy, and anesthesia or motor deficit is often found at the time of presentation.

## Borderline Borderline Leprosy

Borderline borderline (BB) disease is unstable and mostly downgrades toward the lepromatous pole, especially when it is untreated. There are many skin lesions of all shapes and sizes including papules, nodules, plaques, and circinate lesions. Characteristic skin lesions are annular or dimorphic. In annular lesions, the inner edge is abrupt, and the outer edge slopes toward normal skin and has islands of clinically normal-looking skin within the plaque, giving a Swiss cheese appearance. The classic dimorphic lesion is shown in Figure 3.

The face might show infiltration, with occasional nodules over the ears and chin. Because of immunologic instability, the BB state is short-lived, and such patients are evidently rarely seen; the disease usually changes rapidly to borderline lepromatous (BL) or BT leprosy. Many nerves are involved, although not symmetrically as in lepromatous leprosy.

## Borderline Lepromatous Leprosy

There are numerous skin lesions in BL, and they are classically distinct but not so well defined. There occur slightly infiltrated macules variable in shapes in not so symmetric distribution, with areas of apparently normal skin in between. With disease progression, papules, nodules, and plaques can develop, although they usually have sloping margins that merge imperceptibly into normal skin (Figure 4). Associated large lesions and of variable morphology indicate downgrading of disease from a higher spectrum. Eyebrows are not completely lost. Peripheral nerve trunks become thickened and develop corresponding anesthesia and paresis but lack symmetry. Nerves are, however, unlikely to be damaged as quickly as in BB and BT leprosy.

## Lepromatous Leprosy

The early lesions of lepromatous leprosy (LL) are minimally infiltrated macules that are innumerable, widely disseminated, and symmetrically distributed. The edges are indistinct, and their surface is shiny and erythematous rather than hypopigmented. In rapidly progressive cases, they coalesce so that the skin is diffusely involved. The early macules of LL are not anesthetic.

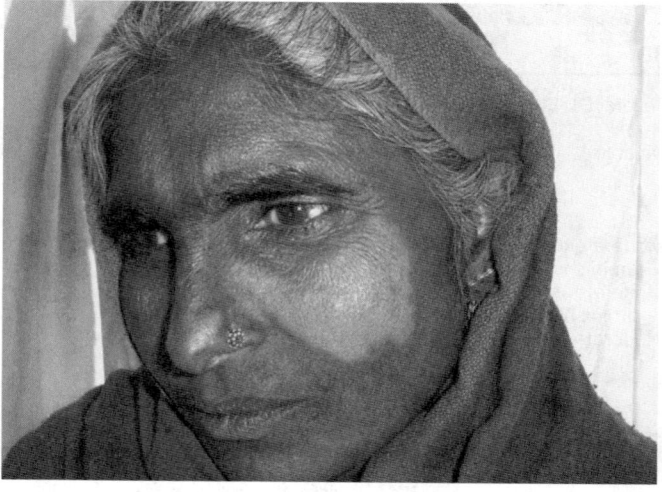

**FIGURE 2.** Borderline tuberculoid leprosy.

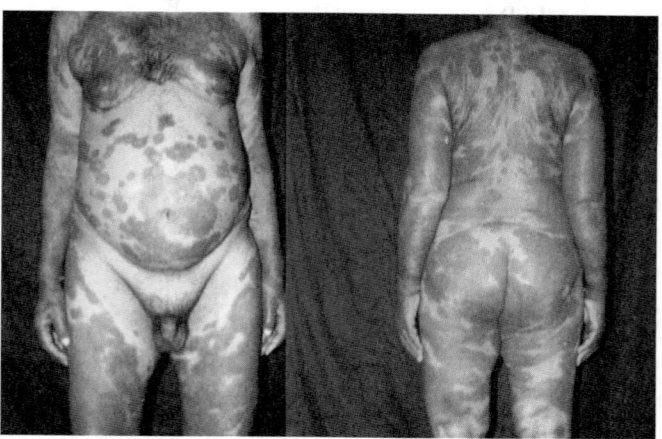

**FIGURE 4.** Borderline lepromatous leprosy.

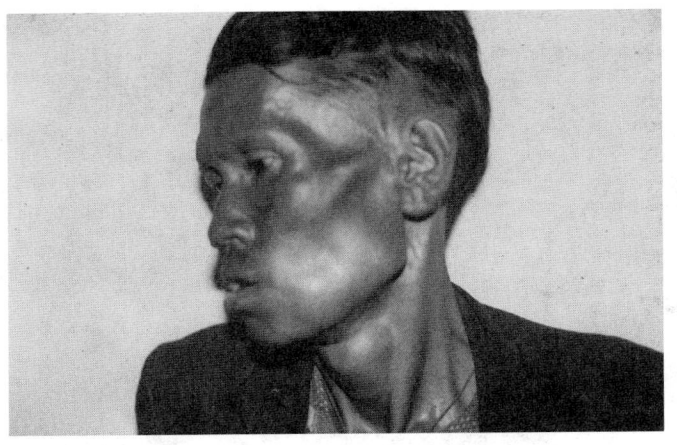

**FIGURE 5.** Lepromatous leprosy (diffuse infiltration).

If the disease is untreated and allowed to progress, the affected skin takes on a waxy appearance and feels full. Thickness of skin is most marked over the face, especially the forehead, earlobes, eyebrows, nose, and malar surfaces (Figure 5). The eyebrows and, ultimately, the eyelashes are lost. The thickened skin accentuates into folds, producing the classic leonine facies. Nodules and even plaques on the face and other areas of the body can follow. By this time, peripheral anesthesia is extensive and is accompanied by anhidrosis, with compensatory hyperhidrosis of the trunk and axillae.

The sensory loss is symmetric and is first detected over the extensors of forearms, legs, hands, and feet, which gradually results in the typical glove-and-stocking distribution. Weakness usually starts in the intrinsic muscles of the hands and feet.

## EXTENT OF INVOLVEMENT

### Nerve Involvement

Nerve damage occurs in two settings: peripheral nerve trunks and small dermal nerves. Small dermal sensory and autonomic nerves are affected in the early part of disease establishment, producing hypoesthesia and anhidrosis within skin lesions. The posterior tibial is the most commonly affected nerve trunk, followed by the ulnar, median, lateral popliteal, and facial nerves. Involvement of these nerves produces enlargement, with or without tenderness, and regional sensory and motor loss. Thickening of the greater auricular nerve is better seen than felt (Figure 6). Rarely, nerve abscess is encountered in peripheral nerve trunks, mostly in the ulnar and lateral popliteal nerves.

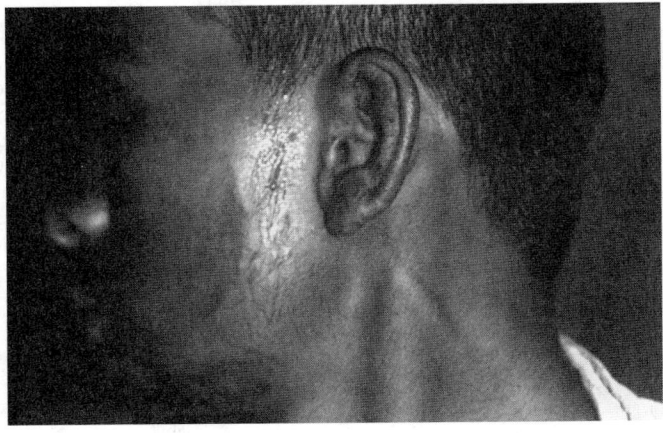

**FIGURE 6.** Nerve involvement (greater auricular nerve thickening).

The morbidity and disability associated with leprosy are secondary to nerve damage. About 25% of leprosy patients have some degree of disability, which is greatest in patients with BL and LL disease. Early recognition and treatment are crucial to prevention of deformities.

### Systemic Involvement

Features of systemic involvement occur usually in longstanding disease and are mainly seen in patients near the lepromatous pole because of bacillary infiltration and the associated granulomatous infiltration that affects various organs, especially the nasal mucosa, eyes, bones, testes, kidneys, lymph nodes, liver, and spleen. Besides the disease, systemic manifestations in the form of such constitutional symptoms as fever, malaise, joint pains, and acute inflammation of eyes, joints, and the reticuloendothelial system (among others) can occur as a part of a type 2 lepra reaction.

## Diagnosis

### CLINICAL DIAGNOSIS

The diagnosis and classification of leprosy have been based on clinical features and skin smears when facilities are available. Clinical diagnosis of leprosy is based on patients having one or more of the three cardinal signs. The cardinal signs are hypopigmented or erythematous skin lesion(s), with definite loss of or impairment of sensations; involvement of the peripheral nerves, as demonstrated by definite thickening, with sensory impairment; and skin smear positive for AFB.

### LABORATORY DIAGNOSIS

Laboratory diagnostic tests such as slit skin smears, histologic examination of involved tissues, serology, and polymerase chain reaction (PCR) studies have been confined to areas where such facilities are available and in academic and research centers.

#### Slit Skin Smears

The diagnostic specificity of skin smears is almost 100%; however, the sensitivity is rarely more than 50% because smear-positive patients represent only 10% to 50% of cases. The inherent problems of skin smears are the logistics and the reliability of the technique of taking, staining, and interpreting the smears. Skin smears help identify patients with MB disease and patients who are experiencing clinical relapse.

#### Skin Biopsies

The biopsy helps to confirm the clinical diagnosis and classification of disease, but it cannot be regarded as the diagnostic gold standard because a number of the histologic features can be nondiagnostic or doubtful. In practice, a clinical and histopathologic correlation may be necessary for resolving a diagnostic difficulty.

#### Serology and Polymerase Chain Reaction

Serology and PCR are rarely used in endemic countries because of their limited availability and lack of uniform diagnostic values across the disease spectrum. The basis of serologic tests is to determine the presence of anti–phenolic glycolipid-1 (PGL-1) antibodies by the *M. leprae* particle agglutination assay (MLPA) and the enzyme-linked immunosorbent assay (ELISA) techniques. The PGL-1 antibody test is specific and more sensitive in patients with MB disease, but unfortunately it is not very helpful in the diagnosis of paucibacillary (PB) disease, and it has low predictive value for diagnosis of early disease. Antibodies to the 35-kD protein of *M. leprae* have been studied for their role in diagnosis of disease with comparable results. PCR for detection of *M. leprae* DNA encoding specific genes is highly sensitive and specific, because it detects *M. leprae* DNA in 95% of MB and 55% of PB patients. Currently, PCR is not used in routine clinical practice.

### Lepromin Test

The lepromin test is not a diagnostic test, but it is helpful for identifying the level of CMI against *M. leprae* in a given patient. It is a nonspecific test of some value in classifying a case of leprosy. It is strongly positive in TL; weakly positive in BT; negative in BB, BL, and LL; and unpredictable in indeterminate leprosy. Lepromin (lepromin A, 160 million bacilli/mL) 0.1mL is injected intradermally, and the reaction is read at 48 hours (Fernandez reaction) and at 3 to 4 weeks (Mitsuda reaction). Neither test is diagnostic, because both may be positive in persons with no evidence of leprosy. However, close contacts of an MB patient who have negative lepromin tests have a greater risk of developing disease.

## Classification Of Disease

Ridley and Jopling (1966) defined five groups on the basis of clinical, bacteriologic, histologic, and immunologic features. These groups are tuberculoid, borderline tuberculoid, midborderline (borderline borderline), borderline lepromatous, and lepromatous leprosy. This is a very useful classification for research purposes, but it is often not feasible in field conditions and primary health centers. This classification does not include the indeterminate and pure neuritic type of leprosy. In general, PB disease is equivalent to indeterminate, tuberculoid, and BT leprosy, and MB disease is equated with BB, BL, and LL disease.

In 1998, the WHO Expert Committee on Leprosy declared skin-slit smears as not essential for institution of MDT. This was necessitated by the unavailability or unreliability of technical expertise for the skin smear in many leprosy-control programs and the potential for transmitting HIV and hepatitis by nonsterile techniques.

Recently, for field workers, WHO has classified leprosy based on the number of skin lesions for treatment purposes. PB leprosy is leprosy with one to five skin lesions. MB leprosy includes more than five skin lesions. If facilities are available, any patient with a positive slit-skin smear should be considered to have MB leprosy.

## Rare Variants

### Lucio Leprosy

Lucio leprosy (LuLp) is a diffuse form of LL. It is common in Mexico and Costa Rica and less common in the Gulf Coast, but it is quite rare in the rest of the world. It manifests as slowly progressive, diffuse, shiny infiltration of skin of the face and most of the body (*lepra bonita*, "beautiful leprosy"). There is loss of eyebrows, hoarseness of voice, and numbness and edema of hands and feet that mimic myxedema. This form of the disease is liable to the most severe of all reactional states, the Lucio phenomenon, in which destructive vasculitis leads to skin necrosis and ulcers.

### Pure Neuritic Leprosy

Pure neuritic leprosy is characterized in the absence of any skin patch by an area of sensory loss along the distribution of a thickened nerve trunk with or without motor deficit. This form is seen most often, but

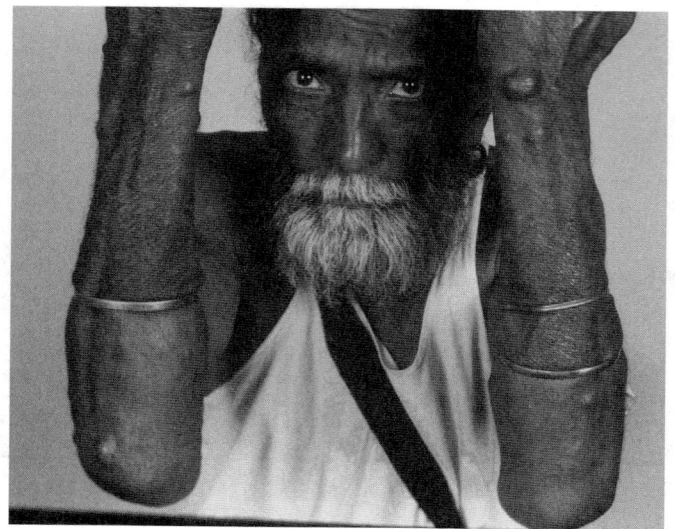

**FIGURE 7.** Histoid leprosy.

not exclusively, in India and Nepal, where it accounts for 5% to 10% of leprosy cases. Histology of a cutaneous nerve might reveal an infiltrate that is characteristic of any type of leprosy.

### Histoid Leprosy

Histoid leprosy, first described in 1960, is now a well-recognized but rarely reported entity. Controversy still remains whether to consider histoid leprosy as a separate entity. It usually occurs in patients who had received irregular or inadequate treatment or dapsone monotherapy or as a spectrum under lepromatous leprosy. It manifests as superficially or deeply fixed cutaneous nodules, plaques, or pads (Figure 7). In a given patient, the number of lesions can vary from a few to a hundred. Histopathologically, the striking feature is predominance of spindle-shaped cells and unusually large numbers of AFB.

## Treatment

The concept of chemotherapy for leprosy has undergone a phenomenal change over the last two decades. The WHO MDT has been successful in eliminating leprosy in many countries. However, the search for new drugs and new drug regimens continues. The goals of advanced therapy include improved patient compliance, alternative agents against clofazimine- and rifampin-resistant bacilli, more efficient killing of persistent bacteria, uniform MDT for all types of leprosy, and supervised short regimens for preventing drug resistance.

### WHO MULTIDRUG THERAPY

The MDT introduced in 1982 has proved to be the most effective tool in controlling leprosy. More than 18 million patients have been cured of the disease, with acceptable cumulative relapse rates of 0.77% for MB and 1.07% for PB disease. MDT as recommended by WHO remains the current and most accepted treatment by all countries with endemic leprosy. A single dose of rifampin (Rifadin)[1] 600 mg plus ofloxacin (Floxin)[1] 400 mg and minocycline (Minocin)[1] 100 mg (ROM therapy) is an acceptable and cost-effective alternative regimen for PB leprosy with one skin lesion, although most still favor the conventional WHO MDT PB regimen.

 **CURRENT DIAGNOSIS**

A case of leprosy is diagnosed in a person who has one or more of the following cardinal signs and who has yet to complete a full course of treatment:

- Hypopigmented or erythematous skin lesion(s) with definite loss or impairment of sensations
- Involvement of the peripheral nerves, as demonstrated by definite thickening with sensory impairment
- Skin smear positive for acid-fast bacilli

---

[1]Not FDA approved for this indication.

# CURRENT THERAPY

**Multidrug Therapy Regimen for Paucibacillary Leprosy (6 months)**

ADULT (50-70 KG)

- Dapsone: 100 mg daily
- Rifampin (Rifadin)[1]: 600 mg once a mo under supervision

CHILD (10-14 Y)

- Dapsone: 50 mg daily
- Rifampin: 450 mg once a mo under supervision

Adjust dose appropriately for a child younger than 10 y. For example, dapsone 25 mg daily and rifampicin 300 mg given once a mo under supervision.

**Multidrug Therapy Regimen for Multibacillary Leprosy (12 months)**

ADULT (50-70 KG)

- Dapsone: 100 mg daily
- Rifampin:[1] 600 mg once a mo under supervision
- Clofazimine (Lamprene): 50 mg daily and 300 mg once a mo under supervision

CHILD (10-14 Y)

- Dapsone: 50 mg daily
- Rifampin[1]: 450 mg once a mo under supervision
- Clofazimine: 50 mg daily and 150 mg once a mo under supervision

Adjust dose appropriately for a child less than 10 y. For example, dapsone 25 mg daily and rifampin 300 mg given once a mo under supervision, clofazimine 50 mg given twice a wk, and clofazimine 100 mg given once a mo under supervision.

## OTHER REGIMENS FOR SPECIAL SITUATIONS

### Drug Substitutions

For adult MB patients who cannot take rifampin, the Seventh WHO Expert Committee on Leprosy recommended daily administration of 50 mg of clofazimine (Lamprene), together with two of the following three drugs: 400 mg ofloxacin,[1] 100 mg minocycline,[1] or 500 mg clarithromycin (Biaxin)[1] once daily for 6 months, followed by daily administration of 50 mg clofazimine plus 100 mg minocycline or 400 mg ofloxacin for at least an additional 18 months. For MB patients who cannot take clofazimine, clofazimine should be replaced with ofloxacin 400 mg daily or minocycline 100 mg daily. Alternatively, the patient may be treated with a monthly administration of a combination consisting of rifampin[1] 600 mg, ofloxacin 400 mg, and minocycline 100 mg (ROM therapy) for 24 months. MB patients who cannot tolerate dapsone should receive only daily clofazimine with no substitution; in PB cases dapsone should be replaced with clofazimine.

### Accompanied Multidrug Therapy

Accompanied MDT (A-MDT) recommended by WHO is an essential element of the "flexible and patient friendly MDT delivery system" suitable to migrant populations, patients living in remote areas, and patients living in areas of civil war. In this policy, the patient is provided the entire supply of MDT drugs at the time of diagnosis: 6 months of medication for a PB patient and 12 months for an MB

---

**Quinolones**

- Clinafloxacin[5]
- Moxifloxacin (Avelox)[1]
- Ofloxacin (Floxin)[1]
- Pefloxacin (Pefocin)[2]
- Sparfloxacin (Zagam)[2]
- Temafloxacin (Omniflox)[2]

**Macrolides**

- Clarithromycin (Biaxin)[1]

**Tetracyclines**

- Minocycline (Minocin)[1]

**Ansamycins**

- KRM-1648[5]
- KRM-1657[5]
- KRM-1668[5]
- Rifabutin (Mycobutin)[1]
- Rifapentine (Priftin)[1]

[1]Not FDA approved for this indication.
[2]Not available in the United States.
[5]Investigational drug in the United States.

---

patient, while asking "someone close or important to the patient" to assume the responsibility of helping the patient complete the full course of treatment. However, poor adherence to self-administration of treatment, a common phenomenon in tuberculosis and leprosy patients, and the associated risk of drug resistance and relapses are to be expected.

### Pregnancy and Lactation

Leprosy is exacerbated during pregnancy, so it is important that the standard multidrug therapy be continued during pregnancy. The standard MDT regimens are safe, both for the mother and the child, and therefore should be continued unchanged during pregnancy and lactation.

### Concomitant Active Tuberculosis

If the patient has both leprosy and active tuberculosis, it is necessary to treat both infections at the same time. Give appropriate antituberculosis therapy in addition to the MDT appropriate to the type of leprosy. Rifampin is common to both regimens, and it must be given in the doses required for tuberculosis.

### Concomitant HIV Infection

The management of a leprosy patient infected with HIV is the same as that of any other leprosy patient without infection with HIV.

### NEWER DRUGS

A few new drugs are available to complement or replace the currently used MDT (Box 1). The objective of the new drugs is not to induce quick clinical regression but to minimize relapses or to address special situations like drug resistance or drug intolerance. Promising bactericidal activity of ofloxacin,[1] clarithromycin,[1] and minocycline[1] against *M. leprae* has been demonstrated in the mouse foot-pad system and then confirmed in clinical trials. Strong bactericidal effects against *M. leprae* of moxifloxacin (Avelox),[1] rifapentine (Priftin),[1] and other derivatives have been identified in in vitro studies. However, no precise recommendation of their use is available yet.

# Reactions

During the course of leprosy, immunologically mediated episodes of acute or subacute inflammation known as *reactions* can occur. Most reactions belong to one of the two major types; reversal reaction (RR or type 1) or erythema nodosum leprosum (ENL or type 2). Reversal reactions can occur throughout the spectrum of leprosy but are more common in patients with borderline leprosy. On the other hand, ENL occurs exclusively in patients with MB disease, especially lepromatous and borderline lepromatous leprosy. Reactions can be disastrous; they cause acute nerve damage resulting in deformities. Almost 30% of MB patients develop reactions during the course of their disease. Reactions may be seen at presentation, during treatment, and even after treatment.

The principles of treatment of reactions are to control the acute inflammation in skin and nerves, ease the pain, halt eye damage, and prevent spread of the disease. Standard antileprosy chemotherapy should be started or continued along with antireaction treatment. Clinical evidence of ongoing neuritis (nerve tenderness, new anesthesia, motor loss) should be carefully sought and, if neuritis is present, corticosteroid treatment should be started immediately.

## TYPE 1 REACTIONS

The type 1 reaction is a type IV hypersensitivity (delayed-type hypersensitivity) reaction, and it typically occurs in borderline disease. It is characterized by acutely inflamed skin lesions or acute neuritis, or both. Existing skin lesions become erythematous or edematous and can desquamate or, rarely, ulcerate. Often, new small lesions also appear at distant sites (Figure 8). Occasionally, edema of face, hands, or feet is the presenting symptom; however, constitutional symptoms are unusual. Although type 1 reactions can occur spontaneously and at any time during the course of the disease, the usual times are after starting treatment and during the puerperium.

Because of the high risk of permanent damage to peripheral nerve trunks, RR needs to be diagnosed as soon as possible and managed adequately. The drug of choice is prednisolone (Delta-Cortef). The usual course begins with 40 to 60 mg daily (up to a maximum of 1 mg/kg), gradually reducing the dose weekly or biweekly and eventually stopping in about 12 weeks. Neural impairment of up to 6 months' duration may be helped by systemic corticosteroid therapy tapered over a period of 4 to 6 months. Adverse effects associated with long-term corticosteroid therapy must be kept in mind.

## TYPE 2 REACTIONS

The type 2 reaction, a type III hypersensitivity reaction (immune-complex mediated) occurs in patients with LL and BL disease. Attacks are often acute in onset but can become chronic or recur over several years. ENL typically manifests as painful, red evanescent nodules on the face and extensor surfaces of the limbs. Rarely, they appear as bullous, pustular, necrotic forms. ENL is often accompanied by systemic symptoms producing fever and malaise, and in severe form it may be complicated by uveitis, dactylitis, arthritis, neuritis, lymphadenitis, myositis, and orchitis.

Acute or subacute neuritis with or without nerve function impairment is one of the major criteria for distinguishing mild and severe ENL. The treatment of ENL should start with general measures as in type 1 reaction. Mild ENL can be treated with analgesics like aspirin. In moderate and severe ENL, corticosteroids or thalidomide (Thalomid) are more useful and may be life saving. Thalidomide (100 mg q8h) has a dramatic effect in controlling ENL, and it may be useful in preventing recurrent ENL, but its teratogenic effects preclude its use in women of childbearing age. Clofazimine (Lamprene) has a useful anti-inflammatory effect in ENL and can be used at 300 mg daily in divided doses as an adjuvant to prednisolone and tapered over several months. Injectable antimonials are often used by Indian leprologists.

### LUCIO'S PHENOMENON

The Lucio phenomenon occurs only in patients with Lucio leprosy. It results from infarction consequent on deep cutaneous vasculitis, causing the appearance of irregularly shaped erythematous patches. The patches sometimes darken and heal, but sometimes they form bullae that necrose, leaving deep, painful ulcers that are slow to heal. The systemic features are severe and can be fatal. Treatment with glucocorticoids (prednisolone) should be instituted at doses of 60 to 80 mg in two equal daily doses supplemented preferably with an augmented daily dose (200-300 mg) of clofazimine.

# Prevention Of Disabilities and Rehabilitation

The socioeconomic impact resulting from the physical and psychological disabilities of leprosy continues to be a burden in endemic countries. Approximately 25% of leprosy patients have some degree of disability, which is greatest in patients with long-standing BL and LL disease.

Preventing patients with nerve damage from progressing to disability and deformity is a challenge that will last for the patient's lifetime. Among the important efforts for prevention are periodic measurement of neural impairment, early and adequate management of reactions, and advice for care of eyes, hands, and feet. Special footwear needs to be provided for patients with foot deformities to prevent ulceration. Early detection and treatment of reactions significantly reduce and prevent such complications as nerve damage with its resultant impairment, eye involvement, and loss of vision. Socioeconomic rehabilitation is another important component of caring for patients.

# Prevention

Large population-based trials in different countries suggest that bacille Calmette-Guérin (BCG) vaccine[1] gives variable protection against leprosy, ranging from 34% to 80%. Therefore, BCG immunization of children for tuberculosis can contribute to leprosy control.

In a recently published large study from India, vaccine containing cultivable mycobacterium, ICRC,[5] provided a protective efficacy of 65% (heat-killed *M. leprae* BCG provided 64% protective efficacy). The role of chemoprophylaxis with bactericidal drugs in contacts of leprosy patients is still debated.

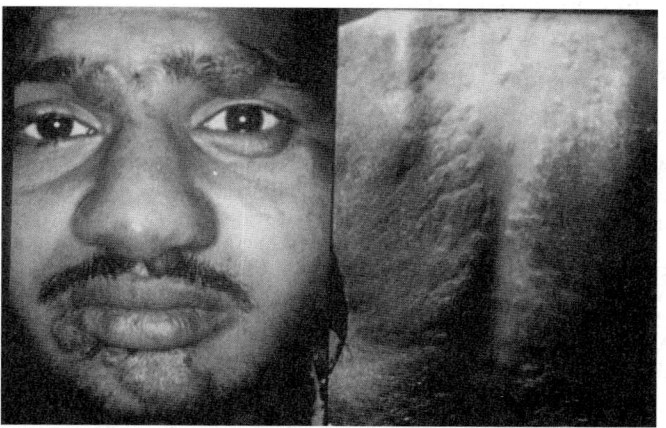

**FIGURE 8.** Borderline tuberculoid leprosy with type 1 reaction.

[1]Not FDA approved for this indication.
[5]Investigational drug in the United States.

## WHO Strategy For 2006 Through 2010

The WHO Technical Advisory Group (TAG) recognizes that new cases will continue to appear in most of the currently endemic countries, and therefore, expertise will have to be maintained at the appropriate level even within an integrated system. The main aim of the strategy is to sustain antileprosy services and the gains made so far. It is expected that by 2010 the disease burden will be further reduced to very low levels through services that would ensure enhancing community awareness, quality diagnosis, adequate management of patients including referral facilities, reduction of stigma, prevention of disabilities, rehabilitation, long-term care of the disabled, and effective partnerships among all stake holders.

### REFERENCES

Abulafia J, Vignale RIA: Leprosy: Pathogenesis updated. Int J Dermatol 1999; 38:321–334.

Bhattacharya SN, Sehgal VN: Reappraisal of the drifting scenario of leprosy multi-drug therapy: New approach proposed for the new millennium. Int J Dermatol 2002;41:321-326.

Britton WJ, Lockwood DN: Leprosy. Lancet 2004;363:1209-1219.

Grosset JH: Newer drugs in leprosy. Int J Lepr Other Mycobact Dis 2001;69 (2 suppl):S14-S18.

Gupte MD: South India immunoprophylaxis trial against leprosy: Relevance of the findings in the context of trends in leprosy. Lepr Rev 2000;71(suppl): S43-S47; discussion S47-S49.

Kumar B, Dogra S, Kaur I: Epidemiological characteristics of leprosy reactions: 15 years experience from North India. Int J Lepr Other Mycobact Dis 2004;72:125-133.

Kumar B, Kaur I, Dogra S, Kumaran MS: Pure neuritic leprosy in India: An appraisal. Int J Lepr Other Mycobact Dis 2004;72:284-290.

Lockwood DN, Kumar B: Treatment of leprosy. BMJ 2004;328:1447-1448.

Naafs B: Current views on reactions in leprosy. Indian J Lepr 2000;72:97-122.

Noordeen SK: Vision beyond 2005. Indian J Lepr 2004;76:171-172.

Pfaltzgraff RE, Bryceson A: Clinical leprosy. In Hastings RC (ed): Leprosy. New York: Churchill Livingstone, 1989, pp 134-176.

WHO Expert Committee on Leprosy: Seventh Report. WHO Technical Report Series No. 874. Geneva: World Health Organization, 1998.

World Health Organization: The Weekly Epidemiological Record 2006; 81(32:309–316. PDF available for download at http://www.who.int/wer/2006/wer8132/en/index.html (accessed May 15, 2007).

# Malaria

Method of
*Paul M. Arguin, MD, and S. Patrick Kachur, MD\**

Malaria is caused by infection with protozoa of the genus *Plasmodium;* it is transmitted by the bite of a female *Anopheles* mosquito, which serves as the vector and definitive host for plasmodia. Rarely, malaria can be transmitted through exposure to infected blood and blood products, injection equipment, or organ transplantation (induced malaria) or by vertical transmission (congenital malaria).

Malaria remains one of the most prevalent infectious diseases in the world. There are an estimated 350 million to 500 million cases every year, and more than 1 million deaths, mostly in children younger than 5 years of age, attributable to this disease. Precise estimates of the burden of the disease are hampered by both massive underreporting from areas lacking adequate health infrastructure and overestimation when liberal case definitions are employed that are not based on laboratory confirmation.

In nonendemic countries, imported malaria (malaria acquired while traveling in an endemic area) is also a significant public health concern. Each year there are about 235 million trips to malaria-endemic countries; about 25 million of these travelers are residents of the United States. As a result, health care providers in nonendemic areas such as the United States must be able to adequately prepare these travelers to help reduce their risk of becoming infected with malaria while traveling and must be alert for the diagnosis in returning ill travelers. In addition, blood banks must also be aware of the travel history of potential donors who may be harboring malaria parasites at the time of donation in order to prevent cases of transfusion-transmitted malaria.

The Centers for Disease Control and Prevention (CDC) receives reports of, on average, 1,300 cases of imported malaria and seven malaria deaths in the United States each year. Each year there are about five cases of malaria reported in persons who do not have a travel history, including cases of congenitally acquired infection, transfusion-transmitted infection, cryptic infection, and occasional instances of locally acquired mosquito-borne infection.

In areas where malaria is not endemic, such as the United States, locally acquired mosquito-borne transmission of malaria (introduced malaria) can occur when a local mosquito acquires the parasite by biting an infected person and then transmits that infection to another person. There have been 11 outbreaks of locally acquired mosquito-borne malaria transmission in the United States since 1992, with the most recent one involving eight cases of *Plasmodium vivax* infection in Florida in 2003. Although the United States was officially recognized as malaria-free in 1970, competent malaria vectors continue to exist in the 48 continental states, Puerto Rico, the Virgin Islands, and Guam. Local transmission can occur whenever infectious persons, competent vectors, conducive environmental conditions, and opportunities for exposure of susceptible persons to mosquitoes come together.

## Etiology

Infection with protozoa of the genus *Plasmodium* causes malaria. Only four species of *Plasmodium* typically cause clinical disease in humans: *P. falciparum, P. vivax, P. ovale,* and *P. malariae.* The life cycle of malaria starts with inoculation of sporozoites into humans from the salivary glands of a female *Anopheles* mosquito during a blood meal (Figure 1) and progresses through an exoerythrocytic phase (tissue schizogany) and an erythrocytic phase (blood schizogany). The development of gametocytes that can be ingested by a subsequent female *Anopheles* mosquito allow the completion of the life cycle.

In *P. vivax* and *P. ovale* infections, some sporozoites might not enter exoerythrocytic schizogony but instead develop into latent hepatic forms, or hypnozoites. These forms can reactivate later and cause acute illness. The resulting infection, which is termed *relapse,* can occur months to years after the initial infection. Persons with *P. vivax* or *P. ovale* infection can have several relapses for up to 4 years and occasionally longer after the primary infection. However, if *P. vivax* or *P. ovale* infections are acquired congenitally or through exposure to blood or blood products, no liver phase occurs and therefore relapses cannot occur. Neither *P. falciparum* nor *P. malariae* has a hypnozoite form. However, if *P. malariae* infection is not treated, symptomatic recrudescences, often associated with splenectomy or immunosuppression, can occur decades after the primary infection.

The incubation period, or the period from infection to the appearance of symptoms, is species dependent. The incubation period is usually 9 to 14 days for *P. falciparum,* 12 to 17 days for *P. vivax,* 16 to 18 days for *P. ovale,* and 18 to 40 days (or longer) for *P. malariae.* Persons taking chemoprophylaxis and those who have acquired partial immunity from repeated exposure to malaria infection can experience a prolonged incubation period.

---

*\*The findings and conclusions in this chapter are those of the authors and do not necessarily represent the views of the Centers for Disease Control and Prevention.*

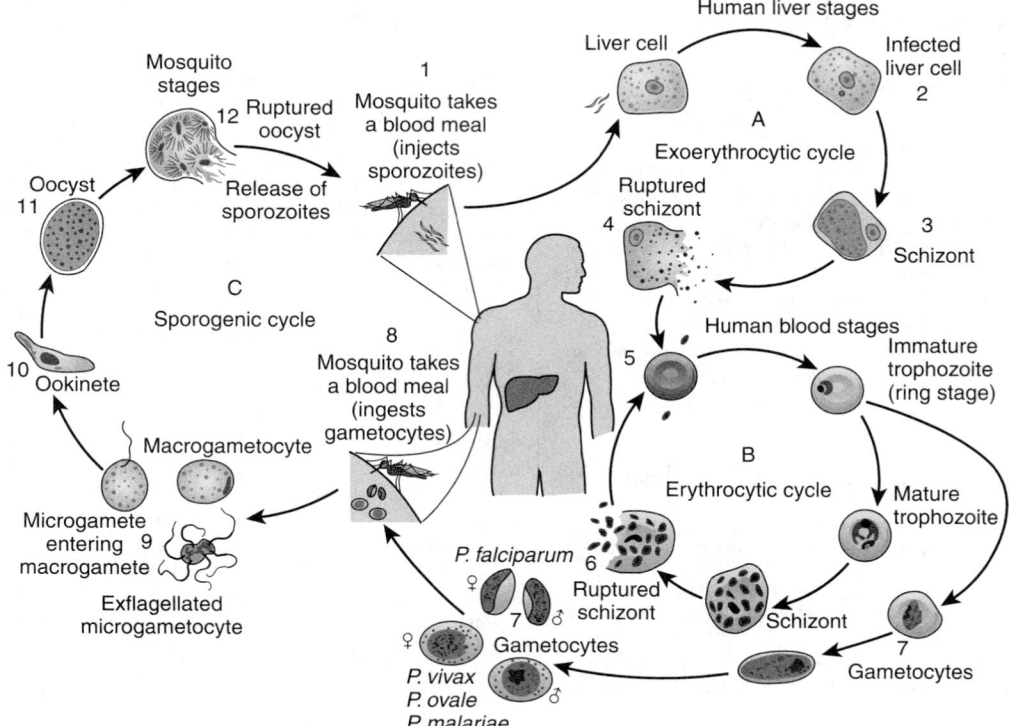

**FIGURE 1.** The malaria parasite life cycle involves two hosts. During a blood meal, a malaria-infected female *Anopheles* mosquito inoculates sporozoites into the human host *(1)*. Sporozoites infect liver cells *(2)* and mature into schizonts *(3)*, which rupture and release merozoites *(4)*. (In *P. vivax* and *P. ovale*, a dormant stage [hypnozoites] can persist in the liver and cause relapses by invading the bloodstream weeks or even years later.) After this initial replication in the liver (exo-erythrocytic cycle or tissue schizogony *A*), the parasites undergo asexual multiplication in the erythrocytes (erythrocytic cycle or blood schizogony *B*). Merozoites infect red blood cells *(5)*. The ring stage trophozoites mature into schizonts, which rupture, releasing merozoites *(6)*. Some parasites differentiate into sexual erythrocytic stages (gametocytes) *(7)*. Blood-stage parasites are responsible for the clinical manifestations of the disease.

The gametocytes, male (microgametocytes) and female (macrogametocytes), are ingested by an *Anopheles* mosquito during a blood meal *(8)*. The parasites' multiplication in the mosquito is known as the *sporogonic cycle (C)*. While in the mosquito's stomach, the microgametes penetrate the macrogametes, generating zygotes *(9)*. The zygotes in turn become motile and elongated (ookinetes) *(10)*, which invade the midgut wall of the mosquito, where they develop into oocysts *(11)*. The oocysts grow, rupture, and release sporozoites *(12)*, which make their way to the mosquito's salivary glands. Inoculation of the sporozoites *(1)* into a new human host perpetuates the malaria life cycle.

# Epidemiology

Malaria is endemic to Africa, South Asia, Southeast Asia, parts of Central Asia and the Caucasus, Oceania, Central America, parts of South America, Haiti and the Dominican Republic, and parts of Turkey and the Middle East. The species-specific geographic distribution is presented in Table 1. *P. falciparum* is the most common species in the tropics and subtropics. *P. vivax* is prevalent in many temperate zones as well as in the tropics and subtropics, making it the species with the widest geographic distribution. Together, *P. falciparum* and *P. vivax* account for more than 90% of clinical malaria illnesses worldwide.

The development of resistance to antimalarial drugs has complicated malaria prophylaxis and treatment. Species-specific resistance patterns are presented in Table 1. Knowledge of species-specific resistance patterns is essential to making appropriate decisions about chemoprophylaxis and treatment. The most up-to-date information about this rapidly evolving process can usually be found on the CDC Web site (www.cdc.gov/malaria) and the World Health Organization (WHO) Web site (www.who/int/topics/malaria).

Among U.S. travelers, the majority of cases of malaria diagnosed each year are acquired in sub-Saharan Africa. Most of these patients report not taking any or one of the recommended drugs for malaria chemoprophylaxis. Also, the most common subgroup of travelers who become infected with malaria are first- and second-generation immigrants who return to their countries of origin to visit friends and relatives (VFR travelers).

# Clinical Features

The clinical presentation of malaria is nonspecific; therefore, clinicians must maintain a high index of suspicion of malaria and routinely elicit a travel history from febrile patients. The clinical presentation of malaria can vary substantially, depending on the infecting species, the level of parasitemia, and the immune status of the patient. The initial clinical symptoms usually include a flu-like prodrome with headache, malaise, and myalgias that is followed by fever. In travelers with these symptoms, the differential diagnosis should include influenza, meningitis, typhoid fever, dengue fever and other arboviral infections, leptospirosis, typhus, and hepatitis.

Malaria paroxysms are produced when infected red blood cells rupture and release merozoites. After a number of cycles of erythrocytic schizogony, the release of merozoites can become synchronized, resulting in classic cyclic fevers. With *P. falciparum*, *P. vivax*, and *P. ovale* infections (tertian malaria), the paroxysms occur in 48-hour cycles, whereas with *P. malariae* infections (quartan malaria), the cycles are 72 hours. However, patients, particularly those with *P. falciparum*, might not develop cyclic paroxysms at all, and so a lack of cyclic fevers should not rule out a diagnosis of malaria.

**TABLE 1** Malaria Species Distribution and Drug-Resistance Pattern

| Species | Known Geographic Distribution | Drug-Resistance Pattern |
| --- | --- | --- |
| *Plasmodium falciparum* | Most malaria-endemic areas except Republic of Korea, China north of Yunnan Province, and some areas of Central Asia and the Caucasus | Chloroquine (Aralen) resistance in nearly all endemic countries with the exception of Haiti, the Dominican Republic, Central America west of the Panama canal, and parts of the Middle East (resistance identified in Oman, Saudi Arabia, and Yemen) Sulfadoxine/pyrimethamine (Fansidar) resistance widespread in South America, Southeast Asia, and Africa Mefloquine (Lariam) resistance in parts of Southeast Asia Reduced susceptibility to quinine in Southeast Asia; longer course of therapy required |
| *Plasmodium malariae* | *Same as for P. falciparum* | No chloroquine resistance is documented |
| *Plasmodium ovale* | Sub-Saharan Africa Reported sporadically in Southern China, Burma, and Southeast Asia | No chloroquine resistance is documented |
| *Plasmodium vivax* | Central and South America, South Asia, Southeast Asia, Oceania, parts of the Middle East, Mexico, North Africa, and Horn of Africa Not common to absent in sub-Saharan Africa, Haiti, and the Dominican Republic | Chloroquine resistance in Papua New Guinea, Indonesia and East Timor Rare instances of chloroquine-resistant *P. vivax* have been reported in Myanmar, India, and Central and South America |

Other symptoms include headache, chills, rigors, myalgias and arthralgias, and abdominal pain. Patients also might complain of diarrhea, vomiting, chest pain, and cough. The presence of gastrointestinal and respiratory symptoms should not lead the physician to exclude malaria as a potential diagnosis. On physical examination, a patient might have jaundice, tachycardia, hypotension (usually secondary to dehydration), and splenomegaly. Laboratory abnormalities in cases of uncomplicated malaria can include mild anemia, an elevated reticulocyte count, thrombocytopenia, lymphopenia, hyperbilirubinemia, and mildly elevated transaminases.

An uncomplicated malaria infection can progress to severe disease or death within hours. Risk factors for severe malaria include delays in treatment, inadequate or inappropriate treatment, a high parasite burden, and lack of acquired immunity. *P. falciparum*, more than any other species of *Plasmodium*, is responsible for the severe disease and death associated with malaria. This tendency has been linked to several features of this species. The tissue and blood schizonts in *P. falciparum* release a larger number of merozoites when they rupture, resulting in a more rapid rise in parasitemia. *P. falciparum*, unlike the other species, can infect both reticulocytes and mature erythrocytes. This destruction of large numbers of red blood cells and suppression of erythropoiesis can produce devastating anemia. In addition, *P. falciparum*–infected erythrocytes adhere to the vascular endothelium of postcapillary venules. It is believed that cytoadherence and severe anemia contribute to tissue hypoxia and end-organ dysfunction. Even the immune response itself contributes to many of the cellular and humoral processes that manifest in severe malaria illness.

Severe malaria caused by *P. falciparum* is associated with a 15% to 20% mortality rate. Signs and symptoms of severe malaria can include impaired consciousness, coma (cerebral malaria), generalized seizures, severe anemia, acute renal failure, pulmonary edema, acute respiratory distress syndrome, hypotension and circulatory collapse, disseminated intravascular coagulation, spontaneous bleeding, metabolic (lactic) acidosis, hypoglycemia, hemoglobinuria, jaundice, and a parasitemia greater than 5%.

Cerebral malaria is characterized by coma that is not attributable to any other cause in a patient infected with *P. falciparum*. It is a life-threatening complication with an estimated 10% to 40% mortality rate. Coma or impaired mental status caused by malaria has to be distinguished from other causes of neurologic symptoms, including hyperpyrexia, hypoglycemia, and concurrent infections.

Signs of cerebral malaria range from disorientation to focal neurologic signs to coma with extensor posturing (including decorticate or decerebrate rigidity) or opisthotonos.

Complications with other species are rare. Splenic rupture has been described in patients who, because of long-standing untreated *P. vivax* infection, have developed massive splenomegaly. With effective chemotherapy, this complication is unusual. Nephritis is a rare complication of persistent *P. malariae* infection but occurs more commonly in children.

## Diagnosis

To provide appropriate therapy, it is essential to identify the infecting malaria species, determine where the infection was acquired, and determine the parasite density. Health care providers evaluating patients for possible malaria must get the results of their malaria smears immediately. Sending these diagnostic tests to offsite laboratories where results are not available for extended periods of time is an unacceptable practice that can result in increased morbidity and mortality from delayed diagnosis and delayed recognition of hyperparasitemia. Initial evaluation of patients with slide-confirmed malaria ideally also should include glucose, a complete blood count, electrolytes, creatinine, urea, and liver function tests. In patients with severe disease or respiratory symptoms, lactate level and arterial blood gases to determine acid-base status should also be obtained.

Malaria should be considered in any febrile patient with a history of travel to an area of malaria transmission regardless of whether the patient gives a history of taking prophylaxis. Information on the location and duration of the trip, the date of return, the history of prophylaxis, and the date of symptom onset enables the physician to assess the risk of malaria and, if necessary, to choose an appropriate course of treatment. Rapid diagnosis and institution of antimalarial treatment can prevent the development of severe morbidity and mortality. A list of key diagnostic points, including elements of the history, physical examination, and laboratory investigations, is presented in the Current Diagnosis box.

A thick and a thin blood smear should be obtained from any patient suspected of having malaria. Blood smears can be used to detect the presence of parasites, identify the species, and determine the parasite density. Initial blood smears may be negative, particularly in

## CURRENT DIAGNOSIS

### History

- Did the patient travel to a malaria-endemic area? (including duration of journey and date of return)
- Which medicine (if any) was prescribed for prophylaxis?
- Was the patient fully compliant with the malaria prophylaxis regimen?
- Is there a history of blood transfusion, organ transplant, intravenous drug use?
- Is there a history of previous malaria infection?
- Has the patient been exposed to mosquitoes?
- Has the patient been around recent visitors from malaria-endemic areas?

### Signs and Symptoms

- Prodrome with headaches, myalgias, and malaise
- Fever
- Chills
- Abdominal pain, nausea, vomiting, diarrhea
- Respiratory distress
- Splenomegaly
- Tachycardia
- Hypotension
- Jaundice
- Seizures
- Altered consciousness, coma

### Initial Laboratory Investigations

- Thick and thin blood smears required for diagnosis; results must be available immediately
  - Thick smear used for parasite detection
  - Thin smear used for species identification and determination of parasite density
- Complete blood count
- Electrolytes
- Blood urea nitrogen and creatinine
- Hepatic transaminases

symptomatic semi-immune persons and those taking prophylaxis. Consequently, a diagnosis of malaria cannot be dismissed on the basis of a single negative smear. Blood smears should be repeated every 12 to 24 hours for a total of 48 to 72 hours before the diagnosis of malaria is excluded. Nearly all patients with clinical symptoms caused by malaria have detectable parasites on well-stained thick blood smears within 48 hours of symptom onset.

Blood smears should he prepared with Giemsa stain and examined under a light microscope. Thick blood smears are more sensitive in detecting malaria parasites, and thin smears are more reliable for identifying species. Both thick and thin smears should be scanned at low magnification and then examined using the $100 \times$ oil-immersion lens. The easiest way to determine the percent parasitemia using the thin smear is to count the parasitized erythrocytes among 500 to 2000 erythrocytes, divide the number of parasitized erythrocytes by the total number of erythrocytes counted, and multiply by 100.

To avoid missing low-density infections, at least 300 high-power fields should be examined before a slide is considered negative. Further details about preparation and interpretation of smears can be found at the CDC Division of Parasitic Diseases diagnostic Internet site (www.dpd.cdc.gov/dpdx).

The severity of malaria can vary with the percent parasitemia. Persons with parasitemia lower than 1% usually have mild disease. Those with 1% to 5% parasitemia can have manifestations of more moderate disease. Although severe malaria can occur even with apparently low parasitemia, persons with greater than 5% parasitemia are at high risk for severe malaria. Thus, it is essential to determine the parasite burden at the time of diagnosis as an assessment of disease severity.

If malaria parasites are detected, blood smears should he repeated every 12 to 24 hours, depending on the severity of illness, until the smears are negative. Sequential smears are useful for monitoring the response to treatment and detecting potential drug failure. Although gametocytes can persist much longer, blood smears should be negative for asexual parasites within 48 to 72 hours after the completion of therapy.

Alternative methods for diagnosis are available. Rapid diagnostic tests (RDTs) detect the presence of parasite antigens by measuring either histidine-rich protein-2 (HRP-2) or parasite enzymes like aldolase and lactate dehydrogenase (pLDH). Determination of parasite density is not possible with these methods. The polymerase chain reaction (PCR) method may be more sensitive for detecting parasites than is microscopy. PCR is particularly valuable for identifying the species of a parasite when species cannot be determined by morphology alone. Currently, PCR is used mostly as a research tool and is available only in reference laboratories. Malaria serology detects antibodies to all four species but cannot be used to diagnose current infections. However, it may be useful for identifying an infective donor in cases of transfusion-related malaria, investigating congenital malaria, assessing the validity of clinical malaria diagnoses in empirically treated nonimmune travelers, and diagnosing tropical splenomegaly syndrome.

## Treatment

### GENERAL INFORMATION

Ideally, treatment for malaria should not be initiated until the diagnosis has been confirmed by laboratory investigations. However, health care providers should not delay treatment when malaria is strongly suspected but the health care system fails to meet the standard of care and provide smear results in a timely manner. Once the diagnosis is confirmed, appropriate antimalarial therapy must be initiated immediately. The choice of treatment should he guided by the degree of parasitemia and the species of *Plasmodium* found, the clinical status of the patient, and the likely drug susceptibility of the infecting species as determined by where the infection was acquired. Although all four species require treatment with a rapidly acting blood schizonticide, patients with *P. vivax* or *P. ovale* also require treatment with primaquine phosphate to decrease the likelihood of a relapse.

Species identification is necessary to distinguish falciparum malaria from nonfalciparum malaria. *P. falciparum* can cause rapid progression of disease and death. Patients with *P. falciparum*, mixed infections with *P. falciparum*, or infections in which the species cannot be identified immediately should he hospitalized and monitored closely to assess for the development of severe malaria and subsequent complications. If the infecting species or probable origin of infection cannot be determined, patients should be treated for multidrug–resistant *P. falciparum* until another species is identified. All patients should have repeat blood smears 12 to 24 hours after initiating treatment to assess for appropriate response.

Using available clinical and laboratory data, physicians must determine whether a patient has uncomplicated or severe malaria. Patients with uncomplicated malaria typically can be treated with oral therapy but might need parenteral therapy if they are unable to take oral medication because of nausea, vomiting, or other reasons. Patients with severe malaria should be immediately started on parenteral malaria therapy.

For detailed treatment information, including doses and frequency of therapy, refer to Table 2.

### ANTIMALARIAL DRUGS

Because of the emergence and spread of drug-resistant strains, the slow rate of development of new antimalarial drugs, and the infrequency with which new drugs that are developed are submitted for FDA

## TABLE 2 Malaria Treatment Recommendations

| Drug | Adult Dose | Pediatric Dose |
|---|---|---|
| Atovaquone-proguanil (Malarone) | Adult tab contains 250 mg atovaquone and 100 mg proguanil<br>4 adult tabs PO as a single daily dose for 3 consecutive d | Pediatric tab contains 62.5 mg atovaquone and 25 mg proguanil<br>Daily dose taken for 3 consecutive d:<br>5-8 kg: 2 pediatric tabs<br>9-10 kg: 3 pediatric tabs<br>11-20 kg: 1 adult tab<br>21-30 kg: 2 adult tabs<br>31-40 kg: 3 adult tabs<br>≥41 kg: 4 adult tabs |
| Chloroquine phosphate (Aralen and generic) | 600 mg base (=1 g salt) PO, then 300 mg base (=500 mg salt) at 6, 24, and 48 h | 10 mg base/kg PO, then 5 mg base/kg at 6, 24, and 48 h |
| Clindamycin oral (Cleocin)[1] | 20 mg base/kg/d PO divided tid for 7 d | 20 mg base/kg/d PO divided tid for 7 d |
| Clindamycin parenteral (Cleocin)[1] | 10 mg base/kg IV followed by 5 mg base/kg IV q8h<br>Switch to oral clindamycin as soon as the patient is able, to complete a 7-d course | 10 mg base/kg IV followed by 5 mg base/kg IV q8h<br>Switch to oral clindamycin as soon as the patient is able, to complete a 7-d course |
| Doxycycline* (Vibramycin and generic)[1] | 100 mg PO or IV bid for 7 d | 2.2 mg/kg PO or IV bid for 7 d* |
| Mefloquine (Lariam and generic)[†] | 750 mg salt (=684 mg base) PO followed by 500 mg salt (=456 mg base) PO 6-12 h after the initial dose | 15 mg salt/kg (=13.7 mg base/kg) PO followed by 10 mg salt/kg (=9.1 mg base/kg) PO 6-12 h after the initial dose |
| Primaquine[‡] | 30 mg base PO qd for 14 d[3] | 0.6 mg base/kg PO qd for 14 d[3] |
| Quinidine gluconate | 6.25 mg base/kg (=10 mg salt/kg) loading dose[§] IV over 1-2 h, then 0.0125 mg base/kg/min (=0.02 mg salt/kg/min) continuous infusion for ≥24 h<br>Alternative regimen: 15 mg base/kg (=24 mg salt/kg) loading dose IV infused over 4 h, followed by 7.5 mg base/kg (=12 mg salt/kg) infused over 4 h q8h, starting 8 h after the loading dose<br>Once parasite density is <1% and the patient can take oral medication, complete treatment with oral quinine | 6.25 mg base/kg (=10 mg salt/kg) loading dose[§] IV over 1-2 h, then 0.0125 mg base/kg/min (=0.02 mg salt/kg/min) continuous infusion for ≥24 h<br>Alternative regimen: 15 mg base/kg (=24 mg salt/kg) loading dose IV infused over 4 h, followed by 7.5 mg base/kg (=12 mg salt/kg) infused over 4 h q8h, starting 8 h after the loading dose<br>Once parasite density is <1% and the patient can take oral medication, complete treatment with oral quinine |
| Quinine sulfate (Qualaquin) | 650 mg salt (=542 mg base) PO tid for 3-7 d[¶] | 10 mg salt/kg (=8.3 mg base/kg) PO tid for 3-7 d[¶] |
| Tetracycline[1],* | 250 mg PO qid for 7 d | 25 mg/kg/d PO divided qid for 7 d* |

[1]Not FDA approved for this indication.
[3]Exceeds dosage recommended by the manufacturer.
*Not indicated for children younger than 8 years.
[†]Because of resistant strains, treatment with mefloquine is not recommended in persons who have acquired infections in parts of Thailand, Burma, Cambodia, Laos, China, and Vietnam.
[‡]All persons who take primaquine should have a documented normal glucose-6-phosphate dehydrogenase (G6PD) level before starting the medication.
[§]Patients should be given a loading dose of quinidine unless they have received more than 40 mg/kg of quinine in the preceding 48 hours or if they received mefloquine treatment within the preceding 12 hours.
[¶]Treat for 7 days if infection was acquired in Southeast Asia; treat for 3 days if infection was acquired in Africa or South America.
*Abbreviation:* tab = tablet.

approval, relatively few drugs are available for prophylaxis and treatment of malaria infections in the United States. For example, resistance to sulfadoxine-pyrimethamine (Fansidar) is widespread in the Amazon River basin area of South America, much of Southeast Asia, other parts of Asia, and, increasingly, in large parts of Africa, rendering this medication largely ineffective for nonimmune travelers. The choice of antimalarial drugs used for treatment should be guided by several factors: the infecting species, where it was acquired (or at least a travel history), drug-resistance patterns, severity of symptoms, and percent parasitemia. The options for antimalarial drugs that can be used for prevention are based on the drug-resistance patterns at the traveler's destination. Additional factors are discussed in more detail in the prevention section.

Antimalarial drugs can be categorized by their ability to kill the organism at various stages in its life cycle (see Figure 1). Drugs that kill malaria parasites infecting liver cells during the exoerythrocytic cycle are referred to as *tissue schizonticides*. Drugs with high levels of tissue schizonticidal activity are useful in preventing relapses from infection with *P. vivax* and *P. ovale*. Drugs that kill malaria parasites that have been released into the bloodstream and are asexually replicating in the erythrocytic cycle are collectively referred to as *blood schizonticides*. Rapidly acting blood schizonticides are the essential components of acute malaria treatment regimens. Drugs can also have activity against the gametocytes, or *gametocytocidal activity*. This activity does not affect a patient's clinical response but can reduce the patient's infectiousness. Currently no medications are available that have activity against malaria sporozoites. Such a drug would have potential usefulness as a chemoprophylactic agent.

Quinine sulfate (oral) (Qualaquin) and its dextroisomer, quinidine gluconate (intravenous), are used to treat malaria. They are blood schizonticides that are effective against the erythrocytic stages of all four species of *Plasmodium* and are also active against the gametocytes of *P. vivax*, *P. ovale*, and *P. malariae*. Common side effects include cinchonism, a syndrome of tinnitus, deafness, headache, nausea, and visual disturbance, as well as hyperinsulinemic hypoglycemia. The longer the duration of therapy, the higher the risk of adverse events.

## CURRENT THERAPY

### Recommended Drugs for Treatment of Specific Types of Malaria*

UNCOMPLICATED CHLOROQUINE-SENSITIVE *P. FALCIPARUM*

- Chloroquine phosphate (Aralen) *or*
- Regimen given for unknown resistance or species

RESISTANCE UNKNOWN OR SPECIES UNKNOWN

- Quinine sulfate* *plus one of the following:*
  - Doxycycline[†] (Vibramycin)[1]
  - Tetracycline[†,1]
  - Clindamycin (Cleocin)[1]
- Atovaquone/proguanil (Malarone)
- Mefloquine[‡] (Lariam)

UNCOMPLICATED *P. MALARIAE*

- Chloroquine phosphate

UNCOMPLICATED *P. VIVAX* OR *P. OVALE* (EXCEPT CHLOROQUINE-RESISTANT *P. VIVAX*)

- Chloroquine phosphate *plus*
- Primaquine phosphate[§]

UNCOMPLICATED CHLOROQUINE-RESISTANT *P. VIVAX*

- Quinine sulfate* *plus one of the following:*
  - Doxycycline[†,1] *plus* primaquine phosphate[§]
  - Tetracycline[†,1] *plus* primaquine phosphate[§]
- Mefloquine[‡] *plus* primaquine phosphate[§]

CHLOROQUINE-SENSITIVE MALARIA DURING PREGNANCY

- Chloroquine phosphate

CHLOROQUINE-RESISTANT *P. FALCIPARUM* DURING PREGNANCY

- Quinine sulfate* *plus* clindamycin[1]

CHLOROQUINE-RESISTANT *P. VIVAX* DURING PREGNANCY

- Quinine sulfate*

SEVERE MALARIA

- Qunindine gluconate *plus one of the following:*
  - Doxycycline[†1]
  - Tetracycline[†,1]
  - Clindamycin[1]

---

[1]Not FDA approved for this indication.
*For dosing, see Table 2.
[†]Not indicated for use in children younger than 8 years
[‡]Because of resistant strains, treatment with mefloquine is not recommended in persons who have acquired infections in parts of Thailand, Burma, Cambodia, Laos, China, and Vietnam.
[§]All persons who take primaquine should have a documented normal glucose-6-phosphate dehydrogenase (G6PD) level before starting the medication.

To shorten the course of therapy, quinine and intravenous quinidine often can be combined with doxycycline (Vibramycin)[1], tetracycline[1], or clindamycin (Cleocin)[1] (see Table 2 for details).

Chloroquine phosphate (Aralen) is approved for preventing and treating malaria, but hydroxychloroquine sulfate (Plaquanil) is approved only for treating malaria. These drugs are blood schizonticides that are active against the erythrocytic stages of all four *Plasmodium* species. They also have gametocytocidal activity against *P. vivax*, *P. ovale*, and *P. malariae*. Chloroquine is the treatment of choice for susceptible strains of *P. falciparum* and *P. vivax*, although chloroquine-resistant forms of both species of malaria have become major public health concerns. Chloroquine is also effective for the treatment of *P. ovale* or *P. malariae* infections. Chloroquine can be taken safely by pregnant women and children. Side effects include gastrointestinal disturbance, dizziness, blurred vision, insomnia, headache, and pruritus. Overdose (ingestion of more than 25 mg base/kg at one time) can lead to acute toxic effects. The toxic effects are predominantly cardiac, leading to cardiac arrest and respiratory failure, usually within 1 to 3 hours after an overdose. For adults, 2.5 to 3 g base may be a fatal dose; for children, 30 to 50 mg base/kg may be fatal.

Atovaquone-proguanil (Malarone), a fixed combination antimalarial drug that is both a blood and tissue schizonticide, can be used for general malaria prophylaxis and for treatment of chloroquine-resistant *P. falciparum*. The tissue schizonticide activity is not sufficient to prevent relapses of *P. vivax* and *P. ovale*. Side effects are rare, but abdominal pain, nausea, vomiting, and headache have been reported. Treatment efficacy, safety, and pharmacokinetic data in children who weigh 5 to 11 kg have recently been extrapolated, allowing prophylaxis doses in these children. Providers should note that this prophylactic dosing for children weighing less than 11 kg constitutes off-label use in the United States. Atovaquone-proguanil should not be used for prophylaxis and treatment in children who weigh less than 5 kg. It is contraindicated in pregnant women, women who are breast-feeding infants who weigh less than 5 kg, and persons with severe renal impairment.

Mefloquine (Lariam) is a long-acting blood schizonticide that is used for preventing and treating malaria. It is effective against the erythrocytic stages of all four species. Side effects include nausea, vomiting, diarrhea, abdominal pain, mild neuropsychiatric complaints (dizziness, headache, somnolence, sleep disorders), myalgia, a mild skin rash, and fatigue. Mefloquine has been associated with rare serious adverse reactions such as seizures and psychoses at prophylactic doses. Although mefloquine can be used to treat chloroquine-resistant *P. falciparum*, adverse reactions are more common at the higher doses used for treatment. Because other options that have fewer adverse events are available for treatment, mefloquine normally is not recommended. Mefloquine is contraindicated in patients with known hypersensitivity to the drug and persons with a history of psychiatric disease. Mefloquine also is contraindicated in persons with a history of seizures (not including febrile seizures in childhood). It should be avoided in patients with cardiac conduction disorders because it prolongs the QTc interval and should be used with caution in persons taking β-blockers. Concomitant administration of mefloquine and quinine or quinidine can produce arrhythmias and increase the risk of seizures. Mefloquine prophylaxis in the second and third trimesters is not associated with an adverse fetal or pregnancy outcome. More limited data suggest that it is probably safe in the first trimester.

Tetracyclines are blood schizonticides that are effective against the erythrocytic stages of all four species of *Plasmodium*. They have some activity against liver schizonts, but not enough to prevent relapses. Because of their relatively slow onset of action, tetracyclines should never be used alone for treatment. Combined with quinine or quinidine, they are effective against chloroquine-resistant *P. falciparum* and *P. vivax*. Doxycycline alone is effective as prophylaxis against chloroquine-resistant and mefloquine-resistant *P. falciparum*. Side effects include gastrointestinal symptoms, *Candida* vaginitis or stomatitis, and idiosyncratic photosensitivity reactions. Tetracyclines should not be used in pregnant women or in children younger than 8 years.

Clindamycin[1] is active against blood schizonts of all four species of *Plasmodium*. Clindamycin can be used in combination with quinine to treat chloroquine-resistant *P. falciparum* infections in people who are not able to take doxycycline. Side effects include diarrhea, nausea, and skin rashes.

---

[1]Not FDA approved for this indication.

[1]Not FDA approved for this indication.

Derivatives of artemisinin (such as artesunate,[2] artemether,[2] and dihydroartemisinin[2]) are compounds derived from the Chinese medicinal plant quinghaosu (*Artemisia annua*) that are active against blood schizonts and gametocytes. Artemisinin and its derivatives are short-acting, highly effective antimalarial drugs for the treatment of uncomplicated multidrug–resistant *P. falciparum* and severe *P. falciparum* infection. These drugs are available in oral, rectal, and intravenous formulations. Although they can be used alone for at least 7 days, combining them with other antimalarial drugs can treat malaria infection effectively and decrease the length of treatment to as little as 3 days. Therefore, using these drugs as a component of combination therapy is recommended for the added efficacy and to safeguard against selecting for drug-resistant parasites. Commonly used artemisinin-based combination therapies (ACTs) include artesunate copackaged with mefloquine (Artequin)[1] and artemether coformulated with lumefantrine (Coartem or Riamet).[1] Although artemisinins and ACTs are not available in the United States, it is anticipated that parenteral artesunate will be available soon for use in treating cases of severe malaria.

Primaquine phosphate, a tissue schizonticide with gametocytocidal activity, is the only drug available to prevent relapse of *P. vivax* and *P. ovale* infections. Primaquine may be used for primary prophylaxis in special situations such as when other prophylactic agents are contraindicated or unavailable. In parts of Southeast Asia and Latin America, short doses of primaquine are used to eliminate gametocyte carriage in patients treated for malaria. Primaquine can cause hemolysis and methemoglobinemia in glucose-6-phosophate dehydrogenase (G6PD)-deficient persons. Before primaquine is used, G6PD deficiency must be ruled out by appropriate laboratory testing. The most common side effect is abdominal pain. Primaquine is contraindicated in pregnant and breast-feeding women.

## DRUG-RESISTANT *P. FALCIPARUM*

For *P. falciparum* infections acquired in chloroquine-resistant areas, there are three treatment options: quinine sulfate plus doxycycline,[1] tetracycline[1], or clindamycin[1]; atovaquone-proguanil alone; and mefloquine alone. Because mefloquine has a higher rate of severe neuropsychiatric reactions at treatment doses, it is not recommended unless the other two options are not available. Also, mefloquine is not recommended for the treatment of *P. falciparum* malaria in persons who acquired the infection in the borders of Thailand with Myanmar and Cambodia, in the western provinces of Cambodia, in the eastern states of Myanmar, on the border between Myanmar and China, in Laos along the borders of Laos and Myanmar, in the adjacent parts of the Thailand-Cambodia border, and in southern Vietnam because of the potential for mefloquine-resistant strains.

## CHLOROQUINE-SENSITIVE *PLASMODIUM* SPECIES

For *P. malariae*, *P. ovale*, chloroquine-sensitive *P. vivax*, and chloroquine-sensitive *P. falciparum* infection, prompt treatment with oral chloroquine phosphate is recommended. In addition, infections with *P. vivax* and *P. ovale* require primaquine to reduce the likelihood of a relapse. Before starting primaquine treatment, patients must be screened for G6PD deficiency.

## DRUG-RESISTANT *P. VIVAX*

Chloroquine-resistant *P. vivax* should he treated with either quinine sulfate plus doxycycline[1] or tetracycline[1] or with mefloquine alone. In addition to either of those regimens, after screening for G6PD deficiency, persons infected with chloroquine-resistant *P. vivax* should be treated with primaquine phosphate to prevent relapse.

[1]Not FDA approved for this indication.
[2]Not available in the United States.

## SEVERE MALARIA

Patients with severe malaria and those who are unable to take oral medications because of depressed sensorium, vomiting, or other reasons should be treated with parenteral antimalarial therapy. Severe malaria is a medical emergency, and treatment with intravenous medication should be initiated immediately (see Current Therapy box and Table 2). Currently in the United States, quinidine gluconate is the only parenteral rapidly acting blood schizonticide available. However, it is anticipated that intravenous artesunate will be available soon.

If possible, the patient should be admitted to an intensive care unit. Continuous blood pressure and cardiac monitoring (to assess the QTc interval) and regular measurements of blood glucose are strongly recommended for patients who receive quinidine therapy. In addition to antimalarial therapy, patients should receive the necessary supportive care. If there is impaired consciousness, the airway should be secured, and breathing and circulation should be assessed. Fluid status, level of consciousness, and vital signs including blood pressure, temperature, and respiratory status should be monitored closely.

Because these patients are at risk for hypoglycemia, severe anemia, renal failure, and acidosis, regular assessment of blood glucose, hemoglobin and hematocrit, creatinine, urea, electrolytes, and acid-base status also is required. Severe anemia requires blood transfusion with packed red blood cells. One should consider exchange transfusion if parasitemia is greater than 10% or if the patient has altered mental status, noncardiogenic pulmonary edema, or renal complications. Dialysis is usually necessary in patients with acute renal failure. Oxygen and other respiratory support may be required in patients with noncardiogenic pulmonary edema.

Corticosteroids should not be used because they have not been shown to provide benefit and have been associated with increased mortality in this setting. Blood smears should be repeated every 12 hours to monitor the therapeutic response. Once parasite density is lower than 1% and the patient is able to eat and drink, the treatment course can be completed with oral medications.

## CONGENITAL AND PREGNANCY-ASSOCIATED MALARIA

Malaria in pregnancy affects both the mother and her fetus. Infection with *P. falciparum* during pregnancy can increase the mother's risk of developing severe disease and anemia and can increase the risk of stillbirth, prematurity, and low birth weight. Babies born to nonimmune mothers with acute malaria are at risk for congenital malaria. If a mother is parasitemic at the time of delivery, blood smears should be performed on the infant. If the blood smears demonstrate malaria parasites, the infant should be treated according to the species present. Primaquine treatment of infants is unnecessary because there is no liver phase with congenital infections. If the infant's blood smear is negative at the time of delivery, health care providers should remain alert for the development of signs and symptoms consistent with malaria and initiate a prompt diagnostic evaluation. Congenital malaria often manifests as fever, anemia, or failure to thrive at 1 to 2 months of age and can be difficult for an unsuspecting clinician to detect.

For pregnant women with uncomplicated malaria caused by *P. malariae*, *P. ovale*, chloroquine-sensitive *P. vivax*, and chloroquine-sensitive *P. falciparum*, prompt treatment with chloroquine is recommended. For pregnant women with chloroquine-resistant *P. vivax*, treatment with quinine for 7 days is recommended. After treatment, all pregnant women with *P. vivax* and *P. ovale* should be given chloroquine prophylaxis for the duration of the pregnancy to prevent relapses; women can be treated with primaquine after delivery if they have a normal G6PD screening test. For pregnant women with uncomplicated chloroquine-resistant *P. falciparum* malaria, prompt treatment with quinine and clindamycin[1] is recommended.

## MALARIA IN CHILDREN

For pediatric patients, treatment options are the same as those for adults except that the drug dose is adjusted by patient weight. The pediatric dose should not exceed the recommended adult dose.

To treat chloroquine-resistant *P. falciparum* in children younger than 8 years, doxycycline and tetracycline should not be used; quinine sulfate given in combination with clindamycin[1] or atovaquone-proguanil alone are the recommended treatment options. Mefloquine can be considered if these options are not available. In rare instances, doxycycline[1] or tetracycline[1] can be used in combination with quinine in children younger than 8 years if other treatment options are not available or are not tolerated and the benefit of adding doxycycline or tetracycline is judged to outweigh the risk.

# Prevention

A combination of personal protective measures and chemoprophylaxis can be highly effective in preventing malaria. Travelers should avoid being outdoors during the peak *Anopheles* biting period between dusk and dawn. When outdoors, travelers should wear clothing that minimizes the amount of exposed skin and apply insect repellents that contain DEET (*N,N*-diethyl-m-toluamide). DEET may be used on adults and children and on infants older than 2 months. Higher concentrations of DEET can have a longer repellent effect, but concentrations greater than 50% provide no added protection. Travelers who are not staying in well-screened or air-conditioned rooms should sleep under insecticide-treated bed nets.

[1]Not FDA approved for this indication.

The choice of prophylactic medication should be made in light of the traveler's destination, length of stay, the presence of resistant strains, and the traveler's age, drug allergies, other medications, and medical history. Health care providers should help travelers make informed decisions about the available chemoprophylaxis options to improve compliance. Often, potential side effects, convenience of the dosing regimen, and cost affect patients' choices of medications. Detailed prophylaxis recommendations are presented in Table 3.

Malaria infection in pregnant women can be more severe than it is in nonpregnant women. Women who are pregnant or likely to become pregnant should be advised to avoid travel to malaria-risk areas. However, pregnant women who choose to travel to these areas should take appropriate antimalarial prophylaxis and use personal protective measures.

Long-term travelers to parts of the world where relapsing forms of malaria (*P. vivax* and *P. ovale*) are present can benefit from presumptive antirelapse therapy, also known as terminal prophylaxis. After returning and completing their standard chemoprophylaxis, persons who are not G6PD deficient can take a 14-day course of primaquine as described in Table 3 to decrease the chance of developing malaria later.

Travelers should be advised that they can contract malaria despite the use of prophylaxis and personal protective measures. Travelers should be aware of the signs and symptoms of malaria and should urgently seek medical care if they develop fever or experience flu-like symptoms. Because many health care providers do not always ask about a history of recent travel, travelers should be advised to specifically inform them of their recent travel to a malaria-endemic country so that the appropriate diagnostic evaluation can be initiated.

## TABLE 3   Malaria Chemoprophylaxis Recommendations

| Drug | Use | Adult Dose | Pediatric Dose | Comments |
|------|-----|-----------|----------------|----------|
| Atovaquone-proguanil (Malarone) | Prophylaxis in areas with chloroquine-resistant or mefloquine-resistant *P. falciparum* | Adult tab contains 250 mg atovaquone and 100 mg proguanil HCl 1 adult tab PO qd | Pediatric tab contains 62.5 mg atovaquone and 25 mg proguanil HCl 5-8 kg:[1] ½ tab qd 9-10 kg:[1] ¾ tab qd 11-20 kg: 1 tab qd 21-30 kg: 2 tabs qd 31-40 kg: 3 tabs qd ≥41 kg: 1 adult tab qd | Begin 1-2 d before travel to malaria-endemic areas. Take daily at the same time each d while in the area and for 7 d after leaving such areas Contraindicated in persons with severe renal impairment (creatinine clearance <30 mL/min) Take with food Not recommended for prophylaxis for children <5 kg or pregnant women. Partial-tab dosages may need to be prepared by a pharmacist and dispensed in individual capsules |
| Chloroquine phosphate* (Aralen and generic) | Prophylaxis only in areas with chloroquine-sensitive *P. falciparum* | 300 mg base (500 mg salt) PO once/wk | 5 mg/kg base (8.3 mg/kg salt) PO once/wk, up to max adult dose of 300 mg base | Begin 1-2 wk before travel to malaria-endemic areas. Take weekly on the same d of the wk while in the area and for 4 wk after leaving such areas. Can exacerbate psoriasis |
| Doxycycline[†] (Vibramycin and generic) | Prophylaxis in areas with chloroquine-resistant or mefloquine-resistant *P. falciparum* | 100 mg PO qd | ≥8 y: 2 mg/kg up to adult dose of 100 mg/d[†] | Begin 1-2 d before travel to malaria-endemic areas. Take daily at the same time each d while in the area and for 4 wk after leaving such areas. Contraindicated in children <8 y and pregnant women |

[1]Not FDA approved for this indication.
*All pregnant women with *P. vivax* and *P. ovale* should be given chloroquine prophylaxis for the duration of the pregnancy to prevent relapses. They can be treated with primaquine after delivery.
[†]Not indicated for children younger than 8 years.

**TABLE 3  Malaria Chemoprophylaxis Recommendations—cont'd**

| Drug | Use | Adult Dose | Pediatric Dose | Comments |
|---|---|---|---|---|
| Hydroxychloroquine sulfate (Plaquenil)[1] | Alternative to chloroquine for prophylaxis only in areas with chloroquine-sensitive *P. falciparum* | 310 mg base (400 mg salt) PO once/wk | 5 mg/kg base (6.5 mg/kg salt) PO once/wk, up to max adult dose of 310 mg base | Begin 1-2 wk before travel to malaria-endemic areas. Take weekly on the same d of the wk while in the area and for 4 wk after leaving such areas |
| Mefloquine (Lariam and generic)[‡] | Prophylaxis in areas with chloroquine-resistant *P. falciparum* | 228 mg base (250 mg salt) PO once/wk | ≤9 kg: 4.6 mg/kg base (5 mg/kg salt) PO once/wk<br>10-19 kg: ¼ tab once/wk<br>20-30 kg: ½ tab once/wk<br>31-45 kg: ¾ tab once/wk<br>≥46 kg: 1 tab once/wk | Begin 1-2 wk before travel to malaria-endemic areas. Take weekly on the same d of the wk while in the area and for 4 wk after leaving such areas.<br>Contraindicated in persons allergic to mefloquine or related compounds (e.g., quinine and quinidine) and in persons with active depression, a recent history of depression, generalized anxiety disorder, psychosis, schizophrenia, other major psychiatric disorders, or seizures.<br>Use with caution in persons with psychiatric disturbances or a previous history of depression.<br>Not recommended for persons with cardiac conduction abnormalities. |
| Primaquine[§] | An option for prophylaxis in special circumstances | 30 mg base (52.6 mg salt) PO qd[3] | 0.6 mg/kg base (1.0 mg/kg salt) up to adult dose PO qd[3] | Begin 1-2 d before travel to malaria-endemic areas. Take daily at the same time each d while in the area and for 7 d after leaving such areas.<br>Contraindicated in persons with G6PD[§] deficiency<br>Contraindicated during pregnancy and lactation unless the infant being breast-fed has a documented normal G6PD level<br>Use in consultation with malaria experts |
| Primaquine | Used for presumptive antirelapse therapy (terminal prophylaxis) to decrease the risk of relapses of *P. vivax* and *P. ovale* | 30 mg base (52.6 mg salt) PO qd, for 14 d after departure from the malaria-endemic area[3] | 0.6 mg/kg base (1.0 mg/kg salt) up to adult dose PO qd for 14 d after departure from the malaria-endemic area[3] | Indicated for persons who have had prolonged exposure to *P. vivax* and *P. ovale* or both<br>Contraindicated in persons with G6PD[§] deficiency<br>Contraindicated during pregnancy and lactation unless the infant being breast-fed has a documented normal G6PD level |

[3]Exceeds dosage recommended by the manufacturer.
[‡]Because of resistant strains, treatment with mefloquine is not recommended in persons who have acquired infections in parts of Thailand, Burma, Cambodia, Laos, China, and Vietnam.
[§]All persons who take primaquine should have a documented normal G6PD level before starting the medication.
*Abbreviations:* G6PD = glucose-6-phosphate dehydrogenase; max = maximum; tab = tablet.

# REFERENCES

Baird JK: Effectiveness of antimalarial drugs. N Engl J Med 2005;352: 1565-1577.

Centers for Disease Control and Prevention: Guidelines for treatment of malaria in the United States. Available at http://www.cdc.gov/malaria/pdf/treatmenttable.pdf (accessed May 15, 2007).

Chen LH, Keystone JS: New strategies for the prevention of malaria in travelers. Infect Dis Clin N Amer 2005;19:185-210.

Guinovart C, Navia MM, Tanner M, et al: Malaria: Burden of disease. Curr Mol Med 2006;6:137-140.

Kitchen AD, Chiodini PL: Malaria and blood transfusion. Vox Sang 2006;90: 77-84.

Leder K, Black J, O'Brien D, et al: Malaria in travelers: A review of the GeoSentinel surveillance network. Clin Infect Dis 2004;39:1104-1112.

Magill AJ: The prevention of malaria. Prim Care 2002;29:815-842.

Newman RD, Parise ME, Barber AM, et al: Malaria-related deaths among U.S. travelers, 1963-2001. Ann Intern Med 2004;141:547-555.

Parise ME, Lewis LS: Severe malaria: North American perspective. In Feldman C, Sarosi GA (eds): Tropical and Parasitic Infections in the ICU. New York: Springer Science, 2005, pp 17-38.

Skarbinski J, James EM, Causer LM, et al: Malaria surveillance—United States, 2004. MMWR Surveill Summ. 2006;55:23-37.

White NJ: The treatment of malaria. N Engl J Med 1996;335(11):800-806.

Whitty CJM, Edmonds S, Mutabingwa TK: Malaria in pregnancy. BJOG. 2005;112:1189-1195.

# Bacterial Meningitis

Method of
*Gary D. Overturf, MD*

Acute bacterial meningitis occurs in all age groups, but predominantly in children younger than 2 years and the elderly (older than 60 years). With the introduction of effective protein conjugate vaccines for *Haemophilus* and pneumococcal infection, the incidence of bacterial meningitis is rapidly declining in children, and adults are now the major population affected. Bacterial meningitis is a medical emergency requiring rapid and decisive action to prevent death or neurologic sequelae. Since the introduction of chloramphenicol (Chloromycetin) in the early 1950s, the mortality has remained between 5% and 40% depending on the age of the patient and the etiology. Of the survivors, 10% to 30% suffer permanent neurologic deficits. Prognosis is affected by the timeliness of therapy, the age of the patient, and the etiology. Presumptive diagnosis and administration of therapy are critical.

## Diagnosis

Acute bacterial meningitis must be considered in the differential diagnosis of persons of any age presenting with fever and headache or signs of meningeal irritation or acute central nervous system dysfunction. Presentations can be subtle at the extremes of age or in patients who have received partially effective antibiotic therapy. The diagnosis of bacterial meningitis requires the examination of the cerebrospinal fluid (CSF), which must be performed as expeditiously as possible. Studies indicate that lumbar puncture may be safely performed on patients who have normal mental status or are without focal neurologic signs or papilledema; clinical impression are predictive of the computed tomography (CT) findings. If there are signs or symptoms suggesting the presence of an intracranial mass (e.g., tumor, cerebral hematoma, or brain abscess), blood cultures should be obtained and empirical antibiotics should be administered prior to the performance of a CT scan.

The CSF findings in bacterial meningitis include a cell count of greater than 500 to 1000 white blood cells (WBC) per mm$^3$ with a predominance of neutrophils, a protein concentration of greater than 150 mg/mL, and a low glucose (e.g., less than 35 to 40 mg/dL). No single value is absolute, and a single value may be normal in up to a third of the cases. The Gram-stained sediment of centrifuged CSF is the critical examination leading to a specific diagnosis. In patients who have not received antibiotics capable of reaching the CSF, the Gram stain is positive in 80% to 90% of culture-confirmed cases. In persons previously treated with antibiotics (e.g., beta-lactam antibiotics, tetracycline, fluoroquinolones), the frequency of positive Gram stains is much reduced (e.g., 60% to 70%), but the cells, cell type, protein, and glucose concentrations are not significantly affected. CSF antigen tests are not reliable, and high false-positive and false-negative rates direct against relying on the use of such tests. Clinical judgment is paramount, and antibiotics should be given in situations of ambiguous results of the CSF examination.

## Antibiotic Selection

The outcome of bacterial meningitis is closely related to the timely use of antibiotics. Hypotension, seizures, an altered mental status, and hypoglycorrhachia at the time of initial antibiotic administration are predictive of higher case fatality and neurologic sequelae. Because prompt administration of antibiotics is critical, the choice of antibiotics usually is made before results of the CSF cultures are known. If organisms are seen on Gram stain, therapy may be directed by the probable bacterial etiology (Table 1). In the event the CSF Gram stain fails to reveal a possible pathogen, empirical antibiotic therapy should be begun based on the age of the patient for those persons who have acquired their infection in the community (Table 2). For those persons who are members of special risk groups, empirical therapy should be based on the likely etiology (Table 3). Once the CSF cultures are completed, therapy can be modified according to results of the culture and sensitivity data.

Antibiotics used in bacterial meningitis should be rapidly bactericidal and achieve high concentrations in the CSF. Antibiotics should be given in maximal doses (Table 4). Because the bactericidal activity of antibiotics in CSF is dose dependent, the fractional CSF-to-serum ratio is very small. Finally, the use of combinations of antibiotics should be minimized to avoid antagonizing the bactericidal activity.

## Special Considerations for Antibiotic Therapy

During the past two decades, resistance to penicillin and some third-generation cephalosporins (e.g., ceftriaxone [Rocephin], cefotaxime

---

### CURRENT DIAGNOSIS

- Patient age and epidemiology:
  - Clinical symptoms: Fever, headache, meningeal signs
  - CSF examination: High opening pressure >300 mm Hg
  - Elevated white blood cell count (>10–>5000)
  - >60% polymorphonuclear cells
- Low CSF glucose (<40 mg/dL or <50% serum glucose)
- High CSF protein (>50–>1.0 g/dL)
- Bacteria present on Gram stain of CSF

*Abbreviation:* CSF = cerebrospinal fluid.

---

### CURRENT THERAPY

- Neonates <2 mo
  - Group B streptococcal infection: cefotaxime (Claforan) or ampicillin
  - Gram-negative rods, other than *Pseudomonas*: cefotaxime
  - *Pseudomonas*: cefepime (Maxipime) or ceftazidime (Fortaz)
  - *Listeria*: Ampicillin + gentamicin (Garamycin)
- Children >2 mo
  - Empirical for unknown etiology: cefotaxime or ceftriaxone (Rocephin)
  - *Streptococcus pneumoniae*: cefotaxime or ceftriaxone
  - *Haemophilus influenza*: cefotaxime or ceftriaxone
  - *Neisseria meningitidis*: ampicillin or cefotaxime
- Older children and adults
  - Empirical for unknown etiology: cefotaxime or ceftriaxone
  - *S. pneumoniae*: cefotaxime or ceftriaxone
  - *N. meningitidis*: ampicillin or cefotaxime
  - Gram negative, postoperative, or *Staphylococcus aureus* (see Tables 1–4)
  - Add vancomycin if at risk for infection with resistant pneumococcus

**TABLE 1 Cerebrospinal Fluid Gram Stain Morphology and Antibiotic Recommendations**

| Morphology | Possible or Probable Pathogens | Treatment Options | Alternative Therapies |
|---|---|---|---|
| Gram-positive cocci, short chains or pairs | Streptococcus pneumoniae, Streptococcus agalactiae (group B streptococci) | Ceftriaxone (Rocephin) or cefotaxime (Claforan) plus vancomycin (Vancocin) | Chloramphenicol (Chloromycetin) |
| Gram-positive cocci, clusters; or gram-positive bacilli | Staphylococcus aureus, Listeria monocytogenes | Vancomycin, ampicillin plus gentamicin (Garamycin) | Nafcillin (Unipen) or Oxacillin, trimethoprim-sulfamethoxazole (Bactrim) |
| Gram-negative diplococci | Neisseria meningitidis | Ceftriaxone or cefotaxime | Ampicillin, Penicillin G, or chloramphenicol |
| Gram-negative coccobacilli | Haemophilus influenzae | Ceftriaxone or cefotaxime | Chloramphenicol |
| Gram-negative bacilli | Escherichia coli, Klebsiella species, Pseudomonas aeruginosa | Cefepime (Maxipime) or ceftazidime (Fortaz) | Imipenem (Primaxin) or meropenem (Merrem) |

[Claforan]) has steadily increased among strains of *Streptococcus pneumoniae*. Currently, approximately 30% to 50% of isolates are either intermediately (inhibitory concentration, 0.1 to 1.0 µg/mL) or fully (inhibitory concentration more than 2.0 µg/mL) resistant to *Penicillin* G and ampicillin. Resistance to ceftriaxone (Rocephin) and cefotaxime (Claforan) may occur as well in 10% to 15% of strains. Vancomycin (Vancocin) is recommended in those regimens for meningitis when pneumococci are considered. However, higher maximal doses are required for vancomycin because of its relatively poor penetration into the CSF. In general, lumbar puncture with CSF culture should be repeated in 48 hours in those cases where vancomycin therapy is the primary drug because of demonstrated penicillin or cephalosporin resistance.

Meningitis caused by gram-negative bacilli such as *Pseudomonas aeruginosa*, *Escherichia coli*, or *Enterobacter cloacae* should be treated with a cephalosporin with an extended spectrum of gram-negative activity, such as ceftazidime (Fortaz) or cefepime (Maxipime). Carbapenem, such as imipenem (Primaxin) or meropenem (Merrem), can also be used for antibiotic-resistant gram-negative enteric and pseudomonas meningitis. Meropenem is associated with less risk of drug-induced seizures and may be a better choice for bacterial meningitis.

Patients with ventriculoatrial and ventriculoperitoneal shunt–associated meningitis and ventriculitis usually require removal of the shunt for cure, as well as the administration of antibiotics to clear the infection. Certain patients with infections caused by organisms of reduced virulence, such as coagulase-negative staphylococci, or those with exquisitely antibiotic-susceptible infections, can be treated with a trial of antibiotics alone.

Because of the extreme sensitivity of *Neisseria meningitidis* to antibiotics, uncomplicated meningitis may be treated with as little as 5 to 7 days of antibiotics. Pneumococcal meningitis may be treated with 10 to 14 days of antibiotics and haemophilus infections are

treated successfully with 7 to 10 days of antibiotics. Gram-negative meningitis was treated in the past with 3 weeks of aminoglycosides, but current experience with newer extended-spectrum cephalosporins (ceftriaxone, cefotaxime, carbapenems) suggests that 2 weeks of therapy is often sufficient in neonates as well as in some elderly patients and postoperative infections.

All patients with bacterial meningitis should be monitored carefully throughout the treatment period. Infectious disease consultation is recommended for most infections of the central nervous system. Repeated lumbar punctures are not routinely recommended for patients with fully susceptible bacterial isolates or in those who show good response to therapy. Repeated sampling of the CSF with lumbar puncture or, when appropriate, shunt or ventricular reservoir puncture should be performed in those with known resistant bacterial isolates, in patients who have an inadequate response, in those patients who deteriorate on therapy, or in those for whom clinical response may correlate poorly with the microbiologic response (shunt infections, neonates, and elderly patients).

## Adjunctive Therapy

Corticosteroids reduce the incidence of permanent neurologic sequelae in children with bacterial meningitis, particularly when caused by *Haemophilus influenza* type b. Data in support of steroids in either pneumococcal or meningococcal infections are less robust. Dexamethasone (Decadron[1]), 0.15 mg/kg every 6 hours for the first

---

[1]Not FDA approved for this indication.

**TABLE 2 Antibiotic Recommendations for Bacterial Meningitis Acquired in the Community, by Age Group and Probable Pathogen**

| Age Group | Probable Pathogens | Empirical Therapy |
|---|---|---|
| Neonate <1 mo | Group B streptococcus; Escherichia coli, or other gram-negative enteric rod; occasionally Listeria monocytogenes | Ampicillin plus cefotaxime (Claforan) |
| Infants 1–3 mo | H. influenzae, N. meningitidis, S. pneumoniae, Group B streptococci | Ceftriaxone (Rocephin) or cefotaxime (Claforan) |
| Children 3 mo–7 y and older children and adults 7–50 y | H. influenzae, S. pneumoniae, N. meningitidis | Ceftriaxone or cefotaxime plus vancomycin (Vancocin) |
| Older adults >50 y | S. pneumoniae, N. meningitidis, and L. monocytogenes | Ceftriaxone plus ampicillin |

**TABLE 3** Antibiotic Recommendations for Presumed Bacterial Meningitis in Persons with Special Risks

| Condition or Risk Factor | Common Pathogens | Antibiotic Recommendations |
|---|---|---|
| Impaired immunity (e.g., HIV, early complement deficiency, agammaglobulinemia) | *Listeria monocytogenes, Streptococcus pneumoniae Haemophilus influenzae* | Ampicillin plus ceftriaxone (Rocephin) or cefotaxime (Claforan) |
| Closed head trauma with CSF leak | *S. pneumoniae, H. influenzae* | Ceftriaxone or cefotaxime plus vancomycin (Vancocin) |
| Asplenia | *S. pneumoniae, H. influenzae* | Ceftriaxone or cefotaxime plus vancomycin |
| Terminal complement deficiency | *Neisseria meningitidis* | Ceftriaxone or cefotaxime |
| Neurosurgical procedures | *Staphylococcus aureus* | Vancomycin plus ceftriaxone or cefotaxime |
| CSF shunt infections | Coagulase-negative staphylococci, gram-negative bacilli | |
| Elderly patients (>65 y) | *S. pneumoniae, Listeria monocytogenes* | Ceftriaxone or cefotaxime plus vancomycin |
| Recurrent bacterial meningitis (see CSF leak) | *Streptococcus pneumoniae* | Ceftriaxone or cefotaxime plus vancomycin |
| Alcoholic patients | *Streptococcus pneumoniae* and gram-negative bacilli | Ceftriaxone or cefotaxime plus vancomycin |

*Abbreviation:* CSF = cerebrospinal fluid.

2 to 4 days of treatment, was evaluated in children older than 2 months with bacterial meningitis. The first dose of dexamethasone should be given before, at the start, or within no later than 12 hours after beginning antibiotics.

Use of corticosteroids in adults is more controversial. Although doses of dexamethasone are recommended by some experts for adults with bacterial meningitis, its efficacy in adult meningitis has not been evaluated in a well-designed prospective trial. A recent study in adults found that corticosteroids significantly reduced the risk for unfavorable outcomes, particularly in patients with pneumococcal meningitis. There has been concern that the anti-inflammatory properties of dexamethasone may decrease the penetration of antibiotics, especially vancomycin, into the CSF. One study in children did not show this to be the case. Dexamethasone[1] should be administered in adults with proven or suspected pneumococcal meningitis, only if it can be given prior to the first dose of antibiotics in a dose of 10 mg every 6 hours for 4 days. In patients with meningitis caused by *Streptococcus pneumoniae* highly resistant to penicillin (minimum inhibitory concentration [MIC] >2.0 µg/mL) or cephalosporins (MIC >4.0 µg/mL), vancomycin should not be used as a single agent if corticosteroids are used.

The addition of rifampin (Rifadin[1]) is often recommended in these situations.

# Chemoprophylaxis for Bacterial Meningitis

Prophylactic antibiotics are recommended in case of meningitis caused by *Neisseria meningitidis* and *Haemophilus influenzae* type b. Prophylaxis is provided to eliminate the carriage of organisms among contacts and prevent spread to hosts susceptible to invasive disease. In cases of meningococcal meningitis, prophylaxis is indicated only for those with household or close intimate contact with the index case. Administration of prophylaxis to large groups (e.g., college students, schoolchildren, or preschool classes) requires a special assessment and

---

[1]Not FDA approved for this indication.

**TABLE 4** Antibiotic Doses for Adults and Children for Treatment of Bacterial Meningitis

| Antibiotic | Daily Adult Dose | Daily Pediatric Dose | Dose Interval |
|---|---|---|---|
| Amikacin (Amikin) | 15 mg/kg | 15–20 mg/kg | 8 h |
| Ampicillin | 12 g | 200–400 mg/kg | 4–6 h |
| Cefotaxime (Claforan) | 12 g | 200–300 mg/kg | 4–6 h |
| Ceftriaxone (Rocephin) | 4 g | 100 mg/kg | 12 h |
| Ceftazidime (Fortaz) | 6 g | 150–200 mg/kg | 8 h |
| Cefepime (Maxipime) | 6 g | 100–150 mg/kg | 8 h |
| Gentamicin (Garamycin) | 5 mg/kg | 7.5 mg/kg | 8 h |
| Meropenem (Merrem) | 6 g | 120 mg/kg | 8 h |
| Nafcillin (Unipen) | 12 g | 200 mg/kg | 4–6 h |
| Penicillin G | 24 million U | 250,000 units/kg | 4 h |
| Tobramycin (Nebcin) | 5 mg/kg | 6–7.5 mg/kg | 8 h |
| Trimethoprim-sulfamethoxazole (Bactrim) | 10-15 mg/kg | 10–20 mg/kg | 8 h |
| Vancomycin (Vancocin) | 2 g | 60 mg/kg | 12 h |

Adapted from Bradley JS, Nelson JD: 2002–2003 Nelson's Pocket Book of Pediatric Antimicrobial Therapy, 15th ed. Philadelphia and New York, Lippincott Williams & Wilkins, 2002.
Gilbert DN, Moellering RC, Sande MA: The Sanford Guide to Antimicrobial Therapy 2005. Hyde Park, Antimicrobial Therapy Inc., 2005.

a recommendation of local or regional health departments. Chemoprophylaxis is not necessary for casual contacts or medical personnel unless there is a direct exposure to respiratory secretions. The recommended dose of rifampin (Rifadin) is 10 mg/kg (600 maximal, adults) twice a day for 2 days; ciprofloxacin (Cipro[1]), 500 mg as single dose, is also effective for adults. Third-generation cephalosporins used in treatment of the index case of meningitis are sufficient to eliminate carriage of the organism.

Chemoprophylaxis for *H. influenzae* type b is recommended for all household contacts of an index case if one of the contacts is an unvaccinated child younger than 4 years. If the index case is treated with ceftriaxone (Rocephin) or cefotaxime (Claforan), prophylaxis is not required, but if treated with ampicillin or chloramphenicol (Chloromycetin), prophylaxis is recommended to eliminate carriage. The recommended regimen for prophylaxis is rifampin,[1] 20 mg/kg (or 600 mg in adults) once a day for 4 days. With the near elimination of invasive infections caused by *Haemophilus influenzae* type b, with the use of routine immunization of children with conjugate haemophilus vaccines, *Haemophilus influenzae* types A, F, and rarely other serotypes have emerged, and the use of prophylaxis is not recommended in these situations because sufficient data are not available to support its efficacy, nor has spread within contacts been documented with any frequency.

## Vaccines for Bacterial Meningitis

The universal recommendation for the use of protein-polysaccharide conjugate *Haemophilus influenzae* type b (HIB) vaccines in 1987 reduced the incidence of bacterial meningitis by this organism by greater than 97%. Three HIB vaccines (PedvaxHIB, ActHIB, HibTITER), licensed in the United States, are routinely given to children in dosage schedules employing three to four doses by 12 to 18 months of age (see www.cdc.gov).

A pneumococcal protein-polysaccharide conjugate vaccine (Prevnar) licensed in 2000 is routinely recommended for children and has markedly reduced the incidence of invasive infections with seven serotypes of pneumococci in children. This vaccine is also recommended for children at high risk of pneumococcal infections (e.g., HIV infection, asplenia, sickle cell disease, and others). A pneumococcal polysaccharide vaccine (Pneumovax 23) is recommended for adults older than 65 years or for those over 50 years with risk factors (e.g., alcoholism, diabetes or other metabolic or renal disease, chronic pulmonary or cardiac disease). Although clear evidence for prevention of bacterial meningitis is lacking, evidence supports its efficacy against invasive pneumococcal diseases, many of which are the preceding infections leading to bacteremia and meningitis.

Currently two vaccines remain available for prevention of meningococcal disease caused by four serotypes, A, C, Y, and W-135. The meningococcal polysaccharide vaccine (Menomune) is recommended for persons older than 2 years at high risk for severe meningococcal infections including adolescents and college students (particularly those residing in dormitories), military recruits, and those with complement deficiencies and asplenia. A quadrivalent protein-polysaccharide conjugate vaccines (Menactra) was licensed in 2005. This vaccine is recommended for routine immunization of all children 11 to 12 years of age and adolescents and college students at high risk as well as those more than 11 to 55 years of age with high-risk factors for meningococcal infection.

### REFERENCES

Anderson EJ, Yogev LR: A rational approach to the management of ventricular shunt infections. Pediatric Infect Dis J 2005;24:557-558.
Andes DR, Craig WA: Pharmacokinetics and pharmacodynamics of antibiotics in meningitis. Infect Dis Clin North Am 1999;13(2):595-618.

De Gans J, van de Beek: Dexamethasone in adults with bacterial meningitis. N Engl J Med 2002;347:1549-1546.
Gray LD, Fedorko DP: Laboratory diagnosis of bacterial meningitis. Clin Microbiol Rev 1992;5:130-145.
Hussein AS, Shafran SD: Acute bacterial meningitis in adults: A 12-year review. Medicine (Baltimore) 2000;79:360-368.
Klinger G, Chin C-Y, Beyene J, et al: Predicting the outcome of neonatal bacterial meningitis. Pediatrics 2000;106:477-482.
Klein JO: Bacterial sepsis and meningitis. In Remington JS, Klein JO (eds): Infectious Diseases of the Fetus and Newborn Infant, 5th ed. New York and Saint Louis, WB Saunders, 2002, pp 943-998.
Odio CM, Faingezicht I, Paris M, et al: The beneficial effects of early dexamethasone administration in infants and children with bacterial meningitis. N Engl J Med 1991;324:1525-1531.
Ronan A, Hogg GG, Klug CL: Cerebrospinal fluid shunt infections in children. Pediatr Infect Dis J 1995;14:782-786.
Schuchat A, Robinson K, Wenger JD, et al: Bacterial meningitis in the United States in 1995. N Engl J Med 1997;337:970-976.
Unhanand M, Mustapha MM, McCracken GH, et al: Gram-negative enteric bacillary meningitis: A twenty-one year experience. J Pediatr 1993;122:15-17.
Van de Beek D, de Gans J, Spanjaard L, et al: Clinical features and prognostic factors in adults with bacterial meningitis. N Engl J Med 2004;351:1849-1858.

# Infectious Mononucleosis

Method of
*Leonard R. Krilov, MD*

Infectious mononucleosis is a clinical illness characterized by fever (typically not higher than 39.5°C [103°F]), sore throat, tender cervical lymphadenopathy, fever, malaise, and anorexia; it occurs most commonly in adolescence and young adulthood. Initially described in the 19th century as glandular fever, the characteristic mononuclear response with atypical-appearing lymphocytes led to the name infectious mononucleosis.

## Etiology

Epstein-Barr virus (EBV) was recognized as the primary cause of infectious mononucleosis in 1968. Other infectious agents such as cytomegalovirus (CMV), toxoplasma, or adenoviruses may cause a minority of cases of mononucleosis (or mononucleosis-like illness).

Epstein-Barr virus is an enveloped, double-stranded DNA virus of the Herpesviridae family. After primary EBV infection, as with other herpesviruses, the virus persists in a latent state throughout the patient's lifetime in a few B lymphocytes and is shed in saliva intermittently.

The virus has also been associated with African Burkitt's lymphoma, nasopharyngeal carcinoma, lymphoproliferative diseases after organ and bone marrow transplantation, and hairy leukoplakia and lymphocytic interstitial pneumonitis in HIV-infected patients. X-linked proliferative disease (Duncan syndrome) is a rare condition in which affected boys develop fulminant uncontrolled lymphoproliferation after acute infectious mononucleosis. Survivors develop severe chronic hypogammaglobulinemia, chronic EBV and enteroviral infections and B-cell lymphomas.

## Epidemiology

Epstein-Barr virus infections occur at a younger age in lower socioeconomic groups; 70% to 90% of such children developing EBV antibodies by age 5 years compared to only 40% to 50% of those from higher socioeconomic groups. For unknown reasons primary infections occurring in adolescence and young adulthood are more likely to manifest as infectious mononucleosis than when initial infection occurs at a younger age. In younger children acute EBV infection is usually clinically inapparent or manifested by a nonspecific, uncomplicated upper respiratory tract infection or pharyngitis. Thus, infectious mononucleosis occurs most commonly among white high school and college students with an annual incidence of approximately 1 in 2500 among such individuals aged 15 to 25 years.

EBV transmission occurs through intimate sharing of saliva (thus, its description as the *kissing disease*) with an incubation period of 20 to 30 days (range 2 to 6 weeks). The efficiency of transmission is low, and outbreaks of disease are rare. Epstein-Barr virus' viral load in whole blood in the acute phase correlates with the severity of symptoms; but viral load in oral secretions is independent of symptoms. There is no seasonality or sex predilection to EBV infections. Post-transfusion development of symptoms of mononucleosis is most often associated with CMV infection.

## Clinical Manifestations

The classic manifestations of infectious mononucleosis are fever, painful exudative pharyngitis, and lymphadenopathy. The enlarged nodes may be limited to the cervical regions (including posteriorly) or generalized. Splenomegaly and frequently hepatomegaly are the other hallmark findings of the illness. Elevated liver function tests are common in the acute phase of disease, but symptomatic jaundice is rare. Eyelid edema (Hoagland sign) has been reported in approximately 25% of cases. The acute symptoms typically resolve over 1 to 4 weeks, but lymphadenopathy and fatigue may last for 2 to 3 months.

Less common clinical manifestations include autoimmune hemolytic anemia (approximately 3%), severe neutropenia to less than 1000/mm³ (approximately 3%), and neurologic involvement in up to 5% of cases. The reported neurologic manifestations of acute EBV infection include meningoencephalitis, Guillain-Barré syndrome, transverse myelitis, facial paralysis, optic neuritis, and metamorphopsia or Alice in Wonderland syndrome with altered perception of sizes, shapes, and spatial relationships.

Most cases of mononucleosis resolve uneventfully. Splenic rupture and the previously cited neurologic complications are the most frequent serious complications of mononucleosis with rare deaths reported.

## Diagnosis

In the presence of the clinical features noted earlier, infectious mononucleosis is diagnosed by the presence of atypical lymphocytosis (>5% to 10% of all leukocytes) frequently in association with a decline in the number of granulocytes and platelets. Additionally, among school-age children and young adults, heterophil or Paul-Bunnell antibodies are detectable in 80% to 90% of cases beginning in the second week of illness and can be detected for up to 6 to 9 months after resolution of symptoms. These IgM antibodies react with horse, sheep, and beef erythrocytes but not guinea pig red cells. They are not EBV-specific and are present in only 50% or fewer of children younger than 4 years of age. Office-based commercial rapid slide kits for detecting heterophil response are 96% to 99% sensitive and give a result in 2 minutes.

## CURRENT DIAGNOSIS

The clinical triad of fever, exudative pharyngitis, and lymphadenitis in association with atypical lymphocytosis and a positive heterophil response makes the diagnosis of infectious mononucleosis. Epstein-Barr virus serologies should be reserved for uncertain cases or to confirm the diagnosis in younger children who may not mount a heterophil response.

Measurement of specific antibodies to EBV can be used to confirm the diagnosis. In the acute phase of illness, IgM and IgG antibodies to the viral capsid antigen (VCA) of EBV are detectable. The IgM response persists for approximately 4 months, whereas the IgG antibodies remain for life. Although the height of the VCA-IgG response decreases as the acute infection resolves, serial measurements of antibody titers are not clinically beneficial as a rule. Antibodies to the EBV nuclear antigen (EBNA) appear several weeks to months after a primary infection and are considered a marker for a past or convalescent infection, but 10% to 20% of individuals never develop detectable levels of EBNA antibodies. More than 80% of patients develop transient antibodies to the early antigen (EA) of the virus as the VCA-IgM clears and EBNA responses develop (Table 1).

## Treatment

There is no effective antiviral therapy for EBV-associated infectious mononucleosis. Rest and supportive care are mainstays of therapy. Corticosteroids are frequently prescribed for severe cases, but critical evaluation of this modality is lacking. Indications include marked tonsillar hypertrophy with upper airway obstruction, neurologic manifestations, and hemolytic anemia. High-dose, short-term courses of steroids (dexamethasone [Decadron][1] [0.25 mg/kg every 6 hours]; methylprednisolone [Solu-Medrol][1] [1 mg/kg every 6 hours]; oral prednisone[1] [40 mg/day]) have been used with dramatic improvement typically noted over 24 to 72 hours.

---

[1]Not FDA approved for this indication.

## CURRENT THERAPY

Rest and supportive care with limitation of physical activity during the first 1 to 4 weeks of illness are the mainstays of managing infectious mononucleosis. Corticosteroids are reserved for severe illness, especially with upper airway obstruction because of tonsillar hypertrophy.

---

**TABLE 1** Infectious Mononucleosis Serological Response Patterns (Typical Patterns)

| | Heterophil Antibody | EBV VCA-IgM | EBV VCA-IgG | EBV EA | EBV EBNA |
|---|---|---|---|---|---|
| No Infection | – | – | – | – | – |
| Acute Infection | + | + | +/+ | +/– | – |
| Past Infection | – | – | + | +/– | + |

*Abbreviations:* EA = early antigen; EBNA = Epstein-Barr (virus) nuclear antigen; EBV = Epstein-Barr virus; VCA = viral capsid antigen.

## REFERENCES

Ambinder RF, Lin L: Mononucleosis in the laboratory. J Infect Dis 2005; 192:1503–1504.

Balfour HH Jr, Holman CJ, Hokanson KM, et al: A prospective clinical study of Epstein-Barr virus and host interactions during acute infectious mononucleosis. J Infect Dis 2005;192:1505–1512.

Barone SR, Krilov LR: Infectious mononucleosis and other Epstein-Barr virus infections. In Hoekelman RA (ed.): Primary Pediatric Care (4th ed.). St. Louis, Mosby, 2001, pp 1573–1577.

Fafi-Kremer S, Morand P, Brion J-P, et al: Long-term shedding of infectious Epstein-Barr virus after infectious mononucleosis. J Infect Dis 2005;191:985–989.

Giffen BE, Xue S: Epstein-Barr virus infections and their association with human malignancies: Some key questions. Ann Med 1998;30:249–254.

Henle G, Henle W, Diehl V: Relation of Burkitt's tumor-associated herpes-type virus to infectious mononucleosis. Proc Natl Acad Sci U S A 1968;59:94–101.

McGowan JE, Chesney PJ, Crossley KB, et al: Guidelines for the use of systemic glucococorticosteroids in the management of selected infections. Working group on steroid use, Antimicrobial Agents Committee, Infectious Diseases Society of America. J Infect Dis 1992;165:1–13.

Paul JR, Bunnell WW: Classics in infectious diseases. The presence of heterophile antibodies in infectious mononucleosis by John R. Paul and W. W. Bunnell. American Journal of the Medical Sciences, 1932. Rev Infect Dis 1982;4:1062–1068.

Sumaya CV, Ench Y: Epstein-Barr virus infectious mononucleosis in children. I. Clinical and general laboratory findings. Pediatrics 1985; 75:1003–1010.

Sumaya CV, Ench Y: Epstein-Barr virus infectious mononucleosis in children. II. Heterophil antibody and viral-specific responses. Pediatrics 1985;75:1011–1019.

# Chronic Fatigue Syndrome

Method of
*James F. Jones, MD*

## Definition

*Chronic fatigue syndrome* (CFS) is the name applied to an illness of unknown origin that at face value resembles unresolved infections, depression, endocrinologic and metabolic disorders, sleep disorders, and many other conditions that include fatigue in their diagnostic criteria.

In the modern era, interest in this illness began with the question of a relationship with a chronic active Epstein-Barr virus infection. Subsequent studies did not support Epstein-Barr virus as the only cause of this syndrome, but several recent studies have found 10% of patients with acute infectious mononucleosis and other infectious diseases might have a similar illness or postinfection fatigue syndrome.

The lack of association with a specific infectious agent led to the generation in 1988 of a definition based on the presence of incapacitating fatigue and varying combinations of signs and symptoms. Any preexisting medical or psychiatric condition was exclusionary. Evaluation of this definition at a number of centers in the United States, Great Britain, and Australia led to the current definition published in 1994 (Box 1). The definition was altered so that preexisting medical conditions that were treated satisfactorily were allowed, as well as certain psychiatric and syndromic diagnoses. Additional changes in the definition included a decrease in the number of symptoms and removal of the signs; signs had been shown to be somewhat arbitrary, and patients could be identified in their absence. The greater number of symptoms in the 1988 version did not allow identification of a specific illness, and they increased the possibility that patients who had primary psychiatric illnesses (e g., somatiform disorders) would be mislabeled with CFS. The 1994 definition still requires more than 6 months of fatigue, but it dropped the 50% level of activity present in

## BOX 1  International Consensus Definition of Chronic Fatigue Syndrome

- Clinically evaluated, unexplained, persistent or relapsing chronic fatigue (lasting more than 6 months) that is of new or definite onset (has not been lifelong); is not the result of ongoing exertion; is not substantially alleviated by rest; and results in substantial reduction in previous levels of occupational, educational, social, or personal activities.
- Four or more of the following symptoms are concurrently present for more than 6 months:
  - Impaired memory or concentration
  - Multijoint pain
  - Muscle pain
  - New headaches
  - Postexertional malaise
  - Sore throat
  - Tender cervical or axillary lymph nodes
  - Unrefreshing sleep
- Exclusionary clinical diagnoses:
  - Any active medical condition that could explain the chronic fatigue
  - Any previously diagnosed medical condition whose resolution has not been documented beyond reasonable clinical doubt and whose continued activity can explain the chronic fatiguing illness
  - Psychotic major depression, bipolar affective disorder, schizophrenia, delusional disorders, dementias, anorexia nervosa, bulimia nervosa
  - Alcohol or other substance abuse within 2 years prior to the onset of the chronic fatigue and at any time afterward

Adapted from Fukuda K. Straus SE, Hickie I, et al: The chronic fatigue syndrome: A comprehensive approach to its definition and study. Ann Intern Med 1994;121:953-959.

the 1988 definition because the requirement was impossible to apply evenly across all patients.

The diagnostic criteria, including exclusion of other illnesses, are described in the Current Diagnosis box. The definition was originally designed as a research tool and included suggestions for unifying the measurement of fatigue and evaluation of the mental status of patients.

## Epidemiology

The prevalence of the syndrome using the 1988 definition is approximately 13 per 100,000, whereas the 1994 definition identified approximately 300 per 100,000. Application of an empiric definition (see later) in a population recruited with unwellness, rather than fatigue, identified a higher prevalence of CFS (Reeves et al, 2007). An increase in CFS cases in an unwell population highlights the need to address illness in general and not just fatigue when considering this diagnosis. One demographic variable that has remained stable is the 3:1 ratio of women to men.

## Diagnosis

Diagnosis of CFS begins with exclusion of other illness processes associated with fatigue and unwellness and subsequent suspicion of the syndrome after taking a history and performing a physical examination and screening laboratory tests (Box 2). It should not be assumed that a patient with fatigue as a presenting complaint has CFS. The history shows whether the illness began acutely or more gradually

## BOX 2  Screening Laboratory Tests

- Alanine aminotransferase
- Albumin
- Alkaline phosphatase
- C-reactive protein
- Complete blood count
- Creatinine
- Electrolytes
- Globulin
- Glucose
- Thyroid-stimulating hormone and free $T_4$
- Total protein
- Urinalysis

*Abbreviation:* $T_4$ = thyroxine.

and whether there are preexisting symptoms. History often provides insight into previously identified factors that influence patient perception of illness. Questioning about typical episodes provides information about cyclic events, possible triggers of symptoms, and possible exposures.

The interviewer gives the patients the opportunity to describe the history of the illness. The interviewer simply guides the patient and tries not to ask leading questions. This process not only gathers information but also serves as an ice breaker between the interviewer and the patient. It allows the interviewer to determine the mental status of the patient, the patient's concentration and memory capabilities, and what may be on the patient's agenda. It usually allows the examiner to determine the kind and scope of prior medical and alternative care evaluations the patients has received.

The diagnosis of CFS should not be made on the first visit. Attempts should be made to determine the duration, the mode of onset, the magnitude, and the consequences of each complaint, although these are not included in the working definition. Only with such thorough questioning will an underlying process responsible for the illness be identified or suspected.

A more recent application of the definition uses three validated questionnaires: the Medical Outcomes Survey Short Form-36 (SF-36), the Multidimensional Fatigue Inventory (MFI), and the CDC Symptom Inventory. These questionnaires provide numeric scores that identify persons with CFS and provide a record of their level of impairment. The Symptom Inventory collects information about the presence, frequency, and intensity of 19 fatigue- and illness-related symptoms during the month preceding the interview; these include all eight CFS-defining symptoms (postexertional fatigue, unrefreshing sleep, problems remembering or concentrating, muscle aches and pains, joint pain, sore throat, tender lymph nodes and swollen glands, and headaches). Perceived frequency of each symptom is rated on a four-point scale (1 = a little of the time, 2 = some of the time, 3 = most of time, 4 = all of the time), and severity or intensity of symptoms is measured on a three-point scale (1 = mild, 2 = moderate, 3 = severe).

The case definition specifies that CFS causes substantial reduction in occupational, educational, social, or recreational activities.

*Substantial reduction* is defined as scores lower than the 25th percentile on the SF-36 using the following four factors: physical function (≤70), or role physical (≤50), or social function (≤75), or role emotional (≤66.67) subscales of the SF-36, related to published norms of the U.S. population according to Ware and Sherbourne. We defined severe fatigue using the Multidimensional Fatigue Inventory as a score of 13 or higher on the general fatigue scale or 10 or higher on the reduced activity scales of the MFI (their respective medians). Finally, because the case definition specifies that characteristic symptoms accompany fatigue, subjects reporting at least 4 symptoms and scoring at least 25 on the Symptom Inventory Case Definition Subscale were considered to have substantial accompanying symptoms.

Routine laboratory evaluations are recommended to address contributory illnesses (see Box 2). Routine testing does not include specific antibody testing, tests of immune function per se, or single-photon emission computed tomography (SPECT) or magnetic resonance imaging (MRI) of the brain. Negative screening test results do not automatically exclude an alternative diagnosis. Specific testing, for example, for a sleep disorder or chronic sinusitis may be necessary. A mental status examination, either informally or by using a standard instrument when indicated, is equally important.

A working diagnosis of CFS may then be made if the evaluation fails to identify an underlying illness. This approach is warranted because the patient's underlying disease might declare itself in the future. Continued adherence to a diagnosis of CFS in the face of an evolving or readily identifiable medical or psychiatric illness is the single most detrimental outcome of a premature or prolonged diagnosis of CFS.

Additional laboratory or other diagnostic testing is based on the individual patient's complaints. The interview techniques listed earlier assist in this process. An additional valuable tool that will lead the interviewer to identify a specific illness or symptoms requiring intervention is simply to ask the patient to list the problems described in decreasing order of magnitude. Which problem causes the most difficulty? Or which problems interfere with the ability to carry out daily functions? Patients often use this exercise to list the consequences of their illness.

## Therapy

Treatment regimens vary with the needs of the individual patient and how he or she perceives the illness. The goals of treatment depend on the person's specific symptoms and eventually the patient's identified needs within a framework of providing reentry into their premorbid condition. Complete return to normal might not be possible immediately, however, nor is this goal appropriate if it is too lofty. In fact, the desire for total immediate recovery can hamper clinical improvement. The patient's adaptation to this new, albeit temporary, state is often a more realistic short-term goal. Therapeutic modalities include education regarding the boundaries and limitations of the diagnosis, development of coping skills, institution of a graduated exercise program when possible, and use of medications to treat symptoms. If the patient is being seen in a multidisciplinary setting, these approaches may be combined into a specific program. If CFS is an infrequent diagnosis in a practice, identifying the problems that cause loss of function becomes critical.

### CURRENT DIAGNOSIS

- Identify duration of fatigue and its consequences.
- Identify primary symptoms.
- Exclude other illnesses/diseases.
- Reconsider the diagnosis on an ongoing basis.
- Chronic fatigue syndrome is a working diagnosis.

### CURRENT THERAPY

- Education regarding the advantages and disadvantages of CFS as a diagnosis
- Development of coping skills
- Cognitive behavior therapy
- Initiation of a graded exercise program
- Symptomatic medication

## EDUCATION

All physicians who make the diagnosis must provide information regarding the illness in general and the specific criteria that allowed recognition of the problem. Just as education regarding asthma and diabetes mellitus is a critical component of therapy for those diseases, education regarding the origin, specific components, and outcome of the syndrome is more critical in this situation.

The literature supports CFS as a condition that is not life threatening or progressive. Lay representations, which are readily available, are often incorrect in painting a uniformly dismal outcome. Physicians should counsel their patients that all illness symptoms should not be attributed to CFS, and patients should seek medical advice when new problems arise or old problems become more prominent. Patients should also be taught that persistent efforts to find a cure via experiences of their acquaintances or the newest information in magazines or on the Internet are not as productive as their participation in a specifically designed program as outlined here. Paramount in this process is their consideration of acceptance of their current, albeit temporary, status. Wanting their lives back and attempting to regain them with a pill are not effective approaches.

A major part of the education and treatment process is the interview process. Giving the patient the opportunity to describe the illness and its consequences in a nonjudgmental situation is critical to gaining the patient's confidence. A physician who makes the diagnosis of CFS literally establishes a contract for long-term care with the patient, and it must be based on mutual trust.

## DEVELOPMENT OF COPING SKILLS

To recommend coping strategies, the provider must know the needs of the patient, another rationale for the patient-generated problem list. If the patient complains of problems with memory and concentration, simple advice regarding using lists and audiotaping activities or needs is logical. If they cannot perform on the job or their behavioral responses to these complaints aggravate the consequences, formal neuropsychological testing or therapy, or both, is required. Assistance with understanding losses is also very important. Depending on the magnitude of the consequences of their illness, patients can lose self-respect and the appreciation of their families, employees, and coworkers. They need to learn that as individuals they are not responsible for these losses but that they are responsible, at least in part, for their recovery. They need to go through a grieving process and then learn how to adapt to their current state. They need to learn to accept and desire incremental levels of progress. Formal psychological therapy may be required to achieve these goals.

The origin of the illness and the character of the fatigue dictate the approach in many cases. If the origin is with an apparent, usually unidentified, flu-like illness that does not resolve, or if the character of the fatigue simulates the malaise of such an illness, the patient needs to know that the symptoms are normal responses. The duration and consequences in the eyes of society and the individual patient are the factors that differentiate a normal resolution of an illness from a prolonged or chronic condition.

The patient also needs to know that resumption of normal activity is not the correct approach. Most patients have symptoms on a daily basis, but they also have days when the symptoms are more or less pronounced (bad and good days). A typical patient performs on the good days as if there were no illness. This action is then followed in 1 or 2 days by an exacerbation of symptoms. Learning to compartmentalize activities and to never exceed their personal limits are critical steps in coping with CFS.

On the other hand, total acceptance of such a program is not appropriate either. Usually, acute-onset patients notice that they can be more active without exacerbation of symptoms regardless of their therapeutic program. This observation usually heralds resolution of the illness. In some instances, the illness is resolving, but the patient perceives the outcome of increased physical activity (e.g., muscle aches and tiredness) as illness symptoms rather than simply the expected consequences of increased activity. The recurrence of the patient's whole syndrome following activity, however, suggests that resolution has not taken place.

## EXERCISE

It seems contradictory to follow the discussion about listening to one's body and avoiding excessive activity with a section that recommends regular exercise. The studies on muscle function show that patients are tired after performing repetitive acts and that there appears to be no primary problem in muscle function. There may a problem in fitness or conditioning, however. Whether this result is a consequence of the illness or the inactivity that accompanies the syndrome is not known.

Lessons from the rehabilitation of patients with cardiac and pulmonary diseases teach us that anaerobic exercise to regain strength should precede exercises to improve aerobic fitness and overall conditioning. A program that includes active stretching followed by range-of-motion contractions and extensions that eventually includes resistance is usually an effective start. Five minutes per day is a typical starting point for a patient who has been totally inactive. The endpoint of each session should be preset by the clock or number of repetitions and should be reached before the patient becomes tired. This endpoint is based on the fact that either tiredness is a trigger for the production of biological changes that are a part of the host's attempt to limit activity or the perception that tiredness triggers illness behavior. At this stage in the understanding of the illness, prevention of activation of either of these pathways and an increase in overall fitness are appropriate goals. This section may be summarized by the adage that no exercise is bad, some is good, and too much exercise is not helpful.

The previous sections on education, coping skills, and exercise provide the kinds of therapy that are offered in cognitive behavior therapy programs.

## SYMPTOMATIC THERAPY

One usually associates symptomatic therapy with medication. Some interventions require alterations in patient habits or changes in biological processes that do not require medication per se.

### Sleep Therapy

The primary example is treatment of sleep problems. A very large percentage of patients presenting for evaluation of fatigue, many of whom carry the diagnosis of CFS, have sleep disorders or disturbances. Some have problems with sleep hygiene. They may read or watch television for prolonged periods (longer than 15 minutes) before trying to go to sleep. This habit can actually allow arousal of the brain within several hours following sleep onset, thus leading to interrupted sleep. Caffeine ingestion after 6 PM and exercise within 4 hours of bedtime can impede getting to sleep.

Patients are often given medication for insomnia that is manifested by going to bed at 11 PM but not being able to get to sleep until 1 or 2 AM, with a waking time of 10 AM. A hypnotic might be prescribed that allows induction of sleep at an earlier time, but the patient might still not experience restorative sleep. One explanation for this series of events is that the patient has a phase-delay syndrome and needs to alter the sleep cycle with prescribed light therapy before improvement is expected. Appropriate use of hypnotics may be important in allowing initial normalization of sleep cycling, but these agents are not sufficient as the sole mode of therapy, nor should they be used for prolonged periods.

Daytime sleepiness is another common problem with multiple origins. Ill-advised symptomatic therapy includes self- or physician-generated use of stimulants. These drugs include caffeine, herbs that contain ephedrine such as Ma huang (Ephedra sinica), and antidepressants that actually serve as stimulants (serotonin and norepinephrine reuptake inhibitors [SNRIs]). These substances might allow short-term improvement in daytime function, but they block identification of the underlying nighttime or daytime origin of the sleep problem.

### Pharmacologic Therapy

Premature treatment can prevent adequate diagnosis and treatment of readily remediated problems. However, symptomatic medications have a definite place in the therapy of CFS. Many CFS patients do not tolerate standard doses of any of the medications used for symptomatic relief.

Classes of drugs that might have beneficial effects for symptom relief include hypnotics of various types, antidepressants of several types if depression is evident, and non-narcotic analgesics. As used in the treatment of fibromyalgia, tricyclic antidepressants and SNRIs are used for symptomatic therapy in the absence of formal depression. Because these classes of medications are being used as adjuncts to the other modes of therapy, they are not always successful. They might need to be changed during the course of the illness.

Often patients come to the physician using a large number of medications. It might not be possible to determine by the history alone whether the patient's symptoms are not at least in part due to the medication regimen. Often the medications need to be tapered and stopped to sort out their influence on the manifesting complaints.

Popular remedies for CFS are discussed primarily to familiarize the practitioner with them and to support previous warnings regarding lack of efficacy. The primary problem with their use is that proof is lacking that such intervention has been uniformly beneficial. This statement is particularly true in cases of parenteral (injectable) repetitious therapy with any substance.

### Alternative Therapies

The effectiveness of diet manipulations and ingestion of herbs, enzymes, amino acids, vitamins, minerals, or hormones, although usually safe, is equally unproven. These agents constitute a large component of the therapeutic armamentarium in use by patients with CFS. Herbs are particularly in vogue. Many of them have medicinal qualities and if taken in excessive amounts may be injurious. Because many of these substances are readily available, they are used by patients who are anxious for improvement in their illness. If the reader has such patients or is such a patient, one must make sure that the remedy in question is safe and that its use is affordable and does not hide illness parameters that require specific identification.

If patients are intent on taking these types of remedies, they should be advised to at least seek the advice of a responsible care provider who is knowledgeable in their use and adverse consequences. Alternative care in many forms is also in vogue and may be helpful if provided in a responsible fashion. Some patients with myalgias and other pain complaints find particular benefit from acupuncture and therapeutic massage.

### Therapeutic Plan

Therapy for CFS patients continues to be directed at relieving symptoms and consequences of the syndrome. It is clear, however, that one approach or one medication is not satisfactory for all patients. Identifying the patient's most problematic symptoms and using a variety of modalities that address those problems in the treatment plan are the most effective ways of assisting the patient. Patients should be reminded not to expect total return to their premorbid state to occur immediately.

Because the use of medications remains arbitrary, failure of one regimen may be followed by successful relief using the more effective modes of therapy, such as cognitive behavior therapy and graduated exercise. Eventually the origins of symptom production will be understood and therapy can be directed with some authority. As it stands now, one must always be careful that whatever the treatment, it must not aggravate the illness.

### REFERENCES

Bazelmans E, Prins JB, Lulofs R, et al; The Netherlands Fatigue Research Group Nijmegen. Cognitive behaviour group therapy for chronic fatigue syndrome: A non-randomised waiting list controlled study. Psychother Psychosom 2005;74(4):218-224.

Jones JF, Maloney EM, Boneva RS, et al: Complementary and alternative medical therapy utilization by people with chronic fatiguing illnesses in the United States. BMC Complement Altern Med 2007;7:12.

Jones JF, Nisenbaum R, Reeves WC: Medication use by persons with chronic fatigue syndrome: Results of a randomized telephone survey in Wichita, Kansas. Health Qual Life Outcomes 2003;1(1):74.

Moss-Morris R, Sharon C, Tobin R, Baldi JC: A randomized controlled graded exercise trial for chronic fatigue syndrome: Outcomes and mechanisms of change. J Health Psychol 2005;10(2):245-259.

Nater UM, Wagner D, Solomon L, et al: Coping styles in people with chronic fatigue syndrome identified from the general population of Wichita, KS. J Psychosom Res 2006;60(6):567-573.

Reeves WC, Jones JF, Maloney E, et al: Prevalence of chronic fatigue syndrome in metropolitan, urban, and rural Georgia. Popul Health Metr 2007;5:5.

Reeves WC, Wagner D, Nisenbaum R, et al: Chronic fatigue syndrome: A clinically empirical approach to its definition and study. BMC Med 2005;3(1):19

Wagner D, Nisenbaum R, Heim C, et al: Psychometric properties of the CDC Symptom Inventory for assessment of Chronic Fatigue Syndrome. BioMed Central Popul Health Metr 2005;3:8.

Ware JE, Sherbourne CD: The MOS 36-item short form health survey (SF-36): Conceptual framework and item selection. Med Care 1992;30:473-483.

Whiting P, Bagnall AM, Sowden AJ, et al: Interventions for the treatment and management of chronic fatigue syndrome: A systematic review. JAMA 2001;286:1360-1368.

# Mumps

Method of
*Joel D. Klein, MD, FAAP*

Mumps is a respiratory viral infection caused by mumps virus, an RNA virus in the family Paramyxoviridae. The virus is spread from human to human through direct contact with airborne droplets.

## Epidemiology

Before the introduction of mumps vaccine, there were large yearly epidemics, usually occurring in the winter and early spring. Infection generally occurred among young children (younger than 15 years), with rare cases in young adults. With the introduction of the mumps vaccine in 1967, there was a dramatic decrease in the number of cases. However, in 1986 and 1987, there was a resurgence of mumps among teenagers and young adults, most of whom were born before routine immunization with the mumps vaccine.

Outbreaks were also seen among some children who had received mumps vaccine, because a single dose of the vaccine did not always confer immunity. In 1989, a second dose of mumps vaccine was recommended to address this issue. Mumps vaccine currently is usually administered as part of a combined vaccine such as measles-mumps-rubella (MMR) or most recently measles-mumps-rubella-varicella (MMRV) (Proquad).

Despite these changes, outbreaks of mumps occasionally occur, usually among college-aged persons. Recent examples include an epidemic in the United Kingdom in the winter of 2004 to 2005 and in the United States in 2006.

## Clinical Manifestations

The incubation period of mumps is 14 to 25 days and involves nonspecific complaints of malaise, low-grade fever, and anorexia. The single most diagnostic physical finding in mumps is unilateral or bilateral parotitis, which occurs in up to 40% of cases. Mumps parotitis can

### CURRENT DIAGNOSIS

- Painful parotid swelling
- Edema of the face in the area of the parotid
- Elevation of serum amylase
- Headache and occasional meningismus
- Viral isolation or serology can confirm diagnosis

## TABLE 1 Complications of Mumps Infection

| Mumps Complications | Incidence of Complications |
| --- | --- |
| Central nervous system | 40%-50% |
| Orchitis and epididymitis | 15%-30% |
| Oophoritis | 7% |
| Pancreatitis | 2%-5% |
| Deafness | 1 in 20,000 reported cases |
| Myocarditis | Rare |
| Arthritis | Rare |
| Thyroiditis | Rare |

occur early in the disease and may be associated with swelling and pain in other salivary glands. There often is erythema of the area and tenderness with palpation of the affected parotid. Patients at times also complain of earache and headache. Swelling over the parotid and related glands can occur rapidly and can result in distortion of the contours of the face, pushing the earlobe upward and outward. Edema can extend to the anterior chest wall as well. Examination of the oral cavity can reveal erythema of the orifice of Stensen's duct without purulent discharge. Parotitis generally resolves within 1 week.

The most commonly reported complications of mumps are aseptic meningitis and encephalitis, which can occur individually or together. Meningitis occurs in 10% to 15% of cases but probably is underreported. There is a typical viral-like pleocytosis in the cerebrospinal fluid (CSF), but the CSF glucose may be low. Encephalitis is rare and is seen in 1 or 2 per 100,000 cases.

Orchitis, either unilateral or bilateral, may be seen in as many as 50% of infected men. This complication can have a rapid onset and can be associated with increased fever, abdominal pain, nausea, and testicular swelling. This complication generally resolves within 1 week and can result in testicular atrophy but rarely infertility. Pancreatitis is sometimes seen, is usually mild, and may be associated with transient hyperglycemia. Table 1 lists the incidence of complications of mumps.

## Diagnosis

Diagnosis of mumps is usually made by clinical examination and history. It should be considered in any patient with sudden onset of parotid swelling and fever. Mumps virus isolation may be attempted on fluids obtained by nasopharyngeal swab and urine. Virus may be excreted for 1 week before and 1 week after the onset of parotitis. When available, PCR may also be used to detect mumps virus in secretions.

Serum amylase determinations, although not specific, may be helpful in situations where mumps is suspected. Serology, which is readily available, may be diagnostic as well. Mumps IgM obtained during the acute infection is usually elevated and diagnostic. Acute and convalescent-paired sera can also be used to retrospectively confirm the diagnosis. Other commonly ordered laboratory tests, including complete blood count (CBC) are not particularly helpful. The CBC might show mild leukopenia with lymphocytosis.

Differential diagnosis of mumps parotitis includes many infections that are listed in Box 1.

## BOX 1 Differential Diagnosis of Mumps Parotitis

- Parainfluenza virus infection
- Enterovirus infection
- Epstein-Barr virus
- Cytomegalovirus infection
- HIV
- Suppurative bacterial infection (Staphylococcus aureus, Streptococcus pneumoniae)
- Nontuberculous mycobacterial infection

## CURRENT THERAPY

- Analgesia for pain
- Warm or cold compresses
- Droplet isolation in the hospital
- Patient may return to school 9 days after the onset of parotid swelling

## Treatment

There is no specific therapy for mumps. Adequate analgesia is important, because many patients are quite uncomfortable. Because most patients are febrile, hydration also plays an important role. This is particularly critical because there may be difficulty swallowing and pain with mastication.

Children with mumps should be excluded from school for 9 days from onset of parotid swelling. Droplet precautions are recommended for patients with mumps admitted to the hospital for a period of 9 days from onset of parotid swelling.

## Prevention

Mumps vaccine should be administered to children at age 12 to 15 months. A second dose should be given at age 4 to 6 years. Patients with HIV who are not severely immunocompromised may receive a combination mumps vaccine. Adults born in 1957 or later, in whom immunity is not known, should receive one dose of a mumps combination vaccine (MMR). Persons born before 1957 are usually considered immune, but they might benefit from immunization during a mumps community outbreak.

## REFERENCES

American Academy of Pediatrics Committee on Infectious Diseases: Mumps. In Pickering LK (ed): Red Book: 2006 Report of the Committee on Infectious Diseases, 27th ed. Elk Grove Village, Ill: American Academy of Pediatrics; 2006, pp 464-468.

Cherry JD: Mumps Virus. In Feigin RD, Cherry JD, Demmler GJ, Kaplan SL (eds). Textbook of Pediatric Infectious Diseases 5th ed. Philadelphia: WB Saunders, 2004 pp 2305-2314.

Gupta RK, Best J, MacMahon E: Mumps and the UK epidemic 2005. BMJ 2005;330:1132-1135.

Litman N, Baum SG: Mumps virus. In Mandell GL, Bennett JE, Dolin R (eds): Principles and Practice of Infectious Diseases, 6th ed. Philadelphia: Churchill Livingstone, 2005, pp 2003-2008.

Maldonado Y: Mumps. In Behrman RE (ed): Nelson Textbook of Pediatrics, 17th ed. Philadelphia: WB Saunders, 2004, pp 1035-1036.

McQuone SJ: Acute viral and bacterial infections of the salivary glands. Otolaryngol Clin North Am 1999;32(5):793-811.

# Plague

Method of
*Douglas A. Drevets, MD, DTM&H*

Plague caused by *Yersinia pestis* is an ancient disease, and historical descriptions indicate that it probably caused Justinian's Plague (AD 541) that led into the first plague pandemic. The second plague pandemic, also known as the Black Death, began in Central Asia in 1347 and then spread to Europe, Asia, and Africa. It killed an estimated 50 million persons. The third and current plague pandemic began in China and then disseminated throughout the world by shipping routes in 1899–1900. *Y. pestis* is a gram-negative, nonmotile, facultatively anaerobic, non-spore-forming coccobacillus that is approximately 0.5 to 0.8 μm in diameter and 1 to 3 μm in length. Genomic sequencing shows that *Y. pestis* is a recently emerged clone of *Y. pseudotuberculosis*.

## Epidemiology

Plague is a zoonosis that is usually spread between mammalian hosts by the bite of infected fleas. The most important enzootic reservoirs are urban and sylvatic rodents; however, domestic cats and dogs also are linked to human disease. Human plague occurs in North and South America, Asia, and Africa. An average of 2547 cases of human plague were reported yearly to the World Health Organization between 1988 and 1997, 76% of which were from Africa, with an overall case fatality rate of 7.1%. In North America, 82% of 295 indigenous cases were from Arizona, Colorado, and New Mexico. Bubonic plague is the most common form in humans, accounting for 97% of cases in a recent outbreak in Madagascar. Similarly, 84% of U.S. cases reported between 1947 and 1996 were the bubonic form, with septicemic and pneumonic plague accounting for 13% and 2%, respectively.

## Modes of Transmission

Most human infections are transmitted from rodent to humans via the bite of an infected flea. Infection also can be acquired by contact with body fluids from infected animals, such as during field dressing of game or by inhalation of respiratory droplets from animals, particularly cats, or humans with pneumonic plague.

## Bioterrorism Threat

Plague was used as an agent of biowarfare by the Japanese in World War II and was a focus of intensive research and development in the former Soviet Union during the Cold War. Primary pneumonic plague is the most likely form of exposure because of biowarfare or bioterrorism.

## Pathogenesis and Clinical Syndromes

Transdermal inoculation of bacilli from the bite of an infected flea ultimately leads to infection of the regional lymph nodes in which massive replication of bacteria creates the bubo (derived from the Greek "bubon" or "groin"), a swollen, erythematous, and painful lymph node in the groin, axilla, or cervical region. Bacteremia and septicemia frequently develop and lead to secondary infection of other organs including lungs, spleen, and the central nervous system. Primary pneumonic plague is a rare natural occurrence and results from the inhalation of respiratory droplets containing *Y. pestis* bacilli from another case of pneumonic plague, usually in humans or in cats. Secondary pneumonic plague results from seeding of the lungs by blood-borne bacteria in the setting of either bubonic or septicemic plague. Septicemic plague also begins with a transdermal exposure but manifests as primary bacteremia/septicemia without the bubo. Less common manifestations include meningitis, pharyngitis, and gastroenteritis.

Bubonic plague is an acute febrile lymphadenitis that develops 2 to 8 days after inoculation. Inflamed lymph nodes are usually 1 to 6 cm and painful. Abrupt onset of fever is an almost universal finding and occurs simultaneously with, or up to 24 hours before, the appearance of the bubo. Headache, malaise, and chills are frequent, along with nausea, vomiting, and diarrhea. Most patients are tachycardic, hypotensive, and appear prostrate and lethargic with episodic restlessness. Leukocytosis with a left shift is typical. Complications include pneumonia, shock, disseminated intravascular coagulation, purpuric skin lesions, acral cyanosis, and gangrene. The differential diagnosis of

## CURRENT DIAGNOSIS

- Travel to a plague endemic area or contact with a case of animal or human plague.
- Abrupt onset of fever and prostration.
- Bubo in groin, axillae, or cervical areas.
- Gram-negative coccobacilli with bipolar staining identified in aspirate from bubo, on blood smear, or from blood-tinged sputum.

bubonic plague includes tularemia and Group A β-hemolytic streptococcal adenitis with bacteremia.

The symptoms of septicemic plague are not distinct from those caused by other gram-negative bacteria, and they are very similar to those of bubonic plague except that abdominal pain is more common in septicemic plague. Septicemic plague must be differentiated from fulminate septicemia caused by other gram-negative bacteria. Primary pneumonic plague has an abrupt onset of fever and influenza-like symptoms 1 to 5 days after inhalation exposure. Symptoms include shortness of breath, cough, chest pain, and bloody sputum with rapid progression to fulminate pneumonia and respiratory failure. Patients with secondary pneumonic infection show respiratory symptoms in addition to those attributed to the bubo or sepsis. Radiographic findings include patchy bronchopneumonia, multilobar consolidations, cavitations, and alveolar hemorrhage and are not pathognomonic of *Y. pestis*. Plague pneumonia must be differentiated from severe influenza, inhalation anthrax, and overwhelming community-acquired pneumonia.

## Diagnosis

Plague is diagnosed by demonstrating *Y. pestis* in blood or body fluids such as a lymph node aspirate, sputum, or cerebrospinal fluid. A tentative diagnosis of bubonic plague can be made rapidly with fluid aspirated from a bubo showing gram-negative coccobacilli with bipolar staining. Serology showing a fourfold rise in antibody titers to F1 antigen or a single titer of more than 1:128 is also diagnostic.

## Treatment

The aminoglycosides gentamicin (Garamycin) and streptomycin, the fluoroquinolones ciprofloxacin (Cipro), levofloxacin (Levaquin), and ofloxacin (Floxin), and tetracyclines (i.e., doxycycline [Vibramycin]) are the first-, second-, and third-line classes of antibiotics, respectively. Typical minimal inhibitory concentrations for 90% ($MIC_{90}$) of tested strains for the fluoroquinolones are less than 0.03 to 0.25 μg/mL compared with less than 1.0 μg/mL and less than 1.0 μg/mL to 4.0 μg/mL for gentamicin and streptomycin, respectively, and less than 1.0 μg/mL for doxycycline. Streptomycin (15 mg/kg up to 1 g intramuscularly [IM] every 12 hours) and gentamicin (5 to 7 mg/kg/day intravenously [IV]/IM in one or two doses daily) are the drugs of choice for severe infection. Standard doses for the fluoroquinolones include ciprofloxacin, 400 mg IV/500 mg orally every 12 hours; levofloxacin, 500 mg IV/orally daily; and ofloxacin, 400 mg IV/orally every 12 hours. Doxycycline is administered at 100 mg IV/orally every 12 hours. Chloramphenicol (25 mg/kg IV/orally every 6 hours) can be

## CURRENT THERAPY

- Prompt administration of gentamicin or ciprofloxacin.
- Aggressive supportive care.
- Respiratory isolation of hospitalized cases.
- Postexposure prophylaxis to close contacts.

used in select circumstances. Antibiotic therapy should be continued for a total of 10 days.

## Prevention and Control

Standard infection control procedures that should be used when caring for patients with suspected plague include a disposable surgical mask, latex gloves, devices to protect mucous membranes, and good hand washing. Hospitalized patients with known or suspected pneumonic plague should be placed in strict isolation for at least 48 hours after appropriate antibiotics are initiated. Postexposure prophylaxis should be given to individuals with close contact (defined as less than 2 meters) with an infectious case or who have had a potential respiratory exposure. The recommended adult antibiotics for prophylaxis are doxycycline or ciprofloxacin in the same doses used for treatment. Postexposure prophylaxis can be given orally and should be continued for 7 days following exposure. Currently, there is no licensed plague vaccine.

## REFERENCES

Butler T: A clinical study of bubonic plague. Observations of the 1970 Vietnam epidemic with emphasis on coagulation studies, skin histology and electrocardiograms. Am J Med 1972;53:268-276.

Boulanger LL, Ettestad P, Fogarty JD, et al: Gentamicin and tetracyclines for the treatment of human plague: Review of 75 cases in New Mexico, 1985–1999. Clin Infect Dis 2004;38:663-669.

Cler DJ, Vernaleo JR, Lombardi LJ, et al: Plague pneumonia disease caused by Yersinia pestis. Semin Respir Infect 1997;12:12-23.

Gage KL, Dennis DT, Orloski KA, et al: Cases of cat-associated human plague in the Western US, 1977–1998. Clin Infect Dis 2000;30: 893-900.

Hull HF, Montes JM, Mann JM: Septicemic plague in New Mexico. J Infect Dis 1987;155: 113-118.

Inglesby TV, Dennis DT, Henderson DA, et al: Plague as a biological weapon: Medical and public health management. Working Group on Civilian Biodefense. JAMA 2000;283: 2281-2290.

Perry RD, Fetherston JD: Yersinia pestis—etiologic agent of plague. Clin Microbiol Rev 1997;10: 35-66.

Prentice MB, Rahalison L: Plague. Lancet 2007;369: 1196–1207.

Ratsitorahina M, Chanteau S, Rahalison L, et al: Epidemiological and diagnostic aspects of the outbreak of pneumonic plague in Madagascar. Lancet 2000;355: 111-113.

Wong JD, Barash JR, Sandfort, RF, Janda JM: Susceptibilities of Yersinia pestis strains to 12 antimicrobial agents. Antimicrob Agents Chemother 2000;44: 1995-1996.

# Anthrax

Method of
*Jon B. Woods, MD*

Anthrax has been a significant disease for both humans and their livestock for millennia. It was the first disease to fulfill Koch's postulates in 1876, as well as the first bacterial disease for which an effective vaccine was developed, for livestock, in 1880. This gram-positive rod-shaped bacillus species differs from the more benign members of its genera in containing two additional plasmids, one encoding for an antiphagocytic poly-D-glutamic acid capsule and the other encoding for two toxins. Three distinct toxin components combine to form two toxins, edema toxin and lethal toxin; the common component, protective antigen (PA), forms a pore through eukaryotic cell walls that allows the other two toxin components, edema factor (EF) and lethal factor (LF), to enter affected host cells. EF is an adenylate cyclase affecting many cell types and is responsible for the edema associated with anthrax infections. LF is a zinc metalloprotease that seems to have its greatest

affect on macrophages; within the cells it cleaves mitogen-activated protein kinase and disrupts the cellular response to infection.

## Background

Anthrax is an enzootic, and occasionally epizootic, disease of grazing animals worldwide. The incredibly durable spores of this bacillus can persist in soil for decades. These spores, when inadvertently ingested by herbivores while grazing, can germinate and then replicate in a rapid progression to bacteremia and subsequent death of the animal. At the time of death these animals can have as many as $10^8$ vegetative bacilli per milliliter of blood. Those bacilli, which are exposed to oxygen upon the animal's death, can sporulate and then reenter the soil to begin the cycle anew.

Human anthrax can take several forms, most commonly cutaneous, but also intestinal, oropharyngeal, and inhalational disease. Naturally occurring human anthrax disease has typically been the result of exposure to infected animals or contaminated animal products such as hair or wool, bone meal, hides, or meat. Less commonly, human cutaneous anthrax has resulted from the bites of flies that have recently fed on infected animals. Gastrointestinal and oropharyngeal anthrax can result from ingestion of the raw or inadequately cooked flesh of an animal infected with anthrax. Endemic inhalational anthrax, or woolsorter's disease, results from inhalation of anthrax spores aerosolized during the manipulation of contaminated animal products, especially hair or wool; this was an exceedingly rare form of disease even prior to the institution of more stringent control measures and closure of most of the U.S. textile mills processing foreign-acquired goat hair by the 1970s. More recently, inhalational anthrax and cutaneous cases have resulted from exposure to spores intentionally processed and disseminated as biologic weapons. The extreme environmental stability of the spores, their ease of production, and their infectivity via the aerosol route are some features that have made *Bacillus anthracis* a top candidate for both nations and terrorists seeking biologic weapons. An apparently accidental aerosol release of dried anthrax spores from a biologic weapons facility in the Soviet city of Sverdlovsk in 1979 resulted in as many as 68 deaths because of inhalational anthrax. More recently, anthrax spores intentionally sent through the U.S. postal system resulted in 11 cases of inhalational anthrax and perhaps as many as 11 cases of cutaneous anthrax.

## Clinical Features

Cutaneous anthrax represents approximately 95% of naturally occurring human anthrax cases. It typically occurs 1 to 7 days after exposure to infected livestock or contaminated livestock products, but rarely it is transmitted to humans by the bites of flies that have recently fed on infected animals. The lesion begins as a painless or mildly pruritic papule at the site of spore inoculation, progressing into an expanding round ulcer by the following day. Over the following several days the ulcer dries to a dark, almost black eschar, which resolves over the ensuing 1 to 2 weeks. The lesion can be surrounded by significant local edema and may be accompanied by regional lymphadenopathy. Treated, cutaneous anthrax is rarely fatal, although without antibiotics, progression to bacteremia and ultimately death can occur in up to 10% to 20% of cases.

Both forms of gastrointestinal anthrax are acquired via ingestion of insufficiently cooked meat from infected animals. The infectious dose is unknown. Intestinal anthrax may be initially misdiagnosed as either gastroenteritis or acute abdomen, typically presenting 1 to 6 days following contaminated meat consumption with fever, nausea, vomiting, and focal abdominal pain. Without prompt initiation of antibiotic therapy, disease can progress to hematemesis, hematochezia or melena, massive serosanguineous or hemorrhagic ascites, and sepsis, with mortality rates greater than 50%. Oropharyngeal anthrax typically presents after a 1- to 6-day incubation period with severe pharyngitis and fever, followed by appearance of pharyngeal or tonsillar ulcers. Gray or tan pseudomembranes can form over the ulcers, which are often accompanied by significant cervical lymphadenopathy and unilateral neck edema. Mortality of oropharyngeal anthrax varies from 10% to 50%.

Inhalation of aerosolized anthrax spores into the pulmonary alveoli can result in inhalational anthrax. The lethal dose via inhalation for 50% of humans ($LD_{50}$) is thought to be between 8000 and 55,000 spores. The alveolar spores are ingested by macrophages and carried to regional lymphatics, where they can germinate and replicate, eventually leading to hemorrhagic mediastinitis. The incubation period is presumably dose dependent, and although typically 1 to 6 days was suspected in at least one human case to be 43 days. Early inhalational anthrax presents suddenly as a nonspecific syndrome consisting of fever, malaise, headache, fatigue, and drenching sweats. Other common symptoms include nausea, vomiting, confusion, a nonproductive cough, and mild chest discomfort. Upper respiratory symptoms are notably absent. Physical findings are nonspecific in the early phase of the disease, but tachycardia is common. Auscultatory lung exam is typically normal at this stage, but dullness to percussion can develop over time in the lower lung fields as hemorrhagic pleural effusions accumulate. These early findings generally persist for 2 to 5 days before progressing fulminantly to tachypnea, cyanosis, shock, and multiorgan system failure. These late findings typically herald impending death within 24 to 36 hours. Gastrointestinal hemorrhage and hemorrhagic meningitis are common at autopsy. Prognosis is poor in the absence of intensive supportive care and early initiation of appropriate antibiotic combinations. Mortality ranges from 45% to more than 85% historically.

## Diagnosis

None of the forms of human anthrax disease can be diagnosed on the basis of clinical findings alone (Table 1). For example, diagnosis of cutaneous anthrax requires the presence of a compatible skin lesion accompanied by confirmatory laboratory studies; an exposure history, or a known risk may also be present. Both forms of gastrointestinal anthrax are typically accompanied by a history of ingestion of the meat of anthrax-infected animals. Early intestinal anthrax can be difficult to differentiate clinically from other causes of gastrointestinal illness to include acute gastroenteritis, dysentery, or even peritonitis. Later in the course of intestinal disease, surgical or autopsy findings may include ileal or cecal ulceration, and bowel edema and necrosis is associated with hemorrhagic mesenteric adenitis and serosanguineous to hemorrhagic ascites. Oropharyngeal anthrax can clinically resemble diphtheria, with pharyngeal lesions and an edematous so-called bull neck. Early inhalational anthrax is a nonspecific febrile syndrome that may be difficult to distinguish clinically from many other infectious diseases. However, the presence of mental status changes, profuse sweating, and absence of upper respiratory symptoms or pneumonia in inhalational anthrax may aid in differentiating it from influenza-like respiratory illnesses.

Gram stain and culture of skin lesions are ideally performed on the fluid of an unopened vesicle and are often positive in the cutaneous anthrax patient who has not received antibiotics. Tissue biopsy can be performed on lesions for immunohistochemical staining in culture-negative patients. Blood culture should be collected in any systemically ill patient suspected of having any form of anthrax disease. *B. anthracis* grows quickly in standard laboratory culture media. Paired acute and convalescent serologic studies may suggest infection in patents that have negative cultures, albeit these studies are not well validated. Stool culture can be positive in intestinal anthrax, although it is only variably so. Peritoneal fluid, pleural effusions, or cerebrospinal fluid (CSF) (when meningitis is present) can potentially demonstrate organisms on Gram stain and culture or may be positive via immunostaining or polymerase chain reaction (PCR) studies.

---

**TABLE 1 Empirical Antibiotic Therapy for Anthrax***

| Cutaneous Anthrax (without Systemic Symptoms) | Inhalational, Gastrointestinal, or Cutaneous Disease with Systemic Symptoms |
|---|---|
| Ciprofloxacin (Cipro[1]) <br>• 500 mg PO twice daily (adults) <br>• 15 mg/kg (up to 500 mg/dose) PO twice daily (children) <br>*or* <br>Doxycycline (Vibramycin) <br>• 100 mg PO twice daily (adults) <br>• 2.2 mg/kg (up to 100 mg/dose) PO bid (children <45 kg) <br>*or (if strain susceptible):* <br>Penicillin G procaine (Bicillin C-R) <br>• 1,200,000 U IM q12h (adults) <br>• 25,000 U/kg (maximum 1,200,000 U) q12h (children) <br>*or* <br>Penicillin V Potassium (Veetids) <br>• 500 mg PO q6h (adults) <br>*or* <br>Amoxicillin (Amoxil[1]) <br>• 500 mg PO q8h (adults and children >40 kg) <br>• 15 mg/kg q8h (children <40 kg) <br>According to CDC recommendations, amoxicillin prophylaxis is appropriate only after 14–21 d of fluoroquinolone or doxycycline and only for populations with relative contraindications to the other drugs (children, pregnancy) | Ciprofloxacin (Cipro IV[1]) <br>• 400 mg IV q12h (adult) <br>• 15 mg/kg/dose (up to 400 mg/dose) q12h (children) <br>*or* <br>Doxycycline (Vibramycin IV) <br>• 200 mg IV, then 100 mg IV q12h (adults) <br>• 2.2 mg/kg (100 mg/dose maximum) q12h (children <45 kg) <br>*or (if strain susceptible):* <br>Penicillin G (Pfizerpen) <br>• 4 million U IV q4h (adults) <br>• 50,000 U/kg (up to 4M U) IV q6h (children) <br>*plus* <br>One or two additional antibiotics with activity against anthrax. Clindamycin (Cleocin[1]) plus rifampin (Rifadin[1]) may be a good empiric choice, pending susceptibilities. Potential additional antibiotics include one or more of the following: clindamycin (Cleocin), rifampin (Rifadin), gentamicin[1] (generic), macrolides (erythromycin [generic], vancomycin (Vancocin[1]), imipenem (Pimaxin[1]), and chloramphenicol[1] (generic). <br>Convert from IV to oral therapy when patient is stable, to complete at least 60 d of antibiotics. <br>**Meningitis** <br>Add Rifampin (Rifadin[1]) 20 mg/kg IV once daily or vancomycin (Vancocin[1]) 1 g IV q12h <br>Oral dosing may be necessary for treatment of systemic disease in a mass casualty situation. |

[1]Not FDA approved for this indication.
*Should be adjusted for susceptibilities.
*Abbreviations:* CDC = Centers for Disease Control and Prevention; IV = intravenous; PO = orally.
Adapted from Woods JB (ed): USAMRIID's Medical Management of Biological Warfare Casualties Handbook, 6th ed. 2005.

**Cutaneous/Oropharyngeal**

- Painless or pruritic lesion beginning 1–7 d after exposure
  - Typical lesion progression from papule to ulcer to dark eschar (see text), often with significant edema

Plus

- Lesion gram stain, culture usually positive if patient has not received antibiotics
  - If negative, punch biopsy of lesion margin for IHC may still be positive
- Blood culture rarely positive in absence of systemic symptoms

Acute and convalescent serology or may give evidence of infection.

**Gastrointestinal**

- Gastrointestinal symptoms (variable) beginning 1–6 d after ingestion exposure.
  - Focal abdominal pain with hematochezia or melena common.
  - Nonspecific bowel wall edema, air–fluid levels, and ascites on radiographs.

Plus

- Stool culture (variably +).
- Blood culture (variably +).
- Acute and convalescent serology or blood sample for PCR may give evidence of infection.
- Ascites: often hemorrhagic.
  - Gram stain and culture, and IHC or PCR, if available, may be positive.

Surgical findings: hemorrhagic mesenteric adenitis, bowel edema, ileal and/or cecal ulcerations.

**Inhalational**

- Nonspecific febrile syndrome beginning abruptly 1–6 (but up to 43) d after aerosol exposure (see text).
  - Absence of upper respiratory findings, no pneumonia.
  - Widened mediastinum ± effusions on CXR or chest CT in *all* cases.

Plus

- Blood culture often positive if patient has not received antibiotics.
- Acute and convalescent serology or blood sample for PCR may give evidence of infection.
- Laboratory studies show hemoconcentration, mildly increased WBC with left shift, mildly increased AST and ALT, hypoalbuminemia.
- CSF (if meningitis) and pleural effusions are hemorrhagic.
- Gram stain and culture often positive.

If negative, IHC or PCR may be positive.

---

*Abbreviations:* AST = serum aspartate aminotransferase (level); ALT = serum alanine aminotransferase (level); CSF = cerebrospinal fluid; CXR = chest radiograph; CT = computed tomography study; IHC = immunohistochemical staining; PCR = polymerase chain reaction (study); WBC = white blood count.

---

For patients with inhalation anthrax during the attacks of 2001, the complete blood count (CBC) revealed a mean white blood cell count of 9800/µL, with a predominance of neutrophils and a mildly elevated hematocrit. Mildly elevated serum sodium, aspartate transaminase (AST), and alanine aminotransferase (ALT) were common, as was hypoalbuminemia.

A widened mediastinum caused by adenitis, as well as pleural effusions, may be visible on chest radiograph in patients with inhalational anthrax. Negative chest radiograph in a patient suspected of inhalational anthrax should prompt a chest computerized tomography (CT) scan. In the 2001 attacks, either the chest radiograph or CT was abnormal in all cases of inhalational disease. Abdominal radiographs in intestinal anthrax may demonstrate any number of nonspecific findings, to include ascites, diffuse air–fluid levels, and bowel edema.

## Treatment

Patient survival for all forms of severe anthrax disease hinges on prompt initiation of appropriate antibiotics. Initial empirical therapy for patients with inhalational anthrax, gastrointestinal anthrax, or cutaneous anthrax with systemic symptoms should include intravenous (IV) ciprofloxacin (Cipro IV) or doxycycline (Vibramycin IV) combined with one or two additional antibiotics effective against anthrax (Table 2). One suggested combination includes a quinolone (ciprofloxacin [Cipro IV]), clindamycin (Cleocin[1]), and rifampin

(Rifadin[1]). Antibiotic choices should be adjusted to reflect the specific susceptibilities of the infecting strain. Rifampin (Rifadin[1]), vancomycin (Vancocin[1]), or chloramphenicol[1] (generic) should be added if meningitis is suspected. IV antibiotics can be switched to oral treatment as the patent's clinical condition improves, to complete at least 60 days of total antibiotic therapy. Specific antidotes for anthrax toxins are in development, including human anthrax immune globulin, which may be available as an investigational therapy for severe anthrax disease through the Centers for Disease Control and Prevention (CDC).

Patients with systemic anthrax disease often require aggressive supportive therapy, including fluid resuscitation, blood products, vasopressor agents, and airway management. Patients may also benefit from drainage of large hemorrhagic pleural or peritoneal fluid accumulations. Although clinical data are lacking, severe edema or meningitis in anthrax disease may benefit from administration of corticosteroids.

Uncomplicated naturally acquired cutaneous anthrax should be treated empirically with 7 to 10 days of either oral ciprofloxacin (Cipro[1]) or doxycycline (Vibramycin). For cutaneous disease thought to have been acquired via exposure to an anthrax aerosol, at least 60 days of antibiotics is recommended.

A licensed anthrax vaccine (BioThrax) has been available in the United States to the armed forces, veterinarians, and textile and laboratory workers since 1970. It is derived from the sterile supernatant of a liquid culture of an attenuated (nonencapsulated) strain of

---

[1]Not FDA approved for this indication.

[1]Not FDA approved for this indication.

**TABLE 2  Anthrax Aerosol Postexposure Prophylaxis***

| Immunized[†] | Not Immunized and Vaccine Available | Not Immunized and Vaccine Not Available |
|---|---|---|
| Ciprofloxacin (Cipro)<br>• 500 mg PO bid for adults<br>• 10–15 mg/kg PO twice daily (up to 1 g/d) for children<br>*or*<br>Doxycycline (Vibramycin)<br>• 100 mg PO bid for adults or children >8 y and >45 kg<br>• 2.2 mg/kg PO bid (up to 200 mg/d) for children <8 y<br>If antibiotic susceptibilities allow, patients who cannot tolerate tetracyclines or quinolone antibiotics can be switched to amoxicillin (Amoxil[1]), 500 mg PO tid for adults and 80 mg/kg divided tid (≥1.5 g/d) in children. | | |
| Continue antibiotics for *at least* 30 d. | Receive at least 3 doses of anthrax vaccine[1] (BioThrax) at 2-wk intervals, and then continue antibiotics for *at least* 1–2 wk after receipt of 3rd dose of vaccine. | Continue antibiotics for *at least* 60 d. |
| Patients should be closely observed after discontinuation of antibiotics.<br>If suspected clinical signs of anthrax disease occur, then resume empirical antibiotics. | | |

[1]Not FDA approved for this indication.
*Unknown antibiotic susceptibilities.
[†]Immunized = completed 6 doses of anthrax vaccine and up to date on boosters, or minimum of 3 doses within past 6 mo. Those who have already received 3 doses within 6 mo of exposure should continue with their routine vaccine schedule.
*Abbreviation:* PO = orally.
Adapted from Woods JB (ed): USAMRIID's Medical Management of Biological Warfare Casualties Handbook, 6th ed. 2005.

*B. anthracis* and is administered subcutaneously in a six-shot primary series over 18 months followed by annual boosters. The vaccine is licensed only for preexposure prophylaxis of persons 18 to 65 years of age but is available investigationally for postexposure and pediatric use.

Individuals exposed to aerosolized anthrax spores should immediately receive postexposure prophylaxis consisting of both oral antibiotics and anthrax vaccine. Oral doxycycline (Vibramycin) or ciprofloxacin (Cipro) are the preferred empiric antibiotics for postexposure prophylaxis. Antibiotics should be continued for variable lengths of time depending on the patient's anthrax immune status and the suspected inhaled dose of anthrax (Table 2). Exposed individuals should also receive the anthrax vaccine[1] (BioThrax) to counter delayed incubation of residual alveolar anthrax after discontinuation of antibiotics.

---

[1]Not FDA approved for this indication.

## CURRENT THERAPY

**Cutaneous Anthrax (without Systemic Symptoms)**

- Oral antibiotics (see Table 2 for details)
  - Doxycycline (Vibramycin), or
  - Ciprofloxacin (Cipro[1])
- Consider nonsteroidal anti-inflammatory agents (NSAIDS) or corticosteroids for severe edema
- Infection control:
  - Contact precautions
Do not debride lesions

**Inhalational, Gastrointestinal, or Cutaneous Disease with Systemic Symptoms**

- Supportive care
  - May need assisted ventilation and/or vasopressors
  - Drain pleural effusions and large peritoneal fluid collections
- Combination IV antibiotics (see Table 2 for details)
  - Doxycycline (Vibramycin IV), or
  - Ciprofloxacin (Cipro IV[1])
Plus
  - One or two additional antibiotics
- Consider corticosteroids for severe edema or meningitis
- Consider human anthrax immune globulin (investigational), if available
- Infection control:
  - Contact precautions (not transmitted by droplet or aerosol)
Avoid autopsy or invasive procedures prior to receipt of antibiotics.

---

[1]Not FDA approved for this indication.

## REFERENCES

Beatty ME, Ashford DA, Griffin PM, et al: Gastrointestinal anthrax, a review of the literature. Arch Intern Med 2003;163:2527-2531.

Centers for Disease Control and Prevention: Notice to readers: Use of anthrax vaccine in response to terrorism: Supplemental recommendations of the Advisory Committee on Immunization Practices. MMWR 2002;51(45); 1024-1026.

Inglesby TV, O'Toole T, Henderson DA, et al: Anthrax as a biological weapon 2002: Updated Recommendations for Management. JAMA 2002;287(17): 2236-2252.

Jernigan JA, Stephens DS, Ashford DA, et al: Bioterrorism-related inhalational anthrax: The first 10 cases reported in the United States. Emerg Infect Dis 2001;7:933-944.

Kuehnert MJ, Doyle TJ, Hill HA, et al: Clinical features that discriminate inhalational anthrax from other acute respiratory illnesses. Clin Infect Dis 2003;36:328-336.

Turnbull PCB: Guidelines for the Surveillance and Control of Anthrax in Humans and Animals, 3rd ed. World Health Organization Report WHO/EMC/ZDI/98.6, 1998.

Woods JB (ed): USAMRIID's Medical Management of Biological Warfare Casualties Handbook, 6th ed. 2005.

# Psittacosis

Method of
*Julian Elliott, MB, BS, FRACP*

## Epidemiology

Psittacosis is the disease caused by infection with the bacterium *Chlamydophila psittaci*, formerly known as *Chlamydia psittaci*. It affects men more than women, and the main age group affected is adults older than 40 years. The main reservoir for psittacosis is birds, particularly psittacine birds (parrots, parakeets, budgerigars, and cockatoos), but other bird species and mammals can be infected. The most common form of acquisition is exposure to infected birds, by breathing in an aerosol of dried feces or from nose or eye secretions.

Risk factors for disease include contact with pet birds—especially a new, sick, or dead bird—and occupational exposure, for example work as a veterinarian, as a zoo keeper, or in a poultry-processing plant. Most cases are sporadic, but outbreaks have occurred associated with pet shops, aviaries, and poultry-processing plants and with mowing lawns in areas with large numbers of psittacine birds. Person-to-person transmission is rare. There is no evidence of infection acquired through ingestion of poultry products.

## Clinical Features

The incubation period varies from 4 to 14 days or longer. The typical presentation of psittacosis is of an influenza-like illness with sudden onset of fever, chills, and prominent headache, but a more gradual onset is also seen. Rigors may be present. Cough is usually later in onset, dry, and not very marked. There may also be diarrhea, pharyngitis, altered mental state, or shortness of breath. Chest examination is usually abnormal, but the findings are often minimal and less prominent than symptoms or x-ray findings would suggest. Pleural effusions are rare.

Patients might present with a fever of unknown origin without obvious respiratory involvement, or the disease can be misdiagnosed as meningitis due to prominent headache, sometimes with photophobia. The degree of illness varies from asymptomatic to life threatening. Elderly persons and pregnant women are susceptible to more severe illness.

Other, less common findings include hemoptysis, proteinuria, hepatosplenomegaly, and encephalitis. Cardiac manifestations include relative bradycardia and rarely myocarditis, culture-negative endocarditis, and pericarditis. Erythema nodosum and other skin manifestations have also been described.

## Diagnosis

Diagnosis depends on eliciting a history of recent bird contact from a patient with a compatible clinical syndrome, most commonly an influenza-like presentation, community-acquired pneumonia (CAP), or fever of unknown origin. The diagnosis should also be considered in a patient with CAP and prominent headache, splenomegaly, or failure to respond to β-lactam antibiotics. If the presentation is of an atypical CAP, the differential diagnosis includes infection with *Legionella* species, *Mycoplasma pneumoniae*, or *Chlamydophila pneumoniae*.

The white cell count is usually normal or slightly elevated, but there is often a left shift or toxic changes. Increases in the C-reactive protein (CRP) and erythrocyte sedimentation rate (ESR) are common. Mildly abnormal liver function tests, hyponatremia, and mild renal impairment are also common. The cerebrospinal fluid sometimes contains a few mononuclear cells but is otherwise normal. The chest x-ray usually shows more than predicted by the examination findings, but is nonspecific. The most common finding is lobar consolidation, but bilateral consolidation or interstitial opacities are also commonly seen.

Culture of *C. psittaci* is difficult and hazardous, so confirmation of diagnosis is more commonly performed using serology. The complement fixation (CF) test is widely used, but it cannot differentiate between *Chlamydia* species. A fourfold rise in titer, using samples collected at least 14 days apart, or a single titer of 1:128 or higher, is interpreted as a positive result. The antibody rise may be delayed or diminished by antibiotic treatment. A microimmunofluorescent (MIF) test is more specific for *Chlamydia* species, with a fourfold rise in titer or an IgM antibody titer of 1:16 interpreted as positive, but this test is not widely available. Polymerase chain reaction (PCR) assays have been developed, but they are not yet available for routine clinical use.

## CURRENT DIAGNOSIS

- The key to successful management of psittacosis is considering it as a possible diagnosis and asking about bird contact.
- The commonest clinical scenarios are influenza-like illness, community-acquired pneumonia, or fever of unknown origin. The typical presentation is sudden onset of fever and chills, with prominent headache. The diagnosis should also be considered in a patient with community-acquired pneumonia and failure to respond to β-lactam antibiotics.
- Nonspecific findings on investigation include a normal or slightly elevated white blood cell count with a left shift or toxic changes, increase in C-reactive protein (CRP) or erythrocyte sedimentation rate (ESR), mildly abnormal liver function tests, hyponatremia, mild renal impairment, and a chest x-ray with more abnormalities than predicted by the examination findings.
- Diagnosis can be confirmed with serology using either the complement fixation test, which is widely used but unable to differentiate between *Chlamydia* species, or the microimmunofluorescent test, which is specific for individual *Chlamydia* species. Either a single high titer or a fourfold rise in titer using samples collected at least 14 days apart are interpreted as positive.

## CURRENT THERAPY

- Empiric therapy should be commenced when the diagnosis is suspected on clinical presentation and initial investigations.
- Tetracyclines are the drugs of choice; for example, doxycycline (Vibramycin) 100 mg bid for 10 to 14 days.
- Macrolides are usually recommended for pregnant women, children, and people with intolerance of tetracyclines, but they are probably less effective.
- Defervescence and improvement in symptoms usually occur within 24 to 48 hours of initiating a tetracycline; subsequent mortality is less than 1%.
- Notification to health authorities facilitates public health investigation and interventions to reduce transmission and control outbreaks.

## Management

When the diagnosis is suspected on clinical presentation and initial investigations, empiric therapy should be commenced. Tetracyclines are the drugs of choice, for example, doxycycline (Vibramycin) 100 mg bid for 10 to 14 days. This class usually leads to defervescence and improvement in symptoms within 24 to 48 hours, and subsequent mortality is less than 1%. Macrolides are usually recommended for pregnant women, children, and patients with intolerance of tetracyclines, but erythromycin (Erythrocin)[1] has been shown to fail in situations where a tetracycline was effective, and there are few clinical data on the efficacy of the other agents in this class. Some data suggest that quinolones may be effective, but further evidence is needed. Tetracycline hydrochloride[2] or doxycycline (4.4 mg/kg/d divided into two infusions) is given intravenously for critically ill patients.

Notification of health authorities is important for initiating public health investigations and interventions to reduce transmission and control of outbreaks.

## REFERENCES

Centers for Disease Control and Prevention: Compendium of measures to control Chlamydia psittaci infection in humans (psittacosis) and pet birds (avian chlamydiosis), 2000. MMWR Morb Mortal Wkly Rep 2000;49 (RR08):1-17.

Crosse BA: Psittacosis: A clinical review. J Infect 1990;21:251-259.

Grayston JT, Thom DH: The chlamydial pneumonias. Curr Clin Top Infect Dis 1991;11:1-18.

Gregory DW, Schaffner W: Psittacosis. Semin Resp Infect 1997;12:7-11.

Hughes P, Chidley K, Cowie J: Neurological complications in psittacosis: A case report and literature review. Respir Med 1995;89:637-638.

Richards M: Psittacosis. UpToDate 2006. Available at http://www.uptodate.com/physicians/pulmonology_toclist.asp (accessed August 18, 2007; subscription required).

Williams J, Tallis G, Dalton C, et al: Community outbreak of psittacosis in a rural Australian town. Lancet 1998;351:1697-1699.

Yung AP, Grayson ML: Psittacosis: A review of 135 cases. Med J Aust 1988;148:228-233.

[1]Not FDA approved for this indication.
[2]Not available in the United States.

# Q Fever

Method of
*Didier Raoult, PhD*

Q fever is widespread zoonosis caused by *Coxiella burnetii*, a small, coccoid, strict intracellular gram-negative bacterium. It lives within the phagolysosome of its eukaryotic host cell at very low pH (4.5-4.8). It had previously been classified in the rickettsial family; however, recent phylogenic data based on study of the 16S rRNA gene sequence have shown that it belongs to *Legionellales* with the *Legionella* species and *Francisella tularensis*.

The bacterium has a spore-like life cycle, which explains its marked resistance to physicochemical agents. In cultures, *C. burnetii* exhibits a phase variation (from virulent phase I to avirulent phase II) caused by a spontaneous chromosome deletion. The avirulent form paradoxically generates high antibody levels in patients, but only patients with chronic infection have high antiphase I immunoglobulin G (IgG) and IgA antibody titers.

*C. burnetii* is a potent biological weapon. The reservoir of *C. burnetii* is wide, and nearly all tested mammals, birds, and ticks can be infected. Outbreaks have also been reported in association with the birth products of mammals (including ungulates and pets), raw milk, slaughterhouses, and farm work. Laboratory outbreaks have been reported. The disease is prevalent everywhere in the world but in New Zealand, but because its clinical spectrum is wide and nonspecific, the observed incidence is directly related to physician interest in Q fever.

## Clinical Features

Q fever is a reportable disease in the United States. In humans, infection is symptomatic in only 50% of patients. Most symptomatic patients experience a flu-like syndrome lasting 2 to 7 days and consisting of severe headaches and cough; 5% to 10% of infected patients may be sick enough to be investigated. They initially have high fever and one or several of pneumonia, hepatitis, meningoencephalitis, rash, myocarditis, and pericarditis. Routine laboratory investigation commonly shows mildly elevated transaminase levels and mild thrombocytopenia.

In special hosts such as immunocompromised patients (specifically those with lymphoma or splenectomy), *C. burnetii* can cause chronic infection. In pregnant women it can lead to recurrent miscarriage, low-birth-weight offspring, and prematurity.

In patients with valvular heart disease and those with arterial aneurysms or a vascular prosthesis, it can cause chronic endocarditis or vascular infection in patients in the two years following primary infection. The clinical picture is that of a chronic blood culture–negative endocarditis; the modified Duke criteria are of diagnostic value in such cases. It is spontaneously fatal in most cases.

## Diagnosis

Because Q fever is pleomorphic, the diagnosis is based mainly on comprehensive serum testing in patients with an unexplained infectious syndrome. Liver biopsy may be of diagnostic value because the typical doughnut granuloma is quasispecific to Q fever. Valves obtained at surgery or autopsy can be used for culture, direct immunostaining, and polymerase chain reaction (PCR).

Three serologic techniques are used. Complement fixation lacks sensitivity, and one third of patients with acute Q fever do not exhibit complement-fixing antibodies within one month after onset of the disease. However, a fourfold increase in antibodies to phase II antigen indicates acute Q fever, and antibody levels against phase I that are higher than 1:200 indicate chronic Q fever. Indirect immunofluorescence assay is the reference method. A single titer of 1:200 for IgG antiphase II associated with a titer of 1:50 for IgM is diagnostic of

TABLE 1

| Q Fever | Recommended Treatment | Alternative Treatment |
|---|---|---|
| Acute | Doxycycline (Vibramyin) 100 mg PO q8h × 14 d | Ofloxacin (Floxin)[1] 200 mg PO q8h × 14 d<br>Cotrimoxazole (Bactrim)[1] 160/800 mg /PO q12h × 14 d |
| Chronic | Doxycycline 100 mg PO q12h *plus* hydroxychloroquine (Plaquenil)[1,2] 200 mg PO q8h × 18 to 36 mo | Doxycycline 100 mg PO q12h *plus* ofloxacin 200 mg PO q8h for 3 y to lifetime |
| Acute in a patient with a valvular lesion | Same as for chronic Q fever for 12 mo | |
| In pregnancy | Cotrimoxazole (Bactrim)[1] 160/800 mg PO q12h until term | |

[1]Not FDA approved for this indication.
[2]Hydroxychloroquine serum level should be 1± 0.2 μg/mL. Doxycycline serum level should be ≥4.5 μg/mL.

acute infection. IgG antibody levels against phase I that are greater than 1:800 and IgA antibody levels greater than 1:50 are highly predictive of chronic infection. Enzyme-linked immunosorbent assay (ELISA) is useful for diagnosing acute infection in detecting IgM antiphase II.

PCR has recently been developed to detect *C. burnetii* DNA in the sera of patients with Q fever. Real-time PCR using multicopy gene *IS1111* is the more sensitive technique. It is positive in the sera of patients with acute Q fever before IgG antibodies to *C. burnetii* become apparent. It is also positive in patients with untreated chronic Q fever. Contamination of PCR can occur, and many unconfirmed results are reported in the literature.

## Treatment

To be active against Q fever, an antibiotic compound has to enter the cell, be effective at an acidic pH (where *C. burnetii* multiplies), and have activity against *C. burnetii*. No antibiotic is bactericidal, but bactericidal activity can be achieved by the addition of hydroxychloroquine (Plaquenil) to doxycycline (Vibramycin).

For acute Q fever, the reference treatment is doxycycline 100 mg orally bid for 2 to 3 weeks. Other compounds have been reported to be effective, such as trimethoprim-sulfamethoxazole (TMP-SMX) (Bactrim),[1] Rifampin (Rifadin)[1] 300 mg bid, and ofloxacin (Floxin)[1] 200 mg bid. In the case of Q fever in pregnant women, one double-strength TMP-SMX[1] tablet (trimethoprim 160 mg, sulfamethoxazole 800 mg) twice daily until delivery prevents fetal death (Table 1).

Chronic endocarditis should be treated for three years, and antibody levels should be monitored. When IgG antiphase I is less than 800 and IgA is less than 50, treatment may be stopped before three years. Two protocols have been evaluated: doxycycline 200 mg daily combined with ofloxacin[1] 400 mg daily for four years to lifetime, and doxycycline combined with hydroxychloroquine[1] for 1.5 to 3 years in an amount to achieve a 1 ± 0.20 μg/mL plasma concentration. Doxycycline serum levels greater than 4.5 μg/mL of serum are associated with a more rapidly favorable outcome. This last regimen is apparently more efficacious in terms of relapse. However, regular ophthalmologic surveillance is critical to detect the accumulation of chloroquine in the retina. Both regimens expose the patient to a major risk of photosensitization.

The combination of doxycycline and hydroxychloroquine for one year has demonstrated efficacy in preventing endocarditis.

## Prevention

Prevention depends on avoiding exposure, particularly by pregnant women and patients with valvulopathy. No vaccine is currently available outside Australia.

[1]Not FDA approved for this indication.

## REFERENCES

Fenollar F, Fournier PE, Raoult D: Molecular detection of *Coxiella burnetii* in the sera of patients with Q fever endocarditis or vascular infection. J Clin Microbiol 2004;42(11):4919-4924.

Klee SR, Tyczka J, Ellerbrok H, et al: Highly sensitive real-time PCR for specific detection and quantification of *Coxiella burnetii*. BMC Microbiol 2006;19:2.

Maurin M, Raoult D: Q fever. Clin Microbiol Rev 1999;12(4):518-553.

Raoult D, Marrie T, Mege J: Natural history and pathophysiology of Q fever. Lancet Infect Dis 2005;5(4):219-226.

Rolain JM, Raoult D: Molecular detection of *Coxiella burnetii* in blood and sera during Q fever. QJM 2005;98(8):615-617.

Rolain JM, Maurin M, Raoult D: Bacteriostatic and bactericidal activities of moxifloxacin against *Coxiella burnetii*. Antimicrob Agents Chemother 2001;45(1):301-302.

# Rabies

Method of
*Alan C. Jackson, MD, FRCPC*

Rabies is an acute infection of the nervous system caused by rabies virus, which is a member of the family Rhabdoviridae in the genus *Lyssavirus*. Other lyssaviruses have only very rarely caused rabies in Europe, Africa, and Australia.

## Pathogenesis

Rabies virus is usually transmitted by bites from rabid animals. Transmission has rarely occurred through an aerosol route (in a laboratory accident or bat cave containing millions of bats) or by transplantation of infected organs and tissues. The virus is in the saliva of the rabid animal and inoculated into subcutaneous tissues or muscles. During most of the long incubation period (lasting 20 to 90 days or longer), the virus is close to the site of inoculation. The virus binds to the nicotinic acetylcholine receptor at the postsynaptic neuromuscular junction and travels toward the central nervous system (CNS) in peripheral nerves by retrograde fast axonal transport. There is rapid dissemination throughout the CNS by fast axonal transport. Under natural conditions, degenerative neuronal changes are not prominent, and it is thought that the rabies virus induces neuronal dysfunction by mechanisms that are not well understood. In rabies vectors, the encephalitis is associated with behavioral changes that lead to transmission by biting. After the CNS infection is established, the virus spreads by autonomic and sensory nerves to multiple organs, including the salivary glands in which the virus is secreted in high titer.

## Clinical Features

In North America, where the bat is the most common rabies vector, a history of an animal bite is usually absent, and there may be no known contact with animals. The incubation period is usually between 20 and 90 days, but it may occasionally last 1 or more years. Prodromal features are nonspecific and include malaise, headache, and fever, and patients may also have anxiety or agitation. Approximately half of patients may experience pain, paresthesias, or pruritus at the site of the wound, which has often healed; this may reflect involvement of local sensory ganglia. Approximately 80% of patients with rabies have encephalitic rabies; approximately 20% have paralytic rabies. In encephalitic rabies, there are characteristic periods of generalized arousal or hyperexcitability separated by lucid periods. Autonomic dysfunction occurs frequently and includes hypersalivation, gooseflesh, cardiac arrhythmias, and priapism. Hydrophobia is the most characteristic feature of rabies and occurs in 50% to 80% of patients; contractions of the diaphragm and other inspiratory muscles occur on swallowing. This may become a conditioned reflex, and even the sight or thought of water can precipitate the muscle contractions. Hydrophobia is thought to be caused by inhibition of inspiratory neurons near the nucleus ambiguus.

In paralytic rabies, prominent muscle weakness usually begins in the bitten extremity and progresses to quadriparesis; typically there is sphincter involvement. Patients have a longer clinical course than in encephalitic rabies. Paralytic rabies is frequently misdiagnosed as the Guillain-Barré syndrome. Coma subsequently develops in both clinical forms. With aggressive medical therapy, a variety of medical complications develop, and multiple organ failure is a frequent occurrence. Survival is very rare and has usually occurred in the context of incomplete postexposure rabies prophylaxis that included administration of some rabies vaccine.

## Epidemiology

Worldwide more than 55,000 human deaths per year are attributed to rabies. The impact is particularly significant in terms of years of life lost because children are frequently the victims. Most human rabies cases occur through transmission from dogs in developing countries with endemic dog rabies, particularly in Asia and Africa. In the United States and Canada, the most common human cases are from insect-eating bats, and often, there is no known history of a bat bite or exposure to bats. A bat bite may not be recognized. The rabies virus variant responsible for most human cases is found in silver-haired bats and eastern pipistrelle bats. These are small bats not frequently in contact with humans. There are a variety of other rabies vectors in North American wildlife, including skunks, raccoons, and foxes, but these species are rarely responsible for transmission to humans. This is likely because of effective postexposure rabies prophylaxis.

## Diagnosis

Most cases of rabies can be diagnosed clinically or the diagnosis strongly suspected, which is particularly important to initiate appropriate barrier nursing techniques and prevent exposures of many health care workers. Some cases may be candidates for an aggressive therapeutic approach. A serum neutralizing titer can be useful in a previously unimmunized individual, but a positive titer may not develop until the second week of clinical illness, and the result of the test may not be readily available. Detection of rabies virus antigen on a skin biopsy obtained from the nape of the neck using a fluorescent antibody technique is a useful diagnostic test. Detection of rabies virus ribonucleic acid (RNA) in saliva using reverse transcription polymerase chain reaction (RT-PCR) amplification is an important recent advance in rapid rabies diagnosis. Rabies virus antigen can be detected in brain tissue obtained by brain biopsy or postmortem.

## Prevention

After recognition of a rabies exposure, rabies can be prevented with initiation of appropriate steps, including wound cleansing and active and passive immunization. After a human is bitten by a dog, cat, or ferret, the animal should be captured, confined, and observed for a period of at least 10 days. The animal should also be examined by a veterinarian prior to its release. If the animal is a stray, unwanted, shows signs, or develops signs of rabies during the observation period, the animal should be killed immediately, and its head should be transported under refrigeration for a laboratory examination. The brain should be examined via an antigen-detection method using the fluorescent antibody technique and viral isolation using cell culture or mouse inoculation.

The incubation period for animals other than dogs, cats, and ferrets is uncertain; these animals should be killed immediately after an exposure, and the head submitted for examination. If the result is negative, one may safely conclude that the animal's saliva did not contain rabies virus and, if immunization has been initiated, it should be discontinued. If an animal escapes after an exposure, it should be considered rabid unless information from public health officials indicates this is unlikely, and rabies prophylaxis should be initiated. The physical presence of a bat may warrant postexposure prophylaxis when a person (such as a small child or sleeping adult) is unable to reliably report contact that could have resulted in a bite.

Local wound care should be given as soon as possible after all exposures, even if immunization is delayed, pending the results of an observation period. All bite wounds and scratches should be washed thoroughly with soap and water. Devitalized tissues should be débrided.

Purified chick embryo cell culture vaccine (RabAvert), rabies vaccine absorbed (RVA), and human diploid cell vaccine (Imovax) are licensed rabies vaccines in the United States and Canada. Other vaccines grown in either primary cell lines (hamster or dog kidney) or continuous cell lines (Vero cells) are also satisfactory and available in other countries. A regimen of five 1-mL doses of rabies vaccine should be given intramuscularly (IM) in the deltoid area (anterolateral aspect of the thigh is also acceptable in children). Ideally, the first dose should be given as soon as possible after exposure, but failing that, it should be given regardless of the length of a delay. Four additional doses should be given on days 3, 7, 14, and 28. Pregnancy is not a contraindication for immunization. Live vaccines should not be given for 1 month after rabies immunization. Local and mild systemic reactions are common. Systemic allergic reactions are uncommon, and anaphylactic reactions may be treated with epinephrine and antihistamines. Corticosteroids may interfere with the development of active immunity. Immunosuppressive medications should not be administered during postexposure therapy unless they are essential. The risk of developing rabies should be carefully considered before deciding to discontinue vaccination because of an adverse reaction. A serum neutralizing antibody determination is necessary only after immunization of immunocompromised patients. Less expensive vaccines, derived from neural

## CURRENT THERAPY

- Details of an exposure determine whether postexposure rabies prophylaxis should be initiated.
- Wound cleansing is very important after a potential rabies exposure.
- Active immunization with a schedule of 5 doses of rabies vaccine at intervals is recommended.
- Passive immunization (if previously unimmunized) consists of human rabies immune globulin infiltrated into the wound and the remainder of the 20 IU/kg dosage given intramuscularly.

tissues, are still used in some developing countries; these vaccines are associated with serious neuroparalytic complications.

Human rabies immune globulin (Imogam or BayRab) should also be administered as passive immunization for protection before the development of immunity from the vaccine. It should be given at the same time as the first dose of vaccine and no later than 7 days after the first dose. Rabies vaccine and human rabies immune globulin should never be administered at the same site or in the same syringe. The recommended dose of human rabies immune globulin is 20 international units (IU)/kg; larger doses should not be given because they may suppress active immunity from the vaccine. After wounds are washed, they should be infiltrated with human rabies immune globulin (if anatomically feasible), and the remainder of the dose should be given IM in the gluteal area. If the exposure involves a mucous membrane, the entire dose should be administered IM. With multiple or large wounds, the human rabies immune globulin may need to be diluted for adequate infiltration of all of the wounds. Adverse effects of human rabies immune globulin include local pain and low-grade fever.

After an exposure, a previously immunized patient should receive two 1-mL doses of rabies vaccine on days 0 and 3, but the patient should not receive human rabies immune globulin.

## Management of Human Rabies

Only six people have survived rabies, and five received rabies vaccine prior to the onset of their disease. The possibilities for an aggressive approach were recently reviewed (see Jackson et al., 2003). There was one survivor in Wisconsin in 2004 who did not receive rabies vaccine. It is now doubtful whether the therapy she received played a significant role in her favorable outcome because a similar approach has failed in many cases. Palliation is an alternative approach and may be appropriate for many patients who develop rabies.

### REFERENCES

Centers for Disease Control and Prevention: Human rabies prevention—United States, 1999: Recommendations of the Advisory Committee on Immunization Practices (ACIP). MMWR 1999;48 (No. RR-1):1-21.

Jackson AC: Human disease. In Jackson AC, Wunner WH (eds): Rabies, 2nd ed. London, Elsevier, Academic Press, 2007, pp 309-340.

Jackson AC: Rabies. Curr Treat Options Infect Dis 2003;5:35-40.

Jackson AC: Rabies: New insights into pathogenesis and treatment. Curr Opin Neurol 2006;19(3):267-270.

Jackson AC, Warrell MJ, Rupprecht CE, et al: Management of rabies in humans. Clin Infect Dis 2003;36:60-63.

Jackson AC, Wunner WH: Rabies, 2nd ed. London, Elsevier, Academic Press, 2007.

World Health Organization: WHO expert consultation on rabies: First report (First Report Edition). Geneva, WHO, 2005.

# Rat-Bite Fever

Method of
*Jean Dudler, MD*

Rat-bite fever (RBF) is a systemic febrile disease caused by infection with *Streptobacillus moniliformis*. As its name implies, it is transmitted by rat bite. However, it can also be transmitted by simple contact with infected rats or even through ingestion of food contaminated with rat excreta. Diagnosis can be difficult, and a high degree of awareness is necessary to make a correct diagnosis. Recognition and early treatment are crucial, because case fatality can be higher than 10% in untreated cases.

## Epidemiology

*S. moniliformis* is part of the normal respiratory flora of the rat. From 50% to 100% of healthy wild, laboratory, and pet rats harbor *S. moniliformis* in the nasopharynx. *S. moniliformis* is also excreted in the urine, and *Spirillum minus* has been demonstrated in conjunctival secretions and blood. Thus, rat-bite fever can be transmitted not only from a bite but also through scratches, handling of dead rats, and even handling of litter material.

Although the rat is the natural reservoir and major vector of the disease, *S. moniliformis* has also been found in other rodents such as mice, squirrels, and gerbils, as well as in other mammals such as weasels and in pets that prey on rodents, such as cats and dogs, which can also act as vectors of the disease.

The major risk factor is exposure to rats, either as an occupational hazard for persons such as laboratory workers, veterinarians, or pet shop employees, or for persons who have rats for pets or feed rats to snakes, especially children. Classically, homelessness and lower socioeconomic status were described as major factors, but most cases reported in the last few years have involved pet rats.

No precise data are available on the true incidence of rat-bite fever because it is not a reportable disease. It appears to be unusual in Western countries, a rarity that could reflect failed diagnosis or a spontaneous recovery in most cases, considering the high percentage of *S. moniliformis* carriage, the frequency of contacts between humans and rats in modern society, and the fairly high risk—estimated around 10%—of developing rat-bite fever after being bitten or scratched.

## Clinical Presentation

Rat-bite fever is a systemic febrile disease. Classically, following a rat bite and a short incubation of 1 to 3 days (but up to 3 weeks), systemic dissemination of the organism is associated with an abrupt onset with intermittent relapsing fever, rigors, myalgias, arthralgias, headache, sore throat, malaise, and vomiting. These symptoms are followed within the first week by the development of a maculopapular rash in 75% of patients. The rash can be pustular, purpuric, or petechial, and it typically involves the extremities, in particular the palms and soles. The bite site typically heals promptly, with minimal inflammation and absent or minimal regional adenopathy.

Up to 50% of infected patients develop an asymmetric migrating polyarthritis, which appears to be exceedingly painful and affects large and middle-sized joints. Joint effusion appears more common in adults. Infection can occur in any tissues. Anemia, meningitis, bronchitis, pneumonia, endocarditis, myocarditis, pericarditis, brain abscess, and infarcts of the spleen and kidneys have been reported as complications of rat-bite fever.

Although most cases seem to resolve spontaneously within 2 weeks, persistence up to 2 years has been reported. The mortality rate in untreated cases is around 10% to 15%, and it rises to more than 50% in the rare cases with cardiac involvement.

Two closely related variants have been described. In Havervill fever, the organism is transmitted by ingestion of contaminated food.

## CURRENT DIAGNOSIS

- The examiner must maintain a high index of suspicion.
- Nonspecific initial symptoms are followed by a maculopapular rash and septic arthritis.
- Exposure to rats is the major risk factor. Transmission can occur with simple contact with infected animals or excreta.
- Notify microbiology laboratory of suspicion (slow growth, 5%-10% $CO_2$ microaerophilic conditions, 20% normal rabbit serum media supplementation, and avoidance of sodium polyanethol sulfonate).

It tends to occur in epidemics and also causes rashes and arthritis, but upper respiratory tract symptoms and vomiting appear more prominent. Sodoku is a rat-bite fever caused by *Spirillum minus;* it is common in Japan. The course is more subacute, arthritic symptoms are rare, and if the bite initially heals, it then ulcerates and is associated with regional lymphadenopathy and a distinctive rash.

## Diagnosis

Diagnosis is difficult, with nonspecific clinical findings, broad differential diagnosis, and difficulties in identifying the responsible organism. Rat-bite fever should not be dismissed in the absence of bite history, because transmission can occur without a bite, and pet lovers or laboratory workers can minimize or forget the bite, especially in the absence of a local reaction.

No reliable serologic test is available, and the definitive diagnosis requires isolation of *S. moniliformis* from the wound, the blood, or the synovial fluid. The microbiology laboratory should be specifically notified of any clinical suspicion because of the hurdles in identification.

*S. moniliformis* is a highly pleomorphic, nonencapsulated, nonmotile gram-negative rod, which may stain positively on Gram stain. It is often dismissed as proteinaceous debris because of its numerous bulbous swellings with occasional clumping (*moniliformis* = "necklace-like"). It grows slowly and requires a microaerophilic environment with 5% to 10% $CO_2$ or anaerobic conditions and media supplementation with 20% normal rabbit serum. Cultures should be held for more than 5 days and should not be dismissed as contamination. *S. moniliformis* is also inhibited by sodium polyanethol sulfonate, a common adjunct in most commercial blood culture media. Identification using polymerase chain reaction amplification and gene sequencing has been used. It can be performed on samples from the patient or animal in question if available.

## Differential Diagnosis

Differential diagnosis is broad and depends on the clinical presentation. Malaria, typhoid fever, and neoplastic disease can cause relapsing fevers, and the presence of a rash and polyarthritis might suggest viral and rickettsial diseases. An asymmetric oligoarthritis points more toward a bacterial etiology, in particular disseminated gonococcal and meningococcal diseases in the context of cutaneous lesions. Lyme disease or secondary syphilis occasionally have such a clinical presentation, but 25% to 50% of patients infected with *S. moniliformis* or *S. minus* have a false-positive VDRL (Venereal Disease Research Laboratory) test. Finally, when classic infectious symptoms such as fever or rash are missing, any causes of polyarthritis, from crystal-related arthropathies to rheumatoid arthritis, can be entertained.

## Treatment

All established cases of rat-bite fever should be treated with antibiotics. Despite being potentially lethal, rat-bite fever is easily treatable by a

## CURRENT THERAPY

**Bite Site**

- Clean and disinfect bite site.
- Local treatment does not prevent further dissemination.
- Administer tetanus toxoid (Td), if indicated.
- Do not give antirabies prophylaxis.

**Established Cases**

- Intravenous penicillin G (Bicillin) 1.2 million U/d for 5 to 7 d, followed by oral penicillin V[1] or ampicillin (Omnipen)[1] 500 mg qid for an additional wk (CDC recommendations).
- Oral tetracycline[1] 500 mg qid or streptomycin[1] 7.5 mg/kg bid IM are alternatives.
- Numerous other antibiotics are reported useful (macrolides, cephalosporins, quinolones)

**Prophylaxis**

- The role of prophylactic antibiotic is unknown. Some authors recommend oral penicillin V.[1]
- Encourage patients with an occupational risk to use protective gloves to handle animals or cages.

simple course of penicillin. The Centers for Disease Control and Prevention recommends intravenous penicillin G 1.2 million units per day for 5 to 7 days followed by oral penicillin V (Pen Vee K)[1] or ampicillin (Omnipen)[1] 500 mg qid for an additional week. For allergic patients, or if an intravenous line cannot be established, oral tetracycline (Achromycin)[1] 500 mg qid or streptomycin[1] 7.5 mg/kg bid intramuscularly are alternatives. Numerous other antibiotics have been reported to be potentially useful, including clarithromycin (Biaxin),[1] cephalosporins, and quinolones, but none has been subjected to any clinical trial.

Typically the bite site heals promptly. It should be cleaned and disinfected, even if local treatment does not appear to prevent further dissemination. Tetanus prophylaxis (Td) administration is indicated as required by the patient's immunization record, but antirabies prophylaxis is usually not required for rodent bite.

The role of prophylactic antibiotics is unknown, but some authors recommend the use of oral penicillin V.[1] Primary prevention by using protective gloves to handle animals or cages should be encouraged for patients with occupational risk.

## REFERENCES

Abdulaziz H, Touchie C, Toye B, Karsh J: Haverhill fever with spine involvement. J Rheumatol 2006;33:1409-1410.

Albedwawi S, LeBlanc C, Show A, Slinger RW: A teenager with fever, rash and arthritis. CMAJ 2006; 175:354.

Berger C, Altwegg M, Meyer A, Nadal D: Broad range polymerase chain reaction for diagnosis of rat-bite fever caused by *Streptobacillus moniliformis*. Pediatr Infect Dis J 2001;20:1181-1182.

Centers for Disease Control and Prevention: Fatal rat-bite fever—Florida and Washington, 2003. MMWR Morb Mortal Wkly Rep. 2005;53:1198-1202.

Holroyd KJ, Reiner AP, Dick JD: *Streptobacillus moniliformis* polyarthritis mimicking rheumatoid arthritis: An urban case of rat bite fever. Am J Med 1988;85:711-714.

Rupp ME: *Streptobacillus moniliformis* endocarditis: Case report and review. Clin Infect Dis 1992;14:769-772.

Schachter ME, Wilcox L, Rau N, et al: Rat-bite fever, Canada. Emerg Infect Dis 2006;12:1301-1302.

---

[1]Not FDA approved for this indication.

Stehle P, Dubuis O, So A, Dudler J: Rat bite fever without fever. Ann Rheum Dis 2003;62:894-896.

van Nood E, Peters SH: Rat-bite fever. Neth J Med 2005;63:319-321.

Washburn RG: *Streptobacillus moniliformis* (rat-bite fever). In Mandell GL, Bennett JE, Dolin R, eds. Mandell, Douglas, and Bennett's Principles and Practice of Infectious Diseases, 4th ed. Philadelphia: Churchill-Livingstone, 2000, pp 2422–2424.

# Relapsing Fever

Method of
*Diego Cadavid, MD*

Relapsing fever is one of several diseases caused by spirochetes. Other human spirochetal diseases are syphilis, Lyme disease, and leptospirosis. Notable features of spirochetes are wavy and helical shapes, length-to-diameter ratios of as much as 100 to 1, and flagella that lie between the inner and outer cell membranes. The spirochetes that cause relapsing fever are in the genus *Borrelia*. Other *Borrelia* species cause Lyme disease, avian spirochetosis, and epidemic bovine abortion. Table 1 shows the main *Borrelia* species of relapsing fever, their vectors, and an estimate of their geographic ranges. In the United States relapsing fever was considered a disease endemic only in the West. However, the recent finding of relapsing fever–like *Borrelia* in ticks and dogs in the eastern United States suggests that the risk of relapsing fever may extend into the East.

## Epidemiology

There are two forms of relapsing fever: epidemic transmitted to humans by the body louse *Pediculus humanus* (louse-borne relapsing fever, LBRF) and endemic transmitted to humans by soft-bodied ticks of the genus *Ornithodoros* (tick-borne relapsing fever, TBRF). In LBRF itching caused by skin infestation with lice leads to scratching, which may result in crushing of lice and release of infected hemolymph into areas of skin abrasion. Louse infestation is associated with cold weather and a lack of hygiene. Migrant workers and soldiers at war are particularly susceptible to this infection. Historically, massive outbreaks of LBRF occurred in Eurasia, Africa, and Latin America, but currently the disease is found only in Ethiopia and neighboring countries. However, immigrants can spread LBRF to other parts of the world.

The main risk factor for TBRF is exposure to endemic areas (Table 1). The risk of infection increases with outdoor activities in areas where rodents nest, like entering caves or sleeping in rustic cabins. *Ornithodoros* ticks are soft-bodied and feed for short periods of time (minutes), usually at night. They can live many years between blood meals and may transmit spirochetes to their offspring transovarially. Infection is produced by regurgitation of infected tick saliva into the skin wound during tick feeding. There are several natural vertebrate reservoirs for TBRF, but most common are rodents (deer mice, chipmunks, squirrels, and rats). In contrast, the body louse *Pediculus humanus* is a strict human parasite, living and multiplying in clothing.

## Clinical Diagnosis

Relapsing fever should be suspected in any patient presenting with two or more episodes of high fever and constitutional symptoms spaced by periods of relative well-being. The index of suspicion increases if the patient has been exposed to endemic areas for TBRF or to countries where LBRF still occurs (Table 1). Whereas LBRF is usually associated with a single febrile relapse, TBRF usually has multiple relapses (up to 13). In LBRF the second episode of fever is typically milder than the first; in TBRF the multiple febrile periods are usually of equal severity. The febrile periods last from 1 to 3 days, and the intervals between fevers last from 3 to 10 days. During the febrile periods, numerous spirochetes are circulating in the blood. This is called spirochetemia and is sometimes unexpectedly detected during routine blood smear examinations. Between fevers, spirochetemia is not observed because the numbers are low. The fever pattern and recurrent spirochetemia are the consequences of antigenic variation of abundant outer membrane lipoproteins of relapsing fever *Borrelia* species that are the target for serotype-specific antibodies.

The mean latency between exposure to ticks in the endemic form or to lice in the epidemic form and onset of symptoms is 6 days (range, 3 to 18 days). Because *Ornithodoros* ticks feed briefly and painlessly at night, patients with TBRF may not be able to recall having been bitten by a tick. The clinical manifestations of TBRF and LBRF are similar, although some differences do exist. Table 2 lists the frequency of the most common manifestations of TBRF. The usual initial presentation is sudden onset of chills followed by high fever, tachycardia, severe headache, vomiting, myalgia and arthralgia, and often delirium. In the early stages, a reddish rash may be seen over the trunk, arms, or legs. The fever remains high for 3 to 5 days, and then it clears abruptly. After an asymptomatic period of 7 to 10 days, the fever and other constitutional symptoms can reappear suddenly. The febrile episodes gradually become less severe, and the person eventually recovers completely. As the disease progresses, fever, jaundice, hepatosplenomegaly, cardiac arrhythmias, and cardiac failure may occur, especially with LBRF. Jaundice is more common at times of relapses. Patients with LBRF are more likely to develop petechiae on the trunk, extremities, and mucous membranes; epistaxis; and blood-tinged sputum. Rupture of the spleen may rarely occur. Multiple neurologic complications can occur as a result of disseminated intravascular coagulation in LBRF and as a result of infection of the meninges and cranial and spinal nerve roots by spirochetes in TBRF. The most common neurologic complications of TBRF are aseptic meningitis and facial palsy. Relapsing fever in pregnant women can cause abortion, premature birth, and neonatal death. Sometimes patients can have nonfebrile relapses, consisting of

**TABLE 1 Relapsing Fever *Borrelia* Species Pathogenic to Humans**

| Relapsing Fever | *Borrelia* Species | Arthropod Vector | Distribution of Disease |
| --- | --- | --- | --- |
| Endemic | B. hermsii | Ornithodoros hermsi | Western North America |
| | B. turicatae | O. turicata | Southwestern North America and northern Mexico |
| | B. venezuelensis | O. rudis | Central America and northern South America |
| | B. hispanica | O. marocanus | Iberian peninsula and northwestern Africa |
| | B. crocidurae | O. erraticus | North and East Africa, Middle East, southern Europe |
| | B. duttoni | O. moubata | Sub-Saharan Africa |
| | B. persica | O. tholozani | Middle East, Greece, Central Asia |
| | B. uzbekistan | O. pappilipes | Tajikistan, Uzbekistan |
| Epidemic | B. recurrentis | Pediculus humanus | Worldwide (recently only in East Africa including immigrants to Europe) |

## TABLE 2  Frequent Clinical Manifestations of Tick-Borne Relapsing Fever

| Sign or Symptom | Frequency (%) |
| --- | --- |
| Headache | 94 |
| Myalgia | 92 |
| Chills | 88 |
| Nausea | 76 |
| Arthralgia | 73 |
| Vomiting | 71 |
| Abdominal pain | 44 |
| Confusion | 38 |
| Dry cough | 27 |
| Ocular pain | 26 |
| Diarrhea | 25 |
| Dizziness | 25 |
| Photophobia | 25 |
| Neck pain | 24 |
| Rash | 18 |
| Dysuria | 13 |
| Jaundice | 10 |
| Hepatomegaly | 10 |
| Splenomegaly | 6 |

periods of severe headache, backache, weakness, and other constitutional symptoms without fever that occur at the time of expected relapses. Delirium may persist for weeks after the fever resolves, and rarely symptoms may be protracted.

Relapsing fever may be confused with many diseases that are relapsing or cause high fevers. These include typhoid fever, yellow fever, dengue, African hemorrhagic fevers, African trypanosomiasis, brucellosis, malaria, leptospirosis, rat-bite fever, intermittent cholangitis, cat-scratch disease, echovirus 9 infection, among others. Relapsing fever *Borrelias* have antigens that are cross reactive with Lyme disease *Borrelias* and inasmuch as the endemic areas of relapsing fever and Lyme disease overlap to some extent, confusion between the two infections can be expected.

## Laboratory Diagnosis

Although the pattern of recurring fever is the clue to diagnosing relapsing fever, confirmation of the diagnosis requires demonstration of spirochetes in peripheral blood taken during an episode of fever. The comparatively large number of spirochetes in the blood during relapsing fever provides the opportunity for the simplest method for

### CURRENT DIAGNOSIS

- There are two forms of relapsing fever: epidemic and endemic.
- Epidemic relapsing fever is transmitted from person to person by the body louse *Pediculus humanus*.
- Endemic relapsing fever is transmitted from rodent reservoirs to humans exposed to endemic areas by soft-bodied ticks of the genus *Ornithodoros*.
- The hallmark of relapsing fever is two or more febrile episodes separated by periods of relative well-being.
- The diagnosis is confirmed by visualization of the etiologic spirochetes in thin peripheral blood smears prepared at times of febrile peaks by phase-contrast or darkfield microscopy or light microscopy after Wright or Giemsa staining.

laboratory diagnosis of the infection, light microscopy of Wright or Giemsa stained thin blood smears or darkfield or phase-contrast microscopy of a wet mount of plasma. The blood should be obtained during or just before peaks of body temperature. Between fever peaks, spirochetes often can be demonstrated by inoculation of blood or cerebrospinal fluid (CSF) into special culture medium (BSK-H with 6% rabbit serum available from Sigma) or experimental animals. Enrichment for spirochetes is achieved by using the platelet-rich fraction of plasma or the buffy coat of sedimented blood. In the United States the most common causes of relapsing fever are *Borrelia hermsii* and *Borrelia turicatae*; both grow in BSK-H medium and in young mice or rats. Whereas direct visual detection of organisms in the blood is the most common method for laboratory confirmation of relapsing fever, immunoassays for antibodies are the most common means of laboratory confirmation for Lyme disease. Although serologic assays have been developed for the agents of relapsing fever, these are not widely available and of dubious utility. The antigenic variation displayed by the relapsing fever species means there are hundreds of different "serotypes." If a different serotype or species is used for preparing the antigen, only antibodies to conserved antigens may be detected. For this reason, a standardized enzyme-linked immunosorbent assay (ELISA) with Lyme disease *Borrelia* as antigen may be the best available serologic assay for relapsing fever. ELISA for *Borrelia burgdorferi* antibodies is routinely done across the United States and Europe. If a positive result for IgM or IgG antibodies is obtained, the Western blot for antibodies to *B. burgdorferi* antigens would be expected to discriminate current or past Lyme disease from relapsing fever, as well as from syphilis, another cause of false-positive Lyme disease ELISA results. Other frequent laboratory abnormalities can occur in relapsing fever but are not diagnostic. These include elevated white blood cell count with increased neutrophils, thrombocytopenia, increased serum bilirubin, proteinuria, microhematuria, prolongation of the prothrombin time (PT) and partial thromboplastin time (PTT), and elevation of fibrin degradation products.

## Treatment

Relapsing fever *Borrelias* are very sensitive to several antibiotics, and antimicrobial resistance is rare. Table 3 summarizes the treatment options for adults and children younger than 8 years. Children older than 8 years can be treated with the same antibiotics as adults, but the doses should be adjusted by weight. Before antibiotics are given, the

### CURRENT THERAPY

- The antibiotic of choice for treatment of relapsing fever is doxycycline (Doryx) except in children or pregnant women. In children <8 y, erythromycin (E-Mycin)[1] or oral penicillin[1] is used instead of tetracycline (Table 3).
- Relapsing fever if severe or complicated with neuroborreliosis requires treatment with the intravenous antibiotics ceftriaxone (Rocephin) or penicillin G (Table 3).
- The louse-borne epidemic form is treated with a single dose, whereas the endemic tick-borne form is treated with multiple doses for at least 1 week (Table 3).
- Antibiotic treatment of relapsing fever results in the Jarisch-Herxheimer reaction in as many as 60% of cases, more often in the epidemic than in the endemic form. It is characterized by the sudden onset of tachycardia, hypotension, chills, rigors, diaphoresis, and high fever. To reduce the risk of the JHR, antibiotics should be started between but not at times of febrile peaks.

[1]Not FDA approved for this indication.

## TABLE 3 Treatment Options for Tick-Borne Relapsing Fever[*]

### Adults
#### Nonsevere forms

1. Doxycycline (Doryx oral), 100 mg PO bid for 1–2 wk[†]
2. Tetracycline (Sumycin), 500 mg PO qid for 1–2 wk
3. Erythromycin (Erythrocin),[1] 500 mg PO tid for 1–2 wk

#### Severe forms

1. Ceftriaxone (Rocephin),[1] 2g IV qd for 1–2 wk
2. Penicillin G parenteral aqueous (Pfizerpen),[1] 4 million U IV q4h for 1–2 wk

### Children (≤8 y)
#### Nonsevere forms

1. Erythromycin suspension oral (EryPed),[1] 30–50 mg/kg/d divided tid for 1–2 wk
2. Azithromycin oral suspension (Zithromax),[1] 20 mg/kg on the first day followed by 10 mg/kg/d for 4 more days
3. Penicillin V (Pen-Vee K),[1] 25–50 mg/kg/d divided qid for 1–2 wk
4. Amoxicillin (Amoxil),[1] 50 mg/kg/d divided tid for 1–2 wk

#### Severe forms

1. Ceftriaxone (Rocephin),[1] 75–100 mg/kg/d IV for 1–2 wk
2. Penicillin G parenteral aqueous (Pfizerpen),[1] 300,000 U/kg/d given IV in divided doses q4h for 1–2 wk

[1]Not FDA approved for this indication.
[*]The same oral agents are used for treatment of louse-borne (epidemic) relapsing fever but given as a single dose.
[†]In general, treatment for 1 wk is recommended in early/milder cases and for up to 2 wk for more severe cases.
Abbreviations: IV = intravenous; PO = orally.

possibility of causing the Jarisch-Herxheimer reaction should be considered (see later). The tetracycline antibiotics are most commonly used for treatment of LBRF and TBRF. The first antibiotic of choice in adults and children older than 8 years is doxycycline (Doryx). In general, shorter treatments are needed for LBRF than for TBRF. Single-dose therapy is usually recommended for LBRF. In contrast, in TBRF even multiple doses of tetracyclines for up to 10 days may fail to prevent relapses, and retreatment can be required. Alternative oral antibiotics to the tetracyclines are erythromycin (E-Mycin),[1] azithromycin (Zithromax),[1] amoxicillin (Amoxil),[1] penicillin,[1] and chloramphenicol (Chloromycetin).[1] However, oral chloramphenicol is no longer available in the United States. Erythromycin, azithromycin, and penicillin do not appear as effective as the tetracyclines; however, they are recommended for children younger than 8 years and for pregnant women. Amoxicillin is another alternative for young children with early Lyme disease; however, it is ineffective for human granulocytic ehrlichiosis, which sometimes occurs as a co-infection with Lyme disease.

Although treatment with antibiotics is usually given orally, they may need to be given intravenously if severe vomiting makes swallowing impractical. If there are symptoms and signs of meningitis or encephalitis without clinical and/or radiologic signs of increased intracranial pressure, the CSF should be examined to rule out central nervous system (CNS) infection. The finding of elevation of CSF cells and protein demands the use of parenteral antibiotics, such as penicillin G or ceftriaxone (Rocephin). Optimally, antibiotic treatment should be started during afebrile periods when the spirochetemia is low. Starting therapy near the peak of a febrile period may induce the Jarisch-Herxheimer reaction, in which high fever and a rise and subsequent fall in blood pressure, sometimes to dangerously low levels, may occur. Dehydration should be treated with fluids given intravenously. Severe headache can be treated with pain relievers such as codeine, and nausea or vomiting can be treated with prochlorperazine.

## Jarisch-Herxheimer Reaction

Antibiotic treatment of relapsing fever causes the Jarisch-Herxheimer reaction (JHR) in as many as 60% of cases. The JHR is more common in LBRF than in TBRF. It is characterized by the sudden onset of tachycardia, hypotension, chills, rigors, diaphoresis, and high fever. Patients with the JHR have said that they felt as if they were going to die. The JHR is caused by the rapid killing of circulating spirochetes 1 to 4 hours after the first dose of antibiotic, which results in the release of large amounts of Borrelia lipoproteins in the circulation followed by massive release of tumor necrosis factor and other cytokines. If possible, patients with the JHR should be transferred to an intensive care unit for close monitoring and treatment. During several hours, the temperature declines and the patient feels better. Large amounts of intravenous fluids (0.9% sodium chloride solution) may be required to treat hypotension. Steroids and nonsteroidal anti-inflammatory agents have no effect on the frequency or severity of the JHR. One study found that pretreatment with anti-TNF-alpha monoclonal antibody (Humira)[1] suppressed the JHR after penicillin treatment for LBRF and reduced the associated increases in plasma cytokines. Death can occur as a result of the JHR secondary to cardiovascular collapse in up to 5% of patients with treated LBRF and much less frequently in TBRF.

## Outcome

Complete recovery occurs in 95% or more of adequately treated patients. The prognosis for untreated cases or if treatment is delayed varies. Mortality as high as 40% is reported in untreated epidemics of LBRF. Relapsing fever also has a high mortality in neonates. Some neurologic sequelae can occur in patients with TBRF complicated with neuroborreliosis.

## Prevention

Prevention of TBRF involves avoidance of rodent- and tick-infested dwellings such as animal burrows, caves, and abandoned cabins. Wearing clothing that protects skin from tick access (e.g., long pants and long-sleeved shirts) is also helpful. Repellents and acaricides provide additional protection. Diethyltoluamide (DEET) repels ticks when applied to clothing or skin, but it must be used with caution. It loses its effectiveness within 1 to several hours when applied to skin and must be reapplied; it is absorbed through the skin and may cause CNS toxicity if used excessively. Picaridin (KBR 3023), which has been used as an insect repellent for years in Europe and Australia, is now available in the United States in 7% solution as Cutter Advanced Repellent (Spectrum Brands). The U.S. Centers for Disease Control and Prevention (CDC) is recommending it as an alternative to DEET. Permethrin Insect Repellent, an acaricide, is more effective than DEET but should not be applied directly to skin. When applied to clothing, it provides good protection for 1 day or more. In LBRF, prevention can be achieved by promoting personal hygiene and by dusting undergarments and the inside of clothing with malathion[1,2] or lindane powder[2] when available. Widespread antibiotic use may be necessary to control epidemics of LBRF, using one or two doses of 100 mg doxycycline given within 1 week of exposure.

[1]Not FDA approved for this indication.

[1]Not FDA approved for this indication.
[2]Not available in the United States.

## REFERENCES

Barbour AG, Hayes SF: Biology of *Borrelia* species. Microbiol Rev 1986;50: 381-400.

Bryceson AD, Parry EH, Perine PL, et al: Louse-borne relapsing fever. Q J Med 1970;39:129-170.

Cadavid D, Barbour AG: Neuroborreliosis during relapsing fever: Review of the clinical manifestations, pathology, and treatment of infections in humans and experimental animals. Clin Infect Dis 1998;26:151-164.

Fekade D, Knox K, Hussein K, et al: Prevention of Jarisch-Herxheimer reactions by treatment with antibodies against tumor necrosis factor alpha. N Engl J Med 1996;335:311-315.

Kazragis RJ, Dever LL, Jorgensen JH, Barbour AG: In vivo activities of ceftriaxone and vancomycin against *Borrelia* spp. in the mouse brain and other sites. Antimicrob Agents Chemother 1996;40:2632-2636.

Melkert PW: Fatal Jarisch-Herxheimer reaction in a case of relapsing fever misdiagnosed as lobar pneumonia. Trop Geogr Med 1987;39:92-93.

Southern P, Sanford J: Relapsing fever. Medicine 1969;48:129-149.

Taft W, Pike J: Relapsing fever. Report of a sporadic outbreak including treatment with penicillin. JAMA 1945;129:1002-1005.

# Lyme Disease

Method of
*Arthur Weinstein, MD, FACP, FACR,
and Shobha Wani, MD*

## Epidemiology

Lyme disease, or borreliosis, is a tick-transmitted infection caused by *Borrelia burgdorferi*. It is the most common insect-borne illness in the United States with more than 20,000 new cases reported annually. It occurs worldwide with hyperendemicity in temperate regions. In the United States, most cases originate from states in the Northeast, mid-Atlantic, upper Midwest, and Pacific coast regions. The life cycle of the Ixodes tick ensures that most cases of human borrelial infection occur from spring to fall. Three genospecies of *B. burgdorferi* account for human disease: *B. burgdorferi sensu stricto*, *B. garinii*, and *B. afzelii*. Although all three are found in Europe and the latter two in Asia, *B. burgdorferi sensu stricto* is the only cause of Lyme disease in the United States. Lyme disease occurs in all age groups with highest frequencies in young children and adults older than 30 years and is equally common in men and women. It often manifests clinically in stages, with exacerbations and remissions in each stage.

## Clinical Features

### EARLY LYME DISEASE

Localized skin infection and early disseminated infection occur within days to weeks after the bite of an infected tick. Erythema migrans (EM) rash, the hallmark of early Lyme disease, occurs in up to 70% to 80% of patients at the site of the tick bite. It usually is macular and asymptomatic but may burn or itch, and it is commonly found at the belt line, inguinal area, or in and around the axilla. It expands over days, often to a very large circumference and with central clearing, giving a bull's-eye appearance. Approximately 10% of patients have multiple skin lesions (disseminated EM), a sign of hematogenous spread of the borrelia. At this early stage, patients may have nonspecific flulike complaints, namely fever, fatigue, myalgia, arthralgia, and headache, resembling a viral syndrome. These symptoms occasionally occur without the rash. In untreated patients, EM resolves spontaneously within days to several weeks after onset, but treatment often accelerates its resolution.

Early disseminated disease occurs days to weeks after the tick bite and may occur without preceding localized EM. Certain subtypes of

## CURRENT DIAGNOSIS

- Erythema migrans is usually asymptomatic and expansile.
- Lyme disease can present with only flulike symptoms: fever, arthralgia, myalgia.
- Antibody testing for borrelial infection is often negative during early infection.
- A two-test strategy (serum ELISA, immunoblot) is recommended for diagnosis.
- IgM antibodies are commonly seen in early infection (4–8 wk) but may persist for many months.
- IgG antibodies are characteristic of late Lyme disease, especially Lyme arthritis.
- Intrathecal antibody synthesis is an important diagnostic marker for neuroborreliosis.
- Clinical symptoms combined with antibody status are of diagnostic importance.

*Abbreviation:* ELISA = enzyme-linked immunosorbent assay.

*B. burgdorferi* are associated with higher frequency of spirochetemia and dissemination to other organs. For instance, in Europe, EM is often an indolent, localized infection, whereas in the United States, it is associated with more intense inflammation and signs that suggest dissemination of the spirochete. The clinical manifestations of dissemination can be highly variable and may include disseminated EM rash and neurologic, cardiac, and musculoskeletal features either alone or in combination. Neurologic features (neuroborreliosis) are seen in approximately 10% of patients and include acute lymphocytic meningitis, cranial neuropathy, especially facial paresis, which may be bilateral, and radiculoneuritis. Neuroborreliosis is more common in Europe where neurotropic subspecies of borrelia (*B. garinii, B. afzelii*) are found. Meningitis usually resolves spontaneously, whereas treatment of other neurologic features can hasten recovery and prevent progression to the later stages of Lyme disease. Carditis, which includes varying degrees of atrioventricular block or mild myopericarditis, may develop in approximately 8% of untreated patients, but early treatment can prevent its occurrence. In more recent series, the incidence of Lyme carditis was reported as less than 1% in the United States. Rheumatic features at this stage consist of migratory, episodic joint, tendon, or bursal pains with or without objective signs of inflammation. Typically there is acute localized pain that lasts days to weeks, remits spontaneously, and then recurs in another region. Inflammatory polyarthritis is not a feature of early or late Lyme disease.

The diagnosis of early Lyme disease relies to a great degree on the clinical presentation. In an endemic area, with a history of possible tick exposure, the presence of a classical EM lesion is sufficient for the diagnosis. With very early infection and isolated EM, laboratory tests for antibodies to *B. burgdorferi* may be negative. Conversely, with disseminated early Lyme disease, antibody testing is frequently positive.

### LATE LYME DISEASE

Late Lyme disease occurs months to years after initial infection (mean, 6 months) and may present de novo without prior features of early Lyme disease. Systemic symptoms are generally minimal or absent. Musculoskeletal complaints, the most common manifestation, are seen in 80% of untreated patients and include intermittent oligoarthritis (50%) and acute or subacute inflammatory arthritis that most often affects one or both knees. This arthritis may begin abruptly with knee pain and a large joint effusion. Synovial fluid is inflammatory with white counts ranging in the thousands or tens of thousands. Radiographs may be normal except for soft-tissue swelling and joint effusion but may also demonstrate osteopenia, bone cysts, and even mild cartilage loss with small erosions. Untreated, these attacks of arthritis generally last many months, recur for several years but eventually may remit. *B. burgdorferi* is not culturable from the synovial fluid of patients with Lyme arthritis, but borrelial DNA can be detected by polymerase chain reaction (PCR) in over 80% of untreated patients. The PCR test is generally negative after appropriate antibiotic therapy.

Neurologic features of late Lyme disease are seen more frequently in Europe because *B. garinii* is the most neurotropic subspecies. There are a wide range of neurologic abnormalities, especially encephalomyelitis and peripheral neuropathy. In the United States, Lyme encephalopathy or polyneuropathy is described with subtle disturbances of memory and concentration, spinal radicular pain, or distal paresthesias. Nerve conduction studies reveal axonal polyneuropathy. Pleocytosis of the cerebrospinal fluid (CSF) is unusual in late neurologic Lyme disease. High CSF protein may be seen, but borrelial organisms by culture or PCR are not commonly found. Important to the diagnosis of neuroborreliosis is the demonstration of increased intrathecal synthesis of borrelia-specific antibodies.

A chronic skin lesion, acrodermatitis chronica atrophicans, caused by *B. afzelii*, is seen most commonly in Europe.

## Laboratory Testing in Lyme Disease

Lyme disease should not be diagnosed purely on serologic tests because false-positive tests are common. Instead, serologic tests should be used to confirm the diagnosis in the appropriate clinical setting. Even a true positive test only confirms recent or past exposure to *B. burgdorferi*, but this must be evaluated in the context of the patient's past and current symptoms.

Despite these methodologic and diagnostic issues, measurement of antibodies to *B. burgdorferi* by enzyme-linked immunoassay (ELISA) is a useful screening test for early and late Lyme disease. This so-called Lyme test is positive in most cases of late Lyme disease and virtually always positive in late Lyme arthritis. It may be negative very early after infection or in those individuals who receive early antibiotic therapy. However, the high rate of false positivity has led to a two-test strategy whereby all sera that show positive or equivocal ELISA tests for borrelial antibodies are tested again by more specific Western (immuno) blotting. In patients with CNS disease, demonstration of intrathecal antibodies by ELISA in relatively higher concentration than serum antibodies is suggestive of neuroborreliosis.

Immunoblotting is usually performed for both IgM and IgG antibodies to borrelial proteins. Although this technique is not as automated or quantitative as ELISA, it is more specific because it identifies the borrelial antigens to which the antibodies are directed. There are recommendations for standardized testing and interpretation of Western blot results. IgM antibodies usually appear 2 to 4 weeks after EM, peak at 6 to 8 weeks, and decline thereafter, although IgM reactivity may occasionally persist for many years. An IgM blot is considered to be positive if two of three specified bands (23, 39, 41 kd) are present. The results of an IgM blot are best interpreted in the first weeks after symptom onset when the true positive rate exceeds the false-positive rate. A positive IgM blot found in a patient with long-standing symptoms should be interpreted with caution because it likely represents a false-positive result. IgG antibodies appear after 4 to 6 weeks, peak at 4 to 6 months, and then remain positive for many years, even decades. An IgG immunoblot is considered to be positive if 5 of 10 specified bands (18, 23, 28, 30, 39, 41, 45, 58, 66, 93 kd) are present. IgG seroconversion, with or without IgM seroconversion, can be taken as presumptive evidence of exposure to *B. burgdorferi* and in the proper clinical context supports the diagnosis of Lyme disease. However, a positive IgG immunoblot does not necessarily mean current or ongoing borreliosis. Conversely, a negative IgG immunoblot is presumptive evidence against the diagnosis of late Lyme disease. An ELISA assay for antibodies to a borrelial-specific surface protein (C6 peptide of VlsE) was demonstrated to be a sensitive and specific single test for the diagnosis of Lyme disease and is commercially available.

Culture of *B. burgdorferi* requires special medium and conditions and takes many weeks. Even so, in expert laboratories the organism can

 **CURRENT THERAPY**

- Early antibiotic therapy hastens resolution of symptoms and prevents late complications.
- In adults, oral therapy with doxycycline (Vibramycin)[1] is preferred for most features of Lyme disease.
- Neuroborreliosis is usually treated with IV ceftriaxone.
- Duration of therapy is generally 2–4 wk.
- Lyme disease is cured after antibiotic treatment (one or two courses) in most patients.
- Some patients with Lyme arthritis develop persistent antibiotic-resistant synovitis, which may be autoimmune and is treated with antirheumatic drugs.
- Patients with chronic fatigue, arthralgia, and myalgia that begins, persists, or recurs after antibiotic treatment for Lyme disease generally have a post–Lyme disease syndrome and not ongoing infection.
- There is no scientific support for prolonged courses of oral or IV antibiotics for Lyme disease.

[1]Not FDA approved for this indication.
*Abbreviation:* IV = intravenous.

be recovered from the EM lesion in a high percentage of patients and from the blood in patients with disseminated early Lyme disease. Risk for spirochetemia starts the day the patient notices the rash and continues for 2 weeks.

*B. burgdorferi* is cultured only rarely from the CSF of patients with neuroborreliosis.

PCR to detect borrelial DNA is also positive with the same or higher frequency as culture from the skin, blood, and CSF. However, it is most useful in the synovial fluid of patients with suspected and untreated Lyme arthritis where it can be positive in more than 80% of patients despite universally negative cultures. PCR analysis of synovial tissue may be more likely to yield positive results than synovial fluid because *B. burgdorferi* associates with connective tissue. However, because virtually all cases of Lyme arthritis are strongly positive by ELISA and immunoblotting for IgG antibodies to *B. burgdorferi*, the diagnosis can usually be made with reasonable certainty using these tests alone.

## Treatment

The goals of treatment of Lyme disease are to resolve the clinical symptoms by eradication of the organism and to prevent late stage disease with early therapy. Although most manifestations resolve spontaneously without treatment, clinical trials demonstrated that treatment with antibiotics hastens resolution and prevents late manifestations of Lyme borreliosis. In most of the trials, treatment of 3 weeks' duration was effective. Revised evidence-based guidelines for treatment have recently been published by the Infectious Diseases Society of America. Generally, early Lyme disease is treated with antimicrobials for 2 to 3 weeks, although studies showed that EM treatment with oral doxycycline for 10 days is as effective as treatment for 20 days. Effective oral medications include doxycycline (Vibramycin),[1] tetracycline, second-generation cephalosporins such as cefuroxime axetil (Ceftin), and amoxicillin (Amoxil).[1] Erythromycin (E-Mycin)[1] and azithromycin (Zithromax)[1] are somewhat less effective. Doxycycline and tetracycline should not be used in children younger than 8 years or in pregnant women. Oral therapy is sufficient for certain clinical features: EM, facial palsy without signs of meningitis, and first-degree

---

[1]Not FDA approved for this indication.

heart block. Oral therapy with doxycycline (Vibramycin) is associated with fewer side effects and is much less expensive than the also employed intravenous (IV) therapy with ceftriaxone (Rocephin).[1] Although amoxicillin and doxycycline appear to be equally efficacious, doxycycline has the distinct advantage of also being effective in treating *Anaplasma phagocytophila* infection, which causes human granulocytic ehrlichiosis (HGE) and is also transmitted by the Ixodes tick. In general, patients with neurologic manifestations, either early or late, other than isolated facial palsy, are treated de novo with IV ceftriaxone (Rocephin)[1] for 3 to 4 weeks, although aqueous penicillin (Penicillin G)[1] is also effective. Carditis with heart block may resolve spontaneously, but patients with higher grades of heart block and with cardiomyopathy are generally treated with IV antibiotics. If the oral regimen fails, as may occur with 20% of patients, parenteral therapy with ceftriaxone or cefotaxime (Claforan)[1] is warranted. In patients with persistent symptoms, a second parenteral regimen is usually administered. There is no need to change the medication because *B. burgdorferi* does not show resistance to any of the antimicrobials recommended.

Oral and parenteral therapies are both used with success in treating Lyme arthritis with treatment duration of 3 to 4 weeks. Occasionally a second month of treatment is needed to eradicate the organism from the joint. Even with successful treatment, the arthritis may resolve quite slowly with synovitis persisting over several months (Table 1).

## PERSISTENT (TREATMENT-RESISTANT) LYME ARTHRITIS

Approximately 10% of patients with Lyme arthritis in the United States are treatment resistant, with recurrent inflammatory effusions, usually in one knee, for months to several years despite appropriate antibiotic therapy. This antibiotic-resistant Lyme arthritis is thought to be related to an intra-articular autoimmune response in predisposed individuals. There is no evidence for persistent infection because borrelial DNA by PCR in synovial fluid or synovial tissue is not found

in these individuals. A genetic predisposition is suggested by the increased frequency of HLA-DR4 and HLA-DRB1*0401, 0101, and related alleles, similar to that seen in rheumatoid arthritis. In this situation, treatment consists of nonsteroidal anti-inflammatory drugs, intraarticular steroid injections, and antirheumatic agents such as hydroxychloroquine (Plaquenil),[1] sulfasalazine (Azulfidine),[1] and even methotrexate (Rheumatrex).[1] In some cases, arthroscopic synovectomy proves effective. This arthritis usually remits after several years.

## POST–LYME DISEASE SYNDROME

Although the long-term prognosis of treated Lyme disease is excellent, some patients develop arthralgia, myalgia, and fatigue, during or soon after infection, which persists despite adequate courses of antibiotics. Other features of this symptom complex include memory and concentration difficulties, neuropathic pains, headache, and unrefreshed sleep. This condition is often called post–Lyme disease syndrome, post-treatment chronic Lyme disease, or chronic Lyme disease. The actual frequency of this condition after Lyme disease is unclear but is likely no more than 5%. Some studies suggested that delay in initiating antibiotic treatment for borrelial infection is more likely to result in post–Lyme disease syndrome. In none of these studies did current serologic status correlate with persistent symptoms. Although these patients have significant somatic complaints and functional disability, they lack objective findings of an inflammatory condition. Although virtually all patients with this syndrome complain of problems with memory and concentration, demonstrable abnormalities on neurocognitive testing are not universally present. The pathogenesis of this chronic post-treatment symptomatic state and its relationship to Lyme disease are unclear. Patients may feel better during antibiotic therapy, but the effect is not durable and relapse is common when antibiotics are discontinued. The symptoms wax and wane, but the overall course is chronic. Controversy has raged as to whether chronic, relatively resistant borrelial infection plays a role and hence whether chronic antibiotic therapy is warranted. However, an important study on post–Lyme syndrome

[1]Not FDA approved for this indication.

---

**TABLE 1  Suggested Treatment of Lyme Disease**

| Clinical Features/Indication | Antibiotic regimen | Regimen | | Duration of Therapy |
|---|---|---|---|---|
| | | Adults | Children | |
| **Early Infection (Local and Disseminated Disease)** | Doxycycline (Vibramycin)[1] | 100 mg bid | <8 y: not recommended >8 y: 1–2 mg/kg bid; maximum 100 mg | 2–3 wk |
| | Tetracycline[1] | 500 mg qid | Not for pregnant women | 2–3 wk |
| | Amoxicillin[1] | 500 mg tid | As above | 2–3 wk |
| | Cefuroxime axetil (Ceftin) | 500 mg bid | 50 mg/kg/d in 3 divided doses | 2–3 wk |
| | Azithromycin (Zithromax)[1] | 500 mg daily | 30 mg/kg/d in 2 divided doses | 7–10 d |
| | Erythromycin[1] | 500 mg qid | 50 mg/kg/d | 2–3 wk |
| **Neuroborreliosis Failure to Respond to Oral Therapy** | Ceftriaxone (Rocephin)[1] Cefotaxime (Claforan)[1] Penicillin G[1] | 2 g IV daily 2 g IV tid 4–5 million U IV q4h | 75–100 mg/kg/d 90–180 mg/kg/d in 3–4 divided doses 2–4 million U IV q4 h | 2–4 wk 2–4 wk 2–4 wk |
| **Carditis** | Oral or IV regimen | | | 2–3 wk |
| **Late Lyme Arthritis** | Oral or IV regimen | | | 4 wk* |
| **Pregnancy** | Amoxicillin Penicillin G Ceftriaxone Cefotaxime | | | 2–4 wk |

*May give another course if poor response.
[1]Not FDA approved for this indication.
*Abbreviation:* IV = intravenous.

patients failed to document the presence of *B. burgdorferi* in the plasma or spinal fluid of these patients by culture or PCR. In addition, a controlled trial failed to show a response to a 3-month course of antibiotics (1 month of IV ceftriaxone [Rocephin][1] followed by 2 months of oral doxycycline[1]). This suggests that chronic infection is not the cause of post–Lyme disease syndrome, that the condition spontaneously waxes and wanes, and that prolonged antibiotic treatment does not result in long-term symptom remission.

## Prevention

The best currently available method for preventing infection with *B. burgdorferi* and other tick-transmitted infections is to avoid tick infested areas through the summer. If exposure is unavoidable, use of protective clothing (shirt tucked into pants and pants tucked under socks) may interfere with attachment by ticks. Wearing light-colored clothing makes it easier to identify ticks. Daily inspection of the entire body to locate and remove ticks also decreases the transmission of infection. Attached ticks should promptly be removed with fine-toothed forceps, if possible. Tick and insect repellent applied to the skin and clothing provides additional protection. The most effective repellent is DEET (diethyltoluamide). Permethrin, a pesticide that kills ticks and mites when applied to clothing, decreases the risk of tick bite. Strategies to reduce the number of ticks may be somewhat effective in decreasing tick-borne illnesses, including the application of acaricides and landscaping to provide desiccating barriers. Although vaccination is available for dogs and a recombinant outer surface protein A (OspA)-based vaccine (LYMErix) is effective and relatively safe in humans, currently no marketed vaccine is available to prevent Lyme disease in humans.

### AFTER TICK BITE

It is not recommended to treat all patients after a tick bite because several prospective studies demonstrated that the risk of drug-associated rash is as great as the risk of developing Lyme disease. Conversely, it may be reasonable to treat persons believed to be at higher risk for the development of borrelial infection prophylactically. Studies showed that transmission of *B. burgdorferi* from tick to host occurs with greater frequency when there has been tick attachment for more than 48 hours resulting in a blood-engorged tick. Because a controlled study demonstrated that a single 200-mg dose of doxycycline[1] effectively prevents Lyme disease when given within 72 hours of a tick bite, the threshold for treating patients after tick bites with this benign regimen is lower than in the past.

### REFERENCES

Klempner MS, Hu LT, Evans J, et al: Two controlled trials of antibiotic treatment in patients with persistent symptoms and a history of Lyme disease. N Engl J Med 2001;345:85-92.

Nadelman RB, Nowakowski J, Fish D, et al: Prophylaxis with single dose doxycycline for the prevention of Lyme disease after an Ixodes scapularis tick bite. N Engl J Med 2001;345:79-84.

Recommendations for test performance and interpretation from the Second National Conference on Serologic Diagnosis of Lyme Disease. MMWR 1995;44:590-591.

Steere AC: Lyme disease. N Engl J Med 2001;345:115-125.

Steere AC, Dhar A, Hernandez J, et al: Systemic symptoms without erythema migrans as the presenting picture of early Lyme disease. Am J Med 2003;114:58-62.

Steere AC, Sikand VK, et al: The presenting manifestations of Lyme disease and the outcomes of treatment. N Engl J Med 2003;348:2472-2474.

Treatment of Lyme disease. The Medical Letter 2005;47:41-43.

Tugwell P, Dennis DT, Weinstein A, et al: Clinical guideline 2: Laboratory evaluation in the diagnosis of Lyme disease. Ann Intern Med 1997;127:1109-1123.

Weinstein A, Britchkov M: Lyme arthritis and post-Lyme disease syndrome. Curr Opin Rheum 2002,14:383-387.

Wormser GP, Dattwyler RJ, Shapiro ED, et al: The clinical assessment, treatment, and prevention of Lyme disease, human granulocytic anaplasmosis, and babesiosis: Clinical practice guidelines by the Infectious Diseases Society of America. Clin Infect Dis 2006;43:1089–1134.

Wormser GP, Ramanathan R, Nowakowski J, et al: Duration of antibiotic therapy for early Lyme disease. A randomized, double-blind, placebo-controlled trial. Ann Intern Med 2003;138: 697-704.

# Rubella and Congenital Rubella Syndrome

Method of
*Susan E. Reef, MD*

Rubella, once thought to be a benign rash illness, gained public health significance when Norman Gregg in 1941 documented the association between rubella during pregnancy and congenital defects. The last pandemic occurred between 1962 and 1965. In the United States, this epidemic resulted in approximately 12.5 million rubella cases, 11,000 fetal deaths (including spontaneous and therapeutic abortions), and 20,000 infants born with congenital rubella syndrome (CRS).

## Background and Epidemiology

Rubella virus is a member of the *Togaviridae* family and the genus *Rubivirus*. It is an enveloped RNA virus with a single antigenic type. Infection is limited to humans. Rubella is transmitted through person-to-person contact or droplets shed from the respiratory secretions of infected persons. The average incubation period is 14 days, with a range of 12 to 23 days. Persons with rubella are most infectious when the rash is erupting, but they can shed virus from 7 days before to 5 to 7 days after rash onset (i.e., the infectious period).

In the prevaccine era, rubella epidemics occurred approximately every 6 to 9 years in the United States. In 1969, live attenuated rubella vaccines were licensed in the United States, and the number of rubella cases decreased from 57,600 cases in 1969 to 223 cases in 1988. With the success of the rubella vaccination program, a goal was established to eliminate indigenous rubella transmission and congenital rubella syndrome (CRS) in the United States by 2000. In 2001 and 2002, fewer than 25 reported rubella cases occurred, and since 2003, 10 or fewer cases have been reported annually.

In October 2004, an independent expert panel was convened to assess progress toward elimination of rubella and CRS in the United States and concluded that rubella is no longer endemic in the United States. Since then, elimination of endemic rubella and CRS has been maintained in the United States. Even though rubella is no longer endemic in the United States, rubella continues to be endemic in many parts of the world. As a result, cases of rubella and CRS related to importation continue to be reported in the United States.

## Clinical Features

The maculopapular erythematous rash of rubella usually starts on the face and neck and progresses downward. The rubella rash occurs in 50% to 80% of rubella-infected persons. The rash, which may be pruritic, usually lasts 1 to 3 days. The rash is fainter than measles rash and doesn't coalesce. However, rubella is sometimes misdiagnosed as measles or scarlet fever. Children usually develop few or no constitutional symptoms, but adults can experience a 1- to 5-day prodrome of low-grade fever, headache, malaise, mild coryza, and conjunctivitis.

Postauricular, occipital, and posterior cervical lymphadenopathy is characteristic and typically precedes the rash by 5 to 10 days.

## Diagnosis

Because many rash illnesses mimic rubella infection and 20% to 50% of rubella infections can be subclinical, laboratory testing is the only way to confirm the diagnosis. Acute rubella infection can be confirmed by the presence of serum rubella immunoglobulin M (IgM), a significant rise in IgG antibody titer in acute and convalescent serum specimens, positive rubella virus culture, or detection of the rubella virus by reverse transcriptase polymerase chain reaction (RT-PCR).

Serologic testing is the most common diagnostic methodology used. Because IgM antibodies might not be detectable before day five after rash onset, a repeat serum should be obtained for a negative rubella IgM in specimens taken before day five. False-positive serum rubella IgM tests have occurred in persons with parvovirus B19 infections, infectious mononucleosis, or a positive rheumatoid factor. To document a significant titer rise in IgG, paired specimens of acute and convalescent sera must be obtained, with the second serum collected about 14 to 21 days after the first specimen. Rubella virus can be isolated from nasal, blood, throat, urine, and cerebrospinal fluid specimens from patients with rubella and CRS. The most frequently positive results come from throat swabs. For viral cultures, the specimen should be obtained by day four after rash onset, which is the time for maximum viral shedding.

Laboratory confirmation of CRS can be obtained by demonstration of rubella-specific IgM antibodies in the infant's cord blood or sera, documentation of persistence of serum rubella IgG titer beyond the time expected from passive transfer of maternal IgG antibody (i.e., rubella titer that does not drop at the expected rate of a twofold dilution per month), isolation of rubella virus, or detection of rubella virus by RT-PCR.

## Complications

Rubella disease is usually mild and results in very few complications. Transient arthralgia or arthritis occurs in up to 70% of women with rubella. Other complications include thrombocytopenic purpura (1 in 3000 rubella cases) and encephalitis (1 in 6000 rubella cases). However, intrauterine rubella infection, particularly during the first trimester, can result in serious consequences such as miscarriage, stillbirth, or the constellation of severe birth defects known as CRS.

---

### CURRENT DIAGNOSIS

- Even though the rubella virus no longer circulates endemically in the United States, rubella is endemic in many parts of the world.
- Rubella and congenital rubella syndrome cases continue to occur in the United States, however, due to importations.
- Diagnosis is based on clinical history and findings, epidemiologic history, and laboratory confirmation.
- Serologic testing is the most common method for diagnosis; viral isolation and reverse transcriptase polymerase chain reaction (RT-PCR) are also available.
- One dose of rubella-containing vaccine is recommended for full protection. Most infants and children receive two doses of rubella vaccine in the MMR (measles, mumps, and rubella) vaccine based on recommendations for measles.

---

## CONGENITAL RUBELLA SYNDROME

For pregnant women infected with rubella during the first 11 weeks of gestation, 90% of the infants born will have CRS; the rate of CRS for infants born to women infected during the first 20 weeks of pregnancy is 20%. The most common congenital defects of CRS are eye defects (e.g., cataracts, congenital glaucoma, pigmentary retinopathy), cardiac defects (e.g., patent ductus arteriosus, peripheral pulmonic stenosis), and hearing impairment. Other clinical manifestations may include microcephaly, developmental delay, purpura, meningoencephalitis, hepatosplenomegaly, low birth weight, and radiolucent bone disease. The pregnant patient with rubella should be counseled about the risks of the congenital defects and her options. Infants with CRS can shed virus from body secretions for up to 1 year and are considered infectious. Persons in contact with these infants (e.g., health care workers, family members) should be immune to rubella either through vaccination or natural infection.

## MANAGEMENT OF EXPOSURE DURING PREGNANCY

As part of routine prenatal care, all pregnant women should be tested for rubella immunity. Women who are IgG positive without recent history of exposure to rubella are considered immune. Reinfection with rubella occurs more often with vaccine-induced immunity than with natural disease; however, the risk of maternal reinfection is rare.

If a pregnant woman is suspected of being exposed to rubella, a blood specimen should be taken as soon as possible and tested for rubella IgG and IgM antibody. The specimen should be stored for possible retesting. A positive IgM regardless of the IgG result can indicate recent or acute infection or may be a false-positive IgM. Therefore, serology should be repeated in 7 to 10 days. Besides repeating the IgM and IgG, additional testing using special tests (e.g., avidity) may be warranted. If the IgM and IgG are negative with the first specimen, a second specimen should be taken 3 to 4 weeks after exposure and tested for IgM and IgG in parallel with the first specimen. Either a positive IgM in the second sera or IgG seroconversion indicates acute infection. As long as the pregnant woman is exposed to rubella, it is important to continue testing for IgG and IgM responses.

## Treatment

There is no proven therapy for rubella. The best strategy is to ensure women are immune by vaccination before pregnancy. Health care providers who treat women of childbearing age should routinely determine rubella immunity and vaccinate those who are susceptible and not pregnant. Women found to be susceptible during pregnancy should be vaccinated immediately postpartum. There is no specific therapy for CRS; however, infants should be evaluated and provided early intervention by specialists who treat the identified CRS defects.

## Rubella Vaccine

In 1969, three live attenuated rubella vaccines were licensed in the United States. In 1979, a new formulation of live attenuated rubella

---

### CURRENT THERAPY

- There is no effective therapy for rubella.
- Vaccination provides excellent protection.
- Pregnant women with rubella should be counseled about the risk of congenital defects.
- Infants with congenital rubella syndrome should be evaluated and treated under the care of appropriate specialists.

---

vaccine (RA 27/3 [Meruvax II]) replaced the other rubella vaccines in the United States, because the RA 27/3 vaccine was found to induce higher antibody titers and to produce an immune response more closely paralleling natural infection than did the other vaccines. Of the persons vaccinated in clinical trials, 95% had serologic evidence of rubella immunity after one dose. From longitudinal studies, rubella vaccine confers immunity for at least 15 years and probably for a lifetime.

A rubella virus–containing vaccine is recommended for persons 12 months old or older unless there is a medical contraindication such as severe immunodeficiency or pregnancy. In the United States, in 2001, the period of time to avoid getting pregnant following a rubella vaccination was shortened from 3 months to 28 days.

Rubella vaccine is available as monovalent formulation (Meruvax II) or in combination with measles and mumps (MMR) or measles, mumps, and varicella (MMRV [ProQuad]). With use of MMR for measles vaccination under the currently recommended two-dose schedule, most children and adolescents now receive two doses of rubella vaccine. The MMR vaccine is recommended at 12 to 15 months of age, with a second dose at 4 to 6 years of age. MMRV vaccine can be given to children aged 12 months to 12 years of age.

Documented evidence of rubella immunity is defined as serologic evidence (e.g., a positive serum rubella IgG), documented immunization with at least one dose of rubella-containing vaccine on or after the first birthday, or birth before 1957 (except women who could become pregnant). Clinical diagnosis of rubella is unreliable and should *not* be considered in assessing immune status.

### REFERENCES

Centers for Disease Control and Prevention: Elimination of rubella and congenital rubella syndrome—United States, 1969-2004. MMWR Morb Mortal Wkly Rep 2005;54:279-282.

Centers for Disease Control and Prevention: Control and prevention of rubella: Evaluation and management of suspected outbreaks, rubella in pregnant women, and surveillance for congenital rubella syndrome. MMWR Recomm Rep 2001;50(RR-12):1-23. Available at http://www.cdc.gov/mmwr/preview/mmwrhtml/rr5012a1.htm (accessed May 15, 2007).

Centers for Disease Control and Prevention: Revised ACIP recommendation for avoiding pregnancy after receiving a rubella-containing vaccine. MMWR Morb Mortal Wkly Rep 2001;50:1117.

Dayan GH, Reef SE, Orenstein WA: Rubella. In Burg FD, Ingelfinger JR, Polin RA, Gershon AA (eds): Current Pediatric Therapy, 18th ed. Philadelphia: WB Saunders, 2006, pp 803-807.

Miller E, Cradock-Watson JE, Pollock TM: Consequences of confirmed maternal rubella at successive stages of pregnancy. Lancet 1982;2:781-784.

Plotkin SA, Reef S: Rubella vaccine. In Plotkin SA, Orenstein WA (eds): Vaccines, 4th ed. Philadelphia: WB Saunders, 2004, pp 707-743.

Watson JC, Hadler SC, Dykewicz CA et al: Measles, mumps, and rubella—vaccine use and strategies for elimination of measles, rubella, and congenital rubella syndrome and control of mumps: Recommendations of the Advisory Committee on Immunization Practices (ACIP). MMWR Recomm Rep 1998;47:1-57.

# Measles (Rubeola)

Method of
*Claude P. Muller, MD, and Jacques Kremer, PhD*

Measles is an acute systemic disease associated with a maculopapular rash, fever, and respiratory symptoms caused by a single-stranded RNA virus of the family of Paramyxoviridae and the genus *Morbillivirus*.

## Epidemiology

With a basic reproduction number of 15, measles virus is the most infectious pathogen. It is transmitted via aerosol to susceptibles (e.g., in kindergarten classes or doctors' offices), and humans are the only natural host. At least 95% of a population must be immune in order to prevent the virus from circulating.

Before the introduction of vaccination, epidemics occurred at regular intervals, and virtually all children had measles during early childhood. Measles induces high levels of antibodies and lifelong protection against the disease. Although vaccine-induced immunity is probably somewhat less robust than immunity after natural infection because of lower and waning antibodies, measles morbidity and mortality have dramatically declined since the introduction of a live-attenuated vaccine in 1963.

As of 2004, endemic circulation of the virus had been interrupted in the Western Hemisphere, as well as in several countries in Europe and the Western Pacific. The success in measles control has encouraged the World Health Organization (WHO) to introduce a timetable for measles elimination in most regions of the world.

In many developing countries, where 98% of global measles deaths occur, measles continues to be a serious condition. Although the 454,000 deaths estimated in 2004 represent a 48% reduction in global measles mortality compared with 1999, measles vaccines are still underused in developing countries.

## Clinical Features

Eight to 14 days after infection, the patient develops characteristic prodromal symptoms including fever and cough, coryza, or conjunctivitis. A maculopapular rash appears 2 to 4 days later (typically on day 12 after exposure) behind the ears and the hairline, spreading from the head to the trunk and the extremities. One or 2 days before the onset of rash, Koplik's spots, the pathognomonic enanthema, appear on the buccal mucosa and fade again as the skin rash evolves.

Uneventful measles lasts about 7 to 10 days, and cough is usually the last symptom to disappear. Patients are infectious from 4 to 5 days before until 4 days after the onset of rash. The course of disease can be complicated by otitis media (3%-9%), bronchitis or bronchopneumonia (1%-6%), and gastrointestinal and neurologic involvement. Postinfectious encephalitis complicates about 1 in 1000 infections, and subacute sclerosing panencephalitis (SSPE) affects approximately 1 in 1,000,000 cases, usually 7 to 10 years after acute measles. Measles also causes immunosupression, facilitating secondary bacterial infections, which are responsible for most measles deaths, especially in developing countries.

Measles outbreaks have sometimes been observed in highly vaccinated populations. A mild, vaccine-modified form of measles, not necessarily covered by the clinical case definition, can occur in vaccinated persons with low-level immunity. In contrast, patients who contracted measles after vaccination with a formalin-inactivated measles vaccine, licensed in 1961 and withdrawn from the market in 1966, suffered from a severe illness referred to as *atypical measles*.

## Diagnosis

The clinical case definition includes any person with fever (>38.3°C), maculopapular rash (≥ 3 d), and at least one of the symptoms of cough, coryza, or conjunctivitis. Laboratory confirmation is based on measles-specific IgM by enzyme-linked immunosorbent assay (ELISA), detected from onset of rash until weeks later. When IgM and IgG are negative early after onset of rash, repeat testing is warranted. The diagnosis can also be confirmed by an increase in measles-specific IgG between paired sera, detection of viral RNA by reverse-transcriptase polymerase chain reaction (RT-PCR), or virus isolation. Nasopharyngeal swabs, oral fluid, peripheral blood mononuclear cells (PBMCs), and the cellular fraction of urine are appropriate specimens for measles RT-PCR and virus isolation, as well as for genotyping of the virus in specialized laboratories. In most countries, confirmed or even suspected cases must be reported to the national health authorities.

## CURRENT DIAGNOSIS

- Fever (>38.3°C) and maculopapular rash (≥3 d) in association with cough, conjunctivitis, or coryza or some combination of these (CDC clinical case definition)
- Pathognomonic Koplik's spots on the buccal mucosa
- Detection of measles-specific IgM or increase in measles-specific IgG in paired sera
- Detection of viral RNA by reverse transcriptase polymerase chain reaction (RT-PCR) in nasopharyngeal swabs, oral fluid, urine, peripheral blood mononuclear cells (PBMCs), (or dried blood spots) with or without virus isolation

## Treatment

There is no specific treatment for acute measles. Supportive therapy includes hydration, antipyretics, bedrest, and protection from light for patients with photophobia. Secondary bacterial infections are treated with antibiotics. Vitamin A supplementation[1] has been shown to improve the clinical outcome in malnourished patients and patients with vitamin A deficiency. Ribavirin (Virazole)[1] and isoprinosin,[2] combined with interferon-α (IFN-α), have been used with limited success in experimental treatments of SSPE.

## Prevention

Measles virus has only one serotype, and current live-attenuated vaccines are effective against all of the 23 known genotypes. Vaccination induces long-lasting protection against the disease even after a single dose. Transplacentally acquired maternal antibodies and immaturity of the infant immune system interfere with seroconversion rates, which, after the first dose, range between 80% and 95% depending on the age of the vaccinee. Improper handling of the vaccine can

[1]Not FDA approved for this indication.
[2]Not available in the United States.

## CURRENT THERAPY

**Treatment**

- There is no specific therapy for treating acute measles.
- Patient care is limited to supportive therapy.
- Secondary bacterial infections are treated with antibiotics.
- Vitamin A supplementation[1] might improve the clinical outcome.

**Supportive Therapy**

- Hydration
- Antipyretics
- Rest
- Protection from light
- Vitamin A[1]
- Treatment for secondary bacterial infections

[1]Not FDA approved for this indication

be another reason for primary vaccine failures. Therefore, two-dose vaccination programs are necessary to achieve a population immunity greater than 95%, which is necessary to interrupt virus circulation.

Measles vaccination is recommended in virtually all countries, but immunization schedules depend on the specific epidemiologic situation of each country. Many industrialized countries use measles-mumps-rubella (MMR) combined vaccines, with a first dose given at 12 to 15 months of age and a second dose at 3 to 6 years of age to catch up children with primary or secondary vaccine failure after the first dose. In many developing countries with large birth cohorts and a higher measles incidence, monovalent measles vaccines (Attenuvax) are administered at 6 to 9 months of age to offset the higher risk of early exposure to wild-type virus and the earlier loss of maternal antibodies. A second dose should be provided as a routine revaccination during early childhood or in follow-up campaigns including broader age groups. Transient fever and rash are observed in 5% to 10% of patients vaccinated with live attenuated strains. Much publicized links to autism or other chronic diseases have never been confirmed by national or international scientific panels.

The vaccine is not recommended for children with primary or acquired severe immunodeficiency, except for children with asymptomatic HIV infection. The disease may be prevented in susceptible persons by hypergammaglobulin given within 6 days or by active immunization within 3 days after exposure. Passive immunization is also recommended in persons with some malignant diseases or deficits in cellular immunity.

## REFERENCES

Bannister BA, Begg NT, Gillespie SH: Childhood Infections: Measles. In Infectious Disease. Oxford: Blackwell Science, 1996, pp 256-260.
Campbell C, Levin S, Humphreys P, et al: Subacute sclerosing panencephalitis: Results of the Canadian Paediatric Surveillance Program and review of the literature. BMC Pediatr 2005;5:47.
Gershon AA: Measles virus. In Mandell GL, Bennett JE, Dolin R (eds): Principles and Practice of Infectious Diseases. New York: Churchill Livingstone, 1995, pp 1519-1525.
Griffin DE: Measles virus. In Knipe DM, Howley PM (eds): Fields Virology. Philadelphia: Lippincott Williams & Wilkins, 2001, pp 1401-1424
World Health Organization: Progress in reducing global measles deaths: 1999-2004. Wkly Epidemiol Rec 2006;81(10):90-94.

# Tetanus

Method of
*Samuel S. Hsu, MD*

Tetanus is a toxin-mediated infectious disease that is acquired from wounds and that results in muscular hyperexcitability and autonomic instability. It has a high mortality rate despite optimal treatment. It is best managed by prevention, which is accomplished with a highly effective low-cost vaccine. Victims are typically inadequately immunized.

## Etiology

The causative agent of tetanus is *Clostridium tetani*, a spore-forming, gram-positive bacillus. The vegetative form is an obligate anaerobe, but the spores remain viable at ambient oxygen concentrations. The spores are ubiquitous in soil, are highly resistant to extremes in temperature and humidity, and can survive indefinitely. When spores enter wounds, they might not germinate immediately if tissue conditions are unfavorable. They can activate well after the wound has healed, which might account for cases of tetanus that have no identifiable source. When conditions are favorable, the spores germinate into mature bacilli, which release the toxin tetanospasmin.

Tetanospasmin is responsible for the clinical manifestations of tetanus. It enters peripheral nerves and travels via retrograde axonal transport to the central nervous system. Tetanospasmin then enters presynaptic neurons and disrupts the release of γ-amino butyric acid (GABA) and glycine, which are inhibitory neurotransmitters. This results in a disinhibition of end-organ neurons, such as motor neurons and those of the autonomic nervous system. Recovery depends on synthesis of new presynaptic components, a process that occurs over 2 to 3 weeks.

## Epidemiology

Most cases occur in developing countries. In 2005, the World Health Organization (WHO) received reports of more than 15,000 cases, two thirds of which occurred in neonates. In contrast, tetanus is a disease of older adults in developed countries. According to the latest data from the Centers for Disease Control and Prevention (CDC), there are an average of 43 cases of tetanus per year in the United States, and the incidence is 0.16 per million population.

Even with optimal treatment, the mortality of tetanus is very high. The global fatality rate is estimated to be 30% to 50%. In the United States, the fatality rate ranges from 11% to 25%. Older adults have a higher mortality, 40% in those older than 60 years compared with 8% in those ages 20 to 59 years.

Lack of immunization is the greatest risk factor for contracting tetanus. The largest groups with the lowest rates of immunization in the United States are older adults and immigrants from Latin America. Serologic surveys show that although 95% of those 6 to 39 years old are adequately immunized, only 74% of those older than 60 years and 59% of those older than 70 years are adequately immunized. Only 75% of Latin American immigrants are adequately immunized. The result is a higher incidence of tetanus in these groups: 0.35 per million adults older than 60 years and 0.38 per million Latin Americans.

## Clinical Features

An acute injury precedes most cases of tetanus, the most common being puncture wounds and lacerations. Nonacute etiologies include chronic wounds, IV drug use, and complications of diabetes. Cases have occurred without a clear etiology. The median time between an injury and onset of symptoms is 7 days, but there have been delayed presentations of up to 3 months. A more rapid onset correlates to a more severe clinical presentation.

There are four clinical forms of tetanus representing the extent and location of neurons involved: generalized, local, cephalic, and neonatal.

In the United States and other developed countries, generalized tetanus is the most common form. The initial symptom in 50% to 75% of cases is trismus ("lockjaw") secondary to masseter muscle spasm. Risus sardonicus, the "ironical smile of tetanus," can occur due to facial muscle contraction. Nuchal rigidity and dysphagia can also be initial complaints. As the disease spreads, generalized muscle spasms occur, either spontaneously or to minor stimuli such as touch or noise. Opisthotonos, a tonic contraction very similar to decorticate posturing, is classically described with tetanus. Severe spasms can result in bone fractures, tendon detachments, and rhabdomyolysis. Mental status is not affected, and spasms are experienced with severe pain.

In the acute phase, death results from acute respiratory failure due to diaphragmatic paralysis or laryngeal spasms. In severe cases, autonomic instability can occur, resulting most importantly in labile hypertension, tachycardia, and pyrexia. Hypotension and bradycardia can also occur. Arrhythmias and myocardial infarction are the most common fatal events. The exact mechanism of this syndrome is unclear but likely involves disinhibition of the sympathetic nervous system.

Local tetanus manifests as persistent muscle rigidity close to a site of injury. The rigidity can linger for weeks to months and often resolves without sequelae. Localized tetanus rarely progresses to generalized tetanus.

## CURRENT DIAGNOSIS

- Tetanus is diagnosed on clinical grounds alone.
- Involuntary muscle spasms are the hallmark of tetanus.
- Generalized tetanus is the most common form. Characteristic features include trismus (lockjaw), risus sardonicus, and opisthotonos.
- Sensory function and mental status are preserved.
- Mimics of tetanus can be excluded by physical findings and select laboratory tests.

Cephalic tetanus is an uncommon variant of localized tetanus that involves the cranial nerves. Cephalic tetanus uniquely results in nerve palsies and muscle spasms. The seventh cranial nerve is most often involved, followed by the sixth, third, fourth, and 12th in decreasing order of frequency. With its predilection for the seventh cranial nerve, it commonly mimics Bell's palsy. Cephalic tetanus also manifests with trismus, but cranial nerve deficits precede the onset of trismus about 40% of the time. Head trauma and otitis media are commonly cited etiologies. About two thirds of cases progress to generalized tetanus.

Neonatal tetanus is generalized tetanus that occurs in newborns around the first week of life. Symptoms begin with nonspecific irritability and poor feeding, and they rapidly progress to generalized spasms. The portal of entry is the freshly cut umbilical cord. The risk of contracting neonatal tetanus is directly related to maternal immunization status, because passive transfer of maternal immunoglobulins is protective. Mortality is very high, 50% to 100%, due to the high load of toxin per body weight in neonates. In the United States, there were three reports of neonatal tetanus in the 1990s, all involving inadequately immunized mothers.

## Diagnosis

The diagnosis of tetanus must be made on clinical grounds alone. There are no laboratory tests that can diagnose or exclude tetanus. Wound cultures rarely yield *C. tetani* and are not available quickly enough to aid diagnosis. Fortunately, the presentation of tetanus is so characteristic that a presumptive diagnosis can be made in most cases. When faced with a potential case of tetanus, it is useful to recall that sensory function and mental status remain normal.

The differential diagnosis is minimal. Most possibilities can be excluded by history, examination, and select laboratory tests. Exact mimics of tetanus occur with strychnine poisoning, which disables glycine release as tetanospasmin does, and hypocalcemia. These are easily excluded by laboratory tests. The differential for trismus includes peritonsillar/odontogenic abscesses and dystonic reactions. Cephalic tetanus without trismus can be easily mistaken for Bell's palsy, central nervous system tumor, or stroke. Neonatal tetanus initially manifests much like a host of other disorders. Once generalized spasms begin, the diagnosis is obvious.

Apte and Karnad describe a bedside test for tetanus in which a spatula is inserted into the pharynx. If the patient gags and tries to expel the spatula, the test is negative for tetanus; if the patient bites the spatula due to reflex masseter spasm, the test is positive for tetanus. The researchers reported 94% sensitivity and 100% specificity.

## Treatment

Treatment involves neutralizing tetanospasmin, removing the source of the toxin, and providing supportive care for muscle spasms, respiration, and autonomic instability. Human tetanus immunoglobulin (hTIG, BayTet) 500 IU IM neutralizes circulating tetanospasmin. It cannot inactivate toxin already within neurons. Its half-life is 25 days; only a single dose is necessary. Doses of hTIG up to 10,000 IU have been used, but the lower dose is effective and has the advantage of

## CURRENT THERAPY

### ACUTE TETANUS

- Human tetanus immune globulin (hTIG, BayTet) 500 IU IM neutralizes tetanus toxin.
- Metronidazole (Flagyl) eliminates reservoirs of *Clostridium tetani*.
- Wounds and abscess must be débrided and drained.
- Benzodiazepines are the drugs of choice to control muscle spasms. In severe cases, paralytics and mechanical ventilation may be required.
- Tetanus immunization must be initiated because surviving tetanus does not confer immunity.

### PROPHYLAXIS IN ACUTE WOUNDS

- Administer tetanus toxoid (Td) if the last booster was more than 10 y ago in non–tetanus-prone or more than 5 y ago in tetanus-prone wounds.
- Administer hTIG 250 IU IM if the patient never completed a primary immunization series and has a tetanus-prone wound.
- Pregnancy is not a contraindication to appropriate use of Td or hTIG.

requiring fewer injections to deliver. This feature is not insignificant, because hTIG is supplied in 250-IU doses, and injections are powerful stimuli for spasms. The adult and pediatric doses are the same. The burden of tetanospasmin, not the patient's size, determines the amount of hTIG needed.

To prevent ongoing production of toxin, antibiotics are needed to eliminate reservoirs of *C. tetani*. Metronidazole (Flagyl) in standard dose is the drug of choice. Penicillin, the historic drug of choice, does not penetrate devascularized wounds and abscesses well. Penicillin also has GABA-antagonist activity, which can potentiate the effects of tetanospasmin. In addition to antibiotics, obviously dirty wounds, abscesses, or devitalized tissue must be cleaned, drained, or excised to decrease the bacterial load.

Benzodiazepines are the drug of choice for muscle spasms because of their GABA-agonist and sedative properties. Daily doses of hundreds or thousands of milligrams have been used to control spasms. For severe cases, paralytics and mechanical ventilation may be needed. Vecuronium (Norcuron)[1] is an ideal agent for immediate and long-term control due to its minimal cardiovascular effects.

Treatment of autonomic instability has been problematic and is the subject of ongoing research. No therapeutic regimen has proved to be universally effective. α-Blockers,[1] β-blockers,[1] clonidine (Catapres),[1] and magnesium[1] have yielded variable success. Fentanyl (Sublimaze)[1] centrally decreases sympathetic outflow and has produced more consistent control of hypertension and tachycardia.

Supportive care includes placing the patient in a quiet, dark environment, minimizing patient manipulation, and treating for complications, most significantly rhabdomyolysis. Importantly, survivors must also receive a tetanus immunization series. The amount of tetanospasmin produced in clinical tetanus is small and partially sequestered in neurons; consequently, an immune response does not occur. Unimmunized survivors of tetanus have become victims a second time.

---

[1]Not FDA approved for this indication.

## Prevention

Tetanus is preventable with proper use of tetanus toxoid and hTIG. Tetanus toxoid is an inactivated form of tetanospasmin. It is available as a single-antigen tetanus toxoid (TT) and combined with diphtheria and pertussis vaccine. The combination vaccines (e.g., Td for adults) are preferable because concurrent immunization is appropriate. The recommended primary immunization schedule is shown in Table 1. Adults should receive boosters every 10 years to maintain immunity.

Common adverse reactions to tetanus toxoid include erythema, swelling, and tenderness at the injection site. Nonspecific systemic effects such as fever, malaise, and anorexia can also occur. Reactions tend to occur more often and more severely if boosters are given more frequently than the recommended schedule. Patients who give a history of "allergy" to tetanus vaccine are most likely referring to a local or nonspecific systemic reaction. These are not contraindications to receiving tetanus toxoid. Other false contraindications include mild, acute illness; fever; and family history of an adverse reaction to vaccination. Anaphylactic reactions, neuropathies, and encephalopathies are rare and constitute the only true contraindications for giving toxoid. Patients who give a history of anaphylaxis should be referred for skin testing because they might no longer be reactive and can receive future vaccinations.

hTIG is derived from human plasma. It is available as 250-IU doses and is approved only for intramuscular use. Intradermal injection cause local irritation due to the concentration of the product and does not represent an allergy to hTIG. Because of this reaction, hTIG should not be infiltrated into the wound. Intravenous injection can cause hypotension. Adverse reactions to properly administered hTIG are rare and consist largely of discomfort at the injection site and slight temperature elevation.

In the setting of an acute injury, the CDC recommendations for tetanus prophylaxis depend on the wound characteristics and the patient's immunization history (Table 2). Many acute wounds can be considered not tetanus prone: recent wounds, linear wounds with sharp edges, well-vascularized wounds, and wounds not obviously contaminated or infected. All other wounds are considered tetanus prone, particularly those resulting from blunt trauma and bites and those that are grossly contaminated or infected.

If the patient has completed primary immunization, a booster is given if the last dose was longer than 5 years ago in a tetanus-prone wound or more than 10 years ago in a non–tetanus-prone wound. Patients with a contraindication to tetanus toxoid must be treated with hTIG alone.

If the patient has not completed primary immunization and the wound is tetanus prone, hTIG 250 IU IM is indicated. hTIG should be given at a site contralateral to the tetanus toxoid to prevent interaction between the two. A tetanus booster is also required, and the patient will need follow-up to complete primary immunization.

### TABLE 1  Tetanus Primary Immunization

| Age | Vaccine | No. of Doses | Schedule |
| --- | --- | --- | --- |
| <7 y | DTaP or DT | 5 | Doses 1-4 at 2, 4, 6, 15 mo<br>Dose 5 between 4 and 6 y |
| >7 y | Td | 3 | First 2 doses more than 4 wk apart<br>Dose 3 at 6 mo after dose 2 |

*Abbreviations:* DT = diphtheria and tetanus (adult); DTaP = diphtheria and tetanus toxoids and acellular pertussis; Td = diphtheria and tetanus (pediatric).
From Immunization Practices Advisory Committee: Diphtheria, tetanus, and pertussis: Recommendations for vaccine use and other preventive measures: Recommendations of the Immunization Practices Advisory Committee (ACIP). MMWR 1991;40(RR-10):1-28.

## TABLE 2  Tetanus Prophylaxis in the Acute Wound

| Wound Status | Primary Immunization | | | |
|---|---|---|---|---|
| | Completed or Last Booster | | | Not Completed |
| | <5 y | >5 y | >10 y | |
| **Clean** | | | | |
| Td* | Yes | No | No | Yes |
| **Tetanus-prone** | | | | |
| Td | Yes | No | Yes | Yes |
| TIG | Yes | No | No | No |

*DTaP or DT for children younger than 7 years.
*Abbreviations:* DT = diphtheria and tetanus (adult); DTaP = diphtheria and tetanus toxoids and acellular pertussis; Td = diphtheria and tetanus (pediatric); TIG = tetanus immune globulin.
Adapted from Immunization Practices Advisory Committee: Diphtheria, tetanus, and pertussis: Recommendations for vaccine use and other preventive measures: Recommendations of the Immunization Practices Advisory Committee (ACIP). MMWR 1991;40(RR-10):1-28.

Due to an aging immune system, in elderly patients tetanus antibodies after vaccination do not form as quickly, do not have as high a peak, and do not persist as long as in younger persons. With low rates of baseline immunity, elderly patients who receive only a tetanus booster can not develop protective levels of antibodies quickly enough in the setting of an acute injury. More liberal use of hTIG in these patients, regardless of primary immunization, may be warranted to ensure protection against tetanus if the last booster was significantly longer than 10 years ago.

Td is safe in pregnancy. Generally, routine immunizations are avoided in the first trimester; however there is considerable evidence that Td is not teratogenic. In the setting of acute wounds, Td should not be withheld if indicated. hTIG is also safe in pregnancy. The main risk with donated biological products is infection, not teratogenesis. Other immune globulin products, such as Rh immune globulin (RhoGam), are commonly used during pregnancy without adverse effects.

## REFERENCES

Ahmadsyah I, Salim A: Treatment of tetanus: An open study to compare the efficacy of procaine penicillin and metronidazole. Br J Med (Clin Res Ed) 1985;291:648-650.

American College of Obstetrics and Gynecology: Immunization during pregnancy. ACOG Committee Opinion No. 282. Obstet Gynecol 2003;101:207-212.

Apte NM, Karnad DR: Short report: The spatula test: A simple bedside test to diagnose tetanus. Am J Trop Med Hyg 1995;53(4):386-387.

Bleck TP, Brauner JS: Tetanus. In Scheld WM, Whitely RJ, Durack DT (eds): Infections of the Central Nervous System, 2nd ed. Philadelphia: Lippincott-Raven, 1997, pp 629-653.

Centers for Disease Control. and Prevention: Diphtheria, tetanus, and pertussis: Recommendations for vaccine use and other preventive measures: Recommendations of the Immunization Practices Advisory Committee (ACIP). MMWR 1991;40(RR-10):1-28.

Centers for Disease Control and Prevention: Tetanus surveillance—United States, 1998-2000. MMWR Surveill Summ 2003;52(SS-3):1-8.

Dietz V, Galazka A, Loon F, et al: Factors affecting the immunogenicity and potency of tetanus toxoid: Implications for the elimination of neonatal and non-neonatal tetanus as public health problems. Bull World Health Org 1997;75(1):81-93.

Sanford JP: Tetanus—forgotten but not gone. N Engl J Med 1995;332(12):812-813.

Silveira CM, Caceres VM, Dutra MG, et al: Safety of tetanus toxoid in pregnant women: A hospital-based case-control study of congenital anomalies. Bull World Health Org 1995;73:605-608.

Talan D, Abrahamian F, Moran G, et al: Tetanus immunity and physician compliance with tetanus prophylaxis practices among emergency department patients presenting with wounds. Ann Emerg Med 2004;43(3):305-314.

# Pertussis

Method of
*Michael E. Pichichero, MD*

Pertussis, or whooping cough, is a highly contagious acute respiratory tract infection caused by *Bordetella pertussis*. It causes prolonged cough illness, without associated fever, characterized by paroxysms of coughing, inspiratory "whoops," and post-tussive vomiting in severe cases and persistent intermittent staccato cough episodes in teenagers and adults. The incidence of pertussis is rising in the United States despite record-high vaccination coverage. In 2004, more cases occurred in adolescents and in adults than children.

## Microbiology and Pathophysiology

*B. pertussis* is a gram-negative coccobacillus that is difficult to grow with standard media. *B. pertussis* does not invade the human host; bacteremia does not occur. The systemic effects of illness are produced by the organism's toxins, especially pertussis toxin. *B. pertussis* attaches to the nasopharynx and tracheobronchial tree with adhesins such as fimbriae, filamentous hemagglutinin, and pertactin where it produces toxins such as pertussis toxin, adenylate cyclase toxin, and tracheal cytotoxin that paralyze the respiratory cilia, resulting in inflammation of the respiratory tract.

## Epidemiology

*B. pertussis* is a human pathogen transmitted from person to person via aerosolized droplets. Pertussis is highly contagious, similar to varicella, infecting 80% to 90% of susceptible contacts. Persons with pertussis are most contagious in the 2 weeks before cough onset and during the first 2 weeks of cough, typically a time frame before medical care is sought or clinicians consider the possibility of the diagnosis.

In 2004, approximately 20,000 cases of pertussis were reported to the Centers for Disease Control and Prevention (CDC); because substantial underreporting is a recognized problem, current estimates of true pertussis incidence per year in the United States probably is in the range of 1 to 3 million cases. A new development is the recognition that pertussis is a disease of adolescents and adults as well as children. Several studies showed that among teenagers and adults who seek care for cough illness of more than 1 week duration, approximately 20% have pertussis.

## Immunity

It has been known for decades that immunity to tetanus wanes over time and boosters are needed approximately every 10 years to sustain protective antibody levels. The phenomenon of waning immunity to pertussis is a newer observation and one of the explanations of the rising incidence of pertussis in the United States. Apparently boosters of pertussis vaccines are also needed, perhaps, like tetanus, approximately every 10 years. Two new adolescent/adult pertussis vaccine formulations that are combined with tetanus and diphtheria vaccines (Boostrix, Adacel) were licensed and recommended for universal use in 2005 to address this problem.

## Clinical Symptoms

Classic pertussis is a 30- to 90-day illness that presents in three stages: catarrhal, paroxysmal, and convalescent. The stages may be shorter in immunized children, adolescents, and adults. Pertussis is most severe when it occurs during the first 6 months of life.

**TABLE 1** Complications From Pertussis in Adolescents and Adults

| Symptoms/Signs | Minnesota | Massachusetts | |
|---|---|---|---|
| | | Adolescents | Adults |
| Paroxysmal cough | 100% | 85% | 87% |
| Whooping | 26% | 30% | 35% |
| Post-tussive emesis | 56% | 45% | 41% |
| Apnea | — | 19% | 37% |
| Cyanosis | — | 6% | 9% |
| Hospitalization | 0% | 1.4% | 3.5% |

In the catarrhal stage, nonspecific symptoms similar to the common cold predominate. The paroxysmal stage is characterized by a persistent cough, sometimes with bursts of numerous rapid coughs. A long inspiratory effort sometimes causes a high-pitched whoop. Typically, the patient is afebrile and, between coughing attacks, usually appears normal. The paroxysmal stage usually lasts 6 weeks. The cough gradually lessens over 2 to 3 weeks during the convalescent period. Milder paroxysms may recur with subsequent respiratory infections for many months following a pertussis infection. Infants may appear very ill and distressed during the paroxysmal stage and require close observation and supportive care. Older children, adolescents, and adults have a prolonged cough with paroxysms but no whoop.

## Complications

Complications occur most commonly among young infants with pertussis. The most common complication is secondary bacterial pneumonia. Hypoxia or effects of pertussis toxin may contribute to neurologic complications including seizures and encephalopathy. In the United States, 90% of deaths occur in children younger than 6 months. Complications from pertussis in adolescents and adults are not uncommon (Table 1).

## Diagnosis

A clinical diagnosis of pertussis is typically made based on the characteristic cough, although patients are often seen several times before the correct diagnosis is considered. Absolute lymphocytosis (>10,000 lymphcytes/mm$^3$) may be seen during the late catarrhal and paroxysmal stages but is less common among adults and immunized children.

### CURRENT DIAGNOSIS

- An illness marked by a staccato cough lasting >7 d in the absence of fever in an adolescent or adult may be pertussis.

Chest radiographs may show peribronchial consolidation, interstitial edema, or variable atelectasis. The presence of fever and consolidation with pertussis suggests a secondary bacterial pneumonia.

Isolation of *B. pertussis* from a culture of nasal secretions remains the gold standard for laboratory diagnosis. A nasopharyngeal specimen is obtained by inserting a small flexible Dacron or calcium alginate swab through the nose to the posterior nasopharynx (attempting to touch the adenoids) where it is held for a few seconds, perhaps inducing a cough. The specimen is transferred to *Bordetella*-specific transport media and subsequently plated on Regan-Lowe charcoal agar or Stainer-Scholte agar. Cultures are usually positive if obtained in the catarrhal or early paroxysmal stage of disease. Success in isolating *B. pertussis* diminishes if patients have received pertussis vaccine or recent antimicrobials or if specimens are obtained beyond the first 2 weeks of cough.

Polymerase chain reaction (PCR) is more sensitive among persons with mild or atypical symptoms and those who have received prior antimicrobial therapy. The CDC recommends using PCR as a presumptive assay in conjunction with culture. Direct fluorescent antibody (DFA) testing has a low sensitivity and variable specificity, requiring experienced laboratory personnel for consistent results. DFA testing should only be performed as a adjunct to culture or PCR. Serologic testing methods have recently emerged as a very valuable diagnostic tool. Single samples of 100 µL of blood can be used to measure pertussis antibodies that are compared to age-specific standards to confirm a clinical diagnosis. These methods are not widely available in hospitals or private laboratories, but state laboratories often can provide this testing.

## Treatment

Infants and children with severe cough paroxysms associated with cyanosis or apnea require hospitalization and intensive care. Infants younger than 3 months should be admitted routinely for observation of their paroxysmal episodes, their need for supportive interventions, and their ability to feed appropriately. Continuous monitoring of heart rate, respiratory rate, and oxygen saturation is indicated.

**TABLE 2** Licensed Vaccines for the Prevention of Pertussis in Infants, Children, Adolescents, and Adults

| Indicated Age Group | Sanofi Pasteur Tripedia infants/children[†] | GlaxoSmithKline Infanrix* infants/children[†] | Sanofi Pasteur Daptacel infants/children[†] | GlaxoSmithKline Boostrix adolescents[‡] | Sanofi Pasteur Adacel adults/adolescents[‡] |
|---|---|---|---|---|---|
| **Antigens** | | | | | |
| PT (µg) | 23.4 | 25 | 10 | 8 | 2.5 |
| FHA (µg) | 23.4 | 25 | 5 | 8 | 5 |
| PRN (µg) | — | 8 | 3 | 2.5 | 3 |
| FIM 2 + 3 (µg) | — | — | 5 | — | 5 |
| D (Lf) | 6.7 | 25 | 15 | 2.5 | 2 |
| T (Lf) | 5 | 10 | 5 | 5 | 5 |

*PEDIARIX also contains these DTaP components.
[†]6 wk to <7 y.
[‡]Boostrix is indicated for 10–18 y; Adacel is indicated for 11–54 y.
*Abbreviations:* D = diphtheria toxoid; FHA = filamentous hemagglutinin; FIM 2 + 3 = fimbrial agglutinogen 2 and 3; PRN = pertactin; PT = pertussis toxoid; T = tetanus toxoid.

## CURRENT THERAPY

- Early treatment of pertussis not only eliminates contagion, it also shortens the illness.
- Macrolides are the treatment of choice; azithromycin (Zithromax) is preferred for ease of dosing, tolerability, and short duration of treatment.

All patients should receive antibiotics. Macrolides are the treatment of choice: erythromycin, clarithromycin (Biaxin),[1] azithromycin (Zithromax),[1] or telithromycin (Ketek).[1] Fluoroquinolones are also effective therapy for pertussis. Trimethoprim-sulfamethoxazole (Bactrim)[1] is an alternative choice although less effective.

## Prevention

Pertussis is a preventable disease by vaccination. Vaccines are available and recommended for universal use in infants, children, adolescents, and selected adult populations (health care workers, adults caring for infants younger than 6 months, and those with chronic respiratory conditions, e.g., chronic obstructive pulmonary disease). Table 2 lists the vaccines licensed in the United States.

### REFERENCES

Farizo KM, Cochi SL, Zell ER, et al: Epidemiological features of pertussis in the United States, 1980–1989. Clin Infect Dis 1992;14(3):708-719.
Lee LH, Pichichero ME. Costs of illness due to *Bordetella pertussis* in families. Arch Fam Med 2000;9(10):989-996.
Pichichero ME, Rennels MB, Edwards KM, et al: Combined tetanus, diphtheria, and 5-component pertussis vaccine for use in adolescents and adults. JAMA 2005;293(24):3003-3011.
Purdy KW, Hay JW, Botteman MF, et al: Evaluation of strategies for use of acellular pertussis vaccine in adolescents and adults: A cost-benefit analysis. Clin Infect Dis 2004;39:20-28.
Skowronski DM, De Serres G, MacDonald D, et al: The changing age and seasonal profile of pertussis in Canada. J Infect Dis 2002;185(10): 1448-1453. Epub 2002 Apr 22.
Strebel P, Nordin J, Edwards K, et al: Population-based incidence of pertussis among adolescents and adults, Minnesota, 1995–1996. J Infect Dis 2001;183(9):1353-1359. Epub 2001 Mar 30.
Yih WK, Lett SM, des Vignes FN, et al: The increasing incidence of pertussis in Massachusetts adolescents and adults, 1989–1998. J Infect Dis 2000;182(5):1409-1416. Epub 2000 Oct 09.

# Office-Based Immunization Practices

Method of
*Robert M. Jacobson, MD*

Routine immunizations represent the cutting edge for consensus-driven, evidence-based practice guidelines in the care of children and adults. Perhaps no other office-based task is so universally accepted and practiced as well as evidenced as immunizations. We should be modeling the rest of our practices on the success that we have enjoyed with immunizations.

---

[1]Not FDA approved for this indication.

## CURRENT DIAGNOSIS

- At each patient contact, practitioners should review the patient's immunization record for vaccines due and overdue.

That is not to say that we are providing immunizations as well as we should; the practice of immunization is difficult, complex, and evolving. Other chapters deal with the specific diseases to which we direct our vaccines. Office practitioners must consider a variety of aspects that go beyond the understanding of the individual vaccine-preventable diseases. These include the adoption of a comprehensive immunization schedule, using a number of immunization-specific practices, and the understanding of common problems associated with immunization in the office.

## The Adoption of a Comprehensive Immunization Schedule

In recent years, we have benefited from efforts made at the national level to harmonize and systematically update recommended schedules for routine immunizations (Table 1). The Advisory Committee on Immunization Practices (ACIP), sponsored by the Centers for Disease Control and Prevention (CDC), works closely with the American Academy of Pediatrics (AAP) and the American Academy of Family Physicians (AAFP) to publish a single set of recommendations for routine immunizations for infants, children, and adolescents younger than 18 years. The Recommended Adult Immunization Schedule is similarly approved by the ACIP, the American College of Obstetricians and Gynecologists (ACOG), and the AAFP. These are published widely in a number of journals as well as on the internet. The harmonized schedules address the use of both individual vaccine components as well as all licensed combination vaccines. The vaccine schedules give ranges of target age ranges for immunization rather than prescribe individual ages. For example, the measles-mumps-rubella combination is to be given from 12 to 15 months of life rather than either 12 months or 15 months. Furthermore, the pediatric schedule includes catch-up schedules for children who did not receive immunizations at the recommended ages. The adult schedule includes common conditions with vaccine-specific recommendations (such as for pregnancy).

Each of the 50 states in the United States has specific immunization requirements for day care, school, and even college attendance. These vary state by state and in some states affect not only initial enrollment but also continued participation in schools. Furthermore, the harmonized schedule mentioned previously has state-specific recommendations for the hepatitis A vaccine recommended for 11 of the 50 states where endemic rates of hepatitis A disease occur at more than 20 cases per 100,000 people.

For your office practice, you are encouraged to adopt a more specific schedule. For example, where the harmonized schedule might give you some latitude with what age to give the dose for the measles-mumps-rubella vaccine, it would be more appropriate for you and your colleagues to pick either 12 or 15 months. When all practitioners sharing an office adopt a uniform practice, they prevent parental and staff confusion and misunderstanding as well as mistakes in vaccine administration and patient scheduling.

## Adoption of Immunization-Specific Practices

### EDUCATION OF SELF AND STAFF

Immunization practices certainly have evolved over the last century, and much of the development has accelerated since the enactment of

## CURRENT THERAPY

- Providing routine immunizations requires an office to organize its educational activities, practice standards, communication methods, and documentation strategies.

the National Childhood Vaccine Injury Act of 1986 (PL 99-660), which established the national Vaccine Injury Compensation Program (VICP), a no-fault alternative to the tort system for resolving vaccine injury claims. This legislation protects vaccine providers and manufacturers from frivolous lawsuits directed against routine childhood immunization. Although in the 1980s it was routine for a child in the first year of life to receive three injections and three oral doses of polio, now the typical infant at 12 months of age may receive 20 separate injections against vaccine-preventable disease. In 2005, two new vaccines were added to the routine childhood schedule: the meningococcal conjugated vaccine (Menactra) and the tetanus-diphtheria-reduced-dose-acellular pertussis (Tdap) vaccine (Boostrix) that replaces the adolescent tetanus-diphtheria (Td) vaccine. Both are to be given routinely at 11 years of age. Such changes require a practitioner's continuing education and practice advancement.

A number of electronic Web sites provide announcements and updates of vaccines in form delivered for health care practitioners; the CDC provides a Web site (www.cdc.gov/vaccines) with information resources for both parents and health care practitioners including sections on updates. In addition, the Immunization Action Coalition, a not-for-profit group dedicated to the dissemination of scientifically correct immunization information, also has a very useful Web site (www.immunize.org). The latter invites practitioners to sign up for routine mailings of updates on immunization practices. Similarly, providers can access the CDC's Morbidity and Mortality Weekly Report (MMWR) online. These provide updates and statements from ACIP. Furthermore, the AAP publishes on its Web site (www.pediatrics.org) its policy statements and recommendation online for members and nonmembers alike.

Paper-based resources are more difficult to keep up to date, but important ones include the paper-based publication *MMWR* published by the CDC and the *Red Book* published by the AAP. The *Red Book* not only does an outstanding job with vaccine-related issues but also includes a host of information for a general practitioner on pediatric and adolescent infectious diseases. The CDC publishes the "Pink Book" both in paper and online. It is formally entitled *Epidemiology and Prevention of Vaccine Preventable Diseases.*

The CDC and the Medical University of South Carolina have sponsored the development of an electronic-based educational program called Teaching Immunization Delivery and Evaluation (TIDE). Its Web site is http://www2.edserv.musc.edu/tide/menu.lasso, and the program is endorsed by the Ambulatory Pediatric Association and the Society of Adolescent Medicine. It is a flexible tool to teach immunization delivery, and it uses clinical scenarios that inspire problem solving. Self-contained modules are available that provide continued education credit.

## ASSESSMENT OF INDIVIDUAL NEEDS

Each patient is unique, but the success of the routine immunization schedule depends on its universality. Precautions and contraindications exist, and the children and adults who most frequently attend health care providers' offices have relatively higher rates of chronic conditions than the general population. These conditions raise questions of contraindications and precautions. Therefore, individuals must be assessed for their individual needs. Even misperceptions of contraindications can lead to delays and require catch-up. Practitioners should be familiar with the routine schedules (Tables 1 and 2) as well as the general precautions of contraindications associated with each vaccine.

One of the most important resources available for the busy practitioner is a chart developed by the CDC organized by condition that specifies which vaccines are contraindicated by that condition. This chart is on the CDC Web site under the tab of Healthcare Professionals. It is entitled "Guide to Contraindications" (www.cdc.gov/vaccines/recs/vac-admin/contraindication).

The CDC has developed survey tools that are available freely to download from its Web site (www.cdc.gov/vaccines). The practitioner can use this with the individual patient to assess vaccine needs. Assessment tools are available online for both adults and children.

## PATIENT EDUCATION

Patient and parent education is incredibly important in applying immunizations. After all, we are giving a form of a biologic with known rates and associations with adverse events to large numbers of persons who are often well and without a medical need or condition. We should inform the patient, and, in the case of a child or adolescent not yet at the age of majority, the parent as best we can about the immunizations, the diseases for which we are vaccinating, the nature of the benefits from the vaccines, as well as the common adverse reactions and possible severe adverse reactions that might occur. The patients and parents should learn for whom the vaccines should be received as well as for whom the vaccines not be received and what they should do in case of an adverse event. This information is complex in depth and breadth, but the National Childhood Vaccine Injury Act of 1986 that created protection for vaccine providers and manufacturers at the same time created regulations with a uniform system of vaccine information statements to be provided. The National Immunization Program publishes brief vaccine-specific statements for all of the routine vaccines given to children and adults. These Vaccine Information Statements (VISs) are published in a highly readable format (www.cdc.gov/vaccines/pubs/vis) and are required by U.S. law to be provided to the parent and recipient before each dose of certain vaccines including those on a routine childhood vaccine schedule. VISs also exist for some of the more exotic vaccines, such as the Japanese encephalitis vaccine, the smallpox vaccine, the typhoid vaccines, the yellow fever vaccine, as well as for the rabies vaccines. The Immunization Action Coalition (www.immunize.org) has partnered with the CDC and has translated the VISs for each vaccine into more than 20 different languages. More detailed information for the vaccines can be obtained from the statements from the ACIP (www.cdc.gov/vaccines/recs/acip), the Food and Drug Administration– approved package inserts, and the AAP's *Red Book.*

## PREVACCINATION PREPARATION

Not only should the parent and recipient of the vaccine be provided the VIS, but efforts should be taken to minimize the discomfort of the recipient. Information plays a large role. A study done at the Mayo Clinic demonstrated that informing the child prior to the visit actually decreased the amount of distress observed at the time of the visit. Furthermore, efforts at the time of the visit including distraction or relaxation techniques can prevent or reduce distress associated with the vaccine. Office staff should learn methods of successful communication, distraction, and relaxation techniques to facilitate routine immunizations.

For some of the vaccines, antipyretics such as acetaminophen (Tylenol) or ibuprofen (Advil) might be administered at the time of immunization and then at regular intervals specific to that drug for the following 24 hours to reduce the occurrence and the severity of fever as well as the local injection pain that might occur with immunization.

The *Red Book* Committee, the Committee on Infectious Diseases of the AAP, recommends that practitioners consider a variety of efforts to minimize the discomfort of immunization including specific injection techniques, the use of multiple vaccinators to immunize simultaneously rather than serially, as well as possibly local anesthetics and nonpharmacologic agents.

## VACCINE DELIVERY

Some vaccines are given intramuscularly (IM) or subcutaneously (SC); still others, via the mouth or nose. IM vaccines should be given deep

**TABLE 1** Recommended Childhood and Adolescent Immunization Schedule

DEPARTMENT OF HEALTH AND HUMAN SERVICES • CENTERS FOR DISEASE CONTROL AND PREVENTION

# Recommended Immunization Schedule for Persons Aged 0–6 Years—UNITED STATES • 2007

| Vaccine▼  Age▶ | Birth | 1 month | 2 months | 4 months | 6 months | 12 months | 15 months | 18 months | 19–23 months | 2–3 years | 4–6 years |
|---|---|---|---|---|---|---|---|---|---|---|---|
| Hepatitis B[1] | HepB | HepB | see footnote 1 | | HepB | | | | HepB Series | | |
| Rotavirus[2] | | | Rota | Rota | Rota | | | | | | |
| Diphtheria, Tetanus, Pertussis[3] | | | DTaP | DTaP | DTaP | | DTaP | | | | DTaP |
| *Haemophilus influenzae* type b[4] | | | Hib | Hib | Hib[4] | Hib | | Hib | | | |
| Pneumococcal[5] | | | PCV | PCV | PCV | PCV | | | | PCV PPV | |
| Inactivated Poliovirus | | | IPV | IPV | | IPV | | | | | IPV |
| Influenza[6] | | | | | | Influenza (Yearly) | | | | | |
| Measles, Mumps, Rubella[7] | | | | | | MMR | | | | | MMR |
| Varicella[8] | | | | | | Varicella | | | | | Varicella |
| Hepatitis A[9] | | | | | | HepA (2 doses) | | | | HepA Series | |
| Meningococcal[10] | | | | | | | | | | MPSV4 | |

Range of recommended ages

Catch-up immunization

Certain high-risk groups

This schedule indicates the recommended ages for routine administration of currently licensed childhood vaccines, as of December 1, 2006, for children aged 0–6 years. Additional information is available at http://www.cdc.gov/nip/recs/child-schedule.htm. Any dose not administered at the recommended age should be administered at any subsequent visit, when indicated and feasible. Additional vaccines may be licensed and recommended during the year. Licensed combination vaccines may be used whenever any components of the combination are indicated and other components of the vaccine are not contraindicated and if approved by the Food and Drug Administration for that dose of the series. Providers should consult the respective Advisory Committee on Immunization Practices statement for detailed recommendations. Clinically significant adverse events that follow immunization should be reported to the Vaccine Adverse Event Reporting System (VAERS). Guidance about how to obtain and complete a VAERS form is available at **http://www.vaers. hhs.gov** or by telephone, **800-822-7967**.

1. **Hepatitis B vaccine (HepB).** *(Minimum age: birth)*
   **At birth:**
   • Administer monovalent HepB to all newborns before hospital discharge.
   • If mother is hepatitis surface antigen (HBsAg)-positive, administer HepB and 0.5 mL of hepatitis B immune globulin (HBIG) within 12 hours of birth.
   • If mother's HBsAg status is unknown, administer HepB within 12 hours of birth. Determine the HBsAg status as soon as possible and if HBsAg-positive, administer HBIG (no later than age 1 week).
   • If mother is HBsAg-negative, the birth dose can only be delayed with physician's order and mother's negative HBsAg laboratory report documented in the infant's medical record.
   **After the birth dose:**
   • The HepB series should be completed with either monovalent HepB or a combination vaccine containing HepB. The second dose should be administered at age 1–2 months. The final dose should be administered at age ≥24 weeks. Infants born to HBsAg-positive mothers should be tested for HBsAg and antibody to HBsAg after completion of ≥3 doses of a licensed HepB series, at age 9–18 months (generally at the next well-child visit).
   **4-month dose:**
   • It is permissible to administer 4 doses of HepB when combination vaccines are administered after the birth dose. If monovalent HepB is used for doses after the birth dose, a dose at age 4 months is not needed.

2. **Rotavirus vaccine (Rota).** *(Minimum age: 6 weeks)*
   • Administer the first dose at age 6–12 weeks. Do not start the series later than age 12 weeks.
   • Administer the final dose in the series by age 32 weeks. Do not administer a dose later than age 32 weeks.
   • Data on safety and efficacy outside of these age ranges are insufficient.

3. **Diphtheria and tetanus toxoids and acellular pertussis vaccine (DTaP).** *(Minimum age: 6 weeks)*
   • The fourth dose of DTaP may be administered as early as age 12 months, provided 6 months have elapsed since the third dose.
   • Administer the final dose in the series at age 4–6 years.

4. ***Haemophilus influenzae* type b conjugate vaccine (Hib).**
   *(Minimum age: 6 weeks)*
   • If PRP-OMP (PedvaxHIB® or ComVax® [Merck]) is administered at ages 2 and 4 months, a dose at age 6 months is not required.
   • TriHiBit® (DTaP/Hib) combination products should not be used for primary immunization but can be used as boosters following any Hib vaccine in children aged ≥12 months.

5. **Pneumococcal vaccine.** *(Minimum age: 6 weeks for pneumococcal conjugate vaccine [PCV]; 2 years for pneumococcal polysaccharide vaccine [PPV])*
   • Administer PCV at ages 24–59 months in certain high-risk groups. Administer PPV to children aged ≥2 years in certain high-risk groups. See *MMWR* 2000;49(No. RR-9):1–35.

6. **Influenza vaccine.** *(Minimum age: 6 months for trivalent inactivated influenza vaccine [TIV]; 5 years for live, attenuated influenza vaccine [LAIV])*
   • All children aged 6–59 months and close contacts of all children aged 0–59 months are recommended to receive influenza vaccine.
   • Influenza vaccine is recommended annually for children aged ≥59 months with certain risk factors, health-care workers, and other persons (including household members) in close contact with persons in groups at high risk. See *MMWR* 2006;55(No. RR-10):1–41.
   • For healthy persons aged 5–49 years, LAIV may be used as an alternative to TIV.
   • Children receiving TIV should receive 0.25 mL if aged 6–35 months or 0.5 mL if aged ≥3 years.
   • Children aged <9 years who are receiving influenza vaccine for the first time should receive 2 doses (separated by ≥4 weeks for TIV and ≥6 weeks for LAIV).

7. **Measles, mumps, and rubella vaccine (MMR).** *(Minimum age: 12 months)*
   • Administer the second dose of MMR at age 4–6 years. MMR may be administered before age 4–6 years, provided ≥4 weeks have elapsed since the first dose and both doses are administered at age ≥12 months.

8. **Varicella vaccine.** *(Minimum age: 12 months)*
   • Administer the second dose of varicella vaccine at age 4–6 years. Varicella vaccine may be administered before age 4–6 years, provided that ≥3 months have elapsed since the first dose and both doses are administered at age ≥12 months. If second dose was administered ≥28 days following the first dose, the second dose does not need to be repeated.

9. **Hepatitis A vaccine (HepA).** *(Minimum age: 12 months)*
   • HepA is recommended for all children aged 1 year (i.e., aged 12–23 months). The 2 doses in the series should be administered at least 6 months apart.
   • Children not fully vaccinated by age 2 years can be vaccinated at subsequent visits.
   • HepA is recommended for certain other groups of children, including in areas where vaccination programs target older children. See *MMWR* 2006;55(No. RR-7):1–23.

10. **Meningococcal polysaccharide vaccine (MPSV4).** *(Minimum age: 2 years)*
    • Administer MPSV4 to children aged 2–10 years with terminal complement deficiencies or anatomic or functional asplenia and certain other high-risk groups. See *MMWR* 2005;54(No. RR-7):1–21.

**Office-Based Immunization Practices**

**151**

The Recommended Immunization Schedules for Persons Aged 0–18 Years are approved by the Advisory Committee on Immunization Practices (http://www.cdc.gov/nip/acip), the American Academy of Pediatrics (http://www.aap.org), and the American Academy of Family Physicians (http://www.aafp.org).
SAFER • HEALTHIER • PEOPLE™

CS103164

*Continued*

DEPARTMENT OF HEALTH AND HUMAN SERVICES • CENTERS FOR DISEASE CONTROL AND PREVENTION

# Recommended Immunization Schedule for Persons Aged 7–18 Years—UNITED STATES • 2007

| Vaccine ▼ | Age ▶ | 7–10 years | 11–12 YEARS | 13–14 years | 15 years | 16–18 years |
|---|---|---|---|---|---|---|
| Tetanus, Diphtheria, Pertussis[1] | | see footnote 1 | Tdap | Tdap | | |
| Human Papillomavirus[2] | | see footnote 2 | HPV (3 doses) | HPV Series | | |
| Meningococcal[3] | | MPSV4 | MCV4 | | MCV4[3] / MCV4 | |
| Pneumococcal[4] | | | PPV | | | |
| Influenza[5] | | | Influenza (Yearly) | | | |
| Hepatitis A[6] | | | HepA Series | | | |
| Hepatitis B[7] | | | HepB Series | | | |
| Inactivated Poliovirus[8] | | | IPV Series | | | |
| Measles, Mumps, Rubella[9] | | | MMR Series | | | |
| Varicella[10] | | | Varicella Series | | | |

Legend:
- Range of recommended ages
- Catch-up immunization
- Certain high-risk groups

This schedule indicates the recommended ages for routine administration of currently licensed childhood vaccines, as of December 1, 2006, for children aged 7–18 years. Additional information is available at **http://www.cdc.gov/nip/recs/child-schedule.htm.** Any dose not administered at the recommended age should be administered at any subsequent visit, when indicated and feasible. Additional vaccines may be licensed and recommended during the year. Licensed combination vaccines may be used whenever any components of the combination are indicated and other components of the vaccine are not contraindicated and if approved by the Food and Drug Administration for that dose of the series. Providers should consult the respective Advisory Committee on Immunization Practices statement for detailed recommendations. Clinically significant adverse events that follow immunization should be reported to the Vaccine Adverse Event Reporting System (VAERS). Guidance about how to obtain and complete a VAERS form is available at **http://www.vaers.hhs.gov** or by telephone, **800-822-7967.**

1. **Tetanus and diphtheria toxoids and acellular pertussis vaccine (Tdap).**
   *(Minimum age: 10 years for BOOSTRIX® and 11 years for ADACEL™)*
   - Administer at age 11–12 years for those who have completed the recommended childhood DTP/DTaP vaccination series and have not received a tetanus and diphtheria toxoids vaccine (Td) booster dose.
   - Adolescents aged 13–18 years who missed the 11–12 year Td/Tdap booster dose should also receive a single dose of Tdap if they have completed the recommended childhood DTP/DTaP vaccination series.

2. **Human papillomavirus vaccine (HPV).** *(Minimum age: 9 years)*
   - Administer the first dose of the HPV vaccine series to females at age 11–12 years.
   - Administer the second dose 2 months after the first dose and the third dose 6 months after the first dose.
   - Administer the HPV vaccine series to females at age 13–18 years if not previously vaccinated.

3. **Meningococcal vaccine.** *(Minimum age: 11 years for meningococcal conjugate vaccine [MCV4]; 2 years for meningococcal polysaccharide vaccine [MPSV4])*
   - Administer MCV4 at age 11–12 years and to previously unvaccinated adolescents at high school entry (at approximately age 15 years).
   - Administer MCV4 to previously unvaccinated college freshmen living in dormitories; MPSV4 is an acceptable alternative.
   - Vaccination against invasive meningococcal disease is recommended for children and adolescents aged ≥2 years with terminal complement deficiencies or anatomic or functional asplenia and certain other high-risk groups. See *MMWR* 2005;54(No. RR-7):1–21. Use MPSV4 for children aged 2–10 years and MCV4 or MPSV4 for older children.

4. **Pneumococcal polysaccharide vaccine (PPV).** *(Minimum age: 2 years)*
   - Administer for certain high-risk groups. See *MMWR* 1997;46(No. RR-8):1–24, and *MMWR* 2000;49(No. RR-9):1–35.

5. **Influenza vaccine.** *(Minimum age: 6 months for trivalent inactivated influenza vaccine [TIV]; 5 years for live, attenuated influenza vaccine [LAIV])*
   - Influenza vaccine is recommended annually for persons with certain risk factors, health-care workers, and other persons (including household members) in close contact with persons in groups at high risk. See *MMWR* 2006;55 (No. RR-10):1–41.
   - For healthy persons aged 5–49 years, LAIV may be used as an alternative to TIV.
   - Children aged <9 years who are receiving influenza vaccine for the first time should receive 2 doses (separated by ≥4 weeks for TIV and ≥6 weeks for LAIV).

6. **Hepatitis A vaccine (HepA).** *(Minimum age: 12 months)*
   - The 2 doses in the series should be administered at least 6 months apart.
   - HepA is recommended for certain other groups of children, including in areas where vaccination programs target older children. See *MMWR* 2006;55 (No. RR-7):1–23.

7. **Hepatitis B vaccine (HepB).** *(Minimum age: birth)*
   - Administer the 3-dose series to those who were not previously vaccinated.
   - A 2-dose series of Recombivax HB® is licensed for children aged 11–15 years.

8. **Inactivated poliovirus vaccine (IPV).** *(Minimum age: 6 weeks)*
   - For children who received an all-IPV or all-oral poliovirus (OPV) series, a fourth dose is not necessary if the third dose was administered at age ≥4 years.
   - If both OPV and IPV were administered as part of a series, a total of 4 doses should be administered, regardless of the child's current age.

9. **Measles, mumps, and rubella vaccine (MMR).** *(Minimum age: 12 months)*
   - If not previously vaccinated, administer 2 doses of MMR during any visit, with ≥4 weeks between the doses.

10. **Varicella vaccine.** *(Minimum age: 12 months)*
    - Administer 2 doses of varicella vaccine to persons without evidence of immunity.
    - Administer 2 doses of varicella vaccine to persons aged <13 years at least 3 months apart. Do not repeat the second dose, if administered ≥28 days after the first dose.
    - Administer 2 doses of varicella vaccine to persons aged ≥13 years at least 4 weeks apart.

**TABLE 2** Recommended Catch-Up Immunization Schedule

# Catch-up Immunization Schedule
## for Persons Aged 4 Months–18 Years Who Start Late or Who Are More Than 1 Month Behind

**UNITED STATES • 2007**

The table below provides catch-up schedules and minimum intervals between doses for children whose vaccinations have been delayed. A vaccine series does not need to be restarted, regardless of the time that has elapsed between doses. Use the section appropriate for the child's age.

| Vaccine | Minimum Age for Dose 1 | Minimum Interval Between Doses | | | |
|---|---|---|---|---|---|
| | | Dose 1 to Dose 2 | Dose 2 to Dose 3 | Dose 3 to Dose 4 | Dose 4 to Dose 5 |
| **CATCH-UP SCHEDULE FOR PERSONS AGED 4 MONTHS–6 YEARS** | | | | | |
| **Hepatitis B**[1] | **Birth** | 4 weeks | **8 weeks** (and 16 weeks after first dose) | | |
| **Rotavirus**[2] | **6 wks** | 4 weeks | 4 weeks | | |
| **Diphtheria, Tetanus, Pertussis**[3] | **6 wks** | 4 weeks | 4 weeks | 6 months | 6 months[3] |
| **Haemophilus influenzae type b**[4] | **6 wks** | **4 weeks** if first dose administered at age <12 months **8 weeks (as final dose)** if first dose administered at age 12-14 months **No further doses needed** if first dose administered at age ≥15 months | **4 weeks**[4] if current age <12 months **8 weeks (as final dose)**[4] if current age ≥12 months and second dose administered at age <15 months **No further doses needed** if previous dose administered at age ≥15 months | **8 weeks (as final dose)** This dose only necessary for children aged 12 months–5 years who received 3 doses before age 12 months | |
| **Pneumococcal**[5] | **6 wks** | **4 weeks** if first dose administered at age <12 months and current age <24 months **8 weeks (as final dose)** if first dose administered at age ≥12 months or current age 24–59 months **No further doses needed** for healthy children if first dose administered at age ≥24 months | **4 weeks** if current age <12 months **8 weeks (as final dose)** if current age ≥12 months **No further doses needed** for healthy children if previous dose administered at age ≥24 months | **8 weeks (as final dose)** This dose only necessary for children aged 12 months–5 years who received 3 doses before age 12 months | |
| **Inactivated Poliovirus**[6] | **6 wks** | 4 weeks | 4 weeks | 4 weeks[6] | |
| **Measles, Mumps, Rubella**[7] | **12 mos** | 4 weeks | | | |
| **Varicella**[8] | **12 mos** | 3 months | | | |
| **Hepatitis A**[9] | **12 mos** | 6 months | | | |
| **CATCH-UP SCHEDULE FOR PERSONS AGED 7–18 YEARS** | | | | | |
| **Tetanus, Diphtheria/ Tetanus, Diphtheria, Pertussis**[10] | **7 yrs**[10] | 4 weeks | **8 weeks** if first dose administered at age <12 months **6 months** if first dose administered at age ≥12 months | **6 months** if first dose administered at age <12 months | |
| **Human Papillomavirus**[11] | **9 yrs** | 4 weeks | 12 weeks | | |
| **Hepatitis A**[9] | **12 mos** | 6 months | | | |
| **Hepatitis B**[1] | **Birth** | 4 weeks | **8 weeks** (and 16 weeks after first dose) | | |
| **Inactivated Poliovirus**[6] | **6 wks** | 4 weeks | 4 weeks | 4 weeks[6] | |
| **Measles, Mumps, Rubella**[7] | **12 mos** | 4 weeks | | | |
| **Varicella**[8] | **12 mos** | **4 weeks** if first dose administered at age ≥13 years **3 months** if first dose administered at age <13 years | | | |

**1. Hepatitis B vaccine (HepB).** *(Minimum age: birth)*
- Administer the 3-dose series to those who were not previously vaccinated.
- A 2-dose series of Recombivax HB® is licensed for children aged 11–15 years.

**2. Rotavirus vaccine (Rota).** *(Minimum age: 6 weeks)*
- Do not start the series later than age 12 weeks.
- Administer the final dose in the series by age 32 weeks. Do not administer a dose later than age 32 weeks.
- Data on safety and efficacy outside of these age ranges are insufficient.

**3. Diphtheria and tetanus toxoids and acellular pertussis vaccine (DTaP).** *(Minimum age: 6 weeks)*
- The fifth dose is not necessary if the fourth dose was administered at age ≥4 years.
- DTaP is not indicated for persons aged ≥7 years.

**4. Haemophilus influenzae type b conjugate vaccine (Hib).** *(Minimum age: 6 weeks)*
- Vaccine is not generally recommended for children aged ≥5 years.
- If current age <12 months and the first 2 doses were PRP-OMP (PedvaxHIB® or ComVax® [Merck]), the third (and final) dose should be administered at age 12–15 months and at least 8 weeks after the second dose.
- If first dose was administered at age 7–11 months, administer 2 doses separated by 4 weeks plus a booster at age 12–15 months.

**5. Pneumococcal conjugate vaccine (PCV).** *(Minimum age: 6 weeks)*
- Vaccine is not generally recommended for children aged ≥5 years.

**6. Inactivated poliovirus vaccine (IPV).** *(Minimum age: 6 weeks)*
- For children who received an all-IPV or all-oral poliovirus (OPV) series, a fourth dose is not necessary if third dose was administered at age ≥4 years.
- If both OPV and IPV were administered as part of a series, a total of 4 doses should be administered, regardless of the child's current age.

**7. Measles, mumps, and rubella vaccine (MMR).** *(Minimum age: 12 months)*
- The second dose of MMR is recommended routinely at age 4–6 years but may be administered earlier if desired.
- If not previously vaccinated, administer 2 doses of MMR during any visit with ≥4 weeks between the doses.

**8. Varicella vaccine.** *(Minimum age: 12 months)*
- The second dose of varicella vaccine is recommended routinely at age 4–6 years but may be administered earlier if desired.
- Do not repeat the second dose in persons aged <13 years if administered ≥28 days after the first dose.

**9. Hepatitis A vaccine (HepA).** *(Minimum age: 12 months)*
- HepA is recommended for certain groups of children, including in areas where vaccination programs target older children. See *MMWR* 2006;55(No. RR-7):1–23.

**10. Tetanus and diphtheria toxoids vaccine (Td) and tetanus and diphtheria toxoids and acellular pertussis vaccine (Tdap).** *(Minimum ages: 7 years for Td, 10 years for BOOSTRIX®, and 11 years for ADACEL™)*
- Tdap should be substituted for a single dose of Td in the primary catch-up series or as a booster if age appropriate; use Td for other doses.
- A 5-year interval from the last Td dose is encouraged when Tdap is used as a booster dose. A booster (fourth) dose is needed if any of the previous doses were administered at age <12 months. Refer to ACIP recommendations for further information. See *MMWR* 2006;55(No. RR-3).

**11. Human papillomavirus vaccine (HPV).** *(Minimum age: 9 years)*
- Administer the HPV vaccine series to females at age 13–18 years if not previously vaccinated.

Information about reporting reactions after immunization is available online at **http://www.vaers.hhs.gov** or by telephone via the 24-hour national toll-free information line 800-822-7967. Suspected cases of vaccine-preventable diseases should be reported to the state or local health department. Additional information, including precautions and contraindications for immunization, is available from the National Center for Immunization and Respiratory Diseases at **http://www.cdc.gov/nip/default.htm** or telephone, **800-CDC-INFO (800-232-4636)**.

**DEPARTMENT OF HEALTH AND HUMAN SERVICES • CENTERS FOR DISEASE CONTROL AND PREVENTION • SAFER • HEALTHIER • PEOPLE**

Office-Based Immunization Practices

CS103164

into a muscle mass. Practitioners should use the anterolateral thigh muscle injections for children younger than 18 months and then move to the deltoid muscle in children older than 18 months when the muscle mass of the deltoid is large enough. SC injections should be given in subcutaneous fat of the anterolateral thigh or triceps with a shorter needle inserted at an angle.

## PREVENTION OF NEEDLE INJURY

For the safety of the patient, parent, and provider, efforts should be made to minimize the exposure to an accidental needle stick. Although the risk of accidental inoculation with the patient's blood is minimal in immunization, as with the use of sharps in any office, employees should examine the safety needles available and choose a safety needle appropriate for minimizing accidental needle sticks. The office should provide a child-proof sharps container that allows for rapid disposal of the needle with a minimal amount of effort. The container should be checked regularly for function and emptied frequently to avoid over-filling during the workday.

## DOCUMENTATION AND RECORDS

All offices should adopt a standard of documentation of immunizations. The physician's or nurse's order for a vaccine should not be used in place of documentation that the vaccine was given. Documentation of the vaccine administered should include the species and the brand name given as well as the lot number. The patient record should also include the location, date, and time. Such a record would be made more useful if all the vaccine-antigens could be viewed at once with regard to series and dates. To best manage combinations currently available as well as future possibilities, the record should be organized by vaccine-antigen and not common vaccine combinations. This requires that a combination vaccine then appear in several antigen categories. Furthermore, the record would be enhanced by clarification when vaccines were not given because of precaution or contraindication as the basis. We have an ongoing problem with the adoption of chickenpox vaccine (Varivax). Those children who previously acquired chickenpox do not need the chickenpox vaccine, but we need to document the occurrence of that disease and its date to prevent overvaccination.

## RECORD SHARING AND REGISTRIES

Vaccine registries at the community level or regional level dramatically reduce the miscommunication and the need for occurrence of both overimmunization as well as empowering physicians and nurses to feel better about taking advantage of missed opportunities in vaccinating children. Most parents whose children are undervaccinated report that their children are "up to date." Records that accurately reflect the child's full vaccine record would better equip the practitioner in best managing those patients.

## VACCINE STORAGE

Storage requirements are much more complex than traditionally practiced. Offices must provide proper refrigeration as well as freezers for vaccines. Certain vaccines require refrigeration, other vaccines require freezing, and some vaccines are more heat labile or cold labile than others. Proper care and maintenance of refrigerator includes the purchase of appropriate dedicated equipment, the monitoring of the temperatures, the purchase of proper containers to be used on the shelves, and adequate space to allow for prevention of errors with storage. Furthermore, the staff must be trained and scheduled to provide oversight in the case of a power or equipment failure.

## ASSESSMENT OF THE OVERALL PROCESS AND ITS OUTCOMES

Assessing an individual's immunization needs, providing the vaccines, and recording them properly in the individual's record is no longer adequate for the assessment of the overall process. Each office should

make efforts to assess its overall practice. Each office must monitor the rates of on-time immunizations as well as up-to-date immunization and look for opportunities to improve these metrics. The effort of collecting this information has led to improvements in rates of on-time vaccination. Immunization practices are evolving and the maintenance of quality as well as the rapid adoption and improvement of practices require regular office meetings of staff. Physicians, nurses, and receptionists must be aware of new changes. Receptionists' misunderstanding of the vaccine needs frequently leads to missed opportunities to vaccinate. Misunderstanding between physicians and other clinicians can also lead to failed attempts. Regular office meetings should occur throughout the year to evaluate the vaccine schedule, the success of vaccinating the panel of patients, and considerations for practice improvements.

## STANDING ORDERS

One of the most successful approaches in the office to make real efforts to improve immunization rates above and beyond that driven by the well child care schedule is to create standing orders that permit nursing staff to provide vaccines to patients without a doctor visit. This is particularly helpful with flu season and for acute care contacts with the patient. Such standing orders need to be written in such a way that they meet state law, facilitate nurse assessment of the patient's vaccine needs, as well as rule out any precautions or contraindications for the child's immunization. Materials exist online at the Immunization Action Coalition (www.immunize.org) that can help in writing such standing orders.

## RECALL REMINDERS AND TRACKING

A second method for improving office vaccination rates are recall reminders and tracking. Providers should develop proactive approaches toward their patient panels to ensure compliance with the routine childhood schedule. Offices should contact patients when vaccines are due. Additional efforts should be made for those subjects who are behind in immunizations. Finally, offices should have systems to identify those children in families for whom the flu vaccine is indicated and make efforts every autumn to contact the families proactively and schedule immunization visits. The broadening of the flu vaccine indications has made this a major issue for office practices who care for either children or adults or both.

## REPORTING ADVERSE EVENTS

The same laws that created the vaccine information statements and the protection for vaccine providers from frivolous lawsuits have also created the Vaccine Adverse Events Reporting System (VAERS). This system, set up by the federal government, collects information on adverse events believed to be related to immunization. These include certain ones required by regulation as well as those temporally associated with the immunizations that strike the provider or family as potentially significant. Vaccine manufacturers and providers are in fact required to report certain adverse events occurring after immunization whether or not they were caused by the immunization.

VAERS has actually led to the discontinuation of certain office-based immunization practices including the use of the tetravalent oral rhesus rotavirus vaccine (RotaShield). It has also helped to protect vaccines from unwarranted claims of harm. Although it has its weaknesses, statistical approaches have made it a powerful tool. Participation for providers of vaccines is required. All office staff, including receptionists, must understand the legal requirements of reporting.

## VACCINES FOR CHILDREN

The U.S. government set up a program entitled Vaccines for Children (VFC) that enables providers to receive free-of-charge vaccines that can be given to patients with certain conditions including those who are younger than 18 years and are Medicaid eligible, uninsured, American Indian or Alaska Native, or whose health insurance benefit plan does not include vaccinations. Some recipients may be charged a vaccine provider fee, which is a limited amount. The federal government purchases vaccine for the VFC program and then distributes it to the state's health departments, which redistributes to the qualified providers. To learn how an office can participate, the VFC program can be contacted at the CDC through its web pages.

# Common Problems

Offices that provide vaccines to their patients struggle with common problems in immunization practice. These include missed or delayed vaccinations, vaccine shortages, catch-ups, change-ups, decisions not to vaccinate, true and false contraindications, multiple providers, and incomplete records. One cannot make these problems disappear, but one can prepare for them, prevent them from happening in many cases, and minimize the harm when they do occur.

## MISSED OR DELAYED VACCINATIONS

Although daycare and school-based requirements have resulted in very high vaccine rates by school entry, on-time immunization is tragically low. Many children do not get their vaccines when due and are left at risk. Although this occurs more frequently among those with multiple providers and those who do not have health insurance, practitioners can change their office practices to reduce the problems in delayed immunizations. First of all, do not relegate routine immunization to the well child visit. Second, be assertive in obtaining the complete vaccine records from your patient's previous providers of health care. Third, create standing order policies to facilitate your office staff providing vaccines without a physician visit.

Furthermore, the practitioner should have charts available in the office explaining how to proceed with a child who has not received vaccines on time. Practitioners cannot be expected to memorize this information. It is complex, age dependent, and vaccine specific. The information must be available for ready reference. With the American Academies of Pediatrics and Family Practitioners, the ACIP has created catch-up schedules (www.cdc.gov/vaccines/recs/schedules). There are two catch-up schedules: one for children 4 months to 6 years of age and one for 7 to 18 years of age (Table 2).

## LOCUS OF RESPONSIBILITY

Providers cannot expect their patients or their patients' parents, to take responsibility for timely vaccination. Patient-held immunization records have failed to improve vaccination rates. Office practitioners must also consider that even in a specialty practice their patients may be expecting them to monitor their immunization needs along with providing them the vaccines that they need. Providers, whether of specialty or primary care, must assess their individual patients and determine who is monitoring the patients' vaccination status and needs. Specialists must never assume that the patient is cognizant of the need or that a primary care provider is actively playing that role. All too often, patients relinquish their relationships with primary care providers once they begin an ongoing relationship with a specialist.

## VACCINE SHORTAGES

Ongoing shortages do occur with vaccine supplies. Most famously are the shortages with the influenza vaccine, but we also have shortages with vaccines when there have been changes in use or recommendations such as the adoption of the adolescent diphtheria/tetanus (Td) at 11 years of age and the rapid acceptance of the pneumococcal conjugate vaccine (Prevar). Manufacturers struggle to produce adequate supplies knowing the expense of creating inadequate supplies actually leads to distrust and anger directed toward the manufacturer as well as difficulties in completing on-time immunizations. Manufacturing too much vaccine can lead to unusable stockpiles of expired vaccine product. Therefore manufacturers seek to reach a balance. Shortages are communicated best to office practices in the United States through the online Web site at the CDC where information is provided for the basis of shortages as well as explanations for what the practitioners should do during this time. In most situations the vaccine providers are expected to record those people who have not received the vaccine on time because of the shortage and are to be called back in a timely manner when vaccine supplies are available.

## CATCH-UP

Catching children up on missed or delayed vaccinations is a major problem. This activity results not just because of shortages but because of parents' delays in immunization. The third and four child in a family often suffer delays in immunizations because of parents' issues with the organization and scheduling of appropriate on-time well child visits. Offices that rely on the well child visit schedules as the only basis for immunization have higher rates of vaccine delays and more problems with catch-up than those who use every opportunity of every visit to assess vaccine status of the child and to vaccinate on time. To make matters worse, the current schedule when on time can call for five injections at once. Imagine the child who has accumulated significant delays and now needs to be caught up. One of the major difficulties of catch-up is the problem of information. I previously mentioned the chart that all vaccine providers should have available to facilitate catching up immunizations (see Table 2).

## CHANGE-UPS

Change-ups are also difficult because the new adoption of a vaccine can lead to some confusion for those who previously received an older moiety. For example, the recipients of the meningococcal polysaccharide vaccine (Menomune) are not due for the meningococcal conjugate vaccine (Menacta), but those who previously received the adolescent tetanus-diphtheria (Td) vaccine may certainly benefit from the new adolescent tetanus-diphtheria-reduced-dose-acellular pertussis vaccine (Tdap, Boostrix).

## DECISIONS NOT TO VACCINATE

There are many reasons why patients may fail to be vaccinated. Common reasons include misunderstandings by the practitioner or parent of contraindications regarding vaccines. These are vaccine specific and complex in language in application. Many more people fail to get vaccines because of contraindications than those who truly have them. Other common reasons include parents' failure to attend to the well-visit schedule and the practitioners' failures to use other visits as the basis for immunization.

Some parents, however, actually consider immunization and choose to refuse. They are suspicious that the vaccines do not work, are not necessary or at least no longer necessary, are not safe, weaken the immune system, provide a poorer immunity than the actual diseases they target, that children receive too many vaccines, and that some vaccine lots are contaminated. Practitioners should be familiar with these concerns and their rebuttals. Two good sources for information on these include CDC (www.cdc.gov/vaccines) and the Immunization Action Coalition (www.immunize.org). The latter organization has actually collected stories of parents who chose not to vaccinate their children and then suffered the consequences of vaccine-preventable disease.

## TRUE AND FALSE CONTRAINDICATIONS

Perhaps one of the most common problems with immunization delivery in the United States with regard to the failure of the provider stems from common misconceptions regarding the presence or absence of contraindication to immunization. Although some contraindications are vaccine specific, certain principles apply. First, family histories of adverse events are never contraindications to immunization. Second, household pregnancy or breast-feeding is never a contraindication to immunization. Third, the presence of an illness or injury by itself is not a contraindication. If the illness is moderate or severe, with or without a fever, then a vaccine's administration may be contraindicated. Although local and systemic adverse reactions do occur with vaccines, these are in general not contraindications to further doses.

It would be impossible for a practitioner to memorize contraindications. The CDC (www.cdc.gov/vaccines) has prepared a user-friendly online table that is indexed by disease and condition to guide the practitioner. This table should be available for ready use throughout the day.

## MULTIPLE PROVIDERS AND INCOMPLETE RECORDS

Both under- and overimmunization occur much more frequently among patients who use more than one provider. Regional registries that allow practitioners to share their vaccine records greatly reduce both missed opportunities to vaccinate as well as the inadvertent administration of unnecessary doses. Practitioners should work with their local and state health departments to develop regional vaccine registries.

For all of the problems we face, for all of the intricacies of practices we must adopt, there is perhaps no one practice more important to the health of the community than the delivery of routine immunizations. Although it is worth the effort, it requires an ongoing commitment to continuing education, practice assessment, and evidence-based improvement of the office practice.

## REFERENCES

American Academy of Family Physicians: AAFP Clinical Recommendations. http://www.aafp.org/x132.xml. Accessed August 7, 2006. This web site provides links to specific AAFP recommendations for immunizations.

American Academy of Pediatrics: American Academy of Pediatrics Policy Statements. http://aappolicy.aappublications.org/Accessed August 7, 2006. This web site provides links to the AAP policies including its online Red Book with its recommendations regarding vaccines and immunizations.

Centers for Disease Control and Prevention: Recommendations of the ACIP (Advisory Committee on Immunization Practices). http://www.cdc.gov/vaccines/pubs/ACIP-list.htm. Last modified on August 13, 2007. Accessed August 19, 2007. This web site provides links to the ACIP recommendations, which are updated annually as new data dictate. All of the documents listed on this page are current, regardless of their publication dates.

Centers for Disease Control and Prevention: Recommended Childhood and Adolescent Immunization Schedule, United States, 2006. http://www.cdc.gov/vaccines/recs/schedules/child-schedule.htm. Last updated August 16, 2007. Accessed August 19, 2007. This web site provides the harmonized 4-page schedule for children and adolescents with informative footnotes and two additional charts for catch-up for children between the ages of 4 months through 6 years and between 7 through 18 years.

Centers for Disease Control and Prevention: Recommended Adult Immunization Schedule by Vaccine and Age Group, United States, October 2005–September 2006. http://www.cdc.gov/vaccines/recs/schedules/adult-schedule.htm. Last updated January 26, 2007. Accessed August 19, 2007. Recommended immunizations for anyone older than 18 years.

Centers for Disease Control and Prevention: Vaccine Information Statements (VIS). http://www.cdc.gov/vaccines/pubs/vis/default.htm. Last updated August 17, 2007. Accessed August 19, 2007. This web page lists links to all of the federally mandated Vaccine Information Statements that practitioners must use in informed parents of the recommended vaccines.

Centers for Disease Control and Prevention: Vaccine Management: Recommendations for Storage and Handling Selected Biologicals. Revised June 2005. http://www.cdc.gov/vaccines/pubs/vac-mgt-book.htm. Last updated on June 12, 2007. Last accessed August 19, 2007. This document provides vaccine-specific instructions on storage of vaccines.

Immunization Action Coalition: State Mandates on Immunization and Vaccine-Preventable Disease. http://www.immunize.org/laws/. Last updated May 31, 2006. Accessed August 7, 2006. This web site provides specific state-by-state rules for school and day-care attendance.

Pickering LK, Baker CJ, Long SS, McMillan JA (eds): Red Book: 2006 Report of the Committee on Infectious Diseases, 27th ed. Elk Grove Village, IL, American Academy of Pediatrics, 2006.

Shefer A, Briss P, Rodewald L, et al: Improving immunization coverage rates: An evidence-based review of the literature. Epidemiol Rev 1999;21(1):96-142. A systematic review of the published studies of interventions to improve vaccines uptake.

# Travel Medicine

Method of
*Cynthia B. Snider, MD, MPH, and*
*William A. Petri, MD, PhD*

Travel medicine is an emerging subspecialty geared toward minimizing the risk of travel-related illness by educating travelers, providing immunization, and providing therapy, if needed, on their return. More than 50 million people from industrialized countries travel to the developing world annually, and 20% to 70% of travelers report some health problem associated with their recent travel. An estimated 4 million people seek medical care for their travel-related symptoms on an annual basis (Box 1).

## Pretravel Counseling

In providing comprehensive medical advice to a patient about to embark on travel, it is important to know the preexisting medical conditions and assess the patient's risk of illness or injury. Pretravel counseling provides an excellent opportunity to review the need for vaccinations and provide general personal precautions. It is essential to obtain a detailed travel itinerary, type of travel, length of stay in each area, and expected activity. Because of the differences in local prevalence of infectious diseases, this information is necessary for determining appropriate chemoprophylaxis. Some activities, such as freshwater exposure, being exposed to wildlife, staying in a village while working for a nonprofit organization, or returning to visit family in rural settings can place travelers at added risk for contracting preventable diseases.

## Travel-Related Infectious Illnesses

### TRAVELER'S DIARRHEA

Traveler's diarrhea is defined as three or more watery stools in less than 24 hours. It is the most common illness to affect travelers. There is a 50% risk of having at least one attack of diarrhea in a 2-week trip. Diarrhea affects 10% to 60% of travelers going to the developing world. In general, children are at greater risk for severe illness and are more susceptible to dehydration.

### Pathogenesis

Traveler's diarrhea is usually contracted from contaminated food. Infection is often due to noninvasive enterotoxigenic *Escherichia coli* (ETEC),

---

**BOX 1  Reducing the Number of Travel-Associated Illnesses**

- Assess the patient's health at baseline prior to travel.
- Understand how the patient's preexisting medical condition can influence the options for chemoprophylaxis or immunizations for preventable diseases.
- Provide guidance and counseling in preparation for travel, including insect-bite and food and water precautions.
- Understand the spectrum of illness and the risk of acquiring certain infectious diseases in areas of travel by reviewing the patient's itinerary.
- Provide guidance regarding when to seek medical evaluation for post-travel illness.

enteroaggregative *E. coli* (EAEC), or strains of *Campylobacter*, *Shigella*, or *Salmonella*. Viruses and parasites are less common causes but should still be considered in patients with chronic diarrhea. Viral threats include hepatitis A, hepatitis E, and Norwalk virus. Protozoa, including *Giardia intestinalis*, *Entomeba histolytica*, and *Cryptosporidium*, can also cause traveler's diarrhea. The cause of diarrhea is often unknown in 20% to 50% of cases.

Patients traveling to areas with poor hygiene should avoid consuming raw vegetables and fruits and unpasteurized dairy products. Pathogens can also be transmitted from contaminated tap water, ice, or improperly cooked foods (Box 2).

## Treatment

Traveler's diarrhea is usually self-limited and lasts approximately 4 days. To minimize the morbidity associated with diarrhea, patients are encouraged to carry oral rehydration salts (CeraLyte) to be mixed with potable water to maintain electrolyte balance, particularly for children and the elderly (Table 1). Antibiotics should be reserved for moderate to severe disease. Up to 80% of patients are cured with a single dose of antibiotics. Drug treatment is summarized in Table 2.

For mild disease, bismuth subsalicylate (Pepto-Bismol) can reduce stool output and minimize the symptoms of diarrhea, nausea, and abdominal pain. Loperamide (Imodium), an over-the-counter synthetic opioid antimotility agent, can also be used. However, loperamide should not be used in patients who have fever or bloody diarrhea. The side effect is constipation.

For moderate to severe diarrhea, as defined by persistent (>3 days) diarrhea or associated symptoms of fever or bloody stool, a short course of antibiotics is warranted. Self-treatment for 1 to 3 days with a fluoroquinolone such as ciprofloxacin (Cipro) is usually recommended.

### TABLE 1 Composition of WHO Oral Rehydration Solution (ORS) for Diarrheal Illness

| Ingredient | Amount | Osmolality |
|---|---|---|
| Sodium chloride | 2.6 g/L | 75 mmol/L |
| Potassium chloride | 1.5 g/L | 20 mmol/L |
| Glucose | 13.5 g/L | 65 mmol/L |
| Trisodium citrate (or sodium bicarbonate) | 2.9 g/L | 10 mmol/L |
| Water | 1 L | 245 (Total) |

Azithromycin (Zithromax)[1] is recommended for patients traveling to Southeast Asia, where there is a high prevalence of fluoroquinolone-resistant *Campylobacter*. Azithromycin can also be used for pregnant women, children, and patients who do not respond to a fluoroquinolone in 48 hours. Patients should see a physician if they do not respond to antibiotics or have bloody stools.

Another alternative is a nonabsorbed oral antibiotic, rifaximin, derived from rifampin. It is FDA approved for treating noninvasive forms of *E. coli* in travelers older than 12 years. Initial studies with travelers in Mexico showed efficacy similar to that of ciprofloxacin but with fewer side effects. It is still not known whether enteric organisms will develop resistance to rifaximin, as seen with rifampin.

Prophylaxis against traveler's diarrhea is not generally prescribed. Patients should be instructed to begin self-treatment if symptoms persist.

## MALARIA

Malaria is a global public health problem. Forty percent of the world's population resides in endemic regions, and malaria causes 300 to 500 million infections each year. Despite taking a large human toll, malaria-related illness and death are largely preventable.

With the increase in international travel to malaria-endemic countries, a growing number of travelers are at risk for contracting this arthropod-borne illness. More than 500,000 travelers require chemoprophylaxis per year. In the United States, the Centers for Diseases Control and Prevention (CDC) reported 1324 malaria cases, including five fatalities, in 2004. In most of these cases, people were not taking the appropriate chemoprophylaxis regimen.

### Epidemiology

In humans, malaria is an arthropod-borne illness transmitted by bites from infected female *Anopheles* mosquitos. It is caused by the parasite *Plasmodium*, with four species in particular: *Plasmodium falciparum*, *P. ovale*, *P. vivax*, and *P. malariae*. *P. falciparum* can cause rapid progressively severe illness with significant mortality.

The risk of acquiring malaria is influenced by geographic patterns. The predominant species of malaria transmitted in sub-Saharan Africa is *P. falciparum*, and there are higher malaria transmission rates in Africa than in other parts of the world. Due to decades of attempted disease eradication, drug-resistance patterns are seen throughout the world. Chloroquine-resistant *P. falciparum* (CRPF) is seen in sub-Saharan Africa and South America. A multi-drug resistant *P. falciparum* is now identified in border areas of Thailand with Cambodia and of Thailand with Myanmar.

Information about malaria risk in specific countries is tracked by various epidemiologic programs, including the CDC and World Health Organization (WHO). The most current information is on their Web sites (CDC travel information at http://www.cdc.gov/travel). The CDC has established a malaria hotline at 770-488-7788.

---

### BOX 2 Preventing Traveler's Diarrhea*

"Boil it, peel it, cook it, or forget it."

- Avoid vegetables or fruits that have not been peeled or cleaned.
- Avoid eating food from street vendors if it is not clear how the food is prepared or cooked.
- Eat food that is hot and cooked thoroughly. Avoid food that has been held at room temperature.
- Hot beverages such as tea and coffee, carbonated drinks, fruit juices, and bottled alcoholic beverages are safe to drink.
- Avoid ice unless is it made with bottled or boiled water.
- If safety of drinking water is questionable, drink bottled water.
- Boiling water for up to 1 minute is the most reliable method of treating possible contaminated water.
- Chemical treatment of water by either iodine or chloride is not effective against *Cryptosporidium* or *Giardia*.
- Filters may be used in some settings, such as hiking. Only the smaller microfilters with 0.1-0.3 μm pores can remove bacteria and protozoa; filters do not remove viruses. Filters with small pores can readily clog with large volumes of water, and they are often not effective for water with large sediment.
- Unpasteurized milk should be boiled before it is consumed.
- Ice cream that might have thawed and refrozen can be a potential source of foodborne illness. If the source is questionable, it should be avoided.

---

*Adapted from CDC information

[1]Not FDA approved for this indication.

**TABLE 2  Self-Treatment for Traveler's Diarrhea**

| Drug | Dosage | Comments |
|---|---|---|
| **Antimotility Medications** | | |
| Bismuth subsalicylate (active ingredient in Pepto-Bismol) | 1 oz liquid or 2 tablets q30min up to 8 doses<br>Not to be used longer than 3 wk | Causes blackening of tongue, stool<br>Not for those with renal insufficiency, anticoagulation therapy, or aspirin allergy<br>Not for children with possible varicella or influenza because it can increase risk for Reye's syndrome |
| Loperamide (Imodium) | 4 mg loading dose, then 2 mg after each loose stool, to a max 16 mg/d | Not for use in children < 2 y<br>Not to be used if patient has fever or bloody stools |
| **Antibiotics** | | |
| Azithromycin (Zithromax)[1] | Adults: 1000 mg once or 500 mg qd for 3 d<br>Children: 10 mg/kg/d | Preferred in children and in women who might be pregnant |
| Ciprofloxacin (Cipro) | 500 mg bid for 1-3 d | Adjust dose for renal insufficiency<br>Can interact with anticoagulation therapy |
| Levofloxacin (Levaquin)[1] | 500 mg qd for 1-3 d | Adjust dose for renal insufficiency<br>Can interact with anticoagulation therapy |
| Rifaximin (Xifaxan) | 200 mg tid for 3 d | No need for renal or hepatic dosage adjustments |

[1]Not FDA approved for this indication.
*Abbreviation:* max = maximum.

## Chemoprophylaxis

Because there are no vaccines that completely guarantee protection against malaria, chemoprophylaxis and personal protection measures play a key role in malaria prevention (Table 3). Travelers should also be reminded that even if they have had malaria before, they can get it again, and so preventive measures are still necessary.

Atovaquone/proguanil (Malarone) is a fixed-combination antimalarial drug that is active on both blood and tissue schizonts. It can be used for both prophylaxis and treatment. Side effects include abdominal discomfort, nausea, vomiting, and headache. This medication is contraindicated in children who weigh less than 11 kg, pregnant women, mothers breast-feeding children who weigh less than 11 kg, patients with severe renal impairment, and patients with known allergies to either atovaquone or proguanil.

Doxycycline (Vibramycin) is effective against the erythrocytic stage of *Plasmodium* species but only minimally effective against liver schzonts, not enough to prevent relapse. It is effective for prophylaxis for chloroquine-resistant and mefloquine-resistant *P. falciparum*. Side effects include nausea, vomiting, abdominal discomfort, and photosensitivity. Patients should be cautioned to use sunscreen when taking doxycycline. Doxycycline can cause yeast infections in female patients and interferes with oral contraceptives. Doxycycline is contraindicated in pregnant women, children younger than 8 years, and patients with known allergies to tetracycline-related drugs.

Mefloquine (Lariam) is effective against the erythrocytic stages of *Plasmodium* species. It is commonly used for prophylaxis but does not prevent *P. vivax* or *P. ovale* relapses. Side effects include headache, nausea, dizziness, anxiety, sleep disturbances, vivid dreams, and visual hallucinations. The severe adverse effects include depression, seizure, and psychosis. Patients with active or recent history of depression, generalized anxiety disorder, schizophrenia, or psychosis should not take mefloquine. It should not be prescribed for those who have underlying seizure disorders or arrhythmias. Mefloquine prophylaxis in the second and third trimesters is not associated with adverse fetal or pregnancy outcome.

In instances where no other antimalarial drug is tolerated, primaquine may serve as an alternative primary prophylaxis. The use of primaquine for malaria chemoprophylaxis should be reviewed by infectious disease physicians or physicians certified in travel medicine. Primaquine can cause severe adverse effects, specifically a fatal hemolysis in those with glucose-6-phosphate dehydrogenase (G6PD) deficiency. Patients must be tested for G6PD deficiency, and normal G6PD levels must be documented before patients take this medication. The side effects include nausea, abdominal discomfort, and vomiting.

Contraindications include G6PD deficiency, pregnancy, breast-feeding of children with unknown G6PD levels, and allergy to primaquine.

### Personal Protective Measures

Personal protective measures (Box 3) also help minimize mosquito exposure. DEET (*N,N*-diethyl-m-tolulamide) is one of the most effective topical insect repellents that can be applied to exposed skin. It repels mosquitoes, fleas, ticks, chiggers, and some flies. Concentrations of 20% to 30% DEET protect for approximately 6 to 12 hours. Higher concentrations do not have higher efficacy rates but do last longer. DEET is not recommended for infants younger than 2 months, but it can be used on children and older infants. Side effects include skin sensitivity and decreased effectiveness of sunscreen. Higher concentrations of DEET are known for dissolving plastic-containing materials.

Permethrin 0.5% (Permanone) is an insecticide spray that can be used on clothing and mosquito nets, tents, and sleeping bags. Pretreated clothing or sleeping bags retain its effects despite multiple launderings, up to 2 or more months.

## Noninfectious Travel Risks

Travelers should be counseled to follow general safety precautions (Box 4). An estimated 5 million people were killed secondary to injuries in 2000. Ninety percent of these injury-related deaths are in middle- to lower-income countries. About 1.2 million fatalities are motor-vehicle related. A study assessing U.S. citizens traveling to Mexico showed 51% injury-related causes of death, 18% of which were motor vehicle related.[17]

Patients should consider purchasing supplemental health insurance policies that include 24-hour access to emergency evacuation and treatment.

### TRAVEL KITS

Travelers should be encouraged to carry their medications with them in the original pharmacy bottles rather than packed in their luggage, in case the luggage is separated from the traveler. In addition, a list of the medications, including generic name, dosage, and reason for taking them, could be useful if the traveler needs to purchase more medication. If the patient uses syringes and needles for a health condition (e.g., diabetes), a medical letter detailing the necessity of these medical supplies can avert interrogation. A patient with a cardiac history should carry a copy of the latest electrocardiogram.

## TABLE 3 Malaria Chemoprophylaxis

| Medication | Adult Dosage | Pediatric Dosage |
|---|---|---|
| **Areas of Chloroquine Resistance: Most of Africa, South America, except Paraguay, Argentina, Chile, Uruguay; parts of the Middle East, India, East Asia, and Southeast Asia** | | |
| Atovaquone-proguanil (Malarone) | 250 mg/100 mg, take 1 tablet daily Begin 1-2 d before entering the area and continue for 7 d after leaving | 11-20 kg: 62.5 mg/25 mg, 1 pediatric tablet daily 21-30 kg: 125 mg/50 mg, 2 pediatric tablets daily 31-40 kg: 187.5 mg/75 mg, 3 pediatric tablets daily >40 kg: 250 mg/100 mg dose, 1 adult tablet daily All doses taken daily, as for adults For >8 y old |
| Doxycycline (Vibramycin) | 100 mg daily, take 1 tablet orally once daily Begin 1-2 d before entering the area, and continue for 4 wk after leaving | 2 mg/kg daily, (max dose, 100 mg/d) |
| Mefloquine HCl (Lariam) | 228 mg base (250 mg salt) 1 tablet once per wk Begin 1 wk before entering area and continue until 4 wk after leaving | <10 kg; 5 mg salt/kg weekly 10-19 kg: one-quarter tablet 20-30 kg: one-half tablet 31-45 kg: three-quarters tablet >45 kg, 1 tablet All doses once/wk, as for adults Can ask pharmacy to compound ingredients into 1 tablet if splitting medication is too difficult for the patient |
| **Areas of Chloroquine Sensitivity: Haiti, the Dominican Republic, Central America west of the Panama Canal, and parts of the Middle East (resistance in Iran, Oman, Saudi Arabia, and Yemen)** | | |
| Chloroquine phosphate (Aralen) | 300 mg base (500 mg salt) 1 tablet once per wk Begin 1 wk before entering area and continue for 4 wk after leaving | 5 mg base/kg body weight (8.3 mg salt/kg), up to adult dose, once/wk |
| **Areas of Mefloquine Resistance: Parts of Southeast Asia, specifically borders between Thailand, Myanmar, and Cambodia** | | |
| Doxycycline | 100 mg daily, take 1 tablet orally once daily Begin 1-2 d before entering the area, and continue for 4 wk after leaving | 2 mg/kg daily, (max dose, 100 mg/d) |
| **Rare Circumstances: Alternative when other prophylactic agents are contraindicated or unavailable** | | |
| Primaquine | 15 mg base daily, 2 tablets orally once daily Begin 1-2 d before entering area and continue until 7 d after leaving | 0.5 mg/kg daily, up to adult dose, as for adults |

## JET LAG

Jet lag is caused by the alteration in circadian rhythm caused by traveling through several time zones. It is more common in travelers going east to west across more than five time zones. Symptoms of jet lag include fatigue, malaise, headache, anorexia, insomnia, and difficulty with concentration. It is alleviated by acclimating to the destination's day and night schedule by not sleeping during daytime hours. Symptoms will dissipate once the biological clock adjusts to the destination time zone. Jet lag generally does not last more than a few days. Good sleep hygiene and hydration promote recovery from jet lag. The use of short-acting hypnotics is controversial. Some research suggests melatonin can reduce effects of jet lag; however, the safety of this remedy has not been scientifically established.

## DEEP VENOUS THROMBOSIS

There are increasing reports of deep venous thrombosis and pulmonary embolism associated with airplane travel. A recent study reports a twofold increase in risk passengers traveling by plane, car, or train longer than 4 hours. The risk is highest in persons with factor V Leiden or body mass index greater than 30. Other risk factors include a prior history of deep venous thrombosis or pulmonary embolism, hypercoagulable states, and pregnancy. Travelers are encouraged to wear elastic stockings and to walk about the plane every 30 to 60 minutes..

## MOTION SICKNESS

Motion sickness is often triggered by an inner ear imbalance. Motion sickness induces nausea, diaphoresis, anorexia, lethargy, and vomiting.

---

### BOX 3 Personal Protective Measures to Prevent Insect Bites

- Malaria-transmitting mosquitoes are most active in the evening. Mosquitoes known to transmit dengue are active in the daytime.
- Sleep in screened areas, and use mosquito nets, preferably permethrin-impregnated nets.
- Wear clothing that covers arms and legs.
- Use insect repellent containing 20%-30% DEET.

*Abbreviation:* DEET = *N,N*-diethyl-m-toluamide.

---

### BOX 4 Preventive Measures to Minimize Accident-Related Injury

- Wear shoes, long sleeves, and pants when engaging in off-road sports or riding on motorcycles.
- Wear safety belts in motor vehicles.
- Wear helmets when riding on motorcycles.
- Minimize driving in the evening when there is poor visibility of road landmarks and increased incidence of drivers under the influence of alcohol.
- Use safety flotation vests when engaging in water activities such as kayaking and rafting.

Motion sickness is aggravated by up-and-down movement of the head and neck and by traveling in small aircraft or cars.

Many medications can remedy the symptoms of motion sickness. Children do best with antihistamines such as diphenhydramine (Benadryl), dimenhydrinate (Dramamine), or promethazine (Phenergan). The side effects of these antihistamines are largely sedation and drowsiness. They are most effective if taken before onset of motion sickness symptoms. Adults can also use these same antihistamine agents, or they may take meclizine (Bonine, Antivert) or scopolamine.

The scopolamine transdermal patch (Transderm-Scop) is effective for 72 hours. The side effects are chiefly anticholinergic, including dry mouth and mydriasis, but it is also known to cause hallucination and delirium in the elderly. The patch is contraindicated for children younger than 12 years and patients with glaucoma or urinary retention.

All of these medications should not be used concomitantly with alcoholic beverages, because alcohol can worsen effects on the sensorium.

## HIGH-ALTITUDE SICKNESS

High-altitude sickness is seen not only in mountain climbers but also in patients traveling to high-altitude destinations. Some patients inquire about their risk of altitude-related illness. It is difficult to predict who will have symptoms, because some patients have mild symptoms at 4000 ft (1200 m). Risks are greatest with abrupt ascent above 9000 ft (2700 m). Minimizing morbidity associated with high-altitude sickness can be achieved through educating travelers to recognize symptoms and seek appropriate medical care.

High-altitude sickness includes the following syndromes: acute mountain sickness (AMS), high-altitude pulmonary edema (HAPE), and high-altitude cerebral edema (HAPE). Symptoms of AMS include headache, fatigue, anorexia, nausea. and vomiting. Symptoms of HAPE include dyspnea on exertion and productive cough, with progression to dyspnea at rest. Symptoms of HACE include altered mental status, severe lethargy, confusion, and truncal ataxia.

AMS can be prevented by acclimating to the specific altitude and not sleeping at a higher altitude if having symptoms of AMS. Drug prevention and treatment include acetazolamide (Diamox) 125 mg twice a day, starting 1 or 2 days before ascent and continuing for 2 or 3 days after reaching maximum altitude. Higher doses of acetazolamide are not proven to be more effective in treating AMS, but they do increase the medication's side effects. Prophylaxis is not routinely recommended.

HAPE and HACE must be urgently evaluated, and rapid descent is critical in managing these syndromes. Medications that can alleviate symptoms include acetazolamide, dexamethasone (Decadron), and nifedipine (Adalat).[1]

# Immunizations

The traveler's recommended immunizations depend on their destination. Some countries require documentation of specific vaccinations, such as certain African countries requiring yellow fever vaccination or Saudi Arabia requiring meningococcal vaccination of travelers during the Hajj. Box 5 shows criteria for recommending immunizations. Table 4 describes the vaccines.

## ROUTINE IMMUNIZATIONS

Travelers should be up to date with routine immunizations including measles, mumps, and rubella (MMR); tetanus, diphtheria, and pertussis (Tdap); varicella; *Haemophilus influenzae* type b and other influenza; polio; and hepatitis B. Adults should have had at least one polio booster (IPV) as an adult. Pneumococcal vaccination should be offered to travelers who are older than 65 years, those who are

---

---

> **BOX 5   Vaccine Advice for Travelers**
>
> Vaccine advice should be based on the following factors:
> - Prevalence of vaccine-preventable disease
> - Risk behavior that can place the patient at risk for acquiring disease
> - Potential side effects of the vaccine
> - Previous vaccination records
> - Underlying health problems that predispose the patient to adverse outcomes from the vaccine, such as immunocompromise, pregnancy, egg allergy

immunocompromised, patients with functional or anatomic asplenia, and those who have chronic illnesses such as diabetes, renal disease, or pulmonary disease. Refer to the CDC National Immunization Program (http://www.cdc.gov/Nip/) for guidelines.

## REQUIRED IMMUNIZATIONS

### Meningitis

Meningococcal vaccine is a quadrivalent vaccine against *Neisseria meningitides*, serogroups A,C,Y, and W135. It does not protect against type B, which represents one third of meningitis cases in the United States. One form (Menactra) is conjugated to diphtheria toxoid. Side effects include headache, fatigue, and malaise, in addition to the pain, induration, and redness at the site of infection. These effects are reportedly more common than with Menomune, but they are similar to those with tetanus toxoid.

Saudi Arabia requires certification of immunization if traveling during the Hajj. It is also recommended for adults and children older than 2 years who are traveling to areas known as the *meningitis belt* in sub-Saharan Africa, from Senegal and Guinea eastward to Ethiopia. The vaccine should also be offered to persons who will have prolonged contact with people from this region or those living in refugee camps and to persons working in the health care settings in these regions.

### Yellow Fever

Yellow fever vaccine (YF-Vax) is a single-dose live, attenuated virus preparation made from the 17D yellow fever virus strain, produced in chick embryo. Historically, it is reported to be one of the safest and most effective live virus vaccines. It should be administered at least 10 days before entering an endemic area, which includes sub-Saharan Africa and tropical South America. Various African countries require an international certification of vaccination or a physician's waiver letter for all entering travelers.

The vaccine can be administered concurrently with hepatitis A and B, typhoid fever, and meningococcal vaccines. Safety of the vaccine during pregnancy is not established, nor is it known if vaccine is excreted in human milk.

Adverse reactions include a vaccine virus–associated encephalitis, which occurs predominantly in infants and immunocompromised patients. Thus, the vaccine is not recommended for infants younger than 9 months, and it is contraindicated in infants younger than 6 months. Travelers with HIV/AIDS, leukemia, lymphoma, or other immunosuppressive disorders and travelers older than 65 years are at greater risk for systemic adverse effects. Risks and benefits of vaccination should be evaluated on a case-by-case basis. A rare risk of viscerotropic disease (estimated at 1 in 400,000 dose administered) is associated with the vaccine, which can result in fatal organ failure.

## RECOMMENDED IMMUNIZATIONS

### Hepatitis

Hepatitis A is the most common vaccine-preventable travel-related illness. Most hepatitis A cases are imported into the United States by travelers to Mexico and Central America. Hepatitis A virus vaccine

## TABLE 4  Travel Immunization Doses

| Vaccine Name | Dosage | Comments |
|---|---|---|
| **Hepatitis A Vaccines** | | |
| Havrix | Age 1–18 y: 720 EU IM (0.5 mL), 2nd dose at 0, 6-18 mo | Two doses provide lifelong immunity<br>Vaqta may be substituted for the 2nd dose<br>Giving the 2nd dose at a longer interval does not interfere with immune response |
| | Age ≥19 y: 1440 EU IM (1.0 mL), 2 doses at 0 and 6-12 mo | |
| Vaqta | Age 1-18 y: 25 U IM (0.5 mL), 2 doses at 0, 6-18 mo | Two doses provide lifelong immunity<br>Havrix may be substituted for the 2nd dose<br>Giving the 2nd dose at a longer interval does not interfere with immune response |
| | Age ≥19 y: 50 U IM (1.0 mL), 2 doses at 0, 6-12 mo | |
| **Hepatitis B Vaccine** | | |
| Engerix-B | Age 0-19 y: 10 µg IM (0.5mL), 3 doses given at 0, 1, 6 mo | No need to restart a series that has been interrupted<br>Engerix-B and Recombivax-HB may be used interchangeably in the 3-dose schedule only |
| | Age ≥20 y: 20 µg IM (1.0mL), 3 doses at 0, 1, 6 mo, or 4 doses at 0, 1, 2, 12 mo | |
| Recombivax-HB | Age 0-19 y: 5 µg, 3 doses at 0, 1, 6 mo | Engerix-B and Recombivax-HB may be used interchangeably in the 3-dose schedule only |
| | Age 11-15 y: 10 µg, 2 doses at 0, 4-6 mo<br>Age ≥20 y: 10 µg, 3 doses at 0, 1, 6 mo | |
| **Hepatitis A and B Vaccine** | | |
| Twinrix | Age ≥18 y: 720 EU or 20 µg IM (1.0 mL), 3 doses given at 0, 1, 6 mo | |
| **Japanese Encephalitis** | | |
| JE Vax | Age 1-2 y: 0.5 mL SC ≥3 y 1.0 mL SC 3 doses given on d 0, 7, 30 | High adverse reactions profile for JE vaccine, including generalized urticaria or angioedema, can occur within min or following vaccination. Most reactions occur in 48 h but can be as late as 17 d after vaccination. Vaccinated persons should be observed for 30 min after vaccination and warned about the possibility of delayed generalized urticaria, often in a generalized distribution or angioedema of the extremities, face, and oropharynx, especially of the lips.<br>They should be advised to remain in areas where they have ready access to medical care and should not embark on international travel within 10 d after receiving a dose of JE vaccine<br>Booster dose: 1 dose at 24 mo, but the full duration of protection is not known |
| **Meningococcal Polysaccharide** | | |
| Menomune (quadrivalent A,C,Y,W-135) | Age ≥2 y: 50 µg SC (0.5mL), 1 dose | May be given for short-term protection against group A to infants 3 mo<br>Revaccination of a single 0.5-mL dose administered subcutaneously may be indicated for persons at high risk for infection, particularly children who were first vaccinated when they were <4 y; such children should be considered for revaccination after 2 or 3 y if they remain at high risk<br>Although the need for revaccination in older children and adults has not been determined, antibody levels decline rapidly over 2-3 y, and revaccination may be considered within 5 y |
| **Meningococcal Polysaccharide Diptheria Toxoid Conjugate** | | |
| Menactra (quadrivalent A,C,Y,W-135) | Age 11-55 y: 4 µg of each antigen IM (0.5 mL) | The need for or timing of a booster dose has not been determined |
| **Rabies** | | |
| Imovax (human diploid cell vaccine) HDCV, RVA (rabies vaccine adsorbed)<br>RabAvert (purified chick embryo cell vaccine [PCEC]) | All ages, 2.5 IU rabies antigen IM (1.0 mL), 3 doses given at 0, 7, and 21 or 28 d | The full course should be given with the same product<br>Travelers who are immunosuppressed should avoid travel to endemic areas and postpone vaccination. If this cannot be avoided, antibody titers should be checked after vaccination<br>If traveler has frequent exposure to rabies (spelunkers, veterinarians, rabies diagnostic laboratory workers, animal control workers in rabies-epizootic areas), check serologic testing for necessary booster doses |

*Continued*

## TABLE 4 Travel Immunization Doses—cont'd

| Vaccine Name | Dosage | Comments |
|---|---|---|
| **Typhoid**<br>Injectable (Typhim V)i<br>Oral live attenuated<br>(Vivotif Berna) | Age ≥2 y: 25 µg IM (0.5 mL)<br>Age ≥6 y: 1 capsule every other d for 4 doses (on d 0, 2, 4, 6) | Booster dose every 2 y if ongoing risk<br>Booster dose: same as the initial four-capsule dose after 5 y<br>Do not take with antibiotics, which kill the attenuated Vivotif bacterium |
| **Yellow Fever**<br>Attenuated virus vaccine (YF-VAX) | Age ≥9 mo: 1 injection 0.5 mL SC | African countries might require evidence of vaccination from all entering travelers, including if only in transit, and some might waive the requirements for travelers staying less than 2 wk who are coming from areas where there is no current evidence of significant risk of contracting yellow fever.<br>The certificate becomes valid 10 d after vaccination with YF-VAX<br>Booster every 10 y if ongoing risk. Avoid in pregnant women, unless high-risk travel. |

Note: Table is based on *Health Information for International Travel 2005-2006,* (http://www.cdc.gov/travel/yb/index.htm). Manufacturer's full prescribing information should be consulted to confirm pediatric doses.

(Havrix, Vagta) is now part of routine childhood immunization in the United States. It recommended to those traveling to countries other than the United States, Canada, Western Europe, Australia, New Zealand, Japan, and South Korea. It consists of two IM injections separated by 6 to 18 months. The initial dose should be given 2 to 4 weeks before departure. Antibodies reach protective levels in more than 95% of vaccinees after the first dose. The second dose confers more than 10 years of immunity. Two hepatitis A vaccines are available in the United States, and they can be used interchangeably.

Immunization is not recommended for children younger than 1 year. Children younger than 1 year and other travelers who cannot receive the vaccine should be given immune globulin (0.02 mL/kg IM if traveling for less than 3 months, or 0.06 mL/kg IM if traveling for longer than 3 months.

Hepatitis B virus vaccine (Engerix-B, Recombivax-HB) is a recombinant hepatitis B surface antigen vaccine composed of three doses taken at 0, 1, and 6 months. It is approved for all ages. It is recommended for travelers possibly engaging in voluntary medical care. It is also available as a combined vaccination with Hepatitis A (Twinrix).

### Typhoid Fever

Typhoid vaccine is available in two formulations: as a live attenuated oral vaccine (Vivotif Berna) and as a purified capsular polysaccharide parenteral vaccine (Typhim Vi). This vaccine is recommended for those traveling to Central and South America, the Indian subcontinent, Africa, and Asia and to those traveling outside routine tourist destinations.

The parenteral formulation is a single IM injection given 2 weeks before departure for children older than 2 years and adults. It confers immunity for 2 to 3 years.

The oral formulation taken every other day for a total of 4 capsules, also administered 2 weeks before departure. It confers immunity for 5 years. The effectiveness of the oral vaccine is reduced if it is taken concomitantly with antibiotics. It is recommended for adults and children older than 6 years. Because the oral formulation is a live attenuated vaccine, it is not recommended for immunocompromised persons.

### Rabies

Rabies is endemic in Africa, Asia, India, and Latin America. Preexposure immunization against rabies (Imovax, RVA, RabAvert) is recommended only for travelers with an occupational risk of exposure and for those planning to have animal exposure in endemic regions where immediate access to medical care might be limited.

After sustaining a skin-penetrating scratch or bite from a potentially rabid animal, the traveler should be seen by a physician for evaluation.

Patients who have received preexposure prophylaxis should promptly receive two additional doses of vaccine on day 0 and day 3. Those who sustain exposure with no prior immunization require treatment with rabies immune globulin (Bayrab) and five doses over the course of 28 days of an approved vaccine.

## Assessing Illness in the Return Traveler

Epidemiologic studies from the 1980s and 1990s estimated 50% of travelers report a health problem (based on 100,000 people traveling to developing countries for 1 month). About 8000 of these patients will seek care, and roughly 300 will be hospitalized for their illness.

The approach to assessing patients returning from international travel is to emphasize clinical manifestations and understand the importance of infectious diseases affecting these returned travelers. A few common infectious causes of illness to returning travelers are discussed here, but the list is by no means complete. Returning travelers should be seen by a physician with a specialty in travel medicine or infectious diseases to be evaluated for their symptoms.

A recent study using GeoSentinel surveillance data from 1998-2004 of 17,300 returned travelers from 230 countries found that two thirds of the diagnoses fell into four major syndromic categories of acute febrile illness, acute diarrhea, dermatologic disorders, and chronic diarrhea. Sixty-four percent presented within 1 month of travel. However, 10% had an indolent course and were not seen until 6 months after their return. Malaria was one of the three most frequent causes of systemic febrile illness and was disproportionately seen in persons traveling to sub-Saharan Africa and Southeast Asia. Acute diarrhea was seen more often in travelers returning from Southeast Asia. Acute diarrhea was predominantly bacterial diarrhea; however, travelers from other areas presented with parasite-induced diarrhea more often than bacterial diarrhea. More dermatologic problems were seen in those visiting Central and South America and the Caribbean (Figure 1).

### FEVER

An estimated 3% of international travelers report new onset of fever. Undifferentiated fever can represent a large differential of diseases, including malaria, enteric fever, rickettsial infections. and meningitis. The potentially most dangerous causes of fever in returning travelers include malaria, typhoid, dengue, leptospirosis, and rickettsial diseases. Travel, incubation period, duration and pattern associated with symptoms, immunizations, and use of chemoprophylaxis for malaria should be carefully assessed.

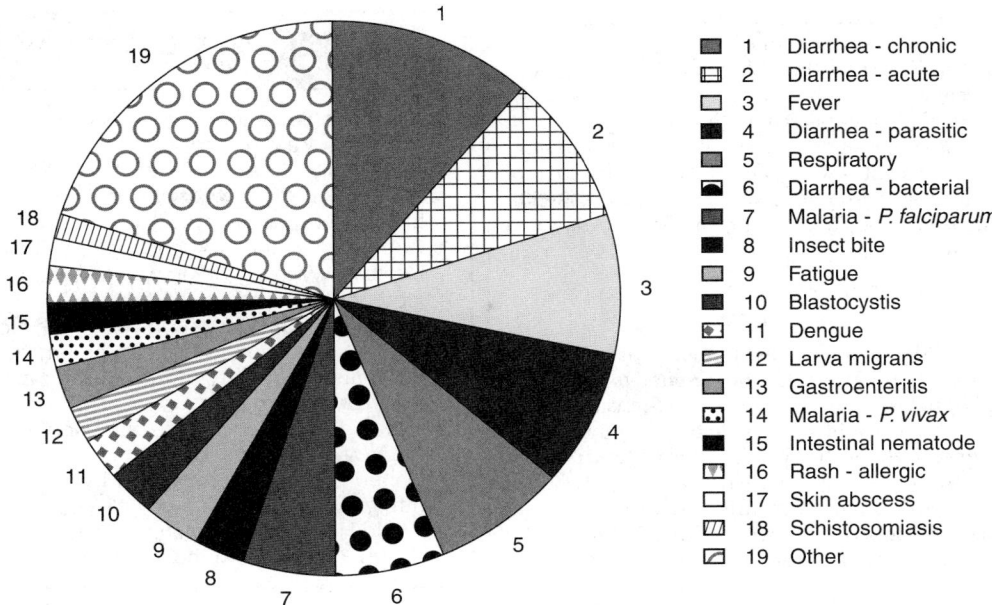

| | | |
|---|---|---|
| 1 | Diarrhea - chronic |
| 2 | Diarrhea - acute |
| 3 | Fever |
| 4 | Diarrhea - parasitic |
| 5 | Respiratory |
| 6 | Diarrhea - bacterial |
| 7 | Malaria - *P. falciparum* |
| 8 | Insect bite |
| 9 | Fatigue |
| 10 | Blastocystis |
| 11 | Dengue |
| 12 | Larva migrans |
| 13 | Gastroenteritis |
| 14 | Malaria - *P. vivax* |
| 15 | Intestinal nematode |
| 16 | Rash - allergic |
| 17 | Skin abscess |
| 18 | Schistosomiasis |
| 19 | Other |

**FIGURE 1.** Illnesses occurring in travelers to the developing world.

## Malaria

Malaria can pose a significant health risk to travelers due to the severity of illness in nonimmune patients. Ninety percent of travelers who contract malaria do not become ill until they return home. The estimated risk of a traveler acquiring malaria will differ depending on region of travel, the time and type of travel, and the intensity of transmission. In epidemiologic surveillance from 1985 through 2002, 11,896 cases of malaria among U.S. civilians were reported to the CDC. The majority, 6961 cases (59%), were acquired in sub-Saharan Africa in comparison with 2237 cases (19%) in Asia and 1672 cases (14%) in the Caribbean and Central and South America. During this period, 76 fatal malaria infections occurred among U.S. civilians; 71 (93%) were caused by *P. falciparum*, of which 52 (73%) were acquired in sub-Saharan Africa.

Studies suggest that the incubation times vary for different malaria species. *P. falciparum* malaria is typically evident within 4 weeks of the traveler's return. *P. ovale* and *P. vivax* malaria, however, can occur much later—as long as 2 to 12 months after the traveler's return. This is significant, because of those late-onset cases of malaria, 60% of the travelers were adherent to their chemoprophylaxis regimen.

Any person who has traveled to malaria-endemic regions and subsequently experiences a fever, chills, headache, nausea, vomiting, or influenza-like symptoms within 3 months of travel should seek immediate medical attention. This syndrome should be considered a medical emergency, and the traveler should report the travel history to the clinician. Thick and thin blood films should be collected as part of the investigations for malaria. The blood films should be repeated every 12 to 24 hours when the patient is symptomatic to catch different levels of blood parasites on stains. Delay in diagnosis and treatment of malaria infections results in serious and, perhaps, fatal outcomes.

Recommendations concerning diagnosis and treatment of malaria can be obtained through the CDC's malaria hotline and from http://www.cdc.gov/malaria/diagnosis_treatment/treatment.htm.

## Dengue Fever

Dengue fever is one of most common causes of systemic febrile illness. It occurs in all regions of travel including sub-Saharan Africa and Central America. However, travelers from sub-Saharan Africa were noted to have more cases of fever caused by rickettsial and tickborne illness versus dengue fever.[8]

Dengue fever, also known as breakbone fever, is a flavivirus transmitted by day-biting mosquitoes, *Aedes aegypti*. There are four serotypes of dengue (DEN1 through DEN4) and no cross immunity among them. No vaccination is available, but repellents are an effective preventive measure.

Seasonal epidemics of dengue infections are common in tropical and subtropical regions. Dengue is endemic to the South Pacific, Asia, the Caribbean, the Americas, and Africa. It is responsible for 12,000 deaths per year. After a 4- to 7-day incubation period, dengue manifests with influenza-like symptoms, including high fevers, headache, myalgias, and arthralgias. Fifty percent of patients report signs of maculopapular rash 3 to 5 days after the onset of fever.

The disease is self-limited. Patients should be encouraged to rest, keep hydrated, and use acetaminophen for fevers. If the disease is a severe form, such as dengue shock syndrome or, rarer, dengue hemorrhagic fever, the patient will need intravenous fluid hydration and supportive care. This disease is diagnosed clinically and by comparison of acute and convalescent serum antibody titers. There is no specific treatment but only supportive care.

## Typhoid Fever

Typhoid fever is caused by *Salmonella enterica typhi*, which produces an acute febrile illness. Typhoid fever is endemic to the Indian subcontinent, Asia, Africa, the Caribbean, and Central and South America. There are an estimated 22 million cases with 200,000 deaths worldwide. The CDC reports 400 cases per year in the United States, and 70% of these cases are associated with travel.

The vaccine does not provide 100% protection. Risks for typhoid fever are minimized by decreasing exposure to fecal-oral contaminated foods and using the "boil it, peel it, cook it, or forget it " strategy (see Box 2).

Typhoid can have an insidious onset, with ongoing fevers, malaise, abdominal discomfort, constipation, and, rarely, diarrhea. If typhoid fever is suspected in a returned traveler, serology assays should be ordered and the patient should be empirically treated with fluoroquinolones or a third-generation cephalosporin.

## Rickettsia

Rickettsial infection is a tickborne illness transmitted by an arthropod vector. African tick typhus, Mediterranean tick typhus, and scrub typhus are a few of the rickettsial infections seen in returned travelers if they come into contact with environments that support these pathogens. Most patients with rickettsial infections recover with timely use of appropriate antibiotic therapy.

Clinical manifestations of rickettsial illnesses can start as a triad of nonspecific symptoms, fever, headache, and myalgias. Specific symptoms include regional lymphadenopathy, rash, and thrombocytopenia. A painless eschar is seen in scrub typhus.

Diagnosis of rickettsial disease is based on the clinical picture and epidemiologic history, isolation of the rickettsial agent by a positive polymerase chain reaction (PCR) test, immunohistologic detection of a microorganism, or by comparison of acute and convalescent serum titers. Patients should be promptly treated with antibiotic therapy and monitored for worsening condition.

## DIARRHEA

Diarrhea in the acute setting is often caused by bacterial organism; however, diarrhea that is persistent and does not respond to antibiotics could be complicated by parasitic infections, antibiotic-resistant bacterial infections, and possibly a postinfectious irritable bowel syndrome. A recent study identified 60% of diarrhea in return travelers to be caused by parasites, except to cases coming from Southeast Asia. Patients with bacterial diarrhea often came from Southeast Asia with *Campylobacter* as one of the main causative organisms. The top causes for parasitic diarrhea include giardiasis and amebiasis. Sensitivities of diagnosis of *Giardia intestinalis*, *Cryptosporidium*, and *Entamoeba histolytica* have improved with use of reverse-transcriptase PCR testing. The key to managing return travelers with diarrhea is to properly investigate their history, especially their antibiotic use, and provide appropriate therapy while conducting investigatory testing to determine the cause of the diarrheal illness (Figure 2).

## DERMATOLOGIC CONDITIONS

Skin lesions and rashes represent up to 8% of illnesses of travelers seeking medical care after recent travel. The etiology of skin lesions can include insect bites, larval infestations, bacterial infections, or drug-related hypersensitivity. The diagnosis of the lesions will depend on identifying the location, their dermatologic pattern and other associated symptoms, and the patient's activity when first noticing the lesion.

Papules are often associated with insect bites, such as scabies. Subcutaneous painful nodules can be seen with myiasis, tungiasis, and furuncles. Myiasis is caused by invading larvae of the tumbu fly in Africa or the botfly in Latin America. Patients often report the sensation of movement under the lesion.

Cutaneous ulcers are often due to pyoderma secondarily infected with *Staphylococcus aureus* or group A streptococci. Painless ulcerative lesions with raised margins and isolated lymphadenopathy should suggest leishmania. Linear or serpiginous lesions, often found on the feet or buttocks, should bring to mind cutaneous larva migrans.

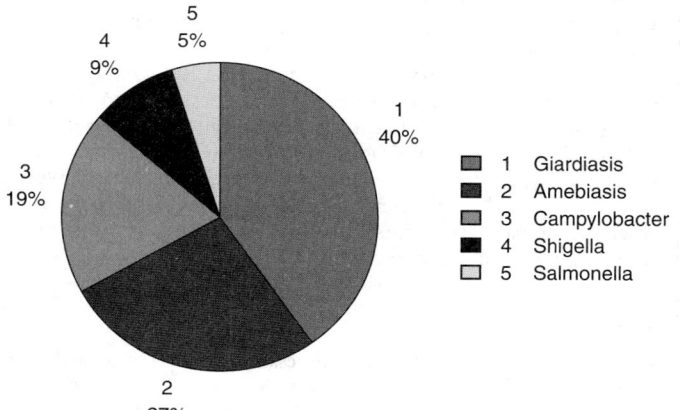

1  40%
2  27%
3  19%
4  9%
5  5%

1  Giardiasis
2  Amebiasis
3  Campylobacter
4  Shigella
5  Salmonella

**FIGURE 2.** Distribution of causes of acute diarrhea in returned travelers.

## Summary

Clinicians who provide medical advice to travelers should be proficient in travel medicine and global epidemiology of infectious diseases. Travel medicine has become specialized, and thus the consultation with a specialist in travel or tropical medicine may be advantageous for travelers who live abroad for any length of time, who have multiple medical problems, who are immunocompromised, who are pregnant, or who are traveling with young children to developing countries. Patients presenting with illness and recent history of travel would also benefit from evaluation by such specialists, because travel medicine specialists have the expertise in seeing various infectious diseases in returning travelers and could expedite the appropriate diagnosis and treatment of the manifesting illness. A listing of travel clinics can be obtained through the American Society of Tropical Medicine and Hygiene. A list of helpful Web sites is given in Box 6.

## REFERENCES

Advice for travelers. Treat Guidel Med Lett 2006;4(45):25-34.

Cannegieter SC, Doggen CJ, Van Houwelingen HC, Rosendaal FR: Related venous thrombosis: Results from a large population-based case control study (MEGA study). PLoS Med 2006;3(8):e307.

Cetron MS, Marfin AA, Julian KG, et al: Yellow fever vaccine. Recommendations of the Advisory Committee on Immunization Practices (ACIP), 2002. MMWR Recomm Rep 2002;51(RR-17):1-10.

Dupont HL, Jiang ZD, Okhuysen PC, et al: Antibacterial chemoprophylaxis in the prevention of traveler's diarrhea: Evaluation of poorly absorbed oral rifaximin. Clin Infect Dis 2005;41:S571-S576.

Eliades MJ, Shah S, Nguyen-Dinh P, et al: Malaria surveillance—United States, 2003. MMWR Surveill Summ 2005;54(2):25-39.

Freedman DO, Weld LH, Kozarsky PE, et al: Spectrum of disease and relation to place of exposure among ill returned travelers. N Engl J Med 2006;354(2):119-130.

Guptill KS, Hargarten SW, Baker TD: American travel deaths in Mexico: Causes and prevention strategies. West J Med 1991;154(2):169-171.

Hill DR, Ericsson CD, Pearson RD, et al: The practice of travel medicine: Guidelines by the Infectious Diseases Society of America. Clin Infect Dis 2006;43(12):1499-1539.

McInnes RJ, Williamson LM, Morrison A: Unintentional injury during foreign travel: A review. J Travel Med 2002;9:297-307.

Peden M, Scurfield R, Sleet D, et al: World Report on Road Traffic Injury Prevention Geneva: World Health Organization; 2004.

Prevention of malaria. Med Lett Drugs Ther 2005;47(1223-1224):100-102.

Ryan ET, Kain KC: Health advice and immunizations for travelers. N Engl J Med 2000;342(23):1716-1725.

Ryan ET, Wilson ME, Kain KC: Illness after international travel. N Engl J Med 2002;347(7):505-516.

Schwartz E, Parise M, Kozarsky P, Cetron M: Delayed onset of malaria: Implications for chemophrophylaxis in travelers. N Engl J Med 2003;349(16): 1510-1516.

Skarbinski J, James EM, Causer LM, et al: Malaria surveillance—United States, 2004. MMWR Surveill Summ 2006;55(SS-04):23-37.

Spira AM: Assessment of travelers who return home ill. Lancet 2003;361: 1459-1469.

Steffen R: Epidemiology of traveler's diarrhea. Clin Infect Dis 2005;41: S536-S540.

Steffen R, Lobel HO: Epidemiological basis for the practices of travel medicine. J Wilderness Med 1994;5:56-66.

Thielman NM, Guerrant RL: Clinical practice: Acute infectious diarrhea. N Engl J Med 2004;350:38-47.

# Toxoplasmosis

Method of
*Thomas T. Ward, MD*

Toxoplasmosis is the disease caused by infection with the obligate intracellular protozoan *Toxoplasma gondii*. Toxoplasmosis is a worldwide zoonosis and causes infection in both birds and mammals. Cats, the definitive hosts for *T. gondii*, are the animals in which the parasite maintains an enteroepithelial sexual cycle. Human beings and domestic animals are secondary hosts and are important in maintaining an extraintestinal asexual cycle of transmission. Although most human infection is asymptomatic, self-limited clinical disease can infrequently occur after primary infection in immunocompetent persons. Because of the persistence of dormant cyst forms, all infection becomes chronic and latent. Primary infection during pregnancy can result in transplacental transmission of infection to the fetus; resultant congenital toxoplasmosis has varied clinical manifestations. Reactivation of dormant cysts is an important cause of infection in immunocompromised patients with defective T-cell–mediated immunity, including those patients with advanced HIV infection, hematologic malignancies, and bone marrow and solid-organ transplants.

*T. gondii* exists in three forms: the oocyst, the tissue cyst, and the tachyzoite. Oocysts are formed only in infected felines; these cats excrete large numbers of cysts for approximately 2 weeks after infection. Oocysts may remain viable in the soil for months and are an important environmental reservoir for infection of incidental hosts. Tachyzoites occur with acute infection in incidental hosts; their presence is required for the histologic confirmation of active disease. Tissue cysts occur after replication of tachyzoites and likely persist for the life of the incidental host. Dormant cysts are most commonly located in skeletal and smooth muscle, heart, brain, and eye. The presence of tissue cysts in histologic sections is indicative of past infection, but by itself it does not signify active infection.

The human incidence of seropositivity for *T. gondii* antibody varies greatly throughout the world. Within the United States, seropositivity increases with age, and the overall seroprevalence is approximately 15%. Within Western Europe, seroprevalence ranges between 50% and 70%. Human transmission occurs by oral exposure to oocysts that have contaminated water sources, vegetables, or other food products or, even more commonly, by ingesting poorly cooked or raw meat that contains tissue cysts. As many as 25% of lamb or pork samples contain tissue cysts.

After human ingestion of either oocysts or tissue cysts, specialized forms of *T. gondii* emerge that penetrate the intestinal mucosa, establish intracellular infection within white blood cells, and enter the blood and lymphatic circulations to result in widespread dissemination throughout the body. Intact cell-mediated immunity leads to clearance of intracellular tachyzoites and the formation of dormant tissue cysts. Impaired cell-mediated immunity leads to either uncontrolled, primary infection (as in the fetus) or reactivation of infection later in life (as in AIDS and other immunosuppressed conditions).

# Diagnosis

The diagnosis of *T. gondii* infection can be established by serologic tests, amplification of specific nucleic acid sequences, or histologic demonstration of the parasite or its antigens. Rarely employed reference or research methods for diagnosis include isolation of the organism, specific IgG avidity tests, various antigen detection tests, and lymphocyte transformation tests.

IgG antibodies appear in immunocompetent individuals within 2 to 3 weeks after infection. A negative IgG test essentially excludes previous or past infection with *T. gondii*. IgG antibody may persist in high titers for years after infection; therefore, a single positive IgG titer does not differentiate whether infection is recently acquired, chronic and latent, or chronic and reactivated. Sequential IgG antibody tests that increase by more than two tube dilutions are consistent with recent infection. Specific IgM and IgA antibody tests are usually positive during the first 6 months after acquisition of infection, and negative tests have a high predictive value for excluding recent infection. A positive IgM test can indicate recent onset of infection; however, both false-positive results and persistently positive IgM antibody test results in chronically infected individuals can occur. When therapeutic decisions will be based on the interpretation of a positive IgM antibody test, confirmatory testing by a reference laboratory should be performed if feasible. Serologic tests can be more difficult to interpret in immunocompromised patients.

Polymerase chain reaction (PCR) for detection of specific *T. gondii* nucleic acid sequences has been successfully employed using vitreous and aqueous humor, bronchoalveolar lavage fluid, peripheral blood buffy coat preparations, cerebrospinal fluid, and amniotic fluid after 18 weeks of gestation. False-positive results on brain tissue PCR tests may occur in patients with HIV infection and suspected toxoplasmic encephalitis.

Specific histopathologic findings on resected lymph nodes can be strongly suggestive of the diagnosis of toxoplasmosis in immunocompetent patients. Demonstration of tachyzoites in tissue is invariably diagnostic of active infection. Although the presence of a single cyst does not differentiate between active and chronic or latent infection, multiple cysts present on cytopathologic examination suggest the presence of active disease. Staining for specific antigens (e.g., immunoperoxidase techniques) is highly specific for active infection when positive, and it is much more sensitive than hematoxylin and eosin or Wright-Giemsa staining alone. Tests employing direct fluorescent antibody tests can be nonspecific and are best avoided.

# Clinical Manifestations

Most patients with acute *T. gondii* infection do not have symptomatic disease. Clinical manifestations of acute infection occasionally occur in immunocompetent adults, as does reactivation of infection within the retina of the eye. Infection during pregnancy results in congenital toxoplasmosis at an incidence of approximately 1 in 8000 live births in the United States; the frequency in which *T. gondii* causes spontaneous abortion is unknown. Reactivation infection from dormant cysts is the cause of toxoplasmic infections in patients with AIDS, patients with bone marrow or solid-organ transplants, and other immunosuppressed hosts. The clinical syndromes in each of the foregoing settings are sufficiently distinct to warrant separate comment.

## ACUTE INFECTION IN IMMUNOCOMPETENT PATIENTS

Approximately 15% of immunocompetent patients who become infected have either regional lymphadenopathy or a mononucleosis-like syndrome characterized by generalized adenopathy and constitutional symptoms. Toxoplasmic lymphadenopathy is largely a self-limited disease in immunocompetent patients, and it rarely requires therapy. Epstein-Barr virus and cytomegalovirus infections are much more common causes of the mononucleosis syndrome. Other causes of lymphadenopathy that need to be considered include cat-scratch disease, lymphoma or metastatic malignancy, sarcoidosis, tuberculosis, and the deep mycoses. Serologic testing and lymph node biopsy are most beneficial in establishing a diagnosis. Infections acquired by blood transfusion or through a laboratory accident may be severe and should be treated.

## OCULAR TOXOPLASMOSIS IN IMMUNOCOMPETENT PATIENTS

Approximately 33% of all cases of chorioretinitis within the Unites States are caused by *T. gondii*. Most cases are believed to result from unrecognized congenital infection that reactivates, most commonly during the second and third decades of life. Retinal clinical findings are highly suggestive of *T. gondii* infection when evaluated by ophthalmologists experienced in managing this infection. Serologic testing is usually positive for prior exposure to toxoplasmosis, but in difficult cases, PCR testing may be performed on samples of aqueous or vitreous humor to confirm the diagnosis. Control of the host inflammatory response by the concomitant use of corticosteroids may be required in some patients receiving therapy for toxoplasmosis. Relapse of infection requiring repeated treatment is not uncommon.

## CONGENITAL TOXOPLASMOSIS

Congenital toxoplasmosis results from transplacental spread of *T. gondii* infection that is asymptomatically acquired either during pregnancy or shortly before the onset of gestation. The risk of fetal infection varies with the stage of trimester; it is highest during the second and third trimesters. Approximately 60% of maternal infections acquired during the third trimester will result in fetal infection. Fetal infection occurring during the first trimester is believed to result frequently in spontaneous abortion. Clinical manifestations of congenital toxoplasmosis are varied. There may be no sequelae, or clinical disease may become manifest at birth or at various times after birth. Children may be born with the nonspecific manifestations of the TORCH (toxoplasmosis, other infections, rubella, cytomegalovirus, and herpes simplex) syndrome, including chorioretinitis, hydrocephalus, intracranial calcifications, hepatosplenomegaly, rash, anemia, and/or jaundice. Other infectious causes such as herpes simplex, cytomegalovirus infection, rubella, and syphilis should be considered and excluded. In those infants born with subclinical congenital infection, studies suggest that most will eventually demonstrate evidence of clinical disease even though they appear normal at birth. Years or decades later, previously subclinically infected children may develop chorioretinitis, seizure disorders, or psychomotor and mental retardation. Early recognition and treatment of congenital infection reduce the likelihood of subsequent sequelae; therefore, congenital *T. gondii* infection should always be treated regardless of whether there are symptoms at birth. Treatment of acute maternal infection diagnosed during pregnancy reduces the risk of fetal infection by approximately 60%.

Because congenital toxoplasmosis occurs almost exclusively in women infected during pregnancy, it is important that such infection be recognized and treated aggressively. In some countries where there is a higher seroprevalence of *T. gondii* infection (e.g., France), routine screening for acquisition of infection during pregnancy is performed. Routine pregnancy screening is not currently advocated in the United States. Women who have IgG antibody but who lack specific IgM antibody are believed to have evidence of past, chronic infection and are not at risk of transmitting congenital infection. A positive IgM test requires further confirmatory testing through a reference laboratory to determine whether infection has been recently acquired. Confirmation of acutely acquired maternal infection during pregnancy mandates testing during and after pregnancy to determine whether fetal or congenital infection has occurred. PCR testing of amniotic fluid at 18 weeks of gestation and beyond is approximately 60% sensitive and 100% specific in diagnosing fetal infection. Diagnosis of congenital toxoplasmosis at birth is usually confirmed by the presence of specific IgA (or IgM) in fetal serum, with careful attention to exclusion of maternal contamination of fetal blood. In children with suspected congenital toxoplasmosis, it is important to perform ophthalmologic evaluation and neuroimaging studies and to examine the cerebrospinal fluid for pleocytosis or elevated protein concentrations.

## TOXOPLASMOSIS IN AIDS AND IMMUNOCOMPROMISED PATIENTS

In immunocompromised patients, toxoplasmosis almost always occurs as reactivation infection. One exception is infection after heart transplantation, in which primary infection can occur when a seronegative host receives a donor heart from a seropositive donor. The central nervous system is the most commonly affected site, resulting in necrotizing focal or multifocal encephalitis and, less frequently, focal spinal cord involvement. Other forms of infection include chorioretinitis, myocarditis, and pneumonia. Active toxoplasmosis in immunodeficient patients can cause significant morbidity and mortality and always requires therapy. The duration of therapy is largely dependent on the degree of chronic immunosuppression, and, on occasion, lifelong maintenance therapy is indicated.

In natural history studies of HIV infection performed before effective antiretroviral therapy, it was observed that approximately one third of toxoplasmosis-seropositive patients with AIDS developed toxoplasmic encephalitis before death. Daily receipt of one tablet of double-strength trimethoprim (160 mg)-sulfamethoxazole (800 mg) (Bactrim DS) largely eliminates the risk of disease. Most episodes of toxoplasmic encephalitis complicating AIDS occur in patients with CD4$^+$ counts of less than 100 cells/mm$^3$, and infection is uncommon if the CD4$^+$ count exceeds 200 cells/mm$^3$. Patients with toxoplasmic encephalitis most commonly present with focal neurologic abnormalities of subacute (weeks) onset, often with fevers, headache, or subtle mental status or memory changes. Motor palsies are the most common focal abnormalities, although cranial nerve abnormalities, visual field defects, and seizure disorders can be the major presenting symptoms. Neuroradiologic imaging is best performed using magnetic resonance imaging, with the most common finding being multiple, ring-enhancing cerebral lesions. Involvement of the basal ganglion area is common. Computed tomography is, in general, less sensitive in defining disease and its extent. Single lesions on magnetic resonance imaging are unusual in toxoplasmic encephalitis and suggest possible central nervous system lymphoma. Multifocal leukoencephalopathy resulting from JC virus can also cause neuroradiologic findings that resemble toxoplasmosis. PCR can be performed on cerebrospinal fluid for Epstein-Barr virus, JC virus, and toxoplasmosis.

A definitive diagnosis of toxoplasmic encephalitis is made by brain biopsy and by the histologic demonstration of tachyzoites. However, to avoid the morbidity associated with brain biopsy, in patients with HIV infection who are toxoplasmosis seropositive and who have consistent neuroradiologic findings, it is now standard practice to treat these patients for toxoplasmosis empirically and to observe the clinical response. Although neuroradiologic resolution is delayed, most patients with toxoplasmic encephalitis demonstrate clinical improvement within 7 days of initiating therapy. Failure to respond clinically to empirical therapy, seronegativity to *T. gondii* antibody, and the presence of a single lesion on magnetic resonance imaging all are findings that suggest the possibility of an alternative diagnosis and warrant consideration of performing a brain biopsy.

Tissue biopsies with histologic examination are usually necessary for diagnosing toxoplasmosis at other sites in immunocompromised patients. PCR testing on bronchoalveolar lavage fluid can be positive in cases of pneumonitis. Endomyocardial biopsy should be performed if toxoplasmosis is a consideration in the seronegative heart recipient of a seropositive donor.

# Therapy

Treatment of toxoplasmosis is summarized in Table 1. Most infections in immunologically normal adults are self-limited and do not require therapy. In ocular, central nervous system, and congenital toxoplasmosis, first-line therapy is the combination of pyrimethamine (Daraprim), and sulfadiazine, with folinic acid (leucovorin, not folic acid). Treatment duration is based on time of clinical resolution, but it is usually approximately 6 weeks in ocular and central nervous system infections and 12 months in congenital infection. In patients with AIDS who have persistently low CD4$^+$ counts (less than 200 cells/mm$^3$), and

**TABLE 1** Therapy of Toxoplasmic Infection

| | Adult Doses | Pediatric Doses |
|---|---|---|
| **Immunologically Normal** | | |
| Acute lymphadenopathy | No treatment | No treatment |
| Acute chorioretinitis | Pyrimethamine (Daraprim) 100 mg PO bid on day 1, then 25 mg PO qd + sulfadiazine 1 g PO qid + folinic acid (leucovorin) 5 mg PO qd | |
| Pregnancy | Spiramycin* 1.0 g PO q8h (see text) | |
| Congenital toxoplasmosis | | Pyrimethamine 2 mg/kg for 2 d, then 1 mg/kg PO qd + sulfadiazine 50 mg/kg PO bid + folinic acid 10 mg 3 × wk PO |
| **AIDS and Immunologically Impaired** | | |
| Encephalitis and other tissue sites of infection | Pyrimethamine 200 mg PO × one dose, then 75 mg PO qd + sulfadiazine 1 g PO qid ?+ folinic acid 5-10 mg PO qd | |

*Not available in the United States except from the FDA (call 301-827-2335).
*Abbreviations:* bid = twice daily; PO = orally; q = every; qd = every day; qid = four times daily.

in other patients with continued profound immunosuppression, long-term maintenance therapy with pyrimethamine– sulfadiazine–folinic acid should be continued at the same doses used for primary therapy. Spiramycin[1,*] (3 g per day) is the drug of choice for pregnant women with acquired primary *T. gondii* infection. Spiramycin should be continued until term if there is no evidence of fetal infection. Spiramycin does not cross the placenta and will not treat infection in the fetus. If fetal infection is demonstrated to be present by amniotic fluid PCR, pyrimethamine– sulfadiazine–folinic acid should be administered during the second and third trimesters. Pyrimethamine is potentially teratogenic and should not be administered during the first 16 weeks of pregnancy.

Allergic reactions to sulfonamides are common in patients with HIV infection. Alternative drugs to sulfadiazine that may be employed in combination therapy include clindamycin (Cleocin),[1] 600 to 1200 mg every 6 hours intravenously or orally; clarithromycin (Biaxin),[1] 1 g every 12 hours orally; atovaquone (Mepron),[1] 750 mg every 6 hours orally; azithromycin (Zithromax),[1] 1200 to 1500 mg per day orally; and dapsone,[1] 100 mg per day orally. Alternatively, increasing experience suggests that trimethoprim-sulfamethoxazole (Bactrim, Septra),[1] 5 mg/kg trimethoprim component every 6 hours orally or intravenously (20 mg/kg per day total), is as effective as the pyrimethamine-containing combination regimens in patients who are not allergic to sulfa agents.

Corticosteroids can be administered to patients with ocular toxoplasmosis in whom a brisk inflammatory response is believed to be contributing to ocular pathology. Similarly, in toxoplasmic encephalitis with cerebral edema or significant mass effect, short-duration corticosteroids may be concomitantly employed with antitoxoplasmic antimicrobial therapy.

## Prevention

Prevention of *T. gondii* infection is of major importance in pregnant women and immunodeficient patients who have not been previously exposed. Risk of primary infection can be reduced by not eating undercooked meat and by taking proper precautions when disposing of or cleaning cat litter material. Cysts in meat are killed at 60°C (140°F) or higher. Hands should be thoroughly washed after soil contamination, and all fruits and vegetables should be washed before they are eaten.

Primary prophylaxis should be administered in patients with AIDS who have CD4+ counts of less than 100 cells/mm³ and who are seropositive for toxoplasmosis antibody. Trimethoprim (160 mg)-sulfamethoxazole (800 mg),[1] one double-strength tablet daily, is highly effective for prevention of toxoplasmosis infection. Alternative prophylactic regimens include either (a) pyrimethamine, 50 to 75 mg orally per week, plus dapsone,[1] 50 mg per day or 200 mg per week; or (b) pyrimethamine-sulfadoxine (Fansidar),[1] three tablets every 2 weeks. Dapsone alone is not effective at preventing toxoplasmosis.

# Cat-Scratch Disease

Method of
*Michael J. Smith, MD*

Cat-scratch disease (CSD), regional lymphadenopathy following a cat scratch or bite, has been described since the 1950s. *Bartonella henselae*, a pleomorphic, facultative intracellular gram-negative bacillus, was not identified as the etiologic agent until 40 years later. As the laboratory detection of *B. henselae* has improved, it has become associated with an increasing number of clinical entities. These have traditionally been divided into typical CSD, the classic finding of unilateral regional lymphadenopathy following a cat scratch or bite, and atypical CSD, which includes all other presentations.

## Epidemiology

As CSD is not a reportable disease, the true incidence remains unknown. However, there are an estimated 24,000 cases in the United States each year. Predominantly a disease of childhood and adolescence, CSD has the highest age-specific incidence rate occurring in children younger than 10 years of age. Although less frequent, CSD does occur in older individuals as well. A recent study found that 6% of patients with confirmed CSD were older than the age of 60 years.

Nearly 90% of patients with CSD have exposure to cats and approximately half recall a definitive scratch or bite. Early epidemiologic evidence suggested an increased risk of CSD in patients with

---

[1]Not FDA approved for this indication.
*Not available in the United States except from the FDA (call 301-827-2335).

---

[1]Not FDA approved for this indication.

kittens as compared to patients with adult cats. It was subsequently shown that kittens have a higher rate of *B. henselae* bacteremia than adult cats. In contrast, adult cats are more likely to have antibodies indicative of past infection. Most bacteremic cats are asymptomatic, so even a healthy-appearing animal can transmit disease.

The cat flea, *Ctenocephalides felis*, has been implicated in the transmission between cats. Consequently, CSD is more prevalent in warm and humid environments that support the growth of fleas with infection occurring primarily in the fall and winter months. To date, no evidence exists for human to human transmission.

## Clinical Manifestations

Typical CSD is the most common form of CSD in immunocompetent patients. Initially, papules develop at the site of inoculation within the first week after a cat scratch or bite. This is followed by the gradual onset of unilateral regional lymphadenopathy over the next several weeks. Occasionally these lymph nodes may suppurate. The location of lymphadenopathy depends on the site of inoculation but most commonly occurs in the axillary, inguinal or cervical chains. In contrast to bacterial lymphadenitis, the lymph nodes are not inflamed. Patients are usually well-appearing and afebrile. Lymphadenopathy gradually resolves over several months without specific therapy.

The most common form of atypical CSD is Parinaud's oculoglandular syndrome (POGS), which occurs when bacteria are inoculated directly into the eye or eyelid. Small papules develop, almost always in the palpebral conjunctiva, in association with ipsilateral preauricular lymphadenopathy. There is also a painless, nonpurulent conjunctivitis. Similar to typical CSD, these symptoms resolve without antimicrobial therapy over several weeks.

Typical CSD and POGS share a similar pathophysiology; direct inoculation followed by a local immune response. In contrast, the other types of atypical CSD are due to systemic infection with *B. henselae*. These include hepatosplenic CSD, osteomyelitis, endocarditis, encephalitis, and neuroretinitis. *Bartonella* has also been implicated in the etiology of fever of unknown origin (FUO). One recent study revealed that 5% of all children with FUO of infectious etiology had antibodies against *B. henselae* indicative of current or recent infection.

In immunocompromised individuals, *B. henselae* can cause life-threatening invasive disease. Bacillary angiomatosis (BA), which is also caused by other *Bartonella* species, is caused by the angioproliferative effects of *Bartonella* and results in multiple vascular tumors in the skin and subcutaneous tissues. Bacillary peliosis (BP) is another form of vasoproliferative disease that leads to the development of blood-filled cysts in the reticuloendothelial element of the liver, spleen, and bone marrow of severely immunocompromised patients.

## Diagnosis

A detailed history and physical examination are essential for the diagnosis of CSD. Any contact with cats or kittens, especially if bites or scratches occurred, should raise suspicion for CSD, regardless of the patient's age and clinical presentation.

*Bartonella* is a fastidious organism that takes several weeks to grow, making culture impractical. Therefore, serologic testing has become the mainstay of diagnosis. Indirect fluorescent antibody testing for IgM and IgG against *B. henselae* is performed by most commercial laboratories as well as the Center for Disease Control. A single elevated titer or a fourfold or greater increase between acute and convalescent titers is diagnostic of CSD.

The combination of history, physical examination, and serologic testing may obviate the need for biopsy in cases of typical CSD. If a node is removed, the characteristic histopathologic finding is the formation of granulomas with microabscesses and central necrosis. Rarely, gram-negative bacilli may be identified using the Warthin-Starry silver stain. These are both non-specific findings, and any patient undergoing biopsy should have samples sent for cytology as well as fungal, mycobacterial, and standard bacterial culture and sensitivity to rule out other etiologies of lymphadenopathy. Polymerase chain reaction (PCR) testing of tissue is emerging as a highly specific diagnostic tool. Sensitivity of PCR testing varies with the specific DNA target used but is usually quite high. It is becoming increasingly available in commercial laboratories.

## Treatment

Treatment of typical CSD is supportive and mainly consists of needle aspiration of suppurative lymph nodes when required. There is no evidence to suggest that treatment with antibiotics significantly alters the course of disease. In the only prospective, randomized, double blinded study of typical CSD, a 5-day course of azithromycin (Zithromax) or placebo was given to 29 patients with clinical CSD. Although the subjects who received azithromycin had a more rapid reduction in lymphadenopathy as measured by ultrasound at 30 days, the long-term outcomes were identical for both groups.

Evidence for the treatment of atypical CSD in immunocompetent patients is limited to case reports and retrospective reviews. Success has been reported using a range of oral antibiotics including trimethoprim-sulfamethoxazole[1] (Bactrim, Septra), rifampin (Rifadin),[1] azithromycin (Zithromax),[1] doxycycline (Vibramycin), and ciprofloxacin (Cipro[1]), as well as intravenous gentamicin (Garamycin).[1] Nevertheless, most cases of atypical CSD are thought to resolve without antibiotic therapy. A notable exception is endocarditis, which requires surgical replacement of the damaged valve in addition to antibiotic therapy. One retrospective review found that treatment of endocarditis with a

---

[1]Not FDA approved for this indication.

## CURRENT DIAGNOSIS

- Suspect CSD in any patient with lymphadenopathy and a history of cat exposure, regardless of age.
- Serologic testing can confirm the diagnosis.
- If biopsy is performed, specimens should be sent for pathology as well as fungal, mycobacterial, and routine bacterial cultures.
- Granulomas with central necrosis are characteristic of CSD but are not specific. When available, PCR is highly specific for CSD.

---

*Abbreviations:* CSD = cat-scratch disease; PCR = polymerase chain reaction.

## CURRENT THERAPY

**Immunocompetent Patients**
- Typical CSD only requires supportive treatment.
- No antibiotics are indicated.
- For atypical CSD there are no definitive treatment recommendations.
- Endocarditis requires surgery and antibiotic therapy, which should include at least 14 days of an aminoglycoside.

**Immunocompromised Patients**
- BA or BP treatment for at least 3 months with either
  - Erythromycin (E.E.S.)[1] 500 mg PO qid or
  - Doxycycline (Vibramycin) 100 mg PO bid.

---

[1]Not FDA approved for this indication.
*Abbreviations:* BA = bacillary angiomatosis; BP = bacillary peliosis; CSD = cat-scratch disease.

regimen that included an aminoglycoside for at least 14 days was significantly associated with a higher rate of survival.

Immunocompromised patients with BA or BP warrant antimicrobial treatment. There have been no controlled studies to determine optimal therapy, but either erythromycin (E.E.S.)[1] or doxycycline (Vibramycin) is effective. Most experts recommend a treatment course of at least 3 months to prevent relapse.

## Prevention

Cat owners should avoid activities that may result in a cat scratch or bite, and should promptly wash any cat-inflicted wounds. Appropriate flea control will also reduce the likelihood of CSD. Because of the risk for invasive disease caused by *B. henselae*, immunocompromised individuals should be specifically warned of the risks of cat exposure. If possible, they should avoid purchasing or adopting kittens.

### REFERENCES

American Academy of Pediatrics: Cat-scratch disease. In Pickering LK (ed.): Red Book: 2003 Report of the Committee on Infectious Diseases (26th ed.). Elk Grove Village, IL, American Academy of Pediatrics, pp 232–234.

Bass JW, Freitas BC, Freitas AD, et al: Prospective randomized double blind placebo-controlled evaluation of azithromycin for treatment of cat-scratch disease. Pediatr Infect Dis J 1998;17:447–452.

Batts S, Demers DM: Spectrum and treatment of cat-scratch disease. Pediatr Infect Dis J 2004;23:1161–1162.

Ben-Ami R, Ephros M, Avidor B, et al: Cat-scratch disease in elderly patients. Clin Infect Dis 2005;41:969–974.

Hansmann Y, DeMartino S, Piemont Y, et al: Diagnosis of cat scratch disease with detection of *Bartonella henselae* PCR: A study of patients with lymph node enlargement. J Clin Microbiol 2005;43:3800–3806.

Jacobs RF, Schutze GE: *Bartonella henselae* as a cause of prolonged fever and fever of unknown origin in children. Clin Infect Dis 1998;26:80–84.

Massei F, Gori L, Machhia P, Maggiore G, et al: The extended spectrum of Bartonellosis in children. Infect Dis Clin North Am 2005;19:691–711.

Raoult D, Fournier PE, Vandenesch F, et al: Outcome and treatment of *Bartonella* endocarditis. Arch of Int Med 2003;163:226–230.

Rolain JM, Brouqui P, Koehler JE, et al: Recommendations for treatment of human infection caused by *Bartonella* species. Antimicrob Agents Chemother 2004;48:1921–1933.

Zangwill KM, Hamilton DH, Perkins BA, et al: Cat scratch disease in Connecticut: Epidemiology, risk factors, and evaluation of a new diagnostic test. N Engl J Med 1993;329:8–13.

# Salmonellosis

Method of
*Arvid E. Underman, MD, FACP, DTMH*

Salmonellosis refers to a group of infections caused by members of the genus *Salmonella*. This genus is named after Salmon, a pathologist who first isolated the organism, later designated as *Salmonella choleraesuis*, from the intestine of pigs with diarrhea. *Salmonellae* are widely distributed throughout nature and are adapted to a myriad of warm and cold-blooded hosts. In humans there are four main clinical presentations:

1. Acute gastroenteritis
2. Bacteremia
3. Focal extraintestinal infection
4. Chronic carriage (Table 1)

## Microbiology

*Salmonellae* are motile, Gram-stain negative, nonspore-forming bacilli that are differentiated from other *Enterobacteriaceae* by inability to

**TABLE 1  Clinical Presentations of Salmonellosis**

Acute gastroenteritis (90%–95% of cases)
Bacteremia (<5% of cases)
- Transient during acute gastroenteritis
- Enteric fever (nontyphoid)
- Persistent or recurrent (especially HIV)
Focal complications following bacteremia
- Bronchopneumonia, empyema, chest wall abscess
- Aortitis with mycotic aneurysm
- Prosthetic graft or valve infection
- Endocarditis, endarteritis
- Osteomyelitis (especially with sickle cell anemia)
- Septic arthritis
- Soft tissue abscess
- Hepatic or splenic abscess
- Meningitis or brain abscess
- Suppurative urogenital disease
Carriage (asymptomatic)
- Convalescent excretors (<2 mo)
- Convalescent carriers (2–12 mo)
- Chronic carriers (>12 mo)

ferment lactose and sucrose while producing acid, hydrogen sulfide, and gas (except *Salmonella typhi*). Members of the genus were more accurately classified into serotypes using the Kauffman-White schema that differentiated and grouped them serologically dependent on their lipopolysaccharide somatic (O) and flagellar (H) antigens.

More recently, DNA analysis has divided the genus into two species. Initially the first of the two species was named *Salmonella choleraesuis* and was divided into six subspecies, each of which was then divided into more than 2400 serotypes (serovars) by Kauffman-White methodology. The second species, *Salmonella Bongori*, is inconsequential. Serotypes were named historically from the host or the geographic locale of the first isolate, such as *Salmonella typhimurium* or *Salmonella dublin*. However, under the new DNA division, *choleraesuis* was both a species and a serotype. To avoid confusion the name *Salmonella enterica* has been widely adopted. The first of the six subspecies (Group I) is also named *enterica*. It contains the more than 1400 serotypes that occur in warm-blooded animals. Using nomenclature employed by the United States Centers for Disease Control and the World Health Organization (WHO), the species and subspecies name is understood; and the serotype is capitalized. Thus, the formal *S. enterica* subspecies *enterica* serotype *typhimurium* becomes simply *S. Typhimurium*, which except for the capital T is where we started!

## Epidemiology

In the last 25 years, the incidence of nontyphoid salmonellosis has increased two- to threefold with approximately 1.5 million cases occurring annually in the United States. This is an underestimate because most cases are sporadic (endemic) and go unreported. Children younger than 5 years of age have the highest incidence of gastroenteritis and constitute the greatest number of cases.

Animals are the source of nontyphoid salmonella infection in humans. Infection occurs from food of animal origin such as meat, poultry, eggs, and dairy products. Contamination may occur during the production, slaughter, processing, or distribution of these products. Outbreaks have been associated with eggs, ice cream, and processed meats. Increasingly there have been outbreaks associated with raw vegetables (e.g., scallions) that are crosscontaminated during growth and distribution. Restaurant or home outbreaks occur in the context of improper preparation, cooking, and refrigeration. Most of the outbreaks can be attributed to centralized mass production and preparation of food along with globalization of the food trade. Novel sources of human salmonella include pet turtles, lizards, iguanas, African hedgehogs, rattlesnakes, and even marijuana contaminated by manure.

Emergence of antibiotic resistant species is a formidable problem. It is believed that resistance is driven worldwide by improper antibiotics use. However, in developed countries it is attributable to widespread use in animal feeds. Large numbers of transferable resistance plasmids have been described. Resistance rates of more than 50% to ampicillin, chloramphenicol (Chloromycetin), and trimethoprim-sulfamethoxazole (TMP-SMZ) (Bactrim) occur in parts of Asia, Africa, and Latin America. One strain of *S. Typhimurium* (DT104) is resistant to five antimicrobials; the three mentioned previously plus tetracycline and streptomycin. This organism has spread widely in livestock throughout the United States, Canada, United Kingdom, Europe, and the Middle East. Likewise, resistance to third-generation cephalosporins is increasing and is mediated by plasmids producing both regular and extended-spectrum beta-lactamases (ESBLs). Even more disturbing is fluoroquinolone resistance caused by mutated DNA gyrase, topoisomerase IV, or efflux pumps. The latter literally expel the quinolone from the bacterium before it can act on its target. Fluoroquinolone resistance is most pronounced in Southeast Asia, Europe, and the Middle East.

## Pathogenesis

Human infection usually requires $10^6$ organisms. Fewer organisms may cause disease in patients who have hypochlorhydria or achlorhydria, have impaired cellular immunity, are at the extremes of age, or are taking certain drugs (Table 2). *Salmonellae* predominately infect the terminal ileum and proximal colon through attachment. Initially host response is by neutrophils followed by lymphocytes and macrophages. Strains vary genetically in their virulence and invasiveness. The organisms can survive intracellularly, thus avoiding antibiotic agents that lack intracellular penetration. Bacteria that are not contained regionally in the gut or lymph nodes may enter the blood. There are many predisposing factors associated with this and subsequent focal complications (see Table 2).

## Clinical Presentation

### GASTOENTERITIS

Acute gastroenteritis is by far the most common clinical presentation of salmonellosis. It should be emphasized that there is considerable

### TABLE 2  Predisposing Factors for Salmonellosis

Gastrointestinal
- Achlorhydria
- Gastric surgery
- Inflammatory bowel disease

Immune or structural compromise
- Age (<6 mo, >60 y)
- Lymphoma
- Splenectomy
- Cirrhosis with portal hypertension
- Diabetes mellitus
- Chronic uremia
- Hemolytic anemia (iron overload)
- Sickle cell (bone infarct, autosplenectomy)
- Systemic lupus
- Atheromata, aortic aneurysm

Infections
- HIV/AIDS (decreased T-cells)
- Malaria
- Bartonellosis
- Schistosomiasis

Drugs
- $H_2$-blockers, $H^+$ proton pump inhibitors
- Antibiotic administration
- Antimotility agents
- Chemotherapy
- Corticosteroids
- Transplant antirejection agents

## CURRENT DIAGNOSIS

- More than 95% of nontyphoid Salmonellosis presents as uncomplicated acute gastroenteritis.
- The clinical presentation of different causes of gastroenteritis and diarrhea overlaps significantly.
- The physician should be familiar with groups of patients at risk for complicated Salmonellosis.
- Specific diagnosis requires culture of the stool or blood.
- Focal complications are always suspect in high-risk patients who are blood culture positive for nontyphoid *Salmonellae* (e.g., aortitis or mycotic aneurysm in patients older than age 60 years with atherosclerosis).

overlap in its presentation with other infectious intestinal pathogens such as *Campylobacter* species. Given this, the incubation ranges from 6 to 96 hours but most commonly occurs between 12 and 48 hours. Initial symptoms include nausea and vomiting, followed by headaches, myalgias, malaise, chills, low-grade fever, abdominal cramps, and diarrhea. High temperatures (40°C [104°F]) should alert the clinician to invasive disease. Stools may be merely loose or profuse and watery. On direct examination, they may or may not contain polymorphonuclear leukocytes or occult blood. The presence of mucus or gross blood in the absence of hemorrhoids or fissures should alert the clinician to organisms causing dysentery such as *Shigella* species. The white count is most often normal or slightly elevated, with a left shift containing 10 to 15 bands. Low white counts with greater numbers of bands should alert the clinician to possible bacteremia or enteric fever. The diagnosis can be confirmed only by stool or blood culture. Serum serology examinations are not helpful. Most healthy adults have a self-limited, uncomplicated course, with resolution of symptoms without treatment within 48 to 72 hours.

## Treatment

### FLUID AND ELECTROLYTE REPLACEMENT

The sine qua non in the treatment of diarrhea is fluid and electrolyte replacement. In most cases increased oral intake of bland juices

## CURRENT THERAPY

- Fluid and electrolyte replacement is of paramount importance.
- The physician should avoid routine empiric antibiotic in acute uncomplicated patients.
- The physician should avoid antimotility agents for diarrhea presenting with fever or with mucus and blood present.
- More than 95% of patients with nontyphoid salmonellosis *will get better* on their own.
- Fluoroquinolone antibiotics should be reserved for when they are truly indicated clinically.
- Increasing resistance mandates sensitivity testing (including tests for ESBL) to guide therapy of bacteremia and its complications.
- Do not prescribe *prophylactic* antibiotics to prevent diarrhea in travellers.
- Stress personal hygiene and prudent food choice with proper preparation.

*Abbreviation:* ESBL = extended spectrum beta lactamases.

coupled with clear broth and temporary elimination of lactose-containing foods will suffice. Commercial electrolyte solutions (Pedialyte) may be useful. Although not readily available in the United States, rehydration salts are widely employed in many developing countries. WHO distributes packets containing its recommended formula of 90 mmol of sodium, 20 of potassium, 80 of chloride, 30 of bicarbonate, along with 111 mmol of glucose to dissolve in 1 L of sterile or boiled water. This mixture should be consumed at a rate sufficient to compensate for diarrheal losses while maintaining an adequate output of dilute appearing urine. Within 24 to 48 hours, the diet can be supplemented with bland, soft foods given in small, frequent feedings. If the patient has profuse vomiting or severe dehydration as determined by orthostatic changes in blood pressure, parenteral rehydration should be used. Frequently, this can be accomplished as an outpatient in an infusion room or with a home agency rather than through admission to hospital. When there is persistent emesis, profuse diarrhea, systemic toxicity, or abnormalities in serum electrolytes, parenteral rehydration in hospital is prudent.

## ANTIMOTILITY AND ANTINAUSEA AGENTS

The use of agents such as atropine-diphenoxylate (Lomotil) or loperamide (Imodium) should be discouraged. Although they may result in symptomatic improvement in cramps and diarrhea, they can increase complications and even predispose to bacteremia. In general, if the patient has a fever and the diarrhea contains blood or mucus, their use should be eschewed. Most pediatricians feel they should never be used in children younger than 5 years of age. An alternative is bismuth subsalicylate (Pepto-Bismol). The adult dose is 1 ounce (2 tablespoons) or 2 tablets (262.5 mg) every 30 minutes for 8 hours. The pediatric dose is 1.1 mL/kg at 4-hour intervals for up to 5 days. Although nausea and vomiting are occasional presenting symptoms with enterocolitis, they rarely persist. Prochlorperazine (Compazine) or trimethobenzamide (Tigan) may be helpful. Both are available in oral, suppository, or parenteral form, even though injectable prochlorperazine (Compazine) has been in short supply. Suppositories usually stimulate further diarrhea. Vomiting may preclude oral administration. A singular muscular injection of prochlorperazine (Compazine) 5 to 10 mg, is often all that is needed. This may be repeated every 4 to 6 hours as needed. Promethazine hydrochloride (Phenergan) is more frequently used in children and may be used orally (0.5 mg/pound or 1 mg/kg every 6 hours) or intramuscularly in the same doses. A 5-HT$_3$ receptor antagonist such as ondansetron (Zofran)[1] is expensive and inefficacious.

## ANTIBIOTICS

The routine empiric use of antibiotics, especially fluoroquinolones, for any and all cases of diarrhea is not only unjustifiable but should be decried. Certainly antibiotics are not needed in the treatment of uncomplicated *Salmonella* gastroenteritis in otherwise healthy children or adults. Studies have shown that they neither shorten the course nor improve symptoms. No doubt some of this usage is patient driven. However, overuse is contributing to the emergence of resistance, and may increase risk of symptomatic and bacteriologic relapse. Indeed antibiotic use may actually prolong the convalescent excretion or contribute to chronic carriage of the organism. Postponing antibiotic therapy until the return of a stool culture often provides the physician with a way to avert the frequent demand for antibiotic therapy. Often patients are better by the time results become available. Nevertheless, high-risk patients, as previously identified (see Table 2), should receive treatment to prevent potential complications from bacteremia. Additionally, if patients are sick enough to require hospitalization, antibiotic therapy should be considered.

Appropriate antibiotic therapy should be guided by susceptibility testing. Initially, TMP-SMZ (cotrimoxazole, Bactrim, or Septra)[1] may be administered to the nonsulfonamide-sensitive patient. The dose is 5 to 8 mg/kg trimethoprim every 12 hours for children or 1 double-strength tablet (160 mg trimethoprim/800 mg sulfamethoxazole) every 12 hours for adults. Although widely used, trimethoprim-sulfamethoxazole has not yet received FDA approval. If the organism is susceptible, ampicillin, 50 mg/kg orally to 100 mg/kg/day intravenously, each in four divided doses for children, or 2 to 4 g/day in four divided doses for adults, may be administered. Amoxicillin (Amoxil)[1] in equivalent oral dosage may be substituted. The duration of therapy is generally 5 days.

Newer fluoroquinolone antibiotics, such as ciprofloxacin,[1] ofloxacin,[1] and norfloxacin,[1] are among the most effective agents with excellent oral bioavailability and intracellular concentration. They are contraindicated in prepubertal children and pregnant women. Adult doses are ciprofloxacin (Cipro), 500 mg twice daily; ofloxacin (Floxin), 400 mg twice daily; or norfloxacin (Noroxin), 400 mg twice daily. It must be emphasized that the trend in the United States to use these agents empirically for all suspected bacterial diarrhea should be vigorously resisted by the thoughtful clinician.

## Bacteremia and Focal Infection

Bacteremia in acute uncomplicated *Salmonella* gastroenteritis is infrequent. Therefore, blood cultures are not routinely necessary except for patients who are in high-risk categories. Shaking chills or high fever (40°C [104°F]) should alert the clinician to possible bacteremia. Focal suppurative infection following bacteremia is also infrequent but may occur at any site. Thus, *Salmonella* has been associated with bronchopneumonia, soft tissue infection, aortic mycotic aneurysms, endocarditis, septic arthritis, splenic or hepatic abscesses, meningitis, and osteomyelitis. The clinician should suspect an endovascular mycotic aneurysm in all blood culture positive patients older than 50 years of age. *Salmonella* should always be suspected in individuals with sickle cell disease in whom bone and joint infection is the most frequent cause of extraintestinal infection. Meningitis occurs primarily in infants younger than 5 months of age. The diagnosis of a *Salmonella* bacteremia in HIV patients will almost always be accompanied by recurrent episodes.

## Treatment

### ANTIBIOTICS

Bacteremia and localized suppurative infection require antibiotic therapy. The choice of effective treatment is less predictable with the emergence of resistance. Therapy must be altered according to the results of susceptibility testing. Therefore the recovery of the organism is extremely important, and adequate cultures of blood or infected material must be obtained before initiation of therapy.

Parenteral ampicillin, 100 to 200 mg/kg/day divided into four doses, or TMP/SMZ,[1] 8 to 10 mg/kg of trimethoprim per day in three divided doses, may be used. In the case of resistance or allergy to the foregoing, third-generation cephalosporins such as cefotaxime (Claforan) or ceftriaxone (Rocephin) have reasonable activity, but intracellular concentrations are not optimal. Cefotaxime, 1 to 2 grams every 6 to 8 hours for adults, or 100 to 200 mg/kg/day in three or four divided doses for children, has been found effective in bacteremia, osteomyelitis, septic arthritis, and a variety of other focal *Salmonella* infections. The use of chloramphenicol (Chloromycetin) is not recommended but a preparation of it in oil (Typhomycine)[2] is in use in developing countries. Ciprofloxacin (Cipro)[1] 7.5 mg/kg intravenously twice daily is becoming a favored agent; not only is it effective but oral bioequivalence facilitates the change to 500 to 750 mg by mouth twice daily. If fluoroquinolone resistance is encountered, imipenem (Primaxin)[1] may be tried. Efficacy data for it or other agents such as azithromycin (Zithromax)[1] are scant.

---

[1]Not FDA approved for this indication.

---

[1]Not FDA approved for this indication.
[2]Not available in the United States

## SURGERY

Focal infection often requires surgery. Often this is as simple as the drainage of localized suppuration or lavage of a septic joint. However, in the case of infected aortic aneurysms, extensive resection and vascular reconstruction are required. Infected prosthetic grafts must be removed in nearly all cases with courses of antibiotics before and after surgery.

The duration of therapy for simple bacteremia is 10 to 14 days. Septic arthritis is usually treated 4 weeks whereas osteomyelitis and endovascular infections require 6 weeks. Oral fluoroquinolones such as ciprofloxacin (Cipro), 500 mg twice daily, may be helpful in treating osteomyelitis. TMP-SMZ (Bactrim)[1] can also be used in this manner. Both have adequate blood levels after oral administration. I have had to use continuous prophylaxis of either TMP-SMZ or ciprofloxacin in several HIV patients to prevent recurrent bacteremia. Because prophylactic TMP-SMZ is used chronically for *Pneumocystis,* it may be preferred.

## Enteric Fever

The clinical picture of nontyphoid *Salmonella* enteric fever is indistinguishable from that of typhoid fever, which is discussed elsewhere in this publication. However, the following discussion also applies to enteric fever caused by nontyphoid *Salmonellae.*

## TREATMENT

The adjunct and antibiotic therapy of nontyphoid enteric fever parallels that of the treatment of typhoid. Antibiotics should be adjusted and altered once the results of susceptibility testing are available. Acceptable regimens include ampicillin, amoxicillin,[1] and TMP-SMZ (Bactrim),[1] along with third-generation cephalosporins and fluoroquinolone antibiotics. My preference was cefotaxime (Claforan)[1] in the same doses as for bacteremic salmonellosis. The duration is 10 to 14 days. Relapse rates are low and is seen within 2 to 6 weeks. Relapse requires an equivalent course of therapy in both dose and duration. Currently, I prefer ciprofloxacin (Cipro)[1] intravenously 7.5 mg/kg every 12 hours continued until the patient is afebrile and clinically able to start it orally. Comparative studies are ongoing using both third-generation cephalosporins, such as ceftriaxone (Rocephin)[1] or cefixime (Suprax),[1] and oral fluoroquinolones in short-course therapy of typhoid as well as nontyphoid enteric fever. Although these show some promise, they are currently not the standard of practice in the United States. Nevertheless, a strong case can be made for oral fluoroquinolones use, with obvious cost saving. Otherwise healthy young adults may be treated orally as outpatients. This advantage, if for no other reason, should *prevent* the physician from prescribing quinolones for uncomplicated gastroenteritis or other self-limited diarrheas of bacterial origin.

Adjunctive measures are of importance, including attention to fluid and electrolyte balance and nutrition. As in typhoid the routine use of corticosteroids is controversial. Use in patients who are steroid dependent or believed to be hypoadrenal is indicated. In those who are delirious, obtunded, comatose, or in shock it may be warranted; but there are little supportive data. It has been my overall impression that nontyphoid enteric fever is somewhat milder than typhoid itself, and complications such as gastrointestinal bleeding or ileal perforation are exceedingly rare.

## Carrier State

Asymptomatic excretion of organisms invariably occurs following clinical *Salmonella* gastroenteritis. It exceeds 8 weeks in 5% to 10% of patients. Chronic carriage, either in the stool or urine, is defined as excretion of the organism for more than 1 year. Its incidence is stated to be 1% in adults and 5% in children younger than 5 years of age. This is somewhat less than that seen with *S. typhi.* Convalescent excreters need only maintain strict personal hygiene to prevent transmission of the organism. Those involved in food preparation or in child and health care should be kept off work until three successive cultures are negative at intervals required by the public health department. It goes without saying that all positive cases of salmonellosis are reportable by law to local public health authorities.

Recently, oral quinolones have been used (ciprofloxacin [Cipro],[1] 500 to 750 mg twice daily for 5 to 14 days), to curtail institutional outbreaks, as in nursing homes or psychiatric facilities. Although this may be expeditious, eliminating or preventing the source of the outbreak in a prospective fashion is preferable. In the case of food handlers and health or child care workers, some feel that quinolone therapy eliminates the problem of convalescent excretion, hence individuals may return to work without delay. The data are debatable and the successive negative stool requirement will not be obviated.

The management of the chronic carriage of nontyphoidal salmonellosis is the same as that of *S. typhi,* which is discussed in detail elsewhere. A 4- to 6-week course of oral antibiotics may be tried when no evidence of gallbladder disease exists. However, if chronic cholecystitis and/or cholelithiasis are present, cholecystectomy is almost always necessary. Despite cholecystectomy, a certain number of individuals will continue to excrete organisms thought to be of hepatobiliary origin. Chronic carriage is seen, albeit rarely, in the United States with either *Schistosoma mansoni* or *Schistosoma haematobium.* When these parasites are treated, subsequent therapy of the *Salmonella* results in termination of the stool or urinary carrier state.

## Prevention

Prevention of salmonellosis has both personal and public health dimensions. Food and leftovers should be rapidly refrigerated. I recommend separate plastic (not wood) cutting boards for meats and vegetables that are washed after each use. Spillage of raw animal juices should be immediately cleaned. All preparation surfaces should be washed and dried after each meal. Detergent rather than antibacterial cleaners should be used; bleach is beautiful.

Public health surveillance is essential with regular inspection of restaurants, food retailers, and industrial food processors. National efforts to coordinate and computerize surveillance systems such as FoodNet should be expanded and fully funded so as to guarantee our food supply. Preservation technologies including irradiation need study.

Finally, the practicing physician should take the time to reiterate to patients with HIV, malignancies or other immune compromised patients (see Table 2) how they can avoid food-borne pathogens.

## REFERENCES

Brenner FW, Villar RG, Angulo FJ, et al: Salmonella nomenclature. J Clin Microbiol 2000;38: 2465–2465.

Fierer J, Swancutt M: Non-typhoid *Salmonella:* A review. In Remington, JS, Swartz, MN (eds.): Current Clinical Topics in Infectious Diseases 20. Boston, Blackwell Science, 2000, pp 134–157.

Herikstad H, Hayes P, Mokhtar M, et al: Emerging quinolone-resistant Salmonella in the United States. Emerg Infect Dis 1997;3:371–372.

Molbak K: Human health consequences of antimicrobial drug resistant *Salmonella* and other foodborne pathogens. Clin Infect Dis 2005;41: 1613–1620.

Sirinivan S, Garner P: Antibiotics for treating Salmonella gut infections. Cochrane Database Sys Rev 2000;93:CD001167.

Su LH, Chiu CH, Chu CS, et al: Antimicrobial resistance in nontyphoid *Salmonella:* A global challenge. Clin Infect Dis 2004;39:546–551.

Voetsch AC, Van Gilder TJ, Angulo FJ, et al: FoodNet estimate of the burden of illness caused by nontyphoidal Salmonella infections in the United States. Clin Infect Dis 2004;38(Suppl 3):S127–134.

---

[1]Not FDA approved for this indication.

[1]Not FDA approved for this indication.

# Typhoid Fever

Method of
*Zulfiqar A. Bhutta, MB, BS, PhD*

Despite vast advances in public health and hygiene in much of the developed world, typhoid fever remains endemic in many developing countries. Probably because of the ease of modern travel, cases are also reported in most developed countries.

## Etiology

Typhoid fever is caused by *Salmonella typhi*, a gram-negative bacterium. A very similar but often less severe disease is caused by *Salmonella* serotype *paratyphi* A. The ratio of disease caused by *S. typhi* to that caused by *S. paratyphi* is approximately 10:1, although the proportion of *S. paratyphi* infections is increasing in some parts of the world. Although *S. typhi* shares many genes with *Escherichia coli* and at least 90% with *Salmonella typhimurium,* several unique gene clusters known as pathogenicity islands and others were acquired during evolution. One of the specific genes is for the polysaccharide capsule Vi. This is present in approximately 90% of all freshly isolated *S. typhi* organisms and has a protective effect against the bactericidal action of the serum of infected patients.

## Epidemiology

Although accurate community-based figures are unavailable, an estimated 16 million cases occur annually, with more than 0.6 million deaths. The vast majority of cases occur in Asia. Given the paucity of microbiologic facilities in developing countries, these figures may largely represent the clinical syndrome. Regional incidence rates vary from 100 to 1000 cases per 100,000 population, and there may be differences in the spectrum of the disorder. Recent population-based studies from south Asia also indicate that, contrary to previous views, the disease may largely affect children younger than 5 years of age. In contrast, data from sub-Saharan Africa and HIV-endemic areas indicate that nontyphoidal *Salmonella* bacteremia far outstrips typhoid fever as a cause of community-acquired bacteremia.

In recent years, typhoid fever is notable for the emergence of drug resistance. Following sporadic outbreaks of chloramphenicol-resistant typhoid, many strains of *S. typhi* developed plasmid-mediated multidrug-resistance to all of the three primary antimicrobials (ampicillin [Chloromycetin], chloramphenicol, and trimethoprim-sulfamethoxazole [Septra]). More troubling, chromosomally acquired quinolone resistance in *S. typhi* was recently described in various parts of Asia and may be a consequence of widespread and indiscriminate use of these agents.

## Pathogenesis

Typhoid fever occurs by the ingestion of the organism, and a variety of sources of fecal contamination are reported, including street vendor foods and contamination of water reservoirs. A larger infecting dose leads to a shorter incubation period and more severe infection. The organism crosses the intestinal mucosal barrier after attachment to the microvilli by an intricate mechanism involving membrane ruffling, actin rearrangement, and internalization in an intracellular vacuole. Once inside the intestinal cells, *S. typhi* find their way into the circulation and reside within the macrophages of the reticuloendothelial system. The clinical syndrome is produced by a release of proinflammatory cytokines (interleukin [IL]-6, IL-1$\beta$, and tumor necrosis factor [TNF]-$\alpha$) from the infected cells. Some 1% to 5% of patients with acute typhoid infection may become chronic carriers of the infection in the gallbladder, depending on age, sex, and treatment regimen.

## Clinical Features

Patients with typhoid fever usually present with high-grade fever and a wide variety of associated symptoms, such as abdominal pain, hepatosplenomegaly, diarrhea, and constipation. In the absence of localizing signs, the early stage of the disease may be difficult to differentiate from other endemic diseases including malaria and dengue fever. The classic stepladder rise of fever is relatively rare, but the presentation of typhoid fever may be tempered by coexisting morbidities and early administration of antibiotics. In malaria-endemic areas and in parts of the world where schistosomiasis is common, the presentation of typhoid may also be atypical.

Although data from South America and parts of Africa suggest typhoid may present as a mild illness in young children, this may vary in different parts of the world. Emerging evidence from south Asia indicates the presentation of typhoid may be more dramatic in children younger than 5 years of age, with comparatively higher rates of complications and hospitalization. Diarrhea, toxicity, and complications such as disseminated intravascular coagulopathy are also more common in infancy, with higher case fatality rates. Some of the other features of typhoid fever seen in adults, however, such as relative bradycardia, are rare, and rose spots may be visible only at an early stage of the illness in fair-skinned children.

It is also recognized that multidrug-resistant (MDR) typhoid is a more severe clinical illness with higher rates of toxicity, complications, and case fatality rates. This may be related to the increased virulence of MDR *S. typhi* as well as a higher number of circulating bacteria. These findings may have implications for treatment algorithms, especially in endemic areas with high rates of MDR typhoid.

## Diagnosis

The mainstay of the diagnosis of typhoid fever is a positive culture from the blood or another anatomic site. But the sensitivity of blood cultures in diagnosing typhoid fever in many parts of the developing world is limited because widespread use of antibiotics may render bacteriologic confirmation difficult. Although bone marrow cultures may increase the likelihood of bacteriologic confirmation of typhoid, these are difficult to obtain and relatively invasive.

The serologic diagnosis of typhoid is also fraught with problems because results of a single Widal test may be positive in only 50% of cases in endemic areas, and serial tests may be required in cases presenting in the first week of illness. Newer serologic tests such as a dot enzyme-linked immunoabsorbent assay (ELISA) (TyphiDot) and the TUBEX tests are promising but require further evaluation in

**CURRENT DIAGNOSIS**

- In the absence of localizing signs, the early stage of the disease may be difficult to differentiate from other endemic diseases such as malaria or dengue fever.
- The presentation and diagnosis of typhoid fever may be tempered by coexisting morbidities and early administration of antibiotics.
- The presentation of typhoid may be more dramatic in children younger than 5 years of age, with comparatively higher rates of complications and hospitalization.
- The sensitivity of blood cultures in diagnosing typhoid fever may be limited in many developing countries because of antibiotic prescribing.
- Multidrug-resistant (MDR) typhoid is a more severe clinical illness with higher rates of toxicity and complications. In particular, recent cases of quinolone-resistant typhoid may be more severe.

large-scale studies in community settings. In much of the developing world, the mainstay of diagnosis of typhoid remains clinical, and several diagnostic algorithms are being evaluated in endemic areas.

## Therapy

An early diagnosis of typhoid fever and institution of appropriate treatment are essential. The vast majority of typhoid patients can be managed at home with oral antibiotics and close medical follow-up for complications or failure to respond to therapy. But patients with persistent vomiting, severe diarrhea, and abdominal distention may require hospitalization and parenteral antibiotic therapy. These are the general principles of typhoid management:

- Adequate rest, hydration, and attention to correction of fluid-electrolyte imbalance
- Antipyretic therapy (acetaminophen, 120 to 750 mg orally every 4 to 6 hours[3]) as required
- Soft, easily digestible diet unless the patient has abdominal distention or ileus
- Antibiotic therapy (the right choice, dosage, and duration)
- Traditional therapy with either chloramphenicol (Chloromycetin) or amoxicillin,[1] associated with relapse rates of 5% to 15% and 4% to 8%, respectively; newer quinolones and third-generation cephalosporins associated with higher cure rates

---

[1]Exceeds dosage recommended by the manufacturer.
[3]Not FDA approved fot this indication.

### CURRENT THERAPY

- The vast majority of typhoid patients can be managed at home with oral antibiotics and close medical follow-up for complications or failure to respond to therapy.
- Although newer quinolones are associated with better cure rates and clinical outcomes, there is insufficient evidence to recommend them as first-line agents in children.
- Recent emergence of quinolone resistance among *S. typhi* isolates requires treatment with alternatives such as third-generation cephalosporins and azithromycin.

Some authorities recommend treatment with second-line agents in all cases of typhoid. Others questioned this on the basis of adequate response to therapy among sensitive cases with first-line agents. Blanket administration of second-line agents such as fluoroquinolones and third-generation cephalosporins in all cases of suspected typhoid is expensive and may lead to the rapid development of further resistance. Table 1 gives the recommended therapy for typhoid fever based on a recent consensus document by the World Health Organization (2003).

## Preventive Strategies for Typhoid

Of the major risk factors for outbreaks of typhoid, contamination of water supplies with sewage is the most important. During outbreaks, therefore, a combination of central chlorination and domestic water

---

**TABLE 1  Treatment of Typhoid Fever Based on Diagnosis, Treatment, and Prevention**

| Susceptibility | Optimal Therapy | | | Alternative Effective Drugs | | |
|---|---|---|---|---|---|---|
| | Antibiotic | Daily Dose (mg/kg) | Days | Antibiotic | Daily Dose (mg/kg) | Days |
| **Uncomplicated Typhoid Fever** | | | | | | |
| Fully sensitive | Fluoroquinolone (e.g., ofloxacin [Floxin][1] or ciprofloxacin [Cipro]) | 15 | 5-7* | Chloramphenicol (Chloromycetin) Amoxicillin[1] TMP-SMX (Bactrim)[1] | 50-75[3] 75-100[1] 8/40 | 14-21 14 14 |
| Multidrug resistance | Fluoroquinolone or Cefixime (Suprax)[1] | 15 15-20[3] | 5-7 7-14 | Azithromycin (Zithromax)[1] Cefixime | 8-10[3] 15-20[3] | 7 7-14 |
| Quinolone resistance[†] | Azithromycin (Rocephin)[1] or Ceftriaxone (Rocephin)[1] | 8-10[3] 75[3] | 7 10-14 | Cefixime[1] | 203 | 7-14 |
| **Severe Typhoid Fever** | | | | | | |
| Fully sensitive | Fluoroquinolone (e.g., ofloxacin)[1] | 15 | 10-14 | Chloramphenicol Ampicillin[1] TMP-SMX | 100[3] 100[3] 8/40 | 14-21 14 14 |
| Multidrug-resistant | Fluoroquinolone | 15 | 10-14 | Ceftriaxone[1] or Cefotaxime (Claforan)[1] | 60[3] 80[3] | 10-14 |
| Quinolone-resistant | Ceftriaxone[1] or cefotaxime[1] | 60[3] 80[3] | 10-14 | Fluoroquinolone | 20[3] | 14 |

[1]Not FDA approved for this indication.
[3]Exceeds dosage recommended by the manufacturer.
*Three-day courses are also effective and are particularly so in epidemic containment.
[†]The optimum treatment for quinolone-resistant typhoid fever is not determined. Azithromycin, the third-generation cephalosporins, or a 10- to 14-day course of high-dose fluoroquinolones is effective.
*Abbreviation*: TMX-SMZ = trimethoprim-sulfamethoxazole.
From World Health Organization (WHO)/Vaccines and Biologicals/03.07.

purification is important. In endemic situations, consumption of street vendor foods, especially ice cream and cut-up fruit, is recognized as an important risk factor. The human-to-human spread by chronic carriers is also important, and attempts should be made to target food handlers and high-risk groups for *S. typhi* carriage screening.

The classic heat-inactivated whole cell vaccine is associated with an unacceptably high rate of side effects. Two newer vaccines that offer protection for school-age children and for adults are the Vi polysaccharide vaccine (Typhim Vi) and the orally administratable, attenuated Ty21a vaccine (Vivotif Berna). Both offer a protective efficacy of 70% to 80% for at least 3 to 5 years. In younger children, the experimental Vi-conjugate vaccine has a protective efficacy exceeding 90% and may offer protection in parts of the world where a large proportion of preschool children are at risk for the disease.

## REFERENCES

Bhutta ZA: Impact of age and drug resistance on mortality in typhoid fever. Arch Dis Child 1996;75:214-217.

Chinh NT, Parry CM, Ly NT, et al: A randomized controlled comparison of azithromycin and ofloxacin for treatment of multidrug-resistant or nalidixic acid-resistant enteric fever. Antimicrob Agents Chemother 2000;44: 1855-1859.

Communicable Disease Surveillance and Response Vaccines and Biologicals, World Health Organization: Treatment of Typhoid Fever. Background Document: The Diagnosis, Prevention and Treatment of Typhoid Fever, 2003, pp. 19-23. Available online at http://www.who.int/entity/vaccine_research/documents/en/typhoid_diagnosis.pdf)

Crump JA, Luby SP, Mintz ED: The global burden of typhoid fever. Bull World Health Organ 2004;82:346-353.

Gasem MH, Keuter M, Dolmans WM, et al: Persistence of salmonellae in blood and bone marrow: Randomized controlled trial comparing ciprofloxacin and chloramphenicol treatments against enteric fever. Antimicrob Agents Chemother 2003;47:1727-1731.

Luby SP, Faizan MK, Fisher-Hoch SP, et al: Risk factors for typhoid fever in an endemic setting, Karachi, Pakistan. Epidemiol Infect 1998;120: 129-138.

Parry CM, Hien TT, Dougan G, et al: Typhoid fever. N Engl J Med 2002; 347:1770-1782.

Sinha A, Sazawal S, Kumar R, et al: Typhoid fever in children aged less than 5 years. Lancet 1999;354:734-737.

Thaver D, Zaidi AK, Critchley J, et al: Fluoroquinolones for treating typhoid and paratyphoid fever (enteric fever) (CD004530.pub2). Cochrane Database Syst Rev 2005;2.

# Rickettsial and Ehrlichial Infections

Method of
*Deverick J. Anderson, MD, and Daniel J. Sexton, MD*

## Rickettsial Infections

### ROCKY MOUNTAIN SPOTTED FEVER

Rocky Mountain spotted fever (RMSF) is the most lethal of several tickborne illnesses that occur in the United States. Between 20% and 25% of infections are fatal if not treated appropriately. *Rickettsia rickettsii*, the obligate intracellular bacterium that causes RMSF, circulates in nature in a complex cycle between ticks and small rodents. Humans are only occasional and accidental hosts for this organism.

### Epidemiology

RMSF is a highly seasonal disease that predominantly occurs in the spring and early summer months; cases occasionally occur in the autumn and even the winter in warmer climates. RMSF occurs with varying frequency in western Canada, much of the continental United States, Mexico, Central America, Brazil, and Colombia. The incidence of RMSF varies by geographic area and, although reporting of cases of RMSF is primarily through passive surveillance, the average reported annual incidence of RMSF is approximately 2.2 cases per 1 million persons.

### Pathogenesis

In the United States, *R. rickettsii* is primarily transmitted by *Dermacentor variabilis* (the American dog tick) in the eastern United States and *Dermacentor andersoni* (the wood tick) in the western United States. Recently, *Rhipicephalus sanguineus* (the common brown dog tick) was recognized as the vector for RMSF in an outbreak in eastern Arizona; this finding is not surprising because this vector also transmits RMSF in Mexico and Central America. Although most infections occur after a tick bite, transmission rarely occurs from crushing or removing infected ticks from humans or animals. Indeed, infection can be experimentally induced with aerosols of infected tick tissues or by mucosal contact. Tick bites are painless and often go unnoticed. Thus, many patients with RMSF have no knowledge of a tick bite prior to the onset of their illness.

### Clinical Features and Diagnosis

After inoculation from a tick bite, *R. rickettsii* proliferates and spreads throughout the body via the bloodstream and lymphatics, as well as by contiguous spread from cell to cell. *R. rickettsii* has a specific tropism for endothelial cells, resulting in widespread vasculitis, increased vascular permeability, edema, and activation of the humoral inflammatory and coagulation mechanisms. Organ dysfunction, hypovolemia, and shock can result from microvascular thrombosis and hemorrhage. Risk factors associated with increased severity and fatal outcomes include increasing age, male gender, diabetes mellitus, glucose-6-phosphate dehydrogenase (G6PD) deficiency, alcohol use, and delay in effective therapy for longer than 6 days after onset of symptoms.

The incubation period for RMSF ranges from 2 to 14 days. Most patients with RMSF develop a rash between the third and fifth days of illness. The typical rash of RMSF begins on the ankles and wrists and spreads both centrally and to the palms and soles. The skin rash often begins as a macular or maculopapular eruption and then usually becomes petechial. As many as 10% of patients do not, however, develop a rash *(spotless RMSF)*. Additionally, the rash can be difficult to recognize in patients with dark skin.

Other symptoms of RMSF are nonspecific and include fever, headache, myalgias, malaise, and anorexia. As the disease progresses and becomes more severe, symptoms such as cough, bleeding, nausea, vomiting, abdominal pain, edema (especially in children), delirium, and focal neurologic symptoms (including seizures) can occur. In the absence of the classic triad of tick bite, fever, and rash, patients with RMSF may be erroneously believed to have an array of other infections such as ehrlichiosis, infectious mononucleosis, viral hepatitis, viral meningitis, measles, influenza, toxic shock syndrome, meningococcemia, leptospirosis, or typhoid fever. Because of shared residence and shared risks for tick exposure, family clusters of infection occasionally occur. When such clusters do occur, assumed person-to-person transmission of a viral or bacterial pathogen may lead to misdiagnosis and delay in treatment. If ineffective antibiotics are prescribed empirically before a typical rash appears, patients with RMSF may be erroneously assumed to have a drug eruption. Such cases can end tragically if the rash is presumed to occur because of (ineffective) drug therapy rather than in spite of it.

Most patients with RMSF have normal white blood cell (WBC) counts. As the severity of illness progresses, thrombocytopenia almost always develops, and WBC counts can become quite low. Although fibrinogen concentrations may be low and fibrin split products can become elevated in patients with RMSF, disseminated intravascular coagulation is uncommon. Other common laboratory abnormalities in patients with RMSF include hyponatremia, elevated serum transaminases, hyperbilirubinemia, and elevated creatinine.

There is no timely diagnostic test for RMSF in the early phase of illness. Thus, it is imperative that therapy be based on individual clinical features and the epidemiologic setting. Patients who have symptoms suggesting RMSF and who present in the spring or summer in an endemic area usually require empiric therapy.

## Treatment

The preferred therapy is doxycycline (Vibramycin) 100 mg orally or intravenously every 12 hours for adults and children who weigh more than 45 kg. For children younger than 8 years or for children older than 8 years but weighing less than 45 kg, the dose is 2.2 mg/kg divided into two doses (maximum dose 200 mg/day).[1] In severe cases, adjunctive therapy such as mechanical ventilation, oxygen therapy, or hemodialysis may be necessary and useful.

The optimal duration of therapy is unknown. Doxycycline can usually be discontinued 2 or 3 days after the patient becomes afebrile. Most clinicians treat patients with RMSF for 7 to 10 days, but this is probably longer than is necessary for cure in all but the most severe cases. Therapy can and should be discontinued within 4 or 5 days in children with RMSF who respond promptly to treatment because the risk of dental staining is minimal when short courses of doxycycline are given. In general, doxycycline use should be avoided in pregnant women. Instead, pregnant women should be given chloramphenicol (Chloromycetin) 500 mg intravenously or orally every 6 hours. Doxycycline may, however, be the preferred agent for treatment of RMSF in pregnant women at the end of pregnancy because chloramphenicol use in such situations can result in the gray baby syndrome, a potentially fatal drug reaction due to chloramphenicol's effect on bilirubin conjugation in term infants.

Although the diagnosis of RMSF can rarely be made in its acute phase by immunohistochemical staining of skin biopsy samples or by polymerase chain reaction, these diagnostic techniques are available only in a few large referral centers. In routine practice, the diagnosis of RMSF is usually proved long after symptoms and treatment have ceased. The mainstay of diagnosis is indirect fluorescent antibody testing, which is available through all state health laboratories. Antibodies typically appear 10 to 12 days after the onset of illness. The optimal time to obtain a convalescent antibody titer is 14 to 21 days after the onset of symptoms. The minimum diagnostic titer in most laboratories is 1:64.

## Prevention

Prevention of many cases of RMSF is impossible because ticks are ubiquitous and many patients with RMSF are unaware of having had a tick bite. Persons with frequent exposure to tick-infested environments should frequently inspect their bodies and clothes for ticks. Early detection and removal of attached ticks can prevent disease transmission. Several hours of feeding are usually required for an infected tick to transmit *R. rickettsii*; thus, RMSF might not occur if infected ticks are removed during this preactivation period. Embedded ticks should be carefully removed by tweezers or by fingers shielded by a cloth, tissues, paper towels, or gloves. Prophylactic antimicrobial therapy is *not* recommended following tick exposure, because only a minuscule percentage of ticks in endemic areas are infected with *R. rickettsii*.

## OTHER RICKETTSIAL INFECTIONS

Rickettsiae other than *R. rickettsii* can also cause human infection. For example, a single case of *Rickettsia parkeri* infection was reported in an otherwise healthy 40-year-old man from coastal Virginia in 2002. *R. parkeri* was first isolated from Gulf Coast ticks in the southern United States more than 60 years ago, but until this Virginia case was recognized, *R. parkeri* was not known to cause infections in humans. The patient presented with symptoms similar to those of RMSF and multiple eschars on his lower extremities. Erythematous papules, which then developed into eschars, preceded the other symptoms by 4 days. The patient failed to respond to other antibiotics but improved with doxycycline therapy. Subsequently, the authors of a serologic study of 15 patients with presumed RMSF reported that four of these 15 patients had higher titers for *R. parkeri* than for *R. rickettsii*, suggesting that infection with *R. parkeri* may be more common than previously realized and that some patients with presumed RMSF actually have *R. parkeri* infection.

# Ehrlichial Infections

*Ehrlichia* and *Anaplasma* are obligate intracellular bacteria that grow within membrane-bound vacuoles in human and animal leukocytes. As yet, there is no clear understanding of the mechanism by which *Ehrlichia* produces disease in humans. Humans infected with *Ehrlichia* do not show tissue necrosis, abscess formation, or a severe inflammatory response. Ehrlichial and anaplasmal infections do not lead to vasculitis, thrombosis, or acute endothelial injury as seen in rickettsial infections. *Ehrlichia* replicates within phagosomes in infected leukocytes and produces intracellular colonies called *morulae*.

Ehrlichiosis typically leads to one of two types of illness in humans: human monocytotropic ehrlichiosis (HME) caused by *Ehrlichia chafeensis* or human granulocytic anaplasmosis (HGA) caused by *Anaplasma phagocytophilum*.

## EPIDEMIOLOGY

Like other tickborne diseases, the actual incidence of ehrlichiosis is difficult to ascertain because reporting is based on a passive surveillance system that undoubtedly fails to detect or report many cases.

The best available evidence suggests that HME has an annual incidence of approximately 0.7 cases per 1 million persons and primarily occurs in the southeastern, south-central, and mid-Atlantic regions of the United States. *E. chafeensis* was first isolated from a soldier in Fort Chaffee, Arkansas, in 1990. Since then, cases of HME have been recognized in New England and the Pacific Northwest as well. First described in 1994, HGA has an annual incidence of approximately 1.6 cases per 1 million persons and has been described in the upper Midwest, California, and almost the entire Atlantic seaboard.

## PATHOGENESIS

The principal vector of *E. chafeensis* is *Amblyomma americanum* (the Lone Star tick); the principal vector of *A. phagocytophilum* is *Ixodes scapularis* (the black-legged tick) in the eastern United States and *I. pacificus* (the western black-legged tick) in the western United States. As opposed to rickettsia, survival of ehrlichia requires horizontal transmission by ticks to and persistent infection in a wild vertebrate host (typically the white-tailed deer or white-footed mouse).

At least two other ehrlichial genogroups cause human disease. Infection of the neutrophils by *E. ewingii* causes mild disease that has mainly been diagnosed in immunocompromised patients in the Midwest. The ehrlichial-like *Neorickettsia sennetsu* group causes a mild mononucleosis-like illness that has never been reported outside East and Southeast Asia.

## CLINICAL FEATURES AND DIAGNOSIS

Both HGE and HMA typically occur from May to September and have similar symptoms. After an incubation period of 7 to 14 days, patients

---

 **CURRENT DIAGNOSIS**

- There are no widely available tests to rapidly and accurately diagnose Rocky Mountain spotted fever (RMSF) in its early phases.
- If morulae are not found in patients with HME or HGA, the diagnosis cannot be established with certainty in the acute phases of these illnesses.

most often present with fever, malaise, myalgias, headaches, and chills. An important minority of patients have nausea, vomiting, arthralgias, cough, or neurologic symptoms including altered mental status or stiff neck. Rash is uncommon in ehrlichiosis, though a faint rash occurs more commonly in patients with HGE than in those with HMA. When a rash is present as a prominent sign, coinfection with another rickettsial or other tickborne pathogen should be suspected. Rarely, patients with severe illness develop meningoencephalitis, septic shock, respiratory insufficiency, congestive heart failure, and acute renal failure.

Mortality rates of 3% for patients with HGE and 1% for patients with HMA have been reported, but these numbers may be inaccurate because many mild cases or cases that are empirically treated with doxycycline escape detection or definitive diagnosis. Immunocompromised patients may have severe illnesses and higher mortality rates.

The most common laboratory abnormalities seen in patients with ehrlichiosis are leukopenia and thrombocytopenia, but elevated serum transaminases, lactate dehydrogenase, and alkaline phosphatase levels also occur commonly. Cerebrospinal fluid abnormalities including pleocytosis are common and can mimic the changes seen in patients with viral or other forms of aseptic meningitis.

Distinguishing between RMSF and ehrlichiosis on the basis of clinical features may be impossible, although the presence of leukopenia and the absence of rash are more typical of ehrlichiosis. There are five methods to diagnose ehrlichiosis:

- Examination of peripheral blood or buffy coat for the presence of characteristic morulae in leukocytes
- Indirect fluorescent antibody (IFA) testing
- Polymerase chain reaction testing of tissues
- Immunochemical staining of erhlichial or anaplasmal antigens in tissue
- Synthesis of the history, clinical, laboratory, and epidemiologic features of individual cases

Culture of *Ehrlichia* is extremely difficult, and laboratories able to perform such cultures are few and often inaccessible to clinicians in daily practice. Although only a minority of patients with ehrlichiosis have morulae detectable in blood smears, a blood film should be examined in all patients with suspected infection; morulae are more commonly seen in patients with HGA than in those with HME.

Convalescent serologic antibody testing should be performed 2 to 3 weeks after onset of symptoms. The minimum diagnostic IFA titer is 1:64, and a fourfold-antibody rise is considered confirmatory of recent infection.

## TREATMENT

As with rickettsial infection, doxycycline[1] is the treatment of choice for ehrlichiosis. Doxycycline can be administered either orally or intravenously at a dose of 100 mg twice per day. For children who weigh less than 45 kg or are younger than 8 years old, the recommended dose is 2.2 mg/kg each day in two divided doses.[1]

There have been no randomized trials of optimal therapy for either HME or HGA, but the consensus of most experienced clinicians is that therapy should be continued for approximately 7 days or for 3 days after defervescence. Defervescence typically occurs within 48 hours of initiation of therapy.

All tetracyclines can cause dental staining, but this risk remains low if a short course is administered. Chloramphenicol[1] has also been used effectively, but, given the higher risk of hematologic toxicity, this medication should be reserved for pregnant patients or patients with adverse reaction to doxycycline. Additionally, some ehrlichia have been shown to be resistant to chloramphenicol in vitro. Thus, doxycycline may be necessary when life-threatening illness occurs in a pregnant patient. Rifampin (Rifadin)[1] has been used to successfully treat a few pregnant patients with HGA, but at present the efficacy of such therapy can only be considered an anecdotal observation; rifampin does not have an FDA approval for this indication.

---

[1]Not FDA approved for this indication.

## CURRENT THERAPY

- In most patients with Rocky Mountain spotted fever (RMSF), human monocytotropic ehrlichiosis (HME), or human granulocytic anaplasmosis (HGA), the cornerstone of management is empiric therapy based on clinical judgment and the epidemiologic setting.
- Doxycycline 100 mg PO or IV bid is the treatment of choice for patients with RMSF, HME, and HGA.
- For children who weigh <45 kg or who are younger than 8 y, the recommended dose of doxycycline is 2.2 mg/kg/d in two divided doses.[1]
- Most clinicians treat patients with RMSF for 7 to 10 d; treatment can usually be discontinued 2 to 3 d after the patient becomes afebrile.
- Treat ehrlichiosis for approximately 7 d or for 3 d after defervescence.
- Chloramphenicol (Chloromycetin) 500 mg IV every 6 h should be used to treat pregnant patients with RMSF and patients with adverse reactions to tetracyclines.
- Alternative therapies for HGE and HMA include chloramphenicol and rifampin (Rifadin),[1] although these should only be used to treat HGE or HMA in pregnant patients or in patients with adverse reaction to doxycycline. Doxycycline, however, may be necessary when life-threatening illness occurs in a pregnant patient.

---

[1]Not FDA approved for this indication.

## REFERENCES

Bakken JS, Dumler JS: Human granulocytic ehrlichiosis. Clin Infect Dis 2000;31:554-560.

Chapman AS, Bakken JS, Folk SM, et al: Diagnosis and management of tickborne rickettsial diseases: Rocky Mountain spotted fever, ehrlichioses, and anaplasmosis—United States: A practical guide for physicians and other health-care and public health professionals. MMWR Recomm Rep 2006;55(RR-4):1-27.

Holman RC, Paddock CD, Curns AT, et al: Analysis of risk factors for fatal Rocky Mountain spotted fever: Evidence for superiority of tetracyclines for therapy. J Infect Dis. 2001;184:1437-1444.

Kaplan JE, Schonberger LB: The sensitivity of various serologic tests in the diagnosis of Rocky Mountain spotted fever. Am J Trop Med Hyg 1986; 35: 840-844.

Kirk JL, Sexton DJ, Fine DP, Muchmore HG: Rocky Mountain spotted fever: A clinical review based on 48 confirmed cases. Medicine (Baltimore) 1990;69:35-45.

Paddock CD, Holman RC, Krebs JW, Childs JE: Assessing the magnitude of fatal Rocky Mountain spotted fever in the United States: Comparison of two national data sources. Am J Trop Med Hyg 2002;67:349-354.

Parola P, Raoult D: Ticks and tickborne bacterial diseases in humans: An emerging infectious threat. Clin Infect Dis 2001;32:897-928.

Pretzman C, Daugherty N, Poetter K, Ralph D: The distribution and dynamics of *Rickettsia* in the tick population of Ohio. Ann N Y Acad Sci 1990;590: 227-236.

Stone JH, Dierberg K, Aram G, Dumler JS: Human monocytic ehrlichiosis. JAMA 2004;292:2263-2270.

# Smallpox

Method of
*Isao Arita, MD*

This chapter discusses the diagnosis and treatment of smallpox. However, in the unlikely event that a patient appears to have smallpox, it is essential to contact your local public health service office to obtain any updates, including vaccination, other methods of preventing further transmission, and protection for yourself and your personnel from the infection.

In 1980, the World Health Organization (WHO) declared that smallpox was eradiated throughout the world and would not return to the human community, and they recommended that smallpox vaccination be discontinued based on their assessment that risk of return of the disease is unlikely. Thus, all the nations in the world discontinued smallpox vaccination, and smallpox virus stocks in laboratories were destroyed except for those in two WHO collaborating centers in the United States and the Soviet Union. These stocks have been maintained to complete necessary research under strict biocontainment measures.

Since then, there has been no smallpox despite continuing global surveillance of the disease. Although the world has been apparently enjoying the benefit of successful smallpox eradication, the terrorist suicide attacks in New York City and Washington D.C. on September 11, 2001 completely altered the situation: Subsequent deliberate delivery of *Bacillus anthracis* from an unknown source alerted the U.S. and global community to the potential threat of bioterrorism, including smallpox as the bioweapon.

These circumstances urgently revived the necessity to remember the experience in smallpox eradication, which was once thought to be the technology of the past and which did not progress much in terms of prevention and treatment. Fortunately, such experience was described in detail and comprehensively by the experts who actually worked in the eradication program in WHO's 1988 publication "Smallpox and Its Eradication." In this section, special efforts are made to describe salient features of such experiences and knowledge for medical professionals at medical facilities, who may employ them in their emergency work for minimizing possible hazard, if smallpox infection occurs.

As in the past, there is no specific treatment for smallpox. In fact, this was one of the reasons international efforts were made to eradicate smallpox. Smallpox was greatly feared because of its 30% case-fatality rate and its ability to spread in any country and in any season. The second reason was that vaccination had been a very effective tool for prevention, but the complications, such as postvaccinal encephalitis, eczema vaccinatum, and progressive vaccinia, were relatively frequent and severe. For example, 10 to 50 persons per 1 million primary vaccinees suffered adverse effects in the United States. These complications prompted a strong consensus that the only way to eliminate such vaccine complications was to eradicate the disease, thereby making vaccination unnecessary.

## Clinical Features

The clinical pictures of smallpox is distinct for diagnosis and surveillance. There is no subclinical infection of epidemiologic significance. If the national security office warns of a possible return of smallpox, the disease ought to be, without much difficulty, suspected by medical personnel, who are concerned about the risk.

Surveillance of deliberate release of smallpox virus will be done by the appropriate national security offices, which require full cooperation by medical professionals. In fact, such cooperation is indispensable. Experience has shown that medical facilities are a common contact point, where persons infected with such severe disease as smallpox will visit, seeking consultation and medical treatment.

## Clinical Course

After the incubation period (usually 10-14 days, ranging rarely 7-19 days), prodromal symptoms begin with fever and malaise. The exanthem develops in a very regular stepwise fashion of macules, papules, vesicles, and pustules (Figure 1). The exanthem is quite characteristic, with uniform features at each step and typical distribution on the body. The lesions are distributed more on the face and extremities, the extensor side is more affected than the flexor side, and there are fewer lesions on the trunk. The appearance is so classic that medical personnel can suspect smallpox once they have seen the good pictures of smallpox exanthems.

Within one week, the skin lesions become pustules, which, in a few days, become confluent and reach maximum size. By the end of the second week, scabbing starts. The scabs fall from the skin, leaving depigmented spots in the affected skin (see Figure 1H). The scabs can persist for as long as 1 month. Within a few months, the depigmented areas become blackish pigmented spots. These are signs with which surveillance identified the presence of transmission retrospectively in the affected community in the recent past, if the surveillance missed the actual presence of smallpox. Finally, the pustules on the face become pockmark scars.

As for the severity of the disease, *Variola major* is the severest type, with a fatality rate of 30%. For smallpox terrorism, *V. major* is the likely strain. *V. minor* causes mild disease, with a fatality rate of a few percent. Intermediate-type disease has been found in some areas, including Africa. The clinical pictures of mild and intermediate smallpox are similar to those caused by *V. major*. Hence, *V. minor* disease should be treated just as *V. major* disease is in practice, when surveillance and control measures are to take place. Only laboratory study can verify the type of *V.* virus. Pregnancy appears to augment the severity of the disease.

History of smallpox vaccination modifies the course of the disease. Vaccinated patients who have smallpox have an accelerated clinical course and fewer skin lesions. This applies to persons vaccinated either before immunization programs ended, when smallpox had not yet been eradicated, or during special containment vaccination programs against the risk of infection. However, the percentage of unvaccinated persons among the global population is rapidly increasing. For clinical diagnosis, it is important to refer to the clinical characteristics, as described earlier.

Meanwhile, in emergency or unexpected circumstances, where the public health service has not yet been ready to organize personnel, persons who were vaccinated in the past may be requested (subject to their agreement to help), after a fresh vaccination, to participate in some emergency activities for surveillance or related activities.

## Differential Diagnosis and Laboratory Studies

During the program of smallpox eradication (1967-1980), surveillance was based on the clinical diagnosis in endemic nations, and only during the last 3 years of the program was laboratory diagnosis practiced by WHO reference laboratories in the United States and the Soviet Union. However, in today's world, it is important to pay special attention to the differential diagnosis, both clinical and laboratory, because a diagnosis of smallpox will necessarily result in a national health emergency including control of traffic, social events, and economic affairs and psychological calamity.

The clinical differential diagnosis includes varicella and other diseases of rash and fever (Table 1). In varicella, the features of the exanthem are different from those of smallpox. The varicella exanthem is a mixture of different types of rash, and the lesions are more abundant on the trunk (Figure 2). For clinicians, it may be difficult to suspect smallpox for the first 2 to 3 days of smallpox rash, because the rash may be mistaken for varicella or some other skin eruption. However, by day 3 to 4, it should be apparent that the rash is smallpox. Human monkeypox is another possible diagnosis, because the type of rash and distribution on the skin are very similar to those of smallpox,

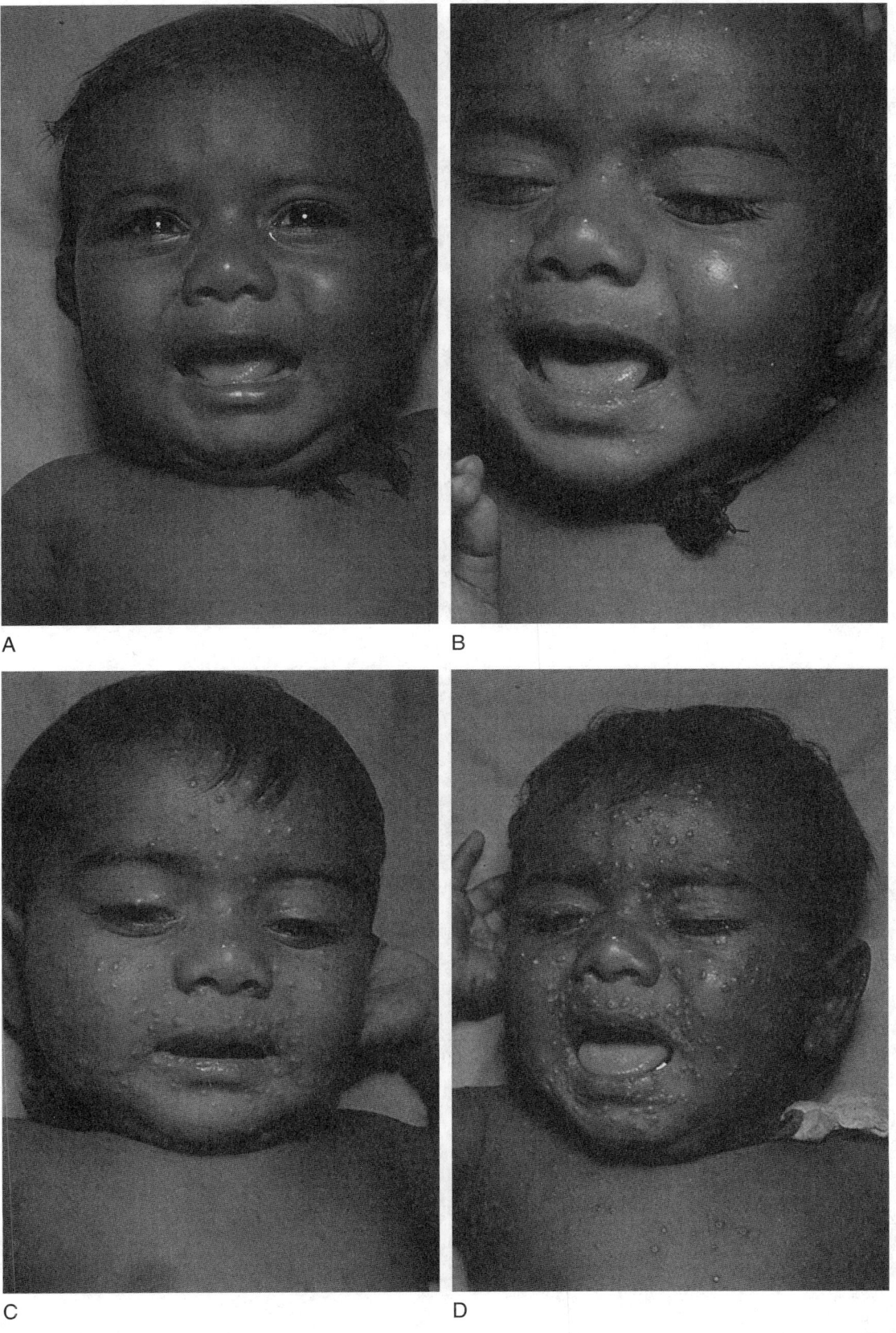

**FIGURE 1.** Lesions of smallpox. **A,** Day 1: The rash appears 1 day after the onset of fever. A few small papules are visible on the face and upper arms. An enanthem is usually present in the oropharynx at this time, but it cannot be seen in this photograph. **B,** Day 3: Additional lesions continue to appear, and some of the papules are becoming obviously vesicular. **C,** Day 4: All lesions have usually appeared by this time. Those that appeared earliest on the face and upper extremities are somewhat more mature than those that appeared later on other parts of the body, but on any specific area of the body all lesions are at approximately the same stage of development. Lesions are present on the palms. **D,** Day 5: Almost all the papules have now become vesicular or pustular, the true vesicular stage usually being very brief. Some of the lesions on the upper arms show early umbilication.

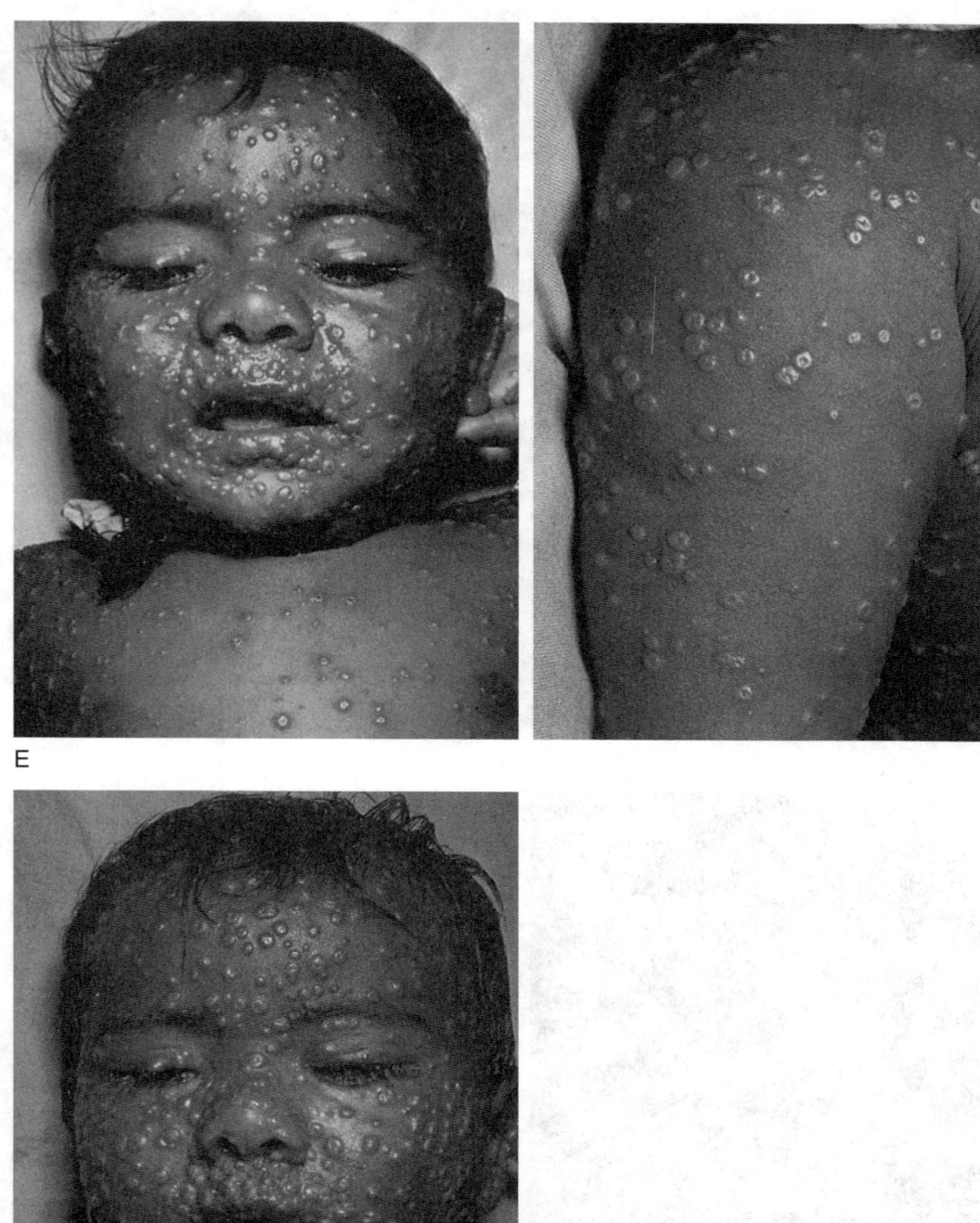

E

F

**FIGURE 1, cont'd E,** Day 6: All the vesicles have now become pustules, which feel round and hard to the touch ("shotty"), like a foreign body. **F,** Day 7: Many of the pustules are now umbilicated and all lesions now appear to be at the same stage of development.

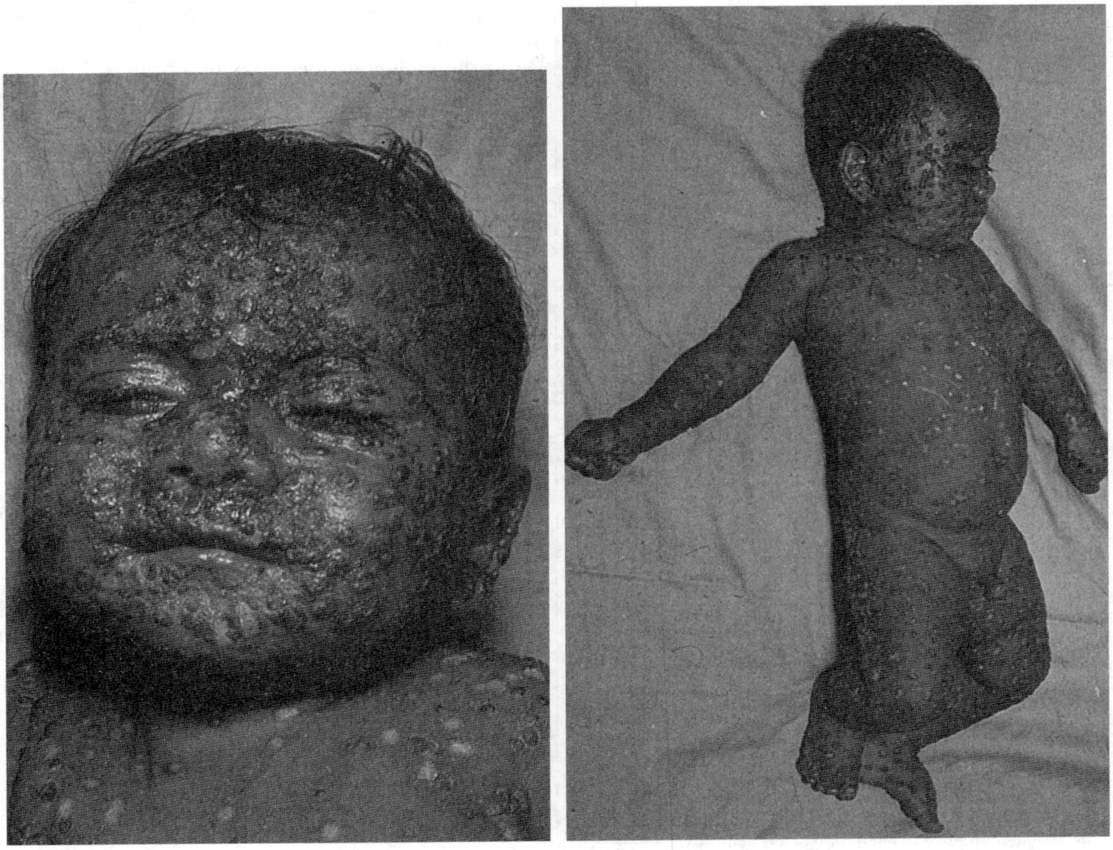

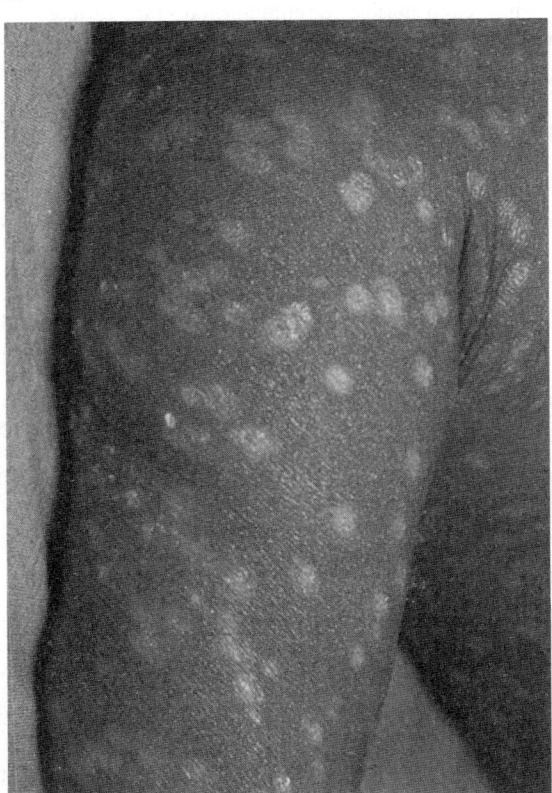

G

H

**FIGURE 1, cont'd G,** Day 13: The lesions are now scabbing, but the eyelids are more swollen than at earlier times. There is no evidence of secondary bacterial infection of the skin lesions. **H,** Day 20: The scabs have separated except on the palms and the soles, leaving depigmented areas. (All photographs from the World Health Organization.)

**TABLE 1**  Alternative Diagnoses in Suspected but Unconfirmed Cases of Smallpox

| | Case Series | | |
| Final Diagnosis | England and Wales, 1946-1948* (Variola major) | India, 1976† (Variola major) | Somalia, 1977-1979‡ (Variola minor) |
| --- | --- | --- | --- |
| Chickenpox | 41 | 53 | 20 |
| Erythema multiforme | 7 | 1 | 0 |
| Allergic dermatitis | 7 | 1 | 1 |
| Drug rash | 6 | 2 | 1 |
| Syphilis | 3 | 4 | 4 |
| Impetigo | 3 | 2 | 0 |
| Scabies | 1 | 1 | 0 |
| Psoriasis | 1 | 1 | 0 |
| Vaccinia | 5 | 0 | 1 |
| Herpes | 2 | 0 | 0 |
| Measles | 2 | 0 | 0 |
| Rubella | 1 | 0 | 0 |
| Molluscum contagiosum | 0 | 0 | 1 |
| Septicemia | 4 | 0 | 0 |
| Skin diseases (various) | 14 | 5 | 0 |
| Other (including no diagnosis made) | 0 | 30 | 1 |
| Total | 97 | 100 | 29 |

*Data from Conybeare ET: Cases in which smallpox was suspected but unconfirmed. Mon Bull Min Health Public Health Lab Serv 1950;9: 56-61.
†During posteradication surveillance in India. Data from Basu RN, Jezek Z, Ward NA: The eradication of smallpox from India. New Delhi: World Health Organization, 1979.
‡During posteradication surveillance in Somalia. Data from Jezek Z, Kriz B, Masar I, et al: [Liquidation of the last foci of variola in the world—Somalia (author's transl)] Cesk Epidemiol Mikrobiol Imunol 1981;30(2):113-124. Czech.
*Source:* World Health Organization.

## CURRENT DIAGNOSIS

- Smallpox was declared eradicated in 1980.
- Smallpox is one of the priority diseases requiring biodefense preparedness.
- Preliminary diagnosis of smallpox should be regarded as a national emergency.
- Smallpox has a characteristic progression of exanthems after prodromal symptoms: macules, papules, vesicles, and pustules. The entire rash is uniform at each stage. The rash lasts about 1 wk after the onset of fever. Check the type of rash on the patient against photos of the exanthems.
- If you suspect smallpox, report it to the local public health service office immediately to get instructions for further emergency action.
- Be prepared to collect specimens from the rash, based on established procedures, and to dispatch them to the designated laboratory.

but the lymphadenopathy (maxillar, inguinal, etc.) is distinctive in monkeypox (Figure 3).

In the differential diagnosis of smallpox, it is important to pay attention to the case history of the patient regarding whether the patient has had contact with a smallpox-like disease. In the case of a smallpox attack, there are two possible scenarios. In the first one, a case of deliberate release of smallpox virus through aerosol or contaminated materials, the case history does not arouse suspicion. The second scenario is a patient with secondary transmission from a primary smallpox patient. In this situation, the case history might show the contact with a smallpox-like disease within 17 days before the onset of rash.

The methods of laboratory diagnosis include electron microscopic test, rapid DNA test, virus isolation, and genetic sequence study. These should be operative services of a laboratory network of either a national reference laboratory or a contracted reference laboratory from another country. WHO should be in a position to assist in these laboratory networks.

The electron microscopic or rapid DNA test can be completed within a day, and virus isolation and genetic sequence tests can be completed in a few days in a designated laboratory in the network. Collection and dispatch of specimens (usually from skin lesions) should be according to the accepted protocol, namely, specimen placed in a leak-proof double container and packed according to the rules of the International Association of Transportation Regulators (IATR) (Figure 4).

The preparedness of the laboratory network is the first priority in any nation that wishes to handle smallpox bioterrorism surveillance properly.

## Treatment

The patient with diagnosed smallpox must be safely transported and admitted to an isolated station or ward for treatment by trained hospital personnel. Patients with suspected smallpox should be also isolated and vaccinated. Patients with suspected smallpox *must not* be treated in the same isolation facilities with smallpox patients.

Currently, there is no effective therapeutic substance licensed for treating smallpox in humans. Before and after the smallpox eradication period (1967-1980), strenuous efforts were made to develop treatment for smallpox, but they have failed. As recently experienced in the United States, immunization of the population as preparedness for biodefense has also failed due to vaccine complications. Most nations, to date, are not in favor of conducting mass vaccination campaigns as preemptive measures. Thus, the research to produce a safer vaccine and the research on an antiviral drug are warranted and continued.

If smallpox reemerges, all patients should receive supportive care. Supportive care can include infection control, such as antibiotics to prevent secondary infection, and intensive rehydration therapy. Ventilator assistance may be needed. In special cases, such as the severe type of hemorrhagic smallpox, patients must also be treated for shock. Attention should be paid to likely renal failure and malnutrition. These medical practices are complicated by the precautions for protection and disinfection that are necessary to prevent smallpox virus contamination of the environment and population.

## CURRENT THERAPY

- We have no specific antiviral drug or treatment of smallpox.
- Provide supportive care as symptoms suggest.
- Consult the local health service office for all the necessary pubic health measures, such as protection for yourself and your staff from infection, disinfection, isolation, vaccination, transport, and other relevant containment methods as required.

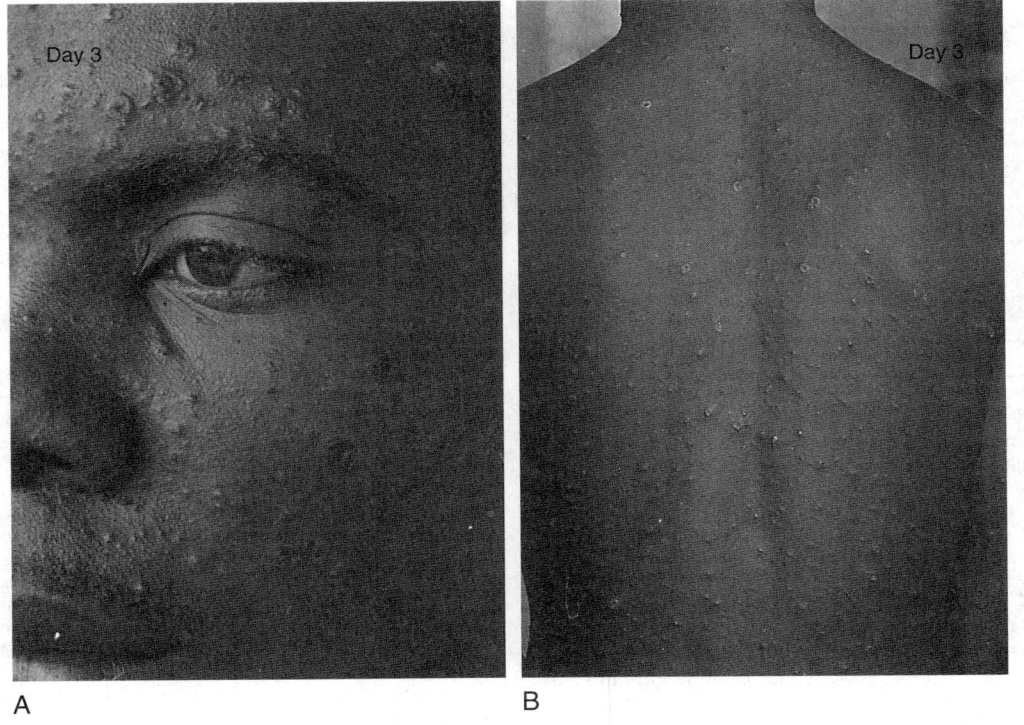

**FIGURE 2.** Chickenpox. **A** and **B**, On the third day of rash, pocks are at different stages of development (papules and vesicles). There are many lesions on the trunk (**B**) and few on the limbs. (Photographs from the World Health Organization.)

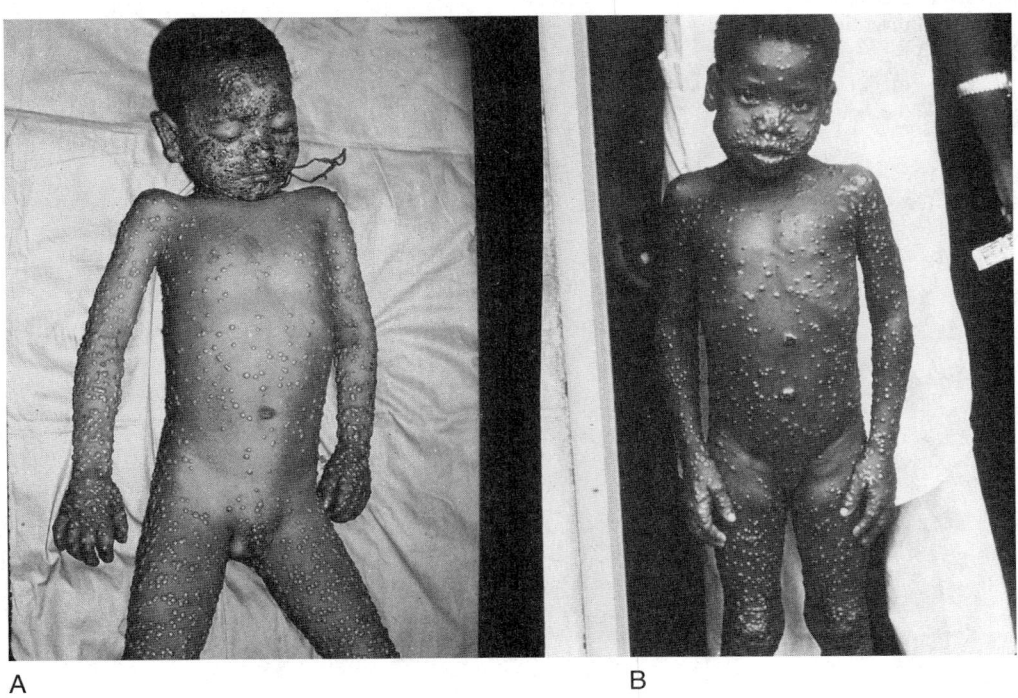

**FIGURE 3.** Similar exanthem in patients infected with smallpox virus (**A**) and monkeypox virus (**B**) on day 7 of exanthem. (Photographs from the World Health Organization.)

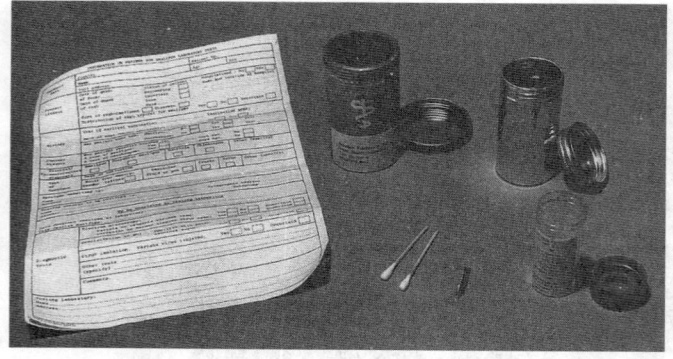

**FIGURE 4.** Container for smallpox specimen collection. Transportation of dangerous pathogens or specimens requires a special double container to ensure safety. (Photograph from the World Health Organization.)

Experience has shown that smallpox vaccination during the incubation period, within 4 to 5 days after the exposure to the infection, can prevent the infection. However, in practice, any person in contact with a smallpox patient or suspected smallpox patient should be vaccinated as soon as possible. Vaccinia immune globulin intravenous (VIGIV) can reduce some complications of vaccination, but there has been no evidence that it is effective for treating smallpox.

Smallpox was once eradicated by the unified efforts of humankind. The strategy was through immunization as a preventive measure, not through curative treatment, which is not available even today, when bioterrorism by smallpox is threatening us. Research is needed to develop a further attenuated vaccine and antiviral drug as well, but use of the vaccine should still play a greater role, as was done in the eradication efforts a quarter century ago.

This article was written in 2006, and because the technical progress will be very rapid, readers are requested to seek updated information that will be available from the World Health Organization (http://www.who.int/csr/disease/smallpox/en/) and the U.S. Centers for Disease Control and Prevention (http://www.bt.cdc.gov/agent/smallpox/index.asp) in 2008.

## Acknowledgments

I am grateful to Dr. D. A. Henderson of Johns Hopkins University, who advised on the preparation of this article and to Ms. M. Nakane of the Agency for Cooperation in International Health (in Japan), who sorted out all important references during the preparation of this article.

## REFERENCES

Arita I: Smallpox vaccine and its stockpile in 2005. Lancet Infect Dis 2005;5(10):647-652.

Breman JG, Henderson DA: Diagnosis and management of smallpox. N Engl J Med 2002;346(17):1300-1308. Available from http://content.nejm.org/cgi/content/full/346/17/1300 (accessed May 30, 2007).

Centers for Disease Control and Prevention: Smallpox response plan and guidelines: Annex 1: Overview of smallpox, clinical presentations, and medical care of smallpox patients. Available from http://www.bt.cdc.gov/agent/smallpox/response-plan/files/annex-1-part1of3.pdf (accessed May 30, 2007).

Centers for Disease Control and Prevention: Smallpox response plan and guidelines: Annex 2: General Guidelines for Smallpox Vaccination Clinics. Available from http://www.bt.cdc.gov/agent/smallpox/response-plan/files/annex-2.pdf (accessed May 30, 2007).

Centers for Disease Control and Prevention: Smallpox response plan and guidelines: Annex 3: Guidelines for Large Scale Smallpox Vaccination Clinics: Logistical Considerations and Guidance for State and Local Planning for Emergency, Large-Scale, Voluntary Administration of Smallpox Vaccine in Response to a Smallpox Outbreak. Available from http://www.bt.cdc.gov/agent/smallpox/response-plan/files/annex-3.pdf (accessed May 30, 2007).

Centers for Disease Control and Prevention: Slides and notes: Smallpox disease and its clinical management. Available from http://www.bt.cdc.gov/agent/smallpox/training/overview/pdf/diseasemgmt.pdf (accessed May 30, 2007).

Centers for Disease Control and Prevention: Smallpox fact sheet: Reaction after smallpox vaccination. Available from http://www.bt.cdc.gov/agent/smallpox/vaccination/pdf/reactions-vacc-public.pdf (accessed May 30, 2007).

Fenner F, Henderson DA, Arita I Jezek Z, Ladnyi ID: Smallpox and Its Eradication. Geneva, Switzerland: World Health Organization, 1988. PDF available at http://whqlibdoc.who.int/smallpox/9241561106.pdf (accessed May 15, 2007).

Institute of Medicine: Assessment of Future Scientific Needs for Live Variola Virus. Washington, DC: National Academies Press, 1999.

University of Pittsburgh Medical Center Center for Biosecurity: Smallpox FAQ, 2005. [on the Internet, cited October 2, 2006] Available from http://www.upmc-biosecurity.org/website/bioagents/smallpox/smallpox_faq_2005.html

# Diseases of the Head and Neck

## Vision Correction Procedures

Method of
*Neil J. Friedman, MD*

Refractive errors are the most common eye disorders. These conditions are characterized by blurred vision because images are not focused properly on the retina. Light rays entering the eye are refracted or bent by the cornea and lens. If eyeglasses or contact lenses are necessary for clear vision, then a refractive error exists.

*Myopia* (nearsightedness) occurs when the power of the eye is too strong, causing images to be focused in front of the retina; *hyperopia* (farsightedness) occurs when the power of the eye is too weak, causing images to be focused behind the retina; and *astigmatism* occurs when the power of the eye is different in different directions, causing images to be focused at more than one location. Astigmatism typically results when the shape of the cornea is more elliptical than spherical (i.e., it is steeper in one meridian than another, like a football rather than a baseball). *Presbyopia* refers to the loss of accommodative power as the eye's natural lens stiffens with age. This generally becomes symptomatic after the age of 40 years, resulting in the need for reading glasses.

In the United States, approximately 25% of the population is nearsighted, 25% is farsighted, and presbyopia eventually develops in everyone. The most common method of correcting refractive errors is with glasses or contact lenses. Surgical correction has also been an option for decades, but many of the earlier procedures failed to achieve wide acceptance because of varying results and safety concerns. Advances in technology and techniques now allow ophthalmologists to provide patients with a variety of procedures for treating their refractive errors. Most of the surgical options are aimed at altering the shape of the cornea. These include incisional, laser, thermal, and implant techniques. Other alternatives involve surgery to insert a lens inside the eye. This article reviews the spectrum of available refractive surgical procedures for vision correction.

## Corneal Refractive Procedures

### INCISIONAL

Cutting the cornea alters its shape, depending on the orientation of the incisions. The most common technique, *radial keratotomy* (RK), consists of creating deep radial incisions with a diamond knife. This procedure to correct low levels of myopia was popular before the advent of laser vision correction. Eighty-five percent of patients achieved 20/40 or better uncorrected visual acuity (UCVA) after the initial procedure. In addition to possible undercorrection and a tendency toward progressive effect (hyperopic drift) with time, adverse events associated with RK include perforation, infection, scarring,

irregular astigmatism, glare or starburst, and fluctuating vision. Therefore, excimer laser techniques, which are safer and more predictable, have essentially replaced RK surgery.

*Astigmatic keratotomy* (AK) is a similar technique in which peripheral arcuate corneal incisions are created to correct astigmatism. However, like RK, AK has largely been replaced by laser procedures. The exception to this trend is a variation of AK known as *limbal relaxing incisions,* which is often performed at the time of cataract surgery to minimize postoperative astigmatism. Relaxing incisions are also commonly used in corneal grafts to reduce astigmatism after corneal transplant surgery.

### EXCIMER LASER

Laser vision correction is currently the most popular surgical method for treating refractive errors. The excimer laser emits a beam of 193-nm wavelength ultraviolet light that can precisely sculpt the cornea. It is a cold laser that breaks molecular bonds to ablate tissue and thereby acts as a laser scalpel to improve the natural focus of the eye. To correct myopia, a central ablation flattens the cornea; for hyperopia, a peripheral ablation steepens the central cornea; and for astigmatism, an elliptical ablation is performed to flatten the steep corneal meridian.

The U.S. Food and Drug Administration (FDA) approved the first excimer laser in 1995 to correct low to moderate levels of myopia. Since that time, lasers have been approved for expanded ranges and combinations of myopia, hyperopia, and astigmatism. Although they are approved for higher amounts, excimer lasers are most effective for treating up to −10.0 D of nearsightedness, +5.0 D of farsightedness, and 4.0 D of astigmatism. To date, more than 10 million laser vision-correction treatments have been performed in the United States alone.

Wavefront technology is now available to measure the higher-order aberrations of an eye, which are the slight optical imperfections in the cornea and lens that degrade the quality of vision. This information produces a unique wavefront map or wavescan for each eye, which is used to guide the laser ablation. Wavefront treatments have resulted in improved visual acuity and contrast sensitivity and have decreased the incidence of nighttime glare and halos. Depending on the level of treatment, 20/20 or better UCVA has been achieved in more than 90% of patients undergoing wavefront procedures. Eye tracking and iris registration software have also improved the results of laser vision correction by ensuring proper alignment of the treatment and significantly reducing the risk of a decentered ablation.

A number of different techniques use the excimer laser. *Photorefractive keratectomy* (PRK), the first procedure for which the laser was FDA approved, refers to laser ablation of the corneal surface after removal of the central epithelium (Figure 1). A soft contact lens is placed on the eye for several days to serve as a bandage until the epithelial defect heals. Therefore, the visual recovery is longer and there is more discomfort than other procedures that preserve the surface epithelium. For high levels of correction, there is also a small risk of superficial haze or scarring, although with newer-generation lasers and

## MYOPIC PHOTOREFRACTIVE KERATECTOMY

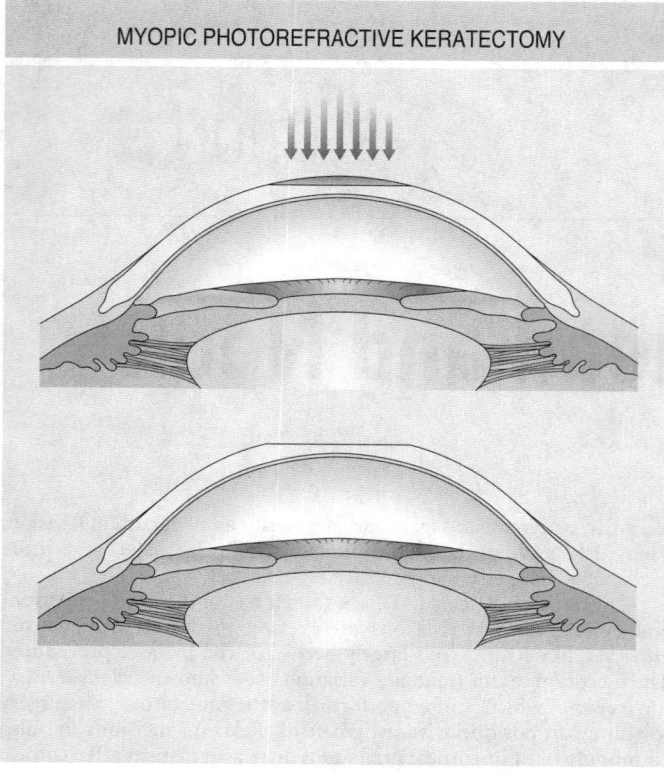

**FIGURE 1.** Photorefractive keratectomy (PRK). After removal of the corneal epithelium, the excimer laser is used to reprofile the anterior curvature of the cornea, which changes its refractive power. (From Yanoff M, Duker JS: Ophthalmology, 2nd ed. St Louis: Mosby, 2003, p 128.)

## LASER *IN SITU* KERATOMILEUSIS

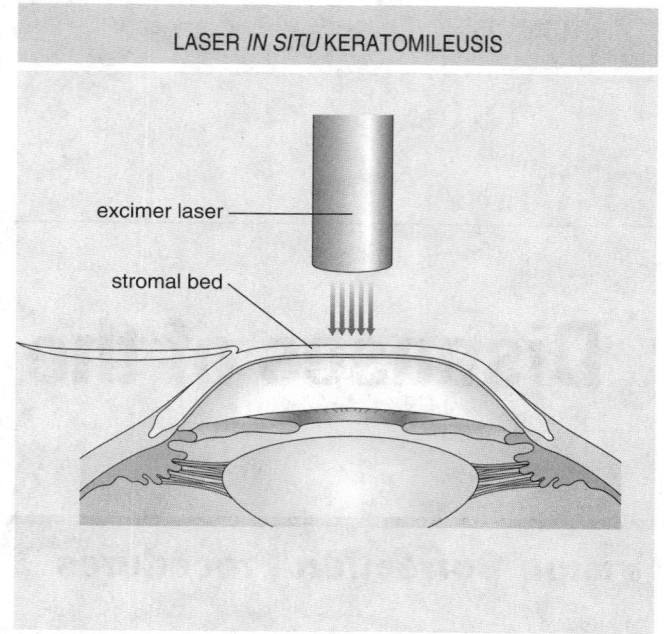

**FIGURE 2.** Laser in situ keratomileusis (LASIK). Excimer laser ablation to the stromal bed after lamellar keratectomy. (From Yanoff M, Duker JS: Ophthalmology, 2nd ed. St Louis: Mosby, 2003, p 175.)

the use of topical antimetabolites (mitomycin C) for high-risk cases, visually significant haze is rare.

*Laser-assisted in situ keratomileusis* (LASIK) is laser ablation of the cornea under a flap (Figure 2). A mechanical or laser keratome cuts a hinged partial-thickness corneal flap that is folded back. Laser energy is then applied to the underlying stromal bed, and the flap is replaced. LASIK allows faster visual recovery and minimal pain after surgery as compared with PRK, but there is an added risk of complications from flap-related problems. These can occur intra- or postoperatively and consist of poor-quality flap, dislocation of the flap, wrinkles in the flap, inflammation under the flap, and epithelial cells growing underneath the flap.

*Laser-assisted subepithelial keratectomy* (LASEK) and *epi-LASIK* (epithelial LASIK) are variations of PRK in which the epithelium is preserved to later cover the treatment area. Alcohol (in LASEK) or a mechanical device (in epi-LASIK) is used to separate an intact flap of epithelium, which is retracted for the laser ablation and then repositioned afterward. Theoretically, these techniques offer the advantages of both PRK and LASIK without the disadvantages, but whether there is any significant difference from PRK is yet to be determined.

Regardless of which laser-correction procedure is chosen, patients experience comparable results in terms of final vision. Safety and predictability are also excellent, but like any surgery, there are potential risks. Fortunately, complications are rare. The computer-controlled excimer laser is extremely precise, ablating approximately 0.25 μm of tissue with each pulse.

The unpredictability in laser vision correction occurs because every person and every eye heals differently. Therefore, the most common sequela is an under- or overcorrection, which can be treated once the eye has stabilized. Glare or halos around lights at night and drier eyes are usually temporary effects, which improve over time. There is a very small risk of infection, scarring, and progressive

corneal thinning (keratectasia). Patients must be carefully screened preoperatively for any ocular or systemic conditions that could interfere with healing. To prevent keratectasia, it is recommended that the residual stromal bed thickness be at least 250 μm after LASIK.

## THERMOKERATOPLASTY

The curvature of the cornea can also be altered by thermal energy, which shrinks stromal collagen. Thermokeratoplasty refers to heating the cornea to change its shape. In *conductive keratoplasty* (CK), a contact probe delivers radiofrequency energy directly to the midperipheral cornea in a ring pattern (Figure 3). This creates a purse-string effect that steepens the central cornea to correct low levels of hyperopia. Studies indicate 95% of patients attain UCVA of 20/40 or better. CK is an extremely safe technique. It also has the advantages of sparing the visual axis and preserving corneal tissue. However, like other forms of hyperopia treatment, regression of effect has been observed.

## IMPLANTS

Inserting various materials and lenses into the cornea has been attempted for decades, but unfortunately there has been limited success with such procedures. *Intrastromal corneal ring segments* (Intacs) are thin plastic 150-degree arc length implants that are placed into deep midperipheral corneal channels (Figure 4). This flattens the central cornea to correct low levels of myopia. These implants spare the visual axis and are reversible and adjustable, but the low range of correction afforded by this technique limits its usefulness. An alternative indication for these inserts may be in patients with keratoconus or keratectasia, as evidenced by studies that demonstrate improvements in vision, stabilizing effect, and ability to alter the degree and location of the corneal protrusion. However, longer follow-up of these patients is necessary.

*Intracorneal inlays* are thin contact lens–like implants that can be placed under a corneal flap. The thickness and shape of the inlay change the corneal curvature to correct the patient's refractive error without removing corneal tissue. Like Intacs, the advantage of this technique is that it is adjustable as well as reversible by exchanging or

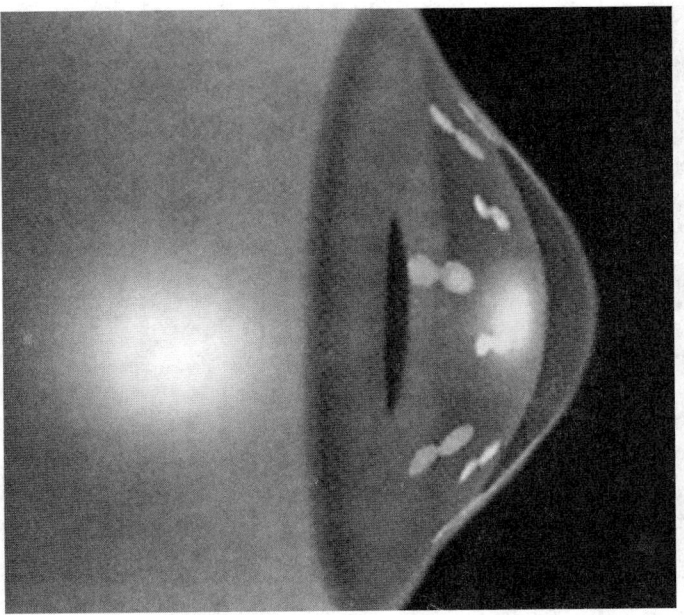

**FIGURE 3.** Side view of the location of a 16-spot thermal kerato-plasty application with the resultant corneal steepening. (From Yanoff M, Duker JS: Ophthalmology, 2nd ed. St Louis: Mosby, 2003, p 204.)

explanting the inlay. Furthermore, there is no tissue removal. However, inserting a device into the cornea has its own set of potential risks. Besides infection and complications in creating corneal channels or flaps, implant decentration or extrusion can occur. Historically, there have been issues with necrosis of the overlying corneal tissue, and the long-term effects of an intracorneal foreign body are unknown.

## Intraocular Refractive Procedures

Intraocular refractive procedures are primarily used to correct higher degrees of myopia and hyperopia in patients for whom laser vision correction is not an option. The main advantages of intraocular surgery are predictability, stability, and preservation of the cornea's natural shape.

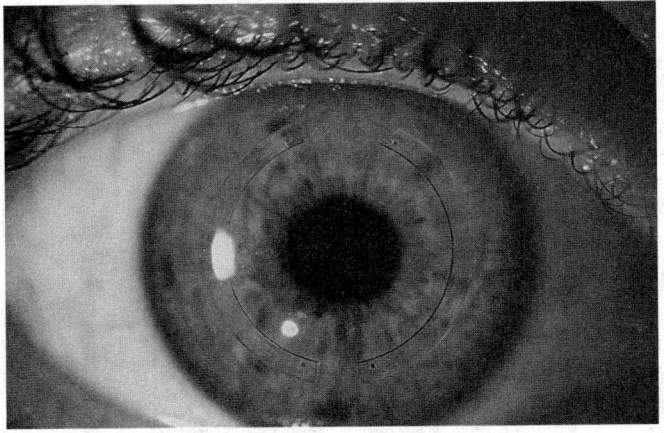

**FIGURE 4.** Intacs (intrastromal corneal ring segments) demonstrating two implants well positioned in the cornea. (From Kaiser P, Friedman N, Pineda R [eds]: Massachusetts Eye and Ear Infirmary Illustrated Manual of Ophthalmology, 2nd ed. Philadelphia: WB Saunders, 2003, p 466.)

## LENS-EXCHANGE SURGERY

*Refractive lens exchange* (RLE) refers to surgically removing the patient's natural lens and replacing it with an intraocular lens (IOL) implant of appropriate power. It is essentially cataract surgery before a cataract has developed. This procedure is extremely accurate and predictable because the requisite measurements and calculations to determine the correct power of lens to implant have been refined from years of experience with cataract surgery. Preexisting astigmatism can also be corrected by implanting a toric IOL, combining the procedure with limbal relaxing incisions, or performing a subsequent laser refractive procedure.

However, lens-exchange surgery is controversial because of the inherent risks of an intraocular procedure (i.e., vision-threatening complications such as intraocular infection or hemorrhage). This is especially true for myopic patients because of the increased risk of retinal detachment. Another disadvantage, particularly for young patients, is the absolute loss of accommodation when the eye's natural lens is removed. Unless a multifocal or accommodating IOL is implanted, the loss of accommodation can be a major concern for patients because their expectation is to reduce their dependence on glasses or contact lenses.

## PHAKIC LENSES

*Phakic intraocular lenses* are lens implants similar to those used for RLE surgery; however, in this procedure the lens implant is inserted into the eye without removing the patient's natural lens. The major benefit of this option is that accommodation is preserved by leaving the patient's own lens in place.

There are three distinct lens designs depending on where the lens is positioned inside the eye. Phakic lenses can be placed in the anterior chamber (Baikoff lens), attached to the iris (Verisyse lens; Figure 5), or positioned in the posterior chamber (Visian lens). The anterior chamber and iris varieties are rigid lenses that require a larger incision, which must be sutured. The posterior chamber style is a foldable lens that can be implanted through a much smaller and sutureless wound.

Up to 95% of patients have UCVA of at least 20/40, and 11% gain two or more lines of best spectacle-corrected visual acuity (BSCVA). For all phakic lenses, it is essential to perform prophylactic peripheral iridotomies prior to surgery to allow proper aqueous flow and prevent angle-closure glaucoma. Similar to RLE, phakic intraocular lens surgery is very accurate, but the additional risks of intraocular complications exist and also include progressive corneal endothelial damage, cataract, glaucoma, and chronic iritis.

## CORRECTION OF PRESBYOPIA

Surgical methods for correcting presbyopia can be divided into two categories: compensatory approaches and restoration of accommodation.

### Compensatory Approaches

#### Monovision

*Monovision* refers to correcting one eye for near and one eye for distance focus. This may be achieved with any of the existing vision-correction procedures by leaving one eye slightly myopic (for near vision) and the other eye emmetropic (for distance vision). Monovision has been most commonly used with presbyopic contact lens wearers, and, because of the high success rate with these patients, similar candidates who subsequently undergo corneal or intraocular refractive surgery often desire monovision as the surgical goal. However, it is essential to undergo a contact lens trial before corrective surgery. In the event that the patient is unhappy with monovision, a second procedure can be performed to correct the residual myopia in the near-focus eye.

A study that evaluated PRK-induced monovision in myopic presbyopes found that postoperatively, none of the monovision patients was using reading glasses, and all of them had binocular acuity of 20/40 or better at distance and 20/30 or better at near. The overall satisfaction level was 86%. The monovision approach preserves BSCVA,

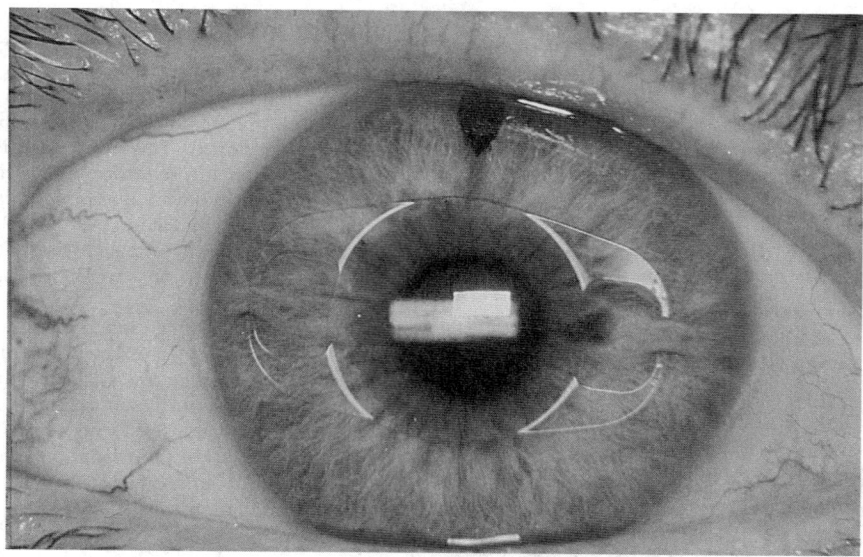

**FIGURE 5.** Phakic intraocular lens demonstrating the Verisyse lens in the anterior chamber attached to the iris at the 3-o'clock and 9-o'clock positions. Note the peripheral iridectomy at the 12-o'clock position to prevent angle-closure glaucoma. (From Kaiser P, Friedman N, Pineda R [eds]: Massachusetts Eye and Ear Infirmary Illustrated Manual of Ophthalmology, 2nd ed. Philadelphia: WB Saunders, 2003, p 459.)

but concerns exist about reduced contrast sensitivity, depth perception, and uncorrected distance vision in the near eye.

### Multifocal Correction

*Multifocal correction* refers to simultaneously correcting near and distance by creating at least two focal points in the eye. Multifocal laser ablation profiles are under development, and corneal inlays may be another option.

This goal can also be accomplished with intraocular surgery by inserting a multifocal IOL implant. Several multifocal IOLs are available for treating presbyopia in patients undergoing cataract and RLE surgery. These lenses have alternating rings of power designated for varying distances (Figure 6). Patient selection is critical in achieving the desired result, and contraindications include ocular and systemic diseases with loss of contrast sensitivity, astigmatism greater than 1 D, pupil size smaller than 2 mm, and age older than 85 years. Efficacy data vary depending on the lens design. Eighty-eight percent of patients given the ReStor lens achieve spectacle independence for distance and near vision, and up to 82% are able to see 20/40 or better at intermediate distances. For the ReZoom lens, spectacle independence for distance, intermediate, and near vision is produced in 93%, 91%, and 67% of patients, respectively. The multifocal approach certainly allows better preservation of binocular function relative to monovision, but there may be a sacrifice in contrast sensitivity, and up to 10% of patients experience glare and ghosting symptoms.

Another implant design for presbyopia is an accommodating IOL. The Crystalens is a flexible hinged monofocal IOL that is presumed to move forward for near focus; however, the actual mechanism has yet to be completely understood (Figure 7). Ninety-four percent of patients enjoy 20/32 or better UCVA at distance, intermediate, and near ranges and can perform most visual functions without spectacles. The advantage of this style of lens over a multifocal IOL is that none of the incoming light is scattered by transition zones, and thus there are no glare effect and no loss of contrast sensitivity.

### Restoration of Accommodation

Surgical methods that attempt to restore accommodation are aimed at creating more space between the ciliary muscle and the lens.

*Anterior ciliary sclerotomy* uses a guarded diamond blade or a laser to create eight partial-thickness radial incisions in the sclera over the ciliary body. Results of small studies showed an unpredictable change in the amplitude of accommodation, and investigators have concluded that this procedure does not work. In addition, the surgery structurally weakens the eye and can produce significant complications including hemorrhage and ocular penetration.

*Scleral expansion* involves inserting four rigid synthetic bands in the sclera just posterior to the limbus to expand the scleral diameter. Theoretically, the effective working distance of the ciliary muscle is restored, increasing the power for accommodation. The procedure is

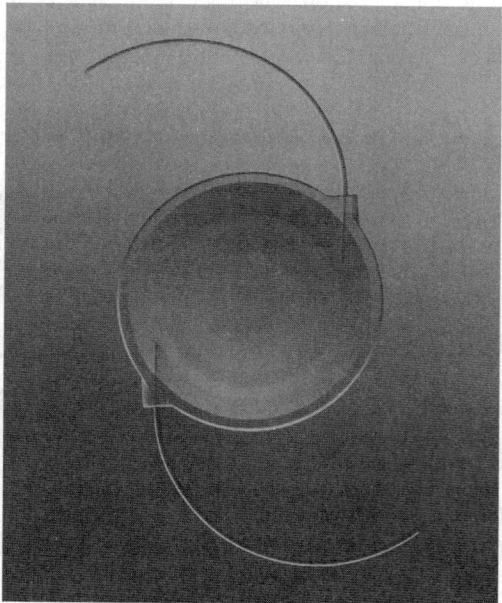

**FIGURE 6.** Foldable silicone multifocal intraocular lens. (From Yanoff M, Duker JS: Ophthalmology, 2nd ed. St Louis: Mosby, 2003, p 319.)

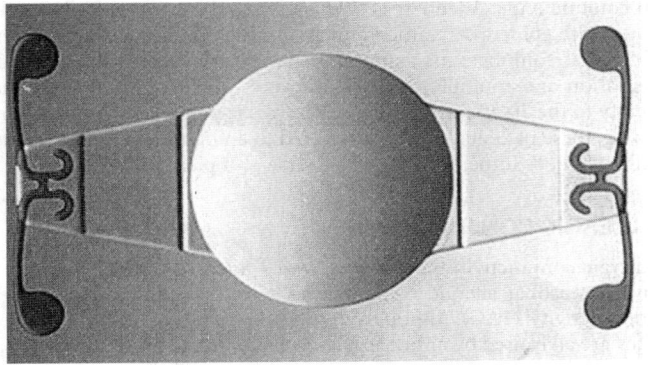

**FIGURE 7.** The Crystalens is essentially a plate haptic lens with a flexible hinge on each side of the central optic. (From Yanoff M, Duker JS: Ophthalmology, 2nd ed. St Louis: Mosby, 2003, p 304.)

reversible, but there is a risk of conjunctival erosion over the bands. Some preliminary work demonstrated that patients undergoing the procedure experienced an improvement in uncorrected near vision and near point of accommodation. However, further studies have yielded inconsistent and disappointing results, with no evidence of accommodation in patients undergoing this treatment.

Presbyopia correction continues to be an exciting area of investigation at the forefront of ophthalmic research. Other innovative strategies that hold future promise for restoring accommodation include truly accommodating IOLs and filling the capsular bag with a substance to mimic the natural crystalline lens.

### REFERENCES

Budak K, Friedman NJ, Koch DD: Limbal relaxing incisions with cataract surgery. J Cataract Refract Surg 2001;27:503-508.

Cumming JS, Slade SG, Chayet A; AT-45 Study Group: Clinical evaluation of the model AT-45 silicone accommodating intraocular lens: Results of feasibility and the initial phase of a Food and Drug Administration clinical trial. Ophthalmology 2001;108:2005-2009.

Guell JL: Are intracorneal rings still useful in refractive surgery? Curr Opin Ophthalmol 2005;16:260-265.

Hamilton DR, Davidorf JM, Maloney RK: Anterior ciliary sclerotomy for treatment of presbyopia: A prospective controlled study. Ophthalmology 2002;109:1970-1976.

Kohnen T, Allen D, Boureau C, et al: European multicenter study of the AcrySof ReSTOR apodized diffractive intraocular lens. Ophthalmology 2006;113:584.

Lin DY, Manche EE: Two-year results of conductive keratoplasty for the correction of low to moderate hyperopia. J Cataract Refract Surg 2003;29:2339-2350.

Qazi MA, Pepose JS, Shuster JJ: Implantation of scleral expansion band segments for the treatment of presbyopia. Am J Ophthalmol 2002;134:808-815.

Sanders DR, Doney K, Poco M; ICL in Treatment of Myopia Study Group: United States Food and Drug Administration clinical trial of the implantable collamer lens (ICL) for moderate to high myopia: Three-year follow-up. Ophthalmology 2004;111:1683-1692.

Vaquero-Ruano M, Encinas JL, Millan I, et al: AMO array multifocal versus monofocal intraocular lenses: Long-term follow-up. J Cataract Refract Surg 1998;24:118-123.

Waring GO, Lynn MJ, McDonnell PJ: Results of the prospective evaluation of radial keratotomy (PERK) study 10 years after surgery. Arch Ophthalmol 1994;112:1298-1308.

Wright KW, Guemes A, Kapadia MS, Wilson SE: Binocular function and patient satisfaction after monovision induced by myopic photorefractive keratectomy. J Cataract Refract Surg 1999;25:177-182.

Yang XJ, Yan HT, Nakahori Y: Evaluation of the effectiveness of laser in situ keratomileusis and photorefractive keratectomy for myopia: A meta-analysis. J Med Invest. 2003;50:180-186.

# Conjunctivitis

Method of
*Arti Sinha, MB, BS, and Ramesh Ayyala, MD*

Conjunctivitis is inflammation of the mucous membrane on the surface of the eye, the conjunctiva.

## Anatomy

The conjunctiva lines the inside surface of the lids and covers the surface of the globe up to the limbus. The portion covering the globe is known as the bulbar conjunctiva; the portion lining the lids is the palpebral conjunctiva. The conjunctiva consists of a nonkeratinized squamous epithelium containing goblet cells and a highly vascularized substantia propria, the site of considerable immunologic activity.

## Symptoms and Signs

Conjunctivitis, a diagnosis of clinical exclusion, should be differentiated from serious red eye–causing conditions such as keratitis, iritis, and angle closure glaucoma. A diagnosis of conjunctivitis should only be made if the vision is normal, with rare exceptions. Focal pathology in the lids such as hordeolum, ulceration, or blepharitis causes a reactive hyperemia and should be excluded in all cases of conjunctivitis.

Classically, patients with all types of conjunctivitis complain of morning crusting and diffuse daytime redness with discharge and 360-degree involvement of the conjunctiva. Other symptoms include a foreign-body sensation, scratching or burning sensation, itching, and photophobia.

The important signs of conjunctivitis include hyperemia (marked redness in the fornix, decreasing toward the limbus), epiphora, exudation, pseudoptosis, papillary hypertrophy, chemosis (edema of the conjunctival stroma), follicles (rounded avascular white or gray lesions), pseudomembranes and membranes, and preauricular adenopathy.

## Types of Conjunctivitis

Conjunctivitis can be classified on the basis of its etiology into bacterial, viral, allergic, and noninfectious forms. The prevalence of each varies. Bacterial conjunctivitis is more common in children than in adults, but most infectious conjunctivitis is viral.

### BACTERIAL CONJUNCTIVITIS

Bacterial conjunctivitis is commonly caused by *Staphylococcus aureus*, *Streptococcus pneumoniae*, *Haemophilus influenzae*, or *Moraxella catarrhalis*. *S. aureus* infection is common in adults, and the others are more common in children. Bacterial conjunctivitis is highly contagious and can spread by direct contact with the patient and his or her secretions or with contaminated objects and surfaces.

Typically, a patient complains of redness and discharge in one eye throughout the day; discharge can also be bilateral. The discharge is thick and globular, usually at the lid margins and in the corners of the eye. It may be yellow, white, or green, and the affected eye is often stuck shut in the morning.

Appropriate first-line treatment for bacterial conjunctivitis includes fluoroquinolones such as ciprofloxacin ophthalmic ointment or drops (Ciloxan). The dose is ½" (1.25 cm) of ointment deposited inside the lower lid or 1 or 2 drops instilled four times daily for 5 to 7 days, tapering with symptomatic relief.

Alternative therapies include bacitracin ointment, polymyxin-bacitracin ointment (Polysporin), or fluoroquinolone drops (ciprofloxacin, ofloxacin [Ocuflox], levofloxacin [Quixin], gatifloxacin

[Zymar], moxifloxacin [Vigamox]). Aminoglycosides, which are toxic to the corneal epithelium, should be avoided. Most bacteria are resistant to erythromycin ointment. The fluoroquinolones are effective and well tolerated and form the treatment of choice for conjunctivitis and for corneal ulcers (especially in contact lens wearers).

### Hyperacute Bacterial Conjunctivitis

Species of *Neisseria*, in particular *Neisseria gonorrhoeae*, can cause a severe and sight-threatening hyperacute bacterial conjunctivitis demanding immediate ophthalmologic referral. Typically, concurrent urethritis coexists because the organism is usually transmitted from the genitalia to the hands and to the eyes.

The infection characteristically manifests with a profuse purulent discharge within 12 hours of inoculation. The other symptoms, comprising redness, irritation, and tenderness to palpation, are rapidly progressive. There is usually marked chemosis, lid swelling, and tender preauricular adenopathy. Left untreated, the infection can progress to keratitis and perforation. A Gram stain of the discharge reveals gramnegative diplococci. These patients require hospital admission for systemic (ceftriaxone 250 mg IM and azithromycin 1 g PO) and topical (fluoroquinolone drops such as gatifloxacin or moxifloxacin) therapy.

### Chlamydial Conjunctivitis

Chlamydia trachomatis, the commonest cause of sexually transmitted genital infections, is the most frequent cause of conjunctivitis in the neonate. Infants delivered through an infected birth canal contract the infection, although birth by cesarean section can also lead to infection, especially if the membranes rupture prematurely. Presentation before 5 days, which can be caused by preterm rupture of the membranes, is unusual; the incubation period is typically 5 to 14 days.

Infection usually results in a watery eye discharge that becomes purulent, with marked swelling of the eyelids and red, thickened conjunctivae. A pseudomembrane or a membrane of granulation tissue (micropannus) can form.

Conjunctival and nasopharyngeal samples should be taken from newborns suspected of chlamydial infection. Because coinfection with *N. gonorrhoeae* is common, the exudate should also be examined with Gram stain.

The treatment of choice for chlamydial conjunctivitis is erythromycin 50 mg/kg/day PO in four divided doses for 14 days. If erythromycin is not tolerated, sulfisoxazole 150 mg/kg/day PO in four to six divided doses PO may be given after the immediate neonatal period. Povidone-iodine solution (Betadine) has been suggested as a cost-effective and a more effective prophylaxis than the currently recommended therapies for chlamydia.

### VIRAL CONJUNCTIVITIS

Viral conjunctivitis is usually caused by adenovirus, with many serotypes implicated. It may be part of a viral prodrome or systemic viral illness, or it may be an isolated manifestation of viral illness. The conjunctivitis typically manifests as injection, watery, or mucoserous discharge, with a burning, sandy, or gritty feeling in one eye. The second eye usually becomes involved within 24 to 48 hours.

On examination there is typically only mucoid discharge in the lower lids, with profuse tearing. The tarsal conjunctiva might have a follicular or bumpy appearance, and an enlarged and tender preauricular node may be present. The symptoms generally get worse for the first 3 to 5 days, with very gradual resolution over the following 1 to 3 weeks. Because there is no specific antiviral drug that resolves the infection, treatment is directed toward symptomatic relief and includes over-the-counter topical antihistamine-decongestants (Naphcon-A, Ocuhist, generics), and artificial tears. Patient education is important because these infections are highly contagious.

### Epidemic Keratoconjunctivitis

Epidemic keratoconjunctivitis is a particularly fulminant form of viral conjunctivitis causing a keratitis (inflammation of the cornea) in addition to conjunctivitis. Adenovirus types 8, 19, and 37 are typically implicated with epidemic keratoconjunctivitis. In addition to the characteristic viral conjunctivitis symptoms, patients develop a foreign-body sensation and multiple corneal infiltrates, which can degrade visual acuity to the 20/40 range. Because keratitis is potentially vision threatening, these patients should be referred to an ophthalmologist for any subsequent treatment involving a course of topical steroids.

### ALLERGIC CONJUNCTIVITIS

Allergic conjunctivitis can be subdivided into acute allergic conjunctivitis, seasonal allergic conjunctivitis (SAC), and perennial allergic conjunctivitis (PAC). Although all three have different clinical courses, they are all caused by airborne allergens binding to an IgE antibody in tears and conjunctiva, resulting in local mast cell degranulation and the release of chemical mediators including histamine, eosinophil chemotactic factors, and platelet-activating factor, among others.

The cardinal symptom of allergic conjunctivitis that distinguishes it from a viral etiology is itching. Symptoms are classified as seasonal if they occur at a particular time of the year and as perennial if they occur year-round. Patients with allergic conjunctivitis often have a history of atopy, seasonal allergy, or specific allergy (e.g., to cats).

Two relatively uncommon types of allergic eye disease, atopic keratoconjunctivitis and vernal keratoconjunctivitis can cause significant damage to the ocular surface if not treated properly, leading to corneal scarring and vision loss.

### Acute Allergic Conjunctivitis

Acute allergic conjunctivitis is an acute hypersensitivity reaction caused by environmental exposure to allergens. It is characterized by intense periods of itching, hyperemia, tearing, chemosis, and eyelid edema. Classically, it resolves in less than 24 hours, irrespective of treatment, and therefore rarely requires long-term treatment. The mainstay of treatment is avoiding the offending allergen.

Topical antihistamines/vasoconstrictors such as naphazoline HCl preparations (Naphcon-A, Vasocon-A, Opcon-A) given up to four times daily are usually sufficient in treating short exacerbation of symptoms. Chronic use (>2 weeks) should be avoided because these drugs can cause rebound hyperemia. For frequent attacks of allergic conjunctivitis (>2 days/mo), a combination drug such as olopatadine (Patanol), consisting of an antihistamine and a mast cell stabilizer, can be used safely up to four times daily[3] for acute exacerbations and twice daily prophylactically. If symptoms remain unresolved, one could try oral antihistamines and combinations of antihistamines and decongestants such as fexofenadine (Allegra), fexofenadine plus pseudoephedrine (Allegra D), loratadine (Claritin), loratadine plus pseudoephedrine (Claritin-D), or cetirizine (Zyrtec). These drugs are best used prophylactically and in combination with artificial tears (due to drying of mucosal surfaces).

### Seasonal and Perennial Allergic Conjunctivitis

Seasonal allergic conjunctivitis, also known as hay fever–type conjunctivitis, is a mild form of ocular allergy commonly associated with rhinitis. It occurs in spring and late summer. It occurs in sensitized persons and is caused by exposure to pollen, grasses, and ragweed. Perennial allergic conjunctivitis is a mild, chronic allergic conjunctivitis related to environmental exposure to year-round allergens such as dust mites and mold.

Both seasonal and perennial allergic conjunctivitis demand frequent, active treatment. Olopatadine (Patanol) is the first-line drug of choice. It should be commenced 2 weeks before the onset of symptoms is anticipated and taken two to four[3] times daily.

Additionally, artificial tears (used at least four times a day) along with oral antihistamines may be helpful. If failed therapy persists for 2 to 3 weeks, a short two-week course of topical steroids such as prednisolone (Pred Mild), fluorometholone (FML), loteprednol (Lotemax),

---

[3]Exceeds dosage recommended by the manufacturer.

or rimexolone[1] (Vexol) two to four times per day might slow the immune response. If control is still not obtained, the patient should be referred to an allergist for consideration of immunotherapy.

## Atopic and Vernal Keratoconjunctivitis

Atopic keratoconjunctivitis a rare, severe, bilateral chronic allergic eye disease. It primarily affects adults older than 40 years and is slightly more prevalent in men than women. Severe itchiness is characteristic and the eyelids are thickened and eczematous. It is commonly associated with blepharitis and occasionally with cataracts and keratoconus.

Vernal keratoconjunctivitis is a severe bilateral allergic eye disease that mainly affects young boys 7 to 10 years old. Patients usually outgrow the disease with the onset of puberty. Exacerbations are common in spring and mainly in warm, dry climates. It is characterized by giant papillae on the upper tarsus, thick mucus discharge, and corneal ulcers. Vernal keratoconjunctivitis is more common in the Mediterranean region, Central America, and South America.

First-line treatment in both syndromes comprises punctal plugs, frequent use of artificial tears, and olopatadine. In fact, olopatadine should be used as daily long-term prophylactic therapy. During exacerbations, pulse therapy with topical steroids may be necessary, with close follow-up with an ophthalmologist. For severe cases, topical cyclosporine emulsion (Restasis) can provide excellent therapy.

## Giant Papillary Conjunctivitis

Giant papillary conjunctivitis (GPC), which might or might not have a true allergic origin, can be described as a reaction to lid movements over foreign materials such as a contact lens, other ocular prosthesis, or exposed suture. As the name suggests, giant papillae characteristically form on the upper tarsus, and the patient complains of a foreign-body sensation. GPC typically occurs in young adults, the same age distribution as contact lens wearers.

GPC usually resolves in less than a week if the mechanical stimulus is removed. Old lenses should be thrown out. All lens solutions should be preservative free, and daily disinfection with 3% hydrogen peroxide is recommended. Lenses should be reintroduced approximately 2 to 3 weeks after symptoms resolve. Frequent use of preservative-free artificial tears may be helpful, and topical antihistamines can relieve acute itching. Topical corticosteroids should be considered only in severe cases of GPC.

## TOXIC CONJUNCTIVITIS

Toxic conjunctivitis, although not an ocular allergy, is a direct and destructive reaction to an offending agent, usually a medicine or a preservative. Successful treatment of this condition depends imperatively on removing the offending agent.

# Diagnosis

## HISTORY

The history should include symptoms and signs and their duration. Are the symptoms and signs potentially related to systemic diseases? Are they unilateral or bilateral? What is the character of the discharge? Determine if the patient has had recent exposure to an infected person, trauma, or contact lens wear. Does the patient have any allergy, asthma, or eczema? What is the patient's use of topical and systemic medications? The history should also include details of any previous episodes of conjunctivitis, previous ophthalmic surgery, and any prior systemic diseases, as well as information about the patient's smoking habits, occupation and hobbies, travel, and sexual activity.

## EXAMINATION

The initial eye examination should incorporate measurement of visual acuity, external examination, and slit-lamp biomicroscopy.

[1]Not FDA approved for this indication.

## CURRENT DIAGNOSIS

**History**

- Symptoms and signs
  - Duration
  - Potentially related to systemic diseases
- Unilateral or bilateral presentation
- Character of discharge
- Recent exposure to an infected person
- Trauma
- Contact lens wear
- Allergy, asthma, eczema
- Use of topical and systemic medications
- Previous episodes of conjunctivitis
- Previous ophthalmic surgery
- Prior systemic diseases
- Smoking habits, occupation and hobbies, travel, and sexual activity

**Examination**

- Measurement of visual acuity
- External examination
  - Skin
  - Abnormalities of the eyelids and adnexa
  - Signs of regional lymphadenopathy
  - Conjunctiva
- Slit-lamp biomicroscopy
  - Eyelid margins
- Eyelashes
- Lacrimal puncta and canaliculi
- Tarsal and forniceal conjunctiva
- Bulbar conjunctiva, limbus
- Cornea
- Anterior chamber, iris
- Dye-staining pattern

The external examination should include in particular the skin, any abnormalities of the eyelids and adnexa, any signs of regional lymphadenopathy, and the conjunctiva. The slit-lamp biomicroscopy should include careful evaluation of the eyelid margins, eyelashes, lacrimal puncta and canaliculi, tarsal and forniceal conjunctiva, bulbar conjunctiva and limbus, cornea, anterior chamber and iris, and dye-staining pattern.

## DIAGNOSTIC TESTS

Cultures of the conjunctiva are indicated in all cases of suspected infectious neonatal conjunctivitis and in adults with bacterial conjunctivitis. Smears for cytology and special stains (e.g., Gram, Giemsa) should also be considered in cases of suspected infectious neonatal conjunctivitis and gonococcal conjunctivitis in any age group.

Conjunctival biopsy is indicated when diseases such as ocular cicatricial pemphigoid or sebaceous gland carcinoma manifest as conjunctivitis.

## COUNSELING AND REFERRAL

When conjunctivitis is associated with a sexually transmitted disease, patients and their sexual partners should be referred to an appropriate medical specialist. In cases of ophthalmia neonatorum caused by gonorrhea, chlamydia, or herpes simplex virus infection, the infant should be referred to a pediatric specialist. If conjunctivitis appears to be a manifestation of a systemic disease, the patient should be referred for evaluation by an appropriate medical specialist.

## CURRENT THERAPY

- Viral and bacterial conjunctivitis are highly contagious, and patients should be warned to avoid contact with family members.
- Frequent hand washing should be encouraged.
- Viral conjunctivitis should be treated conservatively with artificial tears and warm compresses.
- Bacterial conjunctivitis should be treated with fluoroquinolone drops as the first line.
- Gonococcal infections should be treated as an emergency with both topical and systemic antibiotics.
- Allergic conjunctivitis is best treated by avoiding the allergen where possible and with antihistamine, mast cell stabilizers, and a short course of steroids.
- Contact lens wearers who develop red eye should be advised to stop wearing the lens and referred immediately to an ophthalmologist.
- Any patient with decreasing vision, increasing pain, and purulent discharge should be referred to an ophthalmologist.

An evaluation of conjunctivitis warrants prompt referral to an ophthalmologist in the following scenarios:

- Vision loss
- Moderate or severe pain
- Severe, purulent discharge
- Corneal involvement
- Conjunctival scarring
- Lack of response to therapy
- Recurrent episodes
- History of herpes simplex virus (HSV) eye disease.

## Treatment

Viral and bacterial conjunctivitis are highly contagious, and patients should be warned to avoid contact with family members. Frequent hand washing should be encouraged.

Viral conjunctivitis should be treated conservatively with artificial tears and warm compresses. Bacterial conjunctivitis should be treated with fluoroquinolone drops as the first line. Gonococcal infections should be treated as an emergency with both topical and systemic antibiotics.

Allergic conjunctivitis is best treated by avoiding the allergen where possible and with antihistamine, mast cell stabilizers, and a short course of steroids.

Contact lens wearers who develop red eye should be advised to stop wearing the lens and referred immediately to an ophthalmologist.

Any patient with decreasing vision, increasing pain, and purulent discharge should be referred to an ophthalmologist.

### REFERENCES

Frackler CR: Chlamydia trachomatis infections in the newborn, 2005. Available at UpToDate website (subscription with password required).

Garcia-Ferrer FJ, Schwab IR, Shetler DJ: Conjunctiva. In Riordan-Eva P, Whitcher JP (eds): Vaughan & Asbury's General Ophthalmology, 16th ed. New York: McGraw-Hill, 2004, pp 100-128.

Maw R, Reza Dana M: Allergic eye disease, 2005. Available at UpToDate website (subscription with password required).

Schachter J, Grossman M: Chlamydia. In Remington JS, Klein JO (eds): Infectious Diseases of the Fetus and Newborn, 5th ed. Philadelphia: WB Saunders, 2001, pp 769-778.

# Optic Neuritis

Method of
*Andrew G. Lee, MD, and*
*Steven L. Galetta, MD*

Optic neuritis (ON) is the most common cause of acute loss of vision caused by an optic neuropathy in a young adult. In this chapter we use the term *ON* to refer to cases that are idiopathic or demyelinating.

## Clinical Features of Demyelinating Optic Neuritis

The typical patient with ON is a young adult woman presenting with acute, unilateral visual loss associated with pain worsened by eye movement. ON can occur in patients of any age and in either gender, however. The examination shows variable loss of visual acuity (20/20 to no light perception), visual field, or color vision, and an ipsilateral relative afferent pupillary defect (RAPD). The optic nerve typically appears normal at onset (i.e., retrobulbar optic neuropathy) but may be swollen (i.e., papillitis). Optic atrophy may develop over time in a sector or diffuse pattern. In cases with papillitis, the disc edema is typically mild. The presence of retinal hemorrhages, exudates, or cotton wool patches should suggest an alternative optic neuropathy (e.g., anterior ischemic optic neuropathy, inflammatory or infiltrative optic neuropathy).

The Optic Neuritis Treatment Trial (ONTT) was a randomized, controlled clinical trial in the United States that has provided excellent clinical information on ON. Table 1 summarizes the typical features, and Table 2 summarizes the atypical features of ON. Table 3 summarizes the recommendations for ON.

## Clinical Course

The majority (95%) of cases of ON recover vision (20/40 or better). Recurrence of ON is seen in up to 19% of patients in the affected eye and 17% in the fellow eye over a 10-year period. Patients with ON are at risk for the development of multiple sclerosis (MS), and that risk may be predicted by the findings on brain magnetic resonance imaging (MRI). Those patients with white matter lesions typical of demyelinating disease on a baseline MRI have a 56% chance of developing clinically definite MS, whereas those with a normal scan have a 22% chance over a 10-year period.

## CURRENT DIAGNOSIS

- Young (<40 years, often female) patient
- Acute loss of vision
- Pain with eye movement
- Relative afferent papillary defect
- Normal-appearing optic nerve common (retrobulbar optic neuropathy)
- Improvement over time
- Associated with multiple sclerosis

## TABLE 1 Features of Typical Optic Neuritis in Adults

Acute to subacute onset
Usually unilateral loss of visual acuity, contrast, color, or visual field
An ipsilateral relative afferent pupillary defect (RAPD)
Periocular pain (90%), especially with eye movement
Normal (65%) or swollen (35%) optic nerve head
A young adult patient (usually <40 y) but may occur at any age
Eventual visual improvement in majority of patients
Absence of anterior or posterior segment inflammation

Modified with permission from Lee AG, Brazis PW: Clinical Pathways in Neuro-ophthalmology: An Evidence-based Approach, 2nd ed. New York, Thieme, 2003.

## CURRENT THERAPY

- Intravenous methylprednisolone (1000 mg/d) for 3 d followed by oral taper speeds rate of visual recovery but does not change final visual outcome versus placebo.
- Oral steroids in conventional doses (e.g., prednisone, 60 mg/d) increased the rate of new attacks and are contraindicated.
- Immunomodulatory therapy (e.g., interferon β-1a or 1b) may reduce the development of clinically definite multiple sclerosis in patients with monophasic neurologic events including optic neuritis with demyelinating lesions on magnetic resonance imaging studies.

## REFERENCES

Beck RW: The optic neuritis treatment trial: Three-year follow-up results. Arch Ophthalmol 1995;113:136-137.
Beck RW, Arrington J, Murtagh FR, et al: Brain magnetic resonance imaging in acute optic neuritis: experience of the optic neuritis study group. Arch Neurol 1993;50:841-846.
Beck RW, Cleary PA, Anderson MA, et al: A randomized, controlled trial of corticosteroids in the treatment of acute optic neuritis. N Engl J Med 1992;326:581-588.

Beck RW, Cleary PA, Trobe JD, et al: The effect of corticosteroids for acute optic neuritis on the subsequent development of multiple sclerosis. N Engl J Med 1993;329:1764-1769.
Galetta SL, Markowitz C, Lee AG: Immunomodulatory agents for the treatment of relapsing MS: A systematic review. Ann Intern Med 2002;162:2161-2169.
Jacobs LD, Beck RW, Simon JH, et al: Intramuscular interferon beta-1a therapy initiated during a first demyelinating event in multiple sclerosis. CHAMPS Study Group. N Engl J Med 2000;343:898-904.

## TABLE 2 Features of Atypical Optic Neuritis in Adults

Bilateral simultaneous onset of optic neuritis in an adult patient
Painless visual loss
Unusual intraocular findings
    Anterior uveitis*
    Posterior uveitis*
    Retinal exudates (e.g., macular "star figure")
    Retinal infiltrates or retinal inflammation
Markedly swollen optic nerve
Marked retinal hemorrhages (e.g., 360 degrees of peripapillary hemorrhages)
Lack of significant improvement or worsening of visual function after 30 d
Age >50 y
Diagnosis or evidence of other systemic conditions other than multiple sclerosis that might cause an optic neuropathy
Extremely steroid-sensitive or steroid-dependent optic neuropathy
No light perception vision

*Anterior uveitis, pars planitis, and retinal periphlebitis may be seen in optic neuritis associated with multiple sclerosis but should be considered as unusual findings.
Modified with permission from Lee AG, Brazis PW: Clinical Pathways in Neuro-ophthalmology: An Evidence-based Approach, 2nd ed. New York, Thieme, 2003.

All patients in the Optic Neuritis Treatment Trial (ONTT) underwent brain MR scan, laboratory testing (e.g., antinuclear antibody (ANA) for systemic lupus erythematosus, serologic testing for syphilis), and a chest radiograph for sarcoidosis. A lumbar puncture however was optional. None of the laboratory testing proved to be helpful in the diagnosis of ON in typical cases. The lumbar puncture only showed demyelinating disease in cases where the cerebrospinal fluid was abnormal. The cranial MR scan however is a powerful predictor for the development of demyelinating disease.

### Treatment of Optic Neuritis

In the ONTT, there were three treatment groups: oral prednisone, intravenous (IV) methylprednisolone followed by oral prednisone, and oral placebo. The final visual outcome was the same in all of the treatment groups, although IV steroids sped the rate of visual recovery. Oral steroids alone, however, at least in conventional doses, increased the rate of new attacks and therefore are not currently recommended in conventional doses for ON.

### The Controlled High-Risk Subject Avonex Multiple Sclerosis Prevention Study

The Controlled High-Risk Subject Avonex (i.e., interferon β-1a) Multiple Sclerosis Prevention Study (CHAMPS) was a randomized, double-blind, placebo-controlled, clinical trial (n = 383). All patients had an acute clinical demyelinating event (e.g., ON) and demyelinating white matter lesions on brain MR scan. All patients received IV methylprednisolone followed by treatment in one of two treatment arms: weekly intramuscular (IM) injections of 30 μg of IFN β-1a (n = 193) and placebo (n = 190). The treatment group had a 44% reduction in the rate of clinically definite MS after 3 years compared to placebo (p = 0.002); a relative reduction in the volume of brain lesions (p < 0.001); fewer new or enlarging MR lesions (p < 0.001); and fewer gadolinium-enhancing lesions (p < 0.001).
The Early Treatment of Multiple Sclerosis (ETOMS) study was a randomized, placebo-controlled trial (n = 308) of interferon β-1a (Rebif) 22 μg subcutaneously weekly. As in CHAMPS, patients had an initial demyelinating event and demyelinating lesions on MRI. There was a decreased rate of progression to clinically definite MS and a reduction in MRI abnormalities in the treatment group.
Treatment with interferon β-1b also delays the onset of definite MS in patients with clinically isolated neurologic syndromes.

**TABLE 3** Summary of Recommendations for Optic Neuritis

Cranial MRI scan should be strongly considered for all patients with ON.

The cranial MR scan is the most powerful predictor for clinically definite MS.

Even a single attack of ON is a risk factor for developing clinically definite MS.

Neurologic consultation should be considered to discuss the risks of MS and the options for treatment (e.g., interferon β-1a or 1b).

*Abbreviations:* MRI = magnetic resonance imaging; MS = multiple sclerosis; ON = optic neuritis.

Kappos L, Polman CH, Freedman MS, et al: Treatment with interferon beta-1b delays conversion to clinically definite and McDonald MS in patients with clinically isolated syndromes. Neurology 2006;67:1242-1249.

Kaufman DI, Trobe JD, Eggenberger ER, Whitaker JN: Practice parameter: The role of corticosteroids in the management of acute monosymptomatic optic neuritis. Report of the Quality Standards Subcommittee of the American Academy of Neurology. Neurology 2000;54:2039-2044.

# Glaucoma

Method of
*Misha F. Syed, MD, and Nicholas P. Bell, MD*

Glaucoma is a group of disorders with various manifestations linked by a common optic neuropathy, resulting in characteristic, progressive optic nerve atrophy, and visual field loss. Glaucoma was once defined simply as intraocular pressure (IOP) greater than 21 mm Hg, but now this is recognized as only a risk factor. Elevated IOP dilates the optic cup, which subjects the ganglion cells to ischemic pressure forces. Peripheral visual field defects emerge in the areas subtended by the damaged retinal ganglion cells. Central vision loss is typically a late finding.

Glaucoma is classified by the anatomy of the anterior chamber angle, which may be *open* or *closed*. Gonioscopy, a detailed evaluation of the angle using a mirrored lens, is required to differentiate types of glaucoma. Childhood glaucoma may be primary or secondary to developmental ocular abnormalities. Patients who do not meet criteria for diagnosis within one of these groups are followed as glaucoma suspects.

Regardless of etiology, glaucoma is a leading cause of irreversible blindness. Of the 67 million people with glaucoma worldwide, 7 million are bilaterally blind. In the United States, more than 2.5 million people are diagnosed with glaucoma, and it is estimated that as many are undiagnosed. Glaucoma is the second leading cause of blindness in the United States; it is the most frequent cause among African Americans, in whom there is an earlier onset and more aggressive course. In 2000 the prevalence of blindness from glaucoma in the United States was greater than 1:130,000 people.

## Types of Glaucoma

### PRIMARY OPEN-ANGLE GLAUCOMA

The most common glaucoma is primary open-angle glaucoma (POAG). Increased resistance to outflow of the aqueous humor through the trabecular meshwork leads to gradual and painless elevation of IOP; hence, it is typically asymptomatic. It is bilateral but

## CURRENT DIAGNOSIS

- The most common form of glaucoma in the United States is POAG.
- Risk factors for POAG include increasing age, African American race, and a positive family history.
- Screening for POAG is recommended every 2 to 4 years after age 40 years and every 1 to 2 years after age 65 years.
- If risk factors for POAG are present, screening is recommended every 2 to 4 years after age 30 years and every 1 to 2 years after age 65 years.
- 95% of patients with POAG and 5% of normal patients may experience IOP elevation >15 mm Hg while taking steroids; therefore, patients with known glaucoma on long-term steroids (>1 month) need close follow-up with an ophthalmologist.
- Primary angle-closure glaucoma has an acute onset with pain, haloes, red eye, decreased vision, and nausea and/or vomiting. Emergent ophthalmologic referral is required.

*Abbreviations:* IOP = intraocular pressure; POAG = primary open-angle glaucoma.

can be asymmetric. The existence of a subgroup of POAG patients without elevated IOP (normal-pressure glaucoma) suggests that other factors may be significant, such as insufficient vascular flow to the optic nerve head, accelerated programmed cell death (apoptosis), diurnal fluctuations of IOP, and autoimmunity.

Diseases such as diabetes mellitus, systemic hypertension, and vasospastic disorders have been associated with glaucoma but are not clearly linked to the disease. Increasing age is a risk factor, because 8% of the population older than 70 years old and only 0.1% of those younger than 40 years of age are affected. African American patients have a 5 to 15 times greater risk than white patients. Immediate family members of glaucoma patients have a 10- to 15-fold increased risk for developing glaucoma.

The prolonged asymptomatic phase of POAG can only be discovered by ocular evaluation. Complete eye examination is recommended every 2 to 4 years for patients older than 40 years of age and every 1 to 2 years for those older than 65 years. Patients with risk factors (age, race, family history) should be evaluated earlier and more frequently.

Screening in the primary care setting can include a family and medical history, vision (and possibly IOP) screening, and examination of the optic nerve head by direct ophthalmoscopy. Clinical findings may be subtle. Visual acuity is often normal, and decreased central vision secondary to glaucoma suggests advanced disease. Normal confrontation fields do not exclude glaucoma because this examination technique has a very low yield in identifying glaucomatous visual field loss. Formal visual field testing is preferred. Although not diagnostic, intraocular pressure greater than 21 mm Hg warrants thorough evaluation. Dilated fundus examination shows enlarged cupping of the optic nerve head and/or asymmetry between the optic nerves. Focal loss of neural rim tissue (notching) may occur, and flame hemorrhages may be seen at the disc margin, especially in actively progressing disease. If glaucoma is suspected, a patient should be referred for further ophthalmologic evaluation.

Patients with suggestive findings but no definitive glaucomatous damage are classified as glaucoma suspects. The Ocular Hypertension Treatment Study, a recent multicenter randomized, controlled clinical trial, conducted a long-term follow-up of glaucoma suspects with elevated IOP, normal optic nerve appearance, and no visual field defects. This study found that over 5 years, maintaining IOP 20% below baseline reduced the rate of progression to POAG from 9.5% to 4.4%.

## SECONDARY OPEN-ANGLE GLAUCOMA

Secondary open-angle glaucomas result from increased resistance to outflow through the trabecular meshwork because of a preexisting or underlying condition. Examples include pigmentary, pseudoexfoliative, traumatic, and steroid-induced glaucoma.

In pigment dispersion syndrome and pseudoexfoliation syndrome, deposition of iris pigment and fibrillar protein, respectively, in the trabecular meshwork may obstruct aqueous outflow and secondarily elevate IOP, leading to glaucoma. Blunt ocular trauma (often remote) is a common cause of unilateral glaucoma because of structural changes in the trabecular meshwork.

Chronic use of glucocorticosteroids can create resistance to trabecular outflow and IOP elevation, resulting in a glaucoma resembling POAG. Steroid-induced pressure elevation generally correlates with the dose and length of administration. Although most often seen with topical and periocular use, it can also result from systemic or inhaled administration. Steroid responses of greater than 15 mm Hg IOP elevation can develop in 95% of patients with POAG and in only 15% of patients without glaucoma. All patients with a known diagnosis of glaucoma should be evaluated by an ophthalmologist within 1 month of initiating a long-term steroid regimen for systemic diseases.

## PRIMARY ANGLE-CLOSURE GLAUCOMA

Primary angle-closure glaucoma can have an acute, subacute, intermittent, or chronic presentation. Attacks of acute angle closure are ocular emergencies, because irreversible vision loss can occur within hours. Those at risk have an anatomic predisposition with narrow anterior chamber angles. If the pupillary margin of the iris contacts the lens for 360 degrees, which may occur in susceptible eyes when the iris is mid-dilated, flow of the aqueous humor from the posterior to the anterior chamber is blocked. The peripheral iris bows anteriorly and apposes the trabecular meshwork, obstructing outflow. The IOP may rise rapidly to greater than 60 mm Hg.

In Asian populations primary angle-closure glaucoma is more common than open-angle glaucoma. The risk increases with age, with most cases occurring during the sixth and seventh decades. Women have primary angle-closure glaucoma attacks 2 to 4 times as often as men. Environmental circumstances may trigger an acute attack of angle closure in predisposed eyes; these include movie theaters or dark rooms (physiologic mydriasis), sudden anxiety or pain (sympathetic stimulation causing pupil dilation), or medications causing mild mydriasis (anticholinergics and adrenergic stimulants such as sleep and cold medications).

The diagnosis of an acute angle-closure glaucoma attack requires gonioscopic evidence of a closed anterior chamber angle preventing aqueous flow into the trabecular meshwork. Patients may complain of ocular pain, brow ache, rainbow-colored halos around lights, and/or blurred vision. They may experience intense nausea and vomiting, bradycardia, and sweating. Ocular exam reveals elevated IOP, conjunctival vascular injection, a cloudy cornea (if IOP rose acutely and recently), a shallow anterior chamber, a closed angle by gonioscopy, and a globe, which is firm to palpation.

## SECONDARY ANGLE-CLOSURE GLAUCOMA

Scarring and adhesions between the peripheral iris and the anterior chamber angle may block outflow of aqueous. Diabetes mellitus may result in neovascularization of the retina, which can progress to neovascularization of the anterior segment including the iris and angle, blocking aqueous outflow and/or closing the angle. The resultant neovascular glaucoma can be devastating and refractory to treatment. Central retinal vein occlusion, a vascular accident closely linked to uncontrolled hypertension and diabetes, can also lead to retinal neovascularization and a similar process. Uveitis from systemic diseases such as sarcoidosis or autoimmune arthropathies can produce intraocular scarring and secondary angle closure if not controlled.

Sulfonamide-based systemic medications can rarely cause swelling of the ciliary body, which anteriorly displaces the lens and iris. This can produce a secondary acute angle-closure glaucoma, which requires

## CURRENT THERAPY

- Although POAG is typically treated first medically, in select circumstances laser and incisional surgery may be appropriate first-line interventions.
- Glaucoma medications lower IOP by either decreasing production of aqueous humor or increasing its outflow.
- Topical β-blockers have been the traditional primary medical therapy for POAG, but prostaglandin analogues are now emerging as the first-line choice.
- Laser trabeculoplasty increases aqueous outflow through the trabecular meshwork.
- Incisional filtering surgery creates a new outflow drain, which bypasses the dysfunctional trabecular meshwork.
- Primary angle closure attacks require emergent treatment both medically and with laser iridotomy.
- Secondary angle closure glaucoma may be difficult to manage medically and often requires surgery.

*Abbreviations:* IOP = intraocular pressure; POAG = primary open-angle glaucoma.

discontinuation of the medication and urgent lowering of the IOP. This phenomenon has also been reported with topiramate (Topamax).

## CHILDHOOD GLAUCOMA

Congenital or childhood glaucoma develops from aqueous outflow obstruction because of abnormal anatomical development of the angle, ocular inflammation, or trauma. Primary congenital glaucoma often presents in infancy with the classic triad of photophobia, epiphora (tearing), and blepharospasm, but these signs are unnecessary for diagnosis. Buphthalmos (enlarged eye) may occur secondary to increased IOP if the glaucoma develops during the first 3 years of life. Juvenile glaucoma is similar in etiology to POAG and has been linked to several specific genetic loci. Enlargement of the cornea and sclera is not seen in this subtype.

## Treatment

The Glaucoma Preferred Practice Pattern Committee of the American Academy of Ophthalmology suggests a target of 20% to 30% reduction of IOP from the untreated levels. Medical treatment is usually attempted first. Parameters that factor into selection of medications include efficacy in lowering IOP, systemic and localized side effect profiles, ease of compliance, and cost (Table 1). Noncompliance with treatment regimens may be responsible for 10% of visual loss in glaucoma; and in one study, approximately 60% of patients failed to use eyedrops as prescribed. If medications fail to control IOP, changes in optic nerve structure and visual field function may occur. Surgical treatment may become necessary to slow the progression of glaucomatous damage.

## PROSTAGLANDIN ANALOGUES

This newest class of antiglaucoma agents has become a popular initial medical treatment because of the efficacy and lack of major systemic side effects. These medications reduce IOP by increasing aqueous humor outflow. Latanoprost (Xalatan), bimatoprost (Lumigan), and travoprost (Travatan) require only once daily dosing, whereas unoprostone (Rescula) is administered twice daily. Side effects include conjunctival hyperemia during the first several weeks of therapy, eyelash lengthening and thickening, occasional iris and periocular skin hyperpigmentation, and rarely, exacerbation of ocular inflammation.

## TABLE 1

| Topical Medications | Efficacy | Local Side Effects | Systemic Side Effects | Dosing | Cost |
|---|---|---|---|---|---|
| Prostaglandin analogues | + + + | + + | none to + | Once daily | + + + |
| β-Blockers | + + + | + | + + + | bid | + +* |
| α₂ Agonists | + + | + + | + + | bid–tid | + + +* |
| Carbonic anhydrase inhibitors | + + | + + | + to + + | bid–tid | + + +† |

+++ = high
++ = moderate
+ = low
* = generic available
† = systemic form less costly

## BETA-ADRENERGIC ANTAGONISTS

Beta-adrenergic antagonists lower IOP by decreasing the production of aqueous humor. They are very effective at lowering IOP and include timolol (Timoptic, Betimol, Istalol), carteolol (Ocupress), metipranolol (OptiPranolol), and levobunolol (Betagan). Topical formulations may be absorbed into the bloodstream, and potential side effects are similar to systemic β-blockers, including exacerbation of chronic obstructive or reactive pulmonary disease, worsening of heart block or heart failure, bradycardia, systemic hypotension, mood effects/altered mental status, decreased libido, and masking of hypoglycemic symptoms in diabetic patients. Care should be taken in patients already taking systemic β-blockers, because additive side effects may develop. Betaxolol (Betoptic) is a selective β₁ antagonist, which may minimize the pulmonary side effects, but still must be used cautiously in patients suffering from asthma or COPD. Topical β-blockers are dosed once or twice daily, depending on the formulation of the eyedrop.

## α₂ AGONISTS

α₂ Adrenergic agonists such as apraclonidine (Iopidine) and brimonidine (Alphagan) lower IOP by decreasing aqueous humor production. They are dosed 2 to 3 times daily. Major systemic side effects include somnolence and dry mouth. These medications should be used cautiously in infants and young children because of the risk of respiratory depression. α₂ Agonists are contraindicated in patients taking monoamine oxidase (MAO) inhibitors because of potential systemic hypertension. Ocular side effects include allergic follicular conjunctivitis, which may necessitate discontinuation.

## CARBONIC ANHYDRASE INHIBITORS

Carbonic anhydrase inhibitors decrease production of aqueous humor. Systemic carbonic anhydrase inhibitors such as acetazolamide (Diamox) and methazolamide (Neptazane) have been used to treat glaucoma for decades, but up to 60% of patients are intolerant of the side effects. These include metallic taste alteration, loss of appetite, fatigue, confusion, nausea and vomiting, paresthesias, polyuria, urolithiasis, and hearing dysfunction or tinnitus. Rare side effects include Stevens-Johnson syndrome (in patients with sulfonamide allergies) and idiosyncratic aplastic anemia. Oral agents may also lower serum potassium levels, and patients on diuretics or digoxin should be monitored closely. Dorzolamide (Trusopt) and brinzolamide (Azopt) are topical preparations of carbonic anhydrase inhibitors dosed 2 to 3 times daily. Systemic side effects are minimized, but ocular stinging, localized allergic responses, and metallic taste alteration may occur. Systemic carbonic anhydrase inhibitors are more efficacious, but the improved tolerability of the topical agents has made them popular.

## NONSPECIFIC SYMPATHOMIMETICS AND PARASYMPATHOMIMETICS

Nonspecific sympathomimetic and parasympathomimetic drugs have historically been used for the treatment of glaucoma, but with the newer agents available these are no longer commonly prescribed. The mechanism for both classes involves increasing aqueous humor outflow. The sympathomimetic agents include epinephrine (Epifrin) and dipivefrin (Propine). Potential adverse effects include systemic hypertension, headache, cardiac arrhythmias including premature ventricular contractions and tachycardia, and anorexia. Parasympathomimetic medications such as pilocarpine (Pilocar) can cause gastrointestinal cramping, diarrhea, vomiting, syncope, hypotension, increased sweating, and pupillary constriction.

## ACUTE ANGLE CLOSURE

Acute angle closure patients require emergent ophthalmologic referral and treatment to prevent severe permanent sequelae. If this is not immediately possible, treatment should be initiated promptly with a topical β-blocker and a topical α₂ agonist every 30 minutes and a single dose of oral acetazolamide (Diamox) (250 mg × 2 tablets). Oral glycerin (Osmoglyn) or intravenous mannitol (Osmitrol) (1.0 to 1.5 g/kg) may be used if necessary. Pilocarpine should be used cautiously because it may worsen underlying inflammation. Once the attack has been broken medically, the corneal edema will clear and a laser peripheral iridotomy can be made to prevent future attacks. This opening in the peripheral iris allows aqueous flow to bypass any obstruction caused by pupillary block. Prophylactic iridotomy of the other eye is recommended if anatomically at risk. The management of *chronic* angle-closure glaucoma is generally similar to that for POAG.

## LASER

Laser may also be used to treat open-angle glaucomas. Argon laser trabeculoplasty (ALT) or the newer selective laser trabeculoplasty (SLT) lowers IOP by facilitating aqueous outflow. For pigmentary, pseudoexfoliative, and select POAG patients, this may be an effective adjunct to medical therapy.

## SURGERY

Surgical measures to control glaucoma include filtering procedures such as trabeculectomy or aqueous shunt placement, which increase aqueous outflow by creating alternative filtration pathways. After trabeculectomy, patients are warned of an increased lifetime risk for serious ocular infection and must report to an ophthalmologist immediately for any changes, including redness, pain, and/or decrease in vision. For poor surgical candidates with severely advanced disease, cyclodestructive procedures can be performed in the office to decrease aqueous production by ablating the ciliary body.

If glaucomatous damage has left an eye with no vision, the only reason to treat IOP is to control pain. In most cases, topical agents will suffice. If pain becomes frequent and severe, injections of retrobulbar absolute alcohol or even enucleation of the blind, painful eye may be offered.

## REFERENCES

Allingham RR: Shields' Textbook of Glaucoma, 5th ed. Philadelphia, Lippincott Williams & Wilkins, 2005.

American Academy of Ophthalmology Online: Preferred practice patterns: Primary angle Closure glaucoma, primary open angle glaucoma, primary open angle glaucoma suspect 2003. Available at http://www.aao.org/

Kass MA, Heuer DK, Higginbotham EJ, et al: The ocular hypertension treatment study: A randomized trial determines that topical ocular hypotensive medication delays or prevents the onset of primary open-angle glaucoma. Arch Ophthalmol 2002;120:701–713.

Morrison JC, Pollack IP: Glaucoma: Science and Practice, New York, Thieme, 2003.

Tsai JC, Forbes M: Medical Management of Glaucoma, 2nd ed. West Islip, NY, Professional Communications, 2004.

# Otitis Externa

Method of
*Jeffrey T. Vrabec, MD*

Otitis externa is defined as an acute infection originating in or limited to the external auditory canal. This common affliction may occur in any age group and may be caused by a variety of infectious agents.

## Anatomy and Physiology

Functionally, the ear canal serves two purposes. It is important for sound localization and because of resonance effects it improves sound perception in the frequency range from 2500 to 4000 hertz (Hz). The ear canal is approximately 25 mm in length and has a diameter of approximately 7.5 mm. The medial half is an osseous channel formed by the merger of the tympanic bone with the mastoid posteriorly and the squamous portion of the temporal bone superiorly. The lateral half of the canal wall is cartilaginous with a thick squamous epithelium that contains sebaceous glands, sweat glands, and hair follicles. The medial skin covering the bony canal is quite thin, measuring only 0.2 mm in thickness. The medial skin lacks a subcutaneous layer and is in continuity with the outermost layer of the tympanic membrane.

The external canal receives its blood supply from the superficial temporal and posterior auricular branches of the external carotid artery. Venous drainage is to the external jugular vein. The external canal receives sensory innervation via multiple cranial nerves. The trigeminal nerve supplies sensation to the superior and anterior aspect of the canal, the facial nerve supplies the anterior inferior area, and the glossopharyngeal and vagus nerves innervate the inferior and posterior regions. Because of the diverse nerve supply, otalgia may often reflect referred pain from oral cavity, nasal, or pharyngeal sources.

Several anatomic features serve to protect the external canal and tympanic membrane (TM) from injury or infection. The gentle curvature of the canal and the narrowing at the bone–cartilage junction (the isthmus) reduce the probability of large objects penetrating the TM. The hair and cerumen also protect the canal, trapping airborne particles that enter the external meatus. Cerumen has the additional benefit of repelling water. The acidic composition of cerumen lowers the ambient pH of the external canal, making it less hospitable to infectious organisms. The phenomenon of epithelial migration is documented in the ear canal. Surface epithelium moves laterally from the umbo to the annulus of the TM and then laterally to the external meatus. Epithelial movement on the TM proceeds at a rate of 0.05 mm per day and is typically slower in the external canal. Lateral migration helps clear the medial canal of surface epithelium and attached debris. This migratory pattern is arrested in chronic infection of the external canal.

## Diagnosis

Infections develop in the external canal when organisms breach the anatomic barriers. Trauma to the canal skin, excessive removal of the cerumen, and excessive moisture in the canal may all facilitate otitis externa. Presenting symptoms of an external ear infection include pain, itching, and hearing loss. Pain develops rapidly, is typically constant, and may be quite severe. Manipulation of the ear or jaw movement exacerbates the pain. Conductive hearing loss occurs because of accumulation of debris in the external canal and is exacerbated by concurrent edema. Persistent symptoms despite treatment are a matter of great concern and may indicate a developing osteitis. Cranial nerve deficits are ominous symptoms and indicate an advanced osteitis of the temporal bone.

Physical examination findings typically include erythema, edema, and drainage. Differences in examination findings can help distinguish bacterial from fungal infections. Bacterial infections usually produce marked edema of the canal skin, especially in the lateral cartilaginous canal. Drainage is usually scant and may have a mucoid or mucopurulent consistency and often has a foul odor. In contrast, fungal infections typically involve the medial canal skin and produce little edema. Drainage is thick and surface spore formation is evident. Focal granulation tissue develops in areas with invasive disease and TM perforations are occasionally present. Bloody drainage can be seen with either bacterial or fungal infections because of maceration of the canal skin or from granulation tissue formation.

Regional or systemic symptoms are uncommon in otitis externa. Periaural erythema, mild lymphadenopathy, and low-grade fever are possible. The presence of regional symptoms indicates a more virulent infection.

## Treatment

The initial approach to outer ear infections involves aural toilet and avoidance of further trauma or moisture. Topical antibiotics are prescribed in accordance with the likely infectious organism. Many preparations have a rather broad spectrum of efficacy so routine culture of aural discharge is not performed. It is prudent to obtain culture and sensitivity data in recalcitrant cases. Analgesics are prescribed as necessary to control pain. Narcotics are occasionally required. Patients are instructed to avoid or minimize water exposure. With appropriate treatment, symptoms improve rapidly, and complete healing is seen in 2 weeks or less.

The most common organism identified in routine cases of external otitis is *Pseudomonas aeruginosa*. Staphylococcal species are the next most common. Topical fluoroquinolone or aminoglycoside antibiotics are the most appropriate choice for treatment. Preparations that include a steroid are recommended. Drops are instilled three times daily until resolution of the infection, usually 7 to 10 days. When severe edema of the canal skin is present, a wick is inserted into the canal to facilitate drug delivery. Persistent symptoms indicate inadequate treatment, although this may also be because of inappropriate antibiotic, inefficient drug delivery, noncompliance, or progressive infection.

## Differential Diagnosis and Treatment

There are many other infectious disorders of the external canal, although each can usually be distinguished by characteristic clinical findings. Malignancy may also mimic chronic infection. Biopsy is recommended for abnormal tissue that does not quickly resolve with treatment.

### ACUTE INFECTIONS

Furuncles occur at the external meatus in the hair-bearing skin. Erythema and edema are localized, and skin a few millimeters away from the infection has a healthy appearance. Pain can be severe and is

## CURRENT DIAGNOSIS

**Presenting symptoms include:**

- Pain: develops rapidly, typically constant; exacerbated by movement of ear or jaw
- Itching
- Hearing loss: exacerbated by concurrent edema

**Exam findings include:**

- Erythema
- Edema
- Drainage: sometimes bloody
- Bacterial infections: often have edema of the canal skin with minimal drainage that has foul odor
- Fungal infections: involve the medial canal skin with slight edema, thick drainage, evident surface spore formation

exacerbated by pressure or manipulation of the auricle. Furuncles are caused by staphylococcal infection. Spontaneous rupture of the lesion leads to resolution of the infection and pain. If fluctuance is present at presentation, the lesion is drained under local anesthesia. Topical antibiotics (bacitracin, neomycin, or mupirocin [Bactroban] ointment or solution) are a useful adjunct.

The physical findings in otomycosis were outlined earlier. The predominant organisms are *Aspergillus* and *Candida* with considerable variation in prevalence according to geographic region. Fungal infections produce more destruction of the canal skin but less edema. Granulation tissue and TM perforations are not uncommon, although most perforations heal spontaneously after eradication of the infection. Treatment requires meticulous cleaning of debris and topical antifungals. Clotrimazole (Lotrimin) solution is effective for *Candida* species, but eradication of *Aspergillus* species is most efficient with ketoconazole (Nizoral) cream applied directly to the affected skin.

Bullous external otitis is diagnosed based on the characteristic finding of hemorrhagic vesicles in the external canal. Spontaneous rupture of the lesions produces bloody otorrhea. The lesions are quite painful, and lancing the bullae to drain the fluid does not provide relief as is seen in bullous myringitis. Involvement of the medial canal skin is typical. The etiology of this infectious process is unclear. However, the disease responds to a broad spectrum of topical antibiotics. Topical or oral analgesics are a useful adjunctive treatment.

Herpes zoster oticus, or Ramsay Hunt syndrome, occurs because of reactivation of latent varicella zoster virus in the geniculate ganglion. Vesicles may develop in the sensory distribution of the facial nerve. The appearance of skin lesions is characteristic of zoster eruptions. Initially, the vesicles are erythematous with a straw-colored fluid. Spontaneous rupture results in a crusted ulcer that may take several weeks to heal. Facial paralysis, dysgeusia, dizziness, and sensorineural hearing loss are typical in herpes zoster oticus but extremely rare in other infectious diseases of the external ear canal. Treatment of the facial paralysis is the primary objective, necessitating systemic steroids and antivirals. The skin lesions of the ear canal usually heal without incident, but secondary bacterial otitis externa is possible.

## CURRENT THERAPY

- Provide aural toilet and encourage avoidance of further trauma and water exposure.
- Obtain culture and sensitivity data in recalcitrant cases.
- Prescribe topical antibiotics that include a steroid and analgesics (for pain) as needed.

## CHRONIC INFECTIOUS DISORDERS

Skull base osteitis occurs when disease extends from soft tissues of the canal into the temporal bone. Elderly patients, diabetics, and immunocompromised individuals are at increased risk of developing osteitis. The diagnosis is suspected when pain, discharge, fever, and/or granulation tissue persist despite treatment. Progressive involvement of the skull base may lead to cranial nerve palsies, vascular thrombosis, and intracranial infection. Laboratory testing reveals a markedly increased sedimentation rate. Technetium-99m bone scan displays increased uptake throughout the course of the disease and is useful for initial diagnosis. Computed tomography (CT) of the temporal bone displays bone erosion in advanced cases. Magnetic resonance imaging (MRI) is useful to detect soft-tissue and dural involvement. Biopsy of infected tissue or bone may be necessary to identify the responsible organism. Systemic antibiotics are selected according to culture and sensitivity data and should be continued until the sedimentation rate returns to normal. This may require months of treatment.

Osteoradionecrosis is a late complication of temporal bone irradiation. Contemporary stereotactic techniques should significantly reduce the incidence of this problem. The process is typically limited, and symptoms are much less severe than in skull base osteitis. Exposed necrotic bone with slight granulation and purulent drainage is seen on examination. Local débridement and topical antibiotics are usually sufficient to control the infection. Recurrence is common because the irradiated ear canal is highly susceptible to infection after exposure to water or minor trauma.

## MISCELLANEOUS

With the exception of herpes zoster oticus, none of the entities just described typically involves the pinna. Inflammation of the external canal in conjunction with pinna involvement may signify dermatologic disease. Some common entities include eczema, neomycin allergy, relapsing polychondritis, and erysipelas.

## REFERENCES

Clark WB, Brook I, Bianki D, Thompson DH: Microbiology of otitis externa. Otolaryngol Head Neck Surg 1997;116:23-25.

Hawke M, Wong J, Krajden S: Clinical and microbiological features of otitis externa. J Otolaryngol 1984;13:289-295.

Hurst WB: Outcome of 22 cases of perforated tympanic membrane caused by otomycosis. J Laryngol Otol 2001;115:879-880.

Litton WB: Epithelial migration over tympanic membrane and external canal. Arch Otolaryngol 1963;77:254-257.

Lucente FE: Fungal infections of the external ear. Otolaryngol Clin North Am 1993;26:995-1006.

Sreepada GS, Kwartler JA: Skull base osteomyelitis secondary to malignant otitis externa. Curr Opin Otolaryngol Head Neck Surg 2003;11:316-323.

Sweeney CJ, Gilden DH: Ramsay Hunt syndrome. J Neurol Neurosurg Psychiatry 2001;71:149-154.

# Otitis Media

Method of
*J. Scott McMurray, MD*

Ear infections, their complications and sequelae, comprise most patient-clinician interactions. Estimates suggest nearly $3 billion in direct and indirect cost for acute otitis media (AOM) and otitis media with effusion were spent in 1995 alone. In 2000 more than 16 million office visits were made for otitis media and 802 prescriptions per 1000 visits were written for a total of more than 13 million prescriptions. As common as the problem may be, it continues to be a source of confusion and controversy in terms of its diagnosis, treatment, and expectation for outcomes. Recently, there has been a renewed interest in determining the appropriate evaluation and management of these afflicted children, based on evidence-based medicine.

Along with new diagnostic protocols and realigned treatment strategies, there is a realization that children may fall into different at-risk groups and will therefore benefit from different treatment options. In his recent editorial in the International Journal of Pediatric Otolaryngology on a practical classification of otitis media subgroups, Richard Rosenfeld quoted Stanley Hoerr saying, "It is difficult to make the asymptomatic patient feel better." Yet, he added, much of the research on which we base our decisions to treat or not to treat children with otitis media has been formulated on those who would otherwise do well without treatment, the so-called innocent bystander. Children in the at-risk or suffering groups have been excluded from research trials for ethical reasons against withholding treatment. It is possible to group children into four subgroups with otitis media:

1. Innocent bystander
2. Susceptible child
3. At-risk child
4. Suffering child

These different subgroups imply different treatment limbs. The innocent bystander may do well without any therapy and may tolerate careful observation, whereas the suffering child with a similar disease process deserves rapid and intensive medical or surgical treatment or both.

The stratification of children into different subgroups may appear daunting at first glance but after closer reflection answers the problem of conflicting research data and perhaps uses more common sense (confirmed by clinical trials) in determining treatment. Otherwise developmentally and physically healthy children may be closely observed rather than treated medically or surgically for their acute ear infection or middle ear effusion (MEE). Other children who are at risk for developmental delays, physically challenged, or suffering from the effects or side effects of AOM or otitis media with effusion should be treated more aggressively with either the appropriate medical or surgical plan of care. Unfortunately, this increases the number of possible permutations when determining the appropriate treatment for the afflicted child. Fortunately, however, this new paradigm allows more freedom in determining the appropriate treatment option to be followed. Our challenge lies in honing our abilities to make a correct diagnosis and an accurate assessment of risk so that an appropriate treatment protocol with adequate follow-up can be implemented.

In 2004, the American Academy of Pediatrics, the American Academy of Family Practice, and the American Academy of Otolaryngology Head and Neck Surgery combined forces to create two separate clinical guidelines for AOM and otitis media with effusion. These guidelines serve as an excellent frame on which to build a knowledge base and understanding for the treatment of all children with AOM or otitis media with effusion. These references are invaluable and are recommended reading for all who treat children with ear pathology.

## Definitions

Acute otitis media is defined as an abrupt onset of inflammation of the middle ear space. This contrasts with otitis media with effusion, which is fluid in the middle ear without signs and symptoms of inflammation. Otitis media with effusion is much more common than AOM but may be seen as a residual finding of a recently resolved infection. The distinction between the two and the ability of the clinician to distinguish between these disease entities is paramount to decision making and appropriate treatment.

The signs and symptoms of AOM are found in an abrupt onset of fluid in the middle ear with redness or distinct pain. Children suffering with AOM may or may not also exhibit systemic signs of infection, such as fever. Fever, pain, and irritability are seen in 90% of children with AOM, but it is also seen in 76% of children with upper aerodigestive tract viral illnesses as well. History alone may lead to an erroneous conclusions and unnecessary treatment. The distinction lies in the

physical findings of MEE with inflammation. Fullness or bulging of the tympanic membrane, air fluid levels, opacification of the tympanic membrane, or bullous vesicles on the tympanic membrane are signs suggesting AOM when associated with acute inflammation. Visualization of the tympanic membrane and the use of pneumatic otoscopy should confirm the presence of a MEE and inflammation. Tympanometry can confirm suspicion of a MEE, but the clinician should work to be proficient with pneumatic otoscopy.

Otitis media with effusion alone may result from a resolved infection or from eustachian tube dysfunction alone. The physical findings are similar to those described but without the signs of acute inflammation. Although the tympanic membrane may be red in the otherwise healthy child crying at the displeasure of being examined, pain and an effusion are not generally associated with normal health.

## Treatment Recommendations

Children with AOM should have adequate pain management. Acetaminophen, ibuprofen, and occasionally narcotics are useful in treating the pain of AOM. Rarely, myringotomy is required to relieve the discomfort of an acute ear infection.

If an acute bacterial infection in the middle ear is recognized, antibacterial therapy may be used in all age groups. If the diagnosis is uncertain, antibacterial therapy is recommended in the very young, younger than age 6 months. Antimicrobials may also be administered if one is uncertain of the diagnosis, if the illness is severe in those from 6 months to 2 years of age. If the child is older than age 2 years and the diagnosis is uncertain, observation and close follow-up is recommended.

If antibacterial treatment is instituted, amoxicillin at 80 to 90 mg/kg/day is used as a first line of therapy. If severe illness is encountered or if coverage for beta-lactamase–positive organisms such as Haemophilus influenzae or Moraxella catarrhalis is required, amoxicillin-clavulanate (Augmentin) is suggested (90 mg/kg/day of the amoxicillin component).

Children who are allergic to amoxicillin, but not with urticaria or anaphylaxis, may be given cefdinir (Omnicef), cefpodoxime (Vantin), or cefuroxime (Ceftin). Children with type-1 hypersensitivity to amoxicillin may be given azithromycin (Zithromax), clarithromycin (Biaxin), erythromycin-sulfisoxazole (Pediazole), or sulfamethoxazole-trimethoprim (Bactrim). In AOM where the organism is thought to be penicillin resistant Streptococcus pneumoniae, clindamycin is a reasonable choice.

Patients who fail to respond within 48 to 72 hours, whether in the observation or antibacterial therapy group, should be reassessed and treatment changed depending on the findings. Reduction of risk factors for AOM is encouraged for everyone. No recommendations were made regarding the efficacy of complementary and alternative medicine for the treatment of AOM.

Otitis media with effusion is common after resolution of acute otitis. Some children also present with asymptomatic otitis media with effusion as well. Treatment of children with persistent middle effusion

**CURRENT THERAPY**

- Adequate pain management is key in treating AOM.
- If a child has an acute bacterial otitis media, antibiotics are indicated.
- Amoxicillin at 80 to 90 mg/kg/day is the first therapy of choice in nonallergic children.
- Children older than age 2 years may be observed without antibiotic therapy if the diagnosis is uncertain.
- Children younger than age 2 years may be treated with antibiotics if the diagnosis is uncertain.

*Abbreviation:* AOM = acute otitis media.

## CURRENT DIAGNOSIS

- The diagnosis of AOM requires acute signs of illness such as fever and pain along with signs of middle ear inflammation such as fluid and erythema.
- Associated symptoms of AOM include fever, pain, and irritability.
- Visualization of the tympanic membrane and pneumatic otoscopy are required to confirm the diagnosis of AOM.
- Fluid behind the tympanic membrane does not necessarily indicate an infection in the middle ear space.

*Abbreviation:* AOM = acute otitis media.

depends on their at-risk grouping. Children at risk for speech, language, or other learning problems should be treated more promptly than other children not at risk. The at-risk groups include children with a permanent hearing loss independent of the otitis media, suspected or known speech and language delays, autism-spectrum disorder or other pervasive developmental disorder, syndromes or craniofacial disorders, blindness or uncorrectable visual impairment, cleft palate with or without associated syndrome, or developmental delay. The management of the child with otitis media with effusion in these at-risk groups should include hearing tests, speech and language assessment and therapy, hearing aids or other amplification devices for hearing loss independent of the otitis media, tympanostomy tube placement, and assessment of hearing after resolution of the otitis media with effusion to detect underlying hearing loss independent of the middle ear fluid.

Children who do not fall in the at-risk group may be watched for 3 months before intervention. If the MEE persists for longer than 3 months, audiometric assessment of hearing should be obtained. Intervention is then based on the presence of a hearing loss of generally greater than 20 decibels, suspicion of language development delay, or other impending complications related to the MEE. If the hearing loss is mild (21 to 39 decibels), strategies to optimize the listening and learning environment and/or surgical intervention should be suggested. If the hearing loss is greater than 40 decibels, surgical intervention to correct the MEE is indicated and most efficacious.

Initial surgical treatment of a problematic persistent MEE as described earlier is tympanostomy tube placement. Adenoidectomy is reserved for children who have other distinct indications, such as nasal airway obstruction or chronic adenitis, or in whom another set of pressure equalization tubes are necessary. Approximately 20% to 50% of children relapse after their tympanostomy tubes extrude and will require additional tubes. When adenoidectomy is performed with the second set of tubes, the rate of recidivism is decreased by 50%. This advantage is seen in children as young as age 2 years, with the greatest effect seen in children aged 3 years and older, regardless of adenoidal size. Children older than age 4 years may also benefit from adenoidectomy and myringotomy without tube placement. Myringotomy alone without tympanostomy tube insertion and/or tonsillectomy alone solely for the treatment of otitis media with effusion has not been found to be efficacious.

## Conclusion

The key to successful management of a child with AOM or otitis media with effusion, as it is with any medical problem, is based on the clinician's ability to correctly diagnose and stratify at-risk groups. The new recommended clinical pathways developed by the AAP, AAFP, and AAO-HNS for AOM and otitis media with effusion may at first seem to increase complexity of treatment because it increases the number of pathways possible. Closer reflection, however, will reveal an easier paradigm. It is the clinician's responsibility to attain the skills and knowledge set to make the correct initial diagnosis and assessment of risk for the patient. The support from the evidence-based-medicine clinical pathways will then help in the decision making and treatment formulation.

## REFERENCES

American Academy of Family Physicians, American Academy of Otolaryngology Head and Neck Surgery, American Academy of Pediatrics Subcomitee on Otitis Media with Effusion: Otitis media with effusion. Pediatrics 2004; 113(5):1412-1429.

American Academy of Pediatrics Subcomitee on Acute Otitis Media: Diagnosis and management of acute otitis media. Pediatrics 2004; 113(5):1451-1465.

Bell LM: The new clinical practice guidelines for acute otitis media: An editorial. Ann Emerg Med 2005; 45(5):514-516.

Bluestone CD: Epidemiology and pathogenesis of chronic suppurative otitis media: Implications for prevention and treatment. Int J Pediatr Otorhinolaryngol 1998; 42(3):207-223.

Ohlms LA, Chen AY, Stewart MG, Franklin DJ: Establishing the etiology of childhood hearing loss. Otolaryngol Head Neck Surg 1999; 120(2):159-163.

Paradise JL, Campbell TF, Dollaghan CA, et al: Developmental outcomes after early or delayed insertion of tympanostomy tubes. N Engl J Med 2005;353(6):576-586.

Rosenfeld RM: A practical classification of otitis media subgoups. Int J Pediatr Otorhinolaryngol 2005; 69(8):1027-1029.

Rosenfeld RM, Culpepper L, Doyle KJ, et al: Clinical practice guideline: Otitis media with effusion. Otolaryngol Head Neck Surg 2004; 130(5 Suppl): S95-118.

Rosenfeld RM, Lous J, Bluestone CD, et al: Recent advances in otitis media. 8. Treatment. Ann Otol Rhinol Laryngol Suppl 2005; 194:114-139.

# Episodic Vertigo

Method of
*Joseph M. Furman, MD, PhD*

Vertigo occurs when a patient perceives motion that is not real. Vertigo is caused by erroneous neural signals arising from the labyrinth or from abnormal processing of balance signals in the brain.

Strictly speaking, the term *vertigo* should be reserved for an illusory sensation of motion of self or surroundings. In this context, vertigo usually represents the manifestation of a peripheral vestibular disorder, but not always. However, "vertigo" is used by many people to represent a specific diagnosis. This use of the term *vertigo* as a diagnosis, rather than as a symptom, can be counterproductive; the clinician may be lulled into a false sense of security and provide suboptimal or delayed treatment.

Determining the optimal treatment for a patient with episodic vertigo often requires establishing a definitive diagnosis. Fortunately, in many patients with episodic vertigo, a specific diagnosis can be reached. However in a significant number of patients, no specific diagnosis can be reached. When a definitive diagnosis cannot be reached, a clinical assessment often points to either a peripheral (inner ear) or to a central (brain) vestibular disorder, which can be helpful in selecting a treatment. Obtaining a detailed history, performing a physical examination, and, when appropriate, ordering laboratory testing are the principal diagnostic tools for assessing a patient with episodic vertigo.

Obtaining a history from a patient with episodic vertigo is especially important because vertigo is subjective, usually transient, and often unaccompanied by physical findings. It is difficult for many patients to describe their abnormal sensations of motion. Rather than *vertigo*, they might use the terms *dizziness, lightheadedness, giddiness,* or *dysequilibrium*. Regardless of the terminology that the patient uses, it is essential to ask about time course, aggravating factors, and associated symptoms. Some patients with episodic vertigo experience symptoms between as well as during attacks.

Physical examination of the patient with episodic vertigo should include a neurologic and otologic examination and a neuro-otologic

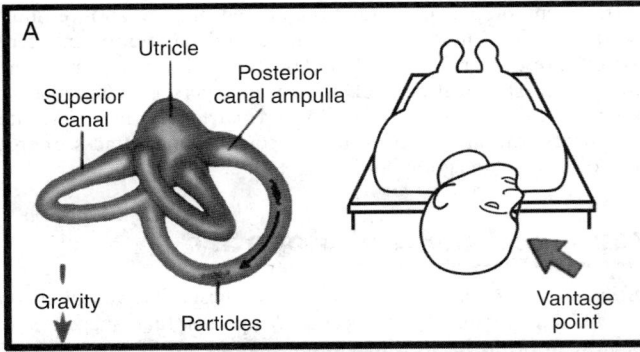

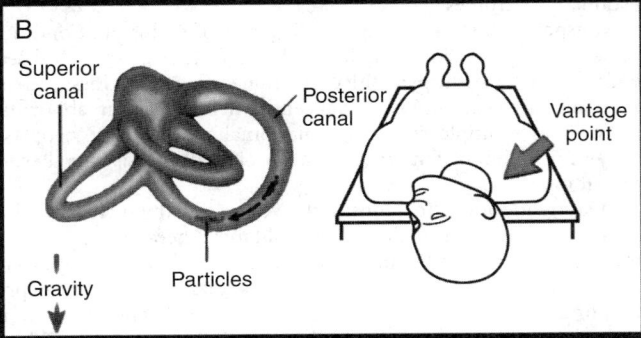

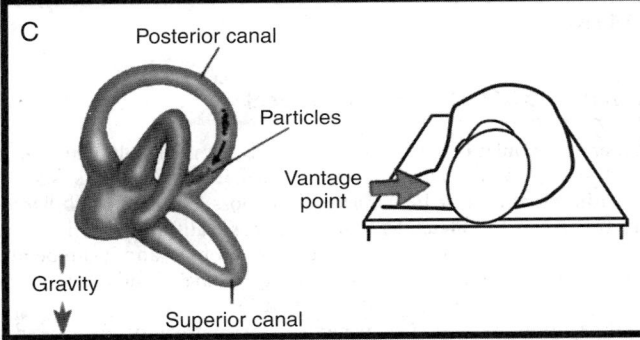

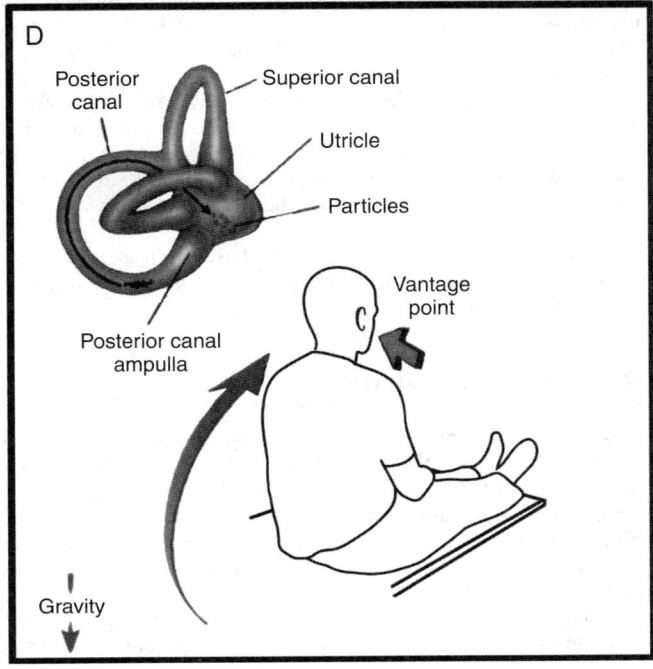

examination that uses several specialized bedside evaluation methods. Laboratory testing of the patient with episodic vertigo may include vestibular laboratory testing, audiometry, and brain imaging.

Some recognized causes of episodic vertigo are relatively common and others are unusual. A few vestibular disorders that cause episodic vertigo are controversial. Some patients suffer from more than one episodic disorder. The Current Diagnosis box lists disorders that cause episodic vertigo.

## Benign Paroxysmal Positional Vertigo

Benign paroxysmal positional vertigo (BPPV) is a well-defined disorder characterized by episodic vertigo induced by rolling in bed and by tipping one's head backward. The disorder is caused by free-floating debris in the posterior semicircular canal.

The preferred treatment is a particle-repositioning maneuver (Figure 1). This treatment is highly successful and provides complete relief for nearly all patients. Some patients cannot undergo a particle repositioning maneuver. For these patients, Brandt-Daroff exercises should be prescribed. Vestibular-suppressant medications may be used early in the disorder, but after several days they should be used sparingly, if at all.

Approximately 15% of patients with one episode of BPPV have a recurrence within 1 year. Home particle repositioning has been advocated for persons with repeated episodes of BPPV. Rarely, surgical procedures are required for patients whose BPPV is refractory to nonsurgical treatments.

## Meniere's Disease

Treatment for this disorder is discussed in depth elsewhere in this volume. The typical manifestation of Meniere's disease includes fluctuating aural fullness, tinnitus, hearing loss, and recurrent bouts of vertigo. Endolymphatic hydrops (swelling of the endolymphatic space) is thought to be the underlying pathophysiologic process of Meniere's disease.

The medical treatment of endolymphatic hydrops includes taking a diuretic and restricting dietary sodium. A combination of hydrochlorothiazide and triamterene (Dyazide) is the diuretic of choice. Dietary sodium should be held below 2 g per day. About 10% to 15% of persons with Meniere's disease eventually fail medical therapy. Surgical treatment options for Meniere's disease, discussed elsewhere in this volume, include chemical labyrinthectomy, endolymphatic sac surgery, labyrinthectomy, and vestibular nerve section.

**FIGURE 1.** Bedside maneuver for treatment of a patient with benign paroxysmal positional vertigo affecting the right ear. The presumed position of the debris within the labyrinth during the maneuver is shown in each panel. The maneuver is a three-step procedure. **A**, The Dix-Hallpike test is performed with the patient's head rotated 45 degrees toward the right ear and the neck slightly extended with the chin pointed slightly upward. This position results in the patient's head hanging to the right. **B**, Once the vertigo and nystagmus provoked by the Dix-Hallpike test cease, the patient's head is rotated about the rostral-caudal body axis until the left ear is down. **C**, The head and body are further rotated until the head is face down. The vertex of the head is kept tilted downward throughout the rotation. The maneuver usually provokes brief vertigo. The patient should be kept in the final, face-down position for about 10 to 15 seconds. **D**, With the head kept turned toward the left shoulder, the patient is brought into the seated position. Once the patient is upright, the head is tilted so that the chin is pointed slightly downward. (Adapted from Furman JM, Cass SP: Benign paroxysmal positional vertigo. N Engl J Med 1999;341[21]:1590-1596.)

---

**BOX 1   Treatment Options for Migraine-Related Dizziness**

- Avoid dietary triggers
- Treat underlying migraine phenomenon
  - Anticonvulsants (e.g., topiramate [Topomax] 25 mg/d to 50 mg bid)
  - Antidepressants (e.g., imipramine [Tofranil][1] 10-100/mg/d or sertraline[1] [Zoloft] 25-75 mg/d)
  - β-Blockers (e.g., propranolol [Inderal] 80-320 mg/d)
  - Calcium channel blockers (e.g., verapamil [Calan] 80-120 mg/d)
- Treat movement-associated disequilibrium with vestibular rehabilitation therapy
- Treat space and motion discomfort with clonazepam (Klonopin)[1] 0.25-0.5 mg bid
- Treat associated anxiety or panic disorder
  - Behavioral therapy
  - Pharmacotherapy
  - Tricyclic antidepressants
- Consider abortive treatment with a triptan for acute migrainous vertigo

---

[1]Not FDA approved for this indication.

---

## Migraine-Related Dizziness

Migraine-related dizziness is a diagnosis of exclusion and should be suspected in patients with nonspecific dizziness or vertigo associated with headache. A past history of migraine headaches or a positive family history of migraine increases the likelihood of this disorder. Patients with migraine-related dizziness almost invariably report exacerbation of symptoms by viewing certain moving visual environments or significant motion sickness sensitivity.

Treatment options for patients with migraine-related dizziness are summarized in Box 1. The patient should be informed about the association between dizziness and an underlying migraine condition and the importance of avoiding dietary triggers such as tyramine-containing foods, alcohol, and caffeine. The underlying migraine condition should be treated with prophylactic antimigraine medications, even if headaches are not currently prominent. If the most prominent vestibular symptom is movement-associated disequilibrium or unsteadiness, vestibular rehabilitation therapy is recommended. If the patient reports severe space and motion discomfort, prescribe low-dose clonazepam[1] (Klonopin) 0.25 mg twice daily. In patients with panic attacks or agoraphobia (migraine-anxiety-related dizziness [MARD]), psychiatric consultation should be obtained, and behavioral therapy and specific medical therapy using antidepressant medications should be considered. Consider triptans to abort episodes of acute migraine-related vertigo.

## Anxiety-Related Dizziness

Anxiety often accompanies dizziness. The cause-and-effect relationship between anxiety and dizziness is uncertain but may be related to a somatopsychic, a psychosomatic, or a common neurologic mechanism. The term *psychogenic dizziness* should be avoided in favor of the term *psychiatric dizziness*. *Psychiatric dizziness* should be used to describe dizziness that occurs exclusively in combination with other symptoms as part of a recognized psychiatric symptom cluster. Hyperventilation is a maneuver that is commonly used to determine whether dizziness is psychogenic, but the test is actually quite nonspecific, and the results of such testing should be interpreted with great caution.

Treatment of patients with a combined anxiety and vestibular disorder should include measures aimed at both conditions simultaneously. The vestibular disorder should be treated in whatever manner is appropriate. The treatment of anxiety disorders includes pharmacotherapy and behavioral therapy. A psychiatric referral is warranted for patients who are suffering from frequent panic attacks or from panic disorder with agoraphobia.

## Nonspecific Vestibulopathy

*Vestibulopathy of unknown origin* and *nonspecific vestibulopathy* describe a complex of nonspecific symptoms that suggest some impairment of the balance system but that do not fit any recognized vestibular syndromes.

Nonspecific vestibulopathy is a diagnosis of exclusion. Conditions that should be considered and ruled out include Meniere's disease (endolymphatic hydrops), BPPV, migraine-related dizziness, anxiety and panic disorders, and potential central nervous system abnormalities such as multiple sclerosis, Chiari malformation, or neoplasm. Follow-up is important because a specific diagnosis can become evident over time.

Treatment options for nonspecific vestibulopathy include medications and a course of vestibular rehabilitation therapy. The choice of treatment depends on the physician's judgment about the importance and predominance of symptoms of nausea, dizziness, anxiety, depression, or a functional impairment of balance. Medications commonly used to decrease dizziness, vertigo, and nausea are listed in Table 1. Sertraline (Zoloft)[1] has been suggested for patients with nonspecific dizziness.

## Bilateral Vestibular Loss

Bilateral vestibular loss most commonly occurs as a result of aminoglycoside-induced ototoxicity. Other pharmaceutical agents such as cisplatin can also cause bilateral vestibular loss. Bilateral vestibular loss can be caused by bilateral Meniere's disease, autoimmune inner ear disease, otosyphilis, or bilateral acoustic neuromas, and it can be idiopathic. The combination of oscillopsia and ataxia (Dandy's syndrome) is pathognomonic for bilateral vestibular loss.

Prevention is the best management for ototoxicity. Treatment for bilateral vestibular loss should include discontinuation of all vestibular suppressant medications and referral for a course of balance rehabilitation therapy. If at all possible, the patient should not receive further ototoxic medications.

Patients should be taught how to use sensory input other than that from the vestibular system, such as from vision and proprioception. A properly fitted cane can provide increased proprioceptive input. The patient should also be cautioned to remove all loose rugs from the home, install night-lights, and install hand rails on stairways and in the bathroom.

Recently, several prosthetic devices have been developed for patients with bilateral vestibular loss. These devices are currently being evaluated for efficacy.

## Acoustic Neuroma

A cerebellopontine angle lesion should be suspected in the setting of dizziness associated with unilateral or asymmetric hearing loss or tinnitus. Diagnostic considerations should include a large acoustic neuroma or meningioma involving the posterior fossa. Large cerebellopontine angle tumors can produce a combination of peripheral and central vestibular abnormalities. Both vestibular nerve and cerebellar function may be impaired.

Management options include observation, microsurgical excision of the tumor, and radiosurgery. Selection of the appropriate treatment

---

[1]Not FDA approved for this indication.

**TABLE 1  Medications Commonly Used to Reduce Dizziness, Vertigo, and Associated Nausea**

| Generic Name (Brand Name) | Class | Dosage | Primary Symptom Being Treated | Side Effects |
|---|---|---|---|---|
| Clonazepam[1] (Klonipin) | Benzodiazepine | 0.25 mg bid | Dizziness | Drowsiness |
| Cyclizine (Marezine) | Piperzine (H$_1$-blocking agent) | 50 mg PO or IM q4-6h | Dizziness | Drowsiness |
| Diazepam[1] (Valium) | Benzodiazepine | 1-10 mg PO, IM, or IV q12h | Dizziness | Lethargy |
| Dimenhydrinate (Dramamine) | Ethanolamine (H$_1$-blocking agent) | 50 mg PO q4-6h | Dizziness | Drowsiness |
| Diphenhydramine (Benadryl) | Ethanolamine (H$_1$-blocking agent) | 25-50 mg PO, IM, or IV q6h | Nausea | Drowsiness |
| Hydroxyzine[1] (Vistaril, Atarax) | Piperazine derivative | 25-100 mg PO[1] q8h | Nausea | Drowsiness |
| Meclizine (Antivert, Bonine) | Piperazine (H$_1$-blocking agent) | 25 mg PO q4-6h | Dizziness | Drowsiness |
| Prochlorperazine Compazine) | Phenothiazine | 10 mg PO or IM q6h or 25 mg PR q12h | Nausea | Extrapyramidal reactions, drowsiness, anticholinergic effects |
| Promethazine (Phenergan) | Phenothiazine | 25 mg PO or PR q6h | Nausea | Extrapyramidal reactions, drowsiness |
| Scopolamine (Transderm Scop) | Amine antimuscarinic | 0.5-mg adhesive skin patches q3d | Dizziness | Dry mouth, blurred vision, drowsiness, disorientation |
| Trimethobenzamide (Tigan) | Substituted ethanolamine | 300 mg PO q6-8h or 200 mg PR or IM | Nausea | Extrapyramidal reactions (unusual) |

[1]Not FDA approved for this indication.

option depends on many factors and should be individualized. Patients should be counseled regarding the possible occurrence of vestibular symptoms following treatment.

## Vertebrobasilar Insufficiency

The blood supply of the vestibular system is derived from the basilar artery. The internal auditory artery arises from the anterior inferior cerebellar artery and gives rise to the anterior vestibular artery, which supplies the vestibular apparatus. Thus, ischemia in the vertebrobasilar artery system can cause vestibular symptoms on the basis of either peripheral vestibular dysfunction, central vestibular dysfunction, or both.

A diagnosis of vertebrobasilar insufficiency should be reserved for patients who have clearly defined episodes of transient neurologic symptoms and signs that can be localized to the posterior circulation. Isolated vertigo, especially if chronic, is rarely a symptom of vertebrobasilar insufficiency.

Management of vertebrobasilar insufficiency includes a thorough cerebrovascular assessment and often an antiplatelet agent.

## Recurrent Vestibulopathy, Recurrent Vestibular Neuritis, and Impaired Compensation

Recurrent vestibulopathy is a clinical syndrome that consists of multiple episodes of vertigo lasting minutes to hours without auditory or neurologic signs or symptoms. Recurrent vestibulopathy is a diagnosis of exclusion. Several other disorders that can cause recurrent vertigo, such as Meniere's disease (endolymphatic hydrops), BPPV, migraine-related dizziness, vertebrobasilar insufficiency, and panic disorder should be excluded before diagnosing recurrent vestibulopathy, which may be a provisional diagnosis and cannot be distinguished clinically from recurrent vestibular neuritis. Treatment for recurrent vestibulopathy is nonspecific and includes antinausea and antiemetic agents (Table 1), which should be prescribed for the patient to have on hand in the event of an episode of acute vertigo.

Most patients who have suffered from a unilateral vestibular loss, such as vestibular neuritis, undergo vestibular compensation, a rebalancing of the neural activity in central vestibular structures that leads to a resolution of the vertigo, nausea, vomiting, blurred vision, and disequilibrium that characterizes an acute unilateral vestibular syndrome. Through compensation, vestibulo-ocular, vestibulospinal, perceptual, and autonomic symptoms and signs of the acute vestibular syndrome largely resolve. Vestibular compensation occurs automatically in persons with a normal central nervous system who have normal vision, normal proprioception, and adequate physical activity. Persistent dizziness that continues following an acute peripheral vestibular ailment may be the result of impaired vestibular compensation.

Failure to compensate for a peripheral vestibular lesion can be the result of fluctuating or aberrant peripheral vestibular activity, a central nervous system abnormality, clinical or subclinical involvement of the contralateral ear, other sensory deficits (especially involving vision and somatosensation), or a sedentary lifestyle. Central nervous system abnormalities that impair vestibular compensation include structural abnormalities and dysfunction caused by certain drugs (e.g., benzodiazepines). Treatment of patients with impaired vestibular compensation includes tapering vestibular suppressant medications and performing a course of vestibular rehabilitation therapy.

## Multiple Sclerosis

Vertigo and imbalance in multiple sclerosis can indicate a lesion in central vestibular structures. A peripheral vestibular abnormality independent of multiple sclerosis should also be considered. Both peripheral and central vestibular symptoms and signs can be seen in patients with multiple sclerosis if they have a lesion that includes the root entry zone in addition to other brainstem structures. A prolonged recovery can be seen in patients with root entry zone lesions caused by multiple sclerosis. Treatment of multiple sclerosis is discussed elsewhere in this volume.

## Mal De Debarquement Syndrome

Normally, a return to stable land after prolonged sea or air travel produces sensations of motion that last for hours to days. In mal de debarquement syndrome, the sensation of motion persists for months or even years. The pathophysiology of mal de debarquement syndrome is probably related to the capability of the vestibular system to adapt to various motion environments that include combinations of vestibular and visual stimuli. Treatments for mal de debarquement syndrome include vestibular suppressants, anxiolytics,[1] antidepressants,[1] and acetazolamide[1] (Diamox). Most cases of mal de debarquement syndrome resolve spontaneously within weeks to months.

## Autoimmune Inner Ear Disease

Autoimmune inner ear disease is a disorder characterized by auditory and vestibular dysfunction that most often is bilateral and is thought to be produced by damage mediated by both cellular and humoral immune mechanisms. Autoimmune inner ear disease is usually bilateral but can begin unilaterally and rapidly progress to involve both sides.

A diagnosis of autoimmune inner ear disease is difficult to confirm. A positive rheumatologic battery or elevated sedimentation rate may be suggestive. Autoimmune inner ear disease is often a diagnosis of exclusion and commonly depends on clinical criteria and response to a trial of corticosteroid therapy.

Treatment of autoimmune inner ear disease usually includes corticosteroids, such as prednisone[1] 1 mg/kg/day for 1 to 2 weeks, followed by a tapering dose and maintenance dose if a positive response has occurred. Cytotoxic agents such as azathioprine[1] (Imuran) and cyclophosphamide[1] (Cytoxan) have also been advocated as an adjunct if the disease stops responding to steroid therapy. Plasmapheresis and intravenous immunoglobulin may be effective.

## Horizontal Semicircular Canal Benign Paroxysmal Positional Vertigo

Horizontal semicircular canal benign paroxysmal positional vertigo is a variant of typical benign paroxysmal positional vertigo. This entity is thought to result from debris in the endolymph of the horizontal semicircular canal rather than in the posterior semicircular canal, as occurs

---

[1]Not FDA approved for this indication.

in typical benign paroxysmal positional vertigo. The diagnosis of horizontal semicircular canal benign paroxysmal positional vertigo can be made by turning a patient's head to the right and to the left while the patient is supine. The patient will become vertiginous for 10 to 30 seconds and a paroxysmal horizontal nystagmus will be observed for as long as the vertigo persists.

Treatment for horizontal semicircular canal benign paroxysmal positional vertigo consists of a particle-repositioning maneuver: The patient is rolled 90 degrees from the supine position toward the unaffected ear, then to the prone position and then to the side-down position with the affected ear down, then back to the seated position.

## Superior Semicircular Canal Dehiscence Syndrome

Superior semicircular canal dehiscence syndrome is a recently described disorder characterized by episodic vertigo induced by loud noises or pressure changes in the external auditory canal. This syndrome can be diagnosed by identifying a thinning (dehiscence) of the superior semicircular canal with careful imaging. Once the syndrome is identified, referral to a neuro-otologic surgeon familiar with the disorder is appropriate because a surgical repair can be helpful.

## Cervicogenic Dizziness

Cervical vertigo is a poorly defined condition that refers to dizziness and disequilibrium thought to be caused by abnormal afferent activity from the neck. Cervical vertigo is a diagnosis of exclusion. A close temporal association of symptoms of dizziness and neck pain following a neck injury should suggest a diagnosis of cervical vertigo. Cervical vertigo can be seen in association with flexion-extension (whiplash) injuries, severe cervical arthritis, herniated cervical disks, and head trauma, especially blunt trauma to the top of the head. Neck muscle spasm and pain are often associated with symptoms of dizziness. Some patients with cervical vertigo experience a vicious cycle of excessive neck muscle activity exacerbating their dizziness, which subsequently exacerbates their neck discomfort.

Treatment of cervical vertigo includes muscle relaxants and physical therapy to improve range of motion of the neck and to reduce neck muscle spasm and discomfort. Use of a cervical collar should be limited to no more than 1 to 2 hours per day.

---

### CURRENT DIAGNOSIS

**Common**

PERIPHERAL VESTIBULAR

- Benign paroxysmal positional vertigo
- Meniere's disease

MIXED

- Anxiety-related dizziness
- Migraine-associated dizziness

UNKNOWN

- Nonspecific vestibulopathy

**Unusual**

PERIPHERAL VESTIBULAR

- Autoimmune inner ear disease
- Bilateral vestibular loss
- Horizontal semicircular canal benign paroxysmal positional vertigo

- Recurrent vestibular neuritis
- Superior semicircular canal dehiscence syndrome

CENTRAL VESTIBULAR

- Mal de debarquement syndrome
- Multiple sclerosis
- Vertebrobasilar insufficiency

MIXED

- Acoustic neuroma

**Controversial Disorders**

PERIPHERAL VESTIBULAR

- Vascular cross-compression syndrome of the eighth cranial nerve

OTHER

- Cervicogenic dizziness

**CURRENT THERAPY**

**Acoustic Neuroma**

- Observation
- Surgical management

**Anxiety-Related Dizziness**

- Antidepressants
- Psychotherapy

**Autoimmune Inner Ear Disease**

- Corticosteroids[1]
- Cytoxic agents (e.g., azathioprine[1] and cyclophosphamide[1])

**Benign Paroxysmal Positional Vertigo**

- Particle repositioning

**Bilateral Vestibular Loss**

- Physical therapy
- Prevention

**Cervicogenic Dizziness**

- Muscle relaxants
- Physical therapy

**Mal de Debarquement Syndrome**

- Acetazolamide (Diamox)[1]
- Antidepressants[1]
- Anxiolytics[1]
- Vestibular suppressants

**Meniere's Disease**

- Hydrochlorothiazide-triamterene (Dyazide)
- Sodium reduction

**Migraine-Related Dizziness**

- Decrease triggers
- Migraine prophylaxis
- Triptans

**Multiple Sclerosis**

- Corticosteroids

**Nonspecific Vestibulopathy**

- Physical therapy
- Sertraline (Zoloft)[1]
- Vestibular suppressants

**Recurrent Vestibulopathy**

- Antiemetics
- Antinausea agents

**Superior Canal Dehiscence Syndrome**

- Observation
- Surgical repair

**Vascular Cross-Compression Syndrome**

- Baclofen (Lioresal)[1]
- Carbamazepine (Tegretol)[1]
- Gabapentin (Neurontin)[1]
- Surgical decompression

**Vertebrobasilar Insufficiency**

- Antiplatelet agents

[1]Not FDA approved for this indication.

# Vascular Cross-Compression Syndrome of the Eighth Cranial Nerve

Vascular cross-compression syndrome of the eighth cranial nerve, which has been called *disabling positional vertigo* and *vestibular paroxysmia*, refers to a cochleovestibular syndrome caused by compression of the eighth cranial nerve by blood vessels within the cerebellopontine angle. The clinical description of vascular compression syndrome of the eighth cranial nerve is controversial, with no agreed-upon set of diagnostic criteria.

Treatment options for vascular cross-compression syndrome of the eighth cranial nerve include pharmacotherapy with carbamazepine (Tegretol),[1] baclofen (Lioresal),[1] or gabapentin (Neurontin).[1] Surgical treatment consists of microvascular decompression. A trial of medical therapy is appropriate before referring a patient for a surgical opinion.

## REFERENCES

Furman JM, Balaban CD, Jacob RG, Marcus DA: Migraine-anxiety related dizziness (MARD): A new disorder? J Neurol Neurosurg Psychiatry 2005;76(1):1-8.
Furman JM, Cass SP: Benign paroxysmal positional vertigo. N Engl J Med 1999;341(21):1590-1596.
Hain TC, Yacovino D: Pharmacologic treatment of persons with dizziness. Neurol Clin 2005;23(3):831-853, vii.

[1]Not FDA approved for this indication.

Minor LB: Clinical manifestations of superior semicircular canal dehiscence. Laryngoscope 2005;115(10):1717-1727.
Radtke A, von Brevern M, Tiel-Wilck K, et al: Self-treatment of benign paroxysmal positional vertigo: Semont maneuver vs Epley procedure. Neurology 2004;63(1):150-152.
Staab JP, Ruckenstein MJ, Amsterdam JD: A prospective trial of sertraline for chronic subjective dizziness. Laryngoscope 2004;114(9):1637-1641.
Tusa RJ: Bedside assessment of the dizzy patient. Neurol Clin 2005;23(3): 655-673, v.
Wall C 3rd, Merfeld DM, Rauch SD, Black FO: Vestibular prostheses: The engineering and biomedical issues. J Vestib Res 2002;12(2-3):95-113.

# Ménière's Disease

Method of:
*Ted A. Meyer, MD, PhD, and Paul R. Lambert, MD*

Ménière's disease is a disorder of fluid balance of the endolymph of the peripheral auditory and vestibular systems. The inner ear contains an endolymph-filled membranous labyrinth housed inside the perilymph-filled bony labyrinth. The sensory receptor cells of the inner ear are contained in the membranous labyrinth. The composition of perilymph is very similar to cerebrospinal fluid (CSF) (high sodium, low potassium), whereas the composition of endolymph is like intracellular fluid (high potassium, low sodium). The uniqueness of endolymph lies in its high positive resting potential (+80 mV). Disturbances in the fluid dynamics of the endolymph appear to be involved in the hearing loss and peripheral vestibular disorders associated with Ménière's disease. The exact mechanism or mechanisms involved in Ménière's disease are not completely understood, but it appears that an overabundance of endolymph, either through overproduction and/or underabsorption, is the pathologic basis of the disease.

## Clinical Presentation

The symptomatology of Ménière's disease was first described almost 150 years ago by the French physician for whom it is named, Prosper Ménière. Patients with Ménière's disease present with unilateral fluctuating sensorineural hearing loss, aural fullness, tinnitus, and spells of disabling vertigo that typically last between 20 minutes and 24 hours. Many patients with Ménière's disease have nonspecific dizziness and imbalance in between spells of vertigo as well. A small percentage of patients develop or present with drop attacks, or spells of Tumarkin. These attacks occur when a patient's vestibular system goes into a crisis and the patient loses extensor tone. Patients often describe an aura followed by a feeling that they are going to fall. Patients do not lose consciousness unless they hit their head. Patients with Ménière's disease may not present with all symptoms, and the severity and progression of hearing loss, tinnitus, and vertigo are variable. For the majority of patients, Ménière's disease occurs in a single ear; however, if patients are followed for a long enough time, the literature reports bilateral Ménière's disease in a wide percentage of patients. Patients with bilateral Ménière's disease whose hearing loss progresses to profound levels are excellent candidates for a cochlear implant.

## Office Evaluation

The majority of patients with dizziness or vertigo present to their primary care physician (PCP) or to the emergency room. Many of these patients are given 25 mg of meclizine (Antivert) and are instructed to take it up to three times a day as needed. When the vertigo spells continue, they are often then referred to an otolaryngologist or otologist. Patients who are regularly taking meclizine as a prophylactic should stop the medication as quickly as possible.

When the patient with dizziness or vertigo presents to the clinic, the diagnosis of Ménière's disease can usually be obtained through the history and physical examination. The patient should give a history of disabling spells of vertigo, aural fullness or a "stuffy ear," fluctuating and progressive hearing loss, and tinnitus. The nature of the vertigo and the duration of the spells aids in the diagnosis. The vertigo is usually severe and can last between 20 minutes and 24 hours. Rarely does a

Ménière's attack last longer than 24 hours. Longer attacks (days) are more consistent with vestibular neuritis. The attacks are not provoked by specific movements, such as the brief spell of benign paroxysmal positional vertigo (BPPV) that lasts seconds to a few minutes often after rolling over in bed. Aural fullness is variable, but when present it is often more pronounced during the attack. The sensorineural hearing loss associated with Ménière's disease is often a low-frequency loss that is fluctuant and progressive. The hearing loss is often worse during the attack; however, some patients are so vertiginous and nauseated during an attack that characteristics of their hearing loss or aural fullness are not appreciated. Tinnitus with Ménière's disease is variable, but many patients describe a low-pitched roaring sound, "like a refrigerator running."

A complete and thorough physical examination should be performed on all patients who present with dizziness or vertigo. The background and expertise of the PCP is different from that of the otologist, and the PCP should evaluate the patient for other causes of dizziness or lightheadedness. The physician should then perform a complete head and neck examination. Otoscopy is usually unremarkable unless the patient has a history of eustachian tube disease. Pneumatic otoscopy should be performed and should not be associated with any vertigo or nystagmus suggestive of a perilymphatic fistula. The cranial nerves and cerebellar function should be assessed. At a minimum, the patient should be evaluated for spontaneous and gaze-evoked nystagmus, and the Dix-Hallpike, Romberg, and Fukuda step tests should be performed. Tuning fork tests should be performed to determine the nature of the hearing loss. Assuming that hearing in the ear not in question is relatively normal, the sound from a tuning fork placed on the center of the head (Weber test) should lateralize to the normal ear. The Rinne test should confirm that hearing by air conduction is louder than bone-conduction hearing.

### AUDIOMETRIC AND VESTIBULAR TESTING

Formal pure-tone and speech audiometry should be obtained on all patients with suspected Ménière's disease. Tympanometry and acoustic reflexes should be obtained as well. Patients usually present with a characteristic asymmetric low-frequency sensorineural loss that may recover to some degree between attacks. Patients with long-standing diagnoses of Ménière's disease rarely demonstrate normal and symmetric hearing. They often present with pure-tone thresholds in the 60-dB range, with diminished word recognition scores.

Vestibular testing is often performed on patients with Ménière's disease. Patients may have relatively normal responses to caloric irrigations in the affected ear; however with long-standing Ménière's disease, caloric responses are usually reduced. The patient should not have spontaneous, positional, or gaze-evoked nystagmus, and ocular motor testing should be unremarkable. Electrocochleography is rarely performed for patients with suspected Ménière's disease anymore.

### LABORATORY AND RADIOLOGIC TESTING

Some otologists believe that Ménière's disease is a clinical diagnosis and when they are confident in the diagnosis, they perform few other tests. With concerns about the exponential increase in the cost of health care, we as health care providers must have accurate data to justify this approach. Other clinicians feel that a battery of tests is warranted for patients who present with the clinical and audiologic manifestations of Ménière's disease, including a magnetic resonance imaging (MRI) scan to search for an acoustic neuroma or other retrocochlear pathology, fluorescent treponemal antibody absorption (FTA-ABS) test for syphilis, and the anti68-kD protein test for autoimmune inner ear disease. The clinician may take a prudent approach when ordering tests for patients with classic symptoms and signs of Ménière's disease and consider ordering more tests when the diagnosis is less clear.

## Treatment

The therapeutic goal of treating patients with Ménière's disease is to prevent or minimize the disabling spells of vertigo. The mainstay of

---

### CURRENT DIAGNOSIS

- Severe and often disabling vertigo lasting minutes to hours
- Fluctuating and progressive sensorineural hearing loss, often low-frequency
- Tinnitus: often low-pitched with roaring quality
- Aural fullness
- Complete neurologic evaluation
- Complete audiometric evaluation
- Consider further testing (MRI, FTA-ABS, tests for autoimmune disorders)

*Abbreviations:* FTA-ABS = fluorescent treponemal antibody absorption (test); MRI = magnetic resonance imaging.

## CURRENT THERAPY

**Medical**

- Low sodium diet (<1500 mg/d)
- Smoking cessation
- Caffeine restriction
- Alcohol restriction
- Diuretic (hydrochlorothiazide, 25 mg, plus triamterene, 37.5 mg qd [Dyazide, Maxzide-25], may increase to bid)
- Vestibular suppressants for acute attacks

**Surgical**

- Hearing preservation:
  - Intratympanic gentamicin
  - Endolymphatic sac decompression/shunt
  - Vestibular nerve section (three approaches)
- Hearing ablative:
  - Labyrinthectomy

---

modern treatment for patients is management of dietary sodium intake and the use of a diuretic. Patients should be instructed to minimize the sodium in their diet. Patients should typically restrict their sodium intake to 1500 mg per day. Many patients consume 5 to 10 g of sodium per day, and a reduction to 1.5 g per day requires a major change in lifestyle. Patients are also asked to decrease their caffeine and alcohol input, and if they smoke, they are told to stop and given information on different options available for smoking cessation. If the patient is not allergic, and there are no medical contraindications, the diuretic of choice is a combination of 25 mg hydrochlorothiazide and 37.5 mg of triamterene (Dyazide, Maxzide-25). Although triamterene is a potassium-sparing diuretic, patients are still encouraged to eat foods containing potassium (bananas, oranges, potatoes) and watch for signs of hypokalemia.

Low-salt diet and diuretic therapy successfully control the spells of vertigo in the majority of patients with Ménière's disease. Before considering another treatment option when low-salt diet and diuretic therapy are not effective, patients should be counseled on maintaining an even more restrictive diet (1000 mg of sodium per day) and if not medically contraindicated, the diuretic can be increased from once to twice daily. For patients who continue to have spells of vertigo despite aggressive medical therapy, other treatment options should be discussed.

## MENIETT

A mechanical device that delivers low-pressure bursts of air to the external auditory canal is now available and shows some promising early results. Patients who consider the Meniett (Xomed) device first undergo a myringotomy and placement of a tympanostomy tube. In an adult, this can often be performed under local anesthesia in the clinic. The Meniett is an expensive device, and many insurance providers do not cover it. However, Medicare currently reimburses for the device.

## OTOTOXIC ANTIBIOTICS

Injecting gentamicin into the middle ear to create a partial chemical labyrinthectomy has become popular in recent years, and it is performed by many general otolaryngologists as well as otologists. The procedure is performed in the office under topical anesthesia. Most otologists use a low-dose titration method in hopes of damaging the vestibular system while causing as little hearing loss as possible. Patients often have vague dizziness or balance problems several days after the procedure, and they normally compensate for this partial chemical labyrinthectomy. Gentamicin is helpful in reducing or halting the

disabling spells of vertigo in the majority of patients who undergo the procedure. The risk of profound hearing loss after a single gentamicin injection is low, but it can occur.

## SURGERY

Three procedures are used for patients with Ménière's disease: endolymphatic sac decompression/shunting, vestibular nerve section, and labyrinthectomy. The procedure is chosen based on the patient's age, overall health, and hearing status. If the patient has good hearing, then an endolymphatic sac decompression/shunt is recommended as the primary surgical procedure. In this outpatient surgery, a mastoidectomy is completed, and the endolymphatic sac is identified. The bone covering the sac is removed to decompress the sac. The sac is opened, and a silastic stent is placed in the sac. The risks of major complications such as facial paralysis or hearing loss are minimized with this procedure. Approximately 65% to 75% of patients undergoing an endolymphatic sac procedure receive substantial benefit.

If the patient continues to have spells of vertigo, the endolymphatic sac decompression can be repeated, or if the hearing is still good, the patient may opt for a vestibular nerve section. The vestibular nerve may be sectioned by one of three approaches (middle fossa, retrosigmoid, or retrolabyrinthine) depending on the surgeon's training and expertise and the age and health status of the patient. These procedures are more involved and in general require an overnight stay in the intensive care unit. There is a slight risk of hearing loss with these procedures from disruption of the blood supply to the cochlea or from damage to the cochlear nerve. More than 90% of patients who undergo vestibular nerve section receive substantial benefit.

If a patient has poor hearing, then a labyrinthectomy is the procedure of choice. A labyrinthectomy is performed via a mastoidectomy. The three semicircular canals are removed and the vestibule is opened to remove the neuroepithelium of the utricle and saccule. Operative risks such as damage to the facial nerve and a CSF leak are low with this procedure. A somewhat less-complete labyrinthectomy can be performed through the external auditory canal. This procedure is typically reserved for an elderly patient. It can be performed while the patient is awake. After a labyrinthectomy, the patient loses all hearing in that ear. Patients undergoing a labyrinthectomy are often acutely vertiginous and many require overnight observation. Control of vertigo after a labyrinthectomy is excellent. Approximately 95% of patients are free from spells of vertigo following this procedure, and the vast majority of patients, even the elderly, recover from this total unilateral vestibular loss quite well.

In summary, Ménière's disease is often misdiagnosed, and despite a great deal of research, it remains poorly understood. Patients must receive proper treatment and be educated about simple methods that can be used to prevent their symptoms. When sodium restriction and diuretics do not control the severe disabling spells of vertigo, patients should be offered one of the treatment options described here.

## REFERENCES

Gates GA Green D: Intermittent pressure therapy of intractable Ménière's disease using the Meniett device: A preliminary report. Laryngoscope 2002;112:1489-1493.

Graham MD, Kemink JL: Transmastoid labyrinthectomy: Surgical management of vertigo in the nonserviceable hearing ear. A five-year experience. Am J Otol 1984;5:295-299.

Harner SG, Driscoll CL, Facer GW, et al: Long-term follow-up of transtympanic gentamicin for Ménière's syndrome. Otol Neurotol 2001;22:210-214.

Lustig LR, Yeagle J, Niparko JK, Minor LB: Cochlear implantation in patients with bilateral Ménière's syndrome. Otol Neurotol 2003;24:397-403.

Schessel DA, Minor LB, Nedzelski J: Ménière's disease and other peripheral disorders. In Cummings CW (ed): Cummings Otolaryngology Head and Neck Surgery. Philadelphia, Mosby, 2005, pp 3209-3253.

Welling DB, Pasha R, Roth LJ, Barin K: The effect of endolymphatic sac excision in Ménière disease. Am J Otol 1996;17:278-282.

# Sinusitis

Method of
*Richard R. Orlandi, MD*

## Classification and Etiologic Factors

Sinus inflammation is reported by more than 30 million adults in the United States and generates nearly 12 million office visits per year and at least $2.4 billion annually in direct medical costs. Loss of productivity likely has an even larger economic impact, with these patients reporting a quality-of-life impairment that is worse than patients with congestive heart failure.

The sinuses are air-filled chambers lined by respiratory epithelium that communicate with the nasal cavity through narrow openings or ostia. Mucus is produced by goblet cells within the respiratory mucosa and is propelled toward the ostia by the surface cilia. This mucociliary clearance is a self-cleaning mechanism for the nose and sinuses. Mucus and trapped particulate matter are transported into the nasopharynx and from there swallowed and eliminated via the gastrointestinal tract. The mucus blanket moves at approximately 8 mm per minute, resulting in a complete turnover every 10 minutes.

The anterior ethmoid and maxillary sinuses drain into a narrow trough within the middle meatus called the ethmoid infundibulum. This narrow system of drainage channels, called the ostiomeatal complex, can become easily blocked if the sinus and nasal mucosa swell because of inflammation, whatever the source. Mucociliary transport is then interrupted, trapping secretions and particulate matter, which can worsen the inflammation. This intensified inflammation can then spread to the frontal sinuses, as well as to the posterior ethmoid and sphenoid sinuses.

Inflammation within the nose has been traditionally referred to as *rhinitis*, whereas that in the paranasal sinuses has been called *sinusitis*. As understanding of the physiology and pathophysiology of the nose and sinuses has improved, it has become clear that the two conditions are interrelated and the term *rhinosinusitis* has been proposed. This disease has been categorized into a number of entities, including acute rhinosinusitis, where signs and symptoms last less than 4 weeks and chronic rhinosinusitis, where they are present for more than 12 weeks. Recurring acute rhinosinusitis, acute exacerbation of chronic rhinosinusitis, and subacute rhinosinusitis are also recognized subcategories.

Rhinosinusitis is an inflammatory condition with multiple etiologic factors. Anatomic variations, allergy, viruses, reflux, chronic bone inflammation (osteitis), fungi, and bacterial superantigens have all been postulated to play a role. Some of these factors, such as allergy or reflux, may create a background inflammation that makes patients more prone to an acute bacterial infection when another etiologic factor is introduced, such as a viral upper respiratory infection (URI). Other factors, such as biofilms, osteitis, fungi, or bacterial superantigens, may perpetuate inflammation in a positive feedback loop and lead to chronic sinus and nasal inflammation. Rarer underlying conditions, such as immunodeficiency, granulomatous diseases, cystic fibrosis, and immotile cilia syndromes, also may predispose patients to acute and chronic rhinosinusitis.

Rhinosinusitis may be a final common pathway of inflammation with multiple etiologies, a constellation of signs and symptoms comprising a syndrome rather than a disease. Acute rhinosinusitis is often a bacterial infection that follows the inflammation of a viral upper respiratory illness. Conversely, chronic rhinosinusitis appears to be a primarily inflammatory condition with acute bacterial exacerbations. Long-term treatment should therefore be anti-inflammatory with antibiotics reserved for acute flares.

## Diagnosis

Diagnosing rhinosinusitis can be challenging. Headache syndromes, allergic and nonallergic rhinitis, nasal septal deviation, esophageal and laryngopharyngeal reflux, and temporomandibular joint disease all share signs and symptoms with rhinosinusitis. Multiple attempts to define one or two key diagnostic criteria have failed, and it appears that the diagnosis of rhinosinusitis rests, instead, on a constellation of signs or symptoms. Some more common ones include facial pain or pressure, a sense of nasal obstruction or congestion, altered sense of smell, discolored nasal discharge, and fever (in acute cases). Minor symptoms include headache, cough, halitosis, fatigue, dental pain, and ear pressure or pain. In children, irritability, fatigue, congestion, and nighttime cough may be the more prominent symptoms.

In differentiating viral upper respiratory infections from acute bacterial rhinosinusitis, the timing and severity of symptoms may be most important. Viral URIs are common in children and adults, and only 1 in 200 such infections progress to acute bacterial rhinosinusitis. When this does occur, symptoms of congestion, facial discomfort, and fever may persist longer than 10 days or worsen within 5 to 7 days of onset. Discolored discharge may be present from the start of the viral URI and does not necessarily correlate with bacterial infection, but rather is a sign of inflammation.

Because the symptoms of rhinosinusitis are nondescript, radiologic imaging may be called upon to make the diagnosis. Plain films of the sinuses have been all but supplanted by computed tomography (CT) because of the much greater information this modality affords. Nevertheless, the CT must be interpreted within the context of the patient's symptoms and prior treatment. Viral upper respiratory conditions generate inflammation within the nasal cavity as well as the sinuses, and CT during a URI will demonstrate changes consistent with "sinusitis." CT does not, therefore, play a prominent role in the diagnosis of acute rhinosinusitis, as it is unable to differentiate viral from bacterial disease. CT is more effective in diagnosing patients with chronic symptoms of rhinosinusitis, especially when performed after a trial of medical therapy and between acute exacerbations. Under these conditions, CT can determine the degree of inflammation and guide additional therapy. Unusual findings on CT mandate further evaluation, including unilateral disease, bone erosion, or sinus expansion. These findings may indicate neoplasia or an impending orbital or intracranial complication. In these cases, magnetic resonance imaging (MRI) may be helpful, but this modality is rarely indicated in

## CURRENT DIAGNOSIS

- Acute rhinosinusitis lasts less than 4 weeks whereas chronic rhinosinusitis is primarily an inflammatory condition, lasting more than 12 weeks.
- Rhinosinusitis shares symptoms with headache syndromes, allergic and nonallergic rhinitis, nasal septal deviation, esophageal and laryngopharyngeal reflux, and temporomandibular joint disease, making diagnosis challenging.
- There are not one or two defining diagnostic characteristics for acute or chronic rhinosinusitis. Instead, the diagnosis is often made using the physician's overall impression.
- Discolored nasal discharge does not necessarily indicate a bacterial infection.
- Imaging cannot differentiate between viral and bacterial rhinosinusitis, making it less helpful in acute disease.
- Symptoms of a viral URI typically resolve within 5 to 7 days. Severe or worsening symptoms during this period, or failure of symptoms to resolve within 7 to 10 days, are more likely to represent an acute bacterial rhinosinusitis.

uncomplicated rhinosinusitis because of its increased expense and lack of specificity.

## Treatment Strategies

Whether the inflammation is acute or chronic, treatment is directed at diminishing the inflammation and re-establishing ostial patency and mucociliary clearance. Antibiotics form the mainstay for treatment of acute bacterial rhinosinusitis. Community-acquired acute bacterial rhinosinusitis is commonly caused by *Streptococcus pneumoniae* or *Haemophilus influenzae* in adults, with the addition of *Moraxella catarrhalis* in children. In acute exacerbations of chronic rhinosinusitis, *Staphylococcus aureus* and other staphylococcal species, as well as gram-negative enteric organisms, play a larger role.

Nearly 70% of patients with acute bacterial rhinosinusitis will improve without antibiotics, but that number goes up to 85% with appropriate antibiotics. The incidence of severe complications from acute rhinosinusitis is low and is not influenced by antibiotic use. Consequently, antibiotics should be prescribed for moderate to severe cases of acute bacterial rhinosinusitis or in immunocompromised individuals who may be more at risk for complications. Uncertain or mild cases of acute bacterial rhinosinusitis may be observed for spontaneous resolution, especially early in the course of disease.

Once the decision is made to prescribe antibiotics, the next complexity is which one to choose. Numerous studies and reviews still support the use of amoxicillin, either in standard or high doses (depending on local resistance patterns). Addition of clavulanate appears to improve the symptom resolution rate but is associated with increased gastrointestinal side effects. Second-line treatment for amoxicillin failures or allergic patients includes respiratory quinolone or macrolide antibiotics.

Adjunctive treatments to reduce inflammation and symptoms include mucolytics/expectorants, nasal saline spray, anticholinergics, and decongestants (both topical and systemic). Topical decongestant therapy should not be continued for more than 5 days because of its propensity to cause a rebound rhinitis medicamentosa. Antihistamines are also indicated in patients with an underlying allergic component.

---

### CURRENT THERAPY

- Treatment of rhinosinusitis is aimed toward decreasing mucosal inflammation and re-establishing patency and mucociliary clearance within the nose and sinuses.
- Acute rhinosinusitis is primarily an infectious condition. Approximately 70% of cases will resolve spontaneously. Antibiotics may be withheld for patients who have mild symptoms or a questionable diagnosis.
- Amoxicillin is the preferred first-line treatment for acute bacterial rhinosinusitis in an immunocompetent patient, with or without clavulanate. Respiratory quinolones or macrolides may be used for first-line treatment failures or for those that are allergic or more likely to suffer complications.
- Adjunctive treatments to reduce inflammation and symptoms in acute disease include mucolytics, nasal saline spray, anticholinergics, and decongestants.
- Chronic rhinosinusitis is primarily an inflammatory disease with secondary acute bacterial exacerbations. Consequently, therapy is principally anti-inflammatory with antibiotics reserved for periodic symptomatic flares.
- Nasal corticosteroids form the mainstay of treatment for chronic rhinosinusitis. Leukotriene inhibitors may play a role, especially in patients with associated asthma, allergic rhinitis, or nasal polyps.

Despite their anti-inflammatory effect, nasal steroid sprays have not been shown to have a clear impact on acute disease.

Because chronic rhinosinusitis is primarily an inflammatory condition with periodic acute bacterial exacerbations, antibiotics play a much smaller role. Nasal corticosteroids instead form the mainstay of treatment for chronic rhinosinusitis. Treatment of underlying allergy, when present, typically also improves the patient's overall sinus and nasal inflammation. Leukotriene inhibitors, effective in treating asthma and allergic rhinitis, may play a role in patients with chronic rhinosinusitis, especially those with nasal polyps. Patients who are not sufficiently responsive to medical therapy often benefit from surgical intervention to widen the sinus drainage pathways, followed by continued medical management.

## Complications of Sinusitis

Complications of sinus disease are rare but potentially serious. The sinuses are separated from the orbit and intracranial cavity by thin bone perforated by venous and lymphatic channels, which can act as conduits for the spread of infection. Intracranial abscess, cerebritis, venous sinus thrombosis, or meningitis may complicate acute sinusitis, typically involving the frontal or sphenoid sinuses. Orbital cellulitis or abscess typically results from ethmoid or maxillary sinusitis and is more common in children. High fever, severe or worsening headache, meningeal signs, altered mental status, infraorbital hypesthesia, significant facial swelling, diplopia, ptosis, chemosis, proptosis, or pupillary or extraocular movement abnormalities should prompt a thorough evaluation, including dedicated imaging and more intensive therapy and observation.

Immunocompromised patients are at special risk for invasive fungal rhinosinusitis, a rare but lethal condition, where weakened host defenses allow tissue invasion and rapid spread of fungus. This disease has a predilection for neutropenic patients, poorly controlled diabetics (particularly during ketoacidosis), and patients undergoing hemodialysis. Early signs may be as subtle as a low-grade fever of unknown origin and can rapidly progress to orbital or cerebral symptoms as a result of extension of the disease to these areas. Therapy is directed toward swift reversal of the underlying immunocompromise, systemic antifungal therapy, and debridement of affected necrotic tissues, which can be disfiguring. Outcomes for this rare condition correlate with the ability to reverse the underlying immunocompromise.

## Summary

Rhinosinusitis represents inflammation of the nose and paranasal sinuses and has many etiologies. The symptoms of rhinosinusitis overlap with many other conditions, making diagnosis somewhat difficult. Imaging may be helpful but must be interpreted in the context of the patient's symptoms. Acute bacterial rhinosinusitis typically follows a viral URI and is an infectious process while chronic rhinosinusitis is primarily an inflammatory process with infrequent bacterial exacerbations. Treatment is therefore primarily anti-infectious in acute disease and anti-inflammatory in chronic disease. As the etiologies and pathophysiology of acute and chronic rhinosinusitis are better defined, improved therapy will likely result.

### REFERENCES

Benninger MS, Ferguson BJ, Hadley JA, et al: Adult chronic rhinosinusitis: definitions, diagnosis, epidemiology, and pathophysiology. Otolaryngol Head Neck Surg 2003;129(3 Suppl):S1-S32.

Lau J, Zucker D, Engels EA, et al: Diagnosis and Treatment of Acute Bacterial Rhinosinusitis. Evidence Report/Technology Assessment No. 9 (Contract 290-97-0019 to the New England Medical Center). Rockville, Md, Agency for Health Care Policy and Research, March 1999.

Orlandi RR, Kennedy DW: Surgical management of rhinosinusitis. Am J Med Sci 1998;316:29-38.

Sinus and Allergy Health Partnership: Antimicrobial treatment guidelines for acute bacterial rhinosinusitis. Otolaryngol Head Neck Surgery 2004;130(1 Suppl):1-45.

# Nonallergic Perennial Rhinitis

Method of
*Claus Bachert, MD, PhD, and
Nicholas Van Bruaene, MD*

Rhinitis is a very common disorder of the nose that is often trivialized although it is the cause of widespread morbidity, increased medical treatment costs, reduced work productivity, and lost school days.

*Rhinitis* strictly means "inflammation of the nasal mucosa," but it can practically be defined as a heterogeneous group of nasal diseases characterized by one or more of sneezing, nasal itching, rhinorrhea, and nasal congestion.

Rhinitis can be roughly divided into infectious, viral (common cold) or bacterial rhinitis, and noninfectious rhinitis. Recently, noninfectious rhinitis has generally been classified as either allergic or nonallergic, depending predominantly on whether or not an allergic etiology can be proven. However, mixed forms can occur.

Allergic rhinitis is the most common type of chronic rhinitis. Underlying pathomechanisms in allergic rhinitis have been comparably well understood, whereas for nonallergic rhinitis, such knowledge is scarce, and there are no specific diagnostic tests available. The term *nonallergic (noninfectious) rhinitis* is commonly applied to any nasal condition in which the symptoms are identical to those seen in allergic rhinitis but for which an allergic etiology has been excluded. Therefore, diagnosis of nonallergic perennial rhinitis is made on exclusion of an identifiable allergy (negative skin prick tests for allergy and a lack of symptoms following allergen exposure), structural abnormality (nasal endoscopy), sinus disease (sinus computed tomography [CT] scan), or other causes as discussed later.

Nonallergic rhinitis can broadly be classified as nonallergic occupational rhinitis, hormonal rhinitis, drug-induced rhinitis, other forms, and idiopathic rhinitis. The "other forms" include nonallergic rhinitis with eosinophilia syndrome (NARES), rhinitis due to physical and chemical factors, food-induced (nonallergic) rhinitis, emotion-induced rhinitis, and atrophic rhinitis. Idiopathic rhinitis is also referred to as vasomotor rhinitis or nonallergic, noninfectious perennial rhinitis (NANIPER).

Although it is difficult to readily diagnose nonallergic rhinitis, it has been suggested that in patients with perennial nonallergic rhinitis this condition persists for more than 3 months per year and produces two or more symptoms, including hypersecretion, blockage, sneezing, and postnasal drip.

Some studies are available on the prevalence of nonallergic rhinitis; however, these data show large variations ranging from around 20% to 50%. This is probably due to difficulties in definition and lack of specific diagnostic tests for nonallergic rhinitis.

## Pathophysiology

Nasal hyperreactivity to various stimuli (e.g., odors, position, temperature, histamine) is a common feature of nonallergic rhinitis, allergic rhinitis, and postinfectious rhinitis and thus does not allow differentiation between allergic and nonallergic causes. Unlike for patients from defined subgroups of nonallergic rhinitis (particularly drug-induced, hormone-induced, and NARES) and patients with allergic rhinitis, the etiology and pathophysiology of nonallergic noninfectious rhinitis remain unknown.

The term *vasomotor rhinitis* has often been used as an equivalent to *rhinitis without clinical evidence for allergy or infection*. However, because allergic rhinitis also is characterized by a vasomotor dysfunction, it has been suggested that *idiopathic rhinitis* is probably a better term than vasomotor rhinitis.

---

> **BOX 1    Agents Causing Nonallergic Occupational Rhinitis**
>
> **Toxic Low-Molecular-Weight Compounds**
> - Aircraft fuel and jet stream exhaust
> - Aldehydes
> - Isocyanates
> - Nonallergenic microbial agents: endotoxin and β-1,3-glycan (compost workers)
> - Solvents
> - Vanadium pentoxide (boiler makers)
>
> **Physical**
> - Long-term exposure to cold, dry air or hot air

## Types of Nonallergic Rhinitis

### NONALLERGIC OCCUPATIONAL RHINITIS

Occupational rhinitis (Box 1) arises in response to an airborne agent present in the workplace. These agents elicit predominantly sneezing, nasal discharge, and blockage and can act via both immunologic (IgE-mediated) and nonimmunologic mechanisms. The nonimmunologic triggers are often irritant or toxic low-molecular-weight compounds such as aldehydes, isocyanates, aircraft fuel and jet stream exhaust, solvents, ninhydrin, pharmaceutical compounds, or chlorine. They can also be physical, such as long-term exposure to cold or dry air.

### HORMONAL RHINITIS

Hormonal rhinitis is known to occur during pregnancy in particular but also during the menstrual cycle, puberty, and in specific endocrine disorders such as acromegaly. Hormonal rhinitis can develop during pregnancy in otherwise healthy women. Neither asthma nor rhinitis is a risk factor for pregnancy rhinitis. Only 2% of patients with nonallergic rhinitis are afflicted with rhinitis due to hypothyroidism or acromegaly. Compared with pregnancy rhinitis, the evidence linking hypothyroidism with nasal pathology is sparse, and the reported increase in nasal secretion associated with thyroid disease is anecdotal.

### DRUG-INDUCED RHINITIS

Several commonly employed medications can induce symptoms of rhinitis when they are administered either topically or systemically (Box 2). The symptoms may be either predictable, as would be the case for known side effects of particular drugs, or unpredictable, based on individual hypersensitivity to certain drugs, in particular aspirin,

> **BOX 2    Medications Causing or Associated with Nonallergic Rhinitis**
>
> - Acetylsalicylic acid
> - Angiotensin-converting enzyme (ACE) inhibitors
> - Antihypertensives
> - β-Blockers
> - Immunosuppressive drugs: Cyclosporine (Neoral, Sandimmune)
> - Methyldopa
> - Nasal topical decongestants: Oxymetazoline (Afrin), naphazoline (Privine), xylometazoline (Otrivin)
> - Nonsteroidal anti-inflammatory drugs (NSAIDs)
> - Oral contraceptives
> - Psychotropic agents: Chlorpromazine, thioridazine, chlordiazepoxide (Librium), amitriptyline (Elavil), perphenazine, alprazolam (Xanax)

which commonly exacerbates rhinitis and asthma. However, intolerance to aspirin or nonsteroidal anti-inflammatory drugs (NSAIDs) predominantly produces rhinorrhea, which may be either isolated or part of a disease complex involving hyperplastic rhinosinusitis, nasal polyps, and asthma. In contrast, intolerance to angiotensin-converting enzyme (ACE) inhibitors, methyldopa, or oral contraceptives, which is less common than aspirin intolerance, leads to predominantly nasal blockage. Overuse of the topical nasal vasoconstrictors (xylometazoline and other α-adrenoceptor agonists) leads to nasal congestion by a mechanism involving a rebound effect hours after the last application. It can also lead to nasal hyperreactivity and hypertrophy of the nasal mucosa, a condition known as *rhinitis medicamentosa.*

## OTHER FORMS OF RHINITIS

### Nonallergic Rhinitis with Eosinophilia Syndrome

NARES was originally characterized on the basis of the presence of greater than 20% eosinophils in nasal smears of symptomatic patients with perennial sneezing attacks, a profuse watery rhinorrhea, nasal pruritus, incomplete nasal obstruction, and occasional loss of smell. In addition to these symptoms, a marked feature of the disease is the lack of evidence of allergy, as indicated by negative skin prick tests or absence of serum IgE antibodies to specific allergens.

Although the specific etiology of NARES is not clear, in view of the features shared by this syndrome and the triad of nasal polyposis, intrinsic asthma, and intolerance to aspirin, and because NARES patients frequently develop nasal polyps and asthma later on in life, it has been suggested that NARES may be an early expression of the triad.

The definition of NARES as a subgroup of nonallergic rhinitis is relevant for therapy because patients seem to respond well to nasal corticosteroids, in contrast to other subgroups of nonallergic rhinitis.

### Rhinitis Due to Physical and Chemical Factors

Nasal symptoms similar to those of rhinitis can be induced by physical and chemical factors in persons with sensitized nasal mucous membranes. Cold, dry air has been shown to lead to a condition known as *skier's nose,* in which acetylcholine-induced rhinorrhea features prominently. Smoke, in particular cigarette smoke, is known for its direct irritating effect on the mucosa of both upper and lower airways. Eosinophil influx, increased IgE-positive cells, and increased interleukin-4 (IL-4) is found in nasal mucosa of smoking adults and passive smoking nonallergic children. Air pollutants derived from liquid petroleum fuels have also been shown to directly exacerbate symptoms of rhinitis in nonallergic persons. Although their effects have generally been extensively investigated and well documented in the lower airways of allergic persons, little information is available about the acute or chronic effects of air pollutants on the nasal mucosa.

### Food-Induced Rhinitis

Certain foods and alcoholic beverages can induce nonallergic rhinitis; the underlying mechanisms are largely unknown. Hot and spicy foods, in particular, which contain capsaicin, lead to a watery rhinorrhea termed *gustatory rhinitis,* probably as a result of the capsaicin stimulating the sensory nerves to release neuropeptides and tachykinins. In contrast, alcoholic beverages are believed to induce symptoms as a result of vasodilation. Dyes, preservatives, and sulfites appear to play a role in a very few cases. Some foods may contain clinically relevant concentrations of histamine or other biogenic amines.

### Emotionally Induced Rhinitis

Although not studied extensively, emotional factors such as stress and sexual arousal have been documented to affect the nose, likely as a result of autonomic stimulation. In patients suffering from postcoital rhinitis, anxiety appears to be a predominant feature, which leads to worsening of the disease.

### Atrophic Rhinitis

Primary atrophic rhinitis is a progressive chronic nasal disease characterized by mucosal atrophy with resorption of the underlying bone of the conchae. It occurs predominantly in women. The atrophy leads to formation of thick crusts, which leave a distinct fetid odor in the nose (ozena). The nasal cavities are enlarged, but there is a sensation of nasal congestion. Although the precise etiology of this condition is not clear, it has been suggested that an infection with *Klebsiella ozaenae* and other bacteria might play a role. It is unknown whether primary atrophic rhinitis is purely an infectious entity or a combination of infectious, hereditary, dietary, and vascular disorders of the paranasal sinuses. However, primary atrophic rhinitis is distinct from secondary atrophic rhinitis, which develops directly as a result of granulomatous nasal infections, chronic sinusitis, excessive nasal surgery, trauma, or irradiation.

## IDIOPATHIC RHINITIS

Once all previously mentioned causes are excluded, a significant percentage of nonallergic noninfectious rhinitis cases still remains. Syndromes of chronic rhinitis with an unknown etiology are categorized under the term *idiopathic rhinitis.*

Idiopathic rhinitis is a diagnosis of exclusion and is solely based on symptoms of nasal blockage, rhinorrhea, and sneezing, although the prevalence of sneezing, conjunctival symptoms, and pruritus is lower than that in allergic rhinitis. Although the subjects have traditionally been classified as either "runners" (those with predominantly rhinorrhea) or "blockers" (those with predominantly nasal congestion and blockage), many patients suffer from more than one type of these symptoms, therefore making it difficult to subdivide the patients into these groups.

# Differential Diagnosis

Allergic rhinitis is the major disease to differentiate from nonallergic rhinitis. It is excluded by appropriate allergy tests. The possibility of a local IgE production within the nasal mucosa may account for some cases in which skin prick tests or IgE antibodies to common allergens are not yet indicative. Several other conditions are known to mimic symptoms of nonallergic noninfectious rhinitis and therefore have to be excluded by careful examination (Box 3).

Anatomic nasal abnormalities not only can cause obstruction but also can block the flow of nasal secretions and lead to rhinorrhea, postnasal drip, and nasal blockage. In children, unilateral congenital choanal atresia can lead to unilaterally reduced nasal airflow and secretions if not diagnosed early in life. Tumors are not very common in the nasal passages, but when established, they can grow rapidly and lead to unilateral nasal obstruction, bleeding, and pain in adults. Rhinorrhea and nasal congestion, in the absence of pruritus, are also characteristic features of nasal mastocytosis, an extremely rare condition in which eosinophils are absent and tests for IgE-mediated disease are negative.

---

**BOX 3  Differential Diagnosis**

- Allergic rhinitis
- Benign and malignant tumors
- Cerebrospinal fluid leakage
- Ciliary defects
- Congenital and acquired abnormalities
  - Adenoid hypertrophy
  - Choanal atresia
  - Nasal septum deviation
  - Nasal turbinate hypertrophy
- Granulomas
- Nasal polyposis
- Sinusitis

## CURRENT DIAGNOSIS

- About one half of rhinitis patients suffer from nonallergic rhinitis or mixed forms.
- There are no clinically useful diagnostic tests for nonallergic rhinitis; it remains an exclusion diagnosis.
- A thorough case history is the best diagnostic tool available and should include drug intake, work exposure, and hormonal as well as emotional status to subdivide the symptoms into subgroups.

In daily clinical practice, the diagnosis of nonallergic rhinitis and its subgroups is mainly based on a thorough case history. If the case history suggests clinically relevant noninfectious rhinitis, other possible diagnoses are excluded in a stepwise fashion:

1. Check possible stimuli, severity, and duration of disease
2. Check drug use (systemic and topical), exposure at the workplace, hormonal status (pregnancy, hypothyroidism, acromegaly), involvement of other organs (asthma, hormonal status)
3. Exclude other nasal disease (nasal rigid endoscopy)
4. Exclude allergy: skin prick test, serum IgE antibodies to the most common inhalant allergens, eventually nasal provocation testing
5. Exclude chronic rhinosinusitis (CT scan)
6. Perform nasal cytology (eosinophilia) and, if shown to be positive, consider performing an oral aspirin challenge

## Management

First, an evaluation of the severity of the disease should be performed to confirm the need for therapy, in connection with counseling on how to avoid nonspecific stimuli. In case of drug-induced, food-induced, or occupational rhinitis, specific avoidance measures are employed as first-line therapy.

### CONVENTIONAL THERAPY

Several treatments (pharmaceutical, nonconventional, and surgical) have been employed for idiopathic nonallergic rhinitis (Box 4). In patients with nasal secretion as the predominant symptom, treatment with intranasal anticholinergics (ipratropium bromide [Atrovent]) has been shown to significantly reduce rhinorrhea, but it has little effect on the other rhinitis symptoms. A topical sympathomimetic provides instant relief of obstruction symptoms. However, it should be avoided or limited to 10 days in view of the risk of developing rhinitis medicamentosa. Systemic sympathomimetics, although commonly used in some countries, seem to have significant side effects when used long term.

## CURRENT THERAPY

- Whenever possible, the treatment should take into account the subgroups of nonallergic perennial rhinitis and lead to avoidance measures.
- In idiopathic rhinitis, although not efficacious in many cases, topical antihistamines and steroids are the two main classes of drugs for treatment. Topical steroids are to be preferred if an inflammatory pathogenesis is suggested.
- Intranasal capsaicin is still considered experimental.
- Surgery is an option in patients with persistent nasal obstruction and secretion not affected by medication.

---

### BOX 4  Treatments for Nonallergic Rhinitis

**Medications Used to Treat Nonallergic Rhinitis**
- Azelastine (Astelin, Allergodil): 2 sprays each nostril qd-bid
- Fluticasone (Flonase, Flixonase AQ): 2 sprays each nostril qd or 1 spray each nostril bid
- Budesonide (Rhinocort AQ): 1 spray each nostril bid to 4 sprays each nostril qd
- Beclomethasone (Beconase AQ, Vancenase AQ): 1-2 sprays each nostril bid

**Symptom-Specific Treatment**
**Nasal Secretion**
- Ipratropium bromide (Atrovent 0.03%): 2 sprays each nostril bid-qid

**Nasal Congestion**
- Xylometazoline, oxymetazoline (Otrivine, Afrin, Nasivine): Dose varies; apply no longer than 1 wk

**Experimental and Nonconventional Therapies**
- Botulinum toxin (Botox)[1]
- Intranasal capsaicin[1]
- Silver nitrate[1]

**Inferior Turbinate Surgery**

---
[1]Not FDA approved for this indication.

---

In contrast to symptom-specific treatment, it is believed that topical steroids and antihistamines are the most appropriate first treatment options because the symptoms of nonallergic rhinitis are often variable and alternate from obstruction and congestion to secretion and rhinorrhea. Of these, fluticasone propionate (Flonase), budesonide (Rhinocort), beclomethasone (Beconase), and azelastine (Astelin) have been approved by the FDA for this indication.

Azelastine nasal spray has been found to be more effective than placebo for the control of rhinorrhea, postnasal drip, sneezing, and nasal congestion in most patients, although its effect on nasal congestion was marginal. Azelastine has a more rapid onset of action as compared with most other antihistamines and intranasal corticosteroids, and thus azelastine spray should be considered as primary therapy for patients who have symptoms of both allergic and nonallergic rhinitis.

Although the efficacy of intranasal steroids in patients with vasomotor rhinitis has been inconsistent, treatment with topical steroids has been mostly useful for treatment of more severe symptoms in patients in whom an inflammatory pathogenesis is a prominent feature of the disease, for example NARES.

### NONCONVENTIONAL THERAPY

Recent evidence suggests that in patients who do not respond to treatment with nasal steroids or antihistamines, treatment with nonconventional therapies such as silver nitrate,[1] botulinum toxin (Botox),[1] and intranasal capsaicin[2] may be beneficial, because these treatments lead to significant reduction in nasal hyperreactivity, nasal airway resistance, and nasal symptom scores. Studies in patients suffering from NANIPER have demonstrated that intranasal capsaicin leads to a significant and long-term reduction in clinical visual analog scale scores compared with placebo. Treatment once daily for 5 weeks with intranasal capsaicin was also shown to significantly improve all

---
[1]Not FDA approved for this indication.
[2]Not available in the United States.

symptoms and produce a larger vascular response throughout a 6-month follow-up period in patients suffering from severe chronic nonallergic rhinitis with nasal vasoconstrictor abuse. Recently, a double-blind randomized application regimen study showed that five treatments of capsaicin on a single day are at least as effective as five treatments of capsaicin in 2 weeks. However, there is no registered drug available for treatment containing capsaicin in whatever form.

## SURGICAL THERAPY

In cases where nasal obstruction and secretion are resistant to medical treatment and the inferior turbinate is hyperplastic, surgical intervention to reduce the size of the turbinate by various procedures has been shown to be useful. Ethmoidal and vidian neurectomies have also been performed by excision, diathermy, and cryotherapy and have produced results with varying degrees and duration of success.

## REFERENCES

Bousquet J, van Cauwenberge P, Khaltaev N, the ARIA Workshop Group: Allergic rhinitis and its impact on asthma—ARIA Workshop Report. J Allergy Clin Immunol 2001;108(5 suppl): S147-S333.
Dykewicz MS, Fineman S, Skoner DP, et al: Diagnosis and management of rhinitis: Complete guidelines of the Joint Task Force on Practice Parameter in Allergy, Asthma and Immunology. American Academy of Allergy, Asthma, and Immunology. Ann Allergy Asthma Immunol 1998;81(5 pt 2): 478-518.
Fokkens WJ: Thoughts on the pathophysiology of nonallergic rhinitis. Curr Allergy Asthma Rep 2002;2:203-209.
Sanico A, Togias A: Noninfectious, nonallergic rhinitis (NINAR): Considerations on possible mechanisms. Am J Rhinol 1998;12:65-72.
van Cauwenberge PB, Wang D-Y, Ingels KJ, et al: Rhinitis: The spectrum of the disease. In WW Busse and ST Holgate (eds): Asthma and Rhinitis, 2nd ed. Oxford: Blackwell Science, 2000, pp 6-13.

# Hoarseness and Laryngitis

Method of
*Michael Johns, MD, and Rupali Shah, MD*

"Hoarseness" is often used broadly to describe any change in voice quality. It is a common manifesting symptom used to describe a variety of complaints including roughness, voice tremor, phonatory fatigue, breathiness, increased vocal effort, restricted pitch range, and other features. More accurately, hoarseness is the result of abnormal flow of air past the vocal folds (or cords). The voice is harsh if there are irregularities of the vocal folds, such as vocal fold nodules, and it is breathy if there is incomplete glottal closure as air passes through the vocal folds, as in unilateral vocal cord paralysis.

Hoarseness can be divided into two broad categories: acute onset and chronic onset. Acute hoarseness is much more common and is often attributed to local inflammation of laryngitis, which is usually self-limited. Chronic hoarseness, on the other hand, may be caused by a variety of processes including laryngopharyngeal reflux, benign polyps, vocal fold nodules, laryngeal papillomatosis, functional dysphonia, tumors, and neurologic etiologies. A malignant etiology should be considered in patients with hoarseness lasting longer than 2 weeks, particularly in those with a history of tobacco or alcohol use.

*Laryngitis* refers to any acute or chronic inflammatory process involving the larynx. Patients can present with dysphonia, odynophonia, dysphagia, odynophagia, cough, dyspnea, or stridor depending on the etiology, affected region, and severity. Evaluation is critical because laryngeal carcinoma can manifest in a similar manner.

## Acute Laryngitis

### DIAGNOSIS

Inflammation of the larynx and vocal fold mucosa lasting less than 2 weeks is typically referred to as *acute laryngitis*, one of the most common pathologies of the larynx. Laryngeal inflammation can result from a variety of causes, including viral, bacterial, or fungal infection, acid reflux, smoking, toxic inhalation, coughing, vocal abuse, direct injury, and allergic reactions. In adults, acute infectious laryngitis is most commonly caused by a viral upper respiratory infection. Patients complain of general viral symptoms such as sore throat, odynophagia, rhinorrhea, postnasal discharge, and congestion along with dysphonia characterized by voice breaks, episodic aphonia, and low vocal pitch. The vocal fold mucosa appear erythematous and edematous. Although rhinovirus is the most likely causative agent, parainfluenza, influenza, and adenovirus have also been associated with the condition.

Fever, sore throat, muffled voice, and dyspnea suggest bacterial laryngitis or acute epiglottitis. Fiberoptic laryngoscopy reveals a swollen, red supraglottis, and lateral neck x-ray demonstrates a swollen epiglottis—the thumbprint sign. The most common pathogen is *Haemophilus influenzae;* however, *Streptococcus pneumoniae, Staphylococcus aureus,* β-hemolytic streptococci, and *Klebsiella pneumoniae* have also been isolated.

Fungal laryngitis clinically resembles leukoplakia and is often misdiagnosed as such; specific fungal stains are required for diagnosis. Systemically or locally immunosuppressed patients (diabetes, HIV, immunosuppressive drugs, malignancy, smoking, inhaled steroids, and chronic oral steroid use) are particularly susceptible to fungal laryngitis.

### TREATMENT

Therapy for acute laryngitis depends on the etiology. Acute viral laryngitis is a self-limited disease. Treatment includes humidification, hydration, cough suppressants, and expectorants. Voice rest or reduced voice use is important because heavy voice use can lead to injury and possibly scarring of the swollen vocal folds.

Antibiotics are reserved for bacterial infection suggested by appropriate symptoms and clinical presentation. In patients with severe bacterial laryngitis, tracheotomy may be necessary if they experience airway compromise. Humidification, hydration, corticosteroids, intravenous antibiotics, and close observation with serial fiberoptic examinations are indicated in less severe cases. Amoxicillin-clavulanate (Augmentin) is often the antibiotic of choice.

An oral antifungal such as fluconazole (Diflucan 200 mg PO the first day followed by 100 mg PO daily to complete at least a 2-week course) can be used to manage fungal laryngitis.

## Chronic Laryngitis

*Chronic laryngitis* is the term often used to describe vocal disturbances lasting longer than 2 weeks. Chronic laryngitis is not a true diagnosis, and an underlying cause should always be sought.

### LARYNGOPHARYNGEAL REFLUX

#### Diagnosis

Laryngopharyngeal reflux (LPR) is the transient retrograde flow of acid into the larynx and pharynx. Direct mucosal injury can manifest as symptoms of hoarseness, dysphagia, chronic cough, postnasal drip, throat clearing, or globus sensation. Gastroesophageal reflux disease (GERD) is defined as mucosal injury of the esophagus and the structures above it due to retrograde flow of gastric contents; common symptoms include heartburn and regurgitation. LPR usually occurs in the upright position during the daytime as opposed to GERD, which is exacerbated in the supine position. Up to 55% of patients with hoarseness are affected by LPR, and approximately one half of these patients do not experience any dyspepsia or classic symptoms of GERD.

Laryngoscopy can reveal a variety of changes within the larynx including erythematous arytenoids with interarytenoid mucosal hypertrophy, subglottic edema, vocal process granulomas, or vocal fold edema, erythema, or ulceration. Diagnosis may be confirmed by ambulatory 24-hour double-probe pH testing, in which probes are placed 5 cm above the lower esophageal sphincter and just above the upper esophageal sphincter. Proximal probe placement is essential to the diagnosis because a single distal probe can produce false negatives.

## Treatment

Appropriate management of LPR disease is multifactorial and encompasses lifestyle modifications and adjuvant medical therapy. Behavioral changes consist of weight loss, smoking cessation, and alcohol avoidance. Important diet adjustments include limiting chocolate, caffeine, red wines, late-night meals, citrus fruits, and fatty foods. Although $H_2$-receptor antagonists, prokinetic agents, and mucosal cytoprotectants are all effective in treating LPR, proton-pump inhibitors (PPIs) such as omeprazole[1] (Prilosec 20-40 mg bid 30-60 min before meals) are considered the mainstay of treatment. Patients with severe cases may be candidates for surgical intervention.

## BENIGN VOCAL FOLD LESIONS

Vibratory collision during phonation imparts maximal stress in the midmembranous vocal fold. Vocal overuse, abuse, or misuse could lead to excessive stress in this area, resulting in tissue remodeling and formation of vocal fold nodules, polyps, and cysts within the superficial layer of the lamina propria. Distinction between these lesions is made by videostrobolaryngoscopy and, sometimes, intraoperative findings.

### Vocal Fold Nodules

Vocal fold nodules are small bilateral lesions that are fairly symmetric, occurring classically at the border of the anterior one third and middle one third of the vocal fold. They occur most commonly in women and young boys and are also associated with vocally demanding occupations. Mild to moderate lesions might only affect the singing voice and go unnoticed in the speaking voice.

Voice therapy aims to maximize singing and speaking efficiency while reducing additional trauma to the lesions and is the first-line treatment for vocal fold nodules. Voice complaints should resolve and nodules should regress with voice therapy alone. Rarely, surgical removal may be considered. Patients should simultaneously receive therapy for other causes of dysphonia, such as laryngopharyngeal reflux and poor vocal hygiene.

### Vocal Fold Polyps

Vocal fold polyps are translucent to red, mobile lesions on the free edge of the anterior one third of the vocal fold. They are usually unilateral sessile or pedunculated lesions that are occasionally large enough to ball-valve into the glottis and cause intermittent respiratory distress. Acute phonotrauma leads to polyp formation by inducing hemorrhage, edema, and leakage of fibrin. Polyps can also be the result of chronic irritation from smoking, GERD, or muscle tension dysphonia.

For small vocal polyps, voice therapy may be adequate. Many cases, however, require adjuvant phonomicrosurgery. The objective of phonomicrosurgery is to achieve reduced dysphonia with minimal disruption of the microarchitecture of the vocal fold, specifically the epithelium and lamina propria, and to promote maximal recovery of normal mucosal vibration. Postoperatively, most surgeons agree that a period of 4 to 14 days of absolute voice rest following surgery allows better healing and phonation.

### Vocal Fold Cysts

There are two types of vocal fold cysts: mucus-retention cysts, caused by an obstructed glandular duct, and epidermoid cysts, which are congenital or secondary to injury. Cysts are usually unilateral but can also be bilateral. They are located just inferior to the vocal fold epithelium or associated with the ligament. Intraoperatively, the cyst is characterized by a distinct capsule.

Voice therapy can improve dysphonia, but it will not cause complete regression of the cyst. The microflap approach is the preferred phonomicrosurgical technique for submucosal pathology; it preserves epithelium and promotes healing by primary intention. In this approach, an incision is made through the epithelium very close to the lesion; the microflap is elevated, exposing the pathology; the lesion is removed; and the microflap is re-draped. Postoperative voice rest and voice therapy are recommended for the best outcome.

## RECURRENT RESPIRATORY PAPILLOMATOSIS

### Diagnosis

Recurrent respiratory papillomatosis (RRP) is the most common cause of hoarseness in children but can occur at any age. These are benign lesions of viral origin that are most commonly associated with human papilloma virus (HPV) types 6 and 11. Respiratory papillomas are of concern because they have the potential to cause respiratory compromise, and they have a small risk of malignant conversion to squamous cell carcinoma. The disease course is highly variable; some patients experience frequent recurrence rates requiring multiple trips to the operating room, and other cases spontaneously resolve.

The papillomas are pink to white, sessile or pedunculated exophytic growths that often arise in clusters. Lesions may be associated with the nose, the soft palate, the epiglottis, the ventricle, the vocal folds, the carina, and bronchial spurs. Areas of transition from ciliated to squamous epithelium are often involved. Symptoms include hoarseness, stridor, obstruction, and, less commonly, chronic cough, pneumonia, failure to thrive, dyspnea, dysphagia, or an acute life-threatening event. History and physical examination are important and include observation for respiratory distress and auscultation for location of obstruction. Diagnosis can be made by fiberoptic nasopharyngoscopy and laryngoscopy.

### Treatment

Currently, no curative measure exists to completely eliminate viral infection. Goals of management should be to remove the mass, create a patent airway, improve voice quality, and reduce frequency of future surgical procedures. Adjuvant therapy reported, but unproven, includes cidofovir (Vistide)[1] injection, interferon-α, acyclovir (Zovirax),[1] and indole 3-carbinol.

## LARYNGEAL CARCINOMA

### Diagnosis

Laryngeal carcinoma accounts for up to 5% of all malignancies diagnosed annually, and it is closely related to smoking and alcohol use. Laryngeal cancer shows a male predominance, with a peak incidence between the sixth and seventh decades. The vast majority are squamous cell carcinomas arising in the glottis. Cure rates for cancers without lymph node metastases approach 95% depending on the site, size, and extent of invasion. The most common manifesting symptom is hoarseness; however, supraglottic tumors can manifest with symptoms of odynophagia, dysphagia, neck mass, or, rarely, referred ear pain. Subglottic carcinomas often manifest late in respiratory distress with biphasic stridor. Full laryngeal examination is indicated in patients with hoarseness lasting longer than 2 weeks.

---

[1]Not FDA approved for this indication.

---

[1]Not FDA approved for this indication.

## Treatment

Laryngeal cancers are staged according to the TNM (tumor, node, metastasis) system of the American Joint Committee on Cancer, which includes factors of tumor size and extent of invasion, nodal involvement, and presence of metastasis. Early cancers, T1 and T2 lesions, may be treated using single-modality therapy by surgical excision or radiation. More advanced cancers, T3 or T4 lesions, require multimodality therapy such as surgery followed by postoperative radiation. Postlaryngectomy speech options include an artificial larynx or electrolarynx, esophageal speech, or tracheoesophageal puncture.

## NEUROLOGIC VOICE DISORDERS

Neurologic voice disorders include hypokinetic disorders, hyperkinetic disorders, and mixed disorders. Diagnosis relies on history and physical examination, and supportive data may be obtained by laryngeal electromyography. Transnasal flexible laryngoscopy is the ideal way to examine movement disorders. Common neurologic causes of dysphonia include Parkinson's disease, essential tremor, and spasmodic dysphonia.

## Parkinson's Disease

The most common movement disorder in the elderly is Parkinson's disease. Classic symptoms include cogwheel rigidity, pill-rolling tremor, mask facies, and shuffling gait. Voice symptoms include a soft voice with a breathy quality. The patient's perception is that the voice is of normal loudness. Patients can also experience vocal tremor, stuttering, or poor articulation.

Lee Silverman voice therapy is the preferred behavioral technique for dysphonia secondary to Parkinson's disease. The goal is to improve physical effort and sensation of one's own voice. Deep brain stimulation and L-dopa have shown little effect on speech. Laryngeal surgery will not affect articulation. Vocal fold augmentation with collagen has been reported in severe cases.

## Essential Tremor

Essential tremor, usually seen in women, commonly manifests as rhythmic motion of the hands and head. Muscles of the larynx, pharynx, and soft palate and the strap muscles of the neck are also commonly involved and influence speech. Voice symptoms are present during all forms of speech, and the tremor is exacerbated by anxiety.

Systemic medications are commonly used with little response. Botulinum toxin (Botox)[1] injection may be useful, but it often does not completely resolve symptoms.

## Spasmodic Dysphonia

Spasmodic dysphonia (SD) is a focal dystonia of adult onset and female predominance that affects the intrinsic muscles of the larynx. There are two major subtypes, abductor SD and, much more commonly, adductor SD. A harsh, strained voice with a strangled quality is typical of adductor SD. These patients experience intermittent breaks during vowel-laden phrases such as "we eat eggs every day." Patients with abductor SD present with a breathy voice and intermittent breaks as they change from voiceless to voiced phonemes such as "she," "he," and "me." The muscle spasms usually affect only the speaking voice; other laryngeal functions, including singing, breathing, swallowing, and coughing, are largely unaffected.

The mainstay of treatment for spasmodic dysphonia has become transcutaneous or transoral botulinum toxin[1] injections. Patients with adductor SD undergo injection of the thyroarytenoid muscles, and patients with abductor SD undergo injection of the posterior cricothyroid muscles. Duration of effect varies from 3 to 6 months, with shorter duration and more variability of effect in abductor SD. Side effects of adductor injections include breathiness and difficulty

---

[1]Not FDA approved for this indication.

 **CURRENT DIAGNOSIS**

- *Laryngitis* is not synonymous with *hoarseness*; *laryngitis* describes any process causing inflammation of the larynx.
- In adults, acute infectious laryngitis is most commonly caused by a viral upper respiratory infection.
- Hoarseness lasting longer than 2 weeks is an indication for laryngeal examination.
- Common symptoms of laryngopharyngeal reflux include hoarseness, cough, throat clearing, or globus sensation. Heartburn and regurgitation are often not present.
- Laryngeal carcinoma is closely related to smoking and alcohol and often manifests with hoarseness. Less common symptoms include dysphagia, neck mass, or biphasic stridor.
- The most common type of laryngeal carcinoma is squamous cell carcinoma of the glottis.
- Neurologic voice disorders are largely diagnosed by history and physical examination; laryngeal electromyography can aid in diagnosis.
- Breathiness, weak voice, weak cough, and difficulty swallowing are all signs of vocal fold paralysis and concern for aspiration.
- Vocal fold paralysis most commonly results from nonlaryngeal carcinoma and iatrogenic causes.

---

swallowing liquids; side effects of abductor injections can include airway compromise secondary to paralysis.

## VOCAL FOLD PARALYSIS

### Diagnosis

A paralyzed vocal fold is laterally displaced, allowing air escape and inadequate glottal closure. The voice disturbance may be vocal fatigue,

 **CURRENT THERAPY**

- Treatment of acute viral laryngitis includes humidification, hydration, cough suppressants, expectorants, and voice rest.
- Antibiotics are reserved for symptoms of bacterial infections (fever, sore throat, muffled voice, and dyspnea).
- Management of laryngopharyngeal reflux includes lifestyle modifications with adjuvant use of a proton-pump inhibitor in most cases; $H_2$-blockers are usually insufficient.
- Vocal fold nodules are treated primarily with voice therapy in most cases.
- Phonomicrosurgery aims to improve vocal function while preserving mucosa; absolute voice rest postoperatively is essential for the best outcomes.
- Surgical excision or radiation is adequate treatment for early laryngeal cancers; late stage cancers require multimodality therapy.
- Intralaryngeal botulinum toxin injections can improve symptoms of spasmodic dysphonia.
- Vocal fold paralysis commonly calls for surgical intervention, which includes injection augmentation or medialization by thyroplasty, without or with arytenoid adduction.

near aphonia, breathiness, or weakness. Patients might also have a weak cough and difficulty swallowing, causing concern for risk of aspiration. Supraglottic hyperfunction is a common compensatory mechanism that can cause the voice to sound improved.

Unilateral vocal fold paralysis can be caused by disruption of vocal fold innervation anywhere along its path. Of the various etiologies, the most common cause of paralysis is nonlaryngeal malignancy, namely bronchogenic carcinoma and skull base tumors. Iatrogenic causes fall closely behind and include surgical procedures (e.g., thyroidectomy, esophagectomy, thymectomy, neck dissection, carotid endarterectomy, anterior cervical spine procedures), endotracheal intubation, or prolonged nasogastric tube placement. Other causes include idiopathic disorders (one third of cases), neck and chest trauma, thoracic aneurysm, stroke, and other neurologic disorders.

In cases where there is a clear temporal relationship between an iatrogenic cause and presentation of paralysis, no further work-up is necessary. If no cause for vocal fold paralysis can be identified, computed tomography (CT) with contrast or magnetic resonance imaging (MRI) from skull base to upper chest is indicated.

## Treatment

Laryngeal electromyography can provide useful prognostic information regarding whether or not a recurrent laryngeal nerve will regain function. A transected nerve or one that has been infiltrated by malignancy will not resume function, whereas a bruised or stretched nerve may be expected to return to normal function within 6 months to 1 year. Speech therapy might help the patient gain compensation from the opposite vocal fold.

Surgical intervention provides excellent rehabilitation. Surgical options include medialization of the affected vocal fold by endoscopic injection of a bulking material such as collagen or fat. Teflon should not be used because long-term fibrotic reactions are noted and irreversible. Injection augmentation is a temporary measure, lasting weeks to months, and may be used to improve the voice while awaiting return of function or another procedure. Thyroplasty, the most common treatment, is a transcervical approach to repositioning the affected vocal fold through placing implant material deep to the thyroid cartilage. Arytenoid adduction is an adjunctive procedure in some cases and consists of placing a suture from the muscular process of the arytenoid to the anterior portion of the thyroid cartilage. This action will simulate adduction and medialize the vocal process.

## REFERENCES

Derkay CS, Darrow DH: Recurrent respiratory papillomatosis. Ann Otol Rhinol Laryngol 2006;115(1):1-11.

Dikkers FG, Nikkels PG: Lamina propria of the mucosa of benign lesions of the vocal folds. Laryngoscope 1999;109(10):1684-1689.

Ford CN: Evaluation and management of laryngopharyngeal reflux. JAMA 2005;294(12):1534-1540.

Johns, MM: Update on the etiology, diagnosis, and treatment of vocal fold nodules, polyps, and cysts. Curr Opin Otolaryngol Head Neck Surg 2003;11:456-461.

Koufman JA: The otolaryngologic manifestations of gastroesophageal reflux disease (GERD): A clinical investigation of 225 patients using ambulatory 24-hour pH monitoring and an experimental investigation of the role of acid and pepsin in the development of laryngeal injury. Laryngoscope 1991;101(53 supp):1-78.

Montgomery WW, Montgomery SK: Montgomery thyroplasty implant system. Ann Otol Rhinol Laryngol 1997;170(supp):1-16.

Pontes P, Avelino M, Pignatari S, Weckx LLM: Effect of local application of cidofovir on the control of recurrences in recurrent laryngeal papillomatosis. Otolaryngol Head Neck Surg 2006;135(1):22-27.

Ramadan HH, Wax MK, Avery S: Outcome and changing cause of unilateral vocal cord paralysis. Otolaryngol Head Neck Surg 1998;118:199-202.

# Streptococcal Pharyngitis

Method of
*John Brusch, MD*

The pharyngitis syndrome (sore throat) is characterized primarily by sore throat with associated fever and myalgias; occasionally with cough. It is responsible for 10% of outpatient visits and an estimated 50% of ambulatory care antibiotic usage. Of adult patients who receive treatment for a sore throat, 73% receive antibiotic treatment when at least 50% of these cases are of viral etiology. The increase in the overall resistance to antibiotics of the oral pharyngeal flora is due, in great part, to this overprescribing of antimicrobial agents. A variety of bacteria and viruses may produce this syndrome. Group A β-hemolytic streptococci (GABHS) is the most common bacterial cause of acute pharyngitis. The diagnosis of "strep throat" has long been a concern of the physician because of its suppurative and nonsuppurative complications. There is such a great deal of overlap in their clinical presentations that the clinician must rely on the laboratory to diagnose GABHS from both other bacteria and viruses as the cause of the sore throat of his/her patient. The correct interpretation of the available diagnostic tests adds to the clinician's burden. For more than 50 years, the appropriate choice of antibiotic and duration of treatment of GABHS pharyngitis has been established. The real challenge of treating streptococcal pharyngitis lies not in the selection of treatment, but in deciding when to institute antibiotic therapy.

## Microbiology

Most sore throats are viral in origin. GABHS is responsible for 10% of cases of adult pharyngitis. Its importance lies in the fact that its treatment can prevent the development of rheumatic fever and local complications. Gonorrheal pharyngitis primarily arises from oral sex, but may be a complication of disseminated gonorrhea. It is usually asymptomatic but may produce a typical sore throat. *Yersinia* pharyngitis, like that of groups C and G streptococci, is foodborne. In United States, *Corynebacterium diphtheriae* pharyngitis occurs primarily among the homeless often in outbreaks. It may not be associated with any systemic symptoms. *Arcanobacterium haemolyticum* is a true mimic of GABHS pharyngitis. This organism is more common in Scandinavia and in the United Kingdom than in other parts of the world. It produces a scarlatiniform rash involving the trunk and extremities (50% of cases) with a vesicular component. Occasionally a membranous exudate, resembling that of diphtheria, occurs. Anaerobic oral pharyngeal overgrowth can produce a severe sore throat (Plaut-Vincent or fusospirochetal angina). It is caused by an anaerobic, nonsporulating gram-negative rod. Infection with this organism classically results in an ulceration of the throat or tonsils that is covered by a grayish membrane. Widespread necrosis of surrounding tissue and sepsis may ensue. The presence of fusospirochetal angina may be a clue to a severe leukopenic state in the host. Cases of *Chlamydia pneumoniae* and *Mycoplasma pneumoniae* sore throat are usually seen with concurrent lung infection. The clinical courses may be quite prolonged. Unresponsiveness to the penicillins provides a useful clue to their presence. Many species of bacteria are commonly cultured from the upper airway. *Staphylococcus aureus*, *Streptococcus pneumoniae*, and *Haemophilus influenzae* are part of the normal pharyngeal flora, especially during the winter. They seldom cause pharyngitis. Their isolation from symptomatic individuals usually represents colonization.

Epstein-Barr virus (EBV) infections of the throat are marked by an exudate pharyngitis with palatal petechiae and a gelatinous uvula. In patients older than 30 years of age, only 25% of EBV pharyngitis presents with the classic picture of diffuse cervical adenopathy, diffuse adenopathy, lymphocytosis, and splenomegaly. These patients often develop a diffuse scarlatiniform rash approximately 5 days into a course of ampicillin or other β-lactam antibiotics ("fifth-day rash"). The pharyngitis of *Cytomegalovirus* and herpesvirus type 6 may present in similar fashion to that of EBV without the fifth-day rash. Primary human immunodeficiency virus (HIV) infection may cause a sore throat that is characterized by a nonexudate pharyngitis fever, diffuse lymphadenopathy, and a maculopapular rash within 1 to 5 weeks of acquisition. Acute retroviral infection is truly a "cannot miss" diagnosis.

## Epidemiology

GABHS pharyngitis primarily affects individuals 5 to 15 years of age. Up to 20% of these are carriers of GABHS. Infection is most commonly spread from human to human by large airborne droplets. The cold weather of winter and early spring produces the highest attack rates as a consequence of the indoor crowding that occurs during these seasons. Symptomatic patients, closeness of contact, and virulent strains are factors that promote spread of the disease. Transmission by both food and water is well documented.

During the acute phase of the illness, M-type streptococci are frequently isolated from the nares and oropharynx. Colonization of the upper airway with these strains can last for several months. Gradually, the streptococci lose their M proteins and with this loss their infectivity. Antibody to the M protein confers type-specific immunity to the host. The carrier state results from the ability of particular strains to penetrate the interior of respiratory epithelial cells. In this location, GABHS is protected from type-specific M protein antibody, from the suppressive effects of the host's oral flora, and from the actions of many types of antibiotics. In the developed world, both suppurative and nonsuppurative complications of GABHS pharyngitis have greatly lessened. This is a result of an overall improvement in living conditions (less crowding) and to the disappearance of M protein from many isolates of GABHS. This decreased pathogenicity has to be factored into any treatment strategy for "strep throat." However, the inner cities of the United States still provide conditions that are conducive to the development of poststreptococcal rheumatic fever.

## Clinical Manifestations

Fever (>100.4°F [38°C]) and sore throat are invariably present in GABHS pharyngitis. The presence of rhinitis, laryngitis, diarrhea, conjunctivitis and bronchitis are inconsistent with this diagnosis and are more characteristic of a viral etiology. Examination reveals pharyngeal erythema or exudative pharyngitis, with or without palatal petechiae, that is associated with significant anterior cervical adenopathy. Untreated, 75% of patients defervesce within 3 days unless there is a local suppurative complication. This may include peritonsillar abscess, suppurative adenitis, and otitis media. Over a few more days, the individual's other signs and symptoms resolve. In the absence of antibiotic therapy, most patients carry streptococci for many months. With appropriate treatment, the carrier state is reduced to between 6% and 29% of patients.

## Diagnosis

Although the diagnosis of GABHS pharyngitis cannot be based solely on clinical signs and symptoms, they have been quite useful in establishing the likelihood of streptococcal infection; especially in adults with an extremely low incidence of "strep throat." Determining the probability of GABHS pharyngitis is essential for establishing indications for diagnostic testing, as well as for interpreting the results of these tests. Several such scoring systems stratifying the importance of physical findings and symptoms have been developed. All are quite similar and include the presence of (a) fever higher than 99.9°F (37.7°C), (b) tonsillar exudate, and (c) anterior cervical adenopathy, and (d) absence of cough. The presence of all four makes the probability of GABHS 56%. When three conditions exist, the likelihood decreases to 32% and plummets to 15% and 6% when there are two and one positive indicators, respectively. If there are no positive indicators, the probability of a positive culture is less than 2.5%. At this level of risk, diagnostic testing is usually not required.

The throat culture remains the diagnostic gold standard. The throat should be swabbed under direct visualization in repeated sweeps extending from each tonsillar fossa and involving the posterior pharynx but avoiding any other area of the mouth. The swabs should be immediately cultured on sheep blood agar incubated in 10% $CO_2$. If there is no growth at 24 hours, the plate is re-incubated for another 24 hours. Sampling errors may cause false negatives in 9% to 12% of patients. Rarely, GABHS will not produce β hemolysis. False positives may be due to β hemolysis produced by non-GABHS organisms.

## CURRENT DIAGNOSIS

| Organism | % of Cases | Comments |
| --- | --- | --- |
| Viral organisms | Total = 40% | Often associated with coryza, laryngitis, and diarrhea |
| Rhinovirus | 20% | |
| Coronavirus | 5% | |
| Herpes simplex | 2% | |
| Retroviruses | ?% | Present in 70% of cases of primary HIV infection |
| Primary Epstein-Barr | ?% | Only 25% exhibit other manifestations of mononucleosis viral infection |
| Coxsackievirus | ?% | Concurrent findings of herpangina and hand, foot, and mouth disease |
| Adenovirus | ?% | Concurrent conjunctivitis |
| Bacterial organisms | Total = ?% | |
| GABHS | 30%-50% in children; 10% in adults | 1%-5% of adults are carriers of GABHS |
| Groups C, G streptococci | 10% | Often foodborne |
| Nonstreptococcal bacteria | 10% | |
| *Neisseria gonorrhoeae* | 1% | May be the only manifestation of gonorrhea; associated with oral sex |
| *Yersinia enterocolitica* | ?% | Often foodborne |
| *Corynebacterium diphtheriae* | ?% | Seen in the homeless; often pharyngitis is the only manifestation |
| *Arcanobacterium hemolyticum* | 0.4% | Causes a diffuse scarlatiniform rash; it is indistinguishable from GABHS pharyngitis |

*Abbreviations:* GABHS, group A β-hemolytic streptococci.

The use of the bacitracin disk controls for this by inhibiting GABHS but not other types of β hemolytic flora. The specificity of the throat culture ranges from 95% to 99% with 88% to 91% sensitivity. When obtained in physicians' offices, the throat cultures are much less sensitive (<75%). The major disadvantage of the throat culture is the diagnostic delay. In adults, this may not be all that significant (see below).

Rapid antigen detection tests (RADTs) were developed to provide useful probability information at the time of the patient's visit. RADTs employ either enzyme or acid techniques to extract streptococcal antigen from the swabs, which is then measured by latex agglutination, coagglutination, or enzyme-linked immunosorbent assay (ELISA) techniques. Overall, the sensitivity of RADTs ranges from 77% to 95%. The higher range of values is associated with the newer optical immunoassay technique, which may approach the sensitivity of a well-performed throat culture. The specificity of the RADT is as high as that of the throat culture. Because of its low sensitivity, a negative RADT in any child or adolescent should be followed by a throat culture. In adults, this approach is not thought to be necessary because of the low incidence of GABHS pharyngitis and rheumatic fever in this population. However, when only an RADT is performed, the opportunity to detect a treatable non-GABHS cause of bacterial pharyngitis is lost.

Both throat culture and RADT are unable to distinguish streptococcal carriers from those whose symptoms are caused by GABHS and not by another organism. Of symptomatic adult patients with positive diagnostic tests, 30% to 50% are not infected with GABHS. Measurement of antibody titers against streptolysin O (ASL-O) or other streptococcal products is the most specific way to diagnose GABHS pharyngitis. Their levels require 2 to 4 weeks to peak and thus are not available to the clinician in a timely fashion.

## Treatment

In the developed world, the reasons why we treat GABHS pharyngitis have markedly changed since the landmark studies that demonstrated such a significant drop in the incidence of poststreptococcal rheumatic fever. This is attributable to the change in epidemiology of the streptococcus (Table 1). In the early days of antimicrobial therapy, it was established that 10 days of treatment with oral penicillin or one intramuscular injection of penicillin G was effective in preventing rheumatic fever if begun within 5 to 9 days after the onset of clinical symptoms of GABHS pharyngitis. It was also demonstrated that for

### CURRENT THERAPY

- Empirically treat all patients with 3 or more clinical predictors of GABHS pharyngitis.
- Optimal treatment still remains 10 days of oral penicillin or one injection of Bicillin.
- Avoid 3-day treatment regimens.
- Avoid trimethoprim-sulfamethoxazole and the tetracyclines (doxycycline). They have little effect on eradicating GABHS.
- Always keep in mind that culture of GABHS from an adult may represent a carrier state and that the pharyngitis is produced by another organism.
- Do not reculture at the end of clinically successful therapy unless the patient has an above-average risk for developing rheumatic fever.
- Always keep in mind the possibility of primary HIV infection as the cause of the pharyngitis.
- Do not culture family members unless there is an epidemic situation of or recurrence of proven GABHS pharyngitis in the family.
- Do not give prophylactic antibiotics to exposed family members.

**TABLE 1 Reasons for Treating Streptococcal Pharyngitis**

| Item | Rationale |
| --- | --- |
| Preventing rheumatic fever | Rheumatic fever occurs in 2.1% of untreated patients and in 0.3% of treated patients |
| Preventing streptococcal glomerulonephritis | No evidence that treatment of streptococcal pharyngitis is effective |
| Preventing scarlet fever | Extremely rare in the antibiotic era |
| Reducing suppurative complications | They accounted for 13% of hospitalizations in the pre-antibiotic era; currently quite unusual |
| Reducing duration and severity of disease | Antibiotics have some mild effect when started early |
| Reducing spread of GABHS | Quite effective in preventing spread; patients become noncontagious after 24 hours of treatment |

*Abbreviation:* GABHS, group A β-hemolytic streptococci.

**TABLE 2 Management Strategies for GABHS Pharyngitis**

| Number of Positive Features | Action |
| --- | --- |
| 0 | No culture; no treatment |
| 1 | Culture; treat positive cultures |
| 2 | Culture; treat positive cultures |
| 3 | No culture or treatment |
| 4 | No culture or treatment |

*Abbreviation:* GABHS, group A β-hemolytic streptococci.

**TABLE 3 Current Therapy**

| Drug | Dose | Duration of Therapy |
| --- | --- | --- |
| Penicillin V (Pen-Vee K) | 1000 mg bid,[3] 25 mg/kg bid* | 10 d |
| Benzathine penicillin (Bicillin) | 1.2 million U, 2500 U/kg* | 1 dose |
| Cephalexin (Keflex) | 500 mg bid, 25 mg/kg bid | 10 d |
| Cefadroxil (Duricef) | 1 g/d, 30 mg/kg/d* | 5 d[†] |
| Cefuroxime (Ceftin) | 250 mg bid, 10 mg/kg bid* | 5 d[†] |
| Amoxicillin-clavulanate (Augmentin)[‡,1] | 250 mg tid, 15 mg/kg tid* | 10 d |
| Azithromycin (Zithromax) | 500 mg first day, then 250 mg qd; 12 mg/kg qd | 5 d[†] |
| Clarithromycin (Biaxin) | 500 mg bid, 8 mg/kg bid* | 10 d |

*For children who weigh less than 40 kg (88 lb).
[†]Only azithromycin is approved by the Food and Drug Administration for less than 10 days of therapy.
[‡]Useful for recurrent GABHS pharyngitis or treatment of the carrier state if necessary.
[1]Not FDA approved for this indication.
[3]Exceeds dosage recommended by the manufacturer.
Abbreviation: GABHS, group A β-hemolytic streptococci.

those patients in whom penicillin failed to eradicate GABHS, the risk of developing rheumatic fever was the same as that of an untreated patient. Table 2 presents the clinical indications for obtaining a throat culture/RADT and beginning antibiotic treatment. I prefer a culture over RADT as it is generally more sensitive and detects other possible pathogens. Its 1- to 2-day delay in receiving final results has little clinical significance. It was recently demonstrated that culture is the most effective and least expensive approach when the prevalence of GABHS pharyngitis is 10% or less. Empirical antibiotic treatment was found to be neither the most clinically useful nor cost-effective strategy for any degree of risk. This stepped approach holds true only for adults in the developed world who have no history of rheumatic fever, immunosuppression, or chronic pharyngitis. It is not applicable during an epidemic of GABHS/rheumatic fever. Eradication of the carrier state is not an indication for treatment unless the patient has a history of rheumatic fever. It is unnecessary to do sensitivity testing of GABHS for any of the β-lactam antibiotics. GABHS remains quite sensitive to penicillin. The administration of oral penicillin for 10 days achieves almost 100% effectiveness in eradicating GABHS. In those who have been treated for 7 days or 5 days, the cure rate decreases to 89% and 50%, respectively.

In penicillin-allergic patients, erythromycin has traditionally been the alternative drug of choice. In the United States, 4% to 5% of isolates are resistant to erythromycin. Resistance to erythromycin is significantly higher in those countries where it is more commonly used as a first-line drug. The other macrolides hold no therapeutic advantage over erythromycin, but are much better tolerated, especially as regards the gastrointestinal tract. In my opinion, clindamycin (Cleocin) rarely should be used because of the significant risk of developing *Clostridium difficile* colitis. The most desirable treatment regimen remains 10 days of penicillin therapy. If compliance is in doubt, one dose of Bicillin is next best. The other β-lactams offer little advantage except for 5-day courses. There is some indication that they may have a somewhat higher clinical and bacteriologic success rate because of their resistance to breakdown by penicillinase-producing oral pharyngeal flora. They have as yet not stood the test of time. Three-day regimens should be avoided because of unacceptably high rates of failure and recurrence. More complete discussions of antibiotic therapy of GABHS pharyngitis are available in the referenced sources (Table 3).

Recurrence of GABHS has increased in the last 20 years from 9% of cases to greater than 30% currently. This has been paralleled by a slight decline in the bacteriologic and clinical success rates, currently 84% and 89%, respectively. Table 4 presents several possible reasons for these trends.

After a successful clinical result, there is no need to repeat the throat culture unless during an outbreak of rheumatic fever or in an individual who has already been stricken by the disease. In the antibiotic era, tonsillectomy for preventing relapse or recurrence is rarely necessary.

## REFERENCES

Bisno AL: Acute pharyngitis. N Engl J Med 2001;344:205.
Bisno JL, Gerber MA, Gwaltney JM, et al: IDSA practice guidelines for the diagnosis and management of group A streptococcal pharyngitis. Clin Infect Dis 2002;35:113.

**TABLE 4 Reasons for Apparent Recurrent GABHS Pharyngitis**

| Cause | Solution |
|---|---|
| Not truly a GABHS pharyngitis (most likely to be of viral origin) | Document infection by culture or RADT (see text) |
| Poor compliance (most frequent cause of recurrence) | Choose 5-day antibiotic regimen or intramuscular benzathine penicillin |
| Repeated exposure to GABHS, especially in families (ping-pong phenomenon) | Culture samples from all family members and treat culture-positive individuals |
| Decreased host immunity to GABHS because of initiation of antibiotic therapy within 48 hours of the onset of symptoms | Delay antibiotic treatment for 48 hours; this does not increase the risk for suppurative or nonsuppurative complications |
| Coexistence of β lactamase-producing bacteria (becoming a more common problem) | Use a β lactamase-resistant antibiotic (cephalosporin or amoxicillin-clavulanate) |
| Patient is carrier for GABHS and pharyngitis is caused by another organism, usually a virus | Confirm by positive culture or RADT in asymptomatic period; also obtain ASL-O titer for weeks after infection (should not show rise in the carrier state); generally no need to treat; if necessary to intervene, use a macrolide or amoxicillin-clavulanate |
| Deep-seated GABHS infection (i.e., tonsillar crypts) | Use intraleukocytic-active antibiotic such as a quinolone or a macrolide |
| Inadequate dose of penicillin | Increase dose or use better-absorbed form (amoxicillin) |

*Abbreviations:* ASL-O, antistreptolysin O; GABHS, group A β-hemolytic streptococci; RADT, rapid antigen detection test.

Gerber MA, Shulman ST: Rapid diagnosis of pharyngitis caused by group A streptococci. Clin Microbiol Rev 2004;17:571.
Komaroff AL: Pharyngitis coryza and related infections in adults. In: Branch WT Jr (ed): Office Practice of Medicine. Philadelphia, WB Saunders, 2003, p. 153.
Stollerman GH: Global changes in group A streptococcal diseases and strategies for their prevention. Adv Intern Med 1982;27:373.

# The Respiratory System

## Acute Respiratory Failure

Method of
*William Henderson, MD, and Sean Keenan, MD*

The maintenance of normal respiration requires adequate oxygen and carbon dioxide ($CO_2$) exchange at the alveolar-capillary interface. For this to occur, there must be adequate minute ventilation, perfusion to capillaries, and appropriate delivery and distribution of gas within the lungs. Failure to properly regulate any of these facets of normal respiration will lead to respiratory failure and, if uncorrected, death.

Respiratory failure is characterized by a failure of oxygenation or ventilation. Therefore, acute respiratory failure is commonly divided into hypoxemic and hypercapnic etiologies.

## Causes of Hypoxic Respiratory Failure

### HYPOVENTILATION

Hypoventilation occurs when there is a central decrease in the drive to breathe, most commonly secondary to medications (e.g., morphine, benzodiazepines). As minute ventilation drops, increased alveolar $CO_2$ displaces oxygen, decreasing the oxygen available for capillary uptake. This occurs because the combined partial pressures of all of the gases within an alveolus must equal atmospheric pressure.

### VENTILATION-PERFUSION MISMATCH

Ventilation-perfusion mismatch is caused by imperfect matching of ventilated and perfused lung units, usually secondary to alveolar injury, infection, or fluid.

### SHUNTS

Shunts may be intracardiac or intrapulmonary. Intracardiac shunts are usually through a patent foramen ovale, but atrial and ventricular septal defects are occasionally seen. Intrapulmonary shunting occurs when blood flows past unventilated alveoli. Whatever the etiology of the shunt, it can be differentiated from ventilation-perfusion mismatching, because it is refractory to increasing alveolar oxygen tension (the application of supplemental oxygen does not relieve the hypoxemia).

### IMPAIRMENT OF DIFFUSION

Impairment of diffusion is caused by short red blood cell transit time through the pulmonary vasculature or because of thickening of the endothelial barrier in the lungs. Diffusion impairment rarely causes hypoxia at rest but can cause hypoxia during exercise.

### DECREASED INSPIRED OXYGEN CONCENTRATION

Decreased inspired oxygen concentration, whether because of high altitude or the presence of other gases, decreases alveolar oxygen tension.

Most patients with hypoxic respiratory failure have a right-to-left intrapulmonary shunt with some ventilation-perfusion mismatch.

## Hypercapnic Respiratory Failure

Arterial $CO_2$ concentrations are inversely proportional to alveolar minute ventilation and are determined by tissue $CO_2$ production and alveolar elimination. Alveolar minute ventilation can be impaired in two ways. First, total minute ventilation can be decreased by extrapulmonary diseases; and second, dead space ventilation may be increased because of lung disease. Dead space ventilation is defined as ventilation that is not delivered to alveoli; in other words it is the ventilation to portions of the airway, such as the trachea, bronchi, and unperfused alveoli, that are not involved in gas exchange.

Primary pulmonary diseases are the most common causes of hypercapnic respiratory failure and are the single greatest cause of admission to the intensive care unit.

## Clinical Presentation

Although dyspnea is the most common symptom associated with acute respiratory failure, the presentation to some degree depends on the precipitating problem. Patients who develop acute hypoxemic respiratory failure will usually have a clear recent history that points to a precipitating cause, such as trauma, pneumonia, sepsis, or pulmonary embolism. Typically, these patients demonstrate significant distress, with tachypnea and agitation as prominent symptoms. Physical examination may reveal signs consistent with the inciting disease, and chest examination will often reveal inspiratory crackles and decreased air entry in affected lung portions.

Patients with predominantly hypercapnic respiratory failure will also exhibit signs and symptoms consistent with the precipitating disease. Patients with recent opioid or benzodiazepine use as a cause of hypoventilation may exhibit a clear troxidone. Those with neuromuscular diseases will typically have a past medical history that points to the cause of their respiratory failure. Most patients with an exacerbation of chronic obstructive respiratory disease (COPD) or of asthma will have a medical history that points to these diseases, and will typically have a recent history that is significant for a gradual and steady worsening of their bronchospastic symptoms. Many of these patients will describe steady and increasing use of bronchodilators over the several days prior to presentation. Physical examination in hypercarbic respiratory failure patients is often helpful in narrowing the differential diagnosis. Patients with a central or toxicologic cause of hypercarbic respiratory failure usually have clear lungs on auscultation and will not exhibit intercostal in drawing or accessory muscle use. Those with an exacerbation of COPD or asthma will often have both of these signs.

## Diagnosis

Initial investigations in the diagnosis of acute respiratory failure include physical examination, pulse oximetry, arterial blood gas analysis and chest radiograph. In some situations, it may be necessary to investigate further through the use of computerized tomography or lung biopsy to establish a diagnosis.

Arterial blood gas analysis is central to the diagnosis and management of acute respiratory failure. Accepted normal values for $PaO_2$ decline with age because of structural changes in the lungs and may be calculated using the formula:

$$PaO_2 = 100.1 - 0.323 \times age$$

While breathing room air, a $PaO_2$ of 55 mm Hg or less is consistent with significant hypoxemic respiratory failure. However, when patients receive supplemental $O_2$, $PaO_2$ may be significantly elevated. It is useful in this situation to calculate a $PaO_2$ to $FIO_2$ ratio (P/F) to account for this increase in alveolar $O_2$ concentration. Patients with normal gas exchange demonstrate a P/F of greater than 500, whereas a P/F of less than 300 is consistent with significant oxygen exchange abnormalities, and less than 200 is consistent with acute respiratory distress syndrome (ARDS).

In healthy patients, the normal range for $PCO_2$ is 35 to 45 mm Hg. Levels higher than this are seen in both chronic and acute hypercarbic respiratory failure. In chronic conditions compensatory reactions increase serum bicarbonate levels to decrease the drop in pH caused by hypercarbia. It is therefore often possible to determine the acuity of the hypercarbia by evaluating the serum bicarbonate level; in chronic hypercarbia, bicarbonate levels will be elevated beyond the normal range, whereas in acute hypercarbia, compensation will not yet have occurred, and bicarbonate levels will be normal.

### CURRENT DIAGNOSIS

- Acute respiratory failure is divided into hypoxemic and hypercapnic etiologies.
- Initial investigations in the diagnosis of acute respiratory failure include physical examination, pulse oximetry, arterial blood gas analysis and chest x-ray.
- Normal values for $PaO_2$ can be calculated using the formula: $PaO_2 = 100.1 - 0.323 \times age$
- On breathing room air, a $PaO_2$ of 55 mm Hg or less is consistent with significant hypoxemic respiratory failure
- In healthy patients, the normal range for $PCO_2$ is 35 to 45 mm Hg. Levels higher than this are seen in both chronic and acute hypercarbic respiratory failure
- In patients with hypoxic respiratory failure, chest radiography often allows the clinician to rapidly narrow the differential diagnosis based on whether the chest x-ray shows normal lung parenchyma, focal abnormalities or diffuse bilateral abnormalities.
- In hypercarbic respiratory failure, the chest x-ray allows the clinician to appreciate the degree of hyperinflation present during exacerbations of COPD or asthma, and may help determine whether an infection has precipitated this exacerbation.

The chest radiograph is an invaluable tool in the diagnosis of respiratory failure. In patients with hypoxic respiratory failure, chest radiography often allows the clinician to rapidly narrow the differential diagnosis based on whether the chest radiograph shows normal lung parenchyma, focal abnormalities or diffuse bilateral abnormalities. In hypercarbic respiratory failure, the chest radiograph allows the clinician to appreciate the degree of hyperinflation present during exacerbations of COPD or asthma and may help determine whether an infection has precipitated this exacerbation. In patients with hypercarbic respiratory failure caused by abnormalities of the central nervous system, the chest radiograph may allow the diagnosis of complicating aspiration pneumonitis.

## Management

The goals of management in acute respiratory failure are to support oxygenation and ventilation, diagnose and treat the underlying cause, and avoid iatrogenic injury.

Maintenance of oxygenation may initially be achieved through the application of supplemental oxygen in an attempt to maintain a $PaO_2$ greater than 65 to 70 mm Hg ($SaO_2 > 92\%$). If this provides insufficient support, consideration should be given to noninvasive positive-pressure ventilation (NPPV) or intubation and mechanical ventilation.

Noninvasive positive-pressure ventilation may be suitable for properly selected patients suffering from acute hypoxic respiratory failure and may decrease the need for mechanical ventilation and decrease morbidity in these patients. However, great caution must be used in the selection of hypoxic patients for NPPV, because it is not an appropriate therapy to use in unstable patients or those with impaired airway protection. Tolerance for NPPV may be improved by using a nasal mask and starting with low inspiratory pressure (e.g., 5 cm $H_2O$).

### CURRENT THERAPY

- Maintain oxygenation with supplemental oxygen in an attempt to maintain a $PaO_2$ greater than 65-70 mm Hg ($SaO_2 > 92\%$).
- β-adrenergic bronchodilators such as albuterol (Ventolin) may decrease bronchospasm in patients with acute exacerbations of COPD or asthma.
- Anticholinergic bronchodilators such as ipratropiurn bromide (Atrovent) may produce added benefit.
- Corticosteroids are used to treat significant exacerbations of diseases associated with bronchospasm and inflammation
- NIPPV has a clear role in the treatment of stable, alert patients with hypercarbic respiratory failure.
- Indications for intubation and mechanical ventilation include: failure of ventilation, failure of oxygenation, failure of airway protection, and inability to manage secretions or pulmonary toilet
- Large tidal volumes during mechanical ventilation worsen lung injury and survival in ARDS patients. In these patients a target tidal volume of no more than 4 to 6 cc/kg predicted body weight may prevent ventilator induced lung injury.
- In hypercarbic respiratory failure caused by exacerbations of COPD or asthma, low levels of PEEP can decrease the work of breathing performed by patients, allowing them to decrease their $CO_2$ production, and decreasing their propensity to develop respiratory muscle failure.
- High levels of PEEP are also associated with barotraumas such as pneumothorax and pneumomediastinum

For patients who are too unstable or who are unable to tolerate NPPV, intubation and mechanical ventilation may be necessary.

In patients with hypoxic respiratory failure secondary to ARDS, careful attention to how ventilatory support is supplied may prevent further lung injury from iatrogenic causes. Recent evidence demonstrates that overly aggressive tidal volumes during mechanical ventilation worsen lung injury and survival in ARDS patients. It is prudent to target a tidal volume of no more than 4 to 6 cc/kg predicted body weight in these patients, and to tolerate lower $PaO_2$ and higher $PCO_2$ than normal in these patients.

Concurrent with support of oxygenation, the treatment of acute hypoxic respiratory failure requires the diagnosis and treatment of the underlying disease. In cases of pneumonia or aspiration, early antibiotic use is recommended, whereas in pulmonary edema, the use of afterload reducing agents (nitroglycerin- or angiotensin-converting enzyme inhibitors) and diuretics such as furosemide (Lasix 20 to 60 mg IV every 6 hours) may be needed. The medical care of patients with pulmonary contusions or alveolar hemorrhage is largely supportive, whereas the management of pulmonary embolism requires anticoagulation, and occasionally, the use of fibrinolytics.

During the treatment of hypercarbic respiratory failure, maintenance of oxygenation is usually less difficult than the maintenance of adequate minute ventilation, clearance of $CO_2$, and prevention of muscular fatigue.

β-Adrenergic bronchodilators such as albuterol (Ventolin) help decrease bronchospasm in patients with acute exacerbations of COPD or asthma. The addition of anticholinergic bronchodilators to β-agonists such as ipratropium bromide (Atrovent) may produce added benefit. Corticosteroids such as hydrocortisone sodium succinate (Solu-Cortef) are used to treat significant exacerbations of diseases associated with bronchospasm and inflammation. These may be given orally (prednisone) or intravenously (methylprednisolone [Solu-Medrol]). Patients with symptoms suggestive of an infectious etiology (e.g., increased sputum, fever, chest radiograph changes) may benefit from antibiotic therapy. NPPV has a clear role in the treatment of stable, alert patients with hypercarbic respiratory failure. When used in this population, NPPV can reduce rates of intubation and intensive care unit (ICU) length of stay. Like other patients who are not adequately supported by or who do not tolerate NPPV, consideration should be given to intubation and mechanical ventilation.

## Mechanical Ventilation

Mechanical ventilation is a powerful tool in the management of acute respiratory failure because it allows the control of minute ventilation, offers opportunities to support oxygenation, and facilitates patient recovery from muscular fatigue. It is important to bear in mind, however, that it does not replace accurate diagnosis and aggressive treatment of the underlying disease.

Indications for intubation and mechanical ventilation include: failure of ventilation, failure of oxygenation, failure of airway protection, and inability to manage secretions or pulmonary toilet. Typically, ventilators in North American ICUs are programmed to deliver a predetermined tidal volume. This occurs unless a clinician-determined airway pressure is exceeded. This mode is called *assist-control* or *volume-control* ventilation. The patient is able to trigger the ventilator, at which time the predetermined tidal volume is delivered. If the patient does not attempt to trigger the ventilator within a specified time period, or is unable to generate sufficient air flow to cause triggering, the ventilator will deliver a minimum number of *mandatory* breaths.

Other less frequently used modes of ventilation include pressure control ventilation, synchronized intermittent mandatory ventilation, bilevel ventilation, and APRV. There is no convincing evidence that one mode improves patient outcomes more than another, but clinical experience suggests that different patients may *prefer* certain modes in terms of comfort and ventilator synchrony.

Positive end-expiratory pressure (PEEP) is a controllable characteristic of both invasive and noninvasive ventilation that is useful in the management of both hypoxic and hypercarbic respiratory failure. During normal breathing in the healthy patient, there is minimal residual pressure (above atmospheric pressure) in the airways at end expiration. The use of mechanical ventilation allows the clinician to artificially exert continuous pressure into the airway and lungs throughout the respiratory cycle, including end expiration. The benefits depend on the clinical scenario. In patients with hypoxic respiratory failure the alveoli are often collapsed because of surfactant abnormalities (ARDS) or flooded with inflammatory cells (pneumonia), edema (left heart failure), blood (alveolar hemorrhage and trauma) or exudates and transudates (ARDS). In these situations PEEP can reinflate atelectatic alveoli and improve oxygenation. In hypercarbic respiratory failure caused by exacerbations of COPD or asthma, low levels of PEEP can decrease the work of breathing performed by patients, allowing them to decrease their $CO_2$ production and their propensity to develop respiratory muscle failure.

Positive end-expiratory pressure, although helpful in acute respiratory failure, may create complications. By increasing intrathoracic pressure, PEEP can impair venous return to the heart and decrease cardiac output, which can cause overt hypotension, or, more subtly, interfere with adequate tissue perfusion (thus preventing the initial purpose of PEEP—improved tissue oxygen delivery). High levels of PEEP are also associated with barotraumas such as pneumothorax and pneumomediastinum.

# Atelectasis

Method of
*Craig Michael Schramm, MD*

The term *atelectasis* refers to the consolidation of an area of lung because of loss of inflating air, rather than displacement by alveolar fluid. It is one of the most common pulmonary abnormalities in patients of all ages. Atelectasis may be characterized by the duration of its presence (i.e., acute or chronic), its location within the lung (central or peripheral, lobar or segmental), or its etiologic mechanisms (Table 1). The term *lobar atelectasis* refers to complete or incomplete collapse of a lobe of lung. *Subsegmental*, *discoid*, and *platelike atelectasis* are synonymous terms indicating collapse at a subsegmental level within a lobe. The presentation and treatment of atelectasis are related to the etiologies involved in its pathogenesis.

## Pathogenesis

The most frequent cause of loss of alveolar gas volume is *resorption atelectasis*, which develops when air is blocked to a lobe, lobar segment, or individual acini. The airway obstruction may result from intrinsic airway lesions such as mucus plugs, foreign bodies, and tumors, extrinsic airway compression, or airway torsion. Alveoli distal to the site of obstruction lose volume because of the passive diffusion of gases from higher partial pressures in the alveoli to lower partial pressures in mixed venous blood. The extent of the resorption atelectasis and the rate by which it develops depend on several factors, including the extent of collateral ventilation in the lung region and the composition of the trapped gas. Complete volume loss occurs within 18 to 24 hours of airway obstruction in a previously healthy lung inflated with room air but within minutes of obstruction during ventilation with 100% oxygen. The loss is also accelerated in the presence of lung disease. In contrast, postobstructive atelectasis is attenuated by collateral ventilation between the obstructed segment and neighboring areas of lung, through accessory ventilatory pathways such as the channels of Martin and pores of Kohn. Obstruction of these pathways by inflammation or lung disease or their incomplete development at birth predisposes an obstructed lung region to develop resorptive atelectasis.

Another common cause of alveolar volume loss is *passive atelectasis* because of the natural propensity of the lung to collapse. Normally, the

## TABLE 1   Etiologies of Atelectasis

**Resorption Atelectasis**
*Intrinsic—airway obstruction*
Mucus plug
Foreign body aspiration
Bronchial granuloma
Bronchial adenoma/tumor
Bronchial stenosis

*Extrinsic airway obstruction*
Hilar adenopathy
Left atrial enlargement
Mediastinal mass
Lung cyst
Airway torsion
Malpositioned endotracheal tube

**Passive Atelectasis**
*Intrapleural—lesions*
Pneumothorax
Pleural effusion or empyema
Diaphragmatic hernia
Chest wall masses

*Hypoventilation*
Postoperative
Neuromuscular weakness
Diaphragm dysfunction

**Dependent Atelectasis**

**Compression Atelectasis**
Peripheral lung mass or cyst
Air trapping in adjacent lung
Bronchial obstruction
Lobar emphysema
Extensive interstitial disease

**Adhesive Atelectasis**
Inadequate surfactant production
Premature infant
Prolonged shallow breathing
Pulmonary embolism
Surfactant destruction
Adult respiratory distress syndrome (ARDS)
Toxic aspiration or inhalation

**Cicatrization Atelectasis**
Pulmonary fibrosis
Pulmonary granulomatous disease

---

inward elastic recoil forces of the lung are balanced by the outward elastic forces of the chest wall. When these opposing forces are uncoupled, as occurs when the intrapleural space is filled with air or fluid, the adjacent lung volume diminishes. Young children are more prone to passive atelectasis than adults because their more compliant chest walls exert less outward forces to balance their lung elastic recoil force. In contrast, adults demonstrate more gravity-dependent effects because of their larger chest dimensions. The weight of blood and tissue in dependent lung regions adds to the opposition of chest wall recoil forces and thereby decreases regional lung volumes. Such gravity-dependent atelectasis may be potentiated by prolonged recumbency as can occur postoperatively or by processes that promote shallow breathing, such as postoperative pain and analgesia or neuromuscular disease. *Compression atelectasis* occurs by a similar mechanism when the expanding forces of the chest wall are countered by compressive forces of a parenchymal lesion, causing the adjacent lung volume to diminish.

Other types of atelectasis include *adhesive atelectasis* and *cicatrization atelectasis*. Alveoli are lined with surfactant to reduce the surface tension at the air–tissue interface. In the absence of surfactant, high surface tensions cause the luminal surfaces of alveolar walls to adhere together. Adhesive atelectasis may result from inadequate surfactant secretion or from excessive surfactant destruction. *Cicatrization atelectasis* refers to the loss of lung volume accompanying pulmonary interstitial fibrosis. Fibrous tissue retracts with time, reducing the

compliance of the lung region and resulting in loss of affected lung volume.

## Diagnosis

The clinical signs of atelectasis depend on its location, extent, and duration. Because of compensatory overdistention of surrounding lung regions, chronic atelectasis presents with fewer signs and symptoms than acute atelectasis. Acute atelectasis of a lobe or lung often is accompanied by tachypnea and dyspnea. Rapid losses of volume may elicit pain in the affected side. Physical examination findings may include ipsilateral shifts in the apical cardiac impulse or the lower extrathoracic trachea because of displacement of the heart and mediastinum to the affected side and dullness to percussion because of increased density in the atelectatic region. Vocal fremitus and breath sounds may be absent when atelectasis is caused by bronchial obstruction but are enhanced when the atelectatic lung is in contact with a patent bronchus. Pectoriloquy and bronchophony may also be appreciated in cases of nonobstructive atelectasis. To be detected, these auscultatory findings usually require at least lobar consolidation to be present, and they are frequently absent in young children because of transmission of sounds from adjacent lung areas. Cyanosis and arterial hypoxemia may be present if there is ventilation–perfusion mismatching in a large area of atelectatic lung.

Although a suspicion of atelectasis may be raised by any of the findings just described, its presence is typically confirmed by chest radiograph. Radiologic signs of atelectasis are variable but include pulmonary opacification, ipsilateral shift of the mediastinum, elevation of the hemidiaphragm, crowding of bronchi and pulmonary vessels, crowding of ribs, displacement of lobar fissures, and compensatory overinflation of the normal lung. Airlessness of an involved lung region usually presents as radiographic opacification; however, some patients with *microatelectasis* have diffuse, distal, passive atelectasis but normal-appearing radiographic lung density. Another type of peripheral lobar collapse can cause *rounded atelectasis*, which is manifest by a round subpleural density often mistaken for a tumor. Air bronchograms within the opacified region are commonly present in atelectasis of all causes other than resorption, where their absence indicates large airway obstruction.

Specific areas of involvement in atelectasis result in distinct radiographic patterns. The right upper lobe tends to collapse superiorly and medially, causing elevation of the right hilum and minor fissure, anterior displacement of the major fissure, and tenting of the juxtaphrenic peak of the diaphragmatic pleura. The left upper lobe usually collapses more anteriorly and superiorly, resulting in anterior displacement of the major fissure and a poorly delineated left perihilar opacity. Compensatory hyperinflation of the superior segment of the left lower lobe may result in an air crescent between the opacified left upper lobe and the mediastinum (the so-called Luftsichel sign). The right middle lobe collapses medially, obscuring the right heart border on a posteroanterior radiograph and resulting in a wedge-shaped triangle or linear band on lateral radiograph demarcated by an inferiorly displaced minor fissure and a superiorly displaced major fissure. Lingular atelectasis obscures the left heart border and has a lateral wedge shape with a more irregular or poorly defined superior border because of the absence of a left minor fissure. Both lower lobes collapse posteriorly and inferiorly, resulting in downward displacement of the hilum, an inferior and medial shift of the major fissure, and blurring of the posterior third of the ipsilateral hemidiaphragm.

## Treatment

The longer that a region of lung remains unexpanded, the more likely it may become infected and eventually develop fibrotic and/or bronchiectatic changes. Successful treatment of atelectasis requires the reestablishment of normal gas volume in the collapsed lung region. In large part, this must entail treating the underlying etiology, ranging from removing an aspirated foreign body in resorptive atelectasis to promoting deep breathing and early ambulation in postoperative passive atelectasis or to administering surfactant in some cases of adhesive atelectasis. In addition, a number of treatment modalities assist in the recruitment of lung volume, either by direct or collateral routes.

Principal among these volume recruitment methods are various types of chest physiotherapy, the most traditional of which are incentive spirometry and chest percussion and postural drainage. Incentive spirometry combines deep inspirations with voluntary coughing. Patients who are unable to perform effort-dependent maneuvers may benefit from administered chest percussion and postural drainage. The delivery of positive pressure either intermittently during inhalation (as with intermittent positive-pressure breathing, or IPPB) or continuously (as with continuous positive airway pressure, or CPAP) may augment lung volume in patients with passive atelectasis because of postoperative sedation, neuromuscular disease, or diaphragmatic dysfunction. Intra- or extrapulmonary applied oscillations may help displace inspissated mucus and reopen plugged airways, particularly if coupled with positive expiratory pressure. Aerosolized β-adrenergic agonists are often administered prior to chest physiotherapy to dilate any constricted airways and facilitate mucociliary clearance, but the efficacy of this practice is unproven. Some patients with mucus plugging may also benefit from mucolytic agents (such as $N$-acetylcysteine [Mucomyst] or recombinant human DNase[1] [Pulmozyme]) delivered either by aerosol or direct intrabronchial lavage.

Flexible bronchoscopy is indicated in patients with respiratory compromise from their atelectasis, in patients with acute atelectasis lasting more than 24 to 48 hours, and in patients with chronic atelectasis refractory to 1 to 2 months of medical management. The bronchoscopy is diagnostic, to look for causes of central airway obstruction. It may be also therapeutic if mucus plugs can be removed by bronchoalveolar lavage; however, nonresorptive types of atelectasis are usually not responsive to lavage. In intubated patients, the bronchoscope may be used as a guide to position the endotracheal tube above the area of atelectasis so that gentle manual insufflation can be delivered directly to the atelectatic region in an attempt to reinflate it.

Occasionally, chronically atelectatic lobes reexpand and function after atelectatic periods of 1 to 2 years. More commonly, however, chronic atelectasis of any etiology progresses to adhesive atelectasis and eventually to a permanently fibrotic lung region. Bronchiectasis may develop in such chronically atelectatic areas, leading to chronic or recurrent purulent infection. If this pattern occurs, surgical resection of the atelectatic lobe may be needed.

## REFERENCES

Fraser RS, Muller NL, Colman N, Pare PD (eds): Fraser and Pare's Diagnosis of Diseases of the Chest, 4th ed. Philadelphia, WB Saunders, 1999, pp 513-562.

Oberwaldner B: Physiotherapy for airway clearance in paediatrics. Eur Respir J 2000;15(1):196-204.

Wallis C, Prasad A: Who needs chest physiotherapy? Moving from anecdote to evidence. Arch Dis Child 1999;80(4):393-397.

Woodring JH, Reed JC: Radiographic manifestations of lobar atelectasis. J Thorac Imaging 1996;11(2):109-144.

# Management of Chronic Obstructive Pulmonary Disease

Method of
*Juan Armando Garcia, MD, and*
*Stephen G. Jenkinson, MD*

Chronic obstructive pulmonary disease (COPD) is characterized by airflow limitation that is not fully reversible. The airflow limitation is usually both progressive and associated with an abnormal inflammatory response of the lungs to noxious particles of gases. Under the direction of the National Heart, Lung, and Blood Institute (NHLBI) and the World Health Organization (WHO), collaborative guidelines on the diagnosis and management of chronic obstructive pulmonary disease (COPD) have been assembled by an expert panel: the Global Initiative for Chronic Obstructive Lung Disease (GOLD). These guidelines define the classifications of COPD on the basis of both severity and type of symptoms and explore all new information on the diagnosis and treatment of COPD. The GOLD initiative aims to improve prevention and management of COPD through a concerted worldwide effort of people involved in all facets of health care policy and to encourage a renewed research interest in this extremely prevalent disease.

To assure that recommendations for management of COPD are based on current scientific literature, the GOLD program established a science committee to update the sections of the report on recommendations for management of COPD each year. Although the update of these sections will occur each year and will be posted on the Web site (http://www.goldcopd.com), the full report will be updated and printed every 5 years. The latest update, including new modifications of management, was published in late 2003.

## Pathophysiology

The pathophysiology of COPD is somewhat different in various patients, and the terms *emphysema* or *chronic bronchitis* were used in the past. Both of these disorders cause airway obstruction. Emphysema is defined pathologically as abnormal permanent enlargement of airspaces distal to the terminal bronchioles, accompanied by destruction of their walls and without obvious fibrosis. This tissue destruction results in enlargement of proximal and distal airspaces and can ultimately form bullae in the lung parenchyma. These bullae result in loss of surface area for gas exchange in the involved lungs. There is also a genetically inherited form of emphysema which is caused by the $\alpha_1$-antitrypsin (AAT) deficiency. This disorder accounts for less than 1% of COPD cases in the United States. AAT is a protease inhibitor produced by the liver that circulates into tissues. Active proteases are released into the lung by lung macrophages, which can contribute to the development of emphysema. When patients smoke cigarettes, they also recruit a neutrophil population into their lungs. These neutrophils release neutrophil elastase (another type of protease) and other toxic molecules, which can destroy alveolar walls and may also contribute to the production of emphysema. AAT offers protection from these effects, but the protection found in normal people is inadequate in patients with AAT deficiency. Patients who develop emphysema despite normal levels of AAT usually develop emphysema in the fifth or sixth decades of life, whereas patients with AAT deficiency can develop emphysema as early as the third or fourth decades of life, depending on the extent of their deficiency and smoking history.

All patients developing emphysema who form bullae before the age of 45 years should be evaluated for AAT deficiency. A normal serum level of AAT is greater than 11 mmol/L (>80 mg/dL). Patients with low levels of AAT should be evaluated by a pulmonologist and may be candidates for AAT replacement therapy.

Chronic bronchitis is defined clinically as the presence of chronic, productive cough for 3 months during each of 2 consecutive years, and

225

---

[1]Not FDA approved for this indication.

for which other causes of chronic cough are excluded. The other most common causes of chronic cough include asthma, gastric reflux, or postnasal drip secondary to sinus disease. The pathologic findings of chronic bronchitis are enlargement of tracheobronchial mucus glands, variable amounts of airway smooth-muscle hyperplasia, inflammation, and bronchial wall thickening. Abnormalities of small airways may be present as well and are accompanied by fibrosis and the presence of a mononuclear inflammatory process. The forced expiratory volume at 1 second ($FEV_1$) of a COPD patient is inversely proportional to the number of inflammatory cells in the airways. Patients with chronic bronchitis also have increased mucus hypersecretion, goblet cell metaplasia, increased submucosal gland formation, and abnormal matrix deposition.

The use of the terms *emphysema* or *chronic bronchitis* is no longer specified in the GOLD definition of COPD. The inflammation seen in COPD is different from that seen in asthma, but some obstructive lung disease patients do have pathologic changes that can be seen in both diseases, so some overlap does occur.

## Epidemiology and Risk Factors

In the United States COPD is presently the fourth leading cause of death and affects more than 21 million people. Death rates have risen more than 22% in the last decade and the disease is responsible for approximately 700,000 hospital stays each year. The disease is now almost equal in men and women because of increasing amounts of tobacco in the female population. The primary risk factor associated with the development of COPD, cigarette smoking increases the death rate and disability caused by COPD and causes lung function to deteriorate over time much more rapidly than in a nonsmoker. Cigar and pipe smokers have greater COPD incidence than nonsmokers. Approximately 20% of smokers will develop COPD. The risk of development of COPD is increased in first-degree relatives of patients with COPD, which suggests the importance of genetic factors, but AAT deficiency is the only proved genetic risk factor in COPD. Exposures other than smoking that have been associated with COPD development include passive smoking, ambient air pollution, occupational dust and chemical exposure, and severe respiratory childhood infections.

## Diagnosis

The diagnosis of COPD is suggested on the basis of symptoms, which may include those caused by the airway irritation (cough and sputum production) and those reflecting altered lung mechanics (dyspnea, wheezing, and occasionally chest pain). Individuals usually experience cough and sputum production years before the development of airflow limitation, while not all individuals with cough and sputum production go on to develop COPD.

Physical examination of individuals with COPD can reveal hyperinflation, wheezing, diminished breath sounds, hyperresonance, or prolonged expiration. Visual inspection during an examination can reveal signs of increased respiratory rate, increased anteroposterior (AP) chest diameter, hyperresonance to chest percussion, and impaired respiratory muscle function. Patients with COPD commonly have a respiration rate greater than 16 breaths per minute, and often this is proportional to disease severity; patients with COPD severe enough to exhibit hypercapnia (partial pressure of arterial carbon dioxide [$PaCO_2$] greater than 45 mm Hg) may have breathing rates of greater than 25 breaths per minute. Absence of wheezing does not exclude COPD. Patients with end-stage COPD may adopt body positions that help relieve dyspnea, such as leaning forward or expiring through pursed lips. Use of accessory muscles for respiration, such as the use of the abdominal rectus muscle on expiration, is a sign of advanced disease. Other signs of hyperinflation may include decreased diaphragm movement, tracheal tug, or pulsus paradoxus greater than 20 mm Hg.

Patients with advanced COPD may also have central cyanosis, peripheral edema, and signs of cor pulmonale associated with right heart failure. Other objective findings often include arterial blood gas

changes demonstrating hypercapnia, severe hypoxemia, compensated respiratory acidosis with elevated carbon dioxide ($CO_2$), tension and a normal pH, and elevated serum bicarbonate level. Morning headaches in COPD patients may be indicative of hypercapnia.

The diagnosis of COPD is confirmed by spirometry. The standard pulmonary function test used to measure airway obstruction is the forced expiratory spirogram. This test assesses the rate of change in volume that occurs as a function of time. Pulmonary functions useful in the evaluation of patients presenting with symptoms of COPD include $FEV_1$, the forced vital capacity (FVC), and the ratio of $FEV_1/FVC$, which is also called the *timed vital capacity*. The FVC provides a measure of lung volume and the $FEV_1$ and $FEV_1/FVC$ both provide a measure of obstruction. In most of these patients, other abnormal lung volumes that may exist include increases in both the total lung capacity (TLC) and the residual volume (RV). These increases in lung volumes are caused by hyperinflation of the lungs.

An $FEV_1/FVC$ less than 70% of predicted confirms the presence of airflow obstruction. The $FEV_1$ serves as a marker of severity of the airflow obstruction. Other pulmonary function tests such as the flow volume loop or diffusing capacity for carbon monoxide ($DL_{CO}$) can help rule out other types of airway obstruction or help quantitate a patient's risk for surgery. Chest radiographs are only helpful for diagnosis in COPD if there are signs of bullous disease or severe hyperinflation or loss of vascular markings. Computed tomography (CT) scanning can show the location of bullous disease which can be helpful in narrowing the differential diagnosis of a patient with airway obstruction and also may be used to help determine if a patient is a candidate for lung reduction surgery.

## COPD Classification

The GOLD committee presented a new classification of COPD. The management of COPD is largely symptom driven, and there is only an imperfect relationship between the degree of airflow limitation and the presence of symptoms. The staging therefore is aimed at practical implementation and should be only regarded as an educational tool, and a general indication of the approach to management. All $FEV_1$ values refer to postbronchodilator $FEV_1$.

This classification includes stages 0 to IV (Figure 1).

*Stage 0: At Risk*—Characterized by chronic cough and sputum production. Lung function, as measured by spirometry, is still normal.

*Stage I: Mild COPD*—Characterized by mild airflow limitation ($FEV_1/FVC$ <70% but $FEV_1$ >80% predicted) and usually, but not always, chronic cough and sputum production. At this stage, the individual may be unaware of abnormal lung function.

*Stage II: Moderate COPD*—Characterized by worsening airflow limitation (<50% $FEV_1$ <80% predicted) and usually the progression of symptoms, with shortness of breath typically developing on exertion. This is the stage at which most patients typically first seek medical attention because of dyspnea or an exacerbation of their disease.

*Stage III: Severe COPD*—Characterized by further worsening of airflow limitation (<30% $FEV_1$ <50% predicted), increased shortness of breath, and repeated exacerbations which have an impact on the patient's quality of life.

*Stage IV: Very Severe COPD*—Characterized by severe air-flow limitation ($FEV_1$ <30% predicted) or the presence of chronic respiratory failure. Patients may have very severe (Stage IV) COPD even if the $FEV_1$ is greater than 30% predicted, if respiratory failure is present. At this stage, quality of life is appreciably impaired and exacerbations may be life-threatening.

## Management of Stable COPD

The general guidelines to management of COPD include the avoidance of risk factors to prevent disease progression and pharmacotherapy as needed to control symptoms. In addition, patient education including counseling about smoking cessation, instruction in physical exercise, and nutritional advice are necessary components of a comprehensive

| | 0: At risk | I: Mild | II: Moderate | III: Severe | IV: Very severe |
|---|---|---|---|---|---|
| Characteristics | • Chronic symptoms<br>• Exposure to risk factors<br>• Normal spirometry | • $FEV_1/FVC < 70\%$<br>• $FEV_1 \geq 80\%$<br>• With or without symptoms | • $FEV_1/FVC < 70\%$<br>• $50\% \leq FEV_1 < 80\%$<br>• With or without symptoms | • $FEV_1/FVC < 70\%$<br>• $30\% \leq FEV_1 < 50\%$<br>• With or without symptoms | • $FEV_1/FVC < 70\%$<br>• $FEV_1 < 30\%$ or $FEV_1 < 50\%$ predicted plus chronic respiratory failure |
| | Avoidance of risk factor(s); influenza vaccination | | | | |
| | | *Add* short-acting bronchodilator when needed | | | |
| | | | *Add* regular treatment with one or more long-acting bronchodilators<br>*Add* rehabilitation | | |
| | | | | *Add* inhaled glucocorticosteroid if repeated exacerbations | |
| | | | | | *Add* long-term oxygen if chronic respiratory failure. Consider surgical treatments |

**FIGURE 1.** Therapy for different stages of COPD

COPD management plan. The goals of management are to relieve symptoms, increase exercise tolerance, improve quality of life, prevent and treat complications, and decrease disease progression.

Smoking cessation is the single most effective (and cost-effective) intervention to reduce the risk of developing COPD and stop its progression. Comprehensive tobacco elimination policies and programs with clear and repeated nonsmoking messages should be delivered through every feasible system possible. Legislation to establish smoke-free schools, public facilities, and work environments should be encouraged by working with government officials, public health workers, and the public. Guidelines for smoking cessation were published by the U.S. Agency for Health Care Policy and Research (AHCPR) in 2000.

There are numerous effective pharmacotherapies for smoking cessation. Except in the presence of special circumstances, pharmacotherapy is recommended when counseling is insufficient. Nicotine replacement therapy in any form (nicotine gum, inhaler, nasal spray [Nicotrol NS], transdermal patch [Nicoderm], sublingual tablet [Nicorette Microtab],[2] or lozenge [Commit]) reliably increases long-term smoking abstinence rates. The antidepressants bupropion (Zyban) and nortriptyline (Pamelor)[1] have also been shown to increase long-term quit rates. The antihypertensive drug clonidine (Catapres)[1] can also be used to help a patient quit smoking, but side effects should be carefully reviewed with each patient. Special consideration should be given before using pharmacotherapy in selected populations including patients smoking fewer than 10 cigarettes per day, pregnant patients, and adolescent smokers.

The overall approach to managing stable COPD should be characterized by a stepwise increase in treatment, depending on the severity of the disease. The management strategy is based on an individualized assessment of disease severity and response to various therapies. Disease severity is determined by the severity of symptoms and airflow limitation (using pulmonary function measurements) and other factors such as the frequency and severity of exacerbations, complications, respiratory failure, co-morbidities (cardiovascular disease and sleep-related disorders), and the general health status of the patient. Different types of pharmacologic agents treat patients with COPD (Box 1). Pharmacologic therapy is used to prevent and control symptoms, reduce the frequency and severity of exacerbations, improve health status, and improve exercise tolerance. Initial use should decrease airway obstruction and decrease dyspnea. None of the existing

medications for COPD had been shown to alter the inevitable long-term decline in lung function that occurs with COPD; however, they can decrease morbidity and may also delay disability and mortality in some patients. Medications may also decrease the number of exacerbations of COPD occurring per year.

Bronchodilators are primary medications for symptomatic management of COPD. Bronchodilator drugs commonly used include anticholinergics (short and long acting), $\beta_2$ agonists (short and long acting), and long-acting methylxanthines. All of these medications have been shown to improve exercise capacity in COPD patients even if the $FEV_1$ is insignificantly changed. Inhaled drugs tend to have fewer side effects than oral drugs. Short-acting bronchodilators on an as-needed basis are recommended for mild (Stage I) COPD. The GOLD guidelines recommend the use of regular daily treatment with bronchodilators for moderate (Stage II) or severe (Stages III and IV) COPD and long-acting bronchodilators are preferred to short-acting drugs because of better compliance because of longer duration of action (Box 1). Regular use of a long-acting anticholinergic (tiotropium [Spiriva]) or a long acting $\beta_2$-agonist (salmeterol [Serevent] or formoterol [Foradil]) improves health status. Theophylline (Theo-Dur) is effective in COPD, but because of its potential toxicity, inhaled bronchodilators are preferred when available. All studies that have shown efficacy of theophylline (Theo-Dur) in COPD were done with slow-release preparations (theophylline [Theo-Dur]). Each of the inhaled bronchodilators requires a delivery device which must be used correctly. Each type of device requires patient education and monitoring, and the GOLD guidelines recommend consideration of the delivery device as part of the selection process for drug treatment in a single patient. As symptoms of COPD worsen, several different types of COPD therapy are given simultaneously, and deletion of drug therapy is usually not possible. In general nebulized therapy for a stable patient is unnecessary unless it has been demonstrated to be more effective than conventional metered dose or dry powder inhaler dose therapy in that patient.

Combinations of bronchodilators with different mechanisms and durations of action tend to increase the degree of bronchodilation in COPD patients with increases in $FEV_1$, $FEV_1/FVC$, and peak expiratory flow (PEF). Changes in pulmonary function are indirectly additive with increasing the number of bronchodilators being administered, but combinations usually increase pulmonary function more than each agent alone. Short-acting $\beta_2$ agonists (SABAs) are quick-relief medications for use only when necessary rather than on a daily, regular schedule. The regular use of a SABA results in twice as much $\beta_2$ agonist use without any noted clinical benefits. Increasing use or daily use of

[1]Not FDA approved for this indication.
[2]Not available in the United States.

## BOX 1  Current Drugs Used to Manage Chronic Obstructive Pulmonary Disease

- SABAs
- Albuterol (salbutamol) (Proventil)
- LABAs
- Formoterol (Foradil)
- Salmeterol (Serevent)
- Short-acting anticholinergics
- Ipratropium (Atrovent)
- Long-acting anticholinergics
- Tiotropium (Spiriva)
- Combination SABA + anticholinergic in 1 inhaler
- Albuterol/ipratropium (Combivent)
- Methylxanthines
- Theophylline (Theo-Dur)
- Inhaled corticosteroids
- Beclomethasone (QVAR)
- Budesonide (Pulmicort)
- Fluticasone (Flovent)
- Triamcinolone (Azmacort)
- Combination LABA + ICS in 1 inhaler
- Formoterol/budesonide (Symbicort)
- Salmeterol/fluticasone (Advair)
- Systemic corticosteroids
- Prednisone
- Methylprednisolone (Medrol)

*Abbreviations:* LABAs = Long-acting $\beta_2$ agonists; SABAs = short-acting $\beta_2$ agonists.

a SABA for rescue indicates the need for additional therapy to achieve long-term control. Inhaled SABAs include albuterol (Proventil, Ventolin), bitolterol (Tornalate), pirbuterol (Maxair), and terbutaline (Brethaire). These medications are effective for 4 to 6 hours after use. Adverse effects of SABAs include palpitations, chest pain, tachycardia, tremor, unstable coronary artery disease or nervousness. Patients with coronary artery disease or cardiac dysrhythmias should also be monitored closely. Use caution in giving these medications to patients receiving monoamine oxidase inhibitors or tricyclic antidepressants. The short-acting anticholinergic agent, ipratropium bromide (Atrovent), causes bronchodilation by competitive inhibition of muscarinic receptors. This agent reverses cholinergically mediated bronchospasm and may decrease mucus-gland secretions. It is effective for 4 to 6 hours after use.

The most recent addition to the long-acting bronchodilators is tiotropium (Spiriva), a long-acting anticholinergic agent that lasts 24 hours, allowing for once-daily administration. Tiotropium (Spiriva) has shown in several recent studies with COPD patients to result in significant improvement in lung function compared with ipratropium (a short-acting anticholinergic) or salmeterol (Serevent, a long-acting $\beta_2$ agonist [LABA]). Inhaled LABAs are highly preferred than the extended-release oral formulation because of longer action and fewer side effects. Salmeterol (Serevent) and formoterol (Foradil) are both long-acting, inhaled $\beta_2$ agonists, and extended-release albuterol (Proventil Repetabs) are long-acting, $\beta_2$ agonists available as oral agents. The long-acting inhaled agents have a slower onset of action and longer duration of action, remaining active for more than 12 hours. The onset of action of formoterol (Foradil) is more rapid than salmeterol (Serevent), but it should not be used for rescue during episodes of acute shortness of breath. It remains a chronic bronchodilator therapy. Like the short-acting inhaled $\beta_2$ agonists, the long-acting agents produce bronchodilation by smooth muscle relaxation as a result of adenylate cyclase activation and increasing cyclic AMP in smooth muscle cells. Combining $\beta_2$ agonists and anticholinergics may increase the effects of these agents. Several studies have shown superior efficacy for either a SABA or LABA in combination with an anticholinergic.

Theophylline (Theo-Dur) inhibits phosphodiesterase action, which causes smooth muscle relaxation and leads to bronchodilation. It also increases central respiratory drive, diaphragm strength, promotes venous pooling in the legs, and may have some mild anti-inflammatory activity. Therapy with theophylline (Theo-Dur) should be individualized, taking into account such factors as drug interactions, current smoking, the patient's age, and the presence of congestive heart failure or liver disease. Serum theophylline (Theo-Dur) concentrations should be maintained at levels between 5 and 15 μg/mL. Dosage adjustment is based on the patient's clinical response, tolerance to the agent, and serum theophylline (Theo-Dur) levels. Some patients metabolize theophylline (Theo-Dur) very rapidly. Although theophylline (Theo-Dur) is not a preferred first line agent in the management of COPD, it may be a second-line agent in patients with severe COPD.

Inhaled corticosteroids (ICSs) are not recommended as single agents for chronic use in COPD management, which is quite different from the recommendations in asthma. They are recommended in combination therapy with other bronchodilators in severe COPD, and the only Food and Drug Administration (FDA)-approved combinations of ICS and a LABA are fluticasone plus salmeterol (Advair) or formoterol (Foradil) plus budesonide (Symbicort)[4] (see Box 1). Systemic steroids are clinically beneficial to patients hospitalized with COPD exacerbations and maximum effects of oral steroids after 3 days of intravenous (IV) steroids are achieved by 2 weeks of therapy. Longer use of oral steroids increases side effects without increasing pulmonary functions. Long-term treatment with oral glucocorticosteroids is not recommended in COPD. There is no evidence of a long-term benefit from this treatment. Moreover, a side effect of long-term treatment with systemic glucocorticosteroid is steroid myopathy, which contributes to muscle weakness, decreased functionality, and respiratory failure in patients with advanced COPD. Oral glucocorticosteroid use for long periods of time can also complicate control of diabetes and hypertension as well as causing bone demineralization.

Other pharmacologic treatments have been evaluated by the GOLD committee with some being beneficial. Use of influenza vaccines can reduce serious illness and death in COPD patients by approximately 50%. Use of the influenza vaccine has also been shown to reduce outpatient visits for influenza and reduces both hospital costs and death. Vaccines containing killed (Fluzone) or live, inactive viruses (FluMist)[1] are recommended and should be given once (in autumn) or twice[3] (in autumn and winter) each year. A pneumococcal vaccine containing 23 virulent serotypes (Pneumovax-23) has been used in an effort to decrease the number of cases of pneumococcal pneumonia in COPD patients but evidence supporting its effectiveness in COPD patients is lacking. An oral vaccine* using a strain of nontypeable *Haemophilus influenzae* has been shown to produce short-lived reduction in the number of exacerbations in some groups of COPD patients. The use of antibiotics, other than in treating infectious exacerbations of COPD or other bacterial infections such as pneumonia, is not recommended. Although a few patients with viscous sputum may benefit from mucolytics, the overall benefit is small. Therefore, the widespread use of these agents cannot be recommended.

Cough, although sometimes a troublesome symptom in COPD, has a significant protective role and the regular use of antitussives is contraindicated in stable COPD. The use of doxapram (Dopram), a nonspecific respiratory stimulant available as an intravenous formulation, is not recommended in stable COPD. Almitrine bismesylate (Duxil) also is not recommended for regular use in stable COPD patients. Narcotics are contraindicated in COPD because of their respiratory depressant effects and potential to worsen hypercapnia. Clinical studies suggest that morphine use to control dyspnea may have serious adverse effects, but it may provide benefits to a few select limited patients. Codeine and other narcotic analgesics should be avoided. Nonsteroidal anti-inflammatory agents (Nedocromil [Tilade]) and leukotriene modifiers have not been adequately tested in COPD

---

*Investigational drug in the United States.
[1]Not FDA approved for this indication.
[3]Exceeds dosage recommended by the manufacturer.
[4]Not yet approved for use in the United States.

patients and are not recommended for use. Alternative healing methods including herbal medicine, acupuncture, and homeopathy are not recommended for treatment in COPD.

Nonpharmacologic management of COPD patients includes pulmonary rehabilitation and long-term oxygen therapy. The principal goals of pulmonary rehabilitation are to improve quality of life, decrease symptoms, and increase physical participation in everyday activities. To accomplish these goals, pulmonary rehabilitation addresses a range of nonpulmonary problems, including exercise deconditioning, relative social isolation, altered mood states (especially depression), muscle wasting, and weight loss. COPD patients at all stages of disease benefit from exercise training programs and improve with respect to both exercise tolerance and symptoms of dyspnea and fatigue. These benefits can be sustained even after a single pulmonary rehabilitation program. Benefits have been reported from rehabilitation programs conducted in inpatient, outpatient, and home settings. Ideally, a comprehensive pulmonary rehabilitation program includes exercise training, nutrition counseling, and education. Baseline and outcome assessments of each participant in a pulmonary rehabilitation program should be made to quantify individual gains and target areas for improvement and include a detailed medical history and physical exam; measurement of spirometry before and after a bronchodilator drug; assessment of exercise capacity; measurement of the impact of breathlessness and/or health status; and assessment of inspiratory and expiratory muscle strength and lower limb strength (e.g., quadriceps) in patients who suffer from muscle wasting.

The long-term administration of oxygen (more than 15 hours per day) to COPD patients with chronic respiratory failure has been shown to increase survival. In studies done in Britain by the Medical Research Council Trial and in the United States in the Nocturnal Oxygen Therapy Trial, patients receiving continuous oxygen therapy had increased survival as compared with patients that did not receive oxygen or received oxygen only at night. Oxygen also has a beneficial impact on hemodynamics, hematologic characteristics, exercise capacity, lung mechanics, and mental state. Oxygen therapy also should be used if the patient has evidence of pulmonary hypertension, peripheral edema suggesting either right- or left-sided heart failure or evidence of polycythemia (hematocrit greater than 55%). Therapy can be given continuously, acutely to combat acute dyspnea, or intermittently during exercise. It is recommended to perform arterial blood gas measurement in patients with $FEV_1$ less than 40% predicted or with clinical findings suggestive of respiratory failure or cor pulmonale.

## Management of Exacerbations

Patients with COPD will have usually two to three exacerbations of symptoms of their disease each year with some requiring hospitalization. The economic and social burden of COPD exacerbations is extremely high. The most common causes of an exacerbation are pulmonary infections (acute bacterial bronchitis) and air pollution. The exact cause of approximately one-third of severe exacerbations cannot be identified and may be related to reactive airway disease. Other conditions that may produce the symptoms of an acute exacerbation of COPD include pneumonia, myocardial ischemia, congestive heart failure, pneumothorax, formation of a pleural effusion, pulmonary embolism, cardiac arrhythmias, esophageal reflux, or noncompliance with medications. The clinical diagnosis of a COPD exacerbation is an increase in amount of sputum production, change in color of sputum, or increase in dyspnea. Exacerbations may also be accompanied by a number of nonspecific complaints such as malaise, insomnia, sleepiness, fatigue, anxiety, depression, confusion, or panic attacks. Patients with exacerbations of COPD may require hospital admission, and some patients will require ICU admission. There is a high incidence of *H. influenzae* infections in patients with a COPD exacerbation caused by infection. Other important bacterial causes include *Streptococcus pneumoniae*, *Moraxella catarrhalis*, and *Pseudomonas aeruginosum*. Hospital admission must be considered in COPD with an exacerbation if they have marked increase in symptoms, failure to respond to outpatient treatment, confusion, lethargy and coma, worsening oxygenation, or development of respiratory

acidosis. Oxygen therapy is usually required in a hospitalized patient with an acute exacerbation of COPD; but this may lead to $CO_2$ retention and acidosis, which in turn could lead to either noninvasive mechanical ventilation, or mechanical ventilation depending on the cause of the exacerbation and the patient's wishes. Hospital mortality for patients with COPD admitted for an acute exacerbation is approximately 10%. Ventilator associated pneumonia is also an important risk in a COPD patient treated with invasive mechanical ventilation.

The primary objectives of mechanical ventilatory support in patients with acute exacerbations of severe COPD are to decrease mortality and morbidity and relieve symptoms. Ventilatory support can be given through an orotracheal or nasotracheal tube or tracheostomy connection, which is referred to as invasive (conventional) mechanical ventilation and is particularly suitable in severe acute exacerbations occurring in patients with end-stage disease. Ventilatory support can also be given through a noninvasive means using either negative or positive pressure devices. Fewer complications occur with noninvasive ventilation, but many patients presenting with severe exacerbations of COPD, including respiratory acidosis, may not be candidates for noninvasive ventilation. Noninvasive positive-pressure ventilation (NPPV) involves using a mechanical ventilator connected by tubing to an interface that allows airflow into the nose or the nose and mouth by using a mask or a mouthpiece. Head straps are used to secure the mask tightly to the patient. NPPV allows ventilation without the use of an endotracheal tube. Use of NPPV in acute respiratory failure has been studied in both uncontrolled and randomized controlled trials. The studies show consistently positive results with success rates of 80% to 85%. Taken together they provide evidence that NPPV increases pH, reduces $PaCO_2$, reduces the severity of breathlessness in the first 4 hours of treatment, and decreases the length of hospital stay. More importantly, mortality and intubation rates are reduced by this intervention. However, NPPV is not appropriate for all patients and invasive mechanical ventilation may still be needed to maximize arterial blood gases values. NPPV can be delivered by different types of ventilators: volume-controlled, pressure-controlled, bilevel positive airway pressure, or continuous positive airway pressure. The use of NPPV together with long-term oxygen therapy has been shown to result in a significant improvement in daytime arterial blood gases, total sleep time, sleep efficiency, quality of life, and overnight $PaCO_2$.

Other treatments that can be useful in COPD patients who must be hospitalized include fluid administration as needed to keep the patient normovolemic; nutrition supplementation as needed with careful attention to the amount of carbohydrates given because excessive amounts can increase $CO_2$ production; and the use of low molecular weight heparin in immobilized patients with or without a history of thromboembolic disease. Manual or mechanical chest percussion and postural drainage may also be beneficial in patients producing greater than 25 mL sputum per day or those with lobar atelectasis.

## Surgical Options

Surgical treatments of COPD include bullectomy, lung volume reduction surgery, and lung transplantation. In carefully selected patients, bullectomy can be effective in reducing dyspnea and improving lung function. A thoracic CT scan, arterial blood gases measurement and comprehensive respiratory function tests are essential before making a decision regarding a patient's suitability for resection of a bulla. Specific large bullae may be removed if they are compressing significant amounts of normal lung tissue.

Lung volume reduction surgery (LVRS) is another option for COPD patients and involves removing 20% to 30% of the upper lobes to improve airway mechanics and increase $FEV_1$. The National Emphysema Treatment Trial (NETT) study was a randomized controlled trial in 1218 patients with severe emphysema who received either LVRS or medical therapy. The results showed no overall survival benefit with LVRS compared with medical therapy, but improved exercise capacity and quality of life. The best outcome of this surgery was in patients with predominantly upper lobe emphysema and initial low exercise capacity. The surgery was prohibitive in patients with an $FEV_1$

of up to 20% and either a homogeneous distribution of emphysema or a concomitant diffusing capacity of lung for carbon monoxide ($DL_{CO}$) of up to 20%.

In appropriately selected patients with very advanced COPD, lung transplantation has been shown to improve quality of life and functional capacity. The average 3-year survival rate is approximately 60% when performed by highly skilled medical or surgical teams that specialize in lung transplantation. Appropriate criteria for lung transplantation recipients include $FEV_1$ of up to 35% of predicted, $PaCO_2$ greater than 55 mm Hg, $PaO_2$ less than 60 mm Hg on room air, or the presence of secondary pulmonary hypertension.

# Cystic Fibrosis

Method of
*Deborah K. Froh, MD*

Cystic fibrosis (CF) is a complex, multisystem chronic illness caused by mutations in the gene for the cystic fibrosis transmembrane conductance regulator (CFTR) protein. Organ systems with exocrine secretory function are affected, most notably the respiratory tract, pancreas, sweat glands, gastrointestinal tract, and male reproductive tract. The treatment burden on patients is high, but median predicted survival is now up to 37 years, and approximately 40% of persons with CF are now adults.

## Genetics

More than 1100 CFTR mutations have been associated with CF. Inheritance is autosomal recessive, with both parents being asymptomatic carriers. In North America, the vast majority of cases occur in whites, in whom the observed incidence is 1 per 3300 births, reflecting a high carrier frequency (1 in 29). However, it also occurs in persons of Latin American (1 in 9500), African (1 in 15,300), and Asian (1 in 32,100) descent.

## Diagnosis

When CF is suspected clinically, a sweat chloride concentration greater than 60 mmol/L is confirmatory. CFTR mutation analysis may be used, but it is not always conclusive due to inability to test for all mutations. Suggestive symptoms include meconium ileus, failure to thrive, steatorrhea or loose frequent stools, rectal prolapse, chronic cough, recurring respiratory symptoms, recurrent sinusitis, and nasal polyps. The median age of symptom-prompted diagnosis is 6 months, but there may be significant delays, and 10% of diagnoses occur in patients older than 10 years. However, newborn screening for CF is expanding rapidly and will result in most cases being diagnosed presymptomatically, within the first month or two of life. Studies have shown this to improve nutritional and possibly pulmonary outcomes.

## Pathophysiology

In CF airways, the combination of impaired chloride secretion through CFTR and excessive sodium absorption through a CFTR-regulated sodium channel (ENaC) results in water loss from the airway-lining fluid, producing severely dehydrated secretions. Ciliary mobility is reduced, airways become obstructed, and pathogens and toxins are poorly cleared. The airway microenvironment in CF favors colonization by specific bacteria such as *Pseudomonas aeruginosa* (Table 1). A high level of chronic neutrophilic airway inflammation has been shown to exist even in presymptomatic, uninfected CF infants.

## TABLE 1 Respiratory Tract Bacteria in Cystic Fibrosis

| Bacterium | Percentage |
|---|---|
| *Pseudomonas aeruginosa* | 56.4% |
| *Staphylococcus aureus* | 51.8% |
| Methicillin-resistant *S. aureus* | 17.2% |
| *Stenotrophomonas maltophilia* | 12.3% |
| *Burkholderia cepacia* complex | 3.1% |

The data show incidence of bacterial pathogens among positive cystic fibrosis respiratory tract cultures reported. Cultures can contain more than one pathogen.

Data from the Cystic Fibrosis Foundation: 2005 National Patient Data Registry Report. Bethesda, Md: Cystic Fibrosis Foundation, 2005, p 12. PDF available at http://www.cff.org/UploadedFiles/research/ClinicalResearch/PatientRegistryReport/2005%20Patient%20Registry%20Report.pdf (accessed May 1, 2007).

## CURRENT DIAGNOSIS

**Diagnostic Features**

- Presence of one or more characteristic phenotypic features *or*
- A history of CF in a sibling *or*
- Positive newborn screening test

*plus*

- Elevated sweat chloride concentrations (chloride >60 mmol/L) *or*
- Identification of two CF associated mutations *or*
- Characteristic abnormalities in ion transport measured across the nasal epithelium

**Characteristic Phenotypic Features:**

- Chronic sinopulmonary disease
    - Chronic cough and sputum production
    - Clinical findings consistent with airway obstruction (wheezing, air trapping)
    - Pansinusitis, nasal polyps
    - Persistent pulmonary infection with typical CF pathogens (*Staphylococcus aureus, Pseudomonas aeruginosa*)
    - Persistent chest radiograph abnormalities (bronchiectasis, atelectasis, infiltrates, hyperinflation)
    - Digital clubbing
- Gastrointestinal and nutritional abnormalities
    - Intestinal: Meconium ileus, DIOS, rectal prolapse
    - Pancreatic: Pancreatic insufficiency (frequent stools), recurrent pancreatitis
    - Hepatic: Focal biliary cirrhosis
    - Nutritional: Protein-calorie malnutrition; hypoproteinemia and edema; complications secondary to fat-soluble vitamin deficiency
- Salt loss syndrome
    - Acute salt depletion
    - Chronic metabolism alkalosis
- Male urogenital abnormalities resulting in obstructive azoospermia.

*Abbreviations:* CF = cystic fibrosis; DIOS = distal intestinal obstruction syndrome.

**CURRENT THERAPY**

- Care at an accredited cystic fibrosis center
- Careful monitoring of pulmonary function, respiratory tract microbiology, and nutritional status
- Daily airway clearance therapies
- Inhaled therapies to thin or hydrate mucus
- Aggressive use of oral, inhaled, and intravenous antibiotics to suppress and treat pathogens and to resolve exacerbations of pulmonary disease
- Control of fat and nutrient malabsorption with exogenous pancrelipase enzymes
- Achievement of normal serum levels of fat-soluble vitamins
- Normal nutritional status (body mass index at 50th percentile), using behavioral feeding therapy, high-calorie diet, oral supplements, night-time gastrostomy feeds, and appetite stimulants as indicated
- Screening for and treatment of complications such as diabetes, decreased bone density, and liver disease
- Patient and family involvement in care planning

Neutrophils release many injurious products, such as neutrophil elastase, and are key contributors to the progression of CF pulmonary disease.

## Management

All persons with CF should be followed at a CF care center accredited by the Cystic Fibrosis Foundation, because this has been demonstrated to result in better outcomes and survival. The multidisciplinary team approach incorporates physicians, nurses, dietitians, respiratory therapists, physical therapists, and social workers trained specifically to care for CF patients. These centers also provide the framework for the myriad clinical research trials now opening to test new therapies.

## PULMONARY DISEASE

It is the triad of airway obstruction, inflammation, and infection that causes damage to the airway walls and surrounding tissue, resulting in bronchiectasis (the signature pathologic change), plugged airways, microabscesses, patchy atelectasis, and areas of chronic pneumonitis. For end stage lung disease, bilateral lung transplantation is an option. With well-managed CF, however, disease progression is slow and pulmonary function can remain excellent for a long time. Frequent CF visits, respiratory tract cultures, and measurement of pulmonary function are essential.

Beginning at diagnosis, airway clearance is initiated as a critical part of daily therapy (Table 2). For infants, this means chest physiotherapy, whereas older children and adults more often use device-based techniques such as high frequency chest wall oscillation (vest), positive expiratory pressure (PEP) mask, or oscillatory positive expiratory pressure (Acapella, Quake, Flutter). Inhaled bronchodilators such as albuterol (Proventil) or levalbuterol (Xopenex) are often used before respiratory therapy. Nebulized dornase alfa (Pulmozyme) provides documented pulmonary benefits and is commonly incorporated into daily therapy early in life; it reduces mucus viscosity by cleaving DNA, which is present in high levels in CF airways from degraded neutrophils. Nebulized hypertonic saline (7%)[1,6] recently was found to improve pulmonary status in CF patients, presumably by inducing mucus hydration and improved secretion clearance.

Managing airway infections is key to preserving lung function, and antibiotics are used heavily for both treatment and suppression of bacterial infection. Prophylactic antibiotics are generally not favored. Programmed chronic cycling of inhaled tobramycin (TOBI) in patients colonized with *P. aeruginosa* has been proved to decrease bacterial load, decrease neutrophilic inflammation, improve pulmonary function, and decrease exacerbations. For acute treatment of airway infection, the choice of oral, inhaled, or intravenous antibiotic therapy depends on the severity of clinical presentation. Signs of pulmonary exacerbation include increased cough and sputum production, dyspnea, decreased energy, weight loss, new findings on chest auscultation or x-ray, and decreased lung function. For mild exacerbations, oral antibiotics along with intensified respiratory therapies may be adequate; if *P. aeruginosa* is known or strongly suspected, ciprofloxacin

---

[1]Not FDA approved for this indication.
[6]May be compounded by pharmacists.

---

## TABLE 2  Common Maintenance Therapies

| Drug or Therapy | Usual Dosage or Frequency |
| --- | --- |
| **Pancreatic Enzymes** Pancrelipase (Creon, Ultrase, Pancrease, Pancrecarb) | 1000-2500 U lipase/kg/meal |
| **Fat-Soluble Vitamins** Vitamins A, D, E, K (AquaDEK, ADEK, ABDEK, Vitamax) | 1 mL liquid or 1 or 2 tabs qd |
| **Nutritional Supplements** High-calorie drinks (Scandishake, Boost Plus, Ensure Plus) | Once or twice daily if needed |
| **Maintenance Respiratory Medications** Albuterol (Proventil) or levalbuterol (Xopenex) Dornase alfa (Pulmozyme) Hypertonic saline, 7%[1,6] Tobramycin for inhalation (TOBI) | 1 nebule or 2-4 puffs bid 1 nebule (2.5 mg) qd 4 mL nebulized qd or bid 1 nebule (300 mg) twice daily, in cycles of 28 d on, 28 d off (*P. aeruginosa*–colonized patients) |
| **Airway Clearance Techniques** Chest PT, high-frequency chest wall oscillation (vest), PEP mask, oscillatory PEP (Acapella, Quake, Flutter) | Twice daily with inhaled therapies |
| **Anti-inflammatory Medication** Azithromycin (Zithromax)[1] | 250-500 mg three times weekly (*P. aeruginosa*–colonized patients) |

[1]Not FDA approved for this indication.
[6]May be compounded by pharmacists.
*Abbreviations:* PEP = positive expiratory pressure; PT = physical therapy.

(Cipro, 15 mg/kg bid for children[1]; 500-750 mg bid for adults) or levofloxacin (Levaquin, 500-750 mg daily) may be selected. When intravenous therapy is needed, typically a combination of a β-lactam and an aminoglycoside is appropriate (Table 3), and prior culture and sensitivity information may guide specific choices.

Other chronic therapies are aimed at airway inflammation. Azithromycin (Zithromax)[1] was recently shown to improve lung function in *P. aeruginosa*–colonized patients. High-dose ibuprofen (Advil)[1] reduced the rate of pulmonary function decline in a major study, but it is not widely used because of potential side effects. Inhaled glucocorticoids[1] are sometimes prescribed but have not been well studied in CF lung disease.

Allergic bronchopulmonary aspergillosis (ABPA) occurs in approximately 10% of CF patients and is usually managed using oral glucocorticoids (prednisone)[1] or antifungal agents such as itraconazole (Sporanox, 200-400 mg daily in two divided doses), or both. Disease activity can wax and wane, and prednisone may be temporarily increased to 1 to 2 mg/kg daily, then tapered down toward low-dose alternate-day therapy (e.g., 10 mg every other day) or stopped for periods.

## NUTRITIONAL MANAGEMENT

There is convincing evidence from the Cystic Fibrosis Foundation Patient Data Registry that better nutritional status is correlated with

---

[1]Not FDA approved for this indication.

better pulmonary function; thus, nutritional goals for these patients are increasingly ambitious. CF patients have elevated energy expenditure, up to 200% of normal. Supplementary snacks and high-calorie drinks and shakes are often recommended. Some patients have a gastrostomy tube to deliver night-time feeds. Occasionally, appetite stimulants such as cyproheptadine[1] (Periactin, 2-4 mg bid or tid) are tried. All patients take supplemental fat-soluble vitamins A, D, E, and K.

Controlling the characteristic fat and nutrient malabsorption is critical to ensuring good nutrition and weight gain. Approximately 85% of patients are pancreatic insufficient due to CFTR-based abnormalities of chloride and bicarbonate transport that lead to plugging of the pancreatic ducts, with subsequent acinar loss and fatty replacement. Exogenous pancreatic enzymes are provided as microtablets or microspheres incorporating lipase, protease, and amylase from animal sources; dosing is individually titrated and most often is 1000 to 2500 units of lipase per kilogram per meal, and less for snacks. Sometimes antacid therapies are added to improve efficiency of enzymes. Controlling pulmonary disease and treating comorbidities such as diabetes are also critical to maintaining nutrition.

## COMPLICATIONS

An essential component of CF care is screening for and managing disease complications (Box 1). An important example is cystic fibrosis–related diabetes, which develops in approximately 25% of patients in the teen to adult years and is increasing along with improved

---

[1]Not FDA approved for this indication.

## TABLE 3   Intravenous Antibiotics for Cystic Fibrosis Exacerbations

| Drug | Dosage* | Comments |
|---|---|---|
| **Aminoglycosides** | | |
| Amikacin (Amikin) | 5-7.5 mg/kg q8h | Peak 25-30 μg/mL, trough 5-10 μg/mL |
| Gentamicin (Garamycin) | 3 mg/kg q8h | Peak 8-12 μg/mL, trough <2 μg/mL |
| Tobramycin (Nebcin) | 3-3.3 mg/kg q8h *or* | Peak 8-12 μg/mL, trough <2μg/mL |
| | 9-10 mg/kg/d q24h | Once-daily dosing validated in adults, less so in children |
| **β-Lactams** | | |
| Aztreonam (Azactam) | 50 mg/kg q8h[3] | Covers *Pa, Hf,* not *Sa* |
| | Adults: 2g q8h | Usually safe for penicillin-allergic patients |
| Ceftazidime (Fortaz) | 50 mg/kg q8h | Covers *Pa, Hf,* some *Bcc,* not *Sa* |
| | Adults: 2g q8h | |
| Cefazolin (Ancef) | 30 mg/kg q8h | Covers *Sa* only |
| | Adults: 1g q8h | |
| Cefepime (Maxipime) | 50 mg/kg q8h | Covers *Pa, Sa,* and *Hf* |
| | Adults: 2g q8h | |
| Imipenem/cilastatin (Primaxin) | 15-25 mg/kg q6h | Covers *Pa, Sa,* and *Hf* |
| | Adults: 500-1g q6h | Administer slowly to avoid adverse effects |
| Meropenem (Merrem) | 40 mg/kg q8h | Covers *Pa, Sa, Hf,* and some *Bcc* |
| | Adults: 1-2g q8h[3] | |
| Nafcillin (Nafcil) | 25-50 mg/kg q6h | Covers *Sa* only |
| | Adults: 1-2g q6h | Dilute to ≤30 mg/mL to decrease risk of phlebitis |
| Piperacillin (Pipracil), and | 100 mg/kg q6h | Dose based on piperacillin content |
| piperacillin/tazobactam (Zosyn) | Adults: 3g q6h | Tazobactam extends coverage to *Sa, Hf,* and *Pa* |
| Ticarcillin (Ticar) and | 100 mg/kg q6h[3] | Dose based on ticarcillin content. |
| Ticarcillin/clavulanate (Timentin) | Adults: 3g q6h | Clavulanate extends coverage to *Sa, Hf, Pa,* and some *S. maltophilia* |
| **Other** | | |
| Ciprofloxacin (Cipro) | 15 mg/kg q12h[1] | Also available as oral suspension or tablet |
| | Adults: 400 mg q12h | |
| Vancomycin (Vancocin) | 15 mg/kg q6h | Peak 25-40 μg/mL, trough 10-15 μg/mL |
| | Adults: 1g q12h | Infuse slowly to avoid histamine release |
| | | Covers only MRSA and *Sa* |

[1]Not FDA approved for this indication in children younger than 18 years.
[3]Exceeds dosage recommended by the manufacturer.
*All doses are for children except where indicated. Calculated antibiotic doses in children should not exceed adult doses. Dosages of most of the antibiotics should be adjusted for patients with renal insufficiency.
*Abbreviations:* Bcc = *Burkholderia cepacia* complex; Hf = *Haemophilus influenzae;* MRSA = methicillin-resistant *Staphylococcus aureus;* Pa = *Pseudomonas aeruginosa;* Sa = *Staphylococcus aureus.*

## BOX 1 Clinical Complications

**Endocrine**
- Cystic fibrosis–related diabetes (CFRD)
- Osteopenia, osteoporosis

**Gastrointestinal**
- Cholelithiasis
- Constipation
- Distal intestinal obstructive syndrome
- Gastroesophageal reflux
- Meconium ileus (neonatal)
- Pancreatitis (in pancreatic-sufficient patients)
- Progressive cirrhosis (rare)
- Rectal prolapse

**Pulmonary**
- Allergic bronchopulmonary aspergillosis
- Atypical mycobacterial infections
- Hemoptysis
- Pneumothorax

**Reproductive**
- Male infertility

longevity of CF patients. Some patients initially have hyperglycemia that is only postprandial or with stress (e.g., pulmonary exacerbations) or steroid therapy. Insulin therapy is typically necessary, but calories and fat should not be restricted. Cystic fibrosis–related diabetes has been associated with worse pulmonary outcomes and survival, but there is recent evidence that good diabetes control can modulate this negative effect.

Notable gastrointestinal complications include distal intestinal obstruction syndrome, usually manifesting as abdominal pain without vomiting or change in bowel movements, often with a right lower quadrant fecal mass. Therapy for distal intestinal obstruction syndrome varies according to clinical severity and includes laxatives, polyethylene glycol (MiraLax, GlycoLax),[1] large volumes of balanced electrolyte solution (GoLytely),[1] or enemas with gastrografin.[1]

Significant liver disease is fortunately rare (<5% of patients), although histologically evident focal biliary cirrhosis is common. Patients who develop severe cirrhosis, portal hypertension, and liver failure may need liver transplantation.

## Future Directions

An effective pipeline of drug development for CF is screening compounds for potential benefit and bringing promising therapies closer to clinical trials. Numerous trials are in progress now, testing new drugs and treatment protocols. Meanwhile, gene therapy remains an active pursuit as well. Current initiatives also stress the importance of continuous quality improvement of clinical care within centers, including patient data tracking, aggressive care, and patient and family involvement.

### REFERENCES

Cystic Fibrosis Foundation: 2005 National Patient Data Registry Report. Bethesda, Md: Cystic Fibrosis Foundation, 2005. PDF available at http://www.cff.org/UploadedFiles/research/ClinicalResearch/PatientRegistry Report/2005%20Patient%20Registry%20Report.pdf (accessed May 1, 2007).

Elkins MR, Robinson M, Rose BR, et al: A controlled trial of long-term inhaled hypertonic saline in patients with cystic fibrosis. N Engl J Med 2006;354(3):229-240.

Gibson R, Burns J, Ramsey B: Pathophysiology and management of pulmonary complications in cystic fibrosis. Am J Respir Crit Care Med 2003; 168(8):918-951.

Grosse SD, Boyle CA, Botkin JR, et al: Newborn screening for cystic fibrosis: Evaluation of benefits and risks and recommendations for state newborn screening programs. MMWR Recomm Rep 2004;53 (RR-13):1-36.

Knoderer CA, Everett JA, Buss WF: Clinical issues surrounding once-daily aminoglycoside dosing in children. Pharmacotherapy 2003;23(1):44-56.

Rosenstein BJ, Cutting GR: Diagnosis of cystic fibrosis: A consensus statement. J Pediatr 1998;132:589-595.

Saiman L, Marshall BC, Mayer-Hamblett N, et al: Azithromycin in patients chronically infected with *Pseudomonas aeruginosa*: A randomized controlled trial. JAMA 2003;290(13):1749-1756.

Stevens DA, Moss RB, Kurup VP, et al: Allergic bronchopulmonary aspergillosis in cystic fibrosis—state of the art. Cystic Fibrosis Foundation Consensus Conference. Clin Infec Dis 2003;37(suppl 3):S225-S264.

# Sleep Apnea

Method of
*Leon Rosenthal, MD*

Obstructive sleep apnea (OSA) is a condition characterized by repetitive episodes of obstruction of the upper airway during sleep. The obstructions may be complete (apnea) or partial (hypopnea), and they result in fluctuations in blood oxygen saturation and disruption of sleep continuity.

By definition, apneic and hypopneic events last a minimum of 10 seconds. The apnea-hypopnea index (AHI) is defined as the total number of apneas and hypopneas during the time asleep divided by the number of hours of sleep. Respiratory effort–related arousal (RERA) is considered an additional type of sleep-related obstructive event. It presents a risk factor for the behavioral morbidity associated with OSA that is as great as those of obstructive apneas and hypopneas. RERAs also by definition last 10 seconds (or longer), reflect a sequence of breaths characterized by increasing respiratory effort, are not associated with oxygen fluctuations, and lead to an arousal from sleep.

In the adult population, the current classification of sleep disorders requires polysomnographic documentation of five or more obstructive respiratory events (obstructive apneas, hypopneas, or RERAs) per hour of sleep to diagnose OSA. To date, the diagnosis is established based on the sleep laboratory assessment using standard polysomnographic techniques. OSA should be suspected based on the clinical assessment, physical examination, and understanding of potential risk factors.

## Epidemiology

The prevalence of OSA (defined as an apnea-hypopnea index of >5/hour) among adults between 30 and 60 years of age has been estimated at 9% for women and 24% for men. The prevalence of the OSA syndrome, which includes symptoms of excessive sleepiness, is estimated at 2% for women and 4% for men. Clearly, male gender represents an independent risk factor for OSA when compared with premenopausal women. The prevalence among women increases with menopause. In regard to ethnicity, African American, Pacific Islander, and Mexican American patients might be at increased risk for OSA.

## Clinical Features

Snoring represents the most common feature of OSA and is usually reported by a bed partner. Many patients are prompted by their spouses to pursue consultation after many years of enduring the disruptive effects of snoring during sleep. The description of periods

---

[1]Not FDA approved for this indication.

of snoring followed by periods of silence, which are terminated by breakthrough snoring make the diagnosis of OSA very likely. In many instances, the patients are described as experiencing stop-breathing episodes during their sleep.

Affected patients might not be aware of any difficulties during their sleep, but some report persistent nocturnal awakenings; some of the awakenings might be associated with a sensation of choking, smothering, or gasping. Nocturnal perspiration, nocturia, and symptoms of nocturnal gastroesophageal reflux are commonly associated with severe OSA. Patients might report awakening unrefreshed, with a dry mouth, and with a headache. Daytime symptoms are commonly encountered; the most frequent complaint is excessive sleepiness, which is a consequence of disrupted sleep.

Increased risk of motor vehicle accidents has been reported among OSA patients, and assessment of the patient's level of sleepiness in the context of their employment and their exposure to driving or operating machinery needs to be established during the clinical assessment. Associated features of excessive sleepiness may be manifested as fatigue, impaired memory and concentration, depression, and changes in personality. Among male patients, impotence due to low testosterone levels has been established in some severe cases of OSA.

Obesity is common in OSA, and a graded increase in OSA prevalence has been documented with increasing body mass index (BMI), neck circumference, and waist-to-hip ratio. However, a potential diagnosis of OSA should not be dismissed in a nonobese patient presenting with symptoms or having risk factors associated with a potential diagnosis of OSA. Physical findings such as a crowded oropharynx with evidence of a redundant soft palate, redundant soft tissue in the oropharyngeal examination, relative macroglossia, and tonsillar hypertrophy are often encountered among patients with OSA. A narrow oropharynx with a high arched palate and short intermolar distance has also been described among some patients with OSA. Retrognathia or micrognathia might also result in narrowing of the retroglossal area, which might increase the risk of OSA when sleeping in the supine position.

OSA has been shown to represent an independent risk factor for systemic arterial hypertension. Thus, difficult to control hypertension should raise the possibility of a diagnosis of OSA. Untreated OSA might also represent a risk factor for stroke; new-onset atrial fibrillation (in particular if triggered during sleep) should raise the clinical suspicion of OSA. Other medical conditions that appear to predispose to OSA include nasal obstruction, nasal septal deviation, hypothyroidism, acromegaly, and congestive heart failure.

Evidence of a potential link between OSA and insulin resistance (and diabetes mellitus) has been reported. Ongoing research is actively pursuing this pathophysiologic pathway, and the increased prevalence of the metabolic syndrome in the general population makes the clinical suspicion of OSA very relevant in these patients because both conditions share a number of clinical characteristics. In fact, it is conceivable that the increased cardiovascular risk conferred by OSA is, at least in part, mediated through the metabolic syndrome.

## Screening and Testing

### LABORATORY SLEEP TEST

The definitive diagnosis of OSA requires an in-laboratory attended sleep test (nocturnal polysomnography), which enables the characterization of multiple physiologic variables. Recording of a limited number of channels in the patient's home can be used for screening purposes (ambulatory oximetry or cardio-respiratory studies, which yield estimates of respiratory disturbance). Although in some cases ambulatory studies might render confirmation of the diagnosis, there is no consensus at present as to the ideal algorithm to be followed to allow the diagnosis of OSA without a sleep laboratory assessment. Ongoing research efforts will likely result in the diagnosis and treatment of some OSA populations without the need for in-laboratory testing.

The in-laboratory sleep test allows characterization of ventilation during sleep. Ventilation includes number of central and obstructive apneas, hypopneas, and RERAs and detailed information on oxygen saturation as well as the depiction of the potentially relevant positional effects on the frequency of respiratory events. Laboratory testing also includes a complete accounting of sleep variables, monitoring of cardiac rhythm, and assessment of possible restless legs syndrome (RLS) or periodic limb movements (PLMs) during sleep. This information enables the clinician to determine the severity of the condition and identifies potentially relevant comorbidities (RLS, PLMs, cardiac arrhythmias).

The split-night protocol during the laboratory assessment allows the clinician to derive the diagnosis of the condition during the first half of the night (ideally 4 hours of diagnostic testing with a minimum of 2 hours if an AHI >40 is confirmed). During the second half of the night, the clinician can titrate continuous positive airway pressure (CPAP), which requires a minimum of 3 hours of sleep. This protocol is a cost-effective use of laboratory resources that allows the clinician to identify therapeutic CPAP settings to help implement therapy at home, and in most instances there is no need for a second sleep study. This protocol is particularly well suited for patients with severe OSA. The possible implementation of CPAP titration should be discussed with the patient in advance, because the initial experience with CPAP is a major determinant of long-term use.

Several algorithms are available to make clinical predictions about the likelihood of a positive diagnosis of OSA. In general, an obese patient with a large neck size (≥17 in for male patients; ≥16.5 in for female patients) and symptoms of excessive sleepiness is likely to be a good candidate for split-night studies. In cases were a diagnostic polysomnography identified a diagnosis of OSA and CPAP is the therapy of choice, a second night in the laboratory for CPAP titration is indicated.

### WHOM TO TEST AND THERAPEUTIC OPTIONS

Clinical signs and symptoms are not necessarily sensitive or specific enough to establish a definitive diagnosis of OSA. Therefore, sleep studies are required for patients who are symptomatic and for others who are asymptomatic but have clinical signs that suggest the diagnosis. Testing allows the examiner to define the severity of the condition, and the results (with adequate clinical correlation) should guide therapeutic intervention.

Epidemiologic data have helped define the index of severity. An AHI of 5 or higher has been shown to represent the minimum threshold value for increased risk of hypertension and an AHI greater than 30 has been associated with a substantial increase in the risk of hypertension. Thus, mild OSA is defined as an AHI of 5 to 15 per hour, moderate OSA is an AHI of 15 to 30 per hour, and severe OSH is an AHI greater than 30 per hour. In addition, a clinically derived index of severity of excessive sleepiness should be determined based on the presence of unwanted sleepiness or involuntary sleep episodes

### CURRENT DIAGNOSIS

**Symptoms and Signs**

- Excessive sleepiness
- Resuscitative snoring or loud snoring
- Witnessed stop-breathing episodes
- Nocturia

**Risk Factors**

- Obesity; large neck circumference (central obesity)
- Sex: men, postmenopausal women
- Age: 30 to 65 years
- Abnormal upper airway (e.g., nasal obstruction, large tongue, redundant soft tissue, large tonsils, retrognathia)
- Family history of obstructive sleep apnea

(mild if the episodes occur during activities that require little attention, moderate if the manifestations are associated with activities that require some attention, and severe if sleepiness is present in activities that require active attention).

Many patients are motivated to pursue treatment because of their desire to eliminate snoring, and others want relief of symptoms of excessive sleepiness. An increasing number of patients understand the potentially negative cardiovascular consequences of untreated OSA and expect therapy if the diagnosis is confirmed. Therapy is justified if the AHI is greater than 5 per hour, and it should not be delayed if the AHI is greater than 30 per hour.

Regardless of the severity of the condition, patients who are overweight should be encouraged to lose weight. In some patients with morbid obesity, bariatric surgery might be a means to enable effective weight loss and likely improvement of ventilation during sleep.

Patients should be counseled to avoid practices that can potentially worsen the severity of OSA. The use of CNS depressants before sleep (alcohol, sleep medications, pain medications) might worsen ventilation during sleep and should be discouraged. In some patients with positional OSA, avoiding the supine position during sleep might suffice in helping normalize ventilation during sleep. However, one needs to question how this can be done effectively over a long time. If upper airway pathology is identified (nasal septum deviation, enlarged tonsils, craniofacial abnormalities), surgical consultation should be pursued. If patients have symptoms of excessive sleepiness, they should be counseled to avoid driving or operating machinery, and the appropriate local laws should be followed regarding the need to notify the relevant administrative authorities.

## Treatment

### CPAP THERAPY

The proper positive airway pressure delivered by a flow generator through an interface of the patient's choice represents the gold standard in the therapy of OSA, because it is almost always successful in maintaining upper airway patency and oxygen saturation, and it improves sleep continuity and architecture. The main barrier to successful therapy is nonacceptance of the therapy or low therapeutic adherence. Treatment is effective as long as the patient uses the device for the entire night, every night. The use of integrated heated humidifiers has minimized issues of upper airway dryness and has helped improve adherence to therapy.

There are many manufacturers of CPAP devices and many interfaces that help maximize comfort with treatment. The clinician should be aware of the characteristics of the specific CPAP unit that is being prescribed to the patient and should monitor the level of comfort of the interface that the patient has selected. Expiratory pressure release (EPR) is available through a couple of CPAP manufacturers. EPR does not seem to compromise the effectiveness of CPAP therapy and improves the patient's sense of comfort with therapy, but it does not seem to systematically improve the level of adherence.

Autotitrating CPAP units are available, and their software has been greatly improved. They have been proved effective in improving ventilation during sleep, but no additional clinical benefits over standard CPAP therapy have been demonstrated.

Bilevel respiratory assist devices deliver alternating levels of positive airway pressure and might be considered as an alternative therapeutic option when standard CPAP is not tolerated or when oxygen saturation is not raised sufficiently with standard CPAP. In some cases of severe OSA (in particular among patients with underlying pulmonary conditions) supplemental oxygen can be used in conjunction with CPAP therapy.

### ORAL APPLIANCE THERAPY

Prostheses worn in the mouth during sleep can help maintain a patent airway. In general, there are two types of appliances, mandibular advancement appliances and tongue-retaining devices. The mandibular advancement appliances are currently used more often and have been more widely studied. They require viable dentition for retention. They are fitted to the maxillary and mandibular dentition to enable the protrusion of the mandible and therefore increase oropharyngeal patency. The most common side effect is excessive salivation, but temporomandibular joint pain might limit the viability of this therapy. Chronic use of the appliance can result in a change of the dental occlusion and lead to discontinuation of therapy. A dentist with expertise in sleep medicine should ideally implement and monitor this type of treatment.

### SURGICAL PROCEDURES

Patients with an identifiable anatomic upper airway (soft tissue) abnormality or craniofacial abnormality might benefit from surgery. There are a variety of soft-tissue procedures that might help stabilize the retropalatal region (the uvulopalatopharyngoplasty), and others are intended to stabilize the retrolingual airway (genioglossal advancement and hyoid myotomy). Office-based procedures have also become available, such as the injection snoreplasty and the pillar procedure, which are intended to stiffen the soft palate and thereby decrease snoring and respiratory events. A substantially more invasive procedure, the maxillomandibular advancement, has been shown very effective in a number of case series. However, it is not possible to predict which patients are likely to have a successful surgical outcome. As a result, many patients undergo a surgical procedure that fails to improve their condition and then require additional surgery or medical treatment of OSA. Surgical consultation with an otorhinolaryngologist or oral surgeon should be pursued for patients who might benefit from this therapeutic approach.

### RESPONSE TO THERAPY

The patient's response to therapy needs to be monitored. In the case of CPAP therapy, monitoring of CPAP adherence is critical, because subjective reports are inaccurate. Resolution of excessive sleepiness is the desired outcome for patients who are symptomatic at baseline. If excessive sleepiness remains problematic despite documentation of desirable CPAP adherence, treatment with modafinil (Provigil) 100 to 400 mg in the morning might be considered.

Other potential conditions affecting sleep need to be monitored and, if needed, treated. Often, other conditions such as poor sleep hygiene, RLS, PLMs, or psychophysiologic insomnia interfere with adequate response to therapy.

For patients who undergo surgery, retesting is indicated. The interval at which retesting should be done depends on the type of surgery that was performed. Retesting 3 months following the surgical intervention is adequate in most cases.

### CURRENT THERAPY

- Continuous positive airway pressure (CPAP) represents the gold standard of therapy.
- Patient education, adequate CPAP settings, and a comfortable interface are critical to achieve a desirable level of treatment adherence.
- Integrated heated humidification minimizes nasal dryness and improves CPAP adherence.
- Clinical follow-up to assess tolerance to CPAP and resolution of symptoms is critical to achieve desired outcomes.
- Improved sleep schedule practices should be encouraged and comorbid conditions should be treated.
- Oral appliance therapy and surgical procedures represent alternative therapeutic options.

## REFERENCES

Dinges DF, Weaver TE: Effects of modafinil on sustained attention and quality of life in OSA patients with residual sleepiness while being treated with NCPAP. Sleep Med 2003;4:393-402.

Gay P, Weaver T, Loube D, et al: Evaluation of positive airway pressure treatment for sleep related breathing disorders in adults: A review by the positive airway pressure task force of the standards of practice committee of the American Academy of Sleep Medicine. Sleep 2006;29:381-401.

Lindberg E, Gislason T: Epidemiology of sleep-related obstructive breathing. Sleep Med Rev 2000;4:411-433.

Mulgrew AT, Fox N, Ayas NT, et al: Diagnosis and initial management of obstructive sleep apnea without polysomnography: A randomized validation study. Ann Intern Med 2007;146:157-166.

Rosenthal L, Bishop C, Guido P, et al: The sleep/wake habits of patients diagnosed as having obstructive sleep apnea. Chest 1997;111:1494-1499.

Rosenthal L, Gerhardstein R, Lumley A, et al: CPAP therapy in patients with mild OSA: Implementation and treatment outcome. Sleep Med 2000;3:215-220.

Sanders M, Givelber R: Overview of obstructive sleep apnea in adults. In Lee-Chiong TF (ed): Sleep: A Comprehensive Handbook. Hoboken, NJ: John Wiley and Sons, 2006, pp 231-240.

Senior B, Rosenthal L, Lumley A, Gerhardstein R, Day R: Efficacy of uvulopalatopharyngoplasty in unselected patients with mild obstructive sleep apnea. Otolaryngol Head Neck Surg 2000;123(3):179-182.

Sleep-related breathing disorders in adults: Recommendations for syndrome definition and measurement techniques in clinical research: The report of an American Academy of Sleep Medicine task force. Sleep 1999;22:667-689.

# Primary Lung Cancer

Method of
*Christopher S. George, MD, and
Teresa M. George, MD*

Lung cancer is a significant health problem in the United States. It is the second most commonly diagnosed cancer in both men and women. Despite not being the most common form of cancer, it has the highest mortality rate of all malignancies, and tumors of the lung and bronchus account for 32% of all cancer deaths in males and for 25% of all cancer deaths in females. In 2007, it was estimated that 213,380 patients would develop lung cancer and that 160,390 deaths would occur. Both men and women have seen increases in mortality over the last 100 years. The mortality in males is finally starting to decrease; in females, there has been a steady rise in mortality over the last 40 years. Only in recent years has this started to level off. Despite advances in diagnosis and treatment, the overall 5-year survival rate is low at 15%.

## Risk Factors

Cigarette smoking remains the major risk factor for the development of lung cancer. It is associated with pulmonary malignancies in more than 80% of cases. The incidence and mortality trends of lung cancer are reflective of the trends of tobacco use of males and females over the last several decades. Both active and passive tobacco exposure have been implicated in the development of lung cancer. Exposure to tobacco other than in cigarettes (e.g., cigar and pipe smoking) has also caused an increase in the incidence of pulmonary cancers, although to a lesser degree than cigarettes. The smoking of marijuana and cocaine has not been studied as much as cigarette use, but it is believed that use of these substances probably increases the risk of lung cancer.

In addition to tobacco, many other environmental and occupational toxins are associated with the development of respiratory cancers. High levels of prolonged exposure to radon, asbestos, haloethers, polycyclic aromatic hydrocarbons, arsenic, and nickel cause lung cancer. Although these increase lung cancer in nonsmokers, the risk appears to be magnified in smokers, demonstrating a synergy between these carcinogens.

Other risk factors for the development of pulmonary malignancies include genetic or familial risk factors. First-degree relatives of patients with lung cancer have a 1.5- to 5-fold increased risk themselves. It should be noted that the exact molecular basis accounting for the increased risk is not well understood.

Patients with certain benign underlying lung diseases may also be at increased risk for the development of lung cancer. In particular, there is an increased risk in patients with pulmonary fibrosis, asbestosis, and possibly even chronic obstructive pulmonary disease (COPD). Increasing numbers of nonsmokers are developing non–small cell lung cancer in this country.

## Clinical Manifestations

Occasionally lung cancer is discovered incidentally with bronchoscopy or chest x-ray; in the majority of cases, patients present with signs and symptoms. The exact clinical presentation depends on the site and spread of the primary tumor (Table 1). Many of the symptoms are nonspecific and may be seen more often in other disease entities. Most commonly, patients present with cough, dyspnea, chest pain, or hemoptysis. Fatigue, weight loss, and bone pain are also seen in patients, especially those with metastatic disease.

There are several distinct syndromes that can be seen with pulmonary malignancies. Some of these are caused by the tumor's spread into the mediastinum or surrounding structures. In the superior vena cava syndrome, patients may exhibit periorbital and facial edema and headaches. In later stages, this may be accompanied by a bluish discoloration and new vessel formation on the anterior chest. Pancoast syndrome results from involvement of the brachial plexus by superior sulcus tumors. Patients may present with shoulder and arm pain with associated sensorimotor changes. If the sympathetic trunk is

## TABLE 1 Clinical Manifestations

| Associated with Primary Lesion | Associated with Intrathoracic Spread | Secondary to Metastases | Paraneoplastic Syndromes |
|---|---|---|---|
| Cough | Pleural effusion | Bone pain | Hypercalcemia |
| Dyspnea | Pericardial effusion | Generalized weakness | Hypertrophic osteoarthropathy |
| Hemoptysis | Hoarseness | Weight loss | SIADH |
| Chest pain | Superior vena cava syndrome | Headache | Cushing's syndrome |
| Weight loss | Pancoast syndrome | Nausea | Eaton-Lambert syndrome |
| Unilateral wheezing | Horner syndrome | Vomiting | Cerebellar ataxia |
| Fever secondary to pneumonia | | Neurologic symptoms | Dementia |
| | | Abdominal pain | Sensorimotor neuropathies |

*Abbreviation:* SIADH, syndrome of inappropriate secretion of antidiuretic hormone.

## CURRENT DIAGNOSIS

- Lung cancer is the second most common cancer in the United States, but has the highest mortality
- Cigarette smoking is the major risk factor
- Most common symptoms are cough, dyspnea, chest pain, and hemoptysis
- Diagnosis is made by cytologic specimen or histologic biopsy
- Staging must be done on all patients and should consist of history, physical examination, laboratory studies, and radiographic examinations
- Preoperative evaluation must be done in patients who are considered for surgery

involved, patients may have Horner syndrome, which is characterized by ptosis, miosis, facial flushing, and anhidrosis on the side affected by the tumor.

In addition to syndromes caused by direct extension of the tumor, patients may also present with syndromes caused by the production of biologically active substances. Some of these are better understood than others. These are collectively referred to as the paraneoplastic syndromes. Examples of paraneoplastic syndromes observed in lung cancer include hypercalcemia from the production of parathyroid hormone-related peptide, hypertrophic osteoarthropathy, syndrome of inappropriate secretion of antidiuretic hormone (SIADH), Cushing's syndrome, and Eaton-Lambert syndrome.

## Diagnosis

Once lung cancer is suspected, pathologic diagnosis must be made (Table 2). The diagnosis can be established based on cytologic specimens or histologic biopsy. Cytologic specimens may consist of sputum, bronchial washings or brushings, transbronchial or transthoracic needle aspirates, or bronchoalveolar lavage. Histologic biopsy can be

**TABLE 2 World Health Organization Histologic Classification of Epithelial Bronchogenic Carcinoma**

| **Malignant** | |
|---|---|
| Squamous cell (epidermal) and spindle cell carcinoma | |
| Small cell | Oat cell carcinoma (lymphocytic-like) |
| | Intermediate cell type |
| | Combined oat cell carcinoma (mixed histologic types, small with squamous cell carcinoma or adenocarcinoma) |
| Adenocarcinoma | Acinar |
| | Papillary |
| | Bronchoalveolar |
| | Mucinous secreting |
| Large cell | Giant cell |
| | Clear cell |
| Adenosquamous carcinoma | Carcinoid |
| | Bronchial gland carcinoma |
| | Adenoid cystic |
| | Mucoepidermoid |
| Others | |

Adapted from World Health Organization: Histologic Typing of Lung Tumors, 2nd ed. Geneva, WHO, 1981.

from endobronchial, transbronchial, transthoracic, or open biopsy procedures. Generally, if the lesion is central, bronchoscopy is recommended for evaluation. If the abnormality is peripheral, use of computed tomography (CT)-guided transthoracic needle aspiration or biopsy is recommended. If the diagnosis is still equivocal, a more definitive open procedure may be needed.

## Pretreatment Evaluation

After a pathologic diagnosis is established, the pretreatment evaluation must be done. This consists of two main parts: complete staging of the tumor so that treatment recommendations can be made (Table 3), and if surgery is a consideration, a preoperative assessment. The primary care physician can take the initial role in both of these evaluations.

Evaluation is needed to determine the stage of the tumor (staging systems for small cell lung cancer [SCLC] and non–small cell lung cancer [NSCLC] are discussed later). A good history and physical examination is the first step in any staging process. Then laboratory studies, including complete blood count, electrolytes, creatinine, calcium, alkaline phosphatase, aspartate aminotransferase (AST), alanine aminotransferase (ALT), bilirubin, and albumin should be done in all patients. The American Thoracic Society recommends that all patients receive CT of the chest with inclusion of liver and adrenals. If pleural effusions are present, patients should undergo evaluation with thoracentesis. Patients with SCLC should also receive bone scan and either CT or magnetic resonance imaging (MRI) of the brain. In patients with NSCLC, a bone scan should only be done in those with

## CURRENT THERAPY

**Non–Small Cell Lung Cancer**

**Stage IA**

- Surgery

**Stage IB**

- Surgery ± chemotherapy

**Stage II**

- Surgery and chemotherapy

**Stage IIIA**

- Surgery ± chemotherapy ± radiation

or

- Chemoradiation ± surgery

**Stage IIIB**

- Chemoradiation ± surgery

**Stage IV**

- Chemotherapy ± VEGF inhibitor, EGFR tyrosine kinase inhibitor, supportive care

**Small Cell Lung Cancer**

**Limited Stage**

- Concurrent chemoradiation ± prophylactic cranial irradiation

**Extensive Stage**

- Chemotherapy
- Palliative radiation
- Clinical trial participation preferred in all stages.

*Abbreviations:* EGFR, epidermal growth factor receptor; VEGF, vascular endothelial growth factor

## TABLE 3 International Staging System for Lung Cancer

| Primary Tumor (T) | Nodal Involvement (N) | Distant Metastasis (M) | Stage Groupings of TNM Subsets |
|---|---|---|---|
| Tx—Primary tumor cannot be assessed or tumor proven by the presence of malignant cells in sputum or bronchial washings but not visualized by imaging or bronchoscopy | Nx—Regional lymph nodes cannot be assessed | M0—No distant metastasis | Occult carcinoma Tx, N0, M0 |
| T0—No evidence of primary tumor | N0—No regional lymph node involvement | M1—distant metastasis present or separate tumor nodules in a different lobe | Stage 0 Tis, N0, M0 |
| Tis—Carcinoma in situ | N1—Ipsilateral peribronchial or hilar nodes involved | | Stage IA T1, N0, M0 |
| T1—Tumor ≤3 cm in greatest dimension, surrounded by lung tissue and no bronchoscopic evidence of tumor proximal to the lobar bronchus | N2—Ipsilateral mediastinal or subcarinal nodes involved | | Stage IB T2, N0, M0 |
| T2—Tumor >3 cm in greatest dimension, or tumor of any size that involves the visceral pleura or is associated with atelectasis extending to the hilum (but not involving the entire lung) and must be ≥2 cm from the carina | N3—Contralateral mediastinal or hilar nodes or scalene or supraclavicular nodes involved | | Stage IIA T2, N1, M0 |
| T3—Tumor involves the chest wall, diaphragm, mediastinal pleura or pericardium, or is <:2 cm from the carina (but does not involve it) | | | Stage IIB T2, N1, M0 T3, N0, M0 |
| T4—Tumor involves the carina or trachea or invades the mediastinum, heart, great vessels, esophagus or vertebrae, or malignant pleural effusion is present, or separate tumor nodules in the same lobe | | | Stage IIIA T3, N1, M0 T1-T3, N2, M0 |
| | | | Stage IIIB Any T, N3, M0 T4, Any N, M0 Stage IV Any T, Any N, M1 |

Adapted from Mountain CF: Revisions in the international staging system for lung cancer. Chest 1997;111:1710-1717.

bone pain or elevated serum calcium or alkaline phosphatase from the bone. Neuroimaging is only recommended in NSCLC patients with signs or symptoms of neurologic disease. Select patients with suspected mediastinal lymph node involvement may require additional procedures such as mediastinoscopy, mediastinotomy, or thoracoscopy for staging. Over the last decade, positron emission tomography (PET) has also become more commonly used in staging. It has been approved by Medicare for the diagnosis, staging, and restaging of NSCLC. The American Society of Clinical Oncologists (ASCO) recommends it for locoregional staging in patients with NSCLC without distant metastatic disease on CT. PET scanning is less clear in the staging of SCLC.

If the patient has limited disease and is recommended for surgery, preoperative assessment must be done. In addition to normal preoperative assessment of cardiovascular risks, pulmonary assessment must be performed as well. The single most useful test is the measurement of forced expiratory volume in 1 second ($FEV_1$). Guidelines from the American College of Chest Physicians state that patients with $FEV_1$ of greater than 2 L generally tolerate pneumonectomy. For lobectomy, an $FEV_1$ of 1 to 1.5 L is recommended. If preoperative $FEV_1$ is less than 2 L, further evaluation with measurement of carbon monoxide diffusion in the lung ($DL_{CO}$), quantitative split perfusion lung scanning, or cardiopulmonary exercise testing may be considered.

## Prognostic Factors

There are several factors that may indicate poorer prognosis in patients with lung cancer. Extent of disease portrays prognosis with those with advanced stages faring worse. Baseline poor performance status and weight loss are also signs of worse prognosis. In SCLC, for an unknown reason, women tend to do better. The presence of paraneoplastic syndromes is a poor prognostic sign. Race, age, and histologic subtype are less important in determining prognosis.

## Treatment

### NON–SMALL CELL LUNG CANCER

#### Stage I

Stage I includes T1 and T2 tumors (see Table 3) without lymph node involvement or distant metastases. Patients undergo mediastinoscopy with frozen section analysis of lymph nodes, followed by resection of the primary tumor. Lobectomy is the typical surgical procedure performed; more proximal tumors may require a pneumonectomy or sleeve resection. Limited surgery, such as a wedge resection, has been associated with inferior results in some series and is generally reserved only for elderly, frail patients, or those with less cardiopulmonary reserve. In these patients, video-assisted thoracic surgery (VATS) may be performed with decreased perioperative morbidity and less postoperative pain. The expected 5-year survival following a lobectomy is 60% to 70% in most series. It has been noted that survival rates are better for patients who have their surgery performed at hospitals that perform higher volumes of this surgery. Also, patients with no or minimal comorbid conditions have better survival rates.

At present, there are limited data for induction or neoadjuvant chemotherapy before surgical resection, and this should be considered experimental. Primary radiation therapy can be used for nonsurgical patients, including those with very poor cardiopulmonary reserve or those who refuse surgery. However, the results are clearly inferior to surgery, with only 15% of patients enjoying long-term survival, as 24% die of other illnesses and 60% succumb to progression of lung cancer. As such, newer radiation techniques are being investigated, such as hyperfractionation and stereotactic radiosurgery.

Postoperative radiation therapy (PORT) remains of unproven benefit. The PORT meta-analysis noted a decrease in survival compared with surgery alone despite potentially reducing local recurrence rates. The cause of this finding is uncertain, but higher rates of cardiopulmonary failure and infections were noted. Outdated radiation therapy techniques may have also contributed. Currently, the routine use of PORT is discouraged as a standard approach. The use of adjuvant chemotherapy was previously thought to be unhelpful, likely because of ineffective chemotherapy developed in the 1980s. Several meta-analyses have shown only 4% to 5% survival benefit. However, several well-conducted international trials have yielded significant results that have changed the standard of care. The Cancer and Leukemia Group B (CALGB) 9633 trial was presented in abstract form in 2004. Three hundred forty-four patients with stage IB were randomized to surgery alone or surgery followed by four cycles of adjuvant carboplatin (Paraplatin[1]) and paclitaxel (Taxol). The 4-year overall survival rate was 59% for the surgery-alone group and 71% for the chemotherapy group. The lung cancer mortality rate decreased from 19.9% to 11%. Importantly, no treatment-related deaths were noted. Unfortunately, the 2006 update only shows a survival advantage for the subset of patients with tumors greater than 4 cm. In 2005, the National Cancer Institute of Canada (NCIC) trial JBR10 was published in the *New England Journal of Medicine*. This study included 482 patients randomized to surgery alone or adjuvant cisplatin (Platinol AQ[1]) and vinorelbine (Navelbine) for four cycles. The patient population was different with both stages IB and II (excluding T3 N0) included. Despite only 50% of patients completing chemotherapy, there was a significant improvement in 5-year overall survival rates of 54% surgery alone compared to 69% surgery plus chemotherapy (p = 0.03). Two treatment-related deaths were noted (0.8%). Median survival was also prolonged at 73 months surgery alone compared to 94 months surgery plus chemotherapy (p = 0.04). In 2006, the Adjuvant Navelbine International Trialist Association (ANITA) published their trial of adjuvant cisplatin (Platinol AQ) and vinorelbine (Navelbine) versus observation after surgery. Seven hundred and ninety-nine patients with stages IB, II, and IIIA disease participated in the study. An absolute overall survival benefit of 8.4% was seen at seven years follow-up. Again, unfortunately only the patients with stages II and IIIA disease appeared to benefit. Thus, adjuvant chemotherapy for stage I patients is controversial and should be limited to those with larger high-risk tumors or administered in the context of a clinical trial. The Japanese have investigated oral uracil plus tegafur (UFT) with a meta-analysis of their six trials showing a 5-year survival benefit of 5%. This drug is currently not available in the United States.

## Stage II

Stage II cancers include those with spread to ipsilateral hilar lymph nodes but no mediastinal nodes or distant metastases. It also includes T3N0 tumors (see Table 3). This stage is the least-common stage. Long-term survival is uncommon without surgical intervention. As with stage I, lobectomy is the standard approach except for proximal tumors that require pneumonectomy. Mediastinal lymph node dissection is associated with a small to moderate survival advantage. The 5-year overall survival rate is 30% to 45% in most studies. Hospital volume appears to influence survival rates. Squamous cell cancers may do better than other tumors. Neoadjuvant chemotherapy studies show encouraging results. Those unfit for surgery have been treated with radiation therapy with 5-year survival rates of 19% to 25%. PORT has not been proven to be helpful in improving long-term survival rates. Adjuvant chemotherapy is the standard approach following surgery as described above.

## Stage III

Stage III is a heterogeneous group that includes patients with ipsilateral or subcarinal nodes (N2) and T3 tumors with N1 nodes for stage IIIA, as well as patients with contralateral nodes (N3) or T4 lesions for stage IIIB (see Table 3). In 1997, the International Staging System removed T3N0 tumors from this group and changed them to stage IIB, making it difficult to interpret results of older studies. The application of prior studies' results to current practice is also limited because of inadequate staging by modern standards.

The treatment of stage III tumors is one of the most controversial aspects of lung cancer care; enrollment in clinical trials is of paramount importance. Patients with nonbulky stage IIIA tumors are generally resected with curative intent. The role of PORT is again unclear. Although no improvement in survival has been noted, radiation can decrease local recurrence (which can be a devastating occurrence) and may be reasonable. The recent adjuvant chemotherapy data from stages I and II combined with the 1995 meta-analysis and recent International Adjuvant Lung Cancer Trial (IALT), suggesting 5% improvement in 5-year survival, also make postoperative chemotherapy a reasonable consideration (whether chemotherapy should be concurrent or sequential is an area needing further investigation). Given the high risk of distant metastases in stage III, induction or neoadjuvant chemotherapy has appeal. The theoretical benefits include decreasing tumor volume, earlier treatment of micrometastatic disease, and better tolerance to the drugs. With all tumors, chemotherapy response rates for the primary tumor is generally higher than with metastatic disease, presumably as a result of less-resistant clones having developed.

PORT alone has been abandoned in favor of chemotherapy or combination radiation and chemotherapy. A recent phase III study by the North American Intergroup reported a significant improvement in progression-free survival with surgery following induction concurrent chemoradiation. The 2005 abstract update also showed no improvement in overall survival as a result of the higher death rate from postoperative complications, including a 29% operative mortality in patients who required a complex pneumonectomy. Despite even trimodality therapy, the 5-year survival rates remain 20% to 25% at most.

Patients with bulky stage IIIA and stage IIIB tumors are generally unresectable and do quite poorly with 5-year survival rates around 5% to 10%. Radiation therapy has been used as a single agent, with local control being a significant problem. Only 17% obtain a complete remission on x-ray. Induction chemotherapy has been repeatedly studied, and has an approximately 10% relative reduction in death or an absolute survival advantage of 2% to 3%. The benefit of this approach seems to disappear after the second year of follow-up. Local failure within the chest remains a significant problem with this approach. Concurrent chemotherapy with radiation offers the potential benefit of improved local and distant control, with chemotherapy adding to local control as a radiation sensitizer and distant control with treatment of micrometastatic disease. The optimal regimen is uncertain and the subject of active investigation. A regimen from the Southwest Oncology Group (SWOG) employing cisplatin (Platinol AQ[1]) and etoposide (VePesid[1]) with radiation followed by docetaxel (Taxotere) has yielded a 5-year overall survival rate of 15%. A regimen with weekly carboplatin (Paraplatin[1]) and paclitaxel (Taxol) is popular in the United States, with phase II data yielding a 4-year survival rate of 16%.

## Stage IIIB with Malignant Pleural Effusion and Stage IV

With rare exceptions, stage IV (see Table 3) patients are incurable with currently available modalities, and the treatment goals are palliation of symptoms and prolongation of survival. Occasionally patients with an

---

[1]Not FDA approved for this indication.

[1]Not FDA approved for this indication.

isolated metastasis, such as that involving the brain, may be cured with surgical resection followed by whole-brain radiation therapy. In the 1970s, when response rates with all chemotherapy were quite low, it was widely held that chemotherapy held no value in the treatment of advanced lung cancer. With the advent of potentially more effective therapies, it has been shown that chemotherapy offers not only some improvement in survival, but also a better quality of life and economic savings because of fewer hospitalizations for symptom management. Although the median survival rates are improved by only 2 to 3 months, with modern therapies, it is expected that 30% to 45% of patients live beyond 1 year, approximately 20% live beyond 2 years, and an occasional patient lives 5 years or longer with metastatic disease. This is in stark contrast to the historical 1-year survival rate of 15% with essentially no 5-year survivors.

The cornerstone of current therapy is platinum-based doublets (two drugs), which is the preferred approach in otherwise healthy patients with preserved functional performance status. Meta-analyses show improved median and 1-year survival response rates compared with single-agent drugs. A large randomized trial comparing four different platinum-containing regimens showed no clear advantage to any. Paclitaxel (Taxol), gemcitabine (Gemzar), vinorelbine (Navelbine), docetaxel (Taxotere), and irinotecan (Camptosar[1]) are among the drugs that can be combined with carboplatin (Paraplatin[1]) or cisplatin (Platinol AQ[1]). The choice of the second agent is somewhat arbitrary at this point, and the decision is often based on the side-effect profile relative to the patient's other medical problems and physician's bias toward a particular regimen. Treatment is generally four to six cycles for those who tolerate the regimen and show clinical and radiographic response. Patients with a poor functional status have (for the most part) been excluded from clinical trials making the optimal treatment of this patient population uncertain. One approach might be to treat those patients debilitated from their cancer with aggressive combination chemotherapy. Those patients disabled by comorbid illnesses may tolerate single-agent chemotherapy better.

Second-line therapy is now available for patients who have progressed after initial treatment. The FDA has approved the single-agent chemotherapy drugs docetaxel (Taxotere) and pemetrexed (Alimta) based on improvement in survival and quality of life.

Recently, there has been a movement toward more targeted drugs in the treatment of lung cancer. Examples are the small-molecule tyrosine kinase-inhibitor erlotinib (Tarceva) and gefitinib (Iressa). Lung cancer growth is dependent on cell surface membrane receptors that regulate intracellular signal transduction pathways. These can affect cell proliferation, apoptosis (programmed cell death), angiogenesis, cell-to-cell adhesion, and motility. In normal cells, these mechanisms are tightly controlled. The malignant cell has transformed and evades these controls allowing uncontrolled malignant growth. One such tyrosine kinase receptor is the epidermal growth factor receptor (EGFR), otherwise known as erbB-1 or HER-1. These inhibitors were developed to regain control of the discussed pathways as mutations in the adenosine triphosphate (ATP)-binding site cleft of the tyrosine kinase domain results in prolonged expression of tyrosine kinase activity in response to the epidermal growth factor. Overall response rates are 10% as second-line therapy. However, certain subgroups appear to have a more favorable response, with bronchoalveolar cell carcinoma patients responding 38% of the time. Women, Asians, and nonsmokers appear to also have a higher response rate. Recently, activating somatic mutations in the tyrosine kinase domain of the EGFR gene have been found to highly correlate to responsiveness to erlotinib (Tarceva) and gefitinib (Iressa). Several studies have addressed the issue of combination therapy with small-molecule tyrosine kinase inhibitors and chemotherapy, but no clinical benefit was found. Consequently, these drugs are currently used as single agents. The vascular endothelial growth factor (VEGF) receptor antagonist bevacizumab (Avastin[1]) provides a survival benefit when combined with carboplatin (Paraplatin[1]) and paclitaxel (Taxol). Lung cancer treatment will probably move further away from traditional nonselective chemotherapy drugs and continue to become more refined with molecularly targeted therapies such as these.

## SMALL CELL LUNG CANCER

Small cell lung cancer accounts for approximately 15% of lung cancers and occurs exclusively in smokers. This malignancy is characterized by rapid growth and early development of widespread metastatic disease. In the 1970s, it was hoped that it would be curable with chemotherapy as most tumors are very sensitive to treatment. Overall, 60% to 80% respond well to chemotherapy, but there is often a concern that tumor lysis syndrome may develop.

Although the primary tumor, regional nodes, *metastases* (TNM staging system as used in NSCLC) also applies (see Table 3), from a practical standpoint patients are classified as limited stage or extensive stage. Patients who have disease that can be encompassed in a single radiation port are classified as limited stage; extensive stage covers those who have widespread disease. The current treatment for limited stage disease involves four cycles of cisplatin (Platinol AQ[1]) and etoposide (VePesid) with concurrent radiation therapy starting with cycle one. The addition of more drugs to the chemotherapy mixture has not resulted in higher cure rates and more toxicity is seen. With the standard approach, 20% to 40% of patients are alive at 2 years; the long-term survival rate is only 10% to 15%. Patients cured of their small cell cancer are at risk for developing non–small cell lung cancers, as well as head and neck malignancies. Isolated brain metastases can also be seen in patients in remission, leading to the concept of prophylactic cranial irradiation. No convincing data exist to definitively prove the benefit of this approach. If offered to patients, a thorough discussion of potential long-term cognitive and neurologic side effects must occur before proceeding.

Patients with extensive stage disease are incurable, but chemotherapy doubles survival with most living 8 to 12 months. A platinum drug (carboplatin or cisplatin) with etoposide (VePesid) for four cycles is first-line therapy. There is no demonstrated benefit to maintenance therapy. Triplet and quadruplet drug therapies have been evaluated but not commonly used because of significant toxicity with minimal benefit. Irinotecan (Camptosar[1]) with cisplatin (Platinol AQ[1]) has shown a survival benefit in a Japanese study, but a recent U.S. study failed to confirm those results. Patients who obtain a radiographic response that is durable beyond 6 months can be retreated with the same regimen on relapse. Other second-line drugs include topotecan (Hycamtin) and paclitaxel (Taxol[1]), but participation in a clinical trial is preferred.

Surgery usually has no role in small cell lung cancer except in the rare patient with a small, solitary, pulmonary nodule. If extensive staging, including mediastinoscopy and bone marrow biopsies, fails to demonstrate widespread disease, the approach includes resection followed by adjuvant chemotherapy.

## Screening

The purpose of any lung cancer screening is to identify asymptomatic individuals with the disease in hopes that screening will detect the cancer at an earlier stage and, as a result, improve overall survival. There have been multiple studies that have looked at lung cancer screening involving thousands of patients. All of these studies were done in males, prior to the lung cancer epidemic in females. Numerous modalities, including plain chest radiography, sputum cytology, and computed tomography, have been evaluated. Despite some suggestion of improvement in stage distribution and resectability, there has been no improvement in mortality. As a result, all of the major advisory organizations have recommended against routine screening for lung cancer even in patients at high risk. In particular, the United States Preventive Services Task Force (USPSTF) states that "the evidence is insufficient to recommend for or against screening in asymptomatic

---

[1]Not FDA approved for this indication.

[1]Not FDA approved for this indication.

persons for lung cancer." This position statement is also upheld by the American Academy of Family Physicians. The case of lung cancer screening is not closed; there are two very large studies under way that may change these recommendations in the future.

Lung cancer remains a major public health problem in the United States. Despite recent advances in treatment, the mortality rate remains quite high. Further research and patient participation in clinical trials will undoubtedly lead to continued progress. Greater impact could be achieved by prevention through smoking cessation programs and by preventing our youth from starting tobacco use in the first place.

## REFERENCES

Albain KS, Swann RS, Rusch VR, et al: Phase III Study of concurrent chemotherapy and radiotherapy (CT/RT) vs CT/RT followed by surgical resection for stage IIIA (pN2) non-small cell lung cancer (NSCLC): Outcome update of North American Intergroup 0139 (RTOG 9309) (abstract 7014). Proc Am Soc Clin Oncol 2005.

Douillard JY, Rosell R, De Lena M, et al: Adjuvant vinorelbine plus cisplatin versus observation in patients with completely resected stage IB-IIIA non-small cell lung cancer (Adjuvant Navelbine International Trialists Association [ANITA]): A randomized controlled trial. Lancet Oncol 2006;7: 719-727.

Jemal A, Siegel R, Ward E, et al: Cancer statistics, 2007. CA Cancer J Clin 2007;57:43-66.

Lung cancer screening: Recommendation statement. Ann Intern Med 2004;140:738.

Lynch TJ, Bell DW, Sordella R, et al: Activating mutations in the epidermal growth factor receptor underlying responsiveness of non-small cell lung cancer to gefitinib. N Engl J Med 2004;350:2129-2139.

Mulshine JL, Sullivan DC: Lung cancer screening. N Engl J Med 2005; 2714-2720.

Sandler A, Gray R, Perry MC, et al: Paclitaxel-carboplatin alone or with bevacizumab for non-small cell lung cancer. N Engl J Med 2006;355:2542-2550.

Shepherd FA, Pereira JR, Ciuleanu T, et al: Erlotinib in previously treated non-small-cell lung cancer. N Engl J Med 2005;353:123-132.

Spira A, Ettinger DS: Drug therapy: Multidisciplinary management of lung cancer. N Engl J Med 2004;350:379-392.

Strauss GM, Herndon J, Maddaus MA, et al: Adjuvant chemotherapy in Stage IB non-small cell lung cancer (NSCLC): Update of Cancer and Leukemia Group B (CALGB) Protocol 9633. J Clin Oncol, 2006 ASCO Annual Meeting Proceedings (Post-Meeting Edition). Vol 24, No 18S (June 20 Supplement), 2006:7007.

Winton T, Livingston R, Johnson D, et al: Vinorelbine plus cisplatin vs. observation in resected non-small cell lung cancer. N Engl J Med 2005;352:2589-2589.

# Coccidioidomycosis

Method of
*Duane R. Hospenthal, MD, PhD\**

Coccidioidomycosis (valley fever) is a fungal infection caused by *Coccidioides* species that produces mild to life-threatening disease. The disease was first described in an Argentinean soldier by Alejandro Posadas, as a medical student, in 1892. Initially, coccidioidomycosis was thought to be a rare, ultimately fatal disseminated infection. It is now known that most infections do not produce apparent disease, and those that do are generally self-limited pneumonias, often mistakenly diagnosed as influenza or community-acquired pneumonia.

*Coccidioides* species are dimorphic fungi that live in the soil as saprobic molds, producing unique structures, spherules, and

---

*Disclaimer: The views expressed herein are those of the author and do not reflect the official policy or position of the Department of the Army, Department of Defense, or the United States government. The author is an employee of the United States government. This work was prepared as part of his official duties and, as such, contains no copyright to be transferred.

endospores in disease. Infection occurs when the infectious particles, the arthroconidia, are inhaled. Previously believed to be a single species, two members of the genus are currently described, *Coccidioides immitis* and *Coccidioides posadasii*. Although this designation has little apparent clinical importance (and differentiating between the species is beyond the scope of most clinical laboratories), it is now known that *C. immitis* causes only the disease localized to California and parts of Arizona.

Coccidioidomycosis is an endemic mycosis localized to the southwestern United States and northern Mexico, with smaller areas of disease located in Central and South America. The endemic niche appears to localize to areas with arid climate and alkaline soils, the lower Sonoran life zone. Disease generally peaks in dry periods following rains, typically in the summer and fall. It has been estimated that about 150,000 infections occur each year, although many think the numbers are much higher. Filipinos and persons of African descent (and perhaps other Asians and Native Americans), pregnant women, and immunocompromised persons are at the highest risk for severe or disseminated disease. Disease typically occurs 7 to 21 days after exposure, and it appears that infection protects persons from subsequent repeat infections.

## Clinical Manifestations

More than one half of coccidioidomycosis infections are asymptomatic and have been identified in past studies by skin testing of persons in the endemic areas. The majority of symptomatic infection is acute pulmonary disease; chronic pulmonary and disseminated disease occur only rarely (<1% of those infected).

### ACUTE PNEUMONIA

Primary respiratory infection typically manifests with nonproductive cough, fever, pleuritic chest pain, malaise, headache, anorexia, myalgia, and often rash. Rash may be faint and diffuse, but may also include erythema multiforme and erythema nodosum. These latter two tend to appear days to weeks after initial pulmonary symptoms and are more common in women. The triad of fever, arthralgias, and erythema nodosum is called *desert rheumatism*. Acute respiratory coccidioidomycosis may be misdiagnosed as influenza or community-acquired pneumonia, but typically it produces longer duration of symptoms than those illnesses. Unlike typical bacterial pneumonias, acute coccidioidomycosis typically remits without therapy, although it may be followed by weeks to months of fatigue.

Severe disease can manifest with protracted symptoms or even a sepsis syndrome. More severe infection (or infection requiring antifungal therapy) is typically defined as that occurring in persons older than 55 years, lasting longer than 2 months, impairing ability to go to work, producing weight loss of more than 10%, night sweats lasting longer than 3 weeks, infiltrates involving more than one half of one lung or both lungs, prominent or persistent hilar lymphadenopathy, or complement fixation (CF) antibody titers greater than 1:16.

### PULMONARY NODULES AND CAVITIES

Following acute infection, pulmonary nodules or thin-walled cavities may be seen in about 5% to 10% of patients. Both of these presentations are often asymptomatic and are found on follow-up or screening chest radiography. Most nodules or cavities do not require specific therapy unless patients are symptomatic. Rupture of a cavity into the pleural space is a rare complication that typically requires both medical and surgical therapy.

### CHRONIC PNEUMONIA

Chronic progressive fibrocavitary pneumonia can develop after primary infection. Most commonly seen in persons with diabetes and preexisting lung disease, this disease is typified by chronic infiltrates and cavitary lesions. This form of coccidioidomycosis can resemble tuberculosis and prove difficult to eradicate.

## CURRENT DIAGNOSIS

- Coccidioidomycosis is a common cause of community-acquired pneumonia in endemic areas.
- Direct examination of sputum, culture, and serologic testing are keys to making the diagnosis in respiratory disease.
- Disseminated infection should be suspected in patients with complement fixation (CF) antibody titers greater than 1:16.
- Peripheral eosinophilia or eosinophils in the cerebrospinal fluid should increase suspicion for coccidioidomycosis in the appropriate clinical setting.

## DISSEMINATED INFECTION

Extrapulmonary dissemination most commonly affects the skin, bones and joints, and meninges, although almost any organ can be involved. Occurring in 0.5% to 1% of those infected, disseminated infection has a much higher incidence (>15%) in the severely immunocompromised (including patients with AIDS, lymphoma, or solid organ transplantation and persons receiving high-dose corticosteroids or tumor necrosis factor α (TNF-α) blocking agents).

Disseminated disease can manifest with localized or widespread involvement. Skin lesions are typically verrucous, but they may be maculopapular or ulcerative. Subcutaneous abscesses are also common. Bone and joint involvement can involve any bone or joint, but the vertebrae are more commonly involved.

Meningitis is the most feared form of coccidioidomycosis. Left untreated, it is typically a fatal infection after a few months. Cure of this infection still eludes modern medicine. Meningitis manifests with chronic symptoms of headache, memory loss, lethargy, and confusion and can be complicated by hydrocephalus and vasculitis.

# Diagnosis

The diagnosis of coccidioidomycosis must begin with awareness of the potential for this infection in the differential. Clinicians in the endemic areas typically include this disease and its many manifestations in their differential diagnosis. Those outside of the endemic areas must remember to obtain a travel history from every patient and to inquire about previous residence if reactivation is suspected in the immunosuppressed. Aside from endemic exposure, peripheral eosinophilia, and rarely eosinophils in cerebrospinal fluid (CSF), can tip clinicians off to the possibility of coccidioidomycosis. Diagnosis is typically made by direct observation or culture of *Coccidioides* or by serologic methods.

Direct examination and culture should be performed on sputum, lesional discharge, biopsy material, and CSF, based on presentation. The spherules and endospores of coccidioidomycosis can be seen with almost every stain (including hematoxylin and eosin [H&E] and Gram stain); typically calcofluor white or KOH is used to examine sputum, aspirates, and CSF. The disease is confirmed on seeing the typical 10- to 80-μm thick-walled rounded structures (spherules) with 2- to 5-μm round endospores inside. Culture is performed by many laboratories; the diagnosis may be made by identifying typical arthroconidia or using the commercially available DNA probe when nondistinct whitish wooly colonies are recovered. *Coccidioides* grows well on most fungal and bacterial culture media, but the diagnostic yield of CSF is not very high. Although the disease is not communicable, the mold form growing in the laboratory (and producing arthroconidia) is highly infectious. Clinicians suspecting coccidioidomycosis should inform the clinical laboratory of their suspicion.

Nonculture diagnosis previously has included skin testing and serology; currently, skin testing reagent is not available. Serologic testing may be done using several commercially available tests. Of these,

## CURRENT THERAPY

- Uncomplicated acute pneumonia in patients not at high risk for complications might not require antifungal therapy.
- Duration of antifungal therapy typically consists of months to years of oral azole (fluconazole [Diflucan][1] or itraconazole [Sporanox][1]): 3-6 months for acute pulmonary disease, 12 or more months for chronic pulmonary disease, years for disseminated disease, and lifelong for meningitis.
- Amphotericin B (Fungizone) is now reserved for rapidly progressive disease, for acute disease with respiratory failure, for treatment failure with azoles, and for use in pregnancy (because of the teratogenicity of the azoles).
- Specialty consultation is warranted for disseminated disease.

---

[1]Not FDA approved for this indication.

---

CF and immunodiffusion testing are most useful. Enzyme-linked immunoassay (EIA) (IgM) and latex agglutination tests are highly sensitive and can be used for initial testing. Because of the potential for false positive results with these tests, confirmation by CF or immunodiffusion testing is suggested. In addition to their use in the diagnosis of coccidioidomycosis, serologic tests should be used to follow the care of persons with chronic or disseminated infections.

Radiology is often key to the diagnosis and management of coccidioidomycosis. Chest x-ray should be performed on all persons suspected to have disease. Chest CT may be useful in chronic pulmonary disease and to follow asymptomatic nodules and cavities. With disseminated disease involving more than one site of infection, bone scan may be useful in discovering the extent of disease and assist in long-term follow-up. Plain x-rays of involved bones or joints and CT or MRI may be useful as well. Neuroradiologic studies may be normal in meningeal disease, but CT or MRI should be included in the diagnosis and management of this disease because hydrocephalus may be present initially or develop subsequently. MRI can also reveal basilar leptomeningeal enhancement.

# Management

## ACUTE INFECTIONS

Untreated, most acute infections resolve spontaneously. Observation may be the treatment of choice for uncomplicated acute pulmonary disease in patients not at higher risk for dissemination or severe disease; some experts think all infected patients should receive antifungal therapy (Table 1). Unfortunately, there are no randomized clinical trials to support treating or not treating in uncomplicated disease in low-risk patients. Immunocompromised patients, those with preexisting lung disease or diabetes, and those at high risk for severe or disseminated disease should receive therapy. Pregnant patients and persons with severe disease should be treated with amphotericin B (Fungizone). Those with respiratory failure can be treated with amphotericin B or high-dose fluconazole (Diflucan).[1] All others may be treated with oral azole therapy (fluconazole [Diflucan],[1] itraconazole [Sporanox],[1] or ketoconazole [Nizoral]) (Table 2). All infected patients, whether treated or not, should be followed up routinely (every 3-6 months) for at least 2 years to ensure that late complications, including dissemination, are not missed.

---

[1]Not FDA approved for this indication.

**TABLE 1 Treatment of Coccidioidomycosis**

| Disease | Primary Therapy | Alternate Therapy | Duration |
|---|---|---|---|
| **Acute Pulmonary Infection** | | | |
| Uncomplicated | | | |
|   Low risk | Observation | Oral azole: Fluconazole (Diflucan),[1] itraconazole (Sporanox),[1] or ketoconazole (Nizoral) 400 mg daily | 3-6 mo |
|   High risk | Oral azole* | Amphotericin B[†] | 3-6 mo |
| Diffuse/severe | Amphotericin B[†] | Oral azoles[‡] | ≥12 mo |
| **Chronic Pulmonary Infection** | | | |
| All infections | Oral azole | Amphotericin B,[†] surgical resection | ≥12 mo |
| **Disseminated Infection** | | | |
| Nonmeningeal | Oral azole[‡,§] | Amphotericin B[†] | Years |
| Meningeal | Oral fluconazole[‡,¶] | Itraconazole,[1] intrathecal[1] amphotericin B | Lifelong |

[1]Not FDA approved for this indication.
*Azoles should not be used in pregnancy.
[†]Patients may be switched to azole therapy once they begin improving clinically.
[‡]High-dose fluconazole (800-1200 mg daily)[1] is often used in severe disease, at least initially
[§]Surgical resection may be used adjunctively.
[¶]Consider early shunting if hydrocephalus is present and corticosteroids if vasculitis is present.

**TABLE 2 Antifungal Agents Used in Coccidioidomycosis**

| Drug | Dose |
|---|---|
| Fluconazole (Diflucan)[1] | 400-1200 mg PO or IV qd |
| Itraconazole (Sporanox)[1] | 200 mg PO or IV bid or tid |
| Ketoconazole (Nizoral) | 200-400 mg PO qd |
| Amphotericin B (Fungizone) | 0.5-1.5 mg/kg qd* |
| Lipid formulations of amphotericin B (Ambisone,[1] Abelcet, Amphotec)[1] | 2-5 mg/kg IV qd |

[1]Not FDA approved for this indication.
*May be given on alternate days to decrease toxicity.

## CHRONIC INFECTIONS

Treatment of chronic pulmonary disease and disseminated disease is generally given for years, sometimes for life. With the currently available drugs, data do not support ever stopping therapy in those with meningitis. Oral azole therapy is typically the treatment of choice for chronic infections, although amphotericin B can be used initially in severe infections, and it may have to be used in patients not responding to azole therapy. Intrathecal[1] amphotericin B is still used by some experts initially in meningitis, and it may be used as a secondary regimen in persons failing azole therapy. In meningeal disease, early shunting should be pursued if hydrocephalus is present, and corticosteroids should be considered if central nervous system vasculitis is suspected. Follow-up of chronic or disseminated disease generally includes interval (typically every 3-6 months) history and physical examination, serologic, and radiologic testing. In meningitis, this follow-up should also include CSF examination.

## REFERENCES

Anstead GM, Corcoran G, Lewis J, et al: Refractory coccidioidomycosis treated with posaconazole. Clin Infect Dis 2005;40:1770-1776.
Galgiani JN: *Coccidioides* species. In Mandell GL, Bennett JE, Dolin R (eds): Mandell, Douglas, and Bennett's Principles and Practice of Infectious Diseases. 6th ed. Philadelphia: Churchill Livingstone, 2005, pp 3040-3051.

[1]Not FDA approved for this indication.

Galgiani JN, Ampel NM, Blair JE, et al: Coccidioidomycosis. Clin Infect Dis 2005;41:1217-1223.
Galgiani JN, Catanzaro A, Cloud GA, et al: Comparison of oral fluconazole and itraconazole for progressive, nonmeningeal coccidioidomycosis: A randomized, double-blind trial. Mycoses Study Group. Ann Intern Med 2000; 133:676-686.
Galgiani JN, Catanzaro A, Cloud GA, et al: Fluconazole therapy for coccidioidal meningitis. Ann Intern Med 1993;119:28-35.
Johnson RH, Einstein HE: Coccidioidal meningitis. Clin Infect Dis 2006; 42:103-107.
Valdivia L, Mix D, Wright M, et al: Coccidioidomycosis as a common cause of community-acquired pneumonia. Emerg Infect Dis 2006;12:958-962.

# Histoplasmosis

Method of
*Linus H. Santo Tomas, MD, MS, and Ralph M. Schapira, MD*

## Etiology and Epidemiology

The causative organism of histoplasmosis, *Histoplasma capsulatum*, is found worldwide, but thrives best in moist acidic soil with high organic content. In the United States, infection is highest in areas of the Ohio, Mississippi, and Missouri River valleys. Bat and avian droppings enhance soil characteristics that augment sporulation. Bats can also be infected, thereby transmitting the fungus in their droppings. *H. capsulatum* is a dimorphic fungus that exists in mycelial form in the environment. The infective spores are introduced to the lungs via inhalation and the organism is transformed to a yeast form in the mammalian host. Most infections are asymptomatic, but immunocompromised hosts and those exposed to large inoculums are more likely to develop progressive or severe disease.

## Pathogenesis

Inhaled spores transform to the yeast form in the alveoli within hours to days. This leads to bronchopneumonia. The organism is ingested by macrophages and may be disseminated hematogenously to regional lymph nodes, liver, spleen, and other organs. Neutrophils, which can also phagocytose the organism and release antifungal proteins and granules, are thought to play an important role in limiting the initial phase of the infection. Yeasts may continue to multiply intracellularly within alveolar macrophages. Maturation of cell-mediated immunity is critical to effective control of the disease. The inflammatory response leads to the development of caseating lesions that heal, forming fibrotic lesions with granulomas. The dense fibrotic lesions frequently calcify. Yeast forms have been identified in these calcified lesions, and although attempts to culture the fungus from these lesions have been unsuccessful, the recrudescence of disease in immunocompromised individuals who are no longer in endemic areas suggests that some organisms may remain viable for years.

## Clinical Manifestations

Most infections are asymptomatic, and in endemic areas it is not unusual for radiologic studies to show evidence of previous infection in the chest and abdomen, which most commonly appear as calcified granulomas in the lung parenchyma or spleen. The incubation period is from 3 to 21 days after exposure. The development of clinical disease is mainly dependent on the immune status of the host and the inoculum load. The more common presentations of the disease are discussed in the following section.

### ACUTE PULMONARY HISTOPLASMOSIS

#### Localized Pulmonary Disease

Sixty percent of those who develop clinical disease present with acute pulmonary histoplasmosis. Initial symptoms are usually nonspecific and consist of fever, chills, fatigue, and cough. The chest radiograph may reveal mediastinal and hilar adenopathy accompanied by patchy pneumonic infiltrates, but may also be normal in some cases. Limited exposure in an immunocompetent host may manifest with a localized pneumonia that may be mistaken for a bacterial pneumonia. Most do not require antifungal treatment unless there is no improvement after a month.

#### Diffuse Pulmonary Involvement

More intense exposure, even in an immunocompetent host, can lead to diffuse pulmonary histoplasmosis. The typical chest radiograph may show bilateral reticulonodular or miliary-type infiltrates. Aside from fever, cough, chest pain, and chills, affected patients can have clinically significant hypoxemia that may require ventilatory support.

### CHRONIC PULMONARY HISTOPLASMOSIS

In persons with underlying pulmonary disease, especially emphysema, the acute exposure can eventually lead to chronic pulmonary histoplasmosis that is characterized by fibrocavitary lesions on chest radiographs. Symptoms include cough, fatigue, fever, weight loss, and night sweats. Patients can also present with hemoptysis and progressive dyspnea. Chronic pulmonary histoplasmosis may mimic progressive mycobacterial disease, particularly tuberculosis.

### GRANULOMATOUS MEDIASTINITIS

Occasionally, lymphadenopathy associated with histoplasmosis may be severe enough to cause compression of the airways, mediastinal vascular structures, and the esophagus. This can lead to cough, chest pain, hemoptysis, dysphagia, and signs of superior vena cava syndrome. Granulomatous mediastinitis has to be distinguished from fibrosing mediastinitis, a rare long-term sequelae of infection. Granulomatous mediastinitis can improve significantly with antifungal and corticosteroid treatment.

## CURRENT DIAGNOSIS

- Because clinical presentation is usually nonspecific, a high index of suspicion is needed to arrive at the diagnosis.
- Histoplasmosis should be considered in nonresolving pneumonia and fever of unknown etiology, especially in endemic areas and immunocompromised hosts.
- For rapid diagnosis, the urine *Histoplasma* polysaccharide antigen detection test has good sensitivity (89%) in disseminated histoplasmosis.
- A combination of tests using different specimen types may be needed to maximize the diagnostic yield and confirm the diagnosis.

### DISSEMINATED HISTOPLASMOSIS

Immunocompromised individuals, whether from extremes of age, debilitating comorbid disease, immunosuppressive medications, or immune deficiency syndromes, are at greater risk for disseminated disease. Symptoms may be nonspecific, and can include fever, chills, and weight loss. Physical examination may reveal pneumonitis, hepatosplenomegaly, and lymphadenopathy. Other manifestations depend on specific organs that may be involved. Five percent to 20% of cases may have central nervous system involvement.

### OTHER MANIFESTATIONS

Less common manifestations of histoplasmosis include pericarditis, rheumatologic syndromes, broncholithiasis, and fibrosing mediastinitis. Pericarditis is thought to be caused by local immunologic response to release of inflammatory substances from adjacent necrotizing lymph nodes. Arthritis or arthralgia is usually polyarticular and symmetric, and is thought to be secondary to a systemic inflammatory response to the infection rather than actual joint invasion.

### DIAGNOSIS

The nonspecific clinical manifestations of histoplasmosis can make diagnosis difficult, and maintaining a high clinical suspicion in the appropriate setting is important. It should be considered as a possible cause of nonresolving pneumonia and fever of unknown origin, especially in endemic areas. A high index of suspicion is also appropriate in immunocompromised hosts. A number of laboratory tests are available for confirmation of suspected disease, each with its own advantages and disadvantages. A combination of these laboratory tests may be needed to maximize the yield of diagnostic tests in less florid infections. Obtaining specimens from respiratory secretions, bronchoalveolar lavage, tissue biopsy, blood, and urine can also increase the overall yield.

### FUNGAL STAINING

Rapid diagnosis of histoplasmosis can be made with identification of *H. capsulatum* with silver-methenamine stain of biologic specimens. The organism may also be identified by Wright stain of peripheral blood smears in individuals with severe disseminated disease. However, these have lower sensitivity compared to antigen detection and culture.

### FUNGAL CULTURE

Blood and bone marrow culture can be positive in 85% to 90% of patients with disseminated and chronic pulmonary disease. The lysis-centrifugation method is best for blood cultures. Analyzing multiple specimens may improve yield. Bronchoalveolar lavage cultures should also be analyzed in patients with pulmonary involvement. The relatively long duration to obtain positive growth on culture limits its usefulness in an acute setting.

## DETECTION OF SERUM ANTIBODIES

Serologic testing for antibodies to histoplasma antigen are positive in 80% to 90% of patients with diffuse pulmonary involvement and disseminated disease. Complement fixation and immunodiffusion assays are available. Precipitins to the M or H antigen may be detected but both have significant false positives as a consequence of cross-reactivity with other fungal infections. Other limitations of the test include false negatives early in the course of disease and reduced sensitivity in immunocompromised hosts.

## POLYSACCHARIDE ANTIGEN DETECTION

The *Histoplasma* polysaccharide antigen can be detected by conventional radioimmunoassay (RIA) or enzyme immunoassay (EIA) in the urine of up to 92% of patients with disseminated disease and in 37% to 39% with self-limited disease. The same test can be used on serum and other body fluids, but the sensitivity may be lower. It is most useful when serologic tests are less likely to be positive, such as in the early phase of an infection or in immunocompromised hosts. Antigen levels correlate with treatment response and recrudescence and can be used to guide treatment of disseminated histoplasmosis.

## Treatment

Most patients who have histoplasmosis recover without treatment. The need for treatment is determined by the type of involvement, the severity and duration of the disease, and the immune status of the patient. Treatment is generally reserved for chronic pulmonary involvement, disseminated disease, or severe acute infections. Such infections most commonly occur in immunocompromised hosts or in those exposed to a large infectious inoculum. Table 1 summarizes the treatment recommendations.

In general, severe disease is initially treated with intravenous deoxycholate amphotericin B (Fungizone) at a dose of 0.7 mg/kg per day. The cumulative dose of amphotericin B depends on the clinical response, but for *Histoplasma* meningitis, completion of a 35-mg/kg course given over 3 to 4 months is recommended. The same cumulative dose of amphotericin B is recommended for other severe forms of histoplasmosis if the patient is unable to take oral medications. A shift from intravenous amphotericin to oral itraconazole (continuation phase) can be considered if there is clinical improvement (i.e., when the patient becomes afebrile, hemodynamically stable, or no longer requires ventilatory support) and is able to take oral medications. The duration of itraconazole (Sporanox) treatment also varies according to the type and severity of histoplasmosis (see Table 1). Monitoring of itraconazole blood levels should be considered if there is concern about absorption or use of medications that may reduce its bioavailability.

The lipid formulations approved for use with invasive fungal infections include amphotericin lipid complex (Abelcet), amphotericin B colloidal dispersion (Amphotec), and liposomal amphotericin B (AmBisome), but only the latter has been studied with histoplasmosis. Recent studies involving AIDS patients suggest that liposomal amphotericin B may lead to better clinical outcomes, including earlier clearance of the fungal burden, as well as improved survival, when compared to deoxycholate amphotericin B and itraconazole for treatment of moderate to severe histoplasmosis. Thus, although liposomal

**TABLE 1 Recommendations for Treatment of Histoplasmosis**

| Type of Histoplasmosis | Treatment Regimen |
| --- | --- |
| **Acute Pulmonary Disease** | |
| Mild to moderate, >4 weeks | Itraconazole (Sporanox) 200 mg, once to twice daily for 6–12 weeks* |
| Severe | Amphotericin B (Fungizone) 0.7 mg/kg/d,[†] then itraconazole 200 mg once to twice daily for 12 weeks |
| | Consider corticosteroids (effectiveness not proven) |
| **Chronic Pulmonary Disease** | |
| Mild to moderate | Itraconazole 200 mg once to twice daily for 12–24 months |
| Severe | Amphotericin B 0.7 mg/kg/d,[†] then itraconazole 200 mg once to twice daily for 12–24 months |
| **Granulomatous Mediastinitis** | |
| Mild to moderate | Itraconazole 200 mg once to twice daily for 6–12 months |
| Severe | Amphotericin B 0.7 mg/kg/d,[†] then itraconazole 200 mg once to twice daily for 6–12 months |
| **Disseminated Disease (without AIDS)** | |
| Mild to moderate | Itraconazole 200 mg once to twice daily for 6-18 months |
| Severe | Amphotericin B 0.7 mg/kg/d,[†] then itraconazole 200 mg once to twice daily for 6–18 months[‡] |
| **Disseminated Disease (with AIDS)** | |
| Mild to moderate | Itraconazole 200 mg once to twice daily for life |
| Severe | Amphotericin B 0.7 mg/kg/d,[†] then itraconazole 200 mg once to twice daily for life |
| Meningitis | Amphotericin B 0.7 mg/kg/d[†] to total 35 mg/kg over 3–4 months, then fluconazole (Diflucan)[1] 800 mg daily[3] for 9–12 months |

*Blood levels may be checked if poor absorption or increased metabolism is suspected.
[†]If amphotericin B is used exclusively, a total course dose of ≤35 mg/kg is recommended. Lipid preparation of amphotericin may be given at 3 mg/kg/d; recent studies in AIDS patients suggest better outcomes compared to deoxycholate amphotericin B (see text).
[‡]Continue treatment until *Histoplasma* urine and serum antigen concentrations <4 units.
[1]Not FDA approved for this indication.
[3]Exceeds dosage recommended by the manufacturer.

## CURRENT THERAPY

- Treatment is indicated in severe acute (diffuse or localized) pulmonary disease, chronic pulmonary disease, granulomatous mediastinitis with obstructive or invasive symptoms, and disseminated infection.
- Mild to moderate acute pulmonary involvement that persists beyond 4 weeks also warrants treatment.
- Intravenous deoxycholate amphotericin B (Fungizone) is the drug of choice for initial treatment of severe disease. Although more expensive, liposomal amphotericin B (AmBisome)[1] may lead to better outcomes in AIDS patients with moderate to severe disease.
- Oral itraconazole (Sporanox) is the drug of choice for initial treatment of mild to moderate disease and in continuation phase therapy of severe disease that has improved after intravenous amphotericin treatment.
- Fluconazole (Diflucan),[1] which is less active than itraconazole against *H. capsulatum*, has special usefulness in continuation phase therapy of meningitis because of its good cerebrospinal fluid penetration.

[1]Not FDA approved for this indication.

amphotericin B[1] may be more costly, it should be considered as an alternative first-line drug for AIDS patients who have moderate to severe disease, especially for those who are at risk for, or who already have, renal insufficiency.

Among the oral agents itraconazole (Sporanox) has the greatest activity against *H. capsulatum*. Ketoconazole (Nizoral) is also active against *Histoplasma* but is less well tolerated than itraconazole. Although fluconazole (Diflucan)[1] is the least active against *Histoplasma*, it has special usefulness in meningitis because of its ability to reach 80% of the blood concentration in the cerebrospinal fluid. To reduce the relapse risk of meningitis, fluconazole 800 mg PO daily[3] is recommended for 9 to 12 months after the full course of intravenous amphotericin is completed. Itraconazole does not enter the cerebrospinal fluid.

Anti-inflammatory treatment, as an adjunct to antifungal therapy, may be considered in certain forms of histoplasmosis. The inflammatory response in diffuse pulmonary histoplasmosis is thought to add to the severity of respiratory dysfunction. In addition to antifungal treatment, a 2-week course of prednisone at 60 mg daily can be considered. Pericarditis may also respond to treatment with corticosteroids or nonsteroidal anti-inflammatory agents. For rheumatologic manifestations, nonsteroidal anti-inflammatory agents can be given for 2 to 12 weeks.

## REFERENCES

Durkin MM, Connolly PA, Wheat LJ: Comparison of radioimmunoassay and enzyme-linked immunoassay methods for detection of *Histoplasma capsulatum* var. *capsulatum* antigen. J Clin Microbiol 1997;35(9):2252-2255.
Johnson PC, Wheat LJ, Cloud GA, et al: Safety and efficacy of liposomal amphotericin B compared with conventional amphotericin B for induction therapy of histoplasmosis in patients with AIDS. Ann Intern Med 2002;137(2):105-109.
Newman SL, Bucher C, Rhodes J, Bullock WE: Phagocytosis of *Histoplasma capsulatum* yeasts and microconidia by human cultured macrophages and alveolar macrophages. Cellular cytoskeleton requirement for attachment and ingestion. J Clin Invest 1990;85(1):223-230.
Newman SL, Gootee L, Gabay JE: Human neutrophil-mediated fungistasis against *Histoplasma capsulatum*. Localization of fungistatic activity to the azurophil granules. J Clin Invest 1993;92(2):624-631.

[1]Not FDA approved for this indication.
[3]Exceeds dosage recommended by the manufacturer.

Sathapatayavongs B, Batteiger BE, Wheat J, et al: Clinical and laboratory features of disseminated histoplasmosis during two large urban outbreaks. Medicine (Baltimore) 1983;62(5):263-270.
Wheat J: Histoplasmosis. Experience during outbreaks in Indianapolis and review of the literature. Medicine (Baltimore) 1997;76(5):339-354.
Wheat J, Sarosi G, McKinsey D, et al: Practice guidelines for the management of patients with histoplasmosis. Infectious Diseases Society of America. Clin Infect Dis 2000;30(4):688-695.
Wheat LJ, Cloud G, Johnson PC, et al: Clearance of fungal burden during treatment of disseminated histoplasmosis with liposomal amphotericin B versus itraconazole. Antimicrob Agents Chemother 2001;45(8):2354-2357.
Wheat LJ, Connolly-Stringfield P, Kohler RB, et al: *Histoplasma capsulatum* polysaccharide antigen detection in diagnosis and management of disseminated histoplasmosis in patients with acquired immunodeficiency syndrome. Am J Med 1989;87(4):396-400.
Wheat LJ, Kauffman CA: Histoplasmosis. Infect Dis Clin North Am 2003;17(1):1-19, vii.
Williams B, Fojtasek M, Connolly-Stringfield P, Wheat J: Diagnosis of histoplasmosis by antigen detection during an outbreak in Indianapolis, Ind. Arch Pathol Lab Med 1994;118(12):1205-1208.

# Blastomycosis

Method of
*Robert Bradsher, MD, and*
*Anupama Menon, MD, MPH*

## Epidemiology

Blastomycosis is caused by infection with the thermally dimorphic fungus *Blastomyces dermatitidis*. The organism grows as a yeast form at 98.6°F (37°C) and as a mycelial form at room temperature. In the environment, the fungus is thought to exist in warm, moist soil associated with decomposing vegetation and decaying wood. In North America, *B. dermatitidis* is endemic along the Mississippi and Ohio River basins, in the regions that surround the Great Lakes, and in a small area of New York and Canada along the St. Lawrence River. Hyperendemic areas with very high rates of blastomycosis have been reported within these endemic regions. Cases outside North America have been described most commonly in Africa, but there have been reports of blastomycosis on several continents.

Infection with *B. dermatitidis* usually occurs via inhalation of aerosolized conidia. Cutaneous inoculation has been reported after inadvertent exposure in the laboratory, at autopsy, and after dog bites. Person-to-person transmission has been described in rare cases of sexual and perinatal transmission. The median incubation period is approximately 30 to 45 days.

## Clinical Manifestations

Approximately 50% of infected individuals may be asymptomatic. Pulmonary disease may be acute or chronic. Acute pulmonary blastomycosis presents similarly to bacterial pneumonia with abrupt onset of fever, chills, pleuritic chest pain, myalgias, arthralgias, and cough that is initially nonproductive but later becomes productive of purulent sputum. Chest radiography demonstrates lobar or segmental consolidation; pleural effusion and hilar adenopathy are unusual. Patients diagnosed with blastomycosis may develop progressive, chronic disease that may involve pulmonary and numerous extrapulmonary sites. Patients with chronic pulmonary blastomycosis present with productive cough, hemoptysis, weight loss, pleuritic chest pain, and low-grade fever. Alveolar or fibronodular infiltrates, mass lesions, nodular lesions, and cavitation are seen on chest radiography. Findings may mimic tuberculosis, other endemic mycoses, or bronchogenic carcinoma. Acute respiratory failure may be seen with miliary disease or diffuse pneumonitis and is associated with a very high mortality.

Hematogenous dissemination to almost any other organ may occur. Manifestations in the skin, bone, or genitourinary tract are the most common and may be seen after clearance of pulmonary manifestations. The skin is the most frequently encountered extrapulmonary site of infection. Lesions are usually characterized as verrucous or ulcerative; they may be mistaken for squamous cell carcinoma, atypical mycobacterial infection, pyoderma gangrenosum, or keratoacanthoma. After the skin, bone is the most frequent site of dissemination. Manifestations include osteolytic lesions with associated soft-tissue abscesses or chronic draining sinuses. Genitourinary disease occurs in some male cases, affecting the prostate and epididymis. Although central nervous system (CNS) infection is reported in only a small number of normal hosts, it is a relatively common complication in immunocompromised patients, in whom it may present as an abscess or meningitis. In a review of AIDS patients with blastomycosis, 40% had CNS involvement. Indeed, blastomycosis is more often disseminated and fulminant in patients with AIDS and other types of chronic immunosuppression; mortality rates of 30% to 40% have been reported in these groups.

# Diagnosis

The definitive diagnosis of blastomycosis is based on isolation of the organism from cultures of clinical specimens. Mycologic media usually demonstrate growth after an incubation period of 2 to 4 weeks. Conversion from the mycelial form to the yeast phase is required for confirmation.

Because isolation of the organism may take weeks, presumptive diagnosis of blastomycosis is established by identification of the characteristic yeast form in clinical specimens. With a compatible clinical picture, treatment should be initiated if round, broad-based budding yeasts with thick, doubly refractile cell walls are seen on a wet mount preparation with addition of 10% potassium hydroxide to digest mammalian cells. In histopathologic specimens, acute suppurative and granulomatous inflammation are found. Visualization in tissue is improved by the use of special stains, such as the Gomori methenamine silver and periodic acid-Schiff stains. Nucleic acid hybridization tests are now commercially available and significantly shorten identification time. Most serologic tests are neither adequately sensitive nor specific to be useful in diagnosing blastomycosis, although newer antigen assays may be more reliable. A recently developed assay detects *Blastomyces* antigen in urine, serum, and other body fluids, including cerebrospinal fluid. The test is most sensitive in urine samples, in which 70% to 80% are positive in disseminated blastomycosis, and almost 100% are positive in pulmonary disease. Antigen is detected in serum in approximately 50% of cases. Cross-reactivity can occur in patients with other endemic mycoses. The assay may be used to monitor response to therapy and to detect recurrence.

# Treatment

Although spontaneous resolution of acute blastomycotic pneumonia has been reported in immunocompetent hosts, most patients with blastomycosis require treatment. Treatment is indicated in all immunocompromised individuals and in all patients with progressive pulmonary disease or extrapulmonary disease. Factors to consider when initiating therapy include the severity and extent of disease, the immune status of the patient, and the toxicities of the antifungal agents.

## PULMONARY DISEASE

For mild to moderate lung disease, itraconazole (Sporanox) is the preferred oral agent because it is efficacious and well tolerated. The initial dose should be 200 to 400 mg daily. Treatment should continue for at least 6 months. Bioavailability of itraconazole capsules is enhanced with food, whereas the oral suspension should be taken while fasting. Attention should be given to the patient's concurrent medications because of the potential for drug–drug interactions. Intravenous itraconazole has not been studied in blastomycosis and has no major benefits to offer. Ketoconazole (Nizoral) at 400 to 800 mg daily is an alternative agent to itraconazole, but it is associated with significant adverse effects, serious drug interactions, and higher rates of relapse. Clinical experience with fluconazole (Diflucan)[1] indicates that this agent is as efficacious as ketoconazole at doses of 400 to 800 mg daily. In patients with life-threatening pulmonary disease, progression of disease while on an azole or inability to tolerate an azole, amphotericin B (Fungizone) remains the agent of choice. A dose of 0.7 to 1.0 mg/kg daily should be administered until a cumulative dose of 1.5 to 2.5 g is completed. Some patients may be switched to oral itraconazole at 200 to 400 mg daily after clinical stabilization with amphotericin B. Lipid formulations of amphotericin B have not been adequately studied, but have been used in patients unable to tolerate conventional amphotericin B.

## NERVOUS SYSTEM DISEASE

CNS infection should be treated with amphotericin B at a dose of 0.7 to 1.0 mg/kg daily to complete a total dose of 2.0 to 2.5 g. Itraconazole and ketoconazole are not recommended because of inadequate CNS penetration; fluconazole at 800 mg daily may be considered if amphotericin B is not tolerated.

## EXTRAPULMONARY DISEASE (WITHOUT CNS INVOLVEMENT)

For mild to moderate disease, itraconazole at 200 to 400 mg daily is recommended for a minimum of 6 months. Patients whose disease

## CURRENT DIAGNOSIS

- Because colonization with *B. dermatitidis* does not occur, identification by culture or histology confirms infection.
- The gold standard for diagnosis is culture of the organism from clinical specimens, which may take up to 4 weeks.
- A presumptive diagnosis may be made by visualization of the typical yeast from clinical specimens in the appropriate setting

## CURRENT THERAPY

- Itraconazole (Sporanox) is the agent used most commonly to treat blastomycosis. It is administered in an oral dose of 200 to 400 mg daily for 6–12 months, depending on the site of infection.
- For life-threatening pulmonary disease (acute respiratory distress syndrome [ARDS]) or severe disseminated disease, amphotericin B (Fungizone) is the drug of choice. After initial improvement, itraconazole may be substituted.
- For CNS blastomycosis, amphotericin is used because itraconazole does not adequately penetrate the CNS. Liposomal amphotericin is used when high doses are needed or adverse effects from amphotericin B are encountered.
- Fluconazole (Diflucan),[1] ketoconazole (Nizoral), and IV itraconazole have lesser roles in the treatment of blastomycosis. Voriconazole (Vfend)[1] has not been studied adequately, but it may hold promise for CNS disease.

[1]Not FDA approved for this indication.

progresses on this agent should be switched to amphotericin B to complete at least 1.5 g. Bone disease should be treated for at least 1 year. For life-threatening disease, amphotericin B at 0.7 to 1.0 mg/kg daily should be administered for a total dose of 2.0 to 2.5 g. In immuno-compromised individuals, many authorities recommend long-term suppressive therapy with itraconazole after a treatment course of amphotericin B. Pregnant women should be treated with ampho-tericin B because the azoles are teratogenic. Data on blastomycosis in children are sparse, but some authorities suggest initial amphotericin B because of a potential unfavorable response to azoles.

## NEW ANTIFUNGAL AGENTS

Voriconazole (Vfend)[1] is active in vitro and in animal models of pulmonary blastomycosis; the in vitro activity against *B. dermatitidis* is similar to itraconazole. Although clinical data in treating blastomyco-sis in humans are inadequate, voriconazole has good CNS penetration based on reports of successful treatment of CNS aspergillosis. Posaconazole (Noxafil),[1] which has recently been licensed in the United States, is also active in vitro and in animal models. Further data are needed before these agents may be recommended for use in blasto-mycosis. The echinocandin class of antifungal agents shows variable activity against *B. dermatitidis* and there are no clinical data to support their use.

## REFERENCES

Bradsher RW: Clinical features of blastomycosis. Semin Respir Infect 1997;12:229-234.

Bradsher RW, Chapman SW, Pappas PG: Blastomycosis. Infect Dis Clin North Am 2003;17:21-40.

Chapman SW. *Blastomyces dermatitidis*. In: Mandell GL, Bennett JE, Dolin R (eds): Principles and Practice of Infectious Diseases. New York, Churchill Livingstone, 2005, pp. 3026-3040.

Chapman SW, Bradsher RW, Campbell GD, et al: Practice guidelines for the management of patients with blastomycosis. Clin Infect Dis 2000;30:679-683.

Chapman SW, Lin AC, Hendricks KA, et al: Endemic blastomycosis in Mississippi: Epidemiological and clinical studies. Semin Respir Infect 1997;12:219-228.

Lemos LB, Guo M, Baliga M: Blastomycosis: organ involvement and etiologic diagnosis. A review of 123 patients from Mississippi. Ann Diagn Pathol 2000;4:391-406.

Pappas PG: Blastomycosis in the immunocompromised patient. Semin Respir Infect 1997;12:243-251

Schutze GE, Hickerson SL, Fortin EM, et al: Blastomycosis in children. Clin Infect Dis 1996;22:496-502.

Sugar AM, Liu X-P: Efficacy of voriconazole in treatment of murine pulmonary blastomycosis. Antimicrob Agents Chemother 2001;45:601-604.

[1]Not FDA approved for this indication.

# Pleural Effusion and Empyema Thoracis

Method of
*Stephen D. Cassivi, MD, MSc, FRCSC, FACS, and
Stephen H. McKellar, MD*

The parietal and visceral pleurae line the inner chest wall and outer surface of the lungs, respectively, within the pleural spaces. One of the functions of the pleurae is to lubricate the pleural spaces by secreting 0.01 mL/kg/hour of serous fluid. Fluid secretion is balanced by the pleura's normal absorptive ability of up to 0.2 mL/kg/hour, normally resulting in only a small amount of residual pleural fluid. Local or systemic illness can affect this balance and result in pleural fluid accumulation, which can serve as a nidus for pleural space infection.

# Pleural Effusion

## CLINICAL FEATURES

Clinically significant pleural effusions often manifest themselves with subtle findings. When symptoms are present, patients often have dysp-nea, pleuritic chest pain, cough or systemic symptoms such as fatigue, fevers, chills, or weight loss. Physical examination often reveals decreased breath sounds, dullness to percussion, and egophony over the affected area. Conventional chest radiographs are often sufficient to confirm the diagnosis of pleural effusion or empyema, particularly when the effusion is large. Subtle, smaller effusions can be recognized by blunting of the costophrenic angles or by decubitus chest radiographs. Ultrasonography and computed tomography (CT) can help character-ize the fluid in terms of loculations and can provide information about the underlying lung parenchyma.

## THORACENTESIS

Thoracentesis can be both diagnostic and therapeutic. Generally, as much fluid as possible should be removed at the time of thoracentesis because the morbidities and risks of the procedure, namely pneumo-thorax, infection, and bleeding, are for the most part unrelated to the volume of fluid removed. In the case of large-volume drainage, consid-eration should be given to the rare but potentially lethal phenomenon of re-expansion pulmonary edema. Rapid re-expansion of compressed lung leads to a rapid increase in blood flow and pulmonary capillary pressure, with resultant extravascular fluid buildup due to a shift across the capillary-alveolar membranes. The first sign of this process is noted when the patient begins to cough uncontrollably during fluid drainage. Usually this occurs when between 800 and 1500 mL of fluid has been acutely drained. If this occurs, the drainage should be temporarily stopped by closing the thoracentesis stopcock off to the patient, with subsequent intermittent drainage until no further fluid is obtainable.

## ETIOLOGY

Diagnosis of the etiology of the effusion begins with inspection of the fluid. Purulent or foul-smelling fluid suggests infection; bloody fluid suggests trauma or malignancy as the underlying cause. Lactate dehy-drogenase, pH, protein, glucose, cell counts with cytology, Gram stain with culture and antimicrobial sensitivities should be ordered for all patients with pleural effusions of indeterminate etiology. Additional laboratory investigations are sought depending on the primary diag-nostic hypotheses. These investigations serve to classify the effusion into one of two categories: transudative or exudative. Common etiolo-gies of pleural effusions are listed in Box 1.

## TREATMENT

Systemic illnesses such as uremia, cirrhosis, and congestive heart fail-ure can lead to transudative effusions. The goal of treatment is to correct or control the underlying systemic pathophysiology.

---

**BOX 1  Common Causes of Pleural Effusions**

**Transudative Pleural Effusion**
Cirrhosis
Congestive heart failure
Nephrotic syndrome
Uremia

**Exudative Pleural Effusion**
Chylothorax
Hemothorax
Infection
Malignancy
Postinfarction syndrome
Subdiaphragmatic source

In contrast, infections and malignancy can cause exudative effusions, which are treated quite differently from transudative effusions. Early infection is treated through adequate drainage and systemic antibiotics (see the empyema section). Malignant effusions, because they usually represent late-stage, unresectable cancer, are treated with palliative intent; relief of dyspnea is the goal.

For patients with malignant pleural effusions or recurrent transudative effusions, the pleural space can be obliterated with sclerosing agents. When the underlying lung is not trapped and able to completely re-expand, our preference is to use thoracoscopic talc pleurodesis. This technique allows thorough examination of the lung and pleural space, permits tissue biopsies, if needed, and facilitates instillation of the sclerosing agents under direct visualization to ensure complete distribution. It is also more expeditious and usually more comfortable for the patient than the alternative strategy of bedside chest tube placement and per tube injection of the sclerosant.

Indwelling, tunneled silastic catheters are becoming an increasingly popular alternative to chemical pleurodesis for palliation in patients with malignant pleural effusions. There is sufficient evidence to support their use based on low morbidity, improved symptoms, and even spontaneous pleurodesis. This technique is a very good alternative in the situation of a trapped, nonexpanding lung, where talc instillation would be futile given the lack of necessary apposition of the two pleural surfaces.

# Empyema Thoracis

## ETIOLOGY

Empyema is defined as the presence of purulent fluid in the pleural space. Pneumonia is the most common cause of empyema, but it can also develop secondary to lung abscess, trauma, bronchopleural fistula, or esophageal perforation or following thoracic surgery. Conceptually, it is best to think of empyema as an infectious continuum but divided into three phases: early/acute exudative, transitional/fibrinopurulent, and late/organized.

---

## CURRENT DIAGNOSIS

Laboratory investigations for the diagnosis of pleural fluid etiology

**Routine Investigations**

- Cell count
- Culture and antibiotic sensitivity
- Cytology
- Glucose
- Gram stain
- Lactate dehydrogenase
- pH
- Protein

**Additional Investigations**

- Acid-fast stain
- Amylase
- Bilirubin
- Chylomicrons
- Creatinine
- Fatty acids
- Triglycerides

Light's criteria for exudative effusion are met if the ratio of pleural fluid to serum protein is >0.5 and the ratio of pleural fluid to serum lactate dehydrogenase is >0.6.

---

## CURRENT THERAPY

| Phase of Empyema | Treatment |
|---|---|
| ■ Early | ■ Intravenous antibiotics<br>■ Drainage with thoracostomy tube |
| ■ Transitional | ■ Intravenous antibiotics<br>■ Thoracoscopy or thoracotomy with drainage and decortication |
| ■ Late | ■ Intravenous antibiotics<br>■ Thoracotomy with drainage and decortication |

---

## TREATMENT

Treatment of empyema depends on when in this continuum the diagnosis is made, because the lung is affected differently in each of the three phases. The overarching principle, however, is adequate drainage of the pleural space to allow re-expansion of the lung.

In the early/acute exudative phase, the lung is not trapped but is surrounded by a layer of purulent fluid. Drainage, either through thoracentesis or tube thoracostomy, accompanied by systemic antibiotics is usually sufficient treatment. Tube thoracostomy is preferred to ensure complete evacuation of the pleural space; evacuation can be confirmed with chest CT.

Empyema in the transitional/fibrinopurulent phase is more challenging to treat due to the loculated nature of the intrapleural fluid. Inadequate drainage procedures are more likely because of the fibrinopurulent adhesions that trap fluid into distinct and noncommunicating collections. Drainage by thoracoscopic guidance or formal decortication are the preferred treatment options because they allow lysis of loculating adhesions and complete drainage of purulent fluid, and, most importantly, they result in re-expansion of the underlying lung.

During the late/organized phase, the lung is usually firmly entrapped beneath a substantial visceral pleural rind. Simple drainage of the usually thin serous effusion at this stage is inadequate because the underlying lung cannot re-expand to fill the space. The resultant residual empty pleural space recurrently fills with fluid that cannot be abated or sterilized until the lung is formally decorticated and allowed to re-expand to fill the pleural space. Expeditious and complete decortication is usually not possible by thoracoscopy at this stage. Open thoracotomy with decortication is the preferred and most common approach. In unfortunate (but rare) cases, the lung does not re-expand fully to fill the space due to either underlying disease or prior resections. In these situations, an open pleural window is sometimes necessary and usually preferable to deforming the chest wall by thoracoplasty.

Postpneumonectomy empyema, usually caused by a bronchopleural fistula, deserves special consideration. As with any pleural infection, the pleural space must be adequately drained, with the additional indication of preventing contralateral soilage of the solitary lung. The fistula must then be closed primarily and should be reinforced with a vascularized pedicle flap. Ultimately, the chest can usually be successfully closed using the procedure described initially by Clagett.

## REFERENCES

Cassivi SD, Deschamps C: Chest tube insertion and management. In Albert RK, Spiro SG, Jett JR (eds): Clinical Respiratory Medicine, 2nd ed. St Louis: Mosby, 2004, pp 175-181.

Clagett OT, Geraci JE: A procedure for the management of postpneumonectomy empyema. J Thorac Cardiovasc Surg 1963;45:141-145.

Owens MW, Milligan SA: Pleuritis and pleural effusions. Curr Opin Pulm Med 1995;1:318-323.

Puskas JD, Mathisen DJ: Treatment strategies for bronchopleural fistula. J Thorac Cardiovascular Surg 1995;109:989-996.

Tremblay A, Michaud G: Single-center experience with 250 tunnelled pleural catheter insertions for malignant pleural effusion. Chest 2006;129:362-368.
Zaheer S, Allen MS, Cassivi SD, et al: Postpneumonectomy empyema: Results after the Clagett procedure. Ann Thorac Surgery 2006;82:279-287.

# Primary Lung Abscess

Method of
*Scott Swanson, MD, and*
*Virginia Litle, MD*

## Definition

A primary lung abscess is defined as a localized collection of pus within the lung parenchyma with associated pulmonary necrosis. Empyema is an extraparenchymal collection of pus within the pleural space. A primary lung abscess can progress to an empyema with a bronchopleural fistula. A secondary lung abscess develops from airway obstruction and suppuration or from extension of another localized infection.

An acute lung abscess has been present for fewer than 6 weeks. An abscess with a longer duration is considered chronic. Most lung abscesses are solitary; but multiple abscesses can occur, especially in immunocompromised patients or in the setting of septic emboli. Primary lung abscesses are more common in the right lung because of the bronchial anatomy and in the posterior segments of the upper lobes and superior segments of the lower lobes of the lungs because they are the dependent segments in the supine patient.

## Cause

The most common cause of a primary lung abscess is aspiration and occurs in patients with impaired level of consciousness from acute alcoholism, drug overdose, seizures, or cerebrovascular accidents. Poor oral hygiene and dentition is a risk factor for primary lung abscess. A necrotizing pneumonia essentially progresses to a primary lung abscess. Cancer, HIV, diabetes mellitus, or organ transplant patients are also at risk of developing a primary lung abscess, as are malnourished and debilitated intensive care unit patients (Table 1).

The secondary lung abscess results from airway obstruction from a benign or malignant tumor, a broncholith, or a foreign body such as an aspirated tooth. A pulmonary infarct can become secondarily infected and result in a secondary lung abscess, whereas an intra-abdominal abscess also can infect the lung across the diaphragm. Infected bronchogenic cysts and bullae are not considered true lung abscesses but radiographically resemble them.

## Signs and Symptoms

A patient typically presents with fever, cough, fatigue, and night sweats. Hemoptysis may be present. An anaerobic infection produces foul-smelling sputum. The patient occasionally has new-onset dyspnea with or without exertion. On exam the patient is tachycardic, tachypneic, and often hypoxemic. Altered mental status, poor dentition, and decreased unilateral breath sounds are common. Erythema or fluctuance of the chest wall suggests an empyema necessitatis, which is not typically associated with a lung abscess.

## Diagnosis and Treatment

The workup involves routine blood work, sputum cultures, blood cultures, and broad-spectrum antibiotics. The degree of leukocytosis will depend on the patient's underlying disease state, but a left shift is present.

**TABLE 1   Risk Factors for Primary Lung Abscess**

- Neurologic impairment
- Alcoholism
- Seizures
- Cerebrovascular accident
- Poor oral hygiene and dentition
- Pneumonia
- Immunodeficiency
- HIV
- Organ transplantation
- Diabetes mellitus
- Chemotherapy
- ICU patient
- Esophageal dysfunction
- Gastroesophageal reflux disease
- Zenker's diverticulum
- Achalasia
- Presbyesophagus
- Esophageal cancer/stricture
- Anemia

*Abbreviation:* ICU = intensive care unit.

There will be an air fluid level on plain chest radiograph. An infected bulla or previously undiagnosed bronchogenic cyst may have similar presentation and study results.

The organisms involved are listed in Table 2. If the specific organism is unknown, empiric intravenous antibiotics traditionally included high-dose penicillin; but with current antibiotic resistance patterns, better choices include single-agent therapy with cefoxitin (Mefoxin), imipenem-cilastatin (Primaxin), piperacillin-tazobactam (Zosyn), or ampicillin-sulbactam (Unasyn).

A noncontrast chest computed tomography (CT) scan is indicated to define the size of the abscess and degree of lobar involvement. A loculated hydropneumothorax on radiographs can also be seen with an empyema with a bronchopleural fistula. The CT may reveal an associated foreign body including a tooth or neoplasm causing obstruction. If the patient has positive blood cultures and multiple, peripheral lung abscesses, an echocardiogram is done to look for an intracardiac source of septic emboli to the lung. Any intravenous or dialysis catheters or chemotherapy ports should be removed.

Flexible or rigid bronchoscopy may then be necessary to relieve airway obstruction, to obtain tissue diagnosis of a neoplasm, or for pulmonary toilet and good sputum samples for culture. Hemoptysis is also an indication for bronchoscopy because the bleeding may be from an endobronchial malignancy, which could be controlled with extraction of the cancer with a rigid bronchoscope or with laser therapy. If there

## CURRENT DIAGNOSIS

Neurologic impairment
- Alcoholism
- Stroke
- Seizure

Poor dentition/oral hygiene
Immunocompromised patient
- Transplant
- Cancer
- HIV
- Diabetic

Fever, productive cough, malaise
Air-fluid level on chest radiograph
CT scan of chest: hydropneumothorax within lung

*Abbreviation:* CT = computed tomography.

## TABLE 2 Organisms Causing Primary or Secondary Lung Abscess

Anaerobic
- *Bacteroides*
- *Peptococcus*
- *Peptostreptococcus*
- *Fusobacterium*
- *Prevotella*
- *Clostridium*

Aerobic
- *Staphylococcus aureus*
- *Klebsiella pneumoniae*
- *Pseudomonas aeruginosa*
- *Streptococcus*
- *Escherichia coli*

is no endobronchial lesion on bronchoscopy, massive hemoptysis (>600 mL/24 hours) from the abscess requires bronchial artery embolization by the interventional radiologists or lung resection to control bleeding.

After initiation of broad spectrum antibiotics, most patients improve. If clinical signs of sepsis continue, more than 90% of cases are successfully treated with CT- or ultrasound-guided drainage of the lung abscess with placement of a pigtail catheter into the cavity and confirmation of the culprit organism to guide antibiotic therapy. Chest tube placement should be avoided because a bronchopleural fistula results.

Risk factors for medical failure include an abscess greater than 6 cm; an immunocompromised patient; or infection with *Staphylococcus aureus*, *Klebsiella pneumoniae*, or *Pseudomonas aeruginosa*. When the abscess persists after 6 weeks of medical treatment or in cases of massive hemoptysis, surgical exploration is indicated. Lung resection can range from a wedge resection to a lobectomy to remove all grossly infected tissue. A pneumonectomy is associated with a high mortality and is rarely indicated or necessary. If lung resection will result in excessive pulmonary compromise, a surgical cavernostomy with rib resection and debridement of infected lung tissue and wound packing with gauze is done. After an average of 2 weeks of dressing changes and optimization of nutrition, the patient undergoes placement of a muscle flap into a clean lung bed and chest closure.

## Prevention

Prevention of impaired consciousness and good oral hygiene prevents development of most primary lung abscesses, especially in the immunocompromised population of cancer, transplant, and HIV patients. Lung abscess incidence should decrease for the patient by maintaining adequate nutrition, elevating the head of the bed more than 30 degrees, and attentive oral care in the intensive care unit (ICU). In ICU patients requiring prolonged endotracheal intubation

## CURRENT THERAPY

Broad-spectrum IV antibiotics
- Second-generation cephalosporin
- A carbapenem
- Third- or fourth-generation penicillin

Continued sepsis
- Percutaneous pigtail drain in abscess
- No chest tube

Persistent abscess after 6 weeks
- Lung resection or rib resection and cavernostomy

*Abbreviation:* IV = intravenous.

(>10 days), a tracheostomy and percutaneous feeding tube also will improve oral hygiene and nutrition and assist with pulmonary toilet to reduce lung abscess risk. Routine pulmonary toilet for all patients with pulmonary abscesses includes chest physiotherapy, postural drainage, incentive spirometry, expectorants, and ambulation.

### REFERENCES

Mansharamani N, Balachandran D, Delaney D, et al: Lung abscess in adults: Clinical comparison of immunocompromised to non-immunocompromised patients. Respir Med 2002;96(3):178–185.

Postma MH, Le Roux RT: The place of external drainage in the management of lung abscess. S Afr J Surg 1986;24(4):156–158.

Refaely Y, Weissberg D: Gangrene of the lung: Treatment in two stages. Ann Thorac Surg 1997;64:970–974.

Rice TW, Ginsberg RJ, Todd TR: Tube drainage of lung abscesses. Ann Thorac Surg 1987;44(4):356–359.

Rowe S, Cheadle WG: Complications of nosocomial pneumonia in the surgical patient. Am J Surg 2000;179(2A):63S-68S.

Tan TQ, Seilheimer DK, Kaplan SL: Pediatric lung abscess: Clinical management and outcome. Pediatr Infect Dis J 1995;14(1):51–55.

Weissberg D: Percutaneous drainage of lung abscess. J Thorac Cardiovasc Surg 1984;87(2):308–312.

# Acute Bronchitis

Method of
*Susan Davids, MD, MPH, and*
*Ralph M. Schapira, MD*

Acute bronchitis is one of the most common diagnoses made by primary care physicians in the United States and accounts for nearly 10 million office visits per year. Acute bronchitis is a transient, self-limited inflammatory process of the upper respiratory tract, specifically the trachea and bronchi. Antibiotics are overprescribed to patients with acute bronchitis; this practice has raised significant concern related to the worldwide rise of antibiotic resistance, which is viewed as one of the world's most pressing public health problems.

Acute bronchitis manifests as an acute respiratory illness of less than 3 weeks' duration, with or without sputum production. Acute bronchitis is a clinical diagnosis and must be distinguished from other respiratory diseases, such as pneumonia, acute exacerbation of chronic bronchitis (episode of worsening of symptoms and expiratory airflow obstruction in patients with chronic obstructive pulmonary disease), and the onset of asthma. Most cases of acute bronchitis occur in the fall and winter. The etiology of acute bronchitis is infectious, and viruses appear to be the cause of most cases. Influenzas A and B are the most common viruses isolated, although a wide variety of infectious agents have been identified, such as adenovirus, coronavirus, parainfluenza virus, respiratory syncytial virus, coxsackievirus, *Mycoplasma pneumoniae*, *Bordetella pertussis*, and *Chlamydia pneumoniae*.

Diagnosis of acute bronchitis is based on findings of a prominent cough that may be accompanied by wheezing and sputum production. Most patients are otherwise healthy and without preexisting respiratory disease. Nonspecific constitutional symptoms may also be part of acute bronchitis. Appropriate management of acute bronchitis is essential because it is one of the most common illnesses that present to physicians in the outpatient setting. Antibiotics are often prescribed unnecessarily for acute bronchitis and other respiratory tract illnesses; these prescriptions may potentially lead to adverse events (i.e., allergic reactions and gastrointestinal side effects) and bacterial resistance. Other medications, such as inhaled bronchodilators and antitussives, are often prescribed for acute bronchitis despite questionable evidence to support their routine use.

Pathophysiology of acute bronchitis involves an acute inflammatory response involving the mucosa of the trachea and bronchi, resulting in injury to the respiratory tract epithelium. Sputum production is increased and bronchoconstriction (potentially resulting in airflow obstruction and wheezing) can occur. Positron emission tomography (PET) of a patient with acute bronchitis confirms that the primary inflammatory changes occur in the trachea and bronchi and not the remainder of the lower respiratory track.

## Diagnosis

Cough, phlegm (which may be purulent as both bacteria and viruses can cause purulent sputum), and wheezing help differentiate acute bronchitis from upper respiratory infections such as pharyngitis and sinusitis. Acute bronchitis must be differentiated from acute bacterial pneumonia. The absence of abnormalities in vital signs (heart rate >100 bpm, respiratory rate >24 breath/min, oral temperature >100.4°F [38°C] and physical examination of the chest) supports the diagnosis of acute bronchitis and makes the need for chest radiography unnecessary in most cases. The treatment and outcome of acute bronchitis and pneumonia are very different; a chest radiograph should always be obtained if there is uncertainty about the diagnosis. Chest radiography will demonstrate no lung infiltrates in a patient with acute bronchitis. In contrast, lung infiltrates are present in pneumonia. Pertussis or whooping cough should be considered in adults with cough in the setting of what appears to be an upper respiratory infection, even in those previously immunized. Typically, the cough of pertussis, unlike acute bronchitis, lasts for longer than 3 weeks. Other respiratory diseases, such as previously undiagnosed asthma, can also mimic acute bronchitis, although several features differentiate asthma from acute bronchitis (see Section 12). Rapid testing to diagnose influenza viruses A and B (the most common causes of acute bronchitis) as a cause of acute bronchitis should be considered given the availability of effective treatment if initiated in the first 48 hours.

## Treatment

### ANTIBIOTICS, INHALED BRONCHODILATORS, AND ANTITUSSIVES

Existing evidence does not support the routine use of antibiotics for uncomplicated cases of acute bronchitis. Although most cases of acute bronchitis are caused by viral infections, upwards of 60% of patients are prescribed antibiotic therapy, which is contributing to the rise of bacterial resistance to commonly used antibiotics. Meta-analyses examining the effectiveness of antibiotic therapy in patients without underlying lung disease suggest no consistent effect of antibiotics on the severity or duration of acute bronchitis. A recent study evaluated children and patients with colored sputum and found that they also did not benefit from antibiotics. This study also found that compared to other populations, the elderly were less likely to benefit from antibiotics. Smokers with acute bronchitis are even more likely to be

prescribed antibiotics. Their response to antibiotics was either equal to or worse than that of nonsmokers.

One possible reason for overuse of antibiotics is the concern by physicians about patient satisfaction. Studies show that patients presenting to the doctor expecting antibiotics were more likely to be prescribed antibiotics; studies also suggest that satisfaction is more related to appropriate patient education than to receiving antibiotics. Patient education should include information regarding the duration of symptoms associated with acute bronchitis. It was found that patients presented on average after 9 days of cough and that the cough persisted for an additional 12 days after the physician visit. This information can impart a realistic expectation of illness duration to the patient.

If influenza is highly suspected and the patient presents within 48 hours of the onset of symptoms, rapid diagnostic testing and treatment should be considered. Both amantadine (Symmetrel) and rimantadine (Flumadine) are effective for influenza A, and neuraminidase inhibitors, inhaled zanamivir (Relenza), and oral oseltamivir (Tamiflu) are effective for influenzas A and B. If these medications are initiated within the first 48 hours of symptoms (and ideally within 30 hours), the duration of illness can be shortened.

The evidence supporting the use of inhaled bronchodilators for the treatment of the symptoms has been variable. Two small trials reported a shorter duration of cough with the use of inhaled β-agonists; another study reported benefit in those with evidence of bronchial hyperresponsiveness. Current recommendations support the use of β-agonists only in patients with evidence of bronchial hyperresponsiveness (wheezing or spirometry demonstrating a forced expiration volume in 1 second [$FEV_1$] <80% of predicted).

Antitussive agents have not been shown to improve the acute or early cough but did show some improvements in cough lasting longer than 3 weeks. The current recommendations are to use antitussives, namely dextromethorphan (Benylin) or codeine, in patients with cough of 2 to 3 weeks' duration.

Acute uncomplicated bronchitis is most often a viral illness in which antibiotics are not routinely indicated. Patients presenting with an acute respiratory illness, who are younger than 65 years old without existing pulmonary disease or other significant comorbid illness, should have a thorough physical examination, including vital signs. If the vital signs are normal and physical examination of the chest is clear, pneumonia can most likely be ruled out. In patients who present within 48 hours of onset of symptoms, influenza should be considered as effective therapy is available for acute bronchitis caused by influenzas A or B. Otherwise, the evidence for treatment with antibiotics does not support their routine use. Bronchodilators should be considered in those with evidence of bronchial hyperresponsiveness; cough suppressants should be considered in those with 2 to 3 weeks of cough. Patient education is an integral part of the treatment, and patients should receive information that provides realistic expectations regarding the duration of cough.

## REFERENCES

Aagaard E, Gonzales R: Management of acute bronchitis in healthy adults. Infect Dis Clin North Am 2004;18:919-937.

Ebell MH: Antibiotic prescribing for cough and symptoms of respiratory tract infection. JAMA 2005;294(3):3062-3064.

Fahey T, Smucny J, Becker L, Glazier R: Antibiotics for acute bronchitis. Cochrane Database Syst Rev 2004;(4):CD000245.

Gonzales R, Sande M: Uncomplicated acute bronchitis. Ann Intern Med 2000; 133:981-991.

Kicska G, Zhuang H, Alavi A: Acute bronchitis imaged with F-18 FDG positron emission tomography. Clin Nucl Med 2003;28(6):511-512.

Little R, Rumsby K, Kelly J, et al: Information leaflet and antibiotic prescribing strategies for acute lower respiratory tract infection. JAMA 2005;293(24): 3029-3035.

Linder JA, Sim I: Antibiotic treatment of acute bronchitis in smokers. J Gen Intern Med 2002;17:230-234.

Martinez FJ: Acute bronchitis: State of the art diagnosis and therapy. Compr Ther 2004;30(1):55-59.

Smucny J, Flynn C, Becker L, Glazier R: Beta$_2$-agonists for acute bronchitis. Cochrane Database Syst Rev 2004;(1):CD001726.

# Bacterial Pneumonia

Method of
*Umur Hatipoğlu, MD, and Israel Rubinstein, MD*

Bacterial pneumonia is a leading cause of mortality and morbidity in the world. Microorganisms gain entry into the lungs via microaspiration of oropharyngeal contents, hematogenous spread, sympathetic spread, or inhalation. Through interaction of factors including virulence of the organism, bacterial burden, and immune system of the host, particularly pulmonary defense mechanisms, alveolar exudation occurs, leading to the clinical symptoms of pneumonia and hypoxemia. Because of differences in microbiology, treatment, and outcome, pneumonia syndromes are separated into two groups: community-acquired pneumonia and hospital-acquired pneumonia. Hospital-acquired pneumonia includes ventilator-associated pneumonia and health care–associated pneumonia.

## Community-Acquired Bacterial Pneumonia

### EPIDEMIOLOGY

Community-acquired pneumonia affects an estimated 5.6 million persons in the United States. Up to 20% of the patients who present with pneumonia from the community require hospitalization. Viral infections—in particular, influenza virus—can predispose to bacterial infections by virtue of impairing pulmonary defense mechanisms. Other predisposing conditions are smoking, alcoholism, underlying lung disease, alteration of mental status, airway obstruction, ciliary dysfunction, cystic fibrosis, immunosuppression, renal failure, and malnutrition. Pneumonia is the most common lethal infectious disease in this country.

### ETIOLOGY

*Streptococcus pneumoniae* is the most commonly implied pathogen in bacterial pneumonia acquired from the community. In most series,

*S. pneumoniae* (pneumococcus) is closely followed by *Mycoplasma pneumoniae*, *Chlamydophila pneumoniae*, and *Haemophilus influenzae*. Group A streptococci—*Streptococcus pyogenes* and *Staphylococcus aureus*, particularly methicillin-resistant strains—are associated with severe pneumonia with high mortality.

Microbiological agents such as *Bacillus anthracis* and *Yersinia pestis* can be used as agents of bioterrorism. Inhalational anthrax was reported in the United States in 2001 when *B. anthracis* was deliberately spread through the postal system in the form of contaminated powder placed in letters.

Usual and some unusual causes of community-acquired pneumonia and suggestive epidemiologic and clinical features are listed in Table 1.

### DIAGNOSIS

Clinical diagnosis of pneumonia can be problematic. There is no single sign or symptom or a constellation of clinical findings that would clinch the diagnosis of pneumonia. Most patients complain of cough productive of sputum, chest pain (pleurisy), and shortness of breath. The fever, rigors, and chills are common signs as well. Extrapulmonary symptoms include nausea, vomiting, diarrhea, and mental status change.

On physical examination, crackles are often heard during auscultation of the lungs. The signs of consolidation, such as bronchial breath sounds, increased vocal fremitus on palpation, whispering pectoriloquy, and dullness to percussion, may be evident.

Chest x-ray finding of consolidation, cavitation, or interstitial infiltration is considered necessary for the diagnosis of pneumonia. However, chest x-ray findings can lag behind clinical findings, particularly in neutropenic or volume-depleted patients. In these cases, we recommend obtaining a follow-up chest x-ray within 24 to 48 hours when clinical suspicion of pneumonia is high. Although CT scan of the chest has higher sensitivity in finding pulmonary infiltration, this costly procedure is warranted only if another underlying pathology is suspected such as an underlying tumor.

In classic texts, pneumonia syndrome is discussed under atypical and typical pneumonia headings. Typical pneumonia has an abrupt onset of hours or days. Affected patients are febrile and produce mucopurulent sputum. Chills and rigors are usually present. The chest x-ray shows lobar consolidation, sometimes accompanied by a pleural effusion. Leukocytosis or leukopenia may be present. Leukopenia can indicate more severe disease. The organisms that cause typical pneumonia syndrome include *S. pneumoniae*, *Moraxella catarrhalis*, *H. influenzae*, *S. aureus*, *S. pyogenes*, gram-negative enterobacteria, and anaerobes. Atypical pneumonia, on the other hand, has a more insidious onset. Cough is not productive. Fever may be low-grade, and malaise is present. Sore throat and earache can be present. Chest x-ray shows patchy or diffuse ground-glass opacities or alveolar interstitial infiltration. Extrapulmonary signs and symptoms such as headache, myalgias, confusion, and electrolyte abnormalities may be more prevalent. Etiologic agents implicated include *M. pneumoniae*, *C. pneumoniae*, *Legionella pneumophila*, and viral infections.

Despite these well-defined clinical syndromes, often there is overlap between the two types and also in the etiologic agents that cause them. Therefore, type of clinical presentation might offer a clue to the etiology; however, it should not interfere with empiric coverage of both atypical and typical agents.

Recently, the Centers for Disease Control and Prevention (CDC) reported 15 cases of methicillin-resistant *S. aureus* (MRSA) community-acquired pneumonia. Disease manifestation was with severe pneumonia, and four of these patients died. Importantly, there was a strong association with previous influenza infection in most cases. Community-acquired MRSA pneumonia should be suspected in severely ill patients during the influenza season.

### LABORATORY TESTING

Usefulness of diagnostic testing to identify specific pathogens has been debated. In only 30% of cases of the community-acquired pneumonia, a specific pathogen is identified via cultures or serologic testing.

## TABLE 1   Characteristics of Select Pathogens in Community-Acquired Pneumonia

| Pathogen | Typical Clinical Features | Mode of Infection | Diagnosis | Treatment |
|---|---|---|---|---|
| *Bacillus anthracis* | Inhalation anthrax: onset similar to flu. Later severe respiratory distress, mediastinal widening on chest x-ray Extrapulmonary: meningitis | Infected animals (goats, sheep, cattle) to humans | Gram stain and culture Serology | Ciprofloxacin (Cipro) 400 mg IV q12h *or* Doxycycline plus one or two other drugs with in vitro susceptibility Anthrax vaccine (Biothrax)* |
| *Chlamydophila pneumoniae* | Sore throat, hoarseness, dry cough Patchy subsegmental infiltrates Extrapulmonary manifestations: meningoencephalitis, pancarditis, arthritis | Person to person | CF, DFA, EIA PCR promising | Macrolides Doxycycline Fluoroquinolones |
| *Chlamydophila psittaci* | Psittacosis: fever, headache, myalgias, arthralgias Bronchopneumonia, interstitial pattern Extrapulmonary: meningoencephalitis, pancarditis, arthritis | Psittacine birds to humans | CF, DFA, EIA PCR promising | Macrolides Doxycycline Fluoroquinolones |
| *Coxiella burnetii* | Q fever: flu-like illness with nonproductive cough and fever Normal WBC, low platelets Interstitial infiltrates Extrapulmonary: endocarditis, hepatitis | Farm animals (cattle, sheep) to humans | PCR | Doxycycline Fluoroquinolones Newer macrolides |
| *Legionella pneumophila* | High-grade fever, cough, headache, bradycardia, diarrhea Extrapulmonary: neuropathy, rhabdomyolysis, glomerulonephritis, hyponatremia, hypophosphatemia, hepatic dysfunction | Inhalation or aspiration of contaminated water | Culture and urinary antigen testing | Macrolides Fluoroquinolones |
| *Mycoplasma pneumoniae* | Young adults and elderly Nonproductive cough, fever, headache, myalgias, URI Bronchopneumonia Extrapulmonary manifestations: bullous myringitis, pericarditis, aseptic meningitis, neuropathy, hemolytic anemia | Person to person | CF for IgM >1:32 Or Fourfold increase in titer | Macrolides Doxycycline (Vibramycin) Fluoroquinolones |
| *Streptococcus pneumoniae* | Acute onset with fever, chills, rigors, and rusty sputum Lobar infiltrate | Person to person | Gram stain and culture of sputum Urinary pneumococcal antigen | β-Lactam antibiotics Macrolides Vancomycin (Vancocin) |

*Available only to military personnel.
*Abbreviations:* CF = complement fixation; DFA = direct immunofluorescence; EIA = enzyme immunoassay; Ig = immunoglobulin; URI = upper respiratory infection; PCR = polymerase chain reaction; WBC = white blood cell count.

### CURRENT DIAGNOSIS

- Clinical diagnosis
  - Fever, cough, purulent sputum
  - Crackles or bronchial breath sounds on auscultation
- Chest x-ray infiltrate might not be present if the patient is dehydrated or neutropenic:
- Elicit history for drug-resistant pathogens and nosocomial pneumonia
- Assess severity of pneumonia using pneumonia severity index calculation

Empiric treatment of pneumonia, particularly in outpatients, is safe and efficacious. However, there is good, although not proved, evidence supporting diagnostic testing in patients who are hospitalized for community-acquired bacterial pneumonia. These include better tailoring of antibiotic therapy based on pathogen identification, preventing increasing antibiotic resistance, cost saving, and identifying reportable causes of community-acquired pneumonia such as *L. pneumophila* and *Mycobacterium tuberculosis* or MRSA, which would require in-hospital measures for containment.

Gram stain and culture of expectorated sputum might prove useful if an adequate sample for interpretation (<10 squamous epithelial cells and >25 white blood cells per high-power field) is obtained and processed by an experienced microbiology technician. Under optimal circumstances, sensitivity of Gram stain for pneumococcal pneumonia can reach 90%. Gram stain and culture of expectorated sputum are particularly valuable in cases of community-acquired pneumonia that do not seem to respond to therapy. This constitutes approximately 10% to 15% of all patients with pneumonia. Because patients are already exposed to antibiotics, microbiological testing at the time of failure to respond to therapy is less likely to yield a specific pathogen. Even with invasive modalities such as bronchoscopy, useful information is available only 40% of the time. We advocate processing of good-quality expectorated sputum for Gram stain and culture on admission to the hospital for this reason. Difficulties in obtaining expectorated sputum should not interfere with administration of empiric therapy.

The American Thoracic Society (ATS) and the Infectious Diseases Society of America (IDSA) recommend obtaining two sets of routine blood cultures in patients with community-acquired pneumonia. However, this modality has a notoriously low yield when applied to the general population of patients with community-acquired pneumonia. Instead, targeted blood cultures for high-risk patients have been recommended. Patients with recent antibiotic therapy, liver disease, low systolic blood pressure, elevated pulse and temperature, elevated blood urea nitrogen (BUN), elevated sodium, and elevated white blood cell count might have higher yields from blood cultures. Our practice is to obtain blood cultures in sicker patients, such as those with Pneumonia Severity Index (PSI) classes IV and V disease. This assessment, however, often meets resistance, because obtaining blood cultures has become a national quality indicator based on association with improved mortality in elderly patients.

Urinary antigen testing for L. pneumophila and S. pneumoniae are now widely available. Because culturing L. pneumophila is difficult and sputum direct fluorescent antibody testing is technically challenging and associated with comparatively low sensitivity, urine testing may be the most practical tool for diagnosis. The test currently detects only L. pneumophila group 1 infection. In North America and Europe, this serotype is responsible for more than 80% of cases. The sensitivity and specificity are particularly good if there is bacteremia. L. pneumophila has higher incidence in sicker patients, such as those admitted to the intensive care unit (ICU). Therefore, the usefulness of the test may be better in this group. Testing for pneumococcal antigen in urine has high sensitivity and specificity. It has been recommended to augment diagnostic testing in community-acquired pneumonia.

When the clinical syndrome of pneumonia is suspected, we order a chest x-ray, complete blood count, sputum Gram stain and culture, and routine chemistry. If patients are febrile (38.4°C), in PSI class IV or V, or received antibiotics recently, urine and blood cultures should be sent for Legionella testing.

When widely available and affordable, nucleic acid amplification tests such as polymerase chain reaction (PCR) are likely to have significant impact on diagnostic testing. High accuracy, rapid turnaround time, and applicability to nonbacterial infectious agents are particularly attractive features of PCR.

## RISK STRATIFICATION AND DECISION TO ADMIT

The first questions that face the clinician after establishing the diagnosis of pneumonia are how ill the patient is and whether the patient needs admission to the hospital or ICU. Assessment of the severity of illness determines not only the need for hospitalization but also the choice of antibiotic therapy. A number of prognostic scoring rules have been published to aid the clinician in making this assessment. However, these are not meant to replace good clinical sense. The patient's social setting, likelihood of compliance with therapy, and ability to take oral medicine are other factors that need to be taken into account.

ATS and IDSA endorse the calculation of the PSI, which was devised by the Pneumonia Patient Outcomes Research Team (PORT). The goal of this prediction rule was to identify patients with community-acquired pneumonia who had a low risk of mortality and adverse outcome. Accordingly, a two-step tool was devised after identifying variables that were associated with increased mortality from a derivation cohort of more than 38,000 adult patients with community-acquired pneumonia.

In the first step, the following variables were queried: age older than 50 years, history of neoplastic disease, congestive heart failure, cerebrovascular disease, renal disease and liver disease, physical findings of altered mental status, pulse 125 beats per minute, respiratory rate 30 per minute, systolic blood pressure less than 90 mm Hg, and temperature less than 35°C or 40°C. If none of these features was present, the patients were assigned to class I and outpatient therapy was recommended. Mortality of patients in class I was 0.1%, and only 5.1% required subsequent hospitalization. If any of these variables was identified, then step 2 of the prediction rule was applied.

In step 2, points were assigned for age, whether the patient was a nursing home resident, above-mentioned coexisting illnesses and physical examination findings, and the additional laboratory and radiographic findings of an arterial pH less than 7.35, BUN 30 mg/dL, sodium less than 130 mmol/L, glucose 250 mg/dL, hematocrit less than 30%, $PaO_2$ less than 60 mm Hg, and the presence of a pleural effusion. Based on point score, four more classes (II-V) are formed, each representing a group with greater morbidity and mortality. Low-risk patients in classes I to III with mortality ranging from 0.1 to 0.9% can be managed as outpatients or with brief in-house observation (class III). Higher-risk patients in classes IV and V, with a mortality risk of 9.3% and 27%, respectively, should be admitted to the hospital.

The PSI has been validated in a number of prospective trials and shown to reduce hospitalization of low-risk patients, resulting in major cost savings without increases in mortality and morbidity. Nevertheless, its calculation (based on 19 variables) has been found to be cumbersome and impractical for busy outpatient settings. Today, simple software programs that can be downloaded from the Internet can help the clinician calculate this index on hand-held computing devices. One such resource is the Agency for Healthcare Research and Quality (http://pda.ahrq.gov/clinic/psi/psicalc.asp), which provides a PSI calculator program that can be downloaded for pocket PC and Palm desktop applications.

Simpler indices have also been proposed such as the CURB (confusion, urea, respiration, blood pressure) and CURB-65. CURB includes coexisting disease, and CURB-65 adds the variable of age older than 65 years. Patients who display two or more of these variables should be considered for admission to the hospital. This scheme is endorsed by the British Thoracic Society as a simple and effective means of stratifying patients into risk groups. In a prospective study, PSI had higher discriminatory power, allowing definition of a greater fraction of patients at low risk compared with the CURB indices.

Studies suggest that incorporation of severity indices into clinical practice would aid in identifying low-risk patients who can be treated as outpatients and translates into major cost savings.

Admission to the ICU of patients with community-acquired pneumonia remains a clinical decision. The American Thoracic Society defined severe community-acquired pneumonia as the presence of one of the two major criteria or the presence of two or three minor criteria. The major criteria are the need for mechanical ventilation and septic shock, and the minor criteria include systolic blood pressure 90 mm Hg or less, multilobar disease, and $PaO_2/FiO_2$ ratio less than 250.

## TREATMENT

Early institution of appropriate treatment for community-acquired pneumonia has been associated with improved outcomes. A number of professional societies have issued guidelines concerning empiric antibiotic treatment. These guidelines emphasize the severity stratification of patients and assessment of the risk of drug-resistant bacteria strains. We will discuss the ATS guidelines that were revised in 2001 and point out some principles that are not covered in the ATS document but covered in IDSA and CDC guidelines.

The ATS guidelines approach antibiotic therapy after stratifying patients into outpatients with and without cardiopulmonary disease or modifying factors (groups 1 and 2), inpatients who are not in the ICU with or without cardiopulmonary disease and modifying factors (groups 3a and 3b), and patients who are admitted to the ICU with or without risk for Pseudomonas aeruginosa (groups 4a and 4b). A list of modifying factors, including risk factors for P. aeruginosa are given in Box 1.

This classification is largely based on the different microbiology observed in each group, and antibiotic coverage is determined accordingly. Patients in group 1 are treated with newer macrolides such as

# CURRENT THERAPY

**Community-Acquired Pneumonia**

GROUP 1 OUTPATIENTS

- Newer macrolides

*or*

- Doxycycline (Vibramycin)

GROUP 2 OUTPATIENTS WITH CPD OR MF

- Oral β-lactam

*plus*

- Oral macrolide or doxycycline

*or*

- Antipneumococcal fluoroquinolone

GROUP 3 INPATIENTS

- CPD or MF
  - Intravenous β-lactam

*plus*

  - Macrolide or doxycycline

*or*

  - Intravenous antipneumococcal fluoroquinolone
- No CPD or MF
  - Intravenous azithromycin
  - (If intolerant, doxycycline plus β-lactam)

*or*

  - Intravenous antipneumococcal fluoroquinolone

GROUP 4 ICU PATIENTS

- No pseudomonal risk
  - Intravenous β-lactam

*plus*

  - Intravenous macrolide or intravenous fluoro-quinolone
- Pseudomonal risk
  - Intravenous antipseudomonal β-lactam

*plus*

- Intravenous antipseudomonal quinolone

*or*

- Intravenous antipseudomonal β-lactam

*plus*

- Intravenous aminoglycoside

*plus*

- Intravenous macrolide

*or*

- Intravenous nonpseudomonal fluoroquinolone

**Hospital-Acquired Pneumonia**

EARLY ONSET

- Ceftriaxone (Rocephin)

*or*

- Levofloxacin (Leaquin), moxifloxacin (Avelox)[1] or ciprofloxacin (Cipro)

*or*

- Ampicillin-sulbactam (Unasyn)[1]

*or*

- Ertapenem (Invanz)[1]

LATE ONSET OR MDR RISK

- Antipseudomonal cephalosporin

*or*

- Antipseudomonal carbapenem

*or*

- β-Lactam–β-lactamase inhibitor

*plus*

- Antipseudomonal fluoroquinolone

*or*

- Aminoglycoside

*plus*

- Linezolid (Zyvox) or Vancomycin (Vancocin)

---

[1]Not FDA approved for this indication.
*Abbreviations:* CPD = cardiopulmonary disease; ICU = intensive care unit; MDR = multidrug resistant; MF = modifiable factors (see Box 1).

---

**BOX 1  Modifying Factors that Increase Risk of Infection**

**Drug-Resistant *Streptococcus pneumoniae***
- Age >65 y
- Alcoholism
- β-Lactam therapy in the past 3 mo
- Exposure to a child in daycare
- Immunosuppression (including corticosteroids)
- Multiple medical comorbidities

**Enteric Gram-Negative Organisms**
- Broad-spectrum antibiotic therapy >7 d in the past month
- Cardiopulmonary disease
- Corticosteroid therapy (>10 mg prednisone daily)
- Malnutrition
- Multiple medical comorbidities
- Nursing home residence
- *Pseudomonas aeruginosa* infection

- Recent antibiotic therapy
- Structural lung disease (e.g., bronchiectasis)

**Multidrug-Resistant Organisms**
- Antibiotic therapy in preceding 90 d
- Chronic dialysis
- Current hospitalization of 5 d or more
- Family member with multidrug-resistant pathogen
- High frequency of antibiotic resistance in the community or in the specific hospital unit
- Home infusion therapy or wound care
- Hospitalization for 2 d or more in the preceding 90 d
- Immunosuppressive disease or therapy
- Nursing home residence
- Presence of risk factors for nosocomial pneumonia

azithromycin (Zithromax) or clarithromycin (Biaxin) or doxycycline (Vibramycin) (patients with allergy or intolerance to macrolides). Patients in group 2 are treated with β-lactam, such as oral cefpodoxime (Vantin), cefuroxime (Ceftin), amoxicillin with or without clavulanate (Augmentin, Amoxil), or parenteral ceftriaxone (Rocephin) followed by oral cefpodoxime, plus a macrolide or doxycycline. An antipneumococcal fluoroquinolone such as levofloxacin (Levaquin), gatifloxacin (Tequin), or moxifloxacin (Avelox) is also considered adequate coverage for patients in group 2.

For patients in group 3a, intravenous azithromycin alone is sufficient. Doxycycline or an antipneumococcal fluoroquinolone can be substituted in patients with macrolide intolerance. For patients in group 3b (cardiopulmonary disease or modifying factors), an intravenous β-lactam antibiotic and intravenous or oral macrolide or doxycycline therapy is recommended. An intravenous antipneumococcal fluoroquinolone alone is also considered sufficient.

For patients in group 4a, combination therapy with an intravenous β-lactam plus either intravenous azithromycin or a fluoroquinolone should be administered. When pseudomonal risk is present (group 4b), an intravenous antipseudomonal β-lactam plus intravenous ciprofloxacin (Cipro) or intravenous antipseudomonal β-lactam plus IV aminoglycoside plus either IV azithromycin or nonpseudomonal fluoroquinolone are appropriate choices. ATS guidelines for empiric treatment of community-acquired pneumonia are summarized in the Current Therapy box, and dosing information for select antibiotics for bacterial pneumonia is given in Table 2.

For suspected aspiration, IDSA guidelines suggest administering amoxicillin-clavulanate for outpatients and fluoroquinolone plus clindamycin (Cleocin) or metronidazole (Flagyl), or a penicillin–β-lactam inhibitor combination. The CDC also issued recommendations with special emphasis on treatment of pneumococcal pneumonia. These guidelines emphasize the use of β-lactam antibiotics, a macrolide, or doxycycline as first-line treatment to avoid fluoroquinolone resistance, which is now a widespread phenomenon with β-lactam and macrolide antibiotics. In addition to these special circumstances, we recommend considering empiric coverage with linezolid (Zyvox) or vancomycin (Vancocin) for MRSA when confronted with severe pneumonia during the influenza season.

Duration of antibiotic therapy has not been firmly determined. Experts recommend 7 to 14 days of treatment for pneumococcal pneumonia and 10 to 21 days of treatment for atypical pneumonia. An alternative approach is to treat the patient with antibiotics until the patient is afebrile for 72 hours. Recent studies have shown that even a 3-day course of antibiotics may be as effective as 8 days of treatment in patients with mild to moderately severe community-acquired pneumonia. Further study is needed to determine the optimal duration of treatment for community-acquired pneumonia. Optimal duration is a course that is short enough to prevent complications of antibiotic therapy and curb cost but also long enough to eradicate the pathogen and prevent complications and bacterial resistance.

As an adjunct to antibiotics, administration of intravenous hydrocortisone (Solu-Cortef)[1] to patients with severe community-acquired pneumonia has been associated with improved mortality. In our severely ill patients admitted to the ICU with community-acquired pneumonia, we begin hydrocortisone infusion at 10 mg/hour after a 200-mg intravenous bolus. We continue infusion until unequivocal clinical improvement is evident or a 7-day course is completed, whichever is sooner.

## CLINICAL COURSE

Symptoms of pneumonia can linger for a long time. In one study, median time to resolution of cough and fatigue was 2 weeks. Patients become afebrile generally by 3 days. Continued fever after 3 days, worsening leukocytosis, or worsening of existing symptoms can signal a complication of pneumonia such as abscess formation, pulmonary gangrene, complicated parapneumonic pleural effusion, or antibiotic failure.

---

[1]Not FDA approved for this indication.

## TABLE 2 Antibiotics Used to Treat Community-Acquired and Hospital-Acquired Pneumonia

| Drug | Dose |
|---|---|
| **Aminoglycosides** | |
| Amikacin (Amikin) | 20 mg/kg/d (trough <4-5 mcg/mL) |
| Gentamicin (generic) | 7 mg/kg/d (trough <1 mcg/mL) |
| Tobramycin (generic) | 7 mg/kg/d (trough <1 mcg/mL) |
| **Antipneumococcal Fluoroquinolones** | |
| Levofloxacin (Levaquin) | 750 mg IV/PO q24h |
| Moxiflocacin (Avelox) | 400 mg IV/PO q24h |
| **Antipseudomonal Cephalosporins** | |
| Cefepime (Maxipime) | 1-2 g q8-12h |
| Ceftazidime (Fortaz) | 2 g q8h |
| **Antipseudomonal Fluoroquinolones** | |
| Ciprofloxacin (Cipro) | 400 mg IV q12h |
| Levofloxacin (Levaquin) | 750 mg IV q24h |
| **β-Lactams (Intravenous)** | |
| Cefotaxime (Claforan) | 1-2 g q8 to12h |
| Ceftriaxone (Rocephin) | 1-2 g q24h |
| **β-Lactams (Oral)** | |
| Amoxicillin (Amoxil, Trimox) | 875 mg PO bid |
| Amoxicillin-clavulanate (Augmentin) | 875 mg PO bid |
| Amoxicillin-clavulanate (1000/62.5 sustained release) (Augmentin XR) | 2 tabs PO q12h |
| Cefuroxime (Ceftin) | 500 mg PO bid |
| Cefpodoxime (Vantin) | 400 mg PO bid |
| **β-Lactam–β-Lactamase Inhibitor** | |
| Piperacillin-tazobactam (Zosyn) | 4.5 g q6h |
| **Carbapenems** | |
| Ertapenem (Invanz) | 1 g IV q24h |
| Imipenem (Primaxin) | 500 mg IV q6h or 1 g IV q8h |
| Meropenem (Merrem) | 1 g IV q8h |
| **Newer Macrolides** | |
| Azithromycin (Zithromax) | 500 mg PO on d 1, 250 mg PO on d 2-5 |
| Clarithromycin (Biaxin) | 500 mg IV q24h 500 mg PO bid |
| Clarithromycin extended release (Biaxin XL) | 1000 mg PO q24h |
| Doxycycline (Adoxa) | 100 mg PO/IV bid |
| **Other** | |
| Linezolid (Zyvox) | 600 mg q12h |
| Vancomycin (generic) | 15 mg/kg q12h |

*Abbreviation:* tab = tablet.

At this stage, it is appropriate to consider alternative diagnoses that can mimic community-acquired pneumonia. These include congestive heart failure, pulmonary embolism, idiopathic interstitial pneumonia (such as cryptogenic organizing pneumonia), malignancy, alveolar hemorrhage, drug-induced lung disease, or pulmonary vasculitis (such as Wegener's granulomatosis). Unusual infections, such as *M. tuberculosis*, *Pneumocystis jiroveci* pneumonia, and fungal infections, should be considered, particularly if suspicion for immunocompromised state such as HIV disease exists.

Pleural effusions often accompany pneumonia. It is strongly recommended that the fluid be sampled to ensure uncomplicated parapneumonic effusion. As a general rule, if the pleural effusion layers by 1 cm from the chest wall on the lateral decubitus film taken with the pleural effusion side down, thoracentesis should be performed. A complicated parapneumonic effusion is said to be present if the pleural fluid pH is less than 7.2. Such effusions require either therapeutic thoracentesis or tube thoracostomy. If frank pus or positive gram stain or culture is present or the pH is less than 7.0, tube thoracostomy is indicated. Aggressive drainage is necessary in these latter two conditions, and failure to do so can result in prolonged illness with distant infectious complications or local problems such as pleural fibrosis and development of restrictive lung defect.

## PREVENTION

Although the efficacy of the polyvalent polysaccharide pneumococcal vaccine (Pneumovax 23) has not been consistently proved, the CDC recommends it for patients aged 19 to 64 years who have cardiovascular disease, chronic pulmonary disease, diabetes mellitus, alcoholism, chronic liver disease, cerebrospinal fluid leaks, and cochlear implants. Patients aged 19 to 64 years living in special environments or social settings such as chronic care facilities are also candidates. Vaccination should be repeated once after 5 years if the initial vaccination was before age 65 years and the patient is older than 65 years. Immunocompromised patients, particularly those with asplenia, should also receive the vaccine and the booster after 5 years.

## BIOLOGICAL WARFARE AGENTS

In a world of growing terrorism threats, physicians need to familiarize themselves with rare causes of pneumonia such as *Y. pestis*, *B. anthracis*, *Francisella tularensis*, *Burkholderia mallei*, and *Burkholderia pseudomallei*, which may be used as agents of biological warfare. The CDC's Web site, http://www.bt.cdc.gov, offers thorough and up-to-date information on biological warfare agents.

### Anthrax

Although ubiquitous in soil, *B. anthracis* rarely causes pneumonia in humans. Most cases are those of cutaneous infections, which occur in persons who handle soil or animals and animal products containing spores of the organism. The disease is called *anthrax* after the Greek word *anthrakos*, which means "coal," because of the black eschar that results from the cutaneous infection. When spores are inhaled, after a variable incubation period (1-60 days), a flu-like illness with headache, myalgias, and fever ensues. A deceptive period of improvement is followed by severe dyspnea, chest pain, cyanosis, and shock. Chest x-ray reveals mediastinal widening.

No person-to-person transmission is documented for inhalational anthrax. However, because its fastidious spores can remain dormant for decades and it causes certain death if not properly treated, *B. anthracis* is considered a potent biological weapon.

The CDC recommends combination therapy with ciprofloxacin 400 mg IV every 12 hours or doxycycline 100 mg IV every 12 hours with the addition of a second antibiotic after in vitro susceptibility testing. Recommended duration is 60 days, including oral treatment when clinically indicated. Treatment is most effective when started early in the course. Anthrax vaccine (Biothrax) was approved by the Food and Drug Administration (FDA) in 1999; however, it is only available to military personnel at this time.

### Plague

Humans are accidental hosts to *Y. pestis*, which is primarily a rodent pathogen. A bite from a flea of an infected rodent causes hemorrhagic lymphadenitis, called *buboes*. When bacteria enter the blood, infection of the lungs and reticuloendothelial system occurs. High fever and coughing fits mark the onset of pneumonic plague. Chest x-ray findings are not specific. Shock and disseminated intravascular coagulation are common causes of death. *Y. pestis* can be transmitted from person to person and has an up to 70% fatality rate, making it a feared biological weapon.

Streptomycin 2 g/day IM or IV in divided doses until the patient is afebrile for at least 3 days is the preferred regimen. However, doxycycline 100 mg IV every 12 hours or gentamicin (Garamycin) 2.5 mg/kg IM every 12 hours for 7 to 10 days are acceptable alternatives.

### Tularemia

Tularemia is a bacterial zoonosis, and small mammals are the usual hosts for the causative organism, *F. tularensis*. Humans are accidental hosts and become ill after handling infectious animal tissues or fluids; direct contact with or ingestion of contaminated food, water, or soil; or inhalation of infective aerosols. After airborne inhalation, hemorrhagic bronchopneumonia, severe pleuritis, and hilar adenopathy develop. Fever with discordant heart rate, chills, dry cough, myalgias, coryza, and sore throat are common symptoms. The fatality rate is not as high as for anthrax or plague; nevertheless, when released airborne, *F. tularensis* can infect a large population.

Preferred treatment is streptomycin 1 g IM every 12 hours or gentamicin 5 mg/kg IM or IV once daily. Doxycycline is considered an appropriate alternative. Duration of treatment is 10 days for streptomycin and gentamicin and 14 to 21 days for doxycycline.

### Melioidosis

Melioidosis (pseudoglanders) is an infectious disease caused by the bacterium *B. pseudomallei*. Melioidosis may be encountered in travelers returning from Southeast Asia. Direct contact with contaminated water and soil results in transmission of the disease. Glanders, a disease caused by *B. mallei*, is contracted by humans from infected domestic animals. Chronic suppurative infections, bacteremia, cutaneous infections, and severe pneumonia can result from infection with either organism. Dry cough or cough productive of clear sputum, high fever, headache, and myalgias are common.

High virulence of these organisms has made them potential candidates for biological warfare. Human-to-human transmission has been reported for both organisms.

Recommended treatment for melioidosis is with ceftazidime (Fortaz)[1] 50 mg/kg up to 2 g IV every 6 hours or imipenem-cilastatin (Primaxin)[1] 25 mg/kg up to 1 g IV every 8 hours for 14 days. Oral eradication therapy with trimethoprim-sulfamethoxazole (Bactrim)[1] up to 3 months may be needed. Experience with glanders is more limited, but similar antibiotics should be effective.

# Hospital-Acquired Pneumonia

Hospital-acquired pneumonia is defined as pneumonia that occurs 48 hours or more after admission and for which there is no evidence of infection on admission. Ventilator-associated pneumonia arises 48 to 72 hours after endotracheal intubation. Nosocomial pneumonia occurs in a patient who was hospitalized in an acute-care hospital for 2 or more days within the past 90 days; who resides in a nursing home or long-term facility; who received recent intravenous antibiotic therapy, chemotherapy, or wound care within the past 30 days of the current infection; or who attended a hospital or hemodialysis clinic. For practical purposes, management of all these entities is the same. However, patients who present from the community might have nosocomial pneumonia that can drastically influence management. Detailed history taking, therefore, is a crucial step for therapeutic decision making.

Hospital-acquired pneumonia remains a major cause of mortality, morbidity, and expenditure for the health care system. Its incidence is approximately five to ten cases per 1000 hospital admissions. Particularly in mechanically ventilated patients, the incidence rises by 3% each day during the first 5 days, 2% during the next 5 days, and 1% per day thereafter. It is estimated that length of stay is prolonged by 8 days and cost increases by $40,000 for each case of nosocomial pneumonia. Although not consistently demonstrated, there is an estimated attributable mortality of 33% to 50%.

Given the burden of these data, it is important to implement measures that reduce the incidence of hospital-acquired pneumonia. To this end, proven preventive strategies include ensuring effective infection control measures such as compliance with hand washing and alcohol-based hand disinfection, avoiding endotracheal intubation whenever

---

[1]Not FDA approved for this indication.

possible by instituting noninvasive positive pressure ventilation, enforcing head of bed elevated at 30 to 45 degrees in all ventilated patients, commencing enteral nutrition after 3 to 5 days with preference over parenteral nutrition, and using a restricted blood products transfusion policy.

Etiologic agents of hospital-acquired pneumonia are varied based on the onset of pneumonia (i.e., early, <5 days after admission, late) and presence of risk factors for multidrug-resistant (MDR) pathogens. These risk factors include antibiotic therapy in the preceding 3 months, current hospital admission of 5 days or more, high frequency of antibiotic resistance in the community or in the hospital, immunosuppressive disease or therapy, having risk factors for nosocomial pneumonia, and having a family member with an MDR pathogen.

Causative agents of early-onset hospital-acquired pneumonia are *S. pneumoniae*, *H. influenzae*, MRSA, *L. pneumophila*, and antibiotic-sensitive enteric gram-negative bacilli such as *E. coli*, *Klebsiella pneumoniae*, and *Enterobacter* species. The pathogens implicated in late-onset hospital-acquired pneumonia are *P. aeruginosa*, *Acinetobacter baumanii-calcoaceticus* complex (ABC), *K. pneumoniae* (extended-spectrum β-lactamase positive), and MRSA. *Acinetobacter* species afflict patients after prolonged hospital stays (average of 26 days) and are particularly troublesome due to multiple antimicrobial resistance patterns.

## DIAGNOSIS

Diagnosis of hospital-acquired pneumonia can be more challenging than diagnosis of community-acquired pneumonia. The presence of a new radiographic infiltrate; purulent respiratory secretions; new-onset leukopenia, leukocytosis, or bandemia; fever higher than 38.4°C; and worsening oxygenation indices such as the $PaO_2$ /$FiO_2$ ratio are highly suggestive but may be oversensitive in the diagnosis of pneumonia. Atelectasis, atypical pulmonary edema, pulmonary embolism with atelectasis or infarction, alveolar hemorrhage, and acute respiratory distress syndrome (ARDS) are the most common mimics of hospital-acquired pneumonia. Nevertheless, the constellation of findings should prompt empiric antibiotic treatment and diagnostic work-up.

The increasing body of clinical evidence indicates that lower respiratory tract sampling, whether invasively or noninvasively, should be undertaken to isolate pathogens. This is particularly important, because MDR pathogens are found in a significant number of cases and require antibiotic adjustment. Moreover, de-escalating antibiotic therapy based on lower respiratory tract cultures has been associated with improved outcomes. Negative lower respiratory tract cultures should also prompt a search for alternative sources of infection such as indwelling line infections, urinary tract infection, *Clostridium difficile* colitis, or intra-abdominal abscess. This strategy also allows health care institutions to establish their specific microbiology of hospital-acquired pneumonia, which in turn is invaluable in tailoring empiric antibiotic therapy. The consensus is that blood cultures are useful as well.

The need to employ invasive methods such as bronchoalveolar lavage (bronchoscopic or blind) and protected specimen brush to sample the lower respiratory tract is still debatable. Semiquantitative cultures of tracheal aspirate are useful if they do not demonstrate the presence of MDR pathogens. Nevertheless, they are not useful in confirming the presence of pneumonia, because pathogens isolated can also represent colonization. Although not strongly recommended, bronchoscopic sampling with quantitative cultures was associated with reduced mortality in one randomized prospective study. This approach might also allow safe discontinuation of antibiotics in patients with hemodynamic stability who have negative quantitative cultures obtained invasively. Empiric antibiotic therapy should not be withheld while waiting for diagnostic studies in clinically unstable patients with hospital-acquired pneumonia.

## TREATMENT

The ATS and IDSA issued joint guidelines for the management of hospital-acquired pneumonia in 2005. The empiric treatment of hospital-acquired pneumonia is based on this document. The empiric treatment of hospital acquired pneumonia addresses the different flora encountered if the pneumonia is early onset or late onset and presence of MDR risk factors.

For early-onset pneumonia with no risk factors for MDR organisms, monotherapy with ceftriaxone (Rocephin), a fluoroquinolone such as levofloxacin (Levaquin) or moxifloxacin (Avelox),[1] ampicillin-sulbactam (Unasyn),[1] or ertapenem (Invanz)[1] is appropriate. If there are MDR risk factors or pneumonia is late onset, combination therapy with an antipseudomonal cephalosporin (such as cefepime [Maxipime] or ceftazidime [Fortaz]) or antipseudomonal carbapenem (imipenem-cilastatin [Primaxin] or meropenem [Merrem][1]) or a β-lactam–β-lactamase inhibitor (piperacillin-tazobactam [Zosyn]) plus an antipseudomonal fluoroquinolone (ciprofloxacin or levofloxacin [Levaquin]) or aminoglycoside (amikacin [Amikin], gentamicin [Garamycin], or tobramycin [Nebcin]) plus linezolid or vancomycin. The duration of treatment is traditionally 10 to 21 days. However, such long courses of therapy can result in newly acquired colonization and antibiotic complications such as *C. difficile* colitis.

A controlled, randomized trial demonstrated that in patients who receive appropriate empiric therapy at the onset of pneumonia, 8 days of therapy was equivalent to 14 days of therapy. The only caveat was that if the initial pathogen was *P. aeruginosa* or ABC, relapses occurred more often with the shorter course.

ABC pneumonia treatment poses special challenges due to the species' MDR nature. Imipenem-cilastatin (Primaxin), colistin (colistimethate [Coly-Mycin M],[1] ampicillin-sulbactam (Unasyn),[1] amikacin (Amikin), rifampin (Rifadin),[1] and tetracycline have been reported active against ABC. Tigecycline (Tygacil)[1] is a new antibiotic in the tetracycline class with satisfactory activity against ABC that is resistant to carbapenems. Like other drugs in its category, however, it is not bactericidal. Combination therapy is advised when treating confirmed or suspected ABC pneumonia.

Response to antibiotic therapy is usually observed within 48 to 72 hours. Therefore, antibiotics need not be changed before this time. No response to treatment can be indicated by continued fever, leukocytosis or leukopenia, worsening chest x-ray infiltrate, and $PaO_2$/$FiO_2$ ratio. These signs suggest an organism not susceptible to the antibiotic regimen chosen (e.g., MDR organisms, *M. tuberculosis*, fungi, and viruses), an alternative diagnosis, or a complication such as empyema formation. Appropriate laboratory tests should be implemented accordingly.

## PREVENTION

Infection-control policies such as hospital-based antibiotic-use guidelines, hand washing, use of alcohol-based disinfectant, and contact isolation for organisms such as MRSA and ABC are strongly recommended. To prevent ventilator-associated pneumonia, semirecumbent positioning in bed at 30 to 45 degrees and aspiration of subglottic secretions are proven strategies. Selective decontamination of the gastrointestinal tract has been shown effective in at least one randomized prospective trial; however, the long-term effects of such a strategy on hospital microbial resistance patterns is unknown.

Despite recent advances in management, bacterial pneumonia remains a significant cause of morbidity and mortality worldwide. A detailed history, application of PSIs, determination of modifying factors, and risk of MDR pathogens are necessary to institute appropriate antibiotic therapy. Physicians should familiarize themselves with the manifestations of pneumonias caused by agents of biological terrorism.

Management guidelines issued by professional societies are practical and have been validated in reducing mortality from bacterial pneumonia. In addition to treatment failure and complications, it is imperative to consider alternative diagnoses to bacterial pneumonia if no clear improvement in clinical condition is evident after 72 hours of antibiotic therapy. Controversial areas include comprehensiveness and invasiveness of the diagnostic work-up to determine the etiology of bacterial pneumonia, duration of antimicrobial therapy, and decision to admit the patient to the ICU.

---

[1]Not FDA approved for this indication.

## REFERENCES

American Thoracic Society; Infectious Diseases Society of America: Guidelines for the management of adults with hospital-acquired, ventilator-associated, and healthcare-associated pneumonia. Am J Respir Crit Care Med 2005; 171:388-416.

Aujesky D, Auble TE, Yealy DM, et al: Prospective comparison of the three validated prediction rules for prognosis in community-acquired pneumonia. Am J Med 2005;118:384-392.

Colice GL, Curtis A, Deslauriers J, et al: Medical and surgical treatment of parapneumonic effusions: An evidence-based guideline. Chest 2000;118: 1158-171.

Confalonieri M, Urbino R, Potena A, et al: Hydrocortisone infusion for severe community-acquired pneumonia: A preliminary randomized study. Am J Respir Crit Care Med 2005;171:242-248.

Craven DE: Blood cultures for community-acquired pneumonia. Am J Respir Crit Care Med 2004;169:327-328.

El Moussaoui R, de Borgie CA, van den Broek P, et al: Effectiveness of discontinuing antibiotic treatment after three days versus eight days in mild to moderate-severe community acquired pneumonia: Randomized, double-blind study. BMJ 2006;332:1355.

File TM: Community-acquired pneumonia. Lancet 2003;362:1991-2001.

Fine MJ, Auble TE, Yealy DM et al: A prediction rule to identify low risk patients with community-acquired pneumonia. N Engl J Med 1997;336:243-250.

Hageman JC, Uyeki TM, Francis JS, et al: Severe community-acquired pneumonia due to *Staphylococcus aureus*, 2003-04 influenza season. Emerg Infect Dis 2006;12:894-899.

Murray CK, Hospenthal DR: Treatment of multidrug resistant *Acinetobacter*. Curr Opin Infect Dis 2005;18:502-506.

Niedermann MS: Review of treatment guidelines for community-acquired pneumonia. Am J Med 2004;117(3A):51S-57S.

Niederman MS, Mandell LA, Anzueto A, et al: Guidelines for the management of adults with community-acquired pneumonia: Diagnosis, assessment of severity, antimicrobial therapy, and prevention. Am J Respir Crit Care Med 2001;163:1730-1754.

# Viral Respiratory Infections

Method of
*Robert C. Welliver, Sr., MD*

Viral infections of the respiratory tract are among the most common infections in humans, and they account for significant morbidity at all ages. Infants and young children can sustain six to eight such infections annually, and adults have an average of nearly two such infections per year.

Rhinoviruses are the most commonly identified etiologic agents and cause illness year-round. Other common causative agents during winter months include influenza viruses and respiratory syncytial virus, and enteroviruses predominate in summer months. The parainfluenza viruses also commonly cause respiratory infection, particularly in autumn (type 1) and late spring or summer (type 3). Coronaviruses, metapneumoviruses, adenoviruses, and other agents are identified less often.

Although each of these agents can cause a common cold, some viral infections are associated with characteristic patterns of respiratory disease. Most of these viruses can also exacerbate asthma, cystic fibrosis, and chronic obstructive pulmonary disease (COPD).

## Common Colds

Colds are the most common of the viral respiratory illnesses. Pharyngitis is usually the earliest sign of a cold, beginning a few days after infection has taken place. Nasal congestion and clear or slightly cloudy rhinorrhea usually follow within 24 to 48 hours. Cough occurs in approximately 30% to 40% of those infected, and fluid can accumulate in middle ear or sinus cavities that have become blocked as a result of mucosal swelling. Ear and sinus cavity infections occur when this fluid is trapped for a week or more. Treatment with antibiotics is ineffective before this time, and they are ineffective especially in the absence of other clinical signs of ear and sinus infections.

Colds are a frequent cause of missed school and work, and even of mild morbidity, but they are rarely serious in otherwise healthy persons. The most appropriate approach to treatment therefore entails rest, with adequate nutrition and hydration. Agents that inhibit the activity of cyclooxygenase probably represent the most effective form of pharmacologic intervention. These compounds include acetaminophen (Tylenol) and the nonsteroidal anti-inflammatory agents (NSAIDs) such as ibuprofen (Motrin). They are effective in reducing fever and, perhaps more importantly in most colds, reducing malaise, headache, and pharyngitis.

Nasal congestion and some rhinorrhea during colds are related to dilation of blood vessels in the nose and sinuses. Vasoconstrictors have therefore been used extensively to attempt to reverse these symptoms. Oral decongestants such as pseudoephedrine (Sudafed) have minimal effect on nasal congestion, and can result in systemic hypertension, anxiety, and difficulty sleeping. The propensity for these compounds to cause cardiac arrhythmias in the very young child has led to recommendations against their use in the first year or two of life. Nasal sprays containing vasoconstricting agents such as oxymetazoline (Afrin) can result in mild temporary relief of nasal obstruction. However, the use of these compounds for more than 3 or 4 days can result in rebound vasodilation and paradoxically increased rhinorrhea.

Numerous investigations have evaluated the role of antihistamines in colds. The release of histamine itself is not associated with fever, cough, or malaise, so effects on these symptoms would not be expected. Furthermore, nasal congestion and discharge may be more related to the release of kinins, and not histamine. Indeed, the administration of antihistamines in adults and, particularly, in children has not demonstrated strikingly positive results. As many as 40% of subjects treated with placebo report beneficial effects. Side effects of histamine use, primarily sedation and dry mouth, are commonly encountered.

Cough can be one of the most irritating symptoms during colds. Cough during colds is principally caused by secretions entering the airway (postnasal drip) and not by inflammation of the airway itself. Therefore, it is not surprising that cough suppressants, especially codeine, have little effect on cough induced by colds. Antihistamines have also been found to be ineffective in relief of cough during colds.

## Influenza-Like Illness

The influenza syndrome is defined as the abrupt onset of fever, headache, and striking degrees of malaise and prostration, often with intense myalgia. Respiratory symptoms can occur concurrently, but they might not be prominent features. The principal cause is, of course, influenza virus, although infection with many other viruses can cause similar (although not as intense) symptoms. The illness is generally self-limited, and most symptoms resolve over 4 or 5 days. Lassitude can persist for up to 2 weeks.

Influenza virus infection and influenza-like illness are best treated symptomatically, relying on rest, adequate intake of fluids and calories,

---

### CURRENT DIAGNOSIS

- Rapid diagnostic kits are available for many common respiratory viruses. These tests are used increasingly to establish that antibiotic therapy is not necessary in many patients with febrile respiratory illnesses or with lower respiratory tract infections.
- The presence of wheezing on physical examination virtually excludes bacterial infection from consideration in subjects with lower respiratory disease.

## CURRENT THERAPY

- The management of most viral respiratory infections consists of rest, adequate caloric and fluid intake, and management of fever and malaise.
- Corticosteroids are essential in the management of croup.
- Specific antiviral therapy is available only for influenza virus infection, and beneficial effects have been more readily achieved in prevention rather than treatment.

and appropriate analgesic therapy. Compounds referred to as *M2 inhibitors* such as amantadine (Symmetrel) and rimantadine (Flumadine) have been approved for therapy. Positive outcomes from therapy with these agents are observed only when therapy is instituted within 48 hours after the onset of symptoms, and benefits are not striking. In recent years, resistance to M2 inhibitors has been commonly observed among circulating epidemic strains of influenza virus.

More recently, inhibitors of the activity of influenza viral neuraminidase have been used in treatment and prevention of influenza virus infection in adults and children. The first such compound released, zanamivir (Relenza,) was administered by inhalation but was unpopular because of its irritating effects on the airway. An oral compound, oseltamivir (TamiFlu), has been used to prevent and to treat influenza virus infection. As with M2 inhibitors, it is believed that treatment should be started within the first 48 hours of symptoms and that prophylaxis should be instituted within 48 hours of exposure. Treatment with oseltamivir shortens the duration of subsequent illness by only about 24 hours. Treatment can prevent some of the complications of influenza infection, including pneumonia. The drug may be more effective as a therapeutic agent, because it may be up to 90% effective in preventing culture-positive symptomatic influenza illness. The recommended dose for adults is 75 mg orally every 12 hours for 5 days. In children, the appropriate dose based on body weight is 30 mg twice daily for children weighing less than 15 kg, 45 mg twice daily for children weighing 15 to 23 kg, 60 mg twice daily for children weighing 23 to 40 kg, and 75 mg twice daily for children weighing more than 40 kg. The principal side effect is nausea, which can be reduced by taking the drug with food.

## Croup

Croup is defined by the occurrence of hoarseness or laryngitis, a deep, brassy or barking cough, and inspiratory stridor. Airway obstruction in croup is caused by constriction in the subglottic area, often noted on radiographs by a steeple-shaped narrowing of the air column in this region. Affected children are usually afebrile and nontoxic in appearance.

Parainfluenza virus type 1 is the primary cause of croup, although infection with many different viruses can produce this illness, and influenza virus can cause a particularly severe form of croup. Bacterial secondary infection occurs uncommonly, but it can result in fever and severe obstruction of the airway. Administration of dexamethasone (Decadron)[1] at 0.6 mg/kg either orally or intramuscularly markedly reduces the rate of hospitalization, admission to the intensive care unit, and intubation for croup.

## Bronchiolitis

Bronchiolitis represents the most common cause for hospitalization of infants in developed countries. Infants present with a history of several days of upper respiratory symptoms, followed by the rapid onset of

[1]Not FDA approved for this indication.

wheezing and labored breathing. Respiratory syncytial virus (RSV) is the most common cause and is the agent found in the most severe cases that result in respiratory failure. Contrasting with asthma, obstruction of the airway in bronchiolitis is a result of plugging of bronchioles with detached epithelium and inflammatory cells. Mucus plugging and constriction of smooth muscle are not prominent. Also in contrast with asthma is the absence of a sustained response to bronchodilators and corticosteroids among infants with bronchiolitis.

Therapy of bronchiolitis primarily consists of administration of supplemental oxygen and replacement of fluid deficits as needed. Ribavirin (Virazole)[1] is a compound with antiviral activity against RSV, but controlled studies have not demonstrated meaningful differences in outcomes between treated and untreated subjects. The compound is quite expensive and must be delivered via a special aerosol generator.

Palivizumab (Synagis), a preparation consisting of a monoclonal antibody against the fusion protein of RSV, has proved to be effective in reducing the rate of hospitalization for RSV infection by approximately 50% when given to high-risk infants. Infants who may be considered candidates for therapy include those with chronic lung disease, those born prematurely, and those with hemodynamically significant congenital heart disease. Doses of palivizumab (15 mg/kg) are given on a monthly basis throughout the local RSV season, usually November through March.

## REFERENCES

Akerlund A, Klint T, Olen L, Runderantz H: Nasal decongestant effect of oxymetazoline in the common cold: An objective dose-response study in 106 patients. J Laryngol Otol 1989;103:743-746.

Buckingham SC, Jafri HS, Bush AN, et al: A randomized, double-blind, placebo-controlled trial of dexamethasone in severe respiratory syncytial virus (RSV) infection: Effects on RSV quantity and clinical outcome. J Infect Dis 2002;185:1222-1228.

Curley FJ, Irwin RS, Pratter MR, et al: Cough and the common cold. Am J Respir Crit Care Med 1988;138:305-311.

Flores G, Horwitz RI: Efficacy of β$_2$-agonists in bronchiolitis: A reappraisal and meta-analysis. Pediatrics 1997;100:233-239.

Johnson DW, Jacobson S, Edney PC, et al: A comparison of nebulized budesonide, intramuscular dexamethasone, and placebo for moderately severe croup. N Engl J Med 1998;339:498-503.

Muether PS, Gwaltney JM Jr: Variant effect of first- and second-generation antihistamines as clues to their mechanism of action on the sneeze reflex in the common cold. Clin Infect Dis 1001;33:1483-1488.

Randolph AG, Wang EL: Ribavirin for respiratory syncytial virus lower respiratory tract infection. Arch Pediatr Adolesc Med 1996;150:942-947.

Tavorner D, Danz C, Economos D: The effects of oral pseudoephedrine on nasal patency in the common cold: A double-blind single-dose placebo-controlled trial. Clin Otolaryngol 1999;24:47-51.

Treanor JJ, Hayden FG, Vrooman PS, et al: Efficacy and safety of the oral neuraminidase inhibitor oseltamivir in treating acute influenza: A randomized controlled trial. US Oral Neuraminnidase Study Group. JAMA 2000;283:1016-1024.

Van Voris LP, Betts RF, Hayden FG, et al: Successful treatment of naturally occurring influenza A/USSR/77 H1N1. JAMA 1981;245:1128-1131.

[1]Not FDA approved for this indication.

# Viral and Mycoplasmal Pneumonias

Method of
*Burke A. Cunha, MD*

Influenza pneumonia is the most important cause of viral pneumonia in adults. Influenza A is the predominant type of influenza found in adults, and influenza B is more common in children. Influenza A has the potential for severe disease, occurs seasonally, and is the predominant type involved in influenza pandemics. *Mycoplasma pneumoniae* community-acquired pneumonia (CAP) was first recognized decades ago as distinctive from bacterial and viral pneumonias. It was originally described by Eaton as "Eaton agent" pneumonia caused by a pleuropneumonia-like organism (PPLO), later shown to be caused by *M. pneumoniae*. *M. pneumoniae* is a common cause of pneumonia in all age groups, but the peak incidence of *M. pneumoniae* CAP is in young adults. *M. pneumoniae* CAP is a common cause of ambulatory CAP.

The term *atypical pneumonia* was first applied to viral pneumonias because the clinical laboratory and radiologic findings were different from those caused by typical bacterial pulmonary pathogens. In influenza pneumonia, the clinical findings are confined to the trachea, bronchi, lung parenchyma, and central nervous system. *M. pneumoniae* CAP is a systemic infection with a pulmonary component. Over the years, atypical pneumonia has come to refer to pneumonia caused by systemic nonviral/nonbacterial pathogen agents that have a pulmonary component. Viral pneumonias are no longer considered atypical pneumonias. Atypical pneumonias may be divided into nonzoonotic and zoonotic atypical CAPs. Nonzoonotic CAPs are most commonly caused by *M. pneumoniae, Chlamydia pneumoniae,* or *Legionella* species; whereas the three most common zoonotic atypical pneumonias are caused by *Chlamydia psittaci* (psittacosis), *Francisella tularensis* (tularemia), or *Coxiella burnetii* (Q fever). All of the atypical pneumonias are distinct clinical entities that may be differentiated on the basis of their characteristic pattern of extrapulmonary organ involvement. Although some viruses may occasionally have extrapulmonary manifestations (i.e., influenza, adenovirus with viral pneumonias), the primary clinical features are confined to the lungs. *M. pneumoniae* is a critical cause of nonzoonotic atypical CAP, particularly in the ambulatory setting. *M. pneumoniae* CAP may be severe in patients with impaired host defenses or those with severe, preexisting cardiopulmonary disease.

# Viral Influenza Pneumonia

Viral influenza pneumonia affects children and adults. Influenza B is the primary type, causing mild influenza in children and adults. Influenza A is primarily an infection of adults that may be mild to severe. Influenza A has the potential for pandemic spread.

Influenza occurs during the winter months, usually peaking in February. Influenza is spread by aerosolized droplet infection from person to person and via fomites. Viral influenza A is classified into subtypes based on neuramidase (N) [YG1] and hemagglutinin (H) surface proteins. An important characteristic of influenza A virus is antigenic drift, which refers to a change in surface protein shift in the neuramidase or hemagglutinin receptors. With influenza A, these surface receptor proteins are important in cellular adherence of the influenza virus and the spread of influenza from respiratory epithelial cells. The vaccine for the flu season most often includes the influenza hemagglutinin and neuramidase types seen at the end of the preceding year's season. Prevention of attachment and spread of the virus is helpful to controlling the spread of influenza; vaccine protection conferred by specific antibody response to influenza A is highly protective (approximately 80% in noncompromised hosts).

During the years when influenza B has been important, vaccines for the subsequent year contain an influenza B component. The prophylactic effects of amantadine (Symmetrel) and rimantadine (Flumadine) are based on preventing viral adherence, thus preventing entry and infection of respiratory epithelial cells. Neuramidase inhibitors have anti-influenza activity.

Clinical manifestations of influenza A in adults varies considerably from mild to fatal infection. Mild infection is usually manifested as an acute febrile illness characterized by headache and myalgias with dry unproductive cough, rhinorrhea, and tracheobronchitis. Mild viral influenza may be a result of influenza A or B and usually resolves in a few days without complications in normal hosts who have good cardiopulmonary function.

Severe viral influenza A occurs in normal healthy adults and may be fatal. The onset of severe influenza A is sudden, and the patient often recalls the exact hour of onset. The patient is febrile with early/extreme prostration rendering the patient bedridden. Fever rapidly rises and may be accompanied by chills. Neck soreness, severe headache, and myalgias are typical. Sore throat, eye pain, conjunctival injection, and hemoptysis are frequently present. Chest pain worsened by deep inspiration is not truly pleuritic but rather reflects influenza A myositis of the intracostal muscles. Shortness of breath is related to the degree of hypoxemia. Severe influenza A causes an oxygen diffusion defect as manifested by an increased A-a gradient (>35). Profound hypoxemia may be accompanied by cyanosis. Hypotension caused by hypoxemia and vascular collapse may follow. The course of severe viral influenza A is fulminant and of short duration.

Physical findings are few in viral influenza (i.e., conjunctival suffusion). Auscultation reveals absolutely quiet lungs because the infectious process is interstitial and not alveolar. Routine blood tests are usually unremarkable except for leukopenia/lymphopenia and, less commonly, thrombocytopenia. Few atypical lymphocytes may be noted, and low titers of cold agglutinins may be present. Cold agglutinins (if present) have low titers less than or equal to 1:16. In severe cases, a pale bluelike hue of the skin may be noted, and there may be bleeding from diffuse intravascular coagulation (DIC) from multiple orifices preterminally. The chest radiograph in uncomplicated viral influenza A is unremarkable or may have minimal perihilar bilateral increased prominence of interstitial markings. In severe influenza A pneumonia, the chest radiograph shows bilateral symmetrical perihilar infiltrates without pleural effusions.

Patients may die from severe influenza A without superimposed bacterial pneumonia. Most deaths during the 1918 pandemic were young military recruits who died of influenza A pneumonia without bacterial superinfection. Viral influenza may be complicated by bacterial pneumonia. Bacterial pneumonias complicating viral influenza may occur concurrently at presentation or may present 1 to 2 weeks after the presentation of viral influenza. Viral influenza A presenting concurrently with a bacterial pneumonia is usually caused by *Staphylococcus aureus*. In contrast to uncomplicated viral influenza, bacterial superinfection is manifested by an increase in fever, shaking chills, leukocytosis, purulent sputum, localized rales on auscultation, bacteremia, and focal/segmental infiltrates on chest radiograph. Alternately, patients with viral influenza A may develop a secondary bacterial infection (same manifestations as noted previously) 1 to 2 weeks later. Secondary bacterial pneumonia is less severe than with concurrent *S. aureus* and is usually caused by *Streptococcus pneumoniae* or *Haemophilus influenzae*.

## ANTI-INFLUENZA THERAPY

Therapy of viral influenza is directed at inhibiting viral replication and preventing further infection of respiratory epithelial cells. The neuramidase inhibitors zanamivir (Relenza) and oseltamivir (Tamiflu) have anti-influenza A and B activity. Neuramidase inhibitors decrease the severity and duration of influenza symptoms by 1 to 2 days. Amantadine (Symmetrel) and rimantadine (Flumadine) are useful prophylactically and therapeutically in influenza. Amantadine and rimantadine have anti-influenza A activity, but no influenza B activity. Amantadine and rimantadine inhibit early M2 protein-dependent replication and prevent adherence of the influenza virus to respiratory epithelial cells, thus preventing progression of infection and minimizing further cell to cell spread. Amantadine and rimantadine also affect peripheral airway dilatation and oxygenation is improved, which is of critical importance because patients with severe influenza A uncomplicated by bacterial superinfection die of severe hypoxemia. Mild influenza A/B may be treated with neuramidase inhibitors. Mild cases of influenza A should be treated at the onset of the illness. For severe influenza A, amantadine or rimantadine in combination[1] with neuramidase inhibitors provide optimal anti-influenza therapy (Table 1). For avian influenza ($H_5N_1$), these antiviral drugs may be ineffective.

---

[1]Not FDA approved for this indication.

**TABLE 1  Adult Anti-Influenza Antivirals**

| Antiviral | Treatment Dose | Prophylactic Dose |
|---|---|---|
| **Mild Influenza A/B** | | |
| Zanamivir (Relenza)[†] | 2 inhalations (5 mg per inhalation) q12h × 5d | No FDA indication |
| **Severe Influenza A** | | |
| Amantadine (Symmetrel)[†] | 200 mg (PO) q24h<br>Persons age 65: 100 mg | 200 mg (PO) q24h<br>Persons age 65: 100 mg |
| | **or** | |
| Rimantadine (Flumadine) | 100 mg (PO) q12h<br>Persons with hepatic/renal failure (CrCl <10 mL/min)<br>or elderly 100 mg (PO) q24h | 100 mg (PO) q12h<br>Persons with hepatic/renal failure<br>(CrCl <10 mL/min) or elderly<br>100 mg (PO) q24h |
| | **plus** | |
| Oseltamivir[1] (Tamiflu)[†] | 75 mg (PO) q12d × 5d* | 75 mg (PO) q24h × 7d |

[1]Not FDA approved for this indication.
*For avian influenza, 150 mg (PO) q12h may be more effective.
[†]Some avian influenza strains may be resistant.

# *Mycoplasma pneumoniae* Pneumonia

*M. pneumoniae* is a common cause of ambulatory CAP. It affects all age groups, and in normal hosts with intact cardiopulmonary function, *Mycoplasma* CAP is usually a mild, self-limiting infection. However, *M. pneumoniae* derives its importance from difficulty in diagnosis, the necessity for non–β-lactam therapy, and because of its effect on peripheral airways.

*Mycoplasma* CAP is one of the nonzoonotic causes of CAP (the others being *Legionella* and *Chlamydia pneumoniae*). *M. pneumoniae* is an atypical pneumonia that is a systemic infectious disease with a pulmonary component. It may be distinguished from other atypical pneumonias by its characteristic pattern of extrapulmonary organ involvement. *M. pneumoniae* CAP most closely resembles *C. pneumoniae* CAP clinically, but is very different from Legionnaires' disease in terms of its epidemiology, age distribution, pattern of extrapulmonary organ involvement, and severity.

Clinically, *M. pneumoniae* presents as a subacute febrile illness. Temperatures rarely exceed 102°F (38.9°C). Rigors are not a feature of *M. pneumoniae* CAP, but patients may complain of chilly sensations. Mild headache and/or myalgias are not uncommon. The most common presenting symptom in *Mycoplasma* CAP is the prolonged, nonproductive dry cough. Patients with *Mycoplasma* CAP often complain of or have mild nonexudative pharyngitis. Rhinorrhea and conjunctivitis are not features of *M. pneumoniae* CAP. Watery diarrhea is commonly present in *Mycoplasma* CAP, but abdominal pain is not a clinical finding. Other extrapulmonary manifestations are uncommon or rare (e.g., meningoencephalitis, pericarditis, hemolytic anemia, glomerular nephritis, Guillain-Barré syndrome, erythema multiforme). *M. pneumoniae* has a distinctive pattern of extrapulmonary organ involvement that does not include cardiac involvement (relative bradycardia) or hepatic involvement, including normal serum glutamate-oxaloacetate transaminase (SGOT) or serum glutamate-pyruvate transaminase (SGPT). The distinguishing laboratory feature of *M. pneumoniae* CAP is elevated cold agglutinin titers. Although a variety of infectious and noninfectious diseases are associated with cold agglutinin elevations, they are usually of low titer (i.e., <1:16). There are no pulmonary infections presenting as CAP that are associated with high elevations of cold agglutinin titers (i.e., ≥1:64). Although elevated cold agglutinins occur early in up to 75% of patients with *M. pneumoniae* CAP, they are still diagnostically important when present. In a patient with CAP and a cold agglutinin titer greater than or equal to 1:64, the diagnosis of *M. pneumoniae* CAP is very likely.

*M. pneumoniae* may be differentiated from the typical bacterial pneumonias because of the presence of extrapulmonary findings, including nonexudative pharyngitis, loose stools or watery diarrhea, erythema multiforme, and high cold agglutinin. Patients with typical bacterial CAP usually have a more acute onset of presentation, a productive cough, and temperatures that may exceed 102°F (38.9°C), often accompanied by chills. Patients with typical pneumonia often have pleuritic chest pain, which is not a feature of *M. pneumoniae* CAP. Among the atypical pneumonias, the zoonotic pneumonias (i.e., tularemia, psittacosis, Q fever) may be eliminated from consideration if there is a recent zoonotic contact history with the appropriate vector.

*C. pneumoniae* resembles closely *M. pneumoniae* CAP. *C. pneumoniae* may be distinguished by the absence of cold agglutinins and the presence of hoarseness, which is a feature of *C. pneumoniae* but not *M. pneumoniae* CAP. Loose stools or watery diarrhea are not usual features of *C. pneumoniae* CAP. The most common clinical problem is differentiating *Legionella* from *Mycoplasma* CAP; this may be done by appreciating the differences in the pattern of extrapulmonary organ involvement with each of these pathogens. *Legionella* may be clinically differentiated from *Mycoplasma* by acuteness of onset or severity, the presence of relative bradycardia, temperatures greater than 102°F (38.9°C), and the presence of abdominal pain. From a laboratory standpoint, highly elevated cold agglutinin titers argue strongly against the diagnosis of *Legionella* and point to *M. pneumoniae*. Nonspecific laboratory tests in a patient with CAP that suggest *Legionella* and argue against *M. pneumoniae* include otherwise unexplained hypophosphatemia, hyponatremia, microscopic hematuria, and increased creatinine. *Legionella* does not affect the upper respiratory tract as does *Mycoplasma* (e.g., nonexudative pharyngitis). Ear findings are not a feature of Legionnaires' disease but are common in *M. pneumoniae* CAP. The finding most likely to cause confusion between *M. pneumoniae* and *Legionella pneumophila* is the presence of loose stools or watery diarrhea, which is found in both.

*M. pneumoniae* may be cultured from the throat in viral culture media, but the diagnosis is usually made serologically. An elevated enzyme-linked immunosorbent assay (ELISA) or enzyme immunoassay (EIA) IgM titer suggests acute or recent infection, but an elevated IgG titer indicates past exposure but not acute infection. Elevated IgG titers regardless of degree of elevation are not diagnostic of current infection with *M. pneumoniae* and only indicate previous antigenic exposure. *M. pneumoniae* ELISA IgM levels may take up to 3 months to decrease. Therefore, clinicians should take into account recent antecedent respiratory illness in order to properly interpret elevated IgM titers, including patients with nonexudative pharyngitis within

## CURRENT DIAGNOSIS

Viral Influenza
- Mild influenza A or B presents acutely with headache, fever, sore throat, plus/minus rhinorrhea.
- Severe influenza A presents with an acute onset (patients often able to name the hour the influenza began) and rapidly become bed bound.
- Headache, myalgias, and prostration are severe.
- Auscultation of the lungs is quiet, disproportionate to the degree of respiratory distress. Influenza is an interstitial process and not alveolar, which explains the absence of rales.
- With severe influenza, patients rapidly become hypoxemic. Hypoxemia is accompanied by an AA gradient (>35), which suggests an interstitial oxygen diffusing defect typical of severe viral influenza pneumonia.
- Severe tracheobronchitis is common and is manifested by hemoptysis.
- Leukopenia/lymphopenia is typical; thrombocytopenia may occur. Low titer elevations of cold agglutinins are not infrequent (≥1:16).
- Patients may have chest pain exacerbated by breathing mimicking pleuritic chest pain. This is the result of direct intracostal muscle involvement with the influenza virus, which results in myositis and pain on inspiration.
- The chest radiograph in early viral influenza, in mild to moderate cases, is normal or near normal, with minimal, if any, increase in perihilar interstitial markings. The chest radiograph in fulminant cases shows symmetrical bilateral patchy infiltrates without pleural effusion in 24 to 48 hours.
- Severe viral influenza A is accompanied by severe hypoxemia or cyanosis, which may be followed by a fatal outcome.
- Influenza pneumonia may present alone without bacterial superinfection. Bacterial infection may accompany or follow.

- Purulent sputum with viral influenza indicates concurrent bacterial pneumonia usually caused by *S. aureus*. Bacterial pneumonia following influenza (after 1 to 2 weeks), is suggested by leukocytosis, focal or segmental pulmonary infiltrates, and purulent sputum; the pathogens are not *S. aureus*, but most commonly are *S. pneumoniae* or *H. influenzae*.
- A laboratory diagnosis may be made by DFA staining of respiratory secretions, viral influenza titers, or viral cultures.

*Mycoplasma pneumoniae*
- In a patient with CAP and a dry nonproductive cough, without severe headache or myalgias, the most likely diagnosis is *M. pneumoniae*. *M. pneumoniae* CAP is commonly accompanied by nonexudative pharyngitis and/or loose stools or watery diarrhea.
- The temperature is usually less than 102°F (38.9°C) and is not accompanied by frank rigors or pleuritic chest pain.
- Relative bradycardia and elevations in the serum transaminases are not features of *M. pneumoniae* CAP.
- Respiratory viruses are often associated with mild elevations of cold agglutinins (≤1:16) but *M. pneumoniae* is the only pathogen causing CAP associated with highly elevated cold agglutinin titers (≥1:64). Elevated cold agglutinin titers occur in up to 75% of patients with *M. pneumoniae*, and occur early and transiently.
- In a patient with CAP, elevated cold agglutinin titers (>1:8) effectively rule out the typical pathogens, as well as *Legionella* species and *C. pneumoniae*.
- Elevated *M. pneumoniae* ELISA IgG titers indicate past exposure/infection and not current infection or co-infection with another pathogen.
- In the absence of an antecedent respiratory tract infection (e.g., nonexudative pharyngitis, otitis, etc., in the preceding 3 months), the presence of an increased *M. pneumoniae* ELISA IgM titer is diagnostic of acute infection.

3 months prior to the presentation of CAP. The combination of an increased *M. pneumoniae* IgM titer and highly elevated cold agglutinin titers is virtually diagnostic of acute infection. Cold agglutinin titers are elevated transiently early and rapidly fall; the simultaneously elevated cold agglutinins and IgM titers of *M. pneumoniae* indicate active or current infection. In patients with CAP caused by another organism (e.g., *S. pneumoniae*), the presence of elevated *Mycoplasma* IgG titers does not indicate co-infection but only preexisting serologic exposure to *M. pneumoniae*.

### THERAPY

*M. pneumoniae* has a predilection for the respiratory epithelial cells and resides literally on their surface. Mycoplasmas have no definite cell wall like the typical pathogens causing CAP. Their position on the surface of the respiratory epithelium and their absence of a cell wall necessitates the therapeutic approach, which includes non–β-lactam antibiotics with the capacity to penetrate into the *Mycoplasma* organisms. Traditionally, macrolides and tetracyclines have been used successfully to treat *M. pneumoniae*. Both CAP tetracyclines and macrolides are effective against *Mycoplasma* because they interfere with intracellular protein synthesis at the ribosomal level. Tetracyclines penetrate intracellularly better than macrolides, with the exception of penetration into the alveolar macrophage, which is relevant in *Legionella*, but not *M. pneumoniae*, infections. Macrolides and tetracyclines are both

active against *Mycoplasma*; the relative lack of penetration by macrolides into respiratory epithelial cells accounts for differences in therapeutic response. Patients treated with macrolides or tetracyclines defervesce rapidly over 24 to 48 hours. Clinical defervescence manifests by an increased feeling of well-being and a decrease in fever. The dry cough persists during and after therapy regardless of the anti-*Mycoplasma* antimicrobial used.

There are important differences in the shedding rates of *Mycoplasma* from respiratory epithelial cells posttherapy when using tetracyclines instead of macrolides. Tetracycline therapy is associated with a more rapid decrease in shedding. Tetracyclines with better ability to penetrate intracellularly, such as doxycycline (Vibramycin), are the most rapid at decreasing *Mycoplasma* shedding, which is an important public health consideration. Mycoplasmas are transmitted by aerosolized droplet infection. Because patients with *Mycoplasma* have a prolonged cough, organisms not eliminated from respiratory epithelial cells may be aerosolized during coughing for weeks following the acute infection, spreading the infection to susceptible individuals via aerosolized droplets. The aim of therapy is to rapidly treat the patient's pneumonia and extrapulmonary sites of involvement. The secondary goal is to rapidly decrease shedding and aerosolization to prevent the spread of *Mycoplasma* to other individuals. An additional therapeutic goal is to decrease the incidence of post-*Mycoplasma* asthma seen in some patients. *M. pneumoniae* CAP may exacerbate preexisting asthma, but may also cause permanent post-CAP asthma in some individuals.

Until recently, doxycycline was the most active antimicrobial to use against *M. pneumoniae*. Currently, the "respiratory quinolones," levofloxacin (Levaquin), gatifloxacin (Tequin), moxifloxacin (Avelox), and gemifloxacin (Factive), are all highly active anti-*M. pneumoniae* antimicrobials. Telithromycin (Ketek), a ketolide antibiotic, also has a high degree of anti-*M. pneumoniae* activity. The respiratory quinolones and telithromycin all penetrate cells efficiently and interfere with intracellular enzymes or protein synthesis of intracellular organisms. Respiratory quinolones and telithromycin are highly effective anti-*Mycoplasma* agents and rapidly decrease shedding of *M. pneumoniae* in respiratory secretions.

Therapy for *M. pneumoniae* is ordinarily 1 to 2 weeks. Patients who have impaired cardiopulmonary disease or compromised host may require 2 full weeks of therapy. In patients with borderline cardiopulmonary function, *M. pneumoniae* as with other relatively low virulence pathogens may present as severe CAP. Antimicrobial therapy for

 ## CURRENT THERAPY

Viral Influenza
- The aim of therapy is to inhibit the influenza virus and prevent its attachment/spread to uninfected respiratory epithelial cells.
- The neuramidase inhibitors shorten the course of influenza by 1 to 2 days and have antiviral activity. These agents are active against both influenza A and B.
  - Amantadine (Symmetrel) or rimantadine (Flumadine) do not have antiviral properties but are important in prevention/therapy.
  - Amantadine and rimantadine prevent the adherence of influenza virus to uninfected upper respiratory epithelial cells, thereby limiting the extent of the infection.
  - Amantadine and rimantadine also have an important therapeutic effect in influenza A by increasing distal airway dilation and increasing oxygen action; their effect on peripheral airways is important in severe influenza A. Amantadine and rimantadine are not active against influenza B.
  - Amantadine and rimantadine should be given for the duration of viral influenza. Used prophylactically, amantadine and rimantadine should be given before, during, and following an outbreak of influenza A.

*Mycoplasma pneumoniae*
- The agents active against *M. pneumoniae* are macrolides, tetracyclines, quinolones, and ketolides. β-Lactam antibiotics are not active against *M. pneumoniae* because the organisms do not contain a bacterial cell wall.
- Goals of therapy of *M. pneumoniae* CAP are to eradicate the infection, decrease the shedding of *Mycoplasma* in respiratory secretions posttherapy, and to prevent posttreatment asthma.
- Therapy is equally efficacious with macrolides, doxycycline (Vibramycin), respiratory quinolones, or telithromycin (Ketek) intravenously, orally, or in combination for 1 to 2 weeks.
- The mode of administration is determined by the severity of the CAP and the setting. Outpatients are usually treated orally. Patients hospitalized with severe CAP are initially treated intravenously and then changed to an oral agent.
- Resistance to *M. pneumoniae* with antimicrobials has not been described and is not a clinical consideration.

**TABLE 2  Antibiotics Effective Against *M. pneumoniae***

| Antibiotic | Dose (Adult) |
|---|---|
| *Mild/Moderate CAP* | |
| Erythromycin | 500 mg (base, estolate, stearate) (PO) q6h |
| Erythromycin lactobionate | 1 g (IV) q6h |
| Clarithromycin (Biaxin) | 500 mg (PO) q12h |
| Azithromycin (Zithromax) | 500 mg (IV) q24h × 2 doses, followed by 500 mg (PO) q24h |
| Gemifloxacin (Factive) | 320 mg (PO) q24h |
| Telithromycin (Ketek) | 800 mg (PO) q24h |
| Doxycycline | 100 mg (IV/PO) q12h |
| *Severe CAP* | |
| Doxycycline | 100 mg (IV/PO) q12h |
| Levofloxacin (Levaquin) | 500 mg (IV/PO) q24h, or 750 mg IV/PO q24h (may allow for shorter duration of therapy) |
| Gatifloxacin (Tequin) | 400 mg (IV/PO) q24h |
| Moxifloxacin (Avelox) | 400 mg (IV/PO) q24h |

typical or atypical CAP should be directed against the presumed pathogen and not based on co-morbidities. Normal healthy hosts are treated with the same antimicrobial as patients hospitalized with severe CAP. Patients hospitalized with compromised cardiopulmonary function severe *Mycoplasma* CAP are most often initially treated intravenously with doxycycline (Vibramycin), a macrolide, or a respiratory quinolone. Most patients with *M. pneumoniae* CAP present in the ambulatory setting, which permits therapy with oral doxycycline, macrolide, a respiratory quinolone, or telithromycin (Ketek) (Table 2).

## REFERENCES

Ali NJ, Sillis M, Andrews BE, et al: The clinical spectrum and diagnosis of *Mycoplasma pneumoniae* infection. Q J Med 1986;58:241-251.
Cunha BA: Influenza and its complications. Emerg Med 2000;2:56-67.
Cunha BA: Hepatic involvement in *Mycoplasma pneumoniae* community-acquired pneumonia. J Clin Microbiol 2003;3:385-386.
Cunha BA: Influenza: Historical aspects of epidemics and pandemics. Infect Dis Clin North Am 2004;18:141-155.
Cunha BA: The atypical pneumonia: Clinical diagnosis and importance. Clin Microbiol Infect 2006;12:12-24.
Cunha BA: Pneumonia Essentials. Royal Oak, MI, Physicians' Press, 2007.
Cunha BA: Urosepsis in the Critical Care Unit. In: Cunha BA (ed): Infectious Diseases in Critical Care Medicine, 2nd ed. New York, NY, Informa Healthcare USA, Inc., pp 527-534.
Cunha BA: Antibiotic Essentials, 6th ed., Royal Oak, MI, Physicians' Press, pp 79-85.
Debré R, Couvreur J: Influenza: Clinical features. In: Debré R, Celers J (eds): Clinical Virology: The Evaluation and Management of Human Viral Infections. Philadelphia, WB Saunders, 1970, pp 507-515.
File TM, Tan JS: *Mycoplasma pneumoniae* pneumonia. In: Marrie TJ (ed): Community-Acquired Pneumonia. New York, Kluwer Academic/Plenum Publishers, 2001, pp 487-500.
Hammerschlag MR: *Mycoplasma pneumoniae* infections. Curr Opin Infect Dis 2001;14:181-186.
Hurt AC, Selleck P, Komadina N, et al: Susceptibility of highly pathogenic A(H5N1) avian influenza viruses to the neuraminidase inhibitors and adamantanes. Antiviral Res 2007;73:228-231.
Louria DB, Blumenfield HL, Ellis JT: Studies on influenza in the pandemic of 1957-1958. II. Pulmonary complications of influenza. J Clin Invest 1959;38:213-265.
Marrie TJ: Empiric treatment of ambulatory community-acquired pneumonia: Always include treatment for atypical agents. Infect Dis Clin North Am 2004;18:829-841.
Murray HW, Masur H, Senterfit LS, Roberts RB: The protean manifestations of *Mycoplasma pneumoniae* infection in adults. Am J Med 1975;58:229-242.
Nisar N, Guleria R, Kumar S, et al: Mycoplasma pneumoniae and its role in asthma. Postgrad Med J 2007;83:100-104.

Schmidt AC: Antiviral therapy for influenza: A clinical and economic comparative review. Drugs 2004;6:2031-2046.

Waites KB, Talkington DF: *Mycoplasma pneumoniae* and its role as a human pathogen. Clin Microbiol Rev 2004;17:697-728.

# Legionellosis

Method of
*Julio A. Ramirez, MD*

In the summer of 1976, an outbreak of approximately 182 cases of pneumonia occurred in persons attending the American Legion convention in Philadelphia. One year later, Dr. McDade reported the identification of *Legionella pneumophila*, the bacterium responsible for the infection. Today, the family of Legionellaceae is composed of more than 40 species, with some species having different serogroups. *L pneumophila* causes approximately 85% of all *Legionella* infections. *L. pneumophila* serogroup 1 is the single most common member of the family causing clinical infections.

## Epidemiology

*Legionella* is an intracellular organism that lives in natural water. In the aquatic environment, the bacteria live and multiply within freshwater amebae. The number of *Legionella* organisms in the water can increase significantly with appropriate local conditions such as warm temperature, lack of biocides, stagnant water, and presence of amebae and other nutrients. These special conditions can be present in artificial water systems such as cooling towers, whirlpools, decorative fountains, and respiratory therapy devices.

The susceptible host acquires the bacteria from water containing the organism. Infection can be acquired by inhaling aerosols containing *Legionella* organisms or by microaspiration of water contaminated with *Legionella*. The hospitalized patient with *Legionella* pneumonia does not require respiratory isolation because legionellosis is not transmitted from person to person.

## Clinical Features

Once *Legionella* organisms reach the respiratory tract, based on the interactions of the organism with the host immune system, the patient can have four possible clinical outcomes: asymptomatic infection, Pontiac fever, legionnaires' disease, or extrapulmonary disease involving the liver, heart, brain, or other organs. Pontiac fever is a nonpneumonic form of disease characterized by fever, headaches, myalgias, and malaise. The patient has an influenza-like illness, with resolution of disease in a few days without specific antimicrobial therapy. Patients with legionnaires' disease present with community-acquired pneumonia associated with high fever, gastrointestinal complaints such as diarrhea, and central nervous system complaints such as headaches or mental status changes. Hospital-acquired pneumonia can occur if *Legionella* is present in the hospital water supply.

## Diagnosis

The currently available laboratory tests for diagnosis of *Legionella* infections include the direct fluorescent antibody stain (DFA), culture, antigen detection in the urine, antibody detection in serum by indirect fluorescent antibody testing (IFA), and DNA amplification using the polymerase chain reaction (PCR). The DFA stain can detect all *L. pneumophila* serogroups, but a large number of bacteria need to be present in sputum for a positive result. *Legionella* can be cultured from respiratory specimens on selective media composed of buffered charcoal–yeast extract agar. The urinary antigen detection has a specificity greater than 95%; the disadvantage is that the test detects only the antigen of *L. pneumophila* serogroup 1. Clinical specimens that have been used to detect *Legionella* by PCR include throat swabs, sputum, tracheal suction, bronchoalveolar lavage fluid, pleural fluid, and lung tissue.

## Treatment

In the pulmonary parenchyma, *Legionella* can infect and multiply inside alveolar macrophages, alveolar epithelial cells, and capillary endothelial cells. The poor clinical outcome with β-lactam antibiotics is due to their lack of penetration into cells. Antibiotics with good intracellular penetration that can be used as monotherapy for *Legionella* infections include macrolides, ketolides, tetracyclines, and quinolones (Table 1). Rifampin (Rifadin)[1] is not used as monotherapy because resistance can rapidly emerge when it is used alone.

Therapy of the patient with severe disease is initiated with intravenous antibiotics. Once the patient reaches clinical stability, the intravenous therapy can be switched to oral therapy. Doses for the most common antibiotics for intravenous and oral therapy are depicted in Table 1. In the nonimmunocompromised patient, the recommended duration of therapy is 7 to 10 days. In immunocompromised patients, because they are at risk for relapsing infection, the recommended duration of therapy is 14 to 21 days.

Several antibiotics have demonstrated clinical efficacy in legionnaires' disease. Data with several in vitro and animal studies comparing different anti-*Legionella* antibiotics indicate that erythromycin (Ery-Tab) is a weak anti-*Legionella* agent. If erythromycin is selected for therapy, it is important to add rifampin to the regimen to increase intracellular killing. From the family of macrolides, azithromycin (Zithromax)[1] is the most active. The best bactericidal activity in the laboratory is achieved with quinolones. Retrospective observational studies indicate that patients treated with levofloxacin (Levaquin) have a shorter time to reach clinical stability and shorter duration of hospital stay. These antibiotics are considered primary anti-*Legionella* agents.

In clinical practice, I treat immunocompromised patients who have severe legionnaires' disease with a combination of an intravenous quinolone plus an intravenous macrolide (e.g., levofloxacin plus azithromycin). This regimen is based only on the theoretical consideration that synergistic killing may be obtained using a quinolone to alter DNA synthesis and a macrolide to alter protein synthesis.

**TABLE 1  Antibiotic Therapy for *Legionella* Infections**

| Antibiotic | Oral Dose | Intravenous Dose |
|---|---|---|
| **Ketolides** | | |
| Telithromycin (Ketek)[1] | 800 mg qd | — |
| **Macrolides** | | |
| Azithromycin (Zithromax)[1] | 500 mg qd | 500 mg qd |
| Clarithromycin (Biaxin)[1] | 500 mg bid | — |
| Erythromycin (Ery-Tab) | 500 mg q6h | 1 g q6h |
| **Quinolones** | | |
| Ciprofloxacin (Cipro)[1] | 750 mg bid | 400 mg bid |
| Levofloxacin (Levaquin) | 750 mg qd | 750 mg qd |
| Moxifloxacin (Avelox)[1] | 400 mg qd | 400 mg qd |
| **Rifamycins** | | |
| Rifampin (Rifadin)[1] | 300 mg bid | 300 mg bid |
| **Tetracyclines** | | |
| Doxycycline (Vibramycin)[1] | 100 mg bid | 100 mg bid |

[1]Not FDA approved for this indication.

# Pulmonary Embolism

Method of
*Victor J. Test, MD, FCCP*

There are estimated to be at least 600,000 episodes of pulmonary embolism (PE) in the United States annually, resulting in between 100,000 and 200,000 deaths. The overwhelming majority of deaths occur when the disease is not suspected or is misdiagnosed. Once the diagnosis is made and effective treatment is initiated, the risk of death diminishes dramatically. The patient who presents with shock has a dramatically higher risk of death from pulmonary embolism.

Pulmonary embolism is closely liked to deep venous thrombosis (DVT). Classically, proximal lower extremity venous thrombosis has been reported to be the source of 90% of emboli, but upper extremity thrombosis and catheter-associated thrombosis are often associated with PE as well. The possibility of thromboembolic disease should be considered in patients who present with chest pain, dyspnea, hemoptysis, syncope, or palpitations. The clinical signs of PE are often quite subtle and can include tachycardia, tachypnea, pleural effusion, jugular venous distention, fever, tricuspid regurgitation, and an increased pulmonic heart tone. Lower extremity findings such as asymmetric edema, leg and calf tenderness, erythema, venous cords, and Homan's signs can indicate a lower extremity DVT.

## Diagnosis

### CLINICAL RISK

The diagnosis of PE and DVT depends on suspicion of the disease. A number of methods can determine the probability that a patient will have a PE. The traditional risk factors have included age greater than 40 years, previous DVT/PE, surgery requiring anesthesia for more than 30 minutes, prolonged immobilization, stroke, heart failure, malignancy (adenocarcinoma and pancreatic carcinoma), fractures of the long bones or pelvis, spinal cord injury, obesity, smoking, pregnancy, estrogen therapy, inflammatory bowel disease, and genetic or acquired thrombophilia. Renal failure, the nephrotic syndrome, central venous catheterization, chronic obstructive pulmonary disease (COPD), and long-distance travel have been identified as risk factors.

### CLINICAL DIAGNOSIS

Traditional tests include arterial blood gas, electrocardiogram, and chest x-ray. Unfortunately, these tests are neither specific nor sensitive. Over the past decade, a bewildering array of diagnostic studies, used alone or in combination, have been evaluated as a means of excluding or confirming the diagnosis of embolism. Patients can be stratified into high-risk, moderate-risk, or low-risk categories by empiric assessment or by using structured clinical prediction rules such as those devised by Wells, which use a point system based on historical factors such as malignancy, hemoptysis, previous DVT/PE, immobilization,

## CURRENT DIAGNOSIS

- The diagnosis of pulmonary embolism is guided by suspicion for the disease.
- Interpretation of the diagnostic testing should be guided by the clinical probability for the presence of pulmonary embolism.
- Multiple diagnostic tests and evaluations may be required for assessment of pulmonary embolic disease.
- In the absence of a contraindication to anticoagulant therapy, therapy should be begun while awaiting confirmatory testing in patients at intermediate or high risk.

recent surgery, tachycardia, clinical evidence of DVT, and absence of an equally likely alternative diagnosis. Clinical prediction rules seem to be less influenced by experience and allow a more standardized approach to the diagnostic process.

Table 1 shows studies that can exclude the diagnosis of embolism at different levels of clinical probability. Table 2 shows studies that can confirm the diagnosis of embolism at different levels of clinical probability.

Often I use a combination of tests to help me rule out the diagnosis of pulmonary embolism. The enzyme-linked immunosorbent assay (ELISA) D-dimer is most useful in ruling out the diagnosis in outpatients at low risk or who have a low pretest probability of pulmonary embolism. In patients who are low risk based on the scoring systems, the incidence of pulmonary embolism at 3 months in the setting of a negative highly sensitive D-dimer assay is extremely low. The sensitivities of the different assays result in a wide variability of sensitivities. In general, intermediate-risk and high-risk patients should receive diagnostic imaging.

As documented in the PIOPED 1 study, a normal ventilation-perfusion ($\dot{V}/\dot{Q}$) scan virtually rules out a pulmonary embolism. A high-probability scan in someone with a moderate or high risk of pulmonary embolism strongly suggests a pulmonary embolism. Unfortunately, the underlying chest x-rays strongly affect the effectiveness of this test. It is still quite useful but is less available because computed tomography (CT) scanning is now the preferred choice in many centers.

The advent of the multislice, multidetector CT scanner has had a substantial impact on the diagnosis of pulmonary embolism. The technology associated with CT scanning has been evolving, whereas the technology associated with $\dot{V}/\dot{Q}$ scanning has been more or less static. The PIOPED 2 study compared CT angiogram (CTA) with CT angiogram with venography (CTA/CTV). The sensitivity of CTA was 83% and the specificity was 96% for PE. The sensitivity of CTA/CTV was 90% and the specificity was 95%. It is clear from this study that clinicians must still use the concept of pretest probability in assessing for PE. Unfortunately, most centers do not use this technology, and I am often forced to use duplex ultrasonography to augment the negative CT to rule out a significant pulmonary embolism.

### TABLE 1 Studies that Exclude the Diagnosis of Embolism

| Test | Clinical Probability | | |
| | Low | Intermediate | High |
| --- | --- | --- | --- |
| Computed tomography | Normal | Normal | — |
| Contrast angiography | Normal | Normal | Normal |
| ELISA D-dimer | Negative | Negative | — |
| V/Q Scan | Normal or low | Normal | Normal |

*Abbreviations:* ELISA = enzyme-linked immunosorbent assay; $\dot{Q}$ = perfusion; $\dot{V}$ = ventilation.

**TABLE 2  Studies that Confirm the Diagnosis of Embolism**

| Test | Clinical Probability | | |
| --- | --- | --- | --- |
| | Low | Intermediate | High |
| Computed tomography | Positive | Positive | Positive |
| Contrast angiography | Positive | Positive | Positive |
| Duplex ultrasound | Positive | Positive | Positive |
| V/Q Scan | — | High | High |

*Abbreviations:* $\dot{Q}$ = perfusion; $\dot{V}$ = ventilation.

The CT angiogram also has the benefit of evaluating for lymphadenopathy and for parenchymal lung disease. The crucial disadvantages are the need to obtain a high-quality and well-timed bolus of contrast to obtain an optimal scan as well as the use of intravenous contrast. CTA typically uses more contrast than standard pulmonary angiography. Pulmonary angiography is the standard imaging procedure but in general has fallen out of use in most centers due to its perceived risk and the increased use of CT scanning. Duplex ultrasonography of the venous system may be used to rule out proximal deep venous thrombosis of the lower extremity.

A radiographic or anatomically massive pulmonary embolism does not always cause hemodynamic instability.

Transthoracic echocardiogram is often used to assess chest pain. In acute pulmonary embolism, the echocardiogram is useful to stratify hemodynamically stable patients to determine which patient is at risk for a poor outcome. The findings of right ventricular dilatation and pulmonary hypertension are poor markers for increased mortality. The echocardiogram may show evidence of right ventricular strain or overload. In addition, the echocardiogram is often used to identify patients at risk for developing hemodynamic decompensation.

## Therapy

Therapy for DVT/PE should be initiated empirically when there is a significant clinical suspicion for the disease and if the risk of systemic anticoagulation is low, because PE is associated with significant mortality. Tests to confirm or exclude pulmonary embolism should be arranged as soon as possible. Supplemental therapies such as oxygen should be employed as indicated by the clinical situation.

---

### CURRENT THERAPY

- If the clinical suspicion is high and there are no contraindications, therapy should begin while confirmatory testing is being arranged
- For hemodynamically stable patients, therapy with dose-adjusted unfractionated heparin or low-molecular-weight heparin is indicated in the absence of complications.
  - Unfractionated heparin: 80 IU/kg ideal body weight bolus; 18 IU/kg/h infusion with monitoring of the aPTT every 4-6 h. Adjust to an aPTT 1.5-3 times control.
  - Low-molecular-weight heparin: Enoxaparin (Lovenox)[1] 1 mg/kg SC twice a d or tinzaparin (Innohep)[1] 175 anti-Xa IU/kg SC once daily
- Warfarin therapy (5 mg/d) should be started on d 1 of therapy with heparin in the absence of contraindications.

---

[1]Not FDA approved for this indication.

### UNFRACTIONATED HEPARIN

Unfractionated heparin (UFH) has been the mainstay of therapy for DVT/PE since the 1970s. Heparin acts by accelerating the activity of antithrombin III. Heparin does not directly dissolve the thrombus, but it prevents the formation of new thrombi. Heparin can be administered subcutaneously or by intermittent intravenous bolus, but is usually given as a constant intravenous infusion to ensure that an adequate therapeutic level has been achieved.

Unfractionated heparin requires monitoring of the activated partial thromboplastin time (aPTT). The typical goal for the aPTT is 1.5 to 3.0 times the control value, which corresponds to a plasma heparin level from 0.3 to 0.7 IU/ mL anti-Xa activity. In certain circumstances, such as the presence of a lupus anticoagulant, anti-Xa levels might have to be monitored.

It is crucial to achieve a therapeutic level of anticoagulation within 12 to 24 hours of starting therapy or the morbidity and mortality will increase. The therapy should begin with a heparin bolus of 80 U/kg followed by a continuous infusion of 18 U/kg /hour. The aPTT should be monitored every 6 hours and adjusted according to a weight-based nomogram until a therapeutic range has been reached; aPTT can then be monitored daily.

The chief complications of unfractionated heparin are bleeding and heparin-induced thrombocytopenia. It is necessary to monitor the platelet count every other day in patients treated with heparin.

### LOW-MOLECULAR-WEIGHT HEPARIN

Low-molecular-weight heparins (LMWHs) are single-molecular-weight heparin molecules that act on factor Xa. They have the advantage of being more predictable in their dose effect. For most patients, the LMWH preparations do not require monitoring of their effect for short-term therapy. Monitoring of the anti-Xa levels should be undertaken with long-term therapy, in obese patients (>150 kg), in very small patients (<40 kg), and in pregnant patients. LMWH has a prolonged half-life in patients with renal insufficiency (creatinine clearance <30 mL/min) and are relatively contraindicated in these patients. There also may be a lower risk of heparin-induced thrombocytopenia, but the platelet count should still be monitored. Enoxaparin (Lovenox) and tinzaparin (Innohep) are currently approved by the FDA for the management of acute deep venous thrombosis with or without pulmonary embolism.

### WARFARIN

Warfarin (Coumadin) is the only vitamin K antagonist available in the United States and is used for the subacute and long-term management of DVT/PE. It prevents the formation of the vitamin K–dependent clotting factors (factors II, V, VII, and IX). It also decreases the levels of protein S and protein C, which are antithrombotic proteins. It can induce hypercoagulability by depleting proteins C and S levels if it is initiated without heparin or LMWH.

Warfarin therapy should begin on the day that anticoagulation is begun with heparin or LMWH unless there is a contraindication to therapy with warfarin. Warfarin is contraindicated in patients who have a known reaction to warfarin, who have a high risk of bleeding, or who are pregnant. In addition, warfarin interacts with many foods and pharmaceutical agents.

The protime (PT) as reflected by the international normalized ratio (INR) should be monitored daily with initiation of therapy. The goal therapeutic INR for most patients is 2.0 to 3.0. The patient should take unfractionated heparin or LMWH for a minimum of 5 days and the INR should be greater than 2.0 for two consecutive days before the unfractionated heparin or LMWH is discontinued.

## ALTERNATIVE AGENTS FOR INITIAL MANAGEMENT

In the setting of a contraindication to the use of heparin, several agents can be used for the initial management of acute DVT/PE. Fondaparinux (Arixtra) is a pentasaccharide that has an anti–factor Xa effect. It has been shown to be effective in the treatment of DVT/PE. It is administered subcutaneously and is cleared renally. It has been demonstrated to be useful in the treatment of DVT/PE. Fondaparinux is now FDA approved for the treatment of DVT and PE, but it is not FDA approved for acute management. Liver enzymes must be monitored. Argatroban (Novastan) and hirudin (lepirudin [Refludan])[1] have been used to manage DVT/PE in the setting of heparin-associated thrombocytopenia.

## LONG-TERM MANAGEMENT

The determination of the duration of therapy for DVT/PE is based on the balance between the risk of bleeding and the risk of recurrence. Patients who have an identifiable reversible risk factor, such as surgery, should receive treatment for 3 months. Patients with an initial episode of idiopathic DVT/PE are at higher risk for recurrence than patients with an identifiable risk factor and should be treated for 6 to 12 months. The exact duration should be determined based on the patient's risk of bleeding. For patients with identifiable risk factors, the duration of treatment is often at least 1 year or longer. In patients with malignancy, long-term therapy with LMWH may be preferable to therapy with warfarin. These patients should be treated for life or until the malignancy is resolved.

## ALTERNATIVE MODES OF THERAPY FOR ACUTE PULMONARY EMBOLISM

### Venocaval Interruption and Inferior Vena Cava Filter Placement

Interruption of the inferior vena cava (IVC) was originally accomplished via surgical ligation of the vena cava or surgical placement of a filter to prevent pulmonary embolism. The IVC filter is now placed percutaneously to prevent recurrence of pulmonary embolism in selected groups. These groups include patients with contraindications to systemic anticoagulation, patients who are undergoing surgical intervention for acute pulmonary embolism, patients with chronic thromboembolic pulmonary hypertension, and possibly patients with limited cardiopulmonary reserve. The IVC filter has been shown to decrease the risk of recurrent pulmonary embolism after placement, but it is associated with an increased risk of venous thrombosis without a survival benefit.

### Thrombolytic Therapy

Thrombolytic agents actively destroy a clot by activating plasminogen. Three agents are FDA approved for acute management of massive PE. These agents are urokinase (Abbokinase), streptokinase (Streptase), and tissue plasminogen activator (TPA; Activase). They have been associated with a significant risk of severe bleeding, including intracranial hemorrhage, and should be used cautiously. They are typically used in patients who are hemodynamically unstable or have suffered sudden death from PE.

Patients with evidence of right ventricular dysfunction by echocardiogram or with substantial elevations of troponin or brain natriuretic peptide (BNP) levels at the time of admission have been demonstrated to be at risk of hemodynamic deterioration. Patients with right ventricular thrombi are at increased risk for hemodynamic decompensation and can benefit from the use of thrombolytic agents. Routine use of thrombolytic agents in this group of patients, which represents approximately 50% of patients with symptomatic emboli, remains controversial.

The use of thrombolytic drugs has been demonstrated to show improvement in right ventricular function by echocardiogram and improvement in lung V/Q scans at 1 to 3 days. At 7 days after therapy, there is no difference in the degree of pulmonary perfusion abnormalities in patients treated with thrombolytics versus those treated with heparin. Thrombolytic agents are contraindicated in patients with intracranial pathology, recent neurosurgery, recent operations, and active bleeding.

## HEMODYNAMIC MANAGEMENT OF HYPOTENSION ASSOCIATED WITH MASSIVE PULMONARY EMBOLISM

Shock is a marker for increased mortality in patients with massive pulmonary embolus. In one study, the mortality rate increased to 31% when the patient presented with shock. Pulmonary embolus should be suspected in patients who ahve cardiac arrest with pulseless electrical activity or who have shock associated with hypoxemia. It is important to maintain an adequate systemic arterial pressure to prevent right ventricular infarction. Intravenous fluids should be used cautiously to prevent overdistention of the overloaded right ventricle. The blood pressure is typically supported with dopamine (Intropin), norepinephrine (Levophed), or phenylephrine (Neo-Synephrine). Inotropic agents such as dobutamine (Dobutrex) can improve cardiac output but can also increase myocardial oxygen consumption and hypotension, so they should be used cautiously.

## INTERVENTIONS FOR MANAGEMENT OF PULMONARY EMBOLISM

The indications for surgical embolectomy include massive pulmonary embolism, persistent shock, and failure of or contraindications to thrombolytic therapy. The morbidity and mortality of surgical intervention in the setting of hemodynamic collapse are significant, and surgery should be performed by experienced teams with readily available cardiopulmonary bypass. Catheter-based embolectomy[1] is available in some centers and is an alternative for some patients.

## REFERENCES

Buller HR, Agnelli G, Hull RD, et al: Antithrombotic therapy for venous thromboembolic disease: The Seventh ACCP Conference on Antithrombotic and Thrombolytic Therapy. Chest 2004;126:4018-4288.

Dalen JE, Alpert JS: Natural history of pulmonary embolism. Prog Cardiovasc Dis 1975;17:257-270.

Elliot CG, Goldhaber SZ, Visani L, De Rosa M: Chest radiographs in acute pulmonary embolism. Chest 2000;118:33-38.

Kearon C, Ginsberg JS, Douketis J, et al: An evaluation of D-dimer in the diagnosis of pulmonary embolism: A randomized controlled trial. Ann Intern Med 2006;144: 812-821.

PIOPED Investigators: Value of the ventilation-perfusion lung scan in acute pulmonary embolism. JAMA 1990;263(20):2753-2759.

PIOPED Investigators: Tissue plasminogen activator for the treatment of acute pulmonary embolism: A collaborative study by the PIOPED Investigators. Chest 1990;97:528-533.

PIOPED II Investigators: Multidectector computed tomography for acute pulmonary embolism. N Engl J Med 2006;354:2317-2327.

Pulido T, Aranda A, Zevallos MA, et al: Pulmonary embolism as a cause of death in patients with heart disease: An autopsy study. Chest 2006;129:1282-1287.

Ryu JH, Olson EJ, Pellikka PA: Clinical recognition of pulmonary embolism: Problem of unrecognized and asymptomatic cases. Mayo Clin Proc 1998;73:873-879.

---

[1]Not FDA approved for this indication.

---

[1]Not FDA approved for this indication.

Sors II, Pacouret G Azarian et al: Hemodynamic effects of bolus vs. 2 hours infusion of alteplase in acute massive pulmonary embolism: A randomized controlled trial. Chest 1994;106:712-717.

Stein PD, Terrin ML, Hales CA, et al: Clinical, laboratory roentgenographic, and electrocardiographic findings in patients with acute pulmonary embolism and no preexisting cardiac or pulmonary disease. Chest 1991;100: 598-603.

Urokinase Pulmonary Embolism Trial. Phase 1 results: A COOPERATIVE Study. JAMA 1970;214:2163-2172.

Wells PS, Anderson DR, Rodger M, et al: Derivation of a simple clinical model to categorize the patients' probability of pulmonary embolism: Increasing the model's utility with the SimpliRED D-dimer. Thromb Haemost 2000;83(3):416-420.

Wicki J, Perneger T, Junod A, et al: Assessing clinical probability of the pulmonary embolism in the emergency ward: A simple score. Arch Intern Med 2001;161:92-97.

Wood KE: Major pulmonary embolism: Review of a pathophysiologic approach to the golden hour of hemodynamically significant pulmonary embolism. Chest 2002;121;877-905.

# Sarcoidosis

Method of
*Surendra K. Sharma, MD, PhD, and*
*Alladi Mohan, MD*

Sarcoidosis is an intriguing multisystem granulomatous disorder of unknown cause(s). Patients often present with bilateral hilar lymphadenopathy, pulmonary infiltration, and ocular and skin lesions. The diagnosis is established when clinical and radiologic findings are supported by histologic evidence of noncaseating epithelioid cell granulomas in the affected organs.

## Etiology

The cause of sarcoidosis has proved tantalizingly elusive. It is also not clear whether sarcoidosis is caused by a single agent, several related agents, or multiple factors. Genetic factors have been thought to play a role in the pathogenesis. It is unlikely that any single gene is involved; probably, genetically predisposed hosts are exposed to antigens that trigger an exaggerated immune response, and this results in the formation of granulomas. Although no significant association has been reported between sarcoidosis and occurrence of HLA phenotypes, the most consistent allele found associated with sarcoidosis has been HLA-B8 in some of the western studies. Presence of DRB1*11 and DRB1*14 and absence of DRB1*07 and DQB1*0201 alleles were independent predictors of sarcoidosis; predominant occurrence of DRB1*14 and its linked DQ alleles were associated with a chronic course with frequent relapses in Indian patients. These observations suggest that ethnic differences in genetic susceptibility to development of and the response to corticosteroid treatment may be important in patients with sarcoidosis.

Observations of community outbreaks and of work-related risk of sarcoidosis for nurses and a study tracing the case contacts on the Isle of Man, suggest a person-to-person transmission or shared exposure to an environmental agent. Exposures to beryllium, clay soil, pine dust, and talc have been implicated, and certain occupations and an association with photocopier use have all been postulated as causes. Wood millers, postal workers, mechanics, firefighters, and health care workers fall into the postulated occupational risk category. Development of sarcoidosis following cardiac and bone marrow transplantation points to an infectious etiology. There are reports associating interferon therapy with the development of sarcoidosis. Recently, it was reported that a patient with clinically silent sarcoidosis who contracted HIV infection became symptomatic with the institution of highly active antiretroviral therapy (HAART).

## Epidemiology

Sarcoidosis has been observed to occur all over the world, affecting both sexes, all races, and all ages. Considerable variation exists in the reported prevalence and clinical presentation by sex, ethnicity, race, and country of origin.

Sarcoidosis is predominantly a disease of adults younger than 40 years and seldom seems to affect children; women have slightly higher disease rates. A second peak has been observed in women older than 60 years from Scandinavian countries and Japan. Late onset by nearly a decade and male preponderance have been described in India. The lifetime risk of sarcoidosis is estimated to be 0.85% and 2.4% for U.S. whites and African Americans, respectively, based on cumulative incidence estimates. Globally, Swedes, Danes, and African Americans appear to have the highest prevalence rates, and the disease is rarely reported from India, Spain, Portugal, Saudi Arabia, or South America.

## Pathogenesis and Pathology

The inciting antigen elicits an inflammatory reaction characterized by the accumulation of activated T cells (predominantly Th1 type) and macrophages, followed by the formation of granulomas. Sarcoid granulomas consist of highly differentiated mononuclear phagocytes, epithelioid cells, giant cells, and lymphocytes surrounded by fibroblasts, mast cells, and extracellular matrix. Sometimes the giant cells contain conch-like (Schaumann bodies), stellate (asteroid bodies), and refractile calcium-containing (residual bodies) inclusions. Classically, these granulomas are noncaseating (non-necrotizing); however, focal coagulative necrosis has occasionally been described. In the lung, the granulomas are most commonly located along the peribronchovascular sheath lymphatics and sometimes in subpleural and interlobular septal lymphatics (lymphangitic distribution). Organ dysfunction in sarcoidosis results when the accumulated inflammatory cells distort the architecture of the affected tissue. If the disease activity is suppressed by spontaneous remission or therapy, sarcoid granulomas resolve by dispersion of the inflammatory cells but can leave behind fibrotic changes.

## Clinical Features

Consistent with the multisystem nature of the disease, patients with sarcoidosis present to various specialists depending on the organs involved. However, the disease is sometimes discovered in an asymptomatic patient when a chest radiograph is incidentally obtained. Sarcoidosis is known to have an acute, subacute, or insidious onset. Two forms of acute sarcoidosis syndromes have been described: Löfgren's syndrome (fever, bilateral hilar adenopathy, erythema nodosum, and arthralgia) and Heerfordt's syndrome (fever, parotid enlargement, anterior uveitis, and facial nerve palsy). The subacute form evolves over a few weeks. The insidious form evolves over several months, and most of these patients eventually develop chronic sarcoidosis. Acute sarcoidosis usually responds best to corticosteroid treatment.

### RACIAL AND ETHNIC VARIATIONS

Although erythema nodosum is often seen in Scandinavian countries and Britain, it is not common in Japan. Ocular involvement is more common in London and Tokyo than in Paris and Los Angeles. Furthermore, African Americans appear to have higher rates of extrapulmonary involvement, chronic uveitis, lupus pernio, cystic bone lesions, and chronic progressive disease, and they have worse long-term prognoses and higher rates of relapse compared with whites, who often present with asymptomatic isolated bihilar adenopathy. Chronic uveitis is more common in African Americans, and lupus pernio is more common in Puerto Ricans. The constitutional symptoms are more common in African Americans and Indians compared with others. In Indian patients with sarcoidosis, the chest radiographs can look startling, but patients can present with minimal symptoms (clinical-radiographic dissociation).

## FAMILIAL CLUSTERING

Familial sarcoidosis has been described, with a rate of at least 19% in affected African American families and 5% in white families. Monozygotic twins have a higher incidence than dizygotic pairs.

# Diagnosis

## CLINICAL

Patients often complain of nonspecific constitutional symptoms such as fever, fatigue, malaise, weight loss, and night sweats. Pulmonary involvement is, by far, the commonest (90%). Patients might complain of cough (which may be nonproductive), dyspnea, and chest pain. Hemoptysis and clubbing are rare. Chest signs on auscultation and airway hyperactivity (<20%), reversible airway obstruction, and clinical presentation mimicking bronchial asthma with seasonal exacerbations are less common. Involvement of the nasal mucosa (<20%) and larynx (<5%) is rare.

Cutaneous involvement (11%-34%) includes erythema nodosum, lupus pernio, plaques, maculopapular lesions, subcutaneous nodules, changes in old scars, alopecia, and hypo- and hyperpigmented areas. Skin lesions seldom cause itching or pain and do not ulcerate.

Ocular involvement (4%-27%) is often present. Uveitis (acute or chronic) is the most common manifestation. Other manifestations include conjunctival follicles, lacrimal gland enlargement, dry eye (keratoconjunctivitis sicca), dacryocystitis, and retinal vasculitis.

Peripheral lymphadenopathy (8%-44%) occurs frequently. Rarely, intra-abdominal lymphadenopathy is present. Bone marrow involvement occurs in 15% to 40% of patients.

Joint symptoms (30%-50%) may be acute and transient or chronic and persistent. Unilateral or bilateral painless parotid gland enlargement (1%-10%) can result in a "chipmunk cheeks" appearance.

Nephrocalcinosis, nephrolithiasis, and renal failure, as well as diabetes insipidus due to hypothalamic or pituitary involvement, can rarely occur. Uncommonly, hypothyroidism, hyperthyroidism, hypothermia, adrenal suppression, and anterior pituitary involvement can occur.

Clinically evident myocardial involvement (5%) includes benign arrhythmias, heart block, and sudden death. The gastrointestinal tract is rarely (<1%) involved. Although granulomas may be found in 50% to 80% of liver biopsy specimens, palpable hepatomegaly (8%-43%) is less often observed. Splenomegaly (2%-27%) is also common. Hepatic involvement rarely causes portal hypertension, hepatic failure, or increased mortality related to liver dysfunction.

Neurosarcoidosis (0.3%-13%) can manifest with cranial nerve involvement (particularly facial palsy), hypothalamic and pituitary lesions, space-occupying mass lesions, and peripheral neuropathy.

## LABORATORY

Because there is no definitive gold standard for the diagnosis, sarcoidosis is essentially a diagnosis of exclusion. Estimation of serum angiotensin-converting enzyme (ACE) activity and gallium scanning have poor specificity; the Kveim-Siltzbach test is not in use currently. Thus, all suspected cases of sarcoidosis must be confirmed by tissue biopsy (see Bronchoscopy, later) to exclude mycobacterial, fungal, and other granulomatous infections and disorders resulting from occupational and environmental causes (inorganic and organic), medication use, or malignant conditions.

Cutaneous anergy is considered to be a cardinal feature of sarcoidosis; tuberculin skin test is often negative in nearly two thirds of the patients. Hematologic abnormalities include anemia, leukopenia, lymphopenia, eosinophilia, and monocytosis and occasionally polycythemia, among others. Hypercalcemia has been reported to occur in 2% to 63% of patients, and hypercalciuria is three times more common than hypercalcemia. Elevated serum aminotransferase, alanine aminotransferase, alkaline phosphatase, and hyperuricemia have also been described.

## RADIOGRAPHIC

The chest radiographs reveal abnormalities in more than 90% of the patients with sarcoidosis at presentation; the characteristic radiologic finding is bilateral hilar lymphadenopathy. Chest radiographic staging of pulmonary sarcoidosis is shown in Table 1. However, these patterns do not represent proper consecutive stages of sarcoidosis. Parenchymal infiltrates that are often bilateral and symmetric involving the upper lobes more often are common. Other patterns include reticular, reticulonodular, or focal alveolar opacities; miliary mottling; and ground-glass appearance. Pleural involvement is rare and includes pleural effusion, thickening, plaques or nodules, and pneumothorax.

Computed tomography (CT) scan of the chest is not routinely required for diagnostic evaluation or follow-up, but it is useful in detecting enlarged lymph nodes or parenchymal infiltrates that are not evident on the conventional chest radiograph in patients with atypical or uncommon manifestations. CT scan of the chest can reveal central bronchovascular thickening and nodularity, miliary nodules, thickening of interlobular septae, luminal irregularity, ground-glass attenuation, architectural distortion, conglomerate masses, honeycombing and cystic destruction, alveolar consolidation, and parenchymal and pleural nodules. CT scan of the abdomen is also useful in identifying lesions in the liver and spleen and retroperitoneal and abdominal lymphadenopathy. CT scan and magnetic resonance imaging (MRI) have been found useful in localizing neurosarcoidosis and sarcoidosis of the bones.

## PULMONARY

The lung function abnormalities of sarcoidosis include decreased lung volume and diffusing capacity. However, these abnormalities are not specific and are typical for interstitial lung disease of any etiology. Pulmonary function abnormalities are present in about 20% of the patients with stage I sarcoidosis, but they occur in 40% to 70% of patients with stage II or III disease. Airway involvement has been observed in about one third of the patients. However, these physiologic abnormalities poorly correlate with the pathologic findings.

## CURRENT DIAGNOSIS

- Sarcoidosis is essentially a diagnosis of exclusion, because there is no definitive gold standard for the diagnosis.
- All suspected cases of sarcoidosis must be confirmed by tissue biopsy to exclude mycobacterial, fungal, other granulomatous infections and disorders resulting from occupational and environmental causes (inorganic and organic), medications, or malignant conditions.
- Specimens must be procured for histopathologic and microbiological examination from the most accessible site with the least invasive method.
- Diagnosis is established when clinical and radiologic findings are supported by histologic evidence of noncaseating epithelioid cell granulomas in the affected organs.

**TABLE 1 Chest Radiographic Staging of Pulmonary Sarcoidosis**

| Stage | Findings |
| --- | --- |
| 0 | Normal chest radiograph |
| I | Bilateral hilar lymphadenopathy without parenchymal infiltrates |
| II | Bilateral hilar lymphadenopathy with parenchymal infiltrates |
| III | Parenchymal infiltrates without hilar lymphadenopathy |
| IV | Advanced fibrosis with evidence of honeycombing, hilar retraction, bullae, cysts, and emphysema |

## BRONCHOSCOPY

Flexible fiberoptic bronchoscopy (FOB) and bronchoscopic techniques such as transbronchial lung biopsy (TBLB), endobronchial biopsy, transbronchial needle aspiration (TBNA), and bronchoalveolar lavage (BAL) have been found useful for studying the disease and procuring tissue for the confirmation of a diagnosis of sarcoidosis. Bronchoscopic appearances of sarcoidosis include nodules, plaques, erythema, and cobblestone appearance. TBLB has a high diagnostic yield because the lesions of sarcoidosis are distributed along the bronchovascular bundle. BAL has very little practical clinical or prognostic usefulness and has been used as a research tool.

Specimens must be procured for testing from the most accessible site (e.g., peripheral lymph node, skin lesions) with the least invasive method. TBLB has a high diagnostic yield (40%-90%) when four or five lung biopsies are carried out. When no peripheral site is accessible and TBLB is inconclusive, mediastinoscopy, video-assisted thoracoscopic surgery (VATS) lung biopsy, and open lung biopsy have all been used. With VATS, lung as well as intrathoracic lymph node material can be procured. Presence of noncaseating epithelioid cell granulomas in tissue biopsy specimens in the appropriate clinical setting confirms the diagnosis of sarcoidosis.

### OTHER INVESTIGATIONS

Endomyocardial biopsy is useful for confirming the diagnosis of cardiac sarcoidosis. Elevated levels of serum ACE have been observed in 40% to 90% of patients with sarcoidosis and are considered a marker of disease activity. Gallium-67 scanning is a useful adjunct in diagnosing sarcoidosis. Increased uptake in bilateral hilar and right paratracheal lymph nodes (lambda sign) and uptake in these lymph nodes as well as parotid and lacrimal glands (panda sign) support the diagnosis but a negative gallium scan does not rule out active sarcoidosis.

## Course and Prognosis

The natural history of sarcoidosis is highly variable. Most patients who present with acute disease are left with no significant sequelae. About one half of all patients have some permanent organ dysfunction, which is usually mild, stable, and nonprogressive. In about 15% to 20% of patients, the disease remains active or relapses are common. Sarcoidosis causes death in less than 10% of patients due to progressive respiratory insufficiency or central nervous system or myocardial involvement.

Adverse clinical prognostic factors in patients with sarcoidosis include older age at onset (>40 years), lupus pernio, chronic uveitis, chronic hypercalcemia, nephrocalcinosis, African American race, progressive pulmonary disease, nasal mucosal involvement, cystic bone lesions, neurosarcoidosis, myocardial sarcoidosis, and chronic respiratory insufficiency.

## Treatment

Not all patients with sarcoidosis require treatment because the disease waxes and wanes. Patients with sarcoidosis who are asymptomatic and those with minimal organ dysfunction should be closely monitored without instituting any treatment. Nonsteroidal anti-inflammatory drugs (NSAIDs) are effective for treatment of musculoskeletal symptoms and erythema nodosum. Inhaled corticosteroids and bronchodilators may be beneficial in patients with airway obstruction. In patients with skin lesions, iritis or uveitis, nasal polyps, or reactive airway disease, topical corticosteroids can be used. Therapy is indicated for patients who are symptomatic, those with deteriorating lung function, and those with serious extrapulmonary disease such as neurologic or cardiac sarcoidosis, hypercalcemia not responding to conventional treatment, and ocular sarcoidosis not responding to topical therapy, among others.

Corticosteroids have been the mainstay of therapy. Although there are reports of short-term improvement, well-controlled clinical trials

## CURRENT THERAPY

- Not all patients with sarcoidosis need to be treated because of the waxing and waning nature of the disease.
- Therapy is indicated for patients with symptoms (e.g., intractable cough, dyspnea), deteriorating lung function, or serious extrapulmonary disease.
- In patients with skin lesions, iritis or uveitis, nasal polyps, or reactive airways disease, topical corticosteroids can be used.
- Corticosteroids have been the mainstay of therapy. However, the appropriate dosage, the value of daily as opposed to alternate-day therapy, and the optimum duration of treatment are still unclear.
- If the patient does not respond to corticosteroid treatment, other agents can be tried. Cytotoxic agents include methotrexate (Rheumatrex),[1] azathioprine (Imuran),[1] cyclophosphamide (Cytoxan),[1] and chlorambucil (Leukeran).[1] Noncytotoxic agents include hydroxychloroquine (Plaquenil),[1] thalidomide (Thalomid),[1] and ketoconazole (Nizoral).[1]

[1]Not FDA approved for this indication.

showing definitive improvement in the long-term outcome with the use of corticosteroids are lacking. Also, the appropriate dosage, value of daily as opposed to alternate-day therapy, and the optimum duration of treatment are also unclear. When indicated, patients with pulmonary sarcoidosis are started on prednisone 0.75 to 1 mg/kg/day for 4 to 6 weeks. Higher doses may be necessary in cardiac sarcoidosis or neurosarcoidosis. Patients are carefully monitored clinically, radiologically, and physiologically. In responders, prednisone is slowly tapered over 2 to 3 months to 5 to 10 mg/day or an every-other-day regimen. Treatment is usually continued for a minimum of 12 months.

Patients should be carefully monitored for the rest of their lives for any recurrences, because re-activation is not uncommon, even after prolonged periods of remission. Even steroid-responsive sarcoidosis has been reported to relapse in about 25% of patients after stopping corticosteroid treatment.

Patients who relapse can again be re-treated with corticosteroids. Some patients require continuous low-dose corticosteroid treatment (<7.5 mg/day) to prevent relapses. If the patient does not respond to corticosteroid treatment, several cytotoxic and noncytotoxic agents have been explored to treat such patients. Cytotoxic treatments include methotrexate (Rheumatrex)[1] 10 to 25 mg/week, azathioprine (Imuran)[1] 50 to 200 mg/day, and cyclophosphamide (Cytoxan)[1] 50 to 150 mg/d orally, 200 to 400 mg/day, or 500 to 2000 mg every 2 weeks intravenously. Noncytotoxic agents include hydroxychloroquine (Plaquenil)[1] 200 to 400 mg/day, thalidomide (Thalomid),[1] and ketoconazole (Nizoral).[1]

Methotrexate and hydroxchloroquine are considered useful not only as steroid-sparing agents but also as replacement therapy, especially in patients with musculoskeletal and cutaneous sarcoidosis. These agents are not safe for use during pregnancy and can cause severe adverse drug reactions that can limit their use. Definitive benefits of these agents are also not established, and treatment should be tailored to the needs of the individual patient only by an experienced clinician. Lung transplantation is reserved for end-stage disease; there is up to a 50% chance of recurrence of sarcoidosis in the transplanted lung.

[1]Not FDA approved for this indication.

## REFERENCES

Alazemi S, Campos MA: Interferon-induced sarcoidosis. Int J Clin Pract 2006;60:201-211.

Almeida FA Jr, Sager JS, Eiger G: Coexistent sarcoidosis and HIV infection: An immunological paradox? J Infect 2006;52:195-201.

American Thoracic Society, the European Respiratory Society, and the World Association of Sarcoidosis and Other Granulomatous Disorders: Statement on sarcoidosis. Am J Respir Crit Care Med 1999;160:736-755.

Baughman RP: Therapeutic options for sarcoidosis: New and old. Curr Opin Pulm Med 2002;8:464-469.

Lynch JP 3rd, Sharma OP, Baughman RP: Extrapulmonary sarcoidosis. Semin Respir Infect 1998;13:229-254.

Sharma OP: Pulmonary sarcoidosis: Management. J Postgrad Med 2002;48: 135-141.

Sharma SK, Balamurugan A, Pandey RM, et al: Human leukocyte antigen-DR alleles influence the clinical course of pulmonary sarcoidosis in Asian Indians. Am J Respir Cell Mol Biol 2003;29:225-231.

Sharma SK, Mohan A: Sarcoidosis: Global scenario and Indian perspective. Indian J Med Res 2002;116:221-247.

Sharma SK, Mohan A: Uncommon manifestations of sarcoidosis. J Assoc Physicians India 2004;52:210-214.

Sharma SK, Mohan A, Guleria JS: Clinical characteristics, pulmonary function abnormalities and outcome of prednisolone treatment in 106 patients with sarcoidosis. J Assoc Physicians India 2001;49:697-704.

Thomas KW, Hunninghake GW: Sarcoidosis. JAMA 2003;289:3300-3303.

# Silicosis and Asbestosis

Method of
*Vinicius C. S. Antao, MD, MSc, PhD, and John E. Parker, MD*

Pneumoconioses are lung diseases caused by the inhalation and deposition of mineral dust. Silica, coal mine dust, and asbestos can lead to pulmonary fibrosis and other types of respiratory diseases.

## Silicosis

Silicosis is the oldest recognized form of pneumoconiosis. Crystalline silica in respirable dust (~0.5-5 μm diameter) can reach the alveolar regions of the lungs and cause fibrosis. The three most important forms of crystalline silica are quartz, tridymite, and cristobalite.

### EPIDEMIOLOGY

Exposure to silica dust occurs in many occupations, such as mining, quarrying, drilling, and tunneling operations. It is also a hazard to stonecutters and to refractory brick, pottery, foundry, and sandblasting workers. Ground silica, which is used in porcelain, cosmetics, and soap, also represents a risk.

Exact information on the incidence and prevalence of silicosis worldwide is unknown, but it seems to be decreasing in industrialized countries due to improvements in working conditions and dust-control measures. Nevertheless, silicosis persists as a serious public health problem, especially in developing countries, where occupational diseases are commonly misclassified and underdiagnosed. In the United States, more than two million workers are exposed to silica and at potential risk of developing the disease.

### PATHOGENESIS

In terms of pathology, the fundamental lesion is a concentric silicotic nodule. The pathogenesis is complex, and four basic mechanisms are involved: direct cytotoxicity, resulting in the local release of enzymes; activation of oxidant production by alveolar macrophages; activation of mediator release from alveolar macrophages and epithelial cells, causing recruitment of polymorphonuclear leukocytes and macrophages and also resulting in production of proinflammatory cytokines and reactive species; and secretion of growth factors from alveolar macrophages and epithelial cells, stimulating fibroblast proliferation. These different mechanisms can lead to eventual cell injury and lung scarring. Many studies have demonstrated that freshly fractured silica particles are more toxic to lung cells than aged silica particles, which can be explained by the presence of free radicals.

### CLINICAL FEATURES

There are four forms of silicosis: chronic, complicated, accelerated, and acute. The form is generally related to the degree or intensity of silica exposure.

Patients with chronic silicosis may be asymptomatic. The radiograph shows small (<10 mm), rounded opacities, mainly in the upper zones, that appear more than 15 years after initial exposure. These parenchymal abnormalities can occur without significant changes in pulmonary function or can lead to mild restriction. An obstructive pattern may be observed on spirometry testing, due to smoking habits or the presence of dust-induced lesions in the small airways. Carbon monoxide diffusing capacity ($DL_{CO}$), which measures the transfer of a diffusion-limited gas (carbon monoxide) across the alveolocapillary membrane, may be decreased due to silicotic changes.

Accelerated silicosis occurs with high levels of exposure after a shorter latency (usually 5-10 years). The radiographic patterns are similar to chronic silicosis, but the progression of disease is more rapid. Patients present with symptoms early, and the lung function deteriorates very quickly, with a rapid decline in forced expiratory volume in one second ($FEV_1$).

Complicated silicosis, also known as progressive massive fibrosis, is a more advanced form of chronic or accelerated silicosis. The most common symptom is exertional dyspnea. Cough can occur due to superimposed infections or chronic obstructive pulmonary disease (COPD). The radiograph is characterized by the presence of large opacities greater than 1 cm in diameter. Spirometry often shows a restrictive pattern caused by fibrosis or a mixed pattern with associated obstruction due to emphysema and dust-related airflow limitation. Carbon monoxide diffusing capacity is reduced. Because of extensive areas of fibrosis and gas exchange abnormalities with hypoxemia, cor pulmonale and respiratory failure can occur in the final stage of the disease.

Acute silicosis can develop within 6 months to 2 years after massive silica exposure. The symptoms are severe dyspnea, weight loss, and weakness. The radiograph shows a pattern completely different from other types of silicosis, with bilateral airspace filling. Pathologically, this pattern is very similar to alveolar proteinosis. Pulmonary fibrosis is not a prominent finding in acute silicosis. The prognosis is guarded and the disease usually progresses, resulting in severe hypoxemia and respiratory failure.

Patients with silicosis are at risk for tuberculosis, nontuberculous mycobacterioses, and bacterial infections, as well as infection-associated bronchiectasis. *Nocardia* infections can occur in patients with acute silicosis.

### DIAGNOSIS

Three important criteria are generally sufficient for a diagnosis of silicosis: a careful occupational history documenting silica exposure with an appropriate latency period; a chest radiograph classified as category 1/0 or greater in accordance with the International Labour Organization (ILO) International Classification of Radiographs of Pneumoconioses; and absence of diseases that can mimic silicosis, such as tuberculosis, sarcoidosis, or pulmonary fungal infections. Lung biopsy typically is not necessary. High-resolution computed tomography (CT) can be useful in achieving more accurate categorization of the parenchymal changes in all types of pneumoconiosis, but the descriptions of the findings are not standardized and the procedure is expensive for medical screening purposes.

**CURRENT DIAGNOSIS**

- Take a detailed medical and occupational history, including all past exposures, with special attention to latency between exposure and onset of disease.
- The chest radiograph shows small, rounded opacities, mainly in the upper zones for silicosis, and small, reticular opacities, mainly in the lower zones for asbestosis.
- Exclude other diseases that can mimic the radiographic appearance of pneumoconiosis.
- Assess severity of disease with lung function tests.

## TREATMENT

### Treatment of Silicosis

All forms of silicosis are irreversible, often progressive (even after the exposure has ceased), and potentially fatal, although they are completely preventable. Many experimental studies have been conducted to establish a treatment for this disease but, because of toxicity and lack of efficacy, they are not generally available for human use.

Tetrandrine,[2] an extract of the root of *Stephania tetranda*, a traditional Chinese medicine, was approved by the State Drugs Administration of China as a drug for the treatment of silicosis. It exhibits anti-inflammatory, antifibrogenetic, and antioxidant effects. Tetrandrine is not available in the United States, and additional research must be conducted to document safety and efficacy. More recently, it has been demonstrated that heme oxygenase-1 (HO-1), a rate-limiting enzyme in heme catabolism, with antioxidative, anti-apoptotic, and anti-inflammatory activities, is persistently expressed in the lung lesions of patients with silicosis. It has been suggested that up-regulation of HO-1 might offer a novel strategy for the treatment of silicosis because it suppresses silica-induced reactive oxygen species (ROS) activity. Nevertheless, this form of treatment is still experimental.

Acute silicosis has been treated with whole-lung lavage to remove the alveolar exudates. The benefits are uncertain, and serious bacterial infections can occur after this procedure. Some reports suggest using prednisone[1] to treat acute silicosis. The initial doses are 40 to 60 mg/day for 1 month. If benefits can be documented, the treatment can be maintained with lower doses (15-20 mg/day) for 6 months. Steroids are potentially dangerous and increase the risk and progression of coexistent tuberculosis or other infections.

After an initial evaluation, based on guidelines for recipient selection, single or bilateral lung or lung-heart transplantation should be considered for select patients with end-stage silicosis. Once a patient is selected as a potential candidate for lung transplantation, further studies, including pulmonary function tests, high-resolution CT scan, complete cardiac evaluation, serologic tests for hepatitis and HIV, and renal and liver function tests, are often required to be performed at the referring center.

Because there is no specific drug to control or reverse the fibrosis, the treatment of silicosis should be focused on alleviating symptoms and preventing and treating the complications of the disease.

### Treatment of Complications

#### Tuberculosis

A common complication of silicosis is pulmonary tuberculosis. Tuberculosis can be present in up to 15% of silicosis patients in some countries. Workers with silicosis or silica exposure for 25 years or more should have tuberculin skin testing. Those who are asymptomatic but have an area of induration greater than 9 mm should receive chemoprophylaxis with isoniazid (INH [Nydrazid]) for 9 to 12 months.

 **CURRENT THERAPY**

- There is no specific treatment for pneumoconiosis.
- Primary prevention is the key to avoid disease.
- Complications such as infections, chronic bronchitis, and cor pulmonale should be recognized and treated promptly.
- A pulmonary rehabilitation program may improve quality of life.
- Lung transplantation is appropriate in select cases.

Clinical symptoms compatible with tuberculosis should prompt rigorous efforts to obtain bacteriologic confirmation of the diagnosis. The current recommended treatment is a course of pyrazinamide (PZA), rifampin (Rifadin), ethambutol (Myambutol), and INH for 2 months, followed by 6 to 7 months of isoniazid and rifampin. Some authors suggest that the two-drug continuation phase of treatment should be prolonged up to 12 months. Long-term follow-up with bacteriologic culture and radiographs is mandatory.

Nontuberculous mycobacteria (NTM), such as *Mycobacterium kansasii* or *Mycobacterium avium-intracellulare*, account for an increasing percentage of mycobacterial diseases in those with silicosis in industrialized countries. Cultures should be done, because treatment needs to be modified according to the type of mycobacterium grown and its drug sensitivity. *Mycobacterium kansasii* usually responds well to a course of rifampin[1] and ethambutol[1] given for 9 months.

### Connective Tissue Disorders

Silicosis is also associated with connective tissue disorders, mainly scleroderma and rheumatoid arthritis.

Treatment of sclerodermatous involvement of the skin and internal organs is a challenge. Immunosuppressive drugs such as prednisone,[1] azathioprine (Imuran),[1] chlorambucil (Leukeran),[1] cyclosporine (Neoral),[1] and many others have been used in attempts to treat this disease. Calcium channel blockers, mainly nifedipine (Procardia),[1] are indicated for treating Raynaud's phenomenon. Some physicians recommend α-adrenergic receptor blockers.

Many drugs are available to control and manage rheumatoid disease, such as corticosteroids, methotrexate (Rheumatrex), or other disease-modifying agents.

Lupus erythematosus has been described in sandblasters with silicosis; pleuritic pain and effusions can occur, and usually there is a significant response to corticosteroids and resolution of effusion within 2 weeks. Spontaneous resolution does not occur. The use of immunosuppressive agents can trigger infections and, although a negative skin test does not rule out infection, tuberculin skin testing must be assessed before treatment.

### Chronic Obstructive Pulmonary Disease

Workers exposed to silica dust are at increased risk for development of COPD. Classification of severity of this obstructive disease can be used as the basis for treatment.

Use of an inhaled short-acting bronchodilator on demand is recommended for all patients with COPD. Long-acting bronchodilators such as formoterol (Foradil) or salmeterol (Serevent), given twice daily, may be used in stage II as continuous medication. Tiotropium bromide (Spiriva) is a long-acting anticholinergic bronchodilator that maintains bronchodilation for at least 24 hours, allowing once-daily administration.

Inhaled steroids (budesonide [Pulmicort], fluticasone [Flovent]) are indicated for severe disease. Systemic corticosteroids can be used

---

[2]Not available in the United States.
[1]Not FDA approved for this indication.

---

[1]Not FDA approved for this indication.

during exacerbations as short-course therapy. Theophylline (Slo-Phyllin) can achieve small improvements in $FEV_1$ with long-term use.

Pulmonary hypertension is the underlying cause of cor pulmonale. If hypoxemia is present, supplemental oxygen is necessary to improve pulmonary hypertension and cor pulmonale. Oxygen therapy should be prescribed when the arterial partial pressure of oxygen ($PaO_2$) is less than 55 mm Hg, arterial oxygen saturation ($SaO_2$) is less than 88%, or $PaO_2$ is 56 to 59 mm Hg with electrocardiographic evidence of P pulmonale, pedal edema, or secondary erythrocytosis. Patients using oxygen for at least 15 hours per day can achieve a decrease in their pulmonary artery pressures and enhanced cardiac output.

More recent advances in the treatment of pulmonary hypertension include phosphodiesterase-5 inhibitors (sildenafil [Revatio]) and endothelin receptor antagonists (bosentan [Tracleer]).

Noninvasive positive-pressure ventilation has a useful role in the treatment of severe COPD exacerbations. Mechanical ventilatory support for respiratory failure is indicated when it is caused by a treatable complication. Pulmonary rehabilitation programs can improve dyspnea and enhance quality-of-life scores.

Episodes of acute bronchitis can occur and are commonly caused by *Haemophilus influenzae*, *Streptococcus pneumoniae*, *Pseudomonas aeruginosa*, and *Moraxella catarrhalis*. Antibiotics should be prescribed for purulent exacerbations. Viral infections and *Mycoplasma pneumoniae* can also be investigated. After dust exposure is controlled, smoking cessation remains the most effective intervention to reduce the risk of COPD and to slow its progression.

### Other Conditions

The International Agency for Research on Cancer (IARC) has classified crystalline silica in occupational exposures as a human lung carcinogen; however, the issue whether silicosis or silica exposure per se is associated with lung cancer remains controversial in the medical literature. Other conditions such as chronic renal disease have also been linked with occupational exposure to silica in a number of populations, although the overall levels of morbidity and mortality probably do not justify medical screening. Pneumothorax can occur spontaneously or may be ventilator related and generally requires urgent placement of a chest tube.

### PREVENTION

In the absence of specific treatment for silicosis, primary prevention is the key to avoiding the disease. Dust controls and a professionally managed respiratory protection program are essential in preventing this disease, combined with specific programs to educate workers regarding the risks of silica dust exposure. Engineering controls such as dust suppression, local exhaust, appropriate general ventilation, and wet techniques have been proved to be effective in reducing exposures when vigorously implemented in workplaces.

Silicosis reporting is required in many states to ensure investigation of possible continuing workplace hazards. National surveillance is also essential to obtain knowledge of the extent and distribution of the disease, thereby facilitating elimination of this disease in the United States.

## Asbestosis

Asbestosis is an interstitial pneumonitis and fibrosis caused by the inhalation of asbestos fibers. In the United States the number of asbestosis deaths increased from 77 (annual age-adjusted death rate: 0.54 per million population) in 1968 to 1493 deaths (6.88 per million) in 2000 as an historical legacy of asbestos exposure; during the same period, deaths for all other pneumoconioses decreased. The geographic distribution of mortality indicates that asbestosis increased particularly in the coastal states, where asbestos was often used in shipbuilding. Other activities with potential risk for asbestosis are mining, insulation application and removal, and use of asbestos-containing materials in construction and manufacturing of cement products.

Other nonmalignant respiratory health effects associated with asbestos are localized pleural plaques, acute pleuritis with effusion,

diffuse pleural thickening, rounded atelectasis, and chronic airflow obstruction. Lung cancer and mesothelioma (a type of pleural cancer) are malignant diseases related to asbestos exposure. The type of fiber, its dimensions (length and diameter), and its biopersistence are important variables in determining the risk of disease, as are dose and latency period. All types of asbestos fibers are potentially fibrogenic and carcinogenic, including chrysotile (the most common type of asbestos) and amphiboles (crocidolite, amosite, and anthophyllite).

The latency period for the development of asbestosis is commonly between 15 to 20 years after initial exposure to this mineral. It usually occurs as an occupational disease related to the intensity of workplace exposure; nevertheless, environmental and nonoccupational exposures to this fiber can cause other types of asbestos-related diseases, such as mesothelioma.

### DIAGNOSIS

The criteria recommended for the clinical diagnosis of asbestosis are a history of asbestos exposure, dyspnea, bibasilar crackles, and pulmonary function showing a restrictive or mixed pattern or reduced lung volumes, plus radiographic abnormalities consistent with small irregular opacities predominant in lower lung fields. In advanced phases of this disease, middle and upper lobes are often affected, and honeycombing can be noted. If findings on routine radiographs are not sufficient to support the diagnosis, high-resolution CT scanning should be performed. An open lung biopsy is occasionally required to establish the diagnosis but only if the history does not clearly document sufficient occupational exposure or the latency period is not compatible with the disease. The presence of asbestos bodies in sputum or bronchoalveolar lavage would be helpful in this differentiation.

### MANAGEMENT

There is no effective treatment for asbestosis, and the disease often progresses after cessation of exposure. Pulmonary hypertension and cor pulmonale can develop, and supplemental oxygen should be provided when indicated (see earlier). Respiratory infections are treated with antibiotics based on the sensitivity of the organism. Mechanical ventilatory support for respiratory failure should be evaluated with careful consideration for the presence of reversible complications or comorbidities.

### PREVENTION

Asbestosis is a preventable disease, and efforts to eliminate it should be vigorous and persistent. Reporting of asbestosis cases to public health authorities is mandatory in some states. According to the Environmental Protection Agency, there is no safe level for asbestos exposure to assure avoidance of asbestos-associated cancer. Engineering controls to eliminate dust in the workplace and material substitution are important preventive measures. Appropriate protective respirators should be selected by an industrial hygienist based on levels of exposure. Smoking cessation is also an important approach to reduce the risk of asbestos-related lung cancer among those with a history of exposure to asbestos, given the synergistic effects of smoking and asbestos on lung cancer.

### REFERENCES

Akira M: High-resolution CT in the evaluation of occupational and environmental disease. Radiol Clin North Am 2002;40:43-59.

American Thoracic Society: Adverse effects of crystalline silica exposure. Am J Respir Crit Care Med 1997;155:761-768.

American Thoracic Society: Diagnosis and initial management of nonmalignant diseases related to asbestos. Am J Respir Crit Care Med 2004;170:691-715.

American Thoracic Society; CDC; Infectious Diseases Society of America: Treatment of tuberculosis. MMWR Recomm Rep 2003;52(RR-11):1-77.

Becklake MR: Occupational exposures: Evidence for a causal association with chronic obstructive pulmonary disease. Am Rev Respir Dis 1989;140: S85-S91.

Castranova V, Vallyathan V: Silicosis and coal workers' pneumoconiosis. Environ Health Perspect 2000;108(Suppl 4):675-684.

Centers for Disease Control and Prevention: Changing patterns of pneumoconiosis mortality—United States, 1968-2000. MMWR Morb Mortal Wkly Rep 2004;53:627-632.

Centers for Disease Control and Prevention: Silicosis screening in surface coal miners—Pennsylvania, 1996-1997. MMWR Morb Mortal Wkly Rep 2000;49:612-615.

Harkin TJ, McGuinness G, Goldring R, et al: Differentiation of the ILO boundary chest roentgenograph (0/1 to 1/0) in asbestosis by high-resolution computed tomography scan, alveolitis, and respiratory impairment. J Occup Environ Med 1996;38:46-52.

Huuskonen O, Kivisaari L, Zitting A, et al: Emphysema findings associated with heavy asbestos-exposure in high resolution computed tomography of Finnish construction workers. J Occup Health 2004;46:266-271.

International Agency for Research on Cancer: Silica and some silicates. IARC Monogr Eval Carcinog Risk Chem Hum 1987;42:1-239.

National Institute for Occupational Safety and Health (NIOSH): Work-Related Lung Disease Surveillance Report 2002. Morgantown, WV: NIOSH, 2003. PDFs available for download at http://www.cdc.gov/niosh/docs/2003-111/2003-111.html (accessed June 1, 2007).

Sato T, Takeno M, Honma K, et al: Heme oxygenase-1, a potential biomarker of chronic silicosis, attenuates silica-induced lung injury. Am J Respir Crit Care Med 2006;174:906-914.

Wagner GR: Screening and Surveillance of Workers Exposed to Mineral Dusts. Geneva: World Health Organization, 1996.

Wilt JL, Parker JE, Banks DE: The diagnosis of pneumoconiosis and novel therapies. In Banks DE, Parker JE (eds): Occupational lung disease. London: Chapman & Hall, 1998, pp 119-138.

Xie QM, Tang HF, Chen JQ, Bian RL: Pharmacologic actions of tetrandrine in inflammatory pulmonary diseases. Acta Pharmacol Sin 2002;23:1107-1113.

# Hypersensitivity Pneumonitis

Method of
*Michael C. Zacharisen, MD*

Hypersensitivity pneumonitis (HP), or extrinsic allergic alveolitis, is an uncommon non-IgE-mediated immunologic inflammatory interstitial pulmonary disease caused by the inhalation of small organic antigens. This disease is seen primarily in adults in relation to occupations or hobbies, but it is reported in children when exposures occur in the residential environment.

## Etiology

Small (less than 5 $\mu m$) organic airborne antigens inhaled into the distal lower respiratory tract can activate alveolar macrophages and induce a cascade of inflammatory cytokines with features of both type III and type IV (antigen-antibody and delayed or cellular type) hypersensitivity reactions. This culminates in an interstitial inflammatory cell infiltration comprised of lymphocytes, plasma cells, and the formation of noncaseating granulomas. The inflammatory cytokines involved are typical of a T helper 1 (TH1) pattern such as $\gamma$-interferon, tumor necrosis factor-$\alpha$ (TNF-$\alpha$), and interleukin-1 (IL-1).

Antigens capable of inducing HP are derived from microorganisms (actinomycetes, bacteria, fungi, amoebae), animal (primarily avian) and plant products, low molecular weight chemicals, and various drugs (Table 1). Cigarette smoking appears to be protective from acute HP by affecting alveolar macrophage function but may worsen the prognosis for chronic HP. Genetic susceptibility is linked to polymorphisms in the promoter region of the TNF-$\alpha$ gene on chromosome 6, and a concomitant viral infection may increase the risk of developing HP.

## Clinical Presentation

Despite the wide variety of causative antigens, clinical presentation is similar and classified as acute, subacute, or chronic. Acute disease is characterized by abrupt onset of nonproductive cough, dyspnea, chest pain, chills, fever, and malaise 4 to 8 hours after exposure. This is typical of occupational HP occurring with exposures at the workplace and is also seen with certain hobbies. The subacute form is characterized by gradual progressive cough and dyspnea without fever and is related to frequent antigen exposure. The chronic form presents with insidious onset of dyspnea with exertion with nonproductive cough and occasional wheezing related to prolonged but low-grade antigen exposure. Fever is lacking, but weakness and weight loss are more common.

## Diagnosis

Acute HP is frequently diagnosed erroneously as infectious pneumonia, and chronic HP may be diagnosed as idiopathic pulmonary fibrosis because of the overlap in clinical findings. No single diagnostic test is available to confirm HP. A combination of elements from the history, physical examination, and basic laboratory, radiographic, and pulmonary function tests establish the diagnosis. Inquiry about home

**TABLE 1 Antigens Capable of Inducing Hypersensitivity Pneumonitis**

| Antigen | Exposure | Dust Source |
|---|---|---|
| Avian | Pigeon, parakeet, dove, duck, chicken, lovebird, goose, owl | Feather bloom or excrement from cage, nest, or coop |
| Bacteria | | |
|   Thermophilic | Farming, compost, building ventilation systems | Moist grain, hay, compost, heating, ventilating and air-conditioning (HVAC) system |
|   Nonthermophilic | Machinists | Metal working fluids* |
| Chemicals | Epoxy resin, plastic, paint | Diisocyanate* |
| Fungi | | |
| Outdoor | Farmers, peat moss workers, woodworkers, grain loaders | Compost, hay, grain, peat moss, wood, bark, sawdust |
| Indoor | Greenhouse, mushroom pickers, sauna water | Moldy airborne mists or disturbed moist soil |
| | Salami, cheese, mushroom, and malt industries | Aerosol mists in food preparation |
| Japan | Trichosporum | Moldy house dust in summer |
| Amoebae | Contaminated water | Residential humidifier |
| Medications | Amiodarone (Cordarone), clozapine (Clozaril), gold, nitrofurantoin (Macrodantin), $\beta$-blocker | Oral administration |
| Unknown | Pet fish food, tap water, mummy wrappings | |

*Also responsible for occupational asthma.

## CURRENT DIAGNOSIS

- History (acute, subacute, chronic):
  - Recurrent or chronic dry cough, dyspnea, chest pain
  - Poor response to asthma therapy and antibiotics
  - Improves with avoidance of offending antigen
- Environment: occupation, home, and hobby
  - Presence of dust, fumes, chemicals, fungi, bacteria, or birds
- Pulmonary function: restrictive defect with or without obstruction with decreased DLCO
- Exercise challenge: hypoxemia with exercise
- Radiologic: chest radiograph and high-resolution computed tomography
  - Interstitial ground glass, reticulonodular, bilateral diffuse infiltrates without lymphadenopathy or pleural fluid
- Laboratory:
  - Precipitating antibodies (indicate significant exposure, not disease)
  - Elevated inflammatory markers: ESR, CRP, LDH, and quantitative immunoglobulins (except IgE)
- Bronchoscopy with alveolar lavage
  - Lymphocytic alveolitis with T-cell subsets CD8+>CD4+ and negative cultures
- Histology: lung biopsy (not required)
  - Noncaseating granulomas and foamy alveolar macrophages, consistent with nonspecific interstitial pneumonitis (NSIP). No vasculitis demonstrated.

*Abbreviations:* CRP = C-reactive protein; DLCO = diffusing capacity of lung for carbon monoxide; ESR = erythrocyte sedimentation rate; LDH = lactate dehydrogenase.

and occupational exposures most often uncovers the sources and nature of the offending antigen.

Diagnostic criteria include the following:
- Symptoms compatible with HP
- Known exposure to an offending antigen
- Recurrent episodes of symptoms 4 to 8 hours after exposure
- Evidence of exposure to the offending antigen by serum precipitins and/or bronchoalveolar lavage fluid (BALF) antibody
- Findings compatible with HP on chest radiograph or high-resolution chest computed tomography (HRCT) scan
- BALF lymphocytosis (if bronchoalveolar lavage [BAL] performed)
- Lung histologic changes compatible with HP
- A "natural challenge" with reproduction of symptoms and laboratory abnormalities after exposure to the suspected environment

Minor criteria include bibasilar rales or crackles, restrictive ventilatory defect on lung function testing, decreased diffusing capacity, and arterial hypoxemia at rest or with exercise. Weight loss is a common finding, especially in children and in the chronic form. Invasive procedures including BAL and open lung biopsy are reserved for difficult cases.

## Treatment

Complete and indefinite avoidance of the causative antigen is most important. Treatment for acute HP includes oxygen, systemic corticosteroids, and antipyretics. For subacute HP, long-term alternate-day steroid therapy may be helpful. A trial of oral steroids for chronic HP is indicated and continued if clinical, radiologic, and pulmonary function parameters improve.

## CURRENT THERAPY

- Avoid offending antigen:
  - Remove/isolate antigen from environment
  - Example: Enclose machining processes, fungicides, biocides, improve ventilation, clean regularly, introduce air purifiers
  - Remove patient from environment
  - Example: change in occupation or hobby
  - Personal respiratory protection
- Oxygen
- Systemic corticosteroids
- Prednisone, 40–80 mg/d with a gradual taper
- Asthma therapy (if obstructive airway defect)

The most important aspect of treatment is avoidance of the offending antigen, whether it is specifically identified or suspected in the environment. Depending on the circumstances (industry versus home environment), intervention may entail personal respiratory protection, enclosing machining processes, changes in the heating, ventilation, air-conditioning process, or even a change of job duties. Changes in occupations and retraining, however, can lead to financial hardship.

Pharmacologic treatment for chronic or recurrent disease is less defined. There are insufficient data on using inhaled corticosteroids at this time. However, one case demonstrated successful treatment with beclomethasone in hydrofluoroalkane (HFA) propellant (QVAR[1]) likely with peripheral airway deposition because of its extrafine aerosol characteristics. Also, a teenager improved with pulse therapy using methylprednisolone (Solu-Medrol) in combination with budesonide inhalation (Pulmicort[1]).

When an obstructive defect is identified, treatment with inhaled corticosteroids, with or without long-acting inhaled bronchodilators, can be started. In challenge studies, albuterol (Proventil) was helpful when there was an acute fall in forced expiratory volume in 1 second ($FEV_1$). Similarly, inhaled cromolyn sodium (Intal[1]) prevented symptoms in the laboratory, but no evidence indicates that it prevents disease during times of natural exposure.

Experimental treatments include cyclosporin A[1] (Neoral) because of its anti-inflammatory effect on inflammatory cytokines produced by alveolar macrophages. Although there are promising in vitro effects of pentoxifylline[1] (Trental) on cytokine production from alveolar macrophages in patients with HP, clinical trials will be necessary to determine clinical efficacy.

## Prognosis

Early treatment of acute and subacute diseases typically results in complete recovery. Patients with the chronic form may experience permanent and progressive symptoms, especially if antigen exposure continues. Although oral steroids may decrease acute symptoms and improve pulmonary function, they do not appear to change the long-term outcome. Findings of pulmonary fibrosis with severe restrictive lung changes portend a poor prognosis. Depending on the antigen, fatalities range from 1% to 10%.

### REFERENCES

Fink JN, Ortega HG, Reynolds HY, et al: Needs and opportunities for research in hypersensitivity pneumonitis. Am J Respir Crit Care Med 2005;71:792-798.

Fink JN, Zacharisen MC: Hypersensitivity pneumonitis. In Adkinson NF, Yunginger JW, Busse WW, et al (eds): Allergy: Principles and Practice, 6th ed. St. Louis, Mosby, 2003, pp 1373-1390.

[1]Not FDA approved for this indication.

Jacobs RL, Andrews CP, Coalson JJ: Hypersensitivity pneumonitis: Beyond classic occupational disease-changing concepts of diagnosis and management. Ann Allergy Asthma Immunol 2005;95:115-128.

Kokkarinen JI, Tukiainen HO, Terho EO: Effect of corticosteroid treatment on the recovery of pulmonary function in farmer's lung. Am Rev Respir Dis 1992;145:3.

Lacasse Y, Selman M, Costabel U, et al: Clinical diagnosis of hypersensitivity pneumonitis. Am J Respir Crit Care Med 2003;168:952-958.

# Tuberculosis and Other Mycobacterial Diseases

Method of

*Surendra Kumar Sharma, MD, PhD, and
Alladi Mohan, MD*

Declared a global emergency in 1993 by the World Health Organization (WHO), tuberculosis (TB) continues to be a major public health problem throughout the world despite relentless global efforts directed at containing the scourge. The HIV infection and AIDS pandemic in the context of increased demographic pressure and poorly run control programs with low case finding and cure rates have been implicated as the cause of the global resurgence of TB.

## Epidemiology

It has been estimated that 2 billion people are infected with *Mycobacterium tuberculosis* globally. There were an estimated 9 million new TB cases and 1.7 million TB deaths in 2004. TB kills more women than all causes of maternal mortality combined.

The WHO African region has the highest estimated incidence rate, but most patients with TB are from the most populous countries of Asia. Current estimates reveal that India, China, Indonesia, Bangladesh, and Pakistan together account for nearly one half the new cases that arise every year. For 2005, a total of 14,093 TB cases (4.8 cases per 100,000 population) were reported in the United States; the TB rate in foreign-born persons in the United States was 8.7 times that of native-born persons. Wide disparities exist in the geographic distribution of cases in the United States.

In 2004, an estimated 13% of all new TB cases (34% in the African region) in adults were attributable to HIV/AIDS, as were 15.5% of the deaths from TB. As a result of HIV/AIDS, incidence of TB in certain countries has gone up by more than 6% per year, crippling the already overburdened health care resources. Despite a decreasing trend observed since 1992, TB still remains a serious public health problem among certain patient populations.

## Natural History

As the natural history of pulmonary TB is understood today, 70% of persons exposed do not get infected and only 30% develop infection. Among those infected, only about 10% develop progressive primary TB, in most cases within 2 years. The infection gets contained in the remaining 90% of the infected subjects, a condition termed *latent TB infection* (LTBI).

The unique ability of *M. tuberculosis* to persist for long periods unrecognized by the human immune system by as yet poorly understood mechanisms results in LTBI. Persons with LTBI are noninfectious and remain symptom free. Immunocompetent patients with LTBI have a 10% lifetime risk of developing reactivation of infection, resulting in postprimary TB; 50% of reactivations occur during the first 2 years of primary infection. In comparison, in HIV-infected persons with LTBI, the risk of reactivation is about 10% per year. Therefore, early diagnosis of persons with LTBI and institution of appropriate antituberculosis treatment can be rewarding, especially in industrialized nations, where prevalence of the active disease is low, because patients with LTBI act as reservoirs to contribute to the pool of active disease. On the other hand, in developing nations, the problem of LTBI might not be an important issue because of high prevalence of the active disease.

Multidrug-resistant tuberculosis (MDR-TB), caused by *M. tuberculosis* that is resistant to both isoniazid (INH, Nydrazid) *and* rifampin (Rifadin) with or without resistance to other drugs, is a phenomenon that is threatening to destabilize global TB control. According to current World Health Organization (WHO) and International Union Against Tuberculosis and Lung Disease (IUATLD) estimates, the median prevalence of MDR-TB has been 1.1% in patients with newly diagnosed disease. The fraction, however, is considerably higher (median prevalence, 7%) in patients who have previously received antituberculosis treatment. Incomplete and inadequate treatment are the most important factors leading to development of MDR-TB, suggesting that it is often a human-made tragedy. MDR-TB is a worldwide problem, being present in virtually all countries that were surveyed.

## Diagnosis

### LATENT INFECTION

The tuberculin skin test (TST) has been the most widely employed tool to detect LTBI. Published evidence suggests that treatment of LTBI results in considerable reduction of active disease. This has prompted the evolution of programs for targeted skin testing and latent tuberculosis treatment in countries such as the United States. In this approach, emphasis is on targeted tuberculin testing among persons at high risk for recent LTBI or with clinical conditions that increase the risk of progression of LTBI to active TB. Infected persons considered to be at high risk for developing active TB are offered treatment of LTBI irrespective of age.

The Mantoux method has been the preferred skin test for detecting LTBI caused by *M. tuberculosis*. It is administered by injecting 0.1 mL

### CURRENT DIAGNOSIS

- It is important to distinguish infection with *M. tuberculosis* from active TB disease.
- Diagnosing latent TB infection by targeted tuberculin skin testing and use of interferon-γ–based assays can facilitate institution of treatment for this condition.
- Patients with active TB disease present with constitutional symptoms such as fever, malaise, anorexia, weight loss, night sweats, and fatigue. They might also present with symptoms related to the organ system(s) involved. The symptoms classically evolve over 4 to 6 weeks.
- Atypical presentation is common in immunosuppressed persons, such as those with late HIV-infection, miliary TB, or occult extrapulmonary TB, resulting in a delay in the diagnosis.
- In patients suspected to have active TB disease, appropriate specimens must be collected for microscopic examination and mycobacterial culture and sensitivity testing and histopathologic examination.
- Diagnosis is established when clinical and radiologic findings are supported by microbiological or histologic evidence of TB.

*Abbreviation:* TB = tuberculosis.

of 5 tuberculin units (TU) of purified protein derivative (PPD) intradermally into the volar or dorsal surface of the forearm. The test is read 48 to 72 hours after administration, and the transverse diameter of induration is recorded in millimeters. Based on the patient scenario, three cut-off levels have been recommended for defining a positive tuberculin reaction: larger than 5 mm (for subjects who are at highest risk for developing TB disease), larger than 10 mm (for subjects with an increased probability of recent infection or with other clinical conditions that increase the risk of TB), and larger than 15 mm of induration (or subjects with no risk factors for TB) (Box 1).

For patients with a negative TST reaction who are subject to repeat TST testing, an increase in reaction size of greater than 10 mm within a period of 2 years should be considered a skin-test conversion suggesting recent infection with *M. tuberculosis*. TST is not contraindicated for persons who have been vaccinated with bacille Calmette-Guérin (BCG), and a positive reaction to tuberculin in BCG-vaccinated persons indicates infection with *M. tuberculosis* when the person tested is at increased risk for recent infection or has medical conditions that increase the risk of disease.

Use of TST for detecting LTBI is hampered by poor specificity in BCG-vaccinated populations and by its low sensitivity in

immunosuppressed persons, who are at highest risk for progression. Recently, blood tests based on detection of interferon-γ (IFN-γ) released by T lymphocytes in response to *M. tuberculosis*–specific antigens have become available, and these tests seem to offer an improvement over the TST. Compared with the TST, the IFN-γ–based assays that use *M. tuberculosis*–specific region of difference 1 (RD1) antigens such as early secretory antigenic target 6 (ESAT6) and culture filtrate protein 10 (CFP10) might have advantages over the TST. The IFN-γ assays are available in enzyme-linked immunosorbent assay (ELISA) (e.g., QuantiFERON-TB and the enhanced QuantiFERON-TB Gold assay) and enzyme-linked immunospot (ELISPOT) (e.g., T SPOT-TB assay) formats. The QuantiFERON-TB Gold assay is available in two formats, a 24-well culture plate format (approved by the FDA) and a newer, simplified in-tube format.[1,2] T SPOT-TB is marketed for use in Europe and is likely to receive FDA approval in the future. Recently, QuantiFERON-TB Gold assay received final approval from the FDA as an aid for diagnosing *M. tuberculosis* infection. These tests are more specific than TST in the BCG-vaccinated population, require no return visit, give results by the next day, and do not have boosting with repeated testing. However, like the TST, IFN-γ assays cannot reliably differentiate infection associated with TB disease from LTBI. The performance of QuantiFERON-TB Gold assay is being evaluated in the United States in certain populations targeted by TB control programs for detecting LTBI.

A chest radiograph (posteroanterior view for adults, with appropriate shielding if the subject is pregnant; posteroanterior and lateral views for children) is indicated for all patients being considered for treatment of LTBI to exclude active pulmonary TB. If the subject does not present with symptoms of active TB disease and the chest radiograph is normal, sputum smear examination for acid-fast bacilli (AFB) is not considered necessary, and the patient should be considered for treatment for LTBI.

## ACTIVE DISEASE

In immunocompetent persons with TB disease, pulmonary involvement occurs in 80% of patients, 15% have isolated extrapulmonary TB, and 5% can have pulmonary and extrapulmonary involvement. In contrast, in immunosuppressed persons such as those with late HIV infection, pulmonary involvement occurs in 30% of patients, 20% have isolated extrapulmonary TB, and 50% can have pulmonary and extrapulmonary involvement.

Patients with active TB disease present with constitutional symptoms such as fever, malaise, anorexia, weight loss, night sweats, and fatigue. They also present with symptoms related to the organ system(s) involved. For example, those with pulmonary TB complain of cough, sputum, and hemoptysis. The symptoms classically evolve over 4 to 6 weeks. However, atypical presentation is common in immunosuppressed patients such as those with late HIV infection, miliary TB, or occult extrapulmonary TB. This results in a delay in the diagnosis and therefore in the institution of specific antituberculosis treatment.

## Treatment

### PRETREATMENT EVALUATION

In many countries, the WHO guidelines that target resource-poor nations that have a high burden of TB are followed in national programs for control of TB. For operational, logistic, and economic reasons, these guidelines differ from those advocated by the guidelines of the American Thoracic Society, Centers for Disease Control and Prevention, and the Infectious Diseases Society of America (ATS/CDC/IDSA guidelines), which are followed in the United States.

In patients suspected to have active TB disease, the ATS/CDC/IDSA guidelines state that appropriate specimens must be collected for microscopic examination and mycobacterial culture and sensitivity testing.

---

---

[1]Not FDA approved for this indication.
[2]Not available in the United States.

## CURRENT THERAPY

- Treatment of TB has been considered the most cost-effective health intervention ever conceived. Antituberculosis treatment aims to kill the tubercle bacilli rapidly, prevent the emergence of drug resistance, and eliminate persistent bacilli from the host's tissues to prevent relapse.
- To accomplish these goals, several antituberculosis drugs must be taken together for a sufficiently long time.
- The decision to initiate antituberculosis treatment should be based on clinical, radiographic, microbiological, and histopathologic information.
- When the patient is seriously ill with a life-threatening condition (such as miliary disease, meningitis) that is believed to be possibly due to TB, treatment using one of the recommended regimens should be initiated promptly, often before AFB smear results are known and usually before mycobacterial culture results have been obtained.
- DOTS is considered an effective way to control TB. Efficiently run TB-control programs based on a policy of DOTS are essential for preventing the emergence of MDR-TB.
- Treatment of patients coinfected with HIV and TB is essentially similar to the treatment of TB in HIV-negative patients. Differences include potential for drug interactions between the rifamycins and antiretroviral agents and immune reconstitution inflammatory syndrome (IRIS) (paradoxical reactions).
- Management of MDR-TB is a challenge that should be undertaken by experienced clinicians at centers equipped with reliable laboratory services for mycobacterial cultures and in vitro sensitivity testing because it requires prolonged use of costly second-line drugs with a significant potential for toxicity.

*Abbreviations:* DOTS = directly observed therapy, short course; MDR = multidrug resistant; TB = tuberculosis.

In patients with suspected pulmonary TB, three sputum specimens must be obtained. If the patient is unable to produce adequate sputum, induction of sputum using hypertonic saline and bronchoscopy may be performed under appropriate infection-control measures. All patients with TB should have counseling and testing for HIV infection. A CD4+ T-lymphocyte count should be obtained for HIV-seropositive patients. These guidelines also suggest serologic testing for hepatitis B and C viruses (in patients with risk factors); baseline measurement of serum aminotransferases, bilirubin, alkaline phosphates, creatinine, and platelet count; and testing of visual acuity and red-green color discrimination if ethambutol (Myambutol) will be used.

## PRINCIPLES OF TREATMENT

Treatment of TB has been considered the most cost-effective health intervention ever conceived. Antituberculosis treatment aims to kill the tubercle bacilli rapidly, prevent the emergence of drug resistance, and eliminate persistent bacilli from the host's tissues to prevent relapse. To accomplish these goals, several antituberculosis drugs must be taken together for a sufficiently long period. WHO recommends the directly observed treatment short-course (DOTS) approach as the only way to control TB globally, and DOTS is the key principle on which many of the TB control programs are run globally. The WHO categorization of patients with TB and the appropriate treatment regimens for each category that is followed in many of the national TB control programs is shown in Table 1. Drugs currently used for treating TB, preparations available currently, the recommend dosage schedule, and regimens described in the ATS/CDC/IDSA guidelines for patients with drug-susceptible TB are listed in Tables 2, 3, and 4 and Box 2.

In the ATS/CDC/IDSA guidelines, the decision to initiate antituberculosis treatment should be based on any clinical, radiographic, microbiological, and histopathologic information that is available. In situations where the patient is seriously ill with a life-threatening condition (such as miliary disease, meningitis) that might be due to TB, treatment using one of the recommended regimens should be initiated promptly, often before AFB smear results are known and usually before mycobacterial culture results have been obtained. A positive smear for AFB provides strong inferential evidence for the diagnosis of TB. However, if clinical suspicion of active TB is high, TST is positive, the initial AFB smears are negative, and no other diagnosis is established, empiric treatment with the appropriate standard treatment regimen should be initiated. If the diagnosis is confirmed by isolation of *M. tuberculosis* or a positive nucleic acid amplification test, there is a clinical or radiographic response within 2 months of initiation of therapy, and no other diagnosis has been established, treatment may be continued to complete a standard course of therapy. If the patient is smear negative, *M. tuberculosis* cannot be isolated, and there is no clinical and radiologic improvement at the end of 2 months, antituberculosis treatment may have to be stopped and an alternative diagnosis must be considered.

In patients with drug-susceptible TB, antituberculosis treatment has two phases: the initial intensive phase, which consists of 2 months of treatment, and the maintenance (continuation) phase, which is usually 4 months. In some patients with potential for relapse, such as those with cavitary disease, and in patients with extrapulmonary disease, the maintenance phase might have to be extended by 3 more months beyond the scheduled 4 months. In TB meningitis, the continuation phase is administered for 10 months. The ATS/CDC/IDSA guidelines advocate the use of corticosteroids in patients with central nervous system TB (including meningitis) and TB pericarditis.

## MONITORING DURING TREATMENT

The patient must be closely monitored clinically, radiographically, and microbiologically at least monthly during the period of treatment to assess the response to treatment and identify possible adverse drug reactions. As per the ATS/CDC/IDSA guidelines, during treatment of patients with pulmonary TB, a sputum specimen for AFB smear and culture should be obtained at monthly intervals until two consecutive specimens are negative on culture. For patients who had positive AFB smears at the time of diagnosis, follow-up smears may be obtained at more frequent intervals until two consecutive specimens are negative. Drug susceptibility tests should be repeated on isolates from patients who have positive cultures after 3 months of treatment. Patients who have positive cultures after 4 months of treatment should be considered to have failed treatment and should be managed accordingly. For patients with extrapulmonary TB, the frequency and kind of evaluation will depend on the site involved and the ease with which specimens can be obtained.

For patients with positive cultures at diagnosis, a repeat chest radiograph at the completion of 2 months of treatment and at the completion of treatment is desirable but is not essential. In patients with negative initial cultures, a chest radiograph is necessary after 2 months of treatment, and a radiograph at the completion of treatment is desirable.

In patients with baseline laboratory abnormalities, liver and renal functions and platelet count might have to be repeated during the course of treatment to ensure that they are not deteriorating. Patients receiving ethambutol according to the standard dosage schedule should be questioned regarding vision symptoms during the monthly visits. If ethambutol is used in a higher dosage or if it is used for more than 2 months, monthly visual acuity and color vision checking must also be done.

Treatment is considered to be completed if the total number of doses are taken in the stipulated duration of treatment. Management of a

**TABLE 1** World Health Organization Standard Regimens for Treating Tuberculosis

| TB Patients | TB Treatment Regimens* | |
|---|---|---|
| | Initial Phase | Continuation Phase |
| **Diagnostic Category I** | | |
| New sputum smear–positive PTB | $2 H_3R_3Z_3E_3$ | $4 H_3R_3$ |
| New smear–negative PTB[†] with extensive parenchymal involvement | 2 HRZE | 4 HR |
| Severe concomitant HIV disease or severe forms of EPTB[‡§] | 2 HRZS | 4 HR |
| **Diagnostic Category II** | | |
| Sputum smear–positive relapse | $2 S_3H_3R_3Z_3E_3$ | $5 H_3R_3E_3$ |
| Sputum smear–positive treatment failure | $1 H_3R_3Z_3E_3$ | 5 HRE |
| Sputum smear–positive after treatment interruption | 2 HRZES/1HRZE | |
| **Diagnostic Category III** | | |
| Sputum smear–negative PTB and EPTB, not severe[¶] | $2 H_3R_3Z_3$ | $4 H_3R_3$ |
| | 2 HRZE | 4 HR |
| | 2 HRZS | 4 HR |
| **Diagnostic Category IV** | | |
| Chronic and MDR-TB cases | Specially designed standardized and individualized regimens will be required | |

*Either daily or three times per week. The number before the letters refers to the number of months of treatment. The subscript number after the letter refers to the number of doses per week.
[†]New sputum smear–negative PTB includes all forms of PTB other than primary complex.
[‡]Severe forms of EPTB include TBM, disseminated/miliary TB, TB pericarditis, TB peritonitis and intestinal TB, bilateral or extensive pleurisy, spinal TB with or without neurologic complications, genitourinary tract TB, and bone and joint TB.
[§]In patients with TBM on Category I treatment, the four drugs used during the intensive phase should be HRZS (instead of HRZE). Continuation phase of treatment in TBM and spinal TB with neurologic complications should be given for 6-7 months, extending the total duration of treatment to 8-9 months.
[¶]Not severe EPTB includes lymph node TB and unilateral pleural effusion.
*Abbreviations:* E = ethambutol (Myambutol); EPTB = extrapulmonary tuberculosis; H = isoniazid (INH); PTB = pulmonary tuberculosis; R = rifampin (Rifadin); S = streptomycin; TB = tuberculosis.; TBM = tuberculosis meningitis; Z = pyrazinamide.
Adapted from World Health Organization: Treatment of Tuberculosis: Guidelines for National Programmes. 3rd ed. Geneva: World Health Organization, 2003.

**TABLE 2** Drugs Used to Treat Tuberculosis

| Drug | Preparations |
|---|---|
| **First-Line Drugs** | |
| Isoniazid (INH, Nydrazid) | Tab: 50 mg,[2] 100 mg, 300 mg |
| | Elixir: 50 mg/5 mL |
| | Aqueous sol'n for IM or IV injection: 100 mg/mL |
| Ethambutol (Myambutol) | Tab: 100 mg, 400 mg, 800 mg,[2] 1000 mg[2] |
| Pyrazinamide | Tab: 500 mg (scored), 750 mg,[2] 1000 mg[2] |
| Rifabutin (Mycobutin)[1] | Cap: 150 mg |
| Rifampin (Rifadin) | Cap: 150 mg, 300 mg, 450 mg,[2] 600 mg[2] (powder may be suspended for PO dosing) |
| | Aqueous sol'n for IV injection[2] |
| | Powder for injection: 600 mg |
| Rifapentine (Priftin) | Tab: 150 mg (film coated) |
| **Second-Line Drugs** | |
| Amikacin[1] (Amikin) | Aqueous sol'n for IM or IV injection: 0.5-g and 1-g vials |
| p-Aminosalicylic acid (PAS) (Paser) | Granules: 4-g packets (can be mixed with food) |
| | Tab: 0.5 g, 1 g (film coated)[2] |
| | Sol'n for IV injection[2] |
| Capreomycin (Capastat) | Aqueous sol'n[2] for IM or IV injection |
| | Powder: 1-g vials for IM or IV injection |
| Cycloserine (Seromycin) | Cap: 250 mg |
| Ethionamide (Trecator-SC) | Tab: 250 mg |
| Gatifloxacin (Tequin)[1] | Tab: 200 mg, 400 mg |
| | Aqueous sol'n for IV injection: 200 mg/20 mL |
| Kanamycin[1] (Kantrex) | Aqueous sol'n for IM or IV injection: 0.5-g and 1-g vials |
| Levofloxacin (Levaquin))[1] | Tab: 250 mg, 500 mg, 750 mg |
| | Aqueous sol'n for IV injection: 0.5-g, 0.75-g vials |
| Moxifloxacin (Avelox))[1] | Tab: 400 mg |
| | Aqueous sol'n for IM or IV injection: 400 mg/250 mL |
| Streptomycin | Aqueous sol'n for IM or IV injection: 0.5-g and 1-g vials[2] |
| | Powder: 1-g vials for injection |

[1]Not FDA approved for this indication.
[2]Not available in the United States.
*Abbreviations:* cap = capsule; sol'n = solution; tab = tablet.

**TABLE 3  Dosage Schedule of First-Line Drugs Used in the Treatment of Tuberculosis**

| | | Dosage Interval | | |
|---|---|---|---|---|
| Drug* | Daily | 2 Days/Week | 3 Days/Week | Important Adverse Effects |
| **Ethambutol (Myambutol)†** | | | | |
| Adults 40-55 kg‡ | 14.5-20.0 mg/kg (800 mg) | 36.4-50.0 mg/kg (2000 mg) | 21.8-30.0 mg/kg (1200 mg) | Ocular toxicity, retrobulbar neuritis |
| Adults 56-75 kg‡ | 16.0-21.4 mg/kg (1200 mg) | 37.3-50.0 mg/kg (2800 mg) | 26.7-35.7 mg/kg (2000 mg) | |
| Adults 76-90 kg‡ | 17.8-21.1 mg/kg (1600 mg)§ | 44.4-52.6 mg/kg (4000 mg)§ | 26.7-31.6 mg/kg (2400 mg)§ | |
| Children | 15-20 mg/kg (1000 mg) | 50 mg/kg (2500 mg) | NA | |
| **Isoniazid (INH)** | | | | |
| Adults | 5 mg/kg (300 mg) | 15 mg/kg (900 mg) | 15 mg/kg (900 mg)¶ | Hepatotoxicity, CNS effects, lupus-like syndrome, hypersensitivity reactions |
| Children | 10-15 mg/kg (300 mg)¶ | 20-30 mg/kg (900 mg) | NA | |
| **Pyrazinamide** | | | | |
| Adults 40-55 kg‡ | 18.2-25.0 mg/kg (1000 mg) | 36.4-50.0 mg/kg (2000 mg) | 27.3-37.5 mg/kg (1500 mg) | |
| Adults 56-75 kg‡ | 20.0-26.8 mg/kg (1500 mg) | 40.0-53.6 mg/kg (3000 mg) | 33.3-44.6 mg/kg (2500 mg) | |
| Adults 76-90 kg‡ | 22.2-26.3 mg/kg (2000 mg)§ | 44.4-52.6 mg/kg (4000 mg)§ | 33.3-39.5 mg/kg (3000 mg)§ | Hepatotoxicity, hyperuricemia, arthralgias, GI tract upset |
| Children | 15-30 mg/kg (2000 mg) | 50 mg/kg (2000 mg) | NA | |
| **Rifabutin (Mycobutin)¹** | | | | |
| Adults | 5 mg/kg (300 mg) | 5 mg/kg (300 mg) | 5 mg/kg (300 mg) | Hepatotoxicity, cutaneous reactions; GI reactions, flu-like syndrome, orange discoloration of bodily fluids, drug interactions, uveitis |
| Children | NA | NA | NA | |
| **Rifampin (Rifadin)** | | | | |
| Adults | 10 mg/kg (600 mg) | 10 mg/kg (600 mg) | 10 mg/kg (600 mg) | Hepatotoxicity, cutaneous reactions; GI reactions, flu-like syndrome, orange discoloration of bodily fluids, drug interactions, uveitis |
| Children | 10-20 mg/kg (600 mg) | NA | 10-20 mg/kg (600 mg) | |

¹Not FDA approved for this indication.
*Maximum dosages are given in parentheses.
†Ethambutol can be used safely in older children, but it should be used with caution in children younger than 5 years, in whom visual acuity cannot be monitored. In younger children, ethambutol may be used at 15 mg/kg/d if there is suspected or proven resistance to isoniazid or rifampin.
‡Based on estimated lean body weight. Children weighing more than 40 kg should receive adult doses.
§Maximum dose regardless of weight.
¶The WHO recommends 10 mg/kg as the dose of isoniazid for adults for the thrice-weekly regimen. The WHO recommends 5 mg/kg as the dose of isoniazid for children for the daily regimen.
Adapted from Blumberg HM, Burman WJ, Chaisson RE, et al: American Thoracic Society, Centers for Disease Control and Prevention, and the Infectious Diseases Society: Treatment of tuberculosis. Am J Respir Crit Care Med 2003;167:603-662; and World Health Organization: Treatment of Tuberculosis: Guidelines for National Programmes, 3rd ed. Geneva: World Health Organization; 2003.
*Abbreviations:* CNS = central nervous system; GI = gastrointestinal; max = maximum; NA = no recommendation.

patient who has interrupted treatment is beyond the scope of this chapter, and the reader is referred to the ATS/CDC/IDSA guidelines for details.

## SPECIAL SITUATIONS

### Latent Infection

Various regimens available for treating LTBI are listed in Table 5. Completion of treatment for LTBI is based not only on the duration of treatment alone but also on the total number of doses administered. For example, the 9-month regimen of daily isoniazid should consist of 270 doses, at minimum, administered within 12 months, allowing for minor interruptions in therapy.

Hepatotoxicity is an important concern when isoniazid, pyrazinamide, and rifampin are being used. Baseline laboratory testing is not routinely indicated for all patients at the start of treatment for LTBI. However, liver function testing should be performed in HIV-positive patients, pregnant women and women in the immediate postpartum period, persons with a history of liver disease, and persons who consume alcohol regularly, among others. All patients receiving treatment should be monitored clinically; laboratory monitoring is indicated for patients whose baseline liver function tests are abnormal and for persons at risk for hepatic disease.

Laboratory monitoring should be used to evaluate possible adverse drug reactions that occur during the course of treatment. A 2-month regimen of rifampin and pyrazinamide regimen was offered in the ATS/CDC/IDSA statement published in 2000. After these guidelines were published, severe liver injury including deaths were reported among 5.8% of 1311 patients treated with the rifampin and pyrazinamide regimen. Revised guidelines recommended that the rifampin and pyrazinamide regimen should generally not be offered to patients with LTBI and that clinicians should choose from the alternative regimens. This regimen definitely should not be used in persons with underlying liver disease, history of alcoholism, or isoniazid-associated liver injury.

**TABLE 4  Treatment Regimens for Patients with Drug-Susceptible Tuberculosis**

| | Intensive Phase | | Maintenance Phase | | |
|---|---|---|---|---|---|
| Regimen | Interval and Doses* (Minimum Duration) | Regimen | Interval and Doses*† (Minimum Duration) | | Range of Total Doses (Minimum Duration) |
| **Regimen 1** RHZE | 7 d/wk for 56 doses (8 wk) *or* 5 d/wk for 40 doses (8 wk)‡ | RH | 7 d/wk for 126 doses (18 wk) *or* 5 d/wk for 90 doses (18 wk)‡ | | 130-182 (26 wk) |
| | | RH | Twice weekly for 36 doses (18 wk)§ | | 76-92 (26 wk) |
| | | RpH | Once weekly for 18 doses (18 wk)¶ | | 58-74 (26 wk) |
| **Regimen 2** RHZE | 7 d/wk for 14 doses (2 wk), then twice weekly for 12 doses (6 wk) | RH | Twice weekly for 36 doses (18 wk)§ | | 62-58 (26 wk) |
| | *or* 5 d/wk for 10 doses (2 wk),‡ then twice weekly for 12 doses (6 wk) | RpH | Once weekly for 18 doses (18 wk)¶ | | 44-40 (26 wk) |
| **Regimen 3** RHZE | Three times weekly for 24 doses (8 wk) | RH | Three times weekly for 54 doses (18 wk) | | 78 (26 wk) |
| **Regimen 4** RHE | 7 d/wk for 56 doses (8 wk) *or* 5 d/wk for 40 doses (8 wk)‡ | RH | 7 d/wk for 217 doses (31 wk) *or* 5 d/wk for 155 doses (31 wk)‡ | | 273-195 (39 wk) |
| | | RH | Twice weekly for 62 doses (31 wk) | | 118-102 (39 wk) |

*When DOT is used, drugs may be given 5 d/wk and the necessary number of doses adjusted accordingly. Although there are no studies that compare 5 with 7 daily doses, extensive experience indicates this would be an effective practice.
†Patients with cavitation on initial chest radiograph and positive cultures at completion of 2 months of therapy should receive a 7-month maintenance phase. The 7-month maintenance phase is 31 weeks, either 217 doses (daily) or 62 doses (twice weekly).
‡5 d/wk administration is always given by DOT.
§Not recommended for HIV-infected patients with CD4+ T lymphocyte count <100/μL.
¶Should be used only in HIV-negative patients who have negative sputum smears at the time of completion of 2 months of therapy and who do not have cavitation on the initial chest radiograph. For patients who started on this regimen and who have a positive culture in the 2-month specimen, treatment should be extended an extra 3 months.
*Abbreviations:* DOT = directly observed therapy; E = ethambutol; H = isoniazid; R = rifampin; Rp = rifapentine; Z = pyrazinamide.
Adapted from Blumberg HM, Burman WJ, Chaisson RE, et al: American Thoracic Society, Centers for Disease Control and Prevention, and the Infectious Diseases Society: Treatment of tuberculosis. Am J Respir Crit Care Med 2003;167:603-662.

---

**BOX 2  Fixed-Dose Combination Preparations**

These preparations are not available in the United States but are listed by the World Health Organization. Quality assurance is essential for ensuring adequate bioavailability while using fixed-dose combinations.

**Daily Regimens**
- Isoniazid + rifampin: 75 mg +150 mg tab, 150 mg +300 mg tab, 30 mg + 60 mg tab, or pack of granules for pediatric use
- Isoniazid + ethambutol: 150 mg + 400 mg tab
- Isoniazid + rifampin + pyrazinamide: 75 mg + 150 mg + 400 mg tab, 30 mg + 60 mg + 150 mg tab, or pack of granules for pediatric use
- Isoniazid + rifampin + pyrazinamide + ethambutol: 75 mg + 150 mg + 400 mg + 275 mg tab

**Thrice-Weekly Regimens**
- Isoniazid + rifampin: 150 mg +150 mg tab, 60 mg + 60 mg tab, or pack of granules for pediatric use
- Isoniazid + rifampin + pyrazinamide: 150 mg + 150 mg + 500 mg tab

*Abbreviation:* tab = tablet.

---

## Coinfection with HIV

Treatment of patients coinfected with HIV and TB is essentially similar to the treatment of TB in HIV-negative persons but with important differences. These include potential for drug interactions between rifamycins and antiretroviral agents and the immune reconstitution inflammatory syndrome (IRIS) (paradoxical reactions), which may be interpreted as clinical deterioration, treatment failure, or drug-resistant TB, among others. Low CD4+ count (<100/μL) at initiation of highly active antiretroviral therapy (HAART) and rapid initial fall in HIV-1 RNA level in response to HAART have been implicated as independent predictors for the development of IRIS.

In HIV-coinfected patients, once-weekly isoniazid-rifapentine (Priftin) should not be used in the continuation phase, and twice weekly isoniazid-rifampin or rifabutin (Mycobutin)[1] should not be used for patients with CD4+ T-lymphocyte counts less than 100/μL because these regimens can result in acquired rifamycin resistance. The optimal time of initiation of antiretroviral treatment in HIV-TB coinfected patients is not known. The ATS/IDSA/CDC guidelines advocate delaying the initiation of HAART until the intensive phase of antituberculosis treatment is completed, if possible. Treatment of HIV-TB coinfected patients must be undertaken by clinicians experienced in this area, and the timing of initiation of HAART should be carefully individualized, weighing the risk of progression of disease, drug interactions, and the benefits from treatment.

[1]Not FDA approved for this indication.

**TABLE 5  Recommended Treatment Regimens for Latent Tuberculosis**

| Drug Regimen | Dosage | | Comments |
|---|---|---|---|
| | Children | Adults | |
| Isoniazid daily for 9 mo | 10-20 mg/kg (max 300 mg) | 5 mg/kg (max 300 mg) | In HIV-infected patients, isoniazid may be administered concurrently with NRTIs or NNRTIs |
| Isoniazid twice-weekly for 9 mo | 20-40 mg/kg (max 900 mg) | 15 mg/kg (max 900 mg) | DOT must be used with twice-weekly dosing |
| Isoniazid daily for 6 mo | 10-20 mg/kg (max 300 mg) | 5 mg/kg (max 300 mg) | Not indicated for HIV-infected persons, those with fibrotic lesions on chest radiographs, or children |
| Isoniazid, twice-weekly for 6 mo | 20-40 mg/kg (max 900 mg) | 15 mg/kg (max 900 mg) | DOT must be used with twice-weekly dosing |
| Rifampin (Rifadin) daily for 4 mo | 10-20 mg/kg (max 600 mg) | 10 mg/kg (max 600 mg) | For persons who are contacts of patients with isoniazid-resistant, rifampin-susceptible TB who cannot tolerate pyrazinamide |

*Abbreviations:* DOT = directly observed therapy; HIV = human immunodeficiency virus; max = maximum; NRTIs = nucleoside reverse transcriptase inhibitors; NNRTIs = non-nucleoside reverse transcriptase inhibitors; TB = tuberculosis.
Data from American Thoracic Society and the Centers for Disease Control and Prevention: Targeted tuberculin testing and treatment of latent tuberculosis infection. Am J Respir Crit Care Med 2000;161(4 Pt 2):S221-S247; and Centers for Disease Control and Prevention (CDC); American Thoracic Society: Update: Adverse event data and revised American Thoracic Society/CDC recommendations against the use of rifampin and pyrazinamide for treatment of latent tuberculosis infection—United States, 2003. MMWR Morb Mortal Weekly Rep 2003;52:735-739.

### Relapse, Treatment Failure, and Drug-Resistant Tuberculosis

A patient who becomes and remains culture-negative while receiving antituberculosis treatment but, at some point after completion of therapy, either becomes culture-positive again or experiences clinical or radiographic deterioration consistent with active tuberculosis is said to have developed *relapse*. Both drug-susceptible and drug-resistant strains can result in relapse. *Treatment failure* is defined as continued or recurrently positive cultures in a patient receiving appropriate antituberculosis treatment. Vigorous microbiological evaluation must be undertaken in patients who present with relapse or treatment failure so that true relapse and drug-resistant TB are identified.

Efficiently run TB control programs based on a policy of DOTS are essential for preventing the emergence of MDR-TB. The management of MDR-TB is a challenge that should be undertaken by experienced clinicians at centers equipped with reliable laboratory services for mycobacterial cultures and in vitro sensitivity testing because it requires the prolonged use of costly second-line drugs with a significant potential for toxicity. Already several countries, with the help of the WHO's Green Light Committee, are rolling out DOTS-Plus, WHO's supplemental strategy to treat MDR-TB, for use in areas with a high prevalence of MDR-TB. The judicious use of drugs; supervised standardized treatment; focused clinical, radiologic, and bacteriologic follow-up; and surgery at the appropriate juncture are key factors in the successful management of these patients.

## Nontuberculous Mycobacterial Disease

The term *nontuberculous mycobacteria* (NTM) is applied to mycobacteria other than *M. tuberculosis* complex that are ubiquitously found in the environment. NTM can cause transient infection, colonize the airways, or contaminate clinical specimens. Classification of NTM recovered from humans is shown in Box 3.

### CLINICAL PRESENTATION AND DIAGNOSTIC CRITERIA

NTM can cause localized pulmonary disease; lymphadenitis; skin, soft tissue, and skeletal infection; infection of bursae, joints, tendon sheaths, and bones; or disseminated disease that may be found in patients with and without AIDS. The diagnosis of NTM infection is suspected based on the clinical presentation and radiographic abnormalities, and

it is confirmed by microbiological characterization. The staining and culture methods, species identification, and susceptibility testing for NTM are beyond the scope of this chapter, and the reader is referred to the ATS 1997 guidelines for details.

### TREATMENT

Treatment of NTM disease requires prolonged administration of multiple drugs. At the time of initial presentation, NTM disease can closely mimic TB, and antituberculosis treatment is often initiated in many of these patients. Thus, by the time the microbiological confirmation is obtained, many patients would have completed the intensive phase of standard antituberculosis treatment. Once laboratory confirmation is obtained, the treatment must be modified to include specific regimens. Direct observation of treatment might not be required in NTM disease because there is no person-to-person transmission and NTM disease does not constitute a public health hazard.

Adult patients with *M. kansasii* pulmonary disease can be treated with a daily three-drug regimen containing isoniazid[1] (300 mg), rifampin[1] (600 mg), and ethambutol[1] (25 mg/kg for 2 mo, then 15 mg/kg) for 18 months. A minimum of 1 year of culture negativity must be ensured. In HIV-positive patients who take protease inhibitors, clarithromycin (Biaxin)[1] or rifabutin[1] will need to be substituted for rifampin.

HIV-negative adults with *M. avium* complex (MAC) pulmonary disease, may be treated with a daily three-drug regimen containing clarithromycin (500 mg twice a day) or azithromycin (250 mg), rifampin[1] (600 mg) or rifabutin (300 mg), and ethambutol[1] (25 mg/kg for 2 months, then 15 mg/kg). Additionally, streptomycin[1] (two to three times per week) can be given for the first 8 weeks. Patients should receive treatment until they remain culture negative for 12 months. Adult HIV-negative patients with disseminated MAC disease should be started on daily clarithromycin (500 mg twice a day) or azithromycin (250 to 500 mg), ethambutol[1] (15 mg/kg /day) and rifampin[1] (600 mg), or rifabutin (300 mg/day). In adult HIV-positive patients with disseminated MAC disease, daily clarithromycin (500 mg twice a day) or azithromycin (250-500 mg), plus ethambutol[1] (15 mg/kg /day) alone may have to be used so that HAART can be administered, avoiding drug interactions with rifamycins. Therapy is considered as long as the cultures remain positive, and discontinuation of treatment can only be considered if the culture remains negative for 12 months. Often patients receive lifetime treatment.

---

[1]Not FDA approved for this indication.

## BOX 3 Classification of Nontuberculous *Mycobacterium* Species Recovered from Humans

**Common Etiologic Species**

**Pulmonary Disease**
- *M. abscessus*
- *M. avium* complex
- *M. kansasii*
- *M. malmoense*
- M. xenopi

**Lymphadenitis**
- *M. abscessus*
- *M. chelonae*
- *M. fortuitum*
- *M. marinum*
- *M. ulcerans*

**Cutaneous Disease**
- *M. abscessus*
- *M. chelonae*
- *M. fortuitum*
- *M. marinum*
- *M. ulcerans*

**Disseminated Disease**
- *M. avium* complex
- *M. chelonae*
- *M. haemophilum*
- *M. kansasii*

**Unusual Etiologic Species**

**Pulmonary Disease**
- *M. asiaticum*
- *M. celatum*

- *M. fortuitum*
- *M. haemophilu*
- *M. shimodii*
- *M. simiae*
- *M. smegmatis*
- *M. szulgai*

**Lymphadenitis**
- *M. avium* complex
- *M. haemophilum*
- *M. kansasii*
- *M. nonchromogenicum*
- *M. smegmatis*

**Cutaneous Disease**
- *M. avium* complex
- *M. haemophilum*
- *M. kansasii*
- *M. nonchromogenicum*
- *M. smegmatis*

**Disseminated Disease**
- *M. abscessus*
- *M. conspicuum*
- *M. fortuitum*
- *M. genavense*
- *M. malmoense*
- *M. marinum*
- *M. simiae*
- *M. xenopi*

285

Adapted from American Thoracic Society: Diagnosis and treatment of disease caused by nontuberculous mycobacteria. Am J Respir Crit Care Med 1997;156(2 Pt 2):S1-S25.

Surgical excision still remains the primary treatment for NTM cervical lymphadenitis, with cure rates of about 95%. In patients with extensive disease or a poor response to surgery, a clarithromycin-containing regimen[1] may be tried. Nonpulmonary disease caused by *M. fortuitum, M. abscessus,* or *M. chelonae* responds to amikacin (Amikin)[1] and clarithromycin,[1] and therapy should be based on in vitro susceptibility tests.

In adults with AIDS who have a CD4[+] T-lymphocyte count of less than 50 cells/μL, especially with a previous history of a opportunistic infection, prophylaxis for disseminated MAC disease must be administered with rifabutin 300 mg/day, clarithromycin 500 mg twice daily, azithromycin 1200 mg once weekly, or azithromycin 1200 mg once weekly plus rifabutin 300 mg daily.

## REFERENCES

American Thoracic Society: Diagnostic standards and classification of tuberculosis in adults and children. This statement was endorsed by the Council of the Infectious Diseases Society of America. (IDSA), September 1999. Am J Respir Crit Care Med 2000;161:1376-1395.

American Thoracic Society: Diagnosis and treatment of disease caused by nontuberculous mycobacteria. Am J Respir Crit Care Med 1997;156(2 Pt 2): S1-S25.

American Thoracic Society and the Centers for Disease Control and Prevention: Targeted tuberculin testing and treatment of latent tuberculosis infection. This statement was endorsed by the Council of the Infectious Diseases Society of America. (IDSA), September 1999. Am J Respir Crit Care Med 2000;161(4 Pt 2):S221-S247.

American Thoracic Society; Centers for Disease Control and Prevention; Infectious Diseases Society of America: Controlling tuberculosis in the United States. Am J Respir Crit Care Med 2005;172:1169-1227.

Blumberg HM, Burman WJ, Chaisson RE, et al; American Thoracic Society, Centers for Disease Control and Prevention, and the Infectious Diseases Society: Treatment of tuberculosis. Am J Respir Crit Care Med 2003; 167:603-662.

Centers for Disease Control and Prevention (CDC): Trends in tuberculosis—United States, 2005. MMWR Morb Mortal Wkly Rep 2006;55:305-308.

Centers for Disease Control and Prevention (CDC): Guidelines for the investigation of contacts of persons with infectious tuberculosis: Recommendations from the National Tuberculosis Controllers Association and CDC. MMWR Morb Mortal Wkly Rep 2005;54:1-47.

Centers for Disease Control and Prevention (CDC); American Thoracic Society: Update: Adverse event data and revised American Thoracic Society/CDC recommendations against the use of rifampin and pyrazinamide for treatment of latent tuberculosis infection—United States, 2003. MMWR Morb Mortal Wkly Rep 2003;52:735-739.

Dye C: Global epidemiology of tuberculosis. Lancet 2006;367:938-940.

Sharma SK, Liu JJ: Progress of DOTS in global tuberculosis control. Lancet 2006;367:951-952.

Sharma SK, Mohan A: Multidrug-resistant tuberculosis: A menace that threatens to destabilize tuberculosis control. Chest 2006;130:261-272.

World Health Organization: Treatment of Tuberculosis: Guidelines for National Programmes, 3rd ed. Geneva: World Health Organization; 2003.

[1]Not FDA approved for this indication.

# The Cardiovascular System

## Acquired Diseases of the Aorta

Method of
*John Byrne, MCh, and*
*R. Clement Darling III, MD*

The management of aortic diseases continues to evolve. The certainties of a decade or two ago have been replaced by questions about new technology. The paradigm shift in general surgery from open to minimally invasive therapy has been mirrored in aortic surgery. Diagnosis now depends more on computed tomography (CT) and magnetic resonance scanning than catheter-based angiography. Treatment has also changed: At the Albany Medical Center, 65% of patients now undergo stenting of their aortic aneurysms; no such stenting was done in 1997. Acquired aortic diseases fall into three categories: aneurysmal disease, occlusive disease, and aortic dissection.

## ANEURYSMAL DISEASES OF THE AORTA

According to Sir William Osler, Canadian physician and educator (1849–1919), "There is no disease more conducive to clinical humility than aneurysm of the aorta." Abdominal aortic aneurysms (AAAs) continue to be a major cause of death. Their first manifestation may be circulatory collapse. They are no respecters of social position or standing: both Charles de Gaulle and Albert Einstein succumbed to ruptured aneurysms. Mortality for elective repair is 2% to 5%. The mortality rate for patients with ruptured AAAs who make it to hospital is 40% or greater. The goal, therefore, is to prevent rupture.

## Definitions

An aneurysm is a permanent focal swelling of an artery. By consensus, an artery is considered to be *aneurysmal* when its diameter increases by 50%. The normal diameter of the male infrarenal aorta is 2.1 cm; the normal female aorta is 1.9 cm. *Ectasia* is diffuse dilation, whereas *arteriomegaly* refers to arteries that are enlarged but not aneurysmal. *Small* AAAs are 3.0 to 5.5 cm by ultrasound; *large* ones are those more than 5.5 cm.

*Inflammatory* aneurysms are AAAs characterized by an intense sterile fibrosis around the aorta and surrounding tissues, often with ureteric obstruction. Mycotic aneurysms are those caused by bacterial infection, most commonly Salmonella. They are never caused by a fungus, despite their name.

## Epidemiology

Approximately 15,000 people die annually in the United States from ruptured AAAs. The incidence of abdominal aortic aneurysms is 36.5 to 49.3 per 100,000 person-years with a male-to-female ratio of 4:1. In men 65 to 80 years of age, 4.3% to 7.1% have an AAA. Thoracic aneurysms have an incidence of 5.9 per 100,000 person-years. They affect the ascending aorta in 40% to 50%, the aortic arch in 10% to 15%, and the descending aorta (including thoracoabdominal) in 35% to 45%.

## Natural History

Aortic aneurysms usually grow at 2 to 3 mm per year. Approximately 20% grow at more than 4 mm per year. There is no means of identifying "rapid growers." The only factor that independently increases growth rate is cigarette smoking. Risk of rupture is directly related to sac diameter. The "small aneurysm" trials have confirmed that the risk of rupture for AAAs less than 5.5 cm in size is 1% or less per annum. Large AAAs measuring 5.5 to 7.0 cm have an annual rupture risk of 6.6%. For an aneurysm larger than 7 cm, the risk rises to 20%. Perhaps owing to their smaller aortas, women have a four times' increased risk of rupture in the 5.0 to 5.9 cm range compared to men, so there may be good reason to intervene at 5 cm in women.

For thoracic aortic aneurysms (TAAs) less than 6 cm in size, the rupture rate at 3 years is 16%. For TAAs larger than 7 cm, the risk is 31%.

## Etiology

AAAs are not simply atherosclerotic, although these patients often have atheroma-related diseases. Patients with low ankle-brachial pressure indexes (ABPIs) indicating peripheral vascular disease have lower rates of expansion than those with normal ABPIs. The two main pathologic processes are proteolysis and inflammation. In AAAs, the adventitia has an intense lymphocytic infiltration, whereas the media is thin with elastin fragments. A subset of enzymes called matrix metalloproteinases (MMPs) are implicated in expansion, specifically MMP-2, MMP-3, and MMP-9. MMPs are normally involved in connective tissue repair. There is also an inherited component to AAAs, as the incidence in first-degree male relatives is six times greater than expected.

Thoracic aortic aneurysms are related to previous aortic dissection, atherosclerosis, collagen vascular diseases (e.g., Marfan's syndrome, autoimmune disorders, Takayasu's arteritis), and syphilis. In some series, chronic dissection accounts for a third of all thoracic aneurysms.

## Diagnosis

Abdominal aortic aneurysms are usually asymptomatic. Back pain indicates either acute expansion of an existing AAA or an inflammatory aneurysm. Rupture is indicated by severe abdominal and back pain and shock. Clinical examination in a thin patient with a large aneurysm is frequently diagnostic. In overweight patients, however, clinical examination can be negative even in the presence of sizable aneurysms. Ultrasound is a reliable and inexpensive diagnostic tool. Many AAAs are picked up incidentally on ultrasound or CT scanning. In patients in whom intervention is planned, a spiral CT scan gives essential additional information.

With thoracic and thoracoabdominal aortic aneurysms, rupture may also be the first indication. Many are discovered incidentally on chest CT or suspected on the basis of an abnormal chest radiograph. Chest, back, and abdominal pain are the most common symptoms. Aortic root dilation may lead to symptoms of congestive heart failure because of aortic insufficiency.

## Treatment

### MEDICAL MANAGEMENT

If risk of rupture of an AAA is related to size, then limiting expansion should prevent rupture. Controlling blood pressure was thought, at one stage, to prevent expansion. However, the only trial of the effects of β-blockers (propranolol) showed no effect on AAA expansion, and there was a large dropout rate because of side effects of the medication. If enzymatic or inflammatory processes are involved, inhibition of these processes ought to prevent expansion. Currently, doxycycline[1] is being evaluated because it is a potent inhibitor of all MMPs.

### SURGICAL TREATMENT

Operative mortality rates are 2% to 5%. The most common approach is a transperitoneal approach to the aorta via a vertical laparotomy incision. A transverse laparotomy incision is sometimes used in patients with pulmonary compromise. An alternative approach, and the one we prefer, is retroperitoneal repair through a left flank incision through the left tenth intercostal space. This affords better access to the proximal neck, results in less pulmonary compromise, and, being extraperitoneal, reduces postoperative ileus. Despite the morbidity involved, open repair is durable and the need for reintervention rare.

Surgery for isolated thoracic aneurysms depends on location and extent. Aneurysms involving the ascending aorta and transverse aorta require cardiopulmonary bypass. The aortic valve is usually replaced with ascending aortic aneurysms, and the arch vessels require implantation with aneurysms of the transverse aorta. Aneurysms confined to the descending aorta traditionally were repaired using a standard Gore-Tex or Dacron tube with reimplantation of the intercostal vessels to reduce the risk of paraplegia. Many of these descending aneurysms are now stented.

Surgery for thoracoabdominal aortic aneurysms is complex and challenging. It is usually performed through a posterolateral thoracotomy incision (fifth and sixth intercostal spaces) using partial cardiopulmonary bypass. Operative mortality is 5% to 10% with paraplegia rates from 5% to 15%.

### ENDOVASCULAR TREATMENT

Endovascular repair involves exposure of the femoral arteries under local, spinal, or general anesthesia. An endograft is then introduced through these groin incisions under radiographic guidance and deployed just distal to the renal arteries. The stent-graft device is then fixed distally in

---

[1]Not FDA approved for this indication.

## CURRENT DIAGNOSIS

**Abdominal Aortic Aneurysms**

- Men > 60 y are most at risk.
- AAAs are usually asymptomatic and often clinically undetected.
- Ultrasound is the test of choice for screening for abdominal aortic aneurysms.

**Aortoiliac Occlusive Disease**

- History and clinical examination are usually diagnostic.
- Pulse volume recordings (PVRs) are usually confirmatory.
- Magnetic resonance angiography (MRA) or contrast angiography is confirmatory.

**Acute Aortic Dissection**

- Awareness of the condition is essential.
- Chest radiographs can point to the diagnosis but are normal in up to 20% of patients.
- Computed tomography and transesophageal echocardiography are the gold standards in diagnosis.

---

the iliacs. The requirements for stenting are a good proximal aortic neck of 1.5 cm or more to fix the device proximally and healthy iliacs to fix the device distally. Exclusion criteria are extreme angulation of the proximal neck or lack of a good proximal neck (juxtarenal AAAs), occluded iliacs precluding delivery of the device to the aorta, or tortuosity of the iliacs. Endovascular aneurysm repair (EVAR) also mandates close CT follow-up to detect graft migration or leakage around the stented graft ("endoleaks"). Approximately 6% of patients per annum require secondary interventions for graft-related problems with current technology. In 2004 and 2005, the results of the first randomized control trials were reported. There were significantly lower mortality rates in patients undergoing EVAR (1.2% to 1.7%) versus open repair (4.6% to 4.7%).

Given the morbidity from open surgery for thoracic aneurysms, EVAR has potential advantages. At our institution, most descending

## CURRENT THERAPY

**Abdominal Aortic Aneurysms**

- There are no proven treatments to prevent AAA expansion.
- Traditional open repair of AAAs has a 2%–5% mortality rate.
- Early data comparing endovascular aneurysm repair (EVAR) with open surgery show EVAR has a significantly lower perioperative mortality.

**Aortoiliac Occlusive Disease**

- Angioplasty and stenting is a good option for high-risk patients or iliac lesions.
- Aortobifemoral bypass is the gold standard treatment but carries a 4%–6% operative mortality.
- Axillobifemoral bypass is reserved for high-risk patients who require surgical bypass.

**Acute Aortic Dissection**

- Stanford type A dissections are treated surgically.
- Medical therapy is preferred for Stanford type B dissections.
- Endovascular therapy is increasingly being used for type B dissections.

thoracic aneurysms are treated this way. Reported mortality rates are 0% to 4% with a 0% to 1.6% paraplegia rate. Thoracoabdominal aneurysms are more difficult to treat, and despite some reports of endovascular treatment, their complexity has led some to question whether they are a "bridge too far" for endoluminal therapy.

## SCREENING

As a screening tool, clinical examination is not useful. Ultrasound is highly sensitive and specific, noninvasive, and cheap—the ideal screening tool. Does it reduce mortality? The largest study enrolled more than 27,000 male patients and showed a 53% reduction in AAA-related mortality in screened versus nonscreened patients. Despite the absence of a national screening program, deaths from ruptured AAAs are decreasing in the United States despite operative mortality remaining constant. This is probably because of the number detected "incidentally" on routine scanning.

# OCCLUSIVE DISEASE OF THE AORTA

René Leriche, a French surgeon (1879–1955), wrote this in 1923: "The ideal treatment [of occlusion of the aortic bifurcation] would be the excision of the occluded part.... and re-establishment of arterial continuity....This ideal will never be achieved."

Atherosclerosis affects both the thoracic and abdominal aorta. When it affects the abdominal aorta, it is primarily occlusive, producing symptoms because of low perfusion. When atherosclerosis affects the thoracic aorta, it is primarily ulcerative and produces embolic disease.

## Definitions

Aortoiliac occlusive lesions are classified according to the TransAtlantic Inter-Society Consensus (TASC) document as types A to D. Type A lesions are single focal stenoses affecting a single iliac artery. The focus of this section is type D lesions, which are those affecting the aorta and usually both iliacs.

Ulcerative atherosclerotic plaques of the thoracic aorta are classified as 1 to 5, with 1 being normal and 5 being the presence of a mobile plaque.

## Epidemiology

Peripheral vascular disease affects 5 million Americans. It is difficult to estimate how many have aortoiliac occlusive disease.

In contrast, the prevalence of aortic atheroma among patients undergoing transesophageal echocardiography (TEE) for routine clinical indications is 8%. It is 38% in those with known carotid disease, and with coronary disease as many as 90% are affected.

## Natural History

From the few natural history studies, patients with lesions confined to the aortic bifurcation tend to be female and have a longer life expectancy than those with more extensive disease.

However, there are many prospective studies of thoracic plaques. High-grade lesions are particularly dangerous. In one study, the risk for cerebral or peripheral events was 33% at 14 months.

## Etiology

As with atherosclerosis elsewhere, the major risk factors are male gender, advancing age, smoking, dyslipidemia, diabetes mellitus, and hypertension. Hyperhomocysteinemia is also now recognized as a significant factor in disease progression. Of these factors, smoking is the factor that is most modifiable.

# Diagnosis

Patients with aortoiliac occlusive disease (AIOD) complain of buttock or thigh claudication or occasionally rest pain. In men, a history of impotence may also point to the diagnosis (Leriche syndrome). Femoral pulses are absent or markedly reduced. Pulse volume recordings (PVRs) show damped or monophasic signals over the femoral arteries. Magnetic resonance angiography (MRA) is noninvasive and accurate and avoids use of nephrotoxic dye. Aortic surgery can be planned on the basis of good-quality MRA images. Formal angiography has long been the gold standard of investigation of occlusive disease. However, in the presence of severe occlusive disease of the aorta and iliacs, patients may need a transaxillary or transbrachial approach. Rarely, AIOD is a source of peripheral atheroemboli producing "blue-toe syndrome."

Thoracic plaques may be asymptomatic or produce emboli resulting in stroke, mesenteric ischemia, or acute extremity ischemia. These lesions are also a source of cerebral emboli when the aorta is manipulated during cardiac surgery. Diagnosis is made by TEE.

# Treatment

## MEDICAL MANAGEMENT

Smoking cessation is key to successful management. All patients should be on low-dose aspirin, and after the Clopidogrel versus Aspirin in Patients at Risk of Ischemic Events (CAPRIE) trial, there is evidence for the addition of clopidogrel (Plavix). All patients should be placed on a statin regardless of cholesterol level. Exercise regimens and oral agents like cilostazol (Pletal) are beneficial. However, aortic disease responds less well to these regimens than infrainguinal disease.

## ENDOVASCULAR TREATMENT

Balloon angioplasty of the abdominal aorta has always been a concern in case of aortic rupture. However, stenting of isolated aortic lesions can be performed safely in selected patients using smaller stents to reduce trauma to the aortic wall. Lesions at the aortic bifurcation and proximal common iliacs have been safely stented for many years using the so-called kissing-stent technique.

## SURGICAL OPTIONS

In patients with aortic atherosclerosis, surgery is often required. The options are aortobifemoral bypass, endarterectomy of the aorta and iliacs, or extra-anatomic bypass with an axillobifemoral bypass or femoro-femoral bypass. Rarely, the thoracic aorta can be used as an inflow source to perform a thoracofemoral bypass. Mortality rates for aortobifemoral bypass are 4% to 6%. This is higher than AAA repair because of coexisting cardiopulmonary and cerebrovascular disease. Patency rates for aortobifemoral bypass are superb, however, with 10-year patency rates in the order of 90%. Axillobifemoral bypass and femoro-femoral bypass have lower morbidities than aortic bypass, but patency rates are only 60% to 80% at 5 years. Therefore, it is reserved for high-risk patients with lower life expectancy.

# AORTIC DISSECTION

"The diagnosis [of aortic dissection]…chiefly depends upon recognition and interpretation of the facts… together with an ever alert suspicion on the part of the physician" (Willius FA, Cragg RW: Mayo Clin Proc, 1941). Acute aortic dissection (AAD) is a catastrophic event. It can be a difficult diagnosis in the emergency setting. In an autopsy study in 2000, acute aortic dissection was the initial clinical impression in only 15% of patients dying from AAD. Awareness of the condition is still paramount in making the diagnosis.

# Definitions

An aortic dissection occurs when an intimal tear allows blood to enter the media. Blood then propagates along the aorta. There are two classification systems: the Stanford and the DeBakey. The Stanford system classifies dissections as type A if the ascending aorta is involved; type B if the descending aorta is affected. In the DeBakey system, type 1 involves the whole aorta and originates in the ascending aorta, type 2 is confined to the ascending aorta, and type 3 includes those distal to the left subclavian artery.

# Epidemiology

Approximately 2000 cases of aortic dissection occur annually in the United States. It is often stated that AAD is the most common aortic catastrophe. This is not quite accurate. Population studies from the Mayo Clinic show the incidence of AAD is 3.5 per 100,000 people. This is identical to that of ruptured thoracic aneurysm but less than that for ruptured AAA (9/100,000). Males are three times more likely than females to have AAD. Half the females affected by AAD are younger than 40 years and often in the third trimester of pregnancy. Interestingly, AAD exhibits chronobiologic variations with a peak onset in the morning and in winter.

# Natural History

Contemporary data show that 21% of patients with aortic dissections die before admission to the hospital. Most natural history studies come from the "pretreatment" era. Untreated type A dissections have a 25% mortality at 24 hours, 70% mortality at 1 week, and 80% mortality at 2 weeks.

# Etiology

The key predisposing factor for AAD is *cystic medial necrosis,* which makes the layers of the aorta less cohesive. Approximately 5% to 10% of AAD patients have an underlying connective tissue disease such as Marfan's or Ehlers-Danlos syndrome. Intimal tears are more likely at points of increased wall stress. The repetitive pulsation of the ascending aorta with each ventricular contraction makes it the most vulnerable area of the aorta. Accordingly, most AADs occur in the ascending aorta (65%). The transverse aorta is affected in 10% and the descending aorta in 25%. Almost 90% of patients are hypertensive. Approximately 15% of patients have no intimal tear but have a spontaneous intramural hematoma because of rupture of vasa vasorum in the aortic wall.

# Diagnosis

Osler stated in 1910 that "a spontaneous tear of the arterial coats is associated with atrocious pain, with symptoms, indeed, in the case of the aorta, of angina pectoris and many instances have been mistaken for it." This remains true. However, if dissection of the transverse aorta occurs, stroke or arm ischemia may be a symptom because of carotid or subclavian occlusion. Involvement of the mesenteric or renal vessels may lead to bowel ischemia or renal failure, and extension to the aortic bifurcation may result in leg ischemia. CT scanning with intravenous contrast is diagnostic. Magnetic resonance angiography and conventional angiography are also useful. TEE determines the site of origin of the dissection, which guides therapy.

# Treatment

## MEDICAL TREATMENT

The goal of medical therapy is to reduce mean arterial blood pressure to 60 to 75 mm Hg. The drugs most frequently used are sodium nitroprusside (Nitropress) and labetalol (Trandate), a combined α- and β-blocker. Patients with Stanford B dissections not involving any of the major aortic branches have a 75% survival rate whether treated medically or surgically. Because many patients with type B dissections are older, medical therapy is more commonly employed. For type A, medical therapy is of little help because of the likelihood of retrograde dissection and cardiac tamponade.

## SURGICAL TREATMENT

For type A dissections, surgery is mandatory. Surgery aims to excise and replace the segment of aorta containing the intimal dissection rather than replace the entire dissected aorta. Even in expert hands, this is associated with mortality rates of up to 20% at 30 days. With type B dissections, emergency surgery is reserved for those patients with visceral, renal, or extremity ischemia.

## ENDOVASCULAR TREATMENT

Because surgery for type B dissections carries at least 11% mortality and the goal of therapy is to seal the "entry point" of the dissection, treatment of AAD by a covered stent-graft seems a plausible idea. Closure of the primary entry tear produces thrombosis of the false lumen that ought to produce a good long-term outcome. However, the walls of freshly dissected aortas are not robust. Despite the absence of controlled trials, initial reports suggest endovascular stenting is at least as good as medical therapy. However, evidence on long-term outcomes is lacking.

The management of acquired aortic diseases is changing. "Doubt is not a pleasant condition, but certainty is absurd," commented Voltaire (1694–1778), the French author and philosopher. The future may bring about advances in medical treatment of AAAs and atherosclerotic disease. Advances in molecular biology may allow for specific targeting of enzymatic defects underlying aneurysmal disease as well as identification of those most at risk. Although there is still a role for open surgery in the management of aortic disease, endovascular therapy will continue to evolve and play an increasing role. There will be further controversies along the way. The only certainty is that the journey is not yet complete.

## REFERENCES

Ashton HA, Buxton MJ, Day NE, et al: Multicentre Aneurysm Screening Study Group. The Multicentre Aneurysm Screening Study (MASS) into the effect of abdominal aortic aneurysm screening on mortality in men: A randomised controlled trial. Lancet 2002;360:1531-1539.

Blankensteijn JD, de Jong SE, Prinssen M, et al: Dutch Randomized Endovascular Aneurysm Management (DREAM) Trial Group. Two-year outcomes after conventional or endovascular repair of abdominal aortic aneurysms. N Engl J Med 2005;352:98-405.

Brewster DC, Cronenwett JL, Hallett JW Jr, et al: Joint Council of the American Association for Vascular Surgery and Society for Vascular Surgery. Guidelines for the treatment of abdominal aortic aneurysms. Report of a subcommittee of the Joint Council of the American Association for Vascular Surgery and Society for Vascular Surgery. J Vasc Surg 2003;37:1106-1117.

CAPRIE Steering Committee: A randomised, blinded trial of Clopidogrel versus Aspirin in Patients at Risk of Ischaemic Events (CAPRIE). Lancet 1996;348:1329-1339.

Clouse WD, Hallett JW Jr, Schaff HV, et al: Acute aortic dissection: Population-based incidence compared with degenerative aortic aneurysm rupture. Mayo Clin Proc 2004;79:176-180.

Collins R, Armitage J, Parish S, et al: Heart Protection Study Collaborative Group. MRC/BHF Heart Protection Study of cholesterol-lowering with simvastatin in 5963 people with diabetes: A randomised placebo-controlled trial. Lancet 2003;361:2005-2016.

Dormandy JA, Rutherford RB: Management of peripheral arterial disease (PAD). TASC Working Group. TransAtlantic Inter-Society Concensus (TASC). J Vasc Surg 2000;31(1 Pt 2):S1-S296.

Greenhalgh RM, Brown LC, Kwong GP, et al: Comparison of endovascular aneurysm repair with open repair in patients with abdominal aortic aneurysm (EVAR trial 1), 30-day operative mortality results: Randomised controlled trial. Lancet 2004;364:843-848.

Johnston KW, Rutherford RB, Tilson MD, et al: Suggested standards for reporting on arterial aneurysms. Subcommittee on Reporting Standards for Arterial Aneurysms, Ad Hoc Committee on Reporting Standards, Society for

Vascular Surgery and North American Chapter, International Society for Cardiovascular Surgery. J Vasc Surg 1991;13:452-458.

Khan IA, Nair CK: Clinical, diagnostic, and management perspectives of aortic dissection. Chest 2002;122:311-328.

Meszaros I, Morocz J, Szlavi J, et al: Epidemiology and clinicopathology of aortic dissection. Chest 2000;117:1271-1278.

# Angina Pectoris

Method of
*John F. Moran, MD*

The diagnosis and management of chest pain remain an important challenge. Although there can be a long differential diagnosis of chest pain to be considered, the diagnosis of angina pectoris is especially important. According to the American Heart Association statistics, chronic stable coronary artery disease is the leading cause of mortality in the United States, accounting for one in five deaths. More than 1.2 million Americans had a myocardial infarction in 2001 out of a total of 13.2 million with coronary disease. Of these 1.2 million patients, 700,000 had a new attack and 500,000 had a recurrent attack.

## Clinical Features

### GENERAL FEATURES

Angina pectoris is associated with myocardial ischemia and left ventricular dysfunction but not necessarily myocardial necrosis. Angina pectoris is usually provoked by exercise and relieved by rest.

Patients give a variety of descriptions of their chest discomfort: strangling, suffocating, chest pressure, chest tightness, or heaviness. Often the patient suffering from effort angina can predict the amount of physical exercise that causes his or her angina and might be a candidate for preventive therapy. The chest discomfort can be characterized in terms of its frequency, duration, and intensity as well as precipitating factors and the time of day that it occurs. The anginal threshold can be influenced by emotional stress, exposure to cold weather, superfluous meals, and cigarette smoking. Angina can last from 10 to 15 minutes and rarely longer. If the chest discomfort lasts for 15 to 30 minutes or more, myocardial necrosis should be suspected. The discomfort can radiate up the left arm along the ulnar aspect, occasionally to the right arm, and occasionally to both arms. Radiation of the discomfort can occur up into the neck and the jaw, shoulders, and back.

Angina pectoris equivalents can consist of exertional dyspnea probably related to diastolic dysfunction or changes in left ventricular compliance that occurs with ischemia. In elderly patients fatigue can be an angina equivalent related to poor cardiac output, when the left ventricle becomes ischemic. Atypical angina has some of these characteristics.

Angina can be classified as stable when its characteristics are unchanged for 60 days. Stable angina pectoris responds to sublingual nitroglycerin (Nitrostat) or rest. Unstable angina pectoris consists of the chest discomfort syndrome, occurring more frequently, lasting longer, and manifesting with lesser degrees of exertion. Unstable angina can occur at rest and at night.

### ANGINA IN WOMEN

There are gender differences reported in the language and the history of angina. Atypical chest pain is more common in female patients. Female patients describe more throat, neck, or jaw discomfort for angina, and the chest discomfort is more likely to occur at rest, during sleep, or with periods of mental stress. Women can have neck and shoulder discomfort. Fatigue, shortness of breath, and nausea with vomiting are often present.

In a recent Finnish study, female patients who use nitrates had increased coronary mortality risks similar in magnitude to those observed in men. This seemed to be true up into the ninth decade of life in their study.

Diagnostic cardiac catheterization is listed as the sixth most commonly performed health care procedure in more than 500,000 women, and total charges exceeded $4 billion. In the Women's Ischemic Syndrome Evaluation (WISE) studies, the data suggest that symptom-driven care is costly even for women with nonobstructive coronary artery disease. They suggested that health conditions may be detected earlier in women because of more frequent use of physician's services.

Five-year rates of hospitalization for women with chest pain and nonobstructive coronary artery disease increased for women with one-vessel to three-vessel coronary artery disease. Similarly, 5-year cardiovascular death or myocardial infarction (MI) rates ranged from 4% to 38% for women with nonobstructive to three-vessel coronary artery disease.

## MANAGEMENT

Because the angina chest pain syndrome is believed to be caused by an imbalance of oxygen supply and demand to the myocardium, management of angina is directed toward increasing the oxygen supply or decreasing oxygen demands. Increasing coronary blood flow with percutaneous interventions or coronary artery bypass graft (CABG) surgery increases oxygen supply to the heart, whereas medication decreases oxygen demand. In any event, the goals of management of angina pectoris include increasing the quantity and quality of life. The American College of Cardiology and the American Heart Association issue periodic updates in guidelines for the management of stable angina pectoris.

## Diagnosis

Box 1 lists the differential diagnosis of chest pain. The diagnosis of angina pectoris presumes a mismatch between myocardial oxygen consumption and oxygen delivery to the myocardium. Angina occurs when there is an area of myocardial ischemia caused by inadequate coronary perfusion and thus insufficient oxygen supply to match oxygen demand. Angina pectoris is a predictable and reproducible anterior chest discomfort after physical activity, or emotional stress. The patient must stop all activities when the chest discomfort occurs. This discomfort is usually relieved within a few minutes of taking nitroglycerin or stopping the activity.

### HISTORY

A successful interview with a potential angina patient requires a consideration of the prevalence of coronary artery disease in that patient. The interpretation of the chest pain is based on a prior probability of disease in that patient, which includes a review of the patient's lifestyle. A likely candidate for coronary artery disease is a man who is older than 60 years and has a history of cigarette smoking.

---

**BOX 1  Differential Diagnosis of Chest Pain**

- Acute aortic dissection
- Acute myocardial infarction
- Acute pericarditis
- Angina pectoris
- Biliary colic
- Costochondritis
- Esophageal motility disorders, reflux
- Idiopathic hypertrophic aortic stenosis
- Musculoskeletal disorders
- Pulmonary embolism
- Severe aortic stenosis
- Severe pulmonary hypertension

Precipitating factors such as anemia or hyperthyroidism should be considered. The differential diagnosis listed in Box 1 is a short list of disorders that can cause chest discomfort, and these can often be differentiated in the history and physical examination.

## TESTING

### Electrocardiogram

After the history and physical examination are completed, a 12-lead electrocardiogram (ECG) is often made. However, it is normal in more than 50% of patients with angina.

### Stress Testing

The next consideration is often the exercise ECG or some noninvasive stress test. This allows an evaluation of ST segment changes. The Duke treadmill score takes ST segment depression, the duration of exercise, and the development of chest discomfort into consideration to increase the sensitivity of the test. The Duke treadmill score allows the patient to be stratified according to the score. A score of 5 or higher carries an annual mortality rate of 0.25%; a high-risk Duke score is −10 or more and carries a 5% annual mortality risk.

The exercise ECG can also be combined with echocardiography or myocardial perfusion scans such as technetium Tc-99m tetrofosmin (Myoview) or thallium. Some patients are unable to walk on the treadmill, and pharmacologic stress testing is available with adenosine (Adenoscan), dipyridamole (Persantine), or dobutamine.[1] Nuclear myocardial perfusion with thallium, myoview, or echocardiography can also be combined with pharmacologic stress.

Electron beam computed tomography (CT) is a technique that identifies calcification of the coronaries, suggesting atherosclerotic disease. The volume of atherosclerotic plaque can also be estimated. Asymptomatic thoracic or abdominal aortic calcifications can also help identify the patient with atherosclerosis and possible coronary artery disease.

A more recent development in diagnostic techniques for coronary artery disease is the 16-detector multislice CT. Studies comparing the multislice CT with coronary angiography have shown positive and negative predictive values of as high at 87% and 99%, respectively. Patients must be able to hold their breath for 20 seconds and have a heart rate less than 70 bpm. β-Blockade usually allows this heart rate. The coronary arteries cannot be assessed well if there is motion artifact, and severe calcification can obscure the coronary lumen. The estimated radiation dose for multislice CT scanning of the coronary arteries can be as high as 13.0 to 16.3 mSv compared with conventional coronary angiography, which has a radiation dose of 3 to 5 mSv.

The specificity of multislice CT scanning can be improved if the test is followed by a dobutamine stress echocardiogram. Cost effectiveness for the diagnosis becomes a factor here. The treadmill and the Duke treadmill scores with or without a myocardial scan might suffice to confirm the diagnosis of angina pectoris and stratify the patient's risk for future cardiac events. ST segment depression alone on the exercise ECG had a sensitivity of 68% and a specificity of 77% in a meta-analysis of 24,074 patients.

In addition to helping to confirm a diagnosis of angina, the ability to walk on the treadmill can stratify patients into a functional class as described by the Canadian Cardiovascular Society (CCS) functional classification. The CCS class I allows patients activity up to 7 metabolic equivalents of exercise (METs). This would be the equivalent of performing 6 minutes of exercise on the Bruce Protocol exercise ECG. CCS class II is any activity of up to 5 METs of exercise. This is the equivalent of completing 3 minutes on the Bruce Protocol test. CCS class III allows any activity up to 2 METs of exercise. This means the patient would not complete the first 3 minutes of the Bruce Protocol exercise test. CCS class IV implies the patient can do less than 2 METs of work; 1 MET is the metabolic equivalent of rest. Clearly, patients with CCS classes II, III, and IV are limited by angina pectoris. Moreover, ST

[1]Not FDA approved for this indication.

segment depression of 1 mm in the first stage of the Bruce Protocol exercise test or 2 mm of ST depression in the second stage of exercise strongly suggest serious coronary artery disease.

In addition to marked ST segment depression and a high-risk Duke treadmill score, other noninvasive tests suggesting high-risk angina include severe left ventricular dysfunction in exercise with an ejection fraction of less than 35%, large perfusion defects on nuclear scanning that are stress induced, and multiple perfusion defects of moderate size with left ventricular dilation or increased pulmonary uptake. Echocardiographic wall motion abnormalities following dobutamine stress that involve more than two segments indicate high risk. In contrast, low-risk noninvasive test results include a low-risk Duke treadmill score, normal wall motion on echocardiography, or a limited resting wall abnormality and a small myocardial perfusion defect on nuclear scanning or a totally normal scan. Intermediate-risk patients fall somewhere between these two.

# Treatment

## STRATEGY FOR MANAGING STABLE ANGINA PECTORIS

Box 2 lists the reasonable strategy for managing patients with angina pectoris. Coronary risk factor reduction fits well with the aggressive management of angina pectoris patients. After precipitating factors for angina are ruled out, lifestyle modifications that include weight control, an exercise program, smoking cessation, and control of diabetes (if it is present) are necessary. Management of hypertension should include a goal that brings blood pressure down in the range of 130/80 mm Hg or lower.

### Blood Pressure

Framingham Heart Study data have indicated the effect of high-normal blood pressure on the risk of cardiovascular disease. The researchers defined high-normal blood pressure as blood pressures ranging from 130/85 to 139/89 mm Hg. An optimal blood pressure was less than 120 mm Hg systolic and less than 80 mm Hg diastolic. The high-normal blood pressure was associated with a risk factor adjusted hazard ratio of 2.5 for women and 1.6 for men. These were not significantly different, but the accrued event rates per 1000 patient-years for

---

**BOX 2   Strategy for Managing Stable Angina Pectoris**

- Identify precipitating factors such as anemia, hyperthyroidism, valvular heart disease (e.g., aortic stenosis, tachyarrhythmias, hypertension).
- Start sublingual nitroglycerin, β-blockers, and aspirin and consider ACE inhibitors.
- Start risk factor modification, statin medication to the ATP III goal of cholesterol <200 mg and LDL cholesterol <100.
- Add a calcium channel blocker if the angina is more frequent than two or three times a week, and consider prophylactic sublingual nitroglycerin before activities.
- Count the use of sublingual nitroglycerin to monitor the success of treatment.
- Use of nitroglycerin patch or ointment at bedtime for nocturnal angina.
- Consider coronary angiography if angina pectoris symptoms are refractory or if the exercise electrocardiogram is abnormal, especially with poor work capacity.

*Abbreviations:* ACE = angiotensin-converting enzyme; ATP III = Adult Treatment Panel III; LDL = low-density lipoprotein

persons younger than 65 years were 4.7 for women and 9.2 for men. The numbers needed to treat (NNT) for patients older than 65 years were estimated to be 24 to 71 men and 34 to 102 women to prevent any cardiovascular events in the 5 years of follow-up.

Although the HOPE (Heart Outcomes Prevention Evaluation) Trial results seem to fit well with this management of blood pressure, overall results of randomized studies of angiotensin-converting enzyme (ACE) inhibitors in patients with coronary artery disease and normal left ventricular function are conflicting. In the HOPE trial, ramipril (Altace) 10 mg/day orally was compared with placebo in 9297 high-risk men and women of at least age 55 years with a history of coronary artery disease, stroke, peripheral vascular disease, or diabetes. In the ramipril group, 14% of the patients died of combined endpoints of MI or stroke; 18% of the patients in the placebo group succumbed to these. In the HOPE trial, blood pressure at entry was 139/79 mm Hg. Both the ramipril and the placebo groups had systolic blood pressures that were in the 130s. The difference in the HOPE Trial endpoint was highly significant. Fewer patients in the ramipril group underwent revascularization, and there were reductions in the new diagnosis of diabetes and in the complications of diabetes in patients who had it.

A recent meta-analysis of seven trials of ACE inhibitors that included a total of 33,960 patients followed for a mean of 4.4 years suggested decreased overall mortality, cardiovascular mortality, MI, and stroke. Of the seven trials studied, five trials enrolled patients with documented coronary artery disease. One trial enrolled patients with coronary disease or patients with diabetes who were 55 years or older, and 80% of that population had documented coronary artery disease. The last trial enrolled patients who had coronary disease, intermittent claudication, or transient ischemic attack. Five different ACE inhibitors were tested, and two of the trials used higher doses than those usually necessary for antihypertensive therapy.

All-cause mortality was lower in the treatment arms compared with the placebo arms in all of the trials except one, and the reduction was significant in HOPE. The cardiovascular mortality was consistently reduced by ACE inhibitors across all trials except CAMELOT (Comparison of Amlodipine versus Enalapril to Limit Occurrences of Thrombosis). The meta-analysis showed a 14% reduction in mortality. In the HOPE Trial, a highly significant 19% reduction was seen in the meta-analysis. In addition, significant reductions in the acute MI were found in both HOPE and EUROPA (European Trial on Reduction of Cardiac Events with Perindopril in Stable Coronary Artery Disease) Trials. There seemed to be no effect on the MI rate in the PEACE (Prevention of Events with ACE Inhibition) Trial, and nonsignificant reductions were observed in the other trials. Overall, there was an 18% reduction in MI with ACE inhibitor therapy. Stroke was less frequent in patients receiving ACE inhibitors in all trials except Part II of the Prevention of Atherosclerosis with Ramipril Trial-2. Overall, there was a 23% relative reduction in the occurrence of stroke in these trials.

In the summary article from the American College of Cardiology/American Heart Association 2002 Guidelines, the use of ACE inhibitors with coronary artery disease or other vascular disease without diabetes or left ventricular dysfunction was a class IIA recommendation. However, the use of ACE inhibitors in all patients with coronary artery disease who have diabetes or left ventricular systolic dysfunction was a class I recommendation.

## Weight and Diet

In addition to blood pressure, other coronary risk factors are important, as is body weight. The ideal body mass index (BMI) goal is 18.5 to 24.9 kg/m². The Lyon Diet Heart Study suggested an increase in survival for patients on the Mediterranean diet, with a reduction of all-cause as well as cardiovascular mortality. MIs were reduced in the treatment group. The Nurses' Health Study follow-up enrolled some 121,700 female registered nurses, and the Health Professionals follow-up recruited 51,529 male health professionals. These studies found that consumption of fruits and vegetables, particularly green leafy vegetables and vitamin C–rich fruits and vegetables, appeared to have a protective effect against coronary heart disease.

## Cholesterol

In addition to diet, lowering the total cholesterol and the LDL cholesterol reduces total mortality by 22% to 30%, coronary events by 24% to 37%, and CABG surgery and angioplasty by 22% to 37%. A recent prospective meta-analysis of 90,056 participants in 14 randomized trials of statins by the Cholesterol Treatment Trialists' (CTT) Collaborators have confirmed these data. In addition, data were available on first strokes after randomization in this meta-analysis. Overall, there was a significant 17% proportional reduction in the incidence of first stroke of any type in the statin group versus control group. In strokes not attributed to hemorrhage and presumed to be ischemic, the overall reduction in stroke reflected a highly significant 19% reduction. The CCT calculations revealed that a reduction in LDL cholesterol of 39 mg/dL (1 mmol/L) sustained for 5 years could produce a reduction in major vascular events of about 23%. This was more than the 21% reductions observed in the weighted analysis. Moreover, a reduction of the LDL cholesterol by 78 mg/dL (2 mmol/L) might be expected to reduce the risk of vascular disease by as much as 40%. In the case of stroke, cohort studies showed no associations between serum cholesterol levels and stroke. However, there is no question that the randomized trials showed that statins reduced the incidence of stroke by about 30%.

Several trials have demonstrated that high-dose aggressive LDL cholesterol lowering therapy can increase benefit to patients. The PROVE-IT (Pravastatin or Atorvastatin Evaluation and Infection Therapy) trial and the MIRACL (Myocardial Ischemia Reduction with Acute Cholesterol Lowering) trial used acute coronary syndrome patients and high-dose (80 mg) atorvastatin (Lipitor). PROVE-IT compared atorvastatin with pravastatin (Pravachol) 40 mg. The IDEAL (Incremental Decrease in Endpoints Through Aggressive Lipid Lowering) study compared 80 mg of atorvastatin with 20 mg of simvastatin (Zocor). Phase Z of the A to Z Trial compared 20 mg of simvastatin with 80 mg of simvastatin. The REVERSAL (Reversing Atherosclerosis with Aggressive Lipid Lowering) trial compared 80 mg of atorvastatin with 40 mg of pravastatin. The TACTICS TIMI 22 trial compared 80 mg of atorvastatin with 40 mg of pravastatin. The ASTEROID (A Study to Evaluate the Effect of Rosuvastatin on Intravascular Ultrasound-Derived Coronary Atheroma Burden) trial used rosuvastatin (Crestor) 40 mg per day.

These trials compared a variety of patients who had hypercholesterolemia. There seemed to be good data to suggest that some patients would be better off with an LDL cholesterol in the range of 75 mg/dL. There clearly was no adverse effect on safety in these trials although there was improved clinical benefit. The meta-analysis data of 90,056 participants lowering the LDL cholesterol by 39 mg/dL with 5 years of statin therapy failed to show any increased risk of any specific nonvascular cause of death or any specific type of cancer. In that meta-analysis of 14 trials, 39,884 patients allocated to a statin, nine patients developed rhabdomyolysis compared with six patients in 39,817 patients allocated to control. The 5-year risk was not significant, with an absolute incidence of 0.01%. High-risk patients would particularly benefit from lowered LDL cholesterol. These patients include those with MI, CABG surgery, or any percutaneous intervention.

The pertinent findings from the Adult Treatment Panel III are presented in Table 1. The goal of an LDL cholesterol of less than 100 mg/dL for coronary artery disease patients might well be reduced with further review by the National Cholesterol Education Program (NCEP). That panel defined diabetes as the equivalent of coronary heart disease even though there may be no symptoms or signs of coronary artery disease in diabetic patients.

## Metabolic Syndrome

The metabolic syndrome requires intensive lifestyle changes as a baseline. The NCEP defined the waist circumference for abdominal obesity for men as greater than 40 inches and for women as greater than 35 inches. They also advocated a higher high-density lipoprotein to 40 mg/dL for men and 50 mg/dL for women. The blood pressure should be in the range of 130/85 mm Hg, and a fasting glucose should be less than 110 mg/dL.

**TABLE 1   Cholesterol Treatment Cutpoints and Targets for Therapy**

| Risk Category | 10-Year Risk* | Cholesterol Goals (mg/dL) | |
| | | LDL | Non-HDL |
|---|---|---|---|
| CAD and CAD equivalent† | >20% | <100 | <130 |
| Multiple risk factors (2+) | 10%-20% | <130 | <160 |
| 0-1 risk factors | <10% | <160 | <190 |

*Based on projections from the Framingham Heart Study for 10-year risk of having a CAD event.
†Diabetes is considered a CAD equivalent, even if the patient has no CAD symptoms.
‡Identifies patients with metabolic syndrome for extensive lifestyle changes.
*Abbreviations:* CAD = coronary artery disease; HDL = high-density lipoprotein; LDL = low-density lipoprotein
Data from the National Cholesterol Education Program Adult Treatment Panel III (ATP III).

The sub-study of the Treating to New Targets (TNT) trial that compared 80 mg of atorvastatin with 10 mg of atorvastatin in 5584 patients with the metabolic syndrome suggested statistically significant benefit with the 80-mg dose. At 3 months, the LDL cholesterol was reduced to 72.6 mg/dL with the 80-mg dose versus 99.3 mg/dL with the low dose of atorvastatin.

For most statin medications the evening dose has a greater effect, probably because of a short biological half-life, and because peak cholesterol synthesis occurs at night. Atorvastatin and rosuvastatin have longer half-lives and do not have this problem. All statin medications lower LDL cholesterol but at different doses. For example, rosuvastatin 5 mg/day, atorvastatin 10 mg/day, and lovastatin (Mevacor) or simvastatin 40 mg/day reduce LDL cholesterol by 35% or approximately 72 mg/dL. Fluvastatin (Lescol) and pravastatin produce smaller reductions even at the higher doses tested. All statins can reach NCEP goals in certain patients.

## Anticoagulants

The antiplatelet aspirin is recommended if not contraindicated. Doses of 75 to 325 mg/day are the usual. The dose of 75 mg/day in the Swedish Angina Pectoris Aspirin Trial (SAPAT) resulted in a 34% reduction in the outcome of MI and sudden death, with a 32% drop in secondary vascular events.

If patients cannot tolerate aspirin or it is contraindicated, clopidogrel (Plavix) 75 mg a day or warfarin (Coumadin) can be used. Clopidogrel was studied in the CAPRIE (Clopidogrel versus Aspirin in Patients at Risk of Ischemic Events) trial; more than 19,000 patients were recruited who had a recent ischemic stroke, MI, or peripheral arterial disease. Clopidogrel and aspirin were compared with aspirin alone. There was a relative risk reduction of 8.7% for the combination of clopidogrel and aspirin against aspirin alone. The greatest benefit and risk reduction were in the peripheral arterial disease patients.

Clopidogrel and ticlopidine (Ticlid) are theinopyridine derivatives. Clopidogrel is favored because of the side effects associated with ticlodipine. Both drugs inhibit platelet aggregation induced by adenosine diphosphate (ADP). In the absence of contraindications, aspirin 75 to 325 mg/day is recommended for routine use in patients with chronic ischemic heart disease.

Combination drug therapy can also help patients reach ATP III goals. Simvastatin and long-acting niacin (Slow-Niacin) reduced major clinical events 90% as compared with a placebo. Statins themselves can significantly lower LDL cholesterol from all pretreatment levels. The absolute reductions were greater in patients with higher pretreatment levels of cholesterol.

## PHARMACOLOGIC THERAPY

### Anti-Anginal Drug Therapy

Nitrates in the treatment of angina pectoris have been a time-honored treatment and are still an important part of therapy. The nitrates seem to work primarily in the venous circulation and reduce preload to the left ventricle. Nitrate preparations are available in sublingual tablets, nitroglycerin spray bottles, ointments, and transdermal nitroglycerin patches. Nitroglycerin ointment or the nitroglycerin patch can be placed at bedtime to prevent nocturnal angina and allow some prevention of angina pectoris in the early morning hours before the patient first awakens.

Isosorbide dinitrate (Isordil) is an anti-anginal agent but has relatively low bioavailability after oral administration. The active metabolite of isosorbide dinitrate is isosorbide mononitrate (Imdur). This is completely bioavailable with oral administration because it does not undergo first-pass hepatic metabolism. Either of these preparations requires a 12-hour nitrate-free interval to avoid nitroglycerin tolerance.

The mechanism of nitroglycerin tolerance is not well understood. Currently the best evidence seems to suggest that there is an impairment of nitrate bioconversion as the mechanism of tolerance induction. Several agents have been suggested to limit or reverse the development of nitrate tolerance, although the evidence is not consistent.

ACE inhibitors have not been associated with amelioration of nitrate efficacy, despite their effects on reversing endothelial dysfunction. Folic acid seems to improve endothelial dysfunction in many situations and can potentiate hemodynamic responses to nitrates. At present, the only management for nitroglycerin tolerance is to allow a nitrate-free interval of at least 12 hours.

A combination of nitrates and sildenafil (Viagra) can cause a prolonged and potentially life-threatening drop in blood pressure. Sildenafil therapy is contraindicated in patients who use nitrates.

### β-Adrenergic Antagonists

β-Blockers, or β-adrenergic receptor blocking agents, are an important part of the therapy for angina pectoris and are often started early in the management of these patients. They can be antihypertensive and antiarrhythmic. Information suggests these medications prolong survival and prevent reinfarction in patients who have had an MI. These agents have different pharmacology, some being selective of β$_1$-receptor block and others being nonselective β-blocking drugs (Table 2). For example, nadolol, pindolol, sotalol, and timolol, all block both β$_1$- and β$_2$-receptors. β-Blockers with less effect on β$_2$-receptors and more effect on β$_1$-receptors are acebutolol, atenolol, metoprolol, and esmolol.

The β$_1$-receptors are primarily found in the heart, and stimulation of these receptors leads to increased atrial ventricular nodal conduction, an increase in heart rate, an increase in contractility, and an increase in norepinephrine release. In contrast, stimulation of β$_2$-receptors causes bronchodilation and vasodilation. Cardioselectivity of β$_1$-blocking drugs disappears as the dose of these drugs increased.

Doses of β-blockers required to control angina might reach a point where they do cause some degree of bronchoconstriction in sensitive patients. Labetolol and carvedilol have α-blocking capabilities as well as β$_1$-blocking capability. Acebutolol and pindolol have some intrinsic sympathomimetic activity. This means they can produce low-grade β-stimulation when sympathetic activity is low, for instance, at rest. For these reasons they might not be as effective in reducing heart rate or the magnitude of ST segment depression in patients with angina.

The gastrointestinal tract does not as readily absorb the β-blockers propanolol, metoprolol, and pindolol. Because of the gastrointestinal absorption, intravenous doses of metoprolol or propanolol can result in much higher concentrations in the bloodstream than oral dosing. Therefore, lower doses of these medications given intravenously will produce an adequate effect (see Table 2).

Barring contraindications, indefinite use of β-blockers in patients with angina pectoris is recommended. Abrupt cessation in patients with angina should be avoided because of the possibility of exacerbation of the angina pectoris.

## TABLE 2 Commonly Used Medications in Angina Pectoris

| Drug | Form | Dose |
| --- | --- | --- |
| **Nitrates** | | |
| Isosorbide dinitrate(Isordil) | Tab | 20-40 mg PO bid |
| Isosorbide mononitrate (Imdur) | Tab | 30-120 mg PO qd |
| Nitroglycerin (Nitrostat) | Sublingual tab | 0.4 mg PO prn |
| Nitroglycerin (Nitrolingual) | Spray | 0.4 mg prn |
| Nitroglycerin (Nitrol) | Ointment | ½-1 inch qid |
| Nitroglycerin (Nitroglyn) | Cap slow release | 2.5 to 13 mg PO bid or tid |
| **β-Blockers** | | |
| Atenolol (Tenormin) | Tab | 50-200 mg PO qd |
| | Soln | 5 mg IV q15min |
| Carvedilol (Coreg) | Tab | 12.5-50 PO mg bid |
| Esmolol (Brevibloc) | Soln | 50-300 μg/kg/min continuous infusion |
| Labetalol (Normodyne, Trandate) | Tab | 200-600 mg PO bid or tid |
| Metoprolol (Lopressor) | Tab | 50-200 mg PO bid |
| | Soln | 5 mg q15min |
| Propranolol (Inderal) | Cap, tab | 20-80 mg PO bid |
| **Calcium Channel Blockers** | | |
| Amlodipine (Norvasc) | Tab | 5-10 mg qd |
| Diltiazem (Cardizem CD) | Tab slow release | 120-480 mg qd |
| Nifedipine (Procardia XL) | Tab slow release | 30-90 mg qd |
| Verapamil (Calan SR) | Caplet slow release | 120-480 mg qd |

*Abbreviations:* cap = capsule; soln = IV solution; tab = tablet.

## Calcium Channel Antagonists

Calcium channel blockers can be considered third-choice agents in the treatment of stable angina pectoris. These medications block the entry of calcium into smooth muscle cells as well as myocytes. Calcium channel antagonists reduce smooth muscle tension in the peripheral vascular bed, producing arterial vasodilation and thereby reducing arterial blood pressure and afterload. They also reduce myocardial contractility. Altogether, they reduce myocardial oxygen consumption. Diltiazem and verapamil reduce the heart rate. Dihydropyridine calcium channel blockers such as nifedipine and amlodipine are among the most potent calcium blocking agents.

Short-acting calcium channel blockers are to be avoided. Only long-acting calcium channel blockers are recommended. Although β-blockers are recommended as first-line treatment for angina pectoris, calcium channel blockers can be used and are equally effective in angina pectoris if β-blockers are not tolerated.

Diltiazem and verapamil depress contractility more than the dihydropyridines, which is a disadvantage. Adverse effects of calcium channel blockers include ankle edema, palpitations, flushing, headaches, and hypotension. These agents can be combined with a β-blocker, especially a long-acting dihydropyridine such as amlodipine or nifedipine XL. These decrease ischemic events and increase exercise time.

Long-acting metoprolol 200 mg/day or nifedipine XL 40 mg/day were more effective when used together than either drug when used separately. The combination showed a greater increase in exercise tolerance over monotherapy with either drug. To avoid complications, the β-blocker should be started first, then the calcium channel blocker should be added for angina control. Dosing is also important. A therapeutic dose of metoprolol is 50 mg twice daily with the goal of bringing the resting heart rate into the 50s. Calcium channel blockers are also effective in the treatment of vasospastic angina.

## BOX 3 Findings in High-Risk Patients

- Hemodynamic instability
- High-risk noninvasive stress testing with depressed ejection fraction, extensive wall motion abnormalities
- Recent revascularization with coronary intervention or coronary bypass graft surgery
- Recurrent ischemia at rest or low levels of activity with medical management
- Recurrent ischemia with heart failure, ventricular gallop, extremes of heart rate, or mitral regurgitation
- Sustained ventricular tachycardia

Even when dosing of these medications is appropriate, most patients with angina pectoris benefit from three agents: nitrates, β-blockers, and calcium channel blockers. Despite these efforts at therapy, many angina patients still fail therapy and continue to have disabling angina classified as class III or IV limitations. The goal of therapy is not only symptomatic relief but also prolonged survival. Probably more than 50% of patients with stable angina will have coronary angiography in an attempt to relieve symptoms. Data show that left main coronary artery disease, triple vessel disease, and double vessel disease involving a proximal left anterior descending coronary artery all benefit from revascularization with prolonged survival. Patients with high-risk noninvasive testing are candidates for angiography (Box 3).

The Asymptomatic Cardiac Ischemia Pilot (ACIP) study randomized patients into three treatment strategies if they were candidates for revascularization. These strategies were angina-guided therapy, angina plus ischemic medications, and revascularization by angioplasty or CABG surgery.

Titrated doses of atenolol with long-acting nifedipine or sustained-release diltiazem and the addition of sustained-release isosorbide dinitrate were used. Mortality rates in the 2-year follow-up in the guided therapy were 6.6% for ischemic-guided therapy, 4.4% for angina plus ischemic medications, and 1.1% for the revascularization strategy. This suggests that revascularization can improve the 2-year prognosis of patients who have objective evidence of ischemia, even if their angina is well controlled on aggressive medical management.

## Future Therapies

Because chronic angina can impair quality of life and is associated with decreased life expectancy affecting 6.4 million Americans, newer therapies are being developed. These current therapies reduce demand-induced myocardial ischemic symptoms but often they are not sufficient. Newer drugs under evaluation include ivabradine[1], omapatrilat[2], fasudil[2], and nicorandil.[1]

Ranolazine (Ranexa) has recently been approved. Ranolazine is an active piperazine derivative with a short half-life of 1.4 to 1.9 hours. Only the prolonged or sustained-release ranolazine is available for patients who still have limiting angina despite triple therapy. Ranolazine should always be used in combination with other medications: amlodipine, β-blockers, or nitrates. It should not be used as an alternative to β-blocker therapy. The therapeutic dose range is 500 to 1000 mg twice a day. This dosage range is generally well tolerated, but constipation, nausea, and dizziness are the most common adverse effects reported.

Ranolazine is extensively metabolized through the CYP3A4 pathway. The medication is contraindicated in patients with hepatic impairment or those with QTc prolongation or who are taking medications known to prolong the QT interval. It is also contraindicated if the patient is taking drugs that are moderately potent CYP3A inhibitors. A baseline ECG to evaluate the QT interval should be performed. At present, ranolazine is only recommended for patients who have failed angina control with triple therapy.

[1]Not available in the United States.
[2]Investigational drug in the United States.

# Other Forms of Angina

## REFRACTORY ANGINA PECTORIS

Despite optimal medical management, angiography with angioplasty, and CABG surgery, many patients still have severe limiting angina. These patents are survivors. There are estimates that as many as 100,000 patients with refractory angina are alive in the United States. For these patients with no options there are methods that will palliate the angina pectoris. The treatment might not affect the basic disease process, but it will decrease the angina pain and increase the patient's quality of life. The prognosis for survival in these patients appears to be low, estimated at a 5% annual mortality.

The OPTIMIST (Options in Myocardial Syndrome Therapies) trial suggested patients with refractory angina have low long-term mortality; during their 3.5-year follow-up period, 11.8% of their patients died. They treated some of their patients with enhanced external counterpulsation (EECP), transmyocardial laser revascularization, and neurostimulation. The international EECP (n = 978 patients) patient registry demonstrated an improvement of at least one angina class in 81% of the patients with class III or IV refractory anginas. Transmyocardial laser revascularization has been shown to reduce cardiac pain, although the information that it affects myocardial ischemia is lacking. Neurostimulation in the form of transcutaneous electrical nerve stimulation (TENS) or spinal cord stimulation has been found useful in relieving pain. Symptom relief with neurostimulation has been found effective in managing patients with refractory angina pectoris.

A recent paper evaluated the prognosis of post-MI patients who had preinfarction stable angina pectoris versus those who did not. Patients who had stable angina pectoris before they developed an MI had less remodeling of the left ventricular volumes. This could improve survival without necessarily improving chest pain.

## UNSTABLE ANGINA PECTORIS

Unstable angina has a changing pattern. The pain or discomfort comes more frequently, lasts longer (perhaps >20 minutes), comes with lesser degrees of exertion, occurs at rest, or occurs at night, and requires additional sublingual nitroglycerin for control. Unstable angina suggests the disruption of a vulnerable atherosclerotic plaque and partial or total closure of a coronary artery as opposed to a fixed atherosclerotic obstruction.

Unstable angina is part of the acute coronary syndrome, which accounts for nearly 1.7 million patients who are hospitalized after presenting to the emergency department in the United States every year. Risk stratification of these patients is performed on the basis of the 12-lead ECG as well as biochemical markers. The acute coronary syndrome also includes ST segment elevation MI and non–ST segment elevation MI or the non–Q wave MI. A rapid evaluation of these patients with acute coronary syndrome is critical. Unstable angina is the part of the acute coronary syndrome where no biochemical marker is elevated. There is no sign of myocardial necrosis.

Much new material on the acute coronary syndrome has been published in the last few years. The data focus on the best treatment for these patients as well as the diagnosis, prognosis, and risk stratification. Biochemical markers such as troponin, creatinine kinase, creatinine kinase MB, B-naturetic peptide, C-reactive protein (CRP), and myoglobin are used. Myoglobin and troponin markers are measured at the onset of the chest pain and at 6 hours and again at 12 hours after admission to the hospital.

### Clinical Findings

Box 3 lists the findings of high-risk patients. They can have accelerating chest pain as well as left ventricular dysfunction or pulmonary edema. New-onset mitral regurgitation, ventricular gallops, hypotension, the extremes of heart rate, and age older than 75 years are all abnormalities found in a high-risk patient. These are usually associated with acute MI and ST segment changes or new-onset bundle branch block. Cardiac enzymes are elevated in these cases. Low-risk chest pain patients have a new-onset or progressive angina and at least a

moderate or perhaps a high likelihood of coronary artery disease based on their history. The ECG may be normal in these patients, and biochemical markers may also be normal.

### Treatment

The problem in the acute coronary syndrome is an abnormal physiology in the vessel wall, that is, plaque, platelets, and thrombus. Therefore, antithrombotic therapy is very important. All patients receive an aspirin, which blocks the thromboxane $A_2$ within 15 to 30 minutes of the oral dose. Clopidogrel is also indicated as an adenosine-mediated platelet blocker, particularly if the patient has an aspirin allergy. Unfractionated heparin is used. Data now suggest a preference for low-molecular-weight heparin. Enoxaparin might have an advantage over unfractionated heparin for patients who have the acute coronary syndrome (ESSENCE).

The results of the CURE (Clopidogrel in Unstable angina to prevent Recurrent Events) trial make clopidogrel a class I indication for the treatment of patients with unstable angina even in patients in whom an early coronary intervention is not considered. The treatment might be continued for 9 months. If a coronary intervention is performed, clopidogrel should be started at 300 mg and continued for at least 3 months at a dose of 75 mg /day. There are trials suggesting that an initial dose of 600 mg clopidogrel can shorten the onset of action.

There are rare cases of thrombotic thrombocytopenic purpura from the use of clopidogrel. These are manifested by thrombocytopenia and microangiopathic hemolytic anemia sometimes associated with neurologic or renal dysfunction. These patients must discontinue clopidogrel and in some instances undergo plasma exchange. Postmyocardial infarction patients who cannot tolerate aspirin or clopidogrel can be given warfarin and titrated to an international normalized ratio (INR) of 2.0 to 3.0. All of these medications have a tendency to increase bleeding, particularly in female and elderly patients. Studies have shown that the risk of bleeding in these patients doubles. However, the risk-to-benefit ratio still favors treatment with these agents.

A platelet glycoprotein (GP) IIb/IIIa inhibitor is also indicated. The GPIIb/IIIa receptors on a platelet number between 60,000 and 80,000 and are regarded as the final common pathway for binding fibrinogen. Table 3 lists the three current drugs that are available: abciximab (Reopro), epitifibatide (Integralin), and tirofiban (Aggrastat). All three of these GPIIb/IIIa receptor blockers have been studied with the simultaneous use of unfractionated heparin and aspirin treatments. Most of the trials of these agents have involved coronary interventions and have shown significant benefits.

A meta-analysis of seven contemporary randomized trials in more than 8000 patients has been reported. Potent antiplatelet therapy and coronary angioplasty with stent placement decreased mortality by 25% at a mean of 2 years of follow-up when compared with a more conservative approach. These data showed that to save one life, 62 patients needed to be treated with invasive therapy. Early invasive therapy also

### TABLE 3  Antithrombotic Drugs

| Drug(s) | Dosing |
|---|---|
| Abciximab (Reopro) with unfractionated heparin and aspirin | 0.25 mg/kg IV bolus followed by an infusion of 0.125 µg/kg/min for 12-24 h up to 10 µg/min |
| Eptifibatide (Integrilin) with unfractionated heparin and aspirin | 180 µg/kg followed by an infusion of 2 µg/kg/min up to 72 h for intervention Max infusion dose 15 mg/h |
| Tirofiban (Aggrastat) with unfractionated heparin and aspirin | 0.4 µg/kg/min for 30 min 0.1 µg/kg/min infusion for 48 h up to 108 hours (PRISM-PLUS) |
| Enoxaparin (Lovenox) | 1 mg/kg SC q 12 h |
| Clopidrogrel (Plavix) | 300 mg initially followed by 75 mg/d |

*Abbreviations:* max = maximum; PRISM-PLUS = Platelet Receptor Inhibition in Ischemic Syndrome Management in Patients Limited by Unstable Signs and Symptoms.

decreased nonfatal infarction by 17% and recurrent unstable angina requiring hospitalization by 31%.

A patient who has thrombocytopenia of less than 100,000 platelets should not be treated with GPIIb/IIIa inhibitors. Tirofiban needs renal adjustment because it is cleared by the kidney. Ideally, abciximab should be administered 10 to 60 minutes before percutaneous intervention. If there is no intervention, abxicimab is not indicated. Tirofiban and eptifibatide are useful in patients with continuing ischemia where no percutaneous intervention in planned. These two medications can also be used in patients with continuing ischemia or other high-risk features in whom a percutaneous intervention is planned.

There are other antithrombin agents, such as lepirudin (Refludin), argatroban (Novostan), and the low-molecular-weight heparin dalteparin (Fragmin). Thrombolytic therapy in the presence of unstable angina is of no benefit to these patients, in contrast to the benefits seen with an acute MI.

### Biomarkers

Much research has been done in the field of biomarkers, and currently several biomarkers are under study. Most experience is with creatinine kinase, creatinine kinase MB, troponin I or T, and myoglobin, but others are under study. Currently available biomarkers include CRP and brain-natriuretic peptide (BNP). BNP has been found to be elevated in patients with congestive heart failure. However, in addition, transient myocardial ischemia can result in an elevation of BNP. This suggests that BNP is linked to ischemic injury in addition to left ventricular dysfunction.

An exercise study using the Bruce protocol evaluated transient myocardial ischemia in 112 patients. If patients had no inducible ischemia, BNP levels were low at baseline (43 pg/mL) and unchanged during and after exercise. If patients developed inducible ischemia by electrocardiographic and technetium Tc-99m tetrofosmin scans, BNP levels rose from a median of 62 to 92 and returned to baseline at 4 hours after exercise. In patients with severe ischemia and median BNP levels (101 pg/mL) at baseline, BNP levels increased to 123 pg/mL and were still elevated at 4 hours after exercise. In that study, patients with no ischemia (43 pg/mL), mild to moderate ischemia (60 pg/mL), and severe ischemia (101 pg/mL) were statistically different. The differences were increased with exercise stress.

Currently, an important inflammatory biomarker is CRP. CRP can identify inflammation, and inflammation predicts the prognosis with acute coronary syndrome. It is also possible that CRP is a marker for atherosclerosis and not necessarily atherothrombosis. One study of 2554 patients with angina but not MI found that CRP significantly correlated with the extent of coronary vascular disease. A high CRP and severe coronary artery disease indicated the highest risk in the 5-year follow-up. There was still a high predictive risk for MI or death in the follow-up regardless of the extent of coronary artery disease if the CRP was elevated. There was a 10-fold difference in the lowest level and the highest level of CRP (2.5% versus 25%). It is likely that more research will result in a panel of biochemical markers that will be useful in stratifying the patients with the acute coronary syndrome in the emergency department.

### Summary

Most patients in the high-risk and intermediate-risk acute coronary syndrome groups receive coronary angiography for the full assessment because of the survival benefit of revascularization. Patients in the low-risk group of unstable angina with no biochemical markers or ECG changes may be considered for a stress test. The abnormal stress tests with echocardiographic or nuclear scans direct further aggressive therapy (see Box 3). Studies in these patients show that an early invasive strategy reduces the incidence of major cardiac events. The data for high-risk acute MI and non–Q-wave MI suggest angiography should be part of the early plan. The data for unstable angina with no biochemical marker elevation are less clear at present.

All patients who present with stable angina or unstable angina should receive aggressive medical management and coronary risk factor reduction. Medication should include β-blockers, lipid-lowering medications, antiplatelet medications, aspirin, and nitrates. Because some studies show a relatively low rate of use of these medications, the American Heart Association has mounted a nationwide effort entitled "Get With the Guidelines." The relative risk reductions for each of the class 1–indicated medications in the study trials vary from 15% to 20% for aspirin, β-blockers, ACE inhibitors, statins, and clopidogrel. It is now clear that the goal of prolonging survival and enhancing the quality of life can only be met by a polypharmacy approach often associated with coronary angiography and revascularization.

### REFERENCES

Baigent C, Keech A, Kearney PM, et al; Cholesterol Treatment Trialists' (CTT) Collaborators: Efficacy and safety of cholesterol-lowering treatment: Perspective meta-analysis of data from 90,056 participants in 14 randomised trials of statins. Lancet 2005;366:1267-1278.

Bavry AA, Kumbhani DJ, Rassi AN, et al: Benefit of early invasive therapy in acute coronary syndromes: A meta-analysis of contemporary randomized clinical trials. J Am Coll Cardiol 2006;48:1319-1325.

Chaitman BR: Ranolazine for the treatment of chronic angina and potential use in other cardiovascular conditions. Circulation 2006;113:2462-2472.

Cohen M, Demers C, Gurfinkel EP, et al: A comparison of low-molecular-weight heparin with unfractionated heparin for unstable coronary artery disease: Efficacy and Safety of Subcutaneous Enoxaparin in Non-Q-Wave Coronary Events Study Group. N Engl J Med 1997;337:447-452.

Danchin N, Cucherat M, Thuillez C, et al: Angiotensin converting enzyme inhibitors in patients with coronary artery disease and absence of heart failure or left ventricular systolic dysfunction: An overview of long-term randomized control trials. Arch Intern Med 2006;166:787-796.

DeJongste M, Tio RA, Foreman RD: Chronic therapeutically refractory angina pectoris. Heart 2004;90:225-230.

Hemingway H, McCallum A, Shipley M, et al: Incidence and prognostic implications of stable angina pectoris among women and men. JAMA 2006;295:1404-1411.

Law MR, Wald NJ, Rudnicka AR: Quantifying the effect of statins on low density lipoprotein cholesterol, ischemic heart disease, and stroke: Systemic review and meta-analysis. BMJ 2003;326:1423.

Nelson GI, Silke B, Ahuja RC, et al: The effect of left ventricular performance of nifedipine and metroprolol singly and together in exercise-induced angina pectoris. Eur Heart J 1984;5:67-79.

Third Report of the National Cholesterol Education Program (NCEP) Expert Panel on Detection, Evaluation, and Treatment of High Blood Cholesterol in Adults (Adult Treatment Panel III) final report. Circulation 2002; 106:3143.

# Cardiac Arrest: Sudden Cardiac Death

Method of
*Robert W. Rho, MD*

Sudden cardiac arrest is the cause of death in up to 250,000 people per year in the United States. This accounts for more than 50% of all cardiovascular deaths. Sudden cardiac arrest is responsible for more deaths in the United States than stroke, breast cancer, and lung cancer combined. Approximately 1 sudden cardiac arrest occurs every 1.5 minutes in the United States. Unfortunately, 80% of cardiac arrests occur outside of the hospital and resuscitation is only attempted in approximately two thirds of these patients. Even in most urban communities, where an organized emergency medical system (EMS) is available, the survival rate of patients who suffer an out-of-hospital cardiac arrest is less than 10%. Approximately 10% to 40% of these patients have severe neurologic impairment at the time of discharge. This chapter provides a contemporary overview of the epidemiology, mechanism, diagnosis, and treatment of cardiac arrest.

## Definitions

- Cardiac arrest: A primary cardiac disorder that results in sudden loss of cardiac output and a resultant loss of end-organ perfusion resulting in death unless the primary cardiac disorder is corrected.
- Sudden death: Death that occurs unexpectedly within a short interval of time from the onset of symptoms. (Definition varies in the literature from 1 hour to 24 hours from the onset of symptoms.)
- Aborted sudden cardiac death: An intervention or spontaneous event that reverses a life-threatening but modifiable cardiac process (malignant arrhythmia, pump failure, or ischemia) that would have otherwise resulted in sudden death.

## Epidemiology

Approximately 250,000–400,000 patients suffer a cardiac arrest annually in the United States. The incidence of cardiac arrest in the United States is estimated to be approximately 1.5 to 2.0 per 1000 subject-years. The incidence of cardiac arrest based on a retrospective review of death certificates in Multnomah County, Oregon, was 1.5 per 1000 subject-years. The incidence of cardiac arrest reported in a population based case-control study in Seattle was 1.9 per 1000 subject-years. The incidence varies across clinical subsets known to be at greater risk of cardiac arrest. In the Seattle study, the incidence in patients with prior myocardial infarction was 13.7 per 1000 subject-years and in those with a history of heart failure was 21.9 per 1000 subject-years.

## Prognosis

Patients who suffer an out-of-hospital cardiac arrest have a poor prognosis. Survival depends on the availability and quality of bystander cardiopulmonary resuscitation (CPR), early defibrillation, and the availability of EMS. In many densely populated urban communities (such as Chicago and New York City), survival to hospital discharge is less than 5%. In smaller urban communities with well-coordinated EMS systems, survival can approach 15% to 20% (Rochester, Minnesota, and Seattle, Washington). The initial rhythm when a defibrillator is available for monitoring has significant prognostic implications. Among patients who have ventricular fibrillation (VF) as their initial rhythm, 10% to 40% survive to hospital discharge. In contrast, patients who are found to be in asystole or pulseless electrical activity (PEA) have a grim prognosis, and less than 5% survive to hospital discharge.

## Etiology

Cardiac arrhythmias account for the vast majority of all causes of cardiac arrests. The remaining minority of patients have cardiac arrest due to nonarrhythmic mechanisms such as left ventricular pump failure and cardiac tamponade.

The majority of patients suffering a cardiac arrest have coronary artery disease (CAD), but other conditions that predispose to cardiac arrest include hypertrophic cardiomyopathy, dilated cardiomyopathy, arrhythmogenic right ventricular cardiomyopathy, myocarditis, drug toxicities (antiarrhythmic agents, cocaine, amphetamines), congenital heart disease (especially tetralogy of Fallot and transposition of the great vessels [after a Mustard or Senning procedure]), ion-channel disorders such as long QT syndrome, Brugada syndrome, and short QT syndrome (Table 1).

Patients with abnormalities in myocardial substrate are predisposed to ventricular tachycardia because of a reentry mechanism. Most patients who suffer a cardiac arrest develop a rapid monomorphic ventricular tachycardia that degenerates to ventricular fibrillation and then ultimately (after 8 to 10 minutes) to asystole (Figure 1).

### TABLE 1  Causes of Cardiac Arrest

1. **Coronary Artery Disease**
   a. Atherosclerotic coronary artery disease
   b. Nonatherosclerotic coronary artery disease
      - Anomalous coronary origin
      - Acute coronary spasm
      - Coronary vasculitis (Kawasaki's disease, connective tissue disease)
      - Aortic dissection
      - Embolic coronary obstruction
2. **Structural Heart Disease**
   a. Ischemic cardiomyopathy
   b. Idiopathic dilated cardiomyopathy
   c. Hypertrophic cardiomyopathy
   d. Arrhythmogenic right ventricular cardiomyopathy
   e. Myocarditis
   f. Prior myocardial infarction
   g. Heart failure exacerbation
3. **Ion Channel Abnormality**
   a. Brugada syndrome
   b. Congenital or acquired long QT syndrome
   c. Short QT syndrome
   d. Idiopathic ventricular fibrillation
4. **Drug Toxicity**
   a. Cocaine
   b. Amphetamines
   c. Antiarrhythmic agents
   d. Digoxin toxicity
   e. Drug-induced long QT syndrome
5. **Metabolic Abnormalities**
   a. Severe hypokalemia or hyperkalemia
   b. Severe hypomagnesemia
   c. Severe acidosis

## Management of Cardiac Arrest

The International Liaison Committee on Resuscitation (ILCOR) published its most recent recommendations for management of patients of cardiac arrest in November 2005. The recommendations from 2000 were updated based on an up-to-date review of resuscitation science between 2000 and 2005. Figure 2 shows the ILCOR universal cardiac arrest algorithm.

The initial rhythm encountered by EMS in patients suffering a cardiac arrest are ventricular fibrillation, pulseless ventricular tachycardia (VT), asystole, and PEA. Most patients who suffer an out-of-hospital cardiac arrest are found to be in ventricular fibrillation, but asystole or PEA has been found to be the initial rhythm in increasing frequency in the more recent literature.

## Acute Management of Cardiac Arrest

Survival from a cardiac arrest depends critically on what the American Heart Association describes as the "chain of survival." The chain of survival includes early recognition and initiation of bystander CPR, activation of the EMS system, early defibrillation (which may include automated external defibrillators), and advanced cardiac life support. Because a bystander may provide three of the four links to the chain of survival, community awareness and education in basic life support is a key element in increasing the likelihood of survival of cardiac arrest victims.

### RECOGNITION

The initial management of patients experiencing cardiac arrest should be focused on the patient's ABCs: airway, breathing, and circulation. Delay in the recognition that a patient is experiencing cardiac arrest

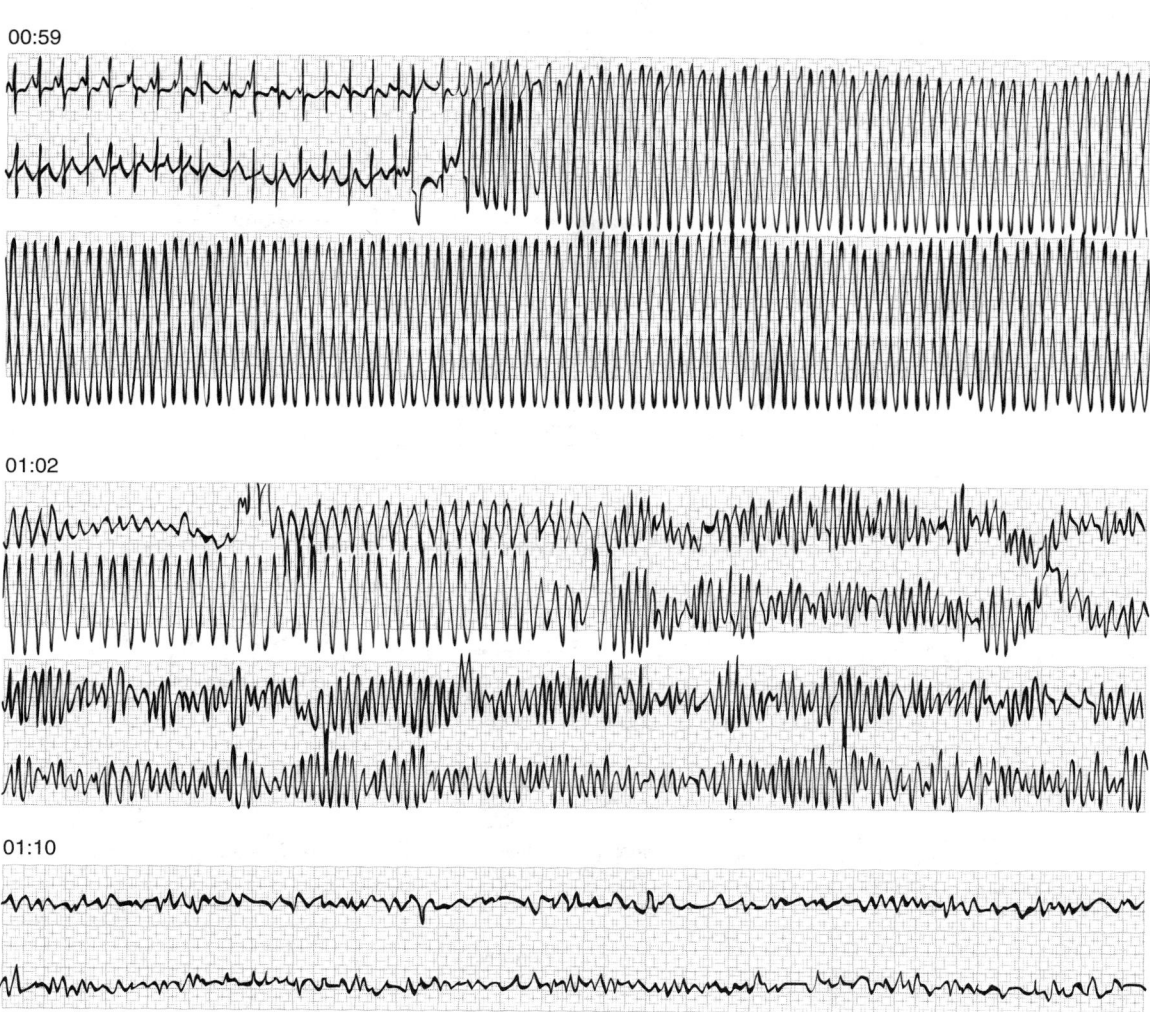

00:59

01:02

01:10

**FIGURE 1.** A Holter tracing of sudden death starting with monomorphic ventricular tachycardia and degenerating into ventricular fibrillation. (From Aziz S, McMahon RF, Garratt CJ: Images in cardiovascular medicine. Sudden cardiac death in arrhythmogenic right ventricular dysplasia. Circulation 2000;101:825-827. Reprinted with permission.)

can waste critical minutes in initiating CPR and providing timely defibrillation. Rescuers should suspect cardiac arrest in any individual who is not moving, not breathing, and unresponsive. Involuntary gasps for air should not be confused for spontaneous respiration because agonal breathing patterns can be present in the early phases of 40% of all cardiac arrests and should not delay initiation of CPR.

## ACTIVATION OF THE EMS SYSTEM

As soon as a patient is recognized to be experiencing a cardiac arrest, the EMS system should be activated. In most communities the system can be activated by calling the universal emergency number 911. The interval of time from onset of the cardiac arrest to arrival of EMS is critical. The shorter this interval of time, the more likely the patient will survive without neurologic injury. Survival is improved in those communities that have a well-organized and well-trained EMS system. Response times can be shortened when other professionals (e.g., firefighters or police officers) trained in CPR and equipped with a defibrillator are employed as first responders.

## AIRWAY

The airway should be opened using a head-tilt, chin-lift technique. If a foreign object is visible, a finger sweep of the oropharynx may be performed. Endotracheal intubation is the optimal means to establish control of the airway. Care must be taken to rule out esophageal

intubation once the tube is inserted. While performing intubation, interruption of CPR must be minimized. Other invasive airway adjuncts have been developed and have proven field success. These include the Combitube and the laryngeal mask airway (LMA).

## BREATHING (VENTILATION)

Ventilation can be achieved by mouth-to-mouth or bag-valve-mask. Each breath should be given a 1-second inspiratory time to achieve a chest rise. A tidal volume of approximately 500 mL to 750 mL should be delivered with a ventilatory rate of 8 to 10 breaths per-minute. When an advanced airway is in place (endotracheal tube or LMA), the rescuer should provide ventilation without interruption in CPR.

## CIRCULATION

The quality of CPR and minimizing interruption of CPR received significant emphasis in the 2005 ILCOR guidelines. Even with optimal chest compressions, the maximum cardiac output achieved is only a third of normal. Chest compressions should be performed with the patient on the floor or with a backboard placed under the patient. The rescuer should place the dominant hand on the lower half of the sternum with the nondominant hand placed over the lower hand. The rescuer should use the weight of his or her torso to compress the chest by 1.5 to 2 cm. After each compression, adequate decompression should be allowed while maintaining a compression-decompression rate of

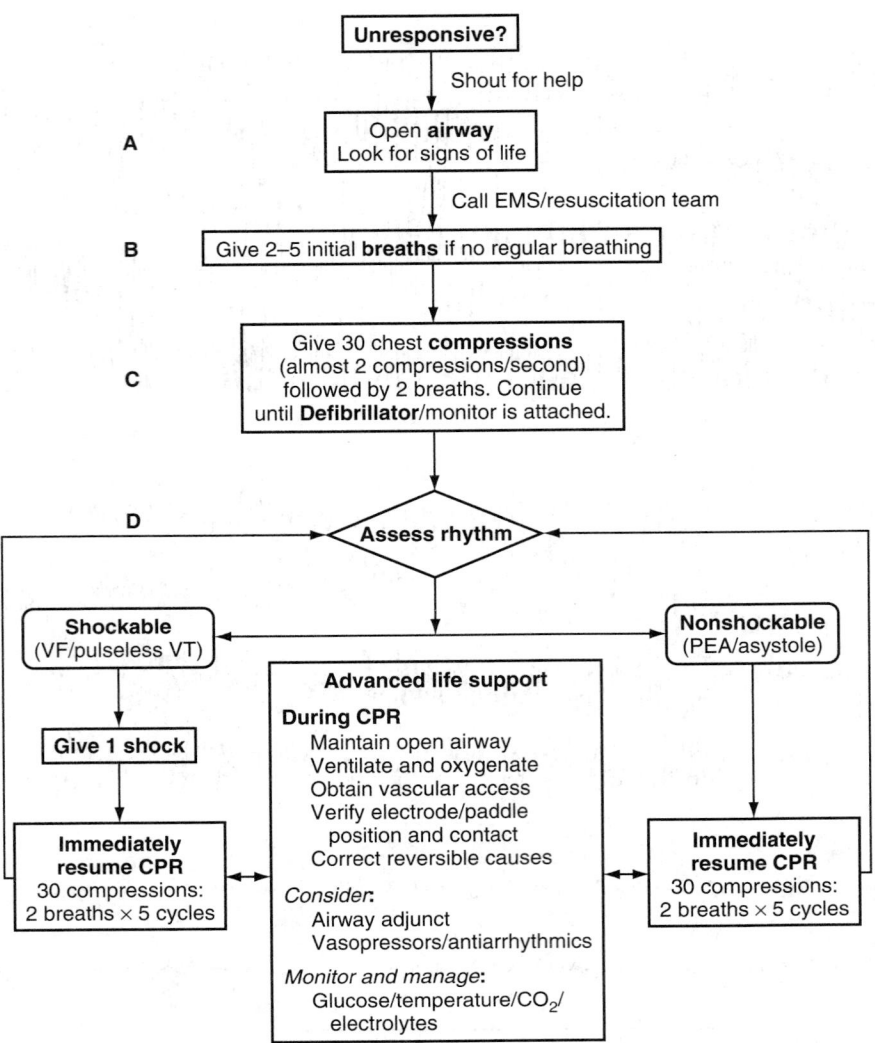

**FIGURE 2.** 2005 ILCOR universal cardiac arrest algorithm. CPR = cardiovascular resuscitation; PEA = pulseless electrical activity; VF = ventricular fibrillation; VT = ventricular tachycardia. (From Circulation 2005;112:1-11. Reprinted with permission.)

100 compressions per minute. The ratio of time for decompression should be at least 50% of the total compression-decompression cycle. Several studies have demonstrated that chest compression rate, depth, and decompression are inadequate even among trained professionals. Inadequate chest compressions may not provide satisfactory hemodynamic support and result in worse survival and neurologic outcome. The quality of CPR (compression, decompression, rate, and depth) should be monitored by all rescuers involved in the resuscitative effort. During prolonged resuscitation, a fatigued rescuer performing CPR should be replaced by a fresh rescuer.

## DEFIBRILLATION

The most critical intervention in patients who have cardiac arrest during ventricular fibrillation or pulseless VT is immediate initiation of chest compressions by a bystander and early defibrillation. In patients with VF, every 1-minute delay in defibrillation reduces the chance of survival by approximately 8% to 10%. The priority of defibrillation and CPR is time dependent. Several studies have demonstrated that when myocardial energy supplies are depleted from prolonged ischemia, coronary perfusion must be achieved before defibrillation. In a study conducted in Seattle, patients who received 90 seconds of CPR before defibrillation had significantly better survival to hospital discharge compared to patients who received defibrillation first. This finding was only significant among patients

who had EMS response times of greater than 4 minutes. In patients with EMS response intervals of less than 4 minutes, there was no difference in survival between the two groups. In a prospective randomized study from Oslo, Norway, 3 minutes of CPR before defibrillation was compared with defibrillation first. In this study, return of spontaneous circulation (ROSC) was observed more frequently in patients who received CPR first compared to defibrillation first (58% vs. 38%; $p < 0.04$) if the EMS response time was more than 5 minutes. There was no difference between the two groups when EMS response time was less than 5 minutes. Survival to hospital discharge was significantly improved in this study in patients who had CPR before defibrillation when EMS response times were more than 5 minutes (22% CPR first vs. 4% defibrillation first; $p = 0.006$). No difference in survival to hospitalization was observed in patients who had EMS response times of less than 5 minutes. These studies demonstrated that CPR prior to defibrillation improved survival in patients who had prolonged VF arrests and did not seem to worsen survival (by delaying defibrillation) in patients who had shorter periods of VF arrest. Based on these data and others, the 2005 ILCOR recommends CPR preceding defibrillation in patients who have an unwitnessed out-of-hospital VF arrest. Furthermore, ILCOR recommends that one shock should be given rather than three successive shocks. This is based on the fact that, in patients who are likely to be successfully defibrillated, the first shock success is very high and a significant interruption in CPR may occur when three successive shocks are delivered because of the time needed to charge the defibrillator, deliver the shock, and check a pulse three times.

When a defibrillator becomes available, the rescuer should continue CPR while the defibrillator is charging. The rescuer should give one shock and continue CPR for five cycles before checking for a pulse. The initial shock energy should be 200 J for a biphasic defibrillator and 360 J for a monophasic defibrillator.

## AUTOMATED EXTERNAL DEFIBRILLATORS

The automated external defibrillator (AED) is a portable device with a battery, capacitor, and a processor that provides an accurate analysis of the cardiac rhythm and an algorithm that instructs the operator if a shock is indicated. The arrhythmia analysis algorithm in the AED has the capacity to interpret complicated cardiac rhythms and to recommend appropriate therapy with a high degree of accuracy. Several studies have demonstrated that AED arrhythmia detection for VF has a 100% sensitivity and specificity. The operation of the AED is simple and involves four steps:

1. Turn on the AED.
2. Connect the pads to the patient.
3. Wait for the AED to analyze cardiac rhythm.
4. Press the shock button (if shock is advised by the AED).

The AED uses voice and text prompts to guide the user through these steps. Because of ease of use, the AED can be safely and reliably operated by a nonmedically trained person.

Since the majority of cardiac arrests occur out of the hospital, the efficacy of AEDs has been tested in a number of conditions. In a 2-year study of AEDs used in a major airline, an AED was used in 200 patients. Of the 15 patients with VF, 6 patients (40%) were successfully defibrillated and survived to hospital discharge. The sensitivity and specificity of VF detection by the AED was 100%.

The efficacy of AEDs was also tested in casinos. This is a unique setting where a large population of patients are monitored by closed-circuit surveillance cameras. In this study, 56 of 105 (53%) patients who suffered a cardiac arrest because of ventricular fibrillation were successfully defibrillated and survived to hospital discharge. The mean time to first shock from the AED in this study was 4.4 minutes, and the mean time for arrival of paramedics was 9.8 minutes. In another study of public access defibrillation (PAD) conducted in Seattle; 475 AEDs were placed in a variety of public settings, and more than 4000 persons were trained in CPR and AED operation. A total of 50 cases of cardiac arrest were treated by PAD before EMS arrival, representing 1.33% of all EMS-treated cardiac arrests in the county. Of the 50 patients treated by PAD, 25 (50%) patients survived to hospital discharge.

## CARDIAC ARREST FROM PULSELESS ELECTRICAL ACTIVITY

PEA is defined by the presence of a heart rhythm that does not generate a pulse. Patients who are found in PEA generally have a poor prognosis but may be successfully resuscitated if a correctable cause is identified and treated promptly. Some correctable causes of PEA include:

1. Hypovolemia
2. Exsanguination
3. Tension pneumothorax
4. Acute pulmonary embolism
5. Cardiac tamponade from a pericardial effusion
6. Hypothermia
7. Hyperkalemia
8. Metabolic acidosis (preexisting)

Patients suspected to be hypovolemic from obvious bleeding should be resuscitated with volume expanders (normal saline, lactated Ringer's) and transfused as soon as blood is available. O negative blood (universal donor) may be transfused in patients in extremis. A tension pneumothorax results from a tear in the pleura that serves as a one-way valve, allowing air to enter but not leave the pleural space.

This results in significant increase in pleural pressure and intrathoracic pressures. It should be suspected in patients with absence of breath sounds and a deviated trachea toward the contralateral lung. A large-bore needle may be inserted at the midclavicular line over the second rib to decompress the affected lung rapidly, followed by insertion of a chest tube. In selective cases an acute pulmonary embolism may be successfully treated with thrombolytic medication. Cardiac tamponade should be treated with a pericardiocentesis. Hypothermia may be treated with rewarming. Hyperkalemia should be treated with intravenous (IV) calcium, insulin and glucose, or sodium bicarbonate. Rapid assessment of these secondary causes and immediate treatment may be life saving in some patients who present with reversible causes of PEA.

## CARDIAC ARREST CAUSED BY ASYSTOLE

Asystole is usually a terminal rhythm in cardiac arrest victims who have had a prolonged episode of hypoxia and ischemic injury. External pacing has demonstrated no improvement in survival in patients who present in the field with asystole. Hyperkalemia is a reversible cause of asystole. Patients who present with asystole because of hyperkalemia may be successfully resuscitated with early bystander CPR and rapid treatment of hyperkalemia.

# Pharmacologic Treatment in Cardiac Arrest

The primary goals in the successful resuscitation of a patient with cardiac arrest is to restore a rhythm that results in adequate perfusion of the two most vulnerable organs to hypoxemia, the heart and the brain, and maintain adequate perfusion to the heart and brain to prevent irreversible injury during the arrest until a rhythm and adequate hemodynamics are restored. To date, no randomized clinical trials have demonstrated an improvement in survival to hospital discharge among patients who have suffered a cardiac arrest attributable to any drugs currently used in advanced cardiac life support.

## Drugs Used to Restore Rhythm

No randomized human studies have demonstrated that the use of antiarrhythmic agents in cardiac arrest improves survival to hospital discharge. Despite the lack of evidence supporting the role of antiarrhythmic agents, these agents are used routinely in shock refractory ventricular arrhythmias.

### AMIODARONE

A randomized, double-blind, placebo-controlled study of IV amiodarone (Cordarone) in out-of-hospital cardiac arrest demonstrated an improvement in survival to hospitalization in patients treated with IV amiodarone versus placebo (44% vs. 34%; $p = 0.03$). This study demonstrated no difference in survival to hospital discharge (13.4% vs. 13.2%) but was not powered to evaluate this endpoint. Furthermore, there was no difference among survivors in the ability to resume independent living activities (55% vs. 50%). In another randomized, controlled study of amiodarone versus lidocaine in out-of-hospital cardiac arrest, amiodarone was superior to lidocaine in survival to hospitalization (22.8% vs. 12%; $p = 0.009$), but there was no difference in survival to hospital discharge.

### LIDOCAINE

No randomized, placebo-controlled studies of lidocaine have been performed in out-of-hospital cardiac arrest. In one study with historical controls, lidocaine was associated with an improvement in return of spontaneous circulation and survival to hospitalization but not in survival to discharge. However, other studies have demonstrated no benefit in survival with lidocaine.

# Drugs Used to Support Blood Pressure

Despite the standard use of vasopressors in cardiac arrest, there is a lack of clinical evidence demonstrating improved survival with these interventions.

## EPINEPHRINE

Epinephrine is a mixed adrenergic agonist and acts on $\alpha$-1, $\alpha$-2, $\beta$-1 and $\beta$-2 adrenergic receptors. It is the $\alpha$ actions of epinephrine that provide the most benefit during resuscitation. Through its $\alpha$ actions, epinephrine increases coronary perfusion pressure and maintains peripheral vascular tone. The beta-adrenergic effects of epinephrine may be detrimental in patients during cardiac arrest. Stimulation of $\beta$-1 receptors results in an increase in myocardial oxygen consumption and decreases subendocardial perfusion.

There are no randomized trials of standard dose epinephrine versus placebo in cardiac arrest. Herlitz et al. compared 417 patients with out-of-hospital VF who received epinephrine (1 mg every 3 to 5 minutes) with 786 patients (historical control) who did not receive epinephrine. Although more patients had return of spontaneous circulation and survived to hospitalization when treated with epinephrine, there was no significant difference in survival to hospital discharge.

Evidence on high-dose epinephrine (5 to 15 mg) in cardiac arrest did not show a benefit in survival in out-of-hospital arrest. Although high-dose epinephrine is associated with a higher rate of return of spontaneous circulation, there is no difference in survival to discharge. These patients who survive to hospitalization are likely to have significant neurologic injury. Most of these patients do not survive to hospital discharge.

Despite the lack of clinical data demonstrating an improvement in survival with epinephrine in cardiac arrest, the ILCOR recommends the continued use of epinephrine at standard dose (1 mg every 3 to 5 minutes) on a routine basis for cardiac arrest. High-dose epinephrine is not recommended.

## VASOPRESSIN

Vasopressin (Pitressin) is an endogenous vasopressor that causes selective vasoconstriction of resistance vessels. Although vasopressin appears to have pharmacologic properties well suited for cardiac arrest (increases vascular tone without $\beta$-adrenergic stimulation), clinical trials comparing vasopressin to epinephrine showed no difference in outcomes. However, in a study of vasopressin versus epinephrine in 1186 patients with cardiac arrest because of VF, PEA, or asystole, vasopressin was superior to epinephrine with the endpoint of survival to discharge in the subset of patients who had asystole (4.7% vs. 1.5%; $p = 0.04$). This study, like others, demonstrated no difference in survival to hospital discharge in the subset of patients who presented with VF or PEA.

The ILCOR concluded that "There is insufficient evidence to support or refute the use of vasopressin as an alternative to, or in combination with, epinephrine in any cardiac arrest rhythm." For the management of cardiac arrest because of VF refractory to defibrillation, asystole, or PEA, a dose of epinephrine (1 mg) IV may be repeated every 3 to 5 minutes. Vasopressin may substitute for the first or second dose of epinephrine. In patients who present with asystole, vasopressin may be preferred over epinephrine. Drugs should be administered without interruption of CPR.

# Alternative Routes for Drug Administration

IV access cannot always be established during a resuscitation attempt. CPR and defibrillation should not be delayed to establish IV access. As an alternative to IV access, resuscitative drugs may be given via the endotracheal tube. Drugs that are absorbed via the trachea can be remembered by the mnemonic *navel*: *n*aloxone, *a*tropine, *v*asopressin, *e*pinephrine, and *l*idocaine. When drugs are administered via the endotracheal tube, two to three times the usual IV dose should be given to achieve the same serum levels.

# Management and Evaluation of Survivors of Cardiac Arrest

The management of survivors of cardiac arrest begins with a continuous effort to identify the cause of the cardiac arrest at the onset of the resuscitation. After return of spontaneous rhythm and circulation, the patient should be monitored in an intensive care setting. During the initial period of hospitalization, the patient is vulnerable to cardiac arrhythmias and hemodynamic and respiratory instability. Patients are also prone to ongoing ischemic neurologic injury. Other issues encountered in the postarrest period include acute renal failure, shock liver, ischemic bowel, sepsis, and acute respiratory distress syndrome. The patients may require antiarrhythmic agents, inotropic support, and ventilatory support during the early period after a cardiac arrest. Frequent monitoring of arterial blood gas and electrolytes should be performed, and abnormalities should be corrected. Recent studies showed an improvement in neurologic outcomes in patients treated with hypothermia (32° to 34° C [90° to 93°F]) for 12 to 24 hours postresuscitation. The ILCOR recommends therapeutic hypothermia in all patients who are unconscious for a period of 12 to 24 hours after a cardiac arrest.

The physician should begin a detailed history and physical examination. Family members should be contacted to see whether the patient had an advance directive. A myocardial infarction should be ruled out with an electrocardiogram (EKG) and serial cardiac enzymes, and a thorough review of available medical records including a complete review of current medications should be performed. Minimum initial workup should include a chest radiograph and laboratory evaluation (electrolytes, arterial blood gas, liver and renal function tests, and toxicology screening). An echocardiogram should be performed to assess the presence or absence of structural heart disease. Because the majority of all cardiac arrests occur in patients with significant coronary artery disease, coronary angiography should be performed in most patients who have suffered a cardiac arrest.

## HISTORY

It is often difficult to obtain any history from the patient. If the patient is awake, he or she may have significant neurologic impairment and retrograde amnesia of events preceding the arrest. History taken from witnesses to the cardiac arrest and family members and friends close to the victim may be valuable. Important information gained from the history would include any recent medications, heart failure symptoms preceding the arrest, angina preceding the arrest, illicit drug use, and a family history of sudden death.

## 12-LEAD ELECTROCARDIOGRAM

A 12-lead EKG may demonstrate signs of myocardial ischemia or injury. Other findings on the 12-lead EKG include the presence of epsilon waves suggesting arrhythmogenic right ventricular cardiomyopathy; incomplete right bundle branch block with ST-segment elevations in the right precordial leads (suggestive of Brugada syndrome); a prolonged or abnormally short (<300 ms) QT segment, which may suggest long QT syndrome or short QT syndrome, respectively; ventricular pre-excitation because of a bypass tract; and severe conduction system disease (bifascicular block or evidence of heart block). The 12-lead EKG should be screened carefully for these abnormalities.

## LABORATORY EVALUATION

Laboratory evaluation should include electrolytes, arterial blood gas, liver and renal function tests, serial cardiac enzymes, complete blood count, and a toxicology screen. The causal role of the abnormalities detected should be interpreted carefully. Hypokalemia may occur because of intracellular shifting of potassium secondary to endogenous catecholamines or epinephrine given during the cardiac arrest. Elevations in myocardial band enzymes of creatine phosphokinase (MB CK) and troponins indicate myocardial infarction; however, mild elevations in cardiac enzymes may result from prolonged CPR and defibrillation and may not be indicative of a primary myocardial infarction.

Other laboratory findings may be helpful in screening for end organ damage. Significant elevations in transaminases and elevated protime may be evidence of ischemic liver injury. Bloody stools and persistent lactic acidosis should increase the suspicion for ischemic bowel. Acute renal failure is commonly seen after an arrest.

## ECHOCARDIOGRAM

An echocardiogram is essential in the workup of patients who have survived a cardiac arrest. The echocardiogram may detect evidence of hypertrophic cardiomyopathy, left ventricular dysfunction, regional wall motion abnormalities, abnormalities in the RV that might be suggestive of arrhythmogenic right ventricular cardiomyopathy, significant valvular disease, and other structural cardiac abnormalities. The presence of left ventricular dysfunction early postarrest may be because of "stunning" (caused by ischemia and defibrillation) and may not be representative of the patient's true left ventricular function.

## CARDIAC CATHETERIZATION

Coronary angiography should be performed in most patients who have suffered a cardiac arrest to rule out significant epicardial coronary artery disease or congenital coronary anomalies.

## ELECTROPHYSIOLOGIC STUDY

Currently, the electrophysiologic study in cardiac arrest victims has a limited role. However, an electrophysiologic study may be useful in a select group of patients: those with ventricular preexcitation (Wolff-Parkinson-White [WPW] pattern) on the EKG because the electrophysiologic study will allow characterization of the anterograde conduction properties of the bypass tract and may offer a curative strategy; patients with suspected bundle branch reentry ventricular tachycardia, which occurs in patients with dilated cardiomyopathy; and provocative drug testing for concealed long QT syndrome (epinephrine), Brugada syndrome (sodium channel blocker), or significant His-Purkinje disease. The electrophysiologic study is not routinely indicated in patients who have suffered a cardiac arrest.

# Neurologic Assessment

Patients who are unconscious after cardiac arrest require an assessment of the degree of irreversible global neurologic injury. Patients should be assessed while normothermic and after all sedation is withheld. Assessment of neurologic status in a comatose patient includes apnea testing and assessment of brainstem reflexes. Absence of reflexes and abnormal apnea testing is associated with a grim prognosis. Additional neurologic testing with excellent predictive accuracy includes a median nerve somatosensory evoked potential (SSEP) and an electroencephalogram (EEG). An abnormal SSEP assessed at 72 hours postresuscitation predicts a poor outcome with 100% specificity. An EEG may also be a useful prognostic tool.

Patients who are conscious may still suffer from varying degrees of amnesia, short term memory loss, and from motor or sensory deficits. They may require physical therapy, occupational therapy, speech therapy, and rehabilitation.

## ROLE OF IMPLANTABLE CARDIAC DEFIBRILLATORS

Currently, most patients who are survivors of a ventricular fibrillation or ventricular tachycardia–related cardiac arrest are treated with an implantable cardiac defibrillator (ICD) even if there is an identifiable

reversible cause. A randomized controlled study of amiodarone versus implantable cardiac defibrillator among cardiac arrest survivors (Antiarrhythmics Versus Implantable Defibrillators [AVID]) demonstrated a survival advantage in patients treated with an ICD. A subset analysis revealed that survival benefit was observed only in patients with ejection fraction (EF) less than 35%. Patients with EF more than 35% had no difference in survival whether treated with an ICD or amiodarone. Patients in AVID with reversible or correctable causes were excluded from and followed in a registry. The mortality among the 278 patients followed in the registry at 3 years was found to be higher than in patients who did not have transient or reversible causes. Contemporary practice is that most patients who have suffered a VT/VF cardiac arrest are treated with an ICD regardless of whether their arrest was because of a transient or reversible cause and regardless of their EF. An important exception are patients with preserved left ventricular function who had a VT/VF arrest within 72 hours of an acute transmural myocardial infarction. These patients have a low recurrence rate of cardiac arrest if they have no evidence of residual ischemia and preserved left ventricular function. Amiodarone is a reasonable option for patients with preserved EF with contraindications for an ICD.

Some situations where an ICD may not be appropriate are patients who have a cardiac arrest less than 72 hours after a transmural myocardial infarction, patients who do not wish to have an ICD, patients who had a cardiac arrest because of rapidly conducting atrial fibrillation via a bypass tract (WPW) that was treated successfully with a radiofrequency ablation procedure, and patients of advanced age and significant co-morbidities (the risks and benefits of ICD implantation should be carefully considered in such patients).

Cardiac arrest is a major public health concern killing hundreds of thousands of people annually in the United States. The cornerstone of treatment of patients suffering a cardiac arrest is early recognition, early activation of EMS, early bystander CPR, early defibrillation, and advanced cardiac life support. Despite our best efforts, the prognosis of cardiac arrest victims remains poor. Recent advances in the science of resuscitation have provided grounds to make some significant changes to the guidelines for resuscitation of cardiac arrest. Communities with a well-established EMS system, public access defibrillation programs, and citizens who are well educated in basic life support have the highest rates of survival for cardiac arrest victims.

## REFERENCES

Antiarrhythmics versus implantable defibrillators (AVID) investigators: A comparison of antiarrhythmic-drug therapy with implantable defibrillators in patients resuscitated from near-fatal ventricular arrhythmias. N Engl J Med 1997;337:1576–1583.

Cobb LA, Fahrenbruch CE, Walsh TR, et al: Influence of cardiopulmonary resuscitation prior to defibrillation in patients with out-of-hospital ventricular fibrillation. JAMA 1999;281:1182–1188.

Connolly SJ, Hallstrom AP, Cappato R, et al: Meta-analysis of the implantable cardioverter defibrillator secondary prevention trials. Eur Heart J 2000;21:2071–2078.

Cully CL, Rea TD, Murray JA, et al: Public access defibrillation in out-of hospital cardiac arrest. Circulation 2004;109:1859–1863.

Dorian P, Cass D, Schwartz B, et al: Amiodarone as compared with lidocaine for shock-resistant ventricular fibrillation. N Engl J Med 2002;346:884–890.

2005 International consensus on cardiopulmonary resuscitation (CPR) and emergency cardiovascular care (ECC) science with treatment recommendations. Circulation 2005;112:1–11.

Kudenchuk PJ, Cobb LA, Copass MK, et al: Amiodarone for resuscitation after out-of-hospital cardiac arrest due to ventricular fibrillation. N Engl J Med 1999;341:871–878.

Page RL, Joglar JA, Kowal RC, et al: Use of automated external defibrillators by a US airline. N Engl J Med 2000;343:1210–1216.

Pepe PE, Fowler RL, Roppolo LP, et al: Clinical review: Reappraising the concept of immediate defibrillatory attempts for out-of-hospital ventricular fibrillation. Crit Care 2004;8:41–45.

Rea TD, Eisenberg MS, Sinibaldi G, et al: Incidence of EMS-treated out-of-hospital cardiac arrest in the United States. Resuscitation 2004; 63:17–24.

Wyse DG, Friedman PL, Brodsky MA, et al: Life threatening ventricular arrhythmias due to transient or correctable causes: high risk for death in follow-up. J Am Coll Cardiol 2001;38:1718–1724.

Zhong J, Dorian P: Epinephrine and vasopressin during cardiopulmonary resuscitation. Resuscitation 2005;66:263–269.

# Atrial Fibrillation

Method of
*Ruth Falik, MD*

Atrial fibrillation (AF), first described in humans in 1906 using the then newly invented electrocardiogram (ECG), is the commonest clinical dysrhythmia for which patients seek treatment. AF is characterized by seemingly disorganized atrial depolarizations without effective atrial contraction. The surface ECG demonstrates an irregular ventricular pattern and the absence of organized atrial activity manifested as an absence of P waves.

## Epidemiology

AF is the most common sustained dysrhythmia in adults. It is a major contributor to cardiovascular morbidity; up to 15% of all strokes in the United States can be attributed to AF. It accounts for one third of hospitalizations for dysrhythmia. The prevalence of AF increases with age from less than 1% in persons younger than 60 years to more than 8% of those older than 80 years. The annual incidence ranges from 0.2% per year for men ages 30 to 39 years and increases to 2.3% per year for men ages 80 to 89 years. The incidence for women is about one half that of men.

Hypertensive, valvular, and ischemic heart disease underlies most cases of chronic AF. Independent risk factors include male gender, hypertension, diabetes, heart failure, and valvular heart disease. Echocardiographic abnormalities predisposing to AF include left atrial dilation, left ventricular hypertrophy, and impaired systolic function.

*Lone atrial fibrillation* describes AF in the absence of demonstrable underlying cardiac disease or a history of hypertension. It is estimated that lone AF occurs in less than 3% of patients with AF. In patients younger than 60 years, lone AF has a benign prognosis; in older patients, there is an increased risk of stroke and death.

Atrial fibrillation is classified according to its duration and temporal pattern. Episodes are *paroxysmal* if they spontaneously terminate, usually within 48 hours of onset. *Persistent* AF does not self-terminate, but it can be electrically or pharmacologically cardioverted to sinus rhythm. *Permanent* AF cannot be cardioverted.

## Pathophysiology

Human mapping studies done in the past 30 years have demonstrated that AF is characterized by multiple wavelets of excitation propagating around the atrial myocardium. Perpetuation of the dysrhythmia is a manifestation of an underlying tissue abnormality. In younger patients and those with paroxysmal AF, there is usually a triggering mechanism. Multielectrode mapping systems have demonstrated that the patterns of activation vary both between patients and between the two atria of individual patients.

AF is the result of multiple reentrant loops continuously circulating in both atria, generating chaotic atrial depolarizations with resultant ineffective atrial contraction. The atrioventricular (AV) node is bombarded with impulses at rates greater than 400 bpm. The refractory period and conductivity of the AV node are determinants of the ventricular rate. Many of the impulses are blocked, and the resultant ventricular rhythm is irregularly irregular.

Shortening of the refractory period of the atria is essential to the perpetuation of AF. Indeed, the longer the duration of AF, the shorter the refractory period; this electrical remodeling of the myocardium explains the adage "atrial fibrillation begets atrial fibrillation." The longer a patient has been in AF, the more difficult it is to reestablish sinus rhythm. At the electrophysiologic level, the consequences of prolonged rapid atrial rate are conduction delay, loss of adaptation of refractoriness to rate, and a dispersion of atrial refractoriness.

Atrial fibrillation results from a complex interaction between initiating triggers and the development of an abnormal tissue substrate capable of maintaining the arrhythmia. Many patients with AF have structural heart disease, but some have no apparent heart disease. These patients tend to be younger and are believed to have a trigger mechanism such as an area of increased automaticity that can be localized to the muscular sleeves of the proximal pulmonary veins.

Prolonged episodes of AF can cause mechanical dysfunction of the atria. With restoration of sinus rhythm, there is a normalization of atrial function over a period of 2 to 4 weeks. Similarly, the tachycardia-mediated left ventricular dysfunction is reversible after rate control is established (generally less than 100 bpm) or sinus rhythm is restored.

## Diagnosis

Patients with AF can present with acute hemodynamic decompensation or they can be entirely asymptomatic. Very often, the diagnosis of AF is an incidental finding during a medical evaluation for other reasons. The diagnosis of AF is based on the history and physical examination and is confirmed with a 12-lead ECG.

Symptoms are determined by multiple factors, including the ventricular rate, underlying left ventricular function, and loss of the atrial kick. Patients might experience severe symptoms such as acute pulmonary edema, angina, or hypotension, or symptoms may be nonspecific, such as fatigue or decreased exercise tolerance.

Physical findings include a slight variation in intensity of the first heart sound, absence of alpha waves in the jugular venous pulse, and an irregularly irregular pulse. When the ventricular rate is fast, there is a difference between the auscultated apical rate and the palpable peripheral pulse rate; this differential is known as a *pulse deficit*.

It is important to identify reversible causes and risk factors including structural heart disease, hypertension, thyrotoxicosis, and excessive alcohol consumption. Mitral stenosis, pericarditis, pneumonia, or pulmonary embolism should be considered and, if present, treated. Echocardiography can provide information regarding mitral valve stenosis, left atrial size (which can predict the likelihood of achieving and maintaining sinus rhythm), and atrial thrombus (see later).

---

 **CURRENT DIAGNOSIS**

- Atrial fibrillation is an irregularly irregular rhythm suspected by history or physical examination and confirmed by 12-lead ECG.
- ECG differentiates between AF and sinus rhythm with frequent atrial premature depolarizations, mutlifocal atrial tachycardia (both of which have an isoelectric baseline and visible P waves), and atrial flutter (flutter waves equal in amplitude and width are seen in most or all leads).
- Symptoms are variable, ranging from none to mild fatigue to cardiac decompensation (hypotension, pulmonary edema, or angina).
- Physical findings include an irregularly irregular pulse, pulse deficit, variable intensity of S1 heart sounds, and no alpha waves in the jugular venous pulse.
- Identify reversible causes and risk factors including structural heart disease, hypertension, thyrotoxicosis, excessive alcohol consumption, pericarditis, and pulmonary embolism.
- Echocardiography can provide information regarding left atrial size, mitral valve structure and function, pulmonary vein size, left ventricular wall dimensions and function, and the presence of atrial thrombus.

---

*Abbreviations:* AF = atrial fibrillation; ECG = electrocardiogram.

Medications including theophylline (Uniphyl) and illicit stimulant drugs should be considered. When possible, it is helpful to determine the duration of the dysrhythmia.

# Treatment

## ACUTE MANAGEMENT

The patient's clinical presentation determines therapy. If the sudden onset of AF with a rapid ventricular rate (RVR) results in chest pain, dyspnea, or hypotension, then immediate electrical (DC) cardioversion is indicated. When there is no evidence of cardiac decompensation, therapeutic decisions should be individualized.

Rate control is essential, as is the prevention of thromboembolic complications, most significantly cerebrovascular. Prolonged episodes of RVR can cause a tachycardia-mediated cardiomyopathy. The approach to patients with AF should be focused on relief of symptoms, control of ventricular rates, and prevention of thromboembolic events.

Whether the patient should be cardioverted to sinus rhythm, either electrically or chemically, is a complicated issue. Most often, symptoms are due to RVR rather than due to the dysrhythmia itself. The exception to this includes patients with significant ventricular diastolic dysfunction (as can be seen in aortic stenosis or hypertensive heart disease) in whom the atrial kick is critical to adequate cardiac output. Atrial kick can contribute as much as 20% to cardiac output.

Hospitalization is not required for all patients. Only those with hemodynamic compromise, those for whom early cardioversion is considered, and those who are severely symptomatic with AF need to be admitted to the hospital. If there is no chest pain, ECG evidence of ischemia, or history of recent myocardial infarction, there is no need for admission to a coronary care unit because ischemic heart disease rarely manifests as AF with no other signs or symptoms. Patients with AF and a rapid, wide-complex ventricular response related to the preexcitation syndrome may also be considered for early electrical cardioversion, because the response to antiarrhythmic medication is difficult to predict and most drugs used for rate control are contraindicated.

If urgent cardioversion is not indicated, then pharmacologic rate control is considered. The atrial rate can exceed 350 bpm in AF, but the ventricular response rate is usually between 110 and 130 bpm. The exception to this is seen in patients with preexcitation, where the ventricular response may exceed 250 bpm or in patients with a hyperadrenergic state such as thyrotoxicosis, fever, or acute blood loss. A slower than expected ventricular rate may be seen in patients with high vagal tone, such as well-conditioned athletes, or in patients with conduction system disease.

Intravenous β-blockers or calcium channel blockers achieve the most consistent and rapid rate control. See Table 1 for the appropriate doses of these drugs. Digoxin (Lanoxin) is of little value in patients in hyperadrenergic states and can be problematic if electrical cardioversion becomes necessary.

Paroxysmal AF is not uncommon. The dysrhythmia-free interval is unpredictable, and it might not be necessary to prescribe ongoing anticoagulation or antiarrhythmic medication. Patients who have had an embolic event should receive long-term anticoagulation even if AF is only paroxysmal. In select patients who do not have ischemic, hypotensive, or heart failure symptoms with their paroxysmal AF, the pill-in-the-pocket approach has been shown to be effective and safe. The use of self-administered oral antiarrhythmic medication—typically flecainide (Tambocor) or propafenone (Rythmol) in a single loading dose—has reduced the number of emergency department visits and hospital admissions.

## ANTICOAGULATION

Nonvalvular AF is the commonest cardiac condition associated with cerebral embolism. The risk of stroke in patients with nonvalvular AF is five to seven times greater than that in controls without AF. Risk factors that predict stroke in patients with nonvalvular AF include a history of stroke or transient ischemic attack, heart failure, a history of hypertension, and age older than 75 years (some consider age 65 years the cutoff). Such patients should be treated with warfarin (Coumadin) anticoagulation to achieve an international normalized ratio (INR) of 2.0 to 3.0 for stroke prevention. Patients with mitral valve stenosis or visualized left atrial clot should be anticoagulated as well. Patients with AF who do not have any of these risk factors have a low stroke risk

## CURRENT THERAPY

- Symptom relief, rate control, and prevention of thromboembolic complications are primary goals of therapy.
- Urgent cardioversion is indicated if the patient is having chest pain, dyspnea, hypotension, or other evidence of cardiac decompensation. In this setting electrical cardioversion is indicated. Parenteral anticoagulation should be started.
- For the vast majority of patients with AF, rate control and anticoagulation are the therapeutic goals; rhythm control has not been shown to be superior in reducing morbidity or mortality.
- Intravenous β-blockers or calcium channel blockers achieve the most consistent and rapid rate control.
- Hospitalization is not required for all patients. When AF is well tolerated, outpatient evaluation and therapy should be considered.
- Anticoagulation for at least 3 weeks prior to elective cardioversion (drug or electrical) is indicated unless one has TEE confirmation that there is no thrombus in the atria.
- Anticoagulation should be continued for at least 4 weeks following successful cardioversion.
- Most patients converted to sinus rhythm should not be given chronic rhythm maintenance drug therapy because the risks outweigh the benefits.

*Abbreviations:* AF = atrial fibrillation; TEE = transesophageal echocardiogram.

**TABLE 1  Drugs for Rate Control in Atrial Fibrillation**

| Drug | Acute Control | Chronic Control |
|---|---|---|
| Digoxin (Lanoxin) | 0.25-0.50 mg IV in repeated doses up to 1.0-1.5 mg over 24 h | Oral maintenance doses range from 0.125-0.5 mg/d* |
| **Calcium Channel Blockers** | | |
| Diltiazem (Cardizem, Dilacor, Diltia, Tiazac) | 0.25 mg/kg IV bolus over 2 min  Repeat after 15 min. with 0.35 mg/kg if no rate control[3]  Maintenance 5-15 mg/h IV for <24 h | Oral controlled release formulation 180-300 mg/d |
| Verapamil (Calan, Covera, Isoptin, Verelan) | 2.5-10 mg IV over 2-3 min  May repeat 5-10 mg. in 15-30 min[†] | Slow-release formula 120-480 mg/d; for doses >240 mg/d, take bid with food |
| **β-Blockers** | | |
| Metoprolol (Lopressor, Toprol[1]) | 5 mg IV bolus  Repeat twice at 2-min intervals* | 25-400 mg/d |

[1]Not FDA approved for this indication.
[3]Exceeds dosage recommended by the manufacturer.
*Doses are reduced in patients with renal failure and when used with drugs known to raise digoxin levels.
[†]No data on maintenance infusion.

## TABLE 2  Pharmacologic Agents Used to Cardiovert Atrial Fibrillation and Maintain Sinus Rhythm

| Drug | Cardioversion Dose | Maintenance Dose | Comments |
|---|---|---|---|
| Amiodarone (Cordarone)[1] | 1200 mg IV in 24 h | 600 mg/d for 2 wk, then 200-400 mg/d | Best for maintaining sinus rhythm |
| Ibutilide (Corvert) | 1 mg IV over 10 min in pts < 60 kg *or* 0.01 mg/kg over 10 min in pts > 60 kg May repeat dose 10 min after end of infusion if no response | Not available (IV only) | Avoid in pts with hypokalemia, prolonged QT interval |
| Quinidine | 200 mg sulfate PO, followed 1-2 h later by 400 mg | 200-400 mg sulfate qid *or* 324-648 mg gluconate tid | Risk of death is increased with long-term therapy |
| Procainamide (Pronestyl) | 100 mg IV q5 min to 1 g (max) | Slow release formulation 1-2 g bid | Long-term use is associated with lupus |
| Propafenone (Rythmol) | 600 mg orally | 150-300 mg tid | Use only in structurally normal heart |
| Sotalol (Betapace) | Not recommended; conversion rate is low | 120-160 mg bid | Need to hospitalize for initiation of therapy to monitor for pro dysrrhythmia effect |

[1]Not FDA approved for this indication.
*Abbreviations:* max = maximum; pt = patient.

---

(2% or less per year), and can be protected with aspirin. Unreliable patients and those with contraindications to anticoagulation (e.g., recent intracranial hemorrhage, thrombocytopenia, increased risk of falling) should also be managed with aspirin.

Patients who have AF longer than 2 days should receive warfarin to achieve an INR of 2.0 to 3.0 for at least 3 weeks before pharmacologic or electrical cardioversion is considered. Alternatively, a transesophageal echocardiogram (TEE) to exclude the presence of an atrial clot identifies patients at low risk for thromboembolic events. These patients are immediately treated with parenteral heparin or low-molecular weight heparin, and this is followed by therapeutic oral anticoagulation with warfarin. Anticoagulation with heparin has been recommended for emergency cardioversion when 3 weeks of anticoagulation or a TEE is not feasible. Anticoagulation should be continued for at least 4 weeks following successful cardioversion because poor atrial contractile function might persist and the risk of AF recurrence is greatest during the first weeks following cardioversion.

### RATE CONTROL VERSUS RHYTHM CONTROL

Rate control with chronic anticoagulation is the recommended strategy for the majority of patients with AF. Rhythm control has not been shown to be superior in reducing morbidity or mortality. This has been demonstrated in large clinical studies (e.g., Atrial Fibrillation Follow-up Investigation of Rhythm Management [AFFIRM], Pharmacologic Intervention in Atrial Fibrillation [PIAF], and Rate Control versus Electrical Cardioversion [RACE]) that demonstrate no advantage to rhythm conversion therapy. In the largest of these studies, AFFIRM, more than 4000 patients with AF were randomized to therapy for either rhythm control with anticoagulation or rate control with anticoagulation. There were no differences in mortality or quality of life between the two groups. In general, patients who are found to be in AF incidentally do well with rate control and anticoagulation.

Symptomatic patients who continue to be symptomatic despite rate control should be considered for electrical or pharmacologic cardioversion. See Table 2 for drugs used to cardiovert AF. Most patients converted to sinus rhythm from AF should not be placed on rhythm maintenance therapy because the risks outweigh the benefits. In a select group of patients whose quality of life is compromised by AF, amiodarone (Cordarone),[1] propafenone (Rythmol), and sotalol (Betapace) are useful for rhythm maintenance. Maintenance of sinus rhythm after cardioversion is influenced by the duration of AF and, for some, left atrial dilation.

### REFRACTORY SYMPTOMATIC ATRIAL FIBRILLATION

The combination of persistent AF and systolic dysfunction can be difficult to rate control without increasing the symptoms of heart failure. Radiofrequency catheter ablation of the atrioventricular node and implantation of a rate-adaptive ventricular pacemaker can provide an alternative to continuing ineffective or poorly tolerated drugs.

For patients in whom AF is triggered by a rapidly firing atrial focus located in the pulmonary veins, the application of radiofrequency energy at the site of the ectopic foci or electrical isolation of the pulmonary vein ostia from the atrium results in a marked reduction in atrial ectopy and the abolition of AF.

Several novel pacing techniques are being investigated for preventing paroxysmal AF. The underlying principle is that inhomogeneous or delayed interatrial or intraatrial conduction times predispose to the development of AF. Both dual-site atrial pacing (high in the right atrium and at the coronary sinus ostium) and biatrial pacing (high in the right atrium and in the mid or proximal coronary sinus) reduce the duration of the P wave and result in a more homogeneous atrial depolarization. For optimal results, pharmacologic therapy has to be combined with pacing therapy.

In patients undergoing open heart surgery for other indications, the Maze procedure, where the atria are dissected into segments and are then rejoined by suturing, thereby reducing the confluent atrial tissue in which wavelets can rotate, had been successful in ablating AF, but it was associated with high mortality rates. More recently, the revised Maze III procedure, using fewer incisions, has dropped mortality to less than 3%, with greater than 95% success in abolishing AF.

### REFERENCES

Alboni P, Botto GL, Baldi N, et al: Outpatient treatment of recent-onset atrial fibrillation with the "pill-in the pocket" approach. N Engl J Med 2004;351(23):2384-2391.

European Heart Rhythm Association; Heart Rhythm Society; American College of Cardiology; et al: ACC/AHA/ESC 2006 Guidelines for the management of patients with atrial fibrillation—executive summary: A report of the American College of Cardiology/American Heart Association Task Force on Practice Guidelines and the European Society of Cardiology Committee for Practice Guidelines (Writing Committee to revise the 2001 Guidelines for the Management of Patients with Atrial Fibrillation). J Am Coll Cardiol 2006;48(4):854-906.

---

[1]Not FDA approved for this indication.

Fye WB: Tracing atrial fibrillation—100 years. N Engl J Med 2006; 355(14): 1412-1414.

McNamara R, Tamariz LJ, Segal JB, Bass E: Management of atrial fibrillation: Review of the evidence for the role of pharmacologic therapy, electrical cardioversion, and echocardiography. Ann Intern Med 2003;139(12): 1018-1033.

Okin PM, Wachtell K, Devereux RB, et al: Regression of electrocardiographic left ventricular hypertrophy and decreased incidence of new-onset atrial fibrillation in patients with hypertension. JAMA 2006;296(10):1242-1248.

Singer DE, Albers GW, Dalen JE, et al: Antithrombotic therapy in atrial fibrillation: The Seventh ACCP Conference on Antithrombotic and Thrombolytic Therapy. Chest 2004;126(3 suppl):429S-456S.

Snow V, Weiss KB, LeFevre M, et al; AAFP Panel on Atrial Fibrillation; ACP Panel on Atrial Fibrillation: Management of newly detected atrial fibrillation: A clinical practice guideline from the American Academy of Family Physicians and the American College of Physicians. Ann Intern Med 2003;139(12):1009-1017.

# Premature Beats

Method of
*Prakash C. Deedwania, MD, and*
*Enrique V. Carbajal, MD*

Premature beats are the most common form of cardiac arrhythmia encountered in clinical practice. Premature beats are one of the most common causes of irregular pulse and palpitations. In many instances, premature beats are not associated with any symptoms. They result from electrical depolarization of myocardium that occurs earlier than the sinus impulse. Premature beats have been referred to by a variety of names, including premature contractions, premature complexes, ectopic beats, and early depolarizations. Although no single term is ideal, most electrophysiologists refer to them as premature complexes because although the term *ectopic beat* denotes the abnormal site of origin of the depolarization, it does not necessarily require the beat to be premature, and, in some cases, ectopic rhythm indeed occurs as an escape phenomenon.

Although premature beats generally occur in patients with organic heart disease, they frequently can be seen in the absence of any structural heart disease, especially in elderly patients. Premature beats can be triggered by, or increase in frequency with, myocardial ischemia and heart failure. Premature beats can be provoked by, or occur in association with, a variety of systemic abnormalities, including electrolyte disturbances, acid-base imbalance, toxins from recreational drug and/or alcohol abuse, metabolic perturbations, systemic illnesses such as thyroid disorders, pulmonary disease, infections, and febrile illnesses, and any condition associated with increased catecholamine levels.

Most premature beats occur as a result of enhanced automaticity, but other electrophysiologic mechanisms, including reentry and triggered activity, might play a role. Based on the corresponding site of origin, premature electrical depolarizations are called *premature atrial complexes* (PACs), *premature junctional complexes* (PJCs), and *premature ventricular complexes* (PVCs). Morphologic features and timing of the premature beat on electrocardiographic (ECG) recording(s) help determine the site of origin and the nature of premature complexes. Premature beats can occur in a repetitive fashion as *bigeminy* (after every other normal beat), *trigeminy* (after each sequence of two normal beats), or *quadrigeminy* (after each sequence of three normal beats). They also can occur as two or three successive premature beats, defined as *couplets* and *triplets*, respectively. In this article, the primary focus is on single premature beats.

## Premature Atrial Complexes

PACs are the most common form of atrial arrhythmias that can originate at any site in the atria. The exact morphology of the atrial

# CURRENT DIAGNOSIS

- Premature beats are identified by their occurrence at times considerably shorter than the regular sinus rhythm cycles.
- The origin of the premature beats is determined by the presence or absence of P waves, morphology of the P wave (when present), QRS configuration, and the presence or absence of a compensatory period.
- The presence of frequent PVCs (≥10 per hour) during the postdischarge evaluation of survivors of acute MI predicts increased risk of arrhythmic death and overall cardiac mortality.

activation (P wave) varies depending on the site of origin of the PAC. Careful and systematic examination of the ECG features of PACs usually can distinguish them from PVCs.

## ELECTROCARDIOGRAPHIC FEATURES

The cardinal features of PACs include their prematurity with reference to sinus beats, abnormal P wave morphology, and, in most cases, QRS morphology that is similar to that of sinus beats. The P wave morphology of the PAC generally differs from the sinus P wave unless the premature complex originates in the high right atrial area adjacent to the sinus node, in which case distinguishing PACs from sinus arrhythmia may be difficult. Although sinus arrhythmias are generally phasic in nature, being influenced by the respiratory cycle, this feature would be helpful in differentiating from high right atrial PACs only when the PACs are frequent and repetitive. When the PAC occurs quite early in the diastolic phase, the P wave may not be obvious on surface ECG because it is often hidden in the preceding T wave and would be evident only by watching carefully for the notched or peaked T wave.

If the PAC is too premature, it might fail to conduct to the ventricles if the atrioventricular (AV) node is refractory owing to conduction of the preceding sinus impulse. Such nonconducted PACs are called *blocked PACs*, and they are important because they can be confused with instances of AV block. Such erroneous interpretation can be avoided by simply remembering a common rule of thumb that requires normal successive P-P intervals for all sinus beats, including the interval for a blocked P wave, before considering the diagnosis of AV block. Although most PACs have a normal or prolonged PR interval, the relationship of the PAC to the subsequent QRS complex depends on the site of origin of the PAC and the prematurity index. For example, a PAC originating in the lower atrial area near the AV node generally has a shorter PR interval, whereas a PAC that is quite premature and originates in the upper left atrial area might have a longer than usual PR interval. In general, the PR interval of a PAC is inversely related to its prematurity.

Because most PACs are able to depolarize the sinus node, they usually can reset the sinus automaticity; therefore, the subsequent pause following most PACs is generally less than compensatory because the sinus node fires earlier than expected. In this case, measurement of the P-P interval between the sinus P wave preceding the PAC and the P wave following the PAC is generally less than twice the basic sinus cycle length. This is in contrast to the full compensatory pause often observed in conjunction with PVCs. In some cases, the PAC collides with the sinus impulse in the perinodal tissue and thus fails to reset the sinus node, thereby resulting in a full compensatory pause.

In general, electrical depolarization below the AV node is normal with PAC and results in an unchanged (baseline) QRS complex. Aberrant conduction, however, may be encountered when the PAC reaches the infranodal tissue during the period when it is still partially refractory. Most frequently, the aberrant conduction usually occurs when a short coupled PAC follows a long pause in patients with sinus bradycardia (long-short cycle). This usually results in a right bundle-branch block pattern and is commonly referred to as the *Ashman phenomenon*.

## CLINICAL FEATURES

Although PACs can occur in normal individuals of all ages, they are quite infrequent except in the elderly. Their frequency increases with age; as many as 50% to 70% of the elderly may have occasional PACs. Some elderly individuals without organic heart disease have frequent PACs and occasionally atrial bigeminy or two to three PACs in a row. Whether the increased frequency of PACs in these individuals is secondary to senile amyloidosis, myocardial fibrosis, or diastolic dysfunction secondary to aging-related changes in the heart is not known. PACs are extremely common in patients with heart disease and in patients with acute as well as chronic respiratory failure. The frequency of PACs can increase markedly during periods of acute febrile illness, shock states, and metabolic disorders, especially in patients with hyperthyroidism and conditions associated with increased catecholamine levels. Use of excessive caffeine, alcohol, tobacco, and recreational drugs can increase the frequency of PACs. In patients with acute myocardial infarction (MI), frequent PACs usually are precursors of atrial fibrillation and occur in association with ventricular failure. In general, the presence of frequent PACs in the setting of acute MI is an indicator of poor prognosis.

In general, PACs are benign except when they are a marker of an underlying cardiopulmonary disorder(s). The major clinical importance of PACs is related to the increased risk of atrial tachyarrhythmias in patients with an established history of such arrhythmias as well as in the elderly who are generally at high risk for atrial fibrillation. As indicated earlier, in rare instances the blocked PACs may be confused with episodes of AV nodal block; however, careful examination of the ECG features described previously easily establishes the correct diagnosis and avoids unnecessary pacemaker implantation.

## TREATMENT

The correction of an underlying structural cardiopulmonary disorder and other precipitating factors (e.g., electrolyte or metabolic abnormalities) usually is all the treatment that is needed. No specific treatment is generally required in most patients because PACs usually are benign except in patients with a history of recurrent atrial tachyarrhythmias, for example, atrial flutter/fibrillation. In such patients, specific treatment may be indicated and could include a β-blocker or a heart rate-modulating calcium channel blocking agent such as verapamil (Calan) or diltiazem (Cardizem). Recent studies have shown that verapamil is quite effective in patients with frequent PACs and multifocal atrial tachycardia in the setting of acute or chronic ventilatory insufficiency. In patients who are at risk for recurrent atrial fibrillation, treatment with a specific antiarrhythmic agent, such as propafenone (Rythmol) or flecainide (Tambocor), may be beneficial; however, these drugs should be used only when the patient has a history of recurrent atrial flutter/fibrillation because of the increased

risk of proarrhythmia, especially in the presence of organic heart disease such as recurrent ischemia or heart failure.

# Premature Junctional Complexes

PJCs are rarely seen in normal individuals and are infrequently encountered even in patients with organic heart disease. When present, PJCs can occur due to abnormal automaticity or reentry phenomenon. Although digitalis toxicity is cited as a common etiologic factor, PJCs also can occur in the setting of MI, myocarditis, and electrolyte/ metabolic disturbances.

## ELECTROCARDIOGRAPHIC FEATURES

The ECG characteristics of PJCs are distinct from those of PACs in that the P wave usually is inverted in the inferior leads (II, III, and aVF) because of retrograde conduction to the atria from the ectopic foci in the junctional area. The second feature of PJCs is that the PR interval almost always is shorter than the normal PR interval because of the proximity of ectopic foci to the AV node and bundle of His. In most cases, the P wave might not even be visible on surface ECGs because it lies hidden within the QRS complex. Rarely, the P wave precedes the QRS complex when the ectopic impulse traverses to the atria before traveling down to depolarize the ventricle. In general, the infranodal conduction of PJCs is normal, and thus the QRS morphology of the conducted PJCs is similar to that noted during sinus rhythm. When the PJC is closely coupled to the preceding sinus beat, aberrant conduction might occur if the impulse traverses down the bundle branch during the relative refractory period (most frequently manifesting as a right bundle-branch block pattern). Because in many instances no obvious P wave accompanies a PJC, aberrantly conducted PJCs may be hard to differentiate from PVCs.

In some instances when PJCs occur during the period when the AV node as well as the infranodal conduction systems both are refractory, the PJC may encounter both retrograde and antegrade blocks for impulse propagation. In such situations, no P wave or QRS complex is related to the PJC. Although the ectopic impulse would be invisible on a surface ECG, it would penetrate a portion of the conduction system and thus make it partially or completely refractory to conduction of the subsequent sinus impulse. This would be manifested as a sudden prolongation of subsequent PR interval in case of partial refractoriness or as an episode of "pseudo AV nodal block" due to the blocked sinus beat if the infranodal tissue were unable to conduct the sinus impulse. Thus, even though some PJCs might not have any surface ECG complexes, their presence can be suspected based on their influence on the conduction of the following sinus beat owing to the electrophysiologic phenomenon described as "concealed conduction."

## CLINICAL FEATURES

PJCs usually are not seen in normal persons and are rarely encountered in cardiac patients except in the setting of digitalis intoxication and infrequently in the setting of MI or myocarditis. In patients with digitalis toxicity, PJCs may lead to junctional tachycardia, occasionally resulting in palpitation, but are rarely associated with hemodynamic compromise. Because in some cases concealed conduction of PJCs might result in periods of varying degrees of pseudo AV blocks, it is clinically important to recognize their presence in order to prevent undue concern and avoid inappropriate pacemaker implantation.

# Premature Ventricular Complexes

PVCs are the most common form of arrhythmia and can be encountered frequently in both healthy individuals as well as in patients with a variety of cardiac disorders. PVCs are often triggered by electrolyte abnormalities, acid-base imbalance, metabolic perturbations, hypoxia, and ischemia.

---

### CURRENT THERAPY

- In general, premature beats in patients without evidence of organic heart disease do not require any specific antiarrhythmic therapy because generally there is no significant increased risk of life-threatening arrhythmia.
- Correction of any underlying structural cardiopulmonary disorder and other precipitating factors (e.g., electrolyte or metabolic abnormalities).
- Suppression of PVCs using currently available antiarrhythmic drugs (except for amiodarone) is not advisable for most patients primarily because of the increased risk of proarrhythmic effects of these drugs.
- In the occasional patient who is disabled by annoying symptoms due to PVCs, a trial of β-blocker therapy should be considered and often is effective in many patients.

## ELECTROCARDIOGRAPHIC FEATURES

PVCs occur as a result of premature depolarization of the ventricles due to ectopic foci in the ventricular myocardium or Purkinje fibers. In general, PVCs result in wide QRS complexes with the T wave axis usually opposite to that of the QRS. In the vast majority of cases, PVCs do not conduct retrogradely and thus do not result in a distinct P wave. The sinus beats may, however, continue uninterrupted and thus manifest as an instance of AV dissociation in conjunction with PVCs. For the same reason, because PVCs usually do not conduct retrogradely and depolarize the atrium and the sinus node, there usually is a full compensatory pause in contrast to the partial compensatory pause generally seen with PACs. In patients with slow sinus rates, however, interpolated PVCs might occur. If the ectopic foci for PVCs are located high in the His-Purkinje system, the resulting premature complexes may have a narrow QRS morphology quite similar to that seen during sinus rhythm. Additionally, if the PVCs occur rather late, in close proximity to the sinus impulse, there may also be a narrow complex QRS because of fusion between the normal depolarization due to sinus impulse and the abnormal activation sequence from the ectopic foci. In the instance of fusion beats, a normal P wave precedes the QRS. The PR interval is shorter, and the QRS morphology may be only partially altered. In some cases, this might give the appearance of an intermittent bundle-branch block or preexcitation (Wolff-Parkinson-White syndrome) pattern.

Based on the morphologic features of PVCs, they have been classified as *uniform* or *multiform;* they also have been referred to as *unifocal* or *multifocal.* Also recommended is classification of PVCs based on their coupling interval with the preceding sinus beat. PVCs with a short coupling interval near or on the previous T wave have been described as showing R-on-T phenomenon; alternatively PVCs may have long coupling intervals. Based on the underlying electrophysiologic mechanism responsible for PVCs, the coupling interval may be *fixed,* as in reentrant beats, or *variable,* as seen with ventricular parasystole. PVCs may have a repetitive pattern, for example, bigeminy or trigeminy, or they may occur in pairs. It is now believed that repetitive PVCs, such as couplets and triplets, are prognostically more important than just the frequency of isolated PVCs.

## CLINICAL FEATURES

PVCs can be recorded frequently in normal individuals, and, similar to PACs, their frequency increases with age. In patients without organic heart disease or without prior evidence of sustained ventricular tachyarrhythmias, the mere presence of frequent PVCs is not considered prognostically important. However, individual exceptions do exist, and the clinician is advised to evaluate each given patient accordingly. In patients with organic heart disease, PVCs are the most common form of arrhythmia and carry significant prognostic importance, especially in survivors of acute MI and patients with recurrent ischemia and advanced heart failure. It has been well established during the past 2 decades that frequent PVCs occurring during the acute phase of MI are associated with an increased risk of sustained ventricular arrhythmias in the initial 48 hours, but they do not predict long-term outcome or risk of arrhythmic events. More recently, it has been shown in patients receiving thrombolytic therapy that PVCs, particularly episodes of nonsustained ventricular tachycardia, increase in frequency but are generally short-lived and represent a sign of myocardial reperfusion. However, the presence of frequent PVCs during the postdischarge evaluation of survivors of MI is indicative of a poor prognosis.

Although as many as 80% to 90% of patients with chronic heart failure have frequent PVCs, the results of several recent studies have shown that only the presence of nonsustained ventricular tachycardia (defined as three or more PVCs in a row) at a rate greater than 100 bpm is strongly predictive of an increased risk of sudden cardiac death in these patients. This is in clear contrast to the findings of several large clinical trials, which showed that more than 10 PVCs per hour in post-MI patients are predictive of a poor prognosis and an increased risk of arrhythmic death.

Overall, the association between PVCs and an increased risk of ventricular tachyarrhythmias and sudden cardiac death appears to be related not only to the frequency and complexity of PVCs but also to the severity of underlying structural heart disease. For example, a patient with mitral valve prolapse and frequent PVCs would be at relatively lower risk for arrhythmic events compared to a patient with advanced heart failure who has repetitive PVCs and episodes of nonsustained ventricular tachycardia. Proper evaluation of the risk of PVCs has become more crucial than ever because most currently available antiarrhythmic drugs have the potential for causing serious adverse reactions, including proarrhythmias, in patients with advanced cardiac disorders.

## TREATMENT

In general, PVCs in patients without evidence of organic heart disease do not require any specific antiarrhythmic therapy because generally there is no significantly increased risk of life-threatening arrhythmia. However, when PVCs are associated with disabling palpitations, reassurance and treatment with β-blockers (atenolol [Tenormin], metoprolol [Toprol-XL]) may help in relieving symptoms. In patients with systemic illness or other provoking factors (e.g., electrolyte abnormalities or acid-base imbalance), immediate correction of the underlying abnormality usually is associated with beneficial effects.

Because of the associated poor prognosis with PVCs in the setting of acute MI, common practice in the past consisted of routine administration of intravenous lidocaine (Xylocaine) in an effort to suppress PVCs during the initial phase of acute MI. However, because recent data suggest that the routine use of lidocaine is not necessary and often can be harmful, lidocaine should be avoided because of the risk of serious adverse reactions, especially central nervous system side effects such as seizures in the elderly. With the ready availability of cardiac monitoring, it now is possible to accurately identify a harbinger of ventricular tachyarrhythmias early in the coronary care unit, so prophylactic use of lidocaine is generally not recommended. Furthermore, results from several studies and their meta-analyses have demonstrated that routine use of prophylactic lidocaine during the acute or healing phase of MI does not alter the overall mortality in patients with acute MI.

In contrast, it is well established that the presence of frequent PVCs (≥10 per hour) during the postdischarge evaluation of survivors of acute MI predicts an increased risk of arrhythmic death and overall cardiac mortality. Numerous trials have been conducted with a variety of different antiarrhythmic drugs. Many of the studies demonstrated that suppression of PVCs with most currently available antiarrhythmic drugs is not beneficial in reducing the increased risk associated with PVCs. The Cardiac Arrhythmia Suppression Trials (CAST I and II) clearly demonstrated that, compared to placebo, treatment with class Ic antiarrhythmic drugs (which primarily work by slowing conduction) was associated with an increased risk of arrhythmic death despite adequate suppression of PVCs. The findings from CAST I and II, as well as several other clinical trials, indicate that although frequent PVCs may be a marker for an adverse event, suppression of PVCs with type I antiarrhythmic agents does not favorably influence the associated increased risk of death. Results from the Canadian Amiodarone Myocardial Infarction Arrhythmia Trial (CAMIAT) and the European Myocardial Infarct Amiodarone Trial (EMIAT) suggest that in patients with frequent PVCs in the post-MI setting, use of amiodarone (Cordarone), a complex drug with predominantly class III antiarrhythmic properties, in combination with β-blockers is associated with improved outcome. However, because of the associated drug toxicity with long-term amiodarone use, it is generally considered suitable only for the high-risk cohort (although many patients with low left ventricular ejection fraction now undergo implantation of an automatic internal cardiac defibrillator).

In general, suppression of PVCs using currently available antiarrhythmic drugs (except for amiodarone) is not advisable for most patients, primarily because of the increased risk of proarrhythmic effects of these drugs. In the occasional patient who is disabled by annoying symptoms due to PVCs, an initial trial of β-blocker therapy should be considered and is effective in many patients. Correction of the provoking factors and appropriate management of any underlying heart disease often are beneficial in managing patients with frequent PVCs.

## REFERENCES

Barrett PA, Peter CT, Swan HJ, et al: The frequency and prognostic significance of electrocardiographic abnormalities in clinically normal individuals. Prog Cardiovasc Dis 1981;23:299.

Boutitie F, Boissel J-P, Connolly SJ, et al, EMIAT and CAMIAT Investigators: Amiodarone interaction with β-blockers: Analysis of the merged EMIAT (European Myocardial Infarct Amiodarone Trial) and CAMIAT (Canadian Amiodarone Myocardial Infarction Trial) databases. Circulation 1999;99:2268.

Brodsky M, Wu D, Denes P, et al: Arrhythmias documented by 24 hour continuous electrocardiographic monitoring in 50 male medical students without apparent heart disease. Am J Cardiol 1977;39:390.

Cairns JA, Connolly SJ, Roberts R, et al: Randomised trial of outcome after myocardial infarction in patients with frequent or repetitive ventricular premature depolarisations: CAMIAT. Lancet 1997;349:675.

Echt DS, Liebson PR, Mitchell B, et al: Mortality and morbidity in patients receiving encainide, flecainide, or placebo. N Engl J Med 1991;324:781.

Fleg J, Kennedy H: Cardiac arrhythmias in a healthy elderly population. Chest 1982;81:302.

Julian DG, Camm AJ, Frangin G, et al: Randomised trial of effect of amiodarone on mortality in patients with left-ventricular dysfunction after recent myocardial infarction: EMIAT. Lancet 1997;349:667.

Morganroth J: Premature ventricular complexes. Diagnosis and indications for therapy. JAMA 1984;252:673.

Romhilt D, Chaffin C, Choi S, et al: Arrhythmias on ambulatory electrocardiographic monitoring in women without apparent heart disease. Am J Cardiol 1984;54:582.

Rosen KM, Rahimtoola SH, Gunnar RM: Pseudo A-V block secondary to premature nonpropagated His bundle depolarizations: Documentation by His bundle electrocardiography. Circulation 1970;42:367.

Ruskin JN: Ventricular extrasystoles in healthy subjects. N Engl J Med 1985;312:238.

Simpson RJ Jr, Cascio WE, Schreiner PJ, et al: Prevalence of premature ventricular contractions in a population of African American and white men and women: The Atherosclerosis Risk in Communities (ARIC) study. Am Heart J 2002;143:535.

# Heart Block

Method of
*Albert A. Del Negro, MD*

The general term *heart block* refers to a group of electrophysiologic disturbances of atrioventricular (AV) conduction. The causes are many, and clinical clues to the significance of AV block as well as mandates for therapy often are deduced from surface electrocardiography (ECG). In other cases, only invasive characterization of heart block with electrophysiologic study provides the direction for therapy.

Starting with Wenckebach and Mobitz, AV block in all its forms remained a descriptive phenomenon until the advent of invasive testing in the 1960s and 1970s; such testing refined our understanding of the significance of the various forms of AV block. In this article, we necessarily start with the anatomy and physiology of the AV conduction system, which serve as a basis for understanding treatment rationales.

## Functional Anatomy of the Atrioventricular Conduction System

The AV node lies at the apex of Koch's triangle, the limits of which in the right heart are the septal portion of the tricuspid valve anteriorly, the ligament of Todaro posteriorly, and the subeustachian isthmus from the inferior septal aspect of the tricuspid valve to the coronary sinus. The AV node itself consists of a mixture of atrial muscle cells, stellate P cells, and transitional cells imbedded in a collagen matrix. On the left side of the ventricular septum, it lies just under the noncoronary sinus of the aortic valve.

The proximal portion of the AV node receives impulses from internodal tracts connecting with the sinus node. These tracts convey impulses using the sodium fast channel. However, in the AV node, conduction is slowed as the sodium fast channel gives way to slow calcium channel-mediated conduction. Sympathetic as well as parasympathetic influences are richly present in the AV node, and these influences have profound effects on automaticity as well as on conduction. The distal portion of the AV node, also known as the *compact AV node*, is somewhat insulated from electrical influences by the surrounding collagen matrix. As the node passes into the transitional area from the atrium to the ventricle, it gives rise to the bundle of His. Data from invasive electrophysiologic testing suggest that the bundle of His is the origin of nodal or junctional rhythm. Furthermore, sympathetic and parasympathetic influences remain strong within this area. Therefore, AV nodal block is not usually associated with cardiovascular collapse because default to the lower-order idiojunctional pacemaker usually sustains cardiac output with a satisfactory heart rate. Furthermore, parasympathetic withdrawal and sympathetic stimulation can speed idiojunctional rhythm and satisfactorily support the heart rate.

Below the area of the bundle of His, however, the major fascicules arise and form the bundle branches. Whereas the right bundle branch fans out throughout the right septum, in most individuals the left bundle branch has at least two major subdivisions. These are the left anterior superior division, a slender division that originates along with the right bundle branch, and the left posterior inferior division, a stout division that originates separately from the right bundle branch and superior division of the left bundle branch. Of major importance is that although sympathetic influences still may have some limited effect on automaticity below the bundle of His, parasympathetic influences that mediate conduction and automaticity are absent. The result of heart block at this level is reliance on idiofascicular or idioventricular pacemakers, which usually are too slow to support the heart rate and hemodynamics satisfactorily. Because of this situation, it is convenient to divide the AV conduction system into two generally different areas: a proximal area (AV node) and a distal area (His bundle, bundle branches, and their divisions).

From the aspect of coronary anatomy, the body of the AV node before the bundle branches (proximal area) is supplied by a branch of the right coronary artery in 90% of individuals, whereas the area of the conduction system below the His bundle (distal area) is fed by branches from the left anterior descending coronary artery in almost 100% of individuals. These facts have implications for the significance of AV block associated with inferior myocardial infarction and anterior myocardial infarction.

## Electrocardiographic Classification of Heart Block

For the purposes of ECG interpretation, the three patterns of AV block are first-, second-, and third-degree AV block. *First-degree AV block* occurs when there is prolongation of the PR interval without failure of conduction of each atrial impulse or P wave. The upper limit of PR conduction time is 0.21 seconds measured in the limb leads of the scalar ECG. Although PR prolongation to greater than 0.21 seconds is generally thought to reflect prolongation of conduction through the AV nodal portion of the conduction system, in reality this may not be the case because PR interval prolongation may reflect delay within the AV node, His bundle, proximal bundle branches, or a combination of the three.

*Second-degree AV block* occurs when some or any P waves fail to propagate to the ventricle. As with first-degree AV block, this pattern does not clearly imply the locus of the block. Second-degree AV block is further divided. In *type I block*, first described by Wenckebach in 1899, there is gradual prolongation of the PR interval until a P wave fails to conduct to the ventricle. This pattern retains his name: *Wenckebach block*. (Part of Wenckebach's genius is that he theorized the electrophysiologic happenings of failed AV conduction without the use of an ECG recording. He used a smoked-drum recorder to record the jugular venous and carotid waves from an individual with second-degree AV block.) Some years later, Mobitz described a second form of second-degree AV block, in which there is no prolongation of the PR interval before loss of conduction. This form is called *Mobitz II*, or *type II, block*. Necessary to the diagnosis of both type I and type II second-degree AV block is the occurrence of at least relatively regular atrial timing, because multiple closely coupled premature atrial beats may fail to conduct even with normal AV conduction.

Although type I second-degree AV block usually implies that the AV node is the locus of the block, especially if the QRS is narrow (<0.120 second), this may not always be the case because the block may occur instead within the bundle of His. If the QRS is wide (bundle branch block), there is at least a 25% to 30% chance that type I block occurs within or below the His bundle.

*High-grade AV block* is a general term for sequentially nonconducted P waves but with some P waves having the ability to conduct; thus, it is a form of second-degree AV block. The diagnosis, as for type I and type II second-degree AV block, requires relatively regular atrial activity. The term implies that fewer than 50% of P waves are able to conduct to the ventricle.

*Third-degree AV block* occurs when no atrial activity is capable of conduction. This results in AV dissociation with the ventricles and atrial beating at different and unrelated rates. Generally speaking, the atrial rate should be faster than the ventricular rate for the diagnosis to be made, because junctional tachycardia (arising from the His-bundle area) may occur at a rate faster than normal sinus rhythm. In such a case, there is AV dissociation but not necessarily AV block because P waves have no chance for conduction owing to the faster usurping junctional rate. Third-degree AV block can occur at the AV nodal level or at the His-Purkinje level; that is, it may be due to either proximal or distal block.

## CLINICAL ASPECTS OF HEART BLOCK

The AV node and the His-Purkinje system have separate embryologic origins, and their failure to unite in development results in congenital AV block. Originally thought to be a benign entity not necessarily requiring pacemaker therapy, the contemporary view is that pacing at an early age is desirable to prevent the development of cardiomyopathy.

Several acquired forms of heart block have varied significance for therapy. Table 1 lists several of the more common causes of AV block. Heart block associated with use of medications generally is reversible with discontinuation of therapy. AV block that is confined to the AV node usually is reversible with time and the course of the clinical entity responsible for it. Even temporary pacing is rarely required because this form of "proximal" block results in preservation of responsive escape mechanisms from the distal AV node and proximal bundle of His that will support the heart rate at physiologic levels. Furthermore,

withdrawal of parasympathetic influences with atropine will speed idiojunctional rhythm to which proximal AV block patients default.

Diseases such as acute diphtheria and acute rheumatic fever provoke first- or second-degree block that resolves with the acute illness. The appearance of AV nodal block in an otherwise healthy young patient without structural heart disease should always suggest the possibility of Lyme disease, a reversible infectious cause of AV block. Often the telltale fever and rash are absent, and AV block may be the first manifestation of the illness. Serologic studies can confirm the diagnosis, and antibiotics can reverse AV block if started early enough. Thiamine deficiency (beriberi), which results in AV nodal block, may not be reversible because scarring within the AV node may permanently impair AV nodal function. Infiltrative diseases causing AV nodal block may cause permanent AV block and lead to the need for permanent pacing. These diseases include sarcoidosis, rheumatoid arthritis, and hemochromatosis, the last of which can also create delay and conduction impairment below the His bundle.

## HEART BLOCK IN ACUTE MYOCARDIAL INFARCTION

Few events in clinical cardiology are more threatening than AV block in acute myocardial infarction. AV block, either second degree or complete third degree, complicates inferior myocardial infarction in approximately 30% of cases. However, because the condition is due to AV nodal block, it almost always is reversible and very rarely requires permanent pacing. Cautious use of atropine can reverse AV block or at least speed idiojunctional rhythm that results from AV nodal block in this setting. Aminophylline[1] also may speed such rhythms and even abolish AV block in this setting because AV block in acute infarction seems to be due to local elaboration of adenosine for which aminophylline is the antidote and not due to the AV nodal infarction itself.

Unlike inferior infarction, acute anterior myocardial infarction rarely provokes AV block. The mechanism of AV block in anterior infarction is necrosis of the proximal fascicles arising from the bundle of His. This is not completely reversible even if conduction block resolves, in marked contrast to inferior infarction. Block at this level results in default of rhythm to so-called idiofascicular or idioventricular rhythm, usually with an inadequate heart rate (20–35 per minute) and subsequent hemodynamic collapse.

An antecedent clue to impending AV block in anterior infarction is the development of bifascicular block (right bundle-branch block and left anterior fascicular block) or new left bundle-branch block. Data suggest the incidence of acute AV block in such patients is upward of 40%. The appearance of such a new conduction abnormality in acute anterior myocardial infarction mandates at least temporary transvenous pacing even before AV block occurs. AV block occurring in anterior infarction with or without antecedent conduction delay, even if transient, also mandates prophylactic temporary transvenous pacing followed by eventual permanent pacing because the natural history of this form of AV block is malignant, and progression to permanent complete AV block is the rule.

Use of positive chronotropic agents for heart rate support in patients with heart block has no role in acute infarction. In the patient with unstable infarction, agents such as dopamine, isoproterenol (Isuprel), and epinephrine have the potential to induce life-threatening tachycardia. Furthermore, prophylactic use of antiarrhythmic agents such as lidocaine and amiodarone (Cordarone) for suppression of potential ventricular arrhythmias in patients with heart block can only worsen AV block in acute infarction. These antiarrhythmic drugs, if necessary for arrhythmia suppression, should be used only after temporary transvenous ventricular pacing has been established.

## ADDITIONAL DIAGNOSTIC AIDS

Table 1 lists the indications for permanent pacing in heart block. Note that type II AV block is an absolute indication for permanent pacing. This is the case because all examples of type II AV block reported in the contemporary medical literature are due to block within or below the His bundle. Invasive cardiac electrophysiologic testing can assist in the differential diagnosis of AV block, that is, whether proximal

## TABLE 1  Clinical Presentation and Indications for Pacing in Acquired Atrioventricular Block

| Etiologies | Locus | Pacing Therapy |
|---|---|---|
| Idiopathic (aging) fibrosis | Distal | Always |
| Sarcoidosis | Proximal | Usually |
| Hemochromatosis | Proximal and distal | Always |
| Lyme disease | Proximal | Always unless reversible |
| β-Blockers, Ca²⁺ channel blockers | Proximal | Never if reversible |
| Na⁺ channel blockers | Distal | Never if reversible |
| Calcific aortic stenosis | Distal | Always |
| Anterior infarction | Distal | Always |
| Inferior infarction | Proximal | Almost never |
| Neuromuscular disorders | Unclear—likely proximal | Always |

(potentially not requiring permanent pacing) or distal (permanent pacing absolutely required). Such testing involves positioning a temporary recording electrode via the femoral transvenous route within the area of the His bundle. Unique ECG recordings from this area easily identify the level of AV block, which has enormous significance for therapy. Furthermore, the recording electrode thereafter can provide temporary transvenous pacing when positioned within the right ventricle. Stressing the conduction system by atrial pacing during invasive electrophysiologic testing in ambiguous cases adds to the clinical decision-making process.

The finding of reversible proximal block does not rule out the use of temporary or even permanent ventricular pacing. Good clinical judgment should assist in the decision about pacing. Pacing is indicated if the heart rate is chronically below 35 bpm or if pauses of 2 seconds or longer occur while the patient is awake, irrespective of the locus of block. Distal block, irrespective of symptoms, should always prompt pacing. In 2002, a joint committee of the American Heart Association, the American College of Cardiology, and the North American Society of Pacing and Electrophysiology (now named the Heart Rhythm Society) set standards for temporary and permanent pacing.

## Pacing Modalities

### TEMPORARY CARDIAC PACING

Table 2 lists the indications for temporary cardiac pacing. Several modalities of temporary pacing exist, and they all are useful. Their utility and applicability depend somewhat on the immediacy of the need for pacing as well as the expertise of the physician in attendance; however, properly executed, each can provide heart rate support for the profoundly bradycardiac patient.

### TEMPORARY TRANSCUTANEOUS PACING

Temporary transcutaneous pacing can be a lifesaving temporary treatment of sudden and unanticipated hemodynamically deleterious bradycardia of any mechanism, including heart block. Passage of current applied from cutaneous large-surface-area electrodes positioned so that the heart is in the path of the current flow will result in cardiac excitation and contraction. Energies of at least 40 to 60 mA are required, but care must be taken not to mistake the contraction of intercostal and pectoral muscles associated with device discharge for cardiac contraction. Verification of a palpable pulse coincident with electrical stimulation is essential. The ECG recorded from modern stimulation devices is filtered to dampen the stimulus of pacing, enabling accurate assessment of cardiac response to the pacing stimulus. Sedation plays an important role in the patient so treated, because associated intercostal or diaphragmatic stimulation can be uncomfortable.

### TEMPORARY PERCUTANEOUS TRANSTHORACIC PACING

In the author's experience, temporary percutaneous transthoracic pacing is little used because it is invasive, involves cardiac puncture, and is seldom effective because it is commonly a last resort applied late in the resuscitative effort. The technique involves passage of a needle from

---

**TABLE 2  Indications for Temporary Pacing in Atrioventricular Block**

Symptomatic second-degree degree AV block
Hemodynamically significant bradycardia due to AV block
Anterior myocardial infarction with new and age-
    indeterminate right bundle-branch block
Third-degree AV block with bradycardia-induced ventricular
    tachycardia/ventricular fibrillation

*Abbreviation:* AV = atrioventricular.

---

the subxiphoid area aiming for the left shoulder until right ventricular blood is aspirated. A J-shaped electrode wire is passed into the right ventricle, and the needle is withdrawn. Recording a unipolar ECG from the needle can verify contact with the right ventricle instead of the right atrium.

### TEMPORARY TRANSVENOUS ENDOCARDIAL PACING

The preferred temporary pacing modality for heart block is temporary transvenous endocardial pacing. Placed from the percutaneous transfemoral, subclavian, or internal jugular route, this technique requires use of fluoroscopy. Complications of the technique include cardiac perforation and the risk of cardiac tamponade. Electrode dislodgment is common unless a temporary active-fixation electrode with a helical coil on the distal portion of the electrode that worms its way into the ventricular wall with rotation of the temporary pacing electrode is used. Currently available electrodes are very flexible and require introduction through a guiding catheter that itself is relatively rigid and that can easily perforate the thin-walled right ventricle. This technique requires an experienced practitioner for safe use.

Positioned from the femoral route, passage into the right ventricular apex is relatively easy. Positioned from the internal jugular or subclavian route, inadvertent passage into the coronary sinus is relatively simple. This is not a satisfactory position from which to pace the heart. This pitfall can be avoided by first passing the pacing catheter from above into the right ventricular outflow tract and into the pulmonary artery, thereafter withdrawing it into the body of the right ventricle and to the right ventricular apex.

After acceptable placement of the temporary pacing electrode, satisfactory parameters of pacing and sensing should be ensured. If the parameters are suitable, 0 silk sutures should be used to secure the electrode to the adjacent skin, coiling the electrode to inhibit traction and dislodgment. Placing a sterile barrier over the assembly at the insertion site will help to ensure impediment to infection. Changing the insertion site at least every 5 days also will prevent problems with infection and venous thrombosis.

Once placed, a temporary pacemaker electrode can facilitate entry of stray electrical currents to the patient's heart. Modern coronary care units are carefully constructed to ensure safe grounding of all electrical devices in the environment. However, the additional measure of placing the connection between the temporary pacing electrode and the temporary pacer cable within a latex or nitrile glove and sealing it with tape will ensure protection against stray currents that can inadvertently induce ventricular fibrillation.

Most patients endure temporary right ventricular pacing well, but those with reduced left ventricular compliance, right ventricular infarct, or postoperative coronary artery bypass surgery may actually deteriorate hemodynamically. The condition results from loss of regular association of the atrium with the ventricle. Temporary dual-chamber pacing will restore hemodynamic balance to such patients. Temporary atrial pacing as well as ventricular pacing is required, and special temporary pacemakers capable of this task are readily available.

Spontaneous electrode dislodgment of temporary pacer electrodes occurs in upward of 20% of patients. This percentage is lower with use of temporary active-fixation electrodes. A rising threshold may be the first clue to impending loss of pacing from dislodgment. The appearance of ventricular ectopy similar in configuration to paced beats signals mechanical stimulation of the myocardium from electrode dislodgment. These events should alert the clinician to re-establish satisfactory parameters of pacing and sensing by repositioning or replacing the pacing electrode.

### PERMANENT PACING

Table 3 lists the indications for permanent cardiac pacing. Percutaneous access of subclavian or axillary veins easily facilitates permanent pacemaker implantation. Cutdown to access the cephalic vein is less common today because the percutaneous route in experienced hands is simple and quick, and the complication of pneumothorax is infrequent and, if promptly recognized, causes little morbidity.

## TABLE 3 Indications for Permanent Pacing in Atrioventricular Block

Symptomatic second-degree AV block at any level
Second-degree AV block within the His-Purkinje system
Third-degree AV block
Mobitz II (type II) AV block
AV block in anterior infarction even if transient
Bilateral bundle branch block (likely distal)

*Abbreviation:* AV = atrioventricular.

Currently, implanters more frequently are cardiologists rather than surgeons because, as devices have become more sophisticated and complicated, the intricacies of pacemaker programming and follow-up are more in the cardiologic than the surgical realm.

After achievement of satisfactory electrode placement verified by measures of sensing and pacing, the operator creates a subcutaneous pocket to accommodate the pacer and its electrode(s). Pacing at high outputs usually confirms the absence of diaphragmatic or intercostal stimulation, which would necessitate electrode repositioning. Individual patient clinical profiles and needs determine programming parameters. These include voltage outputs, parameters of sensing P waves and R waves, and programmed schemes to detect and potentially treat arrhythmias. Modern pacers have the ability to alert the monitoring physician about occult arrhythmias (e.g., ventricular tachycardia or atrial fibrillation) that have a major impact on treatment.

Following implantation, observation in a monitored setting can ensure normal and satisfactory pacemaker function. Early problems include sensing failure, induction of mechanically induced ventricular ectopy, and failure of pacing to capture the heart. Pacing electrode dislodgment is the most frequent cause of these postoperative problems. Although pacemaker programming can overcome several problems, a thorough evaluation postimplantation can assure that repeat surgery to reposition the electrodes is not necessary.

Follow-up of patients with pacemakers has the aim of reducing the energy required of pacing based on office or clinical evaluation of the minimum energy requirement for successful and consistent cardiac pacing (threshold determination). This conservation of battery energy lengthens battery life and reduces the need for frequent surgeries to replace depleted pacer batteries. Frequency of office visits depends on prior performance history and the patient's condition, but visits once yearly are adequate for patients with single-chamber pacers and twice yearly for patients with dual-chamber pacers. Transtelephonic monitoring on a regular basis detects arrhythmias if patients are symptomatic and provides assessment of battery function by recording and verifying pacing rates. A rate reduction when a magnet is placed over the pacer signals the need for device replacement.

## PACING DEFIBRILLATORS

The choice of pacing therapy now embraces an entirely new modality of therapy. The implantable cardiac pacer/defibrillator provides heart rate support with atrial and ventricular pacing, arrhythmia monitoring with reports, and stored and real-time electrograms available to the monitoring physician during clinical interrogation. These devices also provide therapy in the form of antitachycardia pacing and cardioversion/defibrillation shock therapy. These devices not only can treat ventricular arrhythmias, but some models also deliver therapy for atrial arrhythmias. Recent studies of patients with depressed left ventricular function document survival improvement in patients with poor left ventricular function (ejection fraction <35%) treated with implantable cardioverter-defibrillators. This constitutes therapy for primary prevention of sudden cardiac arrest in a highly vulnerable population. These facts make it imperative that preoperative assessment of pacemaker candidates with heart disease, especially those with congestive heart failure, include estimations of ejection fraction. Those on a stable and standard regimen for treatment of heart failure, including β-blockers, angiotensin-converting enzyme inhibitors, or angiotensin receptor blockers and spironolactone (Aldactone) when appropriate, with ejection fractions less than 35% should receive a pacing defibrillator rather than a pacemaker alone even in the absence of demonstrable ventricular arrhythmias.

Chronic cardiomyopathy of any etiology results in suboptimal systolic effort of the left ventricle. Magnifying this problem is the frequent association of cardiomyopathy with left bundle-branch block. Because activation of the left ventricle begins at the interventricular septum and spreads outward to activate the basal-posterior portion of the left ventricle last, the presence of left bundle-branch block results in markedly delayed posterolateral wall activation. This considerable delay promotes left ventricular dyssynchrony, in which two already impaired walls move not as a unit but separately. In patients with left ventricular dysfunction and class II or III heart failure and bundle-branch block, cardiac function and clinical class improve with pacing and cardiac resynchronization therapy. Right ventricular stimulation occurs at the right ventricular apex via the traditionally implanted right ventricular electrode. Left ventricular activation timed with right ventricular activation occurs from an electrode placed within the coronary sinus and advanced through the coronary venous system to the lateral wall on the left ventricular epicardial surface. Resynchronization occurs by attachment of right and left ventricular electrodes to a cardiac resynchronization therapy device that delivers separate but simultaneously timed stimuli to these two places and resynchronizes ventricular activation and contraction.

Studies of heart block and its treatment have progressed considerably in the last several years. The parallel growth in the technology of pacing and the several scientific studies evaluating the natural history of cardiomyopathy of any etiology have resulted in the application of pacing therapy coupled with defibrillator therapy to an increasing number of patients. As time passes and our understanding of conduction system disease increases, the number of patients treated with the various forms of pacing therapy likely will grow exponentially.

## REFERENCES

Bardy GH, Lee KL, Mark DB, et al: Amiodarone or an implantable-cardioverter defibrillator for congestive heart failure. N Engl J Med 2005;352:225-2237.

Bristow MR, Saxon LA, Boehmer J, et al; for the Comparison of Medical Therapy, Pacing, and Defibrillation in Heart Failure (COMPANION) Investigators: Cardiac resynchronization therapy with or without an implantable defibrillator in advanced chronic heart failure. N Engl J Med 2004;350:2140-2150.

Gregoratos G, Abrams J, Epstein AE, et al: ACC/AHA/NASPE 2002 guideline update for implantation of cardiac pacemakers and antiarrhythmia devices. Circulation 2002;106:2145-2161.

Moss AJ, Zareba W, Hall WJ, et al; Multicenter Automatic Defibrillator Implantation Trial II Investigators: Prophylactic implantation of a defibrillator in patients with myocardial infarction and reduced ejection fraction. N Engl J Med 2002;346:877-883.

Young JB, Abraham WT, Smith Al, et al: Combined cardiac resynchronization and implantable cardioversion defibrillation in advanced chronic heart failure: The MIRACLE ICD Trial. JAMA 2003;289:2685-2694.

# Tachycardias

Method of
*Chirag Sandesara, MD, and Brian Olshansky, MD*

Tachycardia is an abnormally rapid heart rate. For adults, tachycardia is defined most commonly as any rhythm exceeding 100 beats/min. Tachycardia may be a normal physiologic response, as in the case of sinus tachycardia. Alternatively, tachycardia may be secondary to a pathologic mechanism that causes a rate inappropriate for physiologic needs.

*Supraventricular tachycardias* require extra electrical tissue above the His bundle for tachycardia to occur, whereas *ventricular tachycardias* require extra tissue at or below the His bundle. Tachycardias can use any cardiac tissue including the sinoatrial node, atria, AV node, or the ventricles. Some tachycardias (e.g., atrial fibrillation) involve extracardiac structures such as the pulmonary veins. The site of tachycardia initiation by premature beats (ectopy) does not identify the tachycardia type but can help disclose the tachycardia mechanism better.

Tachycardias can be regular, regularly irregular, or irregularly irregular. The QRS complex during tachycardia can be narrow (<120 ms), wide (≥120 ms), or both. All narrow QRS tachycardias are supraventricular, but wide complex tachycardias can be supraventricular or ventricular.

Symptoms and patient outcomes depend on the tachycardia type, the rate, and the presence or absence of any concomitant cardiovascular condition. Treatment is geared to reduce symptoms, improve physiologic conditions caused by tachycardias, prevent complications like thromboembolism, and reduce the risk of sudden cardiac death.

## Mechanisms

The mechanisms responsible for tachycardias are automaticity, reentry, and triggered activity. Normal (and enhanced) automaticity generates tachycardias when catecholamines or sympathetic stimulation excite specific tissue. Abnormal automaticity is spontaneous activation of cardiac tissue (nonpacemaker cells) due to partially depolarized and damaged myocardium. Automatic tachycardias are focal even though they can span a relatively large area. Reentry requires an activation pathway (a large or small circuit) where a cardiac impulse continuously reexcites tissue. Requirements for reentry are a zone of tissue that conducts slowly, unidirectional block at the initiation of reentry, and defined activation pathway(s). Triggered activity is due to depolarizations occurring during (early) or immediately after (delayed) action potentials. Afterdepolarizations are oscillations that depend on preceding action potentials.

It may be difficult to discern if a tachycardia is due to triggered activity, automaticity, or reentry, but it is important to understand the mechanism because it can determine therapy. One therapeutic option is to use catheter-based ablation that purposely damages tissue to cure a tachycardia. For a tachycardia emanating from a focal site (such as a tachycardia resulting from an abnormal automaticity or triggered activity), eliminating a single spot with radiofrequency energy cures the tachycardia. For tachycardias involving reentry, part of the reentry circuit must be eliminated. Similarly, drugs are chosen to affect part of a reentry circuit, suppress automaticity, or reduce triggered activity.

Mechanisms of tachycardia may be complex. Atrial fibrillation can initiate from triggered or automatic activity located in pulmonary veins. Complex, unstable reentry circuits can then ensue. Eliminating reentry circuits in atrial fibrillation does not eliminate the inciting cause and does not cure the tachycardia.

## Clinical Features

The sensation of abnormal beating of the heart (palpitations) is the most common symptom of tachycardia. Other symptoms include syncope, dizziness, lightheadedness, a sense of impending doom, diaphoresis, dyspnea, neck tightness, and chest discomfort. Symptoms can be vague, nonspecific, transient, inconsistent or even absent. Cardiac arrest leading to sudden death is an unfortunate outcome of many ventricular and some supraventricular tachycardias, especially in the presence of structural heart disease with impaired ventricular function or when extremely rapid rates ensue.

Symptoms tend to occur at the onset or the termination of the tachycardia, when there is an abrupt change in rate. The situation can be misdiagnosed as panic attack or another condition when the pertinent problem may be tachycardia. Patients with persistent tachycardias can adjust to the tachycardia and develop vague symptoms such as fatigue. This occurs commonly in elderly patients with atrial fibrillation.

## Classification

Supraventricular tachycardias requiring the sinus node are sinus tachycardia, sinus node reentry tachycardia, and inappropriate sinus tachycardia. Supraventricular tachycardias requiring the AV node are AV nodal reentry tachycardia, orthodromic and antidromic AV reentry tachycardia, accelerated junctional tachycardia, nonparoxysmal junctional tachycardia, and junctional ectopic tachycardia. Supraventricular tachycardias requiring only atrial tissue include atrial flutter, atrial tachycardia (unifocal or multifocal), and atrial fibrillation. Atrial fibrillation can involve extracardiac structures (Table 1, Figure 1).

Supraventricular tachycardias can also have a wide QRS complex if there is a preexisting bundle branch block, ventricular preexcitation, or rate-dependent (phase III) aberration. Wide QRS complex tachycardias are commonly assumed to be supraventricular if the patient appears to be tolerating it; in most cases this assumption is incorrect. Any wide QRS complex tachycardia is ventricular tachycardia until proven otherwise.

Most ventricular tachycardias are associated with underlying structural heart disease. Even if they appear stable and well tolerated, they may be life threatening. The most common setting for ventricular tachycardia is ischemic heart disease, where the myocardial scar is the substrate for reentry. Structural heart disease of many types, such as dilated cardiomyopathy, valvular cardiomyopathy, infiltrative diseases (amyloidosis and arrhythmogenic right ventricular cardiomyopathy), and hypertrophic cardiomyopathy can cause ventricular tachycardia (Figure 2).

Monomorphic ventricular tachycardia commonly results from coronary artery disease, valvular cardiomyopathies, and dilated cardiomyopathy. Polymorphic ventricular tachycardias can be due to ischemic and nonischemic cardiomyopathy, but conditions such as congenital channelopathies (Brugada's syndrome, congenital long QT interval syndrome, and catecholaminergic polymorphic ventricular tachycardia), hypertrophic cardiomyopathy, and arrhythmogenic right ventricular cardiomyopathy must be considered. Myocardial ischemia and many drugs can initiate polymorphic ventricular tachycardias.

Polymorphic ventricular tachycardias are similar but are slower than ventricular fibrillation (rate <250 bpm). Polymorphic ventricular tachycardias associated with a long QT interval at tachycardia onset are torsades de pointes (Fig. 3). Torsades de pointes often occurs in paroxysms but can also initiate ventricular fibrillation. Torsades de pointes may be associated with the congenital long QT interval syndrome. In that case, the QT interval remains prolonged. More commonly, torsades de pointes occurs in the setting of a drug-induced or electrolyte-induced condition. Then, the QT interval prolongation is associated with an abrupt slowing in heart rate. Therefore, the QT interval just at the tachycardia onset is prolonged, even if it is not prolonged at other times.

Many drugs can prolong the QT interval and place the patient at risk for torsades de pointes. The patient at highest risk for torsades de pointes is the elderly patient, generally female, who has other cardiovascular comorbidities. Patients who are generally debilitated or who have liver or renal disease are at higher risk. Nevertheless, torsades de pointes can occur in any patient when the QT interval is sufficiently prolonged. No specific QT interval is required for torsades de pointes to occur.

## TABLE 1 Supraventricular Tachycardias Based on Anatomic Location

| Sinus Node | AV Node | Atrial Tissue |
|---|---|---|
| Sinus tachycardia | Nonparoxysmal junctional tachycardia | Atrial fibrillation/flutter |
| Inappropriate sinus tachycardia | Atrioventricular nodal reentrant tachycardia | Atrial tachycardia (multifocal or unifocal) |
| Sinoatrial nodal reentrant tachycardia | Atrioventricular reentrant tachycardia | Wolff-Parkinson-White syndrome |

*Abbreviation:* AV = atrioventricular.

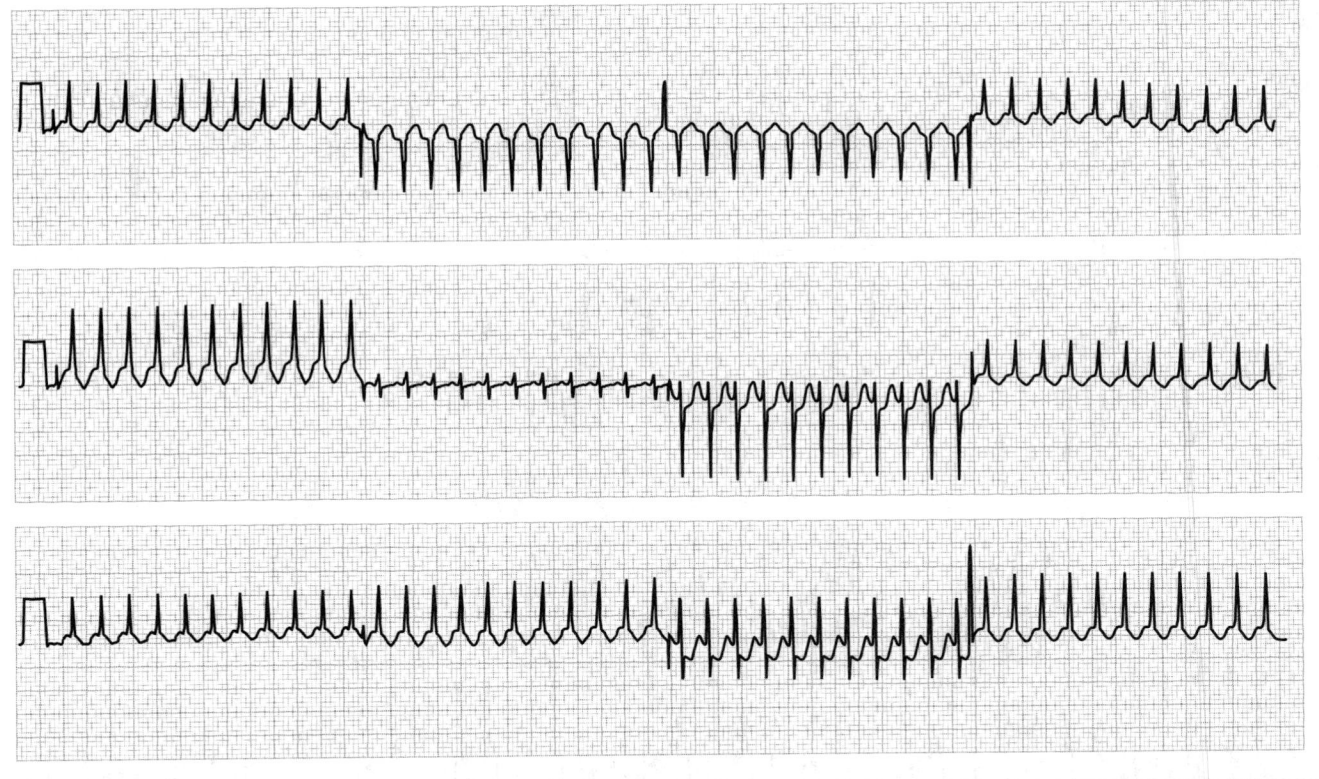

**FIGURE 1.** A 12-lead electrocardiogram of a typical regular narrow QRS complex supraventricular tachycardia with nonspecific ST-T wave changes.

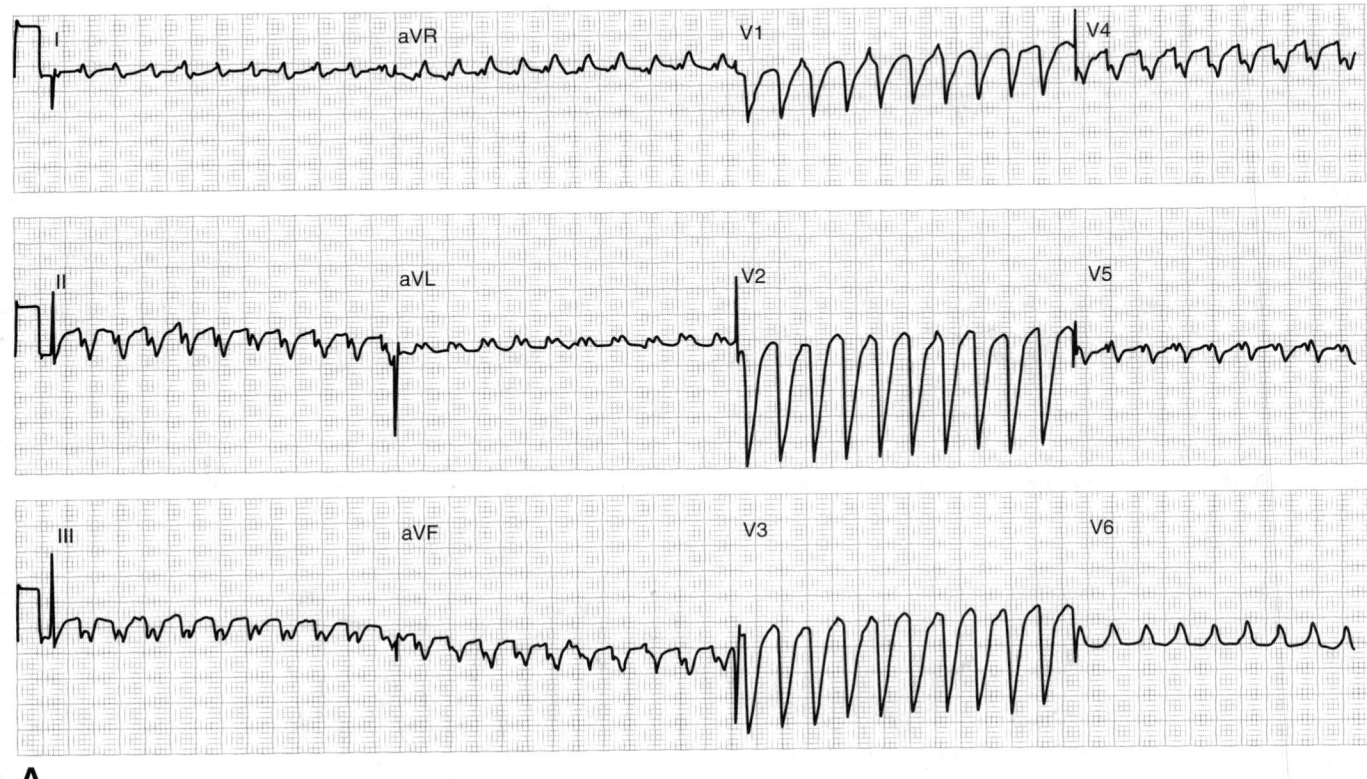

**A**

**FIGURE 2.** **A,** A 12-lead electrocardiogram of ventricular tachycardia. AV dissociation is evident in V1. This wide QRS tachycardia has an unusual axis and near concordance across the precordium.

*Continued*

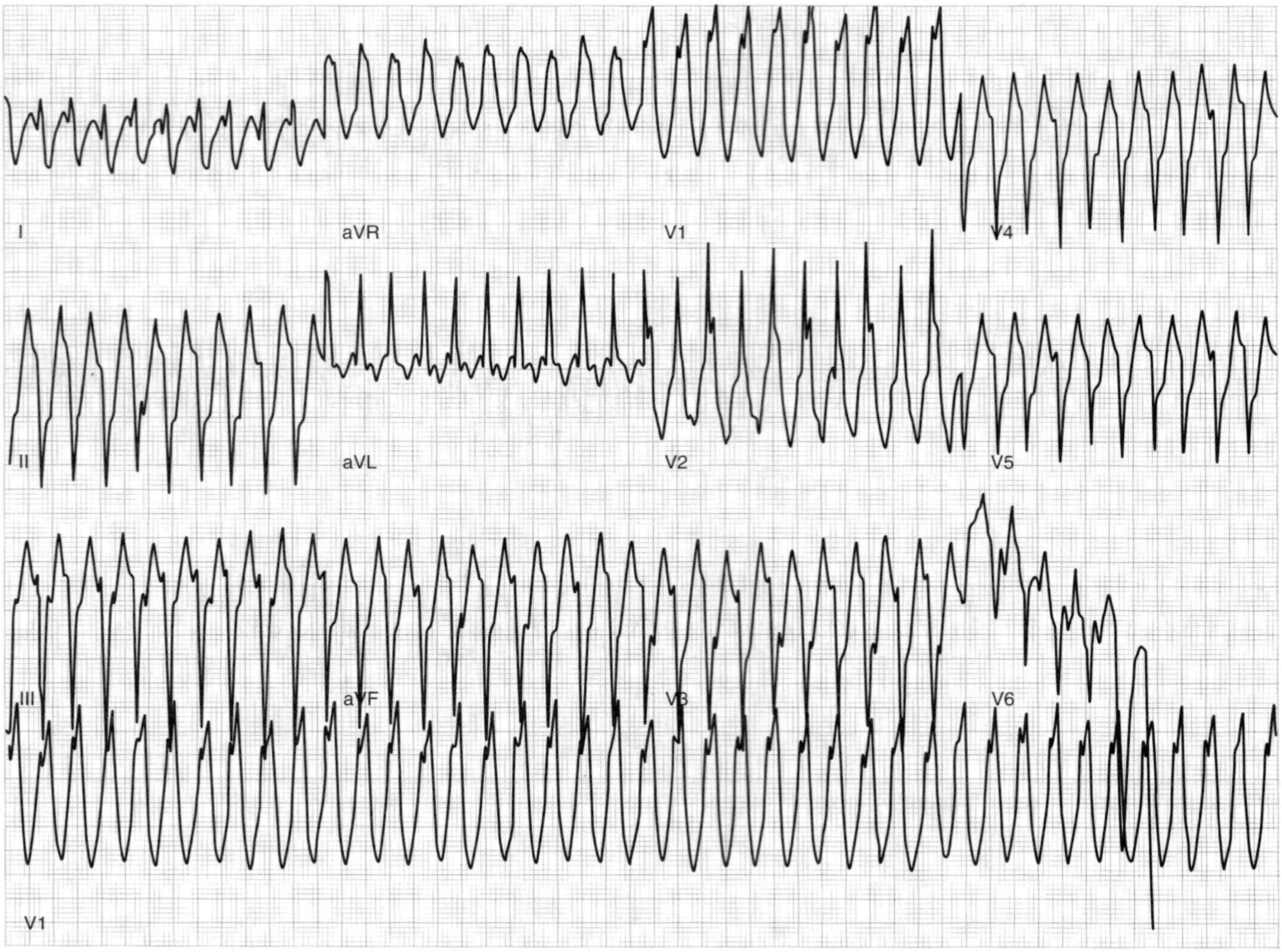

B

**FIGURE 2, cont'd.**  B, Idiopathic left ventricular tachycardia.

A unique form of ventricular tachycardia observed in patients with conduction system disease and dilated cardiomyopathy is termed *bundle branch reentry* and involves the His-Purkinje system. Fascicular tachycardias involving only part of the His-Purkinje system and some ventricular myocardium might have a relatively narrow QRS. These tachycardias are amenable to catheter ablation.

Idiopathic ventricular tachycardia—tachycardia not associated with identifiable structural heart disease—has two common morphologies: right bundle superior axis morphology or left bundle inferior axis morphology. Idiopathic ventricular tachycardia with a right bundle branch block morphology and superior axis involves tissue in the left ventricle near the apical septum, can be verapamil responsive, and is referred to as *Belhassen's tachycardia*. Idiopathic right ventricular tachycardia with a left bundle branch block and an inferior axis commonly originates in the right ventricular outflow tract, the left ventricular outflow tract, or an epicardial location. These outflow tract tachycardias are focal in origin, likely due to triggered activity, and are catecholamine and exercise sensitive. Some forms of right ventricular free wall ventricular tachycardia respond to adenosine. Both common types of idiopathic ventricular tachycardia are readily amenable to ablation (Table 2).

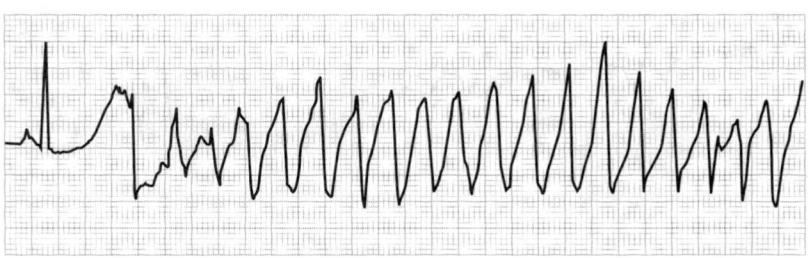

**FIGURE 3.**  Torsades de pointes. Note the "twisting of the points" QRS morphology and the long QT interval at tachycardia initiation.

## TABLE 2  Ventricular Tachycardias

| Type | Description |
| --- | --- |
| Monomorphic | All QRSs have the same shape<br>Can be sustained, nonsustained, or repetitive |
| Polymorphic | QRS shapes vary<br>Can be sustained, nonsustained, or catecholaminergic |
| Accelerated idioventricular rhythm | Ectopic ventricular rhythm with ≥3 consecutive ventricular premature beats occurring at a rate <100 bpm but faster than the normal ventricular intrinsic escape rate of 30 to 40 bpm |
| Ventricular tachycardia storm | Incessant VT, typically present in >50% of a 24-h period |
| Adenosine-sensitive VT | VT terminating with adenosine |
| Verapamil-sensitive VT | VT responsive to verapamil and with RBBB or LBBB morphology |
| Ventricular flutter | A regular ventricular arrhythmia approximately 300 bpm with a monomorphic appearance |
| Ventricular fibrillation | Rapid, usually >300 bpm, grossly irregular ventricular rhythm with marked variability in QRS, morphology, and amplitude |
| Torsades de pointes | VT associated with a long QT or $QT_c$ interval<br>Congenital, acquired (heart block, medications) |
| Brugada's syndrome | RBBB with ST segment elevation in leads V1 through V3 |
| Ventricular arrhythmias associated with short QT syndrome | $QT_c$ ≤300 ms |
| Fascicular tachycardia | Originates from or requires participation of the distal fascicles (right or left bundle branches) |
| Bundle branch reentrant tachycardia | Reentry involving the His-Purkinje system, usually with LBBB morphology |
| Idiopathic RBBB VT | Absence of structural heart disease with RBBB morphology, typically responsive to verapamil |
| Outflow tract VT | Right or left ventricular outflow tract without structural heart disease |

*Abbreviations:* LBBB = left bundle branch block; RBBB = right bundle branch block; VT = ventricular tachycardia.

## Supraventricular or Ventricular?

The QRS morphology, the QRS width, presence of P waves, relationship of P waves to QRS complexes, and tachycardia regularity help clarify the tachycardia type. The electrocardiogram (ECG) is the most useful noninvasive tool to diagnose tachycardias. When a tachycardia is present, if possible and if time permits, it is best to obtain a 12-lead ECG. Sometimes an intervention such as a carotid sinus massage or adenosine administration during electrocardiographic recording aids in the diagnosis.

Regular supraventricular tachycardias can have P waves preceding, within, or following the QRS complex. Sinus tachycardias have a P-wave morphology similar to that in sinus rhythm on the 12-lead ECG. The P wave generally precedes the QRS complex. Typical AV nodal reentry supraventricular tachycardia has the P-wave immediately following, or in, the QRS complex. On the ECG, a pseudo-r′ in lead V1 may be present (Figure 4). In AV reentry supraventricular tachycardia, due to retrograde conduction through an accessory pathway and due to a macro reentry circuit, the P wave follows the QRS complex and is in the ST segment (Figure 5). In sinoatrial reentry tachycardia, the P wave looks the same as in sinus rhythm, but the tachycardia begins and stops abruptly, similar to other supraventricular tachycardias (Figure 6). Atrial tachycardias have P waves that differ from sinus rhythm. The AV interval can be long, short, or variable, and AV block may be present.

If the P-wave morphology is similar beat to beat, but there is irregular AV conduction, the type of supraventricular tachycardia is an atrial tachycardia or atrial flutter. During atrial flutter, there generally is not a flat baseline but evidence of continuous electrical activity, often in a saw-tooth pattern (Figure 7). Atrial flutter tends to have a rate greater than 250 bpm. Atrial tachycardia can be associated with regular P waves but there is generally an isoelectric baseline and the rate tends to be slower than 200 bpm in most cases.

An irregular narrow complex tachycardia associated with variable P-wave morphologies is multifocal atrial tachycardia. If there are no clear-cut P waves and the rhythm is irregularly irregular, the diagnosis is atrial fibrillation. Another example of an irregular narrow complex tachycardia is sinus tachycardia with multiple premature atrial contractions.

Most regular wide QRS complex tachycardias are ventricular tachycardias. Other possibilities include supraventricular (or sinus) tachycardia with rate-dependent (phase III) aberrancy or preexisting bundle branch block. Pacemaker-mediated tachycardia is yet another type of a wide QRS tachycardia.

Several criteria help distinguish supraventricular from ventricular tachycardia when the QRS is wide. The tachycardia is likely to be ventricular tachycardia if the tachycardia is initiated by a premature ventricular beat with a morphology similar to the QRS during tachycardia (Figure 8). Ventricular tachycardia is more likely if the morphology of the QRS is different from the baseline conducted QRS complexes (but a similar morphology does not rule out ventricular tachycardia).

Capture or fusion beats indicate ventricular tachycardia. A capture beat occurs when an atrial beat conducts through the AV node to activate the ventricle before a tachycardia beat. A fusion beat is similar, but it collides and fuses with the ventricular tachycardia, resulting in a beat different from the conducted beat and from the tachycardia. Pseudofusion beats can occur when ventricular tachycardia fuses with a ventricular ectopic beat.

Complete or incomplete dissociation of the atria from the ventricles during tachycardia is a key diagnostic feature of ventricular tachycardia. If the wide complex tachycardia has an unusual morphology atypical for a right or a left bundle branch block, an unusual QRS axis (markedly rightward or superior), and very wide QRS complex (>160 ms with a baseline conducted QRS complex <120 ms) or a markedly delayed intrinsicoid QRS deflection, then the diagnosis is most likely ventricular tachycardia. Any wide QRS tachycardia associated with structural heart disease is likely ventricular tachycardia.

An irregular wide QRS complex tachycardia (especially when it varies beat to beat) can be ventricular tachycardia, but when a tachycardia is

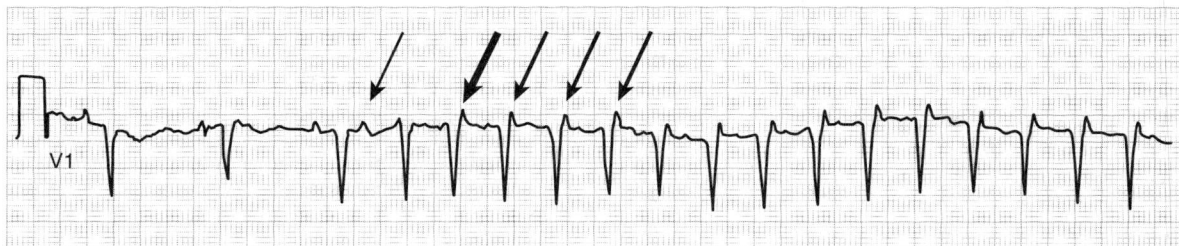

**FIGURE 4.** AV nodal reentry tachycardia started with a premature atrial beat and an associated long PR interval. The *arrows* point to the pseudo-r′ wave in V1. This wave is characteristic of this tachycardia.

## CURRENT DIAGNOSIS

- Tachycardias may be secondary to a normal physiologic response or they may be due to an abnormal automaticity, reentry, or triggered activity.
- Tachycardias can originate in the sinus node, atrioventricular node, His-Purkinje system, atria, ventricles, or pulmonary veins.
- The symptoms of tachycardias are broad and nonspecific and do not predict the type of tachycardia. Patients might or might not be aware of their tachycardia.
- Tachycardias are classified by their location of activity (supraventricular or ventricular) and they are distinguished as either narrow (<120 ms) or wide (>120 ms) QRS complex tachycardia.
- Narrow QRS complex tachycardias always originate at or above the atrioventricular junction, whereas wide QRS complex tachycardias can originate in the atria or the ventricles.
- Clinicians must use a stepwise approach when determining the diagnosis of a tachycardia.

irregularly irregular and there are no visible P waves, atrial fibrillation or flutter with a bundle branch block, with rate-dependent aberrancy or conduction down an accessory pathway (i.e., Wolff-Parkinson-White [WPW] syndrome) is likely. In the case of ventricular preexcitation due to the WPW syndrome, the QRS can vary beat by beat. Polymorphic ventricular tachycardias are wide, rapid, constantly changing, and unassociated with P waves and are tolerated poorly.

## Treatment

### A STEPWISE APPROACH

A stepwise approach to the patient with tachycardia is recommended. Acute management (arrhythmia termination or rate control) differs from chronic management (prevention of tachycardia and its inherent risks). Tachycardia (but *not* sinus tachycardia) causing low blood pressure leading to cognitive impairment, chest pain, or heart failure requires immediate action. The urgency of the approach taken depends on the severity of the physiologic consequence of the tachycardia. The first step is to assess the patient and the severity of the manifesting symptoms and hemodynamics (hypotension, angina, heart failure, or syncope).

## CURRENT THERAPY

- Preexcited atrial fibrillation should not be acutely treated with digoxin, calcium channel blockers, or β-blockers.
- Supraventricular tachycardia can effectively be managed in most instances with catheter ablation.
- The best long-term treatment to prevent death in patients with sustained ventricular tachycardia associated with structural heart disease is an implantable cardioverter defibrillator.
- Patients who have frequent shocks and implantable cardioverter defibrillators might require catheter ablation or antiarrhythmic drug therapy.
- Intravenous magnesium is a first-line therapy for drug-induced torsades de pointes.

The next step is to determine what type of tachycardia is present (Figure 9). The best way to do this is to obtain an electrocardiographic monitoring recording and save it for future evaluation. Ideally, it is best to obtain a 12-lead ECG and compare it with any previously recorded ECGs that may be available. As part of this assessment process, any old records and history of previous therapies that failed to work, or were successful, are crucial for effective acute care treatment. The patient or the family might even know what therapies worked or did not.

The next step is to treat the tachycardia (described later). Immediate electrical cardioversion is indicated for patients not tolerating the tachycardia hemodynamically, except in the case of sinus tachycardia, when the etiology of tachycardia must be considered and can include fever, hypotension, pulmonary embolus, hyperthyroidism, or even heart failure. Well-tolerated wide complex tachycardias causing hemodynamic collapse must be treated as ventricular tachycardia until proven otherwise. Tools to treat tachycardias include electrical cardioversion, antiarrhythmic drugs, β-blockers, calcium channel blockers, adenosine, and even carotid massage, depending on the presumed cause of the tachycardia.

After initial stabilization and treatment, it is important to have a triage plan. Conversion of supraventricular tachycardia does not require hospital admission in an otherwise healthy patient, but patients with ventricular tachycardia or new-onset atrial fibrillation with an uncontrolled ventricular rate require hospitalization. It is best to refer a patient with a tachycardia to a physician who routinely cares for arrhythmias.

Chronic tachycardia management involves prevention, rate control, and reduction in the long-term risk of its recurrence. It is best to attempt to make the diagnosis based on available arrhythmia recordings. All attempts should be made to obtain any arrhythmia recordings, especially the 12-lead ECGs during the tachycardia and at baseline.

After obtaining a 12-lead ECG, ordering an echocardiogram is the next step because it can detect the presence of structural heart disease, cardiac function, ventricular hypertrophy, valvular abnormalities, and chamber size. A young patient with a typical form of supraventricular tachycardia does not require an echocardiogram, but it is required for most other patients, in particular, those with atrial fibrillation or ventricular tachycardia. For these patients, a transthoracic echocardiogram along with further cardiac assessment is advised. A transesophageal echocardiogram can detect atrial clots and is useful to determine the feasibility of cardioversion without risk of stroke in patients with atrial flutter or fibrillation lasting longer than 48 hours and for whom longstanding effective anticoagulation has not been administered.

An electrophysiology test can help identify the mechanism of the tachycardia to further guide therapy, including ablation. Electrophysiology testing should be considered for patients in whom there is evidence of ventricular tachycardia. For a patient with a wide QRS complex tachycardia in whom the diagnosis is not clear, an electrophysiologic study is the best approach to determine the diagnosis with certainty. An electrophysiology test is useful not only for diagnostic purposes but also to potentially cure the tachycardia with ablation. For patients with impaired ventricular function (left ventricular ejection fraction <0.35) and ventricular tachycardia, proceeding directly to an implantable cardioverter defibrillator is ultimately advisable.

Other procedures, such as treadmill stress testing, can help demonstrate the role of ischemia and catecholamines on tachycardia initiation. Some tachycardias, such as catecholamine-dependent idiopathic ventricular tachycardia, might only manifest with stress or exercise.

### ACUTE MANAGEMENT

#### Supraventricular Tachycardia

The initial treatment of a regular supraventricular tachycardia with normal hemodynamics is a vagal maneuver such as a Valsalva, carotid massage, or immersion of the face in ice water (the diving reflex). For these reflexes to be effective, the patient should be supine or in the Trendelenburg position.

Patients with supraventricular tachycardia who do not respond to vagal maneuvers (or those who have mild hypotension) should be given adenosine.

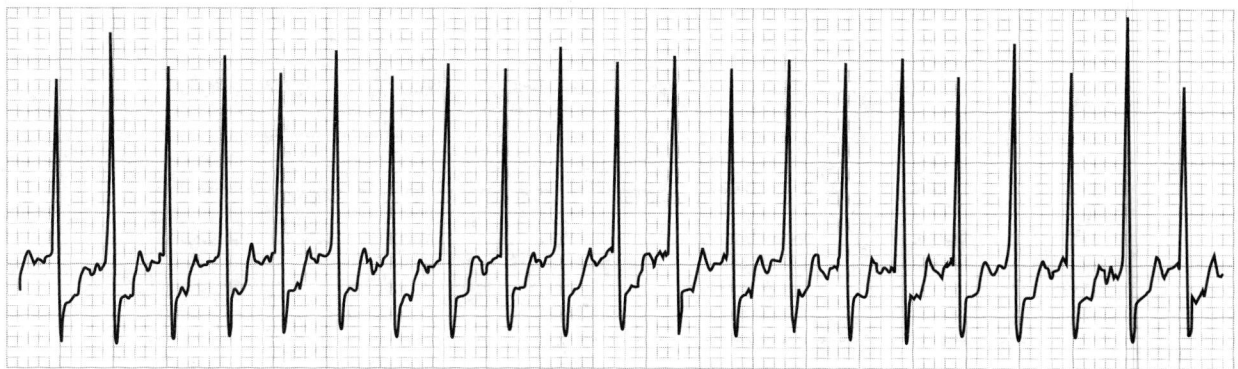

**FIGURE 5.** AV reentry tachycardia caused by retrograde conduction via an accessory pathway. The P wave is buried in the ST segment.

Adenosine is a purinergic AV nodal blocker with a short half-life (9-12 sec), as is indicated for the termination of supraventricular tachycardias involving the AV node. It is 95% effective for this purpose and is the first-line drug for acute conversion of supraventricular tachycardia.

Adenosine is given as a 6-mg rapid intravenous push bolus, and it should be followed by a saline flush. If the first bolus is ineffective, 12 mg is the next dose, and this may be repeated (check to be sure that the IV line is working properly).

Adenosine is ineffective in terminating tachycardias that do not require AV nodal conduction, such as atrial flutter or atrial fibrillation. Adenosine can stop some atrial tachycardias and idiopathic outflow tract ventricular tachycardias. Although adenosine will not stop atrial fibrillation, multifocal atrial tachycardia, and atrial flutter, it can help determine if one of these tachycardias is present (if it is not obvious on the ECG) (Figure 10).

Adenosine is contraindicated in patients with a transplanted heart because it can cause cardiac arrest with prolonged asystole. The effect of adenosine is prolonged markedly with dipyridamole (Persantine). Adenosine may be ineffective in the presence of theophylline (Uniphyl) or large amounts of caffeine. Adenosine is also contraindicated in atrial fibrillation with WPW syndrome because it can increase the ventricular rate. This drug blocks AV conduction in atrial flutter and allows visualization of flutter waves, but it does not convert this rhythm to sinus rhythm. Rarely, adenosine can initiate atrial fibrillation.

Verapamil (Calan) may be required for patients with regular supraventricular tachycardias that recur after adenosine or for those who do not tolerate adenosine. The dose is 5 to 15 mg IV. Verapamil is negatively inotropic and can cause bradycardia and vasodilation. It is contraindicated for acute management of wide complex tachycardias and WPW syndrome. In rare instances, in patients with known idiopathic ventricular tachycardia, verapamil may be useful for converting the tachycardia.

For patients with atrial flutter, atrial tachycardia, and atrial fibrillation with rapid rates (not associated with WPW syndrome), IV β-blockade or calcium channel antagonists (verapamil or diltiazem) can provide rate control. Patients with poorly tolerated supraventricular

tachycardias should be considered for direct current cardioversion (with anesthesia if the patient is awake) but this is rarely required for supraventricular tachycardias and should be used with caution in patients with atrial flutter and fibrillation who may be at risk for stroke with the cardioversion.

## Atrial Flutter and Fibrillation

Acute management involves rate control and prevention of stroke. Acute management of rate control is achieved with intravenous β-adrenergic blocking drugs, calcium antagonists, and digoxin. Need for anticoagulation depends on the length of the episodes, and extensive discussions regarding anticoagulation of atrial fibrillation is beyond the scope of this article.

It may be necessary to cardiovert a patient to normal sinus rhythm, particularly when the atrial fibrillation is not well tolerated or associated with severe hypotension, congestive heart failure, or myocardial ischemia. In these cases, the risk of the rhythm can outweigh the small risk of stroke with cardioversion, and it is best to determine what the risks of stroke are before cardioverting a patient with atrial fibrillation.

Antiarrhythmic drug strategies to treat atrial fibrillation depend on the presence or absence of underlying structural heart disease. Extensive guidelines have been written in this regard. Acutely, caution is advised regarding the necessity to convert a patient back to sinus rhythm due to the substantial risk of stroke if atrial fibrillation has been present for more than 48 hours. Patients with atrial fibrillation or atrial flutter that has lasted less than 48 hours may be cardioverted without anticoagulation. Patients with atrial fibrillation or atrial flutter lasting longer than 48 hours or in whom the length of the episode is unknown should be anticoagulated with warfarin (Coumadin) for 3 to 6 weeks to an international normalized ratio (INR) value of 2.0 or greater before attempting cardioversion. An alternative is to perform a transesophageal echocardiogram to assess for a left atrial clot. Patients may be safely cardioverted with ongoing anticoagulation if there are no left atrial clots even if atrial fibrillation lasted longer than 48 hours

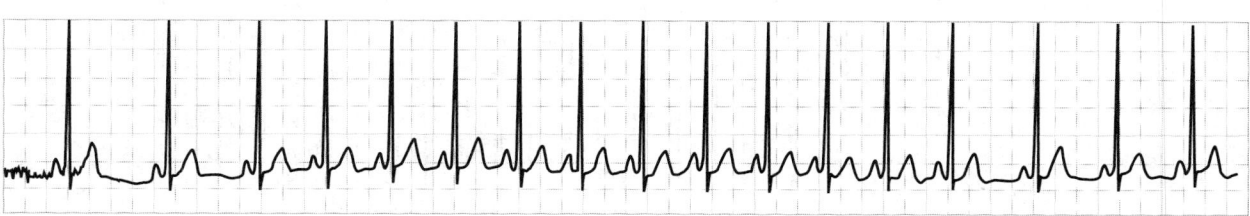

**FIGURE 6.** Sinoatrial reentry tachycardia. The P wave during tachycardia is similar to the sinus P wave. Tachycardia starts and stops abruptly.

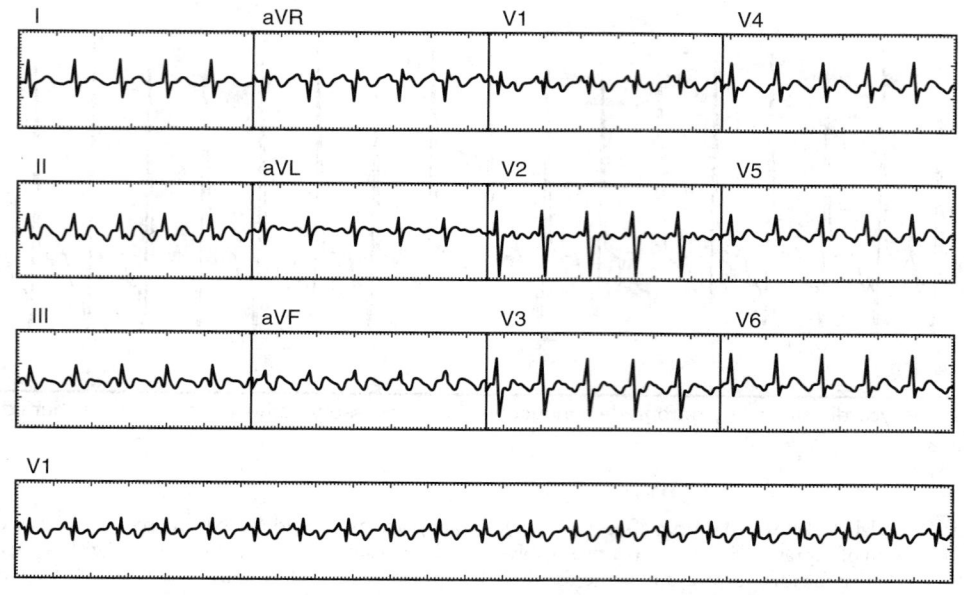

**FIGURE 7.** Atrial flutter with 2:1 conduction. The characteristic saw-tooth pattern is notable in leads II, III, and aVF. Sometimes flutter waves can be missed. Atrial flutter can masquerade as other arrhythmias.

and even if the patient was not well anticoagulated initially. Such a patient, however, would still require anticoagulation with warfarin thereafter for at least 4 weeks.

Pharmacologic therapy of atrial fibrillation and flutter consists of intravenous β-blockers or calcium channel blockers as the first-line approach to control the ventricular rate. The dosing for IV metoprolol (Lopressor) is 5 mg IV every 5 minutes for up to three doses. Alternatively, esmolol (Brevibloc) may be useful because of its short half-life, and it can be easily titrated. IV diltiazem is given as a loading dose of 10 to 20 mg IV followed by 5 to 10 mg/hour titrated to a maximum of 20 mg/hour.[1] One advantage of this drug is that it frequently does not cause severe hypotension.

Digoxin is potentially useful but has now been superseded by calcium channel blockers and β-blockers. It may be useful in conjunction with one of these other two drug classes. Digoxin may be particularly useful in patients presenting with congestive heart failure

and rapid rates in atrial fibrillation in whom there may be concern about the negative inotropic effects of β-blockers and calcium channel blockers. It is given initially as 0.5 mg IV, repeated in 30 minutes. It is then administered 0.25 mg IV every 2 hours until the rate is 80 to 90 bpm. Digoxin should not be given at a dose greater than 1 mg over 24 hours.

Ibutilide (Corvert) 1 mg over 10 minutes and then one more repeat dose at 10 minutes, if necessary, can convert atrial flutter and fibrillation to sinus rhythm, but there is approximately an 8% risk of torsades de pointes. Careful observation of the QT interval is required, and intravenous magnesium sulfate in a 1- to 2-g bolus can reduce the risk of torsades de pointes.

Procainamide (Pronestyl) and amiodarone have also been used to convert atrial flutter and fibrillation but less successfully. The role of procainamide is no longer clear because it is not a first-line drug. Amiodarone (Cordarone)[1] has gained popularity in treating atrial fibrillation, especially in postoperative patients. The drug is loaded as 150 mg IV over 10 minutes followed by 1 mg/minute for 6 hours and 0.5 mg/minute for 18 hours. Amiodarone[1] can be converted to an oral

---

[1]Not FDA approved for this indication.

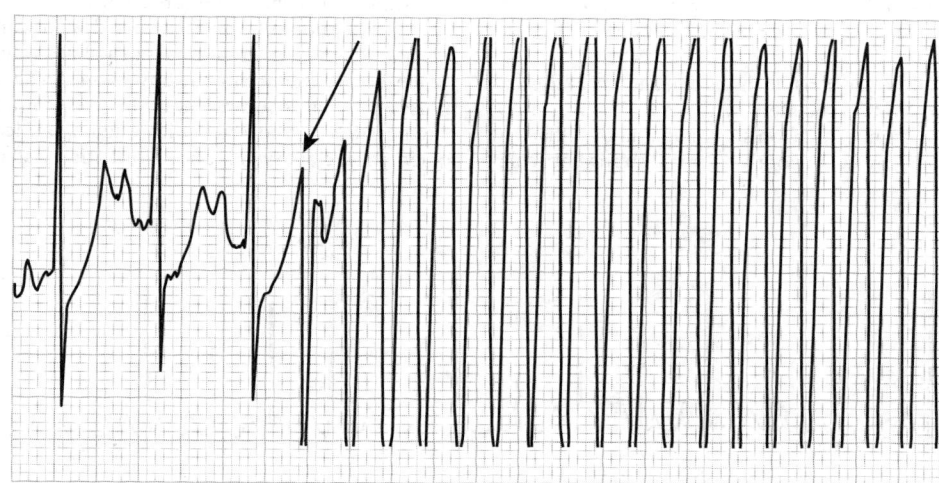

**FIGURE 8.** This rhythm strip is ventricular tachycardia initiated by a premature ventricular beat *(arrow).* This initial beat helps with the diagnosis.

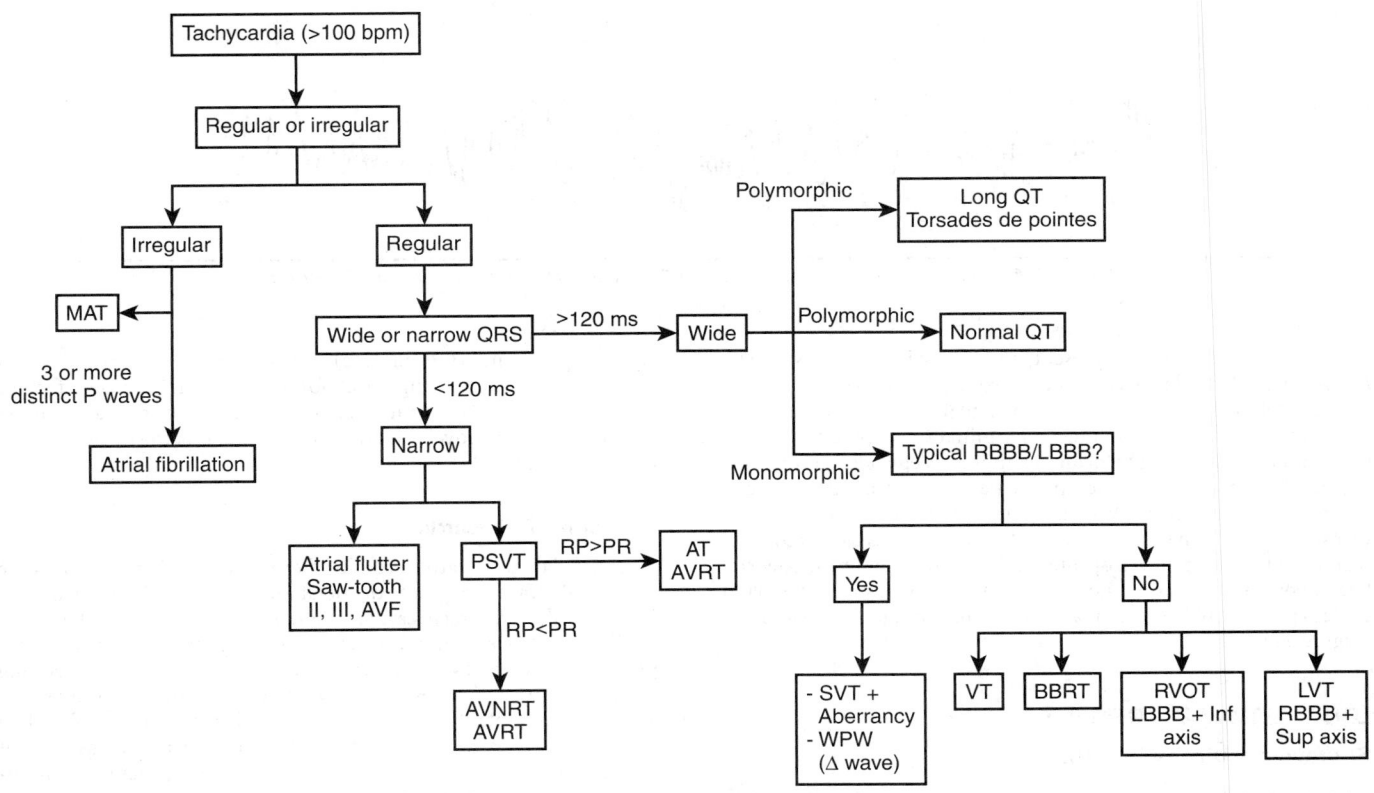

**FIGURE 9.** Step-by-step evaluation of tachycardia. AT = atrial tachycardia; AVNRT = atrioventricular nodal reentrant tachycardia; AVRT = atrioventricular reentrant tachycardia; BBRT = bundle branch reentry tachycardia; Inf = inferior; LBBB = left bundle branch block; LVT = left ventricular tachycardia; MAT = multifocal atrial tachycardia; PSVT = paroxysmal supraventricular tachycardia; RBBB = right bundle branch block; RVOT = right ventricular outflow tract; Sup = superior; SVT = supraventricular tachycardia; VT = ventricular tachycardia; WPW = Wolff-Parkinson-White.

dose starting with 400 mg twice a day and tapering to 200 mg a day over 3 weeks. Amiodarone is more effective for preventing atrial fibrillation after it has been converted to normal sinus rhythm than actually converting the patient to sinus rhythm.

For patients with no structural heart disease or risk of ischemia, the pill-in-the-pocket technique of giving 100 to 200 mg of flecainide[1] (Tambocor) orally or 300 to 600 mg of propafenone (Rhythmol) orally can convert a patient to sinus rhythm.

### Ventricular Tachycardia

For patients with well-tolerated ventricular tachycardia, the initial therapy is drug treatment. This includes intravenous procainamide or amiodarone. The loading time for IV procainamide is long and it can cause hypotension or torsades de pointes. Recent evidence indicates that IV amiodarone may be superior to procainamide to prevent but not convert tachycardia. Amiodarone is the first-line therapy. There is an acute risk of hypotension and bradycardia. If drug therapy is not successful, synchronized cardioversion with

shocks (200, 300, then 360 J with anesthesia as necessary) might correct the rhythm.

Patients who have implantable defibrillators and are having frequent shocks or frequent episodes of tachycardia likely require antiarrhythmic drug therapy. IV amiodarone is the drug of choice, but consultation with an arrhythmia specialist is recommended.

When the rhythm is not well tolerated, ventricular tachycardia must be defibrillated immediately with direct current shock (200, 300, 360 J unsynchronized). For persistent ventricular tachycardia, IV epinephrine or vasopressin[1] (Pitressin) should be given followed by a repeat electrical shock. If ventricular tachycardia persists, amiodarone 300 mg should be given through a widely patent intravenous line followed by repeat defibrillation.

For patients with sustained polymorphic ventricular tachycardia, immediate defibrillation is required. If there are recurrent episodes of polymorphic ventricular tachycardia, intravenous lidocaine should be considered. If the QT interval is not prolonged during underlying sinus rhythm, intravenous amiodarone may be given. Amiodarone should be given with caution or should not be given at all if the QT interval is prolonged because it can exacerbate torsades de pointes. If polymorphic ventricular tachycardia is not due to torsades de pointes, the cause must be understood first, and then the problem may be treated.

---

[1]Not FDA approved for this indication.

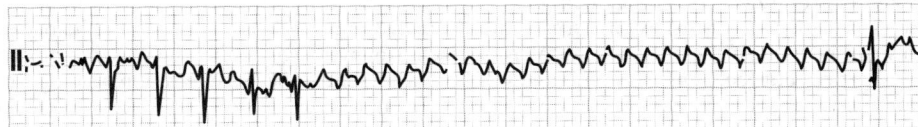

**FIGURE 10.** Adenosine uncovers the underlying cause of the supraventricular tachycardia. It is typical atrial flutter.

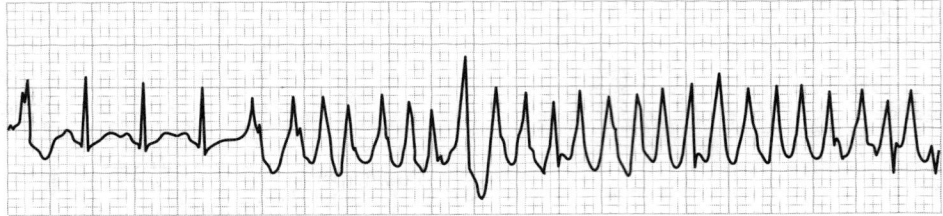

**FIGURE 11.** Polymorphic irregular ventricular tachycardia with a normal QT interval.

If torsades de pointes is present, an understanding of its initiating factors should be clarified. Sustained and poorly tolerated episodes require defibrillation. Atrial or ventricular pacing can reduce the episodes of torsades de pointes if its initiation is pause dependent. Occasionally, lidocaine (Xylocaine) suppresses episodes of torsades de pointes. The mainstay of therapy, however, is removing the inciting cause and administering IV magnesium sulfate. There is no reason to measure baseline magnesium levels because it does not predict who will or will not respond. Isoproterenol (Isuprel) might initially stabilize the patient but should not be used if there is risk of ischemia or if there is polymorphic ventricular tachycardia without QT prolongation (Figure 11).

## LONG-TERM MANAGEMENT

### Supraventricular Tachycardia

Long-term treatment for supraventricular tachycardias includes antiarrhythmic drug therapy, β-blockers, calcium antagonists, digoxin, and catheter ablation. The preferable treatment for episodic supraventricular tachycardia is complete elimination of the problem with radiofrequency catheter ablation. Depending on the cause of supraventricular tachycardia, the chance for a successful curative ablation is between 80% and 98%. For AV nodal reentry and AV reciprocating tachycardias, the success rate of ablation is 95% to 98%. For atrial tachycardias it is somewhat less and for atrial fibrillation it remains about 70% (without adequate controlled data supporting this).

For regular supraventricular tachycardias, when ablation is not an option or is not successful, the need for any treatment must be reconsidered. For patients with symptomatic or recurrent episodes, β-blockers, calcium antagonists, and digoxin, alone or in combination, may be considered as first-line therapies. For atrial tachycardias, atrial flutter, and atrial fibrillation, rate control is a reasonable option with consideration for anticoagulation if ablation is not appropriate or successful. Patients with atrial flutter and atrial fibrillation are at risk for stroke, especially if they are older; have hypertension, diabetes, or congestive heart failure; or have had a previous history of stroke. For these patients, anticoagulation with warfarin is recommended and there is no good substitute for this drug. It is unclear if patients with atrial tachycardia are at a lower risk for stroke compared with those with atrial flutter or fibrillation.

The use of antiarrhythmic drug therapy depends on the symptoms of the patient, the age, and the hemodynamic effects of the rhythm. There is a long list of medications. Class IC antiarrhythmic drugs, such as flecainide and propafenone, are used for patients with no structural heart disease and no evidence of ischemia. For patients with structural heart disease, sotalol (Betapace) and amiodarone[1] are commonly used, but amiodarone is associated with long-term side effects of significance and therefore it is usually not a first-line drug unless the patient has very poor left ventricular function and concurrent congestive heart failure symptoms. Dofetilide (Tikosyn) is another drug that is useful in patients with persistent atrial flutter and fibrillation. The risks and benefits of these drugs and their use are beyond the scope of this article, but each must be considered seriously for its risks before use. Second-line and third-line drugs include quinidine (Quinaglute), disopyramide (Norpace), and procainamide. These drugs are not often used because of their high risk and low benefit ratio. There is no evidence that any antiarrhythmic drug improves survival of patients, but they can improve symptoms (Table 3).

### Ventricular Tachycardia

If ventricular tachycardia results from acute ischemia, an acute myocardial infarction, or a toxic metabolic condition, long-term therapy directed at the tachycardia might not be necessary after acute stabilization. For patients who remain at long-term risk of recurrent episodes of sustained ventricular tachycardia when there is underlying structural heart disease, especially when there is impaired ventricular function, an implantable cardioverter defibrillator is the first-line therapy. Occasionally, antiarrhythmic drug therapy may be useful, but there is no evidence that an antiarrhythmic drug, including amiodarone, will prolong life (even though it may suppress the tachycardia). Antiarrhythmic drugs have a vital role to suppress recurrent ventricular tachycardia in patients who have an implantable cardioverter defibrillator. Ablation can treat recurrent ventricular tachycardia, but ablation is not the first-line therapy for ventricular tachycardia because it is unlikely to reduce the risk of sudden death in patients with structural heart disease. It is highly effective for conditions such as bundle branch reentry. Ablation therapy is useful in patients with idiopathic ventricular tachycardia. An implantable cardioverter defibrillator is not indicated or appropriate for idiopathic ventricular tachycardia.

First-line drug therapy for suppression of ventricular tachycardia includes sotalol and amiodarone. Amiodarone is the best first-line therapy for heart failure patients with implantable cardioverter defibrillators and recurrent ventricular tachycardia in whom β-blockers and other therapies do not appear to be successful in suppressing the episodes. The long-term risks of amiodarone are substantial and include hypothyroidism, hyperthyroidism, optic neuritis, pulmonary fibrosis, liver function abnormalities, neurologic abnormalities, skin problems, bradycardia, and other issues. Other considerations against amiodarone are that the half-life is long and there are important drug–drug interactions.

Sotalol is occasionally considered for patients with recurrent ventricular tachycardia in particular when the ejection fraction is not markedly depressed. Other drugs that are useful for long-term suppression of ventricular arrhythmias include mexiletine (Mexitil), procainamide, and quinidine, but these drugs are associated with long-term risks and side effects, making them less useful and remain as second- and third-line options only when other drugs have failed to be successful or have created problems.

## CONSULTATION

Patients with tachycardia should undergo consultation with an arrhythmia specialist such as a cardiologist or, preferably, a cardiac electrophysiologist. Patients with symptomatic supraventricular tachycardia should have an electrophysiology consultation and should undergo electrophysiologic testing with the possibility of ablation. The management of ventricular tachycardia is highly complex because the patient is at high risk for sudden death. An arrhythmia specialist should undertake long-term management.

---

[1]Not FDA approved for this indication.

**TABLE 3 Antiarrhythmic Drugs**

| Vaughn-Williams Class | Dosing | Indication | Side Effects | Comments |
|---|---|---|---|---|
| **Class IA** | | | | |
| **Na+ channel blocker (prolongs QRS, QT)** | | | | |
| Quinidine (Quinaglute) | PO: 324-648 mg q8-12 h | Prevents SVT | Abdominal cramping, diarrhea, tinnitus | Avoid use in AF because of increased mortality; Closely monitor QTC when initiating therapy |
| Procainamide (Pronestyl) | IV: load = 1g; IV: infusion = 1-4 mg/min; PO: 250-500 mg q6h | Terminates VT or AF; Prevents SVT | Lupus, hypotension, His Purkinje block | Useful to terminate stable pre-excited AF |
| Disopyramide (Norpace) | PO: 200-400 mg bid | Prevents SVT | Anticholinergic, urinary retention, negative inotrope | Useful for SVT therapy in diastolic dysfunction; Hypoglycemia |
| **Class 1B** | | | | |
| **Na+ channel blocker** | | | | |
| Xylocaine (lidocaine) | IV: load 1-2 mg/kg; IV: infusion 1-4 mg/min | Terminates VT; Prevents VT | Seizures, parathesia; Diplopia | Very active and useful during ischemia |
| Mexilitine (Mexitil) | PO: 200-300 mg q8h | Prevents VT | Tremor, seizures | Contraindicated in heart block |
| **Class 1C** | | | | |
| **Na+ channel blocker (prolongs the QRS complex)** | | | | |
| Flecainide (Tambocor) | PO: 50-150 mg q12h | Prevents SVT (flutter and fibrillation) | Heart failure | Use beta blockers to prevent 1:1 atrioventricular conduction |
| Propafenone (Rythmol) | PO: 150-300 mg q8h | Prevents SVT (flutter and fibrillation) | Nausea, metallic taste | Use beta blockers to prevent 1:1 atrioventricular conduction |
| **Class II** | | | | |
| **β-blockers** | | | | |
| (slows rate, prolongs PR) | | | | |
| Metoprolol (Lopressor) | PO: 25-100 mg bid; IV: 1-10 mg | Decreases VR in SVT; Prevents SVT | Bradycardia, hypotension, atrioventricular nodal suppression | Careful initiation and uptitration in symptomatic heart failure |
| Esmolol (Brevibloc) | IV: load = 500 μg/kg | Decreases VR in SVT | Bradycardia, hypotension, atrioventricular nodal suppression | Careful initiation and uptitration in symptomatic heart failure |
| **Class III** | | | | |
| **K+ channel blockers (prolongs QT)** | | | | |
| Sotalol (Betapace) | PO: 80-160 mg bid | Prevents AFL, AF, and VT | Torsades de pointes | Avoid in renal failure |
| Amiodarone (Cordarone) | IV: load = 150 mg × 10 min, then 1 mg/min × 6h, then 0.5 mg/min; PO: 200-400 mg po qd | Terminates VT; Prevents SVT or VT | Optic neuritis, liver disease, Hyper- or hypothyroid, pulmonary fibrosis, skin discoloration | Side effects limit its use in young patients; Increases defibrillation threshold |
| Dofetilide (Tikosyn) | PO: 125-500 μg bid | Prevents AF and AFL | QT prolongation, Torsades de pointes | In hospital initiation, decrease dose in renal failure |
| Ibutilide (Corvert) | IV: 1 mg over 10 min, may repeat in 20 min | Prevents AF; Cardioversion of AF, AFL | QT prolongation, Torsades de pointes | In hospital initiation, observe patients with continuous ECG recording for 4 hours after dosing to assess for QTc prolongation |

Continued

Tachycardias

323

**TABLE 3 Antiarrhythmic Drugs—cont'd**

| Vaughn-Williams Class | Dosing | Indication | Side Effects | Comments |
|---|---|---|---|---|
| **Class IV** | | | | |
| **Ca$^+$ channel blocker** | | | | |
| Verapamil (Calan) | PO: 80-240 tid | Decreases VR in SVT, prevents SVT | Constipation, dizziness, heart failure exacerbation | Avoid use in patients with heart failure or heart block |
| Diltiazem (Cardizem) | IV: bolus 10-20 mg<br>IV: 5-15 mg/h<br>PO: 120-360 mg qd | Decreases VR in AFL, AF | Constipation, dizziness, heart failure exacerbation | Contraindicated in WPW |
| **Miscellaneous** | | | | |
| Digoxin (Lanoxin) | IV: load 0.5 mg,<br>then 0.25 mg q6 h to 1 mg | Decreases VR in AFL, AF | Nausea, vomiting, diarrhea, blurred vision, visual disturbances (yellow-green halos), confusion, depression | Narrow therapeutic window<br>Digitalis toxicity more common with hypokalemia, hypomagnesemia, and hypercalcemia |
| Adenosine (Adenocard) | IV: 6-18 mg rapid IV push | Terminates SVT<br>Allows for visualization atrial arrhythmias | Chest pain and dyspnea during administration | Contraindicated in WPW<br>Adenosine is augmented by dipyridamole and diminished by theophylline<br>Denervated hearts are supersensitive to adenosine<br>Therapeutic and diagnostic<br>Very short half-life |

# Specific Tachycardias

## SINUS TACHYCARDIA

Sinus tachycardia has a warm-up and cool-down phase. The electrocardiographic diagnosis of sinus tachycardia requires a heart rate >100 bpm and upright P waves in I, II, and AVF and negative in AVR. The PR interval can increase with increasing heart rates. The most common cause of sinus tachycardia is exercise to meet physiologic demands or a fight-or-flight response leading to a catecholamine surge. Young athletes can have heart rates approaching 200 bpm with sinus tachycardia. Other common causes of sinus tachycardia include hypotension, fever, hyperthyroidism, anxiety, sepsis, anemia, pulmonary embolism, heart failure, ischemia or infarction, and hypoxia. Caffeine, theophylline, nicotine, cocaine, and methamphetamines can initiate sinus tachycardia. The mainstay of treatment is eliminating or modifying the trigger; no specific therapy is indicated.

Inappropriate sinus tachycardia is an unexpected increase in sinus rate inconsistent with physiologic demands or out of proportion with the level of physical, emotional, pathologic, or pharmacologic stress. It can be persistent or intermittent or paroxysmal. The causes for this condition are not well understood and the diagnosis is one of exclusion. This tachycardia occurs in persons without structural heart disease who have no apparent underlying cause for the tachycardia. Therapy with high doses of β-blockers may be unsuccessful. Catheter ablation to modulate sinus node function is occasionally beneficial, but one caveat is that there is overlap between this condition and postural orthostatic tachycardia syndrome (POTS), a dysautonomic condition that leads to an abrupt increase in heart rate with standing likely due to inappropriate peripheral vasodilation. For POTS, sinus node modification will increase symptoms and worsen hemodynamics.

## SINUS NODE REENTRY

Sinus node reentry tachycardia involves the sinus node and surrounding tissue. This tachycardia has a P wave morphology similar to sinus and is generally slower and more irregular than other supraventricular tachycardias. Sinus node reentry tachycardia responds to vagal maneuvers, adenosine, β-blockers, calcium channel blockers, or digoxin. Ablation is successful.

## ATRIOVENTRICULAR NODAL REENTRY

Atrioventricular nodal reentry tachycardia, the most common form of regular supraventricular tachycardia, accounts for 60% of such tachycardias. The substrate is at least two functionally and anatomically distinct pathways (fast and slow pathways). During atrioventricular nodal reentry tachycardia, the slow pathway is generally the anterograde limb and the fast pathway serves as the retrograde limb of the circuit (slow-fast reentry). Following conduction through the slow pathway to the AV node, rapid conduction proceeds over the fast pathway and then reenters the slow pathway. Atrioventricular nodal reentry tachycardia is commonly associated with a P wave buried in the QRS complex or just after it. A pseudo-r′ may be noted in lead V1 in atrioventricular nodal reentry tachycardia. The R-P duration is less than 40 ms.

AV nodal reentry tachycardias respond to vagal maneuvers, adenosine, β-blockers, calcium channel blockers, or digoxin. Ablation has a more than 95% success rate with a very low risk of AV block (<1%), as opposed to drug therapy, which may be effective only in up to 60% of patients.

## ATRIOVENTRICULAR REENTRY

Atrioventricular reentry tachycardia uses an accessory pathway as part of a macroreentry tachycardia involving the atria, the AV node, the His-Purkinje system, and the ventricles. Generally, the conduction pathway for the accessory limb is from the atria to the ventricle (orthodromic tachycardia; *orthodromic* meaning normal conduction down the AV node). It rarely conducts antegrade to cause an antidromic tachycardia (retrograde conduction through the AV node). The most common form (orthodromic tachycardia) results in a short R-P tachycardia with a P wave in the ST segment rather than in the QRS complex.

AV reentry tachycardia responds to vagal maneuvers, adenosine, β-blockers, calcium channel blockers, or digoxin. Ablation is highly successful (>95%) and depends on pathway location. Complications also depend on pathway location. Heart block occurs in less than 1% of septal accessory pathways, perforation is a risk of left-sided pathways, and there is a small risk of coronary artery damage. The overall incidence of complications is 1% to 4%, with procedural death less than 0.2%. For patients without structural heart disease who do not respond to AV-nodal-blocking drugs or choose not to have catheter ablation, flecainide, propafenone, or sotalol may be effective.

## ATRIAL TACHYCARDIA

Focal atrial tachycardias are usually characterized by regular atrial activation from atrial areas with centrifugal spread, with rates usually between 100 and 250 bpm (rarely 300 bpm). They can arise from right or left atrial sites. Atrial tachycardias without structural heart disease are generally of focal origin. Macroreentry atrial tachycardia is generally associated with structural (often congenital) heart disease. The axis of the P wave depends on the location of the focus of the atrial reentry circuit, and the P wave morphology is different from the sinus. The PR interval is not helpful in making the diagnosis, and AV block may be present. Classes IC and III antiarrhythmic drugs treat atrial tachycardia effectively. Catheter ablation is 70% to 90% successful depending on the tachycardia location and mechanism.

## MULTIFOCAL ATRIAL TACHYCARDIA

Multifocal atrial tachycardia, characterized by three different P-wave morphologies, is commonly associated with pulmonary disease but can result from metabolic or electrolyte derangements (Figure 12). Treatment of the underlying etiology, usually chronic obstructive pulmonary disease, is the best option. AV nodal blockers may be tried, but β-blockers are usually contraindicated due to underlying pulmonary disease. Calcium channel blockers and amiodarone are often used without much supporting data to treat rapid rates and symptoms. There is no role for ablation therapy.

## ATRIAL FIBRILLATION

The actual cause of atrial fibrillation is multifactorial, and the mechanisms responsible are poorly understood. Potential mechanisms include triggered activity from pulmonary veins and multiple atrial reentry circuits. Although atrial fibrillation is associated with increased mortality, the reason to treat is to reduce symptoms, prevent stroke, and reduce the risk of tachycardia-induced ventricular dysfunction. There may be acute triggers (ethanol, dehydration, infection, or surgical intervention).

Therapeutic options include rate control, rhythm control, and anticoagulation. Rhythm control is not mandatory. It has not been shown to be associated with better survival outcomes. For younger symptomatic patients without structural heart disease and without risk for myocardial ischemia, flecainide, propafenone, or sotalol are first-line drugs to control the rhythm. Dofetilide and amiodarone are commonly used in patients with persistent atrial fibrillation who are older and have structural heart disease.

Patients with drug-refractory atrial fibrillation might require catheter ablation for symptom improvement. For older (>75 years), less symptomatic patients, rate control with AV nodal blocking agents and anticoagulation is generally preferred. When heart rate control cannot be achieved, it is reasonable to pursue catheter ablation of the AV node with a permanent pacemaker. It is very useful when rapid ventricular rates decrease cardiac output in patients with atrial fibrillation, even with acceptable medical therapy. Limitations of AV node ablation with pacemaker implantation are the needs for continued anticoagulation and AV dyssynchrony.

For patients who have atrial fibrillation, are older than 60 years, and have no heart disease (lone atrial fibrillation), the risk of thromboembolism is low without treatment. For other patients with atrial fibrillation, the risks of warfarin must be carefully balanced against the benefits. Those who are at greatest risk are older than 75 years; have a history of a stroke, diabetes, or hypertension; or have heart failure.

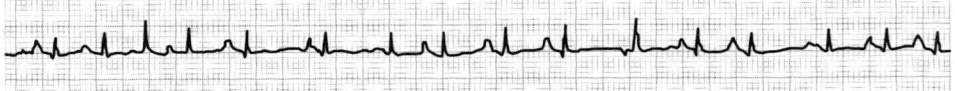

**FIGURE 12.** Multifocal atrial tachycardia. Multiple P-wave morphologies are present.

Pulmonary vein isolation procedures are evolving to treat atrial fibrillation. Success rates are reported to be from 50% to more than 90%, but outcomes are open to scrutiny. Ablation has most promise in younger patients without structural heart disease who have paroxysmal atrial fibrillation.

## ATRIAL FLUTTER

Atrial flutter is a macroreentry tachycardia involving large portions of the atria. Right-sided (typical) atrial flutter is the most common form and requires the isthmus of the right atrium and tissue circumscribing the inferior annulus of the tricuspid valve. The ECG of typical counterclockwise atrial flutter is characteristic of a saw-tooth pattern in leads II, III, and AVF. Atypical right atrial, clockwise, and left atrial flutters are less common. The atrial rate is between 250 and 300 bpm. Atrial flutter can be associated with atrial fibrillation.

Control of the ventricular rate with β-blockers, digoxin, and calcium channel antagonists is possible but more difficult than it is for atrial fibrillation. Risks of stroke are similar to those for atrial fibrillation. Ablation of typical forms of atrial flutter are highly successful (>95%), but atypical forms of atrial flutter are more challenging to ablate, with success rates between 50% and 90%.

## WOLFF-PARKINSON-WHITE SYNDROME

In the WPW syndrome, an extranodal accessory pathway (or pathways) connects the atria to the ventricles. Antegrade conduction from the atria to the ventricles leads to early activation of the ventricles (preexcitation). The initial portion of the QRS is thus slurred (a delta wave is present) and the PR segment is short (typically <120 ms) (Figure 13). Ventricular preexcitation on the ECG is evidence of the presence of an anomalous AV connection, which results in ventricular activation prior to what would have occurred through the normal His-Purkinje system alone.

The delta wave is produced by AV conduction over an accessory pathway. The QRS during sinus rhythm (usually >120 ms) represents fusion of ventricular depolarization over two or more conduction pathways: the accessory pathway(s) and the normal conduction system.

This syndrome is associated with supraventricular tachycardias including AV reciprocating tachycardia and atrial fibrillation. Atrial fibrillation can conduct via the accessory pathway and the AV node leading to ventricular fibrillation and death (Figure 14). The risk of sudden death is small but present, especially in the presence of digoxin and calcium channel blockers because they block the AV node and force conduction through the accessory pathway, allowing a very rapid ventricular rate to develop.

Treatment includes use of antiarrhythmic drugs such as procainamide. Sotalol[1] or amiodarone[1] can effectively block conduction through the accessory pathway and prevent preexcitation. Vagal maneuvers and adenosine can be used to stop acute attacks, but there is a small risk of precipitating atrial fibrillation.

Optimal treatment is ablation of the accessory pathway. Routine use of an electrophysiology test to risk stratify asymptomatic patients with preexcitation is controversial but should be considered for those in high-risk occupations or who engage in competitive physical activity (airline pilots, bus drivers, professional athletes). Asymptomatic patients with intermittent preexcitation who engage in high-risk activity may be considered for ablation. Ablation is indicated for patients who have atrial fibrillation. Ablation also treats the atrial fibrillation. Some advocate ablation of all accessory pathways regardless of symptoms.

## VENTRICULAR TACHYCARDIA

Ventricular tachycardia is potentially life threatening, especially in patients with structural heart disease or underlying channelopathy.

---

[1]Not FDA approved for this indication.

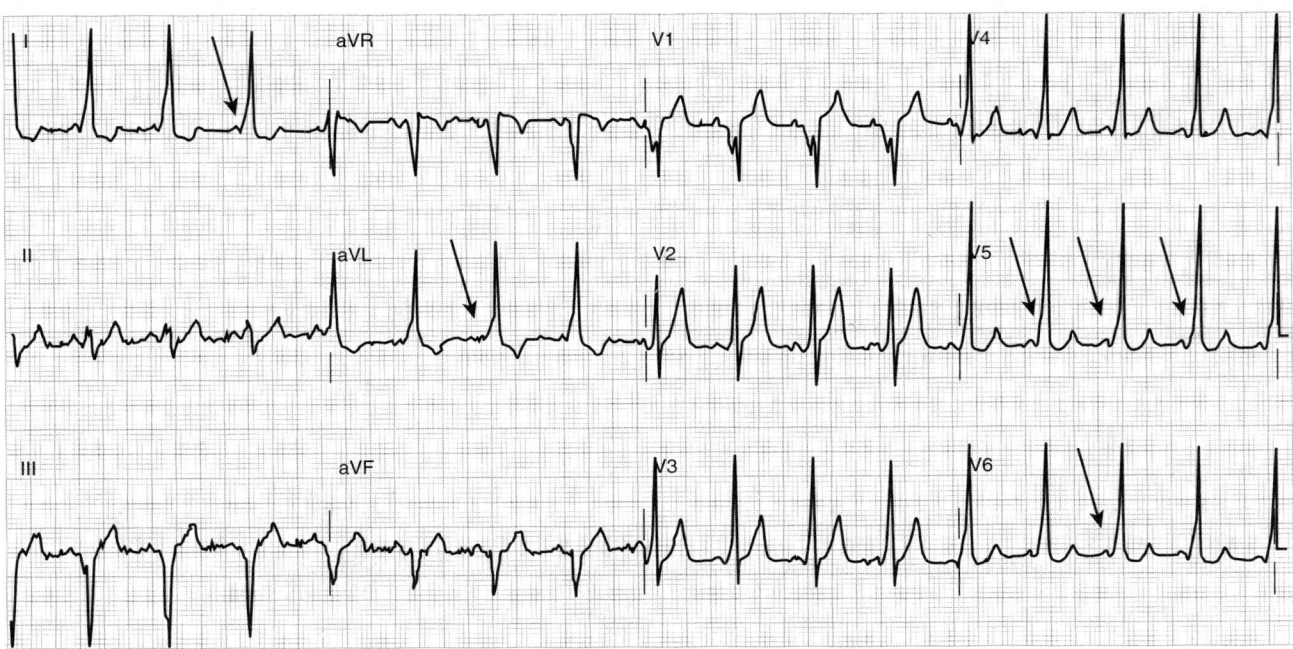

**FIGURE 13.** Wolff-Parkinson-White syndrome. The *arrows* show the slurred upstroke of the QRS complex that is termed the *delta wave*.

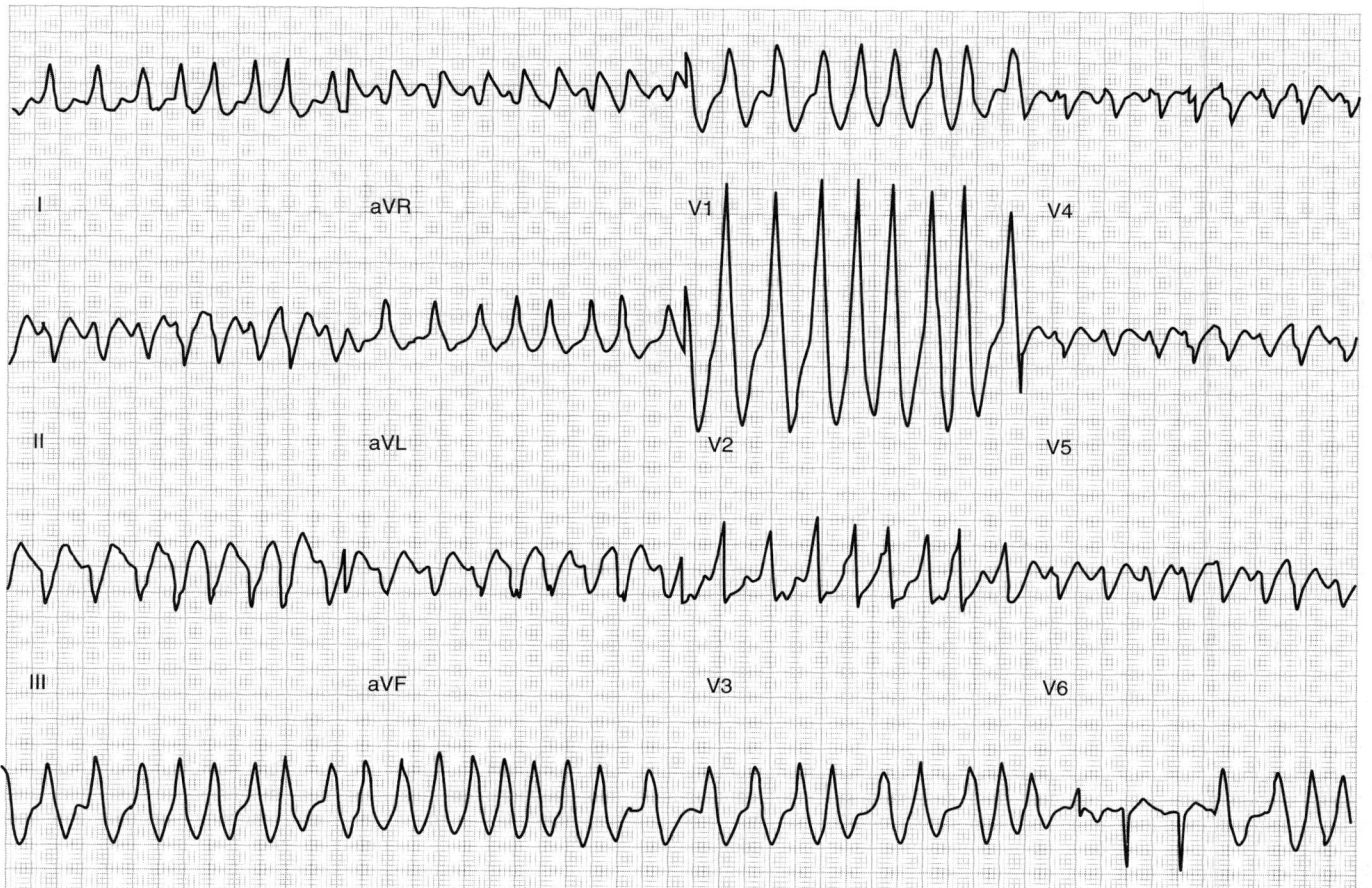

**FIGURE 14.** Atrial fibrillation with Wolff-Parkinson-White syndrome. There are varying degrees of fusion.

The immediate treatment of hemodynamically unstable ventricular tachycardia is direct current cardioversion. For patients with frequent runs of nonsustained and well-tolerated ventricular tachycardia, drug therapies include lidocaine (acutely), mexiletine, quinidine, procainamide (chronically), sotalol (chronically), amiodarone (chronically or acutely), and β-blockers. Drug therapy might not prevent tachycardia recurrence or death. Guidelines now indicate which patients might benefit from an implantable cardioverter defibrillator based on composite information from large multicenter-controlled clinical trials.

Patients who have symptomatic idiopathic ventricular tachycardia (uncontrolled by drug therapy), structural heart disease with frequent tachycardia recurrence leading to implantable cardioverter defibrillator shocks, bundle branch reentry, and incessant ventricular tachycardias should be considered for catheter ablation.

## REFERENCES

American Heart Association ECC Committee, Subcommittees and Task Forces: 2005 American Heart Association Guidelines for Cardiopulmonary Resusci-tation and Emergency Cardiovascular Care. Circulation 2005;112:IV-1—IV-5.

Bardy GH, Lee KL, Mark DB, et al: Amiodarone or an implantable cardioverter-defibrillator for congestive heart failure. N Engl J Med 2005;352:225-237.

Bathina MN, Mickelsen S, Brooks C, et al: Radiofrequency catheter ablation versus medical therapy for initial treatment of supraventricular tachycardia and its impact on quality of life and healthcare costs. Am J Cardiol 1998;82:589-593.

Blomström-Lundqvist C, Scheinman M, Aliot E, et al: ACC/AHA/ESC Guidelines for the management of patients with supraventricular arrhythmias—executive summary. J Am Coll Cardiol 2003;42:1493-1531.

Buxton AE, Calkins H, Callans DJ, et al: ACC/AHA/HRS 2006 key data elements and definitions for electrophysiological studies and procedures. J Am Coll Cardiol 2006;48:2360-2396.

Fuster V, Ryden L, Cannom D, et al: ACC/AHA/ESC 2006 Guidelines for management of patients with atrial fibrillation. J Am Coll Cardiol 2006;48:149-246.

Roden DM: Antiarrhythmic drugs: From mechanisms to clinical practice. Heart 2000;84:339-346.

Vijayaraman P, Kok LC, Rhee B: Wide complex tachycardia: What is the mechanism? Heart Rhythm 2005;2:107-109.

Wellens HJ: Electrophysiology: Ventricular tachycardia: Diagnosis of broad QRS complex tachycardia. Heart 2001;86:579-585.

Wellens HJ, Pappone C, Santinelli V, et al: When to perform catheter ablation in asymptomatic patients with a Wolff-Parkinson-White electrocardiogram. Circulation 2005;112(14):2201-2216.

Zipes D, Cramm A, Borggrefe M, et al: Ventricular arrhythmias and sudden cardiac death: ACC/AHA/ESC 2006 guidelines for management of patients with ventricular arrhythmias and the prevention of sudden cardiac death. J Am Coll Cardiol 2006;48:1064-1108.

Zipes DP, Jalife J: Cardiac Electrophysiology: From Cell to Bedside, 4th ed. Philadelphia: WB Saunders, 2004.

# Congenital Heart Disease

Method of
*Robb L. Romp, MD, and Yung R. Lau, MD*

Congenital heart disease is the most common type of severe congenital malformation, with a prevalence of approximately 8 per 1000 live births. Proper evaluation of patients for congenital heart disease includes reviewing the past medical history, performing a systematic physical examination, and using selective ancillary testing.

The etiology of most congenital heart disease is unknown, but numerous high-risk populations have been identified. Fetal exposure to maternal diabetes, rubella, or teratogens such as ethanol and retinoic acid leads to an increased incidence of cardiac malformation. Certain chromosomal abnormalities, including Down syndrome (trisomy 21), DiGeorge's syndrome (22q11 deletion), and Turner's syndrome (XO) are associated with specific cardiac lesions. Some forms of congenital heart disease carry increased risk for familial transmission.

## Cardiac Evaluation

The physical examination begins with gross inspection for dysmorphic features suggesting syndromes related to congenital heart disease. Next, a thorough review of vital signs including growth parameters, four extremity blood pressures, and oxygen saturation should be conducted. Normal arterial saturations should be greater than 93% in newborns. In the presence of desaturation, a hyperoxia challenge (measuring partial oxygen pressure of blood while breathing 100% oxygen) can be helpful. Infants with pulmonary disease can typically achieve a partial oxygen pressure in excess of 150 mm Hg, whereas infants with intracardiac right-to-left shunting cannot. Respiratory symptoms, including tachypnea and hyperpnea, are frequent findings in cardiac malformations that cause increased pulmonary blood flow. Hepatomegaly is also common in cardiac malformations with important pulmonary overcirculation. The extremities should be evaluated for evidence of impaired perfusion, clubbing, or edema. Abnormal pulses and brachiofemoral pulse delay are markers for certain types of congenital heart disease.

Evaluation of the heart itself includes observing and palpating the location and size of the cardiac impulse on the precordium. Auscultation of cardiac sounds should focus sequentially on the first and second heart sounds and then on murmurs. The first heart sound is typically single in pediatric patients. The second heart sound varies with respiration, with splitting that widens during inspiration and narrows to a single sound during expiration.

Murmurs are described based on intensity from I (quietest) to VI (loudest), and a palpable thrill is present in murmurs of grades IV to VI. The timing and amplitude of murmurs help to identify the cause of the sound. Systolic ejection murmurs have an onset after the first heart sound and a crescendo-decrescendo quality that terminates before the second heart sound. When such murmurs are soft and vibratory and vary with patient position, they are generally benign or innocent. Harsher and louder ejection murmurs are more likely to represent obstructed blood flow, such as valve stenosis.

Holosystolic murmurs have an onset coincident with the first heart sound. These murmurs are caused most commonly by ventricular septal defects but are also associated with mitral or tricuspid valve insufficiency. Continuous murmurs extend from systole through the second heart sound into diastole and represent flow from the systemic arterial circulation into the pulmonary or venous circulation. Diastolic murmurs are isolated in diastole and can be caused by aortic or pulmonary valve insufficiency. Diastolic rumbles can also be caused by excess flow across the tricuspid or mitral valve due to intracardiac left-to-right shunting. The location of the murmur and direction of radiation are helpful in determining the cause of the sound.

Ancillary testing plays an important role in diagnosing congenital heart disease. Chest radiography can help identify the presence of cardiac enlargement and the prominence of the pulmonary vascularity. These findings help determine whether a heart defect is causing increased, normal, or decreased pulmonary blood flow. The electrocardiogram (ECG) can identify conduction abnormalities that are associated with certain congenital malformations. In experienced hands, echocardiography is the primary tool for diagnosis of congenital heart disease. Most malformations of the heart can be delineated completely by transthoracic echocardiography, and fetal echocardiography can be used to diagnose many cardiac abnormalities prenatally. Although cardiac catheterization has, in the past, played a role in defining congenital heart disease, most catheterizations are now performed for interventional purposes, such as closing septal defects, dilating stenotic valves, or stenting open narrowed vessels. Cardiac computed tomography (CT) and magnetic resonance imaging (MRI) are becoming increasingly important noninvasive diagnostic tools for extracardiac vascular abnormalities and patients in whom only limited transthoracic echocardiographic images can be obtained.

Using an evaluation including only the physical examination, oxygen saturation, and chest x-ray, it should be possible to identify patients with significant congenital heart disease and in turn the urgency of an evaluation by a pediatric cardiologist. This same basic evaluation permits patients to be readily categorized based on the presence or absence of cyanosis and the amount of pulmonary blood flow. Acyanotic lesions include those with increased pulmonary blood flow and those with normal pulmonary blood flow but obstruction of flow from the heart. Cyanotic lesions include those with increased or decreased pulmonary blood flow.

---

## CURRENT THERAPY

- Endocarditis prophylaxis is recommended for:
    - Unrepaired cyanotic CHD
    - Recently repaired CHD (< 6 months from surgical or catheterization repair)
    - Repaired CHD with residual defects near prosthetic material
- Catheterization and surgical techniques have improved outcomes for complex congenital heart disease
- Exercise restrictions exist for certain congenital heart disease
- All congenital heart disease patients should have long-term follow-up for complications of disease

---

*Abbreviations:* ASD = atrial septal defect; PDA = patent ductus arteriosus; VSD = ventricular septal defect.

---

## CURRENT DIAGNOSIS

- History and physical examination, including growth parameters, blood pressures, respiratory rate, pulse oximetry, work of breathing, hepatomegaly, and peripheral pulses
- Cardiac examination, including description of murmur and heart sounds
- Ancillary testing, including chest radiograph and electrocardiogram
- Consultation with pediatric cardiologist for:
    - Abnormal examination suggesting congenital heart disease
    - High-risk populations (trisomy 21)

## Acyanotic Lesions with Increased Pulmonary Blood Flow

Acyanotic cardiac defects with increased pulmonary blood flow make up the largest category of congenital heart disease and include ventricular septal defect, atrial septal defect, atrioventricular canal defect, and patent ductus arteriosus. Such defects permit left-to-right shunting, the magnitude of which depends on the size of the defect and the relative resistances of the pulmonary and systemic vascular beds. As the pulmonary vascular resistance falls within the first weeks of life, the quantity of shunting increases substantially. This leads to the typical findings of cardiomegaly and increased pulmonary vascularity on the chest radiograph. Symptoms are related to the magnitude of additional pulmonary flow.

## VENTRICULAR SEPTAL DEFECT

A ventricular septal defect (VSD), an opening in the ventricular septum, is the most common cardiac malformation. It is present as an isolated lesion in one quarter and as a component of a cardiac malformation in one half of all patients with congenital heart disease. The hemodynamic importance and natural history of a VSD are related to its location and size. A VSD located in the muscular septum, remote from the valves, is the most common type and fortunately the most likely to undergo spontaneous closure. Defects of the perimembranous septum can also decrease in size over time, but perimembranous defects are more likely to be associated with other abnormalities and to require surgical closure. Defects of the inlet and outlet portions of the ventricular septum are relatively rare. Large defects (approaching the size of the aortic annulus) are almost certain to cause symptoms from pulmonary overcirculation and to require surgical closure. Moderate-sized defects (about one half the size of the aortic annulus) can cause sufficient symptoms to require medical management but often spontaneously decrease in size to the point where they no longer require surgical or medical intervention. Small defects (less than one half the aortic annulus) are unlikely to cause symptoms or require intervention.

Most often, a newborn with a VSD has no murmur immediately after birth, due to the relatively high pulmonary vascular resistance, which prevents significant left-to-right shunting. As the pulmonary resistance falls in the first few weeks of life, shunting increases. In small and moderate VSDs, a concomitant decrease in right ventricular pressure occurs and a characteristic harsh holosystolic murmur is heard. In a large VSD, there is little restriction of flow, and no holosystolic murmur is present. Patients with pulmonary overcirculation caused by important left-to-right shunts typically develop symptoms in the first weeks to months of life. Tachypnea is often the first sign, followed by poor feeding, diaphoresis, and eventual failure to thrive. The chest x-ray shows increased cardiac size and pulmonary vascular markings in proportion to the size of the shunt. In rare circumstances, a large VSD can lead to persistent elevation of the pulmonary resistance. Though such patients have no murmur and few symptoms, they are at risk for developing pulmonary vascular obstructive disease.

Management of ventricular septal defects depends on the patient's symptoms and the magnitude of shunting permitted by the defect. Symptomatic patients are usually treated with a combination of diuretics, digoxin (Lanoxin), and afterload reduction. Patients who are refractory to medical management and those with large nonrestrictive defects should undergo surgical closure during infancy to prevent the development of irreversible pulmonary vascular obstructive disease. Surgical closure might also be indicated in asymptomatic children with significant shunting that persists, due to long-term risk of pulmonary vascular obstructive disease. Surgical closure is currently the standard of care for defects requiring closure, but trials are under way for catheter-delivered devices that will play an increasingly important role in VSD closure in the future.

## ATRIAL SEPTAL DEFECT

An atrial septal defect (ASD) is an opening in the atrial septum that permits important left-to-right shunting. The magnitude of the shunt depends on the size of the defect and the relative compliance of the ventricles. Despite the increased pulmonary blood flow permitted by a large ASD, such a defect generally does not cause pulmonary hypertension or symptoms during childhood. The increased right ventricular output and flow across the pulmonary valve cause the systolic ejection murmur and widely split second heart sound, which does not narrow during expiration.

If the magnitude of the shunt is substantial, ASD closure should be performed during childhood to avoid the long-term risks of pulmonary vascular disease and atrial arrhythmias. With the exception of large ASDs and some defects located eccentrically within the atrial septum that require surgical closure, most ASDs are now closed using a catheter-delivery system in which a device is positioned within the defect to prevent shunting. Medical therapy is rarely necessary.

## ATRIOVENTRICULAR CANAL DEFECT

Atrioventricular (AV) canal defects are malformations caused by incomplete fusion of the endocardial cushions during embryonic development. These cushions normally fuse to form the tricuspid and mitral valves as well as the adjacent portions of the atrial and ventricular septum. Endocardial cushion defects include a spectrum of abnormalities ranging from an isolated defect in the atrial septum, known as a primum ASD, to a common AV canal defect in which there is a single AV valve in association with a large ASD and VSD. A common AV canal defect permits substantial left-to-right shunting at both the atrial and ventricular levels, which leads to early symptoms from both excess pulmonary blood flow and pulmonary hypertension. Patients typically develop early symptoms of congestive heart failure in the first months of life.

Physical findings include tachypnea and hepatomegaly. The cardiac examination reveals a hyperdynamic precordium and a systolic ejection murmur from increased flow across the pulmonary valve. A holosystolic murmur is likely caused by AV valve insufficiency, which is commonly present, rather than VSD shunting. The chest x-ray shows cardiomegaly and increased pulmonary vascularity. The EGC characteristically reveals left axis deviation.

AV canal defects require surgical repair. Although such patients can benefit from medical treatment with diuretics, digoxin, and afterload reduction, the onset of heart failure symptoms is generally the point at which surgery is considered. Surgical techniques vary and include use of one or two patches (depending on the size of the septal defects) and division of the common AV valve into two separate components.

## PATENT DUCTUS ARTERIOSUS

The patent ductus arteriosus (PDA) is a normal prenatal vessel connecting the pulmonary artery and the aorta that permits the output of the right ventricle to bypass the fetal lungs. The PDA typically constricts and closes within the first days of postnatal life. Persistent PDA is present in one in 1250 live births, with an increasing prevalence in premature infants (as common as 80% for infants with a birth weight of less than 750 g). The presence of a PDA permits left-to-right shunting that is related to the size of the PDA and the relative resistance of the pulmonary and systemic vascular beds. Significant shunting leads to volume overload of the left heart and pulmonary vascular bed that manifest clinically as tachycardia, tachypnea, and widened pulse pressures. A large ductus in a patient with low pulmonary vascular resistance causes a continuous murmur. Often the diastolic component of the murmur is diminished in newborns who might have elevated pulmonary resistance, making clinical diagnosis more challenging.

In the infant, the need for closure of a PDA depends on the clinical significance of the shunt. As a general rule, a PDA that causes symptoms or results in dilation of the left heart should be closed. In an older child, closure of a PDA is advisable if a classic murmur is present in order to eliminate the lifetime risk of endocarditis.

Several options are available to close a PDA. Preterm infants often respond to medical management with prostaglandin inhibitors such as indomethacin (Indocin) or ibuprofen (Motrin). If medical therapy is unsuccessful or contraindicated, surgical ligation of the ductus is performed. In older children, interventional catheterization techniques using several available devices are widely used to occlude the ductus.

# Acyanotic Lesions With Obstruction

Obstruction of blood flow from the heart can be caused by aortic stenosis, pulmonary stenosis, or coarctation of the aorta. These lesions are not associated with cyanosis, except in cases of critically severe obstruction in neonates.

## COARCTATION OF THE AORTA

Coarctation, which has a prevalence of 1 in 3000 live births, is a narrowing of the aortic arch between the origin of the left subclavian artery and the insertion of the ductus arteriosus–ligamentum. Coarctation can manifest in two ways: neonatal critical coarctation and non-neonatal coarctation. Critical coarctation manifests as shock caused by impaired systemic cardiac output when the ductus arteriosus closes spontaneously in the neonatal period. Less severe forms of coarctation cause hypertension in the proximal aorta (best measured in the right arm) and both delayed and diminished pulses in the femoral arteries.

Coarctation should be excluded as the etiology of hypertension in any pediatric patient. The heart sounds are normal unless there is an associated anomaly, such as a bicuspid aortic valve. A continuous murmur may be heard over the back. Chest x-ray findings can include the "3 sign" caused by indentation of the aorta at the point of coarctation and rib notching due to engorged intercostal arteries carrying collateral flow.

Treatment of coarctation depends on the age at presentation. Critical coarctation is initially treated medically with prostaglandin $E_1$ (Alprostadil) to maintain ductal patency. Surgical repair, involving resection of the coarctation site and elongated anastomosis of the proximal and descending ends of the aorta, is the most widely used therapy in infants. After repair, infants can develop re-coarctation from anastomotic scarring, which responds well to balloon angioplasty in the catheterization laboratory. Older children and adults may be candidates for catheterization interventions including balloon angioplasty or stenting of native coarctation as an initial intervention (Figure 1).

## AORTIC STENOSIS

The incidence of aortic stenosis is as great as 1 in 2600 live births. Obstruction most commonly occurs at the level of the valve itself, due to dysplasia or fusion of the valve leaflets, but it can also involve the region below or above the valve. Critical aortic stenosis manifests as shock in the neonatal period, when systemic cardiac output is compromised. Severe aortic stenosis can manifest with exertional chest pain, syncope, or even sudden death. Mild to moderate aortic stenosis is generally asymptomatic.

Cardiac examination reveals an ejection click and a systolic ejection murmur that radiates to the carotids and increases in intensity in relation to severity of stenosis. With moderate to severe stenosis, a thrill may also be palpated in the suprasternal notch. The ECG is normal with mild stenosis but shows evidence of left ventricular hypertrophy and strain with increasingly severe aortic stenosis. Dilation of the ascending aorta may be apparent on chest x-ray.

Aortic stenosis has a tendency to progress over time and therefore requires close follow-up. With higher degrees of severity, exercise restrictions are recommended. For moderate and severe aortic stenosis, balloon valvuloplasty performed in the catheterization laboratory is recommended to reduce the obstruction. Though generally effective in reducing the stenosis, valvuloplasty can cause aortic insufficiency. Surgery is reserved for patients who have aortic stenosis associated with important insufficiency or stenosis caused by a severely dysplastic valve not responsive to balloon dilation.

## PULMONARY STENOSIS

Pulmonary stenosis is a common form of congenital heart disease, with an incidence of 1 in 1250 live births. As in aortic stenosis, the valve leaflets are thickened and they separate incompletely from one another. Critical pulmonary stenosis can result in impaired pulmonary blood flow and cyanosis in newborns (due to right-to-left shunting through the patent foramen ovale), but less severe forms of pulmonary stenosis are generally asymptomatic. An ejection click and systolic ejection murmur are present, with the intensity and duration of the murmur proportional to the severity of stenosis. ECG findings may include right ventricular hypertrophy or strain. Echocardiography can accurately grade the severity of stenosis. Balloon valvuloplasty is the treatment of choice for moderate and severe valvular pulmonary stenosis and provides excellent long-term relief of obstruction.

# Cyanotic Lesions with Decreased Pulmonary Blood Flow

Cyanotic lesions with decreased pulmonary vascularity are caused by obstructed pulmonary blood flow and right-to-left shunting within the heart. The most common lesions are tetralogy of Fallot and

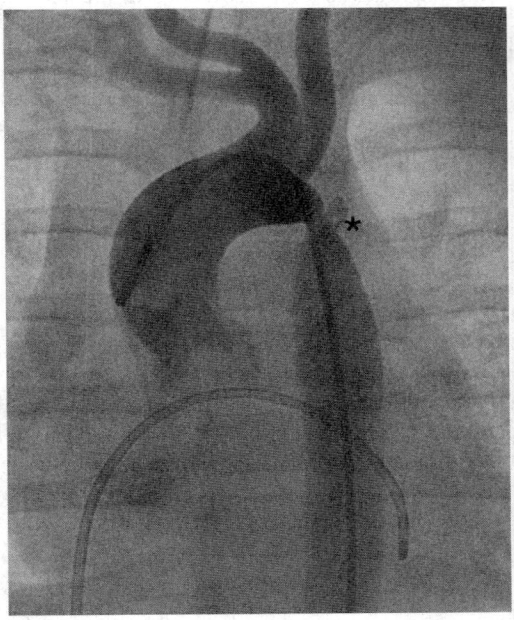
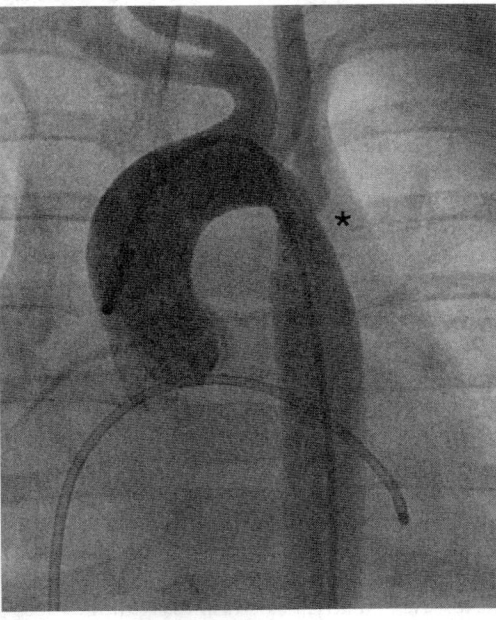

A

B

**FIGURE 1.** Angiography demonstrating aortic coarctation. **A,** There is moderate to severe coarctation with reduced blood flow into the left subclavian artery (*). **B,** Following balloon angioplasty, the obstruction is reduced and filling of the subclavian artery is normalized.

tricuspid atresia. Affected patients have varying degrees of cyanosis. The absence of pulmonary overcirculation prevents the development of tachypnea seen in patients with congestive heart failure.

## TETRALOGY OF FALLOT

Tetralogy of Fallot is the most common form of cyanotic congenital heart disease, with an incidence of about 1 in 3000 live births. Malalignment of the perimembranous ventricular septum leads to the tetralogy, which consists of pulmonary outflow tract obstruction, large ventricular septal defect with aortic override, and right ventricular hypertrophy. The severity of pulmonary outflow tract obstruction dictates the degree of cyanosis, ranging from pulmonary atresia with severe cyanosis to more mild pulmonary stenosis with normal saturations. Hypercyanotic spells are precipitated by spasm of the subpulmonary infundibular muscle, which causes acute worsening of pulmonary outflow tract obstruction and potentially life-threatening cyanosis. Squatting is a maneuver used by older unrepaired patients to increase the systemic vascular resistance and overcome the pulmonary obstruction causing a hypercyanotic spell.

The examination is notable for cyanosis in the case of more severe obstruction of the pulmonary outflow tract. A harsh systolic ejection murmur is present in the pulmonary region. The chest x-ray shows decreased pulmonary vascularity with an absent pulmonary segment and upturned apex of the cardiac silhouette, which gives the classic boot-shaped heart.

Tetralogy does not typically require medical management, and in fact, diuretics and positive inotropes can increase the likelihood of hypercyanotic spells. Hypercyanotic spells are a medical emergency and must be treated aggressively (Box 1). Patients with pulmonary atresia are ductal dependent and require prostaglandin therapy to maintain ductal patency. These patients commonly undergo surgical placement of a modified Blalock-Taussig shunt between the subclavian artery and the pulmonary artery to secure pulmonary blood flow during infancy. Repair of the intracardiac abnormalities can be undertaken as early as the neonatal period, but it is often delayed until later in infancy in the patient with only mild cyanosis.

Surgical repair involves patch closure of the VSD with enlargement of the pulmonary outflow tract by resection of subpulmonary muscle bundles and enlargement of the pulmonary valve with a transannular patch. Lifelong endocarditis prophylaxis is recommended, but most patients require no other long-term medical management. Although the functional outcomes are excellent during childhood, right ventricular dilation and dysfunction are common long-term complications that can require surgical placement of a competent pulmonary valve.

## TRICUSPID ATRESIA

Tricuspid atresia is a rare cardiac malformation with an incidence of 1 in 17,500 live births. In this condition, the tricuspid valve is plate-like and does not permit flow from the right atrium to the right ventricle. Instead, the systemic venous return shunts right to left

---

### BOX 1 Management of Hypercyanotic "Tet" Spells

**Noninvasive Treatments**
Patient in calm environment (mother's lap)
Supplemental oxygen
Swaddled knee-chest position to increase systemic afterload

**Invasive Treatments**
- Morphine or ketamine (Ketalar)
- Volume expansion (packed red blood cells if anemic)
- Phenylephrine (Neo-Synephrine) to increase systemic afterload
- Esmolol (Brevibloc) to relax the infundibular spasm
- Anesthetize and paralyze
- Surgical repair or palliation

---

across an atrial septal defect, mixing with the pulmonary venous return in the left atrium. Blood flow to the lungs is either through a VSD to a hypoplastic right ventricle and thereby to the pulmonary artery or is ductal dependent from the aorta to the pulmonary arteries by way of a PDA.

Patients are severely cyanotic from the time of birth but can have relatively quiet hearts without pathologic murmurs. The ECG is helpful in making the diagnosis due to the presence of left axis deviation. The chest x-ray shows diminished pulmonary vascularity and relatively small heart size, similar to tetralogy of Fallot.

Treatment of tricuspid atresia depends on the degree of flow through the hypoplastic right ventricle. Ductal-dependent patients require prostaglandin to maintain ductal patency until placement of a modified Blalock-Taussig shunt in the neonatal period. All patients eventually undergo cavopulmonary anastomosis by means of a modified Glenn operation (superior vena caval anastomosis to pulmonary artery) during infancy and a modified Fontan operation (inferior vena caval anastomosis to pulmonary artery) during early childhood (Figure 2). The cavopulmonary anastomoses permit the systemic venous return to bypass the heart and flow passively through the lungs, allowing the functional single ventricle to be used as the systemic ventricle. The modified Glenn and modified Fontan operations are used as a common final pathway in most cardiac malformations resulting in a functional single ventricle.

# Cyanotic Lesions with Increased Pulmonary Blood Flow

Cyanosis with increased pulmonary blood flow suggests the presence of an admixture lesion that has both right-to-left and left-to-right shunting. Patients in this category have both cyanosis and early development of tachypnea due to pulmonary overcirculation. The most common lesions include transposition of the great arteries, truncus arteriosus, total anomalous pulmonary venous connection, and hypoplastic left heart syndrome.

## TRANSPOSITION OF THE GREAT ARTERIES

Transposition of the great arteries (TGA) has a prevalence of 1 in 4000 live births. In TGA, the aorta arises from the right ventricle and the pulmonary artery arises from the left ventricle. This arrangement of parallel systemic and pulmonary circulations causes severe cyanosis. Mixing between the systemic and pulmonary circulations depends on the presence of an ASD, which permits shunting of the oxygenated pulmonary venous return to the right heart, where it is pumped to the systemic circulation. Cardiac examination reveals a single second heart sound without pathologic murmurs. The chest x-ray shows cardiomegaly with a narrow superior mediastinum related to the parallel orientation of the great arteries.

Treatment of TGA involves prompt recognition and institution of prostaglandin infusion to maintain ductal patency. If an adequate ASD is not present, a balloon atrial septostomy is performed urgently to enhance mixing of systemic and pulmonary circulations. Repair is done in the first week of life by means of an arterial switch operation, which involves transection and relocation of the great arteries so they arise from the correct ventricle.

## TRUNCUS ARTERIOSUS

Truncus arteriosus is a rare cardiac malformation with a prevalence of about 1 in 25,000 live births. A single great artery is situated above a large VSD, receiving the outputs of both the right and left ventricles. This ascending truncal artery supplies the coronary, pulmonary, and systemic circulations. There is severe pulmonary overcirculation with relatively mild cyanosis but early development of tachypnea and respiratory distress related to severe congestive heart failure. A continuous murmur of flow into the pulmonary arteries is present and there is often a diastolic murmur and ejection click caused by an insufficient and dysplastic truncal valve. The chest x-ray shows cardiomegaly and prominent pulmonary vascular markings.

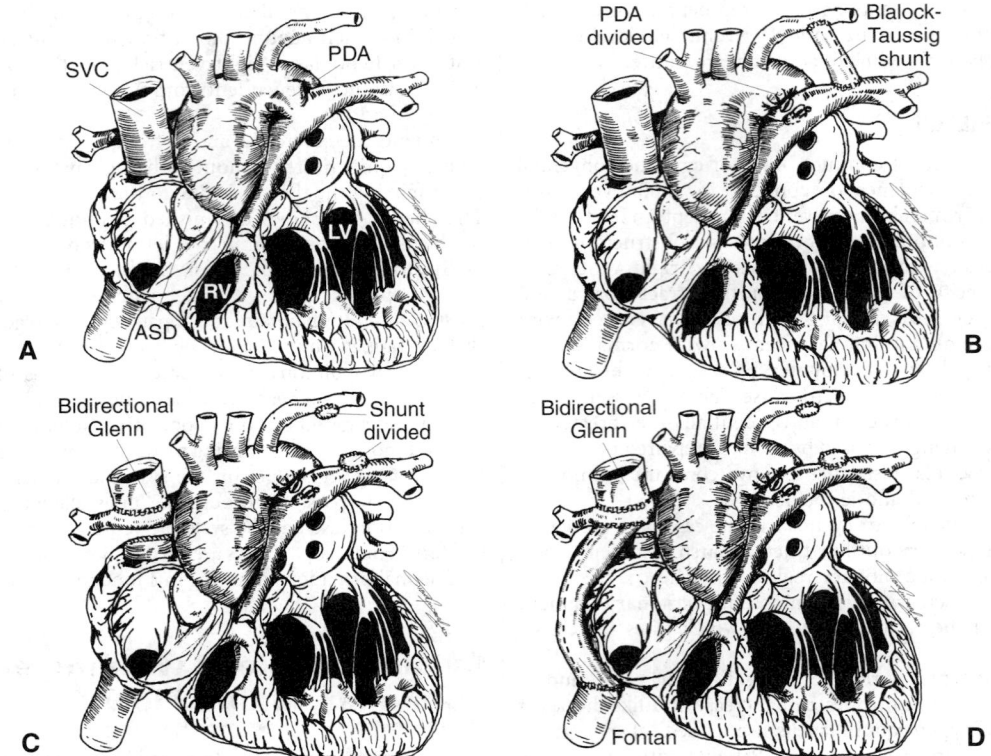

**FIGURE 2.** Illustrations of tricuspid atresia and surgical palliations. **A,** Pulmonary blood flow originates from the patent ductus arteriosus (PDA). **B,** A modified Blalock-Taussig shunt replaces the PDA as the source of pulmonary blood flow. **C,** Pulmonary blood flow is through the bidirectional Glenn connection of the superior vena cava (SVC) to the right pulmonary artery. **D,** Following the modified Fontan connection of the inferior vena cava to the right pulmonary artery, the systemic venous return bypasses the heart, entirely separating the deoxygenated blood from the oxygenated blood. *Abbreviation:* ASD = atrial septal defect.

Medical management with diuretics and digoxin can alleviate symptoms, but definitive treatment involves early surgical repair within days to weeks of diagnosis. The VSD is closed in such a way as to direct blood from the left ventricle to the truncal valve (which serves as the new aortic valve), and a conduit is placed between the right ventricle and the detached pulmonary arteries. Repeat catheterizations and surgical replacement of obstructed conduits are inevitable during childhood.

## TOTAL ANOMALOUS PULMONARY VENOUS CONNECTION

Total anomalous pulmonary venous connection (TAPVC) is a rare form of congenital heart disease, with a prevalence of 1 in 17,500 live births. The pulmonary veins drain to a confluence that connects anomalously to either the innominate vein, the coronary sinus, or below the diaphragm to the inferior vena cava. In all types, the pulmonary venous return mixes with the systemic venous return in the right atrium. The systemic cardiac output is dependent on right-to-left shunting through an ASD. Pulmonary blood flow is increased and the level of cyanosis is generally mild. A systolic ejection murmur is present over the pulmonary valve. The chest x-ray shows cardiomegaly and vascular engorgement. Subdiaphragmatic forms of TAPVC can have obstruction of the anomalous pulmonary venous connection, which can cause respiratory distress and severe cyanosis within hours of birth. Surgical repair is performed in the neonatal period and involves ASD closure and anastomosis of the pulmonary venous confluence to the left atrium.

## HYPOPLASTIC LEFT HEART

Hypoplastic left heart (HLH) is relatively rare, with a prevalence of 1 in 3500 live births. There is hypoplasia of the mitral valve, left ventricle, aortic valve, and ascending aorta to a degree that the left heart is not able to support the systemic circulation. The pulmonary venous return shunts left to right across an ASD to mix with the systemic venous return in the right atrium, and the systemic circulation is dependent on right-to-left shunting across the PDA.

Patients are cyanotic and develop severe pulmonary overcirculation as newborns. Presentation often involves circulatory collapse when the PDA closes, causing impaired systemic perfusion. The examination is notable for cyanosis and a single second heart sound but no important murmurs. The chest x-ray shows cardiomegaly and increased pulmonary vascularity.

Treatment involves early recognition and institution of prostaglandin infusion to maintain ductal patency. Surgical palliation in the first week of life involves the Norwood stage 1 procedure, which has mortality rates approaching 10% at many larger medical centers. Patients require future surgeries during infancy and childhood, including the Glenn and Fontan cavopulmonary anastomoses, which permit passive systemic venous return to the lungs and establish the single right ventricle as the systemic pump. Although such patients have a diminished exercise tolerance and risk of right ventricular failure long term, they can have a reasonable quality of life through childhood.

## REFERENCES

Allen, HD, Gutgesell, HP, Clark, EB, Driscoll, DK (eds): Moss and Adams' Heart Disease in Infants, Children, and Adolescents, 6th ed. Philadelphia: Lippincott Williams & Wilkins, 2001.

Garson, A, Bricker, JT, Fisher, DJ, Neish, SR (eds): The Science and Practice of Pediatric Cardiology, 2nd ed. Baltimore: Williams & Wilkins, 1998.

Johnson, WH, Moller, JH: Pediatric Cardiology. Philadelphia: Lippincott Williams & Wilkins, 2001.

Keane, JF, Lock, JE, Fyler, DC (eds): Nadas' Pediatric Cardiology, 2nd ed. Philadelphia: Saunders, 2006.

Maron, BJ, Zipes, DP: 36th Bethesda conference: Eligibility recommendations for competitive athletes with cardiovascular abnormalities. J Am Coll Cardiol 2005;45(8):1312-1375.

Nichols, DG, Ungerleider, RM, Spevak, PJ, et al (eds): Critical Heart Disease in Infants and Children, 2nd ed. Philadelphia: Mosby, 2006.

Rudolph, AM: Congenital Diseases of the Heart: Clinical Physiological Considerations, 2nd ed. Armonk, NY: Futura, 2001.

# Hypertrophic Cardiomyopathy

Method of
*Ali J. Marian, MD*

## Definition

Hypertrophic cardiomyopathy (HCM) is a primary disease of the myocardium characterized by unexplained cardiac hypertrophy, a hyperdynamic left ventricle with a small cavity, and often dynamic outflow tract obstruction. The pathologic features of HCM include myocyte hypertrophy, disarray, and interstitial fibrosis. Myocyte disarray is considered the pathologic hallmark of HCM.

The current clinical diagnosis of HCM is neither specific nor highly sensitive. For example, the presence of systemic hypertension, per convention, excludes the diagnosis of HCM, despite the possibility of concomitant HCM in hypertensive individuals. "Unexplained cardiac hypertrophy" also can occur in storage diseases, mitochondrial disorders, and triplet repeat syndromes. The presence of a hyperdynamic left ventricle, outflow tract obstruction, and asymmetric hypertrophy favors the diagnosis of true HCM. In contrast, depressed global cardiac systolic function, conduction defects, neurologic abnormalities, and skeletal myopathy favor the possibility of a phenocopy.

## Prevalence

The prevalence of HCM, defined as a wall thickness of 15 mm or greater on echocardiogram in the absence of a secondary cause, is estimated to be 1:500 in individuals 23 to 35 years old. However, the disease probably is more common, as expression of cardiac hypertrophy is age dependent. Many young individuals with the disease-causing mutation may exhibit mild hypertrophy or express cardiac hypertrophy late in life.

## Clinical Manifestations

Clinical manifestations of HCM are variable, ranging from an asymptomatic course to that of severe heart failure and sudden cardiac death (SCD). The majority of patients with HCM are asymptomatic or minimally symptomatic. The most common symptoms are dyspnea, chest pain, palpitations, and lightheadedness. Syncope is an infrequent symptom that often indicates serious cardiac arrhythmias. Atrial fibrillation and nonsustained ventricular tachycardia are the most common cardiac arrhythmias in patients with HCM.

HCM is the most common cause of SCD and often is the first manifestation of the disease in young competitive athletes, accounting for almost half of cases. A history of SCD, syncope, a strong family history of SCD, serious ventricular arrhythmias including frequent episodes of nonsustained ventricular tachycardia, severe cardiac hypertrophy,

## CURRENT DIAGNOSIS

- Cardiac hypertrophy in the absence of known etiology, usually asymmetric with predominant involvement of the interventricular septum
- Hyperdynamic left ventricle with a small cavity size
- Outflow tract obstruction

exertional hypotension, and genetic factors are considered risk factors for SCD. None of the risk factors alone is a reliable predictor; hence, the global risk, which is derived from a combination of multiple risk factors, should be assessed. The overall estimated annual mortality rate of patients with HCM is about 1% in the adult population.

## Molecular Genetics

HCM is a genetic disease with an autosomal dominant mode of inheritance. A family history of HCM can be elicited in approximately half to two thirds of cases. The seminal report by Seidman and colleagues in 1999 of the R403Q mutation in the β-myosin heavy chain (β-MyHC) led to elucidation of the molecular genetic basis of HCM. To date, more than 400 causal mutations in more than a dozen different genes, all encoding the sarcomeric proteins, have been identified. Accordingly, HCM is considered a disease of mutant sarcomeric proteins (excluding HCM phenocopy). Mutations in *MYH7* and *MYBPC3*, which encode β-MyHC and myosin-binding protein-C (MyBP-C), respectively, are the most common, each accounting for approximately 30% of HCM cases. Mutations in *TNNT2* and *TNNI3*, which encode cardiac troponin T and cardiac troponin I, respectively, each accounts for 3% to 5% of HCM cases. The vast majority of causal mutations are missense and private mutations; hence, the frequency of each specific mutation is low.

There is considerable variability in the phenotypic expression of HCM, even among patients with similar or identical causal mutations. Multiple mutations are often associated with more severe phenotypes but are present in only a small fraction of cases. The genetic background of individuals, defined by the presence of single nucleotide polymorphisms, is considered an important determinant of phenotypic

## CURRENT THERAPY

**Asymptomatic**

- Periodic follow-up for symptoms and risk factors assessment for SCD
- ICD implantation in patients at high risk for SCD

**Symptomatic**

- ICD implantation in patients at high risk for SCD
- Medical therapy with β-blockers and calcium channel blockers
- Surgical myectomy, transcoronary septal ablation, and dual-chamber pacing in patients refractory to medical therapy, septal thickness >15 mm, and outflow tract obstruction >50 mm Hg
- Atrial fibrillation
  1. Acute: Cardioversion
  2. Chronic: β-Blockers and amiodarone (Cordarone), anticoagulation, and radiofrequency ablation if refractory to medical therapy
- Syncope
  1. β-Blockers and clonidine in patients with inappropriate vasodilatory response
  2. ICD and antiarrhythmic drugs in patients with ventricular arrhythmias
  3. Antiarrhythmic drugs in patients with supraventricular arrhythmias and radiofrequency ablation for refractory cases
  4. Myectomy or transcoronary septal ablation in patients with severe outflow tract obstruction

*Abbreviations:* ICD = internal cardioverter-defibrillator; SCD = sudden cardiac death.

variability of HCM. In addition, environmental factors, such as isometric exercises, are expected to affect phenotypic expression of HCM.

## GENETIC SCREENING

There is considerable interest in genetic testing for the diagnosis and prognostication of HCM patients. Currently, the primary utility of genetic testing is in families in which the causal mutation is already known, which makes possible the accurate diagnosis of mutation carriers from noncarriers. In families in which the causal mutation is unknown, initial genetic linkage mapping could help to identify the putative candidate gene, followed by mutation screening. Genetic testing in isolated cases of HCM is complicated by the need for extensive genetic screening of a large number of genes and a 30% to 40% chance of not finding the causal mutation. However, advances in rapid and high-throughput screening techniques are expected to change the current approach. The significance of genetic testing in clinical prognostication and identification of individuals at risk for SCD remains to be established. In general, information on the causal genes as well as the modifier genes and the environmental factors will be necessary for accurate prognostication and genetic counseling of HCM patients.

# Pathogenesis

Elucidation of the molecular genetic basis of HCM has provided significant clues to its pathogenesis. The evolution of phenotype can be categorized into three sets: the initial functional phenotype, the intermediary molecular phenotype, and the final morphologic phenotype. The collective results of a large number of in vitro and in vivo mechanistic studies indicate that the initial defects are diverse and encompass reduced ATPase activity of the myofibrils, impaired actomyosin cross-bridging, and enhanced $Ca^{2+}$ sensitivity of myofibrils. The intermediary molecular phenotype occurs in response to the functional phenotype and is largely unknown but is expected to include expression and activation of intracellular signaling molecules. The morphologic and histologic phenotypes are the consequence of the intermediary molecular phenotype and, hence, are considered secondary and potentially reversible.

# Treatment

The goals in the management of patients with HCM are fourfold: to determine the risk of SCD, to reduce the risk of SCD, to alleviate symptoms, and to provide genetic counseling to patients and family members.

## MANAGEMENT ACCORDING TO THE RISK OF SUDDEN CARDIAC DEATH

There is no close correlation between the risk of SCD and the presence of symptoms. Overall, the majority of patients with HCM are at low risk for SCD and are asymptomatic or minimally symptomatic. These individuals require periodic evaluation to determine risk of SCD and to assess symptoms. Accordingly, history, physical examination, electrocardiography, Holter monitoring, and two-dimensional and Doppler echocardiography are performed at least annually. Asymptomatic individuals at high risk for SCD should undergo internal cardioverter-defibrillator (ICD) implantation. Otherwise, no pharmacologic or nonpharmacologic intervention is necessary in asymptomatic patients who are at low risk for SCD.

## MANAGEMENT OF SYMPTOMATIC PATIENTS

Therapeutic options in symptomatic patients include pharmacologic therapy, surgical myectomy, and transcatheter septal ablation; the latter two are options for those with significant outflow tract obstruction. Symptomatic patients at high risk for SCD should undergo ICD implantation in addition to medical therapy. Medical treatment of symptomatic patients is largely empiric and limited to β-blockers,

verapamil hydrochloride[1] (Calan and Verelan), disopyramide[1] (Norpace), low-dose diuretics, and amiodarone[1] (Cordarone and Pacerone[1]). The goals are to improve diastolic function, reduce outflow tract obstruction, and prevent cardiac arrhythmias. β-Blockers such as atenolol (Tenormin[1]) and metoprolol (Lopressor and Toprol XL[1]) are the first line of therapy and are generally well tolerated. β-Blockers with intrinsic sympathetic activity are avoided. β-Blockers are also the preferred choice in patients with sympathetic-driven symptoms, such as exercise-induced dyspnea, outflow tract obstruction, and chest pain. The most common side effect of β-blocker therapy is easy fatigability. Other side effects include excess bradycardia, hypotension, and bronchospasm.

Verapamil and, to lesser extent, diltiazem (Cardizem, Cartia XT, Dilacor, Tiazac[1]) are the most commonly used calcium channel blockers in patients with HCM. They are commonly used in conjunction with β-blockers. Symptomatic relief with calcium channel blockers presumably is achieved through improving left ventricular relaxation and reducing left ventricular filling pressure. Calcium channel blockers impart a negative inotropic effect, which could contribute to reduction of outflow tract obstruction. Nonetheless, the use of verapamil is primarily restricted to patients without an outflow tract obstruction because of concern about the vasodilatory effect inducing hypotension, syncope, and rarely death. The most common side effect of verapamil is constipation. Nifedipine (Adalat and Procardia) is avoided because of its potent vasodilatory effect.

Disopyramide is commonly reserved for patients who do not respond to β-blockers and/or calcium channel blockers, because of the relatively higher rate of anticholinergic side effects with disopyramide. The beneficial effect of disopyramide is mediated through its negative inotropic effect, which results in a significant reduction in left ventricular outflow tract gradient and symptomatic improvement. Diuretics are used judiciously to relieve dyspnea while avoiding intravascular volume depletion. Rapid changes in intravascular volume should be avoided because of enhanced susceptibility to hypotension. Mineralocorticoid receptor blockers may be preferable because of their antihypertrophic and antifibrotic effects in addition to their diuretic effects. Angiotensin-converting enzyme inhibitors and angiotensin-II receptor blockers are not conventionally used. However, experimental data favor their use because of their antihypertrophic and antifibrotic effects.

In a small fraction of patients, HCM evolves into advanced heart failure with systolic dysfunction and a congestive state. These patients are treated, as are those with other forms of systolic heart failure, with β-blockers, angiotensin-converting enzyme inhibitors, angiotensin-II receptor blockers, digoxin, and diuretics.

## MANAGEMENT OF CARDIAC ARRHYTHMIAS

Patients with palpitations should undergo 12-lead electrocardiography, Holter monitoring, and electrophysiologic studies, if needed, to delineate the etiology and to provide appropriate therapy. Chronic or intermittent atrial fibrillation occurs in approximately 20% of patients. Atrial fibrillation with a fast ventricular rate is not well tolerated and often results in severe dyspnea and hypotension, particularly in those with severe cardiac hypertrophy or left ventricular outflow tract obstruction. Electrical cardioversion is indicated in such patients. Electrical or chemical cardioversion is also warranted in patients with new-onset atrial fibrillation (<48 hours in duration) if they are at low risk for intracardiac thrombus. Otherwise, transesophageal echocardiography should be performed to exclude intracardiac thrombi prior to cardioversion. Patients with chronic or intermittent atrial fibrillation require chronic anticoagulation. Medical treatment of atrial fibrillation includes use of β-blockers, verapamil, diltiazem, and amiodarone. Amiodarone is the most effective, but its long-term use is associated with considerable toxicity; therefore, only low-dose amiodarone (up to 200 mg daily) is recommended. Experience with other antiarrhythmic agents, such as flecainide (Tambocor), for treatment of arrhythmias in patients with HCM is limited. Radiofrequency ablation is reserved for patients refractory to medical therapy.

Patients with frequent nonsustained ventricular tachycardia or sustained ventricular tachycardia should undergo ICD implantation

---

[1]Not FDA approved for this indication.

because they are considered at high risk for SCD. In addition, medical treatment with antiarrhythmic drugs such as amiodarone or β-blockers is recommended. Patients with rare episodes of nonsustained ventricular tachycardia should undergo further evaluation to assess the risk of SCD and then treated according to the risk of SCD.

## MANAGEMENT OF SYNCOPE

Recurrent syncope is a serious event in patients with HCM because it often heralds SCD. The most common causes of syncope are malignant ventricular or supraventricular arrhythmias, exercise-induced hypotension, severe outflow tract obstruction, and neurally mediated syncope (vasodepressor syncope). Evaluation of patients with syncope includes Holter monitoring, exercise test, tilt-table testing, and, if needed, electrophysiologic studies. Patients with repetitive bursts of nonsustained ventricular tachycardia and those with sustained ventricular tachycardia are candidates for ICD implantation. Ventricular arrhythmia is the main cause of SCD in individuals with HCM. Implantation of an ICD as a preventive measure reduces the risk of SCD.

Patients with syncope due to supraventricular arrhythmias are treated with antiarrhythmic drugs, and those refractory to medical therapy are treated with radiofrequency ablation. Surgical myectomy and transcoronary septal ablation are considered in patients with syncope due to severe outflow tract obstruction. Treatment of patients with syncope due to an inappropriate peripheral vascular response to exercise includes propranolol (Inderal[1]), clonidine (Catapres[1]), and sometimes paroxetine (Paxil[1]).

## MANAGEMENT OF OUTFLOW TRACT OBSTRUCTION

Left ventricular outflow tract obstruction is a dynamic phenotype that is associated with symptoms of heart failure, but its contribution to the risk of SCD is not well established. Most patients with outflow tract obstruction respond well to medical therapy and remain asymptomatic or mildly symptomatic. Treatment with β-blockers alone may suffice. A subset of patients who exhibit significant resting or exercise-induced outflow tract obstruction (>50 mm Hg) remain in New York Heart Association functional class III and IV despite optimal medical therapy. These patients are candidates for percutaneous transcoronary septal ablation or surgical myectomy. The prerequisite for invasive interventions is an interventricular septal thickness of 15 mm and greater. Otherwise, invasive procedures are not warranted because of a potentially excessive risk-to-benefit ratio. Instead, treatment should focus on diastolic dysfunction.

No prospective randomized studies have compared clinical outcomes after surgical myectomy and percutaneous transcoronary septal ablation. Several observational studies suggest the two interventions are equally effective in reducing the left ventricular outflow tract gradient and alleviating symptoms. However, neither is a curative intervention, and additional treatment usually is necessary.

A. **Surgical Myectomy (Myomectomy):** Surgical myectomy involves resection of a small portion of the interventricular septum, commonly at the base, through a transaortic approach (Morrow procedure). It reduces outflow tract obstruction and results in significant improvement of heart failure symptoms. It is best reserved for symptomatic patients with significant outflow tract obstruction at rest who are refractory to pharmacologic therapy. It is the procedure of choice in patients with concomitant valvular disease and/or coronary artery disease. The recurrence rate of outflow tract obstruction is low, and a second intervention is seldom required. The overall mortality rate of surgical myectomy in experienced centers is 1% to 5%, but the rate is higher among the elderly and those with concomitant cardiac surgeries. Surgical myectomy is associated with excellent short-term and long-term symptomatic relief and survival, and it has a favorable impact on the risk of SCD.

B. **Transcoronary Septal Ablation:** The procedure is performed through percutaneous coronary catheterization and injection of 1 to 3 mL of pure ethanol into the main septal perforators of the left anterior descending artery. Accordingly, focal myocardial necrosis, emulating surgical myectomy, is induced. It reduces the outflow tract gradient significantly and improves symptoms. It is indicated in symptomatic patients who are refractory to medical therapy, have an interventricular septal thickness of 15 mm and greater, and have a significant resting left ventricular outflow tract gradient. In those with significant exertional dyspnea, a provoked exercise-induced gradient can be used as a surrogate phenotype for septal ablation.

Overall, the procedure is well tolerated and has relatively low perioperative morbidity and mortality. The most common complication is the development of advanced atrioventricular (AV) conduction defect requiring permanent pacemaker placement in 15% to 20% of patients. There is a small risk of ventricular arrhythmias arising from the localized myocardial necrosis. Progressive left ventricular remodeling occurs predominantly within the first 6 months. Short-term and intermediary follow-up data show favorable outcome that is largely comparable, but probably not equal, to that of surgical myectomy.

C. **Dual-Chamber Pacing:** Dual-chamber pacing is designed to reduce outflow tract obstruction by inducing dyssynchronized left ventricular contraction. Thus, optimal timing of the AV interval is considered essential. Randomized clinical studies show no significant direct benefit to pacing strategy but rather a considerable placebo effect and no discernible improvement in exercise tolerance. Accordingly, dual-chamber pacing is reserved for occasional symptomatic patients who are refractory to medical therapy and are not candidates for either surgical or transcatheter septal ablation.

## Experimental Pharmacologic Agents

Recent experimental studies have suggested the potential utility of β-hydroxy-β-methylglutaryl-coenzyme A (HMG-CoA) reductase inhibitors (statins), angiotensin-II receptor blockers, aldosterone blockers, and antioxidants in the prevention, attenuation, and reversal of cardiac phenotype in patients with HCM. Clinical studies testing the potential utility of these agents for treatment of patients with HCM are ongoing.

### REFERENCES

Cannan CR, Reeder GS, Bailey KR, et al: Natural history of hypertrophic cardiomyopathy. A population-based study, 1976 through 1990. Circulation 1995;92:2488-2495.

Geisterfer-Lowrance AA, Kass S, Tanigawa G, et al: A molecular basis for familial hypertrophic cardiomyopathy: a beta cardiac myosin heavy chain gene missense mutation. Cell 1990;62:999-1006.

Hess OM, Sigwart U: New treatment strategies for hypertrophic obstructive cardiomyopathy: Alcohol ablation of the septum: the new gold standard? J Am Coll Cardiol 2004;44:2054-2055.

Marian AJ: Pathogenesis of diverse clinical and pathological phenotypes in hypertrophic cardiomyopathy. Lancet 2000;355:58-60.

Marian AJ: Recent advances in genetics and treatment of hypertrophic cardiomyopathy. Future Cardiol 2005;1:341-353.

Maron BJ, Gardin JM, Flack JM, et al: Prevalence of hypertrophic cardiomyopathy in a general population of young adults. Echocardiographic analysis of 4111 subjects in the CARDIA Study. Coronary Artery Risk Development in (Young) Adults. Circulation 1995;92:785-789.

Maron BJ, Shen WK, Link MS, et al: Efficacy of implantable cardioverter-defibrillators for the prevention of sudden death in patients with hypertrophic cardiomyopathy. N Engl J Med 2000;342:365-373.

Maron BJ, Shirani J, Poliac LC, et al: Sudden death in young competitive athletes. Clinical, demographic, and pathological profiles. JAMA 1996;276:199-204.

Ommen SR, Maron BJ, Olivotto I, et al: Long-term effects of surgical septal myectomy on survival in patients with obstructive hypertrophic cardiomyopathy. J Am Coll Cardiol 2005;46:470-476.

Woo A, Williams WG, Choi R, et al: Clinical and echocardiographic determinants of long-term survival after surgical myectomy in obstructive hypertrophic cardiomyopathy. Circulation 2005;111:2033-2041.

[1]Not FDA approved for this indication.

# Mitral Valve Prolapse: The Floppy Mitral Valve, Mitral Valve Prolapse, and Mitral Valvular Regurgitation

Method of
*Charles F. Wooley, MD, and*
*Harisios Boudoulas, MD, PhD*

The floppy mitral valve (FMV) is the central theme in the mitral valve prolapse (MVP) narrative. It has taken 6 decades to reconcile the observations by the pathologists who described the FMV morphology in the 1940s with the role of the FMV in clinical mitral valvular regurgitation (MVR). When the early cardiac surgeons encountered floppy, myxomatous mitral valves at open heart surgery, they described prolapse (MVP) of the FMV into the left atrium and used the FMV terminology for descriptive purposes, a term also used by the early cardiac pathologists. The clinicians initially described, and later recorded, apical systolic clicks and late systolic murmurs, but with a few exceptions they tended to regard these auscultatory findings as extracardiac in origin. When left ventricular angiography became feasible, the pathologic, surgical, and auscultatory phenomena were reconciled and came into clear focus. The nonejection systolic clicks were clearly related to prolapse (MVP) of an FMV into the left atrium, and the mid to late apical systolic murmurs represented a unique form of MVR. At this stage of clinical understanding, the auscultatory, angiographic, surgical, and pathologic correlates were quite distinct.

When the M-mode echocardiogram came into clinical usage, the result was a mixed blessing for diagnostic accuracy in patients with the FMV–MVP–MVR triad. Clinical auscultatory findings were ignored, and the nonspecific echocardiographic criteria produced a prolonged period of diagnostic confusion, elements of which persist to the present. This era was characterized by the separation of MVP from FMV, and the result was grossly exaggerated estimates of the incidence and prevalence of MVP. Gradually, however, with the use of the evolving technologic advances in multidimensional echo-Doppler transthoracic and esophageal techniques, close attention to in vivo mitral valve anatomy, and rigorous clinical conference, reason was restored to the diagnostic process. Revised imaging diagnostic criteria once again were based on fundamental FMV morphology, the mechanisms of MVP, and precise identification and quantification of MVR.

These developmental observations are highly significant because no other valvular lesion has a lineage similar to that of FMV. Thus, recognition and definition of an FMV as a discrete pathologic entity producing mitral valvular dysfunction was the key step to our current understanding (Figure 1). Essential steps in comprehending the clinical significance of the FMV–MVP–MVR triad was the recognition that the mitral valve dysfunction associated with FMV resulted in prolapse of the mitral valve into the left atrium (MVP) and that FMV/MVP resulted in a specific form of mitral valvular regurgitation (MVR).

## Pathologic Observations

Early cardiac pathologists also called attention to the long natural history of patients with FMVs. In 1944 Bailey and Hickam pointed out the discrete nature of FMV and emphasized that this type of valve was a nonrheumatic entity. They noted fibrosis of the mitral valve without rheumatic stenosis, increased valve thickness with histologic evidence of dense acellular connective tissue thickening and basophilic areas of degeneration. The long natural history of the disorder, the susceptibility to infectious endocarditis, and the late onset of rapidly progressive congestive heart failure were important clinical correlates. Subsequent studies of FMV incidence, pathobiology, and complications by Davies and other cardiac pathologists provided clinicians with a new chapter in valvular heart disease. Thus, the natural history of patients with

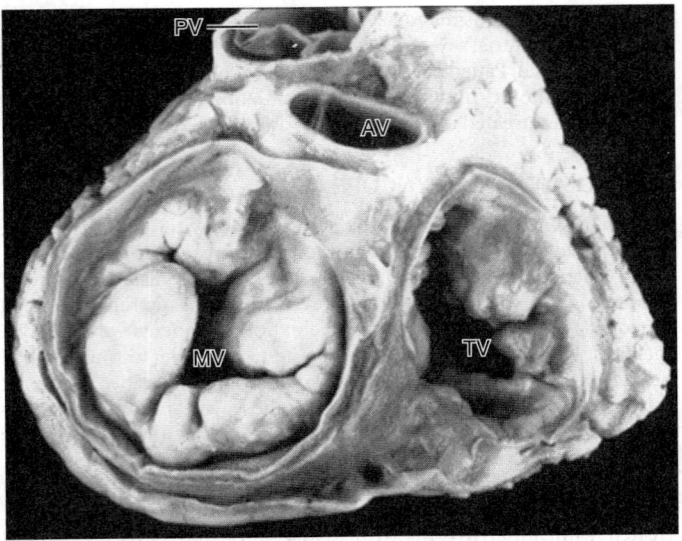

**FIGURE 1.** Floppy mitral valve. *Abbreviations:* AV = aortic valve; MV = mitral valve; PV = pulmonic valve; TV = tricuspid valve. (Photograph courtesy of Dr. William D. Edwards, Mayo Clinic.)

FMVs was reasonably well defined early on; however, the translation of these early observations into the clinical realm took much longer than generally appreciated.

## Surgical Observations

Open heart surgery allowed cardiac surgeons to visualize the mitral valve in the beating heart. In 1965, Read and colleagues used the term *floppy valve syndrome* to describe patients with significant mitral and aortic valvular regurgitation due to myxomatous transformation of the mitral and aortic valves. Valvular regurgitation was related to "valve prolapse" because of loss of valve integrity from structural fatigue, ruptured chordae, or interference with valvular coaptation. Their report was marked by descriptive language—floppy valve for myxomatous changes in valve tissue; dynamic terminology—valve prolapse as a mechanism for valvular regurgitation; and the recognition of connective tissue disorders as the etiology for valvular disease. Subsequently, cardiac surgeons developed FMV reconstructive procedures from careful analysis of FMV morphology and dynamics.

## Clinical Observations

During the 1960s, the clinicians' approach to FMV and MVR, in particular by Barlow, Criley, and their coworkers, resulted from auscultatory–phonocardiographic, hemodynamic, and angiographic studies of patients with apical systolic clicks and apical mid and late systolic murmurs. Apical systolic clicks were shown to be of intracardiac origin, distinct from aortic and pulmonary ejection clicks, and were classified as nonejection clicks; apical mid and late systolic murmurs were related to a unique anatomic type of MVR associated with FMV prolapse into the left atrium (i.e., MVP); and bulging of the mitral leaflets was identified as the angiographic counterpart of the balloon deformity seen at necropsy by Bailey and Hickam in 1944.

MVP postural auscultatory phenomena (i.e., postural exercise hemodynamic abnormalities and changes in timing and intensity of the systolic click–apical systolic murmur) were explained in hemodynamic terms as changes in the timing and extent of MVP, and the time of onset and duration of MVR were related to postural changes in left ventricular volume and contractility (Figure 2). Thus, by the 1970s and 1980s, clinical auscultatory observations, postural auscultatory dynamics, and angiographic definition of FMV characteristics with established pathologic correlates provided a reasonable clinical diagnostic profile for the FMV–MVP–MVR triad.

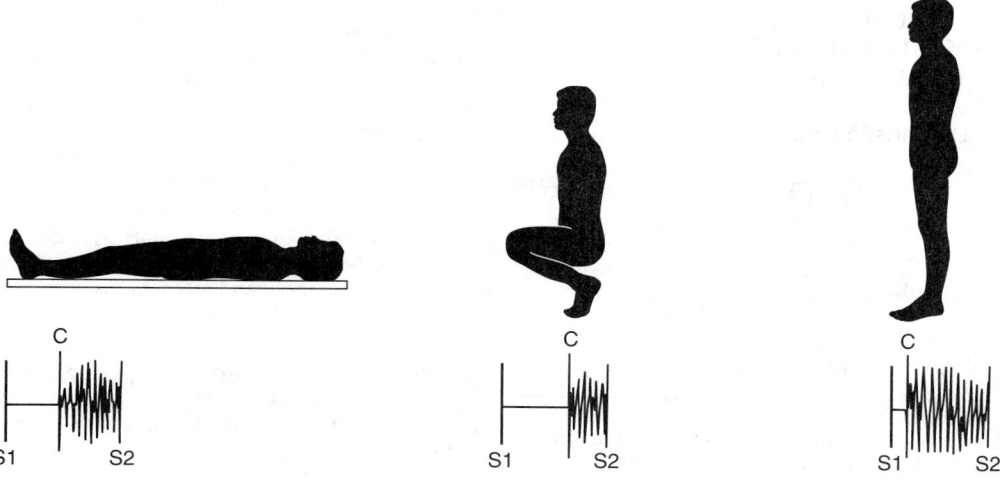

**FIGURE 2.** Floppy mitral valve–mitral valve prolapse–mitral valvular regurgitation: Postural auscultatory complex. *Abbreviations:* C = systolic click; $S_1$ = first heart sound; $S_2$ = second heart sound.

A number of events transpired that obscured this relatively simple diagnostic profile. Clinical phonocardiography virtually disappeared as remuneration for phonocardiograms was halted and production of phonocardiographic equipment ceased. This was followed by an auscultatory "silent spring" phenomenon, when physicians in training were not exposed to the self-critique that phonocardiography imposed on the discipline of auscultation.

Sensitivity and specificity diagnostic criteria suffered, as studies that relied on unproven M-mode echocardiographic criteria proliferated, FMV was uncoupled from MVP, and estimates of MVP incidence and prevalence reached epidemic proportions. Patients or individuals with small, hyperdynamic left ventricles were placed into the same category as patients with the FMV–MVP–MVR triad. When the M-mode echocardiographic prolapse comet swept across psychiatry, individuals with anxiety and panic syndromes were engulfed, and the epidemic became pandemic.

## Historical Perspective

Why introduce the historical perspective? First, recalling the ways in which MVR, FMV, and MVP diagnostic criteria evolved during the past 50 years helps us understand that these clinical entities were moving targets, constantly being defined and redefined by pathologists, surgeons, auscultors, imagers, and epidemiologists, and hence the multitude of names for the clinical entities and the variability of diagnostic criteria. Second, when the FMV–MVP–MVR clinical auscultatory–phonocardiographic–angiographic profile was separated from the prolapse imaging diagnosis that ignored FMV morphology and focused on a 1- to 2-mm disputed zone, cardiologists wandered into areas fraught with difficulties. As the MVP pendulum moved away from the exaggerated incidence/prevalence figures of the past 2 decades, it is apparent that the FMV occupies the high ground and is the central issue in the FMV–MVP–MVR triad (see Figure 1).

## Heritable Disorders of Connective Tissue

FMV may be an inherited lesion, either as an isolated event or as part of the recognized or incompletely defined heritable disorders of connective tissue. FMV–MVP inheritance and phenotypic features have been well described. FMV has gradually become recognized as a common cardiac lesion in the Marfan syndrome. Although FMV–MVP may be genetically determined, clinical manifestations do not usually become evident before childhood. Although children and adolescents with FMV–MVP may have the same symptoms as adults, the frequency of symptoms appears to be less in children. At present, the family history remains the cornerstone in clinical genetic analysis, as FMV genetic diagnostic testing has not entered clinical practice.

## DIAGNOSTIC CONSIDERATIONS

FMV is a common mitral valve abnormality with a broad spectrum of structural and functional changes. Although the pathobiology of FMV has been, and continues to be, re-examined in contemporary terms, we are still dealing with gross structural and morphologic characteristics at the clinical level. Distinguishing between a normal mitral valve with its minor variants and an FMV mitral valve with an intrinsic structural derangement remains a central issue. Thus, it is important to emphasize the necessity for clinical coherence in the FMV–MVP–MVR dialogue.

Tic-tac-toe has its origins in the ancient "three in a row" category of games of strategy. Diagnostic tic-tac-toe avoids the pitfalls of a diagnosis based on a single phenomenon and places emphasis on a multidimensional approach to FMV–MVP–MVR diagnostics similar to our diagnostic approach to any complex cardiac disorder or disease (Figure 3).

We are more comfortable with the FMV–MVP–MVR diagnosis when (1) the clinical auscultatory phenomena are precisely described, preferably recorded, and dynamic auscultation has been performed; (2) the clinical auscultatory phenomena are matched with an imaging procedure that captures and quantitates FMV morphology and function; and (3) the imaging procedure demonstrates MVP and the presence, absence, or quantification of MVR.

Postural auscultation, electrocardiogram, and echocardiogram with Doppler, assessment of orthostasis, dynamic exercise testing, ambulatory

---

 **CURRENT DIAGNOSIS**

- Clinical coherence should exist among the medical history, the physical examination, and the imaging procedure.
- Because the floppy mitral valve–mitral valve prolapse–mitral valvular regurgitation triad is accompanied by dynamic clinical phenomena, dynamic examination procedures may be indicated in individual situations.
- A family pedigree is a vital part of the clinical evaluation.

## MEDICAL HISTORY, PHYSICAL EXAMINATION, LABORATORY

### Diagnostic tic-tac-toe

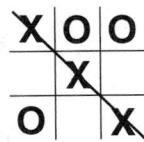

### Multidimensional approach to FMV, MVP, MVR diagnosis

**FIGURE 3.** Diagnostic tic-tac-toe. Emphasis is placed on a multidimensional approach to the diagnosis. *Abbreviations:* FMV = floppy mitral valve; MVP = mitral valve prolapse; MVR = mitral valvular regurgitation.

electrocardiographic or blood pressure monitoring, and dynamic interventional imaging or hemodynamic studies may be required, depending on the patient's symptoms or the specific clinical situation.

### FLOPPY MITRAL VALVE—MITRAL VALVE PROLAPSE—MITRAL VALVULAR REGURGITATION: CLASSIFICATION

The classification of cardiovascular diseases is in constant evolution, and our textbooks and literature do not always reflect the dynamics of this process. At present, we classify patients with the FMV–MVP–MVR triad into two general categories (Table 1). The first category places

---

### TABLE 1 Classification of Floppy Mitral Valve–Mitral Valve Prolapse–Mitral Valvular Regurgitation (FMV-MVP-MVR)

**FMV-MVP-MVR**

Common mitral valve abnormality with a spectrum of structural and functional changes, mild to severe

**The Basis for**

Systolic click; mid-late systolic murmur
Mild or progressive mitral valve dysfunction
Progressive mitral regurgitation, atrial fibrillation, congestive heart failure
Infectious endocarditis
Embolic phenomena
Characterized by long natural history
May be heritable or associated with heritable disorders of connective tissue
Conduction system involvement possibly leading to arrhythmias and conduction defects

**FMV-MVP-MVR Syndrome**

Patients with mitral valve prolapse
Symptom complex; chest pain, palpitations, arrhythmias, fatigue, exercise intolerance, dyspnea, postural phenomena, syncope-presyncope, neuropsychiatric symptoms
Neuroendocrine or autonomic dysfunction (high catecholamine levels, catecholamine regulation abnormality, hyperresponse to adrenergic stimulation, parasympathetic abnormality, baroreflex modulation abnormality, renin-aldosterone regulation abnormality, decreased intravascular volume, decreased ventricular diastolic volume in the upright posture, atrial natriuretic factor secretion abnormality) may provide explanation for symptoms
Mitral valve prolapse—a possible marker for autonomic dysfunction

---

emphasis on the FMV anatomy and pathobiology and includes patients whose symptoms, physical findings, laboratory abnormalities, and clinical course are directly related to the progressive mitral valve dysfunction and complications associated with the FMV–MVP–MVR triad. The second category includes FMV–MVP patients whose symptoms cannot be explained on the basis of the valvular abnormality alone but result from the occurrence, or coexistence, of various forms of neuroendocrine or autonomic nervous system dysfunction. We refer to this group as patients with the FMV–MVP syndrome.

We have found this to be a clinically useful classification, but one that should be subject to revision or modification as we better understand the pathogenesis and mechanisms of symptoms in patients with the FMV– MVP–MVR triad.

### FLOPPY MITRAL VALVE—MITRAL VALVE PROLAPSE—MITRAL VALVULAR REGURGITATION: COMPLICATIONS AND NATURAL HISTORY

Profiles of the natural history of the FMV–MVP–MVR triad have been limited by variations in diagnostic criteria, the nature of the populations studied, and the duration of clinical follow-up.

The FMV–MVP association has well-defined clinical auscultatory correlates; however, the sensitivity and specificity of these clinical phenomena have not been determined with contemporary objective methods. Similarly, the FMV–MVP association has specific imaging correlates, yet these are being constantly redefined as echo-Doppler, magnetic resonance imaging, and angiographic technologies improve and diagnostic criteria are reassessed.

The FMV–MVP association may lead to progressive mitral valvular dysfunction and severe MVR over time; however, the individual patient's natural history may not fully develop for 7 to 8 decades. Hence, studies or evaluations at one point in time have limitations (Figure 4).

Valve surface phenomena occur in patients with FMVs. A FMV is particularly vulnerable to infection and may be a site for infective endocarditis. The pathogenesis is poorly understood, and we currently mask our lack of understanding by using incident-related antibiotic prophylaxis prior to dental, gastrointestinal, and genitourinary procedures. Although guidelines have been evolving, simply stated, infectious endocarditis prophylaxis is indicated for patients with FMVs. Thromboemboli are additional valve surface complications of FMV; however, this is an area that is not well defined.

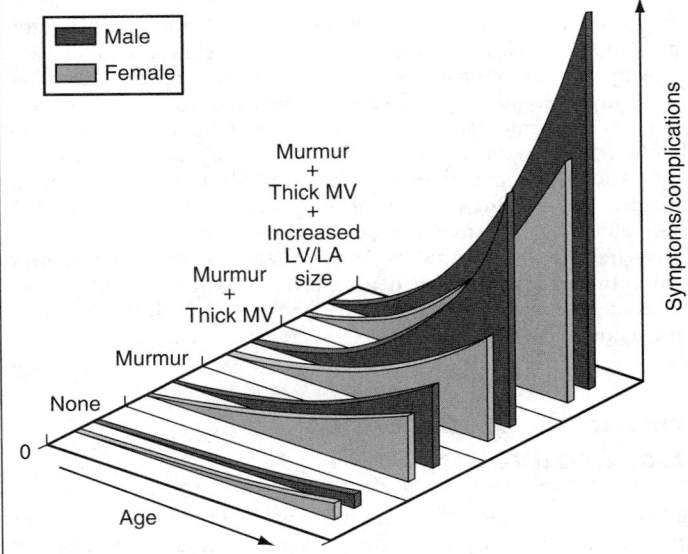

**FIGURE 4.** Floppy mitral valve—mitral valve prolapse—mitral valvular regurgitation: High-risk patient. Symptoms and complications plotted against age. *Abbreviations:* LA = left atrium; LV = left ventricle; MV = mitral valve.

Chordal rupture, progressive MVR, left atrial and left ventricular failures, and atrial and ventricular arrhythmias occur in varying combinations and permutations, usually as late complications in certain patients with FMV. FMVs have been documented as being one of the leading causes of MVR requiring mitral valve surgery. Sudden cardiac death has been reported in a small subset of patients with FMV.

## Therapeutic Implications

Each of the FMV–MVP–MVR complications has implications involving prevention, recognition, and treatment. Individual patient evaluation and management are fundamental considerations, as is the necessity of regular, long-term clinical follow-up.

Individuals with progressive mitral valvular dysfunction require initial and periodic assessment of their hemodynamic status. Individuals with the MVP syndrome as defined earlier whose symptoms may be related to autonomic dysfunction, neuroendocrine abnormalities, volume depletion, or vasoconstriction require investigation and therapeutic approaches aimed at these pathogenetic mechanisms. Both groups require careful explanations of their individual situation, the rationale for regular follow-up, and infective endocarditis prophylaxis.

## High-risk Patients

Individuals with FMV–MVP and thick, redundant mitral valve leaflets are at high risk for developing complications; those older than 50 years with arterial hypertension are at particularly high risk (see Figure 4). A mitral systolic murmur also is a risk factor for complications. Left atrial and left ventricular enlargement and dysfunction in patients with FMV–MVP–MVR have been used as predictors for the need for mitral valve surgery. When two or more of these abnormalities coexist, the possibility of complications increases. In contrast, the absence of all three of these features identifies patients at low risk (see Figure 4). These individuals, whether or not they are symptomatic, may require more sophisticated imaging studies, exercise testing, or hemodynamic and angiographic assessment. Individuals with a history of atrial or ventricular arrhythmias should be evaluated with contemporary electrophysiologic monitoring or testing. Patients who have a history of syncope, lightheadedness, or unexplained collapse or who are postresuscitation require further diagnostic testing.

### SURGICAL CONSIDERATIONS

Decisions regarding surgical intervention (mitral valve repair or replacement) in symptomatic FMV patients have been based on the impact of MVR on left atrial and left ventricular functions expressed in both hemodynamic terms and echocardiographic measurements. Improvements in FMV repair techniques and intraoperative imaging coupled with better echo-Doppler methods of quantitating MVR severity prompted recommendations for earlier intervention extending

into the asymptomatic state. This is another moving target in the FMV–MVP–MVR lineage that requires careful assessment and analysis by thoughtful clinicians.

Patients with MVP syndrome are sensitive to volume depletion and increased adrenergic activity. Thus, prophylaxis for volume depletion before, during, or immediately after physical exercise may be particularly beneficial to patients with low intravascular volume. Removing catecholamine and cyclic adenosine monophosphate stimulation by abstaining from caffeine, tobacco, alcohol, and prescription or over-the-counter drugs containing epinephrine may help. Low doses of β-blocking drugs administered for a short time during stressful periods or in a single dose may be beneficial. Exercise programs are frequently beneficial in patients with the MVP syndrome.

Summing up, the concept of a triad, a group of three closely related things, as expressed in the floppy mitral valve–mitral valve prolapse–mitral valvular regurgitation triad, emphasizes the central role of the FMV in the MVP–MVR lineage. A recent in-depth review of the subject by Hayek, Gring, and Griffin contains clinical wisdom for clinicians involved in the diagnosis, care, and management of patients with the FMV–MVP–MVR triad.

## REFERENCES

Bailey OT, Hickam JB: Rupture of mitral chordae tendineae. Am Heart J 1944;28:578-600.

Barlow JB, Pocock WA, Marchand P, et al: The significance of late systolic murmurs. Am Heart J 1963;66:443-452.

Bashore TM, Grines CL, Utlak D, et al: Postural exercise abnormalities in symptomatic patients with mitral valve prolapse. J Am Coll Cardiol 1988;3:499-507.

Boudoulas H, Wooley CF: Mitral Valve: Floppy Mitral Valve, Mitral Valve Prolapse, Mitral Valvular Regurgitation. Armonk, NY, Futura, 2000.

Carpentier A: Cardiac valve surgery: The "French correction." J Thorac Cardiovasc Surg 1983;3:323-337.

Criley JM, Lewis KB, Humphries JO, et al: Prolapse of the mitral valve: Clinical and cineangiographic findings. Br Heart J 1966;28:488-496.

Davies MJ, Moore BP, Braimbridge MV: The floppy mitral valve. Study of incidence, pathology, and complications in surgical, necropsy and forensic material. Br Heart J 1978;40:468-481.

Enriquez-Sarano M, Avierinos JF, Messika-Zeitoun D, et al: Quantitative determinants of the outcome of asymptomatic mitral regurgitation. N Engl J Med 2005;352:875-883.

Fontana ME, Wooley CF, Leighton RF, Lewis RP: Postural changes in left ventricular and mitral valvular dynamics in the systolic click-late systolic murmur syndrome. Circulation 1975;1:165-173.

Glesby MJ, Pyeritz RE: Association of mitral valve prolapse and systemic abnormalities of connective tissue. JAMA 1989;262:523-528.

Hayek E, Gring CN, Griffin BP: Mitral valve prolapse. Lancet 2005;365:507-518.

Otto CM, Salerno CT: Timing of surgery in asymptomatic mitral regurgitation. N Engl J Med 2005;352:928-929.

Read RC, Thal AP, Wendt VE: Symptomatic valvular myxomatous transformation (the floppy valve syndrome). A possible forme fruste of the Marfan syndrome. Circulation 1965;32:897-910.

# Heart Failure

Method of
*Marc A. Silver, MD*

Heart failure is an epidemic in the United States. Every day, clinicians face the task of caring for more patients with heart failure in all its forms. Heart failure is the primary reason for hospitalization of Americans older than 65 years, and although 6 million Americans are estimated to have symptomatic heart failure, that number is expected to double over the next 7 years. Many millions more have asymptomatic left ventricular dysfunction or existing medical conditions that make it quite likely heart failure will develop and they will die.

It is truly in the hands of primary care physicians, who care for most heart failure patients, as well as those with common precursors of heart failure, to understand heart failure and its natural history better and thereby make an impact on this challenging epidemic. With this concept in mind, heart failure is discussed here from the perspective of understanding its natural history or stages, as well as a chronic disease process amenable to strategic planning.

## Definitions

All clinicians define heart failure differently. Some choose to think about heart failure only when the patient has advanced disease characterized by significant volume overload and exercise limitation. Others consider heart failure to be present only when the left ventricle is dilated. Although broad by intent, *heart failure* is usually defined as a complex clinical syndrome that affects cardiac function (its ability to fill and/or eject blood) and is often preceded by and certainly accompanied by systemic neurohormonal abnormalities that participate in and perpetuate the dysfunction of the heart as well as other target organs, including the vasculature and muscles.

Although a wide range of signs and symptoms may accompany the heart failure syndrome of whatever cause, once symptomatic, patients usually have evidence of dyspnea, fatigue, and sodium and water retention manifested as congestion in the lungs, legs, and gut. It is useful, however, to think about heart failure not only as a symptomatic disease but also as a disease whose development begins decades before the patient crosses the threshold of clinical symptoms.

## Classification and Stages of Heart Failure

Although many clinicians bristle at the concept of prescribed sets of recommendations or guidelines applied to a diverse disease process such as heart failure, these guidelines are frequently a place where available evidence is evaluated in a critical way and balanced with consensus to provide a distillation of what might work when caring for a patient with a disease process.

One of the well-accepted standard guidelines for heart failure recently was revised. Within the 2001 Revision of the American College of Cardiology/American Heart Association Guidelines for the Evaluation and Management of Chronic Heart Failure for the Adult (executive summary and full text available online at http://www.acc.org/clinical/guidelines/failure/ hf_index.htm), aside from detailed information on the testing and therapies currently supported by evidence, appears a new classification for heart failure (Table 1). The classification most clinicians are familiar with is that of the New York Heart Association (NYHA) (Box 1). The NYHA classification is generally applied to patients who at some point become symptomatic. Although they may revert to a symptom-free status (NYHA functional class I), it is still implied the patient has overt heart failure. Even though the NYHA classification is of great value and carries prognostic value, it also tends to allow us to think of a patient with mild or moderate symptoms (i.e., NYHA functional class II to III) as having a mild or moderate disease, but indeed, patients in this category have a markedly shortened life span and by definition less than optimal functional status.

The new classification (Box 2), in contrast, identifies four stages of heart failure based on the spectrum of common clinical syndromes from which they have evolved. By so doing, it is hoped the clinician recognizes the patient's increased risk for the clinical syndrome and then acts aggressively to reduce the risk and/or intervene earlier just as one would with a patient at risk for cancer.

The classification addresses four stages. Unlike the NYHA classification, in which a patient may easily pass back and forth through several functional classes over a period of days to weeks, as the patient passes through each stage of the new classification, there is no longer any hope of reverting to an earlier stage, which should act as an impetus to capture the patient at the earliest stage and prevent progression to the next stage by using the proper diagnostics and therapeutics.

Stage A refers to patients who by virtue of having other common clinical conditions are at increased risk of heart failure ultimately developing. These conditions include hypertension, diabetes mellitus, and coronary artery disease. Similarly, patients with a family history of heart failure have an increased risk. The heart failure syndrome clearly does not develop in all these patients, but acknowledging their at-risk status gives the clinician and the patient fair warning of the potential risk of development of heart failure and may serve as an early warning detection system for the insidious progression to more advanced heart failure. Progression to the next stage is preventable, and disease progression is usually measured in years or decades.

Stage B refers to patients in whom structural and even functional abnormalities in heart function are already developed, but because of enormous cardiac reserve, the signs or symptoms that usually bring these patients to medical attention are not yet developed. This stage has also been referred to as "asymptomatic left ventricular dysfunction." Progression to the next stage may be slowed and again may be measured in years.

Stage C represents most of what is called heart failure today: specifically, a patient who has structural and functional disease but who has now progressed and used up enough cardiac reserve actually to have signs and symptoms of the disease. By looking at heart failure in this perspective, it becomes clear that any symptomatic heart failure indeed represents a serious condition that the clinician must diagnose and treat accordingly. In this stage of the disease, clinicians can intervene to improve symptoms and quality of life, as well as improve, but not completely abolish, the increased mortality. Progression to the next stage is quite variable but is usually measured in months to years.

## TABLE 1   Common Heart Failure Drugs and Their Therapeutic Targets

| Drug | Dose | Comment |
|---|---|---|
| Loop diuretics (expressed as furosemide [Lasix] equivalent units) | 40-100 mg once or twice daily | Many factors affect the doses required, such as patient compliance with dietary restrictions, fluid intake, and associated titration of other medication, including ACE inhibitors and β-blockers. |
| ACE inhibitors (expressed as enalapril [Vasotec] equivalent units) | 10-20 mg twice daily | Higher doses seem to have an impact on hospitalization rates. Be aware of adverse events that will limit use, including hyperkalemia. To allow adequate titration of β-blockers, reduced doses may be used. |
| β-Blockers (expressed as carvedilol [Coreg] equivalent units) | 25-50 mg twice daily | Dependent on body size. Although data suggest clinical improvement and decreased mortality with smaller doses, the target remains full dose. |
| Digoxin | 0.125-0.25 mg daily | Adjustment needed for renal function. Routine measurement of serum levels is not required unless done to confirm toxicity. |

*Abbreviation:* ACE = angiotensin-converting enzyme.

I. Symptoms occur only at a level that would cause
normal individuals to become symptomatic.
II. Symptoms occur with ordinary exertion or moderate
levels of activity.
III. Symptoms occur with less than ordinary degrees of
activity.
IV. Symptoms occur even at rest.

*This classification scheme is generally applied to patients
once they are or have been symptomatic with heart failure
(stages C and D). Note: In general, the classification implies the
patient's worst level of functioning related to a heart failure
symptom (e.g., fatigue, dyspnea, exercise intolerance).

---

Stage D represents very advanced disease in which even standard measures cannot overcome its severity and advanced measures need to be undertaken. During this stage, despite best efforts, patients usually have increased use of resources, decreased quality of life, and progressive limitation. Although many advanced resources are applied during this stage, including heart transplantation and ventricular restraint and assist devices, generally these patients ultimately die of either progressive heart failure or sudden cardiac death.

## Steps for Appropriate Heart Failure Management

Physicians often take a reflex approach to initiating drug therapy in a patient with symptomatic heart failure. For example, a patient who is volume overloaded might be treated with diuretics as monotherapy while overlooking the need not only to treat the current symptoms but also plan a strategy to limit progression of disease. Thus a useful approach in planning patient care involves two broad steps. The first is assessing the information needed to create a management plan, and the second is understanding the therapeutic targets in heart failure treatment.

An assessment of what is known or yet needed to be known to best make the diagnosis and treat a patient with heart failure is a very useful step. This assessment generally involves an understanding of the etiology of the heart failure, the current stage or functional class, and so forth. Even after a detailed history and physical examination and collection of some diagnostic data, however, a gap can remain in the information needed to complete the therapeutic plan. Generally, the clinician can group the areas that need to be completed into three main categories: diagnostics, therapeutics, and prognostics. In fact, these three areas are useful to consider each time a patient is seen in the office or hospital. Even though treatment is often initiated without complete information in each of these areas, not asking what other information is needed often leads to an incomplete understanding of the disease syndrome, as well as suboptimal therapy.

*Diagnostics* refers to any additional information that allows a better understanding of the etiology, status, degree of limitation, and signs and symptoms of a patient. For example, an echocardiogram allows assessment of the nature and degree of left ventricular function and may lead to consideration of myocardial ischemia (wall motion abnormalities) or valvular disease (valvular regurgitation or stenosis) as a therapeutic target. Often in this category are tests that might reveal an easily addressable cause of the heart failure and even a form of heart failure that is potentially reversible (such as hyperthyroidism).

*Therapeutics* refers to the design of the treatment strategy based on what is currently known about the patient and that patient's disease. It is also useful to write down a therapeutic plan, including the one or two next steps that might be taken should the patient's signs or symptoms not abate with the current regimen. For example, the clinician might begin with using angiotensin-converting enzyme (ACE) inhibitors but indicate that if the patient is found to have underlying

**Stage A**
- Patients who are at increased risk for heart failure because of associated medical conditions (e.g., hypertension, coronary artery disease, or diabetes mellitus).
- Heart structure and function: Not yet affected.
- Potential therapies: Treatment of hypertension, smoking cessation, and weight loss; ACE inhibitors in appropriate patients.

**Stage B**
- Patients who have abnormal heart structure and/or function but who have not manifested signs or symptoms.
- Heart structure and function: Abnormal.
- Potential therapies: Same as for stage A, plus ACE inhibitors and β-blockers in all appropriate patients.

**Stage C**
- Patients with symptomatic heart failure. These patients indeed have advanced heart failure. Note that signs and symptoms develop as late phenomena after significant perturbation of many homeostatic mechanisms and the consumption of large cardiac reserves.
- Heart structure and function: Abnormal.
- Potential therapies: Same as for stages A and B, plus ACE inhibitors, β-blockers, and digoxin and diuretics in most patients; also, coronary revascularization and repair of mitral regurgitation in select patients.

**Stage D**
- Patients with extremely advanced heart failure.
- Heart structure and function: Extremely abnormal.
- Potential therapies: Same as for stages A, B, and C, plus consideration of advanced therapies including investigational therapies, consideration for left ventricular assist devices, heart transplantation for appropriate patients, as well as end-of-life counseling and hospice.

*Abbreviation:* ACE = angiotensin-converting enzyme.

---

coronary artery disease, the addition of long-acting nitrates should be considered.

*Prognostics* refers to focusing in on what is known about the patient's heart failure in terms of predicting what might be the path of progression in the near future. Although imperfect, many pieces of information are closely linked to survival and disease progression, including functional status, exercise tolerance, and left ventricular ejection fraction. In considering any additional prognostics, the clinician should always ask what might be done differently given the result. Over the years we have become more willing to intervene earlier with therapeutics, which can alter progression of the disease, and therefore we depend less on a bad set of prognostic markers to make these decisions. Nevertheless, awareness of a low peak oxygen consumption, a low right ventricular ejection fraction, or a markedly elevated neurohormonal marker often serves to alert the physician and the patient and family to review the current therapeutic plan and broaden considerations to include the next level of care and treatment, which might consist of investigational therapies and evaluation for heart transplantation. The role of measurement of B-type natriuretic peptide in this regard is of some interest and may prove to be a prognostic marker against which to target our therapies.

### TREATMENT TARGETS

In designing the drug treatment plan, the following treatment targets for patients with heart failure should be considered: improved survival, improved symptoms, slowing and/or reversal of disease progression, improved functional status and quality of life, avoidance of troublesome adverse events, and decreased use of resources, including hospitalization.

## BOX 3    Nonpharmacologic Therapies for Patients with Heart Failure

**Definitely Helps Reduce Symptoms or Improve Functional Status**
- Salt restriction (target: 2.3 g of salt per day)
- Exercise
- Stress reduction
- Screening for depression
- Smoking cessation
- Weight loss
- Treatment of documented sleep-disordered breathing

**May Be of Use in Selected Patients**
- Fluid restriction
- Avoidance of alcohol

With the recognition that not all these targets are concordant or attainable, the drug regimen reflects these targets and our understanding of the ability of drugs to address them.

In general, patients with symptomatic heart failure are managed with a core group of four drug classes, including diuretics, an ACE inhibitor, a β-blocker, and, usually, digoxin. The former and the latter are generally applied to relieve symptoms or to improve functional status or exercise tolerance, whereas the middle two are also administered with the specific intention of altering disease progression, reversing the structural and/or functional abnormalities of the heart and other target organs, and improving medium- and long-term survival.

Increasing evidence supports the initiation of ACE inhibitors and β-blocker jointly when caring for a symptomatic patient. Diuretics often need to be adjusted up or down, depending on a patient's level of compensation, as well as where they are in terms of other (β-blocker) titration. Target doses for most of the commonly used drugs come from clinical trials suggesting their benefit (ACE inhibitors) or from tradition, as well as from attempts to balance drug efficacy with drug safety (digoxin and diuretics). Target doses are listed in Table 1. Excellent details and practical considerations of implementing and titrating heart failure drugs can be found in recent guidelines (http://www.acc.org/clinical/guidelines/failure/ hf_index.htm).

### NONPHARMACOLOGIC MEASURES

An enormous armamentarium outside routine drug therapy is available to clinicians caring for patients with heart failure. In general, most nonpharmacologic measures should be used in a simultaneous fashion with the initiation and titration of drug therapy. Although most of these therapies either have not or will not undergo rigorous clinical investigation, they nonetheless remain therapeutic cornerstones of complete heart failure care. Dramatic functional improvement can often be observed with more careful attention to nonpharmacologic therapies. Of particular interest is an understanding that sleep-disordered breathing (including obstructive and central forms of sleep apnea) may be present in nearly 40% of heart failure patients. Increasing evidence suggests therapy that includes continuous positive airway pressure may alter symptoms, disease progression, and even survival (Box 3). As far as dietary advice, generally admonitions for avoidance of excessive sodium intake and fluid are given along with specific information on lowering dietary saturated fat. Emerging information is that the patient with heart failure suffers a significant energy imbalance, however, and may well benefit from nutritional assessment, including measurement of nitrogen balance.

## Use of Disease Management and Other Resources

Perhaps one of the greatest tools at hand for clinicians caring for patients with heart failure, as well as for their families, is providing a

## CURRENT DIAGNOSIS

- Determine the etiology. It is critical to determine the underlying cause of a patient's heart failure; common clinical conditions including hypertension, diabetes mellitus, and coronary artery disease increase the risk of developing heart failure.
- Assess a patient's stage and functional class (see text). These are good guides to help recognize disease severity and guide treatment. Symptoms include evidence of dyspnea, fatigue, and sodium and water retention as congestion in the lungs, legs, and gut; these are usually late symptoms.
- Assess the volume status on every patient at every visit. Inability to assess volume carefully often leads to errors in therapeutics.
- Use additional tests and biomarkers such as peak oxygen consumption, ventricular ejection fraction, and elevated neurohormonal markers (B-type natriuretic peptide), which may provide early clues to disease severity.

thorough understanding of the heart failure syndrome and how self-empowered actions may have a significant impact on how they feel, what they can do, and how long they might live. Studies have repeatedly demonstrated the benefits of a structured disease management program in reducing symptoms, improving functional status, and, in particular, reducing heart failure hospitalizations. The clinician frequently can best serve the patient by fostering and supporting a heart failure disease management program. Although not present in all communities yet, the resources required (a physician and/or a nurse champion) are often accessible. Abundant educational patient-oriented books and materials are available to support these programs.

Disease management programs are often part of a larger specialized heart failure center. Within these structures are advanced strategies, including investigational therapies. It is incumbent on clinicians to be

## CURRENT THERAPY

**Targets**
- Improved survival
- Improved symptoms
- Slowing and/or reversal of disease progression
- Improved functional status, quality of life
- Avoidance of adverse events
- Decreased use of resources including hospitalization

**Care for Patients With Heart Failure**
- Treatment of hypertension
- Smoking cessation
- Dietary counseling
- Exercise
- Weight loss
- Treatment of sleep-disordered breathing
- Angiotensin-converting enzyme (ACE) inhibitors (at target doses)
- β-Blockers (at target doses)
- Digoxin and diuretics
- Coronary revascularization
- Repair of mitral regurgitation
- Investigational therapies
- End-of-life counseling and hospice

aware of these local and regional resources and refer patients when appropriate. Even with advanced disease, these centers can often offer improved outcomes and strategies not available to all clinicians.

Another area within the disease management spectrum is the home care programs that exist in most communities. These services frequently provide a link between intensive hospital-based care and infrequent, less intensive office-based care. In addition, for many patients with advanced disease, home care meets the constraints of patients and families.

For patients with advanced disease, physicians often begin discussions surrounding end-of-life issues too late. Patients who have advanced disease requiring frequent hospitalization and treatment generally are aware of their likelihood of death and, in fact, they value regaining some control of their lives through discussion of end-of-life planning and preferences. For some, hospice care is the choice made, whereas for others, referral to specialized centers and participation in emerging therapies through clinical trials might be the correct choice. Understanding comes only with an open and frank discussion with each patient and family.

## Emerging and Emerged New Therapeutic Areas

Because of the intense interest in heart failure, a variety of important additional therapies are undergoing clinical investigation. These therapies include new application of biventricular pacemakers, aggressive mitral valve repair for patients with ongoing mitral valve regurgitation, and the use of left ventricular assist devices as bridges to heart recovery, as well as destination or permanent therapies. Moreover, several new cardiac restraint devices are being applied with some success. Within years, genomic therapies will broaden, as will areas of vascular and myogenic regeneration. Again, although most clinicians are not aware of all these newly emerging therapies, they can offer their patients referrals to specialized centers where suitable therapies can be sought.

## REFERENCES

Gattis WA, O'Connor CM, Gallup DS, et al: Predischarge initiation of carvedilol in patients hospitalized for decompensated heart failure: Results of the Initiation Management Predischarge: Process for Assessment of Carvedilol Therapy in Heart Failure (IMPACT_HF) trial. J Am Coll Cardiol 2004;43:1534-1541.

Hunt SA, Baker DW, Chin MH, et al: ACC/AHA guidelines for the evaluation and management of heart failure in the adult: A report of the American College of Cardiology/American Heart Association Task Force on Practice Guidelines (Committee to Revise the 1995 Guidelines for the Evaluation and Management of Heart Failure), 2001. American College of Cardiology Web site. Available online at http://www.acc.org/clinical/guidelines/failure/hf_index.htm

Konstam MA: Systolic and diastolic dysfunction in heart failure? Time for a new paradigm. J Card Fail 2003;9:1-3.

Pitt B, Remme W, Zannad F, et al: Eplerenone, a selective aldosterone blocker in patients with left ventricular dysfunction after myocardial infarction. N Engl J Med 2003;348:1309-1321.

Poole-Wilson PA, Swedberg K, Cleland JG, et al: Comparison of carvedilol and metoprolol on clinical outcomes in patients with chronic heart failure in the Carvedilol or Metoprolol European Trial (COMET): Randomized controlled trial. Lancet 2003;362:7-13.

Redfield MM: Heart failure—an epidemic of uncertain proportions. N Engl J Med 2002;347:1442-1444.

# Infective Endocarditis

Method of
*Navin M. Amin, MD*

## Epidemiologic Changes

Infective endocarditis denotes microbial infection of the cardiac valves and, less frequently, infection of the mural endocardium or of septal defects. At present, infective endocarditis accounts for 1 case per 1000 hospital admissions. The age of patients with endocarditis has increased. In the preantibiotic era, the average age of patients with endocarditis was 32 to 39 years old; currently more than half the cases occur in patients older than 60 years of age. Men are affected twice as often as women; the ratio increases to 5:1 in men older than 60 years of age.

Three major epidemiologic changes are observed in endocarditis:

1. The pattern of infective organisms has changed. Early in the antibiotic era, group A *Streptococci* (β hemolyticus), *Pneumococci*, *Gonococci*, and *Meningococci* were the predominant pathogens. *Streptococcus viridans*, *Staphylococcus aureus* (methicillin-sensitive [MSSA] or methicillin resistant [MRSA]), coagulase—negative *Staphylococcus epidermidis* or *lugdunensis*—and gram- negative organisms are more common today.
2. Certain signs and symptoms, once characteristic of endocarditis, are seen in less than 5% of cases today: peripheral lesions involving skin, nails, and eyes—petechiae, subungual hemorrhage, Janeway lesions, Osler nodes, or Roth's spots.
3. Surgical procedures can be both a cause and a cure of endocarditis. Prosthetic valves inserted to improve mechanically malfunctioning valves can predispose recipients to endocarditis. But surgery can be lifesaving in patients with refractory congestive heart failure (CHF) or resistant infections.

## Forms of Endocarditis

Endocarditis is classified as acute or subacute on the basis of its clinical course. The acute form, which evolves over days to weeks, is diagnosed within 2 weeks. Invasive organisms such as *Staphylococcus aureus*, *Staphylococcus epidermidis*, *Streptococcus pneumoniae*, group A streptococci, *Neisseria gonorrhoeae*, *Haemophilus influenzae*, *Salmonella*, other Enterobacteriaceae, Serratia, and *Pseudomonas aeruginosa* are usually the cause. Clinically acute endocarditis is associated with high fever, systemic toxicity, and leukocytosis with rapid destruction of the valves. It carries high morbidity and mortality.

Subacute endocarditis has a duration of more than 6 weeks and an indolent course. The most common agents are streptococcal species, with *Streptococcus viridans* the most predominant: *Enterococcus*, HACEK (*Haemophilus, Actinobacillus, Cardiobacterium, Eikenella, Kingella*) organisms, fungi, and *Coxiella burnetii*. Clinically subacute endocarditis is associated with prolonged low-grade fever (fever of unknown origin [FUO]), night sweats, weight loss, and vague symptoms such as generalized weakness, lethargy, and myalgia.

Infective endocarditis can also be grouped into three categories:

1. *Native valve endocarditis* usually develops when there is structural damage to the heart valve. Rheumatic/ syphilitic valvular disease is responsible in 20% to 40% of the cases. The mitral valve is involved in 85%, and the aortic valve is affected in 50% of the cases. In patients older than age 60 years, 30% of cases occur with degenerative cardiac lesions such as calcified mitral valve annulus and calcified nodular lesions secondary to atherosclerosis or postmyocardial infarction thrombus. Twenty percent of cases with mitral valve prolapse (with thickened leaflets or significant mitral regurgitation) and obstructive cardiomyopathy can predispose to endocarditis. In 6% to 25% of cases, congenital heart disease is a risk factor as is evident in ventricular septal defect (VSD), patent ductus arteriosus (PDA),

tetralogy of Fallot, or coarctation of the aorta. It can also occur with a stenotic or regurgitant valve such as bicuspid aortic valve and pulmonary stenosis. Endocarditis is rare in patients with atrial septal defect (secundum type) because of the low-pressure gradient between the atria. Finally is a group of patients without any structural defect who are susceptible to endocarditis. Tricuspid valve endocarditis can develop in intravenous drug abusers and immunocompromised patients (with chronic renal failure, severe burns, chronic active hepatitis, collagen vascular disease, or neoplasm involving the pancreas, lung, or stomach).

2. *Prosthetic valve endocarditis* (PVE) at present constitutes 20% of all cases of endocarditis. It occurs in 2% to 4% of patients with a prosthetic valve. It can be early or late. Early PVE occurs within 60 days of the valve replacement, and predominant organisms are *Staphylococcus epidermidis* and *S. aureus* (MSSA or MRSA). In the case of late-onset endocarditis, which occurs after 2 months, *Streptococcus viridans* is the main offending pathogen.

3. *Nosocomial endocarditis* commonly affects patients older than age 60 years and seriously ill hospitalized patients. These individuals are subjected to invasive procedures such as insertion of central venous pressure, monitoring lines, hyperalimentation catheters, or intracardiac pacemaker wires that represent nidus of infection. Box 1 summarizes the factors predisposing to endocarditis.

## Microbiology

Any microorganism can cause endocarditis (Table 1). Certain pathogens have increased ability to adhere to valvular leaflets, thereby establishing infection. Approximately 70% of the cases are caused by streptococci and staphylococci.

---

### BOX 1   Factors Predisposing to Endocarditis

**Native Valve Endocarditis**
- Structural Damage
  Rheumatic valvular disease
  Syphilitic valvular disease
  Degenerative
    Calcified mitral/aortic valve
    Calcified post-MI thrombus
  Mitral valve prolapse
  IHSS
  Congenital heart disease
    Regurgitant or stenotic valve, bicuspid
      aortic valve, PS, Ebstein's anomaly, Marfan's
      syndrome
    High-pressure shunt, VSD, PDA, coarctation
      of the aorta, tetralogy of Fallot
- No Structural Damage
  Catheter Induced
  IVDA
  Immunocompromised

**Prosthetic Valve Endocarditis**
- Early (<2 mo)
  *Staphylococcus epidermidis*
  *Staphylococcus aureus*
- Late (>2 mo)
  *Staphylococcus viridans*

**Nosocomial Endocarditis**
- Invasive procedures

---

*Abbreviations*: IHSS = idiopathic hypertrophic subaortic stenosis; IVDA = intravenous drug abuse; MI = myocardial infarction; PDA = patent ductus arteriosus; PS = pulmonary stenosis; VSD = ventricular septal defect.
Adapted with permission from Amin NM: Infective endocarditis. Consultant 1994;34(3):319-343.

---

Staphylococci (MSSA or MRSA) are encountered predominantly in intravenous drug abuse (IVDA), in early PVE, in an immunocompromised host, and in nosocomial endocarditis. *S. viridans* is more commonly seen in native valve endocarditis and in late PVE. Gram-negative bacilli commonly cause right-sided endocarditis as in IVDA and in patients with intravascular catheters.

Approximately 10% of patients with endocarditis have a negative blood culture after 48 to 72 hours of incubation. Factors that produce culture-negative endocarditis are (1) antibiotic therapy before cultures are obtained; (2) a low level of bacteremia (common with right-sided and mural endocarditis); (3) infection with fastidious or nutritionally deficient bacteria that require prolonged cultures (2 to 3 weeks) or additional supplements (e.g., pyridoxine) for growth; this group includes HACEK organisms, *Brucella,* and nutritionally deficient streptococci; (4) nonbacterial infectious agents such as fungi, viruses, spirochetes, *Rickettsia, Chlamydia,* or parasites; and (5) noninfectious causes: left atrial myxoma, Libman-Sacks endocarditis, systemic lupus erythematosus, Löffler's hypereosinophilic endocarditis, carcinoid syndromes, and marantic endocarditis associated with malignancies of the pancreas, stomach, or lung.

## Clinical Manifestations

The clinical manifestations of infective endocarditis are extremely diverse and can mimic pulmonary, neurologic, renal, or bone and joint disease. The classic manifestations of fever, heart murmur, splenomegaly, and petechiae of the skin and the mucous membranes help establish the diagnosis.

The onset may be abrupt or insidious. The early manifestations may be vague flulike symptoms that occur within 3 weeks after an invasive procedure. The patient may complain of malaise, fatigue, weakness, myalgia, arthralgia, low-grade fever, night sweats, or weight loss. Anorexia is almost universal. When the onset is acute, as in intravenous (IV) drug abuse, PVE, or nosocomial endocarditis, there may be evidence of severe infection heralded by high fever (90% to 95%), shaking chills and rigors, or, more ominous, symptoms of frank heart failure or embolic phenomena.

In patients older than age 60 years, diagnosis is often delayed because 5% may not have fever or are admitted with diagnosis of cerebral vascular accident (CVA), pneumonia, occult neoplasm, degenerative joint disease, or osteomyelitis. Infective endocarditis should always be considered in patients older than age 60 years who have fever and associated unexplained CHF, CVA, renal failure, weight loss, anemia, new-onset murmur, or confusional state.

In 85% of the cases, cardiac manifestations include a heart murmur. In right-sided endocarditis and mural infection, murmur is absent. A new or changing murmur (usually of aortic regurgitation) occurs in 5% to 10% of patients and is a very helpful diagnostic sign. Persistent or progressive CHF is indicative of a serious complication that carries a high mortality rate.

Peripheral cutaneous manifestations take a variety of forms: skin pallor caused by secondary anemia; petechiae found in 20% to 40% of cases concentrated on the conjunctiva, palate, buccal mucosa, and distal extremities; clubbing of nails in 10% to 20% if infection is long-standing; splinter hemorrhages as linear red-to-brown streaks in the middle of the nail bed of fingers and toes; Osler nodes (5% to 20% cases), which are small painful, tender, purplish subcutaneous nodules in the pads of fingers and toes; and Janeway lesions, which are small macular, painless, erythematous or hemorrhagic plaques on the palms or soles.

Ocular manifestations include Roth's spots, which occur in 5% of the patients and appear as oval or boat-shaped white or pale retinal lesions surrounded by hemorrhage and located near the optic disk. In a few cases there may be presence of cotton-wool exudates, petechiae, or flame-shaped hemorrhages.

Embolization can occur in 15% to 35% of cases. A cerebral emboli may produce hemiplegia, monoplegia, aphasia, or unilateral blindness. Mesenteric emboli can result in acute abdominal pain, ileus, or melena. Splenic emboli may cause left upper quadrant pain that radiates to the left shoulder of the chest with a small pleural effusion or splenic frictional rub. Flank pain with hematuria indicates a

## TABLE 1 Microbiology of Infective Endocarditis

| Type of Infection | Specific Associated Risk Factors |
|---|---|
| **Bacterial** | |
| Gram Positive | |
| Streptococci (40%-60%) | |
| *S. viridans, S. pneumoniae, S. bovis, S. pyogenes,* | NVE, late-onset PVE |
| *S. sanguis* | |
| Enterococci (Group D) (5%-20%) | |
| *S. faecalis, S. faecium, S. durans* | Gastrointestinal malignancies |
| Staphylococci (17%-40%) | IVDA, early PVE |
| *S. aureus* (MRSA), *S. epidermidis* (MRSE), *S. lugdunensis* | |
| Diphtheroids | |
| *Listeria* | IVDA, early PVE |
| Gram Negative | |
| Cultured easily | |
| *Pseudomonas aeruginosa, Serratia marcescens,* | IVDA, immunocompromised, nosocomial endocarditis |
| *Salmonella, Proteus mirabilis, Shigella, Providencia,* | |
| *Enterobacter, Neisseria gonorrhoeae, Escherichia coli* | |
| Difficult to culture | |
| (HACEK) (1%-10%) | |
| *Haemophilus, Actinobacillus, Cardiobacterium,* | |
| *Eikenella, Kingella* | |
| (not HACEK) | |
| *Brucella, Legionella* | |
| **Nonbacterial** | |
| Fungi (2%-4%) | |
| *Candida, Aspergillus, Histoplasma, Coccidioides,* | IVDA, PVE, cardiac surgery, IV catheters, |
| *Blastomyces* | immunosuppressed |
| Viruses | |
| Coxsackie B, adenovirus | |
| Spirochetes | |
| *Borrelia burgdorferi* | Tick bite |
| *Spirillum minus* | Rat bite |
| Rickettsiae | |
| *Coxiella burnetii* | Infected livestock or unpasteurized milk |
| Chlamydia | |
| *C. psittaci* | Infected birds |
| Parasites | |
| *Trypanosoma cruzi* (Chagas' disease) | Kissing bug bite |

*Abbreviations:* IVDA, intravenous drug abuse; MRSA, methicillin-resistant staphylococcus aureus; MRSE, methicillin-resistant staphylococcus epidermidis; NVE, native valve endocarditis; PVE, prosthetic valve endocarditis.
Modified from Amin NM: Infective endocarditis. Consultant 1994;34(3):319-343.

renal infarction. Peripheral arterial emboli may produce pain or gangrene. Large arterial occlusions are frequently seen with fungal endocarditis. Very rarely, emboli to coronary arteries cause acute myocardial infarction, myocardial abscess, or mycotic aneurysm.

Neurologic complications (30% to 40%) include CVA from embolization, mycotic aneurysm causing cerebral of subdural hemorrhage and seizure, and brain abscess or toxic encephalopathy with confusion and nonspecific obtundation.

Renal manifestations are accompanied by microscopic or frank hematuria secondary to renal infarct, diffuse membranoproliferative glomerulonephritis, focal embolic glomerulonephritis, or renal abscess.

Splenomegaly occurs in 25% to 45% of the patients and is more common in subacute than in acute endocarditis.

## Diagnosis

Infective endocarditis may mimic any systemic disorder. For this reason and because of its high morbidity and mortality, the diagnosis should be kept in mind whenever a high-risk patient has an unexplained fever, constitutional symptoms, or multiple systemic involvement with a changing or new heart murmur. A high index of suspicion for endocarditis in certain clinical situations is very helpful:

- Intravenous drug abusers with high fever
- Patients older than age 60 years with nonspecific vague symptoms with a calcified mitral valve annulus
- Unknown source of embolization
- Certain virulent infections caused by organisms such as *Staphylococcus* or *Enterococcus*

A thorough history, complete examination, and laboratory tests should establish the correct diagnosis. Box 2 outlines the various laboratory abnormalities in infective endocarditis.

A baseline electrocardiogram (ECG) is helpful to detect chamber enlargement or possible conduction defect that may indicate underlying valvular or congenital anomalies. Later development of first-degree atrioventricular (AV) block, new bundle branch block, or new ectopic beats may indicate a myocardial abscess, especially in aortic valve endocarditis.

Echocardiography (transesophageal [TEE], M mode, two-dimensional, or Doppler) can confirm the diagnosis, detect complications, and help assess the prognosis. The echocardiogram can detect vegetations larger than 2 to 3 mm on mitral or aortic valves. Sensitivity in detecting vegetations is approximately 87% to 90% with TEE, 30% to 75% with M-mode, 40% to 50% with two-dimensional, and 50% with Doppler echocardiography. False-positive results are seen with old healed vegetations, myxomatous valvular degeneration, arterial myxoma, or a thrombus.

Echocardiogram can detect complications such as torn or perforated valves, ruptured chordae tendineae, myocardial abscess, or pericardial effusion that may require surgical intervention. Large-sized vegetations in the left side of the heart or in the aortic valve, or myocardial abscess, suggest a relatively poor prognosis, and surgery may be indicated.

## BOX 2 Laboratory Abnormalities in Endocarditis

Hematologic
    Leukocytosis
    Anemia of chronic disorder
    Thrombocytopenia (10% SBE)
    Elevated ESR
    Urine analysis
    Hematuria, microscopic
    Proteinuria
Cardiac abnormality
    ECG: chamber enlargement, conduction defect
Chest x-ray
    Cardiomegaly
    Evidence of congestive heart failure
    Nodular infiltrate (staphylococcal endocarditis)
Diagnostic gold standards
    Echocardiography (transesophageal preferred)
    Three sets of blood (embolus) cultures
Immunologic abnormalities
    Rheumatoid factor (disappears after treatment)
    Hypergammaglobulinemia
    Cryoglobulinemia
    Circulating immune complexes
    Low complement levels

*Abbreviations*: ECG = electrocardiogram; ESR = erythrocyte sedimentation rate; SBE = subacute bacterial endocarditis.

Serial blood cultures are required to establish the diagnosis by isolating the offending bacterium or fungus. A minimum of three blood samples should be drawn 30 to 60 minutes apart before initiating empiric antibiotic therapy. If the patient has taken antibiotics in the preceding 2 weeks, two or three additional sets of blood cultures should be taken. Cultures of arterial blood offer no additional advantage over venous blood. Ninety percent of the blood cultures become positive within 7 days of incubation. Negative blood cultures are likely seen in patients who have received prior antibiotics or who have endocarditis caused by fastidious gram-negative (HACEK) bacilli, fungi, or nutritionally deficient streptococci. The microbiology laboratory should be alerted to the suspected endocarditis, and a report for prolonged incubation for 2 weeks included.

In fungal endocarditis, in which there is embolization of large arteries, a culture of the removed embolus can establish the diagnosis. Serologic studies can be helpful in fungal infection (histoplasmosis or coccidioidomycosis) or when rickettsial (Q fever) *Legionella* or *Chlamydia* infections are suspected.

# Treatment of Infective Endocarditis

The main goal is eradicating the infecting pathogens as quickly as possible to reduce the risks of morbidity and mortality. This can be achieved with antibiotic therapy, surgical intervention, or both.

## ANTIBIOTIC THERAPY

In using antibiotics to treat infective endocarditis, the following guidelines are helpful:

- Parental antibiotics are used to sustain bactericidal activity.
- Bactericidal antimicrobials are used for complete eradication of the pathogens. Synergistic bactericidal activity is achieved with combination therapy such as ampicillin and aminoglycosides in treatment of enterococcal endocarditis.
- The drug regimen and appropriate duration of course, 2 to 6 weeks, must be tailored to prevent relapse.
- The bactericidal activity of the antibiotic is monitored by determining the minimum inhibitory concentration (MIC) and the minimum bactericidal concentration (MBC) against the infecting organisms.

## TABLE 2 Antibiotic Regimens for Bacterial Endocarditis

| Infecting Organism | Antibiotic | Dosage, Route, and Frequency | Duration in Weeks |
|---|---|---|---|
| Penicillin susceptible *Streptococcus viridans,* and *S. bovis* (MIC <0.2 µg/dL) | *Preferred Regimen* Penicillin G | 12-16 million U/d IV in 6 divided doses | 4 |
| | or Penicillin G *PLUS* | 12-16 million U/d IV in 6 divided doses | 4 |
| | Gentamicin | 1 mg/kg IM or IV q8h | 2 |
| | or Penicillin G *PLUS* Gentamicin | Dosages same as above regimen | 2 |
| | or Ceftriaxone | 2g IV or IM q24h | 4 |
| | *Alternative Regimen* Vancomycin | 0.5 g IV q6h | 4 |
| Relative penicillin-resistant streptococci (MIC >0.2 µg/dL) | *Preferred Regimen* Penicillin G *PLUS* | 20-30 million U/d IV in 6 divided doses | 4 |
| | Gentamicin | 1 mg/kg IV or IM q8h | 4 |
| | *Alternative Regimen* Vancomycin | 0.5 g IV q6h | 4 |
| *Staphylococcus epidermidis* (MRSE) | *Native Valve* Vancomycin | 0.5 g IV q6h | 4 |
| | *Prosthetic Valve* Vancomycin *PLUS* | 0.5 g IV q6h | 4-6 |
| | Gentamicin | 1 mg/kg IV or IM q8h | 2 |
| | or Rifampin | 300 mg PO/IV q12h | 2 |
| *Enterococcus (S. faecalis, S. faecium, S. durans)* | *Preferred Regimen* Penicillin G *PLUS* | 20-30 million U/d IV in 6 divided doses | 4-6 |
| | Gentamicin | 1 mg/kg IM or IV q8h | 4-6 |

**TABLE 2** Antibiotic Regimens for Bacterial Endocarditis—cont'd

| Infecting Organism | Antibiotic | Dosage, Route, and Frequency | Duration in Weeks |
|---|---|---|---|
| | or Ampicillin *PLUS* | 2g IV q4h | 4-6 |
| | Gentamicin *Alternative Regimen* | 1mg/kg IM or IV q8h | 4-6 |
| | Vancomycin *PLUS* | 0.5 g IV q6h | 4-6 |
| | Gentamicin *Preferred Regimen* | 1 mg/kg IM or IV q8h | 4-6 |
| *Staphylococcus aureus* (methicillin sensitive) | Nafcillin or Oxacillin or | 2 g IV q4h | 4-6 |
| | Oxacillin *PLUS* | 2 g IV q4h | 4-6 |
| | Gentamicin *OR/PLUS* | 1 mg/kg IM or IV q8h | 2 |
| | Rifampin *Alternative Regimen* | 300 mg PO/IV q12h | 2 |
| | Cefazolin or | 2 g IV q6h | 4-6 |
| | Vancomycin | 0.5 g IV q6h | 4-6 |
| *S. aureus* (methicillin resistant [MRSA]) | Vancomycin *PLUS* | 0.5 g IV q6h | 4-6 |
| | Gentamicin *OR/PLUS* | 1 mg/kg IM or IV q8h | 2 |
| | Rifampin[1] | 300 mg PO/IV q12h | 2 |
| HACEK group *(Haemophilus, Actinobacillus, Cardiobacterium, Eikenella, Kingella)* | Ampicillin or | 2 g IV q6h | 4 |
| | Ampicillin *PLUS* | 2 g IV q6h | 4 |
| | Gentamicin or | 1 mg/kg IM or IV q8h | 4 |
| Culture negative | Ceftriaxone Vancomycin *PLUS* | 2 g IV q24h 0.5 g IV q8h | 4 6 |
| | Gentamicin | 1 mg/kg IM or IV q8h | 6 |

*Abbreviations:* MIC = minimum inhibitory concentration
Modified from Amin NM: Infective Endocarditis. Consultant 1994;34(3):319-343.
[1]Not FDA approved for this indication

• Antibiotic therapy is initiated as quickly as possible. When endocarditis is severe and/or complicated, empiric treatment should be instituted immediately with antibiotics effective against *S. aureus* and enterococci. A combination of vancomycin (Vancocin) and gentamicin (Garamycin) is recommended. Once a specific organism is identified, appropriate bactericidal antibiotics should be used.

Most streptococci other than enterococci are exquisitely sensitive to penicillin. If MIC is less than 0.2 μg per mL, high-dose penicillin alone or in combination with either gentamicin (Garamycin) or streptomycin or ceftriaxone (Rocephin) can be used for 4 weeks. If the MIC is below 0.1 μg per mL, treatment should be for 2 weeks. If MIC is greater than 0.2 μg per mL or the MBC to MIC ratio exceeds 10:1, as it occurs in 15% to 20% of cases with *S. viridans* infection, higher dose of penicillin with aminoglycoside should be used. In penicillin-allergic patients, vancomycin is the best alternative with or without aminoglycoside (Table 2).

In enterococcal endocarditis, ampicillin is recommended in combination with an aminoglycoside. Gentamicin is preferred because 40% of the isolates are resistant to streptomycin. In penicillin-allergic patients, vancomycin with an aminoglycoside is the best choice.

In *S. aureus* infection, semisynthetic penicillin or first-generation cephalosporins are the agents of first choice. Addition of gentamicin or rifampin (Rifadin)[1] during the first few days rapidly reduces bacteremia. Vancomycin is recommended for patients allergic to penicillin or if the organism is methicillin resistant (MRSA). Addition of rifampin, although controversial, is recommended in patients demonstrating poor bactericidal activity during therapy with beta-lactams or vancomycin and for patients with suppurative complication, such as a valve ring abscess.

Endocarditis with *S. epidermidis*, which commonly develops on prosthetic valves, is ideally treated with vancomycin and rifampin.[1] An aminoglycoside may be added for 2 weeks.

Gram-negative infections causing high mortality are best treated with broad-spectrum penicillin or, preferably, a third-generation cephalosporin with an aminoglycoside. In most of these patients, valve replacement is necessary.

## SURGICAL INTERVENTIONS

Approximately 25% of patients with severe or complicated endocarditis undergo surgery. The chief indications for surgery are refractory moderate or severe CHF; perivalvular invasion or myocardial abscess as evident by persistent fever despite antibiotics or electrocardiographic changes of conduction defects; systemic or arterial embolization; fungal endocarditis; PVE of early onset; large bulky vegetations that increase risk of CHF; persistent infection (particularly with gram-negative bacilli) that does not respond to 7 to 10 days of antibiotic therapy; and staphylococcal endocarditis in IV drug abusers that does not respond to antimicrobials.

## PREVENTION OF BACTERIAL ENDOCARDITIS

Transient bacteremia that develops after a variety of manipulations or surgical procedures in patients with structural heart defects causes endocarditis. Prophylactic antibiotics in this situation can be highly effective when given before the procedure. Administration of these agents only once is required 30 minutes to 2 hours before the procedure (Table 3).

[1]Not FDA approved for this indication.

**TABLE 3**  Preprocedural Antibiotic Prophylaxis for At-Risk Patients

| Type of Procedure and Situation | Antibiotic | Dosage, Route, and Frequency |
|---|---|---|
| **Dental, oral respiratory tract, and esophageal procedures** | | |
| Standard prophylaxis | Amoxicillin | 2 g PO 1 h before procedure |
| Patient unable to take oral medication | Ampicillin | 2 g IM/IV within 30 min before procedure |
| Patient allergic to penicillin | Clindamycin (Cleocin*) | 600 mg PO 1 h before procedure |
| | *or* | |
| | cefadroxil (Duricef*) | 2 g PO 1 h before procedure |
| | *or* | |
| | cephalexin (Keflex*) | 2 g PO 1 h before procedure |
| | *or* | |
| | azithromycin (Zithromax*) | 500 mg PO 1 h before procedure |
| | *or* | |
| | clarithromycin (Biaxin*) | 500 mg PO 1 h before procedure |
| Patient allergic to penicillin and unable to take oral medication | Clindamycin (Cleocin*) | 600 g IV within 30 min of starting procedure |
| | *or* | |
| | cefazolin (Ancef) | 1 g IV within 30 min of starting procedure |
| | *or* | |
| | vancomycin (Vancocin) | 1 g IV over 1-2 h within 60 min of starting procedure |
| **Genitourinary/gastrointestinal procedures** | | |
| Moderate-risk patient | Amoxicillin | 2 g PO 1 h before procedure |
| | *or* | |
| | ampicillin | 2 g IM/IV within 30 min of starting procedure |
| Moderate-risk penicillin-allergic patient | Vancomycin | 1 g IV over 1-2 h infusion completed within 30-60 min of starting procedure |
| High-risk patient | Ampicillin | 2 g IM/IV given within 30 min of starting procedure |
| | *PLUS* | |
| | gentamicin | 1.5 mg/kg IV given within 30 min of starting procedure |
| | *6 h later* | |
| | Ampicillin | 1 g IM or IV |
| | *or* | |
| | amoxicillin | 1 g PO |
| High-risk penicillin-allergic patient | Vancomycin | 1 g IV over 1-2 h |
| | *PLUS* | |
| | gentamicin | 1.5 mg/kg IV given within 30 min of starting procedure |

Modified from Dajani AS, Taubert KA, Wilson W, et al: Prevention of bacterial endocarditis: Recommendation by the American Heart Association. JAMA 1997;277(22):1794-1801.
*Not FDA approved for this indication

In choosing prophylactic therapy, the following questions (Table 4) are useful:

- Is the patient at increased risk for endocarditis with underlying structural defect?
- Is there a high risk the procedure will produce bacteremia with organisms that cause endocarditis, such as *S. viridans* infection with oral cavity procedures or enterococcal with gastrointestinal or genitourinary procedures?

Antibiotic prophylaxis is recommended for patients with VSD, PDA, pulmonary or aortic stenosis, tetralogy of Fallot, or coarctation of the aorta. Such therapy is needed for patients with rheumatic or syphilitic valvular defects, prosthetic valves, calcified valves, obstructive cardiomyopathy, or mitral valve prolapse with either regurgitant murmur or with thickened mitral valve leaflets.

Endocarditis prophylaxis is not advised for patients with isolated secundum atrial septal defect or those who have undergone surgical repair for VSD or PDA and have no residual defect beyond 6 months. The same is true for those who have coronary artery bypass graft, previous rheumatic fever, or Kawasaki disease without any valve dysfunction. Prophylaxis is not recommended for those who have mitral valve prolapse (MVP) without mitral regurgitation (MR) and for persons with a cardiac pacemaker or implanted defibrillator (Table 5).

Procedures for which antibiotic prophylaxis is needed are those in which transient bacteremia develops when mucosal surfaces colonized with microorganisms are traumatized. For example, bacteremia may occur following dental manipulation in 80% of cases or in 20% of patients after urethral instrumentation. Prophylactic antimicrobials are recommended for high-risk patients who are scheduled to have certain dental, oropharyngeal, gastrointestinal, or genitourinary manipulations.

Standard antibiotic prophylaxis for patients undergoing oral, dental, or upper respiratory tract manipulations include oral amoxicillin. Clindamycin (Cleocin),[1] cefadroxil (Duricef),[1] cephalexin

**CURRENT DIAGNOSIS**

- High index of suspicion
- Febrile patient (temperature >38°C [100.4°F]) with
  Valvular or congenital heart defects
  Intravenous drug abuse
  Prosthetic or vascular access
  New onset or changing cardiac murmur
  Unknown source of embolization
- Positive blood cultures on at least two different specimens.
- Presence of vegetation detected on echocardiography (transesophageal [TEE] preferred)

## TABLE 4 Indications for Endocardial Prophylaxis

| Cardiac Conditions | Procedures |
|---|---|
| **High-risk category**<br>Prosthetic valve<br>Previous endocarditis<br>Complex cyanotic disease<br>   Tetralogy of Fallot, single ventricle<br>Surgically conducted systemic-pulmonary shunt<br><br>**Moderate-risk category**<br>Congenital heart disease: VSD, PDA, AS, PS<br>Acquired valvular dysfunction<br>   Rheumatic/syphilitic<br>Hypertrophic cardiomyopathy<br>MVP with MR or thickened leaflets | **Dental**<br>Dental extraction<br>Periodontal procedures: surgery, scaling, root planing<br>Dental implant replacement<br>Subgingival placement of antibiotic fibers<br>Intraligamentary local anesthetic injection<br>Cleaning of teeth or implants<br><br>**Respiratory**<br>Tonsillectomy/adenoidectomy<br>Rigid bronchoscopy<br><br>**Gastrointestinal**<br>Sclerotherapy<br>Esophageal stricture dilation<br>ERCP with biliary obstruction<br>Biliary tract surgery<br>Surgery involving intestinal mucosa<br><br>**Genitourinary**<br>Prostatic surgery<br>Cystoscopy<br>Urethral dilation<br>Septic abortion |

Abbreviations: AS = aortic stenosis; ERCP = endoscopic retrograde cholangiopancreatography; MVP = mitral valve prolapse; MR = mitral regurgitation; PDA = patent ductus arteriosus; PS = pulmonary stenosis; VSD = ventricular septal defect.
Modified from Dajani AS, Taubert KA, Wilson W, et al: Prevention of bacterial endocarditis: Recommendations by the American Heart Association. JAMA 1997;277(22):1794-1801.

(Keflex),[1] or azithromycin (Zithromax)[1] or clarithromycin (Biaxin)[1] should be given to those who cannot tolerate or are allergic to penicillin.

Parenteral ampicillin is recommended for patients who cannot take oral antibiotics and for those at high risk for infective endocarditis, such as patients with a prosthetic valve, previous endocarditis, or surgical systemic pulmonary shunts. Clindamycin[1] or cefazolin (Ancef) can be used as an alternative. Patients undergoing gastrointestinal or genitourinary instrumentation should be given vancomycin.

As recommended by the American Heart Association, all prophylactic antibiotics should be used only once before the procedure. There is no need for additional antibiotic administration except in high-risk patients who are undergoing gastrointestinal or genitourinary manipulation and who are given an ampicillin and gentamicin combination.

[1]Not FDA approved for this indication.

## TABLE 5 Endocardial Prophylaxis Not Recommended

| Cardiac Conditions | Procedures |
|---|---|
| Isolated secundum ASD<br>Surgical repair of ASD, VSD, PDA (without residue > 6 mo)<br>Previous CABG surgery<br>MVP without valvular dysfunction<br>Functional murmur<br>Kawasaki disease without valvular dysfunction<br>Previous rheumatic fever without valve dysfunction<br>Cardiac pacemaker and implanted defibrillators<br>Cardiac catheterization, balloon angioplasty<br>Coronary stent placement | **Dental**<br>Restorative dentistry<br>Local anesthetic injections<br>Intracanal treatment<br>Postoperative suture removal<br>Oral impression/radiograph<br>Fluoride treatment<br>Shedding of primary teeth<br><br>**Respiratory**<br>Endotracheal intubation<br>Fiberoptic bronchoscopy<br>Tympanostomy tube insertion<br><br>**Gastrointestinal**<br>TEE*<br>Endoscopy with/without biopsy*<br><br>**Genitourinary**<br>Vaginal delivery/hysterectomy*<br>Cesarean section<br>Urethral catheterization<br>Uterine dilation and curettage<br>Insertion/removal of IUD<br>Circumcision |

*Prophylaxis optional for high-risk category.
Abbreviations: ASD = atrial septal defect; CABG = coronary artery bypass graft; IUD = intrauterine device; MVP = mitral valve prolapse; PDA = patent ductus arteriosus; TEE = transesophageal echocardiogram; VSD = ventricular septal defect.
Modified from Dajani AS, Taubert KA, Wilson W, et al: Prevention of bacterial endocarditis: Recommendations by the American Heart Association. JAMA 1997;277(22):1794-1801.

## CURRENT THERAPY

- Empiric antibiotics should be started immediately with vancomycin and gentamicin.
- Specific therapy should be started once the pathogen is identified:
  - Use combination therapy for synergetic activity.
  - Monitor MIC/MBC level whenever possible.
  - Administer therapy for 2 to 6 weeks.
- Surgical interventions should be undertaken for severe, refractory, and complicated endocarditis.
- Prophylactic antibiotics are recommended in patients with structural heart defects undergoing surgical procedures or manipulations that can cause transient bacteremia, as recommended by the American Heart Association.
- Administration of antibiotic is usually once and 30 minutes to 1 to 2 hours before the procedure.

*Abbreviations:* MBC = minimum bactericidal concentration; MIC = minimum inhibitory concentration.

## REFERENCES

Amin NM: Infective endocarditis. Consultant 1994;34(3):319-343.

Bansal RC: Infective endocarditis. Med Clin North Am 1995;79:1205-1220.

Bayer AS, Bolger AF, Taubert KA, et al: Diagnosis and management of infective endocarditis and its complications. Circulation 1998;98:2936-2948.

Bayer AS, Ward JI, Ginzton LE, Shapiro SM: Evaluation of new clinical criteria for diagnosis of infective endocarditis. Am J Med 1994;96:211-219.

Cunha BA, Gill MV, Lazar JM: Acute infective endocarditis. Infect Dis Clin North Am 1996;10(4):811-834.

Dajanai AS, Taubert KA, Wilson W, et al: Prevention of bacterial endocarditis. Recommendations by American Heart Association. JAMA 1997;277: 1794-1801.

Giessel BE, Koenig CJ, Blake RL: Management of bacterial endocarditis. Am Fam Physician 2000;61:1725-1732.

Karchner AW: Infections on prosthetic valves and intravascular infections. In Mandell GL, Bennett JE, Dolin R (eds): Mandell, Douglas and Bennett's Principles and Practice of Infectious Diseases, 5th ed. Philadelphia, Churchill Livingstone, 2000, pp 903-917.

Li JS, Sexton DJ, Mick N, et al: Proposed modification to Duke criteria for diagnosis of infective endocarditis. Clin Infect Dis 2000;30:633-638.

Mylonakis E, Calderwood SB: Infective endocarditis in adults. N Engl J Med 2001;345(18):1318-1330.

# Hypertension

Method of
*L. Michael Prisant, MD*

## Physiologic Variability of Blood Pressure

Like temperature and heart rate, blood pressure is a continuous physiologic variable. Blood pressure progressively increases from birth. The 90th percentile blood pressure for boys in the United States is 87/68 mm Hg at birth and 136/84 mm Hg by 18 years. With aging, progressive fragmentation of elastin occurs in the aorta and other large blood vessels and results in loss of the dampening or buffering function of the aorta. Thus, the recoil or pump function of the aorta diminishes. When the aorta is less elastic, systolic blood pressure is amplified because more blood is delivered to the periphery during systole. The reflected waves from the periphery return to the aortic root before the end of systole and augment systolic blood pressure. Diastolic blood pressure drops because there is less residual stroke volume to be delivered to the periphery during diastole. Thus, the hallmark of the loss of the recoil function of the aorta is a widened pulse pressure, which is the difference between systolic and diastolic blood pressures.

Differences in physiology according to the time of the day, time of the month, or season of the year encompass the discipline of chronobiology. There are daily and seasonal variations in blood pressure. During summer months, blood pressure is lower, and winter months it is higher. With the daily activation of the sympathetic nervous system prior to awakening, blood pressure and heart rate increase (Figure 1). These changes in blood pressure parallel the morning activation in catecholamines, renin, and angiotensin.

The peak blood pressure is between 6 AM and noon. Associated with the morning surge in blood pressure, there is a disproportionately higher rate of myocardial infarction, stroke, aortic dissection, and sudden cardiac death in the morning than other times of the day.

Activity and sleep influence the level of blood pressure throughout the day. Between midnight and 6 AM, blood pressure is generally lowest. The systolic blood pressure normally increases with pain, stress, or dynamic exercise.

Normally, blood pressure declines 10% to 20% from the daytime activity period to the sleep period. Patients with less than a 10% reduction in daytime blood pressure are referred to as *nondippers* and have more target organ damage.

## Definitions

Blood pressure is a continuous physiologic variable associated with vascular disease (Figure 2). Diastolic blood pressure confers risk, but systolic blood pressure is a more potent risk factor. Furthermore, as pulse pressure widens, so does the risk. Although our cutpoint for a normal and an abnormal blood pressure is arbitrary, definitions for a treatment threshold are based on outcome trials.

The current classification of blood pressure is shown in Table 1. For adults aged 18 years and older, a blood pressure less than 120/80 mm Hg is normal, and 140/90 mm Hg or higher is hypertension. A diagnosis of hypertension is based on the average of two or more properly measured blood pressure readings on each of two or more office visits. The higher systolic or diastolic blood pressure from the four or more measurements determines the classification. The stage of hypertension at the initial visit indicates the time frame for follow-up assessment and subsequently the magnitude of therapy required.

Prehypertension is a category that identifies persons at high risk for developing hypertension and alerts patients and clinicians to intervene and prevent or delay disease from developing. The prevalence of prehypertension for adults 20 to 74 years was 37.4% in the 1999-2000 National Health and Nutrition Examination Survey (NHANES). In the Trial of Preventing Hypertension (TROPHY) Study (*N* = 772), despite

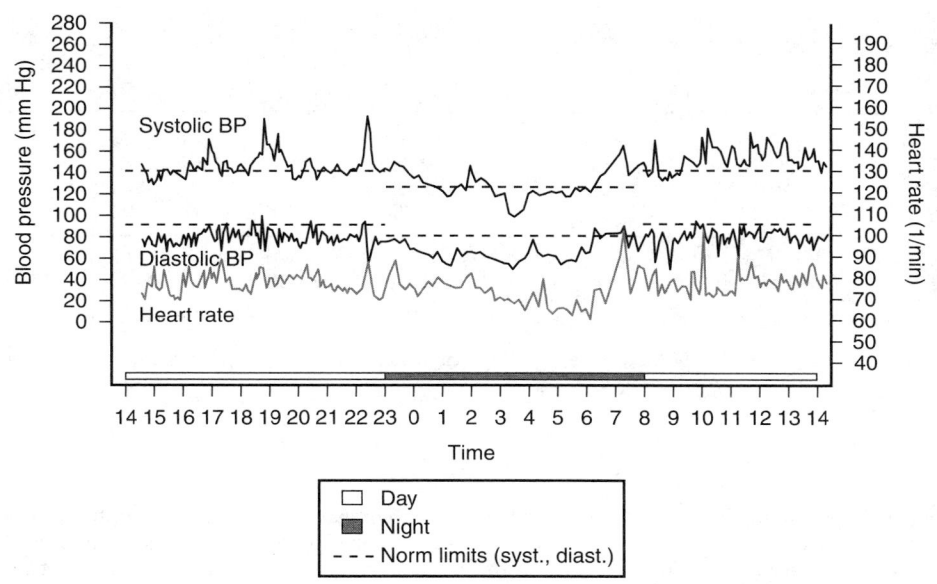

**FIGURE 1.** Ambulatory blood pressure recording. *Abbreviations:* diast = diastole; syst = systole.

nonpharmacologic treatment, 40% of prehypertensive study participants developed hypertension after 2 years and 63% after 4 years. Patients with prehypertension often have the concomitant risk factors of hypercholesterolemia, hypertriglyceridemia, low HDL cholesterol, glucose intolerance, increased waist circumference, and obesity. Furthermore, prehypertension has a higher risk of cardiovascular disease than normal blood pressure.

## PREVALENCE

In the United States among persons 20 years or older, 69.7 million have prehypertension (Figure 3). In 1999 and 2000, there were at least 65.2 million adults with hypertension, a 30% increase from 1988 to 1994, and this condition affects more than 30% of the population. It is the most common medical reason for an office visit. The prevalence of hypertension (Figure 4) is slightly higher among women than men, significantly higher among non-Hispanic blacks compared with whites

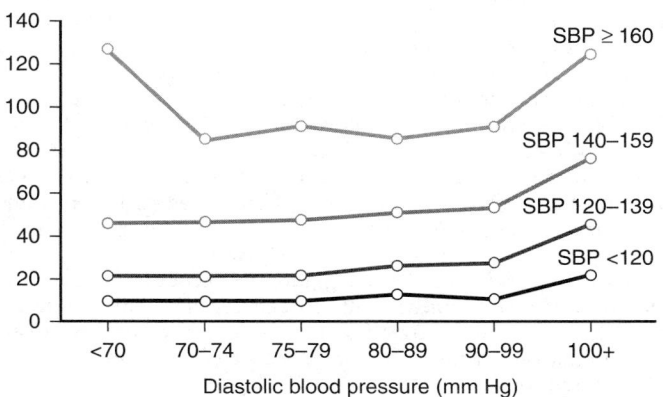

**FIGURE 2.** Age-adjusted coronary heart disease death rates per 10,000 person-years among 316,099 men by level of blood pressure. *Abbreviation:* SBP = systolic blood pressure. Derived from Neaton JD, Wentworth D: Serum cholesterol, blood pressure, cigarette smoking, and death from coronary heart disease. Overall findings and differences by age for 316,099 white men. Multiple Risk Factor Intervention Trial Research Group. Arch Intern Med 1992;152:56-64.

or Latin Americans, and increases with age. As the population becomes more obese, it is likely that hypertension, diabetes mellitus, cardiovascular disease, and end-stage renal disease will escalate.

## VASCULAR RISKS OF HYPERTENSION

Hypertension promotes alteration or rupture of arteries or arterioles in the brain, eyes, heart, and kidneys (hypertensive events) and progressive atherosclerosis involving the aorta or carotid, coronary, iliofemoral, and renal arteries (atherosclerotic events).

The cardiovascular sequelae of hypertension include angina, unstable angina, myocardial infarction, atrial fibrillation, sudden death, left ventricular hypertrophy, and congestive heart failure (both systolic and diastolic). Left ventricular hypertrophy is not only a target organ response to increased afterload, but is also the most potent cardiovascular risk factor. When left ventricular hypertrophy is present, it is associated with a higher prevalence of coronary heart disease, cardiovascular death (including sudden cardiac death), stroke, heart failure, and atrial fibrillation. Even without obstructive coronary disease, left ventricular hypertrophy impedes perfusion of blood from the epicardial to the endocardial surface, promoting angina, myocardial infarction, ventricular ectopy, myocardial fibrosis, and heart failure (Figure 5). Seventy-five percent of all patients with heart failure have antecedent hypertension. Chronic heart failure can occur early in the natural history of the disease due to diastolic filling abnormalities with normal systolic function without a dilated ventricle, or it can occur late due to reduced systolic function with a dilated ventricle. Patients with diastolic or preserved ejection fraction heart failure have a mortality rate similar to that of asymptomatic patients with a reduced ejection fraction. Chronic heart failure is the only cardiovascular disease increasing in incidence and prevalence.

The cerebrovascular consequences of hypertension include stroke, cerebral edema, and dementia. Acute intracerebral hemorrhage is usually due to rupture of a small, penetrating intraparenchymal artery. Ischemic strokes result from obstruction of arterial flow by local atherothrombosis, embolization, or small vessel occlusion. Uncontrolled hypertension is more likely to rupture a berry aneurysm, causing a subarachnoid hemorrhage. Hypertensive encephalopathy results from the consequence of increased blood pressure (accelerated or malignant hypertension) exceeding the confines of cerebral autoregulation. Cerebral edema, microinfarcts, petechial hemorrhages, and fibrinoid necrosis of the arterioles are present. Manifestations of hypertensive encephalopathy include headaches, nausea, vomiting,

**TABLE 1   Classification of Blood Pressure for Adults**

| Classification* | Systolic BP (mm Hg) | | Diastolic BP (mm Hg) | Follow-up Recommended† |
|---|---|---|---|---|
| Normal | <120 | and | <80 | Recheck within 2 y |
| Prehypertension | 120-139 | or | 80-89 | Recheck within 1 y |
| Stage 1 hypertension | 140-159 | or | 90-99 | Recheck within 2 mo |
| Stage 2 hypertension | ≥160 | or | ≥100 | Evaluate or refer to source of care within 1 mo‡ |

*The classification is based on the average of *two or more* properly measured, seated, blood pressure readings on each of *two or more* office visits. The *higher* systolic or diastolic blood pressure from the *four or more* measurements determines the classification.

†Based on initial average blood pressure measurements.

‡For patients with higher blood pressures (e.g., >180/110 mm Hg), evaluate and treat immediately or within 1 week depending on clinical situation and complications.

Modified from Chobanian AV, Bakris GL, Black HR, et al: Seventh report of the Joint National Committee on Prevention, Detection, Evaluation, and Treatment of High Blood Pressure. Hypertension 2003;42:1206-1252.

visual disturbances, seizures, impaired consciousness, and reversible focal neurologic symptoms and signs.

Hypertension is only second to diabetes mellitus as a cause of chronic kidney disease. Hypertensive nephropathy is the consequence of alteration in small arteries and arterioles producing hyaline arteriosclerosis with chronic hypertension and myointimal hyperplasia and fibrinoid necrosis with accelerated or malignant hypertension. Preglomerular arteriolar destruction, glomerular collapse, tubular atrophy, and interstitial fibrosis occur in a progressive fashion. Nephrosclerosis reduces renal blood flow, resulting in early increases of uric acid and progressive excretory failure, characterized by a rising blood urea nitrogen and creatinine. Microalbuminuria (30-300 mg/d) is an incipient manifestation of hypertensive renal disease and a cardiovascular risk factor. Atherosclerotic renal artery stenosis independently causes renal ischemia, excessive renin secretion, and further elevation in blood pressure.

Examination of the retinal vessels provides a window to examine the vascular effects of hypertension. The ocular manifestations of hypertension include retinopathy, optic neuropathy, choroidopathy with retinal detachment, and central or branch retinal vein occlusion. The normal arteriole-to-venule ratio is 2:3. Arteriolar narrowing occurs early in hypertension. Retinal arterioles normally have a yellow-white appearance, but as arteriosclerosis develops, the appearance becomes reddish-brown (copper wiring) and then white (silver wiring). Arterioles and venules share a common adventitial sheath. Arteriosclerosis compresses the venules, causing arteriovenous nicking, a predictor for mortality and stroke. The interruption of venous flow where a retinal artery crosses a vein can result in central or

branch retinal vein occlusion. Uncontrolled severe hypertension causes flame-shaped retinal hemorrhages, cotton-wool spots (retinal infarcts), and blurring of the optic disk margin (papilledema). Retinal hard exudates can indicate prior accelerated or malignant hypertension. They are yellow-white lipid deposits with sharp borders. A macular star, a hard exudate, radiates out from the fovea and is the consequence of retinal edema.

Large artery involvement from hypertension causes dilation or dissection of the thoracic aorta. Hypertension is present in 69% of ascending aortic dissections and 77% of descending aortic dissections. The definition of an abdominal aortic aneurysm is a segment of aorta that exceeds 3 cm in diameter, or the ratio of the abnormal to normal segment of aortic diameter is 1.5 or greater.

Hypertension may be an important factor in the pathogenesis and growth of abdominal aneurysms. Hypertension, diabetes, and cigarette smoking are associated with lower extremity peripheral arterial disease. Hypertension increased the risk of intermittent claudication 2.5-fold in men and 4-fold in women in the Framingham Heart Study. The risk was proportional to the magnitude of high blood pressure. One should remember that lower extremity peripheral arterial disease predicts a high prevalence of coronary disease.

## MEASUREMENT OF BLOOD PRESSURE

Health care providers need to be trained to perform blood pressure measurements correctly to avoid inaccurate labeling (and insurance premium hikes), psychological trauma, and inappropriate medication use. At least two or three measurements at 1-minute intervals should be performed at every visit. My preference is three measurements; the first of these three blood pressure measurements is used to locate the systolic and diastolic blood pressures, and the average of the last two is used for decision making. Initial blood pressure measurements should include measurement in the contralateral arm. A mercury manometer should be used to measure blood pressure because it is the gold standard and the most accurate. If an aneroid or electronic sphygmomanometer is used, it must be calibrated against a mercury manometer every 3 to 6 months using a Y-connection to determine if there is more than 4 mm Hg difference between devices over a range of blood pressures (40-260 mm Hg) for assessment of the accuracy of the nonmercury equipment. White-coat effect can be limited by teaching, monitoring, and retraining office personnel to perform blood pressure measurements according to the standards of the American Heart Association.

The patient should be seated in a quiet room in a chair with the back and arm supported and the legs uncrossed. There should be no talking during the measurements. Abstinence from tobacco use or caffeine ingestion within 30 minutes of the initial measurements of blood pressure is necessary. Subsequent readings are performed after a 5- to 15-minute period of rest. Cuff application is on an uncovered and supported arm at heart level. The length of the cuff bladder should encircle 80% of the arm circumference, and the width of the cuff bladder should be 40% of the arm circumference. Placing a small cuff

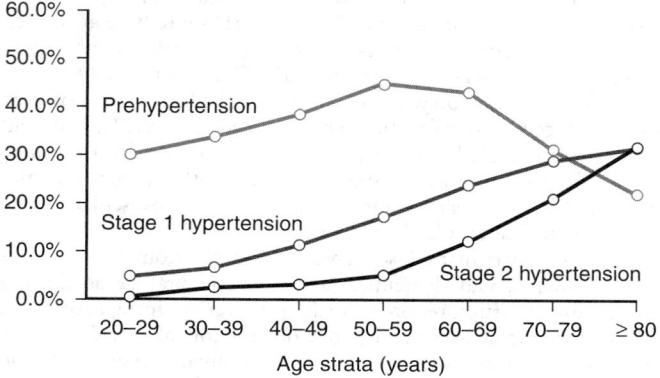

**FIGURE 3.** Prevalence of prehypertension and stages 1 and 2 hypertension by age strata. Derived from Qureshi AI, Suri MF, Kirmani JF, Divani AA: Prevalence and trends of prehypertension and hypertension in United States: National Health and Nutrition Examination Surveys 1976 to 2000. Med Sci Monit 2005;11(9): CR403-CR409.

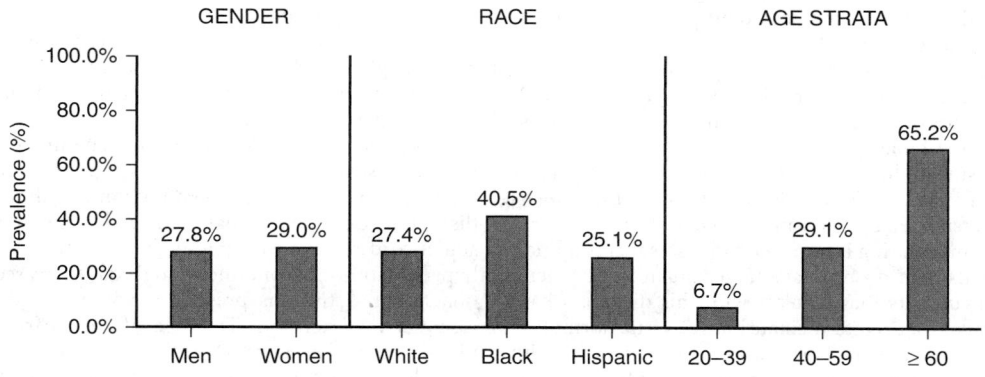

**FIGURE 4.** Prevalence of hypertension by race, gender, and age strata in the United States, 1999-2002. Derived from Centers for Disease Control and Prevention: Racial/ethnic disparities in prevalence, treatment, and control of hypertension—United States, 1999-2002. MMWR Morb Mortal Wkly Rep. 2005;54(1):7-9.

on obese patients is a common cause of pseudohypertension. *Pseudohypertension* refers to falsely elevated blood pressure that is an artifact of measurement.

Radial artery palpation is used to estimate the systolic blood pressure once the cuff is applied snugly and evenly over the brachial artery. The cuff should be distended about 20 to 30 mm Hg above the palpable systolic blood pressure. Radial artery palpation prevents underestimating systolic blood pressure or overestimating diastolic blood pressure, which is associated with the silent period (auscultatory gap) between the systolic and diastolic blood pressures, and prevents the pain of excess cuff inflation pressure that elevates systolic blood pressure. Osler's sign is a palpable pulseless radial artery

present after the cuff is inflated above the systolic blood pressure. This sign, a clue for pseudohypertension from atherosclerosis, is not discriminatory.

The bell of the stethoscope is used to auscultate low-intensity Korotkoff sounds over the brachial artery, and then the cuff is slowly deflated with each heart beat, or 2 to 3 mm Hg per second. The systolic blood pressure is the first faint tapping sound of two successive beats after cuff deflation, and the diastolic blood pressure is the point at which Korotkoff sounds completely cease. If the diastolic blood pressure approaches zero, then the diastolic blood pressure is reported as the period marked by an abrupt muffling sound quality. All values are reported to the nearest 2 mm Hg. If more than 20% of

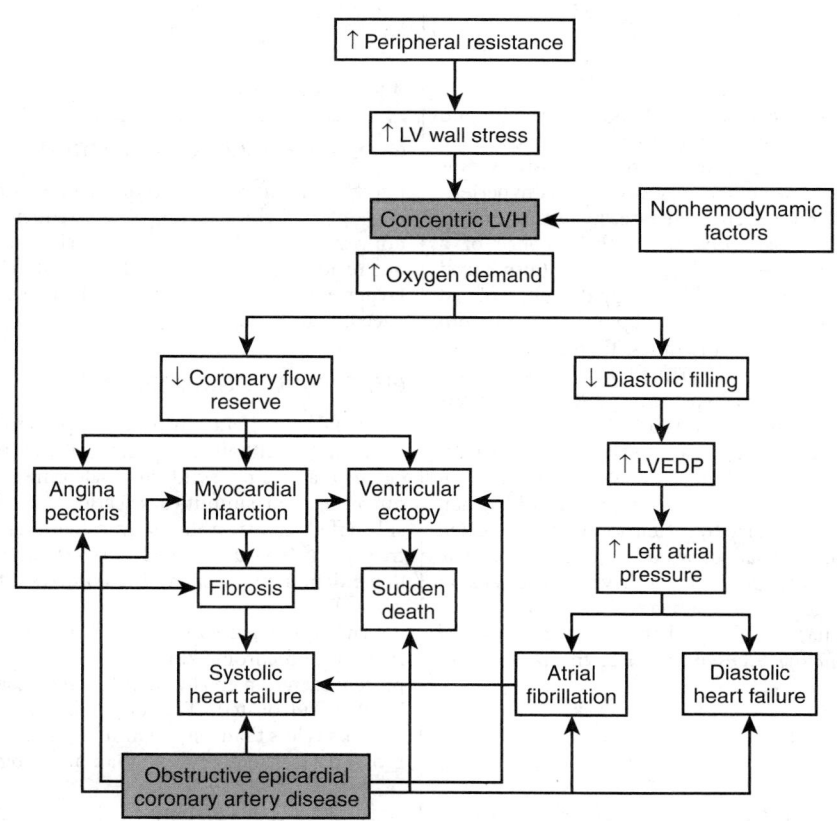

**FIGURE 5.** Hypertensive heart disease. *Abbreviations:* LF = left ventricle; LVEDP = left ventricular diastolic filling pressure; LVH = left ventricular hypertrophy. Reproduced with permission from Prisant LM: Hypertensive heart disease. J Clin Hypertens (Greenwich) 2005;7:231-238. Copyright 2005 by Le Jacq, Ltd.

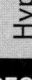

the measurements end in zero, then a zero-digit preference is documented and retraining is necessary.

Blood pressure can decline over subsequent visits even without active drug therapy. This has been referred to as the *placebo effect*. It highlights the importance of not making a diagnosis of hypertension at a single office visit (see Table 1).

Home blood pressure monitoring may be useful for the care of patients. *White coat hypertension* (also called *office hypertension*) refers to elevated blood pressure that occurs in the medical environment. Home blood pressure monitoring is advocated to assess this condition in hypertensive patients who do not have target organ involvement. However, research documents that patients with this diagnosis have target organ involvement that is intermediate between true normotensive and true hypertensive patients. Furthermore, many patients with white coat hypertension develop true hypertension. Another application is masked hypertension, defined as normal office blood pressure and elevated home or ambulatory blood pressure. More research is required, but these patients appear to have increased cardiovascular risk. However, the best argument for the use of home blood pressure measurements is the involvement of patients with their disease.

Many home devices (e.g., wrist devices) are not accurate for decision-making. An objective source of information at http://www.dableducational.com/sphygmomanometers.html helps to guide physician recommendations. The patient should be told to take two seated measurements twice daily after resting for 5 minutes. Values consistently less than 130/80 mm Hg are normal.

Ambulatory blood pressure monitoring provides information on the average 24-hour blood pressure, diurnal variation of blood pressure, and the variability of blood pressure. It is the only means for recording sleep blood pressure. Daytime and sleep blood pressures that exceed 135/85 mm Hg and 120/75 mm Hg, respectively, are abnormal. Medicare currently reimburses ambulatory blood pressure for the diagnosis of white coat hypertension in patients who have three office measurements exceeding 140/90 mm Hg, two out-of-office measurements less than 140/90 mm Hg, and no evidence of target organ damage. However, individual test repeatability is limited.

### OTHER DEFINITIONS

*Labile hypertension* refers to episodically normal and abnormal blood pressures, but *borderline hypertension* is a preferable term because there is no more or less blood pressure variability in normotensive versus sustained hypertensive patients. Secondary hypertension is hypertension of a known cause (e.g., renovascular disease, hyperthyroidism, pheochromocytoma, primary renal disease). In the absence of a secondary cause, the diagnosis of essential hypertension (also called *idiopathic* or *primary hypertension*) is established by default. Isolated systolic hypertension is defined as a systolic blood pressure of 140 mm Hg or greater and a diastolic blood pressure of less than 90 mm Hg.

The presence of resistant, accelerated, or malignant hypertension should provoke suspicion of secondary hypertension. *Resistant hypertension* defines hypertension greater than 160/100 mm Hg despite rational, maximal three-drug therapy in an adherent patient. *Refractory hypertension* refers to a blood pressure greater than 140/90 mm Hg (or greater than 160/90 mm Hg in patients older than 60 years) in patients without secondary hypertension who are treated with maximal doses of two appropriate drugs that are given adequate time to be effective. *Accelerated hypertension* is severe hypertension associated with ongoing target organ damage (e.g., heart failure, kidney failure, unstable angina) and flame-shaped hemorrhages and cotton-wool spots. *Malignant hypertension* requires the presence of papilledema.

## Pathogenesis

There is no single mechanism that explains the genesis of essential hypertension, unlike the mechanisms for secondary hypertension. Essential hypertension is viewed as a polygenic trait with various subsets of genes that are additive. In contrast to first-degree relatives of normotensive patients, first-degree relatives of hypertensive patients are more likely to develop hypertension. African Americans tend to have an earlier onset and more severe hypertension than whites. Excess body weight, psychosocial stress, sodium and potassium ingestion, alcohol consumption, and physical activity modify the level of blood pressure in an individual patient.

Other factors are also important. The impact of the sympathetic nervous system on blood pressure is appreciated in patients who have a cervical spinal cord injury and chronically low blood pressure. The distal portion of the spinal cord retains function, and activation of spinal cord reflexes working independently can result in paroxysmal hypertension or autonomic dysreflexia. Increased sympathetic nervous system activity is present in younger and older persons with essential hypertension. The role of the heart in elevating systolic blood pressure is suggested in high cardiac output states associated with low systemic vascular resistance, such as hyperthyroidism, anemia, and aortic insufficiency. The importance of the kidney is supported by normalization of blood pressure after transplantation of a kidney from a normotensive patient into a patient with renal failure due to hypertension.

### EVALUATION

The goals for the initial evaluation (Box 1) are to document that the patient has a sustained elevation in blood pressure, to identify the presence of hypertensive and atherosclerotic target organ involvement, to screen for other cardiovascular risk factors (diabetes mellitus, dyslipidemia, tobacco use, physical inactivity, obesity, family history), to identify factors (e.g., gout, asthma) that might modify treatment, and to diagnose correctable causes of secondary hypertension. Box 1 lists the components of the physical examination and their implications. Initial tests prior to treatment are a fasting glucose, hematocrit, serum potassium, calcium, creatinine, complete lipid profile, urinalysis, and electrocardiogram. Box 2 lists the components of the laboratory studies and their implications. Additional studies may be needed based on the history, physical examination, and results of the laboratory studies.

## Therapy

### NONPHARMACOLOGIC THERAPY

Lifestyle modification is recommended for all patients with prehypertension and hypertension. Weight reduction, sodium restriction, alcohol restriction, and increased physical activity lower blood pressure, but recidivism is common. The DASH (Dietary Approaches to Stop Hypertension) diet lowered systolic blood pressure 8 to 14 mm Hg in a feeding trial.

### PHARMACOLOGIC THERAPY

There is a proliferation of antihypertensive medications that target different mechanisms. Although the number of pharmacologic agents may seem bewildering, selecting drugs within a class that have outcome data simplifies selection (see Box 2). Dosing frequency, side effects, cost, and many other factors influence adherence to treatment. Low-dose, fixed-dose combination therapy reduces dose-dependent side effects and maximizes attainment of blood pressure control.

The blood pressure goal for hypertensive patients with diabetes mellitus and chronic kidney disease is less than 130/80 mm Hg. With protein excretion greater than 1 g/day, a goal of less than 125/75 mm Hg is often advocated. The target blood pressure for the remaining patients is less than 140/90 mm Hg. To achieve blood pressure control, most patients require more than one drug.

#### Factors in Drug Selection

Characteristics to consider when selecting an antihypertensive drug include mode of action, route of elimination, and potential drug interactions. Assuming a drug within a drug class has a class effect in

**BOX 1** Physical Examination

## Blood Pressure Measurement
### Isolated Increased Systolic Blood Pressure
- Anemia
- Aortic regurgitation
- Arteriovenous fistula
- Atherosclerosis
- Hyperthyroidism

### Inequality of Pressure Between Arms
- Coarctation of the aorta
- Cervical rib
- Dissection of the aorta
- Subclavian atherosclerosis
- Subclavian steal syndrome
- Supravalvular aortic stenosis
- Variability of measurements

### Orthostatic Changes
- Autonomic failure
- Diabetes mellitus
- Hypovolemia
- Pheochromocytoma

## General Appearance
### Angioneurotic Edema
- ACE inhibitor therapy

### Café-au-lait Spots, Neurofibromatosis
- Pheochromocytoma
- Renal artery stenosis

### Central Obesity, Acne, Moon Face, Hirsutism, Thin Skin, Striae, Bruises, Wasted Limbs, Buffalo Hump
- Cushing's syndrome

### Coarse Hair, Thick Lips and Tongue, Puffy Eyelids, Myxedema
- Hypothyroidism

### Exogenous Obesity
- Sleep apnea
- Diabetes mellitus
- Pseudohypertension

### Exophthalmos, Lid Retraction, Tremulousness, Goiter
- Hyperthyroidism

### Gynecomastia
- Adrenal hyperplasia or tumor
- Anabolic steroids
- Calcium channel blockers
- Chronic renal failure
- Cyclosporine (Sandimmune)
- Hyperthyroidism
- Methyldopa (Aldomet)
- Reserpine
- Spironolactone (Aldactone)

### Marfanoid Features, Mucosal Neuromas
- Pheochromocytoma

### Periorbital Edema, Pallor
- Renal disease

### Plethora, Conjunctival Suffusion
- Polycythemia

### Prognathism; Enlarged Tongue, Nose, Hands, and Feet
- Acromegaly

### Webbing of the Neck, Broad Chest, Wide-spaced Nipples, Low Posterior Hairline, Short Stature
- Coarctation of the aorta
- Turner's syndrome

## Fundus
### Arteriole-to-Venule Ratio < 2:3
- Advanced age
- Hypertensive retinopathy

### Arteriovenous Nicking
- Hypertensive retinopathy

### Copper or Silver Wire Reflex
- Advanced age
- Hypertensive arteriosclerosis

### Cotton-wool Spots
- Anemia
- Accelerated hypertension
- Diabetic retinopathy
- Hyperviscosity
- Vasculitis

### Flame-shaped Retinal Hemorrhages
- Accelerated hypertension

### Papilledema
- Hypertensive encephalopathy
- Intracranial hypertension
- Malignant hypertension

## Neck
### Carotid Bruits
- Atherosclerosis of carotid artery

### Jugular Venous Distention
- Right-sided heart failure

### Thyroid Enlargement
- Hyperthyroidism
- Hypothyroidism

## Lungs
### Rales
- Heart failure

### Wheezes
- Asthma
- β-Blocker therapy
- Chronic lung disease
- Heart failure

## Heart
### Tachycardia
- Anemia
- Heart failure
- Hyperthyroidism
- Pheochromocytoma

### Atrial fibrillation
- Hyperthyroidism
- Ischemic heart disease
- Left atrial enlargement

*Continued*

## BOX 1 Physical Examination—cont'd

**Palpable Pulses of Intercostal Arteries of Posterior Thorax**
- Coarctation of the aorta

**Sustained, Enlarged (>3 cm) Apical Impulse**
- Left ventricular hypertrophy

**Apical Impulse Outside Midclavicular Line**
- Left ventricular dilation
- Left ventricular hypertrophy

**Tambour $S_2$**
- Aortic root dilatation

**$S_3$ Gallop**
- Anemia
- Arteriovenous fistula
- Cardiomyopathy
- Heart failure
- Hyperthyroidism
- Regurgitant valvular disease

**$S_4$ Gallop**
- Anemia
- Arteriovenous fistula
- Cardiomyopathy
- Coronary artery disease
- Hyperthyroidism
- Left ventricular hypertrophy

**Basal Systolic Murmur**
- Aortic stenosis
- Benign murmur
- Coarctation of aorta
- Hypertension

**Basal Diastolic Murmur**
- Aortic insufficiency
- Dissecting aorta

**Pericardial Rub**
- Uremic pericarditis

### Abdomen and Genitalia
**Palpable Kidneys**
- Polycystic kidney disease

**Mass with Expansile Pulsation**
- Abdominal aneurysm

**Suprapubic Mass**
- Distended urinary bladder

**Systolic or Systolic-diastolic Bruit**
- Arteriovenous malformation
- Mesenteric artery stenosis
- Renal artery stenosis

**Small Testes or Clitoromegaly**
- Anabolic steroid use

### Extremities
**Decreased Femoral Pulses**
- Aortofemoral atherosclerosis
- Coarctation of the aorta

**Femoral Bruits**
- Aortofemoral atherosclerosis

**Radial-femoral Delay**
- Aortofemoral atherosclerosis
- Coarctation of the aorta

**Peripheral Edema**
- Calcium antagonist therapy
- Chronic renal failure
- Direct vasodilator therapy
- Nephrotic syndrome
- Right-sided heart failure

*Abbreviation:* ACE = angiotensin-converting enzyme.
Modified from Prisant LM: Hypertension. In Conn RB, Borer WZ, Snyder JW (eds): Current Diagnosis 9. Philadelphia: WB Saunders, 1997, pp 349-359.

---

protecting or reducing target organ damage is an error, especially among hypertensive patients who have compelling indications for specific drug classes (Table 2). Age, race, comorbid conditions, and renal function influence initial drug selection. For instance, β-blockers, angiotensin-converting enzyme (ACE) inhibitors, and angiotensin receptor blockers (ARBs) are less effective as initial therapy in African American patients than in whites. Older patients respond better to diuretics and calcium channel blockers (CCBs) than to ACE inhibitors. A diminished glomerular filtration rate requires reduction of the drug dose or avoidance of the drug. The highest priority for drug selection is based on comorbid illness to prevent target organ damage.

A conservation-of-medication approach can be used to treat more than one disease with a single drug and lessen pharmaceutical costs. For instance, a nonselective β-blocker could be used to treat both hypertension and migraine headaches or essential tremor. Another example is treating a patient who has heart failure, diabetes, and hypertension with an ACE inhibitor and a diuretic.

Most patients require more than one drug to achieve their target blood pressure. The current recommendation is to use two drugs from the outset with stage II hypertension. This approach does require caution to avoid hypotension, especially in elderly patients. African Americans, patients with systolic hypertension, hypertensive diabetic patients, and patients with chronic kidney disease need the most drugs.

## Dosing Strategies and Drug Efficacy

Stage I hypertensive or frail, elderly patients are treated initially with a low initial dose. Assessment of efficacy is in 4 to 6 weeks. At that follow-up visit, the patient is questioned about drug-specific side effects. If the medication is tolerated, but the blood pressure is not at goal, then the drug should be titrated or a second drug added. Titrated monotherapy for any drug class is unlikely to achieve a placebo-corrected control rate greater than 50%.

As the dose of a drug is doubled, there is a decrement of additional blood pressure lowering when compared with the previous dose, and drug-induced adverse effects increase. However, not all side effects are dose-dependent. For example, ACE inhibitors have the dose-independent side effects of cough and angioneurotic edema. The balance of blood pressure lowering and unacceptable adverse drug reactions is about two titrations.

Because adherence to therapy decreases if drugs are dosed frequently throughout the day, drugs should be selected that are dosed once or twice daily. Fixed-dose combinations also improve adherence and provide financial advantages for patients. Synchronizing the dosing of antihypertensive medications with other medications can improve overall adherence.

Drugs that combine different pharmacologic mechanisms increase the likelihood of reaching the target blood pressure. Not all

## BOX 2  Laboratory Assessment of Hypertension

**Hypokalemia**
- Cushing's syndrome
- Diuretic use
- Primary hyperaldosteronism

**Hypercalcemia**
- Hyperparathyroidism
- Thiazide diuretics

**Hyperglycemia**
- Acromegaly
- β-Blockers
- Corticosteroids
- Cushing's syndrome
- Diabetes mellitus
- Diuretics
- Pheochromocytoma

**Hypercholesterolemia**
- Anabolic steroids
- Hypercortisolism
- Hyperparathyroidism
- Hypothyroidism
- Nephrotic syndrome
- Primary lipid disorder
- Progestational agents

**Increased serum creatinine**
- Acromegaly
- ACE inhibitor or ARB use
- Avoid renally excreted drugs
- Primary renal disease
- Renovascular hypertension

**Hyperkalemia**
- ACE inhibitor or ARB use
- Chronic renal failure
- NSAIDs
- Potassium chloride supplement
- Potassium-sparing diuretics
- Salt substitutes
- Type IV renal tubular acidosis

**Hyperuricemia**
- Chronic renal failure
- Diuretics
- Early sign of renal disease
- Gout
- Hyperparathyroidism
- Hypothyroidism
- Polycystic kidney disease
- Polycythemia
- Toxemia of pregnancy

**Hypertriglyceridemia**
- β-Blocker use
- Chronic renal failure
- Diabetes mellitus
- Diuretic use
- Estrogen use
- Ethanol abuse
- Liver disease
- Obesity

**Abnormal liver function**
- Avoid hepatically metabolized drugs
- Ethanol abuse
- Hypertriglyceridemia

*Abbreviations:* ACE = angiotensin-converting enzyme; ARB = angiotensin receptor blocker; NSAID = nonsteroidal anti-inflammatory drug.
Modified from Prisant LM: Hypertension. In Conn RB, Borer WZ, Snyder JW (eds): Current Diagnosis 9. Philadelphia: WB Saunders, 1997, pp 349-359.

---

antihypertensive drugs are additive to one another. Diuretics tend to augment the blood pressure–lowering effect of most antihypertensive agents.

## Drug Classes

Hypertension may be treated with diuretics, β-blockers, CCBs, ACE inhibitors, ARBs, α₂-stimulants, α₁-blockers, peripheral sympatholytics, and direct vasodilators. The oral direct renin inhibitor aliskiren, the first of a new class of drugs, was recently released. Endothelin antagonists, selective I1-imidazoline receptor agonists, and vasopeptidase inhibitors may be added to our treatment armamentarium in the future.

α₂-Stimulants, sympatholytics, and direct vasodilators are not used initially for the treatment of hypertension. α₂-Stimulants include clonidine (Catapres), methyldopa (Aldomet), guanabenz (Wytensin), and guanfacine (Tenex); peripheral sympatholytics include reserpine; and direct vasodilators include hydralazine (Apresoline) and minoxidil (Loniten). α1-Blockers (prazosin [Minipress], terazosin [Hytrin], and doxazosin [Cardura]) have fallen out of favor as initial therapy for hypertension but have been safely used for many years. Peripheral

## TABLE 2  Drug Choices for Compelling Indications

| Indication | Aldosterone Antagonist | ACE Inhibitor | ARB | β-Blocker | CCB | Diuretic |
|---|---|---|---|---|---|---|
| Chronic kidney disease | | × | × | | | |
| Diabetes mellitus | | × | × | × | × | × |
| Heart failure | × | × | × | × | | × |
| High coronary disease risk | | × | | × | × | × |
| Prior myocardial infarction | × | × | × | × | | |
| Recurrent stroke | | × | × | | | × |

*Abbreviations:* ACE = angiotensin-converting enzyme; ARB = angiotensin receptor blocker; CCB = calcium channel blocker.
Modified from Chobanian AV, Bakris GL, Black HR, et al; and the National Blood Pressure Education Program: The Seventh Report of the Joint National Committee on Prevention, Detection, Evaluation, and Treatment of High Blood Pressure. JAMA 2003;289:2073-2082.

sympatholytics are not used often, although low-dose reserpine (0.05-0.1 mg daily) with a diuretic is effective for patients who have limited resources.

### Diuretics

There are thiazide or thiazide-like, loop, and potassium-sparing diuretics. Thiazide (e.g., hydrochlorothiazide [Esidrix]) and thiazide-like diuretics (e.g., chlorthalidone [Hygroton], indapamide [Lozol], and metolazone [Zaroxolyn]) increase sodium excretion by inhibiting the sodium-chloride pump in the early segment of the distal convoluted tubule and reduce plasma volume initially. This results in increased plasma renin activity and aldosterone, which facilitates potassium loss. Systemic vascular resistance progressively declines and plasma volume approaches pretreatment levels.

Thiazide or thiazide-like diuretics reduce strokes, heart failure, and total cardiovascular mortality. Diuretics are proven in isolated systolic hypertension and diastolic hypertension trials. Diuretics are especially effective for obese patients, African Americans, the elderly, diabetic patients, patients with systolic heart failure, and patients with excess sodium intake. Thiazides decrease osteoporosis.

Thiazide diuretics enhance the efficacy of other drug classes and are required as a triple component with direct vasodilators. Nonsteroidal anti-inflammatory drugs (NSAIDs) attenuate the antihypertensive effect of diuretics. The side effects of thiazide diuretics include volume depletion, hyponatremia, hypokalemic alkalosis, hypomagnesemia, hypercalcemia, hyperuricemia, gout, sexual dysfunction, and occasionally sulfonamide-related skin eruptions. Glucose intolerance and diabetes mellitus with diuretics are due to hypokalemia. Thiazides must be avoided in patients with severe recurrent gout, hyponatremia, and volume depletion.

Loop diuretics—furosemide (Lasix), bumetanide (Bumex), torsemide (Demadex), and ethacrynic acid (Edecrin)—act at the thick ascending loop of Henle to prevent chloride and sodium reabsorption. They have a rapid onset of action compared with thiazide diuretics. The longest-acting loop diuretic is torsemide. Loop diuretics should not be used for hypertensive patients who have normal renal function. They are required in patients whose serum creatinine exceeds 2.5 mg/dL. For patients who have a true sulfur allergy, ethacrynic acid is the only nonsulfonamide diuretic available. However, permanent ototoxicity occurs at high doses.

The potassium-sparing diuretics—amiloride (Midamor), triamterene (Dyrenium), spironolactone (Aldactone), and eplerenone (Inspra)—are often used in combination with hydrochlorothiazide. They decrease magnesium and potassium excretion. Amiloride and triamterene block the epithelial sodium transport channel, and, unlike aldosterone blockers, they do not lower blood pressure much. Spironolactone is a potent nonselective aldosterone blocker, acting also on androgen and progesterone receptors, and eplerenone is a selective aldosterone blocker. Spironolactone reduces mortality in advanced heart failure, and eplerenone decreases mortality in postinfarction patients with left ventricular dysfunction. Both drugs are effective for resistant hypertension. Hyperkalemia can occur in patients with chronic kidney disease and type IV renal tubular acidosis. Concomitant treatment with potassium supplements, over-the-counter salt substitutes, ACE inhibitors, ARBs, and NSAIDs requires careful monitoring. Spironolactone causes sexual dysfunction, gynecomastia, mastodynia, and menorrhagia at higher doses.

### β-Blockers

β-blockers are a heterogeneous class of drugs. Their antihypertensive mechanism of action is unclear because most β-blockers increase peripheral vascular resistance acutely. However, they inhibit renin release, decrease angiotensin II and aldosterone, and reduce heart rate, cardiac output, and blood pressure. Labetalol and carvedilol also block the $\alpha_1$-receptor and cause vasodilation. Acebutolol, carteolol, pindolol, and penbutolol possess intrinsic sympathomimetic activity, a characteristic that causes vasodilation and stimulates the β-receptor if resting sympathetic activity is low. Nebivolol[2] uniquely has nitric oxide–mediated vasodilating properties. Cardioselective $\beta_1$-blockers—acebutolol, atenolol, betaxolol, bisoprolol, metoprolol tartrate,

metoprolol succinate, and nebivolol[2]—cause less bronchospasm and claudication in low doses. Atenolol, nadolol, betaxolol, and carteolol are hydrophilic β-blockers that are renally eliminated. Intravenous β-blockers include atenolol, esmolol, metoprolol tartrate, and labetalol.

Although β-blockers are no longer endorsed for initial therapy for uncomplicated hypertension, the combination of β-blockers and diuretics reduced total mortality in elderly hypertensive patients. The most important mandatory indications are for myocardial infarction and heart failure patients. Timolol, metoprolol tartrate, propranolol, acebutolol, and carvedilol reduced postinfarction mortality. Bisoprolol, carvedilol, and metoprolol succinate (but not metoprolol tartrate) decrease total mortality in chronic heart failure. In addition, atenolol and bisoprolol diminish cardiovascular events in the perioperative period.

Hypertensive younger patients who are anxious or who have hyperkinetic heart syndrome benefit from β-blocker treatment. Nonselective β-blockers, such as propranolol, are useful in the treatment of essential tremor and migraine headaches because they block the $\beta_2$-receptor. β-Blockers diminish the ventricular response rate of atrial fibrillation and other supraventricular tachycardias. β-Blockers reduce blood pressure less in African Americans compared with whites unless the β-blocker is combined with a diuretic. Cardioselective $\beta_1$-blockers are preferred for bronchospastic pulmonary disease, peripheral vascular disease, and diabetes mellitus, although no β-blocker is selective at large doses. Nonselective β-blockers should not be used with insulin-requiring diabetes mellitus because hypoglycemic symptoms are masked and a hypertensive response to hypoglycemia ensues.

β-blockers are not additive to ACE inhibitors, ARBs, and $\alpha_2$-stimulants to further reduce blood pressure. The use of $\alpha_2$-stimulants and β-blockers together increases blood pressure, and abrupt withdrawal of either drug results in a markedly elevated blood pressure from unopposed α-receptor–induced vasoconstriction. Verapamil or diltiazem with a β-blocker can cause heart failure, extreme bradycardia, and advanced heart block.

Fatigue, weight gain, depression, erectile dysfunction, claudication, and lipid abnormalities are reported as adverse drug reactions to β-blockers. Care must be taken to taper β-blockers over a 14-day period in patients with coronary artery disease.

### Angiotensin-Converting Enzyme Inhibitors

ACE inhibitors inhibit the angiotensin-converting enzyme, blocking the conversion of angiotensin I to angiotensin II and bradykinin breakdown. However, there are other pathways by which angiotensin II is generated, which cause angiotensin II levels to drift toward baseline levels. Other blood pressure lowering effects of ACE inhibitors involve bradykinin, prostacyclin (prostaglandin $I_2$ [$PGI_2$]), nitric oxide, aldosterone, endothelin, the sympathetic nervous system, and venodilation.

Several characteristics differentiate ACE inhibitors: the zinc-binding ligand (carboxyl, phosphoryl, sulfhydryl), which permits attachment of the ACE inhibitor to the angiotensin-converting enzyme; whether or not the drug is a prodrug; tissue ACE inhibition; and lipophilicity. Captopril has a sulfhydryl zinc-binding ligand that can cause a skin rash and taste disturbances, and fosinopril uses a phosphoryl group. Prodrugs remain inactive until converted by the liver, which improves absorption. Captopril and lisinopril are not prodrugs. The prodrug characteristic is not used to select a drug unless the patient has severe hepatic dysfunction. Tissue ACE inhibition and lipophilicity are not proven to be therapeutically important.

Trandolapril, ramipril, perindopril, and lisinopril are the longest-acting ACE inhibitors. Captopril is dosed 2 to 3 times per day. Because most ACE inhibitors require renal excretion, the dose is reduced with chronic kidney disease. However, fosinopril and trandolapril use hepatic and renal excretion. Food reduces the absorption of captopril and moexipril. Enalaprilat is an intravenous formulation.

---

[2]Not available in the United States.

Enalapril is the only ACE inhibitor proven to reduce the total mortality in chronic heart failure. Captopril, lisinopril, ramipril, and trandolapril reduce cardiovascular mortality in patients having left ventricular dysfunction after a myocardial infarction. Ramipril is proven to prevent myocardial infarction, stroke, and cardiovascular death in patients with vascular disease. Benazepril, captopril, and ramipril reduce progression of renal insufficiency.

ACE inhibitors are necessary treatment for heart failure, postinfarction left ventricular dysfunction, recurrent stroke, diabetes mellitus, and chronic kidney disease, and they are required in patients with a high risk of cardiovascular events (see Table 2). Like β-blockers, ACE inhibitors are less effective in African Americans compared with whites unless they are combined with a diuretic. In the African American Study of Kidney Disease (AASK), which researched hypertensive renal insufficiency, ramipril was superior to amlodipine or metoprolol in slowing the rate of glomerular filtration rate decline. ACE inhibitors are also used for scleroderma renal crisis. They also reduce the rate of development of diabetes.

ACE inhibitors are additive with diuretics or CCBs, but not with β-blockers or ARBs. NSAIDs attenuate the blood-pressure–lowering effect of ACE inhibitors.

Hypotension occurs if ACE inhibitors are given to patients who have high renin levels or volume depletion or who are taking diuretics. ACE inhibitors rarely cause cholestatic jaundice and pancreatitis. Side effects of ACE inhibitors are an intractable cough, hyperkalemia, deteriorating creatinine, and angioneurotic edema. ACE inhibitors cause reversible renal insufficiency with bilateral renal artery stenosis, renal artery stenosis in a solitary kidney, or renal artery compression from a polycystic kidney.

Creatinine rises with chronic disease, heart failure, volume depletion, sepsis, and the use of NSAIDs, cyclosporine, and tacrolimus. When the creatinine increase is greater than 30%, the ACE inhibitor should be stopped and the cause determined. NSAIDs, potassium-sparing diuretics, potassium supplements, chronic kidney disease, and type IV renal tubular acidosis elevate potassium in patients treated with an ACE inhibitor. Cough is reported in 10% of patients. Angioneurotic edema can be life threatening if the larynx is involved. The face is most often affected, but edema also can involve the hands, feet, genitalia, and bowel. Angioneurotic edema affects 0.72% of African American versus 0.31% of non African American patients. ACE inhibitors are contraindicated during pregnancy.

## Angiotensin Receptor Blockers

ARBs attach to the type I angiotensin II (AT1) receptor and cause plasma renin, angiotensin I, and angiotensin II to increase. Blockade of the AT1 receptor can stimulate the AT2 receptor to increase nitric oxide production and dilate arterioles.

The ARBs are not as heterogenous as ACE inhibitors and β-blockers. Telmisartan has the longest terminal half-life. Losartan, which is uricosuric, has an active E3174 metabolite that lowers blood pressure. Candesartan cilexetil and olmesartan medoxomil are prodrugs. Food reduces the absorption of valsartan.

ARBs do not reduce blood pressure as much in African American patients as in white patients unless they are combined with a diuretic. Outcomes document a benefit for diabetic nephropathy (losartan and irbesartan), strokes (losartan, candesartan, and eprosartan), heart failure (candesartan and valsartan), postmyocardial infarction with left ventricular dysfunction (valsartan), and left ventricular hypertrophy (losartan). Telmisartan is as effective as enalapril for renoprotection in type 2 diabetes mellitus. Hypertensive diabetic patients with left ventricular hypertrophy had a reduction in total mortality with losartan compared with atenolol. ARBs reduce the rate of development of diabetes. A large outcomes trial is comparing ramipril, telmisartan, or the combination in high-risk patients.

ARBs are additive to diuretics and CCBs; however, there are fewer data on the combination with other antihypertensive agents. The combination of losartan and trandolapril is nephroprotective in nondiabetic renal disease with proteinuria, and candesartan added to an ACE reduces cardiovascular death and heart failure hospitalizations.

The side effects of ARBs are similar to placebo. Angioedema is quite rare. Like ACE inhibitors, ARBs are contraindicated in pregnancy, and increases in serum creatinine and potassium can occur.

## Calcium Channel Blockers

The three classes of CCBs are dihydropyridine (nifedipine and others), benzothiazepine (diltiazem), and phenylalkylamine (verapamil). They block the calcium flux into cells, causing vasodilation. They also cause acute and repetitive natriuresis, inhibit aldosterone, and interfere with $\alpha_2$-stimulated angiotensin II vasoconstriction. The nondihydropyridine CCBs reduce myocardial contractility and alter sinoatrial and atrioventricular conduction. Dihydropyridines have a dose-dependent negative inotropic effect, but this is counterbalanced by systemic vasodilation.

All CCBs have a short duration of action, except amlodipine, and require drug delivery systems to prolong their duration of action. Three CCBs (Covera HS, Verelan PM, Cardizem LA) are chronotherapeutic formulations that are dosed at 10:00 PM and achieve a peak concentration in the early morning hours when most cardiovascular events occur. Intravenous nicardipine is used for hypertensive emergencies without myocardial ischemia. Diltiazem and verapamil can be given intravenously.

CCBs reduce blood pressure in white and African American patients. CCBs are less susceptible to blood pressure attenuation from excessive sodium ingestion and NSAIDs than are other antihypertensive drugs. Nitrendipine decreased strokes in elderly patients with isolated systolic hypertension. The combination of amlodipine and perindopril decreased total mortality when compared with a diuretic and atenolol in an open label, blinded endpoint study.

CCBs are contraindicated in patients with systolic heart failure, acute myocardial infarction, or unstable angina. It is used for cocaine-induced vasospasm and cyclosporine-induced hypertension. Amlodipine offered no protection against hypertensive nephrosclerosis in African American patients or diabetic nephropathy when compared with ARBs or ACE inhibitors. Amlodipine, diltiazem, nicardipine, nifedipine, and verapamil have an indication for stable angina. Diltiazem and verapamil are approved for atrial fibrillation, atrial flutter, and paroxysmal supraventricular tachycardia.

Most drugs are additive to CCBs. The combination of amlodipine and the $\alpha_1$-blocker doxazosin appears to be synergistic. The use of a dihydropyridine and nondihydropyridine CCB is also additive.

Constipation is a dose-dependent side effect of verapamil. Diltiazem can cause sinus bradycardia, peripheral edema, headache, dizziness, asthenia, fatigue, and rash. Dose-dependent peripheral edema with dihydropyridines is not a result of salt and water retention. It is caused by precapillary arterial vasodilation and relative venular constriction and is ameliorated by an ACE inhibitor. Gingival overgrowth and esophageal reflux occur with CCBs.

## $\alpha_1$-Blockers

Norepinephrine interacts with the postsynaptic $\alpha_1$-receptors on vascular smooth muscle cells to cause vasoconstriction. Selective $\alpha_1$-blockers (prazosin, terazosin, and doxazosin) cause venous and arterial dilation. Although tachycardia is unexpected, sodium and water retention can occur. This class of drugs is no longer considered for initial therapy because the Antihypertensive and Lipid-lowering Treatment to Prevent Heart Attack Trial (ALLHAT) observed more heart failure and strokes with doxazosin than with chlorthalidone.

The $\alpha_1$-blockers are additive to most drugs except $\alpha_2$-stimulants. They improve urinary flow with prostatism by lessening urinary sphincter constriction. They reduce LDL cholesterol and triglycerides, increase HDL cholesterol, improve insulin sensitivity, and are unlikely to cause erectile dysfunction.

Volume depletion can produce first-dose hypotension or syncope; thus, slow titration is necessary. If the drug is stopped, retitration is required. Stress urinary incontinence, asthenia, nasal congestion, and priapism are known adverse drug reactions.

### Central α₂-Stimulants

Methyldopa, clonidine, guanabenz, and guanfacine reduce sympathetic outflow from the nucleus tractus solitarii and rostral ventrolateral medulla and decrease norepinephrine and renin. However, high doses paradoxically raise blood pressure by stimulating peripheral α₂-receptors.

This drug class is not recommended as initial therapy for hypertension due to sodium and water retention. These drugs are effective for most patient groups, but they are poorly tolerated. They are ineffective in patients with spinal cord transection. Guanfacine is the longest-acting oral drug. The transdermal clonidine preparation is effective for 7 days, but it requires 3 days initially to achieve adequate blood levels. Methyldopa is safely used for pregnancy-induced hypertension. α₂-Stimulants are additive to diuretics, but they are not additive to α₁-blockers or β-blockers.

Common adverse drug reactions are sedation, erectile dysfunction, dry mouth, dental caries, and periodontal disease. A discontinuation syndrome, characterized by very high blood pressure, tachycardia, tremulousness, and anxiety, is precipitated within 24 to 36 hours after stopping the medication and is magnified with concomitant β-blocker therapy. Bradycardia occurs when used with rate-lowering medications or sick sinus syndrome. Skin irritation or an allergic skin reaction is seen with the transdermal preparation. Hepatotoxicity, Coombs' positive hemolytic anemia, and galactorrhea occur with methyldopa.

### Direct Vasodilators

Hydralazine and minoxidil dilate resistance and capacitance vessels; increase renin, norepinephrine, cardiac output; and cause salt and water retention. Minoxidil is the most potent oral antihypertensive drug and the longest-acting direct vasodilator.

Direct vasodilators are used for refractory hypertension. A diuretic and a heart rate–lowering drug is given as a part of a triple drug regimen. Hydralazine is used safely during pregnancy. The combination of hydralazine and nitrates (BiDil) reduced mortality and heart failure hospitalizations in African Americans with chronic systolic dysfunction.

Hydralazine is inactivated in the liver by acetylation, which has a genetically determined rate. Toxicity is more likely to occur with slow acetylators. The dose is limited to 200 mg/day to avoid a lupus-like reaction, which is characterized by arthralgias, weight loss, splenomegaly, and pleural and pericardial effusions. Minoxidil causes fluid retention, hypertrichosis, and pericardial effusion.

## Other Conditions

### RESISTANT HYPERTENSION

There are a number of reasons why patients fail to achieve blood pressure control with appropriate doses of three antihypertensive drugs. Improper blood pressure measurement from a noncalibrated, inaccurate sphygmomanometer or wrong cuff size is common. Volume overload due to excess sodium intake, excretory failure, and inadequate or improper diuretic dosing are important considerations. Using medications that are not complementary is a common reason for resistant hypertension. Concomitant medications that interfere with antihypertensive drugs or raise blood pressure are listed in Box 3. Consumption of more than 30 grams of ethanol daily raises blood pressure and increases the risk of a stroke. Exogenous obesity and insulin resistance are patient factors associated with resistant hypertension.

Clues to nonadherence are suggested by evasive answers to direct questions about medications, failure to keep appointments, complaints about costs or side effects, and lack of knowledge about medications and their dosing. A simple way to evaluate nonadherence is to bring the patient to the clinic in the morning, observe the patient swallowing the medications, and measure the blood pressure hourly for 5 hours. Assessment of secondary hypertension or noninvasive hemodynamic measurements may be undertaken if the cause of resistant hypertension is not apparent.

---

---

## SECONDARY HYPERTENSION

Age, history, physical examination (see Box 2), severity of hypertension, or initial laboratory studies (see Box 3) provide clues to secondary causes of hypertension. Resistant hypertension, well-controlled blood pressure that increases without explanation, and abrupt-onset hypertension are additional signs.

Chronic kidney disease and renovascular hypertension are the most common etiologies. An abnormal serum creatinine, estimated glomerular filtration rate, or urinary sediment point to renal parenchymal disease. A renal ultrasound may be helpful for further evaluation. Acute or chronic bladder outlet obstruction also elevates blood pressure. In the absence of a family history, onset of hypertension before age 30 years may be from renovascular hypertension due to fibromuscular dysplasia. After age 55 years, atherosclerotic renovascular hypertension should be suspected, especially in tobacco users and with carotid and femoral bruits. Other findings suggestive of renovascular hypertension include an abdominal bruit that has a diastolic component, accelerated hypertension, recurrent flash pulmonary edema, renal failure of uncertain etiology, and acute renal failure precipitated by an ACE inhibitor or

---

 **CURRENT DIAGNOSIS**

- Perform two or three blood measurements on two or more visits to diagnose hypertension.
- Assess the patient with a targeted history, physical examination, and laboratory tests.
- Recognize hypertensive and atherosclerotic target organ involvement.
- Screen for other cardiovascular risk factors.
- Identify comorbid conditions that alter treatment.
- Discover correctable secondary causes of hypertension.

an ARB. A renal arteriogram defines the anatomy of the renal arteries, but it does not say if the anatomic obstruction is causing renovascular hypertension. Captopril renography, duplex Doppler sonography, and magnetic resonance imaging (MRI) are used to screen patients, but they are not always accurate.

There are a number of endocrine causes of hypertension. Hypothyroidism is the most common and causes diastolic hypertension. Hyperthyroidism raises systolic blood pressure. Hyperparathyroidism elevates calcium and parathyroid hormone levels and causes osteopenia and nephrolithiasis. Cushing's syndrome is tested with a dexamethasone suppression test. Increased urinary potassium with low serum potassium suggests hyperaldosteronism. Measuring an elevated 24-hour aldosterone level in a salt-loaded patient and finding suppressed renin levels under conditions of ambulation and sodium depletion locates the defect to the adrenal gland. Paroxysms of hypertension with headache, palpitations, pallor, and perspiration occur in patients with a pheochromocytoma. Orthostatic changes in blood pressure are present. Unless the patient is treated with an α-blocker and is sodium repleted, β-blockers must be avoided because they further elevate blood pressure. Plasma-free metanephrines and fractionated urinary metanephrines are the most sensitive tests. Inaccurate results may be due to comorbid conditions or concomitant medications. MRI can help locate the tumor. [131]I-meta-iodobenzylguanidine concentrates in up to 85% of tumors.

Diminished and delayed pulses in the right femoral artery compared with the right brachial artery, the presence of a systolic murmur over the anterior chest, bruits over the back, and visible notching of the posterior ribs on a chest x-ray are important clues of aortic coarctation. If the obstruction occurs before the left subclavian artery, systolic blood pressure is higher in the right arm than the left arm, and there is a decreased or absent left brachial pulse. A transesophageal echocardiogram can be used to confirm the diagnosis.

## HYPERTENSIVE EMERGENCIES

A hypertensive emergency is defined as a blood pressure greater than 180/120 mm Hg and the presence of ongoing vascular damage. Cardiac causes include unstable angina pectoris, acute myocardial infarction, aortic dissection, and acute pulmonary edema. Cerebrovascular causes are hypertensive encephalopathy, ischemic stroke, intracerebral hemorrhage, and subarachnoid hemorrhage. Eclampsia is another cause.

These patients are admitted to an intensive care unit for continuous monitoring of blood pressure, volume status, urinary output, electrocardiogram, and mental status. Intravenous medication should be titrated to reduce mean arterial pressure 15% to 25%. An attempt to normalize blood pressure can cause coronary, cerebral, and renal ischemia. However, for aortic dissection patients, systolic blood pressure is lowered to 100 mm Hg with sodium nitroprusside after the heart rate is reduced with β-blockers, unless myocardial or cerebral

ischemia limits the goal. The treatment of blood pressure with ischemic strokes is very controversial among neurologists.

Intravenous nitroglycerin is needed for coronary ischemia. Nitroprusside is an ideal agent for most hypertensive emergencies because it is titratable and hypotension resolves within 2 minutes of stopping the infusion. It is given at 0.3 μg/kg/min with the head of the bed elevated. If dosed at < 2 μg/kg/min, cyanide toxicity is unlikely. Fenoldopam, a dopamine-1 receptor agonist, is advocated when renal insufficiency prevents the use of nitroprusside. Esmolol is helpful for aortic dissections and perioperative hypertension. Intravenous hydralazine and magnesium sulfate are given for eclampsia.

Asymptomatic patients with very high blood pressure and no evidence of ongoing vascular damage do not require immediate normalization of blood pressure. Drug therapy is initiated, and the patient is scheduled for an evaluation in 1 week.

## REFERENCES

Calhoun DA, Zaman MA, Nishizaka MK: Resistant hypertension. Curr Hypertens Rep 2002;4:221-228.

Chobanian AV, Bakris GL, Black HR, et al: Seventh report of the Joint National Committee on Prevention, Detection, Evaluation, and Treatment of High Blood Pressure. Hypertension 2003;42:1206-1252.

Pickering TG, Hall JE, Appel LJ, et al: Recommendations for blood pressure measurement in humans and experimental animals: Part 1: Blood pressure measurement in humans: A statement for professionals from the Subcommittee of Professional and Public Education of the American Heart Association Council on High Blood Pressure Research. Hypertension 2005;45:142-161.

Prisant LM (ed): Hypertension in the Elderly. Totowa, NJ: Humana Press, 2005.

Prisant LM: Hypertensive heart disease. J Clin Hypertens (Greenwich) 2005;7:231-238.

Prisant LM: Pharmacology of antihypertensive drugs. In Weir MR (ed): Hypertension. Philadelphia: American College of Physicians, 2005, pp 85-114.

Prisant LM: Nutritional treatment of blood pressure: Major nonpharmacologic trials of prevention or treatment of hypertension. In Berdanier CD (ed): CRC Handbook of Nutrition and Food. Boca Raton, FL: CRC Press, 2002, pp 999-1010.

Taler SJ, Textor SC, Augustine JE: Resistant hypertension: Comparing hemodynamic management to specialist care. Hypertension 2002;39:982-988.

---

### C CURRENT THERAPY

- Choose initial antihypertensive medication based on age, race, target organ damage, and coexisting illnesses.
- Question patients about adverse drug reactions before initiating therapy and during follow-up visits.
- Titrate the initial drug choice once or twice at 4- to 6-week intervals.
- Use additional complementary medications to reach blood pressure treatment goals.
- Target a blood pressure of 130/80 mm Hg for diabetes mellitus and chronic kidney disease and 140/90 mm Hg for all other patients.
- Investigate over-the-counter, herbal, and prescribed (including ophthalmic) medications for possible pharmacokinetic and pharmacodynamic interactions with antihypertensive drugs.

# Acute Myocardial Infarction

Method of
*Kevin A. Bybee, MD,*
*and Stephen L. Kopecky, MD*

During the 20th century, acute myocardial infarction (AMI) became the leading cause of death in the United States and in other developed regions of the world including Europe. Individual mortality rates from AMI have recently decreased in both men and women because of modern therapeutic advances and increasing public awareness of AMI symptoms and the need for emergent evaluation. Despite advances in the diagnosis and treatment of AMI, however, it will likely remain the leading cause of death well into the future, given the aging of the population and the increasing prevalence of type II diabetes mellitus. Information obtained from clinical trials has revolutionized the modern approach to patients with AMI, emphasizing early and accurate diagnosis, early risk stratification, and prompt reperfusion therapy in those with ST-segment-elevation myocardial infarction (STEMI).

## Diagnosis

In 2000 the American College of Cardiology (ACC) and the European Society of Cardiology (ESC) issued a joint recommendation that redefines the diagnosis of AMI, thus replacing the World Health

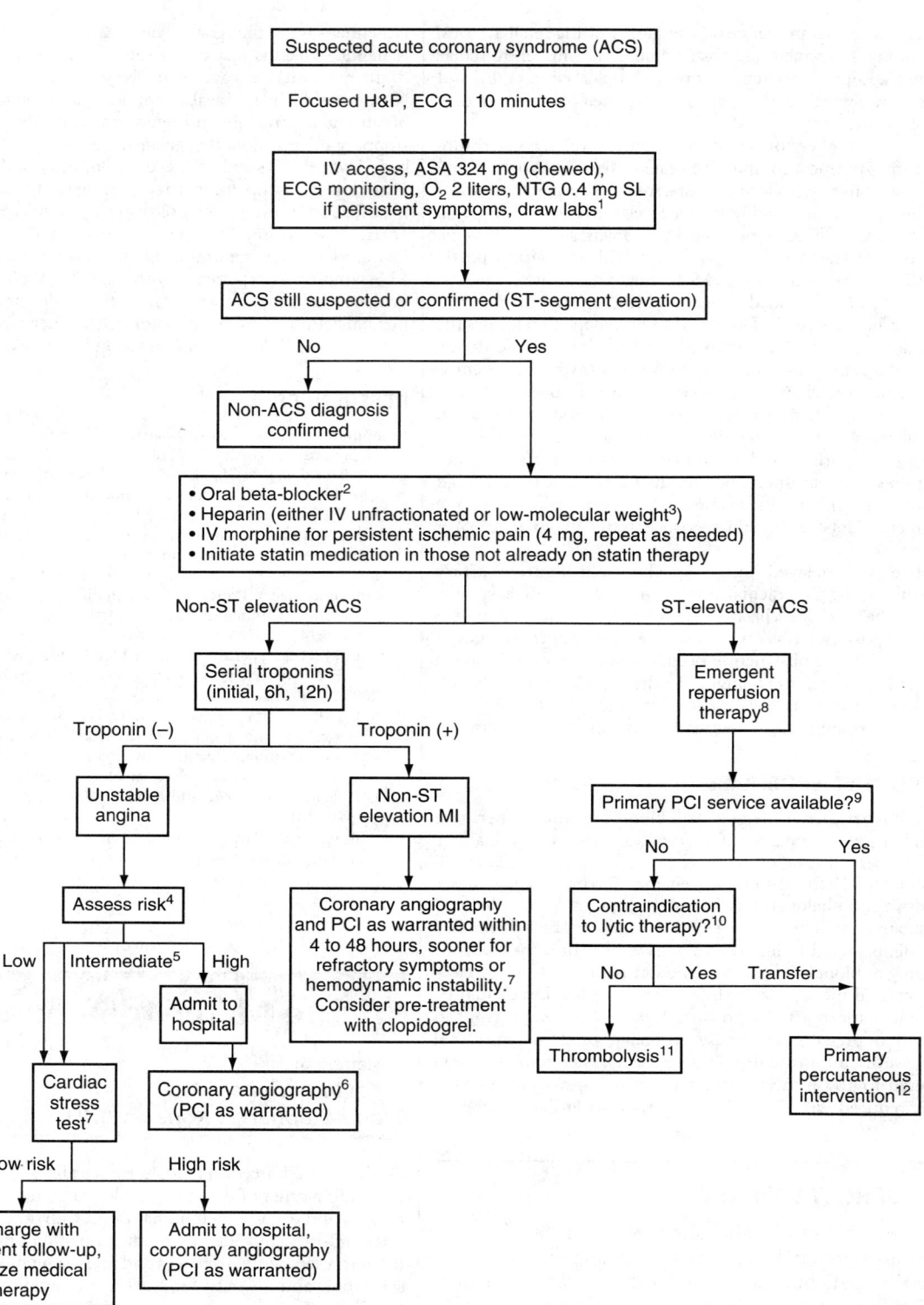

**FIGURE 1.** Algorithm for evaluation and treatment of patients with suspected acute coronary syndromes. ACS = acute coronary syndrome; ALT = alanine amino transferase; ASA = aspirin; CBC = complete blood count; CXR = chest radiograph; ECG = electrocardiogram; H&P = history and physical; IV = intravenous; MI = myocardial infarction; NSTEMI = non-ST-segment-elevation myocardial infarction; NTG = nitroglycerin; PCI = percutaneous coronary intervention; SL = sublingual.

[1]Troponin, CBC , electrolytes, creatinine, ALT, CXR.

[2]Reserve IV beta-blocker therapy for those patients with other indications for IV beta-blocker therapy.

[3]Low-molecular-weight heparin appears superior to IV unfractionated heparin in patients with unstable angina with high risk features and those with NSTEMI. Some interventionists prefer IV unfractionated heparin in patients undergoing coronary angiography/PCI.

[4]See Table 1 for risk assessment.

[5]For intermediate-risk patients, consider risk stratification if the chest pain unit is available.

[6]Consider addition of glycoprotein (GP) IIb/IIIa inhibitor. GP IIa/IIIb inhibitor can be initiated upon admission or just prior to PCI in the cardiac catheterization laboratory.

Organization definition. The ACC/ESC definition requires the typical rise and fall of troponin or more rapid rise and fall of creatinine kinase myocardial band (CK-MB) in addition to one of the following:

- Symptoms consistent with myocardial ischemia
- Electrocardiogram (ECG) changes indicating myocardial ischemia (ST-segment depression or elevation)
- New pathologic Q waves
- Percutaneous coronary intervention (PCI)

Pathologic findings of AMI at autopsy are also considered diagnostic. Additionally, any patient presenting with a clinical history consistent with AMI and new left bundle branch block should be triaged as STEMI. Based on the ACC/ESC guidelines, as well as recommendations issued by the ACC and American Heart Association (AHA) in 2002, differentiating between unstable angina (UA) and non-ST-segment-elevation myocardial infarction (NSTEMI) is based on whether biomarkers of myocardial injury are elevated, denoting myocardial necrosis. Detectable elevations of troponin and CK-MB may not be apparent in those who present within the first 4 to 6 hours following symptom onset. Thus distinguishing between UA and NSTEMI may not be possible at the time of initial evaluation and may require serial measurements of cardiac biomarkers.

## PATHOPHYSIOLOGY

AMI occurs when myocardial necrosis results from prolonged myocardial ischemia. Acute coronary syndromes (ACS) represent a spectrum of clinical presentations including UA, NSTEMI, and STEMI. Despite this spectrum of presentations, the underlying pathophysiologic mechanisms are similar in most cases. The most common initiating mechanism responsible for AMI is acute plaque rupture, with subsequent exposure of thrombogenic substances with the lipid-laden plaque core to circulating blood and consequent coronary thrombus formation. STEMI is almost always a result of complete thrombotic coronary occlusion. Subtotal coronary occlusion often results in UA or NSTEMI. Myocardial necrosis in the setting of NSTEMI may result from transient complete coronary occlusion with spontaneous partial recanalization, persistent near-complete coronary occlusion, and distal embolization of plaque debris and platelet-rich thrombi with associated vascular spasm. Most plaque ruptures involve relatively small, vulnerable nonobstructive coronary plaques. Studies using intravascular ultrasound document the presence of multiple ruptured plaques in many patients presenting with AMI. AMI can also result from endothelial erosion and in situations of prolonged increases in myocardial oxygen demand in the setting of a stable, yet high-grade coronary lesion. Other rare mechanisms of AMI include coronary artery spasm, coronary artery embolism, coronary artery dissection, and coronary injury from trauma.

## HISTORY

Initial assessment of patients with suspected ACS should begin with a focused history, physical examination, and 12-lead ECG (Figure 1). Patients with AMI can present with a variety of symptoms—from crushing substernal chest pain to no pain at all. This variability in symptoms can make initial diagnosis challenging in some patients and reinforces the importance of physicians remaining astute. The discomfort classically associated with AMI is described as a crushing, squeezing, or tightness in the anterior left chest. These symptoms can radiate to the jaw, teeth, shoulders, arms, and back and usually last for at least 20 minutes. Older (age >75 years) patients, diabetics, and female patients are more likely to present with dyspnea as their primary symptom. Patients with AMI usually do not have pleuritic chest pain, which suggests an alternative diagnosis such as pericarditis, pulmonary embolism, pneumothorax, or pneumonia. Patients with tearing pain may have aortic dissection.

## PHYSICAL EXAMINATION

The physical examination usually does not help significantly in the diagnosis of AMI, but it does it aid in the risk stratification of patients with suspected AMI and in an evaluation for non-AMI etiologies responsible for patient symptoms. Hemodynamic stability should be assessed. Evaluation of jugular venous pressure and wave form can give clues to right ventricular infarction and right atrial pressure as well as indirect information about left heart function and intravascular volume status. Lung evaluation should note the presence of rales, indicating left heart failure. Cardiac palpation can give clues to underlying cardiomyopathy. A soft $S_1$ suggests reduced left ventricle (LV) systolic function or first-degree atrioventricular (AV) block. A holosystolic murmur could indicate mitral regurgitation resulting from ischemic papillary muscle dysfunction or ventricular septal defect. An $S_4$ gallop is often present, indicating abnormal left ventricular relaxation, whereas an $S_3$ gallop suggests elevated left ventricular end-diastolic pressure. Hypotension at the time of presentation is usually caused by large areas of ischemic myocardium. Hypotension and rales greater than one third of the lung field are indicators of increased morbidity and mortality during hospitalization. Unstable patients should also be assessed for mechanical complications of AMI such as papillary muscle rupture, ventricular septal defect, and left ventricular free-wall rupture.

Alternative etiologies responsible for the patient's presentation should also be sought during the physical examination. Symmetry of pulses in all extremities and symmetry of blood pressure in both arms should be assessed in evaluating for aortic dissection. A pericardial rub suggests pericarditis, whereas a pleural rub suggests pulmonary embolism or pneumonia. Palpation of the chest wall may be helpful in identifying musculoskeletal etiologies. However, for unclear reasons, patients with documented AMI may have increased pain with chest wall palpation.

## ELECTROCARDIOGRAM

The initial ECG plays an important role in the diagnosis, risk stratification, and management of patients with AMI and should be performed on all patients with chest pain and/or dyspnea immediately upon presentation. Patients presenting with AMI should be classified as non-ST-elevation ACS or ST-segment-elevation ACS. This nomenclature is preferred because ST-segment elevation at the time of presentation indicates ongoing myocardial injury and identifies patients who can benefit from prompt reperfusion therapy. The ECG is normal at the time of presentation in 10% of patients with AMI and therefore should be used as a supportive tool in addition to the clinical history, physical examination, and laboratory evaluation.

---

[7]Exercise electrocardiogram preferred; exercise imaging study if baseline ST changes present or if patient is on digoxin; pharmacologic imaging study if unable to walk on treadmill to acceptable workload.

[8]Administer reperfusion therapy if symptom onset within 12 hours. Refer for coronary angiography if symptom onset more than 12 hours and persistent chest symptoms or hemodynamic instability.

[9]Can consider transport to primary PCI facility if door-to-balloon time still less than 90 minutes.

[10]See Table 2 for absolute and relative contraindications to thrombolytic therapy.

[11]Door-to-needle time should be less than 30 minutes.

[12]Door-to-balloon time should be less than 90 minutes; goal is less than 60 minutes.

## TABLE 1   Infarct-Related Artery and Associated Distribution of Electrocardiographic ST-Segment Elevation

| Location of Coronary Occlusion | Distribution of ST-Segment Elevation | 30-Day Mortality with Successful Reperfusion* |
|---|---|---|
| Proximal LAD (proximal to first septal perforator) | $V_1$-$V_6$, aVL, I, new LBBB common | 19.6% |
| Mid-LAD (distal to first septal perforator and proximal to first large diagonal branch) | $V_1$-$V_6$, aVL, I, | 9.2% |
| Distal LAD (distal to first large diagonal branch) or diagonal branch | $V_1$-$V_4$, or aVL, I, $V_{5-6}$ | 6.8% |
| Right coronary artery | II, III, aVF, $V_{5-6}$ ($V_3$R, $V_4$R with RV infarction) | 6.4% |
| Left circumflex | $V_{5-6}$, III, II, aVF (can have minimal ECG changes) | 4.5% |

*Derived from Global Utilization of Streptokinase and t-PA for Occluded Coronary Arteries-I (GUSTO-I) cohort population of patients receiving successful reperfusion therapy.
*Abbreviations:* ECG = electrocardiogram; LAD = left anterior descending; LBBB = left bundle branch block; RV = right ventricle.

### ST-Segment-Elevation Myocardial Infarction

STEMI is characterized by at least 1 mm of ST-segment elevation in two or more contiguous ECG leads. Reciprocal ST-segment depression may be present in leads remote from those with ST elevation and is associated with higher risk. The distribution of ST-segment elevation on the ECG can give clues to the coronary artery responsible for the ischemia (Table 1). A right-sided ECG should be obtained in all patients with inferior STEMI to evaluate for evidence of right ventricular infarction manifest by ST-segment elevation in lead $V_3$R and/or $V_4$R. Marked ST depression in leads $V_1$ to $V_3$ is the hallmark of acute posterior infarction, which can be confirmed by ST-segment elevation in posteriorly placed leads ($V_7$R to $V_9$R), and should be treated as an STEMI. Patients presenting with symptoms consistent with AMI and a new left bundle branch block should be triaged and managed as an STEMI.

Other disease entities with associated ST-segment elevation should be kept in mind when assessing a patient with suspected STEMI. These include pericarditis, myocarditis, left ventricular aneurysm, early repolarization, coronary artery spasm, intracranial bleeding, head trauma, and transient left ventricular apical ballooning syndrome.

### Non-ST-Segment-Elevation Myocardial Infarction

Patients with NSTEMI can present with marked or minimal ST-segment depression, isolated T wave changes, or with no ST-segment or T wave changes at all. ST-segment depression identifies patients at higher risk who subsequently benefit most from an aggressive management strategy.

### BIOMARKERS OF CARDIAC INJURY

Because of their high sensitivity and specificity for myocardial necrosis, cardiac troponin T and troponin I assays are preferred in the initial evaluation of patients with suspected AMI. Detectable troponin elevations usually occur 3 to 6 hours following onset of myocardial necrosis and thus may not be abnormal at the time of initial presentation. As a result, troponin may not be useful in the early diagnosis of STEMI and is most helpful in discerning UA and NSTEMI. Troponin remains elevated for 7 to 14 days following AMI.

Creatine kinase (CK) and CK-MB are less sensitive and less specific for myocardial necrosis. Elevated CK levels are detectable 4 to 6 hours following AMI and peak around 24 hours following the onset of necrosis. CK concentrations return to normal by 72 hours and thus may be useful in the diagnosis of reinfarction. CK-MB is not entirely specific for myocardial muscle and can be elevated in situations of skeletal muscle, bowel, and prostate injury.

## Risk Stratification

Several characteristics are associated with a worse prognosis in patients with unstable angina (Table 2), NSTEMI, and STEMI, including advanced age, female gender, hemodynamic alterations (hypotension, tachycardia), left heart failure (pulmonary rales, S3 gallop, elevated BNP [brain natriuretic peptide]), cumulative extent of ST-segment deviation, new bundle branch block, proximal or mid-LAD (left anterior descending coronary artery) occlusion, aspirin use at the time of AMI, elevated C-reactive protein, diabetes mellitus, prior myocardial infarction or prior coronary artery bypass grafting, concomitant peripheral vascular disease, and underlying renal insufficiency. The thrombolysis in myocardial infarction (TIMI) risk scores for STEMI and NSTEMI are prognostically useful (Tables 3 and 4). Intermediate-risk UA patients may be risk stratified over 6 to 9 hours with serial biomarkers and an exercise ECG. If biomarkers become positive or the stress test is positive, the patient should be admitted. If negative, the patient should be dismissed with follow-up in 72 hours for re-evaluation and coronary artery disease (CAD) risk factor modification.

## Treatment

The goals of initial treatment of patients presenting with AMI are:

- Obtain intravenous (IV) access and stabilize hemodynamics if unstable.
- Relieve ischemic discomfort using IV morphine and sublingual or IV nitroglycerin.
- Minimize myocardial oxygen supply-and-demand mismatch with IV β-blockers (goal: heart rate less than 70 beats per minute as blood pressure tolerates) and supplemental oxygen.
- Maintain or restore myocardial perfusion using aspirin and heparin (either IV unfractionated or subcutaneous low molecular weight).

Patients with STEMI should receive prompt reperfusion therapy (thrombolysis or primary percutaneous intervention). Table 5 outlines the recommended dosing regimens of medications commonly used in ACS.

### Aspirin

All patients presenting with a proved or suspected AMI should receive 324 mg of aspirin (four 81 mg tablets chewed and swallowed or as a rectal suppository if unable to take orally) and continue at 81 mg daily thereafter. Aspirin significantly reduces mortality in AMI. In patients with STEMI, aspirin reduces mortality to a similar extent as thrombolytic therapy, with additive benefits of both. Aspirin-allergic patients should receive 300 mg of clopidogrel (Plavix).

### Clopidogrel

Clopidogrel (Plavix) blocks the platelet ADP receptor and can be given in place of aspirin in aspirin-allergic patients. A 300-mg loading dose

## TABLE 2  Risk Stratification in Patients With Unstable Angina

| High Risk (20% Event Rate*) | Intermediate Risk (~6% Event Rate*) | Low Risk (~<1% Event Rate*) |
|---|---|---|
| Presence of at least one of the following: | No *high-risk* features but at least one of the following: | No *high intermediate risk* features but may present with one of the following: |
| - Acceleration of ischemic symptoms in last 48 h<br>- Ongoing rest pain > 20 min<br>- Age >75 y<br>- New or worsening MR murmur<br>- Pulmonary edema or evidence of worsening heart failure.<br>- Hemodynamic instability<br>- Rest angina associated with dynamic ST-segment deviation >0.05 mV<br>- New bundle branch block<br>- Ventricular tachycardia | - Known atherosclerotic vascular disease (prior MI/PCI/CABG, peripheral, cerebrovascular)<br>- Rest pain (>20 min) now resolved with moderate or high likelihood of CAD<br>- Rest angina <20 min relieved with NTG<br>- Age >70 y<br>- Prior aspirin usage<br>- T wave inversions > 0.2 mV<br>- Q waves | - New-onset angina within 2 wk to 2 mo<br>- Increasing frequency of exertional angina without rest pain.<br>- Normal or unchanged ECG |

*Risk for death, unfatal MI at 6 months.
*Abbreviations:* CABG = coronary artery bypass graft; CAD = coronary arterial disease; ECG = electrocardiogram; MI = myocardial infarction; MR = mitral regurgitation; MV = millivolt; NTG = nitroglycerin; PCI = percutaneous coronary intervention.

is administered with 75 mg daily administered thereafter. We prefer to administer 600 mg clopidogrel in ACS patients who are expected to have PCI within 6 hours of initial medical contact; otherwise, we give 300 mg on admission. The 600-mg dose of clopidogrel has been shown to shorten the time to attainment of maximal platelet inhibition. Clopidogrel is as efficacious as aspirin in AMI. Clopidogrel is beneficial in those undergoing primary percutaneous intervention for STEMI. Clopidogrel in addition to aspirin, compared with aspirin alone, reduces the risk of cardiovascular death, myocardial infarction, or stroke in patients with NSTEMI who do not undergo percutaneous revascularization (CURE [Clopidogrel in Unstable Angina to Prevent Recurrent Events] trial) and in those who do undergo percutaneous revascularization (PCI-CURE [Percutaneous Coronary Intervention-Clopidogrel in Unstable Angina to Prevent Recurrent Ischemic Events] and CREDO [Clopidogrel for the Reduction of Events During Observation] trials). The decision to give clopidogrel prior to coronary angiography in patients with AMI should take into account the ultimate requirement of coronary artery bypass graft (CABG) in some patients, which would delay CABG for 5 to 7 days following the administration of clopidogrel. Clopidogrel, 75 mg daily, should be continued for at least 9, and preferably, 12 months following percutaneous coronary revascularization in the setting of AMI. If coronary angiography is not anticipated, clopidogrel should be initiated and also continued for 9 to 12 months. A recent study suggests that clopidogrel imparts incremental benefit when given in combination with thrombolytic therapy in the setting of STEMI.

### Heparin

Patients presenting with AMI should be treated with either IV unfractionated heparin (IVUFH) (60 IU/kg bolus, then 12 IU/kg per hour infusion) or subcutaneous low-molecular-weight heparin (LMWH), except for STEMI patients receiving streptokinase. In STEMI, IVUFH is required to maintain vessel patency in those receiving a fibrin-specific thrombolytic agent (alteplase, reteplase, and tenecteplase). The use of LMWH in combination with thrombolytic therapy is still being evaluated in clinical trials and is not currently recommended. Administration of LMWH reduces the risk of death and ischemic events compared with IVUFH in patients with NSTEMI and in unstable angina when high-risk features are present (see Table 2). LMWH appears safe when continued up until the time of coronary angiography and percutaneous intervention; however, individual PCI operator preference should be taken into account. LMWH should not be given to patients with significant renal insufficiency (creatinine clearance less than 30 mL per minute) or morbid obesity.

### β-Blockers

All patients with suspected or confirmed AMI should receive prompt oral β-blocker therapy, which should be continued indefinitely in the absence of contraindications. We prefer metoprolol in the acute setting given its relatively short half-life compared with atenolol. Intravenous β-blockers should be reserved for patients with an urgent indication

## TABLE 3  TIMI Risk Score for Unstable Angina/Non-ST-Segment-Elevation Myocardial Infarction

| One Point for Each of the Following: | Score | Risk of Adverse Event* |
|---|---|---|
| Age ≥65 y | 0/1 | 4.7% |
| Presence of ≥3 CV risk factors[†] | 2 | 8.3% |
| Recent (<24 h) severe angina | 3 | 13.2% |
| Known coronary stenosis ≥50% | 4 | 19.9% |
| ST-segment deviation on admission ECG ≥0.5 mm | 5 | 26.2% |
| Use of aspirin within past 7 d | 6/7 | 40.9% |
| Elevated biomarkers of cardiac injury (troponin, CK-MB) | | |

*Death, MI, or urgent revascularization within 14 days.
[†]Family history of premature coronary artery disease, hypertension, hyperlipidemia, diabetes mellitus, active smoker.
*Abbreviations:* CV = cardiovascular; ECG = electrocardiogram.

## TABLE 4 TIMI Risk Score for ST-Segment-Elevation Myocardial Infarction

| Risk Factor | Points | Score | 30-Day Mortality (%) |
|---|---|---|---|
| Age ≥75 y | 3 | 0 | 0.8 |
| Age 65-74 y | 2 | 1 | 1.6 |
| Systolic BP <100 mm Hg | 3 | 2 | 2.2 |
| Heart rate >100 beats/min | 2 | 3 | 4.4 |
| Killip class >1 | 2 | 4 | 7.3 |
| Anterior MI or LBBB | 1 | 5 | 12.4 |
| Diabetes mellitus, HTN, or angina | 1 | 6 | 16.1 |
| Weight <67 kg | 1 | 7 | 23.4 |
| Symptom onset to treatment >4 h | 1 | 8 | 26.8 |
| | | >8 | 35.9 |

*Abbreviations:* BP = blood pressure; HTN = hypertension; LBBB = left bundle branch block; MI = myocardial infarction.

for intravenous β-blockade such as those with a concomitant supraventicular tachyarrhythmia. Routine intravenous β-blocker administration in those with AMI has been associated with worse outcomes, including higher rates of heart failure. β-Blockers are beneficial in AMI due to their ability to reduce oxygen supply-and-demand mismatch by lowering heart rate, reducing myocardial contractility, and reducing afterload through systemic blood pressure reduction. In addition to reducing mortality in AMI, oral β-blockers also reduce the risk of atrial and ventricular tachyarrythmias and reduce the risk of mechanical complications such as free wall rupture.

### Nitroglycerin

Nitroglycerin can be administered as a sublingual formulation or as an IV infusion and is given if symptoms of ongoing myocardial ischemia persist. Nitroglycerin does not improve prognosis in AMI and should be used with caution in patients with right ventricular infarction that could result in hypotension. Nitroglycerin should not be administered to patients who have taken Viagra or other phosphodiesterase inhibitor within 24 hours.

### Glycoprotein IIb/IIIa Inhibitors

Glycoprotein (GP) IIb/IIIa inhibitors block the GP IIb/IIIa platelet receptor, which functions as the receptor for fibrinogen adherence.

GP IIb/IIIa inhibitors reduce ischemic complications associated with PCI and should be administered in patients for whom an early invasive strategy is planned. It is not clear if upstream GP IIb/IIIa administration upon admission is superior to initiation in the catheterization laboratory just prior to PCI. Benefit is shown with eptifibatide (Integrilin) and tirofiban (Aggrastat) in patients with non-ST-elevation ACS who do not undergo early PCI. This benefit appears isolated to high-risk patients including those with troponin elevation, ST-segment depression more than 0.5 mV, diabetes mellitus, and LV ejection fraction less than 40%. Post hoc analyses suggest a potential differential benefit of GP IIb/IIIa therapy in men versus women, and it is an area of continued investigation.

### HMG-CoA Reductase Inhibitors (Statins)

Early, aggressive statin therapy in patients with AMI has been shown to improve early clinical outcomes. Two large randomized trials have demonstrated a clinical benefit in patients randomized to atorvastain 80 mg soon after presentation with AMI. The PROVE-IT (Pravastatin or Atorvastatin Evaluation and Infection Therapy) trial showed that intensive atorvastatin therapy with 80 mg daily (mean LDL [low-density lipoprotein]: 62 mg/dL) initiated following ACS significantly reduces adverse cardiac events compared with less intensive statin therapy using pravastatin 40 mg daily (mean LDL: 95 mg/dL). A recently published randomized trail (ARMYDA-ACS) demonstrated that

## TABLE 5 Dosage of Medications Commonly Used in the Treatment of Myocardial Infarction

| Medication | Dosing and Administration |
|---|---|
| **Aspirin** | • 324 mg chewed and swallowed (81 mg × 4) upon presentation, then 81 to 325 mg daily.<br>• If unable to take PO, crush and administer via NG tube or as 325-mg rectal suppository. |
| **Clopidogrel (Plavix)** | • 300-mg oral loading dose, then 75 mg PO daily for 9 to 12 mo or indefinitely in high-risk patients. |
| **Heparin**<br>• IV unfractionated | • 60 U/kg IV bolus (max: 5000 U), then 12 U/kg/h (max: 1000 U/h) for 48 h or PCI (goal aPTT 1.5 = 2.5 × control). |
| • Low-molecular-weight<br>  Enoxaparin (Lovenox)<br>  (Dalteparin (Fragmin) | • 1 mg/kg SC Q12 h for 48 to 72 h or until PCI. Initial 30-mg IV bolus can be given.<br>• 120 IU/kg SC (max 10,000 IU) Q12 h. |
| **β-Blockers**<br>• Metoprolol (Lopressor)<br>• Atenolol (Tenormin)<br>• Esmolol (Brevibloc) | • 5 mg IV Q5 min × 3 to goal heart rate 60-65/min or hypotension, then 50 mg PO Q12 h.<br>• 5 mg IV Q5 min × 3 to goal heart rate 60-65/min or hypotension, then 50-100 mg PO daily.<br>• 500 μg/kg IV bolus, then 50 μg/kg/min titrating to HR. |
| **Nitroglycerin** | 0.4 mg sublingual Q5 min × 3 for persistent ischemic pain or IV infusion starting at 5-10 μg/min with up titration for persistent ischemic pain. |
| **Morphine sulfate** | 4 to 6 mg IV; repeat as needed. |
| **GP IIb/IIIa inhibitors**<br>• Eptifibatide (Integrelin)<br>• Tirofiban (Aggrastat)<br>• Abciximab (ReoPro) | • 180 μg/kg IV bolus, then infuse at 2.0 μg/kg/min × 72 h to 96 h<br>• 0.4 μg/kg/min IV for 30 min, then 0.1 μg/kg/min × 48 to 96 h<br>• Use ony if PCI planned or likely; 0.25 mg/kg bolus followed by infusion at 0.125 μg/kg/min (max 10 μg/min) for 12 to 24 h. |

*Abbreviations:* IV = intravenous; HR = heart rate; NG = nasogastric; PCI = percutaneous coronary intervention; PO = by mouth; SC = subcutaneous.

**TABLE 6** Thrombolytic Agents

| Thrombolytic | Dosing/Administration | Fibrin Specific |
|---|---|---|
| Alteplase (t-PA) (Activase) | 15 mg IV bolus, then 0.75 mg/kg over 30 min (max 50 mg), then 0.5 mg/kg over 60 min (max 35 mg) | Yes |
| Reteplase (rPA) (Retevase) | 10 U IV bolus over 2 min, then second 10-U IV bolus 30 min later | Yes |
| Tenecteplase (TNK) (TNKase) | 0.5 mg/kg single IV bolus (max 50 mg), or weight <60 kg, 30 mg; 60-69 kg, 35 mg; 70-79 kg, 40 mg; 80-89 kg, 45 mg; ≥90 kg, 50 mg | Yes |
| Streptokinase (Streptase) | 1.5 million U IV over 60 min | Yes |

*Abbreviation:* IV = intravenous.

pretreatment of ACS patients with atorvastatin 80 mg 12 hours prior to PCI conferred an 88% reduction in 30-day major adverse cardiac events and significantly reduced peri-procedural MI rates. We administer immediate aggressive statin therapy to all patients presenting with suspected ACS/AMI.

## REPERFUSION THERAPY IN ST-SEGMENT-ELEVATION MYOCARDIAL INFARCTION

Patients presenting with STEMI represent a true medical emergency and require accurate, yet expeditious evaluation and treatment directed at reperfusion of ischemic myocardium. Regardless of the modality of reperfusion used, the time from symptom onset to establishment of myocardial reperfusion is the strongest predictor of myocardial salvage, recovery of myocardial function, and reperfusion-mediated improvements in mortality. Patients receiving successful reperfusion within 2 hours of symptom onset derive the greatest benefit from reperfusion therapy.

### Thrombolysis

Thrombolytic therapy is the most commonly utilized method of reperfusion worldwide. The fibrin-specific t-PA derived thrombolytic agents (alteplase [Activase], reteplase [Retavase], and tenecteplase [TNKase]) have proved superior but significantly more expensive than the fibrin-nonspecific agents such as streptokinase. The fibrin-specific agents reduce 30-day mortality rates by 15% compared with streptokinase and appear to provide similar rates of successful reperfusion and mortality reduction. They differ primarily in the manner in which they are given and subsequently the ease of administration (Table 6). Clinically, successful thrombolysis is associated with resolution of chest symptoms and reduction of ST-segment elevation by at least 50%. Patients with persistent symptoms, persistence of ST-segment elevation, and/or hemodynamic instability following thrombolysis should be referred for emergent coronary angiography. The absence of contraindications to thrombolytic therapy should be assured prior to administration (Box 1).

The benefit of routine predischarge coronary angiography in patients with apparent successful thrombolysis has been shown to be beneficial in a recent randomized trial. Patients who successfully reperfuse following thrombolysis and do not undergo in-hospital coronary angiography should undergo a submaximal exercise stress test or pharmacologic stress test prior to hospital discharge. Patients with an abnormal predischarge stress test, recurrent symptoms, or ECG changes, and those with an LV ejection fraction less than 40%, should undergo coronary angiography with PCI as warranted prior to discharge.

### Early Invasive Versus Conservative Therapy in Unstable Angina/Non-ST-Segment-Elevation Myocardial Infarction

Patients with NSTEMI usually do not have complete occlusion of the culprit coronary artery. Thus emergent revascularization is generally not indicated except in patients with hemodynamic instability or persistent symptoms despite initial medical therapy. Whether or not patients with UA/NSTEMI benefit from an early invasive approach (i.e., routine coronary angiography and PCI as indicated during hospitalization) was evaluated in three studies using modern antithrombotic/antiplatelet therapy and current PCI technology. The FRISC II (Fragmin and Fast Revascularization During Instability in Coronary Artery Disease), TACTICS-TIMI 18 (Treat Angina With Aggrastat and Determine Cost of Therapy With Invasive or Conservative Strategy-Thrombolysis in Myocardial Infarction), and RITA 3 (Randomized Intervention Trial of Unstable Angina 3) trials demonstrate improved outcomes with an early invasive strategy in intermediate- and high-risk patients with unstable angina and in patients with NSTEMI. In response to the accumulating data demonstrating a benefit from an early invasive approach using contemporary medical management and modern interventional techniques, the ACC/AHA guidelines now recommend an early invasive approach in patients with NSTEMI.

## ELECTRICAL COMPLICATIONS ASSOCIATED WITH ACUTE MYOCARDIAL INFARCTION

Conduction abnormalities are common in patients with AMI and should be assessed in all patients. Ischemia-mediated alterations in cardiac conduction can manifest as AV block (first, second, and third degree), bundle branch block, and fascicular block.

---

**BOX 1 Contraindications for Thrombolytic Administration**

**Absolute**
- Prior intracranial hemorrhage
- Ischemic stroke within prior 3 mo
- Ongoing active bleeding (not including menses)
- Significant head injury or facial trauma within 3 mo
- Possible or suspected aortic dissection
- Intracranial neoplasm
- Intracranial vascular structural abnormality

**Relative**
- Recent internal bleeding (within 4 wk)
- Major surgery within 3 wk
- History of ischemic stroke
- Traumatic or prolonged (>10 min) CPR
- Pregnancy
- Current use of warfarin (Coumadin) with INR >2.0
- Noncompressible vascular puncture
- Significant hypertension on presentation (SBP >180 mm Hg or DBP >110 mm Hg)
- History of chronic, severe, poorly controlled hypertension
- Active peptic ulcer disease
- Prior streptokinase exposure (for repeat streptokinase administration)

*Abbreviations:* CPR = cardiopulmonary resuscitation; DBP = diastolic blood pressure; INR = international normalized ratio; SBP = systolic blood pressure.

**TABLE 7** Treatment of Ventricular Arrhythmias Associated With Acute Myocardial Infarction

| Arrhythmia | Electrical Shock* | Other Therapeutic Measures |
|---|---|---|
| Sustained polymorphic VT | Yes, 200 J, 300 J, 360 J | As per current ACLS recommendations<br>Normalize electrolyte abnormalities |
| Sustained monomorphic VT: with symptoms or hemodynamic compromise | Yes, 100, 200, 300, 360 | As per current ACLS recommendations |
| Sustained monomorphic VT: without symptoms or hemodynamic compromise | No | Amiodarone (Cordarone), 150 mg IV infused over 10 min, then 360 mg over 6 h (1 mg/min), then 540 mg over 18 h (0.5 mg/min) (max 2.2 g over 24 h) |
| Nonsustained VT (within 48 h of MI) | No | No treatment recommended unless symptomatic or associated with hemodynamic compromise |
| Nonsustained VT (>48 h following MI) | No | Electrophysiology study with programmed stimulation. If sustained VT inducible, then insertion of AICD. |
| Accelerated idioventricular rhythm | No | None |

*Abbreviations:* ACLS = Advanced Cardiac Life Support; AICD = Automatic Implantable Cardioverter Defribrillator; MI = myocardial infarction; VT = ventricular tachycardia.
*Energy is for monophasic defibrillators.

Conduction abnormalities at the AV node level in the setting of inferior AMI are usually transient and usually do not require transvenous pacing, even in the setting of high-grade AV block. AV block as well as new bundle branch block in patients with anterior STEMI portends a worse prognosis and is associated with a high risk of progression to complete heart block. Temporary transvenous pacing should be considered in those with anterior myocardial infarction (MI) and Mobitz 2 AV block, third-degree AV block, or new left bundle-branch block (LBBB).

Ventricular fibrillation can complicate myocardial infarction and should be treated promptly with unsynchronized electrical shock as per current ACLS guidelines. Table 7 lists recommendations for the approach and treatment of ventricular tachycardia in the setting of AMI.

## ADJUNCTIVE THERAPY/HOSPITAL DISCHARGE MEDICATIONS

Aspirin, 81 mg to 325 mg, should be continued indefinitely in all ACS patients. An angiotensin-converting enzyme inhibitor (ACEI) should be started within 24 hours in all hemodynamically stable patients with large anterior infarctions and in patients with LV ejection fraction less than 40%. We prefer starting with a short-acting ACEI such as captopril (Capoten), 3.125 mg by mouth every 8 hours, with titration upward as tolerated. Upon discharge, a longer acting ACEI can be substituted. Statin therapy in the setting of ACS improves short- and long-term outcomes and should be initiated before discharge in all ACS patients regardless of cholesterol levels. Patients should be continued on aggressive statin lipid-lowering therapy with a goal LDL ≤70 mg/dL. All patients with ACS should be discharged on a β-blocker unless a contraindication exists. One randomized trial (COMET [Carvedilol Or Metoprolol European Trial]) suggests that carvedilol (Coreg) at optimal doses is superior to short-acting metoprolol tartrate (Lopressor) in patients with symptomatic chronic heart failure and LV ejection fraction of less than 35%. Patients receiving a drug eluting stent as a part of their AMI treatment need to continue clopidogrel therapy uninterrupted for at least 9 and preferably 12 months due to the risk of acute stent thrombosis. Patients receiving a bare metal stent need to continue clopidogrel for at least 1 month uninterrupted following stent placement. This should be reinforced to the patient as a part of their discharge instructions.

## CARDIAC REHABILITATION/SECONDARY PREVENTION/RISK FACTOR MODIFICATION

All patients should undergo cardiovascular risk factor assessment and modification during and following hospitalization. Blood pressure readings should ideally be lower than 120/80 mm Hg. Smoking cessation should be addressed and glycemic control optimized in diabetic patients. Patients should be instructed on an AHA step II low-fat diet, and statin therapy should be initiated and/or modified to achieve an LDL lower than 70 mg/dL. The goal of cardiac rehabilitation is to help the patient safely return to and maintain normal daily activities and promote secondary prevention measures. This generally includes a staged approach with patients attending monitored exercise sessions for the first 6 to 8 weeks following MI during which levels of exercise are gradually increased. Following an uncomplicated MI, patients are instructed to return to work in 14 to 28 days, with driving allowed within 7 to 14 days. Patients with complicated MI, including those with significant ventricular arrhythmias, require a more gradual return to normal daily activities.

## HOSPITAL FOLLOW-UP VISIT

Patients should generally be seen in follow-up between 3 and 6 weeks following hospital discharge. They should be evaluated for recurrence of symptoms, evidence of heart failure, and medication intolerance or noncompliance. Medications should be reviewed individually and the rationale for each discussed. Modification of cardiovascular risk factors should continue. A transthoracic echocardiogram should be obtained to assess LV function 4 to 6 weeks following discharge. Patients with an LVEF of less than 30% should be considered for prophylactic internal defibrillator insertion. Patients with an LVEF between 31% and 40% should undergo 48-hour Holter monitoring with subsequent referral to an electrophysiologist if nonsustained ventricular tachycardia (VT) is present.

### CURRENT DIAGNOSIS

Acute myocardial infarction is defined as the typical rise and fall of cardiac troponin or creatine kinase myocardial band in addition to one of the following:

- Symptoms consistent with myocardial ischemia
- Electrocardiogram changes indicating myocardial ischemia (ST-segment depression or elevation)
- New pathologic Q waves
- Percutaneous coronary intervention

## REFERENCES

Antman EM, Anbe DT, Armstrong PW, Bates ER, et al: ACC/AHA guidelines for the management of patients with ST-elevation myocardial infarction: A report of the American College of Cardiology/American Heart Association Task Force on Practice Guidelines, 2004. Available at www.acc.org/clinical/guidelines/stemi/index.pdf

Boersma E, Harrington RA, Moliterno DJ, et al: Platelet glycoprotein IIb/IIIa inhibitors in acute coronary syndromes: A meta-analysis of all major randomized clinical trials. Lancet 2002;359:189-198.

Braunwald E, Antman EM, Beasley JW, Califf RM, et al: ACC/AHA 2002 guideline update for the management of patients with unstable angina and non-ST-segment elevation myocardial infarction: Summary article: A report of the American College of Cardiology/American Heart Association Task Force on Practice Guidelines (Committee on the Management of Patients with Unstable Angina). J Am Coll Cardiol 2002;40:1366-1374.

Cannon CP, Weintraub WS, Demopoulos LA, et al: Comparison of early invasive and conservative strategies in patients with unstable coronary syndromes treated with the glycoprotein IIb/IIIa inhibitor tirofiban. N Engl J Med 2001;344:1879-1887.

Cohen M, Demers C, Gurfinkel EP, et al: A comparison of low-molecular-weight heparin with unfractionated heparin for unstable coronary artery disease. Efficacy and Safety of Subcutaneous Enoxaparin in Non-Q-Wave Coronary Events Study Group. N Engl J Med 1997;337:447-452.

Fox KA, Poole-Wilson PA, Henderson RA, et al: Interventional versus conservative treatment for patients with unstable angina or non-ST-elevation myocardial infarction: The British Heart Foundation RITA 3 randomised trial. Randomized intervention trial of unstable angina. Lancet 2002;360:743-751.

Hochman JS, Sleeper LA, Webb JG, et al: Early revascularization in acute myocardial infarction complicated by cardiogenic shock. N Engl J Med 1999;341:625-634.

Schwartz GG, Olsson AG, Ezekowitz MD, et al: Effects of atorvastatin on early recurrent ischemic events in acute coronary syndromes: The MIRACL study: A randomized controlled trial. JAMA 2001;285:1711-1718.

Yusuf S, Zhao F, Mehta SR, et al: Effects of clopidogrel in addition to aspirin in patients with acute coronary syndromes without ST-segment elevation. N Engl J Med 2001;345:494-502.

# Pericarditis

Method of
*Brian D. Hoit, MD*

Although the diagnosis and treatment of pericardial disease is often simple and rewarding, it may offer unexpected challenges and frustrations to both clinician and patient for several reasons. First, the presence of pericardial heart disease may escape detection, often remaining clinically silent, being apparent only during the evaluation of unrelated complaints. In addition, pericardial disease may complicate, and be overshadowed by, extracardiac manifestations from a number of systemic disorders. Second, although guidelines for the diagnosis and management of pericardial diseases are now available, there are few randomized, placebo-controlled trials from which appropriate therapy may be selected and important clinical decisions supported. The physician thus often must rely heavily on clinical judgment because most data originate from small uncontrolled trials and anecdotal experience. Finally, therapeutic options in most cases are limited to nonspecific anti-inflammatory agents, drainage of pericardial fluid, and pericardiectomy. Although there is general agreement on how these measures should be applied in the patient with either very mild or severe disease, there is little consensus on how the large number of cases encountered with clinical manifestations between these two extremes should be managed. With these important caveats in mind, the options available for treating pericardial heart disease are reviewed here.

## Acute Pericarditis

Hospitalization is warranted for most, if not all, patients who present with an initial episode of acute pericarditis to determine an etiology and to observe for the development of cardiac tamponade; close, early follow-up is critically important in the remainder. Table 1 lists the major definable causes of pericardial heart disease; however, in many cases, the etiology of pericardial heart disease is never identified..Features indicative of high-risk pericarditis that warrants hospitalization include fever higher than 38°C (100°F), subacute onset, an immune depressed state, trauma, oral anticoagulant therapy, myopericarditis, large pericardial effusion, cardiac tamponade, and aspirin failure. Establishing the exact cause of acute pericarditis is an important part of management in the high-risk case, but considerable judgment must be exercised when deciding whether and how to investigate suspected acute viral and idiopathic pericarditis.

Acute pericarditis usually responds to oral nonsteroidal anti-inflammatory drugs (NSAIDs), such as ASA, 650 mg every 4 to 6 hours, or ibuprofen, 300 to 800 mg every 6 to 8 hours. Gastrointestinal (GI) prophylaxis with $H_2$ blockers or proton pump inhibitors is often warranted, particularly in those at high risk or who require longer durations of treatment. Selective COX-2 inhibitors are NSAIDs with few adverse GI effects, but they are implicated in adverse cardiovascular events; moreover, they have not been tested in acute pericarditis. Cumulative anecdotal data suggest that colchicine[1] (1 mg/day, with or without a 2 mg loading dose), either as a supplement to the use of NSAIDs or as monotherapy, is effective for the acute episode, well tolerated, and may prevent recurrences. A recent prospective randomized, open-label trial found that colchicine[1] (1 to 2 mg for the first day, followed by 0.5 to 1 mg/day for 3 months) in addition to aspirin was more effective than aspirin alone in reducing symptoms and recurrences. Side effects (diarrhea and nausea) are usually mild and most often do not necessitate withdrawal of the drug.

Chest pain is often alleviated in 1 to 2 days, and the friction rub and ST segment elevation resolve shortly thereafter. The duration of therapy is controversial; a month of NSAIDs (e.g., high-dose aspirin for 7 to 10 days followed by a taper over 3 to 4 weeks) and 3 months of colchicine[1] is a regimen based on evidence. The intensity of therapy is

---

[1]Not FDA approved for this indication.

## CURRENT DIAGNOSIS

| | Acute Pericarditis | Acute Myocardial Infarction |
|---|---|---|
| History | Sharp, retrosternal pain, pleuritic, radiates to trapezius ridge | Dull, precordial chest pain, radiates to neck/arm |
| Physical | Friction rub; may be fever, signs of inflammation, signs of underlying associated diseases | May be murmurs, ventricular gallops; signs of pulmonary congestion |
| EKG | Diffuse; characteristic evolutionary pattern; PR depression; absent Q waves pattern | Indicative ST and Q waves; characteristic evolutionary pattern |
| CXR | May be normal in uncomplicated cases. May be signs of effusion, associated diseases | May be normal in uncomplicated cases. May be large heart, signs of pulmonary congestion |
| Echo | Pericardial effusion confirms clinical suspicion. May be normal | Regional wall motion abnormalities. May identify mechanical complications |
| Laboratory | Nonspecific markers of inflammation; With extensive pericarditis may see isoenzyme changes characteristic of acute MI | Characteristic CK and troponin isoenzymes |

*Abbreviations:* CK = creatine kinase; CXR = chest radiograph; EKG = electrocardiogram; MI = myocardial infarction.

dictated by the distress of the patient, and intravenous (IV) ketorolac (Toradol), 30 mg every 6 hours, or narcotics may be required for severe pain. Although some cases necessitate steroid therapy (prednisone, 60 to 80 mg/day) for a week to control pain (with the dosage tapered carefully on an individual basis thereafter), corticosteroids should be avoided unless there are specific indications (such as connective tissue disease, autoreactive, or uremic pericarditis) because they enhance viral multiplication and may result in recurrences when the dosage is tapered; colchicine[1] may be particularly useful in this situation. Importantly, tuberculous and pyogenic pericarditis should be excluded before steroid therapy is initiated. Intrapericardial instillation of triamcinolone (Kenalog), 300 mg/m$^2$, avoids systemic side effects and is highly effective. Patients in whom pericarditis represents one manifestation of systemic illness (such as sepsis, uremia, connective tissue disease, or neoplasia) should receive therapy directed toward the primary disorder in addition to palliative and supportive treatment.

## Recurrent Pericarditis

Recurrent or relapsing acute pericarditis is one of the most distressing disorders of the pericardium for both patient and physician.

---

[1]Not FDA approved for this indication.

### TABLE 1 Etiology of Pericardial Heart Disease

Idiopathic
Infectious (viral, bacterial, mycobacterial, fungal, protozoal, AIDS)
Neoplastic (breast, lung, melanoma, lymphoma, leukemia; mesothelioma)
Post myocardial infarction
Radiation induced
Nephrogenic (dialytic and uremic)
Traumatic (blunt and penetrating, chylopericardium)
Connective tissue diseases and arteritides (rheumatoid arthritis, systemic lupus erythematosus, scleroderma, polyarteritis nodosa, Takayasu's arteritis, Wegener's granulomatosis)
Myxedema
Iatrogenic (diagnostic and therapeutic procedures, drugs)
Miscellaneous (sarcoidosis, amyloidosis, Whipple's disease, dissecting aortic aneurysm)

Reproduced with permission from Hoit BD: Pericarditis. In Rakel RE, Bope ET (eds): Conn's Current Therapy 2002. Philadelphia, Elsevier, 2002.

Atypical features, such as the absence of physical findings, offer challenges for diagnosis and management and often necessitate close follow-up and rigorous emotional support. Recurrences occur with highly variable frequency over a course of many years; although they may be spontaneous, occurring at varying intervals after discontinuation of drug (i.e., "recurrent"), they are more commonly associated with either discontinuation or tapering of anti-inflammatory drugs (i.e., "incessant").

Painful recurrences of pericarditis may respond to NSAIDs but commonly require additional therapy. A recent prospective, randomized open-label trial compared aspirin (or steroids when necessary) and colchicine[1] (0.5 to 1 mg/day after a 1- to 2-mg load for 6 months) with aspirin alone. This study suggests that colchicine[1] is both efficacious and safe for the prevention of recurrences; moreover, corticosteroid use was an independent risk factor for further recurrences. When necessary, prednisone is begun at a high dose (1 to 1.5 mg/kg/day) for at least 4 weeks and tapered slowly (approximately 5 mg every 3 days) over the next 2 to 3 months. Azathioprine[1] (Imuran) and cyclophosphamide[1] (Cytoxan) are used to prevent recurrent episodes in patients who fail to respond to high-dose corticosteroids or who experience severe corticosteroid side effects; pericardiectomy should be considered only when repeated attempts at medical treatment have clearly failed, especially when there is evidence (e.g., from serial bone density scans) of steroid-induced complications.

## Treatment of Specific Causes of Pericarditis

### PURULENT PERICARDITIS

The incidence and bacterial spectrum of purulent pericarditis have changed because of the increasing frequency of cardiac surgery and instrumentation, selection-induced changes in the flora responsible for hospital-acquired infections, and the prolonged survival of immunocompromised hosts. Bacterial pericarditis is treated with surgical exploration and drainage (pericardiectomy is preferable) and appropriate systemic antibiotics. A high index of suspicion is critical because in the appropriate setting, pericardial involvement is often unrecognized when it complicates systemic infection, and the characteristic features of acute pericarditis are frequently absent. The threshold for echocardiography in the septic patient should be low, and whenever purulent pericarditis is suspected, the pericardial space should be explored. Fibrinolytics may be used to lyse fibrous adhesions, liquefy purulent exudates, and prevent constrictive pericarditis.

## MYCOBACTERIAL AND FUNGAL PERICARDITIS

Tuberculosis is a major cause of pericarditis in nonindustrialized countries but is an uncommon cause of pericarditis in the United States. Nevertheless, its incidence is increasing because of HIV infection. Pericardial fluid should be removed, cultured, and antituberculous therapy begun. Depending on the echocardiographic appearance, subxiphoid drainage may be necessary. Some recommend early pericardiectomy in all cases of tuberculosis pericarditis, but the long-term (16 years) prognosis of patients without cardiac compression during the acute illness who are treated with medical therapy alone is excellent. Multiple drug therapy and corticosteroids are effective in tuberculous pericarditis, whereas atypical mycobacterial infections (especially *Myobacterium avium intracellulare*) may be resistant to treatment. Patients with tuberculous pericarditis should receive triple drug therapy (isoniazid, 5 mg/kg to a maximum of 300 mg; rifampin [Rifadin], 10 mg/kg to a maximum of 600 mg; and either streptomycin, 15 mg/kg to a maximum of 1 g, or ethambutol [Myambutol], 5 to 25 mg/kg to a maximum of 2.5 g) for a minimum of 9 months. Corticosteroids (prednisone, 1 to 2 mg/kg/day) may be useful if pericardial effusion persists or recurs during therapy, and they appear beneficial acutely in reducing morbidity and mortality. Pericardiectomy may be necessary for recurrent cardiac tamponade.

Patients should be observed for constriction because up to half of patients require pericardiectomy; failure to improve or worsening over 1 to 2 months, pericardial thickening, or evidence of constriction requires urgent pericardiectomy. In patients with hemodynamics consistent with effusive-constrictive pericarditis, plans for visceral and parietal pericardiectomy after a few weeks of chemotherapy are advisable.. Persistent hypotension may signify tuberculous adrenal insufficiency.

Pericarditis complicating deep fungal infection with histoplasma or coccidiomycosis may be immunologic, resolve spontaneously, and not require specific therapy. Amphotericin B (up to 2.5 g total), itraconazole (Sporanox), 200 to 400 mg/day, ketoconazole (Nizoral), 200 to 400 mg/day, and fluconazole (Diflucan), 200 to 400 mg/day, are rarely required. Tamponading effusion and constriction require decompression. Surgical decompression and specific antifungal or antimicrobial

therapy may be necessary for disseminated infection with *Candida*, *Aspergillus*, *Actinomycetes*, and *Nocardia*.

## NEOPLASTIC PERICARDITIS

Metastatic neoplasia remains the leading cause of pericardial disease in hospitalized patients, most often in patients with lung or breast cancer, melanoma, lymphoma, and acute leukemia. Many cases are asymptomatic and found only incidentally at autopsy, but others cause symptoms and may progress to cardiac tamponade. The pericardium may be thickened and cause constriction; less commonly, effusive-constrictive pericarditis occurs.

In almost every case, fluid should be removed if large effusions are refractory or if tamponade ensues. The specific approach depends on the patient's expected longevity and medical condition. Pericardiocentesis is associated with a high recurrence rate and does not provide tissue for biopsy. Sclerosing agents, such as tetracycline (500 to 1000 mg in 20 mL of sterile saline), reduce recurrences and can be considered for patients with a poor prognosis. However, sclerosis is painful, does not improve prognosis, and may not be superior to an indwelling catheter alone. Subtotal pericardiectomy is most effective but should only be performed in carefully selected patients. Balloon pericardiotomy avoids the discomfort and risk of surgery in critically ill patients with predictably limited survival.

## PERICARDITIS COMPLICATING MYOCARDIAL INFARCTION

Pericarditis is common in the first few days after myocardial infarction, occurring in as many as 28% to 43% of fatal infarctions, but it is clinically apparent in as few as 7% of cases. Pericardial involvement is related to infarct size and associated with a poor prognosis. An important clinical issue is the extent to which acute pericarditis in myocardial infarction influences management with anticoagulants. A pericardial friction rub occurring in the first 2 or 3 days without an associated pericardial effusion should not influence clinical decisions, but pericarditis occurring later in the course or accompanied by pericardial effusion or tamponade is a contraindication to anticoagulant therapy. Cardiac tamponade seldom occurs, except in patients who receive systemic anticoagulants or have cardiac rupture.

Treatment of infarct pericarditis is seldom indicated, but when symptomatic it responds to ASA; corticosteroids should be avoided because of concerns of impaired infarct healing, steroid dependency, and toxic side effects.

## RADIATION-INDUCED PERICARDIAL DISEASE

Acute pericarditis occurring early during radiation therapy is uncommon and most likely the result of the radiation-induced effects on the tumor rather than a direct toxic effect of the radiation on the pericardium. In this instance, therapy should not be disrupted, although a reduction in dose may be necessary. A delayed (usually less than 1 year, but highly variable) form of pericardial injury may present as acute pericarditis or effusion (often with some degree of cardiac compression); constrictive and effusive-constrictive pericarditis may become manifest only after many years.

Acute radiation-induced pericarditis can be managed symptomatically as acute idiopathic pericarditis. Hemodynamically insignificant pericardial effusion can also be managed conservatively because spontaneous resolution is the rule; however, pericardiectomy should be offered to symptomatic patients with large recurrent pericardial effusions. Constrictive pericarditis requires pericardiectomy unless otherwise contraindicated.

## PERICARDIAL DISEASE IN PATIENTS WITH RENAL FAILURE

Pericarditis complicates both uremia and dialytic therapy (hemo- and peritoneal), and may be clinically silent. The clinical manifestation of nephrogenic pericardial disease may be acute fibrinous pericarditis, pericardial effusion, or cardiac tamponade; classic constrictive pericarditis is rare.

---

### CURRENT THERAPY

| Type | Therapy |
|---|---|
| Acute viral/nonspecific pericarditis | ASA, NSAIDS, colchicine |
| Recurrent pericarditis | Colchicines in addition to ASA/NSAIDs; prednisone* |
| Purulent pericarditis | Specific systemic antibiotics; drainage; fibrinolytics |
| TB pericarditis | Antituberculous therapy; steroids; May require pericardiectomy |
| Neoplastic pericarditis | May require drainage; recurrences reduced by sclerosis, pericardiectomy |
| Postinfarction pericarditis | ASA |
| Nephrogenic pericarditis | Intensification of dialysis; drainage for tamponade and large resistant chronic effusions; instillation of steroids |

*Prednisone should be avoided if possible.
See text for details, specific indications, and doses.
*Abbreviations:* ASA = aspirin; NSAIDS = nonsteroidal anti-inflammatory drugs; TB = tuberculosis.

Although intensification of dialysis is an accepted treatment modality for hemodynamically insignificant disease, considerable controversy exists regarding the optimal management of large, persistent, or recurrent pericardial effusion. Tamponade is an indication for pericardial drainage, and large resistant, chronic effusion warrant pericardiocentesis, but a conservative approach—that is, intensification of dialysis and NSAIDs—may suffice in less severe cases. The instillation of nonabsorbable steroids (triamcinolone, 50 mg every 6 hours[3] for 2 to 3 days) directly into the pericardial space is advocated, but randomized controlled data are absent. If needle drainage is necessary, an indwelling catheter should be left in the pericardial space for at least 2 to 3 days. Dialysis-associated effusive pericarditis usually responds to intensification of dialysis and regional heparinization or by changing to peritoneal dialysis. Pericardiectomy may be necessary for intractable effusions.

## Other Causes of Pericardial Disease

Pericarditis may accompany virtually any connective tissue disease and may present as either acute or chronic pericarditis with or without an effusion.. However, most cases are subclinical and in many instances are recognized only at autopsy. In the absence of tamponading or secondarily infected effusions, NSAIDs and corticosteroids are useful. Myxedema-associated effusions develop slowly and may grow very large; slow resolution usually follows institution of thyroid replacement therapy.

Iatrogenic pericardial disease results from both the calculated complications and the unanticipated misadventures of diagnostic and therapeutic procedures. Importantly, a wide variety of drugs and toxins may cause pericardial heart disease by producing drug-induced lupus (e.g., procainamide, hydralazine, isoniazid), a hypersensitivity or idiosyncratic reaction (e.g., penicillins, thiazides, anthracyclines), pericardial irritation, or hemorrhage (e.g., anticoagulants). Chylous pericardial effusions generally follow traumatic or surgical injury to the thoracic duct but may result from neoplastic obstruction of the thoracic duct, or they may be idiopathic. Failure to respond to either ligation of the thoracic duct and partial pericardiectomy or to a diet rich in medium chain triglycerides warrants implantation of a valved pericardioperitoneal conduit.

## Pericardial Effusion and Tamponade

In the absence of tamponade or suspected purulent pericarditis, there are few indications for pericardial drainage. Persistent large and unexplained effusions (especially when tuberculosis is suspect or when present for more than 3 months) may warrant pericardiocentesis. Occasionally, suspected malignancy or systemic disease may necessitate pericardial drainage and biopsy. However, *routine* drainage of large effusions (20 mm echo-free space in diastole) has a very low diagnostic yield (7%) and no therapeutic benefit. Figure 1 presents an approach to the management of moderate and large pericardial effusions.

It is important to remember that tamponade is a clinical diagnosis and "echocardiographic signs of tamponade" is not by itself an indication for pericardiocentesis. Although the absence of any cardiac chamber collapse has a high negative predictive value (92%), the positive predictive value is substantially reduced (58%).

Removal of small amounts of tamponading pericardial fluid (approximately 50 mL) produces considerable symptomatic and hemodynamic improvement because of the steep pericardial pressure–volume relation. Unless there is concomitant cardiac disease or coexisting constriction (i.e., effusive-constrictive pericarditis), removal of all of the pericardial fluid normalizes pericardial, atrial, ventricular diastolic and arterial pressures, and cardiac output. Mild or low-pressure tamponade (i.e., when the venous pressure is less than 10 cm of water, arterial blood pressure is normal and pulsus paradoxus is

### MANAGEMENT OF MODERATE-LARGE PERICARDIAL EFFUSIONS

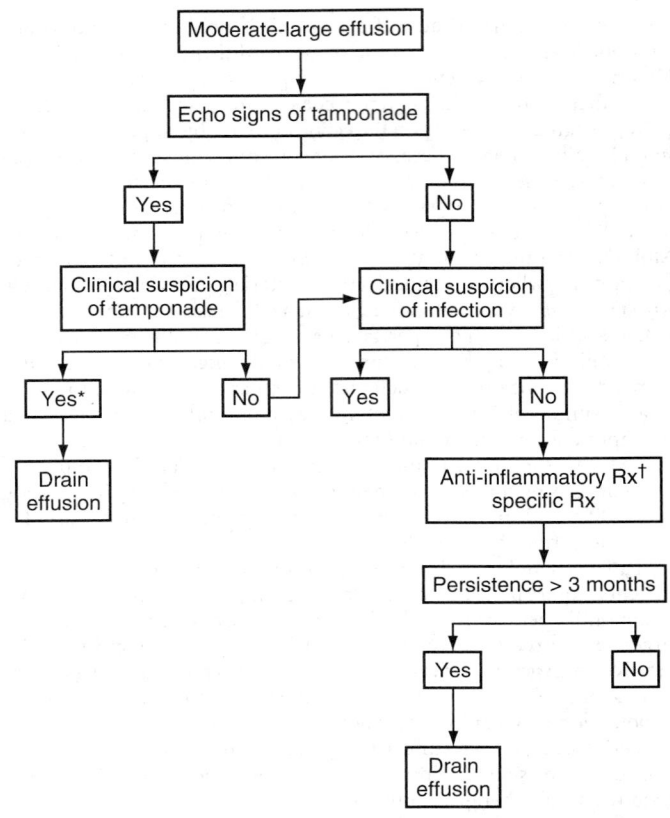

**FIGURE 1.** Algorithm for the management of moderate to large pericardial effusions. *Right heart catheterization may be required. †Anti-inflammatory treatment if there are signs of pericarditis. (Reprinted with permission from Hoit BD: Management of effusive and constrictive pericardial heart disease. Circulation 2002;105: 2939-2942.)

absent), particularly when the etiology is idiopathic, viral, or when responsive to specific therapy (e.g., thyroid hormone), does not require pericardiocentesis. At the other extreme, hyperacute tamponade (usually resulting from cardiac trauma) necessitates immediate pericardiocentesis as an initial triage measure. However, the majority of patients fall between these two extremes and require pericardial drainage. Either surgical means (via subxiphoid incision, video-assisted thoracoscopy, or thoracotomy) or percutaneously (with a needle or balloon catheter) accomplishes pericardial drainage. The choice between needle pericardiocentesis and surgical drainage depends on institutional resources and physician experience, the etiology of the effusion, the need for diagnostic tissue samples, and the prognosis of the patient. Unless the situation is immediately life threatening, experienced staff should perform pericardiocentesis in a facility equipped with radiographic, echocardiographic, and hemodynamic monitoring to optimize the success and safety of the procedure. The safety of the procedure is increased by using 2D echo guidance. Pericardiocentesis is ill advised when there is less than 1 cm of effusion, loculation, or evidence of fibrin and adhesion.

Recurrent effusions may be treated by either repeat pericardiocentesis, sclerotherapy with tetracycline, surgical creation of a pericardial window, or pericardiectomy. Subtotal pericardiectomy is preferred when the patient is expected to survive greater than 1 year. A pleuropericardial window provides a large area for fluid to be reabsorbed and is often performed in patients with malignant effusions. Pericardiectomy may be required for recurrent effusions in dialysis patients. In critically ill patients, a pericardial window may be created percutaneously with a balloon catheter.

# Constrictive Pericarditis

Constrictive pericarditis is a condition in which a thickened, scarred, and often calcified pericardium limits diastolic filling of the ventricles. Although acute pericarditis from most causes may eventuate in constrictive pericarditis, the most common antecedents are idiopathic, cardiac trauma and surgery, mediastinal irradiation, tuberculosis and other infectious diseases, neoplasms (particularly lung and breast), renal failure, and connective tissue diseases. Although it is commonly thought that a normal pericardial thickness excludes the diagnosis of constrictive pericarditis, 28% of 143 surgically confirmed cases had normal pericardial thickness on CT scan, and 18% had normal thickness on histopathologic examination.

Classic chronic constrictive pericarditis is less frequently encountered than in the past, whereas subacute constrictive pericarditis (weeks to months after the inciting injury, e.g., after cardiac surgery) is becoming more common. In this latter group of patients, constriction may be transitory, with a course that may span a matter of weeks to a few months; not surprisingly, pericardial calcification is uncommon. Doppler-detected constrictive physiology resolved without pericardiectomy in 36 of 212 patients studied retrospectively at Mayo Clinic after an average of approximately 8 weeks.

Pericardiectomy is the definitive treatment for constrictive pericarditis but is unwarranted either in very early constriction (occult and functional class I) or in severe, advanced disease (functional Class IV) when the risk of surgery is excessive (operative mortality 30% to 40% vs. 6% to 19%) and the benefits are diminished. It is prudent to give hemodynamically stable patients with subacute constrictive pericarditis a trial of conservative management for 2 to 3 months until it is clear that the constrictive process is permanent before recommending pericardiectomy. Complete or extensive pericardial resection is desirable.

Medical therapy of constrictive pericarditis has a small but important role. In some patients, constrictive pericarditis resolves either spontaneously or in response to various combinations of NSAIDs, steroids, and antibiotics; in the remaining patients, medical therapy is adjunctive.

## REFERENCES

Haley JH, Tajik AJ, Danielson GK, et al: Transient constrictive pericarditis: Causes and natural history. J Am Coll Cardiol 2004;43:271-275.

Imazio M, Bobbio M, Cecchi E, et al: Colchicine as first-choice therapy for recurrent pericarditis: Results of the CORE (COlchicine for REcurrent pericarditis) trial. Arch Intern Med 2005;165:1987-1991.

Imazio M, Bobbio M, Cecchi E, et al: Colchicine in addition to conventional therapy for acute pericarditis: Results of the COlchicine for acute PEricarditis (COPE) trial. Circulation 2005;112:2012-2016.

Imazio M, Demichelis B, Parrini I, et al: Day-hospital treatment of acute pericarditis: A management program for outpatient therapy. J Am Coll Cardiol 2004;43:1042-1046.

Maisch B, Ristic AD, Pankuweit S: Intrapericardial treatment of autoreactive pericardial effusion with triamcinolone; the way to avoid side effects of systemic corticosteroid therapy. Eur Heart J 2002;23:1503-1508.

Maisch B, Seferovic PM, Ristic AD, et al: Guidelines on the diagnosis and management of pericardial diseases executive summary: The task force on the diagnosis and management of pericardial diseases of the European society of cardiology. Eur Heart J 2004;25:587-610.

Merce J, Sagrista-Sauleda J, Permanyer-Miralda G, Soler-Soler J: Should pericardial drainage be performed routinely in patients who have a large pericardial effusion without tamponade? Am J Med 1998;105:106-109.

Talreja DR, Edwards WD, Danielson GK, et al: Constrictive pericarditis in 26 patients with histologically normal pericardial thickness. Circulation 2003;108:1852-1857.

# Peripheral Arterial Disease

Method of
*Jason T. Lee, MD, Maisie M. Fung, MD, and E. John Harris, Jr., MD*

Peripheral arterial disease (PAD) encompasses a wide spectrum of disease entities involving blood vessels outside of the heart and the brain. This includes blood vessels of the upper and lower extremities, the carotid artery, and the aorta. The majority of the clinical manifestations of PAD occur as a consequence of progressive atherosclerotic narrowing of these vessels. Other acquired diseases of arteries are related to aneurysm formation, inflammation, or degenerative disorders. Significant morbidity and mortality results from PAD, and patients can present in very acute or chronic settings. Recognizing the signs and symptoms of these diseases is paramount for the primary care physician to formulate an accurate differential diagnosis. Prompt diagnostic testing and appropriate referral to a vascular surgeon are necessary to provide definitive management and optimize patient outcomes. In the past decade, there have been numerous advances in the diagnosis, management, and treatment of PAD. Less invasive screening tests are supplementing and even replacing traditional angiography, and treatment options with endovascular approaches such as angioplasty and stenting are increasingly available and being shown to be feasible. In this chapter we focus on the most commonly encountered PADs including carotid artery stenosis and lower extremity occlusive disease.

## Carotid Artery Disease

Carotid artery disease most commonly involves atherosclerotic changes in the carotid arteries resulting in stenosis of the vessels around the carotid bifurcation. Diminished flow and irregular plaque formation of the common and internal carotid arteries can lead to embolic or thrombotic events that may cause transient ischemic attacks (TIAs), amaurosis fugax, or stroke. Carotid occlusive disease accounts for 30% to 40% of all reported strokes. Stroke remains the third leading cause of death in the United States (only behind heart disease and cancer). According to the American Heart Association (AHA), 700,000 people in the United States experienced a stroke in 2001, with nearly a third being recurrent. One in 15 deaths in the United States in 2001 was from a cerebrovascular accident. On a positive note, there was a 63% decrease in stroke/death rates from 1970 to 2002. There remains, however, high cost associated with the care of stroke survivors in terms of long-term rehabilitation, diminished productivity, chronic medications, and other co-morbid medical conditions. Risk factors for carotid artery disease include smoking,

## CURRENT DIAGNOSIS

- Routine examination including palpation of extremity pulses and auscultation for bruits of the carotid artery and abdominal aorta should be performed during all health maintenance examinations.
- Duplex ultrasound by an accredited vascular laboratory can accurately measure the degree of carotid disease and determine which patients will benefit from carotid intervention.
- Vascular claudication is described as reproducible pain in the lower extremities brought on by exertion that is relieved by rest and should be evaluated by lower extremity duplex ultrasound evaluation of arterial waveforms with ankle-brachial indexes.

## CURRENT THERAPY

- Carotid endarterectomy is a durable and safe procedure that is indicated for symptomatic carotid stenosis >70% and asymptomatic carotid stenosis >80% to reduce future stroke risk.
- Symptomatic patients who are deemed high risk can be considered for carotid stenting at a high-volume vascular center.
- Aggressive medical management and risk factor modification with a supervised exercise regimen should be instituted for all patients with claudication.
- Critical limb ischemia is a progressive process that requires urgent referral to a vascular surgeon for revascularization by open surgical or endovascular techniques.

diabetes, hypertension, high cholesterol, and family history of disease. Prevention strategies focus on the use of antiplatelet agents, smoking cessation, hypertension control, lipid-lowering medications, diabetes control, and screening for carotid artery disease.

Carotid artery disease can be symptomatic or asymptomatic. Asymptomatic patients may be diagnosed by the primary care physician after a carotid bruit is detected on physical examination, but more commonly no bruit is auscultated and risk factors and/or family history lead to a screening duplex ultrasound. Recently, patients are seeking consultation for confirmation of a carotid duplex examination done as part of a vascular screening series or total body scan outside of the physician's office. Symptomatic patients present with symptoms of stroke or TIAs. TIAs differ from strokes in that they are acute, focal neurologic deficits that resolve completely within 24 hours, whereas strokes involve incomplete recovery. A classic type of ocular TIA is amaurosis fugax, where there is a painless monocular loss of vision caused by retinal artery embolus or thrombus. Patients classically describe a curtain being drawn over the eye that appears and resolves suddenly and completely. Other symptoms associated with TIAs or strokes include motor, sensory, or speech defects. Global symptoms such as dizziness, syncope, or altered mentation are less clearly associated with carotid occlusive disease.

Patients with suspected carotid artery disease should undergo a thorough physical examination including pulse examination, listening for bruits, and neurologic examination. Diagnosis can be confirmed via duplex ultrasound scan of both carotid arteries (Figure 1). This can quantify the degree and location of the stenosis. The degree of stenosis is typically reported as a percentage of narrowing and is based on velocity criteria standardized and validated for each vascular laboratory. Computed tomography (CT) scan or magnetic resonance imaging (MRI) of the brain is necessary when stroke or TIA is suspected. Positive imaging findings within brain parenchyma indicate that an acute event has occurred. The advantage of MRI is that imaging of the neck and brain with magnetic resonance angiography (MRA) can be performed simultaneously to give details regarding carotid and vertebral artery anatomy as well as the intracranial circulation. The degree of stenosis seen on MRA is often overestimated and should be corroborated by a duplex ultrasound. Cerebral arteriography is currently used infrequently in the preoperative phase and reserved for cases in which questions remain unresolved with the other imaging modalities. Improvements in imaging technology also are allowing CT angiography to become more widely available.

Management of carotid artery disease is based on the degree of carotid stenosis measured by the various imaging modalities. Carotid endarterectomy (CEA) remains the most common procedure performed by vascular surgeons in the United States and is one of the most extensively studied operative procedures in the medical literature. Randomized, prospective trials including the North American Symptomatic Carotid Endarterectomy Trial (NASCET), European Carotid Surgery Trial (ECST), and the Veterans Affairs (VA) trial showed an approximately 50% relative risk reduction in symptomatic patients with more than a 70% stenosis who underwent surgery compared with medical treatment with aspirin. In the NASCET trial, the ipsilateral stroke rate at 2-year follow-up was reduced to 9% in the surgically treated patients as opposed to 26% in the medically treated patients, and the study was halted with all patients in the medical arm then offered CEA. The VA trial and ECST provide similar data documenting the benefit of surgical intervention in symptomatic patients with greater than 70% stenosis.

For asymptomatic patients, the Asymptomatic Carotid Atherosclerosis Study (ACAS) showed a 53% relative risk reduction of ipsilateral stroke at 5 years from 11.0% to 5.1% in surgically treated patients with greater than 60% stenosis. This represents, however, only a 1% absolute risk reduction per year, which is certainly less dramatic than the protective effects of intervention on a symptomatic patient. For this reason and with the development of newer antiplatelet agents like clopidogrel (Plavix), surgery at our institution is offered to asymptomatic patients only when they have reached 80% stenosis. Potential complications of surgery for either symptomatic or asymptomatic patients include myocardial infarction, stroke, bleeding, infection, cranial nerve injury, and recurrent stenosis. The possibility of recurrent disease highlights the importance of long-term follow-up after CEA that should include yearly duplex examination.

With the advent of endovascular techniques being driven by industry and patient desires for more minimally invasive interventions, it is no surprise that carotid angioplasty and stenting (CAS) has emerged as an alternative therapy. Recently published data, although sparse, suggests that in high-risk patients, CAS is not worse than traditional open surgery in terms of stroke and death rates. However, the best candidates for these procedures and long-term durability of these approaches are yet to be delineated. High-risk patients are defined differently at various institutions, but typically include those with severe uncontrolled co-morbid coronary symptoms, recurrent disease after previous endarterectomy, or irradiated necks. Currently there are only two FDA-approved devices for use (RX ACCULINK, manufactured by the Guidant Corporation, Indianapolis, Indiana; and Xact, manufactured by Abbott Laboratories, Abbott Park, Illinois). We believe carotid angioplasty and stenting should only be performed in high-volume centers with multidisciplinary expertise and the desire to track patients long term.

For patients who do not yet meet the criteria for surgery as determined by percentage of carotid stenosis, daily aspirin and aggressive risk factor reduction are indicated. These patients should be followed by duplex ultrasounds every 6 months and seen regularly by the vascular surgeon. Any new symptoms or progression of disease to a critical stenosis warrants a more aggressive approach to intervention.

## Lower Extremity Arterial Occlusive Disease

Lower extremity peripheral arterial disease is a broad category of clinical entities that includes aortoiliac occlusive disease and femoropopliteotibial occlusive disease. The most common etiology of these diseases is atherosclerosis causing narrowing within these blood vessels. Risk factors again include smoking, hypertension, diabetes, elevated cholesterol, and family history. Up to 40% of patients also have coexisting coronary artery disease (CAD). Patients typically present with claudication, defined as pain in the lower extremities brought on by a reproducible amount of exercise and relieved only by a short period of rest. Depending on the location of the occlusion, symptoms may involve the buttocks, hip, thigh, or calf, and they can include impotence in men.

Lower extremity claudication is a significant health care issue, with studies documenting that 12% of the population experience claudication. Patients typically describe the pain as a sensation of muscle cramps or fatigue. This leads to chronic pain and health care provider visits, decreased productivity at work, and the possible progression toward a more sedentary lifestyle. The presence of claudication doubles age-specific mortality and decreases life expectancy on average by 10 years, and for this reason, patients should be aggressively

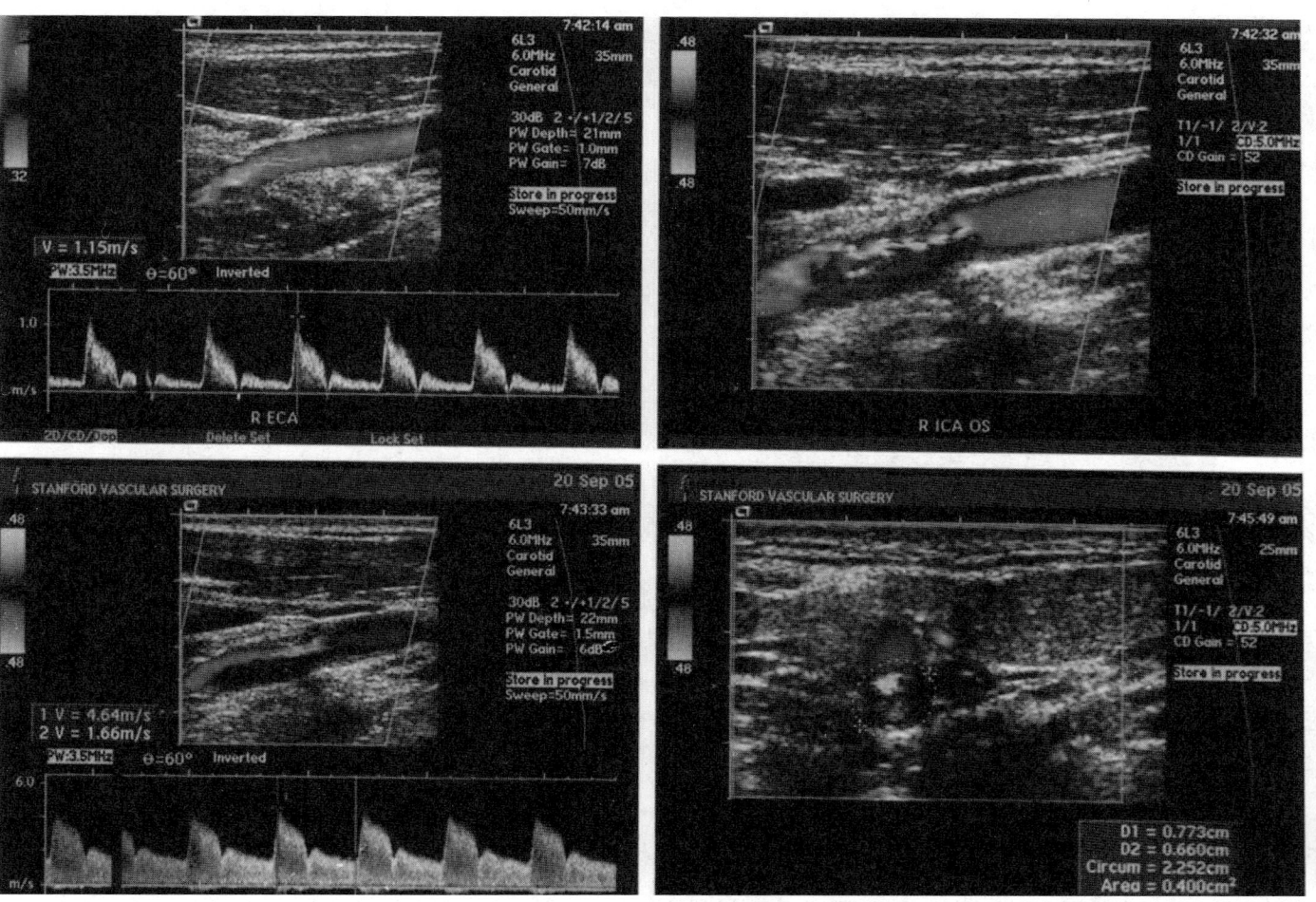

**FIGURE 1.** Duplex ultrasound scan of 51-year-old man with hypercholesterolemia and hypertension found to have a right carotid bruit on examination. Note the severe narrowing of the right internal carotid artery orifice (evidenced by a peak systolic velocity of 4.64 m/s, which corresponds to a stenosis of 80%–89% by velocity criteria). He underwent successful right carotid endarterectomy.

managed medically with selective surgical intervention. It is important to note that the rate of limb loss in patients with claudication is approximately 3% to 6% over 10 years, so preventive care measures instituted by the primary care physician are a vital adjunct to vascular consultation.

Approximately 15% of mild cases of claudication progress to more significant lower extremity ischemia manifested by rest pain and tissue loss; typically seen in diabetic patients who continue to smoke. This indicates more severe atherosclerotic narrowing and the need for more aggressive and urgent management. Patients typically describe pain in the front of the foot occurring at night that is relieved by hanging the foot over the edge of bed or getting out of bed. Careful physical inspection looking for tissue changes is also important to document the severity of lower extremity occlusive disease. Skin atrophy with thickened nails, loss of hair on dorsum of the foot, shiny skin, and toe or heel ulcerations are all signs of significant atherosclerotic disease.

Documentation of pulses is important and can be graded as diminished or absent. Pulse palpation, however, is quite subjective and predisposed to error. When pulses are not easily palpable, a handheld Doppler in the clinic can be used objectively to assess blood flow, especially when ankle blood pressures are obtained. The ankle-brachial index (ABI) is obtained by dividing the systolic pressure at the ankle into that of the arm. Normal ABIs range from 1.0 to 1.2. Patients with claudication usually have an ABI less than 0.7, and patients with tissue loss have an ABI less than 0.5. An ABI less than 0.3 suggests critical ischemia and warrants urgent evaluation and intervention. Caution must be used in interpreting ABIs from diabetic patients because their arteries may be calcified, which leads to falsely elevated ABIs.

The vascular laboratory can provide useful diagnostic information regarding lower extremity blood flow. Referral for formal duplex ultrasound with arterial waveform analysis is extremely helpful in determining the degree and location of stenosis. It is appropriate to obtain vascular consultation for patients with diminished ABIs and symptoms of lower extremity arterial occlusive disease. The decision to obtain more invasive and expensive studies should be made in consultation with the vascular surgeon. Recent advances in imaging technology have allowed CT angiography (Figure 2) and MRA to be a less invasive method of determining the extent of aortic, iliac, and distal occlusive changes. Traditional diagnostic angiography can be performed to delineate further the extent of disease, and it has the advantage of allowing access for percutaneous endovascular treatment of focal occlusive disease in the same setting.

Patients with mild claudication should be treated medically with aggressive risk factor reduction. Emphasis should be placed on smoking cessation, increasing exercise, weight loss, and controlling diabetes, hypertension, and high cholesterol. A strictly supervised exercise regimen is the only consistent therapy that increases pain-free walking distance and maximal walking distance. Numerous studies have looked at various medications for the treatment of claudication, all with conflicting and often short-term success. FDA-approved medications include pentoxifylline (Trental) and cilostazol (Pletal), yet only a 30% response rate is observed in typical claudicants. These agents help lower blood viscosity and inhibit platelet aggregation. Although results with these medications are variable, a trial of 6 to 8 weeks of therapy should be attempted along with the exercise regimen. Long-term population studies have found that approximately 75% of patients experience

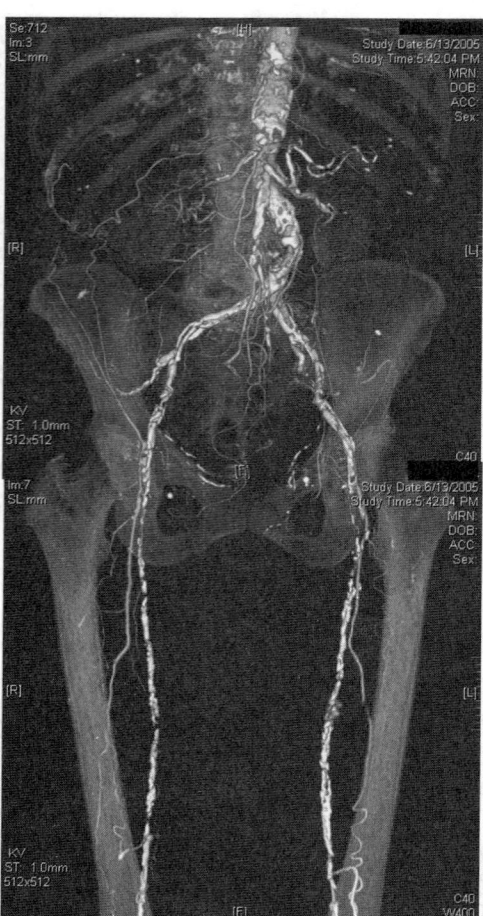

**FIGURE 2.** Computed tomographic (CT) angiography of an 81-year-old woman with severe thigh, buttock, and leg claudication and rest pain and a nonhealing left foot wound demonstrating severe calcified disease of her abdominal aorta and occluded iliac vessels and superficial femoral vessels. She underwent open aortofemoral bypass, which resulted in significant improvement in her walking and healing of her wound.

improvement in symptoms with medical management alone. Sustained symptom relief requires a regular walking regimen.

Patients who do not respond to medical management alone may be candidates for revascularization. Indications for revascularization include claudication that significantly interferes with lifestyle, rest pain, nonhealing wounds, and tissue loss or necrosis. Open surgical options include aortofemoral reconstruction for aortoiliac occlusive disease and femoral-tibial bypasses for more distal disease. Long-term results from these operations are excellent in terms of relief of symptoms and wound healing. Morbidity rates from open surgery are in the range of 2% to 6% with possible complications including myocardial infarction, bleeding, wound infections, graft infection or thrombosis, and limb loss. Careful graft surveillance after bypass with duplex ultrasound is an important adjunct to maintain long-term patency of grafts.

Endovascular interventions of the lower extremities typically include angioplasty, stenting, and atherectomy. These procedures are most successful in cases involving short stenoses of the iliac arteries. As the disease enters the more distal vessels, there is a significant decrease in the durability of traditional angioplasty and stenting. Future improvements in the technology and developments such as drug-eluting stents may improve future use of endovascular interventions in the lower extremities. As with open surgical revascularization, the importance of long-term surveillance with duplex ultrasound allows reintervention when restenosis occurs. In contrast to failed surgical revascularization, failed endovascular revascularizations can lead to worsened and more acute limb ischemia. Although percutaneous methods appear to be less invasive, they are clearly not less risky, and

ideally should be performed by vascular specialists dedicated to caring for all aspects of patients with lower extremity occlusive disease.

## REFERENCES

Jemal A, Ward E, Hao Y, Thun M: Trends in the leading causes of death in the United States, 1970–2002. JAMA, 2005;294:1255-1259.

Moore WS, Barnett MJ, Beebe HE, et al: Guidelines for carotid endarterectomy: A multidisciplinary consensus statement from the Ad Hoc Committee, American Heart Association. Stroke 1995;26:188-201.

The Executive Committee for the Asymptomatic Carotid Atherosclerosis Study: Endarterectomy for asymptomatic carotid artery stenosis. JAMA 1995;273:1421.

Norgren L, Hiatt WR, Dormandy JA, et al: Inter-Society Consensus for the Management of Peripheral Arterial Disease (TASC II). J Vasc Surg 2007;45:S5-S67.

# Venous Thrombosis

Method of
*Paul L. F. Giangrande, MD*

## Air Travel And Thrombosis

The subject of air travel and thrombosis has been the subject of much debate in both the lay and medical press in recent years, although a possible link has been recognized for many years, and the very first report concerned a physician who traveled from Boston to Venezuela in 1946. However, venous thromboembolism is not exclusively associated with air travel, and it has also been documented following long car, bus, and train journeys.

A case-control study of 160 consecutive patients with deep venous thrombosis (DVT) showed that 39 of 160 (24.5%) had recently completed a journey by car, train, or plane of longer than 4 hours; nine of these patients had traveled by air. When the patients with DVT were compared with the control group, a history of recent travel was reported four times more often in the subjects with venous thromboembolism (odds ratio [OR] = 4). This correlation has been confirmed by a recent and much larger case-control study, the Multiple Environment and Genetic Assessment (MEGA) study, from the Netherlands, which confirmed that travel by car, bus, train, or plane is associated with an increased risk of venous thrombosis. Thrombosis associated with flight is also by no means restricted to those in the relatively confined conditions of economy class, and thus the alternative term of "travelers' thrombosis" has been suggested.

It is possible to derive some general conclusions from published cases of venous thromboembolism associated with travel. Thromboembolism is rarely observed after flights of less than 5 hours, and typically, the flights are 12 hours or longer. The risk rises with age, and persons older than 50 years are more at risk, whereas those younger than 40 years are less vulnerable. Symptoms of thromboembolism do not usually develop during or immediately after the flight but tend to appear within 3 days of arrival, when the patient may present far away from the airport, and thus the causal link might not be immediately apparent. Symptoms of thrombosis or pulmonary embolism have been reported up to 2 weeks after a long flight. Pulmonary embolism may also be the first manifestation, without any symptoms in the lower limbs. Although most case reports and studies involve DVT in the lower limbs, there are also reports of cerebral venous thrombosis and arterial thrombosis associated with long flights.

The consequences of venous thromboembolism are not insignificant. Quite apart from the pain and discomfort, which can ruin a holiday or business trip, pulmonary embolism is estimated to develop in approximately 10% of cases. The mortality associated with pulmonary embolism rises with increasing age, but it is in the range of 2% to 15%

of cases. The inconvenience and side effects of warfarin treatment should also not be overlooked.

Approximately 60% of patients develop postphlebitis syndrome (persistent swelling and discomfort of the leg, often associated with ulceration) within 2 years despite appropriate anticoagulant therapy. A history of thrombosis precludes future prescription of hormone replacement therapy (HRT) or oral contraceptive pills (OCPs) for women, and it can make it difficult to secure travel insurance in the future because of the increased risk of recurrence.

## Epidemiology

The precise incidence of thromboembolism in relation to air travel is uncertain, though it has been estimated that at least 5% of all cases of DVT may be linked to air travel. A study based on 56 confirmed cases of pulmonary embolism among 135.3 million passengers passing through one airport in the period between 1993 and 2000 clearly demonstrated an association between duration of travel and risk of pulmonary was significantly higher (1.5 cases per million) for passengers traveling more than 5000 km when compared with a risk of only 0.01 cases per million among passengers traveling less than 5000 km.

Cases of pulmonary embolism clearly only represent the tip of the iceberg of cases of DVT. A recent observational study from New Zealand, based on the study of 878 passengers who traveled extensively (at least 10 hours; mean, 39 hours) reported an incidence of venous thromboembolism of 1%, including four cases of pulmonary embolism and five of DVT. However, the incidence of latent, asymptomatic thrombosis is likely to be even higher. A prospective study of long-haul air passengers older than 50 years reported that 12 of 116 passengers (10%) were found by duplex scanning to have asymptomatic DVT confined to the calf.

## Etiology

The etiology of venous thrombosis is usually multifactorial, with a combination of both constitutional and environmental factors responsible for causing a thrombosis in a patient at a given time. The three underlying causes of thrombosis are classically defined as Virchow's triad: stasis, hypercoagulability of the blood, and vessel wall disease.

Stasis in the venous circulation of the lower limbs is undoubtedly the major factor in promoting the development of venous thromboembolism associated with travel. The potential danger of confinement in cramped conditions has been recognized for some years. An increase in the incidence of fatal pulmonary embolism was reported during the Blitz in London during the Second World War. Simpson recognized that the primary cause was mechanical impairment of venous circulation due to squatting for a prolonged period in air raid shelters, and he recommended that bunks should be installed. The term *economy class syndrome* was coined to describe the phenomenon, and this also emphasizes the role of impaired venous circulation due to prolonged immobility in a cramped position. Ingestion of alcohol also encourages immobility during a flight, and the use of strong sedative medication may also be associated with an increased risk of venous thrombosis.

A number of other risk factors are now also recognized, primarily through clinical experience in the setting of surgery, which predispose to venous thromboembolism. These are listed in Box 1.

The effect of age was highlighted in a recent study from Australia, which concluded that the annual risk of venous thromboembolism is increased by 12% if one long-haul flight is undertaken annually. However, the incidence of thromboembolism was less than 1 per 100,000 arriving passengers younger than 40 years, but it rose steadily to exceed 14 per 100,000 in those aged 75 years or older.

A hematologic abnormality might predispose a person to development of venous thromboembolism. Such disorders include the relatively rare congenital (inherited) deficiencies of natural anticoagulants, such as antithrombin, protein C, or protein S. A recent

study demonstrated that an inherited thrombophilic defect or use of an OCP increased the risk of thrombosis associated with air travel 16-fold and 14-fold, respectively. The MEGA study has also demonstrated that positivity for the factor V Leiden thrombophilic mutation, body mass index greater than 30, height greater than 1.9 or less than 1.6 meters, and use of OCPs are strong susceptibility factors. In one small uncontrolled, retrospective study of patients with flight-related DVT, 6 of 20 (30%) subjects had a thrombophilic defect (factor V Leiden in 5). Four subjects had a history of a previous episode of thrombosis, and other potential risk factors were identified in 10 subjects (including malignancy, leg in plaster cast, use of OCP or HRT). Five of the 20 patients had a negative thrombophilia screen and no other identifiable risk factor.

The value of screening passengers for thrombophilic defects before long-haul flights has been raised. It is generally accepted that routine screening of passengers or screening of pilots as part of their medical screening is not justified or cost-effective. Such screening is not, of course, routinely offered in other circumstances associated with an increased risk of thrombosis (e.g., before starting an OCP, pregnancy, before orthopedic surgery), and no case has yet been established for air travel to be treated differently from current practice for thrombophilia screening in other fields.

Some evidence now suggests that exposure to the mild hypobaric hypoxia encountered in pressurized aircraft might also result in activation of the coagulation and thus encourage thrombosis. Aircraft typically fly at altitudes of between 35,000 and 40,000 feet to avoid turbulence and drag, thus benefiting fuel consumption. The cabin air is derived from the outside atmospheric air, which is drawn in and compressed. The maximum pressure in the cabin at cruising altitude is influenced by the allowable differential pressure across the wall of the cabin. This varies with aircraft design, but the lowest pressure permitted by the regulatory authorities for civil aircraft is equivalent to atmospheric pressure at an altitude of 8000 feet. Although the percentage of oxygen in the cabin remains unchanged at around 21%, the partial pressure of oxygen is reduced to around 74% of the sea level value. The very cold air at this altitude (typically around −50°C) contains only negligible water vapor, and the humidity in the cabin is thus typically very low.

Markers of activation of coagulation were transiently elevated in an uncontrolled study of 20 healthy male volunteers who were exposed to a hypobaric environment designed to simulate the conditions of an airplane cabin. The plasma levels of prothrombin fragments 1 and 2, thrombin-antithrombin (TAT) complex, and activated coagulation factor VII increased significantly, although the D-dimer level remained unchanged. Treatment with heparin inhibited the development of this apparent activation of the coagulation cascade. Another study of eight subjects who ascended rapidly to high altitudes by helicopter in Nepal documented increases in the levels of prothrombin fragments 1 and 2 and PAI-1 (plasminogen activator inhibitor, a key inhibitor of fibrinolysis). Activation of coagulation associated with flight, reflected by an increase in plasma levels of TAT complex, was also demonstrated in a crossover study in which 71 healthy volunteers were studied in the setting of an 8-hour flight, with the same volunteers monitored in two controlled-exposure situations.

Contrary to the widespread belief that passengers on long-haul flights can develop dehydration through increased insensible loss of water across the skin and mucous surfaces, it has been calculated that the maximum possible increase in insensible loss of water over an 8-hour period in such conditions is only around 100 mL. Although systemic dehydration is not a significant factor in healthy persons, the low humidity in an aircraft cabin can certainly lead to dryness of the mucous membranes and a sensation of thirst. Excessive consumption of alcohol or gastrointestinal infections associated with vomiting and diarrhea can also exacerbate dehydration.

## Prevention

A number of general measures may be taken to minimize the risk of thrombosis associated with long flights. Perhaps the most important step is to consider at the outset whether the passenger is actually fit to fly in the first place. For example, it is probably wise to defer long-haul travel after recent major orthopedic surgery. Passengers should be encouraged to carry out leg exercises from time to time while seated (e.g., flexion, extension, and rotation of the ankles help to promote circulation in the lower limbs). However, many airlines discourage unnecessary walking about in the cabin because there is always the possibility of encountering unexpected air turbulence. Hand luggage stowed under seats also restricts movement. Passengers should take advantage of refueling stops on long-haul flights to get off the plane and walk around for awhile. Adequate hydration should be ensured during the flight. It is not necessary to abstain from alcohol, but excessive consumption should be avoided because it promotes diuresis and discourages mobility. Similarly, sedatives are best avoided. Although estrogen-containing OCPs and HRT are recognized risk factors for venous thrombosis, I do not advocate interrupting such hormonal medication for the period of travel.

A recent review of 10 randomized studies for the Cochrane Database has confirmed the value of compression hosiery (flight socks). In the very first study performed, 231 passengers were recruited before long-haul flights and randomized into two groups. Of those who did not wear compression hosiery, 12 of 116 (10%) were found after the flight to have asymptomatic calf DVT with duplex ultrasonography, but none of the 115 who wore compression hosiery was affected. In the LONFLIT-4 study of 372 passengers considered to be at medium to high risk of thromboembolism, none of the 179 subjects wearing compression hosiery developed DVT, but six of 179 (3.35%) controls developed asymptomatic DVT (four DVT, two superficial) (P <0.002). In the subsequent LONFLIT-5 study of 224 high-risk passengers who went on an even longer flight, DVT was observed in six of 102 (5.8%) control subjects and only one of 103 (0.97%) subjects wearing compression hosiery (P <0.0025). Quite apart from reducing the risk of thrombosis, compression hosiery helps to prevent edema of the legs and feet, which can itself cause discomfort after a long flight.

Flight socks have the advantage of being readily available without prescription and are washable and thus reusable. They apply graduated pressure to the leg that is maximal at the ankle, thus encouraging venous return. The usual full-length stockings used in hospitals for prophylaxis of thromboembolism in patients undergoing surgery are not suitable for use in flight because they provide a lower pressure at the ankle (UK Class I standard: 14-17 mm Hg) because they are designed for recumbent patients. It is also important that the patient is provided with the correct type and size of compression stocking; unfortunately, there is no internationally agreed standard with regard to the degree of compression. The stockings also need to be worn correctly, taking care to ensure that there is no constriction in the popliteal area. Stockings are contraindicated in cases of peripheral vascular disease because the additional compression could provoke ischemia.

Aspirin[1] has been advocated by some in the general prophylaxis of thrombosis associated with travel, but any beneficial effect is weak in absolute terms. Aspirin is certainly very effective in preventing arterial thrombosis, because platelets play a major role in thrombosis in the arterial circulation. Arterial thrombi are rich in platelets on histologic examination, whereas thrombi in the venous circulation consist primarily of red cells enmeshed in fibrin strands but contain few platelets. It has been estimated that if the rate of travel-related DVT is 20 per 100,000 travelers, then 17,000 people would need to be treated with aspirin to prevent just one episode of DVT. Furthermore, there is a significant potential for adverse reactions: 13% of subjects taking aspirin in a study to evaluate its potential in preventing venous thrombosis associated with air travel reported gastrointestinal symptoms such as dyspepsia. Heparin may be considered in the relatively few passengers considered to be at particularly high risk for thrombosis (e.g., history of more than one thrombotic episode and an identified thrombophilic abnormality), although many such subjects are already likely to be on long-term oral anticoagulation anyway.

Unfortunately, there are no consensus guidelines yet and it is clear that there is still a wide difference in practice. This was emphasized by the results of a survey of more than 2000 delegates attending an international conference on thrombosis in Australia, which noted that 80% had taken precautions to prevent travel-related thrombosis. Just 17% wore compression hosiery and 21% relied on aspirin either alone or in combination with other measures.

## Summary

It is now generally accepted that there is an association between long-distance air travel as well as other forms of long-distance travel and venous thromboembolism. The risk is largely confined to those with recognized additional risk factors for venous thromboembolism. Leg exercises while seated help to reduce the risk of DVT. There is also clear evidence from prospective and randomized clinical trials to support the use of compression hosiery as a preventive measure. By contrast, there is no firm evidence to support the indiscriminate use of aspirin as a routine prophylactic measure.

## REFERENCES

Ashkan K, Nasim A, Dennis MJ, Sayers RD: Acute arterial thrombosis after a long-haul flight. J R Soc Med 1998;91:324.

Belcaro G, Cesarone MR, Shah SS, et al: Prevention of edema, flight microangiopathy and venous thrombosis in long flights with elastic stockings. A randomized trial: The LONFLIT 4 Concorde Edema-SSL Study. Angiology 2002;53:635-645.

Belcaro G, Cesarone MR, Nicolaides AN, et al: Prevention of venous thrombosis with elastic stockings during long-haul flights: The LONFLIT 5 JAP study. Clin Appl Thromb Hemost 2003;9:197-201.

Bendz B, Rostrup M, Sevre K, et al: Association between hypobaric hypoxia and activation of coagulation in human beings. Lancet 2000;356:1657-1658.

Bendz B, Sevre K, Andersen TO, Sandset PM: Low molecular weight heparin prevents activation of coagulation in a hypobaric environment. Blood Coagul Fibrinolysis 2001;12:371-374.

Cannegieter SC, Doggen CJ, van Houwelingen HC, Rosendaal FR: Travel-related venous thrombosis: Results from a large population-based case control study (MEGA study). PLoS Med 2006;3:e307.

Cesarone MR, Belcaro G, Nicolaides AN, et al: Venous thrombosis from air travel: The LONFLIT 3 study—prevention with aspirin vs. low molecular weight heparin (LMWH) in high risk subjects: A randomized trial. Angiology 2002;53:1-6.

Clarke M, Hopewell S, Juszczak E, et al: Compression stockings for preventing deep vein thrombosis in airline passengers. Cochrane Database Syst Rev 2006;(2):CD004002.

Collins REC, Field S, Castleden WM: Thrombosis of leg arteries after prolonged travel. BMJ 1979;2:1478.

Cruickshank JM, Gorlin R, Jennett B: Air travel and thrombotic episodes: The economy class syndrome. Lancet 1988;2:497-498.

Giangrande PLF: Air travel and thrombosis. Br J Haematol 2002;117: 509-512.

[1]Not FDA approved for this indication.

Hagg S, Spigset O: Antipsychotic-induced venous thromboembolism: A review of the evidence. CNS Drugs 2002;16:765-776.

Homans J: Thrombosis of the deep leg veins due to prolonged sitting. N Engl J Med 1954;250:148-149.

Hughes RJ, Hopkins RJ, Hill S, et al: Frequency of venous thromboembolism in low to moderate risk long distance air travellers: The New Zealand Air Traveller's Thrombosis (NZATT) Study. Lancet 2003;362: 2039-2044.

Kelman CW, Kortt MA, Becker NG, et al: Deep vein thrombosis and air travel: Record linkage study. BMJ 2003;327:1072-1075.

Kuipers S, Cannegieter SC, Middeldorp S, et al: Use of preventive measures for air travel–related venous thrombosis in professionals who attend medical conferences. J Thromb Haemost 2006;4:2373-2376.

Lapostolle F, Surget V, Borron SW,et al: Severe pulmonary embolism associated with air travel. N Engl J Med 2001;345:779-783.

Loke YK, Derry S: Air travel and venous thrombosis: How much help might aspirin be? Med Gen Med 2002;4:4. Available at http://www.medscape.com/viewarticle/441153 (accessed June 1, 2007).

Martinelli I, Taioli E, Battaglioli T, et al: Risk of venous thromboembolism after air travel: Interaction with thrombophilia and oral contraceptives. Arch Intern Med 2006;163:2674-2676.

Mannucci PM, Gringeri A, Peyvandi F, et al: Short-term exposure to high altitude causes coagulation activation and inhibits fibrinolysis. Thromb Haemost 2002;87:342-343.

Nicholson AN: Dehydration and long haul flights. Travel Med Int 1998;16: 177-181.

Pfausler B, Vollert H, Bosch S, Schmutzhard E: Cerebral venous thrombosis: A new diagnosis in travel medicine. J Travel Med 1996;3:165-167.

Rege KP, Bevan DH, Chitolie A, Shannon MS: Risk factors and thrombosis after airline flight. Thromb Haemost 1999;81:995-996.

Rosendaal FR: Venous thrombosis: A multicausal disease. Lancet 1999;353: 1167-1173.

Schreijer AJM, Cannegieter SC, Meijers JCM, et al: Activation of coagulation system during air travel: A crossover study. Lancet 2006;367: 832-838.

Scurr JH, Machin SJ, Bailey-King S, et al: Frequency and prevention of symptomless deep-vein thrombosis in long-haul flights: A randomized trial. Lancet 2001;357:1485-1489.

Simpson K: Shelter deaths from pulmonary embolism. Lancet 1940;11:744.

Teenen RP, MacKay AJ: Peripheral arterial thrombosis related to commercial airline flights: Another manifestation of the economy class syndrome. Br J Clin Prac 1992;46:165-166.

Thomassen R, Vandenbroucke JP, Rosendaal FR: Antipsychotic drugs and venous thrombosis. Br J Psychiatry 2001;179:63-66.

Zornberg GL, Jick H: Antipsychotic drug use and risk of first-time idiopathic venous thromboembolism: A case-control study. Lancet 2000;356: 1219-1223.

# The Blood and Spleen

## Aplastic Anemia

Method of
*Abdo Haddad, MD, and*
*Jaroslaw P. Maciejewski, MD, PhD*

Historically, aplastic anemia (AA) has been the subject of intense investigations that have resulted in the assignment of bone marrow as a site of blood cell production, facilitated the concept of the hematopoietic stem cell, and led to the introduction of allogeneic bone marrow transplantation (BMT) as a therapeutic modality for human hematologic disorders. AA is defined as peripheral blood pancytopenia with obligatory hypocellular bone marrow. The current definition includes a decrease in at least two of three peripheral blood cell lineages. The current definition of AA incorporates severity of blood count depression that clearly correlates with prognosis. If not treated, severe AA is invariably fatal, whereas moderate AA has a good long-term prognosis.

The incidence of AA is estimated to be between two and five cases per million in the West but may be two to five times more frequent in the Far East. Typically, AA is a disease of the young, but the incidence has two peaks: one between the ages of 15 and 25 years and the other after the sixth decade of life. Whether the often described second peak is the result of diagnostic overlap of AA and myelodysplastic syndrome (MDS), which affects older individuals and can mimic AA, especially if marrow is hypocellular, is unclear.

## Pathogenesis

### CLASSIFICATION BASED ON PATHOGENESIS

Based on pathogenesis, AA can be classified as either inherited or acquired. Inherited forms of AA include Fanconi anemia and variants of dyskeratosis congenita, which are related to various mutations in the telomerase complex. Conceptually, acquired AA may evolve as a primary disease, occurring in the form of idiopathic AA, or as a secondary condition related to iatrogenic use of ionizing radiation and cytotoxic therapy, idiosyncratic drug reactions, certain viruses, or in association with autoimmune conditions (Figure 1). Of note, the term "idiopathic" refers to the inability to identify a cause. It is possible that some unknown etiologic agents, such as viruses and certain chemicals, also serve as triggers in idiopathic AA. When iatrogenic causes are excluded, most cases of AA are idiopathic (Table 1).

## ETIOLOGIC FACTORS AND THEIR INVOLVEMENT IN THE PATHOPHYSIOLOGY OF APLASTIC ANEMIA

Injury to the stem cell compartment with a qualitative and quantitative stem cell defect is the ultimate result of various and diverse pathophysiologic mechanisms. Idiopathic AA is likely mediated by the autoimmune attack of T cells leading to proliferation block and apoptosis of progenitor and stem cells. Apart from any infectious and systemic diseases that must be excluded before the diagnosis of idiopathic AA is made, direct or indirect causes of AA include direct chemical hematopoietic injury (see Figure 1). Treatment with cytotoxic chemotherapeutic drugs or irradiation causes direct injury to the bone marrow cells, which may lead to AA. However, a patient with acquired AA rarely has a history of such exposures.

### Direct Chemical Hematopoietic Injury

Treatment with cytotoxic chemotherapeutic drugs can cause direct injury to the bone marrow cells, but a typical patient with acquired AA rarely has a history of such exposures, which would preclude the diagnosis of idiopathic AA.

### Radiation

Both chronic and acute radiation exposure results in dose- and duration-dependent injury to the stem cell compartment. The lethal dose is dependent upon the level of supportive care. If the patient survives the acute phase, bone marrow hypoplasia may be the predominant factor influencing long-term prognosis.

### Direct Effects of Viruses

Viral infections, which include human cytomegalovirus and Epstein-Barr virus, have been implicated in rare cases of AA but do not constitute a typical cause of idiopathic AA.

### Drug-related Aplastic Anemia

Medications may induce AA in the form of an idiosyncratic reaction. Various epidemiologic studies have implicated many drugs. Historically, chloramphenicol was considered the most notorious agent in AA. However, the etiologic fraction of AA attributed to drugs is low, and for most agents the odds ratio shows only a marginally increased risk of AA (i.e., between onefold and 10-fold). Of note, drug-related AA may display a similar course to the typical immune-mediated AA and often responds to immunosuppressive agents (Table 2).

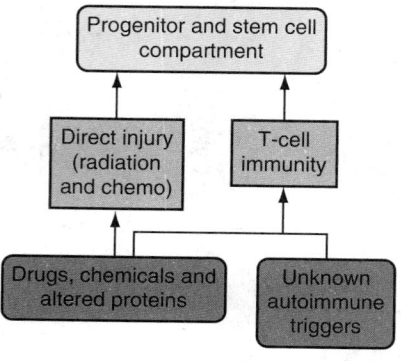

**FIGURE 1.** Stem cell injury in aplastic anemia.

## TABLE 1   Etiology of Aplastic Anemia

| Acquired Aplastic Anemia | Inherited Aplastic Anemia |
| --- | --- |
| Idiopathic aplastic anemia | Fanconi anemia |
| Pregnancy | Dyskeratosis congenita |
| Paroxysmal nocturnal | Reticular dysgenesis |
|   hemoglobinuria | Shwachman anemia |
| Secondary | Genetic primary |
|   **Drugs** |   nonhematologic |
|     Iatrogenic/cytotoxic |   syndromes |
|     Idiosyncratic | |
|       Chloramphenicol | |
|       Nonsteroidal anti- | |
|         inflammatory drug | |
|       Gold | |
|       Antiepileptics | |
|       Others | |
|   **Radiation** | |
|     Iatrogenic | |
|     Accidental | |
|   **Viruses** | |
|     Epstein-Barr virus | |
|     Non-A, non-B, non-C, | |
|       non-G hepatitis | |
|     Parvovirus | |
|     HIV | |
| Pancytopenia of | |
|   autoimmune diseases | |

### Immune-Mediated Marrow Failure

Immune-mediated bone marrow failure is the most common cause of idiopathic AA. This process likely is triggered by viruses (e.g., AA/hepatitis syndrome is likely caused by a currently hypothetic non-A, B, C, D, E hepatitis virus) or by chemicals of altered proteins (e.g., resulting from transcription of mutated genes). Regardless of the inciting agents, the subsequent immunologic reaction may be uniform for various etiologies and includes an autoimmune T cell–mediated attack on hematopoietic progenitor and stem cells.

### PATHOPHYSIOLOGY OF APLASTIC ANEMIA

The pathophysiology of idiopathic AA includes two major components: the stem cell compartment and immune effector mechanisms. Despite intense investigation, bone marrow stroma has not been identified as an important factor in the pathophysiology of AA. Aplastic stroma supports the growth of normal hematopoietic progenitors, and BMT is a successful therapeutic modality in AA, thus favoring the argument that patient's stromal cells can support the maintenance, proliferation, and differentiation of transplanted hematopoietic stem cells of the donor.

### Stem Cells in Aplastic Anemia

A profound defect in the hematopoietic stem cell compartment has been consistently found in AA, as measured by colony-forming assays, long-term culture-initiating cell assays, and flow cytometry. It has been estimated that in AA the number of hematopoietic stem cells is decreased between 10-fold and 1000-fold. Hematopoietic suppression involves all stages of hematopoietic development. Apoptosis of hematopoietic progenitor and stem cells represents the final pathway; it has been consistently found in AA and is thought to be the result of immune effector mechanisms, including direct cell-mediated toxicity and inhibitory cytokines.

### Autoimmune Mechanisms in Aplastic Anemia

Polyclonal T cell responses and increased frequency of activated cytotoxic T (Tc) cells and products, including interferon-γ and Fas ligand, have been found in AA. Although the initial inciting events may be diverse, the subsequent pathophysiologic mechanisms involve expansion of autoimmune clones recognizing antigens displayed by hematopoietic progenitor and stem cells. The effector pathways include direct killing via perforin/granzyme secretion, Fas-mediated killing, as well as effects of cytokines with inhibitory properties on hematopoiesis. Increased levels of interferon γ have been found in AA, likely as a result of altered Th1/Th2 and Tc1/Tc2 balances. Whereas principally T cell responses are polyclonal in AA, immunodominant cytotoxic T cell clones can be detected and can serve as markers of the autoimmune process. Of note, inflammatory signs and markers, such as elevated erythrocyte sedimentation rate or C-reactive protein level, are consistently negative in AA. Patients with AA do not show hypoglobulinemia or hyperglobulinemia. Pathologic B cell responses and humoral immunity have not been conversely implicated in the pathophysiology of AA.

## TABLE 2   Drugs Most Commonly Implicated in Aplastic Anemia

| Dose-Dependent Marrow Cytopenia | Drug That May Associate with Cytopenia | Drugs That Rarely Associate with Cytopenia |
| --- | --- | --- |
| Chemotherapy | Chloramphenicol | Antibiotics |
| | Nonsteroidal anti-inflammatory drugs | Allopurinol (Zyloprim) |
| | Carbamazepine (Tegretol) | Amiodarone (Cordarone), methyldopa |
| | Antithyroids |   (Aldomet), quinidine |
| | Gold, penicillamine (Cuprimine) | Lithium |
| | Sulfonamides | Chlorpromazine |
| | Antidiabetics | Antihistamine |

## Target Antigens

Target antigens are not known, but from the spectrum of hematopoietic inhibition it can be concluded that they are located on immature hematopoietic stem cells. Specific autoantibodies have been only rarely described in AA, and their role remains unclear. The targets of immune recognition of antigens may be altered proteins, autoantigens, or cross-reactive antigens.

# Clinical Presentation and Diagnostic Considerations

## CLINICAL PRESENTATION

Pancytopenia and hypocellular bone marrow are the hallmarks of AA. The most common initial presentation is bleeding (serious bleeding, easy bruisability, petechiae, gum and nose bleeding, and, in females, heavy menstrual flow). Patients are rarely infected at presentation despite a low absolute neutrophil count (ANC). If patients with pancytopenia show systemic symptoms, such as fever, weight loss, pain, anorexia, and night sweats, then the possibility of alternative diagnoses should be entertained. Fatigue, lightheadedness, and shortness of breath are symptoms of anemia. AA patients can present with very low hemoglobin levels that are remarkably well tolerated but suggestive of the gradual decline in hemoglobin value.

## PHYSICAL EXAMINATION

Patients with severe disease may look remarkably well given the levels of cytopenia. Petechiae usually occur over the pretibial surfaces, arm wrists, and occasionally in the oral area. Ecchymoses may present secondary to minor trauma. Retinal hemorrhage, gingival oozing, traces of heme in stool, and vaginal bleeding may occur in AA. Hepatomegaly and splenomegaly are unusual in AA. The examiner should look for physical stigmata of hereditary conditions, such as Fanconi anemia or dyskeratosis congenita. Icterus may indicate an ongoing hemolysis and point toward a diagnosis of paroxysmal nocturnal hemoglobinuria (PNH) or suggest the possibility of hepatitis.

## DIAGNOSIS AND DIFFERENTIAL DIAGNOSIS

Diagnosis of AA requires exclusion of systemic diseases that could mimic AA. The most common causes of cytopenia and marrow hypocellularity are obvious (e.g., history of cytotoxic drug usage); many other possible differential diagnostic considerations are rare (Table 3). All potentially offending medications should be discontinued. Blood cell count may be depressed to various extents; patients show low numbers of reticulocytes. Relative lymphocytosis is common, and most patients show a decrease in ANC and monocyte counts. Hypocellularity of the marrow is an obligatory finding for establishing the diagnosis of AA. Megaloblastic changes in erythroid series are common. The presence of even a few blasts indicates that the diagnosis of AA is unlikely. In typical cases, megakaryocytes are absent or severely diminished. The severity of AA can be described based on peripheral parameters (Table 4). The determination of a reticulocyte count is important for the diagnosis of bone marrow failure and the assessment of the severity of AA. The cytogenetic evaluation should show a normal karyotype. Although it is rational to assume that abnormal karyotyping precludes the diagnosis of AA (is consistent with myelodysplasia), the presence of some unbalanced translocations may be compatible with AA. In children and younger adults, Fanconi anemia should be excluded by appropriate tests. The diagnostic algorithm is outlined in Figure 2. PNH flow cytometry (detection of granulocytes and erythrocytes missing otherwise constitutive glycosylphosphatidylinositol (GPI)-anchored proteins) should be performed to establish baseline levels and rule out AA/PNH syndrome. Of note, 30% of AA patients may harbor subclinical levels of GPI-deficient cells. It is important to distinguish some of the common forms of AA.

**TABLE 3 Differential Diagnosis of Pancytopenia**

| Hypocellular Marrow | Hypercellular Marrow |
|---|---|
| Acquired aplastic anemia | **Primary Bone Marrow Disease** |
| Inherited aplastic anemia | Myelodysplastic syndrome |
| Myelodysplastic syndrome | Paroxysmal nocturnal hemoglobinuria |
| Rare aleukemic leukemia | Myelofibrosis |
| Acute lymphoblastic leukemia | Aleukemic leukemia |
| Lymphomas of the bone marrow | Bone marrow lymphoma |
| | Hairy cell leukemia |
| | **Secondary to Systemic Disease** |
| | Systemic lupus erythematosus |
| | Hypersplenism |
| | Vitamin $B_{12}$, folic acid deficiency |
| | Overwhelming infection |
| | Alcohol |
| | Brucellosis |
| | Ehrlichiosis |
| | Sarcoidosis |
| | Tuberculosis |

### Pregnancy-Associated AA

Pregnancy seems to predispose women to AA, but the mechanism remains unclear, making the nature of the association controversial. AA often resolves with termination of the pregnancy but can recur during subsequent pregnancies. Even if the initial presentation of AA was not associated with pregnancy, women with a recent history of successfully treated AA should be counseled not to get pregnant. Successful pregnancies have been described, and in the majority of cases most women had positive outcomes.

### Seronegative Hepatitis/Aplastic Anemia Syndrome

From 2% to 9% of AA patients have a history of preceding hepatitis. In typical cases, AA evolves 3 to 6 months following a latency interval after initially severe and often fulminant non-A, B, C, D, and E hepatitis. At the time of AA presentation, transaminases may normalize.

### Post-Mononucleosis Aplastic Anemia

In rare instances, Epstein-Barr virus infections are associated with AA. The usual course is severe, and most of the described cases showed negative outcomes. Infectious mononucleosis may present with neutropenia and is clearly distinct from Epstein-Barr virus–associated AA.

**TABLE 4 Severity Classification of Aplastic Anemia by Laboratory**

| Severe Aplastic Anemia | Moderate Aplastic Anemia |
|---|---|
| Bone marrow cellularity <10% Depression of at least two of three hematopoietic lineages: Absolute neutrophil count <500/µL Transfusion dependence with ARC <40,000/µL Platelet count <20,000/µL | Decreased bone marrow cellularity Depression of at least two of three hematopoietic lineages not fulfilling the criteria for severe aplastic anemia |

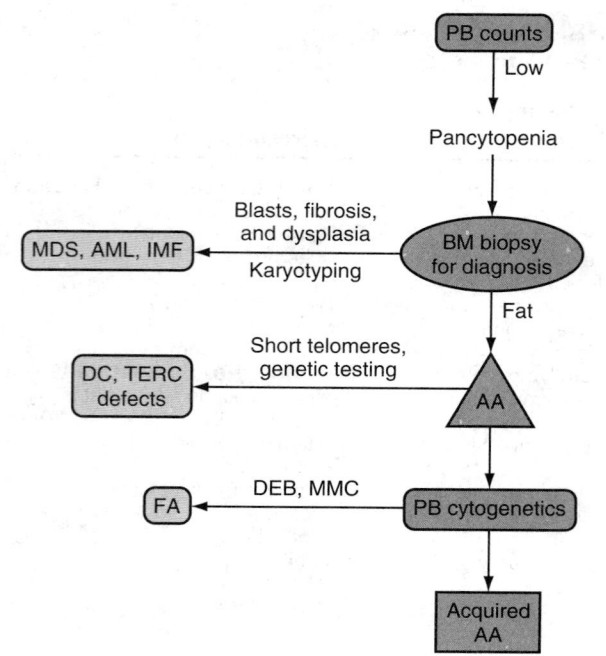

**FIGURE 2.** Diagnostic algorithm in aplastic anemia (AA). *Abbreviations:* AML = acute myeloid leukemia; BM = bone marrow; DC = dyskeratosis congenita; DEB = diepoxybutane; FA = Fanconi anemia; IMF = idiopathic myelofibrosis; MDS = myelodysplastic syndrome; MMC = mitomycin C; PB = peripheral blood; TERC = telomerase RNA component.

### Paroxysmal Nocturnal Hemoglobinuria/Aplastic Anemia Syndrome

There is a strong association between AA and PNH. Manifest PNH can evolve in up to 15% of patients with AA, and GPI anchor–deficient clones are present in a significant proportion of patients with AA. However, AA/PNH syndrome usually displays higher percentages of GPI anchor–deficient blood cells and concomitant bone marrow suppression as indicated by depressed platelet count, ANC, and reticulocyte counts with frequently hypocellular bone marrow. Whereas moderate cytopenia may be consistent with the diagnosis of PNH, AA/PNH syndrome displays a clear crossover between the two diseases.

### Chronic Moderate Aplastic Anemia

Moderate AA may serve as a transition stage of severe AA. However, some patients will maintain moderately depressed blood counts over extended periods (>3 months). Chronic moderate AA may constitute a separate entity, and some inherited marrow failure syndromes likely fall into this category. The response rates to immunosuppressive agents are not established and may be lower than those in severe AA. The therapies may include cyclosporine A (CsA; (Sandimmune[1]), antithymocyte globulin (ATG; Atgam), or anti–interleukin-2 receptor monoclonal antibody (daclizumab [Zenapax[1]], basiliximab [Simulect][1]), especially if patients are transfusion dependent. However, the prognosis is favorable if blood counts remain stable. Many hematologists may elect to approach moderate AA expectantly and treat only if counts worsen.

## Therapy of Aplastic Anemia

### SUPPORTIVE CARE

Consequences of pancytopenia can be life-threatening. AA can be cured by BMT or by immunosuppressive therapy (IS). Advances in

[1]Not FDA approved for this indication.

supportive care likely are reflected in the improved survival rates of patients with AA in general, but especially patients who are refractory to therapies now can survive for extended periods.

Blood product transfusions have improved survival in patients with AA. Modern technology has made red blood cells and platelets available and fairly safe for transfusion. Alloimmunization is a major problem related to platelet transfusion. Alloimmunization can be prevented or delayed by the use of single donor–donor platelet transfusion and leukocyte depletion. The trigger values for platelet transfusions are a subject of controversy, but most hematologists transfuse platelets when levels fall below 10,000 to 20,000/μL. If a transplant from a related donor is planned, transfusions of blood from relatives should be avoided. Individuals who are physically fit may be asymptomatic, with a hemoglobin level higher than 7 g/dL. AA patients with ANC less than 500/μL are at increased risk for infection, and the recommendations for starting an empirical antibiotic therapy are the same as for other causes of prolonged neutropenia. Hematopoietic growth factors usually are ineffective for typical AA. Clearly, a broad-spectrum antibiotic and novel antifungal agent improve outcomes in patients with neutropenic fever.

### CONSERVATIVE THERAPIES

IS with horse or rabbit ATG followed by CsA is the first-line, conservative therapy for severe AA (see Figure 3). Response rates are between 60% and 90%, with long-term survival in 60% to 70% of patients. ATG alone and CsA alone are inferior to the ATG/CsA combination. Refractory patients have poor prognosis. Repeated cycles of ATG/CsA can salvage up to 50% of initial nonresponders. Relapses are common (35%), but they can also be salvaged with repeated cycles of IS. In some patients, the counts remain dependent on chronic CsA therapy. In general, patients with HLA-DR1501 and those with the presence of PNH clones show higher rates of responsiveness to IS. Growth factors such as granulocyte colony-stimulating factor (filgrastim [Neupogen]), erythropoietin,[1] or granulocyte-macrophage colony-stimulating factor (sargramostim [Leukine][1]) do not appear to improve the response rate, and their benefit in conjunction with intense IS is questionable. Typical AA patients will not show response to granulocyte colony-stimulating factor and erythropoietin.

[1]Not FDA approved for this indication.

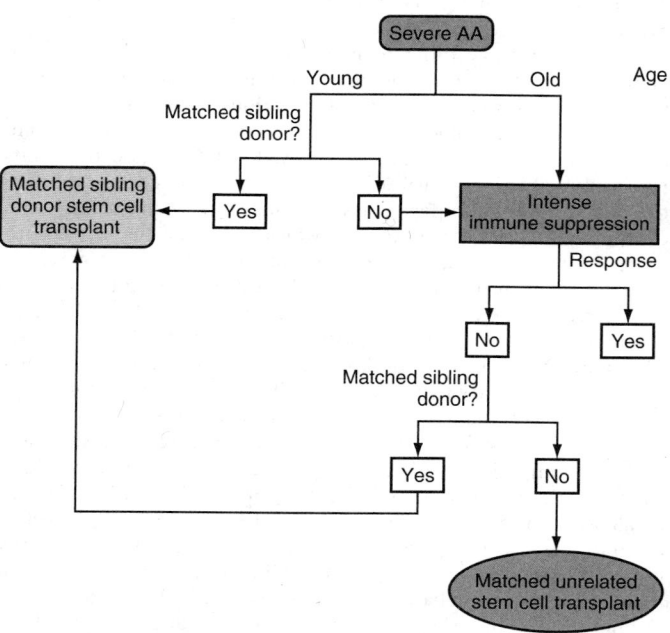

**FIGURE 3.** Severe aplastic anemia (AA) management.

However, prolonged therapy with granulocyte colony-stimulating factor and erythropoietin has been applied as salvage therapy for patients refractory to IS. Corticosteroids are used to alleviate the side effects of serum sickness with ATG but should not be used as the sole agent in severe AA. Historically, androgens have been used as therapy for AA and show significant response rates, but they are clearly inferior to IS and consequently have a role only as a salvage modality.

## BONE MARROW TRANSPLANTATION

Allogeneic BMT can cure AA (see Figure 3). Best results are achieved in children and young adults transplanted with grafts derived from matched sibling donors; survival rates range from 80% to 90%. Most common regimens use bone marrow as a source of stem cells along with cyclophosphamide (Cytoxan)/ATG–based conditioning regimens. BMT remains the treatment of choice for children with severe AA, if an appropriate family donor is available. Patients younger than 20 years have a 20% chance of developing acute graft-versus-host disease (GVHD). The risk of GVHD can be as high as 40% in patients older than 40 years. Methotrexate/CsA combination is used for GVHD prophylaxis. In general, for older patients the resulting overall survival from sibling–donor BMT as a first-line therapy is comparable or even superior to that from IS. Patients refractory to IS will be considered for BMT as second-line therapy. BMT results from a matched unrelated donor are less favorable, with survival ranging between 40% and 60%. Nonmyeloablative approaches are currently under development to improve BMT results in older patients and in those without a matched related donor.

## Complications and Long-term Prognosis

Patients successfully treated with IS have an excellent prognosis, whereas nonresponders who cannot undergo BMT have a poor prognosis. However, in recent years the survival of chronically pancytopenic patients has improved due to advances in supportive care. Conversion of severe AA into moderate disease appears to be sufficient in significantly improving the long-term prognosis of patients. Thus, partial remissions of severe AA are compatible with long-term survival. The most common complications of conservatively treated AA include a high relapse rate, which can be as high as 37% in 10 years, and evolution of clonal disease, including MDS and PNH. The prognosis of relapse is good, with a high rate of success for reinduction IS. Evolution to MDS has poor prognosis, especially if accompanied by aberrations of chromosome 7 or complex cytogenetic abnormalities. The evolution rate is 10% to 20% in 15 years. Manifest hemolytic PNH may develop in another 10% to 20% of patients with AA. Although PNH may be associated with severe morbidity, most patients will show a good long-term survival. Recipients of allogeneic grafts show a different set of long-term complications, including chronic GVHD, cataracts, thyroid disorders, secondary cancers, and avascular bone necrosis.

## REFERENCES

Bacigalupo A, Brand R, Oneto R, et al: Treatment of acquired severe aplastic anemia: Bone marrow transplantation compared with immunosuppressive therapy—The European group for blood and marrow transplantation experience. Semin Hematol 2000;37:69-80.

Bottiger LE: Epidemiology and aetiology of aplastic anemia. Haematol Blood Transfus 1979;24:27-37.

Hoffman R, Benz EJ, Shattil SJ: Hematology Basic Principles and Practice, 4th ed. Philadelphia, Churchill-Livingstone, 2005.

Maciejewski JP, Risitano A: Hematopoietic stem cells in aplastic anemia. Arch Med Res 2003;34:520-527.

Maciejewski JP, Rivera C, Kook H, et al: Relationship between bone marrow failure syndromes and the presence of glycophosphatidyl inositol-anchored protein-deficient clones. Br J Haematol 2001;115:1015-1022.

Maciejewski JP, Selleri C: Evolution of clonal cytogenetic abnormalities in aplastic anemia. Leuk Lymphoma 2004;45:433-440.

Margolis DA, Casper JT: Alternative-donor hematopoietic stem-cell transplantation for severe aplastic anemia. Semin Hematol 2000;37:43-55.

Rosenfeld S, Follmann D, Nunez O, Young NS: Antithymocyte globulin and cyclosporine for severe aplastic anemia: Association between hematologic response and long-term outcome. JAMA 2003;289:1130-1135.

Young NS: Acquired aplastic anemia. Ann Intern Med 2002;136:534-546.

Young NS, Gerson ST, High K: Clinical Hematology, 1st ed. Philadelphia, Mosby-Elsevier, 2006.

Young NS, Maciejewski J: The pathophysiology of acquired aplastic anemia. N Engl J Med 1997;336:1365-1372.

# Iron Deficiency

Method of
*James C. Barton, MD*

Iron deficiency is common worldwide. In developed countries, iron requirements of reproductive-age women (menstruation, pregnancy, lactation) and the increased iron requirements for growth in infants and children often exceed dietary iron availability and absorption. Pathologic blood loss in men and postmenopausal women, especially that from the gastrointestinal tract, is also a common cause of iron deficiency. In less well-developed areas, diets poor in absorbable iron, vegetarianism, intestinal parasitism, chronic diarrhea, and multiparity are common causes of iron deficiency.

Successful treatment of iron deficiency depends on identification and management of its cause(s) and administration of a regimen that takes into account the cause and severity of iron deficiency, comorbid disorders, and concomitant medications.

## Normal Iron Metabolism

Body iron quantities are regulated by controlled absorption that responds to the rate of erythropoiesis and other body demands. Quantities of total body iron in healthy adults are approximately 4.0 g in men and 3.5 g in women. Hemoglobin in men contains about 2.0 g Fe and in women about 1.5 g Fe. Storage sites in men contain about 1.0 g and in women about 0.3 g. The remaining iron, approximately 6% of total body quantities, is incorporated in myoglobin, heme-containing enzymes, transferrin, and other compounds.

Dietary iron typically consists of heme derived from animal products, nonheme ionic iron in vegetable foods, and inorganic iron added to fortify certain foodstuffs. Iron compounds must be soluble for absorption to occur. Heme iron is readily soluble. Absorption of nonheme iron is facilitated by gastric acid, ascorbic acid (vitamin C), and certain amino acids and sugars that maintain iron solubility at acid values of pH. Other substances commonly present in food, such as tannate in tea and phytates in vegetables, inhibit iron absorption.

Iron is absorbed only from the small intestine, especially the duodenum. Transport of nonheme iron across the microvilli of absorptive enterocytes requires its reduction to a soluble ferrous form and binding to DCT1 (divalent cation transporter), quantities of which are increased in iron deficiency. Heme enters enterocytes via a surface receptor and is cleaved thereafter to release iron. Other iron uptake mechanisms also exist in enterocytes. Transport of iron to transferrin in the blood is modulated by ferroportin (an iron export protein), HFE (hemochromatosis) protein, and transferrin receptor at the basolateral surfaces of enterocytes. On average, 5% to 10% of food iron is absorbed daily.

Iron is highly conserved due to phagocytosis and digestion of senescent erythrocytes by macrophages in the spleen, marrow, and liver and by iron storage in ferritin molecules (or degraded ferritin aggregates known as *hemosiderin*). Hepcidin, a liver-derived polypeptide that is a potent regulator of iron absorption and transport, regulates the release of conserved iron into the circulation from macrophages via ferroportin. Iron is delivered by transferrin to erythrocytes and other cells via their surface transferrin receptors. Unavoidable iron losses of about 1.0 mg daily occur due to exfoliation of skin and gastrointestinal tract cells, perspiration, and minor trauma. In menstruating women, additional average daily iron losses average 0.5 to 1.0 mg. Average net iron losses with normal term pregnancies are 700 mg. If insufficient quantities of iron are presented to the gastrointestinal tract in a form acceptable for absorption, or if iron absorptive mechanisms are not intact, iron depletion, iron-deficient erythropoiesis, and iron-deficiency anemia develop sequentially in accordance with the rate of net iron loss.

## Causes of Iron Deficiency

Some infants and adolescents ingest insufficient dietary iron to meet physiologic demands of rapid growth. Many women of childbearing age develop iron deficiency due to the high iron requirements of menstruation, pregnancy, and lactation. Many otherwise healthy regular blood donors and highly trained athletes develop iron deficiency.

Pathologic blood loss from gastrointestinal tract lesions of diverse etiologies is a common cause. These include erosion or ulceration of the esophagus, stomach, or duodenum, malignant neoplasms (particularly those of the colon, esophagus, or stomach), microangiopathy (inherited or acquired), inflammatory disorders (especially Crohn's disease), diverticula, and polyps. Chronic intestinal blood loss due to hookworms is common in tropical regions. Some patients who receive warfarin (Coumadin) or aspirin therapy have chronic gastrointestinal blood loss without demonstrable anatomic lesions. Nonbleeding gastrointestinal causes in patients with few or no gastrointestinal symptoms include atrophic gastritis, celiac disease, and *Helicobacter pylori* gastritis.

Less commonly, there is urinary tract blood loss from lesions within the kidneys, ureters, or bladder or due to conditions that cause hemoglobinuria (e.g., defective heart valve prostheses, paroxysmal nocturnal hemoglobinuria). Chronic blood loss from the respiratory tract is sometimes caused by recurrent epistaxis or hemoptysis (e.g., idiopathic pulmonary hemosiderosis, lung fluke infestation).

Blood loss during major chest operations or with hip or knee replacement can induce iron deficiency that is unapparent until weeks or months later. Patients on chronic hemodialysis develop iron deficiency due to blood retained in dialysis apparatus, hemolysis, and laboratory testing. Antitransferrin antibodies or mutations of the ceruloplasmin gene have been reported as rare causes.

## Signs and Symptoms of Iron Deficiency

Many persons develop weakness, ease of fatigue, or dyspnea with exertion, often before anemia develops. Infants or children can present with retarded motor and intellectual skills.

Pica, the compulsive ingestion of (often) non-nutritive substances, is a distinctive consequence that occurs in approximately one half of persons with iron deficiency, especially women. Ice eating (pagophagia) is the most common form of pica; some patients prefer dirt or clay, salt, sand, paper, cold fruit or lettuce, laundry starch, or other substances.

Some patients report evidence of bleeding. In adults with severe, chronic iron deficiency, sore mouth or tongue, nail and hair changes, dysphagia, paresthesias, and loss of memory and normal affect sometimes occur. Others present with restless legs.

Iron deficiency is diagnosed in a high percentage of children and adults coincidentally when routine physical and laboratory evaluations are performed. The most common physical sign of iron deficiency is pallor, although some patients have angular stomatitis, glossitis, koilonychia, or cricoid or esophageal web.

**TABLE 1** Laboratory Assessment of Iron Deficiency*

| Laboratory Measurement | Diagnostic Result |
|---|---|
| **Depletion of Iron Stores** | |
| Serum ferritin concentration | <50 ng/mL |
| Serum total iron-binding capacity | Increased |
| Stainable marrow iron | Absent |
| **Iron-Deficient Erythropoiesis** | |
| Serum transferrin saturation | <15% |
| Mean corpuscular volume | <80 fL |
| RDW | Increased |
| Free erythrocyte protoporphyrin concentration | Increased |
| Reticulocyte index | Low |
| Serum transferrin receptor concentration | Increased |
| **Iron-Deficiency Anemia** | |
| Hemoglobin concentration | Men: <13.0 g/dL Women: <12.0 g/dL |

*Consult laboratory-specific reference ranges. The differential diagnosis often includes anemia of chronic disease or inflammation, renal insufficiency, or malignancy, in which total iron-binding capacity is usually decreased, serum ferritin concentration is normal or increased, and RDW is normal. These forms of anemia can also occur concomitantly with iron deficiency. In some patients, the differential diagnosis also includes thalassemia minor, hemoglobinopathy E or Lepore hemoglobinopathy, various forms of sideroblastic anemia, anemia of chronic liver disease, anemia of chronic hemolysis, hypoplastic and aplastic anemias, myeloproliferative and myelodysplastic disorders, congenital dyserythropoietic anemias, anemia of myxedema, and megaloblastic anemia.
*Abbreviation:* RDW = red blood cell distribution width.

## Laboratory Abnormalities

Laboratory abnormalities associated with iron deficiency and other forms of anemia in the differential diagnosis are displayed in Table 1. Because iron deficiency is more common in women, many laboratories report lower reference limits for iron measures in women than men. Nonetheless, astute clinicians recognize that serum iron measures characteristic of iron deficiency are equally applicable to men and women. Persons with serum ferritin less than 50 ng/mL often have iron depletion or deficiency by bone marrow examination criteria, regardless of the laboratory's lower reference limit for serum ferritin. Other causes of abnormal serum iron measures or anemia occur in some patients with iron deficiency (see Table 1).

## Principles of Iron Replacement Therapy

Treatment should be undertaken after the diagnosis is established and potential benefits and adverse effects of therapy options have been considered (Table 2). Therapy must be individualized and monitored regularly. Many patients can be treated with oral iron preparations. Hematinic combinations should not be used in lieu of an adequate pretreatment evaluation. There is no indication for administering iron therapy except to treat iron deficiency.

Intravenous iron therapy should be reserved for noncompliant patients, those unable to take oral iron, patients who absorb iron poorly, patients who have not had a satisfactory therapeutic response to oral iron replacement, and patients in whom recurrent bleeding causes iron loss in excess of what can be replaced at an acceptable rate with oral therapy. For chronic hemodialysis patients, intravenous iron administration is the only suitable route of replacement. However, intravenous therapy does not induce a more rapid erythropoietic response than is possible with oral replacement. Intravenous iron

## TABLE 2 Adverse Effects of Iron Replacement Therapy*

| Adverse Effect | Form of Iron Therapy | Relative Frequency | Susceptible Patients |
|---|---|---|---|
| Black discoloration of stools | Iron salts,[†] carbonyl iron[†] | Very common | Children, adults |
| Epigastric pain, nausea, constipation, abdominal cramps, metallic taste | Iron salts[†] (more likely, especially with ascorbic acid), carbonyl iron[†] (less likely), intravenous iron[‡] (unlikely) | Common | Children, adults |
| Acute iron poisoning | Iron salts[†] | Common in children; rare in adults | Children: accidental ingestion Adults: accidental ingestion, suicide attempt |
| Arthralgias, myalgias, bone aches, low-grade fever | Intravenous iron[‡] (likely with doses >500 mg Fe), oral iron (less likely)[†] | Uncommon | Children, adults |
| Decreased absorption of other medications | Iron salts, carbonyl iron[†] | Uncommon | Children, adults |
| Flushing, hypotension | Intravenous iron[‡] | Uncommon with proper administration | Children, adults |
| Skin discoloration due to extravasation | Intravenous iron[‡] | Very uncommon with proper administration | Children, adults |
| Tooth discoloration (temporary) | Liquid oral iron elixir[§] | Very uncommon with proper administration | Children |
| Severe hypersensitivity, anaphylaxis | Intravenous iron[‡] | Very uncommon with proper administration | Children, adults |
| Increased susceptibility to infections with *Vibrio vulnificus* and other *Vibrio* species | Intravenous iron (dose-related)[‡] | Probably uncommon | Hemodialysis patients who consume raw shellfish or are exposed to water from warm seas |
| Iron overload | Intravenous iron (more likely),[‡] oral iron (less likely)[†] | Rare | Adults |

*I do not recommend single intravenous iron doses >500 mg due to risk of post-treatment myalgias, arthralgias, and low-grade fever. I do not recommend intramuscular iron therapy due to risk of severe allergy or anaphylaxis; pain, discoloration, and atrophy of subcutaneous tissues at injection sites; therapy failure due to limitations of iron doses; and rare occurrence of sarcomas at injection sites. Avoid intravenous iron therapy in pregnant women unless the benefit outweighs the potential risk to the fetus. Intravenous iron therapy for children should be undertaken only by pediatricians experienced in such management.

[†]Feosol Ferrous Sulfate Tablets, 65 mg Fe/tablet; Niferex Film Coated Tablets, 50 mg Fe/tablet; Feosol Carbonyl Iron Tablets, 45 mg Fe; ICAR Pediatric Chewables, 15 mg Fe/tablet; ICAR Pediatric Suspension, 15 mg Fe/1.25 mL.

[‡]InFeD, 50 mg Fe/mL; Dexferrum, 50 mg Fe/mL; Venofer, 20 mg Fe/mL; Ferrlecit, 12.5 mg Fe/mL.

[§]Niferex Elixir, 100 mg Fe/5 mL.

therapy should be given only by physicians experienced in such treatment who are prepared to treat hypotension or other hypersensitivity symptoms that sometimes occur. I do not recommend single intravenous iron doses greater than 500 mg (see Table 2).

Increasing the quantity of food iron is important in children with iron deficiency, many of whom have other nutritional deficits. Infants and some children need iron supplements; these should be prescribed by experienced pediatricians. In adults, dietary maneuvers as treatment are often ineffective. Multivitamins that contain "daily" amounts of iron (usually 10-20 mg Fe as inorganic iron salts) are usually inadequate for replacement therapy, and there is no basis for advising patients to take these preparations routinely unless they are premenopausal women, vigorous athletes, chronic blood donors, or vegetarians with uncomplicated iron depletion. Erythrocyte transfusion is indicated to elevate the circulating red blood cell mass in persons with iron-deficiency anemia who have vigorous bleeding or cardiac or respiratory compromise.

## ORAL IRON THERAPY

### Carbonyl Iron

Carbonyl iron consists of microspheres of pure iron precipitated from the gas iron pentacarbonyl; it is widely used for food iron fortification. This is the oral therapy of choice for most persons, because it causes less gastrointestinal toxicity than iron salts and is equally effective in correcting iron deficiency. Increasing the dosage gradually over a few weeks until the target dose is reached can improve tolerance in some patients.

The usual adult dosage is 45 mg three times daily (Feosol Carbonyl Iron tablets, 45 mg Fe/tablet), preferably taken on an empty stomach.

Doses for adolescents (to be divided into three or four equal portions) are higher: For adolescent boys younger than 18 years, the dose is 90 to 135 mg daily, and for menstruating adolescent girls 12 to 18 years, the dose is 45 to 135 mg daily. In preadolescent school-age children, administer up to 6 mg/kg/day (ICAR Pediatric Chewables, 15 mg Fe/tablet); in infants and young children, administer 3 mg/kg/day (ICAR Pediatric Suspension, 15 mg Fe/1.25 mL).

In patients with anemia, the hemoglobin concentration usually increases about 1.0 g/dL weekly. Continue treatment until anemia is corrected and serum ferritin concentration is higher than 50 ng/mL; microcytosis, if present, typically resolves several months after iron stores are replete. In patients who have gastrointestinal symptoms, administer iron with meals or reduce dosing frequency, but expect delayed correction of iron deficiency. Completion of therapy in patients without continuing blood loss typically requires several months.

### Iron Salts

Iron salts are suitable for many children and adults. The most commonly used preparation is ferrous sulfate (Feosol Ferrous Sulfate Tablets, 65 mg Fe/tablet; many generic brands); a polysaccharide-iron complex is also popular (Niferex Film Coated Tablets, 50 mg Fe/tablet).

In adults, the dose is one tablet three times daily, preferably on an empty stomach. In older children, the dose is 5 mg/kg of iron daily as tablets or elixir (administered by an adult).

Rate of response of anemia, monitoring of hemoglobin and ferritin concentrations, and dose adjustments for adverse gastrointestinal symptoms attributed to treatment are similar to those for carbonyl iron therapy. Ferrous gluconate, ferrous fumarate, polysaccharide-iron

## CURRENT DIAGNOSIS

- Weakness, fatigue, pica, and pallor are common.
- Transferrin saturation is usually <15% (decreased serum iron level, normal or elevated total iron-binding capacity).
- Serum transferrin receptor concentration is elevated in most cases.
- Serum ferritin level is typically <20 ng/mL.
- Serum ferritin level is normal or elevated in patients who also have anemia of chronic disease, active liver disease, renal insufficiency, or malignancy.
- Reticulocytopenia and normal or low erythrocyte count are typical.
- Anemia with or without microcytosis is a late development.

complex, and enteric-coated iron preparations can be used similarly. However, they might contain less iron per tablet than ferrous sulfate or be less absorbable, and thus induce therapeutic responses less rapidly. Most are more expensive.

## INTRAVENOUS IRON THERAPY

### Iron Dextran

Iron dextran preparations (InFeD or Dexferrum, 50 mg Fe/mL) are indicated for treatment of iron deficiency in persons with normal renal function who fail to respond to or do not tolerate oral iron supplementation. Iron dextran is safe and effective when administered properly (see Table 2). Each infusion in adults should consist of 500 mg Fe in 250 to 500 mL of normal saline. I recommend premedication with intravenous dexamethasone (Deltasone) (10 mg) plus either diphenhydramine (Benadryl) (25 mg), cimetidine (Tagamet) (400 mg), or famotidine (Pepcid) (20 mg) and giving a test dose of 25 mg Fe or approximately 5 mL over 10 to 15 minutes in a freely flowing intravenous line. If there is no immediate adverse effect, the remaining dose should be infused over 2 to 3 hours. Infusions are repeated every 2 to 3 weeks until anemia is corrected and iron stores are replete, as described for oral iron preparations. Many patients who require intravenous iron dextran for initial management have recurrent bleeding and thus require periodic maintenance infusions.

## CURRENT THERAPY

- Identify and correct causes of inadequate nutrition and blood loss.
- Individualize therapy and monitor outcomes regularly.
- Many patients can be treated with oral preparations; noncompliance is the most common cause of treatment failure.
- Oral therapy often fails in patients who take antacids, H₂ blockers, proton pump antagonists, or calcium supplements.
- Use intravenous therapy for noncompliance or inadequate response to oral iron, severe iron deficiency, recurrent blood loss, malabsorption, or hemodialysis.
- Many patients with nondialysis chronic renal disease, chronic inflammation, or malignancy and all hemodialysis patients require erythropoietin (Epogen, Procrit, Aranesp) therapy to maximize response to iron replacement.

### Iron Sucrose

Iron sucrose (Venofer, 20 mg Fe/mL) is indicated for treatment of iron deficiency in patients undergoing chronic hemodialysis who also receive erythropoietin therapy (epoetin alfa, epoetin beta, or darbepoetin). In previously untreated patients, a test dose should be administered before the first infusion as described for iron dextran. Doses of 200 to 300 mg[1] Fe administered intravenously over 2 hours during hemodialysis are safe and effective. In anemic patients with non–dialysis-dependent chronic kidney disease, oral and intravenous iron therapies yield similar hemoglobin responses, but intravenous iron is more effective in increasing iron stores. Goals of therapy include maintenance of serum transferrin saturation at least 30%, serum ferritin concentration at least 300 ng/mL, and hemoglobin greater than 11.0 g/dL. Most hemodialysis patients require ongoing or recurrent therapy.

### Iron Gluconate

This product (Ferrlecit, 12.5 mg Fe/mL) is also indicated for treating iron deficiency in patients undergoing chronic hemodialysis who are receiving erythropoietin therapy. A test dose should be administered before the first infusion, as described for iron dextran. Typical treatments consist of 125 mg of Fe administered intravenously at each hemodialysis treatment. Adequacy of therapy is monitored in the same manner as for iron sucrose therapy.

## FAILURE OF IRON REPLACEMENT THERAPY

The most common cause of unsuccessful therapy with oral iron supplements is poor compliance due to adverse gastrointestinal effects. Another common cause is unrecognized or uncorrectable chronic or recurrent blood loss associated with angiodysplasia of the gastrointestinal tract or chronic anticoagulant therapy. Some commonly prescribed drugs markedly decrease iron absorption, including antacids, H₂ blockers, proton pump antagonists, calcium supplements, and tetracycline. Gastrectomy, duodenectomy, achlorhydria, celiac disease, and gastric or intestinal bypass are often associated with iron malabsorption. Patients suspected to have suboptimal iron absorption unrelated to medications should be evaluated for additional causes of anemia. Many patients who have inadequate responses to oral iron therapy require intravenous iron replacement. In persons with chronic disease or renal insufficiency and in those receiving anticancer chemotherapy, erythropoietin therapy is often necessary to induce a satisfactory erythropoietic response.

## REFERENCES

Annibale B, Capurso G, Chistolini A, et al: Gastrointestinal causes of refractory iron deficiency anemia in patients without gastrointestinal symptoms. Am J Med 2001;111:439-445.

Barton JC, Barton EH, Bertoli LF, et al: Intravenous iron dextran therapy in patients with iron deficiency and normal renal function who failed to respond to or did not tolerate oral iron supplementation. Am J Med 2000;109:27-32.

Cook JD, Flowers CH, Skikne BS: The quantitative assessment of body iron. Blood 2003;101:3359-3364.

Ferguson BJ, Skikne BS, Simpson KM, et al: Serum transferrin receptor distinguishes the anemia of chronic disease from iron deficiency anemia. J Lab Clin Med 1992;119:385-390.

Hershko C, Bar-Or D, Gaziel Y, et al: Diagnosis of iron deficiency anemia in a rural population of children: Relative usefulness of serum ferritin, red cell protoporphyrin, red cell indices, and transferrin saturation determinations. Am J Clin Nutr 1981;34:1600-1610.

Hershko C, Hoffbrand AV, Keret D, et al: Role of autoimmune gastritis, Helicobacter pylori and celiac disease in refractory or unexplained iron deficiency anemia. Haematologica 2005;90:585-595.

Ioannou GN, Rockey DC, Bryson CL, et al: Iron deficiency and gastrointestinal malignancy: A population-based cohort study. Am J Med 2002;113: 276-280.

---

[1]Not FDA approved for this indication.

Lozoff B, Beard J, Connor J, et al: Long-lasting neural and behavioral effects of iron deficiency in infancy. Nutr Rev 2006;64:S34-S43.

Van Wyck DB, Roppolo M, Martinez CO, et al: A randomized, controlled trial comparing IV iron sucrose to oral iron in anemic patients with nondialysis-dependent CKD. Kidney Int 2005;68:2846-2856.

Yates JM, Logan EC, Stewart RM: Iron deficiency anaemia in general practice: Clinical outcomes over three years and factors influencing diagnostic investigations. Postgrad Med J 2004;80:405-410.

# Autoimmune Hemolytic Anemia

Method of
*Charles J. Parker, MD*

There are three general categories of autoimmune hemolytic anemia (AIHA), and each group has idiopathic and secondary forms (Table 1). In this review, drug-induced immune hemolytic anemia is treated as a subcategory of warm-antibody AIHA.

## Warm-Antibody Autoimmune Hemolytic Anemia

Immune hemolytic anemia should be included in the differential diagnosis of patients with laboratory evidence of hemolysis (Table 2). The criteria for diagnosis of warm-antibody AIHA are shown in Table 3. In addition to the general laboratory signs of hemolysis (see Table 2), patients with warm-antibody AIHA present with two other important laboratory features. First, the peripheral blood film shows microspherocytes; and second, the direct antiglobulin (Coombs) test is positive (see Table 3). In approximately 67% of patients, the Coombs test is positive for both immunoglobulin G (IgG) and complement, in 20% the test is positive for IgG but not complement, and in the remaining 13% the test is positive for complement but not IgG. The indirect Coombs test is positive in approximately 60% of cases. It is uncommon, but not rare, to have cases of "Coombs negative" warm-antibody AIHA (≈5% of cases are Coombs negative). In these cases, patients have laboratory evidence of hemolysis, and the peripheral blood film shows microspherocytes and polychromasia, but the standard Coombs test is negative. The presence of IgG, complement, or both, however, can often be demonstrated using more sensitive assays available in reference laboratories (e.g., radioimmunobinding assays using monoclonal antibodies or enzyme-linked antiglobulin tests). The clinical diagnosis of Coombs negative AIHA is also supported by observing a response to an empirical trial of corticosteroids (see later).

**TABLE 1 Classification of Autoimmune Hemolytic Anemias**

**Warm-Antibody Autoimmune Hemolytic Anemia (Accounts for Approximately 80% of Cases)**
*Idiopathic*
*Secondary* (found in association with chronic lymphocytic leukemia, lymphoma [Hodgkin's and non-Hodgkin's], connective tissue diseases (primarily systemic lupus erythematosus), ulcerative colitis, ovarian cysts, immunodeficiency syndromes [including AIDS], antiphospholipid syndrome)
*Drug-induced*

**Cold Agglutinin Syndrome (Accounts for Approximately 18% of Cases)**
*Idiopathic*
*Secondary* (found in association with *Mycoplasma pneumoniae* infection, infectious mononucleosis, lymphoreticular malignancy, viral infections)

**Paroxysmal Cold Hemoglobinuria (Accounts for Approximately 2% of Cases)**
*Idiopathic* (associated with a chronic autoimmune disease in adults)
*Secondary* (found in association with viral illnesses, typically in children; also associated with syphilis)

**TABLE 2 Laboratory Values That Suggest Hemolysis**

Reticulocytosis >125,000/μL of blood*
Indirect bilirubin concentration between 1 and 5 mg/dL[†]
Haptoglobin concentration <50 mg/dL[‡]
Elevated lactic dehydrogenase concentration[§]

*If automated determination of reticulocyte concentration is unavailable, the value can be derived by multiplying the reticulocyte count (reported in percent) by the red blood cell (RBC) concentration (RBC/μL) and dividing the total by 100. For example, if the reticulocyte count is 1 and the RBC concentration is $5 \times 10^6$/μL, the number of reticulocytes per microliter of blood is 50,000.
[†]Patients with Gilbert disease have an increased indirect bilirubin level in the absence of hemolysis. Unless the patient has underlying liver disease, the direct bilirubin level is rarely elevated in association with hemolysis.
[‡]Haptoglobin is an acute-phase reactant. When hemolysis occurs in association with inflammatory processes or with steroid administration, haptoglobin levels may be within the normal range.
[§]The normal range for lactate dehydrogenase (LDH) depends on the assay and the units of measurement and, therefore, varies among laboratories. LDH is mildly to moderately elevated in cases of extravascular hemolysis. Values are much higher in cases of intravascular hemolysis.

**TABLE 3 Key Diagnostic Points for Warm-Antibody Autoimmune Hemolytic Anemia and Cold Agglutinin Syndrome**

**Warm-Antibody Autoimmune Hemolytic Anemia**
Patient has not been transfused during previous 4 months*
Laboratory evidence of hemolysis[†]
Peripheral blood film shows microspherocytes and polychromasia
Positive direct Coombs test for IgG, complement C3, or both
Absence of a cold agglutinin of high thermal amplitude[‡]
Patient has a warm antibody with broad reactivity in the serum or eluted from the red cell[§]

**Cold Agglutinin Syndrome**
Clinical evidence of hemolytic anemia[†]
Agglutination of erythrocytes observed on blood film or when anticoagulated blood sample is collected at room temperature
Positive Coombs test for complement C3
Negative Coombs test for IgG**
Presence of a cold agglutinin with reactivity up to at least 30°C[¶]

*Patient may still have autoimmune hemolytic anemia, but delayed transfusion reaction should be excluded.
[†]See Table 2.
[‡]Reactivity up to 30°C.
[§]If the antibody is not present in the plasma (indirect Coombs test is negative), it can be eluted from the red cell membrane and its reactivity subsequently characterized.
**Cold agglutinins are almost invariably immunoglobulin M (IgM) antibodies that activate complement.
[¶]The antibody causes agglutination at temperatures up to 30°C.
Abbreviation: IgG = immunoglobulin G.

**TABLE 4  Summary of Current Therapy for Warm-Antibody Autoimmune Hemolytic Anemia**

Prednisone (1.0–1.5 mg/kg/day)*
Splenectomy†
Immunosuppressive therapy‡
Other§

*Patients who do not respond after 3 weeks are considered treatment failures. If patients respond, steroids should be tapered gradually over 3–4 months.
†Indications: (1) failure to respond to steroids; (2) steroid dose required to maintain remission is unacceptably high (10 mg/day or 15 mg/qod).
‡Indications: (1) failure to respond to splenectomy (or a combination of splenectomy and low-dose prednisone); (2) patients who cannot tolerate splenectomy. Cyclophosphamide (Cytoxan; 1.5–2.0 mg/kg/day) or azathioprine (Imuran; 2.0–2.5 mg/kg/day) is recommended. Treatment should continue for at least 3 months. Rituximab (anti-CD20), mycophenolate mofetil (CellCept), alemtuzumab (Campath), and cyclosporin A (Seromycin) have also shown efficacy.
§Plasmapheresis with plasma exchange may be beneficial in emergency situations. Intravenous immunoglobulin G produces a transient response in ≈ 30% of patients. Responses to danazol (Danocrine) and immunoadsorption columns have been reported. Patients should be supplemented with folate 1 mg/day.

The anti–red blood cell (RBC) antibodies of warm-antibody AIHA are almost invariably classified as panagglutinins because they cause agglutination of all of the erythrocytes that are part of the standard test panel used by the blood bank to characterize the reactivity of anti-RBC antibodies. More detailed analysis often shows that the antibodies are directed against antigenic determinants within the Rh system (although many other specificities have been reported).

## MANAGEMENT OF IDIOPATHIC WARM-ANTIBODY AUTOIMMUNE HEMOLYTIC ANEMIA

An approach to treatment of warm-antibody AIHA is given in Table 4. All patients should receive folate supplementation to compensate for the increased utilization resulting from the compensatory enhancement of erythropoiesis. Approximately 80% of patients with warm-antibody AIHA will respond to steroids, and the response is usually rapid (within a few days); however, permanent remissions are observed in less than 20% of cases. The decision to recommend splenectomy should be based on clinical criteria (see Table 4) because splenic sequestration studies using radiolabeled erythrocytes have not proved to be predictive of a response to splenectomy. In patients who relapse after splenectomy, low doses of steroids (≤5 mg/day) may be effective in controlling the hemolytic process. Immunosuppressive therapy (see Table 4) is often beneficial in patients who have not responded to splenectomy. Plasmapheresis with plasma exchange is unconventional therapy but offers the possibility of rapidly ameliorating the hemolysis in emergency situations. In contrast to its effectiveness in the management of immune thrombocytopenia, intravenous immunoglobulin therapy appears to be significantly less efficacious as treatment for AIHA. Approximately 30% of patients respond to intravenous immunoglobulin G, but responses are not durable, and maintenance therapy given every 3 to 4 weeks is usually required. Occasionally patients respond to the synthetic androgen danazol (Danocrine). Anecdotal reports suggest that some patients with AIHA may respond to immunoadsorbent therapy using immobilized protein A from *Staphylococcus aureus*. Response of refractory warm-antibody AIHA to rituximab (Rituxan) has been observed anecdotally and reported in small series.

## MANAGEMENT OF SECONDARY WARM-ANTIBODY AUTOIMMUNE HEMOLYTIC ANEMIA

The approach to management of patients with secondary AIHA is similar to that described for patients with idiopathic AIHA. In the case of patients with chronic lymphocytic leukemia (CLL), it is particularly important to emphasize that treating the underlying disease is unlikely to ameliorate immune-mediated processes (e.g., AIHA or immune thrombocytopenic purpura [ITP]). In fact, treatment of CLL with purine nucleoside analogues, particularly fludarabine, has been associated with the development of AIHA and ITP. Patients who develop AIHA or ITP following fludarabine therapy should never receive additional fludarabine or other purine nucleoside analogues because of reports suggesting that such treatment may exacerbate AIHA or ITP, causing these processes to become intractable. Under these circumstances, morbidity and mortality rates are alarmingly high.

In general, for patients with secondary warm-antibody AIHA, the decision to treat the primary disease should be made separately from the decision to treat the hemolytic anemia. For example, a patient with Rai stage 0 CLL who has AIHA but no other symptoms should receive treatment for AIHA but not for CLL. In some instances, however, secondary AIHA may respond to treatment of the primary disease (e.g., treatment of lymphoma with combination chemotherapy). In other instances, treatment of the primary disease overlaps with treatment of AIHA (e.g., steroid therapy for systemic lupus erythematosus).

### RESPONSE TO THERAPY

A normal hematocrit level is not necessary in order for the patient to be classified as a treatment success. The goal of therapy is to restore the hematocrit to a level that provides adequate oxygen transport capacity (usually >30% unless there are attendant problems). Furthermore, although the titer of the direct antiglobulin (Coombs) test may decrease in response to therapy, it is unusual for the test to become negative. Thus, a goal of therapy should not be normalization of the Coombs test.

It is important to keep in mind that idiopathic warm AIHA is a chronic disease and that relapses are common. Steroids should be tapered very slowly (over several months); however, disease exacerbations during the taper are frequently observed and are frustrating for both patient and physician. Patients requiring more than 10 mg of prednisone every day or more than 15 mg of prednisone every other day for more than a few months are candidates for splenectomy. Patients undergoing splenectomy should receive preoperative vaccinations against pneumococcal and meningococcal disease and against *Haemophilus influenzae* type B. Management of chronic AIHA is challenging, and not unusually patients require a combination of steroids, splenectomy, and immunosuppressive therapy. Patients should be informed that the disease is usually chronic and that relapses are common. Physicians should be prepared to monitor the patient frequently so that relapses can be treated promptly and therapy-related problems prevented. Prolonged use of steroids at unacceptably high levels is the most frequent cause of iatrogenic problems associated with treatment of chronic warm-antibody AIHA.

If the dose of prednisone required to maintain an appropriate hematocrit is unacceptably high after splenectomy, then immunosuppressive therapy should be initiated. In patients younger than 70 years, azathioprine (Imuran) is preferred over cyclophosphamide (Cytoxan) because the former is less leukemogenic than the latter. During the course of treatment, the hematocrit level, reticulocyte count, and lactate dehydrogenase (LDH) should be monitored regularly. A rising hematocrit in association with a falling reticulocyte count and LDH is consistent with a response to therapy. On the other hand, a falling hematocrit in association with a falling reticulocyte count suggests a superimposed bone marrow problem (e.g., parvovirus infection or megaloblastic crisis associated with folate deficiency) that requires further evaluation.

### TRANSFUSION

Transfusion of patients with warm-antibody AIHA should be undertaken with caution. It is important to remember that response to steroid therapy is usually rapid (within a few days). Therefore, in most instances, transfusion can be avoided by reducing oxygen demand, which is accomplished by placing the patient at rest. Nonetheless, in cases of fulminant hemolysis or when a patient at rest becomes symptomatic while awaiting a response to therapy, transfusion can be lifesaving. Careful consideration should be given to the volume of blood infused because overtransfusion can be dangerous for two reasons. First, patients may become volume overloaded, causing further cardiopulmonary embarrassment. Second, the rate of hemolysis of donor red cells is exponentially related to the amount of blood infused. Consequently, problems associated with acute hemolysis are more likely to occur in patients who have received relatively large amounts of blood. Accordingly, the minimum amount of blood required to control the patient's symptoms should be transfused (e.g., 100 mL of packed cells twice per day may be effective in preventing high-output heart failure).

Because the autoantibody is almost always a panagglutinin, it is virtually impossible to find donor cells that are not recognized by the patient's antibody. Therefore, the goal of the blood bank staff is not to find donor cells that are unreactive in the cross-matching studies but rather to ensure that the patient's ABO and Rh phenotypes are properly determined and that the patient does not have an alloantibody in addition to an autoantibody. A detailed history of previous pregnancies and transfusions is important because patients with warm-antibody AIHA who have never been pregnant or been transfused likely would not have become alloimmunized. A number of assays are available that allow identification of a concurrent alloantibody, but these types of studies are not performed routinely. Accordingly, it is important that the blood bank have a level of sophistication and experience that ensures competence in the performance and interpretation of these critical studies.

Some immunohematologists advocate that studies be undertaken to determine the relative specificity of the autoantibody so that donor cells lacking the antigen can be transfused. For example, the antibody may react more strongly with cells that have the "little e" antigen than with those that have the "big E" antigen (E and e are part of the Rh antigen system). In this case, the antibody is said to have relative specificity for "little e." However, data from limited studies suggesting a clinical benefit from transfusing cells that lack the antigen of relative specificity are not compelling. Nonetheless, it seems prudent to determine the relative specificity of the antibody and to avoid transfusing cells that express the antigen, especially if in vitro studies indicate a strong degree of specificity (e.g., if the antibody induces hemolysis of antigen-positive but not antigen-negative cells).

Patients with AIHA who are being transfused should be monitored closely both during and after the infusion. Laboratory studies to document the extent of hemolysis (e.g., LDH, haptoglobin, plasma free hemoglobin, and hemoglobinuria) and the development of renal compromise should be obtained.

## Drug-Induced Immune Hemolytic Anemia

In reviews of drug-induced hemolytic anemia from 30 years ago, methyldopa (Aldomet) was reported to be the responsible agent in the majority of cases. Because the use of methyldopa (Aldomet) as an antihypertensive has markedly declined over the last 20 years, the incidence of drug-induced hemolytic anemia has probably fallen. Nonetheless, drug-induced hemolytic anemia continues to account for a significant proportion of all cases of acquired immune hemolytic anemia, with cefotetan (Cefotan) and ceftriaxone (Rocephin) currently the drugs most commonly involved. At least 12 cyclosporins have been reported to cause drug-induced immune hemolytic anemia.

When evaluating patients with evidence of immune hemolysis, eliciting a detailed drug history is essential. In addition, a temporal relationship between drug administration and the development of hemolysis should be sought. Unfortunately, such relationships are often rendered inconclusive because patients are taking multiple drugs. Although some drugs induce immune hemolytic anemia more frequently than do others, in any one patient, any drug must be considered potentially culpable.

There are three basic mechanisms by which drugs can induce immune hemolytic anemia (Table 5). Prototypic drugs are included for each mechanism, but it is important to keep in mind that these drugs represent the best-characterized examples and that other drugs may induce hemolysis by the same mechanisms. For example, levodopa (Larodopa) and procainamide (Procan) have been reported to induce immune hemolytic anemia in a manner analogous to that of methyldopa (Aldomet). A detailed review of all of the drugs that have been implicated in the production of AIHA is beyond the purview of this article.

Recent reports strongly suggest that quinine can induce the hemolytic uremic syndrome (HUS). Patients present with chills, sweats, nausea and vomiting, abdominal pain, oliguria, and petechiae following exposure to quinine in the form of medications or beverages. Laboratory studies show anemia, severe thrombocytopenia, markedly elevated serum LDH level, and azotemia. Drug-dependent antibodies reactive with platelets, erythrocytes, and granulocytes have been identified. These patients have a favorable outcome when treated with plasmapheresis with plasma exchange and dialysis as indicated. Thus, prompt recognition and appropriate treatment of this clinical entity are imperative.

In an individual patient, almost any drug can produce an idiosyncratic reaction resulting in immune hemolytic anemia. Therefore, for patients with newly diagnosed acquired immune hemolytic anemia, all drugs that are not absolutely essential should be discontinued. Furthermore, any drug implicated by temporal events (and particularly any drug that has been reported to induce immune hemolysis) should be stopped and alternative therapy using a structurally unrelated compound initiated. A causal role for a particular drug can be established by using an in vitro assay. The basis of these types of assays is the indirect Coombs test modified to determine if antibody binding to the red cell is drug dependent. The technical aspects of the test (particularly the concentration of drug to use) can be obtained from published reports if studies of a particular drug have been performed. If a drug that has not been shown to induce immune hemolysis is suspected, experiments to establish the optimal conditions for testing are required. Unfortunately, drug-related antibodies cannot be conclusively demonstrated in many cases in which the clinical suspicion is strong. Adding to the problem is the fact that antibodies may be directed against metabolites rather than to the whole drug. In these cases, ex vivo antigens (present in the serum or urine of the patient) may be required to demonstrate the drug-dependent nature of the antibody.

## Cold Agglutinin Syndrome

Whereas the presence of cold agglutinins in the plasma is relatively common, cold agglutinins that produce clinically significant hemolysis are relatively uncommon. A cold agglutinin titer of less than 1:64 is normal. Patients with cold agglutinin syndrome may complain of Raynaud's phenomenon or of acrocyanosis of the ears, nose tip, fingers, and toes that occurs at cold temperatures and vanishes quickly upon warming. These symptoms arise because as the blood flows through skin capillaries, the intravascular temperature drops to levels at which the cold agglutinin is functional. As a consequence of the agglutination, blood flow through the small vessels is restricted. Hemoglobinuria following exposure to cold may be part of the history, but, in general, this symptom is unusual. Hepatosplenomegaly is not usually prominent, and lymphadenopathy is uncommon. Agglutination of the red cells at room temperature is an obvious consequence of the disease.

The criteria for diagnosis of cold agglutinin syndrome are given in Table 3. It should be emphasized that mere observance of cold agglutination is not diagnostic of cold agglutinin disease. The antibodies of cold agglutinin disease are almost invariably immunoglobulin M (IgM), and, in the vast majority of cases, they are directed against determinants of the I antigen system. In most instances, the cold agglutinin titer in cold agglutinin syndrome is greater than 1:1000, but the titer at 4°C does not correlate well with the hemolytic potential of the antibody. A more useful characterization is determination of the thermal amplitude of the antibody (defined as the highest temperature at which the antibody causes agglutination). The majority of cold agglutinins that produce clinically significant hemolysis have a thermal

## TABLE 5  Characteristics of Drug-Induced Hemolytic Anemias

### Quinidine/Quinine Prototype
**Proposed mechanism**
The drug acts as a hapten after binding to a cell membrane protein. Consequently, antibodies against constituents of the drug–membrane protein complex arise.

**Clinical characteristics**
Small doses of drug induce the process.
Intravascular hemolysis is common; hemolysis may be severe and life-threatening. Can produce HUS.

**Laboratory findings**
Direct Coombs test positive for complement but not IgG.
Antibody may be IgG or IgM.
Positivity of the indirect Coombs test depends on the presence of the drug in the reaction mixture, thus demonstrating the drug-dependent nature of the antibody.

**Therapy**
Discontinue drug.
Supportive care (maintain renal blood flow, transfuse as needed).
In patients with severe hemolysis, an empirical trial of steroids is warranted.
Patients with HUS appear to benefit from plasma exchange. Dialysis is often required.

### Penicillin Prototype
**Proposed mechanism**
Drug binds tightly to red cell. Antidrug antibody binds to drug on red cell surface.

**Clinical characteristics**
Large doses of drug required (10 million units or more per day).
Hemolysis is usually subacute, developing over 1–2 weeks.
Patients may have positive Coombs test without clinical evidence of hemolysis.
In rare instances, the process may be life-threatening.

**Laboratory findings**
Direct Coombs test positive for IgG, rarely positive for complement.
Patient's serum will react in indirect Coombs test with red cells coated with drug.

**Therapy**
Discontinue drug in cases of overt hemolysis.
If hemolysis is clinically insignificant, the drug can be continued while the patient is monitored closely.

### Methyldopa (Aldomet) Prototype*
**Proposed mechanism**
Speculative but may alter the immune system, resulting in a pathophysiologic process similar to that observed in idiopathic autoimmune hemolytic anemia.

**Clinical characteristics**
Dose and time dependent (patient will have taken drug for at least 3 months).
Hemolysis is usually mild and resolves gradually over several weeks after cessation of the drug.
Patients may have positive Coombs test without clinical evidence of hemolysis.

**Laboratory findings**
Direct Coombs test positive for IgG, rarely for complement. When hemolysis is present, indirect Coombs test is invariably positive.
Positivity of Coombs test is not dependent on having the drug in the reaction mixture.
Coombs test may be positive for months after cessation of drug.

**Therapy**
Discontinue drug in cases of overt hemolysis.
If hemolysis is clinically insignificant, the drug can be continued while the patient is monitored closely. However, the availability of other effective agents makes prudent the switch to a structurally unrelated alternative antihypertensive agent.

*Methyldopa (Aldomet) is rarely used in current practice, but the mechanism of drug-induced hemolytic anemia may be applicable to other currently used agents, including levodopa (Larodopa) and procainamide (Procan)
*Abbreviations:* HUS = hemolytic uremic syndrome; IgG = immunoglobulin G; IgM = immunoglobulin M.

amplitude of at least 30°C (if the thermal amplitude is <30°C, the antibody will not fully activate the complement system).

## MANAGEMENT OF COLD AGGLUTININ SYNDROME

Treatment of cold agglutinin syndrome is notoriously difficult because currently available therapeutic modalities (i.e., corticosteroids, splenectomy, and alkylating agents) are relatively ineffective. Fortunately, most patients have a low-grade, compensated anemia that is best managed by general supportive measures (avoiding cold exposure, transfusion if necessary). A minority of patients may benefit from chlorambucil (Leukeran; 0.1–0.2 mg/kg/day) or cyclophosphamide (Cytoxan; 1.5–2.0 mg/kg/day), and these agents should be prescribed if the disease is complicated by severe anemia. Several case reports and a few small series suggest that patients refractory to other treatments may respond to rituximab (Rituxan). This treatment is particularly attractive because of its favorable therapeutic index (generally well tolerated and associated with relatively few adverse effects). In situations where the cold agglutinin syndrome arises in association with an underlying neoplasia, the hemolytic process often ameliorates in response to treatment of the underlying disease. Patients should avoid cold conditions, and in some instances patients may have to move to a warm climate. Inasmuch as the antibody is IgM, plasmapheresis offers the opportunity to lower the antibody concentrations in emergency situations.

## TABLE 6 Secondary Chronic Cold Agglutinin Disease

### *Mycoplasma pneumoniae* Infections
Approximately 50% of patients have elevated cold agglutinin titers, but overt hemolysis is rare.

When it does occur, the hemolytic process begins in the second or third week of the infection and onset is rapid. Fatalities have been reported.

Characteristically the cold reacting antibody is an IgM that recognizes I antigens.

The antibody may cross-react with mycoplasmal antigens.

The hemolysis is self-limited and steroids are ineffective.

### Infectious Mononucleosis
Clinically significant hemolysis occurs infrequently.

Hemolysis occurs 1–2 weeks after onset of infection.

The antibody may be IgM anti-i, IgM anti-I, or IgG anti-i.*

Hemolysis is usually self-limited, but steroids may be of benefit.

Association with reticuloendothelial neoplasia is unusual.

---

*The I antigen is found predominantly on adult red cells, whereas the i antigen is found primarily on fetal red cells. In primary cold agglutinin disease, the antibody is almost invariably IgM anti-I. The cold agglutinins associated with infectious mononucleosis are unusual in that they may have specificity for the i antigen, and they may be IgG.
*Abbreviations:* IgG = immunoglobulin G; IgM = immunoglobulin M.

## TRANSFUSION

The I antigen is present on all adult red cells. Thus, it is not possible to transfuse nonreactive donor cells. Difficulties in establishing ABO and Rh phenotypes and in identifying alloantibodies are usually not encountered, however, because tests can be performed at a temperature above that at which the cold agglutinin is active. The clinical benefit of using in-line blood warmers during transfusion of patients with cold agglutinin disease (or with paroxysmal cold hemoglobinuria [PCH], see later) has not been clearly established. In general, properly crossed-matched blood can be transfused safely if it is warmed to room temperature and infused slowly. In cases of particularly severe cold agglutinin syndrome or PCH, however, use of an in-line warmer seems prudent.

## SECONDARY COLD AGGLUTININ SYNDROME

Although the finding of cold agglutinins in association with infectious processes is relatively common (particularly for *Mycoplasma pneumoniae* infection and infectious mononucleosis), clinically significant hemolysis in this setting is unusual. The association of cold agglutinin disease with lymphoproliferative neoplasias is also uncommon. Some features of secondary cold agglutinin disease are given in Table 6.

# Paroxysmal Cold Hemoglobinuria

PCH is an uncommon disease that can be dramatic in presentation. Patients with PCH (usually children) experience acute attacks of shaking chills, fever, malaise, and aching pains involving the abdomen, back, and legs. Hemoglobin is usually present in the first urine passed after the attack. A history of exposure to cold is usually elicited, although the extent of the exposure may be modest. In rare instances, cold exposure is not part of the presenting history. Often there is a history of a flulike prodromal illness. The anemia is usually moderate to severe at the time of presentation and may be progressive despite keeping the patient warm.

The diagnosis of PCH is made by finding the Donath-Landsteiner antibody in the patient's plasma. This IgG antibody is directed against the P blood group antigen and is identified by using a bithermal assay. First, the patient's serum is incubated with erythrocytes at 4°C. Under these conditions, the cold reacting antibody binds to the red cells. Subsequently, the reaction mixture is warmed to 37°C, and the cells hemolyze as a result of complement activation initiated by the Donath-Landsteiner antibody.

## MANAGEMENT OF PAROXYSMAL COLD HEMOGLOBINURIA

Most patients with PCH require only supportive care because the process is usually transient. The patient should be kept warm at all times. Guidelines for transfusion are the same as those for patients with cold agglutinin syndrome (see earlier). In severe cases, an empiric trial of corticosteroids is warranted. Although the association is now rare, patients with PCH should be evaluated for evidence of syphilis. PCH has also been reported as part of a chronic autoimmune process in adults.

## REFERENCES

Arndt PA, Garratty G: The changing spectrum of drug-induced immune hemolytic anemia. Semin Hematol 2005;42:137-144.

Berentsen S, Ulvestad E, Gjertsen BT, et al: Rituximab for primary chronic cold agglutinin disease: A prospective study of 37 courses of therapy in 27 patients. Blood 2004;103:2925-2928.

Gottschall JL, Elliot W, Lianos E, et al: Quinine-induced immune thrombocytopenia associated with hemolytic uremic syndrome: A new clinical entity. Blood 1991;77:306-310.

Rosse WF, Hillmen P, Schreiber AD: Immune-mediated hemolytic anemia. Hematology (Am Soc Hematol Educ Program) 2004:48-62.

Shanafelt TD, Madueme HL, Wolf RC, Tefferi A: Rituximab for immune cytopenia in adults: Idiopathic thrombocytopenic purpura, autoimmune hemolytic anemia, and Evans syndrome. Mayo Clin Proc 2003;78: 1340-1346.

# Nonimmune Hemolytic Anemia

Method of
*Stella T. Chou, MD, and*
*Mitchell J. Weiss, MD, PhD*

The hemolytic anemias (HAs) are a heterogeneous group of disorders characterized by accelerated erythrocyte destruction. Intrinsic causes of hemolysis are usually inherited and include abnormalities in the erythrocyte membrane, metabolic defects, and altered hemoglobin structure. Extrinsic causes include erythrocyte-directed antibodies, trauma, infections, and toxins. Within these categories, there are virtually hundreds of specific etiologies. Here we address the most common and clinically significant disorders, focusing mainly on the congenital HAs.

## Diagnosis

Anemia with reticulocytosis, hyperbilirubinemia, and an elevated lactate dehydrogenase (LDH) level strongly suggests hemolysis. The family history is often helpful for diagnosis. In particular, the clinician should inquire about ethnic background and family members with anemia, splenectomy, early gallstones/cholecystectomy, or significant neonatal jaundice. Several forms of HA confer protection against *Plasmodium falciparum* malaria. Accordingly, these disorders are relatively common in malaria endemic regions such as Africa, the Mediterranean basin, and Asia because of positive selective genetic pressure. Assessment of erythrocyte indexes and morphology are critical and frequently reveal distinct diagnostic clues (Table 1). Together, these initial data usually point to a specific diagnosis that can be confirmed by directed specialized testing that includes more detailed examination of erythrocytes and DNA analysis.

## CURRENT DIAGNOSIS

- Anemia, reticulocytosis and hyperbilirubinemia suggest hemolytic anemia (HA).
- Reticulocytopenia in the context of chronic HA suggests a Parvovirus-induced aplastic crisis.
- Erythrocyte-intrinsic etiologies for HA are usually inherited abnormalities affecting the erythrocyte membrane, enzymes, or hemoglobin structure.
- Congenital HA can present with severe neonatal jaundice.
- Extrinsic causes for HA include antierythrocyte antibodies, trauma, infection, and toxins.
- History, physical examination, and examination of erythrocyte morphology combined with more specialized testing usually provides a specific diagnosis.
- Paroxysmal nocturnal hemoglobinuria is a clonal somatically acquired hematopoietic disorder characterized by intravascular hemolysis, thromboses, and sometimes cytopenias. Diagnosis is made by flow cytometry demonstrating a population of cells that lack glycosyl phosphatidylinositol (GPI)-anchored membrane proteins.

In addition, patients with primary hemolytic disorders may present during an aplastic episode, most typically from Parvovirus B19 infection. In this case, erythrocyte production stops temporarily resulting in reticulocytopenia and declining hemoglobin.

## Management

Folate replacement is recommended for most patients with moderate to severe congenital hemolytic anemia. Iron from hemolyzed erythrocytes is usually reabsorbed, and supplementation is not necessary.

## CURRENT THERAPY

- Many forms of congenital severe HA are ameliorated by splenectomy.
- Long-term risks of splenectomy include susceptibility to sepsis from encapsulated organisms and possibly increased risk of thrombosis.
- Splenectomized patients should be immunized against *Streptococcus pneumoniae*, *Haemophilus influenzae* type B, and *Neisseria meningitidis*. Daily penicillin prophylaxis is recommended for children.
- Splenectomized patients presenting with fever should receive appropriate parenteral antibiotics until a negative blood culture is documented.
- Aplastic crisis and hyperhemolytic episodes associated with HA are managed with erythrocyte transfusion.
- Folate (folic acid) replacement, 1 mg/d, is recommended for moderate to severe HA.

Formation of gallstones is a common complication of HA, and therefore periodic screening abdominal ultrasounds are warranted. Concomitant Gilbert's syndrome, caused by a variant in the uridine diphosphoglucuronate glucuronosyltransferase 1A (UGT1A) gene promoter, increases the propensity for gallstones. Neonatal jaundice is common in many of the inherited disorders and may necessitate exchange transfusion for severe hyperbilirubinemia. Parvovirus B19–induced aplastic crisis is a life-threatening complication of congenital HA that frequently requires blood transfusion. Therefore, it is essential that patients with known hemolytic disorders be counseled to seek medical attention if they experience symptoms of viral illness, increased pallor, and lethargy.

Splenectomy is an effective treatment for many forms of severe congenital HA. The most significant problem from splenectomy is

---

**TABLE 1  Causes of Nonimmune Hemolytic Anemia**

| Type of Defect | Disease Mechanism | Example | Erythrocyte Morphology |
|---|---|---|---|
| Intrinsic erythrocyte defect | Membranopathy | Hereditary spherocytosis | Spherocytes |
| | | Hereditary elliptocytosis | Elliptocytes |
| | | Hereditary stomatocytosis | Stomatocytes |
| | | Hereditary xerocytosis | Target cells, echinocytes |
| | | Hereditary pyropoikilocytosis | Micropoikilocytes, microspherocytes, fragmented erythrocytes |
| | | Paroxysmal nocturnal hemoglobinuria | Macrocytosis |
| | Enzymopathy | G6PD deficiency | Heinz bodies, bite cells, blister cells, anisocytosis, poikilocytosis |
| | | Pyruvate kinase deficiency | Echinocytes |
| | Hemoglobinopathy | Sickle cell disease | Sickle cells |
| | | Thalassemia | Microcytosis, target cells |
| | | Unstable hemoglobinopathies | Heinz bodies |
| Extrinsic erythrocyte defect | Trauma | Heart valve hemolysis (macrovascular) | Schistocytes |
| | | DIC/TTP/HUS (microvascular) | Schistocytes |
| | Thermal injury | Severe burns | Schistocytes |
| | Chemicals | Arsenic, lead, copper, and chlorates | Varied |
| | Toxins | Bee and wasp stings, spider bites, and snake venom | Schistocytes |
| | Infections | Malaria, *Babesia*, *Bartonella*, clostridia, streptococci, staphylococci, enterococcus, salmonella, mycoplasma, EBV, CMV, HSV, rubeola, influenza A | Intraerythrocytic parasites; Schistocytes with bacterial infections |

*Abbreviations:* CMV = cytomegalovirus; DIC = disseminated intravascular coagulation; EBV = Epstein-Barr virus; HSV = herpes simplex virus; HUS = hemolytic uremic syndrome; TTP = thrombotic thrombocytopenic purpura.

increased risk of life-threatening infections from encapsulated organisms. Prior to splenectomy, patients should be vaccinated against *Streptococcus pneumoniae, Haemophilus influenzae type B,* and *Neisseria meningitidis.* Daily penicillin prophylaxis is recommended postsplenectomy, particularly for children. Splenectomized patients presenting with fever should be managed promptly with physical examination, blood culture, and appropriate parenteral antibiotics.

# Congenital Hemolytic Anemias

## ERYTHROCYTE MEMBRANE ABNORMALITIES

The erythrocyte membrane must be flexible and strong enough to withstand multiple passages through small capillary beds. A specialized membrane composed of a lipid bilayer, integral membrane proteins, and an underlying skeletal network formed by numerous proteins supports these requirements. Erythrocyte membrane proteins include alpha and beta spectrin, ankyrin, protein 4.1, and actin. Inherited mutations in these proteins disrupts the integrity of the membrane to cause HA.

### Hereditary Spherocytosis

Hereditary spherocytosis is the most common cause of nonimmune HA in populations from Northern Europe and North America, with a prevalence of approximately 1 in 2000.

#### Pathophysiology

Hereditary spherocytosis is caused by varying degrees of spectrin loss, usually from deficient or dysfunctional ankyrin, band 3 and/or protein 4.2, or, less frequently, a primary spectrin defect. Disruption of the membrane skeleton destabilizes the lipid bilayer causing splenic removal of microvesicles and subsequent spherocyte formation. The molecular basis of hereditary spherocytosis is heterogeneous. Approximately two thirds of cases are autosomal dominant, with the remaining one third being autosomal recessive or arising from new mutations.

#### Clinical Manifestations and Diagnosis

The severity of hereditary spherocytosis varies from asymptomatic to severe and typically correlates with the degree of spectrin deficiency. Most diagnoses of hereditary spherocytosis are made in childhood, from a positive family history or a clinical presentation of anemia, jaundice, and splenomegaly. New patients occasionally present with a Parvovirus-induced aplastic crisis. In these clinical contexts, an elevated mean corpuscular hemoglobin concentration (MCHC) strongly indicates hereditary spherocytosis. This value reflects a decreased surface-to-volume ratio caused by splenic removal of the erythrocyte membrane. In addition, the red cell distribution width (RDW) reflecting size variation, is elevated. The blood smear demonstrates spherocytes (erythrocytes lacking central pallor). A positive incubated osmotic fragility test, which demonstrates increased susceptibility to hypotonic lysis, supports the diagnosis. However, it is important to note that osmotic fragility is normal in 10% to 20% of hereditary spherocytosis cases. Moreover, other disorders, most notably immune HAs, are also characterized by spherocytes with increased osmotic fragility. A positive direct antiglobulin test (Coombs test) usually distinguishes immune HA from hereditary spherocytosis.

Patients with mild hereditary spherocytosis may have normal or near normal hemoglobin levels, mild reticulocytosis and hyperbilirubinemia, and typically have an uncomplicated course. More severely affected patients experience additional complications including severe neonatal hyperbilirubinemia and hyperhemolytic episodes later in life. The latter are frequently precipitated by viral illness and are characterized by worsening anemia, signs of accelerated hemolysis, and often, splenic enlargement. Rare complications of severe hereditary spherocytosis include leg ulcers, gout, and extramedullary hematopoiesis.

#### Management

Aplastic and hyperhemolytic episodes are supported with erythrocyte transfusions. Although splenectomy improves the anemia and reduces the risk of gallstones by removing the site of erythrocyte destruction, splenectomy should be reserved for patients with severe hemolysis, recurrent life-threatening hyperhemolytic episodes, or growth failure. Most clinicians prefer to treat as needed with transfusions until after 5 years of age when the postsplenectomy infection risk declines. In less severely affected patients, the threshold for recommending splenectomy varies among clinicians. In most centers, splenectomy is performed laparoscopically with very low morbidity and rapid recovery times. Moreover, improved vaccines, particularly pneumococcal, reduce the risk for postsplenectomy sepsis. However, some data indicate that splenectomy increases the long-term risk for venous and arterial thromboses, cardiovascular disease, and pulmonary hypertension. Accessory spleens are relatively common and should be searched for at the time of surgery.

### Hereditary Elliptocytosis and Pyropoikilocytosis

The hereditary elliptocytoses are a heterogeneous group of inherited HAs with oval-shaped erythrocytes. Hereditary elliptocytosis is relatively common in African, Mediterranean, and Asian populations. Hereditary pyropoikilocytosis is a more rare and severe form of HA with erythrocyte fragmentation in which one parent usually has hereditary elliptocytosis.

#### Pathophysiology

Most forms of hereditary elliptocytoses are inherited in an autosomal dominant fashion and are relatively mild. The underlying molecular defects are usually mutations in genes encoding alpha or beta spectrin, band 3, or protein 4.1. These mutations all destabilize the latticework of spectrin organization underlying the plasma membrane to induce an oval or elliptical shape. Assorted hereditary elliptocytoses mutations that qualitatively alter membrane proteins produce subtle variations in cell shape that distinguish different clinical subtypes, which are categorized according to erythrocyte morphology. In hereditary pyropoikilocytosis, the patient usually inherits a common hereditary elliptocytosis mutation from one parent and a milder subclinical defect in spectrin synthesis from the other parent.

#### Clinical Manifestations and Diagnosis

Hereditary elliptocytosis is classified into three subtypes according to morphology: common hereditary elliptocytosis, the most prevalent form, which is characterized by biconcave elliptocytes; spherocytic hereditary elliptocytosis, a phenotype between hereditary spherocytosis and hereditary elliptocytosis; and Southeast Asian ovalocytosis, characterized by oval erythrocytes. Most patients are asymptomatic and diagnosed incidentally with minimal or mild compensated hemolysis. The peripheral smear demonstrates more than 30% elliptocytes. Patients who are homozygous or compound heterozygous have more severe HA. The peripheral blood smear also has budding erythrocytes, fragments, and other poikilocytes. Hereditary pyropoikilocytosis, at the extreme end of this spectrum, causes bizarre fragmented erythrocytes with microspherocytosis and micropoikilocytosis. The mean corpuscular volume is very low (25 to 75 fL), the osmotic fragility is abnormal, and erythrocytes characteristically demonstrate thermal instability. Hereditary pyropoikilocytosis typically presents in newborns or infants with jaundice and anemia.

#### Management

Most hereditary elliptocytoses patients have a mild course and do not require treatment. In cases of severe hemolysis because of homozygous or compound heterozygous hereditary elliptocytosis or hereditary pyropoikilocytosis, splenectomy is indicated.

## Hereditary Stomatocytosis and Xerocytosis

Hereditary stomatocytosis and xerocytosis are rare inherited causes of hemolytic anemia associated with abnormal erythrocyte cation permeability and volume (increased in stomatocytosis and decreased in xerocytosis). Both disorders are autosomal dominant. Hereditary stomatocytosis patients have erythrocytes with a mouth-shaped (stoma) area of central pallor, whereas hereditary xerocytosis patients demonstrate target cells and echinocytes. The clinical courses of these diseases are highly variable, ranging from asymptomatic to moderate hemolysis and subsequent anemia. Most patients do not require treatment. Importantly, splenectomy is contraindicated in hereditary stomatocytosis because of an increased incidence of life-threatening thrombosis.

## ERYTHROCYTE METABOLISM ABNORMALITIES

Erythrocytes rely on two major biochemical pathways: glycolysis for energy to maintain metabolic needs and the hexose-monophosphate shunt for antioxidant pathways. More than 20 enzymes are involved in these two pathways, and defects in each one are associated with various forms of HA. The two most common enzymopathies are deficiencies in glucose-6-phosphate dehydrogenase (G6PD) and pyruvate kinase (PK).

### Glucose-6-Phosphate Dehydrogenase Deficiency

G6PD deficiency is the most common erythrocyte metabolism disorder, affecting as much as 3% of the world's population.

#### Pathophysiology

G6PD is the first enzyme in the hexose-monophosphate pathway, which is required to maintain a high level of reduced glutathione, an important antioxidant. G6PD-deficient erythrocytes undergo increased hemoglobin oxidation leading to hemolysis. G6PD deficiency is an X-linked recessive disorder. More than 300 G6PD genetic variants affect enzyme activity to different extents that determine the severity of HA. Type A⁻ is a genetic variant seen in 10% to 15% of African American males and is associated with mild to moderate G6PD deficiency. Variants causing more severe HA are more prevalent in Mediterranean and Asian populations.

#### Clinical Manifestations and Diagnosis

G6PD deficiency is an X-linked disorder; therefore, hemizygous males and homozygous females are typically affected. Many G6PD variants are associated with neonatal jaundice. Severe forms of G6PD deficiency can cause chronic ongoing HA, but most commonly, affected individuals are asymptomatic in between hemolytic episodes. However, anemia develops rapidly following a precipitating event related to oxidative stress that induces acute intravascular hemolysis with the severity determined by the G6PD variant and the offending agent. Drugs are the most common inciting event in Africans with the A⁻ variant (Table 2). Other precipitating events include mothball (naphthalene) exposure and infections. In some Mediterranean and Asian variants, ingestion of fava beans can cause acute life-threatening hemolysis. Symptoms can include fever, abdominal pain, nausea, diarrhea, and impressive hemoglobinuria, frequently described as Coca-Cola colored. The spleen is often enlarged and tender. Anemia ranges from mild to life-threatening and is normocytic and normochromic. Morphologic abnormalities include anisocytosis, poikilocytosis, "bite cells" (erythrocytes that are partially destroyed in the spleen), and "blister cells" (a thin strip of membrane overlying a bleb of clear cytoplasm). A methyl violet stain to detect Heinz bodies, indicative of denatured hemoglobin, is typically positive. Immediately after an acute hemolytic event, G6PD levels can be deceptively normal because of an elevated reticulocyte count, which can express significant enzymatic activity in some variants. Therefore, G6PD levels should be tested weeks to months later to obtain a true baseline level.

## TABLE 2 Drugs Capable of Precipitating Hemolysis in G6PD Deficiency

| | |
|---|---|
| **Analgesics and Antipyretics** | Acetanilid* |
| | Acetylsalicylic acid (aspirin) |
| **Antibacterials** | Chloramphenicol |
| | Furazolidone (Furoxone)* |
| | Nalidixic acid (NeGram)* |
| | Nitrofurantoin (Furadantin)* |
| | Sulfonamides* |
| | Trimethoprim-sulfamethoxazole (Bactrim) |
| **Antimalarials** | Pamaquine* |
| | Pentaquine* |
| | Primaquine* |
| | Quinacrine |
| **Miscellaneous** | Dimercaptosuccinic acid (Succimer) |
| | Methylene blue* |
| | Phenazopyridine (Pyridium)* |
| | Urate oxidase* |
| | Vitamin K |

*These drugs have an increased tendency to cause clinically significant hemolysis. Most patients with mild G6PD deficiency alleles tolerate drugs that are not marked by the asterisk. For a more comprehensive list of drug–G6PD interactions, see reading by Beutler.
Abbreviation: G6PD = glucose-6-phosphate dehydrogenase.

#### Management

Treatment of the A⁻ variant of G6PD deficiency is mostly preventive by avoiding oxidant stresses. When acute hemolytic episodes result in symptomatic anemia, erythrocyte transfusions are indicated. Rarely, acute renal failure develops secondary to severe intravascular hemolysis. This is managed by vigorous hydration, alkalinization, electrolyte monitoring, and occasionally hemodialysis.

### Pyruvate Kinase Deficiency

Pyruvate kinase (PK) deficiency, which is most commonly seen in Northern European populations, accounts for more than 80% of the HAs due to glycolytic disorders.

#### Pathophysiology

PK deficiency is genetically heterogeneous, with many different mutations impairing enzyme activity to different extents. Pyruvate kinase deficiency causes decreased production of ATP, impairing erythrocyte survival. Inheritance is usually autosomal recessive; simple heterozygotes with 50% enzyme activity are unaffected.

#### Clinical Manifestations and Diagnosis

PK deficiency is extremely heterogeneous, ranging from life-threatening HA to asymptomatic compensated hemolysis. Erythrocyte morphology may be normal or show echinocytes (small dense crenated erythrocytes). Quantitation of erythrocyte enzyme activity is usually diagnostic.

#### Management

General supportive care for chronic hemolysis and supportive erythrocyte transfusions when needed are the mainstays of therapy. Patients with severe hemolysis may benefit from splenectomy, although the response is variable and unpredictable.

## HEMOGLOBINOPATHIES

HA can be caused by mutations that alter the α- or β-like globin proteins that contribute to hemoglobin structure. Quantitative defects that impair globin gene expression comprise the thalassemia syndromes, discussed in the article on thalassemia. Qualitative defects are usually caused by missense mutations that alter hemoglobin structure and stability. The most important examples are the sickle syndromes, discussed in the article on sickle cell disease. Numerous other missense mutations that destabilize hemoglobin also cause HA. In these cases, hemoglobin precipitates may be detected by a Heinz body stain. Unstable hemoglobins can also be detected by hemoglobin electrophoresis or increased precipitation upon exposure to heat or isopropanol. If any of these tests are positive in the context of hemolysis, direct globin gene sequencing can provide a definitive diagnosis.

# Acquired Nonimmune Hemolytic Anemias

## PAROXYSMAL NOCTURNAL HEMOGLOBINURIA

Paroxysmal nocturnal hemoglobinuria (PNH) is a rare acquired disease with chronic HA, thrombosis, and often pancytopenia. The hemolytic anemia results from increased erythrocyte sensitivity to complement-mediated hemolysis.

### Pathophysiology

PNH is an acquired clonal disorder caused by a somatically acquired inactivating mutation in the X-linked phosphatidylinositol glycan, class A (PIGA) gene, which encodes an enzyme involved in the synthesis of glycosyl phosphatidylinositol (GPI) anchor proteins. All blood cells derived from the abnormal clone lack surface proteins that require the GPI anchor. Hemolysis occurs from the deficiency of specific GPI-linked surface proteins that inhibit complement activation. The hypercoagulable state seen in PNH is most likely related to complement-mediated platelet activation and elevated levels of ADP from lysed erythrocytes, leading to platelet aggregation. For unknown reasons, PNH commonly progresses to aplastic anemia.

### Clinical Manifestations and Diagnosis

PNH can present as a primary hemolytic syndrome with chronic intravascular HA, a thrombotic event, or with pancytopenia. Few patients exhibit the classic nocturnal hemoglobinuria, reporting red or brownish urine in the morning. In most patients hemoglobinuria occurs irregularly and is often precipitated by infection or stress. Iron deficiency can occur from urinary loss. Associated thromboses may be venous or arterial and can involve extremities, the hepatic vein (Budd-Chiari syndrome), other intraabdominal veins, and cerebral veins. Hence, PNH can present as severe abdominal pain or headaches. The majority of patients have defective hematopoiesis, ranging from a macrocytic anemia to severe aplastic anemia and pancytopenia. Rarely, PNH can also evolve into a myelodysplastic syndrome or acute leukemia. The median survival for patients diagnosed with PNH is 10 to 15 years.

Laboratory findings include anemia, variable reticulocytosis, leukopenia, and thrombocytopenia. The bone marrow examination typically reveals erythroid hyperplasia or, in the case of associated aplastic anemia, hypocellularity. Urine hemosiderin is typical. Laboratory diagnosis of PNH previously relied on assays that demonstrated abnormal erythrocyte sensitivity to complement (Ham test, sucrose hemolysis test). The current standard is flow cytometry demonstrating the absence of hematopoietic GPI-linked proteins, typically CD55 and CD59, on some or all circulating cells.

### Management

Oral iron supplementation is recommended to replace the urinary losses associated with intravascular hemolysis. Corticosteroids can sometimes improve the hemolysis in the first 24 to 72 hours of a hemolytic episode. A recent phase 3 trial showed that eculizumab, a monoclonal antibody that inhibits activation of the terminal complement complex, is effective for the hemolytic anemia of PNH. Eculizamab was recently FDA-approved and is entering clinical practice. Anticoagulation is indicated for documented thromboses, and thrombolytic therapy can be effective for patients with hepatic vein thrombosis or massive thrombotic events. Short-term prophylactic therapy should be used in the setting of surgery or prolonged immobilization, even if there is no history of thrombosis. HLA-identical bone marrow transplantation is indicated for bone marrow failure associated with PNH. Alternatively, immunosuppressive therapy with antithymocyte globulin and cyclosporine is used for patients without a suitable bone marrow donor.

# Hemolytic Anemia Caused by Erythrocyte Fragmentation

Erythrocyte fragmentation can occur in the macrovascular or microvascular circulations. Shear stress produces fragmented erythrocytes (schistocytes). Macroangiopathic hemolysis can occur with prosthetic surfaces, large thromboses, and aged or damaged heart valves, but it is usually mild. Microangiopathic causes of hemolysis include disseminated intravascular coagulation, thrombotic thrombocytopenic purpura, and hemolytic uremic syndrome, which are discussed in their respective articles.

# Hemolytic Anemia Caused by Chemical and Physical Agents

Arsenic, lead, copper, and chlorates can cause hemolysis through numerous mechanisms. Most notably, hemolytic anemia may be the presenting feature of the copper toxicity of Wilson's disease. Animal toxins associated with intravascular hemolysis include bee and wasp stings, brown recluse spider bites, and snake venom. Severe burns can also cause fragmentation hemolysis from the thermal injury.

# Hemolytic Anemia Caused by Infection

Infections cause hemolysis by direct invasion of the erythrocyte, toxin production, or by immune-mediated mechanisms. Malaria is the most common infectious cause of hemolytic anemia worldwide. *Plasmodium falciparum* invades erythrocytes and is associated with severe hemolysis and hemoglobinuria (blackwater fever). Other parasitic infections associated with hemolysis are *Babesia microti* and *Bartonella bacilliformis*. Bacterial organisms that cause hemolysis via erythrocyte membrane injury and toxins include clostridia, streptococci, staphylococci, enterococcus, and salmonella. Immune hemolysis is associated with *Mycoplasma pneumoniae*, Epstein-Barr virus, cytomegalovirus, herpes simplex, rubeola, and influenza A (see topic in Section 2). Hemolysis improves once the underlying infection resolves.

## REFERENCES

Beutler E: Glucose-6-phosphate dehydrogenase deficiency and other red cell enzyme abnormalities, in Beutler E, et al. (eds): Williams Hematology. New York, McGraw-Hill, 2001, pp 527-545.

Bolton-Maggs PH, Stevens RF, Dodd NJ, et al: Guidelines for the diagnosis and management of hereditary spherocytosis. Br J Haematol 2004; 126(4):455-474.

Gallagher P, Lux S: Disorders of the erythrocyte membrane, in Nathan D, et al (eds): Nathan and Oski's Hematology of Infancy and Childhood. Philadelphia, WB Saunders, 2003, pp 560-684.

Hillmen P, Young NS, Schubert J, et al: The complement inhibitor eculizumab in paroxysmal nocturnal hemoglobinuria. N Engl J Med 2006;355(12): 1233-1243.

Parker C, Omine M, Richards S, et al: Diagnosis and management of paroxysmal nocturnal hemoglobinuria. Blood 2005;106(12): 3699-3709.

Tse WT, Lux SE: Red blood cell membrane disorders. Br J Haematol 1999;104(1):2-13.

Zanella A, Fermo E, Bianchi P, Valentini G: Red cell pyruvate kinase deficiency: Molecular and clinical aspects. Br J Haematol 2005;130(1):11-25.

# Pernicious Anemia and Other Megaloblastic Anemias

Method of
*Eugene P. Frenkel, MD*

Historically, pernicious anemia was the prevalent prototypic megaloblastic anemia. At present, its diagnostic incidence, when appropriately defined, has been overshadowed by many other pathophysiologic mechanisms that produce similar hematologic and neurologic changes.

The term *megaloblastic anemia* identifies peripheral blood findings of red cell macrocytosis (mean corpuscular volume [MCV] >96 fL) associated with macro-ovalocytes and anisocytosis. Because macrocytosis can be seen in many clinical circumstances in the absence of a megaloblastic state (Box 1), the true diagnosis defines defective erythroid maturation in the bone marrow, wherein the red cell precursors have enlarged reticulated nuclear chromatin characteristic of defective DNA synthesis with normal permissive RNA synthesis, resulting in a large cytoplasmic mass. Because the defective DNA

---

**BOX 1   Etiologic and Pathophysiologic Mechanisms for Macrocytosis and Megaloblastosis**

**Nonmegaloblastic Macrocytosis***
These are nonprogressive over time, usually associated with a normal RDW, and banal macrocytes (nonovalocytic macrocytes seen in true megaloblastic states)
- Aplastic anemia
- Chronic alcohol use
- Chronic liver disease
- Myelodysplastic syndromes
- Postsplenectomy states

**Megaloblastic Anemia**
- Deficiency or defects in vitamin $B_{12}$ (cobalamin) metabolism
  - Inadequate diet: Strict vegan patients
  - Inadequate absorption: Lack of intrinsic factor
- Classic pernicious anemia
- Aging stomach
- Intrinsic factor inhibition
- Small intestinal disease/resection
- Abnormal utilization (e.g., nitrous oxide anesthesia, etc.)
- Deficiency or defects in folate metabolism
  - Inadequate intake
  - Altered absorption
  - Abnormal utilization—especially chemotherapeutic drugs, anticonvulsants, alcoholism
  - Increased excretion, renal dialysis

---

*Mean corpuscular volume is usually 96 to 100 $\mu m^3$.

---

synthesis is not exclusive to the red cells, giant metamyelocytes reflect the defect in white cells, and macro-megakaryocytes also occur. Indeed, defective DNA synthesis is seen not only in the bone marrow but also in all proliferating cells (e.g., buccal mucosa, gastrointestinal tract, etc.)

## Etiology

Almost one century after Addison's (1855) annotation of an unusual anemia, termed *pernicious anemia*, Minot and Murphy (1926) showed that the anemia could be "abolished" by (almost) raw liver, and in 1929 Dr. William Castle described an "intrinsic factor" in the stomach, which was required for liver extract to correct the anemia. Then in 1938, Lucy Wills and Barbara Evans described a nutritional anemia in pregnant women that failed to respond to liver extract, thereby posing the conundrum that a second form of megaloblastic anemia existed. Important resolution of this dilemma came when Pfiffner and Stokstad found a relevant growth factor in yeast and green plants, which they named folic acid. In 1948, Karl Folkers identified and crystallized vitamin $B_{12}$, which was subsequently shown to require intrinsic factor for facilitated absorption in the terminal ileum. Absorption was defined in the upper small intestine. Subsequently, the finding of circulating autoantibodies to intrinsic factor in patients with (genetic) pernicious anemia appeared to complete the pathogenesis and clinical picture related to these two moieties.

Almost immediately this simplistic clinical construct began to unravel. As shown in Box 1, vitamin $B_{12}$ (cobalamin) absorption was related to the increasing incidence of megaloblastic anemia with age. The concept of the aging stomach changed the clinical expression of megaloblastic anemia. As we age (after 50 years), the release of vitamin $B_{12}$ from food proteins declines due to reduced pepsin activity at a low pH. The known decrease in gastric acidity with aging may be the most important factor of such decreased extraction of vitamin $B_{12}$ from food, but it is clearly not the only factor. However, such patients have normal absorption of crystalline vitamin $B_{12}$, so that treatment with nonfood vitamin $B_{12}$ results in a physiologic response.

Clearly a very common addition to the effects with aging is the new ubiquitous use of proton pump inhibitors for the treatment of gastric reflux and heartburn. These agents reduce secretion of intrinsic factor as well as pepsin and gastric acid, and they are now recognized as an important factor in decreased vitamin $B_{12}$ absorption.

## Clinical Features

A very important aspect of vitamin $B_{12}$ deficiency is that in addition to the anemia, neurologic deficits are a significant part of the clinical expression. Neurologic deficits are being seen with remarkable frequency, and in the past two decades they are actually the common presenting complaint, often occurring in the *absence* of anemia. These include posterolateral spinal column dysmyelinization with resultant peripheral paresthesias, loss of vibratory and positional sense, decreased deep tendon reflexes, and even ataxia. In addition, classic peripheral neuropathy or even cerebral dysfunction with depression, irritability, and memory loss can occur. Because these signs and symptoms are often present in the absence of anemia, the clinician needs special vigilance to evaluate the neurologic findings and relate them to vitamin $B_{12}$ deficiency. The explanation for the dichotomy of progressive neurologic deficits in the absence of anemia appears to be the increased availability of folate in fortified food, because folate can replace vitamin $B_{12}$ in blood cell production but not in neural function.

Another correlative clinical event has been the recognition of severe and rapid progressive neurologic lesions in patients undergoing nitrous oxide exposure. This has been seen after its use in open heart surgery and even when used for 2 to 3 hours for oral surgery. We now know that nitrous oxide interferes with the two known enzymatic pathways in vitamin $B_{12}$ metabolism. As noted earlier, the methylcobalamin methyltransferase biochemical pathway can be bypassed by folate. However, functional inactivation and interference of the second pathway (methylmalonyl coenzyme–mutase reaction) occur. This alteration

## CURRENT DIAGNOSIS

- Pernicious anemia is the result of autoantibody loss of gastric intrinsic factor, resulting in failure of facilitated absorption of vitamin $B_{12}$ in the terminal ileum.
- Megaloblastic anemia is almost entirely related to deficiency or defective (altered) utilization of vitamin $B_{12}$ or folate.
- Megaloblastic anemia in association with neurologic deficit is due to vitamin $B_{12}$.
- Determination of serum methylmalonic acid and homocysteine are the best, most sensitive, and most specific tests for the etiologic basis of megaloblastic anemia and demonstrate presence of the metabolic defect.
- Repletement of vitamin $B_{12}$ or folate is best defined by identifying the pathophysiologic mechanism for the defect.
- With age, the effective extraction of vitamin $B_{12}$ from food declines, with resultant vitamin $B_{12}$ deficiency.
- Folate supplementation is very important in the first trimester of pregnancy to protect from neural tube abnormalities in the fetus.

cannot be bypassed by folate and has been demonstrated to result in nerve dysmyelinization.

The changing pattern of the causes of megaloblastic anemia is also related to folate metabolism. The FDA-mandated addition of folate to whole grain products beginning in 1998 has remarkably changed the occurrence of folate deficiency in the United States and the development of megaloblastic anemia. It, of course, may be the basis for the prominent increase in the neurologic presentation in vitamin $B_{12}$ deficiency. A very important observation relative to folate metabolism is the clear requirement for supplemental folate during pregnancy. The most important reason is that folate is critical for normal neural tube formation in the first weeks of pregnancy.

## Diagnosis

### LABORATORY DIAGNOSIS OF VITAMIN $B_{12}$ AND FOLATE METABOLIC DEFICIENCIES

Diagnostic value of a low serum vitamin $B_{12}$ value in patients with megaloblastic anemia is well confirmed. However, evaluation of patients with little or no hematologic abnormalities, but with a variety of neurologic or psychiatric changes, particularly in the older age group, has defined a significantly decreased sensitivity and specificity for the serum vitamin $B_{12}$ assay.

Characterization of the only two metabolic pathways for vitamin $B_{12}$ metabolism had long ago provided assays of the intermediates of the two functional coenzymes: methylcobalamin active in the homocysteine-to-methonine pathway and adenosylcobalamine in the salvage pathway. Vitamin $B_{12}$ deficiency results in an increase in serum methylmalonic acid and serum (or plasma) total homocysteine. Normally, serum methylmalonic acid (MMA) is undetectable (commonly defined as <0.4 mmol/L). An increase in serum and urine MMA has been shown to be highly sensitive and specific for the diagnosis of vitamin $B_{12}$ deficiency. It is now clearly the gold standard in the clinical evaluation of suspected vitamin $B_{12}$ deficiency because it defines true tissue depletion. As would be expected, homocysteine is also increased with tissue vitamin $B_{12}$ deficiency.

The laboratory diagnosis of folate deficiency has been even more difficult than that of vitamin $B_{12}$. The serum folate assay has been commonly used. Unfortunately, it is remarkably affected by a short period of dietary deprivation or recent alcohol ingestion, and slight hemolysis will increase the serum value. Red cell folate levels have been considered a more stable site to measure. Because the red cell life span

is 120 days, the red cell folate measurement is a mean of the events over a prolonged period. Unfortunately, it is difficult to perform and is insensitive to issues relating to alcohol ingestion and pregnancy.

By contrast, measurements of homocysteine levels are very sensitive and serve as an excellent assessment of folate deficiency, when the serum MMA is *normal*. The assay of MMA and homocysteine provides approximately a 99% sensitivity and specificity for the diagnosis of vitamin $B_{12}$– or folate-deficient states and are truly the tests of choice.

### PHYSIOLOGIC ISSUES RELATIVE TO VITAMIN $B_{12}$ AND FOLATE

The average American diet contains 5 to 30 μg of vitamin $B_{12}$, and the absorption has been considered to be 1 to 2 μg/day, with a projected daily requirement of 0.5 to 1.0 μg/day. Issues related to the efficiency of the enterohepatic circulation make these numbers far from precise, because it has been projected that 1 to 10 μg of cobalamins are re-cycled daily.

The folate content of the mean American diet is about 280 μg for men and 210 μg for women. Although previous estimates of daily requirements had been 400 μg/day, recent daily recommendations have been 200 μg/day for men and 180 μg/day for women. Tissue stores of folate are limited and levels begin to decline within 2 weeks of deprivation. Indeed, acute clinical deprivation is a recognized event in intensive care units. Studies of this rapid deprivation suggest that our daily needs are closer to 400 μg per day and that the mean tissue storage content is approximately 5000 μg.

## Treatment

### GENERAL PRINCIPLES OF THERAPY

The first and most critical therapeutic concern is the clinical stability of the patient who presents with severe anemia or rapidly progressive neurologic deficit, especially where an impending or pseudo spinal cord transection appears to be developing. However, because megaloblastic anemias usually develop slowly, compensatory cardiopulmonary responses are often associated with only modest symptoms, even when patients present with hemoglobin levels less than 3 or 4 g/dL. Often the impulse is to quickly treat with multiple hematinics while awaiting diagnostic data from the laboratory. The appropriate approach is to recognize that even with specific diagnosis and therapy, the red cell values will not improve for at least 7 to 14 days. The red cell needs must be judged solely on the cardiopulmonary and cerebral functional status of the patient, and if required, cautious transfusion is the urgent treatment of choice. Commonly, only a single unit of packed red cells is needed. Transfusion(s) should be given

## CURRENT THERAPY

- The decision for therapy depends on the determination of the etiology (vitamin $B_{12}$ or folate) and the definition of the pathophysiologic mechanism for the deficiency or altered metabolism.
- The cardiopulmonary status of the patient with anemia determines the therapeutic initiation, because hematologic repair will take 7 to 14 days regardless of the hematinic used. Cautious red cell transfusions should be used to stabilize the cardiopulmonary issues.
- Parenteral vitamin $B_{12}$ is the therapy of choice in classic pernicious anemia.
- Oral vitamin $B_{12}$ (at pharmacologic doses) is very effective in the management of patients with the aging stomach.
- Folate supplementation is essential during the first trimester of pregnancy to protect neural tube development.

slowly (over 3 to 4 hours), because rapid volume shifts can precipitate functional problems related to the precarious hemodynamic status of these patients.

Less commonly, the neurologic deterioration (such as with the nitrous oxide effect) of the patient encourages urgency of therapy. Such rapid progression virtually defines the etiology to be due to vitamin $B_{12}$. Although rare, if progression appears rapid, serum should be collected and treatment with parenteral vitamin $B_{12}$ instituted immediately.

The second important principle is the requirement for a specific etiologic diagnosis, because the pathophysiologic mechanism that produced the defect must be defined to determine reversibility of the cause and the duration of therapy (e.g., short term, lifetime). Thus, (genetic) pernicious anemia will demand a lifetime of vitamin $B_{12}$ replacement therapy, whereas vitamin $B_{12}$ deficiency due to jejunal diverticula can be approached with short-term vitamin $B_{12}$ therapy, antibiotics, and the consideration of surgical repair. Similarly, the aged stomach syndrome can easily be managed with oral vitamin $B_{12}$ supplements.

The third issue relates to an understanding of the rate and pattern of repair of the clinical abnormalities. When the anemia fails to respond in the expected time frame, the question of an incorrect diagnosis or an unrecognized associated lesion must be considered. For instance, iron deficiency is often unrecognized when it is associated with megaloblastosis; it will, however, result in a suboptimal therapeutic response. This can be particularly noteworthy in vitamin $B_{12}$ deficiency, when patients with pernicious anemia have an increased risk of gastric cancer, and the finding of iron deficiency can provide the clue to its diagnostic pursuit.

Fourth, the serial follow-up of patients after therapeutic restitution requires an understanding of the natural history of the underlying disease status. Patients can only be educated about the need for therapy and follow-up when the physician understands the cause and mechanism. This is important, because the ease with which repair can be achieved sometimes belies the significance of the problem. For instance, pernicious anemia patients have an increased incidence of gastric cancer and have the potential to develop endocrinopathies (especially hypothyroidism and hypoadrenalism) secondary to autoantibodies. Thus, they will need a lifetime of therapy and serial clinical evaluation.

Finally, the concept of a therapeutic trial in patients with megaloblastic states does not eliminate the need for a specific diagnosis and determination of the pathophysiologic mechanism. Certainly, an elevated MMA or homocysteine S can be used as a parameter for a trial of therapy; correction of the defect should similarly correct the metabolic abnormality in 10 to 14 days. This allows affirmation of the diagnosis and confirms the presence of tissue deficiency.

### TREATMENT OF VITAMIN $B_{12}$ (COBALAMIN) DEFICIENCY

Normal tissue vitamin $B_{12}$ stores (primarily in liver and bone marrow) range between 7 and 15 mg. Clinically significant deficiency is expressed when tissue stores are reduced to 30% to 50% of normal. The goal of therapy is to replete tissue stores. However, with each dose of vitamin $B_{12}$, the percentage of the given dose retained by tissues declines. In essence, fractional urinary excretion of an administered dose increases as the stores are progressively repleted. Therefore, significantly more must be administered than one would calculate from the amount known to exist in total body tissues. The fractional retention is better when temporal gaps (daily or every few days) are left between doses. These physiologic issues help explain the many repletement schedules found in literature, and further allow the clinician to adopt a sequence most appropriate to the patient and the related clinical issues.

Because most of the mechanisms of vitamin $B_{12}$ deficiency relate to decreased absorption, the initial therapy should begin with cyanocobalamin or hydroxycobalamin 1 mg (1000 μm) given subcutaneously or intramuscularly. This is rapidly absorbed from either site, with peak serum levels in approximately 1 hour after injection. Following this initial dose, approximately 65% will be retained. Intravenous injection produces a much greater urinary loss and should not be used. A simple repletement schedule from that point is 1 mg given daily or every other day during the first 2 weeks and then weekly

for the next month, by which time normal peripheral hematologic values are expected.

Thereafter, the pathophysiologic mechanism of the deficiency will determine the approach to future therapy. For patients in whom gastric intrinsic factor secretion is defective (pernicious anemia), vitamin $B_{12}$ must be given for life. Monthly or bimonthly injections of 1 mg provide simple, inexpensive, and effective therapy that requires no special monitoring. In patients with neurologic deficits, more frequent administration (weekly) of vitamin $B_{12}$ has been used in the first 6 months, a time when neurologic repair is at the maximum. It must be emphasized that such an increased frequency is empiric, with no defined supportive data. Similarly, shortening the interval between injections, often requested by elderly patients who express having an improved sense of well-being with the treatment, is based on specific evidence.

The elderly most often have vitamin $B_{12}$ deficiency due to ineffective liberation of vitamin $B_{12}$ bound to protein in food. In these patients the absorption of crystalline vitamin $B_{12}$ is normal. In such circumstances, as well as in the strict vegan (no dietary animal products) patient, oral vitamin $B_{12}$ can be used. Oral 1 mg (1000 μg) tablets are inexpensive and available for such use and should be given daily. We have successfully treated patients with the aged stomach with oral vitamin $B_{12}$ alone, without initial parenteral repair.

Increased daily vitamin $B_{12}$ requirements occur in pregnancy and lactation, thyrotoxicosis, and liver or renal disease, especially where protein loss is extensive. Because tissue concentrations of vitamin $B_{12}$ are in the milligram range and daily requirements are in the microgram range, the normal stores are adequate for 1 to 3 years in the absence of supplementation. Deficiency is therefore uncommonly associated with such an increased need, except in the pregnant vegan patient.

Side effects from vitamin $B_{12}$ therapy are extremely rare. Patients with the very rare early Leber's disease (hereditary optic nerve atrophy) have been reported in the past to have increased atrophy with institution of high-dose therapy. Rarely, pruritus and skin rash have occurred, and more rarely anaphylactic shock has been reported.

Short-term sequelae of repletement therapy in megaloblastic states can occur regardless of the etiology of the deficiency. These include hypokalemia and hyperuricemia, especially in the first 48 to 72 hours of institution of therapy. Therefore, potassium supplementation is wise when therapy is started.

### TREATMENT OF FOLATE DEFICIENCY

Normal tissue stores of folate are approximately 5000 μg (5 mg) with a projected daily requirement of 200 to 400 μg. These limited stores result in folate deficiency more quickly with dietary deprivation than in vitamin $B_{12}$ deficiency. Because most clinical circumstances of folate deficiency are due to inadequate intake or drug interference, oral repletement is the usual mode, giving 1 mg (or 5 mg[3]) folic acid pills, a commonly available form, per day. In general, 1 mg/day provides a significant excess and allows rapid repletement of tissue stores. In known malabsorption syndromes, the 5 mg[3] daily folic acid oral dose is preferable. Tissue stores can be repleted easily in a few weeks with daily oral therapy, and therefore the duration of therapy is determined on the persistence of the cause.

Folate prophylaxis is very important through pregnancy, where at least 600 μg of folate per day is desirable. However, because of its critical need in neurologic development, doses in the range of 4 mg/day are recommended to prevent neural tube defects. However, these should begin 4 weeks before the pregnancy and continue at least through the first 3 months of gestation. High doses of folate (>500 μg/day) have allegedly reduced zinc absorption; thus, mineral supplementation during pregnancy may be appropriate. Another circumstance that merits folate prophylaxis is in patients on long-standing anticonvulsant therapy, because folate deficiency has been associated with an increased seizure frequency.

It again merits emphasis that empiric folate therapy in a patient with megaloblastic anemia will repair the anemia, but if the correct diagnosis is vitamin $B_{12}$ deficiency, a fulminant neurologic deficit can ensue.

---

[3]Exceeds dosage recommended by the manufacturer.

## REFERENCES

Carmel R: Cobalamin, the stomach, and aging. Am J Clin Nutr 1997:66: 750-759.

Herbert VD, Colman N: Folic acid and vitamin B$_{12}$. In Shils ME, Young VR (eds): Modern Nutrition in Health and Disease, 7th ed. Philadelphia: Lea & Febiger, 1988, pp 388-416.

Lindenbaum J, Healton EB, Savage DG, et al: Neuropsychiatric disorders caused by cobalamin deficiency in the absence of anemia or macrocytosis. N Engl J Med 1988;318:1720-1728.

Stabler SP, Allen RH, Savage DG, et al: Clinical spectrum and diagnosis of cobalamin deficiency. Blood 1990;76:871-881.

# Thalassemia

Method of
*Susan P. Perrine, MD, and*
*Serguei A. Castaneda, MD*

## Pathophysiology: Basic Mechanisms of Hemoglobin Synthesis

The sequential expression of the globin genes results in production of specific types of hemoglobins at different stages of development. At 12 weeks of gestation, a transition from embryonic to fetal hemoglobin ($\alpha_2\gamma_2$) occurs, and at 28 weeks of gestation, increasing amounts of $\beta$-globin and of adult hemoglobin A (Hb A, $\alpha_2\beta_2$) are produced. $\alpha$-Like globin protein must equal $\beta$-like globin proteins for intact hemoglobin tetramers to form. Thalassemia syndromes result from deficiencies in either $\alpha$-globin ($\alpha$-thalassemia) or $\beta$-like globin ($\beta$-thalassemia) chains. The diseases become apparent when the deficient globin is required during development. During gestation, $\alpha$-thalassemia is symptomatic because $\alpha$-globin is required for fetal hemoglobin (Hb F, $\alpha_2\gamma_2$). Because $\beta$-globin is not required in large amounts before birth, $\beta$-thalassemia is asymptomatic until approximately 6 months after birth. Mutations that cause prolonged production of fetal $\gamma$-globin chains may present later, at 2 to 4 years of age.

The major pathologic process in thalassemia is the imbalance of $\alpha$- and non-$\alpha$-globin chain accumulation. The unaffected chains, produced in normal amounts, precipitate during erythropoiesis. In $\beta$-thalassemia, the precipitated $\alpha$-globin chains are particularly toxic, damaging cell membranes and causing rapid cell death (apoptosis). Red blood cell life span is further shortened by removal of abnormal cells in the reticuloendothelial system. Erythropoietin levels increase, causing erythroid hyperplasia. Hypersplenism causes more severe anemia.

In $\alpha$-thalassemic fetuses, the unbalanced fetal ($\gamma$)-globin chains form tetramers ($\gamma_4$, hemoglobin Bart's); excess $\beta$-globin ($\beta_4$, hemoglobin H) accumulates after birth. Hemoglobin Bart's and hemoglobin H result in milder ineffective erythropoiesis but have abnormal oxygen binding. If all four $\alpha$-globin genes are deleted, only hemoglobin Bart's is formed, with a massively left-shifted oxygen dissociation curve that provides no oxygen delivery to tissues and results in a lethal intrauterine condition, hydrops fetalis. Decreased production of $\alpha$-globin from three or four abnormal $\alpha$-globin genes causes moderate hemolytic anemia, hemoglobin H disease. Deletion of one ($\alpha$-thalassemia-2) or two ($\alpha$-thalassemia-1) loci is asymptomatic.

Thalassemia syndromes are graded according to severity of the anemia. Thalassemia major, in which severe anemia manifests during infancy, is caused by inheritance of two severely impaired $\beta$-globin alleles. Such homozygous or doubly heterozygous conditions have milder manifestations when there is an increase in fetal globin chain production or when the co-inheritance of $\alpha$-thalassemia decreases the

## CURRENT DIAGNOSIS

- Microcytic anemia (MCV <80 fL)
- Blood smear: hypochromia, microcytes, target cells, nucleated RBCs
- (Hemoglobin H inclusion bodies) in $\alpha$-thalassemia
- Quantitative hemoglobin electrophoresis
- $\alpha$-Thalassemia: Hb Bart's ($\gamma_4$) in cord blood or Hb H ($\beta_4$) in fresh (not stored) blood specimens
- $\beta$-Thalassemia: elevated Hb F ($\alpha_2\gamma_2$), Hb A$_2$ ($\alpha_2\delta_2$), or both
  - $\beta^{0o}$-Thalassemia: absence of Hb A ($\alpha_2\beta_2$)
  - $\beta$++-Thalassemia: decreased Hb A
- Hb E/$\beta$-thalassemia: Hb E and decreased or absent Hb A
- Molecular mutation analysis demonstrates two mutations in $\beta$-thalassemia major or thalassemia intermedia, and specific deletions in $\alpha$-thalassemia
- Normal iron levels

*Abbreviations:* MCV = mean cell volume; HB = hemoglobin; RBC = red blood cell.

---

net imbalance of $\alpha$-globin to $\beta$-globin. Thalassemia trait (inheritance of a single defective allele) is characterized by mild hypochromic, microcytic anemia and does not require treatment. Thalassemia intermedia causes moderate anemia with total hemoglobin levels of 6.0 to 10.0 g/dL. These patients require occasional transfusions with infections but do not require regular transfusions during childhood. Many thalassemia intermedia patients deteriorate later in life and develop similar complications as in thalassemia major.

## Diagnosis

The diagnosis of severe thalassemia is usually straightforward in ethnic groups at risk (Mediterranean, African, Asian, Middle Eastern, East Indian) but occurs in any group. Thalassemia major and intermedia are marked by severe microcytic anemia; hyperbilirubinemia, elevated lactate dehydrogenase levels, and splenomegaly appear in the first few years of life. Hemoglobin A is absent on hemoglobin electrophoresis in $\beta^o$-thalassemia and decreased in $\beta^+$-thalassemia. Hydrops fetalis ($\alpha$-thalassemia with classic four-gene deletions) presents as polyhydramnios and fetal distress during the second trimester. $\beta$-Thalassemia trait is characterized by mild anemia (hematocrit more than 30), low mean corpuscular volume (less than 75 fL), and erythrocytosis (red blood cell [RBC] count usually more than $5 \times 10^6$ per mm$^3$) with elevated hemoglobins A$_2$ ($\alpha_2\delta_2$) and/or F. $\alpha$-Thalassemia is most easily diagnosed by the presence of hemoglobin Bart's in cord blood. Hemoglobin H is unstable, and electrophoresis of fresh blood is required for its detection. Basophilic stippling, target cells, fragmented cells (schistocytes), and nucleated RBCs are typical of the severe thalassemias. The reticulocyte count may be relatively low because of ineffective erythropoiesis, and mean cell volume (MCV) may become high through skipped cell divisions. Prenatal diagnosis of thalassemia is performed by direct polymerase chain reaction (PCR) analysis of fetal DNA obtained by amniocentesis or chorionic villus sampling.

## Transfusion Therapy

In $\beta$-thalassemia major, RBC transfusion is the mainstay of supportive therapy. Transfusions should maintain a hemoglobin level ideally above 10.5 to 11 g/dL (range, 10.5 to 13 g/dL) to suppress endogenous erythropoiesis, with the least amount of transfused blood required. Regular transfusions are begun for a persistent hemoglobin level below 7 g/dL in children with two $\beta$-thalassemic mutations or with severe

## CURRENT THERAPY

**Thalassemia Major**

- Transfusions: 15 mL/kg PRBCs q3–4wk (to maintain total hemoglobin 10.5–13 g/dL)
- Splenectomy after 4–5 y of age, antibiotic prophylaxis
- Iron chelation: deferoxamine + deferiprone* + deferasirox†

---

*Orphan drug in the United States.
†FDA approved deferasirox in 2005.
*Abbreviation:* PRBC = packed red blood cell.

α-thalassemia diagnosed in utero. A complete genotype of the patient's RBCs should be performed before transfusions are begun, to facilitate identification of involved antigens in the event of isoimmunization. Transfusions of 15 mL/kg of packed RBCs should be given at 3- to 4-week intervals using compatible blood from a limited donor pool and filtered to remove white blood cells. Cytomegalovirus (CMV)-negative preparations should be used for transplantation candidates. Acetaminophen and diphenhydramine before transfusions prevent febrile reactions. Transfusion records should be meticulously maintained to assess mean pre- and posttransfusion hemoglobin levels and annual blood consumption. An increase in transfusion requirements suggests hypersplenism, isoimmunization, or an accessory spleen.

Transfusions can transmit infections, including hepatitis viruses, human immunodeficiency virus (HIV), CMV, and other pathogens. Hepatitis C develops in 30% to 90% of transfused patients and advances to cirrhosis in 85%. Patients should be vaccinated against hepatitis A and B and monitored for elevated transaminase levels and hepatitis C antibodies. Combined treatment with PEG interferon alfa-2a or -2b and ribavirin produces sustained responses in hepatitis C. HIV testing should be performed annually.

Partial exchange transfusion by erythrocytapheresis, in which older red blood cells are exchanged for fresh packed red cells by pheresis, reduces iron accumulation compared to simple transfusion with iron chelation. Partial exchange transfusion by erythrocytapheresis does expose patients to more units of packed RBCs, minor side effects related to citrate, and requires two large vascular catheters for each monthly procedure, which can be limiting.

### SPLENECTOMY

Splenectomy should be performed if a 40% or greater increase in the transfusion requirement occurs during a 1-year period, for a transfusion requirement greater than 200 mL/kg/year of packed RBCs without isoimmunization, or for thrombocytopenia. Splenectomy increases the risk of overwhelming sepsis with encapsulated organisms and *Yersinia* species, especially in young children, and, ideally, is deferred until children are 4 to 5 years of age. New infectious pathogens are a concern. Polyvalent pneumococcal vaccine should be given at least 1 month before splenectomy. Prophylactic oral Penicillin VK should be used in children younger than 10 years and for invasive (dental) procedures. Immediate medical attention should be sought and broad-spectrum antibiotics given emergently for significant fever (more than 38°C [101°F]) because patients are at risk for a fulminant course and death within hours.

### COMPLICATIONS OF TRANSFUSION THERAPY

Approximately 1 mg of iron per mL of packed RBCs is administered in packed RBC transfusions, with no mechanism for elimination. Iron deposition causes dysfunction in the heart, liver, and endocrine organs. Glucose intolerance with insulin-dependent diabetes mellitus, primary hypothyroidism, hypoparathyroidism, delayed puberty, amenorrhea, and osteopenia are common; arrhythmias are often precipitated by cardiac hemosiderosis and hypocalcemia secondary to hypoparathyroidism. Growth retardation may respond to growth hormone before age 13 years. Hepatic iron and hepatitis C lead to fibrosis and cirrhosis.

Cardiac dysfunction is detectable early by cardiovascular magnetic resonance and effective transverse relaxation time (T2*) measurements less than 20 milliseconds (ms) as well as reduced ejection fractions. Presenting symptoms are fatigue, arrhythmias, or pericarditis, advancing to congestive heart failure (CHF), and arrhythmias. Cardiac events are the major cause of death in transfused patients (60%). Other causes are infections (13%) and liver disease, notably hepatitis C complications including hepatocellular carcinoma (6%). Pulmonary hypertension develops in both transfused thalassemia major and untransfused intermedia patients with hemolysis; a tricuspid regurgitation (TR) jet velocity greater than 2 ms is associated with 25% mortality.

Osteopenia occurs in approximately 55% of thalassemia major and intermedia patients, may be severe and cause fractures, and even occurs in transfused patients in early childhood. Affected patients should be maintained on elemental calcium (1500 mg/day) and vitamin D (400 IU per day). Osteoporosis should be treated with bisphosphonates such as pamidronate (Aredia, 30 to 60 mg/month intravenous [IV]) or alendronate (Fosamax, 70 mg/week orally [PO]) and monitored with calcium, phosphate, 1,25-hydroxyvitamin D levels, 24-hour urinary calcium and hydroxyproline, and bone mineral density or dual-energy X-ray absorptiometry (DEXA) measurements annually.

### MONITORING AND TREATMENT OF IRON OVERLOAD (see Table 1)

Although the parenteral iron chelator deferoxamine mesylate (Desferal) was the only first-line iron chelator available for many years, compliance is difficult, and oral iron chelators are better tolerated. Recently, the oral chelator deferiprone (L1) was definitively shown to provide superior chelation of cardiac iron, and it eliminated all cardiac events in patients treated over 8 years. Another oral iron chelator, deferasirox, was approved by the Food and Drug Administration (FDA) in 2005. Deferoxamine can maintain negative iron balance relative to the transfusion burden when administered five to seven times per week as a continuous subcutaneous or IV infusion, or as twice-daily bolus subcutaneous (not intramuscular) injections of the same total dose. Urinary iron excretion is used to adjust the dosage to maintain negative iron balance with deferoxamine. Although deferoxamine has been the only iron chelator available, cardiac failure has been the leading cause of death in thalassemia in the United States. Cardiac failure was eliminated from patients treated with deferiprone (L1) in seven thalassemia centers in Italy. Deferiprone has improved cardiac function in asymptomatic patients with impaired myocardial function and cardiac siderosis.

Iron overload should be documented by a challenge test after 12 to 18 months of regular transfusions because children require iron for growth, and chelation is detrimental for non-iron-overloaded patients. To begin chelation, iron in a 24-hour urine sample after 500 mg of deferoxamine subcutaneously should exceed 1 mg, or the serum ferritin level should consistently exceed 1000 μg/mL. Small infusion pumps are used for deferoxamine (20 to 60 mg/kg/day subcutaneously for 8 to 12 hours per night for 5 to 7 days per week), and it should be infused particularly at the time of blood transfusions, when significant iron is released from older transfused blood cells. Irritation and local reactions can be prevented by increasing the diluent to 2 mL per 500 mg of deferoxamine, hydrocortisone (2 mg/mL), or with topical diphenhydramine. A topical anesthetic cream should be applied 30 to 60 minutes before insertion of the needle. IV administration through an indwelling port device is often more tolerable because such devices can be accessed once weekly without repeated needle sticks. IV chelation is more effective, so fewer treatment days may suffice.

Arrhythmias and congestive heart failure have been reversed with high-dose deferoxamine in some patients (15 mg/kg/hour maximum for 24 hours per day, 7 days per week); the most effective treatment for cardiac iron overload is the combination of deferiprone and deferoxamine. Anaphylactic reactions can be treated with desensitization;

## TABLE 1 Recommended Monitoring of Thalassemia Patients

| Monitoring of Patients Undergoing Regular Transfusions | Cardiac Monitoring After 5 Years of Transfusions | Monitoring of Endocrine and Osteoporosis | Monitoring of Effects of Deferoxamine Therapy |
|---|---|---|---|
| Red blood cell phenotype (before transfusions)<br>History, monthly physical examination<br>Pre- and post-transfusion CBC and record of amounts of each transfusion<br>Indirect antibody screen twice annually or with a positive Coombs test result on crossmatch<br>Liver function studies (ALT, AST, bilirubin, LDH, alkaline phosphatase, albumin, total protein, and ferritin q3mo)<br>Hepatitis A and B panels (before vaccine)<br>Hepatitis C antibody (mRNA by PCR if antibody positive) and HIV test annually<br>INR and PTT annually<br>Liver biopsy, after 5 y of transfusions or with hepatomegaly, to assess iron content and fibrosis<br>T2* and R2* MRI of hepatic and cardiac iron | Echocardiogram, ECG annually<br>T2* (cardiac MRI)<br>24-hour Holter or event monitor (for patients >12 y)<br>Cardiology consultation, stress test (for patients >18 y) | TSH, free $T_4$ parathormone, calcium, inorganic phosphorus, growth hormone levels annually<br>Glucose tolerance test, Cortrosyn stimulation test annually<br>Gonadotropins and estradiol or testosterone after 12 y of age<br>Bone mineral density test or DEXA, bone age annually<br>24-h urine calcium, creatinine, hydroxyproline annually<br>Serum calcium, phosphorus, alkaline phosphatase, 1,25-hydroxyvitamin D level twice annually | Ophthalmologic and hearing evaluation annually<br>Sitting and standing height, weight q4–6mo until 18 y of age<br>Zinc, copper, selenium, vitamin C, and vitamin E levels q4–6mo<br>Urinary iron excretion annually or biannually and dose adjustment |

*Abbreviations:* ALT = alanine aminotransferase; AST = aspartate aminotransferase; CBC = complete blood cell count; ECG = electrocardiogram; GGT = gamma-glutamyltransferase; HIV = human immunodeficiency virus; INR = international normalized ratio; LDH = lactate dehydrogenase; MRI = magnetic resonance imaging; PCR = polymerase chain reaction; PT = prothrombin time; PTT = partial thromboplastin time; TSH = thyroid-stimulating hormone.

idiosyncratic acute respiratory distress syndromes are rare but life-threatening, necessitating rapid recognition and intensive care. Excessive doses of deferoxamine can cause optic and acoustic neuritis, so ophthalmologic and hearing evaluations should be performed annually.

Iron overload causes depletion of vitamin C, which inhibits iron release from reticuloendothelial cells. Sudden availability of vitamin C can cause a massive release of iron and serious cardiotoxicity. Vitamin C (60 to 100 mg per day, to a maximum of 2 mg/kg/day PO) should be given only after the first cycle of deferoxamine in patients with reduced ascorbate levels. Despite deferoxamine therapy, 50% to 60% of transfused thalassemia patients have died of cardiac disease before 35 years of age.

New oral iron chelators offer major advantages. The oral chelator deferiprone (L1, Ferriprox,* 75 to 100 mg/kg/day PO) has been approved in 47 countries outside North America and can be obtained on an individual treatment investigational new drug (IND) basis through the FDA (at the time of this submission) and ideally will be approved in North America soon as a first-line iron chelator.

Deferiprone crosses cell membranes more readily than deferoxamine does and selectively chelates cardiac iron, improves cardiac function, and prevents cardiac events. An international trial demonstrated that deferiprone does not promote hepatic fibrosis.

Another oral chelator deferasirox (Exjade) has shown efficacy in reducing hepatic iron overload at doses of 20 to 30 mg/kg/day PO, taken once daily, and was recently approved in the United States.

The most promising approach to managing iron overload is combined use of two chelators to produce a shuttle effect, using a bi- or tridentate chelator, such as deferiprone* that crosses membranes to mobilize iron from tissue compartments into the bloodstream, to exchange with a hexadentate "sink" such as deferoxamine. Combined use of deferiprone (75 mg/kg/day for 4 days per week) followed by deferoxamine (2 weekend days) produced greater iron excretion and reduced hepatic damage compared to deferoxamine alone and was accepted by patients who refused deferoxamine for 5 to 6 days per week. Other chelators in trials include 40SD02 (S-Desferal[4]), deferoxamine attached to a starch polymer, which can be given once per week IV, and deferritin (GT56-252). Deferasirox, deferiprone,[4] GT56-252,[4] and HBED[4] should all be useful in combination with deferoxamine because individual patients may respond differently to select chelators.

Serial ferritin levels should be followed every 3 to 6 months but *not correlated directly with cardiac iron*. Liver biopsy is used to assess hepatic iron and fibrosis but does not correlate with *cardiac* iron burden. Magnetic resonance imaging is available in selected centers. Myocardial T2* relaxation measurements less than 20 ms indicate ventricular dysfunction and impending failure. R2* correlates inversely with hepatic iron burden. Regularly updated information on medical centers that perform noninvasive imaging, deferiprone (L1) FDA Individual Treatment Use program, and open clinical trials is provided by the Cooley's Anemia Foundation (800-522-7222 or www.cooleysanemia.org).

---

*Orphan drug in the United States.

---

*Orphan drug in the United States.
[4]Not yet approved for use in the United States.

## THALASSEMIA INTERMEDIA

Patients with β-thalassemia who do not develop debilitating anemia should usually not be committed to a lifelong transfusion regimen, particularly when the hemoglobin levels remain above 8 g/dL. These patients generally have good exercise tolerability and feel well unless there is significant facial deformity from marrow expansion or other serious complication. Most specialists avoid regular transfusions at hemoglobin levels above 7 g/dL, particularly when the blood supply predictably transmits hepatitis C.

*Intermittent* transfusions are often necessary with infections and pregnancy and with increasing age. Hypertransfusion can often be avoided by splenectomy. Patients should be monitored for marrow expansion, facial deformity, splenomegaly, growth retardation, endocrinopathies, and osteopenia. Pulmonary hypertension is a recently recognized risk, related to chronic hemolysis in untransfused patients. Tricuspid regurgitation (TR jet of greater than 2 ms) is associated with a 25% mortality, for which transfusions should be instituted. Anemia, particularly in patients with high baseline Hb F levels (more than 65%) and erythropoietin levels (more than 130 mU/mL), often responds to experimental therapies to stimulate fetal globin production. Patients with β+ thalassemia and baseline erythropoietin levels less than 130 mU/mL require erythropoietin and a fetal globin stimulant.

The hyperplastic marrow in thalassemia intermedia stimulates intestinal iron absorption, and eventually, iron overload and endocrine deficiencies occur as in thalassemia major, although more slowly. Cardiomyopathy does not typically develop in untransfused patients. Avoidance of iron-rich meats and regular consumption of tea can reduce iron absorption. Osteopenia occurs in 55% of major and intermedia patients. Hypercoagulability and thromboembolic events may occur particularly in splenectomized patients, with conditions predisposing to thrombosis such as postoperative bedrest. This tendency is likely related to thrombocytosis, abnormalities in levels of coagulation factors, red cell membrane abnormalities that contribute to hypercoagulability, and hepatic dysfunction. Folic acid and antioxidant supplements should be used supportively.

Spinal cord compression syndromes from thoracic or vertebral paraspinal bone marrow masses should be suspected with acute or increasing weakness, numbness, and diminished reflexes in the lower extremities, and it constitutes a medical emergency. Diagnosis is made by magnetic resonance imaging (MRI) or computed tomography (CT); radiation therapy and steroids should be instituted emergently.

## α-THALASSEMIA

The homozygous form of α-thalassemia is classically lethal in utero. Prenatal diagnosis and milder variants have enabled affected fetuses to be supported to term with intrauterine transfusions, followed by regular postnatal transfusions. For milder hemoglobin H disease, only folic acid, antioxidants, and monitoring for severe anemia during infections or with increasing splenomegaly are necessary. Because hemoglobin H is sensitive to oxidant stress, drugs such as sulfonamides should be avoided, particularly with coexistent glucose-6-phosphate dehydrogenase (G6PD) deficiency. Iron status should be monitored.

## TRANSPLANTATION

Allogeneic bone marrow or stem cell transplantation is curative by replacing the patient's hematopoietic stem cells with normal stem cells, which contain normal β-globin genes or one normal and one thalassemic globin gene. Transplantation from a histocompatibility leukocyte antigen (HLA)-identical related donor in patients younger than 8 years, without hepatic fibrosis, and good iron chelation (risk class 1) has an excellent prognosis. The overall mortality rate of transplantation in experienced centers is still approximately 15%, and significant morbidity can result from graft-versus-host disease (GVHD). Unrelated donors and cord blood as sources of donor cells have increased risks of GVHD and graft rejection but provide broader availability. Relapses (graft rejection) occur in 8% of patients receiving related donor transplants.

Because many patients do well clinically even with mixed chimeric states, less myeloablative preparative regimens are being evaluated in patients of higher risk classes to reduce morbidity. The serious risks of this curative treatment modality must be weighed against the lifelong burden of transfusion and chelation. This balance may be shifted with the approval of oral iron chelators.

## STIMULATION OF FETAL GLOBIN GENE SYNTHESIS AND ERYTHROPOIESIS

A large body of evidence shows that reactivating fetal globin to approximately 60% to 70% of α-globin chain synthesis ameliorates anemia in β-thalassemia enough to eliminate transfusion requirements. Chemotherapeutic agents (hydroxyurea and 5-azacytidine or decitabine), short chain fatty acid (SCFA) derivatives, and rHu erythropoietin (EPO) are being evaluated in clinical trials with the highest hematologic responses observed in patients with baseline (untransfused) Hb F levels greater than 50% and erythropoietin levels greater than 130 mU/mL. Combinations of these agents will likely be required to eliminate regular transfusion requirements in severe β-thalassemia patients. Nonmutagenic, noncytotoxic agents are preferable over chemotherapy for lifelong treatment. Sodium phenylbutyrate (Buphenyl*) and arginine butyrate* have increased total hemoglobin by 1 to 4 g/dL above baseline in untransfused patients but require large numbers of tablets or IV infusion, respectively. Patients with β+ thalassemia and baseline EPO levels less than 80 mU/mL have responded best to combined therapy with butyrate and EPO. The long-acting EPO preparation darbepoetin (Aranesp) increases hemoglobin in some. These therapies require supplementation with oral iron to be effective, even in the presence of elevated ferritin levels, because stored iron may not be available for erythropoiesis, and several months of treatment are often required. New oral SCFA derivatives under evaluation appear more tolerable.

# Gene Transfer

Gene therapy for β-thalassemia requires transfer of the fetal (γ) or a normal β-globin gene into repopulating hematopoietic stem cells and high-level expression of transferred genes with their regulatory elements, solely in erythrocytes. This transgene must be integrated at sites that allow high-level expression throughout life, a formidable challenge. Problems that must be surmounted include production of safe, effective vectors for long-term treatment, prevention of silencing of transduced genes, difficulty in transducing rare pluripotent repopulating stem cells, selective expansion of transduced stem cells, and ablative chemotherapy prior to infusion of transfected cells to create space for expansion of transduced stem cells. Progress is being made in all these areas. Clinical trials of gene therapy with limited endpoints, such as mobilization and harvesting of stem cells, are projected to begin in 2006–2007.

## REFERENCES

Aessopos A, Farmakis D, Deftereos S, et al: Thalassemia heart disease: A comparative evaluation of thalassemia major and thalassemia intermedia. Chest 2005;127:1523-1530.

Anderson LJ, Wonke B, Prescott E, et al: Comparison of effects of oral deferiprone and subcutaneous desferrioxamine on myocardial iron concentrations and ventricular function in beta-thalassaemia. Lancet 2002;360: 516-520.

Borgna-Pignatti C, Cappellini MD, DeStefano P, et al: Cardiac morbidity and mortality in deferoxamine- or deferiprone-treated patients with thalassemia major. Online first edition paper in Blood, December 22, 2005.

Cohen AR, Galanello R, Piga A, et al: Safety profile of the oral iron chelator deferiprone: A multicentre study. Br J Haematol 2000;108(2):305-312.

Cunningham MJ, Macklin EA, Neufeld EJ, Cohen AR: Complications of beta-thalassemia major in North America. Blood 2004;104:34-39.

Eldor A, Rachmilewitz EA: The hypercoagulable state in thalassemia. Blood 2002;99:36-43.

---

*Orphan drug in the United States.

Giardina PJ, Grady RW: Chelation therapy in beta-thalassemia: An optimistic update. Semin Hematol 2001;38:360-366.

Hershko C, Cappellini MD, Galanello R, et al: Purging iron from the heart. Br J Haematol 2004;125:545-551.

Pennell DJ, Berdoukas V, Karagiora M, et al: Randomized controlled trial of deferiprone or deferoxamine in beta thalassemia major patients with asymptomatic myocardial siderosis. Online first edition paper in Blood, December 13, 2005.

Piga A, Gaglioti C, Fogliacco E, Tricta F: Comparative effects of deferiprone and deferoxamine on survival and cardiac disease in patients with thalassemia major: A retrospective analysis. Haematologica 2003;88:489-496.

Schrier SL, Angelucci E: New strategies in the treatment of the thalassemias. Annu Rev Med 2005;56:157-171.

Voskaridou E, Terpos E, Spina G, et al: Pamidronate is an effective treatment for osteoporosis in patients with beta-thalassaemia. Br J Haematol 2003;123:730-737.

Wonke B: Clinical management of beta-thalassemia major. Semin Hematol 2001;38:350-359.

# Sickle Cell Disease

Method of

*Mark Layton, MD, and Antonio Almeida, MD*

Sickle cell disease (SCD) is one of the commonest inherited diseases worldwide, affecting mostly persons whose ancestors originated from sub-Saharan Africa, the Eastern Mediterranean basin, the Arabian Peninsula, and the Indian subcontinent. In some West African regions, the incidence of affected children is higher than 19 per 1000 live births. Population migration has resulted in a significant number of affected persons in other regions, especially in the Americas, where almost 1 in 1000 births are affected, concentrated mainly in urban areas. It is estimated that worldwide, 250,000 affected children are born every year.

The inheritance of SCD follows a classic autosomal recessive pattern. The molecular defect that gives rise to SCD is a point mutation in the β globin gene that results in a single amino acid substitution from valine to glutamic acid at position 6 of the β chain. Heterozygotes for this mutation are phenotypically normal, and homozygotes are affected. Compound heterozygotes for sickle/β-thalassemia and sickle/hemoglobin C also suffer from SCD.

The pathophysiology of SCD is a direct consequence of the physical properties of sickle hemoglobin (HbS). This molecule is less soluble than its normal counterpart and polymerizes when the red cell is deoxygenated or dehydrated, forming fibrils and deforming the cells to produce a characteristic sickle shape. This sickling process is initially reversible, but eventually the cells become permanently damaged and are removed from the circulation. Sickling of erythrocytes has two important pathophysiologic consequences:

- The life span of sickled erythrocytes is severely reduced to approximately 15 days, as compared with the normal red blood cell life span of 120 days.
- Erythrocytes deformed by sickling are more rigid and adherent than their normal counterparts and thus block vessels in the microvasculature, especially postcapillary venules, causing tissue ischemia. The mechanism for this process is multifactorial. There is mounting evidence that microvascular occlusion in SCD is also mediated by leukocyte-endothelial adhesion, platelet activation, increased thrombin formation, and damage to endothelial cells.

The multiple clinical manifestations of SCD reflect these two processes. There is, however, a marked heterogeneity in the clinical severity of this disease; a minority of patients are severely affected and incapacitated, and other patients remain relatively asymptomatic throughout life.

Several factors that modify clinical severity have been identified (Box 1). A high hemoglobin F (HbF) level, seen in persons with

**BOX 1 Factors that Predict Severity in Sickle Cell Disease**

- Low hemoglobin F
- High leukocyte count
- Frequent or early-onset painful episodes
- Hemoglobin <7g/dL
- Coinheritance of α-thalassemia

Senegal and Arab-India haplotypes, and the coinheritance of an α-thalassemia mutation have been shown to be protective and improve survival. Polymorphisms of genes associated with cell adhesion, thrombophilia, inflammation, and regulation of blood pressure, such as *VCAM1, MTHFR,* and *NOH1,* have also been associated with SCD clinical variation. Several observational studies have identified leukocytosis, anemia, and a high rate of painful crises as adverse risk factors, but the ability to predict global disease severity is still imperfect.

## Therapeutic Strategies in Sickle Cell Disease

### PREVENTIVE STRATEGIES

#### Screening

Antenatal and neonatal screening programs to detect SCD carriers and affected infants were initially targeted only at those considered to be at risk by virtue of ethnicity. However, issues raised by intermarriage, migration, and equality have led many authorities to abandon selective testing and extend hemoglobinopathy screening programs to the whole population. The purpose of antenatal screening is to offer couples genetic counseling and the opportunity to make informed reproductive decisions, although studies have demonstrated that the majority of at-risk couples decline prenatal diagnosis.

The detection of affected babies by neonatal screening has been shown to reduce mortality. Splenic infarction develops from infancy in SCD and places affected children at high risk for infection with encapsulated bacteria. Early diagnosis permits penicillin prophylaxis and vaccination to prevent pneumococcal sepsis and the education of parents to detect early signs of splenic sequestration and other SCD-related complications.

#### Infection

Hyposplenism due to repetitive vasoocclusive damage renders patients with SCD at greater risk for infection. Vaccination against *Streptococcus pneumoniae, Haemophilus influenzae, Neisseria meningitides,* and influenza in conjunction with prophylactic penicillin or, in those with hypersensitivity, erythromycin is advised to prevent overwhelming sepsis. This is particularly important in children, where fever is common and often not brought to medical attention promptly. Penicillin should be initiated from 3 months of age. Rigorous antimalarial chemoprophylaxis is recommended when visiting areas where malaria is endemic.

### SUPPORTIVE MEASURES DURING ACUTE COMPLICATIONS

#### Hydration, Oxygenation, and Treatment of Infections

Vasoocclusive episodes (crises) may be precipitated by infection, exposure to heat or cold, inadequate fluid intake, and adverse living conditions. Patients should be educated to avoid these factors where possible and seek medical attention early in the course of infection.

The mainstay of therapy for vasoocclusive complications is adequate hydration and oxygenation. Hydration with hypotonic solutions, such as 5% dextrose, can help to reverse erythrocyte dehydration, which favors polymerization of hemoglobin S. Oxygen therapy is often encouraged, although clear evidence of benefit in the absence of hypoxemia is lacking.

It is common practice to increase the dose of penicillin empirically during a crisis. In patients with a clear focus of infection, broad-spectrum antibiotic therapy is indicated.

### Pain Control

Skeletal pain, often intense, is the commonest clinical manifestation of SCD, and its effective control represents one of the greatest challenges in management. As for all pain control, the analgesia ladder should be followed, but in the acute stages, opiate analgesia is often the only effective therapy. In view of their effect on the renal vasculature, prolonged use of nonsteroidal anti-inflammatory agents (NSAIDs) should be avoided, but their judicious use can aid pain control.

Occasionally, weak opiates such as codeine suffice, but the majority of patients with acute painful episodes require potent opiates administered orally or parenterally for effective analgesia. Morphine or diamorphine (heroin)[2] are favored in all but those with true hypersensitivity or intolerance. These may be administered by continuous infusion. The doses required for adequate pain control vary depending on individual tolerance from 10μg/kg/hour to 100μg/kg/hour[3] (equivalent to 1-6 mg/h in an average adult), with intermittent boluses for breakthrough pain. Where there are no facilities for safe continuous infusion, intermittent bolus administration may be used, but this method of administration may be less effective in achieving pain control.

Meperidine (Demerol) should be avoided when at all possible due to the risk of seizures, particularly after prolonged use. In addition, its short half-life and immediate elating effects can contribute drug-seeking behavior encountered in a small minority of SCD patients.

It is essential that respiratory rate, oxygen saturation, and sedation level of patients receiving opiate analgesia are monitored carefully. Aperients, antiemetics, and antihistamines are helpful in reducing undesirable side effects and should be considered when opiates are initiated.

Chronic pain can develop from irreversible bone damage. Prolonged use of NSAIDs is not advisable, and many patients require oral opiates for its control.

In the context of pain control, cognitive behavior therapy has been shown to be effective in reducing rates of hospital admission. Intervention by psychology and pain management specialists can dramatically improve a patient's quality of life and represents an important element of the multidisciplinary model of care for SCD.

### TRANSFUSION

Red cell transfusion is widely used in the management of SCD in an effort to replace sickled erythrocytes with normal red blood cells and thus prevent progression or recurrence of complications. It is estimated that 50% of all patients have received a transfusion in their lifetime and 5% require a chronic transfusion program. Despite its hazards, transfusion plays a vital role in the treatment of acute life-threatening complications of SCD.

There are three main transfusion strategies: top-up transfusions, used mainly to correct anemia of varied etiology; isovolemic exchange transfusion, indicated for severe acute complications, long term-prevention of complications, and (more controversially) to terminate prolonged painful episodes; and hypertransfusion intended to suppress the endogenous production of red cells containing hemoglobin S to prevent long-term complications. The absolute and relative indications for these are detailed in Box 2. Preoperative transfusion is recommended for major orthopedic, abdominal, and chest surgery and for neurosurgery, but its role in other operations is less clear.

---

> ### BOX 2   Indications for Blood Transfusion in Sickle Cell Disease
>
> **Top-up**
> - Aplastic crisis
> - Sequestration syndromes
> - Exchange
> - Acute chest syndrome
> - Hepatic failure
> - Mesenteric syndrome*
> - Multiorgan failure
> - Priapism*
> - Stroke
>
> **Hypertransfusion or Chronic Exchange Program**
> - Chronic lung or cardiac disease
> - Leg ulcers*
> - Recurrent vasoocclusive crises
> - Stroke
>
> ---
>
> *Commonly used but of no proven value.

Preferably, isovolemic exchange transfusion should be performed by automated apheresis, but in the emergency setting, manual exchange transfusion, alternating phlebotomy with transfusion and intravenous fluids to maintain a hematocrit of around 0.30, is effective.

Although widely used, transfusion in SCD has a high rate of complications and should be undertaken only after due consideration. Apart from a similar rate of acute transfusion reactions to that seen in the general population, there is a higher rate of alloimmunization, most commonly against Kell, C, and E antigens, which can be reduced by phenotyping of the transfused cells to avoid sensitization. Blood should be selected from donors who are HbS negative. Occasionally, transfusion precipitates a hyperhemolytic crisis. This potentially life-threatening complication produces rapid and relentless hemolysis of both donor and recipient red cells. Treatment involves immune suppression with high-dose corticosteroids, intravenous immunoglobulin, and judicious transfusion of phenotype-identical red cell units.

Iron overload is the principal long-term complication of chronic transfusion, causing cardiac and hepatic damage and endocrinopathy. The rate of iron accumulation may be limited by exchange transfusion. Chelation with deferoxamine (Desmeral) is extremely burdensome and compliance is often suboptimal. Two oral iron chelators are currently available, deferiprone[2] and deferasirox (Exjade), of which the latter has been shown to be effective in SCD in reducing liver iron content in patients with hepatic siderosis.

### HYDROXYUREA

Hydroxyurea (Hydrea) inhibits vasoocclusion in SCD through a variety of mechanisms: the increased production of γ globin chains, and hence HbF, which reduces HbS polymerization; increased red cell deformability; downregulation of adhesion molecules, which limits cell-endothelium interactions; and reduction in leukocyte count. Its efficacy in preventing recurrence of acute chest syndrome and painful crises is well established, and these remain the only clear indications for the use of hydroxyurea in SCD. It has also been advocated for prevention of stroke, when other strategies, such as transfusion, are not viable. Patients generally achieve the greatest benefit at the maximum tolerated dose, namely, a dose just below that at which cytopenia is seen; blood counts, hemoglobin, and HbF levels should be monitored regularly. There is no evidence that long-term therapy is leukemogenic, but patients should be warned of the theoretical risk and advised strongly against conception while on hydroxyurea. A minority

---

[2]Not available in the United States.
[3]Exceeds dosage recommended by the manufacturer.

[2]Not available in the United States.

of patients fail to respond, and in such cases, therapy should be withdrawn after a trial of 6 months.

## BONE MARROW TRANSPLANTATION

Bone marrow transplantation (BMT) remains the only curative treatment for SCD, but only a small minority of patients are eligible (Box 3). Of patients receiving transplants, overall survival after 5 years is approximately 95%, with approximately 80% disease-free survival. The risks of BMT must be weighed carefully against the potential benefits on an individual basis.

# Manifestations Caused by Reduced Erythrocyte Survival and Increased Turnover

## ANEMIA

A hemoglobin concentration of 6 to 9 g/dL is found in virtually all patients with homozygous SCD or those with S/β-thalassemia. Patients with HbSC are generally less anemic and can have Hb values in the normal range. Like all clinical manifestations of SCD, there is a wide variability among patients, and it is essential to establish each individual patient's steady-state range to accurately interpret the cause of symptoms and avoid unnecessary therapeutic interventions. At steady-state concentrations, anemia is well tolerated and does not produce symptoms. This is explained by the metabolic adaption that accompanies chronic anemia and by the fact that sickle erythrocytes have a lower affinity for oxygen, which maintains adequate tissue oxygenation at lower hemoglobin concentrations.

As in all chronic hemolytic anemias, more nutrients are required for cell replication, particularly folic acid (folate). Supplementation should be encouraged to prevent megaloblastic anemia, especially in children and pregnant women.

## GALLSTONES

Jaundice, of varying degree, is a finding in most patients with SCD and results from the increased rate of heme catabolism. Consequently, there is a high prevalence of gallstones, up to 70% by adulthood. Early surgical intervention in symptomatic patients with biliary colic, cholecystitis, or obstruction is recommended to avert further complications. Coinheritance of Gilbert's syndrome is associated with an increased risk of cholelithiasis.

## APLASTIC CRISIS

The aplastic crisis is a specific complication that occurs in the context of acute infection with parvovirus B19. The infection is self-limited and lasts about 10 days, by which time the virus is eliminated in the presence of normal immunity. One of the main targets of infection is erythroblasts, in which a maturation arrest is observed for the duration of the infection. Given the shortened life span of sickle erythrocytes, even transient arrest in production can lead to profound anemia.

Patients present with anemia without conspicuous icterus, reticulocytopenia, and (not infrequently) vasoocclusive symptoms. In this context, transfusion is normally required. If the patient is febrile, antibiotics may be administered to cover bacterial infection. Patients with aplastic crises may be extremely unwell and develop secondary complications including acute chest syndrome and stroke. Some sources advocate high-dose steroids in such cases in an attempt to dampen the inflammatory response or intravenous immunoglobulin to accelerate viral clearance, but the effectiveness of these approaches is not established.

# Manifestations Caused by Vasoocclusion

## BONE DISEASE

Bone involvement (Box 4) is the commonest manifestation of SCD and takes the form of either acute painful (vasoocclusive) crises or pain due to chronic bone and joint damage, including avascular necrosis. Osteomyelitis can mimic pain syndromes caused by sickling and should always be considered in the differential diagnosis.

### Painful Crisis

Bone marrow infarction, leading to painful, or vasoocclusive, crisis, is the most common manifestation of SCD requiring hospital admission. Patients report intense localized pain and tenderness of acute onset and often precipitated by infection, dehydration, or exposure to cold. When infarction occurs at the epiphyses, reactive arthropathy, which can resemble septic arthritis, can occur. In infants, involvement of the hands or feet (dactylitis) is characteristic.

Treatment of these episodes is conservative, with hydration, adequate oxygenation, and usually opiate analgesia. Administration of opiates using patient-controlled analgesia devices is regarded by many as the preferred mode of delivery, failing which intermittent parenteral administration of opiates is in most cases effective. Acetaminophen (Tylenol) and NSAIDs may be useful adjuncts to opiates. Regular pulse oximetry recording and monitoring of respiratory rate and sedation score are mandatory during opiate administration. Thromboprophylaxis is recommended during periods of immobility. Vasoocclusive crises are generally self-limited, but exchange transfusion may be considered in protracted episodes.

### Dactylitis

In children younger than 7 years, infarction can occur in the phalanges of the hands and feet, which still contain bone marrow at that age.

The acute clinical scenario is painful swelling of one or more digits. Infarction in the epiphyses results in premature fusion, with shortening of the affected digit(s).

## Osteomyelitis

Increased susceptibility to infection, discussed later, coupled with recurrent bone marrow infarction predispose SCD patients to development of osteomyelitis with a prevalence of up to 12% in some studies. Diagnosis may be difficult and, despite advances in imaging techniques, it relies mainly on a low threshold of suspicion and clinical acumen. Staphylococcal species are, as in the general population, the most common organisms isolated, but there is a higher incidence of infection with intestinal flora such as *Salmonella, Enterobacter,* and *Escherichia coli.*

The choice of antibiotic depends on the results of microbial cultures, but for empiric treatment of suspected infection, combination therapy with a third-generation cephalosporin and ciprofloxacin (Cipro) is a rational choice. The duration of therapy depends on clinical response but is usually in the range of 6 weeks to 3 months. A septic abscess can form, requiring surgical drainage.

## Avascular Necrosis

Reported rates of avascular necrosis in SCD vary from 12% to 50%, although the true incidence is difficult to establish due to the significant proportion of silent disease. The most common areas to be affected are the femoral heads followed by the humeral heads. Bilateral disease is usual, as is disease in multiple sites.

When symptomatic, the affected joint is painful even at rest, and there are stiffness and limited range of movement. However, a large percentage of patients have asymptomatic disease. The early stages are radiologically silent and best detected using magnetic resonance imaging (MRI). Untreated, 87% of affected femoral heads collapse within 5 years.

Surgical treatment is almost always required. The only conservative method to prevent deterioration is absolute rest and avoidance of weight bearing, which is usually an unacceptable or unattainable option. Early disease might respond to coring and osteotomy but more advanced disease requires joint replacement. Surgery should be carried out in specialized centers by surgeons experienced in dealing with SCD patients because there are a high incidence of complications and a high failure rate.

## PULMONARY DISEASE

### Acute Chest Syndrome

Acute chest syndrome affects 50% of patients with SCD and is the commonest cause of death in adults. It is often preceded by a painful crisis. The pathogenesis is not yet fully defined, but a variety of possible precipitating factors, such as infection, bone marrow fat embolism, and atelectasis, especially following abdominal surgery, have been identified.

Clinically, acute chest syndrome should be suspected in the presence of fever, shortness of breath, and chest wall pain and tenderness. Tachypnea and hypoxemia are characteristic, often with bilateral signs on auscultation of the chest. Radiologically, new pulmonary infiltrates, often bilateral and involving multiple lobes, are seen. Increased hemolytic rate, with anemia and lactate dehydrogenase greater than steady-state levels and marked hypoxemia of arterial blood, support the diagnosis.

There is a characteristic rapid progression with worsening hypoxemia, sometimes within a few hours, which makes the recognition and treatment of acute chest syndrome a medical emergency.

In the differential, the main diagnoses to be considered are infection and pulmonary embolism. Due to the higher risk in SCD of infection and its role in the development of acute chest syndrome, broad-spectrum antibiotics are recommended. A suitable antibiotic combination based on the pattern of organisms isolated from patients with acute chest syndrome is a third-generation cephalosporin or β-lactam with a macrolide.

Overhydration can precipitate pulmonary edema, and close monitoring of fluid balance is vital. In less severe forms, simple oxygen administration may suffice to maintain normoxemia, failing which escalating respiratory support with PEEP (positive end-expiratory pressure), CPAP (continuous positive airway pressure), or mechanical ventilation may be required. Extracorporeal membrane oxygenation has been used successfully for severe acute chest syndrome refractory to mechanical ventilation. Chest pain contributes to impaired ventilation, and adequate pain control to alleviate this is important. Opiate-induced narcosis must, however, be avoided.

The main strategy in the treatment of acute chest syndrome is transfusion. The aim is to reduce HbS levels to less than 20%. Severely anemic patients may receive simple transfusion, but most require exchange transfusion. Delay must be avoided because of the risk of progressive respiratory failure and death associated with acute chest syndrome. Transfusion often results in a rapid improvement in clinical status and averts a potentially fatal outcome.

Recurrent acute chest syndrome occurs in 80% of those who have had a previous episode. In patients with frequent, severe life-threatening crises, regular transfusion, either simple or exchange, has been used to prevent recurrence. The Multicenter Study of Hydroxyurea in Sickle Cell Anemia showed a 50% reduction in acute chest syndrome in the treatment group, and this is now the recommended therapy to reduce the risk of acute chest syndrome. Although the efficacy of this approach in SCD is well documented, it suffers several detractions, namely, problems of venous access, transfusion hazards, and iron overload.

### Chronic Lung Disease

Chronic pulmonary damage is a common complication in patients with SCD. Pulmonary fibrosis is not unusual in those who have suffered recurrent acute chest syndrome. However, pulmonary hypertension is emerging as a major cause of morbidity and mortality. Its pathogenesis is complex and involves multiple mechanisms that include thromboembolism, asplenia, depletion of nitric oxide due to scavenging by free hemoglobin released through intravascular hemolysis, chronic hypoxia, and vasoocclusion in the pulmonary vasculature. Its diagnosis is challenging because the main symptom is breathlessness on exertion, which may be attributed to chronic anemia. More severe symptoms and signs of right-sided heart failure are uncommon and generally only seen in very advanced disease.

Patients tend to be older, with evidence of increased hemolysis, renal and hepatic dysfunction, and greater lifetime transfusion requirement. Those in whom pulmonary hypertension is suspected are best assessed with the 6-minute walk distance test. A firm diagnosis requires establishment of high pulmonary pressures either by echocardiographic measurement of tricuspid valve regurgitant jet velocity (TRV) or by cardiac catheterization. In pulmonary hypertension associated with SCD, TRV greater than 2.5 m/sec are common, and mean pulmonary arterial pressures tend to be moderately elevated at 30 to 40 mm Hg, with elevated capillary wedge pressures. High pressures correlate with reduced distances in the 6-minute walk test. Lung function tests reveal airway obstruction, restrictive lung disease, and hypoxemia.

Pulmonary hypertension is associated with increased morbidity and mortality and should be sought and treated aggressively. Patients who on screening are found to have TRV greater than 2.5 m/sec should be investigated for other causes of pulmonary hypertension, such as thromboembolism, left ventricular dysfunction, and chronic or nocturnal hypoxemia. Intensification of SCD-specific therapy, in the form of a transfusion program or hydroxyurea, should be considered. Specific vasoactive agents, such as sildenafil (Viagra), prostaglandins, and inhaled nitric oxide, are currently under study.

## CEREBROVASCULAR DISEASE

Stroke is a life-threatening complication in SCD, affecting children more commonly than adults. It is estimated that approximately 300 in 100,000 children with SCD have clinically evident cerebrovascular accidents, but as many as 50% of patients suffer silent brain injury.

This latter group can, in the absence of overt stroke, have measurable neurocognitive impairments and an increased risk of further neurologic progression.

There are few reliable clinical features that predict the occurrence of stroke, although a low pain rate, hypertension, previous seizures, and increased leukocyte count are all associated with higher incidence of stroke. The STOP (Stroke Prevention Trial in Sickle Cell Anemia) study in children with SCD established that an elevated middle cerebral artery flow velocity determined by transcranial Doppler (TCD) predicted future development of overt stroke and the presence of silent cerebral infarcts.

The main cause of infarcts in SCD is stenosis and subsequently occlusion of large to medium-sized cerebral arteries, manifest at an early stage by increased arterial flow velocity. A fragile collateral circulation often develops, which can take the form of moyamoya, and predisposes to later hemorrhagic stroke.

Acute stroke must be treated as an emergency and immediate isovolemic red blood cell exchange transfusion should be carried out, followed by maintenance hypertransfusion or exchange transfusions aiming at maintaining the HbS below 30%. Without such therapy, 70% of children suffer recurrent events. The STOP study also showed the benefit of screening children with TCD: Initiating a prophylactic transfusion program in those with increased flow velocities greatly reduced the incidence of stroke.

The optimal duration of transfusion has not been established, and even after many years up to 50% of patients suffer a further stroke within months of discontinuing transfusion. There is no evidence yet that any other therapy, including hydroxyurea, is as effective as transfusion in preventing stroke.

## SEQUESTRATION SYNDROMES

Sequestration occurs as a result of occlusion of the venous outflow from the liver and spleen. Splenic sequestration occurs predominantly in early childhood and manifests with left upper quadrant pain, anemia, and, if unrecognized, hypovolemic collapse due to sequestration of a large percentage of the blood volume. Therefore, parents should be familiar with the symptoms of splenic sequestration and taught splenic palpation so that prompt medical care can be sought when sequestration is at an early stage. Treatment involves transfusion and maintenance of the intravascular volume. It is controversial whether splenectomy is beneficial after a single episode, but most advocate it following two episodes.

Hepatic sequestration is less common. It manifests with painful hepatic enlargement and elevation of liver enzymes. Treatment is conservative, with fluids and analgesia, but hepatic failure can occur. The value of exchange transfusion in this setting is debatable and is generally reserved for severe cases.

## SICKLE NEPHROPATHY

Virtually all patients with SCD develop hyposthenuria at a young age due to distal tubular impairment secondary to sickling. This increases the likelihood of dehydration and is also responsible for the increased incidence of enuresis among children with SCD. There is no specific therapy, but maintenance of an adequate fluid intake should be emphasized.

Renal papillary necrosis can occur at any age and usually manifests with hematuria and occasionally with colic due to ureteric obstruction by necrotic papillae. Aggressive hydration and analgesia generally suffice as therapy in these cases.

The most worrying renal manifestation of SCD is glomerulonephropathy. This is usually heralded by proteinuria and microscopic hematuria, and glomerular filtration should be formally measured. Angiotensin-converting enzyme (ACE) inhibitors can reduce the rate of progression and should be considered given the significant risk of progression to end-stage renal failure. Treatment of renal failure in SCD does not differ from that in other patients. The lack of endogenous erythropoietin coupled with more frequent transfusions can attenuate painful episodes. Recombinant erythropoietin replacement should be monitored closely to prevent an excessive rise in hematocrit, which can lead to increased vasoocclusive symptoms.

## RETINOPATHY

Ocular complications are common, affecting approximately 20% of patients. These typically resemble diabetic retinopathy, with thinning of the retina and neovascularization. Laser photocoagulation may be required to prevent retinal hemorrhage. Although the role of preemptive intervention is disputed, most experts recommend full ophthalmologic screening be undertaken on a regular basis.

## PRIAPISM

Priapism is due to obstruction of the venous outflow from the penis, resulting in painful sustained erection. The sensitive nature of the problem often leads to underreporting, but it is estimated that 90% of male patients with SCD have at least one episode by the age of 21. Prolonged episodes can lead to permanent impairment of erectile function and should be treated urgently. Surgical drainage and irrigation of the corpora cavernosa and exchange transfusion are most often used to reverse priapism acutely. Most commonly, patients suffer from self-limited or stuttering priapism, which is nevertheless very disruptive. These episodes are generally associated with nocturnal erections. In some cases, simple measures such as emptying the bladder, exercise, a hot bath or shower, and analgesia are sufficient to terminate an attack. Failing this, treatment with vasodilators such as pseudoephedrine (Sudafed) or etilnefrine hydrochloride[1] and, for persistent recurrence, the antiandrogen cipoterone acetate[1] might prove effective in prevention. Recent reports suggest sildenafil is effective in some cases.

## LEG ULCERS

Leg ulcers are a common complication, affecting approximately 10% of patients. They can occur after trauma or spontaneously and are often recurrent, painful, and slow to heal. Several treatment options have been explored with varying rates of success, including topical dressings, compression stockings, zinc supplementation, blood transfusion, hydroxyurea,[2] and topical granulocyte-macrophage colony-stimulating factor (GM-CSF).[2] Hydroxyurea should be used with caution because it has been implicated as a cause of skin ulceration. Clearance of secondary infection is essential to allow the ulcers to heal.

# Novel Therapies in Sickle Cell Disease

In addition to hydroxyurea, other agents have been used to stimulate the production of HbF in SCD. Decitabine (Decogen), a hypomethylating agent, has been shown in preliminary studies to increase HbF production in hemoglobinopathies, and clinical trials are in progress. Histone deacetylase inhibitors, such as butyrate derivatives, show promise by the same mechanism of action.

Reduction of red cell dehydration is another potential therapeutic target. Possible beneficial agents under study include magnesium supplementation, which inhibits the $K^+/Cl^-$ cotransport, and inhibitors of the Gardos channel.

Several agents have been shown to reduce cell adhesion in vitro and might hold clinical promise. Among these is nitric oxide (NO) which, in addition to being a potent vasodilator, inhibits adhesive interactions between blood cells and the endothelium.

As the genetic basis of disease severity is unraveled, more specific targeted therapies for SCD are likely to emerge.

## REFERENCES

Amrolia PJ, Almeida A, Davies SC, Roberts IA: Therapeutic Challenges in childhood sickle cell disease. Part 2: A problem-orientated approach. Br J Haematol 2005;120(5):737-743.

---

[1]Not available in the United States.
[2]Not FDA approved for this indication.

Amrolia PJ, Almeida A, Halsey C, et al: Therapeutic challenges in childhood sickle cell disease. Part 1: Current and future treatment options. Br J Haematol 2003;120(5):725-736.

Charache S, Terrin ML, Moore RD, et al: Effect of hydroxyurea on the frequency of painful crises in sickle cell anemia. Investigators of the Multicenter Study of Hydroxyurea in Sickle Cell Anemia. N Engl J Med 1995;332(20): 1317-1322.

Embury SH: New treatments of sickle cell disease. West J Med 1996;164(5):444.

# Neutropenia

Method of
*Melvin H. Freedman, MD*

An absolute neutrophil count (ANC) is equal to the total white blood cell count per microliter multiplied by the combined percentage of neutrophils and bands. Neutropenia is defined as an ANC below two standard deviations of the normal mean. Normal neutrophil levels can be stratified for age and race. For whites beyond infancy, the lower limit for normal neutrophil counts is 1500/μL. Blacks have somewhat lower neutrophil counts; the lower limit of normal is approximately 1200/μL. Individual patients may be characterized as having mild neutropenia with cell counts of 1000 to 1500/μL, moderate neutropenia with cell counts of 500 to 1000/μL, or severe neutropenia with cell counts less than 500/μL. This stratification is useful for predicting risk because patients with severe neutropenia have increased susceptibility to life-threatening infections.

## Classification

Table 1 is a classification for formulating an informative clinical and laboratory assessment that leads to a specific diagnosis of neutropenia. There are some general points to consider when using this table. Unlike anemia and thrombocytopenia, which can be categorized as being caused by decreased production or increased destruction using marrow morphology and specific laboratory indicators, neutropenia is much more complex to define kinetically and laboratory testing is not as refined. Thus, for practical reasons, the classification in Table 1 is based on the *cellular basis* for neutropenia: either an acquired extracellular cause or a congenital, inherited, or intracellular cause.

Many of the diagnoses are age related. Most of the congenital or inherited diagnoses are detected early in infancy or childhood. In adolescence and adulthood, most of the disorders are acquired, but there is obviously some overlap. Some neutropenic conditions are common, others are rare. Viral-induced marrow suppression is the most common cause of childhood neutropenia, whereas congenital or inherited disorders are very rare. Drug-induced, autoimmune, and nutritional deficiency neutropenias are encountered more frequently in adult patients. There is also a clinical distinction between acute-onset and severe chronic neutropenia. Acute neutropenia can develop if neutrophils are used rapidly when marrow production is impaired.

Drugs used for chemotherapy are particularly likely to induce neutropenia because of their cytotoxic effect on the high proliferative rate of neutrophil precursors and the relatively short half-life of blood neutrophils. Other nonchemotherapeutic drugs can induce severe neutropenia by idiosyncratic or hypersensitivity reactions. These drugs include analgesics, antipsychotic agents, anticonvulsants, antithyroid drugs, cardiovascular drugs, the sulfas, and antibiotics.

*Severe chronic neutropenia* is a general term that describes ANCs less than 500/μL on serial testing for at least 3 months. Because neutrophils are crucial in protecting the body against invasion by bacteria, severe chronic neutropenia regularly predisposes a patient to pyogenic infections. Chronic neutropenia is caused by a variety of hematologic disorders as well as immunologic, metabolic, and infectious diseases. Congenital neutropenia, cyclic neutropenia, and idiopathic neutropenia are three major diagnostic categories of severe chronic neutropenia that respond to granulocyte colony-stimulating factor (G-CSF) therapy (see later).

Some neutropenias are serious with overt symptomatology, whereas others are clinically silent and are discovered in the context of a routine medical examination. Most severe forms of neutropenia ultimately present with one or more of the following: fever of unknown origin (so-called fever neutropenia), chronic oropharyngeal ulcers, gingivitis, periodontal disease, bacterial or fungal septicemia, cellulitis of the skin or perirectal area, abscesses despite the absence of true pus, and other life-threatening infections.

## Clinical and Laboratory Evaluation

A complete medical history is an essential first step. Key historical information about previous blood cell counts may require some detective work. These counts are routinely performed in other physicians' offices for evaluation of other medical problems. This information can provide immediate confirmation that an episode of neutropenia is acquired or of recent onset. By using Table 1, other useful historical data can be generated. A detailed evaluation of infections is needed to determine the type, severity, duration, and recurrences, as well as the age at onset of symptoms to document whether the disorder is congenital or acquired. Antecedent viral infection should be noted; this is by far the most common explanation for neutropenia in young children. Medication usage, including that of nonprescription drugs, should be elicited. Symptoms of other systemic disorders such as autoimmune disease or chronic liver dysfunction that could produce splenomegaly

**TABLE 1  Classification of Neutropenia**

**Acquired or Extracellular Causes**
Viral-induced marrow suppression
Nonviral infection or sepsis
Drug induced:
 Chemotherapy
 Other drugs
Immune mediated:
 Autoimmune disease at all ages
 Neonatal isoimmune
Neonatal neutropenia/maternal hypertension
Neonatal neutropenia/organic acid disorders
Hypersplenism
Nutritional deficiencies (vitamin $B_{12}$, folate, copper)
Pure white cell aplasia
Idiopathic neutropenia

**Congenital, Inherited, or Intracellular Causes**
Congenital neutropenia (agranulocytosis)/Kostmann's syndrome
Cyclic neutropenia
Autosomal dominant familial neutropenia
Dysgamma-/agammaglobulinemia, cellular immunodeficiency syndromes
Shwachman-Diamond syndrome
Glycogen storage disease type 1b
Barth syndrome

**Other Causes**
Fanconi anemia
Myelokathexis
Lazy leukocyte syndrome
Reticular dysgenesis
Cartilage-hair hypoplasia
Dyskeratosis congenita
Pseudo-neutropenia

## CURRENT DIAGNOSIS

- Confirm a sustained ANC below lower limit of normal by serial testing.
- Establish cause by history, physical examination, and laboratory testing in context of *extracellular* versus *intracellular* etiologies (see Table 1).
- Severe chronic neutropenia (ANC <500/µL for >3 mo) requires urgent investigation and close supervision.

*Abbreviation:* ANC = absolute neutrophil count.

## CURRENT THERAPY

- Fever of >38.5°C (101.3°F) with an ANC < 500/µL is a medical emergency and requires immediate blood and urine cultures and stat IV antibiotics based on the following considerations (see text):
  - Start an IV line; give standard fluids at 1.5 times maintenance.
  - If taking medications, stop them.
  - Consider past history of antibiotic resistance of previously cultured organisms.
  - Consider patient's clinical stability or instability or shock.
  - Determine if a significant β-lactam allergy exists or not.
  - Choose appropriate antibiotic combinations based on above.
  - Give IV G-CSF, 5–10 µg/kg (maximum dose, 300 µg)[3] once daily.

[3]Exceeds dosage recommended by the manufacturer.
*Abbreviations:* ANC, absolute neutrophil count; G-CSF = granulocyte colony-stimulating factor; IV = intravenous.

must also be reviewed. The nutritional history should include symptomatology of vitamin $B_{12}$ or folic acid deficiency.

For infants and children with neutropenia, the historical questions are more specific. In neonatal neutropenia, failure to thrive is suggestive of a metabolic disorder. A maternal history of hypertension is an important explanation for neonatal neutropenia. Similarly, in neonates, a family history of previously affected siblings but with non-neutropenic parents suggests an autosomal recessive inheritance pattern as seen in some Kostmann's syndrome patients, some immune deficiency disorders, Shwachman-Diamond syndrome, glycogen storage disease type 1b, and metabolic disorders. A history of a parent with neutropenia with one or more affected offspring implies an autosomal dominant mode of transmission as seen in one form of cyclic neutropenia and in a type of noncyclic severe chronic neutropenia. This history for classic cyclic neutropenia is that of mouth ulcers, periodontal complaints, cervical lymphadenopathy, fever, malaise, or infections every 21 days.

The physical examination is directed to sites of current or recent infections, especially the oral cavity, skin, perineum, and perirectal area. In adults, the focus should also be on signs of nutritional deficiency, collagen vascular disease, and splenomegaly, as well as pallor, bruises, or petechiae, which suggest a more generalized marrow disorder because of replacement or a myelodysplastic syndrome. In infants and children, particular attention is paid to growth and developmental parameters. A detailed evaluation is also performed for the presence of phenotypic abnormalities and skeletal anomalies, which are seen in Fanconi anemia, in Shwachman-Diamond syndrome, and in some of the other disorders listed in Table 1.

In infants and young children, the workup also includes blood cell counts on parents and siblings to unmask an inherited cause; testing for antineutrophil antibodies to diagnose autoimmune neutropenia of infancy; serologic studies for collagen vascular disorders; immunoglobulin quantitation and cellular immunity screening for diagnosis of an immunodeficiency syndrome; serial blood cell counts two to three times a week for 4 to 8 weeks to determine a predictable cyclic pattern; bone marrow aspiration and biopsy for diagnostic morphology coupled with cytogenetic studies on marrow cells to exclude a malignant clonal change; and a polymerase chain reaction molecular analysis of the cells for Epstein-Barr virus, cytomegalovirus, and herpes simplex virus. The marrow morphology can be very specific in diagnosing congenital neutropenia/Kostmann's syndrome (maturation arrest at the myelocyte stage) and myelokathexis (myeloid hypercellularity with degenerative, pyknotic granulocytes).

Specific syndromes listed in Table 1 such as Shwachman-Diamond syndrome, glycogen storage disease type 1b, neutropenia associated with metabolic disorders, and Fanconi anemia require highly specialized diagnostic testing at a subspecialty center. Many of the investigations for infants and younger children are also pertinent for older children and adults. Additional testing for older patients, however, should include determination of serum copper, serum vitamin $B_{12}$, and red blood cell folate levels; an HIV detection study in the appropriate clinical setting; and, if hypersplenism is present, imaging and other diagnostic testing to determine the cause.

## Therapy

### GENERAL MEASURES

Management depends on the degree of the neutropenia, its etiology, and the patient's previous history of infections. In healthy-appearing asymptomatic adults and older children with isolated neutropenia and cell counts greater than 750/µL, clinical observation only without further diagnostic study may be warranted. Medications that may account for the neutropenia should be stopped, if possible. Serial blood cell counts can determine if the neutropenia is transient or persistent. If it persists longer than 4 to 8 weeks, additional workup is needed. If anemia or thrombocytopenia is present at any time, however, bone marrow aspiration or biopsy is the next diagnostic test. Infants, younger children, and patients of all ages with a history of chronic, recurrent, or severe infection with neutrophil counts less than 750/µL, especially less than 500/µL, require further diagnostic testing and a decision about medical intervention.

General preventive measures should include good hand washing, meticulous skin care, and good oral hygiene with regular dental check-ups and professional cleaning. For neutropenic mouth ulcers, a "magic mouthwash" can be prepared by a pharmacist containing equal parts of 2% viscous lidocaine (Xylocaine) and diphenhydramine (Benadryl) in normal saline. A peroxide-based mouthwash can also be used for oral hygiene. Rectal examinations and rectal temperature taking, as well as suppositories and enemas, should be avoided if possible.

Patients who are neutropenic but with ANCs greater than 1000/µL generally exhibit normal defense against infection and can be regarded in the same manner as non-neutropenic patients. For patients with ANCs greater than 500/µL but less than 1000/µL who have recurrent infections, preventive medical therapy is an option. Before the cytokine era, prophylactic antibiotics were sometimes used. The most popular agents were the penicillins and trimethoprim-sulfamethoxazole (Bactrim, Septra). These antibiotics may be effective in diminishing the frequency of infections and can be tried, but there may be significant problems associated with their continuous use. These include gastrointestinal complaints, "selection," and then overgrowth of antibiotic-resistant organisms and allergic reactions.

Patients whose ANC is less than 500/µL are at serious risk of bacterial infection, particularly from pathogens such as *Staphylococcus aureus* and gram-negative organisms. These are often of endogenous origin in the neutropenic host. The onset of fever of greater than 38.5°C (101.3°F) in these patients should be regarded as a medical emergency. By virtue of the low neutrophil counts, they may have few signs of inflammation but they must be hospitalized and empirically treated with antibiotics while awaiting culture results. In my clinic and emergency department, we immediately activate a treatment protocol before admission to avoid any delay in antibiotic therapy. The protocol was developed in our institution for management of patients on chemotherapy who develop fever-neutropenia, but it is equally suitable for any patient with a neutrophil count of less than 500/μL.

## EMERGENCY DEPARTMENT MANAGEMENT

Stop all medications. Start an intravenous (IV) line and give standard fluids at 1.5 times maintenance. Order a chest film, a serum creatinine study, a urinalysis, and obtain cultures of blood and urine and from any apparent focus of infection. When selecting antibiotics, always consider the patient's past history regarding antibiotic resistance of previously cultured organisms as well as the patient's clinical stability. Standard initial antibiotics for the stable patient as described later may not be appropriate for a patient who has had previous serious infection from an antibiotic-resistant organism.

Administer the following antibiotics stat (i.e., they should be given before patient transfer from a clinic or emergency department to a hospital ward and before administration of any blood product):

*For stable patients with no significant beta-lactam allergy, give:*

- Piperacillin-tazobactam (Tazocin): children: 80 mg piperacillin/kg IV every 8 hours; adolescents and adults: maximum dose, 4 g IV every 8 hours
- Gentamicin: children younger than 9 years, 10 mg/kg IV every 24 hours; from 9 to younger than 12 years, 8 mg/kg IV every 24 hours; 12 years or older, 6 mg/kg IV every 24 hours; adults, 1 to 2 mg/kg IV every 8 hours or 4 to 6 mg/kg IV every 24 hours

*If a significant β-lactam allergy exists, give:*

- Ciprofloxacin (Cipro): children, 10 mg/kg IV every 12 hours; adults, 400 mg IV every 12 hours
- Clindamycin (Cleocin): children, 10 mg/kg IV every 8 hours; adults, 600 mg IV every 8 hours
- Gentamicin: dose as above

*If the patient is unstable or in septic shock with no significant beta-lactam allergy, give:*

- Meropenem (Merrem IV): children, 20 mg/kg IV every 8 hours; adults, 1 g IV every 8 hours
- Vancomycin (Vancocin): children, 15 mg/kg IV every 6 hours; adults, 1 g IV every 6 hours
- Gentamicin, dose as above

*If a significant β-lactam allergy exists, give*

- Ciprofloxacin: dose as above
- Vancomycin: dose as above
- Amikacin (Amikin): children, 20 mg/kg[3] IV every 24 hours; adults, 500 mg IV every 12 hours.

## MANAGEMENT AFTER ADMISSION

Vital signs are measured hourly until the patient's condition stabilizes and then every 4 hours or as indicated. If blood cultures are subsequently positive, repeat cultures should be drawn when this result becomes known. Antibiotics specifically directed toward the identified organism should be added to the broad-spectrum therapy if the initial antibiotics do not provide adequate coverage. Broad-spectrum coverage must not be replaced by specific, narrow-coverage antibiotics alone in the neutropenic patient.

[3]Exceeds dosage recommended by the manufacturer.

For patients who become afebrile, with an ANC of greater than 500/μL and with negative cultures, antibiotics can be stopped. For patients who become afebrile and with negative cultures but with neutrophils less than 500/μL, antibiotics can usually be stopped after 48 hours of therapy.

Patients who are persistently febrile but stable should continue to receive the initial empirical antibiotic regimen as described. If the patient's condition indicates an evolving infection at a particular site (e.g., abdominal pain, severe mucositis, pneumonia), antibiotics directed toward possible causative organisms should be added to the broad-spectrum coverage. After 5 to 7 days of persistent fever, consider the addition of amphotericin (Amphocin): for children, 1 mg/kg once a day IV, or, if older than 2 years, caspofungin (Cancidas), 50 mg/m² once a day IV. For adults, give amphotericin, 3 to 4 mg/kg once a day IV, or caspofungin, 70 mg IV once on day 1 followed by 50 mg IV once a day thereafter.

## SPECIFIC AND GROWTH FACTOR TREATMENT

Referring to Table 1, there are several diagnoses of acquired neutropenia that respond to specific treatment. Excluding chemotherapy-induced neutropenia, when a drug is suspected as causing the problem, the product should be stopped and general supportive measures instituted. If neutropenia is severe, administration of growth factor (cytokine therapy) should be started (see later). Autoimmune neutropenia of infancy occurring in the first 3 years of life is clinically benign and self-limited, but the spontaneous resolution may take months to years. No therapy is needed unless a bacterial infection ensues, at which point cytokine therapy is initiated in combination with antibiotics.

Treatment of chronic autoimmune neutropenia in older children and adults is usually supportive if the neutropenia is an isolated manifestation. Cytokine therapy and antibiotics should be used, however, if infection is a problem. A more generalized multisystem autoimmune disorder usually requires specialized management, conventionally starting with corticosteroids. One of these disorders, Felty's syndrome (rheumatoid arthritis, splenomegaly, and neutropenia), is managed with options ranging from splenectomy, antirheumatic therapy, immunosuppression, plasmapheresis, IV immunoglobulin (IVIG), and cytokine therapy.

Isoimmune neonatal neutropenia is the neutrophil equivalent of Rh hemolytic disease of the newborn and lasts an average of 7 weeks postnatally. Therapy is supportive with antibiotics as necessary, but in life-threatening infections, plasma exchange to remove antineutrophil antibodies, transfusion of maternal neutrophils that lack the immunogenetic antigen, IV immunoglobulin, and cytokine therapy can be used individually or in combination. In neutropenic neonates born to mothers with pregnancy-induced hypertension, the condition is characteristically limited to the first 72 hours of life and seldom requires treatment.

"Hypersplenic" neutropenia is seldom severe enough to cause serious infection. Therapy should be directed at correcting the underlying cause of splenomegaly if possible. Splenectomy is a last resort. Replacement therapy for nutritional deficiencies of vitamin $B_{12}$ and folic acid specifically and promptly correct the associated neutropenia. Pure white cell aplasia, in which the bone marrow morphology shows absence of myeloid precursors, occurs in most cases with a thymoma and occasionally with ibuprofen therapy. Thymectomy may be effective in the former situation but usually also requires immunosuppression and/or IV immunoglobulins. With ibuprofen-induced neutropenia, stopping the drug corrects the problem.

For many of the congenital or inherited neutropenias, cytokine therapy is extremely effective in reversing the abnormal hematology. Severe chronic neutropenia was targeted in 1987 for clinical trials with G-CSF (filgrastim [Neupogen]), and more than 95% of patients with congenital, cyclic, and idiopathic forms of neutropenia responded completely. Based on data compiled by the Severe Chronic Neutropenia International Registry (University of Washington, Seattle), G-CSF is now considered the standard first-line treatment for these conditions. A second product, granulocyte-macrophage colony-stimulating factor (GM-CSF, sargramostim [Leukine]), is second-line therapy for severe chronic neutropenia in North America because of less predictable neutrophilic responses. For adults on chemotherapy for nonmyeloid malignancies, pegfilgrastim (Neulasta) can be used to offset severe neutropenia. The product is a long-lasting form of G-CSF that is indicated to decrease the incidence of infection in patients receiving marrow-suppressive antineoplastic agents (see later).

For patients with a neutrophil count of less than 500/μL with congenital neutropenia (encompassing Kostmann's syndrome, Shwachman-Diamond syndrome, glycogen storage disease type 1b, and Fanconi anemia), and for the cyclic and idiopathic forms, G-CSF is started at 5 μg/kg/day subcutaneously. If the ANC rises to 1000 to 5000/μL and plateaus, the same G-CSF dosage is maintained. If the ANC exceeds 5000/μL, the dose is reduced to 3 μg/kg to bring the count to 1000 to 5000/μL. If the ANC still exceeds 5000/μL, the dose is lowered further to 1 μg/kg or to alternate-day dosing, for example, 1 to 2 μg/kg every second day.

If there is no response to the starting dose, the G-CSF is increased to 10 μg/kg/day. If there is still no effect, increments are continued every 2 to 4 weeks to 20 μg/kg/day,[3] then 30 μg/kg/day,[3] and so on, up to a maximum of 120 μg/kg/day[3] (which would require a twice-daily administration or multiple subcutaneous injections at the same time). A patient who fails to respond to 120 μg/kg/day is defined as being refractory to G-CSF treatment. A trial of GM-CSF would then be warranted using a starting dose of 3 to 15 μg/kg/day (250 μg/m$^2$/day) subcutaneously. Another option is a hematopoietic stem cell transplantation if there is an HLA-matched donor.

G-CSF, 5 to 10 μg/kg/day, either IV or subcutaneously, is also indicated for other forms of severe neutropenia, especially those associated with chemotherapy, using the following guidelines that we developed at the Hospital for Sick Children, Toronto:

- For febrile neutropenic patients who have positive blood cultures, have an identified focus of infection, and/or whose vital signs are unstable
- For patients receiving chemotherapy protocols that predictably induce severe neutropenia to increase safety and to ensure that the full course of chemotherapy is administered and given on time. G-CSF should be administered after the first and subsequent cycles of the chemotherapy in these patients
- With antineoplastic dose-escalation protocols that predictably induce severe neutropenia
- For patients enrolled in multicenter chemotherapy protocols that specify the use of G-CSF
- For patients receiving antineoplastic agents in conjunction with large-volume irradiation involving bone marrow

In this setting as a preventive agent, G-CSF can be stopped when neutrophils are more than 1500 μL for 2 consecutive days. When G-CSF is given for fever-neutropenia, or to patients whose condition is unstable or who have a focus of infection or a positive culture, it can be stopped when neutrophils are greater than 1000/μL for 2 days if the patient is clinically improved, the focus has resolved, and the cultures are negative.

For adults receiving Neulasta, the recommended dosage is a single subcutaneous injection of 6 mg administered once per cycle of chemotherapy. It should not be given in the interval between 14 days before and 24 hours after chemotherapy because of the potential for an increase in sensitivity of rapidly dividing myeloid to cytotoxicity.

## REFERENCES

Dinauer MC: The phagocyte system and disorders of granulopoiesis and granulocyte function. In Nathan DG, Orkin SH, Ginsburg D, Look AT (eds): Hematology of Infancy and Childhood, 6th ed. Philadelphia, WB Saunders, 2003, pp 923-1010.

Kowalczyk A (ed): 2005–2006 Drug Handbook and Formulary, Hospital for Sick Children, 24th ed. pp 178-185. To order or for drug information: Telephone: 416-813-6703; e-mail: druginfo@sickkids.ca

Watts RG: Neutropenia. In Greer JP, Foerster J, Lukens JN, et al (eds): Wintrobe's Clinical Hematology, 11th ed. Philadelphia, Lippincott, Williams & Wilkins, 2004, pp 1777-1800.

---

[3]Exceeds dosage recommended by the manufacturer.

# Hemolytic Disease of the Newborn

Method of
*James W. Kendig, MD*

Hemolytic disease of the fetus and newborn refers to a spectrum of problems that were formerly classified as four separate entities: erythroblastosis fetalis, congenital anemia, icterus gravis neonatorum, and hydrops fetalis. Further studies demonstrated that these entities are all manifestations of a single disease caused by red blood cell isoimmunization (alloimmunization).

The major red blood cell surface antigen responsible for this process is the $Rh_o(D)$ antigen. Because there is no corresponding "d" antigen, the term "d" refers only to the absence of the $Rh_o(D)$ antigen. $Rh_o(D)$-negative individuals (dd) have no $Rh_o(D)$ antigens on their red blood cells. $Rh_o(D)$-positive individuals may be homozygous (DD) or heterozygous (Dd) for the $Rh_o(D)$ gene, which is located on the short arm of chromosome 1. In addition to the $Rh_o(D)$ gene, the Rh blood group system includes the related Cc Ee structural gene, which encodes four specific antigens (C, c, E, and e) on the red blood cell surface. Zygosity for $Rh_o(D)$ may be predicted on the basis of classic serologic tests for the antigens C, c, D, E, e, and the known incidence of various phenotypes in different racial and ethnic groups.

$Rh_o(D)$ alloimmunization occurs when fetal $Rh_o(D)$-positive red blood cells (inherited from the father) cross the placenta and enter the circulation of an $Rh_o(D)$-negative (dd) mother. The maternal immune system is stimulated to produce $Rh_o(D)$ antibodies (IgG). ABO incompatibility (mother 0 and fetus A or B) helps to protect against the $Rh_o(D)$ sensitization of the $Rh_o(D)$-negative mother.

The maternal $Rh_o(D)$ antibodies cross the placenta of the current or a subsequent pregnancy and cause the destruction of the $Rh_o(D)$-positive fetal red blood cells. The fetus responds to this hemolytic anemia with extramedullary hematopoiesis involving the liver and spleen. The hepatic production of fetal albumin is compromised, leading to hydrops with edema, ascites, and pericardial and pleural effusions. Bilirubin, produced by the hemolysis of fetal red blood cells, readily crosses the placenta and is excreted by the maternal liver. After delivery, however, neonatal hyperbilirubinemia develops, which may lead to an acute encephalopathy (kernicterus). Other red blood cell antigen–antibody systems (Kidd, Kell, Duffy, the C/c and E/e alleles of the Rh system, and, rarely, the ABO system) may occasionally result in hemolytic disease of the fetus and newborn. In the case of anti-Kell isoimmunization, fetal anemia is caused by a suppression of erythropoiesis in addition to hemolysis.

## Prevention of $Rh_o(D)$ Alloimmunization

The development, commercial production, and widespread use of commercially prepared $Rh_o(D)$ immunoglobulin (RhoGAM) for the prevention of $Rh_o(D)$ alloimmunization are among the greatest scientific and medical achievements of the 20th century. This is an example of passive immunization preventing active immunization, but the precise mechanism by which the administration of the $Rh_o(D)$ antibody blocks the mother's production of the same antibody is still not fully understood. RhoGAM is not beneficial to the $Rh_o(D)$-negative woman after alloimmunization has taken place, and it does not prevent sensitization because of the C/c and E/e antigens of the Rh blood group system. Box 1 gives a list of events and procedures that may lead to the $Rh_o(D)$ alloimmunization of the $Rh_o(D)$-negative woman. An intramuscular dose of RhoGAM (300 μg) should be administered after these events and procedures. In the event of a severe fetal-to-maternal hemorrhage at delivery, more than 300 μg of RhoGAM may be required.

## BOX 1   Reproductive Events and Procedures That Can Lead to Alloimmunization of the Rh₀(D)-Negative Woman

### Events

- Threatened abortion and antepartum hemorrhage
- Spontaneous abortion
- Delivery at any gestational age
- Ectopic pregnancy
- Hydatidiform molar pregnancy
- Abdominal trauma and motor vehicle accidents during pregnancy
- Inadvertent transfusion with Rh-positive blood

### Procedures

- Cordocentesis
- Chorionic villous sampling
- Induced abortion
- Amniocentesis any time during pregnancy
- External cephalic version
- Delivery at any time

Blood type (ABO and Rh₀(D)) and an antibody screen (the indirect Coombs test) should be obtained on the first prenatal visit. The antibody screen detects Rh₀(D) antibodies as well as antibodies directed against the other red blood cell antigens, such as Kell, Duffy, C/c, and E/e. If the antibody screen is positive, alloimmunization has already occurred, and serial titers should be obtained. If the antibody titer is 1:16 or greater by 20 weeks' gestation, further testing is necessary.

### ANTEPARTUM PREVENTION

At 28 weeks' gestation, all Rh₀(D)-negative mothers should have an antibody screen (indirect Coombs test). If the test is negative, a prophylactic intramuscular dose of RhoGAM (300 μg) should be administered, unless the father of the infant is definitely known to be Rh₀(D)-negative (dd). The purpose of this prophylactic antepartum dose is to prevent alloimmunization during the pregnancy. The half-life of this dose is 12 weeks. This antepartum dose may lead to a weakly positive indirect Coombs test in the mother at the time of delivery and a weakly positive direct Coombs test in the infant.

### POSTPARTUM PREVENTION

Every Rh₀(D)-negative mother who has not undergone Rh₀(D) alloimmunization should receive an intramuscular dose of *at least* 300 μg of RhoGAM after the delivery of an Rh₀(D)-positive newborn. This critical step in the prevention of Rh₀(D) disease requires careful communication among the labor and delivery area, the hospital blood bank, and the postpartum floor. These communication issues are particularly important when early discharge from the hospital is being considered and when the birth has occurred outside the hospital.

A single dose of RhoGAM (300 μg) neutralizes approximately 30 mL of Rh₀(D)-positive fetal whole blood or 15 mL of packed fetal red blood cells. If a large fetal-to-maternal transfusion should occur at the time of delivery, a single dose of RhoGAM may be inadequate to prevent alloimmunization. Because of this possibility, the hospital blood bank should check the mother's blood after delivery to determine the presence and the magnitude of a fetal-to-maternal bleed. The rosette test is used to screen maternal blood for the presence of fetal red blood cells, and the Kleihauer-Betke stain is used to evaluate the magnitude of a fetal-to-maternal bleed. This information is used to determine the need for a larger (more than 300 μg) dose of intramuscular RhoGAM. RhoGAM should be administered within 72 hours of delivery. If administration has been inadvertently omitted, it may still

be given up to 4 weeks after delivery. The Rh₀(D)-negative mother who is already Rh₀(D) alloimmunized at the time of delivery will not benefit from the administration of RhoGAM.

## Obstetric Management of the Mother With a Positive Initial Antibody Screen

All pregnant women should have an antibody screen (indirect Coombs test) at the first prenatal visit. If the result is positive, the blood bank identifies the antibody and determines its titer. The blood bank examines the father's red blood cells for the corresponding antigen. If the father's result is negative for the antigen, and if the mother has absolutely no doubts regarding paternity, no further studies are required. If the father's result is positive for the involved antigen, the

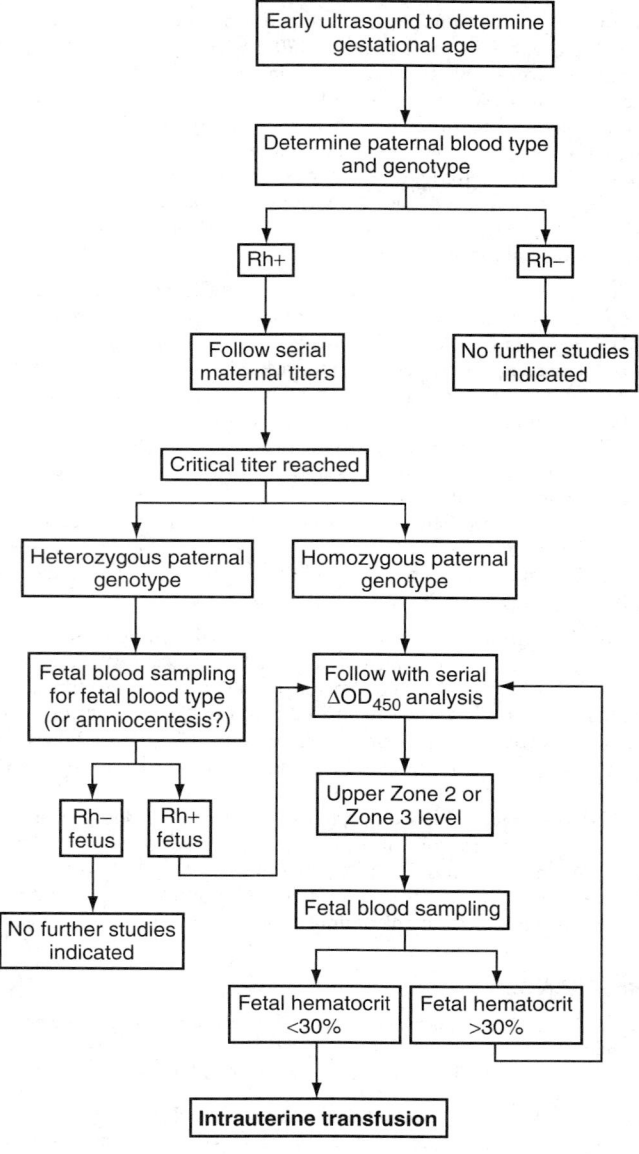

**FIGURE 1.** Algorithm used at Baylor College of Medicine, Houston, for the management of newly diagnosed, red blood cell Rh₀(D) alloimmunization in pregnancy. (From Moise KJ: Changing trends in the management of red blood cell alloimmunization in pregnancy. Arch Pathol Lab Med 1994;118:421-428. Copyright 1994, American Medical Association. Used with permission.)

mother should have serial antibody titers at 1-month intervals. Early ultrasonography should also be done for gestational age assessment. If a critical antibody titer of 1:16 is reached, there is a risk of the development of erythroblastosis fetalis and hydrops, and further investigation and interventions are required (Figure 1).

The $Rh_o(D)$-alloimmunized mother with a history of a previous pregnancy requiring an intrauterine transfusion or a neonatal exchange transfusion is at a high risk for hydrops. With this history, serial $\Delta OD_{450}$ (optical density at 450 nm) evaluations of amniotic fluid are recommended, starting at 20 to 22 weeks' gestation, even if the antibody titer has not reached the critical level of 1:16.

## PATERNAL ZYGOSITY

If the maternal antibody is $Rh_o(D)$, and the father has the corresponding $Rh_o(D)$ antigen, the blood bank determines whether he is homozygous (DD) or heterozygous (Dd). This prediction is based on the classic serologic tests for the C, c, E, and e antigens and the known incidence of various phenotypes in different racial and ethnic groups. If the father is heterozygous, there is a 50% chance that the fetal red blood cells are $Rh_o(D)$-negative (dd) and that the fetus is not at risk for the development of erythroblastosis fetalis. If the father is heterozygous, it is useful to determine the fetal blood type.

## DETERMINATION OF FETAL BLOOD TYPE

Techniques for obtaining samples of fetal blood from the umbilical vessels, using ultrasound guidance, have been perfected and are available at large regional perinatal centers. This procedure, known as cordocentesis, involves obvious risks and should be performed only by specialists experienced in fetal and maternal medicine. Several centers have used the polymerase chain reaction (PCR) to identify the fetal $Rh_o(D)$ genotype. This new technique is based on the amplification of the DNA from a few fetal red blood cells found in a centrifuged sample of amniotic fluid. If the mother has $Rh_o(D)$ antibodies and the fetus is $Rh_o(D)$-negative (by cordocentesis of a fetal blood sample or by PCR of fetal red blood cells from amniotic fluid), no further studies are indicated.

## AMNIOTIC FLUID $\Delta OD_{450}$ MEASUREMENTS

If the maternal antibody titer reaches a critical titer of 1:16 and if there is a possibility that the fetal red blood cells are positive for the corresponding antigen, serial measurements of amniotic fluid $\Delta OD_{450}$ should be done every 10 to 14 days to evaluate the level of bilirubin in the amniotic fluid. These values are plotted on the modified Liley curve (Figure 2).

## INTRAUTERINE FETAL TRANSFUSION

When $\Delta OD_{450}$ values climb to the upper indeterminate zone or anywhere in the $Rh_o(D)$-positive (affected) zone on the modified Liley curve, cordocentesis should be done to measure the fetal hematocrit. If this value is less than 30%, an intravascular fetal transfusion (via cordocentesis) of packed red blood cells should be carried out at a regional perinatal center by specialists experienced in maternal and fetal medicine. For severe hydrops, more than one intrauterine transfusion may be required. The timing of delivery should be based on gestational age estimates and the determination of fetal lung maturity.

# Management of the Newborn With Erythroblastosis Fetalis

## DELIVERY ROOM MANAGEMENT

With advances in the field of maternal–fetal medicine and the use of intravascular fetal transfusions, it is unusual for an infant to be delivered with severe erythroblastosis and hydrops secondary to $Rh_o(D)$. When this does occur, however, three teams of neonatologists, pediatricians, and nurse practitioners must be immediately available to initiate multiple interventions.

One team is responsible for airway management, including intubation, and the initiation of positive-pressure ventilation. This team also monitors the heart rate and initiates chest compressions, if needed. A second team is responsible for securing immediate intravascular access, usually via the umbilical vein. A hematocrit value is obtained

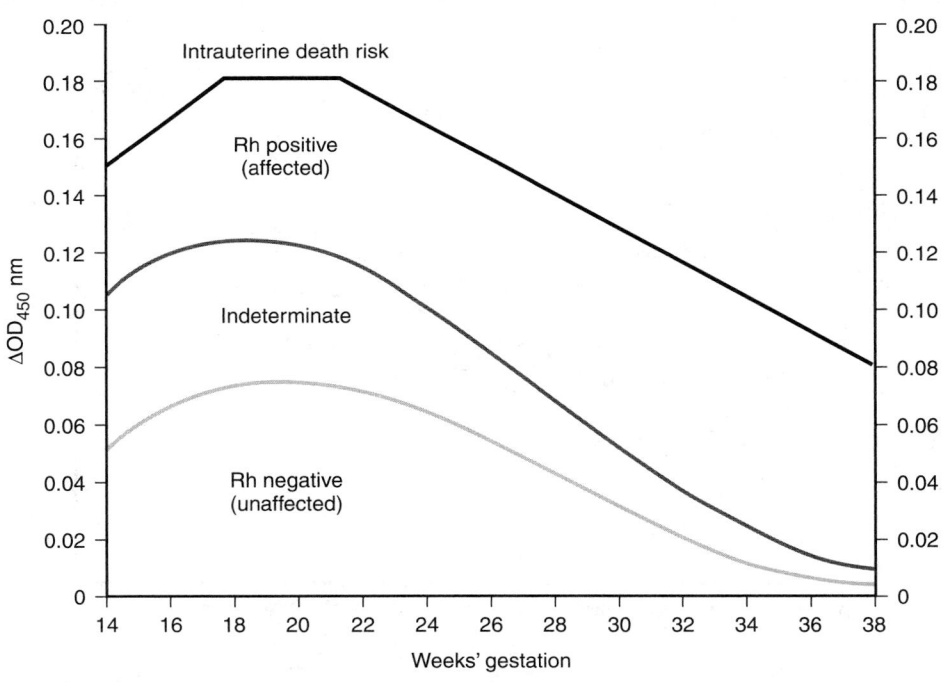

**FIGURE 2.** Amniotic fluid optical density ($\Delta OD_{450}$) zones for management of pregnancy complicated by $Rh_o(D)$ alloimmunization. (From Queenan JT, Tomai TP, Ural SH, King JC: Deviation in amniotic fluid optical density at a wavelength of 450 nm in Rh-immunized pregnancies from 14 to 40 weeks' gestation: A proposal for clinical management. Am J Obstet Gynecol 1993;168:1370-1376. Used with permission.)

immediately, and if it is less than 30%, a partial exchange transfusion using 25 to 80 mL per kg of packed red blood cells is carried out within 30 minutes of birth to raise the hematocrit to 40% or higher. A third team should be available to perform paracentesis and thoracentesis, if needed. With severe hydrops, effective pulmonary ventilation frequently cannot be achieved until large collections of pleural and ascitic fluid have been removed.

Immediately after umbilical cord clamping, the obstetric team should obtain a sample of cord blood, which is sent to the laboratory for a direct Coombs test and determination of hematocrit, reticulocyte count, total and direct bilirubin levels, cord pH, and blood gas tension values.

## INTENSIVE PHOTOTHERAPY

Upon admission to the neonatal intensive care nursery, the infant with erythroblastosis fetalis should be placed immediately under intensive phototherapy. This can be achieved by using multiple banks of special blue fluorescent tubes (e.g., F20T12/BB manufactured by General Electric, Westinghouse, and Sylvania).

Place the full-term infant in a bassinet rather than an incubator, and line the sides of the bassinet with white linens or aluminum foil to maximize surface area exposure.

Obtain serial serum bilirubin values (total and direct) at 2- to 3-hour intervals to establish the rate of rise under intensive phototherapy, and plot the levels, as shown in Figure 3.

## INTRAVENOUS GAMMA GLOBULIN

The administration of intravenous immune globulin (IVIG) (0.5 g/kg over 2 hours) is recommended if the total serum bilirubin is rising in spite of intensive phototherapy or if the total serum bilirubin is within 2 to 3 mg/dL of the exchange level shown in Figure 3.

## NEONATAL DOUBLE-VOLUME EXCHANGE TRANSFUSION

With the widespread use of RhoGAM to prevent the alloimmunization of $Rh_o(D)$-negative women, coupled with advances in fetal intravascular transfusion therapy, neonatal double-volume exchange transfusions

## CURRENT DIAGNOSIS

- Blood type—ABO and $Rh_o(D)$—and an antibody screen (the indirect Coombs test) should be obtained on the first prenatal visit. If the antibody screen is positive, alloimmunization has already occurred, and serial titers should be obtained. If the titer reaches a critical level of 1:16 or greater, additional testing such as determination of paternal zygosity, amniocentesis, and cordocentesis will need to be done by a specialist in maternal–fetal medicine.
- All $Rh_o(D)$-negative mothers who deliver an $Rh_o(D)$-positive infant should be screened with a rosette test or a Kleihauer-Betke test to detect an excessive fetal–maternal hemorrhage. Those mothers with evidence of an excessive fetal–maternal hemorrhage may need more than the standard 1 vial of $Rh_o(D)$-immunoglobulin (RhoGAM).
- There is no single simple test to tell what level of bilirubin is dangerous to any given infant at any given time.
- Following intensive phototherapy and/or exchange transfusion for moderate to severe erythroblastosis fetalis, serial hematocrit values must be followed carefully for 4 to 8 weeks to determine the need for a top-up transfusion of packed red blood cells.

are becoming rare procedures. When neonatal exchange transfusions are required, they should be done by experienced neonatologists and pediatricians working in neonatal centers that are prepared to deal with the various complications of the procedure, which include hypoglycemia, thrombocytopenia, necrotizing enterocolitis, and infection.

After the delivery of an infant with erythroblastosis fetalis, serial serum bilirubin values (total and direct) should be obtained at 2- to 3-hour intervals to establish the rate of rise. A serum indirect bilirubin level that is climbing by more than 0.5 mg per dL per hour indicates that there is a relatively brisk hemolytic process that may require

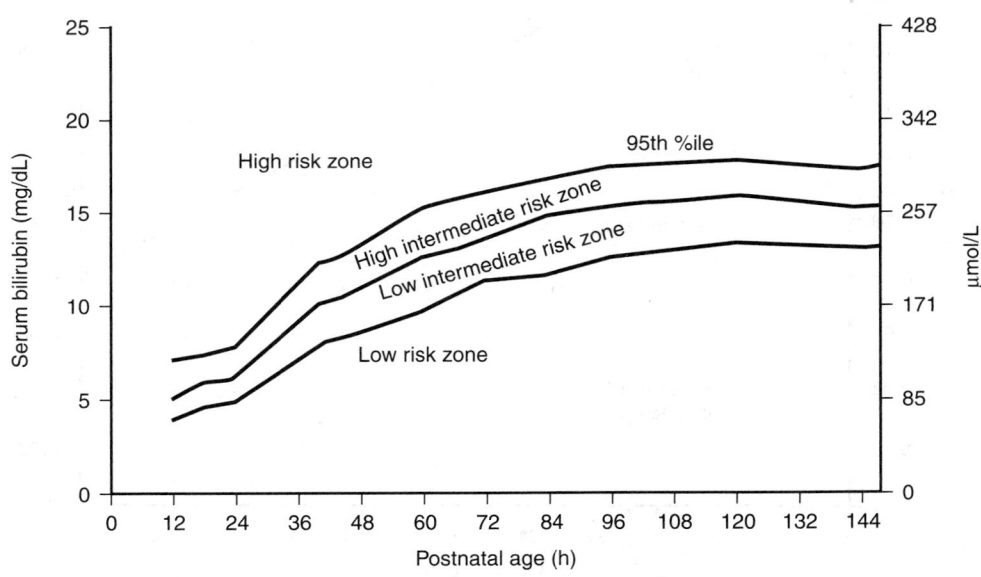

**FIGURE 3.** Nomogram for designation of risk in 2840 well newborns at 36 or more weeks' gestational age with birth weight of 2000 g or more, or 35 or more weeks' gestational age and birth weight of 2500 g or more based on the hour-specific serum bilirubin values. The serum bilirubin level was obtained before discharge, and the zone in which the value fell predicted the likelihood of a subsequent bilirubin level exceeding the 95th percentile (high-risk zone). (From Pediatrics 2004;114(1):297-316, American Academy of Pediatrics. Used with permission.)

## CURRENT THERAPY

■ The unsensitized, $Rh_o(D)$-negative patient should receive prophylactic anti-D immunoglobulin (RhoGAM) at 28 weeks' gestation and again post-delivery at any gestational age if newborn infant is $Rh_o(D)$ positive.

■ The unsensitized, $Rh_o(D)$-negative patient should receive prophylactic RhoGAM after any of the following events and procedures: Ectopic gestation, abruption of placenta, abortion, abdominal trauma, amniocentesis, cordocentesis, chorionic villous sampling, and external cephalic version.

■ The combined use of intensive phototherapy and intravenous immunoglobulin may reduce the need for an exchange transfusion.

a double-volume exchange transfusion within the first 12 hours after birth. Recently published guidelines for exchange transfusions are shown in Figure 3. In addition to lowering the serum bilirubin level, an early double-volume exchange transfusion helps to correct the fetal anemia and removes a significant portion of the antibody-coated red blood cells before they hemolyze. The blood sample for routine metabolic screens for hypothyroidism, inborn errors of metabolism, and hemoglobinopathies should be drawn before the exchange transfusion is performed.

Serial serum bilirubin levels should be continued even if an early double-volume exchange transfusion is not mandated by the rate of rise. It is impossible to determine exactly what level of indirect bilirubin constitutes a risk for encephalopathy (kernicterus on neuropathology) in any given infant at any given time. Prematurity, hypoxia, asphyxia, acidosis, sepsis, and hypoalbuminemia may increase the risk of bilirubin encephalopathy. Various drugs, such as the sulfa preparations and ceftriaxone, displace bilirubin from albumin-binding sites and increase the risk for encephalopathy.

In the otherwise healthy, full-term newborn with hemolytic disease, the indirect bilirubin level should not be permitted to climb above 20 mg per dL. With prematurity and hemolytic disease, lower threshold levels for exchange transfusion, based on gestational age, birth weight, chronologic age in days, and the presence or absence of other risk factors for bilirubin encephalopathy are recommended. Premature newborns with hemolytic disease should be managed by experienced neonatologists working in regional perinatal centers. Phototherapy is used as an adjunct to exchange transfusion, and in the case of mild hemolytic disease, phototherapy alone may be sufficient to control the bilirubin level.

### DELAYED NEONATAL RED BLOOD CELL TRANSFUSIONS

A slow hemolysis frequently continues for up to 6 to 8 weeks after delivery in those infants who received a fetal intravascular transfusion or an exchange transfusion after delivery and in those infants with a mild hemolysis requiring only phototherapy. These infants should be followed up with serial hematocrit determinations at 1- to 2-week intervals during the first 6 to 8 weeks after birth. A transfusion of packed red blood cells (10 to 15 mL per kg) may be necessary to correct severe anemia. With severe hemolytic anemia, particularly in infants who received intrauterine transfusions, fetal and neonatal iron stores are elevated. Neonatal iron therapy should be withheld until the serum ferritin level returns to normal.

### REFERENCES

American Academy of Pediatrics: Clinical practice guidelines for management of hyperbilirubinemia in the newborn infant 35 or more weeks of gestation. Pediatrics 2004;114(1):297-316.

American College of Obstetricians and Gynecologists: Prevention of RhD Alloimmunization. ACOG Practice Bulletin 4. Washington, DC, ACOG, 1999.

Gottstein R, Cooke RWI: Systematic review of intravenous immunoglobulin in haemolytic disease of the newborn. Arch Dis Child Fetal Neonatal Ed 2003;88:F6-F10.

Harkness UF, Spinnato JA: Prevention and management of RhD isoimmunization. Clin Perinatol 2004;31(4):721-742.

Maisels MJ: Why use homeopathic doses of phototherapy? Pediatrics 1996;98:283-287.

McKenna DS, Nagaraja HN, O'Shaughnessy R: Management of pregnancies complicated by anti-Kell isoimmunization. Obstet Gynecol 1999;93:667-673.

# Hemophilia and Related Disorders

Method of
*Wing-Yen Wong, MD*

Hemophilia A and B and von Willebrand's disease (vWd) are the most common causes of bleeding. Less common bleeding disorders also need to be considered in the orderly workup of any coagulopathy. The newborn with prolonged bleeding after circumcision, the toddler with bruises not only on the shins and arms but also in areas not usually subject to direct trauma such as the torso and neck, and the teenager with more than 5 to 7 days of heavy menstrual bleeding all deserve attention. Moderately affected children may not present until toddler age when they are more active. The axiom of joint bleeding as the usual site for the hemophilias and mucosal bleeds for vWd tends to hold true. However, severe vWd can have joint bleeds, and extreme lyonization can result in female carriers of hemophilia presenting with menorrhagia. The important criteria for diagnosis are the patient's medical and family history augmented by age-appropriate interpretation of laboratory tests. This chapter focuses on a practical approach to diagnosis and treatment choices for hemophilia A and B, and vWd.

## Epidemiology and Genetic Transmission

Inheritance patterns are divided into three main groups: hemophilia A and B are X-linked recessive, vWd is usually autosomal dominant, and some vWd and other factor deficiencies are autosomal recessive.

Approximately 30% of hemophilia in boys presents with new mutations and negative family histories. Incidence of hemophilia A is estimated at 1 in 5000 male births and 1 in 30,000 for hemophilia B. There are no geographic or racial differences. Mild hemophilia is often misdiagnosed and therefore may be underrepresented. Carrier and prenatal testing from blood and amniotic samples has more than 90% accuracy if performed at established laboratories, particularly if blood samples from various affected family members are available for DNA linkage studies.

Inversion within intron 22 of the FVIII gene is found in more than 45% of severely affected hemophilia A patients. DNA analysis for this and other mutations is available at certain research laboratories. Testing from chorionic villus sampling can be done at 10 to 12 weeks' gestation if the specific genetic mutation is known, but sampling of fetal blood for FVIII activity cannot be done prior to 16 weeks' gestation.

The incidence of vWd is unknown, and estimates vary from 0.2% to 2.0%. There are no gender or racial differences. The complexity of the various vWd subtypes and the generally mild nature of vWd has not lent itself to easy prenatal testing and hence is not usually performed. A large number of vWd molecular gene defects are identified.

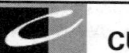

## CURRENT THERAPY

| Bleeds/Procedures | Hemophilia A | Hemophilia B | Type 1 vWd |
|---|---|---|---|
| Minor | 20–30 U/kg/12–24 h × 1–3 doses | 30–50 U/kg/24-48 h × 1–3 doses | Stimate, 1–2 s/d × 1–2 d |
| Major* | 40–50 U/kg /8–12 h | 60–100 U/kg/12–24 h | Humate-P, 30–60 RCoF U/kg/12–24 h |
| Continuous infusion | Load with bolus as above; then 2–5 U/kg/h | Load with bolus as above; then 5–10 U/kg/h | |

*Major bleeds/surgeries: levels should be monitored and maintained at 100% for at least 72 h.
*Abbreviations:* RCoF = ristocetin cofactor; vWd = von Willebrand's disease.

The information can be obtained from online databank sites. DNA testing can be helpful for vWd subtypes such as type 2N, which can be misdiagnosed as hemophilia A because both disorders have low levels of FVIII. In vWd type 2A, both vWf (von Willebrand's factor) and ristocetin cofactor (RCoF) are decreased, whereas hemophilia A has normal vWf and RCoF levels. People with blood type O have slightly lower baseline levels of vWd than type AB.

FXI deficiency is the most common hereditary coagulopathy in patients of Jewish descent. The degree of bleeding is highly variable.

## Disease Classification and Laboratory Testing

The activated partial prothrombin time (APTT) measures most common clotting factor abnormalities associated with bleeding diatheses except for FVII and FXIII. Hemophilia A and B patients with inhibitors have prolonged APTT uncorrected by a 1:1 mixing ratio with normal plasma. FVII deficiency is associated with a prolonged PT, whereas FXIII deficiency has normal prothrombin time (PT), APTT, and thrombin time (TT). Some causes of a prolonged APTT not associated with significant bleeding even with major trauma or surgery include deficiencies of high molecular weight kininogen (HMWK), prekallikrein, and FXII. Exclusion of an inhibitor such as antiphospholipid antibody should also be considered in the face of a prolonged APTT and a benign bleeding history. Excessive fibrinolysis such as α-2-antiplasmin deficiency also causes increased bleeding, but these disorders are rare.

The mechanism of disease in the coagulopathies may involve failure of synthesis of the necessary coagulation factor or synthesis of abnormal proteins with impaired activity. Hence, the functional protein activity may differ from the amount of protein measured.

Hemophilia A and B result in inadequate generation of thrombin for clot formation. The degree of disease severity and onset of symptoms vary with plasma FVIII or FIX activity levels. Boys with less than 1% factor activity have severe disease with early onset of joint and muscle bleeds. Those with hemophilia A have bleeding symptoms earlier in life, usually within the first year, compared to hemophilia B. Moderate and mild disease correlate to factor activity levels of 1% to 5% and more than 5%, respectively. Carrier females have factor levels ranging from 30% to 70%.

In vWd, the mechanism of disease is associated with failure to form an effective primary platelet plug. There are three main types of vWd and numerous subtypes. Type 1 vWd is caused by a partial quantitative deficiency of vWf, type 2 has qualitative variants, and type 3 has marked, sometimes complete, deficiency of vWf. Overall, types 1 and 2 tend to have mild to moderate severity of bleeding, whereas the rarer type 3 tends to have severe disease.

Type 2N has a defective affinity for FVIII, and both FVIII and vWf are markedly decreased. It is critical that physicians, especially gynecologists and obstetricians, consider the workup and diagnosis for vWd in any female with menorrhagia. Diagnosis of vWd can be difficult to ascertain with some affected individuals having near normal or fluctuating von Willebrand's factor antigen (vWf:Ag) and RCoF levels and significant clinical bleeding. Table 1 outlines the main characteristics of hemophilia A and vWd.

## Treatment Options

### HEMOPHILIA A AND B

The hallmark to effective treatment remains replacement of the deficient or abnormal factor as early as possible, at the appropriate dosage and frequency. The ability to self-infuse or have a caregiver administer the factor at home at the first sign of any bleeding has a positive impact on disease outcome. For this approach to be effective, early recognition of bleeding is required. Early symptoms for joint or muscle bleeds include increased warmth, tingling sensations, or a vague feeling at the affected or target joint. Increased irritability in the infant or young child often heralds the onset of a bleed. Patients should not wait for swelling or discoloration to infuse.

Care at a specialty hemophilia treatment center (HTC) significantly improves disease outcome. These facilities have the necessary expertise to coordinate all aspects of diagnosis and care, acute and chronic, as well as a multifaceted team approach. Close telephone contact should be maintained between the family and HTC personnel in the event of any bleeding episode, even when home therapy has been initiated successfully.

For mild hemophilia A, desmopressin (Stimate), a concentrated form of desmopressin acetate (DDAVP), can be used without exposure to blood products. This is particularly helpful in persons avoiding

**TABLE 1 Key Diagnostic Comparison of Hemophilia A and von Willebrand's Disease**

| | Hemophilia A | vWd* |
|---|---|---|
| Inheritance | X-linked | Autosomal |
| Bleeding pattern | Mainly joint, muscle bleeds | Mainly mucous membrane bleeds (e.g., epistaxis, menorrhagia) |
| PTT | ↑ | Nl or ↑ |
| FVIIIa | ↓ | Nl or ↓ |
| vWF:Ag | Nl | ↓ or Nl |
| RcoF | Nl | ↓ or Nl |
| Ivy bleeding time | Nl | ↑ |

*Modifying factors include blood type (type O has decreased vWf), stress, physical activity, estrogen use, and pregnancy. Normal values do not definitively exclude diagnosis of vWd and can vary from time to time within the same individual.
*Abbreviations:* PTT = partial thromboplastin time; RCoF = ristocetin cofactor; vWd = von Willebrand's disease; vWf = von Willebrand's factor; vWf:Ag = von Willebrand's factor antigen.

## TABLE 2 FVIII and FIX Concentrates

| Factor Type | FVIII | FIX |
|---|---|---|
| Recombinant | Helixate FS/ Kogenate-FS ReFacto Recombinate Advate | BeneFix |
| Ultra high purity Plasma derived | Hemofil M Monarc M Monoclate-P | AlphaNine SD Mononine |
| Other plasma derived | Alphanate* SD Humate-P*† Koate-DVI* | Bebulin VH Profilnine SD Proplex-T |

*Contains varying amounts of von Willebrand's factor.
†FDA approved for von Willebrand's disease.

blood products for religious reasons and in decreasing the risk of infectious transmissions. Details of this treatment option are covered later in the section on the treatment of vWd. Stimate should not be used for FIX-deficient patients.

The current treatment of choice for newly diagnosed severely affected individuals with hemophilia A or B is recombinant FVIII or FIX. New products within this category are being added to our armamentarium. Choice of treatment product for previously treated patients largely depends on patient preference and prior rating of clinical efficacy. Studies showed that infusion of ultra-high-purity products is associated with preservation of CD4 counts in HIV-infected individuals.

Table 2 lists the replacement factor choices for hemophilia A and B in categories of purity. With established efficacy, random changes are not advisable unless otherwise clinically indicated. However, because of intermittent product shortages, physicians and patients are sometimes required to substitute proprietary factor concentrates. I attempt to keep within a similar category if at all possible. A product may have two different brand names but can be interchangeable (e.g., Helixate and Kogenate). ReFacto is a recombinant FVIII product that has the B domain deleted and is a slightly smaller molecule. A new longer-acting liposomal-pegylated rFVIII is currently undergoing clinical trials.

## TREATMENT DOSAGE AND FREQUENCY

Dosing regimens are targeted to maintain replacement plasma factor at certain levels based on the severity and site of bleed. FVIII has a shorter half-life than FIX and should be infused every 8 to 12 hours for an acute bleed compared to every 12 to 24 hours for FIX. FXIII has the longest half-life $T_{12}$ and can be replaced monthly for most patients. Mild muscle and soft-tissue bleeds require 30% factor plasma level for 1 to 2 days. Major hemorrhage, surgeries, and gastrointestinal (GI) or central nervous system (CNS) bleeds require more than 90% to 100% levels for at least 72 hours. Continuous infusions are often employed for major surgeries or severe bleeds to achieve consistent plasma factor levels.

Here are the calculations to achieve these targeted levels:

FVIII infusions: number of units required per dose = weight (kg) × % factor level desired × 0.5 (e.g., to achieve 100% in a 50-kg person, number of units required per dose = 50 × 100 × 0.5 = 2500 U)

However, wastage of extra factor above the calculated range is discouraged. Hence, the amount actually given is often rounded up to the closest vial size:

FIX infusions: number of units required per dose = weight (kg) × % factor level desired × 1

BeneFix infusion: number of units required per dose = weight (kg) × % factor level desired × 1.2

Monitoring of plasma levels (at 1 hour pre- and postinfusion) with initial infusions and at times of dosage change would guide dosage adjustment needs.

## TREATMENT IN THE PRESENCE OF INHIBITORS

Inhibitory antibodies to FVIII arise in 30% of those with severely affected hemophilia A and 3% to 5% of children with hemophilia B during the first 15 to 30 infusion exposures. These antibodies develop after exposure to the exogenous protein and therefore tend to occur in those with large gene deletions and severe disease. The presence of inhibitors should be suspected when failure to achieve adequate hemostasis with routine replacement therapy is observed. Inhibitors are measured by the Bethesda assay in Bethesda units (BUs). High-titer or high-responding inhibitors are more than 5 BU. The level of inhibitor activity determines the choice of appropriate management options. Low-titer or low-responding FVIII inhibitors can be managed by using higher doses of factor concentrate. For mild to moderate bleeds, a dose of twice the routine amount usually suffices. For major bleeds, a bolus of 100 to 150 U/kg[3] followed by continuous infusion at 15 to 20 U/kg/hour for 3 to 4 days may be required. Inhibitor titers may rise sharply because of an anamnestic response and need to be monitored for optimum care.

High-responding inhibitors pose a difficult therapeutic challenge. Often continuous infusions fail to achieve and maintain hemostasis, particularly in major bleeds or surgery. Porcine FVIII at a 100 to 150 U/kg starting dose is successful in hemophilia A inhibitor patients. Monitoring antiporcine FVIII antibodies should be performed. Prothrombin complex concentrates (PCCs), a pool of FII, FIX, X, and FVII, can be used at 75 to 100 U/kg of FIX for minor bleeds. The dose can be repeated once or twice every 12 hours. If bleeding is not controlled within two to three doses, alternate treatment should be used. Heparin should be added at 5 to 10 U/mL of the reconstituted PCC. The mechanism of action is unclear. Activated prothrombin complex concentrates (APCCs) can be similarly applied at 50 to 75 U/kg FIX. Both PCCs and APCCs have increased thrombogenic potential, and myocardial infarcts are reported with their use.

However, frequent monitoring of fibrin-split products or d-dimers as signals of thrombosis is of questionable value. The PCCs (Konyne, Proplex-T) and APCCs (FEIBA) are plasma-derived pooled concentrates. They have been the mainstay of inhibitor therapy and demonstrate good efficacy. Recombinant FVIIa (NovoSeven) is available with less thrombogenic effects. Dosage for rFVIIa is recommended at 90 µg/kg for 2 to 4 hours, but optimum dosing is not known. rFVIIa can be used either in the home or hospital setting. PCCs or APCCs should not be administered in close temporal proximity to rFVIIa because that would potentiate the danger of thrombosis, although there are instances of life-threatening bleeds or surgeries in high-titer inhibitor patients where combination of both were used under close monitoring at a HTC setting.

A specific group of FIX inhibitor patients develop anaphylactoid reactions upon infusion of concentrates containing any amount of FIX. The reactions vary from feeling flushed with chest discomfort to coughing, wheezing, and frank hypotension and shock requiring intubation and resuscitative efforts. Vigilance to possible anaphylactoid reactions in hemophilia B patients should be exercised. PCCs and APCCs should be avoided when detected. The use of rFVIIa is a proven safe and effective recourse for these patients.

Long-term management of hemophilia A and B inhibitor patients includes immune tolerance induction (ITI) to eradicate the antibody completely. There are numerous approaches involving the use of an immunosuppressant and daily FVIII. These methods vary with the dose of FVIII, use of intravenous immunoglobulin (IVIg) and/or cyclophosphamide, antibody adsorption column, or steroids. The decision to initiate such therapy should only be taken after serious consideration of the risks of failure (10% to 30%), intercurrent bleeding, and the enormous commitment required. Low pre-ITI inhibitor titer and early intervention is associated with a higher success rate.

---

[3]Exceeds dosage recommended by the manufacturer.

ITI should be performed under the care of an experienced HTC. As such, specific protocols are not outlined in this chapter.

## Acquired Hemophilia

Acquired inhibitors occur later in life and are autoantibodies, predominantly to FVIII. Risk factors include diseases such as systemic lupus erythematosus (SLE), rheumatoid arthritis, malignancies, inflammatory bowel disease, and peripartum. More than 50% of cases have no identifiable cause. An estimated 30% to 40% remit spontaneously, and heroic interventions may not be necessary. When needed, the management of such patients can be difficult, with mortality rates exceeding 20%. A similar approach as outlined earlier for congenital hemophilia patients can be used, including ITI. rFVIIa has had more than 90% efficacy in the surgery setting for this high-risk group.

## Preventive Measures

The primary focus of early intervention is to prevent the onset of chronic sequelae associated with bleeds. To that aim, primary and secondary prophylaxis are advocated. The success of prophylaxis is evidenced by the marked decline in arthropathies and hospitalizations in the past 5 years. Factor infusion at 20 to 40 U/kg two to three times a week, particularly prior to organized sports or physical activity, reduces bleeds. Plasma factor level should be kept within the 1% to 2% range for effective prophylaxis, although beneficial effects are seen even when these levels are not strictly enforced. In the infant and young child, primary prophylaxis is started prior to chronic arthropathy or co-morbidities. This often requires placement of a central venous access with associated risks of infection and thrombosis. Secondary prophylaxis should be encouraged in the older child or teenager and adult. The benefits of decreased bleeds, increased school or work attendance, and general quality of life is well documented.

Routine well child immunizations including hepatitis A and B vaccines should be given. Regular exercise and development of good muscle tone and strength decreases joint and muscle bleeds, not to mention optimizing the development of self-esteem and social interaction. Affected children are encouraged to participate in activities such as swimming and group sports with the proviso of consistent use of protective gear such as helmets and knee/elbow pads.

## Adjunctive Therapy

Antifibrinolytics such as ε-aminocaproic acid (εACA) (Amicar) or tranexamic acid (Cyklokapron) decrease clot lysis. εACA is available in liquid, tablet, and IV forms. The liquid preparation comes in 250 mg/mL, and 50 mg/kg can be used four times daily[1] for 5 to 7 days. It should be used with extreme caution, if at all, in GI or renal bleeds. Antifibrinolytics are used with rFVIIa. Other agents include fibrin sealants, topical thrombin, and microfibrillar collagen, especially in the presence of mucosal bleeds. Adequate analgesia, for example, acetaminophen (Tylenol) with codeine or morphine, may be necessary for pain relief. Anti-inflammatory medications such as steroids are used in some cases to reduce edema in acute hemorrhage or synovitis. However, medications affecting platelet function such as aspirin or ibuprofen should be avoided. The mnemonic RICE—Rest, Ice, Compression, Elevation—should be applied to joint bleeds, although ice is often difficult to maintain on an irritable child. Oral contraceptives may reduce menorrhagia and also increase plasma FVIII and FIX levels.

### GENE TRANSFER

Preliminary clinical trials of various FVIII and FIX gene transfer modalities can produce the target factor but are unable to maintain a sustained factor level. More studies are ongoing, but a detailed discussion is beyond the scope of this article.

## VON WILLEBRAND'S DISEASE

DDAVP (Stimate) is effective in raising FVIII and vWf levels three to four times that of baseline levels in most individuals with mild to moderate hemophilia and vWd. It can be used for dental extractions and minor procedures. Stimate does not raise the level in severely affected individuals adequately to achieve hemostasis (e.g., a 1% baseline vWf level would only increase to 3% to 4% postadministration). Stimate can be administered IV or intranasally. IV dosage is 0.3 μg/kg. Intranasal dosage is 1 squirt (approximately 150 μg) for those less than 50 kg and 2 squirts for patients more than 50 kg. Intranasal administration is more convenient for most patients with faster access to treatment because they can carry the dispenser with them at all times. Side effects include facial flushing, transient blood pressure increases, and fluid retention. Fluid restriction is required to decrease the risk of hypertension, hyponatremia, and seizures. Stimate is contraindicated in neonates and the elderly (older than 75 years). Average time to peak level of FVIII and vWf is 45 minutes after IV and 90 minutes after intranasal administration. With its rapid response, it is most likely that the mechanism of action of Stimate is release of the premanufactured FVIII and vWf from storage sites. Because of depletion of stores from frequent use, Stimate should only be given one to two times a day for a maximum of 3 days consecutively. A trial dose is given at the HTC, and pre- and postdose levels are measured to document an adequate response prior to prescription of the drug for use. Educational sessions on its appropriate use and possible side effects have to be given *prior* to dispensing Stimate. A few patients may respond to the IV route of administration after failing the intranasal trial.

Key points in the use of DDAVP for mild hemophilia A and type 1 vWd are as follows:

- Only the concentrated form (1.5 mg/mL) of DDAVP should be used. The trade name is Stimate. Reference should be made only to Stimate as the appropriate medication to avoid prescription and dispensing errors. DDAVP used for enuresis is ineffective in achieving hemostatic control.
- Fluid should be restricted just prior to and for 12 to 24 hours postadministration.
- The treating physician should be notified if hemostasis is not achieved after the first two doses. Tachyphylaxis and concomitant side effects should be considered.

Treatment for patients with type 2s and 3 vWd require IV factor concentrate replacements containing adequate amounts of vWf. Table 2 lists these preparations that include Humate-P and Alphanate. Dosage for Humate-P can be calculated based on the vWf activity expressed as ristocetin cofactor (vWf:RCoF) units. For minor procedures and bleeding, 40 to 50 IU/kg every 8 to 12 hours for one to two doses is usually sufficient. However, major surgeries and bleeds including suspected intracranial hemorrhage (ICH) would require a loading dose of 60 to 80 IU/kg, then 40 to 60 IU/kg every 8 to 12 hours for a minimum of 5 to 10 days, keeping the vWf:RCoF activity more than 50%. Stimate is used as adjunctive therapy in type 3 vWd but should be avoided in most type 2 and platelet-type vWd patients. Recombinant and high-purity FVIII and FIX concentrates should *not* be used for vWd.

Recombinant vWF is available only at a research level and is being developed for future clinical trials. Adjunctive therapy as listed for hemophilia applies generally to vWd as well, including oral progesterone-containing contraceptives.

## Other Related Disorders

Deficiencies of the other factors are often diagnosed by the APTT, PT, and TT. There are rare cases of familial combined factor deficiencies (e.g., FV + FVIII, FVIII + FIX, FII + VII + IX + X). In the latter case, high doses of vitamin K may be helpful.

---

[1]Not FDA approved for this indication.

Severe FVII deficiency (prolonged PT, less than 1% FVII) can vary in presentation, although most neonates succumb to intracranial hemorrhage (ICH). It would seem rational that the principle of replacing the deficient factor applies in this disease as in hemophilia A and B. rFVII is efficacious in maintaining hemostasis at 20 to 30 µg/kg every 6 to 12 hours. For the rest of the factor deficiencies that present with bleeding, fresh-frozen plasma (FFP) is often effective. Specific factor replacement is usually not available in the United States (e.g., FXI). Fibrinogen (Factor I) abnormalities require cryoprecipitate for effective hemostasis. FXIII deficiency can be treated with FFP or cryoprecipitate. Prophylactic treatment with FFP uses 10 mL/kg, or 1 to 2 U in adults every 4 to 6 weeks, or cryoprecipitate, 1 bag/10 kg body weight. The amount of each factor in FFP and cryoprecipitate varies according to the donor pool. Dosage varies according to the severity of bleeds and the half-life of the plasma factor involved. It is advisable for the overall treatment of any patient with a bleeding diathesis to be carried out at or under the guidance of a HTC.

## REFERENCES

Ewing NP, Sanders NL, Dietrich SL, et al: Induction of immune tolerance of factor VIII in hemophiliacs with inhibitors. JAMA 1988;259:65-68.

Fuente B, Kasper CK, Rickles FR, et al: Response of patients with mild and moderate hemophilia A and von Willebrand disease to treatment with desmopressin. Ann Intern Med 1985;103:6-15.

Lusher JM, Arkin S, Abildgaard CF, et al: Recombinant factor VIII for the treatment of previously untreated patients with hemophilia. N Engl J Med 1993;328:453-459.

Manco-Johnson MJ, Nuss R, Geraghty S, et al: Results of secondary prophylaxis in children with severe hemophilia. Am J Hematol 1994;47:113-117.

Roth DA, Tawa NE, O'Brien J, et al: Non-viral gene transfer of blood coagulation factor VIII in patients with severe hemophilia A. Blood 2000;96:2532 [abstract].

Souci JM, Nuss R, Evatt B, et al: Mortality among males with hemophilia: Relations with source of medical care. Blood 2000;96:437-442.

Tuddenheam EGD, Schwabb R, Seehafer J, et al: Haemophilia A: Database of nucleotide substitutions, deletions, insertions and rearrangements of the factor VIII gene, second edition. Nucleic Acid Res 1994;22:3511-3533.

Warrier I, Koerper MA, DiMichele D, et al: Factor IX inhibitors and anaphylaxis in hemophilia B. J Pediatr Hematol Oncol 1997;19:23-27.

# Platelet-Mediated Bleeding Disorders

Method of
*Suman Sood, MD, and Charles S. Abrams, MD*

Quantitative and qualitative platelet defects are commonly encountered in clinical practice and can result in bleeding diatheses.

## Elements of Platelet Function

The vascular endothelium separates platelets from adhesive substrates in the subendothelial connective tissue. Platelet-mediated hemostasis is initiated by adherence to exposed collagen, fibronectin, and laminin following a breach to the vessel wall. Intracellular signaling cascades lead to secretion of platelet granules, synthesis, and release of thromboxane $A_2$, and a conformational change in platelet surface glycoprotein IIb/IIIa (GPIIb/IIIa) that enables it to bind soluble fibrinogen or von Willebrand's factor (vWF). Release of thromboxane $A_2$ and agonists within the secretion granules, such as adenosine diphosphate (ADP) and serotonin, activate neighboring platelets to perpetuate the process.

Fibrinogen binding to GPIIb/IIIa cross-links the platelets into a hemostatic plug, resulting in platelet aggregation and accumulation at the site of injury. Other signaling pathways initiated by agonists such as thrombin, thromboxane $A_2$, and collagen help promote the process of aggregation. Activated platelet plasma membrane interacts with circulating coagulation factors and provides a surface for assembly and generation of active factor X and thrombin. Secondary hemostasis occurs when the platelet plug is stabilized further by a thrombin-mediated fibrin mesh. The arrest of bleeding in a superficial wound almost exclusively results from the primary hemostatic plug.

Platelet-mediated bleeding disorders are characterized by a prolonged bleeding time, mucocutaneous bleeding, petechiae, and purpura. In contrast, deficiencies in secondary hemostasis result in delayed deep bleeding, such as bleeding into muscles and joints.

## Quantitative Bleeding Disorders

Adequate numbers of platelets are required to achieve primary hemostasis. Thrombocytopenia can result from decreased platelet production by bone marrow megakaryocytes, accelerated platelet removal, or platelet sequestration in an enlarged spleen. The clinical context is essential because there is no easy test to differentiate among these possibilities. Most commonly, thrombocytopenia is caused by accelerated platelet removal.

Hemorrhage following trauma or surgery generally does not occur if the platelet count is more than 50,000/µL. In an otherwise hemostatically normal patient, significant spontaneous bleeding usually does not occur with a platelet count greater than 5000 to 10,000/µL. However, there is no absolute threshold for spontaneous bleeding due to thrombocytopenia, and spontaneous bleeding can occur at higher counts when fever, sepsis, severe anemia, and other hemostatic defects are present or when platelet function is impaired by medication. Notably, a prolonged cutaneous bleeding time does not accurately predict clinical bleeding.

### THROMBOCYTOPENIA DUE TO DECREASED PLATELET PRODUCTION

Decreased platelet production occurs in primary diseases of the bone marrow such as acute leukemia and aplastic anemia; myelophthisic processes in which marrow is replaced by metastatic carcinoma, fibrosis, or multiple myeloma; following chemotherapy or radiation therapy; with ethanol toxicity; and during infections with viruses such as HIV, cytomegalovirus (CMV), Epstein-Barr virus (EBV), and varicella. Thrombocytopenia also occurs when megakaryocyte proliferation is impaired by myelodysplasia.

Overt bleeding in these disorders, when clearly a result of thrombocytopenia, is treated by platelet transfusion. Prophylactic platelet transfusion, however, is an area of controversy and is complicated by the short life span of platelets (10 days), the 5-day shelf life of stored platelets, and platelet immunogenicity. In patients undergoing treatment for acute leukemia, outcome is unchanged when platelet counts of 5,000 to 10,000/µL are used as the threshold for prophylactic transfusion. Single-donor apheresis platelets or platelet donors who are HLA identical to the recipient should be considered to prevent alloimmunization. The multicenter Platelet Dose trial in patients with malignancy is currently accruing and should help clarify these issues.

### THROMBOCYTOPENIA DUE TO INCREASED PLATELET DESTRUCTION

Nonimmune and immune processes can lead to a shortened platelet life span. Nonimmune causes include sepsis, disseminated intravascular coagulation (DIC), thrombotic thrombocytopenic purpura/hemolytic uremic syndrome (TTP/HUS), preeclampsia and eclampsia, cardiopulmonary bypass, and giant cavernous hemangiomas. The thrombocytopenia resolves with treatment of the underlying disorder, and platelet transfusion is rarely necessary. In TTP/HUS, thrombocytopenia is associated with thrombosis rather than bleeding, and controversial reports exist of clinical deterioration following platelet transfusion.

Immune-mediated platelet destruction can occur due to medication, alloimmune sensitization, or autoimmunity. Medications should always be considered a possible cause of thrombocytopenia. The potential list is long, but drugs with strong evidence of antibody-mediated platelet destruction include quinine (Qualaquin), quinidine, sulfonamides, and gold salts. Besides stopping the offending medication, emergent treatment for severe thrombocytopenia with bleeding includes platelet transfusion, and corticosteroids with or without intravenous immunoglobulin (IVIg).

Heparin-induced thrombocytopenia (HIT) is a special case of drug-induced thrombocytopenia associated with arterial and venous thrombosis rather than bleeding. HIT occurs in 2% to 5% of patients given unfractionated heparin by any route for 5 to 10 days. Antibodies develop to a heparin–platelet factor 4 (PF4) complex. HIT must always be considered when thrombocytopenia is detected in a hospitalized patient. If a patient has HIT, all heparin administration should be stopped, and alternative anticoagulation such as the direct thrombin inhibitors recombinant hirudin and argatroban should be instituted, at least until the platelet count normalizes. Warfarin (Coumadin) should not be used in acute HIT because of its delayed therapeutic effect and association with a syndrome of venous limb gangrene. Platelet transfusions in this disease are controversial, because some reports suggest that they can precipitate thrombotic complications.

Alloimmune thrombocytopenia due to sensitization to alloantigens such as Pl$^{A1}$ can result from transfusion (post-transfusion purpura, PTP) or maternal sensitization during pregnancy (neonatal alloimmune thrombocytopenia, NAIT). PTP causes profound thrombocytopenia 7 to 10 days after transfusion and can be treated with IVIg or plasma exchange. NAIT can cause severe thrombocytopenia and bleeding in neonates and is treated with platelet transfusion, corticosteroids, and IVIg.

Autoimmune thrombocytopenia, also known as idiopathic thrombocytopenic purpura (ITP), is caused by circulating antiplatelet autoantibodies. An ITP-like picture can also occur in autoimmune diseases such as systemic lupus erythematosus, in patients with low-grade lymphoproliferative disorders such as chronic lymphocytic leukemia, and in patients with HIV infections. ITP can occur at any age in both sexes and manifests with either mucocutaneous bleeding or unexplained asymptomatic thrombocytopenia. The complete blood count (CBC) is otherwise normal, splenomegaly is absent, and peripheral blood smears are only remarkable for a decreased number of platelets, some of which may be larger than normal. Bone marrow examination is usually not necessary in the absence of other findings suggesting myelodysplasia, but it typically shows normal or increased numbers of megakaryocytes.

Management of ITP is guided by symptoms and platelet count. Asymptomatic patients with platelet counts greater than 30,000/μL can be followed without treatment. With bleeding or a platelet count less than 30,000/μL, treatment with prednisone is initiated. Refractory patients may require splenectomy (60%-75% remission rate), other immunosuppressive medications, or new thrombopoiesis-stimulating agents. Emergent presentation with severe thrombocytopenia (<5000/μL) or internal bleeding should be treated with high doses of pulse corticosteroids or IVIg, or both. Platelet transfusion may be given concurrently with the IVIg for critical bleeding. Anti-D immune globulin may be substituted for IVIg in Rh$^+$ patients who have not undergone splenectomy; however, occasional patients develop severe autoimmune hemolysis.

## THROMBOCYTOPENIA DUE TO HYPERSPLENISM

Approximately 30% of the circulating platelet mass is normally present in the spleen. Additional platelets may be sequestered when the spleen enlarges due to portal hypertension or infiltrative diseases. Platelet counts in patients with hypersplenism generally are not lower than 40,000 to 50,000/μL. Consequently, bleeding due to thrombocytopenia from hypersplenism alone is unusual.

---

 **CURRENT DIAGNOSIS**

- Platelet-mediated bleeding disorders are characterized by a prolonged bleeding time, mucocutaneous bleeding, petechiae, and purpura.
- Thrombocytopenia can result from decreased platelet production, accelerated platelet removal, or platelet sequestration in an enlarged spleen.
- In an otherwise hemostatically normal patient, significant spontaneous bleeding generally does not occur until the platelet count declines to <5000-10,000/μL. A prolonged bleeding time does not predict clinical bleeding.
- Medications are common causes of quantitative and qualitative platelet defects.
- Heparin-induced thrombocytopenia must always be considered when thrombocytopenia is detected in a hospitalized patient.
- Idiopathic thrombocytopenic purpura manifests as otherwise unexplained spontaneous mucocutaneous bleeding or asymptomatic thrombocytopenia and is a diagnosis of exclusion.
- Although many medications impair platelet function in vitro, only a few, including aspirin, ticlopidine (Ticlid), clopidogrel (Plavix), and the glycoprotein IIb/IIIa antagonists induce clinically significant bleeding.
- While hereditary disorders of platelet adhesion and aggregation are rare, hereditary disorders of platelet secretion are not uncommon causes of easy bruising, menorrhagia, and excessive postoperative and postpartum blood loss. Platelet aggregation studies are helpful for diagnosis.

---

# Qualitative Platelet Disorders

## ACQUIRED QUALITATIVE PLATELET DISORDERS

Acquired disorders of platelet function are relatively common but are usually asymptomatic or mild. Nonetheless, they can be of substantial clinical importance when engrafted on another hemostatic abnormality. They are subclassified as resulting from drugs, hematologic diseases, and systemic disorders. Drugs are the most common cause of dysfunction, most notably aspirin, which irreversibly inactivates the enzyme cyclooxygenase-1 (COX-1), thus inducing a permanent blockade in platelet prostaglandin synthesis and consequently thromboxane A$_2$ synthesis. Although the antihemostatic effect is minimal in normal persons, it may be quite prominent in a patient with an underlying bleeding disorder. Nonsteroidal anti-inflammatory drugs (NSAIDs) reversibly inhibit platelet prostaglandin synthesis and generally have little effect on hemostasis. Other medications that interfere significantly with platelet function include clopidogrel (Plavix), ticlopidine (Ticlid), and GPIIb/IIIa receptor antagonists. Numerous other drugs have been implicated in platelet dysfunction in case reports, but the evidence for most of these medications is less well established.

Bone marrow processes that can produce intrinsically abnormal platelets include myeloproliferative disorders, leukemias, myelodysplastic syndromes, and dysproteinemias such as multiple myeloma and Waldenström's macroglobulinemia, in which abnormal plasma proteins impair platelet function. In addition, acquired forms of von Willebrand's disease, a rare disorder that can arise secondary to critical aortic stenosis, multiple myeloma, or other clonal lymphoproliferative disorders, can lead to a bleeding diathesis.

Renal failure is the most prominent systemic disorder associated with abnormal platelet function. The hemostatic defect is generally mild and corrects rapidly with the initiation of dialysis. Intravenous desmopressin (DDAVP), a vasopressin analogue that causes release of von Willebrand's factor (vWF) from tissue stores, is helpful in uremia, shortening bleeding time in 50% to 75% of patients. Dosing may be

## CURRENT THERAPY

- In the absence of bleeding, platelet counts of 5000-10,000/µL are used as the threshold for prophylactic transfusion. Single-donor apheresis platelets should be considered to prevent alloimmunization.

- For hemorrhaging patients or for patients scheduled to undergo delicate operations such as neurosurgery, maintaining the platelet count greater than 75,000 to 100,000/µL is recommended.

- When heparin-induced thrombocytopenia is a possibility, all heparin administration must be stopped and alternative anticoagulation instituted, at least until the platelet count returns to normal.

- Because bleeding in patients with ITP is usually minimal to absent until platelet counts decline to <30,000/µL, asymptomatic patients with platelet counts >30,000 can be followed without treatment.

- Treatment for ITP is initiated with prednisone (1 mg/kg); patients who fail to enter clinical remission are candidates for splenectomy or treatment with immunosuppressive agents including rituximab[1] (Rituxan) and azathioprine[1] (Imuran).

- High doses of corticosteroids (methylprednisolone (Solu-Medrol, 1 g/d for 3 d) or IVIg (1 g/kg/d for 2 d) are indicated for emergency treatment of ITP. Platelet transfusion given concurrently with IVIg can be effective for critical bleeding. Anti-D immune globulin (WinRho) may be used instead of IVIg in Rh+ patients, although this treatment can induce clinically significant hemolysis.

- The platelet dysfunction of uremia is usually corrected by dialysis. Maintaining the hemoglobin above 10 g/dL helps minimize bleeding by increasing interactions between platelets and the blood vessel wall. Intravenous desmopressin (DDAVP) given at a dose of 0.3 µg/kg IV over 15 to 30 minutes shortens the bleeding time in most patients with uremia for approximately 4 hours.

- When necessary, treatment of hereditary disorders of platelet adhesion and aggregation usually requires platelet transfusion.

---

[1]Not FDA approved for this indication.
*Abbreviations:* ITP = idiopathic thrombocytopenic purpura; IVIg = intravenous immunoglobulin.

repeated, although tachyphylaxis can occur. Maintaining the hemoglobin greater than 10 g/dL can optimize the efficiency of platelets by enhancing the interactions between platelets and the blood vessel wall. DIC can also lead to impaired platelet function. Thrombocytopenia is a consistent feature of cardiopulmonary bypass surgery, typically secondary to hemodilution, platelet membrane activation from interaction with the bypass circuit, and fragmentation from hypothermia. It generally resolves spontaneously within several days after bypass, but platelet transfusions may be helpful if bleeding persists.

## HEREDITARY QUALITATIVE PLATELET DISORDERS

Bernard-Soulier syndrome (BSS) and Glanzmann's thrombasthenia (GT) are rare autosomal recessive disorders of the platelet membrane glycoproteins GPIb/IX and GPIIb/IIIa, respectively. They manifest with mucocutaneous bleeding in infancy or childhood. Patients with BSS are also thrombocytopenic and have very large platelets that do not agglutinate when exposed to ristocetin. Platelet counts and

morphology are normal in GT, but the platelets cannot aggregate in response to ADP or thrombin. Reliable treatment of bleeding in both conditions requires platelet transfusion.

Hereditary disorders of platelet secretion are not uncommon causes of mucocutaneous bleeding and can be due to alpha granule deficiency (gray platelet syndrome), the more common dense granule deficiency (δ storage pool disease [δSPD]), or to aspirin-like defects resulting from abnormalities of the platelet secretory mechanism. δSPD may be associated with albinism (Hermansky-Pudlack and Chédiak-Higashi syndromes) or occur in otherwise normal persons. Patients with δSPD have normal platelet counts with prolonged bleeding times and abnormal platelet aggregation studies with a diagnostic increased adenosine triphosphate-to-adenosine diphosphate (ATP/ADP) ratio due to the absence of platelet dense granule ADP. Although bleeding in patients with secretion disorders can be controlled by platelet transfusion, DDAVP sometimes shortens the bleeding times and improves hemostasis.

## REFERENCES

Bennett JS: Novel platelet inhibitors. Ann Rev Med 2001;52:161-184.
Bolton-Maggs PHB, Chalmers EA, Collins PW, et al: A review of inherited platelet disorders with guidelines for their management on behalf of the UKHCDO. Br J Haematol 2006;135:603-633.
Cines DB, Blanchette VS: Immune thrombocytopenic purpura. N Engl J Med 2002;346:995-1008.
Kaw D, Malhotra D: Platelet dysfunction and end-stage renal disease. Semin Dial 2006;19:317-22.
Lind SE: The bleeding time does not predict surgical bleeding. Blood 1991;77:2547-2552.
Mannucci PM: Drug therapy: Treatment of von Willebrand's disease. N Engl J Med 2004;351:683-694.
Nurden AT: Qualitative disorders of platelets and megakaryocytes. J Thromb Hemostasis 2006;3:1773-1782.
Stanworth SJ, Hyde C, Brunskill S, et al: Platelet transfusion prophylaxis for patients with hematological malignancies: Where to now? Br J Haematol 2005;131:588-595.
Warkentin TE: Heparin-induced thrombocytopenia: Pathogenesis and management. Br J Haematol 2003;121:535-555.

# Disseminated Intravascular Coagulation

Method of
*Marcel Levi, MD*

Systemic activation of coagulation can occur in the context of a variety of disorders, most of which are associated with inflammatory activation. This coagulation activation may only be detectable by measuring sensitive molecular markers for activation of coagulation factors and pathways, but it can become clinically manifest as changes in routine coagulation tests occur. The spectrum of clinically manifest coagulation activation ranges from a small decrease in platelet count and subclinical prolongation of global clotting times to fulminant disseminated intravascular coagulation (DIC) characterized by simultaneous widespread microvascular thrombosis and profuse bleeding from various sites.

Another group of syndromes that lead to microvascular obstruction and consequent organ dysfunction is represented by the thrombotic microangiopathies. Thrombotic microangiopathies encompass syndromes such as thrombotic thrombocytopenic purpura (TTP), the hemolytic-uremic syndrome (HUS), severe malignant hypertension, chemotherapy-induced microangiopathic hemolytic anemia, and the HELLP (*h*emolysis, *e*levated *l*iver enzymes, *l*ow *p*latelets) syndrome.

Clinically, these two groups of diseases manifest with similar characteristics, and a common pathologic hallmark of both groups is endothelial cell pertubation and damage, but the etiology and pathophysiology are quite different. Consequently, adequate management of each of these disorders requires a different approach, and thus a proper differential diagnosis is of utmost importance.

## Pathophysiology

### DISSEMINATED INTRAVASCULAR COAGULATION

DIC is not a disease in itself but is always secondary to an underlying disorder. DIC is a syndrome caused by systemic intravascular activation of coagulation, which may be secondary to various underlying conditions. Formation of microvascular thrombi, in concert with inflammatory activation, can cause failure of the microvasculature and thereby contribute to organ dysfunction. Ongoing and insufficiently compensated consumption of platelets and coagulation factors can pose a risk factor for bleeding, especially in perioperative patients or patients who need to undergo invasive procedures.

The trigger for the activation of the coagulation system is nearly always mediated by several of the proinflammatory cytokines expressed and released by mononuclear cells and endothelial cells. Thrombin generation proceeds via the (extrinsic) tissue factor/factor VIIa route. Tissue factor may be expressed on activated and inactivated mononuclear cells and endothelial cells and is capable of binding factor VIIa, which then activates downstream coagulation cascades. Concomitantly, function of inhibitory mechanisms of thrombin generation, such as antithrombin III and the proteins C and S system, is impaired.

Antithrombin appears to be incapable of adequate regulation of thrombin activity in DIC for several reasons. Antithrombin levels are continuously consumed by the ongoing formation of thrombin and other activated proteases that are susceptible to antithrombin complex formation, and antithrombin is degraded by elastase released from activated neutrophils. Liver failure and extravascular leakage of this protease inhibitor occur as a consequence of capillary leakage; because of this, impaired synthesis of antithrombin further contributes to low levels of antithrombin.

There are several reasons for severe injury to the protein C system in DIC. As with antithrombin, enhanced consumption, impaired liver synthesis, and vascular leakage can result in low circulating levels of protein C. Second, activation of the cytokine network, in particular high levels of tumor necrosis factor $\alpha$ (TNF-$\alpha$), results in a marked down-regulation of thrombomodulin on endothelial cells, thereby prohibiting adequate protein C activation. In addition, the anticoagulant capacity of activated protein C is reduced by low levels of the free fraction of protein S. In plasma, 60% of the cofactor protein S is complexed to a complement regulatory protein, C4b binding protein (C4bBP), and increased plasma levels of C4bBP as a consequence of the acute phase reaction in sepsis can result in a relative protein S deficiency.

A third mechanism contributing to the enhanced fibrin deposition in DIC is impaired fibrin degradation, due to high circulating levels of plasminogen activator inhibitor 1 (PAI-1), the main physiologic inhibitor of fibrinolysis. Recent studies have shown that a functional mutation in the *PAI-1* gene, the 4G/5G polymorphism, not only influenced the plasma levels of PAI-1 but also was linked to clinical outcome in sepsis and DIC. In other clinical studies in patients with DIC, a high plasma level of PAI-1 was one of the strongest predictors of mortality.

### THROMBOTIC MICROANGIOPATHIES

A common pathogenetic feature of the thrombotic microangiopathies appears to be endothelial damage, causing platelet adhesion and aggregation, thrombin formation, and an impaired fibrinolysis. The multiple clinical consequences of this extensive endothelial dysfunction include thrombocytopenia, mechanical fragmentation of red cells with hemolytic anemia, and obstruction of the microvasculature of various organs, such as the kidneys and brain (leading to renal failure and neurologic dysfunction, respectively).

Despite this common final pathway, the various thrombotic microangiopathies have different underlying etiologies. TTP is caused by deficiency of von Willebrand's factor cleaving protease (ADAMTS-13), resulting in endothelial cell-attached ultra-large von Willebrand's multimers, which readily bind to platelet surface glycoprotein (GP) Ib and cause platelet adhesion and aggregation. Genetic mutations in the *ADAMTS13* gene associated with lower activity of the protease have been linked to the occurrence of juvenile and familial TTP. Acquired deficiency of ADAMTS13, due to an autoantibody, has been demonstrated to occur in patients with sporadic TTP. The formation of platelet aggregates in the microvasculature subsequently lead to microvascular obstruction, consumption thrombocytopenia, and mechanical hemolytic anemia.

In HUS, a cytotoxin released on infection with a specific serogroup of gram-negative microorganisms (usually *Escherichia coli* serotype O157:H7) is responsible for endothelial cell and platelet activation.

In the case of malignant hypertension or chemotherapy-induced thrombotic microangiopathy, presumably direct mechanical or chemical damage, respectively, to the endothelium is responsible for the enhanced endothelial cell–platelet interaction.

## Differential Diagnosis

Patients with DIC have a low or rapidly decreasing platelet count, prolonged global coagulation tests, low plasma levels of coagulation factors and inhibitors, and increased markers of fibrin formation or degradation, or both, such as D-dimer or fibrin degradation products (FDPs). Coagulation proteins with a marked acute phase behavior, such as factor VIII or fibrinogen, are usually not decreased or might even increase. One of the often-advocated laboratory tests for the diagnosis of DIC, fibrinogen, is therefore not a very good marker for DIC, except in very severe cases, although sequential measurements can give some insight.

There is no single laboratory test with sufficient accuracy for the diagnosis of DIC. However, a diagnosis of DIC may be made using a simple scoring system based on a combination of routinely available coagulation tests (see the Current Diagnosis box). In a prospective

---

 **CURRENT DIAGNOSIS**

**Diagnostic Algorithm for Diagnosing DIC**

1. Score global coagulation test results:
   a. Platelet count:
      $>100 \times 10^9/L = 0$, $<100 \times 10^9/L = 1$, $< 50 \times 10^9/L = 2$
   b. Elevated fibrin-related marker (e.g., fibrin degradation products or D-dimer*):
      No increase = 0, moderate increase = 2, strong increase = 3
   c. Prolonged prothrombin time:
      <3 sec = 0, >3 but <6 sec = 1, >6 sec = 2
   d. Fibrinogen level:
      >1.0 g/L = 0, < 1.0 g/L = 1
2. Calculate score:
   >5: Compatible with overt DIC; repeat scoring daily.
   <5: Suggestive (not affirmative) for nonovert DIC; repeat next 1-2 days.

---

*In the prospective validation studies, D-dimer assays were used, and a value above the upper limit of normal (0.4 μg/L) was considered moderately elevated, whereas a value above 10 times the upper limit of normal (4.0 μg/L) was considered as a strong increase.

validation study, the sensitivity and specificity of this DIC score were found to be more than 95%. Furthermore, this DIC score was found to be a strong and independent predictor of mortality in a large series of patients with severe sepsis, and it identifies patients who will have most benefit from interventions in the coagulation system.

A diagnosis of thrombotic microangiopathy relies on the combination of thrombocytopenia, Coombs'-negative hemolytic anemia, and the presence of schistocytes in the blood smear. Additional information can be achieved by measurement of ADAMTS-13 and autoantibodies toward this metalloprotease and by culture (usually from the stool or urine) of microorganisms capable of producing cytotoxin in case of HUS. Importantly, and as a general distinguishing feature from DIC, patients with thrombotic microangiopathies have no or just minor signs of activation of plasmatic coagulation (normal or only slightly abnormal prothrombin time and activated partial thromboplastin time (PT and aPTT).

## Treatment

### DISSEMINATED INTRAVASCULAR COAGULATION

The basis of DIC treatment is the specific and vigorous treatment of the underlying disorder. However, additional supportive treatment specifically aimed at the coagulation abnormalities may be required.

Low levels of platelets and coagulation factors can increase the risk of bleeding. However, plasma or platelet substitution therapy should not be instituted on the basis of laboratory results alone; it is only indicated in patients with active bleeding and in those requiring an invasive procedure or otherwise at risk for bleeding complications.

Experimental studies have shown that heparin can at least partly inhibit the activation of coagulation in sepsis and other causes of DIC. A recent large trial in patients with sepsis showed a slight benefit of low-dose heparin on 28-day mortality and underscored the importance of not stopping heparin in patients with DIC and abnormal coagulation parameters.

The use of antithrombin III concentrates in patients with DIC has been studied relatively intensively. All trials showed some beneficial effect in terms of improvement of laboratory parameters, shortening of the duration of DIC; however, none of the trials demonstrated a significant reduction of mortality. A large-scale multicenter randomized, controlled trial to directly address this issue also showed no significant reduction in mortality of septic patients who were treated with antithrombin concentrate. Interestingly, the subgroup of patients who had DIC and who did not receive heparin showed a remarkable survival benefit, but this needs prospective validation

Based on the notion that depression of the protein C system can significantly contribute to the pathophysiology of DIC, supplementation of activated protein C[1] (Xigris) might potentially be of benefit. A beneficial effect of recombinant human activated protein C was demonstrated in two randomized, controlled trials. The potential benefit of activated protein C was also shown for duration of mechanical ventilation, shock, and length of ICU stay as well as for days free of systemic inflammatory response. Activated protein C appears to be relatively more effective in patients with more severe disease, and a prospective trial in septic patients with relatively low disease severity did not show any benefit of activated protein C. Also, in the protein C studies, patients with DIC seemed to have the greatest benefit from this treatment.

### THROMBOTIC MICROANGIOPATHIES

For a long time, treatment of TTP by infusion of large volumes of donor plasma or plasmapheresis was known to positively affect the clinical course of patients with the congenital or acquired form of this disease. The rationale for this treatment has now become clear, because with this strategy the deficiency of ADAMTS13 will be corrected. In addition, patients with acquired TTP should receive immunosuppressive regimens, usually including steroids.

---

[1]Not FDA approved for this indication, but approved for sepsis.

## CURRENT THERAPY

The cornerstone of the treatment of DIC is treatment of the underlying disorder.

- Supportive treatment aimed at the coagulation derangement in patients with DIC could include:
  - Transfusion of plasma: Only in case of bleeding or around invasive procedure and if the PT and/or aPTT is prolonged. Recommended dose: 4-6 U/24 h.
  - Transfusion of platelets: Only in case of bleeding and if the platelet count is $<50\times10^9$/L. Recommended dose: 5-10 donor units/24 h.
  - Heparin: As low-dose prophylactic (low-molecular-weight) heparin. Should not be stopped in case of DIC and should not be stopped when treatment with activated protein C is initiated. Should not be combined with antithrombin treatment. Recommended dose: unfractionated heparin 7500 U SC, or enoxaparin[1] (Lovenox) 20 mg, or nadroparin[2] (Fraxiparine) 2850 anti–factor Xa units (all SC).
  - Recombinant human activated protein C (drotrecogin alfa, activated, Xigris) in case of DIC complicating sepsis. Recommended dose: 24 µg/kg/h for 4 days.
  - Antithrombin[1*] (Thrombate) concentrate. Usually considered when antithrombin level is <20%-30%. Recommended dose: 7500 U[3]/24 h.
- Treatment of TTP is based on plasmapheresis (at least 6 units of plasma/24 h) and institution of immunosuppressive therapy (usually high-dose steroids). If no rapid increase in platelet count occurs, treatment should be intensified.
- Treatment of other types of thrombotic microangiopathies is based on adequate treatment of the underlying disorder and supportive treatment aimed at specific organ failures (e.g., renal replacement therapy in case of renal failure).

---

[1]Not FDA approved for this indication.
[2]Not available in the United States.
[3]Exceeds dosage recommended by the manufacturer.
[*]Not EMEA approved for this indication.
*Abbreviations:* aPTT = activated partial thromboplastin time; DIC = disseminated intravascular coagulation; EMEA = European Agency for the Evaluation of Medicinal Products; PT = prothrombin time; TTP = thrombotic thrombocytopenic purpura.

---

Patients with HUS do not benefit from plasma infusion and plasmapheresis, although this treatment is usually instituted awaiting definitive laboratory results excluding TTP. If a diagnosis of HUS has been established, therapy is merely supportive. Obviously, an underlying infection with a verotoxin-producing microorganism requires adequate antibiotic treatment.

Other forms of thrombotic microangiopathies are usually managed by proper treatment of the underlying disorder.

## REFERENCES

Bernard GR, Vincent JL, Laterre PF, et al: Efficacy and safety of recombinant human activated protein C for severe sepsis. N Engl J Med 2001;344(10):699-709.

George JN: Clinical practice: Thrombotic thrombocytopenic purpura. N Engl J Med 2006;354(18):1927-1935.

Levi M: Current understanding of disseminated intravascular coagulation. Br J Haematol 2004;124(5):567-576.

Levi M, van der Poll T, Buller HR: Bidirectional relation between inflammation and coagulation. Circulation 2004;109(22):2698-2704.

Mannucci PM: Thrombotic thromboytopenic purpura: Another example of immunomediated thrombosis. Pathophysiol Haemost Thromb 2006; 35(1-2):89-97.

Moake JL: Thrombotic microangiopathies. N Engl J Med 2002;347(8):589-600.

Taylor FBJ, Toh CH, Hoots WK, et al: Towards definition, clinical and laboratory criteria, and a scoring system for disseminated intravascular coagulation. Thromb Haemost 2001;86(5):1327-1330.

# Thrombotic Thrombocytopenic Purpura

Method of
*James N. George, MD*

Thrombotic thrombocytopenic purpura (TTP) is a multisystem disorder defined pathologically by platelet thrombi occluding arterioles and capillaries of nearly all organs. A review of all patients reported until 1964 described a characteristic pentad of abnormalities: thrombocytopenia, microangiopathic hemolytic anemia, neurologic and renal abnormalities, and fever. In 1991, the Canadian Apheresis Study Group documented the effectiveness of plasma exchange treatment; mortality was 22% compared to 90% in patients reported before 1964. The availability of effective therapy created the urgency for diagnosis; urgency for diagnosis required more limited diagnostic criteria. Current diagnostic criteria are only thrombocytopenia and microangiopathic hemolytic anemia without another apparent etiology.

## Etiologies and Associated Conditions

TTP is a syndrome with multiple etiologies. *Hemolytic uremic syndrome* (HUS), also diagnosed by thrombocytopenia and microangiopathic hemolytic anemia, is the term applied to the childhood illness caused by Shiga toxin-producing bacteria, such as *Escherichia coli* 0157:H7, and manifesting predominant renal failure. Most children with HUS following a prodrome of diarrhea survive with only supportive care. In adults, syndromes described as TTP or HUS are not distinct. Although it is commonly stated that patients with TTP have predominant neurologic abnormalities, whereas patients with HUS have predominant renal failure, some patients may have neither neurologic abnormalities nor renal failure or both. Therefore, among adults a distinction of TTP from HUS has no importance for initial diagnosis and management; the author uses the term TTP for all of the adult syndromes.

Table 1 describes clinical categories of TTP. Among patients with no preceding illness or apparent associated condition, termed *idiopathic TTP*, many have a deficiency of ADAMTS13, a plasma enzyme required for normal processing of von Willebrand's factor to smaller multimers. Acquired deficiency is caused by an autoantibody that inhibits ADAMTS13 activity; absence of ADAMTS13 activity results in abnormally large von Willebrand factor's multimers that facilitate formation of platelet thrombi. Deficiency of ADAMTS13 may not be sufficient to cause an acute episode of TTP. Acute episodes are often triggered by inflammatory conditions or pregnancy. The etiology of idiopathic TTP in patients without severe ADAMTS13 deficiency is not known. Congenital deficiencies of ADAMTS13 are very rare and not addressed here.

Drug-dependent antibodies can cause acute TTP as a result of diffuse endothelial damage resulting in microvascular thrombi. Quinine is the most common etiology. In addition to the characteristic features of TTP, including acute renal failure, quinine-dependent antibodies to diverse tissues can also cause liver toxicity, neutropenia, and disseminated intravascular coagulation. Ticlopidine (Ticlid) and clopidogrel (Plavix) are also associated with TTP. Other drugs, notably cancer chemotherapeutic and immunosuppressive (cyclosporine [Sandimmune], tacrolimus [Prograf]) agents, can cause a chronic, progressive, dose-dependent disorder similar to TTP. Syndromes similar to TTP may also occur in patients following allogeneic hematopoietic stem cell transplantation, but in many patients signs suggesting TTP following stem cell transplantation may actually be caused by systemic infections.

## Diagnosis

The unexpected observation of thrombocytopenia and microangiopathic hemolytic anemia initiates consideration of TTP. However, these minimal criteria are not specific. The most important diagnostic criterion is to exclude alternative etiologies. Thrombocytopenia and microangiopathic hemolytic anemia may also be caused by systemic infections, such as cytomegalovirus, Rocky Mountain spotted fever, and aspergillosis. Disseminated carcinoma causing occlusion of small vessels may mimic TTP. Malignant hypertension can cause all clinical features of TTP. The obstetric disorders of severe preeclampsia, eclampsia, and HELLP (*h*emolysis, *e*levated *l*iver function tests, *l*ow *p*latelets) syndrome may be initially indistinguishable from TTP. Acute flares of autoimmune disorders such as systemic lupus erythematosus may also be indistinguishable from TTP.

---

**TABLE 1   Clinical Categories of Acquired TTP**

| Category | Comments |
|---|---|
| Idiopathic | Defined by absence of the associated conditions described below. Many patients may have severe ADAMTS13 deficiency. Immunosuppressive treatment, in addition to plasma exchange, is appropriate. |
| Shiga toxin | Follows enterohemorrhagic infection with *Escherichia coli* 0157:H7 or other Shiga toxin–producing organism. The etiology for the typical HUS of children, who are treated only with supportive care. In adults, plasma exchange is appropriate. Immunosuppressive treatment unnecessary. |
| Drug-induced immunologic | Quinine most common etiology; may also occur with ticlopidine or clopidogrel. Plasma exchange may be beneficial; immunosuppressive treatment unnecessary. |
| Drug-induced, dose-dependent toxicity | May occur with cancer chemotherapeutic agents (e.g., mitomycin C [Mutamycin], gemcitabine [Gemzar]) or immunosuppressive agents (cyclosporine [Sandimmune], tacrolimus [Prograf]). Insidious onset, often after etiologic agent discontinued. Benefit of plasma exchange uncertain. |
| Hematopoietic stem cell transplantation | A syndrome with clinical features of TTP may occur after allogeneic transplants. In most patients, initially unrecognized systemic infection is the cause of signs that suggested TTP. Benefit of plasma exchange doubtful. |

*Abbreviations:* TTP = thrombotic thrombocytopenic purpura.

**CURRENT DIAGNOSIS**

- Suspicion for the diagnosis of TTP
  - Unexplained thrombocytopenia and anemia
- Support for the diagnosis of TTP:
  - Evidence for microangiopathic hemolysis: fragmented red cells on the peripheral blood smear, elevated levels of serum bilirubin and lactate dehydrogenase (LDH)
  - Presence of neurologic or renal function abnormalities
  - (High fever and chills are evidence against the diagnosis of TTP)
- Confirmation of the diagnosis of TTP:
  - Exclusion of alternative etiologies
    - Malignant hypertension
    - Systemic infection
    - Systemic neoplasm
    - Preeclampsia, eclampsia, HELLP syndrome
    - Autoimmune disorders, such as systemic lupus erythematosus

*Abbreviations:* HELLP = hemolysis, elevated liver enzymes, and low platelets; TTP = thrombotic thrombocytopenic purpura.

Because there are no conclusive diagnostic criteria, the decision to initiate plasma exchange treatment often depends on the severity of illness, progression of the patient's course, and confidence that other etiologies were excluded.

# Treatment

## PLASMA EXCHANGE THERAPY

Plasma exchange is the only treatment with effectiveness documented by a randomized clinical trial. The presence of severe acquired ADAMTS13 deficiency in some patients with TTP leads to the hypothesis that plasma exchange is effective because of removal of anti-ADAMTS13 antibodies and replacement of ADAMTS13 enzyme activity. However, plasma exchange treatment also appears to be effective in patients without ADAMTS13 deficiency. Although plasma exchange is not the standard treatment for children who have a diarrhea prodrome and the suspected etiology of *E. coli* 0157:H7, it may be beneficial in adults with TTP caused by *E. coli* 0157:H7. Plasma exchange may also be beneficial for patients with acute immune-mediated drug-induced TTP. Plasma exchange may not benefit patients whose syndromes are caused by dose-dependent drug toxicity or follow allogeneic hematopoietic stem cell transplantation.

Plasma exchange requires placement of a central venous catheter, similar to the catheters used for hemodialysis. There is substantial risk for critical complications caused by catheter insertion, catheter-related sepsis, and allergic reactions to plasma (Table 2). Therefore, the initial management decision regarding plasma exchange must balance the confidence in the diagnosis of TTP with the risks of the procedure. Plasma exchange is initially performed once daily, exchanging one plasma volume. In patients who are not initially responsive, or who deteriorate after beginning plasma exchange, higher volumes of plasma exchange may be more effective. Cryoprecipitate-poor plasma and routine fresh-frozen plasma are equally effective. Daily plasma exchange is continued until the platelet count returns to normal; further plasma exchange may have no benefit for residual renal or neurologic abnormalities. When plasma exchange is stopped, the signs of TTP may promptly recur, indicating an exacerbation of continued active TTP. In these patients, daily plasma exchange is resumed and adjunctive immunosuppressive therapy is appropriate.

 **CURRENT THERAPY**

- Plasma exchange:
  - Principal treatment for TTP.
  - Initial regimen: one plasma volume exchanged per day. For refractory patients increased exchange volume (1.5 plasma volumes) or increased frequency (one plasma volume twice daily) may be appropriate.
  - Fresh-frozen plasma and cryoprecipitate-poor plasma are equivalent as replacement fluid.
- Glucocorticoids:
  - Indicated for patients with idiopathic TTP and for patients who require prolonged plasma exchange.
  - Regimen may be oral prednisone, 1 mg/kg/d. For severely ill patients, IV methylprednisolone, 250–1000 mg/d for 3 d, may be appropriate.
- Intensive immunosuppression:
  - Indicated for patients with recurrent exacerbations or relapses
  - Regimen may be IV cyclophosphamide (Cytoxan[1]), 1000 mg/m² repeated at 3–4 wk intervals as needed, or rituximab (Rituxan[1]), 375 mg/m²/wk for 4 wk.

[1]Not FDA approved for this indication.
*Abbreviations:* IV = intravenous; TTP = thrombotic thrombocytopenic purpura.

## IMMUNOSUPPRESSIVE THERAPY

Patients with idiopathic TTP related to the frequent autoimmune etiology causing ADAMTS13 deficiency should receive immunosuppressive therapy initially with glucocorticoids. A standard regimen is oral prednisone, 1 mg/kg/day. For more critically ill patients, intravenous methylprednisolone in higher doses, such as 1000 mg/day for 3 days, may be appropriate as initial therapy. Treatment with glucocorticoids may diminish the duration of required plasma exchange and diminish the risk for subsequent exacerbations. In patients who require prolonged and repeated courses of plasma exchange, more intensive immunosuppressive therapy is appropriate, with agents such as cyclophosphamide (Cytoxan[1]) or rituximab (Rituxan[1]). Cyclophosphamide is typically given intravenously in a dose of 1000 mg/m², repeated in 3 to 4 weeks as needed. Rituximab is given intravenously in the standard dose of 375 mg/m²/week for 4 weeks.

[1]Not FDA approved for this indication.

**TABLE 2  Complications of Plasma Exchange Treatment for TTP**

| Complication | Approximate Frequency |
| --- | --- |
| Death | 2% |
| Sepsis | 15% |
| Venous thrombosis requiring anticoagulant treatment | 2% |
| Hypotension or hypoxia requiring intensive care | 7% |

*Abbreviations:* TTP = thrombotic thrombocytopenic purpura.
Data adapted from Howard MA, Williams LA, Terrell DR: Complications of plasma exchange in patients treated for clinically suspected thrombotic thrombocytopenic purpura-hemolytic uremic syndrome. III. An additional study of 54 consecutive patients. Transfusion 2006;46(1):154-156.

## MANAGEMENT DURING REMISSION

Remission of TTP is achieved when there is no evidence of disease for 30 days after plasma exchange treatment is stopped. No treatment has documented effectiveness for maintaining remission and preventing relapses. Relapses may occur in as many as 50% of patients whose TTP is associated with severe ADAMTS13 deficiency; patients with other etiologies have a negligible risk for relapse. Appropriate management is only careful follow-up, with prompt evaluation, including a complete blood count, for any acute symptoms. If TTP recurs, daily plasma exchange is resumed and intensive immunotherapy is appropriate, ideally to achieve a more durable remission. Because pregnancy is associated with the occurrence of acute episodes of TTP and TTP occurs most commonly in young women, the risk of a future pregnancy is a common and serious concern. But in spite of the association of TTP and pregnancy, most subsequent pregnancies are uncomplicated.

## Prognosis

Complete hematologic recovery is expected. In patients with acute renal failure, persistent renal insufficiency is common. Although most patients recover completely with no evidence of sequelae, many patients describe continuing subtle cognitive difficulties. Physicians should be aware of these potential difficulties to counsel and support their patients appropriately.

## REFERENCES

Allford S, Hunt BJ, Rose P, Machin S; Haemostasis and Thrombosis Task Force: Guidelines on the diagnosis and management of the thrombotic microangiopathic haemolytic anemias. Br J Haematol 2003;120:556-573.

Amorosi EL, Ultmann JE: Thrombotic thrombocytopenic purpura: Report of 16 cases and review of the literature. Medicine 1966;45:139-159.

George JN: The association of pregnancy with thrombotic thrombocytopenic purpura-hemolytic uremic syndrome. Curr Opin Hematol 2003;10:339-344.

George JN: Clinical practice. Thrombotic thrombocytopenic purpura. N Engl J Med 2006;354(18):1927-1935.

George JN, Li X, McMinn JR, et al: Thrombotic thrombocytopenic purpura-hemolytic uremic syndrome following allogeneic hematopoietic stem cell transplantation: A diagnostic dilemma. Transfusion 2004;44:294-304.

Howard MA, Williams LA, Terrell DR: Complications of plasma exchange in patients treated for clinically suspected thrombotic thrombocytopenic purpura-hemolytic uremic syndrome. III. An additional study of 54 consecutive patients. Transfusion 2006;46(1):154-156.

Kojouri K, Vesely SK, George JN: Quinine-associated thrombotic thrombocytopenic purpura-hemolytic uremic syndrome: Frequency, clinical features, and long-term outcomes. Ann Intern Med 2001;135:1047-1051.

McMinn JR, George JN: Evaluation of women with clinically suspected thrombotic thrombocytopenic purpura-hemolytic uremic syndrome during pregnancy. J Clin Apheresis 2001;16:202-209.

Moake JL: Thrombotic microangiopathies. N Engl J Med 2002;347:589-600.

Rock GA, Shumak KH, Buskard NA, et al: Comparison of plasma exchange with plasma infusion in the treatment of thrombotic thrombocytopenic purpura. N Engl J Med 1991;325:393-397.

Vesely SK, George JN, Lammle B, et al: ADAMTS13 activity in thrombotic thrombocytopenic purpura-hemolytic uremic syndrome: Relation to presenting features and clinical outcomes in a prospective cohort of 142 patients. Blood 2003;101:60-68.

Vesely SK, Li X, McMinn JR, et al: Pregnancy outcomes after recovery from thrombotic thrombocytopenic purpura-hemolytic uremic syndrome. Transfusion 2004;44:1149-1158.

# Hemochromatosis

Method of
*Lawrie W. Powell, MD, PhD*

When von Recklinghausen coined the name *hemochromatosis* in 1889 (because he believed the pigment in tissues was derived from the blood), he described the advanced disease with gross iron deposition in tissues and organ damage. Cirrhosis, diabetes mellitus, arthritis, cardiomyopathy, and hypogonadotrophic hypogonadism were the classical features. In his definitive monograph of the disease in 1935, Sheldon confirmed and extended this description, concluding that "in spite of its implicit but unproven assumptions it is the best name for the disease." Numerous large series and reviews were subsequently published leading to widespread acceptance of the concept of hemochromatosis as a disease of iron storage in which an inappropriate increase in intestinal iron absorption leads to excessive quantities of iron in tissues with eventual functional impairment of the organs involved, especially the liver, pancreas, heart, and pituitary. Simon and associates' discovery that the inheritance of HH is closely linked to the human leukocyte antigen (HLA)-A locus on chromosome 6 made definite identification of homozygous relatives of affected probands possible, and it eventually led to the identification of the two most common missense mutations, C282Y and H63D, of the major histocompatibility complex (MHC) class I gene on 6p, designated the hemochromatosis gene (HFE).

It is now established that 90% or more of cases of hemochromatosis in subjects of northern European extraction are because of homozygosity for the C282Y mutation in this gene. This is one of the most common genetic mutations in white populations (see later). It is probable, therefore, that von Recklinghausen and Sheldon were referring to this form of HFE-associated hemochromatosis. However, more recently additional mutations in other molecules involved in iron metabolism, notably hepcidin, hemojuvelin, and ferroportin, have been identified, and with the exception of the iron overload disorder resulting from mutations in the cellular iron transporter ferroportin, the resultant clinicopathologic syndrome closely resembles HFE-associated hemochromatosis. This has led to a new classification of iron overload and hemochromatosis that encompasses these newly described forms (Table 1).

Although a very similar clinicopathologic syndrome occurs with iron overload secondary to iron-loading anemia such as thalassemia major or sideroblastic anemia, the term *secondary* or *acquired hemochromatosis* has largely been abandoned in favor of defining the primary disease, that is, thalassemia major with secondary iron overload.

## Iron Homeostasis

Despite the abundance of iron in nature, the solubility of its stable ferric form is extremely low. Living organisms hence were compelled to develop efficient mechanisms for iron transport and storage. There is no mechanism for excreting excess iron, and the inevitable end result of iron absorption exceeding physiologic needs is iron overload.

In recent years a number of key mechanisms have been described that are responsible for adaptation to changing environmental conditions. Production of the iron storage protein ferritin and the transferrin receptor (TfR) protein is reciprocally regulated by a translational mechanism in which the iron regulatory protein (IRP) is reversibly bound to the iron response elements (IRE) of their respective mRNAs. A similar iron-dependent translational mechanism may be responsible for the production of divalent metal transporter 1 (DMT1), which is responsible for the uptake of ferrous iron from the brush border of duodenal enterocytes (Figure 1), and ferroportin (IREG1), which is responsible for the export of ferrous iron through

## TABLE 1 Classification of Iron Overload and Hemochromatosis

1. Primary hereditary hemochromatosis
   HFE-associated hereditary hemochromatosis (type 1)
     C282Y homozygosity
   C282Y/H63D compound heterozygosity
   Non-HFE associated hereditary hemochromatosis
     Juvenile hemochromatosis (type 2) (2A, hepcidin mutations; 2B, hemojuvelin mutations)
   Transferrin receptor 2 mutations hemochromatosis (type 3)
   Ferroportin mutations (autosomal dominant hemochromatosis) (type 4)
2. Acquired (secondary) iron overload
   Iron-loading anemias
     Thalassemia major
     Sideroblastic anemia
     Chronic hemolytic anemia
   Dietary iron overload (African)
   Parenteral iron overload (including multiple blood transfusions)
3. Other causes of iron overload (but rarely to the degree seen in hemochromatosis)
   Long-term hemodialysis
   Chronic liver disease
     Hepatitis C
     Alcoholic liver disease
   Nonalcoholic steatohepatitis
     Porphyria cutanea tarda
   Dysmetabolic iron overload syndrome
   Post-portacaval shunting
   Iron overload in sub-Sahara Africa
   Neonatal iron overload
   Aceruloplasminemia
   Congenital atransferrinemia

# Genetics of Hereditary Hemochromatosis

The inheritance of the disease follows classical Mendelian genetics as an autosomal recessive trait. The most common scenario is thus two parents are heterozygous for the C282Y mutation and 25% of offspring are either normal or homozygous and 50% are heterozygous. Approximately 90% to 95% of HFE-related hemochromatosis in people of northern European extraction can be attributed to homozygous mutations of C282Y. C282Y/H63D compound heterozygotes contribute 4%, whereas H63D homozygotes may have elevated transferrin saturation or serum ferritin levels but do not develop serious iron overload. Rarer forms of non-HFE-linked hemochromatosis are not discussed further here but are well described in a recent review by Pietrangelo (2004).

# Early Clinical Presentation and Diagnosis

Compelling evidence indicates that the classic clinical manifestations of hemochromatosis such as cirrhosis, diabetes, and so on are related to tissue damage by iron because they occur in HFE-associated hemochromatosis, other forms of hemochromatosis described earlier, and also in gross iron loading secondary to the iron-loading anemias. However, with increased clinical awareness and improved diagnostic methodology, hemochromatosis is now frequently recognized at a much earlier stage before complications arise (latent or precirrhotic hemochromatosis). This is best seen in cascade screening in families after the diagnosis of an index case and in population screening. As a result it is perhaps not surprising that the clinical penetrance and frequency of complications of hemochromatosis is a subject of much current controversy. One recent controlled population study concluded that less than 1% of homozygotes for C282Y have advanced disease. Similarly, in the large Hemochromatosis and Iron Overload Screening (HEIRS) population study of 100,000 North Americans, self-reported symptoms of hemochromatosis were not more common in C282Y homozygous subjects than controls except for self-reported liver disease. However, both of these studies were based on self-reported questionnaires and did not include liver biopsy. A study of 672 C282Y homozygotes incorporating detailed clinical evaluation and liver biopsy in approximately 50% of individuals concluded that cirrhosis was present in 5.8% of homozygous men and 1.9% of homozygous women, and all of these subjects were asymptomatic. Further, advanced hepatic fibrosis was present in 25% of subjects and significantly improved after phlebotomy therapy. The logical conclusion

the basolateral members of the same cells. The brush border ferric reductase converts ferric to ferrous iron for use by DMT1, and hephaestin, a transmembrane-bound ferroxidase, converts ferrous to ferric iron, creating a concentration gradient of ferrous iron across the cell membrane facilitating iron egress. At low iron conditions the translation of TfR, DMT1, and ferroportin is enhanced, with the opposite occurring at high iron conditions. In addition, a new protein, hepcidin, was described recently and is probably the most important regulator of iron homeostasis. Hepcidin functions as an inhibitor of iron absorption and release from macrophages. Its production is increased by iron overload and inflammation and is suppressed by iron deficiency.

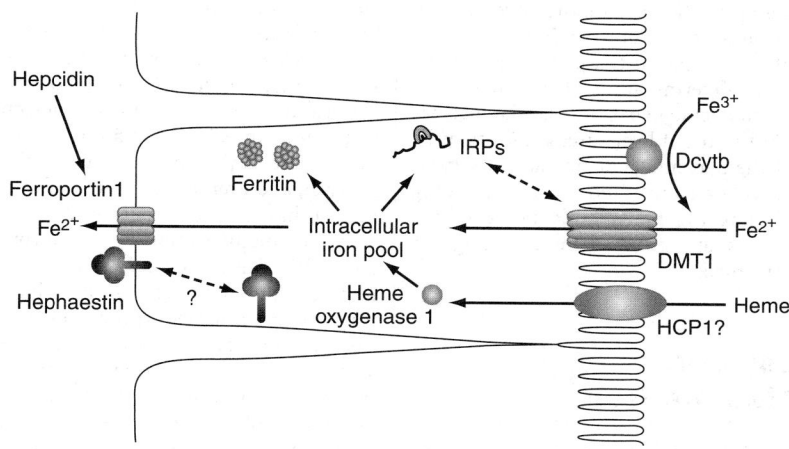

**FIGURE 1.** Cellular control of iron transport in the duodenal enterocyte. Dcytb = duodenal cytochrome b, DMT1 = divalent metal transporter 1, IRPs = iron regulatory proteins, HCP1 = haem carrier protein 1.

is that a significant proportion of C282Y homozygous individuals are asymptomatic but have hepatic fibrosis. The factors that determine whether this progresses to cirrhosis are not well understood, but heavy alcohol intake is identified as a significant factor.

The association of hepatomegaly, skin pigmentation, diabetes mellitus, heart disease, arthritis, and hypogonadism should suggest the diagnosis. A high index of suspicion is needed to make the diagnosis early. Indeed, increasingly, the diagnosis of early hemochromatosis is made at health checkups by primary care physicians or by cascade family screening. There are strong advocates of population screening, but this is controversial at the present time.

As many as 30% of patients are asymptomatic at the time of diagnosis. Furthermore, the presence of asymptomatic cirrhosis in 5% of patients highlights the importance of improving detection rates and screening strategies. The development of cascade screening for family members of affected probands, as well as incidental findings of abnormal iron studies (opportunistic screening often performed to investigate lethargy when the clinician expects to detect iron deficiency), has increased the number of asymptomatic individuals identified with early hemochromatosis. Progression to organ damage as a consequence of iron overload requires in excess of 10 g of parenchymal iron storage and usually occurs after 40 years of age, but heavy alcohol intake substantially increases the risk of cirrhosis at lower body iron levels.

## Laboratory Testing

In the absence of a consensus for population screening, a variety of indications for testing for hemochromatosis currently exist. Clearly patients with symptoms of liver disease and abnormal iron studies should be tested using genetic mutation analysis. In addition, those with type 2 diabetes, early-onset cardiac disease, premature sexual dysfunction, and atypical arthropathy require further evaluation. In the asymptomatic population, first-degree relatives of probands, individuals with abnormal iron studies detected incidentally, and those with clinical, biochemical, or radiologic evidence of liver disease should all be tested for hereditary hemochromatosis.

The transferrin saturation is the best initial phenotypic screening test. It is accepted as an accurate phenotypic marker of the genetic defect in HFE-associated hemochromatosis, but the level at which it should prompt further testing for hemochromatosis is controversial. A fasting transferrin saturation of 45% detected virtually all affected homozygotes, but the specificity increases with higher values.

The serum ferritin concentration is a good index of body iron stores. An increase of 1 μg/L in serum ferritin level reflects an increase of approximately 7 mg in body stores. In most untreated patients with hemochromatosis, the serum ferritin level is greatly increased. However, in patients with inflammation and hepatocellular necrosis, serum ferritin levels may be elevated out of proportion to body iron stores because of increased release from tissues. Importantly, in these situations the transferrin saturation is usually normal. In contrast, the serum ferritin in the absence of inflammation is a good guide to the degree of iron overload. A repeat determination of serum ferritin should, therefore, be carried out after acute hepatocellular damage has subsided (e.g., in drug- or alcohol-induced liver disease). Ordinarily, the combined measurements of the percentage of transferrin saturation and serum ferritin level provide a simple and reliable screening test for hemochromatosis, including the precirrhotic phase of the disease. If either of these tests is abnormal, genetic testing for hemochromatosis should be performed.

## Role of Liver Biopsy and Measurement of Hepatic Iron

The role of liver biopsy has changed since the introduction of the genetic test to one of primarily prognostic value specifically to establish or exclude the presence of cirrhosis. The current indications for liver biopsy are now generally accepted as follows: age older than

40 years, serum ferritin more than 1000 μg/L, abnormal liver function tests, or hepatomegaly, or a combination of these. Absence of severe fibrosis can be predicted with reasonable confidence without the need for liver biopsy. The most significant variable for negative prediction is serum ferritin equal to 1000 μg/L with a prevalence of severe fibrosis of 1% to 3%. Liver biopsy in the setting of C282Y homozygosity or compound heterozygosity is now considered unnecessary if the serum ferritin level is less than 1000 μg/mL and the serum transaminase levels are normal. Similar guidelines cannot be used in the absence of C282Y homozygosity. The serum ferritin level is elevated in iron-loading anemias, chronic hemolysis, blood transfusions, hepatitis C, alcoholism, and steatohepatitis because of hepatic inflammation and also secondary iron overload. Liver biopsy should be considered even in C282Y or H63D heterozygotes with these disorders. Although transferrin saturation is significantly increased in individuals with either homozygosity or heterozygosity of the H63D mutation regardless of gender, serum ferritin is not usually affected and progressive iron overload does not develop. Liver biopsy should also be utilized in those individuals with clinical iron overload and uninformative genetic mutation analysis to firmly establish their diagnosis.

Comparison of usefulness of MRI for the assessment of liver iron burden with liver biopsy was undertaken in recent studies. Use of a highly T2-weighted protocol comparing liver and muscle (L/M) signal intensity produced a 89% sensitivity and 80% specificity using a threshold L/M ratio below 0.88. The investigators were able to detect liver iron concentration down to a threshold of 1.8 mg Fe/g dry tissue. In a second study, the ratio between iron concentration and signal intensity on magnetic resonance imaging (MRI) was calculated and an inverse linear relationship was found. The normal value for liver iron is less than 36 μmol/g. The positive predictive value for hemochromatosis and iron overload, respectively, was more than 85 μmol/g and more than 58 μmol/g, whereas the negative predictive value was 100% at concentrations less than 40 μmol/g and less than 20 μmol/g, respectively.

Several attempts have been made to define serum markers of fibrosis and to determine whether it is possible to stratify subjects further with genetic hemochromatosis who may require liver biopsy. Serum type IV collagen concentrations are significantly increased in hemochromatosis patients when compared with healthy controls. Additionally, correlations between degree of fibrosis and serum type IV collagen concentrations are shown. In contrast, markers such as serum laminin, which is 81% accurate for detecting cirrhosis in alcoholics and those with chronic viral hepatitis, are not as useful in hemochromatosis. Recent claims that a panel of markers can accurately predict hepatic fibrosis are yet to be substantiated.

## Treatment

Hemochromatosis should be treated with once to twice weekly phlebotomy in the first instance. Approximately 1 g of iron is removed with four phlebotomies. Hemoglobin monitoring as well as assessment of serum ferritin after each 1 to 2 g of iron is removed is required. In the absence of contraindications, venesection should be continued until serum ferritin is less than 50 μg/L. Individuals who commence treatment prior to the development of cirrhosis or diabetes have normal survival, and even in the setting of cirrhosis, patients with hemochromatosis have improved survival.

Some manifestations are improved by phlebotomy, including fatigue, malaise, elevated serum transaminase levels, and insulin requirements in diabetes. In addition, exercise tolerance and cardiac function can improve with aggressive iron depletion in patients with cardiac complications. In such cases chelation therapy with desferrioxamine is indicated. Although its progression can be slowed, diabetes is not completely reversed. Hypogonadism, arthropathy, and cirrhosis do not resolve with venesection, and arthropathy may progress after complete iron removal. Treatment is symptomatic, although hip and knee replacement may be required. Hypogonadotrophic hypogonadism may be treated successfully with gonadotrophin therapy with or without parenteral testosterone therapy.

Chelation therapy is only used in rare circumstances when contraindications to venesection exist or in rare instances of cardiac disease as mentioned earlier. Subcutaneous desferrioxamine is the agent used for chelation when it is required. A typical regimen would be 1 to 2 g desferrioxamine in 100 to 200 mL water or saline infused over 10 to 12 hours during sleep. Patients should restrict their intake of iron-rich food and vitamin C. Obviously they should not be prescribed iron supplementation.

A new orally administered iron chelating agent, deferasirox (Exjade) has been approved for use in secondary iron overload and is currently under trial for primary hemochromatosis.

## Liver Transplantation and Hemochromatosis

Much recent interest has been expressed in liver transplantation in subjects with hemochromatosis, both from the viewpoint of effective therapy for end-stage disease but also as to whether it sheds light on the basic pathophysiology of the disease. The results of orthotopic liver transplantation for end-stage hemochromatosis are less impressive than for other liver diseases. This is attributed to late diagnosis (often at the time of transplantation) or the concurrence of primary hepatocellular carcinoma, but also to a high infection rate, possibly related to the effects of gross hepatic iron deposition. Thus, if possible, subjects with end-stage liver disease because of hemochromatosis should undergo intensive deironing by phlebotomy and possibly desferrioxamine before transplantation.

The available evidence indicates that the fundamental metabolic abnormality in hemochromatosis is reversed by successful liver transplantation. Patients do not reaccumulate iron if transplanted with a donor liver from an HFE normal subject, and the transferrin saturation and the serum ferritin levels remain normal in the absence of inflammation. This strongly suggests that the basic defect responsible for HFE-associated hemochromatosis lies within the liver. This is consistent with the findings of Bridle et al., who found that hepcidin RNA levels were low, but not absent functionally, in C282Y homozygous patients with hemochromatosis whether treated or untreated. Gehrke et al. subsequently published similar observations. HFE thus appears to interact with hepcidin within the liver, probably in the hepatocyte, and the C282Y mutation interferes with this, resulting in low hepcidin levels and consequently inappropriately increased intestinal iron absorption leading to progressive hepatic iron overload. The precise elucidation of this interaction will be of great interest.

### REFERENCES

Adams PC, Reboussin DM, Barton JC, et al: Hemochromatosis and iron-overload screening in a racially diverse population. N Engl J Med 2005; 352(17):1769-1778.

Bacon BR, Powell LW, Adams PC, et al: Molecular medicine and hemochromatosis: At the crossroads. Gastroenterology 1999;116(1):193-207.

Beutler E, Felitti VJ, Koziol JA, et al: Penetrance of 845G-A (C282Y) HFE hereditary haemochromatosis mutation in the USA. Lancet 2002; 359:211-218.

Bridle KR, Frazer DM, Wilkins SJ, et al: Disrupted hepcidin regulation in HFE-associated haemochromatosis and the liver as a regulator of body iron homoeostasis. Lancet 2003;361(9358):669-673.

Feder JN, Gnirke A, Thomas W, et al: A novel MHC class I-like gene is mutated in patients with hereditary haemochromatosis. Nat Genet 1996;13(4): 399-408.

Guyader D, Jacquelinet C, Moirand R, et al: Noninvasive prediction of fibrosis in C282Y homozygous hemochromatosis. Gastroenterology 1998;115(4): 929-936.

Pietrangelo A: Hereditary hemochromatosis—a new look at an old disease. N Engl J Med 2004;350(23):2383-2397.

Powell LW, Dixon JL, Ramm GA, et al: Screening for hemochromatosis in asymptomatic subjects with or without a family history. Arch Intern Med 2006;166:294-301.

Sheldon J: Haemochromatosis. London, Oxford University Press, 1935, p 339.

Simon M, Alexandre JL, Fauchet R, et al: The genetics of hemochromatosis. Prog Med Genet 1980;4:135-168.

St Pierre TG, Clark PR, Chua-anusorn W, et al: Noninvasive measurement and imaging of liver iron concentrations using proton magnetic resonance. Blood 2005;105(2):855-861. Epub 2004 July 15.

Tavill AS: Diagnosis and management of hemochromatosis. AASLD practice guidelines. Hepatology 2001;33(5):1321-1328.

von Recklinghausen F, Taggeblet de: Versainumlung Deutsch Naturforsch Arzt Heidelberg 1889;62:324-325.

# Hodgkin's Disease: Chemotherapy

Method of
*David J. Straus, MD*

The use of radiotherapy and chemotherapy for Hodgkin's disease is one of the major success stories in medical oncology. An understanding of the clinical features and course of the disease aided this success. Extended field radiation therapy (EF RT), introduced nearly 40 years ago by Kaplan, was a major advance in the treatment of patients with early-stage Hodgkin's disease. DeVita and colleagues introduced combination chemotherapy to the treatment of advanced stages of Hodgkin's disease in the mid-1960s, which was the second major advance in treatment. Combinations of chemotherapy with radiation therapy were widely used during the past 20 years, and further improvements in outcome were seen with this approach, particularly in patients with early stages of Hodgkin's disease. More recently, chemotherapy alone has been employed for many patients with excellent results. Less late toxicity may be seen in patients cured of their Hodgkin's disease with reduction in the amount of radiation therapy in combination with chemotherapy or its complete elimination when it is not required.

## Histopathology

Currently, the Rye modification of the Lukes and Butler classification is in use throughout the world. The lymphocyte-predominant subtype is characterized by an abundance of small lymphocytes with occasional, often atypical, Reed-Sternberg (R-S) cells of lymphocytic-histiocytic variety (L and H, or so-called popcorn cells) with vesicular, polylobulated nuclei and small nucleoli. Unlike the other forms of Hodgkin's disease, the atypical cells usually have B-cell antigens (CD19, 20, 22, 79a). The growth pattern is usually nodular, although less commonly a diffuse pattern is seen. The classic presentation is in a high cervical node in a young asymptomatic male. It is associated with a favorable prognosis, although late recurrences are reported in some series.

Nodular sclerosis is the most common subtype in North America and Western Europe. There is often abundant fibrosis in the node dividing tumor nodules containing inflammatory cells and the "lacunar cell" variant of R-S cells with a clear area surrounding the cells. The typical presentation is in a young female with mediastinal involvement with or without symptoms. Although it was classically believed to carry a relatively favorable prognosis, this seems to depend on the stage of the disease, the bulkiness of the tumor masses, and the presence or absence of systemic symptoms. The new World Health Organization (WHO) classification of neoplastic diseases of the hematopoietic and lymphoid tissues adds two histologic grades of nodular sclerosis Hodgkin's disease according to the British National Lymphoma Investigation criteria (grade 1, few R-S cells; grade 2, many R-S cells). Some studies demonstrated a worse outcome associated with grade 2 cases, and others showed no difference in outcome. For now, the grading is not required for clinical purposes but should be the subject of future investigations.

Mixed cellularity is characterized by a pleomorphic cellular infiltrate of plasma cells, eosinophils, lymphocytes, histiocytes, and R-S cells. Subdiaphragmatic and extranodal presentations and the presence of B systems may be somewhat more frequent than with the nodular sclerosis subtype. It is the second most common histologic subtype in North America and Western Europe and more common in the poorer parts of the world and among indigent populations. It is also somewhat more common among older patients. It is associated with a worse prognosis than nodular sclerosis, but this may be because of the association of this subtype with the unfavorable clinical prognostic features.

The lymphocyte-depletion subtype has a paucity of cellular elements and an increased reticular network. It is associated with advanced age, systemic symptoms, retroperitoneal lymphadenopathy, and extranodal involvement. It is a diagnosis that is now made infrequently because modern immunophenotyping and molecular genetic studies have demonstrated that many cases formerly thought to be lymphocyte-depletion Hodgkin's disease are actually T-cell non-Hodgkin's lymphomas. Lymphocyte-depletion Hodgkin's disease has the worst prognosis of the four histologic subtypes.

The R-S cells, in the cases of nodular sclerosis, mixed cellularity, and lymphocyte-depletion Hodgkin's disease, carry the CD30 surface antigen, an antigen that is expressed on activated and proliferating lymphocytes. They also stain with antibodies to CD15, more commonly a myeloid marker. Recent cloning of this molecule has enabled its identification as a new member of the tumor necrosis factor (TNF) receptor superfamily. Single cell polymerase chain reaction (PCR) of classic R-S cells literally scraped from slides shows a follicular center B-cell origin for these cells with clonally rearranged but crippled V heavy chain genes presumably leading to a block in apoptosis.

The R-S–like cells in the nodular variant of lymphocyte-predominant Hodgkin's disease are weakly reactive or nonreactive with antibodies to CD30, and, unlike those in the other Hodgkin's disease subtypes, demonstrate a mature B-cell marker phenotype with CD20 and also pan-lymphocyte antigen (CD45, leukocyte common antigen) expression. Molecular genetic studies also have demonstrated the clonal B-cell origin of the nodular variant of lymphocyte-predominant Hodgkin's disease. The R-S cells of the diffuse variant of lymphocyte-predominant Hodgkin's disease have the phenotypic features of classic R-S cells.

## Staging

The current staging classification was established by the Ann Arbor Workshop in 1971. There is both clinical staging (CS), which consists of all staging procedures short of staging laparotomy, and pathologic staging (PS), which refers to the findings at staging laparotomy during which liver biopsies, splenectomy, and excisional biopsies of retroperitoneal nodes are performed. Staging laparotomies are performed infrequently at the present time because fewer patients are treated with radiation therapy alone and more patients with systemic treatment with chemotherapy alone or in combination with radiation therapy.

The Ann Arbor classification divides Hodgkin's disease into four stages: Stage I refers to disease limited to a single lymph node or lymph node group. Stage II refers to disease in two or more noncontiguous lymph node groups and/or spleen on the same side of the diaphragm. Stage III refers to disease in two or more lymph node groups and/or spleen on both sides of the diaphragm. Stage IV refers to disease in extranodal sites, usually lung, liver, bone or bone marrow, and more rarely other sites. Extranodal involvement by extension from lymph node disease to such sites as the lung, bone, pleura, or skin may occur in stages $I_E$ and is not considered to increase the stage to IV. Such disease is designated by a subscript E ($I_E$, $II_E$, $III_E$). For each stage, the absence of systemic symptoms is designated by the suffix A, whereas the presence of unexplained fevers to 38°C (100.4°F) or higher, night sweats, and/or weight loss greater than 10% over 6 months is designated by a B suffix. In general, the prognosis worsens with higher stage, and, within each stage, the presence of symptoms (B) carries a worse prognosis than absence of such symptoms (A). A mediastinal tumor greater than a third of the thoracic diameter or lymph node disease

## CURRENT DIAGNOSIS

- History: Enlarged lymph nodes, fevers to 38°C (100.4°F) (27% of patients), drenching night sweats, weight loss, pruritus, alcohol-induced pain in areas of enlarged lymph nodes (10% of patients), chest pain, cough, dyspnea
- Physical examination: Enlarged nontender lymph nodes (neck, supraclavicular, axillary, inguinal regions), palpable enlarged spleen and liver, signs of pleural effusion
- Laboratory: Anemia (usually normochromic, normocytic), granulocytosis, eosinophilia, thrombocytosis, elevated erythrocyte sedimentation rate, elevated alkaline phosphatase without other indications of liver involvement (other liver enzymes, bilirubin can be elevated in addition with liver involvement), low albumin
- Imaging: Superior or anterior mediastinal mass on chest radiograph, enlarged axillary, supraclavicular, mediastinal, retroperitoneal, inguinal nodes, liver and spleen on computerized tomography, increased radioactive nuclide uptake on gallium or positron emission scans
- Diagnosis: Tissue biopsy (fine-needle aspirate cytology rarely adequate)
- Classic Hodgkin's lymphoma: Reed-Sternberg cells CD30+, CD15+, usually CD20–
    - Nodular sclerosis
    - Mixed cellularity
    - Lymphocyte rich
    - Lymphocyte depleted (rare)
- Nodular lymphocyte-predominant Hodgkin's lymphoma: Reed-Sternberg morphologic variants ("L & H," "popcorn" cells) CD20+, CD30–, CD15–

greater than 10 cm is defined as bulky; a subscript X is added to the numerical stage if such disease is present (e.g., $I_XB$, $II_XA$, $II_XB$, $III_XA$, $III_XB$). Stage IIIA1 refers to subdiaphragmatic disease in spleen and/or high abdominal node, whereas IIIA2 indicates disease in lower retroperitoneal nodes.

Staging procedures include chest radiograph, computerized tomography (CT) of the chest, abdomen, and pelvis with oral and intravenous contrast, complete blood counts with platelet and differential counts, bone marrow aspiration and biopsy, serum liver biochemistries including alkaline phosphatase, and erythrocyte sedimentation rate. The latter test carries prognostic significance. A CT of the abdomen and pelvis will show enlarged retroperitoneal, mesenteric, and pelvic lymph nodes that are involved by disease.

If there are masses in the liver on CT scan, a positron emission tomography (PET) scan or liver-spleen scintigram or, if there are gross abnormalities of serum liver biochemical studies, a liver biopsy should be performed under CT-guided or laparoscopic visualization if the masses are accessible. Slight elevations of serum alkaline phosphatase may be seen without liver involvement.

Gallium-67 scanning is a useful imaging procedure for following mediastinal disease, but it can be associated with false negatives and false positives. It is of value in the decision of whether to biopsy a residual mass following treatment to determine the presence or absence of residual disease. A PET scan provides similar and even more detailed information. [18F]fluoro-2-deoxy-D-glucose (FDG) PET scanning is useful in predicting recurrences in residual masses following treatment for Hodgkin's disease. False-negative studies are less common (the negative predictive value is 95%) than false-positive studies (the positive predictive value is 60%).

A CT scan of the chest may show disease, particularly retrosternal disease, missed by a plain chest radiograph. Also, some patients with bulky mediastinal and hilar nodal disease have peripheral lung nodules that can only be detected by chest CT. Although traditional radiotherapy

## CURRENT THERAPY

- Clinical stages I and II without bulky disease: Four cycles of ABVD with IF RT or six cycles of ABVD alone would both be acceptable. Although the equivalence of the outcome of chemotherapy alone to chemotherapy plus RT is not yet proven definitively, chemotherapy alone would probably reduce the late toxicities of treatment, most of which are related to RT.
- Clinical stages $II_xA/II_xB$: Six cycles of ABVD plus IF RT or Stanford V.
- Clinical stage IIIA: Six cycles of ABVD.
- Clinical stages IIIB and IV: Six cycles of ABVD, Stanford V, or BEACOPP regimens.
- Relapsed/refractory disease: Salvage chemotherapy followed by high-dose chemotherapy with peripheral blood stem cell support for most cases.

---

*Abbreviations:* ABVD = doxorubicin, bleomycin, vinblastine, and dacarbazine; BEACOPP = bleomycin, etoposide, doxorubicin, cyclophosphamide, vincristine, and prednisone; IF RT = involved field radiation therapy; RT = radiation therapy; Stanford V = 12-week chemotherapy program consisting of doxorubicin, vinblastine, bleomycin, nitrogen mustard, vincristine, etoposide,[1] and prednisone followed by RT to bulky sites (adenopathy = 5 cm, macroscopic splenic nodules).

[1]Not FDA approved for this indication.

---

treatment seems rarely affected by these findings, CT does allow for refinements in radiotherapy treatment planning.

## Treatment

### STAGES IA/B AND IIA/B, NONBULKY

The work of Gilbert, Peters, and, later, Kaplan demonstrated that recurrences rarely occur within the treated lymph node areas with doses of radiation therapy (RT) to 3500 to 4500 cGy. The use of the linear accelerator made it possible to deliver these doses to large fields. The mantle port (cervical, supraclavicular, mediastinal, and axillary regions—an area like the mantle on a suit of armor) and the inverted Y port (para-aortic nodes, spleen [if not removed], splenic pedicle, and iliac, inguinal, and femoral nodes) and combinations of the two were developed in the 1960s. Total lymphoid irradiation (TLI) refers to combinations of the two that have also at times included low-dose irradiation of liver and lung. Subtotal lymphoid irradiation (STLI) includes the mantle port with irradiation of para-aortic nodes, splenic pedicle, and spleen if it was not removed.

Local irradiation is probably adequate for high-cervical-stage IA disease and lymphocyte-predominant or nodular sclerosis histology in a young patient. Lymphocyte-predominant Hodgkin's disease is often clinically localized, is usually effectively treated with irradiation alone, and may relapse late (a clinical feature reminiscent of low-grade lymphoma). The 15-year disease-specific survival is excellent (more than 90%).

There is also general agreement that bulky mediastinal disease with a mediastinal mass diameter more than a third of the chest diameter should be treated with combined modality treatment with chemotherapy and RT. Recently some groups have treated selected patients with bulky mediastinal masses whose disease is well defined on CT scan with RT only using ports designed with the aid of the CT scan.

The prognostic importance of contiguous extension of disease from hilar nodes into the lung parenchyma is controversial. Some centers employing radiotherapy only report good results using low-dose irradiation also administered to the entire affected lung aided by thin lung blocks. However, these patients are usually treated with combined chemotherapy and less complex involved field RT (IF RT).

The European Organization for Research and Treatment of Cancer (EORTC) found elevations of the erythrocyte sedimentation rate (ESR) (more than 50 mm/hour for stages IA and IIA, more than 30 mm/hour for stages IB and IIB) to be a powerful adverse prognostic factor among patients treated with RT only. However, this is not an adverse prognostic factor for patients treated with chemotherapy or combined modality treatment.

There are several treatment options for the majority of patients with stages IA and IIA Hodgkin's disease. Subtotal lymphoid irradiation, which can include the spleen, to doses of at least 3500 cGy in 3.5 weeks has resulted in a complete remission (CR) percentage in excess of 90% with a 20% to 40% relapse rate in pathologically staged patients, probably depending on radiotherapy technique and/or patient selection. The likelihood of salvage of these patients into a second durable CR may be in excess of 50%. This approach is rarely employed because of the long-term potential toxicities of extensive RT and the lower relapse rates seen after treatment with combined modality treatment or chemotherapy alone.

Combination chemotherapy alone and when combined with radiotherapy has resulted in a CR percentage greater than 90% with a relapse rate of approximately 10% or less. This was achieved in the past with six cycles of chemotherapy with MOPP (mechlorethamine [nitrogen mustard], vincristine [Oncovin], procarbazine, and prednisone) or similar regimens.

When radiotherapy is also used, fewer cycles of chemotherapy may give similar results. A protocol at Memorial Hospital randomized patients to four cycles of either MOPP or thiotepa, bleomycin, and vinblastine (TBV) combined with modified extended-field RT. The results with a median follow-up time of 65 months (7 to 96 months) were similar in both arms of this trial and also similar to the results achieved with six cycles of MOPP and similar radiotherapy.

Two French studies suggest that three cycles of MOPP may be sufficient in combination with radiotherapy. The H8-F trial of the EORTC demonstrated the superiority of three cycles of a MOPP/Adriamycin (doxorubicin), bleomycin, and vincristine/vinblastine (ABV) hybrid plus IF RT (36 to 40 Gy) (4-year treatment failure-free survival [TTFS] rate 99%) to EF RT at the same dose (TTFS rate 77%; $p < 0.001$) in favorable early-stage Hodgkin's disease.

The Southwest Oncology Group (SWOG) demonstrated a superior failure-free survival for three cycles of doxorubicin and vinblastine plus STLI (94%) as compared to STLI alone (81%; $p < .001$). The German Hodgkin's Lymphoma Study Group HD-7 study compared two cycles of doxorubicin, bleomycin, vinblastine, and dacarbazine (ABVD) plus EF RT (30 Gy)/IF RT boost (10 Gy) to EF RT (30 Gy)/IF RT (10 Gy) in favorable stage I and II patients. The freedom from treatment failure was 96% for combined modality treatment compared to 84% for EF RT alone.

From February 1990 to July 1996, in a randomized trial of patients with clinically staged early Hodgkin's disease (I bulky and/or B; IIA, IIA bulky, and IIEA), a comparison was made of four cycles of ABVD followed by STLI versus the same regimen followed by IF RT. There were 136 patients assessable, with the main characteristics fairly well balanced between the two arms. After a median follow-up of 87 months (range, 8 to 123), treatment outcome was as follows: complete remission 100% after ABVD plus STLI versus 97% after ABVD plus IF RT; FFP 97% versus 94%, and total survival 93% versus 94%, respectively. These results indicate that four cycles of ABVD followed by IF RT can achieve results comparable to the same regimen followed by extensive RT. This effective and safe regimen can be considered to be a standard option for most patients with early-stage Hodgkin's disease.

The results of a randomized trial from Memorial Hospital of chemotherapy with ABVD alone or combined with RT in clinical stages I, II, and IIIA disease without bulky mediastinal or peripheral nodal involvement were reported recently. Although this trial was not statistically powered to show equivalence of the two treatment approaches, no differences in CR percentage, freedom from progression, or overall survival were seen. The results of a randomized phase III trial of standard treatment (STLI, favorable; two cycles of ABVD plus STLI, unfavorable) versus experimental treatment (four to six cycles of ABVD alone) in stage IA and IIA patients without high-risk factors were recently reported from the National Cancer Institute of

Canada Clinical Trial Group (NCIC-CTG) and the Eastern Cooperative Oncology Group (ECOG). The estimated progression-free survival (PFS) was 93% for the patients on the standard treatment arm and 87% for those in the experimental treatment arm, a statistically significant result. There was no difference in overall survival. Somewhat less than 30% of patients on the experimental arm received four cycles of ABVD alone, although it is not clear that an excess of relapses were seen in this group. In view of the high rate of salvageability of patients who might relapse after this type of chemotherapy, and the late morbidity of treatment that is mostly attributable to RT, the clinical meaning of a 6% difference in PFS is unclear. On the basis of these results, chemotherapy alone with six cycles of ABVD alone, which is more standard than four cycles, for nonbulky early-stage Hodgkin's disease, is also a treatment option, although, as mentioned earlier, there may be a slightly higher risk of relapse.

## STAGES II$_X$, III, AND IV

The major advance for patients with advanced Hodgkin's disease came from the use of MOPP by DeVita and colleagues. Eighty-four percent of 188 patients achieved a CR, and 66% of these were free of disease for more than 10 years. Ninety percent of these patients had stage IIIB or IVB disease. There are many modifications of the MOPP regimen that achieved similar results.

The groups at Memorial Hospital and at the National Tumor Institute in Milan pioneered the use of alternating potentially non-cross-resistant drug combinations and low-dose RT. Santoro, Bonadonna, and their colleagues developed the ABVD combination and demonstrated similar CR percentages as seen with MOPP. Also, it was demonstrated that at least some patients relapsing after MOPP could be put into second remissions, although the duration of these remissions is not as long as with primary treatment. They suggested that the ABVD combination might be potentially non-cross-resistant with MOPP in that tumors resistant to MOPP might be sensitive to ABVD.

Following this suggestion, a program of alternating monthly MOPP and ABVD combined with reduced-dose RT was developed at Memorial Hospital. Adjuvant reduced-dose RT to the initially involved bulky lymph node regions was employed to prevent relapses in these areas. A protocol was designed in 1975 in which MOPP and ABVD were alternated monthly for eight cycles in combination with reduced-dose RT to bulky sites. In 1979, a new trial was started in which MOPP/ABVD/RT (eight-drug regimen) was randomized against three alternating potentially non-cross-resistant combinations (ten-drug regimen) and RT. The third combination was lomustine (CCNU), melphalan (Alkeran), and vindesine (DVA), following the demonstration of activity of vindesine alone and in this combination for relapsed patients. The same reduced-dose RT was administered as in the initial trial.

The results for the initial eight-drug/RT protocol and the subsequent eight-drug/RT versus ten-drug/RT protocol were the same. Between 1975 and 1988, 270 patients were treated with either two or three alternating drug combinations and low-dose RT. Two hundred twenty-two patients (82%) achieved a CR, 38 (14%) a PR, and 10 (4%) progressed. At 10 years, the relapse-free survival for the patients achieving a CR was 80%, overall survival was 74%, and progression-free survival was 70%. The relapse-free survival for CS IIB patients was 89% and at 10 years was 73% each for CS IIIB and IV patients.

Similar results were achieved in a number of trials with alternating monthly chemotherapy with or without RT. The cancer and acute leukemia group B (CALGB) conducted a randomized trial in patients with stages IIIA2, IIIB, and IV disease with assignment to MOPP, ABVD, or alternating MOPP/ABVD. Response and failure-free survival rates were superior for both MOPP/ABVD and ABVD as compared with MOPP alone. Similar results were also achieved using a compressed schedule hybrid approach in which the nitrogen mustard and vincristine are given on day 1 along with oral procarbazine, prednisone, doxorubicin, bleomycin, and vinblastine on day 8 (MOPP/ABV hybrid). Recently, the results of an intergroup (CALGB, Southwest Oncology Group [SWOG], ECOG, NCIC-CTG) randomized trial

established ABVD as equivalent in treatment outcome to MOPP/ABV hybrid with less acute toxicity, myelodysplastic syndrome, and leukemia.

A number of short-course, dose-intense chemotherapy regimens combined with RT were introduced over the past decade. The Stanford V is a 12-week chemotherapy program consisting of doxorubicin, vinblastine, bleomycin, nitrogen mustard, vincristine, etoposide,[1] and prednisone followed by RT to bulky sites (adenopathy = 5 cm, macroscopic splenic nodules). In a phase 2 trial conducted by ECOG in 47 patients with bulky mediastinal stage I/II or stages III/IV disease, the FFP was 85% and overall survival 96% at 5 years. Grade 3 or 4 neutropenia was seen in 59% of patients, and there was one acute monocytic leukemia. This regimen is strongly dependent on the RT to achieve maximal results.

The German Hodgkin's Lymphoma Study Group conducted a three-arm randomized trial, using a combination of bleomycin, etoposide, Adriamycin (doxorubicin), cyclophosphamide, vincristine, and prednisone (BEACOPP) versus dose-escalated BEACOPP with the aid of granulocyte colony-stimulating factor (G-CSF) versus cyclophosphamide, Oncovin (vincristine), procarbazine, and prednisone (COPP)/ABVD ($\infty$ 8). After chemotherapy, RT was administered to initially bulky nodal sites or sites of residual disease. The freedom from treatment failure rates at 5 years were 69% for COPP/ABVD, 76% for standard BEACOPP, and 87% for dose-escalated BEACOPP ($p < 0.001$ for COPP/ABVD vs. dose-escalated BEACOPP). The 5-year survival rates were 83% for COPP/ABVD, 88% for standard BEACOPP, and 91% for dose-escalated BEACOPP ($p = 0.002$ for COPP/ABVD vs. dose-escalated BEACOPP). There was a considerable amount of acute toxicity including grade 4 neutropenia in 90% of patients and grade 4 thrombocytopenia in 47% with dose-escalated BEACOPP. The rate of secondary acute leukemias at 5 years was 2.5%, significantly higher than in the other two arms of the trial. The toxicity of this regimen and the possibility of successful salvage of resistant or relapsed patients after ABVD have somewhat tempered the enthusiasm for its use in this country.

However, another randomized trial showed a benefit for a conventional hybrid regimen over a shortened dose-intensified regimen using doxorubicin, cyclophosphamide, etoposide, vincristine, bleomycin, and prednisone (VAPEC-B) versus chlorambucil, vinblastine, procarbazine, prednisone/etoposide, vinblastine, and doxorubicin (ChlVPP/EVA) hybrid: A British and Italian cooperative trial of 225 patients with bulky or stage B I and II or stages III and IV were randomized to either 11 weekly cycles of VAPEC-B or ChlVPP/EVA hybrid. This trial also included RT to initial bulky nodal sites or sites of residual disease after chemotherapy. At a median follow-up time of 25 months, there was almost a three times increased progression rate in the VAPEC-B arm as compared with the ChlVPP/EVA hybrid arm.

Until recently, our policy was to administer adjuvant RT to all initially involved lymph node sites, whether or not they are bulky, in combination with alternating chemotherapy regimens for patients with advanced stages of Hodgkin's disease. The results of a large definitive randomized trial conducted by the EORTC showed no benefit to IF RT in patients achieving a CR after six to eight cycles of MOPP/ABV hybrid in patients with stages III and IV Hodgkin's disease, although a benefit for RT was seen in patients who only achieved a PR. At a median follow-up time of more than 6 years, there was an excess of deaths because of other causes including secondary malignancies approaching statistical significance in the group of patients in CR who received IF RT.

The issue of combined modality treatment as opposed to chemotherapy alone in most patients is being further addressed in a phase III randomized trial of short-course, intensive chemotherapy combined with involved field RT with the Stanford V regimen versus ABVD with RT only to bulky mediastinal sites in patients with locally extensive or stages III/IV Hodgkin's disease that is being conducted by ECOG and CALGB.

Based on the results with alternating chemotherapy with CS IIB, IIIB, and IV patients, a prognostic model was constructed in which five

---

[1]Not FDA approved for this indication.

pretreatment characteristics emerged as having adverse prognostic importance in a multivariable analysis:

1. Low hematocrit
2. High-serum lactic acid dehydrogenase (LDH)
3. Older than 45 years
4. Inguinal node involvement (a reflection of extensive subdiaphragmatic disease)
5. Bulky mediastinal disease greater than 0.45 of the thoracic diameter

Approximately 60% of the patients had none or only one of these adverse factors, and their survival was greater than 95%. Patients with two or more of these factors had a dramatically inferior survival rate. The utility of this model has been confirmed by others.

Hasenclever and Diehl for the International Prognostic Factors Project on advanced Hodgkin's disease published a prognostic model based on a retrospective analysis of 1618 patients from 25 centers. In the final model, seven factors were used:

1. Albumin less than 4 g/dL
2. Hemoglobin (Hgb) less than 10.5 g/dL
3. Male sex
4. Stage IV
5. 45 years of age
6. White blood cell (WBC) count = 15,000 mm$^3$
7. Lymphocyte count less than 600 mm$^3$ or less than 8% of WBC

The worst prognostic group (7% = five, six, or seven factors) had a 5-year overall survival (OS) of 56% and a FFP of 42%. This model does not separate out a group with a very poor prognosis. A recently made comparison of seven prognostic models for Hodgkin's disease was retrospectively applied to 516 patients with advanced Hodgkin's disease. Three models were found to be the most predictive of outcome: the International Prognostic Factors Project Index (employing albumin, hemoglobin, gender, stage, age, WBC, and lymphocyte count); the Memorial Sloan-Kettering Cancer Center model (employing age, lactate dehydrogenase [LDH], hematocrit, inguinal nodal involvement, and mediastinal mass bulk); and the International Database on Hodgkin's disease (employing stage, age, B symptoms, albumin, and gender). Integration of the three models in a linear model improved their predictive power: Between 19% and 25% of patients fell into groups with either a 10% or a 50% risk of failure.

## Salvage Treatment

Because of the high relapse rates seen following conventional salvage chemotherapy after primary chemotherapy, most groups are using high-dose chemotherapy with or without RT depending on the prior treatment with autologous bone marrow or peripheral stem cell rescue. The results are promising in selected patients with more than half the patients achieving remission of varying durations transplanted in second or subsequent remission. Results of high-dose chemoradiotherapy with autologous stem cell transplantation in 65 patients with relapsed or refractory Hodgkin's disease treated between 1994 and 1998 at Memorial Sloan-Kettering Cancer Center were recently reported. At a median follow-up time of 43 months, estimates of the proportion of patients alive are 73% and event free are 58% by intent-to-treat analysis. In a multivariable logistic regression model, there were three adverse prognostic factors: extranodal sites of relapse or refractory disease, complete remission duration of less than 1 year, or refractory disease and B symptoms. Patients with zero or one adverse factor had an OS of 90% and an event-free survival (EFS) of 83%. Patients with two adverse factors had an OS of 57% and an EFS of 27%, and those with three adverse factors had an OS of 25% and an EFS of 10%.

## Toxicity

Most long-term toxicity of chemotherapy seems to be related to alkylating agent and procarbazine-containing regimens of the MOPP type. There is approximately a 3% lifetime risk of acute leukemia following MOPP-type chemotherapy. Among solid tumors, only alkylating agent-based regimens are associated with an increased risk of lung cancer. Azoospermia occurs in approximately 80% of men treated with six cycles of MOPP, and another 10% are rendered oligospermic. Sperm banking with cryopreservation is encouraged for male patients who may wish to have children in the future. Female patients younger than 30 years are less likely to become permanently infertile than those older than 30 years. The risks of infertility and secondary myelodysplastic syndromes or acute leukemias are less with ABVD than with MOPP-type regimens.

Vascular damage to coronary and peripheral arteries is a concern with RT. Carotid stenosis risk is increased after cervical RT. Patients who receive mantle field RT have a threefold increased risk of fatal myocardial infarction. Heart-valve fibrosis requiring surgical replacement and more subtle abnormalities, such as restrictive cardiomyopathy and conduction abnormalities, were also reported following mediastinal RT. The actuarial risk of second malignancies is 22% to 27% at 25 to 30 years following treatment for Hodgkin's disease. Most of this risk seems to be related to RT.

Neuromuscular problems are another late complication related to RT. Neck muscle atrophy resulting in neck pain and difficulty in neck extension occurs in some patients. Symptomatic radiation pulmonary and pericardial fibrosis and brachial plexopathies occur with current RT techniques but less frequently than in the past. Secondary hypothyroidism is usually manageable with thyroid replacement therapy.

Pulmonary toxicity from bleomycin treatment is a problem with the ABVD regimen. The major nonhematologic toxicity is pulmonary and related to bleomycin. In the trial conducted at Memorial Hospital, 33 patients (22%) discontinued bleomycin because of a decrease in DLCO. Ten of the symptomatic patients received brief courses of corticosteroids, and there was one death because of bleomycin during treatment.

## REFERENCES

Adams MJ, Lipsitz SR, Colan SD et al: Cardiovascular status in long-term survivors of Hodgkin's disease treated with chest radiotherapy. J Clin Oncol 22(15);2004:3139-3148.

Aleman BM, Raemaekers JM, Tirelli V, et al: Involved-field radiotherapy for advanced Hodgkin's lymphoma. N Engl J Med 348(24);2003:2396-2406.

Bhatia S, Yasui Y, Robison LL, et al: High risk of subsequent neoplasms continues with extended follow-up of childhood Hodgkin's disease: Report from the Late Effects Study Group. J Clin Oncol 21(23);2003:4386-4394.

Bonadonna G, Bonfante V, Viviani S, et al: ABVD plus subtotal nodal versus involved-field radiotherapy in early-stage Hodgkin's disease: Long-term results. J Clin Oncol 22(14);2004:2835-2841.

Diehl V, Franklin J, Pfreundschuh M, et al: Standard and increased-dose BEACOPP chemotherapy compared with COPP-ABVD for advanced Hodgkin's disease. N Engl J Med 348(24);2003:2386-2395.

Hasenclever D, Diehl V: A prognostic score for advanced Hodgkin's disease. International Prognostic Factors Project on Advanced Hodgkin's Disease. N Engl J Med 339(21);1998:1506-1514.

Horning SJ, Hoppe RT, Breslin S, et al: Stanford V and radiotherapy for locally extensive and advanced Hodgkin's disease: Mature results of a prospective clinical trial. J Clin Oncol 20(3);2002:630-637.

Hull MC, Morris CG, Pipine CJ, et al: Valvular dysfunction and carotid, subclavian, and coronary artery disease in survivors of Hodgkin lymphoma treated with radiation therapy. JAMA 290(21);2003:2831-2837.

Radford JA, Rohatiner AZ, Ryder WD, et al: ChlVPP/EVA hybrid versus the weekly VAPEC-B regimen for previously untreated Hodgkin's disease. J Clin Oncol 20(13);2002:2988-2994.

Straus DJ, Gaynor JJ, Myers J, et al: Prognostic factors among 185 adults with newly diagnosed advanced Hodgkin's disease treated with alternating potentially noncross-resistant chemotherapy and intermediate-dose radiation therapy. J Clin Oncol 8(7);1990:1173-1186.

Straus DJ, Portlock CS, Qin J, et al: Results of a prospective randomized clinical trial of doxorubicin, bleomycin, vinblastine, and dacarbazine (ABVD) followed by radiation therapy (RT) versus ABVD alone for stages I, II, and IIIA nonbulky Hodgkin disease. Blood 104(12);2004:3483-3489.

435

# Hodgkin's Disease: Radiation Therapy

Method of
*Pelayo C. Besa, MD*

Hodgkin's disease is a malignancy of lymph nodes with a predictable pattern of spread. Advances in treatment have made Hodgkin's disease a highly curable cancer with a long-term survival rate of more than 90%. Cure rate, defined as 10-year freedom from relapse, for early-stage disease is in the range of 80% to 90%; for intermediate-stage disease, 70% to 80%; and for advanced disease, 30% to 50%.

Radiation therapy plays a major role in the management of Hodgkin's disease. Treatment planning and patient selection are based on thorough clinical staging and review of the pathology. Most patients afflicted with Hodgkin's disease are less than 30 years old and will be cured; therefore, they will be at risk of late toxicity from treatment. Ideal therapy should provide the highest cure rate with minimal long-term toxicity. With this goal, treatment programs have gradually adjusted therapy to the different clinical settings.

Adequate radiation therapy requires pretreatment simulation and therapy with a linear accelerator with a minimal photon beam energy of 6 MV through parallel opposed fields that deliver a tumoricidal dose in a fractionated fashion. Treatment reproducibility is verified periodically with portal films. After completion of therapy, the patient is observed regularly to detect early relapse and evaluate treatment-related toxicity.

## Patient Evaluation and Staging

To determine the best treatment approach, the patient needs to undergo disease staging. A complete medical history is obtained with special attention to the tumor history, presence of B symptoms (unexplained fever, drenching night sweats, and unexplained weight loss), and general performance status. The physical examination should be thorough, with special attention to all nodal areas, Waldeyer's ring, liver, and spleen. When a single nodal site is involved, the low neck or supraclavicular area is involved in 60% of the cases, the mediastinum in 15%, axillae in 10%, and the inguinal-femoral regions in 10%. The disease progresses with involvement of contiguous nodal regions. Upper abdominal nodes are considered contiguous to the supraclavicular nodes through the thoracic duct. A biopsy must be performed, preferably with sampling from the most clinically suspicious node.

The hematologic assessment should include complete blood cell and platelet counts, erythrocyte sedimentation rate, and screen chemistries, including lactate dehydrogenase and thyroid function studies. An elevated erythrocyte sedimentation rate is associated with high risk of subclinical disease in the abdomen. An abnormal blood cell count and an elevated lactic dehydrogenase level suggest bone marrow involvement. Thyroid function testing must be done as a follow-up study because of a substantial risk of late dysfunction caused by radiation therapy.

Routine imaging studies include chest radiographs and computed tomography (CT) of the chest, abdomen, and pelvis. Magnetic resonance imaging (MRI) is used occasionally to better delineate hilar adenopathy and chest wall and pericardial extension and, in the abdomen, to distinguish unfilled bowel and vessels from adenopathy. Positron emission tomography fused with computed tomography (PET-CT) scans are most useful for distinguishing active disease in enlarged lymph nodes. Treatment response is evaluated with repeated PET-CT.

Bone marrow biopsies are performed in all patients except those with early stage (stage I or II) disease and no B symptoms. The overall frequency of bone marrow involvement in Hodgkin's disease is only 5%. Hodgkin's disease is staged according to the Ann Arbor staging classification system (Table 1). Figure 1 shows the lymphoid regions used in this system. Note that the infraclavicular, cervical occipital, and preauricular areas are a single region.

## Radiation Treatment Technique

Treatment planning starts by reviewing the staging evaluation and pathology report. Clinical and radiologic studies are used to outline the extent of disease. The treatment fields include the known disease areas and adjacent nodal regions. Treatment volume varies according to the treatment plan. The *treatment volumes* are defined as involved field, extended field, and subtotal nodal irradiation. *Involved field irradiation* includes the entire nodal area in which nodes with Hodgkin's disease are noted; for example, if a low neck node is involved, the entire

---

### CURRENT DIAGNOSIS

| History | Tumor history |
| --- | --- |
| | B symptoms (unexplained fever, drenching night sweats, unexplained weight loss) |
| Physical | All nodal areas |
| | Waldeyer's ring |
| | Liver/spleen |
| Laboratory tests | Complete CBC |
| | Erythrocyte sedimentation rate |
| | LDH |
| | Screen chemistries |
| Radiologic studies | CT chest/abdomen/pelvis |
| | PET-CT |
| Pathology | Lymph node or extranodal site |
| | Bone marrow |

*Abbreviations:* CBC = complete blood count; CT = computed tomography; LDH = lactate dehydrogenase; PET-CT = positron emission tomography fused with computed tomography.

---

### TABLE 1   Ann Arbor Staging Classification System

**Stage I**
Involvement of single lymph node region (I) or localized involvement of an extralymphatic organ or site (IE)

**Stage II**
Involvement of two or more lymph node regions on the same side of the diaphragm (II) or localized involvement of an extra lymphatic organ or site and one or more nodal regions on the same side of the diaphragm (IIE)

**Stage III**
Involvement of lymph node regions on both sides of the diaphragm (III), which may be accompanied by localized involvement of an extralymphatic organ or site (IIIE)

**Stage IV**
Diffuse involvement of one or more extralymphatic organs with or without associated lymph node involvement

**Systemic Symptoms**
A: Absence of systemic symptoms defined as B.
B: Unexplained fever with temperatures above 38°C (100°F), unexplained weight loss >10%, body weight, or drenching night sweats

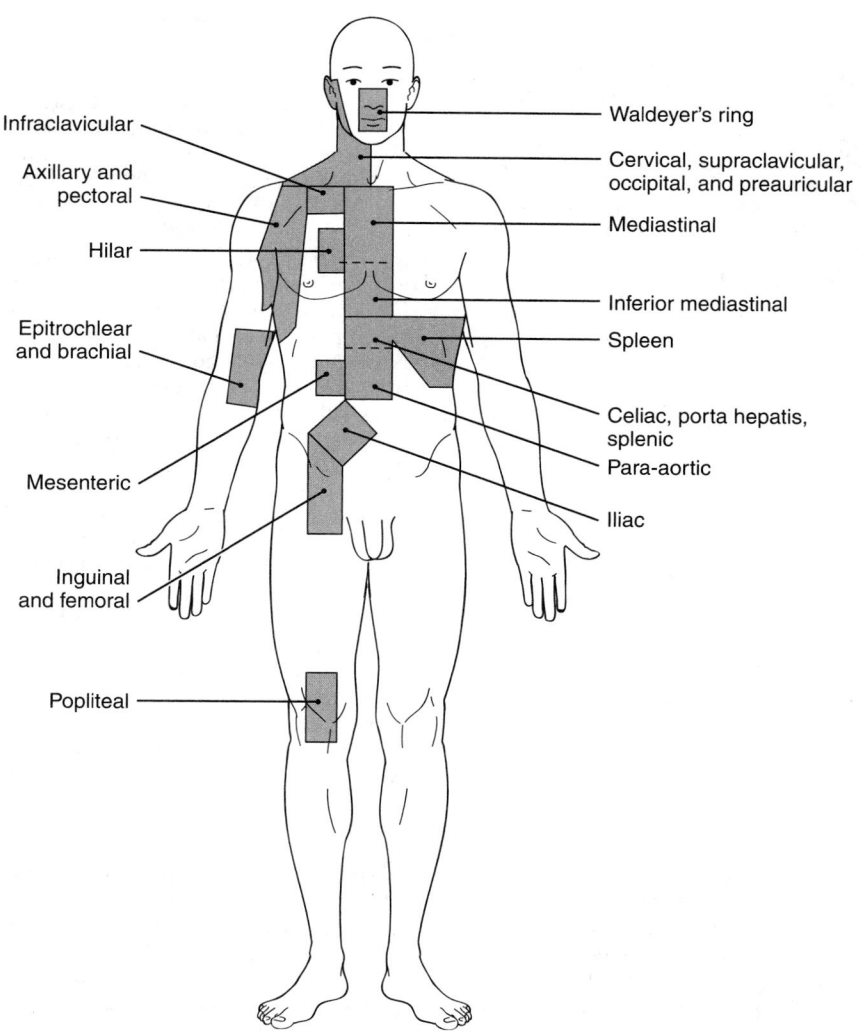

**FIGURE 1.** Lymphoid regions for Ann Arbor staging of Hodgkin's disease.

Infraclavicular

Axillary and pectoral

Hilar

Epitrochlear and brachial

Mesenteric

Inguinal and femoral

Popliteal

Waldeyer's ring

Cervical, supraclavicular, occipital, and preauricular

Mediastinal

Inferior mediastinal

Spleen

Celiac, porta hepatis, splenic

Para-aortic

Iliac

neck and supraclavicular areas are treated. *Extended field irradiation* treats the entire nodal region. *Subtotal nodal irradiation* includes all the regions at risk: the supradiaphragmatic area including neck, supraclavicular, infraclavicular, axillary, mediastinal, and hilar nodes, and the infradiaphragmatic area, including para-aortic nodes, spleen, pelvic, and inguinal-femoral nodes. The nodal areas not included are mesenteric, presacral, popliteal, brachial, and epitrochlear nodes because they are only rarely involved with Hodgkin's disease. These regions are treated in three areas: the mantle for the supradiaphragmatic region, the abdomen, and the pelvis, including inguinal and femoral nodes (Figure 2). The junction between the fields must be placed away from the tumor to prevent underdosing, and normal tissue tolerance must be considered to avoid organ toxicity.

After the treatment plan is determined, the radiation field is simulated and marked on the patient. The simulator is a diagnostic radiography unit that reproduces the geometry of the therapy machine and takes verification films of the treatment fields. CT simulation is used to better outline the treatment areas and protect the normal tissue. CT cuts are used to outline the areas at risk, treatment volume, and the organs. Digital reconstructed images from CT simulation match the verification films from the simulator. To optimize reproducibility of the daily setup, patient immobilization devices are used; for example, a face mask of low-temperature thermal plastic (polycarbolactone) or vacuum body mold can be used for the mantle. Treatment fields include lymphoid regions, and to encompass all these areas, large and irregular fields are necessary.

The treatment volume generated with the CT simulation is used to outline the field to be treated and to design the blocks for the areas to be protected from irradiation. Divergent blocks are constructed from the drawings on the digital reconstructed images using either a low-melting-point alloy such as Lipowitz metal (Cerrobend) or a multileaf collimator, a machine device that shapes the beam with small movable leaves. Typically, the dose is prescribed to be delivered along the central axis at the midplane. The dose is higher for thin areas where diameters are small. To calculate the dose in the different areas, the three-dimensional reconstruction from the CT simulation is used and a dose distribution is obtained. Partial transmission blocks or shrinking field technique are used to compensate for the difference in the diameters and to make the dose homogeneous throughout the treatment field. Better dose distributions are obtained with intensity modulated radiation therapy, using an electronic compensator, which modifies the beam moving the multileaf collimator to block the areas when they reach the prescribed dose.

Patients are treated on a linear accelerator at a 100-cm source-to-surface distance, usually using 6-MV photons for the upper torso and 18-MV photons for the abdomen and pelvis. The patient is seen on the treatment table by the radiation oncologist to verify the proper location of the fields. Machine portal films for verification are taken at the beginning of treatment and weekly thereafter. The dose delivered to the visible tumor areas is 39.6 Gy in 22 fractions over 4.5 weeks. The nodal areas treated prophylactically receive 30.6 Gy in 17 fractions over 3.5 weeks. In general, the treatment field is arranged with parallel

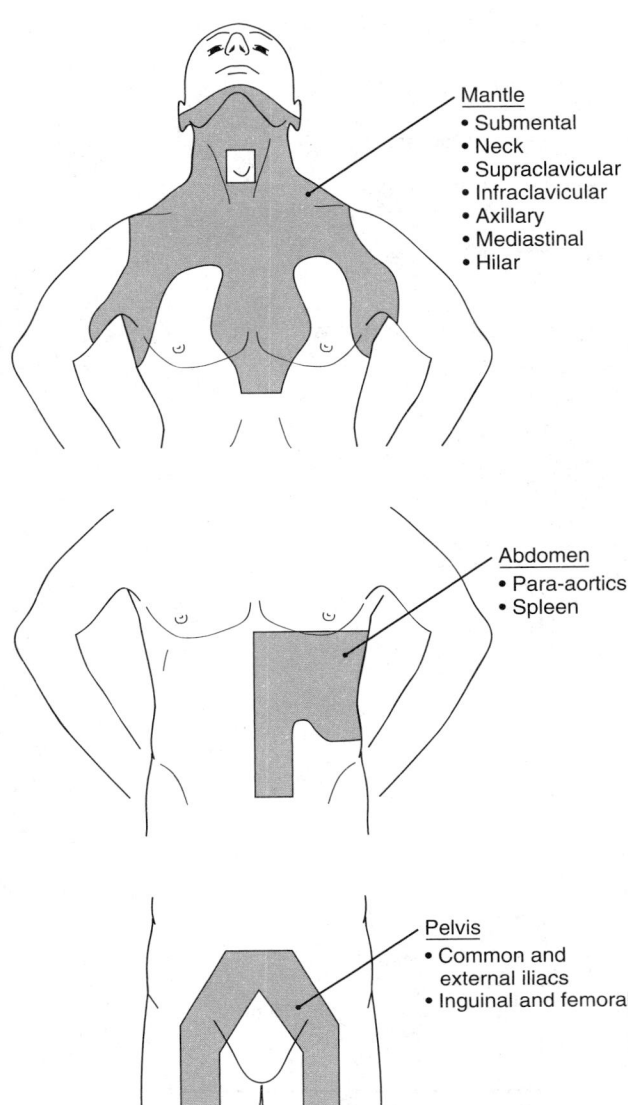

Mantle
- Submental
- Neck
- Supraclavicular
- Infraclavicular
- Axillary
- Mediastinal
- Hilar

Abdomen
- Para-aortics
- Spleen

Pelvis
- Common and external iliacs
- Inguinal and femoral

**FIGURE 2.** Radiation therapy extended fields: supradiaphragmatic: mantle; infradiaphragmatic: abdomen and pelvis.

opposed fields, using even-weighted beams, and all fields are treated daily. When two fields are matched (e.g., mantle and abdomen), special gap calculations are used to avoid overlap. If the adjacent fields overlie the spinal cord, CT simulation is used to computer-generated isodose calculations to determine the dose at the cord.

## Mantle Field Irradiation

Radiation to the mantle field treats the supradiaphragmatic nodal regions. The mantle field extends from the mastoid and base of the mandible to the diaphragm and encompasses the submental, occipital, cervical, supraclavicular, infraclavicular, axillary, mediastinal, and hilar nodes. The patient is treated using parallel opposed anteroposterior fields, with individually contoured lung and heart blocks. Usually, the cervical spine is blocked posteriorly, the larynx anteriorly, and both humeral heads anteriorly and posteriorly. The mantle is treated with equally loaded beams to a dose of 30.6 Gy in 17 fractions. At this point, treatment is stopped for the areas of prophylactic irradiation and continues only for the areas of gross involvement to a dose of 39.6 Gy. Obese patients have a wide mediastinum when they lie on their back and can be treated sitting in a specially designed chair to decrease the amount of normal lung treated.

## Subdiaphragmatic Irradiation

Subdiaphragmatic nodal areas are usually divided into two treatment fields: the abdomen, which includes the para-aortic nodes and spleen, with or without the pelvis, which includes the common and external iliac nodes and the inguinal-femoral regions. If the pelvic field is treated concurrently with the para-aortic field, the term *inverted Y* is used.

The field encompassing the para-aortic and spleen areas extends from the diaphragm to the bottom of the fourth lumbar vertebra; field edges are matched with those of the mantle with an appropriate skin gap; to encompass the para-aortic nodes, the field is drawn to the width of the transverse processes of the lumbar vertebral bodies, provided that the abdominal CT scan does not show nodes in a more lateral position. Radiation is delivered using parallel opposed antero-posterior fields with equally loaded beams that deliver a dose of 30.6 Gy in 17 fractions. An additional 9-Gy boost in five fractions is given to areas with tumor involvement. Individually contoured blocks are made to protect the kidneys and bowel. Often, it is not necessary to treat the pelvic lymph nodes and the radiation treatment stops at the level of the fourth lumbar vertebra. If needed, pelvic treatment is given through parallel opposed anteroposterior fields with 6-MV photons from the front (because the inguinal-femoral nodes are superficial) and 18-MV photons from the back. The pelvic field matches the abdomen field at the level of the fourth lumbar vertebra and extends to encompass the femoral lymph nodes. The nodal areas must be evaluated on the CT scan.

Careful blocking is used to spare the bone marrow as much as possible and, in young women, the ovaries. The ovaries are transposed medially and placed as low as possible behind the uterus to avoid radi-ation-induced amenorrhea and sterility. The ovaries are marked with radiopaque clips to aid in the placement of a double-thickness block. At a distance of 2 cm from the edge of the block, the ovaries receive approximately 8% of the pelvic dose.

## Combined Modality Therapy

Many patients with intermediate or advanced Hodgkin's disease bene-fit from combined chemotherapy and radiation therapy. To reduce the toxicity from the combined modality approach, treatment must be tailored to the extent of disease and the risk of normal tissue injury. Special attention must be paid to the chemotherapy drugs, the number of cycles, the total dose, the time frequency between cycles or intensity, the radiation fields, the volume of tissue irradiated, and doses. Both the medical oncologist and the radiation oncologist must work together from the beginning to tailor the treatment plan.

Most patients with Hodgkin's disease treated with combined modal-ity receive initially four or six cycles of a combination of doxorubicin (Adriamycin), bleomycin (Blenoxane), vinblastine (Velban), and dacar-bazine (DTIC), the ABVD regimen, followed by radiation therapy to the involved areas. For patients with advanced Hodgkin's disease (stage IIIB or IV) or mediastinal masses larger than 15 cm, six cycles of chemother-apy are given, followed by radiation therapy to the involved sites.

PET-CT is used to evaluate the treatment response to chemotherapy. The test is done before chemotherapy begins and, if positive, repeated before radiation is delivered. Patients who become negative have a lower relapse rate.

## Treatment Recommendations and Results

### SUPRADIAPHRAGMATIC FAVORABLE STAGES I AND IIA

Upper torso presentation in patients younger than 40 years, with three or fewer sites of involvement, no large mediastinal mass, no B symptoms, and erythrocyte sedimentation rate less than 50 mm/hour should be treated with radiation therapy alone. Radiation is given to the mantle field and the para-aortic and spleen areas (Figure 2). Patients with mediastinal disease are excluded because they benefit from induction chemotherapy, which reduces the mediastinal mass and decreases

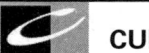

## CURRENT THERAPY

| Disease Extension | Treatment |
|---|---|
| Favorable I–IIA | XRT |
| Unfavorable I–IIB and favorable III | ABVD + IF-XRT |
| Advanced III–IV | ABVD or ABVD + IF-XRT |
| Relapse or refractory | High-dose chemotherapy + IF-XRT |

*Abbreviations:* ABVD = doxorubicin/bleomycin/vinblastine/dacarbazine; IF = Involved field. XRT = radiotherapy.

radiation to normal lung. Freedom from relapse for this group of patients is 80% to 90% (Table 2).

Patients with stage IA nodular lymphocyte predominant Hodgkin's disease are a special subgroup who tend to have disease localized and have a late relapse pattern similar to low-grade nodular lymphomas. These patients must be treated to the involved field (Figure 3).

### SUPRADIAPHRAGMATIC UNFAVORABLE STAGES I THROUGH IIA AND IIB

This group includes all patients with stages I and II disease who do not meet the so-called favorable criteria. These patients have an increased risk of abdominal involvement, approaching 30% according to the laparotomy data. Treatment is with combined modality therapy. Chemotherapy (four or six cycles of ABVD) is given first, followed by radiation therapy to the involved fields. The radiotherapy dose varies according to the chemotherapy response: For complete response 30 Gy is used, and for partial response, 40 Gy. Patients in this group, treated with chemotherapy followed by radiation therapy, have a disease-free survival between 80% and 90% and a survival rate of 90% at 6 years (Table 2).

### STAGES I AND II WITH MEDIASTINAL INVOLVEMENT

Mediastinal involvement in very common in Hodgkin's disease and presents a special challenge to the radiation oncologist because toxicity to the lungs and heart must be avoided. The extent of mediastinal tumor involvement is determined by measuring the maximum single horizontal width of the mediastinum on a standing posteroanterior chest radiograph. Three categories are defined as follows: Tumors less than 7.5 cm are small, those larger than 7.5 cm to less than 15 cm are large or bulky, and those larger than 15 cm are massive.

Patients with mediastinal involvement mass are treated with combined modality therapy. Chemotherapy is administered first to decrease the size of the mediastinal tumor. Patients receive six cycles of combination chemotherapy followed by radiation therapy to the involved field. Bleomycin is stopped after the fourth cycle if mediastinal irradiation is planned. Patients in this group, treated with combination chemotherapy followed by radiation therapy, have a disease-free survival of 80% and an 89% survival rate at 10 years (see Table 2).

### STAGES I AND II: SUBDIAPHRAGMATIC INVOLVEMENT

Fewer than 10% of patients with stage I or II Hodgkin's disease present with disease limited to the subdiaphragmatic areas. CT of the abdomen and pelvis is used to evaluate nodal and spleen involvement, and treatment is adjusted to the extent of tumor involvement.

For stage IA inguinal presentation, radiation is delivered to the involved field. More advanced cases receive combined modality therapy. Radiation therapy fields include the para-aortic nodes, the spleen, the common and external iliac nodes, and the inguinal-femoral regions. Treatment results for these patients are similar to those with supradiaphragmatic presentations.

### FAVORABLE STAGE III

Nodal involvement in patients with stage III disease varies greatly. This heterogeneous group of patients is divided into subgroups according to extent of abdominal disease. Stage III$_1$ includes patients with disease limited to the upper abdomen (involving the celiac region, splenic hilum, and spleen). When the disease extends to the para-aortic region, it is classified as stage III$_2$; and if the pelvis or inguinal region is involved, the classification is stage III$_3$. With the exception of patients presenting with stage III$_3$ disease or IIIB, all patients with stage III receive six cycles of combination chemotherapy (ABVD), followed by radiation therapy to the involved areas (Figure 3). The relapse-free rate for this group is 85% with a cause-specific survival of 80% at 10 years.

### ADVANCED STAGES III AND IV

The majority of patients with stage III$_3$ and many with stage IV receive combined modality therapy. Radiotherapy can be omitted for the patients that achieve a complete response to chemotherapy. Only approximately 35% of patients with advanced-stage disease treated with chemotherapy alone are alive and well at 10 years. Patterns of failure after chemotherapy show that recurrence overwhelmingly occurs in previously involved areas. Patients with stage III$_3$ ant IV Hodgkin's disease are treated initially with six cycles of combination chemotherapy (ABVD), followed by irradiation to the involved sites. With combined modality therapy, relapse-free survival of 85% and overall survival of 85% at 5 years is reported (see Table 2).

For relapsed or refractory Hodgkin's disease, involved field radiotherapy is used after high-dose chemotherapy and autologous bone marrow transplantation, with better local control and probable improved survival. The disease-free survival at 3 years is 66% and the survival is 57%.

## TABLE 2 Treatment Results for Hodgkin's Disease

| Series | Stage | Treatment | Survival % (y) | Freedom from Relapse % (y) |
|---|---|---|---|---|
| EORTC | I—IIA Favorable | XRT | 96 (6) | 81 (6) |
| EORTC | I—II Unfavorable | MOPP/ABV-XRT | 89 (6) | 94 (6) |
| JCRT | I—II large mediastinal mass | MOPP-XRT | 88 (10) | 89 (10) |
| MDACC | III (except III$_3$) | MOPP-XRT | 87 (10) | 83 (10) |
| EORTC | IIIB—IV | MOPP/ABV | 85 (5) | 85 (5) |

*Abbreviations:* ABV = doxorubicin, bleomycin, vinblastine; EORTC = European Organization for Research and Treatment of Cancer; JCRT = Joint Center for Radiation Therapy; MDACC = MD Anderson Cancer Center; MOPP = mechlorethamine, vincristine, procarbazine, prednisone; XRT = radiotherapy.

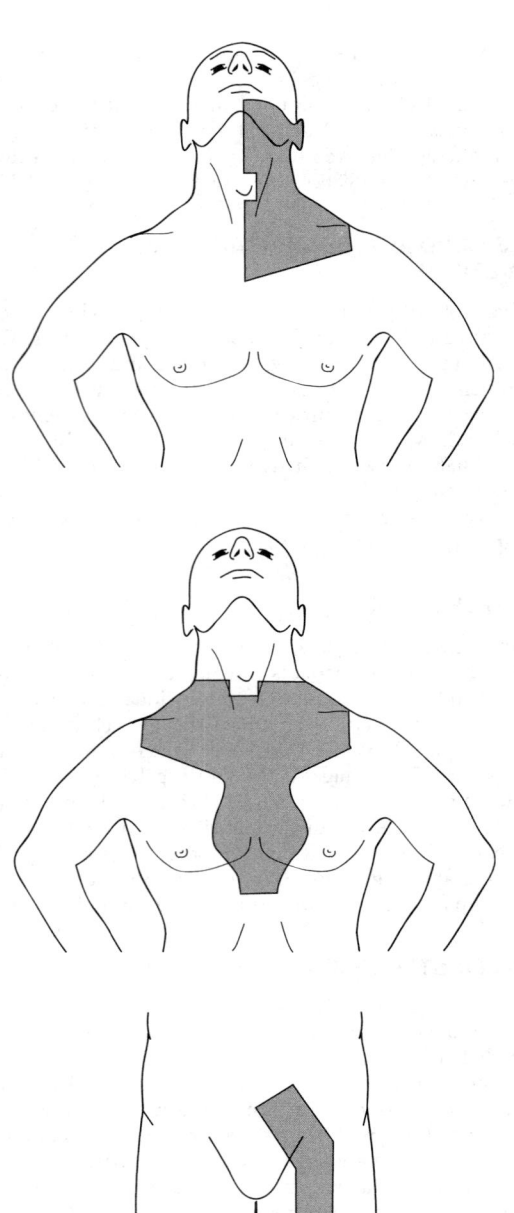

**FIGURE 3.** Radiation therapy involved field examples: neck, mediastinum, and inguinal-femoral.

## Complications

Complications are classified as acute or late. Acute complications occur during or shortly after the course of radiation therapy; they are treated symptomatically and resolve quickly after the completion of treatment. Acute complications include mild skin reactions and hair loss in the irradiated areas, dysphasia, dry cough, nausea, and diarrhea. These complications are treated symptomatically with skin ointments, analgesics, cough suppressants, and antinausea and antidiarrheal agents.

Late complications occur after treatment is complete, months or years later, and tend to be permanent. Late complications include pneumonitis, pericarditis, hypothyroidism, dental caries, and second malignancies. These reported toxicities observed in long-term survivors are clearly associated with treatment techniques that are different from the ones used today; therefore, in the future a decrease in these toxicities is expected.

Radiation pneumonitis occurs infrequently, and its risk is proportional to the volume of lung irradiated, the total dose, and the fraction size. The patient typically presents 6 to 12 weeks after the completion of the radiation therapy with dry cough, shortness of breath, pleuritic chest pain, and fever. The chest radiograph reveals interstitial infiltrates. Severe cases require treatment with high doses of corticosteroids for 4 to 6 weeks, with gradual tapering to avoid recurrence of symptoms.

Pericarditis is rare, occurring 6 to 12 months after treatment and usually after irradiation of the entire heart. Pericarditis presents as an acute episode of chest pain, fatigue, fever, and friction rubs or sometimes with decreased heart sounds because of pericardial effusion. Patients with mild pericarditis are managed with nonsteroidal anti-inflammatory agents, and for severe cases corticosteroids are used. Constrictive pericarditis and pericardial tamponade are rare complications that require surgical correction.

Subclinical hypothyroidism develops in a third of patients treated with mantle field irradiation. Patients are asymptomatic, and the physician is alerted by the elevation in the thyroid-stimulating hormone seen on the routine yearly blood measurement. Thyroid hormone replacement is necessary to avoid development of symptomatic hypothyroidism with weight gain, lethargy, temperature intolerance, irritability, and changes in skin and hair.

*Xerostomia* (mouth dryness) develops during irradiation of the mantle field that treats a portion of the salivary glands. There is minimal risk of clinically significant xerostomia, but partial decrease in saliva produces a favorable environment for dental caries. This complication can be prevented with pretreatment dental evaluation, careful dental care, and the daily use of fluoride.

Serious abdominal complications are extremely rare. An occasional gastric ulcer may occur. Bowel obstruction is related to prior laparotomy. In men, pelvic irradiation with adequate testicular shielding produces only temporary azoospermia. In women, ovariopexy is needed before pelvic irradiation to preserve fertility. The ovaries are meticulously shielded, but even this may not preserve ovarian function, especially in women older than 30 years.

The improved survival of patients with Hodgkin's disease is associated with an increase in the frequency of second malignancies. Leukemias are associated with the use of alkylating agents, and solid tumors are associated with radiation therapy. The most common cancers seen are breast cancer that occurs at a younger age, lung cancer in smokers, thyroid cancer, and non-Hodgkin's lymphoma. Shrink in the irradiation volume, with the use of involved fields, and the decrease in the total dose delivered should reduce the incidence of solid tumors in the future. Workup for early detection of cancer must be included in the yearly follow-up, and recommendations to avoid smoking given to all patients.

## REFERENCES

Berthe MP, Aleman MD, John MM, et al: Involved-field radiotherapy for advanced Hodgkin's lymphoma. N Engl J Med 2003;348;24.

Eich H, Mueller R, Engert A, et al: Comparison of 30 Gy versus 20 Gy involved field radiotherapy after two versus four cycles ABVD in early stage Hodgkin's lymphoma: Interim analysis of the German Hodgkin Study Group Trial HD10. Int J Radiat Oncol Biol Phys 2005;63(S1):S1-S2. Proceedings of the 47th Annual ASTRO meeting.

Hughes-Davies L, Tarbell NJ, Coleman CN, et al: Stage IA-IIB Hodgkin's disease: Management and outcome of extensive thoracic involvement. Int J Radiat Oncol Biol Phys 1997;39(2):361-369.

Noordijk EM, Carde P, Dupouy N, et al: Combined-modality therapy for clinical stage I or II Hodgkin's lymphoma: Long-term results of the European Organisation for Research and Treatment of Cancer H7 randomized controlled trails. J Clin Oncol 2006;24(19):3128-3135.

Poen JC, Hoppe RT, Horning SJ: High-dose therapy and autologous bone marrow transplantation for relapsed/refractory Hodgkin's disease: The impact of involved field radiotherapy on patterns of failure and survival. Int J Radiat Oncol Biol Phys 1996;36(1):3-12.

# Acute Leukemias in Adults

Method of
*Jonathan E. Kolitz, MD*

The acute leukemias are clonal hematopoietic neoplasms that cause death by usurping the bone marrow's ability to produce normal blood elements. The replacement of marrow by primitive progenitor cells (blasts) leads to infection from neutropenia, bleeding from thrombocytopenia and coagulopathies, and anemia. The two major subtypes of acute leukemia are acute lymphoblastic leukemia (ALL) and acute myeloid leukemia (AML). ALL is the predominant acute leukemia of childhood, and the incidence of AML increases with age.

AML may be associated with antecedent hematologic disorders such as the myeloproliferative disorders and the myelodysplastic syndrome (MDS). Such cases of AML, along with those associated with prior exposure to chemotherapy or radiation, are associated with especially poor outcomes.

## Diagnosis

Once acute leukemia is suspected, diagnostic measures must be rapidly undertaken (Table 1). Readily available in most centers are tools that can categorize the acute leukemia in preparation for specific therapy. In addition to morphology, flow cytometry can rapidly establish a diagnosis of acute leukemia by applying combinations of monoclonal antibody stains directed at antigens known as *cluster designation (CD) groups*. A panel of 10 or more antigens is generally studied to properly assign lineage. Acute leukemia with minimal expression of lineage-specific antigens may be difficult to categorize. In addition, an occasional leukemia expresses antigens common to more than one lineage (biphenotypic leukemia) or even manifests as two distinct clonal processes. Most often, the combination of morphologic review and the application of the tests outlined in Table 1 satisfactorily establish a diagnosis.

Cytogenetics has become an essential tool both for categorizing leukemias and for establishing prognosis and detecting minimal residual disease (MRD), the remnant of leukemia that is almost invariably subclinically present when a patient is clinically in complete remission (CR). The eradication of MRD is a principal goal of leukemia therapy.

## CURRENT DIAGNOSIS

- Leukocytosis and increased blasts or leukopenia (aleukemic leukemia)
- Anemia and/or thrombocytopenia
- Adenopathy, organomegaly, bone pain more common in ALL
- Central nervous system and/or testicular involvement more common in ALL
- High LDH, tumor lysis syndrome more common in L3 ALL (Burkitt's leukemia).
- Coagulopathy typical in APL.
- Bone marrow aspirate and biopsy must include routine Wright-Giemsa stain, complete immunophenotype using flow cytometry and immunohistochemistry, and cytogenetics for appropriate diagnostic categorization and for prognostic purposes.

*Abbreviations:* ALL = acute lymphoblastic leukemia; AML = Acute myeloid leukemia; LDH = lactate dehydrogenase; APL = acute promyelocytic leukemia.

## Classification

The categorization of acute leukemia has shifted from the original French-American-British (FAB) classification system, which was based on morphology, to the World Health Organization (WHO) classification scheme (Box 1). The WHO system recognizes the original FAB categories but specifies wherever possible subtypes that have distinct clinical and cytogenetic features. It is hoped that as the molecular understanding of acute leukemia evolves, subsets will be shifted from the original FAB to an expanded WHO classification.

## Prognostic Factors

The prognosis of patients with acute leukemia depends on multiple variables. Outcomes of patients with acute leukemia are strongly influenced by the cytogenetic abnormalities present at diagnosis. Important prognostic factors are outlined in Box 2. Listed in Box 2 are several recently identified gene mutations that have been associated with

## TABLE 1  Diagnostic Tests in Acute Leukemia

| Test | Comment |
| --- | --- |
| Complete blood count and differential | |
| DIC screen | Especially in APL, monocytic leukemias |
| Chemistry profile, including uric acid, phosphorus, LDH | |
| HLA typing | Irrespective of transplantation intent, to identify compatible platelets units if needed |
| Bone marrow aspirate | Dry tap can occur in extensively infiltrated (packed) marrow or in the presence of fibrosis |
| Bone marrow biopsy | Permits determination of cellularity, immunophenotyping |
| Immunohistochemistry | Chemical stains for lineage, monoclonal antibody stains for specific antigens on paraffin sections from biopsy |
| Flow cytometry | Stain blasts with monoclonal antibodies directed at lineage-specific antigens |
| FISH | Rapidly diagnoses suspected subtypes of acute leukemia, especially APL |
| Cytogenetics | Analyzes metaphases for numeric and structural changes in banded chromosomes |
| PCR | Sensitive technique to measure minimal residual disease. Sensitivity is 1 in $10^4$ to $10^6$ leukemic cells. |

*Abbreviations:* APL = acute promyelocytic leukemia; DIC = disseminated intravascular coagulation; FISH = fluorescence-in-situ-hybridization; HLA = human leukocyte antigen; LDH = lactate dehydrogenase; PCR = polymerase chain reaction.

## BOX 1   World Health Organization Classification of the Acute Leukemias

### Acute Myeloid Leukemias
- With recurrent genetic abnormalities
  - AML with t(8;21) (AML-1-ETO)
  - AML with abnormal marrow eosinophils
  - AML with inv(16)(p13q22) or t(16;16)(p13q22) (*CBFβ-MYH11*) [FAB M4Eo]
  - Acute promyelocytic leukemia: AML with t(15;17)(q22q12) (*PML-RARα*) [FAB M3]
  - AML with MLL (11q23) abnormalities
- With multilineage dysplasia
- With or without antecedent myelodysplastic or myeloproliferative disorder
- Therapy-related
  - Alkylating agent related
  - Topoisomerase II inhibitor related
  - Other types
- Not otherwise categorized
  - AML, minimally differentiated [FAB M0]
  - AML without maturation [FAB M1]
  - AML with maturation [FAB M2]
  - Acute myelomonocytic leukemia [FAB M4]
  - Acute monoblastic and monocytic leukemias [FAB M5]
  - Acute erythroid leukemia [FAB M6]
  - Acute megakaryoblastic leukemia [FAB M7]
  - Acute basophilic leukemia
  - Acute panmyelosis with myelofibrosis
  - Myeloid sarcoma

### Acute Leukemias of Ambiguous Lineage
- Undifferentiated acute leukemia
- Bilineal acute leukemia
- Biphenotypic acute leukemia

### Acute Lymphoblastic Leukemia/Lymphoblastic Lymphoma
- Precursor B ALL
- Precursor T ALL

*Note:* FAB classifications are given in square brackets following some classifications.
*Abbreviations:* ALL = acute lymphoblastic leukemia; AML = acute myeloid leukemia; ETO = *ETO* (eight twenty-one) gene; FAB = French-American-British classification system; MLL = mixed lineage leukemia.

## BOX 2   Prognostic Factors in Acute Leukemia

### Favorable
#### *Acute Myeloid Leukemia*
- Age <60 years
- t(15;17), t(8;21), inv(16), t(16;16), t(8;21)
- De novo disease
- Nucleophosmin gene mutation*
- CCAAT/enhancer binding protein mutation*

#### *Acute Lymphoblastic Leukemia*
- Age 2-10 years
- Hyperdiploidy
- Early blast clearance with chemotherapy
- Mature B cell (Burkitt's leukemia) or T cell phenotype
- WBC <30,000/μL
- t(12;21)

### Unfavorable
#### *Acute Myeloid Leukemia*
- Age >70 years
- Chromosome 7 abnormalities, complex karyotypes, t(6;9); inv(3); t(3;3)
- Multidrug resistance gene expression
- WBC >100,000/μL
- Fms-like tyrosine kinase (flt3) mutation
- Brain and leukemia cytoplasmic (BAALC) gene mutation*
- ETS-related gene (ERG) mutation*
- Antecedent MDS or myeloproliferative disorder
- Therapy-related AML

#### *Acute Lymphoblastic Leukemia*
- Age <2 or >10 years
- t(9;22); t(4;11); -7; +8
- Pro-B (very early B lineage) phenotype
- Hypodiploidy
- WBC >30,000/μL
- Time to CR >4-5 weeks
- MLL gene mutation

*Among the approximately 50% of patients with AML and normal cytogenetics
*Abbreviations:* AML = acute myeloid leukemia; CR = complete remission; MDS = myelodysplastic syndrome; MLL = mixed lineage leukemia; WBC = white blood cell.

---

distinct outcomes in the 50% or so of patients with AML who have a normal karyotype, a group regarded as a whole to have an intermediate prognosis.

# Treatment

## ACUTE MYELOID LEUKEMIA

The therapy of acute leukemia is divided into sequential components. For both AML and ALL, induction therapy involves a period of intensive antileukemic therapy generally given in an inpatient hospital setting. Typically, a central venous catheter is placed to ensure the venous access needed for the chemotherapy and vigorous antibiotic and blood product support required during the period of severe myelosuppression.

### Induction

The backbone of induction chemotherapy for AML consists of a combination of 3 days of an anthracycline given by short IV bolus with a 7-day continuous IV (CIV) infusion of cytarabine (Ara-C, Cytosar-U) 100-200 mg/m²/day (3- and 7-day regimens). Anthracyclines include daunorubicin (cerubidine) given at doses between 45 and 90 mg/m², idarubicin (Idamycin) 12 mg/m², and mitoxantrone (Novantrone) 12 mg/m², each given daily for 3 days. There are no conclusive data showing that the choice of anthracycline is fundamentally important. Randomized trials have not compared pharmacologically and pharmacodynamically equivalent doses of these agents. An ongoing randomized trial will help clarify if daunorubicin 45 mg/m² given daily for 3 days differs from twice that dose given in the same manner, both combined with infusional cytarabine, in untreated patients with AML.

Increasing the cytarabine infusional dose from 100 mg/m² to twice that dose has not improved outcomes. Neither has extending the 7-day cytarabine infusion to 10 days. Escalating the dose of cytarabine to 3000 mg/m² (High-Dose Ara-C, or HiDAC) has not increased

---

³Exceeds dosage recommended by the manufacturer.

## CURRENT THERAPY

- AML in patients younger than 60 years and favorable cytogenetics
  - Anthracycline/cytarabine induction
  - High-dose cytarabine consolidation × 3-4 cycles
- AML under age 60, unfavorable cytogenetics, including normal
  - Anthracycline/cytarabine induction followed by either high-dose cytarabine consolidation or stem cell transplantation
- Acute promyelocytic leukemia
  - Anthracycline with or without cytarabine plus all-*trans*-retinoic acid induction
  - Anthracycline consolidation × 2 cycles generally with all-*trans*-retinoic acid
  - Maintenance therapy with all-*trans*-retinoic acid, with or without PO 6-mercaptopurine and methotrexate (role being determined)
  - High-dose cytarabine, mylotarg, and arsenic trioxide in untreated patients being studied
- AML in patients older than 60 years
  - Options as in patients younger than 60 years in select patients
  - Investigational therapies.
- ALL
  - Five-drug induction regimen (see text)
  - Consolidation therapy with high-dose cytarabine and methotrexate, L-asparaginase, 6-mercaptopurine, cyclophosphamide
  - Maintenance therapy with vincristine, steroids, PO 6-mercaptopurine, and methotrexate for 18 months
  - CNS prophylaxis with systemic and intrathecal therapies
  - Cranial radiotherapy is an option but is potentially toxic
- L3 ALL (Burkitt's leukemia)
  - Short-course intensive high-dose cytarabine, methotrexate therapy plus anthracycline, vincristine, cyclophosphamide; intensive systemic and intrathecal CNS prophylactic therapy
  - No maintenance
  - Rituximab[1] (Rituxan) may be effective
- Myeloid growth factors more effective in reducing periods of neutropenia and infectious risk in ALL than in AML.

---

[1]Not FDA approved for this indication.

the incidence of CR when given during induction. Typical schedules of high-dose cytarabine entail once- or twice-daily administration for 5 or 6 days. A phase III trial suggested that even in the absence of improvements in CR, high-dose cytarabine given during induction improved relapse-free survival. Similar data exist for the use of etoposide[1] (VePesid) during induction, an important third class (epidophyllotoxins) of drugs active against acute leukemia, when given at a dose of 75 mg/m² IV daily for 7 days. High-dose cytarabine or etoposide has been used by clinicians during induction but is not considered standard of care at this time, particularly in the elderly.

Typically, in patients undergoing induction, a bone marrow aspirate and biopsy is done 14 days after starting therapy. Residual

---

[1]Not FDA approved for this indication.

leukemia is then treated with a second course of therapy using an abbreviated schedule of the original induction. Therapy may be changed and intensified at that time in select younger patients with minimal evidence of an antileukemic effect, often including high-dose cytarabine.

About 60% to 80% of younger patients with previously untreated, de novo AML achieve CR, most with one course of induction therapy. Therapy-related mortality is between 5% and 10%, with deaths occurring most often as a result of sepsis or hemorrhage, with or without the accompaniment of resistant leukemia.

### Consolidation

Once CR is attained, it is essential for the younger patient to move on to intensive treatments aimed at eradicating MRD. By the time a morphologic CR is attained, the total body leukemic cell burden may have fallen only 3 logs (from $10^{12}$ to $10^9$ cells), so substantial further treatment is needed. Patients with very poor risk karyotypes (complex cytogenetics, chromosome 7 or 3 abnormalities, t(6;9), among others) may be best served by allogeneic transplantation (myeloablative chemotherapy followed by infusion of stem cells from an immunologically matched donor) if a suitable human leukocyte antigen (HLA)-matched donor can be identified.

For most patients, intensive, repeated cycles of chemotherapy are given, usually with high-dose cytarabine alone or a high-dose cytarabine–containing combination. Older patients in CR often receive one or two courses of consolidation using the less-intensive combination of 2 days of an anthracycline and 5 days of infusional cytarabine (2 and 5 regimen). Repeated courses of high-dose cytarabine are especially benefit patients with the favorable cytogenetics of t(8;21), inv(16), and t(16;16), with a cure fraction of more than 50%.

### Stem-Cell Transplantation

For the bulk of the patients (about 50%) with normal cytogenetics, the choice is between several courses of high-dose cytarabine or a similar variant, or an allogeneic or autologous stem-cell transplant (ASCT). ASCT involves collecting stem cells from a patient in CR, which are then infused back to the patient after myeloablative chemotherapy is given.

Prognostic factors are being increasingly described in normal-karyotype AML, but it is premature to make treatment recommendations based on these early data. Several trials have compared intensive chemotherapy with ASCT, and although trends favoring relapse-free survival in patients undergoing ASCT have been seen, only one phase III trial has demonstrated that patients benefited from ASCT given late in their clinical course. The Cancer and Leukemia Group B has shown that ASCT yields results similar to those achieved with four courses of high-dose cytarabine followed by maintenance therapy in patients with normal cytogenetics. It has been suggested that ASCT may be associated with less morbidity than multiple courses of high-dose chemotherapy.

The advantage presented by ASCT, that of administering myeloablative doses of chemotherapy, might be negated by failure to eradicate residual leukemia in the infused stem cells. Attempts to improve outcomes have included intensifying the chemotherapy given prior to stem cell collection (in vivo purging) as well as ex vivo purging of stem cell collections with high doses of cytotoxic agents or monoclonal antibodies (or both). The use of peripheral stem cells reduces the time to hematopoietic engraftment. Whether overall treatment outcomes will improve with the increased use of peripheral blood rather than marrow as a source of stem cells remains to be seen.

Allogeneic transplants are limited to the 30% to 35% or so of eligible patients who have a donor. Although the risk of infusing leukemic cells is eliminated in allogeneic transplants, greater risks exist related to the immunologic effect of infused donor T cells against host tissues (graft-versus-host disease, GVHD). The other important consequence is the development of a direct antileukemic effect called *graft-versus-leukemia* (GVL). In younger patients, especially those younger than 30 years, GVHD tends to be manageable, and outcomes in AML patients receiving transplants in first CR can be excellent. The risk of GVHD and associated complications greatly increases with age.

The high-dose chemotherapy, given with or without total body irradiation, can cause unacceptable toxicities in older patients.

An attempt to counter this problem has been the ongoing exploration of reduced-intensity transplants, in which low doses of immunosuppressive agents such as fludarabine[1] (Fludara), antithymocyte globulin[1] (Atgam, others), alemtuzumab[1] (CamPath), melphalan[1] (Alkeran), or busulfan[1] (Myleran PO or Busulfex IV) are used to suppress host defenses sufficiently to permit engraftment of donor stem cells. This can lead to a curative GVL effect in some patients. The relative safety of the preparative regimen can be negated, however, by the development of severe GVHD. Methodologies to enhance the GVL effect while limiting the sequelae of GVHD are being actively studied. Select patients older than 60 years, and even older than 70 years, have been treated using this approach.

## Maintenance

Unlike in ALL, there is no evidence that lower doses of chemotherapy given for prolonged periods after induction and consolidation (maintenance therapy) improve survival, although time to relapse may be favorably affected. Overall, about 30% of patients with AML younger than 60 years with other than favorable cytogenetics are cured.

## Older Patients

Older patients present a special challenge. Patients older than 60 years, and especially older than 70 years, are more likely to harbor resistant forms of AML associated with poor-risk cytogenetic features and multidrug-resistance phenotypes. Comorbid conditions limit tolerance for severely myelotoxic therapies. Nonetheless, a good performance status predicts a more favorable outcome, even in older patients. The patient's physiologic state must be factored in with other established predictors of outcome in deciding whether or with what to treat older patients with AML.

Several randomized trials suggest that treatment of older patients who have AML can lead to better outcomes with respect to survival than purely supportive or palliative approaches. Ideally, investigational therapies should be evaluated in this high-risk patient population. Select older patients can benefit from intensive therapies used in younger patients, such as the 7- and 3-day regimens described earlier. Depending on performance status and other prognostic factors, the probability of a patient older than 60 years entering CR using conventional induction treatment is 30% to 50%, with therapy-related mortality of 20% to 40%. Only about 10% are long survivors.

For many patients, investigational agents, attenuated doses of conventional induction regimens, or alternative therapies that have been most often used in high-risk MDS may be considered. A non–anthracycline-containing combination of the topoisomerase I inhibitor topotecan[1] (Hycamptin, 1.5 mg/m$^2$/day by CIV) and cytarabine 2 g/m$^2$, each given daily for 5 days, has moderate activity in older patients with AML, as does the non–cytarabine-containing combination of mitoxantrone (Novantrone) 10 mg/m$^2$ and etoposide[1] (Toposar) 100 mg/m$^2$ each given daily IV for 5 days.

Fludarabine[1] 25 to 30 mg/m$^2$ IV daily for 4 days has been combined with high-dose cytarabine and filgrastim (Neupogen) in the non–anthracycline-containing FLAG (fludarabine, cytarabine, granulocyte colony-stimulating factor [G-CSF]) regimen.

Hypomethylating agents that induce the expression of silenced genes such as 5-azacytidine[1] (Vidaza, 75 mg/m$^2$ SC daily for 7 days every 4 weeks) or* decitabine[1] (Dacogen), using various doses and schedules, may have activity in select older patients with AML, as may low doses of cytarabine (10 mg/m$^2$ SC bid for 14-21 days every 28 days). Low-dose cytarabine has also been recently combined with arsenic trioxide[8] (Trisenox) in an investigational regimen for elderly patients with AML.

Clofarabine (Clolar) is a newly developed nucleoside analogue that might have activity in older patients with AML. The optimal dose and schedule remain under study.

The anti-CD33 monoclonal antibody–calicheamycin construct gemtuzumab ozogamycin (Mylotarg) can induce CR in a small fraction (about 20%) of older patients with untreated AML. The approved dose and schedule when used as a single agent is 9 mg/m$^2$ IV on days 1 and 15. Various combinations of this antibody with chemotherapy are being investigated.

The orally available farnesyl transferase inhibitor tipifarnib (Zarnestra)[1] has proven disappointing when used as a single agent.

## Investigational Therapy

Relapsed and refractory disease and AML in the elderly demand the use of investigational therapies. High-dose cytarabine can occasionally induce response in a patient resistant to a conventional anthracycline-cytarabine regimen. For almost all suitable patients, a CR achieved after an initial induction failure or a second CR must be rapidly consolidated with a transplant-based strategy.

Investigational approaches have involved novel agents with inhibitory properties directed against proliferative, differentiation, immunomodulatory, angiogenic, and drug-resistance pathways. Efforts to improve outcomes by inhibiting P-glycoprotein, a transmembrane drug efflux pump that confers multidrug resistance, have had limited success. A partial list of novel agents, most of which are being studied in AML but some of which may be active in ALL, is presented in Table 2. Ongoing efforts are assessing the use of these agents alone and in combination with chemotherapy.

Filgrastim[1] (and sargramostin (Leukine) are myeloid growth factors that have been studied in AML to hasten myeloid recovery as well as to stimulate proliferation of leukemic cells in order to increase their susceptibility to cell cycle–active cytotoxic agents such as cytarabine. Benefits have been, at best, marginal, with some indication that periods of neutropenia and hospital stays are reduced but without clear evidence that survival is increased. Studies looking at cell cycle activation effects have been conflicting but mostly negative.

## ACUTE PROMYELOCYTIC LEUKEMIA

Acute promyelocytic leukemia (APL) represents a paradigm for a malignancy that is yielding to targeted strategies that are not principally dependent on cytotoxic agents. Representing only about 5% to 10% of adult AML, 70% to 80% of patients with newly diagnosed disease can now expect to be cured.

All-*trans*-retinoic acid (ATRA, tretinoin, Vesanoid) induces terminal differentiation and apoptosis in APL cells. It can induce CR in most patients with APL given alone at a dose of 45 mg/m$^2$ PO daily in 2 divided doses for 30 to 45 days, but it cannot eradicate the disease by itself. The combination of anthracycline-based chemotherapy and ATRA induces CR and polymerase chain reaction (PCR, a highly sensitive assay for MRD, see Table 1) negativity in 70% to 80% of patients. A non–anthracycline-containing combination using arsenic trioxide (Trisenox, 0.15 mg/kg IV over 2 hours daily until CR and then repeated for 4 to 6 cycles) with or without ATRA induces similar outcomes, although long-term follow-up is shorter than with chemotherapy-containing regimens.

APL is sensitive to anthracyclines, so consolidation courses consisting, for example, of two courses of daunorubicin 50 mg/m$^2$ IV daily for 3 days, usually given in combination with ATRA, induces a high cure fraction. The results of a phase III North American Intergroup trial in which untreated patients were randomized to receive or not receive two courses of arsenic trioxide in addition to anthracycline-based chemotherapy have shown results favoring the arsenic arm.

Patients with APL who present with high WBC counts (>10,000/μL) have adverse outcomes, and attempts have been made to improve their prognosis using strategies that include gemtuzumab ozogamicin (Mylotarg) (APL strongly expresses CD33) or treatment with high-dose cytarabine.

Maintenance therapy with ATRA for a year, with or without the oral chemotherapy agents methotrexate (Rheumatrex, others) 20 mg/m$^2$

[1]Not FDA approved for this indication.
*Approved for MDS, not acute leukemia.
[8]Orphan drug in the United States.

[1]Not FDA approved for this indication.

## TABLE 2 Investigational Therapies of Acute Leukemia

| Drug | Mechanism of Action |
|---|---|
| Bevacizumab (Avastin)[1] | VEGF inhibitor |
| SU5416 (Semaxanib)[5] | VEGF-R, c-kit, and flt-3 inhibitor |
| SU11248 (Sugen)[5] | VEGF-R, c-kit, and flt-3 inhibitor |
| Tipifarnib (Zarnestra)[5] | Farnesyl transferase inhibitor |
| Lonafarnib (SCH66336)[5] | Farnesyl transferase inhibitor |
| Valproic acid (Depakote)[1] | Histone deacetylase inhibitor |
| SAHA[1] | Histone deacetylase inhibitor |
| PKC412[5] | flt-3 inhibitor |
| MLN518[5] | flt-3 inhibitor |
| CEP701[5] | flt-3 inhibitor |
| Decitabine[1] | DNA methyltransferase inhibitor |
| Imatinib (Gleevec)[1] | *bcr-abl* inhibitor: Ph+ ALL, AML |
| Dasatinib (BMS-354825)* | *bcr-abl*, src inhibitor, Ph+ ALL, AML |
| Oblimersen (Genasense)[5] | *bcl-2* mRNA inhibitor (antisense therapy) |
| Interleukin-2 (Proleukin)[1] | T and NK cell stimulant |
| PR-1[5] | Vaccine for AML |
| Hum-195-Bismuth 213[5] | Radiolabeled monoclonal antibody for AML |
| Alemtuzumab (CamPath)[1] | Monoclonal antibody for ALL |
| VNP40101M (Cloretazine)[5] | Alkylating agent |
| Troxacitabine (Troxatyl)[5] | Purine nucleoside analogue |
| Zosuquidar[5] | Inhibitor of multidrug resistance |
| Cyclosporin A (Sandimmune)[1] | Inhibitor of multidrug resistance |

[1]Not FDA approved for this indication.
[5]Investigational drug in the United States.
*Approved for ALL in 2006.
    http://www.fda.gov/cder/foi/label/2006/022072lbl.pdf
*Abbreviations:* ALL = acute lymphoblastic leukemia; AML = acute myeloid leukemia; NK = natural killer cells; Ph = Philadelphia chromosome; SAHA = suberoylanilide hydroxamic acid; VEGF = vascular endothelial growth factor; VEGF-R = vascular endothelial growth factor receptor.
*Definitions:* bcr-abl = gene product of the Ph (Philadelphia) chromosome translocation t(9;22); c-kit = transmembrane tyrosine kinase (CD117); DNA methyltransferase = inhibition promotes gene transcription; farnesyl transferase = enzyme in ras pathway; flt-3 = fms-like transmembrane tyrosine kinase; histone deacetylase = inhibition promotes histone disassembly and gene transcription; multidrug resistance = major mediator of resistance to anthracyclines, vinca alkaloids, and epidophyllotoxins is a transmembrane drug efflux pump, *p*-glycoprotein, or mdr-1.

orally once per week and 6-mercaptopurine (Purinethol) 60 mg/m² orally daily, has been used to prevent relapse in APL. It may be that patients who are molecularly negative by PCR after completing induction and consolidation do not need maintenance. This question is posed in a planned phase III trial.

ATRA needs to be given intermittently because it can induce its own metabolism. Patients treated with ATRA or arsenic trioxide can develop a differentiation syndrome marked by fever, dyspnea, weight gain, pulmonary infiltrates, pleural effusions, and even death. This can result, in part, from interactions between maturing leukemic promyelocytes and the pulmonary vascular endothelium as well as cytokine release. Most patients respond to interruptions in drug therapy and brief courses of dexamethasone 10 mg IV twice daily.

APL generally manifests with a low WBC count and evidence of coagulopathy, including severe hypofibrinogenemia. ATRA helps to reverse the coagulopathy, but it is critical to maintain the fibrinogen greater than 100 mg/dL and the platelet count higher than the traditional 10,000 to 20,000/μL. Nonrandomized clinical experience suggests that keeping the platelet count higher than 50,000/μL in APL is important until laboratory evidence of disseminated intravascular coagulation (DIC) reverses. There are no convincing data to support the use of low-dose heparin or antifibrinolytic agents in APL.

Relapsed APL is generally approached with an attempt at reinduction using regimens similar to those that were initially effective. ASCT has been an active salvage therapy in APL in second CR,

although an allogeneic transplant could be considered in suitable high-risk patients.

## ACUTE LYMPHOBLASTIC LEUKEMIA

Approximately 30% to 40% of adults with ALL are cured. CR rates are high, approaching 90% in patients younger than 60 years, but relapse rates are substantially higher than in childhood ALL. One important reason for this disparity is that the Ph chromosome is far more common in adults than in children (30%-40% vs. 5%). Also, the favorable t(12;21) is overrepresented in childhood ALL. Furthermore, children with ALL have been treated more intensively than adults, using higher doses of cytotoxic agents with shorter treatment-free intervals and more aggressive use of prophylactic therapy aimed at preventing central nervous system (CNS) relapse.

The backbone of induction therapy for ALL consists of weekly doses of vincristine 2 mg IV weekly for 4 weeks combined with prednisone 60 mg/m² PO daily for 21 days or dexamethasone 6 mg/m² orally daily for 14 to 21 days. Response rates have increased as additional drugs have been added to the induction framework, so that a typical induction regimen for adult ALL often includes cyclophosphamide (600-1200 mg/m² IV once on day 1 or 300 mg/m² IV bid for 3 days in a regimen called HyperCVAD), daunorubicin (45-80 mg/m² IV daily on days 1 to 3 and L-asparaginase (Elspar, 6000 U/m²) SC or IM biweekly for 6 doses. PEG-asparaginase (Oncaspar) 2500 IU/m² IM or IV given twice during induction 2 weeks apart has also been used. A two-drug induction regimen using a high-dose anthracycline (e.g., mitoxantrone 60-80 mg/m² IV[3] given once) with high-dose cytarabine has been studied, which is then followed in patients achieving CR by more traditional anti-ALL regimens. Childhood regimens have intensified further the use of L-asparaginase.

Achieving CR by 4 to 5 weeks after starting induction is prognostically important. For the majority of patients in CR, repeated cycles of multiple agents with both antileukemia effects and the capacity for crossing the blood-brain barrier are given. This is because the CNS is a major sanctuary site in ALL. Efforts are directed early in therapy to identify or eradicate occult disease in the CSF. High doses of methotrexate (1000 to 3500 mg/m² IV). are given, followed by rescue with folinic acid (leucovorin) 25 to 50 mg PO every 6 hours until serum methotrexate levels drop to less than .05 M. High-dose cytarabine (3000 mg/m² IV daily for 2-3 days) is also an active anti-ALL agent that, along with methotrexate, penetrates well into the CSF. Repeated courses using these agents, with or without cyclophosphamide, L-asparaginase, and 6-mercaptopurine, are given over a period of about 6 months, after which about 18 months of lower-dose maintenance therapy is given, usually using monthly courses of vincristine (2 mg IV day 1), and oral pulses of prednisone (60 mg/m²) or dexamethasone (6 mg/m²) on days 1 to 5, daily doses of oral 6-mercaptopurine (60 mg/m²), and weekly doses of oral methotrexate (20 mg/m²). Variants of these regimens are described in the references.

The incidence of CNS disease has been reduced to 5% to 10% using prophylactic therapies as discussed earlier, along with repeated intrathecal instillations of methotrexate (6 mg/m²/dose) and cytarabine (30 mg/m²/dose), alone or in combination, via the lumbar route or intraventricularly using an Omaya reservoir. Commonly, 6 to 12 prophylactic treatments are given during induction and consolidation. Prophylactic cranial irradiation (up to 2400 cGy) has also been used. Because radiotherapy can induce cognitive defects, especially when combined with high-dose antimetabolite-based treatments, attempts are being made to clarify whether or not systemic and intrathecal treatments can suffice to prevent CNS disease, without cranial radiotherapy. In the setting of established CNS disease, most practitioners favor using whole-brain radiotherapy in addition to vigorous intrathecal treatments.

Drug resistance in the significant minority of patients with Ph+ ALL is being countered using targeted therapies that inhibit the specific product of the fusion gene that occurs in that disease (*bcr-abl*). Imatinib[1] (Gleevec) 600 to 800 mg orally daily induces transient remissions in

---

[3]Exceeds dosage recommended by the manufacturer.
[1]Not FDA approved for this indication.

a significant minority of patients with Ph⁺ ALL. Other inhibitors include nilotinib (Tasigna)[1], a more potent *bcr-abl* inhibitor, and dasatinib (Sprycel) which inhibits additional oncogenic pathways besides *bcr-abl*. Ongoing trials are clarifying the efficacy of cytotoxic therapies in combination with imatinib.[1] It is still critical to identify donors for allogeneic transplantation in patients with Ph⁺ ALL entering into CR. ASCT is also being studied in Ph⁺ ALL in conjunction with imatinib[1] and chemotherapy.

T-lineage ALL has been believed to have an inferior outcome to B-lineage ALL, but current intensive adult regimens have yielded outcomes in T-cell disease that are at least as good as those seen in the other ALL subtypes.

Mature B lineage ALL (Burkitt's leukemia or L3 ALL) is a highly proliferative form of acute leukemia, which demands distinct treatment that concentrates on the use of antimetabolites (high-dose methotrexate and high-dose cytarabine as described earlier for consolidation therapy of ALL) early in therapy along with an anthracycline, vincristine, cyclophosphamide, and corticosteroids. The risk of CNS disease is especially high in Burkitt's leukemia, and vigorous prophylactic CNS therapy is needed. Unlike typical ALL regimens, short-term (3 months or less) cyclic therapy without maintenance therapy is curative. Somewhat more prolonged regimens using similar drugs and most recently including the anti-CD20 monoclonal antibody rituximab[1] (375 mg/m² given every 3 weeks) have also been studied. Older patients might better tolerate such less dose-intense regimens. More than 80% of younger adults and perhaps 40% to 50% of older adults are cured. For both typical B lineage ALL and Burkitt's leukemia, judicious use of filgrastim (5 µg/kg/day SC) given daily after chemotherapy cycles will hasten myeloid recovery and reduce infectious risk.

Future directions in treating ALL include improving prognostic factor analysis, studying the more intensive childhood regimens in younger adults (younger than 30 years), continuing to refine CNS prophylactic measures, and evaluating new agents. Alemtuzumab[1] is being studied in the MRD setting in patients with ALL. Clofarabine is active in relapsed ALL and will be studied in earlier patients. Except for very poor risk patients, the role of early allogenic transplant in ALL remains undefined. Nelarabine (Arranon) is a newly approved purine nucleoside analogue. At a dose of 1500 mg/m² IV on days 1, 3, and 5 every 21 days, it is active in relapsed and refractory T-ALL. It is hoped that outcomes in both forms of acute leukemia will improve with the intelligent use of new agents in the context of carefully designed and conducted clinical trials.

## REFERENCES

Kolitz JE: Acute myeloid leukemia and the myelodysplastic syndromes. In Chang AE, Ganz PA, Hayes DF et al (eds): Oncology: An Evidence-Based Approach. New York: Springer, 2006, pp 1151-1172.

Odenike OM, Michaelis LC, Stock W: Acute lymphoblastic leukemia. In Chang AE, Ganz PA, Hayes DF et al (eds): Oncology: An Evidence-Based Approach. New York: Springer, 2006, pp 1173-1201.

Pui CH, Evans WE: Treatment of acute lymphoblastic leukemia. N Engl J Med 2006;354:166-178.

Sanz MA, Tallman MS, Lo-Coco F: Tricks of the trade for the appropriate management of newly diagnosed acute promyelocytic leukemia. Blood 2005;105:3019-3025.

Tallman MS, Gilliland DG, Rowe JM: Drug therapy of acute myeloid leukemia. Blood 2005;106:1154-1163.

---

[1]Not FDA approved for this indication.

# Acute Leukemia in Children

Method of
*Maureen M. O'Brien, MD, and Norman J. Lacayo, MD*

Acute leukemias represent approximately 30% of all malignancies diagnosed in children younger than 15 years and 25% of malignancies in children and adolescents younger than 20 years. Approximately 3250 new cases of leukemia are diagnosed annually in the United States. Acute lymphoblastic leukemia (ALL) accounts for approximately 80% of cases (2500 cases per year). About 20% of cases (800-900 cases per year) are acute myeloid leukemia (AML) and a small fraction (1%) is chronic myeloid leukemia (CML).

There is a sharp peak in ALL incidence among 2- and 3-year-olds (>80 per million), which decreases by ages 8 to 10 years (20 per million). The incidence of ALL among 2- and 3-year-olds is approximately fourfold greater than that for infants and is nearly 10-fold greater than that for 19-year-olds. In contrast, AML rates are highest in the first two years of life, decrease with a nadir at approximately 9 years of age, and slowly increase again during adolescence.

Leukemias are believed to arise from hematopoietic progenitor cells that acquire genetic alterations leading to unchecked proliferation and self-renewal. Over the past 50 years, our understanding of the molecular pathogenesis of acute leukemias has markedly increased. This knowledge, coupled with clinical risk stratification and clinical investigation, has led to substantial improvements in survival for children with acute leukemias. Currently, approximately 75% to 80% of children with ALL and 50% to 60% of children with AML achieve long-term survival.

Ongoing challenges in the care of children with acute leukemias include novel strategies for the treatment of relapsed disease, which has a dismal prognosis, and treatment reduction strategies in children with low-risk disease in whom long-term complications of treatment are becoming more evident. In addition, advances in the supportive care of children during treatment as well as stem cell transplantation have contributed to the improved survival of children with leukemia.

## Diagnosis

Classically, children with acute leukemia present with symptoms of pancytopenia, including pallor and fatigue from anemia and epistaxis, ecchymoses, and petechiae due to thrombocytopenia (75% of children have platelet count <100,000/µL at diagnosis). White blood cell (WBC) count may be elevated (>50,000/µL in 20% of children) or low (<10,000/µL in 50% of children). If they are neutropenic, children can present with significant infection or overwhelming sepsis. Children have lymphadenopathy in 50% of cases. Approximately 25% of children present with bone pain due to bone marrow expansion by malignant blasts and stretching of periosteal nerves. Rarely, extremity pain is also due to malignant joint effusion. Children with mediastinal masses (usually associated with T-cell ALL) can present with cough or other respiratory symptoms, which can be mistaken for pneumonia or asthma. Leukemia within the central nervous system (CNS) can manifest with headache or cranial nerve abnormalities. Uncommonly, ALL manifests as an isolated testicular mass and AML as a soft-tissue mass (chloroma).

However, the presenting signs and symptoms of acute leukemia can be subtle and develop over weeks to months, often beginning with fatigue and decreased energy. Children can develop persistent or intermittent fevers and can present to their pediatrician with these nonspecific complaints, which can be easily attributed to a viral illness. These children require a careful physical examination including evaluation for lymphadenopathy or hepatosplenomegaly. Physical examination abnormalities or persistent nonspecific symptoms that do not resolve within 2 to 3 weeks merit further evaluation with a complete blood

## CURRENT DIAGNOSIS

- History (including family history of blood disorders or cancer) and physical examination
- Complete blood count with a manual white blood cell differential and review of the peripheral smear
- Chest x-ray (PA and lateral views)
- Serum electrolytes, BUN, creatinine, uric acid, calcium, phosphorus, LDH, ALT, bilirubin
- Coagulation studies: PT, PTT, fibrinogen
- Varicella titer (IgG)
- Bone marrow aspirate and biopsy for morphology, blast cell immunophenotype, cytogenetics, and minimal residual disease studies
- Lumbar puncture with CSF cell count, morphology on a spun preparation, protein, and glucose

*Abbreviations:* ALT= alanine aminotransferase; BUN = blood urea nitrogen; CSF = cerebrospinal fluid; IgG = immunoglobulin G; LDH = lactate dehydrogenase; PA = posteroanterior; PT = prothrombin time; PTT = partial thromboplastin time.

count (CBC). Abnormalities of the CBC, such as cytopenias of more than one lineage or the presence of peripheral blasts in blood should result in urgent referral to a pediatric oncology center. These centers provide specialized diagnostic testing including flow cytometry and cytogenetic analysis that is standard in the evaluation of children with leukemia, as well as multidisciplinary treatment and coordination of patient participation in multi-institutional clinical trials.

Evaluation of any child presenting with concerning symptoms or an abnormal CBC should include a chemistry panel, to evaluate for hepatic or renal dysfunction, and elevated uric acid, potassium, and phosphate suggesting tumor lysis syndrome. Determination of prothrombin time (PT), activated partial thromboplastin time (aPTT), and fibrinogen is necessary to evaluate for coagulopathy, which can increase bleeding risk and is common in acute promyelocytic leukemia (APML). Patients should be examined for signs of infection and appropriate cultures (blood, urine, stool) should be drawn in children with fever or concerning symptoms. Chest radiography should be performed to evaluate for the presence of a mediastinal mass, which can complicate management of the patient due to respiratory distress and the inability to sedate the child for invasive procedures (see the Current Diagnosis box).

Ultimately, however, diagnosis depends on the results of bone marrow aspirate and biopsy, which typically reveal replacement of normal hematopoietic precursors with leukemic blasts. Morphologically, these blasts have high nuclear-to-cytoplasmic ratios and can have prominent nucleoli, vacuoles (Burkitt's leukemia), and intracytoplasmic inclusions (Auer rod, M2 AML). The presence of more than 25% blasts in the bone marrow is diagnostic of acute leukemia, and samples are then submitted for morphologic evaluation, flow cytometry, cytogenetic analysis, and further investigational studies. When the diagnosis of acute leukemia is confirmed, further evaluation will also include lumbar puncture and morphologic examination of the cerebrospinal fluid (CSF) for leukemic blasts. In boys, examination for testicular swelling and masses is necessary to determine if leukemic involvement is present; this should be documented by ultrasound evaluation and testicular biopsy if the diagnosis is in question because treatment varies depending on involvement of these sanctuary sites (CNS or testes).

## Classification

Acute leukemia is separated into two major subgroups, ALL and AML. Historically, the FAB (French-American-British) classification has been used in which ALL consists of three subtypes, L1 through L3, and AML consists of eight subtypes, M0 through M7. However, the 1999

WHO classification conference has suggested that for ALL, these FAB terms are not relevant because they do not predict immunophenotype, cytogenetics, or clinical outcome. The exception is L3 lymphoblasts, which are undifferentiated and contain large nucleoli and have deep blue vacuolated cytoplasm. This morphology is synonymous with Burkitt's (mature B-cell) leukemia.

In contrast, the FAB classification for AML remains standard and characterizes blasts by differentiation pathways. In general, M0 and M1 blasts are undifferentiated and lack granules. M2 blasts are more mature, contain cytoplasmic granules, and can have Auer rods (coalesced granules). M3 blasts are found in APML and have prominent granules. M4 blasts occur in acute myelomonocytic leukemia and are a mixture of myeloblasts and monoblasts. One specific subtype, M4eo, shows markedly increased marrow eosinophils and blasts with large, coarse granules. M4eo morphology is strongly associated with the cytogenetic abnormality inversion 16 [inv(16)]. M5 AML (acute monoblastic leukemia) blasts have indented nuclei consistent with monoblastic differentiation. M6 AML (acute erythroid leukemia) blasts show evidence of erythroid lineage, and M7 AML (acute megakaryocytic leukemia) blasts appear undifferentiated. M7 AML is often associated with extensive bone marrow fibrosis, and the diagnosis may be hampered by difficulty aspirating an adequate sample. The biopsy is critical to the correct diagnosis in this case. Children with trisomy 21 (Down syndrome) who develop AML almost exclusively have M7 AML.

## IMMUNOPHENOTYPING

The accuracy of morphologic diagnosis is significantly increased with the incorporation of immunophenotyping of cell surface cluster of differentiation (CD) markers by flow cytometry and cytogenetic analysis for translocations associated with specific subtypes of leukemia. This testing is particularly important for risk stratification in pediatric ALL. In general, ALL is divided into three major subtypes based on immunophenotype: B-precursor (70%-80% of patients), mature B cell (2%-5% of patients), and T cell (15% of patients) blasts. B-precursor blasts express CD10, CD19, and CD20, whereas mature B-cell blasts express these markers in addition to CD22, CD25, and surface immunoglobulin (sIg). In contrast, T cell lineage lymphoblasts express CD2, CD3, CD4, CD5, CD7, and CD8, whereas myeloid blasts express CD11, CD13, CD15, CD33, CD34, and CD65. Usually, lymphoblasts of different lineages can be readily distinguished from each other and from myeloid leukemias, although in some cases the leukemic blasts can aberrantly express a variety of cell surface proteins. Diagnosis in these cases is determined by the predominance of lymphoid versus myeloid markers, and the blasts may ultimately be described as *biphenotypic*.

## ALL CYTOGENETICS AND RISK STRATIFICATION

Leukemic blasts are further classified based on their chromosomal number and cytogenetic profile using standard karyotype analysis as well as molecular techniques to detect specific translocations that have both diagnostic and prognostic significance (Box 1). In B-precursor ALL, modal chromosome number is important in prognosis. Hyperdiploidy (50-60 chromosomes) occurs in 30% of cases and is associated with good prognosis, particularly if combined with trisomies of chromosomes 4, 10, and 17, but hypodiploidy (fewer than 45 chromosomes) is associated with poor outcome.

Specific translocations in ALL lymphoblasts include t(9;22) *bcr/abl* translocation (Philadelphia chromosome [Ph], typically the 185-kD fusion protein), which occurs in about 5% of ALL patients, mainly adolescents, and is associated with poor outcome. The t(4;11) translocation fuses the *MLL* (mixed lineage leukemia) gene on chromosome 11 band q23 to the *AF4* gene on chromosome 4 band q21, forming an *MLL/AF4* fusion gene. This translocation is prevalent in infant ALL (60% of infants) and is associated with poor outcome, as are other *MLL* fusion partner leukemias.

In contrast to these translocations associated with poor outcome, t(12;21)(p12;q22) (*TEL/AML-1*) is the most common genetic lesion in childhood ALL, occurring in 15% to 25% of children with B-precursor ALL and is associated with a good prognosis. The translocation is cryptic and requires specific molecular techniques (reverse-transcriptase polymerase chain reaction [RT-PCR] or fluorescence in situ hybridization [FISH] analysis) for detection. This translocation is generally considered to have good prognosis, with high blast sensitivity to intensive asparaginase therapy, although an association with late relapse has been reported.

Other translocations include t(1;19) *E2A/PBX1* translocation in 5% of B-precursor ALL patients, which is not currently used for risk stratification.

Mature B-cell ALL is characterized by the t(8;14) translocation, which places the *MYC* gene under the control of the immunoglobulin heavy chain promoter. In T-cell ALL, approximately 60% of patients have an abnormal karyotype, often involving chromosomes 14 or 7 at the locations of the T-cell receptor *(TCR)* genes, which become fused to a transcription factor *(LMO2, LYL, TAL1)*. In addition, T-cell ALL lymphoblasts have a high frequency (>50% of cases) of gain of function Notch-1 mutations, which may be associated with improved prognosis.

Treatment of the child with ALL is based on risk-adapted therapy. As cure rates for childhood ALL have improved overall, great interest has developed in risk stratification of patients based on clinical characteristics, immunophenotype, and cytogenetics in order to identify groups of low-risk patients for whom toxic therapy can be minimized and high-risk patients for whom aggressive treatment, including consideration of bone marrow transplant (BMT), is indicated. For example, T-cell ALL patients tend to be male and to have elevated WBC count and extramedullary disease (mediastinal mass, CNS involvement). These patients had historically poor outcome compared with B-precursor ALL patients. However, with current intensive treatment protocols, long-term survival for these patients now approaches 70% to 80%, similar to survival of children with B-precursor ALL.

Important clinical characteristics for risk stratification include WBC count and age at the time of diagnosis, which are independent predictors of prognosis and have been established by the National Cancer Institute (NCI) as the standard criteria for risk assignment at diagnosis in precursor B-cell ALL. Other prognostic factors used for risk assignment during induction therapy include presence of CNS disease and specific cytogenetic abnormalities. European investigators have traditionally used clinical response to a 1-week treatment prophase with prednisone and intrathecal methotrexate to stratify those with poor prednisone response to intensive therapy, because this is an independent predictor of poor clinical outcome.

Response to induction therapy based on bone marrow evaluation is another cornerstone of risk stratification. Rapid responders with an M1 remission marrow (<5% blasts by morphology) by day 8 of induction have excellent outcomes, and slower responders fare worse. In extreme cases, patients who fail induction or have continued presence of overt morphologic leukemia after 4 to 6 weeks of intensive chemotherapy (which occurs in 1% of patients) have extremely poor outcomes and should proceed to BMT if remission is eventually achieved.

New molecular techniques continue to refine risk stratification for children with ALL. Minimal residual disease (MRD) monitoring by multiparameter flow cytometry can detect leukemic blasts at a level of 0.1 to 0.01% even in a morphologically M1 bone marrow aspirate sample. Studies have demonstrated that children with negative blood MRD by day 8 of induction have an excellent prognosis, and those with positive bone marrow MRD by day 29 (end of induction) have high rates of relapse. Current clinical trials for children with leukemia now incorporate MRD monitoring at the end of induction into risk stratification for additional therapy and are evaluating the sensitivity and specificity of MRD in predicting later relapse.

Based on these considerations, at the time of diagnosis, children with ALL are stratified as standard risk (age 1-9.99 years and WBC < 50,000/μL) or high risk (age <1 year or >10 years, WBC >50,000/μL, overt CNS leukemia). Once cytogenetic and induction-response data are available, patients are further stratified into lower risk (trisomies of chromosomes 4, 10, and 17 or TEL/AML1 and translocation), standard risk (unremarkable cytogenetics), high risk (adolescents, infants), or very high risk [induction failure, t(9;22), t(4;11)], and subsequent treatment intensity is based on this classification.

## AML CYTOGENETICS AND RISK STRATIFICATION

Factors with favorable prognostic significance in AML include Down syndrome, the karyotypic abnormalities inv(16) and t(8;21) seen in the core binding factor leukemias, and (15;17) (Box 2). Poor prognostic factors include failure to achieve remission, FLT3 (a member of the receptor tyrosine kinase family) internal tandem duplication (FLT3-ITD), therapy-related AML, AML arising from myelodysplastic syndrome (MDS), FAB subtypes M6 and M7, monosomy 7, del5q (less common), and refractory anemia with excess blasts in transformation (RAEB-T).

Patients without favorable or poor prognostic factors are considered to have an intermediate risk status. Remission induction and long-term survival vary substantially between these subgroups; therefore, accurate risk stratification is critical to identify patients who will benefit from aggressive therapies such as hematopoietic stem-cell transplantation or novel therapies, as well as patients who have good outcome with current regimens.

The use of MRD in pilot studies shows that it can identify a subset of patients at higher risk of relapse. This group of patients can benefit from new therapeutic approaches. As the MRD technology improves, its sensitivity and specificity and positive predictive value for relapse will also improve.

# Treatment

## ACUTE LYMPHOBLASTIC LEUKEMIA

The vast majority of children with ALL are treated in a clinical trial. In the United States and Canada, although a small number of centers treat children on institutional protocols, most pediatric oncology centers are members of the Children's Oncology Group (COG) and enroll children in multicenter national trials. These clinical trials allow adequate patient numbers to determine efficacy of regimens, coordination of biological and molecular studies, and access of any child to the current state-of-the-art standard of care. Informed consent must be obtained for treatment according to the trial protocol as well as the submission of bone marrow or peripheral blood samples for biological studies.

At the time of diagnosis, typically in conjunction with another diagnostic procedure (bone marrow aspirate/biopsy or lumbar puncture), the child should have placement of a central venous catheter (CVC) that can be used for delivering medications and for blood sampling. The type of CVC will depend on the individual institutional practices. In general, implanted catheters (portacaths) are associated with lower infection rates, but external multilumen catheters (Broviac or Hickman) should be placed in small infants and in patients likely to need BMT. In a child with a large mediastinal mass in whom sedation for procedures is not possible, bone marrow aspirate and lumbar puncture might need to be performed with local anesthesia only, and a peripherally inserted central catheter (PICC) may be placed in lieu of a CVC until the mediastinal mass has responded to chemotherapy.

### Treatment Phases

The treatment of ALL is divided into three general phases: remission induction (4-6 weeks), consolidation and delayed intensification (6 months), and maintenance. The total treatment lasts between 24 and 36 months.

### Induction

The induction regimen for standard-risk patients (age 1-10 years, WBC <50,000/$\mu$L) includes three chemotherapeutic agents, daily oral corticosteroid (prednisone or dexamethasone) for 28 days, four doses of weekly intravenous vincristine (Vincasar), and one dose of intramuscular pegylated asparaginase (Elspar). This is combined with CNS prophylaxis and treatment with intrathecal methotrexate. For high-risk patients, an anthracycline (daunorubicin [Cerubidine] or doxorubicin [Adriamycin]) is added to improve the rate of remission induction in this group. Overall, 98% of patients achieve first morphologic remission (M1 marrow defined as <5% bone marrow blasts with recovery of trilineage hematopoeisis and peripheral blood counts) at day 29 of induction with this regimen. Patients with M2 marrow (5%-25% blasts) after 29 days of induction receive 2 additional weeks of therapy, and those who remain M3 (>25% bone marrow blasts) have failed induction. Children who fail to achieve first remission after 6 weeks of induction have a very poor prognosis and should be considered for myeloablative allogeneic BMT if they achieve remission with an alternative regimen.

A number of complications can develop during induction. The majority of these are secondary to chemotherapeutic agents and can be managed with aggressive supportive care. Prolonged use of high-dose steroids can result in hypertension, hyperglycemia, weight gain, mood changes, and gastritis. Perturbation of clotting factors by asparaginase therapy, which interferes with hepatic protein production, can lead to bleeding or thrombosis depending on the balance of procoagulant and anticoagulant factors. Asparaginase therapy can also result in acute anaphylaxis as well as severe pancreatitis, both of which are indications for omission of future asparaginase therapy (except in the case of allergy, when *Erwinia* asparaginase can be substituted). Use of anthracyclines requires monitoring of cardiac function, and vincristine can cause peripheral neuropathy, constipation, and ileus. Finally, the risks of infection and tumor lysis syndrome are highest during induction. Management of these problems is detailed in the section on supportive care.

### Consolidation, Interim Maintenance, and Delayed Intensification

Following achievement of first remission, the intensity of the consolidation, interim maintenance, and delayed intensification phases depends on risk stratification including clinical features, cytogenetics, and response to therapy or MRD. In general, consolidation is characterized by intensive therapy including cyclophosphamide (Cytoxan), cytarabine (Cytosar), 6-thioguanine (Tabloid)[1] or 6-mercaptopurine (Purinethol), asparaginase (Elspar), and vincristine (Vincasar). For lower-risk patients, consolidation may include only vincristine and antimetabolite therapy. Depending on risk stratification, consolidation lasts between 4 and 8 weeks.

Consolidation is followed by interim maintenance, which lasts 8 weeks and includes antimetabolite therapy with daily oral 6-mercaptopurine, weekly oral methotrexate (Trexall), intermittent vincristine, and glucocorticoid pulses as well as continued CNS prophylaxis with intrathecal methotrexate. For higher-risk patients, interim maintenance is augmented with escalating-dose IV methotrexate and asparaginase. This less-intensive phase is then followed by delayed intensification, which includes reinduction and reconsolidation. High-risk patients may then receive second interim maintenance and delayed intensification courses before proceeding to maintenance therapy.

For all patients, an additional goal of this phase of treatment is to target involved sanctuary sites (see the later discussion of CNS prophylaxis). In male patients, the testis is a sanctuary site and requires close monitoring at the time of each physical examination. For patients with testicular mass or swelling at the time of diagnosis, enlargement should be confirmed by ultrasound and then leukemic involvement proved by testicular biopsy. For patients with biopsy-proved testicular disease, treatment includes bilateral testicular irradiation at 2400 cGy in 12 once-daily fractions (200 cGy per fraction).

### Maintenance

Maintenance therapy consists of daily oral 6-mercaptopurine, weekly oral methotrexate, monthly intravenous vincristine, and 5-day pulses of oral dexamethasone. Maintenance continues until total duration of therapy is 2 years from the start of interim maintenance for female patients and 3 years from the start of interim maintenance for male patients. Length of treatment differs because male patients have a poorer prognosis than female patients, which can be improved by prolonged maintenance therapy.

### Therapy for High-Risk Groups

The current very-high-risk ALL COG protocol includes a subset of patients with poor outcomes and an expected 5-year event-free survival (EFS) rate of <45%. This group includes patients with Ph+ ALL [t(9;22)], hypodiploidy, MLL rearrangement with a slow early response to induction chemotherapy, and induction failures (an M3 [>25% blasts] bone marrow at the end of induction therapy or MRD >1%).

---

[1]Not FDA approved for this indication.

In this group of patients, allogeneic BMT is recommended in first remission for those with matched sibling donors. In addition, protocols for patients with t(9;22) now include the *BCR-ABL* tyrosine kinase inhibitor imatinib (Gleevec) in combination with intensive multiagent chemotherapy in an effort to improve outcomes for this subgroup. For infants with MLL rearrangement with rapid induction response, treatment currently consists of intensive chemotherapy on high-risk protocols due to excessive treatment-related mortality in this subgroup during BMT.

## Central Nervous System Prophylaxis

The CNS is a sanctuary site for leukemic blasts due to poor penetrance of the CNS by many chemotherapeutic agents. Historically, it was found that without CNS prophylaxis in patients *without* overt CNS leukemia at diagnosis, these patients would relapse in the CNS at a high rate even while maintaining bone marrow remission. CNS status is determined by a diagnostic lumbar puncture at the time of diagnosis (CNS 1: <5 WBCs, no blasts on cytospin; CNS 2: <5 WBCs, blasts seen on cytospin; CNS 3: ≥5 WBCs with blasts on cytospin or overt signs of CNS leukemia such as facial nerve palsy).

In the past, CNS leukemia prophylaxis was achieved with cranial radiation, which provides effective prophylaxis but with excessive long-term toxicity, including neurocognitive impairment and increased risk of secondary malignancy. As a result, CNS prophylaxis is currently achieved with repeated doses of intrathecal methotrexate throughout all phases of therapy. Research is ongoing to determine the effect of this treatment on long-term neurocognitive function. Patients with CNS 2 status receive additional doses of intrathecal methotrexate during induction and are subsequently treated with the same regimen as CNS 1 patients. Currently, cranial radiation (1800 cGy) combined with intrathecal methotrexate is reserved for patients with documented CNS 3 disease or patients without CNS disease who have high risk of relapse in the CNS (1200-1800 cGy), such as T-cell ALL patients.

## Relapse Treatment

Although the overall outcomes for children with ALL have markedly improved over the past 40 years, the treatment of children who experience relapse remains a significant challenge. The number of children with relapsed acute leukemia equals or exceeds the incidence of most other pediatric tumors. Despite intensive and risk-stratified treatment regimens, 15% to 20% of patients relapse, and the vast majority of these children ultimately die of disease.

The majority of relapses (75%) occur within 3 years from diagnosis, and treatment and prognosis depend on site of relapse (bone marrow or extramedullary), timing of relapse (months from diagnosis), and immunophenotype. For children enrolled in the Children's Cancer Group (CCG) 1900 series trials between 1997 and 2002, 12% of patients experienced bone marrow relapse, 4% experienced CNS relapse, and 1.3% experienced testes relapse. The 3-year survival rates were 28%, 60%, and 60%, respectively. Second remission rates range from 70% to 90% in different series depending on timing and site of relapse, but the 3-year survival rate for patients with marrow relapse within 3 years of diagnosis is less than 10%.

Factors associated with extremely poor outcome include T-cell ALL relapse and early bone marrow relapse (duration of first remission <36 months). Outcomes are somewhat better for isolated CNS or testicular relapse and late bone marrow relapse with B-precursor ALL.

Treatment of early marrow relapse involves intensive reinduction chemotherapy in an attempt to achieve second remission, followed by myeloablative allogeneic BMT for patients with an acceptable donor. For patients without an unrelated donor, intensive chemotherapy with consideration of phase I/II studies of novel agents is indicated given the extremely poor prognosis for this group, many of whom will relapse again before BMT even when a donor is available. For patients with late bone marrow relapse (>36 months from diagnosis), research is currently ongoing to determine the role of BMT versus intensive chemotherapy, although for patients with a matched sibling donor, most oncologists would proceed with BMT if the patient achieves second remission.

Isolated CNS relapse has a more favorable outcome than bone marrow relapse. In terms of risk stratification, early CNS relapse (<18 months from diagnosis) is considered similar in prognosis to late marrow relapse, and patients with late CNS relapse (>18 months from diagnosis) have the most favorable outcome. Patients are treated with weekly intrathecal triple chemotherapy (methotrexate, cytarabine, hydrocortisone) until the CSF is negative for blasts. Craniospinal radiation therapy is also indicated, with a dose of 2400 (cranial)/1500 (spinal) cGy for early CNS relapse and cranial radiation to 1800 cGy for late CNS relapse. In addition, all CNS relapse patients receive intensive systemic reinduction, consolidation, and maintenance chemotherapy because CNS relapse is a harbinger of eventual relapse in the bone marrow. Current studies are ongoing to determine if the cranial radiation dose in children with late CNS relapse can be decreased further to 1200 cGy following 12 months of intensive chemotherapy incorporating agents known to cross the blood-brain barrier (dexamethasone, high-dose methotrexate, asparaginase, and high-dose cytarabine).

Testicular relapse is suspected when testicular swelling or mass is noted on physical examination. Relapse should be confirmed with testicular biopsy and evaluation for concurrent bone marrow and CNS relapse should be undertaken and treated as described earlier. Treatment of isolated testicular relapse (ITR) has historically involved bilateral testicular radiation to 2400 cGy combined with intensive systemic chemotherapy. However, as with isolated CNS relapse, the most significant factor influencing survival following ITR is the length of the first remission. Patients with ITR <18 months from diagnosis have 5-year EFS rates of 45% compared to 60% EFS rate for patients with ITR ≥18 months from diagnosis.

Testicular radiation is effective at eradicating leukemia, but risk of sterility and endocrine late effects following testicular radiation are significant, with a majority of boys requiring hormonal replacement at some stage for induction of puberty, continuing pubertal maturation, or both. Primary germ cell dysfunction is associated with doses of 1200 cGy, and testicular doses of 2400 cGy result in Leydig cell failure, particularly in prepubertal boys.

Current research protocols for patients with late ITR involve the use of intensive systemic chemotherapy including high-dose methotrexate (shown to penetrate the blood-testes barrier) with inclusion of testicular radiation to 2400 cGy only in boys who have persistent biopsy-proven testicular relapse after intensive systemic induction chemotherapy. As in isolated CNS relapse, therapy is combined with intensive systemic chemotherapy for 2 years due to the risk of subsequent bone marrow relapse following ITR.

## ACUTE MYELOID LEUKEMIA

Acute myeloid leukemia (AML) accounts for 20% of new cases of pediatric leukemia each year. AML represents a biologically heterogeneous group of diseases that arises from abnormal myeloid cell progenitors. Despite aggressive therapy, overall cure rates remain at about 50%. The key to improvement in this group of diseases has been identifying different subgroups of patients based on karyotypic and molecular characteristics. The current approach is to further refine risk-stratification and to develop risk-based or molecularly targeted therapies. The therapy outline is modeled after the St. Jude AML 2002 Consortium Study.

### Induction

On completion of a diagnostic work-up and evaluation of eligibility for a clinical trial, the next step is to proceed with informed consent. We advocate enrollment in open clinical trials from the Children's Oncology Group or multi-institutional consortia for all eligible patients with consent from the parents or guardians.

Induction chemotherapy is started as we await molecular and karyotype testing for risk stratification. Due to the intensity of the induction phase of therapy and the need for supportive care we, advocate the early placement of an indwelling central venous catheter if this can be achieved safely. Therapy consists of anthracyclines (usually daunorubicin

---

[1]Not FDA approved for this indication.

or idarubicin [Idamycin]) for 3 days, cytosine arabinosine for 7 to 10 days, and etoposide (Toposar)[1] or thioguanine for 5 days.

Some pilot and front-line studies are using chemotherapy with or without gemtuzumab ozogomycin (Mylotarg). This drug is an anti-CD33 monoclonal antibody conjugated with ozogomycin. It is not known at this time if its use during induction will result in an increased relapse-free survival.

Most induction regimens result in remission rates of 85% to 90% when repeated twice. The use of time-intense induction (timing a second induction during early count recovery after the first induction) usually results in prolonged hospital stay for nearly all patients during the induction phase. This allows timely and intense supportive care in the inpatient setting. Family members and the patient undergo HLA typing because a matched sibling hematopoietic stem cell transplant may be indicated for very high-risk factors (monosomy 7, 7q-, primary induction failures) or high-risk factors (FLT3-ITD, MDS-AML, M6 and M7 subtypes, and RAEB-T). A matched unrelated donor may also be considered for very-high-risk patients.

The FAB-defined APML subtype is the only subtype of AML with molecularly targeted therapy. The induction regimen for this subtype of AML includes all-*trans*-retinoic acid (ATRA) in combination with anthracyclines, cytosine arabinoside, and arsenic.

## Consolidation

With the induction of a remission, the next phase of therapy includes typically three courses of consolidation. Common combination therapies include mitoxantrone (Novantrone) and cytosine arabinoside, high-dose cytosine arabinoside with L-asparaginase,[1] cytosine arabinoside and etoposide,[1] and 2-CdA (2-chlorodeoxyadenosine, Leustatin)[1] with cytosine arabinoside. In this setting, patients with very-high-risk or high-risk factors may proceed with a hematopoietic stem-cell transplant if a matched sibling donor is available. In addition, for very-high-risk patients, a matched unrelated donor transplant may be considered because the outcome on chemotherapy alone is very poor.

## Maintenance

Maintenance therapy fails to demonstrate any benefit following intense induction and consolidation therapy, except in the molecularly targeted APML subtype. ATRA is continued during maintenance.

## Central Nervous System Therapy

Central nervous system prophylaxis is achieved using intrathecal cytosine arabinoside at diagnosis, followed by triple intrathecal therapy (cytosine arabinoside, hydrocortisone, and methotrexate) during each subsequent course of therapy. Intrathecal therapy is used in most protocols because of the historical observation that many patients develop CNS relapse in the absence of CNS prophylaxis.

## Hematopoietic Stem Cell Transplantation

Hematopoietic stem cell transplantation results in a statistically significant survival advantage compared with chemotherapy alone, specifically for patients with high or very high risk factors. Due to the morbidity and mortality associated with transplantation, it is not recommended for patients with good risk factors, such as (inv(16), t(8;21) or t(15;17), even those who have a matched sibling donor. For patients with favorable risk factors, transplantation is reserved for the relapse setting or second remission. In contrast, patients with high- or very-high-risk factors may be candidates for a matched sibling donor transplant in first remission. For patients with very-high-risk factors, a matched unrelated donor in first remission may be indicated due to the inferior outcome using chemotherapy alone. In the relapsed patients, matched and unmatched donor transplantations are less controversial because the outcome with chemotherapy is very poor. The preparative regimens for transplant usually include high-dose chemotherapy (busulfan,[1] cyclophosphamide, cytarabine arabinoside) or total body irradiation with high-dose chemotherapy.

## Relapse Treatment

Most relapses occur in the bone marrow. The prognosis is very poor for those who relapse less than 1 year from remission (~10% survival). Those who relapse longer than 1 year from remission fare better but still with dismal outcomes (~20%-30% survival). The treatment approach is to use chemotherapy to achieve remission and to follow chemotherapy with hematopoietic stem-cell transplantation. Reinduction therapy usually consists of mitoxantrone and etoposide[1] or L-asparaginase[1] with high-dose cytarabine arabinoside.

Once a remission is achieved with chemotherapy, the use of any available matched or mismatched donor is recommended, including cord blood stem cells. Other active agents include 2-CdA[1] or gemtuzumab ozogomycin. Two new drugs that will be available for children with refractory and relapsed AML through the Children's Oncology Group include the combination of clofarabine (Clolar)[1] (a novel nucleoside analogue) with cytosine arabinoside and the combination of lestaurtinib[8] (an FLT3 inhibitor) with idarubicin and cytosine arabinoside.

Relapse in extramedullary sites is less common. CNS relapses will require administration of intrathecal therapy and craniospinal irradiation. It is unclear if systemic therapy and hematopoietic stem cell transplantation result in increased relapse-free survival. For soft-tissue relapses (granulocytic sarcoma), local and systemic therapy followed by a stem cell transplant, similar to the approach for bone marrow relapse, are indicated.

A cornerstone for the success of AML therapy has been the participation of the majority of de novo childhood AML patients in clinical trials. As we better understand the biology of this disease and the number of available targeted agents increase, it will be very important to offer phase I and phase II studies to as many patients as possible so we can further improve the outcomes of all childhood AML patients who relapse.

## Atypical Manifestations

Rarely, AML manifests as congenital leukemia or extramedullary leukemia (skin, gingival, chloromas, or CNS). Congenital leukemia occurs in the first few weeks of life and can manifest as leukemia cutis. The skin lesions might spontaneously disappear, but they usually reappear with bone marrow involvement. Skin and CNS leukemia are more common in infants than in older children. At diagnosis, only 5% to 15% of patients present with CNS disease. They commonly are asymptomatic; however, some present with headache, vomiting, papilledema, or cranial nerve palsy. For patients who present with chloroma (myeloblastomas or granulocytic sarcomas), these are commonly found in the head or neck region. These lesions can result in later bone marrow involvement. All patients with atypical manifestation need systemic therapy as outlined previously. These atypical manifestations can also occur in relapse.

## Acute Complications

Tumor lysis syndrome, hyperleukocytosis, and transfusion support are discussed in the supportive care section.

### Infections

Due to severe and prolonged neutropenia, patients are at risk for bacterial infections (viridans streptococcal infection after high-dose cytarabine arabinoside) and fungal infections (candidemia and aspergillosis). Dental examination and oral hygiene during and after chemotherapy are routinely recommended to prevent β-hemolytic streptococcal infection. Fungal prophylaxis is recommended; agents available include fluconazole (Diflucan) and voriconazole (Vfend). These antifungal drugs should be used with caution due to drug interactions. Routinely, patients are started on trimethoprim-sulfamethoxazole (TMP-SMX; Septra) for

---

[1]Not FDA approved for this indication.

---

[1]Not FDA approved for this indication.
[8]Orphan drug in the United States.

*Pneumocystis jiroveci* pneumonia (PCP; formerly *Pneumocystis carinii* pneumonia) prophylaxis. The dose is 150 mg/m$^2$/day in two divided doses 3 days per week.

### Febrile Neutropenia

The definitions of fever can vary slightly; we use any fever higher than 38.3°C or higher than 38°C that persists for 1 hour with an absolute neutrophil count less than 500. We treat empirically with ceftazidime (Fortaz) and vancomycin (Vancocin) at the commonly recommended doses to treat gram-positive and gram-negative organisms. Extended coverage is strongly recommended if viridans streptococcal sepsis or typhilitis is suspected.

## Supportive Care

Although improved chemotherapy combinations and risk stratification have contributed greatly to better outcomes in childhood leukemias, excellent supportive care and treatment of complications of both the underlying disease and therapy have also played critical roles in the survival of these patients. Important aspects of supportive care include management of hyperleukocytosis, tumor lysis syndrome and metabolic derangements, and infection.

### HYPERLEUKOCYTOSIS

Hyperleukocytosis (WBC >100,000/μL) can lead to clinical symptoms due to leukostasis, a clinicopathologic syndrome caused by the sludging of circulating leukemic blasts in tissue microvasculature due to altered rheology as well as interactions with blood vessel endothelial surfaces. Symptoms are typically neurologic (ranging from confusion and somnolence to stupor and coma) or pulmonary with dyspnea, infiltrates on chest x-ray, and respiratory distress. This syndrome is most common in AML and is rarely seen in ALL, even with markedly elevated WBCs. In general, in an ALL patient, a WBC count greater than 200,000/μL or a WBC count greater than 100,000/μL with clinical symptoms of leukostasis is an indication for intervention. Intervention can include aggressive hydration, cytoreduction with hydroxyurea (Hydrea)[1], or leukopheresis for aggressive removal of circulating blasts until definitive therapy can be initiated. In the AML patient, clinically relevant leukostasis can occur with a WBC of 100,000/μL.

### TUMOR LYSIS SYNDROME

Tumor lysis syndrome (TLS) results from the rapid turnover of malignant lymphoblasts. Cell death leads to release of intracellular contents, leading to hyperkalemia, hyperuricemia with secondary uric acid nephropathy and oliguric renal failure, and hyperphosphatemia with secondary hypocalcemia. In the presence of a high blast burden (WBC >100,000/μL) or extremely rapid cell turnover (Burkitt's leukemia), the ensuing metabolic derangements and uric acid nephropathy can be life threatening, although TLS can occur in any child with acute leukemia.

Therefore, at the time of diagnosis (or suspected diagnosis) of ALL, TLS prophylaxis should be initiated with intravenous hydration at 2400 to 3000 mL/mm$^2$/day to maintain urine output at greater than 100 mL/m$^2$/hour until peripheral blasts and extramedullary disease are reduced. This fluid should be alkalinized to a target urinary pH of 6.5 to 7.5 to facilitate uric acid excretion. Patients at lower risk of significant TLS (low WBC) should receive allopurinol (Zyloprim) 300mg/m$^2$/day orally in three divided doses throughout the first 4 to 7 days of induction therapy because rapid blast lysis with the initiation of treatment can result in TLS. In fact, prior to the use of allopurinol, acute uric acid nephropathy developed in as many as 10% of ALL patients.

In patients at high risk for TLS and subsequent uric acid nephropathy and renal failure, urate oxidase (rasburicase [Elitek]) may be administered intravenously. Urate oxidase rapidly converts uric acid to soluble allantoin; in this case, urinary alkalinization is not necessary. This medication is well tolerated except for infrequent allergic reaction and has markedly reduced the frequency with which Burkitt's leukemia or lymphoma patients require dialysis due to TLS.

In addition to management of hyperuricemia, patients must be closely monitored for hyperkalemia and hyperphosphatemia and treated appropriately with binding agents or dialysis (or both) in severe cases.

### INFECTION

Infection is a major source of morbidity and mortality throughout treatment for leukemia, although it is most prominent during the intensive portions of ALL treatment such as induction and delayed intensification blocks as well as all portions of ALL therapy. In addition to risk of bacterial infection, depression of T–cell mediated immunity can predispose to viral, fungal, and opportunistic infections.

#### Bacterial

The rate of invasive bacterial infection and sepsis increases as WBC, in particular absolute neutrophil count (ANC), falls. Specifically, the risk of serious bacterial infection either with gram-negative rods from the patient's own gastrointestinal tract or gram-positive organisms through damaged oral mucosal surfaces or via central venous catheters, markedly increases when the ANC falls below 500/μL. Because of lack of white blood cells, patients are predisposed to severe infection and might lack the usual clinical signs and symptoms of inflammation (pain, erythema, purulent drainage).

Therefore, the clinician must be vigilant for subtle signs of infection, and broad-spectrum antibiotics should be initiated immediately in neutropenic patients who develop fever (> 38.0°C). Various combinations of antibiotics can be used but most commonly includes an antipseudomonal cephalosporin such as ceftazidime or cefipime. For patients with clinical signs of sepsis such as hypotension or specific symptoms (severe mucositis or abdominal pain), antibiotic coverage should be broadened to include additional gram-negative coverage with an aminoglycoside, gram-positive coverage with vancomycin, and anaerobic coverage with metronidazole or clindamycin. Carbapenems (i.e., meropenem) are indicated in children with penicillin or cephalosporin allergy.

Children receiving high-dose cytarabine therapy (AML and relapsed ALL patients) have a high incidence of life-threatening *streptococcus viridans* bacteremia. Any child who has received this therapy and presents with fever and neutropenia should receive intravenous vancomycin as well as ceftazidime regardless of presence of specific symptoms.

All patients should receive *P. jiroveci* prophylaxis with TMP-SMX at a dose of 5 mg/kg/day divided into three doses on three sequential days per week throughout therapy and continue for 6 months from the completion of treatment. For patients with sulfa allergy or who cannot tolerate TMP-SMX, second-line options include inhaled pentamidine (Pentam), oral dapsone (Aczone),[1] or oral atovaquone (Mepron).

#### Viral

Leukemia patients presenting with a rash suggesting primary varicella or shingles reactivation should be admitted to the hospital for intravenous acyclovir (Zovirax) treatment until the lesions are crusted, due to risk of dissemination. Asymptomatic children exposed to a sick contact with primary varicella should receive prophylactic intravenous immunoglobulin (IVIg) or, if available, VZIg (varicella zoster immune globulin). Other viral infections do not require hospitalization or specific therapy unless complications occur (e.g., respiratory distress with RSV infection). Patients should receive annual influenza vaccination, but in general, children with leukemia can tolerate routine viral respiratory and gastrointestinal illnesses and do not require specific isolation precautions outside of the hospital.

---

[1]Not FDA approved for this indication.

[1]Not FDA approved for this indication.

## Fungal

Fungal infections represent an area of additional concern for patients being treated for leukemia, mainly during periods of prolonged neutropenia such as ALL induction or any intensive block of AML therapy. The most common pathogens include *Candida* and *Aspergillus* species. In neutropenic patients, fever longer than 5 to 7 days despite adequate antibiotic therapy is an indication for the empiric initiation of broad antifungal therapy, usually with liposomal amphotericin B (Ambisome), as well as imaging for occult fungal infection in the sinuses, lungs, liver, or spleen.

Treatment of a probable or confirmed invasive fungal infection often requires long-term multiagent antifungal therapy. Current AML protocols include fungal prophylaxis with either fluconazole or voriconazole due to the high risk of infection in this population and the high rate of morbidity from these infections. Similar prophylaxis should be considered for any child undergoing intensive therapy for relapsed ALL.

## HEMORRHAGE

Prior to the introduction of ATRA, APML induction therapy was associated with significant treatment related mortality due to hemorrhagic complications. Today the use of ATRA* with chemotherapy is usually not complicated by a bleeding diathesis. However, the use of ATRA is associated with the retinoic acid syndrome. This is a syndrome characterized by severe respiratory distress, capillary leak syndrome, and pseudotumor cerebri. This complication is successfully managed with temporary cessation of ATRA and administration of decadron. ATRA is usually restarted at a lower dose once the side effects have resolved.

## TRANSFUSION

Other important aspects of supportive care for children with leukemia include the judicious use of blood component transfusions.

In general, packed red blood cell transfusions are recommended for hemoglobin levels less than 8 g/dL or at higher hemoglobin levels if the child is symptomatic (fatigue, headache, shortness of breath, tachycardia). At the time of diagnosis, children are often severely anemic but minimally symptomatic because the anemia has evolved slowly over time. In this setting, blood transfusion should be administered slowly over hours to avoid volume overload. All transfusions should be irradiated to prevent transfusion-related graft-versus-host disease (GVHD) and to prevent cytomegalovirus (CMV) exposure.

Platelet transfusions are indicated for platelet counts less than 10,000/μL or for bleeding. Platelets should be administered to a platelet count greater than 50,000/μL before diagnostic lumbar puncture to prevent a traumatic tap, which can be difficult to interpret and can introduce peripheral blasts into the spinal fluid.

In general, growth factors such as G-CSF (granulocyte colony-stimulating factor, Neupogen) and erythropoietin (Epogen, Procrit) are rarely administered to children being treated for leukemia due to the theoretical risk of stimulating a malignant clone, although G-CSF is becoming an integral part of some highly intensive relapsed ALL protocols.

## Late Effects of Therapy

The success of leukemia therapy comes at a price. Although treatment-related mortality continues to decrease as we implement better supportive care strategies, an increasing number of survivors suffer from late effects of therapy. The Children's Oncology Group has recently published detailed long-term follow-up guidelines for pediatric oncologists and other physicians (http://www.survivorshipguidelines.org/). These guidelines do not supplant disease-specific follow-up care, but they seek to complement and standardize the care of childhood, adolescent, and young adult cancer survivors. All pediatric oncology centers should establish late effects clinics to provide care for the increasing population of survivors. As the number of long-term effects investigators grows, their experience and expertise are integral parts of clinical trial development. The ultimate objective is to modulate the intensity of therapy to maximize its efficacy and to minimize the short-term and long-term sequelae.

It is necessary for all cancer survivors to have a record of a summary of their cancer therapy. Most leukemia cancer survivors graduate to long-term follow-up within 4 or 5 years after completing therapy. After this, they need follow-up visits once a year. The most concerning toxicity occurs in the CNS from high-dose methotrexate or cytarabine arabinoside and from intrathecal methotrexate with or without craniospinal irradiation. These patients can experience a lower educational attainment due to diminished cognitive functioning and usually experience a greater need for special education services.

Many studies document increased weight and body mass index in survivors of childhood leukemia. There is also now increased awareness of adverse cardiovascular and diabetes risk profiles (the metabolic syndrome) due to leukemia therapy. Patients who receive high cumulative doses of anthracyclines also need yearly follow-up of cardiac function.

Fertility is another issue of concern; this is now more commonly addressed with adolescents and young adults at diagnosis if the planned therapy could result in sterility.

Psychosocial evaluation continues to be an important part of long-term follow-up because many patients deal with issues of assistance to procure educational resources, job placement, and health insurance.

## REFERENCES

Armstrong SA, Look AT: Molecular genetics of acute lymphoblastic leukemia. J Clin Oncol 2005;23:6306-6315.

Bonnet D, Dick JE: Human acute myeloid leukemia is organized as a hierarchy that originates from a primitive hematopoietic cell. Nat Med 1997;3:730-737.

Carroll WL, Bhojwani D, Min D-J, et al: Childhood acute lymphoblastic leukemia in the age of genomics. Pediatr Blood Cancer 2006;46:570-578.

Chessells JM, Veys P, Kempski H, et al: Long-term follow-up of relapsed childhood acute lymphoblastic leukemia. Br J Haematol 2003; 123:396-405.

Creutzig U, Renhardt D, Diekamp S, et al: AML patients with Down syndrome have a high cure rate with AML-BFM therapy with reduced dose intensity. Leukemia 2005;19:1355-1360.

Gaynon PS: Childhood acute lymphoblastic leukemia and relapse. Br J Haematol 2005;131:579-587.

Jones LK and Saha V: Philadelphia positive acute lymphoblastic leukemia of childhood. Br J Haematol 2005;130:489-500.

Kaspers GJ, Creutzig U: Pediatric acute myeloid leukemia: International progress and future directions. Leukemia 2005;19:2025-2029.

Meshinchi S, Alonzo TA, Stirewalt DL, et al: Clinical implications of FLT3 mutations in pediatric AML. Blood 2006;108:3654-3661.

Pui C-H, Relling M, and Downing JR: Mechanisms of disease: Acute lymphoblastic leukemia. N Engl J Med 2004;350:1535-1548.

Pui C-H, Cheng C, Leung W, et al: Extended follow-up of long-term survivors of childhood acute lymphoblastic leukemia. N Engl J Med 2003;349:640-649.

Pui C-H, Evans W: Drug therapy: Treatment of acute lymphoblastic leukemia. N Engl J Med 2006;354:166-178.

Ravindranath Y, Yeager AM, Chang MN, et al: Autologous bone marrow transplantation versus intensive consolidation chemotherapy for acute myeloid leukemia in childhood. Pediatric Oncology Group. N Engl J Med 1996;334:1428-1434.

Rubnitz JE, Razzouk BI, Lensing S, et al: Prognostic factors and outcome of recurrence in childhood acute myeloid leukemia. Cancer 2007;109:157-163.

Sievers EL, Lange BJ, Alonzo TA, et al: Immunophenotypic evidence of leukemia after induction therapy predicts relapse: Results from a prospective Children's Cancer Group study of 252 patients with acute myeloid leukemia. Blood 2003;101:3398-3406.

Tallman MS, Andersen JW, Schiffer CA, et al: All-trans retinoic acid in acute promyelocytic leukemia: Long-term outcome and prognostic factor analysis from the North American Intergroup protocol. Blood 2002;100:4298-4302.

Webb DK, Harrison G, Stevens RF, et al: Relationships between age at diagnosis, clinical features, and outcome of therapy in children treated in the Medical Research Council AML 10 and 12 trials for acute myeloid leukemia. Blood 2001;98:1714-1720.

Woods WG, Neudorf S, Gold S, et al: A comparison of allogeneic bone marrow transplantation, autologous bone marrow transplantation, and aggressive chemotherapy in children with acute myeloid leukemia in remission. Blood 2001;97:56-62.

*FDA approved for APL but not ALL, AML, or CML.

# Chronic Leukemias

Method of
*Helen Enright, MD, and*
*Jonathan Bond, MB, MRCPI*

## Chronic Lymphocytic Leukemia

Chronic lymphocytic leukemia (CLL) is the most common leukemia in the Western world with an incidence of thirty per million per year. Two thirds of patients are male. The median age at presentation is 65 to 70 years of age.

Nearly 50% of patients are asymptomatic at presentation with the diagnosis made incidentally following a routine blood count. Symptomatic presentation relates to consequences of bone marrow failure, lymphadenopathy and/or hepatosplenomegaly, constitutional symptoms, or autoimmune complications such as hemolytic anemia.

### DIAGNOSIS

The presence of peripheral blood lymphocytosis of greater than $5 \times 10^9$/L is required for the diagnosis of CLL. The blood film typically shows small mature lymphocytes in addition to fragile cells damaged in the film-spreading process called smudge cells. Immunophenotyping shows a clonal population of mature B lymphocytes that aberrantly express CD5.

Diagnostic evaluation should include direct Coombs test (DCT) (positive in 35%) and serum immunoglobulin estimation.

Bone marrow aspiration and biopsy is important in delineating the extent and pattern of marrow involvement (nodular, diffuse, or interstitial) and to evaluate response to treatment. Cytogenetic analysis may reveal important prognostic information.

Two main staging systems exist (Box 1). These are based on the extent of disease and degree of bone marrow failure.

### PROGNOSIS

CLL has an extremely variable clinical course. Ideally, prediction of the likely rate of progression of disease would direct therapeutic intervention.

The staging systems of Rai and Binet are the longest-standing means of assessing the prognosis of individual patients with CLL. These have inherent limitations, notably to predict if patients presenting with early stage disease would still have rapid clinical progression.

Recent studies on prognostic indicators have focused on biological and molecular characteristics of leukemic cells.

Adverse cytogenetic features at diagnosis include trisomy 12 and anomalies affecting the tumor suppressor gene p53 on chromosome 17p, the latter predicting a poor response to chemotherapy.

Gene expression profiling has identified two distinct subgroups of disease based on the presence or absence of somatic mutation in the specific immunoglobulin heavy-chain variable region ($IgV_H$) genes in leukemic cells. Although technically difficult to analyze, this information has important prognostic significance, with a median survival of 25 years in *mutated* cases versus 8 years in *unmutated* cases.

Levels of expression of ZAP-70 (which normally functions as a T cell signaling molecule) by CLL cells have been shown to correlate inversely with $IgV_H$ gene mutation status. This is evaluated by flow cytometry and thus could theoretically be available as a prognostic marker in most routine hematology laboratories.

The prognostic significance of levels of CD38 expression, beta$_2$-microglobulin, lactate dehydrogenase (LDH), thymidine kinase, and soluble CD23 remains under investigation.

### INDICATIONS FOR TREATMENT

CLL is a heterogeneous disease with a variable and often indolent course; a proportion of patients never require treatment for their disease. CLL is not curable by conventional treatment approaches, although reports of long-term disease-free survival (DFS) with newer treatment regimens including transplantation have led to some reconsideration of this tenet. The objective of treatment in the majority of cases, however, is disease control and palliation of symptoms.

Indications for treatment were published by the National Cancer Institute (NCI) Working Group in 1996 (Box 2). These include all Binet stages B and C and some stage A patients. Isolated lymphocytosis or hypogammaglobulinemia are not indications for treatment.

#### Supportive Treatment

Regular intravenous immunoglobulin (400 mg/kg every 3 to 4 weeks) should be considered in hypogammaglobulinemic patients with recurrent infections. The incidence of viral and fungal infections in CLL patients increases with the use of more intensive therapy, especially with purine analogues and alemtuzumab (Campath). Prophylaxis against *Pneumocystis carinii* is indicated in these patients. Autoimmune complications are treated in the same manner as in non-CLL associated cases, that is, usually with steroids—most patients will also require treatment of CLL in this setting. Erythropoietin may be useful in anemic patients.

#### Initial Treatment

The traditional first-line option for patients requiring treatment was the alkylating agent chlorambucil (Leukeran), which induces partial responses (PR) in 60% to 70% of patients. Treatment of early-stage disease does not confer a survival benefit, and there appears no difference in effect of continuous compared with intermittent dosing in

---

**BOX 1    The Rai and Binet Staging Systems for Chronic Lymphocytic Leukemia (CLL)**

**Rai System**
- 0: No anemia, thrombocytopenia, or physical signs
- I: Lymphadenopathy only
- II: Splenomegaly and/or hepatomegaly but no anemia or thrombocytopenia
- III: Anemia (Hb < 11.0 g/dL)
- IV: Thrombocytopenia (platelet count <100 × 10$^9$/L)

**Binet System**
- A: 0 to 2 areas* involved—can be further subdivided into A(0), A(I), and A(II)
- B: 3 to 5 areas involved
- C: Anemia (Hb <10.0 g/dL) or thrombocytopenia (<100 × 10$^9$/L)

*Each general lymph node region, the liver, and the spleen constitutes an area.
*Abbreviation:* Hb = hemoglobin.

---

**BOX 2    Indications for Treatment of Chronic Lymphocytic Leukemia (CLL) Suggested by the National Cancer Institute Working Group (1996)**

- Progressive bone marrow failure
- Massive (>10 cm) or progressive lymphadenopathy
- Massive (>6 cm) or progressive splenomegaly
- Progressive lymphocytosis (doubling time <6 months or > 50% rise in lymphocyte count within 2 months)
- Systemic symptoms, e.g., debilitating night sweats, fevers, fatigue, weight loss
- Autoimmune cytopenias

patients needing treatment. There is no demonstrable therapeutic advantage to the addition of prednisone to chlorambucil, whereas combination regimens such as cyclophosphamide, hydroxydaunomycin (doxorubicin), Oncovin (vincristine), and prednisone (CHOP), despite higher overall response rates (ORR), show no relative survival benefit.

More recently, treatment with the purine analogue fludarabine (Fludara) has been shown to result in ORR of 70% to 80% in untreated disease with complete response (CR) rates of 20%, and these results have led to its increased use as a first-line agent. Intravenous treatment is given at a dose of 25 mg/m$^2$ for 5 days, usually for six courses at four weekly intervals. Treatment with the oral formulation of the drug (40 mg/m$^2$) yields comparable response rates.

Comparative studies of fludarabine and alkylator-based regimens have consistently shown increased ORR, CR, and duration of response in fludarabine-treated groups. This has, however, not translated to an increase in overall survival, possibly because of crossover in study designs and high response rates to second-line treatment.

Fludarabine has potent immunosuppressive effects, causing increased susceptibility to serious infections. Defects in lymphocyte function may persist for months and even years after discontinuation of treatment. Transfusion should be with cytomegalovirus (CMV) seronegative and gamma-irradiated blood products. Purine analogues may also trigger autoimmune complications including refractory hemolysis and so are contraindicated in patients with a positive DCT.

Combination treatment with fludarabine with cyclophosphamide (Cytoxan) results in higher CR rates than with fludarabine alone with responses in 40% of cases previously resistant to fludarabine. The combination regimen fludarabine (25 mg/m$^2$) and cyclophosphamide (250 mg/m$^2$) (FCR) for 3 days with the anti-CD20 monoclonal antibody rituximab (Rituxan)[1] (375 mg/m$^2$, day 1 only) has resulted in ORR of more than 90% and CR rates of 70% in previously untreated patients.

### Second-Line Treatment

Most patients who initially respond to first-line therapy have subsequent further progression of CLL requiring retreatment. Alkylating agents may be reintroduced, but responses are usually short-lived. Patients relapsing after initial fludarabine treatment are unlikely to respond to single agent alkylator therapy.

Fludarabine produces impressive results in patients previously treated with chlorambucil with ORR of 60% to 70% in patients responsive to alkylators and 20% to 50% in those previously resistant. Retreatment with fludarabine results in approximately 85% ORR in previously sensitive patients.

Combination treatment with cyclophosphamide, vincristine, and prednisone (CVP)[1] gives ORR in 31% of previously treated patients and is commonly used in patients with bulky disease. There is little evidence that anthracycline-based regimens confer therapeutic advantage over fludarabine in patients with relapsed disease. Responses have been seen, however, in fludarabine-resistant cases, and these may be considered in this setting.

The use of alemtuzumab (Campath), a monoclonal anti-CD52 antibody that specifically targets lymphocytes, has given ORR of 33% to 40% when studied in heavily pretreated patients. The achievement of CR in this setting may be associated with long-term DFS in selected patients. Bulky lymphadenopathy is poorly responsive to this treatment. Alemtuzumab is potently immunosuppressive with a high risk of infective complications, notably CMV reactivation (seen in 10%).

Rituximab (Rituxan)[1] as a single agent has yielded disappointing results. Its use in the combination FCR, however, has shown impressive ORR of greater than 70%, with CR rates as high as 25% reported.

Patients with p53 mutations who are resistant to treatment have a particularly poor prognosis. Responses to both alemtuzumab and high-dose methylprednisolone[1] have, however, been demonstrated in this setting.

## Stem Cell Transplantation

Peripheral blood stem cell (PBSC) and marrow transplant remain experimental in CLL. PBSC mobilization followed by high-dose therapy and stem cell rescue is feasible, although extensive pretreatment with fludarabine may compromise stem cell mobilization and harvesting.

Allogeneic transplant offers the only current potential for cure of CLL, and long-term DFS is possible, even in poor risk patients, with three-year survival rates of 46% reported, although treatment-related mortality (TRM) of 46% is also seen. The encouraging response rates seen with fludarabine-based regimens with much lower attendant morbidity means myeloablative allogeneic transplant is usually reserved for young patients with poor prognostic features.

Attempts have been made to decrease transplant toxicity while harnessing beneficial graft-versus-leukemia (GVL) effects by using nonmyeloablative conditioning regimens. These regimens have resulted in CR rates of approximately 40% with chronic graft-versus-host disease (GVHD) occurring in 75% of patients and TRM of 15% to 20%.

## Richter's Syndrome

Transformation to a high-grade, usually diffuse, large-cell lymphoma occurs in 5% to 10% of CLL. Prognosis is poor with low response rates to therapy and very short survival rates (2 to 8 months).

## T Cell Prolymphocytic Leukemia (T-PLL)

Typically follows an aggressive clinical course with survival usually less than 1 year. It is slightly more common in males with a median age at presentation of 65 years of age. Patients usually have hepatosplenomegaly and lymphadenopathy with skin involvement in 20% of cases. There is typically a marked lymphocytosis ($>100 \times 10^9$/L).

Treatment responses are usually disappointing. Chlorambucil, pentostatin (Nipent), or combination regimens such as CHOP are usually ineffective or give a transient short-lived PR. Recent encouraging responses have been seen with alemtuzumab with ORR of 51% to 76%, although infusion-related adverse events and infective complications are common.

## T Cell Large Granular Lymphocytic (T-LGL) Leukemia

T-LGL leukemia is characterized by a persistent increase in clonal large granular lymphocytes in the peripheral blood that may infiltrate the bone marrow, liver, and spleen.

The median age at presentation is 50 to 60 years of age with males and females equally affected. The commonest clinical presentations relate to neutropenia and splenomegaly (seen in 50% of cases).

The abnormal lymphocytes usually have a mature T cell immunophenotype—expression of natural killer cell markers (e.g., CD56) is associated with a more aggressive clinical course.

Complications of neutropenia and (more rarely) red cell aplasia are believed to be cytokine-mediated. Immunologic abnormalities are common, including clinical and/or serologic evidence of rheumatoid arthritis in 30% of cases.

T-LGL leukemia usually follows an indolent clinical course, and treatment is not indicated in asymptomatic cases. Recurrent infection because of neutropenia is the commonest indication for intervention. Neutropenia may respond to corticosteroids whereas granulocyte colony-stimulating factor (G-CSF) (Neupogen)[1] may be effective in some cases.

Cyclosporine A (Neoral)[1] (5 to 10 mg/kg/day) and low-dose oral methotrexate (Rheumatrex)[1] (usually 7.5 mg/week) are used. Cyclophosphamide (Cytoxan)[1] (100 mg/day) has shown efficacy in pure red (blood) cell aplasia (PRCA).

---

[1]Not FDA approved for this indication.

[1]Not FDA approved for this indication.

Treatment responses in the more aggressive forms of the disease (including combination chemotherapy) have been almost universally disappointing.

## Hairy Cell Leukemia

Hairy cell leukemia is characterized by malignant proliferation of mature B lymphocytes with cytoplasmic projections, giving it a characteristic morphologic appearance. Patients usually present with splenomegaly and/or pancytopenia (with monocytopenia characteristic).

Bone marrow aspiration is typically difficult because of increased fibrosis. Tartrate-resistant acid phosphatase (TRAP) stain is usually positive. The bone marrow biopsy shows an interstitial infiltrate of widely spaced lymphoid cells.

Variant cases have distinct morphology and tend to have a poorer response to treatment.

Cladribine (Leustatin) is the treatment of choice, usually given as a continuous infusion over 7 days at 0.1 mg/kg/day. CR rates of 50% to 91% with progression-free survival (PFS) and DFS at 4 years of up to 84% and 96%, respectively, are reported. Alternative dosing schedules have also been used successfully.

Pentostatin (Nipent) produces ORR of 84% with CR of 64% when given at doses of 5 mg/m$^2$ for 2 days every 2 weeks until maximum response.

Interferon alfa-2a (Roferon-A) (3 million IU/day by subcutaneous injection for 16 to 24 weeks initially) may be considered in cases refractory to purine analogues. Splenectomy may be considered where splenomegaly is the dominant clinical feature and other treatments have failed.

## Chronic Myeloid Leukemia

Chronic myeloid leukemia (CML) is characterized by a specific chromosomal translocation resulting in the generation of an aberrant tyrosine kinase, which fuels proliferation of a malignant clone of myeloid cells.

Most patients present in chronic phase with proliferation of well-differentiated myeloid cells. Some present with more advanced disease or in blast crisis, similar to acute leukemia.

CML has an annual incidence of 1 to 2 cases per 100,000 population (accounting for 15% to 20% of all leukemia) with a slight male preponderance. Typical age of presentation is 40 to 60 years of age.

### CLINICAL FEATURES

Up to 20% to 50% of cases are diagnosed incidentally following blood tests performed for other reasons. Symptomatic presentation includes:

- Systemic symptoms such as sweats, fatigue and malaise
- Symptoms referable to splenomegaly, that is, abdominal discomfort or early satiety
- Rarely, may present with acute gout, priapism, or with symptoms of hyperviscosity because of very high leukocyte counts

### LABORATORY FEATURES

CML usually presents with neutrophil leukocytosis. There is a "left shift" with increased myelocytes and metamyelocytes in the peripheral blood and bone marrow. The differential diagnosis includes a leukemoid reaction to infection, inflammation, or malignancy. There is typically basophilia and often eosinophilia. The platelet count is normal or elevated and mild anemia is common. Biochemical markers of increased cell turnover, such as LDH and urate, are typically elevated.

Bone marrow aspiration and biopsy show myeloid hyperplasia, but dysplastic features are not prominent.

In chronic phase, the blast count is typically less than 5%. The transition to accelerated and blast phases is defined by increasing blast percentages and other hematologic abnormalities (Box 3).

---

**BOX 3   World Health Organization Definitions of Accelerated and Blast Phases of Chronic Myeloid Leukemia (CML)**

**Accelerated Phase (One or more features is required for diagnosis)**
- Blasts 10% to 19% (PB/BM)
- PB basophils > 20%
- Platelet count <100 × 10$^9$/L (unrelated to therapy)
- Platelet count > 1000 × 10$^9$/L
- Increasing splenic size
- Increasing WCC (all unresponsive to therapy)
- Cytogenetic evidence of clonal evolution

**Blast Phase (One or more features is required for diagnosis)**
- Blasts > 20% (PB/BM)
- Extramedullary blast proliferation (i.e., chloromata)
- Large foci or clusters of blasts in bone marrow biopsy

---

*Abbreviations:* BM = bone marrow; CML = chronic myeloid leukemia; PB = peripheral blood; WCC = white cell count.

### PROGNOSIS

The median survival of patients in chronic phase is 4 to 6 years. Patients with more advanced disease have much shorter life expectancy with median survival of less than 1 year in accelerated phase and 3 to 6 months in blast phase.

The classic prognostic scoring system for CML is that of Sokal, devised in 1984, which includes patient age, splenic size, peripheral blood blast percentage, and platelet count at diagnosis. Other scoring systems have also been used that consider parameters such as basophil and eosinophil counts. More recently, there is increasing interest in risk assessment based on the achievement of cytogenetic and molecular responses with treatment.

### MOLECULAR BIOLOGY

CML is characterized by a chromosomal translocation involving chromosomes 9 and 22, which results in the fusion of the *ABL* oncogene on chromosome 9 with the breakpoint cluster region (BCR) of chromosome 22.

In 90% to 95% of cases, this results from a t(9;22) (q34;q11) translocation resulting in the formation of the Philadelphia chromosome (Figure 1). In rare cases, variant translocations involving other chromosomes or cryptic translocations may occur. These anomalies may be detected by conventional karyotyping of metaphase cells, fluorescence in situ hybridization (FISH), or by polymerase chain reaction (PCR) techniques. Rarely, no translocation is detectable and these patients tend to have more rapid disease progression.

The abnormal *BCR/ABL* fusion gene in CML encodes an abnormal tyrosine kinase that is constitutively activated and phosphorylates proteins in signaling pathways involved in cellular proliferation and apoptosis. The resultant inhibition of apoptosis and abnormal proliferation results in the accumulation of excessive myeloid cells in the bone marrow.

### TREATMENT

Nontransplant treatment options in the pre-imatinib era included hydroxyurea, busulphan, and interferon (IFN) with or without cytarabine.

Both hydroxyurea (Hydrea) and busulphan (Busulfex) suppress myeloid hyperplasia with reduction of the leukocyte count, although cytogenetic responses are rare, with no evidence of prolongation of overall survival.

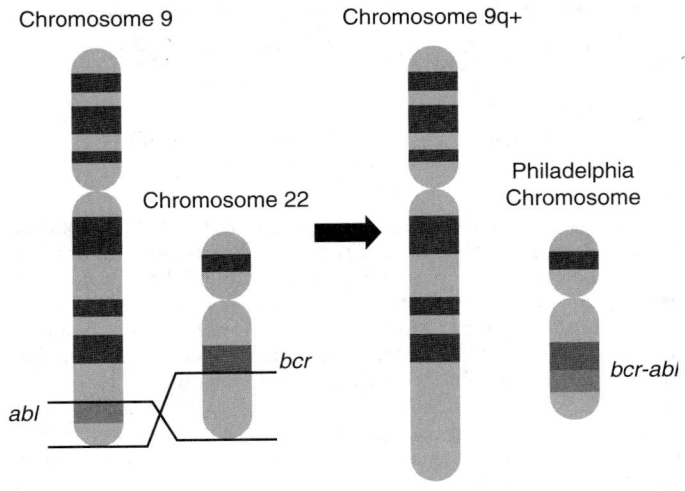

**FIGURE 1.** The Philadelphia chromosome.

## CURRENT DIAGNOSIS

Chronic Myeloid Leukemia
- Neutrophil leukocytosis
- Splenomegaly
- Demonstration of t(9;22) translocation/BCR/ABL by PCR

Chronic Lymphocytic Leukemia
- Lymphocytosis (lymphocytes coexpress CD5 and CD19)
- Lymphadenopathy
- Splenomegaly
- Anemia/thrombocytopenia

*Abbreviation:* PCR = polymerase chain reaction.

Interferon alfa-2a (Roferon-A) (5 million U/m²/day by subcutaneous injection) when used as a single agent produces hematologic responses in a majority of patients with complete cytogenetic remission (CCR) in 13% to 27%. IFN has well-recognized flulike adverse effects at time of injection that frequently limit dose escalation.

The combination of interferon plus cytarabine (Cytosar-U) results in increased rates of cytogenetic response compared with single agent IFN (41% versus 24% major cytogenetic response [MCR] at 12 months in one study), with improved overall survival. This combination was considered the standard of care for initial treatment of CML prior to the introduction of imatinib.

Imatinib (Gleevec) selectively inhibits the tyrosine kinase activity of *BCR/ABL* by binding its ATP-binding site, thereby inhibiting protein phosphorylation by the enzyme and blocking downstream signaling.

Following impressive preclinical and early clinical data, the International Research Information Service (IRIS) study was the first to compare the use of imatinib (400 mg/day) with conventional treatment (IFN and cytosine arabinoside [ara-C] in combination) in previously untreated patients in a randomized controlled setting. Imatinib treatment was superior in newly diagnosed chronic phase patients in several areas, notably achievement of cytogenetic responses (with MCR and CCR of 87% and 76% respectively with imatinib versus 35% and 14% in the combination group), whereas achievement of major molecular response (defined as at least a 3-log reduction in *BCR/ABL* by PCR) was seen in 39% of the imatinib group with only 2% in the combination arm achieving this response.

Significant quality of life benefits were also seen, attributable to the relative ease of administration (oral) and reduced incidence of side effects in the imatinib group. A survival benefit was not demonstrated; perhaps because of the crossover design of the study, a majority of patients in the combination group switched to imatinib treatment.

The latest data after 30 months of treatment show a still impressive MCR rate of 90% with a CCR rate of 82%.

Studies of the use of imatinib in accelerated phase disease have shown CCR in 24% of patients whereas activity has also been demonstrated in blast crisis with ORR of 55% to 70% seen. The incidence and severity of side effects seems consistent across treatment groups. These include nausea, ankle edema, skin rash, and cytopenias, all of which are usually mild to moderate in severity.

Fifteen percent to twenty percent of CML patients exhibit primary resistance to imatinib. Secondary resistance following initially successful treatment is seen in approximately 8% to 15% of chronic phase patients after 18 to 24 months.

Resistance is thought to occur by a number of mechanisms, including enhanced tyrosine kinase activity via chromosome or gene amplification, mutations within the ATP-binding site, or the development of new clonal cytogenetic abnormalities.

Ongoing studies include investigation of optimal dosage (400 mg vs. 800 mg) and the role of imatinib in combination with IFN[1] or ara-C.[1]

## TREATMENT MONITORING

Response to treatment in CML has traditionally been monitored by full blood count and cytogenetic analysis. Latest data from the IRIS study suggest that CCR is associated with a decreased risk of disease progression. In addition, there is good evidence that achievement of a good molecular response as measured by quantitative PCR may result in improved PFS. Monitoring for ABL kinase domain mutations may be useful in determining likelihood of or emergence of resistance.

A broad consensus currently supports three-monthly monitoring of *BCR/ABL* mRNA levels by quantitative PCR with six-monthly assessment of cytogenetic status. A rising *BCR/ABL* level should trigger search for kinase domain mutations.

Stem cell transplantation currently provides the only proven means of achieving long-term DFS in CML. A suitable donor may not, however, be available, whereas medical co-morbidity or advanced patient age may provide unacceptable mortality risks.

Success of allogeneic transplantation is determined by several factors, notably patient age and stage of disease at time of transplant. Chronic phase patients transplanted within a year of diagnosis have significantly improved survival (70% versus 40%) than those transplanted later in the course of disease. Overall, mortality posttransplant approaches 20% in the first 100 days, mainly because of infection and GVHD.

Donor lymphocyte infusion (DLI), by inducing a GVL effect, can reestablish remission in patients relapsing following transplant, often with molecular remission and prolonged survival in responders. This maneuver may be associated with exacerbation or triggering of GVHD, and optimum dosing and scheduling remains under investigation.

Nonmyeloablative transplantation using less intensive pretransplant preparative regimens aims to harness more beneficial GVL effects with reduced transplant-related morbidity, and, to date, mortality has been studied in relatively small series and is currently regarded as suboptimal

---

[1]Not FDA approved for this indication.

## CURRENT THERAPY

- Imatinib is the initial treatment of choice for most patients.
- Other nontransplant approaches include hydroxyurea, busulphan, and interferon (± ara-C).
- Allogeneic transplant should be considered in young patients presenting in chronic phase.
- Autologous and nonmyeloablative transplant remains experimental.

treatment in fit patients where a suitable donor is available. It may be used in patients medically unfit for a myeloablative procedure but remains experimental.

Transplantation using matched unrelated donor (MUD) grafts may be considered for young patients who lack a sibling donor. Improvements in transplant outcome are attributable to improved molecular typing of donors, supportive care, and GVHD prophylaxis. Data from the National Marrow Donor Program show DFS for patients younger than 35 years of age comparable to that seen with sibling donors, although rates of GVHD are higher.

The use of autologous transplant remains largely experimental. Data from UK centers show low morbidity and mortality with a suggestion of increased duration of chronic phase and prolonged survival.

## TREATMENT OPTIONS IN THE IMATINIB ERA

The advent of imatinib has heralded a major change in treatment approaches to CML. This has been accompanied by increased complexity of therapeutic decisions with several ongoing areas of investigation. It is unknown if prolonged prior treatment with imatinib and consequent delayed transplant will compromise transplant outcome. Although CCR is common with imatinib, most patients do not achieve a molecular remission as measured by current techniques. It is as yet unclear if this has meaningful clinical consequences or if prolonged DFS with molecularly positive disease may prove a valid therapeutic target for many patients.

Most centers institute imatinib in all patients older than 50 years of age and most patients older than 40 years of age. Failure of or resistance to treatment may be considered an impetus to transplant in medically fit patients. The use of nonmyeloablative transplant regimens may expand the eligible patient population. The proven efficacy of transplant in younger patients (especially those younger than 30 years of age) with a suitable donor makes this still the preferred treatment option in these patients. MUD transplantation is also a valid option in this group.

Evaluation of patient wishes and expectations with regard to potential morbidity, mortality, and survival benefits is an integral part of the decision-making process. It is hoped that the evolving data on the use of imatinib and ongoing experience with transplant may aid therapeutic decisions and facilitate consistent management approaches in the years to come.

## REFERENCES

Crespo M, Bosch F, Villamar N, et al: ZAP-70 expression as a surrogate for immunoglobulin-variable-region mutations in chronic lymphocytic leukemia. N Engl J Med 2003;348:1764.

Gabor EP, Mishalani S, Lee S: Rapid response to cyclosporine therapy and sustained remission in large granular lymphocyte leukemia. Blood 1996;87:1199.

Gratwohl A, Hermans J, Goldman JM et al: Risk assessment for patients with chronic myeloid leukaemia before allogeneic blood or marrow transplantation. Chronic Leukaemia Working Party of the European Group for Blood and Marrow Transplantation. Lancet 1998;352:1087.

Jaffe ES, Harris NL, Stein H, et al (eds): World Health Organization Classification of Tumours. Pathology and Genetics of Tumours of Haemopoietic and Lymphoid Tissues. Lyon, IARC Press, 2001.

Jehn U, Bortl R, Dietzfelbinger H, et al: An update: 12-year follow-up of patients with hairy cell leukemia following treatment with 2-chlorodeoxyadenosine. Leukemia 2004;18(9):1476.

Keating MJ, O'Brien S, Lerner S, et al: Long-term follow-up of patients with chronic lymphocytic leukemia (CLL) receiving fludarabine regimens as initial therapy. Blood 1998;92:1165.

Kurzrock R, Kantarjian HM, Druker BJ, et al: Philadelphia chromosome-positive leukemias: From basic mechanisms to molecular therapeutics. Ann Intern Med 2003;138:319.

O'Brien SG, Guilhot F, Larson RA, et al: Imatinib compared with interferon and low-dose cytarabine for newly-diagnosed chronic-phase chronic myeloid leukemia. N Engl J Med 2003;348:994.

Paneesha S, Milligan DW: Stem cell transplantation for chronic lymphocytic leukemia. Br J Haematol 2005;128(2):145.

# Non-Hodgkin's Lymphoma

Method of
*Lawrence Rice, MD, and Uday Popat, MD*

Rather than representing a single disease, non-Hodgkin's lymphomas (NHLs) comprise a diverse spectrum of disorders, varying from the most rapidly growing cancer known to the most indolent of neoplasms having no impact on well-being and requiring no treatment. Together these clonal lymphocyte proliferations comprise 5% of all cancers, ranking fifth in incidence, yet their importance is far greater than their frequency. Reasons for this include that lymphomas have critically accelerated scientific understanding of neoplasia, displaying the roles of oncogenic viruses, specific genetic alterations, and the interplay of tumor with host immune factors. Lymphomas are the most common cancers in adolescents and young adults. Regarding therapy, breakthroughs in lymphomas are being applied to curing cancers more generally. The efficacy of the earliest chemotherapy drugs were established in lymphomas; the principles of combination chemotherapy and of curative radiotherapy were gleaned.

## Epidemiology and Genetics

Indolent NHLs are disorders of older individuals (rare younger than age 40 years). Although large B-cell lymphomas are also most common after age 65 years, the incidence curve is much flatter such that they also represent the most common cancer in adolescents and young adults. Other lymphomas have distinctive epidemiologic patterns, such as T-cell lymphoblastic lymphoma occurring mainly in adolescent and young adult men and primary mediastinal large B-cell lymphoma in young women. Burkitt's lymphoma presents as jaw tumors in children in third-world countries related to Epstein-Barr virus (EBV) infection, but presents as abdominal masses or leukemia in young adults in developed Western countries. Hepatitis C increases the risk for several lymphomas, particularly primary splenic marginal zone B-cell lymphoma. Many lymphomas increase with HIV infection, but Burkitt's lymphoma and large B-cell lymphomas with CNS primaries are particularly common. Mucosa-associated lymphoid tissue lymphoma (MALToma) of the stomach is associated with *Helicobacter pylori*.

Lymphomas often display distinctive acquired cytogenetic abnormalities. The abnormal gene products provide clues to pathogenesis and targets for therapy. Examples include Burkitt's lymphoma where translocations involve the c-myc oncogene on chromosome 8 and immunoglobulin heavy- or light-chain genes. Follicular lymphomas have a characteristic t(14;18) affecting BCL-2 gene regulation of cellular apoptosis. In many lymphomas cytogenetic patterns provide prognostic information (e.g., small lymphocytic lymphoma) or can help establish the proper diagnosis, such as (11;14) with cyclin D overexpression in mantle cell lymphoma.

## Classification of Lymphomas and Leukemias

Differentiating lymphomas from lymphoid leukemias is arbitrary and semantic, based on whether a clonal neoplasm presents mainly in lymph nodes and tissues versus prominent peripheral blood involvement. Thus, B-cell chronic lymphocytic leukemia and small lymphocytic lymphoma represent different clinical presentations of the same malignant disorder; disease behavior and treatment principles are identical. Similarly, B-cell (L3 type) acute lymphoblastic leukemia and Burkitt's lymphoma are the same disorder, as are T-cell acute lymphoblastic leukemia and lymphoblastic lymphoma.

A major advance in understanding and managing NHLs emerged 40 years ago with the Rappaport classification system.

## TABLE 1 Proposed World Health Organization Classification Scheme for Non-Hodgkin's Lymphoma

### B-Cell Neoplasms

**Precursor B-cell neoplasm**
Precursor B-lymphoblastic leukemia/lymphoma

**Mature B-cell neoplasms**
B-cell chronic lymphocytic leukemia/small lymphocytic lymphoma
B-cell prolymphocytic leukemia
Lymphoplasmacytic lymphoma
Splenic marginal zone B-cell lymphoma (± villous lymphocytes)
Hairy cell leukemia
Plasma cell myeloma/plasmacytoma
Extranodal marginal zone B-cell lymphoma of the MALT type
Nodal marginal zone B-cell lymphoma (± monocytoid B cells)
Follicular lymphoma
Mantle cell lymphoma
Diffuse large-B-cell lymphoma
   Mediastinal large-B-cell lymphoma
   Primary effusion lymphoma
Burkitt lymphoma

### T-Cell and NK Cell Neoplasms

**Precursor T-cell neoplasm**
Precursor T-lymphoblastic lymphoma/leukemia

**Mature T-cell neoplasms**
T-cell prolymphocytic leukemia
T-cell granular lymphocytic leukemia
Aggressive NK cell leukemia
Adult T-cell lymphoma/leukemia (HTLV-1-positive)
Extranodal NK/T-cell lymphoma, nasal type
Enteropathy-type T-cell lymphoma
Hepatosplenic γδ T-cell lymphoma
Subcutaneous panniculitis-like T-cell lymphoma
Mycosis fungoides/Sézary syndrome
Anaplastic large-cell lymphoma, T/null cell, primary cutaneous type
Anaplastic large-cell lymphoma, T/null cell, primary systemic type
Peripheral T-cell lymphoma, not otherwise characterized
Angioimmunoblastic T-cell lymphoma

*Abbreviations:* HTLV-1 = human T-cell leukemia virus 1; MALT = mucosa-associated lymphoid tissue; NK = natural killer.

Morphologic parameters such as whether malignant cells were large or small and whether they showed a nodular (follicular) growth pattern separated disorders into clinically useful categories predicting disease behavior and responsiveness to therapies. Proliferating alternative classification schemes since have daunted students and clinicians, becoming an object for satires. Nevertheless, modern classification goes beyond morphology, bringing to bear advances in molecular biology, flow cytometry, and cytogenetics to establish homogeneous disease entities that behave more predictably. Optimizing a patient's treatment requires familiarity with up-to-date classification (Table 1).

## Evaluation, Staging, and Prognosis

A thorough history specifically addresses whether the *B symptoms* of fevers, night sweats, and weight loss are present. Physical exam pays extra attention to palpating lymph nodes and abdominal viscera. All patients require a complete blood count (CBC) with differential, blood chemistries including tests of renal function, hepatic function, calcium and lactate dehydrogenase (LD), and chest radiograph. Essential staging procedures are computed tomography (CT) scans (chest, abdomen, pelvis) and bone marrow. Bone marrow biopsy must be obtained but bilateral biopsies are not routinely indicated. Nonroutine tests for certain patients and certain disease subtypes include lumbar puncture and gallium scanning. Positron emission tomography appears promising, and its role is being investigated. The Ann Arbor staging system remains standard: Stage I is involvement of one lymph node region (or IE single extranodal site); stage II, multiple lymph node regions on the same side of the diaphragm; stage III, lymph nodes on both sides of the diaphragm; and stage IV, extralymphatic spread such as to bone marrow, liver or pleura. *A* follows the stage if *B* symptoms are absent.

The most important factors guiding treatment and prognosis are histology and stage. Age and co-morbidities must be considered. An international prognostic index developed for large-cell lymphomas can, with some modification, also be applied to other lymphomas. Scores are generated from five parameters:

1. Age
2. Stage
3. Number of extranodal sites
4. Performance status
5. Serum LD

Another modality applicable to prognostic stratification with diffuse large-cell lymphoma is microarray gene expression profiling, able to separate good risk "germinal center like large-cell lymphoma" from poor risk "activated B-cell lymphoma."

## Treatment of Some Specific Disease Entities

### INDOLENT LYMPHOMAS

The common indolent lymphomas are small lymphocytic lymphoma and grade 1 follicular lymphoma, representing more than one third of NHLs. The great majority (85% to 90%) present with stage III or IV disease; in fact 90% to 100% of small lymphocytic lymphomas and 40% to 90% of follicular lymphomas have bone marrow involvement, marking them stage IV. Patients with apparent localized presentations are candidates for radiotherapy with curative intent (recognizing that two thirds will eventually relapse). Adjuvant chemotherapy is under study for such patients.

Stage III and IV patients cannot be cured with standard therapies, yet median survival for asymptomatic subgroups exceeds 10 years. So, a *watch and wait* approach with no initial therapy is appropriate for most patients, given that the disease is often asymptomatic, indolent in behavior, incurable, and associated with prolonged survival. (One cannot deliver palliative therapy to individuals who are asymptomatic.) Initially untreated patients average 4 years or more before

---

 **CURRENT DIAGNOSIS**

- Precise histologic diagnosis is mandatory.
- Currently, this requires assessment of cell surface markers (e.g., by flow cytometry) and increasingly of cytogenetic and molecular markers.
- Clinical staging requires history of systemic symptoms (weight loss, fever, sweats) and careful palpation of lymph node areas, spleen, and liver.
- Evaluation requires CBC, hepatic and renal function and LD.
- Routine staging is completed by CT scans of nodal areas and bone marrow biopsy.
- Other modalities (lumbar puncture; PET scan) are for select cases or investigational.
- An international prognostic index (age, stage, number of extranodal sites, performance status, serum LD) is clinically useful.

*Abbreviations:* CBC = complete blood count; CT = computed tomography; LD = lactate dehydrogenase; PET = positron emission tomography.

disease progression mandates treatment, with no decrement in survival attributable to treatment delay. Twenty percent of patients with follicular lymphoma, and a greater number with small lymphocytic lymphoma may never require treatment even after more than 10 years of follow-up.

Factors that mandate treatment at presentation or during follow-up are mainly related to emerging cytopenias (e.g., significant anemia) or systemic symptoms. Young age and psychoemotional factors can be reasons for early therapy, but most patients readily accept no initial treatment when the rationale is fully explained. A major problem impacting survival is transformation to more histologically aggressive lymphomas (Richter-like syndrome); this may occur at 5% per year regardless of treatment.

When treatment is warranted, additions to our armamentarium have increased choices, making decisions less clear-cut. Single oral alkylating agents such as cyclophosphamide (Cytoxan) and chlorambucil (Leukeran) were mainstays and remain reasonable choices for many. Response rates are approximately 50%, few complete, but clinical problems may be dramatically reversed for years. These agents are inexpensive, convenient, and most patients experience no side-effects. Potential toxicities are myelosuppression, leukemogenesis emerging after few years (in approximately 1%), and bladder toxicity with cyclophosphamide. Cyclophosphamide (often intravenous) is the backbone of the traditional CVP regimen, with vincristine (Oncovin) and prednisone. Adding doxorubicin (Adriamycin)—the CHOP (cyclophosphamide, hydroxydaunomycin [doxorubicin], Oncovin [vincristine], and prednisone) regimen—adds toxicity without survival benefit in indolent lymphomas. Nucleoside analogues, particularly fludarabine, are active in these disorders. Response rates may exceed those of alkylating agents at the costs of toxicities and inconvenience (several days monthly of intravenous therapy). Beyond myelosuppression, long-lasting immunosuppression creates significant risks for serious opportunistic infection. Newer combinations such as FC (fludarabine, cyclophosphamide) and FND (fludarabine, mitoxantrone [Novantrone], dexamethasone) reduce the fludarabine dose, reducing toxicities. Spectacular remission rates have been observed with these regimens, making them attractive choices both for initial and salvage therapy.

The promise of monoclonal antibody therapy is realized in these disorders. Rituximab (Rituxan), an anti-CD20 monoclonal antibody, can be administered singly or in combination with any chemotherapy regimen, either initially or for salvage. It has rapidly become the world's largest selling antineoplastic agent, even though the only cancers for which it is used are B-cell lymphoproliferative disorders. It is remarkably nontoxic, with fever, chills, and manageable hypotension occurring mainly during the first infusion; infectious risks are low. Understandably, regimens such as FC-R and FND-R are becoming popular. Molecular remissions emerge with these regimens, fueling hopes that curative goals may become realistic. Other monoclonal antibodies for indolent lymphomas are more toxic and used for salvage therapy. These include anti-CD52 alemtuzumab (Campath) for small lymphocytic lymphoma, associated with high opportunistic infection risks, and anti-CD20 antibodies conjugated to radioisotopes. Recurrent or refractory disease is treated with approaches discussed earlier, but rate and duration of response shortens with each subsequent relapse. To re-emphasize, observation without treatment is reasonable for asymptomatic relapse; more harm has resulted from overly aggressive treatment than the reverse. Patients transforming to large-cell lymphoma have a worse prognosis than de novo large-cell lymphoma, but some respond to combination chemotherapy with or without stem cell transplants. Transplants, both autologous and allogeneic, have benefited selected patients, but utility is limited by the age of patients, the anticipation of long survival, and the frequency of bone marrow involvement, which could contaminate autografts. Grade 1 and 2 follicular lymphomas are considered indolent, but grade 3 (follicular large cell) should be treated as diffuse large-cell lymphoma (in the following text), because it progresses more rapidly and because long-lasting remissions can be achieved.

### DIFFUSE LARGE B-CELL LYMPHOMA

This most common lymphoma subtype comprises another one third of cases. Unlike indolent lymphomas, these are clinically aggressive with survival of few months untreated. Alkylating agents or monoclonal antibodies used alone are ineffective. Contrasting with indolent lymphomas, there is a reasonable possibility of cure with appropriate chemotherapy. Localized presentations (Stage I or II) occur in less than 30% of large-cell cases. Nonbulky localized disease is treated with three cycles of CHOP or CHOP-R (cyclophosphamide, hydroxydaunomycin [doxorubicin], Oncovin [vincristine], prednisone, and rituximab) followed by involved-field radiotherapy. A good majority of such patients are cured, as demonstrated in a randomized trial showing progression-free survival of 76% with chemoradiation compared to 67% with eight cycles of CHOP. Patients with stage III or IV disease are given six to eight cycles of CHOP or CHOP-R. Complete response to CHOP will occur in two thirds, and one third will be cured. More intensive regimens like MACOP-B (methotrexate, doxorubicin, cyclophosphamide, Oncovin, prednisone, and bleomycin), ProMACE-CytaBOM (prednisone, methotrexate [with leucovorin rescue], Adriamycin, cyclophosphamide, etoposide, cytarabine, bleomycin, Oncovin, dexamethasone), or m-BACOD (methotrexate, bleomycin, Adriamycin, cyclophosphamide, Oncovin dexamethasone) are more toxic, more difficult to administer, and no more efficacious than CHOP. The addition of rituximab improves the progression-free survival to 54% compared with 30% in patients receiving CHOP without rituximab. Hence, CHOP-R is the standard of care in patients with advanced CD20 positive diffuse large B-cell lymphomas. A baseline echocardiogram is performed because of the potential cardiotoxicity of doxorubicin. Restaging procedures are usually done after four treatment courses. Two additional courses are delivered after remission is confirmed. Prophylactic intrathecal chemotherapy should be strongly considered with involvement of the testis, ovary, breast, sinuses, bone marrow, more than one extranodal site, or a high LD. Recurrent or refractory disease carries a poor prognosis. Cure is still reasonably possible in candidates for autologous stem cell transplantation (those relatively young without serious co-morbidities). It is crucial that they have *chemotherapy-sensitive* relapse; that is, the disease is not progressing during therapy. Common salvage regimens include ICE (ifosfamide, carboplatin, etoposide), ESHAP (etoposide, Solu-Medrol, high-dose ara-C, Platinol), and DHAP (dexamethasone, high-dose ara-C, Platinol), using ifosfamide, platinums, etoposide, cytosine arabinoside, and corticosteroids. Two thirds of patients respond, but longer outlook remains bleak unless stem cell transplant ensues (event-free survival improved from 12% to 46% in a randomized study). Patients refractory to salvage therapy may be candidates for investigational agents, allogeneic transplantation or palliative care.

Peripheral T-cell lymphoma and anaplastic large-cell lymphoma are treated similarly to diffuse large B-cell lymphoma.

### LYMPHOBLASTIC AND BURKITT'S LYMPHOMAS

These represent variant presentations of T-cell and B-cell acute lymphoblastic leukemia, respectively, and they are treated with acute lymphoblastic leukemia (ALL) protocols, which employ vincristine, anthracyclines, cyclophosphamide, cytosine arabinoside, and methotrexate (e.g., Hyper-CVAD [cyclophosphamide, vincristine, Adriamycin, dexamethasone, methotrexate, cytarabine]). Prophylactic CNS therapy is mandatory. Care must be taken to avoid the tumor lysis syndrome (especially with Burkitt's lymphoma) by vigorous hydration, alkalinization of urine, allopurinol, and close monitoring. Approximately one third of patients with these disorders can be cured by chemotherapy (higher in some patient subsets).

### LYMPHOMAS RELATED TO INFECTIOUS AGENTS

HIV predisposes to many lymphomas but particularly to Burkitt's lymphoma and primary CNS large-cell lymphoma. The addition of antiretroviral therapy to chemotherapy improves results. Hepatitis C also predisposes to several lymphomas, particularly primary splenic marginal zone lymphoma. Interferon therapy is highly efficacious for this lymphoma when associated with hepatitis C. (The toxicities of interferon relative to any benefit mitigate against its use in other lymphomas.) With MALToma of the stomach related to *Helicobacter pylori* infection, eradication of the organism with antibiotics results in *spontaneous* regression of the neoplasm in patients with superficial, node-negative, low-grade disease; but others often require chemotherapy or radiotherapy.

## CURRENT THERAPY

- Low-grade (indolent) lymphomas are usually advanced (stage III or IV) and asymptomatic—these can be followed without therapy (*watch and wait*).
- Most common indications for therapy of low-grade lymphomas are emergence of systemic systems, progressive cytopenias, or histologic transformation.
- Most effective therapies for low-grade lymphomas are alkylating agents (cyclophosphamide), nucleoside analogues (fludarabine), monoclonal antibodies (rituximab), or combinations of these.
- Corticosteroids, anthracyclines and analogues, and alkaloids are also effective.
- Large B-cell lymphomas (intermediate to high grade) require moderately aggressive chemotherapy and are potentially curable.
- The regimen of choice for large B-cell lymphomas is CHOP-R.
- High-grade lymphomas (lymphoblastic, Burkitt's) are tissue variants of acute lymphoid leukemias and should be treated with ALL-type regimens.

*Abbreviations:* ALL = acute lymphoblastic leukemia; CHOP-R = cyclophosphamide, hydroxydaunomycin (doxorubicin), Oncovin (vincristine), prednisone, and rituximab.

## LYMPHOMAS RELATED TO IMMUNE SUPPRESSION OR DEFICIENCY

It has been known for decades that lymphomas complicate primary immunodeficiency disorders. Lymphomas with AIDS are addressed above. Post-transplant lymphoproliferative disorder is usually (but not always) a monoclonal proliferation of B-cells expressing large amounts of EBV DNA. Incidence varies from 1% in renal transplant recipients to 2% to 5% in more heavily immunosuppressed organ transplant recipients. The main therapeutic maneuver is to stop or substantially decrease immunosuppressive therapies. This leads to lymphoma resolution in half. Rituximab may be added, but antivirals have not proven beneficial. The prognosis is poor for patients who progress despite these actions, but some respond well to combination chemotherapy. Immunosuppressive drugs also relate to lymphomas apart from transplantation. Withdrawal of methotrexate from rheumatoid arthritis patients can produce *spontaneous* lymphoma regression.

## Other Treatment Modalities

### SURGICAL THERAPY

This has been advocated for isolated extranodal lymphomas, such as stomach or bowel, but its role should be relegated to obtaining biopsy material for diagnosis. Even here, it may be supplanted by needle biopsy with ancillary flow cytometry, histochemistry, and cytogenetics, sometimes allowing definitive diagnosis. (Nonsurgical therapies of gastrointestinal lymphomas do entail a small risk of bowel perforation.)

### STEM CELL (BONE MARROW) TRANSPLANT

Autologous stem cell transplants, now usually collected from peripheral blood by cytapheresis, have been favored for lymphomas. This is the preferred therapy (after cytoreduction) for patients with *chemotherapy-sensitive* relapse where cure remains the goal. *Up-front* use as a form of consolidation intensification for high-risk patients is under investigation. Continuing investigations address the necessity for and means to accomplish purging of tumor cells from autografts. Allogeneic transplants, seeking the advantage of *graft versus tumor* effects, afford a chance of cure for selected patients but with increased risks of toxicity. Toxicities are being reduced by less intensive conditioning regimens.

## FUTURE THERAPIES

Tumor vaccines are in clinical trials and new monoclonal antibodies loom. Molecular advances bring forth agents such as BCL-2 antisense oligonucleotides, currently in clinical trials.

## REFERENCES

A predictive model for aggressive non-Hodgkin's lymphoma. The international Non-Hodgkin's Lymphoma Prognostic Factors Project. N Engl J Med 1993;329:987-994.

Ardeshna KM, Smith P, Norton A, et al: Long-term effect of a watch and wait policy versus immediate systemic treatment for asymptomatic advanced-stage non-Hodgkin lymphoma: A randomised controlled trial. Lancet 2003;362:516-522.

Coiffier B, Lepage E, Briere J, et al: CHOP chemotherapy plus rituximab compared with CHOP alone in elderly patients with diffuse large-B-cell lymphoma. N Engl J Med 2002;346:235-242.

Fisher R, Gaynor E, Dahlberg S, et al: Comparison of a standard regimen (CHOP) with three intensive chemotherapy regimens for advanced non-Hodgkin's lymphoma. N Engl J Med 1993;328:1002-1006.

Horning SJ, Rosenberg SA: The natural history of initially untreated low-grade non-Hodgkin's lymphoma. N Engl J Med 1984;311:1471-1475.

MacManus M, Hoppe RT: Is radiotherapy curative for stage I and II low-grade follicular lymphoma? Results of a long-term follow-up study of patients treated at Stanford University. J Clin Oncol 1996;14:1282-1290.

Marcus R, Imrie K, Belch A, et al: CVP chemotherapy plus rituximab compared with CVP as first-line treatment for advanced follicular lymphoma. Blood 2005;105:1417-1423.

Miller T, Dahlberg S, Cassady J, et al: Chemotherapy alone compared with chemotherapy plus radiotherapy for localized intermediate- and high-grade non-Hodgkin's lymphoma. N Engl J Med 1998;339:21-26.

Philip T, Guglielmi C, Hagenbeek A, et al: Autologous bone marrow transplantation as compared with salvage chemotherapy in relapses of chemotherapy-sensitive non-Hodgkin's lymphoma. N Engl J Med 1995;333:1540-1545.

# Multiple Myeloma

Method of
*Rodger E. Tiedemann, MB, ChB, PhD,*
*and A. Keith Stewart, MB, ChB*

Multiple myeloma is a malignancy of clonal plasma cells that proliferate and accumulate in the bone marrow. The neoplastic plasma cells typically produce a monoclonal immunoglobulin (or M protein) that can be detected in blood or urine. In the United States, myeloma accounts for 15% of hematologic malignancies and for nearly 2% of all deaths due to cancer. The incidence is 4 in 100,000 per year, although African Americans have an incidence twice that of whites. The median age at diagnosis is 65 to 70 years.

Multiple myeloma is often but not always preceded by a premalignant phase known as *monoclonal gammopathy of undetermined significance* (MGUS). MGUS is found in up to 3% of patients older than 50 years, and studies with 30-year follow-ups indicate that approximately 1% of MGUS patients per year progress to myeloma.

Myeloma remains incurable and is associated with a median survival of only 3 to 4 years, although its clinical course can be extremely variable, ranging from indolent disease that progresses only over the space of a decade to aggressive disease causing death within months.

## Diagnosis

### CLINICAL FEATURES

Bone pain, recurrent infection and symptoms of anemia, renal impairment, or hypercalcemia should raise suspicion of a diagnosis of myeloma. These clinical features can result directly from the mass effect of plasma cells lesions (plasmacytoma) or can arise indirectly from the M-protein or cytokines secreted by plasma cells.

## CURRENT DIAGNOSIS

**Multiple Myeloma**

- Monoclonal protein in the serum or urine* *and*
- Bone marrow (clonal) plasmacytosis or soft tissue plasmacytoma *and*
- Evidence of related end-organ damage or tissue injury†

**Smoldering Myeloma**

- Serum monoclonal protein ≥3.0 g/dL *and/or*
- Bone marrow (clonal) plasma cells ≥10% *and*
- *No* related organ or tissue impairment†

**Monoclonal Gammopathy of Undetermined Significance**

- Serum monoclonal protein <3.0 g/dL *and*
- Bone marrow plasma cells <10% *and*
- *No* related organ or tissue impairment† *and*
- *No* evidence of other B cell proliferative disorder or amyloidosis

---

*A monoclonal protein is not detected in approximately 1% of MM patients.
†Myeloma-related end-organ damage can consist of hypercalcemia (>2.75 mmol/L or >0.25 mmol/L above normal limits), renal impairment (serum creatinine>173 mmol/L or >1.96 mg/dL), anemia (hemoglobin <10 g/dL or >2 g/dL below normal limits), or bone lesions (lytic lesions or osteopenia with compression fracture), abbreviated to the acronym CRAB. Based on the International Working Group criteria for multiple myeloma (MM), smoldering myeloma (SMM), and monoclonal gammopathy of undetermined significance (MGUS).

---

Common nonspecific laboratory findings such as an elevated erythrocyte sedimentation rate, normocytic anemia, rouleaux formation, and hypergammaglobulinemia should also prompt consideration of a diagnosis of myeloma, among other possibilities.

## INVESTIGATIONS

### Laboratory

Patients suspected of having myeloma require careful investigation (Box 1). Most patients (98%) with myeloma have an M protein detectable either by serum or urine protein electrophoresis. Serum electrophoresis alone shows a monoclonal band in 80% of cases.

---

### BOX 1  Investigations in Multiple Myeloma

- Serum protein electrophoresis
- 24-Hour urine collection for total and Bence Jones protein quantitation
- Immunoelectrophoresis or immunofixation of serum and urine
- CBC with differential and reticulocyte count
- Serum creatinine, calcium, uric acid, electrolytes, lactic acid dehydrogenase, alkaline phosphatase
- Bone marrow aspirate and biopsy
- Cytogenetics and/or FISH [e.g., for del(13) and t(4;14)] recommended
- Skeletal survey
- $\beta_2$-microglobulin, C-reactive protein, plasma cell labeling index if available
- If indicated: Biopsy of soft tissue masses
- If hyperviscosity is suspected: Serum viscosity
- If indicated: Cryoglobulins, MRI or CT of affected areas, biopsy for amyloidosis

---

*Abbreviations:* CBC = complete blood count; CT = computed tomography; MRI = magnetic resonance imaging; FISH = fluorescence in situ hybridization.

---

The components of the monoclonal immunoglobulin are identified by immunoelectrophoresis and immunofixation. Sixty percent of myeloma patients have a monoclonal immunoglobulin (Ig)G paraprotein, and 20% have a monoclonal IgA. Isolated monoclonal light chain without identifiable heavy chain is detected in another 15% of myeloma patients (commonly known as *light-chain myeloma* or *Bence Jones myeloma*). Monoclonal IgD and biclonal gammopathies are rarer; each accounts for 1% to 2% of myeloma cases. In 1% of cases, malignant plasma cells synthesize but do not secrete immunoglobulin, and an M protein cannot be detected (nonsecretory myeloma).

Bone marrow aspiration and biopsy are essential in the diagnostic process and typically show increased numbers of plasma cells (>10%). Aspiration and biopsy might also reveal abnormal plasma cell morphology or amyloid deposition in the marrow space or within blood vessel walls.

### Radiology

Plain x-rays of the axial skeleton and long bones are used to survey for skeletal evidence of myeloma and to assess for impending pathologic fracture. Magnetic resonance imaging (MRI) (using T1/T2 settings plus STIR [short T1 inversion recovery] sequences) can also be used and is particularly sensitive in detecting less overt patchy plasma cell involvement of the bone marrow. MRI may be especially useful when plain x-ray films are negative but the index of suspicion for myeloma remains high. In patients with confirmed multiple myeloma, the size and number of lesions on MRI correlate with prognosis. Computed tomography (CT) is less sensitive than MRI but is useful in defining lesions when cord compression is suspected and urgent treatment may be required. Because myeloma lesions are *osteolytic*, a nuclear bone scan, which best detects *osteoblastic* lesions, is not generally useful.

### DIAGNOSTIC CRITERIA

Various minimal criteria for the diagnosis of myeloma have been published, most recently those of the International Myeloma Working Group (see the Current Diagnosis box), which has sought to provide standardization.

The presence or absence of myeloma-related end-organ damage and the levels of monoclonal protein and bone marrow involvement by clonal plasmacytosis are keys to distinguishing symptomatic multiple myeloma (MM) from smoldering myeloma (SMM) and MGUS. Myeloma-related end-organ damage can consist of hypercalcemia, *renal impairment, anemia,* or *bone lesions* (CRAB). Other less common criteria for end-organ damage due to myeloma include symptomatic hyperviscosity or recurrent bacterial infections (≥2 in 12 months).

In most MM patients, plasma cells account for more than 10% of nucleated marrow cells; however, rare symptomatic MM patients can present with plasma cells less than 10%, and a lower limit is not specified in the Working Group criteria. Approximately 1% of patients with symptomatic multiple myeloma do not have a detectable monoclonal protein when highly sensitive techniques are employed.

MGUS may be difficult to distinguish from SMM or early stage MM. Features that help to support a diagnosis of myeloma include depression of the normal immunoglobulin levels and high paraprotein concentration (>30 g/L in serum or >1 g/24 h in urine). Although MGUS and SMM do not usually require immediate therapy, it is nevertheless important to distinguish between the two because the prognoses differ.

Primary or immunoglobulin light chain (AL) amyloidosis is a plasma cell neoplasm related to myeloma that secretes an abnormal immunoglobulin that deposits in tissues in a β-pleated sheet conformation. Notably, 20% of AL amyloid patients have overt myeloma, whereas among myeloma patients nearly 15% develop primary amyloidosis. Amyloidosis should be suspected in myeloma patients who develop progressive neuropathy, cardiac dysfunction with hypotension, enlarged tongue, swollen joints, hepatomegaly, or nephrotic syndrome. A needle biopsy of the involved tissue is the most reliable method to yield a diagnosis, but if involved tissue is inaccessible,

**TABLE 1  International Staging System for Myeloma**

| Stage | Criteria | Median Survival* |
|-------|----------|------------------|
| 1 | Serum $\beta_2$ microglobulin <3.5 mg/dL and serum albumin ≥3.5 g/dL | 62 months |
| 2 | Serum $\beta_2$ microglobulin < 3.5 mg/dL and serum albumin <3.5 g/dL<br>*or*<br>Serum $\beta_2$ microglobulin 3.5-5.5 mg/dL (irrespective of serum albumin) | 44 months |
| 3 | Serum $\beta_2$ microglobulin >5.5 mg/dL | 29 months |

*Times reflect median overall survival by International Staging System stage.

blind abdominal fat pad needle aspiration may be helpful. Samples are assessed by Congo red staining for birefringence.

## Staging and Prognosis

Several staging systems are in existence. The Salmon/Durie system, developed in 1975, remains widely used and integrates the results of CBC, serum creatinine, calcium, serum and urine M protein levels, and radiology to correlate approximate tumor mass with survival. More recently, the new International Staging System (ISS) has been derived and validated by the International Myeloma Working Group from a cohort of 11,000 patients with newly diagnosed untreated myeloma. The ISS (Table 1) uses a simple combination of serum $\beta_2$ microglobulin and serum albumin to provide a reproducible and powerful three-stage classification that stratifies patients to groups with median overall survivals of 62, 44, or 29 months.

More sophisticated prognostic tests including tumor cytogenetics and fluorescence-in-situ-hybridization (FISH) are now increasingly recognized as powerful determinants of outcome, and in the near future molecular stratification of tumors may be used to guide therapy. Aberrations such as deletion of chromosome 13, deletion of 17p, or translocation between chromosomes 4 and 14, t(4;14), causing overexpression of fibroblast growth factor receptor 3 *(FGFR3)* and *MMSET* genes, have been associated with significantly poorer survival compared with the absence of any informative abnormality or with t(11;14) translocation or hyperdiploidy.

## Therapy

### OVERVIEW

Although there are many treatment options for patients with multiple myeloma, at present there is no cure. The disease may remain indolent for many years in some patients, particularly in those with smoldering myeloma or in those with low-level M protein (<30 g/L) and absent bone lesions. There is no evidence that early treatment prolongs survival. Therefore, therapy is generally reserved for patients with symptoms. The decision to begin therapy is based on the patient's symptoms and physical status and results of laboratory and radiographic investigations. Those with smoldering myeloma are not usually treated except within clinical trials. Treatment should be initiated in patients with impending complications (such as renal insufficiency or impending pathologic fracture) even if the patient is not yet symptomatic.

Because multiple myeloma is a systemic disorder from the onset, the primary treatment modality is chemotherapy (Box 2). For eligible patients, the physician should consider a treatment strategy that includes high-dose melphalan combined with autologous peripheral blood stem cell transplantation (ASCT). Four randomized trials comparing high-dose therapy (HDT) plus ASCT with conventional chemotherapy have each shown a survival advantage for HDT, on the order of 5 to 13 months (depending on the alternative treatment strategy provided). These randomized trials were all conducted in patients younger than 65 to 70 years; however, occasional patients older than 70 years might also be candidates for HDT and ASCT on the basis of superior physiologic status.

### HIGH-DOSE THERAPY WITH AUTOLOGOUS STEM CELL TRANSPLANTATION

In patients in whom ASCT is planned, induction therapy is used to control the presenting disease before stem cell harvest. Care must be taken to avoid the use of agents excessively toxic to hematopoietic stem cells (e.g., melphalan). Historically, common induction regimens have included high-dose dexamethasone alone or combined with vincristine and doxorubicin (VAD). VAD is generally given as vincristine 0.4 mg/day IV plus doxorubicin 9 mg/m$^2$/day IV on days 1 to 4, and dexamethasone 40 mg orally on days 1 to 4, 9 to 12, and 17 to 20. This is usually repeated every 28 days for four cycles. VAD induces partial remission (PR) in approximately 50% to 70% of patients and complete remission (CR) in 5% to 10% of patients. Dexamethasone alone is only mildly less effective and is useful as initial treatment in patients with severe cytopenia, with renal failure, or requiring extensive radiotherapy.

 **CURRENT THERAPY**

**Transplant Candidate (Often <65-70 Years)**

- Induction therapy:
  - High-dose dexamethasone (HDD), often used in combination with vincristine and doxorubicin (VAD) or with thalidomide (thal/dex). Follow with collection of stem cells
  - High-dose melphalan (HDM) and autologous hematopoietic stem cell transplantation (SCT)
- For relapse or induction failure consider:
  - Thal/dex
  - Lenalidomide (Revlimid)/dexamethasone (rev/dex)
  - Bortezomib (Velcade)/dexamethasone (velcade/dex)
  - Cyclophosphamide/prednisone
- Repeat autologous SCT if first remission is longer than 18-24 months

**Not a Transplant Candidate (Often >65-70 Years)**

- Melphalan/prednisone (MP) ± thalidomide (MPT)
- For relapse or induction failure consider:
  - MPT or thal/dex, if no prior thalidomide
  - Rev/dex
  - Velcade/dex
  - Cyclophosphamide/prednisone

**Select Patients**

- Bisphosphonates, particularly for previous or present bone disease: Zoledronic acid (Zometa) 4 mg IV or pamidronate (Aredia) 60-90 mg IV, repeated every 4-6 weeks
- Erythropoietin for Hb <10 g/dL (caution: should not be used together with thalidomide or lenalidomide due to increased venous thrombosis)

## BOX 2 Chemotherapy Regimens for Multiple Myeloma

### High-Dose Dexamethasone (HDD)
- Dexamethasone (Decadron) 40 mg PO on days 1-4, 9-12, 17-20
- Repeat every 4 weeks

### Thal/Dex
- Thalidomide 100-200 mg PO qd, plus HDD
- Prophylactic anticoagulation required (aspirin 325 mg PO qd or full-dose anticoagulation)

### Rev/Dex
- Lenalidomide (Revlimid) 25 mg PO on days 1-21, plus HDD
- Repeat every 4 weeks
- Anticoagulation required

### VAD
- Vincristine 0.4 mg IV on days 1-4
- Doxorubicin (Adriamycin) 9 mg/m$^2$/day IV on days 1-4
- HDD days 1-4, 9-12, 17-20 all cycles
- Repeat every 4 weeks (typically × 4) (short-infusional regimen)

### High-Dose Melphalan (HDM)
- Melphalan (Alkeran) 200 mg/m$^2$ IV,[3] followed by SCT

### Velcade/Dex
- Bortezomib (Velcade) 1.3 mg/m$^2$ IV on days 1, 4, 8, and 11, plus HDD
- Repeat every 3 weeks (e.g., × 8)

### MP
- Melphalan (Alkeran) 9 mg/m$^2$ PO on days 1-4
- Prednisone 100 mg PO on days 1-4
- Repeat both every 4-6 weeks

### MPT
- Melphalan (Alkeran) 9 mg/m$^2$ PO on days 1-4
- Prednisone 100 mg/m$^2$ PO on days 1-7
- Thalidomide 100 mg PO qd, continuous
- Repeat melphalan and prednisone every 4-6 weeks × 12 cycles
- Requires prophylactic anticoagulation

### Cyclophosphamide
- Cyclophosphamide (Cytoxan) 300 mg/m$^2$ weekly PO or IV
- Often given together with prednisone 100 mg PO on alternate days

---

[3]Exceeds dosage recommended by the manufacturer
*Abbreviation:* SCT = stem cell transplantation.
*Note:* Dose reductions may be necessary for side effects, advanced age, frailty, cytopenias, or impaired renal or liver function.

An alternative oral induction regimen consists of thalidomide (Thalomid) 200 mg daily plus dexamethasone (thal/dex). The dexamethasone is given 40 mg/day on days 1 to 4, 9 to 12, and 17 to 20 on odd cycles and days 1 to 4 on even cycles. Thal/dex produces response rates comparable with VAD and superior to dexamethasone alone. Adverse effects include an increased rate of venous thrombosis (15%), which necessitates prophylactic anticoagulation; neuropathy; somnolence; and constipation.

Use of thalidomide within the induction regimen can limit the efficacy of thalidomide-based regimens at relapse. No overall survival advantage is conferred by using this agent upfront instead of as a de novo agent at relapse. In one large study, approximately 50% of 668 myeloma patients were randomly assigned to receive daily thalidomide starting alongside standard HDT plus ASCT therapy. Incorporation of thalidomide into HDT had no effect on overall survival (OS). Use of thalidomide alongside HDT did result in increased event-free survival (EFS). However, this was balanced by substantially shortened survival following relapse and by higher rates of severe peripheral neuropathy and deep venous thrombosis (DVT).

Combination therapies using newer agents such as bortezomib (Velcade) or lenalidomide (Revlimid) are being investigated as induction regimens. These offer the promise of deeper remissions in greater numbers of patients than current induction treatments. However, their benefit on OS following HDT and ASCT remains to be determined.

Following recovery from induction treatment, peripheral blood stem cells are collected from the patient via a cell separator (apheresis) and are frozen until their reinfusion after high-dose chemotherapy. Stem cell mobilization typically requires pretreatment with cyclophosphamide and granulocyte colony-stimulating factor (G-CSF). High-dose melphalan[2] (Alkeran), 200 mg/m$^2$, is the most common HDT used and in patients younger than 65 years is associated with an upfront mortality rate of approximately 1%.

Unfortunately, many patients continue to have evidence of myeloma after ASCT and all patients eventually relapse. The median time to progression in myeloma patients treated with HDT and ASCT is 18 to 24 months. Pre-relapse maintenance therapy following HDT using various agents (e.g., interferon-α [IFN-α], steroids, thalidomide, or combination chemotherapy) is being tested in several clinical trials; however, evidence of significant benefit in OS is currently lacking.

Tandem sequential ASCTs have been reported to improve OS compared with single ASCT. This benefit was not seen within the first 2 years of follow-up; however, it was subsequently observed up to 7 years after ASCT. The benefits of early tandem transplantation are unlikely to be universal; advantages appear to accrue primarily in patients who fail to achieve satisfactory remission following their first ASCT procedure.

There is no clear standard of treatment following relapse after HDT. Treatment with standard alkylating agents or newer agents, repeat HDT plus ASCT, entry into a clinical trial, or allogeneic transplantation can each be considered.

## ALLOGENEIC TRANSPLANTATION

An allogeneic transplant uses stem cells obtained from an HLA-matched donor, usually a sibling, to repopulate the bone marrow following chemotherapy. Allogeneic transplantation can theoretically provide an immunologic graft-versus-myeloma effect that can lead to significant reductions in tumor mass and prolonged remission. However, this potential benefit is balanced by high rates of transplant-related mortality (TRM) and a risk of troublesome graft-versus-host disease (GVHD). Less than 10% of myeloma patients are eligible for intensive myeloablative allogeneic protocols because 90% are aged 50 years or older, and only one third have an HLA-compatible donor. Nonmyeloablative (mini) allogeneic transplantation may be achievable in greater numbers of patients and offers a lower risk of early TRM. However, this approach is again associated with significant risk of GVHD (45% acute GVHD, 55% chronic GVHD reported), and we believe it should be considered primarily in the setting of well-planned clinical trials.

## STANDARD ALKYLATING AGENT THERAPY

For elderly patients or those who do not want, or cannot tolerate, aggressive therapy, various oral chemotherapy regimens may be used. Oral melphalan plus predisone (MP), given as melphalan 9 mg/m$^2$ plus prednisone 100 mg daily for 4 days at 4- to 6-week intervals, is the gold standard in this setting and induces objective responses in 50% to 60% of patients and a median OS of 2 to 3 years. Because melphalan

---

[3]Exceeds dosage recommended by the manufacturer.

absorption is reduced by food, it should be given in the morning on an empty stomach. Dose reduction should be considered in the elderly and for renal insufficiency. Melphalan doses are titrated to induce mild midcycle cytopenia. A mild neutropenic nadir ($1.0$-$1.5 \times 10^9/L$) or thrombocytopenia ($<100 \times 10^9/L$) is often targeted to ensure maximal efficacy. Severe cytopenia should be avoided by delaying treatment in weekly increments if significant cytopenias persist at follow-up and by reducing subsequent melphalan dosing in 2- to 4-mg/day decrements. MP is generally continued until maximal reduction in the M protein has occurred plus 2 to 4 months (plateau), or for approximately 1 year. At this point, treatment is stopped because cumulative melphalan exposure can result in late development of myelodysplastic syndrome or leukemia. Objective responses can occur slowly, and unless rapidly progressive disease occurs, treatment should not be abandoned until at least three cycles of treatment can be assessed.

Addition of thalidomide to MP (MPT) has recently been shown to improve the results of MP therapy. MPT is given as melphalan 4 mg/m$^2$ for 7 days, prednisone 40 mg/m$^2$ for 7 days, and thalidomide 100 mg daily continuously, repeated every 4 weeks for six cycles. Use of MPT in patients older than 65 years resulted in an increased response rate (76%) compared with MP (48%), more complete responses or near-complete responses (28 vs. 7%), and longer EFS (33 vs. 14 months). These gains were balanced, however, by increased toxicity (grade 3-4 toxicity: 49% vs. 25%) and by the need for concurrent anticoagulation (e.g., enoxaparin [Lovenox] 40 mg SC daily). In patients who tolerated six cycles of MPT, there was a trend to survival advantage at 3 years compared with patients treated with similar doses of MP (80 vs. 64%; hazard ratio [HR], 0.68; $P = 0.19$), even when MP patients were permitted to cross over and receive thalidomide following disease progression.

Cyclophosphamide (Cytoxan) can be used as an alternative to melphalan in select patients with a weekly dose of 400 to 500 mg orally or intravenously. Cyclophosphamide is less likely to suppress thrombopoiesis and has less myelosuppressive potentiation in renal failure. It is often administered in conjunction with prednisone 100 mg orally on alternate days.

Multidrug regimens using combinations of vincristine, anthracyclines, melphalan, BCNU [1,3 bis(2-chloroethyl)-1-nitrosourea], cyclophosphamide and corticosteroids can provide a faster onset of action than MP and may be useful in patients with high tumor loads or acute complications. Significantly, however, a large meta-analysis of more than 6000 patients indicates that conventional multiagent chemotherapy regimens do not improve overall survival beyond that achieved with standard MP, even in poor-risk patients.

## REFRACTORY MYELOMA AND NOVEL AGENTS

All patients with multiple myeloma who initially respond to treatment subsequently relapse. If relapse occurs more than 6 months after treatment response, a repeat trial of the previous treatment should be considered. Similarly, for patients who have experienced lasting remission (several years) after HDT, repeat HDT and ASCT may be useful. Myeloma patients often continue to show useful responses to prior therapies, although the quality and duration of response generally diminish with repeated exposure.

Patients who become refractory to alkylating agents typically respond poorly to ensuing chemotherapy and traditionally have had a poor prognosis. Dexamethasone often continues to be useful in relapsed patients. Unfortunately, complications of corticosteroids such as depression or agitation, infection, diabetes, hypertension, osteoporosis, and osteonecrosis can limit long-term use.

Importantly, thalidomide has been found to induce response rates of 30% to 35% in patients with relapsed or refractory myeloma when used as a single agent, with a median progression-free survival of 5 months. A greater response rate of approximately 55% is seen when thalidomide is used in combination with corticosteroids, with an improved median time to progression of 12 months and median OS of 27 months, providing a statistically significant advantage over conventional salvage chemotherapy in relapse. Most studies using thalidomide have used a dose of at least 200 mg daily; however, lower doses of 50 to 100 mg daily might also be effective. Adverse effects of thalidomide,

which can influence the maximum obtainable dose, include sedation, constipation, and peripheral neuropathy. Rash, venous thrombosis, and the risk of birth defects are also problematic.

Lenalidomide (Revlimid, CC-5013), a derivative of thalidomide with greater potency and less toxicity, has shown promising activity in relapsed or refractory and untreated myeloma. In preliminary studies, lenalidomide 25mg daily on days 1 to 21, repeated every 4 weeks, plus dexamethasone (rev/dex), caused objective responses in 91% of patients with newly diagnosed myeloma, including CR in 6%, and very good PR in 32%. In relapsed patients, rev/dex has been shown to be superior to dexamethasone alone in a multicenter randomized trial of more than 350 patients with progressive myeloma, achieving an overall response rate of 58% (versus 22% for dexamethasone alone) and a median time to progression of 13.1 months (versus 5.1 months for dexamethasone). Other trials have demonstrated lenalidomide efficacy in patients refractory or intolerant to thalidomide. Head-to-head randomized comparisons with thalidomide are awaited at the time of writing.

Bortezomib (Velcade, PS-341), a first-in-class proteosome inhibitor, is an FDA-approved novel antimyeloma agent. When given intravenously at a dose of 1.3 mg/m$^2$ on days 1, 4, 8, and 11 on a 21-day schedule for eight cycles, followed by a lower intensity 35-day maintenance schedule, bortezomib resulted in objective responses in 46% of relapsed patients, including CR or near CR in 13%. Notably, the APEX (Assessment of Proteasome Inhibition for Extending Remissions) trial has shown bortezomib to be superior to single-agent dexamethasone as a salvage therapy for relapsed patients, 99% of whom have been exposed to prior corticosteroid therapy. Bortezomib provided an OS at 1 year of 80%, versus 66% for dexamethasone ($P = 0.003$), and median time to disease progression of 6.2 months, compared with 3.5 months for dexamethasone. In patients who do not respond to bortezomib alone, cotreatment with dexamethasone can result in additional partial or minimal responses in 15% to 20%. Notable toxicities of bortezomib include fatigue, gastrointestinal disturbance, painful peripheral neuropathy, and thrombocytopenia.

A multitude of clinical trials evaluating thalidomide, lenalidomide, or bortezomib, in combination with conventional therapies or with each other, are now accruing patients worldwide. These might result in rapid changes in the approach to myeloma treatment in coming years.

## SUPPORTIVE THERAPY

### Renal Failure

Approximately 20% of patients with myeloma have significant renal dysfunction, with serum creatinine >2.0 mg/dL at diagnosis. Common causes include cast nephropathy, dehydration, hypercalcemia, infection, use of nephrotoxic drugs, or amyloid deposition. Cast nephropathy involves deposition of amorphous nonfibrillary material (monoclonal immunoglobulin, usually light chain—thus *light chain deposition disease* or *myeloma kidney*) in the distal tubules and differs from renal amyloidosis in its distribution, absence of β-pleated sheet structure, and absence of Congo red staining. Additionally, the nephrotic syndrome is rare in myeloma kidney and should raise a suspicion of amyloidosis.

Adequate hydration and prompt chemotherapy are pivotal to management and can reverse mild dysfunction in 50% of patients. Allopurinol (Zyloprim) 300 mg daily (or less, according to creatinine clearance) is useful for controlling or preventing secondary hyperuricemia. Nonsteroidal anti-inflammatory drugs (NSAIDs) and nephrotoxic antibiotics should generally be stopped or avoided in the presence of renal impairment. Severe renal failure can require hemodialysis support in order to administer chemotherapy. In addition, plasmapheresis to reduce the plasma M protein can help limit acute renal damage and perhaps reduce the risk of long-term dialysis. However, randomized trials are lacking.

### Hypercalcemia

Aggressive hydration with isotonic saline (150-200 mL/h) and steroid therapy (prednisone 100 mg/day) generally leads to rapid resolution of hypercalcemia. Treatment directed at the myeloma should then be instituted. Intravenous bisphosphonates such as pamidronate (Aredia) 60 to 90 mg or zoledronic acid (Zometa) 4 mg, are also commonly employed after resolution of coexisting renal dysfunction and can provide additional bone protection.

## Anemia

Most patients with myeloma develop anemia, whose etiology is often multifactorial. Where anemia is caused primarily by marrow infiltration, specific antimyeloma therapy (with or without transfusion) may be beneficial. Recombinant erythropoietin (Eprex)[2] may be helpful in severe anemia (Hb ≤80 g/L), even in the absence of renal failure, because myeloma patients often have decreased levels or impaired response to endogenous erythropoietin. Doses of 150 U/kg three times weekly have led to hematologic responses in up to 70% of patients. Lower doses may be effective in patients with renal failure.

## Skeletal Lesions

Bone lesions causing pain or impending pathologic fracture should be treated early. Skeletal imaging should be performed and repeated at regular intervals if pain develops. Internal fixation of impending long bone fractures (usually indicated when >50% cortical erosion is present) can prevent the significant pain and immobility associated with fracture. Advanced bone lesions that threaten fracture or are painful and unresponsive to systemic chemotherapy are best managed with localized radiation (20-30 Gy). Adequate analgesia is vital and often requires narcotics. Vertebroplasty or kyphoplasty can help decrease pain caused by compression fractures of the spine.

All myeloma patients with active bone disease, including those with significant osteopenia, should be treated with intravenous bisphosphonates unless contraindications exist. Pamidronate 90 mg over 2 hours or zoledronic acid 4 mg over 15 minutes IV every 4 weeks show equal efficacy. Common side effects include flulike symptoms such as fatigue, anorexia, nausea, and bone pain; these can last 3 to 5 days but generally diminish with repeated exposure. More problematic is the recently reported association between prolonged bisphosphonate therapy and osteonecrosis of the mandible. Most cases have been reported in patients also receiving chemotherapy and corticosteroids who had undergone a dental procedure such as tooth extraction. A dental examination with preventive intervention should be considered before bisphosphonate therapy, and invasive dental procedures should, if possible, be avoided in patients receiving bisphosphonate treatment. Because hypocalcemia, renal impairment, and proteinuria can occur in patients receiving bisphosphonates, regular monitoring of serum calcium, electrolytes, creatinine, and urine protein is recommended.

## Hyperviscosity Syndrome

Impaired vision, cognitive changes, mucosal bleeding, and congestive heart failure can occur as a consequence of increased serum protein concentration. Symptoms generally do not occur with serum viscosities less than 4.0 Cp (viscosity of water = 1 Cp, normal serum viscosity is 1.4-1.8 Cp), although the relationship between clinical signs and measured viscosity is imprecise. Hyperviscosity is most commonly seen in disorders associated with elevated IgM and is more common in IgA myeloma than in IgG myeloma. Plasmapheresis is used to acutely reduce the level of M protein, and myeloma chemotherapy should be instituted to decrease paraprotein production.

## Spinal Cord Compression

Compression of the spinal cord or nerve roots can result from expansion of an extradural soft tissue plasmacytoma or from vertebral collapse and is a medical emergency. Lower back or radicular pain is a typical manifesting symptom. Leg weakness, urinary retention, incontinence, or obstipation can indicate impending cord damage. Urgent MRI or CT

scanning is indicated to identify the extent of compression. To prevent permanent paraplegia, high-dose steroids (dexamethasone 16-96 mg/day) should be started immediately to reduce cord edema, and local irradiation (25-30 Gy) should be administered.

## REFERENCES

Attal M, Harousseau JL, Facon T, et al: Single versus double autologous stem-cell transplantation for multiple myeloma. N Engl J Med 2003;349:2495-2502.

Barlogie B, Tricot G, Anaissie E, et al: Thalidomide and hematopoietic-cell transplantation for multiple myeloma. N Engl J Med 2006;354:1021-1030.

Dimopoulos MA, Zervas K, Kouvatseas G, et al: Thalidomide and dexamethasone combination for refractory multiple myeloma. Ann Oncol 2001;12:991-995.

Durie BG, Kyle RA, Belch A, et al: Myeloma management guidelines: A consensus report from the Scientific Advisors of the International Myeloma Foundation. Hematol J 2003;4:379-398.

Fonseca R, Blood E, Rue M, et al: Clinical and biologic implications of recurrent genomic aberrations in myeloma. Blood 2003;101:4569-4575.

Greipp PR, San Miguel J, Durie BG, et al: International staging system for multiple myeloma. J Clin Oncol 2005;23:3412-3420.

Harousseau JL, Attal,M: The role of stem cell transplantation in multiple myeloma. Blood Rev 2002;16:245-253.

International Myeloma Working Group: Criteria for the classification of monoclonal gammopathies, multiple myeloma and related disorders. Br J Haematol 2003;121:749-757.

Kyle RA, Therneau TM, Rajkumar SV, et al: A long-term study of prognosis in monoclonal gammopathy of undetermined significance. N Engl J Med 2002;346:564-569.

Palumbo A, Bringhen S, Caravita T, et al: Oral melphalan and prednisone chemotherapy plus thalidomide compared with melphalan and prednisone alone in elderly patients with multiple myeloma: Randomised controlled trial. Lancet 2006;367:825-831.

Rajkumar SV, Hayman SR, Lacy MQ, et al: Combination therapy with lenalidomide plus dexamethasone (rev/dex) for newly diagnosed myeloma. Blood 2005;106:4050-4053.

Reece DE: An update of the management of multiple myeloma: The changing landscape. Hematology (Am Soc Hematol Educ Program), 2005; 353-359.

Richardson PG, Sonneveld P, Schuster MW, et al: Bortezomib or high-dose dexamethasone for relapsed multiple myeloma. N Engl J Med 2005;352:2487-2498.

# Polycythemia Vera

Method of
*Michael Kroll, MD, and Jennifer Wright, MD*

Polycythemia vera (PV) is a clonal disorder of myeloid progenitors resulting in erythrocytosis and varying degrees of thrombocytosis and leukocytosis. The erythrocytosis persists in spite of low levels of erythropoietin.

A mutation in the Janus kinase 2 *(JAK2)* gene is observed in most cases of PV. This mutation results in a substitution of phenylalanine for valine at amino acid residue 617 (V617F). This substitution in a critical binding partner of the cytoplasmic domain of the erythropoietin receptor leads to proliferation signals in the absence of erythropoietin binding. The presence of the mutation assists in diagnosis by distinguishing PV from secondary causes of erythrocytosis and it provides a potential target for new therapies.

## Clinical Presentation

Patients with PV are usually identified by abnormal blood counts obtained for unrelated reasons, although some visit a physician with complaints related to arterial or venous thrombosis. The median age at diagnosis is 60 years. Male and female patients are equally affected.

---

[2]Not available in the United States.

As many as 40% of PV patients suffer some form of thrombosis. The first thrombotic event might occur prior to the diagnosis of PV. In a large retrospective review by the Italian Polycythemia Study Group of 1213 PV patients evaluated over 20 years, 20% received the diagnosis at the time of their first thrombosis and 14% reported a history of thrombosis, mainly within the 2 years preceding a diagnosis of PV. Arterial thromboses, such as ischemic stroke and myocardial infarction, outnumber venous thrombosis by two to one. Sites of venous thrombosis may be unusual, such as hepatic vein thrombosis (Budd-Chiari syndrome), and the presence of an unusual venous thrombosis should prompt an evaluation for PV. PV patients older than 60 years or with a prior thrombosis are at increased risk for PV-associated thromboses.

Bleeding is also a problem. It is most likely to occur with extreme thrombocytosis (platelet counts >1,000,000-1,500,000/μL). GI bleeding, often associated with aspirin use, can occur with lower platelet counts and is sometimes the chief complaint leading to a diagnosis of PV. Bleeding might bring the hematocrit to within normal limits, thereby confusing the clinical picture. One should think of the possibility of PV when normal red cell counts are maintained in the face of iron deficiency.

Other symptoms that could prompt medical attention are erythromelalgia (painful inflammation in the distal extremities), pruritis (especially after a hot bath or shower), and discomfort or early satiety from splenomegaly.

## Natural History

The median survival for PV patients is 15 to 20 years, although it is considerably shorter in patients whose PV is undiagnosed or untreated. Even with appropriate treatment, however, PV carries with it a slight increase in mortality as compared with age-, sex-, and comorbid condition–matched controls. Decreased survival is due mainly to thrombosis.

There is a higher incidence of acute leukemia among PV patients, particularly when they have been treated with an alkylating agent or radioactive phosphorous ($^{32}$P). The development of myelofibrosis also complicates the clinical course of PV, perhaps more often in patients with uncontrolled thrombocytosis. Overall, about 4% of all PV patients suffer at some time from a hematologic transformation, with myelofibrosis occurring in about 2.5% and an acute myeloid leukemia occurring in about 1.5%.

## Diagnosis

The initial goal in the evaluation of a patient with a persistently elevated hematocrit is to determine whether the erythrocytosis is absolute or relative. This goal is accomplished by measuring an elevated red cell mass accompanied by a normal plasma volume. Relative (or apparent) erythrocytosis, which is defined as a normal red cell mass with a low plasma volume, includes a heterogeneous group of benign and reversible conditions, such as diuretic use or smoker's polycythemia. With long-term follow-up, nearly one third of those with apparent erythrocytosis have normalization of the hematocrit following routine interventions, such as changing medications or quitting smoking.

Levels of hemoglobin or hematocrit are sometimes used as surrogates for red cell mass measurements, but one must be aware of their limitations. PV patients often have normal hemoglobin concentrations. For example, in one study only 35% of men and 63% of women with PV had elevated hemoglobin (defined as >18.5 g/dL for men and >16.5 g/dL for women). This is the reason for using several additional diagnostic elements when making the diagnosis of PV. These diagnostic elements are broadly described as the clinicopathologic features that are associated with erythrocytosis in PV patients (rule-in criteria) and those that are associated with secondary erythrocytosis (rule-out criteria).

A medical history should identify most causes of secondary erythrocytosis. A history of cyanotic congenital heart disease, chronic lung disease, kidney transplantation, or medications such as androgens

## CURRENT DIAGNOSIS

Diagnosis requires both absolute criteria plus one major criterion or two minor criteria.

### Absolute Criteria

- Elevated red cell mass
    - >25% predicted *or*
    - Hb >18.5 or Hct >60 in male patients *or*
    - Hb >16.5 or Hct >56 in female patients
- No secondary erythrocytosis
    - No elevation of erythropoietin
    - Normal arterial oxygen saturation
    - Carboxyhemoglobin levels normal

### Major Criteria

- Splenomegaly on examination
- *JAK2* V617F mutation or other evidence of clonality (excluding *bcr/abl*)

### Minor Criteria

- Thrombocytosis
- Leukocytosis
- Low serum erythropoietin
- Spontaneous erythroid colony growth

---

Adapted from Campbell PJ, Green AR: Management of polycythemia vera and essential thrombocythemia. Hematol Am Soc Hematol Educ Program 2005;201-208; McMullin MF, Bareford D, Campbell P, et al: Guidelines for the diagnosis, investigation and management of polycythaemia/erythrocytosis. Br J Haem 2005;130:174-195; and Michiels JJ, De Raeve H, Berneman Z, et al: The 2001 World Health Organization and updated European clinical and pathological criteria for the diagnosis, classification, and staging of the Philadelphia chromosome-negative chronic myeloproliferative disorders. Semin Thromb Hemost 2006;32(4):307-340.

or exogenous erythropoietin excludes PV as the cause of erythrocytosis. Smoking elevates hematocrit not only by inducing lung injury and hypoxemia but also by increasing carboxyhemoglobin concentrations and decreasing plasma volume. One must also be aware of rare inherited polycythemias, and a lifetime personal or family history of erythrocytosis should prompt an evaluation for high oxygen affinity hemoglobin or some other syndrome of hereditary erythrocytosis.

Hypoxemia-induced erythrocytosis is evaluated by measuring arterial oxygen saturation. Oxygen saturation is unaffected by carboxyhemoglobin, however, and normal $O_2$ saturation does not eliminate a diagnosis of smoker's polycythemia. Patients with obstructive sleep apnea can have normal saturations during the day and yet suffer a secondary erythrocytosis because of nighttime hypoxemia. Renal cell carcinoma and benign renal disease (such as hydronephrosis and polycystic kidneys) can stimulate erythropoietin production and cause erythrocytosis. Nonrenal neoplasms, such as hepatocellular carcinoma and uterine leiomyoma, also lead to pathologic elevations of serum erythropoietin levels directing elevated red cell counts. Elevated levels of erythropoietin rule out PV and point to a diagnosis of secondary erythrocytosis.

A low serum erythropoietin level is consistent with a diagnosis of PV. Normal levels are not helpful because they are seen in PV, secondary erythrocytoses, and apparent erythrocytoses. Other laboratory abnormalities observed in PV include elevated serum vitamin $B_{12}$ and leukocyte alkaline phosphatase. Iron deficiency may be present because iron is being consumed by the hyperproliferative erythron or because of GI bleeding or therapeutic phlebotomy. Neutrophilia and thrombocytosis often occur and are useful diagnostic adjuncts. The bone marrow typically shows trilineage hyperplasia, varying amounts of reticulin, and absent or low iron, and it is the best test for excluding a diagnosis of myelofibrosis. Erythroid colonies can be cultured from PV blood or bone marrow without adding erythropoietin, and erythropoietin-independent erythroid colony formation is sometimes used as a diagnostic test.

An activating mutation has been identified in the JAK2 protein that associates with the cytoplasmic tail of the erythropoietin receptor. This mutation—V617F—is found in patients with all myeloproliferative disorders, but it is most commonly associated with PV. The mutation leads to continual activation of genes usually signaled when erythropoietin binds to its receptor. These genes drive erythropoiesis totally independent of the influence of erythropoietin. The *JAK2* mutation has been identified in 65% to 97% of patients with PV. Detection of the *JAK2* V617F mutation requires only a simple polymerase chain reaction–based test. A positive test is a major criterion for making the diagnosis of PV.

## Treatment

Morbidity and mortality associated with PV are reduced by lowering the risk of thrombosis and by controlling bleeding and other symptoms.

### THROMBOSIS

The hematocrit (Hct) correlates with the risk of thrombosis, and higher rates of thrombosis are seen at Hct levels greater than 0.45. The cornerstone of treatment is to maintain the Hct below this level using phlebotomy. Moderate iron deficiency should emerge, if it is not present initially, but it does not pose any threat. Patients should be cautioned against taking iron supplements. If iron is required, the hemoglobin (Hb) or Hct should be monitored closely.

 **CURRENT THERAPY**

**Hematocrit <45%**

- Phlebotomy
- Cytoreduction with hydroxyurea (Hydrea)[1] beginning at 500 mg PO daily
    - Intolerance to phlebotomy
    - Thrombocytosis develops
    - Symptomatic splenomegaly

**Platelets <450,000/μL**

- Cytoreduction with hydroxyurea[1]
    - Age ≥60
    - Prior thrombosis
- Anagrelide (Agrylin) beginning at 0.5 mg PO bid if the patient is hydroxyurea intolerant
- Interferon-α-2 (Roferon, Intron A)[1]
    - During pregnancy
- Prevent thrombosis
    - Daily baby (81 mg) aspirin
- Control reversible cardiovascular risks
    - Smoking
    - Diabetes
    - Hyperlipidemia
    - Hypertension
    - Obesity
- Control bleeding
    - Plateletpheresis for extremely high platelet counts (≥1,000,000/μL)
    - Stop aspirin

---

[1]Not FDA approved for this indication.

Some patients cannot tolerate phlebotomy, and therefore chemotherapy is required to control the Hct. Hydroxyurea (Hydrea)[1] is effective at reducing both the hematocrit and the platelet count. Adverse effects include pancytopenia, leg ulcers, and gastrointestinal complaints. Although there has been concern about a potential increased risk of leukemia associated with hydroxyurea, this risk has not been demonstrated conclusively. Other agents such as busulfan (Myeleran)[1] or [32]P, however, are clearly associated with a significant risk of leukemic transformation. These agents are very rarely used today, although oral busulfan, because it can be given intermittently, is sometimes employed for patients who are unable to comply with daily hydroxyurea dosing. Interferon-α-2 (Roferon or Intron A)[1] is also effective at controlling the Hct, carries no increased risk of leukemia, and is the recommended treatment for pregnant PV patients who cannot tolerate phlebotomy. Flulike symptoms and fatigue are common side effects of interferon-α-2.

Platelets contribute to thrombotic risk. The European Collaboration on Low-Dose Aspirin in Polycythemia Vera trial demonstrated in a prospective, randomized fashion that daily low-dose aspirin effectively reduces the risk of thrombosis without significantly increasing the risk of major bleeding episodes. Therefore, unless there is a clear contraindication, low-dose aspirin should be included in the treatment of all PV patients, including pregnant women. Reduction of the platelet count to normal also reduces the risk of thrombosis. Hydroxyurea[1] is used to reduce the platelet count when thrombocytosis develops, especially if other risk factors for thrombosis are present. Anagrelide (Agrylin) selectively reduces the platelet count and is an FDA-approved alternative to hydroxyurea.

Other known risk factors for cardiovascular disease, such as smoking, dyslipidemia, hypertension, diabetes, and obesity, should be identified and treated.

### BLEEDING

Extremely high platelet counts, high doses of aspirin, or a history of gastrointestinal bleeding increases the risk of hemorrhagic events. Bleeding is typically mucocutaneous and from the gastrointestinal tract. Management of bleeding depends on the clinical severity of the event. It is usually first managed by stopping aspirin. If the platelet counts are extremely high (>1,000,000- 1,500,000/μL), plateletpheresis is used to control bleeding. It works by rapidly reducing the platelet count and thereby reversing a hemostatic defect resulting from platelets absorbing plasma von Willebrand's factor (causing an acquired von Willebrand's syndrome).

### OTHER SYMPTOMS

Erythromelalgia often resolves with aspirin therapy. Higher (anti-inflammatory) doses of aspirin may be required initially, but reduction of the dose to 81 mg/day is usually possible after symptoms are controlled. Pruritus usually improves when the Hct is controlled, but H$_2$-blockers or selective serotonin reuptake inhibitors[1] can help those with more severe or intractable itching. Symptoms of splenomegaly are improved by hydroxyurea.[1]

### REFERENCES

Campbell PJ, Green AR: Management of polycythemia vera and essential thrombocythemia. Hematol Am Soc Hematol Educ Program 2005;201-208. Available at http://asheducationbook.hematologylibrary.org/cgi/content/full/2005/1/201 (accessed May 27, 2007).

Coretlazzo s, Finazzi G: Hydroxyurea for patients with essential thrombocythemia and a high risk of thrombosis. N Engl J Med 1995;332:1132-1136.

Gruppo Italiano Studio Policitemia: Polycythemia vera: The natural history of 1213 patients followed for 20 years. Ann Intern Med 1995;123:656-664.

James C, Ugo V, Le Couedic JP, et al: A unique clonal *JAK2* mutation leading to constitutive signaling causes polycythaemia vera. Nature 2005;434:1144-1148.

---

[1]Not FDA approved for this indication.

Johansson PL, Safai-Kutti S, Kutti J: An elevated venous hemoglobin concentration cannot be used as a surrogate marker for absolute erythrocytosis: A study of patients with polycythaemia vera and apparent polycythaemia. Br J Haem 2005;129:701-705.

Kralovics R, Passamonti F, Buser AS, et al: A gain-of-function mutation of *JAK2* in myeloproliferative disorders. N Engl J Med 2005;352:1779-1790.

Landolfi R, Marchioli R, Kutti J, et al: Efficacy and safety of low-dose aspirin in polycythemia vera. N Engl J Med 2004;350:114-124.

Marchioli R, Finazzi G: Vascular and neoplastic risk in a large cohort of patients with polycythemia vera. J Clin Oncol 2005;23:2224-2232.

McMullin MF, Bareford D, Campbell P, et al. Guidelines for the diagnosis, investigation and management of polycythaemia/erythrocytosis. Br J Haem 2005;130:174-195.

Michiels JJ, De Raeve H, Berneman Z, et al: The 2001 World Health Organization and updated European clinical and pathological criteria for the diagnosis, classification, and staging of the Philadelphia chromosome-negative chronic myeloproliferative disorders. Semin Thromb Hemost 2006;32(4):307-340.

Pearson TC, Wetherley-Mein G: Vascular occlusive episodes and venous haematocrit in primary proliferative polycythaemia. Lancet 1978;2:1219-1222.

Schafer AI: Molecular basis of the diagnosis and treatment if polycythemia vera and essential thrombocythemia. Blood 2006;107:4214-4222.

Spivak JL: Polycythemia vera: Myths, mechanisms, and management. Blood 2002;100:4272-4290.

# Porphyria

Method of
*Herbert L. Bonkovsky, MD,*
*and Manish Thapar, MD*

The porphyrias are metabolic disorders caused primarily by inherited defects in heme synthesis (Table 1). They manifest clinically in two major ways: with neurovisceral symptoms and signs (including abdominal pain, constipation, and weakness) and with cutaneous symptoms and signs. In hereditary coproporphyria and variegate porphyria, patients can present with both kinds of symptoms; in the other forms of porphyria, patients have one or the other kind of clinical presentation.

## Classification

In considering therapy for the porphyrias, it is useful to classify them into two major categories: acute or inducible porphyrias and chronic cutaneous porphyrias (see Table 1). Regardless of the specific form of acute porphyria or associated enzymatic defect, all of the acute porphyrias produce similar neurovisceral manifestations and should be managed in a similar manner. Management of cutaneous porphyria, although more specific to the particular type, also involves application of some general principles.

## Diagnosis

A complete discussion of the diagnosis of porphyria is beyond the scope of this article. However, a correct and definitive diagnosis at the outset is of paramount importance. Box 1 and Table 2 give the recommended approach to diagnosis. Because of the complicated and unfamiliar tests often required for diagnosis, it is recommended that physicians without special training in the porphyrias discuss possible patients with, or refer patients to, physicians who have such expertise. See http://www.porphyriafoundation.com/index.html or call 713-266-9617 for an updated listing. Resources with descriptions on how to diagnose or exclude porphyrias are listed in the references.

## Treatment

### ACUTE HEPATIC PORPHYRIAS
#### Management of Acute Attacks

The cardinal symptom of acute porphyria is severe colicky abdominal pain. Nausea, vomiting, constipation, and pain or paresthesias in the extremities are present in about one half of patients. Tachycardia and dark urine are the most common signs. The pathogenesis of acute porphyric attacks involves a deficiency of hepatic heme and induction of hepatic 5-aminolevulinic acid (ALA) synthase by stressors, with resultant overproduction of ALA, which is neurotoxic.

**TABLE 1 Classification and Major Features of Human Porphyrias**

| Disease | Primary Enzymatic Defect | Autosomal Inheritance | Clinical Features | |
| | | | Neurovisceral Symptoms | Photosensitivity Dermatosis |
|---|---|---|---|---|
| *Acute or Inducible Porphyrias* | | | | |
| ALA-D deficiency porphyria | ALA dehydratase | Recessive | + | − |
| Acute intermittent porphyria | PBG deaminase | Dominant | + | − |
| Hereditary coproporphyria | Coproporphyrinogen oxidase | Dominant | + | + |
| Variegate porphyria | Protoporphyrinogen oxidase | Dominant | + | + |
| *Chronic Cutaneous Porphyrias* | | | | |
| Congenital erythropoietic | Uroporphyrinogen III (co)-synthase | Recessive | − | ++ |
| Hepatoerythropoietic porphyria | Uroporphyrinogen decarboxylase | Recessive | ± | + |
| Porphyria cutanea tarda | Uroporphyrinogen decarboxylase | Dominant (acquired variant exists) | − | + |
| Protoporphyria | Ferrochelatase | Recessive | −* | + |

*Abbreviations*: ALA = 5-aminolevulinic acid, the first intermediate in the heme biosynthetic pathway; ALA-D = ALA dehydratase; PBG = porphobilinogen, the second intermediate in the heme biosynthetic pathway.
*A neurovisceral syndrome reminiscent of those observed in the acute porphyrias has been described in a few patients with protoporphyria and hepatic failure around the time of orthotopic liver transplantation.

## BOX 1   Key to Diagnosis: Screening Tests for Porphyrias

Urinary PBG (porphobilinogen) is substantially elevated in all patients with acute attacks of AIP, HCP, and VP and often during latent periods as well, a finding that occurs in no other medical condition. Urinary PBG offers both sensitivity and specificity in diagnosing the acute porphyrias. PBG is not increased in ADP; diagnosis of this rare condition requires measurement of ALA.

If serum or urine ALA and/or PBG are increased, second-line testing is done to determine the precise disorder of porphyrin metabolism, although treatment (which is the same regardless of the type of acute porphyria) should not be delayed pending these results.

A simple test of considerable value for diagnosis and differential diagnosis of the cutaneous porphyrias is the plasma porphyrin fluorescence pattern. In this test, the fluorescence emission spectrum of diluted plasma is measured. The exciting wavelength is the Soret band (400-410 nm). Uroporphyrin and coproporphyrin, which accumulate in PCT and HCP, have a peak at 618 nm, and protoporphyrin, which accumulates in PP, has a peak at 636 nm. A protein-porphyrin complex unique to VP has a peak at 626 nm. The latter is nearly always present in postpubertal VP patients, and it is the simplest and most reliable method for making a presumptive diagnosis of VP.

*Abbreviations:* AIP = acute intermittent porphyria; ALA = 5-aminolevulinic acid; CEP = congenital erythopoietic porphyria; EPP = erythopoietic protoporphyria; HEP = hepatoerythopoietic porphyria, HCP = hereditary corproporphyria; PBG = porphobilinogen; PCT = porphyria cutanea tarda; VP = variegate porphyria

## CURRENT DIAGNOSIS

**Suspected Acute Porphyria**

- In suspected acute porphyria, the screening test of choice is random spot urine for qualitative or quantitative porphobilinogen and creatinine. Urinary porphobilinogen is markedly (>10× ULN) increased.
- Mild to moderate increases of urinary porphyrins, with normal urinary ALA and PBG are *not* diagnostic of porphyria but more likely due to secondary porphyrinurias.
- The most useful test for diagnosis of variegate porphyria is the emission fluorescence of plasma excited by the Soret band (excitation wavelength ~ 400 nm). Peak emission at 626 nm is pathognomic of variegate porphyria.

**Suspected Cutaneous Porphyria**

- Typical skin lesions of CEP, PCT, or HEP are vesicles and bullae on the hands and face.
- Typical skin lesions of EPP are solar urticaria, acute burning and itching.
- The single most useful screening test is plasma porphyrin and fluorescence emission pattern.
- In clinically manifest cutaneous porphyria, plasma porphyrins are increased and the fluorescence emission pattern is helpful in the differential diagnosis (with excitation light of ~400 nm, peak emission wavelengths are ~618 nm in CEP, HEP, PCT, HCP; 626 nm in VP; and 634 nm in EPP).
- In EPP, urinary porphyrins and porphyrin precursors are completely normal.

*Abbreviations:* ALA = 5-aminolevulinic acid; CEP = congenital erythopoietic prophyria; EPP = erythopoietic protoporphyria; HCP = hereditary coproporphyria; HEP = hepatoerythopoietic porphyria, PBG = prophobilinogen; PCT = porphyria cutanea tarda; ULN = upper limit of normal; VP = variegate porphyria

General measures should include parenteral hydration and pain control with meperidine (Demerol) 50 to 150 mg or morphine 3 to 10 mg. Addition of a phenothiazine (e.g., chlorpromazine [Thorazine], 25 to 50 mg) enhances the analgesic and sedative effects of the narcotic. Propranolol (Inderal) may be given for control of severe tachycardia or arterial hypertension. The dose should be titrated carefully because of the risk of serious bradycardia and hypotension from propranolol. Frequent checks (every 6 hours) of neuromuscular function, looking for developing weakness of crucial muscles such as the diaphragm, by measuring the vital capacity are recommended.

Specific treatment is directed at correcting the deficiency of hepatic heme and decreasing activity of ALA synthase. The treatment

of choice of an acute attack requiring hospital admission is intravenous heme.

Heme is administered intravenously at a dose of 3 to 4 mg/kg/day for 4 days; it is taken up primarily by the liver and replenishes the depleted heme pool. Heme should be started early for most attacks. At this time in the United States, only one FDA-approved form of

## TABLE 2   Further Testing to Confirm the Diagnosis of Acute Porphyrias

| Type of Porphyria | RBC PBG Deaminase | Urinary Porphyrins | Fecal Porphyrins | Plasma Porphyrins | Peak of Porphyrin Emission Fluorescence (nm) |
|---|---|---|---|---|---|
| Acute intermittent (AIP) | Low: <50% | Markedly increased (uroporphyrins) | Normal or slightly Increased | Normal or slightly increased | 618 |
| Variegate porphyria (VP) | Normal | Markedly increased (coproporphyrins) | Markedly increased (copro- and protoporphyrin) | Markedly increased | 626 |
| Hereditary coproporphyria (HCP) | Normal | Markedly increased (coproporphyrins) | Markedly increased (coproporphyrins) | Mostly normal | 618 |
| ALA dehydratase porphyria | Normal | Increased (5-aminolevulinic acid and coproporphyrin) | Normal or slightly increased | Increased | 618 |

*Abbreviations*: PBG = porphobilinogen; RBC = red blood cell.

## CURRENT THERAPY

### Acute Porphyria

- Remove inciting factors: Alcohol, drugs, toxins and chemicals (see Box 2)
- Nutritional supplementation: ≥300 g glucose/day may be given enterally if tolerated
- Intravenous heme: 3-5 mg/kg/d for 3-5 days
- Frequent checks of neurologic status: Especially watch for development of paresis of muscles of respiration
- Monitor for hypokalemia, hypomagnesemia, or hyponatremia and treat vigorously, if found
- Parenteral meperidine (Demerol) 50-150 mg or morphine 3-10 mg q4-6h for pain
- Chlorpromazine (Thorazine) 25-50 mg q4-6h for nausea and agitation
- Propranolol (Inderal) 10-40 mg q6h for tachycardia and hypertension
- Magnesium sulfate, gabapentin (Neurontin), and/or vigabatrin (Sabril)[2] for seizures
- All cases should undergo hepatocellular carcinoma screening every 6 months even in the absence of cirrhosis.
- All first-degree family members should be screened for porphyria

### Cutaneous Porphyria

- General measures: Protect skin from light and trauma; treat secondary skin infections
- Congenital erythropoietic porphyria: Oral activated charcoal; hypertransfusion to suppress erythropoiesis; heme infusion; splenectomy for hemolysis; glucocorticoid trial for anemia; bone marrow transplantation (gene therapy in the future)
- Hepatoerythropoietic porphyria: Uncertain; probably the same as for congenital erythropoietic porphyria (phlebotomy and antimalarials are not effective)
- Porphyria cutanea tarda: Stop ethanol, estrogen, or other precipitating chemicals; iron depletion by phlebotomy; treat chronic hepatitis C, if present; chloroquine (Aralen)[1] or hydroxychloroquine (Plaquenil)[3]; urinary alkalinization
- Protoporphyria: β-Carotene; adequate iron; oral charcoal; cholecystectomy for gallstones; plasmapheresis; intravenous heme; hypertransfusion; liver transplantation; (gene therapy in the future)

---

[1]Not FDA approved for this indication.
[2]Not available in the United States.
[4]Not yet approved for use in the United States.

---

heme is available: heme hydroxide or hematin (Panhematin, Ovation Pharmaceuticals, Deerfield, IL; www.ovationpharma.com). Each vial of hematin contains 313 mg of heme, supplied as a lyophilized powder that also contains sodium carbonate. The manufacturer recommends dissolving the powder in sterile water. In this form, the resultant hematin solution is unstable and must be administered within 1 hour of preparation. It is also irritating to veins, often producing thrombophlebitis, and causes a mild coagulopathy due to adverse effects on clotting factors and platelets.

It is now recommended that lyophilized hematin be reconstituted with human albumin (1:1 molar complex), which increases its stability and decreases unwanted side effects. To prepare such a solution, add 132 mL of 25% human serum albumin (33 g) to a vial containing lyophilized hematin and mix gently. Heme given in this form has biochemical and clinical effects on porphyria that appear equivalent to those of freshly prepared aqueous solutions of hematin and are superior to those of aged aqueous solutions of hematin. Hematin can be delivered within a few hours to anywhere in the United States by calling the 24/7 Ovation hotline at 1-888-514-5204.

In some other countries, another effective form of heme is available: heme arginate (Normosang).[2] This preparation consists of heme complexed to arginine and is supplied as a solution that usually is also diluted in approximately 5% human serum albumin just before administration. Usual doses are as for Panhematin.

Another way to decrease ALA synthase is to administer glucose or other readily metabolized carbohydrates, taking advantage of the phenomenon of carbohydrate repression of the enzyme, the so-called glucose effect. This may be used for mild attacks or when awaiting IV hematin. At least 300 g of glucose per day is given, enterally if tolerated or as a 10% infusion. Some patients have elevations of antidiuretic hormone (ADH) and can rapidly develop profound symptomatic hyponatremia and hypomagnesemia, especially when dextrose in water is given intravenously. As a rule, it is best to give dextrose in half-normal saline. Serum electrolytes including magnesium should be checked every 12 hours for the first few days. Hypokalemia or hypomagnesemia should be corrected promptly.

Many drugs and chemicals are known to exacerbate acute porphyrias, and many others are theoretically risky because they induce hepatic cytochrome P-450, deplete hepatic regulatory heme, and induce ALA synthase, especially in animals with a partial block in heme synthesis (Box 2). Among dangerous drugs, the worst offenders are barbiturates, ethanol excess, hydantoins, and sulfonamides. These drugs are absolutely contraindicated in patients with acute porphyric attacks; others, listed in the first two sections of Box 2, should be avoided if possible. The last section of Box 2 lists drugs believed to be safe; however, a wise practice is to use as few systemically absorbed drugs as possible.

### Therapy of Seizures in Patients with Acute Porphyria

Treatment of seizures in porphyric patients has been particularly problematic because most of the commonly used anticonvulsants also induce cytochrome P-450 and can precipitate or worsen acute attacks (see Box 2). Seizures in acute attacks can also occur due to hyponatremia or hypomagnesemia. Seizures in patients with acute porphyria have been treated with bromides, which are effective and do not exacerbate porphyria, but they have a narrow therapeutic window. High doses of magnesium sulfate (3 g loading dose; then 1 g/h in 0.15 M NaCl, with or without 5% dextrose) have been of benefit. A suggested therapeutic range for serum magnesium level is 4 to 8 mEq/L. Clonazepam (Klonopin) has helped some patients, but in large doses it has made others worse. High doses of clonazepam must be considered a potential hazard, because it induces cytochrome P-450 and ALA synthase in cultured hepatocytes (see Box 2).

The safety of newer anticonvulsant medications has been studied in cultured liver cells. Phenobarbital, felbamate (Felbatol), lamotrigine (Lamictal), or tiagabine (Gabitril), but not gabapentin (Neurontin) or vigabatrin (Sabril),[2] increased levels of porphyrins and the mRNA of ALA synthase, the first and rate-controlling enzyme of porphyrin synthesis. Vigabatrin[2] or gabapentin is therefore recommended in patients with acute porphyria and seizures. Administration of gabapentin should be individualized; the usual dose range for adults is 900 to 1800 mg/day, given in three divided doses.

### Management of Frequent Recurrent Attacks

Some unfortunate women suffer attacks of acute porphyria nearly every month during the luteal phase of their menstrual cycles. Some are helped by oral contraceptives, which are believed to act by interrupting their endogenous cyclic production of sex hormones. However, such therapy is a double-edged sword, because exogenous estrogens and progestogens can induce ALA synthase (see Box 2). Minimal effective doses should be used, and patients should be followed closely, particularly in the first few months. Regular infusions of heme have also been

---

[2]Not available in the United States.

## BOX 2  Some Drugs and Chemicals in Acute Hepatic Porphyrias

**Reported to Exacerbate Disease**

Aminoglutethimide (Cytadren)
Antipyrine
Aminopyrine
Barbiturates
Barbamazepine
Carbamazepine (Tegretol)
Carisoprodol (Soma)
Chloramphenicol (Chloromycetin)
Clindamycin (Cleocin)
Danazol (Danocrine)
Dihydralazine
Diclofenac (Voltaren)
Erythromycin
Estrogens
Ethanol excess
Fosphenytoin (Cerebyx)
Griseofulvin (Grifulvin)
Hydralazine
Hydantoins
Hydroxyzine (Vistaril)
Indinavir (Crixivan)
Ketoconazole (Nizoral)
Ketamine (Ketalar)
Lidocaine
Lynestrenol
Medroxyprogesterone (Provera)
Methyldopa (Aldomet)
Metoclopramide (Reglan)
Norethisterone (Micronor, Aygestin)
Nitrofurantoin (Microdantin)
Oral contraceptives
Orphenadrine (Norflex)
Phenylbutazone
Phenytoin (Dilantin)
Primidone (Mysoline)
Progestogens
Pyrazinamide
Rifampicin (Rifadin)
Sulfonamides
Spironolactone (Aldactone)
Tamoxifen (Nolvadex)
Testosterone
Theophylline and its derivatives
Trimethoprim
Valproic acid (Depakote)

**Theoretically Risky**

Amlodipine (Norvasc)
Amiodarone (Cordarone)
Amitriptyline (Elavil)
Azathioprine (Imuran)
Amphetamines
Atorvastatin (Lipitor)

Bosentan (Tracleer)
Buspirone (Buspar)
Clonidine (Catapres)
Clonazepam (Klonopin) (large doses)
Ceftriaxone (Rocephin)
Cervistatin (Baycol)
Cetirizine (Zyrtec)
Diazepam (Valium)
Diltiazem (Cardizem)
Diphenhydramine (Benadryl)
Econazole (Spectazole)
Ethosuximide (Zarontin)
Felodipine (Plendil)
Fluconazole (Diflucan)
Fluvastatin (Lescol)
Glibenclamide (Diabeta)
Glipizide (Glucotrol)
Guaifenesin (Robitussin)
Heavy metals
Halothane
Hyoscyamine (Levsin)
Imipramine (Tofranil)
Isoniazid
Itraconazole (Sporanox)
Lansoprazole (Prevacid)
Lamotrigine (Lamictal)
Lamivudine (Epivir)
Metronidazole (Flagyl)
Montelukast (Singulair)
Nortriptyline (Pamelor)
Nifedipine (Adalat)
Oxytetracycline
Oxcarbazepine (Trileptal)
Pioglitazone (Actos)
Probenecid
Quinine (Qualaquin)
Rabeprazole (Aciphex)
Rosiglitazone (Avandia)
Sulfonylureas
Simvastatin (Zocor)
Telithromycin (Ketek)
Tetracycline
Topiramate (Topamax)
Tramadol (Ultram)
Verapamil (Calan)
Voriconazole (VFEND)
All agents known to induce
  cytochrome P-450 or to increase
  hepatic heme turnover

**Believed to be Safe**

Acetaminophen (Tylenol)
Allopurinol (Zyloprim)

Aspirin
Atropine
Azithromycin (Zithromax)
Bisacodyl (Dulcolax)
Bromides
Cimetidine (Tagamet)
Chlorpromazine
Cephalexin (Keflex)
Ciprofloxacin (Cipro)
Candesartan (Atacand)
Captopril (Capoten)
Dopamine
Digoxin (Lanoxin)
Enalapril (Vasotec)
Ezetimibe (Zetia)
Furosemide (Lasix)
Fondaparinux (Arixtra)
Gabapentin (Neurontin)
Glucocorticoids
Gemfibrozil (Lopid)
Heparin
Hydrochlorothiazide (Microzide)
Ibuprofen (Motrin, Advil)
Insulin
Iron
Irbesartan (Avapro)
Labetalol (Trandate)
Lisinopril (Prinivil, Zestril)
Lithium (Lithobid)
Meperidine (Demerol)
Morphine
Nicotinic Acid (Niaspan)
Nystatin (Mycostatin)
Naproxen (Naprosyn)
Ofloxacin (Floxin)
Ondansetron (Zofran)
Penicillin and its derivatives
Phenylephrine
Phenylpropanolamine
Propranolol (Inderal)
Quinapril (Accupril)
Ramipril (Altace)
Streptomycin
Tetanus toxoid
Thiamine (vitamin $B_1$)
Tobramycin (Tobrex)
Valsartan (Diovan)
Vancomycin (Vancocin)
Vitamins A, B, C, D, and E
Vigabatrin (Sabril)[2]

[2]Not available in the United States.
Refer to http://www.porphyriafoundation.com/ and http://www.porphyria-europe.com/ for more detailed lists.

of benefit but require frequent IV access. Also, chronic heme therapy can lead to iron overload, because heme is about 8% iron by weight.

For most women with cyclic attacks of acute porphyria, the treatment of choice is a luteinizing hormone-releasing hormone (LHRH) analogue. Leuprolide (Lupron)[1] has been used most often. The usual daily dose is 1 mg (0.2 mL), subcutaneously, although higher doses are occasionally required. LHRH analogues can produce initial worsening of porphyric symptoms due to partial agonist effects, followed by improvement due to chronic antagonist effects. Therapy with LHRH analogues is usually continued for at least 1 year and sometimes longer. The use of bisphosphonates to minimize development of osteoporosis is advised when prolonged therapy with LHRH analogues is undertaken.

[1]Not FDA approved for this indication.

## Prevention of Attacks

Patients should be counseled not to use ethanol and avoid drugs not known to be safe (see Box 2). The use of herbal remedies and alternative therapies is also to be discouraged because many such preparations are likely to contain porphyrogenic compounds. Patients should also avoid very-low-calorie diets or prolonged periods of fasting and should receive prompt and vigorous management of intercurrent illnesses or other stressors. Pregnancy does not usually cause acute porphyria to worsen, and termination of pregnancy is not usually indicated on medical grounds, even if both mother and fetus have acute porphyria.

A small fraction of patients with frequent attacks require chronic infusions of heme. In some, the heme needs to be given weekly or even twice weekly. These patients need to be watched for the development of iron overload and can require iron-reduction therapy by therapeutic phlebotomies if serum ferritin exceeds 1000 ng/mL.

Relatives at risk should be evaluated thoroughly and all probands and relatives found to be carriers should be educated and encouraged to wear medical alert bracelets and to carry medical alert cards.

In a rare patient with recalcitrant and unremitting disease, consideration may be given to orthotopic liver transplantation. Liver transplantation has been described in case reports as resulting in biochemical and clinical remission.

Studies have shown a 60- to 70-fold increased prevalence of hepatocellular carcinoma in patients with hepatic porphyrias even in the absence of cirrhosis or steatohepatitis. This lends credence to periodic screening for hepatocellular cancer in this patient population.

## CHRONIC CUTANEOUS PORPHYRIAS

Porphyrin accumulations in the skin, red cells, and hepatocytes are responsible for the pathophysiologic changes of the chronic porphyrias. The general principles of therapy of chronic cutaneous porphyrias are to decrease the overproduction and increase the excretion of porphyrins as much as possible. Protection of the skin from light (opaque sunscreens and/or clothing) and physical trauma should also be recommended. Oral activated charcoal or cholestyramine (Questran) can improve symptoms by absorbing porphyrins and hastening their excretion in the urine. In several diseases, the chronic blistering and ulcerating skin lesions are prone to secondary infection, which requires prompt treatment to minimize further damage.

### Congenital Erythropoietic Porphyria

Congenital erythropoietic porphyria (CEP; Günther's disease) is a rare autosomal recessive disorder that manifests in infancy with red urine, erythrodontia, anemia, and a severe blistering dermatosis. The marked overproduction of uroporphyrin I characteristic of CEP arises from erythroid precursors. Elevated levels of porphyrins have been improved by large oral doses of activated charcoal (30-60 g every 6 hours), by hypertransfusion, and by infusions of heme. Unfortunately, long-term therapy with any of these is difficult, and chronic transfusions exacerbate iron overload, which is often a preexisting problem related to ineffective erythropoiesis and increased iron absorption. Some patients with hemolysis have responded to splenectomy, and glucocorticoids have also been reported to improve anemia. Because of the rarity and phenotypic heterogeneity of CEP, a consensus regarding therapy has not emerged. A few patients have been cured by bone marrow transplantation. In the future, gene replacement therapy will deserve serious consideration for treatment of severely affected patients.

### Hepatoerythropoietic Porphyria

Hepatoerythropoietic porphyria (HEP) is even rarer than CEP, which it resembles clinically. HEP is due to homozygous or compound heterozygous defects, leading to severe deficiency of uroporphyrinogen decarboxylase. Infants present with severe skin fragility and extensive vesicle and bulla formation, leading to scarring and mutilation of sun-exposed skin. They also present with hypertrichosis, erythrodontia, anemia, and hepatosplenomegaly.

The general and specific measures outlined earlier for therapy of CEP are rational in HEP as well, although none has been shown clearly effective in HEP. HEP shows no response to therapeutic phlebotomy, unlike porphyria cutanea tarda, even though both share a defect in uroporphyrinogen decarboxylase.

### Porphyria Cutanea Tarda (PCT)

Porphyria cutanea tarda (PCT) is the most common type of porphyria. It is characterized by an inherited or acquired defect in activity of hepatic uroporphyrinogen decarboxylase. In the common inherited form(s) of PCT, there is a 50% decrease in activity of the decarboxylase, usually identifiable in nonliver tissues as well as in the liver. A defect in the decarboxylase is not sufficient to produce clinical manifestations; other factors, such as iron overload, chronic hepatitis C, ethanol abuse, estrogens, and porphyrogenic toxins, are important pathogenic elements. The typical patient is a middle-aged man with a vesiculobullous eruption on the dorsa of the hands. Patients usually abuse ethanol and have evidence of modest iron overload and liver injury. In some parts of the world, including the United States, most patients with PCT also have chronic hepatitis C.

Patients with mild PCT often respond simply to the general measures and removal of the precipitating agent such as estrogen, ethanol, or halo-aromatic chemical exposure. For those with more severe disease, the treatment of choice is phlebotomy for depletion of hepatic iron stores. The initial treatment regimen should be removal of a pint of blood each week, continued until the patient has developed a mild degree of anemia with decreased serum ferritin, transferrin saturation, and erythrocytic mean corpuscular volume (MCV). Although most patients with PCT have moderate iron overload (~3-4 g), phlebotomy therapy is effective even when hepatic iron stores are not increased.

Unfortunately, the response to iron removal or other therapy of PCT is slow, and evidence of improvement in the skin might not appear for months. It is important to let patients know this and to encourage them to persist in therapy, for it will eventually succeed. Patients should not take medicinal iron and are encouraged to decrease their intake of red meats, which contain relatively large amounts of heme iron, a form of iron particularly well absorbed.

Recent results from our center and others showed that most patients with active PCT also have chronic hepatitis C infection and one or both of the mutations of the *HFE* gene associated with HLA-linked hereditary hemochromatosis. All patients with PCT should be screened for hepatitis C infection and for *HFE* gene mutations (C282Y and H63D).

Chloroquine (Aralen)[1] and hydroxychloroquine (Plaquenil)[1] form water-soluble complexes with uroporphyrin, increasing porphyrin removal from tissue stores and excretion in the urine. However, in previously untreated PCT, the doses of these drugs usually used for other disorders can cause acute hepatic injury with fever, jaundice, and right upper quadrant pain. This is due to excessively rapid mobilization of porphyrin from the liver. For this reason, such drugs should be started slowly at low doses (125 mg 2-3 times per week) with gradual increase to 500 mg/day. Monitoring for possible retinal damage is advisable whenever chronic chloroquine or hydroxychloroquine therapy is used.

PCT can occur in association with end-stage renal disease. Because the chloroquine-porphyrin complex is poorly dialyzable, chloroquine is ineffective. Because of anemia, phlebotomy is relatively contraindicated in such patients. However, administration of recombinant human erythropoietin (Epogen, Procrit) stimulates iron mobilization for red cell production sufficient to support therapeutic phlebotomyies.

### Protoporphyria

Also called erythopoietic protoporphyria (EPP), protoporphyria (PP) is a disorder with highly variable clinical expression. Infants and children develop intense burning pain of sun-exposed skin following brief exposure in the spring and summer. A few hours later, erythema,

---

[1]Not FDA approved for this indication.

edema, and itching become prominent. Vesicles only develop with prolonged exposure. With chronic and repeated exposure, involved skin can become leathery and hyperkeratotic. This is especially prominent in a malar butterfly distribution on the face and over the knuckles of the hands. Diagnosis of PP requires demonstration of increased amounts of protoporphyrin, without increased coproporphyrin, in the stool, red cells, or both. It is the only form of clinically manifested porphyria in which urinary heme precursors are normal. A common complication of PP is development of pigment gallstones, which contain a high content of protoporphyrin. A rare, but serious, complication is development of severe liver disease, due to precipitation of protoporphyrin in hepatocytes and biliary radicles. Such disease can progress and produce liver failure with all its usual complications.

In addition to the usual general measures, PP is treated with β-carotene (Solatene). The usual adult dose is 120 to 180 mg/day. The recommended therapeutic serum β-carotene level is 600 to 800 μg/dL. Drugs or chemicals that can increase protoporphyrin production or decrease its utilization should be avoided. Griseofulvin (Grifulvin) is the most obvious example, because it can cause a protoporphyric condition in mice. Any drug or toxin (e.g., excess alcohol) that produces cholestasis is a risk, because protoporphyrin must be excreted through the bile. Patients should be immunized against hepatitis A and B unless they clearly are immune. Avoidance of iron deficiency is important, because iron deficiency can exacerbate overproduction of protoporphyrin. Oral cholestyramine and activated charcoal have been suggested as treatments to prevent the enterohepatic circulation of protoporphyrin, which appears to be substantial. Patients with symptomatic gallstones are best treated by cholecystectomy, as long as they do not have severe liver disease or other contraindications to surgery.

Patients with evidence of liver disease require regular and frequent monitoring, because decompensation can occur quickly. Those with abnormal liver chemistries or very high red cell (>1500 μg/dL) or plasma (>150 μg/dL) protoporphyrin concentrations should undergo liver biopsy. Patients with liver injury must avoid ethanol or other hepatotoxins that can act synergistically to accelerate liver damage. Liver transplantation is an option for those with advanced liver disease, although it does not correct the biochemical abnormality because ferrochelatase deficiency in the bone marrow persists.

Unfortunately, some patients with PP who have undergone liver transplantation have redeveloped pigmentary fibrosis quite rapidly. Thus, transplantation of bone marrow before, during, or after liver transplantation is considered. In the future, gene therapy (the normal ferrochelatase gene targeted to the bone marrow stem cells) will be a major advance. Transient improvements in PP have been achieved by plasmapheresis followed by intravenous heme infusions. The dose of heme used has been 3 to 5 mg/kg/day. Such therapy is recommended, particularly as a way to stabilize hepatic function while transplantation is awaited or to decrease plasma protoporphyrin concentrations just prior to transplantation. Without such therapy, several patients have suffered severe neuromuscular complications, requiring prolonged and expensive convalescence.

## REFERENCES

Anderson KE, Bishop DF, Desnick RJ, Sassa S: Disorders of heme biosynthesis, In Scriver CR, Beaudet AL, Sly WS, Valle D (eds): The Metabolic and Molecular Bases of Inherited Disease, 8th ed. New York: McGraw-Hill, 2001, pp 2991-3042.

Anderson KE, Bloomer JR, Bonkovsky HL, et al: Recommendations for the diagnosis and treatment of the acute porphyrias. Ann Intern Med 2005;142:439-450.

Anderson KE, Bonkovsky HL, Bloomer JR, Shedlofsky SI: Reconstitution of hematin for intravenous infusion. Ann Intern Med 2006;144: 537-538.

Bonkovsky HL, Barnard GF: Diagnosis of porphyric syndromes: A practical approach in the era of molecular biology. Semin Liver Dis 1998;18:57-65.

Bonkovsky HL, Barnard GF: The hepatic porphyrias. In Brandt L (ed): Clinical Practice of Gastroenterology. Philadelphia: Current Medicine, 1998, pp 947-960.

Bonkovsky HL, Healey JF, Lourie AN, Gerron GG: Intravenous heme-albumin in acute intermittent porphyria: Evidence for repletion of hepatic hemoproteins and regulatory heme pools. Am J Gastroenterol 1991;86: 1050-1056.

Bonkovsky HL, Poh-Fitzpatrick M, Pimstone N, et al: Porphyria cutanea tarda, hepatitis C, and HFE gene mutations in North America. Hepatology 1998;27:1661-1669.

Chemmanur AT, Bonkovsky HL: Hepatic porphyrias: Diagnosis and management. Clin Liver Dis 2004;8:807-838.

McGuire BM, Bonkovsky HL, Carithers RL Jr, et al: Liver transplantation for erythropoietic protoporphyria liver disease. Liver Transpl 2005;11: 1590-1596.

# Therapeutic Use of Blood Components

Method of
*Peter A. Millward, MD, and*
*Mark E. Brecher, MD*

The transfusion of blood was the first successful transplantation of living tissue in humans. Today, transfusion is so commonplace that it is rarely thought of as a transplant. In 2001, for allogeneic transfusions within the United States alone, it is estimated that 13,898,000 units of whole blood or red blood cells, 2,614,000 units of whole blood–derived platelets, 1,264,000 units of apheresis platelets, and 3,926,000 units of plasma were administered. For red blood cell–containing products alone, this equates to 1 unit transfused every 2.3 seconds. A basic understanding of indications for blood component therapy is essential to optimally treat patients.

## Red Blood Cells

Red blood cells are collected via whole blood donation or automated erythrocytapheresis. Both collection techniques employ a sterile closed system for blood collection. The blood is collected into plastic blood bags containing a sufficient formulation of anticoagulant and preservative solution.

The components of the anticoagulant solution determine the maximum shelf life (ranging from 21 to 35 days) of collected blood and blood components. The solution can contain citrate (trisodium citrate and citric acid), dextrose, phosphate (monobasic sodium phosphate), and adenine. Citrate is for anticoagulation, dextrose and adenine are for metabolic energy, and phosphate is for buffering pH.

Shelf life of red cells may be extended to 42 days with the addition of an preservative-additive solution, such as Adsol (AS-1), Nutricel (AS-3), or Optisol (AS-5). This additive solution must be added within 72 hours from primary collection. Additive solution contains dextrose, adenine, and sodium chloride and contains either monobasic sodium phosphate or mannitol.

Even with anticoagulant and preservative-additive solutions, biochemical changes, called storage lesions, develop with stored red blood cells. These biochemical changes are decreased pH, adenosine triphosphate (ATP), and 2,3-diphosphoglycerate (DPG) and increased plasma potassium and plasma hemoglobin (Hb). Even in massively transfused patients, storage lesions do not routinely cause significant clinical consequences when transfused.

The standard collection volume for a whole blood donation is 450 mL ± 45 mL. Because whole blood is rarely indicated, centrifugation is used to separate a whole-blood donation into various components, which maximizes this limited resource. One red blood cell (RBC) unit, also known as *packed RBCs*, is made by removing a significant portion of plasma from a whole-blood donation. Using apheresis technique, one or two RBC units can be specifically collected with each donation. With either technique, an RBC unit volume is approximately 300 mL. Based on the preservative-additive solution used, an RBC unit averages a hematocrit of 60% to 80%.

After initial processing of whole blood, an RBC unit is composed of RBCs, white blood cells (WBCs), platelets, and plasma. An erythrocytapheresis RBC unit is composed of RBCs with decreased platelets and plasma and are *leukocyte reduced* ($<5 \times 10^6$ leukocytes per component) due to intraprocedural leukocyte filtration.

RBC units can be further modified for specific needs of the patient to leukoreduced RBCs, washed RBCs, irradiated RBCs, and frozen deglycerolized RBCs.

## LEUKOREDUCED RED BLOOD CELLS

In the United States, a leukoreduced RBC unit must have less than 5 million leukocytes per unit. This decrease in leukocytes is achieved using a leukocyte filter that extracts leukocytes based on their relative larger size and propensity to adhere to certain fiber types. Current leukoreduction filters remove between 3 and 5 log of leukocytes in an RBC unit. Leukocyte filtration can occur during or immediately after collection (prestorage leukocyte reduction) or at the time of transfusion (poststorage leukocyte reduction).

Common indications for leukoreduced RBCs are multiple febrile, nonhemolytic transfusion reactions (FNHTR), prevention of HLA alloimmunization, and reduction of cytomegalovirus (CMV) transmission.

An FNHTR is defined by a greater than 1°C (2°F) temperature rise occurring up to 2 hours after transfusion and unexplained by the patient's underlying medical condition; it may be accompanied by chills, rigors, nausea, vomiting, malaise, and headache. Two mechanisms of FNHTR with RBC transfusion have been proposed: recipient anti-HLA or antigranulocyte antibodies react with donor leukocytes and induce cytokine release, or donor leukocytes form an antigen-antibody complex resulting in recipient monocytes to release cytokines. Both mechanisms depend on the presence of donor leukocytes, and therefore leukoreduction effectively decreases the incidence of FNHTR associated with red blood cell transfusions.

The formation of HLA antibodies (also known as HLA alloimmunization) can lead to platelet transfusion refractoriness, which is especially problematic for patients requiring substantial platelet transfusion support (e.g., hematology-oncology patients). All potential candidates for bone marrow (BMT) or solid organ transplantation should receive leukoreduced RBCs to minimize the formation of HLA antibodies.

Transfusion-transmitted CMV (TT-CMV) infections in high-risk populations, such as CMV-negative neonates, AIDS patients, and BMT candidates or patients, are associated with considerable mortality and morbidity. CMV is latent in leukocytes, specifically in the monocyte-macrophage lineage. Based on Bowden and colleagues' findings in 1995, leukoreduced RBCs offer a CMV-safe blood product that is an equivalent alternative to providing blood from a CMV-seronegative donor. These findings and other confirming studies led to numerous institutions using leukoreduced RBCs as their sole method for providing CMV-safe blood products and abandoning a CMV-seronegative inventory. Recently, Nicholas and colleagues questioned the equivalence of leukoreduced blood products versus CMV-seronegative blood products and called for further investigation.

## WASHED RED BLOOD CELLS

The objective of washing RBCs is to effectively remove 99% of antibodies, plasma proteins, and electrolytes contained within the RBC component. The washing process involves repetitive steps of infusion of normal (0.9%) saline and centrifugation, with final resuspension of washed RBCs in normal saline. Because this process is an open system and the anticoagulant-preservative solution is removed, washed red cells must be transfused within 24 hours. This process can be automated or achieved with a manual technique, leading to up to 20% red cell loss. Approximately 20% to 90% of the platelets and 90% of the leukocytes are removed during this procedure. This decrease in leukocytes is not effective enough to render the component leukoreduced ($<5 \times 10^6$ leukocytes per unit).

Common indications for washed RBCs are recurrent severe allergic reactions not controlled with antihistamines and immunoglobulin A (IgA) deficiency. Washed RBCs also reduce the potassium load of the product. IgA-deficient patients can develop anti-IgA antibodies that react to donor IgA in plasma and lead to anaphylaxis. Potassium accumulates in the plasma during storage of the RBC unit or following irradiation.

## IRRADIATED RED BLOOD CELLS

The goal of irradiation is to prevent proliferation of transfused immunocompetent T lymphocytes. This goal is accomplished by using cesium-137 or cobalt-60 as a radiation source, which administers a dose of 2500 cGy (25 Gy or 2500 rad) to the central portion of the RBC unit and a minimum of 1500 cGy to all other areas of the component. Due to decreased survival and viability of the RBCs and increased potassium leakage, irradiated RBCs expire on their original assigned outdate or 28 days after irradiation, whichever occurs first.

The only indication for the irradiated RBCs is to prevent transfusion-associated graft-versus-host disease (TA-GVHD). TA-GVHD is a rare, fatal complication (mortality >90%) caused by the engraftment and proliferation of donor T lymphocytes in the transfused recipient. Irradiated RBCs are indicated for patients receiving hematopoietic stem cell or bone marrow transplantation, patients with congenital immunodeficiency syndromes, intrauterine transfusions, neonates, HLA-matched platelet transfusions, patients with Hodgkin's disease, and patients with chronic lymphocytic leukemia treated with purine analogues (e.g., fludarabine [Fludara]).

Patients receiving transfusions from first-degree relatives require irradiation because of the increased risk of TA-GVHD due to HLA similarity of donor and recipient.

## FROZEN RED BLOOD CELLS

The purpose of frozen RBCs is to store units with rare blood types and autologous units for extended periods of time (routinely up to 10 years, but storage may be extended for certain circumstances). Before freezing the RBCs, glycerol, a cryoprotective agent, is added to the system, which allows freezing of the red cells without damage. Based on the concentration of glycerol used (~20% or ~40%), the storage temperatures vary. Most commonly in the United States, 40% glycerol is used, and therefore the frozen RBCs are stored at −65°C.

Frozen RBCs must be deglycerolized before transfusion. Washing the product in saline solutions of progressively decreasing osmolarity achieves glycerol removal. During the process, 99.9% of the plasma along with the vast majority of WBCs and platelets are removed. Depending on the technique used to deglycerolize the RBCs, once deglycerolized, these units have a 24-hour (open system) or 14-day (closed system) shelf life.

Frozen RBCs are indicated for heavily alloimmunized patients (e.g., multiple clinically significant RBC antigens) who require rare phenotypic RBCs for compatible transfusions.

Due to the multiple washing steps in the deglycerolized procedure, these units can be considered equivalent to a washed RBC unit.

## INDICATIONS FOR RED BLOOD CELL TRANSFUSION

The purpose of RBC transfusions is to provide oxygen-carrying capacity and to maintain tissue oxygenation when the intravascular volume and cardiac function are adequate for perfusion. In a 70-kg recipient, 1 unit of transfused RBCs should increase the hemoglobin by 1 g/dL and the hematocrit by 3%. To obtain the same expected response in a pediatric patient, the RBC transfusion dose should be 15 mL/kg. RBC transfusions should only be used when time or underlying pathophysiology precludes other management (e.g., iron, erythropoietin, folic acid [folate]). Criteria for administering RBC transfusions include:

- Hb <8 g/dL in an otherwise healthy patient
- Hb <11 g/dL in cases of increased risk of ischemia (e.g., pulmonary disease, coronary artery disease, cerebral vascular disease)
- Acute blood loss >15% of total blood volume (e.g., 750 mL in 70-kg man) or with evidence of inadequate oxygen delivery (e.g., electrocardiographic signs of cardiac ischemia, tachycardia, cyanosis)

- Symptomatic anemia in a normovolemic patient (e.g., tachycardia, mental status changes, electrocardiographic signs of cardiac ischemia, angina, shortness of breath, lightheadedness or dizziness with mild exertion)
- Regular predetermined therapeutic program for severe hypoplastic or aplastic anemia or for bone marrow suppression for hemoglobinopathies

The post-transfusion hemoglobin should not exceed 11.5 g/dL (12.5 g/dL in cases of increased risk of organ or tissue ischemia). Attempts to increase wound healing or merely to take advantage of available predonated autologous blood without a valid medical indication are not acceptable uses for RBC transfusions.

# Platelets

Platelets are often a limited resource because of their relatively short shelf life and the inability to stockpile this product through freezing techniques. Temperature, pH, and gas exchange are critical issues for platelet viability and function, and they all determine the storage shelf life. Platelets remain viable for up to 7 days after collection, but the current 5-day shelf life has been instituted because of increased rates of clinically significant bacterial contamination on days 6 and 7. At a temperature lower than 20°C, platelets can be damaged and become nonfunctional. Platelets must be maintained at room temperature (20°-24°C) with gentle agitation in gas-permeable bags. Gas-permeable bags are required for platelet storage to ensure proper oxygenation and facilitate removal of carbon dioxide buildup. Constant gentle agitation is required to facilitate this gas exchange.

At present, two methods to obtain platelets are employed in the United States. First, platelets may be prepared from whole blood donations via centrifugation separation. These platelets are commonly referred to as *platelet concentrates, random donor platelets*, or *whole blood–derived platelets*. One platelet concentrate can be manufactured from a single whole blood donation. This platelet concentrate should have $5.5 \times 10^{10}$ platelets per unit in 40 to 70 mL of plasma. One platelet concentrate should increase the platelet count by 7 to $10 \times 10^9/L$ in a 70-kg recipient. Therefore, general platelet-concentrate dosing consists of a pool of 4 to 6 platelet concentrates, also known as a *four-pack* or *six-pack*, respectively. Second, platelets may be prepared using apheresis technology. These products are called *apheresis platelets, single-donor platelets*, or *platelet pheresis*.

Due to current apheresis technology, most apheresis platelets are leukoreduced at the time of collection. Apheresis platelets should have $3.0 \times 10^{11}$ platelets per unit in 300 to 500 mL of plasma. One apheresis unit should increase the platelet count by 40 to $60 \times 10^9/L$ in a 70-kg recipient.

One apheresis platelet product has an equivalent dose of a six-pack of platelet concentrates. In the United States, the use of apheresis platelets has been increasing annually. In 2004, it was estimated that 77% of all therapeutic doses of platelets transfused were apheresis platelets.

Once a platelet component is collected, it may be further modified in the same manner as RBCs: leukoreduced, washed, or irradiated.

## LEUKOREDUCED PLATELETS

As with leukoreduced RBCs, common indications for leukoreduced platelets are multiple FNHTRs, prevention of human leukocyte antigen (HLA) alloimmunization, and reduction of CMV transmission. The proposed mechanisms by which leukoreduction prevents these conditions are discussed in the leukoreduced RBCs section. These mechanisms are the same with one exception. FNHTRs with RBCs are associated with an active release of cytokines induced by leukocyte-antibody interaction. The mechanism of FNHTR with platelets differs and is due to passively transfused cytokines. At room temperature, residual donor leukocytes release cytokines that accumulate during storage. Therefore, prestorage leukocyte reduction is the only effective way to prevent FNHTR with platelet transfusions because the leukocytes are removed before releasing their cytokines.

It has been determined that cytokine accumulation does not occur if a blood product is refrigerated, which explains why both prestorage and poststorage RBC leukoreductions prevent FNHTRs.

## WASHED PLATELETS

As with RBCs, the goal of washing platelets is to effectively remove 99% of antibodies, plasma proteins, and electrolytes contained within the component. The process involves washing platelets with normal saline or saline buffered with ACD-A (acid citrate dextrose) or citrate. This process can be achieved via automated or manual technique, leading to approximately 33% platelet loss. Once a platelet component is washed, it must be transfused within 4 hours because it is now an open system with removed anticoagulant-preservative solution at room temperature. This differs from washed RBCs that have a 24-hour shelf life after washing.

The two most common indications for washed platelets are recurrent severe allergic or anaphylactic reactions and IgA-deficiency in patients with IgA antibodies.

## IRRADIATED PLATELETS

As with RBCs, the objective of irradiating platelets is to prevent immunocompetent T lymphocytes from proliferating and leading to TA-GVHD in the transfused recipient. The current dose (2500 cGy to the central portion of the unit and 1500 cGy to other portions of the unit) inactivates the T lymphocytes within the product and achieves this goal without significantly altering platelet function during their maximum shelf life.

Indications for irradiated platelets are the same as for irradiated RBCs: hematopoietic stem cell or BMT patients, congenital immunodeficiency syndrome patients, intrauterine transfusions, neonates, HLA-matched platelet transfusions, Hodgkin's disease patients, and chronic lymphocytic leukemia patients treated with purine analogues (e.g., fludarabine).

Patients receiving transfusions from first-degree relatives require irradiation because of the increased risk of TA-GVHD due to HLA similarity of donor and recipient.

## INDICATIONS FOR PLATELET TRANSFUSION

Criteria for instituting a platelet transfusion include:

- Platelet count $<10 \times 10^9/L$ for prophylaxis in a stable, nonfebrile patient
- Platelet count $<20 \times 10^9/L$ for prophylaxis with fever or instability
- Platelet count $<50 \times 10^9/L$ in a patient with documented hemorrhage or rapidly decreasing platelet count or planned invasive or surgical procedure
- Diffuse microvascular bleeding in a patient with disseminated intravascular coagulation or following a massive blood loss (>1 blood volume) with a platelet count not yet available
- Bleeding in a patient with platelet dysfunction

It is unacceptable to empirically transfuse platelets for a massively transfused patient not exhibiting a clinical coagulopathy or for extrinsic platelet dysfunction (e.g., renal failure, hyperproteinemia, or von Willebrand's disease). Platelet transfusion is contraindicated in thrombotic thrombocytopenic purpura (TTP), hemolytic-uremic syndrome (HUS), or idiopathic thrombocytopenic purpura (ITP) unless the patient is experiencing life-threatening bleeding or coagulopathy.

## PLATELET REFRACTORINESS

Both nonimmune and immune causes lead to poor platelet increment following transfusion. To accurately assess response to platelet transfusion, a post-transfusion platelet count should be obtained 10 to 60 minutes after the transfusion is complete. If the patient does not respond appropriately, platelet refractoriness must be considered.

Platelet refractoriness is defined as failure to achieve an appropriate post-transfusion response on more than one occasion. A post-transfusion corrected count increment (CCI) can be calculated to more accurately assess refractoriness. The CCI is calculated as follows:

$$CCI = \frac{(\text{post-transfusion count} - \text{pretransfusion count}) \times \text{body surface area}}{\text{platelets tranfused} \times 10^{11}}$$

where platelet counts are in microliters and body surface area is in square meters. A CCI less than 5000 (using a 10- to 60-minute post-transfusion platelet count) on two separate occasions is consistent with platelet refractoriness.

The most common causes for poor platelet increments are nonimmune causes, including splenomegaly, bleeding, fever, sepsis, and disseminated intravascular coagulation (DIC). If refractoriness is determined to be nonimmune in etiology, management often consists of increasing the dose or frequency (or both) of transfused platelets. HLA alloimmunization is the primary cause of immune-mediated platelet refractoriness. Other immune-mediated causes for poor platelet increment are anti–platelet-specific antibodies, drug-induced antibodies, and immune or idiopathic thrombocytopenia purpura (ITP). If HLA alloimmunization is the cause, three common treatment options can be employed:

- Give platelets that are platelet crossmatch compatible with recipient plasma
- Provide HLA antigen-negative platelets (for the identified HLA antibodies)
- Give HLA matched (class I: HLA A and HLA B) platelets

## Plasma

### FROZEN PLASMA

Platelet-poor plasma is obtained by centrifugation and separation of a whole-blood donation or direct collection with apheresis technique. If this plasma is frozen at −18°C within 8 hours of original collection, the product contains adequate levels of all labile (factor V and factor VIII) and nonlabile coagulation factors and is called *fresh frozen plasma* (FFP). If this plasma is frozen at −18°C for more than 8 hours but within 24 hours from original collection, the product contains adequate levels of all nonlabile and decreased levels of labile coagulation factors and is called *plasma frozen within 24 hours*. Both types of plasma units have a volume of approximately 220 mL, and both can be stored for 12 months at −18°C.

These products are indicated for the correction of multiple or specific coagulation factor deficiencies or for the empiric treatment of TTP or HUS. The usual starting dose is 5 to 15 mL/kg (2 to 4 units in a 70-kg recipient).

### INDICATIONS FOR PLASMA TRANSFUSION

Criteria for implementing a plasma infusion include:

- Treatment or prophylaxis of multiple or specific coagulation factor deficiencies (PT and/or PTT >1.5 times the mean normal value)
- Congenital coagulation factor deficiencies (antithrombin III; factors II, V, VII, IX, X, and XI; plasminogen; antiplasmin)
- Acquired coagulation factor deficiencies related to warfarin (Coumadin) therapy, vitamin K deficiency, liver disease, massive transfusion (>1 blood volume in 24 h), and disseminated intravascular coagulation
- Patients with a suspected coagulation deficiency (PT/PTT pending) who are bleeding, or at risk of bleeding, from an invasive procedure

Unacceptable criteria are empiric use during massive transfusion in which the patient does not exhibit clinical coagulopathy, nutritional supplementation, or volume replacement. There is little evidence to support prophylactic plasma infusion in patients with mild prolongation of the prothrombin time (<1.5 times the mean normal value).

### CRYOPRECIPITATE

Cryoprecipitate is a cold insoluble fraction of FFP that precipitates when FFP is thawed at 4°C. A unit of cryoprecipitate contains approximately 10 mL, which can be stored for 12 months at −18°C. Each unit contains approximately 80 to 100 U of factor VIII and 250 mg of fibrinogen, along with factor XIII, von Willebrand's factor, and fibronectin.

The usual starting dose is one unit per 7 to 10 kg, and therefore multiple units must be pooled for a therapeutic dose. Once pooled, cryoprecipitate must be transfused within 4 hours. In a 70-kg man, 14 units would be expected to raise the fibrinogen 100 mg/dL. Cryoprecipitate (2-4 units) may also be applied topically, with an equal volume of bovine thrombin, taking advantage of its adhesive, hemostatic, and sealant properties.

Appropriate indications for cryoprecipitate include:

- A bleeding patient with congenital or acquired hypofibrinogenemia, dysfibrinogenemia, or afibrinogenmia (fibrinogen <150 mg/dL)
- Treatment or prevention of bleeding associated with certain known or suspected clotting factor deficiencies (factor VIII, von Willebrand's, factor XIII, or factor I)
- Treatment of surface oozing and maintenance of tissues in tight apposition to each other or sealing of leaking spaces (fibrin glue)

Rather than cryoprecipitate, factor concentrates are mostly used to treat hemophilia A and type I von Willebrand's disease. Desmopressin acetate (DDAVP) may be used as an alternative treatment for these patients and for patients with certain platelet dysfunctional disorders.

## Granulocytes

Using apheresis techniques, granulocytes contain approximately 20 to $30 \times 10^9$ granulocytes per collection, 200 to 400 mL of donor plasma, 10 to 30 mL of donor RBCs, and some donor platelets. Like platelets, this product is stored at room temperature but without agitation. Granulocytes have a 24-hour shelf life, but they should be transfused as soon as possible because of rapid decline of function and viability of the leukocytes.

There are several special considerations for this product. Granulocytes must be ABO compatible with the recipient because of significant RBC contamination. This is an Rh-specific product for female patients of childbearing age. CMV-negative donors must be used for CMV-negative recipients because the product cannot be leukoreduced. It is an HLA-matched product for alloimmunized patients. Granulocytes should be irradiated to prevent TA-GVHD.

Granulocyte infusions are indicated for adult neutropenic patients (granulocyte count <500/μL) who have fever for 24 to 48 hours due to bacterial or fungal sepsis that is unresponsive to appropriate antibiotic or antifungal treatment. In infants, granulocyte therapy should be considered in bacterial septicemic patients with a granulocyte count less than 3000/μL. Daily granulocyte transfusion should be continued until infection resolves or the granulocyte count remains greater than 500/μL for 48 hours.

### REFERENCES

Bowden RA, Slichter SJ, Sayers M, et al: A comparison of filtered leukocyte-reduced and cytomegalovirus (CMV) seronegative blood products for the prevention of transfusion-associated CMV infection after marrow transplant. Blood 1995;86:3598-3603.

Brecher ME (ed): Technical Manual, 15th ed. Bethesda, MD: American Association of Blood Banks, 2005.

British Committee for Standards in Haematology, Blood Transfusion Task Force: Guidelines for the use of platelet transfusions. Br J Haematol 2003;122:10-23.

Development Task Force of the College of American Pathologists: Practice parameters for the use of fresh frozen plasma, cryoprecipitate and platelets. JAMA 1994;271:777.

Goodnough LT, Brecher ME, Kanter MH, AuBuchon JP: Transfusion medicine. First of two parts—blood transfusion. N Engl J Med 1999;340:438-447.

Goodnough LT, Brecher ME, Kanter MH, AuBuchon JP: Transfusion medicine. Second of two parts—blood conservation. N Engl J Med 1999;340:525-533.

Menitove JE, McElligott MC, Aster RH: Febrile transfusion reaction: What blood component should be given next? Vox Sang 1978;5:101-106.

Nichols WG, Price TH, Corey L, Boeckh M: Transfusion-transmitted cytomegalovirus infection after receipt of leukoreduced blood products. Blood 2003;101:4195-4200.

Strauss R: Neutrophil (granulocyte) transfusions in the new millennium. Transfusion 1998;38:710-712.

The Trial to Reduce Alloimmunization to Platelets Study Group: Leukocyte reduction and ultraviolet B irradiation of platelets to prevent alloimmunization and refractoriness to platelet transfusions. N Engl J Med 1997;337:1861-1869.

Wandt H, Frank M, Ehninger G, et al: Safety and cost effectiveness of a $10 \times 10^9$/L trigger for prophylactic platelet transfusions compared with the traditional $20 \times 10^9$/L trigger: A prospective comparative trial in 105 patients with acute myeloid leukemia. Blood 1998;91:3601-3606.

# Adverse Effects of Blood Transfusion

Method of
*Chelsea A. Sheppard, MD,*
*and Christopher D. Hillyer, MD*

Although blood transfusion is a beneficial and not uncommonly life-saving therapy, it carries inherent risks or adverse effects. These adverse effects are commonly classified either as *transfusion reactions* (Table 1), which occur immediately or shortly following the transfusion event, or as *transfusion-related complications*, which can occur up to many years following transfusion. These latter complications are commonly divided into *infectious* (Table 2) and *noninfectious* (Table 3) categories. Indeed, 0.5% to 3% of all transfusions result in an adverse event; however, the majority of these are minor reactions with no long-term sequelae.

Herein we describe a large number of adverse events so that the physician can determine if his or her patient has had an adverse effect from a transfusion, assign a diagnosis, and consider if an intervention is needed. For a complete discussion of all of the adverse events related to transfusion, as well as more detailed references, the reader is referred to *Blood Banking and Transfusion Medicine* (see References).

## Transfusion Reactions

When a patient experiences an immediate reaction to a transfusion, the most important question to answer is whether hemolysis is occurring. Thus, transfusion medicine specialists usually classify transfusion reactions as either *hemolytic* or *nonhemolytic*.

Hemolytic reactions are caused by recipient antibodies targeted against donor red cell antigens and the resultant response, which attempts to destroy or clear those foreign cells. These antibodies may be naturally occurring (e.g., a recipient with group A blood has antibodies to B-group red cells) or they can occur after exposure to foreign blood from past transfusion, pregnancy, or transplantation. This process is termed *alloimmunization*.

Nonhemolytic reactions occur via a variety of mechanisms usually involving recipient response to donor leukocytes or their byproducts, including inflammatory cytokines.

### HEMOLYTIC TRANSFUSION REACTIONS

#### Acute Hemolytic Transfusion Reaction

##### Clinical Description

Arguably, the most devastating transfusion reaction is an acute hemolytic reaction caused by the mistransfusion of ABO incompatible blood. *Mistransfusion* is defined as failure to give the right blood product to the right person at the right time and for the right reason. The severity of the reaction is dose dependent; however, infusion of even a small amount of incompatible blood can cause intravascular hemolysis, resulting in a range of signs and symptoms including pain at the infusion site, back, or flank; fever; chills or rigors; hemoglobinuria or hemoglobinemia; chest pain; circulatory collapse or shock; vasoconstriction with resultant end organ ischemia; and activation of the coagulation system, resulting in microangiopathic thrombosis.

The annual incidence of ABO-mismatched transfusion according to observed errors in the New York State database and the FDA database of transfusion-associated fatalities has been reported at between 1 in 12,000 and 1 in 19,000 transfused units. The fatality rate ranges from 1 in 800,000 to 1 in 2,000,000 transfused units. However, these numbers do not take into account the large number of near misses, which have been reported to be as common as 1 in 3000 to 4000 units transfused per year.

##### Diagnosis

The first signs of an acute hemolytic transfusion reaction (AHTR) are usually fever and pain. However, a decrease in blood pressure, tachycardia, and hemoglobinuria may be the only signs in an anesthetized patient.

Laboratory studies can help confirm a diagnosis of intravascular hemolysis. Red cell abnormalities including schistocytes on peripheral smear, increased indirect bilirubin and jaundice, and decreased haptoglobin are signs of increased red cell destruction. Elevated lactate dehydrogenase (LDH) and reticulocyte count indicate increased red cell turnover. It is important to maintain adequate renal function; therefore, it is necessary to monitor blood urea nitrogen (BUN), creatinine, and urine output.

Occasionally, patients with severe intravascular hemolysis can develop disseminated intravascular coagulation (DIC). Serial measurements including prothrombin time (PT), activated partial thromboplastin time (aPTT), D-dimer, fibrinogen, antithrombin, and platelet count can be used to evaluate for the presence of an ongoing consumptive process. After the transfusion is stopped, the unit itself and a post-transfusion sample should be immediately sent to the blood bank for further analysis. The blood bank will perform a clerical check for correct patient identification, look for the presence of visible hemolysis in the post-transfusion plasma, and compare direct Coombs' test results from the pre- and post-transfusion samples for evidence of in vivo antibody adsorption on the red cells.

##### Treatment and Prevention

If an acute hemolytic transfusion reaction is suspected, the transfusion should be stopped immediately. Intravenous fluids should be given to maintain an adequate blood pressure and to aid the kidneys in expelling circulating hemoglobin. Some experts recommend furosemide (Lasix) or mannitol (Osmitrol) to induce diuresis; however, this has not been studied in a randomized fashion. A patient who develops signs of shock should be treated accordingly. Vasopressors and mechanical ventilation may be required in cases of circulatory collapse and respiratory failure.

Most cases of mistransfusion are the result of human error. More than one half of these errors occur from misidentification of the patient at the bedside. Approximately one third of these errors occur in the blood bank as a result of either a clerical misprint or the misidentification of a specimen. Despite strict transfusion procedures and protocols, the use of hospital identification wrist bands, and multiple redundant check systems, mistransfusions still occur at an alarming rate. Therefore, systems including the use of bar codes, barrier technology (Blood-Loc), and radiofrequency identification (RFID) systems are under investigation.

#### Delayed Hemolytic Transfusion Reaction

##### Clinical Description

Red blood cell antibodies acquired through exposure to foreign antigen can cause a delayed hemolytic transfusion reaction (DHTR). These patients can develop signs and symptoms of intra- or extravascular hemolysis approximately 2 weeks after transfusion due to the

## TABLE 1 Transfusion Reactions

| Type | Frequency | Common Signs and Symptoms | Laboratory Diagnosis | Therapy |
|------|-----------|---------------------------|----------------------|---------|
| **Hemolytic** | | | | |
| AHTR | Rare | Pain at the infusion site, back, or flanks<br>Fever, chills, rigors<br>Hemoglobinuria or hemoglobinemia<br>Chest pain<br>Circulatory collapse and shock<br>Vasoconstriction resultant end organ ischemia<br>Activation of the coagulation system, resulting in microangiopathic thrombosis | Schistocytes on peripheral smear<br>Indirect bilirubinemia and jaundice<br>Decreased haptoglobin<br>Elevated LDH and reticulocyte count | Stop the transfusion<br>Maintain IV fluids (1 L NS over 1-2 h) to maintain urine flow >1mL/kg/h<br>Diuresis with furosemide or mannitol<br>Support cardiovascular and respiratory function with vasopressors<br>Intubate if necessary |
| Bacterial contamination | Rare | Fever, chills, rigors<br>Hypotension<br>Intravascular hemolysis | Positive blood cultures<br>Similar organism found in product and recipient | Antibiotics<br>Treat shock if appropriate |
| DHTR | Rare | Intra- or extravascular hemolysis | Same as AHTR, with spherocytes on peripheral smear if hemolysis is predominantly extravascular | Monitor renal function; forced diuresis or dialysis may be required to support renal function if extravascular hemolysis is severe<br>Transfuse with antigen-negative blood if anemia is symptomatic |
| **Nonhemolytic** | | | | |
| Allergic | Common | Itching, urticaria, generalized flushing or rash, angioedema<br>Wheezing, cough | No abnormal laboratory tests | Diphenhydramine 25-50 mg PO or IV<br>May premedicate for future transfusions if recurrent |
| Anaphylactic | Rare | Shortness of breath, vasomotor instability, bronchospasm | No abnormal laboratory tests | Epinephrine 1:1000 0.3 mL IM<br>Secure airway |
| FNHTR | Common | Fever, chills, rigors<br>Absence of hemolysis | No abnormal laboratory tests<br>R/o hemolysis | Acetaminophen 650 mg PO if not contraindicated<br>May premedicate for future transfusions if recurrent |
| TA-GVHD | Rare | Fever, mucositis, dermatitis, hepatitis, enterocolitis, pancytopenia | Low blood counts, low reticulocyte count, elevated liver enzymes, elevated inflammatory markers | Treatment is usually ineffective<br>High dose steroids, OKT3, cyclosporine A, and antithymocyte globulin may be helpful<br>Irradiate blood for high-risk patients to prevent TA-GVHD |
| TRALI | Rare | Noncardiogenic pulmonary edema with dyspnea, acute hypoxemia, hypotension, occasionally fever<br>Bilateral infiltrates on CXR<br>Signs of congestive heart failure (increased jugular venous pressure and/or a third heart sound) absent<br>Normal pulmonary capillary wedge pressure. | HLA/HNA antibody or antigen cognates between recipient and donor can support diagnosis | Respiratory support<br>High-dose steroids<br>Avoid diuretics in hypotensive patients |

*Abbreviations:* AHTR = acute hemolytic transfusion reaction; CXR = chest x-ray; DHTR = delayed hemolytic transfusion reaction; FNHTR = febrile nonhemolytic transfusion reaction; HLA = human leukocyte antigen; HNA = human neutrophil antigen; LDH = lactate dehydrogenase; NS = normal saline; OKT3 = muromonab CD3; r/o = rule out; TA-GVHD = transfusion-associated graft-versus-host disease; TRALI = transfusion-related acute lung injury.

formation of a de novo alloantibody. Alternatively, symptoms appearing 3 to 4 days after transfusion support previous exposure to the antigen and a robust amnestic response on reexposure to antigen-positive blood.

### Diagnosis

Patients with a history of a recent transfusion and signs and symptoms of hemolysis should be evaluated for a possible DHTR. Laboratory studies for intra- and extravascular hemolysis are described earlier.

However, in delayed hemolytic transfusion reactions, extravascular hemolysis is more common; thus, spherocytes rather than schistocytes may be the predominant abnormal morphologic red cell type on peripheral smear.

Alloantibodies are usually detected during the antibody screen carried in blood banks as a "type and screen." If the screen is positive, the specificity of the antibody is determined. For patients with multiple antibodies, this can significantly lengthen the time it takes for the pretransfusion work-up. If the patient has not recently received a transfusion, antibody titers may be too low to be detected at the time

**TABLE 2 Infectious Complications of Transfusion**

| Type | Risk of Transfusion Transmitted Infection from Screened Units |
|---|---|
| **Viruses** | |
| CMV | Leukoreduction has made transfusion transmission rare (~1% remaining risk) |
| EBV | Rare |
| HAV | Rare |
| HBV | ~1:200,000 |
| HCV* | ~1:2 million |
| HHV | |
| HIV* | ~1:2 million to 4 million |
| HTLV | <1:3 million |
| WNV* | Rare |
| **Parasitic Infections** | |
| Babesia spp. | Rare |
| Plasmodium spp. | 1:4 million |
| Trypanosoma cruzi | Rare |
| **Prions** | |
| CJD, BSE | Rare |

*Risk after nucleic acid testing was implemented.

Abbreviations: BSE = bovine spongiform encephalopathy; CJD = Creutzfeldt-Jakob disease; CMV = cytomegalovirus; EBV = Epstein-Barr virus; HAV = hepatitis A virus; HBV = hepatitis B virus; HCV = hepatitis C virus; HHV = human herpesvirus; HTLV = human T-cell lymphotropic virus; WNV = West Nile virus.

of screening. However, if the patient is rechallenged with the antigen, an amnestic antibody response can cause destruction of the transfused cells. Intravascular and extravascular hemolysis can be severe and life threatening.

### Treatment and Prevention

Treatment of intra- and extravascular hemolysis is discussed under acute hemolytic transfusion reactions.

The inherent immunogenicity of the antigen, antigen concentration per erythrocyte, transfused cell dosage, and individual patient factors determine the rate of alloimmunization. Patients with sickle cell disease are at greater risk, and immunosuppressed patients may be at less risk. Highly immunogenic antigens such as Kell, Duffy, and Kidd are generally associated with more severe reactions. These antigens are also commonly implicated in hemolytic disease of the newborn because these antibodies can cross the placenta.

Antibody screening is required before transfusion in any patient who has received a transfusion or been pregnant in the last 30 days; thus, it is important to take a thorough transfusion history. Additionally, hospitalized patients receiving transfusions should be rescreened every 3 days because antibodies that are initially too low in titer to be detected might be identified later.

### Bacterial Contamination of Blood Products

#### Clinical Description

Bacterial contamination at the time of collection usually occurs through one of three mechanisms: asymptomatic donor bacteremia, introduction of skin flora to the unit, or manufacturing processes and manipulation of the unit. Initially, the amount of bacteria present is low; however, during storage the bacteria can proliferate to levels of $10^6$/mL or greater. This amount of bacteria transfused over a short time can result in a spectrum of clinical signs and symptoms including bacteremia, fever, chills, hypotension, nausea, vomiting, diarrhea, and oliguria, which can progress to sepsis and ultimately multisystem organ failure and death.

#### Pathophysiology

The most common bacteria identified in 70% to 80% of contaminated platelets are gram-positive skin flora introduced to the unit during collection; however, 40% to 80% of fatalities are due to endotoxin-producing gram-negative organisms. The severity of the reaction depends on the species of bacteria present, the inoculum, the rate of bacterial propagation, and patient factors including underlying disease, including leukocyte count, the status of the immune system, and use of concomitant antibiotics in the recipient.

#### Diagnosis

Blood cultures should be obtained both from the recipient (cultures should not be drawn from the same line used for the transfusion) and from the blood product in question. Confirmation requires that the same organism be cultured from both sites. False negatives can occur in patients taking antibiotics. False-positive cultures are common due to improper collection of the sample.

Additional laboratory tests can help evaluate for end-organ damage including tests of renal and liver function. Endotoxin-induced DIC is a common complication; therefore, serial measurements of the PT, APTT, D-dimer, fibrinogen, antithrombin, and platelet count may be useful in evaluating for the presence of an ongoing consumptive process.

#### Treatment and Prevention

Sepsis caused by transfusion of a bacterially contaminated unit can be fatal. Antibiotics should be given empirically as soon as symptoms appear. The patient can develop septic shock and should be treated accordingly.

Bacterial contamination is the third most common cause of transfusion-associated fatality reported to the FDA. Improved phlebotomy practices (strict arm preparation standards and diversion of the first 10 mL containing the skin plug), donor questioning for recent illnesses or travel to endemic areas, better materials used in product collection and storage, and implementation of platelet culturing have helped reduce the incidence of fatality as a result of bacterial contamination of blood products. Red cell units and plasma, which are stored refrigerated or frozen, are less often implicated in bacteria-related transfusion reactions. However, platelets, which are stored at room temperature in a large volume of plasma and in a bag that allows oxygen diffusion, are most commonly implicated.

Prior to 2004 and the implementation of American Association of Blood Banks (AABB) Standard 5.1.5.1, which charged blood banks with the responsibility of limiting and detecting bacterial contamination, the infectious risk of receiving a contaminated unit was estimated at 1 in 2000 to 1 in 3000 platelet units per year. Risk of death was 1 in 60,000 to 1 in 85,000 units transfused. Since implementation of the AABB standard, many of the nation's blood collection systems have begun culturing platelet units using automated systems, which detect $CO_2$ generation or $O_2$ consumption by bacteria for 24 hours prior to hospital distribution. Despite a marked reduction in the number of cases of transfusion-transmitted bacterial infections, rare fatal consequences have been reported.

Pathogen reduction technology aims at eradicating pathogens without harming the blood cells or generating toxic chemical agents. Several methods under investigation include a number of photodynamic processes that use psoralen-based chemicals, phenothiazine dyes (methylene blue [urolene blue]), or riboflavin (vitamin $B_2$) followed by ultraviolet light to inactivate bacteria and viruses by degrading nucleic acids. Other methods include solvent-detergent treatment and treatment with FRALEs (frangible anchor linker effectors). The appeal of pathogen reduction is that it is proactive and may be able to prevent new and emerging infections. Nonetheless, serious regulatory hurdles remain before these methods are approved for use in the United States.

**TABLE 3 Noninfectious Complications of Transfusion**

| Type | Frequency | Common Signs and Symptoms | Laboratory Diagnosis | Therapy |
|------|-----------|---------------------------|----------------------|---------|
| **Massive Transfusion Reactions** | | | | |
| Coagulopathy | Common in massive transfusion | Hemorrhage usually described as mucosal bleeding or oozing from suture lines | Prolonged PT, PTT Fibrinogen <100 mg/dL Rapidly decreasing platelet count and antithrombin level | Replace clotting factors with FFP In massive transfusion, RBC/FFP ratio should be 1:1-2 If fibrinogen <100 mg/dL transfuse 1 cryoprecipitate pool and recheck fibrinogen Transfuse platelets if count <50,000/μL |
| Citrate toxicity | Rare | Muscle cramping, shortness of breath secondary to bronchospasm, tetanic contractions, distal extremity numbness, tingling sensations, seizures | Decreased ionized calcium Monitor for hypomagnesemia | Calcium gluconate 2 g/250 mL NS Replete magnesium if indicated |
| Hyperkalemia | Rare | Generalized fatigue, weakness, paresthesias, paralysis, palpitations ECG changes: peaked T waves, shortened QT interval, ST segment depression | Elevated serum potassium Monitor for evidence of metabolic alkalosis Monitor for ECG changes | Replete with oral or IV potassium preparations if indicated |
| Iron overload | Rare | Iron deposition with end-organ damage in heart, liver, lungs, pituitary, thyroid, adrenals, exocrine pancreas | Elevated iron, ferritin (~10-20 g in patients with SCD are typical), and transferrin saturation | Phlebotomy or iron chelators if indicated |
| **Transfusion-Related Immunomodulation** | | | | |
| Platelet refractoriness (HLA) | Occasional in highly sensitized patients | FNHTR No response or inadequate response to platelet transfusion | Corrected count increment (see text), flow cytomtery, or ELISA screen for anti-HLA antibodies or platelet-specific antibodies | Consider appropriateness of HLA-matched or crossmatched platelets, contact transfusion medicine specialist |
| Post-transfusion purpura (HPA) | Rare | Severe thrombocytopenia 5-10 d after transfusion Bruising and petechiae Can result in severe hemorrhage | Flow cytomtery or ELISA screen for anti–platelet-specific antibodies Must r/o other causes of thrombocytopenia, including HIT and DIC | Self-limited IVIg Efficacy of antigen-negative platelets is controversial |
| **Other** | | | | |
| Volume overload | Common | Cardiogenic pulmonary edema with dyspnea, acute hypoxemia, hypertension Bilateral infiltrates on CXR Signs of congestive heart failure, increased jugular venous pressure, and/or absent third heart sound Elevated pulmonary capillary wedge pressure. | BNP can help distinguish volume overload from TRALI | Diuresis If transfusion is required, slow the rate |

*Abbreviations:* BNP = brain natriuretic peptide; CXR = chest x-ray; DIC = disseminated intravascular coagulation; ECG = electorcardiogram; ELISA = enzyme-linked immunosorbent assay; FNHTR = febrile nonhemolytic transfusion reaction; FFP = fresh frozen plasma; HIT = heparin-induced thrombocytopenia; HLA = human leukocyte antigen; HPA = human platelet antigen; IVIg = intravenous immunoglobulin; NS = normal saline; PT = prothrombin time; PTT = partial thromboplastin time; RBC = red blood cells; r/o = rule out; SCD = sickle cell disease; TRALI = transfusion-related acute lung injury.

## NONHEMOLYTIC TRANSFUSION REACTIONS

### Transfusion-Related Acute Lung Injury

#### Clinical Description

Transfusion-related acute lung injury (TRALI) has now become the most common cause of transfusion-associated death *reported* to the FDA, with an incidence that ranges widely from 1 case per 432 whole blood units transfused to 1 case per 557,000 red blood cell units transfused. Because it was not until 2004 that standardized criteria were widely accepted for defining and diagnosing TRALI, these previous figures might not reflect current incidence, and thus most authorities agree that the true incidence of TRALI is unknown. Nonetheless, it is becoming increasingly clear that platelets and FFP are the most commonly implicated blood products due to the large plasma volume of these products and the likelihood of alloantibodies being passively transferred (see later).

TRALI is a clinical syndrome characterized by noncardiogenic pulmonary edema with dyspnea, acute hypoxemia, hypotension, and occasionally fever. Bilateral infiltrates in a white-out pattern are commonly described on chest x-ray. Signs of congestive heart failure (increased jugular venous pressure and/or a third heart sound) are usually absent. The pulmonary capillary wedge pressure is typically normal. Symptoms usually appear 1 to 6 hours after transfusion and resolve in 96 hours.

#### Diagnosis

Until recently, accepted criteria allowing standardized diagnosis of TRALI were lacking, thus complicating the ability to make accurate diagnoses and hindering attempts at determining true incidence rates. In April 2004, a consensus conference convened in Toronto, Ontario, and attempted to further adapt and improve previously proposed definitions of TRALI. The consensus panel recommended criteria for *TRALI* and *possible TRALI*.

*TRALI* was defined as a new occurrence of acute-onset acute lung injury (ALI) with hypoxemia and bilateral infiltrates on chest x-ray, but no evidence of left atrial hypertension. The ALI cannot have been preexisting, but it must emerge during or within 6 hours of the end the transfusion and have no temporal relation to an alternative ALI risk factor. *Possible TRALI* included cases in which there was a temporal association with an alternative ALI risk factor.

These proposed definitions continue to suffer the limitations inherent in the American-European Consensus Conference definition of ALI (including the subjectivity of certain findings, including chest x-ray and volume status and the influence of PEEP on measurements of the $PaO_2/FiO_2$ ratio). Brain natriuretic protein (BNP) might help to distinguish cardiogenic from noncardiogenic pulmonary edema.

#### Pathophysiology

The events and mechanisms that cause TRALI are incompletely understood. They have been described as antibody-mediated and non–antibody-mediated. Antibody-mediated mechanisms implicate alloantibodies directed toward human leukocyte antigen (HLA) or human neutrophil antigen (HNA) on leukocytes or lung tissue, which lead to granulocyte activation and pulmonary injury. In approximately 90% of TRALI cases where antibodies are identified, the antibodies are of donor origin and react with recipient leukocyte epitopes. Multiparous women and recipients of previous transfusions are more likely to be alloimmunized. Many investigators have suggested that a number of hits may be required to cause a full-blown case of TRALI.

The two-hit model of TRALI may be antibody- or non–antibody-mediated. In this model, the first hit is usually described as an underlying illness that primes recipient pulmonary endothelial cells and leukocytes. *Priming* refers to the development of a heightened stage of (cellular) activation. The second hit is delivered by the transfusion, which contains factors (either antibodies or biological response modifiers [BRMs], such as cytokines or certain lipids) capable of inducing complete activation of the presequestered primed neutrophils in the recipient's lungs. This results in the release of cytotoxic compounds in the pulmonary vasculature, leading to endothelial damage, capillary leak, and noncardiogenic pulmonary edema, namely, TRALI.

#### Treatment and Prevention

Treatment is primarily respiratory support until the injury resolves (usually in 24-96 hours); however, high-dose intravenous steroids may be beneficial. Approximately 20% of patients with TRALI require 1 week or more to fully recover. Death is estimated to occur in 6% to 23% of cases; survivors have no permanent sequelae.

Without a simple laboratory test to prospectively eliminate high-risk blood products, recommended strategies to prevent TRALI are currently based on deferral of donors implicated in TRALI cases. The United Kingdom has preemptively deferred all women from donating plasma. In the United States, the use of male-only plasma is under consideration, as is the testing of all plasma and platelet units for anti-HLA or anti-HNA antibodies.

### Febrile Nonhemolytic Transfusion Reaction

#### Clinical Description

Febrile nonhemolytic transfusion reaction (FNHTR) is defined as an increase in the recipient's temperature of at least 1°C or 2°F during transfusion in the absence of another cause of fever. Some patients develop chills or rigors. FNHTRs are very common, occurring in 0.1% to 0.5% of all leukodepleted transfusions occurring per year in the United States. The incidence is significantly higher in nonleukoreduced blood products. Additionally, transfusion reactions such as FNHTRs and allergic reactions are believed to be underreported in patients with frequent febrile episodes due to underlying diseases such as cancer and sepsis. Other causes for transfusion-associated fever, including hemolysis or bacterial contamination, must be excluded before a diagnosis of FNHTR can be made.

#### Pathophysiology

FNHTRS are attributed to white blood cells (WBCs) in blood products that synthesize and release proinflammatory cytokines during storage. Preformed recipient antibodies that target donor WBCs can also lead to cytokine release after transfusion.

#### Treatment and Prevention

Antipyretics are often used to treat these reactions. Patients prone to FNHTRs can require premedication with antipyretics. Many transfusion medicine services have implemented universal leukoreduction protocols to prevent FNHTRs.

### Allergic Reactions

#### Clinical Description

Allergic transfusion reactions are very common. Allergic reactions are variably severe and result in a spectrum of clinical signs and symptoms. Uncomplicated or simple reactions manifest as itching, urticaria, generalized flushing or rash, or local swelling, also known as *angioedema*. However, recipients can also develop anaphylactoid reactions in which wheezing, cough, shortness of breath, vasomotor instability, and bronchospasm are typically observed. IgA-deficient patients with circulating anti-IgA antibodies can develop life-threatening anaphylaxis and cardiovascular collapse requiring emergent therapy. Most reactions are afebrile. The incidence of uncomplicated allergic reactions is 1% to 3%; however, anaphylactic reactions are very rare (0.002%-0.005% of all transfusions).

#### Pathophysiology

Simple allergic reactions occur when donor plasma proteins are targeted by preformed IgE antibodies on recipient mast cells, leading to histamine release. More severe reactions have been attributed to antibodies against IgA, C4 determinants, or other nonbiological elements (ethylene oxide used for sterilization of tubing sets). The presence of anti-IgA antibodies in IgA-deficient patients cannot predict the occurrence of allergic reactions.

### Treatment and Prevention

Most simple allergic reactions can be treated with antihistamines or anticholinergic medications (e.g., diphenhydramine). Patients with more severe reactions can require IV steroids or epinephrine. Patients with respiratory failure require supportive therapy. In patients with recurrent allergic reactions, prophylactic antihistamine therapy administered 30 minutes before transfusion may be helpful. In patients with simple allergic reactions involving only the skin, the transfusion may be restarted 15 to 30 minutes after the administration of antihistamines; however, transfusions should never be restarted in patients with more severe reactions.

## Transfusion-Associated Graft-Versus-Host Disease

### Clinical Description

Transfusion-associated graft-versus-host disease (TA-GVHD) is a rare but uniformly fatal complication of blood transfusions in severely immunosuppressed patients in which donor lymphocytes escape immune clearance in the recipient and engraft. Following clonal expansion, these cells cause immune destruction of host tissues including the skin, gastrointestinal (GI) tract, liver, and bone marrow. These patients develop fever, mucositis, dermatitis (starting as a blistering rash on the palms, soles, and face, which then can generalize), hepatitis, enterocolitis with large volumes of secretory diarrhea, and pancytopenia, 1 to 2 weeks after transfusion. Infections are the most common cause of death, which generally occurs within 3 to 4 weeks of the transfusion.

The degree of immunosuppression and the dose of T lymphocytes are factors in determining an individual patient's risk of developing TA-GVHD. Patients with hematologic malignancy, patients with congenital immunodeficiency, premature infants weighing less than 1200 g, bone marrow transplant recipients, and patients receiving fludarabine (Fludara) (see Box 1 for a complete list) are susceptible. Patients with HIV, healthy newborns, and patients who are neutropenic due to sepsis are generally considered to be at low risk. There is a minimally increased risk associated with solid tumor transplants (especially heart and liver) or solid tumor malignancies. There have been reports of TA-GVHD associated with neuroblastomas, rhabdomyosarcomas, bladder tumors, and small cell lung cancer. It is possible that more immunosuppressive and myeloablative chemotherapy protocols are responsible for these cases.

The degree of HLA similarity between the donor and recipient is also an important determinant of a patient's risk of developing TA-GVHD. These patients may be immunocompetent heterozygotes of an HLA haplotype for which the donor is homozygous. Therefore, patients receiving transfusions from first-degree relatives or populations in which there is a great deal of HLA homology (including some Asian populations) might also require irradiated blood products.

### Treatment and Prevention

The mortality rate of TA-GVHD approximates 100%. Currently, there is no effective treatment; however, high-dose steroids, muromonab-CD3 (OKT-3), cyclosporine A (Neoral, Sandimmune) and antithymocyte globulin (Atgam, Thymoglobin) have been used with few successes.

Prevention of TA-GVHD via irradiation of blood products in at-risk populations is absolutely required. A minimum dose of 25 Gy delivered to the midline of the container (with a minimum of 15 Gy to the distal parts of the bag) cross-links the DNA of T cells, thereby preventing replication and potential engraftment and expansion.

---

### BOX 1 Risk Factors for the Development of TA-GVHD

**Significantly Increased Risk**
- Bone marrow transplantation
  - Allogeneic and autologous
  - HLA-matched platelet transfusions
  - Hodgkin's disease
  - Intrauterine transfusions
  - Patients treated with purine analogue drugs
  - Transfusions from blood relatives
- Congenital immunodeficiency syndromes

**Minimally Increased Risk**
- Acute leukemia
- Exchange transfusions
- Non-Hodgkin's lymphoma
- Preterm infants (<1200 g)
- Solid organ transplant recipients
- Solid tumors treated with intensive chemotherapy or radiotherapy

**Perceived but No Reported Increased Risk**
- Healthy newborns
- Patients with AIDS

---

*Abbreviations:* HLA = human leukocyte antigen; TA-GVHD = transfusion-associated graft-versus-host disease. Modified from Schroeder ML: Transfusion-associated graft-versus-host disease. Br J Haematol 2002;117:275-287.

---

## Transfusion-Related Complications

### INFECTIOUS COMPLICATIONS

#### Viral Transmission

##### Clinical Description

A large number of viruses, including HIV-1 and HIV-2; hepatitis A, B, and C (HAV, HBV, HCV); human T-lymphotrophic viruses (HTLV) 1 and 2; cytomegalovirus (CMV); and West Nile virus can be transmitted via transfusion. These viruses, with the exception of CMV, are acquired from cellular and noncellular blood and blood products including plasma-derived clotting factors, intravenous immunoglobulin (IVIg), and anti-D immunoglobulin. CMV remains latent in monocytes and is essentially therefore transmitted only in cellular products. Other viruses that are potentially transmitted via transfusion are HAV, transfusion-transmitted virus (TTV), Epstein-Barr virus (EBV), human herpesvirus 8 (HHV 8), and parvovirus B19.

##### Hepatitis

Hepatitis viruses (especially B and C) are readily transfusion transmissible. About 70% of patients infected with HCV develop chronic infections resulting in chronic active hepatitis, cirrhosis, or hepatocellular carcinoma (HCC). A smaller but significant fraction of patients infected with HBV develop chronic disease proceeding to cirrhosis. Hepatitis viruses A and E are rarely transmitted through blood transfusion. Hepatitis G, TTV, and SEN viruses emerged as candidates for non–A to E type post-transfusion hepatitis, but no clear association has been demonstrated.

##### Human Immunodeficiency Virus

The annual risk of transfusion-transmitted HIV with the addition of nucleic acid testing is reported to be less than 1 in 2,000,000 units in the United States (1:4,000,000 in Canada). However, despite the implementation of this very sensitive testing, cases of transfusion-transmitted HIV have been reported. The average survival after diagnosis for adults and children with transfusion-transmitted HIV is approximately 5.6 months and 13.7 months, respectively.

### West Nile Virus and Other Flaviviruses

In 2002, there was an emergence of West Nile virus in the United States, and several cases of transfusion-transmitted disease were identified. Infected elderly and immunocompromised patients developed a severe flulike illness rarely resulting in death. Other flaviviruses including dengue are transfusion transmissible and could threaten the blood supply if an epidemic were to emerge in the United States.

### Parvovirus B19

Parvovirus B19 has been transmitted through plasma-derived products including clotting factors. Immunocompromised patients can develop erythema infectiosum, arthralgias, and aplastic crises with chronic anemia after infection with parvovirus B19.

### Cytomegalovirus

Transfusion transmission of CMV to immunocompetent patients usually causes an asymptomatic infection or rarely an infectious mononucleosis. However, in seronegative immunocompromised patients, transfusion transmission can lead to lethal CMV disease. Seronegative immunocompromised patients include premature low-birth-weight infants (<1500 g) born to seronegative mothers and seronegative recipients of autologous or seronegative allogeneic bone marrow or peripheral blood stem cell transplantation.

Following primary infection, CMV remains latent and can reactivate, with subsequent production of progeny virus in macrophages. Transfusion-transmitted CMV can be mitigated through the transfusion of leukoreduced or seronegative blood. The rate of infectivity with either leukoreduced or seronegative blood is approximately the same (1%). Box 2 lists the indications for which many hospital blood banks dispense CMV seronegative blood or leukoreduced blood.

### Parasitic and Emerging Infections

#### Clinical Description

*Trypanosoma cruzi*, *Plasmodium* spp., and *Babesia* spp. can be transmitted by blood transfusion. *T. cruzi* can cause fatal cardiac and GI disease (Chagas' disease). Malaria, the disease caused by *Plasmodium*, can cause fatal intravascular hemolysis and DIC. Human babesiosis generally causes a mild flulike syndrome, but it can be lethal in the elderly and in immunocompromised patients. At the time of this writing, no agent is tested for in the United States, but it appears likely that tests for *T. cruzi* will commence by early 2007.

---

**BOX 2  Indications for CMV Seronegative or Leukoreduced Blood**

- Intrauterine transfusions
- Premature low-birth-weight infants (<1500 g) born to SN mothers
- SN recipients of autologous bone marrow or peripheral blood stem cell transplantation
- SN recipients of seronegative allogeneic bone marrow or peripheral blood stem cell transplantation
- SN recipients of solid organ transplants from SN donors

*Abbreviations:* CMV = cytomegalovirus; SN = seronegative.

---

### TRYPANOSOMA CRUZI

There have been fewer than 10 cases of transfusion-transmitted *T. cruzi* reported in the United States and Canada since 1990. Many of these patients were immunocompromised as a result of hematologic malignancy, AIDS, or bone marrow transplantation. Some of these recipients received platelets only, others received multiple blood products. A majority of the patients developed Chagas' disease. At least one case was fatal. Others did respond to nitrofurtimox[2] (Nifurtimox), interferon-γ[1] (Actimmune), and benznidazole,[1] followed by itraconazole[1] (Sporanox) and fluconazole[1] (Diflucan). In endemic areas, transfusion transmission of Chagas' disease is more common. No screening is currently done for these parasites in blood donors. In the United States, 1 in 25,000 donors are estimated to be seropositive, and as many as one half of these donors are actively parasitemic.

### PLASMODIUM SPECIES AND BABESIA SPECIES

Annually, approximately two cases of transfusion-transmitted *Plasmodium* infections are reported in the United States. Donors who have traveled to malaria-endemic countries are deferred from donation for a period of 1 year. Red cell exchange may be helpful in patients with high parasitemia loads and intravascular hemolysis; however, this is controversial.

There have been more than 50 cases of transfusion-transmitted *Babesia* infections in the world. Currently, there are no licensed tests for screening the blood supply. Human babesiosis is treated with antibiotics.

### PRIONS

The agent of variant Creutzfeldt-Jakob disease (vCJD), a novel human prion disease that results in a rare and fatal human neurodegenerative condition, can be transmitted via blood transfusion. Although this agent has no nucleic acids, the transmission results in the conversion of normal prion protein to the abnormal β-sheet amyloid responsible for the clinical disease.

Since 2003, it has been established that prion infection could be transmitted via blood transfusion in animals. Additionally, in 2003 the first case of probable transfusion-transmitted vCJD was reported. The recipient received a transfusion in 1996 from a donor now known to have been incubating vCJD. The recipient died in 1996 from complications of vCJD.

In 2006, the National CJD Surveillance Unit (NCJDSU) and the UK Blood Services (UKBS) released the Transfusion Medicine Epidemiology Review (TMER), a look-back investigation that confirmed three separate incidents of probable transfusion transmission of vCJD infection. Two of these patients died less than 7 years after infection. At this time, sporadic CJD and familial CJD have still not been shown conclusively to be transfusion transmitted.

To date there is no known treatment for transmissible spongiform encephalopathy. The AABB Standard 5.4.1A Requirements for Allogeneic Donor Qualification states that donors with a risk of vCJD as defined by the FDA Guidance for Industry (January 2002) should be indefinitely deferred from giving blood. Currently those donors include anyone who has traveled to or resided in the United Kingdom for a cumulative period of 3 or more months between 1980 and the end of 1996, those with a history of 5 or more years of cumulative residence or travel in France since 1980, and current and former U.S. military personnel, civilian military personnel, and their dependents who were stationed at European bases for 6 months or more between 1980 and 1996.

## NONINFECTIOUS COMPLICATIONS

### Transfusion-Related Immunomodulation

#### Clinical Description

Transfusion-related immunomodulation (TRIM) describes the immunosuppression that occurs after transfusion. TRIM was first recognized in the 1960s and 1970s in renal allograft recipients who had

---

[1]Not FDA approved for this indication.
[2]Not available in the United States.

less rejection and improved graft survival after receiving blood transfusions from their donors. Since then, TRIM has been implicated in the development of postoperative infections, the recurrence of resected malignancies (especially colorectal cancer), spontaneous abortions, and inflammatory bowel disease. TRIM has been suggested to cause reactivation of latent viruses such as CMV.

## Pathophysiology

Most authorities agree that TRIM exists, although the mechanisms and magnitude are unclear. However, it is believed that donor WBCs, BRMs, and soluble HLA antigens that have accumulated during storage exert an effect on cell-mediated immunity. TRIM appears to be dose dependent, and thus conservative transfusion triggers might decrease the incidence.

## Treatment and Prevention

There is no known treatment for TRIM. Leukoreduction and washing might reduce the incidence of TRIM.

## Alloimmunization

Alloimmunization is the development of an antibody to a foreign donor antigen after exposure through blood transfusion, pregnancy, or transplantation. These antibodies, if directed against RBC antigens, can cause DHTRs and AHTRs. Anti-HLA antibodies can cause FNHTRs and platelet refractoriness. These patients may be difficult to match for bone marrow or solid organ transplants. Thrombocytopenia can result in patients who develop platelet-specific antigens either in utero (neonatal alloimmune thrombocytopenia) or after transfusion (post-transfusion purpura).

## Refractoriness to Platelet Transfusions

Patients who become refractory to platelet transfusion can do so by several different mechanisms including immune-mediated and non–immune-mediated mechanisms. Immune-mediated refractoriness occurs in highly sensitized patients with anti-HLA or anti–platelet-specific antibodies to donor-specific antigens. Alternatively, patients with sepsis, DIC, fever, splenomegaly, or portal hypertension and persons taking certain drugs can also appear refractory to platelet transfusion due to the sequestration or accelerated clearance of the transfused platelets.

## Diagnosis

The expected corrected count index (CCI) can help distinguish between immune-mediated and non–immune-mediated platelet refractoriness. The CCI is calculated 15 minutes to 1 hour after transfusion using the following equation:

$$CCI = \frac{(\text{Post-transfusion platelet count} - \text{Pretransfusion platelet count}) \times \text{Body surface area}}{\text{Number of platelets tranfused} \times 10^{11}}$$

A CCI less than 5000 after two sequential platelet transfusions suggests immune-mediated platelet refractoriness. These patients should be screened for anti-HLA and anti–platelet-specific antibodies if other causes of non–immune-mediated refractoriness have been excluded.

## Pathophysiology

HLA antibodies are not routinely tested for in most clinical laboratories and blood banks. Additionally, because platelets are not crossmatched prior to transfusion, the only clue to a significant HLA antibody may be FNHTR or the lack of response to a platelet transfusion. Patients who develop multiple HLA antibodies can become refractory to platelet transfusion. Rarely, patients develop platelet-specific antibodies, causing platelet refractoriness.

## Treatment and Prevention

Treatment depends on the etiology of platelet refractoriness. Patients with non–immune-mediated refractoriness (including those with splenic sequestration, sepsis, or DIC) require treatment of the underlying disease. If an immune-mediated mechanism is more likely, HLA-matched or crossmatched platelets can be supplied on request. Leukoreduction can potentially reduce HLA-alloimmunization.

## Post-transfusion Purpura

Post-transfusion purpura (PTP) is a rare disorder caused by alloantibodies to platelet-specific glycoprotein, most commonly human platelet antigen (HPA)-1a, resulting in destruction of both transfused platelets and the patient's own platelets, leading to severe thrombocytopenia and risk of life-threatening hemorrhage. Thrombocytopenia can last 1 to 2 weeks after transfusion. IVIg is the first-line treatment. The use of washed antigen-negative platelets is controversial.

## Volume Overload

### Clinical Description

The development of cardiogenic pulmonary edema and other signs of congestive heart failure after transfusion suggest volume overload. The annual reported incidence in the United States of volume overload secondary to transfusion is greatly variable, anywhere from 1 in 100 to 1 in 15,000 units, and largely depends on patient population. The elderly and newborn, as well as patients with cardiac disease, renal insufficiency, and anemia with expanded plasma volumes, are at greater risk for developing volume overload, especially with massive transfusions.

### Diagnosis

Diagnosis depends on establishing a cardiac etiology for the resulting dyspnea and pulmonary edema. Elevated central venous pressures or pulmonary wedge pressures, chest x-ray consistent with pulmonary edema, and response to diuretics are used to confirm the suspected diagnosis. It is important to rule out TRALI and other etiologies of acute respiratory distress syndrome (ARDS). BNP may be a useful adjuvant marker in establishing a diagnosis of volume overload secondary to transfusion.

### Treatment and Prevention

Some patients respond simply to slowing the rate of the transfusion. Others require diuretics and supportive therapy.

## Massive Transfusion Coagulopathy

### Clinical Description

Massive transfusion is usually defined as transfusion of 10 or more units of RBCs in less than 24 hours. Massive transfusion usually occurs in the setting of trauma and can be complicated by coagulopathy secondary to dilution of clotting factors and platelets, hypothermia, and hypofibrinogenemia. Patients often receive crystalloid fluids and numerous uncrossmatched group O packed red cells in transit to the hospital or in the emergency department to correct hypovolemia before receiving plasma (which requires at least 30 minutes' thawing time) or platelets. This results in dilution of platelets, clotting proteins, and fibrinogen. Additionally, as the patient's blood pressure is normalized, bleeding becomes brisker resulting in further losses of platelets and clotting factors.

### Treatment and Prevention

Ideally, patients with massive bleeding are transfused with whole blood, thereby minimizing the complications of dilution. Additionally, current guidelines are based on whole-blood transfusion and wash-out equations, simple mathematical models that calculate exponential decay of blood components during bleeding, assuming that the blood volume of the patient is stable and the replacement rates are constant and equal. Blood volumes and bleeding rates are usually quite variable, and replacement tends to lag behind blood loss; therefore, these guidelines and equations tend to underestimate needs. Computer modeling has demonstrated that patients with penetrating traumas have generally lost 2500 mL (or one half the average blood volume) by the time they arrive in the emergency department, 3200 mL (or two thirds the average blood volume) by the start of surgery, and 11,000 mL (or more than two blood volumes) at the end of surgery. PT will be prolonged (>1.5 times normal) after a loss of less than one blood volume. Fibrinogen is next, dropping below 0.8 g/L, in a little over one blood volume. Platelets stay above $50,000 \times 10^9$/L until after losses of more than two blood volumes.

Various massive transfusion protocols have been reviewed extensively in the literature. Early plasma replacement at higher plasma–to–red cells ratios (~1:1) is gaining popularity in this clinical setting despite the fear that some patients may be overtransfused. However, there are few studies comparing conservative with liberal plasma and platelet transfusion with regard to outcome.

Hypothermia due to massive transfusion of refrigerated and recently thawed products contributes to the coagulopathy associated with massive transfusion. For this reason, many products are transfused through blood warmers. The use of cryoprecipitate for fibrinogen replacement is often necessary and more efficient than use of plasma.

## OTHER ADVERSE EVENTS

Less frequent adverse events of transfusion include hypocalcemia due to large infusions of citrate anticoagulant, hyperkalemia due to RBC leakage during storage, mechanical hemolysis, and iron overload. These events are rare and typically affect infants receiving large amounts of old blood or patients receiving chronic transfusions; thus they are outside of the scope of this article. However, it is important to be aware of their existence and to monitor patients accordingly for signs of their development.

## REFERENCES

Allain JP, Bianco C, Blajchman MA, et al: Protecting the blood supply from emerging pathogens: The role of pathogen inactivation. Transfus Med Rev 2005;19(2):110-126.

Blumberg N: Deleterious clinical effects of transfusion immunomodulation proven beyond a reasonable doubt. Transfusion 2005; 45(suppl):33S-39S.

Blumberg N, Heal JM, Gettings KEJ: WBC reduction of RBC transfusions is associated with decreased incidence of RBC alloimmunization. Transfusion 2003;43:945-952.

Dodd RY, Notari IV, Stramer SL: Current prevalence and incidence of infectious disease markers and estimated window-period risk in the American Red Cross blood donor population. Transfusion 2002;42(8):975-979.

Goldman M, Webert KE, Arnold DM, et al; TRALI Consensus Panel: Proceedings of a consensus conference: Towards an understanding of TRALI. Transfus Med Rev 2005;19(1):2-31.

Hillyer CD, Silberstein LE, Ness PM, et al (eds): Blood Banking and Transfusion Medicine, 2nd ed. Philadelphia: Churchill Livingstone, 2007.

Hirschberg A, Dugas M, Banez EI, et al: Minimizing dilutional coagulopathy in exsanguinating hemorrhage: A computer simulation. J Trauma 2003;54: 454-463.

Kleinman S, Caulfield T, Chan P, et al: Toward an understanding of transfusion-related acute lung injury: Statement of a consensus panel. Transfusion 2004;44(12):1774-1789.

Lee D: Perception of blood transfusion risk. Transfus Med Rev 2006; 20(2): 141-148.

Linden JV, Wagner K, Voytovich AE, Sheehan J: Transfusion errors in New York State: An analysis of 10 years' experience. Transfusion 2000;40:1207-1213.

Luban NC: Transfusion safety: Where are we today? Ann N Y Acad Sci 2005; 1054:325-341.

Schroeder ML. Transfusion-associated graft-versus-host disease. Br J Haematol 2002;117:275-287.

Sheppard CA, Roback JD, Hillyer CD: Transfusion-transmitted cytomegalovirus infection: Consideration toward an optimal plan for its mitigation. Blood Ther Med 2005;5(1):6-14.

Zhou L, Giacherio D, Cooling L, Davenport RD: Use of B-natriuretic peptide as a diagnostic marker in the differential diagnosis of transfusion-associated circulatory overload. Transfusion 2005;45:1056-1063.

Zou S, Dodd RY, Stramer SL, Strong DM, for the Tissue Safety Group: Probability of Viremia with HBV, HCV, HIV and HTLV among tissue donors in the United States. N Engl J Med 2004;351(8):751-759.

# The Digestive System

## Cholelithiasis and Cholecystitis

Method of
*Grant R. Caddy, MD*

## Cholelithiasis

Gallstones affect 10% to 12% of people in Western populations, and the prevalence increases with age. The majority of patients with gallstones (approximately 80%) remain asymptomatic. The risk of complications, mainly that of acute cholecystitis, occurs in around 2% of patients with symptomatic gallstones.

Gallstones can be classified depending on their composition. The commonest stones are cholesterol or cholesterol-predominant stones (mixed stones), which make up around 80% to 85% of all gallstones. Mixed stones can be multiple, of varying sizes, and faceted. Most are radiolucent but 10% are radiopaque. Pure cholesterol stones are commonly solitary but may be multiple and are radiolucent. Pigment stones are less common in Western populations and are associated with hemolytic disorders such as hemolytic anemias, malaria and cirrhosis.

Risk factors for cholesterol-predominant stone formation are shown in Box 1. Female patients have a 2 to 8 times greater risk of developing gallstones than male patients. This increased risk appears

### BOX 1  Risk Factors for Developing Gallstones

- Age >50 years (relative risk, 2.5; *P* <.001)
- Bile salt loss (e.g., terminal ileal disease)
- Diabetes mellitus
- Female gender
- First-degree relative with symptomatic gallstone disease
- Gallbladder dysmotility and stasis
- Genetic factors
- High intake of carbohydrates and high glycemic load
- Hyperlipidemia
- Overweight and obesity
- Positive family history of previous cholecystectomy in a first-degree family member
- Pregnancy
- Starvation
- Total parenteral nutrition

to decline following menopause. High intake of carbohydrate, high glycemic load, and high glycemic index foods increases the risk of symptomatic gallstone disease by approximately 1.5 times. Other risk factors include a high body mass index (BMI), rapid weight loss (>1.5 kg/week), and history of dieting or gastric bypass surgery. In a 10-year follow-up study, patients who were overweight (defined as BMI >25) were approximately twice as likely to develop gallstones compared with controls. It has also been documented that following antiobesity surgery, 20% to 35% of patients develop gallstones in the postoperative period.

Complications of symptomatic gallstones are shown in Box 2.

## Acute Cholecystitis

Acute cholecystitis is suspected when patients present with pain localized to the right upper quadrant (RUQ), pain aggravated by palpation in the RUQ (with or without a positive Murphy's sign), and an inflammatory response (e.g., fever and elevation in white blood cell count, C-reactive protein, and/or erythrocyte sedimentation rate). The exact mechanism of acute cholecystitis is uncertain, but blockage of the cystic duct in addition to irritation to the gallbladder mucosa result in further recruitment of inflammatory mediators such as prostaglandins (PG) $I_2$ and $E_2$. Secondary infection develops in approximately 20% of patients, usually with *Escherichia coli*, *Klebsiella* species, or *Streptococcus faecalis*. Mild elevations in bilirubin, aspartate aminotransferase (AST), alkaline phosphatase (ALP), and γ-glutamyl transpeptidase (GGT) are not uncommon (in up to one third of patients), but high levels often indicate concomitant choledocholithiasis, cholangitis, or Mirizzi's syndrome (see later).

### DIAGNOSIS

First-line radiologic investigation should be a transabdominal ultrasound (TUS), which has a high specificity for cholecystitis (>98%). In addition

### BOX 2  Complications of Gallstones

- Acalculous cholecystitis
- Acute cholecystitis
- Biliary colic
- Cholecystoenteric fistulas
- Choledocholithiasis ± ascending cholangitis
- Chronic cholecystitis
- Gallstone ileus
- Gallstone pancreatitis
- Gangrenous gallbladder and gallbladder perforation
- Mirizzi's syndrome

## CURRENT DIAGNOSIS

- The majority of patients with gallstones (approximately 80%) remain asymptomatic. The risk of complications, mainly acute cholecystitis, occurs in around 2% of patients with symptomatic gallstones.
- Mild elevations in bilirubin, AST, ALP, and GGT occur in approximately one third of patients but high levels often indicate concomitant choledocholithiasis or cholangitis.
- TUS has a high specificity for cholecystitis (>98%). A HIDA scan has a sensitivity of >95% and a specificity of 90%.
- Approximately 10% to 18% of patients undergoing cholecystectomy have coexisting bile duct stones.
- In choledocholithiasis, TUS is particularly sensitive if there is biliary dilatation (sensitivity is 96%) but is less sensitive in detecting stones within the duct (sensitivity is 63%).
- EUS, MRCP, and ERCP are equivalent in accuracy rates for detecting choledocholithiasis, but because of the complication rate of ERCP, this procedure should be reserved for patients with a high probability of choledocholithiasis.

*Abbreviations:* ALP = alkaline phosphatase; AST = aspartate aminotransferase; ERCP = endoscopic retrograde cholangiopancreatography; EUS = endoscopic ultrasound; GGT = γ-glutamyl transpeptidase; HIDA = hepatobiliary iminodiacetic acid; MRCP = magnetic resonance cholangiopancreatography; TUS = transabdominal ultrasound.

## CURRENT THERAPY

- Patients with symptomatic gallstones should undergo laparoscopic cholecystectomy if there is no contraindication.
- For acute cholecystitis, first-line treatment is supportive care with intravenous hydration, analgesia (NSAIDs), and antibiotics. If there are no contraindications, patients should undergo laparoscopic cholecystectomy within 72 hours.
- Percutaneous cholecystostomy is an alternative option in patients with acalculous cholecystitis who are too unwell to undergo cholecystectomy.
- Treatment options for patients with choledocholithiasis include ERCP and stone removal followed by laparoscopic cholecystectomy or, in patients with an intact gallbladder, cholecystectomy and bile duct exploration. Overall, there are no differences in morbidity and mortality between the two procedures.
- There is a limited role for other techniques such as extracorporeal shockwave lithotripsy and endoscopic laser lithotripsy or oral dissolution therapy.

*Abbreviation:* ERCP = endoscopic retrograde cholangiopancreatography.

---

to identifying gallstones, gallbladder thickening (>4-5 mm), edema, adjacent pericolic fluid, and tenderness with the transducer strongly suggest cholecystitis. Hepatobiliary iminodiacetic acid (HIDA) scan should be reserved for second-line investigation if the diagnosis remains in doubt. If the cystic duct is patent, HIDA will be taken up by the gallbladder and will be evident on scanning the abdomen after 1 hour. A positive test fails to detect any localization of HIDA within the gallbladder due to obstruction of the cystic duct. The test has a sensitivity of greater than 95% but a specificity of 90%.

## TREATMENT

Patients should receive supportive care as first-line treatment with intravenous hydration and analgesia. There is evidence that non-steroidal anti-inflammatory drugs (NSAIDs) have additional benefits other than their analgesic properties, due to their antagonist effect on prostaglandins, which are central to the inflammation of cholecystitis. NSAIDs reduce intraluminal pressure in the gallbladder, which is increased in acute cholecystitis. In addition, NSAIDs have been shown to reduce the rate of progression of biliary colic to acute cholecystitis. Due to the risk of secondary infection, antibiotics such as cephalosporin (Zinacef) and metronidazole (Flagyl) are generally recommended, but in uncomplicated cholecystitis, the routine use of antibiotics does not appear to reduce the risk of gallbladder empyema.

Laparoscopic cholecystectomy remains the most common surgical treatment for acute cholecystitis and is considered the treatment of choice for most patients. The advantages of laparoscopic cholecystectomy over open cholecystectomy are well documented and include reduced mortality, reduced postoperative pain, better cosmetic result, and a reduction in hospital stay. Studies investigating the optimal timing of laparoscopic cholecystectomy following acute cholecystitis suggest that early cholecystectomy (within 72 hours) compared with delayed cholecystectomy results in a reduction in hospital stay and readmission rate but no overall differences in operation time, conversion rate, or complication rates. Patient symptom scores (diarrhea, indigestion, and abdominal pain) at 4 weeks are significantly better in patients undergoing early cholecystectomy versus supportive treatment followed by delayed cholecystectomy.

There is evidence supporting mini-laparotomy cholecystectomy (usually defined as open cholecystectomy through an incision of 4 to 7 cm) with similar overall results to laparoscopic cholecystectomy. In one prospective study, laparoscopic cholecystectomy took a longer time to perform but produced a slightly shorter postoperative hospital stay and a smoother postoperative course than mini-laparotomy. The choice of which operation to perform is often determined by the experience of individual surgical centers.

## COMPLICATIONS

### Emphysematous Cholecystitis

Acute emphysematous cholecystitis is characterized by the presence of gas within the wall or lumen of the gallbladder caused by the gas-forming organisms (e.g., *Clostridium welchii* or *E.coli*). Symptoms can be identical to those of acute cholecystitis. In contrast to acute cholecystitis, emphysematous cholecystitis occurs more commonly in elderly and diabetic patients. Its importance lies in the increased rates of early gangrene and perforation of the gallbladder. Treatment is with empiric antibiotic therapy and early cholecystectomy.

### Gangrenous Cholecystitis

Gangrenous cholecystitis occurs in 2% to 20% of patients admitted with acute cholecystitis. The risk factors for gangrenous cholecystitis is increased in male patients older than 50 years; in patients with diabetes, history of cardiovascular disease, or white blood cell count greater than 15,000/mm³; and in those who delay seeking medical treatment. The risk of gallbladder perforation and mortality is increased with gangrenous cholecystitis. Treatment is with empiric antibiotic therapy and early cholecystectomy.

### Gallbladder Perforation

Gallbladder perforation can occur following gangrenous cholecystitis. It is estimated to occur in 3% to 10% of patients with acute cholecystitis. Like gangrenous cholecystitis, patients with gallbladder perforations have similar characteristics including older age and cardiovascular disease. In addition, perforations were associated with more postoperative complications that required more ICU admissions and longer hospital stays. Perforations may be localized, resulting in a pericholecystic abscess, or, less commonly, free perforations may occur into the peritoneum. Diagnosis is often difficult preoperatively.

### Acalculous Cholecystitis

Acalculous cholecystitis occurs in 5% to 10% of cases of cholecystitis. It is often associated with critically ill patients, severe trauma, burns, and cardiovascular surgery but is also associated with patients who have diabetes, cardiovascular disease, or AIDS and in patients on total parenteral nutrition or opiates. Without treatment, the mortality rate is 30% to 50%.

Characteristic features on TUS are thickened gallbladder wall, absence of gallstones, gallbladder distension, Murphy's sign induced by probe, and emphysematous cholecystitis with or without perforation. Treatment is initially with supportive therapy with antibiotics and urgent referral for laparoscopic cholecystectomy. In patients with high operative risk, percutaneous cholecystostomy (insertion of a drain into the gallbladder) under radiologic guidance is an alternative treatment.

Other complications of cholelithiasis include gallstone ileus, cholecystoenteric fistulas, and Mirizzi's syndrome (obstruction of the bile duct secondary to extrinsic compression from an impacted stone in the cystic duct)

### Acute Cholecystitis in Pregnancy

Overall acute cholecystitis in pregnancy is relatively uncommon. The optimal treatment remains controversial. Conservative management of a pregnant patient results in resolution of symptoms in approximately 90% of patients. However, up to 60% of patients have recurrent symptoms (readmission with acute cholecystitis, biliary colic, and premature delivery). Due to concerns of fetal loss, a conservative approach is often adopted. However, studies have supported the role of laparoscopic cholecystectomy as a safe procedure in pregnant patients with acute cholecystitis, resulting in decreased hospital stay, reduced rate of labor induction, and reduced preterm deliveries.

## Chronic Cholecystitis

Chronic cholecystitis refers to recurrent episodes of gallbladder inflammation usually due to stones. These episodes may be asymptomatic but they can also result in recurrent episodes of pain. However, there does not appear to be any correlation of symptoms and degree of fibrosis and thickening of the gallbladder wall. Patients with symptomatic gallstones with recurrent biliary colic should be referred for laparoscopic cholecystectomy.

## Biliary Sludge

Biliary sludge is usually diagnosed on ultrasonography. Its appearance on ultrasonography is of layered echoes in the dependent portion of the gallbladder, with no associated acoustic shadows. It is often made up of cholesterol crystals and calcium salts.

Precipitating factors include total parenteral nutrition, rapid weight loss, pregnancy, prolonged fasting, bone marrow and solid organ transplants, and drugs such as octreotide (Sandostatin) and ceftriaxone (Rocephin). In one study, 50% of patients presenting with symptomatic biliary sludge had complete resolution of gallbladder sludge on repeat imaging. In the remaining group, in 50% the sludge remained but patients were asymptomatic and in 50% further symptoms developed.

The management of biliary sludge should be managed similar to gallbladder stones. Asymptomatic sludge should be managed conservatively. Symptomatic patients should be considered for laparoscopic cholecystectomy.

# Choledocholithiasis

### PRESENTATION

Approximately 10% to 18% of patients undergoing cholecystectomy have coexisting bile duct stones. The symptoms of choledocholithiasis are varied and include biliary colic, jaundice, cholangitis, and pancreatitis. Conversely, a portion of patients with choledocholithiasis are asymptomatic, with a prevalence estimated to be up to 12%. In patients who present with symptoms of retained bile duct stones, the risk of subsequent symptoms is up to 50%, and the risk of complications is up to 25% if the stones are left untreated.

Patients with choledocholithiasis often present with biliary colic—pain that is often located in the RUQ and lasting between 30 minutes and several hours. There is often associated nausea and vomiting. If there is partial or complete obstruction of the common bile duct, then patients develop jaundice with associated pale stools and dark urine. Infection often occurs, resulting in a cholangitis. Approximately three fourths of patients with cholangitis have Charcot's triad of jaundice, fever, and pain. However, in 10% of patients pain may be the only feature of cholangitis. Due to bacterial translocation from the bile duct to the bloodstream, 20% of patients with cholangitis have a bacteremia, usually with gram-negative organisms.

Smaller bile duct stones (up to 8 mm) are more likely to pass spontaneously through the ampulla into the duodenum. However, it is the passage of smaller stones through the ampulla that is more likely to result in gallstone pancreatitis compared with larger stones. For example, one study found that patients who presented with gallstone pancreatitis had a mean stone diameter of 4 mm compared with patients presenting with obstructive jaundice, who had a mean stone diameter of 9 mm.

### DIFFERENTIAL DIAGNOSIS

The differential of choledocholithiasis will depend on the clinical presentation. Differentials are shown in Box 3.

### DIAGNOSIS

Patients presenting with symptomatic choledocholithiasis often have elevations in serum GGT and ALP (increased in 94% and 91% of cases, respectively). Bilirubin levels may be increased depending on if obstruction of the bile duct has occurred.

TUS is the commonest method of imaging the gallbladder and biliary tree in choledocholithiasis. TUS is particularly sensitive if there is biliary dilation (sensitivity up to 96%). It is less sensitive in detecting stones within the duct (sensitivity up to 63%) but has high specificity (specificity 95%). Therefore, a negative TUS does not rule out suspected choledocholithiasis.

Other radiologic investigations include computed tomography (CT), endoscopic ultrasound (EUS), magnetic resonance cholangiopancreatography (MRCP), and endoscopic retrograde cholangiopancreatography (ERCP). A National Institutes of Health (NIH) consensus statement found that EUS, MRCP, and ERCP were equivalent in accuracy rates. However, due to the risks of ERCP (pancreatitis, bleeding, perforation, infection), ERCP is recommended in patients with a high probability of choledocholithiasis. In patients with an intermediate probability, other imaging modalities, such as MRCP or EUS, should be considered.

### TREATMENT

Generally, patients with symptomatic choledocholithiasis should be offered treatment because of the high risk of recurrent symptoms and complications if stones are left in situ as already discussed. In some special circumstances, adopting a conservative approach may be appropriate such as severe end-stage dementia or severe comorbid factors that make removal hazardous.

The two main methods of bile duct stone removal are at ERCP or, in patients with an intact gallbladder, laparoscopic cholecystectomy and bile duct exploration (LC+BDE). Current practice in choosing between the two methods depends on center preference and local

## BOX 3  Differential Diagnosis of Choledocholithiasis by Presentation

### Jaundice with or without Pain

- Alcoholic liver disease
- Benign stricture
- Bile duct injuries
- Drug induced
- Malignant stricture
- Parasitic infection of the biliary tree
- Primary biliary cirrhosis
- Sclerosing cholangitis
- Viral hepatitis

### Biliary Colic

- Acute pancreatitis
- Cholecystitis
- Duodenitis
- Esophageal spasm
- Inferior myocardial infarction
- Peptic ulcer disease
- Sphincter of Oddi dysfunction

### Pancreatitis

- Appendicitis
- Biliary colic
- Dissecting aneurysm
- Diverticulitis
- Ectopic pregnancy
- Hematoma of abdominal muscles
- Inferior myocardial infarction
- Mesenteric infarction
- Perforated gastric or duodenal ulcer

### Cholestatic Liver Function Tests

- Alcoholic liver disease
- Ampullary carcinoma
- Biliary strictures
- Drugs
- Granulomatous hepatitis
- Malignant infiltration of the liver
- Nonalcoholic fatty liver disease (NAFLD)
- Primary biliary cirrhosis
- Sclerosing cholangitis

expertise in laparoscopic bile duct exploration. A recent Cochrane Database of systematic review comparing LC+BDE and ERCP found that both methods were equally effective, with no significant difference in morbidity and mortality. However, shorter hospital stay was achieved in patients undergoing LC+BDE.

There is a limited role for other techniques, such as extracorporeal shockwave lithotripsy and endoscopic laser lithotripsy, and these techniques should be reserved for bile duct stones that cannot be removed at ERCP or LC+CBE due to technical or safety reasons.

### REFERENCES

Al-Waili N, Saloom KY: The analgesic effect of intravenous tenoxicam in symptomatic treatment of biliary colic: A comparison with hyoscine N-butylbromide. Eur J Med Res 1998;3(10):475-479.

Field AE, Coakley EH, Must A, et al: Impact of overweight on the risk of developing common chronic diseases during a 10-year period. Arch Intern Med 2001;161(13):1581-1586.

Johansson M, Thune A, Blomqvist A, et al: Impact of choice of therapeutic strategy for acute cholecystitis on patient's health-related quality of life. Results of a randomized, controlled clinical trial. Dig Surg 2004;21(5-6):359-362.

Lau H, Lo CY, Patil NG, Yuen WK: Early versus delayed-interval laparoscopic cholecystectomy for acute cholecystitis: A meta-analysis. Surg Endosc 2006;20(1):82-87.

Lu EJ, Curet MJ, El-Sayed YY, Kirkwood KS: Medical versus surgical management of biliary tract disease in pregnancy. Am J Surg. 2004;188(6):755-759.

Martin DJ, Vernon DR, Toouli J: Surgical versus endoscopic treatment of bile duct stones. Cochrane Database Syst Rev 2006;(2):CD003327.

Miller K, Hell E, Lang B, Lengauer E: Gallstone formation prophylaxis after gastric restrictive procedures for weight loss: A randomized double-blind placebo-controlled trial. Ann Surg 2003;238(5):697-702.

NIH state-of-the-science statement on endoscopic retrograde cholangiopancreatography (ERCP) for diagnosis and therapy. NIH Consens State Sci Statements. 2002;19(1):1-26.

Papi C, Catarci M, D'Ambrosio L, et al: Timing of cholecystectomy for acute calculous cholecystitis: A meta-analysis. Am J Gastroenterol. 2004;99(1):147-155.

Ros A, Gustafsson L, Krook H, et al: Laparoscopic cholecystectomy versus minilaparotomy cholecystectomy: A prospective, randomized, single-blind study. Ann Surg 2001;234(6):741-749.

Thornell E, Nilsson B, Jansson R, Svanvik J: Effect of short-term indomethacin treatment on the clinical course of acute obstructive cholecystitis. Eur J Surg 1991;157(2):127-130.

Tsai CJ, Leitzmann MF, Willett WC, Giovannucci EL: Dietary carbohydrates and glycaemic load and the incidence of symptomatic gall stone disease in men. Gut 2005;54(6):823-828.

# Cirrhosis

Method of
*Richard K. Sterling, MD, Wissam E. Mattar, MD, and Paul Y. Kwo, MD*

Cirrhosis is defined as the development of fibrosis of the liver with the formation of regenerative nodules. Typically it follows a chronic injury to hepatocytes that activate the perisinusoidal stellate cells by cytokines, which transforms them into myofibroblasts capable of proliferating and depositing collagen type 1. Progressively the normal liver histology is replaced by the fibrotic, distorted architecture. It is the resultant impairment in the synthetic, metabolic, and hemodynamic functions of the liver that defines cirrhosis clinically.

## Common Clinical Manifestations

In addition to the particular expression of every etiology, most cirrhotic patients have little or no clinical features in the early stages, and many are already being followed up for abnormal liver panels before the development of cirrhosis. Patients may present with fatigue, weakness, nausea, abdominal discomfort, loss of appetite with weight loss, and pruritus. On physical examination, there may be jaundice, skin hematomas, spider angiomas, palmar erythema, gynecomastia, testicular atrophy, and caput medusae. The spleen and the liver could be palpable with tenderness in the right upper quadrant. Attention should also be given to the so-called seven hand signs of cirrhosis: palmar erythema, Dupuytren's contracture, telangiectasias, thenar wasting, leukonychia or Terry's nails, clubbing, and asterixis. As liver function decompensates, the more specific clinical manifestations of complications appear. Ascites, spontaneous bacterial peritonitis (SBP), hepatic encephalopathy (HE), esophageal varices, hepatorenal syndrome (HRS), hepatopulmonary syndrome (HPS), portopulmonary hypertension, and hepatocellular carcinoma (HCC), as well as other less apparent complications such as hematologic disturbances and hepatic osteodystrophy, are problems to address in the decompensated stage (Table 1).

## TABLE 1 Key Current Diagnoses

| | |
|---|---|
| Ascites | Shifting dullness on physical exam, abdominal ultrasound, diagnostic paracentesis |
| SBP | Ascitic fluid: PMN cells count above 250/mm³, positive gram stain, positive cultures |
| Esophageal/ gastric varices | EGD |
| HE | Neuropsychiatric abnormalities; rule out other etiologies, search for precipitating factors |
| HRS I | Decrease of >50% in creatinine clearance or doubling of serum creatinine in less than 2 wk; rule out other etiologies of ARF |
| HRS II | Progressive renal failure, refractory ascites |
| Hepatopulmonary syndrome | Hypoxia, intrapulmonary vascular dilations, contrast-enhanced echocardiography or technetium-labeled macroaggregated albumin scanning |
| Portopulmonary hypertension | Pulmonary hypertension without secondary etiologies other than portal hypertension |
| Hepatocellular carcinoma | Lesion >2 cm with arterial enhancement or AFP >400 µg/mL, FNA in other suspicious lesions |

*Abbreviations:* AFP = alpha-fetoprotein; ARF = acute renal failure; EGD = esophagogastroduodenoscopy; FNA = fine-needle aspiration; HE = hepatic encephalopathy; HRS = hepatorenal syndrome; PMN = polymorphonuclear neutrophil (leukocyte).

## Common Laboratory and Imaging Findings

Frequently, tests confirm the clinical suspicion of cirrhosis in the presence of the characteristic physical findings of advanced liver disease. Laboratory studies could help establish the etiologic diagnosis and screen or confirm complications. In general, alanine aminotransferase (ALT) and aspartate aminotransferase (AST) are elevated but can be in the normal range. In the absence of chronic alcohol use, cirrhosis may be indicated by a higher AST than ALT. Bilirubin often increases only in advanced stages. High alkaline phosphatase pinpoints to a cholestatic component. Albumin trends to lower levels and the prothrombin time (PT) or international normalized ratio (INR) increases with the severity of the synthetic disturbance. Cytopenias, especially thrombocytopenia,

 **CURRENT DIAGNOSIS**

- Symptoms: fatigue, weakness, nausea, abdominal discomfort, loss of appetite with weight loss, pruritus
- Physical exam (general): jaundice, skin hematomas, spider angiomas, palmar erythema, gynecomastia, testicular atrophy, caput medusae, Dupuytren's contracture, thenar wasting, leukonychia or Terry's nails, clubbing, splenomegaly
- Physical exam (in decompensation): ascites, hepatic encephalopathy (asterixis)
- Complications: spontaneous bacterial peritonitis, esophageal/gastric varices, portal hypertensive gastropathy, hepatorenal syndrome, hepatopulmonary syndrome, portopulmonary hypertension, hepatocellular carcinoma

are common. A low platelet count is often the only initial laboratory finding.

Imaging studies such as abdominal ultrasound (US), computed tomography (CT) scan, and magnetic resonance imaging (MRI) can suggest the diagnosis by revealing abnormalities in size, shape, and contour of the liver. However, they are not perfect, and liver biopsy remains the gold standard. Liver imaging can be helpful for the evaluation of portal hypertension and biliary tree abnormalities and to look for complications of advanced liver disease such as ascites, vascular thombosis, and HCC.

## Diagnosis

Obtaining adequate tissue from the liver confirms the diagnosis of cirrhosis. Biopsies could be obtained percutaneously except in the presence of a prolonged PT more than 3 seconds, thrombocytopenia of less than 60,000 to 80,000, or the presence of ascites. In these instances, an open biopsy or a transjugular approach can be used.

## Severity of Cirrhosis

Multiple scores have been created to categorize the severity of disease. The Child-Pugh score is the most widely used (Table 2). It incorporates three laboratory values (PT, bilirubin, and albumin) and two clinical features (ascites and encephalopathy). Class A patients have an 85% 2-year survival, compared with 60% and 35% for classes B and C, respectively. The MELD (Model for End-stage Liver Disease) score has now supplanted the Child-Pugh classification for listing the patient for liver transplantation (Table 2) and is calculated by a formula that includes bilirubin, creatinine, and the INR instead of PT.

## Causes

The etiologies that could lead to cirrhosis are very diverse and can be categorized into toxins and drugs, viruses, autoimmune diseases, biliary disease, metabolic, vascular and idiopathic (Table 3).

## Treatment

There are limited treatments to reverse advanced fibrosis, but controlling the etiology preferably before end-stage disease ensues is highly

## TABLE 2 Classification of Cirrhosis

| | Child-Pugh Points | | |
|---|---|---|---|
| | **1** | **2** | **3** |
| Bilirubin (mg/dL) | <2.0 | 2.1–3.0 | >3.0 |
| Prothrombin time (seconds prolonged) | <4 | 4–6 | >6 |
| Albumin (g/L) | >3.5 | 2.8–3.5 | <2.8 |
| Ascites | None | Mild–moderate | Severe |
| Encephalopathy | None | Mild–moderate | Severe |

Child's class A: 5–6, Child's class B: 7–9, Child's class C: 10–15.

| MELD Score | 3-mo Mortality |
|---|---|
| <10 | 2%–8% |
| 10–19 | 6%–29% |
| 20–29 | 50%–76% |
| 30–39 | 62%–83% |
| ≥40 | 100% |

*Abbreviation:* INR = international normalized ratio; MELD = Model for End-stage Liver Disease. MELD Score = 11.2 ln (INR) + 3.78 ln (bilirubin) + 9.57 ln (creatinine) + 6.43

**TABLE 3   Common Causes of Cirrhosis**

| Etiology | Diagnostic Test |
| --- | --- |
| Alcohol | History, AST-to-ALT ratio >2, liver biopsy |
| Viral hepatitis B | Surface antigen, E antigen, HBV DNA |
| Viral hepatitis C | HCV antibody, HCV RNA, HCV genotype |
| Autoimmune hepatitis | ANA, ASMA, A-LKM |
| Primary biliary cirrhosis | AMA |
| Primary sclerosing cholangitis | P-ANCA, ERCP, MRCP |
| Alpha 1 antitrypsin deficiency | A$_1$AT level, phenotype |
| Wilson's disease | Ceruloplasmin, serum Cu, Kayser-Fleischer rings |
| NASH | Liver biopsy, history of metabolic syndrome |
| Budd-Chiari syndrome | Duplex of the hepatic vein |
| Cryptogenic | Diagnosis of exclusion |

*Abbreviations:* A-LKM = anti–liver/kidney microsome; ALT = alanine aminotransferase; AMA = antimitochondrial antibody; ANA = antinuclear antibody; ASMA = antismooth muscle antibody; AST = aspartate aminotransferase; Cu = copper; ERCP = endoscopic retrograde cholangiopancreatography; HBV = hepatitis B virus; HCV = hepatitis C virus; MRCP = magnetic retrograde cholangiopancreatography; NASH = nonalcoholic steatohepatitis; P-ANCA = perinuclear antineutrophil cytoplasmic antibody.

## CURRENT THERAPY

**Procedure/Reason**

- Upper endoscopy: Screen for varices.
  - If moderate or large, primary prophylaxis with nonselective β-blocker to prevent bleeding.
  - If none, then repeat q2y.
- Liver imaging (ultrasound or CT): screen/surveillance for hepatocellular carcinoma.
  - Repeat q6–12 mo.
- Alpha fetoprotein: Screen/surveillance for hepatocellular carcinoma.
  - Repeat q3–6 mo.
- Diagnostic paracentesis: Send fluid for WBC, differential, albumin, and total protein.
  - Exclude SBP (PMN <250).
  - Calculate SAAG.
- Hepatitis A and B serology: Vaccinate if negative.
- Diet: Low sodium:
  - 2 g/d if ascites.
  - 3–5 g if no ascites.
  - Avoid protein restriction unless uncontrolled encephalopathy.
- Medications: Avoid NSAIDs.
- Avoid aminoglycosides.
- Liver transplant referral/evaluation: if hepatic decompensation, variceal bleeding, or hepatocellular carcinoma.

*Abbreviations:* NSAIDs = nonsteroidal anti-inflammatory drugs; PMN = polymorphonuclear neutrophil (leukocyte); SAAG = serum ascites-albumin gradient; SBP = spontaneous bacterial peritonitis; WBC = white blood cell count.

recommended. Treatment of the complications of cirrhosis could be lifesaving or palliative.

# Treatment of the Etiologies

## CHRONIC VIRAL HEPATITIS

More information can be obtained from the article on viral hepatitis in this volume.

## ALCOHOL

Alcohol abuse could lead to a spectrum of liver disease states that range from asymptomatic fatty liver to cirrhosis. The average total intake to develop cirrhosis is 80 g of ethanol per day for 20 years. Lesser doses in women, chronic viral hepatitis, and hemochromatosis could lead to higher risks of developing cirrhosis.

History, physical examination, and laboratory features can be specific for alcoholic hepatitis. An AST value more than two times the level of the ALT (related both to the deficiency in pyridoxal-6-phosphate and the direct mitochondrial toxicity of alcohol) suggests alcohol as the culprit of liver injury. If this ratio is less than 2, alcohol is unlikely to be the cause of liver injury. Aminotransferases usually do not exceed 500 UI/L. If they do, other coexisting etiologies, such as acetaminophen or acute viral hepatitis, should be excluded. Elevations in gamma glutamyl transferase (GGT) and carbohydrate-deficient transferase (CDT) could also suggest alcohol as the etiology of hepatitis. Thrombocytopenia and anemia with macrocytosis are classical findings but not specific. In acute alcoholic hepatitis (AH), alkaline phosphatase and GGT are typically and persistently elevated. Approximately 10% of the cases of AH are atypical or unclear, and in these a liver biopsy is required. A rapid bedside screening by looking for encephalopathy and ascites could evaluate the severity of alcohol-induced liver injury. If one or both are present, then calculating the MELD score and the discriminant function (DF), 4.6 × (PT patient – PT control) + bilirubin in mg/dL, help assess the mortality risk and the subsequent management plan. A DF value greater than 32 predicts a 50% mortality in 1 month in those with acute alcoholic hepatitis.

The best treatment for alcoholic liver disease is total abstinence. Progression of disease and accelerated mortality are likely in patients who continue to drink. It should be emphasized that nutritional needs are to be addressed (protein 1 to 1.5 g/kg/day with caloric needs being 1.2 to 1.4 × resting energy expenditure divided as 50% from carbohydrate and 30% from fat mainly unsaturated). If dietary intake is insufficient, supplements are indicated. A nighttime snack is encouraged. The administration of 50 to 100 mg/day of thiamine along with intravenous (IV) glucose, 100 mg/day of pyridoxine (vitamin B$_6$), and 1 mg/day of folic acid is often required. Supplementation with phosphorus, magnesium, and potassium are necessary if serum levels are low. Colchicine[1] has no benefits and should not be prescribed. Pentoxifylline (Trental),[1] at a dose of 400 mg every 8 hours for 4 weeks, showed significant survival benefit equivalent to those reported with corticosteroids. Infliximab (Remicade)[1] with corticosteroids increased mortality from infectious complications in one study and should not be administered in acute alcoholic hepatitis.

In acute AH with a DF of 32 or with hepatic encephalopathy, it is recommended to administer 40 mg of prednisone or 32 mg of methylprednisolone for 28 days, which can increase survival. A MELD score of 21 is suggested as a cutoff for beginning treatment with steroids. Predictors of the response to corticosteroids are decreasing DF, MELD score, and creatinine and bilirubin levels after 1 week of treatment. If these improvements are not seen, continued steroids are of little benefit. Liver transplantation is the best treatment for advanced alcoholic liver disease. Alcohol abstinence for 6 months is routinely required before transplantation in alcoholics. This time frame can be changed on an individual basis.

[1]Not FDA approved for this indication.

## AUTOIMMUNE HEPATITIS

The exclusion of replicating hepatitis virus infection together with female sex, hypergammaglobulinemia, and response to immunosuppressive treatment are the hallmarks of an accurate diagnosis of autoimmune hepatitis (AIH). A score based mainly on gender, liver chemistries, immunoglobulins titers, histology, absence of viral hepatitis, and alcohol abuse was created to predict the chance of diagnosing AIH. Liver biopsy, which is helpful for diagnosis, management, and prognosis, shows characteristically an increase in plasma cells with interface hepatitis.

AIH can be divided into two categories. In type 1, antibodies to nuclei (ANA) and/or to smooth muscle (SMA) are present. In type 2, anti–liver/kidney microsome-1 (ALKM-1) antibodies are most common. Untreated disease has a mortality rate of 50% at 5 years. Two fundamental goals are distinguished: induction of remission and maintenance of remission. Treatment is guided by the American Association for the Study of Liver Diseases (AASLD) guidelines, which recommend treating active disease and observing closely milder forms; severe disease is considered when aminotransferases are 10 times the normal limit, or five times the normal limit with gammaglobulins that are twice the normal, or if on histology central necrosis or bridging fibrosis is present. Some authors recommend treatment of any symptomatic patient.

The AASLD recommends treatment by corticosteroids alone or in combination with azathioprine (Imuran)[1] for its steroid-sparing effects in patients who are susceptible to the side effects of steroids. For initial induction, adults who are on prednisone alone should be on 60 mg/day and then the dose tapered by 10 mg/week to a dose of 15 to 20 mg/day by 6 months. Prednisone at 20 to 30 mg/day is sufficient if given with azathioprine[1] at a dose of 50 mg/day. Prednisone can be reduced to 15 mg/day in 5-mg decrements every 2 weeks. Once the liver panel is normalized, azathioprine[1] at 50 to 75 mg/day and prednisone at 10 to 20 mg/day are continued, and then prednisone can be decreased to 10 mg/day by 2.5 mg every 3 months. Remission is defined by a decrease by half of the aminotransferase levels and normalization of the bilirubin and the gammaglobulin levels with improvement of the histologic features. In addition to the blood work including immunoglobulins, a liver biopsy, although not required to stop therapy, is essential to confirm complete remission and is helpful in the decision process. Most patients require both drugs for a year, at which time prednisone could be tapered. Ninety percent are responders to this regimen. However, recurrence rates after stopping treatment are as high as 90% and are inversely correlated with the pathology findings. It is for this reason that many patients remain on long-term azathioprine[1] at a dose of 0.5 mg/kg/day.

## PRIMARY BILIARY CIRRHOSIS

Primary biliary cirrhosis (PBC) is an autoimmune disease affecting middle-aged women. PBC results in progressive granulomatous destruction of the bile ducts. Manifestations classic of the disease are fatigue, pruritus, osteoporosis, hypercholesterolemia and skin xanthomas, sicca syndrome, vitamin deficiencies, and recurrent urinary tract infections. Most patients with PBC when discovered have no symptoms, and it is often suspected when alkaline phosphatase is elevated. Bilirubin stays in the normal range until late in the progression and is strongly correlated with prognosis. The AMA (antimitochondrial antibody) is positive in 95% of the cases. SMA and ANA can be positive in a third of the patients with PBC. Diagnosis is made by the constellation of cholestatic picture, exclusion of extrahepatic disease, positivity for AMA, and a compatible liver biopsy with granulomatous nonsuppurative cholangitis.

The first-line treatment is ursodeoxycholic acid (UDCA). It is a safe drug that lowers toxic bile acid levels and has a protective effect on the membranes of the liver cells. It is administered at a dose of 13 to 15 mg/kg/day. Cholestatic enzymes can fall to normal or near normal levels, and UDCA can delay disease progression and increase survival.

It is a second-line agent for unresponsive pruritus. Although immunosuppressive therapy with methotrexate[1] at 0.25 mg/kg/week and colchicine[1] at 0.6 mg twice daily needs more verification, some authors use it in advanced stages of PBC. Their association with UDCA was additive in some reports.

Pruritus is difficult to manage; in mild cases, skin hydration (emollients and warm baths) with hydroxyzine (Atarax), 25 mg, or cyproheptadine (Periactin), 4 mg every 8 hours, can be sufficient. The first-line therapies for moderate to severe pruritus are cholestyramine (Questran) and colestipol (Colestid). Cholestyramine is taken apart from any other medication. The dose is 4 g before breakfast and dinner, with extra doses to be taken before lunch or bedtime. Second-line therapies for severe pruritus include rifampin (Rifadin),[1] at 300 to 600 mg/day twice daily, phenobarbital,[1] at 120 mg/day, opioid antagonists like naltrexone (ReVia)[1] 10 to 50 mg/day which can lead to significant decrease in the perception of pruritus. In patients who fail to respond, methotrexate,[1] colchicine,[1] sertraline (Zoloft)[1] at 75 mg/day, paroxetine (Paxil)[1] at 20 mg/day, or phototherapy (UVB) could be tried. Because plasmapheresis is inconvenient it is only used when none of the treatments just cited work because it will only give temporary relief. Liver transplantation is the only definitive treatment for severe pruritus.

Hypothyroidism and sicca syndrome associated with PBC should be addressed. Because of chronic cholestasis, fat-soluble vitamin deficiencies (A, D, and K) may occur in PBC. For osteoporosis, the only proven treatment is liver transplant, but vitamin D at 50,000 U/week can prevent osteopenia and is indicated with calcium at 1 to 1.5 g/day if osteopenia is documented. If levels of 25-hydroxy vitamin D are low, supplementation at a dose of 20 µg/day is ideal. Hormone replacement therapy (HRT) is recommended in postmenopausal women. Calcitonin (Miacalcin) or alendronate (Fosamax) are considered if osteoporosis is documented. If vitamin A, which correlates to retinol-binding protein and albumin and inversely to bilirubin, is low, then 15,000 UI/day should be used; otherwise 5000 UI/day is considered as the maintenance regimen. Vitamin E at a regular dose of 400 IU/day can be supplemented. Vitamin K at 5 to 10 mg/day is only supplemented if the patient has bleeding tendencies that are obvious, which only is present if the patient is on cholestyramine or has advanced liver disease. If the patient has a steatorrhea of more than 40 g/day, then restriction of fat is indicated, with replacement by medium chain fatty acids up to a dose of 60 mL/day (medium-chain triglycerides [MCT] oil, 1 tablespoon three to four times a day).

## PRIMARY SCLEROSING CHOLANGITIS (PSC)

PSC is an uncommon disease characterized by progressive diffuse inflammation of the intra- and extrahepatic bile ducts. An estimated 70% to 90% of the patients are men older than 20 years. These ducts are intermittently strictured and dilated. Up to 90% of the cases have ulcerative colitis, less commonly Crohn's disease. PSC harbors a 15% lifetime risk for developing cholangiocarcinoma. No screening for cholangiocarcinoma in patients with PSC is beneficial.

Suggestive symptoms of PSC include right upper quadrant pain, fatigue, pruritus, and jaundice; 25% are asymptomatic. Typically liver tests demonstrate a cholestatic pattern with transaminases less than 300 IU/L. Perinuclear antineutrophil cytoplasmic antibodies (P-ANCA) are associated with 70% of PSC and of inflammatory bowel disease and can be helpful in the diagnosis in difficult cases. Endoscopic retrograde cholangiopancreatography (ERCP) and magnetic resonance cholangiopancreatography (MRCP) confirm the diagnosis by showing the intra- and/or extrahepatic bile strictures, beading, and dilations and ruling out secondary causes of stenosis. Liver biopsy supports the diagnosis and determines the severity of the disease but is unnecessary to make the diagnosis. Typical findings include ductopenic and periductal fibrosis.

Treatment is limited and there are no approved therapies for PSC. Ursodiol (UDCA) at standard doses (12 to 15 mg/kg/day) is not effective and unlike in PBC, UDCA did not show survival improvement in

---

[1]Not FDA approved for this indication.

[1]Not FDA approved for this indication.

this condition. In the presence of a dominant stricture anywhere in the biliary tree, cytologic brushing should be performed to rule out cholangiocarcinoma. Endoscopic or radiologic dilation or stent placement should be attempted while knowing that the risk of restenosis is 30% to 50% with the same failure rate for reintervention; no survival benefit is shown, but jaundice, pruritus, and liver tests improve significantly. It is recommended to administer antibiotics 1 hour before any hepatobiliary procedure for cholangitis prophylaxis. The treatment of choice for advanced PSC is liver transplantation with 70% to 80% survival at 5 years. Treatment of pruritus, osteoporosis, steatorrhea, and fat-soluble vitamin deficiencies are the same as those for PBC. No test is recommended for cholangiocarcinoma screening; in suspicious cases, percutaneous guided-needle biopsy is the procedure of choice.

## NONALCOHOLIC STEATOHEPATITIS

The majority of cryptogenic cirrhosis is caused by nonalcoholic steatohepatitis (NASH), which presents almost identically as alcoholic hepatitis, with the exception that the patient drinks less than 40 g of alcohol per week. NASH is correlated to obesity and central obesity, insulin resistance, type II diabetes, hyperlipidemia; it is now called the metabolic syndrome. Drugs like corticosteroids, estrogens, tamoxifen, and amiodarone are also associated with NASH. Total parenteral nutrition, rapid weight loss, and starvation can induce NASH. It is often suspected in patients with constantly enlarged liver, unexplained increased levels of aminotransferases, and the presence of a fatty liver on imaging studies. NASH is diagnosed on liver biopsy when steatosis and inflammation are present and after the exclusion of alcoholic, viral, metabolic, and autoimmune hepatitis by their respective laboratory tests. It is now recognized that NASH can progress to cirrhosis in a fourth of the cases. Diabetes, high body mass index (BMI), and fibrosis on diagnosis are predictors of progression. Usually ALT and AST levels are elevated, and unlike in alcoholic liver disease, ALT is the same or greater than AST.

The first-line treatment of NASH is always related to the underlying cause if present. Essentially lowering insulin resistance, which is universal in NASH, targets all components of the metabolic syndrome. Diabetes should be controlled. Weight reduction and exercise are correlated with improvement in liver enzymes. Rapid weight loss, especially after bypass surgeries, is ill advised in those with fibrosis/ cirrhosis because it may precipitate liver failure by necroinflammation, portal fibrosis, and bile stasis. Although there is no proven medical therapy for NASH, some small studies encourage the use of insulin-sensitizing agents and antioxidants, either alone or in combination. However, until results from ongoing clinical trials are available, these agents cannot be recommended.

## HEMOCHROMATOSIS

Hemochromatosis (HC) is defined as an excessive deposition of iron in major organs such as the liver, kidneys, heart, endocrine glands (pancreas and pituitary), and joints. The main etiology, hereditary HC, results from a genetic mutation on the short arm of chromosome 6. Most patients with clinical HC are homozygous for C282Y, whereas those with only H63D mutations are not at increased risk of liver disease. Most patients are in their 40s or 50s, and cirrhosis develops in more than 60% of the cases. Screening is recommended in persons who are symptomatic (e.g., liver disease, skin pigmentation, diabetes), who are first-degree relatives of patients with hemochromatosis, or who have abnormal iron studies. Fasting iron saturation (total iron-binding capacity [TIBC]) and ferritin levels are the first tests to be done; then genotyping is required if the iron studies are suggestive (TIBC more than 45%) or if the patient is a first-degree relative of a C282Y homozygous patient. In patients who are homozygous and older than 40 years, have signs of liver disease, or have ferritin levels above 1000 μg/mL, a biopsy is recommended to exclude cirrhosis. A patient with a serum ferritin less than 1000 μg/mL without hepatomegaly and a normal AST is unlikely to have cirrhosis. Conversely, patients with a ferritin greater than 1000 μg/mL, a platelet count less than 200,000, and an elevated AST have a high probability of cirrhosis. Biopsy rules out secondary causes of iron overload (like alcohol or HCV) and assesses the fibrotic changes, which determine the prognosis.

An effective treatment of HC is serial phlebotomies. It is recommended to withdraw 1 U of blood, which contains 200 to 250 mg of iron every week and, if not tolerated, one phlebotomy every 2 to 4 weeks until the patient adapts to blood withdrawal. Once iron stores return to normal, reflected by a serum ferritin level of less than 50 μg/mL and a transferrin saturation of less than 50%, maintenance phlebotomy every 2 to 6 months is done. Hemoglobin should be monitored to avoid anemia. Levels of approximately 10 to 12 g/dL are acceptable.

HC patients must be regularly screened for hepatocellular carcinoma. Most foods are not restricted, except for iron and vitamin C supplements. Vitamin C increases iron absorption and can induce arrhythmias, but fruits and vegetables should not be limited. Daily alcohol consumption is ill advised because it will increase iron absorption, but occasional drinking is permitted in those without advanced liver disease. Liver transplantation is the definitive therapy, but cardiac involvement should be carefully evaluated. Even in acceptable candidates, survival following liver transplantation is reduced compared to most other indications.

## WILSON'S DISEASE

Wilson's disease (WD), an autosomal recessive disorder, is the inability to excrete copper into bile properly and to incorporate it into ceruloplasmin (CP), leading first to inappropriate copper accumulation in the liver and later in the eyes, kidneys, and central nervous system. Liver abnormalities in WD are particular for their association with psychiatric and neurologic symptoms like dystonia, tremor, unsteady gait, slurred speech, and drooling because of the involvement of the basal ganglia. Recurrent or chronic low-grade hemolysis can be a presenting manifestation in approximately 10% of the patients.

Diagnosis of WD is confirmed when Kayser-Fleischer (KF) rings are present along with a CP level of less than 20 mg/dL. A ceruloplasmin level under 5 mg/dL or a basal 24-hour urinary copper excretion of more than 100 μg is a strong evidence of WD. If KF rings are absent or CP levels are normal, a liver biopsy should be done. Abnormal liver tests with a 24-hour urinary copper excretion of more than 40 μg with a decreased ceruloplasmin level are also an indication for liver biopsy. On quantitative copper measurement, levels greater than 250 μg/g of dry liver weight are indicative of WD. Neurologic evaluation and MR imaging are recommended prior to treatment in all patients. Screening of first-degree relatives by clinical and biologic means is indicated.

The chelating agents D-penicillamine (Cuprimine) or trientine (Syprine) are initially given at 250 to 500 mg per day, then increased to 1 to 1.5 g a day in four divided doses. Improvement appears 2 to 12 months later, and monitoring is obtained by the 24-hour urinary copper excretion, which should stay above 200 μg. Nonceruloplasmin-bound copper concentration and aminotransferases should normalize with successful treatment. The maintenance regimen is approximately 750 to 1000 mg per day. Supplementation with 25 to 50 mg of pyridoxine is required with D-penicillamine, and iron should not be administered with trientine. Many severe hypersensitivity reactions could limit their use; thus blood counts, liver function tests, creatinine, and urinalysis should be obtained regularly. Zinc gluconate, which eliminates copper from the gut, is given at 50 mg three times a day. It is the first choice for maintenance therapy and can be used in presymptomatic patients. Urinary copper excretion is required for monitoring and should be less than 75 μg in 24 hours. Maintenance therapy is lifelong. Liver and shellfish are the only banned food for patients on initiation of treatment; during maintenance therapy once a week ingestion of these foods is acceptable.

## ALPHA₁-ANTITRYPSIN DEFICIENCY

Liver damage is caused by the accumulation of the mutant $A_1AT$ in the hepatocytes. An estimated 10% to 15% of individuals with the homozygous form PiZZ (protease inhibitor phenotype ZZ) eventually develop cirrhosis with older age, Male gender and obesity are the only known predisposing factors. Most patients with liver damage are children. After excluding the most common causes of cirrhosis, diagnosis is done by phenotyping the $A_1AT$ protein and not by measurement of the total $A_1AT$ protein in the serum. Patients with chronic disease should be screened for hepatocellular carcinoma. An effective treatment is liver transplantation with a 5-year survival rate of 80%. Hepatocyte transplantation holds promise in this disease.

## Treatment of Complications

Many patients with cirrhosis have no serious outward complications from the disease that are clinically evident. These patients are described as having compensated cirrhosis (Child's class A). For the remaining patients, several classic complications may occur, and this is described as the decompensated state. The onset of the decompensated state may herald a clinical decline with reduced survival compared to the compensated state. The major complications include ascites, bleeding from esophagogastric varices, and hepatic encephalopathy. Other common and serious complications include SBP, hepatorenal syndrome, and hepatocellular carcinoma (Table 4).

### ASCITES

Ascites is the most common complication of cirrhosis. In 50% of those with compensated cirrhosis, ascites will develop within 10 years (30% in 5 years). The onset of ascites is associated with a poor prognosis, with ascites associated with a 50% mortality rate at 1 to 2 years, compared to a 10% mortality rate at 1 year in those with compensated cirrhosis. In diuretic responsive ascites, there is a 50% 2-year survival rate, but in those with diuretic-resistant ascites, there is increased mortality with a 50% 6-month survival and a 25% 1-year survival.

Portal hypertension is a prerequisite for the formation of ascites. In response to portal hypertension, there is vasodilation of the arterioles

### TABLE 4 Key Current Treatments

| | |
|---|---|
| Ascites and peripheral edema | Sodium restriction, spironolactone and furosemide, therapeutic paracentesis with and without albumin infusion, TIPSS, OLT |
| SBP | Cefotaxime, ceftriaxone, ofloxacin, albumin infusion, discontinue diuretics |
| SBP prophylaxis | TMP-SMX, norfloxacin, ciprofloxacin |
| Hepatic encephalopathy | Treat precipitating etiologies, lactulose or Lactinol, metronidazole, rifaximin, or vancomycin, low-protein diet |
| Bleeding from esophageal/gastric varices | Hemodynamic stabilization, balloon tamponade, vasopressin, octreotide, nitroglycerin, band ligation, sclerotherapy, TIPSS |
| Esophageal/gastric varices prophylaxis | Propranolol or nadolol, nitrates, sclerotherapy, band ligation, TIPSS, OLT |
| HRS I | Treat precipitating etiologies, OLT, antibiotics, albumin, midodrine, octreotide, terlipressin, TIPSS |
| HRS II | Serial paracentesis, diuretics, TIPSS, OLT |
| Portopulmonary hypertension | Calcium channel blockers, bosentan, isoproterenol |
| Hepatopulmonary syndrome | OLT |
| Hepatocellular carcinoma | Surgical resection, OLT, chemoembolization, radiofrequency, irradiation |

*Abbreviations:* HRS = hepatorenal syndrome; OLT = orthotopic liver transplantation; SBP = spontaneous bacterial peritonitis; TIPPS = transjugular intrahepatic portosystemic shunt; TMP-SMX = trimethoprim-sulfamethoxazole.

of the splanchnic bed that is mediated by nitric oxide. In response to this vasodilation with decreased effective arterial blood volume, and as a compensatory mechanism, there is activation of the renin-angiotensin system. This leads to significant sodium retention, which, when coupled with an increase in hydrostatic pressure in the portal system and a decrease in oncotic pressure caused by hypoalbuminemia, leads to accumulation of ascitic fluid in the abdomen with ascitic fluid primarily weeping off the surface of the liver into the peritoneal cavity. The formation of ascites secondary to cirrhosis is one of the considerations for liver transplantation.

Clinical examination is unreliable in detecting small amounts of ascites (less than 2 L), especially in obese patients. Therefore US is the ideal test to detect small amounts of peritoneal fluid (as low as 100 mL) and can also be used to determine patency or thrombosis of the hepatic and portal vasculature. A paracentesis should be performed for newly diagnosed ascites and the fluid examined for total protein, cell count, cultures (inoculated at the bedside), and albumin. The serum ascites-albumin gradient (SAAG), determined by subtracting the ascitic fluid albumin from the serum albumin determined at the same time, confirms the presence of portal hypertension as having a role in the development of ascites with more than 97% accuracy if the gradient is greater than 1.1g/dL. If the total protein in the ascitic fluid is less than 1.1 g/dL, this suggests the patient is at high risk for spontaneous bacterial peritonitis, and prophylaxis should be considered. A polymorphonuclear neutrophil (leukocyte) (PMN) count of greater than $250/mm^3$ is essential for diagnosing SBP. Paracentesis carries a small risk of bowel perforation and abdominal wall hematoma (less than 1 in 1000 patients).

Ascites may be graded in severity and treatment can be tailored based on this grade. In 15% of the patients who have mild ascites, sodium restriction to 3 to 5 g/day may be sufficient if they have the ability to excrete this sodium load. For those patients with higher-grade ascites, sodium restriction to 2 g/day is recommended, as well as the initiation of diuretics. Oral spironolactone (Aldactone) is effective in 20% to 50% when used alone; additive effect is obtained when used with furosemide (Lasix). Initial doses are 100 mg and 40 mg daily, respectively, and are given once in the morning. Painful gynecomastia may result from spironolactone, and if this occurs, amiloride (Midamor), 5 to 20 mg/day, or triamterene (Dyrenium), 50 to 100 mg/day, may be substituted. Amiloride is less effective than spironolactone in reducing ascites. The dosage of furosemide and spironolactone can be increased in case of resistance every 3 to 5 days up to a maximum of 160 mg/day for furosemide and 400 mg for spironolactone or 40 mg for amiloride. Tense ascites should be treated first with therapeutic paracentesis followed by administration of diuretics and salt restriction.

A key indicator of response to diuretics is a random spot urine test to see if the ratio of sodium to potassium concentration is greater than 1. If so, then it is 90% certain that the patient is excreting a satisfactory amount of sodium (minimum 78 mmol/day). Urine sodium of less than 10 mEq/day is considered a diuretic-resistant state. A 24-hour urinary sodium more than 78 mmol is the best indicator of adequate natriuresis. The ideal weight loss should be 0.5 kg/day in patients without edema, and 1 kg/day in those with lower extremity edema. If it is observed that there is no weight loss, but patients have a good sodium clearance, then the compliance with sodium restriction must be considered and reviewed with the patient. Inpatient treatment is indicated with significant encephalopathy, bacterial infections, or gastrointestinal (GI) hemorrhage. If patients do not have these complications and are steadily losing weight, they may be followed as outpatients. Fluid restriction to 1.5 L/day may be required with development of severe (sodium less than 125 mmol/L) or symptomatic hyponatremia.

In 10% of cases of ascites, patients do not respond to diuretic therapy, reaccumulate fluid rapidly after paracentesis, or have a contraindication to the use of diuretics (encephalopathy, hyponatremia with the fluid restriction, or a creatinine more than 2 mg/dL). Then two other methods are available: serial paracentesis and transjugular intrahepatic portosystemic stent shunt (TIPSS) placement. Large-volume paracentesis is highly effective and should be followed by diuretics, which lengthen the period of reaccumulation of fluid, and should always be accompanied by cell counts to rule out SBP. Circulatory disturbance and hepatorenal syndrome are potential complications that could be prevented by the infusion of 5 to 10 g of albumin for every liter of ascites drained when removing volumes larger than 5 L.

TIPSS is a radiologically placed shunt that relieves portal hypertension by shunting blood between the portal vein and the hepatic vein. TIPSS is effective in approximately 66% of patients with refractory ascites and has the same survival benefit as serial paracentesis with a decrease in the incidence of HRS. TIPSS is recommended when it becomes necessary to draw fluid more than two times in a month or when it is impractical. The major complication of TIPSS is hepatic encephalopathy (up to 60%); thus it should be recommended with caution in those with Child-Pugh class C or in those with a MELD greater than 19. Other requirements for the successful placement of TIPSS is relatively preserved cardiac function without significant elevation of right-sided heart pressures, patency of the portal vein, and the absence of severe hepatic encephalopathy. Liver transplantation is the definitive treatment for refractory ascites and may be considered for all appropriate candidates. Another treatment for patients ineligible for transplant, TIPSS, and serial paracentesis are peritoneovenous shunts, although infection and long-term patency with these remain a problem.

## SPONTANEOUS BACTERIAL PERITONITIS

SBP is the spontaneous proliferation of bacteria in the ascitic fluid in the absence of intra-abdominal source of infection. Hospitalized patients with decompensated cirrhosis have a 10% to 30% chance of having SBP. Once it occurs there is a 20% mortality rate per treated episode (90% if untreated), and SBP recurs in approximately 70% of patients at 1 year. In patients with cirrhosis and ascites, with sudden onset of fever, encephalopathy of unclear etiology, abdominal pain, renal failure, acidosis, or peripheral leukocytosis, there should be high clinical suspicion for SBP, and they should receive immediate antibiotic therapy before the data from the paracentesis and cultures are available. Cirrhotic patients with SBP may also remain clinically silent. All patients with an ascitic fluid with PMN counts above 250/mm³ must receive empirical antibiotic therapy and be tested in their ascitic fluid for total protein, lactate dehydrogenase (LDH), glucose, and Gram stain to differentiate it from secondary peritonitis. Culture-negative neutrocytic ascites are treated as SBP. Blood and urine cultures should be done, and ascitic fluid cultures should always be in blood culture bottles at the patient's bedside. Aerobic gram-negative organisms account for 70% of the cases, with *Escherichia coli* and *Klebsiella* species predominating. Gram-positive cocci are present in 30% of the cases, with streptococci dominating. Anaerobic organisms are rare, and when isolated they should raise the suspicion of secondary peritonitis from a perforated viscus.

The treatments of choice for SBP are the third-generation cephalosporins cefotaxime (Claforan), at a dose of 2 g IV every 8 hours, and ceftriaxone (Rocephin), at 1 g every 12 hours for 5 days. Aminoglycosides should not be used because of increased nephrotoxicity. For atypical presentations a paracentesis should be considered after 48 hours and a PMN count performed again. In SBP, the PMN count should be 50% of its previous level, whereas in other sources of peritonitis, the PMN count may be higher or unchanged. Alternatively, the patient may take oral ofloxacin (Floxin) if the patient has no vomiting, shock, or hemorrhage, has a creatinine of less than 3 mg/dL and no or mild encephalopathy. Albumin infusion at a rate of 1.5 g/kg of body weight within 6 hours after starting antibiotic treatment and readministered on the third day of treatment at 1 g/kg decreases mortality after an episode of SBP. All diuretics should be stopped during infection.

The incidence of recurrent SBP may be reduced by administration of prophylactic antibiotics. Norfloxacin (Noroxin),[1] at 400 mg/day, or trimethoprim-sulfamethoxazole (TMX) (Bactrim), at one double-strength tablet daily for 5 days a week, are indicated for prophylaxis in patients who already had an episode of SBP and those who have ascitic protein levels less than 1 g/dL on diagnostic paracentesis. Norfloxacin prophylaxis has reduced SBP occurrence by 60% and is highly cost effective. Ciprofloxacin (Cipro), at a dose of 750 mg once weekly, is also efficacious. For patients admitted to the hospital for cirrhosis and GI hemorrhage, norfloxacin,[1] at 400 mg twice a day, ofloxacin, 400 mg/day or TMX, one tablet twice a day for 7 days, decreases infection rates and prolongs survival.

## ESOPHAGEAL VARICES

Patients with cirrhosis should be screened for varices when first diagnosed and then every 3 years until found. Refer to the article on esophageal varices in this volume for more information.

## ENCEPHALOPATHY

HE is characterized by neuropsychiatric abnormalities that are primarily caused by nitrogenous products, endogenous ligands for benzodiazepines, and other unknown toxins released by bacteria from the colon that are incompletely metabolized by the cirrhotic liver or bypass the liver because of portal hypertension and portosystemic shunting. HE can develop in 28% of cirrhotic patients within 10 years of the diagnosis of cirrhosis and portal hypertension. Older age and severity of cirrhosis are the only known factors to predict the risk of developing HE. HE has five stages for its severity: Stage 0 is normal or only features abnormal results on psychometric tests, referred to as minimal HE, and stage 4 represents the most severe form with deep coma (Table 5).

Precipitating causes of HE include infection (usually urinary tract, pneumonia, or SBP), renal insufficiency, GI bleed, hypokalemia, excess protein in the diet, use of sedatives such as benzodiazepines and other tranquilizers and sedatives, constipation or noncompliance with lactulose, portal vein thrombosis, further hepatic parenchymal damage, hepatocellular carcinoma, and recent TIPSS placement. When assessing a mental status change in a patient with cirrhosis, other causes of motor and mental disturbance other than hepatic encephalopathy should be investigated. CT of the head must be obtained if there is any neurologic sign concerning an intracranial lesion.

Most cases of HE are preventable, and recognition of the precipitating causes just described will help prevent this complication. Lactulose (Cephulac), at 30 to 60 g/day, titrated to achieve a goal of three to four soft bowel movements a day with a pH less than 6, is effective in 90% of the patients. Lactinol is slightly better tolerated. Excessive use leading to diarrhea is to be avoided because it can lead to prerenal azotemia and other electrolyte imbalances. In patients who have profound HE and are unable to take medications orally, Lactinol and lactulose can be administered via a nasogastric tube or as enemas at a dose of 300 mL in 700 mL of tap water two to three times a day with a response in 4 to 6 hours. Opiate analgesics, calcium, and iron supplements can all exacerbate HE and should be avoided. Also oral nonabsorbable antibiotics such as metronidazole (Flagyl),[1] at 250 mg three times a day, rifaximin (Xifaxan),[1] at 400 mg two to three times a day, and vancomycin (Vancocin),[1] at 2 g/day, can help alleviate HE in the remaining 10% of cases resistant to disaccharides. Because of renal toxicity, neomycin should be avoided. In severe HE, oral intake should be held. In milder forms, protein intake should be titrated by increasing the protein intake by 10 g/day over 3 to 5 days starting from 20 g/day to a maximum dose of 80 g/day depending on individual tolerances. Avoidance of negative nitrogen balance is crucial. An infusion of dextrose helps decrease protein catabolism. For chronic HE, lactulose and moderate protein restriction to 0.8 g/kg/day are recommended.

## HEPATORENAL SYNDROME

Approximately 40% of patients with cirrhosis and ascites will develop HRS within 5 years. This complication occurs when there is avid continuous sodium retention with dilutional hyponatremia and activation of the renin-angiotensin system, in the setting of ineffective arterial blood flow because of splanchnic vasodilation. Initially, renal perfusion is maintained because of renal vasodilatation that is mediated by prostaglandins. With progressive disease, renal vasoconstriction

---

[1]Not FDA approved for this indication.

[1]Not FDA approved for this indication.

**TABLE 5  Grades and Clinical Manifestations of Hepatic Encephalopathy**

| Encephalopathy Grade | Level of Consciousness | Mental Status | Neurologic Signs | EEG Abnormalities |
|---|---|---|---|---|
| 0 | Normal | Normal | None | None |
| Subclinical | Normal | Normal | Psychometric tests may be abnormal | None |
| 1 | Day-night reversal, restlessness | Forgetful, mild confusion, Irritable | Tremor, apraxia, impaired handwriting | Triphasic waves (5 cycles/s) |
| 2 | Lethargy | Disorientation to time, inappropriate behavior | Asterixis, ataxia, dysarthria | Triphasic waves (5 cycles/s) |
| 3 | Somnolent, confused | Disorientation to time, inappropriate behavior | Asterixis, hyperreflexia, Babinski signs | Triphasic waves (5 cycles/s) |
| 4 | Coma | None | Decerebration | Delta activity |

*Abbreviation:* EEG = electroencephalogram.

occurs in response to arterial vasodilation, leading to reduction of renal blood flow and the glomerular filtration rates with subsequent hepatorenal syndrome. A common precipitant of HRS is the use of nonsteroidal anti-inflammatory drugs (NSAIDs). Patients with ascites should scrupulously avoid other nephrotoxic agents such as aminoglycosides. Other precipitants are aggressive use of diuretics with volume depletion, large-volume paracentesis without albumin infusion, SBP, and sepsis. In the diagnosis of HRS, several key criteria are almost always present (Table 6).

There are two clinical types of hepatorenal syndrome, type I and type II. In type I there is a decrease of more than 50% in creatinine clearance to less than 20 mL/minute or a doubling of the creatinine level to more than 2.5 mg/dL in 2 weeks. The prognosis for type I HRS is dismal, with 80% mortality within 2 weeks after diagnosis. Type II is a more progressive form and can evolve into type I. In type II the renal deterioration does not fulfill the criteria for type I and it presents in the form of refractory ascites. Survival is 50% in type II after 6 months.

Clinical management of these patients includes an investigation for a precipitating cause, including infection such as SBP, bacteremia, or catheter-related bacteremia, and appropriate cultures should be sent. Broad-spectrum antibiotics should be started irrespective of proof of infection.

The most successful treatment for HRS is liver transplantation, with survival rates greater than 80% over 1 year. The next most effective treatment for type I HRS is albumin infusion (20 to 40 g/day for 20 days) with concomitant arterial vasoconstrictors. Midodrine (ProAmatine), titrated to 7.5 to 15 mg three times a day for 20 days, to achieve an increase in mean arterial blood pressure of 15 mm Hg in combination with octreotide (Sandostatin),[1] at a dose of 100 to 300 µg subcutaneously three times a day, improves renal function in selected patients with type 1 HRS in small uncontrolled trials. Similarly, terlipressin,[2] a synthetic analogue of vasopressin, infused at 0.5 to 2 mg over 4 to 6 hours for 15 days, increases the glomerular filtration rate (GFR) in up to 75% of the patients. TIPS can improve creatinine clearance and survival in well-selected patients with MELD scores less than 18. It is reasonable in patients not eligible for or awaiting liver transplantation. TIPSS in combination with midodrine, octreotide,[1] and albumin may have some benefit in HRS patients. Type II HRS is treated as refractory ascites in an outpatient setting.

## HEPATOPULMONARY SYNDROME

HPS is defined in patients with cirrhosis as the increase in the alveolar-arterial gradient on room air and the documentation of intrapulmonary vascular dilations, which cause right to left shunting corrected partially by oxygen at 100%. It is associated with spider angiomata and presents as platypnea and orthodeoxia. Diagnosis is confirmed by contrast-enhanced echocardiography or technetium-labeled macroaggregated albumin scanning. The only treatment in highly selected populations is liver transplantation.

## PORTOPULMONARY HYPERTENSION

Portopulmonary hypertension (PPHTN) is characterized by a mean pulmonary artery pressure measured by cardiac catheterization above 25 mm Hg on rest with a pulmonary capillary wedge pressure less than 15 mm Hg, a pulmonary vascular resistance (PVR) greater than 120 dynes/second/cm-5, and the presence of portal hypertension without any other secondary cause of pulmonary hypertension. Clinical manifestations are similar to those with primary PHTN. Treatment with calcium channel blockers is indicated if the patient has more than 20% reduction in mPAP during the trial with vasodilators on cardiac catheterization. Bosentan (Tracleer), at 62.5 mg per day for 4 weeks, increased thereafter to 125 mg daily, improves symptoms and exercise capacity. Preoperatively, Epoprostenol (Flolan) is given at 10 to 28 µg/kg/mm³ for a few months to decrease the mPAP to levels acceptable for liver transplantation. Liver transplantation may reverse minor or moderate degrees of pulmonary hypertension but is contraindicated in patients with pulmonary hypertension above 40 to 45 mm Hg because of high postoperative mortality related to cardiac failure.

## HEPATOCELLULAR CARCINOMA

Patients with cirrhosis, regardless of etiology, have an increased risk for the development of HCC. An estimated 10% to 15% of patients with

---

[1]Not FDA approved for this indication.

---

**TABLE 6  Diagnostic Criteria for Hepatorenal Syndrome as Proposed by the International Ascites Club**

1. Serum creatinine >1.5 mg/dL indicating low glomerular filtration rate
2. Exclusion of shock, volume depletion, bacterial infection, nephrotoxic drugs
3. Failure to improve with discontinuing diuretics, volume expansion with 1.5 L normal saline
4. No evidence of proteinuria, obstruction, parenchymal renal disease

---

[1]Not FDA approved for this indication.
[2]Not available in the United States.

cirrhosis develop HCC after 10 years of diagnosis with a median survival of 6 to 20 months. Selected patients who successfully undergo orthotopic liver transplantation (OLT) for HCC have survival rates equal to those without HCC.

Screening for HCC is best accomplished by measuring serum alpha fetoprotein (AFP) and abdominal US every 6 months. Because of a sensitivity ranging between 20% and 65% (depending on the cutoff value), AFP is not proven to improve the outcome in cirrhotics from HCC. The positive predictive value for AFP levels above 20 or for a suspicious lesion on ultrasound is low; therefore imaging with triple-phase helical CT, MRI, or magnetic resonance angiography is indicated if any one of these two situations is present. These imaging modalities can reliably diagnose HCC if tumors are greater than 2 cm and there is an arterial enhancing lesion seen on two of the imaging tests just cited or seen on one test with an AFP level above 400 µg/mL. In these cases a biopsy is not required. Suspicious lesions between 1 and 2 cm should be biopsied by fine-needle aspiration (FNA), which does not worsen the outcome from tumor seeding along the needle tack, and tumors less than 1 cm should be monitored by repeat scanning every 3 months until they grow above 1 cm. Des-gamma-carboxy prothrombin (DCP) and lectin reactive AFP (AFP-L3)-to-AFP ratio are tumor markers that are measured alone or in combination with AFP and can increase the sensitivity and specificity of HCC screening.

Treatment of HCC is approached in an algorithmic fashion with surgery the ultimate goal because it is the only curative treatment. A tumor is resectable when it is confined to the liver and shows no vascular invasion and no portal hypertension. Size alone should not influence the decision. General performance of the patient, tumor stage, and assessment of liver function determine if the procedure is practical (Child's class A) or not (Child's class B/C). Prior to resection, a search for metastatic disease should be undertaken. Ninety percent of cirrhotic patients with HCC have decompensation of their cirrhosis, which contraindicates surgical resection. With earlier detection of HCC there is greater likelihood of successful outcomes with transplantation. To be a candidate for liver transplantation, the patient must have no vascular invasion, no metastatic disease, no lymphatic spread, and no more than three suspected lesions in the liver. If there are multiple lesions in the liver, all must be less than 3 cm in diameter; if only one lesion is present, it must be less than 5 cm in diameter. A major drawback of liver transplantation is long waiting times for cadaveric donor matching.

Other alternative therapies include chemoembolization, ethanol or acetic acid injection into the tumor, radiofrequency ablation, and irradiation with intra-arterial yttrium-tagged microspheres. All patients should be considered candidates for some kind of intervention. These therapies should be considered palliative, although survival for radiofrequency ablation and percutaneous ethanol injection may approach survival in surgical resection for tumors less than 3 cm. Any approach can be considered in nonresectable tumors depending on the team preferences and/or local expertise. Chemotherapy is only indicated in the context of a clinical trial.

Prevention of the development of HCC is also possible: Hepatitis B vaccine has decreased the incidence of HCC by a third in highly infected areas. Also in clinical trials for the treatment of chronic hepatitis C with interferon-based therapies, studies have suggested that patients with compensated liver cirrhosis, whether or not they have a sustained response, may have reduction of their risk of HCC.

## Other Considerations

### VACCINATION

Hepatitis A and B vaccines should be given to all patients with chronic liver disease who are found to be nonimmune to these viruses. Pneumonia and SBP because of streptococcal pneumonia are very common in cirrhotic patients; thus all patients in this population should receive a single dose of the polyvalent pneumococcal vaccine. An annual injection of the influenza vaccine protects against influenza.

## LIVER TRANSPLANTATION

Liver transplantation (LT) is the definitive treatment for a variety of irreversible problems associated with chronic liver disease. Patients with Child's class B, and those with complications from cirrhosis such as refractory ascites, variceal bleeding, and any other condition that is irreversible and progressive should be referred early for liver transplantation evaluation. HRS type 1 and HPS should expedite the referral for transplantation. The MELD score was developed to replace the Child-Pugh score as a disease severity score. A score of more than 10 is an indication for referral to a transplantation center. The MELD score (for calculation, visit www.unos.org/resources/MeldPeldCalculator.asp?index=98) is designed to improve the organ allocation system, so that available organs are directed to patients based on the severity of their liver disease rather than on the total time on the waiting list. Contraindications for liver transplantation depend on the local approach, but universal contraindications are high perioperative risk (e.g., severe cardiac failure), uncontrolled malignancies within the previous 5 years, and active alcohol or drug abuse. LT offers an overall 5-year survival rate of greater than 60% to 70%.

### REFERENCES

Boyer TD, Haskal ZJ: The role of transjugular intrahepatic portosystemic shunt in the management of portal hypertension. Hepatology 2005;41:386-400.

Cardenas A, Gines P: Management of complications of cirrhosis in patients awaiting liver transplantation. J Hepatology 2005;42:S124-S133.

Czaja AJ, Freese DK: Diagnosis and treatment of autoimmune hepatitis. Hepatology 2002;36:479-497.

D'Amico G, Luca A, Morabito A, et al: Uncovered transjugular intrahepatic portosystemic shunt for refractory ascites: A meta-analysis. Gastroenterology 2005;129:1282-1293.

Levitsky J, Mailliard ME: Diagnosis and therapy of alcoholic liver disease. Semin Liver Dis 2004;24:233-247.

Moore KP, Wong F, Gines P, et al: The management of ascites in cirrhosis: Report on the consensus conference of the International Ascites Club. Hepatology 2003;38:258-266.

Murray KF, Carithers RL Jr: AASLD Practice Guidelines: Evaluation of the patient for liver transplantation. Hepatology 2005;41:1407-1432.

Runyon BA: Management of adult patients with ascites due to cirrhosis. Hepatology 2004;39:841-856.

Sanyal AJ: AGA technical review on nonalcoholic fatty liver disease. Gastroenterology 2002;123:1705-1725.

Tavill AS: Diagnosis and management of hemochromatosis. Hepatology 2001;33:1321-1328.

# Bleeding Esophageal Varices

Method of
*Gary C. Chen, MD, and Rome Jutabha, MD*

Esophageal variceal bleeding, which is a consequence of portal hypertension, is one of the most dreadful complications of liver cirrhosis. It accounts for approximately one third of diagnoses in patients presenting with upper gastrointestinal (GI) bleeding. Despite the significant advances and improvements in the early diagnosis and treatment for esophageal variceal bleeding, the mortality rate of first episode of esophageal variceal bleeding remains very high (20% to 35%). In patients with liver cirrhosis, the prevalence of esophageal varices is approximately 60%, but newer studies with better endoscopic assessment and longer periods of follow-up suggested the prevalence could be as high as 80% to 90%. Cirrhotic patients with esophageal varices without previous variceal bleeding have a 25% to 40% chance of first variceal hemorrhage when they do not receive effective prophylactic treatment. The risk of first variceal bleeding is significantly related to the patient's Child-Pugh class, the size and wall thickness of the varices, the presence of red markings of varices observed at the time of endoscopy, and the hepatic venous pressure gradient (HVPG) or intravariceal pressure. Management of patients with esophageal varices includes prevention of the first bleeding episode (primary prophylaxis), control of actively bleeding esophageal varices, and the prevention of recurrent esophageal variceal bleeding (secondary prophylaxis).

The Child-Pugh classification system is a scoring index of liver dysfunction in cirrhotic patients (Table 1). This classification is based on the measurement of serum bilirubin level, serum albumin level, prothrombin time, and the presence of ascitic fluids and encephalopathy. For example, a patient with Child-Pugh class C cirrhosis who has red marking on large-size varices has an estimated 60% likelihood of variceal bleeding over a 2-year span. In contrast, a patient with Child-Pugh class A cirrhosis, no or small size varices, and esophageal varices without red markings would be at a much lower risk of developing variceal bleeding.

Elevated pressure within the portal venous system also increases the risk of variceal bleeding. Normal portal vein pressure is less than 10 mm Hg because the vascular resistance in the hepatic sinusoids is low. An elevated portal venous pressure distends the veins proximal to the site of the block and increases capillary pressure in organs drained by the obstructed veins. The HVPG is used to directly and accurately measure the portal venous pressure. This measurement is obtained by using a pressure-sensitive balloon-tipped catheter usually inserted via the transjugular route to measure pressures within the hepatic veins. The HVPG can serve as an important factor for predicting variceal bleeding. Normal HVPG is 2 to 6 mm Hg. Patients with HVPG greater than 12 mm Hg are considered having portal hypertension. A study that followed 87 patients with cirrhosis and large-size esophageal varices but without previous history of bleeding esophageal varices over a 1-year period found that 72% of the patients with HVPG greater than 16 mm Hg developed variceal bleeding. However, in patients who have presinusoidal portal hypertension such as portal or splenic vein thrombosis and schistosomiasis, HVPG can underestimate the portal venous pressure. Furthermore, measurement of the HVPG requires an invasive technique; hence, it is not commonly adopted in the clinical setting.

Nonetheless, the combination of these clinical predictors can be used to classify a patient's risk of developing bleeding esophageal varices. The mortality rate of patients with bleeding esophageal varices is 20% to 30% within 1 year after the initially hemorrhagic episode. Furthermore, there is a 70% chance of a second episode of bleeding from esophageal varices in patients who have had an episode of variceal bleeding within 1 year of the bleeding episode if left untreated. In other words, once a patient develops variceal bleeding, the risks of recurrent variceal bleeding and mortality increase. Therefore, it is logical to screen for and offer the high-risk cirrhotic patients safe and effective medical or endoscopic treatments to prevent the first episode of esophageal variceal bleeding.

## TABLE 1  Child-Pugh Classification System of Liver Disease Severity Index

| Parameter | Points | | |
|---|---|---|---|
| | 1 | 2 | 3 |
| Serum bilirubin, mg/dL | ≤ 2 | 2–3 | > 3 |
| Serum albumin, g/dL | > 3.5 | 2.8–3.5 | < 2.8 |
| Prothrombin, sec | 1–3 | 4–6 | > 6 |
| Ascites | Absent | Slight | Moderate |
| Encephalopathy | None | Grade 1–2 | Grade 3–4 |

5–6 points = Grade A (compensated liver disease, 1-year survival is 100%).
7–9 points = Grade B (significantly functional compromised liver disease, 1-year survival is 80%).
10–15 points = Grade C (decompensated liver disease, 1-year survival is 45%).

# Acute Bleeding From Esophageal Varices

Bleeding esophageal varices is one of the common causes of upper GI hemorrhage. It accounts for an estimated one third of diagnoses in patients presenting with upper GI bleeding. In 1985 the diagnosis of bleeding esophageal varices accounted for approximately 62,000 total hospital days in nonfederal, short-stay hospitals in the United States and was without a doubt the most expensive of all GI disorders in terms of average daily cost of hospitalization ($1091/day). Patients with bleeding esophageal varices tend to present with hematemesis and melena. Often there is evidence of large amount volume of bleeding because the high portal pressures precipitate the rupture of esophageal varices. Relevant history of chronic liver disease and thorough physical examination yielding the stigmata of liver cirrhosis can help guide clinicians toward the correct diagnosis. However, clinicians must remember that although esophageal varices are the most common cause of upper GI bleeding in cirrhotic patients requiring emergent endoscopy, peptic ulcer disease, gastric varices, Mallory-Weiss tears, and portal hypertensive gastropathy are also frequent causes of upper GI bleeding in this group of patients. In patients with active bleeding esophageal varices, only approximately half of the patients stop bleeding spontaneously, which is significantly lower than other forms of upper GI bleeding. In addition, more than 50% of the patients will have recurrent bleeding within the first week of the initial bleeding episode.

Because bleeding esophageal varices is a life-threatening medical emergency, patients with bleeding esophageal varices require immediate medical attention with admission to the hospital. All patients with hemodynamic instability (shock, orthostatic hypotension, decrease in hematocrit of at least 6%, or transfusion requirement more than 2 units of packed red blood cell (RBCs) or active bleeding (manifested by hematemesis, bright red blood per nasogastric tube, or hematochezia) should be admitted to the intensive care unit for resuscitation and close monitoring with automated blood pressure monitoring, ECG monitoring, and pulse oximetry. Because signs such as hypotension and/or tachycardia are often found in the patient, hemodynamic resuscitation is the vital first step in the treatment process. Endotracheal intubation should be considered for the severely encephalopathic, uncooperative, or unconscious patient, if the airway could be compromised, to provide adequate ventilation and prevent aspiration. Nasogastric or orogastric tube lavage should be performed to remove particulate matter, fresh blood, and clots to facilitate anticipated endoscopy examination and to decrease the risk of aspiration. Two large-bore intravenous (IV) catheters that are at least 18 gauge in size should be established. For hypotensive patients the IV catheters should be running wide open; and a central catheter should be established as well, in case pressor medications need to be initiated. It is important to remember that the initial hematocrit level poorly reflects the degree of blood loss if the bleeding is acute. Therefore, estimating the patient's volume loss could be more useful in assessing an acutely bleeding patient. Blood loss should be aggressively replaced by packed RBCs to maintain hematocrit above 30%. Patient's hemoglobin and hematocrit should be followed every 2 to 6 hours depending on the status of the patient. Platelet count should be kept above 50,000/mm³ while the patient is actively bleeding. Desmopressin acetate (DDAVP), which is a synthetic analogue of vasopressin, can be considered in patients with concurrent renal failure in which uremia can lead to platelet dysfunction. End-stage liver disease patients often have at least some degree of coagulopathy, so transfusion of clotting factors with fresh frozen plasma should be performed if necessary. The goal is to maintain international normalized ratio (INR) less than 1.5 in these patients. Small-scale studies have suggested that recombinant human factor VIIa could assist in the treatment of coagulopathy by enhancing the normalization of serum prothrombin time. Subcutaneous (SC) administration of vitamin K can be considered if the patient is at risk for vitamin K deficiency, if the bleeding episode does not stop acutely, or if the patient has abnormal prothrombin time. It should be given at 5 to 10 mg SC/day. Three doses of vitamin K administration should adequately replenish a patient's vitamin K supply. It is also important to hold all nonsteroidal anti-inflammatory medications, anticoagulants, sucralfate, antacids, iron supplements, and food during the bleeding episode.

A synthetic and long-acting analogue of somatostatin, IV octreotide should be given if bleeding esophageal varices is suspected to assist in the reduction of portal venous pressure by indirectly causing splanchnic vasoconstriction and decreased portal flow. It can stop variceal bleeding in up to 80% of the cases. Intravenous octreotide is given as an initial 50 μg bolus followed by continuous infusion of 50 μg/hour. A higher dose of octreotide does not appear to further the lowering of portal venous pressure and perhaps could lead to elevation of systemic venous pressure. Its safety profile is generally excellent with abdominal discomfort and elevated serum glucose that can occasionally occur in patients receiving this medication. Intravenous vasopressin is an alternative medication that reduces portal pressure by directly constricting the mesenteric arterioles and decreasing portal venous inflow. It is administered by an IV bolus of 0.4 U followed by 0.4 to 0.8 U/minute infusions. Unfortunately, vasopressin is associated with potential serious side effects including myocardial, bowel, and limb ischemia because of its systemic vasoconstrictive effects. Administering nitroglycerin by IV is recommended concurrently along with vasopressin to counter the vasopressin-induced systemic vasoconstriction effect. It is administered at a rate of 10 to 40 μg/minute. We use octreotide over vasopressin in the setting of acute bleeding esophageal varices because of the lower risk of adverse events. The optimal duration of octreotide or vasopressin is unclear, but we recommend either drug to be continued for 2 to 3 days after the esophageal variceal bleeding episode is adequately controlled. Because patients with bleeding esophageal varices are at risk of having concurrent peptic ulcer disease or developing stress-induced peptic ulcers, administration of proton pump inhibitor medication is also recommended.

Another important aspect of managing this group of patients is to prevent and decrease the impact of complications associated with bleeding esophageal varices. A patient likely could achieve hemostasis but only to succumb to the associated complications such as infections including aspiration pneumonia, bacterial peritonitis, urinary tract infection, sepsis; hepatic encephalopathy; and renal failure because of acute tubular necrosis or hepatorenal syndrome. Cirrhotic patients who are hospitalized with a GI hemorrhage tend to be at high risk for developing infections. Therefore, it is reasonable to provide prophylactic antibiotic coverage in this group of patients. Most experts tend to use a fluoroquinolone class antibiotic such as ciprofloxacin or levofloxacin for 5 to 7 days total, initially administered by IV and followed by oral route. However, physicians should take the local patterns of antibiotic resistance into consideration when choosing the antibiotic regimen. Furthermore, it is important to elevate the head of the patient's bed to more than 30 degrees to decrease the risk of aspiration. Hepatic encephalopathy should be treated with lactulose to induce three loose bowel movements each day. Close monitoring of the stool output of patients with hepatic encephalopathy is important because too much watery diarrhea from lactulose can deplete these patients intravascularly, whereas too few bowel movements can worsen the encephalopathy. In terms of renal failure, it can be minimized by adequate hydration of the patient as well as avoidance of nephrotoxic drugs.

Esophagogastrodudenoscopic therapy is the definitive treatment of choice for bleeding esophageal varices; therefore, this procedure should be performed once the patient is hemodynamically stable for endoscopy exam. Endoscopy is also highly sensitive and specific for locating and identifying bleeding lesions in the upper GI tract. Modern endoscopic therapies can achieve hemostasis in up to 90% of the cases. Combining endoscopic and pharmacologic therapies has made great strides in decreasing the mortality of esophageal variceal bleeding. A complete and thorough endoscopic examination is necessary to rule out other etiologies of upper GI hemorrhage. Bleeding esophageal varices are confirmed on endoscopy if there is active bleeding from esophageal varices, a platelet plug is found on the surface of the varix, or varices are present and no other source of hemorrhage is found. Two types of endoscopic treatments can be carried out: endoscopic band ligation (Figure 1) and endoscopic sclerotherapy (Figure 2), with endoscopic band ligation as the recommended treatment option. Endoscopic band ligation is carried out by placing elastic rubber bands around the esophageal varices located in the distal portion of

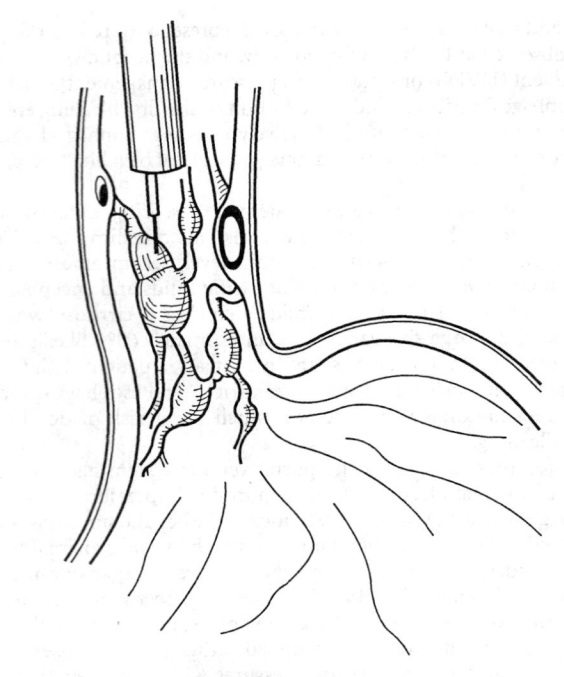

**FIGURE 1.** Endoscopic band ligation performed with a flexible endoscope. A varix is aspirated into the device using endoscopic suction and ensnared with an elastic band. (From Schaefer J. In GI/Liver Secrets. Philadelphia, Hanley and Belfus, 1996, p 355. Reprinted with permission.)

the esophagus. Endoscopic sclerotherapy involves the injection of a form of sclerosant into the esophageal varices. Both types of treatment measures have similar efficacy in terms of achieving hemostasis, but one study suggested band ligation has better long-term outcome. Sclerotherapy's advantages are that it is easy to use, more widely available, and a less costly procedure to perform. However, endoscopic band ligation is the preferred method mainly because it has lower risk of procedural associated complications. The potential complications of endoscopic sclerotherapy include local ulceration or bleeding, esophageal stricture formation, esophageal perforation, mediastinitis,

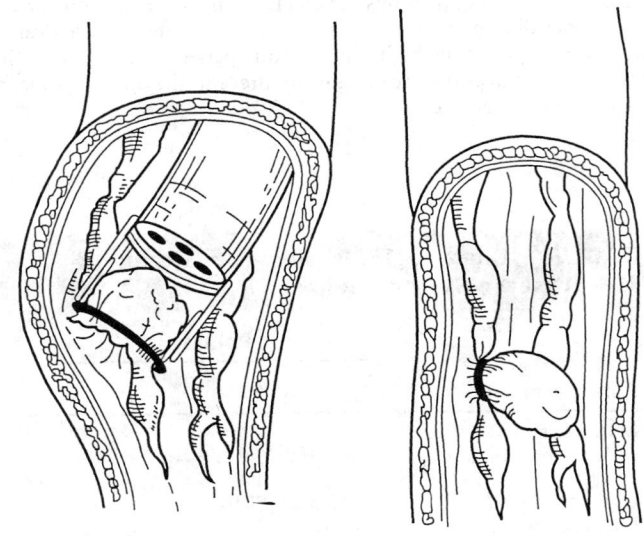

**FIGURE 2.** Endoscopic sclerotherapy performed with a flexible endoscope. A flexible injection needle is used to inject sclerosant into the varix. (From Schaefer J. In GI/Liver Secrets. Philadelphia, Hanley and Belfus, 1996, p 355. Reprinted with permission.)

and aspiration pneumonia. However, some endoscopists still prefer endoscopic sclerotherapy because of the ability to visualize bleeding sites, and because the application of band ligation can sometimes make the endoscopic field difficult to visualize. Endoscopists should also evaluate whether the patient has evidence of portal hypertensive gastropathy, because both treatments could potentially worsen this condition and increase the risk of bleeding from the stomach.

Unfortunately, emergent endoscopic therapy fails to control acute esophageal variceal bleeding in 15% to 20% of patients. Furthermore, early rebleeding can occur after a bleeding-free period of at least 24 hours. In these circumstances the patient may require a transjugular intrahepatic portosystemic shunt (TIPS) or, in rare cases, surgical intervention to decrease portal venous pressure to control bleeding. The TIPS procedure is performed by inserting an expandable wire mesh stent into the hepatic vein via the jugular vein and advancing to the intrahepatic part of the hepatic vein, creating a portosystemic shunt from the portal vein to the hepatic vein without the need for general anesthesia or major surgery. In 80% to 90% of the patients, TIPS can control acute bleeding esophageal varices. However, there is a 30% increased risk of developing new or worsening hepatic encephalopathy after placement of TIPS. In addition it could precipitate liver failure in the patient. Hence, TIPS should solely be reserved for patients who have failed pharmacologic and endoscopic therapies. There are two main types of emergent surgical interventions available: portosystemic shunt surgery and devascularization procedures such as distal esophageal transection. They both seem effective in controlling bleeding. However, both types of surgical procedures require experienced surgeons, have a wide variety of complications, and have high intraoperative and postoperative mortality rates.

Another option for patients who are unresponsive to endoscopic and pharmacologic therapies is balloon tamponade, which is a temporary measure to control acute hemorrhage. Sengstaken-Blakemore and Minnesota tubes are the most common types of balloons used in practice. Balloon tamponade can provide temporary cessation of active bleeding in 30% to 90% of the cases, with rebleeding occurring in 50% of the cases after the balloon is deflated. The balloon typically has three parts: a gastric balloon, an esophageal balloon, and a gastric suction port. Once the tube is inserted into the patient, the gastric balloon is inflated first, once the tube reaches the stomach, and drawn up against the gastroesophageal junction and secured in place. If this maneuver still does not control bleeding, the esophageal balloon is inflated with tension applied to the tube to directly tamponade the esophageal varices. A nasogastric tube should be placed concurrent with this procedure to prevent tracheal aspiration. This procedure requires experienced endoscopists to perform, because it is associated with significant complications including esophageal rupture, esophageal perforation, local ulceration, tracheal aspiration, and accidentally misplacing the tube into the airway. Given the high risk of complications, patients should have endotracheal intubation and mechanical ventilation support before undergoing the balloon tamponade procedure. Balloon tamponade should only be a temporary measure, and patients should have TIPS or surgical interventions performed as soon as possible (Figure 3).

## Prevention of Recurrent Esophageal Variceal Bleeding

A history of bleeding esophageal varices is the best predictor of future esophageal variceal bleeding. The risk of rebleeding is 60% to 70% without further therapy after the initial bleeding episode is controlled. The risk of rebleeding is the highest in the first 6 weeks after cessation of active bleeding. The clinical predictors used to classify a patient's risk of developing initial bleeding esophageal varices mentioned earlier can also be used to predict the risk of recurrent bleeding. Therefore, secondary prophylaxis is important to decrease the risk of rebleeding. Several treatment options are available to prevent recurrent bleeding including pharmacologic, endoscopic, surgical, TIPS, and orthotopic liver transplantation. Nonselective β-blockers such as nadolol and propranolol can decrease portal pressure and variceal blood flow. Patients who can tolerate nonselective β-blockers may start propranolol at 20 mg twice a day, or nadolol at 40 mg once a day, gradually titrating the

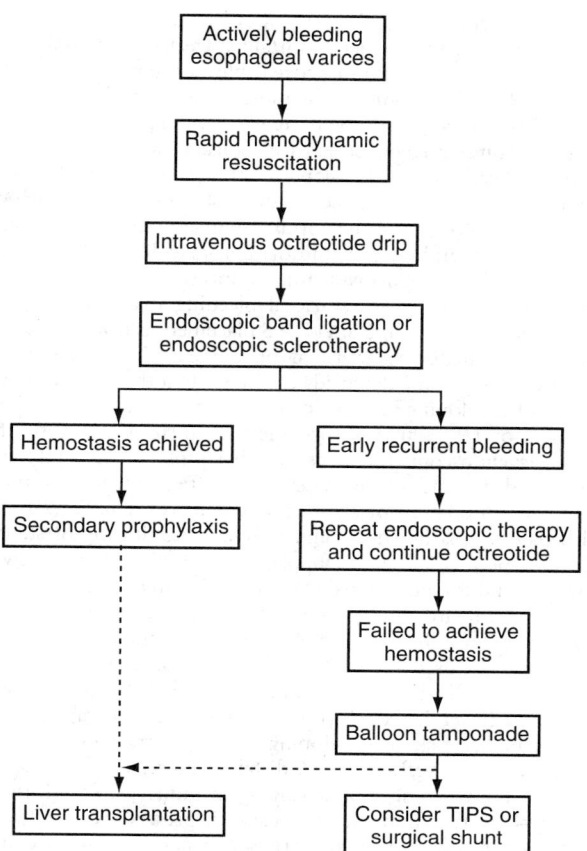

**FIGURE 3.** Recommended algorithm for the management of acute bleeding esophageal varices. TIPS = transjugular intrahepatic portosystemic shunt.

medication dosage up until heart rate decreases by 20% to 30% or reaches 55 to 60 beats per minute. Nadolol has the advantage of being once-a-day dosing, because patient compliance can be an issue in some cirrhotic patients; however, it is a more expensive medication and less widely available. Titrating the dosage of nonselective β-blockers based on the HVPG has been evaluated by studies and appeared more effective than titration of the dosage based on heart rate alone. Unfortunately, adverse side effects and poor compliance are significant problems in achieving sustained benefit with the nonselective β-blockers. Long-acting nitrates such as isosorbide mononitrate also reduce portal pressure, but no study has demonstrated that it can decrease recurrent bleeding or mortality as a monotherapy. The mechanism of nitrates appears to be its ability to cause a decrease in outflow resistance in the portal system. Combining nonselective β-blockers and long-acting nitrates has been more effective and better tolerated than using nonselective β-blockers alone to reduce recurrent bleeding.

Endoscopic band ligation is the treatment of choice at most institutes to prevent recurrent esophageal variceal bleeding. Endoscopic band ligation appears to be at least as equally effective as sclerotherapy in preventing recurrence of bleeding and has a better complication profile. Serial endoscopic band ligation treatments are performed on an outpatient basis at 14-day intervals until varices in the distal esophagus are obliterated. Achieving complete obliteration usually requires three to four endoscopy sessions, after which follow-up endoscopy should be performed every 3 to 6 months to evaluate for any recurring varices. The main downside of band ligation is that small varices can be difficult to band and might be hard to obliterate with this technique. Patients treated with endoscopic band ligation alone have approximately 20% to 40% risk of rebleeding from the esophageal varices. However, if sclerotherapy is performed, it should be repeated 3 to 7 days after the initial session, followed by sessions at 1 to 2 weeks until all varices are completely obliterated. Treatment with sclerotherapy can reduce the risk of recurrent bleeding by 50% at 1 year, but data have not shown its ability to reduce patient mortality. Treatment combining endoscopic band ligation and nonselective β-blockers has an estimated 25% chance of rebleeding. Combination of nonselective β-blockers and sclerotherapy does not appear to be more effective than sclerotherapy alone. Whether combining nonselective β-blockers with long-acting nitrates is more effective than endoscopic therapy in decreasing the risk of rebleeding is still to be determined by future studies.

Procedures that decompress the portal system are recommended in patients who failed endoscopic and/or pharmacologic therapies. Transjugular intrahepatic portosystemic shunt is more effective at preventing recurrent esophageal variceal bleeding than endoscopic therapies. The risk of rebleeding after TIPS placement is 8% to 18% at 1 year. It also eliminates the risks of operative and postoperative complications. However, the downside of TIPS is that there is the 30% increased risk of developing new or worsening hepatic encephalopathy after placement of TIPS. Furthermore, there is no survival benefit of using TIPS over endoscopic therapies. Another problem with TIPS is that stenosis and dysfunction of the shunt are frequent. As a result, endoscopic balloon dilation or stent replacement is often needed to re-establish patency of the shunt, and frequent monitoring of stent patency is often performed using Doppler ultrasound. Unfortunately, Doppler ultrasound is neither sensitive nor specific in detecting shunt patency. All these potential problems of TIPS can lead to a significantly higher amount of overall cost. Therefore, given all these considerations, TIPS should be used as a bridge to liver transplantation.

Rebleeding occurs in 10% to 20% of patients treated with surgical shunts, which is lower in comparison to endoscopic therapies but also carries a higher risk of developing new or worsening hepatic encephalopathy. Selective shunts (e.g., distal splenorenal shunt) have lower risk of hepatic encephalopathy than nonselective shunts (e.g., portacaval interposition shunt) because it preserves better liver function. However, selective shunts are somewhat less effective in preventing rebleeding. Yet, although nonselective shunts are more effective at decompressing the portal system, it is associated with higher risk of operative and postoperative complications. Decompressive surgical shunt procedures tend to be considered in noncompliant patients, patients who are ineligible for liver transportation, Child-Pugh A and B patients, and for patients who have failed endoscopic therapies. Selective shunt is the preferred method of the two types of shunt surgeries; the nonselective shunt should only be considered in emergency situations in the hands of an experienced surgeon. Nonetheless, the choice of surgical treatment should be individualized with consideration of the surgeon's expertise, patient compliance, and severity of cirrhosis in the patient.

Of course, the best and ultimate treatment option for cirrhotic patients with history of bleeding esophageal varices is liver transplantation. Every cirrhotic patient should be evaluated for liver transplant eligibility. Nonetheless, most of the patients with Child-Pugh A and B can be managed with the treatment measures discussed earlier until liver diseases further deteriorate, whereas more severe patients should be treated adequately to control esophageal variceal bleeding in the pretransplant phase. Clinicians should follow all patients with cirrhosis closely, and patient compliance issues should be emphasized.

## Primary Prophylaxis for Bleeding Esophageal Varices

The annual risk of cirrhotic patients developing varices is approximately 6%. Because of the high mortality rate from bleeding esophageal varices, prevention of the initial bleeding episode is desirable. Therefore, endoscopy screening looking for evidence of esophageal varices is often recommended. We recommend endoscopic screening for the following subgroups of patients: all newly diagnosed cirrhotic patients and all other cirrhotic patients who are medically stable, motivated and willing to be treated prophylactically, and would benefit from medical or endoscopic therapies. Patients who are unlikely to benefit from prophylactic treatments and those with short life expectancy should be excluded from screening endoscopy. Low-risk cirrhotic patients, such as the ones that have no or small esophageal varices, may not require prophylactic treatment and a repeat screening endoscopy may be performed in 2 years. The newly developed PillCam ESO video capsule endoscope (Given Diagnostic System, Yoqneam, Israel) is equipped with miniature cameras on both ends, is approximately the size of a multivitamin, and takes approximately 20 minutes to perform with little patient discomfort; it might be a useful screening tool for monitoring esophageal varices in the near future. Study has already demonstrated PillCam ESO video capsule endoscope to be a sensitive diagnostic modality for visualization of esophageal mucosal pathology and may provide an effective method to evaluate patients for esophageal disease.

Both pharmacologic and endoscopic treatments are available for primary prophylaxis for bleeding esophageal varices. The aim in using pharmacologic therapy in this setting is, again, to reduce portal pressure and, in turn, intravariceal pressure. Nonselective β-blockers and long-acting nitrates are the main categories of medications that have been used for this purpose. In most randomized studies of prophylactic β-blocker therapy compared with control, β-blockers decreased the risk of first esophageal variceal hemorrhage and the risk of death associated with GI bleeding. In a meta-analysis of nine randomized trials comparing prophylactic β-blockers with no active treatment (i.e., placebo) to prevent first esophageal variceal bleeding, the incidence of bleeding was significantly reduced with β-blocker therapy versus control. This effect was more pronounced in patients with large- or medium-sized varices or in those with varices and an HVPG greater than 12 mm Hg. However, adverse side effects and poor compliance were significant problems in achieving sustained benefit with β-blockers. Nevertheless, prophylactic therapy with propranolol or nadolol is the standard of care for the prevention of a first esophageal variceal bleeding episode. Combination therapy with propranolol and long-acting nitrate such as isosorbide mononitrate may be superior to using β-blocker alone in the primary prevention of variceal bleeding. Unfortunately, because many patients with advanced cirrhosis often have blood pressure on the lower side, it can be difficult for them to tolerate both β-blocker and nitrate at the same time. Because of the potential to cause systemic vasodilation, nitrates should not be used as monotherapy in cirrhotic patients.

However, endoscopic band ligation is an effective endoscopic treatment of active variceal bleeding and secondary prevention of esophageal variceal bleeding. A recent randomized study compared endoscopic band ligation and propranolol to prevent initial variceal

---

**CURRENT DIAGNOSIS**

- Esophageal varices commonly occur in cirrhotic patients because of portal hypertension.
- A significant portion of patients with esophageal varices will develop upper GI bleeding episodes that can lead to a high mortality rate if left untreated.
- The diagnosis of esophageal varices is established by upper endoscopy but the recently developed PillCam ESO video capsule endoscope has the potential to perform rapid screening measure.

*Abbreviation:* GI = gastrointestinal.

---

**CURRENT THERAPY**

- Hemodynamic resuscitation is the first step that needs to be performed in patients with actively bleeding esophageal varices.
- Combination therapy with pharmacologic and endoscopic treatments should be performed in patients with acute bleeding esophageal varices.
- Primary prophylaxis and secondary prophylaxis are important objectives in preventing initial bleeding episode and recurrent bleeding, respectively.

hemorrhage in cirrhotics with high-risk esophageal varices and concluded that prophylactic propranolol had a significantly higher treatment-failure rate than endoscopic banding. This study also concluded that propranolol was not significantly safer than banding but was associated with arithmetically more frequent severe adverse events requiring discontinuation of therapy. The direct costs of the propranolol group were not significantly less than banding. Therefore, the results of this study suggested that prophylactic banding seems to be a more promising treatment than propranolol for preventing initial variceal bleeding for compliant patients who are at high risk of initial variceal hemorrhage and who are candidates for liver transplantation. So, endoscopic band ligation perhaps should be considered as frontline for the primary prophylaxis of bleeding esophageal varices. No studies have addressed the efficacy of the effectiveness in preventing initial variceal bleeding of combining endoscopic band ligation with β-blocker treatment. Primary prophylaxis with sclerotherapy leads to a higher mortality rate than placebo or β-blocker therapy and should not be performed.

## Conclusions

Bleeding esophageal varices occurs frequently in cirrhotic patients and can lead to significant mortality, disability, productivity, and costs. Because of the poor outcomes that can result once the initial bleeding episode occurs, primary prophylaxis should be carried out. It is the responsibility of clinicians to screen out the patients at risk of developing and having esophageal varices. For patients who already had a bleeding episode, secondary prophylaxis is vital in preventing future bleeds. At the present moment, combination therapies appear to be more effective for the prevention and treatment of bleeding esophageal varices. However, patient education and awareness are also important objectives that clinicians must not forget.

### REFERENCES

Brown DM, Everhart JE: Cost of digestive diseases in the United States. In Everhart JE (ed.): Digestive Diseases in the United States: Epidemiology and Impact. US Department of Health and Human Services, Public Health Service, National Institutes of Health, National Institute of Diabetes and Digestive and Kidney Diseases. (NIH Publication no. 94–1447.57–82). Washington, DC, US Government Printing Office, 1994.

Ejlersen E, Melsen T, Ingerslev J, et al: Recombinant activated factor VII (rFVIIa) acutely normalizes prothrombin time in patients with cirrhosis during bleeding from oesophageal varices. Scand J Gastroenterol 2001; 36:1081.

Eliakim R, Sharma VK, Yassin K. A prospective study of the diagnostic accuracy of PillCam ESO esophageal capsule endoscopy versus conventional upper endoscopy in patients with chronic gastroesophageal reflux diseases. J Clin Gastroenterol 2005;39:572-578.

Everhart JE: Overview. In Everhart JE (ed.): Digestive diseases in the United States: Epidemiology and Impact. US Department of Health and Human Services, Public Health Service, National Institutes of Health, National Institute of Diabetes and Digestive and Kidney Diseases. (NIH Publication no. 94–1447.3–53). Washington, DC, US Government Printing Office, 1994.

Imperiale TF, McCullough AJ: Prophylactic beta-blocker therapy: Clinical implications of an aggregate analysis. Hepatology 1992;15:354-356.

Jutabha R, Jensen DM, Martin P: Randomized study comparing banding and propranolol to prevent initial variceal hemorrhage in cirrhotics with high-risk esophageal varices. Gastroenterology 2005;128:870-881.

Kovacs TOG, Jensen DM: Therapeutic endoscopy for upper gastrointestinal bleeding. In Taylor MB, Gollan J, Peppercorn MA, et al (eds.): Gastrointestinal Emergencies (2nd ed.). Baltimore: Williams & Wilkins, 1997, pp 181-198.

Nevens F, Bustami R, Scheys I, et al: Variceal pressure is a factor predicting the risk of a first variceal bleeding: A prospective cohort study in cirrhotic patients. Hepatology 1998;27:15.

Stiegman GV, Goff JS, Michaletz-Onody PA, et al: Endoscopic sclerotherapy as compared with endoscopic ligation for bleeding esophageal varices. N Engl J Med 1992;326:1527.

Thabut D, de Franchis R, Bendsten F, et al: Efficacy of activated recombinant factor VII (RFVIIA; Novoseven®) in cirrhotic patients with upper gastrointestinal bleeding: A randomized placebo-controlled double-blind multicenter trial (abstract). J Hepatol 3;38(Suppl):13.

# Dysphagia and Esophageal Obstruction

Method of
*Philip O. Katz, MD, and Girish Anand, MD*

*Dysphagia* refers to a subjective sensation of the delayed passage of food from the mouth through the esophagus to the stomach. It derives its origin from Greek *dys* meaning "difficulty" and *phagia* meaning "eat."

Dysphagia has been reported in about 2% of healthy adults older than 65 years. The incidence increases to 12% to 13% in the hospitalized elderly. Dysphagia has been reported in about 50% to 60% of patients in nursing homes and other chronic care facilities.

There may be associated pain with swallowing (odynophagia) if there is coexistent inflammation. Most patients describe dysphagia as a feeling of food getting "stuck" or "not going down right." The history plays an important role in understanding the anatomic location and the severity of the symptoms. Key questions like the exact location where the food is getting stuck, associated regurgitation, types of foods causing dysphagia, and presence of weight loss or heartburn are crucial in assessing the symptom of dysphagia.

## Pathophysiology

In the swallowing process, the oropharyngeal and esophageal phases transport solid or liquid boluses rapidly from the mouth to the stomach. *Primary peristalsis* is the classic coordinated motor pattern of the esophagus, combined with almost simultaneous upper and lower esophageal sphincter relaxation initiated by the act of swallowing. The food bolus is transferred by a progressive pharyngeal contraction through the relaxed upper esophageal sphincter (UES) into the esophagus. The UES closure is followed by a progressive circular contraction beginning in the upper esophagus and proceeding distally along the esophageal body to propel the bolus through the relaxed lower esophageal sphincter (LES), which subsequently closes with a prolonged contraction.

*Secondary peristalsis* is a progressive contraction in the esophageal body occurring in response to its distention by stimulation of sensory receptors in the esophageal body. It usually begins at or above a level corresponding to the location of the stimulus and is limited to the esophagus. A local intramural mechanism can at times take over as a reserve mechanism to produce peristalsis in the smooth muscle segment of the esophagus. This has been called *tertiary peristalsis*.

Any problem with either the strength or coordination of the musculature causes difficulty with movement of food, leading to obstruction. Similarly, any narrowing in the path of transit causes obstruction and distention of the lumen, leading to the sensation of dysphagia. The motility abnormalities might not be constant, thus giving intermittent dysphagia. The extent of luminal obstruction guides the diagnosis. Partial obstruction might initially give only solid food dysphagia related to large food boluses (e.g., steak). When the extent of obstruction progresses to near total occlusion, the symptoms involve both solid and liquid dysphagia. The extent of associated inflammation (esophagitis) determines whether or not odynophagia is an associated symptom.

## Diagnosis

A careful history helps to localize the site of abnormality, and this forms the basis of further work-up. The evaluation of dysphagia begins with a complete history. A problem initiating a swallow and associated coughing or choking indicates a more proximal or oropharyngeal cause for the symptoms. Pure solid food dysphagia suggests a structural lesion, stricture, ring, or malignancy. A problem initially with solids progressing later to liquids suggests a benign or malignant stricture.

Rapidly progressive dysphagia is concerning for malignancy. The presence of other medical problems such as stroke or scleroderma might point to a systemic cause of the symptoms. A careful history of medications is important, because many drugs have been implicated in pill esophagitis and can cause dysphagia as well as odynophagia. The history can also differentiate dysphagia from globus sensation (feeling of a lump in the throat), which has a different evaluation from dysphagia.

Dysphagia for all practical purposes can be classified into oropharyngeal and esophageal dysphagia.

## OROPHARYNGEAL DYSPHAGIA

Difficulty in transferring a food bolus from the hypopharyngeal area to the esophageal body across the upper esophageal sphincter gives rise to the suspicion of oropharyngeal or transfer dysphagia. Several clues in the patient's history help to establish the cause.

The onset of symptoms in oropharyngeal dysphagia is almost immediate. The patient describes the feeling of choking or coughing on initiation of swallowing and frequently points to the cervical region as the site of dysphagia. Patients might describe regurgitation of food, aspiration, or halitosis, which can point to a structural abnormality such as a Zenker's diverticulum.

Patients might have to resort to certain physical maneuvers, such as extending their arms and neck and using their fingers to move the bolus. There may be associated speech abnormalities such as hoarseness, nasal quality, or dysarthria, which points to a neuromuscular cause for the oropharyngeal dysphagia. The various causes of oropharyngeal dysphagia are listed in Box 1.

In patients with oropharyngeal dysphagia, the oral cavity, head, and neck should be carefully examined. Special attention should be paid to the neurologic examination, especially the nerves involved in the act of swallowing, namely cranial nerves V, VII, IX, X, XI, and XII. Clues in the physical examination might suggest polymyositis or dermatomyositis as the cause of symptoms.

Video fluoroscopy (barium swallow) is a good first test that permits visualization of the swallowing mechanism. It can identify aspiration, pooling, and abnormal motor activities. This examination concentrates on the cervical esophageal region. A barium swallow can delineate the anatomic anomalies and also can show the remainder of the esophagus. The study starts with liquid barium, progressing to a solid phase. Different consistencies of food are used to assess the oropharynx, UES, and proximal esophagus.

A structural abnormality found on the barium examination generally requires an endoscopy for confirmation or treatment. Endoscopy is not the first test to use to evaluate oropharyngeal dysphagia, because the chances of missing an abnormality in the upper part of esophagus are higher than in the distal esophagus.

A nasopharyngeal laryngoscopy performed by the otolaryngologist provides detailed information of the hypopharynx, larynx, and oropharynx. It also allows a clear visualization of the vocal cords, valleculae, and the pyriform sinuses to assess any pooling of secretions.

Patients with oropharyngeal dysphagia who have an unrevealing barium study or endoscopy might need an esophageal manometry study with careful attention to the UES. Incoordination between UES opening and pharyngeal contractions can cause relaxation (opening) or shortening opening may be associated with dysphagia as well.

Zenker's diverticulum is an outpouching of the mucosa through an area of muscular weakness between the transverse fibers of the cricopharyngeus and the oblique fibers of the lower inferior constrictor. These generally occur in older adults and can show symptoms of pulmonary aspirations, gurgling, or regurgitation. Rarely, they become large enough to manifest as a mass and even cause esophageal obstruction.

## ESOPHAGEAL DYSPHAGIA

Esophageal dysphagia occurs either from mechanical or motility causes. The abnormality lies within the body of the esophagus or the lower esophageal sphincter. Patients often complain of symptoms localizing to the upper epigastric region or lower sternum although the association is less significant than in oropharyngeal dysphagia. The type of food producing symptoms and its temporal progression help to identify the cause of symptoms. Dysphagia progressing from solids to liquids usually indicates a mechanical cause, and dysphagia to both solids and liquids from the outset favors a motility disorder. Symptoms of associated heartburn, weight loss, anemia, and regurgitation further narrow the differential diagnosis. Other medical conditions such as radiation therapy and medication use may be associated with dysphagia, as may infectious esophagitis. Both are often associated with odynophagia as well. Opportunistic infections—especially in the setting of HIV disease and AIDS—such as candida, cytomegalovirus, and herpes virus, are the most common and can be managed adequately with medical therapy.

The various causes of esophageal dysphagia are listed in Box 2.

The most common initial diagnostic approach to esophageal dysphagia is to perform endoscopy. In addition to the diagnostic value, endoscopy affords an opportunity to obtain tissue samples and do therapeutic intervention. A barium swallow with a solid bolus challenge is a reasonable alternative, especially with patients in whom oropharyngeal causes are a possibility or when the history suggests

## BOX 2 Causes of Esophageal Dysphagia

**Structural (Mechanical)**

*Intrinsic*
- Benign tumors
- Carcinoma: Adenocarcinoma and squamous cell cancer
- Diverticula
- Eosinophilic esophagitis
- Esophageal rings and webs: Schatzki's ring
- Foreign body
- Infections: Herpes, CMV, EBV, MAI, *Candida, Pneumocystis*
- Peptic strictures
- Pill esophagitis
- Radiation strictures or esophagitis

*Extrinsic*
- Cervical osteophytes
- Mediastinal masses
- Vascular compression: Dysphagia lusoria

**Motility (Neuromuscular)**
- Achalasia
- Diffuse esophageal spasm (DES)
- Hypertensive lower esophageal sphincter
- Ineffective esophageal motility disorder
- Nutcracker esophagus
- Secondary causes like scleroderma, Sjögren's syndrome, Chagas' disease

**Functional**
- Functional dysphagia

*Abbreviations:* CMV = cytomegalovirus; EBV = Epstein-Barr virus; MAI = *Mycobacterium avium-intracellulare.*

---

and anorexia. The staging of esophageal cancer involves CT scanning of the chest and abdomen and endoscopic ultrasonography (EUS). EUS provides the most accurate estimate of disease stage and assists with management decisions. The 5-year survival rate for patients with advanced esophageal cancer continues to be less than 5%.

Eosinophilic esophagitis is seen more often as a cause of dysphagia, particularly in young adults. Extensive diffuse eosinophilic infiltration (>20 per high power field), particularly in the proximal esophagus, is seen. The disease can manifest for the first time as a food impaction requiring emergency endoscopic therapy. Feline esophagus, concentric mucosal rings, or ringed esophagus is the classic endoscopic description of eosinophilic esophagitis.

Pill-induced esophagitis has been shown to occur with a variety of medications including bisphosphonates, doxycycline, potassium chloride, quinidine, nonsteroidal anti-inflammatory drugs (NSAIDs), aspirin, and iron preparations.

Vascular anomalies such as double aortic arch or aberrant right subclavian artery can cause dysphagia.

## MOTILITY CAUSES

Patients reporting both solid and liquid dysphagia are more likely to have a motility disorder. Achalasia is a disease in which there is a loss of peristalsis in the distal esophagus and a failure of LES relaxation. These patients complain of chest pain, regurgitation, heartburn, and weight loss in addition to dysphagia. A barium swallow is the primary screening test when achalasia is suspected and manometry is confirmatory. The characteristic features on manometry include elevated resting LES pressure, incomplete LES relaxation, and aperistalsis.

Spastic motility disorders also manifest with dysphagia and often associated chest pain. The group of spastic motility disorders includes distal esophageal spasm, nutcracker esophagus, and hypertensive LES. The clinical relevance of these abnormalities identified during esophageal manometry is debated, and their management can be challenging.

505

---

a complex stricture or achalasia. An endoscopy is required if a structural abnormality is discovered on the barium study.

## STRUCTURAL CAUSES

Patients reporting only solid food dysphagia typically have a mechanical cause for their symptoms. This can progress to both solid and liquid dysphagia in cases of a high-grade obstruction. These patients tend to develop food impaction and might regurgitate. Benign causes for these symptoms include an esophageal web or a distal esophageal ring. The rings, also called Schatzki's rings, are smooth, thin mucosal structures at the gastroesophageal junction covered by squamous mucosa above and columnar epithelium below. Muscular rings, on the other hand, are characterized by hypertrophic esophageal musculature and are generally located about 2 cm above the gastroesophageal junction. Nonprogressive, episodic dysphagia is a characteristic of esophageal rings. Dysphagia becomes prominent when the diameter is smaller than 13 mm. Rings can manifest with acute dysphagia associated with impaction of a piece of meat, often referred to as "steakhouse syndrome." Esophageal webs, often asymptomatic, have been associated with iron deficiency anemia (Plummer-Vinson syndrome).

Peptic strictures occur in 8% to 10% of patients with symptomatic gastroesophageal reflux disease (GERD). Peptic strictures are associated with a long duration of reflux symptoms, male sex, and older age. Symptoms of dysphagia occur when the luminal diameter narrows to 13 mm or less.

Radiation-related strictures or esophagitis are seen in persons undergoing radiotherapy for thoracic or head or neck tumors. In the acute setting esophagitis is the predominant finding and can progress to fibrosis and strictures in the chronic phase.

Malignancy is the primary concern in patients with rapidly progressive solid food dysphagia associated with weight loss

## Treatment

### OROPHARYNGEAL DYSPHAGIA

Surgical and endoscopic therapeutic options are available, and these should be based on the patient's age and surgical risk. Surgery has been the mainstay of symptomatic Zenker's diverticulum. These involve cricopharyngeal myotomy with or without diverticulectomy or diverticulopexy. The efficacy of myotomy has been observed to be in excess of 80%. More recently, endoscopic techniques involving coagulation or cutting of the bridge, especially the cricopharyngeal muscle, between the esophagus and the diverticulum have been used. This approach is especially good for patients who are poor surgical risks and is now being used widely by experts in this technique.

Botulinum toxin injection might be an alternative to cricopharyngeal myotomy, although results are variable. Injection is usually performed under electromyographic guidance and has been shown to relieve dysphagia in small trials.

---

 **CURRENT THERAPY**

- Treat the underlying disorder (e.g., GERD).
- Dilatation and antireflux therapy manage most peptic strictures.
- Multimodality therapy should be considered for malignant dysphagia.
- Achalasia can be effectively treated with pneumatic dilatation or surgery.
- Swallowing rehabilitation is helpful for oropharyngeal dysphagia following stroke.

The presence of other structural abnormalities such as proximal strictures, can require endoscopic measures such as dilatation. A neoplasm requires appropriate intervention with surgical resection, chemotherapy, or radiation therapy.

If the oropharyngeal dysphagia is believed to be from nonstructural causes, swallowing rehabilitation may be the best option available. Swallowing rehabilitation is carried out by trained speech and language therapists, who teach patients maneuvers to overcome the risks of aspiration and improve dysphagia. These can involve proper positioning of the head and neck during swallowing, oral motor exercises, and deliberate multiple swallows. Certain diet modifications can improve swallowing and prevent aspirations.

The risk of malnutrition or recurrent aspiration can require placement of gastrostomy tubes for managing long-term nutritional needs.

## ESOPHAGEAL DYSPHAGIA

The treatment of peptic strictures can involve dilatation, biopsies to rule out malignancy, and medical therapy for reflux. Proton pump inhibitor therapy has been shown to reduce the development of these strictures and the need for future dilatation.

Radiation-related strictures or esophagitis may be difficult to treat and require frequent esophageal dilatation.

The treatment of esophageal cancer depends on the stage of the cancer at the time of diagnosis. The various options available include surgery, chemotherapy, radiation therapy, palliative intraluminal stenting, and, more recently, photodynamic therapy.

Eosinophilic esophagitis is treated with topical steroid therapy with fluticasone[1] (Flovent), oral methylprednisolone, or montelukast in

---

[1]Not FDA approved for this indication.

addition to dietary restrictions. These treatments have been studied in small series and have been shown to be beneficial. Dilatation may be helpful but must be done with care.

Treatment of pill-induced esophagitis involves stopping the offending agent and dilatation of strictures as needed.

Treatment modalities for achalasia include pneumatic dilatation of the LES, laparoscopic myotomy, botulinum toxin injection, and medical therapy with nitrates and calcium channel blockers. Medical therapy should be considered only for people who are not candidates for other modalities. Good to excellent relief of dysphagia can be achieved in patients with achalasia whether treated with pneumatic dilatation or myotomy. Many patients require multiple approaches and should be managed by experts in the field. Minimally invasive (laparoscopic or thoracoscopic) myotomy is gaining popularity, and in some centers it has become the procedure of choice.

Proposed treatments for distal esophageal spasm, nutcracker esophagus, and hypertensive LES include proton pump inhibitors, nitrates, calcium channel blockers, phosphodiesterase inhibitors, and tricyclic antidepressants or selective serotonin reuptake inhibitors.[1] Botulinum toxin[1] application and endoscopic dilatation have been tried in small series with varying results.

## Summary

This review outlines the various causes and management of dysphagia. A careful history and examination with use of certain diagnostic tests help in establishing the reason for the symptom of dysphagia. Most of the conditions can be managed by medical therapy, endoscopic therapy, or surgery. A possible approach is outlined in Figure 1.

### REFERENCES

Cook IJ, Kahrilas PJ: AGA technical review on management of oropharyngeal dysphagia. Gastroenterology 1999;116(2):455-479.

Katz PO, Gilbert J, Castell DO: Pneumatic dilatation is effective long-term treatment for achalasia. Dig Dis Sci 1998;43(9):1973-1977.

Khazanchi A, Katz PO: Strategies for treating severe refractory dysphagia. Gastrointest Endosc Clin N Am 2001;11(2):371-386, viii.

Spechler SJ: American Gastroenterological Association medical position statement on treatment of patients with dysphagia caused by benign disorders of the distal esophagus. Gastroenterology 1999;117(1):229-233.

Trate DM, Parkman HP, Fisher RS: Dysphagia: Evaluation, diagnosis and treatment. Prim Care 1996;(3):417-432.

Tutuian R, Castell DO: Esophageal motility disorders (distal esophageal spasm, nutcracker esophagus, and hypertensive lower esophageal sphincter): Modern management. Curr Treat Options Gastroenterol 2006;9(4):283-294.

Yan BM, Shaffer EA: Eosinophilic esophagitis: A newly established cause of dysphagia. World J Gastroenterol. 2006;12(15):2328-2334.

---

[1]Not FDA approved for this indication.

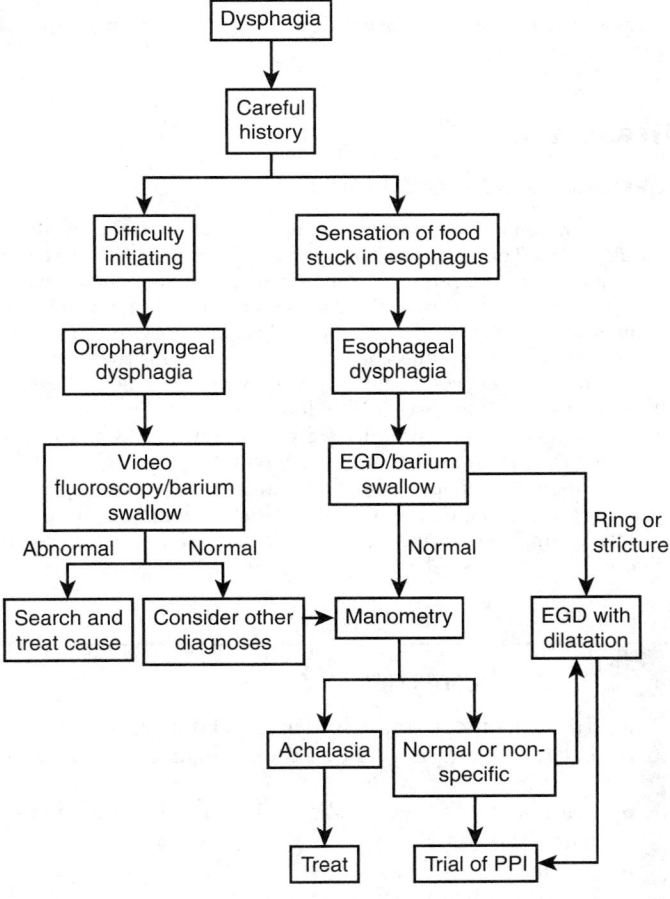

**FIGURE 1.** Diagnostic algorithm for patients with dysphagia. *Abbreviations:* EGD = esophagogastroduodenoscopy; PPI = proton pump inhibitor.

# Diverticula of the Alimentary Tract

Method of
*Harris R. Clearfield, MD*

Diverticula are often asymptomatic but may produce symptoms if they distend with food or liquid and compress the lumen (Zenker's and epiphrenic diverticula), harbor sufficient organisms to produce a bacterial overgrowth syndrome (jejunal diverticula), or become inflamed or bleed (Meckel and colonic diverticula).

# Esophageal Diverticula

## HYPOPHARYNGEAL DIVERTICULA

The hypopharyngeal diverticulum (Zenker's diverticulum) is found in approximately 2% of patients presenting with dysphagia, and the majority of cases occur in patients beyond the seventh decade of life. The diverticulum generally protrudes between the cricopharyngeus muscle (superior esophageal sphincter) and the inferior constrictor muscles as a result of high pressure produced by transient inadequate or uncoordinated relaxation of the superior esophageal sphincter during swallowing. Because the cervical spine prevents posterior extension, the diverticulum enlarges laterally, usually to the left side. Small diverticula are asymptomatic, but progressive enlargement can occur as a result of food-induced stretching. The opening of the diverticulum may become larger than the lumen of the esophagus, so that food and liquid can preferentially enter the diverticulum and subsequently spill over into the lumen of the esophagus. The progressively enlarging diverticulum may exert sufficient pressure on the esophagus to produce dysphagia and perhaps aspiration. Symptoms include cervical dysphagia, coughing while eating, bad breath from the fermenting food, a swelling in the neck (usually during meals or liquid ingestion) caused by the enlarging diverticulum, and nocturnal wheezing resulting from aspiration. Medications may also accumulate in the diverticulum causing erratic absorption. The symptoms may be suggestive, but barium upper gastrointestinal (GI) tract radiographic films usually establish the diagnosis. If a Zenker's diverticulum is suspected, upper endoscopy, if necessary, should be accomplished by inserting the instrument under direct vision to reduce the likelihood of perforation.

### Treatment

No treatment is required for asymptomatic diverticula, but those producing symptoms often require surgery. Although external surgery such as diverticulectomy and myotomy of the superior sphincter is an effective therapy, the use of endoscopic staple diverticulotomy has become increasingly popular. It can be accomplished on an outpatient basis with a more rapid convalescence and a lower rate of complications as compared to external surgery, although there is a recurrence rate of approximately 12%.

## MIDESOPHAGEAL DIVERTICULA

Midesophageal diverticula were once thought to result from a fibrotic "pull" or "traction" from an adjacent mediastinal inflammatory reaction, such as tuberculosis. This theory was largely replaced by the observation that many diverticula are associated with motility abnormalities such as achalasia or esophageal spasm. The diverticula are usually small and wide mouthed, so that food trapping rarely occurs and symptoms are unusual. If chest pain is associated with these diverticula, esophageal motility studies should be performed. No treatment is usually required for the diverticula.

## EPIPHRENIC DIVERTICULA

Epiphrenic diverticula occur in the distal esophagus and are thought to result from high pressure generated by a motility disorder of the lower esophageal sphincter or distal esophagus, such as achalasia, esophageal spasm, or hypertensive lower esophageal sphincter. Most diverticula are asymptomatic, but an occasional diverticulum may progressively distend and begin to trap food and secretions, leading to dysphagia, substernal discomfort, or vomiting (often nocturnal). The diagnosis is usually established by barium upper GI studies, but upper endoscopy also reveals the lesion.

### Treatment

No treatment or evaluation is required for small asymptomatic outpouchings, but detailed esophageal motility studies should be performed for larger diverticula. Symptomatic diverticula associated with a motility disorder are treated with calcium channel blockers, but medical therapy is usually ineffective. If surgery is required, myotomy of the lower esophageal sphincter down to the cardia of the stomach and proximal to the mouth of the diverticulum may suffice for relatively small diverticula, but diverticulectomy plus myotomy is best for large diverticula. The procedure is most commonly performed by an "open" approach, but increasing evidence supports a laparoscopic approach. Either type of surgery should be combined with an antireflux procedure to prevent reflux resulting from loss of the lower esophageal sphincter's competence.

# Small Intestinal Diverticula

## DUODENAL DIVERTICULA

Duodenal diverticula are noted in approximately 5% of patients studied with barium upper GI radiographs and in 10% to 20% of patients studied by endoscopic retrograde cholangiopancreatography (ERCP). They are the most common small bowel diverticula and are exceeded in frequency only by colonic diverticula. They usually occur within the "C loop," often adjacent to the ampulla of Vater (referred to as juxtapapillary diverticula), and are rarely found on the lateral wall of the duodenum. The diverticula increase in frequency with advancing age. They are usually composed of mucosa without muscle fibers, which suggests they are the result of duodenal pressure, but congenital diverticula may also occur. There appears to be no increased incidence of colonic diverticula in patients with duodenal diverticula, thus negating the concept of a general GI predisposition to diverticular formation.

The ERCP endoscope, which is side viewing, is best suited for the detection of juxtapapillary diverticula, but they may be observed by standard upper endoscopy and barium radiographs. Because imaging studies are usually obtained related to upper GI symptoms, it is tempting to ascribe such symptoms to the presence of the diverticula. However, it is difficult to establish a correlation between these occasionally encountered diverticula and a variety of dyspeptic or aerophagic complaints. Nevertheless, there does appear to be a correlation between the presence of juxtapapillary diverticula and infected bile, common duct stones, and gallstones. This raises the possibility that the diverticula may compromise flow in the common bile duct by exerting extrinsic pressure, thus promoting stasis and common duct calculi formation. Dysfunction of the sphincter of Oddi is ascribed to the presence of adjacent diverticula and could lead to reflux of duodenal contents and bacteria into the biliary tree. Rare cases of pancreatitis are thought to be secondary to juxtapapillary diverticula. The presence of juxtapapillary diverticula may complicate diagnostic and therapeutic ERCP procedures.

### Treatment

Duodenal diverticula rarely produce symptoms and therefore usually require no therapy. Resection should be considered if studies suggest that external pressure on the common bile duct is causing obstruction or stone disease. Upper GI tract bleeding, brisk rather than occult, may rarely arise from these diverticula, but efforts should be made to define some other, more likely etiology. A causal relationship between duodenal diverticula and bleeding should be established only with convincing endoscopic or angiographic findings. The management of the bleeding is similar to that of other causes of upper GI tract hemorrhage, but emergency excision of the diverticulum could be required if supportive measures are unsuccessful. Diverticular perforation and abscess are even more uncommon and would prompt computed tomography (CT) scan, ultrasonography, or surgical exploration to establish the diagnosis. Diverticulectomy would be required for such patients.

## JEJUNAL AND ILEAL DIVERTICULA

Jejunal and ileal diverticula are uncommon and are thought to be primarily of the acquired type. They tend to occur on the mesenteric border of the small bowel where blood vessels penetrate from the serosal surface, thus creating a potential weakness in the musculature.

Multiple large diverticula, usually jejunal, may permit sufficient bacterial overgrowth to result in a malabsorption syndrome. This complication may be associated with a more generalized bowel motility disorder, such as scleroderma. The symptoms are those of other malabsorption syndromes and include megaloblastic anemia secondary to vitamin $B_{12}$ or folate deficiency, steatorrhea, diarrhea, weight loss, and fat-soluble vitamin deficiency. Jejunal diverticula are also associated with intestinal pseudo-obstruction, although the retrospective nature of the published reports does not permit an estimate of the frequency of this relationship. The diverticula appear to be a manifestation of the pseudo-obstruction rather than the cause. The generalized nature of the small bowel motility disorder in these patients is illustrated by such associated findings as esophageal dysmotility, the CREST syndrome (calcinosis cutis, Raynaud phenomenon, esophageal dysfunction, sclerodactyly, and telangiectasia), and degenerated smooth muscle cells consistent with a visceral myopathy. Large small bowel diverticula have caused volvulus and are also complicated by hemorrhage and perforation (diverticulitis).

## Treatment

The bacterial overgrowth of small bowel diverticulosis often responds to antibiotic therapy. Tetracycline, 250 mg four times daily, or other broad-spectrum antibiotics for 7 to 10 days may be effective. Unfortunately, relapse is common and some patients benefit from 1 week of antibiotic therapy each month. A promotility agent such as metoclopramide[1] 250 mg or 500 mg can be taken 30-60 minutes before meals in an attempt to decrease small intestinal stasis. Vitamin $B_{12}$, folic acid, and fat-soluble vitamins should be provided, and dietary fat and milk products should be reduced. Resection of the small bowel containing the diverticula is suggested for patients with chronic symptoms, but this may prove to be ineffective if the diverticula are the result of a generalized neuropathic or myopathic process. Surgery should be reserved for acute complications such as bleeding, diverticulitis, or volvulus. It is therefore important to consider an associated motility disturbance in patients with symptomatic small bowel diverticula.

## MECKEL'S DIVERTICULUM

Meckel's diverticulum, which is present in 1% to 3% of the population, represents the failure of the intestinal end of the primitive yolk duct (vitelline duct) to close completely. The diverticula usually occur on the antimesenteric surface of the ileum, approximately 60 to 80 cm from the ileocecal valve, but they may occur as far as 200 cm proximal to the valve. The diverticulum is usually several centimeters in size, but diverticula measuring up to 10 cm are described. The majority of the diverticula are asymptomatic. The major complications of bleeding, inflammation, and obstruction are seen most commonly in infants and young children (60%), with a male predominance. Adult males are also more likely to develop complications from the diverticula. The most common presenting complication in adults is bleeding, whereas the most common childhood presentation is obstruction. Bleeding generally results from the presence of ectopic gastric mucosa within the sac, a finding in approximately 50% to 70% of symptomatic patients. The acid production leads to ulceration and bleeding from within or adjacent to the diverticulum. The bleeding is more frequently maroon or red than tarry and is more likely to be brisk than occult. Obstruction, with or without a fibrous attachment to the umbilicus, can result from volvulus or intussusception and may be of the closed-loop type. Inflammation of the diverticulum (diverticulitis) is less common than appendicitis because of the diverticular wide neck that permits the fecal stream to exit easily. The motility of the ileum decreases the likelihood that the inflammation will be sealed off, increasing the possibility of perforation should diverticulitis occur. The presence of painless, massive lower GI tract bleeding in an infant or child should suggest the possibility of Meckel's diverticulum. Bowel obstruction or peritonitis in this age group should also raise this suspicion. Although less common, the preceding complications can also occur in adults.

The diagnosis of Meckel's diverticulum is rarely made by barium small bowel examination, although this study (or small bowel enema) may be useful in selected patients to exclude other disorders. The $^{99m}Tc$ pertechnetate isotope is taken up by Meckel's diverticula containing gastric mucosa and may be helpful for establishing the diagnosis, but a negative examination does not exclude the possibility (many diverticula do not contain gastric mucosa, and even those that have the heterotopic gastric mucosa may not be visualized). Sensitivity is enhanced somewhat by pretreating patients with acid-suppressive therapy prior to isotope scanning. CT scanning has been helpful in diagnosis and should be performed if Meckel diverticulum is suspected, but false negatives also occur. The wireless videocapsule is helpful in a case report, but caution should be exercised if the process is Meckel's diverticulitis because the capsule may become lodged in an area of edema and narrowing. Mesenteric angiography may be useful during an active bleeding episode; intestinal obstruction is diagnosed on the basis of clinical and radiographic criteria; and peritonitis in an infant or child should suggest appendicitis or diverticulitis.

## Treatment

The treatment of symptomatic Meckel's diverticulum requires blood replacement, localization of the bleeding point if possible by isotope scan, CT scan, angiography, or videocapsule. Diverticulectomy is advised if the symptomatic diverticulum is identified, but one study suggested that the distribution of the heterotopic gastric mucosa may be at the base of short diverticula and thus could require localized small bowel resection.

Laparoscopic resection for Meckel's diverticula in adults is reported. Occasionally patients, both young and old, may bleed intermittently posing diagnostic difficulties if the preceding localizing efforts prove unrewarding. Bowel obstruction requires immediate surgery, and Meckel's diverticulitis usually requires exploration. There is some controversy as to the management of an asymptomatic Meckel's diverticulum discovered during surgery for some other disorder. An analysis of 1476 patients at the Mayo Clinic could not support or reject the recommendation that all Meckel's diverticula found incidentally be removed. Some of the criteria that could be used for selective resection include male sex, patient younger than 50 years, and diverticular length more than 2 cm.

# Diverticular Disease of the Colon

In diverticular disease of the colon, diverticula occur in two rows on either side of the colon, with a distinct clustering in the sigmoid colon. Although diverticula may also be observed in the proximal colon, it is most unusual for patients to have right-sided or transverse colonic diverticula in the absence of sigmoid involvement. The frequency of diverticula formation is almost directly related to age and increases to approximately 50% of individuals in their ninth decade. Although diverticula are uncommon before 40 years of age, complications from diverticular disease do occur in young people.

The diminished frequency of diverticula among individuals from Africa, Asia, and certain areas of South America is attributed to a high-fiber diet, which tends to decrease transit time in the gut, to increase stool frequency, and to result in softer, larger stools. This is an attractive hypothesis, but it is difficult to distinguish healthy persons from those with diverticulosis on the basis of stool weight and frequency. Another theory regarding the cause of colonic diverticula is related to the high sigmoid pressure observed in patients with the irritable bowel syndrome or those who strain during defecation. This is the basis of the supposition that increased intraluminal pressure forces the mucosa to protrude through the relatively weak areas of the colonic musculature adjacent to the blood vessels that penetrate from the serosal surface. This explanation seems reasonable, but diverticula are found in patients with no history of irritable bowel symptoms or chronic constipation. Stool weight and sigmoid pressure remain the primary explanations, but there is presently no convincing and unifying explanation for the development of colonic diverticula.

---

[1]Not FDA approved for this indication.

## DIVERTICULOSIS

Uncomplicated diverticula do not produce symptoms, but in patients with the irritable bowel syndrome, colonic diverticula may be revealed by barium enema examination or colonoscopy. Treatment, therefore, should not be directed to the diverticula but should focus on the predominant symptoms, such as pain, diarrhea, or constipation. Consider therapy with a high-fiber diet, psyllium preparations (Metamucil, Konsyl), or methyl cellulose (Citrucel) for constipation. Crampy pain or diarrhea may respond to antispasmodic medications (Bentyl, Levbid) or antidiarrheal agents such as loperamide (Imodium) or diphenoxylate (Lomotil). Patients with diverticula and the irritable bowel syndrome should not be informed that they have diverticular disease or diverticulitis because these labels may induce added anxiety and create confusion for physicians who may subsequently evaluate the patients.

## DIVERTICULAR BLEEDING

Diverticula are one of the major causes of massive colonic hemorrhage. The bleeding is usually painless and rarely accompanies clinical diverticulitis. It is thought to result from the presence of an inspissated diverticular fecalith that erodes or ulcerates into an adjacent penetrating artery. The close relationship of the diverticula to these arteries explains why bleeding is often more severe from diverticula than encountered from an arteriovenous malformation (AVM). Although right-sided diverticula are occasionally cited as the most common cause of diverticular bleeding, colonoscopy examinations suggest that the AVM is a more common etiology of right colon bleeding. The bleeding site (but not the cause) may be established by a technetium isotope bleeding study (often an initial study) or by angiography, but these studies must obviously be performed during the bleeding episode if localization is to be made with confidence. Cleansing of the colon with a lavage solution (GoLYTELY, Colyte) can be accomplished in selected patients during the bleeding episode if hemodynamic stability can be achieved, permitting a colonoscopic examination that may determine the site of bleeding and the cause (diverticula, AVM, or neoplasm). However, colonoscopy is most often performed after bleeding ceases.

### Treatment

It is more important to determine which segment of the colon is the site of brisk bleeding (sigmoid, left, transverse, or right colon) than to identify the specific diverticulum or other etiology. Hemodynamic stability should be achieved before time-consuming diagnostic studies are initiated. The most common cause for death resulting from GI hemorrhage is inadequate transfusions. An isotope bleeding study may demonstrate the area of colonic bleeding but is helpful only if the patient is bleeding actively during the study window. Angiography permits the most precise localization of bleeding points if active bleeding is present. If a bleeding diverticulum is identified, angiographic embolization can be performed or vasopressin infusion may result in sufficient local vasoconstriction to permit cessation of bleeding. Colonoscopy during a colonic hemorrhage can be achieved if the patient is stable and capable of tolerating the cleansing preparation. The examination may show evidence of vascular lesions, "oozing" from a presumably culpable diverticulum, or neoplasm (benign polyps rarely bleed massively). It is useful to remember that one of the causes of lower GI bleeding is upper GI bleeding, suggesting that an upper endoscopy or enteroscopy should be considered if a colonic site is not definitely shown. If major bleeding continues and the diagnostic strategies just outlined are unrewarding, a subtotal resection with ileorectal anastomosis should be considered. A "blind" left-sided colectomy in patients with known diverticular disease may be disastrous if the bleeding originates from the right colon. If diverticular bleeding stops with conservative measures, elective surgery need not be immediately considered because there is a reasonable possibility that bleeding will not recur. Recurrent bleeding should be approached surgically if the site is identified.

## DIVERTICULITIS

Diverticulitis results from a microperforation of a single diverticulum, usually into pericolic tissues. The inflammatory reaction is generally walled off by surrounding omentum or adjacent bowel loops but may progress to an abscess or phlegmon (marked cellulites without pus). If the inflammatory process is not sealed, a free perforation may rarely occur. Diverticulitis usually involves the sigmoid colon, but instances of right-sided diverticulitis are encountered.

The patient usually complains of left lower quadrant or suprapubic pain that may be accompanied by back pain, nausea, vomiting, dysuria, or fever. Gross rectal bleeding is unusual. Physical examination generally reveals tenderness over the left lower quadrant, suprapubic area, or both. Muscle guarding or rebound tenderness may be elicited.

An elevated white blood cell count has little localizing value but can be useful in distinguishing between the irritable colon (normal count) and diverticulitis (leukocytosis is common). A urinalysis may reflect the presence of cystitis secondary to an adjacent inflammatory reaction or a true colovesical fistula (ask the patient about the passage of gas during urination). An obstruction series may provide little information, but a sigmoid obstruction secondary to edema and inflammation may be noted, or a partial small bowel obstruction may result from a segment of distal jejunum or proximal ileum that becomes surrounded by the pericolonic inflammatory reaction. A CT scan provides the most useful information, such as an abscess, pericolonic inflammation, or air in the bladder if a fistula is present. The CT scan may not demonstrate these findings if obtained very early in the inflammatory process. Blood cultures should be obtained in febrile patients.

Sigmoidoscopy and colonoscopy should be avoided during the acute process so that free perforation secondary to air insufflation can be avoided. Contrast radiographic films of the colon are ordinarily deferred for the same reason, but early imaging may be required if the clinical picture is atypical, perhaps raising the possibility of ischemia, acute colitis, or perforated neoplasm. In such circumstances, meglumine diatrizoate (Gastrografin) administration given without air insufflation is usually sufficient to outline the pathology. A CT scan should be considered. This may show a fistula, partial obstruction, or evidence of an extrinsic mass effect on the colon. Colonoscopy is less useful for the diagnosis of recent diverticulitis but can be helpful in the differential diagnosis.

The differential diagnosis may include the irritable bowel syndrome, but the presence of fever, leukocytosis, and/or peritoneal signs should suggest an inflammatory reaction. Ovarian pathology, appendicitis (the appendix may extend down into the pelvis), inflammatory bowel disease, and ischemic colitis should be considered. A confined perforation of a colonic carcinoma is more difficult to exclude during the acute process. Even the surgeon may have problems making that distinction during emergency exploration because the surrounding inflammatory reaction may be intense.

Complications include fistulas to the bladder (less common in women because the uterus "protects" the bladder), small bowel, or vagina. Free perforation, which is rare but significantly increases the morbidity and mortality rate, abdominal abscess, partial or complete obstruction of the small or large bowel, and septicemia may occur. Another serious complication of diverticulitis is spread of the bacteria through the portal vein to the liver leading to pyelophlebitis (pus in the portal vein) and pyogenic liver abscess.

### Treatment

Mild cases of diverticulitis with low-grade fever, tenderness without peritonitis, and modest leukocytosis may be treated on an ambulatory basis with clear liquids and a combination of oral levofloxacin (Levaquin) and metronidazole (Flagyl). If the fever subsides and clinical improvement is noted in 72 hours, the diet can be gradually increased. Immunocompromised patients should be treated earlier and more aggressively. More severe cases require hospitalization. The bowel should be kept at rest and intravenous (IV) fluids given. Nasogastric suction should be used if peritonitis or obstruction is present. Parenteral broad-spectrum antibiotic coverage against aerobes

## CURRENT DIAGNOSIS

- Cervical dysphagia associated with bad breath and a swelling in the neck during eating strongly suggests Zenker's diverticulum.
- Although most duodenal diverticula are asymptomatic, those adjacent to the ampulla of Vater can cause pressure on the bile duct resulting in stasis and common duct calculi.
- The most common presenting complication of Meckel's diverticulum in adults is bleeding, whereas the most common childhood presentation is obstruction.
- Patients with the irritable bowel syndrome may present with severe left lower quadrant pain and tenderness, but diverticulitis should be suspected if there is fever, leukocytosis, or peritoneal findings.
- A negative Meckel's pertechnetate isotope scan does not exclude the diverticulum because many do not contain heterotopic gastric mucosa.
- Colonic bleeding from diverticular disease is usually more severe than that encountered from arteriovenous malformations, polyps, or neoplasms.

and anaerobes is given. Single-therapy agents include piperacillin/tazobactam (Zosyn), ticarcillin/clavulanate (Timentin), or imipenem/cilastatin (Primaxin). Combination IV therapy could include levofloxacin (Levaquin) plus metronidazole or ampicillin/sulbactam (Unasyn) plus metronidazole. Percutaneous CT-guided aspiration of

## CURRENT THERAPY

- Symptomatic Zenker's diverticulum requires resection, most recently performed by an endoscopic staple diverticulotomy.
- Small symptomatic epiphrenic diverticula can be treated with lower esophageal myotomy, but large diverticula may also require diverticulectomy plus myotomy. Both procedures should be accompanied by an antireflux wrap procedure.
- There is controversy regarding the removal of asymptomatic Meckel's diverticula. Factors that may support excision of such diverticula include size larger than 2 cm, male sex, and patients <50 y.
- If major and continued diverticular bleeding cannot be localized by imaging studies, a subtotal colectomy is preferable to a "blind" left colectomy. If bleeding ceases, elective resection is not necessarily required.
- Moderate diverticulitis (fever, abdominal pain and tenderness, and a modest WBC elevation without other complications) may be treated on an outpatient basis with clear liquid diet and a broad-spectrum oral antibiotic plus metronidazole (Flagyl).
- Severe episodes of diverticulitis (peritoneal signs and marked WBC elevation and/or mass or abscess) require hospitalization with IV fluids and IV antibiotics.
- Elective surgery for acute diverticulitis is not necessarily required for recurrent episodes if the events are relatively mild.

*Abbreviations:* IV = intravenous; WBC = white blood cells.

a pericolonic or pelvic abscess, especially if 4 cm or larger, may hasten resolution of the process and perhaps permit a one-stage resection and anastomosis if surgery is subsequently required.

If the patient fails to improve, as judged by the white blood cell count, fever status, and abdominal findings, surgical intervention may be required. A one-stage procedure with resection of the inflamed bowel and reanastomosis is more often performed, but a staged procedure with a diverting colostomy is preferable if significant peritonitis or infection is present in the area of the planned anastomosis or if the anastomosis cannot be accomplished without tension. Laparoscopic sigmoid resection, with its attendant shorter hospital stay, is an alternative to open sigmoid resection.

If the patient responds to medical therapy, diet is gradually advanced, but the patient is instructed to avoid small hard particles such as seeds, nuts, corn, and fish bones to prevent their entrapment in diverticula (this advice seems reasonable but is not evidence based). It is also prudent to avoid constipation by increasing the fiber content of the diet, using either bran cereals, psyllium products such as Metamucil or Konsyl, or Citrucel. Elective resection of the sigmoid colon after the diverticulitis has resolved with medical therapy was once advocated, but current experience indicates that approximately 50% of patients have no further symptoms. Although some would advise surgery for a recurrent episode of diverticulitis, a prompt response to medical therapy could suggest that surgery should be deferred. Elective resection should be considered after a first attack in patients younger than 50 years (their recurrence rate appears to be higher) and in those patients who have experienced a particularly severe first attack.

## REFERENCES

Chang CY, Payyapilli RJ, Scher RL: Endoscopic staple diverticulotomy for Zenker's diverticulum; Review of literature and experience in 159 consecutive patients. Laryngoscope 2003;113:957-965.
Gonzalez R, Smith CD, Mattar SG, et al: Laparoscopic vs. open resection for the treatment of diverticular disease. Surg Endosc 2004;18:276-280.
Janes S, Meagher A, Frizelle FA: Elective surgery after acute diverticulitis. Br J Surg 2005;92:133-142.
Levy AD, Hobbs CM: From the archives of the AFIP. Meckel's diverticulum: Radiologic features with pathologic correlation. Radiographics 2004;24: 565-587.
Maggard MA, Chandler CF, Schmit PJ, et al: Surgical diverticulitis: Treatment options. Am Surg 2001;67:1185-1189.
Matthews BD, Nelms CD, Lohr CE, et al: Minimally invasive management of epiphrenic esophageal diverticula. Am Surg 2003;69:465-470.
Park JJ, Wolff BG, Tollefson MK, et al: Meckel diverticulum: The Mayo Clinic experience with 1476 patients (1950–2002). Ann Surg 2005;241:529-533.
Salem L, Anaya DA, Flum DR: Temporal changes in the management of diverticulitis. J Surg Res 2005;124:159.
Siewert B, Tye G, Kruskal J, et al: Impact of CT-guided drainage in the treatment of diverticular abscesses: Size matters. Am J Roentgenol 2006;186:680-686.
Zoepf T, Zoepf DS, Benz D, Riemann JF: The relationship between juxtapapillary duodenal diverticula and disorders of the biliopancreatic system, analysis of 350 patients. Gastrointest Endosc 2001;54:56-61.

# Inflammatory Bowel Disease

Method of
*Mark A. Peppercorn, MD, and Alan C. Moss, MD*

Inflammatory bowel disease (IBD) describes the spectrum of chronic intestinal inflammation from Crohn's disease to ulcerative colitis. This condition is currently thought to occur as a consequence of a persistent and inappropriate immunologic response to gut luminal antigens. The absence of enteric parasites in developed societies and defects in mucosal innate defenses are recent additions to the many hypotheses on the pathogenesis. Irrespective of the cause, Crohn's disease (CD) and ulcerative colitis (UC) respond to a similar range of anti-inflammatory and immunomodulator therapy in inducing and maintaining remission.

Both CD and UC are characterized by mucosal ulceration, which is patchy in CD but continuous in UC. In CD the focal areas (skip lesions) of transmural inflammation and ulceration can penetrate the gut wall, leading to fistulous tracts. In 80% of patients the terminal ileum is involved, and half of these have both ileal and colonic disease. These patients typically present with crampy abdominal pain, diarrhea, and evidence of weight loss or fevers. Up to a third of patients develop peri-anal disease, characterized by fistulas or abscesses during their life span. Patients may also present with mouth ulcers, gastric ulceration, or skin manifestations such as erythema nodosum. These clinical patterns are dynamic, with more than 60% of patients having a change in clinical behavior over 10 years. For small intestinal disease, computed tomography (CT) with contrast is the investigation of choice, with a sensitivity of 95% in most studies. A small bowel series has advantages over CT in early disease and fistula and sinus tract delineation; magnetic resonance imaging (MRI) is superior in perianal disease. Assessment of colonic disease and tissue diagnosis is best performed with full colonoscopy and terminal ileum intubation; this allows staging of the condition and exclusion of other causes of terminal ileum inflammation such as tuberculosis (TB) or *Yersinia* infection. There are no diagnostic blood tests for CD per se, although erythrocyte sedimentation rate (ESR), C-reactive protein (CRP), and complete blood count (CBC) are useful markers of disease activity. CRP elevation is positively associated with clinical and endoscopic activity and severe histologic disease. Anti-*Saccharomyces cerevisiae* antibodies (ASCA) are positive in 40% to 70% of patients with CD, with a reported specificity of 95%; this may be useful in patients where the clinical pattern of colitis is nondiagnostic. In patients with a family history of CD, polymorphisms in the NOD2 gene confer an increased risk of ileal disease and fibrostenotic disease. These mutations can be found in up to 30% of patients with CD, depending on ethnic group. However, 3% of the population may also harbor such mutations, limiting their role at the diagnostic level.

UC, in contrast, is characterized by continuous inflammation proximally from the rectum; two thirds of patients have disease limited to distal to the splenic flexure at presentation, and the rest have more extensive disease. The geography of the disease is usually described in terms of its extent: proctitis (rectum), distal colitis (rectum to descending), left-sided colitis (to splenic flexure), extensive colitis (beyond splenic flexure), and pancolitis (to cecum). UC usually causes bloody diarrhea, urgency, and lower abdominal pain, progressing to fecal incontinence and nocturnal symptoms in severe disease. Up to 30% of patients progress from distal to pancolitis over 10 years. Colonoscopy remains the investigation of choice in mapping disease geography and confirming tissue diagnosis. Similar to CD, inflammatory markers such as ESR and CRP are useful to confirm clinical disease activity and predict those likely to require surgery. Antineutrophil cytoplasmic antibodies (P-ANCA) can be detected in 50% to 70% of patients with UC but in only 5% to 10% of patients with CD. These patients tend to have more aggressive disease, leading to early surgery. The main diagnoses to exclude are infective colitides, such as infection with *Clostridium difficile*, *Campylobacter*, *Shigella*, or *Salmonella*. Ischemic colitis and nonsteroidal anti-inflammatory drug (NSAID)-induced colitis can also mimic UC.

The natural history of IBD is of frequent flares of the condition in response to unknown triggers. In CD, for example, 75% of patients have a chronic intermittent course, 15% have chronically active disease, and 10% remain in remission. The management of active disease can be divided into pharmacologic therapy, surgery, and nonpharmacologic interventions. Agents are usually described in terms of obtaining remission during flare-ups and maintaining remission in the medium to long term. We describe each of these in detail and then specifically in relation to disease subtypes.

## Pharmacologic Therapy

### AMINOSALICYLATES

Sulfasalazine (Azulfidine), the original aminosalicylate compound, consists of sulfapyridine (an antibiotic) and 5-aminosalicylic acid (5-ASA) (an anti-inflammatory) bound with an azo bond. After ingestion, sulfasalazine reaches the colon practically unabsorbed, where the enzymatic action of colonic bacteria cleaves the azo bond to release the active 5-ASA from sulfapyridine. Because the sulfapyridine moiety is the cause of most of the adverse effects of sulfasalazine, most modern aminosalicylates contain 5-ASA alone or combined with an inert carrier via the azo bond. For the purposes of this discussion, we refer to the nonsulfa aminosalicylates, such as mesalamine (Asacol), balsalazide (Colazal), and olsalazine (Dipentum), as "5-ASA." The exact mechanism of action of aminosalicylates is unclear, but they appear to orchestrate a broad range of anti-inflammatory properties within the intestinal mucosa. At a molecular level they inhibit arachidonic acid metabolism and are free-radical scavengers, two pathways through which local inflammation and necrosis occurs in the intestine. They inhibit activation of peripheral and intestinal lymphocytes and their release of immunoglobulin and proinflammatory cytokines. The therapeutic effects of these alterations are dose dependent and can take up to 14 days to reach their peak clinical response. Doses of more than 2 g/day of 5-ASA are required to obtain benefit in inducing remission, occurring in 40% to 80% of patients after 4 to 8 weeks of treatment in UC. In the longer term, sulfasalazine and the 5-ASA preparations maintain remission in 60% to 80% of these patients.

---

### CURRENT DIAGNOSIS

- Diagnosis should only be based on a combination of clinical, radiologic, endoscopic, and histologic features.
- Exclude tuberculosis, *Yersinia* infection, and NSAID use in suspected Crohn's disease.
- Exclude *Clostridium difficile*, *Campylobacter*, *Shigella*, and *Salmonella* infection, NSAID use, and ischemic colitis in suspected ulcerative colitis.
- Distinction between Crohn's disease and ulcerative colitis has implications for surgical interventions and prognosis.
- Nocturnal diarrhea, bloody diarrhea, weight loss, and low energy levels suggest severe disease.
- CBC, ESR, CRP, and albumin levels are useful in distinguishing disease exacerbations from functional symptoms.

*Abbreviations:* CBC = complete blood count; CRP = C-reactive protein; ESR = erythrocyte sedimentation rate; NSAID = nonsteroidal anti-inflammatory drug.

---

### CURRENT THERAPY

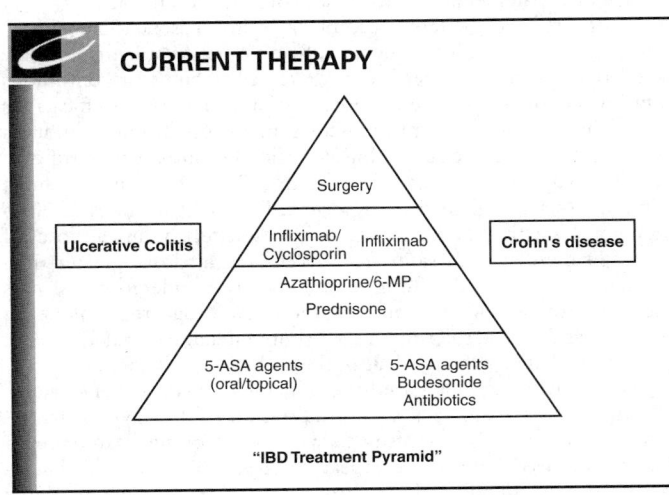

"IBD Treatment Pyramid"

A number of oral 5-ASA are preparations available. Asacol and Salofalk (in Canada) contain mesalamine coated with a pH-sensitive acrylic polymer that dissolves above pH of 6/7, typically releasing mesalamine in the terminal ileum and colon. Pentasa contains mesalamine microspheres that release 5-ASA throughout the gastrointestinal (GI) tract as these microspheres become hydrated and diffuse out of the capsule; this potentially makes it suitable for treatment of proximal small bowel disease. Olsalazine (Dipentum) contains two 5-ASA molecules joined by an azo bond that is cleaved by colonic bacteria. Balsalazide (Colazal) consists of 5-ASA bound by an azo bond to an inactive molecule, which also requires bacterial digestion to release the active 5-ASA molecules. In addition to oral therapy, topical preparations in the form of suppositories, foam, and enemas are widely used in treating distal disease. Mesalamine enemas (Rowasa) reach up to the proximal sigmoid, foam extends to the midsigmoid, whereas mesalamine suppositories (Canasa) reach the first 10 to 12 cm of the rectosigmoid region only. Patients with proctitis often find the foam preparations less irritating and easier to retain than enemas. The side-effect profile of topical therapy is superior to oral 5-ASAs in patients with distal disease. Recent data have demonstrated efficacy of topical 5-ASAs even in patients with pancolitis when used in conjunction with oral therapy.

Adverse effects from the aminosalicylate compounds are uncommon, but a number of potentially severe effects can occur. The majority of side effects occur more commonly in patients treated with sulfasalazine. The most common adverse events reported are headache, fever, and rash in up to 10% of patients. These are generally dose dependent and can be ameliorated by reducing the dose. In some patients (1% to 2%), 5-ASA can ironically cause an intolerance syndrome marked by severe diarrhea and abdominal pain; this should be considered in any patients whose symptoms worsen with therapy. Rare hypersensitivity side effects of sulfasalazine and 5-ASA include pancreatitis, nephritis, pneumonitis, pericarditis, and hepatitis. Agranulocytosis is a severe but rare side effect of sulfasalazine, which typically occurs within the first 8 weeks of therapy; it usually responds to discontinuation of sulfasalazine within 2 weeks. Infertility may also occur because of sulfasalazine in male patients by causing a reversible reduction in sperm function and number. This effect is dose dependent and can be avoided by using nonsulfa-containing 5-ASAs in these patients.

## CORTICOSTEROIDS

Corticosteroids have long been used, and continue to be used, in the acute management of flares of IBD. Their exact mechanism of action is unclear, although they are a potent inhibitor of cytokine release by inducing inactivation of NFkB. This leads to a reduction in lymphocyte recruitment to inflamed areas, reduced vascular permeability, and inhibition of cytokine-mediated tissue necrosis. Although oral corticosteroids are absorbed rapidly, their biologic anti-inflammatory effects take 4 to 9 hours to take effect, regardless of mode of delivery. There appears to be no difference in the benefits of oral steroids when compared to parenteral steroids in rates of remission in IBD.

Methylprednisolone (Solu-Medrol) or hydrocortisone (Solu-Cortef) can be given parenterally in patients with severe disease or in those unable to tolerate oral intake. They are given either as bolus or continuous infusion, although no evidence indicates that either is more efficacious in obtaining remission. Intramuscular methylprednisolone induces response faster than oral prednisolone in the outpatient setting in patients with moderately active colitis. Prednisone is the most commonly used oral corticosteroid in IBD, usually at doses of 30 to 60 mg as a starting dose. The dose-response effect occurs at doses of 20 to 60 mg/day, with side effects occurring at doses greater than 40 mg. It is absorbed within 30 minutes and undergoes first-pass metabolism in the liver to produce the active drug prednisolone. In both UC and CD, steroids induce a response in approximately 80% of patients, and approximately half of these obtain remission.

These corticosteroids have little mineralocorticoid or androgenic effects, but the main risk is of suppression of the hypothalamic-pituitary-adrenal axis and Cushing's syndrome. Chronic steroid use for less than 3 weeks does not appear to suppress the hypothalamic-pituitary axis, significantly, regardless of dose. Patients receiving steroid therapy for IBD for longer than this period should have any future reduction in steroid dose undertaken slowly (e.g., 5 mg weekly) to prevent hypoadrenalism. The main other side effect of concern is osteoporosis because up to 25% of patients with IBD have osteoporosis on bone density scans. Corticosteroid use is a major risk factor for vertebral fractures in these patients. Adequate calcium (1200 mg/day) and vitamin D (800 IU/day) are essential for patients receiving chronic steroids in IBD.

Such adverse effects with conventional synthetic steroids may be reduced with use of newer steroids such as budesonide (Entocort EC) and beclomethasone. Budesonide capsules are designed to release the active drug in the distal small bowel, where there is rapid mucosal uptake. Because of extensive hepatic metabolism, less than 10% becomes systemically available, thus reducing side effects. Beclomethasone also has high mucosal absorption with minimal systemic bioavailability.

## AZATHIOPRINE/6-MERCAPTOPURINE

Azathioprine (Imuran, Azasan)[1] is a prodrug that is converted into 6-mercaptopurine[1] (6-MP, [Purinethol]) by glutathione in red blood cells. The 6-MP product is subsequently metabolized to both 6-methylmercaptopurine (6-MMP) by the TPMT enzyme, and to 6-thioguanine (6-TG) by a series of enzymatic alterations. The incorporation of 6-TG into activated lymphocytes results in activation of apoptotic pathways and inhibition of cytokine release, thus inhibiting the role of lymphocytes in IBD. These therapeutic effects take approximately 8 to 12 weeks to manifest in clinical response, which reflects the chronic inflammatory role of activated lymphocytes in IBD. Both azathioprine[1] and 6-MP (Purinethol)[1] are used in inducing and maintaining remission in both CD and UC, with efficacy rates of 60% to 70%. Azathioprine is equivalent to 6-MP in efficacy because 88% of azathioprine is metabolized to 6-MP. In practice, 6-MP is usually underdosed, whereas azathioprine is overdosed by clinicians. Full dose is 1.5 to 2.5 mg/kg for azathioprine and 1.5 mg/kg for 6-MP, although most gastroenterologists begin at a lower dose and titrate upward if no adverse effects are noted.

Side effects occur in up to 25% of patients on azathioprine[1]/6-MP,[1] but these are usually mild. Nausea and vomiting is common soon after initiation of azathioprine therapy, but in most cases this subsides or requires a trial of 6-MP instead. Bone marrow suppression and pancreatitis are two more serious adverse effects seen in patients with IBD. Leukopenia is usually dose dependent and should be prevented by monitoring CBC. We check the CBC weekly for 1 month, then every 2 weeks for 1 month, then every 3 months. Pancreatitis occurs more commonly in patients with CD and appears to be idiosyncratic. Hepatitis in the form of elevated aspartate transaminase/alanine transaminase (AST/ALT) may also occur, but this usually responds to dose reduction. There is a theoretical increased risk of infections and neoplasia in patients on immunomodulators such as azathioprine/6-MP. Meta-analysis of cohort studies reported an increased risk of lymphoma in patients with IBD treated with azathioprine/6-MP, but risk-benefit models suggest the benefits of such therapy still outweigh this risk.

In recent years it was recognized that an individual's level of the TPMT enzyme influences the amount of the active 6-TG metabolite they produce during azathioprine[1]/6-MP therapy.[1] Patients with low TPMT levels because of genetic polymorphisms, approximately 1 in 300 of population, produce higher levels of 6-TG and are at higher risk of leukopenia. In theory, the measurement of TPMT levels prior to commencement of therapy might identify individuals at high risk of toxicity. However, integration of TPMT testing in patients with IBD has produced mixed results in preventing toxicity; prospective data have only shown a correlation between TPMT levels and early leukopenia in patients with IBD.

## METHOTREXATE

Methotrexate (MTX)[1] is a folate analogue that prevents conversion of folic acid to folinic acid, its active intracellular metabolite. This action

---

[1]Not FDA approved for this indication.

leads to accumulation of adenosine, a potent anti-inflammatory that inhibits the production of a number of cytokines from neutrophils, macrophages, and lymphocytes. MTX also causes inhibition of proliferation and induction of apoptosis in activated T-lymphocytes. Similar to azathioprine, this effect takes up to 12 weeks to manifest clinically, and is therefore often used in patients who are steroid dependent or have failed azathioprine[1]/6-MP therapy.[1] MTX given intramuscularly shows results in 40% to 65% of patients in inducing and maintaining remission in CD. Trials using oral MTX failed to show a benefit over placebo, possibly because of variable absorption.

The main adverse effects of MTX are hepatotoxicity, myelosuppression, pneumonitis, infertility, and teratogenicity. Myelosuppression is uncommon in those receiving MTX for more than 1 year, but they should be screened for by checking the CBC every 1 to 3 months. The hepatic toxicity of MTX is well documented in other conditions where it is used at high doses, such as psoriasis. Series of IBD patients taking MTX show low prevalence of liver fibrosis with accumulated dosage greater than 2.5 g. Patients who receive MTX should have CBC and liver function tests (LFTs) frequently and further investigation if serial abnormalities appear. Folic acid supplementation is recommended in all patients who receive MTX, at least 4 hours after MTX administration.

## ANTICYTOKINE THERAPY

Anticytokine therapy refers to the development of antibody therapy targeted against specific cytokines that play a role in the pathogenesis of CD, including TNF, IL-12, IL-6, and IL-8. Only anti-TNF is accepted so far into mainstream therapy based on clinical trials. Infliximab (Remicade) is a chimeric antibody (75% human, 25% mouse) against the TNF-α molecule, which leads to induction of apoptosis in activated lymphocytes. It also appears to reduce the number of inflammatory cells at the site of mucosal inflammation, possibly by inhibiting leukocyte migration. Infliximab induces and maintains remission in patients with luminal and fistulizing CD and recently induced remission in active UC. It is given as an intravenous (IV) infusion over 2 hours at 0, 2, and 6 weeks, and 8 weeks thereafter to maintain remission. In patients with CD, approximately 60% of patients respond within 2 weeks, and 30% to 50% of responders maintain response for up to 1 year. Patients who do not smoke, are also taking immunomodulators, and have nonstricturing disease achieve the best response to this therapy in CD. Recent trials in ulcerative colitis reported response rates of 70% in patients with pancolitis refractory to steroids and immunomodulators.

Adverse effects to infliximab primarily relate to immunologic reactions to the TNF antibody, which is mouse derived. Up to 60% of patients receiving infliximab develop anti-infliximab antibodies, which may cause infusion reactions and flulike illness after subsequent therapy. Thankfully these are usually mild and can be prevented by using prednisone and antihistamines prior to infusions. In the longer term up to 50% of patients may require a higher dose or shorter interval between doses to overcome loss of efficacy. More serious side effects such as reactivation of TB, cardiac events in patients with congestive cardiac failure, demyelination, and lymphoma are reported. Reactivation of latent TB occurs with an incidence of 0.46 per 1000 patient-years; therefore all patients should undergo a purified protein derivative (PPD) test and chest radiograph prior to commencement of therapy. The use of infliximab in patients with intra-abdominal collections and strictures is relatively contraindicated.

In the area of TNF inhibition, preliminary data suggest the humanized anti-TNF antibody Adalimumab (Humira)[1] and the humanized pegylated anti-TNF fragment certolizumab (Cimzia)[2] are effective in induction of response and remission in active CD. The advantage of these agents over infliximab is that they are administered subcutaneously and appear to induce fewer antibodies. Further data will be required to establish their role in CD.

## CYCLOSPORINE

Cyclosporine (Neoral)[1] inhibits cytokine production primarily in activated T-helper cells by binding to calcineurin and inhibiting proinflammatory transcription factors. Its role in UC is mainly in steroid-refractory patients (no response to 72 hours of high-dose steroids) with severe colitis. It has a response rate of 80% when administered as an IV infusion for a mean of 7 days in clinical trials. However, up to 60% of responders relapse within 6 months, and by 7 years approximately 60% will have required a colectomy. The relapse rate may be reduced by immunomodulator therapy. Tacrolimus (Prograf),[1] which acts via similar pathways, shows a similar response, up to 80% in severe colitis in small studies. Cyclosporine has a number of side effects, including renal impairment, hyperkalemia, tremor, hypertension, and hirsutism. Patients with low magnesium or cholesterol are at risk of seizures. In addition there is a risk of *Pneumocystis* pneumonia, aspergillus, and cytomegalovirus (CMV) infection because of immunosuppression. Data from Europe reported mortality rates as high as 3% in patients receiving cyclosporine, although this would not be the U.S. experience.

## ANTIBIOTICS/PROBIOTICS

Because the intestinal microflora plays a role in the pathogenesis of intestinal inflammation, manipulating the composition of this environment would be expected to ameliorate the disease process in IBD. Recent advances in the understanding of IBD suggest an impaired mucosal bacterial sensing, leading to invasion by the microflora and sustained immune response. It appears certain bacteria may be phenotype specific in the inflammatory response they elicit.

In UC, oral vancomycin (Vancocin), tobramycin (Nebcin), ciprofloxacin (Cipro), and rifaximin (Xifaxan) all improve response rates in the short term in patients with moderate to severe disease activity. IV metronidazole and tobramycin also show better response rates than placebo. These responses are not maintained in the longer term in clinical trials, however, and in the majority of trials patients were also on steroids. In practice, antibiotics are often administered to patients with severe disease requiring hospitalization as an adjunct to immunosuppressive therapy. The role of the novel nonabsorbed antibiotic rifaximin remains to be determined in active colitis and pouchitis.

The results in CD are more impressive with antibiotic therapy. Metronidazole (Flagyl) has intracellular activity against anaerobes and parasites primarily. In clinical trials it reduced colonic disease activity compared to sulfasalazine and placebo. Metronidazole is most successful in treating perianal disease, with demonstrated complete healing of chronic fistulas and symptom improvement. Finally, in patients who have undergone resection for CD, metronidazole taken for 12 weeks reduces the recurrence of endoscopic lesions at 3 months and clinical recurrence for up to 1 year. The chronicity of therapy requires close monitoring for peripheral neuropathy, the most serious adverse effect. This is unlikely to occur at daily doses less than 1 g. Patients who develop paresthesia should initially have dose reduction, followed by cessation if symptoms persist. Ciprofloxacin also produces clinical response, with 72% of patients with CD achieving complete or partial remission in recent trials. The combination of metronidazole and ciprofloxacin produces results similar to both steroids and mesalamine in patients with active disease and is a commonly used alternative to steroids. Ciprofloxacin also provides synergistic results when administered with infliximab for CD fistulas. Many gastroenterologists use antibiotic therapy in colonic and perianal CD as adjunctive therapy or as an alternative to steroids. Broad-spectrum antibiotics are also the mainstay of therapy for patients with CD who present with localized peritonitis because of a microperforation or bacterial overgrowth secondary to chronic strictures.

At the opposite end of the bacterial spectrum, probiotics have more recently been used to treat IBD. Probiotics are viable bacteria that induce beneficial therapeutic effects in intestinal mucosa. The rationale is that laboratory studies suggest that a balance between beneficial

---

[1]Not FDA approved for this indication.
[2]Not available in the United States.

---

[1]Not FDA approved for this indication.

and aggressive commensal enteric microflora determines mucosal immune response in genetically susceptible individuals. Patients with IBD tend to have higher concentrations of adherent and invasive strains of bacteria such as *Bacteroides*, *Enterococci*, and *Escherichia coli*. The most studied probiotics in controlled trials to date are *Saccharomyces boulardii*, *E. coli Nissle 1917*, *Lactobacillus GG*, and a combination of eight species (*VSL#3*). In CD these randomized controlled trials produced mixed results, with some benefit demonstrated in small trials in maintenance of medically induced remission but no benefit in preventing postoperative recurrence. In ulcerative colitis, *E. coli Nissle 1917* was equal to mesalamine, and *Bifidobacteria*-fermented milk superior to placebo, in maintaining medically induced remission. No randomized controlled trials have been published in obtaining remission in patients with active disease, although a combination of bacteria showed benefit in a recent open trial. The most impressive results to date emerged in treatment of patients with pouchitis, inflammation in the ileo-anal pouch that is constructed after colectomy in patients with ulcerative colitis. *VSL#3*, a combination of eight bacterial species, is superior to placebo in preventing the development of pouchitis after pouch closure and maintaining remission after a treated episode of pouchitis. Thus, at present, the evidence suggests a definite role for probiotics as an alternative to standard therapy in prevention of pouchitis and maintenance of remission in ulcerative colitis. A number of topics in our understanding of probiotics remain to be elucidated, such as their exact anti-inflammatory mechanisms, and which probiotic strains are best suited to which conditions. A more rigorous comparison of different strains to each other and standard therapy is required. An additional approach is to stimulate the growth of an individual's commensal bacteria through dietary substances, such as oligosaccharides, inulin, and psyllium. These so-called prebiotics may tip the balance of enteric growth in favor of *Lactobacilli*, which alter luminal pH and impair invasion of disease-associated species. Some evidence indicates a potential role for this strategy in mild to moderate UC.

## EXPERIMENTAL THERAPIES

As with many chronic conditions, IBD treatment still lacks a therapy that can induce high remission rates that are sustained in the long term without significant side effects. In particular, ileal CD and pancolitis that do not respond to standard therapy can prove problematic for clinicians. A high placebo response rate in CD trials (up to 50%) can make it difficult to judge the benefits of novel therapies. In response, molecular approaches targeted against specific inflammatory mediators are used with mixed effects in IBD. These include IL-11 (Oprelvekin [Neumega]),[1] thalidomide,[1] anti-IL12,* growth hormone,[1] and bone marrow transplantation. Antibodies against integrins (MLNO2, natalizumab [Tysabri]),[1] which promote translocation of lymphocytes into inflamed mucosa, improve response and remission rates in active IBD. However, the development of JC virus-related progressive multifocal leukoencephalopathy (PML) in a number of patients treated with natalizumab has raised concerns about anti-integrin therapy at present. MLNO2, which inhibits integrins specific to the gut, may avoid this rare complication. Two alternative approaches include removal of leukocytes using apheresis columns or administration of granulocyte colony-stimulating factor in patients with CD. Although many of these agents demonstrated efficacy in small trials, they are not used routinely in practice or are not licensed for treatment of IBD.

## NUTRITIONAL SUPPORT

Patients with IBD tend to have a high prevalence of protein-calorie malnutrition; up to 80% in some series. This tends to develop gradually in patients with small bowel CD but more rapidly in patients with UC during severe attacks. In addition to general malnutrition, specific deficits in calcium, vitamin D, vitamin B12, folate, iron, zinc, and selenium are common in patients with IBD. Calcium/vitamin D depletion, in conjunction with steroid use and chronic inflammation, can

lead to osteopenia in 40% to 50% of patients and to osteoporosis in up to 25%. This is associated with a 40% greater relative risk of fractures in these patients. Folate deficiency has an epidemiologic association with colorectal cancer, and supplementation may have a protective effect against dysplasia in ulcerative colitis. Zinc deficiency impairs mucosal healing, especially fistula closure, whereas selenium depletion can lead to cardiomyopathy.

Nutrition in IBD can be divided into general supportive nutrition and nutrition as primary therapy. All patients should be encouraged to maintain a balanced healthy diet without restrictions. Patients with strictures should adhere to a low-residue diet, and patients with overlap irritable bowel syndrome should avoid high-fiber foods. Calcium (1200 mg/day) and vitamin D (800 IU/day) should be taken by all patients if dietary calcium is inadequate. Folate deficiency should be sought and corrected if found. These approaches are yet to be validated in controlled trials. There is a high prevalence of lactose intolerance (40%) in patients with CD, and this should be considered and excluded if diarrhea persists despite minimal inflammatory activity. In patients with malnutrition, enteral nutrition is the preferred option as general nutritional support in most cases. Total parenteral nutrition (TPN) is associated with higher costs, greater length of stay, and more complications than enteral nutrition and should be restricted on a short term to patients with bowel obstruction or perforation, toxic megacolon, preoperatively, or for postoperative fistulas. Rarely home TPN may be required in the longer term for short-bowel syndrome after multiple resections.

Enteral nutrition as primary therapy in CD has been examined in a number of trials since the early 1980s. Systematic review of these trials concluded that enteral nutrition is superior to placebo but inferior to steroids in inducing remission in active Crohn's ileitis. Elemental diets do not appear to differ from nonelemental diets in this regard. The main problem with enteral nutrition is that it can take up to 4 weeks to demonstrate an effect, which can be difficult to comply with for these patients. Additionally, factors such as palatability, motivation, and resources can limit its use in adults. However, it remains a viable option to avoid or reduce steroids in patients with intestinal CD. There are no data to support use of enteral nutrition in ulcerative colitis, but it may be required in patients with severe colitis to supplement calorific intake.

# Surgery

In the era of biologic therapy for IBD, surgery still remains an important therapeutic option for patients. In patients with UC, toxic megacolon, fulminant colitis, steroid-refractory disease, high-grade dysplasia, and cancer are all indications for colectomy. Where possible, panproctocolectomy and ileal pouch–anal anastomosis (IPAA) is the procedure of choice. This has a technical success rate of up to 95%, with the advantage of removing the diseased organ and thus cancer risk. Most patients defecate from six to eight times per day after IPAA because of the lack of colonic reservoir. Postoperative impotence in men and dyspareunia in women occurs in less than 5% of patients. In addition there is a 15% risk per year of pouchitis in the long term, which can be problematic in some patients. Hospitalized patients with severe pancolitis who do not respond to IV steroids within 72 hours should either be referred for surgery or started on cyclosporin (Neoral)[1] or infliximab (Remicade) based on current evidence. It is worthwhile for all patients with refractory UC to meet an experienced colorectal surgeon and ostomy nurse during the course of the illness to prepare them psychologically for possible surgery.

For patients with CD, indications for surgery include strictures, inflammatory collections or abscesses, fistulas, perforation, and neoplasia. Up to 70% of patients require surgery during their lifetime. Those patients who smoke or have NOD2 mutations are more likely to require surgery during the course of their disease because they are more associated with penetrating and/or stricturing disease. Local surgical therapy, such as stricturoplasty, seton placement, and limited resection, are preferred in CD because of the high rate of postoperative

[1]Not FDA approved for this indication.
*Investigational drug in the United States.

[1]Not FDA approved for this indication.

recurrence; approximately 50% at 5 years. Immunomodulators, such as 6-MP, and 5-ASA appear to reduce this risk and should be offered to all patients postoperatively. In those who have terminal ileum resection, bile salt diarrhea is common postoperatively and can be treated with cholestyramine. Vitamin $B_{12}$ deficiency may occur and should be prevented with regular $B_{12}$ injections or intranasal therapy.

## Alternative Therapy

It is recognized that approximately half of all patients with IBD try nonconventional therapies during the course of their illness. The majority of these have not been assessed in randomized controlled trials or even reported in the medical literature. However, there are a number of alternative treatments we recommend to patients with mild to moderate disease who do not wish to advance to immunomodulators or biologic therapy. These are not evidence based but rather experience and anecdote based.

Aloe vera[1] has established healing properties, particularly in skin disorders. A single randomized clinical trial (RCT) in patients with mild to moderate ulcerative colitis reported that oral aloe vera gel for 4 weeks produced a significant clinical and histologic response in a small trial of 44 patients. The dose used was 100 mL of aloe vera gel taken orally per day.

Short-chain fatty acid (SCFA)[1] enemas administered daily show some promise in subsets of patients with proctitis, including those with diversion and radiation proctitis. SCFAs are an important component of mucosal nutrition, hence the rationale for their use. RCTs in ulcerative colitis reported mixed results, but they remain an option in proctitis and distal colitis that is refractory to conventional therapy.

Finally, dietary manipulation, in the form of the "Specific Carbohydrate Diet,"[1] has been used by a number of our patients. This involves minimizing the dietary intake of carbohydrates to monosaccharides, in an attempt to reduce the carbohydrates available for pathogenic gut bacteria. It is a restrictive diet that requires motivation. The efficacy of this dietary manipulation has not been reported in RCTs.

## Management Strategies: Ulcerative Colitis

Management of UC depends on the disease geography and severity, based on prior endoscopy and symptoms. The Simple Colitis Activity Index can be used to assess disease severity in the office without laboratory results (Walmsley, 1998).

### MILD TO MODERATE DISEASE

Aminosalicylates are the agents of choice for inducing remission in patients with mild to moderate UC. Patients with proctitis obtain the best response with topical therapy such as mesalamine suppositories (Canasa), 1 g once a day, whereas distal disease requires enemas (Rowasa), 4 g per day. Topical therapy is associated with a more rapid clinical response than oral 5-ASAs alone and a greater efficacy than topical steroids. Up to 80% of patients should be in remission by 6 weeks. We advise patients to insert the enema at bedtime to increase its retention. In the event of poor response or difficulty with the rectal route, oral 5-ASAs should be used. In addition, the combination of oral and topical 5-ASA agents produces better clinical results than either alone. Because the topical therapy can take up to 2 weeks to produce a clinical response, topical steroids (Cortifoam) may be used concomitantly for this period in patients who are particularly symptomatic.

In patients with left-sided extensive pancolitis, oral sulfasalazine (Azulfidine), at 2 to 4 g/day, and 5-ASA agents, at 2 to 4.8 g/day[3] should be prescribed because lower doses are not effective in inducing remission. Doses of 5-ASAs up to 4.8 g are usually well tolerated and

produce clinical response in 60% of patients by 3 weeks and up to 80% in remission by 8 weeks. The dose used is probably more important than the 5-ASA agent used because there has been little comparison between the agents. Sulfasalazine has similar response rates but at a higher risk of adverse events than the other aminosalicylates, and it should be avoided in men considering fatherhood. It is significantly less expensive than the other 5-ASA agents, however, and thus more cost effective given its low absolute risk of side effects. Once remission is achieved, the same 5-ASA dose should be continued to maintain remission. As many as 90% of patients remain in remission at 1 year. Other than steroids, little evidence supports other therapies in mild to moderate disease; antibiotics, probiotics, or aloe gel may be tried in patients who cannot tolerate 5-ASAs.

### SEVERE DISEASE

Approximately 9% of patients present with severely active disease, requiring supplementary therapy to 5-ASAs. It is worth excluding surreptitious NSAID use, concomitant infection by stool culture, and 5-ASA intolerance, prior to proceeding to more potent agents. In particular, *Clostridium difficile* infection in those recently hospitalized or on antibiotics, and CMV infection in those receiving steroids can cause severe colitis.

The mainstay of induction of remission in severe disease is an oral steroid. Prednisone at a dose of 40 to 60 mg/day is highly effective in inducing remission in patients with moderate to severe disease. Approximately 80% of patients respond, and 54% are in remission at 1 month. No studies have compared the efficacy of oral to IV administration. Hydrocortisone (Solu-Cortef), at 100 mg IV every 6 hours, or methylprednisolone (Solu-Medrol), 40 mg/day IV, can be used in the few patients who do not respond or have difficulty with oral absorption. Hyperglycemia occurs commonly and should be monitored for, especially in those receiving IV steroids. In those patients who respond to steroids, the aim should be to begin a steroid taper after approximately 2 weeks of high-dose therapy. The dose should be reduced by 5 mg weekly until either the steroids are withdrawn or the patient develops recurrence of symptoms. If patients are not already on 5-ASAs, they should be started during the steroid taper as maintenance therapy. If patients cannot be withdrawn from steroid therapy because of recurrence of symptoms (steroid dependent), azathioprine (Imuran, Azasan),[1] at a dose of 1.5 to 2.5 mg/kg, or 6-MP (Purinethol),[1] at a dose of 1.5 mg/kg, should be started as maintenance therapy. As discussed previously, it may take 12 weeks for full effect, and patients should have their AST, ALT, and CBC checked regularly for adverse effects. The strategy here is to remove the steroids gradually as the therapeutic effect of azathioprine/6-MP manifests. Once in remission, treatment should continue indefinitely because patients who later have their maintenance drugs stopped have a higher rate of relapse. These agents can be used for induction of remission also, but the long time to clinical effect is usually too long when patients have severe disease.

In those cases with severe colitis where steroids do not induce a clinical response, the options then are cyclosporine (Neoral),[1] infliximab (Remicade), or surgery at present. Steroids are usually given for 72 hours to determine their response before proceeding to these options, although surgery is indicated sooner for toxic megacolon, fulminant colitis, or hemorrhage. One study demonstrated that those patients with a bowel frequency of more than eight times per day or a CRP greater than 45 have an 85% chance of colectomy after 3 days of medical therapy. Cyclosporine,[1] at a dose of 2 to 4 mg/kg/day by infusion, produces a response in up to 80% of patients after 8 days of therapy. Recent data suggest the response from 2 mg/kg is similar to 4 mg/kg with less adverse events. Renal function, blood pressure, magnesium levels, cholesterol, and cyclosporine levels should be monitored during treatment. Magnesium less than 0.5 mg/dL or a cholesterol level less than 120 mg/dL increases the risk of seizures. Opportunistic infections such as *Pneumocystis* pneumonia (PCP) and *Aspergillus* should be considered if patients develop respiratory symptoms.

---

[1]Not FDA approved for this indication.
[3]Exceeds dosage recommended by the manufacturer.

---

[1]Not FDA approved for this indication.

We routinely prescribe prophylaxis against PCP with sulfamethoxazole/trimethoprim (Bactrim) because deaths from this infection are reported in patients receiving cyclosporine for ulcerative colitis. Patients usually respond within 4 days of treatment; in this case they can be switched to oral cyclosporine[1] at a dose of 5 to 7 mg/kg/day, with maintenance of serum trough levels between 150 and 250 µg/mL.

The other medical option is infliximab (Remicade) at a dose of 5 mg/kg by IV infusion. In patients with severe ulcerative colitis who are hospitalized, this halves the risk of colectomy at 90 days. For patients with moderate to severe UC, infliximab produces response in 65% and puts approximately 30% of patients into remission at 30 weeks if given at 0, 2, 6 weeks, and at 8 weeks thereafter. The precautions and side effects are similar to its use in CD. All patients should have a PPD and chest radiograph (CXR) prior to instigation of therapy, and infusion reactions can be prevented with prednisone or IV hydrocortisone. No comparison between cyclosporine and infliximab has been made in these patients to date. If these medical options do not improve individual cases, surgery will be required.

# Management Strategy: Crohn's Disease

At any one time, approximately 50% of patients with CD will be in remission or have mild disease that is responsive to therapy. Of the rest, 40% will be postsurgery and 10% will have severe or treatment-refractory disease.

## MILD TO MODERATE DISEASE

In patients with ileocolonic disease, there are three initial treatment options: antibiotics, 5-ASAs, or budesonide (Entocort EC). Evidence from clinical trials and clinical experience differs as to which agent to use, but all three show moderate efficacy in this setting. There is significant controversy among IBD experts about which agent should be used as first-line therapy. We generally use mesalamine (Asacol, Pentasa, Salofalk) first for ileal disease, followed by ciprofloxacin (Cipro) or metronidazole (Flagyl) in nonresponders. For ileocolonic disease we use sulfasalazine (Azulfidine) as first-line therapy, followed by the other 5-ASAs. Other experts in the field start with budesonide (Entocort EC), whereas we reserve this for nonresponders to initial therapy.

Metronidazole, at doses of 500 mg three times daily, and ciprofloxacin, at 500 mg twice daily, produce a moderate clinical response in patients with ileal and colonic disease and more marked improvements in those with perianal disease. Therapy should continue for at least 3 months to maximize the therapeutic benefit, and the development of paresthesia should warrant dose reduction or discontinuation of metronidazole. Patients on ciprofloxacin should be warned about the risk of tendon rupture. In the event of a partial response to one agent, the combination of metronidazole and ciprofloxacin is often used prior to proceeding to steroids. Antibiotic resistance does not seem to be a problem in our practice, despite prolonged therapy.

Budesonide (Entocort EC), at 3 mg three times daily, is as effective as prednisone and superior to mesalamine with fewer side effects in ileitis and ileocolonic disease. Patients who respond may be continued at a maintenance dose of 6 mg/day because this reduces relapse rates. For colonic disease, 5-ASAs are first-line therapy in CD. Mesalamine at 4 g/day or sulfasalazine (Azulfidine) at 3 g/day produces a clinical response in 50% to 60% of patients. This response takes up to 2 weeks to develop and requires adequate doses of 5-ASA. The role of 5-ASAs in maintaining remission once achieved is controversial, although probably worthwhile if patients have responded. Regardless of which agent is used to induce remission, if therapy cannot be tapered without worsening of symptoms, immunomodulator therapy should be initiated. Azathioprine (Imuran[1]), 6-MP (Purinethol[1]), and methotrexate[1] should be started in this setting.

## SEVERE DISEASE

The selection of more aggressive therapy for CD should be individualized for each patient because this area is rapidly evolving. As in UC, oral steroids are highly effective first-line therapy for severe CD. Approximately 60% to 80% of cases respond to prednisone, 40 to 60 mg/day, and this should be tapered once the clinical status stabilizes. In this setting, azathioprine,[1] 1.5 to 2.5 mg/kg, or 6-MP,[1] 1.5 mg/kg, may be started during the steroid taper period or withheld until further episodes. Patients treated with immunomodulator maintenance therapy have a reduced risk of relapse in the medium term.

If patients do not respond to steroids, or they are concerned about their adverse effects, the next options are infliximab or methotrexate. Infliximab should be administered at a dose of 5 mg/kg at 0, 2 and 6 weeks initially. Patients usually notice a response within 1 to 2 weeks in the 60% of patients who respond. The development of infusion-related reactions can be prevented on subsequent doses by slowing the rate of infusion or administering prednisone, 50 mg twice daily, on the day before administration, or hydrocortisone, 200 mg IV, prior to the infusion. In those who respond to infliximab, repeated infusions every 8 weeks maintain approximately 30% to 40% in remission in the medium term. If this response wanes with time, either increase the dose to 10 mg/kg or shorten the duration between infusions. It is debatable whether the addition of azathioprine[1] or 6-MP[1] to infliximab produces major benefits in clinical efficacy, but it may increase the risk of adverse effects of immunosuppression.

An alternative to infliximab in steroid-refractory disease is methotrexate.[1] Induction of remission with 25 mg IM weekly, followed by 15 mg IM weekly, induced remission in approximately 40% of patients treated and maintained 65% in remission in clinical trials at 1 year. All patients should have their AST/ALT and CBC monitored and take folic acid supplementation. This therapy is teratogenic so should be discussed prior to its use in women of child-bearing age or women intending to conceive.

Strictures that do not respond to medical therapy require surgical intervention because some of these will be "cold" stenotic strictures without mucosa inflammation. Draining fistulas are primarily treated with antibiotics as above or infliximab with azathioprine[1]/6-MP[1] in more resistant cases. Deep perianal fistulas can be treated with seton placement and superficial ones with fistulotomy.

# Pregnancy

Pregnancy often raises questions about both pregnancy and disease outcomes and about drug therapy for women with IBD. There is a small increased risk of low birth weight and premature delivery in women with IBD, especially those with CD. The risk of a child of an affected parent developing UC is 2% to 5% and developing CD is 5% to 10% over their lifetime. Patients in remission at the time of conception are no more likely to develop a relapse than at other times of life, although if this occurs it is most often in the first trimester. Many cases of relapse in disease activity are actually because of discontinuation of maintenance therapy once the pregnancy is confirmed. In general, patients in remission with IBD have better pregnancy outcomes than those with active disease; therefore continuation of suitable maintenance medications is important in this setting. Apart from methotrexate, most drugs used for management of IBD can safely be used during pregnancy. This includes 5-ASAs, steroids, azathioprine,[1] 6-MP,[1] cyclosporine,[1] infliximab, and metronidazole (after the first trimester). As with all drugs, the benefits need to be weighed against potential adverse effects that are unknown. Drugs that should be avoided if possible during breast-feeding include olsalazine (Dipentum), azathioprine[1]/6-MP,[1] methotrexate,[1] cyclosporine,[1] and infliximab[1] if possible. Apart from the 5-ASA agents and steroids, there is little experience documented in breast-feeding with these drugs; women in this situation should consult with their pediatrician.

---

[1]Not FDA approved for this indication.

[1]Not FDA approved for this indication.

## Colon Cancer Surveillance

The risk of colorectal cancer (CRC) is increased in patients who have colitis for greater than 8 years; the excess risk is 19.2 for those with pancolitis and 2.8 for those with left-sided disease. At 20 years since onset of diagnosis, patients have an 8% risk of cancer. In particular, patients with primary sclerosing cholangitis and UC have a 31% risk of CRC at 20 years.

Surveillance for CRC should begin at 8 years after diagnosis for patients with disease beyond the descending colon and continue every 2 years. In patients with distal colitis and Crohn's colitis, the ideal surveillance intervals are more difficult to determine because the risk may be similar to more extensive colitis. Our personal practice is to perform surveillance on all those with UC above the rectum or extensive colonic CD after 8 years of disease. Because of the higher risk of CRC, all patients with primary sclerosing cholangitis should have surveillance regardless of their duration of UC or CD. Those patients in whom dysplasia or adenomas are detected require more intensive surveillance or consideration of colectomy. The finding of high-grade dysplasia or dysplasia-associated lesion or mass (DALM) is an indication for colectomy. However, when low-grade dysplasia is found, the risk of neoplasia progression is controversial, varying between 5% and 50%. We most often recommend colectomy for patients with long-standing colitis and low-grade dysplasia.

In those at high risk of CRC (e.g., family history of CRC, long disease history, primary sclerosing cholangitis [PSC], extensive colitis), chemoprophylaxis should be advised. 5-ASA at doses of 1.5 to 2 g/day in some case-control studies reduced CRC risk by at least 50%. Folic acid supplements, calcium, and NSAIDs such as aspirin reduce the risk of CRC in the general population. It is not known whether a combination of these produces an additive benefit, and they have not specifically been studied in IBD.

## REFERENCES

Aberra FN, Lichtenstein GR: Review article: Monitoring of immunomodulators in inflammatory bowel disease. Aliment Pharmacol Ther 2005;21:307-319.

Banerjee S, Peppercorn MA: Inflammatory bowel disease. Medical therapy of specific clinical presentations. Gastroenterol Clin North Am 2002;31:185-202.

Campieri M: New steroids and new salicylates in inflammatory bowel disease: A critical appraisal. Gut 2002;50(Suppl 3):III43-III46.

Farrell RJ, Peppercorn MA: Ulcerative colitis. Lancet 2002;359:331-340.

Ferrero S, Ragni N: Inflammatory bowel disease: Management issues during pregnancy. Arch Gynecol Obstet 2004;270:79-85.

Hanauer SB, Korelitz BI, Rutgeerts P: Postoperative maintenance of Crohn's disease remission with 6-mercaptopurine, mesalamine, or placebo: A 2-year trial. Gastroenterology 2004;127:723-729.

Jain SK, Peppercorn MA: Inflammatory bowel disease and colon cancer: A review. Dig Dis 1997;15:243-252.

Loftus EV Jr, Schoenfeld P, Sandborn WJ: The epidemiology and natural history of Crohn's disease in population-based patient cohorts from North America: A systematic review. Aliment Pharmacol Ther 2002; 16:51-60.

Rutgeerts P, Van AG, Vermeire S: Optimizing anti-TNF treatment in inflammatory bowel disease. Gastroenterology 2004;126:1593-1610.

Thukral C, Travassos WJ, Peppercorn MA: The role of antibiotics in inflammatory bowel disease. Curr Treat Options Gastroenterol 2005;8:223-228.

Velayos FS, Terdiman JP, Walsh JM: Effect of 5-aminosalicylate use on colorectal cancer and dysplasia risk: A systematic review and metaanalysis of observational studies. Am J Gastroenterol 2005;100:1345-1353.

Walmsley RS, Ayres RC, Pounder RE, Allan RN: A simple clinical colitis activity index. Gut 1998;43:29-32.

# Irritable Bowel Syndrome

Method of
*Michael P. Jones, MD*

## Definition

When confronted with a symptomatic patient, traditionally trained physicians are taught to search for a disease so that a specific diagnosis and therapy can be instituted. Unfortunately, in the clinical arena, this is most often not the case. In fact, an organic explanation for symptoms in the primary care setting occurs in less than 20% of cases.

When the evaluation of a patient's digestive complaints fails to identify a disease, the patient is considered to have a *functional gastrointestinal disorder* (FGID). The pathophysiology of FGID is unknown and multifactorial. These conditions are believed to result from dysregulation of sensory or motor function of the digestive tract and from abnormalities in the central nervous system (CNS) regulation of digestive function and visceral sensory processing. Purported pathophysiologic mechanisms are listed in Box 1.

Because FGIDs lack defined pathophysiology, they are diagnosed using symptom-based criteria. Although the term *irritable bowel syndrome* (IBS) is often misused in clinical practice to define any digestive complaint that eludes specific diagnosis, it should be kept in mind that IBS is actually one of 28 adult and 17 pediatric FGIDs. An abbreviated listing of adult FGID is shown in Box 2. The diagnostic criteria for IBS are given in Box 3.

Patients with IBS can be further categorized based on predominant bowel pattern as either constipation, diarrhea, mixed, or untyped. This subcategorization on relies patients' reports of stool consistency rather than frequency or defecatory sensations or efforts. Although these subcategories may be helpful in directing therapy, many patients experience changes in bowel pattern over the course of their illness, which makes these subcategories of limited utility.

Symptoms consistent with IBS are common in the community, with a reported prevalence of 10% to 15%. Only about 25% of people with IBS seek care for their symptoms. IBS consulters differ from nonconsulters in having more severe pain, greater health worries, more recent adverse life events, greater psychological comorbidity, and less-adaptive coping skills or illness behavior. These factors must be assessed and addressed to achieve optimal outcomes.

## Diagnostic Evaluation

The diagnosis of IBS is based on positive symptom criteria and the exclusion of underlying conditions that might cause similar symptoms. The presence of alarm features (advanced age, gastrointestinal bleeding or anemia, weight loss, fever, family history of inflammatory bowel disease or digestive malignancy, abnormal findings on physical examination) identifies patients in need of further diagnostic testing. In the absence of alarm features, diagnostic evaluation is employed as needed to exclude other conditions that have reasonably entered the differential diagnosis for a given patient. Patients without alarm features who fulfill diagnostic criteria for IBS are unlikely to have another explanation for their symptoms. Colonoscopy performed in these patients rarely discovers significant pathology. Colon cancer is found in less than 1%.

Similarly, although laboratory studies (complete blood count [CBC], chemistry panel, erythrocyte sedimentation rate [ESR]) are often obtained in patients meeting diagnostic criteria for IBS and having no alarm features, the utility of these studies is unproven. Thyroid function testing has been advocated because thyroid disorders are associated with changes in bowel function. However, thyroid dysfunction has the same prevalence in patients with IBS as in the general population. Recently, screening for celiac disease has been advocated and several studies report a higher prevalence of celiac sprue

## BOX 1  Pathophysiologic Alterations in Functional Gastrointestinal Disorders

### Genetic Predisposition

- Monozygotic twins are significantly more likely than dizygotic twins to have a concordant diagnosis of IBS.
- Preliminary evidence suggests lower levels of certain cytokines, serotonin transport proteins, and other signaling proteins may be present in some patients with FGID.

### Early Family Environment

- Children of parents with IBS are more likely to seek care for both digestive and nondigestive complaints.

### Psychosocial Factors

- Psychological stress can both induce and exacerbate digestive symptoms in healthy subjects and in patients with FGID.
- Psychosocial factors influence illness experience and illness behavior.

### Abnormal Digestive Motility

- Abnormal motor responses or patterns are commonly seen but correlate poorly with symptoms.

### Abnormal Digestive Sensation

- Patients with FGID might have lower thresholds for visceral pain (hypersensitivity) or perceive normal digestive sensations as unpleasant (allodynia).
- Hypervigilance can modify gut perception.

### Inflammation

- Increased inflammatory cells and cytokines are seen in a subset of patients, particularly those with persistent symptoms after enteric infection.

### Bacterial Flora

- Symptoms and cytokine patterns in patients with IBS can improve following supplementation with *Bifidobacterium infantis*.
- Bacterial overgrowth may be a factor in some patients with IBS.

*Abbreviations:* FGID = functional gastrointestinal disorder; IBS = irritable bowel syndrome.

## BOX 2  Functional Gastrointestinal Disorders*

- Functional esophageal disorders
  - Functional heartburn
  - Functional chest pain
  - Functional dysphagia
- Functional gastroduodenal disorders
  - Functional dyspepsia
  - Belching disorders
  - Nausea and vomiting disorders
  - Rumination syndromes
- Functional bowel disorders
  - Irritable bowel syndrome
  - Functional bloating
  - Functional constipation
- Functional abdominal pain syndrome
- Functional gallbladder and sphincter of Oddi disorders
- Functional anorectal disorders
  - Functional fecal incontinence
  - Functional anorectal pain
  - Functional defecation disorders

*Abbreviated listing of the Rome III classification scheme.

they are in the general population. Additionally, most patients with true carbohydrate maldigestion have little difficulty recognizing it. Symptoms induced by fatty foods are often mistaken for lactose intolerance because many dairy products are also often high in fat. Finally, an assessment of eating behavior may be of greater usefulness than a search for malabsorption syndromes. Patients with IBS may have maladaptive eating behavior, which can include hurried fast food meals eaten in the office, fad diets, or even true eating disorders.

Radiographic or endoscopic evaluation of the lower digestive tract is not routinely required in the absence of alarm features.

## Treatment

### INITIAL MANAGEMENT

Treatment is aimed at relieving symptoms and restoring quality of life. Given the absence of globally efficacious therapies in IBS and the often

in patients with IBS than in matched controls. Although the usefulness of this recommendation requires further study, it currently seems reasonable, particularly in IBS patients with diarrhea.

Perhaps of greater usefulness than serologic assessment for celiac disease is a careful diet history. In the absence of highly effective pharmacologic therapies, identifying symptom triggers becomes much more important. Although much is made of lactose and fructose intolerance, these conditions are not more prevalent among patients with IBS than

### CURRENT DIAGNOSIS

- Irritable bowel syndrome (IBS) is a symptomatically defined diagnosis of exclusion.
- Patients meeting diagnostic criteria for IBS who do not have alarm features can be generally be safely managed without further diagnostic evaluation.
- Patients with alarm features or those failing to respond to initial empiric management should undergo evaluation targeting a symptom-based differential diagnosis.

## BOX 3  Diagnostic Criteria for Irritable Bowel Syndrome

Rome III criteria for the irritable bowel syndrome are listed along with supportive symptoms. Supportive symptoms are not part of the diagnostic criteria.

- Recurrent abdominal pain or discomfort at least 3 days per month in the last 3 months associated with two or more of the following:
  - Improvement with defecation
  - Onset associated with a change in frequency of stool
  - Onset associated with a change in form (appearance) of stool.
- Supportive symptoms:
  - Abnormal stool frequency (>3 bowel movements/day or ≤3 bowel movements/week)
  - Abnormal stool form
  - Straining during defecation
  - Urgency (having to rush to have a bowel movement)
  - Feeling of incomplete bowel movement
  - Passing mucus (white material) during a bowel movement
  - Bloating

## CURRENT THERAPY

- There is no irritable bowel syndrome (IBS) pill or IBS diet.
- Effective management of patients with IBS is best achieved using a biopsychosocial approach rather than simply focusing on digestive anatomy and physiology.
- Effective management of IBS primarily involves identifying dietary and psychosocial triggers that cause or exacerbate symptoms.
- Effective management of IBS involves understanding and addressing the patient's agenda and concerns as well as providing adequate education and reassurance.
- Pharmacologic and dietary management of IBS is empiric and symptom driven.

chronic nature of the condition, strategies that avoid overreliance on pharmacologic interventions are preferred.

Establishing an effective physician–patient relationship is an important outcome determinant. Efforts should be made to address illness concerns, reduce symptom-associated anxiety, and provide adequate education and reassurance. Symptom triggers, both dietary and situational, should be identified. Specific issues that the physician should evaluate include recent major life events (e.g., marriage, divorce, family death, relocation, job change), diet or medication changes, illness worries, psychiatric comorbidity, impairment in daily function (e.g., recent inability to work or socialize), and complicating treatment factors (e.g., a history of narcotic or laxative abuse, pending disability or litigation).

Realistic treatment goals and relationship boundaries need to be set. The patient should be involved in the care, and the framework for a long-term relationship with the physician needs to be established.

### Dietary Therapy

There is no specific IBS diet. Identifying specific foods that trigger symptoms is an important therapeutic step, but caution should be taken to avoid excessive dietary restriction. Patients might experience symptoms as a generalized response to eating, and for these persons, dietary therapy is not effective. Although supplemental dietary fiber has traditionally been employed, there is little evidence to suggest its efficacy in IBS. In fact, although supplemental fiber can improve simple constipation, it often worsens bloating and pain in patients with IBS.

### Antispasmodics

Antispasmodics inhibit intestinal contractions and can help treat crampy abdominal pain and bloating. The most commonly used agents are dicyclomine (Bentyl) and hyoscyomine (Levsin). The anticholinergic effects of these agents relieve symptoms but can also lead to adverse effects that limit their use. Peppermint oil has mild calcium channel blocking activity, which inhibits intestinal contractions. Peppermint oil capsules have demonstrated efficacy in treating pain and bloating.

### Antidiarrheals

Loperamide (Imodium) is effective in relieving diarrhea and improving global symptoms. It slows intestinal transit and improves anal sphincter tone. Importantly, it does not cross the blood-brain barrier, which limits side effects compared with other opioids. Cholestyramine may be helpful in patients with diarrhea after cholecystectomy and for the rare patient with bile acid malabsorption.

### Laxatives

In patients with simple constipation, supplemental fiber (25 g/day) has been shown to be efficacious in improving bowel habits. The efficacy of fiber in constipation-predominant IBS is at best mixed. For patients either not responding to or made worse by fiber, osmotic laxatives are reasonable. These include sorbitol, milk of magnesia, or polyethylene glycol preparations.

## Follow-Up

### EVALUATION OF THE PATIENT FAILING INITIAL MANAGEMENT

Patients not responding to education, reassurance, and initial medical management might require more specialized diagnostic evaluation. For patients with severe constipation, tests for pelvic floor dysfunction and intestinal transit may be useful. The former can involve anorectal manometry and magnetic resonance or fluoroscopic defecography. Colonic transit is most commonly assessed using radiopaque markers (Sitzmarks).

For patients with persistent diarrhea, consideration should be given to stool studies and serum chemistries looking for evidence of malabsorption (increased fecal fat, stool osmotic gap suggesting laxative use, hypoalbuminemia or proteinemia along with electrolyte disturbances). Serologic studies for celiac disease should be obtained and consideration given to obtaining biosies of the small bowel. Testing for carbohydrate intolerance (particularly lactose and fructose) should be considered. This can be accomplished using breath hydrogen testing, which avoids phlebotomy. Colonoscopy into the terminal ileum and with random biopsies can also be considered, looking for Crohn's disease as well as microscopic and collagenous colitis.

In patients with severe bloating or abdominal pain, plain abdominal radiographs at a minimum or abdominopelvic computed tomography (CT) scan should be considered. A more careful psychosocial assessment with attention to affective disorders, somatoform disorders, a history of abuse, recent adverse life events, and maladaptive pain beliefs or coping behavior can be quite helpful.

### TREATMENT OF THE PATIENT FAILING INITIAL MANAGEMENT

#### Constipation-Predominant IBS

Identification and treatment of pelvic floor disorders and dysynergic defecation have a high likelihood of success. About three fourths of patients with obstructive defecation respond to physical therapy. Tegaserod, a partial 5-HT$_4$ agonist, has been approved for treating chronic constipation and constipation-predominant IBS in women. Although generally well tolerated, the agent is expensive, its long-term efficacy and safety are unknown, and its usefulness beyond standard therapies for constipation has never been critically evaluated. Selective serotonin reuptake inhibitors (SSRIs) have been shown to significantly accelerate intestinal transit and might be useful in patients with abdominal pain or affective disorders and constipation. Behavioral therapies, particularly relaxation techniques and gut-directed hypnotherapy, are effective in treating refractory constipation.

#### Diarrhea-Predominant IBS

Tincture of opium and paregoric have been used to treat chronic refractory diarrhea for years and are efficacious. These agents must be used carefully because of the potential for dependency and abuse. Tricyclic antidepressants[1] are useful to treat visceral pain, and their anticholinergic effects also help treat diarrhea. Alosetron (Lotronex), a 5-HT$_3$ antagonist, was approved to treat women with diarrhea-predominant IBS. Unfortunately, this drug is expensive and associated with severe constipation and ischemic colitis. It is available only through a restricted access protocol.

---

[1]Not FDA approved for this indication.

### Pain-Predominant IBS

Tricylcic antidepressants[1] are effective for treating visceral pain syndromes, and analgesia is achieved with lower doses than are used to treat depression. The most widely used agents are amitriptyline (Elavil)[1] and nortriptyline (Pamelor).[1] The initial dose for these agents is 10 mg at bedtime, titrating up as needed. Fatigue and anticholinergic effects often limit their use. SSRIs are being used with increasing frequency but are incompletely studied. Paroxetine (Paxil)[1] is the best-studied agent and has been shown to improve quality of life and decrease the number of days with pain.

### Newer and Nontraditional Therapies

A variety of psychotherapies have been shown to reduce abdominal pain, improve bowel habits, and improve quality of life. These treatments include cognitive behavior therapy, hypnosis, and stress management and relaxation therapy. In general, these treatments are effective comparable or superior with standard pharmacologic therapy. Their efficacy does not depend on the presence of concomitant affective disorders.

Emerging evidence suggests that probiotics may be helpful in treating IBS. Probiotics containing *Bifidobacterium infantis* have been shown to significantly reduce symptoms, potentially by modifying cytokine profiles. Bacterial overgrowth in the small intestine has recently attracted attention as a potential cause of IBS symptoms, but further support for this hypothesis is needed.

Peppermint oil was discussed above. Ginger[7] has been used as an antiemetic but has not been shown superior to placebo in several trials. Aloe is used to treat constipation. Its efficacy is unknown and it does contain stimulant anthraquinones.

### REFERENCES

Creed F, Fernandes L, Guthrie E, et al: The cost-effectiveness of psychotherapy and paroxetine for severe irritable bowel syndrome. Gastroenterology 2003;124:303-317.

Drossman DA, Camilleri M, Mayer EA, Whitehead WE: AGA technical review on irritable bowel syndrome. Gastroenterology 2002;123:2108-2131.

Drossman DA, Toner BB, Whitehead WE, et al: Cognitive-behavioral therapy versus education and desipramine versus placebo for moderate to severe functional bowel disorders. Gastroenterology 2003;125:19-31.

Longstreth GF, Thompson WG, Chey WD, et al: Functional bowel disorders. Gastroenterology 2006;130:1480-1491.

O'Mahony L, McCarthy J, Kelly P, et al: Lactobacillus and bifidobacterium in irritable bowel syndrome: Symptom responses and relationship to cytokine profiles. Gastroenterology 2005;128:541-551.

Spanier JA, Howden CW, Jones MP: A systematic review of alternative therapies in the irritable bowel syndrome. Arch Intern Med 2003;163:265-274.

[1]Not FDA approved for this indication.
[7]Available as a dietary supplement.

# Hemorrhoids, Anal Fissure, and Anorectal Abscess and Fistula

Method of
*Neil H. Hyman, MD*

Anal canal diseases such as hemorrhoids, anal fissures, anorectal abscesses, and fistulas are very common. Although these conditions seldom cause life-threatening complications, they are a major cause of patient discomfort, morbidity, and diminished quality of life. Because most anorectal disorders are diagnosed and treated in the outpatient setting, physicians receive little exposure to them during their medical training. Further, relatively little attention is given to anorectal disease in most medical and surgical textbooks. Therefore, misperceptions and misdiagnoses are extremely common, leading to considerable unnecessary suffering.

The vast majority of the time, the diagnosis is readily made based on the patient's symptoms. An accurate history is the key to appropriate diagnosis and successful management.

## History

Patients most often ascribe any perianal symptom to a "hemorrhoid" problem. When using this term, the patient might mean that there is a palpable perianal lesion, anal itching, pain, rectal bleeding, or abnormal discharge, to name a few common anorectal symptoms. However, the correct diagnosis and treatment often are unrelated to hemorrhoidal disease.

Two of the most common complaints are pain and bleeding (Table 1). Pain that occurs with defecation, often associated with bright red blood on the toilet tissue, is typical for an anal fissure. Constant pain of acute onset is most often caused by a thrombosed external hemorrhoid or a perianal abscess. Anal outlet bleeding is characterized by bright red blood that appears on the toilet tissue or perhaps drips into the toilet water. This type of bleeding associated with pain on defecation strongly suggests an anal fissure. Painless bleeding of this type is typical for internal hemorrhoids.

## Physical Examination

An accurate patient history is usually sufficient to make the diagnosis. The physical examination is usually confirmatory, especially when a patient is having pain and only a brief physical examination is possible. The practitioner needs to know what he or she is looking for.

## Hemorrhoids

The anal cushions consist of redundant rectal mucosa, arterioles, venules, and arteriovenous malformations that are supported by elastic connective tissue and smooth muscle fibers. These can be found in all patients, classically in the right anterior, right posterior, and left lateral position. In this light, hemorrhoids really are normal anatomic structures. When there is weakening of the supportive tissue and these cushions prolapse, or there is erosion into the submucosal vascular plexus and there is bleeding, one uses the term *hemorrhoids*.

Internal hemorrhoids occur above the dentate line, where there is typically columnar or transitional epithelium. Common symptoms include prolapse or bleeding. Internal hemorrhoids are typically classified on the basis of the degree of prolapse (Table 2).

The external hemorrhoidal plexuses lie below the dentate line and are prone to thrombosis. Perianal skin tags are often called external hemorrhoids. Numerous symptoms are often ascribed to these skin tags because they are readily apparent to the patient. Most often, these skin tags are an incidental finding and not the cause of the patient's symptoms.

### TABLE 1  Differential Diagnosis of Anal Lesions

| Lesion | Pain | Bleeding |
|---|---|---|
| Anal fissure | With defecation | Yes |
| Internal hemorrhoids | Usually not | Yes |
| Thrombosed external hemorrhoid | Constant | Only if ulcerated |
| Perianal abscess | Constant | Mixed with pus |

**TABLE 2  Classification of Internal Hemorrhoids**

| Grade | Physical Findings |
|-------|-------------------|
| I | Prominent hemorrhoidal vessels, no prolapse |
| II | Prolapse with Valsalva and spontaneous reduction |
| III | Prolapse with Valsalva, requires manual reduction |
| IV | Chronically prolapsed, manual reduction ineffective |

## EVALUATION

A targeted history and physical examination is the most important determinant of the need for further evaluation and treatment. Painless bleeding is a common symptom from internal hemorrhoids. Physical examination should typically include visual inspection of the anal canal, a digital rectal examination, and often anoscopy. Generally speaking, patients older than 50 years, those with a family history of colorectal neoplasm, and those with more worrisome symptoms (e.g., blood mixed in with the stool, change in stool caliber, abdominal pain) typically require full colonic evaluation with colonoscopy. Most other patients require at most a flexible sigmoidoscopy to evaluate their bleeding. Colonoscopy does not cure bleeding hemorrhoids!

External hemorrhoids or skin tags are usually an innocent finding. However, external hemorrhoids can cause pain owing to acute thrombosis or can present anal hygiene problems when stool collects on them, making cleansing difficult. Although anal itching is often ascribed to the skin tags, the tags are usually the result of irritation and scratching rather than the cause.

## TREATMENT

Dietary management consisting of adequate fluid and fiber supplementation is the primary treatment for most patients with hemorrhoids. Patients should also be instructed to avoid excessive straining during defecation.

Patients with significant prolapse (typically grade 3 or 4) require a more aggressive treatment modality. The vast majority can be treated with office-based procedures such as hemorrhoid banding. The aim of these treatments is to decrease vascularity, diminish hemorrhoidal volume, and increase fixation of the fibrovascular cushion to the rectal wall. Rubber band ligation has been associated with a 65% to 85% success rate but often requires repeating. Surgical hemorrhoidectomy should be reserved for patients whose hemorrhoids are refractory to less-invasive procedures, patients who are unable to tolerate office-based procedures, and patients with large combined internal and external hemorrhoids.

Thrombosed external hemorrhoids may be treated conservatively with sitz baths, avoidance of constipation, and analgesics. However, if the pain is increasing or excessive, or conservative management fails, then excision is warranted. Thrombosed external hemorrhoids should be excised, and simple enucleation of the clot is generally inadequate. The most painful aspect of the treatment is the injection of local anesthesia; excising the hemorrhoid does not increase the morbidity. Simple enucleation of the clot often leads to repeat thrombosis within the next 24 to 48 hours. Large skin tags that create significant hygiene problems can also be readily excised on an outpatient basis with local anesthesia.

## Anal Fissures

An anal fissure is a crack or tear in the richly innervated squamous lining of the anal canal between the anal verge and the dentate line. The classic symptoms are ripping or tearing with defecation, which is associated with blood on the toilet tissue. Patients often feel like they are passing glass or sharp objects in their stool and have a sensation that the anal canal is too small to allow passage of the stool. Anal fissures can be agonizingly painful. They are commonly associated with extremes of bowel function such as excessively hard and large stools or frequent diarrhea, which abrades the anoderm.

## EVALUATION

The diagnosis is typically readily made on the basis of the characteristic history. An effort should be made to identify the cause of the patient's fissure (e.g., constipation or diarrhea) and manage it appropriately. Because fissures are so often painful, physical examination is necessarily limited. Simply spreading the buttocks to observe the anal canal is often very uncomfortable. Most fissures occur in the posterior midline, and this is where attention should initially be directed. Chronic anal fissures are often associated with secondary findings such as an external skin tag and a hypertrophied anal papilla. It is the sentinel anal tag that explains why patients with a fissure most often think they have a hemorrhoid. The true culprit, an anal fissure, is usually lurking at the cephalad aspect of the anal tag. Digital examination is often impossible owing to the pain and sphincter spasm.

Most anal fissures are associated with very high pressures in the anal canal. In fact, the pressures can exceed those of systemic blood pressure, impairing perfusion to the fissure and preventing healing. Most fissures are elliptic and located in the midline. Fissures with an atypical appearance, those not associated with sphincter hypertonia, or those in a lateral position suggest an alternative pathogenesis such as Crohn's disease or a sexually transmitted disease.

## TREATMENT

Acute anal fissures typically respond to conservative measures. This includes fluid and fiber supplementation, sitz baths, and possibly stool softeners if the patient has hard stools. Adjunctive measures such as topical anesthetics may be used for patient comfort.

Topical nitrates[1] have been associated with pain relief and a marginal improvement in fissure healing rates. However, the principal side effect has been headaches, which are dose related. Topical calcium channel blockers such as nifedipine (Adalat, Procardia)[1] appear to be at least equally efficacious and are associated with fewer side effects. Botulinum toxin (Botox)[1] injections have been used for anal fissures that fail to respond to these conservative measures; however, even if the injections are effective, recurrence rates over time appear to be high.

Patients with symptoms that are refractory to conservative measures should be considered for surgery. The treatment of choice is usually a lateral internal sphincterotomy; this corrects the markedly elevated anal canal pressures that are associated with an anal fissure and leads to healing in well over of 90% of cases. The very low morbidity and almost immediate pain relief make this procedure among the most effective of any surgical intervention. However, surgical sphincterotomy is associated with a small risk of minor fecal incontinence.

## Anorectal Abscess And Fistula

Most perianal abscesses arise from cryptoglandular obstruction. Specifically, the duct of an anal gland becomes occluded, with subsequent bacterial overgrowth and retrograde infection. Fortunately, at least one half of anorectal abscesses resolve after adequate drainage. However, many patients develop a persistent epithelialized tract from the infected gland inside the anal canal to the external drainage site (anal fistula).

## EVALUATION

Patients with an anorectal abscess typically present with acute pain. Often there are systemic signs of infection such as malaise and fever.

There are relatively few causes of acute anorectal pain. Pain that occurs with defecation is typically caused by an anal fissure. Thrombosed external hemorrhoids are also readily apparent on physical examination. Most patients with an anorectal abscess present with

---

[1]Not FDA approved for this indication.

an obvious red, tender, fluctuant mass. However, more deep-seated abscesses can manifest in a far more subtle manner.

Physical examination typically consists of only visual inspection. If the abscess is identified, no further evaluation is really required at that time. Patients with pain who do not have a discernible abnormality should undergo a careful digital examination; in some patients, this examination requires a formal anesthetic. Imaging studies such as computed tomography (CT) or magnetic resonance imaging (MRI) are only required in select ambiguous circumstances.

In the chronic phase, patients typically present with an external opening on the perianal skin that drains purulent material. Quite often, the patient describes a cycle of perianal pain followed by drainage and relief of symptoms. This sequence repeats itself over and over again. Alternatively, the patient might seem to be abscess prone; specifically, the patient presents every few months with an acute abscess requiring drainage. All of these clinical scenarios suggest an anal fistula.

## TREATMENT

A perianal abscess should be adequately drained. Lack of fluctuance is not an appropriate reason to delay timely drainage. Perianal erythema typically indicates that the abscess will be found deeper in the anal canal or ischiorectal fossa. Outside of unusual circumstances or specific immunocompromised states, perianal cellulitis does not occur.

Most abscesses are readily localized and easily drained in the outpatient setting under local anesthesia. Packing the abscess cavity is typically painful and usually unnecessary. Rather, a cruciate incision should be made that is adequate to facilitate complete drainage of the abscess cavity. An inadequate incision often leads to recurrent abscess formation.

Patients with diffuse erythema, in whom precise localization is not possible, commonly require drainage under anesthesia. Similarly, patients who appear toxic or are immunocompromised might need drainage in the operating room to ensure there are no loculations.

Antibiotics are an unnecessary addition to routine incision and drainage of uncomplicated perianal abscesses. Similarly, a culture is not required in most cases. The addition of antibiotics does not improve healing times or reduce recurrences. However, in patients with immunosuppression, diabetes, prosthetic devices, or excessive cellulitis, adjunctive antibiotic therapy should be considered.

An anal fistula denotes the chronic phase of anorectal sepsis and is the natural history in up to 50% of perianal abscesses. A fistula is believed to arise from persistent sepsis or the development of an epithelialized tract. Anal fistulas are characterized based on their location relative to the sphincter muscles. Fortunately, most anal fistulas involve a relatively small amount of muscle and can be readily treated by fistulotomy, or unroofing of the anal fistula tract. However, complex fistulas can be among the most difficult and frustrating problems for patient and colorectal surgeon alike. Generally speaking, patients with deep tracts involving considerable portions of this sphincter muscle or patients with preexisting fecal incontinence require an alternative approach. These might include injection of fibrin glue, endoanal advancement flap repair of the internal opening, or perhaps placement of a biological plug. These techniques appear to have a substantially lower success rate than fistulotomy.

## REFERENCES

Boyum J, Hyman N: Fissure-in-ano. Semin Colon Rectal Surg 2003;14:107-110.
Cataldo P, Ellis N, Gregorcyk S, Hyman N, et al: Practice parameter for the management of hemorrhoids. Dis Colon Rectum 2005;48:189-194.
Hyman NH: Anorectal abscess and fistula. Prim Care 1999;26:69-80.
Hyman N: Incontinence after lateral internal sphincterotomy: A prospective study and quality of life assessment. Dis Colon Rectum 2004;47:35-38.
Keighley MR, Buchmann P, Minervium S, et al: Prospective trials of minor surgical procedures and high fibre diet for haemorrhoids. BMJ 1997;2: 967-969.
Orsay C, Rakinic J, Perry B, et al: Practice parameter for the management of anal fissures. Dis Colon Rectum 2004;47:2003-2007.
Nelson R: Operative procedures for fissure in ano. Cochrane Database Syst Rev 2005;(2):CD002199.

Richard CS, Gregoire R, Plewes EA, et al: Internal sphincterotomy is superior to topical nitroglycerin in the treatment of chronic anal fissure: Results of a randomized, controlled trial by the Canadian Colorectal Surgical Trials Group. Dis Colon Rectum 2000;43:1048-1057.
Whiteford M, Kilkenny J, Hyman N, et al: Practice parameter for the treatment of perianal abscess and fistula-in-ano. Dis Colon Rectum 2005;48: 1337-1342.

# Gastritis and Peptic Ulcer Disease

Method of
*Sripathi R. Kethu, MD, and Steven F. Moss, MD*

Gastritis is by definition a histopathologic diagnosis, and peptic ulcer disease (PUD) is an endoscopic or radiologic diagnosis. Neither of these conditions has a specific symptom complex to help the clinician arrive at a diagnosis. Instead, physicians encounter patients with symptoms of dyspepsia that might or might not be secondary to gastritis or PUD. Thus, for the primary care provider, the discussion of gastritis and PUD must be prefaced by first considering the approach to the patient with dyspeptic symptoms.

## Dyspepsia

*Dyspepsia* refers to pain or discomfort centered in the upper abdomen, which may be intermittent or continuous and might or might not be related to meals. The symptoms may be described by several other terms, including *bloating, fullness, belching*, and *nausea* or simply as *indigestion*.

The prevalence of uninvestigated dyspepsia in the general population is not well documented. However, up to 25% of people in the community each year report chronic or recurrent pain or discomfort in the upper abdomen, and approximately 2% to 5% of family practice consultations are for dyspepsia.

### ETIOLOGY AND DIFFERENTIAL DIAGNOSIS

Dyspepsia can result from an identifiable cause such as peptic ulcer disease, malignancy, gastroesophageal reflux, or the use of specific medications. Other rare causes include pancreatic-biliary disease, gastroparesis, celiac disease, lactose intolerance, and parasitic diseases such as giardiasis. Patients who have no definite structural or biochemical explanation for their symptoms are considered to have functional dyspepsia (nonulcer dyspepsia). There is a subset of patients in whom dyspepsia might coexist with a microbiological or structural abnormality such as *Helicobacter pylori* gastritis or duodenitis or with gallstones, but a causal relation between these abnormalities and dyspepsia may be unclear.

The patient's age is one of the most important factors in tailoring the management of patients with dyspepsia because of the very low probability of stomach cancer in younger patients (typically this cutoff is arbitrarily fixed at 55 years). Thus, if a patient older than 55 years presents with new-onset upper abdominal complaints, or patients younger than this age develop alarm symptoms (anemia, anorexia, weight loss >10% of body weight, early satiety, dysphagia, or gastrointestinal (GI) bleeding either overt or occult), prompt endoscopic evaluation is required to detect the cause before administering empiric therapy.

In a primary care setting, the patient's history is crucial in elucidating the cause of dyspepsia. Peptic ulcer disease is an important consideration in the differential diagnosis of dyspepsia, accounting for up to 15% of cases. Although it is impossible to distinguish gastric and duodenal ulcers by symptoms alone, the pain of gastric and duodenal ulcers is typically epigastric, episodic, and often worse at night. Symptoms are often temporarily relieved with food or antacids in duodenal ulcer; in contrast, food can precipitate gastric ulcer pain. Associated symptoms such as anorexia, nausea, or vomiting can point toward the diagnosis of gastric ulcer or pyloric stenosis. Patients with gastric malignancy, which accounts for less than 2% of all cases of dyspepsia, can also present with similar symptoms.

Gastroesophageal reflux disease (GERD) may be the underlying disorder in 10% to 15% of patients with dyspepsia. Other typical symptoms in GERD include heartburn or a retrosternal burning pain or a feeling of regurgitation of food or acid. However, about 20% of patients with GERD present with epigastric pain alone, thereby creating a diagnostic problem. If medications are responsible for dyspepsia, generally a temporal relationship can be established between the medication intake and the onset of dyspeptic symptoms. Nonsteroidal anti-inflammatory drugs (NSAIDs) are the most common offending agents; other medications that cause dyspepsia are corticosteroids, iron preparations, digitalis, potassium supplements, bisphosphonates, niacin, and antibiotics, particularly erythromycin and ampicillin.

Functional, or nonulcer, dyspepsia accounts for up to 60% of all cases of dyspepsia. Functional dyspepsia and PUD share many symptoms, thus making the distinction by history alone impossible. By definition, the cause of functional dyspepsia is obscure; the putative pathophysiologic abnormalities that have been proposed to cause or to be associated with functional dyspepsia are gastric acid hypersecretion, *H. pylori* infection, gastroduodenal dysmotility, visceral hyperalgesia, and psychological distress including physical or sexual abuse. Although functional dyspepsia is a benign condition, it is the hardest to treat given the uncertain interplay between numerous pathogenic mechanisms.

## EVALUATION

Currently the best test in the evaluation of dyspepsia is upper endoscopy. Barium meal radiographs are less sensitive and specific.

In a younger patient (age < 55 years), in the absence of alarm symptoms, and after excluding other causes such as GERD and NSAID use by history, an *H. pylori* test and treat strategy, followed by proton pump inhibitor (PPI) treatment if the patient remains symptomatic or is not infected by *H. pylori*, is the management strategy of choice. The justification for this approach is that among patients with uninvestigated dyspepsia who are *H. pylori* positive, a substantial number have peptic ulcers, and a few without ulcers can improve symptomatically following eradication of *H. pylori*. Whether this strategy is suitable for affluent populations in the United States who have a very low prevalence of *H. pylori* is debatable because it can result in the diagnosis of almost as many false-positive *H. pylori* infections and lead to inappropriate eradication therapy. Furthermore, the cost benefits of the test and treat approach over one with early invasive testing remains unproven in practice. In other populations, noninvasive testing for *H. pylori* either by stool antigen test or urea breath test is reasonable. These tests are relatively less expensive compared with either upper endoscopy or indefinite empiric acid-suppressive therapy and are more accurate than serology.

If symptoms persist after *H. pylori* eradication therapy, or if empiric acid-suppressive therapy in *H. pylori*–negative patients fails, upper endoscopy should be undertaken. Ultrasonography is not recommended as a routine next step unless the history or biochemical tests suggest pancreatic-biliary disease. In patients with diabetes or a history suggesting autonomic neuropathy, a gastric emptying scan (scintigraphy) may be considered to document gastroparesis. Even though functional dyspepsia should be considered a diagnosis of exclusion, clinicians should use their judgment on a case-by-case basis to limit the use of numerous invasive and expensive investigations whenever possible.

## MANAGEMENT

Once the cause of dyspepsia is established, management involves treating the underlying cause. The most challenging task is managing patients with functional dyspepsia. *H. pylori* eradication therapy for patients who do not have an ulcer can result in symptomatic improvement in a small minority, approximately in 15% of patients, at best, over placebo. However, most patients remain symptomatic after eradication therapy, thus requiring other therapies.

Reassurance and explanation are important first steps in management. Proving that the symptoms do not represent a malignancy may be sufficient. Patients should be educated to avoid any obvious offending agents, such as coffee, alcohol, smoking, NSAIDs, and spicy and fatty foods; this helps relieve symptoms in some patients. Precipitant psychosocial factors including anxiety and depression should also be explored and treated appropriately. Pharmacologic therapy is not always required, and if required, it should be individualized. No single drug has been clearly shown to be beneficial over the long term, and the results of pharmacologic therapy are disappointing overall.

First-line therapies usually involve a therapeutic trial of either antisecretory agents such as $H_2$-receptor antagonists ($H_2$-RAs) or PPIs. A prokinetic agent such as metoclopramide (Reglan) 10 mg 1 hour after meals and at bedtime for 4 to 6 weeks may be useful as an alternative therapy. A drug holiday during therapy can help determine if the medication is still needed. The benefits of individual drugs should be weighed against the side-effect profile and cost. Metoclopramide, for example, is associated with neuropsychiatric complications and therefore cannot be recommended for the long term. Antidepressants such as amitriptyline (Elavil)[1] 150 mg at bedtime or antispasmodics such as dicyclomine (Bentyl)[1] 20 to 40 mg every 6 hours, can be tried as a next step, but the results are marginal at best. Alternative therapies such as acupuncture, cognitive behavior therapy, and hypnotherapy have been anecdotally reported to be beneficial.

# Gastritis

Exposure of the gastric mucosa to various insults can lead to epithelial damage and regeneration with minimal or no inflammation (gastropathy), or the epithelial damage may be associated with significant inflammation (gastritis). For an endoscopist, gastritis usually means petechiae or erosions of the gastric mucosa. These endoscopic findings might not have a good correlation with the presence of inflammatory cells on biopsy. Strictly speaking, gastritis is a histopathologic diagnosis associated with the presence of inflammatory cells. Gastritis and gastropathy can be categorized according to the histologic features and the etiology (Box 1).

## ACUTE EROSIVE AND HEMORRHAGIC GASTROPATHY

The most common causes of acute erosive and hemorrhagic gastropathy include NSAIDs, alcohol, and stress due to critical illness. Clinically, the patient might present with nonspecific complaints such as epigastric pain, nausea, or vomiting and occasionally with upper bleeding alone. Upper endoscopy usually reveals erythema or erosions.

---

[1]Not FDA approved for this indication.

---

**BOX 1  Classification of Gastritis**

- Acute erosive and hemorrhagic gastropathy
- Chronic gastritis
  - *Helicobacter pylori* gastritis (may be atrophic or nonatrophic)
  - Pernicious anemia–associated atrophic gastritis (type A gastritis or autoimmune gastritis)
- Others
  - Eosinophilic gastritis
  - Infectious (Cytomegalovirus, Herpes virus)
  - Granulomatous gastritis (Crohn's disease)
  - Portal gastropathy

Histologically, there is usually no or minimal inflammation, hence the term *gastropathy* instead of *gastritis*. Stress gastritis, most likely due to chronic gastric ischemia, can lead to gastric ulceration, usually multiple small ulcers involving the proximal part of the stomach.

Management of symptomatic gastropathy caused by NSAIDs or alcohol involves minimizing or avoiding the offending agents or taking the NSAIDs with food. A short course of H₂-RAs or PPIs is recommended if the patient has persistent symptoms despite conservative measures. Long-term acid-suppression therapy with PPIs may be necessary for patients believed to be at high risk for bleeding but in whom chronic NSAID use is necessary. The development of cyclooxygenase-2 (COX-2) selective NSAIDs has diminished but not eliminated clinically important gastroduodenal bleeding, and the benefit of these agents should be weighed against their reported risk of cardiovascular complications.

Endoscopy is recommended only for patients with risk factors for developing an ulcer (see the section on peptic ulcer disease). Many critically ill hospitalized patients develop superficial erosions ("stress gastritis) from chronic gastric ischemia, but this rarely leads to clinically significant gastric bleeding. Two risk factors that are associated with a high risk of clinically significant bleeding are mechanical ventilation and a coagulopathy. In the absence of these two risk factors, the risk of significant bleeding is less than 0.1%. Preventing stress gastritis and ulcers with the use of acid-suppression medications is strongly recommended in all critically ill patients, particularly if they have the previously mentioned risk factors. The superiority of oral or intravenous PPIs over H₂-RAs in this setting has not been definitely established.

## CHRONIC *HELICOBACTER PYLORI* GASTRITIS

*H. pylori* is a gram-negative spiral bacterium acquired in childhood that colonizes the gastric mucosa and usually causes an antral-predominant gastritis. In the developed world, infection is more prevalent in the elderly, the poor, and immigrants from high-incidence regions such as Asia, Africa, and Central and South America.

Inflammation associated with chronic *H. pylori* colonization may be confined to the superficial mucosa or can extend deeper into the gastric glands, leading in some cases to gastric atrophy (atrophic gastritis) and intestinal metaplasia of the gastric epithelium. The majority of all gastric and duodenal ulcers are caused by *H. pylori*; approximately 10% of all patients with chronic gastritis due to *H. pylori* eventually develop peptic ulcer disease.

A more uncommon consequence of *H. pylori* infection is adenocarcinoma of the stomach, typically developing after many decades of infection and after histologic progression from atrophic gastritis through intestinal metaplasia and dysplasia. *H. pylori* infection is associated with a threefold to sixfold increased risk of distal gastric cancer, leading to its designation by the World Health Organization as a carcinogen. It is also a major risk factor for the relatively rare mucosa-associated lymphoid tissue (MALT) gastric B-cell lymphoma. (See the section on peptic ulcer disease for detailed discussion of diagnosis and management of *H. pylori*.)

Factors believed to be important determinants of individual clinical outcome following *H. pylori* infection include host genetics, nutritional and general health status, and specific *H. pylori* virulence genes.

## PERNICIOUS ANEMIA–ASSOCIATED ATROPHIC GASTRITIS

Pernicious anemia–associated atrophic gastritis (type A gastritis or autoimmune gastritis) is an autoimmune disorder characterized by antiparietal cell antibodies leading to parietal cell destruction. The disease is more common in women and in persons of northern European descent. Parietal cell destruction in the gastric fundus leads to achlorhydria, and the impaired intrinsic factor production results in vitamin B₁₂ malabsorption. Generally, patients are asymptomatic until extreme vitamin B₁₂ deficiency causes anemia leading to neurologic syndromes. Patients are at increased risk for developing carcinoid tumors (secondary to prolonged hypergastrinemia) and adenocarcinoma of the stomach. Treatment involves vitamin B₁₂ supplementation even if the serum vitamin B₁₂ level is not low. The usefulness of

periodic endoscopic screening to detect carcinoma or carcinoid tumors is controversial in this condition.

# Peptic Ulcer Disease

*Peptic ulcer disease* is a generic term used to indicate a mucosal defect in the stomach or duodenum. As opposed to an erosion, which is a superficial lesion, an ulcer has a perceivable depth extending through the submucosa. PUD is believed to occur when factors aggressive to the gastric mucosa dominate (such as *H. pylori* infection or gastric acid hypersecretion) or when mucosal defense mechanisms are impaired (by NSAIDs, for example), or both.

The lifetime risk of PUD in the United States is approximately 10%, with a male-to-female ratio of 1.3:1 for a duodenal ulcer and 1:1 for a gastric ulcer. Duodenal ulcer occurs more commonly between ages 25 and 55 years, whereas gastric ulcer affects a slightly older population (ages 40-70 years). NSAID use or *H. pylori* infection increases the peptic ulcer risk by about 20-fold. Cigarette smoking not only increases the ulcer risk (by twofold), but also retards ulcer healing and increases the risk of bleeding. Despite popular beliefs, alcohol and dietary factors have no established relation with the cause of ulcers or their healing. Psychological stress can play some role in idiopathic ulcers.

## ETIOLOGY

Depending on their etiology, ulcers can be classified in four groups: *H. pylori*–associated ulcers, NSAID-induced ulcers, idiopathic (non–*H. pylori*, non-NSAID) ulcers, and Zollinger-Ellison syndrome (discussed later). Other less-common causes include ulcers secondary to drugs other than NSAIDs (e.g., potassium chloride, bisphosphonates), stress ulcers due to a critical illness, ulcers of Crohn's disease, and infectious causes (*Cytomegalovirus* ulcers in HIV patients, *Herpes simplex*).

### *Helicobacter pylori*–Associated Ulcers

*H. pylori* infection is responsible for the majority of peptic ulcers. *H. pylori* is believed to be transmitted from person to person, probably via the fecal–oral route. The prevalence of *H. pylori* is between 20% and 50% in the Western world, including the United States. However, *H. pylori* is much more prevalent in developing nations, affecting as many as 90% of the population. In the United States, the prevalence is higher in the elderly, probably reflecting the poor sanitary conditions that existed in the early part of the century, and is more common in those of African American or Latin American ethnicity. *H. pylori* is also more prevalent in persons of low socioeconomic status, possibly related to crowded childhood living conditions.

Initial studies reported that *H. pylori* was present in about 90% of patients with duodenal ulcers and 60% of patients with gastric ulcer. More recent estimates show slightly lower prevalence of *H. pylori* in both duodenal ulcer and gastric ulcer, probably reflecting the relative increase in NSAID-associated ulcers. Approximately 10% of all persons infected with *H. pylori* develop PUD over their lifetime.

The exact pathophysiologic mechanism(s) by which *H. pylori* causes either duodenal or gastric ulcer and why only a minority of infected persons develop clinically overt disease is not known. Generally, duodenal ulcer is a disease of acid hypersecretion and gastric ulcer is associated with states of low acid secretion. *H. pylori* can potentially cause both of these secretory abnormalities. Gastric acid hypersecretion in duodenal ulcer occurs secondary to increased gastrin release by a healthy acid-secreting gastric body mucosa (Figure 1). In contrast, when *H. pylori*–associated gastritis affects the proximal stomach too, this results in loss of gastric glands (atrophic gastritis) and hypochlorhydria with impaired mucosal defense, leading to gastric ulceration and even gastric cancer.

### NSAID-Induced Ulcers

NSAIDs are among the most prescribed medications in the United States. The incidence of ulcers in chronic NSAID users is approximately

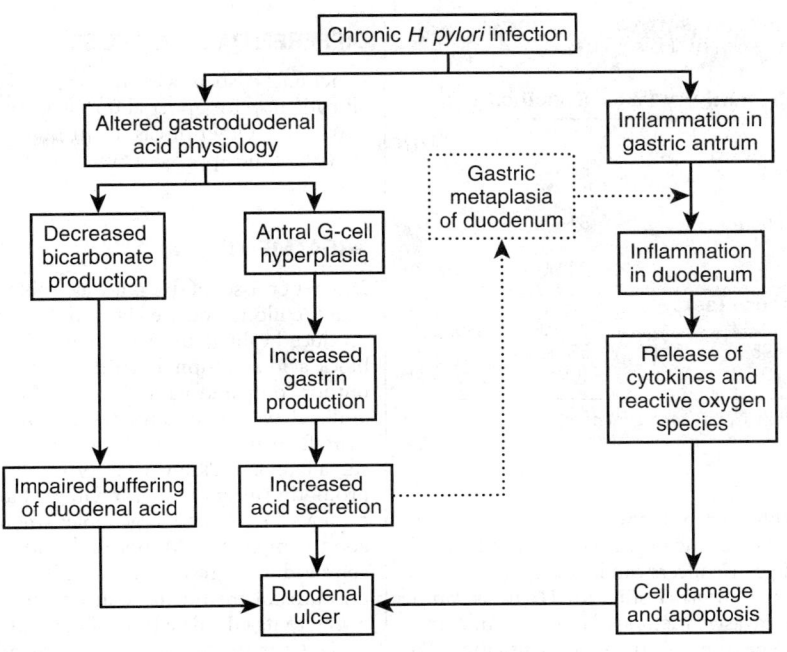

**FIGURE 1.** Proposed pathogenic mechanisms leading to *Helicobacter pylori*–induced duodenal ulcer.

15% to 20%. The risk of NSAID-induced ulcers increases dramatically with the presence of specific risk factors (particularly with age >60 years and a prior history of peptic ulcer) and also with high doses of NSAIDs and concurrent use of either anticoagulants or high-dose corticosteroids. NSAIDs cause gastric ulcers much more commonly than duodenal ulcers. Up to 40% of these persons remain asymptomatic, and patients commonly present with complications.

The most important mechanism by which NSAIDs cause ulcers is by indirectly decreasing prostaglandin production via the inhibition of COX-1. Prostaglandins are important in maintaining mucosal integrity by producing mucus, stimulating bicarbonate production, decreasing acid production, and maintaining mucosal blood flow. The analgesic and anti-inflammatory effects of NSAIDs result from the inhibition of the COX-2 isoenzyme. Nonselective NSAIDs cause inhibition of both COX-2 and COX-1, resulting in considerable GI toxicity. The more recently developed selective COX-2 inhibitors, such as celecoxib (Celebrex), as the name implies, inhibit COX-2 to a much greater extent than COX-1, leading to their better GI safety profile. However, recent reports of cardiovascular complications attributed to COX-2 inhibitors have severely restricted their use.

### Idiopathic Ulcers

In a specific subgroup of patients who develop ulcers, all the known etiologic factors are excluded. This subgroup should not be confused with patients who have unexplained ulcers, 60% of whom have a history of surreptitious NSAID use. The true incidence of idiopathic ulcers is hard to assess in various studies as a result of false-negative *H. pylori* tests or surreptitious use of NSAIDs, and the exact pathogenic mechanism that causes these idiopathic ulcers remains unknown. Various abnormalities including genetic predisposition, defective mucosal defense mechanisms, and increased acid production have all been postulated.

## CLINICAL FEATURES

Clinical signs and symptoms are unreliable and are not specific enough to make a diagnosis of a peptic ulcer. Upper abdominal pain (dyspepsia) is present in more than 80% of patients; however, only 15% of patients with dyspepsia have PUD. Pain is typically epigastric, described as burning and nonradiating. Food or antacids can relieve duodenal ulcer pain. Nausea or anorexia can occur with gastric ulcers.

Nocturnal symptoms awaken patients in two thirds of duodenal ulcer and one third of gastric ulcer cases. Symptoms usually wax and wane over a period of months. The physical examination is usually normal in PUD patients. Epigastric tenderness may be present on palpation, but it is an unreliable sign with a positive predictive value of less than 50%. Stool tests for occult blood may be positive in one third of patients.

## DIAGNOSTIC WORK-UP

Routine laboratory studies are not helpful in establishing a diagnosis of PUD. Upper endoscopy is the gold standard in making a diagnosis of peptic ulcer. Endoscopy has the advantage of taking biopsies for the presence of *H. pylori* infection and, in the case of gastric ulcer, to rule out malignancy. However, endoscopy is more expensive and invasive. In the absence of alarm symptoms, double-contrast barium radiography may be a suitable second choice. If barium radiography shows an ulcer (gastric or duodenal), *H. pylori* must be tested noninvasively. Treatment can be instituted with acid-suppression therapy with or without antibiotics depending on the presence of *H. pylori*. Gastric pH and fasting gastrin levels should be obtained only if there is clinical suspicion for gastrinoma (see the section on Zollinger-Ellison syndrome).

 **CURRENT DIAGNOSIS**

- In the majority of cases of dyspepsia, no structural abnormality can be identified after investigation.
- Patients with dyspepsia who are older than 55 years or who have alarm symptoms (anemia, anorexia, weight loss, early satiety, dysphagia, or gastrointestinal bleeding) should undergo upper endoscopy.
- *Helicobacter pylori* infection and NSAIDs are the two most common causes of peptic ulcer disease.
- Endoscopic biopsy, urea breath test, and stool antigen testing are the most accurate ways to diagnose active *H. pylori* infection.
- Zollinger-Ellison syndrome should be suspected if there are multiple duodenal ulcers, ulcers that are refractory to treatment, or peptic ulcers associated with diarrhea.

## TABLE 1  Diagnostic Tests for *H. pylori*

| Diagnostic Test | Sensitivity (%) | Specificity (%) |
|---|---|---|
| **Noninvasive Tests** | | |
| Serum ELISA test for antibody | 85 | 80 |
| Urea breath test ($^{14}C$ or $^{13}C$) | 95-100 | 91-98 |
| Stool antigen test | 91-98 | 94-99 |
| **Invasive (Endoscopy-Based) Tests** | | |
| Rapid urease test | 93-97 | 95-100 |
| Histology | >95 | 98-99 |
| Culture | 70-80 | 100 |

*Abbreviation:* ELISA = enzyme-linked immunosorbent assay.

For gastric ulcers, it is advisable to repeat the endoscopy after 6 to 8 weeks of therapy to confirm the healing of the ulcer and re-biopsy if it is not healed, because 5% of gastric ulcers can be malignant.

Many tests are available for *H. pylori*. Testing for *H. pylori* can be made by either noninvasive or invasive methods (Table 1). An appropriate test should be chosen depending on the clinical situation. For example, testing for serologic antibodies against *H. pylori* may be appropriate for the initial testing for *H. pylori* though it is not as accurate as breath or stool tests. Also, serology is not useful to check for eradication after therapy, because it will not distinguish current active infection from prior infection that was treated (antibody levels fall slowly and unpredictably). Office-based qualitative antibody tests are cheaper compared with enzyme-linked immunosorbent assay (ELISA) test done in the laboratory but not as accurate, and they have been superseded by stool antigen and breath testing. Patients with alarm symptoms and all patients older than 55 years who have dyspeptic symptoms should undergo endoscopy, at which time *H. pylori* testing can be done by biopsy if an ulcer is found. Confirmation of the eradication of *H. pylori* should be considered after treating this infection in ulcer patients, by either the stool antigen test or the urea breath test, depending on the local resources. Confirmation of eradication by gastric biopsy is only recommended if endoscopy is performed for another reason, for example, to confirm healing of a gastric ulcer.

## DIFFERENTIAL DIAGNOSIS

Functional dyspepsia is a major differential diagnostic consideration in all patients with upper abdominal pain (see the section on functional dyspepsia). Other diseases that mimic the symptoms of PUD include cancers of the upper gastrointestinal tract, biliary colic, and mesenteric ischemia.

## TREATMENT

Different classes of drugs are available to treat PUD (Table 2). Antacids heal the ulcers and are cheap but are relatively ineffective, are slow to produce healing, and have many side effects. Both PPIs and $H_2$-RAs block acid secretion, but PPIs inhibit more than 90% of the 24-acid output compared with 65% with $H_2$-RAs; hence, PPIs heal the ulcer and relieve symptoms faster. Ulcer-healing rates of sucralfate (Carafate) are similar to those for $H_2$-RAs. The mechanism of action of sucralfate is unknown; it probably coats the ulcer base, thereby promoting ulcer healing, and might have other effects too. The frequent dosing schedule and large tablet size of sucralfate is not conducive to good compliance. Misoprostol (Cytotec) is a prostaglandin analogue approved for preventing NSAID-induced ulcers. Compliance with misoprostol treatment is also a problem, particularly at high doses, owing to its GI side effects of abdominal cramping and diarrhea.

*H. pylori* eradication is recommended in all ulcer patients who are *H. pylori* positive, but *H. pylori* infection should not be assumed without a documented positive test. *H. pylori* eradication heals ulcers and reduces the ulcer recurrence dramatically, to less than 20% after 2 years. Select *H. pylori* eradication regimens are summarized in Table 3. Confirmation of eradication is mandatory for complicated ulcer associated with bleeding, perforation, or obstruction and is recommended in all ulcer patients receiving *H. pylori* therapy. Treatment of idiopathic ulcers is difficult and often requires indefinite maintenance antisecretory therapy, particularly for a complicated ulcer.

## PREVENTION

Ulcers can recur either with continued use of NSAIDs or with *H. pylori* infection that persists after the initial antibiotic course. The incidence of antibiotic resistance to *H. pylori* is rising all over the world. In the United States, approximately 30% of *H. pylori* strains are now resistant to metronidazole (Flagyl), and 10% to 12% are resistant to

## TABLE 2  Treatment Options for Peptic Ulcers*

| Pharmacologic Agent | Active Ulcer (Gastric or Duodenal)† | Prevention of NSAID-Induced Ulcer Recurrence |
|---|---|---|
| **Antisecretory Agents** | | |
| ***H₂-Receptor Antagonists*** | | |
| Cimetidine (Tagamet) | 400 mg bid or 800 mg qhs | Double the dose indicated for active ulcer[1] |
| Famotidine (Pepcid) | 20 mg bid or 40 mg qhs | |
| Nizatidine (Axid) | 150 mg bid or 300 mg qhs | |
| Ranitidine (Zantac) | 150 mg bid or 300 mg qhs | |
| ***Proton Pump Inhibitors*** | | |
| Esomeprazole (Nexium) | 40 mg qd | 40 mg qd[1] |
| Lansoprazole (Prevacid) | 30 mg qd | 30 mg qd[1] |
| Omeprazole (Prilosec) | 20 mg qd | 20 mg qd[1] |
| Pantoprazole (Protonix) | 40 mg qd | 40 mg qd[1] |
| Rabeprazole (Aciphex) | 20 mg qd | 20 mg qd[1] |
| **Mucosal Protectants** | | |
| Misoprostol (Cytotec) | 200 µg qid | 200 µg qid or 400 µg bid |
| Sucralfate (Carafate) | 1 gm qid | Not effective |

[1]Not FDA approved for this indication.
*All patients should be tested for *H.pylori* and treated if positive.
†Duration of treatment for duodenal ulcer is 4 weeks with proton pump inhibitor (PPI) and 6 weeks with $H_2$-receptor antagonist. Duration of treatment for gastric ulcer is 8 weeks with either PPI or $H_2$-receptor antagonist.

## TABLE 3 Select FDA-Approved *Helicobacter pylori* Eradication Regimens

| Drug Combination | Dosing Schedule |
| --- | --- |
| PPI* (omeprazole 20 mg or lansoprazole 30 mg) + amoxicillin 1 g + clarithromycin 500 mg | Each bid for 10-14 d |
| Esomeprazole* 40 mg qd + amoxicillin 1 g bid + clarithromycin 500 mg bid | For 10 d |
| PPI* (omeprazole 20 mg or lansoprazole 30 mg) + amoxicillin 1g + metronidazole 500 mg | Each bid for 10-14 d |
| Rabeprazole* 20 mg + amoxicillin 1 g + clarithromycin 500 mg | Each bid for 7 d |
| Bismuth subsalicylate 525 mg + metronidazole 250 mg + tetracycline 500 mg[†] | Each qid for 2 wk plus $H_2$-RA for 4 wk |

*Although not yet approved, pantoprazole (Protonix) can be substituted.
[†]In patients with penicillin allergy, this regimen can be used. Alternatively, PPI + clarithromycin + metronidazole can be used.
*Abbreviations:* FDA = U.S. Food and Drug Administration; PPI = proton pump inhibitor.

clarithromycin (Biaxin), which decreases the cure rates by as much as 50% and 37%, respectively. If the patient has persistent symptoms after therapy, eradication failure should be strongly suspected and noninvasive testing for *H. pylori* should be performed. If the initial diagnosis of the ulcer was made by radiography, endoscopy is the next reasonable test. Drugs that are clearly shown to be superior to placebo in preventing NSAID-induced ulcers are PPIs and misoprostol (Cytotec). Double the standard doses of $H_2$-RAs used for active ulcers are significantly better than placebo in preventing NSAID-induced gastroduodenal ulcers (see Table 2). PPIs are generally preferred over $H_2$-RAs given the simplicity of the dosing schedule and comparable cost. Elderly patients who require long-term NSAID therapy should receive *H. pylori* eradication therapy if they are infected with this bacterium.

## COMPLICATIONS

### Hemorrhage

Gastrointestinal bleeding is the most common complication of PUD. Approximately 10% to 20% of ulcer patients develop significant GI bleeding, with overall mortality of up to 10%. Patients generally present with either melena or hematemesis. Endoscopy is indicated for diagnosis, risk stratification, and therapy in all patients with significant bleeding. High-dose oral or intravenous PPIs should be instituted before endoscopy if upper bleeding is suspected. All *H. pylori*–positive patients must have confirmation of eradication after therapy.

### CURRENT TREATMENT

- In patients with dyspepsia who are younger than 55 years, a *Helicobacter pylori* test-and-treat strategy, followed by PPI treatment (if the patient remains symptomatic or is not infected by *H. pylori*) is the management strategy of choice.
- Long-term acid-suppression therapy with PPIs may be necessary for patients believed to be at high risk for bleeding but in whom chronic NSAID use is necessary.
- PPIs inhibit more than 90% of the 24-acid output compared with 65% with $H_2$-RAs; hence PPIs heal peptic ulcers and relieve symptoms faster.
- Elderly patients who require long-term NSAID therapy should receive *H. pylori* eradication therapy if they are infected with this bacterium.
- Triple therapy (PPI plus amoxicillin and clarithromycin) is the most widely used treatment strategy for *H. pylori* in the United States.

*Abbreviations:* $H_2$-RA = $H_2$-receptor antagonist; NSAID = nonsteroidal anti-inflammatory drug; PPI = proton pump inhibitor.

### Perforation

Perforations occur in approximately 5% to 7% of ulcer patients. The incidence has not changed in spite of decreasing prevalence of *H. pylori*, because the use of NSAIDs continues to increase. The decision whether to manage operatively or nonoperatively should be made on a case-by-case basis.

### Obstruction

Duodenal bulb or pyloric channel ulcers cause scarring and gastric outlet obstruction in approximately 2% of patients with PUD. Patients then present with early satiety, vomiting, and weight loss. Management involves *H. pylori* eradication and acid suppression along with endoscopic dilatation. Surgery is reserved for patients who do not respond to endoscopic therapy.

## Zollinger-Ellison Syndrome

Less than 1% of PUD is caused by Zollinger-Ellison syndrome (ZES). This syndrome results from a gastrin-producing neuroendocrine tumor (gastrinoma), two thirds of which are malignant. PUD is caused by increased acid production from very high serum gastrin levels. Most gastrinomas arise in the gastrinoma triangle, bounded by the porta hepatis, neck of the pancreas, and third portion of the duodenum. The pancreas and the duodenum are the two organs most commonly involved. Approximately one quarter of gastrinomas are part of the multiple endocrine neoplasia type 1 (MEN-1) syndrome, which is associated with parathyroid hyperplasia, pituitary tumors, and pancreatic endocrine tumors.

Gastrinomas commonly manifest between ages 30 and 50 years and have a male-to-female ratio of 2:1. The clinical features include peptic ulcers (90%), diarrhea (60%), and GERD (20%), all of which are due to gastric acid hypersecretion. The majority of ulcers occur in the duodenum. ZES should be suspected if the ulcers are multiple, in unusual locations, refractory to treatment, or associated with diarrhea.

Diagnosis is made by measuring fasting gastrin levels and gastric pH. If the gastrin levels are elevated to more than 1000 pg/mL in the right clinical setting, the diagnosis of ZES is established. Hypochlorhydria secondary to gastric atrophy from *H. pylori* or autoimmune gastritis, or due to acid suppression therapy by $H_2$-RAs and PPIs, can increase gastrin levels. Therefore, gastrin levels should be measured after $H_2$-RAs are held for 24 hours and PPIs for 1 week.

The gastric pH should be measured to distinguish ZES from hypochlorhydria. Gastric pH is less than 2 in ZES, whereas in achlorhydria secondary to gastric atrophy, gastric pH is greater than 2.

Provocative tests, such as the secretin test, can also be used to diagnose gastrinoma. Intravenous administration of secretin can decrease or slightly increase gastrin levels in normal patients and in patients with antral G-cell hyperplasia. In cases of gastrinoma, gastrin levels are significantly increased (>200 pg/mL) from the basal levels.

Tumor localization should be investigated by somatostatin receptor scintigraphy (Octreoscan), computed tomography, magnetic resonance imaging, and endoscopic ultrasound.

Treatment involves medical therapy with a high-dose PPI titrated against symptoms, gastric pH, and endoscopic findings. Surgical resection of isolated hepatic metastasis will decrease symptoms and prolongs survival.

## REFERENCES

Chan FK, Graham DY: Review article: Prevention of non-steroidal anti-inflammatory drug gastrointestinal complications: Review and recommendations based on risk assessment. Aliment Pharmacol Ther 2004;19(10): 1051-1061.

Chan FK, Leung WK: Peptic-ulcer disease. Lancet. 2002;360(9337):933-941.

Stollman N, Metz DC: Pathophysiology and prophylaxis of stress ulcer in intensive care unit patients. J Crit Care 2005;20(1):35-45.

Suerbaum S, Michetti P: *Helicobacter pylori* infection. N Engl J Med 2002; 347(15):1175-1186.

Talley NJ; American Gastroenterological Association: American Gastroenterological Association medical position statement: Evaluation of dyspepsia. Gastroenterology 2005;129(5):1753-1755.

Talley NJ, Vakil N; Practice Parameters Committee of the American College of Gastroenterology: Guidelines for the management of dyspepsia. Am J Gastroenterol. 2005;100(10):2324-2337.

# Acute and Chronic Hepatitis

Method of
*Mamta K. Jain, MD, MPH, and*
*Daniel M. Brailita, MD*

Viral hepatitis is the most common cause of acute and chronic liver disease worldwide. Given the increasing number of new diagnoses and the risk of chronic liver disease, cirrhosis, and hepatocellular carcinoma, viral hepatitis is a serious health care problem. This article focuses on the epidemiology, diagnosis, prevention, and, in some cases, therapies that are available.

Several viruses are considered hepatotropic because viremia is associated with elevation of serum aminotransferases. However, *viral hepatitis* refers to infections caused by hepatitis viruses A through E. Hepatitis A (HAV) and E (HEV) viruses have a fecal-oral transmission route and do not produce chronic infection; hepatitis B (HBV), C (HCV), and D (HDV) viruses have a parenteral transmission route and can lead to chronic liver disease, hepatocellular carcinoma, and cirrhosis.

Other viral infections, which can involve the liver as one manifestation of a systemic infection, include HIV, Epstein–Barr virus (EBV), cytomegalovirus (CMV), herpes simplex virus (HSV), and varicella-zoster virus (VZV). These viruses can cause acute hepatitis, which can be fatal, especially in immunocompromised patients. Only hepatitis A, B, C, D, and E viral infections (characteristics are outlined in Table 1) are discussed in this article.

## Acute Hepatitis Versus Chronic Hepatitis

### ACUTE HEPATITIS

Acute hepatitis can be either symptomatic or asymptomatic. Generally, asymptomatic disease occurs in younger children. Symptomatic clinical disease is often seen in adolescents and adults. In the prodromal phase, a person can experience flulike illness with malaise, fever, anorexia, nausea, vomiting, and mild abdominal pain. During the icteric phase, jaundice appears, often accompanied by dark-brown urine and acholic or clay-colored stools. However, these signs may be seen in some persons without jaundice. Less frequent symptoms include arthralgias, rash, diarrhea, and lymphadenopathy.

Typical laboratory tests show high elevations of liver enzymes including alanine aminotransferase (ALT) and aspartate aminotransferase (AST) (often in the 1000 IU/mL range), an increase in bilirubin, and sometimes an increase in alkaline phosphatase. Fulminant hepatic failure, a rare complication, can be seen, with prolongation of prothrombin time (PT), coagulopathy, encephalopathy, and jaundice.

Patients with fulminant hepatic failure, because of the high mortality rate, should be managed in specialized centers with access to liver transplantation and close monitoring of coagulopathy, volume status, and neurologic status.

### CHRONIC HEPATITIS

HBV and HCV can cause acute infection, either symptomatic or asymptomatic, and can progress to chronic liver disease. Most patients with chronic viral hepatitis are asymptomatic or complain of mild fatigue only; progression to cirrhosis, hepatocellular carcinoma, and end-stage liver disease is possible. The clinical examination can be normal or stigmata of chronic liver disease may be observed, such as spider angiomas, palmar erythema, testicular atrophy, and gynecomastia. The laboratory tests might show mild to moderate transaminitis in the chronic phase. The degree of ALT and AST elevation might not reflect the severity of liver fibrosis. Often, patients with cirrhosis have normal ALT and AST levels. The degree of fibrosis in chronic liver disease is based on histologic findings on liver biopsy.

Cirrhotic patients can develop portal hypertension leading to an enlarged spleen, variceal bleeding, ascites, and encephalopathy. Other clinical parameters that indicate progressive liver disease include: decrease in serum albumin and platelet count, rise of serum bilirubin, and prolongation of PT. In these patients, transplantation may be necessary. Cirrhotic patients are also at increased risk for developing hepatocellular cancer (HCC) and should be screened by alpha fetoprotein (AFP) and abdominal ultrasound every 6 months. In addition, these

## TABLE 1  Characteristics of Hepatitis A through E

| Virus | HAV | HBV | HCV | HDV | HEV |
|---|---|---|---|---|---|
| Family | Picornaviridae | Hepadnaviridae | Flaviviridae | Deltavirus (no separate family) | Hepeviridae |
| Size | 27 nm | 42 nm | 50-55 nm | 36 nm | 32 nm |
| Nucleic acid | ssRNA | dsDNA | ssRNA | ssRNA | ssRNA |
| Transmission | Fecal-oral | Vertical, percutaneous, sexual | Blood products, percutaneous, sexual | Mainly percutaneous | Fecal-oral |
| Incubation | 15-45 d | 1-6 mo | 7 wk | 3-20 wk | 15-60 d |
| Chronic infection? | No | Yes | Yes | Yes | No |
| Vaccine available? | Yes | Yes | No | No | Experimental |

*Abbreviations:* HAV = hepatitis A virus; HBV = hepatitis B virus; HCV = hepatitis C virus; HDV = hepatitis D virus; HEV = hepatitis E virus; ss = single-stranded; ds = double-stranded.

**TABLE 2** Vaccination Schedules for Hepatitis Vaccines Licensed in the United States

| Vaccine | Type | Dose | Schedule |
|---|---|---|---|
| **Hepatitis A Virus** | | | |
| Havrix (GlaxoSmithKline) | Inactivated HAV | 12 mo-18 y: 0.5 mL (720 EL.U)<br>>18 y: 1 mL (1440 EL.U) | 0 and 6-12 mo |
| Vaqta (Merck) | Inactivated HAV | 12 mo-18 y: 0.5 mL (25 U)<br>>18 y: 1 mL (50 U) | 0 and 6-18 mo |
| **Hepatitis A and B Viruses** | | | |
| Twinrix (GlaxoSmithKline) | Inactivated HAV and recombinant HBV | >18 y: 1 mL | 0, 1, and 6 mo |
| **Hepatitis B Virus** | | | |
| Recombivax-HB (Merck) | Recombinant HBV | 0-19 y: 0.5 mL (5 µg) | Infants: birth, 1-4, and 6-18 mo<br>Older children: 0, 1-2, and 4 mo |
| | | >20 y: 1 mL (10 µg) | 0, 1, and 6 mo |
| Engerix-B (GlaxoSmithKline) | Recombinant HBV | 0-19 y: 0.5 mL (10 µg) | Infants: birth, 1-4, and 6-18 mo<br>Older children: 0, 1-2, and 4 mo |
| | | >20 y: 1 mL (20 µg) | 0, 1, and 6 mo |
| | | Dialysis patients: double adult dose | 0, 1, 2, and 6 mo. |
| Comvax (Merck) | Recombinant HBV, HiB | Approved for 6 wk-4 y of age: 1 dose | 2, 4, and 12-15 mo |
| Pediarix (GlaxoSmithKline) | Recombinant HBV, DTaP, IPV | Approved for 6 wk- 6y of age.: 1 dose | 2, 4, and 6 mo |

*Abbreviations:* DTaP = diphtheria, tetanus toxoids, and acellular pertussis vaccine; EL.U = enzyme-linked immunosorbent assay units of HAV antigen; HiB = *Haemophilus influenzae* group B vaccine; IPV = inactivated polio vaccine; U = units of HAV antigen.

patients are at risk for fulminant hepatitis due to other viruses and should be vaccinated for vaccine-preventable infections. For example, patients with HCV-related cirrhosis should be vaccinated for HAV and HBV. Vaccination schedules are shown in Table 2.

# Hepatitis A

## EPIDEMIOLOGY

HAV is the leading cause of acute viral hepatitis worldwide and is a reportable disease in the United States, but significant shifts in HAV epidemiology have been seen since the introduction of licensed vaccines from 1995 to 1999. In 2004, an estimated 56,000 new infections occurred in the United States, which represents a historically low rate; to compare, more than 356,000 infections occurred in 1995. Higher prevalence of HAV is seen in children in less developed countries where sanitation is poor and infection occurs at an early age.

The virus is transmitted mainly by the fecal–oral route via contaminated food or water. In industrialized countries, like the United States, sporadic cases are more common and the prevalence of acute HAV is higher in adults. Populations at risk include children in daycare centers, close contacts of viremic patients, persons with substandard hygiene habits, or eating undercooked food, travelers in endemic areas, and men who have sex with men (MSM). Waterborne outbreaks are rare in developed countries but can be seen in less developed countries.

## CLINICAL FEATURES

Infection with HAV does not lead to chronic liver disease. Acute infection is asymptomatic in most children, especially children younger than 2 years, but it is symptomatic in children older than 5 years. Symptomatic illness occurs after an incubation of 15 to 45 days. The viral prodrome before the onset of jaundice (see acute hepatitis) typically lasts 2 to 7 days. Hepatomegaly is possible. Typically, significant improvement occurs by the end of the third week, with normalization of ALT and AST, fading jaundice, and resolution of hepatomegaly.

The clinical patterns include asymptomatic infection without jaundice, symptomatic infection with jaundice but with a limited 8-week course, cholestatic infection with jaundice with usually a longer course, relapsing infection with two or more episodes over a 6- to 10-week period, and, rarely, fulminant hepatic failure. Complete recovery is achieved in most persons by 6 months. The prognosis is excellent, with no progression to chronic disease. Mortality, occurring in less than 0.4%, is more common in the extremes of age (infants and the elderly, especially those with diabetes).

## DIAGNOSIS

Acute HAV infection is diagnosed by detecting anti-HAV immunoglobulin M (IgM) (see Table 3) in the acute serum sample, which appears before the onset of clinical symptoms and persists for 3 to 6 months. Anti-HAV IgG appears after IgM and persists for years, indicating immunity. Although different variants of HAV have been identified, only one serotype is responsible for cross-reactivity to all variants. HAV antigen is detectable in the stool 1 to 2 weeks before the onset of symptoms, disappears before jaundice, and reappears during relapses. ALT and AST are typically very high and recover in 3 weeks. Bilirubin peaks at 12 to 30 mg/dL and starts declining in 2 to 3 weeks. The patient is no longer infectious 1 week after the onset of jaundice.

## TREATMENT AND PREVENTION

The treatment of HAV is supportive. Hygiene is important in prevention of infection.

Persons with documented HAV immunity (previous infection) do not need passive or active prophylaxis. Active prophylaxis, obtained by HAV vaccines, offers prolonged immunity. Prevaccination testing of children is not indicated due to low incidence of infection in the United States, but it may be cost-effective in select adult populations. Currently in the United States three licensed vaccines are available: Havrix, Vaqta, and the combination HAV/HBV vaccine Twinrix.

**TABLE 3** Serologic Parameters for Hepatitis A Virus

| Type | Anti-HAV IgM | Anti-HAV IgG |
|---|---|---|
| Acute | + | − |
| Exposed | ± | + |
| Immunized | ± | + |

*Abbreviation:* anti-HAV = antibodies to hepatitis A; HAV = hepatitis A virus; Ig = immunoglobulin.

## CURRENT DIAGNOSIS

- Acute hepatitis is self-limited and does not cause progressive liver disease.
- Chronic hepatitis can lead to cirrhosis and end-stage liver disease.
- Hepatitis A is a vaccine-preventable disease, but sporadic outbreaks still occur.
- Travelers to less developed countries should be vaccinated for hepatitis A.
- Hepatitis B can cause both acute and chronic liver disease. In most cases, infection resolves through natural immune clearance. For patients with chronic infection, several therapies exist.
- Hepatitis B is a vaccine-preventable disease.
- Hepatitis C is a leading cause of chronic liver disease.
- Combination therapies for hepatitis C with pegylated interferon and ribavirin are available but are only effective in 50% of patients.
- Hepatitis E is a self-limited disease seen mostly in less developed countries. Travelers should drink bottled or boiled water in endemic countries to avoid infection.
- Mortality is high in pregnant women who acquire hepatitis E.
- Hepatocellular cancer is a complication of chronic liver disease and should be screened for regularly.

The vaccines are highly effective if used appropriately. Immunity occurs in 1 month.

HAV vaccine should be given to all children ages 1 to 18 years, travelers to endemic areas, MSM, recreational drug users, those with chronic liver disease, persons with clotting factor disorders, and persons at risk for occupational exposure. During outbreaks, unvaccinated children should receive both active and passive prophylaxis.

Passive prophylaxis, obtained by administration of pooled immunoglobulins (Ig), offers limited protection, but it is important during HAV outbreaks in daycare centers and among food handlers, household contacts of patients with acute HAV, and persons traveling to HAV-endemic areas within 4 weeks from the first dose of HAV vaccine. A 0.02 mL/kg Ig dose is 80% to 90% effective as postexposure prophylaxis if given within 2 weeks, but it also attenuates the clinical disease if given after 2 weeks. A 0.06 mL/kg Ig dose given before travel confers immunity for 3 to 5 months. (See Table 2 for the vaccination schedules.)

# Hepatitis B

## EPIDEMIOLOGY

Worldwide, the number of HBV infections exceeds 350 million. In the United States, an estimated 1.25 million people are chronically infected. The number of acute infections in the United States has decreased from 260,000 per year in the 1980s to 60,000 per year in 2004. The decline is largely due to the routine use of HBV vaccine.

In areas of high prevalence, such as Southeast Asia, China, and Africa, the most common route of transmission is vertically from mother to child and horizontally among children. However, in the United States and other Western countries, which are considered low-prevalence areas, horizontal spread among adults is the most common, especially through sexual contact or through injection drug use. The virus is transmitted by passage of infectious bodily fluids through percutaneous routes or disrupted mucosal membranes. HBV is 100 times more infectious than HIV and approximately 8 to 10 times more infectious than HCV.

Routine testing for HBV should be offered to persons with multiple sexual partners, MSM, parenteral drug users, household contacts of infected persons, children born to infected mothers or to immigrants from highly endemic areas, hemodialysis patients, pregnant women, HIV-positive persons, and health care and public safety workers.

## CLINICAL FEATURES

Acute HBV infection occurs after an incubation period of 30 to 180 days. The age and immune status of the exposed person are correlated with the outcome of the acute infection, but why some patients ultimately clear the viral infection is not known. Acute HBV is subclinical in 90% of young children but 30% to 80% of adults have anicteric or icteric forms (see the discussion of acute hepatitis). Resolution of jaundice generally occurs within 1 to 3 months. Eighty percent of acute HBV resolves with disappearance of hepatitis B surface antigen (HBsAg) by 12 to 24 weeks. As in HAV, less than 1% of the cases progress to fulminant hepatic failure, which generally occurs within 4 weeks of onset of symptoms.

Chronic hepatitis following acute infection develops in 90% of infants born to hepatitis B e antigen (HBeAg)-positive mothers, 30% of children infected at 1 to 5 years of age, and 6% of those infected after 5 years of age. Immunosuppressed persons are more likely to develop chronic infection. From 15% to 25% of the chronically infected patients die from complications of HBV including cirrhosis and HCC.

Extrahepatic manifestations are common in both acute and chronic HBV infection. Arthritis-dermatitis is manifested with fever, arthralgia, rash, and edema. Polyarteritis nodosa (PAN), a systemic necrotizing vasculitis, is a serious complication of HBV infection. Glomerulonephritis occurs with several different glomerular lesions and can manifest with the nephrotic syndrome. Essential mixed cryoglobulinemia is not seen as commonly as in HCV and is often asymptomatic.

## DIAGNOSIS

The diagnosis of acute HBV infection (Table 4) is made by the presence of HBsAg and antibodies to hepatitis B core antigen (anti-HBcAg). During the replicative phase of the infection, HBV DNA and HBeAg, a marker of viral replication, are also positive. HBsAg appears first, before the onset of symptoms, and disappears 3 to 6 months after the infection in persons who recover without chronic infection. Hepatitis B surface antibodies (anti-HBs) are protective and appear after the clearance of HBsAg. Anti-HBs also appear after successful vaccination. The persistence of HBsAg longer than 6 months usually indicates chronic infection; however, clearance after 6 to 12 months is possible. There is a serologic window between the disappearance of HBsAg and the appearance of HBsAb when the diagnosis of acute infection is only possible by detection of anti-HBcAg IgM. Anti-HBcAg is detectable throughout the course of disease (IgM is replaced by IgG in chronic infection), but it does not give protection and its presence means natural infection.

HBeAg seroconversion, referring to loss of HBeAg and development of antibodies to HBeAg (anti-HBe), can occur through immune clearance during acute infection or through antiviral therapies in chronic infection. However, mutations in the precore and basal core promoter regions of HBV can give rise to HBeAg mutants in which patients are HBeAg-negative, but produce HBV DNA and can develop progressive liver disease.

Inactive carriers are persons who have evidence of HBV DNA by highly sensitive polymerase chain reaction (PCR) methods and also have normal serum aminotransferases. Long-term follow-ups of these persons suggest that they do not develop progressive liver disease. Liver function tests may need to be monitored every 6 to 12 months. Active carriers have evidence of HBV DNA by non-PCR methods and elevated or intermittently elevated serum aminotransferases.

## TREATMENT

Treatment goals include HBeAg seroconversion, significant decrease in HBV DNA or viral suppression, normalization of aminotransferases,

**TABLE 4  Serologic Parameters for Hepatitis B Virus**

| Type | HBsAg | Anti-HBs | HBeAg | Anti-HBe | Anti-HBc | HBV DNA |
|------|-------|----------|-------|----------|----------|---------|
| Acute | ± | − | + | − | IgM | + |
| Immune clearance (recovered) | − | + | − | + | IgG | −* |
| Chronic | + | − | ± | ± | IgG | + |
| Vaccination | − | + | − | − | − | − |

*May have detectable HBV DNA by more sensitive assays.
*Abbreviations:* anti-HBc = antibodies to hepatitis B core antigen; anti-HBe = antibodies to hepatitis B e antigen; anti-HBs = antibodies to hepatitis B surface; HBeAg = hepatitis B e antigen; HBsAg = hepatitis B surface antigen; HBV = hepatitis B virus.

and improvement of fibrosis on liver biopsy. Patients with more than $10^4$ copies/mL of HBV DNA and abnormal liver function tests may need to be considered for therapy, especially if they are cirrhotic (see Table 5 for guidelines). A specialist should evaluate those who do not meet the guidelines outlined in Table 5 but have detectable HBV DNA levels to determine risk of disease progression.

Older therapies such as interferon-α-2b (IFN-α-2b) (Intron A) given three times weekly for 4 months have been replaced with the newer pegylated IFN-α-2a (Pegasys) once-weekly treatment given for 12 months (see Table 5), in which one third of patients who are HBeAg-positive at baseline obtain HBeAg loss. Interferon is more effective in patients with high ALT and low HBV DNA.

Lamivudine (Epivir), adefovir (Hepsera), and entecavir (Baraclude) are oral agents directed against viral replication. They have few adverse effects in comparison with interferon-based therapies (see discussion of HCV for side effects) but HBeAg loss rates are not as high as with interferon therapies. Lamivudine is also safe for use in decompensated liver disease. For lamivudine, response rates in HBeAg-positive patients have been 16% to 18% in loss of antigen and 49% to 56% in histologic improvement; higher ALT predicted better response. In HBeAg-negative patients, good response rates were offset by the greater than 90% relapse rate after 1 year. Over time, lamivudine resistance (70% with 5 years of therapy) can develop, making lamivudine ineffective.

Adefovir can be used either initially in treatment-naive persons or as second-line treatment for those with lamivudine resistance. Long-term therapy with adefovir has revealed development of resistance in 3% with 2 years of therapy and 30% with 5 years of therapy. The relapse rate is high if medication is stopped.

Entecavir can suppress HBV replication significantly and is active for both lamivudine- and adefovir-resistant mutations. Entecavir is administered at two doses depending on whether the drug is being used in a naive or treatment-experienced patient. Telbivudine has also received FDA approval for the treatment of chronic HBV, however resistance can develop in one-third of patients after one year.

Several other agents including tenofovir (Viread)[1] and emtricitabine (Emtriva)[1] (used in HIV infection) also have activity against HBV.

## PREVENTION

Vaccination against HBV with newer DNA recombinant vaccines has changed the epidemiology of the disease and significantly decreased the number of new infections. The currently available HBV vaccines are Engerix-B and Recombivax HB (see Table 2 for vaccine schedule

---

[1]Not FDA approved for this indication.

**TABLE 5  Current Therapies for Chronic Hepatitis B and C Viruses**

| Virus and Type | Treatment Decision Factors | Treatment Strategy | Therapy Options |
|----------------|---------------------------|--------------------|------------------|
| HBV, HBeAg-positive* | HBV DNA >20,000 copies/mL, elevated ALT† | Treat until HBV DNA is undetectable and HBeAg seroconversion plus 6 additional mo | Lamivudine (Epivir) 100 mg PO qd<br>Adefovir (Hepsera) 10 mg PO qd<br>Entecavir (Baraclude) 0.5 mg PO qd for naive, 1 mg PO qd for experienced<br>Telbivudine (Tyzeka) 600 mg PO qd<br>IFN-α-2b (Intron A) 10 million units SC 3 ×/wk for 16 wk<br>PEG-IFN-α-2a (Pegasys) 180 µg SC weekly for 48 wk |
| HBV, liver cirrhosis | Decompensated | Combination therapy with lamivudine or entecavir *plus* adefovir; place on transplant list | Adefovir *plus* entecavir or lamivudine (dose as for HBeAg-positive)<br>Interferon therapy is contraindicated |
|  | Compensated | If HBV DNA >2000 copies, treat long term with adefovir or entecavir | Adefovir or entecavir (dose as for HBeAg-positive) |
| HCV, genotype 1 | If no contraindications | Treatment for 48 wk<br>Discontinue if no virologic response at 12 wk | PEG-IFN-α-2a (Pegasys) 180 µg SC weekly *or* PEG-IFN-α-2b (PEG-Intron) 1.5 µg/kg SC weekly *plus*<br>Ribavirin (Rebetol, Ribasphere, Copegus) 1200 mg (>75 kg) or 1000 mg (<75 kg) in 2 divided doses |
| HCV, genotype 2 and 3 | If no contraindications | Treatment for 24 wk | PEG-IFN (dose as for genotype 1) *plus* Ribavirin 800 mg PO qd in 2 divided doses |

*HBeAg-negative, threshold for treatment >2000 copies/mL.
†Normal ALT may need to have liver biopsy to determine if treatment is necessary
*Abbreviations:* HBV = hepatitis B; HBeAg = hepatitis B e antigen; HCV = hepatitis C; IFN = interferon; PEG = pegylated.

and dose). Combination vaccines effective against both HAV and HBV are available (see the discussion of hepatitis A).

Due to the high risk of vertical transmission, all infants born to HBsAg-positive mothers should receive a first dose of HBV vaccine and passive prophylaxis with hepatitis B immune globulin (HBIg) 0.5 mL IM, in a separate site from the vaccine, in the first 12 hours after delivery. Vaccination of all other stable infants before hospital discharge is now recommended. All children and adolescents are currently included in a catch-up vaccination program.

Vaccination is also recommended for health care workers, persons with chronic liver disease, and all persons considered at risk (i.e., persons recommended to be screened for HBV). Generally, a postvaccine HBsAb titer of greater than 10 IU/mL is considered protective, but postvaccination testing is necessary only for health care workers. Boosting is indicated for hemodialysis patients. The vaccine is more than 95% efficacious in immunocompetent patients.

# Hepatitis C

## EPIDEMIOLOGY

Worldwide, an estimated 3% of persons have HCV antibodies and more than 170 million people are chronically infected. No available HCV vaccine exists. In the United States, as well as most developed countries, the number of new infections has decreased significantly due to screening of blood products. However, the number of new diagnoses continues to rise, with an estimated burden of 3.2 million chronic infections in the United States; most of these persons were infected through intravenous drug use or receipt of blood products decades ago. Transmission from mother to child is also possible. In 1992, a commercial assay became available for HCV testing and has been used to test blood products since then. Other routes of transmission include tattoos, especially if occurring during incarceration, and intranasal cocaine use. Sexual transmission is rare among heterosexual couples. The Centers for Disease Control and Prevention (CDC) does not recommend changes in sexual practices in monogamous couples. However, risk of sexual transmission might be increased in persons with multiple sexual partners or MSM.

The CDC and the American Association for the Study of Liver Diseases (AASLD) recommend HCV testing for parenteral drug users, hemophiliacs, and other persons receiving blood products or organ transplants before 1992, HIV-positive persons, hemodialysis patients, health care workers with occupational exposure to HCV-positive blood, children born to infected mothers, partners of HCV-positive patients, and persons with unexplained liver function test abnormalities. HCV-positive persons should be counseled about how to avoid transmitting the disease to others.

## CLINICAL FEATURES

There are six major genotypes of HCV, and they have a geographic distribution. In the United States, 60% to 70% of persons are infected with genotype 1, whereas genotypes 2 and 3 are more common in Europe. In Egypt, the predominant genotype is 4. The importance of genotype lies in its predictive value for treatment response to combination therapy with PEG-IFN and ribavirin.

Following an incubation period averaging 7 weeks, acute hepatitis C usually is asymptomatic; it manifests as a flulike illness or rarely as a mild icteric disease. Following acute infection, 50% to 85% of the patients develop chronic infection. Of these, 70% progress to chronic liver disease. Overall, 1% to 5% of infected persons die of HCV-related complications.

Progression to HCC occurs in the setting of cirrhosis, and all HCV-infected cirrhotic patients should be screened for HCC regularly. Extrahepatic manifestations are rare during acute infection but common in chronic infection. Well-described extrahepatic manifestations are essential mixed cryoglobulinemias, membranoproliferative glomerulopathy, leukocytoclastic vasculitis, immune arthropathies, and porphyria cutanea tarda. There may be an increased incidence of non-Hodgkin's lymphoma in HCV-infected patients.

## DIAGNOSIS

The diagnosis (Table 6) is based on detection of antibodies against HCV (anti-HCV). HCV antibodies are not protective and only serve as a marker of infection. The third-generation enzyme immunoassay (EIA) has 97% sensitivity in detecting total antibodies and can be confirmed by direct detection using HCV RNA. If the HCV RNA is negative, a recombinant immunoblot assay (RIBA) can be performed; if RIBA is negative, EIA is a false positive. If the EIA and RIBA are positive but HCV RNA is repeatedly negative, prior infection and natural immune clearance have occurred, which can be seen in 15% to 50% of acute infections, and no further testing is required.

The quantitative HCV RNA assays have lower sensitivity than the qualitative assays. A quantitative assay is obtained to confirm infection (presence of virus) and determine the level of viremia; however, the actual RNA level is only important as a prognostic factor for treatment response. It does not correlate with severity of liver disease. A genotypes should also be ordered because it affects the treatment duration and predicts therapeutic response.

Qualitative HCV RNA assays are available with limits of detection of 50 UI/mL. The only FDA-approved quantitative test is Bayer's Versant HCV RNA 3.0, with limits of detection of 615,000 to 7,700,000 copies/mL, but other quantitative assays are available. The same quantitative test should be used to monitor treatment response.

## TREATMENT

The goal of treatment is eradication of infection and prevention of complications from chronic HCV infection such as end-stage liver disease. Sustained virologic response (SVR) is defined as an undetectable HCV RNA by qualitative assays (<50 IU/mL) 6 months after completion of HCV treatment. Follow-up studies in patients who have achieved an SVR were unable to detect reemergence of HCV RNA up to 5 years after therapy. Currently, the treatment of choice is combination therapy with pegylated interferon (Pegasys or PEG-Intron) and ribavirin (Rebetol, Ribasphere, or Copegus). Pegylated interferon, a synthetic compound with weekly subcutaneous dosing, is used in combination with oral ribavirin (see Table 5 for treatment options).

Patients with genotype 1 and high HCV viral loads achieved a SVR of 41% with pegylated interferon–ribavirin combination therapy, and the SVR in genotype 1 patients with low viral loads was 56%; genotypes 2 and 3 achieved higher rates, of 74% and 81%, respectively. Race appears to affect treatment response in genotype 1 African Americans, who respond less often (<20%) compared with whites (~50%). HIV-infected persons with genotype 1 also respond less often (~30%).

Treatment can be considered in patients who do not have uncontrolled depression, thyroid disease, diabetes, or heart disease; transplant recipients; pregnant or lactating women; patients with autoimmune diseases; and patients with malignancies. Side effects of pegylated interferon include flulike symptoms, thrombocytopenia, leukopenia, anemia, depression, thyroid dysfunction, fatigue, and alopecia. Ribavirin, a teratogen, is contraindicated in renal failure and often causes anemia and a rash. Determining candidates for therapy is an individualized decision based on HCV genotype, degree of fibrosis, HCV RNA level, and other comorbid illnesses. For genotype 1 patients, treatment should be given for 48 weeks; treatment should be discontinued if there is no evidence of response by week 12. For genotypes 2 and 3 patients,

**TABLE 6  Serologic Parameters for Hepatitis C Virus**

| HCV | Anti-HCV | HCV RNA |
| --- | --- | --- |
| Acute | + | + |
| Chronic | + | + |
| Past Infection | + | − |

*Abbreviations:* anti-HCV = antibodies to hepatitis C; HCV = hepatitis C.

treatment should be given for 24 weeks. Retreatment is not indicated in patients who have failed the combination therapy using pegylated interferon.

Treatments targeting the HCV genome transcriptions and translation, currently under evaluation, may be a new therapeutic option for genotype 1 patients in the near future.

# Hepatitis D

HDV is a defective virus only found in HBV-infected persons. It consists of an RNA genome and a hepatitis delta antigen (HDAg); the viral envelope is composed of HBsAg. HDV depends on HBV to acquire the HBsAg needed for viral envelope assembly and transport into the hepatocyte, which is the only target cell. The HDV genome can replicate independently, and nonencapsulated particles circulate in the blood of the infected persons, but because they lack HBsAg, these forms are not pathogenic.

## EPIDEMIOLOGY AND CLINICAL FEATURES

The distribution of HDV is variable but is estimated to infect 5% of those with chronic HBV. The prevalence rate is highest in South America and the Mediterranean basin. Prevalence rates in northern Europe and North America are low, and the population at risk seems to be confined to injection drug users. There are two forms of acquisition: coinfection (simultaneously with HBV) and superinfection (in previously HBV-infected persons). In coinfection, seen primarily in injection drug users, HDV is usually self-limited because acute HBV infection generally resolves, but chronic HDV infection can develop in 5% of patients who are coinfected. A biphasic elevation in liver enzymes may be seen in coinfection because of delay in HDV replication, but it is not seen in acute HBV infection alone. Coinfected persons may be at increased risk for fulminant HBV. HDV superinfection occurs in the setting of chronic liver disease and should be suspected in any HBsAg-positive patient with an acute flare of hepatitis or decompensation of preexisting liver disease. HDV superinfection develops into chronic HDV infection in 70% of patients characterized by persistent HDV viremia.

## DIAGNOSIS AND TREATMENT

The most useful test for diagnosis is the HDV IgM or total anti-HDV (both IgM and IgG) (Table 7). In chronic HDV infection, anti-HDV IgM can persist for some time and is a marker of serious liver disease. Anti-HDV IgG develops over time and can persist, but detection of anti-HDV IgG does not indicate chronic disease and may be seen in patients who have recovered. HDV RNA testing is available mainly for treatment follow-up.

The only treatment option available for chronic infection is interferon therapy. High doses are needed for up to 48 weeks. Nucleoside therapy is not effective for HDV infection. The success rate is controversial but the relapse rate is low. Vaccination against HBV is the most effective prevention.

# Hepatitis E

## EPIDEMIOLOGY

HEV causes an acute, icteric, self-limited hepatitis. HEV is endemic in Southeast and Central Asia, North Africa, and, most recently, Iraq. Epidemic outbreaks of HEV occur, affecting hundreds to thousands of persons. Attack rates are lower in children (0.2%-10%) but higher in adults (3%-30%). A high mortality rate is seen in pregnant women (5%-25%) who acquire HEV. Transmission is through the fecal-oral route and is associated with contaminated water. Recurrent epidemics are seen in countries where sanitation is poor. Person-to-person transmission is unlikely in epidemics. Sporadic HEV in endemic areas accounts for up to 50% to 70% of acute hepatitis but less than 1% in nonendemic areas.

## CLINICAL FEATURES

The incubation period is 15 to 60 days. HEV can be detected in the stool approximately 1 week before clinical disease appears and up to 2 weeks after onset of clinical symptoms. The prodromal phase typically lasts 1 to 4 days, followed by an icteric phase and clinical signs and symptoms typical of any viral hepatitis.

## DIAGNOSIS, TREATMENT, AND PREVENTION

Diagnosis is made by detection of anti-HEV IgM (Table 8) that can be detected at onset of illness; it is unclear if HEV antibodies confer immunity. Treatment is supportive. Because no vaccine is available, travelers to endemic areas should drink boiled or bottled water.

# Hepatocellular Carcinoma Screening

Both HBV and HCV are associated with hepatocellular carcinoma, with higher incidence in cirrhotic patients. By contrast, HDV appears to lower the chance of HBV-infected patients to develop HCC. AASLD guidelines recommend screening with a AFP and liver ultrasound every 6 months in all HBV carriers at risk for HCC, such as adults older than 45 years, cirrhotic patients, and patients with a family history of HCC. Computed tomography or magnetic resonance imaging studies are more sensitive but more expensive methods of screening for HCC. Routine screening of HBV carriers from endemic areas without other known risk factors may be performed although there is no proven benefit. Based on current clinical data, all HCV-positive cirrhotic patients should be screened because the HCC incidence is 2% to 8% per year in this group.

# HIV Coinfection

Patients coinfected with HIV and hepatitis B or C are difficult to manage. The treatment options should be carefully weighed and an experienced physician should help manage them. Several drugs are active against both HIV and HBV, and their value in treating coinfections is under evaluation. All chronic hepatitis patients should be tested for HIV because of shared transmission routes.

**TABLE 7** Serologic Parameters for Hepatitis D Virus

| HDV | HBsAg | Anti-HBc | Anti-HDV | HDV Ag |
|---|---|---|---|---|
| Coinfection | + | IgM | IgM | + |
| Superinfection | + | IgG | IgM | + |
| Chronic Infection | + | IgG | IgM/IgG | + |

*Abbreviations:* anti-HDV = antibodies to hepatitis D; HDV = hepatitis D; HDV Ag = hepatitis D antigen.

**TABLE 8** Serologic Parameters for Hepatitis E Virus

| HEV | Anti-HEV |
|---|---|
| Acute | IgM |
| Recovered | IgG |

*Abbreviations:* anti-HEV = antibodies to hepatitis E; HEV = hepatitis E.

## REFERENCES

Chang T, Gish R, De Man RA, et al: A comparison of entecavir and lamivudine for HBeAg-positive chronic hepatitis B. N Engl J Med 2006;354: 1001-1010.

Dienstag JL, Schiff ER, Wright TL, et al: Lamivudine as the initial treatment for chronic hepatitis B virus in the United States. N Engl J Med 1999;341: 1256-1263.

Emerson SU, Purcell RH: Running like water: The Omnipresence of hepatitis E. N Engl J Med 2004;351:2367-2368.

Erhard A, Gerlich W, Starke C, et al: Treatment of chronic hepatitis delta with pegylated interferon alfa-2b. Liver Int 2006;26(7):805-810.

Fiore AE., Wasley A, Bell BP: Prevention of hepatitis A through active or passive immunization. Recommendations of the Advisory Committee on Immunization Practices (ACIP). MMWR Recomm Rep 2006;55(RR-07):1-23.

Fried MW, Shiffman ML, Reddy KR, et al: Peginterferon-alfa 2a plus ribavirin for chronic hepatitis C virus infection. N Engl J Med 2002;347(13):975-982.

Hadziyannis SJ, Sette H, Morgan TR, et al: Peginterferon alfa 2a (40 kilodaltons) and ribavirin combination therapy in chronic hepatitis C: Randomized study of the effect of treatment duration and ribavirin dose. Ann Intern Med 2004;140:346-355.

Keeffe EB, Dieterich DT, Han SH, et al: A treatment algorithm for the management of chronic hepatitis B virus infection in the United States: An update. Clin Gastroenterol Hepatol 2006;4(8):936-962.

Lok A, McMahon B: Chronic hepatitis B: Update of recommendations. AASLD Guideline. Hepatology 2004;39:857-861.

Manns MP, McHutchinson JG, Gordon SC, et al: Peginterferon alfa-2b plus ribavirin compared with interferon alfa-2b plus ribavirin for initial treatment of chronic hepatitis C: A randomized trial. Lancet 2001;358:958-965.

Marcellin P, Chang TT, Lim SG, et al: Adefovir dipivoxil for the treatment of hepatitis B e antigen–positive chronic hepatitis B. N Engl J Med 2003;348: 808-816.

Strader BD, Wright T, Thomas DL, et al: Diagnosis, management, and treatment of hepatitis C. AASLD Practice Guideline. Hepatology 2004;39(4):1147-1171.

# Malabsorption

Method of
*Lawrence R. Schiller, MD*

Every day the average human being consumes 2000-3000 kcal of food, much of it in the form of polymers or other complex molecules that must be digested and absorbed by the gut. The processes of digestion and absorption are complex and are readily disturbed by pathologic processes. More than 200 conditions have been described that can adversely affect nutrient absorption.

Strictly speaking, *maldigestion* refers to impaired hydrolysis of nutrients, usually due to lack of luminal factors, such as bile acids and pancreatic enzymes, and *malabsorption* refers to impaired mucosal transport. For clinical purposes, "malabsorption" is used to describe both processes.

Malabsorption can be generalized (panmalabsorption) or limited to a specific category of nutrients. Generalized malabsorption is usually due to maldigestion or to extensive mucosal dysfunction. Specific malabsorption occurs when a single transporter is disabled.

The causes of malabsorption can be divided into three categories: impaired luminal hydrolysis, impaired mucosal function (mucosal hydrolysis, uptake, packaging, and excretion), and impaired removal of nutrients from the mucosa (Box 1).

## Diagnosis

### SYMPTOMS AND SIGNS

Most patients with panmalabsorption have changes in their stools (Box 2). Steatorrhea (excess fat in stools) is characterized by pale color, bulkiness, greasiness, and a tendency to float (probably because of incorporated gas). Occasionally patients with malabsorption present

---

### BOX 1   Causes of Malabsorption or Maldigestion

- Impaired luminal hydrolysis or solublization
  - Bile acid deficiency
  - Impaired mucosal hydrolysis, uptake, or packaging
  - Pancreatic exocrine insufficiency
  - Postgastrectomy syndrome
  - Rapid intestinal transit
  - Small bowel bacterial overgrowth
  - Zollinger-Ellison syndrome
- Brush border or metabolic disorders
  - Abetalipoproteinemia
  - Glucose-galactose malabsorption
  - Lactase deficiency
  - Sucrase-isomaltase deficiency
- Mucosal diseases
  - Amyloidosis
  - Chronic mesenteric ischemia
  - Crohn's disease
  - Celiac sprue
  - Collagenous sprue
  - Eosinophilic gastroenteritis
  - Immunoproliferative small intestinal disease (IPSID)
  - Lymphoma
  - Nongranulomatous ulcerative jejunoileitis
  - Radiation enteritis
  - Systemic mastocytosis
- Infectious diseases
  - AIDS enteropathy
  - *Mycobacterium avium-intracellulare*
  - Parasitic diseases
  - Small bowel bacterial overgrowth
  - Tropical sprue
  - Whipple's disease
- After intestinal resection
- Chronic mesenteric ischemia
- Impaired removal of nutrients
  - Lymphangiectasia

---

### BOX 2   Symptoms and Signs of Malabsorption or Maldigestion

- Changes in stool characteristics
  - Floating stools
  - Pale, bulky, greasy stools
  - Watery diarrhea
- Increased colonic gas production
  - Abdominal distention
  - Borborygmi
- Vitamin and mineral deficiencies
  - Anemia
  - Cheilosis
  - Glossitis
  - Dermatitis
  - Neuropathy
  - Night blindness
  - Osteomalacia
  - Paresthesia
  - Tetany
- Ecchymosis
- Fatigue, weakness
- Edema
- Weight loss, muscle wasting

## CURRENT DIAGNOSIS

- Recognize the presence of generalized malabsorption by the combination of typical symptoms: diarrhea, greasy stools, flatulence, weight loss, fatigue, edema.
- Recognize the presence of specific malabsorption by associated symptoms and those symptoms particular to deficiency states of the malabsorbed substance: flatus, diarrhea, anemia, dermatitis, glossitis, neuropathy, paresthesias, tetany, ecchymosis.
- Documentation of generalized malabsorption is best done by stool analysis demonstrating steatorrhea and acid stools (reflecting carbohydrate malabsorption). Diagnosis depends on visualization of the small bowel by endoscopy or radiography and small bowel biopsy. Additional tests may be needed.
- Documentation of specific malabsorption is best done by demonstrating low blood levels of the malabsorbed substance or by tests designed to measure absorption of that substance. Diagnosis depends on studies designed to identify the likely diagnosis for a given situation.

with watery stools due to the osmotic effects of unabsorbed carbohydrates and short-chain fatty acids.

Abdominal distention and excess flatus also commonly occur due to fermentation of unabsorbed carbohydrate by colonic bacteria. This can occur not only with panmalabsorption but also with specific malabsorption of carbohydrate (e.g., lactase deficiency).

Weight loss is typical with severe panmalabsorption, but it might not be very prominent with lesser degrees of malabsorption due to compensatory hyperphagia. Weight loss is most prominent early in the course of the illness, but body weight usually stabilizes as calorie absorption and body weight come into balance again. This is in contrast to illnesses like cancer or tuberculosis that produce continuing weight loss. If a patient with malabsorption has continuing weight loss, inflammatory bowel disease or lymphoma should be considered.

Abdominal pain is usually not present with malabsorption, although some cramping may be associated with diarrhea. Severe pain should bring chronic pancreatitis, Zollinger-Ellison syndrome, lymphoma, Crohn's disease, or mesenteric ischemia to mind.

Constitutional symptoms of fatigue and weakness commonly occur, even early in the course. In contrast, appetite is impaired only late in the course of most malabsorption states. Edema is uncommon until late in the course unless protein-losing enteropathy is present.

Vitamin and mineral deficiencies can lead to several symptoms or signs. Glossitis and cheilosis are common in patients with water-soluble vitamin deficiencies. Florid beriberi, pellagra, and scurvy are not commonly seen unless malabsorption has been particularly severe or long-lasting. Fat-soluble vitamin deficiencies also are unlikely to develop except when malabsorption has been long-standing because of substantial body stores.

Miscellaneous findings occasionally seen in patients with malabsorption can provide clues to the diagnosis. Aphthous ulcers in the mouth may be seen with celiac disease, Behçet's syndrome, or Crohn's disease. Hyperpigmentation is seen in Whipple's disease, and dermatitis herpetiformis (pruritic, blistering skin lesions) is seen in celiac disease. Scleroderma can manifest with tight skin, digital ulceration, nail changes, and Raynaud's phenomenon. Chronic sinusitis, bronchitis, and recurrent pneumonia suggest cystic fibrosis or IgA deficiency. Several systemic diseases can be associated with malabsorption syndrome (Box 3).

## TESTS

### Routine Laboratory Tests

Routine laboratory tests (Box 4) commonly are abnormal in patients with established malabsorption syndrome. Anemia is common but

---

### BOX 3  Systemic Diseases Associated with Malabsorption or Maldigestion

**Endocrine Diseases**
- Addison's disease
- Diabetes mellitus
- Hypoparathyroidism
- Hyperthyroidism, hypothyroidism

**Collagen-Vascular and Miscellaneous Diseases**
- AIDS
- Amyloidosis
- Scleroderma
- Vasculitis (systemic lupus erythematosus, polyarteritis nodosa)

---

not universal. Iron deficiency anemia may be the only finding in some patients with celiac disease. Microcytic anemia may be present in Whipple's disease (due to occult blood loss) and in lymphomas manifesting with malabsorption. Macrocytic anemia due to folate or vitamin $B_{12}$ deficiency can occur in short bowel syndrome, small bowel bacterial overgrowth, or ileal disease. Lymphopenia may be present in patients with AIDS or lymphangiectasia.

Electrolyte abnormalities may be due to a combination of poor intake and excess loss in stool. Renal function usually is well maintained in malabsorption syndrome, but blood urea nitrogen may be low due to poor protein absorption, and serum creatinine concentration may be low due to depletion of muscle mass. Serum calcium levels may be low due to malabsorption, vitamin D deficiency, or intraluminal complexing of calcium by fatty acids. Hypomagnesemia can produce hypocalcemia or hypokalemia that is resistant to intravenous repletion. Serum phosphorus, cholesterol, and triglyceride levels may be reduced due to poor intake or malabsorption. Liver tests may be abnormal due to fatty liver. Serum protein and albumin levels are well preserved in patients with malabsorption unless protein-losing enteropathy or an acute illness is present.

Prothrombin time is normal unless vitamin K malabsorption (typically associated with steatorrhea), anticoagulant therapy, antibiotic therapy, or colectomy is present.

Assays are available for several potentially malabsorbed substances, including iron, vitamin $B_{12}$, folate, 25-hydroxyvitamin D, and β-carotene. Malabsorption tends to lower blood levels, but substantial body stores of many of these can mitigate the reduction in concentration that otherwise might occur. Thus, the sensitivity and specificity of these assays for malabsorption are poor.

### Tests for Malabsorption

#### Fat Malabsorption

The simplest test for fat malabsorption is a qualitative microscopic examination of stool using a fat-soluble stain, such as Sudan III. The finding of more than 5 stained droplets per high power field is abnormal and correlates well with quantitative measurement of fecal fat excretion. The test is subject to false-positive results with some drugs and food additives, such as mineral oil, orlistat, and olestra.

## CURRENT THERAPY

- Once a diagnosis is reached, therapy can be directed toward that specific problem:
    - Gluten-free diet for celiac disease
    - Antibiotics for bacterial overgrowth
    - Lactose-free diet for lactase deficiency

## BOX 4   Laboratory Tests for Evaluation of Malabsorption or Maldigestion

**Routine Blood Tests**
- Complete blood count
- Hemoglobin/hematocrit
- Platelet count
- WBC differential count

**Biochemistry Tests**
- Blood urea nitrogen
- Potassium
- Prothrombin time
- Serum albumin
- Serum calcium
- Serum creatinine

**Blood Levels of Potentially Malabsorbed Substances**
- Fat absorption
- Qualitative fecal fat
- Quantitative fecal fat
- Serum iron, vitamin $B_{12}$, folate, 25-OH vitamin D, carotene

**Protein Absorption and Protein-Losing Enteropathy**
- $\alpha_1$-Antitrypsin clearance
- Fecal nitrogen excretion

**Carbohydrate Absorption**
- Osmotic gap in stool water
- Quantitative excretion (anthrone)

- Stool pH <5.5
- Stool reducing substances
- D-Xylose absorption test
- Oral glucose, sucrose, and lactose tolerance tests
- Breath hydrogen tests

**Vitamin $B_{12}$ Absorption**
- Schilling test with intrinsic factor

**Bile Acid Malabsorption**
- $^{14}$C-glycocholic acid breath test
- Fecal bile acid excretion
- Radiolabeled bile acid excretion
- $^{75}$SeHCAT retention

**Small Bowel Bacterial Overgrowth**
- $^{14}$C-glycocholic acid breath test
- $^{14}$C-xylose breath test
- Glucose breath hydrogen test
- Quantitative culture of jejunal aspirate

**Exocrine Pancreatic Insufficiency**
- Dual-labeled Schilling test
- Secretin/CCK test
- Stool chymotrypsin concentration

**Serologic Testing for Celiac Disease**
- Anti-tissue transglutaminase antibody (IgA)
- Anti-endomysial antibody (IgA)

*Abbreviations:* CCK = cholecystokinin; SLE = systemic lupus erythematosus; $^{75}$SeHCAT = selenium-75-labeled taurohomocholic acid.

---

A more precise estimate of fat absorption is obtained by a quantitative analysis of a timed stool collection (48 or 72 hours). During the collection, a diary of dietary intake should be maintained so that fat excretion can be assessed as a percentage of intake. Normal fat excretion is <7% of intake when stool weight is normal, but it can be twice as high due to voluminous diarrhea without indicating defective mucosal transport of fat. Thus, fat excretion must be judged against stool weight. Stool fat concentration (grams of fat per 100 grams of stool) also is of value. Pancreatic exocrine insufficiency is associated with high fecal fat concentration (>10g/100g stool) because unlike hydrolyzed fat, unhydrolyzed fat does not stimulate colonic water and electrolyte secretion that would dilute fecal fat concentration.

### Protein Malabsorption

Fecal nitrogen excretion can be employed as a marker of protein malabsorption, but is not often used in clinical medicine because it adds little to the evaluation. If protein-losing enteropathy is suspected, an $\alpha_1$-antitrypsin clearance study can be done. In this study, *fecal* excretion of $\alpha_1$-antitrypsin, a serum protein that is relatively resistant to hydrolysis by luminal enzymes, is divided by *serum* concentration of $\alpha_1$-antitrypsin, and the volume of serum leaked into the lumen can be calculated. Values of more than 180 mL/day are associated with hypoalbuminemia.

### Carbohydrate Malabsorption

Carbohydrate malabsorption is difficult to measure directly because fermentation of malabsorbed carbohydrate by colonic bacteria reduces the amount of intact carbohydrate that can be recovered in stool. Indirect estimates of carbohydrate malabsorption can be made by examining fecal pH (<5.5 with carbohydrate malabsorption) or fecal osmotic gap (>100 mOsm/kg with osmotic diarrhea). Oral carbohydrate

tolerance tests may be used to evaluate absorption of sugars, such as lactose or fructose. Following an oral load of a given sugar, blood glucose levels are monitored; failure of blood glucose to increase suggests malabsorption.

Another test for carbohydrate malabsorption is the D-xylose absorption test. In this test, a 25-gram dose of D-xylose is given orally; blood xylose levels are measured 1 and 3 hours later, and urinary excretion of xylose is measured for 5 hours. Failure of blood xylose to rise above 20 mg/dL at 1 hour or above 22.5 mg/dL at 3 hours or failure of urinary excretion to exceed 5 g in 5 hours suggests malabsorption. In addition, because xylose does not require pancreatic enzymes or bile acids for absorption, an abnormal D-xylose test suggests a mucosal problem as the cause for malabsorption. The results of this test can be misleading if the patient is dehydrated or has ascites, if renal function is compromised, or if bacterial overgrowth is present in the upper small bowel.

Breath hydrogen testing is another method to assess carbohydrate absorption. If substrates such as lactose or sucrose are not absorbed in the small intestine, they pass into the colon, where bacterial fermentation produces hydrogen gas. The hydrogen is absorbed into the bloodstream and then is exhaled. The concentration of hydrogen in exhaled breath can be measured easily; a rise of more than 10 to 20 ppm after ingestion of a specific substrate is consistent with malabsorption. False-positive results can be seen in patients with small bowel bacterial overgrowth, and false-negative results can be seen in patients who lack hydrogen-producing flora or who have been on antibiotics recently.

### Vitamin $B_{12}$ Malabsorption

The Schilling test can be used to measure vitamin $B_{12}$ absorption. For purposes of a malabsorption evaluation, part II of the Schilling test (measurement of radiolabeled $B_{12}$ absorption *with* intrinsic factor) is all that is needed. Recovery of less than 9% of the radiolabel in the urine is abnormal and suggests ileal dysfunction. The test may be falsely positive in patients with pancreatic exocrine insufficiency, small bowel bacterial overgrowth, or renal failure.

### Bile Acid Malabsorption

Tests for bile acid malabsorption are not widely available in the United States. Direct measurement of bile acid excretion has been used mainly in research studies. Retention of a radioactive taurocholic acid analogue (SeHCAT, selenium-75-labeled taurohomocholic acid) is used in Europe to assess bile acid malabsorption. A breath test using $^{14}$C-glycocholic acid has been used for evaluating small bowel bacterial overgrowth, but it may have application for assessing bile acid malabsorption as well.

### Small Bowel Bacterial Overgrowth

The gold standard method used to test for small bowel bacterial overgrowth in the upper intestine is quantitative culture of jejunal fluid. The sample can be obtained during endoscopy and sent to the laboratory with instructions to quantitate the aerobic and anaerobic flora. Finding more than $10^5$ bacteria per mL confirms bacterial overgrowth. Breath tests using glucose, $^{14}$C-xylose, and lactulose also have been described for this purpose.

### Pancreatic Exocrine Insufficiency

Tests for pancreatic exocrine insufficiency are not commonly used. The gold standard test is a secretin test. This study requires duodenal intubation, injection of secretin, and measurement of bicarbonate output. A tubeless test, the bentiromide test, had average clinical utility; it is no longer available in the United States. Measurement of fecal chymotrypsin or elastase activity is only moderately useful in predicting the presence of exocrine pancreatic insufficiency. For most situations, a therapeutic trial using a high dose of pancreatic enzymes with monitoring of the effect on steatorrhea is the best that can be done.

## Evaluation of Suspected Malabsorption

When malabsorption is suspected because of the history, physical findings, and setting, the physician must decide if the malabsorption involves a specific nutrient or represents a generalized process (Figure 1).

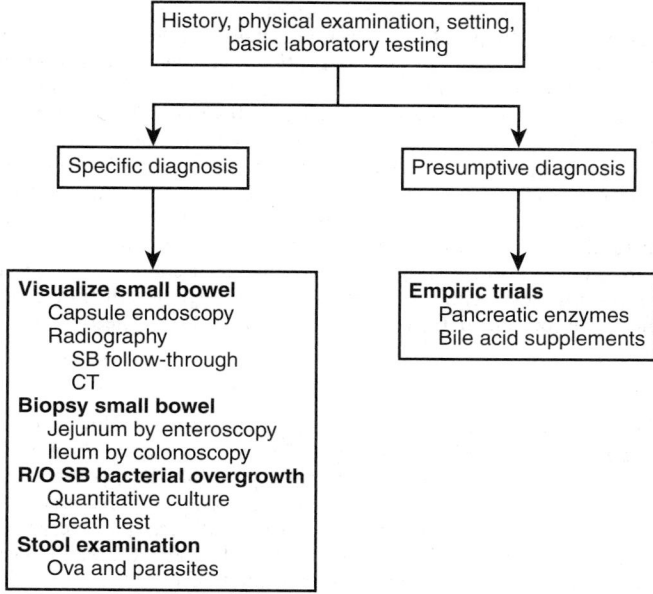

**FIGURE 1.** Flow chart for evaluation of malabsorption or maldigestion. *Abbreviations:* CT = computed tomography; R/O = rule out; SB = small bowel.

If the malabsorption seems to be specific, a diet and symptom diary, breath tests using the presumptively malabsorbed substrate, and stool pH to identify acid stools seen with carbohydrate malabsorption are reasonable diagnostic maneuvers.

Suspected generalized malabsorption requires a more intense evaluation. Steatorrhea should be confirmed with either a qualitative fecal fat test (e.g., Sudan stain) or a quantitative stool collection for measurement of fat excretion. If steatorrhea is confirmed, the small bowel should be visualized with either capsule endoscopy or radiography (small bowel follow-through examination or computed tomography) and biopsied from above by enteroscopy and from below by colonoscopy. During enteroscopy, an aspirate of small bowel contents can be obtained for quantitative culture to look for small bowel bacterial overgrowth. An alternative method to detect small bowel bacterial overgrowth is breath testing (see earlier). Stool samples also should be examined with microscopy or immunoassay for the presence of parasites that may be associated with malabsorption.

This sequence of evaluation often leads to a specific diagnosis. When it does not, empiric trials of pancreatic enzyme replacement or bile acid supplementation can lead to a presumptive diagnosis of pancreatic exocrine insufficiency or bile acid deficiency. Hard endpoints (e.g., quantitative fat excretion) should be used to assess the effectiveness of these empiric trials.

## Specific Disorders Associated with Malabsorption

### MALABSORPTION OF SPECIFIC NUTRIENTS

#### Disaccharidase Deficiency

Ingested disaccharides such as lactose and sucrose and starch-digestion products such as maltotriose and α-limit dextrins must be hydrolyzed by brush border enzymes into monosaccharides for absorption by the mucosa. If these brush border enzymes are not active or if the brush border is damaged, malabsorption of the specific carbohydrate substrate results. This can result in gaseousness or osmotic diarrhea when those substrates are ingested. This rarely occurs on a congenital basis, but it commonly occurs as an acquired disorder.

Lactase deficiency is the most common acquired disaccharidase deficiency. Infant mammals all rely on lactose as the carbohydrate source in milk, but lactase activity is shut off after weaning in most species. Most human populations lose lactase activity during adolescence as a normal part of maturation. Members of the northern European gene pool might maintain lactase activity into adult life, but lactase activity declines gradually in many. At some point the amount of lactose ingested might exceed the ability of the remaining enzyme to hydrolyze it, resulting in lactose malabsorption and symptoms. This also can occur with acute conditions such as gastroenteritis that can disturb the mucosa and temporarily reduce lactase activity. Patients might not recognize lactose ingestion as a cause of their problem because they have not had difficulty tolerating lactose in the past. Restriction of lactose in the diet (or use of products that have predigested lactose) mitigates symptoms. Use of exogenous lactase as a tablet may only be partially effective because of incomplete hydrolysis of ingested lactose.

#### Transport Defects at the Brush Border

Glucose-galactose malabsorption is a rare congenital disorder resulting from an inactive hexose transporter in the brush border. Hydrolysis of lactose is intact, but transport across the apical membrane of the enterocyte fails to occur. Fructose absorption, which is mediated by a different carrier, is unaffected.

In all human beings the ability to absorb fructose is limited by the availability of carriers in the brush border and may be overwhelmed when excess fructose is ingested. This can occur relatively easily nowadays, because high-fructose corn syrup is used frequently as a sweetener in commercial products such as soda pop. Limiting the amount of fructose ingested will reduce symptoms.

Abetalipoproteinemia is a rare condition that prevents absorption of long-chain fatty acids due to failure to form chylomicrons. Use of medium-chain triglycerides that do not require transport in chylomicrons can bypass this defect.

Pernicious anemia develops when failure to secrete intrinsic factor in the stomach prevents vitamin $B_{12}$ absorption by the ileal mucosa. Parenteral replacement with cyanocobalamin by injection (Cyanoject) or nasal spray (Nascobal) is necessary.

## GENERALIZED MALABSORPTION

### Celiac Disease

Celiac disease (also known as celiac sprue) is a disorder in which the mucosa of the small bowel is damaged due to activation of the mucosal immune system by ingestion of gluten, a protein component found in wheat, barley, and rye. People who have HLA-DQ2 or DQ8 are susceptible to this condition because these specific antigen-presenting proteins produce particularly strong reactions by interacting with a unique peptide digestion product of gluten. Tissue transglutaminase, an enzyme produced in the mucosa, is an important cofactor in pathogenesis by amplifying the immunogenicity of gluten peptide fragments and is the target of autoantibodies that are characteristic of this disease. The condition produces generalized malabsorption by destroying the villi of the small intestine, reducing the surface area available for absorption.

In addition to malabsorption syndrome with diarrhea and weight loss, celiac disease can produce a host of nonspecific symptoms, including abdominal pain, fatigue, muscle and joint pains, and headaches and seemingly unrelated problems such as iron deficiency anemia, abnormal liver tests, and osteoporosis. These protean manifestations mean that celiac disease must be considered in the differential diagnosis of many conditions. The clinical course is quite variable, with symptoms coming and going. Symptoms can develop during childhood and produce growth retardation or first become manifest in adulthood.

Testing for celiac disease has been simplified by the development of an assay for anti–tissue transglutaminase antibodies. This test largely supplants measurement of antigluten antibodies, although these remain of some use in evaluating adherence to a gluten-free diet. IgA antibodies are the most useful for diagnosis, but IgA deficiency is common enough that an IgA level should be measured concomitantly.

Although serologic tests have high sensitivity and specificity, the implications of adhering to a gluten-free diet are so extreme that the diagnosis of celiac disease should be confirmed whenever possible by small bowel mucosal biopsy, now obtained routinely by endoscopy. An empiric trial of a gluten-free diet may be difficult to interpret because many persons with gastrointestinal symptoms improve with dietary carbohydrate restriction. Wheat starch is particularly hard to digest (due to gluten coating wheat starch granules), and ordinarily 20% of wheat starch are not absorbed by the small bowel and enter the colon.

Treatment of celiac disease at present involves strict lifetime exclusion of gluten from the diet. This is a difficult regimen that excludes most processed foods. Assistance of a dietitian is most helpful. The prognosis with effective treatment is very good. Symptoms should respond to the diet within weeks; failure to do so should prompt an examination of compliance with the diet or reconsideration of the diagnosis. Failure to respond may be seen when lymphoma or adenocarcinoma complicate the course of celiac disease or in cases of "refractory sprue" or "collagenous sprue" which can have a different autoimmune basis from classic celiac disease and which might respond to immunosuppressive drugs such as corticosteroids or azathioprine (Imuran)[1]. Persistent diarrhea may be observed in patients with celiac disease who have concomitant microscopic colitis, another condition that is linked to HLA-DQ2 and HLA-DQ8.

### Inflammatory Diseases

Diseases that produce extensive mucosal damage by inflammation cause generalized malabsorption by reduction of mucosal surface area, by promotion of small bowel bacterial overgrowth, by ileal dysfunction,

---

[1]Not FDA approved for this indication.

or by development of enteroenteric or enterocolic fistulas. Examples include jejunoileitis due to Crohn's disease, nongranulomatous ulcerative jejunoileitis, radiation enteritis, and chronic mesenteric ischemia. With Crohn's disease, previous resection can add to the problem (see later). Therapy aimed at the underlying process can improve absorption; in some cases (e.g., radiation enteritis) no effective therapy is available for the underlying problem, and symptomatic management is all that is possible. This includes use of antidiarrheal drugs to prolong contact time between luminal contents and the small bowel mucosa, ingestion of a reduced fat diet to reduce steatorrhea, and use of vitamin and mineral supplements to prevent deficiency states.

### Infiltrative Disorders

Several conditions involve infiltration of the intestinal mucosa with cells or extracellular matrix that impede absorption or modify mucosal function by secretion of cytokines and other regulatory substances. These include eosinophilic gastroenteritis, systemic mastocytosis, immunoproliferative small intestinal disease (IPSID), lymphoma, and amyloidosis. These conditions are diagnosed by mucosal biopsy, but special stains might have to be employed to identify the infiltrating cells or matrix accurately.

Treatment of the underlying processes can improve absorption, but it is not uniformly effective. For eosinophilic gastroenteritis, a hypoallergenic (elimination) diet and corticosteroids may be useful. Mild systemic mastocytosis is treated with the mast cell-stabilizer sodium chromoglycate, $H_1$- and $H_2$-receptor antagonists, and low-dose aspirin. More advanced disease might respond to interferon or cytotoxic chemotherapy. IPSID initially is treated with antibiotics because small bowel bacterial overgrowth may be a causative factor. Once malignant change has occurred, it is treated like lymphoma with cytotoxic chemotherapy. Amyloidosis affecting the gut is not amenable to therapy and is usually fatal.

### Infectious Diseases

#### Small Bowel Bacterial Overgrowth

Small bowel bacterial overgrowth in the jejunum can produce generalized malabsorption. It can occur whenever the mechanisms that reduce overgrowth are compromised. These situations include achlorhydria or hypochlorhydria, motility disorders of the small intestine (e.g., diabetes mellitus or scleroderma), and anatomic alterations (e.g., diverticulosis, gastrocolic fistula, or blind loops postoperatively). Fat malabsorption is attributed to bacterial deconjugation of bile acid. Bacterial toxins or free fatty acids can produce patchy mucosal damage, leading to less efficient carbohydrate and protein absorption. Bacteria also can compete with the mucosa for uptake of certain nutrients such as vitamin $B_{12}$.

Diagnosis of small bowel bacterial overgrowth can be difficult (see earlier). Treatment consists of antibiotic therapy unless a surgically correctable anatomic defect is discovered. Tetracycline is no longer uniformly effective; amoxicillin–clavulinic acid (Augmentin), cephalosporins, ciprofloxacin (Cipro), metronidazole (Flagyl), and rifaximin (Xifaxan) may be employed. Therapy should be given for 1 to 2 weeks initially and then discontinued. It should be restarted when symptoms recur. If this occurs quickly, longer treatment periods should be considered. Continuous antibiotic therapy is needed rarely.

#### Tropical Sprue

Tropical sprue is a progressive, chronic malabsorptive condition occurring in both the indigenous population and in visitors residing in certain tropical countries for extended periods. The prevalence of tropical sprue seems to be decreasing for uncertain reasons. The disease starts as an acute diarrheal disease that becomes a persistent diarrhea associated with substantial weight loss and typically megaloblastic anemia. Villi become shortened and thickened (partial villous atrophy), but the flat mucosa of celiac disease is not usually present. Enterocytes have disrupted brush borders and can have megaloblastic changes; the submucosa has a chronic inflammatory infiltrate. Intestinal biopsy is required for diagnosis.

Currently, tropical sprue is believed to represent a form of bacterial overgrowth with organisms that secrete enterotoxins. Most patients have evidence of excessive gram-negative bacterial colonization of the jejunum. The declining prevalence of tropical sprue may be due to improved nutrition, better sanitation, or prompt treatment of acute diarrhea with antibiotics. Treatment consists of pharmacologic doses of folic acid (folate) (5 mg daily[3]), injection of cyanocobalamin (if deficient), and antibiotic therapy for 1 to 6 months. Tetracycline 250 mg four times a day or sulfonamide is the treatment of choice. Newer antibiotics have not been tested extensively in this condition. Improvement should be noted after a few weeks. The prognosis with treatment is excellent; without treatment, tropical sprue can be fatal. Recurrence can occur.

## Whipple's Disease

Whipple's disease is a rare chronic bacterial infection with multisystem involvement. The small bowel typically is heavily infiltrated with foamy macrophages containing periodic acid–Schiff (PAS)-positive material, distorting the villi. Small bowel biopsy with special stains or electron microscopy or a specific polymerase chain reaction (PCR) is diagnostic. Foamy macrophages and bacteria can be found outside the intestine in lymph nodes, spleen, liver, central nervous system, heart, and synovium. Accordingly, symptoms are protean. The bacterium has been identified as *Tropheryma whippelii*, a relative of *Acinetobacter*. It does not appear to be very contagious, and no direct person-to-person transmission has been demonstrated. Presumably differences in host resistance allow proliferation within macrophages without clearance of the bacteria.

Whipple's disease occurs mainly in older white men, but women and all ethnic groups are susceptible. Patients can present with malabsorption syndrome or with symptoms related to the extraintestinal disease (arthritis, fever, dementia, headache, or muscle weakness). Gross or occult gastrointestinal bleeding can occur. Protein-losing enteropathy may be present.

Treatment with any of several antibiotics (penicillin, erythromycin, ampicillin, tetracycline, chloramphenicol, or trimethoprim-sulfamethoxazole (TMP-SMX) produces excellent symptomatic responses within days to weeks, but it should be continued for months to years. Even with protracted courses, relapses are common.

## Other Infections

*Mycobacterium avium–intracellulare* is another chronic bacterial infection that can cause malabsorption, particularly in patients with AIDS. Mucosal biopsy with special stains to distinguish it from Whipple's disease is essential. Antibiotic therapy can reduce the intensity of infection; clearance depends on immunologic reconstitution with antiretroviral therapy. Clarithromycin (Biaxin) and ethambutol (Myambutol) are recommended as initial therapy.

Parasitic diseases can produce malabsorption by competing for nutrients and causing mechanical occlusion of the absorptive surface and epithelial damage. Protozoa that may be associated with malabsorption include *Giardia lamblia*, *Isospora belli*, *Cryptosporidium*, and *Enterocytozoon bieneusi*. Tapeworms associated with malabsorption include *Taenia saginata* (beef tapeworm), *Hymenolepis nana* (dwarf tapeworm), and *Diphyllobothrium latum* (fish tapeworm).

*Giardia lamblia* is a cosmopolitan parasite acquired from contaminated water or from another person by fecal-oral transmission. Cysts are relatively hardy, and ingestion of as few as 10 cysts is sufficient to establish infection. Patients with dysgammaglobulinemia (especially IgA deficiency) are likely to become infected. Diagnosis depends on finding the organism (cysts or trophozoites) in stool by microscopy (sensitivity ~50% for a single specimen), or detection of giardia antigens by immunologic testing of stool (sensitivity >90%), or discovery of the organism on small bowel biopsy.

Therapy consists of a single dose of tinidazole (Tindamax) (2 g), metronidazole (Flagyl)[1] (250 mg three times a day for a week),

nitazoxanide (Alinia) (500 mg twice a day for three days), or quinacrine[2] (100 mg three times a day for a week).

*Isospora belli* and *Cryptosporidium* spp. are coccidia, protozoa that disrupt the epithelium by intracellular invasion (*Isospora*) or by attaching to the brush border, destroying microvilli (*Crptosporidium*). Stool examination or small bowel biopsy can identify the organism. *Cryptosporidium* antigen can be discovered by immunoassay on stool with excellent sensitivity. *Isospora* can be treated with TMP-SMX[1] or furazolidone.[2] *Cryptosporidium* can be treated by nitazoxanide.

Microsporidia are intracellular organisms now believed to be most closely related to fungi and are implicated in diarrhea and malabsorption in patients with AIDS and other immunodeficiency states. Small bowel biopsy can show partial villous atrophy, and electron microscopy displays characteristic changes. Stool examination occasionally is helpful. No treatment is of proven value.

Tapeworms compete with their hosts for nutrients in the lumen. *Diphyllobothrium latum* can produce vitamin B[12] deficiency. The others can result in more extensive nutritional deficiencies. Diagnosis is based on stool examination, and treatment depends on the particular organism identified.

## Luminal Problems Causing Malabsorption

### Pancreatic Exocrine Insufficiency

Pancreatic exocrine insufficiency is the most common luminal problem that results in maldigestion. Patients develop symptoms of malabsorption when pancreatic enzyme secretion is reduced by >90%. There are several clinical features that distinguish pancreatic exocrine insufficiency from mucosal disorders, such as celiac disease. When fat is not digested, it is transported through the gastrointestinal tract as intact triglyceride, which can appear as oil in the stool. In contrast, if fat is digested but not absorbed, it is in the form of fatty acids that can produce secretory diarrhea in the colon, resulting in more voluminous, even watery stools. This has two important ramifications: Fecal fat concentration is lower with mucosal disease (typically <9% by weight), and hypocalcemia due to formation of soaps (calcium plus 2 fatty acids) is seen with mucosal disease but not with pancreatic exocrine insufficiency. In addition, patients with mucosal disease tend to have more problems with water-soluble vitamin deficiencies than those with pancreatic exocrine insufficiency. In some patients with pancreatic exocrine insufficiency, carbohydrate malabsorption can produce substantial bloating, flatulence, and watery diarrhea.

Tests to document pancreatic exocrine insufficiency are not widely available or are nonspecific (see earlier), and so diagnosis usually hinges on a consistent history, demonstration of anatomic problems in the pancreas (calcification or abnormal ducts), and documentation of a response of steatorrhea to empiric treatment with a large dose of exogenous enzymes.

### Bile Acid Deficiency

Bile acid deficiency is a less common cause of maldigestion, and malabsorption in this setting is limited to fat and fat-soluble vitamins. The usual setting is a patient with an extensive ileal resection (see later), but this also occurs in certain cholestatic conditions in which bile acid secretion by the liver is markedly compromised, such as advanced primary biliary cirrhosis, or complete extrahepatic biliary obstruction. As with pancreatic exocrine insufficiency, stools tend to have high fat concentrations (>9% by weight) when bile acid secretion is limited by hepatic or biliary disorders.

### Zollinger-Ellison Syndrome

Zollinger-Ellison syndrome produces several abnormalities that can affect absorption. High rates of gastric acid secretion produce persistently low pH in the duodenum, which precipitates bile acid and inactivates

---

[1]Not FDA approved for this indication.
[3]Exceeds dosage recommended by the manufacturer.

[1]Not FDA approved for this indication.
[2]Not available in the United States.

pancreatic enzymes. In addition, excess acid can damage the absorptive cells directly.

## Postoperative Malabsorption

Substantial malabsorption can result from gastric surgeries. Weight loss can result from inadequate intake due to early satiety or symptoms of dumping syndrome. Malabsorption can result from impaired mechanical disruption of food, mismatching of chyme delivery and enzyme secretion, rapid transit, or small bowel bacterial overgrowth due to loss of the gastric acid barrier. In addition, gastric surgery sometimes brings out latent celiac disease.

Short intestinal resections are well tolerated, but more extensive resections produce diarrhea and malabsorption of variable severity. When these symptoms are associated with weight loss or dehydrating diarrhea, short bowel syndrome is said to exist. In general, nutrient absorptive needs can be met if at least 100 cm of jejunum are preserved, but fluid absorption will be insufficient and diarrhea may be profuse. The process of intestinal adaptation permits improved absorption with time; it depends on exposure of the absorptive surface to nutrients. Absorption of specific substances, such as bile acids or vitamin $B_{12}$, is reduced permanently by resection of the terminal ileum.

Malabsorption in short bowel syndrome is not due solely to loss of absorptive surface area. Gastric acid hypersecretion, bile acid deficiency, rapid transit (due to loss of the ileal brake), and bacterial overgrowth may be present. These conditions are amenable to treatment and therapy with antisecretory drugs, exogenous bile acids, opiate antidiarrheals, or antibiotics can produce substantial improvement. Injection of growth hormone in combination with glutamine and a special diet has been approved as treatment for short bowel syndrome; it can reduce the volume of parenteral fluid or nutrients required. Results with small bowel transplantation are improving with the use of better immunosuppressive regimens, and it remains the only cure for select patients with postresection malabsorption.

Attention to nutrition is vital in any patient with malabsorption. If adequate nutrition cannot be maintained by oral intake, nutritional therapy is needed. Because of impaired bowel function, success with enteral nutrition may be impossible; parenteral nutrition may be needed. It is important to distinguish between the need for supplemental fluid and electrolytes and the need for nutrients; total parenteral nutrition is not a good choice for patients who only require fluids and electrolytes.

## REFERENCES

Bai JC, Mazure RM, Vazquez H, et al: Whipple's disease. Clin Gastroenterol Hepatol 2004;2:849-860.

Culliford AN, Green PH: Refractory sprue. Curr Gastroenterol Rep 2003;5: 373-378.

Green PH, Jabri B: Celiac disease. Annu Rev Med 2006;57:207-221.

Gupta V, Toskes PP: Diagnosis and management of chronic pancreatitis. Postgrad Med J 2005;81:491-497.

Horslen SP: Optimal management of the post-intestinal transplant patient. Gastroenterology 2006;130(2 suppl 1):S132-S137.

Jeejeebhoy KN: Management of short bowel syndrome: Avoidance of total parenteral nutrition. Gastroenterology 2006;130(2 suppl 1):S60-S66.

Nath SK: Tropical sprue. Curr Gastroenterol Rep 2005;7:343-349.

O'Keefe SJ, Buchman AL, Fishbein TM, et al: Short bowel syndrome and intestinal failure: Consensus definitions and review. Clin Gastroenterol Hepatol 2006;4:6-10.

Petroniene R, Dubcenco E, Baker JP, et al: Given capsule endoscopy in celiac disease. Gastrointest Endosc Clin N Am 2004;14:115-127.

Schiller LR: Nutrition management of chronic diarrhea and malabsorption. Nutr Clin Pract 2006;21:34-39.

Simren M, Stotzer PO: Use and abuse of hydrogen breath tests. Gut 2006;55: 297-303.

Singh VV, Toskes PP: Small bowel bacterial overgrowth: Presentation, diagnosis, and treatment. Curr Gastroenterol Rep 2003;5:365-372.

Swallow DM: Genetics of lactase persistence and lactose intolerance. Annu Rev Genet 2003;37:197-219.

# Acute and Chronic Pancreatitis

Method of
*Carmen C. Solorzano, MD, and
Richard A. Prinz, MD*

## Acute Pancreatitis

Acute pancreatitis is an inflammatory process of the pancreas, with variable involvement of adjacent regional tissues or remote organ systems. The clinical manifestations of acute pancreatitis are heterogeneous but usually are of rapid onset. Most patients have epigastric pain, which can range from very mild to severe with associated hemodynamic instability. Early diagnosis and staging are necessary to provide appropriate treatment.

### INCIDENCE AND ETIOLOGY

The incidence of acute pancreatitis has been reported to be as high as 38 per 100,000 population per year and appears to be increasing. Around 15% to 20% of patients will develop severe life-threatening complications requiring prolonged intensive care support at considerable cost.

Gallstones and alcohol abuse are the leading causes of acute pancreatitis in the United States, accounting for up to 80% of cases. Acute alcoholic pancreatitis may occur after binge drinking, but in most cases the patient has a minimum 5- to 7-year history of regular, heavy ethanol ingestion. Controversy exists as to whether alcohol alone, without prior gland injury, can cause the condition, as only a minority of alcoholics ever develop acute pancreatitis, implying multifactorial causation. A gallstone in the common bile duct (choledocholithiasis) may incite acute pancreatitis as it passes through the sphincter of Oddi en route to the duodenum. It does so, at least in principle, by transiently obstructing pancreatic duct flow and perhaps also by promoting reflux of bile into the pancreatic duct. As with alcoholic acute pancreatitis, the exact mechanisms remain uncertain. Perhaps 10% of attacks remain "idiopathic" in spite of thorough investigation. Other infrequent causes of acute pancreatitis are listed in Table 1.

### PATHOGENESIS

Although the etiologic factor is known in 85% of patients with acute pancreatitis, the pathologic basis for the condition is incompletely understood. Most patients have a mild form of acute pancreatitis, which is associated with minimal organ dysfunction and an uneventful recovery. These patients respond to appropriate fluid administration, with rapid normalization of physical signs and laboratory values. The predominant pathologic finding in mild acute pancreatitis is interstitial

---

### TABLE 1   Causes of Acute Pancreatitis

Biliary tract disease (gallstones and microlithiasis)
Alcohol abuse
Drug reaction
Pancreatic or ampullary tumors
Ampullary stenosis
Congenital anomalies of the pancreatic or biliary anatomy
Hypertriglyceridemia
Hypercalcemia
Trauma (external or iatrogenic)
Infection (mumps...)
Bites (scorpion, spiders, Gila monster)
Tropical pancreatitis
Idiopathic

edema with occasional parenchymal necrosis. On the other hand, 10% to 15% of patients have severe acute pancreatitis, which is associated with organ failure and/or local complications, such as acute fluid collections, necrosis, abscess, and pseudocyst formation.

In most experimental models of acute pancreatitis, secretion of digestive enzymes from the acinar cell is disturbed. Inappropriate activation of the proteolytic enzyme trypsin outside the gastrointestinal tract leads to inflammation and autodigestion. Tissue destruction results in an influx of leukocytes and macrophages, which, together with the pancreas itself, elaborate numerous inflammatory mediators leading to systemic inflammatory response syndrome. This is thought to be the first step in the development of pancreatitis. Trypsinogen is activated through hydrolysis of an N-terminal peptide called *trypsinogen-activating peptide*. Several natural mechanisms prevent pancreatic autodigestion by activated trypsin. These include: production of serine protease inhibitor Kazal type 1 (SPINK1), also known as *pancreatic secretory trypsin inhibitor* (PSTI), which reversibly inhibits activated trypsin; trypsin-activated trypsin-like enzymes that degrade trypsinogen; and bicarbonate-rich secretions, which are dependent on the normal production of the cystic fibrosis transmembrane conductance receptor (CFTR). SPINK1 mutations have been identified in familial pancreatitis and in children with idiopathic chronic pancreatitis. Because SPINK1 mutations are more common than is pancreatitis, they are thought to be modifiers or promoters rather than the cause of the disease.

The cationic trypsinogen gene that causes hereditary pancreatitis was discovered in 1996. Its mutation leads to a conformational change in the structure of the trypsinogen–SPINK1 complex and may lead to an impaired SPINK1-mediated defense mechanism against activated trypsin. Hereditary pancreatitis is an autosomal dominant condition with clinical and pathologic manifestations identical to those of sporadic pancreatitis. It has an 80% penetrance and is manifested by recurrent episodes of acute pancreatitis, progression to chronic pancreatitis, and development of pancreatic cancer. Many of these mutations have also been noted in patients with idiopathic pancreatitis.

## DIAGNOSIS

The predominant symptom of acute pancreatitis is severe, constant epigastric pain. The onset is rapid, although not as sudden as that of perforated duodenal ulcer. The pain frequently radiates through to the back and may be partially diminished by sitting and leaning forward, or by lying curled in a fetal position. The signs of Cullen and Grey-Turner, periumbilical and flank bruising, respectively, are rare. Nausea and vomiting are frequent. These symptoms cause most patients to seek medical attention within 6 to 12 hours of the onset of pancreatitis, although delay is often seen among inebriated patients. Patients appear acutely ill, and they are usually tachycardic. Hypotension denotes a severe attack. The abdomen is quiet, tender, and full to palpation in the epigastrium.

The simplest laboratory test that suggests the diagnosis of acute pancreatitis is an elevated serum amylase level. Acute acinar cell injury causes a rapid rise in serum amylase level. Normal kidneys efficiently clear amylase, so typically the serum amylase level returns toward normal by the third or fourth day of the attack. A number of acute abdominal surgical emergencies cause hyperamylasemia, such as perforated duodenal ulcer, but rarely to the level of elevation seen with acute pancreatitis. The severity of pancreatitis does not correlate with the degree of amylase elevation. Patients with acute biliary pancreatitis tend to have very high amylase levels, even during a mild attack, presumably because the pancreas was completely normal at the outset. A lesser elevation of serum amylase is usually observed in acute alcoholic pancreatitis, especially during a second or subsequent attack. Serum lipase concentration rises within 4 to 8 hours and returns to normal after 8 to 14 days, making it a useful method for patients presenting late. Lipase elevation may be more sensitive than amylase elevation in patients with alcoholic pancreatitis and is more specific as a marker of acute pancreatitis than is elevated amylase.

Plain abdominal radiographs are useful mainly to exclude other conditions, such as perforated peptic ulcer and mechanical small-bowel obstruction. Ultrasound of the abdomen may disclose edema of the pancreatic parenchyma. However, this finding is often obscured by overlying bowel gas, which acts as an acoustic barrier. Ultrasound is most useful for diagnosing gallbladder stones. It can also accurately calibrate the common bile duct diameter, suggesting choledocholithiasis if distended. A contrast-enhanced abdominal computed tomography (CT) scan (although often unnecessary) more reliably diagnoses acute pancreatitis. The severity of the attack and its outcome can be graded and correlated to the CT appearance of the pancreas and parapancreatic tissues (see next section).

## QUANTIFICATION OF SEVERITY

Between 70% and 80% of all attacks of acute pancreatitis are mild, resulting in little short- or long-term morbidity and virtually no mortality. The remainder are severe attacks, involving a variable fraction of pancreatic necrosis, extensive short- and long-term morbidity, and a mortality rate between 10% and 30%. Predicting severe pancreatitis soon after hospital admission allows early triage to intensive care for supportive treatment. To this end, several systems of severity measurement have been developed and correlated with outcome. Of these systems, the best known is the scoring system devised by Ranson and associates (Table 2). They identified 11 "criteria," five of which were determined on admission and six others at 48 hours after admission, which correlated with ultimate risk of morbidity and mortality. Patients exhibiting two or fewer of the prognostic criteria are likely to survive a relatively mild attack, those with three to six criteria have progressively more severe disease and a greater probability of death, and those with seven or more criteria will almost certainly not survive. The Ranson prognostic score has the advantages of strong clinical correlation and a simple, universally available data set. Its disadvantages are that it requires 48 hours to complete, and it is not useful after 48 hours. It was originally developed to grade acute alcoholic pancreatitis. The Acute Physiology and Chronic Health Evaluation (APACHE) II evaluates 12 prognostic variables that cover all organ systems. Scores greater than 13 in acute pancreatitis have been associated with poor prognosis. An advantage of APACHE II is that it can be used at any time during the hospital course. The Balthazar Score predicts severity of acute pancreatitis based on CT appearance of the pancreas, including presence or absence of pancreatic necrosis. According to these criteria, if 30% of the pancreas is nonperfused, the chances are high that the patient will progress to complicated acute pancreatitis. The Atlanta Classification defines severe acute

---

## CURRENT DIAGNOSIS

**Acute Pancreatitis**

CLINICAL MANIFESTATIONS

- Severe constant epigastric pain
- Pain radiates to the back
- Nausea and vomiting
- Mild pancreatitis responds to supportive treatment with no organ failure

RADIOLOGIC AND LABORATORY TESTS

- Flat and upright plain abdominal film to rule out small-bowel obstruction, perforated ulcer
- Serum amylase and lipase levels
- Ultrasound of the abdomen, with attention to the right upper quadrant (gallbladder, bile ducts, pancreas)
- Contrast-enhanced computed tomography

EVALUATE SEVERITY OF PANCREATITIS

- Ranson criteria
- Acute Physiology and Chronic Health Evaluation (APACHE) II
- Degree of pancreatic necrosis on contrast-enhanced computed tomography

## TABLE 2 Ranson Criteria of Severity of Acute Pancreatitis*

| On Admission | At 48 Hours |
|---|---|
| 1. Age >55 years | 6. Hematocrit fall >10%[†] |
| 2. White blood cell count >16,000 cells/mm³ | 7. Serum calcium <8 mg/dL |
| | 8. Base deficit >4 mEq/L |
| 3. Serum glucose >200 mg/dL | 9. Blood urea nitrogen increase >5 mg/dL[†] |
| 4. Serum lactate dehydrogenase >350 IU/L | 10. Arterial Po₂ <60 mm Hg[‡] |
| | 11. Fluid sequestration >6L[‡] |
| 5. Aspartate transaminase >250 U/dL | |

*Criteria are modified slightly for gallstone pancreatitis.
[†]Compared to admission values.
[‡]Fluid volume infused minus urine and nasogastric tube output.

pancreatitis using standard clinical manifestations, three or more Ranson criteria or an APACHE II score of eight or more, evidence of organ failure, and intrapancreatic pathologic findings such as necrosis (Table 3).

## MANAGEMENT OF MILD ACUTE PANCREATITIS

Although recovery without specific treatment is the rule, all patients are watched closely in a hospital setting because rapid deterioration is not always predictable. Management consists of nothing by mouth, hydration with intravenous crystalloid solution, and analgesia as needed. Prophylaxis against deep venous thrombosis with low-dose subcutaneous heparin and/or sequential calf compression should be routine. Alcoholic patients must be assessed for risk of alcohol withdrawal syndromes. Laboratory tests on admission should include either an arterial blood gas measurement or oxygen saturation measured by pulse oximetry. Oral intake of liquids is resumed when the abdomen is soft and nontender, which usually correlates with a normalized serum

## TABLE 3 Atlanta Symposium Clinically Based Classification System for Acute Pancreatitis*

**Mild Acute Pancreatitis (75%)**
Clinical manifestations (abdominal tenderness, vomiting, hypoactive bowel sounds)
Lacks features of severe pancreatitis
Patients respond appropriately to fluid administration
Minimal organ dysfunction
Contrast enhancement of pancreatic parenchyma is usually normal
Intrapancreatic pathology: Interstitial edema rarely necrosis

**Severe Acute Pancreatitis (25%)**
Clinical manifestations (abdominal tenderness, vomiting, hypoactive bowel sounds)
Ranson ≥3, Acute Physiology and Chronic Health Evaluation (APACHE) II ≥8
Organ failure
Intrapancreatic pathology: Necrosis, less commonly interstitial edema

**Pancreatic Necrosis**
Nonenhanced parenchyma on contrast-enhanced computed tomography >3 cm or involving >30% of the gland
Pathology: Macroscopic focal or diffuse areas of devitalized pancreatic tissue and peripancreatic fat necrosis

*Adapted from Arch Surg 1993;128:586-990.

amylase level. If the liquids do not exacerbate the attack, the diet can be advanced as tolerated. A right upper quadrant ultrasound is performed in all patients, even alcoholic patients, because they too may harbor gallstones. Nasogastric suction is indicated if ileus and vomiting are present because of the risk of aspiration. Likewise, gastric antisecretory agents are given only if there is concern about peptic ulcer or stress gastritis.

## MANAGEMENT OF SEVERE ACUTE PANCREATITIS

Severe acute pancreatitis is usually evident on initial clinical assessment; if not, the grave situation declares itself within the subsequent 24 to 48 hours. Early mortality from severe acute pancreatitis results from cardiovascular and/or respiratory failure. Thus, patients are managed in an intensive care unit, with urinary, central venous pressure, and arterial catheters, cardiac and pulse oximetry monitoring, and close observation. Profound and ongoing intravascular volume loss results from fluid sequestration within the retroperitoneum as well as a diffuse capillary leak, which causes generalized edema. Intravascular volume is maintained by crystalloid infusion, titrated to maintain adequate tissue perfusion. Inotropic cardiac support is used as needed once intravascular volume repletion is achieved. Packed red blood cells are transfused as needed to maintain adequate oxygen-carrying capacity. Respiratory function frequently worsens precipitously in the first 24 hours, requiring endotracheal intubation and ventilatory support. Analgesia and sedation are liberally administered, as is stress ulcer prophylaxis.

At present, no pharmacologic therapy dependably ameliorates the severity of the pancreatitis or decreases the risk of systemic complications. Neither octreotide (Sandostatin),[1] a somatostatin analogue that inhibits pancreatic exocrine secretion, nor various protease inhibitors have improved mortality. Newer therapies targeting mediators of the pancreatic and systemic inflammatory response could in theory improve outcome, especially if administered very early in the attack. One such agent, a platelet-activating factor antagonist called *lexipafant*, showed promise in initial laboratory investigations but did not prove beneficial in clinical trials. Because retroperitoneal and peritoneal exudates contain activated digestive enzymes and a host of other vasoactive and inflammatory mediators, peritoneal dialysis might logically improve the condition of patients with severe acute pancreatitis. Indeed, several trials report amelioration of the cardiovascular collapse associated with a severe attack, although overall hospital mortality due mainly to late infectious sequela was not altered. Finally, operation has almost no role early in the course of severe acute pancreatitis (first 14 days), except to rule out another suspected cause of the acute abdomen or to resect gangrenous bowel, which has developed as a complication of the severe pancreatitis.

---

[1]Not FDA approved for this indication.

 **CURRENT THERAPY**

**Acute Pancreatitis**

MILD ACUTE PANCREATITIS

- Supportive therapy: Intravenous fluids, pain control, diet as tolerated
- If gallstones: Cholecystectomy and cholangiogram during same hospitalization or shortly thereafter

SEVERE ACUTE PANCREATITIS

- Admission to intensive care unit
- Supportive therapy: Intravenous fluids, pain control, antibiotics, enteral or parenteral nutrition
- Surgical treatment of infected pancreatic necrosis
- Surgical or endoscopic treatment of pseudocyst

## NECROSIS AND INFECTION

The presence of pancreatic necrosis can be detected by dynamic CT scanning or by serum markers, if available. The probability of complications and of death correlates with the amount of pancreas that is necrotic. When 20% or less of the gland undergoes necrosis, secondary pancreatic infection is rare, and survival is expected. If 50% or more of the gland is necrotic, secondary infection becomes very probable, and mortality is as high as 50%. Secondary infection of necrotic pancreatic and peripancreatic tissues is relatively common and is the principal cause of mortality from severe acute pancreatitis. Infecting organisms are usually enteric gram-negative bacilli, but infection with gram-positive organisms and fungi is now recognized as well. A trend toward reduced pancreatic infection (as well as other systemic infection) has been shown following the prolonged use of newer antibiotics, which effectively penetrate pancreatic tissue. However, infections that develop in patients treated with prophylactic antibiotics tend to involve resistant organisms. One standard prophylactic antibiotic regimen gaining acceptance uses imipenem-cilastatin (Primaxin) started soon after admission and continued for at least 2 weeks. These patients have many intravenous and invasive monitoring catheters, which are potential portals for entry of gram-positive organisms that can secondarily infect the pancreas. Rigid adherence to appropriate infection control measures is required to minimize this risk.

Infected pancreatic necrosis is the most dreaded and lethal complication of severe acute pancreatitis. The condition becomes apparent most frequently during the third and fourth weeks of hospitalization and is marked by fever, increasing pain, tenderness, and fullness in the upper abdomen. The patient usually appears septic. Contrastenhanced CT may reveal extraluminal retroperitoneal gas, which is a radiographic hallmark of infected necrosis. Percutaneous image-guided fine-needle aspiration of the pancreas, with immediate gram stain and culture of the aspirate, can reveal the presence of organisms, which is diagnostic of infected necrosis. Infected pancreatic necrosis is almost always fatal without aggressive débridement and drainage of the retroperitoneum. The standard for wide débridement is an open laparotomy, although laparoscopic, endoscopic, and percutaneous techniques are being described and developed. Surgical strategy ranges from débridement with closed suction and irrigation of the retroperitoneum to multiple planned operative débridements every 2 to 3 days until all necrotic material is removed. All approaches are time and labor intensive, but they offer the only chance for survival of the majority of patients.

Sterile pancreatic necrosis is associated with severe acute pancreatitis but, unlike infected pancreatic necrosis, is usually managed without the need for urgent operation. Acute peripancreatic fluid collections frequently arise. They may include reactive serous effusions but likely represent secondary or even main pancreatic ductal disruption, with resultant leak of pancreatic juice into the lesser peritoneal sac or other anatomic spaces surrounding the pancreas. These acute collections often resorb spontaneously, requiring no specific treatment. If infection of the fluid is suspected or if pain and tenderness are increasing, the collections may be percutaneously aspirated or even drained. In some centers, endoscopically placed transpapillary drains are inserted into the pancreatic duct, occasionally through the disruption into the fluid collection, to accomplish drainage. Finally, if such collections do not spontaneously disappear and do not require early drainage, they may evolve into a pancreatic pseudocyst.

A few patients with sterile pancreatic necrosis fail to improve in spite of optimal, protracted conservative care. These patients deserve operative exploration and pancreatic débridement on the grounds of failed nonoperative treatment, coupled perhaps with the suspicion that a smoldering, occult infection has eluded discovery. The operation is delayed as long as is practical, to allow areas undergoing necrosis to demarcate and liquefy. This makes the débridement technically easier. The pancreas and adjacent tissues are débrided and drained, provision for enteric feeding is established, and the abdomen is closed with the expectation that the need for reoperation will be likely.

### BILIARY (GALLSTONE) PANCREATITIS

Gallstone pancreatitis is caused by transient obstruction of the pancreatic duct at the ampulla of Vater. The offending gallstone need not be large; "biliary sludge" and even biliary "microlithiasis" appear to be capable of provoking acute pancreatitis. As a rule, patients with gallstone pancreatitis have multiple small gallstones within the gallbladder, a comparatively wide cystic duct (promoting passage into the common bile duct), and a distinct "common channel" of the bile and pancreatic ducts.

Nonalcoholic patients with acute pancreatitis very likely have biliary lithiasis as the underlying cause. The presence of gallstones within the gallbladder virtually makes the diagnosis. A distended common bile duct seen by ultrasound further suggests the recent passage of a stone. Serum bilirubin and/or alkaline phosphatase levels may be mildly elevated, but often both are normal. If the ultrasound fails to reveal gallbladder stones or sludge and other rare causes are excluded, an endoscopic ultrasound may identify sludge or microlithiasis in a stable patient. Endoscopic ultrasound can also complement the pancreatic anatomic findings on CT. If endoscopic ultrasound is not available or is inconclusive, the next diagnostic step includes endoscopic retrograde cholangiopancreatography (ERCP). A sample of bile can be obtained to examine for microscopic crystals (this can be achieved by duodenal drainage as well), and small stones or anatomic anomalies may be identified.

Gallstone pancreatitis is usually mild, resolving clinically within 2 to 4 days. Serum bilirubin and alkaline phosphatase levels are typically normal or return to normal within this period, suggesting a low probability of persistent stone(s) within the common bile duct. Cholecystectomy eliminates the source of further stones and thus prevents recurrent pancreatitis; it should be performed during the same hospitalization or shortly thereafter. An intraoperative cholangiogram is performed, unless it has been undertaken preoperatively. If pancreatitis resolves but liver function tests suggest a persistent stone in the bile duct, then preoperative ERCP with papillotomy and stone extraction is appropriate, followed by prompt cholecystectomy.

If the intraoperative cholangiogram shows choledocholithiasis, a laparoscopic or open common bile duct exploration or a postoperative ERCP with papillotomy with stone removal can be performed, depending on the available expertise. Severe gallstone pancreatitis is managed like severe pancreatitis of any cause. Usually, the inciting stone has passed, leaving the bile and pancreatic ducts unobstructed; therefore, routine, early ERCP is not warranted. However, if a stone is persistently obstructing the ampulla of Vater, if the patient has jaundice, or if the patient has signs of cholangitis, urgent ERCP and stone extraction may be necessary.

# Chronic Pancreatitis

Chronic pancreatitis (CP) is an irreversible, progressive inflammatory disease of the pancreas characterized by pain, fibrosis, and progressive loss of exocrine and/or endocrine function. The early course of this disease may often manifest as repeated attacks of acute pancreatitis. It occurs in men more frequently than in women. Excessive alcohol consumption is usually the cause in developed countries.

### INCIDENCE

In several Western industrialized countries, the estimated prevalence of CP is approximately 10 to 15 per 100,000 population, with an annual incidence of 3.5 to 4 per 100,000 population. These rates may actually underestimate the problem because the diagnosis of CP is not based on advanced diagnostic tools such as ERCP and CT scan. In a recent report from Japan using CT and ERCP, the incidence of CP is 12 per 100,000 and prevalence is 45 per 100,000 population, which are much higher than in Western countries. In southern India, the prevalence of CP has been estimated to be 125 per 100,000 with the majority being calcific pancreatitis. The cause of this tropical pancreatitis is thought to be dietary. According to estimates of the Commission on Professional and Hospital Activities, CP ranks as the 27th most common digestive disease in the United States, with a threefold higher prevalence in the black male population.

The majority of care for CP is directed toward ameliorating pain, but a substantial amount of resources is also spent on treating complications. More than half of CP patients will develop pancreatic diabetes;

one third of these patients will be insulin dependent, and nearly 50% will eventually require surgical intervention for pain or other complications. Optimal care of the patient with CP relies on supportive medical management of endocrine and exocrine insufficiency and of pain. Surgical intervention is generally reserved for intractable pain and specific complications such as pseudocyst and biliary or intestinal obstruction. As many as half of all patients will die within 20 years of their diagnosis of CP, a rate much higher than their age-matched population.

## ETIOLOGY AND PATHOGENESIS

CP appears to be a multifactorial process involving both a genetic predisposition and environmental factors (see Table 4). Alcohol use is by far the number one cause of CP in the Western world, accounting for an estimated 70% of the cases in the United States and Europe. About 10% of chronic alcoholics will develop CP, roughly the same percentage of alcoholics who develop hepatic cirrhosis. Average age at diagnosis of alcoholic pancreatitis is 35 to 45 years with an 11- to 18-year history of 150 to 175 g of alcohol ingestion daily.

Ingested alcohol results in direct damage to the acinar cell with increased concentration of protein secretion, decreased production of bicarbonate, and decreased fluid volume as demonstrated in experimental models and in patients with alcoholic pancreatitis. This combination appears to result in protein and calcium precipitation within the pancreatic duct system, subsequent ductal obstruction, activation of pancreatic enzymes, and autodigestion of the gland. Over time, a fibrotic response results in permanent ductal abnormalities, calcification, and stone formation.

Dietary factors, such as high-fat and high-protein intake and trace mineral insufficiency, seem to be epidemiologically associated with CP. Another theory suggests the presence of an acinar cell product, lithostatin or pancreatic stone protein, that prevents calcium precipitation. Decreased concentrations of lithostatin and decreased levels of lithostatin messenger RNA have been found in the pancreatic juice and acini of patients with chronic calcific pancreatitis, suggesting a genetic component of risk for developing the disease. Alcohol-induced derangement of lipid metabolism has also been postulated as inducing the periacinar fibrosis and changes associated with alcoholic pancreatitis. The range of experimentally identified abnormalities supports the multifactorial nature of the disease.

Another form of CP, tropical pancreatitis, may be caused by protein malnutrition and cyanogens found in cassava root. The clinical and histologic features of tropical pancreatitis are nearly identical to those of alcoholic CP. Obstructive pancreatitis results from both congenital and acquired ductal obstruction, as in pancreas divisum, congenital and acquired strictures, and neoplasia. Unlike alcoholic pancreatitis, the obstructed pancreas shows uniform inflammatory changes with preserved ductal epithelium and rare protein plugs. The hypothesis that high intraductal pressure results in pancreatitis has been proposed based partly on the demonstration of high intraductal pressures in these patients.

Additional causes of CP include hypercalcemia, hyperlipidemia, autoimmune diseases, and genetic alterations, as seen in hereditary and idiopathic pancreatitis (see section on acute pancreatitis). The mechanism by which pancreatitis develops in these situations is unclear.

## TABLE 4   Causes of Chronic Pancreatitis

| | |
|---|---|
| Alcohol | Toxic Substances |
| Obstruction | Tropical pancreatitis |
|   Pancreas divisum | Hypercalcemia |
|   Congenital strictures | Hyperlipidemia |
|   Acquired strictures | Genetic |
|   Acute pancreatitis | Autoimmune |
|   Trauma | Idiopathic |
|   Endoscopic retrograde | |
|     cholangiopancreatography | |
|   Neoplasm | |
|   Pancreatic | |
|   Periampullary | |

## DIAGNOSIS

Patients with CP typically present with persistent midepigastric pain, often with a thoracolumbar component. The pain may be exacerbated by eating and by alcohol consumption. Nausea, vomiting, and hemodynamic instability are less frequent than with acute pancreatitis. Examination often reveals upper abdominal fullness and tenderness with frequent associated signs of malnutrition and occasionally jaundice. The classic triad of CP—pancreatic calcification, diabetes mellitus, and steatorrhea—occurs in fewer than 25% of cases, although two thirds of patients will have an abnormal glucose tolerance test at the time of presentation. Because of the difficulty of obtaining pancreatic tissue for histologic analysis, CP is usually diagnosed by pancreatic imaging with or without tests of exocrine function. Radiologic evidence of pancreatic calcification is pathognomonic and is present in only 30% to 50% of patients.

Pain is present in 75% of patients. Initially the pain is characterized by recurrent attacks but tends to become persistent with variable periods of remission. Occasionally it will "burn out" over time. The etiology of pain is uncertain. Table 5 lists some of the proposed factors. The most recent theory suggests hypoxia and damage to local sensory nerves with exposure to inflammatory irritants such as histamine, prostaglandins, and pancreatic enzymes.

Laboratory values are of limited value in evaluating CP. Pancreatic enzyme levels (amylase, lipase) may be elevated in acute exacerbations but are not a good measure of chronic disease, pancreatic function, or pancreatic reserve, nor do they correlate with symptoms. Functional studies are cumbersome and are rarely required to diagnose CP. However, stimulated pancreatic secretions collected from the duodenum (amylase, lipase, trypsin, chymotrypsin, and bicarbonate), urine tests (nitroblue tetrazolium–*para*-aminobenzoic acid [NBT-PABA] test, and pancreolauryl test), or serum studies (P-isoamylase and trypsin), provide reliable estimates of pancreatic functional reserve and can be useful in evaluating treatment strategies. Serum liver enzyme levels and leukocyte counts may provide important information regarding complications of the disease.

### Imaging

Plain abdominal radiographs reveal pancreatic calcification in less than 50% of patients and are otherwise nonspecific in CP. Transabdominal ultrasound can determine the size and consistency of the gland, characteristics of the biliary tree, and the presence of complications. A skilled ultrasonographer may achieve 70% sensitivity in diagnosing the disease.

   **CURRENT DIAGNOSIS**

**Chronic Pancreatitis**

CLINICAL MANIFESTATIONS

- Persistent midepigastric pain exacerbated by eating or alcohol consumption
- One or more present: Malnutrition, steatorrhea, glucose intolerance

RADIOLOGIC AND LABORATORY TESTS

- Computed tomography scan of the pancreas may show calcifications, pancreatic duct dilation, and/or pseudocyst formation
- Endoscopic retrograde cholangiopancreatography is the gold standard diagnostic test but is used only when computed tomography is not sufficient to make the diagnosis or clarify anatomy
- Amylase and lipase levels are not useful
- Functional pancreatic studies are cumbersome and rarely required

**TABLE 5  Proposed Factors Producing Pain in Chronic Pancreatitis**

Ductal hypertension
Autodigestion
Parenchymal ischemia
Perineural inflammation

CT approaches 90% sensitivity and greater than 90% specificity in diagnosing CP and should be considered in all suspected patients to classify their disease and determine the presence of complications and surgically correctable lesions. CT scan is the best radiologic modality for detecting calcifications, pancreatic ductal dilation, and pseudocysts and may be the only imaging study necessary in most cases.

ERCP remains the gold standard for diagnosis and staging of CP, with a sensitivity up to 95% and specificity greater than 90%. The small but finite incidence of serious complications related to ERCP should limit its use to those patients who require anatomic definition not provided by other imaging studies and in patients suspected of ampullary or ductal obstruction amenable to ERCP treatment.

Magnetic resonance imaging (MRI), magnetic resonance cholangiopancreatography (MRCP), and CT cholangiopancreatography/angiography are rapidly evolving and can replace diagnostic ERCP in most situations. This technology provides definition of soft tissues and ductal anatomy but remains institutional and operator dependent. Likewise, endoscopic ultrasound is becoming more available and may play a role in the early diagnosis of CP.

## MEDICAL TREATMENT

Medical treatment of CP consists primarily of supportive care. Pain relief, metabolic and nutritional support, as well as pancreatic endocrine and exocrine support, are the mainstays of medical therapy. Pain control is difficult, often requiring opiate analgesics. Abstinence from alcohol must be the initial goal, as alcohol consumption predicts recurrent pain even after surgical intervention. Oral pancreatic enzyme supplementation and octreotide[1] may provide modest pain relief, probably due to reduced pancreatic secretion. Because opiate addiction increases in proportion

---

[1]Not FDA approved for this indication.

---

## CURRENT THERAPY

### Chronic Pancreatitis

#### MEDICAL TREATMENT

- Abstinence from alcohol
- Pain control, preferably with nonopioid analgesics, pancreatic enzymes, octreotide
- Nutritional support: Low-fat foods, adequate protein and vitamins
- Management of diabetes
- Management of exocrine insufficiency with pancreatic enzymes

#### SURGICAL TREATMENT

- Indications: Pain refractory to medical management, inability to exclude malignancy, biliary or enteral obstruction, pseudocyst, pancreatic ascites, pancreatic fistula
- Dilated pancreatic duct: Internal drainage procedure
- Nondilated pancreatic duct: Resection
- Pseudocyst: Internal surgical drainage or endoscopic techniques

---

to duration of disease, nonsteroidal anti-inflammatory drugs should be prescribed early and chronically. Opiates should be reserved for exacerbations and intractable pain. Some authorities recommend surgical intervention prior to the chronic administration of opiates.

Malnutrition is common due to fear of pain after eating, as well as poor dietary habits and nutritional problems, in the alcoholic population. Attention should be directed at providing a low-fat diet with adequate protein and calories and vitamin supplementation. Parenteral or jejunal feedings may be required in certain situations, such as preoperative preparation and episodes of acute exacerbation.

Pancreatic exocrine insufficiency necessary to produce protein malabsorption does not occur until 90% of acinar mass has been lost. However, steatorrhea, or fat malabsorption, is a common and often troublesome problem in patents with CP. In addition to lipase from the pancreas, digestion of lipids depends on salivary and gastric hydrolysis, alkalinization in the duodenum, and adequate bile acid concentrations, all of which may be diminished in alcoholics. Pancreatic exocrine enzyme replacement is indicated to ameliorate steatorrhea. Present enzyme preparations include enteric-coated and encapsulated forms to aid delivery of active enzymes and decrease the volume of administration. Gastric acid suppression may also be necessary to provide an adequate pH environment for enzyme activity.

Endocrine insufficiency in CP is primarily manifested as pancreatic diabetes. Its treatment is similar to that for other forms of diabetes in that it may be controlled by diet, oral hypoglycemic agents, or insulin.

## SURGICAL TREATMENT

The first line of therapy in CP should be noninjurious; surgical intervention should be reserved for intractable disease. Additional indications for surgical intervention are listed in Table 6. The choice of operation depends on the anatomic findings in each patient (Table 7). Pancreatic and biliary duct anatomy should be carefully evaluated preoperatively. Improvements in perioperative preparation and care have enabled routine performance of surgical procedures on the pancreas, with very low mortality and morbidity. Contemporary series of operations for CP demonstrate mortality rates less than 3% and complication rates less than 30%, comparable to the rates of other major intra-abdominal operations.

In a minority of patients, stenosis or stricture of the ampulla of Vater can be treated with simple sphincterotomy or sphincteroplasty. Initial results with this technique revealed improvement in pain, but the results were short lived and correlated with alcohol abstinence. Although these procedures have been successful in limiting recurrent acute bouts of pancreatitis in pancreas divisum, no benefit has been realized for patients with CP. This experience suggests that sphincterotomy and pancreatic duct stenting will have little effect on the long-term management of CP from other etiologies.

The pancreatic duct in CP usually is either dilated diffusely or in a beaded ("chain-of-lakes") pattern. A dilated pancreatic duct is best treated with internal drainage of the pancreatic duct into a Roux-en-Y limb of jejunum. Historically, 8 mm was considered the lower limit of dilation amenable to internal drainage, but the procedure has proved tenable and successful in relieving pain in patients with duct dilation

---

**TABLE 6  Indications for Surgery in Chronic Pancreatitis**

Pain refractory to medical management
Inability to exclude pancreatic malignancy
Complications
Pseudocyst
Biliary obstruction
Duodenal obstruction
Splenic vein thrombosis
Pancreatic fistula
Colonic obstruction
Pancreatic ascites
Pancreatic abscess

**TABLE 7  Selection of Operation for Chronic Pancreatitis**

| Disease limited to tail of gland | Distal pancreatectomy |
|---|---|
| Obstruction in head of gland | |
|     Dilated pancreatic duct | LR-LPJ |
|     Nondilated pancreatic duct | Whipple, DPPHR |
| No obstruction in head of gland | |
|     Dilated pancreatic duct | LPJ |
|     Nondilated pancreatic duct | Distal resection (40%–95%), total pancreatectomy |
| Unable to tolerate major operation | Neurolysis? |
| Failure of primary drainage/ resection | Additional drainage/ resection, neurolysis |
| Inability to rule out malignancy | Resection |

*Abbreviations:* DPPHR = duodenal preserving pancreatic head resection; LR-LPJ = local resection–longitudinal pancreaticojejunostomy.

of greater than 5 mm. The Partington-Rochelle modification of the Puestow operation (lateral pancreaticojejunostomy) has resulted in good to excellent relief of pain in 70% to 80% of patients. Concomitant procedures to address complications such as pseudocyst and biliary obstruction can be incorporated into the jejunal limb. There is no evidence that surgery improves pancreatic function, as was hoped by the pioneers of ductal drainage procedures.

The Frey procedure is based on the concept that the head of the pancreas and uncinate process may not be completely drained by longitudinal pancreaticojejunostomy. This procedure entails a "coring out" or local resection of the head of the gland combined with lateral pancreaticojejunostomy. Results have been promising; only 13% of patients have reported no pain relief. Another proposed mechanism for the success of this operation is the reversal of ischemia or ductal hypertension that irritates sensory nerves in the head of the gland.

When the pancreatic duct is not dilated, decompressing procedures are not feasible. However, patients may obtain relief of pain with pancreatic resection. Debate continues on the merits and complications of partial (40%–80%) distal pancreatectomy, subtotal (95%) distal pancreatectomy (Child's procedure), pancreaticoduodenectomy (Whipple's procedure), and total pancreatectomy. Duodenum-preserving pancreatic head resection (Beger's procedure) performed in the 10% to 30% of CP patients with an inflammatory mass in the head of the gland has shown excellent pain relief, comparable to that of a Whipple procedure. Pancreatic insufficiency resulting from resection procedures is generally proportional to the extent of resection, with severe exocrine insufficiency and a particularly brittle and difficult to control form of pancreatic diabetes at the extreme. Attempts at autologous pancreatic islet cell transplantation at the time of pancreas resection were initially promising, but enthusiasm for the technique has waned because of less than satisfactory long-term results.

Several approaches to nerve ablation have been proposed based on the theory that the pain of CP is related to inflammatory involvement of the splanchnic nerves. Extraperitoneal, intraperitoneal, thoracic, and thoracoscopic splanchnicectomy as well as complete denervation procedures have been attempted to treat the pain of CP. Results have been unpredictable, often unconfirmed, and with limited follow-up. Neurotomy may be considered in patients who have not obtained relief of pain after surgical drainage or resection procedures.

## PANCREATIC PSEUDOCYST

Pancreatic pseudocysts are walled-off collections of fluid and debris resulting from disruption of the pancreatic duct and are most commonly associated with acute and chronic pancreatitis. Pseudocysts will develop in up to 10% of patients after an episode of acute alcoholic pancreatitis. They may also occur after trauma or in association with a neoplasm. The wall is vascularized inflammatory tissue without an epithelial lining and may contain pancreatic parenchyma. Pseudocysts may occur in any region of the gland and are multiple in 10% to 15%

of patients. Fluid collections occurring within 3 weeks of an acute episode of pancreatitis are considered acute fluid collections, and 30% to 40% of these collections will resolve spontaneously.

The most common presentation is abdominal pain, present in 90% of patients. Physical examination often reveals a tender abdominal fullness or mass. Nonspecific complaints of nausea, vomiting, early satiety, and weight loss are common. More dramatic presentations may result from free intraperitoneal rupture, intracystic hemorrhage or infection, gastric variceal bleeding resulting from splenic or portal vein thrombosis, or intraperitoneal hemorrhage from adjacent pseudoaneurysm rupture. Laboratory findings are nonspecific, although persistent amylase elevation is common. Imaging with CT is preferable, but ultrasound is nearly as sensitive and can be recommended for follow-up to determine interval changes in size.

Sampling of a postpancreatitis fluid collection is rarely indicated. However, if there has not been a preceding episode of pancreatitis, fluid cytology and chemistry can help differentiate a pseudocyst from a more likely mucinous or serous cystic neoplasm.

The natural history of asymptomatic pseudocysts reveals that nearly half remain stable, decrease in size, or completely resolve at 1-year follow-up, irrespective of size. However, pseudocysts larger than 6 cm are more likely to require operation during follow-up. Pseudocysts present for more than 12 weeks almost never resolve spontaneously and have a high rate of complications. Therefore, current management of pancreatic pseudocysts takes into account the presence or absence of symptoms, the age and size of the pseudocyst, and the presence or absence of complications. Postpancreatitis fluid collections that are asymptomatic in a stable patient can be followed with monthly imaging to evaluate resolution, stability, and enlargement. Failure to resolve and evidence of enlargement are indications for intervention. If, on the other hand, the pseudocyst is symptomatic, early intervention should be considered. Generally, a period of 6 weeks is desired prior to surgical intervention to assure adequate maturation of the cyst wall.

The preferred operative management of a pseudocyst is internal drainage into the gastrointestinal tract. This can be accomplished by anastomosis of the opened cyst wall to the stomach (cystogastrostomy), duodenum (cystoduodenostomy), or a Roux-en-Y limb of jejunum (cystojejunostomy), depending on the location of the pseudocyst. Multiple pseudocysts can be addressed simultaneously by connecting the pseudocysts and draining them as one, separately draining each cyst into a Roux-en-Y jejunal limb, or a combination of the internal drainage procedures. A lateral pancreaticojejunostomy should be added when the pancreatic duct is dilated. The cyst wall should be biopsied on all occasions, as cystic neoplasms of the pancreas can mimic a pseudocyst. Infected pseudocysts are generally treated as pancreatic abscesses.

Simple aspiration of pseudocysts will fail to resolve the fluid collection in as many as 80% of patients. Prolonged catheter drainage has demonstrated better resolution rates but may take months of drain maintenance. New endoscopic techniques that place an endoprosthesis through the intestinal lumen into the pseudocyst and that bridge the pancreatic duct disruption with a pancreatic duct stent are currently being analyzed.

## ENDOSCOPIC THERAPY

Endoscopic approaches to ductal decompression have been attempted in CP. These include endoscopic clearance of the main pancreatic duct with pancreatic sphincterotomy and basketing of stones for removal, extracorporeal shock wave lithotripsy, transpapillary drainage of pseudocysts, and dilation and stenting of ductal strictures. Various endoscopic series have reported success rates of 50% to 70% for clearing the pancreatic duct and 60% to 80% for long-term pain relief. The risk of complications is approximately 10%. The early results of endoscopic therapy are comparable with those of surgery, but all endoscopic reports have been case series, some with little long-term follow-up. Randomized controlled studies using adequate and constant methods for evaluating and reporting results and comparing endoscopic, medical, and surgical treatment modalities are now required.

## REFERENCES

Balthazar EJ, Robinson DL, Megibow AJ, Ranson JH: Acute pancreatitis: Value of CT in establishing prognosis. Radiology 1990;174:331-336.

Baron TH, Morgan DE: Acute necrotizing pancreatis. N Engl J Med 1999; 340:1412-1417.

Bradley EL 3rd: A clinically based classification system for acute pancreatitis. Summary of the International Symposium on Acute Pancreatitis, Atlanta, Ga, September 11 through 13, 1992. Arch Surg 1993;128:586-590.

Howare J, Idezuki Y, Ihse I, Prinz RA: Surgical Diseases of the Pancreas, 3rd ed. Baltimore, Williams & Wilkins, 1998.

Mitchell RM, Byrne MF, Baillie J: Pancreatitis. Lancet 2003;361:1447-1455.

Tandon RK, Sato N, Garg PK; Consensus Study Group: Chronic pancreatitis: Asia-Pacific consensus report. J Gastroenterol Hepatol 2002;17:508-518.

Triester SL, Kowdley KV: Prognostic factors in acute pancreatitis. J Clin Gastroenterol 2002;34:167-176.

Uhl W, Warshaw A, Imrie C, et al; International Association of Pancreatology: IAP guidelines for the surgical management of acute pancreatitis. Pancreatology 2002;2:565-573.

Working Party of the British Society of Gastroenterology; Association of Surgeons of Great Britain and Ireland; Pancreatic Society of Great Britain and Ireland; Association of Upper GI Surgeons of Great Britain and Ireland: UK guidelines for the management of acute pancreatitis. Gut 2005;54 (Suppl. 3):iii1-iii9.

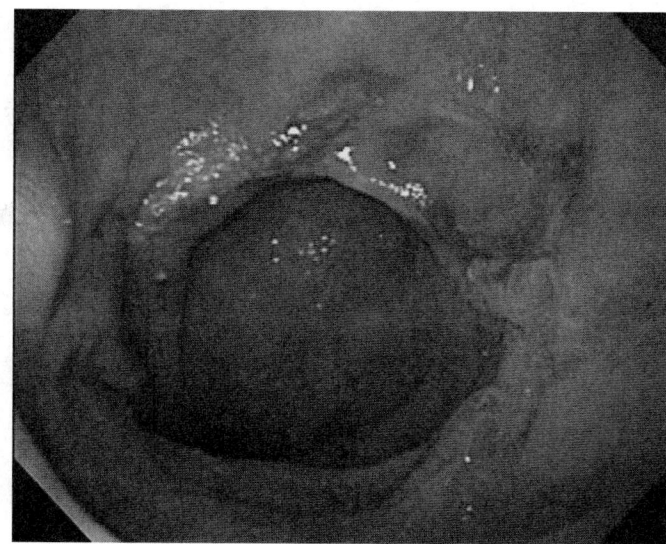

**FIGURE 1.** Endoscopic image of erosive esophagitis (Los Angeles grade C).

# Gastroesophageal Reflux Disease

Method of
*Sachin Wani, MD, and Prateek Sharma, MD*

Gastroesophageal reflux disease (GERD) includes a broad spectrum of upper gastrointestinal (GI) manifestations caused by the reflux of stomach contents. It affects around 20% to 50% of adults in Western countries, and more than 15 million Americans experience heartburn on a daily basis. The annual direct cost for managing this disease is estimated to be more than $10 billion in the United States. Afflicted persons have a significantly decreased quality of life that deteriorates as the severity of GERD symptoms increase. The last two decades have seen major advances in the diagnosis and pathophysiology of GERD combined with a burgeoning use of pharmacologic, surgical, and endoluminal therapies for managing GERD.

## Definitions and Classification

A universally accepted definition of GERD and its various symptoms and complications is lacking, and the use of varied definitions and terminology for GERD is often a source of confusion. Such definitions have made a pragmatic distinction between persons whose reflux-induced symptoms justify the diagnosis of GERD and the many persons in the general population who experience a clinically insignificant level of reflux-induced symptoms.

A recent international consensus group defined GERD as a condition that develops when the reflux of stomach contents causes troublesome symptoms or complications. Determination of whether symptoms were troublesome should be patient centered; mild symptoms occurring 2 or more days a week and moderate or severe symptoms occurring more than once a week are often considered troublesome by patients.

Based on the findings at upper endoscopy, GERD patients are categorized into those with erosive esophagitis and those with nonerosive reflux disease (NERD). Less than 50% of patients with typical GERD symptoms have endoscopic evidence of erosive esophagitis characterized by mucosal breaks (Figure 1). *NERD* describes patients who have no mucosal breaks and who have reflux symptoms with or without abnormal esophageal acid exposure during ambulatory 24-hour esophageal

pH monitoring. Recently, a conceptual change in the classification of GERD-related disease manifestations has been proposed (Box 1). This allows symptoms to define the disease but also permits further characterization if mucosal injury is identified. It is aimed at improving disease management, making studies more generalizable and ultimately assisting patients and physicians to manage the disease.

---

**BOX 1  Clinical Spectrum of Gastroesophageal Reflux Disease**

**Esophageal Syndromes**
***Symptomatic Syndromes***
- Reflux chest pain syndromes
- Typical reflux syndrome (heartburn, regurgitation)

***Syndrome with Esophageal Injury***
- Barrett's esophagus
- Esophageal adenocarcinoma
- Reflux esophagitis
- Reflux stricture

**Extraesophageal Syndromes**
***Established Associations***
- Reflux asthma syndrome
- Reflux cough syndrome
- Reflux dental erosion syndrome
- Reflux laryngitis syndrome

***Proposed Associations***
- Idiopathic pulmonary fibrosis
- Pharyngitis
- Recurrent otitis media
- Sinusitis

---

Adapted from Vakil N, van Zanten SV, Kahrilas P, et al: The Montreal definition and classification of gastroesophageal reflux disease: A global evidence-based consensus. Am J Gastroenterol 2006;101:1900-1920 (with permission).

# Epidemiology

According to U.S. population surveys, 44% of all Americans experience heartburn at least once a month, 14% at least once a week, and up to 7% daily. In a recent population-based study in Sweden, reflux symptoms were reported by 40% and erosive esophagitis was diagnosed in nearly 16%. There appears to be little difference between the prevalence of GERD in North America and in Europe. Data suggest that the prevalence of GERD is on the rise in several Asia-Pacific regions that were once considered a zone of low prevalence of GERD.

Although there is a lack of epidemiologic data for GERD in the pediatric age group, it is increasingly clear that symptoms suggesting GERD are not uncommon in children. GERD appears to affect about 7% of all infants during the first year of life to the extent that they are brought to medical attention. Data on the incidence of GERD are limited.

Genetic factors have been implicated, because the prevalence of reflux symptoms is high in the parents of affected patients, and concordance of reflux disease is higher in monozygotic than in dizygotic twins. The relation between age and GERD is unclear, although data suggest that advancing age is a risk factor for severe esophagitis and fewer reflux symptoms. Male gender is a risk factor for erosive esophagitis, and men typically have more severe reflux disease.

Lifestyle factors associated with GERD include obesity and consumption of tobacco, alcohol, coffee, chocolate, mint, citrus fruits and juices, carbonated beverages, fatty foods, and high-calorie late meals. The data on these factors are not conclusive in spite of some evidence linking them to the main mechanism of the disease, transient relaxation of the lower esophageal sphincter. A high body mass index (BMI) has been associated with an elevated risk of GERD and a specific dose-response relationship between increasing BMI and GERD prevalence has been demonstrated.

Studies have found little or no overall effect of *Helicobacter pylori* eradication on GERD. Some studies, especially from East Asia and in patients with chronic atrophic gastritis, have shown a negative association between *H. pylori* and GERD.

# Pathophysiology

The structure and function of the lower esophageal sphincter (LES) are of paramount importance in GERD. The LES is a segment of smooth muscle in the distal esophagus that maintains a pressure of at least 15 mm Hg above the intragastric pressure by tonic contractions. The main pathophysiologic mechanisms that contribute to the development of GERD are frequent transient relaxation of the LES, impaired clearance of regurgitated gastric acid, hiatal hernia, and delayed gastric emptying. Obesity is believed to increase the risk of GERD by imposing mechanical stresses on the esophagogastric junction by increased intragastric pressure and anatomic disruption of the esophagogastric junction, which results in a hiatal hernia. Hiatal hernia has broad pathophysiologic implications in GERD pathogenesis: increased incidence of strain-induced reflux, reduced threshold for distention-induced transient LES relaxations, swallow-induced reflux, reduced LES pressure, and impaired acid clearance. Key factors in removing refluxed material (esophageal peristalsis) and neutralizing acid (salivary secretions, esophageal epithelium, and bicarbonate secretion), as well as the characteristics and quantity of gastric fluids, are believed to play roles in the pathogenesis of GERD.

# Clinical Features

Heartburn and acid regurgitation are well established classic or typical symptoms of GERD. *Heartburn* is defined as a burning sensation in the retrosternal area, and *regurgitation* is defined as the perception of flow of refluxed gastric content into the mouth or hypopharynx. Upper abdominal or lower retrosternal symptoms such as bloating or abdominal pain are not definitive for GERD and are grouped under the umbrella of the current definition of dyspepsia. Other possible symptoms include globus (lump in the throat) and water brash (excessive salivation).

---

> **BOX 2   Alarm Symptoms of GERD that Require Prompt Referral for Upper Endoscopy**
>
> - Gastrointestinal bleeding (occult or overt)
> - Iron deficiency anemia
> - Pain while swallowing (odynophagia)
> - Persistent vomiting
> - Progressive difficulty swallowing (dysphagia)
> - Unintentional weight loss
> - Anorexia
>
> ---
>
> *Abbreviation:* GERD = gastroesophageal reflux disease.

In addition to these symptoms, many manifestations of GERD involve extraesophageal organs (extraesophageal syndromes), and established associations include chronic cough, laryngitis, bronchial asthma, and dental erosions. The proposed associations are pharyngitis, sinusitis, idiopathic pulmonary fibrosis, and recurrent otitis media. Alarm symptoms include dysphagia, odynophagia, progressive unintentional weight loss, GI bleeding, anemia, anorexia, and persistent vomiting (Box 2). In the presence of alarm symptoms, prompt endoscopy is strongly indicated.

# Diagnosis

## SYMPTOM ASSESSMENT

Symptom pattern evaluation, by structured interview or validated questionnaires, is the single most important diagnostic step, because a

---

 **CURRENT DIAGNOSIS**

- Heartburn and acid regurgitation are well-established cardinal symptoms of GERD. Several ear, nose, and throat, respiratory, and sleep disorders; oral diseases; and symptoms such as chest pain have been associated with GERD (extraesophageal syndromes).
- Complications of GERD are esophageal strictures, ulcers, Barrett's esophagus, and esophageal adenocarcinoma.
- Alarm symptoms that prompt urgent endoscopy include dysphagia, odynophagia, progressive unintentional weight loss, gastrointestinal bleeding, anemia, anorexia, and persistent vomiting.
- There is no gold standard for the diagnosis of GERD.
- Symptom pattern evaluation, by structured interview or validated questionnaires, is the single most important diagnostic step because endoscopy does not diagnose a high percentage of reflux disease.
- Based on the findings at upper endoscopy, GERD is categorized into two groups: erosive esophagitis and nonerosive reflux disease.
- The identification of erosive esophagitis at endoscopy is highly specific (90%-95%) for the diagnosis of GERD, but endoscopy per se has a low sensitivity.
- Empiric treatment with proton pump inhibitors (PPIs) in patients with a history suggesting typical or uncomplicated GERD is recommended. Alleviation of symptoms serves as an adequate diagnosis.
- Esophageal pH monitoring may be useful for patients with atypical symptoms or in patients who respond poorly to an adequate trial of acid-suppression therapy.

high percentage of patients with reflux disease are not recognized by endoscopy. Diagnosis, treatment, and assessment of outcomes rely heavily on symptom evaluation. Symptom severity has no consistent relation to the severity of mucosal injury, and hence endoscopic findings cannot be used as a surrogate for determining symptom severity.

## UPPER GASTROINTESTINAL ENDOSCOPY

The identification of erosive esophagitis at endoscopy is highly specific (90%-95%) for the diagnosis of GERD; however, endoscopy itself has a low sensitivity. The Los Angeles classification is used to categorize the extent of mucosal injury (Box 3). Upper endoscopic evaluation is recommended for evaluating alarm symptoms to look for complications such as esophageal ulcers, strictures, or malignancy. It is only indicated in patients who do not respond to adequate acid-suppression therapy and for screening for Barrett's esophagus (although this indication is controversial). At present, routine esophageal biopsies are not recommended for the assessment of GERD.

Several recent advances have improved the diagnostic yield of endoscopy in GERD. These include magnification endoscopy, magnification chromoendoscopy, video capsule endoscopy, and narrow band imaging. Currently, these are being evaluated in clinical trials and are not established options in routine clinical practice. Reliability of histologic assessment, especially in NERD patients (increases in polymorphonuclear and mononuclear white cells, basal cell hyperplasia, papillary elongation, and dilated intercellular spaces), has been explored and appears promising.

## EMPIRIC TREATMENT WITH ACID-SUPPRESSION THERAPY

If the patient's history appears to be typical of uncomplicated GERD, alleviation of symptoms with an initial trial of empiric acid-suppressive therapy is recommended and can serve as an adequate diagnosis. Proton pump inhibitors (PPIs) are effective in healing esophagitis and controlling symptoms; thus, a poor response to a trial of empiric therapy should prompt referral for further investigations, and an alternative diagnosis should be considered.

## AMBULATORY ESOPHAGEAL pH MONITORING

Twenty-four-hour esophageal pH monitoring is not an appropriate initial diagnostic method because diagnosis can be reached with a high level of accuracy without pH monitoring. Although initially proposed as a gold standard for diagnosiing GERD, it is probably not a gold standard because sensitivity does not exceed 75%. It is also relatively expensive, inconvenient, uncomfortable, and not widely available. It is useful for the minority of patients with atypical symptoms or in patients who poorly respond to an adequate trial of acid-suppression therapy. Multichannel intraluminal impedance monitoring with pH sensors can detect acidic, weakly acidic, and nonacidic reflux; its usefulness in the clinical setting needs further research and validation.

## BARIUM ESOPHAGRAM

The barium esophagram has a low diagnostic yield in the diagnosis of GERD and should not be used in patients with typical GERD symptoms without dysphagia. It can detect severe cases of erosive esophagitis and is useful for the initial evaluation of patients with dysphagia. It can identify esophageal strictures, esophageal motor abnormalities, and diverticula.

# Treatment

The goals of treatment are to relieve symptoms, promote healing, and prevent complications.

## LIFESTYLE MODIFICATIONS

Experts typically recommend lifestyle modifications in patients with GERD, although supporting data are sparse. Lifestyle changes that have been recommended include smoking cessation; weight loss; avoiding late-evening meals; avoiding foods such as citrus fruits, coffee, chocolate, mint, spicy foods, and fatty foods; avoiding alcohol; and sleeping with the head of the bed elevated. Lifestyle interventions should not be recommended as the primary treatment in patients with bothersome

## CURRENT THERAPY

- Lifestyle changes such as smoking cessation, weight loss, avoidance of late-evening meals, avoiding foods such as chocolate, avoiding alcohol, and sleeping with the head of the bed elevated can play an adjunctive role with acid-suppression therapy or antireflux surgery, but evidence is sparse.
- Pharmacologic options include antacids, histamine type 2–receptor antagonists ($H_2$-RAs), and proton pump inhibitors (PPIs).
- PPIs are unequivocally the most cost-effective pharmacologic agents for treating GERD and have become the mainstay of medical GERD management.
- GERD is predominantly a chronic relapsing disorder, and most patients with healed erosive esophagitis (80%-90%) relapse within 6 to 12 months without treatment.
- The fraction of patients with nonerosive reflux disease (NERD) responding to a standard dose of PPI is approximately 20% to 30% lower than has been documented in patients with erosive esophagitis, along with a longer lagtime to sustained symptom response.
- Most patients with severe esophagitis (Los Angeles grade C or D) or with nocturnal or extraesophageal manifestations of GERD probably require long-term maintenance therapy.
- PPIs may be suitable for intermittent and on-demand therapy in patients with uncomplicated symptomatic GERD (NERD and Los Angeles grade A or B).
- Antireflux surgery may be appropriate for young, otherwise healthy patients in whom medical management is not tolerated or who refuse to take medications chronically.

---

### BOX 3 Los Angeles Classification of Esophagitis

**LA Grade A**
- One mucosal break (or more) no longer than 5 mm
- Does not extend between the tops of two mucosal folds

**LA Grade B**
- One mucosal break (or more) more than 5 mm long
- Does not extend between the tops of two mucosal folds

**LA Grade C**
- One mucosal break (or more) that is continuous between the tops of two or more mucosal folds
- Involves less than 75% of the circumference

**LA Grade D**
- One mucosal break (or more) that involves at least 75% of the esophageal circumference

---

*Abbreviation:* LA = Los Angeles.

GERD symptoms, but they can play an adjunctive role with acid-suppression therapy or antireflux surgery.

## PHARMACOLOGIC THERAPY

Pharmacologic options include over-the-counter medications such as antacids, histamine type 2–receptor antagonists ($H_2$-RAs), and PPIs. Systematic reviews have confirmed that PPIs, by blockade of the gastric acid proton pump—$H^+$,$K^+$-ATPase (adenosine triphosphatase)—are more effective than $H_2$-RAs at healing esophagitis and maintaining remission from mucosal injury and symptoms. PPIs are unequivocally the most cost-effective pharmacologic agents for treating GERD and have become the mainstay of medical GERD management. The management plan should acknowledge that GERD is predominantly a chronic relapsing disorder in most patients and usually reoccurs once treatment is discontinued. Most patients with healed erosive esophagitis (80%-90%) relapse within 6 to 12 months without treatment. Most patients with nocturnal or extraesophageal manifestations of GERD are likely to require long-term maintenance therapy.

Several guidelines have been published for the management of GERD. Current evidence lends support to initial therapy with a PPI once daily for 4 to 8 weeks. When initial therapy fails to control symptoms, either the diagnosis is incorrect or the chosen treatment has not been sufficiently effective. Treatment needs to be intensified if, on review of the patient, it is concluded that reflux disease is still the most likely diagnosis. Doubling the dose of PPI may be required. If severe erosive esophagitis (Los Angeles grade C or D) has been documented, full-dose PPI therapy is indicated.

If symptoms resolve, stopping therapy can be considered, although the chances for relapse are present. This approach is not recommended in patients with severe erosive esophagitis. If symptoms persist despite PPI use, endoscopy followed by 24-hour esophageal pH monitoring should be considered. Factors associated with lack of response to PPIs include inadequate compliance or dosing, incorrect diagnosis, and nonacid reflux.

The goal of long-term treatment is to step down management to the lowest level of medical therapy that controls symptoms. Recent data suggest that PPIs may be suitable for intermittent and on-demand therapy in patients with uncomplicated symptomatic GERD (NERD and Los Angeles grade A or B). This is not recommended in patients with severe esophagitis, complicated GERD (e.g., esophageal stricture, ulcer, or Barrett's esophagus), nocturnal GERD, or extraesophageal manifestations. Such therapy has been shown to be a cost-effective therapeutic option in symptomatic GERD patients, but patients who relapse should resume the dose that controlled their symptoms previously. The management algorithm is shown in Figure 2.

Other medications such as baclofen have been studied in the management of GERD. It acts by inhibiting transient LES relaxation via the γ-aminobutyric acid B receptor (GABA-B) and has been shown to reduce reflux. However, the side effects of this drug limit its application for treating GERD.

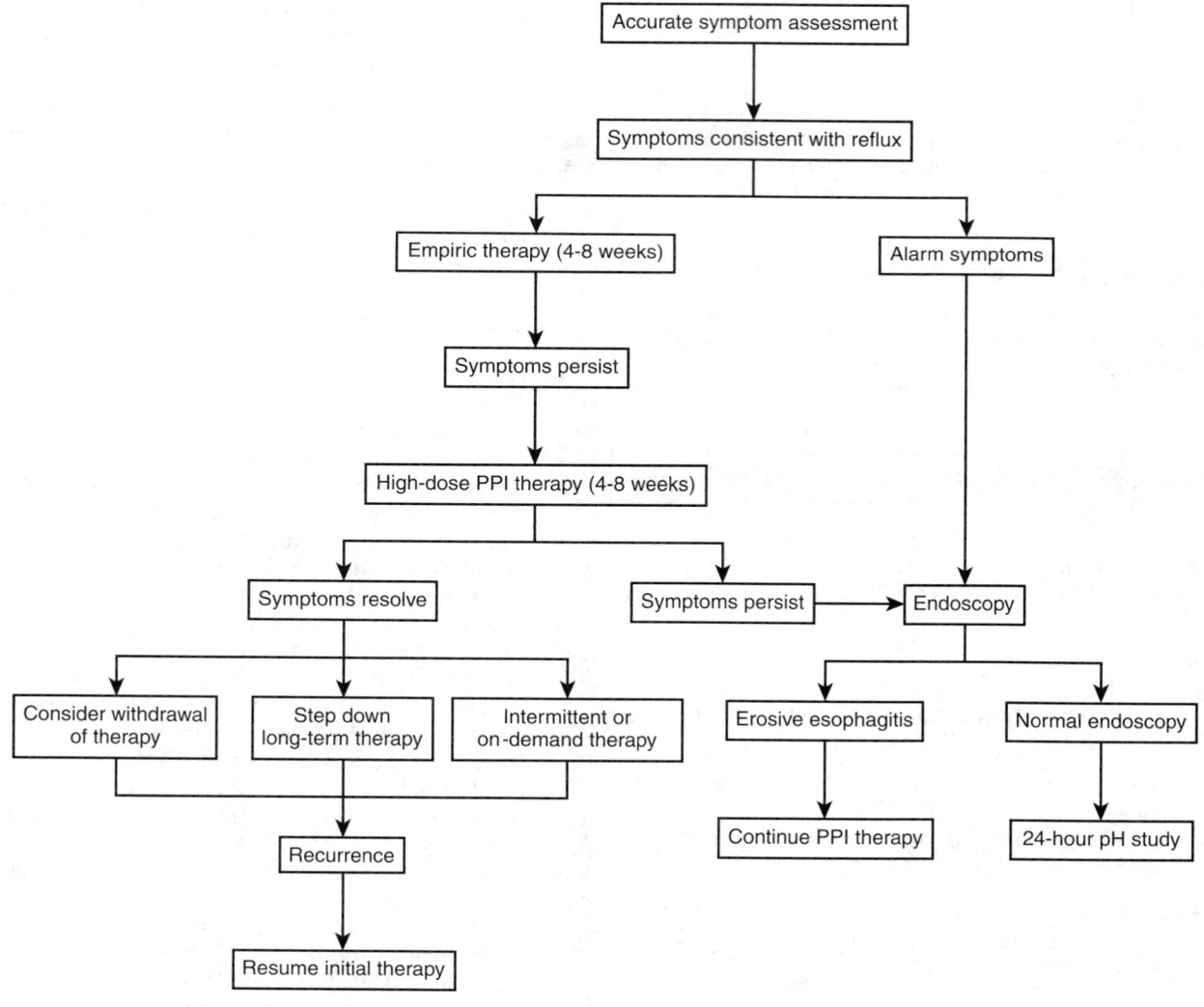

**FIGURE 2.**  Management pathway for patients with typical reflux symptoms. *Abbreviation:* PPI = proton pump inhibitor.

## SURGICAL MANAGEMENT

Antireflux surgery augments the reflux barrier by a full or partial wrap of the gastric fundus (fundoplication) around the lower esophagus and can be performed laparoscopically. Recent reports confirm that laparoscopic antireflux surgery has similar outcomes to the open procedure. Antireflux surgery has an operative mortality rate of 0.5% to 1%; mortality is reduced with laparoscopic surgery and the experience of the surgeon.

Some patients managed with surgery still require acid-suppression therapy, and there is no convincing evidence that fundoplication reduces the risk of esophageal adenocarcinoma in the long term. Nevertheless, antireflux surgery may be appropriate for young, otherwise healthy patients in whom medical management is not tolerated or who refuse to take medications chronically. It is imperative to confirm a diagnosis of GERD before subjecting a patient to this procedure. Combinations of diagnostic tools like endoscopy, 24-hour pH monitoring, and manometry can identify patients who are likely candidates for surgery.

## ENDOSCOPIC ANTIREFLUX PROCEDURES

Endoscopic techniques have been developed to treat GERD because long-term PPI therapy is expensive and does not affect the main abnormality in reflux disease: abnormal relaxation of the LES. Endoscopic procedures can be divided into three main approaches: endoscopic application of radiofrequency to the lower esophagus, suturing devices for the LES, and injection or implantation of inert material into the muscle layer of the distal esophagus. Results have been inconsistent with regard to symptom relief, PPI use, and effects on 24-hour pH results. Several endoscopic antireflux devices (Enteryx, Gatekeeper technique, endoscopic suturing device) have recently been withdrawn from the market for safety reasons or insufficient efficacy. Prolonged follow-up is required, and future devices and studies should be rigorously conducted with endpoints including efficacy, safety, and cost-effectiveness. Currently, these procedures are not advocated in routine practice.

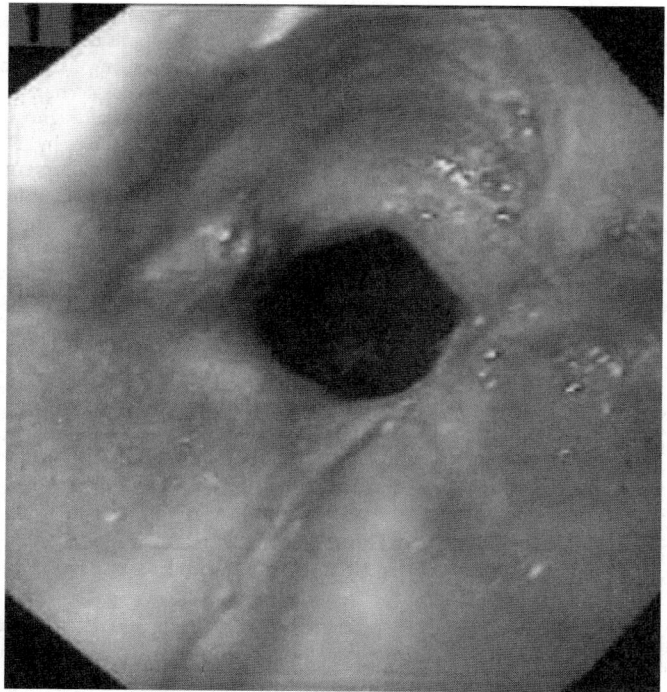

**FIGURE 3.** Esophageal stricture secondary to chronic gastroesophageal reflux disease.

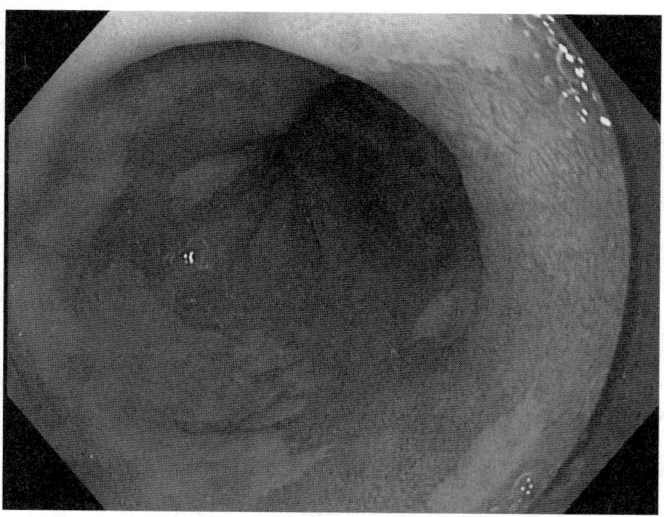

**FIGURE 4.** Endoscopic image of Barrett's esophagus.

## Complications

Complications that could develop in GERD patients include esophageal strictures, esophageal ulceration, Barrett's esophagus, and rarely esophageal adenocarcinoma. Esophageal strictures (Figure 3) and ulcers have a prevalence of approximately 0.1% and 0.05%, respectively. Both are associated with white race, male gender, and increasing age.

Barrett's esophagus is an acquired condition resulting from chronic GERD and is a well-recognized premalignant condition leading to esophageal adenocarcinoma (Figure 4). It is estimated that 10% to 15% of patients with GERD have Barrett's esophagus. It is characterized by a metaplastic transformation of the squamous epithelium to a columnar type highlighted by the presence of goblet cells appreciated on histologic evaluation. The condition entails a 30- to 50-fold greater risk of developing esophageal adenocarcinoma and has an incidence of development of adenocarcinoma that approaches 0.5% annually.

Endoscopic screening of patients with chronic GERD symptoms has been proposed as a method for detecting Barrett's esophagus and early cancer. Patients with Barrett's esophagus are then typically enrolled in surveillance programs to monitor the lesion for progression. Although data in support of screening and surveillance are lacking, the practice is widespread and endorsed by many international gastroenterologic societies, with the ultimate aim of preventing deaths from esophageal adenocarcinoma. Epidemiologic studies suggest that patients with more frequent, severe, and long-lasting symptoms of reflux are at the greatest risk for development of Barrett's esophagus.

## REFERENCES

Donnellan C, Sharma N, Preston C, Maoayyedi P: Medical treatments for the maintenance therapy of reflux oesophagitis and endoscopic negative reflux disease. Cochrane Database Syst Rev 2004;4:CD003245.

DeVault KR, Castell DO; American College of Gastroenterology: Updated guidelines for the diagnosis and treatment of gastroesophageal reflux disease. Am J Gastroenterol 2005;100:190-200.

Dent J, Armstrong D, Delaney B, et al: Symptom evaluation in reflux disease: Workshop background, processes, terminology, recommendations, and discussion outputs. Gut 2004;53(suppl 4):iv1-24.

Kaltenbach T, Crockett S, Gerson LB: Are lifestyle measures effective in patients with gastroesophageal reflux disease? An evidence-based approach. Arch Intern Med 2006;166(9):965-971.

Klinkenburg-Knol EC, Jansen JM, Festen HP, et al: Double-blind multicentre comparison of omeprazole and ranitidine in the treatment of reflux oesophagitis. Lancet 1987;1:349-351.

Lagergren J, Bergström R, Lindgren A, Nyrén O: Symptomatic gastroesophageal reflux as a risk factor for esophageal adenocarcinoma. N Engl J Med 1999; 340:825-831.

Lundell LR, Dent J, Bennett JR, et al: Endoscopic assessment of oesophagitis: Clinical and functional correlates and further validation of the Los Angeles classification. Gut 1999;45:172-180.

Sampliner RE; Practice Parameters Committee of the American College of Gastroenterology: Updated guidelines for the diagnosis, surveillance, and therapy of Barrett's esophagus. Am J Gastroenterol 2002;97:1888-1895.

Shaw MJ, Talley NJ, Beebe TJ, et al: Initial validation of a diagnostic questionnaire for gastroesophageal reflux disease. Am J Gastroenterol 2001;96:52-57.

Spechler SJ, Lee E, Ahnen D, et al: Long-term outcome of medical and surgical therapies for gastroesophageal reflux disease: Follow-up of a randomized controlled trial. JAMA 2001;285:2331-2338.

Vakil N, van Zanten SV, Kahrilas P, et al: The Montreal definition and classification of gastroesophageal reflux disease: A global evidence-based consensus. Am J Gastroenterol 2006;101:1900-1920.

Wiklund I, Carlsson J, Vakil N: Gastroesophageal reflux symptoms and well-being in a random sample of the general population of a Swedish community. Am J Gastroenterol 2006;101:18-28.

# Tumors of the Stomach

Method of
*Scott A. Hundahl, MD*

## Gastric Adenocarcinoma

From earliest cancer registry activity through World War II, adenocarcinoma of the stomach ranked number one among solid organ neoplasms in the United States. Since that time, both incidence and mortality have declined. Worldwide, however, gastric adenocarcinoma remains a common neoplasm, eclipsed only by lung cancer in incidence and mortality.

Several pathology classification schemes have been proposed for gastric adenocarcinoma, including the Borrmann morphologic classification, the Broder differentiation classification, the histologic World Health Organization (WHO) classification, the Nagayo-Komagome classification, the Ming classification, and the Goseki classification. None is more widely used than the 1951 Jarvi-Lauren (aka "Lauren") classification, which divides gastric adenocarcinoma into intestinal-type (gland-forming tumors) and diffuse-type (discohesive) tumors.

The Jarvi-Lauren classification, when combined with epidemiologic information, identifies three main histoepidemiologic patterns:

1. Intestinal-type tumors arising from the distal stomach, associated with preexisting atrophic gastritis and intestinal metaplasia (*Helicobacter pylori*–associated),
2. Diffuse-type tumors involving the body of the stomach (*H. pylori*–associated) but usually not associated with significant intestinal metaplasia, and
3. Intestinal-type tumors of the gastroesophageal junction

In high-incidence regions of the world, such as Japan and Korea, up to two thirds of gastric adenocarcinomas are of the first type and are strongly associated with chronic multifocal atrophic gastritis and intestinal metaplasia from chronic *H. pylori* infection. The process usually begins at the antral-corpus junction along the lesser curvature and predisposes to cancers of the intestinal type occurring in the sixth and seventh decades of life. The second type of gastric adenocarcinoma, also associated with *H. pylori*, afflicts younger individuals in the fourth and fifth decades of life. The last type, seen in lower-incidence regions of the world, such as the United States, is associated with chronic gastroesophageal reflux and Barrett's esophagitis.

It has been estimated that 42% of gastric adenocarcinomas worldwide can be attributed to chronic *H. pylori* infection. Strains containing the cagA gene appear more dangerous. The infection usually starts by the second or third decade and, unless successfully treated, gives rise to chronic inflammation, atrophic gastritis, and eventually intestinal metaplasia, which is a premalignant histologic condition. Dietary factors, such as high-salt and high-nitrate intake, can accentuate this progression. As the condition progresses, acid-producing oxyntic mucosa is progressively eliminated, gastric pH increases, and bacterial overgrowth with non–*H. pylori* bacteria is facilitated. The original *H. pylori*, which requires an acid environment to thrive, often disappears at this point. Once intestinal metaplasia is established, dietary factors become particularly important in mitigating the risk of cancer development. Protective factors include intake of vitamin C, fresh fruits and vegetables, and antioxidants. The association of *H. pylori* infection with the development of intestinal metaplasia suggests that early detection and elimination of this infection might prevent gastric cancer. Unfortunately, in high-incidence areas, reinfection from contaminated water supplies and other sources is common, thus undermining the strategy. In addition, in prevention trials to date, any benefit is restricted to the subgroups without preexisting intestinal metaplasia.

General risk factors for gastric cancer include low socioeconomic status, smoking, a diet deficient in fresh fruits and vegetables or high in salt-preserved, nitrate-laden foods, previous gastric ulcer, ionizing radiation, family history, and previous gastric resection. Blood group A is associated with higher risk of developing a diffuse-type tumor. Predisposing genetic conditions include the Lynch syndrome (i.e., hereditary nonpolyposis colorectal cancer, a condition with microsatellite instability due to deficient DNA repair enzymes) and, for diffuse tumors, specific germline mutations in the E-cadherin gene, as first detected in certain New Zealand Maori kindreds.

In Western populations, by the time gastric cancer causes symptoms, the disease is often relatively advanced. In a large National Cancer Data Base survey of U.S. patients, presenting ascribable symptoms included weight loss (62%), abdominal/epigastric pain (52%), nausea (34%), anorexia (32%), early satiety (32%), dysphagia (26%), and melena (18%).

Mass screening combining upper GI series, endoscopy, and serum pepsinogen I/II ratio have proven beneficial in high-incidence areas, such as Japan, but cannot be justified in the United States, where incidence is low. However, for defined risk groups, such as those with established atrophic gastritis and established intestinal metaplasia, a strong family history, or hereditary nonpolyposis colorectal cancer syndrome, surveillance screening should definitely be considered.

In the United States, diagnosis is usually made by upper endoscopy. One should be aware that diffuse-type cancers presenting as linitis plastica are often associated with minimal visible mucosal changes, and deep biopsies are often required for establishing the diagnosis. Furthermore, small, "early" gastric cancers ("early" defined by the Japanese as in situ and T1 cancers, with or without node involvement) can be associated with particularly subtle mucosal changes, presenting a challenge for even the most experienced endoscopist.

Extent-of-disease studies for gastric adenocarcinoma include endoscopic ultrasound, which is good for estimating depth of tumor and visualizing immediately adjacent nodes, and helical CT scanning,

---

 **CURRENT DIAGNOSIS**

- Chronic *Helicobacter pylori* infection gives rise to atrophic gastritis and intestinal metaplasia, which predispose to cancer. Surveillance issue.
- Mucosal changes in diffuse-type gastric cancer presenting as linitis plastica can be minimal. Deep mucosal biopsies are required.
- Helical computed tomography, endoscopic ultrasound, and minilaparotomy or laparoscopy for pretreatment staging of gastric cancer.
- In early growth, gastrointestinal stromal tumors are rarely associated with mucosal changes.

## CURRENT THERAPY

- For local-regional cancer, complete surgical resection remains the key component of curative treatment.
- Total gastrectomy and splenectomy/pancreatectomy should *not* be routine but performed only when required for negative-margin resection.
- Surgical goal with respect to node dissection for cancer is a low Maruyama index operation (see references).
- For fit patients with good postoperative caloric intake, postoperative adjuvant chemoradiation is considered standard for all but stage IA cases.
- Node dissection is not required for gastrointestinal stromal tumors.

which is good for evaluating extraluminal extent of disease, intra-abdominal and/or mediastinal extension/spread, and liver/lung metastases. Because even high-resolution CT scanning can miss small peritoneal implants, extraregional nodal spread, and small liver metastases, staging laparoscopy and minilaparotomy are valuable adjuncts and should be considered mandatory if any preoperative treatment is considered.

Although a long-established, much-modified Japanese staging system, the "General Rules," finds widespread use in many areas of the world, the American Joint Committee on Cancer and the Union Internationale Contre le Cancer (AJCC/UICC) TNM system is by far the dominant staging system used. T stage is defined a bit differently than for colorectal cancer: muscularis propria penetration short of serosal penetration is still considered T2 disease; a serosal breach is required for T3 disease; and a T4 designation requires direct involvement of adjacent structures. Optimally accurate nodal "N" designation requires that more than 15 nodes be examined by the pathologist. N1 disease means metastases in one to six regional nodes, N2 disease means metastases in 7 to 15 regional nodes, and N3 disease means metastases in more than 15 nodes. Any N3 disease, any node-positive T4 disease, any M1 distant metastatic disease, and any involved extraregional M1 nodes translate in the staging matrix to stage IV disease. The reader is referred to the AJCC staging manual referenced at the end of this article.

Curative treatment of gastric cancer involves, as main therapy, complete negative-margin surgical resection of disease. Various experts have shown endoscopic mucosal resection and minimally invasive techniques to be appropriate for some selected in situ and T1 tumors, but most tumors in the United States are discovered at a stage where formal open surgery is required. To secure a negative intramural margin of resection, a gross margin of 2 cm is usually adequate for exophytic, noninfiltrating tumors, and a margin of at least 6 cm of grossly normal tissue is recommended for ulcerated or infiltrating tumors or diffuse histology. Closest mural margins are generally checked by frozen section at the time of surgery to confirm adequacy of resection. Total gastrectomy is not indicated as a routine procedure, except in linitis plastica, but is warranted whenever required for a negative-margin resection.

Routine splenectomy for treatment of gastric cancer, as well as routine distal pancreatectomy (performed in the past to clear splenic nodes), should be avoided unless definitely required for complete resection of visible/palpable disease.

The extent of lymph node dissection in this disease has generated—and continues to generate—international controversy. Although several prospective, randomized trials of non-Asian populations—none perfect—fail to demonstrate that routine extensive lymphadenectomy increases survival, insufficient lymphadenectomy has also been shown to definitely compromise survival. A prospectively planned analysis of a large U.S. adjuvant chemoradiation trial and a blinded reanalysis of a large Dutch surgical trial have shown that the adequacy of lymphadenectomy for a given case can be quantified using the "Maruyama index of unresected disease" (the Maruyama index), and that this measure independently correlates with survival in a "dose-response" proportional fashion. Prospectively using the Maruyama Computer Program to predict the extent of nodal spread for a given cancer case is one way to assure a low Maruyama index surgical resection.

Sentinel node biopsy, an established technique for treatment of other cancers, has failed to win support for cancer of the stomach, because of the organ's lymphatic complexity and the relatively high reported false-negative rates.

A large North American prospective, randomized trial of postoperative adjuvant 5-fluorouracil (5-FU)–based chemoradiation in completely resected gastric cancer revealed a significant increase in disease-free and overall survival with this treatment. The postoperative nature of this trial thwarted implementation of surgical guidelines, and the extent of node dissection for most patients in the trial was minimal, with survival compromise for such patients demonstrated. Practitioners in some countries, such as Japan, dismiss the necessity of adjuvant postoperative adjuvant chemoradiation with the (unproven but reasonable) argument that this is only a salvage technique for inadequate surgery. A separate Korean chemoradiation series has shown benefit even for radically treated cases, however. For patients with good postoperative performance status, good organ function, and adequate nutrition, postoperative adjuvant chemoradiation therapy is considered standard in North America.

Recently, survival data from a U.K. study of preoperative plus postoperative epirubicin, *cis*-platinum, and continuous-infusion 5-FU (ECF) chemotherapy versus surgery alone have shown encouraging results. However, results of other preoperative chemotherapy studies have been negative. This approach, although promising, is still considered investigational in North America.

In Korea, a positive trial of adjuvant perioperative intraperitoneal chemotherapy has been reported. Considerable morbidity and mortality are associated with this adjuvant treatment, however, and this therapy likely will not be implemented without refinement and independent duplication of results.

For localized disease deemed not resectable to negative margins, chemotherapy and chemoradiotherapy have been used to convert such tumors to potentially resectable status. With successful, negative-margin resection, some of these patients survive long term. Without any surgery, administration of 5-FU–based concomitant chemoradiotherapy to patients with residual, unresected local-regional disease can also result in some degree of 5-year survival (reported in excess of 10%).

## Other Gastric Tumors

*Gastrointestinal stromal tumors* (GISTs) present as submucosal spindle cell tumors in the sarcoma family. In contrast to leiomyosarcomas and other spindle cell sarcomas, they express the antigen CD117 and most (>80%) tumors have activating mutations of c-*kit*. Formerly considered rare, approximately 5000 of these tumors per year are now diagnosed in the United States. Owing to the pattern of growth in the gastric wall, deep to the mucosa, early symptoms are unusual, and these tumors will often grow to massive size before mucosal ulceration and hemorrhage (or other major symptoms) finally develop. GISTs are classified as sarcomas. Treatment of localized primary tumors consists of complete surgical resection, which usually can be accomplished with a 2-cm margin of grossly normal tissue. Specific lymph node dissection is not indicated for this histology. Surgical series indicate that approximately 50% of primary gastric tumors will metastasize and recur within 5 years, with risk factors including size greater than 5 cm and more than one mitosis per high-power field. For patients with widespread metastases, generally located in the peritoneal cavity or the liver, first-line therapy is now the well-tolerated oral agent imatinib mesylate (Gleevec or STI-571) at an initial dose of 400 mg daily, which generates partial responses in more than 50% of cases and stable disease in an additional 25% of cases. Side effects are minimal, and 1-year survival in treated patients is approximately 85%.

*Carcinoid tumors* of the stomach have a similar behavior to small-bowel carcinoids. When small (i.e., <1 cm) and unassociated with invasion of the muscularis propria, local excision to negative margins is generally deemed sufficient. For such tumors, endoscopic resection has an established role. However, even small tumors can metastasize to lymph nodes. Wider gastrectomy with lymph node dissection is generally recommended for gastric tumors larger than 1 cm. Many of these tumors are associated with serum hypergastrinemia; those without this finding tend to be more aggressive. When metastatic to the liver or other organs, surgical cytoreduction (or other means of tumor ablation) can offer considerable palliation to those with carcinoid syndrome, and this technique should always be considered. Octreotide therapy now represents a palliative mainstay in all patients with carcinoid syndrome.

*Gastric lymphomas* encompass most of the lymphoma subtypes, but low-grade, mucosa-associated B-cell lymphomas, so-called B-cell mucosa-associated lymphoid tissue (MALT) lymphomas, deserve special mention because they are strongly associated with *H. pylori* infection. Indeed, localized cases can be controlled simply by treating the *H. pylori* infection. In such cases, however, molecular studies indicate persistence of the offending lymphoid clone in about half of cases. In particular, if *H. pylori* infection recurs, the lymphoma in such cases returns. For further information on this and other gastrointestinal lymphomas, see the article on lymphoma.

## REFERENCES

Dematteo RP, Heinrich MC, El-Rifai WM, Demetri G: Clinical management of gastrointestinal stromal tumors: Before and after STI-571. Hum Pathol 2002;33:466-477.

Greene FL, Page DL, Fleming ID, et al (eds): AJCC Cancer Staging Manual. New York, Springer, 2002.

Hartgrink HH, van de Velde CJ, Putter H, et al: Extended lymph node dissection for gastric cancer: Who may benefit? Final results of the randomized Dutch gastric cancer group trial. J Clin Oncol 2004;22:2069-2077.

Hundahl SA, Macdonald JS, Benedetti J, Fitzsimmons T: Surgical treatment variation in a prospective, randomized trial of chemoradiotherapy in gastric cancer: The effect of undertreatment. Ann Surg Oncol 2002;9:278-286.

Kim S, Lim DH, Lee J, et al: An observational study suggesting clinical benefit for adjuvant postoperative chemoradiation in a population of over 500 cases after gastric resection with D2 nodal dissection for adenocarcinoma of the stomach. Int J Radiat Oncol Biol Phys 2005;63:1279-1285.

Macdonald JS, Smalley SR, Benedetti J, et al: Chemoradiotherapy after surgery compared with surgery alone for adenocarcinoma of the stomach or gastroesophageal junction. N Engl J Med 2001;345:725-730.

Modlin IM, Lye KD, Kidd M: Carcinoid tumors of the stomach. Surg Oncol 2003;12:153-172.

Peeters KCMJ, Hundahl SA, Kranenbarg EK, et al: Low Maruyama index surgery for gastric cancer: Blinded reanalysis of the Dutch D1-D2 trial. World J Surg 2005;29:1576-1584.

# Tumors of the Rectum and Colon

Method of
*Dana M. Hayden, MD, MPH,*
*and Marc Brand, MD*

## Epidemiology And Etiology

Colorectal cancer is a serious public health issue, because it remains the second most common cancer diagnosis and cause of cancer death in the United States. In 2005, approximately 100,000 persons received a new diagnosis of colon cancer and 40,000 persons received a new diagnosis of rectal cancer. From 1992 to 2002, decreases in incidence and mortality have been seen as well as increases in screening; however, these trends are modest and have not been seen consistently among all ethnic or racial groups in the United States. Physicians and public health activists must continue to raise awareness and increase the availability of screening in order to continue this recent impact.

The etiology of colorectal cancer includes environmental and genetic factors. Cancer rates vary widely by geographic region, and diet appears to be a major contributor. High rates of colorectal cancer are associated with diets rich in processed, high-fat, low-fiber foods. It is believed that this diet slows intestinal transit time, thus prolonging the colonic exposure to carcinogenic metabolites that may be present secondary to bacterial digestion. Environmental effects are also evidenced by retrospective migrant studies. When migrating populations move from a region with lower rates to one with higher rates of colorectal cancer, these groups adopt the risk prevalent in their new region. Other environmental factors, including smoking and alcohol consumption, also contribute to colorectal cancer risk.

Genetics also plays a significant role in etiology. Although approximately 90% of cases are sporadic, about 10% of U.S. adults have a first-degree relative with colorectal cancer. Somatic mutations on the *APC* gene have been found in familial clusters, and about one third of patients with familial colorectal cancer have an affected family member. Hereditary nonpolyposis colon cancer (HNPCC) is an autosomal dominant inherited disorder accounting for about 5% to 10% of colon and rectal cancer cases. Another autosomal dominant syndrome, familial adenomatous polyposis (FAP), accounts for only 1% of colon and rectal cancer; however, cancer is inevitable if polyps are present. In addition to these inherited syndromes, inflammatory bowel disease also increases the risk of colorectal cancer.

Most colorectal tumors are believed to develop from adenomatous polyps. This adenoma-carcinoma progression has been well studied, and several mutations involving the activation of oncogenes and inactivation of tumor suppression genes have been identified. Deletions on chromosomes 5q, 17p, and 18q as well as mutations of the *ras* protooncogene and p53 gene have been found in patients with benign adenomas, carcinomas, and FAP. It appears that accumulation of these mutations leads to the progression from adenoma to invasive carcinoma. Also, DNA mismatch repair gene mutations on multiple chromosomes, including 2p, have been identified in HNPCC patients. These breakthroughs have enabled genetic testing for family members at risk for FAP and HNPCC.

## High-Risk Colorectal Syndromes

Hereditary nonpolyposis colon cancer confers a lifetime risk of cancer of approximately 80%. There are minimal physical findings and few polyps. The diagnosis should be suspected with early age at cancer diagnosis, proximal location of tumors, and high rate of synchronous and metachronous lesions. To diagnose HNPCC, the patient must meet several requirements (Amsterdam criteria) or be found to have mismatch repair gene mutations (Box 1). Colorectal tumors are believed to develop more quickly in HNPCC than in sporadic cases, and these patients also have an increased risk of noncolorectal cancers: endometrial, ovarian, small intestinal, renal, and gastric cancers.

Familial adenomatous polyposis is more easily diagnosed than HNPCC (see Box 1). More than 100 adenomatous polyps must be present in the colon, and diagnosis does not depend on family history. Severe polyposis may be found (>1000 polyps) or an attenuated FAP variant (20-100 polyps). Unfortunately, the development of colorectal cancer is certain. Patients also suffer from noncolorectal manifestations, such as osteomas and desmoid tumors in Gardner's syndrome, brain tumors in Turcot's syndrome, and duodenal adenomas. Less stringent criteria are used to diagnose at-risk relatives: one or more polyps found at early age (<50 years) or presence of extracolonic manifestations.

Ulcerative colitis and Crohn's colitis also confer a high risk of colorectal cancer. This risk increases with extent and duration of disease. Colorectal cancer risk begins to increase after 10 years of symptomatic colitis and increases approximately 1% per year thereafter. Higher cancer rates are also associated with pancolitis.

---

**BOX 1  Guidelines for Diagnosis of Hereditary Nonpolyposis Colon Cancer and Familial Adenomatous Polyposis Syndromes**

**Hereditary Nonpolyposis Colon Cancer**
*Amsterdam Criteria (3-2-1-0 Rule)*
- At least three relatives with histologically confirmed colorectal cancer, at least one being a first-degree relative of the other two
- Colorectal cancer involving at least two generations
- At least one case of colorectal cancer diagnosed before age 50 years
- FAP syndrome excluded

*Bethesda Guidelines*
- Amsterdam criteria met
- Patient with colorectal cancer *and* first-degree relative with colorectal cancer diagnosed before age 45 years *or* extracolonic HNPCC-related cancer diagnosed before age 45 years *or* colorectal adenoma found before age 45 years
- Patient with two HNPCC-related cancers, two synchronous or metachronous colorectal tumors, or one colorectal tumor and one HNPCC-related cancer

- Patient with signet-ring cells or right-sided undifferentiated colorectal cancer
- Patient with endometrial cancer diagnosed before age 45 years
- Patient with colorectal adenoma present before age 40 years
- If any of these criteria are met, proceed with genetic counseling

**Familial Adenomatous Polyposis**
- Multiple colonic adenomas (classic FAP >100, attenuated 20-100)
- Not based on family history
- At-risk relatives identified for FAP if one or more adenomas are found before age 50 years or with extracolonic manifestations
- Genetic testing is useful if FAP is an attenuated form or if diagnosis is unclear (80% FAP patients test positive for a genetic marker)

*Abbreviations:* FAP = familial adenomatous polyposis; HNPCC = hereditary nonpolyposis colon cancer.

---

# Screening And Diagnosis

## AVERAGE RISK

Colorectal cancer has a premalignant phase that is easily diagnosed and treatable; thus, a well-defined screening protocol is both feasible and necessary. Adults are considered to have average risk if they have no family history of colorectal cancer, no evidence of a genetic syndrome, and no symptoms suspicious for cancer. Screening for the average-risk person should begin at the age of 50 years (Table 1). One screening option is annual fecal occult blood testing (FOBT) coupled with a flexible sigmoidoscopy every 5 years. This combination significantly

---

**TABLE 1  Screening Protocols for Colorectal Cancer**

| Screening Test | Age to Begin | Interval |
| --- | --- | --- |
| **Average-Risk Patients** | | |
| Air-contrast barium enema | 50 y | 5-10 y |
| Colonoscopy | 50 y | 10 y |
| Fecal occult blood test | 50 y | Annually |
| Flexible sigmoidoscopy | 50 y | 5 y |
| **High-Risk Patients** | | |
| *Personal History of Polyps* | | |
| Colonoscopy | | 3 y for high risk (3 or more, unfavorable) |
| | | 5-10 y lower risk |
| *Familial Colorectal Cancer* | | |
| Colonoscopy | 10 y earlier than age at diagnosis of youngest relative | 5 y |
| *Ulcerative or Crohn's Colitis* | | |
| Colonoscopy | 8-12 y after symptoms | 1-2 y from onset |
| | | Multiple random 4-quadrant biopsies |
| *Hereditary Nonpolyposis Colorectal Cancer** | | |
| Colonoscopy | At least age 20-25 y or 10 y before age of youngest affected relative | 1-3 y before age 30 y, 2 y before age 40 y, annually after age 40 y |
| Endometrial and ovarian cancer screening | | |
| Transvaginal ultrasound, endometrial aspirate biopsy, CA-125 | Age 30-35 | Annually |
| If genetic testing negative | Average risk screening protocol | |
| *Familial Adenomatous Polyposis** | | |
| Rigid/flexible sigmoidoscopy | Age 10 | Annually |
| Colonoscopy | if 1 polyp found | Annually |
| Duodenal polyposis | | |
| Upper endoscopy | Age 25 | Surveillance based on Spigelman classification |

*Genetic testing "+," not informative or not done.

decreases mortality, increases 5-year survival, and reduces the rate of metastasis found at diagnosis. FOBT must be handled correctly to maintain the sensitivity and specificity at approximately 90%. The patient must refrain from eating red meat and horseradish and from taking nonsteroidal anti-inflammatories or vitamin C for 2 days before the test. Samples must be taken from two different areas of three consecutive stools, they must be stored at room temperature, and they must be rehydrated and tested within 4 days of collection.

Flexible sigmoidoscopy should be performed every 5 years. Advantages include a simple bowel preparation (saline laxative enema an hour before the procedure), the ability to biopsy and remove polyps, visualization of polyps smaller than 1 cm, and no need for sedation. Endoscopists can visualize the entire sigmoid colon in approximately 90% of patients. The examination is relatively sensitive, identifying two thirds of patients with adenomas as well as approximately 40% to 60% of adenomas that are visualized during complete colonoscopy.

Flexible sigmoidoscopy every 5 years may also be combined with air-contrast barium enema (ACBE) every 5 to 10 years. This examination is less invasive than endoscopy, but it does require effort on the parts of the patient and the radiologist. Barium enema can evaluate the entire colon in approximately 90% to 95% of cases. Sigmoidoscopy is added to increase this test's sensitivity because it better visualizes the rectosigmoid mucosa. Positive results for screening include a single positive FOBT window, a polyp or mass seen on barium enema, one or more polyps larger than 1 cm, or other mucosal abnormalities visualized during endoscopy. If any of these examinations reveal positive findings, a follow-up colonoscopy should be performed.

Complete colonoscopy every 10 years is the most sensitive option for screening. However, the patient must endure complete bowel preparation and sedation, and there is a small risk of bowel perforation. The greatest benefit of colonoscopy is the ability to examine the entire colon. Complete evaluation to the cecum is achieved in approximately 95% of patients, although this varies with the endoscopist's experience. The interval of evaluation is based on research indicating that polyps have a dwell time extending more than 10 years before progressing to cancer. The other screening tools require more frequent follow-up due to their decreased sensitivities and lack of complete colonic evaluation.

### HIGH RISK

Screening protocols for high-risk patients must adjust to the increased likelihood of disease and earlier age at onset. These patients include persons with a personal history of polyps, persons with symptoms suspicious for cancer, persons with a family history of colorectal cancer (especially a first-degree relative), patients with ulcerative or Crohn's colitis, and patients who have FAP or HNPCC or who are members of FAP or HNPCC families (see Table 1). Symptoms suspicious for cancer include bleeding, change in bowel habits or caliber of stool,

and obstruction. Hemorrhoids should not be diagnosed in persons with rectal bleeding until a complete colonoscopy is performed and cancer or another source of bleeding is excluded.

## Treatment

### PREOPERATIVE EVALUATION

Once a diagnosis of colorectal cancer is confirmed, the patient should undergo a thorough preoperative evaluation, including a history and physical, routine blood tests and a carcinoembryonic antigen (CEA) level, chest x-ray, and complete evaluation of the colon with either barium enema or colonoscopy. Knowledge of the patient's symptoms is also important. If the patient is anemic or obstructed, preoperative admission for transfusion or resuscitation and careful bowel preparation may be necessary.

Preoperative staging is controversial for colon cancer but it is essential for rectal tumors. Rigid proctoscopy most accurately measures tumor distance from the anal verge, and endorectal ultrasound evaluates the depth of tumor invasion and the presence of enlarged lymph nodes. If ultrasound reveals evidence of invasion into perirectal fat or adjacent organs or the presence of metastatic nodes, preoperative chemotherapy and radiation treatment should be administered. Recent studies indicate several benefits of neoadjuvant therapy: downstaging rectal tumors, decreasing size of bulky tumors, allowing less-morbid operations (including sphincter-preserving resection), and decreasing rates of local recurrence.

One final preoperative consideration is the decision to perform laparoscopic versus open surgery. Laparoscopic surgery for colon tumors is becoming more common; however, laparoscopy for rectal cancer is still controversial. Concerns about port site recurrences and adherence to oncologic principles continue to be raised. Several trials are currently under way, yet it still remains unclear if the laparoscopic approach provides advantages over traditional open surgery in regard to cost, operative time, recovery, or duration of hospitalization. However, these studies do indicate that laparoscopy is at least as safe and feasible as open surgery if performed by an experienced laparoscopic surgeon.

### SURGICAL CONSIDERATIONS

#### Tumors of the Colon

During cancer resection, initial exploration of the abdomen for evidence of peritoneal spread, adjacent organ involvement, or liver metastasis is essential because positive findings can alter the surgical plan. Based on

### CURRENT DIAGNOSIS

- Screening of average-risk patients should begin at age 50 years.
- Follow-up colonoscopy should be performed if any of the screening tests are positive, including positive fecal occult blood test or polyp larger than 1 centimeter found on barium enema or sigmoidoscopy.
- Patients with symptoms suspicious for colorectal cancer should have colonoscopy.
- Patients with known high-risk colorectal syndromes including ulcerative or Crohn's colitis, hereditary nonpolyposis colon cancer, and familial adenomatous polyposis or persons with a family history of colorectal cancer should have earlier and more frequent endoscopic surveillance.

### CURRENT THERAPY

- Laparoscopic or open segmental resection for colonic tumors
- Postoperative chemotherapy for stage III colonic tumors or stage II tumors with unfavorable characteristics
- Transanal, local excision for small, superficial, well-differentiated rectal tumors
- Formal resection of rectum with sphincter preservation, if possible, for larger, locally invasive tumors or if nodal metastasis is present
- Preoperative chemotherapy and radiation if a rectal tumor is locally invasive or if nodal metastasis is present
- Postoperative chemotherapy and radiation for stages II and III rectal tumors or if preoperative treatment is given
- Follow-up surveillance includes frequent history and physicals, CEA levels, CT scans of the chest and abdomen, and endoscopy during the first 3 to 5 years postoperatively

*Abbreviations:* CEA = carcinoembryonic antigen; CT = computed tomography.

oncologic principles, tumors of the colon should be resected en bloc along with their vascular and lymphatic supplies. Concern about local recurrence and lymphatic spread guides distal resection, and the tumor's vascular supply dictates the proximal margin to prevent systemic spread.

For a lesion in the cecum or ascending colon, a right hemicolectomy is performed, creating an anastomosis between the terminal ileum and the proximal transverse colon. For a transverse lesion, an extended right hemicolectomy is performed. Tumors involving the splenic flexure or descending colon require a left hemicolectomy, connecting the midtransverse colon to the proximal rectum. Sigmoid tumors are treated by resection of the sigmoid colon followed by anastomosis between the descending colon and proximal rectum.

Wide excision of the resected segment's mesentery is essential. Sampling the greatest number of nodes provides the most accurate tumor staging.

## Tumors of the Rectum

Unlike colon cancer, there are several options available for treating rectal tumors. The two main approaches include transanal local excision of the tumor and formal resection of the rectum. Lesions may be amenable to transanal excision if the tumor is accessible and preoperative evaluation reveals that the cancer is well differentiated and confined to the mucosa or submucosa with no evidence of lymphatic or vascular invasion (T1N0). If possible, transanal excision is preferable because it avoids the morbidity of an abdominal operation. Newer methods such as transanal endoscopic microsurgery (TEM) can reach more proximal rectal tumors and allow excision of larger lesions.

If the rectal tumor is not accessible transanally or there is evidence of local invasion or nodal metastasis (T3 or N1), preoperative chemotherapy and radiation followed by formal resection should be performed. A sphincter-preserving low anterior resection (LAR) is preferred if the rectal tumor has an adequate distal margin and the sphincteric muscles are not involved. However, an abdominoperineal resection (APR) with permanent colostomy is generally required if the lower edge of the tumor is palpable within 2 cm of the anorectal junction. Significant morbidities associated with this operation include sexual dysfunction, delayed perineal wound healing and infection, bladder dysfunction, and a permanent ostomy.

## Obstructive Cancer

Treatment for obstructing colorectal cancer differs from an elective resection due to the acuteness of the obstruction and the patient's extent of debilitation. Most patients are treated with resection of the obstructing cancer and creation of an ostomy.

Critically ill patients may have a proximal diversion and colostomy and return later for tumor resection. A new alternative to these two-stage approaches is endoscopic placement of a colonic stent. This procedure relieves the obstruction and allows the patient to recover before undergoing definitive surgery.

Other single-surgery approaches include resection with intraoperative lavage and primary anastomosis or subtotal colectomy with ileorectal anastomosis, both of which have been shown to be safe alternatives.

## Cancer Related to High-Risk Colorectal Conditions

In patients with high-risk colorectal conditions, surgical treatment is based on cancer prevention as well as treatment. Patients with severe ulcerative or Crohn's colitis or HNPCC may consider prophylactic surgery. However, if suspicious polyps or severe polyposis are found in FAP patients, surgery is indicated.

Surgical options include a total proctocolectomy with ileal pouch–anal anastomosis or ileostomy or a total abdominal colectomy with ileorectal anastomosis. Aggressive surveillance of the preserved rectal mucosa or ileal pouch must be performed because cancer risk is not completely eliminated. Because HNPCC carries risks of endometrial and ovarian cancers, total abdominal hysterectomy with bilateral salpingo-oophorectomy should be considered if the patient is postmenopausal or has completed childbearing.

# Postoperative Management

## STAGING AND POSTOPERATIVE THERAPY

Staging of the tumor allows the surgical and oncologic teams to provide a prognosis for the patient as well as determine the necessity of additional therapy. Several staging systems and guidelines have been established and revised. Dukes staging and the TNM system stage colorectal tumors according to depth of tumor invasion and presence of nodal involvement and distant metastasis (Table 2).

Chemotherapy is generally advised for patients with node-positive disease (stage III) or those with rectal cancer who received preoperative treatment. Studies have shown for stage III and, less evidently, for stage II disease, postoperative chemotherapy and radiation in combination with surgery decrease rates of systemic spread, local recurrence, and mortality. The current chemotherapy given for colorectal cancer is 5-fluorouracil (5-FU, Adrucil), an inhibitor of thymidylate synthase,

**TABLE 2  Staging of Colorectal Cancer**

| Features | Stage | TMN | Dukes | Aster-Coller | ACPS |
|---|---|---|---|---|---|
| **Depth of Invasion** | | | | | |
| Lamina propria, muscularis mucosa | 0 | T0/Tis | — | A | O |
| Submucosa | I | T1 | A | B1 | A |
| Muscularis propria | I | T2 | A | B1 | A |
| Subserosa, pericolic fat | II | T3 | A | B1 | B |
| Adjacent organs, tumor perforation | II | T4 | B | B2 | B |
| **Nodal Involvement** | | | | | |
| None | III | N0 | — | — | — |
| 1-3 nodes | III | N1 | C1,C2 | C1,C2 | C |
| >3 nodes | III | N2 | C1,C2 | C1,C2 | C |
| **Distant Metastases** | | | | | |
| Absent | IV | M0 | — | — | — |
| Present | IV | M1 | — | — | D |

*Abbreviations:* ACPS = Australian clinicopathological staging system; AJCC = American Joint Committee on Cancer; Tis = tumor in situ; TMN = tumor, node, metastasis.
*Staging systems:* ACPS, 1983; AJCC TMN system, 1997; Aster-Coller system, 1954; Dukes staging system, 1934.

combined with levamisole (Ergamisol)[2] or leucovorin. Newer adjuvant therapies, including antibodies and immunomodulatory agents, are under investigation. Postoperative radiation is reserved for stage II and III rectal tumors.

## POSTOPERATIVE SURVEILLANCE

The American Society of Clinical Oncology recommends a surveillance strategy that includes appropriate frequency of history and physical examinations, serum CEA levels, CT scans, and endoscopic surveillance (Box 2). These guidelines are based on studies that show the risk of colon and rectal cancer recurrence extends approximately 3 and 5 years after primary therapy, respectively. Revision of the guidelines has also occurred secondary to more recent studies evaluating the effects of follow-up intensity on survival and recurrence. Although the results have been mixed, it appears that aggressive surveillance does improve survival and allows reoperation in patients with stages II and III disease.

## REFERENCES

Brand MI, Church JM: High risk premalignant colorectal conditions. In Saclarides TJ, Millikan KW, Godellas CV (eds): Surgical Oncology: An Algorithmic Approach. New York: Springer-Verlag, 2003, pp 346-363.

Brand MI: Colon cancer. In Saclarides TJ, Millikan KW, Godellas CV (ed) Surgical Oncology: An Algorithmic Approach. New York: Springer-Verlag, 2003, pp 332-345.

Desch CE, Benson AB, Somerfield MR, et al: Colorectal cancer surveillance: 2005 update of an American Society of Clinical Oncology Practice Guideline. J Clin Oncol 2005;23:8512-8519.

Edwards BK, Brown ML, Wingo PA, et al: Annual report to the nation on the status of cancer, 1975-2002, featuring population-based trends in cancer treatment. J Clin Oncol 2005;97:1407-1427.

Fearon ER, Vogelstein B: A genetic model for colorectal tumorigenesis. Cell 1990;61:759-767.

Itzkowitz SH, Present DH; Crohn's and Colitis Foundation of America Colon Cancer in IBD Study Group: Consensus conference: Colorectal cancer screening and surveillance in inflammatory bowel disease. Inflamm Bowel Dis 2005;11:314-321.

Centers for Disease Control and Prevention: Recent trends in mortality rate of four major cancers, by sex and race/ethnicity—United States, 1990-1998. MMWR Morb Mortal Wkly Rep 2002;51:49-53.

Saclarides TJ: Rectal cancer. In Saclarides TJ, Millikan KW, Godellas CV (ed) Surgical Oncology: An Algorithmic Approach. New York: Springer-Verlag, 2003, pp 364-373.

Sample CB, Watson M, Okrainec A, et al: Long-term outcomes of laparoscopic surgery for colorectal cancer. Surg Endosc 2006;20:30-34.

# Intestinal Parasites

Method of
*Douglas W. MacPherson, MD, MSc (CTM)*

Intestinal parasites represent an important group of infectious agents. They are less commonly appreciated as clinical causes of infectious gastrointestinal (GI) illnesses in North America, in particular compared with diseases associated with bacterial, viral, and microbial toxins, but they still represent a significant burden of disease in North America and globally, due to associated case morbidity and mortality. Intestinal parasites are often associated with economically less-developed regions that have low levels of environmental sanitation (food and water) and where high standards of personal hygiene may be challenging to maintain. Intestinal parasites are also important personal and public health disease agents in economically advanced countries. When the diagnosis of intestinal parasites is delayed or missed, both the patient and society suffer increased losses of economic productivity and quality and duration of life.

Parasites are classified as protozoan or metazoan. The protozoa are single-celled animals. Typically they can replicate within the host and there is no set limit to the duration of infection. They are further classified by their organ of locomotion as being flagellate (*Giardia lamblia*), ciliate (*Balantidium coli*), amoeboid (*Entamoeba histolytica*), or no apparent organ of locomotion (*Cryptosporidium* spp). The metazoans are multicellular animals. Typically they reproduce but, with few exceptions, do not replicate in the host, and they have a limited period of infection without reinfection determined by their own life span. They are also classified by their morphologic appearance (flat or round) and the presence of segmented bodies: flat, segmented (cestodes or tapeworms such as *Taenia saginata* or the beef tapeworm); flat, nonsegmented (trematodes or flukes such as *Fasciola hepatica*); round, nonsegmented (nematodes or roundworms such as *Ascaris lumbricoides*); and round, segmented (annelids or earthworms and leeches). Leeches can attach to the upper airway or mouth of a human host, but this group of worms does not generally affect the intestines.

This approach to parasite classification is of more than taxonomic and diagnostic significance because it correlates with therapeutic options as well (Tables 1 and 2).

For the clinician, knowing the distinction between clinically significant parasites, parasites that are not parasitic (nonpathogens or commensals), and intestinal parasites that have their major clinical manifestations outside of the GI tract is important because it leads to the appropriate clinical and diagnostic assessments and promotes good management outcomes. Many intestinal parasites have complex life cycles and intermediary hosts, and some have humans only as accidental hosts. The complexity of parasite interactions with human hosts is beyond the consideration of this article.

Parasites that are not parasitic can be very challenging to clinicians and to the person found to be carrying the agent. Excessive secondary investigation or exposure to unnecessary treatment of nonpathogens

## TABLE 1 Treatment of Intestinal Protozoa

| Drug[3] | Adult Dose | Pediatric Dose |
|---|---|---|
| **Balantidium coli** | | |
| Tetracycline (Sumycin) or | 500 mg PO qid × 10 d | 10 mg/kg PO qid × 10d, max 2.0 g/d |
| Metronidazole (Flagyl)[1] or | 750 mg tid × 10 d | 35-50 mg/kg/d in 3 doses × 5 d |
| Iodoquinol (Yodoxin)[1] | 650 mg PO tid × 20 d | 40 mg/kg/d in 3 doses × 20 d, max 2.0 g/d |
| **Cryptosporidium spp.*** | | |
| Nitazoxanide (Alinia) | 500 mg PO bid × 3 d | 1-3 y: 100 mg PO bid × 3d |
| | | 4-11 y: 200 mg PO bid × 3d |
| **Cyclospora cayetanensis*** | | |
| TMP-SMX (Bactrim) | 160 mg TMP/800 mg SMX[1] (1 DS tab) PO bid × 7-10 d | 5 mg/kg TMP/25 mg/kg SMX PO bid × 7-10 d |
| **Dientamoeba fragilis[†]** | | |
| Iodoquinol or | 650 mg PO tid × 20d | 30-40 mg/kg/d in 3 doses × 20 d, max 2.0 g/d |
| Paromomycin (Humatin)[1] or | 25-35 mg/kg/d in 3 doses × 7 d | 25-35 mg/kg/d in 3 doses × 7 d |
| Tetracycline or | 500 mg PO qid × 10 d | 10 mg/kg PO qid × 10 d, max 2.0 g/d |
| Metronidazole | 500-750 mg tid × 10 d | 20-40 mg/kg/d in 3 doses/d × 10 d |
| **Giardia lamblia** | | |
| **Preferred Regimens** | | |
| Metronidazole[1] or | 250 mg PO tid × 5 d | 5 mg/kg tid × 5 d |
| Metronidazole[1] or | 2.0 g PO qhs × 3 d | |
| Nitazoxanide or | 500 mg PO bid × 3 d | 1-3 y: 100 mg PO bid × 3 d |
| | | 4-11 y: 200 mg PO bid × 3 d |
| Tinidazole (Tindamax) | 2.0 g PO × 1 dose | 50 mg/kg PO × 1 dose |
| **Alternative Regimens** | | |
| Paromomycin[1] or | 25-35 mg/kg/d PO in 3 doses × 7 d | 25-35 mg/kg/d PO in 3 doses × 7 d |
| Furazolidone (Furoxone)[2] or | 100 mg PO qid × 7-10 d | 1.5 mg/kg PO qid × 7-10 d |
| Quinacrine[2] | 100 mg PO tid × 5 d | 2 mg/kg PO tid × 5 d, max 300 mg/d |
| **Entamoeba histolytica** | | |
| **Luminal Disease** | | |
| Iodoquinol or | 650 mg PO tid × 20 d | 10 mg/kg PO tid × 20 d, max 2.0 g/d |
| Paromomycin or | 25-35 mg/kg/d in 3 doses × 7 d | 25-35 mg/kg/d in 3 doses × 7 d |
| Diloxanide furoate[2] | 500 mg PO tid × 10 d | 7 mg/kg PO tid × 10 d |
| **Extraluminal Disease: Treatment for Luminal Disease plus:** | | |
| Metronidazole or | 500-750 mg PO tid × 7-10 d | 35-50 mg/kg/d in 3 doses × 7-10 d |
| Tinidazole | 2.0 g PO qd × 3-5 d | 50 mg/kg/d × 3-5 d, max 2.0 g/d |
| **Isospora belli** | | |
| TMP-SMX[1] | 160 mg TMP/800 mg SMX (1 DS tab) PO bid × 7-10 d | 5 mg/kg TMP/25 mg/kg SMX PO bid × 7-10 d |
| **Intestinal microsporidiosis:*** | | |
| **Enterocytozoon bieneusi** | | |
| Fumagillin[2] | 60 mg/d PO × 14 d | |
| **Encephalitozoon intestinalis** | | |
| Albendazole (Albenza)[1] | 400 mg PO bid × 21 d | |

[1]Not FDA approved for this indication.
[2]Not available in the United States.
[3]First drug listed is the drug of choice.
*Cryptosporidium and Cyclospora infection is often self-limited without treatment in immunocompetent hosts; intestinal microsporidiosis is clinically rare in immunocompetent hosts. In HIV-infected patients, use HAART.
[†]Evidence of pathogenicity of Dientamoeba fragilis is controversial. Results of treatment on parasite clearance and clinical symptoms are inconsistent.
Abbreviations: DS = double strength; HAART = highly active antiretroviral therapy; tab = tablet; TMP-SMX = trimethoprim-sulfamethoxazole.

can be reduced if the diagnostic facility does not report clinically insignificant findings. Another challenge to diagnostic facilities, clinicians, and patients is associated nonparasitic laboratory findings in stool examinations. For example, the finding of Charcot-Leyden crystals, believed to be the breakdown elements of eosinophils, has generated considerable debate in enteric parasitology circles on interpretation and whether finding them has any diagnostic relevance to intestinal parasitic infection. Another example is the finding of *Blastocystis hominis* in stools examined for parasites. Although the taxonomic classification of this organism has been hotly debated, it certainly is not a protozoan parasite. Its role as a bowel pathogen is uncertain, and the effects of therapeutic interventions on its persistence in the GI tract and impact on clinical symptoms are also unclear.

The third group of parasitic diseases occur when the infectious parasitic agent is ingested but they do not have their major clinical manifestation in the GI tract. These diseases include toxoplasmosis (*Toxoplasma gondii*), trichinellosis (*Trichinella spiralis*), toxocariasis (*Toxocara canis*),

cystercercosis (tissue larval infestation due to *Taenia solium*), and many other infections that occur in North America or that are potentially imported by returning international travelers, immigrants, or illegal aliens. These diseases are not discussed further in this chapter.

The index of clinical and diagnostic suspicion must be very high when addressing less prevalent conditions or diseases that are not endemic and only arrive through importation. Special populations such as pediatric, elderly, pregnant, and immunocompromised patients and migrants of all kinds, particularly those transiting from areas with endemic high parasitic transmission and areas with poor environmental hygiene, are at particular risk for parasitic infestation of the GI tract and resulting disease. These groups also require a higher index of suspicion for clinical management in diagnosis and treatment. Certain community environments can also represent risk environments for parasitic intestinal infections where maintaining high levels of personal hygiene may be difficult (e.g., daycare centers, refugee camps, detention centers) or where commonality of water or

## TABLE 2 Treatment of Intestinal Metazoa

| Treatment[4] | Adult Dosing | Pediatric Dosing |
| --- | --- | --- |
| **Ancylostoma canium** | | |
| Albendazole[1] or | 400 mg PO once | 400 mg PO once |
| Mebendazole (Vermox) or | 100 mg PO bid × 3 d | 100 mg PO bid × 3 d |
| Pyrantel pamoate (Reese's Pinworm)[1] or | 11 mg/kg once, max 1.0 g | 11 mg/kg once, max 1.0 g |
| Endoscopic removal | — | — |
| **Anisakis sp.** | | |
| Endoscopic or surgical removal | — | — |
| **Ascaris lumbricoides** | | |
| Albendazole[1] or | 400 mg PO once | 400 mg PO once |
| Ivermectin (Stromectol)[1] or | 150-200 µg/kg once | 150-200 µg/kg once |
| Mebendazole or | 100 mg PO bid × 3 d | 100 mg PO bid × 3 d |
| Mebendazole | 500 mg[23] PO once | 500 mg[23] PO once |
| **Capillaria philippinensis** | | |
| Mebendazole[1] or | 200 mg[3] PO bid × 20 d | 200 mg[3] PO bid × 20 d |
| Albendazole[1] | 400 mg PO qd × 10 d | 400 mg PO qd × 10 d |
| **Enterobius vermicularis** | | |
| Pyrantel pamoate or | 11 mg/kg base, single dose; repeat in 14 d; max 1.0 g | 11 mg/kg base, single dose; repeat in 14 d; max 1.0 g |
| Albendazole[1] or | 400 mg PO once; repeat in 14 d | 400 mg PO once; repeat in 14 d |
| Mebendazole | 100 mg PO once; repeat in 14 d | 100 mg PO once; repeat in 14 d |
| **Flukes (intestinal and liver)** | | |
| **Clonorchis sinensis** | | |
| Praziquantel (Biltricide) or | 75 mg/kg in 3 doses in 1 d | 75 mg/kg in 3 doses in 1 d |
| Albendazole[1] | 400 mg PO once | 400 mg PO once |
| **Fasciola hepatica** | | |
| Triclabendazole[2] or | 10 mg/kg once or twice | 10 mg/kg once or twice |
| Bithionol[5]r | 30-50 mg/kg on alternate d × 10-15 doses | 30-50 mg/kg on alternate d × 10-15 doses |
| ***Fasciolopsis buski, Heterophyes heterophyes, Metagonimus yokogawai, Metorchis conjunctus, Opisthorchis viverrini*** | | |
| Praziquantel | 75 mg/kg in 3 doses in 1 d | 75 mg/kg in 3 doses in 1 d |
| **Nanophyetus salmincola** | | |
| Praziquantel | 60 mg/kg in 3 doses in 1 d | 60 mg/kg in 3 doses in 1 d |
| **Schistosomiasis** | | |
| **S. haematobium** | | |
| Praziquantel | 40 mg/kg in 2 doses in 1 d | 40 mg/kg in 2 doses in 1 d |
| **S. japonicum** | | |
| Praziquantel | 60 mg/kg in 3 doses in 1 d | 60 mg/kg in 3 doses in 1 d |
| **S. mekongi** | | |
| Praziquantel | 60 mg/kg in 3 doses in 1 d | 60 mg/kg in 3 doses in 1 d |
| **S. mansoni** | | |
| Praziquantel or | 40 mg/kg in 2 doses in 1 d | 40 mg/kg in 2 doses in 1 d |
| Oxamniquine[1] | 15 mg/kg once | 20 mg/kg/d in 2 doses in 1 d* |
| **Hookworm: *Ancylostoma duodenale, Necator americanus*** | | |
| Albendazole[1] or | 400 mg PO once | 400 mg PO once |
| Mebendazole or | 100 mg PO once | 100 mg PO once |
| Pyrantel pamoate[1] | 11 mg/kg base × 3d; max 1.0 g | 11 mg/kg base × 3d; max 1.0 g |
| **Strongyloides stercoralis** | | |
| Ivermectin or | 200 µg/kg/d × 2 d | 200 µg/kg/d × 2 d |
| Albendazole[1] or | 400 mg PO bid × 7 d | 400 mg PO bid × 7 d |
| Thiabendazole (Mintezol) | 50 mg/kg/d in 2 doses × 2 d, max 3 g/d | 50 mg/kg/d in 2 doses × 2 d, max 3 g/d |
| **Tapeworms (intestinal)** | | |
| ***Diphyllobothrium spp., Taenia spp.,[†] Dipylidium caninum*** | | |
| Praziquantel[1] or | 5-10 mg/kg once | 5-10 mg/kg once |
| Niclosamide[2] | 2 gm once | 50 mg/kg once |
| **Hymenolepis nana** | | |
| Praziquantel[1] or | 25 mg/kg once | 25 mg/kg once |
| Nitazoxanide[1] | 500 mg bid × 3d | 1-3 y: 100 mg bid × 3 d |
| | | 4-11 y: 200 mg bid × 3d |
| **Tapeworms (larval)** | | |
| **Echinococcus granulosus** | | |
| Albendazole | 400 mg PO bid × 1-6 mo | 15 mg/kg/d (max 800 mg) × 1-6 mo |
| **E. multilocularis** | | |
| Surgical excision[6] | — | — |
| ***Cysticercosis (T. solium) (drug therapy is controversial)*** | | |
| Albendazole or | 400 mg PO bid × 8-30 d | 15 mg/kg (max 800 mg/d) in 2 doses × 8-30 d; repeat as needed |
| Praziquantel | 50-100 mg/kg/d in 3 doses × 30 d | 50-100 mg/kg/d in 3 doses × 30 d |
| **Trichuris trichiura** | | |
| Mebendazole or | 100 mg PO bid × 3 d | 100 mg PO bid × 3 d |
| Albendazole[1] or | 400 mg PO × 3 d | 400 mg PO × 3 d |
| Ivermectin[1] or | 200 µg/kg × 3 d | 200 µg/kg × 3 d |
| Mebendazole | 500 mg[3] PO once | 500 mg[3] PO once |

[1]Not FDA approved for this indication.
[2]Not available in the United States.
[3]Exceeds dosage recommended by the manufacturer.
[4]First drug/treatment listed is the drug/treatment of choice.
[5]Investigational drug in the United States.
[6]In surgically untreatable cases albendazole is recommended (see dosing for *E. granulosis*).
* *S. mansoni* treatment with oxamniquine in Africa: 40-60 mg/kg over 2-3 d.
[†]Speciation of *Taenia* spp. can be made on passage of a tape segment or identification of the head (scolex) of the adult worm. This can assist in the clinical management of the patient.
*Abbreviations:* max = maximum; tab = tablet; TMP-SMX = trimethoprim-sulfamethoxazole.

food sources and environmental management can result in mass exposure due to parasite contamination.

# General Laboratory Diagnostic Considerations

Specific requests for appropriate laboratory referral, management, and diagnosis are required to diagnose intraintestinal parasites. Fecal samples for routine parasitology testing are collected into a fixative-preservative solution. Several different stool ova and parasite (O&P) solutions are available, and the choice of these does have some significance in laboratory proficiency performance. However, it is probably equally important for the clinician and patient to have highly trained, diagnostically experienced, dedicated, and certified parasitology technologists performing the specimen examination in a laboratory that meets modern quality-management practices for diagnostic services.

A single examination of a fixed-preserved stool specimen finds most relevant parasites in highly proficient parasitology laboratories. Exceptions to a single-examined specimen can occur when there are very low parasite burdens or when the specimen is less than ideal due to collection errors (e.g., contamination with water or urine, stool mixed with interfering substances such as barium, patient use of antimicrobials), preservation errors, freezing or overheating the specimen, delays in transportation and examination, or professional or laboratory diagnostic challenges. In all cases of diagnostic laboratory testing, the provision of clinically relevant epidemiologic information, such as travel history or foreign exposure, comorbid medical conditions, environmental or occupational exposures, outbreak information, or even the suspected parasite can help the laboratory provide better diagnostic service to the patient and clinician.

Some intestinal parasites are best diagnosed by a combination of techniques, such as serology with or without stool examination, tissue pathology, or other tests. Direct detection of passed entire worms or worm segments by collection on a pinworm paddle or by placing detected worm elements into normal saline and one of the stool preservatives for O&P is ideal for many of the intestinal worm infections. Extremely rarely, parasite stool culture is required to isolate the parasite through augmentation by growth and replication. The stool culture techniques are usually only available in specialized diagnostic facilities or research laboratories. Other laboratory techniques, including blood serology, stool antigen detection, or polymerase chain reaction, have not yet become a standard of laboratory management, but they can have a complementary and future role in clinical and outbreak management of parasitic intestinal infections.

# Protozoan Intestinal Infections

Common intestinal protozoan infections and the associated clinical features are shown in Table 3.

## FLAGELLATES

### Giardia lamblia

*Giardia lamblia* (also known as *Giardia intestinalis*) is probably the most common sporadic intestinal parasitic infection in North America. It is directly transmitted by fecally contaminated water and possibly food as the environmentally stable cysts. Once the cysts are ingested and in the stomach, the intraluminal trophozoite form of the parasite is released. It feeds in the upper regions of the small bowel. Although it attaches to the small bowel wall, *Giardia lamblia* does not invade submucosally.

Giardiasis is classically associated with upper and lower intestinal bloating and foul gas, abdominal cramping, and loose to watery diarrhea. Bloody stool is not a feature of giardiasis. Significant weight loss can occur with *Giardia* infections. Low-grade and chronic GI symptoms can also occur due to persistent infections or the development of malabsorption syndrome or lactose intolerance due to the original infection. These symptoms can continue for months to years.

Small bowel intubation, aspiration, or the use of entero tests or string tests is rarely required for diagnosis, and the techniques of preserved-fixed stool examination should be pursued first for diagnosis. Serologic testing for giardiasis is of little to no value. Both cysts and trophozoites can be found in the stool, but only the cysts survive in the environment to infect the next host. Humans are not the only hosts for *Giardia lamblia*, so other animal sources of contaminated water and potentially food can occur.

Young children are the most commonly infected patient with *Giardia*, but all age groups are at risk. International travelers, campers in wilderness areas who use ground water potentially fecally contaminated by other campers or wild animals, and persons whose social behavior creates exposure to feces, such as coprophagia and oral-anal contact, are at increased risk for infection. A rare cause of chronic giardiasis is congenital hypogammaglobulinemia. Asymptomatic infections are also very common, particularly in high-transmission areas including the tropics and some group-care settings. Some have debated if asymptomatic infections with *Giardia lamblia* need to be treated, but because of the ease of person-to-person transmission, a supportable argument can be made from a public health perspective to treat symptomatic and asymptomatic infected persons (see Table 1).

### Dientamoeba fragilis

*Dientamoeba fragilis* has no recognized cystic form and is found only in the flagellated trophozoite form in stool. Its mode of transmission is uncertain but is presumed to be fecal-oral, with perhaps an intermediary carrier host or an unrecognized environmentally stable form to bridge passage from the host to infecting the next victim. Whether *D. fragilis* is an intestinal pathogen or not is very controversial. An association with abdominal complaints, particularly in young children, is claimed, but treatment has inconsistent outcomes in both parasite clearance and in clinical improvement.

## AMEBAS

*Entamoeba histolytica* is the causative agent of amebiasis, which can be asymptomatic or can cause abdominal pain, diarrhea, and constitutional symptoms of fever, malaise, and weight loss. Invasive amebiasis is associated with bowel wall ulcerations, bleeding, and a dysentery syndrome with a diffuse colitis. Systemic invasion with the parasite causes luminal abscesses (amebomas) that can mimic constricting lesions of the colonic wall (strictures and malignancies), amebic peritonitis, and liver abscesses. The liver abscesses are remarkable for the lack of inflammatory host response (hence, a misnomer of "abscess"), can be multiple, and can rupture through the liver capsule, abdominal wall, or diaphragm into the pleural space or lung. The drainage from the abscess, described as *anchovy paste*, consists of necrotic liver cells and the parasite.

Aside from the classic morphology of the cysts and trophozoites of *E. histolytica*, on staining only the trophozoites of *E. histolytica* ingest red blood cells, which can be seen within the parasite. The clinicodiagnostic challenge is that several *Entamoeba* species are morphologically similar to *E. histolytica* but do not cause clinical illness. These species include *E. dispar*, *E. moshcovskii*, and the smaller *E. hartmanni*. Routine tests to distinguish these cysts and trophozoites in stool specimens are generally not available. As an estimate, 90% to 95% of what appears to be *E. histolytica* in North America are nonpathogenic species.

The clinical presentation, parasite intracellular red blood cells, finding *E. histolytica* trophozoites in a bowel ulcer, positive ameba serology, and typical radiologic and pathologic findings definitively characterize a case of invasive amebiasis. Fortunately, invasive *E. histolytica* is not endemic to most of North America, and clinical cases of invasive disease are rare. Mexico and parts of Latin America, southern Africa, and India are endemic areas for the invasive parasite. Immigrants, international travelers, and those in contact with a fecal carrier of *E. histolytica* are at risk for clinical disease from this parasite.

Although nonpathogenic *Entamoeba* species do not require treatment, even asymptomatic *E. histolytica* should be treated to reduce the risk of future invasive disease and prevent person-to-person

**TABLE 3**  Diagnosis of Intestinal Protozoa

| Parasitic Organism | Clinical Notes | Comments |
|---|---|---|
| **Protozoans** | | |
| *Balantidium coli* | Can cause a dysentery syndrome similar to amebic colitis | Large ciliated parasite of pigs, rarely affects humans |
| *Cryptosporidium* spp. | Self-limited diarrhea to profuse watery diarrhea, particularly in immunocompromised hosts (HIV/AIDS) | Requires specific staining or other diagnostic techniques on stool |
| *Cyclospora cayetanensis* | Similar illness to cryptosporidiosis | Has been associated with imported fresh fruit and international travel |
| *Dientamoeba fragilis* | Nonspecific intestinal symptoms; pathogenicity uncertain | Clinical response to treatment and parasite clearance inconsistent |
| *Entamoeba histolytica* | Asymptomatic to diarrhea, dysentery, and invasive tissue disease | Must be distinguished from morphologically identical nonpathogens |
| *Giardia lamblia* | Secretory and malabsorptive diarrhea | Cosmopolitan; fecal-oral |
| Intestinal microsporidiosis | Secretory, watery diarrhea | Most clinically severe in immunocompromised patients (HIV/AIDS) |
| **Metazoans** | | |
| *Enterobius vermicularis* | Pinworm: puritus ani, vulvitis, and vaginitis | Common infection in children; easily transmitted; autoinfection |
| *Trichuris trichiura* | Whipworm: intestinal irritation; rarely frank blood | Common infection in children |
| Hookworms | Microscopic blood loss, anemia | In addition to specific treatment, iron replacement is important |
| *Stronglyoides stercoralis* | Chronic, persistent infection; Risk of hyperinfection and disseminated disease with steroid use and immune compromise | High index of suspicion based on epidemiology and risk of exposure; Serologic screening for infection; Stool and body tissues or fluids for disease |
| *Taenia saginata* and *Diphyllobothrim* spp. | Nonspecific intestinal complaints; Passing of segments | Noninvasive giant tapeworms; Fish tapeworm associated with vitamin B$_{12}$ deficiency |
| *Taenia solium* | Similar symptoms to other giant adult tapeworms; Larval disease (neuro-cystercercosis) occurs in humans | Differential diagnosis from other *Taenia* spp. is essential for proper management of intestinal infection and consideration of tissue complications |
| Other intestinal tapeworms | Minor and usually nonspecific intestinal symptoms | Unusual infections in humans |
| *Ecchinococcus* spp. | Larval infection in humans; Endemic areas in rural and northern North America; No direct intestinal symptoms usually | *E. granulosis*: Cystic liver and other organ disease; *E. multilocularis*: Invasive cystic liver disease in Arctic regions of North America |
| Flukes | Few endemic infections in North America; largely imported | Nonspecific intestinal or biliary disease symptoms; An incidental, but clinically important stool O&P finding (also urine and rarely pulmonary), usually in immigrants |

*Abbreviation:* O&P = ova and parasites.

transmission (see Table 1). Except for the pathogenic *Entamoeba* species, intestinal ameba of human beings are nonpathogens and do not require treatment.

## INTESTINAL PARASITES WITH NO ORGAN OF LOCOMOTION

### Cryptosporidium Species

*Cryptosporidium* species infections cause acute and generally self-limited watery diarrhea syndromes. These infections occur commonly in young children who are in group-care settings, international travelers, and persons infected with HIV in whom cryptosporidiosis is an acquired immunodeficiency syndrome–defining condition. In the immunocompromised host, the volume of diarrhea stool losses can be life threatening. Cryptosporidiosis has also been associated with large urban water system fecal contamination and significant outbreaks in the United States. *Cryptosporidium* is very easily spread person-to-person, particularly in household contact situations with an affected child.

Specific treatment is generally not required in immunocompetent hosts. Supportive care and hydration for all patients, and antibiotics

(see Table 1) for immunosuppressed hosts, are indicated. Diagnosis requires special acid-fast staining of stools processed for O&P. The parasite can also be detected in bowel biopsies.

### Cyclospora cayetanensis

*Cyclospora cayetanensis* infections clinically follow a similar pattern to cryptosporidiosis, with watery diarrhea that is usually self-limited. The age distribution of affected persons extends to adulthood. Initial outbreaks in North America were associated with imported fresh food products from Latin America. Sporadic cases and cases in returned international travelers are also seen. This parasite is variably acid-fast staining, and oocysts autofluoresce under ultraviolet light microscopy. See Table 1 for treatment options.

### Isospora belli

Symptomatic infections with *Isospora belli* requiring medical care are unusual in immunocompetent hosts (see Table 1). As with most protozoan bowel infections, a short duration of diarrhea is the usual course, but chronic remittent diarrhea with abdominal cramps can also occur.

## Microsporidians

The microsporidian agents (*Enterocytozoon bieneusi, Encephalitozoon intestinalis*, and others) are obligate intracellular parasites of humans and cause diarrhea most notably in significantly immunocompromised patients. Other human hosts may be infected and can carry the parasite for a time, but prolonged intestinal illness, except in immunocompromised patients, does not occur with this parasite. Symptomatic care and management of the underlying immunocompromise condition, such as HIV/AIDS with antiretroviral treatment, is the most effective treatment approach (see Table 1).

## CILIATES

*Balantidium coli* is the only ciliated protozoan pathogen of human beings. Its natural host in North America is the domestic swine, and it rarely affects humans. The clinical presentation extends from asymptomatic to low-grade and chronic abdominal discomfort with diarrhea. In its most severe form, balantidiasis is very similar to bowel invasive amebiasis with a dysentery syndrome. Diagnosis is by stool O&P examination where the large ciliated organism is unique in diagnostic parasitology. See Table 1 for treatment options.

# Metazoan Intestinal Infections

The metazoan bowel infections represent the true worms affecting human beings. Most of these infections are associated with fecal contamination of the environment and involve either direct oral ingestion through food or water or an intermediary host for oral ingestion, but some are acquired by specific food consumption. A few of these parasites are not acquired through the ingestion route. Due to the generally high standards of both environmental and personal hygiene in North America, these infections are usually acquired by transmission under predictable conditions of poverty, close human contact, or international travel, or they are imported by migration from higher-prevalence areas of the world.

In addition to their morphologic and taxonomic differences, the intestinal worms often differ clinically from the protozoan infections by having complex life cycles limiting the potential for autoinfection. They have a defined life expectancy in the human host, and unless the host is reinfected, they can have a self-limited duration of infection due to tissue phases in development. They may be associated with host blood eosinophilia. Many, because of the size of the adult worms, are visible to the naked eye when passed by the host.

## THE ROUNDWORMS (NEMATODES)

### Enterobius vermicularis

*Enterobius vermicularis* (pinworm) is a cosmopolitan parasitic infection of the lower bowel, commonly affecting young children and their caregivers. Almost unique among the geohelminths, *E. vermicularis* eggs can be infectious immediately on passing in the stool. The adult worms pass out the anal verge to lay their eggs on the perianal skin, resulting in puritus ani. The eggs are taken up on the skin of the host's hands and fingernails during scratching, and if introduced into the mouth, they reinfect the affected person or infect anyone else that the infected person is in contact with. This has implications for clinical and therapeutic management approaches.

This parasite is also associated with vulvitis and vaginitis. Unlike other parasites, direct examination of the perianal area can reveal adult worms, which tend to be most active at night. Collection of specimens from the perianal area (pinworm paddles) may be most effective at confirming the diagnosis, because eggs are not plentiful in the stool O&P collection. See Table 2 for treatment options.

### Ascaris lumbricoides

*Ascaris lumbricoides*, also known as the round worm, is endemic in only a few areas of North America because it requires a period of soil incubation to be infectious to the next human host. Transmission is feces to soil contamination to oral route. Before establishing itself in the intestines, the fertilized egg releases its larva in the upper gut, where it migrates through the bowel wall to the lung and is aspirated back to the gut, where it completes its development into the adult worm. The pulmonary phase of the infection may be associated with cough, wheeze, or asthma-like symptoms, pulmonary infiltrates, and peripheral blood eosinophia.

Once in the intestines, the adult ascaris worm may be asymptomatic but due to its size (6-8 in × 0.25 in), a single worm in the wrong place (bile or pancreatic duct, appendix), migrating up the esophagus, or passed in the stool can cause significant attention or severe clinical illness. Although it is rare to have a large number of *Ascaris* adults, a ball of worms can block the gut lumen and manifest as an acute intestinal obstruction. See Table 2 for treatment options.

### Trichuris trichura

*Trichuris trichura* infections are also known as the *whipworm* due to the shape of the adult parasite. As for other geohelminths, it is also more common in children than in adults. It attaches to the lower intestine wall in feeding from luminal contents, causes bowel irritation, and can cause frequent stooling. Adult worms can be seen in the stool, but this infection is also easily diagnosed with stool O&P examination. See Table 2 for treatment options.

### Hookworm

Hookworm infection is one of the most common and debilitating helminth infections of humans due to the chronic blood loss and anemia associated with both of the most common hookworms, *Necator americanus* and *Ancylostoma duodenale*. The eggs passed in feces incubate in moist soil, where the larval forms penetrate through the skin and pass through the pulmonary tree before maturing to adulthood in the intestines. Although intestinal symptoms are often minor or even asymptomatic, iron deficiency, particularly in childhood and in pregnancy, has significant morbidity associated with it, including negative impact on intellectual development and increased fetal and maternal mortality. Aside from specific treatment (see Table 2), iron replenishment can prevent the sequelae of chronic anemia in affected children and women. Animal hookworms do not mature in the human host but can cause skin eruptions known as *cutaneous larval migrans*.

### Strongyloides stercoralis

*Strongyloides stercoralis* is another human hookworm but is capable of autoinfection in the human gut, and as a result can cause persistent infections lasting decades. It can also cause disseminated infection of larval forms when the human host becomes immunosuppressed by steroid use, age, or other illnesses such as human T-cell lymphotropic virus, type I. Hyperinfection is associated with larval worms penetrating into all visceral and cutaneous compartments. Diagnosis of chronic strongyloidiasis is challenging because eggs are rarely seen in stools, the larvae are in scarce numbers until hyperinfection occurs, and the adults live in the submucosal gut. In the right epidemiologic setting, strongyloides serology is diagnostic of infection. Eosinophilia is nonspecific and often is absent when the host is immunosuppressed. During hyperinfection, larval forms of several stages can be readily found in stool and in all body fluids and tissues. It is essential to think of this diagnosis based on epidemiologic risks (age, comorbid disease, and exposure in Asia, southern Europe, and parts of the United States) and the significant risks associated with immune suppression and disseminated disease, because treatment failure is common in advanced infections. See Table 2 for treatment options.

### Other Nematodes

Other nematode intestinal infections in humans are rare but are occasionally seen in patients in North America. *Angiostrongylus* species, *Capillaria phillipinensis*, and *Anasakis* species are three of the more common and important infections. See Table 2 for treatment options.

# THE TAPEWORMS (CESTODES)

## Beef Tapeworm

*Taenia saginata* (beef tapeworm) is acquired by ingesting the larval form in undercooked beef. It is most commonly acquired in sub-Sahara Africa and the Middle East. The adult worm matures in the upper gut of the human host by extensions from the head (scolex) and neck of segments of the tape-like worm. Adult *Taenia* species can reach several meters in length. Nonspecific abdominal symptoms are common with the giant tapeworms. The segments, which at maturity are filled with eggs (all *Taenia sp.* eggs are morphologically similar), can break off from the main body of the worm and can be passed singly or in chains. These segments can also be motile, causing the sensation of motion in the perianal area or in the undergarments. The proglottids or the head of the adult worm can be speciated in the parasitology laboratory. In the environment, the eggs are hardy and stable. Once ingested by a grazing cattle beast, the larval forms encyst in the muscle tissues, to be passed on to the next human host. Beef tapeworm does not cause invasive disease in humans. See Table 2 for treatment options.

## Pork Tapeworm

*Taenia solium* (pork tapeworm) occurs in areas of swine raising and human fecal contamination of the environment. Endemic zones include Mexico and much of Latin America, the Middle East, sub-Saharan Africa, and southern and Southeast Asia. Humans can serve as the definitive host (adult worm) by ingesting undercooked infected pork meat and as an intermediary host (larval forms) through ingestion of eggs passed in human feces or regurgitation and swallowing of eggs from an internal adult worm. The adult worms can manifest in a similar manner to the beef or fish tapeworm, but larval disease (cystercercosis) is much more severe due to larvae in neural tissue (brain, eyes). Diagnosis of intestinal infection is by examination of the stool O&P for *Taenia* spp. eggs or a proglottid or the head of the tapeworm.

## Fish Tapeworm

*Diphylobothrium latum* or *Diphylobothrium pacificum* (fish tapeworm) infections are acquired from eating infected and undercooked, raw, or pickled fish flesh. Infections are cosmopolitan but particularly common in fish-processing and fish-eating areas of the world. Humans are the definitive host for the adult worm, which can reach lengths of more than 5 meters. Symptoms of the adult fish tapeworm are similar to those for the *Taenia* species infections (see Table 2 for treatment options). The fish tapeworm can compete with the human host for absorption of vitamin $B_{12}$, resulting in pernicious anemia.

## Other Tapeworms

Other tapeworms affecting the human intestinal tract include the rat-associated *Hymenolepis nana* (dwarf tapeworm) and *Hymenolepis diminuta* (rat tapeworm) and the dog tapeworm (*Dipyllidium cannum*). *H. nana* is another worm whose eggs are infectious on passing from the human host, allowing autoinfection or person-to-person transmission. See Table 2 for treatment options.

*Ecchinococcus granulosis*, *E. multilocularis*, and other species do not have intestinal manifestations or findings of the parasite in stool specimens. Although the infections are acquired via ingestion and the gut, their major manifestations are hepatic or extraintestinal.

# THE FLUKES (TREMATODES)

*Schistosoma haemtobium*, *S. japonicum*, *S. mansoni*, and other human schistosome species are not endemically transmitted in North America.

However, they are important due to importation in international travelers and immigrants.

All species are acquired through contact with freshwater larvae that penetrate the skin. This phase of the infection is usually asymptomatic, but exposure to avian schistosome is associated with a cercarial rash. As the parasites mature and migrate through the human host, there is a systemic and pulmonary phase associated with fever and skin rash (Katayama fever) occurring several weeks to months before the eggs of the adult can be found in the stool or urine. This clinical diagnosis can be confirmed by serologic testing.

The adult worms settle in a venous plexus, where they mate and release eggs into the local tissues (liver, intestines, or urinary bladder). As the eggs pass through the tissues they cause an inflammatory reaction and form granulomata. Because the adult pairs can live and produce eggs for many decades, the total worm burden is important in determining the outcome of chronic infection.

Hepatitic fibrosis with venous hypertension, protein-wasting enteropathies, structural urinary tract abnormalities leading to chronic, recurrent bacterial infections, urinary tract outflow obstruction, hematuria, and bladder carcinoma are consequences of chronic schistosome infection. Other syndromes due to atypical deposition of schistosome eggs with granulomas can occur.

Morphologically diagnostic eggs can be found in the relevant specimen (stool, urine) or in tissue biopsies, where they are associated with granuloma formation. Treatment can clear the adult infections (see Table 2), but the consequences of the eggs in tissues and the secondary effects on the tissues are only diminished by early treatment and clearance of the adult worm burden.

Other trematode infections of humans are rare in North America. *Paragonimus westermani* (lung fluke), *Fasciola hepatica*, *Fasciola gigantica*, *Clonorchis* and *Opistorchis* species (liver flukes), *Fasciolopsis bruski*, *Heterophyes* species (intestinal flukes), and others can excrete their eggs in sputum (lung fluke) or stool (all three). See Table 2 for treatment options.

# REFERENCES

Centers for Disease Control and Prevention, Division of Parasitic Disease: *Blastocystis hominis* infection. Available at: http://www.dpd.cdc.gov/dpdx/HTML/Blastocystis.htm (accessed June 17, 2007).

Drugs for parasitic infections. Med Lett Drugs Ther 2004;46(1189):1-12.

Herwaldt BL, Beach MJ: The return of *Cyclospora* in 1997: Another outbreak of cyclosporiasis in North America associated with imported raspberries. Cyclospora Working Group. Ann Intern Med 1999;130:210-220.

Lee MB, Keystone JS, Kain KC: The cost implications of reporting non-pathogenic protozoa. Clin Infect Dis 2000;30:401-402.

Morris RD, Naumova EN, Griffiths JK: Did Milwaukee experience waterborne cryptosporidiosis before the large documented outbreak in 1993? Epidemiology 1998;9:264-270.

Pietrzak-Johnston SM, Bishop H, Wahlquist S, et al: Evaluation of commercially available preservatives for laboratory detection of helminths and protozoa in human fecal specimens. J Clin Micro 2000;38:1959-1964.

Pillai DR, Keystone JS, Sheppard DC, et al: *Entamoeba histolytica* and *Entamoeba dispar*: Epidemiology and comparison of diagnostic methods in a setting of nonendemicity. Clin Infect Dis 1999;29:1315-1318.

Redlinger T, Corella-Barud V, Graham J, et al: Hyperendemic *Cryptosporidium* and *Giardia* in households lacking municipal sewer and water on the United States–Mexico border. Am J Trop Med Hyg 2002;66:794-798.

Senay H, MacPherson DW: Blastocystis hominis: Epidemiology and natural history. Clin Infect Dis 1990;162:897-890.

Senay H, MacPherson DW: Parasitology: Diagnostic yield of stool examination. CMAJ 1989;140:1329-1331.

Wilson ME: A World Guide to Infections: Diseases, Distribution, Diagnosis. New York: Oxford University Press, 1991.

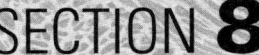

# Metabolic Disorders

## Diabetes Mellitus in Adults

Method of
*Anthony L. McCall, MD, PhD, and*
*J. Terry Saunders, PhD*

## Epidemiology

The Centers for Disease Control and Prevention (CDC) estimated that in 2005 the prevalence of diabetes in the United States was 20.8 million. Diabetes is diagnosed in 14.6 million persons and undiagnosed in 6.2 million. Type 2 diabetes mellitus (T2DM) is 90% to 95% of prevalent diabetes, and type 1 diabetes (T1DM) is about 5% to 10%. There are fewer persons with secondary or monogenic forms of diabetes, called *maturity-onset diabetes of the young* (MODY). About 41 million people in the United States are believed to have prediabetes.

The focus of this article is T2DM because it is the most prevalent form and is increasing rapidly in the United States and worldwide. A few comments are made on adult T1DM. This chapter emphasizes both lifestyle and pharmacologic treatments.

## Diagnosis and Classification of Diabetes and Prediabetes

### DIAGNOSIS

Most diabetes is diagnosed by random or fasting glucose (Table 1). Symptoms should be present if random glucose criteria are used, but surprisingly, many people with diabetes are relatively asymptomatic. In the elderly, cognitive changes can occur and atypical symptoms such as prostatism can appear. The American Diabetes Association (ADA) screening recommendations suggest screening every 3 years starting at age 45 for the general population, but they suggest earlier and more frequent screening in those with high risk.

Patients from diabetes-prone ethnic groups (e.g., Latin Americans, African Americans, Native Americans) or with a strong family history, polycystic ovary syndrome (PCOS), or gestational diabetes should have early and frequent screenings. High-risk persons include those with prediabetes (impaired glucose tolerance, impaired fasting glucose) or who meet the National Cholesterol Education Program (NCEP) criteria for the metabolic syndrome or its individual components (dyslipidemia, hypertension, central obesity, prediabetes). The metabolic syndrome as defined by the NCEP is criticized as flawed, but

such critique does not reduce the importance of fully documenting and treating cardiometabolic risk components in those with or at risk for T2DM. The metabolic syndrome concept is useful to teach patients and clinicians about these risks and the response of the overweight and sedentary to a healthier lifestyle.

### CLASSIFICATION

The classification of diabetes into its two most prominent types (T1DM and T2DM) seems straightforward in theory but in practice is increasingly confusing as more Americans become overweight. Although T1DM patients are traditionally lean, many now are overweight and some have metabolic syndrome characteristics. About 80% to 90% of persons with T2DM are overweight or have metabolic syndrome characteristics, but some are leaner and more active and do not have the metabolic syndrome. C-peptide measurements are not very helpful for those who are difficult to classify, but measuring three antibodies—including IA-2 (islet cell antigen 512), anti-GAD$_{65}$ (glutamic acid decarboxylase), and anti-insulin antibodies in high titers—can clarify a diagnosis of latent autoimmune diabetes. Age at onset, body habitus, severe loss of glycemic control with or without ketonemia, and weight loss all suggest insulin deficiency but might not be definitive.

## Pathophysiology

The primary causes of most adult diabetes are insulin resistance and lack of compensatory insulin secretion. Insulin resistance is typically longstanding and begins at a young age because of heredity combined with environmental causes (sedentary lifestyle and calorie overconsumption with resultant overweight). Insulin secretory defects usually start about 10 years before diagnosis, and no therapy is proven so far to prevent progressive loss of insulin secretion. A few patients develop diabetes associated with malnutrition, but this is much less common. Longstanding insulin resistance is associated with dyslipidemia, central obesity, hypertension, and hyperglycemia. This long prodrome accounts for the common coexistence of cardiovascular disease and diabetes.

### CARDIOVASCULAR RISK MANAGEMENT

Cardiovascular risk management in diabetes starts with lifestyle counseling and education. It is paramount that patients understand the intimate and direct links among diabetes, glycemic control, and cardiovascular disease. Drug interventions are ultimately needed for glycemia, lipid risks, and blood pressure in most patients. Women have higher relative risk and similar overall risk as men and are often undertreated. Specific recommended targets of therapy for diabetes

**TABLE 1**  Diagnosis and Classification of Diabetes and Prediabetes

| Diagnosis | Glucose Test | Diagnostic Level | Comments |
|---|---|---|---|
| Diabetes | Random | ≥200 mg/dL | Plus classic symptoms* |
| Diabetes | Fasting | ≥126 mg/dL | 8-hour fast; need confirmation |
| Diabetes | Postglucose load (75 g in nonpregnant adults) | ≥200 mg/dL at 2 h | Need confirmation |
| Prediabetes IFG | Fasting | ≥100 mg/dL | Decreased insulin secretion |
| Prediabetes IGT | Postglucose load (75 g) | 140-199 mg/dL at 2 h | Increased insulin resistance |

*Polyuria, polydipsia, unexplained weight loss.
*Abbreviations:* IFG = impaired fasting glucose; IGT = impaired glucose tolerance

in glycemia, blood pressure, dyslipidemia, and lifestyle are shown in Box 1.

## DOCUMENTING AND FOLLOWING COMPLICATIONS

Patients should have a thorough examination and evaluation for complications at the time of diabetes diagnosis. About one half of patients with newly diagnosed T2DM have established chronic complications, indicating delayed recognition of this disorder.

Neuropathy and circulatory signs and symptoms on foot examination should be assessed. Risk of ulcer and amputation can be gauged by 10-g Semmes-Weinstein monofilaments that test for severe neuropathy and attendant risk of ulceration. Retina examinations should be done by skilled eye professionals likely to pick up significant eye disease.

High-risk patients (poor glycemic control, established retinopathy, especially if preproliferative or worse) should be referred promptly to an eye specialist. Pregnancy counseling should be given to all women of childbearing age with diabetes. Microalbumin-to-creatinine ratio in the urine should be assessed and kidney function (serum creatinine and blood urea nitrogen [BUN]) should be tracked yearly.

Home glucose monitoring should be taught to patients so they understand the effects of food, stress, and exercise on glycemic patterns. Diabetes education should be arranged for all patients, preferably by a diabetes educator. Diabetes is unique in being a self-managed condition where patient knowledge and skills are critical to avoiding complications.

## Treatment

### BEHAVIORAL SELF-MANAGEMENT

Self-management of behavioral factors, including eating, physical activity, and psychological stress, is essential to good diabetes self-care. Ideally, professional support for behavioral self-management should be a coordinated, multidisciplinary effort involving expertise appropriate to a given patient from the areas of nutrition, nursing, exercise

---

**BOX 1**  Summary of Goals for Treatment

**Lifestyle**
***Medical Nutrition Therapy (individualized)***
- Appropriate calories
- Low saturated and *trans* fats
- Moderate, consistent carbohydrates (whole grains, vegetables, fruits)
- Healthy fats and proteins

***Activity***
- Consistent, regular activity tailored to complications and safety

**Glycemia**
- Best possible without frequent or severe hypoglycemia
- HbA1c <7% minimally; 6% or less if possible

**Self-Monitored Blood Glucose**
- Preprandial 90-130 mg/dL; <110 ideally
- Postprandial (1 to 2 h) <180 minimal; <140 ideally

**Lipids**
- LDL <100 mg/dL; optional <70 mg/dL (ACS, clinical ASCVD)
- Non-HDL <130 mg/dL; optional <100 mg/dL
- HDL >40 mg/dL (men); > 50 mg/dL (women)
- Triglycerides <150 mg/dL

**Blood Pressure**
- Systolic <130 mm Hg
- Diastolic < 80 mm Hg

*Abbreviations:* ACS = acute coronary syndrome, ASCVD = atherosclerotic cardiovascular disease (also multiple severe risk factors that are difficult to control); HDL = high-density lipoprotein; LDL = low-density lipoprotein.

---

 **CURRENT DIAGNOSIS**

- Screening for diabetes should be done in high-risk populations, especially:
  - Those with prediabetes or the metabolic syndrome.
  - High-risk ethnic groups (e.g., Native American, Latino American, African American).
  - Gestational diabetes.
- Patients might present with atypical symptoms.
- Most diabetes is type 2 in adults, but type 1 does occur in adults, and delayed diagnosis is common.
- Cardiovascular risk should be aggressively screened for and treated.
- Complications should be documented and tracked.
  - Check fasting lipids.
- Check renal function and albuminuria yearly.
  - Have a low threshold for stress testing, with imaging for all patients.
  - Refer for yearly eye examinations.
  - Check feet for sensation, deformity, and circulation at regular visits.
- All patients should receive an educational assessment and training in self-management and self-monitoring of blood glucose.
- Take a diet history; this is especially important for patients on insulin.
- Get a baseline HbA1c and repeat 2 to 4 times per year.

## CURRENT THERAPY

- Diabetes requires nutrition and behavioral self-management counseling as well as drug therapy.
- Repeatedly encourage healthy eating and an active lifestyle.
- Prediabetes diagnosis represents an opportunity for behavioral and drug interventions.
- Metformin (Glucophage) is usually the first drug therapy.
- Don't expect one drug to do the job for very poorly controlled glycemia.
- Dual defects (insulin resistance and secretion) should be addressed in most patients.
- Very insulin resistant patients might need a dual insulin resistance strategy.
- Therapy goals for both HbA1c and self-monitored blood glucose can be achieved in most patients.
- Cardiovascular risk reduction therapy is a very high priority.
- When patients have not met goals on dual oral agent therapy, basal insulin is often the most appropriate choice, particularly when patients are not near glycemic goals.
- For oral agent therapy, add don't switch unless side effects require it.
- When adding basal insulin, continue oral agent therapies.
- Threatening patients with insulin therapy is counterproductive.
- Follow the 3F rule: Fix the fasting glucose first, especially in patients with poor glycemic control.
- Prompt recognition of the need for meal insulin is critical to achieve glycemic goals.
- Balance meal and basal insulin.

training, and behavioral counseling. The provider should develop a referral network of available multidisciplinary resources and make regular use of any appropriate community-based resources (e.g., weight loss programs, fitness programs, diabetes support groups). Unfortunately, multidisciplinary resources are often in short supply or difficult to pay for. Therefore, it is essential that the provider develop basic skills and techniques for working with patients on behavior change.

Behavior change is slow and is inherently a multisession activity. Quick, one-shot interventions seldom change longstanding patterns of behavior. Initial sessions should be scheduled closely together (1-2 weeks), then further apart as the patient gains momentum and confidence. If multiple one-on-one sessions are impossible, other options such as group meetings, telephone support, or e-mail messaging should be considered.

Behavior change interventions should be highly individualized and specific. General advice about diet and exercise does not address the life experience or problems of a given patient and is often perceived as insensitive or unhelpful. Arriving at individualized objectives for behavior change can be accomplished using a simple three-step process composed of initial assessment, setting behavioral objectives, and follow-up and reassessment.

### Initial Assessment

Initial assessment includes identifying salient features of social and family history that can affect efforts to change behavior. A nutrition assessment should be performed, including an appraisal of usual food intake, the patient's perception of problem eating behavior, and weight history. A physical activity assessment should also be conducted, focusing on past and current physical activity, preferences, perceived barriers,

and general attitudes. Readiness to make changes in behavior should be assessed by asking how important a patient thinks it is to change a given area of behavior and how confident she or he can succeed in making changes (on a 1 to 10 scale). Discussion of specific objectives for behavioral change should occur in areas where the patient indicates a definite readiness to begin. Other areas of change should be discussed, but not forced or driven by the provider. Finally, ask patients about current levels and sources of stress. Because depression is common with diabetes, patients should be screened for possible depression.

### Behavioral Objectives

Setting behavioral objectives is initiated and facilitated by the provider, but the patient is responsible for selecting his or her own behavioral objectives. Resist the temptation to take over responsibility for this function. Objectives should be FIRM: *f*ew (1-3 at a time is plenty), *i*ndividualized to the patient's specific behavioral challenges, *r*ealistic (beware of trying to make big strides quickly), and *m*easurable. For measurement, the patient should be given a tracking form (such as the example in Figure 1) to use in recording daily progress on each objective. Note that although the patient might have long-term goals in the areas of weight loss, calorie intake, or general fitness, specific behavioral objectives such as eating a bowl of cereal for breakfast or walking one-half hour on five mornings each week are the means to achieving those outcomes. The primary focus of provider-patient discussions of progress should be on behavioral objectives, not outcomes.

### Follow-up and Reassessment

Follow-up and reassessment occur during each return visit, following a period of patient efforts to carry out mutually agreed on behavioral objectives. Reassessment focuses on the behavioral records kept by patients as well as on their verbal reports of difficulties and successes. Praise and encouragement are the order of the day. Efforts to initiate behavior change are highly responsive to external positive reinforcement, and the patient will need maximum external reinforcement until new behavior becomes self-sustaining. After review and discussion of patient records, new behavioral objectives or incremental changes in existing objectives are selected by mutual agreement, with the patient taking the lead.

A modest weight loss of 5% to 10% has a positive impact on cardiovascular risk factors and progression of diabetes. Reassure patients that medical goals for weight loss are achievable and worth the effort.

When discussing changes in eating with patients, distinguish dieting from gradual behavioral changes that result in a lasting pattern of healthy eating. Diets are impermanent and run the risk of large weight losses followed by even larger weight gains. Gradual behavioral changes offer the possibility of permanent lifestyle changes.

Prohibiting or demonizing foods is counterproductive. It leads patients to think of food in moral extremes (e.g., "sugar is bad for my diabetes") rather than along a continuum of nutritional benefit and blood glucose control. Food prohibition also casts the provider as withholding and overly controlling. These traps can be avoided by exploring very small changes that are not perceived as significant losses.

Patients may be extremely confused about the role of carbohydrates in weight loss and weight maintenance because of popular myths about sugar and the controversy surrounding low-carbohydrate diets. Low-carbohydrate diets (<130 g/day) are not recommended as an approach to weight loss. Carbohydrates should be included as an important part of a healthy diet for people with diabetes. Recommendations for limiting carbohydrate consumption at meals are based on controlling postprandial blood glucose (<180 mg/dL 1 to 2 hours after beginning a meal). Carbohydrate counting and blood glucose pattern management are complicated and time consuming to teach. Referral to a dietitian for medical nutrition therapy (MNT) or nutrition education through an ADA-recognized diabetes patient education program is recommended.

The best place to begin setting behavioral objectives for nutrition and exercise is where the patient is currently. Obtaining a 3-day food

**My Behavioral Goals**

To take better care of my diabetes and improve my health, I will:
(Write your behavioral goal in the blank spaces below and track your daily progress in the boxes on the tracking form. Make notes about your successes and challenges.)

Walk for 30 minutes, 5 days per week

Circle the day you will start and mark your progress every day with a check or number.

| Monday | Tuesday | Wednesday | Thursday | Friday | Saturday | Sunday |
|--------|---------|-----------|----------|--------|----------|--------|
|        |         | (20)      | 10       | 25     | 30       | 25     |
| 0      | 30      |           |          |        |          |        |
|        |         |           |          |        |          |        |

| Date | My Successes |
|------|--------------|
| 11/30 | Finally did 30 minutes on Saturday! |
|      |              |
|      |              |
|      |              |
|      |              |

| | My Challenges |
|------|---------|
|      |         |
|      |         |
|      |         |
|      |         |
|      |         |

**FIGURE 1.** Example of a behavioral goals tracking form.

record (2 work days and one nonwork day) and a baseline for activity (we generally use a week of daily steps measured with a pedometer) provide a solid baseline for setting objectives.

An irregular pattern of eating often underlies unhealthy food choices. For example, staying up late encourages late-night snacking, which in turn can suppress interest in eating breakfast. Eating tends to be deferred to the afternoon or evening, perpetuating the cycle.

A modest reduction in caloric consumption of around 250 to 500 kcal/day and moderate physical activity on the order of at least 150 minutes a week are the recommended approaches to weight loss. Reducing calories through decreased food consumption is more effective for weight loss than increasing energy expenditure through physical activity. Box 2 contains a checklist of healthy eating behaviors that can be used to stimulate patients' thinking about places they might like to make changes. Physical activity plays an important role in weight maintenance, but higher levels of activity (200 min/week) may be required to prevent long-term weight regain. Box 3 lists ways that patients can become more active. It is worth repeating that the point of these and other suggestions is not to direct patients but to expand their thinking about what might work for them.

Stress reduction is important in controlling blood glucose, but it can also play a role by helping patients achieve a mental focus on their behavior-management efforts. We encourage patients to sit calmly for a period of 5 to 10 minutes each day, focusing on slow deep breathing and muscle relaxation. Activities such as yoga or tai chi also reduce stress and support awareness of body and mind. Box 4 contains suggestions for coping behaviors that may be useful to patients in dealing with stress.

## PHARMACOLOGIC THERAPY

### Overview

Eventually, most patients with T2DM require drug treatment, often with multiple agents (combination therapy). Progressive insulin secretory loss probably is the primary explanation for the need to advance treatment. A resultant general rule with all therapies is *add, don't switch*. Table 2 lists major types of pharmacotherapeutic interventions with their usual hemoglobin (Hb) A1c lowering, balance of preprandial versus postprandial effects, and some comments on their actions and side effects. Table 3 lists classes of drugs, commonly used agents, and typical doses.

Recently the ADA and European Association for the Study of Diabetes (EASD) have issued a joint consensus algorithm on controlling hyperglycemia in T2DM. In our practice, we similarly initiate behavioral self-management along with medication, typically metformin unless there are contraindications or intolerance. Commonly, ineffective early attempts by physicians to change behavior (e.g., giving general advice) lead to abandonment of this therapy. A second oral medication may be initiated if patients cannot achieve glycemic goals. Commonly, we favor insulin secretagogues especially glimepiride (Amaryl) or extended-release glipizide (Glucotrol XL) for their relatively low risk of hypoglycemia, convenient once-daily dosing, and low expense. An alternative treatment strategy for heavier, more insulin-resistant patients is use of a thiazolidinedione, effectively a dual insulin-resistance strategy (see thiazolidinediones).

More reliably effective is the use of basal insulin treatment as a second agent to achieve control. Insulin initiation should be preceded

---

## BOX 2  Checklist of Healthy Eating Behaviors

☑ **Eat meals and snacks at set times to promote health.**

*Examples:*
- I will eat breakfast within 1 hour of getting up.
- I will not skip meals.
- Other: ...............................................
...............................................

☑ **Eat healthy carbohydrates.**

*Examples:*
- I will avoid regular soft drinks and choose water or diet soft drinks instead.
- I will eat 5-7 servings of fruits and vegetables every day.
- I will choose whole-grain breads and cereals.
- Other: ...............................................
...............................................

☑ **Decrease serving sizes.**

*Examples:*
- I will keep a record of the food I eat and drink.
- I will know what counts as a serving size.
- When I am eating out, I will share or split an entrée and eat a salad.
- Other: ...............................................
...............................................

☑ **Eat less fat and choose healthy fats.**

*Examples:*
- I will bake, broil, roast, grill, or boil instead of fry food.
- I will have a meatless meal at least once a week.
- I will choose fried or high-fat foods no more than once a week.
- I will drink fat-free or low-fat milk.
- I will use healthy oils (olive oil, canola oil) and buy tub margarine.
- Other: ...............................................
...............................................

☑ **Make other healthy choices.**

*Examples:*
- I will drink plenty of fluids (at least 8 glasses of water or low-calorie fluid per day).
- I will limit how much alcohol I drink. (Women should drink no more than 1 alcoholic drink per day. Men should drink no more than 2 alcoholic drinks per day.)
- Other: ...............................................
...............................................

*Unpublished source:* Virginia Center for Diabetes Professional Education, University of Virginia; Virginia Diabetes Council.

---

by an open discussion of the patient's attitudes, beliefs, and possible fears regarding insulin. Insulin therapy should never be used as a threat or possible negative consequence for failure to carry out behavioral management. Many patients associate insulin with serious diabetes complications and mortality. A positive attitude about the value of insulin therapy and a reassuring, educational approach can help to reduce initial fears enough to begin. Self-demonstration of injection technique using saline is also useful in overcoming fear of injections. Improvement in blood glucose control with insulin generally makes patients feel better, which further reinforces its perceived value.

## Oral Agents

### Secretagogues

These drugs enhance insulin secretion. There are first- and second-generation oral sulfonylureas; the latter are most commonly used. They are inexpensive, are moderately effective, and often can be dosed once daily. First-generation agents such as tolbutamide, chlorpropamide (Diabenese), and tolazamide (Tolinase) are less often used than the second-generation agents glyburide (Diabeta, Glynase), glipizide (Glucotrol), and glimepiride (Amaryl).

---

## BOX 3  Checklist for Physical Activity

☑ **Do something that you enjoy.**

*Examples:*
- I will take the stairs.
- I will park my car farther away and walk.
- I will walk.
- I will swim or do water exercises.
- I will ride a bike.
- I will use an exercise video.
- I will do yoga.
- Other: ...............................................
...............................................

☑ **How often?**

*Examples:*
- ❏ Every day
- ❏ 3x/week
- ❏ 5x/week
- ❏ ..............

☑ **How long?**

*Examples:*
- ❏ 10 minutes
- ❏ 15 minutes
- ❏ 20 minutes
- ❏ 30 minutes
- ❏ 60 minutes
- ❏ __ minutes

☑ **Limit inactivity.**

*Examples:*
- I will watch no more than 1 hour of television per day.
- I will spend no more than 2 hour(s) per day on the computer.
- Other: ...............................................
...............................................

*Unpublished source:* Virginia Center for Diabetes Professional Education, University of Virginia; Virginia Diabetes Council.

The dose-response characteristics of sulfonylureas suggest that one half the approved maximum dose achieves maximum HbA1c lowering, typically 1 to 1.5 percentage points. If the patient is not at goal with half-maximum doses, it is more effective to add a second agent than raise the dose. Common side effects include hypoglycemia, weight gain of about 2 kg, and, more rarely, hematologic or skin reactions.

Rapid secretagogues, the glinides (repaglinide [Prandin] and nateglinide [Starlix]), are more expensive and should be considered for patients who are sulfonylurea allergic, extremely erratic in eating, or at high risk for hypoglycemia.

### Biguanides

Metformin is the only available agent in this class. It is useful in both obese and normal weight T2DM patients. HbA1c lowering is typically about 1.5 percentage points in monotherapy or in combination therapy. Maximum efficacy is achieved with 2000 mg daily. The sustained-release preparation will last 24 hours if given with the evening meal.

Metformin's hypoglycemic mechanism is primarily by reduction of liver glucose production. It is cleared by the kidney, and the risk of lactic acidosis, a rare side effect with 50% mortality, may be increased in renal dysfunction. Serum creatinine should be less than 1.4 mg/dL in women and less than 1.5 mg/dL in men, and glomerular filtration rate (GFR) should be assessed in patients 80 years and older. It is also an increased lactic acidosis risk in patients with drug-treated congestive heart failure (CHF) or respiratory insufficiency. Intravascular contrast administration should prompt holding the drug for 24 to 48 hours until renal function is assured to be adequate. GI side effects are common initially and are dose dependent but wane; they can require gradual titration. Sustained-release preparations have fewer GI side effects. Weight gain is less with this drug than with many others for diabetes. The United Kingdom Prospective Diabetes Study (UKPDS) found that risk of MI and death was reduced, making it a first choice for pharmacotherapy in most patients.

## TABLE 2 Overview and Characteristics of Therapy Interventions

| Drug Type | HbA1c Lowering (Percentage Points) | Effect on Glycemia Levels | | Actions | Side Effects |
|---|---|---|---|---|---|
| | | Preprandial | Postprandial | | |
| SUs and non-SU rapid secretagogues | 1.5-2 | ++ | + | Direct and indirect secretagogue | Hypoglycemia, weight gain |
| Biguanides | 1.5-2 | +++ | 0 | ↓ hepatic glucose output | GI, lactic acidosis, weight neutral |
| Thiazolidinediones | 0.7-1.5 | +++ | 0 | ↑ muscle insulin sensitivity | Edema, CHF |
| Incretin agonists | 0.9-1.1 | + | ++ | Strong GLP-1 effects ↑ insulin ↓glucagon | Nausea, vomiting, weight loss |
| DPP-4 inhibitors | 0.6-0.8 | + | ++ | Moderate GLP-1 effects ↑ insulin ↓ glucagon | Weight neutral |
| Basal insulin | 1.5-2.5 | +++* | 0* | ↓ hepatic glucose output, ↑ muscle glucose disposal | Hypoglycemia, weight gain |
| Meal insulin | 1.0-2.0 | 0-+* | ++* | ↓ hepatic glucose output, ↑ muscle glucose disposal | Hypoglycemia, weight gain |
| Inhaled insulin | 1.5-2.5 | ++ | ++ | ↓ hepatic glucose output, ↑ muscle glucose disposal | Hypoglycemia, weight gain, cough, altered PFTs |
| Pramlintide | 0.5-0.7 | 0-+ | ++ | ↑ insulin ↓ glucagon | Nausea, vomiting |

*Abbreviations:* CHF = congestive heart failure; DPP = dipeptidyl peptidase; GI = gastrointestinal; GLP = glucagon-like peptide; Hb = hemoglobin; PFT = pulmonary function test; SU = sulfonylurea.

**TABLE 3 Dosing Used for Various Agents**

| Agent | Dose |
| --- | --- |
| **Thiazolidinediones** | |
| Pioglitazone (Actos) | 15, 30, 45 mg |
| Rosiglitazone (Avandia) | 2, 4, 8 mg |
| **α-Glucosidase inhibitors** | |
| Acarbose (Precose) | 25, 50, 100 mg ac |
| Miglitol (Glycet) | 25, 50, 100 mg ac |
| **Biguanides** | |
| Metformin (Glucophage) IR | 500, 850, 1000 mg |
| Metformin SR | 500, 750 mg |
| **Glinides** | |
| Nateglinide (Starlix) | 60-120 mg ac |
| Repaglinide (Prandin) | 0.5-4 mg ac |
| **Sulfonylureas (Second Generation)** | |
| Glimepiride (Amaryl) | 1-4 mg |
| Glipizide (Glucotrol) IR | 2.5-20 mg |
| Glipizide SR | 2.5-10 mg |
| Glyburide (Glynase) | 1.25-10; 1.5-6 mg |
| **Incretins** | |
| Exenatide (Byetta) | 5, 10 μg |
| Sitagliptin (Januvia) | 100 mg |
| Vildagliptin (Galvus)[4] | 50, 100 mg |
| **Amylin Agonists** | |
| Pramlintide (Symlin) | 15, 30, 60, 90, 120 μg |
| **Insulin** | |
| Aspart (Novolog) | No dose limit |
| Detemir (Levemir) | No dose limit |
| Glargine (Lantus) | No dose limit |
| Glulisine (Apidra) | No dose limit |
| Inhaled powder insulin (Exubera) | No dose limit |
| Lispro (Humalog) | No dose limit |
| NPH | No dose limit |
| Regular | No dose limit |

[4]Not yet approved for use in the United States.
*Abbreviations:* ac = before meals; IR = immediate release; NPH = neutral protamine Hagedorn; SR = sustained release.

### Thiazolidinediones

Two drugs of the thiazolidinedione (TZD) class are available, rosiglitazone (Avandia) and pioglitazone (Actos). Both have similar glycemic-lowering effects and side effects. These drugs work by increasing the sensitivity of muscle tissue and fat to insulin action, probably through action of adipokines like adiponectin and muscle effects on adenosine monophosphate–activated protein kinase (AMPK), a fuel sensor enzyme. HbA1c lowering varies considerably, dependent on whether patients are very insulin resistant (central adiposity, often hypertriglyceridemia) and whether there is adequate endogenous insulin secretion (short diabetes duration or secretagogues) or insulin is given.

Diabetes may be prevented with rosiglitazone, and this is being tested for pioglitazone. Both TZDs can precipitate edema, weight gain due to obesity, and occasionally congestive heart failure even absent a prior heart failure history. It is thus wise to track weight in all patients and limit it to 5 or 6 pounds. The risk of heart failure is increased when TZDs are combined with insulin. Both TZDs have beneficial effects on some lipid parameters, but pioglitazone appears more effective in reducing hypertriglyceridemia. Recent analyses suggest, but do not prove, increased coronary ischemic events with rosiglitazone. Pioglitazone studies suggest reduced ischemic risk (stroke or myocardial infarction). Both medicines may increase heart failure, and new studies suggest more self-reported fractures in women, which will need further study.

### Incretins

Incretins are gut hormones that enhance food-induced insulin secretion. Incretin drugs either are receptor agonists (e.g., exenatide) for glucagon-like peptide-1 (GLP-1), perhaps the most important incretin, or they enhance endogenous levels for both GLP-1 and gastrointestinal insulinotropic polypeptide (GIP).

Exenatide (Byetta) is the only available GLP-1 receptor agonist. Its actions increase meal insulin, decrease meal hyperglucagonemia, decrease rate of stomach emptying, and suppress appetite, which may cause a moderate weight loss. It works immediately on injection. It has substantial GI side effects including nausea, vomiting, and diarrhea in a large minority of patients. Despite this, many patients favor it, probably because the side effects generally wane within weeks and there can be substantial weight loss in some very overweight patients. Typically, exenatide is given in doses of 5 μg twice daily at meals, advancing after a month to 10 μg twice daily. Patients might report that nausea is more tolerable if they have a little food in their stomach at the time of dosing.

Because incretin drugs all have a glucose-dependent insulin secretion and glucagon suppression, there is little tendency for hypoglycemia used alone or when they are combined with metformin and TZDs in comparison with sulfonylureas. HbA1c lowering with exenatide has been 0.9 to 1.1 percentage points.

### Dipeptidyl Peptidase-4 Inhibitors

Dipeptidyl peptidase-4 (DPP-4) is the peptidase that normally rapidly degrades the incretins GLP-1 and GIP to inactive proteolytic products. Inhibitors of DPP-4 have been shown to enhance GLP-1 and GIP levels to high physiologic levels and thereby reduce HbA1c concentrations, typically about 0.6 to 0.8 percentage points. At this writing, one of two drugs, sitagliptin (Januvia), has been approved and appears to be effective in doses of 100 mg once daily. This drug is excreted by the kidney largely unchanged and therefore should be given in lower doses (50 mg once daily) for those with moderate renal insufficiency (GFR 30-50 mL/min) and further reduced (25 mg) for those with severe renal dysfunction (GFR <30 mL/min).

Vildagliptin (Galvus)[4] has been studied in once- or twice-daily dosing studies in the range of 50 to 200 mg daily. It appears to have HbA1c lowering similar to sitagliptin's. Vildagliptin doses need not be adjusted with renal dysfunction. Because both DPP-4 inhibitors are oral, they may be preferred to the injectable exenatide. The side effects for these drugs are relatively minor and cause little nausea, vomiting, or diarrhea. They also do not cause significant weight loss but, like metformin, appear to be weight neutral.

### Amylin Agonists

Insulin is cosecreted with another beta cell hormone called amylin. The effects of amylin appear to be to help lower glycemia, reduce excess glucagon levels, curb appetite, and possibly reduce the rate of gastric emptying. A synthetic analogue of amylin, pramlintide (Symlin), is available as an injectable agent for treating both T1DM and T2DM as an adjunct to insulin. It lowers HbA1c about 0.5 to 0.7 percentage points. It also appears to have some weight loss effect, typically around 1 to 2 kg. Its action primarily controls glucose postprandially. Nausea and vomiting can occur in patients with either T2DM or T1DM but are worse in T1DM patients who require low doses at first (15 μg or less with meals) and slower titration. Those with T2DM usually start with 60 μg and can usually advance to 90 to 120 μg at meals.

### Insulin

#### Barriers to Insulin Use

Insulin deficiency underlies the genesis of both T1DM and T2DM. Progression of therapy to use of insulin typically with oral agents in T2DM also seems predicated on progressive loss of insulin secretion. Nonetheless, it is often started too late, and patients often are in very poor control when this is done. Reluctance by patients and physicians alike might underlie this. Physicians should understand that

---

[4]Not yet approved for use in the United States.

exogenous insulin in T2DM is needed, does not negatively alter life quality, and is more likely to achieve therapeutic targets. Moreover, exogenous insulin does not worsen insulin resistance, does not cause excess cardiovascular disease, and has a low frequency of severe hypoglycemia, especially when used relatively early in the disease. Table 4 lists common insulin preparations and some notes about kinetics and timing.

### Starting Insulin: Use of Basal Insulin in Type 2 Diabetes

How should insulin be started? Practitioners should use temporary insulin for patients whose glycemia is initially poorly controlled or when patients temporarily have worse control due to illness or medications, such as glucocorticoids. It is unwise to use insulin as a threat because it creates a sense of personal failure and dread of insulin use. When therapy progresses but there is failure to achieve glycemic goals after one or two oral medications, use of basal insulin is often the best way to achieve euglycemia, especially if patients are much more than 1 percentage point from HbA1c goal (< 7%).

The Treat-to-Target Trial offers a good example of how to initiate insulin therapy. In this study, as often in our practice, patients start with a basal insulin either with NPH insulin or insulin glargine (Lantus). Insulin detemir (Levemir) represents another new option to be used similarly. Insulin is instituted as 10 U once daily, commonly in the evening near bedtime, followed by weekly increases between 2 and 8 units depending on proximity to glucose goals, focusing on the fasting glucose.

This strategy is sometimes called the *fix the fasting first* rule. Average doses in that study were around 45 to 50 units for patients whose BMI was about 31 kg/m². An alternative initial dosing might be 0.2 U/kg body weight, but whatever the starting dose, a forced titration guided by patient self-monitoring with clear communication of target fasting glucose (90-130 mg/dL), size of increment (or decrement in case of hypoglycemia; usually 10%-20% of dose), and frequency of change (every 3-7 days) is necessary to get most patients to overall glycemic (HbA1c) goal. This strategy is referred to as *pattern management*. The intent is to use monitoring to adjust the insulin dose likely to affect the fasting glucose for basal insulin therapy. NPH and detemir usually can be used once daily, typically at bedtime. Patients using glargine may choose any time of the day as long as it is reasonably consistent, usually within an hour. Occasionally, twice-daily NPH or detemir is used.

At some point, basal insulin therapy alone may be insufficient for glycemic control for T2DM patients. Usually this is a consideration in patients whose HbA1c values are over 9% to 9.5% or where the fasting goal is met but HbA1c remains elevated. The need for meal insulin is particularly likely to occur with larger meals, such as supper. Diagnostically, what is important is to have patients check either both before and after large meals or, if they are unwilling to check frequently, simply check about 2 to 3 hours after meals. Self-monitored glucose values that exceed even minimum postprandial glycemic guidelines (<180 mg/dL) indicate the need for meal insulin. A common mistake made in practice is to treat fasting hyperglycemia only with increases in basal insulin, when in some patients, the cause is overeating or lack of meal insulin the previous evening. This can be discerned by observing the pattern of glycemia, with lows often between meals or overnight and highs occurring after meals or at bedtime.

## FIXED-RATIO COMBINED INSULINS

A commonly employed strategy is to use fixed-ratio combination short-acting (either regular or rapid analogue) insulin combined with

---

### TABLE 4  Insulin Preparations

| Insulin Type | Pharmacokinetics | | | Comments |
|---|---|---|---|---|
| | Onset (h) | Peak (h) | Duration (h) | |
| **Basal Insulin** | | | | |
| NPH (Humulin N, Novolin N) | 0.5 | 4-10 | 18 | Kinetics is dose dependent; Peak effects exert meal action; Dose at breakfast, hs, supper* |
| Glargine† (Lantus) | 2-4 | none | 24* | Up to 1/3 of C-peptide-negative T1DM need bid administration; Dose can be given at any time of day if consistent |
| Detemir† (Levemir) | | Less peak activity than NPH | | Kinetics is dose dependent; Dose at breakfast, hs, supper* |
| **Meal Insulin** | | | | |
| Regular (Humulin R, Novolin R) | 15-30 | 2-3 | 5-8 | Give 1/2 hour before meals |
| Lispro (Humalog) | 0.1-0.2 | 1.5-2.0 | 4 | Dose at mealtime or immediately after |
| Aspart (Novolog) | 0.1-0.2 | 1.5-2.0 | 4 | Dose at mealtime or immediately after |
| Glulisine (Apidra) | 0.1-0.2 | 1.5-2.0 | 4 | Dose at mealtime or immediately after |
| **Mixed Preparations** | | | | |
| NPH/regular (Humulin, Novolin) | 70/30 dual kinetics based on components | | | Dosing 1/2 hour before meals; Should not be dosed at hs |
| Lispro/NPLispro (Humalog Mix75/25, | 25/75 dual kinetics | | | Dosing at mealtime; should not be dosed at hs |
| Lispro/NPLispro Humalog Mix 50/50) | 50/50 dual kinetics | | | Dosing at mealtime; should not be dosed at hs |
| Aspart/NPAspart (NovoLog Mix 70/30) | 30/70 dual kinetics | | | Dosing at mealtime; should not be dosed at hs |
| Inhaled insulin (Exubera) | 0.1-0.2 | 1.5-2.0 | 6-8 | Meal insulin dosing with substantial basal insulin effects |

*Bedtime dosing may be preferred for some patients, especially those on low doses.
†Should not be mixed with other insulins or used in the same syringe that other insulin has been in.
*Abbreviations:* hs = bedtime; NPH = neutral protamine Hagedorn.

intermediate insulin (NPH or neutral protamine modified rapid analogue that mimics NPH timing). Examples of these preparations include 70/30 NPH and regular insulin, 75/25 neutral protamine lispro and lispro insulin (Humalog), and 70/30 neutral protamine aspart and aspart insulin (Novolog). These have the advantage of being able to achieve control very conveniently in T2DM patients who have quite poor control (HbA1c of 9.5% or more) with a simple twice-daily injection regimen. They also offer the advantage of greater dosing accuracy, especially when used with insulin pens. Important to the success of these formulations is consistent eating and carbohydrate intake with meals. Unfortunately, when such consistency is not advised or followed, patterns of glycemia can be erratic and hypoglycemia can be significantly increased due to both components of the combination. Patients who skip meals are poor candidates for such treatments and should either switch to individual dosing of an insulin mixture or, even safer, use a basal bolus insulin regimen.

## INHALED INSULIN

Recently approved and marketed is the first available dry-powder inhaled insulin (Exubera), which is absorbed by pulmonary capillaries. The kinetics of this agent are unique and it is always dosed only at mealtimes. It has a rapid onset similar to that of rapid analogues, but because it is regular insulin, its duration of action is 6 to 8 hours, which presumably accounts for substantial lowering of fasting glucose levels (50 mg/dL or more) in some studies. Dosing in milligrams (not units) is initially suggested based on weight, and doses of blister packs are administered by a fairly large inhaler (11.5 inches when open) that patients must be taught to use. Blister packs are available in 1-mg and 3-mg strengths. Patients weighing 66 to 87 lbs should start with a 1-mg pack at meals, and patients who weigh more than 308 lbs should use up to two 3-mg packs plus a 1-mg pack, which are taken sequentially.

Cough and changes in pulmonary function tests may occur. Although these appear to be mostly mild and reversible, they require screening with an forced expiratory volume at 1 second (FEV$_1$), and it is recommended also to consider testing for dissociation of pulmonary diffusing capacity (DLCO) before treatment. Exubera should not be used if either of these two lung tests are less than 70% of predicted. An American Thoracic Society–approved spirometer should be used to evaluate lung function. Repeat testing is suggested at 6 months, 1 year, and yearly thereafter following treatment initiation.

## ADULTS WITH TYPE 1 DM

A significant minority of patients with a diagnosis of T2DM actually have a late onset of T1DM and typical autoimmunity (IA-2 antibodies, GAD-65 antibodies, and insulin antibodies). The diagnosis should certainly be suspected in patients who rapidly fail combination oral agent therapy. Nonobese body habitus, marked weight loss, extremely elevated glucose values, or a family or personal history of autoimmune disease (e.g., Hashimoto's or Graves' thyroid problems) should lead to diagnostic evaluation for such signs of autoimmunity.

T1DM patients need combined mealtime and basal insulin therapy. Although it is tempting to do so in a convenient fashion with combined preparations such as those with analogue fixed ratios, it usually is far preferable to use a better basal insulin, such as glargine or detemir combined with a rapid-acting analogue (separately injected) before meals. Sometimes an insulin pump is the best way for patients who have frequent hypoglycemia or marked variability to achieve good glycemic control safely. T1DM patients should preferably be seen by an endocrine specialist or other practitioner with extensive experience in T1DM management. Ready access to diabetes educators is an important key to success with both T1DM and T2DM.

## ADULTS WITH TYPE 2 DM

Many T2DM patients eventually need mealtime insulin. For those on insulin alone, incretin mimetics[1] can be successfully used for mealtime

control, because they effectively lower prandial hyperglycemia. If using exenatide, then additional injections will be required at the two major meals of the day. If using an incretin-enhancer drug such as sitagliptin, injections are not required. There are no published data yet to provide guidelines for this strategy, but we have occasionally used this approach with exenatide in patients who need to lose weight, who gain considerable weight with meal insulin, or who experience poor control despite attempts to regulate meal glycemia with short-acting insulins.

## REFERENCES

American Diabetes Association: Diagnosis and classification of diabetes mellitus. Diabetes Care 2006;29(Suppl. 1):S43-S48.

Diabetes Prevention Program Research Group: The Diabetes Prevention Program (DPP): Description of lifestyle intervention. Diabetes Care 2002;25:2165-2171.

Grundy SM, Cleeman JI, Daniels SR, et al: Diagnosis and management of the metabolic syndrome. An American Heart Association/National Heart, Lung, and Blood Institute Scientific Statement. Executive summary. Circulation 2005;112:2735-2752.

Kahn R, Buse J, Ferrannini E, Stern M: The metabolic syndrome: Time for a critical appraisal. Joint statement from the American Diabetes Association and the European Association for the Study of Diabetes. Diabetes Care 2005;8:2289-2304.

Knowler WC, Barrett-Connor E, Fowler SE, et al: Reduction in the incidence of type 2 diabetes with lifestyle intervention or metformin. N Engl J Med 2002;346:393-403.

Monnier L, Lapinski H, Colette C: Contributions of fasting and postprandial plasma glucose increments to the overall diurnal hyperglycemia of type 2 diabetic patients: Variations with increasing levels of HbA1c. Diabetes Care 2003;26:881-885.

Nathan DM, Buse JB, Davidson MB, et al: Management of hyperglycemia in type 2 diabetes: A consensus algorithm for the initiation and adjustment of therapy. A consensus statement from the American Diabetes Association and the European Association for the Study of Diabetes. Diabetes Care 2006;29:1963-1972.

Nesto RW, Bell D, Bonow RO, et al: Thiazolidinedione use, fluid retention, and congestive heart failure. A consensus statement from the American Heart Association and American Diabetes Association. Diabetes Care 2004;27:256-263.

Pihoker C, Gilliam LK, Hampe CS, Lernmark A: Autoantibodies in diabetes. Diabetes 2005;54:S52-S61.

Riddle MC, Rosenstock J, Gerich J: The treat-to-target trial: Randomized addition of glargine or human NPH insulin to oral therapy of type 2 diabetic patients. Diabetes Care 2003;26:3080-3086.

# Diabetes Mellitus in Children and Adolescents

Method of
*Lori M. B. Laffel, MD, MPH,
and Jamie R. S. Wood, MD*

Diabetes mellitus is a group of metabolic disorders that have hyperglycemia as a common feature caused by inadequate insulin secretion, insulin action, or both. Chronic hyperglycemia and its numerous downstream effects lead to micro- and macrovascular complications involving the eyes, kidneys, nerves, and blood vessels. Childhood and adolescent years are periods of rapid physical growth and psychosocial change, and these two factors make the care of children and adolescents with diabetes both challenging and rewarding. The health care professional must balance the important goals of optimal glycemic control and normal growth and development along with the risks of hypoglycemia and the challenges of expected glycemic excursions during childhood. Multidisciplinary care is the hallmark of successful diabetes management for the child and adolescent with diabetes and for family members.

---

[1]Not FDA approved for this indication.

The American Diabetes Association (ADA) classifies diabetes mellitus into four main types: type 1 diabetes (T1D), type 2 diabetes (T2D), other specific types, and gestational diabetes mellitus (Table 1). T1D is caused by insulin deficiency, which results from the autoimmune destruction of the pancreatic β cells. There are multiple genetic loci in the major histocompatibility region of chromosome 6 that predispose (DR 3/4, DQ 0201/0302, DR 4/4, and DQ 0300/0302) or protect against (DQB1*0602, DQA1*0102) the development of T1D. T2D is caused by the combination of insulin resistance and relative insulin deficiency.

Genetic forms of diabetes include maturity-onset diabetes in the young (MODY), mitochondrial diabetes, and certain syndromes of insulin resistance. MODY is characterized by young age of onset, autosomal dominant inheritance, the lack of association with obesity, and a variable phenotype. The most common disease of the exocrine pancreas that causes diabetes in children and adolescents is cystic fibrosis. Glucocorticoids used in the treatment of systemic illnesses are also commonly associated with hyperglycemia and diabetes. Certain genetic syndromes, such as Down syndrome, Klinefelter's syndrome, and Turner's syndrome, increase the risk for diabetes.

## Diagnosis

The diagnosis of T1D in children and adolescents is typically straightforward. The classic symptoms of polyuria, polydipsia, polyphagia, and weight loss over a several-week period are common. A thorough history and physical exam may reveal perineal candidiasis or thrush. Such symptoms may be followed by nausea, abdominal pain, vomiting, lethargy, and Kussmaul respirations if diabetic ketoacidosis (DKA)

and lactic acidosis develop. The presentation of T2D in children and adolescents can be more subtle and sometimes even clinically silent. However, approximately a third of adolescents with T2D have ketosis and a quarter have ketoacidosis at presentation.

The Current Diagnosis box outlines the diagnosis of diabetes mellitus. In the asymptomatic child or adolescent, diabetes is diagnosed when a fasting plasma glucose is 126 mg/dL or more, a 2-hour plasma glucose during an oral glucose tolerance test (OGTT) is 200 mg/dL or more, or a random plasma glucose is 200 mg/dL or more with confirmation on a second day. The symptomatic child or adolescent with a random plasma glucose of 200 mg/dL or more does not need repeat testing to confirm the diagnosis. Measurement of islet cell autoantibodies consistent with T1D (GAD, insulin, IA2) at diagnosis may help distinguish between type 1 and T2D. Care must be taken to avoid delay in the diagnosis and initiation of treatment because of the risk of rapid metabolic deterioration with insulin deficiency.

## Initial Management

The goals of initial management of the child or adolescent newly diagnosed with diabetes mellitus are to correct fluid and electrolyte imbalances, reverse hepatic gluconeogenesis and ketogenesis by halting lipolysis with insulin replacement, and begin the process of diabetes education. The location of this initial management depends on the severity of the clinical presentation, the age of the patient, the psychosocial assessment of the child or adolescent and caregiver, and the diabetes-related resources available in the family's geographic location (availability of an outpatient education program).

## Diabetic Ketoacidosis

Approximately 30% of children with newly diagnosed T1D present with diabetic ketoacidosis (DKA). Children who are younger (less than 4 years), without a first-degree relative with T1D, and from a family of lower socioeconomic status are at higher risk of DKA at onset of T1D. The majority of DKA episodes occur in patients with established diabetes, not in those newly diagnosed. Children or adolescents with established T1D are at higher risk for DKA if they are in poor metabolic control, have had a previous episode of DKA, are peripubertal/adolescent girls, have a psychiatric disorder, or are from a disadvantaged background.

---

### TABLE 1   Classification of Diabetes Mellitus*

Type 1 diabetes
Type 2 diabetes
Other specific types:
- Genetic defects of β-cell function
  - MODY 1: chromosome 20, HNF-4α
  - MODY 2: chromosome 7, glucokinase
  - MODY 3: chromosome 12, HNF-1α
  - MODY 4: chromosome 13, IPF-1
  - MODY 5: chromosome 17, HNF-1β
  - MODY 6: chromosome 2, NeuroD1
  - Mitochondrial diabetes
- Genetic defects in insulin action
  - Leprechaunism
  - Rabson-Mendenhall syndrome
- Diseases of the exocrine pancreas
  - Pancreatitis
  - Cystic fibrosis
  - Pancreatectomy
- Endocrinopathies
  - Acromegaly
  - Cushing's syndrome
  - Glucagonoma
  - Pheochromocytoma
- Drug or chemical induced
  - Glucocorticoids
- Infections
  - Congenital rubella
  - Cytomegalovirus
- Other genetic syndromes associated with diabetes
  - Down's syndrome
  - Klinefelter's syndrome
  - Turner's syndrome
Gestational diabetes mellitus (GDM)

---

*Table is not all inconclusive and gives examples of each subtype of diabetes mellitus. For complete list, see American Diabetes Association: Diagnosis and classification of diabetes mellitus. Diabetes Care 2005;28 (Suppl 1):S37-S42.
*Abbreviations:* MODY = maturity-onset diabetes in the young.

---

### CURRENT DIAGNOSIS

**ADA Recommendations for the Diagnosis of Diabetes**

- Symptoms (polyuria, polydipsia, unexplained weight loss) and a casual plasma glucose (any time of day without regard to time since last meal) ≥200 mg/dL (11.1 mmol/L) *or*
- Fasting (no caloric intake for at least 8 h) plasma glucose ≥126 mg/dL (7.0 mmol/L) *or*
- 2-hour plasma glucose ≥200 mg/dL (11.1 mmol/L) during an oral glucose tolerance test (glucose load of 75 g anhydrous glucose dissolved in water or 1.75 g/kg body weight if weight <43 kg).

---

Note: Criteria 2 and 3 should be confirmed on a second day if child/adolescent is asymptomatic. The OGTT is not recommended for routine clinical use and should be reserved for the asymptomatic child with incidental glucosuria/hyperglycemia or in the child with suspected diabetes but normal fasting plasma glucose.
Adapted from American Diabetes Association: Care of children and adolescents with type 1 diabetes. Diabetes Care 2005;28(1):186-212.

Management of DKA in children and adolescents is based on the same principles used in adults and therefore is covered in a separate chapter in this book. The development of cerebral edema, however, warrants discussion because this complication is seen primarily in children and is associated with both high morbidity and mortality. Risk factors for the development of cerebral edema include lower initial partial pressure of carbon dioxide, higher initial serum urea nitrogen concentrations, treatment with bicarbonate, and an attenuated rise in measured serum sodium concentrations during therapy. In addition, children who are younger (less than 5 years), have new-onset T1D, and longer duration of symptoms may also be at an increased risk. A high index of suspicion is needed with mannitol (Osmitrol) at the bedside to allow for timely intervention.

## Initiation of Insulin Replacement Therapy

Subcutaneous insulin is initiated in the patient who does not present in DKA or following intravenous insulin therapy in the child with resolved DKA who is tolerating oral intake (pH of $\geq 7.3$, tCO$_2$ $\geq 18$, anion gap $12 \pm 2$ mEq/L). The starting dose of insulin replacement therapy depends on the age, weight, and pubertal status of the patient, as well as the presence or absence of DKA. For the prepubertal child without DKA, the starting dose is usually 0.25 to 0.5 U/kg/day. For the prepubertal child with resolved DKA, the usual starting dose is 0.5 to 0.75 U/kg/day. For the pubertal child without DKA, the starting dose is 0.5 to 0.75 U/kg/day and for the pubertal child with resolved DKA, 0.75 to 1 U/kg/day. This total daily dose (TDD) of insulin is typically divided into either two or three injections per day, with the latter the preference toward implementation of intensive therapy (Figure 1). The twice-daily regimen may be selected for the younger (less than 4 years) child or if the psychosocial assessment determines that fewer injections per day would be beneficial. The use of an insulin pump at diagnosis remains within the research realm currently.

When the patient is metabolically stable, the focus turns to the psychosocial assessment of the child or adolescent and caregiver(s) and the initiation of diabetes education. A licensed social worker or other mental health professional evaluates each family and screens for circumstances that might complicate diabetes management: family composition, alternative caregiver(s), financial concerns, lack of health insurance, psychiatric or medical illness in a family member, or severe emotional distress of caregiver secondary to the diabetes diagnosis.

Diabetes education is provided by a certified diabetes nurse educator (DNE) and focuses on the set of essential skills needed to keep a child or adolescent with diabetes safe at home and school. These survival skills include techniques of blood glucose monitoring, urine or blood ketone measurement, drawing up and administration of subcutaneous insulin and glucagon, recognition and treatment of hypoglycemia and hyperglycemia, basics of sick day management, and indications for and methods of contacting the child's diabetes team. In addition to the survival skills, the child or adolescent and family should meet with a registered dietician who will assist them in developing an individualized meal plan and introduce the family to the concept of carbohydrate counting or exchanges. Once the child or adolescent (if developmentally appropriate) and caregiver(s) demonstrate the knowledge and skills needed, they are discharged with the expectation of daily phone contact with a member of their diabetes team to further titrate insulin doses and answer questions. When available and clinically indicated, a visiting nurse may assist with ongoing home-based education and support in the short term.

## Outpatient Diabetes Care

The management of children and adolescents with diabetes requires a multidisciplinary team approach. Members of this team include either a pediatric endocrinologist or pediatrician with training in diabetes, a pediatric DNE, a dietician, and a mental health professional (social worker and psychologist). Members of this team need to be easily accessible to the family in times of illness or metabolic crisis. Another member of the child/adolescent's team is a pediatrician or family doctor who will continue to provide routine well child care including anticipatory guidance, immunizations, and general medical care.

In the first few months of outpatient diabetes care, patients are seen frequently by members of the diabetes team to assess the family's adaptation to the new diagnosis, reinforce skills and knowledge learned during the first few days, and expand on the skills and knowledge needed for intensive diabetes management. Patients are subsequently seen at a minimum frequency of every 3 months, alternating between their DNE and their pediatric endocrinologist. Visits with the dietician are recommended yearly or more frequently if circumstances warrant (e.g., young child or toddler, desired weight loss, initiating pump therapy, etc.).

## Diabetes Education

Diabetes education is an ongoing process with continuous need for review of previously learned material and introduction of new concepts as the family develops a more sophisticated understanding of intensive diabetes management. The educator should evaluate the patient and his or her caregiver's knowledge and skills regularly. In addition, age-appropriate issues need to be discussed as the patient matures (e.g., driving guidelines, issues related to alcohol and smoking, etc.).

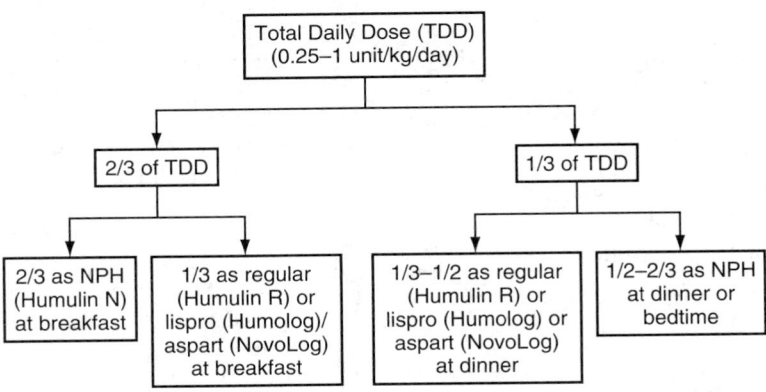

**FIGURE 1.** Initiation of Insulin Replacement Therapy. Two thirds of the total daily dose (TDD) is given at breakfast and further divided into NPH (two thirds) and short/rapid-acting insulin (one third). The remaining one third is either given in one injection at dinner (in a twice-daily regimen) or divided between dinner and bedtime (in a thrice-daily regimen), and should also be divided into NPH (two thirds) and short/rapid-acting insulin (one third). Short/rapid-acting insulin can be regular (Humulin R), lispro (Humalog), or aspart (NovoLog).

Diabetes education needs to be tailored to each family taking into account their educational level and cultural practices. The educator must be sensitive to the age and developmental stage of the child or adolescent, and shift his or her educational efforts from the caregiver(s) to the adolescent when it is developmentally appropriate. Continued parental involvement and supervision of the adolescent with diabetes is crucial to good metabolic control.

The health care provider should complete a focused interval history at each visit that includes recent illnesses, visits to the emergency department, hospitalizations, medications prescribed other than insulin, types of insulin and current doses, daily routine including meal plan and activity level, self-care behaviors and identifying who performs them, episodes of hypoglycemia and their precipitants, school performance, emotional health, and a review of systems focusing on symptoms of hyperglycemia (polyuria, polydipsia, polyphagia, weight loss, candidal infections) and the possible development of other autoimmune disorders. If appropriate, a history of tobacco, alcohol, recreational drugs, and sexual activity should be elicited. A focused physical examination that includes measurement of blood pressure and heart rate, weight, height, body mass index (BMI), and examination of the thyroid gland, sites of blood glucose monitoring, and insulin injections should be completed at each visit. A more thorough physical examination including Tanner staging should be performed once per year or more frequently if indicated.

The hemoglobin A1C, the fraction of hemoglobin that has glucose attached to it, is a measure of the average level of blood glucose over the preceding 2 to 3 months. It should be measured every 3 months and serves as an objective measure of blood glucose control. A discrepancy between the hemoglobin A1C and the average blood glucose levels from self-monitoring records suggests that the patient needs to monitor at different times of day, may benefit from a review of blood glucose monitoring technique and equipment, or there may be fabrication of results. Obtaining computer downloaded data helps eliminate the latter possibility.

## Goals of Therapy

The Diabetes Control and Complications Trial (DCCT) demonstrated that the incidence of microvascular complications was reduced with improved blood glucose control (hemoglobin A1C approximately 7%). The reduction in complications, however, was accompanied by an increased risk of severe hypoglycemia. Because young children are more vulnerable to hypoglycemia (reduced catecholamine response to hypoglycemia, decreased ability to communicate symptoms of hypoglycemia, and risk for neuropsychologic impairment from hypoglycemia), the ADA has developed age-specific glycemic targets (Table 2).

**TABLE 2 Blood Glucose and A1C Goals for Type 1 Diabetes by Age Group**

| Age Group | Plasma Blood Glucose Range (mg/dL) | | A1C |
|---|---|---|---|
| | Before Meals | Bedtime/ Overnight | |
| <6 y | 100–180 | 110–200 | 7.5%–8.5% |
| 6–12 y | 90–180 | 100–180 | <8% |
| 13–19 y | 90–130 | 90–150 | <7.5% |

Goals should be individualized; lower goals may be reasonable and achievable without hypoglycemia.
Goals should be higher in patients with frequent hypoglycemia or hypoglycemia unawareness.
Adapted from American Diabetes Association: Care of children and adolescents with type 1 diabetes. Diabetes Care 2005;28(1):186-212.

## Insulin Therapy

The ideal insulin replacement therapy would be one that mirrors the basal and prandial insulin secretion in individuals without diabetes. Numerous insulin preparations are available that vary in time to onset, peak, and duration of action (Table 3). No single regimen is superior to another; thus individualization of the insulin regimen to the child or adolescent and family remains a major determinant. Important factors for consideration include blood glucose monitoring frequency, number of daily injections the family can perform, the need for flexibility in meal planning, and the unique family schedule. Regimens range in intensity from twice-a-day injections with a set dose of premixed insulin to intensive diabetes management with multiple injections per day of two or more types of insulin or use of an insulin pump (continuous subcutaneous insulin infusion [CSII]).

The typical regimen that children or adolescents begin at diagnosis was described previously (Figure 1). Some centers initiate a basal-bolus regimen in which insulin is replaced in a manner that attempts to mimic physiologic insulin release. Basal-bolus regimens include the insulin pump and glargine (Lantus) given once a day with rapid-acting insulin (lispro [Humalog] or aspart [NovoLog]) before each meal/snack and as needed for correction of hyperglycemia. The school-age child who hopes to avoid an injection at lunch often benefits from a regimen of glargine (Lantus) at dinner or bedtime, along with NPH (Humulin N) and a rapid-acting insulin at breakfast, plus a rapid-acting insulin at dinner. The peak of the NPH covers carbohydrate intake at lunch. The use of basal insulin analogue glargine (Lantus) in the evening is associated with less nocturnal hypoglycemia.

Patients on a basal-bolus regimen determine their insulin doses based on an insulin-to-carbohydrate ratio and a correction factor or sensitivity index (CF or SI). The insulin-to-carbohydrate ratio is the number of grams of carbohydrate covered by 1 U of insulin (roughly 450 divided by TDD) for each meal and snack. The CF/SI is the expected decrement in glucose following 1 U of rapid-acting insulin

**CURRENT THERAPY**

**Examples of Insulin Regimens**

Injections bid:
- Insulin mixtures (70/30, 75/25) given at breakfast and dinner
- NPH and rapid- or short-acting insulin given at breakfast and dinner

Injections tid:
- NPH and rapid- or short-acting insulin given at breakfast, rapid- or short-acting insulin given at dinner, and NPH given at bedtime
- NPH and rapid- or short-acting insulin given at breakfast, rapid- or short-acting insulin given at dinner, and NPH or glargine (Lantus) given at bedtime

Injections qid:
- NPH and rapid-acting insulin given at breakfast, rapid-acting insulin given at lunch and dinner, and rapid-acting insulin and NPH given at bedtime
- NPH and rapid-acting insulin given at breakfast and lunch, rapid-acting insulin given at dinner, and NPH given at bedtime
- Rapid-acting insulin given at breakfast, lunch, and dinner, and glargine (Lantus) given at breakfast, dinner, or bedtime

Continuous subcutaneous insulin infusion (CSII)
- Rapid-acting insulin given for basal requirements and as bolus at every meal/snack and periodically to correct hyperglycemia (no more frequent than q2–3h)

**TABLE 3** Insulin Analogues

| Insulin Preparation | Onset of Action | Peak Action | Effective Duration |
|---|---|---|---|
| **Rapid Acting** | | | |
| Insulin lispro | 5–15 min | 30–90 min | 2–4 h |
| Insulin aspart | 5–10 min | 60–180 min | 3–5 h |
| Insulin glulisine* | 5–15 min | 30–90 min | 3–5 h |
| **Short Acting** | | | |
| Regular (soluble insulin) | 30–60 min | 2–3 h | 3–6 h |
| **Intermediate Acting** | | | |
| Lente (insulin zinc preparation)† | 3–4 h | 4–12 h | 12–18 h |
| NPH (isophane insulin) | 2–4 h | 4–10 h | 10–16 h |
| **Long Acting** | | | |
| Ultralente (extended insulin zinc preparation)† | 4–6 h | 8–20 h | 20–24 h |
| Insulin glargine | 1.1 h | None | 24 h |
| Insulin detemir* | 2–3 h | 6–14 h | 16–24 h |
| **Insulin mixtures** | | | |
| 70/30 human mix‡ (70% NPH, 30% regular) | 30–60 min | dual | 10–16 h |
| 70/30 aspart analogue mix (70% intermediate, 30% aspart)‡ | 5–15 min | dual | 10–16 h |
| 75/25 lispro analog mix‡ (75% intermediate, 25% lispro) | 5–15 min | dual | 10–16 h |
| 50/50 human mix (50% NPH, 50% regular) | 30–60 min | dual | 10–16 h |

*FDA approved for adult use only.
In many countries, including the United States, insulin preparations contain 100 U/mL and are referred to as U-100 insulin. Highly concentrated U-500 short-acting insulin is available and used primarily in adults with severe insulin resistance.
†Recently discontinued by manufacturer (Lilly); estimated to be available until end of 2005.
‡Typically used in fixed doses in twice-a-day insulin regimens.
Profiles for each insulin preparation are reasonable estimates only, based on data from adult study participants. There is variation between individuals, and time of onset, peak, and duration are also affected by size of dose, site and depth of injection, dilution, exercise, and temperature.

(roughly 1650 divided by TDD). The CF/SI is applied no more than every 2 to 3 hours to lower an elevated blood glucose toward the target range to avoid so-called stacking of insulin action and subsequent hypoglycemia. For patients on a combination of intermediate-acting insulin (NPH) and rapid- or short-acting insulin, meals typically contain a certain amount of carbohydrates (e.g., 60 g or 4 carbohydrate exchanges) and require consistency in timing to avoid hypoglycemia.

The CSII, otherwise known as insulin pump therapy, comes the closest to mimicking the basal and prandial insulin secretion of an individual without diabetes. The insulin pump is steadily becoming a commonly used method to replace insulin, especially in the pediatric population. There are many advantages to the insulin pump including the elimination of multiple daily injections, increased flexibility in meal planning, ease of decreasing insulin for physical activity, fewer hypoglycemic events, and the ability to deliver very small amounts of insulin. The disadvantages are more frequent blood glucose monitoring, always being tethered to the pump, and increased risk for the development of DKA. Because only rapid-acting insulin (lispro [Humalog] or aspart [NovoLog]) is used in the insulin pump, discontinuation of insulin delivery can result in ketone production within hours. Increased vigilance, therefore, is necessary to ensure proper functioning of the insulin pump with frequent blood glucose monitoring and checking for ketones if hyperglycemia develops.

## Self-Monitoring

One of the main goals of diabetes education is to teach and empower the patient and family in the self-management of diabetes. Self-management of diabetes includes measuring blood glucose and blood/urine ketone levels, recording the results along with amount of carbohydrate intake and amount of insulin administered, and the ability to make insulin dosing decisions based on the interpretation of these records. Monitoring blood glucose four or more times daily is recommended in children with T1D. Additional monitoring may be necessary postprandially, overnight, or during periods of increased physical activity to help optimize control and prevent severe hypoglycemia. Preschool or early school-age children may require more frequent monitoring because of their inability to recognize symptoms or to communicate during episodes of hypoglycemia. In addition, children and adolescents using the insulin pump typically check their blood sugar six or more times per day. Ketone measurements should be done whenever the blood glucose is greater than 250 to 300 mg/dL and/or if the patient is ill, especially with nausea, vomiting, or abdominal pain. Ketones can be measured either in the urine (acetoacetate and acetone) or blood (β-hydroxybutyric acid). Measurement of blood ketones is now available on a home meter and is the preferred method in the current era stressing blood glucose monitoring. The key to successful intensive diabetes management is frequent blood glucose monitoring, good record keeping, and communication of these results with the diabetes team at frequent intervals so that timely modifications can be made to the insulin regimen and/or meal plan.

## Medical Nutrition Therapy

The meal plan remains an important component of management aimed at good glycemic control, although it is often the most difficult aspect of intensive diabetes management for families. A dietician trained in pediatric nutrition and diabetes should meet with the family at the time of T1D diagnosis and periodically thereafter. The dietician should help develop a meal plan that is individualized to the patient's daily schedule, food preferences, cultural influences, and physical activity. The meal plan is more likely to be successful if it is designed to fit into the family's already established schedule and preferences. The patient and family should also be instructed on carbohydrate counting so that either carbohydrate exchanges or insulin-to-carbohydrate ratios can be used. Like the child without diabetes, the total number of recommended calories follows the child's growth requirements along with consideration of the need for weight gain or loss. Growth velocity, weight gain, and BMI should be monitored at every visit to ensure that the meal plan is sufficient to meet the energy requirements of the patient. Unexpected weight loss or poor weight gain should prompt consideration of suboptimal metabolic control, as well as eating disorders, thyroid dysfunction, or gastrointestinal disease.

The ADA does not have pediatric specific guidelines for medical nutrition therapy, but the recommendations for adults can be extrapolated to children. The ADA recommends that carbohydrates provide 45% to 65% of total calories, with protein and fat contributing 15% and 30%, respectively. The patient and family should be educated to avoid foods high in cholesterol, saturated fat, and concentrated sweets and select foods high in complex carbohydrate and dietary fiber.

All children and adolescents are recommended to have three meals per day. If they receive intermediate-acting insulin preparations, they should also receive three snacks per day (morning, afternoon, and bedtime) to match anticipated peaks of insulin action. If the child or adolescent is on a basal-bolus regimen, snacks are optional and require insulin coverage based on insulin-to-carbohydrate ratios.

## Exercise

Exercise, or periods of sustained physical activity, can be beneficial to the patient by contributing to a sense of well-being, helping achieve the recommended BMI, improving glycemic control (exercise enhances insulin sensitivity), improving the lipid panel (increasing HDL), and lowering blood pressure and improving cardiovascular fitness. All children and adolescents, especially those with diabetes, should be encouraged to participate in routine physical activity.

The child or adolescent with diabetes needs to take precautions to avoid hypoglycemia during periods of increased physical activity. The patient and family need to check blood glucose before the initiation of activity, every hour during sustained activity, and at the completion of physical activity. For the first several days of increased activity, the child should also check his or her blood sugar frequently during the 12-hour postexercise period because there is often a delayed drop in the blood glucose following exercise (i.e., the lag effect). Some children require additional carbohydrate before, during, and after activity; lower insulin doses on the days of increased physical activity; or both. It is suggested that the child take 5 to 15 g of carbohydrates, depending on age and exercise intensity, before exercise if the blood sugar is below target, and repeat the 5 to 15 g of carbohydrate for every 30 minutes of sustained activity. Rapid-acting carbohydrate should be readily available, and coaches and trainers should be aware of the diagnosis of diabetes and trained in the treatment of hypoglycemia.

## Psychosocial Support

The mental health professional is an important member of the diabetes team. A thorough family assessment generally accompanies the diabetes diagnosis with appropriate referrals for additional services as needed. Thereafter, children or adolescents should be referred back to a mental health professional if social, emotional, or economic barriers to the achievement of good glycemic control are identified. Family conflict, especially conflict over diabetes care, can be associated with deterioration in glycemic control. Encouragement of ongoing family teamwork in the management of childhood diabetes promotes successful outcomes with respect to glycemic control, reducing diabetes-specific conflict, and preventing acute complications and emergency assessments.

## Sick Day Management

The goals for the management of children and adolescents during sick days are never omit insulin, prevent dehydration and hypoglycemia, monitor blood glucose frequently (every 2 to 4 hours), monitor for ketosis, provide supplemental rapid- or short-acting insulin doses (5% to 20% of TDD) depending on degree of hyperglycemia and ketosis,

treat underlying illness, and have frequent contact with the diabetes team. The majority of DKA among children or adolescents with established diabetes is caused by insulin omission or errors in administration of insulin. Inadequate insulin therapy in the context of an intercurrent illness accounts for the remaining small percentage. Although it is more common for children to require more insulin during illnesses, some children require a reduction of the basal and/or rapid-acting insulin dose if he or she is unable to eat and the blood glucose is less than 200 mg/dL.

Families need to be educated about symptoms that warrant immediate medical attention, including signs of dehydration (dry mouth, sunken eyes, cracked lips, weight loss, dry skin), persistent vomiting for more than 2 to 4 hours, persistence of blood glucose levels greater than 300 mg/dL or ketones for more than 12 hours, or symptoms of DKA (nausea, abdominal pain, chest pain, vomiting, ketotic breath, hyperventilation, or altered consciousness). It is helpful for the diabetes team to review sick day management annually with the family (can accompany flu immunization) to avoid metabolic decompensation during intercurrent illness.

## Hypoglycemia

Fear of hypoglycemia can be a common occurrence in the management of childhood diabetes, especially among caregivers, and can be a barrier to optimal glycemic control. Recognition and treatment of hypoglycemia are important topics for diabetes education. Families are trained to treat hypoglycemia with 10 to 15 g of rapid-acting carbohydrate, recheck blood glucose in 15 minutes, repeat treatment with 10 to 15 g if blood sugar remains below target, and follow with a protein-containing snack if a meal will not follow within 1 to 2 hours. This technique avoids the natural tendency to overtreat low blood glucose levels. Caregivers should also receive glucagon training (20 to 30 µg/kg; maximum 1 mg) for severe hypoglycemia and low-dose glucagon (1 U on an insulin syringe for every year of life up to 15 years) for impending hypoglycemia, for example, in the context of a gastrointestinal illness or inadvertent insulin administration (lispro given instead of NPH). A member of the diabetes team should assess frequency, treatment, awareness, and circumstances of hypoglycemia at each visit.

## Screening for Diabetes-Related Complications

Patients, families, and caregivers worry about the risk of diabetes-related complications, and therefore the diabetes team must educate families and screen for complications with sensitivity and optimism, emphasizing prevention of complications and the maintenance of health. Screening for nephropathy, hypertension, dyslipidemia, and retinopathy are indicated.

Microalbuminuria (MA) is the first sign of diabetic nephropathy, and patients who develop persistent MA are at increased risk of progression to macroalbuminuria. Poor glycemic control, smoking, and a family history of essential hypertension are risk factors for the development of MA and nephropathy. Identification of persistent MA provides an opportunity for intervention and prevention of progressive renal disease through improvements in glycemic control and/or therapy with angiotensin-converting enzyme (ACE) inhibitors. There are currently no pediatric data on the use of angiotensin receptor blockers (ARBs). Table 4 outlines definitions, screening recommendations, and treatment.

Hypertension is an important predictor of the progression of diabetic nephropathy to end-stage renal disease. Hypertension in children and adolescents may go unrecognized because providers are not familiar with the gender-, age-, and height-specific definitions. Blood pressure should be measured every 3 months with standardized technique, using the proper size cuff. If elevated blood pressures are detected and confirmed, the first step is to exclude causes not related to diabetes. Table 4 outlines the definitions, screening recommendations, and treatment.

**TABLE 4  Screening for Diabetes-Related Complications**

| Complication | How to Screen | Definition | When to Screen | Therapy |
|---|---|---|---|---|
| Microalbuminuria | Spot urine sample timed overnight or 24-h collection | Spot urine albumin/creatinine ratio 30–299 µg/g or AER 20–199 µg/min from timed collection | Annual screening begins at 10 y or after ≥5 y duration of diabetes | Optimize glucose control, smoking cessation, normalize BP |
| Persistent microalbuminuria | | 2/3 of urine samples meet above criteria | | Above, plus addition of ACE inhibitor |
| High-normal BP | Manual BP measurement with standard technique | Systolic or diastolic BP within the 90th–95th percentile for age, gender, and height | At every clinic visit | Dietary intervention, weight control, and exercise; if target BP not reached within 3–6 mo, then initiate pharmacologic therapy |
| Hypertension | | Systolic or diastolic BP above the 95th percentile for age, gender, and height, or >130/80 on ≥3 occasions (whichever is lower) | | Above, plus pharmacologic therapy titrated to achieve target BP |

*Note:* Urine collection should not be performed following vigorous exercise, during an acute infection, during a female patient's menstrual cycle, or following an episode of severe hypoglycemia. Once angiotensin-converting enzyme (ACE) inhibitor is started, microalbumin excretion should be monitored q3–6 mo. Target BP is <130/80 or <90th percentile for age, gender, and height. Initial drug treatment is ACE inhibition.
*Abbreviations:* AER = albumin excretion rate; BP = blood pressure.

Dyslipidemia and diabetes are established risk factors for cardiovascular disease, and recent research suggests that a significant proportion of adolescents with diabetes already have evidence of atherosclerosis. Low-density lipoprotein (LDL) cholesterol is most closely associated with cardiovascular disease, and therefore, the ADA has developed guidelines for LDL cholesterol. Screening may be delayed until puberty if family history is negative for cardiovascular disease. A lipid profile should be performed on prepubertal children with diabetes who are older than 2 years if there is a positive family history of cardiovascular disease or if the family history is unknown. If the LDL cholesterol is less than 100 mg/dL, screening can be repeated every 5 years. The mainstay of therapy for dyslipidemia is dietary management (saturated fat less than 7% of calories and less than 200 mg/day of cholesterol). Children with levels between 130 and 159 mg/dL should be started on medication if diet and lifestyle modification are unsuccessful after 6 months or if the child has additional risk factors for cardiovascular disease, such as obesity or hypertension. Pharmacotherapy is recommended if the LDL cholesterol is more than 160 mg/dL. The LDL goal for children with diabetes is less than 100 mg/dL.

Diabetic retinopathy is a feared complication because it is the leading cause of vision loss. According to the ADA, the first ophthalmologic exam should be requested when the child is 10 years or older and has had diabetes for more than 3 to 5 years. Examinations with an eye care professional with expertise in diabetic retinopathy should occur early.

## Screening for Other Autoimmune Diseases

Children and adolescents with T1D are at an increased risk for other autoimmune diseases and should be screened accordingly. Approximately 15% of patients with T1D also have autoimmune thyroid disease. All children and adolescents should be screened for autoimmune thyroid disease at the time of diabetes diagnosis once

**TABLE 5  Risk Factors and Screening for Type 2 Diabetes in Children**

| Criteria | Age of Initiation | Frequency | Method |
|---|---|---|---|
| Overweight (BMI >85th percentile for age and gender), weight for height >85th percentile, or weight >120% of ideal for height<br>Plus 2 of the following risk factors:<br>Family history of T2D in 1st- or 2nd-degree relative<br>Race/ethnicity (American Indian, African American, Hispanic, Asian/Pacific Islander)<br>Signs of or conditions associated with insulin resistance (acanthosis nigricans, PCOS, HTN, dyslipidemia) | 10 y or at pubertal onset if puberty occurs at a younger age | q2y | Fasting plasma glucose |

*Note:* Clinical judgment should be used to test for diabetes in high-risk patients who do not meet these criteria.
*Abbreviations:* BMI = body mass index; T2D = type 2 diabetes; HTN = hypertension; PCOS = polycystic ovarian syndrome.
Adapted from American Diabetes Association: Type 2 diabetes in children. Diabetes Care 2000;23(3):381-389.

**TABLE 6  Medications to Treat Type 2 Diabetes**

| Class | Mechanism of Action | Adverse Effects |
|---|---|---|
| Biguanides (metformin)* | Decrease hepatic glucose production Increase peripheral glucose disposal | Gastrointestinal upset Lactic acidosis |
| Sulfonylureas (glimepiride, glyburide, glipizide) | Insulin secretagogues | Hypoglycemia Weight gain |
| Meglitinides (repaglinide, nateglinide) | Insulin secretagogues | Hypoglycemia Weight gain |
| α-Glucosidase inhibitors (acarbose) | Decrease gut carbohydrate absorption | Gastrointestinal upset |
| Thiazolidinediones (rosiglitazone and pioglitazone) | Decrease hepatic glucose production Increase peripheral glucose disposal | Weight gain Edema Increased liver enzymes Anemia |

*Metformin (Glucophage) is the only medication with FDA approval for use in children.

metabolic control is established. TSH measurement is a useful initial screen, with and without measuring the presence of thyroid autoantibodies. Screening should be repeated yearly or if there is any clinical suspicion of thyroid disease (abnormal growth rate, symptoms of hypo- or hyperthyroidism, goiter on examination, erratic blood glucose control).

Another commonly associated disorder is celiac disease. Nearly 6% of patients with T1D have elevated levels of circulating autoantibodies to tissue transglutaminase. Celiac disease can cause diarrhea, weight loss or failure to gain weight, abdominal pain, fatigue, and unexplained hypoglycemia or erratic blood glucose secondary to malabsorption. Patients with T1D should be screened with circulating IgA autoantibody to tissue transglutaminase. A quantitative serum IgA level should be drawn at the same time to rule out IgA deficiency as a cause for falsely low IgA tissue transglutaminase levels. Positive antibodies should be confirmed with a second measurement, and if positive, a referral should be made to a gastroenterologist for small bowel biopsy. If the diagnosis is confirmed, celiac disease is treated with a gluten-free diet with recommendations and support from a registered dietician with pediatric expertise in diabetes and celiac management.

# Type 2 Diabetes Mellitus in Youth

With the increasing prevalence of childhood obesity during the last two decades, there is an increased occurrence of T2D in youth. Based on National Health and Nutrition Examination survey data, the prevalence of overweight children (defined as a body mass index greater than the 95th percentile for children and youth) increased from 5% in the 1970s to more than 15% by 1999. The epidemic of obesity follows the increased consumption of fast foods, increased consumption of soft drinks, increased sedentary behavior with more television watching, and decreased physical activity. Mirroring this epidemic of childhood obesity is the occurrence of T2D in children and adolescents. Before 1990, T2D in youth was a rare occurrence. By 2000, between 8% and 45% of all newly diagnosed cases of childhood diabetes were caused by T2D. T2D occurs most commonly in those with a family history of T2D; individuals from certain racial and ethnic minority groups including Native Americans, Hispanics, African Americans, and Asian and Pacific Islanders; those with obesity falling above the 85th percentile for BMI based on age and gender; and in association with markers of insulin resistance (Table 5). Markers of insulin resistance include the occurrence of acanthosis nigricans and polycystic ovarian syndrome (PCOS). In addition, other well-known risk factors include hypertension and hyperlipidemia.

As noted earlier, the diagnosis of T2D is based on fasting plasma glucose (FPG), 2-hour glucose value during an OGTT, or a casual glucose level. Because T2D often goes without symptoms, individuals who are overweight, have a positive family history of T2D, come from one of the high-risk racial and ethnic minority groups, and/or have markers of insulin resistance warrant screening for T2D. Screening can be performed with a FPG or OGTT when clinical concerns are high and the FPG is normal.

Currently one oral medication is approved for the treatment of T2D in youth. This medication is metformin (Glucophage), which is also available in a liquid formulation. The maximum recommended daily dose of metformin (Glucophage) in youth is 2000 mg/day divided as 1000 mg twice daily. Often patients with T2D present in ketoacidosis and require initial insulin therapy. The goal of management of the child with T2D is initial stabilization often with insulin therapy, metformin (Glucophage) directed at managing the insulin resistance, and education. Once glucose levels are stabilized, insulin dosage may be lowered along with continued treatment with metformin (Glucophage) and approaches to lifestyle management. Lifestyle management involves a healthy diet, increasing exercise, and decreasing sedentary behaviors.

Other medications used to treat T2D include second-generation sulfonylureas, meglitinides, thiazolidinediones, and α-glucosidase inhibitors, none of which is currently approved for use in pediatric patients. There is ongoing studies to assess the efficacy and safety of these medications (Table 6).

## REFERENCES

American Diabetes Association: Diagnosis and classification of diabetes mellitus. Diabetes Care 2005;28 (Suppl 1):S37-S42.

American Diabetes Association: Type 2 diabetes in children. Diabetes Care 2000;23(3):381-389.

Barroso I: Genetics of type 2 diabetes. Diabet Med 2005;22:517-535.

Dunger DB, Sperling MA, Acerini CL, et al: ESPE/LWPES consensus statement on diabetic ketoacidosis in children and adolescents. Arch Dis Child 2004;89:188-194.

Fox LA, Buckloh LM, Smith SD, et al: A randomized controlled trial of insulin pump therapy in young children with type 1 diabetes. Diabetes Care 2005;28:1277-1281.

Glaser N, Barnett P, McCaslin I, et al: The Pediatric Emergency Medicine Collaborative Research Committee of the American Academy of Pediatrics. N Engl J Med 2001;344(4):264-269.

Goodwin G, Volkening LK, Laffel LM: Younger age at onset of type 1 diabetes in concordant sibling pairs is associated with increased risk for autoimmune thyroid disease. Diabetes Care 2006;29(6)1397-1398.

Hannon TS, Rao G, Arslanian SA: Childhood obesity and type 2 diabetes mellitus. Pediatrics 2005;116(2):473-480.

Hirsch IB: Insulin analogues. N Engl J Med 2005;352:174-183.

Laffel LM, Vangsness L, Connell A, et al: Impact of ambulatory, family-focused teamwork intervention on glycemic control in youth with type 1 diabetes. J Pediatr 2003;142(4):409-416.

Rosenbloom AL: Cerebral edema in diabetic ketoacidosis and other acute devastating complications: Recent observations. Pediatr Diabetes 2005;6:41-49.

Silverstein J, Klingensmith G, Copeland K, et al: American Diabetes Association: Care of children and adolescents with type 1 diabetes. Diabetes Care 2005;28(1):186-212.

Wysocki T, Harris MA, Mauras N, et al: Absence of adverse effects of severe hypoglycemia on cognitive function in school-aged children with diabetes over 18 months. Diabetes Care 2003;26(4):1100-1105.

# Diabetic Ketoacidosis and Hyperglycemic Hyperosmolar Syndrome

Method of
*Robert A. Kreisberg, MD, and*
*Elizabeth D. Ennis, MD*

Hyperglycemic crisis includes the disorders of diabetic ketoacidosis (DKA) and the hyperglycemic hyperosmolar syndrome (HHS). They are often severe and life threatening, requiring prompt and appropriate therapy. Both are characterized by hyperglycemia and moderate to severe deficits of water, electrolytes, and minerals. They differ in the severity of the hyperglycemia and ketoacidosis and in the deficits of water and electrolytes. Patients often have features of both syndromes so that classification as one or the other might not be possible (Figure 1). Successful treatment of these disorders requires an understanding of their pathophysiology, appropriate use of insulin, correction of volume and electrolyte deficiencies, and a compulsive approach to patient management.

Although mortality from hyperglycemic crisis may be declining, there are still about 2500 deaths per year attributable to these disorders, with an overall age-adjusted rate of 23.8 per 100,000 people with diabetes.

The profiles of patients with DKA and HHS have changed. Although many with DKA continue to be young patients with type 1 diabetes (T1DM), a new group of patients with DKA has emerged. Many patients from minority ethnic groups who have type 2 diabetes (T2DM) present with DKA (a presentation sometimes referred to as *type 1.5 diabetes*). This group constitutes as much as 40% to 50% of minority patients with DKA and is characterized by severe obesity. After recovering from decompensated diabetes, these patients can often achieve subsequent control with diet, with or without oral agents. The average age for DKA is 43 years, emphasizing the changing demographics of this disorder. Young patients can also present with HHS.

## Precipitating Factors

Decompensated diabetes invariably occurs as a result of intercurrent illness, omission or discontinuation of insulin, or new-onset diabetes.

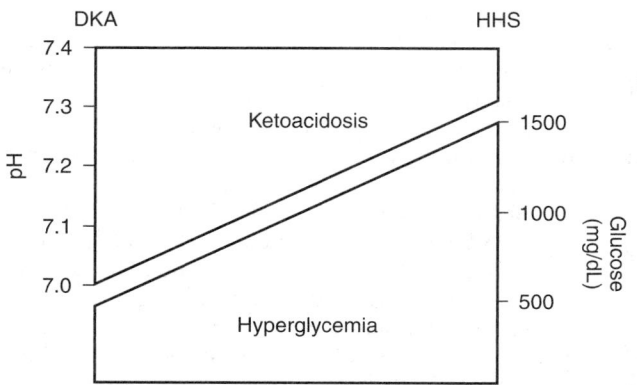

**FIGURE 1.** Severity of hyperglycemic and ketoacidosis in diabetic ketoacidosis (DKA) and hyperglycemic hyperosmolar syndrome (HHS). Classic metabolic profiles are expressed at the extreme left and right of the diagram. A continuum of combinations of hyperglycemia and ketoacidosis is possible, which is consistent with the observation that approximately 33% of patients with decompensated diabetes mellitus have features of both syndromes. (Redrawn with permission from LeRoith D, Taylor SI, Olefsky JM: Diabetes Mellitus: A Fundamental and Clinical Text, 3rd ed. Lippincott Williams & Wilkins, 1996.)

Acute intercurrent illness is an important precipitant for both DKA and HHS. In the elderly with HHS it may be difficult to know if myocardial infarction, stroke, mesenteric thrombosis, intestinal obstruction, or other conditions are the cause of HHS or are the effect of the predisposition to thrombosis that occurs as a result of the severe hemoconcentration.

Numerous drugs are associated with DKA and HHS, many of which include newer psychiatric agents. Thus, all medications should be reviewed for their potential to precipitate clinical diabetes mellitus or diabetic decompensation.

## Pathophysiology

A relative or absolute deficiency of insulin, in the presence of increased levels of glucose counterregulatory hormones (cortisol, catecholamines, glucagon, and growth hormone) that occur with intercurrent illness, stress, or just severely decompensated diabetes, sets the stage for DKA and for HHS. This loss of balance between insulin and glucagon coupled with predicted changes in glucose counterregulatory hormones leads to glycogenolysis, protein breakdown, gluconeogenesis, lipolysis, increased levels of free fatty acids, and ketogenesis. Free fatty acids released from adipose tissue and amino acids released from body protein stores provide the substrates for ketogenesis and gluconeogenesis. Hydrogen ion, due to ketoacid production, titrates bicarbonate and other body buffers, leading to acidosis.

It is not entirely clear why patients with decompensated diabetes and HHS have less intense ketogenesis and milder ketoacidosis than those with DKA. The less severe ketoacidosis has been attributed to lower concentrations of glucose counterregulatory hormones, less severe insulin deficiency, and reduced responsiveness of tissues to insulin deficiency and glucose counterregulatory hormone excess as a consequence of age. DKA and HHS, often discussed as two separate entities, constitute ends of a continuum of severe diabetic decompensation and hyperglycemia (see Figure 1). Patients with severe decompensation can have features of both disorders. The older age of patients with HHS probably contributes to alterations in central nervous system (CNS) function.

The sequence of events leading to presentation differs depending on the rates of ketogenesis. Those with accelerated ketogenesis (characteristic of DKA) quickly become acidemic, leading to an earlier presentation (usually within 1-3 days), because the acidosis makes them ill. If the rates of ketogenesis are low, the prodrome is more protracted (7-10 days), allowing greater water and electrolyte loss and the development of more severe hyperglycemia. In HHS there is greater hyperosmolality due to the very high glucose levels and to the normal or increased serum sodium levels. When the effective osmolality ($E_{Osm}$) is 320 mOsm/L or more, mental function declines and patients are often lethargic, confused, obtunded, or comatose. Effective osmolality is calculated with the following equation:

$$E_{Osm} = 2(Na^+ + K^+) + (plasma\ glucose/18)$$

where $Na^+$ and $K^+$ are in mEq/L and glucose is in mg/dL. Urea is omitted from the calculation, because urea is distributed in total body water and does not contribute to the osmotic gradient.

The initial response to the increase in extracellular osmolality due to hyperglycemia is for intracellular water to follow the osmotic gradient and shift into the extracellular compartment. This accounts for the mild hyponatremia characteristic of DKA. This increase in the extracellular volume leads to an increase in glomerular filtration rate (GFR) and enhanced excretion of water in the urine due to the osmotic diuresis from glucosuria. The early presentation of patients with DKA dictates a smaller loss of free water. However, only about two thirds of patients with DKA have classic hyponatremia, and one third has normal or high serum sodium concentrations consistent with greater free water loss, which is characteristic of HHS.

The evolution of changes in the serum sodium concentration in decompensated diabetes is dynamic and is influenced by the duration of the hyperglycemia and access to free water. Older patients, often in nursing homes, are at particular risk. It is no surprise that their water needs are often unmet as a consequence of an age-related blunting of thirst and their dependency on others to meet their free water requirements. As the duration of decompensation lengthens, the initial early shift of free water into the vascular compartment and resultant hyponatremia disappears and the serum sodium concentration returns to normal. When the prodrome is prolonged there is volume contraction, reduced filtration, and excretion of glucose in the urine and the development of hypernatremia. The increased effective osmolality in HHS is primarily due to hyperglycemia, but hypernatremia can also contribute to this finding.

The classic anion-gap acid-base abnormalities in DKA are due to the loss of bicarbonate and its replacement by ketoacid anions (acetoacetate and β-hydroxybutyrate). However, many patients with DKA also have a hyperchloremic component, particularly if fluid intake has been maintained during the prodrome. This leads to enhanced filtration and loss of ketoacid anions in the urine and increased tubular reasborption of chloride. On admission, only about one half of the patients with DKA have a classic anion-gap acidosis and another 40% have a mixed acidosis (a combination of anion-gap ketoacidosis and hyperchloremic metabolic acidosis). In these patients the increase in the anion gap accounts for only 0.4 to 0.8 of the reduction in bicarbonate concentration.

Classically, patients with HHS are much less acidemic (by definition, pH ≥7.30 and bicarbonate >15 mEq/L). Urinary ketones are only weakly positive and the degree of ketoacidosis is generally defined as mild. Often, the acidosis is attributed to coexisting renal dysfunction or lactic acidosis occurring in the setting of severe intravascular volume depletion. Relatively little is known about the extent of ketoacidosis in HHS because these patients often have concomitant metabolic alkalosis due to preceding treatment with diuretic agents and because the frequency of concomitant extreme hypovolemia compromises oxygen delivery, leading to lactic acidosis and preferential formation of β-hydroxybutyrate. Because β-hydroxybutyrate is not detected by the qualitative nitroprusside reagents used for detecting ketone bodies, the degree of ketoacidosis is often underestimated. Direct measurement of β-hydroxybutyrate could be helpful in resolving this question and in the management of DKA.

# Diagnosis

The diagnostic features of DKA and HHS are shown in Table 1. The glucose concentration is not a defining characteristic of DKA. Euglycemic DKA (glucose <300-325 mg/dL) can be observed in pregnant women with type 1 diabetes with coexistent alcoholism, type 1 diabetes, and malnutrition. DKA can be further defined as mild, moderate, or severe based on pH and bicarbonate levels:

- Mild: pH 7.25-7.30; $HCO_3^-$ 15-18 mEq/L
- Moderate: pH 7.00-7.24; $HCO_3^-$ 10-14 mEq/L
- Severe: pH ≤7.00; $HCO_3^-$ <10 mEq/L

Patients with DKA and HHS have substantial deficits of water, sodium, chloride, potassium, magnesium, calcium, and phosphorus (Table 2). These deficits are usually obscured on presentation because of the water deficit, and these important deficits appear during therapy. The average serum sodium in DKA is 128 mEq/L, as compared with

## TABLE 1  Diagnostic Features of DKA and HHS

| Measurement | DKA | HHS |
| --- | --- | --- |
| Glucose (mg/dL) | ≥300 | ≥600 |
| $E_{Osm}$ (mOsm/kg) | <320 | ≥320 |
| pH | ≤7.30 | ≥7.30 |
| $HCO_3^-$ (mEq/L) | <18 | ≥15 |
| Ketones (absent to +++) | ++ to +++ | Negative to + |
| Dehydration (absent to +++) | + to ++ | ++ to +++ |

*Abbreviations:* DKA = diabetic ketoacidosis; $E_{Osm}$ effective osmolality; HHS = hyperglycemic hyperosmolar syndrome.

## TABLE 2  Average Deficits of Water and Electrolytes in DKA and HHS

| Water and Electrolytes | DKA | HHS |
| --- | --- | --- |
| Water (mL/kg) | 100 | 100-200 |
| $Na^+$ (mEq/kg) | 7-10 | 5-13 |
| $Cl^-$ (mEq/kg) | 3-5 | 3-7 |
| $K^+$ (mEq/kg) | 3-5 | 5-15 |
| $PO_4^{2-}$ (mmol/kg) | 1-2 | 1-2 |
| $Ca^{2+}$ (mEq/kg) | 1-2 | 1-2 |
| $Mg^{2+}$ (mEq/kg) | 1-2 | 1-2 |

*Abbreviations:* DKA = diabetic ketoacidosis; $E_{Osm}$ effective osmolality; HHS = hyperglycemic hyperosmolar syndrome.
Data from Ennis ED, Kreisberg RA: Diabetic Ketoacidosis and the hyperglycemic hyperosmolar syndrome. In LeRoith D, Taylor SI, Olefsky JM (eds): Diabetes Mellitus: A Fundamental and Clinical Text. Philadelphia: Lippincott Williams & Wilkins, 2004, pp 627-642; and Matz R: Hyperglycemic hyperosmolar syndrome. In Porte D, Sherwin RS, Baron A (eds): Ellenberg and Rifkin's Diabetes Mellitus. New York: McGraw-Hill, 2003, pp 587-600.

the average serum sodium in HHS of 143 mEq/L. The difference of 15 mEq/L is consistent with a much greater deficit of water in HHS.

Serum amylase and lipase, which might suggest pancreatitis or other intra-abdominal disease, are usually abnormal in patients with DKA or HHS. However, in the vast majority of patients these abnormalities are due to the metabolic acidosis that accompanies DKA and HHS and are not due to pancreatitis or an intra-abdominal catastrophe, although the potential of intra-abdominal disease to precipitate decompensated diabetes should not be overlooked. To confound the

## CURRENT DIAGNOSIS

- Determine whether diabetes is new or established. If it is established, document therapy used and whether it was discontinued or the doses of agents used were reduced.
- Look for precipitating factors such as infection, myocardial infarction, intra-abdominal disease, CNS disease, and other medical illnesses. Document other medications being used and their potential for precipitating decompensation.
- Perform a careful physical examination with particular emphasis on the abdomen, chest, perineal area, and legs, looking for infection or cellulitis.
- Obtain CBC, urinalysis, metabolic profile (BUN, creatinine, electrolytes, liver tests), amylase, lipase, troponin (if myocardial infarction is a possibility), serum ketones, osmolality, and ABG. Obtain ECG, chest and abdominal films, and other imaging studies as dictated by the clinical findings. Obtain a urine culture and other cultures, as indicated, if empiric antibiotic therapy is used.
- Altered mental status in DKA is unusual. If DKA is present, consider CNS imaging techniques and a lumbar puncture. In HHS the $S_{Osm}$ typically exceeds 340 mOsm/kg in patients who have CNS alterations due to diabetic decompensation. In obtunded HHS patients with $S_{Osm}$ <340 mOsm/kg, other causes of CNS dysfunction should be aggressively sought.

*Abbreviations:* ABG = arterial blood gas; BUN = blood urea nitrogen; CBC = complete blood count; CNS = central nervous system; DKA = diabetic ketoacidosis; ECG = electrocardiogram; HHS = hyperglycemic hyperosmolar syndrome

issue, patients without abdominal pain can have elevated levels of amylase and lipase, and other patients with abdominal symptoms have normal levels of amylase and lipase. Abdominal symptoms and findings usually regress as the DKA and HHS are effectively treated. Persistence or appearance of abdominal symptoms or findings in the presence of elevated levels of amylase and lipase require further careful investigation.

The serum potassium in DKA is normal or elevated in approximately 80% of patients and is low in about 20% of patients. Hyperkalemia occurs despite a potassium deficit of 3 to 5 mEq/kg in DKA and 5 to 15 mEq/kg in HHS. This is consistent with the longer HHS prodrome and the fact that many elderly patients are using potassium-wasting diuretics. Hypokalemia on admission indicates severe potassium deficiency and requires treatment before starting insulin.

## Treatment

The treatment of DKA, HHS, and combinations of these disorders requires correction of hyperglycemia, electrolyte deficiencies, and acidosis by aggressive management with insulin, fluid, and electrolyte replacement as well as being aware of important pitfalls that can develop during therapy.

### ADMINISTER INSULIN

Ten units of regular or rapid-acting insulin should be administered intravenously followed by an insulin infusion of 0.1 U/kg/hour.

Normal saline (1 L/hour for 2-3 hours) followed by normal or half-normal saline (250-500 mL/hour) should be administered (see the Current Therapy box for details). With appropriate fluid and insulin therapy, the glucose concentration should decrease at a rate of 50 to 100 mg/dL/hour. Considering the average glucose level in DKA, it should take 4 to 6 hours for the glucose concentration to fall to the range of 250 to 300 mg/dL. It will take longer for the glucose concentration to reach this level in HHS. During the first 1 to 2 hours of therapy, the decrease in glucose concentration is primarily due to fluid administration. If the subsequent rate of decrease is less than 50 mg/dL/hour, the hourly infusion rate of insulin should be doubled. When using higher than usual insulin doses, hypokalemia should be anticipated.

### ADMINISTER DEXTROSE

When the glucose concentration reaches 250 to 300 mg/dL, intravenous fluids should be adjusted to incorporate 5% dextrose. The insulin dose should not be reduced until the pH is at least 7.3 or the $HCO_3^-$ is at least 18 mEq/L. This takes twice as long as the correction of hyperglycemia (8-12 hours). Thus, the addition of glucose in sufficient amounts to maintain the blood glucose at an acceptable level (250-300 mg/dL) is required while insulin therapy continues in order to correct the underlying acidosis.

### FLUID REPLACEMENT

Suboptimal correction of fluid deficits leads to persistently high levels of glucose counterregulatory hormones and insulin resistance.

---

## CURRENT THERAPY

- Insert a urinary catheter to monitor hourly urine output if the patient is unable to void or is obtunded.
- Insert a nasogastric tube if the abdomen is distended or bowel sounds are abnormal.
- Place an intravenous line and start fluids; initially use 0.9% saline (1000-1500 mL/h) to restore intravascular volume and effect hemodynamic stability, followed by 0.45% or 0.9% saline (250-500 mL/h) as determined by an assessment of intravascular volume, urine output, and clinical status. Remember, the water deficit can be variable. Replace approximately 50% of the perceived water deficit in 8 hours and 100% by 24 hours unless circumstances dictate otherwise.
- Add potassium to intravenous fluids when the adequacy of urine output has been established. The amount of potassium needed is dictated by the initial serum potassium level and usually varies between 20 and 40 mEq/L of fluid. No potassium should be administered if the potassium level is ≥5.5 mEq/L. The serum potassium should be maintained between 4 and 5 mEq/L.

- With effective therapy of hyperglycemia and ketoacidosis, the potassium nadir is at 4 to 6 hours.
- Insulin should be administered promptly except when the serum potassium is <3.3 mEq/L. Give 10 U of regular insulin as an IV bolus, followed by a continuous insulin infusion at a dose of 0.1 U/kg/h. In overweight or obese patients the use of insulin on the basis of weight may be inaccurate or impossible to accurately determine. In such patients, larger boluses and infusion doses may be necessary, but do not initially use more than 15 U for either of these. The subsequent insulin dose should be adjusted based on the glucose, $HCO_3^-$, and pH responses. Do not reduce insulin until the pH is ≥7.30 and the $HCO_3^-$ is ≥18 mEq/L.
- Bicarbonate is not usually necessary in patients with DKA, but its use should be individualized. If the pH is <7.0-7.1, 50 mmol bicarbonate can be infused over 1 hour, and 100 mmol bicarbonate can be infused over 2 hours. Effective therapy with fluids and insulin should make subsequent bicarbonate therapy unnecessary.

- Check the blood glucose every hour and electrolytes every 2 to 4 hours until the patient is stable.
- The glucose should decrease at a rate of 50-100 mg/dL/h. When the glucose reaches 250 to 300 mg/dL, glucose should be added to the infusion fluids (0.9% or 0.45% saline with 5% dextrose) to prevent or slow the further reduction of glucose level; usually 5 to 10 g/h of glucose is required.
- It takes twice as long for the bicarbonate to reach 18 mEq/L or the pH ≥7.3 than for the glucose to reach 250 to 300 mg/h. Continue the initial insulin infusion rate until these targets are reached before reducing the infusion to 2 to 3 U/h. Continue this infusion rate until subcutaneous insulin has been initiated and is effective.
- The subcutaneous insulin dose should be determined from prior insulin doses in patients with preexisting diabetes; the dose of insulin in new diabetics should be estimated by providing 0.4 to 0.5 U/kg, one half administered as intermediate or long-acting insulin once or twice daily and one half as rapid-acting insulin before meals and snacks.

Optimal insulin administration is necessary to reverse ketoacidosis, but reversal of hyperglycemia is primarily due to fluid replacement, dilution, and increased excretion of glucose in the urine.

## ADMINISTER POTASSIUM

Potassium, as the chloride or phosphate, should be administered at a rate to keep the serum concentration within normal limits. If the potassium is less than 3.3 mEq/L, potassium should be replaced before starting insulin. If the serum potassium is greater than 5.5 mEq/L, potassium administration should be withheld until the serum potassium is within the normal range and there is adequate urine output. Insulin corrects the acidosis and promotes potassium entry into cells, independent of its effects on glucose. Correction of fluid deficits during treatment increases the urinary excretion of potassium (about one half of the administered potassium is excreted in the urine). If the patient is oliguric, potassium supplementation is still needed, but the rate of potassium administration should be reduced by at least 50% and the serum potassium should be followed carefully.

## FURTHER ADJUSTMENTS

Hyperchloremia is common after treatment of DKA. There are multiple reasons for this. The base deficit is much greater than the availability of ketones to regenerate bicarbonate. The sodium-acquisitive kidney reabsorbs sodium with the most available anion, chloride, which during treatment has been given in large amounts. There is increased excretion and loss of ketones in the urine as a consequence of correction of volume deficits, thereby further limiting substrate for bicarbonate regeneration. There is no evidence that the mild hyperchloremic metabolic acidosis, which often develops during the therapy of DKA and HHS, is detrimental.

Hyperventilation reverses slowly, so systemic pH may be normal at lower than normal bicarbonate concentrations.

In patients with severe hyperosmolality and hypernatremia, the serum sodium concentration can further increase as the glucose concentration decreases unless free water is replaced. The final serum sodium concentration that occurs after correction of the hyperglycemia can be calculated by correcting the sodium for the hyperglycemia. The usual correction factor is 1.8, that is, the serum sodium increases by 1.8 mEq/L for each 100 mg/dL decrease in glucose. This correction is based on hypothetical conditions. More recently, replication of the effects of hyperglycemia in vivo in humans suggests that a correction factor of 2.4 is more accurate.

Changes in the serum sodium concentration during treatment should influence subsequent treatment decisions. The sodium level can be expected to increase during therapy of DKA and return to or toward the normal range. Should the serum sodium remain unchanged or decrease as the hyperglycemia of DKA is corrected, the patient is receiving excess free water, and normal saline should be substituted for half-normal saline. This may be important in treating DKA in children because hyponatremia and hypo-osmolality have been associated with the development of cerebral edema in children. An increasing serum sodium in HHS, where pretreatment levels are already normal or high, is expected as hyperglycemia is corrected and water moves from the extracellular to the intracellular compartments. An increasing serum sodium level during therapy should be an indication to switch from normal to half-normal saline if the patient is hemodynamically stable.

The concentration of all electrolytes will decrease with therapy. The nadir of the serum potassium and phosphorus occurs at 4 to 6 hours. No replacement of phosphorus is necessary unless the concentration of phosphate is less than 1.0 mg/dL. Occasionally, patients require replacement of magnesium and calcium if tetany occurs, although tetany usually occurs with excessive phosphorus administration.

## REFERENCES

American Diabetes Association: Hyperglycemic crises in diabetes. Diabetes Care 2004;27:S94-S102.

Androgue HJ, Wilson H, Boyd AE, Eknoyau G: Plasma acid-base patterns in diabetic ketoacidosis. N Engl J Med 1982;26:1603-1610.

Bhowmick SK, Levens KL, Rettig KR: Hyperosmolar hyperglycemic crisis: An acute life-threatening event in children and adolescents with type 2 diabetes mellitus. Endocr Pract 2006;11(1):23-29.

Ennis ED, Kreisberg RA: Diabetic ketoacidosis and the hyperglycemic hyperosmolar syndrome. In Porte D, Sherwin RS, Baron A (eds): Ellenberg and Rifkin's Diabetes Mellitus. New York: McGraw-Hill, 2003, pp 573-586.

Ennis ED, Kreisberg RA: Diabetic ketoacidosis. In Porte D, Sherwin RS, Baron A (eds): Ellenberg and Rifkin's Diabetes Mellitus. New York: McGraw-Hill, 2003, pp 573-580.

Glaser N, Barnett P, McCaslin I, et al: Risk factors for cerebral edema in children with diabetic ketoacidosis. N Engl J Med 201;644:254-269.

Hillier TA, Abbott RD, Barrett EJ: Hyponatremia: Evaluating the correction factor for hyperglycemia. Am J Med 2000;108(2):180-181.

Kitabchi AE: Ketosis-prone diabetes—A new subgroup of patients with atypical type 1 and type 2 diabetes? J Clin Endocrinol Metab 2003;88:5087-5089.

Kitabchi AE, Umpierrez GE, Murphy MD, Kreisberg RA: Hyperglycemic crisis in adult patients with diabetes mellitus: A consensus statement from the American Diabetes Association. Diabetes Care 2006;29:2739-2748.

Matz R: Hyperglycemic hyperosmolar syndrome. In Porte D, Sherwin RS, Baron A (eds): Ellenberg and Rifkin's Diabetes Mellitus. New York: McGraw-Hill, 2003, pp 587-600.

Wang J, Williams DE, Narayan KMV, Geiss LS: Declining death rates from hyperglycemic crisis among adults with diabetes, U.S., 1985-2002. Diabetes Care 2006;29:2018-2022.

# Hyponatremia

Method of
*Gregory Proctor, MD, and Moshe Levi, MD*

Hyponatremia is defined as plasma sodium ($Na^+$) concentration of less than 135 mEq/L. It is a common finding in the hospitalized patient, with an estimated inpatient incidence of 10% to 15%.

Hyponatremia arises when water intake exceeds the kidney's ability to excrete free water. Normal renal excretion of electrolyte free water requires that three processes be intact. First, glomerular filtration must occur with delivery of ultrafiltrate to the tubular lumen. Second, solute removal must occur in the thick ascending limb and distal tubule, where tubular fluid can be diluted. Third, circulating levels of antidiuretic hormone (ADH) must be appropriately low, minimizing tubular aquaporin channel expression and water reabsorption. When all three processes are intact, minimally dilute urine of 50 to 60 mOsm/kg is excreted. Therefore, a patient who excretes a normal dietary solute intake of 600 to 900 mOsm/day can excrete a maximum urine volume of 10 to 18 L/day. Most cases of hyponatremia are due to a renal impairment in water excretion arising from high circulating levels of ADH. The remainder of cases result from water intake in excess of renal water excretory capacity limited by renal solute abundance or glomerular filtration rate (GFR).

## Approach to Hyponatremia

Preliminary evaluation of hyponatremia should begin with measurement of the serum osmolality and classification into hypo-osmolar, normo-osmolar, or hyperosmolar hyponatremia (Box 1).

Hyperosmolar hyponatremia is most commonly caused by severe hyperglycemia as seen in diabetic ketoacidosis (DKA) or uncontrolled type 2 diabetes mellitus. It may also be seen during hypertonic infusion of mannitol (Osmitrol) used to treat intracranial hypertension. High serum concentrations of glucose resulting from insulinopenic states in types 1 and 2 diabetes mellitus cause water movement out of the intracellular space into the extracellular space, leading to dilution of the serum sodium ($S_{Na}$). For every 100 mg/dL increase in serum glucose, the serum sodium decreases by approximately 1.6 mEq/L. Treatment of hyperglycemia with insulin rapidly moves glucose into

## BOX 1 Causes and Classification of Hyponatremia

### High Plasma Osmolality
- Hyperglycemia
- Hypertonic mannitol

### Normal Plasma Osmolality (Pseudohyponatremia)
- Hyperlipidemia
- Hyperparaproteinemia

### Low Plasma Osmolality
#### High Circulating ADH
- Cirrhosis
- Drugs
- ECV depletion
- Glucocorticoid deficiency
- Heart failure
- Hypothyroidism
- Pregnancy
- Severe hypoalbuminemia
- SIADH
- True volume depletion

#### Low Circulating ADH
- Acute or chronic renal failure
- Low solute intake (beer potomania)
- Primary polydipsia

*Abbreviations:* ADH = antidiuretic hormone (vasopressin); CKD = chronic kidney disease; ECV = effective circulating volume depletion; SIADH = secretion of inappropriate antidiuretic hormone.

cells followed by water movement in the same direction, resulting in correction of the hyponatremia.

Normo-osmolar hyponatremia, also known as pseudohyponatremia, occurs when a component of the solid phase of plasma is increased, as seen in severe hypertriglyceridemia or paraproteinemia. Normo-osmolar hyponatremia is a laboratory artifact resulting in falsely low serum sodium. It occurs when flame photometry methods are used to measure sodium concentration in whole plasma and does not occur when serum is analyzed with direct potentiometry, which measures actual serum sodium concentration.

Hypo-osmolar hyponatremia is by far the most common form of hyponatremia and is the focus of the remainder of this chapter.

## HYPO-OSMOLAR HYPONATREMIA: ASSESSMENT OF VOLUME STATUS

Following measurement of serum osmolality and exclusion of pseudohyponatremia and hyperosmolar hypernatremia, the next step in the evaluating hyponatremia is assessing the patient's volume status (Figure 1). A careful physical examination should be performed to determine the patient's effective circulating volume (ECV) and net total body sodium. This allows classification of the patient into one of three categories: hypovolemic hyponatremia (with a deficit in total body sodium), hypervolemic hyponatremia (with excess total body sodium), or euvolemic hyponatremia (with near-normal total body sodium).

Patients with *hypovolemic hyponatremia* have a deficit in total body sodium causing low ECV and nonosmotic release of antidiuretic hormone (ADH). High circulating ADH levels stimulate excessive renal water reabsorption and subsequent development of hyponatremia. Physical examination typically shows flat neck veins, absence of edema, dry mucous membranes and axillae, orthostatic hypotension, and tachycardia. When volume losses are nonrenal (due to hemorrhage, diarrhea, dermal losses, or third spacing of fluids as in pancreatitis or peritonitis), the spot urine sodium concentration ($U_{Na^+}$) is low, typically

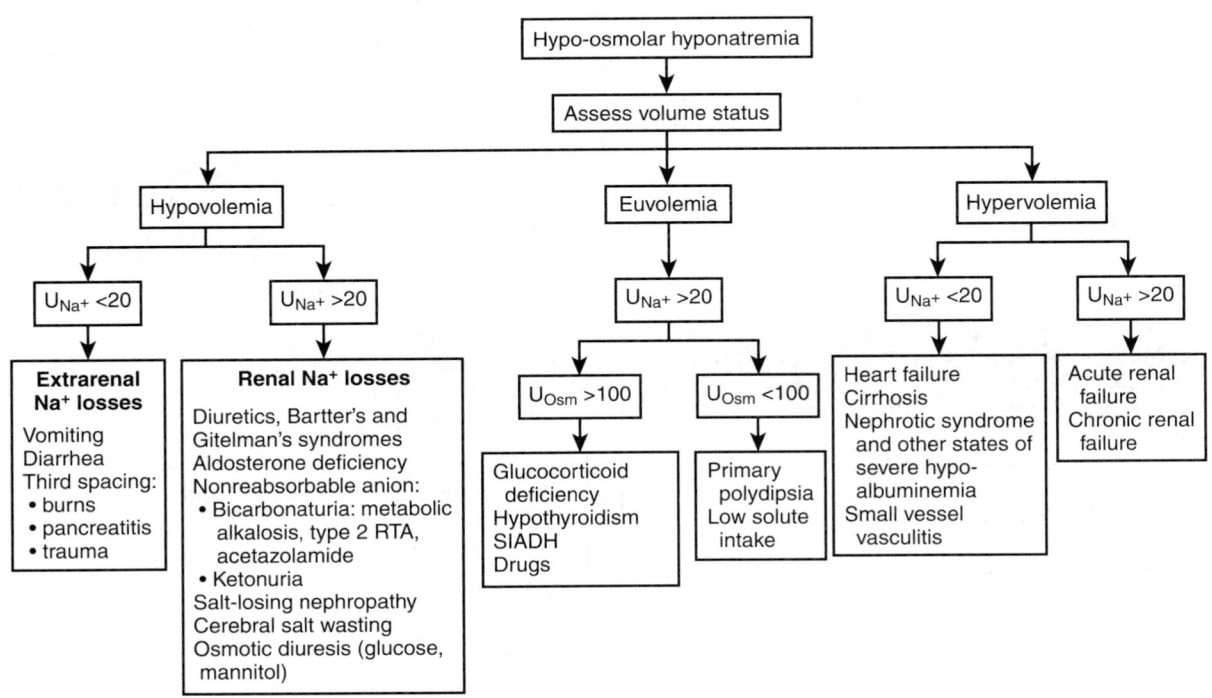

**FIGURE 1.** Diagnostic approach to hypo-osmolar hyponatremia. *Abbreviations:* RTA, renal tubular acidosis; SIADH, syndrome of inappropriate antidiuretic hormone secretion; $U_{Na^+}$, urinary sodium concentration (mEq/L); $U_{Osm}$, urine osmolality (mOsm/kg water).

less than 20 mEq/L (see Figure 1). When volume losses are due in part to renal sodium wasting, the $U_{Na^+}$ is greater than 20 mEq/L. Such renal sodium wasting may be seen in the presence of active diuretics, mineralocorticoid deficiency, osmotic diuresis, salt-losing nephropathy, bicarbonaturia (most commonly from vomiting), and ketonuria.

*Hypervolemic hyponatremic* patients have excess total body sodium manifested by edema. These patients have low ECV secondary to heart failure, cirrhosis, or severe hypoalbuminemia (as may be seen in the nephrotic syndrome). Low ECV stimulates nonosmotic release of vasopressin, renal water reabsorption, and subsequent hyponatremia. Spot urinary sodium is very low (often <10 mEq/L) due to avid renal sodium retention. Physical examination demonstrates any combination of peripheral edema, ascites, pulmonary congestion, and jugular venous distention. Hypervolemic hyponatremia may also be seen in acute or chronic renal failure where appropriate renal excretion of sodium and water is greatly decreased. In such situations, hyponatremia is dilutional, occurring as a result of water intake in excess of sodium intake. It is a common finding in patients with end-stage renal disease (ESRD) who cannot excrete large dietary water intake. The $U_{Na^+}$ may be greater than 20 mEq/L in these cases because of either appropriate sodium excretion in the setting of high ECV or sodium wasting from frank tubular dysfunction.

*Euvolemic hyponatremia* is commonly seen in hospitalized patients. These patients have normal ECV and manifest no signs of edema or hypovolemia. They are in sodium balance and therefore have spot urinary sodium concentrations that reflect excretion of dietary intake ($U_{Na^+}$ >20 mEq/L). Causes of euvolemic hyponatremia are hypothyroidism, glucocorticoid deficiency, acute emotional stress or psychosis, certain drugs, secretion of inappropriate ADH (SIADH), primary polydipsia, or very low solute intake. Circulating ADH levels are high in all these disorders except for primary polydipsia and low solute intake. High ADH levels are reflected by less than maximally concentrated urine ($U_{Osm}$ >100 mOsm/kg). ADH levels are appropriately low in primary polydipsia and low solute intake as reflected by $U_{Osm}$ less than 100 mOsm/kg. Drugs associated with euvolemic hyponatremia are believed to act largely by stimulating release of ADH from the posterior pituitary gland (Box 2) but can act to potentiate the effect of ADH on the distal tubule. SIADH may be caused by a wide variety of central nervous system (CNS) and pulmonary disorders as well as carcinomas of the lung, pancreas, and duodenum (Box 3).

## SYMPTOMS

Symptoms of acute hyponatremia occur directly as a result of water movement into the brain and the development of cerebral edema. Early symptoms are anorexia and nausea and may occur even with mild reductions in serum sodium concentration. As hyponatremia worsens, depressed sensorium, seizures, coma, and death from cerebral herniation may occur. These symptoms cam occur even with mild

## CURRENT DIAGNOSIS

- Determine if hyponatremia is hypo-osmolar, normo-osmolar or hyperosmolar.
- If a hypo-osmolar state exists, perform a careful physical examination to establish the patient's volume status (presence of edema, jugular venous distention, ascites, orthostatic hypotension, dry mucous membranes).
- Then measure the urine sodium and osmolality to further narrow the differential diagnosis.

reductions in serum sodium in young patients and constitute a medical emergency.

## CEREBRAL ADAPTATION TO HYPONATREMIA

Cerebral adaptation to hypotonicity involves early movement of water (within 1-3 hours) out of cells into the CSF, followed by shunting into the systemic circulation. Next, brain cells adapt by losing cellular potassium, organic solutes, and then other organic osmolytes such as phosphocreatine, myoinositol, and amino acids. This adaptation requires 48 to 72 hours and is very effective in reducing brain swelling. Thus, when hyponatremia occurs slowly, allowing time for adaptation to occur, patients can present with few or no symptoms. When hyponatremia develops acutely, in less than 48 hours, adaptation has not had time to occur and patients are at high risk for developing cerebral edema and intracranial hypertension. Whereas patients with acute hyponatremia are particularly at risk for cerebral edema, those with chronic, asymptomatic hyponatremia (in whom cerebral adaptation has occurred) are at risk for osmotic demyelination syndrome if correction occurs too rapidly.

# Treatment

Treatment of hyponatremia is dictated by presence or absence of symptoms and acute versus chronic development (Figure 2). Hyponatremia that develops in less than 48 hours is considered acute.

---

**BOX 2 Medications Associated with Euvolemic Hyponatremia**

- Amitriptyline (Elavil)
- Antidepressants (especially SSRIs)
- Carbamazepine (Tegretol)
- Chlorpropamide (Diabinese)
- Clofibrate (Atromid-S)[2]
- Cyclophosphamide (Cytoxan)
- DDAVP (Desmopressin)
- Haloperidol (Haldol), thioridazine, thiothixene (Navane)
- Nonsteroidal anti-inflammatory drugs
- Oxytocin (Pitocin)
- Vincristine (Vincasar)

[2]Not available in the United States.
*Abbreviation:* SSRI = selective serotonin reuptake inhibitor.

---

**BOX 3 Causes of SIADH**

- Acute emotional stress, psychosis, or physical pain
- Pulmonary disease
  - Pulmonary abscess
  - Tuberculosis
  - Viral, bacterial, or fungal pneumonia
- CNS disease
  - Brain abscess
  - Brain trauma
  - Encephalitis
  - Guillain-Barré syndrome
  - Intraparenchymal, subarachnoid, or subdural hemorrhage
  - Ischemic CVA
  - Meningitis
- Carcinomas
  - Duodenum
  - Lung
  - Pancreas

*Abbreviations:* CNS, central nervous system; CVA, cerebral vascular accident; SIADH = secretion of inappropriate antidiuretic hormone.

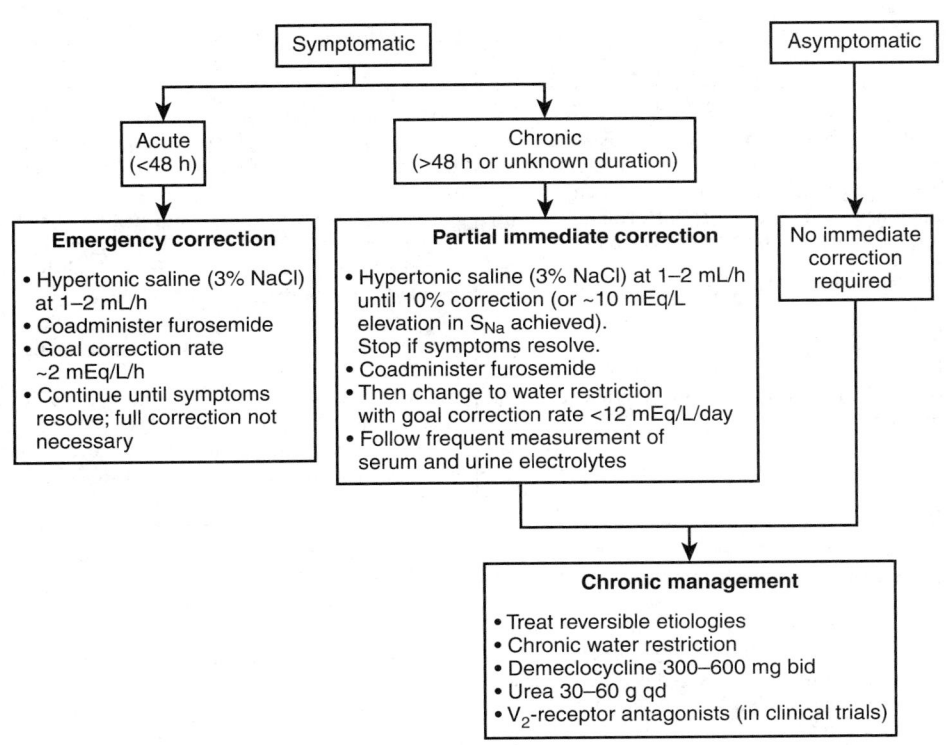

**FIGURE 2.** Treatment algorithm for severe euvolemic hyponatremia: serum sodium ($S_{Na}$) <125 mEq/L.

If the time course is greater than 48 hours *or if the time-course is unknown,* then hyponatremia is considered chronic.

## ACUTE HYPONATREMIA

Acute symptomatic hyponatremia should be treated promptly because of the high morbidity associated with acute cerebral edema. Serum $Na^+$

## CURRENT THERAPY

- Symptomatic acute hyponatremia (<48 h duration) warrants immediate correction with hypertonic saline (3% NaCl) infused at 1-2[3] mL/kg/h with coadministration of furosemide (Lasix) until symptoms resolve.
- Symptomatic chronic hyponatremia (>48 h duration) warrants immediate partial correction of approximately 10% of the sodium deficit (~10 mEq/L elevation in $S_{Na^+}$) using hypertonic saline (3% NaCl) infused at 1-2[3] mL/kg/h coadministered with furosemide, followed by slower correction not faster than 1-1.5 mEq/L/h or 12 mEq/L/day.
- Asymptomatic hyponatremia requires no immediate intervention and may be treated with correction of the underlying etiology (e.g., discontinuation of drugs that cause hyponatremia, hormone replacement in hypothyroidism or cortisol deficiency, 0.9% saline in hypovolemic hyponatremia, diuresis, inotropes and water restriction for heart failure, water restriction for SIADH and cirrhosis.

[3]Exceeds dosage recommended by the manufacturer.
*Abbreviations:* $S_{Na^+}$ = serum sodium, SIADH = secretion of inappropriate antidiuretic hormone.

should be raised by 2 mEq/L/hour until symptoms resolve by infusing hypertonic saline (3% NaCl) at 1 to 2[3] mL/kg/hour. The rate of correction should aim for approximately 2 mEq/L/hour. Full correction is probably safe but is not necessary. In the setting of antidiuresis, where spot urinary sodium ($U_{Na}$) and potassium ($U_K$) concentrations sum to greater than 150 mEq/L ($U_{Na} + U_K$ > 150 mEq/L), administration of furosemide (Lasix) with hypertonic saline ensures electrolyte-free water excretion and correction of hyponatremia.

## CHRONIC HYOPNATREMIA

Chronic symptomatic hyponatremia must be handled with care. Promptly increase the serum $Na^+$ concentration by 10% (or by approximately 10 mEq/L). After completing this initial rapid correction, further correction should not exceed a rate of 1.0 to 1.5 mEq/L/hour or 12 mEq/L/24 hours.

Chronic asymptomatic hyponatremia is treated conservatively, because these patients are at risk for osmotic demyelination syndrome if correction is too rapid. No immediate intervention is needed. The underlying cause of hyponatremia should be carefully sought. If hypothyroidism or cortisol deficiency is present, then hormone replacement is indicated followed by close observation of the serum sodium. Likewise, if the cause is congestive heart failure, gentle diuresis and a trial of inotropes can improve myocardial function and ECV leading to improvement in hyponatremia. If the cause is hypovolemic hyponatremia, careful restoration of ECV by administration of 0.9% saline with careful observation of serum sodium is indicated. In general, if the underlying cause of hyponatremia cannot be identified or corrected (as in end-stage liver or heart disease, severe nephrotic syndrome, and some forms of SIADH) several approaches are available.

### Fluid Restriction

Fluid restriction is usually successful if the patient is compliant. The degree of fluid restriction can be estimated by two methods.

[3]Exceeds dosage recommended by the manufacturer.

Division of the daily osmolar load by the minimal urine osmolality approximates the maximal urine volume and hence the daily fluid allowance. The daily osmolar load in a North American diet is estimated at approximately 10 mOsm per kilogram of body weight, and the minimal urine osmolality is obtained directly by measurement of the patient's urine osmolality. Therefore, fluid restriction (liters) is less than the daily osmolar load (mOsm/day)/$U_{Osm}$ (mOsm/L). The second method employs simultaneous measurement of spot urinary sodium, potassium, and serum sodium concentrations and a calculation of:

$$\text{Urine osmolality} = \frac{(U_{Na} + U_K)}{S_{Na}}$$

If the value is < 0.5, then fluid is restricted to a maximum of 1 L/day. If the value is 0.5 to 1.0, fluid is restricted to a maximum of 500 mL/day. If the value is greater than 1.0, then fluid restriction alone might not be sufficient to raise the serum sodium concentration.

## Pharmacologic Therapy

Pharmacologic agents include demeclocycline, urea, daily sodium chloride tablets plus low-dose furosemide, and $V_2$-receptor antagonists, which inhibit vasopressin-mediated water reabsorption. One IV formulation, conivaptan (Vaprisol), has been approved for treatment of euvolemic hyponatremia, and several oral $V_2$ antagonists are undergoing clinical trials for approval by the U.S Food and Drug Administration. $V_2$-receptor antagonists will likely become the first-line treatment for euvolemic and hypervolemic hypernatremia.

Until broad clinical experience with $V_2$ antagonists is obtained, demeclocycline (Declomycin),[1] a drug that inhibits renal tubular responsiveness to ADH, leading to increased water excretion, is currently the agent of choice. Onset is 3 to 6 days. Demeclocycline is prescribed in doses of 300 to 900 mg/day with unrestricted water intake. Furosemide 40 mg/day in combination with 2 to 3 grams of sodium chloride tablets will force increased urine volume and allow a patient to consume more water. Finally, prescription of urea (Ureaphil)[1] 30 to 60 g/day increases urinary solute, and hence water excretion is limited by unpalatable taste and gastrointestinal symptoms.

## REFERENCES

Berl T, Schrier RW; The patient with hyponatremia or hypernatremia. In Schrier RW (ed): Manual of Nephrology, 6th ed. Philadelphia: Lippincott Williams & Wilkins, 2005, pp 21-36.

Kumar S, Berl T: Sodium. Lancet 1998;352:220-228.

Thurman J, Halterman R, Berl T: Therapy of dysnatremic disorders. In Brady N, Wilcox C (eds): Therapy of Nephrology and Hypertension. Philadelphia: WB Saunders, 2003, pp 335-348.

[1]Not FDA approved for this indication.

# Hyperuricemia and Gout

Method of
*Brian F. Mandell, MD, PhD*

Gouty arthritis is the most common cause of attacks of acute inflammatory arthritis. The occurrence and the demographics of gout can be explained by the presence of hyperuricemia in patients who experience gouty arthritis, tophaceous deposits of uric acid, and uric acid nephrolithiasis. Urate begins to precipitate in biological fluids at levels greater than 6.8 mg/dL. The major predictor of urate levels in a given patient is the ability of that person's kidneys to efficiently excrete uric acid. Several factors influence the renal transport and excretion of uric

acid, including genetically determined expression and properties of uric acid transporters in the proximal tubules including urate-transporter-1 (URAT-1), hormonal (estrogen) influences on expression of URAT-1, the glomerular filtration rate (GFR), and the presence of alcohol, medications, and endogenous anions and other substances that can affect the efficiency of uric acid secretion from blood into the urine.

Most of the urate load that must be excreted comes from metabolism of endogenous purines. Dietary intake of purine precursors to uric acid can raise the serum urate slightly in some patients if their kidneys cannot efficiently excrete the extra uric acid load. Humans do not have the enzyme *uricase*, which in other species directly metabolizes urate to the more soluble compound allantoin. Thus, urate must be excreted via renal and to a lesser extent gastrointestinal disposal mechanisms. The genetic, hormonal, medication, and to a certain extent behavioral (alcohol intake) effects on uric acid excretion explain to a large part the familial occurrence of gout. These effects also explain the predilection of gout to affect men, postmenopausal women, and patients with hypertension and renal disease. However, as discussed later, hyperuricemia may also contribute to the development of hypertension, other vascular diseases, and progression of renal insufficiency.

The constant bathing of tissues in levels of urate above the potential saturation point of 6.8 mg/dL can result in the deposition of urate crystals. Urate crystals can be directly toxic to cells via membranolytic effects, but they also can invoke an extremely vigorous acute neutrophil inflammatory response triggered through components of the innate immune system. Chronic crystal deposition can result in a granulomatous inflammatory reaction that is far less dramatic than acute gouty attacks.

Although a significant percentage of the population in Western countries has a level exceeding 6.8 mg/dL, it is only the minority who develop acute and chronic gouty arthritis. The explanation for this is not entirely clear, likely reflecting our limited understanding of the factors controlling the nucleation of urate into crystals and factors in addition to pH, temperature, and concentration that can influence tissue deposition. In patients with chronic biological hyperuricemia (>6.8 mg/dL), sudden fluctuations, up or down, of the serum urate level can provoke acute attacks of gout. Such fluctuations can be caused by many things including alcohol ingestion, starvation, fluid shifts during surgery, medications, and interventions specifically directed at lowering the serum urate level.

## Acute and Chronic Arthritis

Acute gouty arthritis typically occurs in men from the third decade onward and in postmenopausal women. However, due to the myriad of reasons, including genetic enzymopathies, that patients can become chronically hyperuricemic, it can occur in patients of both sexes at all ages. Generally, patients are exposed to several years of serum urate levels greater than 6.8 mg/dL before the first attack of gout. Initial attacks are often extremely acute in onset and are dramatic in terms of the degree of pain and signs of inflammation. Some patients recall multiple twinges of discomfort before the first attack. Initial attacks often involve the lower extremities, including the base of the great toe, midfoot, or knee, but virtually any joint, tendon sheath, or bursa can be involved. Attacks can occur during the night or first appear during the day, and it is not uncommon that patients attribute the first attack to twisting their ankle or stepping off a curb wrong and self-medicate without seeing a physician.

Attacks are self-limited; the initial attacks can last 3 to 10 days even without anti-inflammatory therapy. Perhaps 10% of patients do not have another attack for many years or never again. However, the overwhelming majority of patients experience recurrent attacks, although not necessarily at the same anatomic site. Over years, if hyperuricemia persists and the patient is not on an anti-inflammatory medication to prevent attacks, gouty flares can occur more frequently, involve more joints, and persist for longer periods if not treated. Tophaceous nodules, usually asymptomatic, can appear around joints, at areas of friction or microtrauma, and particularly within the olecranon bursae, along the ulnar aspect of the forearms, around bunions, along the Achilles tendons, and within the finger pads.

Gout occasionally evolves into a chronic polyarthritis that is characterized by multiple deformed joints. There is often asymmetric joint involvement in these patients, with a nodular component to the joint swelling that is greater than that observed in rheumatoid arthritis. Involvement of the distal interphalangeal joints of the hands, particularly in postmenopausal women with osteoarthritis and Heberden's nodes, also distinguishes this from rheumatoid (but not psoriatic) arthritis. Chronic gouty polyarthritis tends to occur with less severe pain than acute attacks, but it has chronic discomfort, stiffness, and loss of joint mobility.

Patients who have received organ transplants and are on chronic therapy with calcineurin antagonists (e.g., cyclosporine), are prone to develop particularly aggressive, rapidly progressing tophaceous gout. They can develop gout in the upper extremities, fingers, shoulders, and tendon sheaths earlier than is normally expected.

Patients with acute gouty arthritis often have fever, especially if the attack involves more than a single joint. Although the pain may be more severe in gout, it is impossible to distinguish with certainty gout from septic arthritis (or pseudogout) on the basis of history, symptoms, physical findings, or laboratory results other than synovial fluid analysis and culture.

The definitive diagnosis of gouty arthritis is made by identifying negatively elongating birefringent needle-shaped crystals in the synovial fluid of an inflamed joint, with the exclusion of infection by fluid culture. Routinely, in the appropriate setting consistent with an acute gout attack in the absence of a concurrent or antecedent bacterial infection or exposure, the finding of urate crystals is sufficient to warrant specific treatment for crystal-induced arthritis. However, crystals can persist for years in joints that have been previously affected by a gout attack unless the serum urate has been lowered. These joints rarely become infected, with crystals still evident in the fluid. Thus, full clinical assessment is warranted, looking for any clues that heighten concern for bacteremia or locally acquired bacterial infection. It is never inappropriate to send inflammatory synovial fluid for microbiological culture while treating the patient for gout based on a positive crystal analysis. If crystals are not seen, the diagnosis of gout should not be made until cultures return as negative and reaspiration identifies crystals.

Although the first episodes of gout should be documented by synovial fluid analysis if at all possible, at times it may be impossible to aspirate fluid due to the location of the apparent attack (e.g., midfoot) or the logistics of the examination (patient refusal for reaspiration, dry aspirates, or inadequate equipment). In these cases, especially with a prior history of documented attacks of gout and no special concern for infection, it may be appropriate to treat empirically for crystal-induced arthritis, with close follow-up and communication with the patient.

## Hyperuricemia

A longstanding asymptomatic serum urate level higher than 6.8 mg/dL is almost invariable in patients as a prodrome to gouty arthritis, and hyperuricemia is the strongest independent risk factor for the development of gout. However, the urate level may be lower than this at the time of an acute attack. This can occur either because something has transiently lowered the urate level (often a medication, crash diet, or intravenous fluid) and thus precipitated the attack, or cytokines such as interleukin-6 released during an acute attack have lowered the serum urate level due to effects on urinary excretion of uric acid.

Whether hyperuricemia is an independent direct contributor to the risk of atherosclerotic cardiovascular disease (ASCVD) is controversial. Up until the past few years the prevalent perspective was that asymptomatic hyperuricemia is benign, and that the epidemiologic association of hyperuricemia with ASCVD was on the basis of shared comorbidities (diuretic use, hypertensive renal disease, insulin-resistance syndromes, and high red meat Western diet). However, analysis of several large patient registries and the data from large ASCVD intervention trials using multiregression analyses suggest that hyperuricemia may be an independent risk factor for cardiovascular events.

In parallel with these analyses there is increased recognition of potential pathophysiologic links between urate levels and vascular disease. Data from a rat model of acute mild hyperuricemia strongly suggest a direct link between hyperuricemia and renin-related hypertension and endothelial dysfunction. Other studies, also in rats, indicate that dietary fructose–induced hyperuricemia can directly induce resistance to some of the effects of insulin, thus leading to the development of components of the metabolic syndrome. Hyperinsulinemia also can directly perpetuate hyperuricemia via suppression of renal uric acid excretion.

At present there is not enough evidence or adequate interventional outcome data in humans to support the treatment of asymptomatic hyperuricemia with the hope of reducing cardiovascular events or progression of renal disease, congestive heart failure (CHF), or ASCVD.

## Treatment

### ANTI-INFLAMMATORIES

The treatment of patients with gout can be conceptually and practically divided into three discrete areas: treating the acute attack, preventing the next attack with anti-inflammatory therapy (prophylaxis), and treating the underlying root cause of gout, hyperuricemia. Although the management of these three areas overlaps, it is useful to specifically address and periodically reevaluate each one at every gouty patient's visit.

Acute gout can be extremely painful and can severely hamper the patient's ability to pursue normal activities. Fortunately, attacks respond fairly quickly to high-dose anti-inflammatory therapy. Pure analgesic therapy is less effective. Attacks generally respond to any one of several classes of medications; the choice of therapeutic agent is usually dictated by the patient's comorbidities (Box 1) and relative contraindications to the different medications. Many experienced clinicians believe, although no controlled trials or high-quality observational data have been collected, that patients respond more rapidly to therapy the earlier in an attack that therapy is initiated. Thus, many clinicians advise patients who suffer from recurrent (documented) gout attacks to initiate therapy at the first *twinge* of what they recognize as an attack. Difficulty in completely resolving an acute attack is often the result of using a too-low dose of anti-inflammatory therapy, discontinuing it as soon as the patient begins to experience relief, or failing to recognize that changes in the serum urate level at the time of the attack can predispose the patient to rebound flares unless some form of continued anti-inflammatory therapy is provided.

---

### CURRENT DIAGNOSIS

- Gouty arthritis is characterized by the acute onset of articular and/or periarticular pain accompanied by objective signs of inflammation.
- Initial attacks of gout are often monoarticular, in the lower extremities, self-limited, and very responsive to high-dose anti-inflammatory therapy.
- Diagnosis is ideally made by documenting the presence of urate crystals in the affected joint or bursal fluid. The serum urate level should not be relied on as a diagnostic test for acute gout.
- Hyperuricemia may be clinically significant when it is >6.8 mg/dL; this is the approximate level at which urate begins to precipitate in biological fluids.
- Some patients with years of inadequately treated gout develop chronically swollen painful arthritis and tissue deposits of uric acid (tophi), which can resemble rheumatoid arthritis.

## BOX 1 Therapy of Acute Gouty Arthritis

- Confirm the diagnosis by arthrocentesis if possible; exclude septic arthritis.
- Avoid changes in drugs that affect the serum urate level, if possible.
- Any nonsteroidal anti-inflammatory drugs (NSAIDs) may be prescribed in high doses. Relative and absolute contraindications include dyspepsia or prior history of treated PUD (can consider using with a PPI), renal insufficiency, thrombocytopenia or platelet dysfunction, recent gastric ulcer with bleed (absolute contraindication), coumadin therapy (strong contraindication), and uncontrolled CHF. Some options include:
  - Indomethacin (Indocin) 50 mg tid (avoid in elderly patients, particularly gastric toxic; decreases renal blood flow and increases confusion in the elderly)
  - Diclofenac (Voltaren) 75 mg bid or 50 mg tid
  - Naproxen (Naprosyn) 500 mg bid
  - Ibuprofen (Motrin) 600-800 mg qid (can negate effect of cardioprotective aspirin)
  - Celecoxib (Celebrex) 200-400[1] mg bid (off label at the higher dose; has no antiplatelet effect; not totally GI safe)
- Colchicine 0.6 mg hourly until relief or GI intolerance, maximum 6 pills. Not generally recommended since diarrhea is extremely common with this regimen. Avoid in setting of renal insufficiency or biliary dysfunction.
- Corticosteroids can be given by oral, parenteral, or intra-articular route, for example:
  - Prednisone 40-60 mg PO once daily until several days of total relief, then slow taper to off (or to baseline dose) over 10 d
  - Methylprednisolone 40-60 mg IV or IM daily as above.
  - ACTH (corticotropin) 40 IU q12-24h as above.
  - Intraarticular methylprednisolone acetate (Depo-Medrol 80 mg/mL) 80 mg into a knee, 8-16 mg into first MTP, 40 mg into ankle or wrist.

---

[1]Exceeds dosage recommended by the manufacturer.
*Abbreviations:* CHF = congestive heart failure; GI = gastrointestinal; MTP = metatarsophalangeal joint; NSAID = nonsteroidal anti-inflammatory drug; PPI = proton pump inhibitor; PUD = peptic ulcer disease.

## CURRENT THERAPY

- Acute gouty arthritis responds to treatment with high-dose anti-inflammatory therapy: nonsteroidal anti-inflammatory drugs, systemic corticosteroids, intra-articular corticosteroids, or colchicine.
- Choice of therapy for acute gout must take into consideration the patient's specific comorbidities and potential drug side effects and interactions.
- The serum urate level should not be manipulated at the time of an acute attack.
- The serum urate level is most effectively treated with drugs inhibiting xanthine oxidase (i.e., allopurinol), which should be titrated to a dose that decreases the serum urate to <6 mg/dL.
- If hypouricemic therapy is initiated, patients should also receive an anti-inflammatory drug to reduce the likelihood of inducing a gout attack with the sudden drop in serum urate.
- Hyperuricemia is a risk factor for the development and progression of cardiovascular disease, but there currently are no data documenting the benefit of treating asymptomatic hyperuricemia.

## CORTICOSTERIODS

Patients with gout often have contraindications to NSAID therapy. Corticosteroids provide an alternative without significant gastric or renal risk, and they do not interact significantly with coumadin. Oral or parenteral therapy may be used, often prednisone 40 mg or approximate equivalent orally or parenterally; once daily is sufficient. The dose should not be tapered until there is a complete response, and therapy should be continued (with tapering) for several days after complete resolution.

Intraarticular corticosteroid is effective, but this is frequently limited by the comfort of the physician with performing the injection, and some clinicians are reluctant to administer a long-acting deposit steroid without excluding the possibility of joint infection (particularly in hospitalized patients).

Parenteral ACTH (H.P. Acthar Gel) administration is favored by some clinicians, and there are experimental data suggesting that it is effective both due to the stimulation of adrenal corticosteroids as well as a direct peripheral anti-inflammatory effect. It is more expensive than prednisone, must be given parenterally in repeated doses, and may be associated with more sodium and fluid retention than prednisone.

## COLCHICINE

Colchicine historically has been said to be a specific therapy for crystal-induced arthritis. Although not proven in human trials, this remains the clinical impression. Colchicine, given in an oral regimen of continued dosing until pain is relieved or side effects develop, has been proved to be effective. However, diarrhea and GI intolerance are almost invariable and can occur before onset of therapeutic efficacy. Thus, the regimen of taking a 0.6-mg colchicine tablet at the onset of the attack and every hour afterward until pain is relieved or side effects appear is less frequently used. Intravenous colchicine is available on some formularies, and a single 2 mg[3] dose is quite often effective. However, because deaths from multiorgan failure have been reported from the intravenous use of colchicine (although usually in inappropriately high doses), some have advocated that the use of this formulation

Likely, a full dose of any nonsteroidal anti-inflammatory drug (NSAID) will be effective. Some response may be noticeable at 4 to 6 hours after the first dose. Treatment ideally should be continued until several days after the attack has completely resolved.

Concerns with using NSAID therapy in this fashion include gastric damage, potentially serious interactions with medications (warfarin, diuretics, aspirin, and nephrotoxins), decreased renal blood flow, fluid retention, and confusion (indomethacin). Cotreatment with a proton pump inhibitor (PPI) should provide some gastric protection, but this protection is likely insufficient to permit NSAID use in the setting of a recent bleed or gastric ulcer. Parenteral administration of an NSAID offers no safety advantage. A selective COX-2 NSAID (etoricoxib)[2] has been shown to be effective, and thus high-dose celecoxib (Celebrex) will also likely be effective. Celecoxib, because it does not affect platelet function, may have some safety advantage in the patient at risk for bleeding due to recent surgery or reduced platelet number or function. Gastric safety advantage in this setting has not been evaluated; it has no renal safety advantage.

---

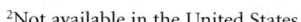

[2]Not available in the United States.

[3]Exceeds dosage recommended by the manufacturer.

be banned. I believe that appropriately dosed, it has value in occasionally encountered clinical situations.

Following an acute attack, patients often suffer additional episodes. This may be due to discontinuation of the therapeutic anti-inflammatory drug prior to complete resolution of the attack or to lack of stabilization of the factors that precipitated the attack. Use of low-dose (0.6 mg once or twice daily) colchicine as a prophylactic agent can be effective in reducing the likelihood of another flare. This can be continued for many weeks or even months if hypouricemic therapy is also initiated (see later). Colchicine is excreted into the biliary system and renally excreted; thus, with renal or biliary disease the drug can accumulate in myeloid, muscle, gastrointestinal, and other tissues. Drug interactions (macrolide antibiotics, most statins, and some calcium channel antagonists) also can promote toxic drug accumulation. Potential side effects include (reversible) leukopenia, axonal neuropathy, vacuolar myopathy, and cardiomyopathy. The axonal and myotoxicity can be acute and associated with myalgias, dysesthesias, and elevated serum creatine phosphokinase (CPK).

## HYPOURICEMIC THERAPY

Because hyperuricemia (>6.8 mg/dL) is necessary for gout to develop, and because chronic reduction of the serum urate to levels below this have been shown to reduce the frequency of gout attacks and detectable urate deposits (tophi), it is reasonable to consider hypouricemic therapy in all patients with gout. However, because some significant complications are associated with hypouricemic therapy (<8% frequency of allergic or hypersensitivity reactions to allopurinol), physicians have been appropriately conservative in their decision to institute this lifelong therapy.

Some patients are otherwise healthy and have no tophi and only extremely infrequent attacks that can be easily managed with short-term NSAID use. Some are quite elderly and do not wish to take another medication in hope of preventing long-term sequelae. In these patients it may be quite appropriate to simply treat attacks if and when they occur. In younger patients with recurrent attacks, those who have relative contraindications to the use of medications used to treat the acute attacks, and those who do not wish to take the chance of missing any functional time due to acute attacks, use of chronic hypouricemic therapy should be considered.

Uricosuric drugs (probenecid) are available in the United States and may be effective and safe in those without a history of stone disease, renal insufficiency, or high levels of excretion of uric acid (>800 mg on a standard diet). Allopurinol, a xanthine oxidase inhibitor of urate synthesis, is generally used to lower the level of serum urate.

There is no set dose of allopurinol. As with the use of antihypertensive medications, which are dosed based on the target BP response, allopurinol dosing should be adjusted to reach the target urate level (often recommended at approximately 6 mg/dL). In clinical practice, it has been inappropriately assumed that 300 mg is the correct dose of allopurinol; however only 20% to 47% of patients (in different studies) attain an appropriately lowered serum urate level with 300 mg dosing. Guidelines have been offered suggesting that the dose of allopurinol should be reduced based on renal function; however, this is an opinion based recommendation based on drug levels, not on prospective dosing observational studies.

It is reasonable to initiate allopurinol at a dose of 50 to 100 mg/day, checking the serum urate and increasing the dose of allopurinol by 100-mg increments every 3 to 4 weeks (still in once-daily dosing). Unfortunately, in many practices it seems that urate levels are not repetitively measured and allopurinol doses are not adjusted; in one study, doses were appropriately measured and adjusted in less than 30% of patients! Allopurinol labeling permits dosing to 800 mg daily, but many clinicians increase the dose above this if necessary in select patients, with appropriate monitoring for any safety concerns.

In patients taking allopurinol, any new rash must be promptly evaluated because a rare but potentially life-threatening complication of therapy with this drug is the Stevens-Johnson reaction. Rare patients also develop a systemic hypersensitivity reaction (fever, hepatitis, vasculitis, rash, and eosinophilia). Extreme care must be exercised when starting allopurinol in patients taking azathioprine, because the active metabolite of azathioprine can rapidly increase and cause toxicity.

Patients started on any hypouricemic therapy are at high risk for developing an acute attack of gout; this can occur in about 30% of patients, accompanying the acute lowering of serum urate level. Thus, it is appropriate before lowering the urate level to initiate a prophylactic anti-inflammatory regimen to protect against an acute gout attack. Colchicine 0.6 mg once or twice daily is a commonly used regimen, NSAIDs can also be used; the choice should be dictated by patient tolerance and comorbidities. Prophylaxis should be continued for many months, if tolerated.

Twenty-four-hour urine collections are used to detect patients with increased production of urate as the etiology for their hyperuricemia. Hyperproduction as the primary contributor to hyperuricemia is rare (enzymopathies) in the absence of readily recognized proliferative disorders. Unless a uricosuric agent is to be used as the primary hypouricemic drug, a 24-hour collection is not usually required because allopurinol is equally effective in the setting of hyperproduction or inefficient uric acid excretion (likely >90% of the time). If a 24-hour collection is required, it can be done on a standard diet, but should be done at least twice. If hyperproduction is documented, collection should be repeated while the patient is on a purine-restricted diet. Losartan (Cozaar),[1] an angiotensin receptor blocker, has some uricosuric activity, as does fenofibrate (Tricor)[1]; these medications can be useful adjuncts in appropriate patients.

In rare patients with extremely severe tophaceous gout and in whom traditional therapy is not tolerated or inefficacious, intravenous uricase therapy is available (rasburicase [Elitek]) off label, but it might not be tolerated on repeat dosing. Current trials are under way with pegylated uricase[5] preparations that may be tolerated on a chronic intermittent basis. These drugs can drop the serum urate to less than 1 mg/dL and dramatically dissolve urate deposits.

Education is a critically important part of the management of gouty arthritis. Once gouty arthritis has been confirmed, patients should know to take an anti-inflammatory medication (NSAID; steroid; colchicine tablets taken one per hour up to a predefined number that does not cause diarrhea in the patient) at the first sign of an attack. Patients and their physicians should recognize the risk factors for gout (beer and mineral spirit ingestion, excess weight, eating a diet with high nonvegetable purine content), and hospitalization for surgical or medical problems.

Current data indicate that hyperuricemia and gout are strongly associated with ASCVD and the metabolic syndrome. Although insufficient information exists to warrant hypouricemic therapy in an effort to reduce this risk, at the least the diagnosis of gout warrants a full evaluation for, and aggressive treatment of, known modifiable risk factors including diabetes, hyperlipidemia, hypertension, smoking, and physical inactivity.

## REFERENCES

Baker JF, Krishnan E, Chen L, Schumacher HR: Serum uric acid and cardiovascular disease: Recent developments, and where do they leave us? Am J Med 2005;118:816-826.

Becker MA, Schumacher HP, Wortmann RL, et al: Febuxostat compared with allopurinol in patients with hyperuricemia and gout. N Engl J Med 2005;353:2450-2461.

Borstad GC, Bryant LR, Abel MP, et al: Colchicine for prophylaxis of acute flares when initiating allopurinol for chronic gouty arthritis. J Rheumatol 2004;31:2429-2432.

Choi HK, Mount DB, Reginato AM: Pathogenesis of gout. Ann Intern Med 2005;143:499-516.

Craig MH, Poole GV, Hauser CJ: Postsurgical gout. Am Surgeon 1994 (Feb):56-59.

Hande KR, Noone RM, Stone WJ: Severe allopurinol toxicity: Description and guidelines for prevention in patients with renal insufficiency. Am J Med 1984;76:47-56.

Johnson RJ, Feig DI, Herrera-Acosta J, Kang D-H: Resurrection of uric acid as a causal risk factor in essential hypertension. Hypertension 2005;45:18-20.

---

[1]Not FDA approved for this indication.

[5]Investigational drug in the United States.

Nakagawa T, Hu H, Zharikov S, et al: A causal role for uric acid in fructose-induced metabolic syndrome. Am J Physiol Renal Physiol 2006;290: F625-F631.

Nuki G: Treatment of crystal arthropathy—history and advances. Rheumatic Dis Clin North Am 2006;32:333-357.

Sarawate CA, Brewer KK, Yang W, et al: Gout medication treatment patterns and adherence to standards of care from a managed care perspective. Mayo Clin Proc 2006;81:925-934.

Stamp L, Searle M, O'Donnell J, Chapman P: Gout in solid organ transplantation: A challenging clinical problem. Drugs 2005;65:2593-2611.

# Dyslipoproteinemias

Method of
*Peter P. Toth, MD, PhD*

The complications of atherosclerotic disease remain the number one cause of death and disability for men and women in industrialized nations. Atherosclerosis is a complex, chronic disease with a multifactorial etiology. Considerable investigation demonstrates an unequivocal relationship between disturbances in cholesterol and lipoprotein metabolism and risk for atherogenesis within the coronary, peripheral, renal, and cerebral vasculature. Dyslipoproteinemias frequently develop in response to genetic and environmental factors and are modifiable through pharmacologic intervention and lifestyle changes. As demonstrated in the Framingham Study, Multiple Risk Factor Intervention Trial and the Seven Countries Study, when serum levels of cholesterol increase, the lifetime risk for developing coronary artery disease (CAD) rises steadily. Consequently, cholesterol is one of the most important endogenous and exogenous toxins that humans are exposed to. The identification and aggressive management of dyslipidemias in both the primary and secondary prevention settings is pivotal to continued efforts to significantly reduce the prevalence of atherosclerotic disease and its clinical sequelae in populations throughout the world.

## Lipoprotein Metabolism and Atherogenesis

Although it is pathogenic, cholesterol is also a critical modulator of cell membrane fluidity and is a precursor for steroid hormone biosynthesis. Consequently, a pool of cholesterol must be available for a variety of physiologic functions. Cholesterol, monoglycerides, free fatty acids, and phospholipids are absorbed from micelles in the intestinal lumen via a series of translocators located within the brush border of jejunal enterocytes. Absorbed cholesterol and lipid are assimilated with apolipoprotein (apo) B48 into chylomicrons. Chylomicrons are released into the lymph and ultimately transported to the central circulation via the thoracic duct. In serum, the triglycerides in chylomicrons are hydrolyzed by lipoprotein lipase. This lipolytic reaction produces chylomicron remnant particles that are taken up by the low-density lipoprotein (LDL) receptor-related protein and metabolized by the liver. The liver secretes very-low-density lipoprotein (VLDL), a lipoprotein enriched with triglycerides, cholesterol, and apoprotein B100. As the triglycerides in VLDL are hydrolyzed by lipoprotein lipase, the size of the lipoprotein particle decreases, eventually forming LDL. LDL particles are concentrated with cholesterol and cholesterol esters and relatively depleted of triglycerides. As the VLDL is progressively converted to LDL, it releases constituents from its surface coat (apoproteins AI, AII, and phospholipids) that are used to form high-density lipoprotein (HDL) in serum.

Patients with hypertriglyceridemia can have elevations in either serum chylomicron or VLDL levels, or both. Patients who consume very high fat diets or who are hyperabsorbers of dietary fat can be hyperchylomicronemic. In contrast, patients with excessive fat storage depots (most notably visceral adiposity) can develop elevated VLDL. Naturally occurring mutations in lipoprotein lipase and an insulin-resistant state can yield hypertriglyceridemia secondary to reduced lipolysis of chylomicrons and VLDL. Reduced lipolysis results in the formation of incompletely digested chylomicrons and VLDL, or "remnant particles" that are widely believed to be atherogenic. Patients with hypertriglyceridemia tend to have reduced serum levels of HDL because:

- There is a decreased release of surface coat constituents from chylomicrons and VLDL.
- As HDL becomes progressively more enriched with triglyceride, it becomes a better substrate for hepatic lipase, an enzyme that catabolizes HDL.

Serum VLDL remnant particles and LDL function as delivery vehicles of cholesterol to peripheral tissues, including blood vessel walls. These lipoproteins are atherogenic because they can traverse the endothelial cell barrier. Macrophages resident within the subendothelial space exposed to LDL oxidized by such enzymes as lipoxygenase or myeloperoxidase upregulate the expression of scavenger receptors (SR-A, CD-36) on their surface and actively take up excessive amounts of cholesterol. This process promotes foam cell and fatty streak development—events that precede atheromatous plaque formation. The activation of macrophages also promotes an inflammatory response with the elaboration of cytokines, interleukins, C-reactive protein, cell mitogens, matrix metalloproteinases, and reactive oxygen species that facilitate lesion progression and instability. LDL and VLDL remnants not taken up by peripheral tissues can be cleared from the circulation by hepatic LDL receptors. Therapies targeted at the upregulation of hepatic LDL receptors are antiatherogenic by virtue of their ability to reduce circulating levels of atherogenic lipoproteins.

HDL particles appear to protect the vasculature from progressive injury and atherogenesis. With few exceptions, in prospective epidemiologic and case-control studies conducted throughout the world, high HDL levels are protective against the development of CAD. For instance, patients with familial hypoalphalipoproteinemia (low HDL) have increased risk for premature CAD, whereas patients with familial hyperalphalipoproteinemia are relatively resistant to atherosclerotic disease. In contrast to LDL, which promotes cholesterol delivery to, and uptake by, vessel wall macrophages, HDL extracts excess cellular cholesterol and delivers it back to the liver for elimination through the gastrointestinal tract in a process referred to as "reverse cholesterol transport." HDL does the following:

- Reduces endothelial cell adhesion molecule (vascular cell adhesion molecule-1, intercellular adhesion molecule-1) expression
- Augments endothelial nitric oxide and prostacyclin production
- Reduces oxidized fatty acid components of LDL
- Decreases platelet aggregability
- Inhibits endothelial cell apoptosis

Recent studies suggest that among the elderly, low HDL is a better predictor of risk for cardiovascular disease than is high LDL. An HDL greater than 60 mg/dL is a negative risk factor. The higher the level of serum HDL, the lower the risk for CAD. Therapeutic maneuvers should not be undertaken to reduce circulating levels of HDL.

## Identification of Lipoprotein Targets

Dyslipoproteinemias constitute a highly prevalent and heterogeneous class of disorders. Derangements in circulating levels of specific lipoprotein classes can be the result of abnormalities in gastrointestinal absorption, enzyme activities, and/or receptor expression. A complete fasting (12 to 14 hours) lipoprotein profile should be obtained from any patient being evaluated for dyslipidemia. Because of the relationship between specific lipoprotein fractions and risk for CAD, a total cholesterol level has little practical clinical utility.

**TABLE 1** Low-density Lipoprotein Cholesterol Goals and Thresholds for Initiating Lifestyle Change and Pharmacologic Intervention

| Risk Category*,† | LDLC Goal | LDLC Level at Which to Initiate TLC | LDLC Level at Which to Consider Drug Therapy |
|---|---|---|---|
| CHD or CHD risk equivalents (10-year risk >20%) | <100 mg/dL (optional goal <70 mg/dL)‡ | ≥100 mg/d all patients regardless of LDL | ≥130 mg/dL (100-129 mg/dL: drug optional) ≥100 mg/d§ (<100 mg/dL: drug optional) |
| 2+ risk factors (10-year risk 10%–20%) | <130 mg/dL (optional goal <100) | ≥130 mg/d all patients regardless of LDL | ≥130 mg/dL (<100 mg/dL: drug optional§) |
| 2+ risk factors (10-year risk 5-10%) | <130 mg/dL | ≥130 mg/dL | ≥160 mg/dL |
| 0-1 risk factor (10-year risk 0-5%) | <160 mg/dL | ≥160 mg/dL | ≥190 mg/dL (160-189 mg/dL: LDL-lowering drug optional) |

Modified from Grundy SM, Cleeman JI, Merz CN, et al: Implications of recent clinical trials for the National Cholesterol Education Program Adult Treatment Panel III guidelines. Circulation 2004;110(2):227-239.
*CHD risk equivalents include diabetes mellitus, peripheral vascular disease, carotid artery disease, abdominal aortic aneurysm and 10 yr Framingham risk >201.
†Risk factors included in Framingham risk evaluation are age, systolic blood pressure, total cholesterol, HDLC, and smoking status.
‡The optional goal of <70 mg/dL is particularly targeted at patients who are "very high" risk, i.e., patients with a recent acute coronary syndrome, poorly controlled diabetics with multiple risk factors, etc.
§When initiating statin therapy in these patients, the goal for LDLC reduction should be 30% to 40% from baseline.
*Abbreviations:* CHD = coronary heart disease; HDLC = high-density lipoprotein cholesterol; LDLC = low-density lipoprotein cholesterol; TLC = therapeutic lifestyle change.

The National Cholesterol Education Program Adult Treatment Panel III (NCEP ATPIII) has systematically defined risk-stratified target levels for atherogenic serum lipoproteins based on the best available evidence to date (Table 1). Risk stratification is performed by evaluating a patient's cardiovascular risk factor burden (number of risk factors) and, if two or more risk factors are present, calculation of the Framingham risk score. Among patients being treated for primary prevention, low risk is defined as a 0-1 risk factor. Moderate and moderately high risk are defined as 2 or more risk factors and a 10-year Framingham risk of less than 10% and 10% to 20%, respectively. In the high-risk category, patients either have CAD (defined as a history of myocardial infarction [MI], stable/unstable angina, revascularization with coronary artery bypass grafting, or percutaneous angioplasty) or a CAD risk equivalent (defined as diabetes mellitus, peripheral vascular disease, significant carotid artery disease [transient ischemic attack or stroke from carotid origin or greater than 50% obstructive atheromatous plaque in a carotid artery], abdominal aortic aneurysm, and a 10-year Framingham risk that exceeds 20%). Among patients with multiple risk factors and no history of CAD or a CAD risk equivalent, it is important to calculate the Framingham risk score so as to differentiate moderate, moderately high, and high risk. An electronic version of a Framingham risk calculator for men and women can be downloaded at www.nhlbi.nih.gov/guidelines/cholesterol. Risk factors recognized by NCEP are summarized in Box 1.

In ATPIII, the NCEP also instituted the following important changes:

- An optimal low-density lipoprotein cholesterol (LDLC) is defined as less than 100 mg/dL for all patients.
- An HDL less than 40 mg/dL is now defined as a categorical risk factor for CAD.
- It introduced target levels for non-high-density lipoprotein cholesterol (HDLC). Non-HDLC (total cholesterol – HDLC) is a measure of the burden of atherogenic lipoproteins in serum (LDL + VLDL).

The risk-stratified target for non-HDLC is the LDLC target plus 30. LDLC remains the primary target of antilipidemic therapy. However, in patients with baseline triglyceride levels greater than 200 mg/dL, non-HDL is the secondary priority for therapy.

Although it is well known by the majority of health care providers that a patient with CAD or a CAD risk equivalent should have an LDLC less than 100 mg/dL, a number of studies show that only 18% to 25% of these patients actually attain this target. An increasing amount of clinical trial evidence is demonstrating that, when it comes to LDLC

reduction and CAD, "the lower, the better." In a recent addendum to ATPIII, the NCEP recommends that physicians consider lowering LDLC to less than 70 mg/dL in very high risk patients. Very high risk patients are defined as patients with established coronary artery disease and: multiple major risk factors, especially diabetes; severe and poorly controlled risk factors, especially cigarette smoking; multiple risk factors for the metabolic syndrome, especially triglycerides ≥200 mg/dL, non–HDLC ≥130 mg/dL, and HDLC < 40 mg/dL; or history of acute coronary syndromes. Other therapeutic options recommended by the ATP III include:

- Initiation of pharmacologic intervention and therapeutic lifestyle change if baseline LDLC is greater than 100 mg/dL in patients with moderately high and high risk.
- Among patients at high risk with baseline LDLC less than 100 mg/dL, further reduction of LDLC by 30% to 40% with medication.

Such stringent criteria for LDLC and non-HDLC reduction require the institution of intensive lifestyle and pharmacologic interventions to ensure therapeutic success.

---

**BOX 1** National Cholesterol Education Program Risk Factors

**Negative**
HDLC > 60 mg/dL

**Positive**
Cigarette smoking
HDL < 40 mg/dL
Hypertension (blood pressure > 140/90 mm Hg or use of antihypertensive agents)
Family history of premature coronary artery disease (CAD in male first-degree relative < 55 yrs; CAD in female first-degree relative < 65 yrs)
Age (men ≥ 45 yrs; women ≥ 55 yrs)

*Abbreviations:* CAD = coronary artery disease; HDL = high-density lipoprotein; HDLC = high-density lipoprotein cholesterol.

# Therapeutic Lifestyle Change

Therapeutic lifestyle change (TLC) constitutes front-line therapy for all patients at risk for CAD. It is recommended that patients who smoke achieve smoking cessation. Smoking is associated with endothelial cell dysfunction as well as increased levels of oxidized LDLC and reduced serum HDLC. The amount of daily ingested cholesterol should not exceed 200 mg. The amount of saturated fat in the diet should be less than 7%, and the total fat intake should not exceed 25% to 35% of calories (Table 2). The distribution of calories from other nutrients should be as follows: 15% protein, 50% to 60% carbohydrates, 10% polyunsaturated fat, and 20% monounsaturated fat. Reductions in saturated fat and increased ingestion of mono- and polyunsaturated fats are associated with reductions in serum LDLC. The ingestion of plant stanols and viscous fiber reduce cholesterol absorption. Patients should be encouraged to exercise for 20 to 30 minutes five times weekly. Exercise facilitates weight loss, which helps to relieve visceral adiposity and insulin resistance. These changes are associated with reduced serum triglycerides and elevations in HDLC.

Although many types of weight loss diets were introduced in recent years, the optimal long-term approach to weight reduction and maintenance is for patients to continue to exercise and restrict fat consumption to within recommended ranges (Table 3). Consultation with a dietitian increases the likelihood of success. For patients who are morbidly obese, bariatric surgery is emerging as an important therapeutic alternative when aggressive lifestyle and pharmacologic interventions fail. Bariatric surgery facilitates significant weight reduction and relieves insulin resistance, reduces blood pressure, and improves lipoprotein profiles. In the Swedish Obese Subjects Study, gastric bypass surgery was associated with a weight loss of 20 kg (44 lb) and decreased the incidence of new-onset type 2 diabetes mellitus by 81% compared to the usual standard of care over 8 years of follow-up. Once adequate weight loss is achieved, it can only be maintained if the patient remains in an isocaloric state through sustained lifestyle modification.

Therapeutic lifestyle change is a particularly important intervention in patients with the metabolic syndrome. Metabolic syndrome develops secondary to the effects of insulin resistance and obesity and is characterized by a set of five risk factors (Table 2). The diagnosis of metabolic syndrome is made when a patient has any three or more of these defining clinical features. Although the metabolic syndrome significantly increases risk for atherosclerotic disease and diabetes mellitus, it is not defined as a CAD risk equivalent. The Framingham risk score should be calculated on all of these patients. LDL and non-HDL goals should be defined by risk stratification. If triglycerides remain elevated (200 to 499 mg/dL) after the LDL goal is reached, then consideration is given to the addition of a triglyceride lowering drug. If triglycerides are greater than 500 mg/dL, patients should be treated

## TABLE 2 NCEP ATP III Criteria for Diagnosing the Metabolic Syndrome*

| Risk Factor | Defining Level |
|---|---|
| **Abdominal Obesity** | |
| Men | Waist > 40 inches |
| Women | Waist > 35 inches |
| **Triglycerides** | ≥150 mg/dL |
| **HDLC** | |
| Men | <40 mg/dL |
| Women | <50 mg/dL |
| **Blood Pressure** | ≥130/≥85 mm Hg |
| **Fasting Glucose** | ≥100 mg/dL |

*Patients having any three of the five risk factors meet criteria for the diagnosis of the metabolic syndrome.

## TABLE 3 Dietary Recommendations for Therapeutic Lifestyle Change

| Dietary Component | Recommendation Allowance |
|---|---|
| Polyunsaturated fat | Up to 10% of total calories |
| Monounsaturated fat | Up to 20% of total calories |
| Total fat | 25%–35% of total calories |
| Carbohydrate | 50%–60% of total calories |
| Dietary fiber | 20–30 g/day |
| Protein | Approximately 15% of total calories |
| Dietary cholesterol | <200 mg/day |

aggressively with triglyceride-lowering medication and a very low fat diet with less than or equal to 15% of calories derived from fat to prevent the development of pancreatitis. Although the NCEP has not defined target levels for HDL, it is recommended that an effort be made to raise low HDL (<40 mg/dL in men, <50 mg/dL in women) through lifestyle modification and drug therapy. The Expert Group on HDL suggests that HDL be raised to greater than 40 mg/dL in patients at high risk or with metabolic syndrome. The American Diabetes Association recommends that HDL be raised to more than 40 mg/dL in diabetic men and to more than 50 mg/dL in diabetic women.

# Pharmacologic Interventions

## STATINS

The statins are reversible, competitive 3-hydroxy-3-methylglutaryl coenzyme A (HMG-CoA) reductase inhibitors. HMG-CoA reductase is the rate-limiting step for cholesterol biosynthesis. The statins provide the most potent means currently available by which to reduce serum levels of LDLC. In addition to reducing cholesterol biosynthesis, the statins augment the clearance of atherogenic apoB100-containing lipoproteins (VLDL, VLDL remnants, and LDL) by upregulating the expression of the LDL receptor on the surface of hepatocytes. These drugs stimulate apoA-I expression and hepatic HDL secretion secondary to weak peroxisomal proliferator-activated receptor-$\alpha$ (PPAR-$\alpha$) agonism.

The statins exert benefit distinct from their ability to alter circulating levels of lipoproteins through their "pleiotropic effects." Statins inhibit the post-translational modification and activation of small G-proteins (Rho and Ras) by blocking the production of such isoprenoids as farnesyl-pyrophosphate and geranylgeranyl-pyrophosphate. This is associated with reductions in the production of a large number of atherogenic stimuli (C-reactive protein, reactive oxygen species, tissue factor, interleukins, adhesion molecules, monocyte chemoattract protein-1, angiotensin-II receptor, and endothelin-1), decreased platelet reactivity and smooth-cell proliferation, and a reversal of endothelial dysfunction, among other effects. Consequently, statins appear to modulate inflammation, oxidative status, vasodilation, thrombotic tendency, and the capacity of a variety of cell types in vessel walls to interact and drive atherogenesis.

The statins are highly efficacious medications. In a growing number of large-scale, placebo-controlled clinical trials, these agents significantly reduced rates of myocardial infarction, stroke, and coronary and all-cause mortality in both the primary and secondary prevention settings. Statins also decrease the frequency of stable and unstable angina and reduce the rate of atheromatous plaque progression and even stimulate some degree of plaque resorption. Statins reduce event rates in men and women, diabetics, smokers, hypertensives, as well as patients older than 70 years of age. Much of the risk reduction achieved with statin therapy is attributable to LDLC reduction. Studies now show that the greater the magnitude of LDLC reduction, the greater the reduction in acute coronary events, especially among patients with CAD or a recent acute coronary syndrome. The benefits of statin therapy are widely assumed to be a class effect.

Six different statins are currently available. These drugs differ by potency and a variety of pharmacokinetic properties. The specific choice of a statin is dictated by the magnitude of LDLC reduction required (baseline versus risk-stratified NCEP target). The LDLC reducing capacity of the statins is as follows:

1. Rosuvastatin (Crestor), 45% to 63% (5 to 40 mg daily)
2. Atorvastatin (Lipitor) 26% to 60% (10 to 80 mg daily)
3. Simvastatin (Zocor) 26% to 47% (10 to 80 mg daily)
4. Lovastatin (Mevacor) 21% to 42% (10 to 80 mg daily)
5. Fluvastatin (Lescol) 22% to 36% (10 to 80 mg daily)
6. Pravastatin (Pravachol) 22% to 34% (10 to 80 mg daily).

Each doubling of the statin dose yields an additional 6% reduction, on average, in serum LDLC (the rule of 6s). The statins provide dose-dependent reductions in serum triglyceride levels (typically 10% to 25%) and elevations in serum HDLC (2% to 14%). Atorvastatin has a tendency to be less and less effective at raising HDLC as the dose is titrated to higher levels. In patients with high baseline triglycerides (>300 mg/dL), the statins increase HDLC significantly more than in patients who are normotriglyceridemic. For instance, simvastatin and rosuvastatin can raise HDLC up to 18% and 22%, respectively, in these patients.

The statins have different pharmacokinetic profiles. Because of their relatively short half-lives (1 to 4 hours), lovastatin, pravastatin, fluvastatin, and simvastatin should be taken in the evening in order to intercept the peak activity of HMG-CoA-reductase that occurs around midnight. Atorvastatin and rosuvastatin can be taken at any time during the day because of their relatively long half-lives (approximately 14 and 19 hours, respectively). The coadministration of cytochrome P450 3A4 inhibitors (azole type antifungals [ketoconazole, itraconazole], HIV protease inhibitors, macrolide antibiotics [erythromycin, clarithromycin], nefazodone [serzone], more than 1 quart of grapefruit juice daily, and cyclosporine) with simvastatin, lovastatin, and atorvastatin should be avoided as these statins are dependent on this P450 isozyme for metabolism. Concomitant dosing can lead to increased risk for toxicity. The dose of simvastatin should not exceed 20 mg daily in patients receiving verapamil or amiodarone.

The benefits of statin therapy significantly outweigh the risks. Hepatotoxicity is defined as an alanine aminotransferase elevation greater than or equal to 3 times the upper limits of normal (ULN), on two occasions at least one month apart. The average risk of this on statin therapy approximates 1%, but risk increases as a function of dose. Mild elevations in serum transaminases are relatively common, and they tend to spontaneously resolve. If transaminitis or hepatotoxicity develops, statin therapy should be discontinued until transaminase levels normalize and a different statin can be started at a lower dose. The most dreaded complication of statin therapy is rhabdomyolysis with skeletal muscle breakdown, myoglobinuria, and renal failure. The risk of this is less than 0.1%, but patients must be counseled about the possibility as well as warning signs for rhabdomyolysis (escalating muscle pain, proximal weakness, brownish-red discoloration of urine). Statins can induce myalgia. However, myalgias in general are common throughout the population. In the Heart Protection Study, among 20,536 patients randomized to either placebo or simvastatin, 40 mg daily, the incidence of myalgia was nearly identical in the two groups of patients. If a patient is experiencing significant myalgia or muscle weakness a serum creatine kinase level can be obtained. Myopathy is defined as a creatine kinase level that exceeds 10 times ULN. Statins are contraindicated in pregnant and nursing women.

## EZETIMIBE

Dietary and biliary sources of cholesterol contribute substantially to circulating levels of this sterol. Although plant sterols and stanols can block cholesterol absorption, Ezetimibe (Zetia) is the first member of lipid-lowering drugs known as cholesterol absorption inhibitors. Ezetimibe inhibits a sterol transporter in the brush border of the jejunal enterocyte identified as Niemann-Pick C1 Like-1 protein that internalizes cholesterol and phytosterols from the intestinal lumen. After being glucuronidated, ezetimibe undergoes enterohepatic recirculation with negligible systemic exposure. The half-life of ezetimibe is

approximately 22 hours and is dosed at 10 mg once daily. Ezetimibe reduces serum LDLC on average by 20%, but up to 24% of patients experience a reduction of greater than or equal to 25%. Ezetimibe also decreases triglycerides by up to 8% and raises HDLC by up to 4%. Ezetimibe does not decrease the absorption of bile acids, steroid hormones (ethinyl estradiol, progesterone), or such fat-soluble vitamins as vitamins A, D, E, or α- and β-carotenes.

The risk of hepatotoxicity with ezetimibe is nearly identical to placebo (0.5% vs. 0.3%), and there is no documented evidence of increased risk for myopathy. Fixed-dose ezetimibe is also available in combination with increasing doses of simvastatin (Vytorin; 10/10; 10/20; 10/40; 10/80 mg daily). Ezetimibe can also be safely used in combination with other statins and provides additive changes in lipoprotein levels to that observed with statin therapy. The addition of ezetimibe to a statin regimen substantially reduces the likelihood of having to titrate the statin.

## BILE ACID BINDING RESINS

The bile acid sequestration agents (BASAs) are orally administered anion exchange resins that bind bile acids in the gastrointestinal tract and prevent them from being reabsorbed into the enterohepatic circulation. These drugs reduce serum LDLC by two mechanisms: (1) increased catabolism of cholesterol secondary to the upregulation of 7-α-hydroxylase, the rate-limiting enzyme for the conversion of cholesterol into bile acids; and (2) increased expression of LDL receptors on the hepatocyte surface that augments the clearance of apoB100-containing lipoproteins from plasma. At maximum doses, the BASAs can reduce serum LDLC by 15% to 30% and increase HDLC by 3% to 5%. It is recommended that these drugs be used in conjunction with a statin whenever possible because BASA therapy increases HMG-CoA reductase activity in the liver, which leads to increased hepatic biosynthesis of cholesterol, thereby offsetting the effects of the BASAs over time.

There are currently three different BASAs available. These include cholestyramine (Questran; 4 to 24 g daily in two to three divided doses daily), colestipol (Colestid; 5 to 30 g in two to four divided doses daily), and colesevelam (WelChol; 1250 mg two to three times daily). The development of constipation, flatulence, and bloating are relatively frequent, though colesevelam has the most favorable side-effect profile of the three available BASAs. Increasing water and soluble fiber ingestion ameliorates some of the difficulty with constipation. The BASAs bind negatively charged molecules in a nonspecific manner. Consequently, they can decrease the absorption of warfarin (Coumadin), phenobarbital, thiazide diuretics, digitalis, β-blockers, thyroxine, statins, fibrates, and ezetimibe. These medications should be taken 1 hour before or 4 hours after the ingestion of a BASA. The BASAs can reduce the absorption of fat-soluble vitamins.

## FIBRATES

The fibrates are fibric acid derivatives that exert a number of effects on lipoprotein metabolism. These agents reduce serum triglycerides by 25% to 50% and raise HDLC by 10% to 20%. Fibrates activate lipoprotein lipase by reducing levels of apoprotein CIII (an inhibitor of this enzyme) and increasing levels of apoprotein CII (an activator of lipoprotein lipase). This stimulates the hydrolysis of triglycerides in chylomicrons and VLDL. Fibrates increase HDLC by two mechanisms. First, the fibrates are PPAR-α agonists and stimulate increased hepatic expression of apoproteins AI and AII. Second, by activating lipoprotein lipase, surface coat mass derived from VLDL is ultimately used to assimilate HDL in serum. In some patients, fibrate therapy may be associated with an increase in serum LDLC (the "β" effect) secondary to increased enzymatic conversion of VLDL to LDL. This effect may diminish over time as the patient increases the expression of hepatic LDL receptors.

The fibrates are particularly valuable for treating dyslipidemia in patients with a combination of hypertriglyceridemia and low HDLC. In this patient type, post-hoc evaluations of data from two studies (the Helsinki Heart Study and the Bezafibrate Infarction Prevention Study) have demonstrated substantial cardiovascular event rate reductions using fibrate therapy. In the Veterans Affairs High-Density Lipoprotein

**CURRENT DIAGNOSIS**

- Dyslipidemia is a highly heterogeneous class of metabolic disorders with an etiology that can depend on abnormalities in the gastrointestinal absorption of cholesterol and lipids and mutations in cell surface receptors and enzymes in pathways regulating lipid metabolism.
- Dyslipidemia is a widely prevalent risk factor for CAD and is associated with elevations in serum LDLC and non-HDLC and low levels of HDLC.
- When making the diagnosis of dyslipidemia, it is important to rule out and treat secondary causes of dyslipidemia, such as thyroid dysfunction, alcoholism, diabetes mellitus, and nephrotic syndrome, among others.
- A complete fasting lipoprotein profile should be performed on anyone undergoing screening for dyslipidemia.
- The diagnosis of dyslipidemia requires comprehensive, global cardiovascular risk evaluation. Target levels for LDLC and non-HDLC are risk stratified. An HDLC of less than 40 mg/dL is a categorical risk factor for CAD.

*Abbreviations:* CAD = coronary artery disease; HDLC = high-density lipoprotein cholesterol; LDLC = low-density lipoprotein cholesterol.

 **CURRENT THERAPY**

- Dyslipidemia is a modifiable risk factor.
- Lifestyle modification is first-line therapy for all patients with dyslipidemia.
- The intensity of pharmacologic intervention depends upon risk-stratified, NCEP targets for LDLC and non-HDLC. In patients with low HDLC, therapeutic effort should be made to raise the level of this lipoprotein as much as possible.
- Dyslipidemia can be treated with statins, fibrates, niacin, and combinations thereof. These drug classes have a substantial amount of end-point driven clinical trial data supporting their use.
- In patients unable to achieve their LDLC target with lifestyle modification and statin therapy, consider adding ezetimibe.
- Patients with severe hypertriglyceridemia unable to adequately reduce serum triglycerides with a low-fat diet and a fibrate likely have a lipoprotein lipase deficiency. These patients can benefit from the addition of orlistat to their pharmacologic regimen.
- The treatment of dyslipidemia in the context of both primary and secondary prevention must be coupled with the aggressive identification and management of all risk factors patients present with, including hypertension, diabetes mellitus, obesity, cigarette smoking, as well as nephropathy and chronic kidney disease.

*Abbreviations:* HDLC = high-density lipoprotein cholesterol; LDLC = low-density lipoprotein cholesterol. NCEP = National Cholesterol Education Program.

Intervention Trial (VA-HIT), men with CAD and low HDL (mean 31 mg/dL) were treated with either gemfibrozil (Lopid) 600 mg orally twice daily or placebo over a 5-year-follow-up period. With a 6% elevation in HDL, no change in LDL, and a 31% decrease in triglycerides, gemfibrozil therapy resulted in a 22% reduction in the composite endpoint of all-cause mortality and nonfatal MI compared to placebo. Gemfibrozil therapy also reduced the risk of stroke and transient ischemic attacks by 31% and 59%, respectively. In addition to lowering the incidence of nonfatal MI and the need for hospitalization for angina, the Fenofibrate Intervention and Event Lowering in Diabetes (FIELD) study demonstrated that the administration of fenofibrate to patients with type 2 diabetes mellitus resulted in significant reductions in endpoints related to microangiopathy, including a 38% reduction in the need for lowering extremity amputation, a 30% reduction in need for laser therapy for proliferative retinopathy, and a 14% reduction in the progression of albuminuria.

Among the diabetic patients in VA-HIT treated with gemfibrozil, there was a 32% reduction in the combined endpoint (41% in CHD death and 40% in stroke). Fibrates have been shown to exert many of the same pleiotropic effects as statins and reduce atheromatous plaque progression in native coronary vessels and in coronary venous bypass grafts.

Like the statins, fibrates are associated with a low incidence of myopathy and mild elevations in serum transaminases. Fibrate therapy can increase the risk for cholelithiasis and can raise prothrombin times by displacing warfarin from albumin binding sites. The periodic monitoring of serum transaminases (6 to 12 weeks after initiating therapy and twice annually thereafter) is recommended. The two most commonly used fibrates are gemfibrozil (Lopid; 600 mg twice daily) and fenofibrate (Tricor; 54 or 160 mg daily). Bezafibrate (Bezalip)[2] is available in Europe and is dosed at 400 mg daily. The use of therapies combining a statin and fibrate is becoming more commonplace in clinical practice, especially as the incidence of complex dyslipidemias increases. Gemfibrozil significantly reduces the glucuronidation of statins, which decreases their elimination. This increases the risk for myopathy/rhabdomyolysis and hepatotoxicity.

When used in combination with gemfibrozil, the doses for simvastatin (Zocor), and rosuvastatin (Crestor), should not exceed 10 mg daily. In general, when embarking on combination therapy, fenofibrate is a safer choice, as it does not adversely impact the glucuronidation of the statins. There are no clinical trial data yet available to assess the effect of statin-fibrate combination therapy on cardiovascular morbidity and mortality.

Among patients in whom serum triglycerides do not normalize in response to a low-fat diet and fibrate therapy, consideration should be given to the addition of other agents. Patients with severe hypertriglyceridemia frequently possess mutations in lipoprotein lipase that reduce the lipolytic activity of this enzyme. In this scenario, the addition of orlistat (Xenical; 120 mg with meals) can reduce the absorption of dietary fat and hence the circulating levels of chylomicrons and triglycerides. Fish-oil capsules enriched with omega-3 (eicosapentaenoic acid) and omega-6 (docosahexaenoic acid) fatty acids can reduce serum triglyceride and VLDL levels and raise HDLC in a dose-dependent manner. Omecor is a fish oil capsule highly enriched with EPA (465 mg) and DHA (375 mg). Omecor is indicated at 4.0 g daily to treat hypertriglyceridemia > 500 mg/dL. In patients with CAD, the American Heart Association recommends that patients take 1.0 g of purified fish oil daily (irrespective of whether or not they have hypertriglyceridemia) or consume two oily fish meals weekly.

## NIACIN

Niacin or nicotinic acid is a B vitamin that exerts multiple beneficial effects on lipoprotein metabolism. In contrast to statins and fibrates, niacin does not stimulate hepatic biosynthesis of HDL. Niacin appears to block HDL particle uptake and catabolism by hepatocytes without adversely impacting reverse cholesterol transport. This helps to increase circulating levels of HDL. Niacin reduces hepatic VLDL and

[2]Not available in the United States.

triglyceride secretion according to two mechanisms: (1) decreasing the flux of fatty acids from adipose tissue to the liver by inhibiting lipase activity; (2) inhibiting triglyceride formation within hepatocytes by inhibiting diacylglycerol acyltransferase. Niacin also reduces serum LDLC concentrations by increasing the catabolism of apoB100. Consequently, niacin beneficially impacts all components of the lipoprotein profile.

When used as monotherapy at 3.0 g daily, crystalline niacin (Niaspan) significantly reduced the incidence of MI and stroke in patients with established CAD in the Coronary Drug Project. In the HDL-Atherosclerosis Treatment Study (HATS) combinations of high-dose niacin (2 to 4 g with simvastatin) reduced cardiovascular morbidity and mortality by up to 90% compared to placebo. This combination therapy also induced atheromatous plaque stabilization over a follow-up period of 3 years. Niaspan should be started at a low dose and gradually titrated upward based on the results of follow-up lipid panels. When evaluated as a function of dose (500 to 2000 mg daily), Niaspan induces the following changes in serum lipid levels: LDLC, 3% to 16% reduction; triglycerides, 5% to 32% reduction; HDLC, 10% to 24% elevation.

Niacin therapy is associated with a number of side effects. The most common side effect with niacin is cutaneous flushing. The incidence of this can be reduced by taking a 325-mg tablet of aspirin one hour before taking niacin. The flushing is prostaglandin mediated. Limiting fat intake for 2 to 3 hours before taking niacin also helps, as fat is a source of arachidonic acid, the substrate for cyclooxygenase. Niaspan is a sustained-release preparation of niacin associated with less flushing. Other side effects include bloating, pruritus, acanthosis nigricans, transient disturbances in glycemic control, and increased serum concentrations of uric acid. Niacin appears to increase rates of proximal tubular reuptake of urate from the glomerular ultrafiltrate. Niacin is available as a combination pill with lovastatin (Advicor; 500/20 mg, 750/20 mg, 1000/20 mg, and 2000/40 mg), and the two drugs give additive changes in the levels of serum lipoproteins.

## Conclusion

Dyslipidemia is a widely prevalent risk factor for CAD. Specific target levels for atherogenic lipoprotein fractions are defined by the NCEP. The treatment of dyslipidemia with lifestyle modification and pharmacologic intervention is associated with significant reductions in cardiovascular morbidity and mortality. It is assumed that health care providers will treat all cardiovascular risk factors (dyslipidemia, hypertension, diabetes or impaired glucose tolerance, obesity, etc.) to nationally defined guideline levels. In support of this, the Clinical Outcomes Using Revascularization and Aggressive Drug Evaluation (COURAGE) trial clearly showed that among patients with CAD and stable angina, aggressive, comprehensive risk factor management with mean attained LDLC of 71 mg/dL, triglycerides of approximately 130 mg/dL, HDLC of 41 mg/dL, blood pressure of 120/70 mm Hg, smoking cessation, and hemoglobin A1c of approximately 7.0% achieved outcomes identical to patients treated with angioplasty combined with aggressive, comprehensive risk factor management.

## REFERENCES

American Diabetes Association: Dyslipidemia management in adults with diabetes. Diabetes Care 2004;27:S68-S71.

Boden WE, O'Rourke RA, Teo KK, et al: Optimal medical therapy with or without PCI for stable coronary disease. N Engl J Med 2007;356:1503-1516.

Brown G, Albers JJ, Fisher LD, et al: Regression of coronary artery disease as a result of intensive lipid-lowering therapy in men with high levels of apolipoprotein B. N Engl J Med 1990;323:1289-1298.

Cannon CP, Braunwald E, McCabe CH, et al., for the Pravastatin or Atorvastatin Evaluation and Infection Therapy–Thrombolysis in Myocardial Infarction 22 Investigators: Comparison of intensive and moderate lipid lowering with statins after acute coronary syndromes. N Engl J Med 2004;350:1495-1504.

Expert Panel on Detection, Evaluation, and Treatment of High Blood Cholesterol in Adults: Executive summary of the third report of the National Cholesterol Education Program (NCEP) Expert Panel on Detection, Evaluation, and Treatment of High blood Cholesterol in Adults (Adult Treatment Panel III). JAMA 2001;285:2486-2497.

Grundy SM, Cleeman JI, Merz CN, et al: Implications of recent clinical trials for the National Cholesterol Education Program Adult Treatment Panel III guidelines. Circulation 2004;110(2):227-239.

Heart Protection Study Collaborative Group: MRC/BHF Heart Protection Study of cholesterol lowering with simvastatin in 20,536 high-risk individuals: A randomised placebo-controlled trial. Lancet 2002;360:7-22.

Mosca L, Appel LJ, Benjamin EJ, et al: Evidence-based guidelines for cardiovascular disease prevention in women. Circulation 2004;109:672-693.

Ridker PM, Bassuk SS, Toth PP: C-reactive protein and risk of cardiovascular disease: Evidence and clinical application. Curr Atheroscler Rep 2003; 5:341-349.

Robins SJ, Collins D, Wittes JF, et al. VA-HIT Study Group. Veterans Affairs High-Density Lipoprotein Intervention Trial. Relation of gemfibrozil treatment and lipid levels with major coronary events. JAMA 2001;285: 1586-1589.

Sacks FM and The Expert Group on HDL Cholesterol: The role of high-density lipoprotein (HDL) cholesterol in the prevention and treatment of coronary heart disease: Expert group recommendations. Am J Cardiol 2002; 90:139-143.

Sever PS, Dahlöf B, Poulter NR, et al., for the ASCOT investigators: Prevention of coronary and stroke events with atorvastatin in hypertensive patients who have average or lower-than-average cholesterol concentrations, in the Anglo-Scandinavian Cardiac Outcomes Trial—Lipid Lowering Arm (ASCOT-LLA): A multicentre randomised controlled trial. Lancet 2003:361:1149-1158.

Sjostrum CD, Peltonen M, Wedel H, et al: Differentiated long-term effects of intentional weight loss on diabetes and hypertension. Hypertension 2000;36:20-25.

Toth PP: Clinician update: HDL and cardiovascular risk. Circulation 2004;109:1809-1812.

Toth PP: Low-density lipoprotein reduction in high risk patients: How low do you go? Curr Atheroscler Rep 2004;6:348-352.

# Obesity

Method of
*Christopher D. Still, DO, and
Gordon L. Jensen, MD, PhD*

Obesity is a heterogeneous disease that has reached epidemic proportions in the United States. For most individuals, it is chronic, relapsing, and multifactorial in origin. It encompasses genetic, environmental, socioeconomic, psychological, and behavioral factors. According to the National Health and Nutrition Examination Survey (NHANES), the prevalence of obesity in the United States has increased from approximately 25% to 33% over a single decade, and obesity now affects nearly 26 million men and 32 million women. Unfortunately, obesity does not spare children or adolescents. NHANES data indicate that approximately 30% of children are overweight (more than 10 million).

The magnitude of obesity differs widely among gender and ethnic groups. There is a marked increase in the prevalence of obesity among females of African American and Mexican American ethnic groups. Some studies estimate nearly 70% of this population is overweight.

Health care providers can no longer view obesity as simply a cosmetic issue caused by a lack of willpower. They need to have an appreciation of its complexity and the related multiple co-morbid medical problems. This chapter discusses the epidemiology, definitions, and assessment of obesity with an emphasis on its clinical consequences and the current techniques in evaluating and treating the obese patient.

## Definition and Assessment

The definition of obesity has always been quite ambiguous. The once widely used determination of so-called ideal body weight based on

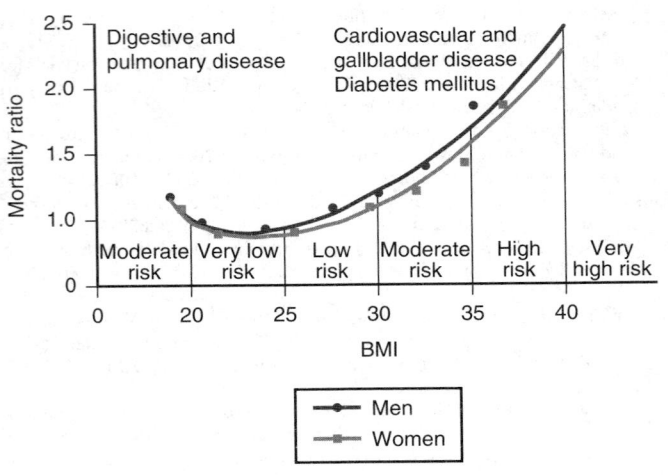

**FIGURE 1.** Correlation between mortality risk and increasing body mass index (BMI). As BMI increases to higher than 25, the risk for mortality from all causes increases. (Adapted with permission from Gray DS: Diagnosis and prevalence of obesity. Med Clin North Am 1989;73:1.)

standard height/weight tables such as the Metropolitan Life Insurance Table has fallen out of favor. Experts now recommend the routine use of the body mass index (BMI). The BMI is defined as the ratio of body weight in kilograms to the height in meters squared (kg/m²). The BMI correlates with body fat and morbidity and mortality (Figure 1).

The BMI differentiates between overweight and obesity. Moreover, as the BMI increases, so does the risk of mortality. A so-called desirable weight individual has a BMI between 20 and 24.9 kg/m². The National Heart, Blood and Lung Institute defines overweight as a body mass index between 25 and 29.9 kg/m². Obesity, therefore, is defined as a BMI more than 30. Patients with a BMI more than 27 with a co-morbid medical problem, such as diabetes mellitus, hypercholesterolemia, hypertension, or sleep apnea, are also at a higher risk of overall mortality and, therefore, more aggressive treatment options may be warranted (Table 1).

In addition to the BMI, waist circumference is another useful tool in assessing the overweight individual. A waist circumference is measured at the smallest area between the xiphoid process and the iliac crest. A waist circumference more than 35 inches in women and more than 39 inches in men reflects an android or visceral fat distribution. This visceral fat upper body distribution puts one at greater risk for developing co-morbid medical problems such as diabetes, heart disease, lipid dyscrasias, insulin resistance, and possibly cancer. In contrast, the gynoid or lower body weight obesity of the hips and buttocks is mainly subcutaneous adipose tissue that is cardioprotective and not associated with adverse sequelae.

## Etiology and Pathophysiology of Obesity

Several etiologic factors classify obesity. Neuroendocrine disorder and single gene deletion syndromes include Cushing's, polycystic ovarian, gonadal failure, Prader-Willi, Cowen's, Carpenter's, and Bardet-Biedl.

 **CURRENT DIAGNOSIS**

- Height, weight, and body mass index
- Waist circumference
- Exclusion of co morbid medical problems such as diabetes, obstructive sleep apnea, and hypercholesterolemia

---

**TABLE 1  Clinical Use of the Body Mass Index (BMI)**

BMI = ratio of weight in kilograms or weight in pounds to (height in meters)² or (height in inches)²
Obesity is defined as BMI >30. If risk factors such as heart disease, hypertension, or elevated serum cholesterol levels are present, more aggressive intervention may be warranted for a BMI >27.

Commonly prescribed medications may also promote weight gain. These include, but are not limited to, classes of drugs such as antidiabetics, antipsychotics, antidepressants, antiepileptics, steroids, hormones and adrenergic agonists (Table 2). It is always important to take a thorough medication history to ensure that no medications, either prescription or over the counter, are taken that promote weight gain.

## Medical Consequences of Obesity

Obesity and its multiple medical co-morbidities are associated with a profound increase in morbidity and premature mortality. With increasing BMI there is an increased prevalence of metabolic syndrome/insulin resistance, diabetes mellitus, hypertension, coronary artery disease, lipid and cholesterol dyscrasias, gallbladder disease, respiratory compromise, degenerative joint disease, infertility, and some cancers. The major complications associated with obesity are addressed next.

### INSULIN RESISTANCE/METABOLIC SYNDROME

The fundamental pathophysiologic defect that often leads to non-insulin-dependent diabetes mellitus (NIDDM) is insulin resistance. It is estimated that 25% of the population is insulin resistant, which is especially prevalent in individuals with the android type of weight distribution. Hyperinsulinemia results from compensatory pancreatic cell hypersecretion and therefore serves as a biologic and laboratory marker of insulin resistance. After prolonged hypersecretion, the insulin secretory capacity of the β cells diminishes, possibly because of the accumulation of amyloid deposits in the islet cells and eventually decompensation of insulin resistant to overt hyperglycemia. In addition, undetermined genetic factors and acquired factors such as aging, sedentary lifestyle, and obesity all contribute to insulin resistance.

---

**TABLE 2  Prescription Medications That May Promote Weight Gain**

| Class of Medication | Examples |
| --- | --- |
| Antidiabetics | Insulin, thioglitazones, sulfonylureas |
| Antipsychotics | Risperidone (Risperdal), clozapine (Clozaril), olanzapine (Zyprexa) |
| Antidepressants | Amitriptyline (Elavil), imipramine (Tofranil), doxepin (Sinequan), lithium desipramine (Norpramin), trazodone (Desyrel), tranylcypromine (Parnate) |
| Antiepileptics | Valproate (Depakote), carbamazepine (Tegretol) |
| Steroids | Glucocorticoids |
| Antihistamines | Astemizole[2] |

[2]Not available in the United States.

Clinically, this syndrome can be associated with abdominal obesity (android adiposity), hypertension, hypertriglyceridemia, high-density lipoprotein/low-density lipoprotein (HDL/LDL) cholesterol abnormalities, hyperuricemia, fluid retention, polycystic ovarian syndrome, hypofibrinolysis, acanthosis nigricans, and skin tags. Studies revealed that treatment options in this patient population favor complex carbohydrate modification, reduced fat intake, regular exercise, and possibly the use of medications, such as metformin, that increase insulin sensitivity.

## DIABETES MELLITUS

Undoubtedly, the increasing prevalence of obesity is associated with the growing prevalence of NIDDM in the United States. Some 70% to 80% of patients with NIDDM are overweight. NHANES data clearly reveal a strong correlation between the relative risk of development of NIDDM and increasing body mass index beyond 27 kg/m². Moreover, there exists a 10-fold increase in the prevalence of obesity in individuals with a BMI more than 40 kg/m². Additional individual risk factors for the development of diabetes mellitus, regardless of gender, include increasing age, family history of NIDDM, and central adipose distribution. What must be emphasized, however, is that even a modest weight loss (5% to 10% of presenting weight) can have tremendous benefit on glycemic control as well as curtailing the development and progression of the multiple co-morbidities associated with diabetes mellitus.

## HYPERTENSION

Hypertension is a common, chronic disease affecting millions of individuals worldwide. A strong correlation exists between hypertension and obesity, with obesity associated with approximately 30% to 50% of the hypertension in the United States. In addition to a reduction in blood pressure, left ventricular mass, which is often associated with longstanding hypertension, has been shown to be reduced with a modest weight loss (5% to 10% of presenting weight). Moreover, a modest weight loss often leads to reduction or elimination of the need for hypertensive pharmacotherapy.

## CORONARY HEART DISEASE

Until recently, obesity was considered only a minor contributor to coronary artery disease (CAD). However, in response to the emerging body of scientific, medical, and behavioral data about the link between excess adiposity and CAD, the American Heart Association reclassified obesity as a major, modifiable risk factor for CAD. In addition to obesity alone, studies suggest when other co-morbidities are present (such as hypertension, elevated LDL cholesterol, diabetes mellitus, and elevated serum triglycerides), obese individuals are at even greater risk for the development of CAD, and more aggressive treatment options may be warranted.

## LIPID DYSCRASIAS

Blood lipid abnormalities are common in the obese individual. Obese individuals who possess the upper body, android, visceral adiposity often have lower HDL cholesterol leading to an increased risk of the development of CAD. On the contrary, individuals who possess the lower body, gynoid, more subcutaneous adiposity often are predisposed to an elevated HDL cholesterol concentration that is cardioprotective. Overweight and obese individuals routinely have normal or slightly elevated total or LDL cholesterol levels. Therefore, individuals with a random total cholesterol level greater than 200 mg/dL warrant a fasting lipid profile.

Unlike cholesterol, obesity predisposes individuals to higher triglyceride levels compared to normal weight individuals. Although hypertriglyceridemia alone and its association with increased morbidity and mortality have been controversial, increased portal free fatty acid availability and hyperinsulinemia increase the synthesis of very low density lipoprotein (VLDL), which is a risk factor for CAD. Pharmacologic intervention is often required when obese individuals exhibit Frederickson class IV or V hyperlipidemia.

## PULMONARY ABNORMALITIES

Severe respiratory insufficiency, commonly known as pickwickian syndrome, may develop in patients with morbid obesity. Obstructive sleep apnea syndrome and obesity hypoventilation syndrome are two primary breathing disorders of the pickwickian syndrome. With obstructive sleep apnea, the tongue obstructs the glottis during sleep impeding air entry to the trachea. In moderately and morbidly obese individuals, obstructive sleep apnea is very common and often misdiagnosed. Symptoms of obstructive sleep apnea include snoring, apneic episodes, excessive daytime somnolence, memory loss, irritability, fatigue, and erectile dysfunction. Nocturnal hypoxemia, a consequence of sleep apnea, may contribute to arrhythmias, pulmonary hypertension, and right-sided heart failure. The most important and first-line intervention should be weight reduction. Moderate weight loss as a result of modified caloric intake improves oxygenation and sleep apnea in obese subjects. The most likely mechanism of improvement after a modest weight loss results from an increase in airway size or from changes in ventilatory drive, which increases upper airway muscle activity.

# Treatment Options

Successful comprehensive weight management programs combine the use of nutritionally balanced, mildly hypocaloric diet regimens, modest regular activity, behavior modification techniques and, when indicated, pharmacotherapy. High rates of recidivism are seen in programs not proportionally balanced or requiring drastic dietary modification.

## INITIAL EVALUATION

Individuals should undergo a comprehensive history and physical examination before initiating any diet and exercise program. Secondary causes of obesity such as Cushing's syndrome, hypothyroidism, and diabetes mellitus should be considered in the initial evaluation. In addition, contraindications to weight reduction such as pregnancy, lactation, unstable mental illness, and medical conditions such as unstable angina or uncontrolled blood pressure should all be evaluated prior to initiation. Eating disorders such as anorexia and bulimia must also be considered. The physical examination should include both the BMI and waist circumference. These are critical to stratify patients to predict and guide various treatment options (Figure 2).

| BMI category | Health risk based on BMI |
|---|---|
| <25 | Minimal–low |
| 25–<27 | Low–moderate |
| 27–<30 | Moderate–low |
| 30–<35 | High–very high |
| 35–<40 | Very high–extremely high |
| >40 | Extremely high |

| Health risk | Treatment options |
|---|---|
| Minimal and low | Healthful eating<br>Increased physical activity<br>Life style changes |
| Moderate | All of the above plus caloric restriction |
| High + very high | All of the above plus pharmacotherapy |
| Extremely high | All of the above plus surgical considerations |

**FIGURE 2.** Determination of health risk based on body mass index (BMI) and various treatment options. (Adapted from the National Institute of Health: Practical Guide to the Identification, Evaluation, and Treatment of Overweight and Obesity in Adults, 1998.)

## CURRENT THERAPY

- Diet, exercise, and behavior modification
- Pharmacotherapy
- Bariatric surgery

Initial blood chemistry studies including complete blood cell count, liver function studies, fasting lipid profile, determination of thyroid-stimulating hormone concentration, fasting glucose level, and renal panel should be considered as well as an electrocardiogram in appropriate individuals.

### DIET

Once any secondary causes of obesity (hypothyroidism, Cushing's syndrome, etc.) are ruled out, determination of what diet regimen to best fit the overweight or obese individual is critical. The implementation of drastic, unrealistic dietary limitations makes long-term compliance difficult.

Popularized in the 1970s, very low calorie diets (VLCDs) were widely used to promote initial rapid weight loss. VLCDs are drastically limited in energy, usually between 600 and 800 calories per day, resulting in significant but usually short-term results.

VLCDs can be beneficial in the instance where rapid weight loss is needed for a specific procedure to be performed (i.e., cardiac catheterization) or life-threatening obstructive sleep apnea where rapid weight loss can significantly reduce the frequency and duration of apneic episodes. Individuals on VLCDs should be closely monitored, and additional supplementation of at least 1500 mL of water, multiple vitamins, calcium, magnesium, and potassium are usually required. VLCDs should be used as an initial step to a less drastic conventional balance deficit meal plan.

Contraindications to VLCDs include recent myocardial infarction, unstable angina, malignant arrhythmias, type I diabetes mellitus, and pregnancy. Medications such as insulin, sulfonylurea hypoglycemics, and antihypertensives must be carefully monitored and often tapered as weight loss ensues.

Popular commercial liquid diet preparations usually contain approximately 10 to 15 g of protein, 30 to 45 g of carbohydrate, and 2 to 3 g of fat. The vastly protein-rich supplements contribute to caloric energy levels and usually range between 180 and 250 calories per serving. Rates of recidivism remain quite high with most commercial diet preparations. This is mostly because of the failure of liquid diets to provide an opportunity for the patient to alter fundamental eating and lifestyle behaviors needed for sustained weight loss.

Over the last several years, low-carbohydrate ketogenic diets such as the Atkins diet have been popular in the lay press. Although initially one may see increased satiety and rapid weight loss because of fluid loss, long-term studies on cardiovascular risk reduction and sustained weight loss over other diet options are ongoing.

What is probably most beneficial for the majority of overweight and obese individuals is a less drastic hypocaloric and balanced meal plan. These typically provide 1200 to 1800 calories per day, 20% to 30% of calories from fat, 50% to 55% from carbohydrates, and 15% to 20% from protein. These conventional diets should result in losses of approximately 1 to 2 lbs per week or 4 to 8 lbs per month. These less drastic meal plans allow individuals to make lifestyle changes, ideally long term.

To recommend a caloric concentration adequately, one must determine the caloric requirement to maintain a patient's weight upon presentation. This is crucial so unrealistic goals are not placed on individuals, setting them up for failure. For instance, in most instances it is unrealistic for a 275-lb man to adhere to 1200 calories per day. As a general rule, a 500-calorie per day deficit promotes a weight loss of 1 lb per week. A moderate degree of restriction is better tolerated, and long-term compliance should be superior to more restrictive caloric plans.

In addition to calories consumed by eating, it is also important to discern how many calories individuals are drinking. Individuals can drink thousands of calories per day and not equate them to "total calories consumed per day." Maintaining blood volume by drinking at least 64 oz of water per day and limiting or avoiding liquids with calories (i.e., regular sodas, juices, alcoholic beverages) has proven beneficial.

### BEHAVIOR MODIFICATION

Behavior modification must be an integral part of any diet plan to promote the best chance of success. Several controlled trials have validated the effectiveness of behavioral techniques. However, in a busy primary care office this can be time consuming. A concise and comprehensive manual that provides specific monthly goals for the practitioner to review with patients is the Learn Program for Weight Control from the American Health Publishing Company in Dallas, Texas. This provides excellent behavior modification lessons for the patient to work through between office visits.

### EXERCISE

In reviewing national weight loss registries in patients who have lost a significant amount of weight and kept it off for greater than 1 year, regular exercise is the most common denominator for weight maintenance. Unfortunately, exercise is the most difficult component of a comprehensive weight management program, partly because of unrealistic expectations placed on obese individuals. Many experts agree that 30 minutes a day, 5 days a week, of aerobic activity is the minimum exercise prescription required for weight loss and maintenance. However, it is unrealistic to expect an obese individual to sustain himself or herself, at least initially, for 30 minutes and therefore, compliance drops precipitously.

A more reasonable starting point is an occurrence type of activity program several times per day. For instance, 3 to 5 minutes of aerobic activity five to six times a day is much better tolerated by a patient, and long-term compliance is greatly enhanced. The use of a pedometer can objectively measure one's number of steps, and goals of 8000 to 10,000 steps per day should be recommended. Also, common everyday activities such as walking up stairs rather than taking the elevator or escalator, parking farther away from an entrance, or not using the television remote control add up to small but meaningful periods of increased activity, thereby increasing energy expenditure. Increased exercise, however, increases muscle mass, which weighs more than adipose tissue. Once a patient progresses to 30 minutes of occurrence exercise, 5 days per week, studies have determined a greater than 50% chance of achieving weight maintenance.

### PHARMACOTHERAPY

During the 1990s, there were great ups and downs in the development of pharmacotherapy for the treatment of obesity. What must be emphasized, however, is that if pharmacotherapy is considered, it must be used as an adjunct to diet, behavior modification, and exercise to attain the best results for patients.

One of the oldest medications that is still available and used is phentermine (Ionamin). Phentermine is adrenergic medication that mildly increases norepinephrine release. This medication was popularized in the early 1990s when Weintraub studied the efficacy of phentermine used in combination with fenfluramine[1,2] or the so-called fen-phen combination. Phentermine, used alone, is not associated with cardiac valvular defects and remains available for use as a single agent for short-term use (3 months). It is available as phentermine HCl and phentermine resin. The resinate, when compared to HCl, is absorbed more slowly and blood levels reach a lower, later, and flatter peak, which is likely to result in more consistent and sustained blood levels. Potential side effects of phentermine include dry mouth, palpitations, tachycardia, hypertension, insomnia, or overstimulation.

---

[1]Not FDA approved for this indication.
[2]Not available in the United States.

Early in 1998, the Food and Drug Administration (FDA) approved the use of sibutramine (Meridia) for the treatment of obesity. Sibutramine is a beta-phenylethylamine that acts as a reuptake inhibitor for both norepinephrine and serotonin. Unlike fenfluramine and dexfenfluramine, sibutramine does not possess any releasing ability of serotonin. It is the potent releasing ability of dexfenfluramine and fenfluramine that has been suggested to be the cause of the valvular heart disease and pulmonary hypertension associated with these medications. To date, there have been no reports of any valvulopathies or primary pulmonary hypertension with the use of sibutramine.

Most common side effects associated with sibutramine include dry mouth, insomnia, and constipation. In addition, tachycardia and hypertension (mean blood pressure increase of 2 to 3 mm Hg and increase in pulse rate by four to five beats per minute) are reported. Therefore, pulse and blood pressure should be monitored when initiating sibutramine. Efficacy studies using sibutramine revealed an approximate 8% weight loss at the end of 12 months when used in combination with diet. Contraindications to sibutramine include use with any monoamine oxidative inhibitors or selective serotonin reuptake inhibitors or in patients with severe renal or hepatic impairment. In addition, it is contraindicated for patients with a history of CAD, congestive heart failure, arrhythmias, stroke, glaucoma, or uncontrolled hypertension.

In May 1999, the FDA approved another medication for the treatment of obesity, orlistat (Xenical). Orlistat tetrahydrolipstatin is a selective inhibitor of pancreatic lipase and thus is a novel approach to weight loss medications. Orlistat is the first nonsystemically acting medication that acts locally in the gastrointestinal tract to block gastric and pancreatic lipase and results in decreased fat absorption. Orlistat inhibits lipases for approximately 90 minutes after ingestion. Approximately a third of digested fat is excreted in the stool by patients taking orlistat. Recently, orlistat has been approved, at the 60-mg dose, for over-the-counter use under the name Alli.

Certain adverse events can be predicted from the mode of action of orlistat including steatorrhea, oily spotting, flatulence with discharge, and fecal urgency. Fat-soluble vitamins A, D, E, and K as well as beta carotene may be modestly decreased in individuals taking orlistat; therefore, multivitamin supplementation is recommended daily. Efficacy studies after 2 years revealed an approximate 9% weight loss when used in combination with a mildly hypocaloric meal plan.

The use of pharmacotherapy as an adjunct to diet, exercise, and behavior modification is indicated for individuals with a BMI more than 30 kg/m$^2$ or more than 27 kg/m$^2$ with a co-morbid medical problem relating to their obesity such as diabetes, hypercholesterolemia, or hypertension. Pharmacotherapy alone is neither indicated nor recommended. Table 3 summarizes commonly prescribed medications for the treatment of obesity.

## BARIATRIC SURGERY

Bariatric surgery for the treatment of obesity, despite impressive outcomes, should be considered for patients suffering from morbid obesity. The surgical candidates who can benefit the most include patients who have failed medical management and who have a BMI more than 40 kg/m$^2$ or have a BMI 35 kg/m$^2$ and also suffer from diabetes, hypertension, obstructive sleep apnea, cardiovascular disease, gastroesophageal reflux disease, degenerative joint disease, or steatohepatitis (fatty liver). Amelioration of those common medical problems should be the prominent reason for considering bariatric surgery.

Contraindications to bariatric surgery include untreated major depression/psychosis, certain personality disorders, active alcohol or drug abuse, and noncompliance with preoperative medical, nutritional, and psychological management. Age greater than 65 years is no longer an absolute contraindication to bariatric surgery, but the risk may outweigh the benefits for patients older than 70 years.

Bariatric surgery for children and adolescents remains highly controversial. However, surgery on patients between 12 and 18 years of age who have significant medical problems relating to their obesity (diabetes mellitus, obstructive sleep apnea, reactive airway disease, steatohepatitis, and metabolic syndrome) has resolved their co-morbidities.

## PREOPERATIVE EVALUATION

A comprehensive team approach is supported and recommended by most physicians and insurance carriers. An ideal program would encompass a minimum of four components: medical, nutritional, psychological, and surgical. This multidisciplinary team is involved in evaluating the patient before surgery and in the education and treatment after surgery. This team ensures optimal medical, nutritional, and psychological care and ensures good insight into the lifelong lifestyle changes after bariatric surgery.

## SURGICAL ASSESSMENT

Once the patient completes the preoperative medical, nutritional, and psychological evaluation and has achieved adequate metabolic control of any medical problems, he or she can be referred to the bariatric surgeon. The surgeon evaluates the patient's motivation and expectations, discusses the risks and benefits of the different surgical interventions, and chooses the most appropriate surgery for each individual patient.

# Most Common Surgical Options

## RESTRICTIVE PROCEDURES: GASTRIC BANDING AND THE ADJUSTABLE LAPAROSCOPIC BAND

Gastric banding has been popular in Europe, but until the 1980s did not receive much attention in the United States. Initial stapling procedures (Figure 3A) were complicated by staple-line ruptures. This has given rise to the more commonly performed vertical-banded gastroplasty (VBG) (Figure 3A). The VBG separates the stomach, forming a small pouch that joins the rest of the stomach through a small channel. This channel is banded, so to speak, with a ring of nonexpandable material that prevents the opening from enlarging. This procedure is relatively easy to perform and involves no bypass of the intestines. The VBG is not routinely performed any longer and has since been replaced by the laparoscopic adjustable band (Figure 3B).

| TABLE 3 Commonly Prescribed Medications for the Treatment of Obesity | | | |
|---|---|---|---|
| **Generic Name** | Phentermine | Sibutramine | Orlistat |
| **Trade Name** | Ionamin<br>Fastin<br>Adipex-P | Meridia | Xenical |
| **Mechanism of Action** | Adrenergic agonist | Norepinephrine and serotonin inhibitor | Lipase inhibitor |
| **Dose** | 15–30 mg<br>37.5 mg | 5–15 mg | 120 mg |
| **Side Effects** | CNS<br>CV | CNS<br>CV | GI |

*Abbreviations:* CNS = central nervous system; CV = cardiovascular; GI = gastrointestinal.

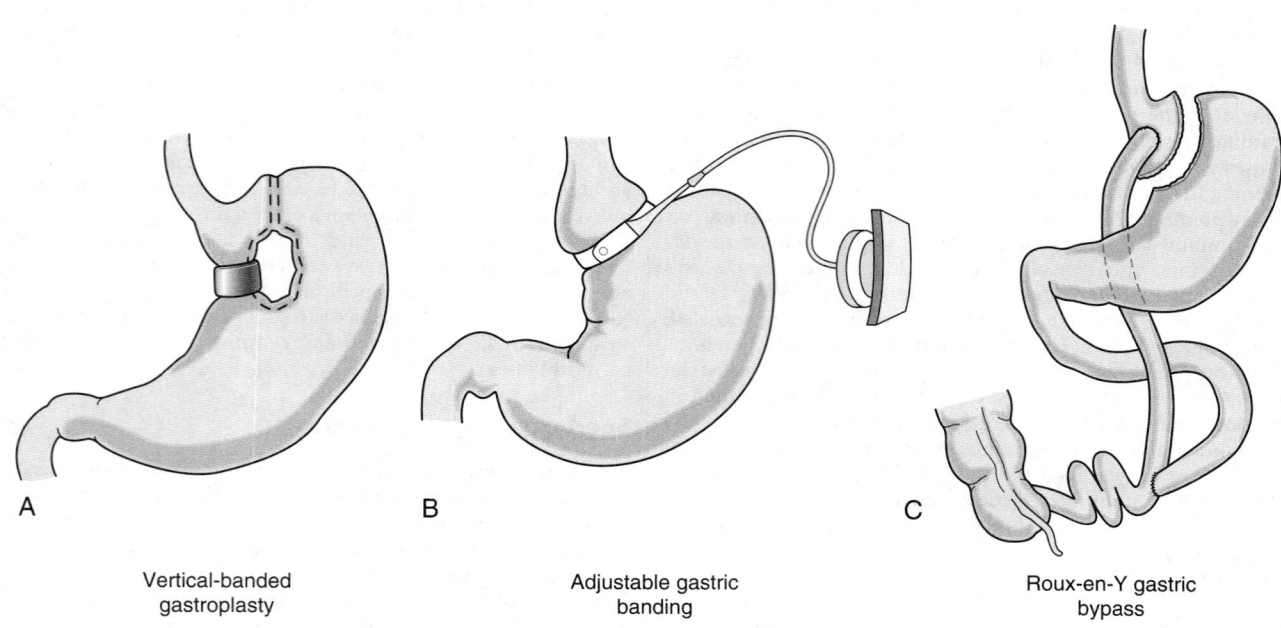

A  Vertical-banded gastroplasty

B  Adjustable gastric banding

C  Roux-en-Y gastric bypass

**FIGURE 3.**  Techniques commonly used for the surgical treatment of obesity: vertical-banded gastroplasty (**A**), adjustable laparoscopic band (**B**), Roux-en-Y gastric bypass (**C**).

The adjustable laparoscopic band is also a purely restrictive and relatively noninvasive procedure that requires no malabsorption. These restricted procedures are generally best suited for patients who eat large quantities of protein and carbohydrates because surgery prevents entry of a large quantity of food. Weight loss may be less adequate in patients who consume high-calorie soft foods and liquids (such as cakes, milkshakes, and ice cream) because these can rapidly pass through the banded channel. Expected weight loss with the adjustable lap band approximates 40% to 60% of excess body weight in properly selected individuals. However, with patients that consume soft foods and liquid calories, long-term weight loss (3 to 5 years postoperatively) may be somewhat variable.

### COMBINED RESTRICTIVE AND MALABSORPTIVE PROCEDURES: ROUX-EN-Y GASTROPLASTY

The Roux-en-Y gastroplasty combines stomach restriction with a bypass procedure and modest malabsorption of a vast majority of the stomach and the first part of the small intestine called the duodenum. This procedure prevents entry of large amounts of food at one time while bypassing the duodenum, where calories are normally absorbed (Figure 3C).

In most instances, the malabsorptive procedures are more effective than VBG and the adjustable lap band for causing and maintaining weight loss. The expected weight loss for the malabsorptive procedures are approximately 70% to 80% of a patient's excess body weight 3 years following surgery and continued maintenance 50% to 60% of excess body weight after 10 years depending on which procedure. Most importantly, co-morbid medical problems relating to obesity such as diabetes, high cholesterol, obstructive sleep apnea, fatty liver, and high blood pressure diminish or resolve after malabsorptive bariatric surgery.

All of the bariatric procedures just discussed are relatively safe, with an overall mortality of less than 2% when performed by an experienced surgeon who has performed at least 75 surgeries.

Pregnancy should be avoided for at least 12 to 18 months after undergoing malabsorptive bariatric surgery. With changes in absorption of iron/vitamins, vitamin $B_{12}$/folate, and protein along with rapid weight loss, women are at higher risk for spinal cord defects and other pregnancy complications. As with other medications during this period, adequate blood levels of oral birth control pills cannot be assured, and additional measures of birth control using barrier methods, patches, or injections are necessary.

## Benefits of Modest Weight Loss

What is often overlooked in the obese individual with multiple co-morbid medical problems is the benefit of a modest weight loss. As health care providers, of primary importance is managing, not curing, the co-morbid medical problems of obese patients (e.g., blood sugar control, reducing cholesterol, etc.). Modest (10% to 15%) weight loss is documented in several studies to produce significant benefit in glucose control, blood pressure, and lipid management. A goal of metabolic fitness, as defined as the absence of biochemical risk factors associated with obesity, such as elevated fasting concentration of cholesterol, triglycerides, glucose, or elevated blood pressure, should be sought. Although in many instances achieving metabolic fitness still leaves patients obese by many practitioners' standards, there is tangible benefit in health risk reduction, increase in quality of life, and improved physical function.

## Future Treatment Options for Obesity

Over the last decade, great advancements have been made in the treatment of obesity. This is related in part to a better understanding of appetite regulation on the neural-hormonal level, discovery of various human obesity genes, molecular targets for obesity treatment as well as various signals that regulate food intake and energy homeostasis. Characterization of obesity-associated gene products has revealed new biochemical pathways and molecular targets for potential pharmacologic intervention that will likely lead to new treatments into the millennium.

Although great strides have been made in the discovery of various hormones, genes, and gene products to develop the ideal antiobesity agent, it is likely that pharmacologic treatments will require combination therapy likely tailored to phenotype and genotype; each requiring a distinct mechanism of action. Optimism remains high for a magic bullet for the cure of obesity; however, one cannot lose sight of the fact that diet, exercise, and behavior modification will remain the cornerstone for any potential future pharmacotherapy

In conclusion, obesity in the United States has reached epidemic proportions, leading to a significant health crisis. Health care providers can no longer view obesity as a social issue but rather they must acknowledge it as a chronic medical condition, like diabetes, requiring long-term treatment. A realistic goal set at the outset to achieve metabolic fitness via a comprehensive weight management program consisting of prudent dietary changes, behavior modification, and regular aerobic exercise, with or without the adjunctive use of pharmacotherapy and/or surgery, will provide the best chance for modest weight loss and maintenance. This will be most rewarding, not only for patients, but also for health care providers managing the multiple comorbid medical problems relating to obesity.

## REFERENCES

Apovain C: The medical management of obesity and the role of pharmacotherapy: An update. Nutr Clin Pract 2000;15:5-12.

Brownell KD, Wadden TA: The Learn Program for Weight Control. Dallas, Tex, American Health Publishing Company.

Buchwald H, Avidor Y, Braunwald E, et al: Bariatric surgery: A systematic review and meta-analysis. JAMA 2004;292(14):1724-1737.

Kushner RF: Roadmaps for Clinical Practice: Case Studies in Disease Prevention and Health Promotion—Assessment and Management of Adult Obesity: A Primer for Physicians. Chicago, American Medical Association, 2003.

National Institutes of Health; National Heart, Lung and Blood Institute: North American Association for the Study of Obesity: The Practical Guide to the Identification, Evaluation, and Treatment of Overweight and Obesity in Adults. Bethesda, Md, National Institutes of Health, 2000.

National Task Force on the Prevention and Treatment of Obesity: Overweight, obesity and health risk. Arch Intern Med 2000;160:898-904.

NIH Consensus Development Conference Panel: Gastrointestinal surgery for severe obesity. Ann Intern Med 1991;115:956-961.

Still C: Geisinger Frequently Asked Questions: Weight Management in Adults: Decker Publishing Company, Hamilton, Ontarió, Canada.

# Osteoporosis

Method of
*Bart L. Clarke, MD, and Sundeep Khosla, MD*

Osteoporosis is defined by the World Health Organization (WHO) as a systemic skeletal disease characterized by compromised bone strength predisposing to increased risk of fracture, where bone strength reflects the integration of bone density and bone quality. Bone quality reflects bone architecture, bone turnover, bone microfracture accumulation, and bone mineralization.

## Etiology

Osteoporosis results from changes in the bone remodeling process that occur during the skeletal life cycle. Postmenopausal osteoporosis generally results from high-turnover bone loss due to estrogen deficiency in the early menopause, in which osteoblasts fail to completely fill in resorption pits formed by osteoclasts, resulting in minor deficits with each bone remodeling cycle. Over time, this results in significant bone loss. Osteoblast precursors and osteoblasts synthesize and secrete receptor activator of nuclear factor (NF)-κB ligand (RANKL), which stimulates receptor activator of NF-κB (RANK) on osteoclast precursors to differentiate and begin resorbing bone. Osteoblast precursors

and osteoblasts also synthesize and secrete osteoprotegerin, which serves as a decoy receptor for RANKL. The balance between RANKL and osteoprotegerin in the local bone environment determines osteoclast activity.

A variety of changes occur in bone mineral density (BMD) measured by dual energy X-ray absorptiometry (DXA) with age in women. Girls experience a rapid increase in BMD starting shortly before puberty. This increase continues until the late teenage years, at which time the rate of increase slows down, until peak BMD is achieved in the late 20s to mid-30s. After about age 35 years, women lose 0.5% to 1.0% of their lumbar spine BMD each year until menopause. Beginning shortly before menopause, women lose as much as 1% to 3% of their lumbar spine BMD each year for the next 5 to 10 years. Postmenopausal women lose BMD less rapidly at other skeletal sites. After this period of rapid bone loss during the early menopause, late postmenopausal women continue to lose lumbar spine BMD at 0.5% to 1.0% each year indefinitely and BMD at other skeletal sites less rapidly.

Men experience the same BMD changes with age as women (except, of course, for the period of rapid bone loss around the time of menopause). Men generally have greater peak areal BMD and bone strength than women due to the larger diameter of their bones, which is a major reason that bones in older men fracture less frequently than older women. Men with osteoporosis often have abnormal gonadal sex steroid levels.

Recent studies using peripheral quantitative computed tomography (CT) scanning, which can distinguish between cortical and trabecular bone loss, show that women and men begin to lose trabecular bone beginning in their 20s, whereas cortical bone loss doesn't start until the mid-50s. With normal aging, women lose greater amounts of trabecular bone than men, whereas men have greater trabecular thinning than women.

## Epidemiology

About 44 million persons in the United States are estimated to be affected by low bone mass, based on the 2000 U.S. Census and projections from the third U.S. National Health and Nutritional Examination Survey (NHANES III). Roughly two thirds of these patients meet current WHO criteria for low bone density and one third for osteoporosis. Eighty percent of those with low bone mass are women, but about 20% are men.

### RISK FACTORS

A variety of risk factors for osteoporosis are recognized. Female gender, postmenopausal status, nulliparity, late onset of menarche, and early menopause from any cause increase risk of bone loss. Women of northern European or Asian background are at higher risk for osteoporosis, as are those with a positive family history for osteoporosis or fracture, regardless of ethnicity. It is estimated that genetic inheritance explains about 60% to 70% of the variance in BMD within populations.

Environmental and dietary factors play key roles in a patient's risk for osteoporosis. Low calcium or vitamin D intake, alcohol abuse, cigarette smoking, and high-protein, high-caffeine, or high-sodium diets all increase risk of bone loss. U.S. National Health and Nutrition Examination Survey III data show that total daily elemental calcium intake in the United States averages 500 to 600 mg for women from age 20 to 90 years and 600 to 700 mg for men in the same age range. Certain medications, such as glucocorticoids, anticonvulsants, or excess thyroid hormone replacement, may cause bone loss. Lack of regular physical exercise, defined as 30 minutes of weight-bearing exercise each day at least 5 days each week, and a slender body frame, with an average adult weight of less than 127 lb, increase the risk of developing osteoporosis.

Risk factors for osteoporotic fracture include a positive family history of osteoporotic fracture, previous personal history of osteoporotic fracture, propensity to fall, and use of medications predisposing to falls (e.g., sedatives, hypnotics, antihypertensives, narcotics).

Patients with significant bone loss are often completely asymptomatic until they experience a fracture. Patients with clinical fractures are easily identified, but the significance of their fractures may be overlooked, because both patients and physicians might believe that fractures that have occurred are a normal part of the aging process. Osteoporotic fractures by definition occur with minimal trauma, often with falls from standing height or less.

## FRACTURES

The average 50-year-old white woman in the United States has a 40% remaining lifetime risk of clinically recognized fracture, with the risk of vertebral, hip, and wrist fractures about equal (16% for each). The estimated remaining lifetime fracture risk increases to more than 50% if asymptomatic vertebral compression fractures are included in this estimate. The average 50-year-old white man has a 4.6% remaining lifetime risk of clinically recognized fracture.

Each year, an estimated 1.5 million fractures occur due to osteoporosis in the United States. Fracture rates are highest in whites and Asians and lower in Latin Americans, Native Americans, and African Americans. The economic cost of these fractures was estimated to be between $12 billion and $18 billion per year in 2002, with 63% of the total cost due to hospital services and 28% due to long-term rehabilitation and nursing home care.

In the United States, more than 250,000 hip fractures result from osteoporosis, with an estimated 20% excess mortality within the first year after fracture and significant functional loss for those who survive. The overall prevalence of hip fracture exceeds 15% by age 80 years and 25% by age 90 years. By age 90 years, 31% of women and 17% of men have had a hip fracture. Hip fractures account for 63% of the total direct costs of osteoporosis. More than 500,000 vertebral fractures occur annually, with resultant loss of height and chronic back pain. It is estimated that more than 25% of women older than 65 years have a vertebral fracture and that as many as 40% of these are asymptomatic. More than 200,000 distal forearm fractures and more than 300,000 other limb fractures occur annually. Limb fractures double every 5 to 8 years after the fifth decade in women, but they do not occur frequently in men until after the seventh decade.

## Diagnosis

### CLINICAL AND LABORATORY DIAGNOSIS

Men or postmenopausal women found to have significant bone loss, with or without fractures, should undergo physical examination and laboratory evaluation to assess for secondary causes of bone loss. Serum total calcium, phosphorus, alkaline phosphatase, creatinine, aspartate aminotransferase (AST), sensitive thyroid-stimulating hormone (TSH), erythrocyte sedimentation rate (ESR), serum protein electrophoresis, and appropriate x-rays (e.g., spine films), should be obtained to rule out the majority of the recognized secondary causes of osteoporosis, if not checked within the 6 months preceding evaluation. Serum parathyroid hormone, 25-hydroxyvitamin D, urine protein electrophoresis, and serum or urine protein immunoelectrophoresis should be assessed when appropriate. Twenty-four-hour urine calcium and creatinine are helpful to establish that patients are taking and absorbing adequate calcium and to make sure they do not have idiopathic hypercalciuria. The most common secondary causes of bone loss found in postmenopausal women are vitamin D insufficiency or deficiency, hyperparathyroidism, hyperthyroidism in women taking L-thyroxine replacement therapy, and hypercalciuria.

### BONE MINERAL DENSITY

Low bone density remains the single most accurate predictor of increased fracture risk. For every 1.0 standard deviation decrease in BMD below the mean for young adults of the same sex and ethnicity, fracture risk roughly doubles at the spine and hip.

BMD should be checked, preferably by DXA, in all patients with a history of osteoporotic fractures or suspected low bone density to quantify the severity of bone loss. All women older than 65 years should undergo bone density testing if it was not done earlier. BMD testing by any technique may be done to confirm the presence and severity of bone loss, but DXA is required to assess bone loss over time and to monitor effects of therapy. Medicare-approved indications for BMD testing include osteoporotic fractures of the hip, spine, wrist, or other bones; x-ray evidence of vertebral deformity or fracture suggesting osteoporosis; postmenopausal estrogen-deficient women at clinical risk for osteoporosis; monitoring osteoporosis therapy with an FDA-approved drug; primary hyperparathyroidism; and glucocorticoid therapy equivalent to or greater than prednisone 7.5 mg/day for more than 3 months or if the expected duration of therapy is more than 3 months.

The BMD T-score, representing the number of standard deviations above or below the young adult mean for persons of the same sex and ethnicity, is currently used to diagnose osteoporosis and low bone density. The WHO currently defines low bone density as a BMD T-score of $-1.0$ to $-2.5$ and osteoporosis as a BMD T-score of less than $-2.5$. A WHO working group is currently developing models to predict individual 10-year fracture risk using a combination of BMD and risk factors.

Biochemical markers of bone turnover are not a substitute for bone density as a means of diagnosing osteoporosis. Several markers of bone resorption have been described, including urine amino- or carboxy-telopeptide of type I collagen (NTx or CTx) and urinary pyridinoline and deoxypyridinoline. Several markers of formation have also been described, including serum bone-specific alkaline phosphatase, osteocalcin, and procollagen type I extension peptides (e.g., procollagen type I intact N-terminal propeptide [PINP]). Bone markers are currently used to monitor the response to treatment with anticatabolic agents and might predict the response to treatment with these drugs better than bone density changes.

## Differential Diagnosis

The differential diagnosis for low bone density and osteoporosis is shown in Box 1.

## Treatment

Treatment of osteoporosis begins with maximizing acquisition of bone mass during growth and development and preventing bone loss after peak bone mass is achieved. All patients should be encouraged to make healthy lifestyle choices in childhood, adolescence, and their young adult years that are likely to maximize their peak BMD in their late 20s to mid-30s and to follow practices later in life known to minimize

---

**BOX 1  Differential Diagnosis of Low Bone Density or Osteoporosis**

- Celiac disease or other malabsorptive disorders
- Chronic liver disease
- Chronic kidney disease
- Endogenous or exogenous glucocorticoid excess
- Hypercalciuria
- Hyperparathyroidism
- Hyperthyroidism
- Hypogonadism of any cause
- Multiple myeloma
- Osteomalacia
- Prolonged heparin therapy
- Prolonged immobilization
- Systemic mastocytosis
- Type 1 diabetes mellitus
- Vitamin D insufficiency or deficiency

## CURRENT DIAGNOSIS

- Serum calcium
- Serum phosphorus
- Serum bone alkaline phosphatase
- Serum creatinine
- Serum AST
- Serum TSH
- Serum 25-hydroxyvitamin D
- Serum PTH
- 24-Hour urine calcium, creatinine, and sodium
- 24-Hour urine NTx or CTx

*Abbreviations:* AST = aspartate aminotransferase; CTx = Carboxyterminal cross-linking telopeptide of bone collagen; NTx = aminoterminal cross-linking telopeptide of bone collagen; PTH = parathyroid hormone; TSH = thyroid-stimulating hormone.

bone loss. Patients with known bone loss should decrease their subsequent likelihood of fracture by minimizing their fall risk and avoiding high-risk activities likely to cause fracture. Modifiable risk factors should be addressed to assist in preserving bone density.

### EXERCISE

Patients with bone loss should perform weight-bearing exercise for a minimum of 3 hours each week to help preserve or increase their BMD and reduce their fall risk. Moderate or higher impact activities, or weight lifting, can help preserve BMD in younger persons.

### CALCIUM

Calcium supplementation can help prevent bone loss, cause mild increases in BMD in some women, and prevent hip fracture in postmenopausal women compliant and persistent with treatment. Women with low BMD or osteoporosis should optimize their total daily elemental calcium intake to 1000 mg until age 50, and then increase this to 1500 mg after age 50. Men should optimize their total daily elemental calcium intake to 1000 mg until age 50, and then increase this to 1500 mg after age 50. The 1997 U.S. National Academy of Sciences dietary reference intakes were established to preserve bone health in healthy adults without osteoporosis or bone loss, and they call for healthy adults to take 1000 mg elemental calcium daily until age 50, and to increase this to 1200 mg/day at age 50 and older.

## CURRENT THERAPY

**Nonpharmacologic Therapies**

- Adequate calcium intake
- Adequate exercise
- Adequate protein intake
- Adequate vitamin D intake
- Low sodium intake

**Pharmacologic Therapies**

- Alendronate (Fosamax)
- Calcitonin nasal spray (Miacalcin)
- Hormone therapy
- Ibandronate (Boniva)
- Raloxifene (Evista)
- Risedronate (Actonel)
- Teriparatide (Forteo)

Healthy men younger than 50 years should take 1000 mg elemental calcium per day, and healthy men older than 50 years should take 1200 mg/day. The Women's Health Initiative (WHI) study showed that calcium 1000 mg/day and vitamin D 400 IU/day does not prevent fractures in noncompliant patients, but it does prevent hip fractures in those who comply with recommendations.

### VITAMIN D

Vitamin D supplementation might prevent loss of BMD or cause mild increases in BMD. Vitamin D stimulates intestinal absorption of calcium and phosphorus. Although adequate sunlight exposure can maintain normal vitamin D levels in some persons, vitamin D 400 IU/day, in the form of one multivitamin or vitamin D capsule daily, is typically recommended for postmenopausal women and men older than 50 years. Patients taking prednisone at more than 10 mg/day should take vitamin D 800 IU/day. Recent meta-analyses of vitamin D clinical trials show that vitamin D can prevent falls and fractures at doses of 700 to 800 IU/day.

### ANTICATABOLIC AGENTS

Bisphosphonates are currently the most potent oral antiresorptive agents available to prevent or treat osteoporosis. Approved oral bisphosphonates include alendronate (Fosamax), risedronate (Actonel), and ibandronate (Boniva). The only approved intravenous bisphosphonate is ibandronate. Bisphosphonates block bone resorption by inhibiting osteoclast activity by several mechanisms, with long-term incorporation into bone. Less than 1% of a dose of an oral bisphosphonate is normally absorbed via the intestine. Oral alendronate and risedronate are proven to decrease bone turnover and reduce vertebral and hip fractures by 50% to 60% in postmenopausal women, whereas oral ibandronate reduces vertebral fractures by 50% to 60%, but it has not yet been proved to reduce nonvertebral, including hip, fractures. Intravenous ibandronate has been shown to prevent bone loss but not fractures. Alendronate 35 or 70 mg once a week is approved for prevention or treatment, respectively, of postmenopausal osteoporosis. Alendronate is also approved for treatment of glucocorticoid-induced osteoporosis and male osteoporosis. Risedronate 35 mg once a week is approved for prevention and treatment of postmenopausal osteoporosis as well as for prevention and treatment of corticosteroid-induced osteoporosis and male osteoporosis.

The first head-to-head comparison trial of oral bisphosphonates recently showed alendronate to be slightly more effective than risedronate at increasing BMD over 24 months, with no difference in side effects. Fracture data are not available from this trial. Patients who stop alendronate after several years of therapy lose bone beginning about 6 months after stopping the drug, but the rate of bone loss is slower than in subjects who had never taken alendronate, and fracture risk does not increase during the first 2 years off the drug. Alendronate appears to be safe when taken for up to 10 years of continuous therapy and risedronate for up to 7 years of continuous therapy.

Patients with hypocalcemia, hypersensitivity to medication, or esophageal irritation or strictures should avoid oral bisphosphonates. Patients with renal insufficiency should not take alendronate if their creatinine clearance is less than 35 mL/min and should not take risendronate if their creatinine clearance is less than 30 mL/min. Patients with malignancy treated with high doses of intravenous bisphosphonates appear to have a significant risk of developing osteonecrosis of the jaw (ONJ), particularly following dental procedures, but the risk of ONJ appears to be extremely low with the oral bisphosphonates at doses used to treat osteoporosis.

Raloxifene (Evista) is the first marketed selective estrogen receptor modulator (SERM), and is approved for prevention or treatment of osteoporosis at 60 mg/day. Raloxifene has been shown to decrease vertebral fractures, but not hip fractures. Raloxifene interacts with estrogen receptor (ER)-α and ER-β similar to estrogen, but it causes a different ligand-receptor conformational change that results in tissue-specific effects. Raloxifene is contraindicated in patients with a history of deep venous thrombosis or pulmonary embolus due to increased clotting risk, and it can worsen vasomotor symptoms. Raloxifene has been shown to reduce the risk of breast cancer, but it does not increase or decrease the risk of cardiovascular disease.

Salmon calcitonin nasal spray (Miacalcin) is approved for treatment of osteoporosis at 200 IU in alternating nostrils each day. Salmon calcitonin nasal spray prevents bone loss and vertebral fractures but not nonvertebral fractures, and it can decrease postvertebral fracture pain. The main side effect of nasal spray salmon calcitonin is rhinitis in 12% of treated patients.

The role of hormone therapy remains controversial. The WHI clinical trial showed that estrogen alone, or combination estrogen and progesterone, decreased bone turnover, bone loss, and fractures as expected, but that heart attack, stroke, venous thromboembolism, and invasive breast cancer occurred more frequently. Hormone therapy is currently approved for prevention, but not treatment, of osteoporosis. The FDA advises using hormone therapy in postmenopausal women in doses as low as possible, for as short a time as possible, before stopping therapy. The WHI study showed benefit of hormone therapy in preventing hot flashes, but not in preventing age-related memory loss or improving quality of life.

## ANABOLIC AGENTS

Recombinant human parathyroid hormone analogues are potent bone anabolic agents. Teriparatide (Forteo) is the first anabolic agent approved for treating women who have severe postmenopausal osteoporosis and high risk of fracture and for treating men who have primary or hypogonadal osteoporosis and high risk of fracture. Teriparatide is given as 20 μg subcutaneously injected once a day for up to 2 years of therapy. Teriparatide might increase bone density more potently than oral bisphosphonates, and it reduces vertebral fractures by 65% and nonvertebral fractures by 53%. Teriparatide used in combination with alendronate is less effective than teriparatide alone, but raloxifene does not appear to impair teriparatide effects on bone. However, it is clear that following 2 years of teriparatide therapy, treatment with an anticatabolic agent, such as a bisphosphonate, is necessary in order to maintain gains in BMD.

Side effects of teriparatide include lightheadedness, dizziness, nausea, or pain at the injection site. Risk of postinjection hypercalcemia is not sufficient to warrant routine monitoring of serum calcium. Teriparatide is contraindicated in patients with a history of osteogenic sarcoma, Paget's disease of bone, unexplained hypercalcemia, history of skeletal radiation exposure, or age less than 18 years. Other anabolic parathyroid hormone analogues are under development.

## FRACTURES

Patients with hip or wrist fractures often require surgical treatment, whereas patients with vertebral fractures usually require pain medication and supportive therapy. Vertebroplasty or kyphoplasty can help with pain relief in patients with significant pain due to vertebral fracture. Patients with vertebral fractures and kyphosis can benefit from a lumbar or other support brace. Patients with fractures should be evaluated for secondary causes of bone loss to make sure that therapy will be effective when it is given. Medications used to treat osteoporosis after fracture are identical to those used to treat or prevent osteoporosis before fracture. The occurrence of a fracture on therapy does not necessarily mean patients have failed therapy, because patients on therapy still have a 20% to 65% chance of fracturing, depending on the therapy selected.

## REFERENCES

Cranney A, Guyatt G, Griffith L, et al: Meta-analyses of therapies for postmenopausal osteoporosis. IX: Summary of meta-analyses of therapies for postmenopausal osteoporosis. Endocr Rev 2002;23:570-578.

Epstein S: The roles of bone mineral density, bone turnover, and other properties in reducing fracture risk during antiresorptive therapy. Mayo Clin Proc 2005;80:379-388.

Hodsman AB, Bauer DC, Dempster DW, et al: Parathyroid hormone and teriparatide for the treatment of osteoporosis: A review of the evidence and suggested guidelines for its use. Endocr Rev 2005;26:688-703.

Khosla S, Melton LJ 3rd, Robb RA, et al: Relationship of volumetric BMD and structural parameters at different skeletal sites to sex steroid levels in men. J Bone Miner Res 2005;20:730-740.

Khosla S, Riggs BL: Pathophysiology of age-related bone loss and osteoporosis. Endocrinol Metab Clin North America 2005;34:1015-1030, xi.

Khosla S, Riggs BL, Robb RA, et al: Relationship of volumetric bone density and structural parameters at different skeletal sites to sex steroid levels in women. J Clin Endocrinol Metab 2005;90(9):5096-5103.

Mauck KF, Clarke BL: Diagnosis, screening, prevention, and treatment of osteoporosis. Mayo Clin Proc 2006;81:662-672.

National Osteoporosis Foundation: America's Bone Health: The State of Osteoporosis and Low Bone Mass in Our Nation. Washington, DC: National Osteoporosis Foundation, 2002.

NIH Consensus Development Panel on Osteoporosis Prevention, Diagnosis, and Therapy. JAMA 2001;285:785-795.

Raisz LG: Pathogenesis of osteoporosis: Concepts, conflicts, and prospects. J Clin Invest 2005;115:3318-3325.

Riggs BL, Hartmann LC: Selective estrogen-receptor modulators—mechanisms of action and application to clinical practice. N Engl J Med 2003;348:618-629.

Riggs BL, Melton JL III, Robb RA, et al: Population-based study of age and sex differences in bone volumetric density, size, geometry, and structure at different skeletal sites. J Bone Miner Res 2004;19:1945-1954.

Sambrook P, Cooper C: Osteoporosis. Lancet 2006;367:2010-2018.

Tanaka S, Nakamura K, Takahasi N, Suda T: Role of RANKL in physiological and pathological bone resorption and therapeutics targeting the RANKL-RANK signaling system. Immunol Rev 2005;208:30-49.

# Paget's Disease of Bone

Method of
*Paul D. Miller, MD*

## Diagnosis

Paget's disease is characterized by excessively high bone turnover in the involved skeletal site(s). Although the bone may appear "osteosclerotic" on radiographic evaluation, the bone strength is actually compromised and may easily fracture. Paget's disease may present with pain in the involved skeleton, or it may be asymptomatic and suspected when a patient is discovered to have either an elevated total serum alkaline phosphatase level or an unexplained elevated bone resorption marker (e.g., urine or serum collagen cross-link of type I collagen: *N*- or *C*-telopeptide). If a physician discovers an unexplained elevated total alkaline phosphatase level, then the source of this elevated enzyme must be differentiated as either hepatic or bone (assuming the patient is not pregnant because the placenta also produces alkaline phosphatase). If the alkaline phosphatase originates from bone, differential diagnosis of the possible causes of an elevated bone-specific alkaline phosphatase (BSAP) level is as follows:

1. Paget's disease
2. Metastatic cancer in bone

---

**CURRENT DIAGNOSIS**

- No known cause.
- Diagnosed by radiography, not by bone scan or magnetic resonance imaging.
- Often asymptomatic.
- May be active with normal biochemical markers of bone turnover: collagen cross-links or bone-specific alkaline phosphatase.

3. Recent large bone fracture
4. Osteomalacia
5. Hyperthyroidism
6. Hyperparathyroidism
7. Medication induced (antiseizure drugs, parathyroid hormone used for treatment of osteoporosis)
8. Immobilization/space travel
9. Vitamin D deficiency without osteomalacia

Many of these potential causes of an elevated BSAP level can be differentiated clinically and by laboratory testing. In patients who still have an elevated BSAP level of undeterminable etiology, a total body bone scan is required to locate any "hot spots" that could suggest Paget's disease. I always simultaneously order a routine radiograph of any hot spots seen on a radioisotope bone scan because Paget's disease is a radiographic, not a bone scan, diagnosis. The one radiographic finding that can be confused with Paget's disease is metastatic prostatic carcinoma. However, metastatic prostatic cancer is associated with an elevated prostate-specific antigen level and other clinical findings of prostatic abnormalities. Given any radiographic finding that one has difficulty distinguishing between Paget's disease and prostatic cancer, a magnetic resonance image is more distinctly abnormal in metastatic cancer to bone, or, if necessary, a bone biopsy is definitive.

Painful Paget's disease requires treatment. Bisphosphonates are the treatment of choice because of their exceptional efficacy and safety when used appropriately in Paget's disease. Bisphosphonates may have the potential of "curing" Paget's disease or, at least, putting the disease into very prolonged and sustained biochemical and clinical remission.

Asymptomatic Paget's disease should also be treated. Although the proportion of patients with asymptomatic Paget's disease who progress to become symptomatic is not known, progression does occur in many patients, and who might or who might not progress cannot be predicted from the initial assessment. Because progression can lead to bony deformities, fractures, hearing loss, neurologic complications (spinal cord compression, nerve entrapment), high-output congestive heart failure, and osteogenic sarcoma, asymptomatic patients merit strong consideration for treatment. To reiterate, because the bisphosphonates are very safe, especially when required only intermittently in Paget's patients, and can be administered either by the oral or intravenous route, they should not be withheld in asymptomatic Paget's patients.

A few patients with Paget's disease may have normal BSAP but elevated bone resorption (NTX/CTX) markers. In my opinion, this combination of disassociated bone formation versus bone resorption markers may be seen in two circumstances: very early Paget's disease—classic or type 1 Paget's disease, and type 2 Paget's disease, in which the BSAP level never becomes elevated despite sustained elevation of the bone resorption markers.

Paget's disease is a disease of the osteoclasts, the cells that induce bone resorption. In pagetic bone biopsies, these osteoclasts are larger, have many more nuclei, and are increased in number compared to osteoclasts seen in normal patients or in patients with osteoporosis. The initial pathophysiologic process in Paget's disease is excessive bone resorption. Thus, the first radiologic defect seen is an osteolytic lesion (a "black" hole) in bone. Hence, early in the pagetic process, an increase in bone resorption markers is seen before the bone formation markers increase. Owing to the normal coupling process between the bone cell lines (increasing or decreasing bone resorption is followed by a directional increase or a decrease in bone formation), bone formation will, in time, also increase, and the BSAP level will ultimately rise. As the BSAP level rises, the osteolytic lesion begins to develop sclerosis and fill in with the white-appearing honeycombed pagetic features. This is the classic sequence in most pagetic patients.

Type 2 Paget's disease looks just like type 1 on radiography: the initial osteolytic lesion is present. The difference between the two forms of Paget's disease is that the osteolytic lesion persists: the bone resorption markers remain elevated without a rise in BSAP or filling in of the osteolytic lesion. There is something different about this very uncommon form of Paget's disease that both I and my colleagues, who see many Paget's patients, have observed in clinical practice. The normal coupling between bone cell lines seems to be absent. It is possible that these patients started out with a low BSAP level, and that it did increase but never above the upper limits of the normal reference range. It may also be true that type 2 Paget's disease is a different disease from a pathophysiologic point of view than type 1 Paget's disease. It is important, however, to stress that even if the BSAP level never becomes elevated, the high NTX/CTX ratio confers enough evidence of high bone turnover of a sufficient magnitude to warrant treatment because these persistent osteolytic pagetic lesions are highly prone to fracture. Multiple myeloma is another clinical condition characterized by high bone resorption and elevated bone resorption markers without an increase in either bone formation or in the bone formation markers BSAP. Despite the presence of many osteolytic lesions in patients with advanced multiple myeloma, the BSAP level never becomes elevated. Hence, myeloma represents another situation in which there is uncoupling between bone resorption and bone formation, as may be seen in type 2 Paget's disease.

Do the two different forms of Paget's disease respond differently to treatment? Probably not, although the proportion of patients with type 2 Paget's disease is small and insufficient for a head-to-head study with type 1 disease to determine any differences in treatment response.

## Treatment

The Food and Drug Administration (FDA)–approved therapies for treatment of Paget's disease are calcitonin and bisphosphonates. Off-label use of gallium nitrate (Ganite)[1] or pliamycin[2] is available for the very rare recalcitrant patient. I have not needed to use either gallium nitrate or pliamycin for more than 20 years because of the exceptional response rate to bisphosphonates. In addition, the response rate seems far greater with bisphosphonates than with calcitonin, which for Paget's disease must be given parenterally and has a high nausea side-effect profile.

Injectable calcitonin has been used for more than 25 years as therapy for Paget's disease and may be considered an option in patients who might not be able to tolerate or to be given a bisphosphonate.

---

[1]Not FDA approved for this indication.
[2]Not available in the United States.

---

 **CURRENT THERAPY**

- Bisphosphonates are the treatment of choice.
- Bisphosphonates should be used in asymptomatic patients who have elevated bone turnover markers.
- May be mono-ostotic (single bone involvement) or polyostotic (more than one bone involved). Once the patient is diagnosed with either mono-ostotic or polyostotic Paget's disease, those bones will be the only ones ever involved. Paget's disease does not spread from one bone to another.
- Recent data suggest that the greater the magnitude of normalization of the total or bone-specific alkaline phosphatase level achieved with treatment, the longer the duration of remission.
- Prevalence is highly variable throughout the world: estimated to be 2% of the white population of North America, declining in northern England, and very rare in China. However, the accuracy of prevalence data must be interpreted in the context that many asymptomatic patients are radiographed, and population radiographic studies that assessed prevalence radiographed only specific skeletal sites, so some involved areas could have been missed.

Subcutaneous administration of 100 IU/day[3] often leads to an average 50% reduction in bone turnover markers 3 to 6 months after therapy. The nasal spray formulation of calcitonin (Miacalcin) is not FDA approved for Paget's disease.

The bisphosphonates available for treatment of Paget's disease are: etidronate (Didronel), alendronate (Fosamax), risedronate (Actonel, oral formulations), and pamidronate (Aredia). Zolendronic acid[4] is currently under review by the FDA for registration for Paget's disease.

The bisphosphonates alendronate and risedronate have the most robust data showing an exceptional positive effect in the treatment of Paget's disease. Alendronate (Fosamax) at a dose of 40 mg/day for 6 months or risedronate (Actonel) at a dose of 30 mg/day for 2 months can rapidly normalize the NTX/CTX ratio or BSAP level in the majority of patients. No head-to-head clinical trials have compared the efficacy of these two bisphosphonates in Paget's disease, although a head-to-head study did compare etidronate to risedronate in active Paget's disease. Risedronate was clearly more effective in reducing the BSAP level and inducing a longer remission than was etidronate. Selection between the two aminobisphosphonates (alendronate and risedronate) probably is based on physician preference, tolerability, and costs. With either bisphosphonate, bone turnover marker should be measured at the end of the treatment period. If the BSAP level has not normalized, either a second course of the oral bisphosphonate or a change to an intravenous bisphosphonate should be considered. As previously stated, normalization of the BSAP level is the goal of treatment, and the lower the BSAP level, the greater the probability of a longer duration of remission.

Recently, clinical trial data on the efficacy of intravenous zolendronic acid[4] in the treatment of Paget's disease were published. The study showed that 5 mg of intravenous zolendronic acid given over 15 minutes induced a more rapid therapeutic response along with a larger proportion of patients who responded with normalization of BSAP level than was seen with risedronate. In addition, in the 6-month posttreatment follow-up, a greater proportion of patients who received zolendronic acid were still in remission than those who had received risedronate. This finding is consistent with the observations suggesting that the duration of remission is related to the magnitude of suppression of BSAP.

Zolendronic acid[4] has also been shown to have a greater effect on alkaline phosphatase than pamidronate, the other available intravenous nitrogen-containing bisphosphonate.

Hence, with highly effective oral and intravenous bisphosphonates available for treatment of Paget's disease, the clinician must choose which one to use. In my practice, all Paget's disease patients who have pain receive an intravenous bisphosphonate because the pain reduction or elimination is very fast. On the other hand, for asymptomatic Paget's patients, I often use an oral bisphosphonate, saving the intravenous formulations for recalcitrant patients or for patients with relapses. This approach may change as the data evolve, confirming that the duration of remission is prolonged with greater suppression of BSAP. Certainly, costs may become a consideration in the choice, as will upper gastrointestinal conditions that could make an oral bisphosphonate risky. On the other hand, in the zolendronic acid versus risedronate clinical trial, more patients receiving zolendronic acid experienced the acute-phase reaction (fever, muscle pain), which was transient and without sequelae. Nevertheless, intravenous formulations may not be preferred in some patients.

Resistance to bisphosphonates may develop in Paget's disease. After repeated doses of a particular bisphosphonate, some patients stop responding to that particular bisphosphonate but do respond to a different bisphosphonate. The reason for resistance development is unknown because it has not been described in patients treated with bisphosphonates for osteoporosis. Another unexplained phenomenon in Paget's patients who develop resistance to a particular bisphosphonate is that often they again become responsive to the bisphosphonate to which they had become unresponsive after a period of not receiving that specific bisphosphonate.

Finally, there are a few instances in the treatment of Paget's disease in which the clinician must use extra diligence. One is the patient with a painful osteolytic lesion in the proximal femur. Bisphosphonate administration will often relieve the pain promptly, which may encourage the patient to increase activity and weight bearing, and then the hip may fracture. In these circumstances, the patient should be cautioned about this potential and provided with a cane to support the leg until the osteolytic lesion fills in (several months). Another area of caution is the patient who does not respond to any treatment, who relapses quickly and has a rapidly progressive radiographic pagetic change, or develops more pain, swelling, and redness over the pagetic bone. Osteogenic sarcoma could be a distinct possibility, and the lesion may require biopsy. Finally, a third area of caution is the patient in whom neurologic impairment may be related to pagetic bone encroachment, spinal cord compression with long-tract signs, spinal stenosis, or basilar skull invagination with neural compromise. Close consultation with a neurosurgeon is needed to help decide on a possible surgical intervention through a highly vascular pagetic bone. Administration of intravenous bisphosphonate 1 to 2 days before surgery might mitigate bleeding because bisphosphonates reduce blood flow in highly vascular areas for a period of time.

Paget's disease is manageable and may be put into very long-term remission by normalization of the biochemical markers of bone turnover. Asymptomatic patients with high bone turnover should be treated to prevent potential long-term complications. Treatment in these patients is very reasonable given the evidence that the newer aminobisphosphonates are highly effective and very safe when used appropriately.

### REFERENCES

Altman RD, Bloch DA, Hochberg MC, Murphy WA: Prevalence of pelvic Paget's disease of bone in the United States. J Bone Miner Res 2000;15:461-465.

Miller PD, Brown JP, Siris ES, et al: A randomized, double-blind comparison of risedronate and etidronate in the treatment of Paget's disease of bone. Am J Med 1999;106:513-520.

Reid IR, Miller PD, Lyles K, et al: Comparison of a single infusion of zolendronic acid with risedronate for Paget's disease. N Engl J Med 2005;353:22-32.

Reid IR, Nicholson GC, Weinstein RS, et al: Biochemical and radiologic improvement in Paget's disease of bone treated with alendronate: A randomized, placebo-controlled trial. Am J Med 1996;101:341-348.

# Parenteral Nutrition in Adults

Method of
*Jeffrey Jim, MD, MS, and Darryl T. Hiyama, MD*

Parenteral nutrition (PN) is the infusion of a hypertonic solution containing carbohydrates, amino acids, lipids, essential vitamins, and trace minerals. Before the 1960s, PN was limited to isotonic or minimally hypertonic solutions infused through peripheral veins. This caused difficulty with volume overload, loss of peripheral access, and inadequate nutrition. Following the development of central venous access, the field of PN has evolved extensively and PN is in common use.

## Indications

Malnutrition itself has been shown to adversely influence physiologic functions and patient survival. Numerous randomized, controlled trials have demonstrated that nutritional support favorably influences patient outcomes by minimizing the consequences of malnutrition (increased infection, poor wound healing, delayed rehabilitation, and mortality). In various diseased states, a clear association between

---

[3]Exceeds dosage recommended by the manufacturer.
[4]Not yet approved for use in the United States.

malnutrition and poor clinical outcome has been well documented. Nutritional support is initiated in patients who have prolonged periods of no nutritional intake, preexisting malnutrition, long duration of illness, or significant multiorgan system failure and during times of increased metabolic demand, such as in the postoperative period and trauma.

As a general rule, enteral feeding through the gastrointestinal tract is preferred over PN. Comparisons with enteral feeding have consistently demonstrated more complications in PN, usually infection related. However, enteral feeding is not always possible. Several societies (including the American Gastroenterology Association and American Society of Parenteral and Enteral Nutrition) have developed guidelines for the indications and recommendations for the use of PN (http://www.nutritioncare.org/publications/2002guidelines.pdf). The primary acute indications for PN are in critically ill patients suffering from malnutrition, sepsis, or acute trauma or when the gastrointestinal tract cannot be used for enteral feeding. The complete dependence on PN for survival is termed *total parenteral nutrition* (TPN).

## Contraindications

Hemodynamic instability and metabolic derangement are absolute contraindications to initiating PN. Patients with good nutritional status or functioning gastrointestinal tracts should not receive PN. If PN is needed, enteral supplementation should be considered. Administration of PN to patients with fatal diseases remains controversial. There are no studies that demonstrate chronic home PN prolongs survival or enhances the quality of life in patients with AIDS or metastatic cancer. The decision to initiate PN in these situations presents a difficult clinical and ethical dilemma.

## Formulation

In most institutions, there is a standard formulation for PN. In addition, health care providers such as dietitians and pharmaceutical services are usually able to assist in determining the appropriate PN solution. Several metabolic and nutritional measurements need to be taken to calculate the appropriate solution for a patient. The total fluid requirement (in mL/day) can be calculated with the following formula: 1500 mL for the first 20 kg, then an additional 20 mL/kg thereafter. Once the total fluid need is calculated, caloric, protein, and electrolyte requirements are determined.

Indirect calorimetry is the optimal method for determining a patient's total caloric needs. However, this technique is neither cost-effective nor readily accessible in most hospitals. The estimated basal metabolic rate (BMR) in normal healthy persons is roughly 25 kcal/kg/day, and more precise values can be calculated using the Harris-Benedict equation (Box 1). Pathologic processes and stress result in significantly elevated BMR. The elevation can be slight (e.g., mild peritonitis or orthopedic trauma) to severe (e.g., significant surface area burns). A rough estimate of caloric needs can also be

### TABLE 1 Daily Protein Requirements

| Patient Condition | Requirement (g/kg/d) |
| --- | --- |
| Normal healthy | 0.8 |
| Hospitalized, mild stress | 1-1.2 |
| Moderate stress | 1.2-1.5 |
| Severe stress | 1.5-2 |
| Renal failure (with dialysis) | 1-1.5 |
| Renal failure (without dialysis) | 0.6-1 |
| Hepatic failure (with encephalopathy) | 0.6-1 |
| Hepatic failure (without encephalopathy) | 1-1.5 |

based on ideal body weight (IBW) calculations. In hospitalized patients, the caloric need to maintain body weight is approximately 33 kcal/kg IBW and to rebuild tissue is 40 kcal/kg IBW.

Protein requirements are met with infusion of an amino acid mixture. The recommended daily allowance of protein in healthy patients is 0.8 grams/kg IBW (Table 1). However, for most hospitalized patients, the requirement is 1.0 to 1.5 g/kg. The maximum daily dose of protein is 2 g/kg (often used in cases of protein-losing enteropathy, open wounds, or high-output fistulas). In cases of renal failure or hepatic encephalopathy, the protein supplementation might need to be reduced to prevent azotemia or encephalopathy.

Electrolytes, trace elements and vitamins are also added to the PN solution. Again, standard solutions are easily prepared, but components can be adjusted based on a patient's metabolic profile (Table 2). Daily monitoring of serum electrolytes should be undertaken once PN has been initiated. Supplementation and adjustments to PN solutions should be made as needed. Consideration should be given to patients with renal insufficiency, with special care to monitor for hyperkalemia, hypercalcemia, and hyperphosphatemia. The chloride and acetate concentrations are balanced in standard solutions, but they can be adjusted depending on the clinical situation. If there is excess loss of chloride (as in high gastric output in proximal fistulas or nasogastric decompression), then the chloride concentration can be increased. If the patient is acidotic, the acetate component is maximized because this molecule is metabolized to bicarbonate. Because vitamin K is not present in commercially prepared solutions, it has to be supplemented on a weekly basis (except in cases of anticoagulation with warfarin [Coumadin]).

Lipid solutions are often administered separately from the standard PN solutions. The calories derived from lipids should constitute approximately 20% to 30% of total energy needs and should not exceed 60%. Commercially available 20% soybean oil emulsion solution is often used, and this provides 2 kcal/mL. Lipids should not be infused for longer than 12 hours per day. This recommendation was made by the Centers for Disease Control and Prevention (CDC),

### BOX 1 Formulas for Calculating Total Caloric Needs

**Harris-Benedict Equation**
Basal metabolic rate (BMR) (kcal/d)
- Male: 66 + (13.7 × weight in kg) + (5 × height in cm) − (6.8 × age in y)
- Females: 665 + (9.6 × weight in kg) + (1.7 × height in cm) − (4.7 × age in y)

**Ideal Body Weight (IBW) (kg)**
- Male: 48 kg + (2.7 × inches over 5 feet)
- Female: 45 kg + (2.3 × inches over 5 feet)

### TABLE 2 Sample Electrolytes in Central Parenteral Nutrition Solutions

| Additive | Usual Concentration (mEq/L) | Usual Concentration Range (mEq/L) |
| --- | --- | --- |
| Acetate | 55 | 70-220 |
| Calcium | 5 | 0-10 |
| Chloride | 35 | 0-150 |
| Magnesium | 10 | 0-15 |
| Phosphate | 10 | 0-80 |
| Potassium | 30 | 0-80 |
| Sodium | 35 | 0-150 |

## BOX 2  Sample Calculations for Central Total Parenteral Nutrition

**Patient: 70-kg female, short gut from resection, unable to tolerate oral/enteral nutrition**

### Requirements

- Fluid: 2500 mL/day
- Calories: 70 kg × estimated 35 kcal/kg/day = 2450 kcal/d
- Protein: 70 kg × 1 g/kg/d = 70 g/d
- Lipid calories: 2450 kcal/d × 25% = 613 kcal
- Protein calories: 70 g/d protein × 4 kcal/g = 280 kcal from proteins
- Remaining 1557 kcal/d from dextrose

### Composition

Using standard 70% dextrose (3.4 kcal/g), 10% amino acid, 20% intralipid (2 kcal/mL)
- Lipid: 613 kcal/d ÷ 2 kcal/mL = 307 mL/d
- Dextrose: 1557 kcal/d ÷ 3.4 kcal/g ÷ 70% = 654 mL/d
- Protein: 70 g/d ÷ 0.1 = 700 mL/d
- Supplements: Approximately 100 mL
- Should include 10 U insulin, standard electrolyte profile
- Sterile water: 739 mL sterile water
- Total volume: 2500 mL/d

**Patient: 80-kg male, diabetic, moderate stress, renal failure with dialysis**

### Requirements

- Fluid: Minimize due to renal failure, otherwise would be 2700 mL/d
- Calories: 80 kg × estimated 35 kcal/kg/d = 2800 kcal/d
- Protein: 80 kg × 1.25 g/kg/d = 100 g/d
- Lipid: 2800 kcal/d × 25% = 700 kcal
- Protein calories: 100 g/d protein × 4 kcal/g = 400 kcal from proteins
- Remaining 1700 kcal/d from dextrose

### Composition

Using concentrated solutions of 70% dextrose (3.4 kcal/g), 15% amino acid, 30% intralipid (3 kcal/mL)
- Lipid: 700 kcal/d ÷ 3 kcal/mL = 233 mL/d
- Dextrose: 1700 kcal/d ÷ 3.4 kcal/g ÷ 70% = 714 mL/d
- Protein: 100 g/d ÷ 0.15 = 667 mL/d
- Supplements: Approximately 100 mL
- Should include at least 10 units insulin; minimize sodium, potassium, phosphate
- Total volume: 1714 mL/d (no additional fluid to prevent volume overload in renal patient)

---

because longer infusion times have been associated with increased infectious complications. The lipid emulsion solution should also be hung higher than other fluids because it has a low specific gravity and can run up other lines.

Additives such as $H_2$-antagonists and insulin can also be placed into PN solutions. The initial dose should be 10 units of regular insulin per liter of PN solution and can be adjusted as necessary (Box 2).

Newer developments have led to consideration for the role of other amino acids, particularly glutamine and arginine. Although these molecules are traditionally considered nonessential amino acids, they are often now considered conditionally essential in times of stress. Although their role in improving outcome is still largely undetermined, they deserve brief consideration. Glutamine is not routinely included in standard amino acid preparations because of its instability in aqueous solutions. However, glutamine is an important precursor in nucleotide synthesis and is an important energy source for intestinal epithelial cells. Although some clinical trials using glutamine supplementation have demonstrated improved healing and lower complication rates, other studies have failed to produce similar results. Arginine is a nitrogen-dense amino acid with important roles in growth as well as in nitrogen and ammonia metabolism. However, studies of supplementation in humans remain inconclusive.

## Initiating Parenteral Nutrition

Before PN is started, the patient should be evaluated for candidacy for nutritional support. Careful attention should be made to assess for adequate circulation and tissue oxygenation, especially in acutely ill patients. Starting nutritional support before optimizing cardiorespiratory function and correcting metabolic disturbances, acid-base disorders, and electrolyte abnormalities can prove detrimental. Baseline laboratory studies should be obtained before initiating PN. These should include a complete blood count, metabolic panel including electrolytes and liver function studies, nutritional laboratories such as albumin and prealbumin, and triglyceride level. The patient should be weighed and there must be accurate intake and output records. Once PN is initiated, the rate of PN infusion should be slowly advanced to the goal rate over 2 to 3 days.

For centrally delivered PN, hypertonic solutions (>1900 mOsm/kg) are infused through a central catheter placed directly into the superior vena cava, where the solution is rapidly diluted. Infusion of such hypertonic solutions through the peripheral veins leads to pain, thrombophlebitis, and venous thrombosis. A variety of central catheters may be used. A peripheral inserted central catheter (PICC) line inserted in an antecubital vein may be placed at the bedside. Although many consider this type of access to be temporary, it can be used for several months if properly maintained. For long-term PN administration, a tunneled catheter with a subcutaneous cuff or a catheter with a subcutaneous port is preferred. However, these require placement with angiographic guidance by interventional radiology or in the operating room by surgery.

## Peripheral Parenteral Nutrition

For peripheral PN, infusions can begin through a peripheral large-bore IV. However, the tonicity of the nutritional formula is limited. Peripheral PN is usually limited to an osmolarity of approximately 600 to 900 mOsm/kg. This formula can be prepared using commercially available solutions of 10% glucose and 5% amino acid. However, these mixtures have a low calorie density (approximately 0.3 to 0.6 kcal/mL) and do not provide sufficient calories unless large volumes are used. With this in mind, peripheral PN is ideal for situations where supplementation is needed for inadequate enteral nutrition. A new peripheral site should be used every 48 to 72 hours to minimize venous complications.

## Monitoring

Once PN has been initiated, the physician and other health care providers need to provide ongoing evaluation to prevent complications associated with PN (Table 3). This often entails frequent laboratory monitoring during the initial period. Diligent care has to be undertaken to reduce catheter-associated complications.

Because hyperglycemia and glucosuria are the most frequent complications associated with PN, optimal blood glucose levels should be maintained. Hyperglycemia can occur if hypertonic solutions are infused too rapidly. In addition, patients with glucose intolerance (latent diabetics or critically ill and stressed patients with peripheral insulin resistance) also develop hyperglycemia. Large randomized, controlled

## TABLE 3 Monitoring While on Parenteral Nutrition

| Laboratory Study | Initial Period | Maintenance* |
|---|---|---|
| Weight | Daily | Daily |
| CBC with platelet count | Daily | Weekly |
| Electrolytes (Na, K, Cl, CO₂, BUN, Cr, Ca, Mg, P) | Daily | Weekly |
| Triglycerides | Daily | Weekly |
| Nutritional (albumin, prealbumin) | On initiation | Weekly |
| Liver function (AST, ALT, T/D bilirubin, ALP) | On initiation | Weekly |
| Urinanalysis | Daily | Weekly |
| Ammonia, ABG | As needed | As needed |

*Maintenance period is defined as stable composition of parenteral nutrition solution.
Abbreviations: ABG = arterial blood gases; ALP = alkaline phosphatase; ALT = alanine aminotransferase; AST = aspartate aminotransferase; BUN = blood urea nitrogen; CBC = complete blood count; Cr, creatinine; T/D = total and direct.

trials have demonstrated that maintaining strict glucose control (80-110 mg/dL) significantly reduced mortality in ICU patients. Urinalysis should also be performed to detect for glucosuria. Blood glucose has to be checked frequently and insulin administered as necessary. In many cases, continuous insulin infusion (insulin drip) is necessary; glucose administration should not exceed 5 mg/kg/min. As the insulin requirement is determined, the amount of insulin added to the PN solutions for the next day is increased. If PN is suddenly stopped (e.g., dislodgement of central venous catheter or PN solution becomes unavailable), 10% dextrose should be infused at the equivalent rate to prevent hypoglycemia.

Because ill patients often develop severe electrolyte abnormalities, serum values should also be monitored daily. Low levels of electrolytes can be replenished through separate infusions and adjustments made to the PN solutions. Although most commercially prepared fat emulsion formulas are generally well tolerated, triglyceride levels should be monitored and infusion held if serum levels become too elevated (>500 mg/dL) to prevent acute pancreatitis. Adequate nitrogen balance can also be monitored through serum biomarkers.

Once tight glucose control has been achieved and electrolytes are within an acceptable range, the duration between laboratory studies can be lengthened. Nutritional laboratories studies (such as albumin and prealbumin levels) and weight should be obtained at least weekly to assess the adequacy of PN. Liver functions studies should also be obtained to monitor for hepatic complications.

Another common and serious complication associated with PN is catheter-related infections. Infection control can be provided by diligent surveillance and following strict PN administration protocols. Once PN is initiated, the access line should remain dedicated to administering PN. Using the same line for infusion of medications, blood draws, or central venous pressure monitoring increases the risk of catheter-associated complications. Meticulous care of the catheter sites should be undertaken to prevent catheter-related infections. The catheter entrance should be inspected as needed and on a regular basis (every 2-3 days). The entrance site should be cleaned, topical antibiotic or antiseptic ointment should be applied, and a new sterile dressing should be placed. Infusion tubing should be discarded after every use. Catheter tips should be covered and kept dry and clean.

## Complications

The complications associated with PN can be divided into four categories: technical problems, infection, metabolic problems, and changes associated with long-term PN.

Technical complications are related to central venous access and are most often encountered during placement of the catheter.

Insertion of a central catheter is an invasive procedure, and possible complications include pneumothorax, hemothorax, vascular injury, cardiac arrhythmia, embolism, and death. Although a dislodged or damaged catheter must be replaced, an occluded catheter can often be remedied with medical intervention. Long-term need for multiple central catheters can also lead to difficulty with venous thrombosis and access.

One of the most serious complications associated with PN is catheter-related infection. Even in studies evaluating strict care of catheters, the incidence of infection was more than 5%. Multilumen catheters and femoral vein location are associated with higher rates of infection. Local superficial infections sometimes can be treated successfully with antibiotics alone. However, if a catheter becomes infected, immediate and aggressive intervention must be undertaken before sepsis develops. Early signs of infection may be subtle and can manifest as glucose intolerance or low grade fever. If a trial of parenteral antibiotics fails to resolve symptoms and no other source of infection is identified, the catheter should be removed and cultured for organisms. A new replacement catheter should be placed at a different site and only after a delay and evidence that bacteremia is absent.

Refeeding syndrome can develop in patients who are moderately to severely malnourished and have limited substrate reserves, as seen in chronic starvation or chronic alcohol abuse. With initiation of PN and delivery of a large nutrient load, the serum levels of potassium, phosphorous, calcium, and magnesium significantly decrease because of compartment shifts due to sodium and fluid retention. The resulting electrolyte abnormalities can manifest with respiratory distress and cardiac arrthymias. This is a medical emergency and is potentially fatal. This is countered by initiating PN with a lower caloric goal with an initial solution that includes ample amounts of electrolytes.

In patients with congestive heart failure, PN can lead to severe fluid overload. Fluids have to be carefully monitored with daily weights and attention to total intake and urine output.

Overfeeding a patient has also been shown to be harmful because excess calories can lead to carbon dioxide retention and respiratory insufficiency. Excess carbohydrates can also lead to excess glycogen deposition and cholestasis. Systemic immunosuppression has been demonstrated with PN administration. When using lipid emulsions, serum triglyceride levels should be checked 4 hours after the first two or three emulsion infusions to ensure that there is adequate clearance of lipids from the circulation.

Long-term administration of PN is also associated with various complications. The incidence of gallstones is high and especially prevalent in patients with short bowel. The alteration in hepatoenteric circulation of bile salts likely contributes to this process. Chronic cholestasis can lead to fibrosis and hepatic insufficiency. In addition, some studies have demonstrated that long-term PN has led to bone loss. The mechanism of this phenomenon is not clear. With lack of stimulation, intestinal atrophy has also been demonstrated in patients undergoing long-term TPN. The clinical significance of an altered mucosal barrier is unclear, although animal studies demonstrated higher rates of bacterial translocation.

## Guidelines For Diseases

### FLUID RESTRICTION

In situations when fluid restriction is required (congestive heart failure), carbohydrates in higher concentrations (30%-35%) in combination with lipid emulsions can be used to deliver adequate calories with lower fluid volumes. Hyperglycemia may be more common in these situations, and hyperlipidemia can also occur.

### BOWEL REST

Several disease processes are often treated with bowel rest. In cases of severe acute pancreatitis and inflammatory bowel disease, a period of bowel rest can reduce abdominal symptoms of pain, bloating, and diarrhea. For enterocutaneous fistulas, fasting reduces output by 30% to 50%. The spontaneous closure rate of intestinal fistulas is more than 50%, but it depends on the patient's overall condition, amount of output (considered high if >500 mL/day), and nutritional status.

There is no consensus that outcomes in these conditions are improved with bowel rest and TPN. In fact, in comparison with enteral feeding, PN results in more complications, such as hyperglycemia, infection, and sepsis. For these reasons, PN should not be routinely started. However, despite the lack of supportive trials, it does seem prudent to initiate PN if a patient cannot tolerate oral or enteral nutrition after 7 to 10 days, to prevent malnutrition. PN lipid administration is safe in patients with acute pancreatitis. For patients with proximal jenunal fistulas, enteral feeding can lead to further complications from malabsorption, and PN is suggested.

## COMPROMISED BOWEL FUNCTION

In patients who have undergone major intestinal resection, short gut syndrome can develop if the remaining functional length of the small bowel is less than 100 cm (<50 cm if the ileocecal valve and colon are present). Enteral nutrition often fails, and patients can develop profuse diarrhea with resultant electrolyte abnormalities. Likewise, patients with normal bowel length can develop functional abnormalities from conditions such as malabsorption from radiation enteritis, sprue, hypoproteinemia, or chronic severe bowel obstruction.

PN should be started, and in certain cases, TPN dependence is permanent and lifelong. Provision of home TPN has been shown to be cost-effective, and patients have an improved quality of life. Early enteral feeding should be attempted due to the trophic nature of feeds to the gut mucosa. After PN is initiated, a portion of patients (about 30%) can be treated with an oral diet and nutritional supplements, and home PN can be stopped.

## SURGERY

Overall, PN during the perioperative period has not been shown to improve surgical outcome or to prevent complications. Therefore, PN should not be administered routinely. Its use remains controversial in certain situations. Select studies have demonstrated reduced major postoperative complications in major hepatic resection and surgery for esophageal and stomach cancers. In addition, in subgroup analysis, preoperative PN reduced postoperative complications in patients with diagnosed malnutrition. Unless a patient has a clear diagnosis of malnutrition or an extended period of bowel dysfunction is anticipated (e.g., prolonged postoperative ileus), oral feeding and enteral supplementation remain the recommendations for the postoperative period.

## RENAL FAILURE

The ability to excrete nitrogen is severely compromised in renal failure. With this in mind, clinical trials have administered PN in which the source of nitrogen is limited to essential amino acids in order to reduce urea production. However, the results have demonstrated no improvement in survival. The only indication to start PN in renal failure patients is the diagnosis of malnutrition when enteral supplementation is contraindicated. The fluid intake should be minimized and the protein requirement should be adjusted based on dialysis dependence. The PN solutions should have a high calorie density (2 kcal/mL), and total sodium intake should be limited to 40 to 70 mmol/day. Concentrated (70% dextrose, 15% amino acid, 30% lipid) macronutrient substrates can be used to compose the appropriate PN solutions. In the event that the patient is undergoing hemodialysis, standard formulations and fluid volumes can be used. As long as the patient is dialyzed, the protein dose can be normal.

## HEPATIC FAILURE

Hepatic metabolism of amino acids is significantly restricted in advanced liver disease. Historically, the protein supplementation in hepatic failure patients was significantly restricted to limit ammonia production. However, severe restriction can lead to malnutrition and worsening liver function. Later studies have shown that patients with severe alcoholic hepatitis can tolerate 75 g/day of supplemental protein.

## CURRENT DIAGNOSIS

- Discuss symptoms and medical and surgical history (abdominal surgeries and venous access).
- Obtain a medication list.
- Obtain a nutritional history (weight pattern, dietary intake, output, fluid status).
- Perform a thorough physical examination, including height and weight.
- Obtain laboratory studies.
- Determine the level of stress and comorbidities (renal and liver disease).
- Determine existing venous access and patency of central veins.

The development of encephalopathy has been demonstrated to be associated with decreased levels of branched chain amino acids (BCAA) and increased aromatic amino acids. Studies using BCAA compared with standard solutions have shown improvements in hepatic encephalopathy, shorter hospital stay, and lower mortality. However, the high expense of BCAA solutions precludes their widespread use.

If a patient with hepatic failure is unable to tolerate enteral nutrition, then PN can be initiated with a standard solution with attention to minimize fluid intake (<1500 mL/day) and sodium intake (20 mmol/day). The protein requirement is decreased and a BCAA solution should be considered in cases of severe and refractory hepatic encephalopathy.

# Special Consideration: Home Parenteral Nutrition

For ease of administration, PN can be administrated by cyclic infusion over 12 to 14 hours. Once a stable PN solution has been established, the total infusion time can be tapered down to 12 hours. This is done by administering the same total volume of PN progressively over a shorter time (e.g., 20 hours for 2 days, then 16 hours for 2 days, then 12 hours thereafter). To avoid periods of hypoglycemia and hyperglycemia, cyclic infusion requires a slow tapering up to goal rate at the

## CURRENT THERAPY

- Evaluate for indications for parenteral nutrition (malnutrition, long illness, multiorgan disease, failed oral or enteral nutrition).
- Obtain secure central venous catheter access.
- Determine the patient's weight and assess comorbidities.
- Estimate the total caloric needs (approximately 35 kca/kg/day).
- Estimate the fluid requirement (1500 mL for the first 20 kg, then 20 mL/kg thereafter).
- Calculate the parenteral nutrition formulation:
- Determine the protein requirement (0.6 to 2 g/kg/day based on the patient's condition)
  - Determine the lipid requirement (approximately 25% of total caloric needs)
  - Supplementation based on electrolyte profile, acid-base status, renal status
  - Additional sterile water if there is no other fluid intake source
  - Monitor for hyperglycemia, laboratory studies, volume status, catheter care.

beginning of PN administration and slow tapering down at the end. Although patient education and participation are important in the success of home PN, qualified nursing visits should be arranged to ensure proper administration and troubleshooting to allow long-term success. There should be a low threshold for intervention if there is a suspicion of catheter-related complications.

## Summary

Parenteral nutrition is a valuable adjunct in the care of patients. Despite the intuitive sentiment that any nutrition is better than no nutrition, starting PN has associated risks and can negatively affect patient morbidity and mortality. However, in carefully selected patients and with diligent monitoring and an awareness of complications, PN can be administered safely, for a prolonged period, and to the overall benefit of patients.

### REFERENCES

ASPEN Board of Directors and the Clinical Guidelines Task Force: Guidelines for the use of parenteral and enteral nutrition in adult and pediatric patients. JPEN J Parenter Enteral Nutr 2002;26(1 suppl):1SA-138SA. PDF available at http://www.nutritioncare.org/publications/2002guidelines.pdf (accessed June 15, 2007).

Forbes A: Parenteral nutrition. Curr Opin Gastroenterol 2006;22(2):160-164.

Howard L: Home parenteral nutrition: Survival, cost and quality of life. Gastroenterology 2006;130(2 suppl 1):S52-S59.

Koretz RL, Lipman To, Klein S; American Gastroenterological Association: AGA technical review on parenteral nutrition. Gastroenterology 2001; 121(4):970-1001.

Veterans Affairs Total Parenteral Nutrition Cooperative Study Group: Perioperative total parenteral nutrition in surgical patients. N Engl J Med 1991; 325(8);525-532.

# Parenteral Fluid Therapy for Infants and Children

Method of

*Jeremy N. Friedman, MB, ChB, and Carolyn E. Beck, MD, MSc*

One could dedicate an entire textbook to the subject of parenteral fluid therapy for infants and children. For the purposes of this article we have chosen to focus on three main issues that confront us, as clinicians, on a daily basis. The first question is what types of intravenous fluids are most appropriate to provide maintenance requirements in children? The second question is how best to assess dehydration. This is extremely common in pediatrics and absolutely critical if appropriate fluid therapy is to be instituted. Finally, when and how should intravenous fluid be used in the management of the dehydrated patient? Unfortunately, many of these issues remain controversial and have not been satisfactorily resolved. As general pediatricians we provide you with some practical, simple, and general principles to guide your approach to parenteral fluid therapy.

## Maintenance Fluids

### FLUID REQUIREMENTS

Hospitalized children often require intravenous fluids, necessitating that physicians have an approach to their requirements—both fluid composition and volume—at their fingertips. While seemingly second

**TABLE 1 Maintenance Fluid Requirements***

| Weight (kg) | 100/50/20 Rule (Daily Requirements) | 4/2/1 Rule (Hourly Requirements) |
|---|---|---|
| 0-10 | 100 mL/kg/d | 4 mL/kg/h |
| 11-20 | 1000 mL + 50 mL/kg/d for every kg 11-20 | 40 mL + 2 mL/kg/h for every kg 11-20 |
| >20 | 1500 mL + 20 mL/kg/d for every kg >20 | 60 mL + 1 mL/kg/h for every kg >20 |

*Assuming normal renal function and usual insensible losses.

nature to many clinicians, the prescription of IV fluids is in fact complex and requires a solid foundation for safe and effective practice.

Maintenance fluid requirements are deep-rooted in pediatric history, dating back to calculations proposed by Holliday and Segar in 1957. These requirements are based on their study of caloric expenditure in healthy children, resulting in the "100/50/20" rule (closely approximated by the "4/2/1" rule) commonly cited today (Table 1). Applying these rules, a 12-kg toddler requires 1100 mL per day by the 100/50/20 rule, or 44 mL per hour by the 4/2/1 rule, values which are almost equivalent.

Maintenance fluids are designed only to replace, or input, naturally occurring output when oral fluids are contraindicated or not tolerated. Output includes urinary losses, in addition to insensible water loss from the skin and lungs. If renal function is abnormal, maintenance fluids by definition do not apply; in this case, fluid requirement is better estimated by calculating insensible water loss (Table 2) and adding it to urine output and any other significant losses (e.g., diarrhea, nasogastric suction). Similarly, factors such as raised body temperature increase insensible water losses and need to be considered when determining appropriate fluid volume.

### ELECTROLYTE REQUIREMENTS

#### Sodium

In the same 1957 paper, Holliday and Segar proposed maintenance sodium requirements for children to be 30 mmol/L. This requirement translates to the use of a hypotonic saline solution for maintenance fluids, equivalent to 0.2% NaCl in 5% dextrose in water ($D_5W$). Although this solution, or similar hypotonic composites, continues to be widely used in pediatric practice, there is good reason to question its appropriateness.

Holliday's water requirements were based on caloric expenditure in healthy children, and electrolyte composition was derived from that of human and cow's milk. The recommended sodium concentration is less than the average dietary salt intake, and the guideline fails to account for impaired water excretion, an important factor in hospitalized children. Several case reports have raised concern about the routine use of hypotonic solutions in hospitalized children, because reports of potentially fatal hyponatremia have come to light. Factors implicated in the development of hyponatremia include the action of

**TABLE 2 Insensible Fluid Losses by Body Surface Area**

| Insensible Losses | Body Surface Area (m²) |
|---|---|
| 400 mL/m² BSA/d (spontaneously breathing) 300 mL/m² BSA/d (ventilated) 500-600 mL/m² BSA/d (neonates) | $\sqrt{\dfrac{Height\,(cm) \times Weight\,(kg)}{3600}}$ |

Abbreviation: BSA = body surface area.

## TABLE 3  Source of Electrolyte-Free Water

| IV Solution | Tonicity | Na (mmol/L) | EFW (%) |
|---|---|---|---|
| D$_5$W/0.9% NaCl | Isotonic | 154 | 0 |
| D$_5$W/0.45% NaCl | Hypotonic | 77 | 50 |
| D$_5$W/0.2% NaCl | Hypotonic | 34 | 78 |

*Abbreviation: EFW = electrolyte-free water.*

antidiuretic hormone (ADH) preventing water excretion as well as the input of electrolyte-free water (EFW).

There are several reasons for ADH secretion to be elevated in hospitalized children. Apart from osmotic forces, stimuli for ADH release include malignancies, central nervous system disorders (including meningitis), pulmonary disorders (including pneumonia), and several medications, including commonly used drugs such as morphine sulfate (morphine). Additionally, nonspecific symptoms such as pain, nausea, and stress, as well as a postoperative state and hypovolemia, all result in an increase in ADH. Given the illness of hospitalized children in the 21st century, it is rare to care for a patient who does not have at least one of these risk factors for elevated ADH, making water retention an essential consideration in the prescription of IV fluids.

With respect to EFW, the routine use of hypotonic maintenance fluids provides the major source for hospitalized patients. There is 154 mmol/L of sodium in 0.9% NaCl (normal saline), which is isotonic with respect to the cell membrane. Ringer's lactate provides a similar sodium concentration. Solutions with less sodium content are hypotonic (Table 3). Holliday's historic prescription of 0.2% NaCl contributes a large degree of EFW (78%). This contribution of free water via IV fluids, compounded by an impaired ability to excrete water, place the hospitalized child at risk for developing acute hyponatremia. Consequently, IV solutions that are less hypotonic, or even isotonic, are starting to be used in pediatric hospital wards.

Potential risks of using isotonic fluids as maintenance solutions include fluid overload in children with an impaired ability to excrete sodium and hypernatremia in patients with renal concentrating defects, significant water loss, or prolonged fluid restriction. In the absence of these factors, the risks of isotonic fluids are largely theoretical.

### Potassium

Maintenance potassium requirements have similarly been derived at 20 mmol/L. In most clinical situations, maintenance potassium should be added to the IV solution. Exceptions include uncertainty regarding the patient's renal function, poor urine output, or any other risk factors for hyperkalemia. In these scenarios, the addition of potassium is not advised, and renal function and electrolytes should be closely monitored. Ongoing losses of potassium (e.g., diarrheal losses) or other reasons for hypokalemia (e.g., prolonged use of albuterol (salbutamol [Ventolin]) can require higher concentrations of potassium, along with appropriate electrolyte monitoring.

### GLUCOSE

Dextrose should routinely be added to maintenance fluids as a carbohydrate source when children are in a fasting state in order to provide some calories (albeit minimal) and prevent ketosis. Generally, a child with normal glucose metabolism requires a 5% dextrose solution (D$_5$W), which can be safely combined with either hypotonic or isotonic solutions. Unlike sodium, glucose can freely cross the cell membrane and thus does not contribute to the osmotic force.

### METHOD FOR PRESCRIBING MAINTENANCE FLUIDS: A PRACTICAL APPROACH

No prospective studies have evaluated the risks or benefits of hypotonic versus isotonic IV fluids. Clearly, the routine use of 0.2% saline requires reconsideration, and it is likely inappropriate for use in

pediatric wards. A case-control study by Hoorn and colleagues, the most rigorous on the topic to date, recommends that isotonic fluids be used perioperatively as well as in children with a plasma sodium less than 138 mmol/L.

Practically, a decision regarding IV fluid composition must be made on a case-by-case basis. The choice may be viewed as a prescription, taking details about the patient, the clinical scenario, and the baseline laboratory values into account, and monitoring and reevaluating the child's fluids and electrolytes on a regular basis. Rather than following strict rules, judgment is required for each patient. The following scenarios provide some guidance about IV fluid composition.

A normal sodium value (≥136 mmol/L) in a patient who is relatively well should lead one to consider half-normal saline (0.45% NaCl) in D$_5$W a good choice. This solution provides more sodium (and contributes less EFW) than 0.2% saline while still providing the patient with some free water. A second patient with the same sodium value, however, might require a different fluid prescription. For example, a child with a low-normal sodium of 137 mmol/L in the clinical context of severe pain, meningitis, or pneumonia—all risk factors for elevated ADH—is likely a good candidate for an isotonic solution such as 0.9% NaCl in D$_5$W. If this same patient presented with a sodium of 132 mmol/L, 0.9% NaCl in D$_5$W should almost certainly be instituted. In any of these solutions, 20 mmol/L of potassium could be added provided that the patient's urine output is appropriate and no other risk factors for hyperkalemia are present.

With respect to the surgical patient, the recent literature would suggest that isotonic fluids (0.9% NaCl in D$_5$W, Ringer's lactate) be routinely used in the perioperative period. Postoperatively, approximately 1% of patients develop a serum sodium less than 130 mmol/L. The development of hyponatremia in this clinical context is not surprising, given the multiple factors placing these patients at risk for increased ADH secretion, namely, pain, nausea, stress, narcotic medications, and volume depletion.

### A NOTE ABOUT VOLUME

Provided that a patient has normal renal function and usual insensible losses, maintenance fluid guidelines may be followed, estimated by the rules noted in Table 1. It is crucial to note, however, that in studies examining the question of IV fluids in children, excess fluid volume—greater than maintenance requirements—was an important factor associated with development of acute hyponatremia. Often clinicians prescribe maintenance IV fluids when the child is unwell and not taking anything by mouth. In most cases, when the patient's clinical condition improves, oral intake is initiated. Be mindful that oral fluid is hypotonic and can add significantly to the patient's free water load. To prevent the development of hyponatremia and its significant clinical consequences in these children, IV fluid prescriptions should be reevaluated on a regular basis, taking oral intake into account and adjusting the IV volume to maintain an appropriate total fluid intake.

## Rehydration

### ASSESSMENT OF DEHYDRATION

#### Gastroenteritis and Dehydration

Acute gastroenteritis accounts for more than 1.5 million outpatient visits, 10% of all pediatric hospitalizations (200 000), and approximately 300 deaths per year in the United States. This pales in comparison with the estimated 30% of worldwide deaths among infants and toddlers, amounting to 8000 children younger than 5 years dying per day, from diarrhea and dehydration in the developing world. Young children with diarrhea are more prone to dehydration than older children and adults because of their higher body surface–to–volume ratio, a higher metabolic rate, and smaller fluid reserves. In addition, they are often dependent on others to provide fluid. Viruses, primarily rotavirus, are responsible for 70% to 80% of infectious diarrhea in the developed world. There are also many other causes of dehydration not

**TABLE 4 Signs Associated with Dehydration**

| Symptom | Minimal or No Dehydration (<3% Loss of Body Weight) | Mild to Moderate Dehydration (3%-9% Loss of Body Weight) | Severe Dehydration (≥10% Loss of Body Weight) |
|---|---|---|---|
| General appearance | Normal | Thirsty, restless or lethargic, but irritable when touched | Drowsy, limp, cold, sweaty ± comatose |
| Urine output | Normal | Decreased | Minimal |
| Breathing | Normal | Normal to increased | Deep and increased |
| Heart rate | Normal | Increased | Increased |
| Systolic blood pressure | Normal | Normal or low | Low |
| Mucous membranes | Moist | Sticky | Dry |
| Eyes | Normal | Slightly sunken | Very sunken |
| Tears | Normal | Decreased | Absent |
| Skin turgor | Instant recoil | <2 sec | >2 sec |
| Capillary refill | Normal | Normal to prolonged | Prolonged >2 sec |

involving diarrhea, including poor oral intake (e.g., stomatitis), increased insensible losses (e.g., fever, tachypnea), and renal losses (e.g., diabetes mellitus, diabetes insipidus).

## Classification of Dehydration

The American Academy of Pediatrics (AAP) classifies dehydration as mild (3%-5% fluid deficit), moderate (6%-9%), and severe (≥10%). The first signs of dehydration are believed to appear when the fluid deficit is 3% to 4%. Dehydration can be further classified based on the serum sodium concentration. Isotonic dehydration (Na 130-150 mmol/L) accounts for the vast majority, and hypotonic (Na <130 mmol/L) and hypertonic (Na >150 mmol/L) dehydration account for less than 5% of the total cases. Inaccurate assessment of dehydration can result in permanent injury and death if fluid deficits are underestimated, and overestimation likely leads to unnecessary interventions and inappropriate use of resources.

## Accuracy of Historic Factors and Physical Examination

Traditional teaching regarding the assessment of dehydration is empiric and based on clinical experience (Table 4). The gold standard for measuring dehydration is considered to be acute body weight change over the course of the illness. Unfortunately, this information is seldom available due to a lack of an accurate pre-illness weight.

Steiner and colleagues recently performed a systematic review of the literature on the precision and accuracy of history, physical examination, and laboratory tests in identifying dehydration in children younger than 5 years. They found that historic factors have only moderate sensitivity as a screening test for dehydration. Duration, frequency, and quantity of vomiting, diarrhea, and urination only give a rough estimate of the risk of dehydration. Signs of dehydration (see Table 4) on physical examination are generally imprecise and tend to show only fair to moderate agreement among examiners. Capillary refill time had the best measurement properties, with a sensitivity of 0.60 (95% CI, 0.29-0.91) and specificity of 0.85 (95% CI, 0.72-0.98) for detecting 5% dehydration. The absence of sunken eyes and dry mucous membranes was also found to be potentially clinically useful in decreasing the likelihood of 5% dehydration.

A prospective cohort study by Gorelick and colleagues in an urban U.S. pediatric emergency department evaluated 10 clinical signs of dehydration and found that any two or more of four factors:

- Capillary refill >2 sec
- Dry mucous membranes
- Absent tears
- Abnormal general appearance

indicate a fluid deficit of at least 5%. This subset of four factors predicted dehydration as well as the entire set.

In addition, a clinical dehydration scale has been developed by Friedman and coworkers using formal measurement methodology. A score of 0 reflects no dehydration, and a maximum score of 8 reflects severe dehydration as per Table 5.

## Eliciting Signs of Dehydration

As is true in the physical examination of any young child, *opportunism* is the operative word! Start with the least-invasive part, which involves observing the child's overall appearance and interaction with the caregiver. This also allows you to record the respiratory rate over a 30-second period, looking for hyperpnea suggesting a metabolic acidosis. To assess capillary refill time, sufficient pressure should gradually be applied to blanch the palmar surface of the distal fingertip, and then immediately released. Less than 1.5 to 2 seconds for restoration of normal color is considered normal. The examining room should be at a warm ambient temperature. Autonomic nervous system abnormalities or extremes in patient temperature can affect measurement. Dryness of the mucous membranes is best assessed by examination of the tongue because the lips are often dry in mouth breathers and in children with conditions other than dehydration. If the child does not cry during your examination, the presence of tears may need to be inquired about on history. Skin turgor is usually assessed by pinching a small skin fold on the lateral abdominal wall at the level of the umbilicus. This is then released, and return to its normal position is classified as immediate, slightly delayed, or prolonged. False negatives can be seen in hypernatremia and obese children, and malnutrition can cause false positive results. Although decreased blood pressure and severe tachycardia

**TABLE 5 A Dehydration Score**

| Characteristic | 0 | 1 | 2 |
|---|---|---|---|
| General appearance | Normal | Thirsty, restless, lethargic, but irritable when touched | Drowsy, limp, cold, sweaty, ± comatose |
| Eyes | Normal | Slightly sunken | Very sunken |
| Mucous membranes (tongue) | Moist | Sticky | Dry |
| Tears | Present | Decreased | Absent |

should be examined for, they are late signs and only tend to become evident in severe dehydration.

Remember that the degree of dehydration may be underestimated in hypertonic dehydration as a result of the movement of water from the intracellular to the extracellular space, which helps to preserve the intravascular volume. In hypotonic dehydration the opposite occurs, and an overestimation of dehydration can result.

### Usefulness of Blood Tests

There is a tendency to want to use blood test results to help in the assessment of dehydration because they are perceived to be more reliable than the features on history and physical examination. Unfortunately their usefulness has not been supported by data in the literature. In his systematic review, Steiner reviewed six studies that looked at blood urea nitrogen (BUN), BUN–to–serum creatinine ratio, and acidosis in children. The only laboratory measurement that seemed to be helpful was serum bicarbonate. A normal serum bicarbonate concentration of more than 17 mEq/L reduced the likelihood of 5% dehydration.

Why are the laboratory findings so unhelpful? A number of reasons have been suggested. In cases of isolated vomiting or nasogastric drainage, either a metabolic alkalosis can result from gastric acid losses or a metabolic acidosis can result from volume contraction and lactic acidosis. Volume depletion without renal insufficiency should cause a disproportionate rise in the BUN with little or no change in creatinine. This is caused by increased passive reabsorption of urea in the proximal tubule as a result of appropriate renal conservation of sodium and water. But BUN results may be misleading because children with gastroenteritis can have decreased protein intake during their illness, which can cause hypouremia. Not knowing the child's baseline BUN means that it could double but still remain in the normal range. Finally, if dehydration is rapid, BUN, which is a waste product that builds up gradually with decreased renal excretion, might not have the chance to increase significantly.

### What Are the Lessons for the Clinician?

Acute change in weight is the best indicator of dehydration. If a child was seen the day before with a weight of 10 kg and returns the next day with a weight of 9 kg, then by definition the child is 10% dehydrated. Unfortunately, this information is not often available, and based on current data, the empiric classification systems suggested in the past are not particularly accurate or reliable. There are more than 30 different potential tests for assessing dehydration but no conclusive way to approach this.

A general classification of a child's dehydration status as none (<3% fluid deficit), some (mild to moderate—3%-9% fluid deficit), or severe (≥10%) is a useful starting point. Having some awareness of the diagnostic usefulness of individual tests allows you to focus on those that have been shown to correlate best with the presence (or absence) of dehydration. Signs of dehydration start to become evident at 3% to 4% fluid deficit. As a single sign, delayed capillary refill seems to have the highest predictive value but can be influenced by a number of factors, including the examination technique and ambient temperature. Groups of signs can simplify and even improve diagnostic precision. For example, any two out of abnormal capillary refill, abnormal general appearance, dry mucous membranes, and reduced tears increase the likelihood of moderate dehydration sixfold.

Commonly obtained laboratory tests are generally not particularly helpful and therefore not usually indicated unless severe dehydration is suspected or other diagnoses requiring testing are being entertained. Of the laboratory tests, a serum bicarbonate greater than 17 mEq/L is the most useful because it means that the child is approximately one fifth as likely to have moderate dehydration. Intuitively, it makes sense that blood tests (e.g., bicarbonate, electrolytes, BUN, creatinine, glucose) should be drawn at the time of IV placement in children with dehydration sufficiently severe to require IV rehydration or in those whose assessment or diagnosis remains unclear after a complete history and physical examination, when they can be used as an adjunctive tool. Current AAP guidelines do not recommend blood tests as part of the assessment of children with diarrhea and mild dehydration.

## FLUID MANAGEMENT OF THE DEHYDRATED CHILD

A number of decisions need to be made by the clinician once the degree of dehydration has been assessed. The first decision is whether to try oral rehydration therapy (ORT) or move immediately to placement of an IV line for parenteral therapy. The next decision is exactly how much fluid and how fast to give it. Finally, if using parenteral therapy, which is the most appropriate solution?

### Does the Child Require Intravenous Therapy?

Quantifying the extent of a child's dehydration accurately is critical in deciding whether the child is safe to be managed at home, requires observation during ORT, or needs to receive immediate IV fluid therapy. Mild or moderate dehydration caused by gastroenteritis can be treated with ORT if the child is able to orally replace fluid losses. Parenteral fluid therapy (or on occasion, ORT by nasogastric tube) is recommended for children with severe dehydration or those who cannot replace the estimated fluid deficit or ongoing losses orally, for example, because of ongoing vomiting. Although ORT is the recommended treatment for acute gastroenteritis with dehydration, it is used in less than 30% of cases in the United States for which it is indicated. Three quarters of pediatric emergency medicine providers, who classified themselves as very familiar with the AAP recommendations for ORT, reported nearly exclusive use of IV fluids for moderately dehydrated children. Some feel that ORT is too time consuming in a busy outpatient setting, and others feel that rapid IV rehydration therapy might break the vomiting cycle more quickly, allowing more rapid discharge home.

### Management with Oral Rehydration Therapy

Absorption of water in the small bowel is mediated by the cotransport of sodium and glucose. Different varieties of ORT are available, based on slight variations in the composition of sodium, chloride, carbohydrate, and osmolality. They have been shown in numerous randomized, controlled trials to be as effective as IV rehydration and to have fewer complications in the management of children with diarrhea and dehydration. Fruit and bubblegum flavors have been added to combat the salty taste, and frozen flavored ice pops are also available. Vomiting is not a contraindication to the use of ORT, and children who are truly dehydrated seldom refuse to drink it.

Children who have no or minimal signs of dehydration can continue with their regular age-appropriate diet, with ORT to compensate for ongoing diarrhea or vomiting losses. Using ORT in mildly to moderately dehydrated children requires 50- to 100 mL/kg given quickly over 3 to 4 hours until the child appears clinically rehydrated. Fluid can be given by spoon, syringe, or cup beginning with 5 mL every few minutes and gradually increasing as tolerated. Gut rest is not indicated, with the goal to quickly return the child to an age-appropriate unrestricted diet after rehydration has been accomplished. Breast-feeding should not be interrupted, and full-strength formula is usually tolerated. Fluid losses from vomiting and diarrhea need to be recorded and replaced on an ongoing basis. An empiric amount of 5 to 10 mL/kg for each watery stool or 2 mL/kg for each emesis has been suggested.

The nasogastric route is an option that should be considered if a slow, steady rate would be helpful (e.g., if the child is vomiting) or if there is refusal to drink (e.g., stomatitis). Children who are not improving with ORT and those who have extremely high losses need to be reassessed carefully on an ongoing basis and remain under careful observation. These children and those who do not tolerate ORT, have a poor suck, have depressed mental status, or are severely dehydrated group require IV rehydration.

Studies of mortality caused by acute diarrhea in the United States have identified prematurity, young maternal age, black race, and rural residence as risk factors for suboptimal outcome. This should be factored in when deciding on length and degree of observation before discharge.

### Intravenous Therapy for Dehydration: How Much and How Fast?

The total volume of fluid required has three components: rehydration requirements to replace the deficit of salt and water, maintenance requirements to maintain euvolemia, and replacement of ongoing losses.

#### Rehydration Requirements (Deficit Therapy)

Step 1 is to restore cardiovascular stability with a rapid bolus of 20 mL/kg over 10 to 30 minutes. Different from providing maintenance fluids, rehydration should always be achieved using isotonic fluids (normal saline or Ringer's lactate), to effectively restore the extracellular fluid volume. Always remember to order fluid on a per-kilogram basis, which differs from the practice in adults, where it may be safe to order by the liter. The child with mild dehydration might not need a bolus, but the severely dehydrated child might require multiple boluses until the pulse, perfusion, and mental status return to normal. Generally, if a child is continuing to show signs of dehydration after 60 mL/kg of isotonic fluid resuscitation, a critical care unit should be consulted and the institution of inotropic therapy considered. Serum electrolytes, bicarbonate, BUN, creatinine, and glucose are usually drawn at the time of the IV start, although rehydration should commence immediately because the laboratory results will not change the initial fluid management.

Step 2 is to calculate the child's fluid deficit based on weight loss or your clinical assessment of dehydration (see previous section). AAP guidelines recommend using a formula of 50 mL/kg deficit for mild dehydration (3%-5% fluid deficit) and 100 mL/kg for moderate dehydration (6%-9% fluid deficit). Subtract the amount of fluid given by bolus from the total amount of rehydration fluid required in 24 hours. In isotonic (Na 130-150 mmol/L) and hypotonic (Na < 130 mmol/L) dehydration, you can give one half of this volume divided over 8 hours, with the other one half over the next 16 hours, or simply divide the total amount required by 24 for a simplified continuous IV rate. Either way, you should aim to rehydrate over 24 hours. As an example, a 10-kg infant who is believed to be 10% dehydrated will require 1000 mL over 24 hours. The baby receives 200 mL as a bolus and then needs 400 mL over the next 8 hours and a further 400 mL over the following 16 hours to account for the rehydration requirement.

For most patients, half-normal saline in $D_5W$ with KCl 20 mEq/L is an appropriate fluid to use. Potassium is usually not included in the intravenous fluids until the child voids. In the less common scenario of hypertonic dehydration (Na >150 mmol/L), the rehydration period should be extended over 48 hours so as not to decrease the serum sodium concentration by more than 0.5-1 mmol/hour, to minimize the risk of cerebral edema. Repeated serum sodium measurements will initially be required every 4 to 6 hours until normalizing.

#### Maintenance Requirements

Step 3 is to calculate maintenance requirements as described earlier and add to the rehydration requirement to come up with an hourly rate. As an example, the 10-kg child previously described requires 40 mL/hour of maintenance fluids, which would be added to the initial rehydration requirement of 50 mL/hour (400 mL over 8 hours) for a total of 90 mL/hour in the first 8 hours. For the next 16 hours this is decreased to 40 mL/hour plus 25 mL/hour (400 mL over 16 hours) for a total of 65 mL/hour. Following return to a euvolemic state, and assuming no ongoing losses, normal maintenance fluid volume may be resumed. Remember to account for oral fluid intake as the patient improves.

#### Replacement Requirements

Step 4 is to calculate replacement requirements. If ongoing stool losses are a factor, they must be accounted for in the IV fluid prescription.

## CURRENT DIAGNOSIS

- Acute change in weight is the best indicator of dehydration, hence the importance of frequent monitoring of weight in children with potential dehydration.
- Signs of dehydration are generally imprecise but start to become evident at 3% to 4% fluid deficit.
- Delayed capillary refill (>2 seconds) seems to have the highest predictive value for dehydration. Any two or more out of delayed capillary refill, dry mucous membranes, absent tears, and abnormal general appearance increases the likelihood of moderate dehydration sixfold.
- Laboratory values are generally unhelpful in assessing dehydration and are not indicated unless IV rehydration is necessary. Of the laboratory tests, the most useful is the serum bicarbonate; a normal bicarbonate (>17 mEq/L) decreases the likelihood of moderate dehydration approximately fivefold.

Volume of stool loss is normally about 5 mL/kg/day. With diarrhea this can increase dramatically to 200 mL/kg/day or more. It is easy to see how rapidly a small infant can become dehydrated if these ongoing losses are not being consistently recorded and replaced. If possible, the stool losses should be measured by weighing the diaper and replacing with 1 mL of fluid for each 1 mL of stool. If this is not possible to record, then an estimate of 5 to 10 mL/kg per stool has been suggested as a rough guide. Depending on how rapidly the losses are occurring, this can be calculated every 4 to 6 hours. As an example, if our dehydrated child had three stools over 4 hours for a total of 200 mL, then a further 50 mL/hour (200 divided by 4) is added to the 90 mL/hour (which comprises the rehydration and maintenance components) for a total of 140 mL/hour.

### A Note on Rapid Rehydration

The preceding approach to the dehydrated child requiring IV fluids adheres to classic pediatric teaching, where circulation is restored via an isotonic fluid bolus, and electrolyte abnormalities are corrected and deficits replaced over a 24-hour period. There is an increasing interest

## CURRENT THERAPY

- Individualize IV orders for children based on the clinical scenario, baseline laboratory results, and frequent reassessments, with particular attention to the concentration of sodium in your prescribed solution. The traditional use of 5% dextrose in 0.2% NaCl is increasingly being questioned, with consideration required for the use of 5% dextrose in half-normal saline or normal saline in certain scenarios.
- Mild or moderate dehydration can be treated with oral rehydration therapy (ORT), which is currently underused in this setting in the United States.
- Appropriate IV therapy for dehydration requires separate consideration of rehydration and maintenance requirements, as well as replacement of ongoing losses.
- IV fluid therapy calculations are really just approximations, and the child's clinical response is far more important. It is therefore imperative to have regular monitoring of clinical signs, urine output, weight, overall fluid balance, and in certain cases serum electrolytes.

in an alternative approach, termed *rapid rehydration*. The principle here is to rapidly and fully restore the extracellular fluid volume, usually using 40 to 60 mL/kg of an isotonic solution over a few hours. Theoretically, hospital admission is averted because the patient is discharged home with oral feedings successfully resumed in an 8- to 24-hour period. Although potentially an important method, rapid rehydration has not yet been prospectively studied and should be used with appropriate caution. Its safety and efficacy, including patients' urine and serum electrolytes, hydration, and accompanying clinical status, have yet to be determined. Further study is needed to clarify the optimal rapid rehydration regime, as well as its safety.

## Monitoring Requirements

It is essential to remember that the fluid therapy calculations for maintenance IV therapy, rehydration, and replacement are all approximations. There is no formula that works in all cases, so therapy must be individualized. The clinical response to therapy is far more important than any calculations, and there is no substitution for frequent clinical and laboratory monitoring. Regular monitoring of any patient on IV fluids should include:

- General appearance, signs of dehydration, heart rate, respiratory rate, blood pressure
- Urine output, urine specific gravity
- Overall fluid balance
- Daily weights
- Electrolytes (if initially abnormal or at risk, e.g., significant ongoing losses)

Euvolemic patients receiving maintenance fluids should maintain their weight and urine output, achieve a balanced fluid status, and have normal electrolytes, with particular attention to the serum sodium.

A previously dehydrated child who is clinically improving demonstrates weight gain, a positive fluid balance, and increasing urine output with decreasing urine specific gravity. In this patient, consideration should be given to decreasing the intravenous fluids and moving toward ORT and normalizing the diet. Conversely, if the steps are followed as outlined and the child still looks dehydrated, continues to lose weight, remains in negative fluid balance, or has poor urine output, then consider further bolus therapy and increasing the intravenous fluid rate.

## REFERENCES

Centers for Disease Control and Prevention: Managing acute gastroenteritis among children: Oral rehydration, maintenance, and nutritional therapy. MMWR Recomm Rep 2003;52(No. RR-16):1-8.

Friedman, JN, Goldman RD, Srivastava R, Parkin PC: Development of a clinical dehydration scale for use in children between 1 and 36 months of age. J Pediatr 2004;145:201-207.

Gorelick MH, Shaw KN, Murphy KO: Validity and reliability of clinical signs in the diagnosis of dehydration in children. Pediatrics 1997;99(5):E6.

Halberthal M, Halperin ML, Bohn D: Acute hyponatraemia in children admitted to hospital: Retrospective analysis of factors contributing to its development and resolution. BMJ 2001;322:780-782.

Holliday MA, Segar WE: The maintenance need for water in parenteral fluid therapy. Pediatrics 1957;19:823-832.

Hoorn EJ, Geary D, Robb M, et al: Acute hyponatremia related to intravenous fluid administration in hospitalized children: An observational study. Pediatrics 2004;113:1279-1284.

Steiner MJ, Dewalt DA, Byerley JS: Is this child dehydrated? JAMA 2004;291:2746-2754.

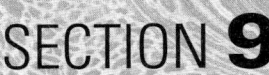

# The Endocrine System

## Acromegaly

Method of
*Mary Lee Vance, MD*

Acromegaly is an uncommon disease that affects the entire body and causes substantial morbidities and the risk of premature mortality if it is not diagnosed and treated promptly and successfully. Delay in diagnosis, an average of 8 years after onset of symptoms, remains a problem. This delay is attributed to the gradual physical changes that can result in marked facial deformity and the lack of recognition of the associated clinical features by physicians. Many patients are treated for hypertension, diabetes, carpal tunnel syndrome, osteoarthritis with joint replacement, sleep apnea, colon polyps, dental malocclusion, and renal stones long before the diagnosis of acromegaly is ascertained.

## Diagnosis

If acromegaly is a consideration, the best screening test is measurement of the serum insulin-like growth factor 1 (IGF-1) level. IGF-1 is an integrated measure of overall growth hormone (GH) secretion. Serum IGF-1 varies according to age, reflecting the decrease in GH secretion with increasing age. Although women produce more GH than men, the levels of IGF-1 are not substantially different between the sexes. Commercial laboratories usually report age-adjusted serum IGF-1 ranges. A falsely elevated IGF-1 level is observed during pregnancy, reflecting placental production of a GH-variant that stimulates IGF-1 production. A random or fasting GH level may be misleading because it is often normal (<10 µg/L) because GH is secreted in pulses, and determination of the pulsatile pattern of GH secretion (e.g., measurement of serum GH every 5 minutes for 24 hours) is not practical in the clinical setting.

The definitive test for acromegaly is the oral glucose test (75 g or 100 g glucose) with measurement of GH every 30 minutes for 2 hours. A normal response is a nadir GH level of less than 1.0 µg/L using a radioimmunoassay (RIA). With more sensitive GH assays (immunoradiometric assay [IRMA] or enzyme-linked immunosorbent assay [ELISA]), a normal GH response has been reported to be less than 0.4 µg/L, but this criterion has yet to be tested widely. Currently, a serum GH of 1.0 µg/L or greater after oral glucose is considered diagnostic of acromegaly.

In addition to assessing GH production, serum prolactin should be measured, because 20% to 40% of patients have concomitant hyperprolactinemia (a consequence of interference with dopamine inhibition of prolactin by a macroadenoma or an adenoma that produces both GH and prolactin). Additionally, assessment of the need for glucocorticoid or thyroid hormone replacement should be determined before treatment.

The best imaging study is specific pituitary magnetic resonance imaging (MRI) without and with gadolinium administration. Because of the delay in diagnosis, the majority of patients (approximately 60%) have a pituitary macroadenoma (>1.0 cm), often with invasion of surrounding structures (bone, dura, cavernous sinus) or compression of the optic chiasm or an optic nerve (requiring an ophthalmologic evaluation, including automated visual field testing). The pretreatment MRI is also useful to assess the probability of the need for adjunctive therapy after surgical removal of as much of the adenoma as possible. The patient should be informed of the possible need for adjunctive therapy after surgery if there is a large tumor.

## Treatment

### TRANSSPHENOIDAL ADENOMECTOMY

The first treatment of choice is resection of the adenoma, preferably by the transsphenoidal route, by an experienced pituitary neurosurgeon. Reported surgical remission rates range between 23% and 83%, depending on the size of the adenoma; patients with a macroadenoma have a lower probability of remission. Because a substantial number of patients have persistent excessive GH secretion, adjunctive therapy is required.

Postoperative evaluation, usually 6 to 8 weeks after surgery, should include measurement of the GH after oral glucose, with measurement of serum glucose and GH every 30 minutes for 120 minutes (normal response: GH <1.0 µg/L) and a serum IGF-1 level as a new baseline (IGF-1 is protein bound and cleared slowly, and it might not decline to normal for up to 3 months after successful surgery). Need for hormone replacements (glucocorticoid, thyroid hormone, gonadal steroid, desmopressin) should also be determined.

Measurement of an early morning serum cortisol and adrenocorticotropic hormone (ACTH) (off of glucocorticoid for 2 days) may be adequate to determine the need for cortisol replacement if cortisol and ACTH levels are low. A stimulation test (most rigorous is insulin hypoglycemia [ITT]; less rigorous is the ACTH [Cortrosyn] stimulation test) may be necessary, particularly if there are other hormone deficits after surgery. A limitation of the ACTH stimulation test is that if it is performed soon after the operation, the cortisol response may be normal, leading to a false conclusion that the hypothalamic-pituitary-adrenal axis is intact.

619

## CURRENT DIAGNOSIS

- Screening studies: serum IGF-1, prolactin, free $T_4$, ACTH, cortisol (AM preferred), LH, FSH, testosterone (men)
- Definitive test: Oral glucose, 75 or 100 g: measure glucose and GH at 0, 30, 60, 90, and 120 minutes
- MRI of pituitary without and with gadolinium

*Abbreviations:* ACTH = adrenocorticotropic hormone; FSH = follicle-stimulating hormone; GH = growth hormone; LH = luteinizing hormone; MRI = magnetic resonance imaging; $T_4$ = thyroxine.

For glucocorticoid replacement, a short-acting preparation is preferred to avoid an adverse effect on bone metabolism (excessive bone resorption) and possible iatrogenic Cushing's syndrome. Hydrocortisone, 15 mg on awakening and 5 mg in late afternoon (some patients do well with 10 mg on awakening and 5 mg at 6 PM) or prednisone 5 mg on awakening (some patients require a late afternoon dose, suggest: 2.5 mg) is usually adequate. The patient should be instructed to double the dose of glucocorticoid in the event of intercurrent illness such as influenza or urinary tract infection. Patients should always wear a bracelet or necklace that identifies adrenal insufficiency.

The need for thyroid hormone replacement is determined by measuring serum free thyroxine (free $T_4$), not thyroid-stimulating hormone (TSH), because the TSH may be in the normal range but not adequate to stimulate normal thyroid hormone secretion. The levothyroxine (Synthroid, Levoxyl) starting dose depends on the patient's age and history of coronary artery disease. If the patient is elderly or has a history of coronary artery disease, begin with a dose of 0.012 or 0.025 mg/day and titrate every 6 weeks to achieve a normal serum free $T_4$ level. Most adults achieve a normal serum free $T_4$ with a dose of 0.088 to 0.125 mg/day.

The need for gonadal steroid replacement in premenopausal women is based on menstrual history after surgery; a serum estradiol may be helpful, but it might not be diagnostic, depending on the time of the menstrual cycle. In men, the history of libido, erectile function, and measurement of a morning serum testosterone are needed. Measurement of a serum prostate-specific antigen (PSA) level is recommended before beginning testosterone replacement.

Assessment of possible diabetes insipidus can be determined clinically and does not usually require a water-deprivation test. If the patient is urinating frequently at night (e.g., hourly) and has resolution of nocturia with a bedtime dose of desmopressin (DDAVP, 0.1 mg), the diagnosis is obvious. The need for a twice daily dose of desmopressin is determined by the frequency of urination during the day and oral fluid intake; the patient is usually aware of when the dose from the prior evening no longer controls polyuria.

## ADDITIONAL THERAPIES

Medical treatment can decrease serum GH and IGF-1 or IGF-1 levels to normal. No medical therapy results in permanent remission of acromegaly. Radiation to the pituitary and residual tumor offers the possibility of definitive treatment; the effect is not immediate and can take several years to result in a normal serum IGF-1 level. For this reason, medical therapy is administered to control hormone hypersecretion while awaiting a beneficial effect of pituitary radiation.

## CURRENT THERAPY

Transsphenoidal surgery is the first choice
- Medical therapy for persistent disease: dopamine agonist, somatostatin analogue, growth hormone receptor antagonist
- Radiation for persistent disease: focused (gamma knife, proton beam, cyber knife, linear accelerator), conventional fractionated
- Medical therapy while awaiting delayed effect of radiation

## Medical Therapy

Three classes of drugs have been used to treat acromegaly: dopamine agonists, somatostatin analogues, and a GH receptor antagonist. Dopamine agonist drugs (cabergoline [Dostinex],[1] bromocriptine [Parlodel]) lower IGF-1 to normal in less than 20% of patients. The advantage of these drugs is oral administration and lower cost than other drugs. The most common side effects of a dopamine agonist include nausea, vomiting, headache, and nasal stuffiness; cabergoline[1] has been reported to produce fewer side effects than bromocriptine. A 3-month trial of a dopamine agonist is a reasonable treatment; if the IGF-1 does not decrease to normal, another medication should be recommended.

The somatostatin analogues, short-acting octreotide (Sandostatin) and long-acting octreotide (Sandostatin LAR or Lanreotide,[2] act directly on the tumor to inhibit GH secretion, lower GH and IGF-1 levels, and, in approximately one third of patients, reduce tumor size. Achievement of a normal serum IGF-1 level with a somatostatin analogue occurs in 50% to 65% of patients. The response to a somatostatin analogue depends on the intrinsic nature of the tumor, namely, the number of somatostatin receptors and binding affinity of the drug to the receptor. Short-acting octreotide is self-administered as a subcutaneous injection every 6 to 8 hours daily; the long-acting drug is administered in the physician's office as a once-monthly intramuscular injection in the buttock. Side effects of somatostatin analogues include transient abdominal pain and diarrhea, which usually diminish with time. The long-term side effect is an 18% risk of developing gallbladder sludge or gallstones, which are often asymptomatic.

The GH receptor antagonist pegvisomant (Somavert) acts on the liver to inhibit generation of IGF-1; IGF-1 is reduced to normal in up to 98% of patients. Because this drug is a modified GH molecule that inhibits GH binding to its receptor, measurement of serum GH is not recommended, because commercial GH assays measure the drug and result in very elevated GH levels. Only serum IGF-1 should be measured to assess efficacy. This medication is self-administered as a subcutaneous injection daily, beginning with a dose of 10 mg daily and titrating up to 30 mg daily, depending on the serum IGF-1 concentration. Because this drug does not act at the pituitary level, there is a risk of continued growth of the pituitary adenoma, especially if the patient has not received pituitary radiation. If the patient has not received pituitary radiation, it is imperative that pituitary anatomy be monitored closely with serial MRI studies (recommended every 6 months). Side effects of pegvisomant are elevated liver enzymes: γ-glutamyl transferase (γ GT), aspartate aminotransferase (AST), alanine aminotransferase (ALT), and bilirubin. Serum liver enzymes should be measured before and monthly for the first 6 months after beginning this drug, and they should be measured if the patient develops fatigue or jaundice. If liver enzymes become abnormal, pegvisomant should be discontinued and not restarted.

## Pituitary Radiation

Fractionated radiation to a pituitary tumor (daily treatment for 4 to 5 weeks) has been employed for more than 50 years. Ultimately, radiation treatment can result in lowering the GH and IGF-1. However, GH and IGF-1 are usually not restored to normal levels after conventional fractionated radiation for at least 5 years, and normalization can take 20 years or more. The persistently high IGF-1 levels present an ongoing risk of morbidity and premature mortality in the absence of medical therapy to lower IGF-1 to normal. Additionally, long-term follow-up has shown increased risks of cerebrovascular disease and mortality in patients treated with conventional fractionated radiation.

More recently, focused methods of radiation delivery have been developed; these include the gamma knife, proton beam, linear accelerator, and cyber knife. Unfortunately, there has been no comparison of the efficacy or complications among these forms of radiation delivery. Focused radiation delivery is theoretically attractive because normal brain tissue receives less radiation. However, all forms of radiation

---

[1]Not FDA approved for this indication.
[2]Not available in the United States.

Melmed S, Casanueva F, Cavagnini F, et al: Consensus statement: Medical management of acromegaly. Eur J Endocrinol 2005;153(6):737-740.
Van der Lely AJ, Hutson RK, Trainer PJ, et al: Long term treatment of acromegaly with pegvisomant, a growth hormone receptor antagonist. Lancet 2001;358:1754-1759.

## BOX 1 Long-Term Follow-up

- Response to pituitary radiation every 6 mo: serum IGF-1 (off of long-acting octreotide (Sandostatin LAR) for 2 mo, off of pegvisomant (Somavert) for 3 to 4 wk)
- New pituitary hormone deficiency every 6 mo after radiation: morning serum ACTH, cortisol, free thyroxine, testosterone (men), menstrual history in premenopausal women
- Imaging: MRI every 12 mo or every 6 mo as indicated clinically (visual disturbance, headache)

delivery affect the normal pituitary tissue, with the potential for development of new pituitary hormone deficiency. Another concern is the potential for development of a secondary brain tumor; this risk is very small, but it cannot be ignored and requires regular monitoring with an MRI study.

The risk of new pituitary hormone deficiency is up to 50% in patients who received conventional fractionated radiotherapy for a nonfunctioning pituitary adenoma, and similar results have been reported in patients with a secretory adenoma. The risk of new pituitary hormone deficiency with the gamma knife (one treatment, focused radiation delivery) is approximately 30%, but this risk will likely increase with longer follow-up. The risk of hypopituitarism with linear accelerator or cyber knife has not been studied adequately, but there is no reason to expect that development of new hormone deficiency will be different from what occurs with other methods of radiation delivery, because radiation cannot discriminate between an adenoma and normal pituitary tissue. Thus, all patients are at risk for developing pituitary insufficiency.

If the patient is to undergo gamma knife treatment, a somatostatin analogue should not be administered at the time of treatment and should be delayed for at least 6 weeks afterward, because several studies have shown a delayed effect of gamma knife response in patients receiving a somatostatin analogue at the time of treatment.

If a patient undergoes pituitary radiation and medical therapy to lower the IGF-1 level, the medication should be discontinued every 6 months and the IGF-1 level should be measured to determine if the radiation therapy is beneficial. Long-acting octreotide therapy should be discontinued 2 months before measuring IGF-1, because the biological action of this drug persists beyond 1 month. Pegvisomant should be discontinued for 3 to 4 weeks before measurement of the IGF-1. At the same time, the need for hormone replacements (cortisol, thyroid hormone, gonadal steroid) should be conducted by measuring a morning serum cortisol, ACTH, free thyroxine; testosterone should be measured in men and the menstrual history should be obtained in premenopausal women. A single ACTH and cortisol level is helpful if the values are very low, indicating the need for glucocorticoid replacement. However, a normal ACTH and cortisol level is not adequate to assess hypothalamic-pituitary-adrenal reserve during stress; an insulin hypoglycemia test is the most reliable method to determine the need for glucocorticoid treatment during the stress of intercurrent illness.

## Summary

The diagnosis of acromegaly is straightforward once the possibility of this disease is entertained. Successful treatment might require a multimodality approach in many patients, with the goal of reducing serum IGF-1 to normal and reducing the risks of ongoing morbidity and premature mortality.

### REFERENCES

Guistina A, Barkan A, Casanueva F, et al: Criteria for cure of acromegaly: A consensus statement. J Clin Endocrinol Metab 2000;85:526-529.
Kreutzer J, Vance ML, Lopes MBS, Laws ER Jr: Surgical management of GH-secreting pituitary adenomas: An outcome study using modern remission criteria. J Clin Endocrinol Metab 2001;86: 4072-4077.

# Adrenocortical Insufficiency

Method of
*Carl D. Malchoff, MD, PhD*

Adrenal insufficiency is a life-threatening disorder that is 100% treatable by timely therapy. Because the clinical presentation is nonspecific and the prevalence is low (about 120 per 1 million persons in Western countries), the diagnosis may be overlooked. Recognition of clinical settings that predispose to adrenal insufficiency can alert the astute physician to consider this disorder when confronted with the nonspecific clinical presentation. The diagnosis is confirmed by biochemical testing that exploits endocrine physiology.

*Adrenal insufficiency* refers to decreased cortisol (hydrocortisone) production. Aldosterone production is low in primary adrenal insufficiency and normal in secondary adrenal insufficiency. Isolated aldosterone deficiency most often occurs in hyporeninemic hypoaldosteronism and is not discussed in this article.

## Endocrine Physiology

The adrenal cortex produces both cortisol (a glucocorticoid) and aldosterone (a mineralocorticoid). Cortisol maintains cardiac output, vascular resistance, and hepatic glucose output. Shock and death can occur without adequate glucocorticoids. Aldosterone modulates renal sodium reabsorption in exchange for potassium excretion. Hyperkalemia is caused by aldosterone deficiency.

Cortisol production is controlled by a simple closed feedback loop. The anterior pituitary gland secretes adrenocorticotropic hormone (ACTH), which stimulates adrenal cortisol production. Cortisol inhibits ACTH release to complete the closed feedback loop. A more complex feedback loop controls aldosterone production, which is stimulated directly by angiotensin II. Angiotensin II is generated from angiotensin I, which itself is a proteolytic product of angiotensin substrate that has been cleaved by the enzyme renin. The juxtaglomerular complex of the kidney releases renin in response to low blood pressure. Aldosterone stimulates the distal tubule to transport sodium from the glomerular filtrate back into the vasculature in exchange for potassium. Water accompanies sodium, producing increases in vascular volume and blood pressure that complete the closed feedback loop.

## Etiology

In primary adrenal insufficiency the adrenal glands are no longer capable of producing adequate amounts of cortisol and aldosterone (Box 1). In secondary adrenal insufficiency, the pituitary gland or hypothalamus is damaged, and decreased cortisol production is secondary to decreased ACTH release from the anterior pituitary. A familiarity with the causes of primary and secondary adrenal insufficiency will help the physician recognize the settings in which adrenal insufficiency can occur.

In developed countries, primary adrenal insufficiency is most commonly caused by autoimmune destruction of the adrenal glands. The leading cause in underdeveloped countries might still be tuberculosis.

Autoimmune polyglandular syndrome (APS) type 2 is most familiar to physicians treating adult patients. This disorder tends to be familial, although the genetics are complex (polygenic). It is associated with type 1 diabetes and Hashimoto's disease. Other autoimmune disorders occur

## BOX 1  Etiology of Adrenal Insufficiency

- Adrenal disorders (primary adrenal insufficiency)
- Autoimmune disorders: Autoimmune polyglandular syndromes types 1 and 2
- Infections with granulomatous response (tuberculosis, histoplasmosis, others)
- Adrenal hemorrhage
  - Meningococcemia and, less commonly, in other causes of sepsis
  - Anticoagulation
  - Severe stress
  - Antiphospholipid syndrome
- Adrenoleukodystrophy
- Amyloidosis
- Congenital adrenal hyperplasia
- Adrenal hypoplasia (developmental disorders)
- AIDS-associated infections: Cytomegalovirus
- Pharmaceuticals: Metyrapone (Metopirone), mitotane (Lysodren), aminoglutethimide (Cytadren), etomidate (Amidate), ketoconazole (Nizoral)

with lower frequency, and autoimmune hypoparathyroidism is not associated with adrenal insufficiency in APS type 2, as it is in APS type 1.

APS type 1 is a mendelian disorder with recessive inheritance caused by mutations of the *AIRE* gene that can regulate immune tolerance in the adrenal cortex and parathyroid tissues. Nearly all patients develop the triad of adrenal insufficiency, hypoparathyroidism, and mucocutaneous candidiasis before adulthood. Other less common manifestations include malabsorption, primary hypogonadism in female patients, and alopecia.

Primary adrenal insufficiency was first described in the mid 1800s in the setting of tuberculosis, and infiltrative destruction of the adrenal glands was observed at autopsy. Other infectious disorders that can infiltrate and destroy the adrenal glands include histoplasmosis, cryptococcosis, and blastomycosis. Hemorrhagic adrenal destruction may be caused by meningococcemia or sepsis from other bacterial infections, by anticoagulation, by the antiphospholipid syndrome and even by severe physical stress alone. Malignancies such as breast, kidney, and lung cancers often metastasize to the adrenal glands, where they manifest as large adrenal masses on imaging studies. However, metastases to the adrenal glands usually do not impair adrenal function, although this should be confirmed by biochemical testing.

Inherited disorders causing adrenal insufficiency can cause hyperplasia or hypoplasia of the adrenal gland or they can cause gradual adrenal gland destruction due to failure to metabolize toxic substances. Adrenal insufficiency with adrenal hyperplasia is caused by defects in the enzymes that convert cholesterol to cortisol and usually manifests in the neonatal period. These disorders are collectively referred to as *congenital adrenal hyperplasia*; increased ACTH production causes the adrenal glands to become hyperplastic, even though they produce inadequate amounts of cortisol. Deficiency of the 21-hydroxylase enzyme is the most common cause, although defects can occur at any step in cortisol synthesis. Neonatal adrenal hypoplasia occurs when genes required for normal adrenal development are defective.

Adrenoleukodsytrophy is an X-linked recessive disorder caused by the failure to oxidize long-chain fatty acids. Both neurologic deficits and adrenal insufficiency progress over time due to the toxicity of long-chain fatty acid accumulation. Metyrapone (Metopirone), aminoglutethimide (Cytadren), and mitotane (Lysodren) are used to treat cortisol excess and can produce adrenal insufficiency. In addition, high-dose ketoconazole (Nizoral) can cause adrenal insufficiency.

Secondary adrenal insufficiency is usually permanent when caused by tumors of the pituitary gland, pituitary irradiation, or traumatic section of the pituitary stalk. However, the defect may be partial. Reversible secondary adrenal insufficiency is commonly caused by long-term high-dose glucocorticoid therapy that suppresses the hypothalamus and pituitary gland. However, this is a slow process, and complete recovery takes about 1 year. Hypophysitis can spontaneously resolve.

## Clinical Presentation

Adrenal insufficiency can manifest as an acute crisis or as a slowly progressive illness. In either case, the presentation is often nonspecific, and the clinical context can alert the physician to the diagnosis. It has been suggested that sepsis and other severe illnesses commonly cause a relative adrenal insufficiency, but this remains controversial.

Acute adrenal crisis manifests with hypotension and often fever. It can occur in a patient with untreated adrenal insufficiency who is subjected to physical stress. Although it is well known to occur in meningococcemia, it can also occur in the setting of sepsis caused by other organisms. Severe illness alone can cause adrenal hemorrhage and adrenal crisis. Adrenal insufficiency should be considered in any patient in the intensive care unit with the sudden onset of fever and hypotension.

The presentation of chronic adrenal insufficiency includes anorexia, weight loss, fatigue, abdominal pain, diarrhea, hyperpigmentation, orthostatic hypotension, hyponatremia, and hyperkalemia. Nearly 100% of subjects have anorexia and weight loss, although there are rare exceptions. Weight gain due to hypothalamic obesity can occur following resection of a craniopharyngioma or other hypothalamic lesion, even in the setting of adrenal insufficiency. The differential diagnosis of unexplained weight loss should include adrenal insufficiency. Electrolyte abnormalities are a useful clue but are not always present. Hyperkalemia occurs in about 60% of subjects with primary adrenal insufficiency and does not occur in secondary adrenal insufficiency. Hyponatremia occurs in about 80% of subjects with primary adrenal insufficiency and 60% of subjects with secondary adrenal insufficiency. Although hypoaldosteronism contributes to hyponatremia in primary adrenal insufficiency, antidiuretic hormone (ADH) is the major cause of hyponatremia. Both hypotension and low cortisol concentrations stimulate its production. Hyperpigmentation occurs only in primary adrenal insufficiency.

It has been proposed that relative adrenal insufficiency occurs frequently in sepsis and other severe illnesses. This is controversial. The increase in serum cortisol concentration following stimulation with cosyntropin (Cortrosyn) is often diminished in sepsis and other severe illnesses, suggesting a relative adrenal insufficiency. Alternatively, this finding can indicate that cortisol production is already maximally stimulated in the sickest patients.

One large multicenter study sought to distinguish between these possibilities by random prospective assignment of septic patients to treatment with stress doses of glucocorticoids plus mineralocorticoids versus placebo. Although there was a small statistical benefit of glucocorticoid treatment in subjects with a diminished response to cosyntropin, the study was flawed by the use of etomidate (Amidate) to sedate some patients. Etomidate is a short-acting anesthetic that inhibits cortisol production. When letters brought this to the attention of the study's authors, they declined the opportunity to reanalyze their results with the etomidate-treated subjects excluded from the analysis. Therefore, it is possible that the benefit of glucocorticoids was limited to subjects with iatrogenic adrenal insufficiency.

No general recommendation can be made concerning the use of stress doses of glucocorticoids in patients with sepsis, and this decision is left to the discretion of the treating physician. The exception is in the patient with meningococcemia, who should always receive stress doses of glucocorticoids, because meningococcemia carries a significant risk of adrenal hemorrhage. Glucocorticoid doses that exceed stress doses may be harmful in sepsis.

After the diagnosis of adrenal insufficiency is established, it is necessary to distinguish between primary and secondary adrenal insufficiency. The 8:00 AM plasma ACTH concentration is greater than 100 pg/mL (22 pmol/L) in primary adrenal insufficiency. If a diagnosis of primary adrenal insufficiency is made, then the adrenal glands should be imaged to help determine the cause, and in boys and young men the diagnosis of adrenoleukodystrophy should be excluded by measuring circulating very-long-chain fatty acids. In secondary adrenal insufficiency the pituitary gland and hypothalamus should be imaged by magnetic resonance imaging (MRI).

## Biochemical Diagnosis

Biochemical confirmation of adrenal insufficiency often requires dynamic testing (Box 2). The normal responses to these tests are established in healthy persons and might not be completely applicable to critically ill patients, especially those with low cortisol-binding globulin.

Although unstimulated serum cortisol concentrations are usually not diagnostic, an 8:00 AM serum cortisol concentration less than 3 µg/dL (83 nmol/L) is diagnostic of adrenal insufficiency, and a random serum cortisol concentration greater than 23 µg/dL excludes adrenal insufficiency.

Dynamic testing with insulin-induced hypoglycemia is generally considered the gold standard for diagnosing adrenal insufficiency. However, the test requires skill and experience to perform, is contraindicated in ill patients, and is relatively contraindicated in patients older than 50 years, in patients with coronary artery disease, and in patients with seizure disorders. Dynamic testing with synthetic $ACTH_{1-24}$ (cosyntropin) is rapid, safe, and usually accurate. It will diagnose primary adrenal insufficiency and long-standing secondary adrenal insufficiency. There are two versions of this test: a standard (high-dose) test that employs a 250-µg cosyntropin dose and a low-dose test that employs a 1-µg cosyntropin dose. There is debate as to which version has greater sensitivity and specificity, but generally they lead to similar conclusions.

Unfortunately, the normal stimulated ranges for each of the different cortisol assays are not well established in most laboratories. Studies have shown considerable variations between different assays for cortisol being performed in the same laboratory. Therefore, the normative data developed in one laboratory might not be applicable to another. A cortisol response of 20 µg/dL (550 nmol/L) or greater at 1 hour following intravenous or intramuscular administration of 250 µg of cosyntropin generally is believed to indicate adequate adrenal function, although the lower normal limit may be 23 µg/dL (635 nmol/L). Various normal values are given for the 1-µg cosyntropin test, and some clinicians have attempted to normalize the cosyntropin response at 30 minutes following the injection rather than 60 minutes.

No test is perfect, and it may be useful to have an experienced endocrinologist assist with the interpretation of borderline results. It is generally considered unnecessary to obtain a basal cortisol concentration, but some, especially those who argue that there is a relative adrenal insufficiency of severe illness, contest this.

For persons with suspected adrenal crisis, it is appropriate to begin dexamethasone (Decadron) before testing for adrenal reserve. Dexamethasone does not cross-react in the immune-based cortisol assays, and, for the first 72 hours of therapy it will not influence the maximum cortisol response to cosyntropin stimulation.

## Treatment

The treatment of adrenal insufficiency depends on the presentation (Box 3). It is usually divided into the extremes: treatment of hypotensive adrenal insufficiency crisis and treatment of otherwise healthy persons with adrenal insufficiency. Some patients fall between these two extremes.

Hypotensive adrenal crisis is treated with stress doses of intravenous glucocorticoids, intravenous normal saline with 5% dextrose, vasoconstricting agents necessary to maintain blood pressure, plus antibiotics if infection is suspected. Maximum cortisol production is about 200 mg/day, so that replacement with 50 to 100 mg hydrocortisone (Solu-Cortef) IV every 6 hours is appropriate. Because hydrocortisone is an effective mineralocorticoid at these high doses and because there are no intravenous mineralocorticoids available, this is the treatment of choice in hyperkalemic patients. In critically ill patients, treatment with stress doses of glucocorticoids should not be withheld pending the results of adrenal function tests. If the patient is not hyperkalemic, then treatment with IV dexamethasone is

---

### BOX 2 Biochemical Testing

**Standard High-Dose ACTH Stimulation Test**

The serum concentration of cortisol is measured 60 min following IV or IM administration of 250 µg cosyntropin (Cortrosyn). Although the normal response is probably >23 µg/dL (635 nmol/L), adrenal function is considered adequate if the response is >20 µg/dL (550 nmol/L).

**Low-Dose ACTH Stimulation Test**

The serum cortisol concentration is measured 60 min following IV administration of 1 µg cosyntropin diluted in normal saline. The minimum normal response is reported by various investigators to be 18-22 µg/dL (500-600 nmol/L).

**Insulin-Induced Hypoglycemia Test**

This test is more sensitive than cosyntropin testing in the setting of recent-onset secondary adrenal insufficiency. Under the supervision of an endocrinologist or other experienced physician, regular insulin (0.1-0.15 U/kg) is administered intravenously. Serum glucose and cortisol concentrations are measured at 0, 10, 20, 30, 45, 60, and 90 min following the injection. If adequate hypoglycemia is attained (serum glucose <40 mg/dL; 22 mmol/L), then the serum cortisol concentration will increase to 20 µg/dL (500 nmol/L) or greater in normal persons.

---

### BOX 3 Treatment of Adrenal Insufficiency

**Adrenal Crisis**
- Administer 1 L normal saline with 5% dextrose IV as fast as possible, and then continue as long as necessary to maintain blood pressure and urine output.
- Immediately administer stress doses of glucocorticoids IV, either hydrocortisone (Solu-Cortef) 50 mg q6h or dexamethasone (Deltasone) 2 mg q12h.
  - Use hydrocortisone to treat hyperkalemia.
  - Use dexamethasone if diagnostic testing will be performed.
- Vasoconstrictors are administered as necessary to maintain blood pressure.

**Adrenal Insufficiency in an Otherwise Healthy Patient**
- Glucocorticoids
  - Hydrocortisone at 20 mg/d or the lowest tolerated dose divided two to four times a d *or* prednisone at 5 mg/d or the lowest tolerated dose divided one to two times a d.
  - Dexamethasone at 0.5 mg/d is usually avoided due to variable metabolism. However, it may be useful for poorly compliant patients.
- Mineralocorticoid
  - Fludrocortisone (Florinef) 0.1 mg/d and titrated to maintain the plasma renin activity in the normal range
- Androgen
  - Dehydroepiandrosterone (DHEA)[7] at 50 mg/d to women, although not all experts agree that it is necessary.
  - Indications for continued use are improved sense of well-being and improved sexual satisfaction.

[7]Available as a dietary supplement.

## CURRENT DIAGNOSIS

- Acute adrenal insufficiency with crisis manifests with hypotension and often fever.
- Chronic adrenal insufficiency without crisis manifests with weight loss and anorexia.
- Primary adrenal insufficiency develops in the setting of disorders affecting the adrenal glands. These include autoimmune disorders, granulomatous diseases, meningococcemia, anticoagulation, and certain pharmaceutical agents.
- Secondary adrenal insufficiency develops in the setting of pituitary disorders.
- Hyponatremia occurs in both primary and secondary adrenal insufficiency.
- Hyperpigmentation occurs in primary adrenal insufficiency but not in secondary adrenal insufficiency.
- Dynamic testing is often necessary to establish the diagnosis. The insulin-induced hypoglycemia test is the gold standard, but this cumbersome test can often be avoided by use of a cosyntropin stimulation test.
- Both the standard high-dose (250 μg) cosyntropin stimulation test and the low-dose (1 μg) stimulation test are useful.
- Some experts contend that a relative adrenal insufficiency in sepsis and other acute illnesses occurs commonly, but this has not been proved.

## CURRENT THERAPY

- Acute adrenal insufficiency with hypotensive crisis should be treated with IV glucocorticoids at stress doses, normal saline with 5% dextrose, plus vasoconstrictors as needed to maintain blood pressure. If necessary, initiate therapy before establishing the diagnosis.
- A stress dose of hydrocortisone (Solu-Cortef) is 50-100 mg q6h, and a stress dose of dexamethasone is 2 mg q12 h. The former should be used in the setting of hyperkalemia, and the latter should be used if diagnostic testing will be performed.
- Glucocorticoid therapy of chronic adrenal insufficiency in an otherwise healthy patient is approximately 20 mg/d hydrocortisone (Cortef) divided in 2 to 4 doses, or prednisone 5 mg/d divided in 1 to 3 doses. The dose is titrated to the lowest tolerated by the patient.
- Dexamethasone (Decadron) has a variable half-life and is difficult to dose correctly for chronic use.
- In primary adrenal insufficiency, fludrocortisone (Florinef) is titrated to a normal upright plasma renin activity, and this is usually about 0.1 mg/dL.
  - A medical alert tag serves as an important reminder to emergency medical personnel of this potentially fatal disorder.
  - Dehydroepiandrosterone (DHEA) may be helpful in women with adrenal insufficiency.

appropriate at 2 mg IV every 12 hours, and dynamic testing can be performed during therapy.

Glucocorticoid therapy for otherwise healthy subjects with adrenal insufficiency is titrated to the lowest glucocorticoid dose at which the patient feels well. This is often a total of 20 mg/day of hydrocortisone divided into two to four doses a day. For convenience reasons, some patients prefer prednisone. The equivalent total daily dose of prednisone is about 5 mg/day as a single dose or divided into two doses a day. Dexamethasone has a half-life that varies between patients and with other medications taken by the patients. It should be avoided unless poor patient compliance is the overwhelming reason for choosing an agent with a long half-life. Patients with mild or partial adrenal insufficiency due to pituitary disease might not require glucocorticoid therapy daily, but only at times of stress.

Mineralocorticoid replacement is required for primary adrenal insufficiency but not for secondary adrenal insufficiency. Fludrocortisone (Florinef) is the only agent available, and it is not available in a parenteral preparation. The replacement dose is titrated to that which maintains the upright plasma renin activity in the normal range, and this is usually about 0.1 mg/day.

The patient should wear a medical alert tag that indicates the diagnosis of adrenal insufficiency.

Dehydroepiandrosterone (DHEA)[7] at doses of about 50 mg/day has been used to treat women with adrenal insufficiency. Dehydroepiandrosterone is a weak, naturally occurring adrenal androgen that is available without prescription. Some, but not all, double blind prospective studies suggest that it increases sexuality and a feeling of well-being in women with adrenal insufficiency. Potential complications include androgen-dependent hair growth and acne.

During minor illness, less than maximal glucocorticoid doses are usually satisfactory. The glucocorticoid dose is usually doubled when a patient develops a viral syndrome with a fever greater than 38.5°C (101°F). Increased glucocorticoid replacement doses are not required during pregnancy, but they are used transiently at delivery. Parenteral glucocorticoids are indicated for adrenal insufficiency patients with vomiting.

## REFERENCES

Abdu TAM, Elhadd TA, Neary R, et al: Comparison of the low dose short synacthen test (1 mg), the conventional dose short synacthen test (250 mg), and the insulin tolerance test for the assessment of the hypothalamo-pituitary-adrenal axis in patients with pituitary disease. J Clin Endocrinol Metab 1999;84:838-843.

Annane D, Sebille V, Charpentier C, et al: Effect of treatment with low doses of hydrocortisone and fludrocortisone on mortality in patients with septic shock. JAMA 2002;288:862-871.

Annane D, Sebille V, Troche G, et al: A 3-level prognostic classification in septic shock based on cortisol levels and cortisol response to corticotropin. JAMA 2000;283:1038-1045.

Dickstein G, Shechner C, Nicholson W, et al: Adrenocorticotropin stimulation test: Effects of basal cortisol level, time of day, and suggested new sensitive low dose test. J Clin Endocrinol Metab 1991;72:773-778.

Mayenknecht J, Diederich S, Bahr V, et al: Comparison of low and high dose corticotropin stimulation tests in patients with pituitary disease. J Clin Endocrinol Metab 1998;83:1558-1562.

Minneci PC, Deans KJ, Banks SM, et al: Meta-analysis: The effect of steroids on survival and shock during sepsis depends on the dose. Ann Int Med 2004;141:47-56.

Oelkers W: Adrenal insufficiency. N Engl J Med 1996;335:1206-1243.

Oelkers W. Diedrich S, Bahr V: Diagnosis and therapy surveillance in Addison's disease: Rapid adrenocorticotropin (ACTH) test and measurement of plasma ACTH, renin activity, and aldosterone. J Clin Endocrinol Metab 1992;75:259-264.

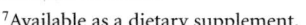

[7]Available as a dietary supplement.

# Cushing's Syndrome

Method of
*Kathryn G. Schuff, MD*

The diagnosis of Cushing's syndrome is one of the most difficult but potentially most important that can be made in a patient. The consequences of pathologic hypercortisolism are significant, and excess mortality and morbidity improve with cure of the disease. Although the evaluation and management often involve specialty referral, the primary care provider plays a pivotal role in suspecting the diagnosis and initiating the workup.

## Clinical Presentation

Although traditionally considered a rare disease with an incidence of 1 to 2 per 100,000, more recently Cushing's syndrome has been reported to occur in up to 3% to 4% of the obese, uncontrolled diabetic population. The classic presentation (moon facies, purple striae, central obesity) is uncommonly seen, and the presentation more commonly overlaps that of polycystic ovary syndrome, the metabolic syndrome, and depression. Given the nonspecific presentation, health care providers should have a low threshold for screening patients for the disease. More specific features (Table 1) that should prompt evaluation include difficult-to-control diabetes mellitus or hypertension, unexplained osteoporosis, and menstrual irregularities. In addition, physical signs that are disquieting include facial rounding, plethora, supraclavicular fat pad filling, central obesity, thin skin (including spontaneous ecchymoses), and proximal muscle weakness, particularly if a change in appearance can be demonstrated. Children exhibit poor linear growth, generalized obesity, and menstrual irregularities. The etiologies of hypercortisolism are varied (Box 1) and include both pathologic etiologies causing subclinical and overt Cushing's syndrome as well as pseudo-Cushing's syndrome, which is temporary, nonpathologic hypercortisolemia caused by concurrent medical or psychiatric illness.

### SUBCLINICAL CUSHING'S SYNDROME

Subtle hypothalamic-pituitary-adrenal (HPA) axis abnormalities and autonomy have been demonstrated in 5% to 20% of patients with incidentally discovered adrenal masses. These patients do not exhibit frank signs, symptoms, or biochemical abnormalities of Cushing's syndrome, and thus this entity is termed subclinical Cushing's syndrome. However,

### BOX 1 Etiologies of Hypercortisolism

- Pseudo-Cushing's syndrome (nonpathologic hypercortisolism)
  - Acute/chronic medical illness
  - Psychiatric illness
  - Alcoholism
- Subclinical Cushing's syndrome (subtle hypercortisolism without features of overt Cushing's syndrome)
  - Adrenal adenoma (incidentaloma)
  - Adrenal macronodular hyperplasia (rare)
  - Pituitary corticotroph adenoma (rare)
  - Aberrant receptor expression (rare)
- Cushing's syndrome (pathologic hypercortisolism)
  - Exogenous glucocorticoid use
  - Oral glucocorticoids (prednisone, dexamethasone [Decadron], hydrocortisone [Cortef])
  - Topical glucocorticoids (inhaled, intranasal, dermal)
  - Injected glucocorticoids (articular, periarticular, intramuscular)
  - Naturopathic preparations
  - Endogenous glucocorticoid production
    - ACTH-dependent
      - Pituitary corticotroph adenoma
        - MEN1 (rare, also includes hyperparathyroidism and pancreatic islet cell tumors)
      - Pituitary corticotroph hyperplasia (some because of ectopic CRH)
      - Ectopic ACTH syndrome
        - Oat-cell lung carcinoma
        - Foregut carcinoid tumors (bronchial, thymic, splenic)
        - Pheochromocytoma
        - Medullary thyroid carcinoma
        - Islet cell tumors
    - ACTH-independent
      - Adrenal adenoma
      - Adrenocortical carcinoma
      - Rare: micronodular hyperplasia
      - Macronodular hyperplasia
        - Aberrant receptor expression (gastric inhibitory peptide–food responsive, 5-hydroxytryptamine, angiotensin II, interleukin-1, luteinizing hormone and human chorionic gonadotropin, vasopressin, β-adrenergic)
      - Pigmented micronodular hyperplasia (Carney's triad)
      - Adrenal rests
      - McCune-Albright (activating mutations)

*Abbreviations:* ACTH = adrenocorticotropic hormone; CRH = corticotrophin-releasing hormone; MEN1 = multiple endocrine neoplasia, type 1.

there are higher rates of hypertension, impaired glucose tolerance, and diabetes in these patients, which often improve with removal of the lesion, and a higher prevalence of cardiovascular dysfunction. Although this syndrome is considered a very mild form of Cushing's syndrome, there appears to be a low rate of progression to overt Cushing's syndrome, and therapeutic decisions must be individualized.

## Diagnostic Evaluation

### EXOGENOUS GLUCOCORTICOIDS

Cushing's syndrome caused by exogenous glucocorticoid use can be obvious, but careful investigation for unsuspected or surreptitious use must be undertaken in all patients. Infrequently recognized culprits are intraarticular, epidural, topical (inhaled, intranasal, and dermal), and naturopathic

### TABLE 1 Clinical Features of Cushing's Syndrome (In Order of Decreasing Specificity)

| Feature | Sensitivity (%) | Specificity (%) |
|---|---|---|
| Hypokalemia (K⁺ <3.6) | 25 | 96 |
| Ecchymoses | 53 | 94 |
| Osteoporosis | 26 | 94 |
| Weakness | 65 | 93 |
| Diastolic blood pressure ≥105 mm Hg | 39 | 83 |
| Red or violaceous striae | 46 | 78 |
| Acne | 52 | 76 |
| Central obesity | 90 | 71 |
| Hirsutism | 50 | 71 |
| Plethora | 82 | 69 |
| Oligomenorrhea | 72 | 49 |
| Generalized obesity | 60 | 38 |
| Abnormal glucose tolerance | 88 | 23 |

preparations. Variations in the metabolic clearance of synthetic glucocorticoids can lead to markedly prolonged glucocorticoid exposure and development of Cushing's syndrome. Detection of the synthetic glucocorticoid may require tandem mass spectrometry evaluation.

## ENDOGENOUS HYPERCORTISOLISM

Evaluation of suspected endogenous hypercortisolemia must follow a stepwise approach (Figure 1). The first step is to make the diagnosis of Cushing's syndrome. The second step is to determine if the abnormal cortisol secretion is adrenocorticotropic hormone (ACTH)-dependent (from either a pituitary adenoma (Cushing's disease) or the ectopic

ACTH syndrome) or ACTH-independent (primary adrenal disease). Finally, in ACTH-dependent Cushing's syndrome, the health care provider must distinguish pituitary sources of ACTH from the ectopic ACTH syndrome. Proceeding in the evaluation in a stepwise approach is critical for correct interpretation of test results because the premise of many of the tests is that preliminary biochemical diagnoses have been confirmed. For example, Cushing's syndrome must be confirmed before the ACTH level can be interpreted. In addition, because of the high prevalence of incidental pituitary and adrenal lesions and the finding of nodular adrenal disease in some cases of Cushing's disease caused by pituitary adenomas, imaging should not be performed until the biochemical diagnoses have been established. Finally, as many as

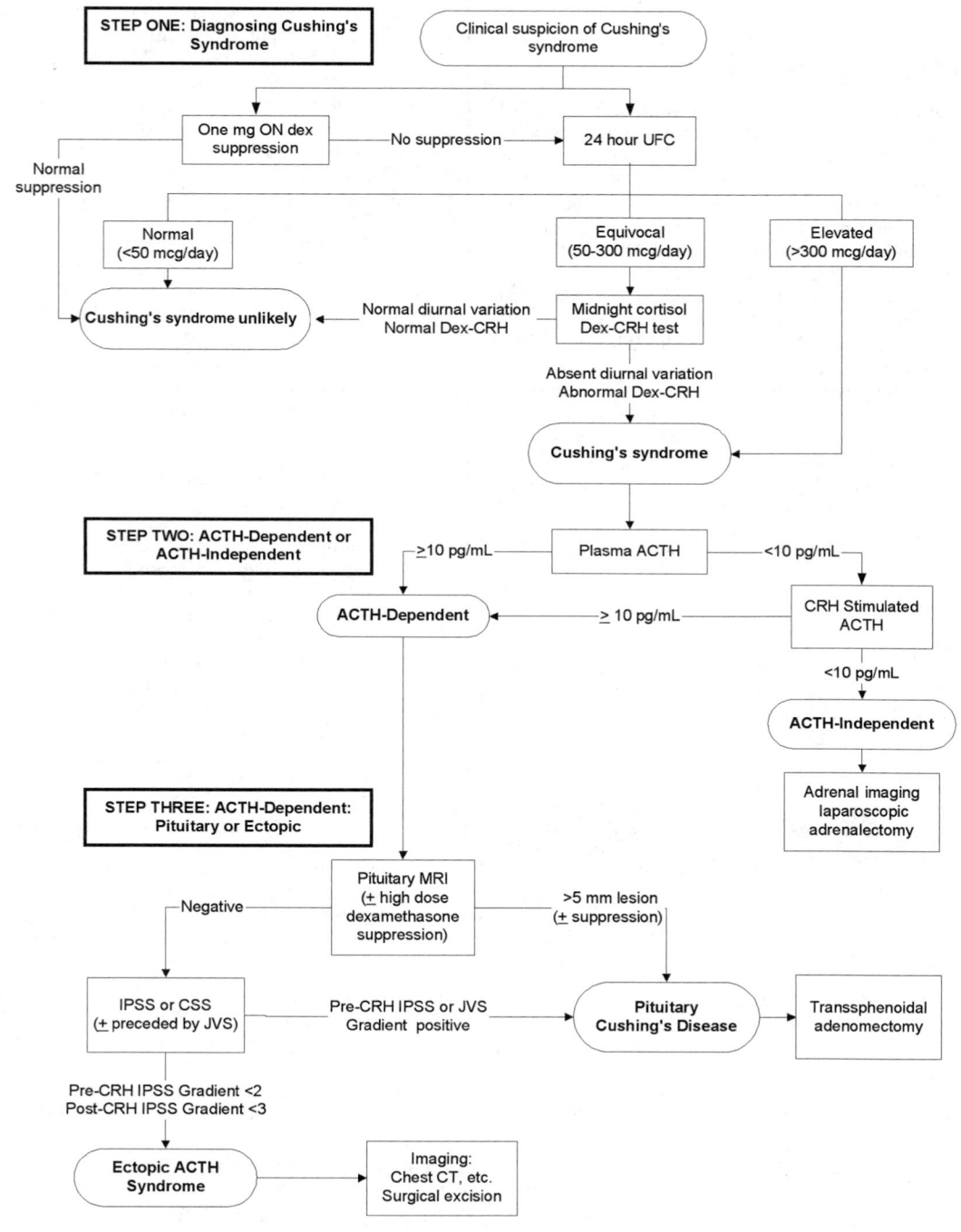

**FIGURE 1.** Stepwise approach to the diagnosis and differential diagnosis of Cushing's syndrome. ACTH = adrenocorticotropin; CRH = corticotrophin-releasing hormone; CSS = cavernous sinus sampling; CT = computed tomography; dex = dexamethasone; IPSS = inferior petrosal sinus sampling; JVS = jugular venous sampling; MRI = magnetic resonance imaging; ON = overnight; UFC = urine-free cortisol.

15% of patients with Cushing's syndrome will have intermittent hypercortisolemia, and care must be taken that the evaluation is performed when the patient is symptomatic or has documented hypercortisolism.

## STEP ONE: DIAGNOSE CUSHING'S SYNDROME

The first step in the evaluation is to establish the diagnosis of Cushing's syndrome by demonstrating pathologic hypercortisolism, either by measuring cortisol overproduction, abnormal HPA regulation, or absent diurnal variation. We recommend four tests for this purpose: the 1 mg overnight dexamethasone suppression (1 mg ON dex) test, measurement of 24-hour urine-free cortisol (24-hour UFC) excretion, assessment of diurnal variation with a midnight serum or salivary cortisol level, and the dexamethasone-suppressed corticotrophin-releasing hormone stimulation (dex-CRH) test.

### One Milligram Overnight Dexamethasone Suppression Test

The 1 mg ON dex test has sensitivity sufficiently high to exclude the diagnosis of Cushing's syndrome; however, it lacks sufficient specificity to confirm the diagnosis, with false-positive rates from 5% to 30%. The test is simple to perform and involves administering 1 mg of dexamethasone (Decadron) by mouth at 11 PM. The serum cortisol at 8 AM the next morning should be less than 5 μg/dL; more strict criteria require suppression to less than 2.5 or 3 μg/dL. A simultaneous dexamethasone (Decadron) level can detect false positives that occur in patients taking medications that accelerate dexamethasone (Decadron) metabolism (phenytoin [Dilantin], phenobarbital [Luminal], rifampin [Rifadin], and primidone [Mysoline]). False positives may also be seen with estrogen therapy and tamoxifen (Nolvadex).

### Measurement of 24-Hour Urine-Free Cortisol Excretion

Because of the high false-positive rate, an abnormal 1 mg ON dex test must be confirmed, usually by measurement of 24-hour UFC excretion. Alternatively, a 24-hour UFC measurement may be the initial step in the evaluation. As shown in Figure 1, marked elevations in 24-hour UFC (>300 μg/day) confirm the diagnosis, but intermediate levels require additional evaluation. Because of potential problems with incomplete collections and intermittent hypercortisolemia, creatinine should be measured in the specimen, and normal 24-hour UFC excretion

should be demonstrated on 2 or 3 occasions before the diagnosis of Cushing's syndrome is excluded. Acute medical illness can cause marked elevations in 24-hour UFC, false positives can occur with high urine volumes, and carbamazepine (Tegretol) can cross-react in the high-pressure liquid chromatography (HPLC) assay.

### Midnight Serum or Salivary Cortisol Levels

Loss of the diurnal rhythm in cortisol secretion is a characteristic feature in Cushing's syndrome (Figure 2). Demonstration of a midnight serum cortisol greater than 7.5 μg/dL distinguishes patients with Cushing's syndrome from normal and pseudo-Cushing's patients with high sensitivity and specificity. More recent improvements in the salivary cortisol assay allow collection of a saliva sample at home, avoiding the logistic difficulties in arranging a blood draw at night. Cut-off values for salivary cortisol measurements vary by assay, but normal suppression is generally between less than 0.2 and 0.55 μg/dL.

### Dexamethasone-Suppressed Corticotropin-Releasing Hormone Stimulation Test

The dex-CRH test detects the relative resistance to dexamethasone (Decadron) suppression and over-responsiveness to ovine corticotropin-releasing factor (oCRH [Acthrel]) in various tumors. It improves on the poor specificity of the 1 mg ON dex test with a higher dose of dexamethasone (Decadron), 0.5 mg by mouth every 6 hours starting at 12 PM and ending at 6 AM on the second day. Because this dose of dexamethasone (Decadron) will suppress many pituitary adenomas, sensitivity of the test is retained by administration of oCRH (Acthrel)[1] 100 μg intravenously at 8 AM on the final day followed by cortisol and ACTH levels every 15 minutes for 1 hour. A plasma cortisol greater than 1.4 μg/dL distinguishes patients with Cushing's syndrome from those with pseudo-Cushing's with high accuracy.

## STEP TWO: ACTH-DEPENDENT OR ACTH-INDEPENDENT DISEASE

Once the diagnosis of Cushing's syndrome has been established, the next step is to determine if the abnormal cortisol secretion is dependent

---

[1]Not FDA approved for this indication.

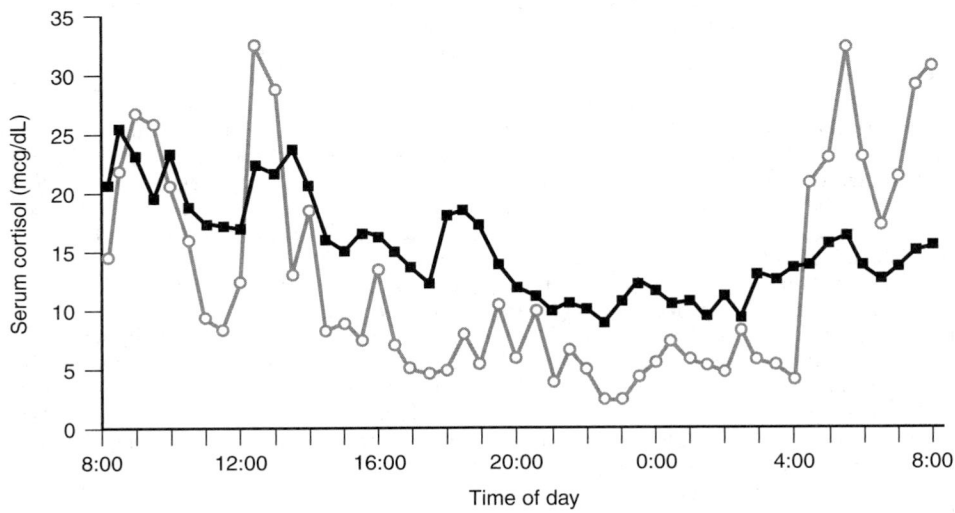

**FIGURE 2.** Diurnal rhythm of cortisol secretion is lost in Cushing's syndrome. Serum cortisol levels were measured every 30 minutes over 24 hours in a patient with proven Cushing's syndrome *(closed squares)* and a patient with pseudo-Cushing's syndrome *(open circles)*. Urine free cortisol (UFC) was mildly elevated in both patients (Cushing's syndrome, 75 μg/day; pseudo-Cushing's syndrome, 76 μg/day). Loss of diurnal variation in cortisol secretion is seen in the patient with Cushing's syndrome, whereas the patient with pseudo-Cushing's syndrome demonstrated normal diurnal variation with low serum cortisol levels (2.2 μg/dL) at midnight. (Data courtesy of Dr. Mary H. Samuels.)

on ACTH. A random ACTH level greater than 10 pg/mL confirms ACTH-dependent disease. However, because ACTH is secreted in a pulsatile, episodic fashion and is rapidly degraded, a low ACTH level must be confirmed by lack of stimulation to more than 10 pg/mL by oCRH (Acthrel),[1] 100 μg intravenously. When ACTH independent disease is confirmed, we then proceed with adrenal imaging, usually with high-resolution (3- to 5-mm sections), computed tomography (CT) to evaluate primary adrenal disease.

## STEP THREE: DISTINGUISH PITUITARY FROM ECTOPIC SOURCES OF ACTH

Once ACTH-dependent disease has been confirmed, the health care provider must determine the source of excess ACTH secretion. Approximately 90% of patients have a pituitary corticotroph adenoma as the source of ACTH. A number of biochemical tests exist to distinguish pituitary from ectopic sources, the most accurate of which is the high-dose dexamethasone suppression test. This test involves comparison of a baseline 24-hour UFC with one collected during the second day of dexamethasone (Decadron) 2 mg by mouth every 6 hours for eight doses. Although failure to suppress more than 90% from the baseline UFC has been reported to have 100% specificity for identifying ectopic tumors, the sensitivity of this test is poor, and there have been subsequent reports of lower specificity. Because of this, we do not rely on biochemical testing. Rather, once ACTH-dependent disease is confirmed, we perform magnetic resonance imaging (MRI) of the pituitary gland. In approximately one half of patients, a definite tumor is identified, and we then proceed with transsphenoidal adenomectomy. However, another reasonable strategy is to proceed with pituitary surgery only if both MRI and high-dose dexamethasone testing suggests a pituitary tumor.

If a tumor is not definitely identified, inferior petrosal or cavernous sinus sampling with oCRH stimulation is required to localize the ACTH source. Finding a central (cavernous sinus or petrosal sinus) to peripheral ratio of more than 2.0 before oCRH or greater than 3.0 after oCRH is highly accurate for identifying a pituitary source of ACTH. In addition, a pre-oCRH lateralization (right to left or left to right) ratio more than 1.4 suggests the intrapituitary location of the tumor. Sampling must be performed by experienced personnel, and the accuracy of the test is highly dependent on oCRH administration, symmetric catheter placement, symmetric flow through the venous sinuses, and hypercortisolemia at the time of testing. In addition, it is critical that the diagnosis of Cushing's syndrome and ACTH-dependence be confirmed before proceeding with sampling. Normal individuals and patients with pseudo-Cushing's syndrome have inferior petrosal sinus sampling (IPSS) results that falsely suggest a pituitary tumor. Patients with ACTH-independent disease (primary adrenal disease) with low but measurable ACTH levels can have IPSS results that falsely suggest either a pituitary tumor or the ectopic ACTH syndrome.

Recently, internal jugular venous sampling has been evaluated as a less invasive alternative to petrosal sinus sampling. A jugular to peripheral ratio of greater than 1.7 before oCRH or more than 2.5 after oCRH indicate a pituitary source with high accuracy. Nondiagnostic ratios are unreliable and should be further evaluated with inferior petrosal or cavernous sinus sampling.

If sampling suggests an ectopic source of ACTH, imaging is then performed to locate the tumor, starting with high resolution CT or MRI of the chest. If those areas are unrevealing, neck, abdomen, and pelvis CT are performed. Octreotide scanning may be helpful but only rarely identifies an abnormality not already seen on anatomic imaging. Often, the culprit lesion is not seen at initial imaging, but becomes apparent on serial studies performed every 6 to 12 months.

Although IPSS is highly accurate, occasional false-negative and rare false-positive results have been reported. In situations where IPSS ratios indicate the ectopic ACTH syndrome but no ectopic tumor can be found, distinguishing a truly occult ectopic ACTH-producing tumor from a false-negative IPSS is extremely difficult. Review of the response of peripheral ACTH levels to oCRH stimulation should be done, because pituitary adenomas have significantly more robust responses than ectopic tumors. Repeat IPSS and consideration of

pituitary exploration are appropriate, particularly if the ACTH response to oCRH, biochemical testing, and/or MRI are consistent with a pituitary adenoma.

# Therapeutic Interventions

## EXOGENOUS GLUCOCORTICOID USE

Once identified, the treatment for iatrogenic Cushing's syndrome is straightforward but often difficult because of the therapeutic benefit of pharmacologic glucocorticoids. Tapering the steroid needs to occur gradually, with close monitoring of the underlying disease process and optimization of nonsteroid therapeutics. Alternate-day dosing regimens may assist in HPA axis recovery but may be limited by the underlying disease process. Patients should wear Medic Alert identification until the taper is completed and normal HPA function is demonstrated.

## ENDOGENOUS CUSHING'S SYNDROME

The therapeutic intervention in essentially all etiologies of endogenous Cushing's syndrome is surgical resection of the autonomous tumor or tissue, except for the case of lung carcinomas causing the ectopic ACTH syndrome, where therapy is tailored to the stage of the cancer. Postoperatively, all patients are treated with stress doses of glucocorticoids, tapering quickly to doses approximately twice physiologic replacement, usually hydrocortisone (Cortef)[1] 20 mg by mouth twice or three times daily. Further slow taper is done over the next several months as tolerated by cortisol withdrawal symptoms and recovery of the HPA axis. A morning serum cortisol level less than 2 μg/dL on the second postoperative day is highly predictive of surgical cure; patients with low but detectable serum cortisol levels, such as less than 5 μg/dL, have varying cure rates. Periodic morning cortisol levels and cosyntropin (Cortrosyn)[1] stimulation testing assess recovery of the HPA axis during and after the glucocorticoid taper.

### Cushing's Disease

Transsphenoidal adenomectomy is recommended for the vast majority of patients with pituitary tumors, except where extensive cavernous sinus involvement indicates a transfrontal approach. Intraoperative ultrasound or MRI can assist in the localization of tumors. If a tumor is not identified at surgery, hemihypophysectomy based on preoperative MRI and/or IPSS or CSS lateralization ratios may result in cure. Often, tumors are not identified on pathology, because they are semiliquid and "lost" during suctioning.

Mortality and morbidity are generally low in experienced centers, but complications can include cerebrospinal fluid leaks, meningitis, visual impairment, hypopituitarism, hemorrhage, venous thromboembolism, and death. Careful monitoring for abnormalities in vasopressin secretion postoperatively is required, both for diabetes insipidus and the syndrome of inappropriate antidiuretic-hormone secretion. Testing of pituitary function including free T4, IGF-1 with possible growth hormone stimulation testing and testosterone levels or menstrual history is performed at 6 weeks postoperatively.

Even in experienced hands, long-term cure of hypercortisolemia is difficult, with initial success rates reported from 68.5% to 91% and relapse rates of up to 15% over a 10-year period. Cure rates are worse for macroadenomas or invasive tumors and second surgeries, reported at 40% to 55%. Even with biochemical cure and improvement in symptoms, studies show persistent compromise in quality of life.

### Primary Adrenal Disease

The laparoscopic approach has essentially replaced open surgery with similar mortality, morbidity, and operative times; and shorter postoperative recovery, hospital stays, and decreased acute and chronic pain.

---

[1]Not FDA approved for this indication.

[1]Not FDA approved for this indication.

## TABLE 2  Drugs Used in the Medical Therapy of Cushing's Syndrome

| Medication | Mechanism of Action | Typical Dosage | Reported Efficacy | Common Toxicities |
|---|---|---|---|---|
| **Steroid Biosynthesis Inhibitors** | | | | |
| Ketoconazole (Nizoral)[1] | Blocks multiple steps in cortisol synthesis | 200-1200 mg/d | 70% | Hepatotoxicity, gynecomastia, nausea, edema, rash |
| Metyrapone (Metopirone)[1] | Blocks 11β-hydroxylase | 500-6000 mg/d | 85% | Hirsutism, acne, lethargy, dizziness, ataxia, edema, nausea, rash |
| Aminoglutethimide (Cytadren) | Blocks cholesterol to pregnenelone conversion | 750-2000 mg/d | >60% Useful additive to metyrapone | Lethargy, somnolence, dizziness, rash, fever, nausea, anorexia, hyopthyroidism |
| Mitotane (o,p′-DDD, Lysodren)[1*] | Blocks side-chain cleavage Adrenolytic | 500-12,000 mg/d | 83% | Gastrointestinal, impaired mentation, dizziness, hyperlipidemia, gynecomastia, transient rash, hepatotoxicity |
| **ACTH Release Inhibitors** | | | | |
| Cyproheptadine (Periactin)[1] | Impairs ACTH secretion | 24 mg/d | 30%-50% | Somnolence, hyperphagia, weight gain |
| Bromocriptine (Parlodel)[1] | Impairs ACTH secretion | 3.75-30 mg/d | 25%-42% | Nausea, dry mouth, postural hypotension |
| Octreotide (Sandostatin)[1] | Inhibits ACTH release | 100-600 μg/d | Limited experience, additive to ketoconazole | Diarrhea, gallstones |
| Valproic acid (Depakene)[1] | Potentiates GABA inhibition of CRH and ACTH release | 1-2 g/d | Limited experience, additive to metyrapone | Sedation, nausea, hepatotoxicity, pancreatitis |
| **Glucocorticoid Receptor Antagonist** | | | | |
| Mifepristone (RU-486, Mifeprex)[1] | Glucocorticoid receptor antagonist | 10-25 mg/kg/d | Limited experience | Nausea, vomiting, irregular menses |

[1]Not FDA approved for this indication.
*FDA approved for treatment of adrenocortical carcinoma.
*Abbreviations:* ACTH = adrenocorticotropic hormone; CRH = corticotropin-releasing hormone; GABA = gamma-aminobutyric acid.

The laparoscopic approach is not used in cases of adrenocortical carcinoma or patients with coagulopathy, previous surgery or trauma. Lesion size was previously a limitation, but with increasing experience appears to no longer be a significant factor. Unilateral adrenalectomy is indicated for adrenal adenomas and adrenocortical carcinomas; the rare nodular hyperplasias are treated with bilateral surgery. Adrenalectomy is curative for adrenal adenomas and hyperplasia, but carcinomas are often advanced at presentation and generally have a poor prognosis. Adrenolytic therapy with mitotane (Lysodren) may be necessary to control hypercortisolemia and tumor growth in carcinomas postoperatively.

## Secondary Therapy for Failed Pituitary Surgery or Occult Ectopic Tumors

If transsphenoidal surgery fails to resolve the hypercortisolemia, patients can be offered pituitary irradiation. If a lesion can be targeted, stereotactic radiosurgery with a linear accelerator (LINAC) system, gamma-knife system, or proton beam system offers lower radiation exposure to surrounding normal tissue and theoretically more effective higher doses to the residual tumor than conventional fractionated radiation therapy. Time to control of hypercortisolemia is variable, reported from 6 to 36 months, requiring interim control of hypercortisolemia by either medical therapy or adrenalectomy. Complications of radiation therapy include hypopituitarism, rare optic neuropathy, and rare (and debated) induction of second tumors and brain necrosis. The risk of Nelson's syndrome (rapid and aggressive growth of corticotroph tumors after adrenalectomy) may be lessened with radiation therapy.

Alternatively, and in the cases of ectopic tumors remaining occult, bilateral adrenalectomy can be performed offering immediate control of hypercortisolemia. Both glucocorticoid and mineralocorticoid (fludrocortisone [Florinef] 0.1 mg by mouth once or twice daily)

replacement are generally required. Glucocorticoids are tapered as described above to physiologic doses of hydrocortisone (Cortef)[1] 20 to 30 mg by mouth daily in single or divided doses. Continued surveillance with imaging is required, because of the risk of development of Nelson's syndrome and the occasional, locally invasive, and rarely metastatic potential of ectopic tumors.

## Medical Management of Hypercortisolemia

Medical management of hypercortisolemia has an inadequate efficacy and side-effect profile for primary or long-term use. However, it has a very important role in temporizing the pathologic effects of long-standing Cushing's syndrome in preparation for surgical treatment and while awaiting definitive cure from radiation therapy. Strategies include medications (Table 2) that block glucocorticoid synthesis, inhibit pituitary ACTH secretion, or block glucocorticoid action. None of the agents that inhibit ACTH release is very effective but might be useful in combination therapy. The most effective medications are those that block glucocorticoid synthesis including ketoconazole[1] (Nizoral), metyrapone[1] (Metopirone), and mitotane[1*] (o,p′DDD, Lysodren). These are usually dosed to partially block cortisol production, suppressing it into the normal range. Alternatively, complete adrenal blockade with replacement hydrocortisone can be attempted. Finally, very limited experience with blockade of the glucocorticoid receptor with mifepristone (Mifeprex)[1] has shown clinical efficacy. Because glucocorticoid levels are unaffected, titration of this medication must be done on clinical grounds.

---

[1]Not FDA approved for this indication.
*FDA approved only for adrenocortical carcinoma.

## CURRENT DIAGNOSIS

- The clinical presentation of Cushing's syndrome is nonspecific and overlaps that of other more common diseases such as polycystic ovary syndrome, the metabolic syndrome, and depression.
- Signs and symptoms more specific for Cushing's syndrome include unexplained osteoporosis, muscle weakness, spontaneous ecchymoses, hypokalemia, central obesity, and plethora. Children present with growth failure, generalized obesity, and menstrual irregularities.
- A stepwise approach to the diagnosis helps avoid pitfalls in the interpretation of diagnostic tests. The first step is to confirm the diagnosis of Cushing's syndrome. The second step is to determine if the patient has ACTH-dependent or ACTH-independent disease. The final step is to determine if the ACTH source is eutopic (from the pituitary gland) or ectopic (the ectopic ACTH syndrome).
- The 1 mg ON dex test is easy to perform and has good sensitivity for diagnosing Cushing's syndrome. However, because of its poor specificity, confirmatory testing with measurement of urine free cortisol, midnight serum or salivary cortisol or the dex-CRH test is required.
- Random or CRH-stimulated ACTH levels greater than 10 pg/mL indicate ACTH-dependent disease.
- Biochemical testing is inadequate for distinguishing pituitary tumors from the ectopic ACTH syndrome. Jugular venous sampling has a high positive predictive value, but if negative, inferior petrosal or cavernous sinus sampling with CRH stimulation is required.
- Pituitary MRI is positive in only approximately one half of patients with corticotroph adenomas.

---

*Abbreviations:* ACTH = adrenocorticotropic hormone; CRH = corticotrophin-releasing hormone; dex = dexamethasone; MRI = magnetic resonance imaging; 1 mg ON dex test = 1 mg overnight dexamethasone suppression test.

## CURRENT THERAPY

- Treatment for Cushing's syndrome is primarily surgical and targeted to the pathologic lesion.
- Transsphenoidal adenomectomy is recommended for pituitary-dependent Cushing's disease, but has a long-term success rate of only 60% to 80%.
- Laparoscopic adrenalectomy has replaced open approaches in the management of primary adrenal lesions except for adrenocortical carcinoma, and for second-line treatment after failed pituitary surgery or failure to localize an occult ectopic tumor.
- Definitive secondary treatments for failed pituitary surgery include pituitary irradiation and bilateral adrenalectomy.
- Medical therapy for Cushing's syndrome is difficult, and reserved for surgical failures awaiting benefit from radiation therapy or in preparation for surgical therapy.

## REFERENCES

Bochicchio D, Losa M, Buchfelder M: Factors influencing the immediate and late outcome of Cushing's disease treated by transsphenoidal surgery: A retrospective study by the European Cushing's disease survey group. J Clin Endocrinol Metab 1995;80:3114-3120.

Hammer GD, Tyrrell JB, Lamborn KR, et al: Transsphenoidal microsurgery for Cushing's disease: Initial outcome and long-term results. J Clin Endocrinol Metab 2004;89:6348-6357.

Ilias I, Chang R, Pacak K, et al: Jugular venous sampling: An alternative to petrosal sinus sampling for the diagnostic evaluation of adrenocorticotropic hormone-dependent Cushing's syndrome. J Clin Endocrinol Metab 2004;89:3795-3800.

Leinung MC, Zimmerman D: Cushing's disease in children. Endocrinol Metab Clin North Am 1994;23:629-39.

Mahmoud-Ahmed AS, Suh JH: Radiation therapy for Cushing's disease: A review. Pituitary 2002;5:175-180.

Nieman LK: Medical therapy of Cushing's disease. Pituitary 2002;5:77-82.

Oldfield E, Doppman J, Nieman L, et al: Petrosal sinus sampling with and without corticotropin-releasing hormone for the differential diagnosis of Cushing's syndrome. N Engl J Med 1991;325:897-905.

Papanicolaou DA, Mullen N, Kyrou I, Nieman LK: Nighttime salivary cortisol: A useful test for the diagnosis of Cushing's syndrome. J Clin Endocrinol Metab 2002;87:4515-4521.

Reincke M: Subclinical Cushing's syndrome. Endocrinol Metab Clin North Am 2000;29:43-56.

Yanovski J, Cutler G, Chrousos G, Nieman L: Corticotropin-releasing hormone stimulation following low-dose dexamethasone (Decadron) administration. JAMA 1993;269:2232-2238.

# Diabetes Insipidus

Method of
*Jennifer Kelly, DO, and Arnold M. Moses, MD*

## General Principles of Treating Central (Neurogenic) Diabetes Insipidus

The hormonal treatment of diabetes insipidus is accomplished using the synthetic nanopeptide desmopressin (1-deamino [8-D-arginine] vasopressin; DDAVP). Arginine vasopressin (AVP) is the natural hormone of humans. Desmopressin is a synthetic analogue of AVP that does not constrict smooth muscle and has a longer antidiuretic action than does the natural hormone. Because of its lack of vasoactivity, desmopressin can be used without precipitating angina, abdominal cramps, or headaches. It can also be used to treat diabetes insipidus during pregnancy because it resists inactivation by placental vasopressinase. The available preparations of vasopressin are listed in the table above. The durations of antidiuretic responses to the different preparations are listed in Table 1.

For most patients with diabetes insipidus, the treatment of choice is intranasal desmopressin (100 µg/mL). Two delivery systems are available: a nasal (rhinal) tube, which the patient uses to blow measured amounts (0.05–0.2 mL) into the nose, and a compression pump system, which delivers 0.1 mL (see Current Therapy). Treatment is usually initiated with 10 µg of intranasal desmopressin. Patients are instructed to repeat this dose when polyuria recurs. Some patients respond better if the hormone is administered on a more defined schedule. The dose administered can be increased or decreased in accordance with the patient's response. Patients should be told to drink only when they are thirsty.

Some patients prefer to start therapy with oral desmopressin; others can be switched to the oral preparation when absorption of the intranasal form is decreased in the presence of nasal congestion. The starting dose of the tablet is usually 0.05 mg (half of a 0.1-mg tablet) twice per day. The maintenance dose is gradually adjusted to provide an adequate limitation of water turnover. The daily oral dose may

## CURRENT DIAGNOSIS

Central diabetes insipidus (DI) can be diagnosed as follows:
1. Ensure urine volume is increased to ≥3 L/day in adults.
2. Rule out glycosuria (dipstick will suffice).
3. Measure serum sodium concentration during ad libitum fluid intake.
4. If the serum sodium concentration is *above* normal while urine osmolality is *less than* 300 mOsm per kilogram of water, injection of desmopressin (DDAVP) at least doubles the urine osmolality in patients with central DI. If the urine osmolality response is less, the patient may have nephrogenic DI.
5. If the serum sodium concentration is *normal* while urine osmolality is *less than* 300 mOsm per kilogram of water, additional procedures, including a water deprivation or saline infusion test, may be required. Refer to an experienced specialist.
6. Magnetic resonance imaging to detect the presence or absence of the pituitary hyperintense signal may be helpful in differentiating central DI from primary polydipsia. Plasma arginine vasopressin levels do *not* differentiate these two polyuric conditions.

range from 0.1 to 1.2 mg in divided doses. We do not currently recommend the use of nonhormonal agents such as chlorpropamide (Diabinese),[1] clofibrate,[1,2] or carbamazepine.[1]

In the uncooperative or unconscious patient with diabetes insipidus, desmopressin should be injected subcutaneously, usually starting with 0.5 or 1.0 µg (see Table 1 for duration of action). Subcutaneous AVP is sometimes used in patients with acute onset of diabetes insipidus after head trauma or neurosurgical procedures. Its short duration of action might help prevent water intoxication in patients receiving poorly monitored intravenous fluids. As with desmopressin, it is safest to administer subsequent doses of AVP when polyuria reappears.

As long as untreated patients with diabetes insipidus are conscious, retain normal thirst, and have enough fluid to drink, they seldom become dehydrated. However, severe dehydration with extremely high serum sodium concentrations may occur acutely when patients with untreated diabetes insipidus do not receive adequate fluids (orally or intravenously).

The most common and important problem in the hospitalized patient with diabetes insipidus is iatrogenic hyponatremia. Particularly when it occurs rapidly, hyponatremia may cause severe neurologic problems. Hyponatremia in this setting is caused by overhydration (only rarely does sodium loss contribute) in patients receiving vasopressin and can be prevented by allowing patients to self-regulate their oral intake of fluids whenever possible. When such self-regulation is not

[1]Not FDA approved for this indication.
[2]Not available in the United States.

## CURRENT THERAPY

| Trade Name | Chemical Composition | Concentration | Size | Pharmaceutical Company |
|---|---|---|---|---|
| **Intranasal Preparations** | | | | |
| Desmopressin Rhinal Tube | Desmopressin acetate | 100 µg/mL | 2.5-mL bottle with rhinal tube delivering sprays of 10–20 µg | Ferring |
| DDAVP Rhinal Tube | Desmopressin acetate | 100 µg/mL | 2.5-mL bottle with rhinal tube delivering sprays of 10–20 µg | Aventis |
| DDAVP Nasal Spray | Desmopressin acetate | 100 µg/mL | 5.0-mL bottle with spray pump delivering 50 sprays of 10 µg each | Aventis |
| **Oral Preparation** | | | | |
| DDAVP Tablets | Desmopressin acetate | Not applicable | 0.1-mg, 0.2-mg tablets | Aventis |
| **Injectable Preparations (Subcutaneous, Intravenous)** | | | | |
| DDAVP Injection | Desmopressin acetate | 4 µg/mL | 1.0, 10.0 mL/vials | Aventis |
| Pitressin Injection | Arginine vasopressin | 20 U/mL | 1 mL/vial | Monarch |
| Arginine Vasopressin Injection | Arginine vasopressin | 20 U/mL | 0.5, 1, and 10 mL/vials | American Regent |

*Caution:* Stimate Nasal Spray (desmopressin acetate) is marketed by Aventis Pharmaceuticals in a 2.5-mL nasal spray bottle. It is designed for treating bleeding disorders and contains 1.5 mg/mL desmopressin. Stimate can be confused easily with the less concentrated preparations of desmopressin acetate that are used for treating diabetes insipidus.

**TABLE 1   Mean Time That Urine Remains Hypertonic in Adults with Diabetes Insipidus***

| Route of Administration | Amount Administered | Mean Duration of Action (hr) |
|---|---|---|
| Intranasal desmopressin | 10 µg (0.1 mL) | 12 |
| | 15 µg (0.15 mL) | 16 |
| | 20 µg (0.2 mL) | 20 |
| Subcutaneous or intravenous desmopressin | 0.5 µg | 10 |
| | 1.0 µg | 14 |
| | 2.0 µg | 18 |
| | 4.0 µg | 22 |
| Oral desmopressin | 0.1 mg | 6–8 |
| | 0.2 mg | 8–12 |
| | 0.4 mg | 16–20 |
| Subcutaneous arginine vasopressin | 5 U | 4 |

*Note: Onset of antidiuretic action of subcutaneous or intravenous preparation is 30–45 minutes. Onset of antidiuretic effect of tablets is about 60 minutes.

feasible because the patient is obtunded, has a defective thirst mechanism, or cannot drink, extreme care must be taken in ordering intravenous fluids to prevent hyponatremia. The patient can be maintained in an antidiuretic state by giving vasopressin when the urine becomes dilute. The intravenous fluid should consist largely of 5% dextrose in water with amounts of normal saline gauged to replace daily urinary sodium losses. The volume of intravenous fluid for every 8-hour period should replace 8-hour urine volumes plus estimated 8-hour insensible losses and fluid losses through perspiration and other routes. The amount of intravenous fluid should be adjusted according to plasma sodium, blood urea nitrogen, and creatinine levels. If hypernatremia occurs, the amount of intravenous fluids should be increased accordingly.

If a major decrease in serum sodium concentration occurs, intravenous fluids should be temporarily discontinued, and, if necessitated by clinical manifestations, the patient should be given 200 to 300 mL of 3% saline, perhaps with 40 mg of furosemide (Lasix) intravenously. Temporary discontinuation of vasopressin should also be considered. To emphasize, the patient with central diabetes insipidus whose fluid intake is maintained intravenously presents a major medical problem and must be followed up carefully to maintain normonatremia.

Pregnancy is associated with significant alterations in water metabolism. The osmotic threshold for secretion of vasopressin is lowered and the threshold for thirst reduced, with a resulting decrease in plasma osmolality by about 10 mOsm per kilogram of water. A deficiency of plasma vasopressin can also result from increased degradation of the hormone by placental vasopressinase. This disorder is referred to as *gestational diabetes insipidus* because the symptoms of diabetes insipidus occur only during pregnancy and remit soon after delivery. An underlying subclinical deficiency in vasopressin secretion may also be involved. Gestational diabetes insipidus is treated successfully with desmopressin, which is not degraded by vasopressinase. The dose of desmopressin should be about the same as that used in the nonpregnant state, but the normal range for serum sodium is about 5 mEq/L lower.

## Principles of Treating Specific Problems

### THE ALERT PATIENT WITH INTACT THIRST

When antidiuretic therapy is initiated in the alert patient with diabetes insipidus, the patient must consciously avoid excessive drinking for at least several days. By that time, the thirst mechanism usually adapts to the more normal urine volume. However, some patients must be reminded to avoid excessive drinking, which causes the syndrome of inappropriate antidiuresis. Thirst may be perceived with normal or low serum sodium concentration because of a dry mouth, as might occur with mouth breathing, anticholinergic drugs, β-adrenergic blockers, or cigarette smoking. An occasional patient is hyperdipsic because of increased circulating angiotensin II levels or from hypothalamic involvement, as may occur with sarcoidosis involving the hypothalamus. Use of ice may help limit fluid intake.

### THE ALERT PATIENT WITH ADIPSIA

The alert patient with adipsia presents a difficult management problem in the hospital and particularly after the patient is discharged from the hospital. Because of the loss of thirst perception, normal serum sodium concentration is maintained only with great difficulty. The patient and family must closely and continuously monitor the patient's intake and output of fluids, body weight, and vital signs. Serum sodium concentration and blood urea nitrogen, uric acid, and creatinine levels should be checked often. Such a patient must always relate fluid intake to volume of urine plus fluid losses through perspiration and the gastrointestinal tract. Failure to properly monitor these patients may allow their condition to go unrecognized until they develop severe dehydration. This may require the infusion of normal saline to restore pulse and blood pressure and then water orally or dextrose in water intravenously. Appropriate antidiuretic therapy should be instituted along with the fluids.

### THE CONFUSED, OBTUNDED, OR UNCONSCIOUS PATIENT

When confused, obtunded, or unconscious, such as postoperatively or after head trauma, the patient with diabetes insipidus is monitored in the same ways described for the alert patient with adipsia. The only major difference is that vasopressin must be given by injection or infusion and the fluids given intravenously. In the presence of hypernatremia and associated hypovolemia, normal saline is required to help restore pulse and blood pressure to normal. Otherwise, patients with hypernatremia should be treated with dextrose in water (see later) while antidiuretic therapy is instituted and maintained.

Postoperative hypernatremia should be prevented by the early recognition of diabetes insipidus before, during, and after surgery and by avoidance of osmotic diuretic use during surgery. The patient should be switched to oral fluids as soon as possible, and the adequacy of the patient's thirst mechanism to control fluid intake appropriately should be evaluated. Diabetes insipidus that occurs postoperatively or after head trauma may be variable (biphasic or triphasic), and frequently the diabetes insipidus is transient. Therefore, hormonal treatment should be withheld periodically to determine whether the symptoms of diabetes insipidus recur. After 6 months of diabetes insipidus, remission is very unlikely.

## Special Problems of Fluid Balance

### THE HYPERNATREMIC PATIENT

Hypernatremia in patients with diabetes insipidus is usually associated with normal total body sodium. The hypernatremia is due to loss of free water by way of the kidneys, but losses from the skin and lungs can aggravate the problem. Alterations in the composition of water and solutes in the brain cells may contribute to the symptoms of hypernatremia. An abrupt increase in plasma sodium concentration causes more severe symptoms than does a gradual rise to the same sodium level.

The goal of treating hypernatremia in patients with diabetes insipidus is restoration of normal plasma volume and tonicity. Desmopressin should be injected to maintain concentrated urine. If the patient has circulatory disturbances due to hypovolemia, isotonic saline should be given until systemic hemodynamics are stabilized. In fact, isotonic saline is relatively hypotonic to plasma in patients with severe hypernatremia and simultaneously corrects both volume and water deficits. After volume deficits are corrected, the hypernatremia can be treated intravenously with 5% dextrose in water, or water can be given by mouth if the patient is able to drink.

The water deficit in these patients can be calculated on the basis of the serum sodium concentration and on the assumption that 60% of body weight is water. For example, if the patient's usual weight is 75 kg, total body water would normally be 75 kg × 0.6 = 45 L. If the serum sodium value is 154 mEq/L, the patient has a 10% deficit of water (154 − 140) ÷ 140 and theoretically requires 4.5 L of water to correct the deficit. Continuing losses of water must also be replaced. Despite inaccuracies, including the assumption that body water is always 60% of the body weight and the postulate that water is lost uniformly throughout all body cells, this approach provides an approximate value that can be used in planning therapy. The major problem is determining the appropriate rate at which to lower serum sodium concentration to normal. Because seizures or even fatal cerebral edema may occur when serum sodium concentration is lowered rapidly, the best recommendation is to correct the hypernatremia over 48 to 72 hours and at a rate not exceeding 0.5 to 2.0 mEq/L/hr. As total body water expands, the serum sodium concentration may fall proportionately. Serum electrolyte values should be monitored frequently to ensure an appropriate response.

Treatment of the hypernatremia due to water loss, as occurs in untreated patients with diabetes insipidus, must also address associated electrolyte abnormalities and underlying medical and surgical conditions. An example is the patient with diabetes insipidus with coexisting hyperglycemia. In this case, the "corrected" serum sodium concentration should be used to calculate the water deficit. Slightly low or abnormal serum sodium concentrations in the presence of high serum glucose often result, when corrected, in hypernatremic values. The corrected serum sodium concentrations can be calculated by increasing the sodium concentration by 1.5 mEq/L for every 100 mg/dL increment in the serum glucose concentration above 100 mg/dL. For example, in a patient with a sodium level of 138 mEq/L and a glucose level of 700 mg/dL, the corrected serum sodium concentration is 138 + (1.5 × 6), or 147 mEq/L.

## THE HYPONATREMIC PATIENT

Hyponatremia in diabetes insipidus occurs almost exclusively in patients who are overhydrated orally or parenterally while they are being treated with desmopressin. The severity of hyponatremia correlates closely with the magnitude of fluid overload. The amount of excessive body water can be calculated using the same approach as described for hypernatremia. Rarely, the hyponatremia is aggravated by large amounts of sodium in the urine, probably related to increased levels of atrial natriuretic peptide and glomerular filtration rate and inhibition of aldosterone. The hyponatremia due to natriuresis in the water-overloaded patient can be corrected only partially with saline infusions, because the natriuresis continues until the hypervolemic state is corrected. Hyponatremia can be caused or aggravated by adrenal or thyroid insufficiency.

A large body of literature on the appropriate rate at which to correct hyponatremia is available. Rapidly occurring (acute) and marked hyponatremia can be lethal and should be treated urgently. Under these conditions, and when neurologic symptoms are severe, initial therapy should raise the serum sodium concentration by 1 to 2 mEq/L/hr regardless of the duration of the electrolyte abnormality. Most authorities agree that the rate of change in serum sodium concentrations should not exceed 12 to 20 mEq/L/day. However, in patients with chronic hyponatremia, correction of serum sodium concentration approximating this rate occasionally causes serious, even fatal complications by inducing central pontine myelinolysis.

Fluid restriction is adequate for treatment of the asymptomatic mildly hyponatremic patient. Urine should be analyzed every 4 to 8 hours for volume and osmolality, and fluid replacement should be ordered in relation to *urine volume*. Remember that insensible fluid losses of about 600 mL of free water per day occur in the usual adult. It is *NOT* appropriate to write for a fixed amount of fluid replacement. Plasma sodium concentration should be checked frequently and fluid replacement adjusted according. The complaint of thirst by a water-restricted patient should not be ignored. Long-term management is usually less disrupted by adjusting fluid intake than by discontinuing hormonal therapy and allowing the patient to "break through." Alternatively, when the patient has symptomatic or severe hyponatremia (serum sodium concentration <115 mEq/L in chronic hyponatremia or 125 mEq/L in acute hyponatremia), intravenous furosemide (Lasix), may help by causing the excretion of urine that is lightly hypotonic or isotonic. After injection of 40 mg or more of furosemide, 100 mL of 3% saline should be infused in the first hour. This rate should be decreased or discontinued subsequently if symptoms have ameliorated or if the plasma sodium concentration has increased by more than 2 mEq/L in that hour. Infusion of more than a total of 250 mL of 3% saline is rarely necessary.

## PREPARATION FOR DIAGNOSTIC TESTS OR TREATMENT

Special care must be taken when patients with treated diabetes insipidus are subjected to certain "standard protocols" associated with many diagnostic and therapeutic procedures. These protocols require the patient to be either fluid restricted, as for preparation for intravenous pyelography, or hydrated, as for intravenous administration of chemotherapy. Tests requiring that a patient receiving no oral fluids should be performed with adequate intravenous hydration matched to the patient's urine output. Intravenous fluids should be started from the time the patient is no longer able to take oral fluids and can be discontinued when oral fluids are again allowed. In contrast, patients receiving antidiuretic therapy for diabetes insipidus should not be made to "force fluids" beyond the amounts determined by thirst or be subject to hydration orders at rates not related to urine output. If high urine flow rates are needed, the patient's antidiuretic therapy must be discontinued. Oral or intravenous fluids can then be given to match the large urine volumes. Sometimes, it may be appropriate (to obtain more precise timing of a diuresis) to continue antidiuretic therapy and administer intravenous furosemide. Close monitoring of serum sodium levels will greatly assist in determining the status of fluid balance in these situations.

# Nephrogenic Diabetes Insipidus

Nephrogenic diabetes insipidus is characterized by resistance of the kidney to the antidiuretic action of vasopressin. This disorder is often hereditary, caused by inactivating mutations of the V2 receptor or of the vasopressin-regulated water channel protein aquaporin 2. Standard doses of desmopressin or AVP do not decrease the polyuria. The urine volume can be decreased by 25% to 40% by severe solute restriction and by further inducing hypovolemia with thiazide diuretics. Rarely, very high doses of desmopressin may be effective in females. Occasionally, acquired nephrogenic diabetes insipidus resolves by eliminating the underlying cause (i.e., treating the hypercalcemia or hypokalemia or discontinuing lithium therapy). Nephrogenic diabetes insipidus due to long-term lithium therapy may persist after discontinuation of lithium. Treatment of lithium-induced nephrogenic diabetes insipidus is limited to a low-sodium diet and possibly diuretics. Treatment may reduce urine volume by up to 30% or 40%. Caution must be taken because solute restriction, especially with a diuretic, may lead to lithium toxicity.

## REFERENCES

Adrogue HJ, Madias NE: Hypernatremia. N Engl J Med 2000;342:1493-1499.

Gross P: Treatment of severe hyponatremia. Kidney Int 2001;60:2417-2427.

Moses AM, Clayton B, Hochhauser L: Use of T1-weighted MR imaging to differentiate between primary polydipsia and central diabetes insipidus. AJNR Am J Neuroradiol 1992;13:1273-1277.

Moses AM, Moses LK, Notman D, Springer J: Antidiuretic responses to injected desmopressin, alone and with indomethacin. J Clin Endocrinol Metab 1981;52:910-913.

Moses AM, Scheinman SJ, Oppenheim A: Marked hypotonic polyuria resulting from nephrogenic diabetes insipidus with partial sensitivity to vasopressin. J Clin Endocrinol 1984;59:1044-1049.

Rose BD, Post TW: Clinical Physiology of Acid-Base and Electrolyte Disorders, 5th ed. New York, McGraw-Hill, 2001, pp 716-719, 764-775.

# Primary Hyperparathyroidism and Hypoparathyroidism

Method of
*John P. Bilezikian, MD*

## Primary Hyperparathyroidism

### INCIDENCE AND GENERAL CHARACTERISTICS

Primary hyperparathyroidism (PHPT) is a relatively common endocrine disease with an incidence as high as 1 in 500 to 1 in 1000. The high visibility of PHPT today marks a dramatic change from several generations ago when it was considered rare. The increased incidence is undoubtedly due to widespread use of the multichannel autoanalyzer. PHPT occurs in individuals of all ages but occurs most frequently in the sixth decade of life. Women are affected more often than men by a ratio of 3:1. PHPT in children is an unusual event. It might be a component of one of several endocrinopathies with a genetic basis, such as multiple endocrine neoplasia (MEN), type I or II. PHPT is caused by excessive secretion of parathyroid hormone (PTH) from one or more parathyroid glands. A benign, solitary adenoma is found in 80% of patients. Less commonly, in 15% to 20% of subjects, all four glands are hyperplastic. Four-gland parathyroid disease may occur sporadically or in association with the MEN syndromes. The most uncommon presentation of PHPT is parathyroid cancer, occurring in less than 0.5% of patients with PHPT.

### DIFFERENTIAL DIAGNOSIS

The major diagnostic distinction to be made is between PHPT and malignancy, the other most common cause of hypercalcemia. These two etiologies account for more than 90% of all patients with hypercalcemia (Table 1). A much longer, complete list of potential causes of hypercalcemia is considered after these two etiologies are ruled out or if there is reason to believe that a different cause is likely. Today, PHPT presents most often as an asymptomatic disorder. In contrast, malignancy-associated hypercalcemia is usually found at a later stage of the malignant process and is associated with symptoms. Besides a major difference in clinical presentation between these two most common causes of hypercalcemia, the PTH immunoassay is a helpful distinguishing point. In patients with PHPT, the PTH level will be elevated or in the upper range of normal, whereas in malignancy, the PTH level is invariably suppressed.

### PATHOPHYSIOLOGY, MOLECULAR GENETICS, AND PATHOLOGY

The pathophysiology of PHPT relates to the loss of normal feedback control of PTH by extracellular calcium. Why the parathyroid cell loses its normal sensitivity to calcium is not known. Genetic abnormalities that could be linked to sporadic parathyroid tumors have been described. A rearrangement of the cyclin D1/(PRAD1) proto-oncogene has been seen in some patients with PHPT. The rearrangement associates the PTH gene with the growth promoter cyclin D1. Only a small number of parathyroid tumors have been demonstrated to harbor this defect. Tumor suppressors, such as the gene associated with MEN-I, have generated interest, as have potential abnormalities in the gene for the calcium-sensing receptor. Although the gene for the calcium receptor has been implicated in familial hypocalciuric hypercalcemia and neonatal severe hyperparathyroidism, there is little evidence for this genetic abnormality in the sporadic form of PHPT. Even the vitamin D receptor has been implicated in pathogenetic abnormalities associated with parathyroid neoplasia.

The typical parathyroid adenoma is an enlarged, oval-shaped, smooth, red-brown gland. A visible rim of normal yellow-brown parathyroid tissue is sometimes seen. The typical parathyroid adenoma is between 300 and 500 mg, much larger than a normal gland that generally weighs 35 to 50 mg. Microscopically, the parathyroid adenoma consists of a network of cells arranged alongside a capillary network, resembling classic endocrine microanatomy. Fat cells are reduced or absent. The form of PHPT characterized by four-gland hyperplasia is seen grossly as enlarged glands that may be of equal size. Microscopically, solid masses of chief cells are seen in the absence of fat cells. In contrast to the adenoma, in which a rim of normal tissue can sometimes be seen, normal tissue is absent in hyperplastic disease.

### SIGNS AND SYMPTOMS

PHPT is associated classically with skeletal and renal complications. In severe cases, the skeleton can be involved in a process called *osteitis fibrosa cystica*. Subperiosteal resorption of the distal phalanges, tapering of the distal clavicles, a "salt and pepper" appearance of the skull, bone cysts, and brown tumors of the long bones are all overt manifestations of hyperparathyroid bone disease. This form of hyperparathyroid bone disease is now most unusual, occurring in fewer than 5% of patients with PHPT. Much less severe, but nevertheless significant, skeletal involvement in PHPT is detected by dual energy x-ray absorptiometry (see later). Similar to the reduced incidence of gross skeletal disease, the kidney is also involved in PHPT much less commonly than before. From an incidence of approximately 33% in the 1960s, most series place the incidence of nephrolithiasis now to be no more than 15% to 20%. Nephrolithiasis, nevertheless, is still the most common complication of PHPT. Other renal features of PHPT include diffuse deposition of calcium–phosphate complexes in the parenchyma (nephrocalcinosis). The frequency of this complication is unknown. Hypercalciuria (daily calcium excretion of >250 mg in women or >300 mg in men) is seen in 30% to 40% of patients. PHPT may be associated with a reduction in creatinine clearance, in the absence of any other cause. Classic associations exist between PHPT and other organs, such as the neuromuscular system, the gastrointestinal tract, and the cardiovascular and articular systems, but such panopleistic features of PHPT are rarely seen today. More vexing are nonspecific elements associated with PHPT, such as easy fatigability, a sense of weakness, and a feeling that the aging process is advancing faster than it should be. This is sometimes accompanied by an intellectual weariness and a sense that cognitive faculties are less sharp. Whether these nonspecific features of PHPT are truly part of the disease process, reversible upon successful parathyroid surgery, remains under active investigation.

### CLINICAL FORMS OF PRIMARY HYPERPARATHYROIDISM

Asymptomatic PHPT with serum calcium levels within 1 mg/dL above the upper limits of normal is the most common clinical presentation. Most patients do not have specific complaints and do not show evidence of any target organ complications. In parts of the world where severe vitamin D deficiency is common, more symptomatic PHPT is seen. Unusual clinical presentations of PHPT include MEN-I and MEN-II, familial PHPT not associated with any other endocrine disorder, familial cystic parathyroid adenomatosis, jaw tumor syndrome, and

## TABLE 1   Differential Diagnosis of Hypercalcemia

Primary hyperparathyroidism
Malignancy
Other endocrinopathies
   Hyperthyroidism
   Pheochromocytoma
   Adrenal insufficiency
   VIPoma
Medications
   Lithium
   Thiazides
   Thyroid hormone
   Vitamin D
   Vitamin A
Granulomatous diseases
Familial hypocalciuric hypercalcemia
Immobilization

neonatal PHPT. A new presentation of PHPT is being described, namely, in individuals with normal serum calcium concentrations but elevated PTH levels. Potential secondary causes of elevated PTH levels are considered but have not been found. It is considered likely that these patients represent the earliest stage of PHPT, when there is glandular overproduction of hormone, before hypercalcemia becomes evident.

## DIAGNOSIS AND EVALUATION

Hypercalcemia and elevated levels of PTH establish the diagnosis. The serum phosphorus concentration tends to be in the lower range of normal. Serum alkaline phosphatase activity may be elevated. More specific markers of bone formation (bone-specific alkaline phosphatase, osteocalcin) and bone resorption (urinary deoxypyridinoline, N-telopeptide of collagen) tend to be in the upper range of normal. In some patients, the actions of PTH in altering renal acid-base handling leads to a small increase in the serum chloride concentration and a concomitant small decrease in the serum bicarbonate concentration. Urinary calcium excretion, when elevated, is not generally excessively high. The circulating 25-hydroxyvitamin D concentration is low, and the 1,25-dihydroxyvitamin D concentration is high in some patients.

## ROLE OF BONE MASS MEASUREMENT

Dual-energy x-ray absorptiometry shows a pattern of skeletal involvement that is consistent with the physiologic actions of PTH, that of eroding cortical bone while sparing cancellous sites. The typical patient with PHPT shows reductions in bone density that are most marked in the distal third of the forearm, a cortical site, with much less involvement of the lumbar spine, a cancellous site. The hip region, a mixture of cortical and cancellous bone, shows changes that are intermediate between changes in the forearm and the lumbar spine.

## TREATMENT

### Localization Tests Prior to Surgery

Imaging of abnormal parathyroid tissue is accomplished most accurately with technetium-99m sestamibi. Sestamibi is taken up by both thyroid and parathyroid tissue, but it persists in the parathyroid glands. Various approaches to the use of technetium-99m sestamibi include using the imaging agent alone, and thereby depending upon a difference in uptake kinetics between thyroid and parathyroid tissue, or in combination with iodine 123 ($^{123}$I). Some believe that use of dual isotopic methods provides better definition of the thyroid from which the image obtained with sestamibi can be subtracted. Even more sophisticated approaches have been developed using sestamibi imaging with single-photon emission computed tomography. Ultrasound, computed tomography, and magnetic resonance imaging are also used

## CURRENT DIAGNOSIS

### Primary Hyperparathyroidism

- Most common cause of hypercalcemia.
- Diagnosis established by elevated serum calcium concentration and parathyroid hormone level that is frankly elevated or is in the upper range of normal.
- In some patients, the parathyroid hormone level is elevated but the serum calcium concentration is normal.

### Hypoparathyroidism

- Much less common than primary hyperparathyroidism.
- Most often due to destruction or removal of the parathyroid glands.
- Diagnosis is established by hypocalcemia and low parathyroid hormone levels.

## CURRENT THERAPY

### Primary Hyperparathyroidism

- When symptoms are present, parathyroid surgery is indicated.
- In the absence of symptoms, surgery is recommended if any one of five criteria are met (see Table 2).
- Preoperative localization testing prior to surgery has become routine.
- Medical management is reserved generally for those who do not meet surgical criteria.
- Prudent use of calcium, hydration, and ambulation is encouraged.
- Pharmacologic agents, such as bisphosphonates and calcimimetics, show promise.

### Hypoparathyroidism

- Acute management of hypocalcemia is a medical emergency and requires intravenous administration of calcium.
- Chronic treatment is based upon adequate calcium, vitamin D, and, in some cases, the active vitamin D metabolite 1,25-dihydroxyvitamin D.

to localize abnormal parathyroid tissue. Invasive localization tests with arteriography and selective venous sampling for PTH are used when noninvasive studies have not been successful. In the past, parathyroid imaging was reserved for patients who had undergone neck surgery. With greater success in parathyroid imaging and the increasing popularity of minimally invasive parathyroid surgery, preoperative imaging is becoming routine in all patients.

## SURGERY

PHPT is cured when abnormal parathyroid tissue is removed. Asymptomatic patients are advised to have surgery if they meet current guidelines (Table 2). Symptomatic patients are always advised to undergo parathyroid surgery. At the present time, a number of different surgical procedures can be performed. The standard four-gland parathyroid gland exploration is performed under general or local anesthesia. The single adenoma is removed, and the other glands are ascertained to be normal but not removed. In the case of multiglandular disease, the approach is to remove all tissue except for a remnant that is left in situ or autotransplanted in the nondominant forearm. A popular recent advance in parathyroid surgery is the minimally invasive parathyroidectomy. This procedure depends upon preoperative localization by an imaging technology and confirmation of the success of parathyroid surgery with intraoperative PTH measurements. The circulating PTH level should fall to less than 50% of the preoperative value within minutes after removal of the parathyroid adenoma.

| TABLE 2  Guidelines for Surgical Management of Asymptomatic Primary Hyperparathyroidism* |
| --- |
| Serum calcium >1 mg/dL above normal |
| Hypercalciuria >400 mg/day |
| Reduced creatinine clearance by >30% |
| Reduced bone density below T score of −2.5 at any site |
| Age <50 years |

*These guidelines are meant only for asymptomatic patients with primary hyperparathyroidism. For patients who are symptomatic (i.e., kidney stones, fractures), surgery is recommended unless there are extenuating medical circumstances.

## MEDICAL MANAGEMENT

In patients who do not meet surgical guidelines or who, for other reasons, will not undergo parathyroid surgery, the following medical principles apply. Adequate hydration and ambulation are always encouraged. Thiazide diuretics are to be avoided because they may lead to worsening hypercalcemia. Dietary intake of calcium should be moderate, avoiding both high- and low-calcium diets. Low-calcium diets theoretically could fuel abnormal parathyroid tissue to secrete more PTH. High-calcium diets could be detrimental by worsening hypercalcemia, especially if the 1,25-dihydroxy vitamin D level is elevated. Monitoring with biannual measurements of the serum calcium and annual measurement of bone mass by dual-energy x-ray absorptiometry are recommended. In patients whose 25-hydroxyvitamin D level is low, careful replacement seems reasonable. The serum calcium concentration must be monitored to guard against the potential for worsening hypercalcemia in some patients.

Oral phosphate will lower the serum calcium concentration in PHPT by approximately 0.5 to 1 mg/dL, but concerns about ectopic calcium–phosphate deposition limit its utility. Prior to the results of the Women's Health Initiative, estrogen was an option in postmenopausal women. The serum calcium concentration would fall by about 0.5 mg/dL; estrogens are no longer advised for this specific reason. Preliminary observations suggest that raloxifene, a selective estrogen receptor modulator, may have calcium-lowering effects similar to those of estrogen in postmenopausal women with PHPT.

The bisphosphonate alendronate (Fosamax) has shown promise in patients with PHPT. Lumbar spine bone density improves by as much as 5% in the first year of therapy. Neither the serum calcium concentration nor the PTH level falls significantly. Patients who will not undergo parathyroid surgery but in whom lumbar spine bone density is reduced may benefit from bisphosphonate therapy.

An early clinical experience with hyperparathyroid postmenopausal women has shown that, in principle, a calcimimetic can significantly reduce PTH and serum calcium levels in patients with the disease. By binding to a site on the calcium-sensing receptor, the calcimimetic increases the affinity of the calcium receptor for extracellular calcium. The result is an increase in intracellular calcium and thus reductions in PTH synthesis and secretion. Even though the drug has not yet been approved for use for PHPT in the United States, early data are promising. The serum calcium concentration typically becomes normal and remains within normal limits for as long as the drug is used. Interestingly, the serum PTH level falls only modestly and continues to be elevated despite correction of the hypercalcemia by the drug.

## Hypoparathyroidism

Hypoparathyroidism is much more uncommon than is PHPT. It results from the destruction, removal, or dysfunction of all parathyroid tissue.

### ETIOLOGY

The most common causes of hypoparathyroidism are neck surgery and an autoimmune process (Table 3). Surgical hypoparathyroidism can follow the operation by many years and can occur after any neck surgery. Autoimmune destruction of the parathyroid glands can occur in an isolated fashion or in connection with a variety of polyglandular syndromes. The two major forms are type I (multiple endocrine gland failure along with candidiasis, pernicious anemia, and/or alopecia) and type II (with adrenal or thyroid failure and/or diabetes mellitus). Activating mutations of the calcium-sensing receptor or of the parathyroid gene itself can be associated with hypoparathyroidism. Parathyroid gland destruction is rarely due to infiltration of the glands by iron, copper, granulomas, or malignancy. In severe magnesium deficiency, parathyroid secretion is impaired along with a peripheral resistance to the actions of PTH. Mild hypoparathyroidism can become symptomatic in the presence of a potent bisphosphonate such as alendronate.

---

**TABLE 3  Causes of Hypoparathyroidism**

Parathyroid gland destruction
Postsurgical
Autoimmune
Sporadic
Polyglandular syndromes
Activating antibodies against the calcium-sensing receptor
Infiltration
Iron, copper
Malignancy
Granulomatous
Genetic
Activating mutations of the calcium-sensing receptor
Inactivating mutations in the PTH gene
DiGeorge syndrome
Impaired secretion and/or action of PTH
Hypomagnesemia
Pseudohypoparathyroidism

*Abbreviation:* PTH = parathyroid hormone.

---

## CLINICAL FEATURES

Increased neuromuscular irritability is the clinical hallmark of hypoparathyroidism. Features of hypoparathyroidism can range from mild paresthesias around the mouth, fingers, and toes to muscle cramping, and, at their worst, carpal, pedal, or laryngospasm. Central nervous system seizure activity is also seen as a severe manifestation of hypocalcemia. These symptoms are due, in part, to the actual serum calcium level but also to the rate at which the serum calcium level falls. Rapid declines in the serum calcium concentrations are more likely to be associated with symptoms than to situations in which the serum calcium concentration has fallen gradually. If respiratory or metabolic alkalosis is present, symptoms can worsen because the partition between bound and free calcium is shifted to the bound state when the blood pH rises. Signs of hypocalcemia include the Chvostek sign (evoked facial nerve irritability), the Trousseau sign (carpal spasm when the blood pressure cuff is inflated to pressures above systolic), and a prolonged QT interval on the electrocardiogram. When severe hypocalcemia is present, impaired cardiac contractility, unresponsive to inotropic agents until the hypocalcemia is corrected, has been reported. Pseudopapilledema and subcapsular cataracts can be seen. In some individuals, hypoparathyroidism is detected only by an asymptomatic reduction in the serum calcium concentration. Pseudohypoparathyroidism is a group of genetic disorders of the PTH receptor/G-protein transduction system responsible for PTH action. In the type I variant, subjects have a classic phenotype (Albright's hereditary osteodystrophy) with short stature, brachydactyly, subcutaneous and basal ganglia calcifications, rounded facies, shortened neck, seizures, and below-average intelligence. Other endocrine glands, such as the thyroid and gonads, can also be dysfunctional. In the type II form of pseudohypoparathyroidism, PHT resistance is present in the absence of the clinical phenotype.

## DIAGNOSIS

Hypocalcemia and an elevated serum phosphorus concentration in association with absent PTH levels confirm the diagnosis of hypoparathyroidism. In pseudohypoparathyroidism, PTH levels are elevated, reflecting the PTH-resistant state, but otherwise the biochemical findings of hypocalcemia and hyperphosphatemia are similar to those of hypoparathyroidism. The urinary calcium concentration is usually not elevated because the filtered load of calcium is low, but actually renal handling of calcium is impaired in this setting because of the lack of PTH. Such individuals have an increase in urinary calcium for the given filtered calcium load, even though the actual amount of urinary calcium excretion might not be excessive.

## TREATMENT

The goals of treatment are to establish a serum calcium concentration that is not associated with symptoms or signs and to prevent long-term complications of hypocalcemia. Acute, symptomatic hypocalcemia is a medical emergency and must be treated urgently. The management of chronic hypocalcemia follows a different set of guidelines.

### Acute Management

The initial approach is to infuse intravenously 1 to 2 ampules of calcium gluconate (90–180 mg of elemental calcium), diluted in 50 to 100 mL of 5% dextrose over a 10- to 15-minute period. If the acute symptoms are not quickly ameliorated, another 1 to 2 ampules can be administered. To raise the serum calcium concentration further, but more gradually, an infusion of 15 mg/kg of calcium gluconate in 1 L of 5% dextrose over 8 to 10 hours will raise the serum calcium concentration by 2 to 3 mg/dL. Because 1 ampule of calcium gluconate contains 90 mg of elemental calcium, 9 to 11 ampules of calcium gluconate are required for an average-size adult (60–70 kg). The serum calcium concentration should be monitored frequently. If the hypocalcemia is due to magnesium deficiency, these measures are also appropriate while magnesium is being replaced. Acute administration of magnesium without calcium will not immediately correct hypocalcemia because peripheral resistance to PTH, one component of hypocalcemia induced by magnesium deficiency, is not corrected for several days. Intravenous replacement of magnesium is 2.4 mg/kg, up to 180 mg, over a 10-minute period or a continuous infusion of 576 mg of magnesium over 24 hours.

### Chronic Management

Oral calcium supplementation is required in virtually all patients. The amount varies but is generally in the range of 1 to 3 g in divided doses. The carbonate or citrated form of calcium is most commonly used. Calcium carbonate is generally preferred because it contains the highest amount of elemental calcium. When calcium preparations are given with meals, both the carbonate and the citrated form of calcium are equally bioavailable. The presence of food obviates the need for gastric acid when calcium carbonate is used.

Most patients also require vitamin D. The amount of ergocalciferol (vitamin D$_2$) or cholecalciferol (vitamin D$_3$) ranges from 25,000 to 200,000 IU daily (1.25–10 mg). These large amounts are required because the absence of PTH and hyperphosphatemia both limit the amount of vitamin D that ultimately is converted to 1,25-dihydroxy- vitamin D, the active metabolite in the kidney. Because activation of vitamin D is impaired, much more vitamin D is required. There is no impairment of the first activation step in the liver, namely, from vitamin D to 25-hydroxyvitamin D, the storage form. Because there is no impairment in this step, large amounts of 25-hydroxyvitamin D can accumulate in fat tissues. At times and unpredictably, these stores can be mobilized and lead to hypercalcemia. Sometimes, the hypercalcemia is severe, requiring emergent treatment. Other times, a simple adjustment in the amount of calcium and/or vitamin D is sufficient. In any event, patients receiving large doses of vitamin D should always be regularly monitored for serum calcium concentrations approximately every 3 to 6 months.

Although many patients with hypoparathyroidism can be adequately managed with oral calcium and vitamin D, other patients also require therapy with 1,25-dihydroxyvitamin D, the active metabolite of vitamin D. 1,25-Dihydroxyvitamin D is used in addition to, but not in place of, vitamin D because 1,25-dihydroxyvitamin D alone does not provide for smooth control. Perhaps this is because 1,25-dihydroxyvitamin D is not stored to any appreciable extent in fat tissue. The half-life of 1,25-dihydroxyvitamin D is as short as 6 hours. Therefore, patients managed without parent vitamin D but with 1,25-dihydroxyvitamin D as the only source of vitamin D are more likely to have unpredictable fluctuations in serum calcium concen-tration. The amount of 1,25-dihydroxyvitamin D ranges from 0.5 to 1.0 μg/day. Some patients require more. Enhanced gastrointestinal absorption of calcium with 1,25-dihydroxyvitamin D can lead to hypercalciuria because in hypoparathyroidism there is no PTH to facilitate calcium reabsorption in the renal tubule. Urinary calcium should be checked on a regular basis. If hypercalciuria occurs, the dose of 1,25-dihydroxyvitamin D and/or vitamin D should be adjusted downward. In this situation, a thiazide diuretic such as hydrochlorthiazide[1] can be used to reduce urinary calcium excretion. In pseudohypoparathyroidism, hypercalciuria is less likely to occur because PTH is present and does have some renal effects in reabsorbing filtered calcium.

Another reason for variability in the control of serum calcium concentration in hypoparathyroidism is a change in medications. For example, if a thiazide or loop diuretic is started for hypertension, the serum calcium concentration may increase or decrease, respectively. Glucocorticoids can lead to a reduction in the serum calcium concentration because glucocorticoids interfere with vitamin D action in the gastrointestinal tract. Bile-sequestering resins can interfere with vitamin D absorption. Midcycle changes in estrogen levels in premenopausal women can lead to altered control.

Hypoparathyroidism is one of the few endocrine disorders for which the replacement hormone, namely, PTH, is not yet available, but it is being studied in some clinical trials.

### REFERENCES

Arnold A, Shattuck TM, Mallya SM, et al: Molecular pathogenesis of primary hyperparathyroidism. J Bone Miner Res 2002;17(Suppl. 2):N30-N36.

Bilezikian JP, Silverberg SJ: Management of asymptomatic primary hyperparathyroidism. N Engl J Med 2004;350:1746-1751.

Bilezikian JP, Silverberg SJ: Primary hyperparathyroidism. In Favus M (ed): Primer on the Metabolic Bone Diseases and Disorders of Calcium Metabolism, 5th ed. Washington DC, American Society for Bone and Mineral Research, 2003, pp 230-235.

Bilezikian JP, Brandi ML, Rubin M, Silverberg SJ: Primary hyperparathyroidism: new concepts in clinical, densitometric, and biochemical features. J Int Med 2005;257:6-17.

Bilezikian JP, Potts JT, El-Hajj Fuleihan G, et al: Summary statement from a workshop on asymptomatic primary hyperparathyroidism: A perspective for the 21st century. J Bone Miner Res 2003;17(Suppl. 2):N2-N11.

Khan AA, Bilezikian JP, Kung AWC, et al: Alendronate in primary hyperparathyroidism: a double-blind, randomized, placebo-controlled trial. J Clin Endocrinol Metab 2004;89:3319-3325.

Marx SJ: Hyperparathyroid and hypoparathyroid disorders. N Engl J Med 2000;343:1863-1875.

Miller PD, Bilezikian JP: Bone densitometry in asymptomatic primary hyperparathyroidism. J Bone Miner Res 2002;17(Suppl. 2):N98-N102.

Peacock M, Bilezikian JP, Klassen PS, et al: Cinacalcet hydrochloride maintains long-term normocalcemia in patients with primary hyperparathyroidism. J Clin Endocrinol Metab 2005;90:135-141.

Silverberg SJ, Bilezikian JP: Clinical presentation of primary hyperparathyroidism in the United States. In Bilezikian JP, Marcus R, Levine MA (eds): The Parathyroids, 2nd ed. San Diego, CA, Academic Press, 2001, pp 349-360.

Silverberg SJ, Bilezikian JP: "Incipient" primary hyperparathyroidism: A "forme fruste" of an old disease. J Clin Endocrinol Metab 2003;88:5348-5352.

Stock JL, Marcus R: Medical management of primary hyperparathyroidism. In Bilezikian JP, Marcus R, Levine MA (eds): The Parathyroids, 2nd ed. San Diego, CA, Academic Press, 2001, pp 459-474.

# Primary Aldosteronism

Method of
*William F. Young, Jr., MD, MSc*

Hypertension, suppressed renin, and increased aldosterone secretion characterize the syndrome of primary aldosteronism, which was first described in 1955. Bilateral idiopathic hyperaldosteronism (IHA) and aldosterone-producing adenoma (APA) are the most common subtypes of primary aldosteronism (Box 1). A much less common

---

[1]Not FDA approved for this indication.

## BOX 1   Forms of Primary Aldosteronism

- Aldosterone-producing adenoma (APA)
- Aldosterone-producing adrenocortical carcinoma
- Bilateral idiopathic hyperplasia (IHA)
- Ectopic aldosterone-secreting tumors
- Familial hyperaldosteronism
  - Familial hyperaldosteronism type I: Glucocorticoid-remediable aldosteronism
  - Familial hyperaldosteronism type II: APA or IHA or both
- Primary (unilateral) adrenal hyperplasia

form, unilateral hyperplasia or primary adrenal hyperplasia, is caused by zona glomerulosa hyperplasia of predominantly one adrenal gland. Two forms of familial hyperaldosteronism (FH) have been described: FH type I and FH type II. FH type I, or glucocorticoid-remediable aldosteronism (GRA), is autosomal dominant in inheritance; it is associated with varying degrees of hyperaldosteronism and suppresses with exogenous glucocorticoids. FH type II refers to the familial occurrence of APA or IHA or both. Very rarely, excessive aldosterone may be secreted by a neoplasm outside of the adrenal gland (e.g., ovary).

## Diagnosis

### CASE FINDING

In the past, clinicians did not consider the diagnosis of primary aldosteronism unless the patient presented with spontaneous hypokalemia, and then the diagnostic evaluation required discontinuing antihypertensive medications for 2 weeks. The spontaneous hypokalemia and no antihypertensive drug diagnostic approach resulted in predicted primary aldosteronism prevalence rates of less than 0.5% of hypertensive patients. However, it is now recognized that most patients with primary aldosteronism are not hypokalemic and present with asymptomatic hypertension, which may be mild or severe. When hypokalemia does occur, it may be associated with nocturia, polyuria, muscle cramps, or palpitations.

Case finding can be completed with a simple morning (8-10 AM) blood test (plasma aldosterone concentration [PAC] to plasma renin activity [PRA] ratio) in a seated ambulant patient. The patient may take any antihypertensive drugs except mineralocorticoid-receptor antagonists (spironolactone [Aldactone] and eplerenone [Inspra]) or high-dose amiloride (Midamor). Hypokalemia is associated with false-negative ratios, and any potassium deficit should be corrected before testing. Although there is some uncertainty about test characteristics and lack of standardization, the PAC/PRA ratio is widely accepted as the case-finding test of choice for primary aldosteronism. Spironolactone, eplerenone, and amiloride should be discontinued 4 to 6 weeks before testing for primary aldosteronism.

The use of the PAC/PRA ratio as a case-finding test followed by aldosterone suppression confirmatory testing has resulted in much higher prevalence estimates (5%-13% of all hypertensives) for primary aldosteronism. The prevalence of primary aldosteronism approaches 20% in patients with resistant hypertension. Patients with hypertension and hypokalemia, treatment-resistant hypertension, hypertension and adrenal incidentaloma, onset of hypertension at a young age (<20 y), severe hypertension, or whenever considering secondary hypertension should undergo testing for primary aldosteronism with a PAC/PRA ratio (cutoff is laboratory dependent) (Figure 1). A high PAC/PRA ratio is a positive screening test result, a finding that warrants confirmatory testing.

### CONFIRMING THE DIAGNOSIS

Confirmatory testing is completed with aldosterone suppression testing (oral sodium loading, saline suppression test, or fludrocortisone [Florinef] suppression testing; see references for details on these testing protocols). At the Mayo Clinic, we prefer the high-sodium diet for 3 to 4 days with 24-hour urine collection (days 3 to 4) for aldosterone,

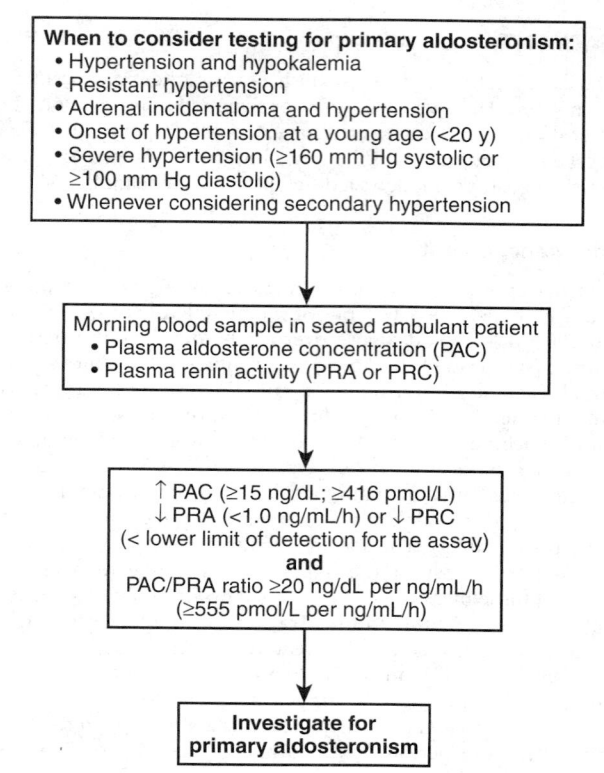

**When to consider testing for primary aldosteronism:**
- Hypertension and hypokalemia
- Resistant hypertension
- Adrenal incidentaloma and hypertension
- Onset of hypertension at a young age (<20 y)
- Severe hypertension (≥160 mm Hg systolic or ≥100 mm Hg diastolic)
- Whenever considering secondary hypertension

Morning blood sample in seated ambulant patient
- Plasma aldosterone concentration (PAC)
- Plasma renin activity (PRA or PRC)

↑ PAC (≥15 ng/dL; ≥416 pmol/L)
↓ PRA (<1.0 ng/mL/h) or ↓ PRC
(< lower limit of detection for the assay)
**and**
PAC/PRA ratio ≥20 ng/dL per ng/mL/h
(≥555 pmol/L per ng/mL/h)

**Investigate for primary aldosteronism**

**FIGURE 1.** In patients with suspected primary aldosteronism, case-finding can be accomplished by measuring a morning (preferably 8 AM) ambulatory paired random PAC and PRA. This test may be performed while the patient is taking antihypertensive medications and without posture stimulation. Spironolactone (Aldactone), eplerenone (Inspra), and high-dose amiloride (Midamor) are the only medications that absolutely interfere with interpretation of the ratio. *Abbreviations*: PAC = plasma aldosterone concentration; PRA = plasma renin activity; PRC = plasma renin concentration.

sodium, and creatinine. When the 24-hour urinary sodium is greater than 200 mEq (confirming adequate sodium loading), patients with primary aldosteronism demonstrate autonomous aldosterone production with urinary aldosterone levels greater than 12 μg/24 hours. During the oral sodium loading, it is important to monitor serum potassium and blood pressure daily and increase potassium supplementation and antihypertensive medications as indicated.

### EVALUATING THE SUBTYPE

Unilateral adrenalectomy in patients with APA or PAH results in normalization of hypokalemia in all; hypertension is improved in all and is cured in approximately 30% to 60% of these patients. In IHA, unilateral or bilateral adrenalectomy seldom corrects the hypertension. IHA and GRA should be treated medically. Therefore, for patients who want to pursue a surgical cure, accurate distinction between the subtypes of primary aldosteronism is a critical step (Figure 2). The subtype evaluation can require one or more tests, the first of which is imaging the adrenal glands with computed tomography (CT) (see Figure 2). When a small, solitary, hypodense macroadenoma (>1 cm and <2 cm) and normal contralateral adrenal morphology are found on CT in a young patient (<40 years) with primary aldosteronism, unilateral adrenalectomy is a reasonable therapeutic option. However, in many cases, CT can show normal-appearing adrenals, minimal unilateral adrenal limb thickening, unilateral microadenomas (1 cm), or bilateral macroadenomas. We have recently found in 203 patients, who were evaluated with both CT and adrenal vein sampling, that CT accurately distinguished APA from IHA in only 53% of patients.

Patients with APAs have more severe hypertension, more frequent hypokalemia, and higher plasma levels (>25 ng/dL; >694 pmol/L) and urinary levels (>30 μg/24 h; >83 nmol/d) of aldosterone, and they are

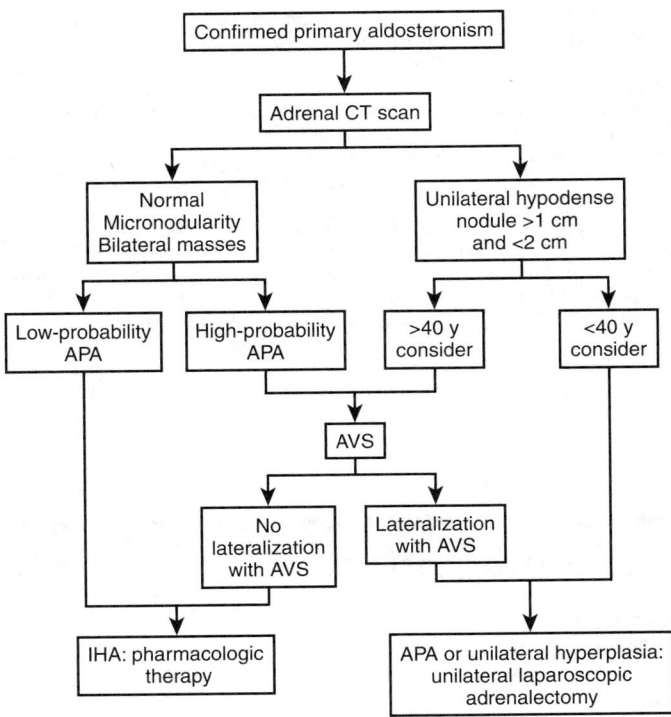

**FIGURE 2.** Subtype evaluation of primary aldosteronism. See text for details. *Abbreviations*: APA = aldosterone-producing adenoma; AVS = adrenal venous sampling; CT = computed tomography; GRA = glucocorticoid-remediable aldosteronism; IHA = idiopathic hyperaldosteronism. (Modified and adapted from Young WF Jr, Hogan MJ: Renin-independent hypermineralocorticoidism. Trends Endocrinol Metab 1994;5:97-106.)

younger (< 50 years) than those with IHA. Patients fitting these descriptors are considered to have a high probability of APA (see Figure 2). However, these factors are not absolute predictors of unilateral versus bilateral adrenal disease. With the addition of adrenal venous sampling (AVS), we have found unilateral APAs in 36% of patients with clinically high-probability APA who had normal findings or unilateral adrenal limb thickening on CT. AVS is essential to direct appropriate therapy in patients who have primary aldosteronism and who want to pursue a surgical treatment option.

# Treatment

## PRINCIPLES

The treatment goal is to prevent the morbidity and mortality associated with hypertension, hypokalemia, and cardiovascular damage. Determining the cause of the primary aldosteronism helps to determine the appropriate treatment. Normalization of blood pressure should not be the only goal in managing the patient who has primary aldosteronism. In addition to the kidneys and colon, mineralocorticoid receptors are present in the heart, brain, and blood vessels. Excessive secretion of aldosterone is associated with increased cardiovascular morbidity. Therefore, normalization of circulating aldosterone or mineralocorticoid receptor blockade should be part of the management plan for all patients with primary aldosteronism.

## SURGERY

Unilateral laparoscopic adrenalectomy is an excellent treatment option for patients with APA or unilateral hyperplasia. Although blood pressure control improves in nearly 100% of patients postoperatively, average long-term cure rates of hypertension after unilateral adrenalectomy for APA range from 30% to 60%. Persistent hypertension following

- Most patients with primary aldosteronism are not hypokalemic and typically present with asymptomatic hypertension, which may be mild or severe.
- Case finding can be completed with a simple morning (8-10 AM) blood test (PAC/PRA ratio) in a seated ambulant patient.
- A high PAC/PRA ratio is a positive screening test result, a finding that warrants confirmatory testing.
- The subtype evaluation can require one or more tests, the first of which is imaging the adrenal glands with computed tomography.
- Adrenal vein sampling is essential to direct appropriate therapy in patients with primary aldosteronism who want to pursue a surgical treatment option.

*Abbreviations*: PAC = plasma aldosterone concentration; PRA = plasma renin activity.

adrenalectomy is correlated directly with having more than one first-degree relative with hypertension, use of more than two antihypertensive agents preoperatively, older age, increased serum creatinine, and duration of hypertension and is most likely due to coexistent primary hypertension.

Laparoscopic adrenalectomy is the preferred surgical approach and is associated with shorter hospital stays and less long-term morbidity than the conventional open approach. To decrease the surgical risk, hypokalemia should be corrected with spironolactone or eplerenone preoperatively; treatment with these drugs should be discontinued postoperatively. PAC should be measured shortly after the operation. For the first few weeks postoperatively, serum potassium levels should be monitored weekly and a generous sodium diet should be followed to prevent the hyperkalemia of hypoaldosteronism that can occur because of chronic suppression of the renin-angiotensin-aldosterone axis. Typically, the hypertension resolves in 1 to 3 months postoperatively. It has been found that adrenalectomy for APA is significantly less expensive than long-term medical therapy alone.

## PHARMACOLOGIC TREATMENT

IHA and GRA should be treated medically. APA patients may be treated medically if the medical treatment includes mineralocorticoid receptor blockade. A sodium-restricted diet (<100 mEq/day of sodium), maintenance of ideal body weight, tobacco avoidance, and

- Because of aldosterone-related cardiovascular toxicity, normalization of circulating aldosterone or mineralocorticoid receptor blockade should be part of the management plan for all patients with primary aldosteronism.
- Unilateral laparoscopic adrenalectomy is an excellent treatment option for patients with aldosterone-producing adenoma or unilateral hyperplasia.
- Patients with bilateral IHA and GRA should be treated medically with a mineralocorticoid receptor antagonist (e.g., spironolactone [Aldactone] or eplerenone [Inspra][1]).

[1]Not FDA approved for this indication.
*Abbreviations*: GRA = Glucocorticoid-remediable aldosteronism; IHA = idiopathic hyperplasia.

regular aerobic exercise contribute significantly to the success of pharmacologic treatment. There have been no placebo-controlled, randomized trials evaluating the relative efficacy of drugs in the treatment of primary aldosteronism.

Spironolactone has been the drug of choice to treat primary aldosteronism for more than 4 decades. It is available in 25-, 50-, and 100-mg tablets. The dosage is 25 mg/day initially and is increased to 400 mg/day if necessary to achieve normokalemia without the aid of oral potassium chloride supplementation. Hypokalemia responds promptly, but hypertension can take as long as 4 to 8 weeks to be corrected. After several months of therapy, this dosage often can be decreased to as little as 25 to 50 mg/day; dosage titration is based on a goal serum potassium level in the high-normal range. Serum potassium should be monitored frequently during the first 4 to 6 weeks of therapy (especially in patients with renal insufficiency or diabetes mellitus). Spironolactone can increase the half-life of digoxin (Lanoxin), and for patients taking this drug, the dosage might need to be adjusted when treatment with spironolactone is started. Concomitant therapy with salicylates should be avoided because they interfere with the tubular secretion of an active metabolite and decrease the effectiveness of spironolactone. Unfortunately, spironolactone is not selective for the mineralocorticoid receptors. For example, antagonism at the testosterone receptor in men can result in painful gynecomastia and impotence. Agonist effects at the progesterone receptor in women can result in menstrual irregularity.

Eplerenone is a new steroid-based antimineralocorticoid, which acts as a competitive and selective mineralocorticoid receptor antagonist. It was approved by the FDA for treating uncomplicated essential hypertension in late 2003. The 9,11-epoxide group in eplerenone results in a significant reduction of the molecule's progestational and antiandrogenic actions compared with spironolactone. Treatment trials comparing the efficacy of eplerenone with spironolactone for treating primary aldosteronism have not been published. Presumably, eplerenone[1] will be the superior drug if it is shown to be as effective as spironolactone for treating mineralocorticoid-dependent hypertension and if it lacks the limiting antiandrogen side effects of spironolactone.

Patients with IHA often require a second antihypertensive agent to achieve good blood pressure control. Hypervolemia is a major reason for resistance to drug therapy, and low doses of a thiazide diuretic (e.g., 12.5-50 mg of hydrochlorothiazide daily) are effective in combination with the mineralocorticoid-receptor antagonist. Because these agents often lead to further hypokalemia, serum potassium levels should be monitored.

## SPECIAL TREATMENT INDICATIONS

### Glucocorticoid Remediable Aldosteronism

Before initiating treatment, GRA should be confirmed with genetic testing. Genetic testing for GRA should be considered in patients with a family history of primary aldosteronism, onset of primary aldosteronism at a young age, or stroke at a young age. In the GRA patient, chronic treatment with physiologic doses of a glucocorticoid (just as patients with congenital adrenal hyperplasia are treated) normalizes blood pressure and corrects hypokalemia. However, treatment with spironolactone in these patients is just as effective and avoids the potential disruption of the hypothalamic-pituitary-adrenal axis and risk of iatrogenic side effects.

### Aldosterone-Producing Adrenal Malignancies

It is difficult to make the diagnosis of adrenal malignancy on the basis of microscopic examination. The only absolute criteria are local invasion or metastatic lesions. Surgical excision is the treatment of choice. Mitotane (Lysodren, o,p′-DDD) is used in patients with persistent tumors.

### REFERENCES

Lim PO, Young WF, MacDonald TM: A review of the medical treatment of primary aldosteronism. J Hypertens 2001;19:353-361.

Montori VM, Young WF Jr: Use of plasma aldosterone concentration-to-plasma renin activity ratio as a screening test for primary aldosteronism: A systematic review of the literature. Endocrinol Metab Clin North Am 2002;31:619-632.

Mulatero P, Stowasser M, Loh K-C, et al: Increased diagnosis of primary aldosteronism, including surgically correctable forms, in centers from five continents. J Clin Endocrinol Metab 2004;89:1045-1050.

Sawka AM, Young WF Jr, Thompson GB, et al: Primary aldosteronism: Factors associated with normalization of blood pressure after surgery. Ann Intern Med 2001;135:258-261.

Sywak M, Pasieka JL: Long-term follow-up and cost benefit of adrenalectomy in patients with primary hyperaldosteronism. Br J Surg 2002;89:1587-1593.

Young WF Jr: Minireview: Primary aldosteronism: Changing concepts in diagnosis and treatment. Endocrinology 2003;144:2208-2213.

Young WF Jr: Primary aldosteronism: Management issues. Ann N Y Acad. Sci 2002;970:61-76.

Young WF Jr, Stanson AW, Thompson GB, et al: Role for adrenal venous sampling in primary aldosteronism. Surgery 2004;136:1227-1235.

# Hypopituitarism

Method of
*Mary Lee Vance, MD*

## Definition

Hypopituitarism is target endocrine gland failure because of insufficient hypothalamic or pituitary hormone stimulation of the target gland or tissue. Loss of hypothalamic or pituitary hormone production may cause secondary adrenal insufficiency, secondary hypothyroidism, secondary gonadal failure, growth hormone (GH) deficiency, and/or diabetes insipidus (DI), alone or in combination. Regardless of the etiology, replacement of glucocorticoid and thyroid hormone is necessary to sustain life; replacement of gonadal steroids, GH, and antidiuretic hormone is necessary for normal function and for prevention of morbidity. Loss of all pituitary function is termed *panhypopituitarism;* loss of one or more pituitary hormones is termed *partial hypopituitarism.*

## Etiology

The most common cause of hypopituitarism is a pituitary lesion (pituitary adenoma, craniopharyngioma, Rathke's cleft cyst) or infiltrative disease (lymphocytic hypophysitis, sarcoidosis, metastatic tumor) (Table 1). In general, the larger the pituitary lesion, the greater the likelihood of loss of pituitary function. Infiltrative disease often causes permanent loss of pituitary function. Selective removal of a pituitary adenoma, taking care to avoid damage to remaining normal pituitary tissue, may result in recovery of pituitary function.

Hypopituitarism also occurs as a result of any type of pituitary radiation for a pituitary lesion, total brain radiation for a brain lesion, or head and neck radiation for carcinoma (the radiation field often involves the pituitary gland). Head trauma may cause loss of pituitary function, occurring in up to 36% of patients studied. Less commonly, developmental defects of the hypothalamus or pituitary cause loss of pituitary function.

## Diagnosis

The diagnosis of pituitary deficiency is often straightforward but sometimes requires a definitive stimulation test to assess hypothalamic-pituitary-adrenal function and GH reserve. In a patient who presents with a large pituitary lesion, the most critical determination is the need for glucocorticoid and thyroid hormone replacement before recommending surgical resection or medical treatment (macroprolactinoma). A subnormal morning serum cortisol or subnormal free thyroxine (FT$_4$)

## TABLE 1 Causes of Hypopituitarism

**Hypothalamic Disease**
- Histocytosis
- Eosinophilic granuloma
- Sarcoidosis
- Hypothalamic tumor (gangliocytoma, hamartoma, optic nerve glioma, third-ventricle tumor)
- Metastatic tumor
- Congenital midline defects

**Pituitary Disease**
- Pituitary adenoma
- Craniopharyngioma
- Rathke's cleft cyst
- Pilocytic astrocytoma
- Infiltrative disease (giant cell granuloma, sarcoidosis, lymphocytic hypophysitis, lymphoma, plasmacytoma, metastatic tumor)
- Chordoma with pituitary involvement
- Parasellar/suprasellar meningioma
- Pituitary apoplexy (hemorrhage into pituitary adenoma, postpartum hemorrhage)
- Congenital pituitary hypoplasia

**Radiation**
- Cranial
- Pituitary
- Head/neck

**Infection**
- Tuberculosis
- Mycoses

**Miscellaneous**
- Head trauma
- Empty sella
- Carotid-cavernous aneurysm

## CURRENT DIAGNOSIS

- Diagnosis is biochemical in association with clinical features. Diagnosis may require a stimulation test to determine the need for replacement of glucocorticoid, growth hormone, or both.
- Initial patient evaluation should include measurement of concentrations of early-morning serum cortisol, adrenocorticotropic hormone (ACTH), $FT_4$, gonadotropins (luteinizing hormone [LH], follicle-stimulating hormone [FSH]), insulin-like growth factor-1 (IGF-1), and testosterone (in men); menstrual history should be obtained from premenopausal women.

low or in the normal range. A normal morning serum cortisol concentration does not provide information regarding the ACTH-cortisol response to stress; the definitive study is an insulin hypoglycemia test in which the serum glucose concentration decreases to 40 mg/dL or less and the serum cortisol concentration increases to 18 µg/dL or greater to exclude secondary impaired hypothalamic-pituitary-adrenal reserve. This test is also the most rigorous test of GH reserve to determine the need for GH replacement (stimulated serum GH concentration <5 ng/mL indicates GH deficiency). Cortisol stimulation with ACTH (Cortrosyn stimulation test) may be misleading in patients with recent ACTH deficiency in whom the cortisol response is normal but the ACTH response to stress is impaired. For this reason, an ACTH stimulation test should not be performed in the immediate postoperative period. It is prudent to wait 4 to 6 weeks after surgery before performing this test.

A subnormal serum $FT_4$ concentration, often in the setting of a "normal" serum thyroid-stimulating hormone (TSH) concentration (not normal for a low $FT_4$), indicates the need for thyroid hormone replacement.

### SECONDARY GONADAL FAILURE

The diagnosis of secondary gonadal failure is straightforward. Chronic amenorrhea in a premenopausal woman indicates gonadotropin insufficiency. In premenopausal women, serum LH and FSH concentrations are typically either low or "normal"; the estradiol level is usually low or in the follicular phase range. In men, a low serum testosterone concentration indicates gonadal insufficiency; a low serum testosterone concentration but LH and FSH concentrations within the "normal" range indicate secondary gonadal failure.

### GROWTH HORMONE DEFICIENCY

The diagnosis of GH deficiency is more complicated, usually requiring a stimulation test. In a patient with three or four other pituitary hormone deficiencies, the probability of GH deficiency is 96% and 99%, respectively. Three or four pituitary hormone deficiencies and a serum IGF-1 concentration less than 84 µg/L reliably predicted GH deficiency in more than 95% of patients. Despite this finding, many third-party payers (insurance companies) require the results of a stimulation test confirming GH deficiency because of the cost and misuse of GH. The most rigorous test for determining GH deficiency is the insulin hypoglycemia test; the next "best" test is the arginine–growth hormone-releasing hormone test. Other tests of GH reserve, such as arginine or clonidine, are less reliable.

## Treatment

Treatment of hypopituitarism requires replacement of all hormone deficiencies with adjustment of hormone doses based on both hormone levels and clinical response. Optimal hormone replacement is the goal. Optimal hormone replacement often requires a great deal of time and effort; "one dose" is not suitable for all patients.

concentration indicates the need for immediate replacement. In a patient who has undergone pituitary surgery, it is important to review the operative note to assess the amount of resection and to make an estimate of remaining pituitary gland (unfortunately, this estimate is not always mentioned in the operative report).

A history of frequent nocturia, polyuria, and excessive thirst is indicative of DI. Diabetes insipidus most commonly occurs in patients with a craniopharyngioma, Rathke's cleft cyst, or infiltrative disease such as lymphocytic hypophysitis or sarcoidosis. An extensive surgical resection in a patient with one of the aforementioned lesions involving the pituitary stalk indicates a high probability of permanent DI. Extensive surgical resection may also damage the pituitary stalk and cause DI. Serum sodium concentration is usually normal in these DI patients who have normal thirst sensation. Serum osmolality usually is normal; urine osmolality usually is low. The diagnosis of DI is made clinically for a patient with a pituitary lesion and does not usually require a formal water deprivation test. A subnormal morning serum cortisol or $FT_4$ level concentration requires prompt glucocorticoid or thyroxine replacement.

A patient who has a large pituitary lesion commonly has loss of some or all anterior pituitary hormone production. This loss is less common in a patient with a small pituitary lesion but requires evaluation and replacement as indicated. In general, a stimulation test to assess for hypothalamic-pituitary-adrenal function to determine the need for cortisol replacement and for GH deficiency should be conducted after surgical removal of the lesion. Recovery of pituitary function after surgical removal of the lesion may occur but is not common; approximately 6% of patients have recovery of some pituitary function after surgery. Postoperative or postradiation assessment should include clinical history (menses in premenopausal women, sexual function in men, symptoms of hypothyroidism, adrenal insufficiency, DI) and basal and dynamic endocrine testing.

A subnormal morning serum cortisol concentration (without administration of steroid for 2–3 days) is usually adequate to diagnose secondary adrenal insufficiency; the serum ACTH concentration may be

## CURRENT THERAPY

- All hormone deficiencies require replacement. Optimal replacement often requires dose adjustments.
- Dose adjustments should be made at appropriate intervals (e.g., after 6 weeks of thyroid hormone or GH replacement).
- Dose adjustments may be necessary in pregnancy (thyroid hormone) or with addition of estrogen (growth hormone).
- Growth hormone replacement is not approved during pregnancy.

Glucocorticoid replacement exemplifies the "art of medicine": no blood test accurately assesses the adequacy or insufficiency of a glucocorticoid dose. In general, a daily dose of hydrocortisone (Cortef) 15 mg on awakening and 5 mg at 6 PM or prednisone 5 mg on awakening and 2.5 mg at 6 PM should be adequate replacement. However, patients who gain weight on this regimen may feel well with a lower dose of hydrocortisone 10 mg on awakening and 5 mg at 6 PM or only 5 mg of prednisone on awakening. Rarely, a patient receiving hydrocortisone replacement requires dosing three times daily. Glucocorticoid replacement with dexamethasone is discouraged because of the long biologic half-life and cumulative effect causing symptoms of Cushing's syndrome and bone loss. Mineralocorticoid therapy (fludrocortisone [Florinef]) is not required in a patient with secondary adrenal insufficiency because mineralocorticoid (aldosterone) secretion is not regulated chronically by pituitary ACTH secretion. Patients should be instructed to double the glucocorticoid dose during intercurrent illness (such as flu, urinary tract infection) and to always wear a medical alert necklace or bracelet.

### THYROID HORMONE REPLACEMENT

Thyroid hormone replacement with L-thyroxine (Synthroid, Levoxyl) should be monitored by measuring $FT_4$, not TSH. Because the TSH level in patients with hypopituitarism is often low, basing hormone replacement therapy on TSH level could result in an inappropriate reduction of the thyroid hormone dose. In healthy patients with no history of coronary artery disease or angina, a beginning dose of 0.088 or 0.1 mg daily is reasonable, with dose adjustment after 1 month of therapy according to the serum free $T_4$ concentration and clinical response. Thyroid hormone replacement in the elderly or in patients with coronary artery disease should be initiated with a small dose (e.g., 0.025 mg/day) and gradually increased to achieve a normal serum $FT_4$ concentration.

### GONADAL STEROID REPLACEMENT

Gonadal steroid replacement in men is most often accomplished physiologically with either a testosterone gel (AndroGel) or a testosterone patch (Androderm) that delivers a physiologic dose over 24 hours. Intramuscular testosterone, testosterone enanthate (Delatestryl), and testosterone cypionate are not physiologic and often result in supraphysiologic levels soon after injection and subphysiologic levels before the next injection. Depending on the interval after injection, intramuscular testosterone may cause mood swings, including irritability and depression. This formulation may cause erythrocytosis and elevated hemoglobin and hematocrit levels. If the patient must use the intramuscular formulation, hemoglobin and hematocrit levels should be monitored periodically. A buccal formulation of testosterone (Striant) is available and requires multiple daily doses; irritation of the gums may occur. Men should undergo a prostate examination and determination of serum prostate-specific antigen concentration yearly. Testosterone replacement does not cause prostate cancer but may promote growth of an undiagnosed carcinoma. Premenopausal women should receive cyclic estrogen and progesterone replacement for its beneficial effect on bone physiology and libido and for prevention of hot flashes. This can be accomplished with an oral contraceptive or cyclic estradiol and progesterone treatment. Annual gynecologic and breast examinations are necessary.

## HORMONE REPLACEMENT FOR DIABETES INSIPIDUS

Hormone replacement for DI with desmopressin acetate (DDAVP) can be administered as an oral formulation or as a nasal spray. Because the duration of biologic activity varies among patients, the beginning dose should be low (0.1-mg tablet at bedtime), and dose frequency should be changed according to the duration of activity. Some patients are controlled with a single bedtime dose, whereas others require dosing two or three times daily. The patient can sense when the effect of desmopressin wears off because of frequent urination and return of increased thirst.

## GROWTH HORMONE REPLACEMENT

Growth hormone (Genotropin, Humatrope, Norditropin, Nutropin) replacement is indicated in GH-deficient adults. The recommendation is to begin with a small dose (0.3 mg/day by subcutaneous injection) and then titrate the dose every 4 to 6 weeks according to the serum IGF-1 level and symptoms. An optimal serum IGF-1 level is at the middle or a little above the middle of the age-adjusted normal range. Women usually require a higher final dose than do men, and women receiving oral estrogen replacement usually require a higher final dose to achieve an optimal serum IGF-1 level than do women not receiving oral estrogen. Patients should be informed that a beneficial effect on energy, endurance, body composition, and serum lipid levels may not be noted for several months (6 months or more). Patients receiving GH replacement should be monitored every 6 months with a serum IGF-1 measurement, to determine the adequacy of the dose, and yearly serum lipid measurements.

## Summary and Conclusions

Loss of pituitary function is common in patients with a hypothalamic or pituitary lesion, resulting either from the lesion or the treatment; these patients require regular monitoring and treatment as indicated. Patients who have undergone pituitary or cranial radiation therapy are always at risk for developing a new pituitary deficiency. Knowing if, or when, a new pituitary deficiency will occur is not possible, thus emphasizing the need for regular endocrine assessment. Optimal hormone replacement is similar to the best possible management of a patient with diabetes mellitus—frequent monitoring and adjustment of hormone doses based on hormone measurements and clinical response. The goal is accurate diagnosis and optimal replacement to prevent risk of premature mortality. With hormone replacement, a patient can lead a normal and productive life.

### REFERENCES

Cook DM, Ludlam WH, Cook MB: Route of estrogen administration helps to determine growth hormone (GH) replacement dose in GH-deficient adults. J Clin Endocrinol Metab 1999;84:3956-3960.

Hartman ML, Crowe BJ, Biller BM, et al: Which patients do not require a GH stimulation test for the diagnosis of adult GH deficiency? J Clin Endocrinol Metab 2002;87:477-485.

Kelly KF, Gonzalo IT, Cohan P, et al: Hypopituitarism following traumatic brain injury and aneurysmal subarachnoid hemorrhage: A preliminary report. J Neurosurg 2000;93:743-752.

Lieberman SA, Oberoi AL, Gilkison CR, et al: Prevalence of neuroendocrine dysfunction in patients recovering from traumatic brain injury. J Clin Endocrinol Metab 2001;86:2752-2756.

Vance ML: Hypopituitarism. N Engl J Med 1994;330:1651-1662.

# Hyperprolactinemia

Method of
*Joumana T. Chaiban, MD, and Baha M. Arafah, MD*

Hyperprolactinemia is a commonly observed entity that can have significant health implications. Approximately 10% of women with amenorrhea and 75% of those with galactorrhea have some degree of hyperprolactinemia. Similarly, hyperprolactinemia was observed in 10% to 20% of women presenting with infertility and in nearly 10% men presenting with erectile dysfunction. The prevalence of hyperprolactinemia in the general population is more than 4%. It may be caused by a variety of conditions ranging from physiologic states such as stress to pathologic conditions such as prolactin-secreting pituitary adenomas.

## Physiology of Prolactin Secretion and Function

Dopamine, secreted by the hypothalamus, is the main modulator of prolactin secretion by the pituitary. Unlike other anterior pituitary hormones, prolactin is under predominantly inhibitory influence by the hypothalamus. Dopamine, transported from the hypothalamus through portal vessels to the anterior pituitary, tonically inhibits prolactin synthesis and secretion by pituitary lactotrophs. In addition to the dominant inhibitory influence of dopamine, other factors are also involved in regulating prolactin release, such as the stimulatory influence of estrogen, the hypothalamic hormone, thyrotropin-releasing hormone (TRH), and, to a lesser extent, serotonin.

In most patients, prolactin circulates predominantly as a 23-kD monomer, with trace amounts of polymers of the monomeric form as a 60-kD species. In addition, prolactin circulates as a high-molecular-weight form termed *big big prolactin* or *macroprolactin*. The latter molecular forms of prolactin have minimal biological activity but are measured in the serum assay systems. Recognizing this entity is important because some patients have an increase in the percentage of circulating macroprolactin and are often confused with patients with true hyperprolactinemia. Prolactin secretion is pulsatile and is often increased by physiologic stimuli such as sleep and emotional and physical stressors. Serum prolactin levels are generally less than 25 µg/L in women and less than 20 µg/L in men.

The main physiologic function of prolactin is to stimulate lactation. Other hormones (e.g., estrogen) are also necessary for prolactin to induce lactation. There is a 10-fold increase in prolactin secretion during pregnancy and lactation, such that serum prolactin levels reach nearly 500 µg/L by the third trimester, with gradual decline to high normal values in the postpartum period. Serum prolactin levels continue to be elevated, with periodic surges in the level during suckling, thus maintaining lactogenesis. The persistence of hyperprolactinemia for more than 1 year after normal delivery and cessation of breast-feeding, or its occurrence in the absence of pregnancy, is generally considered inappropriate and should raise concern for pathologic states of hyperprolactinemia.

## Causes of Hyperprolactinemia

Although hyperprolactinemia can be a normal transient response to physiologic events such as pregnancy, it is often a manifestation of a pathologic entity or drug intake (Box 1). Physiologic causes of hyperprolactinemia are usually self-evident and, with the exception of pregnancy, are associated with mild and transient elevations in serum prolactin levels. Recognizing the dominant inhibitory effects of dopamine on prolactin secretion makes it easier to understand why hyperprolactinemia is a common feature in patients receiving drugs that are dopamine antagonists (e.g., antipsychotics) or others that interfere with dopamine synthesis. Similarly, estrogen stimulates pituitary lactotrophs and causes increased prolactin secretion. Although the mechanism is unknown,

## BOX 1 Causes of Hyperprolactinemia

**Physiologic States**
- Lactation
- Pregnancy
- Sleep
- Stress
- Suckling

**Drugs**
- Dopamine receptor antagonists
- Estrogens
- Inhibitors of dopamine synthesis or release
- Monoamine oxidase inhibitors
- Verapamil

**Pathologic Conditions**
*Pituitary Diseases*
- Compression of pituitary stalk or portal vessels by a perisellar mass
- Nonsecreting adenomas
- Prolactin-secreting pituitary tumors

*Hypothalamic Diseases*
- Cranial irradiation
- Granulomatous diseases
- Infiltrative diseases
- Tumors: Primary or metastatic
- Other

*Neurogenic Disorders*
- Breast or nipple stimulation
- Chest wall injury
- Spinal cord lesions
- Suckling

*Miscellaneous Conditions*
- Chronic renal failure
- Idiopathic
- Macroprolactin
- Polycystic ovary disease
- Primary hypothyroidism

verapamil (Calan) is one of the calcium channel blockers that was recently associated with development of hyperprolactinemia.

Less than one third of patients with severe long-standing primary hypothyroidism have mild elevations (up to 25-40 µg/L) in their serum prolactin levels that return to normal with physiologic thyroxine therapy. It is postulated that the increased hypothalamic secretion of TRH that accompanies primary hypothyroidism is responsible for the mild hyperprolactinemia in such cases. Decreased clearance of prolactin and alterations in hypothalamic dopamine regulation are the postulated mechanisms for hyperprolactinemia in patients with renal failure.

In light of the dominant inhibitory influence of hypothalamic hormones on prolactin secretion, it would not be surprising to know that hyperprolactinemia is a common feature of hypothalamic diseases and of perisellar mass lesions (e.g., meningiomas, pituitary tumors) that obstruct the flow through portal vessels. These instances of hyperprolactinemia are often associated with varying degrees of deficiencies in other anterior pituitary hormone functions (hypopituitarism).

## Hyperprolactinemia and Pituitary Tumors

As shown in Table 1, several potential pathophysiologic mechanisms can account for the occurrence of hyperprolactinemia in patients with pituitary adenomas. In such instances, prolactin can be

**TABLE 1  Causes of Hyperprolactinemia in Patients with Pituitary Tumors**

| Tumor Type | Mechanism | Expected Serum Prolactin Levels |
|---|---|---|
| **Functioning Tumors** | | |
| Pure prolactin-secreting | Secretes prolactin only | >100 µg/L |
| Mixed-cell tumors | Secretes prolactin and other hormones (e.g., growth hormone) | 30-100 µg/L |
| Non–prolactin-secreting | Prolactin is secreted by the normal pituitary through compression of portal vessels and pituitary stalk | 25-75 µg/L |
| **Other Pituitary Tumors** | | |
| Nonfunctioning tumors | Prolactin is secreted by the normal pituitary through compression of portal vessels and pituitary stalk | 25-75 µg/L |
| Functioning and non-functioning tumors | Prolactin is secreted by the normal pituitary through other mechanisms (e.g., dopamine antagonists, estrogen) | 25-75 µg/L |

secreted autonomously by the tumor itself, and the serum levels are usually very high (>100 µg/L). Alternatively, prolactin can be secreted by the normal pituitary gland through different mechanisms (see Table 1), and the associated serum levels will be lower, depending on the cause. In patients with pituitary tumors, the manifestations of hyperprolactinemia can vary depending on the type and size of the tumor under discussion. For example, patients with large pituitary tumors often have headaches and visual deficits in addition to signs and symptoms of hypopituitarism. Prolactinomas vary in size at presentation. Most women with prolactinomas present with microadenomas, oligomenorrhea and/or amenorrhea, and galactorrhea. Men often present with macroadenomas and erectile dysfunction.

## Clinical Features

When produced in excessive quantities, prolactin has effects in addition to its influence on lactation. Hyperprolactinemia causes inhibition of the pulsatile gonadotropin-releasing hormone (GnRH) release from the hypothalamus, leading to decreased gonadotropin release and subsequently to impaired gonadal steroidogenesis and infertility. Other effects of significant hyperprolactinemia include possible loss of bone mineral greater than what can be attributed to the associated hypogonadism.

From a pathophysiologic standpoint, clinical manifestations of hyperprolactinemia can be classified as either signs and symptoms from the hyperprolactinemia itself, regardless of its cause, or those related to the underlying causes of the hyperprolactinemia.

In women, symptoms and signs resulting from the hyperprolactinemia include amenorrhea or oligomenorrhea, galactorrhea, diminished libido, hypogonadism (vaginal dryness and dyspareunia), and infertility. In men, signs and symptoms of hypogonadism (diminished libido and potency) predominate, although up to 20% of men also have galactorrhea. With prolonged hyperprolactinemia and hypogonadism, osteoporosis is an additional feature of hyperprolactinemia in both men and women.

In patients whose hyperprolactinemia is caused by primary hypothyroidism there are significant signs and symptoms related to the primary diagnosis (hypothyroidism).

## Diagnosis

The diagnostic significance of hyperprolactinemia is determined, to a large extent, by the degree of elevation in serum prolactin levels and the associated clinical presentation. Although it is safe to conclude that a serum prolactin level of greater than 200 µg/L is almost certainly due to a small or larger prolactin-secreting pituitary adenoma (prolactinoma), many other potential diagnostic possibilities exist when the level is minimally (25-50 µg/L) or moderately (50-100 µg/L) elevated. Similarly, serum prolactin levels that are greater than 100 µg/L are most often caused by prolactinomas, although other possibilities can be associated with such levels.

Particularly in patients whose serum prolactin level is less than 100 µg/L, one needs to integrate all available clinical data to achieve a working diagnosis. Some patients have multiple causes of hyperprolactinemia. In general, drug-induced hyperprolactinemia (e.g., antipsychotic dopamine antagonists) is associated with serum prolactin levels of 40 to 100 µg/L. In such patients, an additional cause for hyperprolactinemia (e.g., estrogen therapy) might be associated with serum prolactin levels of 100 to 150 µg/L and thus overlap with the potential possibility of a prolactinoma. The same argument can be made in patients with other diseases or illnesses independently associated with hyperprolactinemia.

A major diagnostic challenge is a patient with mild hyperprolactinemia (25-75 µg/L) who also has clinical symptoms such as those that can be associated with partial or complete loss of pituitary function (hypopituitarism). In such patients, two distinct possibilities should be considered, and both require a magnetic resonance imaging (MRI) scan of the sella turcica. The first possibility includes a nonsecreting pituitary tumor or parasellar mass (e.g., meningioma, pituitary tumor, hypothalamic mass) that is compressing the pituitary stalk and portal vessels and thus results in hyperprolactinemia and loss of all other pituitary function. The second possibility includes prolactinomas that exhibit the

**CURRENT DIAGNOSIS**

**History and Physical Examination**

- Review the medication list
- Look for signs and symptoms related to specific causes of hyperprolactinemia: Pregnancy, renal failure, hypothyroidism, pituitary or hypothalamic disease.
- Look for subtle features of hypopituitarism
- Inquire about symptoms and signs caused by hyperprolactinemia: Hypogonadism, osteoporosis, galactorrhea.

**Testing**

- Laboratory: prolactin, renal and thyroid function tests, anterior pituitary hormones in cases of pituitary adenomas
- Be aware of the pitfalls in serum prolactin measurements:
  - The hook effect in patients with pituitary macroadenomas and moderate hyperprolactinemia
  - The possibility of macroprolactinemia in patients without significant symptoms or signs
- MRI of the sella with and without gadolinium enhancement should be done in patients with significant hyperprolactinemia, those who have evidence for other pituitary hormone deficits, and others without an obvious cause for hyperprolactinemia.

hook effect. In such patients, measurements of prolactin level in a serially diluted (1:10, 1:100) serum sample address that possibility. A common feature of either of these possibilities is the associated presence of headaches and visual symptoms.

It is important to incorporate the clinical picture in deciding the extent of the work-up for hyperprolactinemia. Whereas an MRI of the sella is necessary in practically all patients with a prolactin level higher than 100 μg/L, an MRI is also important in patients with even mild degrees of hyperprolactinemia when they have headaches, visual complaints, or symptoms or signs suggesting other pituitary hormone abnormalities. Similarly, an MRI of the sella might be necessary in patients who have no obvious reason for the hyperprolactinemia (regardless of its degree), especially when they have symptoms. Caution should be exercised in asymptomatic patients who have mild hyperprolactinemia and are recently discovered to have pituitary microadenomas. In such instances, the microadenoma might be an incidental finding and therefore requires no treatment but only continued follow-up.

An incidentally discovered mild hyperprolactinemia without any obvious known cause and without other clinical signs or symptoms (particularly reproductive), is likely the benign entity, macroprolactinemia. Macroprolactinemia accounts for 10% of all cases of hyperprolactinemia, and it can be followed without any intervention. Laboratory studies used to identify patients with macroprolactinemia include gel filtration or precipitation by polyethylene glycol before the measurement is made.

# Treatment

Patients with no signs and symptoms related to hyperprolactinemia might not require treatment even when the cause is a microprolactinoma. These microadenomas rarely grow, and thus, in the absence of symptoms, no treatment is indicated, but continued follow-up is warranted.

The ultimate goal of therapy is to restore gonadal function and fertility. In patients with pituitary adenomas, an additional goal of therapy is to eliminate the mechanical effects of the tumor on surrounding tissue. Eliminating or treating the underlying cause of hyperprolactinemia is the primary approach in managing patients with this biochemical abnormality. For example, treating an underlying hypothyroid state or eliminating an implicated medication corrects the hyperprolactinemia. In most instances of drug-induced hyperprolactinemia, one can treat the symptoms caused by hyperprolactinemia (estrogen in women and testosterone in men) even though the serum prolactin level after such therapy might increase even further.

---

## CURRENT THERAPY

- The decision to treat the hyperprolactinemia should be based on the cause and associated symptoms.
- Treat and/or eliminate the probable underlying cause whenever possible.
- Treatment of the hyperprolactinemia:
  - Dopamine agonists are the first and best approach for treating prolactin-secreting pituitary adenomas. Therapy works, regardless of the cause. Cabergoline (Dostinex) (best available option), pergolide (Permax), quinagolide (Norprolac),[1] bromocriptine (Parlodel) (least-favored option).
  - Resection of a hypothalamic or pituitary lesion, if applicable
  - Adjunctive radiation therapy for tumors that are invasive or unresectable and others that are not responsive to surgery or medical therapy, if applicable

---

[1]Not FDA approved for this indication.

Treatment of idiopathic hyperprolactinemia can follow the same approach outlined for the management of microprolactinomas.

At times, antipsychotic dopamine antagonists cannot be easily discontinued because of significant psychiatric illness. Furthermore, patients receiving antipsychotic drugs might experience worsening of their psychiatric symptoms when given dopamine agonists to correct the hyperprolactinemia. In such instances, clinical judgment should be exercised as to which is more clinically beneficial for the patient's well-being.

Treatment is indicated for all patients with symptoms, particularly those with hypogonadism. Patients with no signs or symptoms might not require treatment unless their adenoma is large. They should be followed carefully because they are likely to present with symptoms at some point.

## PHARMACOLOGIC THERAPY

Most authorities in the field believe that dopamine agonists are the treatment of choice for patients with prolactinomas. Patients with macroprolactinomas are managed in a manner similar to that for patients with microadenomas.

Currently, three dopamine agonists are available for clinical use: bromocriptine (Parlodel), pergolide (Permax),* and cabergoline (Dostinex). These agents are effective in their ability to decrease serum prolactin levels and shrink tumor sizes. However, theoretically and practically, cabergoline is believed to be the most effective because it has more D2-receptor specificity and a longer half-life. The three dopamine agonists have different half-lives, and consequently the frequency of their administration is different for optimal benefit. Bromocriptine has to be used three or four times daily (5-30[3] mg/day; average dose, 7.5 mg), pergolide can be used once or twice daily (0.05-0.25 mg/day; average dose, 0.1 mg), and cabergoline is used two to four times weekly (0.5-2.0[3] mg/week).

A recent study suggested that of the three dopamine agonists, cabergoline was the most effective in reducing tumor size. Although cabergoline was effective in all patients, it appears to be most effective in those who never received dopamine agonists previously. In most patients, tumor shrinkage occurs over several months, although rapid changes were reported in occasional patients.

Serum prolactin levels are normalized over several weeks in approximately 80% to 90% of patients given any of the three dopamine agonists at optimal dosing schedules. Of these patients, shrinkage of the tumor can be noted in about 70% within 3 to 6 months. In 30% to 40% of patients, the adenoma can no longer be visualized on imaging studies. Patients with persistent hyperprolactinemia should be given the highest tolerable dose recommended. The dose of the dopamine agonist can be increased every 6 to 8 weeks until the serum prolactin level is normal or until adverse effects are encountered.

One can use serum prolactin levels to monitor and follow patients being treated without having to do frequent MRIs. However, infrequently, patients develop cystic changes in their tumors with dopamine therapy and therefore might have an increase in size of the pituitary mass despite low serum prolactin levels. For these reasons, a follow-up MRI is necessary in all patients with dopamine therapy, especially those who presented with macroadenomas. We usually do not get the MRI until the serum prolactin level is normal or, alternatively, when patients have mechanical symptoms such as headaches and visual disturbances.

Common side effects from all dopamine agonists include nausea, vomiting, constipation, dizziness, postural hypotension, and nasal congestion. These side effects can be minimized by introducing the drug very slowly and mixing it with food. In using cabergoline, we prefer to distribute the total weekly dose so that the drug is given on a daily or every-other-day schedule.

Duration of therapy in patients with prolactin-secreting pituitary microadenomas is still not clear. We recommend at least 5 to 6 years of continuous therapy before the therapy can be slowly tapered and discontinued. If during that period a rise in serum prolactin level is observed, the dose can be increased and treatment prolonged.

Even in patients with suprasellar extension and chiasmal compression, dopamine agonist therapy is the treatment of choice in patients

---

[3]Exceeds dosage recommended by the manufacturer.
*Recently withdrawn from the U.S. market.

with macroprolactinomas. Patients should be monitored carefully to ensure tumor regression with medical therapy.

## SURGICAL THERAPY

Patients with chiasmal compression who do not respond to medical therapy within the first 3 to 4 months should have surgery to debulk the tumor and alleviate pressure from the optic chiasm.

## RADIATION THERAPY

Although radiation therapy was commonly used in the past as an alternative treatment, it is now reserved for patients with tumors that cannot be controlled medically or surgically. Only a small number of patients require radiation treatment.

## Follow-up

Regardless of the therapeutic choice, patients need to be followed up regularly and for indefinite periods. Occasional patients whose tumors are resistant to dopamine agonists and radiation require multiple surgical procedures, including transfrontal craniotomy.

## Prolactinomas and Pregnancy

A potential area of concern in patients with prolactinoma is pregnancy. It is commonly known that once serum prolactin decreases, fertility is restored in men and women within a few weeks. It is important for women to use contraception to avoid pregnancy. Initially, patients interested in getting pregnant are asked to use mechanical contraception for several months until two or three menstrual cycles are reported. This helps patients recognize the possibility of potential pregnancy once mechanical contraception is discontinued. The rationale for this approach is to minimize the use of dopamine agonists during pregnancy. In addition, it is advisable, but not necessarily essential, for patients to switch to bromocriptine[1] from the newer, longer-acting agents during the time from when mechanical contraception is discontinued until pregnancy.

Bromocriptine[1] has been used during all stages of pregnancy to suppress compressive symptoms. Bromocriptine crosses the placenta and suppresses pituitary prolactin secretion, but it has not been associated with increased fetal abnormalities. Although other agents such as pergolide and cabergoline were occasionally used during pregnancy without side effects, the experience with bromocriptine is more extensive, and thus it is the preferred drug during pregnancy if treatment with dopamine agonists becomes necessary. In the absence of any form of contraception, patients often get pregnant before menses are resumed.

Because estrogens normally stimulate lactotrophs, it was initially believed that a prolactinoma might increase in size during pregnancy. This, however, was not found to be a clinically relevant issue in most patients. It is estimated that less than 5% of microadenomas slightly increase in size during pregnancy. The risk is somewhat higher in patients with macroadenomas, especially with suprasellar extension, and is estimated to be 15%. Measurement of serum prolactin during pregnancy in these patients is not helpful in identifying those with potential tumor growth. In women who had a minimal to moderate decrease in tumor size with initial medical therapy, some authorities use a surgical debulking procedure before pregnancy to decrease the chance of tumor expansion during pregnancy. If compressive symptoms develop during pregnancy, and surgery is not recommended, bromocriptine[1] is an effective agent in such instances.

## Summary

Hyperprolactinemia is often reported in the general population and its cause is often easy to recognize. Identifying the pathophysiologic basis

of hyperprolactinemia and its associated clinical presentation should precede any therapeutic intervention. Eliminating the offending drug or treating the primary cause is effective and rewarding. The most significant cause of hyperprolactinemia is prolactinoma, and these are effectively treated with dopamine agonists. Such treatments lower serum prolactin levels to normal and shrink existing tumors so that surgical therapy is not often used in these patients. Surgical resection can be an alternative approach in the small percentage of patients who are resistant to dopamine agonists' therapy and in the few who are unable to tolerate these drugs.

## REFERENCES

Arafah BM: Reversible hypopituitarism in patients with large nonfunctioning pituitary adenomas. J Clin Endocrinol Metab 1986;62:1173-1179.

Arafah BM, Nasrallah M: Pituitary tumors: Pathophysiology, clinical manifestations and management. Endocr Relat Cancer 2001;8:287-305.

Barlier A, Jaquet P: Quinagolide: A valuable treatment option for hyperprolactinemia. Eur J Endocrinol 2006;154:187-195.

Gibney J, Smith TP, McKenna TJ: Clinical relevance of macroprolactin. Clin Endocrinol (Oxf) 2005;62:633-643.

Gillam MP, Molitch ME, Lombardi G, Colao A: Advances in the treatment of prolactinomas. Endocr Rev 2006;27:485-534.

Honbo KS, Van Herle AJ, Kellett KA: Serum prolactin levels in untreated primary hypothyroidism. Am J Med 1978;64:782-787.

Schlechte JA: Prolactinomas. N Engl J Med 2003;349: 2035-2041.

Sievertsen GD, Lim VS, Nakawatase C, Frohman LA: Metabolic clearance and secretion rates of human prolactin in normal subjects and patients with chronic renal failure. J Clin Endocrinol Metab 1980;50:846-852.

# Hypothyroidism

Method of
*John T. Nicoloff, MD, and
Jonathan S. LoPresti, MD, PhD*

Diagnosis and treatment of hypothyroidism is an extremely rewarding experience both for the patient and clinician because lifelong restoration of a euthyroid state can be safely and economically achieved with the appropriate use of oral L-thyroxine ($T_4$) replacement therapy. Although there are many potential causes for hypothyroidism (Table 1), autoimmune thyroiditis (chronic thyroiditis, lymphocytic thyroiditis, Hashimoto's thyroiditis) represents most spontaneously occurring cases of primary hypothyroidism. The initial phases of the disease often start in early adolescence; the incidence of hypothyroidism often reaches its peak in older patient populations in which some degree of biochemical hypothyroidism becomes demonstrable in approximately 8% of males and 20% of females by the age of 70 years. This pattern is the result of the inherently slow, progressive, and unremitting nature of the underlying destructive autoimmune process. Unfortunately, establishing a clinical diagnosis of hypothyroidism generally is a difficult task, especially during the early stages of the disease. The insidious character of thyroid destruction and the lack of specific symptoms that raise suspicion in either the patient or physician make the diagnosis of hypothyroidism problematic. However, this diagnostic limitation can be overcome by establishing the presence of what is most often termed *biochemical* or *subclinical* or *mild* hypothyroidism as defined by consistent elevations in serum thyroid-stimulating hormone (TSH) concentrations when serum free thyroxine ($FT_4$) levels still remain within the normal range. This diagnosis may be further bolstered by the additional findings of detectable serum antithyroperoxidase (anti-TPO) antibodies and the presence of a small, firm goiter. Therefore, the diagnosis of hypothyroidism secondary to chronic autoimmune thyroiditis can definitively be diagnosed at the earliest stages of the disease before the development of significant morbidity occurs. Furthermore, advances in technology have both reduced the cost and improved the accuracy

---

[1]Not FDA approved for this indication.

## TABLE 1  Etiology of Hypothyroidism

**Primary Hypothyroidism**
- Chronic autoimmune thyroiditis (Hashimoto's, lymphocytic)
- Iatrogenic: $^{131}$I therapy, thyroidectomy, external radiation
- Drugs: methimazole (Tapazole), PTU, perchlorate, lithium, amiodarone
- Immune modulators: interferon-$\alpha$, interleukins, postpartum period
- Congenital: complete or partial thyroid gland absence, peroxidase deficiency
- Severe dietary iodine deficiency
- Thyroid infiltrative diseases (rare): lymphoma, Riedel's struma, amyloidosis, hemochromatosis

**Central Hypothyroidism**
- Pituitary TSH deficiency (secondary hypothyroidism): Sheehan's syndrome, pituitary tumors, hypophysitis, trauma (surgery, radiation, head injury), empty sella syndrome
- Hypothalamic TRH deficiency (tertiary hypothyroidism): tumor, craniopharyngioma, Sheehan's syndrome, infiltrative diseases (sarcoidosis, tuberculosis, histiocytosis, lymphoma, eosinophilic granuloma)

**Transient Hypothyroidism**
- Subacute thyroiditis
- Postpartum thyroiditis

**Congenital Thyroid Hormone Resistance (Genetic)**
- Peripheral variant
- Central variant

*Abbreviations:* $^{131}$I = iodine-131; PTU = propylthiouracil; TRH = thyrotropin releasing hormone; TSH = thyroid-stimulating hormone.

of serum TSH measurements, thereby making it possible to perform cost-effective serum TSH screening on large *at-risk* populations. Therefore, the challenge for the clinician is to identify populations that are likely to be *at risk* for developing hypothyroidism, establish a diagnosis of subclinical disease, and initiate oral $T_4$ therapy before overt signs and symptoms of hypothyroidism become clinically apparent.

## Etiology

### PRIMARY HYPOTHYROIDISM

Chronic autoimmune thyroiditis is responsible for most spontaneously occurring cases of thyroid gland failure. As its name implies, chronic autoimmune thyroiditis results from an immunologic process characterized by the insidious, cell-mediated destruction of the thyroid gland. Lymphocytic thyroiditis and Hashimoto's thyroiditis represent specific pathologic terms that describe histologic variants of this autoimmune thyroid gland destruction. The disorder is characterized by progressive infiltration of the thyroid by lymphocytes, lymphoid follicles, and other inflammatory cells over many years, ultimately producing a remnant scar where the gland was located. The onset of the disease commonly occurs in early adolescence and primarily in females (5:1 female-to-male ratio) who display a small, irregular, firm, nontender goiter (so-called adolescent goiter) in an otherwise healthy young adult. Even in this initial phase of the disease, serum TSH concentrations can become persistently elevated; and serum anti-TPO antibodies are frequently detectable. The former is responsible for the compensatory goiter formation, and the latter serving as a nonspecific marker of the underlying thyroid autoimmunity. With advancing age, the cumulative incidence of hypothyroidism gradually rises in both females and males with the female-to-male ratio declining from an initial value of 5:1 to a 2:1 ratio by age 70 years. This latter finding is consistent with the concept of a genetic predisposition for developing autoimmune thyroiditis with thyroid dysfunction displayed earlier in the female population. It is noteworthy that this same age/sex pattern is commonly observed with other autoimmune diseases as well. Exposure to iodine-containing drugs such as intravenous (IV)

contrast dyes and to immune modulating agents such as interferon can precipitate or exacerbate this underlying autoimmune process in susceptible individuals, occasionally producing an abrupt onset of thyroid gland failure and development of hypothyroidism. However, on withdrawal of these agents, thyroid function usually returns to the pretreatment status. In a similar context, postpartum thyroiditis represents a transient autoimmune exacerbation of thyroid dysfunction occurring during early postpartum in women with either preexisting or the genetic tendency for autoimmune thyroid disease. Although most of these women subsequently experience a spontaneous resolution of this mild and transient form of biochemical hypothyroidism within a few weeks, they should be considered to be an at-risk population for developing spontaneous hypothyroidism in the future.

### UNCOMMON CAUSES OF PRIMARY HYPOTHYROIDISM

Severe dietary iodine deficiency, surgical thyroidectomy, iodine-131 ($^{131}$I) ablation, and excessive antithyroid drug administration represent obvious and anticipated causes of primary hypothyroidism and therefore should not represent either a diagnostic or therapeutic problem for the clinician. Approximately one third of patients with subacute thyroiditis will experience a mild to moderate primary hypothyroidism from 6 weeks to 6 months following the onset of this virally mediated destruction of the thyroid. However, in contrast to chronic autoimmune thyroiditis, this form of hypothyroidism is transient in character; eventual full recovery of thyroid gland function and histology is the norm. Neonatal hypothyroidism, or cretinism, represents a rare but important treatable cause of infant mental retardation. Although clinically difficult to recognize at birth, the widespread use of neonatal thyroid screening testing and early $T_4$ replacement therapy has essentially abolished this form of hypothyroidism in medically advanced countries. Fortunately, thyroid neonatal screening programs are also rapidly spreading to the underdeveloped regions of the world to address this treatable form of hypothyroidism.

### CENTRAL HYPOTHYROIDISM

Central hypothyroidism is a rarely encountered entity representing less than 1% of all cases of hypothyroidism. It results from a wide variety of pathologic conditions that impair pituitary TSH, secondary hypothyroidism, and/or hypothalamic thyrotropin-releasing hormone (TRH), tertiary hypothyroidism production, or secretion resulting in a decline in function of the thyroid gland. Common causes of central hypothyroidism include pituitary tumors, empty sella syndrome, trauma, postpartum pituitary necrosis (Sheehan's syndrome), hypophysitis, whole-brain radiation, and a variety of infiltrative diseases (see Table 1). Of considerable diagnostic importance is that the biologic properties of the TSH secreted in secondary hypothyroidism are often altered (because of impaired TRH action on TSH formation) resulting in forms of TSH that have markedly reduced bioactivity while retaining normal immunoactivity. This phenomenon often results in falsely normal TSH values reported in patients who are otherwise biochemically and clinically hypothyroid. Therefore, the utility of serum TSH measurements by immunoassay in accurately assessing thyroid status is essentially lost either for establishing the initial diagnosis or monitoring the adequacy of $T_4$ replacement therapy in patients with secondary hypothyroidism.

## Diagnosis

The clinical diagnosis of hypothyroidism is inherently difficult to establish because the classic features of this condition only become fully evident in the latest stages of the disease. Furthermore, the classic signs and symptoms of hypothyroidism such as weight gain, hypertension, dry skin, hair loss, cold intolerance, chronic fatigue, constipation, and fluid retention are nonspecific in character and commonly occur in populations without hypothyroidism. Only the presence of an asymptomatic, small, firm goiter and delayed deep tendon reflexes provide findings of some diagnostic utility and specificity. However,

## CURRENT DIAGNOSIS

- Hypothyroidism presents with nonspecific signs and symptoms. Therefore, hypothyroidism requires biochemical diagnosis.
- Screening of all adults older than 35 years of age should be considered.
- Definitive indications for screening include a positive family history and/or the presence of a goiter on exam.
- Routine screening tests include a serum TSH level and anti-TPO titer.
- Primary hypothyroidism is confirmed by elevated serum TSH levels and low $T_4$ values.
- Secondary hypothyroidism is diagnosed by low serum $T_4$ levels.
- Subclinical hypothyroidism is defined as a normal $T_4$ and a minimally elevated TSH level.

*Abbreviations:* anti-TPO = antithyroperoxidase; $T_4$ = L-thyroxine; TSH = thyroid-stimulating hormone.

these signs are usually not routinely assessed unless a suspicion that the patient is at risk for developing hypothyroidism is present. Common risk factors include a positive family history of thyroid or other autoimmune diseases and the detection of an elevated serum TSH value with routine blood tests.

### AT-RISK POPULATIONS FOR PRIMARY HYPOTHYROIDISM

Because the propensity for the development of autoimmune diseases is strongly influenced by genetic factors, it is not surprising to find that hypothyroidism secondary to chronic thyroiditis is a familial disorder. Therefore, eliciting a family history either of an *underactive* or *overactive* thyroid condition, the use of thyroid medications, or the presence of a goiter all point toward the possibility of the patient harboring an occult thyroid disorder. If any of these conditions are present in the family, undertaking of a more careful neck examination palpating for a goiter, eliciting deep tendon reflexes evaluating for a slow relaxation phase, and measuring serum TSH and anti-TPO levels can be justified. A positive family history for other autoimmune disorders such as vitiligo, pernicious anemia, myasthenia gravis, Addison's disease, and type 1 diabetes mellitus increases the risk of developing autoimmune hypothyroidism. The discovery of such a history of familial autoimmunity is considerably useful because it raises the probability of detecting subclinical hypothyroidism.

### LABORATORY DETECTION OF SUBCLINICAL HYPOTHYROIDISM

Measurement of serum TSH levels occupies a central role in establishing the laboratory diagnosis of primary hypothyroidism, especially in its earliest subclinical stage. Because thyroxine secretion declines as a result of the progressive destruction of the thyroid gland from chronic thyroiditis, even a small decrease in serum $FT_4$ concentration within the normal range promptly produces a reciprocal increase in the serum TSH value. Importantly, the relative magnitude of this serum TSH rise far exceeds the fall in $FT_4$ resulting from an *amplified* hypothalamic–pituitary negative feedback response, for example, a two-fold change in $FT_4$ produces a 100-fold change in TSH. Therefore, this isolated elevation in serum TSH not only serves as an early marker for impending thyroid gland failure but also acts to stimulate the preferential secretion of more biologically active triiodothyronine ($T_3$) by the thyroid gland, thereby masking the onset of the signs and symptoms of hypothyroidism. This latter phenomenon helps, in part, to explain the subclinical character of this syndrome. When such an isolated elevation in serum TSH is detected, the serum TSH determination

should be repeated along with a serum anti-TPO measurement for diagnostic verification and as an indicator of the underlying autoimmune nature of the process. If not already performed, complete a careful family history, as characterized earlier; a careful neck examination for the presence of a goiter; and an assessment of deep tendon reflexes.

### WHEN ARE SERUM THYROID-STIMULATING HORMONE ELEVATIONS SIGNIFICANT?

In ambulatory, clinically well individuals, any persistent serum TSH elevation should be considered as strong evidence for the presence of primary hypothyroidism, even when the serum $FT_4$ values remain within the normal range. With a normal reference range of serum TSH concentration of 0.5 to 3.5 mU/L, individuals displaying TSH increases from 3.5 to 10 mU/L or even higher are often remarkably free of hypothyroid symptoms, particularly in younger patients. However, bolstered by the additional findings of detectable anti-TPO antibodies, a positive family history for thyroid or other autoimmune diseases as well as the presence of a small firm goiter, this suspicion evolves into the realm of diagnostic certainty, even with modest rises in serum TSH levels. If, however, these additional confirmatory findings are absent but serum TSH elevations persist, some clinicians may choose to defer making a diagnosis of primary hypothyroidism, especially if the rise in serum TSH is minimal (less than 10 mU/L). In this case, the physician should continue to monitor serum TSH concentrations at 6- to 12-month intervals to ascertain the persistence and progression of hypothyroidism rather than to initiate lifelong oral $T_4$ therapy. Keep in mind, however, that many patients with mild subclinical hypothyroidism may experience unexpected symptomatic benefit as well as lowering of serum lipid levels following the initiation of $T_4$ replacement therapy. In this sense, *subclinical* hypothyroidism may represent a misnomer.

### TRANSIENT SERUM THYROID-STIMULATING HORMONE ELEVATIONS ASSOCIATED WITH SYSTEMIC ILLNESSES

In contrast to the relatively stable serum TSH values encountered in healthy ambulatory populations, serum TSH values can become quite labile with acute illnesses where serum TSH values are commonly in the range characteristic of both hyper- and hypothyroidism. Generally, as the illness worsens, serum TSH concentrations become suppressed whereas during recovery they can rebound to elevated values. Obviously, these transient changes in serum TSH levels greatly impair the utility of serum TSH determination as a diagnostic tool. Therefore, greater reliance must be placed on serum $FT_4$ measurements in sick patients. Interestingly, the therapeutic use of both glucocorticoids and dopamine will also cause dramatic transient reductions in serum TSH levels during their acute administration, followed by rebound elevations when these agents are withdrawn. It is believed that this results from direct inhibitory action on the release of TSH from the pituitary. Presumably, a similar inhibitory action from the endogenous cortisol increase on TSH secretion in response to major stress is responsible for the spontaneous decline in serum TSH in acute illness. When such transient changes in serum TSH occur in ambulatory patient populations, acute therapeutic glucocorticoid administration most often proves to be the culprit, such as asthma therapy. However, when chronic glucocorticoid therapy is employed, serum TSH concentrations generally remain in the normal range in the euthyroid patient.

### THYROID-STIMULATING HORMONE SCREENING OF ADULT POPULATIONS

Serum TSH screening of adult populations is cost effectively performed because of technological advances made in the automation of TSH assay methods. This fact has led the American Thyroid Association to recommend screening of the entire population for thyroid disease starting at age 35 years and at 5-year intervals thereafter if initial screening results are normal. Other more restrictive population screening recommendations include testing the entire prenatal population and all the adult population starting at age 60 years. Certainly, all individuals providing a familial history of thyroid or other autoimmune diseases also make up a logical group deserving of TSH screening, as well. In the final analysis, it comes down to what is perceived to be the cost-to-benefit ratio of such an undertaking. Presently, a broad consensus in the medical community on this subject has not yet been formed regarding screening for thyroid disease in the population.

## Treatment

### ORAL L-THYROXINE ALONE AS THE SOLE FORM OF THYROID HORMONE REPLACEMENT THERAPY

The advantages of employing oral $LT_4$ (Synthroid) as the sole thyroid replacement therapy are many and include the following:

- The availability of several well-standardized, competitively priced brands of synthetic oral $LT_4$ (Table 2)
- A long biological half-life approximating 7 days, thereby making day to day compliance less critical
- Production of remarkably stable circulating levels of $FT_4$, which can be easily and accurately measured by routine laboratory testing methods
- Production of stable physiologic circulating levels of triiodothyronine ($T_3$), the active form of thyroid hormone, derived from the peripheral tissue conversion from $T_4$
- Allows the physiologically adaptive regulation of $T_4$ to $T_3$ conversion to occur in response to alterations in nutrition and stresses associated with illness and injury

In contrast, the use of oral $LT_3$ (Cytomel) alone or in combination with $LT_4$ possesses none of these important advantages and therefore is not recommended for use as standard hormone replacement therapy.

### INITIATION AND MAINTENANCE OF OPTIMAL LT₄ REPLACEMENT THERAPY IN PRIMARY HYPOTHYROIDISM

It is important to initiate oral $LT_4$ replacement therapy slowly, starting with a $LT_4$ dose of 25 µg daily and subsequently increasing the dose by 25 µg every 6 weeks until the serum $FT_4$ levels reach the midnormal range. A total daily $LT_4$ dose ranging between 50 and 125 µg usually is required to achieve this goal of a normal $FT_4$ value (a daily dose of 125 µg of $LT_4$ is needed for full replacement in an adult with no residual thyroid function). This deliberate treatment approach is essential to allow sufficient time for the myriad of metabolic alterations produced by $T_4$ therapy to take place. After achieving this initial goal of normal serum $FT_4$ levels, serial serum TSH levels can be measured to achieve an optimal individualized TSH target value ranging between 0.5 to 2.0 mU/L. However, with each $LT_4$ dosage adjustment, it is important to allow a period of at least 6 weeks for a new metabolic equilibrium to be achieved before serum TSH is remeasured. As noted, this $LT_4$ titration process requires that considerable time and patience be practiced by both by the clinician and patient. Once the final optimal serum TSH level is achieved, this daily oral $LT_4$ dose requirement rarely changes as long as the patient remains compliant and the brand of $T_4$

### TABLE 2  Thyroid Hormone Preparations

| Generic Name | Brand Name |
|---|---|
| Levothyroxine sodium ($LT_4$) | • Levothroid<br>• Levoxyl<br>• Unithroid |
| Liothyronine sodium ($LT_3$) | Cytomel |
| Liotrix ($LT_4$ and $LT_3$ combination) | Thyrolar |
| Thyroid USP ($LT_3$ and $LT_4$ extract) | Armour Thyroid |

*Abbreviations:* $LT_4$ = levothyroxine; $LT_3$ = liothyronine.

## CURRENT THERAPY

- Treatment of choice for hypothyroidism should be a nongeneric levothyroxine preparation.
- Interchanging of brands is contraindicated because each levothyroxine preparation has a unique absorption profile.
- Levothyroxine sodium (Synthroid) dosing should start at 25 µg daily and be increased slowly until the ideal dose is reached as determined by a serum TSH level.
- Goal of levothyroxine therapy in primary hypothyroidism is a serum TSH value between 0.5 mU/L and 2.0 mU/L.
- Goal of therapy in secondary hypothyroidism is a normal $T_4$ level.
- Treatment of subclinical hypothyroidism should be determined on a case-by-case basis.

*Abbreviations:* $T_4$ = L-thyroxine; TSH = thyroid-stimulating hormone.

medication is not altered. One possible exception to this rule is that a slight reduction in $LT_4$ dose requirement often occurs after the age of 60 years presumably in association with a general slowing of overall metabolism.

### TREATMENT OF CENTRAL HYPOTHYROIDISM

The initiation of oral $LT_4$ therapy in patients with central hypothyroidism is essentially the same as detailed previously for primary hypothyroidism. However, before starting $LT_4$ therapy, special care must be exercised to ensure adequate glucocorticoid replacement as thyroid hormone may accelerate glucocorticoid disposal and thereby may precipitate an Addisonian crisis. Additionally, because the measurement of serum TSH concentrations cannot serve as a useful therapeutic end-point in patients with central hypothyroidism, the adequacy of $LT_4$ replacement therapy must then rely on normalizing serum $FT_4$ values.

### COMMON PITFALLS IN OPTIMAL ORAL L-THYROXINE THERAPY

The clinician should become suspicious that a problem likely exists in the management of $LT_4$ therapy when marked variability in serum TSH values occurs on a fixed $LT_4$ maintenance dose. The three most likely causes for this phenomenon are as follows:

1. Noncompliance: Poor compliance represents the most commonly encountered problem causing suboptimal $LT_4$ maintenance therapy. The principal reason for noncompliance usually relates to the fact that patients do not experience any immediate change in their state of health when stopping $LT_4$ therapy. This often results in patients missing their daily $LT_4$ dose or when they run out of their $T_4$ supply, not promptly replacing it. To compound the problem, when the patients are asked, "Are you taking your thyroid medication?" they can honestly say, "Yes," because they may have recently restarted therapy in anticipation of the next physician visit. Therefore, one might ask, "How often do you forget to take your thyroid medication?" to remove the stigma from noncompliance. Patients often look puzzled when queried in such a manner but they then rapidly understand when their physician reassures them, "We all forget to take our medication at some time—I certainly do." Experience indicates that such misinformation is the most common cause for physicians inadvertently prescribing excessive dosages of oral $LT_4$ therapy

2. Drugs and other factors altering $T_4$ absorption and metabolism: Table 3 lists some of the most common causes leading to a need for

an increase in oral LT$_4$ dose requirements. Drugs or conditions that reduce gastric acidity also decrease T$_4$ absorption because the hormone is more readily absorbed in its acidic form. Because T$_4$ is highly lipophilic, drugs that interfere with fat absorption also will impair thyroxine absorption, as well. Still other drugs act to accelerate hepatic T$_4$ disposal by the so-called hepatic "first pass effect." Administering oral LT$_4$ separately in the morning before taking drugs that interfere with GI absorption can mitigate this problem. Otherwise, compensatory increases in the oral LT$_4$ dosing schedule will be required.

3. Switching oral LT$_4$ brands: The T$_4$ content of oral thyroxine preparations is well standardized and carefully monitored by the FDA. However, variations in tablet dissolution characteristics and other features of the tablet structure appear to influence the efficiency of T$_4$ gastrointestinal absorption. These facts make it desirable not to switch the brand of an oral LT$_4$ preparation once the optimal dose has been ascertained for any given patient. For the same reason, generic T$_4$ brands should be avoided because the source of the T$_4$ tablets may vary over time.

## Special Situations

### PREGNANCY

Women with hypothyroidism who become pregnant usually require substantial increases in their oral LT$_4$ maintenance dose. Such upward dose adjustments must be performed very early in pregnancy because normal fetal brain development in the first 12 weeks of gestation depends on maternal thyroxine as its source of thyroid hormone. Furthermore, there is strong circumstantial evidence that a deficiency in maternal T$_4$ at this stage of pregnancy is associated with a subsequent reduction in intelligence quotient in the offspring. It is noteworthy that one possible cause for this increased oral LT$_4$ requirement results from the concurrent use of oral iron supplements, which interfere with T$_4$ absorption (Table 3). To reduce this effect of iron on T$_4$ absorption, it is advisable to take the oral LT$_4$ dose and the iron at separate times.

### SURGICAL PROCEDURES

Surgery usually does not present a special problem for hypothyroid patients who have received adequate preoperative oral LT$_4$ replacement therapy. The failure to receive oral medications for a few days postoperatively also is not a therapeutically important problem by virtue of the long 7-day half-life of thyroxine. However, in rare cases of prolonged restriction of oral intake, LT$_4$ can then be administered as a 500 µg IV bolus every 5 days until oral intake can be restarted. In the untreated or inadequately treated hypothyroid patient requiring elective surgery, surgery should be deferred until a euthyroid state is restored with LT$_4$ therapy to significantly reduce operative and postoperative morbidity. In those instances of surgical emergencies or in

patients with severe coronary artery disease, surgery should proceed because such surgery is reasonably well tolerated if IV LT$_4$ therapy is administered in the immediate postoperative period.

## MYXEDEMA COMA

Myxedema coma is a somewhat imprecise term in that this syndrome should be more appropriately termed *decompensated* hypothyroidism. Myxedema coma does not simply represent the natural progression of severe hypothyroidism but signifies an instance where intervening illness or events are responsible for precipitating a significant deterioration in mental status (i.e., acute psychosis, confusion, stupor, and coma) and producing cardiovascular collapse in the patient. The key to therapy is determining the precipitating cause and promptly initiating appropriate therapy. Occult infection and sepsis represent the most common etiologies of decompensation, but a long list of primary and contributing causes includes blood loss, excessive use of diuretics, carbon dioxide retention, oversedation with medications, overuse of tranquilizers and narcotics, and so forth. The use of IV LT$_4$ at an initial dose of 500 µg undoubtedly plays a positive role in marshalling an improved host response but is only useful in conjunction with the identification and reversal of the precipitating event(s).

## REFERENCES

Foley TP Jr.: Hypothyroidism. Pediatr Rev 2004;25: 94-100.
Green WL: New questions regarding bioequivalence of levothyroxine preparations: A clinician's response. AAPS J 2005;7:54-58.
LoPresti JS: Thyroid function tests. In Shindo M, Singer P (eds.): *Clinics in Otolaryngology*. WB Saunders, Philadelphia, pp 557-576, 1996.
LoPresti JS, Nicoloff JT: Myxedema coma: A form of decompensated hypothyroidism. In Ober KP (ed.): Endocrinology and Metabolism Clinics of North America. WB Saunders, Philadelphia, 1993, pp 279-290.
Roberts CG, Ladenson PW: Hypothyroidism. Lancet 2004;363:1558-1594.
Surks MI, Goswami G, Daniels GH: The thyrotropin reference range should remain unchanged. J Clin Endocrinol Metab 2005;90:5489-5496.
Wartofsky L, Dickey RA: The evidence for a narrower thyrotropin reference range is compelling. J Clin Endocrinol Metab 2005;90:5483-5488.

---

# Hyperthyroidism

Method of
*Peter A. Singer, MD*

Hyperthyroidism encompasses a heterogeneous group of disorders, all of which have two features in common. Firstly, all of the types of hyperthyroidism include a β-adrenergic–mediated symptom complex of varying degrees of severity characterized by symptoms of nervousness, heat intolerance, irritability, palpitations, and increased bowel motility, with frequency of movements. Secondly, hyperthyroidism is associated with the catabolic effects of excess circulating levels of thyroid hormone; such effects can include weight loss, fatigue, muscle weakness, increased appetite, and bone loss. The symptoms and signs of hyperthyroidism depend on a number of variables, including levels of circulating thyroid hormone, duration of disease, the age of the patient, and concurrent illnesses.

Hyperthyroidism can be classified according to the capacity of the thyroid gland to trap radioactive iodine (Box 1). Disorders with increased radioiodine uptake have thyroid gland autonomy (with the exception of thyroid-stimulating hormone [TSH]-secreting pituitary tumors) and require specific treatment, whereas those with suppressed radioiodine uptake include conditions that are usually self-limited and might require only symptomatic treatment.

Physical examination of the hyperthyroid patient generally reveals a person who is somewhat anxious and has a rapid pulse. In the elderly, atrial fibrillation is common, and many elderly patients have widened pulse pressure, warm skin, and palpable thyroid gland findings,

---

### TABLE 3 Common Causes Requiring Oral Levothyroxine Dosage Adjustment

**Increased LT$_4$ Administration Required**
- Poor compliance
- Decreased gastrointestinal absorption: oral iron, lipid-binding drugs, sucralfate, calcium carbonate, achlorhydria, proton-blocking drugs
- Altered T$_4$ metabolism: phenobarbital, phenytoin, carbamazepine, rifampin, HAART
- Pregnancy
- Nephrotic syndrome

**Decreased LT$_4$ Administration Required**
- Aging

*Abbreviations:* HAART = highly active antiretroviral therapy; LT$_4$ = levothyroxine; T$_4$ = L-thyroxine.

depending on the underlying etiology. Examination of the eyes in all types of hyperthyroidism might show eyelid retraction, which is mediated by β-adrenergic stimulation. Infiltrative ophthalmopathy is seen almost exclusively in patients with thyrotoxic Graves' disease.

## Diagnosis

Because many of the symptoms of hyperthyroidism may be compatible with some nonthyroid disorders, such as anxiety or the perimenopausal state, TSH, should be measured in patients in whom hyperthyroidism is suspected. TSH suppressed in hyperthroidism, although in patients with rare TSH-secreting pituitary tumors, TSH levels may be normal or even slightly elevated. TSH levels may be suppressed in hospitalized patients, especially those who are seriously ill or who are receiving pharmacologic doses of glucocorticoids or dopamine, thus limiting the usefulness of serum TSH measurements in such patients.

A suppressed TSH level in patients suspected to have hyperthyroidism should be complemented with a serum free thyroxine ($T_4$) or its estimate to confirm the diagnosis. Patients with normal thyroid hormone levels and suppressed TSH concentrations have what is termed *subclinical hyperthyroidism*, a disorder usually free of overt symptoms of hyperthyroidism.

After the diagnosis of hyperthyroidism is confirmed, its etiology should be determined by obtaining a thyroid radioactive iodine uptake. Patients with obvious Graves' disease (such as those with infiltrative ophthalmopathy or large goiters with bruits), may forgo the radioactive iodine uptake test. It is important, however, to differentiate between Graves' disease and low radioactive iodine uptake conditions, which usually are self-limited.

In addition to the radioactive iodine uptake, a scan may be helpful in establishing the diagnosis in patients with suspected toxic multinodular goiter, a condition encountered more commonly nowadays due to increasing immigration into the United States from endemic goiter regions.

## Treatment

Because approximately 80% of patients with hyperthyroidism in the United States have thyrotoxic Graves' disease, most of the comments in this article pertain to that disorder. Among patients with high radioactive iodine–uptake hyperthyroidism, only Graves' disease may be associated with remission following the use of thionamide drugs.

## CURRENT DIAGNOSIS

**Symptoms of Graves' Hyperthyroidism**
- Emotional lability
- Eye irritation, photophobia, diplopia
- Fatigue
- Heat intolerance
- Increased appetite
- Increased frequency of bowel movements
- Increased perspiration
- Menstrual irregularities
- Muscle weakness
- Nervousness
- Palpitations
- Shortness of breath
- Sleep disturbances
- Weight loss

**Signs of Graves' Hyperthyroidism**
- Diffuse goiter
- Eye stare
- Hyperreflexia
- Infiltrative dermopathy (~5%)
- Proptosis
- Proximal muscle weakness
- Systolic hypertension
- Tachycardia
- Thyroid bruit
- Warm, smooth skin
- Widened pulse pressure

### DEVELOPING A TREATMENT STRATEGY

#### General Measures and Patient Education

Essential in the early management of Graves' hyperthyroidism is emphasizing to the patient that strict adherence to the treatment regimen is essential in alleviating symptoms and restoring health. Persons with hyperthyroidism commonly tend to be impatient, likely due to their symptoms, and it must be stressed that compliance with treatment advice is essential for a successful outcome. If family members or friends accompany the patient to the appointment, it is helpful to make them familiar with the treatment plan as well.

#### Initial Treatment of Symptoms

Because many of the symptoms of hyperthyroidism are related to enhanced β-adrenergic stimulation, I routinely employ β-adrenergic–blocking drugs, although mild symptoms might not warrant their use. I prefer propranolol (Inderal),[1] even though it must be given approximately every 6 hours to be completely effective. Propranolol's relatively short half-life makes this agent preferable, because patients learn to titrate their own medication, depending on their symptoms. As patients improve during the course of thionamide therapy (see later), they can omit more doses of propranolol.

The usual starting dose of propranolol[1] is between 20 and 40 mg approximately every 6 hours (or four times a day), and the desired target heart rate is approximately 80 beats per minute. Some physicians prefer longer acting β-blockers, such as atenolol (Tenormin),[1] which may be given as a single daily dose. In patients in whom compliance may be problematic, or in those who prefer once-daily dosing, atenolol 50 to 100 mg a day is an excellent alternative. Other long-acting β-blockers are nadolol (Corgard)[1] and metoprolol (Lopressor).[1]

---

[1]Not FDA approved for this indication.

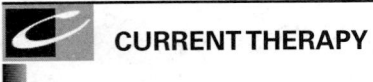
| Treatment Modality | Advantages | Disadvantages |
| --- | --- | --- |
| Thionamide drugs | Chance of remission<br>Relatively inexpensive | Relapse (40%)<br>Side effects (5-10%) |
| Surgery | Rapid, permanent cure | Surgical complications (hypocalcemia, recurrent nerve injury ~1%-3%)<br>Hypothyroidism |
| Radioactive iodine | Permanent cure | Expensive<br>Hypothyroidism |

Long-acting β-blockers are cardioselective and are not contraindicated in patients with coexisting asthma, as propranolol is.

In my experience, patients who are treated with adequate doses of β-adrenergic blocking drugs have significant relief of symptoms within a few days after the medication is initiated.

### Reduction of Serum Thyroid Hormone Levels

Unfortunately, there have been few advances in the management of hyperthyroidism in recent years. Treatment basically consists of lowering the concentrations of serum thyroxine ($T_4$) and triiodothyronine ($T_3$), which may be accomplished either with thionamide drugs or with ablative therapy, either radioiodine or surgery. In the United States, radioiodine ablation with $^{131}$I is the preferred method of treatment of most practicing endocrinologists. Indeed, in a survey of thyroid experts completed in 1991, 69% of respondents chose radioiodine as the primary form of therapy for a prototypic 43-year-old woman with uncomplicated Graves' disease. Only 1% of physicians recommended surgery, and 30% selected thionamide drugs as the primary form of therapy. The responses were in sharp contrast to thyroid experts in both Europe and Japan, where a similar survey revealed that the majority of physicians favored thionamide drugs as the primary form of therapy. The rationale provided by physicians in the United States who selected radioiodine therapy was the fact that the remission rate following 1 to 2 years of thionamide drugs was only approximately 30%.

Before recommending a specific type of therapy for a patient with Graves' disease, it is essential that the patient be aware of the benefits and pitfalls of each type of treatment.

### THIONAMIDE DRUG THERAPY

#### Initial Treatment

Currently, there are two thionamide drugs available for clinical use in the United States, methimazole (MMI, Tapazole) available in 5-mg and 10-mg tablets, and propylthiouracil (PTU) available in 50-mg tablets. Both agents inhibit the synthesis of thyroid hormone by blocking organification of iodine. PTU also inhibits peripheral conversion of $T_4$ to $T_3$, although clinically this may be more of a theoretical than a practical advantage.

I generally prefer MMI, rather than PTU, because of its longer biological half-life and its potency. For uncomplicated hyperthyroidism, MMI may initially be given 2 to 3 times a day in a total dose of 20 to 30 mg, whereas PTU is usually administered 3 to 4 times a day in a total dose of 300 to 400 mg. When biochemical euthyroidism is achieved, usually after 6 to 8 weeks of therapy, MMI may be given once a day, or PTU twice a day, and the total dose may be halved. The relative simplicity of using MMI versus PTU can render it more suitable for patients in whom compliance may be difficult. It must be stressed to the patient that omitting medication doses can result in a rebound of the hyperthyroid state, because the intrathyroid deficiency of iodine produced by thionamide drugs results in more avid trapping of exogenous iodide.

In general, I obtain serum $T_4$ and $T_3$ levels about 6 to 8 weeks after initiating thionamide drug therapy to ensure adequacy of treatment response. If there has been little clinical or biochemical improvement, the likeliest scenario is that doses of medication are being omitted. A serum TSH provides no additional information at this point, because TSH suppression is common for up to 3 or 4 months after euthyroidism has been achieved. Patients with very large goiters and fairly severe hyperthyroidism often take somewhat longer than 6 to 8 weeks to become euthyroid and can require larger doses of MMI (e.g., 40 mg/day) or PTU (e.g., 400-600 mg/day).

I stress to patients that any improvement with thionamide drugs can take several weeks, and I recommend that they defer, if possible, making definitive decisions regarding long-term thionamide versus ablative therapy until they have improved to the extent that they are better able to make more reasoned choices. I always discuss the various forms of treatment of hyperthyroidism with patients during our first appointment, however, and reiterate the options after they have improved.

Although the overall remission rate of patients treated with thionamide drugs in the United States is approximately 30%, some patients are more likely than others to go into remission. Patients with mild hyperthyroidism, small goiters, and a negative family history for hyperthyroidism are more likely to respond favorably, as are patients who respond quickly to thionamide drugs in terms of thyroid gland shrinkage and biochemical improvement. Conversely, patients with severe thyrotoxicosis and those with a strong family history of Graves' disease infrequently go into remission. Some clinicians have advocated serologic markers, such as thyroid-stimulating immunoglobulin or anti-TPO antibodies, to predict the likelihood of remission, but there has been no confirmation of their usefulness for such a purpose.

#### Continuing Treatment

I reevaluate patients taking thionamide drugs approximately every 3 months, and in addition to the clinical examination, I obtain a serum free $T_4$ (estimate) and TSH. If hypothyroidism occurs while on medication, I often add levothyroxine (Synthroid) rather than reduce the dose of thionamide drug. Most patients can be maintained euthyroid on 20 mg of MMI and 0.1 mg of levothyroxine taken in a single daily dose. If PTU is employed, it usually must be given twice daily.

Combined therapy with thionamide drugs and levothyroxine resulted in a considerable amount of controversy several years ago, following the publication of an article from a Japanese group of researchers who reported that 98% of patients taking both MMI and levothyroxine achieved remission. The researchers maintained serum TSH levels in the suppressed range and theorized that TSH inhibition with levothyroxine resulted in less stimulation of antigen release. Unfortunately, their findings have not been confirmed in subsequent studies, either in Japan or elsewhere. Some physicians, however, have reported improved remission rates following longer durations of thionamide administration, of up to 10 years. The practical aspects of such prolonged therapy however, might be open to question.

#### Side Effects of Thionamide Drugs

The most common allergic side effects of thionamide drugs range from mild maculopapular rashes to urticarial eruptions and occur in approximately 5% of patients. Allergic reactions usually do not occur

---

[1]Not FDA approved for this indication.

until 2 to 4 weeks after initiation of therapy. Mild symptoms may be managed with antihistamines, although complete resolution of itching and rash is uncommon. Therefore, I routinely switch patients from the type of medication they are taking (e.g., MMI) to PTU. Approximately 20% of patients are also allergic to the other thionamides, preventing their continued use.

The most serious side effect of thionamide drugs is agranulocytosis, and although it is rare (0.2%-0.5% of patients), it is potentially fatal. It is usually manifested by fever and symptoms of infection, such as a severe sore throat. Patients must be instructed that if they develop fever and signs and symptoms of infection, they must stop the thionamide drug and call their physician immediately. A white blood cell count and differential must be performed, and if agranulocytosis is diagnosed, hospital admission is required. Successful reversal of agranulocytosis, sometimes employing granulocyte colony stimulating factor (G-CSF), should occur within a few days to a week.

Some physicians obtain periodic white blood cell (WBC) counts, although this practice is probably unnecessary because the WBC does not predict agranulocytosis. Nevertheless, before initiating therapy with thionamide drugs, it is helpful to have a baseline WBC because leukopenia is common in patients with Graves' disease, and if a subsequent WBC is obtained, it is useful for comparison.

Other potential side effects of antithyroid drugs include arthralgias and, rarely, hepatitis. Hepatitis is also potentially fatal.

### Stopping Antithyroid Drug Therapy

If therapy with thionamide drugs is used to induce remission, an endpoint of therapy should be determined. I usually treat for 12 to 18 months and then discontinue the thionamide agent. Patients are reevaluated approximately 4 to 6 weeks later, and a serum TSH is obtained. If the serum TSH is suppressed during thionamide therapy, the likelihood of remission is poor. If the patient is euthyroid at 4 to 6 weeks, the next visit is scheduled for approximately 3 months later and at increasing intervals thereafter, but at intervals no longer than 1 year.

Most relapses of hyperthyroidism occur within the first year after stopping thionamide drugs, but they can occur at any time. If relapse occurs, a second course of thionamide drugs does not appear to increase the likelihood of remission, and ablation with radioiodine is then recommended. Some patients, however, prefer to take antithyroid drugs for several, or even many years and often can be maintained on a very small dose of thionamide drug (e.g., 2.5-5 mg/day of MMI). Although such extended therapy is not my preference, there is no absolute contraindication to it. Patients on such a regimen need to be instructed that periodic follow-up, perhaps every 3 to 6 months, is necessary.

### RADIOACTIVE IODINE THERAPY

Therapy with radioiodine ($^{131}$I) is the preferred method of treatment for hyperthyroidism among other thyroid specialists practicing in the United States. Radioiodine has distinct advantages: It is effective, relatively inexpensive, and predictable, and it appears to be free of side effects other than the development of hypothyroidism. Radioiodine has been used to treat hyperthyroidism for approximately 45 years in the United States, and careful follow-up has failed to show an increased incidence of cancer in patients so treated or in genetic defects in offspring of $^{131}$I-treated patients. Radioiodine is contraindicated during pregnancy, which should be ruled out in women of childbearing age before its administration. In addition, women who are breast-feeding should not be treated with radioiodine, because the isotope can recirculate in breast milk for up to several weeks after administration.

### Selection of Radioiodine Dose

Some clinicians advocate administering a $^{131}$I dose that is sufficient to control hyperthyroidism without resulting in hypothyroidism. Various strategies have been employed over the years in an effort to achieve this goal, but they generally have failed. Therefore, I prefer administering a dose large enough to result in hypothyroidism, which usually occurs within 3 to 6 months after $^{131}$I administration. A dose of 15 mCi of $^{131}$I is usually sufficient to achieve this goal, but the appropriate dose depends on the radioactive iodine uptake and size of the thyroid gland. A 24-hour radioactive iodine uptake should be measured before the treatment dose is administered to ensure that adequate quantities of $^{131}$I will be absorbed by the thyroid. A dose of 100-150 fCi/g of thyroid tissue is generally an adequate ablative dose. Some patients are resistant to an initial dose of $^{131}$I and require a second or even third treatment. In my experience, male patients, Asians, and patients with large goiters appear to require larger or additional doses. If patients continue to be hyperthyroid 6 months after an initial treatment with $^{131}$I, a second dose is administered.

Before administering radioiodine, I usually pretreat patients with thionamide drugs until they are euthyroid, because depletion of thyroid hormone from the thyroid prevents release of excess of thyroid hormone from the gland, thereby preventing exacerbation of hyperthyroidism. This is especially important for older patients or those with cardiovascular risk factors. Antithyroid drugs should be discontinued 3 to 5 days before radioiodine treatment. Patients receiving $^{131}$I without having been pretreated with antithyroid drugs (for example, patients who are allergic to thionamides) benefit from administration of propranolol[1] or other β-blockers after treatment, because their underlying hyperthyroidism may be transiently exacerbated by $^{131}$I-induced thyroiditis.

### Follow-up after Radioiodine Treatment

I usually evaluate patients approximately 6 weeks following radioiodine administration in order to assess the clinical and biochemical responses. If the thyroid gland has not decreased in size by 6 weeks, a beneficial response from radioiodine is unlikely. If patients are euthyroid at 6 weeks, they return 4 to 6 weeks later, and if they are hypothyroid by that time, levothyroxine therapy is begun. If patients are still euthyroid (or hyperthyroid) 3 months after therapy, they are reevaluated in another 3 months. Nearly all patients are hypothyroid by 6 months after radioiodine treatment, and those who are still hyperthyroid require another treatment dose.

As experience with radioiodine has increased over the years, age limits for patients believed to be appropriate for treatment have decreased. It appears to be safe to treat teenagers with radioiodine, although I defer treatment in those who have not completed linear growth. There is little concern for developing thyroid nodularity in teenagers following $^{131}$I treatment provided ablative doses are administered.

### Radioiodine Treatment and Graves' Ophthalmopathy

Some clinicians think the administration of $^{131}$I to patients with Graves' ophthalmopathy can worsen the eye disease and administration of pharmacologic amounts of glucocorticoids for a period of one month to 6 weeks following radioiodine treatment will lessen the likelihood of this occurrence. The data concerning efficacy of steroids are not conclusive, however. I believe that patients with moderate symptoms and signs of eye disease should be evaluated by an ophthalmologist with expertise in Graves' ophthalmopathy before administration of $^{131}$I. Indeed, it is often helpful to involve the ophthalmologist in the care of patients with ophthalmopathy, regardless of the type of treatment for hyperthyroidism.

### SURGERY

Surgery for Graves' hyperthyroidism is infrequently employed in the United States. Candidates for such treatment include children and teenagers, especially those who have difficulty complying with antithyroid drugs. Other indications include patients with very large goiters, especially those likely to be resistant to radioiodine because of large goiter size. In addition, surgery is the only choice for patients who are allergic to thionamide drugs and who refuse to take radioiodine. Surgery is also indicated for pregnant patients who are allergic to

---

[1]Not FDA approved for this indication.

thionamide drugs (see later). Patients who have a coexistent thyroid nodule suspicious for cancer on fine-needle aspiration should be treated surgically.

Before surgery, it is preferred to render the patient euthyroid with thionamide drugs. Some surgeons prefer to administer exogenous iodides for 10 days before surgery. Exogenous iodides produce benefit both by inhibiting thyroid hormone release and by decreasing thyroid gland vascularity. Potassium iodide or Lugol's solution, 10 drops in a glass of water daily for 10 days, is sufficient.

Patients electing to undergo thyroidectomy should be made aware that permanent hypothyroidism will most likely result and that they will require the same type of follow-up as those treated with radioiodine. If insufficient thyroid tissue is removed, persistent or recurrent hyperthyroidism will result, which will necessitate radioiodine ablation.

Although surgery has the advantage of being rapidly curative, it also has potential complications. One is injury to the recurrent laryngeal nerve and the other is the possibility of permanent hypoparathyroidism. In skilled hands, these complications occur no more than 1% to 3% of the time, yet these potential risks must be explained fully to the patient beforehand.

## Other Forms of Hyperthyroidism

### TOXIC NODULAR GOITER

Toxic multinodular goiter increases in prevalence with increasing age. In elderly persons it is a more common cause of hyperthyroidism than is Graves' disease. The diagnosis should be documented with a radioactive iodine uptake and thyroid scan. Patients with toxic multinodular goiter will not go into remission on thionamide drugs, limiting definitive treatment to either radioiodine or surgery.

Before radioiodine is employed in elderly patients, thionamide drugs should be administered to minimize the risk of exacerbating hyperthyroidism. Radioiodine is the treatment of choice for most patients with toxic multinodular goiter, although surgery may be preferred for patients with especially large glands or with symptoms of compression who are good operative risks. If radioiodine is used for treatment of toxic nodular goiter, the dose required is usually greater than that employed for Graves' disease.

A single thyroid nodule producing hyperthyroidism occurs much less often than toxic multinodular goiter, and it generally occurs in persons younger than those with multinodular goiter. Although radioiodine is commonly employed for such patients, surgery is usually recommended for patients younger than 25 to 30 years.

### HYPERTHYROIDISM AND PREGNANCY

Hyperthyroidism during pregnancy can lead to adverse outcomes both for mother and fetus. Adequate control of hyperthyroidism during pregnancy is essential. Either MMI or PTU may be used during pregnancy, but most clinicians favor PTU because it does not cross the placenta as easily as does MMI. For hyperthyroidism that is difficult to control, or if the patient is allergic to antithyroid drugs, thyroidectomy should be performed during the second trimester. β-Adrenergic blocking agents may be given safely during pregnancy to control symptoms.

Patients who continue to be treated with thionamide drugs during pregnancy should have a thyroid-stimulating immunoglobulin level drawn during the last trimester to predict the possible occurrence of neonatal hyperthyroidism. Hyperthyroid pregnant patients should be followed carefully at least every 4 to 6 weeks, and close communication should be maintained between the endocrinologist and obstetrician. It is advisable to use the lowest dose of thionamide drug that maintains maternal euthyroidism.

### THYROID STORM

Thyroid storm (or crisis) is characterized by severe manifestations of hyperthyroidism, fever, and altered mental status. The disorder is usually precipitated by a concurrent illness.

Early recognition and treatment of thyroid storm are essential because it is life threatening. Patients must be managed in the intensive care unit, and, in addition to general supportive measures and treatment of concurrent illness, aggressive pharmacologic management of the hyperthyroidism is necessary. Either MMI or PTU may be used, although PTU has the potential advantage of reducing production of $T_3$ from $T_4$. A dose of 150 mg of PTU every 6 hours or 15 to 20 mg of MMI every 8 hours is usually sufficient. For patients unable to take medication orally, MMI may be crushed and given by nasogastric tube or may be prepared by the pharmacy as a rectal suppository.

In addition to thionamide drugs, exogenous iodides should be administered. Iopanoic acid may be used for this purpose, because it not only inhibits thyroid hormone release but also has the advantage of being a potent inhibitor of $T_4$ to $T_3$ conversion. A dose of 500 mg to 1 g orally daily is sufficient. However it is not currently available in the United States. Alternatively, iodine can be administered in the form of Lugol's solution or saturated solution of potassium iodide, 10 drops in water three times daily, or sodium iodide, 500 mg intravenously every 12 hours. It is essential to administer the first dose of thionamide drug a few hours before administration of iodides to prevent further organification of iodide with resultant additional thyroid hormone production. Some clinicians also use pharmacologic doses of glucocorticoids to further inhibit $T_4$ to $T_3$ conversion, although the clinical efficacy of this treatment has not been shown convincingly.

β-Blocking agents, preferably propranolol,[1] are essential in the management of thyroid storm and may be given either orally or intravenously. If the latter route is used, 1 mg every 5 to 10 minutes is given intravenously until the heart rate is less than 100 bpm. Once adequate control of the heart rate is achieved, oral propranolol may be given, and doses of 160 mg or more every 6 hours are not uncommon. Heart failure, which may be due in part to uncontrolled tachycardia, must be treated with adequate digitalis. If diuretics[1] are used, they must be administered very cautiously, because patients with thyroid storm are peripherally vasodilated and can suffer vascular collapse if conventional doses of diuretics are given. Plasmapheresis has been described as a treatment for thyroid storm, although I have neither used it nor seen it employed.

## REFERENCES

Auer J, Scheibner P, Mische T, et al: Subclinical hyperthyroidism is a risk factor for atrial fibrillation. Am Heart J 2001;142:838-842.

Baldini M, Gallazzi M, Orsatti A, et al: Treatment of benign nodular goiter with mildly suppressive doses of L-thyroxine: Effects on bone mineral density and on nodule size. J Intern Med 2002;251:407-414.

Bauer DC, Ettinger B, Nevitt MC, Stone KL: Risk for fracture in women with low serum levels of thyroid-stimulating hormone. Ann Intern Med 2001;134:561-568.

Charkes ND: The many causes of subclinical hyperthyroidism. Thyroid 1996;5:391-396.

Cooper DS: Antithyroid drugs. N Engl J Med 1984;311:1353-1362.

Cooper DS: Antithyroid drugs and radioiodine therapy: A grain of (iodized) salt. Ann Intern Med 1994;121:612-614.

Cooper DS: Treatment of thyrotoxicosis. In Braverman LE, Utiger RD (eds): Werner and Ingbar's The Thyroid: A Fundamental and Clinical Text, 7th ed. Philadelphia, Lippincott-Raven, 1996, pp 708-734.

Cooper DS: Antithyroid drugs for the treatment of hyperthyroidism caused by Graves' disease. Endocrinol Metab Clin North Am 1998;27:225-247.

Franklyn JA: The management of hyperthyroidism. N Engl J Med 1994;130:1731-1738.

Franklyn JA: Drug therapy: The management of hyperthyroidism. N Engl J Med 1994;330:1731-1738.

Klein I, Becker D, Levey G: Treatment of hyperthyroid disease. Ann Inter Med 1994;121:281-288.

Klein I, Ojamaa K: Cardiovascular manifestations of endocrine disease. J Clin Endocrinol Metab 1992;75:339-342.

McIver B, Morris JC: The pathogenesis of Graves' disease. Endocrinol Metab Clin North Am 1998;27:73-89.

Mestman JH: Hyperthyroidism and pregnancy. Best Pract Res Clin Endocrinol Metab 2004;18:267-288.

Motomura K, Brent GA: Mechanisms of thyroid hormone action. Endocrinol Metab Clin North Am 1998;27:1-23.

---

[1]Not FDA approved for this indication.

Papi G, Pearce EN, Braverman LE, et al: A clinical and therapeutic approach to thyrotoxicosis with thyroid-stimulating hormone suppression only. Am J Med 2005;118:349-361.

Roti E, Minelli R, Salvi M: Management of hyperthyroidism and hypothyroidism in the pregnant woman. J Clin Endocrinol Metab 1996;81: 1679-1682.

Sawin CT: Thyroid dysfunction in older persons. Adv Intern Med 1991;37: 223-249.

Sawin CT, Geller A, Wolf P, et al: Low serum thyrotropin concentrations as a risk factor for atrial fibrillation in older persons. N Engl J Med 1994;331:1249-1252.

Singer PA, Cooper D, Levy E, et al: Treatment guidelines for patients with hyperthyroidism and hypothyroidism. JAMA 1995;273:808-812.

Surks, MI, Chopra I. Mariash C, et al: American Thyroid Association guidelines for use of laboratory tests in thyroid disorders. JAMA 1990;263:1529-1532.

Torring O, Tallstedt L, Wallin G, et al: Graves' hyperthyroidism: Treatment with antithyroid drugs, surgery, or radioiodine a prospective, randomized study. J Clin Endocrinol Metab 1996;81:2986-2993.

Wing DA, Millar LK, Koonings PP, et al: A comparision of propylthiouracil versus methimazole in the treatment of hyperthyroidism in pregnancy. Am J Obstet Gynecol 1994;170:90-95.

# Thyroid Cancer

Method of

*Marlon A. Guerrero, MD, and Nancy D. Perrier, MD*

Thyroid cancer is the most common endocrine malignancy and accounts for approximately 2% of all cancers. The incidence of thyroid cancer has increased more than 50% since 1975, but mortality remains relatively constant at 0.5 deaths per 100,000 persons annually. In 2006, approximately 30,180 new cases of thyroid cancer were diagnosed in the United States—an 8% increase from 2005. Thyroid cancer has a female predominance, and the lifetime risk of developing thyroid cancer is 1.02% for women and 0.36% for men. Thyroid cancer accounts for 3% of malignancies in women and is now the seventh most common cancer among women.

## Classification

Thyroid cancer is classified according to the cells of origin as either follicular or parafollicular. Cancers originating from follicular cells are further subdivided into differentiated and undifferentiated cancers. Papillary (PTC) and follicular (FTC) thyroid carcinomas are of follicular origin and are collectively referred to as *differentiated thyroid cancers*. They account for 90% of thyroid cancers (80% PTC and 10% FTC). The aggressive Hürthle cell variant (HCC) of FTC constitutes 3% of thyroid cancers; 8% of HCCs are found to have anaplastic differentiation. Undifferentiated anaplastic thyroid carcinomas (ATC), also of follicular cell origin, have a particularly poor prognosis but fortunately account for only 2% of thyroid cancers.

Medullary thyroid carcinoma (MTC) is a neuroendocrine tumor of parafollicular cell origin and accounts for 5% of thyroid cancers. Two forms have been identified: sporadic (80% of MTC) and hereditary (20%). The hereditary form occurs in association with multiple endocrine neoplasia (MEN) types 2a and 2b and as familial (non-MEN) MTC. All hereditary forms are autosomal dominant and are associated with early C-cell hyperplasia and a germline mutation in the *RET* proto-oncogene. Approximately 50% of patients with MTC present with regional lymph node disease, and an additional 13% have distant metastases.

Another rare cancer of the thyroid is lymphoma, which represents less than 1% of all thyroid cancers. Its development is closely associated with Hashimoto's thyroiditis. The majority of cases are the non-Hodgkin's B-cell type.

# Clinical Presentation and Evaluation

Thyroid cancer typically manifests as an asymptomatic solid thyroid nodule. The work-up of a thyroid nodule commences with a detailed history. The clinician must be cognizant of the risk factors associated with thyroid cancer (Box 1). The greatest risk is exposure to ionizing radiation during childhood (90% of radiation-induced thyroid cancers are PTC). A strong family history or a personal history of thyroid cancer also increases the risk. Several familial syndromes are associated with thyroid cancer. Differentiated cancers can occur as part of a constellation of diseases in familial adenomatous polyposis, Gardner's syndrome, and Cowden disease. MTC is known to occur as part of MEN-2a (MTC, pheochromocytoma, and hyperparathyroidism) and MEN-2b (MTC, pheochromocytoma, marfanoid habitus, and mucosal neuromas).

A complete physical examination should entail meticulous examination of the head and neck region and lymphatic basins. A firm, fixed thyroid nodule that moves vertically with swallowing is suspicious for cancer. An enlarging nodule or cervical lymphadenopathy also suggests malignant disease. Though rare, obstructive symptoms such as dysphagia, hoarseness, stridor, and pain may be evident at initial presentation. This uncommon presentation occurs predominantly with ATC or advanced disease.

The recommended tests for patients with a dominant, solid thyroid nodule are outlined in Figure 1. In general, only incidentally identified nodules larger than 1 cm or those clinically palpable should be evaluated. Evaluation for nodules smaller than 1 cm may be considered in patients considered at high risk (see Box 1). All patients should undergo evaluation of thyroid function by measurement of serum thyroid-stimulating hormone (TSH). A low TSH level (suggesting hyperthyroidism) should be assessed with either an iodine-123 ($^{123}$I) or technetium-99m ($^{99m}$Tc) scan. A hot nodule (with high radiotracer uptake) denotes autonomous thyroid function (hyperthyroidism) and is more likely to be benign. On the other hand, a cold nodule (with radiotracer uptake less than the surrounding thyroid tissue) is more likely to be malignant. A patient with a normal or elevated TSH level or a cold thyroid nodule should be further evaluated with neck ultrasonography, usually followed by fine-needle aspiration (FNA). Nodules larger than 1 cm or those with suspicious ultrasound findings should undergo FNA.

Ultrasonography increases the diagnostic accuracy of FNA compared with palpation-guided FNA, permits identification of solid

---

## BOX 1  Risk Factors for Thyroid Cancers

**Differentiated Carcinoma**
- Cowden disease (multiple hamartomas)
- Familial adenomatous polyposis
- Familial nonmedullary thyroid cancer
- Gardner's syndrome (gastrointestinal polyps, osteomas, soft tissue tumors)
- Ionizing radiation

**Anaplastic Carcinoma**
- Differentiated thyroid cancer
- Endemic goiter
- Previous or concurrent thyroid disease

**Medullary Carcinoma**
- Familial (*RET* proto-oncogene mutation)
- MEN-2a (pheochromocytoma, hyperparathyroidism, MTC)
- MEN-2b (pheochromocytoma, MTC, mucosal neuromas, marfanoid habitus)

*Abbreviations:* MEN = multiple endocrine neoplasia; MTC = medullary thyroid cancer.

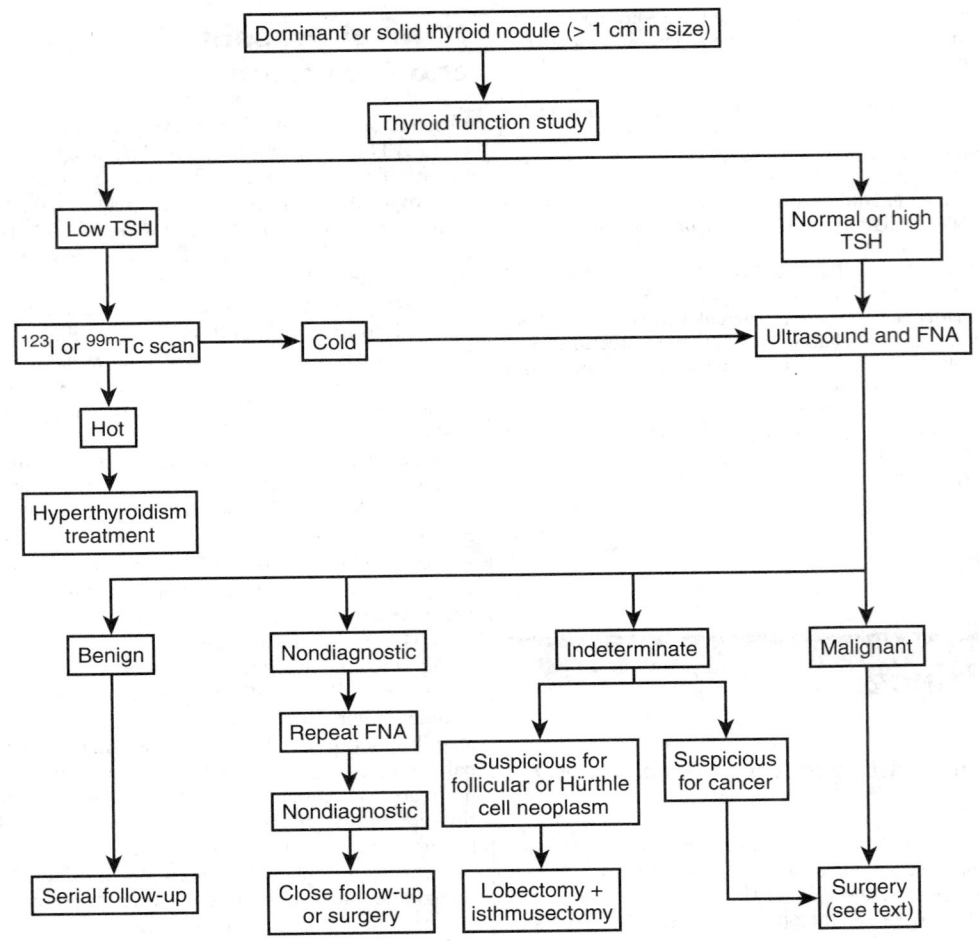

**FIGURE 1.** Tests recommended for thyroid nodules. *Abbreviations:* <sup>123</sup>I, iodine-123; FNA, fine-needle aspiration; <sup>99m</sup>Tc, technetium 99m; TSH, thyroid-stimulating hormone.

components within a cystic nodule, allows simultaneous assessment of cervical lymph nodes, and identifies characteristics suspicious for malignancy (irregular border, microcalcifications, tissue invasion, and increased vascularity).

The finding of MTC on FNA warrants a full preoperative evaluation to identify MEN-2a or 2b. Serum calcitonin and carcinoembryonic antigen (CEA) are usually elevated in MTC, and levels should be checked before surgical intervention so that the values can be used as markers for follow-up care. It is also imperative to check serum levels of calcium and parathyroid hormone and plasma metanephrines (to rule out coexisting pheochromocytoma) to identify MEN.

Positive results or a high suspicion of MEN-2a or MEN-2b is an indication for *RET* proto-oncogene testing. For MEN-2b patients, the stereotypic phenotype of mucosal neuromas or marfanoid facies should prompt suspicion of the disease and a full work-up. Genetic testing should also be offered to even those with seemingly sporadic disease because of the possibility of carrying a germline *RET* proto-oncogene mutation. If the gene is found, then family members should be screened because there is a 50% penetration of this autosomal dominant gene. The specific *RET* proto-oncogene mutation is further stratified by codon mutations into incrementing levels of clinical importance (low, moderate, high risk) to direct timing of intervention in otherwise asymptomatic carriers.

Computed tomography of the chest, abdomen, and pelvis is indicated to evaluate for pheochromocytoma or pancreatic tumors. If pheochromocytoma is identified, it should be surgically treated before addressing the thyroid disease.

Thyroid cancer is staged using the TNM classification system (Table 1). ATCs are almost universally fatal. Because of this lethality, all are categorized as stage IV in the TNM classification system.

# Cytology

The cytologic results of FNA are classified as benign, malignant, indeterminate, or nondiagnostic. FNA is 95% accurate in diagnosing PTC, ATC, and MTC. Indeterminate cytology is found in 15% to 30% of FNA specimens. Approximately 10% to 20% of FNA results are nondiagnostic. This can result from inadequate sampling, areas of necrosis or calcification, or cystic degeneration. Repeat aspiration is warranted, specifically under ultrasound guidance. Nodules with a continual nondiagnostic FNA warrant close observation. Surgery should be strongly considered if the nondiagnostic nodule is solid. Occasionally, ATC is confused with lymphoma. Core-needle biopsy with immunohistochemical staining and flow cytometry is used to exclude lymphoma if differentiation cannot be made by FNA.

A cytologic finding consistent with PTC is a monolayer sheet of cells forming papillae, with occasional calcifications (psammoma bodies). The nuclei are typically enlarged, irregular, and overlapping, with peripheral margination of the chromatin (Orphan Annie eyes), nuclear grooves, and inclusion bodies.

Unlike the other thyroid cancers, follicular thyroid cancer (FTC) and Hürthle cell carcinoma (HCC) cannot be diagnosed by FNA and can only be designated as "neoplasms" on cytologic assessment. An assembly of hypercellular follicular cells with minimal colloid favors FTC, but distinction from an adenoma cannot be made by FNA alone. Capsular or vascular invasion must be identified on permanent histologic sections following surgical resection for both neoplasms to be diagnosed as malignant. Hürthle cell carcinoma is typically found to have large polygonal follicular cells with eosinophilic cytoplasm. The overall rate of malignancy associated with these indeterminate thyroid lesions on permanent histology is 20%.

## TABLE 1 AJCC TNM Staging System for Thyroid Cancer

| Stage | Characteristic |
|-------|----------------|
| **Tumor (T)** | |
| TX | Primary tumor cannot be assessed |
| T0 | No evidence of primary tumor |
| T1 | Tumor 2 cm or less in greatest dimension limited to the thyroid |
| T2 | Tumor more than 2 cm but not more than 4 cm in greatest dimension limited to the thyroid |
| T3 | Tumor more than 4 cm in greatest dimension limited to the thyroid or any tumor with minimal extrathyroidal extension |
| T4a | Tumor of any size extending beyond the thyroid capsule to invade subcutaneous soft tissues, larynx, trachea, esophagus, or recurrent laryngeal nerve. Intrathyroidal anaplastic carcinoma—surgically resectable |
| T4b | Tumor invading prevertebral fascia or encasing carotid artery or mediastinal vessels. Extrathyroidal anaplastic carcinoma—surgically unresectable |
| **Regional Lymph Nodes (N)** | |
| NX | Regional lymph nodes cannot be assessed |
| N0 | No regional lymph node metastasis |
| N1 | Regional lymph node metastasis |
| N1a | Metastasis to level VI (pretracheal, paratracheal, and prelaryngeal/Delphian lymph nodes) |
| N1b | Metastasis to unilateral, bilateral, or contralateral cervical or superior mediastinal lymph nodes |
| **Distant Metastasis (M)** | |
| MX | Distant metastasis cannot be assessed |
| M0 | No distant metastasis |
| M1 | Distant metastasis |

## TABLE 2 Staging of Papillary or Follicular Carcinoma

| Stage | Classification <45 Years | ≥45 Years |
|-------|--------------------------|-----------|
| I | Any T, any N, M0 | T1, N0, M0 |
| II | Any T, any N, M1 | T2, N0, M0 |
| III | | T3, N0, M0 |
| | | T1, N1a, M0 |
| | | T2, N1a, M0 |
| | | T3, N1a, M0 |
| IVA | | T4a, N0, M0 |
| | | T4a, N1a, M0 |
| | | T1, N1b, M0 |
| | | T2, N1b, M0 |
| | | T3, N1b, M0 |
| | | T4a, N1b, M0 |
| IVB | | T4b, Any N, M0 |
| IVC | | Any T, Any N, M1 |

The diagnosis of ATC is confirmed by identifying numerous mitotic figures and marked cellular pleomorphism on FNA. In ATC, three histologic patterns have been identified: spindle cell, giant cell, and squamoid. In addition, high mitotic activity, vascular invasion, necrosis, and paucity of staining for thyroglobulin are also common. Anaplastic cells do not transport iodine or produce thyroglobulin and do not contain thyrotropin receptors.

A cytologic finding of eosinophilic cells interspersed with amyloid and a vascular stroma is representative of MTC. Immunohistochemical staining for calcitonin confirms the diagnosis of MTC.

# Treatment and Follow-up

## DIFFERENTIATED THYROID CANCERS

A preoperative neck ultrasound to evaluate the entire thyroid and bilateral cervical lymph nodes should be performed for proper staging (Table 2). Total thyroidectomy is the surgical treatment of choice for differentiated thyroid cancer.

## Surgery

### Papillary Thyroid Cancer

There is no consensus, but some suggest that lobectomy with isthmusectomy is acceptable for minimally invasive PTC less than 1 cm, particularly in cases in which the lesion was noted incidentally (e.g., after lobectomy for an autonomous functioning toxic thyroid nodule).

If PTC is identified before surgery, however, a total thyroidectomy should be performed regardless of tumor size. The rationale for total thyroidectomy is that up to 80% of PTCs are multicentric, 30% are multifocal, and 5% to 10% of recurrences after lobectomy occur in the contralateral thyroid lobe. Three additional benefits are afforded by a total thyroidectomy compared with a lesser operation: radioactive iodine

($^{131}$I) may be used to ablate residual disease, the specificity of $^{131}$I for detecting recurrence or metastasis is increased, and serum thyroglobulin levels may be used as a sensitive marker for persistent or recurrent disease.

A central neck dissection in conjunction with a total thyroidectomy is recommended for PTC given that microscopic cervical lymph node involvement is present in 35% of patients at initial diagnosis. The morbidity of reoperative surgery in the cervical region justifies extirpation of potential microscopic disease, as part of initial treatment, to prevent recurrence (40-year local recurrence rate is 35%). If lateral cervical lymphatic involvement is present (clinically, radiographically, or by FNA during preoperative staging) on the side of disease, an ipsilateral compartment-oriented neck dissection is also performed at the time of total thyroidectomy and central neck dissection.

### Follicular Thyroid Cancer and Hürthle Cell Cancer

The surgical approach to FTC and HCC differs from that for PTC because these tumors cannot be definitively diagnosed by FNA. Because only 20% of indeterminate lesions on FNA harbor a malignancy and multifocality is not common in FTC or HCC, an initial lobectomy and isthmusectomy are recommended in patients with indeterminate lesions to provide a specimen for histologic evaluation. Intraoperative frozen-section analysis is not used because it is unreliable in assessing capsular or vascular invasion. If final pathology results indicate an adenoma, no further treatment is needed.

The diagnosis of follicular carcinoma or Hürthle cell carcinoma on final pathologic evaluation necessitates a completion thyroidectomy. Central node dissection is considered for the Hürthle cell variant, but it is not always necessary for pure follicular disease because the principal route of dissemination is hematogenous. If lymphatic involvement is present, however, a lymph node dissection is warranted.

### Radioiodine Ablation

Small residual disease after surgical intervention can be treated by radioiodine ablation in patients with differentiated thyroid carcinomas. Radioiodine scanning (1-3 mCi) may be performed to detect residual disease 4 to 6 weeks after surgical intervention if the extent of the thyroid remnant cannot be determined. Following thyroidectomy and before radioiodine ablation, patients are placed on a low-iodine diet (< 50 µg/day). Thyroid hormone suppression is normally delayed until after radioiodine ablation therapy in order to maximize iodine uptake ablation therapy. A low dose (25-75 µg/day) of liothyronine (Cytomel) may be used to alleviate hypothyroid symptoms before $^{131}$I scanning.

The drug must be discontinued at least 2 weeks before ablation. Levothyroxine (Synthroid, Levoxyl) may be used as an alternative to

Cytomel but must be discontinued a minimum of 4 weeks before ablation because of its longer half-life. As an alternative to withdrawing the thyroid hormone, 0.9 mg of recombinant TSH (Thyrogen)[1] may be administered intramuscularly daily for 2 days before [131]I scanning. This regimen eliminates the requirement of being hypothyroid before ablation because recombinant TSH stimulates [131]I uptake. With all methods, the goal is to increase serum TSH concentrations to levels greater than 30 mU/L.

Radioiodine ablation is typically performed on patients with stage III or IV disease and stage II disease in those younger than 45 years. [131]I is taken up into cells and then undergoes β decay, releasing high-energy electrons that induce cytotoxicity. The minimum dose to achieve ablation is 30 to 100 mCi. Locally invasive, residual, or metastatic disease may be treated with 100 to 200 mCi. A post-therapy [131]I whole-body scan should be performed 5 to 8 days after the ablation. Patients with uptake identified only in the thyroid bed should be followed routinely. Uptake outside the thyroid bed merits a full metastatic work-up. Low-risk patients with undetectable serum thyroglobulin and a negative cervical ultrasound on follow-up do not require subsequent whole-body scans.

## Thyroid Hormone Supplementation

Following radioiodine ablation, lifelong thyroid hormone supplementation is recommended to suppress TSH to less than 0.1 mU/L for high-risk patients (macroscopic tumor invasion, residual disease, distant metastases, or [131]I uptake outside the thyroid bed) and 0.1 to 0.5 mU/L for low-risk patients. Levothyroxine is started at 100 to 200 mg/day, but doses greater than 2 μg/kg/day may be required for adequate suppression. The potential side effects of TSH suppression include atrial fibrillation, cardiac dysfunction, and acceleration of osteoporosis.

## Follow-up

Initial post-treatment evaluation involves measuring serum thyroglobulin during TSH suppression and a cervical ultrasound at 6 months. Patients with a negative ultrasound and serum thyroglobulin levels less than 1 ng/mL should have thryoglobulin levels measured again after discontinuing levothyroxine or using recombinant TSH (see earlier). Continued surveillance is warranted if serum thyroglobulin levels are less than 2 ng/mL. Serum thyroglobulin levels between 2 and 5 ng/mL after recombinant TSH or less than 10 ng/mL after thyroid hormone withdrawal should be followed up routinely. A concerning ultrasound finding, steadily rising thyroglobulin (more than twofold), or a serum thyroglobulin 5 ng/mL or higher after recombinant TSH or 10 ng/mL or higher after thyroid hormone withdrawal should prompt a metastatic work-up.

Routine surveillance after a negative 6-month evaluation consists of a physical examination and measurement of serum TSH and thyroglobulin at 6- to 12-month intervals. A cervical ultrasound to evaluate the thyroid bed and nodal compartments should be performed at 12 months after surgery, then annually for 3 to 5 years. One limitation to thyroglobulin measurements is the presence of anti–thyroglobulin antibodies in 25% of thyroid cancer patients; these antibodies result in falsely lowered thyroglobulin concentrations. Anti–thyroglobulin antibodies should be assessed during every thyroglobulin measurement.

## ANAPLASTIC THYROID CANCER

Undifferentiated ATC is the most aggressive thyroid malignancy and is associated with a disease-related mortality rate of nearly 100%, and therefore all are categorized as stage IV (Table 3). More than 90% of those affected are older than 50 years. The majority of patients present with advanced disease that is nearly always inoperable. At the initial evaluation, nearly 40% of patients have cervical lymph node disease, more than 70% have local tissue invasion, and more than 50% have distant metastases, with the lung being the most common site (80%).

---

[1]Not FDA approved for this indication.

### TABLE 3   Staging of Anaplastic Carcinoma

| Stage | Classification |
| --- | --- |
| IVA | T4a, any N, M0 |
| IVB | T4b, any N, M0 |
| IVC | Any T, any N, M1 |

Doxorubicin (Adriamycin) is the chemotherapeutic drug most commonly used for ATC, but when used alone, doxorubicin does not prolong survival. The addition of cisplatin (Platinol),[1] bleomycin (Blenoxane),[1] paclitaxel (Taxol),[1] and other drugs has not affected survival either. However, an improved short-term survival rate has been demonstrated with a combination of radiation and chemotherapy. The standard treatment regimen for ATC is thus chemoradiation. External-beam radiation therapy improves local disease control, and chemotherapy improves radiosensitivity. Current chemoradiation protocols use radiation dosages between 30 and 60 Gy with chemotherapy.

Owing to the advanced stage at which most ATC are diagnosed, surgery is usually palliative, and aggressive surgical resection (radical neck dissection) or debulking is discouraged because it has no impact on survival. Surgery may be undertaken if the tumor responds to chemoradiation or in the rare instance that the tumor is small and localized. Prophylactic tracheostomy has not improved survival and is associated with high morbidity. Thus, the sole indication for tracheostomy is impending airway obstruction.

## MEDULLARY THYROID CANCER

A total thyroidectomy with bilateral central lymph node dissection (level VI) is the operation of choice for MTC. A compartment-oriented modified neck dissection is performed for tumors greater than 1 cm and for patients with pathologically involved lymph nodes identified during central neck dissection or with suspicious lymph nodes found on preoperative ultrasonography. MTC staging is shown in Table 4.

In contrast to the treatment of differentiated thyroid cancers, radioiodine ablation has no role in MTC. External-beam radiation therapy is indicated in patients with bulky cervical disease, residual disease, microscopically positive margins, soft tissue invasion, or lymph node metastasis. This is typically given at a dosage of 40 Gy in 20 fractions over 4 weeks and is directed at the cervical, supraclavicular, and upper mediastinal lymph nodes. A subsequent dosage boost of 10 Gy in 5 fractions may then be directed solely to the thyroid bed.

Patients with inherited MTC should undergo total thyroidectomy and central node dissection. If the disease is diagnosed early, patients identified as risk level III (high risk; codons 883, 918, 922 *RET*) should undergo surgery during the first year of life. Those who are stratified

---

[1]Not FDA approved for this indication.

### TABLE 4   Staging of Medullary Carcinoma

| Stage | Classification |
| --- | --- |
| I | T1, N0, M0 |
| II | T2, N0, M0 |
| III | T3, N0, M0 |
| | T1, N1a, M0 |
| | T2, N1a, M0 |
| | T3, N1a, M0 |
| IVA | T4a, N0, M0 |
| | T4a, N1a, M0 |
| | T1, N1b, M0 |
| | T2, N1b, M0 |
| | T3, N1b, M0 |
| | T4a, N1b, M0 |
| IVB | T4b, any N, M0 |
| IVC | Any T, any N, M1 |

## CURRENT DIAGNOSIS

### Presentation

- Asymptomatic solitary solid thyroid nodule (most common presentation)
- Cervical lymphadenopathy
- Compressive symptoms (dysphagia, stridor, hoarseness, pain)

### Work-up

- Ultrasonography of cervical region
- Fine-needle aspiration
- If medullary thyroid cancer, evaluate for multiple endocrine neoplasia by obtaining:
  - Serum levels of calcitonin, calcium, parathyroid hormone, and plasma metanephrine
  - Genetic testing and family screening

## CURRENT THERAPY

### Papillary Thyroid Cancer

- Total thyroidectomy and central lymph node dissection
- Unilateral compartment oriented modified neck dissection if positive lateral lymph node disease
- Postoperative radioiodine ablation for residual, locally invasive, recurrent, or metastatic disease
- Lifelong thyroid hormone suppression
- Thyroglobulin monitoring

### Follicular Thyroid Neoplasm

- Initial lobectomy and isthmusectomy
- Completion thyroidectomy if cancer on final pathology
- Consider postoperative radioiodine ablation for residual, locally invasive, recurrent, or metastatic disease or for uptake in the thyroid bed on whole-body $^{131}$I scanning
- Lifelong thyroid hormone suppression
- Thyroglobulin monitoring

### Medullary Thyroid Cancer

- Total thyroidectomy and bilateral central lymph node dissection
- Consider compartment-oriented modified neck dissection
- Consider external-beam radiation with residual disease, soft tissue invasion, positive margins, or recurrence
- Long-term serial serum calcitonin and carcinoembryonic antigen monitoring
- Annual ultrasound of the neck

### Anaplastic Thyroid Cancer

- Chemoradiation is the mainstay treatment modality.
- Consider surgical intervention after chemoradiation only if the tumor is resectable.
- Perform tracheostomy only if the airway is compromised.

---

into risk level II (moderate risk; codons 609, 611, 618, 620, 630, 634 *RET*) should have surgery by the age of 5 years. Patients with risk level I (low risk; codons 731, 768, 790, 804, 891 *RET*) codon mutations should have an annual calcium provocative calcitonin test, and surgery may be deferred until tests become abnormal after the age of 5 years.

Routine follow-up includes calcitonin and CEA measurements at 2 months and then every 6 to 12 months. A physical examination and cervical ultrasonography are performed annually. Calcitonin levels of 250 pg/mL or greater should prompt a metastatic work-up with ultrasonography of the neck and computed tomography of the chest and abdomen. Calcitonin levels less than 250 pg/mL are rarely associated with radiographic evidence of recurrence or metastasis but merit close follow-up. Postoperative calcitonin elevation without identifiable disease is not an indication for external-beam radiation therapy.

## Prognosis

Most differentiated thyroid cancers manifest at an early stage and are associated with an excellent outlook. PTC is associated with a 10-year overall survival rate of up to 93%, and FTC has an 85% 10-year overall survival rate.

Approximately 30% of differentiated thyroid cancers recur, two thirds during the first decade after treatment. The risk of recurrent disease has a bimodal distribution, with the risk increased in patients younger than 20 years and older than 60 years. The majority of recurrences are local (68%), and only 32% of recurrences are distant metastases. The type of recurrence greatly affects prognosis. Local recurrences are associated with a 12% 30-year disease-related mortality rate, compared with 43% for distant recurrences.

Other factors associated with an increased mortality rate are male gender, age 40 years and older, local tumor invasion, regional lymph node metastases, and delay in therapy more than 12 months after initial diagnosis. HCC is a more aggressive variant of FTC and is associated with a 10-year overall survival rate of 76%.

The majority of ATC patients present with advanced disease. Long-term survival is rare, and the 10-year overall survival rate is only 14%. The median survival is less than 1 year.

The prognosis is intermediate for MTC, with an associated 10-year overall survival rate of 75%. Though cervical disease is present in up to 50% of patients at diagnosis, the addition of compartment-oriented lymph node dissection decreases the rate of cervical recurrence to 13%. The hereditary form of MTC tends to have a better prognosis than the sporadic form. This may be due in part to earlier diagnosis as a result of genetic screening. Within the hereditary MTC category, familial MTC has the best prognosis, and MEN-2b has the worst.

## REFERENCES

Al-Brahim N, Asa SL: Papillary thyroid carcinoma: An overview. Arch Pathol Lab Med 2006;130:1057-1062.

Are C, Shaha AR: Anaplastic thyroid carcinoma: Biology, pathogenesis, prognostic factors and treatment approaches. Ann Surg Oncol 2006;13:453-464.

Blankenship DR, Chin E, Terris DJ: Contemporary management of thyroid cancer. Am J Otolaryngol 2005;26:249-260.

Cooper DS, Doherty GM, Haugen BR, et al; The American Thyroid Association Guidelines Taskforce. Management guidelines for patients with thyroid nodules and differentiated thyroid cancer. Thyroid 2006;16(2):109-142.

Greene FL, Page DL, Fleming ID, et al: Thyroid. In Greene FL, Page DL, Fleming ID, et al (eds): AJCC Cancer Staging Manual, 6th ed. New York: Springer, 2002, pp 77-87.

Jemal A, Siegel R, Ward E, et al: Cancer statistics 2006. CA Cancer J Clin 2006;56:106-130.

Kouvaraki MA, Shapiro SE, Lee JE, Evans DB, Perrier ND: Surgical management of thyroid carcinoma. J Natl Compr Canc Netw 2005;3:458-466.

Lopez-Penabad L, Chiu AC, Hoff AO, et al: Prognostic factors in patients with Hürthle cell neoplasms of the thyroid. Cancer 2003;97:1186-1194.

Mazzaferri EL, Jhiang SM: Long-term impact of initial surgical and medical therapy on papillary and follicular thyroid cancer. Am J Med 1994;97:418-428. Erratum in Am J Med 1995;98:215.

National Comprehensive Cancer Network: Thyroid carcinoma. Clinical practice guidelines in oncology, version 2.2007. PDF available at http://nccn.org/professionals/physician_gls/PDF/thyroid.pdf (accessed June 15, 2007).

Sherman SI: Thyroid carcinoma. Lancet 2003;361:501-511.

Yen TW, Shapiro SE, Gagel RF, et al: Medullary thyroid carcinoma: Results of a standardized surgical approach in a contemporary series of 80 consecutive patients. Surgery 2003;134:890-899.

# Pheochromocytomas

Method of
*Pierre-François Plouin, MD*

Pheochromocytomas (PHs) and functional paragangliomas (PGLs) are neoplasms of chromaffin tissue that synthesize catecholamines. Most of these tumors appear in the adrenal medulla (PH proper), but 10% to 20% arise in extra-adrenal chromaffin tissue (PGL). In descending order of frequency, functional PGL can develop in the Zuckerkandl body (located at the root of the upper mesenteric artery), the sympathetic plexus of the urinary bladder, the kidneys, and the heart, sympathetic ganglia in the mediastinum, the head, or the neck. Most head and neck PGLs are nonfunctional. Patients with familial diseases can have bilateral PH or PH plus functional or nonfunctional PGL.

The prevalence of PH and functional PGL is about 0.1% in patients with hypertension and 4% in patients with incidentally discovered adrenal masses or incidentalomas. Their incidence in the general population is less than 1 per 100,000 persons per year. The lifetime incidence of PH and PGL is high in familial syndromes affected by these tumors: 1% to 5% in neurofibromatosis type 1 (NF1), 15% to 20% in von Hippel–Lindau (VHL) disease, 30% to 50% in multiple endocrine neoplasia type 2 (MEN-2), and probably more than 50% in *SDHB* and *SDHD* gene mutation carriers.

## Presentation

The increase in catecholamine production in patients with PH and functional PGL causes symptoms (mainly headaches, palpitations, and excessive sweating) and signs (mainly hypertension, weight loss, and diabetes) that reflect the effects of catecholamines on α- and β-adrenergic receptors. Signs and symptoms are varying and often paroxysmal due to the variable and disorderly release of catecholamines by the tumor. The typical presentation is a combination of variable hypertension with paroxysmal symptoms, either occurring spontaneously or provoked by abdominal pressure during anteflexion, micturition, or defecation.

The diagnosis of PH or PGL can be delayed for several reasons. First, these tumors are rare. Second, hypertension may be absent for long periods because active catecholamines can be converted into biologically inactive metanephrines within the tumor. Third, the symptoms and signs are nonspecific and are common to both the tumoral (in PH and PGL) and neuronal (during stress) release of catecholamines. For these reasons, the mean time from the onset of hypertension, when present, to diagnosis of the tumor exceeds 3 years. Indeed, the tumor is often discovered fortuitously during diagnostic testing for symptoms or clinical conditions not related to adrenal disease.

Presymptomatic diagnosis during the exploration of incidentalomas currently accounts for 25% of all cases. Presymptomatic diagnosis is also possible in patients with phenotypic evidence or a family history of a genetic disease associated with PH or PGL.

## Diagnosis

### LABORATORY TESTING

Biochemical investigation for PH or PGL is offered to hypertensive patients reporting bouts of headaches, palpitations, and sweating, those with hypertension resistant to treatment, and those with incidentalomas or with a familial disease conferring a predisposition to PH or PGL (Figure 1). The positive diagnosis of PH and functional PGL is based on the quantification of plasma or urinary metanephrines (metanephrine itself and normetanephrine), because this test is more sensitive than the quantification of urinary vanillylmandelic acid excretion or plasma concentrations of catecholamines, neuropeptide Y, or chromogranin A. The relative merits of the various determinations of plasma and urinary metanephrines are summarized in Table 1.

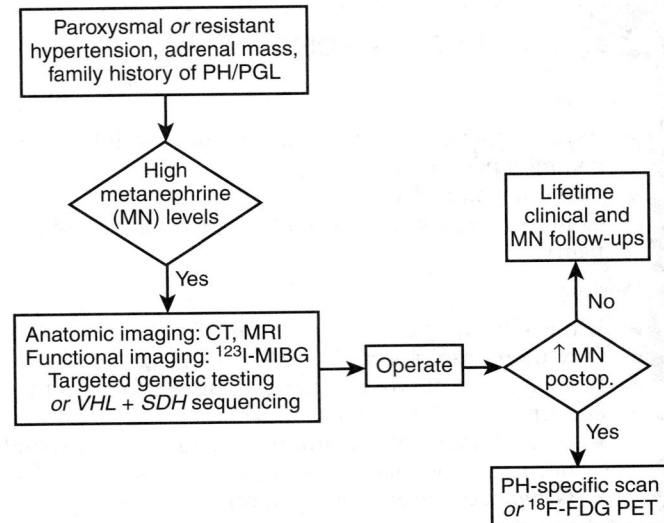

**FIGURE 1.** Algorithm for the initial management and long-term follow-up of patients with pheochromocytomas (PH) and secreting paragangliomas (PGL). *Abbreviations:* CT = computed tomography; $^{18}$F-FDG PET = $^{18}$F-fluorodeoxyglucose positron-emission tomography; MIBG = $^{123}$I-metaiodobenzylguanidine; MRI = magnetic resonance imaging.

Patients undergoing biochemical tests for PH or PGL should be given instructions enabling them to obtain an accurate 24-hour sample of acidified urine (for urine testing) and should be told to avoid tricyclic antidepressants and acetaminophen (paracetamol, Tylenol) for 5 days, because these drugs can cause false-positive results in plasma metanephrine tests. Because accurate plasma or urinary metanephrine assays are readily available, there is no need to subject patients to the hazards of pharmacologic provocative or suppression tests.

### IMAGING

Preoperative imaging tests are designed to locate the tumor and to determine whether it is single or multiple, adrenal or ectopic, benign or malignant, and isolated or present with other neoplasms in the context of familial syndromes. The combination of anatomic imaging studies based on computed tomography (CT) or magnetic resonance imaging (MRI) and radionuclide imaging studies yields a sensitivity of almost 100% for the diagnosis of catecholamine-producing tumors. CT is the most commonly used anatomic imaging technique, but MRI is preferred for children and pregnant patients.

Functional imaging with $^{123}$I-metaiodobenzylguanidine (MIBG) should be carried out when possible, because $^{131}$I-MIBG scintigraphy is less sensitive. Labetalol (Trandate, Normodyne) and antipsychotic drugs should be withdrawn for several days before the investigations because they reduce MIBG uptake. If no MIBG uptake is observed, mostly in cases of nonfunctional PGL, additional investigations by scintigraphy with nonspecific ligands such as somatostatin receptor scintigraphy or $^{18}$F-fluorodeoxyglucose positron-emission tomography ($^{18}$F-FDG PET) should be carried out.

In addition to the primary tumor, imaging tests can disclose lymph node, bone, liver, or pulmonary metastases, thereby establishing the presence of malignant PH or PGL.

## Differential Diagnosis

Catecholamine-secreting tumors mimic paroxysmal conditions with hypertension or cardiac rhythm disorders, particularly panic attacks, in which sympathetic activation linked to anxiety reproduces the signs and symptoms of PH. Plasma and urinary metanephrine concentrations are usually normal in these conditions. Acute cardiovascular events, such as myocardial infarction, pulmonary edema, and stroke,

**TABLE 1** Advantages and Limitations of Determining Metanephrine and Normetanephrine in Urine or Plasma

| Determinations* | Advantages | Limitations |
|---|---|---|
| Urinary-free and conjugated MN and NMN | Easy determination, widely available<br>Integration of 24-h secretion<br>Sensitivity enhanced by use of the MN+NMN-to-creatinine ratio | Need for an acidified 24-h urine collection |
| Plasma-free and conjugated MN and NMN | Long half-life, high concentration (25× higher than free MN and NMN) | Includes sulfate-conjugated MN and NMN produced in the GI tract<br>High in cases of renal failure |
| Plasma-free MN and NMN | Reflects tumor release of MN and NMN and the conversion of epinephrine and norepinephrine into MN and NMN<br>Provides the best combination of sensitivity and specificity | Unstable, low concentration, technically demanding<br>Acetaminophen-containing drugs can give false-positive results |

*All these tests have sensitivities exceeding 90%.
*Abbreviations:* GI = gastrointestinal; MN = metanephrine; NMN = normetanephrine.

also induce an increase in catecholamine levels that may be sustained for several days and are associated with an increase in plasma or urinary metanephrine concentration. The diagnosis of PH or secreting PGL is excluded in these cases by the normalization of metanephrine levels 10 days after the onset of the event.

## Genetic Counseling

Before 2000, three different familial and syndromic diseases were known to result in PH or PGL: MEN-2 due to *RET* gene mutations, VHL disease due to *VHL* gene mutations, and NF1 due to *NF1* mutations. The overall incidence of familial PH or PGL was estimated at 10%. The recent identification of mutations in the *VHL*, *SDHB*, and *SDHD* genes in patients with apparently sporadic tumors has increased estimates of the incidence of an underlying genetic disease in patients with PH or PGL to 20% to 25%. Familial cases are more likely to be bilateral and recurrent than sporadic cases. Carriers of *SDHB* mutations have a high risk of malignant primary tumor or metastatic recurrence. Genetic screening should therefore be offered to most patients with PH or PGL (Figure 2).

Targeted genetic testing should be offered to patients with phenotypic signs consistent with or a family history of MEN-2, VHL disease, or hereditary PGL. Phenotypic signs of MEN-2 include medullary thyroid cancer and hyperparathyroidism, signs of VHL disease include hemangioblastomas and renal or pancreatic tumors, and signs of hereditary PGL include head and neck PGLs and family history in the paternal branch. In patients with an apparently sporadic PH or PGL, priority should be given to analysis of the *VHL*, *SDHB*, and *SDHD* genes. In patients with bilateral PH, the *RET* and *VHL* should be analyzed first. Identification of a causative mutation in one affected

patient should lead to presymptomatic genetic testing of the family, because early detection of small tumors in persons deemed to be at risk can reduce the morbidity of the disease. Screening for *NF1* gene mutations is feasible but rarely carried out, because the NF1 phenotype (multiple café-au-lait spots, neurofibromas, Lisch nodules, and axillary and inguinal freckling) is sufficiently clear for diagnosis of the condition in adults.

## Treatment

### TREATMENT OBJECTIVES

PH and functional PGL carry risks of hypersecretion and tumor growth. Surgery aims to eliminate both risks. The consequences of hypersecretion should be carefully managed before and during surgery. Primary tumor resection does not eliminate the risk of tumor persistence (in malignant tumors) or tumor recurrence (mostly in genetic diseases).

### PREOPERATIVE MANAGEMENT

Blood pressure (BP) should be normalized, whenever possible, before surgery, because the incidence of perioperative complications has been consistently linked to preoperative BP. Given the variability of BP in PH or PGL, it may be useful to determine 24-hour ambulatory BP. Antihypertensive regimens aim to reduce mean office BP to less than 140/90 mm Hg or 24-hour ambulatory BP to less than 125/80 mm Hg. However, the total abolition of hypertensive paroxysms is not currently possible, and patients should undergo surgery after 1 to 2 weeks of preparation.

BP control requires α- and β-adrenergic antagonists. Because most PHs and PGLs secrete predominantly norepinephrine, an α-agonist, α-adrenergic antagonists are the cornerstone of hypertensive control. Noncompetitive α-blockers, such as phenoxybenzamine (Dibenzyline), bind covalently to α-receptors, causing an irreversible blockade. They allow stable BP control, but they increase the risk of hypotension during tumor removal and the immediate postoperative period. Competitive α-blockers, such as prazosin (Minipress) are more suitable. The initial dose of prazosin can induce a sharp drop in BP, so the dose should be gradually increased from 0.5 to 5 mg three times a day. α-Adrenergic blockade generally gives rise to tachycardia secondary to catecholamine β-receptor stimulation. This requires the subsequent addition of a β-blocker, such as 25 to 100 mg atenolol (Tenormine) daily.

If adrenergic blockade proves insufficient to control BP, then a dihydropyridine may also be administered. Arrhythmia prevention is based on β-blockade and the careful correction of hypokalemia: The chronic excess of catecholamine causes secondary hyperaldosteronism, resulting in an increase in potassium loss. The sodium intake of patients should not be restricted and diuretics should not be used.

GENETIC DIAGNOSIS IN PH/PGL

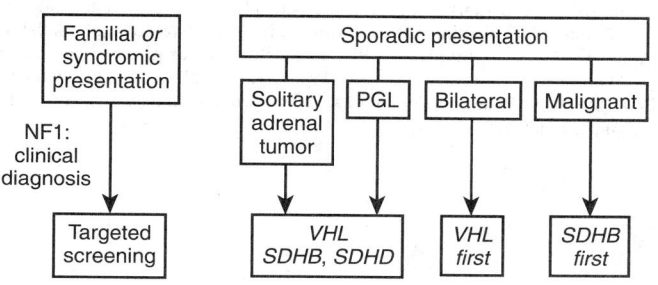

**FIGURE 2.** Suggested genetic screening in patients with pheochromocytomas (PH) and secreting paragangliomas (PGL). *Abbreviation:* NF1 = neurofibromatosis type 1.

## CURRENT DIAGNOSIS

- Most patients with symptomatic PH or functional PGL are hypertensive. Blood pressure typically rises when symptoms are present (mostly headaches, palpitations, and sweating).
- Presymptomatic diagnosis has become common in patients with incidentally discovered adrenal masses (incidentalomas) and in relatives of patients with symptomatic PH.
- The diagnosis of PH or functional PGL is based on the determination of metanephrines.
- Most catecholamine-secreting tumors arise in the adrenal glands (PH proper) and are easily detected by computed tomography or magnetic resonance imaging. Patients might also harbor extra-adrenal primary tumors (PGL) or distant metastases. Adrenal imaging should therefore be combined with whole-body metaiodobenzylguanidine scintigraphy.
- One in four patients with PH or PGL has germline mutations conferring a predisposition to catecholamine-secreting tumors. The identification of a causative mutation should lead to presymptomatic genetic testing in the family.

*Abbreviations:* PGL = paraganglioma; PH = pheochromocytoma.

## ANESTHESIA AND SURGERY

Anesthesia and surgery in patients with PH or PGL may be complex and involve large and acute variations in BP and heart rate. Almost every possible anesthetic technique has been advocated. Perioperative safety relies primarily on correct preoperative pharmacologic control and the referral of patients to centers with extensive experience in treating the disease.

Large variations in BP and heart rate can occur during induction, intubation, peritoneal incision, and tumor handling and devascularization. Radial artery pressure and the electrocardiogram (ECG) should be monitored continuously. I generally use intravenous infusions of nicardipine (Cardene) 0.1 to 1[3] mg/min to control BP and intravenous esmolol (Brevibloc) loading infusion of 0.5 mg/kg/min over 1 minute to control arrhythmia.

[3]Exceeds dosage recommended by the manufacturer.

## CURRENT THERAPY

- Patients with catecholamine-secreting tumors should be referred to centers with extensive experience in the anesthetic and surgical management of the disease.
- Blood pressure should be normalized before surgery, using α-adrenergic and possibly β-adrenergic antagonists.
- Most PHs and many PGLs can be resected laparoscopically.
- Adrenal cortex–sparing surgery is feasible in patients with bilateral PH.
- PH and PGL can recur. Patients should be subject to lifelong follow-up, with checkups at least yearly, including blood pressure measurement and metanephrine determination.

*Abbreviations:* PGL = paraganglioma; PH = pheochromocytoma.

Laparoscopic surgery has supplanted open surgery in the management of most cases of PH and intra-abdominal PGL. Adrenal cortex–sparing surgery may be carried out by laparoscopy in patients with hereditary forms of PH.

# Postoperative and Long-term Follow-up

Plasma or urinary metanephrine concentration should be determined 10 days after surgery, to check for normalization. If metanephrine concentrations remain high, [123]I-MIBG scintigraphy should be performed. This technique can detect distant metastases whose MIBG uptake was masked by the primary tumor's higher metabolic activity before surgery. No MIBG uptake might occur in dedifferentiated metastases, and nonspecific radionuclide imaging may be required (see Figure 1).

Because PH and PGL can recur, patients undergoing surgery for PH or PGL should have lifelong follow-up, with checkups at least once yearly, including BP measurement and plasma or urinary metanephrine determination. In a cohort of patients undergoing surgery for PH or PGL, the 10-year probability of recurrence—defined as the reappearance of the disease after eradication of the tumor had been confirmed by negative biochemical and imaging tests—was 16%. Patients with recurrences were younger, had larger tumors, and were more likely to have familial disease or bilateral or extra-adrenal PGL than patients with no recurrence. Recurrences were malignant in one in two patients.

Malignant PH or PGL is compatible with prolonged survival, with symptom-free intervals lasting from months to decades. In 54 patients with malignant PH or PGL followed at my center, the 5-year and 10-year probabilities of survival were 0.75 and 0.52, respectively.

In cases of small recurrences with an accessible vascular pedicle, surgical excision may be preceded or replaced by therapeutic embolization. In cases in which soft-tissue or skeletal metastases are too widespread for surgery or embolization, several palliative therapies may be considered. Pharmacologic treatment aimed at the long-term blockade of catecholamine synthesis with α-methyl-*p*-tyrosine (Demser) 1 to 4 g/day in divided doses can improve the patient's quality of life, but it has no effect on tumor progression. Conventional radiotherapy can provide effective palliation in cases of painful metastases. Metabolic radiotherapy with [131]I-MIBG and chemotherapy can provide clinical, hormonal, and, in some cases, tumoral improvement.

## REFERENCES

Diner EK, Franks ME, Behari A, et al: Partial adrenalectomy: The National Cancer Institute experience. Urology 2005;66:19-23.
Eisenhofer G, Bornstein SR, Brouwers FM, et al.: Malignant pheochromocytoma: Current status and initiatives for future progress. Endocr Relat Cancer 2004;11:423-436.
Ilias I, Pacak K: Current approaches and recommended algorithm for the diagnostic localization of pheochromocytoma. J Clin Endocrinol Metab 2004;89:479-491.
Lenders JW, Pacak K, Walther MM, et al: Biochemical diagnosis of pheochromocytoma: Which test is best? JAMA. 2002;287:1427-1434.
Plouin PF, Duclos JM, Soppelsa F, et al: Factors associated with perioperative morbidity and mortality in patients with pheochromocytoma: Analysis of 165 operations at a single center. J Clin Endocrinol Metab 2001;86:1480-1486.
Plouin PF, Gimenez-Roqueplo AP: The genetic basis of pheochromocytoma: Who to screen and how? Nat Clin Pract Endocrinol Metab 2006;2:60-61.
Prys-Roberts C: Phaeochromocytoma: Recent progress in its management. Br J Anaesth 2000;85:44-57.

# Thyroiditis

Method of

*Katherine Hughes, MB, ChB,*
*and Mark W. J. Strachan, MD*

The term *thyroiditis* describes any disorder in which there is an inflammatory infiltrate into the thyroid gland. There are numerous potential causes of thyroiditis including autoimmunity, infection, chemical and biological agents, and radiation. By far the commonest forms of thyroiditis are Hashimoto's (chronic lymphocytic) thyroiditis and Graves' disease, both of which have an autoimmune etiology. They are discussed in detail elsewhere in this book.

## Autoimmune

### SILENT (PAINLESS OR SUBACUTE LYMPHOCYTIC) THYROIDITIS

Silent thyroiditis is characterized by inflammatory destruction of the thyroid tissue leading to over-spill of preformed thyroid hormones into the circulation. This can occur following viral infection or in persons with underlying autoimmune disease. As thyroid hormone stores are depleted, 50% of patients progress from the hyperthyroid phase to a temporary period of hypothyroidism. The period of thyrotoxicosis typically lasts for some 4 to 6 weeks, and the hypothyroidism usually resolves within 6 to 12 months, once the follicular cells have recovered. Characteristically there is low radioiodine uptake, erythrocyte sedimentation rate is normal or near-normal, and low-titer thyroid antibodies appear transiently in the serum. A history of L-thyroxine (Synthroid, Levoxyl) or iodine ingestion must be excluded.

Treatment of mild hyperthyroidism is not required. If the patient has prominent adrenergic symptoms, a β-adrenergic receptor–blocking drug, for example propranolol 40 to 80 mg/day (Inderal), should be prescribed. Antithyroid drugs are not effective. In the hypothyroid phase, treatment is not required unless the patient is symptomatic or there is a prolonged period before recovery of thyroid function. If required, the patient can be treated with L-thyroxine 50 to 100 μg/day. This should be withdrawn after approximately 6 to 12 months so thyroid function can be reassessed for recovery. The presence of autoantibodies in high titer suggests an underlying autoimmune pathology and a high risk of recurrence and progression to permanent hypothyroidism.

### POSTPARTUM THYROIDITIS

Postpartum thyroiditis is a destructive inflammatory process of the thyroid tissue, very similar to silent thyroiditis, which typically occurs within 2 to 6 months of delivery. It develops following 5% to 10% of all pregnancies in iodine-replete areas, but is three times more common in women with type 1 diabetes. Anti–thyroid peroxidase (TPO) antibodies are usually positive, and indeed the presence of anti-TPO antibodies in early pregnancy predicts a 30% to 50% chance of developing postpartum thyroiditis. The most common clinical presentation is with hypothyroidism, but in one third of cases isolated hyperthyroidism occurs, and in a further one quarter there is a period of hyperthyroidism followed by hypothyroidism.

Symptoms such as fatigue, anxiety, and low mood are common in postpartum women, and so the diagnosis of thyroiditis is easily missed. Thyroid function tests should, therefore, be performed as a matter of routine at 6 to 8 weeks postpartum in women with type 1 diabetes, positive TPO antibodies, goiter, or a previous history of postpartum thyroiditis (because recurrence is likely). There should also be a low threshold to perform thyroid function tests at any stage in postpartum women with nonspecific symptoms that suggest thyroiditis.

In postpartum thyroiditis, the thyroid is painless, often there is no goiter, and the erythrocyte sedimentation rate is not elevated. In women whose initial presentation is with thyrotoxicosis, the main differential diagnosis is Graves' disease. In the absence of specific clinical features of Graves' disease, the underlying cause of thyrotoxicosis might not be immediately apparent. Thyroid receptor antibodies are positive in up to 25% of women with postpartum thyroiditis and may be negative in a small fraction with Graves' disease. Thyroid scintigraphy is the key discriminatory test, but it necessitates the temporary cessation of breast-feeding. The thyrotoxicosis of postpartum thyroiditis is usually mild and self-limited, and so severity and persistence are often the most useful guides.

Treatment of the hyperthyroid phase is the same as for silent or painless thyroiditis, namely with long-acting β-adrenergic blockade in symptomatic women. The hypothyroid phase is treated with L-thyroxine if patients are symptomatic or if a further pregnancy is planned for the near future. L-Thyroxine should be reduced or discontinued after 6 to 12 months to determine if the thyroid gland has recovered from the episode. Hypothyroidism that persists longer than 12 months is usually permanent.

## Infection

### DE QUERVAIN'S (SUBACUTE) THYROIDITIS

De Quervain's thyroiditis often follows an upper respiratory tract infection and is believed to be viral in origin. It is more common in summer months. Disruption of the thyroid follicles leads to discharge of preformed thyroid hormone into the circulation, leading to hyperthyroidism. This hyperthyroid state usually lasts 4 to 8 weeks. Occasionally it persists for longer. Transient hypothyroidism can develop as stores of thyroid hormone in thyroid tissue are depleted.

Clinically, the affected patient presents with fever, asthenia, malaise, thyroid pain, and tenderness radiating to the ear. Patients also might report dysphagia and symptoms of thyroid hormone excess. Clinically the thyroid gland is firm and very tender on palpation. Supporting investigations include elevated erythrocyte sedimentation rate and low radioiodine uptake.

Prominent adrenergic symptoms are controlled with β-adrenoreceptor blocking drugs, such as propanolol (Inderal) 40-80mg/day. Nonsteroidal anti-inflammatory drugs (NSAIDs) such as ibuprofen 400 mg up to 4 times daily can be used for thyroid pain. Glucocorticoids, such as prednisolone 40 to 60mg/day, in a tapering course of 4 to 6 weeks, can be used if NSAIDs fail to provide pain relief. Hypothyroidism is usually transient and mild and does not require treatment, but L-thyroxine may be instituted in symptomatic patients. Hypothyroidism persisting longer than 1 year is usually permanent.

### ACUTE SUPPURATIVE (PYOGENIC) THYROIDITIS

Acute suppurative infections of the thyroid are extremely rare and usually indicate underlying immunocompromised status, thyroid pathology, or an anatomic defect. In children, the commonest underlying cause is an internal fistula extending from the piriform sinus to the thyroid. Agents causing acute suppurative thyroiditis include bacteria, fungi, mycobacteria, and parasites. The inoculation of the thyroid usually occurs after pyogenic infection at a distant site.

Clinically, the patient has a painful, tender thyroid, with swelling, erythema, possible abscess, and constitutional symptoms. Pain may be referred to the pharynx or ears. Inflammatory markers are markedly elevated and thyroid function is usually normal, although hyper- and hypothyroidism can develop. Fine-needle aspiration and culture should be performed. Treatment is with targeted antimicrobial therapy and excision and drainage of any abscess. There is usually recovery of thyroid function.

## Drugs and Radiation

### AMIODARONE

A 200 mg tablet of amiodarone (Cordarone) contains 75 mg of iodine of which approximately 10% is deiodinated (compared with a daily dietary requirement of just 125 μg), and so up to 20% of treated patients develop thyroid dysfunction. All patients should have thyroid function testing before commencing amiodarone, and thyroid function should be monitored every 6 months while on treatment. Amiodarone persists in the body for many months after cessation, and so thyroid function should continue to be monitored for up to 12 months after it is discontinued. Hypothyroidism is more common in iodine-rich areas and is due to the precipitation of thyroid autoimmunity or the direct blockade and destruction of thyroid tissue by iodine. It may be treated with L-thyroxine, although higher doses are often required compared with other causes of hypothyroidism; amiodarone can continue to be administered if clinically necessary.

Amiodarone-induced thyrotoxicosis (AIT) is more common in iodine-deficient areas. Amiodarone impairs peripheral conversion of thyroxine ($T_4$) to triiodothyronine ($T_3$) and so it is important that $T_3$ and thyroid-stimulating hormone (TSH) concentrations are measured in patients with suspected AIT, because it is not uncommon to find normal concentrations of $T_3$ despite markedly elevated $T_4$ concentrations.

Two forms of AIT are described. Type 1 AIT is more likely to occur in patients with preexisting subclinical thyroid disorders and is due to iodine-induced synthesis and release of thyroid hormone. Type 2 AIT is a destructive thyroiditis that results in release of preformed thyroid hormone. Discrimination of the two forms is not straightforward, because radioiodine uptake might not be elevated in the type 1 form due to the high iodine load. Color-flow Doppler ultrasonography and measurement of serum interleukin 6 (IL-6) may be useful, because there is a typical pattern of increased vascularity of the thyroid gland and not substantially elevated concentrations of IL-6 in the type 1 form and the reverse pattern in the type 2 form. However, these investigations might not be available routinely, and mixed patterns are observed, so often it is not possible to subclassify the etiology of AIT.

If possible, amiodarone should be discontinued in AIT, but because of the prolonged period of elimination, additional therapy will invariably be required for several months. Type 1 AIT should, in theory, respond to antithyroid drugs, such as methimazole (Tapazole) 40 to 60mg/day. If the patient fails to respond, or if the thyrotoxicosis is severe, potassium perchlorate 1g/day should be commenced and continued until the patient is euthyroid. Perchlorate inhibits the entry of iodide into the thyroid cells and so facilitates its discharge from the gland. A complete blood count should be checked every few weeks to detect any blood dyscrasias.

Treatment of type 2 AIT is with systemic glucocorticoids, such as prednisolone 30 to 40mg/day for 3 months. The dose of steroid should be gradually reduced to minimize recurrence. Iopanoic acid may be an alternative in type 2 AIT when glucocorticoids are contraindicated. Triple therapy with a glucocorticoid, a thionamide, and potassium perchlorate is sometimes required, particularly when a definitive classification of AIT cannot be made and a rapid therapeutic response is required, such as due to a precarious cardiovascular status. If amiodarone therapy cannot be discontinued, total thyroidectomy may be required.

## LITHIUM

Lithium therapy, usually for bipolar depression, is associated with an increased risk of hypothyroidism. Female sex and commencing lithium therapy at an older age are the main risk factors, and up to 50% of women older than 65 years who are treated with lithium have hypothyroidism. Lithium, like iodide, inhibits thyroid hormone release and it also can promote the development of thyroid autoimmunity. Treatment is with L-thyroxine, and there is usually no requirement to discontinue the lithium. Lithium-induced thyrotoxicosis is substantially less common and is usually caused by a silent thyroiditis precipitated by direct toxicity of lithium on the thyroid cells.

## CYTOKINE THERAPY

Interferon-α (IFN-α) and interleukin-2 (IL-2) activate the immune system and so can induce or activate autoimmune disease. Fifteen

## CURRENT DIAGNOSIS

**Silent, Painless, Subacute Lymphocytic**
- Transient mild hyperthyroidism followed by hypothyroidism
- Painless

**Postpartum**
- Transient thyroid dysfunction 2-6 months postpartum
- Common in women with type 1 diabetes and/or positive thyroid antibodies

**De Quervain's, Subacute**
- Pain in neck, radiating to ears; constitutional upset
- Biochemical hyperthyroidism, elevated ESR, and low RAI uptake

**Acute Suppurative, Pyogenic**
- Painful, erythematous neck, with fever and marked systemic symptoms
- Elevated inflammatory markers
- Fine-needle aspiration with culture of pyogenic material

**Amiodarone (Cordarone)-Induced Thyrotoxicosis**
- Elevated $T_4$ *and* $T_3$; suppressed thyrotropin
- Type 1 AIT: Preexisting subclinical thyroid disease, hypervascular thyroid on Doppler ultrasound, normal IL-6
- Type 2 AIT: Reduced blood flow on Doppler ultrasound, elevated IL-6.

**Lithium**
- Usually hypothyroidism

**Cytokines (IFN-α, IL-2)**
- Destructive thyroiditis with hyperthyroidism and hypothyroidism

**Radiation**
- Thyroid pain and transient hyperthyroidism after external radiation treatment or RAI

**Reidel's**
- Rare
- Fibrosis may extend into other neck structures
- Diagnosis with open biopsy

*Abbreviations:* AIT = amiodarone-induced thyrotoxicosis; ESR = erythrocyte sedimentation rate; IL = interleukin; RAI = radioactive iodine; $T_3$ = triiodothyronine; $T_4$ = thyroxine.

percent of patients treated with INF-α develop abnormal thyroid function, and this may be either thyrotoxicosis or hypothyroidism. The thyroid pathology encountered includes a destructive thyroiditis, Graves' disease, or autoimmune hypothyroidism. Patients with preexisting thyroid antibodies are at increased risk and should be monitored regularly during therapy.

Thyroiditis usually occurs in the first few weeks of therapy and occurs at a similar time to the development of thyroid antibodies. The hyperthyroidism is usually mild and takes weeks to months to resolve. If hyperthyroidism is mild, treatment is not required; if it is severe, a β-adrenoreceptor blocking drug can be used. Thyroid pain is treated with NSAIDs or corticosteroids. Hypothyroidism can require therapy with L-thyroxine if it is symptomatic or persistent. Thyroid function usually returns to normal after treatment is discontinued.

## CURRENT THERAPY

**Silent, Painless, Subacute Lymphocytic**

- β-Blockers if hyperthyroid
- Consider L-thyroxine if hypothyroid

**Postpartum**

- β-Blockers if hyperthyroid
- Short course of L-thyroxine if hypothyroid

**De Quervain's, Subacute**

- NSAIDs or corticosteroids

**Acute Suppurative, Pyogenic**

- Antimicrobial therapy and abscess drainage

**Amiodarone (Cordarone)-Induced Thyrotoxicosis**

- Stop amiodarone (Cordarone) if possible
- Type 1 AIT: antithyroid drugs and potassium perchlorate
- Type 2 AIT: Glucocorticoids; ioponoic acid if steroids are contraindicated

**Lithium**

- L-Thyroxine if hypothyroid

**Cytokines (IFN-α, IL-2)**

- NSAIDs or corticosteroids if painful
- β-Blockers if hyperthyroid

**Radiation**

- NSAIDs or corticosteroids if painful
- β-Blockers if hyperthyroid
- L-Thyroxine if hypothyroid

**Reidel's**

- Corticosteroids, tamoxifen (Nolvadex), and surgery

---

*Abbreviations:* AIT = amiodarone-induced thyrotoxicosis; IL = interleukin; NSAID = nonsteroidal anti-inflammatory drug.

## RADIATION

Both radioiodine therapy and external beam radiation can cause radiation-induced thyroiditis. There may be associated thyroid pain and transient hyperthyroidism because of release of thyroid hormones. Treatment options include short courses of NSAIDs, corticosteroids, and β-blockers. Subsequent hypothyroidism should be treated with L-thyroxine, although hypothyroidism developing within 6 months of radioiodine therapy might not be permanent.

## Unknown Etiology

Riedel's (fibrous) thyroiditis is an extremely uncommon condition where an invasive fibrotic process occurs in the thyroid gland. The fibrosis may be unilateral or diffuse and extend into adjacent neck structures. Riedel's thyroiditis is also associated with mediastinal and retroperitoneal fibrosis. The thyroid gland is moderately enlarged and stony hard. Inflammatory markers are not elevated, but hypothyroidism and hypoparathyroidism can occur. Diagnosis is by open biopsy. The main differential diagnosis is fibrotic Hashimoto's thyroiditis or undifferentiated cancer. L-Thyroxine is indicated for hypothyroidism, it but does not alter the disease process. Progressive esophageal and tracheal compression can occur, necessitating partial thyroidectomy. Anecdotal reports have suggested that systemic glucocorticoid therapy or tamoxifen (Nolvadex)[1] can induce regression.

### REFERENCES

Bogazzi F, Bartalena L, Cosci C, et al: Treatment of type II amiodarone-induced thyrotoxicosis by either iopanoic acid or glucocorticoids: A prospective, randomized study. J Clin Endocrinol Metab 2003;88(5):1999-2002.

Carella C, Mazziotti G, Amato G, et al: Interferon-α related thyroid disease. J Clin Endocrinol Metab 2004;89:3656-3661.

Martino E, Bartalena L, Bogazzi F, Braverman LE: The effects of amiodarone on the thyroid. Endocr Rev 2001;22:240-254.

Pearce EN, Farwell AP, Braverman LE: Current concepts: Thyroiditis. N Engl J Med 2003;348:2646-2655.

Stagnaro-Green A: Postpartum thyroiditis. J Clin Endocrinol Metab 2002; 87(9):4042-4047.

---

[1]Not FDA approved for this indication.

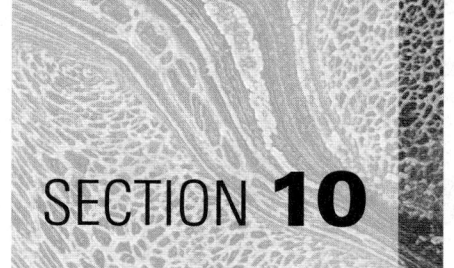

# The Urogenital Tract

## Bacterial Infections of the Urinary Tract in Males

Method of
*Brian A. VanderBrink, MD, and*
*Robert M. Moldwin, MD*

### Epidemiology

The incidence of urinary tract infections (UTIs) in males follows a bimodal distribution with peaks in infancy and after 50 years of age likely secondary to the presence of foreskin and the effects of prostatic enlargement, respectively. Urinary tract infections in males of all ages are traditionally classified as *complicated* because of the high incidence of associated urologic abnormalities, including incomplete emptying, urolithiasis, and obstruction.

### Infant Evaluation

Early diagnosis and treatment of a febrile UTI in the male infant is critical to preserve renal function of the growing kidney and to prevent progression to life-threatening septicemia. A history of vesicoureteral reflux (VUR) in a sibling suggests up to a 34% risk of VUR in the patient. When a UTI is suspected, obtaining a reliable urine culture, preferably by sterile urethral catheterization, is crucial to confirm the diagnosis. Once therapy is completed, a course of prophylactic antibiotics should begin to prevent further infections while evaluation continues. Further evaluation entails both ultrasound and voiding cystourethrogram to assess if obstruction or reflux exists, respectively.

Although epidemiology suggests the presence of foreskin is associated with a higher risk of neonatal UTI, recommending circumcision for prevention of recurring UTIs remains controversial. The benefits of circumcision may be more profound later in life because recent observational studies have demonstrated a protective effect of circumcision against HIV infection in high-prevalence regions.

### Epididymitis

Bacterial infection of the epididymis is typically the result of sexual activity or bladder outlet obstruction, and the causative agent may differ dependent on the mechanism of inoculation. In males younger than 35 years of age with acute epididymitis, the most common isolated organisms include *Neisseria gonorrhoeae*, *Chlamydia trachomatis*, and *Ureaplasma urealyticum*, which are transmitted during unprotected sexual intercourse. Homosexual men who practice unprotected anal intercourse have a higher incidence of coliforms as the causative agent.

In males older than 35 years of age, *Escherichia coli* is the most frequent cause of epididymitis. Epididymitis is also potentiated by elevated intravesical pressures generated in patients with bladder outlet obstruction, there by resulting in urethral-vasal reflux of enteric organisms. Tuberculosis is a rare but important cause of epididymitis that assumes a greater relative importance in high-prevalence regions.

Scrotal pain is present in all cases of epididymitis but is not pathognomonic, and the clinician must remember that the pain may be referred in origin. The significant findings on physical exam include preservation of cremasteric reflexes, a normal vertical lie of the testicle without foreshortening of the spermatic cord, and tender scrotal contents with particular tenderness and induration of the epididymis. A *reactive* hydrocele may be present, which precludes a complete physical examination of the scrotal contents. Doppler ultrasound is a useful adjunct to the history and physical examination, helping to differentiate acute epididymitis from surgical emergencies such as acute testicular torsion or an incarcerated inguinal hernia. Ultrasound may also be useful to diagnose scrotal abscess or guide scrotal drainage.

### Prostatitis

Most forms of prostatitis are associated with pelvic, perineal, penile, and/or scrotal pain, but frequently no overt microbial etiology can be identified; hence, in 1995 the National Institutes of Health workshop on prostatitis classified prostatitis into four main categories:

1. Acute bacterial
2. Chronic bacterial
3. Chronic pelvic pain syndrome
4. Asymptomatic inflammatory prostatitis

The hallmark features of category 1 prostatitis usually include those of acute bacterial cystitis and constitutional symptoms such as fever and chills. Acute urinary retention, progression to prostatic abscess, and frank sepsis is more common in diabetic and other immunocompromised patients. Category 2 prostatitis is typified by recurring urinary tract infections yet constitutes a small percentage of chronic prostatitis patients. In one study only 7% of 656 patients seen in a urology clinic for evaluation of prostatitis symptoms had bacteriologically proven category 2 disease.

Historically, categorization of prostatitis has been based on leukocyte and bacterial localization studies (from urine and expressed prostatic secretions) originally described in 1968 and simplified in 1997. However, even these *gold-standard* localization studies have been called into question with recent studies showing comparable rates of uropathogenic bacteria in both expressed prostatic secretions and postmassage urine cultures from men with chronic prostatitis/chronic pelvic pain syndrome and asymptomatic controls (8.0% versus 8.3%, respectively).

## Key Treatment

Clinical presentation dictates medical care of the male presenting with UTI. For example, category 1 prostatitis may be associated with urinary retention for which Foley catheter or suprapubic drainage is required. Radiographic imaging to exclude abscess should be contemplated in the category 1 prostatitis or epididymitis patient with unremitting infection despite *adequate* antibiotic therapy.

Patients who appear nontoxic and are able to tolerate oral medications can be safely treated as outpatients. Empirical selection of the antibiotic and its duration is influenced by a number of variables including site of infection, antibiotic tissue penetration, patient allergy profile, patient current medications, and co-morbidities. Trimethoprim-sulfamethoxazole (TMP-SMZ) (Bactrim) is effective against most uropathogens with the notable exception of *Enterococcus* and *Pseudomonas* species; however, resistance to community-acquired organisms continues to grow. Because of their broad spectrum of activity and excellent tissue penetration, such as prostate and kidney, fluoroquinolones are an attractive class of antibiotics for outpatient therapy, especially in areas where TMP-SMZ resistance is high. Patients requiring hospitalization may require intravenous antibiotics to provide broad spectrum coverage while awaiting urine and blood culture and sensitivities.

Urinary tract infections in males are almost always characterized as complicated and therefore require 7 or more days of antibiotic therapy. With reference to duration of antibiotic therapy, no standard of care has been developed for genitourinary infections that are not associated with bacteremia. Common practice has been 10 to 14 days of antimicrobial therapy for epididymitis and 4 to 6 weeks of therapy for category 2 prostatitis (chronic bacterial prostatitis). Prophylactic antibiotic therapy should be considered for patients who frequently relapse. In male patients who have a chronic indwelling catheter, bacteriuria should only be treated if acute symptoms referable to urinary tract are present (i.e., flank, suprapubic, or scrotal pain) or before genitourinary tract procedures.

## REFERENCES

Berger RE, Alexander ER, Harnisch JP, Paulsen CA: Etiology, manifestations and therapy of acute epididymitis: Prospective study of 50 cases. J Urol 1979;121:750-754.

Craig JC, Knight JF, Sureshkumar P, et al: Lack of circumcision increases the risk of urinary tract infection in young men. J Pediatr 1996;128:23-27.

Griebling TL: Urologic diseases in America project: Trends in resource use for urinary tract infections in men. J Urol 2005;173: 1288-1294.

Kass EJ, Kernen KM, Carey JM: Pediatric urinary tract infection and the necessity of complete urological imaging. BJU Int 2000;86: 94-96.

Krieger JN, Nyberg L Jr, Nickel JC: NIH consensus definition and classification of prostatitis. JAMA 1999;282:236.

Meares EM, Stamey TA: Bacteriologic localization patterns in bacterial prostatitis and urethritis. Invest Urol 1968;5:492-518

Nickel JC, Alexander RB, Schaeffer AJ, et al: Leukocytes and bacteria in men with chronic prostatitis/chronic pelvic pain syndrome compared to asymptomatic controls. J Urol 2003;170:818-822.

Nickel JC: The Pre and Post massage Test (PPMT): A simple screen for prostatitis. Tech Urol 1997;3:38-43.

Noe HN: The long-term results of prospective sibling reflux screening. J Urol 1992;148:1739-1742.

Reynolds SJ, Shepherd ME, Risbud AR, et al: Male circumcision and risk of HIV-1 and other sexually transmitted infections in India. Lancet 2004;363: 1039-1040.

Ulleryd P, Zackrisson B, Aus G, et al: Selective urological evaluation in men with febrile urinary tract infection. BJU Int 2001;88:15-20.

Weidner W, Schiefer H-G: Inflammatory disease of the prostate: Frequency and pathogenesis. In Garraway M (ed.): Epidemiology of Prostate Disease. New York, Springer, 1995, pp 85-93.

# Urinary Tract Infections in Women

Method of
*Burke A. Cunha, MD*

## General Concepts

Urinary tract infections (UTIs) are common in adult women. The two major clinical manifestations of UTIs in adult women are cystitis or pyelonephritis. Young adult women may also present with so-called dysuria pyuria syndrome (abacteriuric cystitis), previously known as acute urethral syndrome, as outpatients. Hospitalized compromised female hosts with cystitis may be complicated by bacteremia or ascending infection. Renal abscess may complicate pyelonephritis in normal or compromised female hosts.

## Cystitis Versus Pyelonephritis

The therapeutic approach to UTIs in adult women depends on accurate localization of the site of infection in the urinary tract. The most common clinical problem is differentiating cystitis from pyelonephritis. Patients with acute bacterial cystitis present with dysuria and frequency, which may or may not be accompanied by suprapubic discomfort or lower back pain. The fever accompanying cystitis is ≤ to 38.9°C (102°F) and is not usually associated with chills. The clinical manifestation of cystitis is confirmed by finding pyuria and significant bacteriuria, (i.e., ≥$10^6$ CFU/mL) in such patients. The urinalysis in acute cystitis is not usually accompanied by microscopic hematuria.

*Staphylococcus saprophyticus* is the only uropathogen in the ambulatory setting that is responsible for the majority of cases of UTIs accompanied by microscopic hematuria. Microscopic hematuria in a urinalysis in a patient with an apparent UTI should be carefully observed and should disappear after therapy of the UTI. If the microscopic hematuria disappears, then the physician can safely assume it was related to the UTI. Particularly in elderly patients, if the microscopic hematuria persists after eradication of the UTI, then the patient should be investigated for a bladder or renal source of the microscopic hematuria.

## Dysuria-Pyuria Syndrome

In sexually active young women, dysuria-pyuria syndrome manifests with the symptoms of cystitis but with negative urine cultures, or if organisms are cultured, they are present in low numbers (i.e., *E coli*) (≤$10^3$ CFU/mL). Most cases of dysuria-pyuria syndrome are caused by *Chlamydia trachomatis*. In patients with dysuria-pyuria syndrome, if the urine is cultured for *Chlamydia*, cultures are frequently positive.

## Catheter-Associated Bacteriuria (CAB)

Hospitalized patients with indwelling Foley catheters often acquire bacteriuria as a function of time that the Foley catheter is in place. Pyuria is often in the urine of patients with indwelling Foleys because the catheter elicits inflammation of the urinary tract. The presence of pyuria and bacteriuria in a patient with an indwelling Foley suggests either UTI or CAB. The majority of such patients are asymptomatic and afebrile. More than 95% of the time these patients have colonization of the urinary tract without infection. The urinalysis in patients with indwelling Foley catheters is helpful if either bacteria without pyuria or pyuria without bacteria is demonstrated. Bacteriuria without pyuria signifies colonization of the urinary tract, whereas pyuria without bacteriuria indicates inflammation of the urinary tract. In non–Foley catheter patients, the presence of pyuria plus significant bacteriuria is diagnostic of a UTI. This is not the case with CAB. As mentioned in the setting of the Foley catheter, bacteriuria plus pyuria almost always represents colonization and not a UTI.

## Benign Bacteriuria of the Elderly

In elderly female patients, varying degrees of relaxation of the pelvic musculature are common. Patients often have varying degrees of cystocele of rectocele, which changes anatomic relationship and the angularity of the urethra as it enters the bladder and predisposes to colonization of the bladder urine by the introital flora, such as coliform flora derived from the colon. For this reason, elderly female patients often have bacteriuria with few or no symptoms of a UTI. The presence of bacteriuria/pyuria is often discovered on a routine urinalysis obtained as part of either admission laboratory work or an outpatient workup/screening test battery. The presence of bacteriuria/pyuria in an elderly female patient without underlying genitourinary (GU) disease or impaired host defenses has been appropriately termed *benign bacteriuria of the elderly*; it has been shown that these patients do not go on to have symptomatic UTIs, ascending infection (e.g., pyelonephritis/renal abscess), or bacteremia from the urinary tract.

## Recurrent Urinary Tract Infections: Reinfection Versus Relapse

Most UTIs in women are acute. CAB is often incorrectly considered a chronic UTI because in most cases it represents colonization rather than infection. Recurrent UTIs are chronic in the sense that they persist over a long period of time, but are really episodic infections. However, the approach to recurrent UTIs is based on determining whether the recurrence is on the basis of reinfection or relapse. The reinfection variety of recurrent UTIs is defined as a recurrent UTI because of different organisms being cultured during each UTI episode. The relapse form of recurrent UTIs is defined as demonstrating the same organism during repeated bouts of UTIs. The reinfection form of recurrent UTIs is usually because of rapid colonization of the vaginal introitus/entry into the urethra, usually following sexual intercourse. The relapse variety of recurrent UTI by the same organism recovered during each episode suggests an underlying structural abnormality of the GU tract. The correct diagnostic approach to recurrent UTIs because of relapse is a thorough investigation of the GU tract from the urethra to the kidneys, which determines a possible source for the focus for the organisms to periodically reappear as a relapsing UTI. Relapse UTIs cannot be successfully approached therapeutically without correcting the underlying condition predisposing to relapse (i.e., bladder calculi, kinked ureters, renal stones, renal abscesses).

## Acute Pyelonephritis

Acute pyelonephritis is most common in pregnancy and as a complication of an ascending infection from cystitis/GU instrumentation. An acute episode of pyelonephritis may occur in patients who have chronic pyelonephritis; the acute episode is superimposed on the chronic condition. Renal abscess may complicate acute and chronic pyelonephritis. Renal cortical abscesses are often caused by gram-positive cocci (e.g., staphylococci acquired hematogenously), whereas medullary abscesses are usually caused by aerobic gram-negative bacilli (e.g., coliforms or enterococci).

Acute pyelonephritis may be differentiated from cystitis by the presence of unilateral costovertebral angle (CVA) tenderness (otherwise unexplainable) and a temperature of $\geq 38.9°C$ (102°F). Bilateral pyelonephritis is unusual, and the presence of bilateral CVA tenderness should suggest an alternative diagnosis. Pyelonephritis is often bilateral pathologically, but clinically it is almost always unilateral in its presentation with CVA tenderness. The urinalysis in pyelonephritis is the same as in cystitis, for example with significant pyuria/ bacteriuria in addition to the findings suggestive of pyelonephritis. The clinical presentation of renal abscess may resemble pyelonephritis if CVA tenderness is present, but this is not an invariable finding. The urinalysis in renal abscess may reveal pyuria and bacteria if the abscess is medullary but only pyuria if the renal abscess is cortical. Renal imaging studies are usually unnecessary in cystitis or pyelonephritis. If there is confusion regarding the presence or absence of chronic pyelonephritis, then a computed tomography/magnetic resonance imaging (CT/MRI) scan of the abdomen or renal ultrasound is appropriate.

## Chronic Pyelonephritis

Chronic pyelonephritis results in shrunken and distorted kidneys with a distorted collecting system. If the patient presents with *chronic pyelonephritis* and has kidneys of normal or large size, then an alternate explanation should be sought. The only way to diagnose a renal abscess with certainty is with renal imaging studies. For this purpose, the CT/MRI of the kidneys is vastly superior in picking up small lesions than is the renal ultrasound. For the purposes of excluding a renal abscess, a negative renal ultrasound should never be used to rule out the diagnosis. A negative renal ultrasound should always be followed with a renal CT/MRI of the kidneys if a renal abscess is in the differential diagnosis.

## Therapeutic Considerations

### ACUTE CYSTITIS

The initial episode of acute complicated cystitis in a normal host without GU abnormalities/preexisting renal disease need not be treated with antimicrobial therapy. Usually treatment with phenazopyridine (Pyridium), which has no antibacterial effect, is sufficient to relieve bladder spasm and the relative urine obstruction because of the bladder spasm, and the bacteria will spontaneously clear itself without antimicrobial therapy. Repeated episodes of acute cystitis should have appropriate diagnostic studies, for example a urinalysis and urinary culture with sensitivities with each episode to differentiate reinfection from relapse. If cystitis occurs in a nonleukopenic compromised host (e.g., with diabetes mellitus, systemic lupus erythematosus, multiple myeloma, cirrhosis, etc.), then a seven-day course of therapy is recommended with an oral agent such as nitrofurantoin (Macrodantin), trimethoprim-sulfamethoxazole (TMP-SMX) (Bactrim), or amoxicillin (Amoxil). Ampicillin should be avoided because of its resistance potential with coliform bacteria.

### DYSURIA-PYURIA SYNDROME

The dysuria-pyuria syndrome because of *Chlamydia* should be treated with a two-week course of doxycycline (Vibramycin). Patients unable to tolerate doxycycline (Vibramycin) may be treated with a macrolide for the same period of time. A grossly hemorrhagic cystitis suggests a viral etiology for which no specific therapy is available. Patients with cystitis and microscopic hematuria are often infected with *S. saprophyticus.*

Fortunately, *S. saprophyticus* is susceptible to a wide range of antibiotics and virtually any agent selected to treat a UTI will be effective. Antimicrobial resistance has not been a problem in *S. saprophyticus* UTIs. Chronic interstitial cystitis is not an infectious disorder and therefore antimicrobial therapy is unnecessary.

## CATHETER-ASSOCIATED BACTERIURIA

CAB in hospitalized patients who are normal hosts without structural abnormalities need not be treated, because virtually all of these patients are colonized and not infected. CAB in nonleukopenic compromised hosts (with diabetes mellitus, systemic lupus erythematosus, multiple myeloma, cirrhosis, and so forth), should be treated to prevent ascending infection/bacteremia from the lower urinary tract. Such individuals should be treated with an oral agent such as amoxicillin (Amoxil), nitrofurantoin (Macrodantin), or TMP-SMX (Bactrim) for 1 to 2 weeks.

Nonleukopenic compromised hosts with enterococci CAB are best treated with oral nitrofurantoin (Macrodantin), which is effective against enterococcal strains such as *E. faecalis* (non-vancomycin-resistant *Enterococcus* [non-VRE]) as well as *E. faecium* [VRE]). *Enterococcus faecalis* strains may also be treated with oral amoxicillin (Amoxil). These instances represent prophylaxis/early therapy because the majority of patients who are nonleukopenic-compromised hosts will have colonization of the urinary tract prior to catheterization or rapidly develop it soon thereafter. Therefore, prevention of ascending infection/bacteremia is the primary aim of therapy in patients with CAB who are compromised on the basis of their host defenses or GU tract abnormalities (e.g., ureteral stents).

## ACUTE PYELONEPHRITIS

Acute pyelonephritis may be caused by aerobic gram-negative bacilli, such as coliforms or enterococci (almost always *E. faecalis*). The empirical treatment of pyelonephritis is based on a Gram stain of the urine,

---

## CURRENT DIAGNOSIS

- Acute uncomplicated cystitis is the most common type of UTI in adult women.
- The initial peak incidence of cystitis occurs with sexual intercourse and gradually increases through adulthood.
- Cystitis may occur as a single event or may be recurrent because of reinfection or relapse.
- Cystitis is usually caused by coliform or enterococci from the fecal flora or by *Staphylococcus saprophyticus* from the skin flora.
- Clinically, cystitis is marked by low-grade fever (≤38.9°C [102°F]) with lower abdominal/ suprapubic discomfort, and/or dysuria.
- *Staphylococcus aureus, Streptococcus pneumoniae,* groups A, C, G streptococci, and *Bacteroides fragilis* are not uropathogens in cystitis.
- In elderly women, *cystitis* manifests as pyuria and bacterluria without fever or dysuria, which is termed *benign bacteriuria of the elderly.*
- A variant of cystitis, the so-called *dysuria/pyuria syndrome,* is also known as *abacteriuric cystitis.*
- Dysuria/pyuria syndrome, most common in young adult women, manifests as cystitis, but urine cultures are negative for bacteria or uropathogens such as *Escherichia coli* are present in low numbers. *Chlamydia trachomatis* is frequently isolated if the urine is cultured for *Chlamydia.*
- Pyelonephritis in women may occur as an uncommon complication of cystitis or during pregnancy.
- It is not possible to predict the uropathogen of cystitis from clinical features except for *S. saprophyticus.*
- *S. saprophyticus* cystitis is characterized by a fishy urine odor, microscopic hematuria, and an alkaline urinary pH.
- Cystitis with alkaline urine suggests infection secondary to *S. saprophyticus, Ureaplasma urealyticum,* or a struvite stone with associated infection caused by a urea-splitting organism such as *Proteus.*
- Microscopic hematuria is common with *S. saprophyticus* cystitis but is uncommon with other uropathogens. If a patient with cystitis and microscopic hematuria fails to promptly resolve with antimicrobial therapy, work up the patient for a bladder/renal neoplasm or renal TB.

- The diagnosis of cystitis in women is made by demonstrating pyuria and significant bacteriuria (≥ $10^6$ col/mL) in the setting of cystitis symptoms.
- Cystitis symptoms with gross hematuria should suggest a viral hemorrhagic cystitis or a renal lesion.
- Pyuria without bacteriuria indicates urinary tract inflammation. Persistent pyuria without bacteriuria should suggest interstitial cystitis or renal TB.
- With cystitis, the specific gravity of the urine is not decreased in contrast to pyelonephritis where the specific gravity is decreased.
- Urinary concentration returns to normal with treatment in pyelonephritis.
- Pyelonephritis may be differentiated from cystitis by the presence of fever ≥38.9°C (102°F) and otherwise unexplained unilateral CVA tenderness.
- The urine analysis/culture findings in pyelonephritis and cystitis are the same. Bacteremia frequently occurs with pyelonephritis but is not a feature of cystitis in normal hosts.
- Nonleukopenic compromised hosts, such as diabetes mellitus, systemic lupus erythematosus, multiple myeloma, cirrhosis, and so on, with cystitis may be complicated by pyelonephritis or bacteremia.
- Pyelonephritis is caused by the same uropathogens that cause cystitis; however, *S. saprophyticus* occurs only in cystitis.
- Acute pyelonephritis clinically improves unless complicated by renal abscess.
- Clinically, pyelonephritis is almost always unilateral, but pathophysical findings may be bilateral.
- Bilateral CVA tenderness should suggest an alternate diagnosis.
- In pyelonephritis, radiologic studies typically show unilateral renal involvement characterized by cortical scarring, medullary abnormalities, and renal shrinkage.
- Bilateral, normal-sized, or enlarged kidneys should suggest an alternate diagnosis to pyelonephritis.

*Abbreviations:* CVA = costovertebral angle; TB = tuberculosis; UTI = urinary tract infection.

## CURRENT THERAPY

- Virtually all cases of initial uncomplicated cystitis will resolve spontaneously with or without treatment. No urine analysis/culture is needed with the initial episode of cystitis.
- For the dysuria of cystitis, phenazopyridine (Pyridium), which has no antibacterial properties but relieves pain and relative urinary obstruction from muscle spasm, may be used. Relief of spasm promptly clears the bacteriuria.
- Recurrent cystitis of the reinfection variety is because of different uropathogens with each episode that the urine is cultured. Reinfection is related to vaginal introital colonization following sexual intercourse and may be treated with a postcoital/HS of an appropriate antibiotic.
- Although the initial attack of cystitis resolves in virtually all patients without treatment, those who prefer to treat may use single-dose therapy with nitrofurantoin (Macrodantin), TMP-SMX (Bactrim), or amoxicillin (Amoxil).
- Cystitis in a nonleukopenic compromised host (discussed previously) should be treated for 1 to 2 weeks to prevent bacteremia/ascending infection, such as pyelonephritis/renal abscess.
- Ampicillin should be avoided because of its high resistance potential. Amoxicillin should be used instead, which has not been associated with resistance and is effective against the common coliforms and enterococci (*Enterococcus faecalis*).
- Nitrofurantoin has no resistance potential, is effective against all common uropathogens and all enterococci, such as *E. faecalis* (non-VRE) and *Enterococcus faecium* (VRE).

- Nitrofurantoin (Macrodantin) is useful in cystitis or catheter-associated bacteremia but is not to be used in pyelonephritis/bacteremia.
- Recurrent UTI of the relapse variety is caused by the same uropathogen with each occurrence. The problem in relapse UTIs is not therapeutic but diagnostic. Relapsing UTIs have an underlying structural abnormality or ureteral shunts that do not permit antimicrobial therapy to be effective.
- The treatment of pyelonephritis is with IV or PO antibiotics, depending on the severity of the clinical manifestation. Treatment is for 2 to 4 weeks with an effective antibiotic.
- For pyelonephritis, parenteral agents useful against coliforms are cephalosporins, aztreonam (Azactam), aminoglycosides, TMP-SMZ (Bactrim), or renally eliminated quinolones. Against enterococci (most of which are non-VRE), parenteral ampicillin, antipseudomonal penicillins, and meropenem (Merrem) are useful.
- Oral antibiotics useful against coliform causes of pyelonephritis include renally eliminated quinolones, amoxicillin (Amoxil), antipseudomonal penicillins, or TMP-SMZ (Bactrim).
- Linezolid (Zyvox) may be used for pyelonephritis caused by enterococci (non-VRE), amoxicillin (Amoxil), or for VRE.
- Patients with acute pyelonephritis become afebrile/nearly afebrile within 72 hours with or without treatment. Persistence of high fevers for greater than 72 hours should be considered as representing a renal abscess until proved otherwise.

*Abbreviations:* HD = half dose; IM = intramuscular; IV = intravenous; TMP-SMZ = trimethoprim-sulfamethoxazole; UTI = urinary tract infection; VRE = vancomycin-resistant *Enterococcus*.

671

which, if the diagnosis is pyelonephritis, will show significant pyuria and a single predominant organism. In a patient with presumed pyelonephritis, the absence of bacteria in the Gram stain of the urine in an acutely ill patient essentially eliminates the diagnosis of pyelonephritis from further consideration, and an alternate explanation for the patient's fever and CVA tenderness should be sought (e.g., renal imaging studies).

Because acute pyelonephritis is often accompanied by bacteremia (urosepsis), parenteral agents may be used initially followed by oral agents; or in mild-to-moderate cases, oral agents may be used for the entire course of therapy. The parenteral agents useful in the treatment of acute pyelonephritis because of aerobic gram-negative bacilli include aminoglycosides, aztreonam (Azactam), antipseudomonal penicillin (e.g., ticarcillin [Ticar]), piperacillin (Pipracil), or a renally excreted respiratory quinolone. Patients presenting with acute pyelonephritis, who have streptococci in the Gram stain of the urine indicating enterococci, may be treated empirically with ampicillin and antipseudomonal penicillin, ticarcillin (Ticar), piperacillin (Pipracil), or meropenem (Merrem). In the rare instance where there is enterococcal urosepsis complicating acute pyelonephritis because of VRE, then linezolid (Zyvox), quinupristin-dalfopristin (Synercid), or daptomycin (Cubicin) may be used. In patients presenting with acute pyelonephritis where a Gram stain is unobtainable or unavailable, then empirical coverage for both aerobic gram-negative bacilli and enterococci (*E. faecalis*), may be achieved with antipseudomonal penicillins, nonrenally eliminated respiratory quinolones, or meropenem (Merrem). After the organism responsible for the pyelonephritis is subsequently identified by urine/blood culture, then the patient may be switched to one of the agents mentioned. Similarly, if the patient is shown to have enterococci as the cause of the urosepsis, it may be

treated initially as non-VRE, as indicated previously in the article. Patients with pyelonephritis are usually treated for 1 to 2 weeks.

Particularly in critically ill patients, initial therapy is often started parenterally. Patients may be switched to an oral agent as soon as the patient clinically defervesces or treated entirely by an oral agent for the duration of therapy. The ideal oral antibiotic has the same spectrum as its parenteral counterpart and has excellent bioavailability; blood/tissue levels are approximately the same after intravenous/oral (IV/PO) administration. For example, by giving 1 g of amoxicillin (Amoxil) every 8 hours, the same blood/tissue levels are achieved as by giving ampicillin by intramuscular injection (IM). Nonrenally eliminated respiratory quinolones, such as levofloxacin (Levaquin) and gatifloxacin (Tequin), achieve the same blood and tissue levels when given either by the IV or PO route. This permits completion of therapy at home and does not require 2 to 4 weeks of inpatient hospitalization for intravenous drug therapy. There is some rationale for treating acute pyelonephritis for an extended period, such as 2 to 4 weeks, to prevent chronic pyelonephritis.

## CHRONIC PYELONEPHRITIS

Patients with chronic pyelonephritis are a therapeutic challenge because of the distorted intrarenal architecture and decreased blood supply to the kidney, which limits access of white blood cells (WBCs), impairs host defenses, and limits penetration of the antibiotic into the infected/diseased areas of the kidney. Treatment of chronic pyelonephritis should be based on susceptibility testing of the isolates that are present in the urine. In chronic pyelonephritis, bacteriuria is intermittent but is present over a long period of time and will persist after short or inadequate treatment. The antibiotic selected should be effective against the isolate recovered from the urine in patients with chronic pyelonephritis and possess the ability to penetrate into diseased kidneys. The ideal oral agents for therapy are TMP-SMX (Bactrim), doxycycline (Vibramycin), or a nonrenally eliminated respiratory quinolone.

## RENAL ABSCESS

Acute pyelonephritis treated appropriately results in a rapid defervescence of temperature and decrease in CVA tenderness within 72 hours. If the temperature does not decrease after 72 hours of appropriate therapy, suggest a renal abscess until proved otherwise. Renal abscesses should be treated for the presumed organism based on the location of the abscess by renal imaging studies. If sensitivities from an isolate available from the urine or percutaneous aspiration of the abscess are unavailable, then empirical treatment directed against aerobic gram-negative bacilli for medullary abscesses is indicated. Treatment is the same as for pyelonephritis except is more prolonged and should be given until the abscess is drained or it resolves. For cortical abscesses in the absence of culture and sensitivity data, antibiotic therapy should be directed against *Staphylococcus aureus* and *E. faecalis*, and treated in the same manner as pyelonephritis but for an extended period of time. Acute pyelonephritis with or without acteremia is usually treated for 7 days.

## RECURRENT UTIs

Reinfection may be treated with nitrofurantoin (Macrodantin), TMP-SMX (Bactrim), or amoxicillin (Amoxil) as a single postcoital dose. Therapeutic approach to relapse is to remove the underlying condition responsible for perpetuating the bacteriuria. Antimicrobial therapy may be selected based on the susceptibility of the organism, but antimicrobial therapy alone will not eradicate the relapsing form of recurrent UTI.

## REFERENCES

Cunha BA: Clinical concepts in the treatment of urinary tract infections. Antibiotics for Clinicians 1999;3:88-93.

Cunha BA: Nosocomial catheter-associated urinary tract infections. Hosp Physician 1986;22:13-16.

Cunha BA: *Staphylococcus saprophyticus* urinary tract infections. Intern Med 1985;6:82-89.

Cunha BA: Single-dose therapy of urinary tract infections. Hosp Physician 1983;19:35-37.

Cunha BA: Urosepsis in the Critical Care Unit. In: Cunha BA (ed): Infectious Diseases in Critical Care Medicine, 2nd ed. Informa Healthcare USA, Inc., New York, NY, pp. 527-534.

Cunha BA: Antibiotic Essentials, 6th ed., Physicians Press, Royal Oak, MI, pp. 79-85.

Cunha BA: Urinary tract infections: Therapy. Postgrad Med 1981;70:149-157.

Hooton TM: The current management strategies for community-acquired urinary tract infection. Infect Dis Clin North Am 2003;17:303-332.

Kahan E, Kahan NR, Chinitz DP: Urinary tract infection in women—Physician's preferences for treatment and adherence to guidelines: A national drug utilization study in a managed care setting. Eur J Clin Pharmacol 2003;59:663-668.

Kraft JK, Stamey TA: The natural history of symptomatic recurrent bacteriuria in women. Medicine (Baltimore) 1977;56:55.

Meiland R, Geerlings SE, Hoepelman LI: Management of bacterial urinary tract infections in adult patients with diabetes mellitus. Drugs 2002;62:1859-1868.

Miller LG, Tang AW: Treatment of uncomplicated urinary tract infections in an era of increasing antimicrobial resistance. Mayo Clin Proc 2004;79:1048-1053.

Nicolle LE: Urinary tract infection: Traditional pharmacologic therapies. Am J Med 2002;113(Suppl 1A):35S-44S.

Nicolle LE, Ronald AR: Recurrent urinary tract infection in adult women: Diagnosis and treatment. Infect Dis Clin North Am 1987;1:793.

Ronald AR, Conway B: An approach to urinary tract infection in women. Infection 1992;20(Suppl 3):S203.

Schaeffer AJ, Stuppy BA: Efficacy and safety of self-start therapy in women with recurrent urinary tract infections. J Urol 1999;161:207.

Wong ES, McKevitt M, Running K, et al: Management of recurrent urinary tract infections with patient administered single-dose therapy. Ann Intern Med 1985;102:302.

# Bacterial Infections of the Urinary Tract in Girls

Method of
*Candice E. Johnson, MD, PhD*

Urinary tract infections (UTIs) are bacterial infections of any mucosal surface of the urinary tract including the urethra, the bladder, the ureters, and the renal calyces, as well as the renal parenchyma (Box 1). The best indicator for differentiating clinical pyelonephritis from cystitis is fever higher than 38.5°C (101.3°F). The classification of UTIs by anatomic location is complicated by the ascending nature of virtually all these infections. Thus, a girl with pyelonephritis usually has cystitis and urethritis simultaneously. Box 2 gives the colony count criteria generally accepted for clinical use, although research studies are usually more stringent.

## Epidemiology and Pathogenesis

Approximately 2.2% of girls will have a UTI in the first 24 months of life. In the first year of life, most UTIs in females are febrile and may be hard to diagnose. Because of this difficulty, girls younger than 36 months with no source of fever should have a urine culture and urinalysis obtained. Unfortunately, the sensitivity of a standard urinalysis is only 82%, although it is 92% specific. For unknown reasons, the prevalence of UTI is much higher in white compared with African American girls, with Hispanics having a rate between the two groups.

Risk factors for UTI include:

- A history of recurrent UTI in the mother
- Family history of vesicoureteral reflux (VUR)
- Dysfunctional voiding patterns
- Constipation

Cleanliness and methods of wiping with toilet paper are not risk factors. In girls, an "unstable bladder" is the main cause of dysfunctional voiding. An unstable bladder has strong contractions at volumes 50% to 75% of capacity. These contractions cause both frequency and incontinence, and girls may sit on their feet to attempt to prevent voiding (Vincent's curtsy). In the most severe cases the girl tightens the external sphincter during bladder contraction, and this leads to high

---

**BOX 1  Classification of Urinary Tract Infections**

- **Urethritis:** Dysuria, frequency or enuresis, accompanied by pyuria, but colony count of $10^3$/mL of urine or less.
- **Cystitis:** Afebrile UTI. Dysuria, frequency or enuresis with colony count of at least $10^4$/mL of urine. Hematuria may be present, but casts, flank pain, temperature more than 38.5°C (101.3°F) and systemic toxicity are absent.
- **Clinical pyelonephritis:** Febrile UTI (≥38°C [100.4°F]), usually accompanied by flank and abdominal pain. The colony count is usually greater than or equal to $10^5$/mL of urine except with *Staphylococcus saprophyticus* or enterococci. Cystitis symptoms may also be present.
- **Proved pyelonephritis:** Shows evidence of acute inflammation on radiologic evaluation by CT, ultrasound, or radionuclide scan.

*Abbreviations*: CT = computed tomography; UTI = urinary tract infection.

bladder pressure. A thickened and trabeculated bladder often occurs as well as VUR.

## Diagnosis

A high index of suspicion is needed to diagnose all UTIs, especially those in infants and toddlers. In addition to fever, manifesting symptoms include anorexia and emesis, abdominal pain, fussiness, neonatal jaundice, poor weight gain, enuresis, and hematuria.

Urine should be collected only by catheter or suprapubic aspiration until the child is toilet trained, because urine bags have contamination rates of up to 50%. Box 2 shows the colony counts that best differentiate real UTIs from contamination.

Urinalysis continues to be performed in most laboratories by a dipstick combined with spun urine sediment. This continues despite studies since 1983 showing that unspun urine counted in a hemocytometer is more sensitive and specific. In a private office, the dipstick results for leukocyte esterase, nitrites, and hematuria are sufficient to decide on empirical treatment of girls. Urine cultures should still be sent, even with a negative dipstick, because, unlike adult women, radiologic workups may be needed for confirmed UTIs in girls.

## Treatment of Afebrile Urinary Tract Infection

Treatment of a girl with an afebrile UTI (cystitis or lower tract) is straightforward, requiring only a knowledge of national and local antibiotic resistance rates. *Escherichia coli* causes more than 90% of cystitis in girls, with other Enterobacteriaceae and *Staphylococcus saprophyticus* comprising the remainder. *E. coli* is resistant to amoxicillin (Amoxil) more than 50% of the time, so this is not appropriate initial therapy. Rates of resistance to trimethoprim (Proloprim) and sulfonamides are highest in the Pacific Coast states, and rates of first-generation cephalosporin resistance vary widely. Drugs that retain high sensitivity rates are the second- and third-generation cephalosporins and nitrofurantoin (Macrodantin). Box 3 provides doses of commonly used drugs, and amoxicillin is preferred if the organism is sensitive.

## Treatment of Febrile Urinary Tract Infection

Unlike the majority of viral and bacterial infections, a single kidney infection may cause permanent damage (i.e., renal scarring) if not treated rapidly and with effective antibiotics. In 1999, outpatient management of febrile UTIs was demonstrated to be effective in a study of 306 children under 24 months of age. A 2004 study in Montreal of 291 patients who were 3 months to 5 years of age showed that at least 75% of febrile children with UTI could be managed in a day treatment center (DTC). These children had a mean of 3.5 visits to

the DTC for intravenous gentamicin (Garamycin), followed by an oral antibiotic to complete 10 days of treatment. Successful treatment was seen in 97% of the UTI episodes, and all first UTIs were evaluated by renal sonography and cystography at the DTC.

Because the DTC concept is not widely available for children in the United States, Figure 1 shows a suggested decision tree that does not use a DTC. Inpatient management is recommended for infants younger than 8 weeks as they do not absorb oral antibiotics predictably. Box 4 lists other variables to consider in deciding on inpatient versus outpatient treatment. Antibiotic choices are given in Box 3. Duration of symptoms before presentation is very important, because renal scarring was seen in British studies after as few as 5 days of delayed diagnosis.

Once on antibiotic therapy, defervescence may be expected in approximately 68% of children younger than 2 years by 24 hours and in 89% by 48 hours. The 11% who remain febrile at 48 hours were no more likely to have renal abscesses or hydronephrosis than the others, and they may be discharged after sensitivities are known. It is convenient to the family to perform the cystogram, if indicated, during hospitalization and it greatly improves compliance.

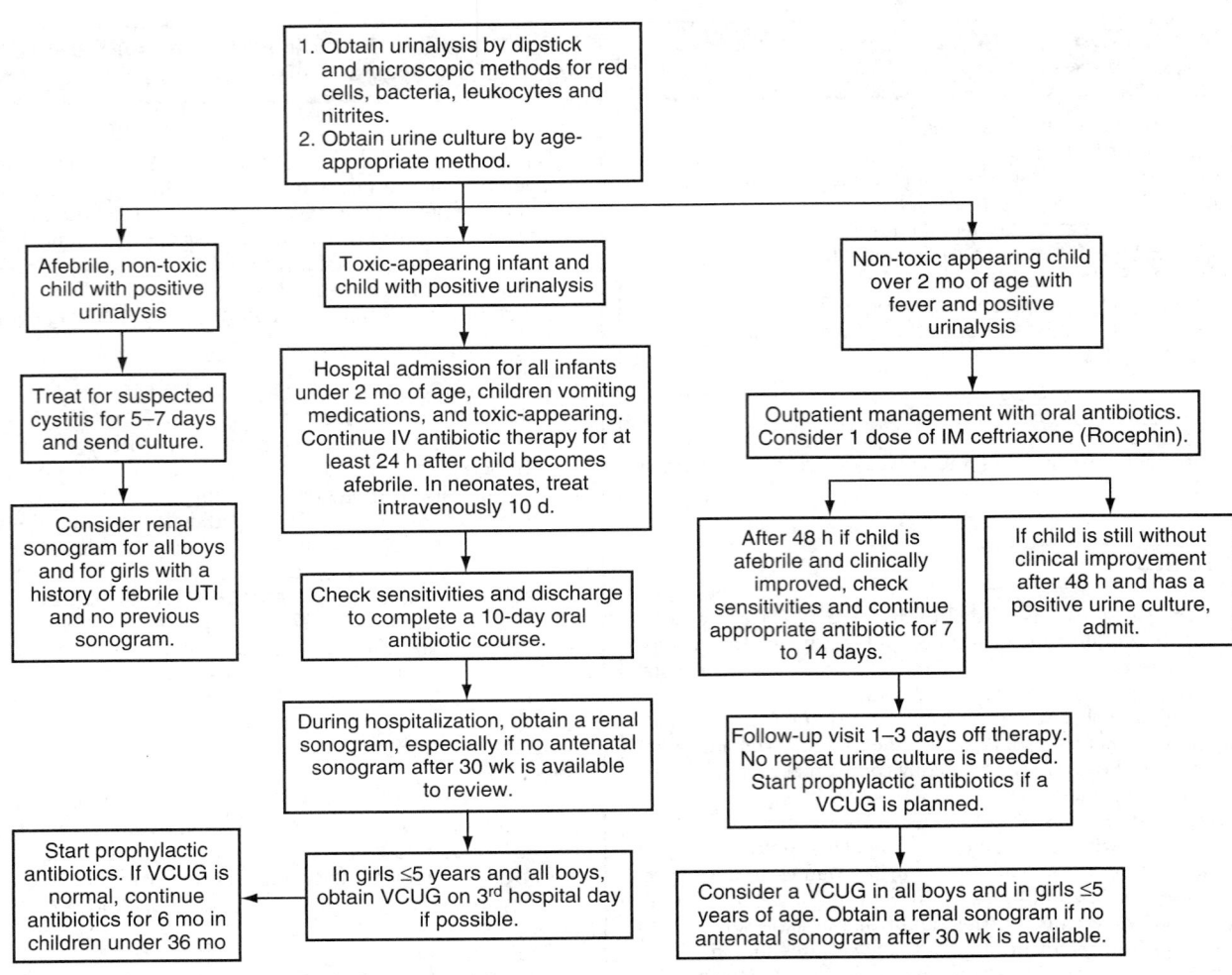

**FIGURE 1.** Treatment of suspected urinary tract infection in children younger than 13 years old.

## Prophylaxis

There is expert agreement that further prospective studies of antibiotic prophylaxis for childhood UTI are needed. In adult women, the cost-to-benefit ratio favors prophylaxis with three or more UTIs per year. In children, because young age is the major risk for renal scarring, studies are lacking, but expert opinion favors 6 months of prophylaxis after

a febrile UTI, with or without VUR. Guidelines from the American Urological Association also suggest prophylaxis for all children with VUR, but the Swedish experts suggest stopping at age 24 months in boys and 5 years in girls. Table 1 lists suggested agents. Unfortunately, the choice of antibiotic is becoming limited as trimethoprim (Proloprim) resistance rates rise.

---

**BOX 4  Proposed Criteria for Hospitalization of Children With Febrile Urinary Tract Infection**

- Sufficient emesis is present to prevent oral therapy.
- Family is judged likely to be noncompliant with antibiotics or follow-up appointments.
- Toxic or ill-appearing child which is suggestive of sepsis.
- Age is younger than 2 months.
- Prolonged duration of symptoms exists (>5 days).
- Renal scarring or impaired renal function is known to be present.
- Diabetes, AIDS, sickle cell, or other serious chronic disease is present.

---

### CURRENT DIAGNOSIS

- A high level of suspicion is required in all febrile infants.
- Boys outnumber girls 10:1 in the neonatal period.
- Girls are at highest risk for UTI when younger than 12 months of age and again at 3 to 5 years of age.
- Urine for culture should not be obtained with a bag, but requires a catheterization or suprapubic aspiration, if the child is not toilet trained.
- The colony count cutoff to define a UTI differs with the method used for collection.
- With a negative urinalysis, febrile UTI becomes much less likely, but an afebrile UTI cannot be ruled out.

*Abbreviations:* UTI = urinary tract infection.

## TABLE 1 Prophylactic Antibiotics for Childhood Urinary Tract Infections

| Drug | Dose | Timing | Side Effects |
|------|------|--------|--------------|
| Trimethoprim-sulfamethoxazole (TMP-SMX) (Bactrim) | 2 mg/kg of TMP component (up to 40 mg) | Bedtime | Rash in ~6% |
| Nitrofurantoin (Macrodantin capsules 25, 50, or 100 mg preferred over oral suspension) | 1-2 mg/kg/d up to 100 mg | Bedtime | Vomiting, abdominal pain |
| Trimethoprim (Primsol oral solution 50 mg/mL or 100 mg tablets) | 2 mg/kg up to 40 mg | Bedtime | Rash in ~1% |

## Radiologic Evaluation

No area of childhood UTI evaluation is as controversial as determining which children merit sonography, radionuclide scans, and cystograms. Two recent studies have helped clarify these issues, and several professional academies have agreed on guidelines for febrile children younger than 2 years of age (Pediatrics, Family Practice, Emergency Physicians, Urological, and College of Radiology). These associations recommend a renal sonogram and a voiding cystogram soon after the first febrile UTI. Figure 2 indicates that the initial cystogram should be a standard fluoroscopic examination to permit accurate grading of VUR. Follow-up cystograms may be radionuclide studies, which carry less risk of gonadal radiation.

Hoberman and colleagues also question the value of the initial renal sonogram. In a cohort of 309 febrile children who had paired dimercaptosuccinic acid (DMSA) radionuclide renal scans and sonography performed within 48 hours of diagnosis, neither study changed management. All had had an antenatal sonogram after 30 weeks of gestation, and anomalies were presumably corrected before UTI could occur. The argument in favor of doing this painless and medically safe study is that children with "dilating reflux" (i.e., grades III-V) would be identified, and the doctor could track down these children if they fail to

keep an appointment for a cystogram. In other words, in the absence of a cystogram, a sonogram with hydronephrosis or pelvic caliectasis *will* change management. In the patient with no health insurance who

### CURRENT THERAPY

- Outpatient therapy of febrile UTIs is usually appropriate in infants older than 2 months of age.
- A single dose of intramuscular ceftriaxone (Rocephin) will cover the first 24 hours after diagnosis when emesis is most likely to occur and antibiotic sensitivities are unknown.
- Febrile girls should be seen between 36 and 48 hours after diagnosis to assess clinical improvements and check urine culture results.
- A voiding cystogram remains essential for febrile girls younger than 5 years of age and all boys.

*Abbreviations:* UTI = urinary tract infection.

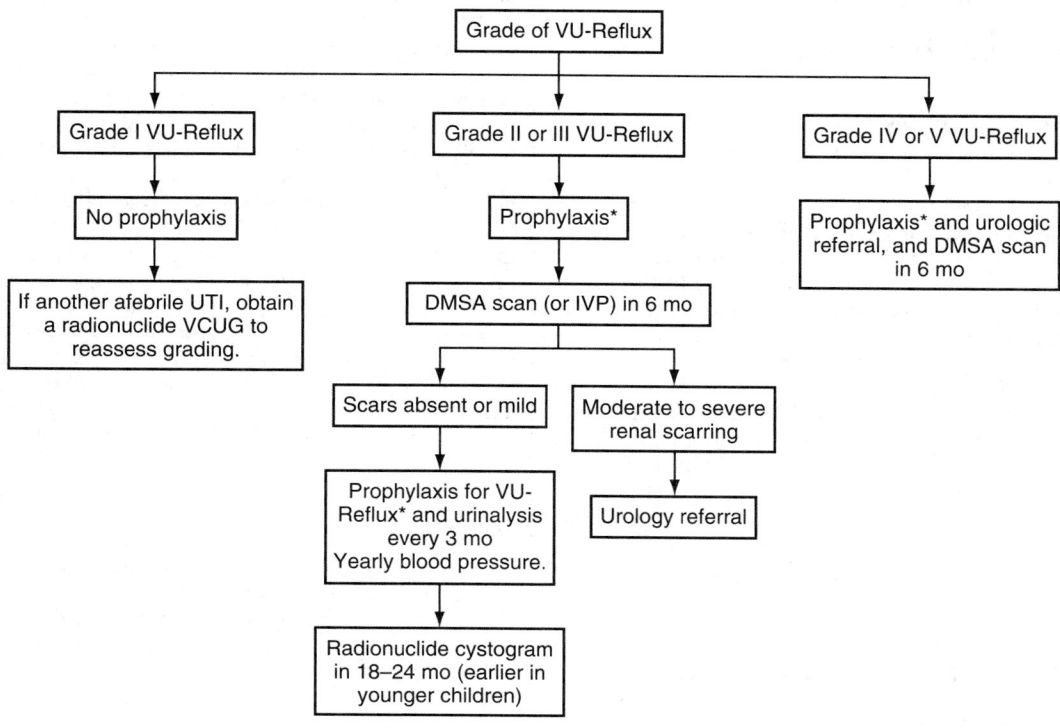

*Trimethoprim (Primsol) (1–2 mg/kg/d at bedtime) or nitrofurantoin (Macrodantin) (same dosage)

**FIGURE 2.** Radiologic management of a child with vesicoureteral reflux.

cannot afford both studies, the more important study is the voiding cystogram, not the sonogram.

## REFERENCES

Abelson Storby K, Osterlund A, Kahlmeter G: Antimicrobial resistance in *Escherichia coli* in urine samples from children and adults: A 12 year analysis. Acta Paediatr 2004;93:487-491.

Bollgren I: Antibacterial prophylaxis in children with urinary tract infection. Acta Paediatr 1999;(Suppl 431):48-52.

Gauthier M, Chevalie I, Sterescu A, et al: Treatment of urinary tract infections among febrile young children with daily intravenous antibiotic therapy at a day treatment center. Pediatrics 2004;114: 469-476.

Hellerstein S: Urinary tract infections in children. Infections in Medicine 2002;19:554-560.

Hoberman A, Charros M, Hickey RW, et al: Imaging studies after a first febrile urinary tract infection in young children. N Engl J Med 2003;348(3):195-202.

Hoberman A, Wald ER, Hickey RW, et al: Oral versus initial intravenous therapy for urinary tract infections in young febrile children. Pediatrics 1999;104(1)79-86.

Jakobsson B, Esbjorner E, Hansson S: Minimum incidence and diagnostic rate of first urinary tract infection. Pediatrics 1999;104(2 Pt):222-226.

Johnson CE: Dysuria. In: Kliegman RM, Greebaum LA, Lye PS, (eds): Practical Strategies in Pediatric Diagnosis and Therapy, 2nd ed. Philadelphia, WB Saunders, 2004, pp 397-411.

Lin D-S, Huang F-Y, Chiu N-C, et al: Comparison of hemocytometer leukocyte counts and standard urinalysis for predicting urinary tract infections in febrile infants. Pediatr Infect Dis J 2000;19:223-227.

Lowe LH, Patel MN, Gatti JM, Alon US: Utility of follow-up renal sonography in children with vesicoureteral reflux and normal initial sonogram. Pediatrics 2004;113:548-550.

Roberts KB: A synopsis of the American Academy of Pediatrics' practice parameter on the diagnosis, treatment, and evaluation of the initial urinary tract infection in febrile infants and young children. Pediatr Rev 1999;20(10):1-4.

Rushton HG: Urinary tract infections in children: Epidemiology, evaluation, and management. Pediatr Clin North Am 1997;44(5):1133-1169.

# Childhood Enuresis

## Method of
## Frank R. Cerniglia, Jr., MD

In general, *enuresis* is associated with purely nighttime wetting. The term, however, means involuntary wetting (day or night) beyond the age of anticipated control. Childhood enuresis includes both day (diurnal) and night (nocturnal) wetting. The latter is further subdivided into primary and secondary nocturnal enuresis. Enuresis is one of the most common problems seen by the pediatric primary care physician and is referred to the pediatric urologist.

The problem, which dates back to as early as 1500 BC, has been the subject of many dissertations on diagnosis, causes, and remedies. Childhood wetting problems, or voiding dysfunctions, affect 5% to 10% of school-aged children and can be a profound source of distress for the child and family as a whole. The number of potential causes for abnormal voiding include anatomic, neuropathic, and functional disorders. Most children who present with day and/or nighttime wetting have a non-neurologic functional voiding abnormality requiring no complex evaluation or invasive study.

## Development of Bladder Control

Urinary continence develops in an ordered process of sequenced maturation that requires no teaching. To attain continence, one needs a low-pressure storage vessel surrounded by smooth muscle to "squeeze" out the urine from the bladder, an "involuntary" internal sphincter, and a complex external sphincteric mechanism with intertwined smooth and skeletal muscle that is under voluntary control. These three mechanisms work in accord to accomplish bladder emptying. The neonate voids by reflex through the sacral spinal cord. The bladder reaches a functional capacity stretch point, and afferent signals are sent to the spinal cord to activate sympathetic outflow to the bladder and urethra. The result is relaxation of the external sphincter and contraction of the detrusor; bladder emptying ensues.

Urinary frequency, incontinence, and nocturnal enuresis are all normal occurrences in the very young child. Infants are asleep approximately 60% of the time with 40% of their voiding episodes occurring during sleep. In year 1 of life, the child voids approximately 20 times per day. During the next 2 years, voiding frequency decreases by as much as 50% while the voided volumes (and bladder capacity) increase by as much as three to four times. Beginning at age 2 years, conscious sensation of bladder fullness develops, although control is not yet mastered. By 4 years, most children have achieved an adult pattern of voiding in which micturition can occur at less than total bladder capacity or be postponed until absolute functional bladder capacity is reached. For the transition to this pattern, three separate events must occur:

1. Capacity of bladder must increase so it can function as a reservoir.
2. The child must gain control over the external sphincter so urination can be allowed or terminated at will.
3. Direct voluntary control over the voiding reflex must develop to allow the child to initiate or inhibit bladder contraction voluntarily.

Simply put, urinary control is obtained when the bladder fills under low pressure to an adequate capacity and then can be emptied, with a detrusor contraction coordinated with complete relaxation of the external sphincter. However, one needs to understand this happens on a continuum. Nocturnal bowel control occurs first, followed by daytime bowel control, daytime urine control, and finally nighttime dryness. Most, but not all, children achieve these functions by the 4th year.

## Evaluation

Pure voiding dysfunction is urinary incontinence without any underlying structural or obvious neurologic abnormality. On the whole, patients with an anatomic abnormality usually have leaked their entire lives, unable to gain continence at any point. The incontinence, instead of being diurnal or nocturnal only, is a combination of both. Children with suspected anatomic defects should be evaluated with imaging of both the kidneys and bladder by ultrasound and voiding cystogram with or without a fluoroscopic urodynamics study. Children with voiding dysfunction are able to gain continence for a varying period of time followed by incontinence.

It is important during history taking to ask the child's primary caregiver for valuable insight into the general aspects of the child's voiding habits. One should ask precise questions, understandable to the child, in order to get accurate answers. This information can be augmented with a voiding diary because many parents may not be totally aware of the specifics and finer points of the child's voiding habits.

### ONSET

At what age was the child toilet trained? If the child was trained, at what point did he or she start wetting? Were there any occurrences in the child's life coinciding with the onset of wetting? Has the child ever been able to be toilet trained? Is the wetting new over the last few days, weeks, or months?

### FREQUENCY

Voiding diaries can be very helpful in diagnosing and treating voiding abnormalities. They can be kept over a 3- to 4-day period and include voiding times, volumes, wet versus dry, and any associated symptoms.

Appropriate volumes can be calculated as age (in years) plus 2 oz. One should determine if the volumes are less than expected. Does the child void infrequently with larger-than-anticipated amounts? How many voids per day? How many accidents per week? Does the child wet multiple times during the day or only at night?

## CHARACTER OF VOIDING

Does the male child compress his urethra while or after voiding? Does he sit or stand to void? Can the parent hear him voiding (good forceful stream) or does he dribble? Does the little girl void with her legs tightly closed? Does she sit back on the toilet or perch on the edge of the seat to help maintain balance (causing pelvic contraction)? Is the child in a rush? Does he or she delay voiding? Is there posturing (squatting, crossing legs)?

## DEGREE

Does the child wet enough to require clothes to be changed, or does the wetting consist of only spotting in the underwear? Is the wetting before voiding (unstable bladder) or after voiding (vaginal pooling)?

Two other important aspects of the history are bowel habits and family history of wetting. Any bowel dysfunction must be corrected before one can treat any wetting abnormality successfully. One should obtain a family history because it is now evident that a genetic component is linked to conditions such as primary nocturnal enuresis. One should also ask about other associated urologic, neurologic, or nephrologic conditions (valves, reflux, renal insufficiency) or any previous surgeries.

## Physical Examination

Once the history is taken, the physical examination should be performed, taking into account not only vitals (height, weight, blood pressure), as a basic starting point, but the general appearance of the child. Uncleanliness, poor hygiene, or poor dentition may suggest neglect or abuse. An abdominal examination should seek to identify masses, a palpable bladder, or stool in the colon. Careful inspection of the child's back for occult spinal dysraphisms includes looking for lipomas, scoliosis, hair patches, cutaneous lesions, sacral or coccygeal defects, or gluteal asymmetry. A basic neurologic examination is essential and should include such points as gait, reflexes, and brief examination room maneuvers to substantiate that no nerve deficits are contributing to the incontinence. Examination of the rectal area is important, but often passed over, and should incorporate assessing sphincter tone, ruling out pelvic masses, and looking for signs of fecal soiling. Additionally, one should inspect the external genitalia to diagnose labial adhesions in young girls, female epispadias (causing total incontinence), and signs of vaginal pooling (butterfly "rash" and irritation of the labia and perineal and perianal areas). In boys, one should look for narrowing or inflammation of the meatus, unretractable foreskin, hypospadias, or epispadias. If the physician can observe the child void, valuable information can be gained about the quality and pattern of the urinary stream.

## Laboratory/Radiograph Examination

A urinalysis should be performed to check for infection, glucosuria, and proteinuria. A specific gravity test can exclude polyuria as a cause for incontinence and indicates if the kidneys concentrate properly. If indicated, a urine culture should be done. If all of the tests just mentioned are normal, no further testing is needed at this initial stage. After the history, physical examination, and urinalysis, the abnormality is classified as anatomic, functional, or neurogenic. When an anatomic problem is suspected, imaging of the upper tract as well as the bladder is needed. Usually a renal ultrasound and voiding cystourethrogram is performed. The same is required if the urine is infected, a neurologic disorder is diagnosed, or there is history of either. More complex testing (magnetic resonance imaging [MRI] or computed tomography [CT] scan) may need to be done if abnormal physical findings of the lower spine or sacrum are found. Although urodynamics testing may be invasive and is not done routinely as a screen, it may be valuable in those select patients with severe symptoms refractory to standard treatment or in the child with a neurologic lesion.

## Diurnal Enuresis

Daytime wetting, or diurnal enuresis, is much more troubling to the school-aged child and adolescent because it is often obvious to family, friends, and peers as well as being socially unacceptable and a source of embarrassment and ridicule. Children who are wet during the day generally experience urge and urge incontinence and may be wet at night as well. They may posture, and when the urine volume is measured, a small bladder capacity may be found. Children generally outgrow daytime wetting as they mature, but until that time treatment can be offered, which parents generally expect. Initial treatment measures are usually directed toward placing the child on a timed voiding schedule (every 2 to 3 hours to empty the bladder before the child has an uninhibited bladder contraction), practicing good hygiene, and, of utmost importance, correcting constipation with stool softeners and a high-fiber diet.

The next step commonly is pharmacologic treatment of the voiding dysfunction. This must be tailored to the type of abnormality and whether there is associated infection or vesicoureteral reflux. For many years, the drug of choice has been oxybutynin (Ditropan) because the mainstay of treatment has been long-term anticholinergic use. Once the underlying bladder overactivity or instability is quashed and the overactivity of the external sphincter lessened, the result is diminished or eliminated elevated intravesical pressure. Another preparation used recently is tolterodine (Detrol).[1] Both of these drugs are now available in once-a-day long-acting formulations (Ditropan XL, Detrol LA). Both have been reported to have side effects in varying degrees such as facial flushing, dry mouth, diminished sweating, occasional blurred vision, and constipation. Other drugs, which have been used with varying levels of success, include hyoscyamine sulfate (Levsin),[1] propantheline (Pro-Banthine),[1] and dicyclomine hydrochloride (Bentyl).[1]

The child who fails initial treatment may need a further workup with fluoroscopic urodynamics studies to assess bladder function, filling pressure, and sphincter coordination with voiding.

## Nocturnal Enuresis

Nocturnal enuresis (NE) has been described in early literature dating back to the Ebers papyrus with various documented causes and remedies across the centuries. It continues to be a very common problem affecting 15% to 20% of school-aged children. The prevalence falls to 5% at 10 years old and affects 1% of 15-year-old teenagers. Fifteen percent of children with monosymptomatic primary nocturnal enuresis experience spontaneous resolution each year. NE can have a serious impact on the child, leading to shame, guilt, and diminished self-esteem. Only about one third of parents seek medical attention; about the same number punish the child for wetting, mistakenly thinking laziness or purposeful behavior has caused the problem. It is therefore incumbent on anyone who treats young children to screen for bed-wetting, educate the parents, and offer treatment if appropriate.

There is no one isolated cause for bed-wetting. It has been attributed to a multifactorial maturational delay in arousal to a full bladder, a delay in maturation of the bladder resulting in a diminished nocturnal bladder capacity, and a diminished circadian rhythm of

---

[1]Not FDA approved for this indication.

## CURRENT DIAGNOSIS

- Obtain a good voiding history, including family history of wetting, history of all elimination habits, and dietary history.
- Do a thorough physical examination, including neurologic and rectal if appropriate and indicated.
- Educate the family and debunk any myths about wetting.
- Give the family multiple treatment options, both pharmacologic and nonpharmacologic, including observation.

antidiuretic hormone production. Even a genetic component is implicated because bed-wetting has been shown to run in families.

Although bed-wetting is considered benign from a physical standpoint, because of the previously described negative impact, treatment options should be offered to the child age 6 years and older. The focus of the physician treating NE should be to ensure the child has no physical abnormality causing the bed-wetting. The child who has pure monosymptomatic nocturnal enuresis needs no further evaluation than a good history and physical examination and a urinalysis.

Treatment should be first directed at treating constipation or any daytime frequency or wetting component, which can be a benign association in 15% to 25% of cases. Treatment measures should include patient education because once the child (and parents) have an understanding of the mechanisms behind bed-wetting, compliance and success of treatment often improve. Initial therapy should also center on evening fluid restriction, avoidance of caffeine and artificial dyes (particularly red number 40), and motivational therapy with rewards and praise for dry nights. The child has no control over wet nights and should never be punished for a wet bed.

If the parents decide treatment is desirable, they can choose between pharmacologic and nonpharmacologic options. For those wishing to avoid medication, conditioning therapy with a moisture-sensitive alarm is an option. Several enuresis alarms are available on the market, all with the goal of awakening the child at or shortly after the time of micturition. The first drops of urine complete a circuit, activating a buzzer designed to awaken the child. It is important for a family member to be involved in the process to ensure the child wakes up and completes the voiding process in the toilet. Over time a conditioned response develops, and the child awakens voluntarily to a full bladder without help from the alarm. This process can take weeks to months, therefore requiring a patient and dedicated family and child to achieve success. The overall success rate has been stated as 50%, but with family involvement and proper use it can be as high as 70% to 90%.

Additional nonpharmacologic treatments offered include motivational therapy, bladder training exercises, hypnotherapy, bladder training, night wakening, and fluid restriction and diet therapy. All except motivational therapy have shown disappointing results.

The alternative to the alarm is pharmacologic treatment. The most commonly used drug now is desmopressin acetate (DDAVP) in tablet form and less commonly nasal spray. Desmopressin acetate is a synthetic analogue of vasopressin, a potent antidiuretic hormone produced by the pituitary gland. Desmopressin acetate tablets are

## CURRENT THERAPY

- Treatment of constipation is the initial measure.
- Children should not be punished for wet nights.
- For the bed-wetting alarms to be effective, family involvement is critical.
- Patience and understanding of the process are important for compliance with therapy and attaining success.

dosed starting at 0.2 mg 1 hour before bed (food and drink should be withheld 1 hour before dosing) and increased by one tablet per week up to 0.6 mg or until dryness is achieved at a lower dose. Success rates increase with higher doses and can be as high as 60% to 70%. Side effects are rare even at the higher doses. If a child responds, that dose is continued for 3 to 6 months before structured weaning by one less tablet a night per week. The drug can also be used long term without reservation. Another advantage is its ability to be used intermittently in situations like nightly or weekend sleepovers at a friend's house or overnight trips.

Another acceptable alternative is imipramine (Tofranil), a tricyclic antidepressant that has generalized effects on the bladder including weak α-adrenergic and anticholinergic effects. It weakly increases arousal and additionally may have some antidiuretic properties. Dosage begins at 25 mg at bedtime and is increased if necessary to 50 mg at bedtime in preadolescents and 75 mg per night in adolescents. There has been some hesitancy recently using imipramine because of certain profound side effects that have been observed. These include insomnia, weight loss, extrapyramidal symptoms, anxiety, and personality changes. Fatal cardiac dysrhythmias have been reported with overdosage. If dosed properly, imipramine can be an effective and safe drug. If effective, medicine is dosed for 6 months before attempts to wean.

## REFERENCES

Cendron M: Primary nocturnal enuresis: Current concepts. Am Fam Physician 1999;59(5):1205-1214, 1219-1220.

Hinsl KK, Hurwitz RS: Urol Clin North Am 1991;18(2):283-293.

Roth DR: Enuresis. In Rakel RE, Bope ET (eds): Conn's Current Therapy 2003, 55th ed. Philadelphia, Elsevier Science, 2003.

Rushton HG: Wetting and functional voiding disorders. Urol Clin North Am 1995;22(1):75-93.

Rushton HG, Belman AB: Enuresis and voiding dysfunction: A national kidney foundation guide to the child who wets. Washington, DC, Children's National Medical Center, 1999.

# Urinary Incontinence

Method of
*E. Ann Gormley, MD*

Urinary incontinence is a significant problem that affects millions of Americans. Patients may not report incontinence to their primary care providers because of embarrassment or misconceptions regarding treatment. Because incontinence is often treatable, it behooves the health care professional to identify patients who might benefit from treatment. Given that the treatment of incontinence varies depending on the etiology, the aim of evaluation is to identify the etiology.

## Etiology

Urinary incontinence is generally the result of either bladder or urethral dysfunction (Table 1). Incontinence also may result from a nonurologic cause and is usually reversible when the underlying problem is treated (Table 2). More uncommon causes of incontinence are urinary fistulae and ectopic ureteral orifices.

### BLADDER DYSFUNCTION

Bladder dysfunction causes urge or overflow incontinence. *Urge incontinence* occurs when the bladder pressure is sufficient to overcome the sphincter mechanism. Elevated bladder or detrusor pressure tends to open the bladder neck and urethra. An elevation in detrusor pressure

## TABLE 1 Etiology of Incontinence

**Bladder Dysfunction**
1. Urge incontinence
   - Detrusor overactivity
     - Idiopathic
     - Neurogenic origin
   - Poor compliance
2. Overflow incontinence

**Urethral Dysfunction**
3. Stress incontinence
   - Anatomic
   - Intrinsic sphincter deficiency

may occur from intermittent bladder contractions (detrusor overactivity) or because of an incremental rise in pressure with increased bladder volume (poor compliance). Detrusor overactivity may be idiopathic, or it may be associated with a neurologic disease (detrusor overactivity of neurogenic origin). Detrusor overactivity is common in the elderly and may be associated with bladder outlet obstruction. Poor bladder compliance results from loss of the viscoelastic features of the bladder or because of a change in neuroregulatory activity. The patient with urge incontinence may appreciate a sudden sensation to void but then is unable to suppress the urge fully. In severe cases, the patient may not be aware of the sensation of needing to void until he or she is actually leaking. The amount of leakage in patients with urge incontinence is variable, depending on the patient's ability to suppress the contraction. Patients with urge incontinence will often have frequency and nocturia in addition to urgency and urge incontinence. They may also have nocturnal enuresis.

*Overactive bladder* is a newer term that describes patients with frequency and urgency with or without urge incontinence.

*Overflow incontinence* occurs at extreme bladder volumes or when the bladder volume reaches the limit of the bladder's viscoelastic properties. The loss of urine is driven by an elevation in detrusor pressure. Overflow incontinence is seen in the case of incomplete bladder emptying caused by either obstruction or poor bladder contractility. Obstruction is rare in women but can result from severe pelvic

prolapse or following surgery for stress incontinence. Patients with overflow incontinence complain of constant dribbling, and they may also describe extreme frequency.

### URETHRAL-RELATED INCONTINENCE

*Urethral-related incontinence*, or *stress incontinence*, occurs because of either urethral hypermobility or intrinsic sphincter deficiency (ISD). Incontinence associated with urethral hypermobility has been called *anatomic incontinence* because the incontinence is due to malposition of the sphincter unit. Displacement of the proximal urethra below the level of the pelvic floor does not allow for transmission of abdominal pressure that normally aids in closing the urethra. Some women with mobility of the bladder neck or urethra do not experience incontinence. ISD was initially believed to occur after failure of one or more operations for stress incontinence. Other causes of ISD include myelodysplasia, trauma, and radiation. Some authors have theorized that all incontinent patients must have an element of ISD in order to actually leak. The patient with stress incontinence leaks urine with any sudden increase in abdominal pressure. In patients with severe ISD, the increase in abdominal pressure required to cause leakage is small, so patients may leak urine with minimal activity.

## Evaluation of the Incontinent Patient

The evaluation of the incontinent patient includes a history, physical examination, laboratory tests, and possibly urodynamic testing. The onset, frequency, severity, and pattern of incontinence should be sought, as well as any associated symptoms such as frequency, dysuria, urgency, and nocturia. Incontinence may be quantified by asking the patient if he or she wears a pad and how often the pad is changed. Obstructive symptoms, such as a feeling of incomplete emptying, hesitancy, straining, or weak stream, may coexist with incontinence, particularly in males and in female patients with previous incontinence procedure, cystoceles, or poor detrusor contractility. Female patients should be asked about symptoms of pelvic prolapse, such as recurrent urinary tract infection, a sensation of vaginal fullness or pressure, or the observation of a bulge in the vagina. All incontinent patients

## TABLE 2 Transient Causes of Incontinence (*DIAPPERS*)

| Cause | Comment |
| --- | --- |
| Delirium | Incontinence may be secondary to delirium and will often stop when acute delirium resolves. |
| Infection | Symptomatic infection may prevent a patient from reaching the toilet in time. |
| Atrophic vaginitis | Vaginitis may cause the same symptoms as an infection. |
| Pharmacologic | |
| • Sedatives | Alcohol and long-acting benzodiazepines may cause confusion and secondary incontinence. |
| • Diuretics | A brisk diuresis may overwhelm the bladder's capacity and cause uninhibited detrusor contractions, resulting in urge incontinence. |
| • Anticholinergics | Many nonprescription and prescription medications have anticholinergic properties. Side effects of anticholinergics include urinary retention with associated frequency and overflow incontinence. |
| • α Adrenergics | Tone in the bladder neck and proximal sphincter is increased by α-adrenergic agonists and can cause urinary retention, particularly in men with prostatism. |
| • α Antagonists | Tone in the smooth muscles of the bladder neck and proximal sphincter is decreased with α-adrenergic antagonists. Women treated with these drugs for hypertension may develop or have an exacerbation of stress incontinence. |
| Psychological | Depression may be occasionally associated with incontinence. |
| Excessive urine production | Excessive intake, diabetes, hypercalcemia, congestive heart failure, and peripheral edema can all lead to polyuria, which can lead to incontinence. |
| Restricted mobility | Incontinence may be precipitated or aggravated if the patient cannot get to the toilet quickly enough. |
| Stool impaction | Patients with impacted stool can have urge or overflow urinary incontinence and may also have fecal incontinence. |

From Resnick NM: Urinary incontinence in the elderly. Med Grand Rounds 1984;3:281-290.

## CURRENT DIAGNOSIS

### Urge Incontinence

Symptoms
- Urgency
- Frequency
- Nocturia
- Unable to reach the toilet with urge

### Stress Incontinence

Symptoms
- Leakage with physical activity

Signs
- Bladder neck mobility
- Positive stress test

### Mixed Incontinence

Symptoms
- Urgency
- Frequency
- Nocturia
- Unable to reach the toilet with urge
- Leakage with physical activity

Signs
- Bladder neck mobility
- Positive stress test

### Overflow Incontinence

Symptoms
- Frequency
- Nocturia
- Urgency
- Leakage with physical activity

Signs
- High postvoid residual

---

should be asked about bowel function and neurologic symptoms. Response to previous treatments, including drugs, should be noted. Important features of the history include previous gynecologic and urologic procedures, neurologic problems, and past medical problems. A list of the patient's current medications, including over-the-counter medications, should be obtained.

Although the history may define the patient's problem, it may be misleading. Urge incontinence may be triggered by activities such as coughing, so according to the patient's history, he or she seems to have stress incontinence. A patient who complains only of urge incontinence may also have stress incontinence. Mixed incontinence is very common; at least 65% of patients with stress incontinence have associated urgency or urge incontinence.

A complete physical examination is performed, with emphasis on the neurologic assessment and on the abdominal, pelvic, and rectal examinations. In females, the condition of the vaginal mucosa and the degree of urethral mobility are determined. Simple pelvic examination with the patient supine is sufficient to determine if the urethra moves with straining or coughing. The degree of movement is not as important as the determination of whether movement occurs. The presence of associated pelvic organ prolapse should be noted because it can contribute to the patient's voiding problems and may have an impact on diagnosis and treatment. A rectal examination in both males and females includes the evaluation of sphincter tone and perineal sensation.

A urinalysis is performed to determine if there is any evidence of hematuria, pyuria, glucosuria, or proteinuria. A urine specimen is sent for cytologic examination if there is hematuria and/or irritative voiding symptoms. The urine is cultured if there is pyuria or bacteriuria. Infection should be treated prior to further investigations or interventions. Hematuria consisting of more than three red cells per high-power field warrants further investigation.

A postvoid residual (PVR) should be measured either with pelvic ultrasound or directly with a catheter. A normal PVR is less than 50 mL, and a PVR greater than 200 mL is abnormal. A significant PVR urine may reflect either bladder outlet obstruction or poor bladder contractility. The only way to distinguish outlet obstruction from poor contractility is with urodynamic testing.

Urodynamic testing is used to accurately diagnose the etiology of a patient's incontinence; however, many patients can be successfully treated without urodynamic testing. The purpose of urodynamic testing is to examine compliance, diagnose stress incontinence, and rule out obstruction as a cause of either overflow or urge incontinence. Urodynamic testing should ideally be performed prior to invasive therapies and certainly in patients who are undergoing repeat procedures following failed procedures.

# Treatment of Urinary Incontinence

### URGE INCONTINENCE

Patients with urge incontinence need to understand that they leak urine because their bladder contracts with little or no warning. The first line of treatment is timed voiding. Often, reminding patients to void every 1 to 2 hours during the day, before they get an urge to void, will result in them staying dry. Other behavioral interventions, such as modification of fluid intake, avoidance of bladder irritants, and bladder retraining, where the patient attempts to consciously delay voiding and to increase the interval between voids, may also have a role in the treatment of urge incontinence.

Anticholinergics are the mainstay of medical therapy in achieving continence. The side effects of anticholinergics include urinary retention, dry mouth, constipation, nausea, blurred vision, tachycardia, drowsiness, and confusion. They are contraindicated in patients with narrow-angle glaucoma. Anticholinergics are also used to decrease bladder pressure in patients with poor compliance. Anticholinergics are combined with clean intermittent catheterization in patients who have a significant PVR prior to treatment and in patients who develop retention while taking anticholinergics.

Patients with intractable detrusor overactivity may require surgical intervention, consisting of neuromodulation with a sacral nerve stimulator or various forms of bladder augmentation.

The primary goal in caring for the patient with poor compliance is treating the high bladder pressure. Complete bladder emptying with clean intermittent catheterization combined with anticholinergics will often lower bladder pressure to a safe range. Some patients may require a combination of anticholinergics and α agonists. Bladder augmentation is required when medical management fails.

### OVERFLOW INCONTINENCE

Overflow incontinence is treated by emptying the bladder. If the cause of overflow is obstruction, then relieving the obstruction should lead to improved emptying. Anatomic obstruction in males derives from either urethral stricture disease or prostatic obstruction. Depending on the severity of urethral stricture disease, the patient may require urethral dilation, internal urethrotomy, or urethroplasty. Prostatic obstruction may be treated in a variety of ways, but transurethral resection remains the gold standard. If a woman is obstructed from previous surgery or from pelvic prolapse, she may benefit from urethrolysis or surgical correction of the prolapse. Clean intermittent catheterization is an option in the obstructed patient who does not want or could not tolerate further surgery.

The patient with overflow incontinence secondary to poor detrusor contractility is best treated with clean intermittent catheterization.

## CURRENT THERAPY

**Urge Incontinence**

Behavioral Changes
- Avoidance of bladder irritants
- Timed voiding
- Pelvic muscle exercises

Anticholinergics—Antimuscarinics—Nonselective for M3 Receptor
- Propantheline (Pro-Banthine)[1] 7.5 to 30 mg orally, three to five times daily
- Tolterodine (Detrol LA) 4 mg orally, daily
- Trospium (Sanctura) 20 mg orally, two times daily
- Solifenacin (Vesicare) 5–10 mg orally, daily

Anticholinergics—Antimuscarinics—Selective for M3 Receptor
- Darifenacin (Enablex) 7.5–15 mg orally, daily

Anticholinergics—Antimuscarinics/Smooth Muscle Relaxants
- Oxybutynin
- Regular (Ditropan) 2.5–5 mg orally, one to three times daily
- Extended-release (Ditropan XL) 5–30 mg orally, daily
- Transdermal (Oxytrol) 3.9-mg patch, twice per week
- Hyoscyamine (Levsin) 0.125–0.375 mg orally, two to four times daily

Anticholinergics/α Agonist—For Urge or Mixed Incontinence
- Imipramine (Tofranil)[1] 10–25 mg, once to three times daily

**Stress Incontinence**

Behavioral Changes
- Weight loss
- Quitting smoking
- Pelvic muscle exercises

α Agonists
- Pseudoephedrine (Sudafed)[1] 30–60 mg, up to four times daily

Surgery
- Anatomic
  - Retropubic suspensions
    - Burch
    - Marshall-Marchetti-Krantz
  - Slings
  - Pubovaginal
  - Midurethral
  - Obturator
- Intrinsic Sphincter Deficiency
  - Slings
    - Pubovaginal
    - Midurethral
    - Obturator
  - Artificial sphincter
- Submucosal Injections with Bulking Agents
  - Collagen (Contigen)
  - Carbon-coated zirconium oxide beads (Durasphere)
  - Ethylene vinyl alcohol copolymer (Tegress)

---

[1]Not FDA approved for this indication.

Indwelling catheters are not an optimum treatment modality for treatment of incontinence. All patients with indwelling catheters will have infected urine, which predisposes them to bladder calculi and ultimately to squamous cell carcinoma of the bladder. Any foreign object in the bladder can cause or exacerbate elevated bladder pressure that is associated with hydronephrosis, ureteral obstruction, renal stones, and eventually renal failure.

## STRESS INCONTINENCE

The amount of incontinence and how it affects the patient often determines the aggressiveness of treatment. The patient who is severely restricted because of severe leakage with minimal movement may not want to try medical therapy but may opt for surgical treatment, whereas the patient who leaks small amounts infrequently may choose conservative treatment. Pelvic floor exercises can improve anatomic stress urinary incontinence by augmenting closure of the external urethral sphincter and by preventing descent and rotation of the bladder neck and urethra. To benefit from the exercises, women must be taught to do the exercises properly, and they must do them. Adjuncts to learning pelvic floor exercises include weighted vaginal cones, a perineometer, and electrical stimulation.

α Agonists such as phenylpropanolamine[1] and pseudoephedrine (Sudafed)[1] can be used for treatment of stress incontinence. The bladder neck and proximal urethra have abundant α receptors. Activation of these receptors by α agonists leads to an increase in smooth muscle tone. The usual dose is twice daily, but some women who are incontinent with exercise may benefit from taking an α agonist 1 hour before exercise. Tricyclic antidepressants, such as imipramine (Tofranil),[1] have both α-agonist and anticholinergic properties.

Surgical therapy for stress incontinence is indicated when a patient does not wish to pursue nonsurgical therapy, or if such therapy has failed. The type of surgical therapy depends on the diagnosis. Patients who have anatomic stress incontinence can benefit from a variety of surgical repairs that restore the bladder neck to its normal retropubic position or improve urethral support. Patients with ISD usually have a well-supported bladder neck. These patients require a procedure that will close or coapt the proximal urethra. Coaptation may be achieved with a variety of bulking agents that are injected into the bladder neck or proximal urethra. A pubovaginal sling is the ideal procedure for the patient with both ISD and anatomic stress incontinence, as a sling will coapt the proximal urethra and restore the bladder neck to its normal location.

Synthetic midurethral slings are ideal for the patient with anatomic stress incontinence who wishes surgery with minimal recovery time. In one of the rare randomized surgical trials for stress incontinence, the result with tension-free vaginal tape has been shown to be comparable to that of a Burch colposuspension at 6, 12, and 24 months. The newest sling is a transobturator sling that is placed transversely underneath the urethra from one obturator foramina to the other. The advantage of this sling is that the retropubic space is avoided, with low risk of bladder, bowel, and major vessel injury.

Randomized trials comparing midurethral or transobturator slings to pubovaginal slings have not been performed.

## MIXED INCONTINENCE

Stress and urge incontinence often coexist. Burgio et al. advocate pelvic muscle exercises with biofeedback for treatment of stress and urge incontinence. Behavioral therapy can result in a reduction in incontinence episodes and patient-perceived improvement.

Imipramine (Tofranil)[1] is beneficial in patients with mixed (stress and urge) incontinence. The recommended dose is 10 to 25 mg, three times daily.

---

[1]Not FDA approved for this indication.

Seventy percent of patients with combined incontinence (stress and urge) will be relieved of urge incontinence following a procedure for stress incontinence. Patients whose urge incontinence does not respond to anticholinergics preoperatively may have a good response to anticholinergics once their stress incontinence is treated. Box 1 provides an overview of treatments.

## REFERENCES

Blaivas JG, Groutz A: Urinary incontinence: Pathophysiology, evaluation, and management overview. In Walsh PC, Retik AB, Vaughan ED Jr, Wein AJ (eds): Campbell's Urology, vol 2, 8th ed. Philadelphia, WB Saunders, 2002, p 1027.

Burgio KL, Locher JL, Goode PS, et al: Behavioral vs drug treatment for urge urinary incontinence in older women: A randomized controlled trial. JAMA 1998;280:1995-2000.

Leach GE, Dmochowski RR, Appell RA, et al: Female Stress Urinary Incontinence Clinical Guidelines Panel summary report on surgical management of female stress urinary incontinence. The American Urological Association. J Urol 1997;158:875.

Ward KL, Hilton P: A randomized trial of colposuspension and tension-free vaginal tape (TVT) for primary genuine stress incontinence: 2 year follow-up. Int Urogynecol J Pelvic Floor Dysfunct 2001;12[Suppl. 2]:S7-S8.

# Epididymitis

Method of
*John N. Krieger, MD*

Epididymitis is the inflammatory reaction of the epididymis to infection or to local trauma. Epididymitis causes major morbidity, accounting for more than 600,000 visits to physicians per year in the United States. Acute epididymitis is responsible for more days lost from military service than any other disease and is responsible for 20% of urologic admissions in the military. A survey of ambulatory patients documented epididymitis as a cause of 1 in 345 visits (0.3%), representing the fifth most common urologic condition, after prostatitis, urinary tract infections, urinary stones, and sexually transmitted infections.

## Clinical Presentation

Painful swelling of the scrotum is the characteristic clinical presentation. In most patients the pain and swelling are unilateral. The onset may be acute over 1 or 2 days or more gradual. Pain can radiate along the spermatic cord or into the lower abdomen. Symptoms of cystitis or urethritis are common. Dysuria or irritative lower urinary tract symptoms are characteristic. Many sexually active men have a urethral discharge. Thus, particular attention should be directed to eliciting a history of genitourinary tract disease or sexual exposure. Some men may have only a nonspecific finding of fever or other signs of infection. This is especially common in hospitalized men who have had urinary tract manipulation or catheterization and may be obtunded by medication.

Tender swelling can occur in the posterior aspect of the scrotum. Usually, the swelling is unilateral and is often accompanied by erythema of the scrotal skin. Early in the course, swelling may be localized to one portion of the epididymis. However, the swelling often progresses to involve the ipsilateral testis, producing an epididymo-orchitis. At this point it is difficult to distinguish the testicle from the epididymis within the inflammatory mass. Scrotal examination reveals the characteristic inflammatory hydrocele caused by secretion of fluid between the layers of the tunica vaginalis. Urethral discharge may be apparent on inspection or on stripping of the urethra.

Ideally, evaluation for urethritis should be done before the patient voids because micturition can make mild urethritis difficult or impossible to detect. The nursing staff should be taught to instruct patients with urogenital tract complaints not to void until after the physical examination. This is a common problem when we are asked to consult on patient management in the emergency department or in primary care settings. Patients with no sexual risk factors or evidence of urethritis should have microscopic evaluation of their midstream urine.

## Pathogenesis

Acute epididymitis occurs when uropathogens overcome the host defenses of the male lower genitourinary tract to establish infection of the epididymis. Most cases result from retrograde ascent of organisms through the urethra, prostate, ejaculatory duct, and vas deferens to reach the epididymis. Structural or functional abnormalities of the lower urinary tract increase the risk of epididymitis.

The risk factors for epididymitis vary substantially in different patient populations. In children and older men, anatomic abnormalities are critical risk factors for development of epididymitis. These include congenital anatomic abnormalities, such as an ectopic ureter draining into the vas deferens in children, and acquired anatomic abnormalities, such as bladder outflow obstruction in older men. In contrast, most sexually active younger men with epididymitis have normal urinary tracts. Thus, urologic investigations are indicated in children and older men with epididymitis but are seldom needed for management of epididymitis in young sexually active men.

Infections of the urethra, bladder, or prostate are important risk factors for development of epididymitis. In children and older men, the most common organisms are the typical bacteria that cause urinary tract infections, especially *Escherichia coli*, other enterics, and pseudomonads. In sexually active men, the most common pathogens are *Chlamydia trachomatis* and *Neisseria gonorrhoeae*. Men who practice insertive anal intercourse are also at risk for epididymitis caused by *E. coli* and other enteric bacteria. In addition to the usual causative organisms, immunocompromised patients are at higher risk for epididymitis caused by mycobacteria and fungi.

## Diagnosis and Treatment

### ACUTE EPIDIDYMITIS

Most patients with acute epididymitis can be considered in two categories, nonspecific bacterial epididymitis or sexually transmitted epididymitis. Unusual patients develop epididymitis after genital trauma or with disseminated infections.

## CURRENT DIAGNOSIS

**History**

- Exposure to sexually transmitted infection
- Urologic abnormalities or genitourinary tract instrumentation
- Symptoms of dysuria or urethral discharge

**Physical Examination**

- Pain or swelling on palpation of the epididymis
- Inflammatory hydrocele
- Scrotal skin erythema
- Urethral discharge
- Abnormal genitourinary tract anatomy
- Elevated temperature

**Laboratory Studies**

- Urethral swab specimen or first-void urine for pyuria
- Midstream urine for evidence of bacteriuria or pyuria
- Urine culture and sensitivity testing
- Samples for evaluation of sexually transmitted infections, as appropriate
- Doppler scrotal ultrasound may be helpful to differentiate epididymitis from testicular torsion or tumor

Clinical evaluation begins with a history, with specific attention to eliciting recognized risk factors, and a thorough physical examination. Initial laboratory tests include urinalysis, culture, and sensitivity testing for men with presumed nonspecific bacterial epididymitis. Men at risk for sexually transmitted epididymitis should also have a

## CURRENT THERAPY

**Age Younger than 35 Years with No History of Allergy**

- Ceftriaxone (Rocephin) 250 mg IM once
  *plus*
- Doxycycline (Vibramicin) 100 mg PO bid for 10 days
  *or*
- Azithromycin (Zithromax) 1 g PO as a single dose

**Age Older than 35 Years or Patient with a History of Allergy to Cephalosporins or Tetracyclines**

- Ofloxacin (Floxin) 300 mg PO bid for 10 days
  *or*
- Levofloxacin (Levaquin) 500 mg PO qd for 10 days

**All Patients**

- Anti-inflammatories
- Decreased activity
- Scrotal elevation
- Pain control

**Follow-up**

- Failure to improve within 3 days: Reevaluate initial diagnosis and therapy
- For persistent swelling and tenderness after therapy, consider:
  - Testicular tumor
  - Abscess
  - Testicular infarction
  - Tuberculosis
  - Fungal epididymitis

gram-stained urethral smear, culture for *N. gonorrhoeae*, and testing for *C. trachomatis*. In the latter group, serologic testing is also recommended for syphilis and for HIV infection.

## NONSPECIFIC BACTERIAL EPIDIDYMITIS

Infection with coliform or *Pseudomonas* species is the most common cause of epididymitis in men older than 35 years. In most series, gram-negative rods caused more than two thirds of cases of bacterial epididymitis. However, gram-positive cocci are also important pathogens and constituted the most common organisms in other reports.

Patients with bacterial epididymitis often have underlying urologic pathology or have a history of genitourinary tract manipulation. Epididymitis can occur weeks or rarely months after genitourinary tract surgery or urethral catheterization. Epididymitis constitutes a special risk for men who undergo urinary tract surgery or instrumentation while they are bacteriuric. Acute and chronic bacterial prostatitis represent other important predisposing conditions for development of bacterial epididymitis.

Medical management is appropriate for most patients with bacterial epididymitis. Typical patients are managed as outpatients. Initial empiric treatment is initiated with agents appropriate for both gram-negative rods and gram-positive cocci pending urine culture and sensitivity results. Fluoroquinolones represent our first choice for management of nonspecific epididymitis in outpatients. Agents of choice include ofloxacin (Floxin) and levofloxacin (Levaquin). Ciprofloxacin (Cipro) represents a reasonable alternative quinolone. In areas where the rate of bacterial resistance is low, trimethoprim-sulfamethoxazole (TMP-SMX; Bactrim, Septra) represents another reasonable alternative. Initial empiric therapy may be changed, if necessary, after culture results are available. A standard course of therapy is 10 days. More prolonged therapy may be needed for select patients such as those with evidence of bacterial prostatitis, whose antimicrobial therapy is continued for 6 to 12 weeks.

Indications for hospitalization include systemic symptoms, such as leukocytosis and fever, complications, or associated medical conditions. In these severe cases, parenteral antimicrobial therapy is used until the patient defervesces. Choices for empiric therapy of severe cases include the combination of an aminoglycoside plus either a β-lactam agent or a third-generation cephalosporin. After resolution of the acute systemic infection, therapy is continued with oral agents, guided by the culture and sensitivity results.

Nonspecific measures are worthwhile, including bedrest, scrotal elevation, analgesics, and local ice packs. A spermatic cord block with bipuvicaine (Marcaine) may be helpful for managing severe pain. We recommend urologic evaluation, because structural or functional abnormalities are common among men and boys with nonspecific bacterial epididymitis.

## SEXUALLY TRANSMITTED EPIDIDYMITIS

Sexually transmitted epididymitis is most common in young men. *C. trachomatis* and *N. gonorrhoeae* are the major pathogens. In most series, chlamydia was identified as the most common cause of epididymitis in younger, sexually active populations. For example, in our institution, *C. trachomatis* infections were documented in 17 (50%) of 34 cases of epididymitis in men younger than 35 years but in only 1 (6%) of 16 cases of epididymitis in men older than 35 years. In the past, these patients were considered to have "idiopathic" nonspecific epididymitis. Sexually transmitted *E. coli* infection also occurs among men who are the insertive partners during anal intercourse.

Often patients with chlamydial epididymitis do not complain of urethral discharge. However, 11 (65%) of 17 patients with epididymitis caused by *Chlamydia* had demonstrable discharge. In most cases, the discharge was scant and watery, characteristic of nongonococcal urethritis. The median interval from the last sexual exposure was 10 days and ranged from 1 to 45 days. Thus, urethral *C. trachomatis* may be carried for long periods before overt epididymitis develops.

In the preantibiotic era, epididymitis occurred in 10% to 30% of men with gonococcal urethritis. However, in current series, *N. gonorrhoeae* was identified in 16% of men with epididymitis in military populations and in 21% of men with epididymitis in civilians younger than 35 years. Many patients with epididymitis do not have a history of urethral discharge, and a discharge may be demonstrable in only 50% of such patients. Diagnosis depends on a high index of clinical suspicion, evaluation for presence of urethritis (which may be asymptomatic), appropriate cultures, or antigen detection tests.

Empiric therapy is recommended before culture results are available. Appropriate therapy includes coverage for both *N. gonorrheae* and *C. trachomatis* infections. The first choice regimen is the combination of ceftriaxone (Rocephin) plus doxycycline (Vibramycin) for 10 days. Allergic patients are treated with one of the quinolone regimens described earlier. Alternatives for coverage of *N. gonorrhoeae* include cefixime (Suprax), ciprofloxacin, ofloxacin, levofloxacin, or spectinomycin (Trobicin). Azithromycin (Zithromax) represents an effective alternative for coverage of *C. trachomatis*. Nonspecific measures are helpful, including bedrest, scrotal elevation, analgesics, and local ice packs. A spermatic cord block with bipuvicaine can reduce the need for analgesics in men with severe pain.

Patients should be evaluated for other sexually transmitted infections, and treatment of sexual partners is important. Patients should be instructed to avoid intercourse until symptoms have resolved completely and to refer all sex partners within the previous 60 days for evaluation and treatment. Underlying genitourinary tract abnormalities are uncommon in this population. Thus, a complete urologic work-up is indicated rarely for patients with uncomplicated sexually transmitted epididymitis.

## UNCOMMON CAUSES

Tuberculous epididymitis is the most common manifestation of genital tuberculosis in men, with orchitis and prostatitis less common. The usual symptom is heaviness or swelling. Scrotal swelling with bead-like enlargement of the vas deferens is characteristic. Chronic draining scrotal sinuses can occur. The systemic mycoses rarely cause epididymitis; blastomycosis is the most common pathogen and can also cause a draining sinus through the scrotal wall. Men with HIV infection and uncomplicated epididymitis should receive the same treatment as those without HIV. However, fungal and mycobacterial causes of epididymitis are more common among patients who are immunocompromised.

In the pediatric population, epididymitis can occur with congenital anatomic abnormalities, such as ectopic ureter or posterior urethral valves. Epididymitis occasionally occurs after testicular trauma. Many of these men have evidence of genitourinary tract infections with organisms outlined earlier, but occasional men develop traumatic epididymitis that is not associated with positive cultures or inflammation. We also described an unusual syndrome of noninfectious epididymitis associated with amiodarone (Cordarone) therapy for refractory ventricular arrhythmias. Rare patients develop epididymitis as a complication of collagen vascular disorders, such as Wegener's granulomatosis or Behçet's disease.

## Differential Diagnosis

Severe inflammation can lead to an enlarged indurated epididymis that is indistinguishable from the testicle. This can present difficulties in the differential diagnosis of epididymitis from testicular torsion or testicular cancer. Normally, the epididymis lies posterior to the testis. This demarcation is often preserved in cases of epididymitis. Reactive hydrocele formation can render palpation of intrascrotal structures difficult. Although transillumination often identifies hydroceles, color-flow Doppler ultrasonography is my preferred imaging study when the diagnosis is in doubt.

Acute epididymitis must be distinguished from testicular torsion at the initial evaluation because uncorrected torsion results in testicular death within 24 hours. Men with swelling and tenderness that persist after completing therapy should be reevaluated for testicular cancer, tuberculosis, or fungal epididymitis.

## Complications

Most patients experience relief of their symptoms within 48 hours. However, swelling and discomfort can persist for weeks or months following eradication of the infecting organism. In some cases, the epididymis remains enlarged or indurated indefinitely. Such men can develop chronic epididymitis, which is characterized by pain and occasionally by recurrent swelling.

Bacterial epididymitis may be an important focus of organisms causing both local morbidity and bacteremia in men with indwelling transurethral catheters. Genitourinary tract complications of acute epididymitis include testicular infarction, scrotal abscess, pyocele of the scrotum, a chronic draining scrotal sinus, chronic epididymitis, and infertility. Ultrasonography, particularly color-flow Doppler ultrasonography, is useful for the differential diagnosis of complicated cases. Surgery may be necessary for complications of acute epididymal infections.

## REFERENCES

Centers for Disease Control and Prevention: Sexually transmitted diseases treatment guidelines, 2006. MMWR Morb Mortal Wkly Rep 2006;55:1-94.

Collins MM, Stafford RS, O'Leary MP, Barry MJ: How common is prostatitis? A national survey of physician visits. J Urol 1998;159:1224-1228.

Furuya R, Takahashi S, Furuya S, et al: Is seminal vesiculitis a discrete disease entity? Clinical and microbiological study of seminal vesiculitis in patients with acute epididymitis. J Urol 2004;171:1550-1553.

Karmazyn B, Steinberg R, Kornreich L, et al: Clinical and sonographic criteria of acute scrotum in children: A retrospective study of 172 boys. Pediatr Radiol 2005;35:302-310.

Krieger JN: Sexually transmitted diseases. In Tanagho EA, McAninch JW (eds): Smith's Urology, 16th ed.. New York: Lange Medical Books/McGraw-Hill, 2004, pp 245-255.

Mittemeyer BT, Lennox KW, Borski AA: Epididymitis: A review of 610 cases. J Urol 1966;95:390-392.

Naber KG, Bergman B, Bishop MC, et al: EAU guidelines for the management of urinary and male genital tract infections. Urinary Tract Infection (UTI) Working Group of the Health Care Office (HCO) of the European Association of Urology (EAU). Eur Urol 2001;40:576-588.

Nickel JC, Siemens DR, Nickel KR, Downey J: The patient with chronic epididymitis: Characterization of an enigmatic syndrome. J Urol 2002;167:1701-1704.

Nickel JC, Teichman JM, Gregoire M, et al: Prevalence, diagnosis, characterization, and treatment of prostatitis, interstitial cystitis, and epididymitis in outpatient urological practice: The Canadian PIE Study. Urology 2005;66:935-940.

Stehr M, Boehm R: Critical validation of colour Doppler ultrasound in diagnostics of acute scrotum in children. Eur J Pediatr Surg 2003;13:386-392.

# Primary Glomerular Diseases

Method of
*Manuel Praga, MD, and Enrique Morales, MD*

## Clinical Presentation And Diagnosis

The clinical manifestations of primary glomerular diseases are very variable, ranging from asymptomatic urinary abnormalities to severe forms of rapidly progressive glomerulonephritis. The different clinical presentations are summarized and defined in Box 1.

Most milder forms of glomerular diseases are diagnosed by a positive dipstick test for microhematuria or proteinuria. All these patients should have quantitative estimations of proteinuria (24-hour proteinuria or protein-to-creatinine ratio in a random sample of urine),

## BOX 1  Clinical Presentations of Glomerular Diseases

### Nephrotic Syndrome
- Proteinuria >3.5 g/d in adults and >40 mg/h/m$^2$ in children
- Hypoalbuminemia
- Hyperlipidemia
- Edema

### Nephritic Syndrome
- Hypertension
- Oliguria
- Edema
- Hematuria (usually macroscopic)
- Red cell casts
- Non-nephrotic proteinuria
- Mild and nonprogressive GFR decrease

### Rapidly Progressive Glomerulonephritis
- Acute or subacute progressive worsening of renal function
- Hematuria (usually macroscopic)
- Red cell casts
- Proteinuria (usually <3.5 g/d)
- Blood pressure often normal

### Persistent Asymptomatic Urinary Abnormalities
- Non-nephrotic proteinuria (<3.5 g/d in adults and <40 mg/h/m$^2$ in children)
- Persistent microscopic hematuria

### Recurrent Macroscopic Hematuria
- Bouts of gross hematuria, usually triggered by infections
- Persistent microhematuria between the episodes of gross hematuria

### Chronic Renal Insufficiency
- Persistent proteinuria and/or microhematuria
- Hypertension
- Small kidneys

### Hypocomplementemia
The C3 and C4 fractions of serum complement are characteristically reduced in some types of glomerular diseases. This is an important clue for diagnosis

---

*Abbreviation:* GFR = glomerular filtration rate.

---

adults (except cases attributed to diabetic nephropathy) and steroid-resistant nephrotic syndrome in children, rapidly progressive nephritis, persistent nephritic syndrome with deteriorating renal function, and, usually, recurrent macroscopic hematuria. The need for renal biopsy in patients with asymptomatic urinary abnormalities should be individualized. The most characteristic pathologic findings of the main primary glomerulonephritis are summarized in Box 2, and their commonest clinical presentations are summarized in Box 3.

## BOX 2  Main Histologic Findings of Primary Glomerular Diseases

### Minimal Change Disease
- Normal glomeruli on light microscopy
- Negative immunofluorescence and diffuse effacement of epithelial foot processes on electron microscopy

### Focal and Segmental Glomerulosclerosis
- Focal (some glomeruli) and segmental (parts of affected glomeruli) scarring of the glomerular tuft

### Membranous Nephropathy
- Thickening of glomerular capillary walls with projections of glomerular basement membrane ("spikes")
- Subepithelial immune deposits detected by immunofluorescence and electron microscopy

### Membranoproliferative Glomerulonephritis
- Increase of mesangial cells and mesangial matrix
- Widening (double contoured appearance) of capillary loops
- IgG, C3, and IgM on immunofluorescence and subendothelial (type I) or intra-GBM (type II) deposits on electron microscopy

### IgA Nephropathy
- Predominant deposition of mesangial IgA on immunofluorescence
- Proliferation of mesangial cellularity and mesangial matrix on light microscopy
- Mesangial electron-dense deposits on electron microscopy

### Acute Postinfectious (Diffuse Proliferative) Glomerulonephritis
- Marked hypercellularity due to mesangial and endothelial cell proliferation and glomerular influx of neutrophils
- Hump-like subepithelial dense deposits on electron microscopy

### Crescentic Glomerulonephritis
- Cellular or fibrocellular crescents in a variable percentage of glomeruli
- Immunofluorescence pattern distinguishes the main three types:
  - Type I: Linear IgG staining of the GBM (anti-GBM disease)
  - Type II: Granular deposits along GBM (immune complex deposition)
  - Type III: Negative immunofluorescence (pauci-immune glomerulonephritis)

---

*Abbreviations:* GBM = glomerular basement membrane; Ig = immunoglobulin.

---

urinary microscopic examination, and serum creatinine. Glomerular disorders can be the renal manifestation of systemic diseases of different causes (e.g., malignancies, infections, autoimmune disorders), as discussed later. Therefore, medical history and physical examination should carefully investigate data suggesting such diseases. In addition to general laboratory analysis and assessment of renal morphology (renal echography), more specific determinations should be performed in all patients with suspected glomerular diseases: protein electrophoresis, serum levels of immunoglobulins, serum complement fractions C3 and C4, antinuclear antibody (ANA), anti-DNA antibodies, antineutrophilic cytoplasmic antibodies (ANCA), and tests for hepatitis B virus (HBV), hepatitis C virus (HCV), and HIV infections.

Renal biopsy is the conclusive method for establishing the diagnosis and classification of primary glomerular disorders. Indications for renal biopsy include the nephrotic syndrome in

## CURRENT DIAGNOSIS

- Clinical presentations of glomerular diseases range from asymptomatic urinary abnormalities (proteinuria, microhematuria) to severe forms of rapidly progressive glomerulonephritis (gross hematuria, edema, acute renal function worsening, hypertension).
- Secondary causes of glomerular disease should be excluded by means of history, physical examination, and appropriate laboratory tests.
- Renal biopsy establishes the diagnosis and classification of primary glomerular diseases.

# Treatment

## CONSERVATIVE THERAPY

Hypertension is a common finding in patients with primary glomerulonephritis. Current guidelines recommend blood pressure targets lower than 130/80 mm Hg in these patients and lower than 125/75 mm Hg in patients with proteinuria greater than 1 g/24 hours. Any antihypertensive drug or drug combinations are useful, and they should be selected on the basis of the patient's characteristics. However, blockade of the renin-angiotensin system either with an angiotensin-converting enzyme inhibitor (ACEI) or an angiotensin receptor blocker (ARB)

---

| BOX 3 | Commonest Presentations of the Main Primary Glomerular Diseases |
|---|---|

**Minimal Change Disease**
- Nephrotic syndrome

**Focal and Segmental Glomerulosclerosis**
- Nephrotic syndrome in more than two thirds of patients
- Non-nephrotic proteinuria in the remaining patients
- Renal insufficiency (20%-40%), hypertension (50%), and microhematuria (40%)

**Membranous Nephropathy**
- Nephrotic syndrome in >80% of patients
- Non-nephrotic proteinuria in the remaining patients

**Membranoproliferative Glomerulonephritis**
- Nephrotic syndrome in 50%
- Nephritic syndrome in 20%-30%
- Asymptomatic urinary abnormalities in 20%-30%
- Hypocomplementemia is common.

**IgA Nephropathy**
- Asymptomatic urinary abnormalities (microhematuria ±proteinuria) in >75%
- Intercalated recurrent or isolated episodes of macroscopic hematuria in >40%
- Nephritic or nephrotic syndrome in <10%

**Acute Postinfectious Glomerulonephritis**
- Nephritic syndrome
- Hypocomplementemia

**Crescentic Glomerulonephritis**
- Rapidly progressive glomerulonephritis

*Abbreviation:* Ig = immunoglobulin.

---

## CURRENT THERAPY

- Appropriate treatment should be instituted as early as possible.
- Blood pressure should be lower than 130/80 mm Hg (<125/75 mm Hg in patients with proteinuria >1 g/24h).
- Angiotensin-converting enzyme inhibitors and angiotensin receptor blockers are indicated in most cases of chronic proteinuric glomerular diseases due to their antiproteinuric, antihypertensive, and renoprotective effects.
- Specific therapy of primary glomerular diseases includes steroids, anticalcineurinic agents, and cytotoxics. Due to the potential risks of these therapies, the likelihood of progression and the presence of chronic irreversible parenchymal damage must be carefully assessed.
- Primary or idiopathic glomerular diseases comprise a wide variety of glomerular histologic lesions, with different clinical presentations and variable prognosis. Although some entities portend a favorable long-term prognosis, a considerable fraction of untreated patients who have other glomerular entities reach end-stage renal failure.

should be the main basis of antihypertensive treatment because of their demonstrated renoprotective effect (slowing or preventing loss of renal function) in patients with chronic renal diseases. The beneficial effects of ACEIs and ARBs appear to be similar and are also observed in proteinuric patients with normal blood pressure. Renal protection induced by ACEIs and ARBs is closely related to the significant reduction in proteinuria that these agents induce. The level of proteinuria is the best way to monitor the efficacy of ACEIs and ARBs. Recent studies in primary glomerular diseases have shown that a combination of ACEI and ARB is more beneficial in terms of renal protection and proteinuria decrease than either drug alone. Serum creatinine and potassium should be monitored after ACEI and ARB therapy is initiated, particularly in patients with reduced renal function.

Hyperlipidemia is a common finding in patients with glomerular diseases, particularly in those with the nephrotic syndrome. Prospective clinical studies have demonstrated that treatment of hyperlipidemia decreases proteinuria and prevents renal function loss. Statins such as atorvastatin (Lipitor) (10-40 mg after the evening meal) are the most commonly used lipid-lowering drugs. A level of LDL cholesterol lower than 100 mg/dL is recommended. Weight loss in obese patients induces a significant reduction in proteinuria, and smoking should be strictly forbidden, because smoking is associated with a more rapid progression toward renal failure in any type of renal disease.

All these measures (blood pressure lowering, treatment with ACEIs and ARBs, treatment of hyperlipidemia, weight loss, cessation of smoking) are also beneficial for the global cardiovascular risk that is significantly higher in proteinuric patients (mainly in those with renal insufficiency) than in the normal population.

The complications of the nephrotic syndrome require specific treatment. Edema is usually managed with a low-sodium diet plus furosemide (Lasix) in doses carefully adjusted to the severity of edema. Daily weight measurement is very important, because excessive diuretic doses can lead to volume depletion and functional worsening of renal function. In resistant cases, combinations of different types of diuretics (furosemide plus a thiazide diuretic, or furosemide plus a potassium-sparing diuretic such as spironolactone [Aldactone] in patients with hypokalemia) are needed. More severe cases require albumin infusions followed by high-dose intravenous furosemide (although intravenous albumin [Albuminar][1] increases proteinuria)

---

[1]Not FDA approved for this indication.

## BOX 4   Immunosuppressive Treatment of Primary Glomerular Disease

### Minimal Change Disease
**First Line**
- Steroids

**Second Line**
- Cytotoxics (frequent relapsers)
- Anticalcineurinics or mycophenolate mofetil (CellCept)[1] (steroid-dependent)

### Focal Segmental Glomerulosclerosis
**First Line**
- Steroids
- ACEIs
- ARBs

**Second Line**
- Anticalcineurinics
- Mycophenolate mofetil[1]

### Membranous Nephropathy
**First Line**
- Anticalcineurinics
- Steroids plus cytotoxics
- ACEIs
- ARBs

**Second Line**
- Mycophenolate mofetil
- Intramuscular ACTH (Synacthen)[1,2]
- Rituximab (Rituxan)[1]

### Membranoproliferative Glomerulonephritis
- Steroids
- ACEIs
- ARBs

### IgA Nephropathy
**First Line**
- ACEIs
- ARBs

**Second Line**
- Steroids
- Fish oil
- Cytotoxics

### Acute Postinfectious Glomerulonephritis
- Conservative therapy

### Crescentic Glomerulonephritis
**Type I (anti-GBM)**
- Steroids
- Cyclophosphamide (Cytoxan)[1]
- Plasmapheresis

**Types II and III**
**Induction**
- Steroids
- Cyclophosphamide[1]
- Plasmapheresis in severe acute renal failure

**Maintenance**
- Low-dose steroids
- Azathioprine (Imuran)[1]

[1]Not FDA approved for this indication.
[2]Not available in the United States.
*Abbreviations:* ACEI = angiotensin-converting enzyme inhibitor; ACTH = adrenocorticotropic hormone; ARB = angiotensin receptor blocker; GBM = glomerular basement membrane; Ig = immunoglobulin.

or even removal of fluids by hemodialysis. Nephrotic patients are at increasing risk for thrombotic events. Prophylactic treatment (subcutaneous low-molecular-weight heparin) is indicated in conditions of high risk, such as immobilization.

## SPECIFIC THERAPY

Box 4 summarizes the immunosuppressive treatment of primary glomerular diseases.

### Minimal Change Disease

Minimal change disease (MCD) is most common in children but also causes 10% to 15% of nephrotic syndrome in adults. Corticosteroid therapy is a very effective treatment for MCD. For children, the dose of prednisone is 60 mg/m$^2$/day and for adults 1 mg/kg/day (up to 80 mg/day). About 75% of patients respond (complete proteinuria disappearance) within 2 weeks, and more than 90% respond within 8 weeks, but adults show in general a slower response than children. Initial steroid dose is continued for 4 weeks and then changed to alternate-day prednisone (40 mg/m$^2$ on alternate days) or to daily prednisone, slowly tapering off over 6 to 10 weeks. Keeping patients on steroids for more than 3 months is associated with a lower 1-year relapse rate.

Up to 75% of children and many adults have nephrotic syndrome relapses. Isolated relapses are re-treated with steroids as in the first episode. Frequent relapsers (two or more relapses within a 6-month period)

are treated with a low-dose steroid course plus cyclophosphamide (Cytoxan) (1.5-2 mg/kg/day) or chlorambucil (Leukeran)[1] (0.1-0.2 mg/kg/day) in an 8-week course. After these short-term cytotoxic courses, a considerable fraction of patients remain free of proteinuria for prolonged periods, with a low rate of serious complications. Longer or repeated courses can induce severe side effects and are not recommended.

The response of steroid-dependent patients (reappearance of the nephrotic syndrome during or immediately after steroid withdrawal) to cytotoxics is poorer than that of frequent relapsers. Steroid-dependent patients and frequent relapsers unresponsive to cytotoxics are commonly treated with cyclosporine (Neoral)[1] given in an initial dose of 3-4 mg/kg in two divided doses, then adjusting for serum levels of 100-175 ng/mL. Most steroid-dependent patients transform into cyclosporine-dependent, and the risk of cyclosporine-induced nephrotoxicity should be considered. Mycophenolate mofetil (MMF, CellCept)[1] (600 mg/m$^2$/12 h in children, 500-1000 mg/12 h in adults) is a very useful alternative. Rates of response and relapse are similar to those of cyclosporine, but tolerance is better and there is no risk of nephrotoxicity. Therapy with cyclosporine or MMF if the patient responds is continued for up to 12 months before slow and careful tapering.

Less than 10% of MCD patients are steroid resistant. Because most of them subsequently have focal segmental glomerulosclerosis (FSGS) on biopsy, their therapeutic approach is the same as for FSGS.

[1]Not FDA approved for this indication.

[1]Not FDA approved for this indication.

## Focal and Segmental Glomerulosclerosis

Causes of secondary FSGS (obesity, reflux nephropathy, reduction in renal mass) should be carefully excluded. Treatment with an ACEI or ARB (or both) is the first option in patients with non-nephrotic proteinuria or in patients with nonaggressive nephrotic syndrome (proteinuria <5 g/day, serum albumin >3 g/dL, normal renal function), mainly if hypertension coexists. Patients with severe nephrotic syndrome or nephrotic proteinuria after ACEI or ARB introduction should be treated with prednisone 1 mg/kg/day. Several retrospective studies have shown that steroid treatment maintained for at least 6 months is followed by more than 50% partial or complete remissions. However, in responsive patients, proteinuria starts to decrease after 2 to 3 months of treatment.

If proteinuria did not show significant changes within this period, introduction of an anticalcineurinic agent together with steroid tapering is recommended. Cyclosporine (doses and blood levels as in MCD) has been the most commonly used drug, and prospective studies have shown more than 70% partial or complete remission after 6 months of treatment. Tacrolimus (Prograf)[1] (0.05-0.10 mg/kg/day in two divided doses, then adjusted for serum levels of 4-7 ng/mL) is proved to be effective in some cyclosporine-resistant FSGS cases.

In patients with complete or partial response to cyclosporine or tacrolimus, these drugs should be maintained at the lowest effective doses for at least 1 year before slowly tapering off. In some patients resistant to steroids and cyclosporine, or in those with mild degrees of renal insufficiency, MMF[1] (same doses as in MCD) has decreased proteinuria and stabilized renal function for prolonged periods. Sirolimus (Rapamune)[1] has induced complete (19%) or partial (38%) remission in a series of 21 steroid-resistant FSGS patients in a recent open-label trial.

About 20% to 25% of children with aggressive forms of FSGS have mutations in the genes coding for several podocyte proteins, mainly podocin. Most of these patients are unresponsive to any kind of treatment.

## Membranous Nephropathy

More than one third of MGN patients have a spontaneous remission, and most remissions take place during the first 2 years of the disease. Conservative therapy should be maintained during the first 9 to 12 months, unless renal function starts to deteriorate. ACEIs or ARBs, or both, can induce partial remission (non-nephrotic proteinuria) in a considerable percentage of cases.

In patients with an aggressive presentation (massive nephrotic syndrome and deteriorating renal function) a 6-month course of alternating monthly prednisone 0.5 mg/kg/day with a month of chlorambucil[1] 0.2 mg/kg/day is recommended. Other clinicians simultaneously use prednisone starting with 1 mg/kg/day and tapering off over 6 months plus chlorambucil 0.15 mg/kg/day for 14 weeks. Another regimen is prednisone 0.5 mg/kg/day every other day for 6 months plus cyclophosphamide[1] 1.5 mg/kg/day for 12 months.

In patients maintaining normal renal function and persistent nephrotic proteinuria beyond 9 to 12 months, immunosuppressive therapy should be initiated, mainly in the presence of markers of poor outcome, which include male gender, older age, and proteinuria persistently higher than 8 g/day after ACEI or ARB treatment. Alternating prednisone and chlorambucil (as indicated earlier), prednisone and cyclophosphamide, and cyclosporine[1] 3-4 mg/kg/day, targeting blood levels of 100-175 ng/mL are beneficial, inducing complete or partial remission in most patients.

Side effects (diabetes, bone necrosis, infections) are more serious with steroids plus cytotoxic treatments; trimethoprim-sulfamethoxazole (TMP-SMX, Bactrim) (80 mg/400 mg/day) should be concurrently administered for *Pneumocystis jiroveci* prophylaxis. Cyclosporine, administered for 6 months, is followed by approximately 50% of recurrences after drug withdrawal.

No studies comparing anticalcineurinic and cytotoxics have been published for MGN. Tacrolimus,[1] another anticalcineurinic agent, can also induce partial response in more than 80% of treated patients, although recurrence after withdrawal is the same (50%) as with cyclosporine. A recent randomized pilot trial reported that tetracosactide (Synacthen),[1,2] an analogue of ACTH (1 mg IM twice a week for 1 year) induced remissions in the same percentage as a regimen of steroids plus cyclophosphamide.

Uncontrolled studies reported that MMF[1] (1000-2000 mg/day) reduced proteinuria and stabilized renal function in some MGN patients unresponsive to other therapies. Rituximab (Rituxan),[1] a monoclonal antibody against CD20 B-lymphocytes, has reduced proteinuria in a pilot study.

## Membranoproliferative Glomerulonephritis

The incidence of idiopathic membranoproliferative glomerulonephritis (MPGN) has progressively decreased over the last decades, being currently an uncommon disease in developed countries. Most cases of MPGN are now secondary to HCV infection and concurrent cryoglobulinemia. No prospective studies about the treatment of idiopathic MPGN have been carried out in the last several years. Uncontrolled series of patients suggested that prolonged (>2 years) prednisone treatment is beneficial in terms of proteinuria reduction and renal survival. Prospective randomized trials with aspirin[1] and dipyridamole (Persantine)[1] showed a significant reduction in proteinuria some decades ago, but later analysis did not demonstrate long-term benefits on renal survival.

Conservative therapy, including ACEIs and ARBs, should be prescribed in all cases. In patients with the nephrotic syndrome after an observation period or in those with more aggressive presentations (deteriorating renal function, crescents), a 6- to 12-month course of prednisone could be indicated. Some small series of patients suggested that cyclophosphamide[1] is effective in aggressive cases of MPGN, but conclusive evidence is lacking.

## Immunoglobulin A Nephropathy

As in all types of primary glomerular diseases, the aggressiveness of therapeutic approaches in patients with immunoglobulin A (IgA) nephropathy should be graded according to the severity of the presentation. In patients with microhematuria and normal renal function, only regular follow-up is required. If slowly increasing proteinuria appears, an ACEI or ARB, or a combination of both drugs, should be started, even in the absence of hypertension, targeting for proteinuria less than 1 g/day and blood pressure lower than 125/75 mm Hg.

In patients with increasing proteinuria greater than 1-1.5 g/day in spite of these measures, other therapies should be contemplated. Steroids were proven to be beneficial in patients with normal renal function and proteinuria greater than 1 g/day in a prospective randomized trial: methylprednisolone (Solu-Medrol) pulses, 1 g/day for 3 days in the beginning of months 1,3, and 5, and oral prednisone 0.5 mg/kg every other day for 6 months reduced proteinuria and increased renal survival in comparison with untreated patients.

Treatment with fish oil supplements[1] in this type of patient remains controversial. Although eicosapentaenoic acid (1.8 g/day) or docosahexaenoic acid (1.2 g/day) demonstrated beneficial effects in some trials, these effects were not reproduced in others.

In patients with more aggressive presentations (proteinuria and deteriorating renal function), a prospective trial demonstrated that prednisone 40 mg/day tapering to 10 mg/day within 2 years plus cyclophosphamide[1] 1.5 mg/kg/day for 3 months followed by azathioprine (Imuran)[1] 1.5 mg/kg/day for at least 2 years significantly improved renal survival in comparison with untreated patients.

After initial suggestions of the benefits of MMF[1] 1000 to 2000 mg/day in IgA nephropathy patients unresponsive to other therapies, recent prospective and controlled trials have failed to demonstrate these good results, although the number of study subjects was small and many of them had advanced renal insufficiency.

## Acute Postinfectious (Diffuse Proliferative) Glomerulonephritis

As in MPGN, the incidence of diffuse proliferative glomerulonephritis has drastically decreased in recent years in developed countries. The prognosis is generally good, and signs and symptoms of the disease (nephritic syndrome) resolve sporadically within 2 to 6 weeks in a great majority of cases. Treatment should be focused on adequate control of blood pressure, salt restriction, and diuretics to prevent fluid excess and the risks of cardiac failure. The triggering infection should be investigated and treated if it has not disappeared spontaneously.

Some patients present with more aggressive courses, developing progressive renal insufficiency. In these cases, crescents involving a large proportion of glomeruli can be observed in a second biopsy. No controlled studies have been carried out in these aggressive cases, but some series of patients recommend high-dose intravenous pulse steroid, followed by oral prednisone 1 mg/kg/day, tapering off over 2 to 3 months. There is no evidence that more aggressive immunosuppressive therapy is beneficial.

## Crescentic Glomerulonephritis

Treatment of crescentic glomerulonephritis (CGN) should be promptly instituted because of the rapid transformation of cellular crescents into irreversible fibrotic crescents that collapse the glomerular tufts. Prognosis of type I (anti-GBM disease) CGN is poorer than that of types II and III, particularly in the presence of oligoanuria, dialysis requirement, or a large fraction of glomeruli with crescents.

Treatment of type I CGN includes steroids, cyclophosphamide,[1] and plasmapheresis. Pulse intravenous methylprednisolone (500-1000 mg daily for 3-4 days) is followed by oral prednisone (1 mg/kg/day for 3-4 weeks, then slowly tapering off over 6 months). Oral cyclophosphamide (2 mg/kg/day) is usually maintained for 2 to 3 months. Plasmapheresis (daily or alternate-day 4-liter exchanges) using albumin as replacement fluid or fresh frozen plasma if bleeding risk is high, is usually performed for 2 to 3 weeks. The duration of plasmapheresis, as well as the intensity and the duration of immunosuppressive therapy, should be guided by the clinical status and the titers of anti-GBM antibodies. In patients without pulmonary hemorrhage and with very advanced renal involvement (massive presence of glomerular fibrotic crescents), aggressive immunosuppression is not indicated.

The precise etiology of type II CGN (e.g., systemic lupus erythematosus, cryoglobulinemia) should be identified and the therapy guided by the diagnosis. If no apparent diagnosis is available, treatment is similar to that for type III (pauci-immune) CGN.

Induction treatment of type III CGN consists of steroids (oral prednisone, 1 mg/kg/day for 3-4 weeks, slowly tapered to a maintenance dose of 10-20 mg), and intravenous monthly pulses of cyclophosphamide (initial dose 0.5 to 1 g/m$^2$, adjusted for renal function and age), which has proved to be as effective and less toxic than oral administration. Once remission is achieved (recovery of renal function, absence of extrarenal symptoms), usually within 3 to 6 months, cyclophosphamide is replaced by azathioprine[1] 1 to 2 mg/kg/day for 12 to 18 months plus prednisone 5 to 10 mg daily or every other day. Positive titers of ANCA, particularly p-ANCA, can indicate more prolonged, low-dose, maintenance treatment, because the risk of recurrence is high. Plasmapheresis (similar to that in type I CGN) is proven to add benefits in type III CGN manifesting with severe renal failure. Although not tested in prospective trials, MMF[1] (1500-3000 mg/day) has been shown effective and well tolerated, even as induction therapy in some series of patients.

---

[1]Not FDA approved for this indication.

## REFERENCES

Cattran DC, Appel GB, Hebert LA, et al: A randomized trial of cyclosporine in patients with steroid-resistant focal segmental glomerulosclerosis. Kidney Int 1999;56:2220-2226.

Cattran DC, Appel GB, Hebert LA, et al: Cyclosporin in patients with steroid-resistant membranous nephropathy: A randomized trial. Kidney Int 2001;59:1484-1490.

Jayne D, Rasmussen N, Andrassy K, et al: A randomized trial of maintenance therapy for vasculitis associated with antineutrophil cytoplasmic autoantibodies. N Engl J Med 2003;349:36-44.

Nakao N, Yoshimura A, Morita H, et al: Combination treatment of angiotensin-II receptor blocker and angiotensin-converting-enzyme inhibitor in non-diabetic renal disease (COOPERATE): A randomized controlled trial. Lancet 2003;361:117-124.

Ponticelli C, Altieri P, Scolari F, et al: A randomized study comparing methyl-prednisolone plus chlorambucil versus methylprednisolone plus cyclophosphamide in idiopathic membranous nephropathy. J Am Soc Nephrol 1998;9:444-450.

Pozzi C, Bolasco PG, Fogazzi GB, et al: Corticosteroids in IgA nephropathy: A randomised controlled trial. Lancet 1999;13:883-887.

Praga M, Gutiérrez E, González E, et al: Treatment of IgA nephropathy with ACE inhibitors: A randomized and controlled trial. J Am Soc Nephrol 2003;14:1578-1583.

Torres A, Domínguez-Gil B, Carreño A, et al: Conservative versus immunosuppressive treatment of patients with idiopathic membranous nephropathy. Kidney Int 2002;61:219-227.

# Pyelonephritis

Method of
*Patricia D. Brown, MD*

Acute pyelonephritis (APN) is a urinary tract infection (UTI) that involves the renal parenchyma, also referred to as *upper tract UTI*. Most episodes of APN occur as a result of ascending infection from the bladder; patients with APN might or might not have symptoms of concomitant cystitis. Rarely, pyelonephritis occurs secondary to hematogenous seeding of the kidney as a result of infection elsewhere, most commonly endocarditis due to *Staphylococcus aureus* or disseminated fungal infection.

## Epidemiology

Surprising little is known about the epidemiology of APN. Similar to cystitis, APN (and hospitalization for APN) is more common in women than men; men have been reported to have higher in-hospital mortality. In contrast to cystitis, risk factors for pyelonephritis are not well defined. One recent study of nonpregnant women 18 to 49 years of age found risk factors for APN included factors known to be risk factors for acute cystitis, including frequency of sexual intercourse, recent UTI, diabetes, and maternal UTI history. The incidence of bacteremia in patients with APN is reported to be 11% to 53% in various studies; risk factors for bacteremia are not well established.

Similar to lower UTI, APN can be further classified into complicated or uncomplicated infection. The factors that make an episode of APN a complicated UTI are outlined in Box 1.

## Clinical Presentation

The classic presenting features of APN include abrupt onset of fever, flank pain, and costovertebral angle tenderness with or without symptoms of lower UTI including dysuria, urgency, and frequency. Unfortunately, there is no single constellation of signs or symptoms that is pathognomonic for APN. When localization studies have been performed on patients with symptoms of acute cystitis, 30% to

## BOX 1   Factors Associated with Complicated Pyelonephritis

- Diabetes
- Foreign body (catheter, stent)
- Health care–associated infections
- Immunocompromise
- Incomplete voiding (detrusor muscle dysfunction due to neurologic disease or medications)
- Infections due to multidrug-resistant pathogens
- Obstruction (including stones)
- Pregnancy
- Recent history of instrumentation
- Renal transplant recipient
- UTI in a male patient
- Vesicoureteral reflux

*Abbreviation:* UTI = urinary tract infection.

## CURRENT DIAGNOSIS

- Abrupt onset of fever, flank pain, and costovertebral angle tenderness with or without symptoms of cystitis are classic presenting features.
- Patients with lower UTI symptoms or laboratory evidence of UTI accompanied by flank pain, fever, or signs of systemic toxicity such as GI complaints should be managed as having APN.
- Urinalysis with microscopic examination should be performed in all patients with suspected APN. Absence of pyuria is strong evidence against the diagnosis.
- A urine culture should be obtained in all patients with APN. Blood cultures should be obtained in those who are hospitalized.
- Patients should be categorized into those with uncomplicated and those with complicated infections.

*Abbreviations:* APN = acute pyelonephritis; GI = gastrointestinal; UTI = urinary tract infection.

50% have been shown to have APN. Women who present with symptoms that have been present more than 7 days and those with a recent history of UTI are more likely to have APN. Flank pain is reported in approximately one half of patients with APN but also occurs in almost 20% of patients with cystitis. Fever is present in one half of patients with APN, but less than 5% of patients with cystitis. Nausea, vomiting, and diarrhea occur commonly in patients with APN, and gastrointestinal (GI) symptoms can dominate the presenting complaints.

In general, patients who present with lower urinary tract symptoms or laboratory evidence of urinary tract infection accompanied by fever, flank pain or tenderness, or signs of systemic toxicity, such as GI symptoms, should be treated for APN.

The diagnosis can be particularly challenging in the frail elderly patient, because symptoms such as frequency, urgency, and incontinence are often chronic in this patient population and unrelated to active UTI. Change in mental status may be the only presenting complaint. Because the prevalence of bacteriuria in this patient population is high, particularly among those with chronic indwelling catheters, UTI must be a diagnosis of exclusion.

Acute pelvic inflammatory disease can have a presentation similar to APN. Pelvic examination should be performed on all sexually active women to exclude this diagnosis.

The differential diagnosis of APN is outlined in Box 2.

## Diagnosis

Urinalysis, ideally with microscopic examination, using a clean-catch, midstream specimen, should be performed in all patients with suspected APN. Pyuria is a key finding in the diagnosis of UTI, and the

## BOX 2   Differential Diagnosis of Acute Pyelonephritis

- Appendicitis
- Cholecystitis
- Diverticulitis
- Gastroenteritis
- Herpes zoster
- Musculoskeletal pain, including vertebral disorders
- Ovarian cysts, tumors
- Pancreatitis
- Perforated viscus
- Pelvic inflammatory disease
- Pneumonia
- Renal stones, renal vein thrombosis, renal infarction

absence of pyuria is strong evidence against a diagnosis of APN. Direct microscopic examination under high power of the urinary sediment from a centrifuged specimen should reveal more than 10 leukocytes per high-powered field. The presence of white blood cell (WBC) casts is highly specific for localization of the infection to the kidney, but it is inadequately sensitive to exclude the diagnosis of APN. The dipstick test for leukocyte esterase is used as a rapid screening test to detect significant pyuria; the sensitivity is reported to be 75% to 96%, with a specificity of 94% to 98%. Because of the lower range of the reported sensitivity of the dipstick test, microscopic examination to exclude significant pyuria should be obtained in patients with suspected APN.

The presence of nitrite in the urine, detected by a dipstick test, has a reported sensitivity of 35% to 85% and a specificity of 92% to 100% for UTI. Microscopic examination of a Gram-stained, centrifuged urine specimen revealing at least one bacterium per oil-immersion field correlates with more than $10^5$ colony-forming units (cfu)/mL of bacteria, with a sensitivity of 95%. Although this is the standard definition of significant bacteriuria, it has been shown that women with UTI can have levels of bacteriuria as low as $10^2$ cfu/mL.

Although the microbiology of APN has remained predictable, significant changes in antimicrobial susceptibility patterns have occurred. Therefore, in contrast to recommendations for acute uncomplicated cystitis, a urine culture should be obtained in all patients with suspected APN. The need to obtain blood cultures has been debated, because blood cultures rarely yield a pathogen different from what was isolated from the urine. Bacteremia has been reported in 11% to 53% of patients hospitalized with APN. Bacteremic patients have a longer length of stay, and one recent report suggests that this is due to a longer time to resolution of fever. Many experts continue to recommend that blood cultures be obtained as part of the diagnostic evaluation of patients who are ill enough to require hospitalization; blood cultures are not necessary for those who will be managed as outpatients.

The role of diagnostic imaging in the management of APN is discussed later. In some cases with an atypical presentation, imaging may be helpful to confirm the diagnosis of APN. In this setting, pre- and postcontrast computed tomography (CT) is the imaging procedure of choice in adults.

## Microbial Etiology

Most cases of APN are caused by *Escherichia coli*. Other enterobacteriaceae, including *Klebsiella* species and *Proteus* species, are also occasionally implicated. Other gram-negative pathogens such as *Pseudomonas*, *Serratia*, *Enterobacter*, and *Acinetobacter* should be considered in health care–associated infections. *Enterococcus* is an uncommon pathogen in community-acquired infections, but it must be considered in health care–associated infections, including vancomycin-resistant enteroccoci. Other gram-positive pathogens include *Streptoccocus agalactiae* and *Staphylococcus* species. Although a common cause of acute cystitis in young women, *Staphylococcus saprophyticus* is a rare cause of pyelonephritis; the finding of *Staphylococcus aureus* in a urine culture should always prompt a search for an extrarenal source of infection that might have served as a source of hematogenous seeding. A Gram stain of the urine is a simple and rapid test to exclude a gram-positive pathogen as the etiology of APN and guide the initial selection of empiric therapy.

The emergence of resistance to trimethoprim-sulfamethoxazole (TMP-SMX [Bactrim]) among *E. coli* has had a major impact on the approach to initial empiric antimicrobial therapy for APN. It is clear that the prevalence of resistance varies depending on geographic region, and clinicians often do not have access to meaningful local resistance data. Recent reports of increasing fluoroquinolone resistance among uropathogens are of great concern, although overall resistance rates in North America remain low.

## Treatment

The first decision in the management of patients with APN is whether or not the patient requires hospitalization. Although prospective randomized trials are lacking, several retrospective studies as well as several prospective nonrandomized trials suggest that outpatient management is safe for many patients. Hospitalization should be considered for patients who cannot tolerate oral intake or who have severe pain or signs of severe sepsis. A strategy of initial management in the emergency department or an observation unit with an initial dose of parenteral antibiotic therapy, intravenous fluids, and symptomatic treatment of nausea and pain may be used in select patients to avoid hospital admission. Patients who will be treated as outpatients should have a stable social situation and the ability to contact the physician and return promptly if their symptoms worsen. Hospitalization is generally recommended for patients with complicated infections. Most experts believe that pregnant women with APN should always be hospitalized.

There are surprisingly few prospective randomized trials of the treatment of pyelonephritis. For patients who require hospitalization, parenteral therapy with an aminoglycoside, a third-generation cephalosporin, or a fluoroquinolone is recommended. At my institution, we discourage fluoroquinolones for this indication because there are other effective alternatives and we wish to minimize the use of these very broad-spectrum agents in the hospital setting. Although

resistance to TMP-SMX among uropathogenic *E. coli* appears to have leveled off and might actually be decreasing, this agent should not be used for empiric therapy of APN.

If a gram-positive pathogen is suspected or suggested by the results of urine Gram stain, ampicillin or ampicillin-sulbactam (Unasyn) with or without an aminoglycoside can be used. Patients should receive intravenous therapy until they are clinically improving and able to reliably tolerate oral intake; oral therapy can be chosen based on the results of urine culture and susceptibility data. TMP-SMX, a fluoroquinolone, and ampicillin are all potential candidates for oral switch therapy. The narrowest spectrum, least expensive agent to which the isolated pathogen is susceptible should be chosen. Despite in vitro susceptibility data, first- and second-generation cephalosporins have a poor track record in the treatment of APN and are generally not recommended, with the exception of pyelonephritis in pregnancy.

Bacteremic patients might take longer to respond but do not require more prolonged parenteral therapy. The total duration of therapy for pyelonephritis is generally 14 days. Seven days of therapy with a fluoroquinolone for uncomplicated APN has been shown to be effective. Longer courses of therapy may be required for select patients with complicated pyelonephritis. For outpatients, initial empiric therapy with a fluoroquinolone is recommended, with adjustment of therapy, if needed, based on the results of urine culture. All of the currently available fluoroquinolones can be used, with the exception of moxifloxacin (Avelox), which does not achieve adequate levels in the urine. Although it is useful in the treatment of cystitis, norfloxacin (Noroxin) is not recommended for the treatment of APN because it does not achieve sustained tissue or serum levels. Suggested antimicrobial dosing regimens for APN are outlined in Box 3.

## Imaging

Imaging is generally not needed in patients with uncomplicated APN. For patients with complicated infections (e.g., history of stones, prior renal surgery), renal ultrasound with abdominal plain films is considered an acceptable alternative to excretory urography. For patients with diabetes or other immunocompromise and for patients who fail to respond after 72 hours of appropriate antibiotic therapy, pre- and postcontrast CT is the imaging procedure of choice.

## Follow-up

Most patients will respond to appropriate antibiotic therapy. Follow-up urine cultures to document microbiological response are not recommended in patients who have responded clinically.

---

### CURRENT THERAPY

- Hospitalization is recommended for patients unable to tolerate oral intake, those with severe pain, and those with signs of severe sepsis. Hospitalization is generally recommended for patients with complicated infections and for all pregnant women.
- Parenteral regimens for hospitalized patients include an aminoglycoside, third-generation cephalosporin, or fluoroquinolone, with oral switch therapy selected on the basis of culture and susceptibility data.
- Initial empiric therapy for outpatients is a fluoroquinolone.
- Imaging is not recommended for patients with uncomplicated infections. Pre- and postcontrast computed tomographic scans should be obtained in those who fail to respond within 72 hours to appropriate antibiotic therapy.

---

### BOX 3 Antimicrobial Therapy for the Management of Acute Pyelonephritis

**Parenteral Regimens**
- Ampicillin 2 g q4h-q6h
- Ampicillin-sulbactam (Unasyn) 3 g q6h
- Ceftriaxone (Rocephin) 1-2 g q24h
- Ciprofloxacin (Cipro) 400 mg q12h
- Gentamicin (Garamycin) 3-5 mg/kg q24h
- Levofloxacin (Levaquin) 250-500 mg q24h

**Oral Regimens**
- Amoxicillin 500 mg q8h
- Ciprofloxacin 500 mg q12h
- Ciprofloxacin XR 1000 mg q24h
- Levofloxacin 250 mg q24h
- Trimethoprim-sulfamethoxazole DS (Bactrim DS) 160/800 mg q12h

## REFERENCES

Foxman B, Klemstine KL, Brown PD: Acute pyelonephritis in US hospitals in 1997: Hospitalization and in-hospital mortality. Ann Epidemiol 2003; 13:144-150.

Pappas PG: Laboratory in the diagnosis and management of urinary tract infections. Med Clin North Am 1991;75:313-325.

Sandler CM, Amis ES Jr, Bigongiari LR, et al: Imaging in acute pyelonephritis. American College of Radiology. ACR appropriateness criteria. Radiology 2000;215(suppl):677-681.

Scholes D, Hooton TM, Roberts PL, et al: Risk factors associated with acute pyelonephritis in healthy women. Ann Intern Med 2005;142:20-27.

Talan DA, Stamm WE, Hooton TM, et al: Comparison of ciprofloxacin (7 days) and trimethoprim-sulfamethoxazole (14 days) for acute uncomplicated pyelonephritis in women: A randomized trial. JAMA 2000;283:1583-1590.

Warren JW, Abrutyn E, Hebel JR, et al: Guidelines for antimicrobial treatment of uncomplicated acute bacterial cystitis and acute pyelonephritis in women. Clin Infect Dis 1999;29:745-758.

# Trauma to the Genitourinary Tract

Method of
*Noel A. Armenakas, MD, and*
*J. James Bruno II, MD*

Injuries to the genitourinary tract often occur in conjunction with injuries to other organs in a polytraumatized patient. Only after the assessment of the "ABCs" (*A*irway, *B*reathing, *C*irculation) should attention be directed to specific organ injuries. Priorities include treatment of life-threatening injuries, control of major hemorrhage and their sequelae (e.g., coagulopathy, hypothermia, metabolic disturbances), and management of intra-abdominal contamination. The urologic consultation is frequently requested after the initial emergency or operating room resuscitation. Overall, genitourinary injuries occur in 10% to 15% of abdominal and pelvic traumas. Of all civilian genitourinary traumas, the kidneys have the highest incidence of involvement, followed by the bladder, urethra, genitals, and ureters (Figure 1).

## Renal Trauma

### ETIOLOGY

Kidney trauma in the civilian population accounts for 60% to 70% of all genitourinary organ injuries. The majority of renal injuries (85%–90%) result from blunt abdominal trauma, including motor vehicle accidents, falls, and assaults. Most blunt renal injuries are low grade. Occasionally, blunt abdominal injuries result in renovascular injuries, usually from rapid deceleration. The most frequently associated injuries occur to the head and central nervous system and less frequently to the abdomen, with splenic and liver injuries prevailing. Penetrating renal injuries most frequently result from gunshot wounds. These are associated with multisystem injuries, most commonly involving the liver, bowel, and spleen.

### DIAGNOSIS

A renal injury is diagnosed by combining a carefully performed history and physical examination with the appropriate laboratory and radiologic evaluations. This comprehensive evaluation allows for accurate staging and appropriate treatment selection. The historical details of the injury can provide significant information regarding potential renal involvement. For example, deceleration injuries from high-speed motor vehicle accidents and falls from heights may be associated with

SITES OF GENITOURINARY TRAUMA

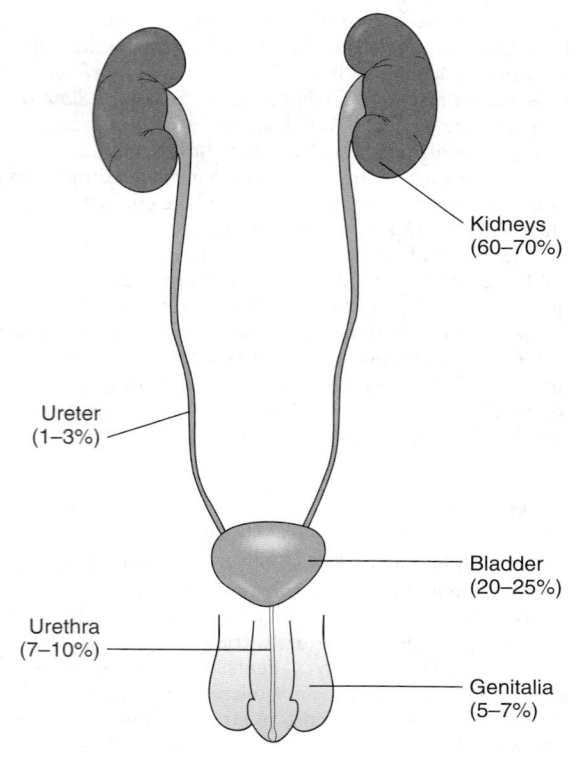

**FIGURE 1.** Genitourinary injuries.

major vascular and/or parenchymal renal damage. On the physical examination, flank contusions, seatbelt marks, lower rib or lumbar vertebral fractures, and upper abdominal or flank tenderness are all clinical indicators of a potential renal injury. Initial blood pressure should be noted because patients with renovascular injuries often present in shock. Any penetrating injury to the flank or upper abdomen suggests the possibility of renal trauma, although the site of injury

## CURRENT DIAGNOSIS

- Renal Trauma
  - History and physical examination
  - Laboratory evaluation (urinalysis, hematocrit)
  - Radiographic assessment
- Ureteral Trauma
  - Radiographic evaluation
  - Intraoperative inspection
- Bladder Trauma
  - History and physical examination (including pelvic and rectal examinations)
  - Urinalysis
  - Cystogram
- Genital Trauma in Males
  - History and physical examination
  - Scrotal sonogram
  - Retrograde urethrogram
- Urethral Trauma
  - History and physical examination (inability to void, pelvic fracture, blood at the meatus, or vaginal introitus)
  - Urinalysis
  - Retrograde urethrogram

(i.e., abdomen, flank, back) does not reliably predict its extent. Weapon and ballistics information (e.g., gun type and caliber, knife length) can be helpful in assessing the depth of penetration and potential débridement requirements.

Urine should be obtained and evaluated for hematuria by either dipstick or microscopic analysis. It is important to collect the first voided or catheterized specimen to avoid false-negative results from dilution after intravenous hydration. The presence of hematuria, defined as more than five erythrocytes per high-power field in adults, is the primary laboratory indicator of a renal injury. However, the amount of hematuria does not correlate with the degree of renal trauma, and its absence cannot exclude a major parenchymal or vascular injury. Other important laboratory tests include a complete blood count and chemistry profile.

Radiographic imaging enables the extent of injury to be defined and should be considered once the patient has been stabilized. The need for radiographic renal imaging is determined by the presence of any of the following criteria:

1. Any *penetrating* injury to the abdomen, flanks, back, or lower chest
2. Any *blunt* injury presenting with either (a) gross hematuria, (b) microscopic hematuria and an initial blood pressure less than 90 mm Hg, or (c) any clinical indicator of renal injury

In adult patients who sustain blunt trauma and are hemodynamically stable with only microscopic hematuria, a clinical diagnosis of a low-grade renal injury can be accurately made without the need for radiographic renal assessment. This recommendation is based on results from several large series that have documented the rarity of an isolated high-grade renal injury in this subgroup. Historically, pediatric patients sustaining blunt abdominal trauma who present with any degree of hematuria, irrespective of hemodynamic stability, have been evaluated radiographically. Newer data confirm that children can be evaluated with the same guidelines as used for adult patients providing the urinalysis shows *fewer than 50* erythrocytes per high-power field. Children who present with blunt abdominal trauma and more than 50 erythrocytes per high-power field should be evaluated radiographically.

Radiographic imaging is undertaken to define the extent and type of renal injury and to complete the staging process accurately. The appropriate imaging study should determine the presence and function of the contralateral kidney and delineate the renal parenchyma and collecting system on the involved side. Currently, computed tomography (CT) is the preferred imaging modality to evaluate renal injuries. If CT is unavailable, a complete excretory urogram (intravenous pyelogram [IVP]) can be obtained. Ultrasonography has a limited role in the acute evaluation of renal trauma because of its inability to differentiate blood from urine, but it can be used for follow-up. Angiography is rarely necessary simply for diagnostic purposes but can have an important therapeutic role in vascular embolization. Magnetic resonance imaging is comparable to CT in identifying renal injuries, but it is more expensive and less readily available, which limits its use.

On the basis of the information obtained radiographically or clinically, renal injuries are classified according to severity into five grades (Figure 2):

Grade I:      Renal contusion or subcapsular hematoma
Grade II:     Less than 1-cm parenchymal (cortex) laceration
Grade III:    Greater than 1-cm parenchymal (cortex and medulla) laceration *without* urinary extravasation
Grade IV:     Parenchymal laceration through renal cortex, medulla, and collecting system *with* urinary extravasation or a contained vascular injury
Grade V:      Shattered kidney or avulsion of renal hilum

In cases in which the patient's instability precludes a complete abdominal radiographic assessment, prior to renal exploration,

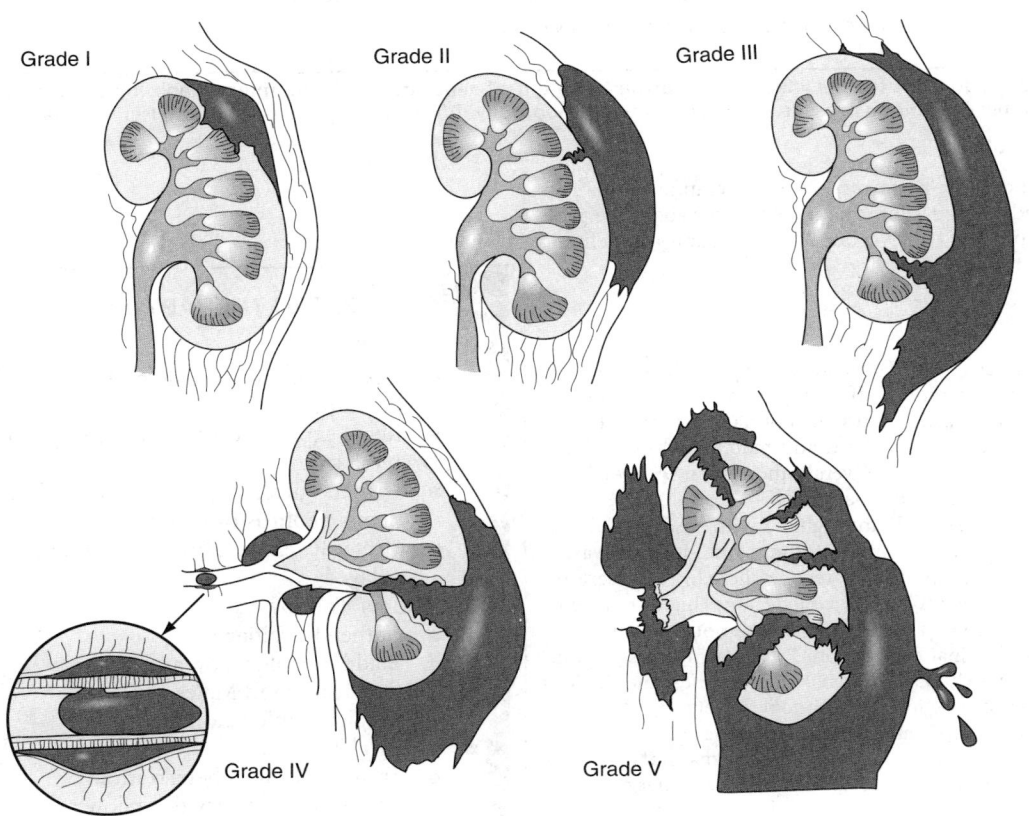

Grade I    Grade II    Grade III

Grade IV    Grade V

**FIGURE 2.** Classification of renal injuries by grade. (Modified from Organ Injury Scaling Committee of the American Association for the Surgery of Trauma. Copyright © 2003, Elsevier Science (USA). All rights reserved.)

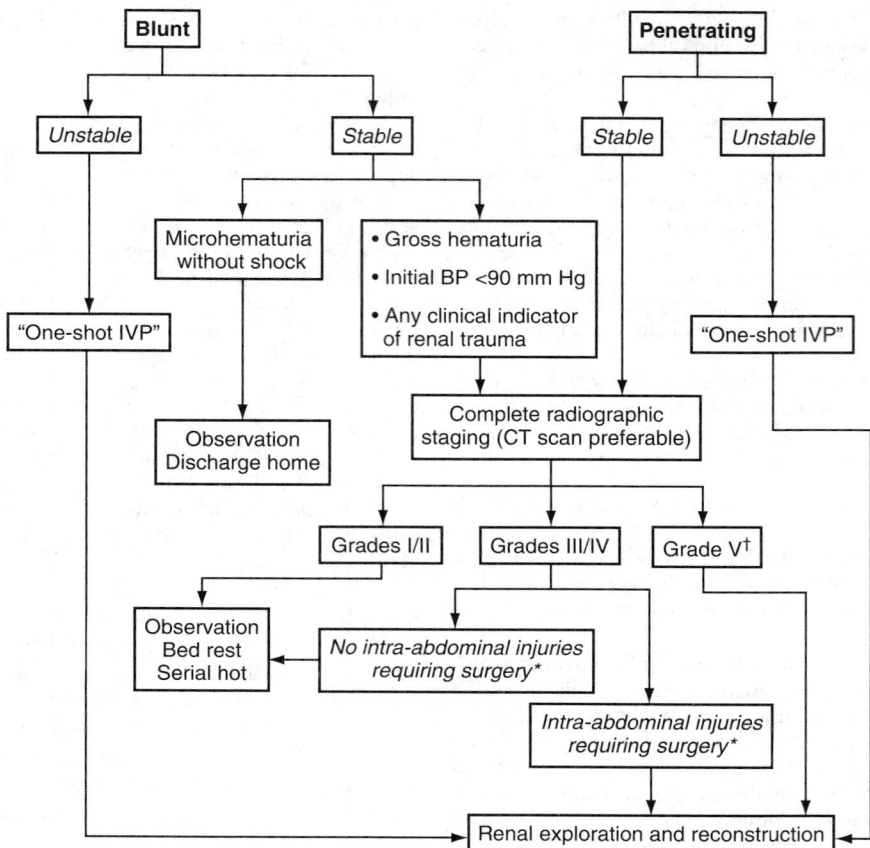

**FIGURE 3.** Algorithm for the diagnosis and management of renal trauma (abdominal, flank, back, or chest injury). *Abbreviations:* BP = blood pressure; CT = computed tomography; IVP = intravenous pyelogram; Hct = hematocrit.

a "one-shot" IVP should be performed in the operating room. This limited imaging study provides information primarily about the presence and function of both kidneys, but it lacks accuracy in defining anatomic details of the injury (Figure 3).

## MANAGEMENT

Low-grade renal injuries (I and II), whether blunt or penetrating, can be managed safely nonoperatively. If they present only with microscopic hematuria, hospitalization is usually not required. Patients with gross hematuria should be hospitalized and maintained on bed rest until the hematuria visibly clears. Overall, more than 95% of blunt renal injuries can be managed nonoperatively.

High-grade renal injuries (III through V) with associated intra-abdominal organ injuries requiring laparotomy and most renovascular injuries are best explored and reconstructed. Nonoperative management can be chosen for *select accurately staged* high-grade renal injuries, providing the patient is stable and does not have any other injuries requiring abdominal exploration. By following these recommendations, approximately 55% of renal stab wounds and 25% of renal gunshot wounds can be managed nonoperatively.

Absolute indications for renal exploration include an expanding or pulsatile retroperitoneal hematoma and hemodynamic instability from renal hemorrhage. Relative indications include urinary extravasation, nonviable renal parenchyma with a major laceration, a renovascular injury in a solitary kidney, persistent bleeding (>2 U packed red blood cells per 24 hours), incomplete radiographic staging, and laparotomy for associated injuries. The presence of more than one

## CURRENT THERAPY

- Renal Trauma
  - Observation with close monitoring of vital signs and hematocrit
  - Renal exploration and attempted reconstruction
- Ureteral Trauma
  - Urinary diversion (via a ureteral stent or percutaneous nephrostomy tube)
  - Ureteral exploration and repair (immediate or delayed)
- Bladder Trauma
  - Catheter drainage
  - Bladder exploration and repair
- Genital Trauma in Males
  - Surgical exploration and repair
- Urethral Trauma
  - Transurethral catheterization
  - Suprapubic urinary diversion
  - Endoscopic realignment
  - Urethral suturing

relative indication often warrants surgical treatment. The selective embolization of hemorrhage via interventional radiology, used more commonly in splenic and hepatic injuries, is a promising new modality for nonoperative management of select renal injuries.

Operative renal exploration is performed through a midline transperitoneal abdominal approach. The renal vessels are identified prior to opening Gerota's fascia. Vascular control becomes important when confronted with deep renal parenchymal or vascular bleeding. Once the kidney is exposed and all injuries are identified, the appropriate reconstructive technique can be performed. Simple lacerations can be managed with renorrhaphy. Polar injuries are best treated by partial nephrectomy. Attempts at vascular repair should be made provided these injuries are discovered promptly.

## OUTCOME

Aggressive accurate staging of renal trauma and careful attention to reconstruction are paramount in avoiding renal loss. Although most renal injuries can be managed nonoperatively, renal salvage can be expected in approximately 70% to 90% of cases requiring exploration. Early complications of renal trauma include bleeding, infection, abscess formation and persistent urinary extravasation. Late complications include hypertension and decreased renal function. Hypertension occurs in approximately 5% of cases and is believed to be caused by mechanisms that activate the renin-angiotensin system. It usually manifests within the first few months of injury, but further delayed onset has been documented. Blood pressure should be measured regularly for the first year and annually thereafter.

## Ureteral Trauma

### ETIOLOGY

Ureteral injuries from external trauma constitute approximately 1% to 3% of all genitourinary injuries. The ureter's mobility and anatomic characteristics protect it from trauma; its narrow diameter and retroperitoneal location between the spine, major muscle groups, and the peritoneal contents make it an unlikely target. Most external ureteral injuries occur from gunshot wounds. The bullet need not physically transect the ureter to cause significant damage. If the bullet's path is simply near the ureter, the temporary cavitation created by the missile can cause significant tissue destruction and delayed necrosis. Such injuries can be difficult to identify initially and often present with delayed sequelae. Penetrating ureteral injuries are almost always associated with multiple organ injuries. The most common sites, in order of decreasing frequency, are the small bowel, colon, liver, and iliac vessels. Ureteral injuries from blunt trauma are rare. They usually occur in children during rapid deceleration, causing excessive hyperextension of their flexible vertebral column with disruption at the ureteropelvic junction. Blunt ureteral injuries also are associated with multiple organ injuries, most commonly to the liver, spleen, and skeletal system.

Iatrogenic ureteral injuries are the most common. They most frequently occur during ureteroscopy, hysterectomy, low anterior colon resection, vaginal surgery, and abdominal aneurysm repair and usually involve the lower ureteral segment.

## DIAGNOSIS

Prompt diagnosis is the first step toward a successful outcome. This may be complicated by the presence of multiple organ injuries and the absence of clinical and laboratory findings specific for ureteral trauma. Indeed, hematuria, which is a reliable indicator of renal trauma, is absent in 30% to 45% of ureteral injuries. These limitations frequently result in delayed recognition manifested by fever, flank pain, urinoma, fistula formation, and eventually sepsis. To avoid this additional morbidity, it is imperative that the evaluating physician maintain a high index of suspicion based on the injury mechanism and location.

Essentially any patient with penetrating abdominal trauma should be suspected of having a ureteral injury and evaluated radiographically. Similarly, children with significant blunt abdominal trauma and multiple associated injuries should undergo radiographic ureteral assessment regardless of findings on urinalysis. Urinary tract imaging can be obtained using either a CT scan or an IVP. Extravasation of contrast is the sine qua non of a ureteral injury. On CT, the extravasated contrast usually will be confined to the medial perirenal space. With complete ureteral disruption, no contrast material will be seen in the distal ureter on delayed images. Extravasation may be seen on an IVP, but frequently the findings are more subtle, such as delayed renal function or mild ureteral dilation or deviation. If the results of the CT or IVP are inconclusive, a retrograde ureterogram can be performed. Although this is the most accurate ureteral imaging test, it is often impractical in the acute trauma setting.

Most penetrating ureteral injuries are diagnosed intraoperatively during the initial exploratory laparotomy performed for management of the associated abdominal injuries. In this setting, direct visual inspection is the most reliable method for assessing ureteral integrity. Intravenous or intraureteral injection of indigo carmine or methylene blue may aid in injury recognition (Figure 4).

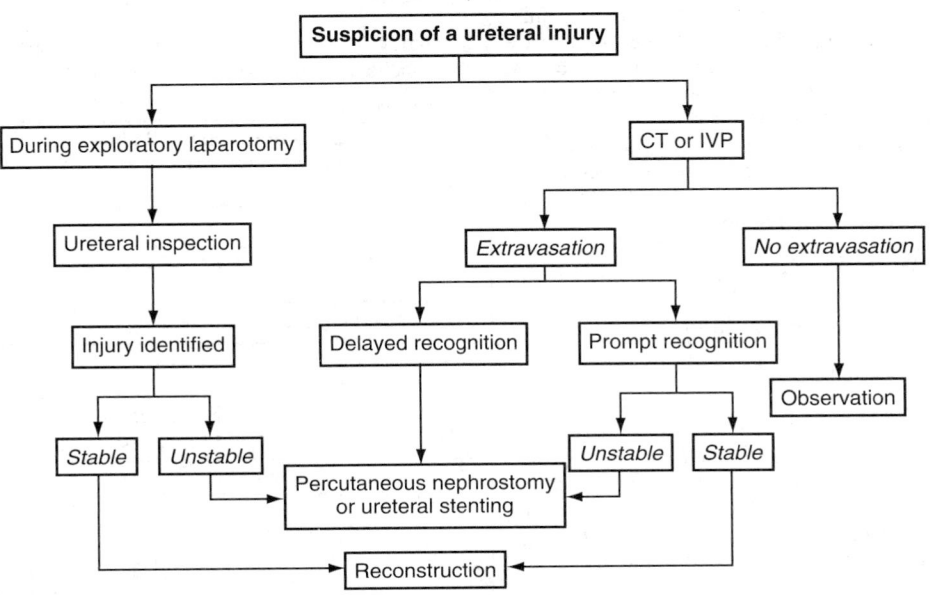

**FIGURE 4.** Algorithm for the diagnosis and management of ureteral trauma (abdominal or rapid deceleration injury). *Abbreviations:* CT = computed tomography; IVP = intravenous pyelogram.

Iatrogenic ureteral injuries are usually discovered more than 24 hours after the insult. Often they present with signs of acute infection from prolonged urinary extravasation or with incisional urinary leakage.

## MANAGEMENT

Selection of the appropriate management of a ureteral injury depends on the patient's condition, the site and extent of injury, and the time of diagnosis. Most patients with ureteral injuries from external trauma require prompt operative exploration for management of the associated abdominal injuries. Concomitant intra-abdominal organ or vascular injuries should not preclude ureteral reconstruction in a stable patient. Ureteral repair can be performed using a variety of reconstructive techniques, depending on the level and length of the injured segment. Regardless of the location, successful surgical repair includes the use of healthy ureteral segments (taking thermal effect into consideration) and a watertight, tension-free anastomosis. Injuries to the distal lower third of the ureter are best managed by bladder reimplantation. For injuries involving the entire lower third of the ureter, a psoas hitch can be used. However, in patients with insufficient bladder capacity or with severe pelvic scarring, a transureteroureterostomy can be fashioned. Injuries encompassing the lower half of the ureter are best managed with an anterior bladder wall (Boari-Ockerblad) flap. Short mid or upper ureteral defects can be bridged with a primary ureteroureterostomy. Complete ureteral avulsions are managed with an ileal interposition or renal autotransplantation.

Ureteral injuries in a patient in whom diagnosis was significantly delayed or in an unstable patient are best managed initially by percutaneous nephrostomy drainage or endoscopic ureteral stenting. Definitive repair can be scheduled electively, if necessary. Approximately 50% of iatrogenic ureteral injuries heal simply with temporary urinary diversion.

## OUTCOME

Early diagnosis and careful reconstruction of ureteral injuries are important in minimizing complications and preserving renal function. Complications are rare but include prolonged extravasation, infection, fistula formation, and stricture.

# Bladder Trauma

## ETIOLOGY

The bladder is second to the kidneys in frequency of injury, accounting for 20% to 25% of all genitourinary injuries. Bladder injuries are caused by either blunt or penetrating trauma to the lower abdomen, pelvis, or perineum. Blunt trauma is the more common mechanism, usually by a severe external force such as a motor vehicle accident, fall, or crush injury. Associated injuries include pelvic and long bone fractures as well as central nervous system and chest injuries. Factors that contribute to bladder rupture include pelvic fracture, bladder distention, and any previous pelvic surgery. The location of the bladder deep within the bony pelvis protects it from most penetrating trauma; however, the possibility of bladder trauma should be considered with any lower abdominal gunshot or stab wound.

Iatrogenic bladder injuries usually occur during transurethral or gynecologic procedures.

## DIAGNOSIS

A bladder injury should be suspected after any external lower abdominal or pelvic trauma. The patient usually complains of abdominal pain and distention and may be unable to urinate. Hemodynamic instability is common because of extensive blood loss in the pelvis. Physical examination should include carefully performed pelvic and rectal examinations.

Gross hematuria occurs in 95% of bladder ruptures from blunt injuries; the remainder have microscopic hematuria. With penetrating injuries, most patients present with microscopic hematuria. Urine is best obtained by urethral catheterization, which must be performed only after inspection of the urethral meatus. *Blood at the meatus is a contraindication to urethral catheterization* because this finding strongly suggests a urethral injury and requires confirmation by retrograde urethrography.

Cystography is the most accurate imaging test to diagnose a bladder injury. With conventional cystography, a plain film of the pelvis is first obtained and then 350 mL of water-soluble contrast material is infused through a catheter by gravity to distend the bladder; anteroposterior and drainage films should be taken. Alternatively, CT cystography can be used, provided the bladder is filled in a retrograde manner (via a transurethral catheter). In most cases, extravasation of contrast is not seen, and the injury is classified as a contusion. Such injuries result in damage to the mucosa or muscularis without loss of bladder wall continuity. With extravasation of contrast material, the distinction between an extraperitoneal and intraperitoneal bladder rupture must be made. Extraperitoneal bladder ruptures are more common. On cystography, these injuries are characterized by extravasation confined to the perivesical soft tissues. With intraperitoneal bladder ruptures, the contrast extravasates in the peritoneal cavity, outlining the bowel loops. Although cystography can accurately diagnose bladder injuries, the amount of contrast extravasated does not correlate with the extent of injury (Figure 5).

## MANAGEMENT

The choice of management depends on the overall status of the patient, the type of bladder injury sustained, and the extent of associated injuries. Bladder contusions can be treated by transurethral catheter drainage alone, which should be maintained until the hematuria completely resolves. Extraperitoneal bladder ruptures in patients who do not require laparotomy can also be managed nonoperatively, provided the urine is sterile at the time of injury and the existing hematuria does not obstruct catheter drainage. Usually the catheter can be removed after approximately 10 to 14 days after a repeat cystogram shows adequate healing. Extraperitoneal ruptures that involve the bladder neck or drain with difficulty should be surgically repaired. All intraperitoneal bladder ruptures require surgical exploration. This is accomplished through a midline infraumbilical incision, avoiding dissection of the pelvic hematoma. The peritoneum is opened and the abdominal viscera inspected; the bladder injury is then repaired from within the bladder lumen, and a transurethral catheter is maintained for 7 to 10 days.

## OUTCOME

Mortality in patients with bladder trauma approaches 20% and is due to the associated injuries rather than the bladder rupture. Short-term

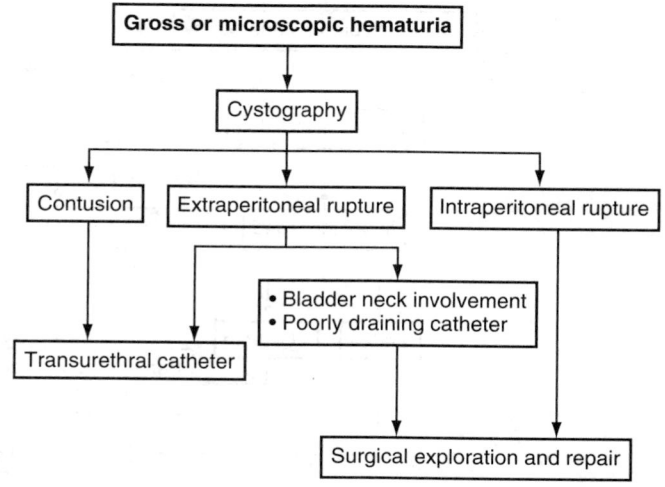

**FIGURE 5.** Algorithm for the diagnosis and management of bladder trauma (lower abdominal or pelvic injury).

complications of the bladder injury include persistent bleeding, urinary extravasation, and infection. Long-term complications are rare but can include fistula formation, urinary incontinence, and bladder instability.

# Genital Trauma in Males

## ETIOLOGY

Injuries to the male genitalia constitute 5% to 7% of all civilian genitourinary injuries. However, in some wartime series, they were the most common genitourinary injuries (60%). This high incidence was the result of the widespread use of ground-level explosives during combat.

Genital injuries include those occurring to the testes, scrotum, and penis. Most testicular injuries result from blunt trauma and are usually unilateral; penetrating testicular injuries from gunshot and stab wounds are less common. Similarly, scrotal trauma from gunshot or stab wounds occurs infrequently; most scrotal injuries occur as a consequence of burns or avulsions. Penile injuries have diverse mechanisms, including ruptures (usually occurring during sexual intercourse), amputations (usually self-inflicted or from entrapment of clothes by heavy machinery), and strangulations (usually from constricting penile rings used to enhance erections). Penetrating injuries (mostly gunshot wounds) can occur, although they usually cause little tissue destruction apart from the entrance and exit wounds.

## DIAGNOSIS

Accurate determination of the extent of a testicular injury by clinical means alone may be difficult; the diagnosis is enhanced by scrotal ultrasonography. A heterogeneous intratesticular echo pattern is the most common ultrasonographic finding of a testicular rupture. In addition, extruded testicular tissue or disruption of the tunica albuginea can be seen occasionally but is not a required sonographic criterion to confirm a rupture. Penile and scrotal injuries can be accurately diagnosed by visual inspection in conjunction with a thorough history. Any patient with trauma to the penis should undergo a retrograde urethrogram because the incidence of a concomitant urethral injury approaches 80%, depending on the mechanism of injury (Figure 6).

## MANAGEMENT

All penetrating testicular injuries and any blunt testicular injury suggestive of a rupture should be surgically explored. Attempts at testicular repair should be made, with orchiectomy limited to extensive unreconstructable injuries. Similarly, penile ruptures and penetrating injuries should be explored promptly and the defect repaired, sparing unnecessary débridement, which could further compromise valuable erectile tissue. Penile amputations should be managed by microsurgical reimplantation, provided the amputated segment is viable. The management of scrotal burns or avulsions requires surgical excision of all nonviable tissue and meticulous wound care. Techniques for delayed scrotal closure include split-thickness skin grafts, rotational thigh flaps, and tissue expanders.

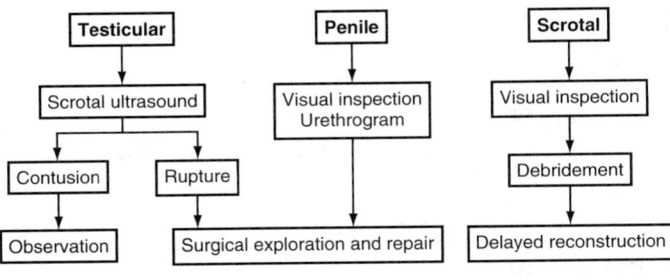

**FIGURE 6.** Algorithm for the diagnosis and management of genital trauma.

## OUTCOME

Genital injuries usually can be diagnosed easily and should be managed promptly. The goal is preservation of genital function and maintenance of cosmesis. Untoward sequelae can be minimized by limiting excessive débridement of penile and testicular tissues and instituting prompt aggressive local wound care with scrotal trauma. Complications of penile and testicular injuries include erectile and reproductive dysfunction, infection, tissue necrosis, and urethral stricture.

# Urethral Trauma

## ETIOLOGY

Urethral injuries compose approximately 7% to 10% of all genitourinary injuries. These injuries are anatomically subdivided into posterior and anterior injuries. In males, the posterior urethra is proximal and the anterior urethra distal to the external (striated) sphincter. Only the posterior urethra exists in females.

Injuries to the posterior urethra occur almost exclusively with pelvic fractures. Specifically, with a crush or deceleration-impact injury, the severe shearing forces necessary to fracture the pelvis are transmitted to the prostatomembranous junction, the weakest portion of the urethra. Overall, the male posterior urethra is injured in up to 10% of all pelvic fractures and the female urethra in up to 4% of all pelvic fractures.

In contrast to posterior urethral trauma, injuries to the anterior urethra are not associated with pelvic fractures. External anterior urethral injuries result from blunt or penetrating trauma. Blunt injuries are more common and are caused by vehicular accidents (often bicycles), falls (straddle-type injuries), and direct blows to the perineum or penis. Penetrating anterior urethral injuries, usually from gunshot wounds, are less frequent but often occur in conjunction with penetrating penile or testicular trauma.

Iatrogenic urethral injuries are by far the most frequent cause of urethral trauma. Examples include inadvertent Foley catheter balloon inflation in the urethra and traumatic lower urinary tract endoscopy (cystoscopy, transurethral surgery). These injuries are often minor and tend to be underreported.

## DIAGNOSIS

The diagnosis of urethral trauma should be suspected from the history. A pelvic fracture or any external penile or perineal injury can be suggestive of urethral trauma. In a conscious patient, a thorough voiding history should be obtained to establish the time and characteristics of the last urination. A urinalysis is an important laboratory adjunct.

The following clinical indicators of urethral trauma warrant a complete urethral evaluation:

1. *Blood at the urethral meatus.* This is the most consistent and accurate clinical indicator of urethral trauma. Its presence should preclude any attempts at urethral instrumentation until the entire urethra is adequately imaged.
2. *Blood at the vaginal introitus.* In female patients following pelvic fracture, this finding is highly suggestive of a urethral injury.
3. *Hematuria.* Although this finding is nonspecific, it is a reliable indicator of urethral trauma. All patients who are able to urinate after a urethral injury will have some degree of hematuria on a first-voided specimen.
4. *Pain on urination or inability to void.* Painful urination occurs after urethral trauma from edema or urinary extravasation. The inability to void suggests urethral disruption.
5. *High-riding prostate.* This may be palpated after a posterior urethral injury because of superior displacement of the prostate, but it is not a very reliable finding.

Assessment of concomitant rectal and genital injuries is mandatory in every case of external urethral trauma. All patients should have a rectal examination with stool Hemoccult testing. In addition, a complete pelvic examination should be performed on female patients.

Retrograde urethrography is the cardinal diagnostic procedure in male patients suspected of having sustained urethral trauma. This must be performed prior to any attempt at transurethral catheterization. Urethroscopy should not be used in the initial diagnosis of urethral trauma in males. In females, however, the short urethra precludes adequate imaging with retrograde urethrography, making urethroscopy the diagnostic modality for identification and staging of these injuries.

Urethral injuries are simplistically classified as follows:

1. *Contusion*, whereby the urethral mucosa remains intact
2. *Partial disruption*, with segmental maintenance of mucosal continuity
3. *Complete disruption* with separation of both urethral ends

The distinction is made by retrograde urethrography. Although any degree of urethral disruption will result in contrast extravasation, the absence of contrast material in the bladder suggests a complete disruption (Figure 7).

## MANAGEMENT

The goal of initial treatment of any urethral trauma is avoidance of any maneuver that can potentiate the injury. Only urethral contusions can be managed safely with transurethral catheterization. With a urethral disruption, the blind passage of a transurethral catheter should be avoided because this can extend the urethral tear, introduce infection, and disrupt a pelvic hematoma. Urinary diversion by means of a suprapubic cystostomy is the easiest and safest option for the initial management of any urethral disruption (partial or complete). After the patient has adequately recovered from the associated injuries and the urethral injury has stabilized, the urethra can be thoroughly evaluated radiographically and the appropriate reconstructive procedure planned when necessary. Immediate repair of the acutely traumatized urethra by means of endoscopic realignment or urethral suturing is technically more difficult than suprapubic cystostomy placement. In select cases, however, it may be successful in minimizing the need for subsequent extensive reconstructive surgery by limiting scar formation. Examples in which primary urethral repair may be considered include most penetrating urethral injuries (by suturing), urethral injuries associated with penile fractures (by suturing), and select partial posterior urethral disruptions (by realignment).

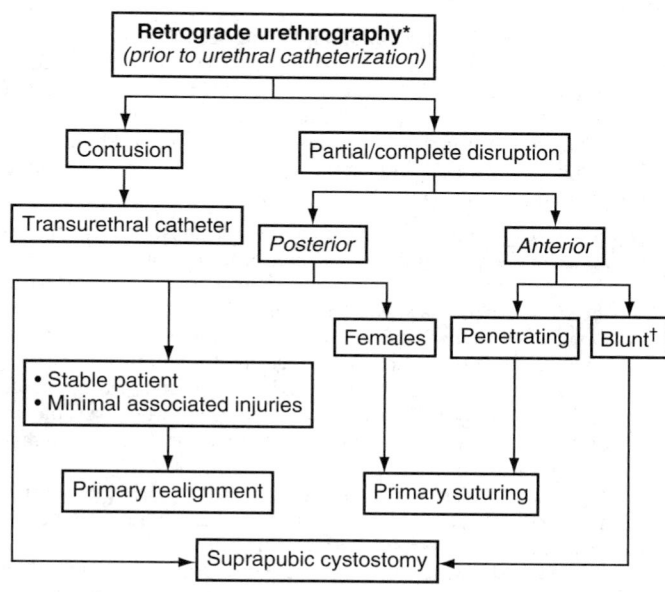

* In females only, proceed to urethroscopy.
† Except in association with penile fractures.

**FIGURE 7.** Algorithm for the diagnosis and management of urethral trauma (penile or perineal injury, pelvic fracture).

A urethral disruption in a female requires immediate surgical repair because any tear involving the short female urethra likely will extend to the bladder neck and disrupt the sphincteric mechanism. Prompt urethral and bladder neck reconstruction is necessary in order to limit posttraumatic incontinence.

## OUTCOME

Urethral injuries from external trauma are some of the most devastating and difficult genitourinary injuries. Major long-term complications, which include urinary incontinence, erectile dysfunction, stricture formation, and recurring infections, are often a result of the initial injury. Adhering to the principles outlined earlier can minimize additional complications.

## REFERENCES

Brandes S, Coburn M, Armenakas NA, McAninch JW: Diagnosis and management of ureteric injury: an evidence-based analysis. BJU Int 2004;94: 277-289.

Chapple C, Barbagli G, Jordan, G, et al: Consensus statement on urethral trauma. BJU Int 2004;93:1135-1202.

Gomez RG, Ceballos L, Coburn M, et al: Consensus statement on bladder injuries. BJU Int 2004;94:27-32.

Morey AF, Metro MJ, Carney KJ, et al: Consensus on genitourinary trauma: External genitalia. BJU Int 2004;94:507-515.

Santucci RA, Wessells H, Bartsch G, et al: Evaluation and management of renal injuries: Consensus statement of the renal trauma subcommittee. BJU Int 2004;93:937-954.

# Prostatitis

Method of
*Andrea Gallina, MD, and Pierre I. Karakiewicz, MD*

The clinical entity termed *prostatitis* affects 2% to 10% of men during their lifetime. Moreover, prostatitis symptoms are the most common cause for urologic consultation in men 50 years of age. The definition of prostatitis includes a large variety of clinical and nonclinical entities with a common underlying background. To standardize the diagnostics and the therapeutic approaches, the National Institutes of Health (NIH) proposed a classification system of prostatitis syndromes. It consists of four categories that reflect the wide variety of clinical manifestations of this syndrome (Box 1).

---

**BOX 1  National Institutes of Health Classification of Prostatitis**

**Category I**
- Acute bacterial prostatitis

**Category II**
- Chronic bacterial prostatitis

**Category III**
- Chronic nonbacterial prostatitis/chronic pelvic pain syndrome (CP/CPPS)
  - III A: Inflammatory CP/CPPS
  - III B: Noninflammatory CP/CPPS

**Category IV**
- Asymptomatic inflammatory prostatitis

# Category I: Acute Bacterial Prostatitis

Acute bacterial prostatitis affects 2% to 5% of prostatitis patients. It typically represents an ascending infection of the prostate with uropathogenic bacteria (*Escherichia coli*, *Klebsiella* spp., *Enterobacter* spp., *Serratia marcescens*, *Pseudomonas aeruginosa*). The classic presentation includes systemic (fever, chills and malaise) and local symptoms. Local symptoms consist of dysuria and perineal and prostatic pain, and they may be associated with complete or partial bladder outlet obstruction (urinary frequency, incomplete emptying, urgency, hesitancy, or retention). The onset may be sudden. The severity of systemic symptoms determines the need for hospitalization.

On history, recent urinary tract infections and urologic instrumentation (e.g., prostate biopsies, urinary catheters) should be ruled out. A gentle digital rectal examination (DRE) (to avoid local or systemic exacerbation of symptoms) assesses the extent of tenderness (acute infection), and rules out masses (abscess formation or associated prostatic or nonprostatic lesions). Postvoid residual is best assessed ultrasonically, because passage of catheters should be avoided. Presence of significant residual (>20% of voided volume) represents a relative indication for catheter drainage. Size 14 F or smaller catheters represent a valid alternative for suprapubic drainage. Urinalysis, midstream specimen for urine culture, and blood cultures (if systemic symptoms are present) complete the assessment.

Patients with systemic symptoms usually require hospitalization. Intravenous antibiotics (ampicillin and gentamicin) and hydration represent the mainstay of therapy. Ciprofloxacin and levofloxacin are alternatives if allergies or other contraindications exist. Once the patient is afebrile for 24 hours or according to blood culture results, oral fluoroquinolones or trimethoprim-sulfamethoxazole (TMP-SMX) may be initiated. Persistent fever and symptoms after 48 hours of IV antibiotic therapy can indicate an abscess formation, which may be identified with computed tomography (CT), magnetic resonance imaging (MRI), or transrectal ultrasonography. Antibiotic-refractory prostatic abscesses might require drainage with transurethral prostatic resection. Periprostatic abscesses may be drained transrectally.

Category I prostatitis represents a complicated urinary tract infection (UTI). Once symptoms have subsided and antibiotic therapy has been completed, a careful investigation of the upper and lower urinary tract is in order to identify any potentially predisposing causes. Imaging studies (ultrasound, CT, MRI), cystoscopy, and urodynamic studies can reveal an underlying cause, such as prostatic hypertrophy with urinary retention, bladder stone or diverticulum, or urethral stricture, among others.

# Category II: Chronic Bacterial Prostatitis

NIH category II prostatitis is defined as a chronic or persistent pathogenic infection (culture proven) of the prostate without systemic symptoms. It accounts for 2% to 5% of patients with prostatitis. It is characterized by intermittent episodes of cystitis-like urinary symptoms, which only rarely involve appreciable discomfort or pain. Recurrent infectious episodes are highly suggestive of chronic bacterial prostatitis, especially if the same pathogen is documented in either a midstream urine specimen or a postprostatic massage urine specimen. *E. coli* (which represents 80% of the infectious agents), *Klebsiella* species, *P. aeruginosa*, and *Proteus* species represent the most commonly seen pathogens.

History and physical and laboratory examinations are virtually the same as those for category I prostatitis. The more protruded nature of category II prostatitis requires 4 to 8 weeks of antimicrobials (fluoroquinolones or TMP-SMX). This therapy is effective in 60% to 80% of patients. However, in cases of recurrent infections, long-term (3-6 months) antibiotic therapy is an alternative treatment. Other modalities have been investigated (for example intraprostatic injection of antibiotics) but have met with limited success.

# Category III: Chronic Nonbacterial Prostatitis/Chronic Pelvic Pain Syndrome

Category III prostatitis (CP/CPPS) accounts for 90% to 95% of prostatitis cases and is the most challenging subgroup. Symptoms include pelvic or perineal (or both) pain or discomfort, as well as urinary or ejaculatory symptoms. Pain may be perineal, suprapubic, coccygeal, rectal, urethral, or testicular or scrotal. Urinary frequency, dysuria, urgency, or incomplete emptying and ejaculatory pain affect a significant proportion of patients. Ejaculatory pain suggests worse prognosis. Presence or absence of inflammatory cells in the ejaculate distinguishes between category IIIA (inflammatory) and category IIIB (noninflammatory) prostatitis. However, the clinical presentation and therapeutic approaches are the same for these two groups, and the reliability of this distinction is suboptimal. Only in up to 5% of patients is a pathogen successfully isolated from urine or semen.

The clinical heterogeneity of category III prostatitis and the absence of a diagnostic marker add complexity to the classification and treatment of this syndrome. A multifactorial etiology, which includes infectious, traumatic, inflammatory, hormonal, neurologic, and psychological triggers, is the most likely cause.

## DIAGNOSIS

The evaluation of patients with category III prostatitis should include a detailed history (focusing on previous infections, trauma, surgery, or neurologic problems). It should be complemented with the NIH Chronic Prostatitis Symptom Index (NIH-CPSI) questionnaire, which is a standardized assessment of the type and severity of symptoms. Physical examination should include the same elements as in categories I and II prostatitis. Urine analysis and midstream culture

## CURRENT DIAGNOSIS

**Category I (Acute Bacterial Prostatitis)**

- History
- Physical examination (including gentle DRE)
- Urinalysis
- Urine culture
- Blood cultures (if systemic symptoms are present)
- Postvoid residual

**Category II (Chronic Bacterial Prostatitis)**

- History
- Physical examination
- Urinalysis
- Urine culture
- Postprostatic massage urine culture
- Evaluation of complicated UTI (optional)

**Category III (Chronic Pelvic Pain Syndrome)**

- History
- Physical examination
- NIH-Chronic Prostatitis Symptom Index (NIH-CPSI) questionnaire
- Urinalysis
- Midstream culture
- Optional tests (cytology, urine flow, postvoid residual, etc)

**Category IV (Asymptomatic Inflammatory Prostatitis)**

- No further evaluation

*Abbreviations:* DRE = digital rectal examination; NIH = National Institutes of Health; UTI = urinary tract infection.

are mandatory. Urinary cytology is recommended to rule out irritative symptoms of bladder cancer. Urine flow rate and residual urine determination can also help in the diagnostic work-up. In rare instances, abdominal, pelvic, or neurologic imaging, urodynamic studies, cystoscopy, or prostate-specific antigen testing may be useful.

In most men, the disease has a protracted natural history. Symptom severity predicts recurrence in 30% of men, and previous symptoms predict recurrence in 50% of men. Unfortunately, in most category III prostatitis patients, the cause of pelvic pain cannot be identified. Thus, the diagnosis of CP/CPPS remains a diagnosis of exclusion.

## TREATMENT

Several treatments have been investigated and studied for category III prostatitis, with mixed results (Figure 1). These include α-blockers, antibiotics, nonsteroidal anti-inflammatory drugs (NSAIDs), and pentosan polysulfate, among others.

Mehik's group tested the efficacy of an α-blocker, alfuzosin (Uroxatral)[1] 5 mg, against placebo for symptom relief in 70 patients. At 6 months, the pain score was lower in the alfuzosin group ($P = 0.02$). Similar results were obtained by Cheah and colleagues in a cohort of 86 patients treated with terazosin (Hytrin),[1] with dose escalation from 1 to 5 mg/day compared with placebo. The α-blocker significantly improved the quality of life and significantly reduced pain at 14 weeks ($P = 0.03$). Nickel and colleagues randomized 58 men younger than 55 years to 0.4 mg tamsulosin (Flomax)[1] or placebo. At 45 days, tamsulosin significantly reduced symptoms. However, these benefits were not always replicated, especially in pretreated men.

A 4- to 6-week trial of antibiotics is one of the key management options for patients with category III prostatitis, despite absence of benefit in placebo-controlled trials. Lack of efficacy at 6 and 12 weeks was shown by Nickel's group, who randomized 80 patients with category III prostatitis to either levofloxacin or placebo for 6 weeks. Alexander's group recapitulated these findings with ciprofloxacin.

NSAIDs were tested in a placebo-controlled trial of 161 patients. Rofecoxib (Vioxx) (50 mg) significantly improved pain and NIH-CPSI scores. It has been withdrawn from the market.

Pentosan polysulfate (Elmiron)[1] was tested in a placebo-controlled, randomized trial of 100 men. Three daily 100-mg doses of Elmiron for 16 weeks resulted in a significant improvement in NIH-CPSI quality-of-life scores.

Several other therapeutic approaches are available. These include prostatic massage, which should be considered once or twice weekly, in men who report some degree of symptom relief. Finasteride (Proscar)[1] 5 mg daily and phytotherapy (e.g., cernilton[7] and quercetin[7]) showed some, albeit limited, efficacy. Tricyclic antidepressants (amitriptyline [Elavil][1]), anticholinergics (oxybutynin [Ditropan][1]), anticonvulsants, lifestyle changes (e.g., nutrition, stress reduction), biofeedback, pelvic

[1]Not FDA approved for this indication.
[7]Available as dietary supplements.

## CURRENT THERAPY

**Category I (Acute Bacterial Prostatitis)**

- Admission
- Intravenous antibiotics (ampicillin or gentamicin)
- Bladder drainage, if urinary retention
- Oral antibiotics for 3 to 4 weeks (fluoroquinolones or TMP-SMX)

**Category II (Chronic Bacterial Prostatitis)**

- Outpatient treatment
- Antibiotics for 4 to 8 weeks (fluoroquinolones or TMP-SMX)
- Long-term antibiotic therapy

**Category III (Chronic Pelvic Pain Syndrome)**

- Antibiotics for 4 to 6 weeks (fluoroquinolone or TMP-SMX)
- α-Blockers (e.g., tamsulosin [Flomax],[1] alfuzosin [Uroxatral],[1] terazosin [Hytrin][1])
- Anti-inflammatory medications
- Finasteride (Proscar),[1] pentosan polysulfate (Elmiron),[1] and phytotherapies (e.g., cernilton,[7] quercetin[7])
- Nonpharmacologic therapies (biofeedback, pelvic floor training, thermal treatments)
- Repeat treatment if relief is noted.
- Combine therapies if partial relief is noted.

**Category IV (Asymptomatic Inflammatory Prostatitis)**

- No treatments

[1]Not FDA approved for this indication.
[7]Available as dietary supplements.
*Abbreviation:* TMP-SMX = trimethoprim-sulfamethoxazole.

floor training, and thermal therapy reduced symptoms in some category III prostatitis patients. The multitude of trials addressing CP/CPPS patients emphasizes the high failure rate (~66%) of sequential monotherapy. It suggests the need for structured assessment of multimodality approaches.

## Category IV: Asymptomatic Inflammatory Prostatitis

Category IV prostatitis is defined as incidental observation of leukocytes in prostatic secretions or tissue obtained during evaluation for

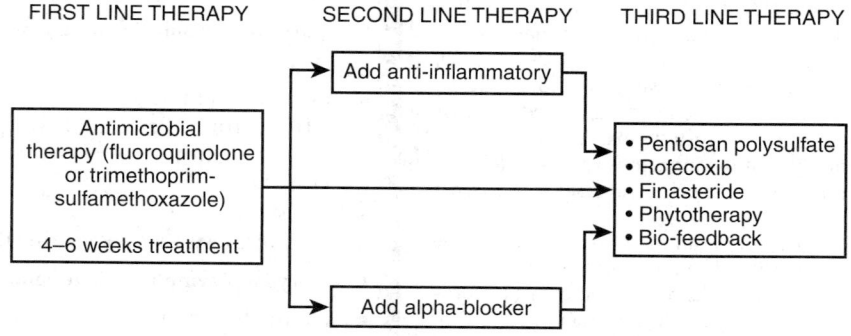

FIRST LINE THERAPY    SECOND LINE THERAPY    THIRD LINE THERAPY

Add anti-inflammatory

Antimicrobial therapy (fluoroquinolone or trimethoprim-sulfamethoxazole)

4–6 weeks treatment

- Pentosan polysulfate
- Rofecoxib
- Finasteride
- Phytotherapy
- Bio-feedback

Add alpha-blocker

**FIGURE 1.** Management of NIH category III prostatitis.

other disorders, (e.g., leukocytes noted in prostate biopsies performed for elevated prostate-specific antigen [PSA]). Epidemiologic studies estimate the prevalence of category IV prostatitis to be as high as 32.2% in a population of men with elevated PSA levels. Category IV prostatitis needs no further evaluation or treatment.

## Acknowledgments

Pierre I. Karakiewicz is partially supported by the Fonds de la Recherche en Santé du Québec, the Centre hospitalier de l'Université de Montréal (CHUM) Foundation, the Department of Surgery, and Les Urologues Associés du CHUM.

## REFERENCES

Clemens JQ, Meenan RT, O'Keeffe-Rosetti MC, et al: Prevalence of prostatitis-like symptoms in a managed care population. J Urol 2006;176(2):593-596.

Dimitrakov JD, Kaplan SA, Kroenke K, et al: Management of chronic prostatitis/chronic pelvic pain syndrome: an evidence-based approach. Urology 2006;67(5):881-888.

Fowler JE Jr: Antimicrobial therapy for bacterial and nonbacterial prostatitis. Urology 2002;60(6 Suppl):24-26.

Habermacher GM, Chason JT, Schaeffer AJ: Prostatitis/chronic pelvic pain syndrome. Annu Rev Med 2006;57:195-206.

Krieger JN, Egan KJ, Ross SO, et al: Chronic pelvic pains represent the most prominent urogenital symptoms of "chronic prostatitis." Urology 1996;48(5):715-721.

Krieger JN, Nyberg L Jr, Nickel JC: NIH consensus definition and classification of prostatitis. JAMA 1999;282(3):236-237.

Krieger JN, Ross SO, Riley DE: Chronic prostatitis: Epidemiology and role of infection. Urology 2002;60(6 Suppl):8-12.

Litwin MS, McNaughton-Collins M, Fowler FJ Jr, et al: The National Institutes of Health chronic prostatitis symptom index: Development and validation of a new outcome measure. Chronic Prostatitis Collaborative Research Network. J Urol 1999;162(2):369-375.

Pontari MA, Ruggieri MR. Mechanisms in prostatitis/chronic pelvic pain syndrome. J Urol 2004;172(3):839-845.

Rothman I, Stanford JL, Kuniyuki A, Berger RE: Self-report of prostatitis and its risk factors in a random sample of middle-aged men. Urology 2004;64(5):876-879.

Schaeffer AJ, Datta NS, Fowler JE Jr, et al: Overview summary statement: Diagnosis and management of chronic prostatitis/chronic pelvic pain syndrome (CP/CPPS). Urology 2002;60(6 Suppl):1-4.

Wagenlehner FM, Weidner W, Sorgel F, Naber KG. The role of antibiotics in chronic bacterial prostatitis. Int J Antimicrob Agents 2005;26(1):1-7.

# Benign Prostatic Hyperplasia

Method of
*Gopal H. Badlani, MD,*
*and Matthew E. Karlovsky, MD*

## Epidemiology

Bladder outlet obstruction (BOO) secondary to benign prostatic hyperplasia (BPH) is one of the most common medical conditions in older men and represents up to a 40% clinical risk for urinary retention in a man's lifetime. It is the most prevalent condition in the aging male, affecting 14 million men in the United States, with an annual cost of $4 billion to treat. Age and normal androgenic function are two of the better established risk factors. Whereas BPH is rare before the age of 40, the prevalence of histologic BPH at autopsy is 50% by 60 years of age and 90% by 85 years of age. Approximately 40% of males 70 years of age or older have lower urinary tract symptoms (LUTS) secondary to BPH, and with age, the prevalence increases. Symptomatically, approximately 25% of 55-year-old men experience

decreased urinary flow rate and other symptoms of BPH. By 75 years of age, the appearance of this symptom increases to 50%. Age, however, is not a causative factor of BOO. Although the risk for developing symptoms from BPH doubles for each decade of life between 60 and 90 years of age, clinical symptoms of the individual patient do not necessarily progress with age. BPH is more commonly diagnosed because of increased life expectancy and a greater tendency today to seek medical advice at an earlier disease stage.

Normal androgenic function is required for development of BPH. Both androgenic and estrogenic hormonal stimulation can induce prostatic hypertrophy. Other factors, such as race, sexual activity, smoking, socioeconomic status, vasectomy, alcohol intake, and diet, have been implicated in BPH development. Identifying men at clinical risk for BPH and its progression has clinical usefulness in selecting the appropriate intervention when necessary.

## Pathophysiology

The pathophysiology of BPH is poorly understood because no direct correlation can be made between prostatic glandular enlargement and the symptomatology of BPH. Because the condition is rare in those younger than 40 years of age and does not develop in castrated men, it is accepted that BPH development requires aging and functional testes for androgen production. BPH is believed to originate in the transitional zone of the prostate, which surrounds the prostatic urethra between the bladder neck and the verumontanum, and is progressive.

Both a static and a dynamic component are involved in BPH development. The static component relates to epithelial and stromal cell proliferation in the prostatic transitional zone (TZ); enlargement is evident as median or lateral lobe hypertrophy. Proliferation is induced by testosterone and its biologically active conversion product, dihydrotestosterone. Conversion of testosterone to dihydrotestosterone occurs via the enzyme $5\alpha$-reductase. Two forms of this enzyme have been described, type 1 and type 2. Type 1 is present in liver, skin, and other organs. Type 2 is present in urogenital tissues. Individuals lacking $5\alpha$-reductase type 2 do not develop genitalia and prostates.

Conversely, the dynamic component relates to prostatic smooth muscle. High concentrations of $\alpha_1$-adrenergic receptors occur in the prostatic capsule and bladder neck. An increase in smooth muscle tone is responsible for increased urethral resistance and pressure. Pharmacologic blockade with $\alpha_1$ antagonists blocks prostatic smooth muscle contraction and decreases urethral resistance and pressure, subsequently relaxing the dynamic component of BPH.

## Symptoms

The diagnosis of BPH is presumptive, based on symptoms. These symptoms, commonly referred to as lower urinary tract symptoms (LUTS), are not specific for BPH. LUTS include frequency, retention, intermittency, decreased force of stream (FOS), straining, urgency, and nocturia. Individuals with LUTS should be carefully assessed to determine the cause, to confirm diagnosis of BPH, and to exclude other bladder and prostate processes. Normal prostate size on digital rectal examination (DRE) does not rule out a diagnosis of BPH because palpable prostate size does not correlate with degree of obstruction or severity of LUTS. However, the odds of having moderate to severe symptoms are five times higher for men with enlarged prostates compared with those with normal prostates. Symptoms of BPH are difficult to assess and quantify, yet they are the keys to proper diagnosis and treatment. Because the vast majority of procedures performed for BPH are to provide symptomatic relief, it is necessary to quantify the level of interference in the quality of life of the patient. Assessment of interference on quality of life can be reliably accomplished using the well-validated International Prostate Symptom Score (IPSS) (Figure 1). Symptoms based on overall score are classified as mild (0 to 7), moderate (8 to 19), and severe (20 to 35). The subjective impact of these symptoms on overall quality of life must also be taken into account. The patient with a severe-range IPSS may feel the symptoms are less bothersome than a patient with a lower IPSS, and this subjective impact on quality of life can direct therapeutic options.

Name:                                    Date:

| | Not at all | Less than 1 time in 5 | Less than half the time | About half the time | More than half the time | Almost always | Your score |
|---|---|---|---|---|---|---|---|
| **Incomplete emptying**<br>Over the past month, how often have you had a sensation of not emptying your bladder completely after you finish urinating? | 0 | 1 | 2 | 3 | 4 | 5 | |
| **Frequency**<br>Over the past month, how often have you had to urinate again less than two hours after you finished urinating? | 0 | 1 | 2 | 3 | 4 | 5 | |
| **Intermittency**<br>Over the past month, how often have you found you stopped and started again several times when you urinated? | 0 | 1 | 2 | 3 | 4 | 5 | |
| **Urgency**<br>Over the past month, how difficult have you found it to postpone urination? | 0 | 1 | 2 | 3 | 4 | 5 | |
| **Weak stream**<br>Over the past month, how often have you had a weak urinary stream? | 0 | 1 | 2 | 3 | 4 | 5 | |
| **Straining**<br>Over the past month, how often have you had to push or strain to begin urination? | 0 | 1 | 2 | 3 | 4 | 5 | |

| | None | 1 time | 2 times | 3 times | 4 times | 5 times or more | Your score |
|---|---|---|---|---|---|---|---|
| **Nocturia**<br>Over the past month, how many times did you most typically get up to urinate from the time you went to bed until the time you got up in the morning? | 0 | 1 | 2 | 3 | 4 | 5 | |

| **Total IPSS score** | |
|---|---|

| **Quality of life due to urinary symptoms** | Delighted | Pleased | Mostly satisfied | Mixed— about equally satisfied and dissatisfied | Mostly dissatisfied | Unhappy | Terrible |
|---|---|---|---|---|---|---|---|
| If you were to spend the rest of your life with your urinary condition the way it is now, how would you feel about that? | 0 | 1 | 2 | 3 | 4 | 5 | 6 |

**FIGURE 1.** International prostate symptom score (IPSS).

# Diagnosis

Diagnosis of BPH relies on an accurate medical history eliciting the specific voiding complaints, as well as quantification of these symptoms using the IPSS. Other possible causes of LUTS also must be ruled out, including urinary tract infection (UTI), urolithiasis, diabetes, urethral stricture, overactive or neurogenic bladder, prostate/bladder cancer, or congestive heart failure. Medications that can exacerbate obstructive symptoms include tricyclic antidepressants, anticholinergic agents, diuretics, narcotics, and first-generation antihistamines and decongestants. Physical examination should include DRE for prostatic abnormalities, such as palpable nodules, induration or irregularities of malignancy, or infection. On DRE, the posterior lobes, not the transition zone, are palpable. Abdominal examination may detect a suprapubic or low abdominal mass in a patient with BPH-induced retention.

The American Urological Association and the American Cancer Society recommend all men older than age 50 receive an annual prostate-specific antigen (PSA) serum level to screen for prostate cancer. In black men or men with a family history of prostate cancer in a first-degree relative, PSA screening should begin at 40 years of age or younger. The normal range for PSA is up to 4.0 µg/mL. Other valuable laboratory data include urinalysis to rule out infection or hematuria, a serum creatinine level to determine renal function, and urine cytologic studies if irritative voiding symptoms are present. More sophisticated studies, such as urinary flow rate, postvoid residual, and pressure flow urodynamic studies, are appropriate for evaluation of men with more severe symptoms (IPSS >8) or with more complex comorbidities. These tests are often used to determine baseline function prior to initiation of therapy or to determine subsequent response to therapy. In patients who fail medical therapy, urodynamic pressure-flow studies and cystoscopy may be appropriate to evaluate the need for operative intervention and to rule out other urologic pathologies. Cystoscopy is also reserved for situations in which invasive treatment is strongly considered. If watchful waiting or noninvasive therapies are appropriate, invasive diagnostic tests are usually not necessary. The variables of importance of disease progression in an artificial neural network analysis were PSA, obstructive symptom score, and transitional zone volume. The Olmsted County study showed risk progression of acute urinary retention (AUR) with age. Overall, a 60-year-old man has a 23% chance of AUR if he survives the next 20 years. The average annual change in prostate volume was 1.6% for all ages. The annual increase was not significantly related to baseline age but was significantly related to baseline prostate volume.

## Treatment

### WATCHFUL WAITING

Indications for treatment of BPH rely, in large part, on the subjective nature of the symptoms. For the majority of patients with BPH, symptoms are not severe or bothersome enough to warrant long-term medical or surgical intervention. Men with an IPSS of less than 8 are usually treated with expectant management. Advising the patient toward lifestyle modifications, such as minimizing evening fluid intake, avoiding caffeine, and avoiding decongestants, anticholinergics, and other medications that impair voiding, often provides an effective resolution of symptoms. In a study of 556 men with moderate symptoms of BPH comparing outcomes following transurethral resection of the prostate (TURP) with watchful waiting for more than 3 years, 8% of men randomized to TURP and 17% of men with watchful waiting failed treatment. Treatment failure with watchful waiting was mostly because of high postvoid residuals and significant increases in IPSS symptoms. Patients who respond poorly to watchful waiting have multiple medical and surgical options for treatment of BPH.

### $\alpha_1$-ADRENERGIC BLOCKING AGENTS

The $\alpha_1$-adrenergic antagonists have been shown in numerous randomized placebo-controlled trials to be safe and effective in the treatment of BPH. The most commonly prescribed $\alpha_1$-adrenergic blockers appear to have similar safety profiles and clinical efficacy and are the common first approach for urologists. Terazosin (Hytrin) and doxazosin (Cardura) were the first $\alpha$ antagonists available for treatment of BPH; however, orthostatic hypotension was a significant concern, requiring careful dose titration. Tamsulosin (Flomax), a highly selective $\alpha$-blocker, does not induce orthostatic hypotension and so does not require dose titration. Overall, the most common side effects include headaches, dizziness, asthenia, and drowsiness. Sexual side effects are limited to retrograde ejaculation. Alfuzosin (Uroxatral), a newer nonspecific $\alpha$-blocker, has minimal vasoactive or retrograde ejaculation side effects. Table 1 provides a list for medication dosing and schedules.

### 5$\alpha$-REDUCTASE INHIBITION

Finasteride (Proscar) and dutasteride (Avodart) are 5$\alpha$-reductase inhibitors (type 1 and type 1/2, respectively) that block conversion of testosterone to dihydrotestosterone, the androgen involved in development of BPH. These medications represent the paradigm for androgen suppression of BPH. They have their greatest therapeutic effect in men with prostates greater than 40 g, and treatment for 6 months or more is usually required for a clinical response. The first randomized, multicenter, double-blind, placebo-controlled trial investigating the efficacy of finasteride demonstrated significant improvements in maximum flow rate and decreased prostatic volume. Since then, further studies have confirmed a reduced risk of acute urinary retention and surgical intervention with finasteride use. Finasteride can reduce BPH-associated hematuria. It is effective as adjuvant therapy, following other treatments, and as neoadjuvant therapy prior to minimally invasive therapy. Adverse effects include decreased libido, ejaculatory dysfunction, and gynecomastia. In the patient being monitored for prostate cancer with PSA testing, finasteride therapy must be taken into account when interpreting PSA values; finasteride decreases PSA values by 50%, leading to a false-negative result.

## Efficacy of Medical Therapy

The Medical Therapy of Prostate Symptoms (MTOPS) study evaluated the efficacy of doxazosin and finasteride to determine if medical therapy delays or prevents disease progression. At 4 years, combination therapy was most effective for reducing risk of clinical progression (AUR) and improving symptom score and urinary flow rate. Finasteride and combination therapy significantly reduced the risk of AUR and invasive therapy over 4 years. Monotherapy with either medication reduced symptom score and improved flow significantly, but to a lesser degree than combination therapy. Doxazosin delayed time to progression of AUR and invasive therapy but not the risk. Without treatment, the risk of BPH progression was 20% more during the trial. Risk factors for progression include baseline prostate volume (>40 g) and higher serum PSA value (>2 μg/mL).

## Phytotherapy

Saw palmetto (*Serenoa repens*)[1,2] extract is the most popular phytotherapeutic agent. Its likely mechanism is inhibition of 5$\alpha$-reductase. A recent meta-analysis of numerous randomized trials using saw palmetto described a mild to moderate improvement in flow and LUTS; however, because of small study sample, varying products, short treatment times, and varying outcomes, these study conclusions are difficult to interpret. Other popular preparations are African plum (*Pygeum africanum*)[1,2] and South African star grass (*Cynodon nlemfuënsis*).[1,2] The former has been shown to have several in vitro effects, such as antiestrogen effects, leukotriene blockade, and inhibition of fibroblast growth factors. The latter has been shown in vitro to increase plasminogen activators, as well as to stimulate release of transforming growth factor-β, an inducer of apoptosis, yet these in vitro effects have not been shown to occur in vivo. A meta-analysis of four clinical trials of South African star grass extract, β-sitosterol, concluded that β-sitosterol improved urologic symptoms and flow rates in men.

[1]Not FDA approved for this indication.
[2]Available as a dietary supplement.

---

**TABLE 1** Common Medications for Benign Prostatic Hyperplasia

| Medication | Class | Dose | Schedule |
| --- | --- | --- | --- |
| Alfuzosin (Uroxatral) | α-1 Blocker | 10 mg | Once daily |
| Doxazosin (Cardura) | α-1 Blocker | 1-8 mg, titrated | Once daily at bedtime |
| Tamsulosin (Flomax) | α-1a Blocker | 0.4 mg | Once daily |
| Terazosin (Hytrin) | α-1 Blocker | 1-10 mg, titrated | Once daily at bedtime |
| Dutasteride (Avodart) | 5-α Reductase inhibitor | 0.5 mg | Once daily |
| Finasteride (Proscar) | 5-α Reductase inhibitor | 5 mg | Once daily |

There is no standard of care for management of patients using phytotherapy. Nor have the long-term safety effects been established. Patients should be cautioned that doses, efficacy, side effects, and drug interactions with phytotherapy are unknown. For the patient refusing medical therapy of α-blockers and 5α-reductase inhibitors, phytotherapy may be attempted as long as the patient understands the limitations of these agents. If retention, UTI, calculi, or decreased renal function occurs, phytotherapy should be discouraged and more aggressive medical and surgical management undertaken.

## Minimally Invasive Therapies

The most commonly employed surgical procedure, and the gold standard for BPH, is transurethral resection of the prostate (TURP), involving endoscopic resection of the obstructive component of the prostate. TURP is highly effective, improving symptoms in up to 95% of patients. Common complications include inability to void postoperatively, clot retention, incontinence, impotence, and retrograde ejaculation. A number of new minimally invasive therapies have been developed to reduce the complications associated with TURP, as well as provide alternatives for the unfavorable surgical candidate. Most minimally invasive therapies use energy, such as radio waves, laser, ultrasound, microwaves, or electrical current.

Transurethral incision of the prostate (TUIP) involves endoscopic placement of one to two incisions into the prostate and capsule to reduce urethral constriction. This procedure is highly effective on prostate glands less than 30 g and is well documented and safe, with efficacy comparable with TURP. TUIP is associated with a 78% to 83% improvement of symptoms. Because TUIP is associated with fewer retrograde ejaculations, less morbidity, and a reoperation rate of less than 1% in 10 years, this procedure is the treatment of choice for small gland BPH in men concerned with fertility and ejaculation.

In transurethral needle ablation (TUNA), low-level energy is transferred by radiofrequency to the prostate, creating a well-defined necrotic lesion within the prostatic parenchyma while preserving the urethral mucosa. A cystoscope-like instrument with two needles set at 90 degrees from each other ablates tissue in 3 to 5 minutes when needles reach temperatures of 27° to 38°C (80° to 100°F). Urethral and rectal temperatures are also vigorously monitored as the device adjusts. Preliminary studies show an increase in peak flow and a decrease in symptom score following TUNA, with no major complications. Transient urinary retention is reported in 10% to 40% of patients. In a prospective study, TURP was superior to TUNA in increasing flow rates but demonstrated comparable improved symptoms at 1 year postoperatively. Transurethral microwave thermotherapy (TUMT) heats prostatic transitional zone tissue to between 60° and 80°C (140° to 176°F), inducing tissue damage. Thermotherapy preferentially destroys smooth muscle by coagulative necrosis while water-conductive cooling of the urethral mucosa preserves periurethral tissues. Although prospective studies indicate that TURP produces more pronounced urinary improvements versus TUMT, thermotherapy consistently improves symptom scores by 75% and increases peak flow rates by 75%. Furthermore, TUMT is a procedure done under local anesthesia. Retrograde ejaculation and urinary retention with prolonged catheterization occurs in greater than one third of patients.

Ultimately, therapeutic decisions depend in large part on symptom scores. Men with low symptom scores without bother are appropriately managed through watchful waiting. As scores increase, or if progression with clinical morbidity develops, more aggressive management is appropriate.

## REFERENCES

Bhargava S, Canda AE, Chapple CR: A rational approach to benign hyperplasia evaluation: Recent advances. Curr Opin Urol 2004;14:1-6.

Djavan B, Waldert M, Ghawidel C, Marberger M: Benign prostatic hyperplasia progression and its impact on treatment. Curr Opin Urol 2004;14:45-50.

Fong YK, Milani S, Djavan B: Role of phytotherapy in men with lower urinary tract symptoms. Curr Opin Urol 2005;15:45-48.

Hoffman RM, MacDonald R, Monga M, Wilt TJ: Transurethral microwave thermotherapy vs. transurethral resection for treating benign prostatic hyperplasia: A systematic review. BJU Int 2004;94:1031-1036.

Walsh PC, Retik A, Vaughan D (eds): Campbell's Urology, 8th ed. Philadelphia, Saunders Elsevier Science, 2002.

# Erectile Dysfunction

Method of
*Luciano Kolodny, MD*

The term *erectile dysfunction* (ED) is relatively new, having replaced *impotence* approximately a decade ago. ED is defined as the "inability of the male to attain or maintain an erection sufficient for satisfactory sexual intercourse." ED affects millions of men worldwide with implications that go far beyond sexual activity alone. ED is now recognized as a sentinel event in cardiovascular disease, diabetes mellitus (DM), and depression. It can also be damaging to interpersonal relationships and self-esteem.

## Epidemiology

The Massachusetts Male Aging Study is one of the pivotal studies on the prevalence of ED. Between 1987 and 1989, men between the ages of 40 and 70 years received questionnaires inquiring about several aspects of their sexual health. Of the 1790 men who received the questionnaires, 1290 responded. They revealed that 52% of them had some degree of dysfunction, 17% with minimal, 25% with moderate, and almost 10% with complete absence of erectile function. It also showed the extremely detrimental link between coronary artery disease (CAD), DM, and ED. A few years later another group used the same patient database and followed up on these subjects. The risk of ED was 26 cases per 1000 men annually, which increased with age, lower education, DM, heart disease, and hypertension.

## Physiology of Erection

The penile erection requires intact vascular, neuronal, and hormonal systems. The intricate details of this process are beyond the scope of this article, but in summary, after any sensorial stimulation, which can be visual, tactile, auditory, or olfactory, nitric oxide (NO) and other neurotransmitters are released at the cavernous nerve terminals. The endothelial cells then release vasoactive relaxing factors, which lead to vasodilatation of the penile blood vessels and increased blood flow. As blood flow increases, compression of the subtunical venular plexuses will substantially decrease venous outflow and finally cause the penis to change from flaccid to erect (Figure 1).

NO is the principal neurotransmitter involved in penile erection, but other vasoactive substances such as vasoactive intestinal peptide, neuropeptide Y, calcitonin gene-related peptide (CGRP), substance P, and serotonin also play roles. High levels of intrapenile NO facilitate the relaxation of intracavernosal trabeculae, thereby maximizing blood flow and penile erection. Nonadrenergic, noncholinergic neurons have been found to release NO, leading to increased production of cyclic guanosine monophosphate (cGMP). Through a series of reactions, cGMP will lead to relaxation of the smooth muscle, directly impacting the ability to go from a flaccid to an erect penile state. The return from erect to flaccid requires the hydrolysis of cGMP to guanosine monophosphate (GMP) by phosphodiesterase 5 (PDE5) (see Figure 1).

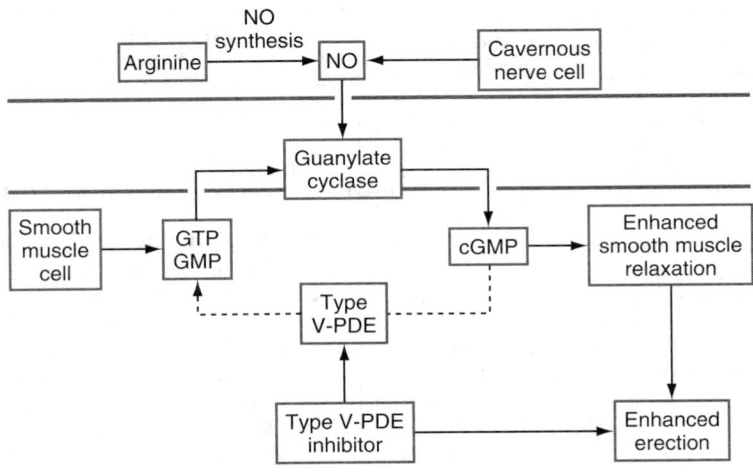

**FIGURE 1.** The biochemical process involved in erections and the mechanism of action of sildenafil citrate (Viagra). The cavernous nerves (S2-S4) innervate the penis and release NO. NO stimulates the production of cGMP in the smooth muscle cells of the penis. cGMP is directly responsible for increasing smooth muscle relaxation, which leads to increased arterial inflow and an erection. When cGMP is metabolized by PDE5, the penis undergoes detumescence. Sildenafil citrate (Viagra) inhibits PDE5 and increases the available cGMP, thereby leading to an enhanced erection. cGMP = cyclic guanosine monophosphate; NO = nitric oxide; PDE5 = phosphodiesterase 5.

## Testosterone and Erectile Function

Testosterone provides intrapenile nitrous oxide synthase (NOS), which has an important role in enhancing the production of NO, subsequent local vasodilatation, and penile erection. There is no correlation between serum testosterone levels and the degree of ED. However, hypogonadal men may experience significantly reduced libido. Hypogonadism is associated with decreased self-esteem, depression, osteoporosis, insulin resistance, increased fat mass, decreased lean body mass, and cognitive dysfunction.

## Pathophysiology of Erectile Dysfunction

ED can be classified as psychogenic, organic (hormonal, vascular, drug-induced, or neurogenic), or mixed psychogenic and organic. Up to 80% of ED cases have an organic origin. The most common cause of ED is vascular disease (Box 1).

Atherosclerosis is the most common cause of vasculogenic ED, whereas endothelial damage is the most common mechanism. Aging is a well-known risk factor for ED, and it is hypothesized that there are alterations in the levels of NO that occur as a consequence of the aging endothelium. Additionally, chronic illness, depression, and lack of a sexual partner are all prevalent in this age population.

Chronic tobacco use is a major risk factor for the development of vasculogenic ED because of its effects on the vascular endothelium. Additionally, blood nicotine levels rise after smoking, which increases sympathetic tone in the penis and leads to nicotine-induced, smooth-muscle contraction in the cavernosal body. Chronic smoking also leads to decreased penile NOS activity and neuronal NOS content.

DM is a major risk factor for ED. In the Massachusetts Male Aging Study, the diabetic subset had a threefold increased prevalence of ED compared with nondiabetic subjects (28% versus 9.6%). In the same study, the overall incidence rate of ED was 26 cases per 1000 man-years in nondiabetics and 50 cases per 1000 man-years in the diabetic population. The pathogenesis of ED in the diabetic patient is related to accelerated atherosclerosis, alterations in the corporal erectile tissue, and neuropathy.

Hypertension is another major risk factor for ED. Whether ED in patients with hypertension is related to the disease itself or to the use of antihypertensive medications has been debated for years. In a study

---

**BOX 1  Classification of Erectile Dysfunction**

**Endocrine**
- Hypogonadism
- Hyperprolactinemia

**Drug Induced**
- β-Blockers
- Calcium channel blockers
- Alcohol
- Nicotine
- Antiandrogens
- Cocaine
- Heroin
- Marijuana
- Cimetidine
- Metoclopramide
- Antidepressant medications
- Antipsychotic medications

**Vascular**
- Coronary artery disease
- Peripheral vascular disease
- Hypertension
- Diabetes mellitus

**Psychogenic**
- Depression
- Performance anxiety

**Neurogenic**
- Spinal cord injury
- Neuropathy (diabetic, hypertensive)
- Cerebrovascular disease
- Radical prostatectomy
- Pelvic surgery

**Multifactorial**
- Aging
- End-stage renal disease
- Pelvic trauma (neurogenic and vasculogenic)
- Diabetes mellitus (neurogenic, vasculogenic, drug induced)

looking at 104 subjects, the differences in incidence or severity of ED were minor between distinct types of antihypertensive medications or the number of agents being used simultaneously. This favors the concept that antihypertensive agents as well as the disease itself contribute to the appearance of ED. There are, however, classes of antihypertensive medications that are notorious for their negative impact on erectile function such as thiazides and β-blockers. The only β-blocker not associated with significant incidence of ED is carvedilol (Coreg).

Hyperlipidemia is another etiologic factor for ED. It is believed to contribute to ED by its relationship to endothelial dysfunction. One study showed that decreasing total cholesterol to less than 200 mg/dL by using atorvastatin (Lipitor) led to significant improvement of ED as measured by the International Index of Erectile Function (IIEF).

ED may be a sentinel manifestation of vascular disorders. In a study of 980 subjects seeking ED advice, 18% were suffering from undiagnosed hypertension, 16% had DM, 5% had ischemic heart disease, 15% had benign prostatic hyperplasia, 4% had prostate cancer, and 1% had depression. ED can itself be an independent marker for CAD. In addition, the extent of CAD correlates with the prevalence of ED.

# Quantification of the Severity of Erectile Dysfunction and Improvement

There are several tools designed to assess the severity of ED, as well as to measure the efficacy of different treatments. We discuss three different measures, the IIEF, the Sexual Encounter Profile (SEP), and the Global Assessment Question (GAQ) (Box 2).

## PATIENT HISTORY

When assessing sexual dysfunction, it is important to inquire about a number of issues:

1. Differentiate between decreased libido and ED: assess whether the patient has one or both
2. Tobacco use: type, amount, duration
3. Alcohol intake
4. History of depression or anxiety disorder
5. Presence of social/relationship stressors
6. Ability to have erections while masturbating versus when with partner
7. List of all prescription, over-the-counter, and herbal medications
8. Knowledge of whether nocturnal erections are present
9. History of drug use: marijuana, cocaine, other recreational drugs
10. History of genitourinary trauma
11. History of prostatic disease, or possible related symptoms
12. History of hypertension, hyperlipidemia, CAD, peripheral vascular disease, cerebrovascular disease
13. History of DM
14. History of spinal cord injury
15. History of penile plaques: possible Peyronie's disease
16. Frequency of intercourse or attempted intercourse
17. Ability to ejaculate

## PHYSICAL EXAMINATION

The physical examination should include a careful testicular examination to assess testicular size, asymmetries, presence of hernias, or varicoceles. Additionally, a digital rectal examination to assess the prostatic size, consistency, and presence of nodules is warranted. Penile inspection and palpation should be performed, with special attention to possible fibrotic plaques. Palpation and auscultation of femoral arteries for possible bruits is another important part of the examination.

## LABORATORY STUDIES

Laboratory workup on a patient with ED should include total and bioavailable testosterone levels drawn in the morning, prolactin,

---

**BOX 2   Tools Used to Quantify Erectile Dysfunction Severity**

Tools used in the quantification of the severity of erectile dysfunction (ED) include the International Index of Erectile Function (IIEF), the Sexual Encounter Profile (SEP), and the Global Assessment Question (GAQ).

**International Index of Erectile Function**

The IIEF is a standardized questionnaire designed to measure ED and detect treatment-related changes. It is a 15-item questionnaire addressing five different domains: erectile function, orgasmic function, sexual desire, intercourse satisfaction, and overall satisfaction. The IIEF is the most frequently used efficacy measurement employed in ED drug trials. Using a scale from 1 (never/almost never) to 5 (almost always/always), men grade each domain. It is very sensitive and specific, and has been validated in 20 languages to assess treatment-related changes in sexual function. The questions 1-5 and 15 are used to quantify erectile dysfunction severity and are as follows:

1. How often were you able to get an erection during sexual activity?
2. When you had erections with sexual stimulation, how often were your erections hard enough for penetration?
3. When you attempted sexual intercourse, how often were you able to penetrate (enter) your partner?
4. During sexual intercourse, how often were you able to maintain your erection after you had penetrated (entered) your partner?
5. During sexual intercourse, how difficult was it to maintain your erection to completion of intercourse?
15. How do you rate your confidence that you could get and keep an erection?

And it is scored as follows:

| | |
|---|---|
| 26-30 | Normal ED |
| 22-25 | Mild ED |
| 17-21 | Mild to moderate ED |
| 11-16 | Moderate ED |
| ≤10 | Severe ED |

**Sexual Encounter Profile**

SEP is a five-question survey provided to patients with ED in clinical studies of oral therapies. The survey is completed after each sexual attempt. The questions are as follows:

1. Were you able to achieve at least some erection?
2. Were you able to insert your penis into your partner's vagina?
3. Did your erection last long enough to have successful intercourse?
4. Were you satisfied with the hardness of your erection?
5. Were you satisfied with the overall sexual experience?

Answers to questions 2 and 3 are the ones most often used in the literature.

**Global Assessment Questions**

GAQ is usually administered at the end of the treatment period during efficacy studies.
Question 1: Has the treatment taken during the study improved your erections?
Question 2: If yes, has the treatment improved your ability to engage in sexual activity?
This is very subjective, and its responses tend to be valued less than SEP and IIEF.

prostate-specific antigen, fasting glucose, and fasting lipid panel. Further studies may be warranted depending on the results of the aforementioned.

# Management of Erectile Dysfunction

The landscape of ED was revolutionized with the introduction of sildenafil citrate (Viagra), the first oral medication for the treatment of this condition. Since then, oral agents have become the preferred mode of treatments by patients in surveys worldwide. There are three oral agents that inhibit PDE5 currently on the market:

1. Sildenafil citrate (Viagra)
2. Vardenafil (Levitra)
3. Tadalafil (Cialis)

All three drugs work by inhibiting PDE5, which maintains intracavernosal levels of cGMP, subsequently producing vasodilatation and penile erection (see Figure 1).

## SILDENAFIL CITRATE (VIAGRA)

Sildenafil citrate (Viagra) is an orally active, potent, and selective inhibitor of cGMP-specific PDE5. The predominant phosphodiesterase isoform in the penile tissue is type 5. The selectivity of sildenafil citrate (Viagra) for PDE5 is approximately 4000-fold greater than its selectivity for phosphodiesterase 3 (PDE3), the isoform involved in the control of cardiac contractility. Sildenafil citrate (Viagra) is absorbed rapidly after oral administration, with an absolute bioavailability of 40%. The time of maximal (T-max) plasma after oral dosing in the fasting state is between 30 and 120 minutes. A high-fat meal increases the time to peak plasma concentration by 60 minutes and reduces the peak plasma concentration by 29%. The half-life of the drug is from 3 to 5 hours. Sildenafil citrate (Viagra) is metabolized by hepatic microsomal cytochrome P450 isoenzyme 3A4 for the most part. Cytochrome P450 3A4 inhibitors, cimetidine (Tagamet), erythromycin, ketoconazole (Nizoral), and protease inhibitors may retard the metabolism of sildenafil citrate (Viagra).

The recommended dose is from 25 to 100 mg as needed approximately 1 hour before sexual activity. In some individuals, the onset of activity may be seen as early as 11 to 19 minutes, but this is not the norm. The usual starting dose is 50 mg.

The maximum recommended dose is 100 mg, and the maximum dosing frequency is once daily. A starting dose of 25 mg can be considered for patients older than age 65 years as well as for patients with severe hepatic cirrhosis or severe renal impairment.

There are more than two dozen, randomized, double-blind, placebo-controlled studies involving this agent. It produces positive results regardless of the etiology of ED. It has been studied in patients with DM, CAD, postcoronary artery bypass graft (post-CABG), spinal cord injury, depression, hypertension, prostate cancer post-prostatectomy, benign prostate enlargement post-transurethral resection of the prostate (TURP), patients on hemodialysis, as well as recipients of renal transplants. Results vary according to the underlying condition causing ED in the first place, ranging from 50% to 85%.

The most common side effects of sildenafil citrate (Viagra) include vasodilatory effects such as headaches, flushing, and nasal congestion caused by hyperemia of the nasal mucosa, as well as dyspepsia. Up to 30% of patients may get at least one side effect. Another side effect that presents on occasion is blurred or blue-green vision because of inhibition of phosphodiesterase 6 (PDE6) in the retina. It is absolutely contraindicated in men taking long-acting or short-acting nitrate drugs, and men taking any form of nitrates should be informed about the dangerous interaction.

Do not prescribe sildenafil citrate (Viagra) to patients with unstable CAD who need nitrates. Assess the need for ordering treadmill testing in select patients. Initial monitoring of blood pressure (BP) after the administration of sildenafil citrate (Viagra) may be indicated in men with complicated congestive heart failure (CHF). α-Blockers should not be used in combination with sildenafil citrate (Viagra) because of possible orthostatic hypotension.

## VARDENAFIL (LEVITRA)

Vardenafil (Levitra) is a highly potent inhibitor of PDE5. It was approved for use in the United States in late 2003. It is a more selective PDE5 inhibitor than sildenafil citrate (Viagra). The absorption of vardenafil (Levitra) is delayed by a fatty content of more than 30% in a meal. However, that does not seem to affect its effectiveness in different trials. The half-life of vardenafil (Levitra) is 4.4 to 4.8 hours, and the clinical effectiveness may be as long as 12 hours. The time for maximum plasma concentration is between 42 and 54 minutes. The first trial using the agent included 580 patients, excluding patients with spinal cord injury, radical prostatectomy, hypogonadism, thyrotoxicosis, or DM.

The successful rates of intercourse were 71% to 75% on patients taking 5 or 10 mg at a time. Those taking 20 mg had a success rate of 80%. The placebo groups had an average success rate of 30%.

Vardenafil (Levitra) has been tested in patients with type 2 DM; 452 patients were enrolled in a double-blind, placebo-controlled trial. The success rate in the vardenafil (Levitra) group ranged from 57% to 72%.

In a different study involving 736 subjects including men with DM and stable CAD, the success rates were 28% for the placebo group, 65% for those taking 5 mg, 80% for those taking 10 mg, and 85% for the 20-mg group.

Patients who were unresponsive to sildenafil citrate (Viagra) at a dose of 100 mg on several attempts were given vardenafil (Levitra) in doses of 10 and 20 mg (proved in trial). Vardenafil (Levitra) produced statistically and clinically significant results compared with placebo in men who were historically unresponsive to sildenafil citrate (Viagra). The dose that offers the best clinical results is 20 mg. It should not be taken more than once every 24 hours. Safety studies have shown no deleterious effects with long-term daily use of this drug for up to 12 months.

The most common side effects include headaches (10% to 21%), flushing (5% to 13%), rhinitis (9% to 17%), and dyspepsia (1% to 6%) because vardenafil (Levitra) does not inhibit PDE6. Unlike sildenafil citrate (Viagra), it does not produce problems of blurred vision or blue-green visual disturbances. The same warning regarding the use of nitrates as sildenafil citrate (Viagra) applies to vardenafil (Levitra). Patients taking vardenafil (Levitra) may use α-blocking agents with caution.

## TADALAFIL (CIALIS)

The third oral agent of this class is tadalafil (Cialis). It has a half-life of 17.5 hours, with two thirds of patients experiencing clinical benefits of this drug up to 36 hours after its use. The clinical onset of action occurs in less than 1 hour. There is no interaction between food and alcohol on the absorption of the drug.

There have been numerous phase II and III studies in Europe, Canada, and the United States using doses of 2, 5, 10, and 25 mg of the drug in comparison with placebo. The average success rates on these studies averaged 17% for placebo, 51% for the 2-mg dose, and 80% for the other doses, as well as up to 88% on the 25-mg dose in one study. In one study looking at 216 subjects with type 2 DM, improved erections were reported in 56% to 64% of the patients.

A recent article looking at all the previously published patient data showed that among 2102 men studied in 11 randomized placebo-controlled trials lasting 12 weeks, each mean improvement in IIEF at 20 mg of tadalafil (Cialis) was 8.6. Mean positive Sexual Encounter Profile Diary Question 3 (SEP3) response was 68% versus 31% in placebo groups. Mean GAQ was 84% versus 33% in placebo group.

In a multicenter, randomized, double-blind, crossover study looking at 181 men who received either sildenafil citrate (Viagra) or tadalafil (Cialis), 73% (132) preferred tadalafil (Cialis) at 20 mg instead of sildenafil citrate (Viagra) at 50 or 100 mg.

The most clinically effective dose of tadalafil (Cialis) is 20 mg. It should be taken at least 30 minutes before intercourse. It may be used with caution in patients using α-blocking agents. Nitrates are absolutely contraindicated for use in patients taking tadalafil (Cialis). The most common side effects include headaches, dyspepsia, back pain, rhinitis, and flushing. There are no visual side effects reported.

## APOMORPHINE (UPRIMA)[1]

Apomorphine (Uprima)[1] is a potent emetic that acts on central dopaminergic receptors. The stimulation of central dopaminergic receptors transmits excitatory signals down the spinal cord to the sacral parasympathetic nucleus, stimulating activity of the sacral nerves supplying the penis. It has been used successfully in up to 67% of patients when administered through a sublingual preparation. Subcutaneous injections[2] of apomorphine (Uprima)[1] produce almost a 100% erectile response, but nausea and vomiting are limiting factors to this mode of administration.

The most common side effects are headache, nausea, and dizziness. Rare syncopal episodes have been reported.

## PHENTOLAMINE (REGITINE)

Phentolamine (Regitine) is an $\alpha_1$- and $\alpha_2$-adrenergic receptor antagonist.

The sympathetic system via the release of noradrenaline (NA) is the primary determinant of cavernosal smooth muscle contraction and detumescence. A relative predominance of NA-induced contraction over NO-induced smooth muscle relaxation may contribute to ED.

In large phase III studies, 55% to 59% of patients receiving 40 and 80 mg were able to achieve vaginal penetration. Adverse effects include nasal congestion (10%), headaches (3% to 5%), dizziness (3% to 5%), tachycardia (3%), and nausea.

## TRAZODONE (DESYREL)[1]

Trazodone (Desyrel)[1] is a serotonin reuptake inhibiting agent. Its action in ED is believed to be the result of central serotonergic and peripheral $\alpha$-adrenolytic activity. The efficacy of trazodone is poorly demonstrated; however, it may have a place in those with performance anxiety. Side effects include drowsiness, insomnia, headaches, and weight loss.

## DIETARY SUPPLEMENTS AND ERECTILE DYSFUNCTION

Yohimbine[1] is an $\alpha_2$-adrenoreceptor antagonist with short duration of action. It is administered orally, and it is believed to have a central effect at adrenergic receptors in brain centers associated with libido and penile erection. A meta-analysis of seven studies established that it is superior to placebo, although results can be very erratic. Side effects include palpitations, tremors, and anxiety. Yohimbine should *not* be recommended as part of the management of ED.

A study with 60 patients who had failed papaverine[1] injections (50 mg or less) were treated with an extract of *Ginkgo biloba*, 60 mg for 12 to 18 months. After 6 months, 50% of the patients reported improvement in erectile function. A placebo-controlled randomized trial using 240 mg of *Ginkgo biloba* extract daily for 24 weeks in patients with vasculogenic ED did not demonstrate significant differences between the groups.

L-Arginine[1] is an amino acid that is the precursor to NO. Three small studies are looking at this drug. There are encouraging results in one study.

Zinc is found in high concentrations in seminal fluid. Anecdotal reports of improvement in ED.

## ALPROSTADIL (PROSTAGLANDIN E1, CAVERJECT, MEDICATED URETHRAL SYSTEM FOR ERECTION)

Prostaglandin E1 ($PGE_1$) exerts a number of pharmacologic effects including systemic vasodilatation, inhibitory actions on platelet aggregation, and relaxation of smooth muscle. $PGE_1$ binds to PGE receptors and causes a relaxation response mediated by cyclic adenosine monophosphate (cAMP). It can be administered intracavernosally or intraurethrally.

---

[1]Not FDA approved for this indication.
[2]Not available in the United States

---

It has been used in combination with papaverine,[1] and the combination was superior to $PGE_1$ alone. The intracavernosal administration seems to be more effective than transurethral (medicated urethral system for erection [MUSE]). MUSE should be administered in 1-mg doses, applied intraurethrally. Responses to intracavernosal injections (Caverject) as high as 80% may be expected in patients with organic ED with a dose of 20 $\mu g$, and much lower to MUSE (35% to 43%). Injections are given with 27- to 30-gauge needles. The administration of $PGE_1$ is usually relegated as an alternative in patients who have contraindications to the use of phosphodiesterase 5 (PDE5) inhibitors. The possible side effects include penile fibrosis, priapism, urethral bleeding, hypotension, or syncopal episodes.

Papaverine[1] is a nonspecific phosphodiesterase inhibitor that increases cAMP and cGMP levels in penile erectile tissue. It produces smooth muscle relaxation and vasodilatation. It decreases the resistance to arterial inflow and increases the resistance to venous outflow. It is highly effective in psychogenic and neurogenic ED but not vasculogenic. It has been commonly used in combination with phentolamine (Regitine). Major side effects include priapism, corporeal fibrosis, and possible elevation of liver transaminases.

Moxisylyte chlorohydrate[2] is an $\alpha$-blocking agent. In a study where 156 subjects received either alprostadil or moxisylyte in a dose-escalating fashion, alprostadil had much better success rates (46% versus 81%).

Chlorpromazine (Thorazine)[1] is useful when given in combination with alprostadil or papaverine. It has $\alpha$-blocking properties, and it is cheaper than phentolamine (Regitine).

Decreased concentration of vasoactive intestinal polypeptide (VIP)* has been reported in the penile tissue of men with ED. VIP is believed to play a role in the erectile process. It is ineffective when administered alone but can be quite effective in combination with phentolamine (Regitine). In a small study of 52 subjects with organic ED, 100% of them achieved an erection sufficient for intercourse. Further studies into the effectiveness of VIP may be needed.

## PENILE PROSTHESES

This surgical approach used to be quite common before the advent of oral agents. The use of prostheses is still a suitable alternative for those who are unresponsive to less invasive treatments. Prostheses can be classified as rod, one-piece inflatable, two-piece inflatable, and three-piece inflatable. Postsurgical infections and malfunctions are the most common complications. Patients are usually satisfied with the results of prosthetic placement.

---

[1]Not FDA approved for this indication.
[2]Not available in the United States
*Investigational drug in the United States.

---

 **CURRENT DIAGNOSIS**

- The risk factors for ED include tobacco, alcohol, and drug use, as well as DM, hypertension, hyperlipidemia, and prostate disease.
- ED is widely prevalent, and incidence sharply increases with age.
- ED is a cardiovascular sentinel event, and its occurrence warrants a cardiac workup.
- The workup of ED should include checking testosterone levels, prolactin, glucose, and lipid levels.
- First-line therapies include the use of PDE5 inhibitors such as sildenafil citrate (Viagra), vardenafil (Levitra), and tadalafil (Cialis).

*Abbreviations:* DM = diabetes mellitus; ED = erectile dysfunction; PDE5 = phosphodiesterase 5.

## CURRENT THERAPY

- PDE5 Inhibitors
  Sildenafil citrate (Viagra) 25-100 mg
  Vardenafil (Levitra) 10-20 mg
  Tadalafil (Cialis) 10-20 mg
- Alprostadil ($PGE_1$)
  Intracavernosal injections (Caverject) 20 µg
  Intraurethral application (MUSE) 1-mg pellet
- Papaverine injections[1] 30-60 mg
- Agents not yet approved for use by the FDA:
  Apomorphine (Uprima)[1] 3, 4, 6 mg
  Phentolamine (oral)[1] 40, 60, 80 mg

---

[1]Not FDA approved for this indication.
*Abbreviations:* MUSE = medicated urethral system for erection; PDE5 = phosphodiesterase 5; $PGE_1$ = prostaglandin E1.

## Vacuum Constrictive Device

Vacuum constrictive device is a plastic cylinder that is placed over the penis and connected to a pump that creates a partial vacuum. After achieving penile rigidity, a band is placed around the base of the penis to maintain the erection. This is a safe, noninvasive, and effective method of treating ED. It requires an understanding partner and the quality of the erection is not ideal; but patients are usually satisfied.

## Testosterone

Patients who have low testosterone levels may benefit substantially from replacement. Men may expect significant improvements in libido, self-esteem, and overall energy levels. Additionally, testosterone is necessary for NO generation in the penile tissue.

The different testosterone preparations include injections such as testosterone enanthate (Delatestryl), cypionate (Depo-Testosterone) given as an intramuscular (IM) injection in doses of 100 to 200 mg, every 2 weeks on average. They also include transdermal testosterone patches (Androderm and Testoderm, 5 mg/d) or transdermal gel (AndroGel 5-g packets, one daily; or Testim 1% testosterone gel, one packet daily). Testosterone gel preparations provide physiologic replacement of testosterone and are preferred more than depot IM injections.

## Future Trends

In the next few years we will see a sharp rise in the use of combination drugs, such as PDE5 inhibitors and apomorphine (Uprima),[1] PDE5 inhibitors and phentolamine (Regitine), and combinations of PDE5 inhibitors and intraurethral and intracavernosal agents. ED will be recognized universally as a cardiovascular sentinel event and also as a risk factor for vascular disease in general.

## REFERENCES

Archer SL: Potassium channels and erectile dysfunction. Vascul Pharmacol 2002;38:61-71.
Burchardt M, Burchardt T, Baer L, et al: Hypertension is associated with severe erectile dysfunction. J Urol 2000;164(10):1188-1191.
Carson CC, Rajfer J, Eardley I, et al: The efficacy and safety of tadalafil: An update. BJU Int 2004;93:1276-1281.
Crowe SM, Streetman DS: Vardenafil treatment for erectile dysfunction. Ann Pharmacother 2004;38:77-85.
Feldman HA, Goldstein I, Hatzichristou DG, et al: Impotence and its medical and psychosocial correlates: Results of the Massachusetts Male Aging Study. J Urol 1994;151(1):54-61.

---

[1]Not FDA approved for this indication.

Jackson G, Betteridge J, Dean J, et al: A systematic approach to erectile dysfunction in the cardiovascular patient: A consensus statement—Update 2002. Int J Clin Pract 2002;56(9):663-671.
Jaynat D, Shepherd MD: Evaluation and treatment of erectile dysfunction in men with diabetes mellitus. Mayo Clin Proc 2002; 77(3):276-282.
Johannes CB, Araujo AB, Feldman HA, et al: Incidence of erectile dysfunction in men ages 40 to 69 years old: Longitudinal results from the Massachusetts Male Aging Study. J Urol 2000;163(2): 460-463.
Kirby M, Jackson G, Betteridge J, et al: Is erectile dysfunction a marker for cardiovascular disease? Int J Clin Pract 2002;55(9): 614-618.
Lue TF: Drug therapy: Erectile dysfunction. N Engl J Med 2000; 342(24): 1802-1813.
Michelakis E, Tymchak W, Archer S: Sildenafil: From the bench to the bedside. CMAJ 2000;163(9):1171-1175.
NIH Consensus Development Panel on Impotence: Impotence (NIH Consensus Conference). JAMA 1993;270(1):83-90.
Padma-Nathan H: Intra-urethral and topical agents in the management of erectile dysfunction. In Carson CC III, Kirby RS, Goldstein I (eds): Textbook of Erectile Dysfunction. Oxford, Isis Medical Media, 1999, pp 323-326.
Rhoden EL, Teloken C, Mafessoni R, et al: Is there any relation between serum levels of testosterone and the severity of erectile dysfunction? Int J Impot Res 2002;14:167-171.
Shokeir AA, Alserafi MA, Mutabagani H: Intracavernosal versus intraurethral alprostadil: A prospective randomized study. BJU Int 1999;83:812-815.
Spahn M, Manning M, Juenemann KP: Intracavernosal therapy. In Carson CC III, Kirby RS, Goldstein I (eds): Textbook of Erectile Dysfunction. Oxford, Isis Medical Media, 1999, pp 345-353.
Sullivan ME, Thompson CS, Dashwood MR, et al: Nitric oxide and penile erection: Is erectile dysfunction another manifestation of vascular disease? Cardiovasc Res 1999;43:658-665.

# Acute Renal Failure

Method of
*Steven D. Weisbord, MD, MSc,
and Paul M. Palevsky, MD*

## Definition, Epidemiology, and Outcomes of Acute Renal Failure

Acute renal failure (ARF) is a clinical syndrome broadly defined as an abrupt decline in renal function over a period of hours to days. Its clinical characteristics relate to the retention of nitrogenous and metabolic waste products and of extracellular fluid resulting from a reduction in the glomerular filtration rate (GFR). Although the initial manifestation of ARF may be decreased urine output, urine volume may remain normal or even increase, with the decline in renal function manifested by increases in blood urea nitrogen and serum creatinine concentrations. Despite a clear conceptual understanding of the syndrome, a universally accepted, operational definition of ARF does not exist, leading to the use of a variety of definitions in clinical studies and confounding efforts to characterize its epidemiology. Definitions have been based on absolute or proportional changes in the serum creatinine concentration, as direct measurement of GFR in the clinical setting is technically difficult. Commonly used definitions have included absolute increases in serum creatinine concentration of 0.5 to 1.0 mg/dL and relative increases of 25% to 100% over 1 to several days. Although expert panels have been convened to develop consensus definitions, the lack of sensitive and easily measured biomarkers of early renal damage has limited such efforts.

The reported incidence of ARF is dependent on both the patient population studied and the definition of renal failure used. ARF develops in as many as 7% of hospitalized patients and complicates up to 30% to 50% of admissions to intensive care units. Its incidence among ambulatory patients is substantially lower. Unfortunately, outcomes associated with ARF have changed little over the past several decades. In-hospital mortality rates in excess of 50% continue to be reported in critically ill patients with ARF despite technologic advances in renal replacement therapies and other supportive care. Multiple studies have identified demographic and clinical factors that portend adverse outcomes from ARF. Older age, male gender, and respiratory, liver, and hematologic failure have all been directly correlated with in-hospital mortality, whereas serum creatinine and urea nitrogen concentrations (presumably reflecting nutritional factors) as well as urine output have inverse relationships with in-hospital mortality. Whereas associated comorbidities contribute to the high mortality associated with ARF, multiple studies have demonstrated that the development of ARF, in and of itself, is a strong predictor of mortality independent of concomitant comorbid conditions. The impact of a change in renal function on hospital outcomes is underscored by a recent study that found that even very small elevations in serum creatinine concentration (0.1–0.2 mg/dL) following cardiac or thoracic aortic surgery were associated with increased 30-day postoperative mortality.

## Classification of Acute Renal Failure

ARF can be broadly classified into prerenal, postrenal, and intrinsic renal etiologies (Table 1). Prerenal ARF is the most common cause of acute renal dysfunction, resulting from hemodynamically mediated reductions in renal blood flow. The hallmarks of prerenal azotemia are the absence of demonstrable pathologic damage to the renal parenchyma and the prompt restoration of renal function following correction of the hemodynamic abnormality.

The second broad category of ARF is postrenal, which is characterized by obstruction of the urinary collecting system. ARF may develop with obstruction of either the lower urinary tract (bladder or urethra) or the upper urinary tract (ureters and kidneys). Upper tract obstruction must, however, be bilateral or affect a solitary functioning kidney in order to cause ARF.

Intrinsic ARF involves renal parenchymal injury. The most common form of intrinsic ARF is acute tubular necrosis (ATN), which develops as the result of nephrotoxic, ischemic, or septic injury to the kidney. With ATN there is renal tubular epithelial cell injury, apoptosis and necrosis of the tubular epithelium, denuding of the epithelial basement membrane, and obstruction of tubular lumens by sloughed epithelial cells and debris. Glomerular histology is preserved, and the decline in renal function is mediated by a combination of intrarenal vasoconstriction, back-leak of glomerular ultrafiltrate across the denuded epithelium, and tubular obstruction. Acute interstitial nephritis, acute glomerulonephritis, rapidly progressive GN, and macrovascular- and microvascular-mediated injury are less common forms of intrinsic ARF.

ARF can also be categorized based on urine volume as nonoliguric, oliguric, or anuric. Oliguria is defined as daily urine output less than 400 mL and anuria as daily urine output less than 50 mL, the latter most commonly encountered in the setting of bilateral urinary tract obstruction or severe ATN associated with shock. In general, nonoliguric ARF is associated with a better prognosis than is oliguric or anuric disease, reflecting lesser degrees of renal injury.

## Diagnostic Features of Specific Syndromes of Acute Renal Failure

### PRERENAL ACUTE RENAL FAILURE

Prerenal ARF results when hemodynamic factors lead to renal hypoperfusion. Prerenal ARF may occur in the setting of true hypovolemia, as may result from diarrhea, vomiting, decreased oral intake, and overly aggressive use of diuretics, or it may occur in relation to clinical conditions associated with decreased effective circulating volume, such

## TABLE 1  Classification of Etiologies of Acute Renal Failure

**Prerenal Acute Renal Failure**
- Decreased Absolute Blood Volume
  - Blood loss: Hemorrhage
  - Cutaneous losses: Burns, sweating
  - Gastrointestinal losses: Diarrhea, vomiting, drainage from intestinal, pancreatic or biliary fistulas
  - Renal losses: Diuretics, osmotic diuresis
- Decreased Effective Blood Volume
  - Heart failure
  - Cirrhosis
  - Nephrotic syndrome
- Intrarenal Hemodynamic Effect
  - Nonsteroidal anti-inflammatory drugs

**Postrenal Acute Renal Failure**
- Upper Tract Obstruction: Bilateral obstruction or unilateral obstruction with single functioning kidney
  - Intrinsic: Nephrolithiasis, papillary necrosis, blood clot, transitional cell carcinoma
  - Extrinsic: Retroperitoneal or pelvic malignancy, retroperitoneal adenopathy, retroperitoneal fibrosis, endometriosis, abdominal aortic aneurysm
- Lower Tract Obstruction
  - Transitional cell carcinoma of the bladder, prostate cancer, benign prostatic hypertrophy, urethral stricture, neurogenic bladder, bladder stones

**Intrinsic Acute Renal Failure**
- Acute Tubular Necrosis
  - Ischemic
  - Nephrotoxic
    - Exogenous: Radiocontrast media, aminoglycosides, amphotericin B (Fungizone), cis-platinum (Platinol), acetaminophen (Tylenol)
    - Endogenous: Rhabdomyolysis, hemolysis
  - Sepsis
- Acute Interstitial Nephritis
  - Medications: Penicillins, cephalosporins, sulfonamides, rifampin (Rifadin), phenytoin (Dilantin), furosemide (Lasix), nonsteroidal anti-inflammatory drugs
  - Infections: Bacterial, viral, rickettsial, mycobacterial
  - Autoimmune disorders: Systemic lupus erythematosus, Sjögren's syndrome, sarcoidosis
- Acute Glomerulonephritis
  - Poststreptococcal glomerulonephritis
  - Postinfectious glomerulonephritis
  - Endocarditis-associated glomerulonephritis
  - Vasculitis/autoimmune disease
  - Thrombotic microangiopathy (hemolytic uremic syndrome, thrombotic thrombocytopenic purpura)
  - Rapidly progressive glomerulonephritis
- Acute Vascular Syndromes
  - Large-vessel disease: Bilateral renal artery thromboembolism or dissection, bilateral renal vein thrombosis
  - Small-vessel disease: Atheroembolic disease
- Intratubular Obstruction
  - Crystals: Calcium oxalate, uric acid, acyclovir (Zovirax), indinavir (Crixivan)
  - Protein: Light-chain nephropath

as congestive heart failure and chronic liver disease. Clinical findings of volume depletion may include absolute or relative hypotension, orthostatic changes in pulse and/or blood pressure, decreased jugular venous pressure, dry mucous membranes, and tenting of the skin. However, many of these physical findings are nonspecific, especially in the elderly and in chronically ill patients. The utility of these physical findings may be diminished in patients with cardiac or liver disease, in whom effective circulating volume may be decreased despite extracellular volume overload with edema.

Assessment of urine chemistry may be helpful in the diagnosis of prerenal azotemia. The urine sodium concentration is usually low (<20 mEq/L), with a fractional excretion of sodium [$FE_{Na}$ (excreted sodium divided by filtered sodium) calculated as $(U_{Na}/P_{Na}) \div (U_{Cr}/P_{Cr})$, where $U_{Na}$ and $P_{Na}$ are the urine and plasma concentrations of sodium, respectively, and $U_{Cr}$ and $P_{Cr}$ are the urine and plasma concentrations of creatinine, respectively] of less than 1% as the result of avid tubular reabsorption of filtered sodium. However, in patients taking diuretics or having underlying chronic kidney disease with impaired sodium conservation, the urinary sodium and fractional excretion of sodium may be elevated. In such cases, a low fractional excretion of urea (<35%) supports the diagnosis of prerenal ARF. Other possible urinary findings are evidence of urinary concentration (urine osmolality >300 or specific gravity >1.015) and a bland urine sediment without casts. In prerenal states, the ratio of blood urea nitrogen to serum creatinine may be increased to greater than 20:1 as a result of increased tubular reabsorption of urea. Table 2 provides a summary of diagnostic findings associated with various etiologies of ARF.

Nonsteroidal anti-inflammatory drugs (NSAIDs) are commonly used medications that can precipitate or exacerbate prerenal ARF. In settings of decreased absolute or effective circulatory volume, local synthesis of vasodilatory prostaglandins opposes the vasoconstrictive effects of angiotensin II on the afferent (preglomerular) arteriole in order to maintain GFR. In settings in which the renin-angiotensin axis is activated, inhibition of prostaglandin synthesis by the kidney results in unopposed vasoconstriction, markedly diminishing GFR. NSAID use, particularly in the setting of chronic kidney disease, older age, concomitant use of angiotensin-converting enzyme inhibitors, use of angiotensin receptor blockers or diuretics, and clinical conditions associated with decreased effective circulating volume (e.g., heart failure and advanced liver failure), is associated with a markedly increased risk of prerenal ARF and an increased risk of developing ATN.

## POSTRENAL ACUTE RENAL FAILURE

The second broad category of ARF is postrenal or obstructive disease, which is characterized by obstruction of the urinary collecting system. ARF develops only when obstruction affects both kidneys or with unilateral upper urinary tract obstruction in the setting of a solitary functioning kidney. The disorders that cause postrenal ARF are usually categorized by the level of urinary tract obstruction. Obstruction to the lower urinary tract (bladder outlet and urethra) commonly results from benign or malignant prostate disease, bladder cancer, or urethral stricture. Obstruction to the upper urinary tract commonly stems from pelvic and retroperitoneal malignancy, retroperitoneal lymphadenopathy, transitional cell carcinoma of the renal pelvis and ureters, bilateral kidney stones, or retroperitoneal fibrosis.

The clinical findings depend on the degree and level of obstruction to urinary flow. Anuria can be seen with complete obstruction, whereas normal urine volume, polyuria, or fluctuating urine output may occur with partial obstruction. Gender-related anatomic differences, notably a longer urethra and periurethral prostatic tissue, make postrenal ARF more common in men. Careful abdominal examination may reveal a tender, distended bladder, suggesting the presence of bladder outlet obstruction. The gold standard diagnostic test is the renal ultrasound, which demonstrates dilation of the renal collecting system (hydronephrosis and/or hydroureter). However, in up to 20% of cases, particularly early in the clinical course or in cases associated with intravascular volume contraction or retroperitoneal fibrosis, ultrasound may fail to demonstrate hydronephrosis despite the underlying presence of obstructive ARF. Documentation of a postvoid bladder urine volume of at least 100 mL by bedside ultrasound or catheterization suggests lower urinary tract obstruction. Outcomes with postrenal ARF depend greatly on the duration and degree of obstruction. With complete obstruction, the likelihood of recovery of renal function decreases after approximately 1 week. Recovery from partial obstruction is more difficult to predict and depends on the severity and duration of obstruction along with other complicating factors.

**TABLE 2  Diagnostic Findings in Acute Renal Failure**

| | BUN/Cr Ratio | $U_{Na}$ (mEq/L) | $FE_{Na}$ | Urinalysis | Other Findings |
|---|---|---|---|---|---|
| Prerenal Acute Renal Failure | >20:1 | <20 | <1% | Normal or hyaline casts<br>Specific gravity >1.015 | $FE_{Urea}$ <35% |
| Intrinsic Acute Renal Failure | | | | | |
| Acute tubular necrosis | 10:1 | >40 | >2%* | Muddy-brown casts, tubular epithelial cells<br>Specific gravity ~1.010 | $FE_{Urea}$ >50% |
| Acute interstitial nephritis | | >20 | >1% | Hematuria, WBCs, WBC casts, eosinophils | Eosinophilia |
| Acute glomerulonephritis | | <20 | <1% | Dysmorphic RBCs, RBC casts | — |
| Intratubular obstruction | | Variable | Variable | Crystalluria or Bence-Jones proteinuria† | Monoclonal paraprotein on electrophoresis |
| Acute vascular syndromes | | >20 | Variable | Hematuria | Elevated lactate dehydrogenase with renal infarction |
| Postrenal Acute Renal Failure | >20:1 | >20 | Variable | Variable | Fluctuating urine output |

*Fractional excretion of sodium ($FE_{Na}$) can be low in cases of radiocontrast nephropathy and pigment nephropathy.
†Calcium oxalate crystals with ethylene glycol intoxication; uric acid crystals with uric acid nephropathy; Bence-Jones proteins, associated with multiple myeloma, can be detected using the sulfosalicylic acid test of urine.
*Abbreviations:* BUN = blood urea nitrogen; Cr = creatinine; $FE_{Urea}$ = fractional excretion of urea; $U_{Na}$ = urine concentration of sodium; RBC = red blood cell; WBC = white blood cell.

## INTRINSIC RENAL DISEASE

### Acute Tubular Necrosis

Most cases of ATN can be linked to renal ischemia, use of nephrotoxic agents, or sepsis. Unlike prerenal azotemia, ATN is characterized by tubular epithelial cell injury leading to impaired reabsorption of sodium with a urine sodium concentration greater than 40 mEq/L and a fractional excretion of sodium greater than 2%. Urine in patients with ATN is typically isosthenuric (isotonic with plasma), with a specific gravity of approximately 1.010. The urine sediment typically demonstrates "muddy brown" coarse granular casts on microscopic analysis. The blood urea nitrogen concentration usually rises in proportion to the serum creatinine concentration, leading to maintenance of the normal ratio of approximately 10:1.

### Radiocontrast-Associated Acute Tubular Necrosis

The administration of intravascular radiocontrast media results in one of the most common forms of ATN, accounting for approximately 10% of hospital-acquired ARF. The administration of intravascular radiocontrast often results in a transient and clinically insignificant (0.1–0.2 mg/dL) rise in the serum creatinine concentration. Radiocontrast nephropathy (RCN) develops when more pronounced reductions in kidney function follow radiocontrast administration. The pathogenesis of RCN is multifactorial and is mediated by both renal vasoconstriction, particularly affecting the renal medulla, and direct epithelial cell toxicity. Clinically, RCN manifests as an abrupt decline in kidney function 24 to 72 hours after radiocontrast administration. The serum creatinine concentration typically peaks within 3 to 5 days and returns to baseline by 7 to 10 days. Several clinical factors increase the risk for RCN, including preexisting chronic kidney disease, diabetes mellitus with or without diabetic nephropathy, congestive heart failure, volume depletion, and increasing dose of radiocontrast media. In contradistinction to other forms of ATN, the fractional excretion of sodium may be low in RCN.

### Aminoglycoside-Associated Acute Tubular Necrosis

Aminoglycoside antibiotics are associated with nephrotoxicity in 10% to 15% of patients. Aminoglycosides are actively taken up and accumulate in proximal tubular cells, leading to toxicity as intracellular concentrations rise. ARF usually develops 7 to 10 days after the initiation of therapy. Because aminoglycosides are renally excreted, dosing of these agents is central to their nephrotoxicity. Aminoglycoside-induced ATN is typically nonoliguric, and near-complete or full recovery of renal function is common, although the course of ARF may be protracted.

### Myoglobinuric Acute Tubular Necrosis

Rhabdomyolysis develops from injury to skeletal muscle and results in the release of cellular constituents, such as creatine phosphokinase and myoglobin, into the systemic circulation. When myoglobin is filtered in large quantities by the kidney, tubular damage and ATN can ensue. Although the classic description of rhabdomyolysis involves severe trauma with crush injuries, an increasing number of cases are linked to nontraumatic etiologies, including use of medications, such as statins, and use of illicit drugs, primarily cocaine. Typical symptoms include muscle soreness and weakness. A dramatically elevated creatine phosphokinase level is the sine qua non of this condition. Commonly, hyperphosphatemia, hyperuricemia, and hyperkalemia complicate rhabdomyolysis due to release of the respective components from damaged muscle. Additionally, hypocalcemia may occur, resulting primarily from calcium deposition in the injured muscle. Subsequent release of deposited calcium during the recovery phase may result in hypercalcemia. Urine findings include heme-pigmented casts and a positive dipstick for heme pigment in the absence of red blood cells on microscopic examination.

### Postoperative Acute Renal Failure

ARF is a relatively common complication following vascular, cardiac, and major abdominal surgical procedures and is associated with particularly high mortality rates. Its development can usually be linked to perioperative episodes of hypotension and/or sepsis. Depending on the definition of ARF and the risk profile of the patient population, ARF develops in 1% to 40% of patients undergoing cardiac surgery, with 1% to 7% of these patients requiring dialysis. Specific clinical factors that increase the risk for ARF following cardiac surgery include cardiogenic shock, decreased baseline renal function, emergent surgery, left ventricular dysfunction, age greater than 70 years, peripheral vascular disease, and left main coronary artery disease. Additionally, valve surgery, particularly of the aortic valve, is associated with greater risk than is coronary artery bypass surgery, with the greatest risk in patients undergoing combined procedures.

### Acute Interstitial Nephritis

Acute interstitial nephritis (AIN) results from inflammatory damage to the renal interstitium. Antibiotics and NSAIDs are the most common etiologic agents, although the list of drugs that can precipitate AIN is extensive. Less commonly, infections and autoimmune diseases lead to AIN. Eosinophilia, fever, and rash classically accompany AIN, although the presence of this complete triad is seen in only approximately one third of patients. Examination of the urine reveals hematuria and sterile pyuria with or without white blood cell casts. Although eosinophiluria is associated with AIN, the sensitivity and positive predictive value of this finding are poor. In contrast, the negative predictive value of this finding is high, making the absence of eosinophiluria a useful test for ruling out AIN. The clinical features of AIN typically develop several days to weeks after exposure to the offending agent, and recovery is common following discontinuation of the agent.

### Acute Glomerulonephritis

Acute GN and rapidly progressive GN are uncommon causes of ARF that can result from myriad conditions and are characterized by primary injury to the glomerulus. The hallmark findings of GN-associated ARF are dysmorphic red blood cells and red blood cell casts on microscopic examination of the urine sediment. The prototypic form of acute GN is poststreptococcal GN; however, acute GN may also develop in the setting of endocarditis and other infections, systemic vasculitis, and autoimmune disease, or it may present as an idiopathic renal-limited disease. Serologic assays for complement levels (C3 and C4), hepatitis markers, antistreptococcal antibodies (ASO), antinuclear antibodies (ANA), antiglomerular basement membrane antibodies (anti-GBM), and antineutrophil cytoplasmic antibodies (ANCA) may be helpful in making a diagnosis; however, renal biopsy is commonly required to determine the specific etiology.

### Intratubular Obstruction

Intratubular obstruction to the flow of urinary filtrate can occur in certain clinical settings and result in an acute decline in renal function. The obstruction may result from precipitation of either crystals or protein within the tubular lumen. Ethylene glycol ingestion is associated with intratubular precipitation of calcium oxalate crystals. This diagnosis should be suspected when ARF develops in the setting of acute intoxication and high anion-gap metabolic acidosis and is usually accompanied by a preponderance of calcium oxalate crystals on examination of the urine sediment. *Tumor lysis syndrome* is a term applied to a constellation of metabolic and clinical findings that may occur after treatment of rapidly proliferative neoplastic disorders, usually of hematologic origin. Marked hyperuricemia leads to intratubular precipitation of uric acid crystals in the distal nephron. Other associated findings include hyperphosphatemia, hyperkalemia, and hypocalcemia. This form of ARF is typically oliguric or anuric. The urine sediment usually demonstrates abundant uric acid crystals or amorphous urates in the setting of an acidic urine. Characteristically, the ratio of urine uric acid to creatinine is greater than 1 in acute uric acid nephropathy, compared to values of less than 0.6 to 0.75 in ARF of other etiologies. Intratubular precipitation of acyclovir and indinavir is the major mechanism of ARF with use of these drugs. Tubular obstruction is also one of the well-recognized complications of multiple myeloma. Monoclonal immunoglobulins and/or light chains precipitate in distal tubules, leading to intratubular obstruction and ARF.

## Acute Vascular Syndromes

Acute vascular syndromes that cause ARF can be broadly divided into large-vessel disease and small-vessel disease. Although uncommon, etiologies for large-vessel disease include bilateral thromboembolism, renal vein thrombosis, and large vessel vasculitis leading to renal infarction. More common is small-vessel disease resulting from atheroemboli that involve the distal renal vasculature. Cholesterol crystals released from atheromatous plaques deposit in small arteries and arterioles. Although nonobstructive, these emboli induce an inflammatory reaction that ultimately leads to fibrosis and obliteration of vessels. Acute and/or subacute renal failure are common sequelae. Along with renal involvement, cutaneous manifestations such as livedo reticularis, abdominal pain from intestinal ischemia and pancreatitis, myositis, and neurologic involvement from emboli to the central nervous system and spinal cord can complicate the clinical picture. Renal atheroemboli should be suspected in any case of ARF that occurs subsequent to instrumentation of the vasculature. Laboratory clues to the diagnosis include eosinophilia, eosinophiluria, and hypocomplementemia, although these findings are not universally present.

# Prevention and Treatment of Acute Renal Failure

## PRERENAL ACUTE RENAL FAILURE

Treatment of prerenal azotemia is directed at augmenting renal perfusion. With true hypovolemia, administration of intravascular isotonic fluid is the primary therapy. Treatment directed at the cause of volume loss, such as diarrhea or vomiting, should also be implemented. In cases of overdiuresis, diuretics should be discontinued and judicious intravascular volume expansion provided. With severely decompensated heart failure, renal perfusion can be optimized using intravenous inotropic agents, although this is usually only a temporizing measure. Cautious intravascular volume expansion can be beneficial in prerenal azotemia in advanced liver disease; however, this must be balanced against the risk of total body volume overload. No data support the routine use of intravenous albumin for expansion of the intravascular space in the majority of patients with advanced liver disease. However, use of intravenous albumin has proved beneficial in preventing renal dysfunction in the treatment of spontaneous bacterial peritonitis and in patients undergoing large volume paracentesis. Prevention of NSAID-related prerenal azotemia hinges on avoiding these agents in patients with chronic kidney disease or other factors that predispose to renal underperfusion. To prevent the evolution of NSAID-associated prerenal ARF into ischemic ATN, prompt discontinuation of the offending NSAID, along with other potentially nephrotoxic agents, is essential.

## POSTRENAL ACUTE RENAL FAILURE

Treatment of postrenal ARF hinges on the prompt relief of obstruction. Placement of a bladder catheter provides relief of functional or anatomic bladder outlet obstruction. Upper tract obstruction requires the placement of ureteral stents or percutaneous nephrostomy tubes.

## INTRINSIC ACUTE RENAL FAILURE

### Acute Tubular Necrosis

#### General Therapeutic Considerations

In the majority of patients, the development of ARF is unpredictable. For this reason, with the exception of specific clinical settings discussed later, preventive measures are limited to broad recommendations for avoidance of nephrotoxic agents when possible, for cautious dosing of such agents when they must be used, particularly in the elderly and in patients with underlying chronic renal insufficiency, and for avoidance

of hypovolemia and hypotension. Similarly, the pharmacologic management of established ATN is ineffective. Although multiple agents, including diuretics, renal vasodilators, natriuretic peptides, and growth factors, have shown promise in animal models and preliminary clinical trials, none has proved to be clinically effective when rigorously evaluated.

The role of loop diuretics in the management of ATN has been controversial. It was hypothesized that decreased oxygen demand resulting from inhibition of sodium transport might reduce the extent of renal injury; however, this benefit has not been substantiated in clinical trials. In addition, diuretics have been used to convert oliguric to nonoliguric ARF in the hope that this will improve prognosis. Although the increased urine volume simplifies fluid management, there is no evidence that the conversion to a nonoliguric state actually impacts outcomes. Rather, the response to diuretics merely identifies patients with less severe renal injury. A recent observational study suggested that diuretic use was associated with an increased risk of death and with nonrecovery of renal function, although these findings were not confirmed in a subsequent trial. Nevertheless, these findings highlight the concern that diuretic therapy may result in delays in initiation of renal replacement therapy. Therefore, we believe that a trial of high-dose furosemide (Lasix; 160–200 mg intravenously) or an equivalent dose of other loop diuretics is reasonable in oliguric patients who are not intravascularly volume depleted, but that diuretic therapy should not be used to delay the initiation of otherwise indicated renal replacement therapy. Repeated dosing of diuretics is not warranted in patients who do not respond.

Dopamine (Intropin) increases renal plasma flow, GFR, and sodium excretion when administered at doses of 0.5 to 2 $\mu$g/kg/min. Although such "renal-dose" dopamine has been widely used in the management of ARF, clinical trials have not established any benefit with regard to survival or need for renal replacement therapy with this agent. Given the risk of complications, especially cardiac tachyarrhythmias, there is no role for low-dose dopamine in the management of ARF. Similarly, there is no established role for fenoldopam mesylate[1] (Corlopam), a selective dopamine-1 receptor agonist, in the management of ARF.

### Renal Replacement Therapy

In the absence of effective pharmacologic therapy, renal replacement therapy remains the primary treatment of severe ARF, providing an effective means for managing hyperkalemia, metabolic acidosis, volume overload, and uremic manifestations. Multiple forms of renal replacement therapy, including intermittent hemodialysis, continuous renal replacement therapy, newer hybrid forms of slow hemodialysis such as sustained low-efficiency dialysis, and peritoneal dialysis, can be used in patients with ARF. Only limited data are available to guide selection of modality of renal replacement therapy. Specifically, no data support improved outcomes associated with continuous renal replacement therapy compared to intermittent hemodialysis, although continuous renal replacement therapy and sustained low-efficiency dialysis both are associated with less hemodynamic instability and more effective volume removal than is intermittent hemodialysis. Therefore, selection of modality should be based on local capabilities and expertise.

Generally accepted indications for initiation of renal replacement therapy in patients with ARF include volume overload, hyperkalemia, metabolic acidosis, and overt uremic manifestations such as encephalopathy and pericarditis. An optimal threshold for initiation of therapy based on level of azotemia is not established, although preemptive initiation of therapy prior to the development of uremic symptoms is well recognized to be associated with improved outcomes. Therefore, it is generally accepted that, in the absence of other indications, renal replacement therapy should be initiated when the blood urea nitrogen concentration reaches approximately 90 to 100 mg/dL, although some data suggest that earlier initiation of therapy may be associated with improved outcomes.

Despite substantial technologic advancements in the dialysis apparatus, the optimal dose of renal replacement therapy in ARF

---

[1]Not FDA approved for this indication.

remains uncertain. Although daily intermittent hemodialysis was associated with improved survival compared to alternate-day dialysis in a prospective study, several methodologic issues related primarily to the relatively low dose of dialysis provided with each treatment raise questions regarding the applicability of the results of this study to general practice. Similarly, although two single-center randomized controlled trials have demonstrated improved survival with increased intensity of continuous renal replacement therapy, results have not been consistent across all studies. It is hoped that ongoing clinical trials will resolve this issue in the near future.

### Therapeutic Considerations for Specific Etiologies of Acute Tubular Necrosis

**RADIOCONTRAST NEPHROPATHY.** Most radiographic procedures that utilize intravascular radiocontrast are planned in advance, making RCN one of the forms of ARF most amenable to preventive measures. Three strategies have been conclusively shown to decrease the risk for RCN in high-risk patients. First is intravascular volume expansion with intravenous fluids. Volume expansion with isotonic saline (1 mL/kg/hr for 12 hours before and 12 hours after the administration of radiocontrast) is more effective than the same volume of hypotonic saline. Several recent studies have suggested that administration of isotonic sodium bicarbonate may be superior to sodium chloride for the prevention of radiocontrast nephropathy. However, confirmation of these results across broader populations of patients and in larger studies is required before the superiority of sodium bicarbonate can be definitively established. Second, low-osmolar radiocontrast agents are associated with less nephrotoxicity than are older high-osmolar agents, and additional protection may be provided by the use of iodixanol (Visipaque), an iso-osmolar radiocontrast agent, in high-risk patients, particularly in patients with chronic kidney disease and diabetes mellitus. Third, minimizing the dose of radiocontrast decreases renal damage.

Along with these measures, the administration of *N*-acetylcysteine[1] (Mucomyst), an antioxidant agent, may be associated with protection from RCN. Although clinical trials have yielded conflicting results and meta-analyses have failed to conclusively demonstrate a beneficial effect, this agent is inexpensive and free of deleterious side effects. Therefore, use of *N*-acetylcysteine (600-1200 mg orally twice daily on the day before and on the day of the procedure) is not inappropriate, albeit not in lieu of proven preventive strategies. Similarly, with the well-recognized relationship between intravascular volume depletion/renal underperfusion and risk for RCN, discontinuation of diuretics and NSAIDs prior to radiocontrast administration is advisable. Mannitol,[1] dopamine[1] (Intropin), fenoldopam[1] (Corlopam), calcium channel blockers, and human β-type natriuretic peptide[1] (Natrecor) are not effective and have no role in the prophylaxis of RCN. Likewise, prophylactic intermittent hemodialysis and continuous hemofiltration have no role in the prevention of RCN. An algorithm for the prevention of RCN is shown in Figure 1.

**AMINOGLYCOSIDE-ASSOCIATED ACUTE TUBULAR NECROSIS.** Based on the observation that proximal tubule uptake of aminoglycosides is saturable, use of once-daily dosing of these antimicrobial agents may be less nephrotoxic than multiple-daily dosing schemes. Although conclusive data are lacking, a series of studies and meta-analyses support the use of once-daily dosing. Therefore, it is not unreasonable to consider once-daily dosing in clinically appropriate circumstances to reduce the risk of ARF. Additional preventive strategies that should be implemented include monitoring of drug levels, discontinuing concomitant nephrotoxic agents, limiting the duration and total dose of therapy, and switching to non-nephrotoxic agents guided by antibiotic sensitivities.

**MYOGLOBINURIC ACUTE RENAL FAILURE.** Rhabdomyolysis is associated with sequestration of large volumes of fluid in the injured muscle. Because the risk of ARF in rhabdomyolysis is associated with intravascular

---

[1]Not FDA approved for this indication.

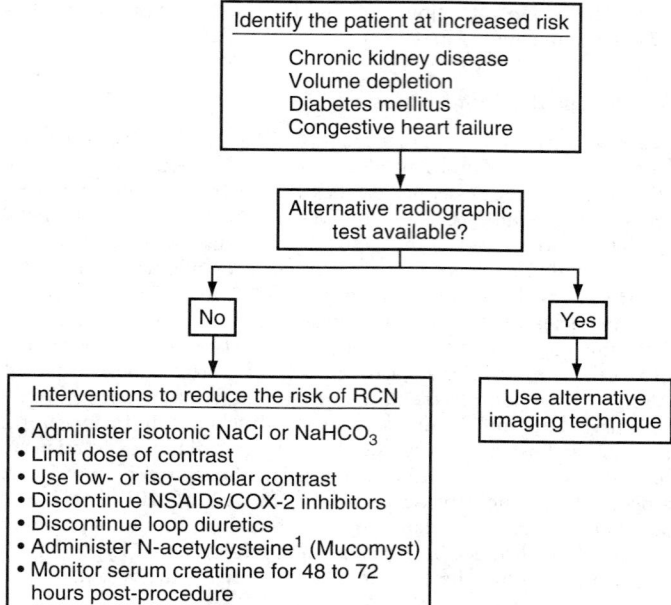

**FIGURE 1.** Management algorithm for the prevention of radiocontrast nephropathy (RCN). [1]Not FDA approved for this indication. *Abbreviations:* COX-2 = cyclooxygenase-2; NaCl = sodium chloride; NaHCO2 = sodium bicarbonate; NSAIDs = nonsteroidal anti-inflammatory drugs.

volume depletion, patients with rhabdomyolysis should be aggressively administered large volumes of isotonic electrolyte solutions to maintain intravascular volume. In patients with crush injuries, the use of aggressive fluid resuscitation with administration of normal saline at 1 L/hr has been shown to minimize the risk of ARF. Optimally, this strategy should be initiated in the field, prior to extraction of the patient. Although use of mannitol as an osmotic diuretic and urinary alkalinization with bicarbonate have been recommended, data supporting the superiority of these agents over isotonic saline alone are inconclusive. Hypocalcemia should not be treated unless the patient is symptomatic because calcium administration increases the risk of hypercalcemia during the recovery phase of rhabdomyolysis.

**POSTOPERATIVE ACUTE RENAL FAILURE.** No specific therapies have been demonstrated to be effective for the prevention or treatment of postoperative ATN.

### Acute Interstitial Nephritis

The primary treatment of AIN is discontinuation of the offending agent. In most patients, renal function recovers, although this can take several weeks. Use of glucocorticoids for treatment of AIN remains controversial. Although case series have suggested a potential benefit of glucocorticoids, their use has not been evaluated in prospective randomized trials. Nonetheless, a trial of glucocorticoids is a reasonable therapeutic option in patients with biopsy-proven AIN in whom renal function fails to improve after discontinuation of the offending drug.

## ACUTE GLOMERULONEPHRITIS

Therapy for acute GN is dependent upon the specific diagnosis. The treatment of poststreptococcal GN is supportive. In patients with endocarditis-associated GN and other forms of infection-associated GN, treatment is directed at the underlying infection. Plasma exchange should be initiated in patients with hemolytic uremic syndrome and thrombotic thrombocytopenic purpura. High-dose glucocorticoids and cytotoxic or immunosuppressive therapy are usually required in patients with vasculitis-associated GN and rapidly progressive GN. In patients with anti-GBM disease, plasmapheresis is often required in addition to high-dose glucocorticoids and cytotoxic therapy.

## INTRATUBULAR OBSTRUCTION

### Oxalate Nephropathy

Fomepizole (Antizol), a competitive inhibitor of alcohol dehydrogenase, and intravenous ethanol[1] are the primary therapies for ethylene glycol intoxication. By inhibiting formation of oxalate, these therapies can prevent the development or arrest the progression of acute oxalate nephropathy. Maintenance of high urinary flow rates with intravenous fluids may help minimize calcium oxalate precipitation. Mannitol can be used as an osmotic diuretic to maintain urine flow rates. Intravenous sodium bicarbonate may be necessary to treat the metabolic acidosis that commonly complicates this form of ARF. Dialysis may be beneficial for rapidly lowering plasma ethylene glycol levels and acutely decreasing the concentrations of plasma oxalate and other metabolites.

### Acute Uric Acid Nephropathy

Tumor lysis syndrome and acute uric acid nephropathy characteristically develop after the initiation of chemotherapy, allowing initiation of treatment to prevent this form of ARF. Volume expansion with intravenous saline to maintain high urine flow rates minimizes the intratubular precipitation of uric acid crystals and is the mainstay of therapy. The role of urinary alkalinization with intravenous sodium bicarbonate is less certain. Although the solubility of uric acid is increased in alkaline urine, the benefit of alkalinization compared to saline alone has not been demonstrated, and it may promote the deposition of calcium phosphate in patients with concomitant hyperphosphatemia. Allopurinol (Zyloprim; 600–900 mg/day) should be initiated in advance of chemotherapy to inhibit xanthine oxidase and block the generation of uric acid. In patients unable to take oral medications, an intravenous form of allopurinol (200–400 mg/m$^2$/day) is available. Alternatively, rasburicase (Elitek; 0.15–0.2 mg/kg/day), a recombinant form of uricase, rapidly metabolizes uric acid to the more soluble allantoin and is approved for use in children. Rasburicase is contraindicated in patients with glucose-6-phosphate dehydrogenase deficiency. In patients who develop ARF, hemodialysis may rapidly lower uric acid concentrations and facilitate recovery of renal function.

### Multiple Myeloma

Acute light-chain nephropathy should be treated with aggressive intravascular volume expansion. Concomitant hypercalcemia, which increases the risk of acute nephropathy, should be treated. Chemotherapy should be initiated to decrease the light-chain burden. Plasmapheresis may be of benefit in some patients by rapidly lowering the filtered light-chain burden. Although it has previously been suggested that plasmapheresis is of benefit in some patients with light-chain nephropathy by rapidly lowering the filtering light-chain burden, this has not been borne out by a more recent multicenter study. For this reason, plasmapheresis is no longer recommended in this setting.

### Atheroembolic Disease

No specific therapy for atheroembolic disease exists. Treatment with antiplatelet agents, steroids, and iloprost[1] (Ventavis), a prostacylin analogue, have all been investigated, with no definitive benefit seen. Supportive care, including the withdrawal of anticoagulants, avoidance of additional intravascular manipulation, and therapy to lower serum cholesterol concentrations with statins, may improve outcomes. Overall mortality from renal atheroembolic disease remains greater than 60% to 80% in some series, underscoring the importance of primary prevention.

## Complications and Additional Therapeutic Considerations

### Electrolyte and Acid-Base Complications

Hyperkalemia is a common complication of ARF, developing as a result of decreased renal excretion, particularly in patients with oliguric ARF. If severe, hyperkalemia can lead to life-threatening arrhythmias. Therapy depends on the degree of elevation of the serum potassium concentration, with severe hyperkalemia requiring urgent therapy. In patients with electrocardiographic changes of hyperkalemia, the initial therapy is intravenous calcium (10–20 mL of 10% calcium gluconate or 10 mL of 10% calcium chloride). This should be followed by intravenous insulin (10–20 U regular insulin), combined with an infusion of dextrose (250 mL of 20% dextrose in water over 1 hour) to prevent hypoglycemia and inhaled albuterol[1] (Proventil) (10–20 mg by nebulizer) to translocate potassium from the extracellular to intracellular compartments. Potassium removal from the body can be achieved by administration of oral or rectal polystyrene sulfonate (Kayexalate) or by initiation of dialysis. In patients with serum potassium concentrations greater than 6 mEq/L but without electrocardiographic changes, intravenous calcium is not required, and treatment should begin with insulin/glucose and/or albuterol to translocate potassium into the intracellular compartment, followed by dialysis or potassium-binding resin. Less severe degrees of hyperkalemia need only be treated with dialysis or binding resins.

Metabolic acidosis is another frequent complication of ARF, manifested initially by a decline in serum bicarbonate concentration. Concomitant pulmonary disease may result in the development of mixed acid-base disorders; hence, confirmation of the presence of acidemia by blood gas analysis is necessary prior to initiation of therapy. The role of bicarbonate therapy in patients with anion-gap metabolic acidosis remains controversial. Although severe acidemia (pH <7.1) may be associated with decreased cardiac function and impaired response to catecholamines, studies of bicarbonate therapy have failed to consistently demonstrate beneficial effects and have suggested potential deleterious consequences from the associated sodium load. Renal replacement therapy usually provides highly effective correction of metabolic acidosis.

Hyperphosphatemia is common in patients with ARF and, if severe, warrants the use of oral binding agents. In severe hyperphosphatemia (>7 mg/dL), short-term administration of aluminum hydroxide[1] (Alu-Cap) rapidly lowers the serum phosphate concentration. Once the serum phosphate concentration is less than 7 mg/dL, calcium-based binders should be used (calcium acetate [PhosLo] 667–1364 mg or calcium carbonate[1] [Tums] 0.5–1.0 g administered with meals). Sevelamer (Renagel), a newer non–calcium-containing polymer that binds intraintestinal phosphate, can be used in patients with hypercalcemia or an elevated calcium-phosphate product. Hemodialysis and renal replacement therapy are highly effective in lowering the plasma phosphate concentration and may lead to hypophosphatemia.

Hypermagnesemia can occur with ARF and is usually due to exogenous magnesium administration in the setting of impaired renal excretory capacity. Extreme caution should be used when administering magnesium to patients with severely decreased GFR. Hemodialysis can be used in severe cases to lower the serum magnesium level.

### Hematologic Complications

ARF can result in platelet dysfunction, predisposing to bleeding complications. The uremic platelet defect is manifested by prolongation of the bleeding time in the setting of a normal platelet count, normal prothrombin time (PT), and normal activated partial thromboplastin

---

[1]Not FDA approved for this indication.

[1]Not FDA approved for this indication.

time (aPTT). This defect is usually corrected, at least in part, by dialysis. If the platelet dysfunction is severe and is complicated by active bleeding, administration of 1-deamino (8-D-arginine) vasopressin (DDAVP[1]; 0.3 μg/kg intravenously) may be of benefit; however, tachyphylaxis usually develops after two to three doses. Intravenous estrogens (conjugated estrogen[1] [Premarin] 0.6 mg/kg) administered daily for 5 days has been shown to correct the platelet defect for up to 14 days. Pooled cryoprecipitate is of benefit but is associated with risk of transmission of viral diseases. Anemia is a common occurrence with ARF; however, the role of recombinant human erythropoietin[1] (Procrit) and other erythropoietic agents in the management of this complication is not well characterized.

## Infectious Complications

Infection is a common comorbidity in patients with ARF. Intravascular and bladder catheters frequently serve as routes of infection. Whenever possible, bladder catheters should be removed and intermittent bladder catheterization used. Temporary dialysis catheters are a frequent source of bacteremia. To reduce the risk of infection, femoral dialysis catheters should be avoided whenever possible and should remain in place for as brief a duration as possible. In patients with prolonged ARF, the use of tunneled dialysis catheters will decrease the risk of infection. In a single small clinical trial, use of antibiotic-impregnated dialysis catheters was associated with a reduced risk of catheter-associated bacteremia. Additional studies confirming these results are needed before this approach can be recommended.

Early recognition and initiation of systemic antimicrobial therapy for blood-borne infections related to central venous catheters are essential, as is the appropriate dosing of antibiotics in the setting of reduced GFR. Removal of central venous catheters in the setting of bacteremia is highly dependent on the clinical status of the patient, the pathogenic organism, and the need for short-term vascular access.

## Cardiopulmonary Complications

Cardiac and pulmonary problems are protean in patients with ARF. Arrhythmias, hypertension, pericarditis, and pericardial effusion can be seen with ARF. Pericarditis, which can be life-threatening, should be treated with intensification of renal replacement therapy. Pulmonary vascular congestion or overt pulmonary edema resulting from impaired diuresis and natriuresis may precipitate the need for renal replacement therapy. In patients with acute lung injury or the acute respiratory distress syndrome who are mechanically ventilated using low-tidal volumes as a lung-protective strategy, the dialysis prescription may require adjustment to provide adequate control of the acidemia resulting from hypercapnia.

## Nutritional Management

The optimal approach to nutritional therapy in the setting of ARF remains a matter of debate. ARF is usually a catabolic state. Although caloric and protein requirements should be individualized based on the overall clinical condition of the patient, protein intake should not be restricted and generally should range from 1.2 to 1.6 g/kg/day, with a minimum daily caloric intake of 30 kcal/kg. Enteral routes of nutritional supplementation are greatly preferred. Renal replacement therapy can be associated with loss of proteins and amino acids, necessitating adjustments in the nutritional prescription. Among nondialysis patients, close attention should be paid to limit intake of potassium (<60 mEq/day) and phosphate (<1.0 g/day).

## REFERENCES

Chertow GM, Levy EM, Hammermeister KE, et al: Independent association between acute renal failure and mortality following cardiac surgery. Am J Med 1998;104:343-348.

Friedrich JO, Adhikari N, Herridge MS, Beyene J: Meta-analysis: Low-dose dopamine increases urine output but does not prevent renal dysfunction or death. Ann Intern Med 2005;142:510-524.

Lassnigg A, Schmidlin D, Mouhieddine M, et al: Minimal changes of serum creatinine predict prognosis in patients after cardiothoracic surgery: A prospective cohort study. J Am Soc Nephrol 2004;15:1597-1605.

Mehta RL, Pascual MT, Soroko S, Chertow GM: Diuretics, mortality, and nonrecovery of renal function in acute renal failure. JAMA 2002;288:2547-2553.

Merten GJ, Burgess WP, Gray LV, et al: Prevention of contrast-induced nephropathy with sodium bicarbonate: A randomized controlled trial. JAMA 2004;291:2328-2334.

Mueller C, Buerkle G, Buettner HJ, et al: Prevention of contrast media-associated nephropathy: Randomized comparison of 2 hydration regimens in 1620 patients undergoing coronary angioplasty. Arch Intern Med 2002;162:329-336.

Nash K, Hafeez A, Hou S: Hospital-acquired renal insufficiency. Am J Kidney Dis 2002;39:930-936.

Pannu N, Manns B, Lee H, Tonelli M: Systematic review of the impact of N-acetylcysteine on contrast nephropathy. Kidney Int 2004;65:1366-1374.

Ronco C, Bellomo R, Homel P, et al: Effects of different doses in continuous venovenous haemofiltration on outcomes of acute renal failure: A prospective randomised trial. Lancet 2000;356:26-30.

Schiffl H, Lang SM, Fischer R: Daily hemodialysis and the outcome of acute renal failure. N Engl J Med 2002;346:305-310.

Stone GW, McCullough PA, Tumlin JA, et al: Fenoldopam mesylate for the prevention of contrast-induced nephropathy: A randomized controlled trial. JAMA 2003;290:2284-2291.

Tepel M, van der Giet M, Schwarzfeld C, et al: Prevention of radiographic-contrast-agent-induced reductions in renal function by acetylcysteine. N Engl J Med 2000;343:180-184.

Uchino S, Doig GS, Bellomo R, et al: Diuretics and mortality in acute renal failure. Crit Care Med 2004;32:1669-1677.

# Chronic Renal Failure

Method of
*Jeffrey A. Kraut, MD*

Chronic renal failure is defined as a reduction in glomerular filtration rate (GFR) below the normal values of approximately 120 to 130 mL/minute developing over months to years. Its incidence has increased significantly over the last several years, but this probably reflects more accurate estimations of GFR. However, there is an increased prevalence of type II diabetes mellitus, a frequent cause of renal disease, in Western societies that could contribute to a higher incidence of chronic renal failure. When renal failure is severe (GFR <10 mL/minute), renal replacement therapy, either dialysis or renal transplantation, is required to preserve life. However, even before several renal failure ensues, the presence of chronic renal failure has an important impact on organ function and can contribute to the development of significant electrolyte derangements, important hormonal abnormalities, and anemia. Also, its presence can alter the metabolism and therefore the blood concentrations and tissue concentrations of drugs administered for the treatment of various diseases. Moreover, a reduced GFR is associated with an increased risk of death, increased incidence of cardiovascular events, and hospitalizations independent of known risk factors or a history of cardiovascular diseases. Finally, the mortality of several surgical procedures is substantially increased by the presence of chronic renal failure. Therefore, detecting and treating patients with chronic renal failure is extremely important.

## Causes of Chronic Renal Failure

Many disorders can cause chronic renal failure. However, epidemiologic studies indicate that diabetes mellitus and hypertension account for the majority of cases (>60%). Chronic glomerulonephritis,

---

[1]Not FDA approved for this indication.

polycystic kidney disease, obstructive uropathy, and ischemic nephropathy caused by atherosclerotic renal artery stenosis are less common, but important causes of renal impairment. The latter disorder is postulated to be more frequent than previously believed and is an important undiagnosed cause of chronic renal impairment.

Recent studies have indicated that a reduction in GFR occurs with aging in the absence of factors known to produce renal injury such as hypertension or diabetes. Indeed, the average GFR of subjects in the 8th decade of life in one large study was 40 to 50 mL/minute. Pathologic examination of these individuals, when available, may reveal only benign nephrosclerosis.

Importantly, because a majority of individuals older than 60 years of age have lower muscle mass, the reduced GFR is not accompanied by a rise in serum creatinine concentration. Therefore, renal failure is not detected unless the physician considers other variables such as the patient's age and muscle mass in assessing GFR (see the following section).

## Approach to the Diagnosis of Chronic Renal Failure

The first step in the diagnosis of chronic renal failure is, of course, to detect a reduction in GFR. In the past, estimations of GFR were based on the measurement of serum creatinine concentration alone. In adults, the normal serum creatinine ranges between 0.6 and 1.3 mg/dL. Individuals with values greater than this are said to have renal failure. However, there is a wide range of normal values. Also, creatinine production, which is dependent on muscle mass, is a critical variable affecting serum creatinine concentration. Thus, a large group of individuals with reduced muscle mass can have serum creatinine values within the normal range, but a decreased GFR. The most common situation in which this paradox is encountered is in the elderly and in individuals with malignancy or chronic liver disease.

Precise measurement of GFR is accomplished by calculating the clearance of creatinine in a timed urine collection, generally 24 hours in duration:

$$\text{Creatinine clearance (mL/minute)} = \text{Ucr (mg/dL)}$$
$$\times \text{volume (mL)}/\text{Scr(mg/dL)}/1440.$$

where Ucr = urine creatinine concentration,
Scr = plasma creatinine concentration

However, timed urine collections are often inaccurate because of errors in collection. Moreover, as renal function progresses and serum creatinine rises, or in the presence of nephrotic range proteinuria, GFR tends to be overestimated by creatinine clearance. Most recently, formulas derived from studies of large groups of patients—such as those by Cockroft and Gault and the Modification of Diet in Renal Disease (MDRD) in which GFR was correlated with other factors (e.g., body weight, age, and serum albumin)—are sufficiently accurate to use for clinical purposes:

Cockroft-Gault: CrCl (mL/minute) = {(140 − age) × wt × [1 − (0.15 × gender)]}/(0.814 × Scr)

MDRD: GFR = $170 \times [\text{PCr}]^{-0.999} \times [\text{Age}]^{-0.176} \times [0.762 \text{ female}] \times [1.180 \text{ if patient is black}] \times [\text{SUN}]^{-0.170} \times [\text{Alb}]^{+0.318}$

Once renal function is depressed, the physician determines whether this represents acute or chronic renal failure, When previous measurements of GFR are available, it is relatively easy to determine if the renal failure is chronic in nature. However, if these studies are not available, demonstration that the kidneys are small in size (less than 8 to 9 cm when they are normally approximately 10 to 12 cm) by renal ultrasound will confirm the chronicity of the disease. Evidence of increased echogenicity reflecting augmented fibrous deposits is also suggestive of chronic disease. However, several disorders associated with chronic renal failure have normal kidney size such as diabetes mellitus, polycystic kidney disease, and amyloidosis. Therefore, normal kidney size does not exclude chronic renal failure. If individuals have normal kidney size, the presence of anemia and/or certain abnormalities of divalent ion metabolism can also suggest the disease is chronic in nature.

Once impaired renal function is recognized, measurements of blood urea nitrogen (BUN), sodium, potassium, chloride, bicarbonate, hemoglobin and hematocrit, and calcium and phosphorus are obtained. A urinalysis is obtained looking for increased excretion of protein, presence of blood in the urine, and abnormal cellular elements. In patients with diabetes, studies to find microalbuminuria (albumin urine concentrations less than 300 mg per day) are important to detect the early stages of renal disease. A 24-hour or spot urine protein and creatinine determination to assess the urine's protein-to-creatinine ratio is obtained to quantitate the amount of protein being excreted. Urine protein excretion in excess of 3.5 g daily indicates the presence of glomerular pathology, whereas interstitial disease is characterized by values below 2 g. However, urine protein excretion can vary with glomerular disease so values below 3.5 g are still consistent with this diagnosis. Assessment of urine protein excretion is important for diagnostic purposes, but also because urine protein excretion is often followed to assess effectiveness of therapy.

Obstruction uropathy, an important cause of chronic renal failure and exacerbation of renal failure, can be excluded in the majority of cases by ultrasound of the kidneys. Doppler ultrasound of the renal arteries performed at the same time is helpful in excluding obstruction of the renal arteries. The necessity of obtaining other diagnostic studies such as measurement of serum complement, blood and urine eosinophils, serum and urine and protein electrophoresis, antiglomerular basement membrane antibodies, anti–double-stranded DNA (dsDNA) antibodies, hepatitis B and C antibodies, sedimentation rate, and HIV studies depends on the context of the renal failure.

Finally, a renal biopsy may be required in certain situations to make a definitive diagnosis. Because treatment of specific diseases can vary, making a precise pathologic diagnosis can be extremely important for proper management. Unfortunately, once the renal failure is moderate to severe in nature, renal pathologic examination may not always be helpful in determining the cause.

---

 **CURRENT DIAGNOSIS**

The following lists the optimal care of patients with chronic kidney disease:

- Test for albuminuria and estimate glomerular filtration rate using MDRD formula yearly for early diagnosis and stratification of CKD.
- If possible, determine cause of kidney disease.
- Initiate treatment to delay or prevent progression of disease including use of converting enzyme inhibitors and/or angiotensin receptor blockers to reduce BP to less than 130/80 mm Hg and urine protein excretion to as low as possible but at least less than 1 g/24 hours.
- Control or prevent biochemical or clinical abnormalities including those of serum potassium, serum bicarbonate, serum phosphorus, parathyroid hormone, and hemoglobin.
- Evaluate patients for presence of and treat important co-morbid conditions, particularly heart disease.
- If the GFR is less than 30 mL/min, consider referral to a nephrologist.

---

*Abbreviations:* BP = blood pressure; CKD = care of patients with chronic kidney disease; GFR = glomerular filtration rate; MDRD = modification of diet in renal disease.

# Clinical and Laboratory Abnormalities in Chronic Renal Failure

Because the kidney plays a critical role in the regulation of the serum concentrations of sodium, potassium, bicarbonate, chloride, calcium, and phosphorus as well as the levels of hemoglobin and hematocrit, blood pressure and extracellular volume, chronic renal injury can lead to derangements in these parameters as summarized in Table 1.

## HYPONATREMIA AND HYPERNATREMIA

The kidney plays an essential role in excreting water by producing a dilute urine (less than 1/6 plasma osmolality) or retaining water by producing a concentrated urine (three to four times plasma osmolality). The ability to concentrate or dilute the urine in the majority of cases is usually retained until GFR falls to less than 30% of normal, and therefore hyponatremia or hypernatremia are uncommon until that time. If the disease is primarily interstitial in nature, alterations in urine concentrating ability can appear prior to significant reductions in GFR. However, even with higher levels of GFR the patient can be at risk for either of these electrolyte abnormalities should they ingest large quantities of fluid or be deprived of appropriate fluid intake.

## HYPERKALEMIA

The kidney plays the most critical role in the regulation of potassium balance. Adaptive changes in renal tubular function and possible colonic function enable the kidney to maintain serum potassium within the normal range until GFR falls below 20% to 25% of normal (serum creatinine of 4 mg/dL or greater). Recent studies indicate a tendency for elevations in serum potassium to appear at even modest reductions in GFR (<60 mL/min). When disease of the kidney involves the medullary portion or hormonal derangements such as hyporeninemic hypoaldosterinism are present, hyperkalemia can be observed prior to significant declines in GFR. In addition, patients with even moderate renal failure have a reduced reserve to eliminated potassium and therefore can develop hyperkalemia if potassium load is increased dramatically.

## METABOLIC ACIDOSIS

A fall in plasma bicarbonate concentration in association with a reduced blood pH (metabolic acidosis) is frequently observed when GFR falls below 20% to 25% of normal. The acidosis results from acid excretion falling below acid production leading to positive proton balance.

## TABLE 1  Clinical and Electrolyte Abnormalities Noted With Chronic Renal Failure

| Clinical or Laboratory Disorder | GFR or Stage of Renal Failure* |
|---|---|
| Hypertension | GFR <60 mL/min (stage 3) |
| Hyponatremia or hypernatremia | GFR <30 mL/min (stage 4) |
| Hyperkalemia* | GFR <30 mL/min (stage 4) |
| Hyperphosphatemia* | GFR <30 mL/min (stage 4) |
| Metabolic acidosis | GFR <30 mL/min (stage 4) |
| Anemia | GFR <60 mL/min (stage 3) |
| Uremic symptoms | GFR <15 mL/min (stage 5) |
| Nausea, vomiting, disturbances in sleep | |

*Descriptions of the various stages are presented in the text. These electrolyte abnormalities can be seen at higher levels of GFR.
*Abbreviations:* GFR = glomerular filtration rate.

Recent studies have documented that a tendency to the development of metabolic acidosis can be seen with mild reductions in GFR (<60 mL/min).

The electrolyte pattern seen with the metabolic acidosis of renal failure is often of the high anion gap variety, but frequently a hyperchloremic (normal anion gap) or combined anion gap and hyperchloremic pattern can be observed. The degree of acidosis is usually mild to moderate with plasma bicarbonate concentration ranging from 12 to 22 mEq/L. Of interest, at any given level of GFR, the acidosis is often not progressive, but plasma bicarbonate concentration remains stable unless renal function declines further or there is an increment in acid production.

## ABNORMAL DIVALENT IN METABOLISM

Serum phosphorus is regulated by the kidney but in most cases remains within the normal range until GFR falls below 20% to 25% of normal. This stabilization of serum phosphorus is attributed to increased tubular excretion of phosphorus as a result of increased parathyroid hormone secretion. As with potassium and bicarbonate, recent studies demonstrate a tendency for elevation in serum phosphorus can be observed with mild renal failure (<50 to 60 mL/min). Serum calcium is usually in the normal range, but varies reciprocally with serum phosphorus. Because of derangements in divalent ion metabolism bone disease with increased tendency to fractures and disordered soft tissue structures can be observed.

Hyperparathyoridism is a common occurrence in patients with renal failure, the values usually being higher with a greater degree of renal impairment. The elevated PTH values are usually induced by hypocalcemia, although increased serum phosphorus concentrations independent of serum calcium values can also play a role. The increased parathyroid hormone levels can induce damage to bone and soft tissue structures, but also may affect other functions such as cardiac function and the production of red blood cells.

## ANEMIA

The kidney is the source of erythropoietin, the hormone that regulates bone marrow production of red blood cells. Thus, with the development of renal impairment, there is a fall in red blood cell production. A fall in red cell survival also contributes to development of anemia. Anemia generally appears when GFR falls below 60 mL/minute. There is a rough correlation between the severity of renal failure and the degree of anemia: the more severe the renal failure the greater the degree of anemia. However, this relationship is not invariable, and many patients have only mild reductions in hemoglobin and hematocrit.

Anemia initially was believed to contribute only to changes in oxygen delivery. However, recent studies show that anemia can contribute to the genesis of left ventricular hypertrophy and other cardiomyopathies noted with chronic renal failure and can raise mortality in patients with chronic renal failure.

## HYPERTENSION

Recent studies emphasize the importance of the kidneys in the regulation of blood pressure, and the bulk of patients with diabetes or other glomerular disease will develop hypertension in the course of their renal failure. In many instances, hypertension does not develop until GFR is below 40% to 50% of normal. The type of renal disease underlying chronic renal failure appears to be important, as hypertension is less common with pyelonephritis. Hypertension might be observed earlier in the course of renal failure, however, in patients with polycystic kidney disease or ischemic nephropathy. Because hypertension is one of the most critical factors in the genesis of cardiovascular disease and can accelerate the progression of renal failure, careful attention of control of hypertension is important.

## VOLUME OVERLOAD

Salt retention often accompanies chronic renal failure even when GFR is not severely compromised. The degree of salt retention can be profound if significant albuminuria with resultant hypoalbuminemia is seen and is more severe as GFR falls below 20% to 25% of normal. Salt retention is a critical factor in the development of hypertension and can promote congestive heart failure.

## Symptoms and Signs of Renal Failure

Patients with chronic renal failure are often asymptomatic with little evidence of disease other than laboratory abnormalities until late in the course of renal failure. If anemia is present, patients may complain of fatigue; and if significant elevations in parathyroid hormone levels are noted, bone pain, ruptured tendons or other disorders of soft tissue structures can be noted. Once moderate to severe renal failure appears, symptoms of the electrolyte abnormalities can be observed. Hyperkalemia, if severe, can lead to arrhythmias or heart block and muscle weakness. Metabolic acidosis can contribute to fatigue. Anemia can contribute to fatigue and changes in mentation and physical stamina. Weight loss related to metabolic acidosis and or retention of various uremic toxins may occur. Sexual dysfunction characterized by reduced libido and reduced fertility are common with moderate to severe renal failure.

Once severe renal failure develops (stage 4 or 5), the uremic syndrome can be observed characterized by a decreased appetite, nausea, vomiting, and subtle changes in mental status including changes in sleep patterns. However, even with severe renal failure many patients feel surprisingly well.

## Management of Chronic Renal Failure

### STAGING OF CHRONIC RENAL FAILURE

As noted earlier, within the last several years, a great deal of effort has been expended into developing guidelines for the evaluation, monitoring, and treatment of patients with chronic renal failure. To this end, experts working with the National Kidney Foundation have divided chronic renal failure into different states based on measurements or estimations of GFR. The value of staging to the physician is that the studies necessary to monitor patients and the complications of chronic renal failure are often different depending on the stage of renal failure.

### Stage 0 (GFR Greater Than 90 mL/minute With Risk Factors for Renal Disease)

Patients at stage 0 have increased risk for development of chronic renal failure, such as those with diabetes or hypertension but who have GFR greater than 90 mL/minute in the absence of proteinuria or urinary sedimentary abnormalities. These patients should have their blood pressure and diabetes controlled. Estimates of GFR should be obtained approximately every 6 months from measurement of serum creatinine, and qualitative tests for urine protein excretion should be obtained. In diabetics measurement of microalbumin should also be obtained. Because control of disease may forestall progression glycosylated hemoglobin (HbA1C) values should also be obtained.

### Stage 1 (GFR Greater Than 90 mL/minute With Albuminuria)

Once evidence of renal damage is obtained, as reflected by microalbuminuria or proteinuria, but GFR is either normal or increased, patients are said to be in stage 1. These individuals should be monitored more closely and strict attention must be given to maintain blood pressure below 130/80. Furthermore, angiotensin converting enzyme inhibitor (ACEI) or angiotensin receptor blocker (ARB) should be given to prevent evolution of microalbuminuria to full-blown proteinuria (see the following). No clinical or laboratory abnormalities are observed at this stage.

### Stage 2: Mild Renal Failure (GFR 60 to 90 mL/minute)

When GFR is mildly reduced to values from 60 to 90 mL/minute, patients are in stage 2. These patients should also be carefully monitored and blood pressure tightly controlled. If diabetes is present, strict attention to maintaining HbA1C within recommended guidelines should be given. Again, it is rare at this stage for any significant clinical abnormalities other than hypertension to be present.

### Stage 3: Moderate Renal Failure (GFR 30 to 59 mL/minute)

When GFR ranges between 30 to 59 mL/minute, patients are in stage 3. At this point hypertension may appear, mild abnormalities in serum phosphorus might be observed, and anemia can be seen. Also in some patients an elevation in serum potassium can be noted, particularly if they are ingesting a relatively high potassium diet. These patients need to be followed more closely, and it is recommended that patients at the lower end of this stage (i.e., close to 30 mL/min) be monitored by a nephrologist.

### Stage 4: Moderate to Severe (GFR from 15 to 29 mL/minute)

Once GFR falls to values from 15 to 29 mL/minute, patients have severe renal failure, or stage 4 disease. At this level of GFR, significant electrolyte abnormalities such as metabolic acidosis, hyperkalemia, and hyperphosphatemia are frequent. Anemia is common and the patient may begin to note reductions in appetite and have a fall in muscle mass. However, there is great variability in the appearance of symptoms or laboratory derangements.

### Stage 5: Severe (GFR Less Than 15 to 29 mL/minute)

When GFR falls below 15 mL/minute, severe electrolyte abnormalities are often present, anemia is common. Clinical symptoms can develop. Renal replacement therapy, either dislysis or transplantation, is usually required at this stage.

Recommendations for treatment of patients are summarized below. The frequency of patient visits, of course, largely depends on the complications of renal disease present and co-morbid conditions. Therefore, these are only general recommendations for frequency of examination.

When patients are in stage 0, they should be seen once per year for renal evaluation. When GFR remains normal or elevated, but proteinuria is present, renal evaluation should be performed every 6 months. When stage 3 develops, we usually repeat renal evaluation every 3 months. Patients in stage 4 are seen more frequently, usually at the minimum of once per month. Patients with end-stage disease require renal replacement therapy.

### GENERAL APPROACH TO TREATMENT OF CHRONIC RENAL FAILURE

Treatment of chronic renal failure can be divided into the modalities that are specific to the underlying disorder and those that are used to treat all patients with chronic renal failure. Thus, patients with systemic lupus erythematosus or other immune-mediated or inflammatory disease may benefit from treatment with steroids and immunosuppressive agents. Treatments specific for individual disorders are beyond the scope of this article.

The physician treating the patient with renal failure has two goals: preventing or delaying progression of renal failure, and alleviating the electrolyte and hormonal abnormalities that can lead to symptoms or complications of the disease. Understanding the methods to accomplish the former requires knowledge of those factors that are integral to progression of the disease.

# FACTORS CAUSING PROGRESSION OF CHRONIC RENAL FAILURE

It has been recognized for several years that once renal failure has developed, renal function can decline at a predictable rate in the absence of further insults to the kidney. Essential to the optimal approach used to treat chronic renal failure, therefore, is an understanding of those factors that can cause progression of renal failure, including:

- Systemic and intraglomerular hypertension
- Glomerular hypertrophy
- Intrarenal precipitation of calcium and phosphorus
- Hyperlipidemia
- Altered metabolism of prostanoids
- Metabolic acidosis
- Anemia
- Tubulointerstitial disease
- Proteinuria

## Intraglomerular Hypertension and Glomerular Hypertrophy

As nephrons are lost, changes are induced in the kidney to preserve GFR such as renal vasodilatation, an increase in glomerular capillary pressure, and an increment in size of individual glomeruli raising wall stress. These adaptive mechanisms probably induce damage by causing endothelial cell damage with detachment of epithelial cells allowing enhanced flux of water and solutes that might cause narrowing of capillary lumens. Also, strain on mesangial cells causes them to produce cytokines and extracellular matrix with resultant expansion of the mesangium and glomerular sclerosis.

## Proteinuria

Although proteinuria has traditionally been a marker of glomerular injury, with greater amounts of urinary protein excretion being associated with more severe injury, recent studies indicate that proteinuria, can induce mesangial and tubular damage. Therefore, treatments to reduce proteinuria, may be beneficial in limiting further renal damage.

## Tubulointerstitial Disease

Some component of tubulointerstitial disease is generally found in individuals with chronic renal failure even when the primary process affects the glomerulus. It has been postulated that the tubulointerstitial disease can produce atrophy of tubules or obstruction destroying individual nephrons. Even when tubular inflammation is treated, progressive scarring can continue unabated. Thus, treatments designed to reduce interstitial fibrosis may be important for preventing progression of disease. At present, only experimental drugs not available for human use have been examined for this purpose.

## Hyperlipidemia

Hyperlipidemia is frequently observed in disorders associated with nephrotic range proteinuria, but is also noted in a large percentage of the general population without renal disease. Experimental evidence obtained from animal studies shows hyperlipidemia can promote progression of renal failure. Thus, loading with cholesterol augments renal injury and treatment with cholesterol-lowering drugs slows the rate of progression. This effect is synergistic to that achieved by lowering blood pressure.

The mechanisms underlying the effects of lipids are not well understood, but possible explanations include mesangial lipid deposition leading to glomerular injury or tubular injury. A few studies performed in human subjects have demonstrated benefit from lipid lowering on the progression of renal injury, although they are not conclusive. Because patients with chronic renal failure have a high prevalence of cardiovascular disease, it is reasonable to inititate therapy with statin drugs to lower serum cholesterol and lipid levels.

## Calcium-Phosphate Deposition

A rise in serum phosphorus, usually seen at the later stages of renal failure, can lead to precipitation of calcium phosphate in the renal interstitium. The deposits can then induce an inflammatory response producing interstitial fibrosis and tubular atrophy. Some have indicated that the deposits may form prior to detectable elevations in serum phosphorus concentrations.

## Increased Glomerular Prostaglandin Production

An increment in glomerular prostaglandin production has been found in several studies of chronic renal failure. The increased prostanoids produce renal vasodilatation and a rise in intraglomerular pressure, factors that augment progression of disease.

# METABOLIC ACIDOSIS

Metabolic acidosis commonly develops in the course of chronic renal failure. In response to the acidosis, ammonia production per residual functioning nephron is augmented. It has been postulated that the increased local production of ammonia in some way induces tubulointerstitial damage. This issue remains controversial, as some studies do not support this possibility.

# SPECIFIC TREATMENT MEASURES

Treatment of patients with chronic renal failure should be designed to ameliorate those factors that can cause progression of renal injury, treat or prevent important complications, and normalize important laboratory abnormalities that contribute to symptoms of the disease.

# Measures Designed to Reduce the Rate of Progression of Renal Failure

## CONTROL OF SYSTEMIC AND INTRAGLOMERULAR HYPERTENSION

Experimental and human studies demonstrate that control of systemic hypertension can slow the rate of progression of renal disease substantially. Recent evidence indicates that target blood pressure levels should be lower than recommended for the general population (<130/80). Control of hypertension with the use of myriad agents can benefit the patient with renal failure. However, as indicated previously, reduction in intraglomerular hypertension may be the most important factor underlying the benefits from blood pressure control. Therefore, when possible, treatment with ACEIs, ARBs, or the combination of these agents should be first-line antihypertensive therapy in these patients. Patients who do not tolerate these drugs might benefit from administration of non-dihydropyridine calcium channel blockers. In patients with proteinuria, even if blood pressure is controlled or they are normotensive, the doses of ACEIs or ARBs should be raised to levels even greater than recommended to reduce urine protein excretion to levels less than 500 mg. This reduction in proteinuria is the most optimal in protecting the kidney.

Potentially serious complications with ACEIs or ARBs include acute reduction in GFR and hyperkalemia. If these complications occur, a reduction in dose or even discontinuation of these agents might be required. It is recommended that these agents be continued even when GFR is less than 20 mL/min. Given the potential severity of these complications, patients should be monitored closely.

## PROTEIN RESTRICTION

The benefits of protein restriction in preventing progression are unclear, but it has suggested that reducing protein intake to 0.8 to 1.0 g/kg body weight of high biologic value is beneficial. Others have indicated that 0.6 g/kg body weight should be used. In patients with

## CURRENT THERAPY

The recommendations for the treatment of patients with renal failure is as follows:

| Recommendation | Goal |
|---|---|
| Control BP | 130/80 mm Hg |
| Reduce proteinuria by administering angiotensin converting enzyme inhibitors or angiotensin receptor blockers. In some cases both agents may have to be given concomitantly. | Decrease urine protein excretion as low as possible but at least less than 1 g per day. |
| Control phosphate concentrations with phosphate binders with noncalcium containing binders when possible. | Serum phosphate <4.5 mg/dL |
| Prevent hyperparathyroidism with vitamin D or calcimimetics. | Maintain PTH <150 pg/mL |
| Correct anemia with erythropoietin and iron replacement as needed. | Maintain Hg between 11 and 12 mg/dL |
| Administer diuretics to control hypertension and volume overload. | Maintain euvolemia when possible |
| Control serum potassium with dietary restriction, diuretics, and/or potassium exchange resin as necessary. | Maintain serum potassium <5.0 mEq/L |
| Keep protein intake at 0.6 to 0.8 g/kg body weight per day. | Slow progression of renal disease while preventing protein depletion |
| Control metabolic acidosis with administration of sodium citrate (Citra pH). | Maintain serum HCO$_3$ >20 mEq/L |

*Abbreviations:* BP = blood pressure; HCO$_3$ = bicarbonate; Hg = mercury; PTH = parathyroid hormone.

substantial proteinuria, the quantity of protein recommended will have to be adjusted to prevent hypoalbuminemia. Once patients reached later stage 4, protein restriction may be useful to prevent expression of uremic symptoms. Reducing protein intake will have the added benefit of decreasing acid, potassium, and phosphate production.

## CONTROL OF LIPIDS

Control of cholesterol with statins may help prevent progression and should reduce the burden of cardiovascular disease, which remains the most lethal disorder for patients with chronic renal failure. Adherence to the newly proposed aggressive recommendation appears reasonable.

# Measures Designed to Treat Significant Laboratory Abnormalities

### ANEMIA

Patients with renal anemia should be treated with erythropoietin (Procrit). Although this requires subcutaneous injection once per week, newer, long-lasting forms (darbepoetin [Aranesp]) enable patients to be treated every 3 weeks. Because iron stores need to be repleted for anemia to be successfully treated, these should be monitored and iron given. Because of the vagaries of ferritin measurements, we use serum iron and iron binding capacity with the goal of maintaining saturation above 20% and near 30%. At present, the target hemoglobin and hematocrit varies between 11 mg/dL and 12 mg/dL 33 and 36, respectively.

### METABOLIC ACIDOSIS

Controversy exists as to the target value of bicarbonate for patients with chronic renal failure. Some experts recommend raising plasma bicarbonate to levels above 20 mEq/L, whereas others recommend complete normalization of plasma bicarbonate. To properly raise plasma bicarbonate concentration, the deficit should be calculated from the formula:

$$\text{Desired} - \text{prevailing level of plasma bicarbonate} \times 50\% \text{ body weight} = \text{Total bicarbonate deficit.}$$

The deficit should be corrected slowly over several days.

Because patients experience gas when the base is given as bicarbonate, the base is usually administered as Shohl's solution sodium citrate,* the citrate being metabolized to bicarbonate in the liver. Each milliliter of Shohl's solution represents 1 mEq of the base.

### DIVALENT ION METABOLISM

Serum phosphorus is controlled by administration of phosphate binders usually starting with calcium citrate (Citracal) or acetate (PhosLo). If these are not successful or if patients have elevated serum calcium levels, then sevelamar (Renagel) or lanthanum (Fosrenol) can be used alone or in combination with calcium binders. Physicians should aim to maintain serum phosphorus levels below 5 mg/dL and keep serum calcium phosphorus product below 60.

Parathyroid hormone (PTH) levels should be maintained below 150 pg/mL, or less depending on stage; levels associated with proper bone remodeling but not to values observed in patients without kidney disease. Suppression of parathyroid hormone secretion can be achieved by administration of various vitamin D analogues. The recent recognition of the calcium-sensing receptor and development of calcimimetic drugs that are extremely effective in lowering PTH secretion may make using vitamin D compounds obsolete in the future.

### HYPERKALEMIA

As this is the most serious electrolyte disorder encountered, patients should be monitored closely. Serum potassium concentrations should be maintained below 5 mEq/L. If hyperkalemia develops during treatment with ACEIs or ARBs, the doses of these agents should be reduced or discontinued. Diuretic administration, often given for control of hypertension, can help control hyperkalemia, but if it should develop, particularly when GFR falls below 20% of normal, it can be treated with the potassium exchange resin, sodium polystyrene sulfonate (Kayexalate).

*Investigational drug in the United States.

## ELEVATED BLOOD UREA NITROGEN CONCENTRATION

The precise solutes that are retained, which are important for the pathogenesis of the uremic syndrome, are not clear. However, BUN is a marker for other retained solutes and is roughly correlated with development of uremic symptoms. When the BUN is greater than 100 mg/dL and serum creatinine concentration is greater than 8 mg/dL uremic symptoms may develop. These symptoms will often abate merely with protein restriction and reduced production of these compounds. Protein restriction is usually not instituted until GFR is less than 15% to 20% of normal. Prior to that time, it is important to maintain protein intake to keep serum albumin within the normal range.

## VOLUME OVERLOAD

Because salt retention is an essential component of the development of hypertension and underlies volume overload, diuretic administration is usually necessary in the treatment of chronic renal failure. Thiazides frequently used in the treatment of hypertension or volume overload in subjects with normal renal function may not be efficacious once GFR is less than or equal to 33% of normal. Therefore, loop diuretics, such as furosemide (Lasix) or a combined loop and proximal tubule diuretic such as metolozone (Zaroxolyn), are generally indicated. Because the effectiveness of both agents requires access to the tubule lumen, the effective dose is often higher than in those with normal renal function. Once patients are in stage 4 renal failure, use of diuretics is hampered by worsening of renal failure and often must be used cautiously.

## REFERENCES

Beco JA, Bansal VK: Medical nutrition therapy in chronic kidney failure: Integrating clinical practice guidelines. J Am Diet Assoc 2004; 104:404-409.

Clase CM, Garg AX, Kiberd BA: Prevalence of low glomerular filtration rate in nondiabetic Americans: Third National Health and Nutrition Examination Survey (NHANES III). J Am Soc Nephrol 2002;13.

Cleveland DR, Jindal KK, Hirsch DJ, et al: Quality of pre-referral care in patients with chronic renal insufficiency. Am J Kidney Dis 2002;40:30-36.

Curtin RB, Becker B, Kimmel PL, Schatell D: An integrated approach to care for patients with chronic kidney disease. Semin Dial 2003;16:399-402.

Djamali A, Kendziorski C, Brazy PC, Becker BN: Disease progression and outcomes in chronic kidney disease and renal transplantation. Kidney Int 2003;64:1800-1807.

KDOQI Clinical practice guidelines and clinical practice recommendations for diabetes and chronic kidney disease. Am J Kidney Dis 2007;49:S1-S154.

Kopple JD: National Kidney Foundation K/DOQI clinical practice guidelines for nutrition in chronic renal failure. Am J Kidney Dis 2001;37:S66-S70.

Maschio G, Alberti D, Janin G, et al: Effect of the angiotensin-converting-enzyme inhibitor benazepril on the progression of chronic renal insufficiency. N Engl J Med 1996;334:939-945.

Tonelli M, Gill J, Pandeya S, et al: Slowing the progression of chronic renal insufficiency. Can Med Assoc J 2002;166:906-907.

# Malignant Tumors of the Urogenital Tract

Method of
*Michael S. Cookson, MD,
and Sam S. Chang, MD*

## CARCINOMA OF THE PROSTATE

Carcinoma of the prostate is the most common solid malignancy in men and the second leading cause of male cancer mortality in the United States. In 2005, it was estimated there would be 232,090 new cases and 30,350 deaths from prostatic cancer alone. The incidence of prostatic carcinoma increases with age, and this is anticipated to continue to increase for the next 25 years in direct relationship to the aging U.S. population. A familial pattern is identified, and prostatic carcinoma is more common in African Americans than in the white population. A high-fat diet is implicated as a contributing factor in some studies. Hereditary prostatic carcinoma has been identified in approximately 9% of patients and may account for as much as 40% of the early age of onset cancers. In fact, the hereditary prostate cancer gene (HPC1) was identified on the long arm of chromosome 1 and is thought to be intimately related to the development of carcinoma of the prostate.

## Diagnosis

More than 95% of prostatic cancers are adenocarcinomas. Prostatic carcinoma can be identified at autopsy in more than 75% of individuals older than 80 years, yet clinically the risk of being diagnosed is estimated at one in six men. Thus, there is a large discrepancy between the microscopic presence of the disease and clinically significant disease. Most men with early-stage prostatic cancer have no disease-related symptoms. Prostatic cancer and benign prostatic hypertrophy (BPH) may occur simultaneously, but there is no apparent causal relationship. Obstructive voiding symptoms or hematuria may be present. Patients with advanced disease may present with pelvic pain, ureteral obstruction, or bone pain from distant metastasis.

Early detection has allowed more patients to be identified with lower stage clinical disease, and as a result, such men have had higher recurrence-free survival rates after treatment. Recommendations from groups such as the American Urologic Association and American Cancer Society generally include annual screening with serum prostate-specific antigen (PSA) determination and a digital rectal examination (DRE) for all men older than 50 years and for all African American men and men with a family history of prostatic cancer starting at 40 years of age. These recommendations are not uniformly accepted; the U.S. Public Health Service Task Force does not endorse screening for prostatic cancer because of a lack of convincing prospective data that screening has an impact on the prostatic cancer death rate. The goal of screening is to detect clinically significant prostatic cancer in individuals with at least 10 years of life expectancy.

Serum PSA is specific for the prostate but is secreted by both benign and malignant prostatic epithelial cells. PSA may be elevated in men with prostatitis, BPH, or prostatic cancer. PSA values differ somewhat depending on the assay used. In general, a level of less than 4.0 µg/mL is considered normal, and in younger men, a value of greater than 2.5 ng/mL may be considered abnormal. Approximately 25% of prostatic carcinoma may occur despite what is considered a

**CURRENT DIAGNOSIS**

**Carcinoma of the Prostate**

- Average-risk patient offered screening with PSA and DRE at 50 years of age
- High-risk patients with strong family history or African Americans at age 45 years
- Patients with an elevated PSA or abnormal DRE referred for discussion regarding risks, benefits, and alternatives to biopsy of the prostate
- Diagnosis made with transrectal ultrasound-guided biopsy of the prostate
- Staging with bone scan for patients with high-grade tumors (Gleason grade 4 or 5), PSA levels >20 µg/mL, elevated alkaline phosphatase levels, or bone pain

*Abbreviations:* DRE = digital rectal examination; PSA = prostate-specific antigen.

normal PSA level, and in some studies, the incidence of prostatic carcinoma is 15% even when the PSA is less than 2 μg/mL.

Serum PSA occurs in several forms, with the majority bound to a alpha-1-antichymotrypsin and another portion that is unconjugated or free in serum. The relative proportion of the two forms can be used to improve the specificity of PSA testing. A greater proportion of free PSA is seen in men with BPH compared to those with prostatic cancer. In general, the lower the percentage of free fraction, the more likely it is to reflect a diagnosis of cancer, with a percentage of less than 25% most commonly associated with prostatic cancer as compared to higher percentages. Newer tests such as complexed PSA are being used to improve the specificity of PSA testing.

Most often, transrectal ultrasonography (TRUS) is used for imaging and as a guide for biopsy of the prostate. TRUS can distinguish the zonal anatomy of the prostate and is an accurate measure of the size of the prostate. Prostatic cancers typically are located in the peripheral zone and may have a hypoechoic pattern. Because of its lack of sensitivity and specificity, TRUS is not used as a screening test.

The grading of prostatic carcinoma is based on the degree of differentiation of the tumor. This provides important prognostic information. Most often, the Gleason grading system is used. Tumors with a Gleason score of 2 to 4 are usually considered to be well differentiated; 5 to 7, moderately differentiated; and 8 to 10, poorly differentiated. Prognosis is strongly linked to grade and Gleason score. Most cancers found through early detection or screening programs are of an intermediate grade (Gleason score 5 to 7).

Staging of prostatic cancer defines the local, regional, and distant extent of disease. The TNM staging system is used to allow categorization of nonpalpable tumors detected because of PSA or ultrasound abnormalities (stage T1c). The primary staging modality for local disease is DRE. Serum PSA levels correlate only roughly with disease extent. However, bone metastasis is quite uncommon in patients with a PSA of less than 20 μg/mL. Radionucleotide bone scanning is the most sensitive method for detection of bone metastases. Bone scan in the absence of symptoms is not required routinely if the PSA value is less than 10 μg/mL and a Gleason sum of less than or equal to 7. Computed tomography (CT) scanning is not routinely used because grossly positive nodes are detected rarely with clinically localized tumor.

Lymph node staging is important in selecting patients for therapy. CT scanning may show enlarged lymph nodes in patients with high-volume or high-grade primary tumors. Laparoscopic pelvic lymphadenectomy is feasible and can provide adequate sampling of the pelvic lymph nodes among those patients not selecting surgery. More commonly, lymph node dissection is performed through an open incision immediately prior to radical prostatectomy.

## Treatment

The optimal therapy for localized prostatic cancer is controversial and must be individualized. For men with a life expectancy of less than 10 years, observation alone may be appropriate. Also, some men choose active surveillance rather than initial treatment but later opt for treatment when clinical evidence indicates worsening disease. Surgery and radiation therapy are the most commonly used treatments. For organ-confined tumors, the 15-year disease-free survival rates are greater than 90% for patients treated with surgery. Moreover, the survival outcome is similar after radiation therapy or surgery; however, randomized comparisons among similarly staged patients are lacking. Brachytherapy involves the use of radioactive seeds (iodine 125 or palladium 103) placed into the prostate. This is also a valid option, with similar long-term disease-free survival in low- and intermediate-risk patients. High-dose radiation (HDR) therapy is also an emerging treatment option that allows high doses of radiation therapy to be administered in a relatively short period of time. Cryotherapy (i.e., freezing of the prostate) is also approved in the treatment of men with prostatic carcinoma, but long-term outcomes are not available.

Radical prostatectomy (RP) may be performed via an open surgical approach or by a laparoscopic technique. Most commonly, it is

## CURRENT THERAPY

### Carcinoma of the Prostate

- Treatment is generally offered to men with at least a 10-y life expectancy.
- Treatment options for clinically localized T1c and T2 tumors include active surveillance/watchful waiting, radiation therapy (both external and brachytherapy), and surgery (open and laparoscopic).
- Treatment for locally advanced tumors T3/T4 include surgery and external radiation in combination with androgen-deprivation therapy (ADT).
- Treatment for patients with metastatic disease N1–2 or M1 is generally palliative with ADT.
- Follow-up includes symptom checks with history, physical examination, and PSA monitoring every 6 months for 2 years and then annually. Any abnormalities may be more fully evaluated with appropriate imaging.

*Abbreviations:* PSA = prostate-specific antigen.

performed via open surgery through a retropubic approach, although some are performed through a perineal incision. Laparoscopic and robot-assisted RPs are being performed with a reduction in blood loss and seemingly comparable oncologic results as compared to open surgery. These minimally invasive techniques may have the potential for improved functional outcomes. In patients who were sexually active before therapy, potency can be retained in nearly 40% to 70% by preservation of the neurovascular bundles. In patients with organ-confined disease, there is an excellent prognosis, with a life expectancy similar to men without prostatic cancer. In patients with positive surgical margins or positive lymph nodes, adjuvant radiation and hormonal therapy may be used, respectively.

Serum PSA should be undetectable after radical prostatectomy because all PSA-producing cells are removed. After radiation therapy, superior results are achieved in patients in whom the PSA level decreases to less than 1 μg/mL. An increasing serum PSA is evidence of tumor recurrence. There is controversy about when to initiate hormonal therapy in men with a rising PSA level after treatment, although several studies suggest early hormonal therapy may be of benefit among those with more aggressive tumors.

Prostatic cancer is a partially androgen-dependent disease. Therefore, the primary treatment for metastatic carcinoma of the prostate is androgen deprivation. Suppression of serum testosterone can be achieved by orchiectomy. Alternatively, medical therapy may be considered. Luteinizing hormone-releasing hormone (LHRH) analogues effectively suppress testosterone to the castrate range within 1 month of administration. LHRH analogues are associated with few serious side effects but do cause vasomotor hot flashes in approximately two thirds of patients. Loss of libido and impotence are also a consequence of treatment.

The median response to hormonal therapy in patients with metastatic disease is approximately 18 to 24 months. After that time, disease progression often occurs and ultimately progresses to death. Once the cancer fails to respond to hormonal therapy, the patient usually dies of the disease, although survival rates of greater than 40 months are reported. Recently, published trials have documented improved survival with docetaxel (Taxotere) chemotherapy among patients with androgen-independent prostatic cancer (AIPC) treatments. In addition, mitoxantrone (Novantrone) is now approved for palliative relief for symptomatic bone pain from AIPC. Radiation can also be effective palliation for isolated sites of bone metastasis. The mechanisms through which prostatic carcinoma escapes hormonal control and achieves androgen independence is an area of intense research.

# TUMORS OF THE RENAL PARENCHYMA

Malignant tumors of the renal parenchyma are either primary or metastatic. Among the primary renal lesions, the tumors may be either malignant or benign. The most common malignant tumor is renal cell carcinoma (RCC), whereas other tumor types such as papillary, collecting duct carcinoma, medullary carcinoma, and sarcomas occur infrequently. The most common benign renal tumors are angiomyolipomas and oncocytomas, the latter of which is often indistinguishable from malignant lesions on radiographic imaging. Metastatic lesions such as lung, breast, and ovary may occur, and lymphoma may be present in the kidney.

# RENAL CELL CARCINOMA

RCC is the most common primary neoplasm of the kidney and accounts for greater than 85% of all primary renal cancers. In the United States, an estimated 36,160 new cases are diagnosed, and approximately 12,660 patients die of the disease each year. Renal cell carcinoma represents approximately 3% of all adult malignancies. It is a tumor that usually occurs in adults between 40 and 60 years of age, although it is reported in younger age groups. It has a 2:1 male-to-female preponderance and a well-documented association with von Hippel-Lindau disease.

RCCs arise from the proximal convoluted tubules. The most consistent chromosomal changes in RCC are deletions and translocations of the short arm of chromosome 3. No specific agent is implicated as the cause of RCC. Tobacco smoking poses an approximately twofold relative risk for developing kidney cancer. Patients with end-stage renal disease (ESRD) with acquired cystic disease of the kidney (ACDK) have an increased risk of RCC as well. Of these patients, RCC develops in 1% to 2%, with younger dialysis patients having the greatest risk. Renal ultrasound is recommended in these patients annually, with CT scans for more complex cysts.

## Diagnosis

Hematuria is the single most common sign associated with renal cell carcinoma; it occurs in 29% to 60% of cases. Flank pain and a palpable mass occur next most frequently, but the classic triad of hematuria, flank pain, and a palpable abdominal mass is reported in only 10% of cases. Other common signs and symptoms are fever, anemia, and elevated sedimentation rate. Although serum lactate dehydrogenase and alkaline phosphatase may be elevated, there are no reliable tumor markers for RCC. RCCs can present only with nonspecific symptoms such as weight loss, fever, or weakness. Most, however, are asymptomatic and are detected incidentally on radiographic imaging.

TNM staging is currently the most commonly used system to determine the extent of the primary lesion, involvement of contiguous structures, vascular involvement, and whether the tumor has metastasized.

## CURRENT DIAGNOSIS

**Renal Cell Carcinoma**

- Hematuria is the single most common sign; occurring in up to 60% of cases. Flank pain and palpable mass occur next most frequently, but the classic triad of hematuria, flank pain, and a palpable abdominal mass occurs in only 10%. Other common signs and symptoms are fever, anemia, and elevated sedimentation rate.
- Most are asymptomatic and detected incidentally on radiographic imaging (renal ultrasound, computed tomography scan, or magnetic resonance imaging).

It allows for a distinction between venous involvement and nodal invasion and stratifies the extent of each stage. RCCs often involve the renal vein and vena cava and may even extend into the right atrium. Five-year survival rates for stages T1N0M0 (less than 7 cm) and T2N0M0 (more than 7 cm) are 80% to 90%, for stages T3N0M0 40% to 60%, and N1–3 and M1 are 10% to 20%.

## Treatment

Radical nephrectomy is the primary treatment of RCC. This classic procedure removes the kidney en bloc within Gerota's fascia along with the ipsilateral adrenal gland and lymph nodes. Radical nephrectomy traditionally is performed as an open procedure (flank, transabdominal, or thoracoabdominal incision). Radical nephrectomy has evolved, with adrenalectomy performed for upper pole tumors, very large tumors, or lesions that directly extend into the adrenal gland. If the RCC extends into the inferior vena cava, open as compared to laparoscopic nephrectomy is usually the preferred approach. Rarely, cardiopulmonary bypass is needed to remove the entire tumor thrombus, which is particularly important for those thrombi that extend above the level of the diaphragm. Laparoscopic radical nephrectomy, both hand assisted and pure laparoscopic, is equally efficacious as compared to open surgery and is potentially less morbid, allowing patients a faster recovery.

A partial nephrectomy is performed in patients with solitary kidneys, in those with bilateral RCC, and in patients with compromised renal function. It is also generally agreed that partial nephrectomy or tumor enucleation may be used in patients with lesions 4 cm or less and a normal contralateral kidney, with local recurrence rates less than 5%. Like radical nephrectomy, laparoscopic techniques are emerging as viable alternatives to open surgical removal. In addition, there is an emergence of minimally invasive approaches that will likely compete with partial nephrectomy in the near future. These include radiofrequency ablation and cryotherapy, which may effectively treat smaller lesions under radiologic guidance, thus reducing or eliminating the need for surgery.

Up to 25% of patients initially seen with symptoms have metastatic disease. Sites of metastasis in decreasing frequency include the

## CURRENT THERAPY

**Renal Cell Carcinoma**

- Treatment for resectable masses is almost always surgical—either radical or partial nephrectomy. Both radical and partial nephrectomy may be done via an open or laparoscopic approach.
- Partial nephrectomy is performed in patients with solitary kidneys, bilateral renal cell carcinoma, and compromised renal insufficiency. Partial nephrectomy or enucleation may be used in patients with lesions ≤4 cm and a normal contralateral kidney, with local recurrence rates of <5%.
- Minimally invasive approaches that are emerging include radiofrequency ablation and cryotherapy, which may effectively treat smaller lesions under radiologic guidance, thus reducing or eliminating the need for surgery.
- Up to 25% of patients have metastatic disease at diagnosis. Sites of metastasis in decreasing frequency include the lungs, lymph nodes, liver, bone, and adrenal gland.
- Chemotherapy and radiation have little to no survival benefit, with radiation only palliating painful metastasis.
- The mainstay of treatment is immunotherapy with 5-year survival rates of 10%–20%.
- Emerging evidence suggests an improved survival for those undergoing nephrectomy prior to immunotherapy.

lungs, lymph nodes, liver, bone, and adrenal gland. Chemotherapy and radiation have little to no survival benefit, with radiation only palliating painful metastasis. The mainstay of treatment is immunotherapy, with 5-year survival rates of 10% to 20%. Emerging evidence suggests an improved survival in those undergoing nephrectomy prior to immunotherapy.

# BENIGN RENAL TUMORS

Benign solid tumors of the kidney are encountered occasionally. An angiomyolipoma can usually be diagnosed by the characteristic appearance of fat within the lesion on CT scan. An angiomyolipoma may occur as an isolated phenomenon or in association with tuberous sclerosis. Tuberous sclerosis is a disease characterized by mental retardation, epilepsy, and adenoma sebaceum. Approximately 50% of patients with tuberous sclerosis develop angiomyolipomas, and many are bilateral and multifocal. The management of angiomyolipomas is controversial. In asymptomatic lesions smaller than 4 cm, observation with annual imaging is reasonable. In patients with an acute bleeding episode, angioinfarction may be used to stabilize the patient. In symptomatic lesions or lesions greater than 4 cm, surgical excision is considered the standard therapy.

Oncocytomas are benign renal tumors that account for between 5% and 10% of solid renal lesions. Renal oncocytomas are more difficult to differentiate from RCCs but usually are round, of uniform density, and may have a central scar or spoke-wheel appearance on CT scan. From a practical standpoint, renal oncocytomas are a pathologic diagnosis, and characteristic masses should be considered to be malignant until proven otherwise. Histologically, they are characterized by eosinophilic granular cells. The cell of origin is thought to be that of distal renal tubules.

## Metastatic Renal Lesions

Lung cancer is the most common solid tumor to metastasize to the kidney, although lymphoma and ovarian, bowel, and breast tumors are also seen. Lymphoma of the kidney is almost always a metastatic manifestation of a systemic disease, and therefore surgical treatment is rarely indicated in the absence of symptoms. However, approximately 15% of renal lymphomas present as solitary masses. It is a challenge to differentiate these tumors from renal cell carcinoma preoperatively.

 **CURRENT DIAGNOSIS**

**Benign Renal Tumors**

- Angiomyolipomas are diagnosed by the characteristic appearance of fat within the lesion on computed tomography (CT) scan.
- Angiomyolipomas may occur as an isolated phenomenon or in association with tuberous sclerosis.
- Tuberous sclerosis is characterized by mental retardation, epilepsy, and adenoma sebaceum. Approximately 50% of patients with tuberous sclerosis develop angiomyolipomas, and many are bilateral and multifocal.
- Oncocytomas are benign renal tumors that account for between 5% and 10% of solid renal lesions.
- Oncocytomas are more difficult to differentiate from RCC but usually are round and of uniform density; they may have a central scar or spoke-wheel appearance on CT scan.
- Oncocytomas are a pathologic diagnosis characterized by eosinophilic granular cells. These masses should be considered malignant until proven otherwise.

 **CURRENT THERAPY**

**Benign Renal Tumors**

- The management is controversial. In asymptomatic lesions <4 cm, observation with annual imaging is reasonable.
- In patients with acute bleeding, angioinfarction may stabilize the patient. In symptomatic lesions or lesions >4 cm, surgical excision is considered standard therapy.

# TUMORS OF THE RENAL PELVIS/URETER

Tumors of the renal pelvis account for approximately 10% of all renal tumors and approximately 5% of all urothelial tumors. Ureteral tumors are even less common, representing approximately 25% of upper tract urothelial tumors. Ureteral tumors are three times more common in men than in women and twice as common in whites as in blacks. Cigarette smoking is strongly associated with an increased risk of developing upper tract transitional cell carcinomas. Additionally, analgesic abuse and cyclophosphamide are associated with an increased risk.

The risk of upper tract tumors is approximately 4% among patients with bladder cancer. However, in patients with carcinoma in situ and high-grade urothelial lesions, the risk may approach 20% with long-term follow-up. Conversely, patients with upper tract tumors have a 40% to 70% risk of developing bladder cancer. Therefore, patients with upper tract tumors should undergo periodic surveillance cystoscopy. The incidence of bilateral upper tract tumors is 2% to 5%. In addition to

 **CURRENT DIAGNOSIS**

**Tumors of the Renal Pelvis/Ureter**

- Renal pelvic tumors account for 10% of all renal tumors and approximately 5% of all urothelial tumors.
- Ureteral tumors are even less common, occurring approximately 25% of the incidence of renal pelvic tumors.
- These tumors are three times more common in men than in women.
- Cigarette smoking is strongly associated with an increased risk. Additionally, analgesic abuse and cyclophosphamide are implicated.
- Most common presenting symptom is hematuria.
- Diagnostic workup usually includes an IVP and cytologic examination of the urine followed by cystoscopy.
- Cytologic examination of the urine may give a false-negative result in up to 85% of patients with a low-grade lesion.
- 50%–75% of patients have a filling defect on IVP. The differential diagnosis includes a tumor, blood clot, fungal ball, sloughed papilla, and radiolucent stone.
- The risk of upper tract tumors is approximately 4% among those patients with bladder cancer. In patients with CIS and high-grade lesions, the risk may approach 20%.
- Patients with upper tract tumors have a 40%–70% risk of developing bladder cancer.

*Abbreviations:* CIS = carcinoma in situ; IVP = intravenous pyelogram.

transitional cell carcinomas, squamous cell carcinomas and adenocarcinomas are included in the differential diagnosis; particularly in a patient with a history of recurrent urinary tract infections or staghorn calculi.

## Diagnosis

As with renal cell carcinomas, the most common presenting symptom of tumors of the renal pelvis/ureter is hematuria. In patients with normal renal function, the diagnostic workup usually includes an intravenous pyelogram (IVP) and urine cytologic examination followed by cystoscopy. However, it must be kept in mind that a voided urine cytologic examination may be falsely negative in up to 85% of patients with a low-grade lesion. Approximately 50% to 75% of patients have a filling defect on IVP. The differential diagnosis includes a tumor, blood clot, fungal ball, sloughed papilla, and radiolucent stone. A retrograde ureteropyelogram may be helpful in documenting the persistence of the filling defect; however, ureteroscopy with biopsy or brushings may be diagnostic. In renal pelvic defects, a noncontrast CT scan with 3-mm cuts through the kidney is usually able to differentiate a stone from a soft-tissue mass because even radiolucent stones on standard urography are opaque on CT scan. The TNM system is recommended for staging.

## Treatment

Patients with low-grade, low-stage lesions do well with conservative or radical treatment. Patients with intermediate- or high-grade tumors are best managed with aggressive surgical resection. Solitary low-grade and low-stage upper ureteral tumors may be managed with segmental resection. Similar distal ureteral tumors can be managed with distal ureterectomy and ureteroneocystostomy. Treatment of high-grade and high-stage tumors is nephroureterectomy with removal of a cuff of the bladder at the ureteral orifice because of the high incidence of ipsilateral ureteral orifice and bladder involvement. This can be accomplished through a single extended flank or midline incision but is often performed through two incisions. Currently, hand-assisted laparoscopic nephroureterectomy is the preferred surgical approach, allowing for complete tumor removal through a single incision and offers the advantage of quicker convalescence. Successful endoscopic management including percutaneous and retrograde approaches is reported in selected cases.

# CARCINOMA OF THE BLADDER

## Transitional Cell Carcinoma of the Bladder

Bladder carcinoma is the fifth most common malignancy in the United States with more than 63,210 new cases annually. It is almost three times more common among men than women, in whom it is the fourth most common cancer. Because of frequent recurrences, particularly among patients with superficial tumors, bladder cancer is the second most prevalent cancer. Bladder cancer is the fifth most common cause of cancer deaths among men. It is approximately four times more prevalent among cigarette smokers and is associated with known carcinogens including occupational exposures such as those of rubber and oil refinery workers. In addition, patients treated with cyclophosphamide (Cytoxan) have up to a ninefold increased risk of developing bladder cancer. This is believed to be secondary to acrolein, a urinary metabolite of cyclophosphamide.

Approximately 90% of bladder malignancies are transitional cell carcinomas. Of these, 70% of tumors are papillary, 10% are sessile, and 20% are mixed. Approximately 20% to 25% of noninvasive tumors progress to muscle invasion during follow-up. However, of patients with muscular invasive bladder cancer, approximately 80% to 90% have invasion at the time of initial presentation. A strong correlation exists between tumor grade and stage; most well-differentiated tumors are superficial and most poorly differentiated tumors are invasive. Carcinoma in situ (CIS) is a poorly differentiated transitional cell carcinoma that is confined to the urothelium. CIS may be found as a solitary or multifocal process and is found in association with invasive carcinoma in approximately 25% of cases. It is associated with a poor prognosis. Between 10% and 20% of patients treated with cystectomy for diffuse CIS are found to have microscopic muscle-invasive disease.

## Diagnosis

Gross painless hematuria is a common presenting sign of bladder cancer. However, approximately 20% of patients may present with only microscopic hematuria. Irritative voiding symptoms such as frequency and urgency may also suggest a malignancy, particularly CIS. Patients suspected of bladder cancer should undergo an evaluation of their upper tracts (IVP or CT scan), cystoscopy, and cytologic examination of the urine. Transurethral biopsy or resection confirms the diagnosis.

# Treatment

Management of bladder carcinoma depends on tumor stage. The TNM system is recommended for staging. For most superficial bladder carcinomas, transurethral resection of the tumor is often the only treatment required. However, for CIS or high-grade superficial tumors, tumors that involve the lamina propria (stage T1), and rapidly recurrent tumors, treatment with intravesical agents such as thiotepa (Thioplex), doxorubicin (Adriamycin), and mitomycin C (Mutamycin)[1] or intravesical bacillus Calmette-Guérin (BCG, Tice) may be indicated.

---

[1]Not FDA approved for this indication.

---

 **CURRENT THERAPY**

**Carcinoma of the Bladder**

- Treatment depends on tumor stage.
- Superficial bladder (Ta) cancers are managed with transurethral resection.
- CIS or high-grade stage Ta, tumors that involve the lamina propria (stage T1), and recurrent tumors are managed with transurethral resection and intravesical therapy such as thiotepa (Thioplex), doxorubicin (Adriamycin), and mitomycin C (Mutamycin)[1] or intravesical bacillus Calmette-Guérin (BCG, Tice).
- Bladder surveillance is mandatory because the recurrence rate in the bladder may be as high as 50% at 5 years.
- Surveillance protocols include cystoscopy and urinary cytologic examinations every 3 months for the first year, every 4 months for the second year, semiannually in year 3, and annually thereafter.
- Periodic evaluation of the upper tracts should be performed as well.
- In superficial tumors that progress in stage or fail conservative therapy and in those that invade the bladder muscle (stages T2–3), a radical cystectomy and urinary diversion is the treatment of choice.
- Urinary diversion may be either incontinent (conduit) or continent (orthotopic or continent cutaneous).
- Five-year survival rates are 85%–60% after cystectomy for stages T2a and T2b, respectively. For stage T3a and T3b tumors, the 5-year survival decreases to 60% and 40%, respectively, whereas patients with node-positive disease have a 5-year survival of <30%.
- Patients with T2–T4 disease may be offered either neoadjuvant or adjuvant chemotherapy. There have been reports of modest survival advantages (<10%) using MVAC in the neoadjuvant setting.
- Patients with M1 disease are generally treated with chemotherapy as well.
- The standard regimen over the past decade has been methotrexate (Trexall),[1] vinblastine (Velban),[1] doxorubicin (Adriamycin), and cisplatin (Platinol) (MVAC); however, durable complete response rates are <15%.
- Newer agents such as gemcitabine (Gemzar) along with cisplatin appear to offer similar response rates and reduced toxicity.

---

[1]Not FDA approved for this indication.
*Abbreviations:* CIS = carcinoma in situ.

MVAC

---

Bladder surveillance is mandatory because the recurrence rate in the bladder may be as high as 50% at 5 years. Surveillance protocols include cystoscopy and urinary cytologies every 3 months for the first year, every 4 months for the second year, semiannually in year 3, and annually thereafter. Periodic evaluation of the upper tract should be performed to rule out the presence of carcinoma of the bladder in that area.

The risk of progression to muscle invasive disease is relatively low (less than 10%) for stage Ta tumors but increases as tumor stage advances (stage T1) or with high-grade lesions. For superficial tumors that progress in stage or fail conservative therapy, and in those that invade the bladder muscle (stage T2 to T3), a radical cystectomy is the treatment of choice. In addition, a thorough lymphadenectomy is performed at the time of surgery; there have been reports of improved survival based on the completeness of the dissection.

Each year there are an estimated 13,180 deaths in the United States from bladder cancer. Five-year survival rates are approximately 85% to 60% after cystectomy for stages T2a and T2b, respectively. For stage T3a and T3b tumors, the 5-year survival decreases to 60% and 40%, whereas patients with node-positive disease have a 5-year survival of less than 30%. Adjuvant chemotherapy is generally offered to patients at high risk for failure (pathologic stages T3b, T4, and N1/2 disease). The standard regimen over the past decade has been methotrexate (Trexall),[1] vinblastine (Velban),[1] doxorubicin (Adriamycin), and cisplatin (Platinol) (MVAC); however, durable complete response rates have been less than 15%. There have been recent reports of modest survival advantages (less than 10%) using MVAC in the neoadjuvant setting. Newer agents such as gemcitabine (Gemzar)[1] along with cisplatin appear to offer similar response rates and reduced toxicity.

Urinary diversion may be accomplished with an ileal or colon conduit, which requires wearing a collection appliance. A continent cutaneous diversion may be created; most often using the right colon with a tapered and a catheterizable efferent limb of ileum (Indiana pouch) or with creation of a nipple valve (Koch pouch). Approximately 50% of cystectomy patients undergo continent diversion. An orthotopic neobladder allows creation of a reservoir using detubularized ileum or colon with direct anastomosis to the urethra. With the development of orthotopic urinary diversion, functional status and quality of life among patients following cystectomy has improved significantly.

## Adenocarcinoma of the Bladder

Adenocarcinomas account for less than 2% of bladder cancers. They are classified into three groups: primary bladder, urachal, and metastatic. Most adenocarcinomas are poorly differentiated and invasive. They are commonly associated with cystitis glandularis rather than CIS. Adenocarcinomas also are found in association with bladder augmentations. Adenocarcinoma is the most common type of cancer in patients with bladder exstrophy. Radical cystectomy with pelvic lymphadectomy is the treatment of choice.

## Squamous Cell Carcinoma of the Bladder

Squamous cell carcinoma accounts for approximately 6% of bladder cancers in the United States but more than 75% of bladder cancers in Egypt. Chronic bladder inflammation, as occurs with chronic indwelling Foley catheters, recurrent bladder infections, or bladder diverticula, is associated with an increase risk of squamous cell carcinoma. Approximately 80% of squamous cell carcinomas in Egypt are associated with *Schistosoma haematobium* infestation. These cancers are known as bilharzial bladder cancers and occur in patients 10 to 20 years younger than those affected with transitional cell carcinoma. The prognosis for squamous cell carcinoma is generally poor, and radical cystectomy is the standard treatment for patients who are surgical candidates. Chemotherapy, particularly regimens used in transitional cell carcinoma, is not effective in squamous cell carcinoma. The benefit of neoadjuvant radiation therapy prior to radical cystectomy is unproved in patients with squamous cell carcinoma with the possible exception of bilharzial cancers.

# URETHRAL CARCINOMA

## Diagnosis

Urethral carcinoma is the only urologic malignancy that is more common in women than men. It usually occurs after 60 years of age. Although the etiology remains undetermined, approximately 50% of cases are associated with urethral stricture. A patient should be evaluated for urethral carcinoma when a urethral mass is palpable, obstruction does not respond to conventional stricture management, a urethral abscess and/or fistula occurs, hematuria is present, or inguinal adenopathy becomes evident. The treatment of the primary tumor is surgical excision. Urethrectomy is performed via a perineal incision. Proximal tumors of the bulbar urethra are managed with cystoprostatectomy and en bloc urethrectomy.

Although the etiology of female urethral carcinoma remains obscure, there is an association with urethral malakoplakia and urethral caruncles. Most patients are white and older than 50 years. The usual presenting symptom is a papillary or fungating urethral mass and hematuria.

## Treatment

For tumors of the proximal urethra or in cases of extension into adjacent structures, cystectomy with en bloc urethrectomy and anterior vaginectomy along with pelvic lymphadenectomy are usually required. Radiation therapy also provides local control in selected cases. In advanced cases, multimodality treatment with chemotherapy and either surgical excision or radiation therapy provides the best chance for cure, although to date no specific regimen has emerged as standard treatment.

# PENILE CANCER

## Diagnosis

Penile cancer is relatively rare in the United States. Poor personal hygiene and retained phimotic foreskin are implicated in the etiology of penile carcinoma. Penile cancer is extremely rare in men circumcised at birth. Squamous cell carcinoma of the penis occurs most commonly in the sixth decade. The symptoms are related to ulceration, necrosis, suppuration, and hemorrhage of the penile lesion. The clinical evaluation of patients with penile cancer includes physical examination with palpation of the inguinal region, liver function tests, chest radiograph, CT of the abdomen and pelvis, and bone scan.

## Treatment

The TNM stage is based primarily on depth of invasion and usually dictates treatment. Small penile cancers limited to the prepuce can be treated by circumcision alone. Partial penectomy with at least a 1-cm margin of normal tissue is used to treat smaller (2 to 5 cm) distal penile tumors. The remaining penis should be long enough to permit voiding in the standing position. The 5-year cure rate for patients treated with partial penectomy is 70% to 80%. Larger distal penile lesions or proximal tumors require total penectomy and perineal urethrostomy. If the scrotum, pubis, or abdominal wall is involved, radical en bloc excision may be necessary.

Many patients have inguinal lymphadenopathy at presentation. However, inguinal lymph node enlargement before excision of the primary tumor may be the result of infection and not metastatic disease. Clinical assessment of the inguinal region thus should be delayed 4 to 6 weeks during which time the patient is treated with antibiotics. If inguinal lymphadenopathy persists or develops, there is a high likelihood of metastatic disease, and ilioinguinal lymphadenectomy should be performed. However, if inguinal lymphadenopathy resolves, prophylactic lymph node dissection may not be necessary. Radiation of the primary tumor and regional lymph nodes is an alternative to surgery in patients with small (2 cm or less) low-stage tumors.

# TESTICULAR CANCER

Malignant disease of the testes can be divided into germinal neoplasms, which includes seminomatous and nonseminomatous germ cell tumors (NSGCTs) and secondary neoplasms. Ninety-five percent of tumors originating in the testis are germ cell tumors. Fewer than 10% of all germ cell tumors arise from extragonadal primary sites. The mediastinum and retroperitoneum are the most common extragonadal sites. Testicular cancer, although relatively rare, represents the most common malignancy in men in the 15- to 35-year-old age group, with 8010 new cases occurring annually.

Testicular cancer has become one of the most curable solid neoplasms and serves as a paradigm for the multimodal treatment of malignancies. The dramatic improvement in survival resulting from the combination of effective diagnostic techniques, improved tumor markers, effective multidrug chemotherapeutic regimens, and modifications of surgical technique has led to a decrease in patient mortality from greater than 50% before 1970 to less than 10% currently.

Germ cell tumors are seen principally in the white population. Recent data show a ratio of approximately 5:1 in white versus black individuals, and a report from the U.S. military showed a relative incidence of 40:1. The cause of germ cell tumors is unknown. Familial clustering is observed, particularly among siblings. Cryptorchidism and Klinefelter's syndrome are predisposing factors in the development of germ cell tumors arising from the testis and mediastinum, respectively. Orchidopexy performed before puberty may not reduce the risk of germ cell tumors but improves the ability to observe the testis.

## Diagnosis

A painless testicular mass is pathognomonic of a primary testicular tumor. This occurs in a minority of patients. The majority of testicular tumors present with diffuse testicular pain, swelling, hardness, or some combination of these findings. Because infectious epididymo-orchitis is more common than a testicular tumor, a trial of antibiotics is often undertaken. If testicular discomfort does not abate or the findings do not revert to normal within 2 to 4 weeks, testicular sonography is indicated. A radical inguinal orchiectomy with ligation of the spermatic cord at the internal ring is required for all patients with suspected testicular tumors.

Regional metastasis first appears in the retroperitoneal lymph nodes below the renal vessels. Right testicular tumors usually metastasize to nodes between the aorta and inferior vena cava (interaortocaval nodes), and left testicular tumors to nodes lateral to the aorta (para-aortic). Left supraclavicular adenopathy and pulmonary nodules may occur with or without retroperitoneal disease. CT scan of the abdomen and pelvis and chest radiography are required. Lymph nodes in the

## CURRENT DIAGNOSIS

**Testicular Cancer**

- Testicular cancer, although relatively rare, represents the most common malignancy in males in the 15- to 35-year-old age group, with 8010 new cases annually.
- Usually presents as a painless enlarging testicular mass.
- Malignant disease of the testes can be divided into germinal neoplasms, which includes seminomatous and nonseminomatous germ cell tumors, and secondary neoplasms.
- 95% of tumors originating in the testis are germ cell tumors. Fewer than 10% of all germ cell tumors arise from extragonadal primary sites. The mediastinum and retroperitoneum are the most common extragonadal sites.
- Testicular cancer is one of the few neoplasms associated with accurate serum markers, β-hCG, and AFP.

primary lymphatic drainage areas (landing zones) of their respective affected testicle that measure between 1 and 2 cm are involved by germ cell tumors in approximately 70% of cases. CT imaging of the chest is required if mediastinal, hilar, or lung parenchymal disease is suspected.

## Treatment

Testicular cancer is one of the few neoplasms associated with accurate serum markers, human β-chorionic gonadotropin (β-hCG), and α-fetoprotein (AFP). These accurate tumor markers allow careful follow-up and intervention earlier in the course of disease. AFP production is restricted to NSGCTs, specifically embryonal carcinoma and yolk sac tumor. Patients with an increased AFP and the finding of pure seminoma on pathologic examination of the orchiectomy specimen should be treated as a NSGCT. Increased serum concentrations of β-hCG may be observed in both seminomatous and nonseminomatous tumors. Increased concentrations of β-hCG are seen in 40% to 60% of patients with metastatic NSGCT and 15% to 20% of patients with metastatic seminomas. A third serum marker, lactate dehydrogenase, is less specific but has independent prognostic value in patients with advanced germ cell tumors. Serum lactate dehydrogenase concentrations are also increased in approximately 60% of patients with NSGCT and 80% of those with seminomatous germ cell tumors.

Increased concentrations of α-fetoprotein, β-hCG, or both without radiographic or clinical findings imply active disease and are sufficient reason to initiate treatment if likely causes of false-positive results are ruled out. The serum half-lives of α-fetoprotein and β-hCG are 5 to 7 days and 30 hours, respectively. Slow clearance suggests residual active disease.

Histologically, seminoma is the most common germ cell tumor, and it is initially considered to be good risk because of its favorable response to treatment. Therapy for low-stage (stages 1, 2a, or 2b) seminomas following radical inguinal orchiectomy is irradiation to the retroperitoneal and ipsilateral pelvic lymph nodes. Relapse recurs in approximately 4% of patients with stage 1 seminomas and 10% of patients with stage 2a or 2b seminomas. Chemotherapy cures more than 90% of patients who have a relapse after radiation therapy. Thus, approximately 99% of patients with low-stage seminomas are cured.

NSGCTs include embryonal cell carcinoma, choriocarcinoma, yolk sac carcinoma, teratoma, and mixed germ cell tumors. The rate of cure for patients with NSGCTs in clinical stage 1 exceeds 95%. Twenty percent of patients with stage 1 tumors with no lymphatic or vascular invasion or invasion into the tunica albuginea, spermatic cord, or scrotum are discovered to have regional lymph node or distant metastasis. Surveillance and nerve-sparing retroperitoneal lymph node dissection

## CURRENT THERAPY

### Testicular Cancer

- A radical inguinal orchiectomy with ligation of spermatic cord at the internal ring is required for all patients with suspected testicular tumors.
- Once a diagnosis is made, serum tumor markers are determined before, during, and after treatment.
- Radiographic staging is performed with a CT scan of the chest/abdomen/pelvis.
- Histologically, seminoma is the most common germ cell tumor, and is initially considered good risk because of its generally favorable response to treatment. Therapy for low-stage (stage 1, 2a, or 2b) seminomas following radical inguinal orchiectomy is irradiation to the retroperitoneal and ipsilateral pelvic lymph nodes. Relapse occurs in approximately 4% of patients with stage 1 seminomas and 10% of patients with stage 2a or 2b seminomas. Chemotherapy cures >90% of patients who have a relapse after radiation therapy. Thus, approximately 99% of patients with low-stage seminomas are cured.
- NSGCTs include embryonal cell carcinoma, choriocarcinoma, yolk sac carcinoma, teratoma, and mixed germ cell tumors. The rate of cure for patients with NSGCTs in clinical stage 1 exceeds 95%.
- Surveillance and RPLND are both standard treatment options for this group of patients. Twenty percent of clinical stage 1 NSGCT patients have lymph node involvement, and those with vascular invasion or predominance of embryonal cell carcinoma are at increased risk (50%).
- RPLND is a major abdominal operation in which lymph nodes from the retroperitoneum are removed from the renal hilum down to the level of the common iliac artery, with lateral margins being confined by the ureters.
- Patients found to have node-positive disease are generally recommended for chemotherapy with usually two cycles.
- Patients with persistently increased concentrations of AFP, β-hCG, or both but without other clinical evidence of disease following orchiectomy usually have systemic disease and are treated with chemotherapy.

### Testicular Cancer

- Initial chemotherapy is required in approximately one third of patients with germ cell tumors. Because relapse is frequent in patients with clinical stage 2c disease or in patients with primary retroperitoneal or mediastinal seminomas who receive radiation alone, these patients are treated initially with chemotherapy. Patients also receive initial chemotherapy if they have stage 3 NSGCTs or multifocal retroperitoneal lymph node involvement, lymph nodes >3 cm in diameter, or tumor-related back pain.
- Postchemotherapy RPLND is usually reserved for residual masses (>3 cm) in patients after treatment for seminoma. In NSGCT, the need for postchemotherapy RPLND is controversial. Some advocate surgery in all patients with initial bulky retroperitoneal disease, whereas others advocate observation rather than surgery in patients with >90% shrinkage of retroperitoneal nodes, no residual nodes >1.5 cm, and no teratomatous elements in the primary tumor.
- Owing in part to the multimodality approach to these tumors, 90%–95% of patients are ultimately cured of their disease.

---

*Abbreviations:* AFP = α-fetoprotein; β-hCG = β-chorionic gonadotropin; CT = computed tomography; NSGCT = nonseminomatous germ cell tumor; RPLND = retroperitoneal lymph node dissection.

(RPLND) are both standard treatment options for this group of patients. If patients have stage 1 disease confined to the testes, attention must be paid to the surgical pathology. In any patient with embryonal histology or the presence of lymphovascular invasion or extension beyond the tunica albuginea, RPLND is recommended. The rationale for this treatment stems from a 30% relapse rate in stage 1 patients with these findings.

RPLND is a major abdominal operation in which lymph nodes from the retroperitoneum are removed from the renal hilum down to the level of the common iliac artery, with lateral margins confined by the ureters. In the past, this procedure resulted in lack of ejaculation and infertility in 100% of patients. By performing a modified-template RPLND, the contralateral area of aorta below the inferior mesenteric artery is not manipulated. This maneuver serves to preserve the confluence of sympathetic fibers along the aorta that are responsible for ejaculation, with a 60% to 88% rate of preservation of ejaculation and no reports of recurrence for stage 1 disease. Patients with persistently increased concentrations of α-fetoprotein, β-hCG, or both but without other clinical evidence of disease following orchiectomy usually have systemic disease. These patients should undergo three or four cycles of standard chemotherapy rather than surgery.

Patients with stage 2 NSGCTs are treated initially with either RPLND or chemotherapy depending on the extent of the disease, serum tumor marker concentrations, and the presence or absence of tumor-related symptoms. Asymptomatic patients with solitary retroperitoneal lymph nodes less than 3 cm in diameter as assessed by CT imaging generally undergo retroperitoneal lymph node dissection, whereas bulky stage 2 disease (more than 5 cm) undergo initial chemotherapy. Recurrences within the retroperitoneum are rare after a properly performed operation.

Adjuvant chemotherapy is an important consideration when any lymph node is more than 2 cm in diameter, at least six nodes are involved, or there is extranodal invasion. The majority of patients in this group who relapsed did not receive adjuvant chemotherapy. Although the rate of cure is the same when chemotherapy is withheld until relapse, patients who received adjuvant therapy require fewer cycles of chemotherapy and avoid additional surgery.

Initial chemotherapy is required in approximately one third of patients with germ cell tumors. Because relapse is frequent in patients with clinical stage 2c disease or in patients with primary retroperitoneal or mediastinal seminomas who receive radiation alone, these patients are treated initially with chemotherapy. Patients also receive initial chemotherapy if they have stage 3 NSGCTs or multifocal retroperitoneal lymph node involvement, lymph nodes more than 2 cm in diameter, or tumor-related back pain.

Postchemotherapy RPLND is usually reserved for residual masses (more than 3 cm) in patients after treatment for seminoma. In NSGCT, the need for postchemotherapy RPLND is controversial. Some groups advocate surgery in all patients with initial bulky retroperitoneal disease, whereas others advocate observation rather than surgery in patients with greater than 90% shrinkage of retroperitoneal nodes, with no residual nodes greater than 1.5 cm, and with no teratomatous elements in the primary tumor. There is no debate, however, concerning the need for removal of any significant postchemotherapy residual mass.

The first combination chemotherapy regimens containing cisplatin (Platinol), vinblastine (Velban), and bleomycin (Blenoxane) resulted in complete remission in 70% to 80% of patients with metastatic germ cell tumors. Subsequent studies show that prolonged maintenance chemotherapy was unnecessary, and vinblastine was replaced by etoposide (Vepesid), which is less toxic and probably more efficacious. Serious adverse effects of combination chemotherapy include neuromuscular toxic affects, death from myelosuppression for bleomycin-induced pulmonary fibrosis, and Raynaud's phenomenon.

Leydig cell tumors make up between 1% and 3% of all testicular tumors. Although the majority of cases are recognized in men between 20 and 60 years of age, approximately a fourth are reported before puberty. The prognosis for Leydig cell tumors following radical inguinal orchiectomy is good because of their generally benign nature.

Gonadoblastoma is a rare tumor occurring almost exclusively in patients with some form of gonadal dysgenesis. Gonadoblastomas constitute approximately 0.5% of all testicular neoplasms and occur in all age groups from infancy to beyond 70 years, although the majority occur in individuals younger than 30 years. Radical orchiectomy is the first step in therapy. The high incidence of bilaterality (50%) mandates a contralateral gonadectomy when gonadal dysgenesis is present. The prognosis is excellent for patients with gonadoblastoma.

The most common secondary neoplasm of the testis and the most frequent of all testicular tumors in patients older than 50 years is lymphoma. The median age is approximately 60 years of age. As with lymphomas elsewhere, patients with poorly differentiated lymphocytic types tend to survive longer than those with the histocytic type. Survival is poor with bilateral disease and among patients presenting with lymphoma at other sites who later experience a testicular tumor relapse. However, among those patients with disease apparently confined to the testis, survival appears to be good.

## REFERENCES

Carver BS, Sheinfeld J: Germ cell tumors of the testis. Ann Surg Oncol 2005;12:871.

Cohen HT, McGovern FJ: Renal-cell carcinoma. N Engl J Med 2005;353:2477.

Cooperberg MR, Moul JW, Carroll PR: The changing face of prostate cancer. J Clin Oncol 2005;23:8146.

Jemal A, Murray T, Ward E, et al: Cancer statistics, 2005. CA Cancer J Clin 2005;55:10.

Stein JP, Lieskovsky G, Cote R, et al: Radical cystectomy in the treatment of invasive bladder cancer: Long-term results in 1,054 patients. J Clin Oncol 2001;19:666.

# Management of Urethral Stricture Disease*

Method of
*Andrew C. Peterson, MD*

Urethral strictures are defined as an area of narrowing in the urethra, usually occurring from scar tissue formation. The strictures may occur anywhere in the urethra from the bladder to the meatus of the penis. They are well documented in ancient literature dating from the Greek and Egyptian period. Urethral stricture disease is relatively common today, mostly acquired from injury or infection. Recently, iatrogenic causes, including urologic instrumentation and placement of indwelling catheters, that cause strictures anywhere in the urethra are the most common cause.

The urethra is commonly described as having two sections: the posterior urethra (starting at the bladder neck, including the prostatic urethra and membranous urethra) and the anterior urethra (starting at the bulbar urethra, including the pendulous urethra and the fossa navicularis and meatus). Posterior urethral strictures are commonly caused by trauma with pelvic fractures and concomitant urethral injuries. Anterior urethral injuries commonly result from direct, blunt penile or perineal trauma, instrumentation, catheterization, and infections.

## Diagnosis and Preoperative Evaluation

Obstructive voiding symptoms are the most common complaints causing patients to seek medical attention, including decreased force of stream, hesitancy, urgency, nocturia, and sometimes acute urinary retention.

---

*The views expressed in this article are those of the author and do not reflect the official policy or position of the United States Army, Department of Defense, or the U.S. government.

## CURRENT DIAGNOSIS

- Young men with recurrent so-called prostatitis and epididymitis should be considered for workup of urethral stricture disease.
- Obstructive voiding symptoms are the most common complaints causing patients to seek medical attention for urethral stricture disease.
- The retrograde urethrogram is the key diagnostic study for evaluation of urethral stricture disease.

Urinary tract infections, urethral bleeding, and, rarely, urethrocutaneous fistula and periurethral abscess may develop. Young men diagnosed with recurrent epididymitis and so-called prostatitis should be completely evaluated for urethral strictures because this is often a missed diagnosis in these cases.

Retrograde urethrography (RUG) is the study of choice for diagnosis. An antegrade voiding study through a previously placed suprapubic tube combined with a RUG often helps define the length and complexity of the stricture. Penile ultrasound may also help define the extent of spongiofibrosis and aid in planning for a surgical reconstruction.

Cystourethroscopy allows for identification of the true caliber of a urethral stricture, and a small flexible ureteroscope may be used to determine the length of the stricture and the quality of the proximal urethra. It may be important to examine the bladder through a suprapubic tract as well for concomitant injury and bladder calculi.

Magnetic resonance imaging (MRI) studies can be invaluable in some cases of posterior urethral strictures after pelvic fracture. This is an important study to define the post-traumatic anatomy, allowing the surgeon to plan the reconstructive approach. MRI should always be used in conjunction with RUG and cystogram and not as a sole technique for evaluation.

## Management

After the final diagnosis and staging of the urethral stricture are completed, the choice of treatment depends heavily on location, etiology, and length. Treatment options for urethral strictures continue to include simple dilation, incision of the urethral stricture using endoscopes (urethrotomy), the UroLume stent, and a wide spectrum of reconstructive surgical techniques that include possible use of skin flaps, skin grafts, and more complex reconstructive techniques. Although no single procedure is appropriate for all strictures, dilation and urethrotomy continue to be most commonly employed. However, these interventions have high recurrence rates, and many patients eventually progress to surgical repair.

## CURRENT THERAPY

- Office/clinic dilation of urethral stricture continues to be the most common initial treatment and is often the first treatment attempted.
- Both dilation and internal urethrotomy have equivalent long-term outcomes for the treatment of short urethral strictures.
- Surgical options for urethral stricture disease are based primarily on the location and length of the stricture.
- In treatment of lichen sclerosis, all of the native surrounding genital skin is subject to this disease so the entire affected urethra must often be excised and replaced with extragenital tissue for reconstruction

## DILATION AND URETHROTOMY

Office/clinic dilation of urethral stricture continues to be the most common initial treatment and is often the first treatment attempted. Techniques used in the office include filiforms and followers, serial dilators, and balloon dilation under endoscopic control. Afterward, patients can be taught self-calibration with a soft catheter for ongoing management. Few patients, however, accept this option in the long term.

Visual internal urethrotomy is performed using local, spinal, or general anesthesia and is ideally aided by a guidewire placed through the stricture under direct vision. The incision is made at either the 12 o'clock or at the 3 and 9 o'clock positions with a cold knife, laser, or cautery. Urethrotomy is especially suited for short strictures in the bulbar urethra and has high failure rates for long strictures associated with significant spongiofibrosis and those located in the pendulous urethra.

Although both of these procedures may be curative, most often the patient requires retreatment. Both dilation and internal urethrotomy have equivalent long-term outcomes for the treatment of short urethral strictures. In those who ultimately require formal operative repair, there is not a higher failure rate if that patient first underwent a prior endoscopic treatment. Therefore, this practice of initial treatment of short urethral strictures with repeat dilations or internal urethrotomies may be reasonable.

## UROLUME STENTS

The UroLume stent (American Medical Systems, Minnetonka, MN) is a permanent, self-expanding metal stent that is FDA approved for the treatment of bulbar urethral strictures. Enthusiastically introduced in 1988, postplacement problems, including postvoid dribbling, perineal pain, erectile pain, and recurrent stricture, significantly limited the use of this device. It is helpful to manage recalcitrant anastomotic bladder neck contracture following radical prostatectomy and in the very elderly who may not be able to tolerate an open operative repair of a urethral stricture.

## SURGICAL INTERVENTION

Surgical options for urethral stricture disease are based primarily on the location and length of the stricture. Tissue, including local grafts or flaps from the penis or scrotum and grafts from remote sources such as mouth, thigh, and preauricular areas, often are needed to reconstruct the urethra. Buccal graft harvested from the mouth currently has the most support.

# Management of Strictures in the Pendulous Urethra

Optimal management of strictures of the pendulous urethra consists of onlay flap repairs using penile skin as described by Orandi, Quartey, McAninch, Turner-Warwick, and Mundy. Strictures from lichen sclerosis, however, require significantly different treatment (see later). The stricture is opened on the ventral side of the penis and the incision carried into healthy urethra on either side. It is then patched with an island of skin carried on a vascular pedicle. Although the ideal skin consists of hairless penile skin, island flaps can be made in the longitudinal or a transverse orientation and may reach up to 15 cm in length and 2 cm in width. Even circumcised men invariably have ample penile skin for these flaps.

# Bulbar Strictures

Historically, flap-based repairs and tubularized single-staged graft urethroplasties were often performed for these strictures. However, these had a failure rate up to 56%, and currently the interest has shifted to excision of tight segments of the stricture and use of grafts (ideally buccal) to augment the anastomosis or to address the stricture in its entirety.

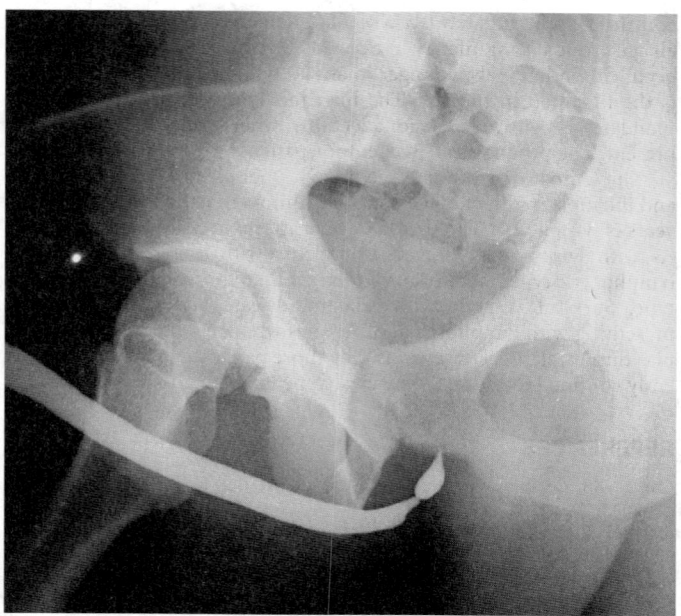

**FIGURE 1.** Retrograde urethrogram showing a short bulbar urethral stricture amenable to excision with primary anastomosis.

For strictures less than 2 cm long, stricture excision and primary reanastomosis remains the ideal procedure with excellent reported long-term results exceeding 90% success rates (Figure 1). For strictures measuring 2 to 4 cm, the latest evolution is the excisional augmented anastomotic urethroplasty. In this procedure, the worst section of the stricture is excised and the repair is augmented with a buccal graft or other onlay (Figure 2). Long strictures where segmental excision is not feasible are best managed with a dorsal onlay alone without excision (Figure 3). Occasionally, very long and dense strictures require a staged repair. Depending on the clinical situation, the entire urethra may need

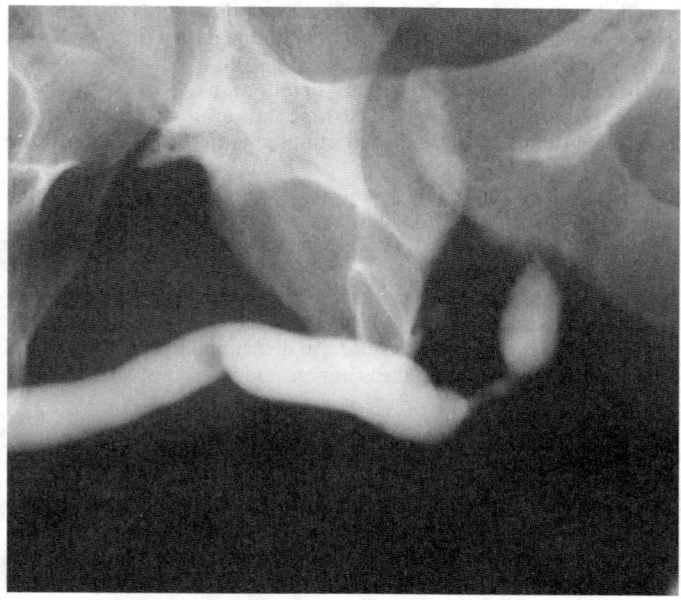

**FIGURE 2.** Retrograde urethrogram showing a longer, more complex, bulbar urethral stricture needing excision of the most significant area of stricture and onlay of the remaining stricture: the excisional, augmented anastomotic urethroplasty.

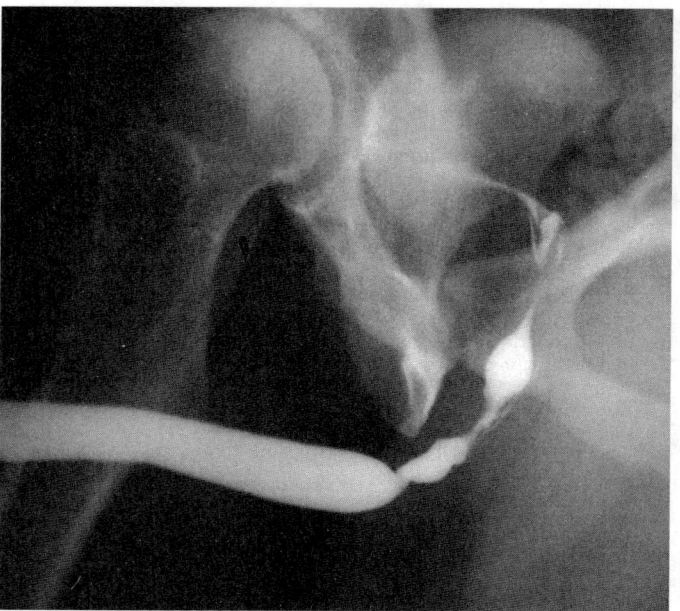

**FIGURE 3.** Retrograde urethrogram showing a very long and complex stricture needing repair with dorsal onlay.

to be excised, replacing with a flat grafted area of buccal mucosa tissue, split-thickness skin graft from the thigh or other areas such as preauricular skin, and rarely bladder or rectal mucosa. The graft is allowed to heal for 6 to 12 months after which the patient is brought back to the operating room for tubularization.

## Strictures from Lichen Sclerosis (Balanitis Xerotica Obliterans)

Balanitis xerotica obliterans, first described in 1928, is a form of lichen sclerosis (LS) and occurs in up to 1 in 300 men. The cause is unclear, and changes from LS most commonly occur in the glans penis and prepuce, causing phimosis with more extensive disease affecting the urethra as far back as the midbulb (Figure 4).

Management includes medications and surgery. Topical steroids, such as clobetasol (Temovate),[1] 0.05% cream applied two to four times daily, may cause significant regression of the scarring process. Surgical therapy ranges from extended simple meatotomy for distal strictures to complex staged repairs for more extensive disease. Because all of the native surrounding genital skin is subject to progression of LS, the entire affected urethra must often be excised and replaced with extragenital tissue for reconstruction. These can be morbid procedures fraught with complications and high failure rates up to 71%. Placement of a perineal urethrostomy may provide a good alternative to complex staged repair (Figure 4).

## Posterior Urethral Strictures

Traumatic injury to the prostatomembranous urethra occurs in approximately 10% of pelvic fractures. This injury may range from urethral elongation without tearing of the urethra to complete transection. With any suspicion of urethral injury in a pelvic trauma patient, a RUG should be performed. If no extravasation is seen, a Foley catheter may be inserted and a cystogram or upper tract study performed as indicated.

---

[1]Not FDA approved for this indication.

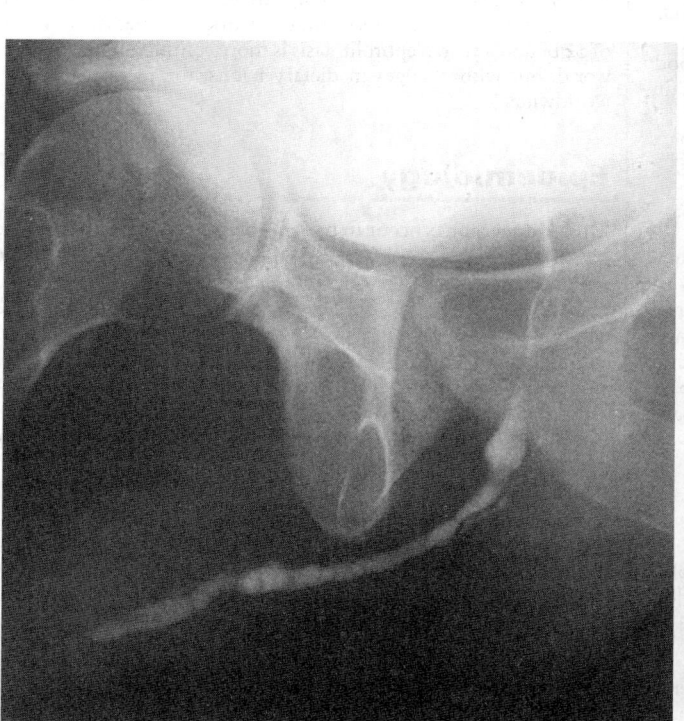
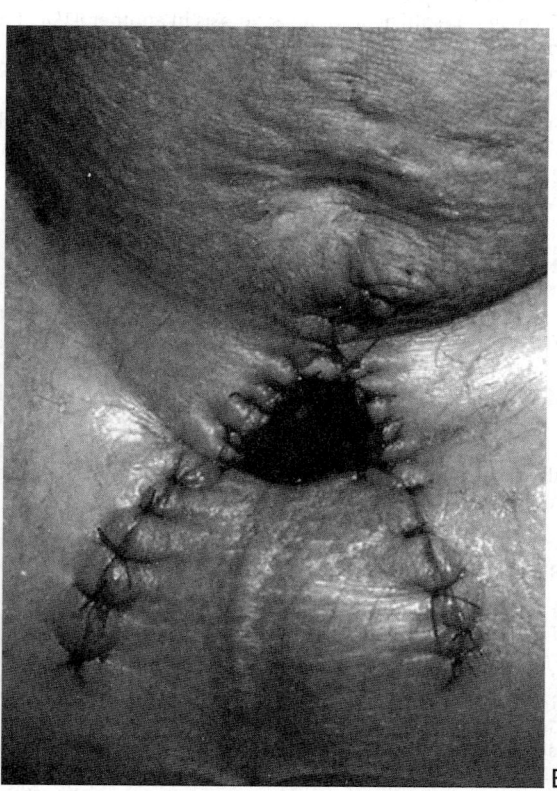

**FIGURE 4.** Retrograde urethrogram (**A**) showing a pan-pendulous urethral stricture from lichen sclerosis. These may be repaired with complex staged reconstruction. However, a simple perineal urethrostomy (**B**) may be appropriate for some patient populations.

When a catheter cannot be placed into the bladder through the urethra because of a posterior urethral injury, bladder drainage should be managed acutely with a suprapubic (SP) catheter. Definitive treatment after 3 to 6 months of recovery allows resolution of hematoma and shortening of the defect. Acute surgical intervention is indicated only in the uncommon situations where there is an associated rectal, bladder, or bladder neck injury or when there is another indication for laparotomy.

*Immediate (primary)* realignment is performed without the preceding indications using a variety of techniques. All involve the acute placement of a catheter across the urethral defect with magnetic guides, interlocking guides, or an open surgical procedure. Long-term restricturing occurs in 50% to 100% of patients, requiring additional future endoscopic procedures, intermittent catheterization, or reconstruction.

*Delayed (primary)* management is an alternative in cases whose recovery allows for return to the operating room 5 to 10 days after injury. An SP tube is placed acutely and realignment accomplished endoscopically when the patient is stable. An antegrade placed flexible endoscope negotiates the bladder neck and emerges in the injured area. A second retrograde endoscope is placed through the urethra to allow for hematoma irrigation, visualization of the defect, and antegrade passage of a stenting catheter across the defect.

*Delayed (secondary)* repair is delayed for 3 or more months following the injury; in the interim the patient is managed by SP catheter drainage. Most of these defects can be repaired with a one-stage perineal anastomotic urethroplasty. This remarkably versatile procedure manages long obliterative strictures well in more than 95% of cases.

The progressive perineal anastomotic repair involves the mobilization of the urethra with transection at the point of obliteration. The bulbar urethra is then reconnected to the prostatomembranous urethra proximal to the obliteration. Depending on the length of the repair needed, one to four of the following well-described sequential steps are used to accomplish a tension free anastomosis:

1. Circumferential mobilization of the distal urethra provides 2 to 3 cm of length sufficient for anastomosis in 8% of cases.
2. Separation of the proximal corporal bodies shortens the distance by 1 to 2 cm and is sufficient for anastomosis in another 41% of cases.
3. Inferior pubectomy with resection of a wedge of bone from the inferior surface of the pubis further shortens the defect by 1 to 2 cm, facilitating anastomosis in another 28% of cases.
4. Rerouting the urethra around the lateral surface of a corporal body provides another 1 to 2 cm of length and is needed for the remaining 23% of cases.

## Future Trends

The current evolution is pointing toward development and acceptance of artificial tissue replacements, allografts, and xenografts for the urethra, obviating the need for graft harvesting. These include Apligraf, a bioengineered product composed of a bovine-collagen fibroblast-containing matrix integrated with a sheet of stratified human epithelium that is similar to human skin. Also, many are currently developing a promising off-the-shelf collagen matrix based on cultured human cadaveric bladder mucosa.

## REFERENCES

Attwater HL: History of urethral stricture. BJU Int 1943;15:39.
Barbagli G, Palminteri E, Lazzeri M, et al: Long-term outcome of urethroplasty after failed urethrotomy versus primary repair. J Urol 2001;165(6 Pt 1):1918-1919.
Barbagli G, Selli C, Tosto A, Palminteri E: Dorsal free graft urethroplasty. J Urol 1996;155(1):123-126.
Depasquale I, Park AJ, Bracka A: The treatment of balanitis xerotica obliterans. BJU Int 2000;86(4):459-465.
El Kassaby AW, Retik AB, Yoo JJ, Atala A: Urethral stricture repair with an off-the-shelf collagen matrix. J Urol 2003;169(1):170-173.
Flynn BJ, Delvecchio FC, Webster GD: Perineal repair of pelvic fracture urethral distraction defects: Experience in 120 patients during the last 10 years. J Urol 2003;170:1877-1880.
Glass RE, Flynn JT, King JB, Blandy JP: Urethral injury and fractured pelvis. Br J Urol 1978;50(7):578-582.
Guralnick ML, Webster GD: The augmented anastomotic urethroplasty: Indications and outcome in 29 patients. J Urol 2001;165(5):1496-1501.
Iselin CE, Webster GD: Dorsal onlay graft urethroplasty for repair of bulbar urethral stricture. J Urol 1999;161(3):815-818.
Kane CJ, Tarman GJ, Summerton DJ, et al: Multi-institutional experience with buccal mucosa onlay urethroplasty for bulbar urethral reconstruction. J Urol 2002;167(3):1314-1317.
McAninch JW: Reconstruction of extensive urethral strictures: circular fasciocutaneous penile flap. J Urol 1993;149(3):488-491.
Orandi A: One-stage urethroplasty. Br J Urol 1968;40(6):717-719.
Quartey JK: One-stage penile/preputial island flap urethroplasty for urethral stricture. J Urol 1985;134(3):474-475.
Santucci RA, Mario LA, McAninch JW: Anastomotic urethroplasty for bulbar urethral stricture: Analysis of 168 patients. J Urol 2002;167(4):1715-1719.
Steenkamp JW, Heyns CF, de Kock ML: Internal urethrotomy versus dilation as treatment for male urethral strictures: A prospective, randomized comparison. J Urol 1997;157(1):98-101.
Venn SN, Mundy AR: Urethroplasty for balanitis xerotica obliterans. Br J Urol 1998;81(5):735-737.
Webster GD, Ramon J: Repair of pelvic fracture posterior urethral defects using an elaborated perineal approach: Experience with 74 cases. J Urol 1991;145(4):744-748.
Webster GD, Sihelnik S: The management of strictures of the membranous urethra. J Urol 1985;134(3):469-473.

# Renal Calculi

Method of
*Sujeet S. Acharya, MD, and Glenn S. Gerber, MD*

Nephrolithiasis is a common condition affecting 5% to 10% of the U.S. population. Roughly 2 million patients a year present with kidney stones on an outpatient basis, an increase of 40% from 1994. Stone disease results in pain, loss of time at work, and medical costs in excess of $2 billion a year. Nephrolithiasis is more common in the industrialized world, but with changes in dietary habits, the incidence is increasing worldwide.

## Epidemiology

Most kidney stones occur in patients between 20 and 50 years old, with peak onsets of disease between the third and fifth decades of life. Patients with recurrent stones often have their first case of nephrolithiasis in their teens or 20s. The recurrence rate of urinary calculi is roughly 50% within 5 years.

In general, male patients are more commonly affected with kidney stones than female patients by a ratio of 2:1. Stones due to infection (struvite stones), however, are more common in women than in men. About 6% of men have onset of disease after age 50 years, compared with 25% in female patients. Stones caused by metabolic or hormonal defects and stone disease in children occur equally between the sexes.

Kidney stones are more prevalent in whites, Latin Americans, and Asians than in African Americans and Native Americans. Geographic variation influences frequency as stones are more common in hot and dry areas.

## Pathophysiology

Supersaturation of urine by constituents such as calcium oxalate and uric acid is necessary for stone formation. If the concentration of an ion reaches a level beyond which it is not soluble, it has reached the level of supersaturation. Crystals and foreign bodies in the bladder serve as nidi for ions from the supersaturated urine to form microscopic lattice structures. These then increase in size by crystal growth and aggregation. Three quarters of renal calculi contain calcium. The majority of the rest contain uric acid. Cystine, struvite, and other stones occur less often.

Although geography, fluid intake, and diet influence the rate of calculi formation, metabolic derangements and heredity are the major causes of kidney stones. Hypercalciuria, whether absorptive, resorptive, or renal, is the most commonly noted metabolic abnormality. Absorptive hypercalciuria is the most common of the three forms of hypercalciuria. Severe (type 1) absorptive hypercalciuria has excess calcium in the urine independent of diet, whereas the calciuria of mild (type 2) absorptive hypercalciuria normalizes on a calcium-restricted diet. Renal hypercalciuria is caused by impaired renal tubular reabsorption of calcium. To balance calcium losses from urine, parathyroid function increases and eventually causes further mobilization of calcium from bone and increased intestinal absorption. As a result, patients with renal hypercalciuria have normal serum calcium. Resorptive hypercalciuria results from primary hyperparathyroidism, causing both serum and urine calcium levels to be high (Table 1).

Other causes of calcium stones include hyperuricosuria (dietary causes, overproduction), hyperoxaluria (enzyme defects, increased vitamin C, inflammatory bowel disease [IBD], bowel resection), gout, and decreased urine levels of the stone inhibitors citrate and magnesium.

Urate stones result from hyperuricosuria (malignancy, myeloproliferative states, glycogen storage disease) and from the net alkali deficit and dehydration during chronic diarrhea states. Cystine stones result from an autosomal recessive disorder in cystine metabolism, leading to cystinuria. Struvite stones result from urinary tract infection with urea-splitting organisms such as *Proteus* and *Klebsiella* species. These cause the formation of magnesium-ammonium-phosphate crystals, which can rapidly coalesce to form stones.

# Diagnosis

## HISTORY AND PHYSICAL EXAMINATION

Patients with urinary calculi present with pain, fever, dysuria, or hematuria. Stones passing into the ureter cause acute obstruction, with proximal urinary tract dilation and are associated with renal colic. Renal colic is marked by cramping, severe flank pain, nausea, and vomiting. While the stone moves distally through the ureter, pain moves from the flank to the abdomen, then to the groin, and finally the scrotal or labial area.

Staghorn calculi are kidney stones occupying the renal pelvis and the calyceal system. These stones are often asymptomatic, and when they do manifest it is usually with hematuria and infection rather than

## CURRENT DIAGNOSIS

- Nephrolithiasis affects 5% to 10% of the U.S. population, male patients more than female patients.
- The majority of renal calculi contain calcium.
- Patients usually have pain, nausea, vomiting, fever, dysuria, or hematuria.
- Physical findings include costovertebral angle and/or abdominal tenderness.
- Laboratory tests should include urinalysis, complete blood count, and chemistry profile.
- Recurrent stone formers should undergo metabolic evaluation including a 24-hour urine collection. This helps in classifying their nephrolithiasis and directs their long-term therapy.
- The standard means to evaluate for a suspected kidney stone is noncontrast computed tomography.

with acute onset of pain. Uncommonly, patients with asymptomatic bilateral obstruction present with renal failure.

During the history it is important to ask about the quality, location, and duration of pain. Prior history of urinary tract infections, urinary calculi, and their management should be noted as well. Other areas useful in stone management include past medical history (hyperparathyroidism), dietary habits, fluid consumption, medications, family history of calculi, loss of renal function, and history of solitary or transplanted kidney.

On physical examination, significant costovertebral angle tenderness is quite common and often moves to the abdomen as the stone migrates. Patients rarely present with peritoneal signs, which is important in distinguishing renal colic from other sources of flank and abdominal pain.

## LABORATORY STUDIES

The initial studies useful for stone patients include urinalysis (with or without culture), complete blood count (CBC), and a chemistry profile. Urinalysis evaluates the urine for hematuria and infection and can also assess for pH and crystals (Table 2). An elevated white blood cell (WBC) count indicates renal or systemic infection. A decreased red blood cell (RBC) count and hemoglobin indicate a chronic disease state or significant ongoing hematuria.

A chemistry profile including serum electrolytes, creatinine, calcium, phosphorus, uric acid, and PTH is necessary to assess a patient's renal and metabolic functions. Acidosis and elevations in serum calcium or urate can help reveal the etiology of the stone(s). The same can be said for alterations in PTH or phosphorus. Finally, an acute significant rise in creatinine from baseline can indicate urgent or emergent surgical intervention to relieve obstruction. This is especially true in patients with a solitary kidney or baseline renal dysfunction.

### TABLE 1  Hypercalciuric States

| Test | Type 1 AH | Type 2 AH | RH | Resorptive |
|------|-----------|-----------|-----|------------|
| **Serum** | | | | |
| Calcium | Normal | Normal | Normal | Elevated |
| Phosphorus | Normal | Normal | Normal | Low |
| PTH | Normal | Normal | Elevated | Elevated |
| 1,25(OH)$_2$D$_3$ | Normal | Normal | Elevated | Elevated |
| **Urinary Calcium** | | | | |
| Fasting urine | Normal | Normal | Elevated | Elevated |
| 24-h restricted* | Elevated | Normal | Elevated | Elevated |
| Post-Ca$^{2+}$ load† | Elevated | Elevated | Elevated | Elevated |

*Urine while patient is on a diet restricted in calcium (400 mg/day) and sodium (10 mEq/day).
†Four-hour urine collection after an oral bolus of 1 g calcium.
*Abbreviations:* 1,25(OH)$_2$D$_3$ = vitamin D$_3$; AH = absorptive hypercalciuria; PTH = parathyroid hormone; RH = renal hypercalciuria.

### TABLE 2  Crystal Shapes in Kidney Stones

| Stone Crystal | Shape under Microscope |
|---------------|------------------------|
| Calcium oxalate dihydrate | Envelope or bipyramidal |
| Calcium oxalate monohydrate | Dumbbell or hourglass |
| Calcium phosphate apatite | Amorphous |
| Cystine | Hexagonal |
| Struvite | Coffin lid |
| Uric acid | Rhomboid |
| | Irregular plates or rosettes |
| | Amorphous |

## TABLE 3  Classification of Nephrolithiasis

| Category | General Features | Urine Study Findings |
|---|---|---|
| **Hypercalciuria** | | |
| Absorptive hypercalciuria | Normal serum calcium<br>Normal serum phosphorus | Hypercalciuria: Urine calcium > 200 mg/24 h<br>Type 1: Hypercalciuria independent of diet<br>Type 2: Normocalciuria with low-calcium diet |
| Renal hypercalciuria | Normal serum calcium<br>Normal serum phosphorus<br>Increased PTH and Vitamin D (2°<br>  hyperparathyroidism) | Hypercalciuria independent of diet |
| Resorptive hypercalciuria | Hypercalcemia<br>Hypophosphatemia<br>Increased PTH and Vitamin D (1°<br>  hyperparathyroidism) | Hypercalciuria independent of diet |
| **Other Causes** | | |
| Cystinuria | | Urine cystine > 250 mg/d |
| Gouty diathesis | Calcium, uric acid, or mixed stones | Persistently acidic urine (pH <5.5) |
| Hyperoxaluria | Main cause is enteric<br>Dehydration and low urine citrate due<br>  to acidosis contribute | Urine oxalate >45 mg/d<br>Oxalate >80 mg/d: primary or enteric<br>Oxalate 45-80 mg/d: dietary causes |
| Hyperuricosuria | Normal serum calcium | Urine uric acid >600 mg/24 h<br>Normal urinary calcium and oxalate<br>Normal fasting and calcium load responses<br>Calcium stones with urine pH >5.5 |
| Hypocitraturia | Associated with distal RTA<br>Complete and incomplete forms<br>Associated with calcium stones | Urine citrate <640 mg/d<br>Hypercalciuria |
| Hypomagnesuria | Often dietary | Urine magnesium <50 mg/d<br>Associated with hypocitraturia, low urine volume |
| Infection stones | | Alkaline urine due to bacterial urease<br>Often hypercalciuria, hypocitraturia |
| Low urine volume | | Urine volume <1 L/d<br>Stone formers should aim for >2 L/d |
| No abnormality | 3%-5% of stone population<br>Normal serum calcium<br>Normal serum PTH | Normal urine volume, pH, calcium, citrate, uric acid,<br>  magnesium, and oxalate |

*Abbreviations:* PTH = parathyroid hormone; RTA = renal tubular acidosis.

Patients who are recurrent stone formers and high-risk first-time stone formers (patients younger than 30 years and those with renal failure, struvite stones, multiple stones, intestinal disease, or solitary or transplanted kidney) warrant a more extensive laboratory evaluation, including a 24-hour urine collection. The 24-hour urine collection measures calcium, uric acid, creatinine, sodium, oxalate, citrate, pH, and volume. Elevation of the 24-hour excretion rate of calcium, oxalate, or uric acid indicates predisposition to stone formation. Other tests include the 24-hour urine collection after 1 week of a diet restricted in calcium, sodium, and oxalate; the fasting urine study; and the calcium load study (Table 3).

### IMAGING STUDIES

Several imaging modalities can evaluate patients with kidney stones. The plain abdominal x-ray is very useful in assessing total stone burden, size, shape, and location of urinary calculi. On these films, calcium-containing stones are radiopaque, but pure uric acid, indinavir-induced, and cystine calculi are relatively radiolucent.

A renal sonogram not only determines the presence of a stone but also detects the presence of hydronephrosis and hydroureter. A stone seen on ultrasound, but not on radiograph, may be a uric acid or cystine stone.

Intravenous pyelogram (IVP) is the standard study for determining size and location of calculi, as well as providing anatomic and functional information. Disadvantages of an IVP are that it is labor intensive, it involves injection of contrast, and it requires bowel preparation for optimal results.

A helical computed tomography (CT) scan without contrast is the most sensitive imaging technique for kidney stones and is at present the standard means for evaluating patients suspected to have calculi. Even stones radiolucent on plain films (except indinavir-induced stones) are seen on a CT scan. Advantages of a CT scan are that it can identify other pathologies, it is a quick study, and it avoids administration of contrast. Disadvantages of a CT scan are that it cannot evaluate renal function and that it is relatively more expensive than IVP.

The renal tomogram is helpful in finding small stones in the kidneys, especially in obese patients.

## Treatment

### MEDICAL CARE

Medical care encompasses emergency management of renal calculi and long-term therapy to dissolve stones and to prevent stones from forming. Once renal colic is diagnosed in the emergent setting, it is important to evaluate for obstruction and infection. Obstruction in the absence of infection can be managed with analgesics (narcotics or nonsteroidal anti-inflammatory drugs [NSAIDs]) and other forms of medical expulsive therapy. Infection in the absence of obstruction can initially be managed with antibiotics. If neither obstruction nor infection are present, then a trial of analgesics and other medical measures to assist in stone passage can be started. NSAIDs such as ketorolac (Toradol), α-blockers like tamsulosin (Flomax),[1] and calcium channel blockers such as nifedipine (Procardia)[1] have ureter-relaxing effects, but their results in published studies are mixed (Table 4).

---

[1]Not FDA approved for this indication.

## TABLE 4  Summary of Medical Expulsive Therapy

| Medicine | Dose |
|---|---|
| **Analgesic** | |
| Hydrocodone w/acetaminophen (Vicodin) | 1-2 tablets (5/500 mg) PO q4-6h prn pain |
| Ibuprofen (Advil, Motrin) | 600-800 mg po q8h prn pain |
| Ketorolac (Toradol) | 30 mg IV q6h prn pain |
| Morphine sulfate | 1-2 mg IV q2-4h prn pain |
| **Antiemetic** | |
| Metoclopramide (Reglan)[1] | 10-20 mg PO or IV q6h prn nausea[3] |
| Prochlorperazine (Compazine) | 5-10 mg PO q6-8h prn nausea |
| **Ureteral Relaxation** | |
| Nifedipine extended release (Procardia XL)[1] | 30 mg PO qd |
| Tamsulosin (Flomax)[1] | 0.4 mg PO qd |
| Terazosin (Hytrin)[1] | 4 mg PO qd |

[1]Not FDA approved for this indication.
[3]Exceeds dosage recommended by the manufacturer.

Stones are more likely to pass if their diameter is 5 mm or less. Patients should increase fluid intake to increase their urine output, and they should be prescribed antiemetics as necessary. Limit medical expulsive therapy to 10 days, and if outpatient treatment fails, refer the patient to a urologist. If obstruction and infection coexist, then the upper urinary collecting system must be decompressed.

In preventing stones from recurring, the most important factor is for the patient to increase fluid intake so that urine output is at least 2 L per day. Excessive salt, oxalate, and protein intake should be avoided. Dietary calcium should only be restricted if indicated by 24-hour urine

## CURRENT THERAPY

- In the absence of infection and upper urinary tract obstruction, a kidney stone can be managed by analgesics, anti-inflammatory medicines, and antiemetics.
- Drugs that allow ureteral relaxation, such as tamsulosin (Flomax),[1] facilitate passage of stones 5 mm or smaller.
- The most important factor in preventing stone recurrence is to increase fluid intake so urine output is at least 2 L/day.
- Dietary restrictions, thiazide diuretics, and potassium citrate therapy depend on the type of stone being treated.
- Minimally invasive methods of treating kidney stones such as extracorporeal shock-wave lithotripsy, ureteroscopy, and percutaneous nephrostolithotomy are employed more often than open surgery.

[1]Not FDA approved for this indication.

collection and metabolic evaluation. Empiric dietary restriction of calcium is not necessary in most patients, and it can have adverse effects on bone mineralization, especially in women and in patients with osteoporosis.

In the absence of sufficient intestinal calcium to bind oxalate, oxalate absorption and hyperoxaluria increase. This can, in fact, increase stone formation in patients with calcium oxalate calculi. Dietary calcium should be restricted to 600 to 800 mg/day in patients with diet-responsive hypercalciuria who form calcium stones. For stone-specific management, see Table 5.

[1]Not FDA approved for this indication.

## TABLE 5  Summary of Medical Treatment by Stone Type

| Treatment | Dose | Comments |
|---|---|---|
| **Absorptive Hypercalciuria** | | |
| Diet restriction | | May be sufficient for type 2 AH |
| Thiazide diuretic (e.g., hydrochlorozide [Hydrodiuril]) | Various doses | Not ↑ intestinal absorption<br>Causes hypercalciuria<br>Inexpensive<br>Effect decreases with time<br>Give potassium supplement |
| Sodium cellulose phosphate (Calcibind) | 10-15 g PO qd | Binds calcium in gut<br>Can also cause hypomagnesemia (binds in gut) and 2nd-degree hyperoxaluria) |
| **Renal Hypercalciuria** | | |
| Thiazide diuretic (e.g., hydrochlorozide [Hydrodiuril]) | 50 mg PO bid | Increase calcium reabsorption in distal tubule<br>↓ extracellular volume →↑ proximal tubule reabsorption<br>2nd-degree hyperparathyroidism corrected, thus normalizing intestinal calcium reabsorption |
| Chlorthalidone (Hygroton)[1] | 50 mg PO qd | Avoid triamterene (Dyrenium) because of risk of triamterene stones |
| **Resorptive Hypercalciuria** | | |
| Parathyroidectomy | | Best chance for improvement of disease<br>Thiazides are contraindicated because they worsen hypercalcemia |
| **Hyperuricosuria** | | |
| Diet restriction | | Restriction of purines |
| Allopurinol (Zyloprim) | 200-600 mg PO qd | |
| Potassium citrate (Urocit-K) | 30-90 mEq/d divided tid-qid with food | Complexes calcium and inhibits urate-induced crystallization |
| **Gouty Diathesis** | | |
| Potassium citrate | 30-90 mEq/d divided tid-qid with food | Increase urinary pH to >5.5<br>Avoid increasing urinary pH to >7.0 or risk calcium phosphate stones |

*Continued*

**TABLE 5   Summary of Medical Treatment by Stone Type—cont'd**

| Treatment | Dose | Comments |
|---|---|---|
| **Hyperoxaluria** | | |
| Calcium citrate | 150 mg PO qd | Binds oxalate in gut, preventing absorption<br>Raises urinary pH and urine citrate levels<br>Add thiazide if hypercalciuria develops |
| **Hypocitraturia** | | |
| Potassium citrate | 30-90 mEq/d divided tid-qid with food | Same therapy whether hypocitraturia is due to distal RTA or chronic diarrhea or is idiopathic<br>Large doses (120 mEq/d[3]) may be needed for severe acidosis |
| **Cystinuria** | | |
| High fluid intake | | Try to reduce urine cystine to <200-300 mg/L |
| Potassium citrate | 30-90 mEq/d divided tid-qid with food | Aim to increase urine pH to >6.5-7.0 |
| D-Penicillamine (Cuprimine) | 125 mg PO qod | Increases cystine solubility<br>Associated with the nephrotic syndrome, dermatitis, and pancytopenia |
| **Infection Stones** | | |
| Various antibiotics | | Control infection |
| Acetohydroxamic acid (Lithostat) | 250 mg PO tid | Works by inhibiting urease of struvite stone-forming organisms |

[1]Not FDA approved for this indication.
[3]Exceeds dosage recommended by the manufacturer.
*Abbreviations:* AH = absorptive hypercalciuria; HCTZ = hydrochlorothiazide; RTA = renal tubular acidosis.

## SURGICAL CARE

The indications for surgery are pain, infection, and obstruction. Contraindications to definitive stone manipulation include uncorrected bleeding diathesis and pregnancy (relative contraindication). Treatment for most renal calculi is noninvasive (e.g., lithotripsy); open surgical excision is limited to isolated atypical cases. In an obstructed and infected collecting system secondary to a stone, emergent relief of obstruction is necessary by ureteral stent or percutaneous nephrostomy placement.

Nearly 85% of kidney stones requiring intervention are treated with extracorporeal shock-wave lithotripsy (ESWL). Shocks are generated via an electrohydraulic, electromagnetic, or piezoelectric source and are focused on the calculus. As the stone is hit by the shockwave, it breaks into smaller fragments that can pass in the urine. ESWL is less successful if the stone is larger than 1.5 cm or is in the lower pole of the kidney. In these cases, fragmentation does take place, but due to either the large volume of fragments or their location, the fragments do not pass completely. Cystine stones do not fragment well with ESWL. Do not perform ESWL in pregnant patients or if there is ureteral obstruction distal to the stone.

Ureteroscopic management is the second most common management option. Either a flexible or rigid endoscope is passed into the bladder and up the ureter to visualize the stone. The stone is either extracted with a grasper or basket device or is fragmented via laser, ultrasonic, or electrohydraulic lithotripsy. Commonly, a ureteral stent is placed at the end of the procedure to prevent obstruction secondary to ureteral spasm or edema.

Percutaneous nephrostolithotomy (PCNL) affords fragmentation and removal of large stones from the kidney and ureter, particularly after failed ESWL. Percutaneous access to the kidney is achieved, and a sheath with a 1-cm lumen allows use of larger and more powerful lithotrites. Due to its morbidity, PCNL is generally reserved for large or complex stones that are refractory to management by ureteroscopy or ESWL.

## CONSULTATIONS

Consultation with a urologist is recommended when stones are present in the settings of infection and obstruction. Referral is required when medical management fails, for stones refractory to outpatient management, and for stones that do not pass spontaneously.

# Follow-up

The postoperative course after minimally invasive stone removal usually consists of discomfort, which is best handled with oral pain medications. If pain continues or worsens, it is important to evaluate for complications such as infection, ureteral obstruction, and hemorrhage. Repeat urine cultures and imaging should be performed to assess for ureteral obstruction or perforation. Antibiotic choice is dictated by urine culture results.

A follow-up examination with abdominal x-ray is often sufficient after uncomplicated stone removal. In patients with stones having unusual characteristics and after difficult or complicated procedures, imaging evaluating renal drainage (IVP, ultrasound, CT scan) may be important.

In patients older than 40 years who have a single stone that passed either spontaneously or after intervention, follow-up for recurrent stones is generally not necessary. These patients have a low recurrence risk, especially if they maintain increased fluid intake. For patients at risk for recurrence, annual radiograph or ultrasound and 24-hour urine analyses are adequate.

## REFERENCES

Menon M, Resnick MI: Urinary lithiasis: Etiology, diagnosis, and medical management. In Walsh PC, Retik AB, Vaughan ED, et al (eds): Campbell's Urology, 8th ed. Philadelphia: WB Saunders, 2002, 3229-3305.

Preminger GM: Medical management of urinary calculus disease. Part 1: Pathogenesis and evaluation. AUA Update Series, lesson 5. 1995;14:37-44.

Preminger GM: Medical management of urinary calculus disease. Part 2: Classification of metabolic disorders and selective medical management. AUA Update Series, lesson 5. 1995;14:45-52.

Stoller MLS, Bolton DM: Urinary stone disease. In Tanagho EA, McAninch JW (eds): Smith's General Urology, 15th ed. New York: McGraw-Hill, 2000, pp 291-321.

# The Sexually Transmitted Diseases

## Chancroid

Method of
*Stanley M. Spinola, MD*

Chancroid is caused by the gram-negative bacillus *Haemophilus ducreyi*. Chancroid is endemic in resource-poor countries in Africa, Asia, South America, and the Caribbean and occurs in sporadic outbreaks in industrialized nations. The annual global prevalence of chancroid is estimated to be 6 million cases, but diagnostic tests for *H. ducreyi* are not routinely performed and its epidemiology is poorly defined. The male-to-female ratio ranges from 3:1 to 25:1. Lack of circumcision is associated with infection in men. Like other agents of genital ulcer disease (GUD), *H. ducreyi* facilitates both acquisition and transmission of HIV-1, and chancroid contributes substantially to the HIV-1 pandemic in Asia and sub-Saharan Africa.

*H. ducreyi* has a short duration of infection, and chancroid can be perpetuated only by highly sexually active populations such as commercial sex workers (CSWs). Infected men usually report intercourse with CSWs. In the United States, chancroid is now rare; less than 100 cases were reported annually from 2000 to 2004. However, outbreaks occurred as recently as 1995 in New Orleans and Jackson, Mississippi. In these outbreaks, additional risk factors for infection included crack cocaine use, exchange of drugs for sex, or sex with a partner who used crack. Elimination of chancroid from CSWs controls outbreaks and reduces endemic disease.

---

### CURRENT DIAGNOSIS

- Patients usually develop 1–4 soft painful ulcers with ragged edges on the foreskin or at the entrance of the vagina. Infected women may also have painless internal vaginal and cervical ulcers. Regional lymphadenitis occurs in 10%–50% of cases.
- Infected men have usually had contact with CSWs.
- Diagnosis is typically made by culture after exclusion of HSV and syphilis.

*Abbreviations:* CSWs = commercial sex workers; HSV = herpes simplex virus.

## Diagnosis

*H. ducreyi* enters the skin through breaks in the epithelium that occur during sex, and erythematous papules form at each entry site within hours to days. Papules evolve into pustules in 2 to 3 days. After several weeks, the pustules ulcerate, and patients usually develop one to four soft painful ulcers with ragged edges. The ulcer may be covered by a yellow or gray purulent exudate and frequently bleeds when scraped. The most frequent sites of the ulcer are the foreskin and the entrance of the vagina. Internal vaginal and cervical ulcers may be painless and go unnoticed by infected women. Suppurative inguinal lymphadenopathy occurs in up to 50% of patients with ulcers. The classic presentation of chancroid occurs in a minority of patients, and chancroid cannot be reliably distinguished from syphilis or herpes on clinical grounds. Mixed infections with *H. ducreyi*, *Treponema pallidum*, and herpes simplex virus (HSV) are common, occurring in approximately 17% of proven chancroid cases. Mixed infection may account for the variable clinical presentations of chancroid and treatment failures.

Confirmation of chancroid is difficult because culture is at best 80% sensitive. A highly sensitive multiplex polymerase chain reaction assay for GUD was developed but not marketed. Culture is the only reliable diagnostic test available for most settings. In practice, the diagnosis of chancroid is typically made by exclusion of HSV and syphilis. If patients with GUD and inguinal lymphadenitis or treatment failures for presumed primary syphilis appear in a community, public health authorities should be notified and diagnostic testing initiated.

## Treatment

*H. ducreyi* is usually resistant to ampicillin, chloramphenicol (Chloromycetin), tetracyclines, trimethoprim (Proloprim), and sulfonamides and is susceptible to macrolides, quinolones, and third-generation cephalosporins. The Centers for Disease Control and Prevention (CDC) recommends single-dose azithromycin (Zithromax), 1 g orally, or ceftriaxone (Rocephin[1]), 250 mg intramuscularly (IM), ciprofloxacin (Cipro[1]), 500 mg orally twice a day for 3 days, or erythromycin base,[1] 500 mg orally three times a day for 7 days. Low-dose erythromycin (250 mg three times a day for 7 days) may be as effective as the standard 500 mg regimen. Single-dose oral ciprofloxacin, 500 mg, may be as effective as the single-dose azithromycin and multiple-dose ciprofloxacin regimens.

---

[1]Not FDA approved for this indication.

## CURRENT THERAPY

- CDC recommends single-dose azithromycin (Zithromax), 1 g orally, or ceftriaxone (Rocephin[1]), 250 mg IM, ciprofloxacin (Cipro[1]), 500 mg PO bid for 3 days, or erythromycin base,[1] 500 mg PO tid for 7 d.
- Low dose erythromycin (250 mg tid for 7 d) may be as effective as the standard 500 mg regimen.
- Single-dose oral ciprofloxacin, 500 mg, may be as effective as single-dose azithromycin and multiple-dose ciprofloxacin regimens.
- Even if *H. ducreyi* is successfully treated, ulcers may persist if HSV or syphilis is present and not treated.
- Recommend HIV testing and syphilis serology at time of presentation and 3 mo later if initial tests are negative.

[1]Not FDA approved for this indication.
*Abbreviations:* IM = intramuscularly; HSV = herpes simplex virus; PO = orally.

Within 1 week of treatment, there should be no purulence and the ulcers should be less tender. Most ulcers heal in 2 weeks, but large ulcers may take 4 weeks to heal. Patients co-infected with HIV and *H. ducreyi* may have a greater number of ulcers that do not heal as quickly as patients infected with *H. ducreyi* alone. However, the antibiotic treatment efficacy of single-dose azithromycin or ciprofloxacin for chancroid in HIV seropositive and seronegative patients is similar. When evaluating the response to treatment, one must distinguish between bacteriologic and clinical cure. Even if *H. ducreyi* is successfully treated, ulcers may persist if HSV or syphilis is present and not treated. Fluctuant buboes may be treated by incision and drainage or needle aspiration; the former lessens the need for repeated procedures. All patients with chancroid should undergo testing for HIV at the time of presentation and 3 months later if the initial test is negative. All sexual contacts should be examined and treated even if GUD is not present.

## REFERENCES

Ballard RC, Ye H, Matta A, et al: Treatment of chancroid with azithromycin. Int J STD AIDS 1996;7(Suppl 1):9-12.

Bong CTH, Bauer ME, Spinola SM: Haemophilus ducreyi: Clinical features, epidemiology, and prospects for disease control. Microbes Infect 2002;4:1141-1148.

Ernst A, Marvez-Valls E, Martin D: Incision and drainage versus aspiration of fluctuant buboes in the emergency department during an epidemic of chancroid. Sex Transm Dis 1995;22(4):217-220.

Kimani J, Bwayo JJ, Anzala AO, et al: Low dose erythromycin regimen for the treatment of chancroid. East Afr Med J 1995;72:645-648.

Lewis DA: Diagnostic tests for chancroid. Sex Transm Infect 2000;76:137-141.

Malonza IM, Tyndall MW, Ndinya-Achola JO, et al: A randomized, double-blind, placebo-controlled trial of single-dose ciprofloxacin versus erythromycin for the treatment of chancroid in Nairobi, Kenya. J Infect Dis 1999;180:1886-1893.

Martin DH, Sargent SJ, Wendel GD, Jr., et al: Comparison of azithromycin and ceftriaxone for the treatment of chancroid. Clin Infect Dis 1995;21:409-414.

Moodley P, Sturm PDJ, Vanmali T, et al: Association between HIV-1 infection, the etiology of genital ulcer disease, and response to syndromic management. Sex Transm Dis 2003;30:241-245.

Trees DL, Morse SA: Chancroid and *Haemophilus ducreyi*: An update. Clin Microbiol Rev 1995;8:357-375.

Tyndall MW, Agoki E, Plummer FA, et al: Single dose azithromycin for the treatment of chancroid: A randomized comparison with erythromycin. Sex Transm Dis 1994;21:231-234.

# Gonorrhea

Method of
*David M. Bamberger, MD*

Gonorrhea is a common sexually transmitted disease of epithelial tissue that usually causes urethral infection in men and cervical infections in women. Conjunctival infections, proctitis, and pharyngeal infections are also observed. *Neisseria gonorrhoeae* is a gram-negative, aerobic, piliated but nonmotile coccus that grows in pairs with adjacent, flattened sides.

## Epidemiology

In 2005, 339,353 cases of gonorrhea were reported in the United States. The rate of 115.6 per 100,000 people reflects a large decrease in incidence from 1976 to 1996 but only a small decrease from 1996 to 2005. Infection rates are much higher in the southeastern states. Rates among women and men are almost equal. The highest rates are observed among women 15 to 19 years of age and men 20 to 24 years of age. Rates among blacks are higher than in whites, Hispanics, Asian/Pacific Islanders, or American Indians/Alaskan natives. Although rates are highest among blacks and those living in the South, the rates have been declining over the past 5 years in these populations and have been increasing among whites and those living in the West. Rates in developing countries are estimated to be substantially higher than in the United States. An estimated 60 million cases of gonorrhea occur worldwide every year.

Cases reported to state and local health departments are underreported. On the basis of a population-based study performed in 2001–2002 in adults 18 to 26 years of age, the prevalence of gonococcal infections was 0.43%. This rate was approximately 10-fold less than for chlamydial infections, the other common cause of urethritis and cervicitis. The population-based study confirmed the substantially higher rate among blacks than whites and a lower rate in the West compared to the South. Most men and women with gonococcal infections in the survey were asymptomatic.

Rates of gonococcal infection are also high among men who have sex with men, lower socioeconomic and educational attainment, users of illicit drugs, and commercial sex workers. Among men having sex with men, the rate of infection increased between 1999 and 2003, particularly from western U.S. cities. Acquisition of infection is more related to differences in sex partner networks, societal factors, and access to health care than the number of sexual partners. Transmission usually occurs among those with no or minimal symptoms. The risk of transmission from a single sexual encounter from an infected woman to her male partner is approximately 20% and is approximately 50% from an infected man to his female partner. The U.S. Preventive Services Task Force recommends that clinicians screen all sexually active women under the age of 25, including those who are pregnant, for gonorrhea infection if they have a history of sexually transmitted infections, new or multiple sex partners, inconsistent condom use, sex work, or drug use.

## Clinical Manifestations

In men, the usual incubation is 2 to 5 days, followed by a urethral discharge that is typically purulent, as opposed to the clear or whitish discharge of chlamydial urethritis. Extragenital infections, such as proctitis or pharyngitis, are more likely to be asymptomatic. Symptoms of proctitis may include tenesmus, rectal discharge, and pain. Acute epididymitis is the most common complication of urethral infection.

In women, the usual symptoms are vaginal discharge or pruritus and dysuria. Pelvic pain is often because of ascending infection. On cervical exam, a mucopurulent discharge is often observed. Vaginal involvement, including periurethral (Skene's) glands and involvement of the Bartholin ducts, is more common in postmenopausal women and prepubertal girls. Rectal involvement is often asymptomatic and caused by contamination with cervicovaginal secretions. Pelvic inflammatory disease (PID) (see the appropriate article) is estimated to occur in 10% to 20% of women with cervical infections. Perihepatitis (Fitz-Hugh-Curtis syndrome) is caused by involvement of the liver capsule. Pharyngeal involvement in both men and women may be a source of transmission and is usually asymptomatic. Autoinoculation of the eye is the usual cause of adult gonococcal conjunctivitis.

Bacteremic dissemination is estimated to occur in 0.5% to 3% of patients, but these estimates may be high because of declining prevalence in strains associated with dissemination (serotype IA, auxotype AHU, failure to express outer membrane protein II). It occurs more often in women or in men who have sex with men; in women it is associated with menstruation or pregnancy, and it may be associated with deficiencies in the terminal components of complement. During the initial phase of illness, patients usually develop fever and polytenosynovitis of the knees, elbows, wrists, and joints of the hands and feet. Discrete papulopustular skin lesions on an erythematous base occur. As the illness continues, septic arthritis manifests in one or two joints, typically the knees, elbows, ankles, or wrists.

## Microbiology and Diagnosis

In men with symptomatic purulent urethritis, a Gram stain of the purulent discharge revealing intracellular gram-negative diplococci is both sensitive and specific. The use of a Gram stain in the diagnosis of cervical infection has lower sensitivity and specificity. Cultures of urethral specimens from men and cervical specimens from women should be plated directly onto media to improve yield and transported promptly to the microbiology laboratory. A special medium such as Thayer-Martin, which inhibits the growth of contaminating organisms, is used for nonsterile sites such as the urethra, cervix, rectum, or pharynx. Plates are incubated at 35°C to 36°C (95°F to 97°F) in 3% to 5% carbon dioxide ($CO_2$).

Nonculture methods are increasingly replacing cultures in the diagnosis of gonococcal infections. Three commercially available nucleic acid amplification tests are currently marketed: the polymerase chain reaction (PCR) assay (Amplicor, Roche), a transcription mediated amplification assay (Aptima, Gen-Probe), and the DNA strand displacement assay (Probe-Tec, Becton Dickinson). These assays are highly sensitive and specific in testing male urethral, female cervical, and male urine specimens. An important advantage of the assays is their utility in testing urine specimens from both men and women and self-collected vaginal specimens from women. The PCR assay was only 55% to 65% sensitive when testing urine samples from women. The strand displacement and transcription mediated amplification assay are moderately more sensitive in testing female urine specimens but sensitivity remains less than 95%. Although most of the current nonculture assays have a specificity of approximately 99%, there is a suboptimal positive predication if testing a population with very low prevalence.

Cultures are still considered the gold standard test in forensic settings and offer the advantage of preserving the specimen for antimicrobial testing, which has become increasingly important in an era of increasing antimicrobial resistance. Cultures remain the only approved diagnostic testing methodology for pharyngeal and rectal specimens.

## Treatment

Treatment for gonococcal infections is best provided at the time of initial presentation with a regimen that is highly effective with single-dose therapy. Adherence with therapy wanes with prolonged outpatient treatment courses. Antimicrobial resistance rates are increasing, and susceptibility testing results are generally not available at the time treatment is provided. In the U.S. Gonococcal Isolate Surveillance Project (GISP) report in 2005, 19.6% of isolates were resistant to penicillin, tetracycline, or both, and 10.5% of isolates demonstrated resistance to ciprofloxacin (Cipro). Chlamydial infection is detected in approximately 20% of men and 42% of women with laboratory-documented gonococcal infections, necessitating the need for co-treatment of *Chlamydia trachomatis* (see Obstetrics and Gynecology section) in patients with gonococcal infections, unless a nucleic acid amplification test is negative for the presence of chlamydia at the time of treatment. Patients with gonococcal infections should also be screened and counseled regarding other sexually transmitted diseases, including HIV and syphilis, and offered hepatitis B vaccination.

An ideal treatment regimen for gonococcal infections of the urethra, cervix, or rectum is inexpensive, well-tolerated, and a single dose. Ceftriaxone (Rocephin), 125 mg given intramuscularly (IM) as a single dose, is highly efficacious for urogenital and rectal infections. It may be reconstituted in 1% lidocaine (Xylocaine) to reduce injection site pain. The 2007 Update to the 2006 *STD Treatment Guidelines* from the Centers for Disease Control and Prevention (CDC) includes only cefixime (Suprax) at 400 mg as a recommended oral regimen. Manufacture of cefixime (Suprax) as an oral tablet ceased in 2002 but may be reintroduced. An oral suspension (100 mg/5 mL) is marketed. Since 2002 quinolone resistance has increased. Several countries in Southeast Asia have rates of fluoroquinolone resistance that exceed 50%. Within the United States, data from the GISP in 2005 indicated a rate of greater than 5% resistance in most Western U.S. cities, and in Atlanta, Philadelphia, New Orleans, and Miami. Outside of the GISP, high rates of fluoroquinolone resistance are also reported in Massachusetts, Michigan, New York, and New Hampshire. The rate of fluoroquinolone resistance in men who have sex with men is 29% compared with 3.8% in heterosexuals. Because of the higher rates of fluoroquinolone resistance, the CDC no longer recommends use of fluoroquinolones for the treatment of gonococcal infections and associated conditions, such as pelvic inflammatory disease. Consequently, only cephalosporins are recommended and available.

---

### CURRENT DIAGNOSIS

- Urethral discharge in men and vaginal discharge and dysuria in women are the common symptoms of gonococcal infections, but many women and some men have asymptomatic or minimally symptomatic infections.
- Urethral Gram stain is an inexpensive sensitive and specific test in men but not women.
- Newer generation nucleic acid amplification tests are highly sensitive and specific in cervical specimens in women and in urethral and urine specimens in men, but some lack sensitivity in urine specimens from women. Nucleic acid amplification tests should not be used in testing specimens from pharyngeal or rectal sources.

---

### CURRENT THERAPY

- Uncomplicated urethritis, cervicitis, or rectal infections should be treated with a single dose of:
- Ceftriaxone (Rocephin), 125 mg IM or Cefixime (Suprax), 400 mg PO
- Alternative therapies include:
  - Azithromycin (Zithromax), 2 g PO
  - Cefpodoxime (Vantin), 200–400 mg PO
- Patients should be treated for concomitant chlamydial infection with
  - Azithromycin (Zithromax), 1 g PO *or*
  - Doxycycline (Vibramycin), 100 mg PO bid for 7 d
- Sexual partners of infected patients should be evaluated and treated for gonorrhea and chlamydia and evaluated and counseled for other sexually transmitted diseases.

Oral cefpodoxime (Vantin) is an alternative to cefixime but is slightly less active in vitro. At a dose of 200 mg, the efficacy is 96.5% (95% confidence interval [CI], 94.8 to 98.9) and is approved for urethritis in males and females and rectal infections in females by the FDA, but not recommended by the CDC because the lower limit of the 95% CI was less than 95%. Use of a 400 mg oral dose is recommended by some state health departments as an alternative, but published efficacy data are limited. A 2 g single oral dose of azithromycin (Zithromax) is highly efficacious but associated with more gastrointestinal intolerance, and azithromycin resistance is increasing and occurs among 2.9% of isolates. Spectinomycin (Trobicin), given as a single 2 g IM dose, is another alternative to ceftriaxone (Rocephin) in patients with a history of allergy to cephalosporins or anaphylaxis to penicillin, but is not available in the United States as of May 2007.

Pharyngeal infections are generally less responsive to treatment. Recommended treatment is 125 mg IM ceftriaxone (Rocephin). A 2-g dose of oral azithromycin (Zithromax) is an alternative in documented cases of cephalosporin allergy. Conjunctival infections in adults are treated with a single dose of 1 g IM ceftriaxone (Rocephin); ophthalmia neonatorum is treated with 25 to 50 mg/kg, not to exceed 125 mg, of intravenous (IV) or IM ceftriaxone. All neonates should receive ocular prophylaxis against gonococcal ophthalmia with 0.5% erythromycin (Ramycin), or 1% tetracycline.

Sexual partners of infected patients should be evaluated and treated for gonorrhea and chlamydia and evaluated and counseled for other sexually transmitted diseases. Expedited partner therapy involves a strategy in which patients deliver treatment and counseling information with medication or a prescription to their partner. This strategy reduces recurrent infections. Operational issues regarding the patient–physician relationship with uncertain current legal status in some states are a barrier in the use of this strategy.

Patients who have uncomplicated gonorrhea and are treated with any of the CDC-recommended regimens do not need to return for a confirmation of cure testing. Patients who have symptoms that persist after treatment should be evaluated by culture for *N. gonorrhoeae*, and any gonococci isolated should be tested for antimicrobial susceptibility.

Disseminated gonococcal infection is treated with 1 g of ceftriaxone (Rocephin) daily, and once a response has occurred may be switched to oral therapy with cefixime (Suprax) or cefpodoxime (Vantin) at 400 mg orally twice daily to finish one week of therapy. Fluoroquinolones may be an alternative treatment option if antimicrobial susceptibility can be documented by culture. Gonococcal endocarditis is treated with 4 weeks of ceftriaxone (Rocephin), and meningitis with 10 to 14 days of ceftriaxone (Rocephin). Treatment of PID is described in the appropriate article.

## REFERENCES

Centers for Disease Control and Prevention. Sexually transmitted diseases treatment guidelines 2006. MMWR Recomm Rep 2006;55(No. RR-11): 42-49.

Centers for Disease Control and Prevention: Update to CDC's Sexually Transmitted Diseases Treatment guidelines, 2006: Fluoroquinolones No Longer Recommended for Treatment of Gonococcal Infections, 2007. MMWR Wkly Rep 2007;56:332-336.

Centers for Disease Control and Prevention: Sexually transmitted disease surveillance 2003 Supplement: Gonococcal Isolate Surveillance Project (GISP) annual report—2005. Atlanta, Ga, U.S. Department of Health and Human Services, January 2007.

Centers for Disease Control and Prevention: STD Surveillance 2004: Accessed December 2, 2004, at http://www.cdc.gov/std/stats/04pdf/NatProfileAll.pdf

Cook RL, Hutchison SL, Ostergaard L, et al: Systematic review: Noninvasive testing for *Chlamydia trachomatis* and *Neisseria gonorrhoeae*. Ann Intern Med 2005;142:914-925.

Golden MR, Wrightington WLH, Handsfield HH, et al: Effect of expedited treatment of sex partners on recurrent or persistent gonorrhea or chlamydial infection. N Engl J Med 2005;352:676-685.

Miller WC, Ford CA, Morris M, et al: Prevalence of chlamydia and gonococcal infections among young adults in the United States. JAMA 2004;291: 2229-2236.

# Nongonococcal Urethritis

Method of
*John N. Krieger, MD*

Urethritis is defined as inflammation of the urethra and is commonly caused by urogenital infection. Urethritis is classified as either gonococcal, in patients whose inflammation is caused by *Neisseria gonorrhoeae*, or nongonococcal (NGU), in patients with inflammation that is not related to infection with *N. gonorrhoeae*.

## Clinical Presentation

More than 4 million NGU cases are estimated to occur among men in the United States every year. Urethritis is characterized by symptoms of urethral discharge and dysuria, often accompanied by increased urinary frequency or pruritis. Signs of urethritis include urethral discharge that can occur spontaneously or after stripping of the urethra, erythema, and urethral tenderness.

Although the clinical presentation varies, the incubation of NGU averages 7 to 14 days from exposure to an infected partner. Typically the onset is gradual, with mild dysuria and mucoid discharge. In some high-risk populations, up to 50% of infections are asymptomatic.

## Etiology

NGU should be considered infectious until proven otherwise. Most infectious cases of urethritis are sexually transmitted.

*Chlamydia trachomatis* remains the most important pathogen, accounting for 15% to 40% of NGU cases. The prevalence of *C. trachomatis* is lower in older patients and in referral populations. Other infectious causes of NGU include *Mycoplasma genitalium*, *Trichomonas vaginalis*, and herpes simplex virus. The etiologic roles are less well defined for other infectious agents including *Ureaplasma urealytimum*, enteric bacteria, anaerobes, and *Candida* species. Occasionally, patients with other urologic conditions (e.g., prostatitis, urethral stricture disease, or, rarely, bacterial urinary tract infection) present with symptoms of NGU. Other unusual causes of NGU include chemical, allergic, and autoimmune processes.

## Diagnosis

It is important to document the presence of urethral inflammation. This may be done by finding mucoid or mucopurulent discharge on physical examination or by diagnostic testing. The Gram stain is the preferred rapid diagnostic test. Urethral inflammation may also be documented by a positive leukocyte esterase test on first-void urine or by finding pyuria on microscopic examination of the first-void urine sediment.

Diagnostic testing for both *N. gonorrhoeae* and *C. trachomatis* organisms is strongly recommended. Specific etiologic diagnosis may guide therapy and can improve compliance and partner notification. These infections are both reportable to state health departments. Patients at risk for *N. gonorrhoeae* and *C. trachomatis* should receive appropriate counseling and should receive testing for HIV and syphilis. Clinical evaluation and treatment of sex partners are critical for preventing complications and interrupting sexual transmission. Pathogens responsible for NGU are associated with cervicitis, pelvic inflammatory disease, and tubal infertility.

The Gram stain is the preferred rapid diagnostic test for evaluating urethritis because it provides high sensitivity and specificity. Gonococcal infection can be established by documenting the presence of white blood cells (WBCs) containing intracellular gram-negative diplococci. Presence of gram-negative rods should raise the suspicion for enteric bacteria.

## CURRENT DIAGNOSIS

- Documenting urethral inflammation is critical for diagnosis of urethritis. One or more of the following techniques can provide documentation:
  - Physical examination showing urethral discharge, either present spontaneously at the meatus or after stripping the urethra. This discharge may be either mucoid or purulent in character.
  - Gram stain of urethral exudate showing five or more WBCs per oil immersion field (×1000). The Gram stain is the preferred rapid diagnostic test.
  - Urine leukocyte esterase dip stick test positive on first-void urine
  - First-void urine sediment microscopic examination demonstrating 10 or more WBCs per high-power field (×400).

*Abbreviation:* WBC = white blood cell.

Confirmatory tests should be employed to identify a specific etiology. *N. gonorrhoeae* and *C. trachomatis* can be detected using culture, DNA hybridization tests on a urethral specimen, or nucleic acid amplification tests on a urethral or urine specimen. Because of their increased sensitivity, nucleic acid amplification tests are recommended for diagnosing chlamydial infection. For urine testing, 10 to 15 mL of first-void urine is collected then evaluated using nucleic acid amplification testing.

Diagnostic tests for the genital mycoplasmas (*M. genitalium*, *U. urealyticum*, and other genital mycoplasmas) are available in research settings. Such tests are usually unavailable for routine clinical use. *T. vaginalis* may be cultured, but specific media are necessary for isolation. To increase sensitivity, cultures of both a urethral swab sample and a urine specimen are recommended.

## Treatment

If gonorrhea cannot be ruled out by Gram stain of urethral secretions, potentially noncompliant patients should be treated for both gonorrhea

## CURRENT THERAPY

**Recommended Regimens**

- Azithromycin (Zithromax) 1 g PO in a single dose
- Doxycycline (Vibramycin) 100 mg PO bid × 7 days

**Alternative Regimens**

- Erythromycin base (E-Mycin, ERYC, E-Base) 500 mg PO qid × 7 days
- Erythromycin ethylsuccinate (EES) 800 mg PO qid × 7 days
- Ofloxacin (Floxin) 300 mg PO bid × 7 days
- Levofloxacin (Levaquin)[1] 500 mg PO qd × 7 days
- If an erythromycin regimen is the only possibility and the patient cannot tolerate high-dose schedules, then one of the following regimens should be considered.
- Erythromycin base (E-Mycin, ERYC, E-Base) 250 mg PO qid × 14 days
- Erythromycin ethylsuccinate (EES) 400 mg PO qid × 14 days

[1]Not FDA approved for this indication.

and chlamydial infection. Both azithromycin (Zithromax) and doxycycline (Vibramycin) are highly effective for treating chlamydial NGU. Azithromycin also provides convenient single dosing and the opportunity for directly observed therapy. Doxycycline is inexpensive but requires twice-daily dosing for a full week. Alternatives include erythromycin and fluoroquinolones regimens.

For patients with erratic health care–seeking behavior in whom poor compliance is anticipated, azithromycin offers the easiest administration. Further, *M. genitalium* appears to respond better to macrolides than to tetracyclines. Patients should be advised to abstain from sex until therapy is completed, symptoms have resolved, and sex partners have been treated.

## Follow-up

Routine follow-up is not recommended for patients whose symptoms resolve after therapy. Patients with persistent or recurrent symptoms should return for reevaluation.

Symptoms alone should not prompt a second course of therapy unless the patient has documented urethritis or a positive test for a urogenital pathogen. Patients should return for evaluation and treatment if their symptoms persist or recur after completion of therapy. Patients with NGU should refer all sex partners in the past 60 days for evaluation and treatment.

## Chronic Urethritis

Chronic urethritis is defined as persistent or recurrent urethritis within 6 weeks following treatment. An estimated 20% to 40% of NGU cases do not respond to first-line therapy. Although up to 20% of men with chlamydial NGU have chronic urethritis, up to 50% of men with non-chlamydial NGU have chronic urethritis. Noncompliance and reinfection are important considerations. Other causes include organisms that do not respond to the standard treatment regimens, such as *T. vaginalis*, tetracycline-resistant mycoplasmas, viral etiologies, and other bacteria.

Up to 30% of NGU has no identifiable infectious etiology. These cases can involve allergy and postinfectious immunologic responses. Before administering therapy, presence of urethral inflammation should be documented. Patients with persistent or recurrent urethritis who did not comply with therapy or who had exposure to an untreated sex partner should be re-treated with the initial drug regimen. Otherwise, recommended treatment regimens include metronidazole (Flagyl),[1] 2 g orally in a single dose, plus either erythromycin base (E-Base), 500 mg orally four times a day for 7 days, or erythromycin ethylsuccinate (EES), 800 mg orally four times a day for 7 days.

## Complications

For infected men, complications of untreated NGU include epididymitis in less than 3% of cases and, rarely, Reiter's syndrome. Patients with a history of NGU also appear to be at increased risk for developing chronic prostatitis/chronic pelvic pain syndrome.

Female sex partners are at risk for pelvic inflammatory disease, tubal infertility, and ectopic pregnancy. Prompt and appropriate therapy and treatment of sexual partners decrease the risk of complications substantially.

### REFERENCES

Aydin D, Kucukbasmaci O, Gonullu N, Aktas Z: Susceptibilities of *Neisseria gonorrhoeae* and *Ureaplasma urealyticum* isolates from male patients with urethritis to several antibiotics including telithromycin. Chemotherapy 2005;51:89-92.

Bradshaw CS, Tabrizi SN, Read TR, et al: Etiologies of nongonococcal urethritis: Bacteria, viruses, and the association with orogenital exposure. J Infect Dis 2006;193:336-345.

[1]Not FDA approved for this indication.

Centers for Disease Control and Prevention: Screening tests to detect *Chlamydia trachomatis* and *Neisseria gonorrhoeae* infections. MMWR Recomm Rep 2002;51(RR-15):3-19.

Centers for Disease Control and Prevention: Sexually transmitted disease treatment guidelines 2002. MMWR Recomm Rep 2002;51(RR-6):30-42.

Deguchi T, Yoshida T, Miyazawa T, et al: Association of *Ureaplasma urealyticum* (biovar 2) with nongonococcal urethritis. Sex Transm Dis 2004;31:192-195.

Falk L, Fredlund H, Jensen JS: Symptomatic urethritis is more prevalent in men infected with *Mycoplasma genitalium* than with *Chlamydia trachomatis*. Sex Transm Infect 2004;80:289-293.

Geisler WM, Yu S, Hook EW 3rd: Chlamydial and gonococcal infection in men without polymorphonuclear leukocytes on Gram stain: Implications for diagnostic approach and management. Sex Transm Dis 2005;32:630-634.

Jensen JS: *Mycoplasma genitalium:* The aetiological agent of urethritis and other sexually transmitted diseases. J Eur Acad Dermatol Venereol 2004;18:1-11.

Kaydos-Daniels SC, Miller WC, Hoffman I, et al: The use of specimens from various genitourinary sites in men, to detect *Trichomonas vaginalis* infection. J Infect Dis 2004;189:1926-1931.

Leung A, Eastick K, Haddon LE, et al: *Mycoplasma genitalium* is associated with symptomatic urethritis. Int J STD AIDS 2006;17:285-288.

O'Mahony C: Adenoviral non-gonococcal urethritis. Int J STD AIDS 2006; 17:203-204.

Ozgül A, Dede I, Taskaynatan MA, et al: Clinical presentations of chlamydial and non-chlamydial reactive arthritis. Rheumatol Int 2006;26:879-885.

Pontari MA, McNaughton-Collins M, O'Leary P, et al: A case-control study of risk factors in men with chronic pelvic pain syndrome. BJU Int 2005;96:559-565.

Swygard H, Sena AC, Hobbs MM, Cohen MS: Trichomoniasis: Clinical manifestations, diagnosis and management. Sex Transm Infect 2004;80:91-95.

Taylor SN: *Mycoplasma genitalium.* Curr Infect Dis Rep 2005;7:453-457.

Taylor-Robinson D, Gilroy CB, Thomas BJ, Hay PE: *Mycoplasma genitalium* in chronic non-gonococcal urethritis. Int J STD AIDS 2004;15:21-25.

Yasuda M, Maeda S, Deguchi T: In vitro activity of fluoroquinolones against *Mycoplasma genitalium* and their bacteriological efficacy for treatment of *M. genitalium*–positive nongonococcal urethritis in men. Clin Infect Dis 2005;41:1357-1359.

# Syphilis

Method of
*Mrunal Shah, MD*

One of the oldest infections known, syphilis dates back more than 500 years. It was known as "The Great Pox" because of its skin manifestations; in contrast to the "small pox" seen around the same time. Studies were done before the use of antibiotics, which is where most of our natural history information comes from. The most recent epidemic occurred in 1990 (20.3 cases per 100,000 population) and has fallen steadily each year since. In the year 2000, the rate was at an all time low of 2.2 cases per 100,000 population. This was a 9.6% drop since 1999. The Centers for Disease Control and Prevention (CDC) hopes to eradicate the disease completely by 2005, but this may be difficult.

Peak ages are 30 to 39 years of age in men and 20 to 24 years of age in women. African Americans have always had higher incidences than whites. In the 1990s, it was 60:1, but the incidence has since declined to 30:1.

## Microbiology

*Treponema pallidum* is the bacterium responsible for causing syphilis. It is very small and cannot be detected by ordinary microscopy, a feature that complicates diagnosis. The organism can be seen with darkfield microscopy, a technique that uses a special condenser to cast an oblique light. This allows visualization of a corkscrew-shaped organism with tightly wound spirals. This organism is extremely sensitive to penicillin, as is discussed later in the article.

It has a very slow doubling rate, therefore requiring longer courses of treatment.

## Pathophysiology

*T. pallidum* initiates infection when it gains access to subcutaneous tissues through microabrasions that can occur during sexual intercourse. Even though it has a slow doubling time (30 hours), it escapes host immune defenses and leads to the initial ulcerative lesion, the chancre. These can be seen anywhere around the genitalia including the cervix, perianal and rectal areas, and the oral mucosa. Regional lymphadenopathy also can be seen. As the host immune system fights the initial infection, *T. pallidum* is disseminated throughout the host. This is known as latency, as the patient will have no symptoms. There is also vertical spread in utero or during delivery, which is why prenatal panels include screening tests for syphilis.

## Clinical Manifestations

The initial clinical manifestation is also called *primary* syphilis. This usually consists of a painless chancre at the site of inoculation. Primary syphilis represents a local infection, but it quickly becomes systemic with widespread dissemination of the spirochete. Because it is painless, most people do not seek medical attention. Even without treatment, the chancre will resolve in 4 to 6 weeks. It is this painlessness that helps separate it from herpes simplex virus (genital herpes) and *Haemophilus ducreyi* (chancroid).

In approximately weeks to months after the resolution of the chancre, patients will develop *secondary* syphilis, which includes systemic symptoms of rash, fever, headache, malaise, anorexia, and diffuse lymphadenopathy. The rash typically involves the palms and soles but can also include mucosal surfaces. Many patients do not realize that they had these lesions. These symptoms usually resolve spontaneously but can relapse for up to 5 years.

After symptoms resolve, and for up to many years later, the disease goes into *latent* syphilis, which is characterized by a lack of symptoms but seropositive test results. This can be separated into early and late latent phases based on being potentially infectious in the early phase. This is defined by the United States Public Health Service (USPHS) as infection of 1 year's duration or less. Anything longer is late latent.

Finally, for the next 1 to 30 years, untreated patients have a 25% to 40% risk of developing *late* or *tertiary* syphilis. It may involve many tissue types, so the spectrum of disease can be very confusing. Moreover, patients need not have had symptoms of primary or secondary syphilis prior to developing late syphilis. Tissues involved include cutaneous (gumma formation), cardiovascular (aortic disease), and central nervous system (CNS) (tabes dorsalis, meningitis, neurosyphilis) diseases (Table 1).

## Diagnosis

The quickest, most direct method of diagnosing primary and secondary syphilis is direct visualization of the spirochete of moist lesions by means of darkfield microscopy. This is difficult and requires using laboratories that perform a high volume of sexually transmitted disease analyses. In general, a moist lesion should be cleaned with saline (not iodine because of bacteriocidal effect). Then, using gauze, the lesion should be unroofed. Any serosanguineous material should be collected on a dry slide for examination.

More common is serologic testing that can be done in most laboratories. The two most common screening tests are rapid plasma reagin (RPR) and the Venereal Disease Research Laboratory (VDRL) test. These tests are designed to test for IgM and IgG antibodies against a cardiolipin-cholesterol-lecithin antigen. Positive tests are reported as a dilutional titer. False positives are less than 1:4, whereas higher titers (1:16 to 1:128) are found in secondary and early latent syphilis. This titer is important as a benchmark to follow treatment. Lack of expected decreases in titer

TABLE 1  Clinical Manifestations and Treatment of Syphilis

| Stage | Clinical Manifestation | Treatment |
|---|---|---|
| Primary | Painless ulcer (chancre), adenopathy | Benzathine penicillin G (Bicillin LA), 2.4 million U IM × 1 |
| Secondary (weeks to months) | Rash, mucocutaneous lesions, adenopathy, hepatitis, arthritis, glomerulonephritis, condyloma lata | Benzathine penicillin G, 2.4 million U IM × 1 |
| Latent | Asymptomatic | |
| Early (<1 year) | | Benzathine penicillin G, 2.4 million U IM × 1 |
| Late | | Benzathine penicillin G, 2.4 million U IM weekly × 3 |
| Tertiary (late) 1-30 years | | |
|   Cutaneous | Gummatous lesions | Benzathine penicillin G, 2.4 million U IM weekly × 3 |
|   Cardiovascular | Aortic aneurysm, aortic insufficiency | Benzathine penicillin G, 2.4 million U IM weekly × 3 |
|   CNS | Neurosyphilis, tabes dorsalis, Argyll-Robertson pupils, paresis, seizures, subtle psychiatric manifestations, dementia; may be asymptomatic | Aqueous crystalline penicillin G, 18-24 million U/d given as 3-4 million units IV q4h for 10-14 days or Procaine penicillin (Wycillin), 2.4 million U qd with probenecid 500 mg PO qid for 10-14 days |

*Abbreviations*: CNS = central nervous system; IM = intramuscularly; IV = intravenously; PO = orally; qd = daily; qid = 4 times per day.
Adapted from the CDC: Guidelines for the treatment of STDs. MMWR Morb Mortal Wkly Rep 2002;51(RR-06):1-80.

indicate inadequate treatment, false-positive result, re-infection, or late-stage therapy.

Before treatment, a positive screening test needs to be confirmed with specific *T. pallidum* antigen testing, such as the fluorescent treponemal antibody absorption test (FTA-ABS). These tests are expensive and have a high false-positive rate, making them unsuitable as screening tests. They also remain positive for life in most people.

Newer molecular tests include the use of polymerase chain reaction (PCR), which can be used to detect multiple organisms. It has high sensitivity and specificity and can distinguish among *H. ducreyi*, herpes simplex virus, and *T. pallidum*. This test is very expensive and is likely to be available only in specialized laboratories, for now.

The most significant morbidity of syphilis occurs during the tertiary phase and includes neurosyphilis. *T. pallidum* can be found in the cerebrospinal fluid (CSF) during primary and secondary phases, but it usually resolves on its own. Those patients who have an abnormal CSF during the latent phase are at higher risk for symptomatic neurosyphilis, making it helpful to distinguish asymptomatic neurosyphilis. The CDC recommends that CSF testing be done whenever there is clinical evidence of neurosyphilis or vision changes, active tertiary syphilis, treatment failure, or HIV infection. CSF-VDRL is highly specific, but, unfortunately, very insensitive (as low as 30%) and therefore can rule in but cannot exclude neurosyphilis.

Although the HIV epidemic showed a resurgence of syphilis, it is controversial as to what diagnostic changes occurred in testing. Several studies show contradictory information; one shows that there was an increase in the false-positive rates, whereas a second study showed a decrease in true-positive rates, and a third study showed higher false negatives. In any case, testing should still be performed as in non-HIV patients and followed accordingly.

Pregnancy poses only increased risk, including perinatal death, premature delivery, low birth weight, congenital anomalies, and active congenital syphilis of the neonate. Physical examination and serologic testing should be performed in any female considering pregnancy or during initial antepartum testing at least. Treatment, discussed below, should be given as if the patient is not pregnant.

## Treatment

In all stages, the main reason for treatment is to prevent progression and spread of the disease. Historic treatments included mercury, salvarsan (an arsenic derivative), fever therapy, and malarial injection. Today's treatment has been in use since 1943, since the introduction of penicillin. Because there has been no reported resistance, penicillin remains the treatment of choice, so much so that penicillin-allergic patients have undergone desensitization therapy in order to receive it. Although penicillin G, given parenterally, is the preferred drug, the preparation used (benzathine, procaine, crystalline), dosage, and duration of therapy depend on stage and clinical manifestations (see Table 1). Oral penicillin is not considered appropriate for treatment. Alternative treatments could include doxycycline (Vibramycin), tetracycline, erythromycin, or ceftriaxone (Rocephin).[1]

Once treatment is started, physicians should be aware of a potential complication called the Jarisch-Herxheimer reaction. It is an acute, febrile reaction accompanied by headache and myalgias, which represents treponemal cell death and release of toxins. It peaks within 2 hours and subsides within 24 hours, and is most common in primary and secondary disease.

## Follow-up of Treated Patients

Any patient with syphilis diagnosed at any stage should get testing for HIV and should be retested in 3 to 6 months if a member of a high-risk population. After treatment, repeat serologic testing should be done at 6 and 12 months and titers at 24 months. If there is not at least a fourfold decrease in 6 months, there is likely treatment failure. A lumbar puncture should be done to rule out neurosyphilis, and retreatment with three weekly injections of 2.4 million units of benzathine penicillin (Bicillin LA) is recommended unless there is evidence of neurosyphilis.

Partners of patients with syphilis should also be notified and treated. In primary disease, any partner within the previous 3 months should be identified. Empiric treatment is recommended unless there is good follow-up and serologic surveillance.

---

[1] Not FDA approved for this indication.

# Contraceptive Methods

Method of
*Lama L. Tolaymat, MD, MPH, and
Andrew M. Kaunitz, MD*

Each year, nearly 2% of U.S. women of reproductive age have an induced abortion. This sobering statistic underscores the importance of women and couples having access to the effective hormonal, intrauterine, and surgical methods of contraception described here.

 **CURRENT THERAPY**

- Two percent of U.S. women of reproductive age have an induced abortion annually.
- Noncontraceptive benefits of oral contraceptive include decreasing the risk of endometrial cancer, ovarian cancer, ectopic pregnancy, and pelvic inflammatory disease as well as treatment of dysmenorrhea, menorrhagia, and acne.
- Combination estrogen-progestin birth control methods (pills, patch, and ring) are contraindicated in women who are smokers >35 y and those with a history of DVT, with cardiovascular disease, or with active liver disease.
- Progestin-only birth control methods (pills, injections, or the progestin-releasing IUD) represent appropriate contraceptive options for women who have medical problems contraindicating combination birth control methods.
- Women with menorrhagia or dysmenorrhea may benefit from extended-cycle oral contraceptive pills (Seasonique and Seasonale).
- Plan B, a progestin-only formulation, is the only oral formulation currently marketed for emergency contraception. Although package labeling indicates it should be taken within 72 hours, effective postcoital contraception is provided if Plan B is taken up to 5 d following unprotected intercourse.
- Copper and progestin-releasing IUDs offer users convenient birth control as effective as sterilization yet completely reversible.
- The copper IUD (ParaGard) may increase menstrual flow and thus may not be a good method for women with menorrhagia.
- Use of the progestin (levonorgestrel)-releasing IUD (Mirena) is associated with noncontraceptive benefits including reduction in heavy menstrual flow because of fibroids or adenomyosis and decreased pain in women with endometriosis.
- Surgical tubal sterilization is associated with a 10-y cumulative failure rate of 1.8%–3%.
- A device for occlusion of the fallopian tubes using hysteroscopy (Essure) was approved for use in the United States in 2002.
- The failure rate associated with vasectomy is 0.94% at 1 y and 1.1% at 5 y, representing pregnancy rates higher than previously reported.

*Abbreviations:* DVT = deep vein thrombosis; IUD = intrauterine device.

# Estrogen/Progestin Combination Oral Contraceptive Pills

Oral contraceptive (OC) use is safe for the majority of users with many noncontraceptive benefits, such as decreasing the risk of endometrial cancer, ovarian cancer, ectopic pregnancy, and pelvic inflammatory disease and treating dysmenorrhea, menorrhagia, and acne. Although OCs represent a highly effective birth control method for correct consistent users, inconsistent or incorrect use accounts for the annual failure rate of 8% experienced overall by OC users.

OCs are usually initiated on the first day of menses or the first Sunday after menses starts. In these cases, a backup method of contraception is not needed. It is helpful to associate pill taking with a daily routine such as tooth brushing to improve compliance.

Conventional combination OC formulations include 21 active and 7 inactive tablets. The progestin component of the OCs suppresses the pituitary secretion of luteinizing hormone (LH), preventing ovulation. The estrogen component (ethinyl estradiol) suppresses secretion of follicle-stimulating hormone (FSH) and enhances cycle control (regular withdrawal bleeding with minimal unscheduled or so-called breakthrough bleeding). If 1 or 2 tablets are missed, the patient should take 1 tablet as soon as possible. Then 1 tablet should be taken twice a day until all the missed tablets are taken. Breast tenderness and nausea, common OC side effects, are related to the estrogen dose. Accordingly, if these side effects persist for more than several cycles, changing to a lower estrogen dose (e.g., switching from a 30- to 35-μg to a 20- to 25-μg) formulation may be useful.

Breakthrough (unscheduled) bleeding and spotting occurs more often in women taking 20-μg estrogen OCs than in those taking 30- to 35-μg formulations. Box 1 lists medical contraindications to all estrogen-progestin contraceptives.

# Combination Oral Contraceptives with Reduced Pill-Free Intervals and/or Extended Cycles

OC formulations with reduced pill-free intervals appear to achieve superior cycle control (less unscheduled or breakthrough bleeding/spotting) despite use of very low doses of estrogen and may achieve higher contraceptive efficacy than conventional 21/7 OC formulations. Three 28-day OC formulations are formulated with 20 μg ethinyl estradiol and have fewer than 7 hormone-free days. One (Mircette), formulated with the progestin desogestrel, includes 2 days of inactive tablets and 5 ethinyl estradiol tablets in place of the 7 inactive tablets. Two recently approved formulations contain 24 active tablets followed by 4 days of inactive pills. One (Yaz) is formulated with the progestin drospirenone. Yaz has been approved by the FDA for

---

**BOX 1   Contraindications to Combination Hormonal Methods**

- Smokers: ≥35 y
- Hypertension: Uncontrolled or ≥35 y
- Diabetes: Vascular disease or ≥35 y
- Migraines: Focal neurologic symptoms or ≥35 y
- Vascular disease: Associated with systemic lupus erythematosus
- Personal history of breast cancer or thromboembolism
- Coronary artery or cerebrovascular disease
- Acute or chronic hepatocellular disease with abnormal liver function
- Cholestatic jaundice with prior pregnancy or contraceptive use

Adapted from http://www.arhp.org/healthcareproviders/cme/onlinecme/wellwoman/TOC.cfm?ID=336

the treatment of premenstrual dysphoric disorder. The other (Loestrin 24) is formulated with the progestin norethindrone acetate and has a shorter duration of withdrawal bleeding than other OCs.

The first extended-cycle OC (Seasonale) to be marketed in the United States includes 84 (12 weeks) of active pills followed by 7 placebo pills, rather than the conventional 21 active tablets followed by 7 placebos. Each active pill contains 150 µg of levonorgestrel and 30 µg of ethinyl estradiol. Over time, this extended approach to OC leads to 4 rather than 13 withdrawal bleeding episodes each year. Women considering extended OC use should be counseled to expect an initially higher rate of breakthrough bleeding and spotting, which declines over time. Women with a history of menorrhagia or dysmenorrhea may be candidates for extended-cycle OC use. In the future, extended-cycle OC formulations with no hormone-free days may become available. A recently approved OC (Seasonique) is identical to Seasonale but substitutes 10 µg of estrogen in place of the 7 placebo tablets that follow the 12 weeks of active tablets in each pack. Breakthrough bleeding and spotting appear to occur less frequently with the use of Seasonique than with Seasonale

## Progestin-Only Oral Contraceptives

Also known as minipills, the progestin-only OC formulation (Micronor) contains even lower doses than combination OCs. The documented rates of failure for progestin-only pills are comparable to those of combination OCs in women who are meticulous about taking the pill at the same time every day. If one pill is taken 3 or more hours late, backup contraception is needed for 48 hours. Most commonly in the United States, minipills are used by lactating women who intrinsically have low fecundability; in this subgroup of women, contraceptive failures with progestin-only OC use are not common.

## Emergency Contraception

With the manufacturer no longer making a dedicated combination emergency contraception (EC) formulation (Preven) as of summer 2004, the only dedicated EC formulation currently available is the progestin-only formulation (Plan B), which consists of two levonorgestrel 750 µg tablets.

Progestin-only EC is more effective and causes less nausea and emesis than combination EC. Package labeling for Plan B indicates that 1 tablet should be taken within 72 hours of unprotected intercourse, followed 12 hours later by a second tablet. Taking the 2 tablets together, however, may be as effective in preventing pregnancy as dividing the dose. Furthermore, Plan B may retain its efficacy in pregnancy prevention when taken up to 5 days after unprotected intercourse. EC is available over the counter at pharmacies for those 18 years of age and older and is also available by prescription for women of any age.

## Injectable Contraception

### PROGESTIN ONLY

Depomedroxyprogesterone acetate (DMPA) (Depo-Provera) is an injectable contraceptive that provides long-acting reversible birth control, as effective as sterilization. The standard dose is 150 mg (1 mL) of DMPA intramuscularly every 3 months (or every 12 to 13 weeks). As with combination OC use, DMPA suppresses ovulation and ovarian estradiol production. In contrast with combination OC use, DMPA includes no estrogen component. Therefore, bone mineral density (BMD) declines during prolonged use of DMPA. In 2004, the FDA placed a black box in DMPA package labeling warning of the risk of significant loss of bone density during DMPA use. Fortunately, in adolescents as well as adult users, BMD rapidly recovers after discontinuation of DMPA, and no evidence indicates that DMPA use causes postmenopausal osteoporosis or fractures. The short-term impact that DMPA has on BMD appears analogous to that of lactation (which also lowers background estrogen levels). Lactation is not a risk factor for osteoporosis later in life. Skeletal health concerns should not restrict

use of DMPA in adults or teens, nor should use of DMPA be considered by itself an indication for testing BMD.

Although concerns regarding weight gain may discourage some women, small randomized clinical trial data found that DMPA did not cause weight gain or increased appetite in short-term users. A subcutaneous DMPA formulation that should facilitate self-administration became available in 2005 and is approved both for contraception and treatment of pain associated with endometriosis.

## Combination Patch

Ortho Evra is a once-a-week transdermal contraceptive patch applied for 3 consecutive weeks, followed by a patch-free week during which withdrawal bleeding is anticipated. The patch can be applied to the lower abdomen, upper outer arm, buttock, or upper torso (except for the breast). The patch delivers a daily systemic dose of 150 µg of norelgestromin and 20 µg of ethinyl estradiol. In a randomized clinical trial, the contraceptive efficacy of the patch was comparable to that of oral contraception. If the patch is detached for greater than 24 hours, the user should start a new patch cycle and use a backup contraceptive method (such as condoms) for 1 week. A recent randomized pharmacokinetic trial found that serum ethinyl estradiol exposure was lower in the users of the vaginal contraceptive ring compared to oral contraceptives and the transdermal patch. This led to the concern that the risk of venous thromboembolus may be higher in women using the transdermal patch. Findings of epidemiologic studies have conflicted regarding whether the risk of venous thromboembolism is higher with the contraceptive patch than with OCs.

## Combination Vaginal Ring

NuvaRing is worn for 3 weeks, then removed for 1 week, during which withdrawal bleeding is anticipated. The ring is composed of a flexible ethylene vinyl acetate copolymer, which releases approximately 120 µg of etonogestrel and 15 µg of ethinyl estradiol per day. The ring is self-inserted and removed. In comparative clinical trials, rates of breakthrough bleeding and spotting were lower with the ring than with OCs. As with the patch, contraceptive efficacy of the ring is similar to that of combination OCs in clinical trials. Backup contraception is needed for 7 days if the ring remains outside of the vagina for more than 3 hours.

## Intrauterine Devices

Intrauterine devices (IUDs) offer users convenient birth control as effective as sterilization yet completely reversible. In women in the United States, use of IUDs has declined from approximately 10% in the mid-1970s to 1% today. Concerns among clinicians and women that IUDs cause salpingitis and tubal infertility account for much of this decline. A systematic review found that if any increased risk in salpingitis is associated with IUD use, it is small and appears confined to the first month postinsertion. Likewise, use of an IUD is not associated with a subsequent increased risk of tubal infertility.

The copper IUD (ParaGard) is approved for up to 10 years of use. It is appropriate for women who prefer regular cycles. Because use of the copper IUD can increase flow and cramps, it is appropriate for women who have no excess menstrual flow or cramps at baseline. The Food and Drug Administration (FDA) approved liberalized safety labeling revisions for the copper IUD in 2005. The revised labeling states that although the IUD may now be used in women with a history of pelvic inflammatory disease (PID) or sexually transmitted disease, it is contraindicated in those with acute PID or current behavior suggesting a high risk thereof. The prior language discouraging use of the IUD in nulliparous women was likewise removed.

The levonorgestrel-releasing IUD (Mirena) is approved for up to 5 years of use. It releases 20 µg of levonorgestrel a day. This progestin-releasing IUD reduces menstrual flow and is therefore appropriate for women who would like their birth control method to reduce flow. Women interested in using the levonorgestrel-releasing IUD should be

## BOX 2   Noncontraceptive Health Benefits of the Levonorgestrel-Releasing Intrauterine Device

- Reduces menorrhagia, including when caused by uterine fibroids or adenomyosis and as an alternative to endometrial ablation or hysterectomy
- Relieves pain caused by endometriosis
- Prevention of endometrial hyperplasia in menopausal women using estrogen therapy; also, treatment of endometrial hyperplasia/cancer
- Prevention of endometrial proliferation and polyps in patients taking tamoxifen (Nolvadex)

aware, however, that initial irregular spotting or bleeding is common after insertion of this device. Hormonal side effects, including acne and ovarian cysts, also occur in some users. Box 2 details the important noncontraceptive benefits associated with use of the levonorgestrel IUD.

## Progestin-Releasing Implants

Progestin-releasing contraceptive implants provide highly effective, convenient birth control. Although Norplant and Jadelle are approved by the FDA, neither is currently marketed in the United States.

Norplant levonorgestrel consists of six capsules and provides contraception up to 5 years. The difficulty with insertion and, in particular, removal of the six capsules, along with frequent complaints of irregular bleeding among users, explains why U.S. clinicians, women, and the manufacturer lost interest in this contraceptive system, which initially was in great demand when introduced in 1991.

Jadelle consists of an implant of two rods each containing 150 mg of levonorgestrel. A single-rod progestin (Etonogestrel) implant (Implanon) is easier and quicker to insert and remove than Norplant, and its use is associated with less bleeding. This highly effective single-rod implant system received FDA approval in 2006.

## Female Sterilization

Tubal sterilization involves using rings (Falope), clips (Filshie or Hulka), electrocautery, or ligature/segmental excision (Pomeroy) to interrupt the patency of the fallopian tubes surgically. In the United States, approximately 700,000 tubal sterilizations are performed annually. Approximately half of them follow delivery, and half of these are performed as outpatient interval procedures. Sterilization is associated with a 10-year cumulative failure rate of 1.8% to 3%. The failure rate is higher in women younger than 28 years. Although sterilization can be reversed in some women and assisted reproductive technology can also be used to achieve pregnancy in many women following sterilization, this procedure should nonetheless be considered permanent.

Hysteroscopic tubal occlusion (Essure) is a device developed and approved for use in the United States in 2002. This device (2 mm in diameter and 4 cm long) is made of titanium, stainless steel, and nickel, and it contains Dacron fibers that induce an inflammatory reaction and fibrosis in the tubal lumen. A hysterosalpingogram is recommended following placement of the Essure device to confirm bilateral tubal occlusion.

## Male Sterilization

Vasectomy involves interruption of the vas deferens, preventing passage of sperm into seminal fluid. This office-based surgical procedure does not interfere with male sexual performance. After vasectomy, couples should use backup contraception until the sperm count reaches zero. According to Jamieson, recent data indicate the failure rate following vasectomy is 9.4 per 1000 procedures at 1 year and 11.3 at 5 years, higher than the previously estimated failure rate.

## REFERENCES

Anderson FD, Gibbons W, Portman D: Safety and efficacy of an extended-regimen oral contraceptive utilizing continuous low-dose ethinyl estradiol. Contraception 2006;73(3):229-234.

Anderson FD, Hait H: A multicenter, randomized study of an extended cycle oral contraceptive. Contraception 2003;68:89-96.

Audet MC, Moreau M, Koltun WD, et al: Evaluation of contraceptive efficacy and cycle control of a transdermal contraceptive patch vs. an oral contraceptive: A randomized controlled trial. JAMA 2001; 285:2347-2354.

Bjarnadottir RI, Tuppurainen M, Killick SR: Comparison of cycle control with a combined contraceptive vaginal ring and oral levonorgestrel/ethinyl estradiol. Am J Obstet Gynecol 2002;186:389-395.

Cole JA, Norman H, Doherty M, Walker AM: Venous thromboembolism, myocardial infarction, and stroke among transdermal contraceptive system users. Obstet Gynecol 2007;109(2 Pt 1):339-346.

Edelman AB, Koontz SL, Nichols MD, Jensen JT: Continuous oral contraceptives: Are bleeding patterns dependent on the hormones given? Obstet Gynecol 2006;107(3):657-665.

Hubacher D, Lara-Ricalde R, Taylor DJ, et al: Use of copper intrauterine devices and the risk of infertility among nulligravid women. N Engl J Med 2001;345:561-567.

Jain J, Jakimiuk AJ, Bode FR, et al: Contraceptive efficacy and safety of DMPA-SC. Contraception 2004;70:269-275.

Jamieson DJ, Costello C, Trussell J, et al: US Collaborative Review of Sterilization Working Group: The risk of pregnancy after vasectomy. Obstet Gynecol 2004;103:848-850.

Jensen JT: Don't forget the other benefits of the levonorgestrel IUS. Contemp OB/GYN 2007;50:46-50.

Jick SS, Kaye JA, Russmann S, Jick H: Risk of nonfatal venous thromboembolism in women using a contraceptive transdermal patch and oral contraceptives containing norgestimate and 35 micrograms of ethinyl estradiol. Contraception 2006;73(3):223-228.

Jones RK, Darroch JE, Henshaw SK: Contraceptive use among U.S. women having abortions in 2000–2001. Perspect Sex Reprod Health 2002;34:294-303.

Kaunitz AM: Revisiting progestin-only OCs. Contemp OB/GYN 1997;42:91-108.

Kaunitz AM: Beyond the pill: New data and options in hormonal and intrauterine contraception. Am J Obstet Gynecol 2005;192:998-1004.

Kaunitz AM: Depo-Provera's black box: Time to reconsider? Contraception 2005;72:165-167.

Ubeda A, Labastida RM, Dexeus S: Essure: A new device for hysteroscopic tubal sterilization in an outpatient setting. Fertil Steril 2004;82:196-199.

Van den Heuvel MW, Van Bragt AJ, Alnabawy AK, Kaptein MC: Comparison of ethinyl estradiol pharmacokinetics in three hormonal contraceptive formulations: The vaginal ring, the transdermal patch and an oral contraceptive. Contraception 2005;72(3):168-174.

Westhoff C: Depot-medroxyprogesterone acetate injection (Depo-Provera): A highly effective contraceptive option with proven long-term safety. Contraception 2003;68(2):75-87.

Westhoff C: Emergency contraception. N Engl J Med 2003;349:1830-1835.

Westhoff C, Davis A: Tubal sterilization: Focus on the U.S. experience. Fertil Steril 2000;73:913-922.

Yonkers KA, Brown C, Pearlstein TB, et al: Efficacy of a new low-dose oral contraceptive with drospirenone in premenstrual dysphoric disorder. Obstet Gynecol 2005;106(3):492-501.

# Diseases of Allergy

## Anaphylaxis and Serum Sickness

Method of
*Stephen F. Kemp, MD*

## Anaphylaxis

Anaphylaxis, an acute and potentially lethal multisystem allergic reaction, is virtually unavoidable in medical practice. Health care professionals must be able to recognize the signs of anaphylaxis, treat an episode promptly and appropriately, and be able to provide preventive recommendations. Epinephrine, which should be administered immediately, is the drug of choice for acute anaphylaxis.

Anaphylaxis is not a reportable disease, and both its morbidity and mortality are probably underestimated. A variety of statistics on the epidemiology of anaphylaxis have been published, but the lifetime risk per person in the U.S. is presumed to be 1% to 3%, with a mortality rate of 1%.

There is no universally accepted definition of anaphylaxis. An international and interdisciplinary group of representatives and experts from thirteen professional, governmental, and lay organizations proposed the following working definition: "Anaphylaxis is a serious allergic reaction that is rapid in onset and may cause death." Clinically, anaphylaxis is considered likely to be present if any one of the following three criteria is satisfied within minutes to hours: Acute onset of illness with involvement of skin, mucosal surface, or both, and at least one of the following: respiratory compromise, hypotension, or end-organ dysfunction; two or more of the following occurring rapidly after exposure to a likely allergen: involvement of skin or mucosal surface, respiratory compromise, hypotension, or persistent gastrointestinal symptoms; hypotension develops after exposure to a known allergen for that patient: age-specific low blood pressure or decline of systolic blood pressure of greater than 30% compared with baseline. In clinical practice, however, waiting until the development of multiorgan symptoms is risky because the ultimate severity of anaphylactic reaction is difficult to predict from the outset.

Anaphylaxis has varied clinical presentations, but respiratory compromise and cardiovascular collapse cause the most concern because they are the most frequent causes of fatalities. Urticaria and angioedema are the most common manifestations (more than 90% in retrospective series) but may be delayed or absent in rapidly progressive anaphylaxis. The previous severity of anaphylaxis is not predictive of the severity of a future reaction. The more rapidly anaphylaxis occurs after exposure to an offending stimulus, the more likely the reaction is to be severe and potentially life threatening. Anaphylaxis often produces signs and symptoms within 5 to 30 minutes, but reactions sometimes may not develop for several hours.

### PATHOPHYSIOLOGY

The chemical mediators that cause anaphylaxis are preformed and released from granules (histamine, tryptase, and others) or are generated from membrane lipids (prostaglandin $D_2$, leukotrienes, and platelet-activating factor) by the activated mast cell or basophil.

Tryptase is concentrated selectively in the secretory granules of all human mast cells. Its plasma levels during mast cell degranulation correlate with the clinical severity of anaphylaxis but need not be elevated in all forms of anaphylaxis (e.g., food-associated anaphylaxis).

Histamine exerts its pathophysiologic effects via both $H_1$ and $H_2$ receptors. Erythema (flushing), hypotension, and headache are mediated by both $H_1$ and $H_2$ receptors, whereas tachycardia, pruritus, bronchospasm, and rhinorrhea are associated with $H_1$ receptors alone.

Increased vascular permeability during anaphylaxis can produce a shift of 50% of intravascular fluid to the extravascular space within 10 minutes. This shift of effective blood volume causes compensatory catecholamine release, activates the renin-angiotensin-aldosterone system, and stimulates production of endothelin-1.

Mast cells accumulate at sites of coronary plaque erosion and rupture and they may contribute to coronary artery thrombosis. Because antibodies attached to mast cells can trigger mast cell degranulation, some investigators suggest that anaphylaxis may promote plaque rupture.

### CURRENT DIAGNOSIS

- Cutaneous: urticaria, angioedema, diffuse erythema, generalized pruritus
- Respiratory: tachypnea, bronchospasm, laryngeal or tongue edema, dysphonia
- Cardiovascular: tachycardia, bradycardia, hypotension, angina, cardiac arrhythmias
- Gastrointestinal: nausea, emesis, diarrhea, abdominal cramps, dysphagia
- Other: rhinitis, conjunctivitis, uterine cramps, headache, dizziness, syncope, blurred vision, seizure

## AGENTS THAT CAUSE ANAPHYLAXIS

Cause and effect often is confirmed historically in subjects who experience recurrent, objective findings of anaphylaxis upon inadvertent reexposure to the offending agent. Diagnostic testing, where appropriate, may confirm the presence of specific IgE and/or the degranulation of mast cells and basophils.

Virtually any agent capable of activating mast cells or basophils may potentially precipitate anaphylactic or anaphylactoid reactions. Table 1 lists common causes of anaphylaxis classified by pathophysiologic mechanism. Idiopathic anaphylaxis, anaphylaxis with no identifiable cause, has accounted for approximately a third of cases in most retrospective studies of anaphylaxis. However, of 601 patients evaluated more than two decades in a university-affiliated practice (the largest retrospective series), 59% of subjects were deemed to have idiopathic anaphylaxis.

Idiopathic anaphylaxis remains a diagnosis of exclusion, however. Serial histories and diagnostic tests for foods, spices, and vegetable gums occasionally identify a specific culprit in subjects previously presumed to have idiopathic anaphylaxis. The most common identifiable causes of anaphylaxis are foods, medications, insect stings, and immunotherapy injections. Anaphylaxis to peanuts and/or tree nuts causes the greatest concern because of its life-threatening severity, especially in subjects with asthma, and the tendency for subjects to develop lifelong allergic responsiveness to these foods.

## RECURRENT ANAPHYLAXIS

Depending on the report, recurrent (biphasic) anaphylaxis occurs in 1% to 20% of subjects who experience anaphylaxis. Signs and symptoms experienced during the recurrent phase of anaphylaxis may be equivalent to or worse than those observed in the initial reaction and may occur 1 to 78 hours (most within 8 hours) after apparent remission. Thus, it may be necessary to monitor subjects up to 24 hours after apparent recovery from the initial phase. Observation periods after apparent recovery from the initial phase should be individualized and based on such factors as comorbid conditions and distance from the patient's home to the closest emergency facility, particularly because there are no reliable predictors of biphasic anaphylaxis

## DIFFERENTIAL DIAGNOSIS

Several systemic disorders share clinical features with anaphylaxis. The vasodepressor (vasovagal) reaction probably is the condition most commonly confused with anaphylactic reactions. In vasodepressor reactions, however, urticaria is absent, dyspnea is generally absent, the blood pressure is usually normal or elevated, and the skin is typically cool and pale. Tachycardia is the rule in anaphylaxis. Bradycardia may be underrecognized in anaphylaxis, however. Brown and others conducted sting challenges in 19 subjects known to be allergic to jack jumper ants (*Myrmecia*). All eight subjects who became hypotensive developed bradycardia after an initial tachycardia.

Systemic mastocytosis, a disease characterized by mast cell proliferation in multiple organs, usually features urticaria pigmentosa (brownish macules that transform into wheals upon stroking them) and recurrent episodes of pruritus, flushing, tachycardia, abdominal pain, diarrhea, syncope, or headache. Other diagnostic considerations include myocardial dysfunction, pulmonary embolism, foreign body aspiration, acute poisoning, and seizure disorder.

## MANAGEMENT OF ANAPHYLAXIS

Table 2 outlines a sequential approach to management. Assessment and maintenance of airway, breathing, circulation, and mentation are necessary before proceeding to other management steps. Subjects are monitored continuously to facilitate prompt detection of any treatment complications. The recumbent position is strongly recommended. In a retrospective review of prehospital anaphylactic fatalities in the United Kingdom, the postural history was known for 10 individuals. Four of the 10 were associated with assumption of an upright or sitting posture and postmortem findings consistent with "empty heart" and pulseless electrical activity.

Epinephrine is the treatment of choice for acute anaphylaxis. Aqueous epinephrine 1:1000 dilution, 0.2 to 0.5 mL (0.01 mg/kg in children; maximum dose, 0.3 mg) administered intramuscularly every 5 minutes, as necessary, should be used to control symptoms and sustain or increase blood pressure. Comparisons of intramuscular injections to subcutaneous injections during acute anaphylaxis are not available. However, absorption is more rapid and plasma levels are higher in asymptomatic individuals who receive epinephrine intramuscularly in the anterolateral thigh.

All subsequent therapeutic interventions depend on the initial response to epinephrine and the severity of the reaction. Development of toxicity or inadequate response to epinephrine injections indicates that additional therapeutic modalities are necessary.

The α-adrenergic effect of epinephrine reverses peripheral vasodilation, which alleviates hypotension and also reduces angioedema and urticaria. It may also minimize further absorption of antigen from a sting or injection. The β-adrenergic properties of epinephrine increase myocardial output and contractility, cause bronchodilation, and suppress further mediator release from mast cells and basophils.

Fatalities during witnessed anaphylaxis usually result from delayed administration of epinephrine and from severe respiratory and/or cardiovascular complications. *There is no absolute contraindication to epinephrine administration in anaphylaxis.*

Oxygen should be administered to subjects with anaphylaxis who require multiple doses of epinephrine, receive inhaled β₂ agonists, have protracted anaphylaxis, or have preexisting hypoxemia or myocardial dysfunction.

Antihistamines (H₁ and H₂ antagonists) support the treatment of anaphylaxis. However, these agents act much slower than epinephrine and should never be administered alone as treatment for anaphylaxis. Antihistamines thus should be considered as *second-line* treatment.

Systemic corticosteroids have no role in the acute management of anaphylaxis because even intravenous administration of these agents may have no effect for 4 to 6 hours after administration. Although corticosteroids traditionally are used in the management of anaphylaxis,

---

### TABLE 1 Representative Agents That Cause Anaphylaxis

IgE dependent:
- Foods (such as peanuts, tree nuts, and crustaceans)
- Medications (such as antibiotics)
- Venoms (fire ants, yellow jackets, others)
- Allergen extracts
- Latex
- Exercise (where food or medication dependent)
- Hormones

IgE independent:
- Nonspecific degranulation of mast cells and basophils
  - Opioids
  - Muscle relaxants
  - Idiopathic
  - Physical factors
    - Exercise
    - Cold, heat
- Disturbance of arachidonic acid metabolism
  - Aspirin and other nonsteroidal anti-inflammatory drugs (NSAIDs)
- Immune aggregates
  - Intravenous immunoglobulin
- Cytotoxic
  - Transfusion reactions to cellular elements (IgM, IgG)
- Multimediator complement activation/activation of contact system
  - Radiocontrast media
  - Angiotensin-converting enzyme (ACE) inhibitor administered during renal dialysis with selected dialysis membranes
  - Protamine (possibly)

Psychogenic

Modified and abridged from Kemp SF, Lockey RF: Anaphylaxis: A review of causes and mechanisms. J Allergy Clin Immunol 2002;110:341-348.

## TABLE 2 Management of Anaphylaxis

Immediate intervention:
- Assessment of airway, breathing, circulation, and adequacy of mentation.
- Administer aqueous epinephrine 1:1000 dilution, 0.2–0.5 mL (0.01 mg/kg in children; maximum dose, 0.3 mg) *intramuscularly* q5min, as necessary, to control symptoms and blood pressure.

Possibly appropriate, subsequent measures depending on response to epinephrine:
- Place subject in recumbent position and elevate lower extremities.
- Establish and maintain airway.
- Administer oxygen.
- Establish venous access.
- Use normal saline IV for fluid replacement.

Specific measures to consider after epinephrine injections, where appropriate:
- An epinephrine infusion might be prepared. Continuous hemodynamic monitoring is essential (see reference for specific details).
- Diphenhydramine (Benadryl). Note: In the management of anaphylaxis, a combination of diphenhydramine and ranitidine (Zantac)[1] is superior to diphenhydramine alone.
- For bronchospasm resistant to epinephrine, use nebulized albuterol (Proventil).
- For refractory hypotension, consider dopamine (Intropin), 400 mg in 500 mL D$_5$W, administered IV at 2–20 µg/kg/min titrated to maintain adequate blood pressure. Continuous hemodynamic monitoring is essential.
- Where use of β-blockers complicates therapy, consider glucagon,[1] 1–5 mg (20–30 µg/kg; maximum: 1 mg in children), administered IV over 5 min followed by an infusion, 5–15 µg/min. Aspiration precautions should be observed.
- For patients with a history of asthma and for those who experience severe or prolonged anaphylaxis, consider methylprednisolone (Solu-Medrol) (1.0–2.0 mg/kg/d).
- Consider transportation to the emergency department or an intensive care facility.

Interventions for cardiopulmonary arrest occurring during anaphylaxis:
- High-dose epinephrine and prolonged resuscitation efforts are encouraged, if necessary, because efforts are more likely to be successful in anaphylaxis where the subject (often young) has a healthy cardiovascular system (see reference for specific details).

Observation and subsequent outpatient follow-up:
- Observation periods after apparent resolution must be individualized and based on such factors as the clinical scenario, co-morbid conditions, and distance from the patient's home to the closest emergency department. After recovery from the acute episode, patients should receive epinephrine syringes (EpiPen or TwinJect) and be instructed in proper technique. Everyone postanaphylaxis requires a careful diagnostic evaluation in consultation with an allergist-immunologist.

[1]Not FDA approved for this indication.
*Abbreviation:* IV = intravenous.
Modified from Lieberman P, Kemp SF, Oppenheimer J, et al (chief eds). Joint Task Force on Practice Parameters. The diagnosis and management of anaphylaxis: An updated practice parameter. J Allergy Clin Immunol 2005;115:S483-S523.

their effect has never been evaluated in placebo-controlled trials. Corticosteroids administered during anaphylaxis might provide additional benefit for patients with asthma or other conditions recently treated with corticosteroids.

Numerous cases of unusually severe or refractory anaphylaxis are reported in subjects receiving β-blocking agents. Greater severity of anaphylaxis observed in usual doses of epinephrine administered during anaphylaxis to subjects taking β-blockers may not produce the desired clinical response. In such situations, both isotonic volume expansion and glucagon[1] administration are recommended. Glucagon may

potentially reverse refractory hypotension and bronchospasm because it bypasses the β-adrenergic receptor and directly activates adenyl cyclase.

Persistent hypotension despite epinephrine injections should first be treated with intravenous crystalloid solutions. Saline is generally preferred. One to 2 L of normal saline might need to be administered to adults at a rate of 5 to 10 mL/kg in the first 5 minutes. Children should receive up to 30 mL/kg in the first hour. Large volumes (e.g., 7 L) are often required.

Vasopressors should be administered if epinephrine injections and volume expansion fail to alleviate hypotension. Dopamine (Intropin) frequently increases blood pressure while maintaining or enhancing renal and splanchnic perfusion. These agents would not be expected to work as well in patients already maximally vasoconstricted by their internal compensatory response to anaphylaxis.

## PREVENTION OF ANAPHYLAXIS

Table 3 outlines the basic principles for the prevention of future anaphylactic episodes in high-risk individuals. An allergist-immunologist can provide comprehensive professional advice on these matters.

All subjects at high risk for recurrent anaphylaxis should carry epinephrine syringes and know how to administer them. An EpiPen (Dey Laboratories) is a spring-loaded, pressure-activated syringe with a single 0.3 mg dose (1:1000 dilution) of epinephrine. It is easy to use and injects through clothing. An EpiPen Jr, which delivers 0.15 mg (1:2000 dilution) epinephrine, is appropriate for children weighing less than 30 kg. The TwinJect (Verus Pharmaceuticals) is a prefilled, pen-sized, epinephrine auto-injector with two doses of either 0.3 or 0.15 mg.

# Serum Sickness

Serum sickness is a clinical syndrome of fever, malaise, and urticarial and/or morbilliform cutaneous eruption that is often preceded by generalized erythema and pruritus. Arthralgias or arthritis (mainly large joints), neuropathy, lymphadenopathy, nephritis, abdominal pain

---

[1]Not FDA approved for this indication.

## TABLE 3 Preventive Measures for Subjects with Anaphylaxis

General measures:
- Obtain thorough history to diagnose life-threatening food or drug allergy.
- Identify cause of anaphylaxis and those individuals at risk for future attacks.
- Provide instruction on proper reading of food and medication labels, where appropriate.
- Patient should avoid exposure to antigens and cross-reactive substances.
- Manage asthma and coronary artery disease optimally.

Specific measures for high-risk subjects:
- Individuals at high risk for anaphylaxis should carry self-injectable syringes of epinephrine (EpiPen or TwinJect) at all times and receive instruction in proper use with placebo trainer.
- Individuals should wear a Medic Alert bracelet or chain.
- Other agents for β-adrenergic antagonists, angiotensin-converting enzyme (ACE) inhibitors, tricyclic antidepressants, and monoamine oxidase inhibitors should be substituted whenever possible.
- Agents suspected of causing anaphylaxis should be administered slowly, supervised, and orally if possible
- Where appropriate, use specific preventive strategies, including pharmacologic prophylaxis, short-term challenge and desensitization, and long-term desensitization.

Modified from Kemp SF: Anaphylaxis: Current concepts in pathophysiology, diagnosis, and management. Immunol Allergy Clin N Am 2001;21:611-634.

(emesis or melena are possible), or vasculitis (cutaneous or systemic) may occur in some cases. Cutaneous vasculitis, also known as hypersensitivity vasculitis, is often manifested by palpable purpura, which most commonly are found on the lower extremities of ambulatory individuals or on the sacral or gluteal region of patients with restricted mobility. These purpura reflect vascular leakage from inflamed postcapillary venules. Systemic vasculitis may occur in association with autoimmune diseases, infection, or malignancy.

Many agents may produce serum sickness or serum sickness–like reactions (Table 4). *Serum sickness* classically refers to the immune complex syndrome caused by immunization with heterologous serum proteins (often equine or murine). The most frequent cause is immune complex-mediated drug hypersensitivity. A serum sickness–like drug reaction generally develops 6 to 21 days after the culprit medication is started, but it can occur within 12 to 48 hours in previously sensitized individuals.

## PATHOGENESIS AND LABORATORY ABNORMALITIES

Healthy individuals regularly generate low levels of circulating immune complexes, which are either excreted by the kidneys or extracted in the liver and spleen by monocytes and macrophages. It is hypothesized that serum sickness results when a drug (hapten) binds to plasma protein and antibodies are generated in response to the drug-protein complex. Complement activation occurs when large quantities of soluble antigen-antibody (immune) complexes fix to vascular endothelial receptors. Complement fragments attract and activate neutrophils, which release proteases that induce tissue injury. The urticaria in serum sickness probably results from immune complex necrotizing vasculitis and complement activation that induces mast cell degranulation. IgE-dependent mechanisms likely are also contributory in some individuals. Laboratory abnormalities include elevated erythrocyte sedimentation rate, leukopenia (acute phase), occasional plasmacytosis, and decreased total hemolytic complement (CH50), C3, and C4. Slight albuminuria, hyaline casts, and microscopic hematuria may also occur.

## TREATMENT

Stoppage of the culprit agent, when identified, is recommended. Serum sickness is usually self-limited and rarely life threatening when the offending drug or protein is stopped or removed. Symptoms generally improve over 2 to 4 weeks as patients clear their immune complexes. Evidence-based treatment recommendations for serum sickness are very limited. Long-acting, less-sedating H₁ antihistamines such as cetirizine (Zyrtec), desloratadine (Clarinex), fexofenadine (Allegra), or loratadine (Claritin) generally control urticaria. Systemic corticosteroids (e.g., prednisone, 0.5 to 1.0 mg/kg/day) may help severe symptoms. Fever and arthralgias typically resolve within 48 to 72 hours of treatment, and the formation of new cutaneous eruptions usually ceases within the same time frame. Antihistamine therapy is continued for 1 week after apparent resolution of symptoms and then slowly discontinued. Skin testing with heterologous antisera is performed routinely to avoid anaphylaxis to future administration of heterologous serum.

---

### TABLE 4 Representative Agents That Cause Serum Sickness

Medications: β-lactam antibiotics, sulfonamides, ciprofloxacin (Cipro), metronidazole (Flagyl), rifampin (Rifadin), allopurinol (Zyloprim), carbamazepine (Tegretol), phenytoin (Dilantin), fluoxetine (Prozac), bupropion (Wellbutrin), methimazole (Tapazole), propylthiouracil, thiazide diuretics, captopril (Capoten), propranolol (Inderal), verapamil (Calan), streptokinase (Streptase), others
Heterologous (animal-derived) antisera:
• Horse: snake and spider venom, tetanus, botulism, diphtheria
• Horse or rabbit: anti-lymphocyte globulin
Mouse: monoclonal antibodies (muromonab-CD3 [Orthoclone OKT3], rituximab [Rituxan], infliximab [Remicade])
Homologous (human-derived) antisera: cytomegalovirus, hepatitis B, rabies, tetanus, perinatal RH₀(D)

---

## REFERENCES

American Heart Association in collaboration with International Liaison Committee on Resuscitation: 2005 American Heart Association guidelines for cardiopulmonary resuscitation and emergency cardiovascular care. Anaphylaxis. Circulation 2005;112(Suppl 4):143-145.
Brown SGA, Blackman KE, Stenlake V, Heddle RJ: Insect sting anaphylaxis: Prospective evaluation of treatment with intravenous adrenaline and volume resuscitation. Emerg Med J 2004;21:149-154.
Kemp SF, Lockey RF: Anaphylaxis: A review of causes and mechanisms. J Allergy Clin Immunol 2002;110:341-348.
Lieberman P: Biphasic anaphylactic reactions. Ann Allergy Asthma Immunol 2005;95:217-226.
Lieberman P, Kemp SF, Oppenheimer J, et al. (chief eds). Joint Task Force on Practice Parameters. The diagnosis and management of anaphylaxis: An updated practice parameter. J Allergy Clin Immunol 2005;115:S483-S523.
Project Team of the Resuscitation Council (UK): Emergency medical treatment of anaphylactic reactions. J Accid Emerg Med 1999;16:243-247.
Pumphrey RSH: Fatal posture in anaphylactic shock. J Allergy Clin Immunol 2003;112:451-452.
Pumphrey RSH: Fatal anaphylaxis in the UK, 1992–2001. Novartis Found Symp 2004;257:116-128.
Sampson HA, Muñoz-Furlong A, Campbell RL, et al: Second symposium on the definition and management of anaphylaxis: Summary report—second National Institute of Allergy and Infectious Disease/Food Allergy and Anaphylaxis Network symposium. J Allergy Clin Immunol 2006;117:391-397.
Simons FER, Gu X, Simons KJ: Epinephrine absorption in adults: Intramuscular versus subcutaneous injection. J Allergy Clin Immunol 2001;108:871-873.
Simons FER, Roberts JR, Gu X, Simons KJ: Epinephrine absorption in children with a history of anaphylaxis. J Allergy Clin Immunol 1998;101:33-37.
Wener M: Serum sickness and serum sickness-like reactions. In: Rose BD (ed): UpToDate, www.uptodateonline.com, Version 15.1 (current through December 2006), Wellesley, Ma.

---

# Asthma in Adolescents and Adults

Method of
*Michael Schatz, MD, MS*

---

Asthma is an extremely common chronic medical condition that causes substantial morbidity among its sufferers. In addition to discomfort, asthma can cause sleep disruption, missed school and work, limitations of recreational activities, and acute episodes requiring emergency hospital care. Although the past 30 years have seen the introduction of increasingly effective and convenient medications, recent surveys continue to suggest that asthma remains suboptimally controlled in the majority of patients. The purpose of this article is to describe an approach to assessment and therapy that leads to optimal asthma control. It is based on the recently released National Asthma Education and Prevention Program (NAEPP) Expert Panel Report 3: Guidelines for the Management of Asthma (http://www.nhlbi.nih.gov/guidelines/asthma/asthgdln.pdf).

## Diagnosis

The first step in evaluating a patient with asthma is to confirm the diagnosis. This is particularly important in patients with atypical symptoms or a poor response to asthma therapy. Asthma is confirmed by the demonstration of reversible airways obstruction, which most commonly is an increase in forced expiratory volume in 1 second (FEV₁) by 12% or more and at least 200 cc after an inhaled bronchodilator. For some patients, 2 to 4 weeks of chronic inhaled asthma therapy or 2 weeks of oral corticosteroid therapy is necessary to demonstrate reversibility. The latter is particularly important in adults with a history of smoking in whom chronic obstructive pulmonary disease (COPD) is a diagnostic consideration. In patients with normal pulmonary function, asthma can also be confirmed by means of methacholine (Provocholine) or exercise challenge.

Particularly important masqueraders of asthma include vocal cord dysfunction, panic attacks, hyperventilation, and cough due to postnasal drip, reflux, or angiotensin-converting enzyme (ACE) inhibitor therapy. All of these can also coexist with asthma, so their presence does not exclude asthma. Even when these conditions coexist with asthma, their diagnosis and appropriate therapy usually reduce the patient's respiratory symptoms.

## Assessment

Assessment of asthmatic patients involves assessment of past severity, identification of aggravating factors, and definition of current status regarding treatment and clinical severity or control.

### PAST SEVERITY

Asthma can be a mild, infrequent illness or a daily severe one. Certain severity markers identify patients who are more likely to experience severe exacerbations or to have symptoms that are more difficult to control and who thus require more careful surveillance. These include histories of asthma hospitalization, especially requiring intensive care or intubation, past requirement for oral corticosteroids, and exacerbation by aspirin or other NSAIDs. In patients with prior severe exacerbations, the rapidity of the onset of the exacerbation should be ascertained.

### AGGRAVATING FACTORS

Factors that appear to trigger asthma symptoms should be assessed because they may be targets for avoidance therapy. Certain aspects of the patient's *environment* that can contribute to asthma triggering should be specifically ascertained, including occupational exposures, age of the home, pets, carpeting, visible mold, passive smoke, and cockroach exposure. Patients with persistent asthma should have in vitro or skin tests to identify *allergic sensitization* to pollens, house dust mites, mold spores, animal dander, and cockroaches that can contribute to the maintenance of asthma inflammation or can trigger episodes. The presence of *comorbidities* that can aggravate asthma, including cigarette smoking, obesity, rhinitis, sinusitis, reflux, and COPD, should be identified and treated. Finally, *psychosocial factors* to assess include a history or symptoms of anxiety or depression, attitudes toward asthma and asthma therapy, adherence to therapy, and social support. These may be targets for therapy or may be necessary to understand in order to create an effective therapeutic plan and therapeutic alliance.

### CURRENT STATUS

Assessment of the current therapy the patient is actually taking is necessary for understanding the asthma's severity and to appropriately initiate or change therapy. It is particularly important to determine if the patient is taking long-term control medications, such as inhaled corticosteroids, long-acting β-agonists, leukotriene modifiers, cromolyn (Intal), nedocromil (Tilade), or theophylline (Theo-Dur). If the patient is not taking controllers, *severity* should be assessed, as described in Table 1, based on symptom frequency, nocturnal awakenings, rescue therapy use, activity limitation, spirometry, and exacerbation history. If the patient is already taking controllers, *control* should be assessed (Table 2). Normal $FEV_1/FVC$ (forced vital capacity) by age is shown in Table 3.

**TABLE 1** Classifying Asthma Severity and Initiating Treatment in Patients 12 Years and Older Not Currently Taking Long-Term Control Medications

| Components of Severity | Classification of Severity | | | |
| --- | --- | --- | --- | --- |
| | | Persistent | | |
| | Intermittent | Mild | Moderate | Severe |
| **Impairment** | | | | |
| Symptoms | ≤2 d/wk | >2 d/wk but not daily | Daily | Throughout the d |
| Nighttime awakenings | ≤2×/mo | 3-4×/mo | >1×/wk but not nightly | Often 7×/wk |
| Short-acting β₂-agonist use for symptom control (not prevention of EIB) | ≤2 d/wk | >2 d/wk but not daily, and not more than 1 time on any d | Daily | Several times per d |
| Interference with normal activity | None | Minor limitation | Some limitation | Extremely limited |
| Lung function† | Normal FEV₁ between exacerbations FEV₁ >80% predicted FEV₁/FVC normal | FEV₁ >80% predicted FEV₁/FVC normal | FEV₁ >60% but <80% predicted FEV₁/FVC reduced 5% | FEV₁ <60% predicted FEV₁/FVC reduced >5% |
| **Risk** | | | | |
| Exacerbations requiring oral systemic corticosteroids | 0-1/y‡ | ≥2/y‡ | | |
| | Consider severity and interval since last exacerbation. Frequency and severity may fluctuate over time for patients in any severity category. | | | |
| | Relative annual risk of exacerbation may be related to FEV₁. | | | |
| **Recommended Step for Initiating Treatment§** | | | | |
| Initiation | Step 1 | Step 2 | Step 3¶ | Step 4 or 5¶ |
| Follow-up | In 2-6 wk, evaluate level of asthma control and adjust therapy accordingly. | | | |

*Level of severity is determined by assessment of both impairment and risk. Assess impairment domain by patient's/caregiver's recall of previous 2-4 weeks and spirometry. Assign severity to the most severe category in which any feature occurs.
†See Table 3 for normal FEV₁/FVC.
‡At present, there are inadequate data to correspond frequencies of exacerbations with different levels of asthma severity. In general, more frequent and intense exacerbations (e.g., requiring urgent, unscheduled care, hospitalization, or ICU admission) indicate greater underlying disease severity.
   For treatment purposes, patients who had ≥ 2 exacerbations requiring oral systemic corticosteroids in the past year may be considered the same as patients who have persistent asthma, even in the absence of impairment levels consistent with persistent asthma.
§See Table 6 for treatment steps. The stepwise approach is meant to assist, not replace, the clinical decision making required to meet individual patient needs.
¶And consider short course of oral systemic corticosteroids.
*Abbreviations:* EIB = exercise-induced bronchospasm; FEV₁ = forced expiratory volume in one second; FVC = forced vital capacity; ICU = intensive care unit.

**TABLE 2   Assessing Asthma Control and Adjusting Therapy in Patients 12 Years and Older**

| Components of Control | Classification of Control* | | |
| --- | --- | --- | --- |
| | Well Controlled | Not Well Controlled | Very Poorly Controlled |
| **Impairment** | | | |
| Symptoms | ≤2 d/wk | >2 d/wk | Throughout the d |
| Nighttime awakenings | ≤2×/mo | 1-3×/wk | ≥4×/wk |
| Short-acting β₂-agonist use for symptom control (not prevention of EIB) | ≤2 d/wk | >2 d/wk | Several times per d |
| Interference with normal activity | None | Some limitation | Extremely limited |
| FEV₁ or peak flow | >80% predicted or personal best | 60%-80% predicted or personal best | <60% predicted or personal best |
| **Validated Questionnaires[b]** | | | |
| ACQ | ≤0.75[†] | ≥1.5 | N/A |
| ACT | ≥20 | 16-19 | ≤15 |
| ATAQ | 0 | 1-2 | 3-4 |
| **Risk** | | | |
| Exacerbations requiring oral systemic corticosteroids | 0-1/y | ≥2/y[a] ⟶ | |
| Progressive loss of lung function | Evaluation requires long-term follow-up care | | |
| Treatment-related adverse effects | Medication side effects can vary in intensity from none to very troublesome and worrisome. The level of intensity does not correlate to specific levels of control, but it should be considered in the overall assessment of risk. | | |
| Recommended action for treatment[‡] | Maintain current step  Regular follow-up at every 1-6 mo to maintain control  Consider step down if well controlled for ≥3 mo | Step up 1 step and reevaluate in 2-6 wk  For side effects, consider alternative treatment options | Consider short course of systemic oral corticosteroids  Step up 1-2 steps and reevaluate in 2 wk  For side effects, consider alternative treatment options |

*The level of control is based on the most severe impairment or risk category. Assess impairment domain by patient's recall of previous 2-4 weeks and by spirometry or peak flow measures. Symptom assessment for longer periods should reflect a global assessment, such as inquiring whether the patient's asthma is better or worse since the last visit.

†ACQ values of 0.76-1.4 are indeterminate regarding well-controlled asthma.

[a]At present, there are inadequate data to correspond frequencies of exacerbations with different levels of asthma control. In general, more frequent and intense exacerbations (e.g., requiring urgent, unscheduled care, hospitalization, or ICU admission) indicate poorer disease control.
For treatment purposes, patients who had ≥ 2 exacerbations requiring oral systemic corticosteroids in the past year may be considered the same as patients who have not-well-controlled asthma, even in the absence of impairment levels consistent with not-well-controlled asthma.

[b]Validated questionnaires for the impairment domain (the questionnaires do not assess lung function or the risk domain). Minimal important difference: 0.5 for the ACQ, 1.0 for the ATAQ, not determined for the ACT.

‡See Table 3 for treatment steps. The stepwise approach is meant to assist, not replace, the clinical decision making required to meet individual patient needs. Before a step up in therapy, review adherence, inhale technique environmental control, and comorbid conditions. If an alternative treatment option was used in a step, discontinue it and use the preferred treatment for that step.

*Abbreviations:* ACQ = Asthma Control Questionnaire; ACT = Asthma Control Test; ATAQ = Asthma Therapy Assessment Questionnaire; EIB = exercise-induced bronchospasm; FEV₁ = forced expiratory volume in one second; N/A = not applicable.

## CURRENT DIAGNOSIS

- Confirm the diagnosis by demonstrating an increase in FEV₁ by 12% or more after asthma therapy.
- Assess past severity by a history of exacerbations requiring hospitalization, intubation, or oral corticosteroids.
- Identify environmental exposures, allergic sensitization, and comorbidities that may be aggravating asthma.
- Assess current *severity* in patients not taking long-term control medications and assess *control* in patients who are taking long-term control medications based on symptom frequency, nocturnal awakenings, rescue therapy use, activity limitation, spirometry, and recent exacerbation history.

*Abbreviation:* FEV₁ = forced expiratory volume in 1 second.

# Long-Term Management

The goals of long-term management are to achieve and maintain well-controlled asthma. Both nonpharmacologic and pharmacologic therapy must be considered.

## NONPHARMACOLOGIC THERAPY

The first tenet of nonpharmacologic therapy in the long-term management of asthma is *education*. Patients need to understand the inflammatory pathophysiology of asthma and the relationships among airway inflammation, bronchospasm, and symptoms. Patients should be informed that the cause of asthma is unknown and there is no cure but that triggers can be identified and asthma can be controlled. They should receive education regarding self-assessment, either based on symptoms or peak flow monitoring, and regarding the recognition of early signs of an impending exacerbation.

The next step is to discuss and agree on the *goals of therapy*. The NAEPP has defined the following goals:

- Prevent chronic and troublesome daytime and nighttime symptoms.
- Maintain optimal pulmonary function for that patient.
- Maintain normal activity, including work, school, leisure activity, and exercise.
- Prevent recurrent exacerbations, especially those requiring urgent medical visits.
- Provide pharmacotherapy with minimal or no adverse effects.
- Achieve patient and family satisfaction with asthma care.

The physician should let the patient know that these are the expectations of optimal management and confirm that those are the patient's goals as well.

## TABLE 3  Normal FEV₁/FVC by Age

| Age Range (y) | Normal FEV$_1$/FVC (%) |
|---|---|
| 8-19 | 85 |
| 20-39 | 80 |
| 40-59 | 75 |
| 60-80 | 70 |

*Abbreviations:* FEV$_1$ = forced expiratory volume in one second;
FVC = forced vital capacity.

A very important component of nonpharmacologic therapy is reduction of relevant *environmental triggers*. Information should be given regarding environmental control of pollen, mite, mold, animal dander, and cockroach antigens (Box 1) that appear to be relevant based on the history and results of skin or in vitro specific IgE tests. Inhalant allergen *immunotherapy* should be considered for patients who have persistent asthma when there is clear evidence of a relationship between symptoms and exposure to an allergen to which the patient is sensitive.

Finally, *psychosocial* issues should be considered and addressed. For many patients, the education and therapeutic alliance described earlier adequately addresses psychosocial concerns. For other patients, poor past adherence requires identifying the barriers to adherence and finding solutions together. Resources for patients with poor social support should be identified. Clinically significant anxiety or depression that can make asthma harder to control should be treated.

## PHARMACOLOGIC STEP THERAPY

The main principle of asthma pharmacologic step therapy is to add therapy in steps until control is achieved (step up) and decrease therapy in reverse steps (step down) to established the lowest effective dose necessary to maintain control.

There are two types of asthma medications: quick-relief medications (Table 4) and long-term control medications (Table 5). Systemic corticosteroids can be used either short-term to treat an exacerbation (see Table 4) or as long-term maintenance therapy for patients with severe disease (see Table 5). The generally recommended steps of pharmacologic therapy are shown in Table 6. Definitions of low, medium, and high dose inhaled corticosteroids for each of the available preparations are given in Table 7. At each therapeutic step level, the NAEPP Expert Panel has indicated *preferred* medications, which generally identify medications with the best balance of efficacy and safety in clinical trials for patients at that level of severity. However, these recommendations are based on population data and must be tailored to individual patient needs, circumstances, and responsiveness to therapy.

All patients with asthma should have an action plan that describes their pharmacologic self-management. Aspects of pharmacologic self-management include the maintenance medication schedule, rescue therapy doses for increased symptoms, when and how to increase control medication therapy, when and how to use prednisone, how to recognize a severe exacerbation, and when and how to seek urgent or emergency care. Control medications should be increased with an upper respiratory infection or with symptoms requiring more than two doses of rescue therapy in 12 hours. Although doubling the dose of inhaled corticosteroids does not appear to generally be sufficient to provide clinical benefit under these circumstances, higher-fold increases may be effective (e.g., three- or fourfold increases). The increased dose of control medications should be maintained at least until increased symptoms resolve. Prednisone is usually needed for patients with incomplete or temporary responses to adequate doses of β-agonists (4 puffs with a spacer, waiting at least 1 minute between puffs), substantial interference with sleep every night, requirement for 12 or more puffs of β-agonist in a 24-hour period, or a peak flow less than 60% predicted. Home treatment of exacerbations is further discussed later.

For patients not on long-term control medications, assess *severity* and select the level of treatment that corresponds to the patient's level of severity (see Table 1). Persistent asthma is most effectively

## BOX 1  Measures to Control Environmental Factors that Can Make Asthma Worse

### Allergens

Reduce or eliminate exposure to the allergen(s) the patient is sensitive to:

### Animal Dander

- Remove animal from house or, at a minimum, keep animal out of the patient's bedroom and keep the bedroom door closed.

### House-dust Mites

- Recommended
  - Encase mattress in a special dust-proof cover
  - Encase pillow in a special dust-proof cover or wash it weekly in hot water.
  - Wash sheets and blankets on the patient's bed in hot water weekly. Water must be hotter than 130°F to kill the mites. Cooler water used with detergent and bleach can also be effective.
- Desirable
  - Reduce indoor humidity to 60% or less.
  - Remove carpets from the bedroom.
  - Avoid sleeping or lying on cloth-covered cushions or furniture.
  - Remove carpets that are laid on concrete.

### Cockroaches

- Keep all food out of the bedroom.
- Keep food and garbage in closed containers.
- Use poison baits, powders, gels or paste (e.g., boric acid). Traps can also be used.
- If a spray is used to kill cockroaches, stay out of the room until the odor goes away.

### Pollens (from Trees, Grass, or Weeds) and Outdoor Molds

- Try to keep windows closed
- If possible, stay indoors, with windows closed, during periods of peak pollen exposure, which are usually during the midday and afternoon.

### Indoor Mold

- Fix all leaks and eliminate water sources associated with mold growth.
- Clean moldy surfaces.
- Dehumidify basements if possible.

### Tobacco Smoke

- Advise patients and others in the home who smoke to stop smoking or to smoke outside the home.
- Discuss ways to reduce exposure to other sources of tobacco smoke, such as from daycare providers and the workplace.

### Indoor and Outdoor Pollutants and Irritants

- If possible, do not use a wood-burning stove, kerosene heater, fireplace, unvented gas stove, or heater
- Try to stay away from strong odors and sprays, such as perfume, talcum powder, hair spray, paints, new carpet, or particle board.

## TABLE 4  Usual Dosages for Quick-Relief Medications for Patients 12 Years and Older

| Medication | Dosage Form | Adult Dose | Comments |
|---|---|---|---|
| **Inhaled Short-Acting β₂-Agonists (SABA)** | | | |
| *Metered-Dose Inhaler* | | ***Applies to all four SABAS*** | |
| Albuterol CFC | 90 µg/puff, 200 puffs/canister | 2 puffs 5 min before exercise | An increasing use or lack of expected effect indicates diminished control of asthma. |
| Albuterol HFA (Proventil, Ventolin) | 90 µg/puff, 200 puffs/canister | *or* | Not recommended for long-term daily treatment. Regular use exceeding 2 d/wk for symptom control |
| Pirbuterol CFC (Maxair) | 200 µg/puff, 400 puffs/canister | 2 puffs q4-6h prn | (not prevention of EIB) indicates the need for additional long-term control therapy |
| Levalbuterol HFA (Xopenox) | 45 µg/puff, 200 puffs/canister | | Differences in potencies exist, but all products are essentially comparable on a per puff basis. |
| | | | May double usual dose for mild exacerbations. |
| | | | Should prime the inhaler by releasing 4 actuations prior to use. Periodically clean HFA activator, as drug may block/plug orifice. |
| | | | Nonselective agents (epinephrine [Primatene Mist], isoproterenol [Isopro Aerometer], metaproterenol [Alupent]) are not recommended due to their potential for excessive cardiac stimulation, especially in high doses. |
| *Nebulizer Solutions* | | | |
| Albuterol (Accuneb, Proventil) | 0.63 mg/3 mL 1.25 mg/3 mL 2.5 mg/3 mL 5 mg/mL (0.5%) | 1.25-5 mg in 3 mL saline q4-8h prn | May mix with budesonide (Pulmicort) inhalant suspension, cromolyn (Intal) or ipratropium (Atrovent) nebulizer solutions. May double the dose for severe exacerbations. |
| Levalbuterol (R-albuterol) (Xopenex) | 0.31 mg/3mL 0.63 mg/3mL 1.25 mg/0.5 mL 1.25 mg/3mL | 0.63 mg- 1.25 mg q8h prn | Compatible with budesonide (Pulmicort) inhalant suspension. The product is a sterile-filled, preservative-free, unit-dose vial. |
| **Anticholinergics** | | | |
| *Metered-Dose Inhalers* | | | |
| Ipratropium HFA (Atrovent) | 17 µg/puff, 200 puffs/canister | 2-3 puffs q6h | Multiple doses in the emergency department (not hospital) setting provide additive benefit to short-acting beta agonists |
| | | | Treatment of choice for bronchospasm due to beta blocker |
| | | | Dose not block EIB |
| | | | Reverses only cholinergically mediated bronchospasm; does not modify reaction to antigen |
| | | | May be alternative for patients who do not tolerate short-acting beta-agonist |
| | | | Evidence is lacking for anticholinergics producing added benefit to β₂ agonists in long-term control asthma therapy. |
| Ipratropium with albuterol (Combivent) | 18 µg/puff of ipratropium bromide and 90 µg/puff of albuterol 200 puffs/canister | 2-3 puffs q6h | |
| *Nebulizer Solutions* | | | |
| Ipratropium bromide | 0.25 mg/mL (0.025%) | 0.25 mg* q 6 h | |
| Ipratropium bromide with albuterol (DuoNeb) | 0.5 mg/3 mL ipratropium bromide and 2.5 mg/3 mL albuterol | 3 mL q4-6h | Contains EDTA to prevent discoloration of the solution. This additive does not induce bronchospasm. |
| **Systemic Corticosteroids** | | | |
| Methylprednisolone (Medrol) | 2, 4, 6, 8, 16, 32 mg tab | Short course (burst): 40-60 mg/d as single or 2 divided doses for 3-10 d | Short courses (bursts) are effective for establishing control when initiating therapy or during a period of gradual deterioration. Action may be begin within an hour. The burst should be continued until symptoms resolve. This usually requires 3-10 d but can require longer. There is no evidence that tapering the dose following improvement prevents relapse in asthma exacerbations. |
| Prednisolone (Delta-Cortef, Prelone) | 5 mg tabs, 5 mg/5 mL, 15 mg/5 mL | | |
| Prednisone (Deltasone, Orasone) | 1, 2.5, 5, 10, 20, 50 mg tabs; 5 mg/mL, 5 mg/5 mL | | |
| *Repository Injection* | | | |
| Methylprednisolone acetate (Depo-Medrol) | 40 mg/mL 80 mg/mL | 240 mg²† IM once | May be used in place of a short burst of oral steroids in patients who are vomiting or if adherence is a problem. |

²Exceeds dosage recommended by the manufacturer.
*0.5 mg per package insert.
†80-120 mg per package insert.
*Abbreviations:* CFC = chlorofluorocarbon; EIB = exercise-induced bronchospasm; HFA = hydrofluoroalkane; PEF = peak expiratory flow; tab = tablet;.

## TABLE 5  Usual Dosages for Long-Term Control Medications for Patients 12 Years and Older

| Medication | Dosage Form* | Adult Dose | Comments |
|---|---|---|---|
| **Systemic Corticosteroids** | | | |
| Methylprednisolone (Medrol) | 2, 4, 8, 16, 32 mg tab | 7.5-60 mg qd in a single dose in AM or qod as needed for control | For long-term treatment of severe persistent asthma, administer single dose in AM either daily or on alternate d (alternate-day therapy may produce less adrenal suppression). |
| Prednisolone (Delta-Cortef, Prelone) | 5 mg tab 5 mg/5 mL, 15 mg/5 mL | Short-course (burst) to achieve control, 40-60 mg/d as single or 2 divided doses for 3-10 d | Short courses (bursts) are effective for establishing control when initiating therapy or during a period of gradual deterioration. There is no evidence that tapering the dose following improvement in symptom control and pulmonary function prevents relapse. |
| Prednisone (Deltasone, Orasone) | 1, 2.5, 5, 10, 20, 50 mg tab 5 mg/mL, 5 mg/5 mL | | |
| **Inhaled Long-Acting β₂-Agonists** | | | Should not be used for acute symptoms relief or exacerbations. Use only with ICS. |
| Salmeterol (Serevent) | DPI 50 µg/blister | 1 blister q12h | Decreased duration of protection against EIB may occur with regular use. |
| Formoterol (Foradil) | DPI 12 µg/single-use capsule | 1 cap q12h | Each cap is for single use only; additional doses should not be administered for at least 12 h. Caps should be used only with the Aerolizor inhaler and should not be taken orally. |
| **Inhaled Combined Medications** | | | |
| Fluticasone and salmeterol (Advair) | DPI 100 µg/50 µg, 250 µg/50 µg, or 500 µg/50 µg HFA 45 µg/21 µg 115 µg/21 µg 230 µg/21 µg | 1 inhalation bid; dose depends on level of control | 100/50 DPI or 45/21 HFA for patients not controlled on low-to-medium dose ICS 250/50 DPI or 115/21 HFA for patients not controlled on medium-to-high dose ICS |
| Budesonide and formoterol (Symbicort) | HFA MDI 80 µg/4.5 µg 160 µg/4.5 µg | 2 inhalations bid; dose depends on level of control | 80/4.5 for patients not controlled on low-to-medium dose ICS 160/4.5 for patients not controlled on medium-to-high dose ICS |
| **Inhaled Cromolyn and Nedocromil** | | | |
| Cromolyn (Intal) | MDI 0.8 mg/puff Nebulizer 20 mg/ampule | 2 puffs qid 1 amp qid | One dose before exercise or allergen exposure provides effective prophylaxis for 1-2 h. Not as effective for EIB as SABA. 4-6 wk trial of cromolyn or nedocronil may be needed to determine maximum benefit Dose by MDI may be inadequate to affect hyperresponsiveness Once control is achieved, the frequency of dosing may be reduced. |
| Nedocromil (Tilade) | MDI 1.75 mg/puff | 2 puffs qid | |
| **Leukotriene Modifiers** | | | |
| *Leukotriene Receptor Antagonists* | | | |
| Montelukast (Singulair) | 4 mg or 5 mg chewable tab 10 mg tab | 10 mg qhs | Montelukast exhibits a flat dose-response curve. Doses >10 mg do not produce a.greater response in adults |
| Zafirlukast (Accolate) | 10 or 20 mg tab | 40 mg/d (20 mg tab bid) | For zafirlukast: Administration with meals decreases bioavailability; take at least 1 h before or 2 h after meals. Zafirlukast is a microsomal p450 enzyme inhibitor that can inhibit the metabolism of warfarin and theophylline. Doses of these drugs should be monitored accordingly Monitor for signs and symptoms of hepatic dysfunction. |
| *5-Lipoxygenase Inhibitor* | | | |
| Zileuton (Zyflo) | 600 mg tab | 2400 mg daily (600 mg qid) | Monitor hepatic enzymes (ALT). Zileuton is a microsomal p450 enzyme inhibitor that can inhibit the metabolism of warfarin and theophylline. Doses of these drugs should be monitored accordingly |
| **Methylxanthines** | | | |
| Theophylline (Slophyllin, Theobid, TheoDur) | Liquids, sustained-release tab, cap | Starting dose 10 mg/kg/d up to 300 mg max Usual max 800 mg/d | Adjust dosage to achieve serum concentration of 5-15 µg/mL at steady-state (≥48 h on same dosage). |

*Continued*

## TABLE 5 Usual Dosages for Long-Term Control Medications for Patients 12 Years and Older—cont'd

| Medication | Dosage Form* | Adult Dose | Comments |
|---|---|---|---|
| **Methylxanthines—cont'd** | | | Due to wide interpatient variability in theophylline metabolic clearance, routine serum theophylline level monitoring is essential. Patient should be told to discontinue if they experience symptoms of toxicity Various factors (diet, food, febrile illness, age, smoking, and other medications) can affect serum concentration |
| **Immunomodulators** Omalizumab (Anti-IgE) | Subcutaneous (SQ) injection 150 mg/ 1.2 mL following reconstitution with 1.4 mL sterile water for injection | 150-375 mg SQ every 2-4 wk, depending on body weight and pretreatment serum 1gE level | Do not administer more than 150 mg per injection site Monitor patient following injections; be prepared and equipped to indentify and treat anaphylaxis that may occur Whether patients will develop significant antibody titers to the drug with long-term administration is unknown |

*See Table 7 for estimated comparative daily dosages for inhaled corticosteroids.
*Abbreviations:* ALT = alanine aminotransferase; amp = ampule; cap = capsule; DPI = dry powder inhaler; EIB = exercise-induced bronchospasm; HFA = hydrofluoroalkane; ICS = inhaled corticosteroid; LABA = long-acting $\beta_2$-agonist; max = maximum; MDI = metered-dose inhaler; SABA = short-acting $\beta_2$-agonist; tab = tablet.

controlled with daily long-term control medications, specifically anti-inflammatory therapy. For patients receiving long-term control medications, identify their current *step of therapy*, based on what they are actually taking (see Table 6), and their level of *control* (see Table 2). In general, step up one step for patients whose asthma is not well controlled. For patients with very poorly controlled asthma, consider increasing by two steps, a course of oral corticosteroids, or both. Before increasing pharmacologic therapy, consider adverse environmental exposures, poor adherence, or comorbidities as targets for intervention. For patients with troublesome or debilitating side effects from asthma therapy, explore a change in therapy.

## TABLE 6 Stepwise Approach For Managing Asthma in Patients 12 Years and Older[a]

| Step | Preferred Therapy | Alternative Therapy |
|---|---|---|
| 1 | Short-acting β-agonist prn. | — |
| 2 | Low-dose ICS | Cromolyn (Intal), LTRA, nedocromil (Tilade), theophylline (Theo-Dur) |
| 3 | Low-dose ICS *plus* LABA *or* Medium-dose ICS | Low-dose ICS *plus* LTRA *or* theophylline *or* zileuton (Zyflo) |
| 4 | Medium-dose ICS *plus* LABA | Medium-dose ICS *plus* LTRA *or* theophylline *or* zileuton |
| 5 | High-dose ICS *plus* LABA Consider omalizumab (Xolair) for patients who have allergies | — |
| 6 | High-dose ICS *plus* LABA *plus* oral corticosteroid[b] Consider omalizumab for patients who have allergies | — |

*Abbreviations:* ICS = inhaled corticosteroid; LABA = long-acting β agonist; LTRA = leukotriene receptor antagonist.
[a]The stepwise approach is meant to assist, not replace, the clincal decision making required to meet individual patient needs.
[b]In step 6, before oral corticosteroids are introduced, a trial of high-dose ICS +LABA+either LTRA, theophylline or zilecton may be considered, although this approach has not been studied in clinical trials.

## Follow-up

Patients whose asthma is not controlled should be seen every 2 to 6 weeks (depending on their initial level of severity or control) until control is achieved. Once control is achieved, follow-up contact at 1- to 6-month intervals is recommended. These checkups should ensure continued control, identify other changes in the patient's status, and update the patient's action plan.

When well-controlled asthma has been maintained for at least 3 months, a step down in therapy can be considered to determine the minimal amount of medication required to maintain control or reduce the risk of side effects. Reduction in therapy should be gradual because asthma can deteriorate at a highly variable rate and intensity. Doses of inhaled corticosteroids may be reduced about 25% to 50% every 3 months to the lowest dose possible to maintain control. Most patients with persistent asthma relapse if inhaled corticosteroids are totally discontinued.

Patients should be encouraged to contact their asthma physician for signs of loss of asthma control, such as nocturnal symptoms, increasing β-agonist use, or activity limitation. The Expert Panel recommends consultation with an asthma specialist if the patient has difficulties achieving or maintaining control of asthma, immunotherapy or omalizumab (Xolair) is being considered, the patient requires step 4 care or higher, or the patient has had an exacerbation requiring hospitalization.

## CURRENT THERAPY

- Nonpharmacologic therapy includes asthma education (especially regarding inhaler technique, self-monitoring, and self-management), reduction in environmental triggers, addressing any relevant psychosocial issues, and immunotherapy for select patients.

- Preferred step therapy for long-term asthma management is (in order): low-dose inhaled corticosteroids; medium-dose inhaled corticosteroids or low-dose inhaled corticosteroids plus long-acting β-agonists; medium-dose inhaled corticosteroids plus long-acting β-agonists; high-dose inhaled corticosteroids plus long-acting β-agonists; and oral prednisone.

- Asthma exacerbations should be treated with high-dose inhaled β-agonists and early use of systemic corticosteroids.

**TABLE 7** Estimated Comparative Daily Dosages for Inhaled Corticosteroids for Patients 12 Years and Older

| Drug | Dosage Form | Daily Dose | | |
|------|-------------|------------|---|---|
| | | Low (μg) | Medium (μg) | High (μg) |
| Beclomethasone HFA (QVAR) | 40 or 80 μg/puff | 80-240 | >240-480 | >480 |
| Budesonide DPI (Pulmicort) | 90,180, or 200 μg/inhalation | 180-600 | >600-1,200 | >1,200 |
| Flunisolide (AeroBid) | 250 μg/puff | 500-1,000 | >1,000-2,000 | >2,000 |
| Flunisolide HFA (AeroSpan) | 80 μg/puff | 320 | >320-640 | >640 |
| Fluticasone-HFA (Flovent HFA, Flovent Diskus) | MDI: 44, 110, 220 μg/puff | 88-264 | >264-440 | >440 |
| | DPI: 50, 100, 250 μg/inhalation | 100-300 | >300-500 | >500 |
| Mometasone DPI (Asmanex) | 200 μg/inhalation | 200 | 400 | >400 |
| Triamcinolone acetonide (Azmacort) | 75 μg/puff | 300-750 | >750-1500 | >1500 |

*Abbreviations:* DPI = dry powder inhaler; HFA = hydrofluoroalkane.

## Treatment of Exacerbations

Asthma exacerbations are acute or subacute episodes of progressively worsening shortness of breath, cough, wheezing, or chest tightness associated with decreases in expiratory airflow.

### HOME MANAGEMENT

Patients' action plans should direct their home therapy of asthma exacerbations according to the following recommendations.

Initial therapy should be with inhaled short-acting β-agonists (2-6 puffs by metered-dose inhaler [MDI] or nebulizer). This may be repeated in 20 minutes. With a good response (minimal or no symptoms and peak expiratory flow (PEF) ≥80% predicted or personal best), the patient may continue β-agonists every 3 to 4 hours for 24 to 48 hours. If repeated β-agonists are needed, a short course of oral corticosteroids should be considered.

With an incomplete response to initial therapy (persistent wheezing and dyspnea and PEF 50% to 79% predicted or personal best), oral corticosteroids should be added, β-agonists should be repeated, and the clinician should be contacted that day.

With a poor response (marked wheezing and dyspnea at rest, PEF <50% predicted or personal best), oral corticosteroids should be added, the β-agonist should be repeated immediately, and the patient should call the clinician and usually proceed to the emergency department. For signs of severe distress (e.g., difficulty talking in full sentences, diaphoresis, drowsiness, confusion, or cyanosis), 911 should be called. Patients with histories of rapid-onset severe exacerbations should have self-injectable epinephrine (Epipen)[1] at home to use at the onset of increased symptoms.

### EMERGENCY DEPARTMENT AND HOSPITAL MANAGEMENT

Assessment should rapidly determine the severity of the exacerbation based on intensity of symptoms, signs (heart rate, respiratory rate, use of accessory muscles, chest auscultation), peak flow (unless the patient is too dyspneic to perform), and pulse oximetry. Treatment should begin immediately following recognition of an exacerbation severe enough to cause dyspnea at rest, peak flow less than 70% predicted or personal best, or pulse oximetry oxygen saturation less than 95%. While treatment is being given, a brief focused history and physical examination pertinent to the exacerbation can be obtained.

In patients with *mild-moderate exacerbations* (PEF >40% predicted), initial therapy is oxygen to achieve oxygen saturation greater than 90% and inhaled short-acting β-agonist by nebulizer or MDI (4-8 puffs) with holding chamber, which may be repeated up to three times in the first hour. Oral corticosteroids (prednisone 40-80 mg) are recommended if there is no immediate response to therapy or if the patient had been recently treated with oral corticosteroids.

In patients with *severe exacerbations* (PEF <40% predicted), initial therapy is oxygen as above, inhaled high-dose short-acting β-agonist (e.g., albuterol 5 mg) and ipratropium (0.5 mg) by nebulizer every 20 minutes or continuously for 1 hour, and oral or intravenous corticosteroids (prednisone or methylprednisolone 80 mg).

Repeated assessments of symptoms, signs, PEF, and oxygen saturation determine the responsiveness of the exacerbation to therapy. Such assessments should be made in patients presenting with severe exacerbations after the initial bronchodilator treatment and in all patients after three doses of bronchodilator therapy (60-90 min after initial treatment). In patients who are improving, short-acting β-agonists may be repeated every hour until a good response is achieved (no distress, PEF >70%). When this response is sustained at least 60 minutes after the last treatment, the patient may usually be discharged on a course of oral corticosteroids (generally prednisone 40-60 mg for 5-10 days), initiation or continuation of medium-dose inhaled corticosteroids, and arrangement for outpatient follow-up.

In patients who are not improving with the above therapy, adjunctive therapy, such as with intravenous magnesium sulfate[1] (2 g) or heliox, may be considered. Intubation and mechanical ventilation may be required for patients with respiratory failure in spite of treatment.

## Summary

Asthma is a very common problem with the potential to cause substantial interference with quality of life. Although there is no cure for asthma, asthma can be well controlled in the majority of patients with proper management and an effective patient-physician relationship. I hope that the method described herein for assessing and managing asthma will help physicians help their patients to achieve well-controlled asthma.

---

[1] Not FDA approved for this indication

# Asthma in Children

Method of
*Gerald B. Kolski, MD, PhD, FAAAAI, FAAP*

Asthma is the most common cause of significant childhood morbidity. This includes school absenteeism, hospitalizations, emergency department visits, and acute care visits. Its prevalence has been increasing throughout the 1990s and into this century. An estimated 5 million children younger than 15 years have asthma as identified by the National Health Interview Survey of 2003. According to this survey, the prevalence of asthma in the general population is somewhere between 6% and 10%. Prevalence in inner-city populations and especially in African Americans is closer to 14% to 15%. Pediatricians and family practitioners are often reluctant to make the diagnosis because of difficulty with giving prognostic information to parents. Wheezing during the first few years of life can often be associated with acute viral infections, especially respiratory syncytial virus (RSV). Longitudinal studies suggest there are three patterns to wheezing in children. There are a group of children who wheeze during infancy associated with viral infections, a second group that wheeze during infancy and also as they get older, and a third group that only develops wheezing later after sensitization with allergens. Because of these groups it is oftentimes difficult to give prognostic information to parents until you have seen the pattern that a child will follow.

Despite tremendous improvement in medications and treatments for asthma, deaths from asthma continue to occur. Most recently, however, the mortality rates seem to have leveled off or decreased slightly.

One theory for the high prevalence of asthma is the "hygiene hypothesis." Studies done in homogeneous populations in Europe and Scandinavian countries have noted less asthma and allergies in rural populations versus those that live in urban environments. Attempts have been made to correlate this with endotoxin exposure during infancy and/or infections during this period of time that turn on immune responses that do not promote allergies. This concept favors an immune response, which postulates that certain infections and endotoxin exposure promote a $T_H1$ T cell response in which interferon gamma and interleukin(IL)-2 predominate, whereas a lack of these infections promotes a $T_H2$ response where there is an IL-4, IL-13, and IL-5 predominance with increased IgE production.

## Pathophysiology

Over the last several decades the idea that reversible bronchoconstriction is the main element in asthma has changed. It has become apparent that in addition to bronchoconstriction there is considerable inflammation involving increased mucus production, inflammatory cell infiltrates, and airway thickening. With longitudinal studies it has become apparent that there may in fact be some fibrosis that leads to "airway remodeling." The increased inflammatory infiltrates lead to increasing airway reactivity characterized by hyperresponsiveness to various stimuli. The inflammatory cell infiltrates can include eosinophils, lymphocytes, basophils, neutrophils, and macrophages depending on the stimulus. Unchecked inflammation is believed to be the cause of the fibrosis. Clearly it is important to try and identify the triggers in an individual patient that are causing the inflammation as well as treating the inflammation.

## Differential Diagnosis

Determining the cause of wheezing in infancy can often be difficult. During the first year of life if the wheezing is associated with a viral infection, a diagnosis of bronchiolitis is often made. A clinical response to bronchodilators might be helpful in assessing whether this is going to be a child with asthma. Recurrent wheezing in an atopic child with a strong family history of asthma would strongly suggest that the child has underlying asthma. An association with eczema and/or other allergic manifestations might also be suggestive of asthma. Because of the difficulty in doing pulmonary functions during the first few years of life, clinical assessment is the key. In addition to asthma, Table 1 lists the other diagnoses that have to be considered. Cystic fibrosis, gastroesophageal reflux disease, and foreign body aspiration probably are the

### TABLE 1  Differential Diagnosis of Wheezing

| Infants | Older Children |
|---|---|
| Laryngomalacia | Asthma |
| Tracheomalacia | Cystic fibrosis |
| Vascular rings | Gastroesophageal reflux disease |
| Subglottic stenosis | Foreign body aspiration |
| Airway congenital masses | Airway tumors |
| Gastroesophageal reflux | Viral infections (RSV, adenovirus) |
| Bronchiolitis | Tuberculosis |
| Pneumonia | |

*Abbreviations:* RSV = respiratory syncytial virus.

most common diagnoses that have to be entertained. Recurrent infiltrates should make you worry about immune deficiencies including hypogammaglobulinemia and ciliary defects such as immotile cilia syndrome.

Diagnostic tests such as a sweat test, immunoglobulins, skin or radioallergosorbent assay test (RAST), barium swallow, bronchoscopy, or chest radiograph may be indicated.

In older children asthma may be diagnosed by doing pulmonary functions. Spirometry can often be done in the office and can be a reproducible way to measure the extent of airway disease in known asthmatics as well as diagnostic by looking at pre- and postbronchodilator responses. The forced expiratory volume at 1 second ($FEV_1$) is often thought to be a measure of large airway obstruction. The $FEF_{25-75}$ or expiratory flow between the 25th and 75th percentile of the forced vital capacity (FVC) is often thought to be a measure of small airway disease. A 15% increase in $FEV_1$ pre- and postbronchodilator or 25% increase in $FEF_{25-75}$ is thought to be diagnostic of asthma. Inhalation challenges with methacholine (Provocholine) or histamine are often used to measure airway reactivity in experimental studies. Bronchoconstriction with these inhalation challenges can determine the degree of airway hyperreactivity. Similar results can also be obtained with exercise challenges or cold air challenges. These tests are often used to diagnose asthma in children whose pulmonary functions at baseline are not significantly depressed. In children with asthma, peak expiratory flow rates (PEFRs) are often used to monitor the asthma as well as the management. This test is effort dependent.

## Key Diagnostic Points Consistent with Asthma

- Recurrent wheezing responding to bronchodilators
- Coughing or wheezing shortly after exercise
- Pulmonary functions that show obstruction responding to bronchodilators
- Strong family history of asthma
- Associated allergic symptoms including seasonal rhinitis, eczema, or urticaria

## History

Once a diagnosis of asthma is made, it is important to determine the trigger for this individual's asthma symptoms or exacerbations. The history is very important in determining treatment. Box 1 lists the most common causes for asthma exacerbations.

The most common perennial allergens are dust mites, cockroaches, mold, and pets. In the inner cities, cockroaches and dust mites are very common causes for allergic sensitization. They are extremely common and very difficult to control. Dust mites need moisture and thus are much more common in humid areas. With increased humidity, molds also can play a significant role. Children are often treated with humidifiers or vaporizers for upper respiratory infections, which may exacerbate dust mite and mold exposure. In drier climates, pets, especially indoor animals, are often exacerbating causes. Recent studies have indicated that more than two or three pets decreased the likelihood of sensitization, whereas an isolated pet is more likely to be associated with the development of allergy. This may have to do with endotoxin and the previously discussed hygiene hypothesis.

### BOX 1  Asthma Triggers

- Allergies: perennial or seasonal
- Viral infections
- Irritants, especially cigarette smoke and air pollution
- Exercise
- Weather changes
- Gastroesophageal reflux
- Medications including aspirin and nonsteroidal anti-inflammatory drugs (NSAIDs)
- Sinusitis

Children who only have difficulty with their asthma in the spring and fall may have sensitization to the pollens. This is very regional and often associated with being outdoors. Pollination and dissemination is most problematic with dry windy days. Keeping the windows closed at night as well as air conditioning may benefit individuals with seasonal allergies. These children may need medications at particular times of the year but not throughout the year. Airway reactivity often continues even 4 to 6 weeks after the allergen is no longer present.

Children who have trouble with viral infections may also have increased reactivity from perennial or seasonal exposures that exacerbate the asthma with infection. It is often helpful to reduce allergy exposure in these individuals so as to reduce their response to viral infections. Parents may be alerted to signs of upper respiratory infection so that they can increase asthma treatment at those times.

At all times cigarette smoke causes increased mucus production as well as decreases mucociliary clearance. Children with asthma thus are especially prone to having difficulty around cigarette smoke. During infancy, cigarette smoke exposure is associated with a two- to threefold increase in risk of asthma as well as upper respiratory infections, ear infections, and pneumonia. Smoking during pregnancy is also associated with a sustained decrease in infant pulmonary functions. Smoke is a form of indoor air pollution. Outdoor air pollution, especially small particles, ozone, nitrogen dioxide, and sulfur dioxide, all can be exacerbating factors in asthma.

Exercise is associated with asthma exacerbations because of the inhalation of cold dry air. Exercise is often associated with mouth breathing. The nose normally moisturizes, filters, and warms the air. Nasal congestion secondary to allergies, viral infections, or nasal obstruction can all lead to more difficulty with exercise as well as with breathing cold dry air at any time.

Weather changes are often a problem secondary to what is in the air or the changes in temperature of the air. Children who have trouble with weather changes are often responding to changes in pollen distribution or other allergens or irritants.

Children who have reflux as the exacerbating cause of their asthma often have difficulty at night when they lie down, shortly after meals, or when ingesting very acidic substances. Often there will be considerable coughing and if the child is old enough to talk some significant heartburn. Reflux is often worse when the asthma is a problem because the lower esophageal sphincter tone decreases with hyperinflation at that time.

Children with sensitivity to aspirin or nonsteroidal anti-inflammatory drugs (NSAIDs) often have associated sinusitis, nasal polyps, and profuse rhinorrhea with aspirin exposure. It often goes undiagnosed until adulthood. Nasal polyps should always raise this possibility in addition to a diagnosis of cystic fibrosis.

Sinusitis can be associated with significant exacerbations of asthma. Often treating the sinusitis treats the asthma exacerbation. Purulent nasal discharge for 5 to 7 days associated with significant coughing and maxillary tenderness may be suggestive of underlying sinusitis. In children with allergic rhinitis, complications of sinusitis often occur.

In all children with asthma it is very important that you try and assess severity of disease. There should be questions asked about whether the patient has ever been intubated or had an intensive care unit admission. In addition questions about recent use of oral corticosteroids should be asked to determine the recent course of asthma. Children with underlying seizure disorders are also important to identify because they are at greater risk for mortality. Signs of mental illness or depression should also be noted because this predisposes children to significant morbidity and mortality.

## Physical Examination

In examining a patient with asthma, the complete physical is extremely helpful. Children with skin findings of eczema or hives associated with an exacerbation of asthma may often lead to a search for an allergy exposure that is responsible for symptoms. Nasal examination may show boggy turbinates suggestive of allergy or erythematous turbinates suggestive of infection. Purulent discharge associated with sinus tenderness may suggest sinusitis. Nasal polyps should also be looked for to ascertain whether the patient may have underlying cystic fibrosis or aspirin-sensitive asthma. Enlarged tonsils and adenoids may predispose to mouth breathing and exacerbate underlying asthma. Examination of the chest may show whether there is a pectus suggesting chronic disease or whether there is hyperinflation with a barrel chest. Supraclavicular, intercostal, and subcostal muscular activity give information as to the work of breathing. The cardiac examination should focus on heart rate as well as any sign that might indicate this is cardiac wheezing instead of asthma. Abdominal examination is important to evaluate any signs of liver or spleen enlargement that might indicate evidence of pulmonary hypertension or cardiac disease. Examination of the extremities is important to look for clubbing and/or cyanosis. The neurologic exam is especially important acutely to ascertain whether the patient is having any change in mental status secondary to hypoxia.

## Treatment

Treatment for asthma has changed considerably since the mid 90's. The chronic management of asthma has focused on assuring that the patient functions as normally as possible with the following goals of asthma management:

- No nocturnal asthma
- Full exercise activity
- No emergency department visits or hospitalizations
- No lost time from school or work
- No or minimal side effects from medication

Asthma treatment has focused on the anti-inflammatory nature of the disease to eliminate long-term damage to the lungs. Asthma treatment has followed the National Heart, Lung, and Blood Institute (NHLBI) guidelines with assessment of asthma severity and management based on the classifications (Table 2). We developed a color-coded questionnaire that gives an indication of asthma control.

## Medications

Asthma medications are classified according to medications that are used for acute relief of symptoms called *relievers* and those that are used for chronic control of symptoms characterized as *controllers*. This classification was established to give patients a better understanding of the role of their individual medications. It is also a better way to educate patients as to why they have to continue to take medications even when they are not having symptoms. It is important to discuss these individual classifications and medications for both acute and chronic management.

### RELIEVERS

Various bronchodilators are used for acute management of asthma. These bronchodilators are predominantly β-agonists such as albuterol (Proventil) and terbutaline (Brethine) that are selective for $\beta_2$-receptors. Table 3 gives the generic as well as trade names for these medications. The short-acting β-agonists are used for acute relief in most circumstances. In children anticholinergics such as ipratropium bromide (Atrovent) are often used in the emergency department and hospital setting acutely but are rarely given chronically. Chronic use of β-agonists is avoided because of a decrease in effectiveness as well as an increase in airway reactivity with their chronic use. With chronic use there is also a decrease in both the number and affinity of β-receptors for these bronchodilators. The affinity as well as number of β-receptors is increased with the use of corticosteroids.

- **Severe:** ABCs, oxygen, monitors, POX, IV, isotonic fluids to maintain volume.

**Start with (consider SC epinephrine if really tight):**

- Albuterol, 0.5% inhalation solution, 0.5 mL (<20 kg), 0.75 mL (>20 kg) q20min × 3 (may give as mini-Nebs or start continuous at 2–3 mL/h). After initial stabilization patient will likely need q2h Nebs or continuous albuterol.
- Methylprednisolone (Solu-Medrol), 2 mg/kg IV (maximum, 125 mg) then start 1 mg/kg q6h (maximum, 80 mg/dose).
- Ipratropium bromide (Atrovent), 250 μg (<5 y), 500 μg (>5 y) × 2, then q4h.

**If minimal improvement:**

- Magnesium sulfate,[1] 45 mg/kg IV over 20 min (maximum, 2 g).

**If still severe, consider terbutaline drip:**

- Terbutaline (Brethine), 2–10 μg/kg loading dose, then start infusion at 0.1–0.4 μg/kg/min (maximum, 6 μg/kg/min). **Needs pediatric intensive care unit (PICU).**

**At any time if minimal air entry, use:**

- Epinephrine (1:1000), 0.01 mL/kg SC (maximum, 0.3 mL) or
- Terbutaline, 0.01 mg/kg SC (maximum, 0.25 mg)

Note: Adequate volume can be critical in maintaining circulatory volume (preload), so use volume freely. Also buffering with THAM for severe acidosis can be useful. These two strategies may help you avoid intubation.

**If you really need to intubate** (impending respiratory failure), use atropine, 0.02 mg/kg IV (minimum), 0.1 mg (maximum, 1 mg); ketamine (Ketalar), 1–2 mg/kg IV; or vecuronium (Norcuron), 0.1–0.2 mg/kg IV.

- **Moderate:** ABCs, POX, oxygen, monitors. ± IV

**Start with**

- Albuterol, 0.5 mL (<20 kg), 0.75 mL (>20 kg) q20min × 3 (may start with mini Nebs or continuous). Then patient will likely need q2h Nebs or continuous albuterol (2 mL/h <10 kg, 3 mL/hr >10 kg)
- Ipratropium bromide, 250 μg (<5 y), 500 μg (>5 y) × 2, then q4h
- Prednisone, 2 mg/kg (maximum, 80 mg) if tolerating PO
  or
- Methylprednisolone, 2 mg/kg (maximum, 80 mg) (continue steroids for 5 d, 2 mg/kg/d)

**If minimal improvement:**

Consider magnesium sulfate as above.

- **Mild:** ABCs, POX

**Start with**

- Albuterol Nebs or MDI with spacer q2–4h
- Prednisolone, 2 mg/kg loading dose (maximum, 80 mg), then 2 mg/kg/d divided bid × 5 d

For mild to moderate exacerbation, discharge home may be considered if patient shows good improvement, is no longer dyspneic or hypoxic, tolerates Nebs q4h, and has good supervision at home.

**CXR:** Consider for a first-time wheezer; a condition other than asthma (i.e., FB); a febrile child with clinical signs of pneumonia; or no clinical improvement or worsening condition (pneumothorax, pneumomediastinum).

**Continuous albuterol:** To calculate the total amount of albuterol and normal saline, remember that the total amount of solution per hour must equal 30 mL.

**Example:** For a child >10 kg, the albuterol dose for continuous Nebs is 3 mL/h so you need to add 27 mL of NSS to run for 1 h (to set it up for 4 h, total mL = 120 with 12 mL albuterol + 108 mL NSS).

---

[1]Not FDA approved for this indication.

*Abbreviations:* ABCs = airway, breathing, and circulation; CXR = chestradiograph; FB = foreign body; IV = intravenous ; Nebs = nebulized; NSS = normal saline solution; POX = pulse oximter; SC = subcutaneous; THAM = tromethamine.

---

In the management of acute episodes of asthma, an algorithm is used (see Current Therapy box). β-agonists are given either by nebulizer or inhaler. In addition to albuterol, a selective stereoisomer levalbuterol (Xopenex) is also available but is more expensive. This isomer may cause fewer side effects and have a slightly longer duration of action. In the acute setting, treatments are often given every 20 minutes times three and then are continued every 2 to 3 hours for hospitalized patients. In critical situations, albuterol may also be given continuously. It is during the acute situation where ipratropium bromide is beneficial for the first 24 to 48 hours of treatment. It can be given by nebulizer every 4 to 6 hours.

Injectable epinephrine is still recommended especially in the acute attack if it is thought to be secondary to allergies or anaphylaxis. It also can be used in the acute situation to make sure that inhaled drugs can reach the lower airway.

Magnesium sulfate[1] is used intravenously in severe asthmatics for its bronchodilator properties to prevent intubation or respiratory failure. This is outlined again in the acute management algorithm (Current Therapy box).

Theophylline (Theolair) was often the mainstay of asthma management in the 1980s, but its toxicity and the difficulty in having to monitor levels has reduced its use. Nausea, vomiting, abdominal pain, and an increase in hyperactivity often lead to noncompliance. With the selective β-agonists their use has been minimal. They can be used for chronic management in patients to decrease corticosteroid need.

Oral or systemic corticosteroids are always indicated in acute management of episodes of asthma exacerbation. The usual recommended starting dose is 2 mg/kg and should be continued during the episode. Prolonged use of corticosteroids may require a taper, but a short course of 4 to 5 days does not usually require a taper. Any patient who was admitted for an acute exacerbation of asthma should go home on a controller with an action plan for future attacks.

In the chronic management of asthma, albuterol is still the mainstay of acute attacks, pre-exercise, and for any reduction in peak flow or pulmonary functions. Albuterol (Proventil) is usually given by metered-dose inhaler and for most patients it is recommended that it be given with a spacer. Spacers increase the deposition in the lower airway and increase the effectiveness of inhaled drugs. In the chronic management of asthma, the NHLBI guidelines recommend that if albuterol is being used more than two or three times a week a step up in controller medications is suggested (Table 2).

## CONTROLLERS

Inhaled corticosteroids are established as the mainstay of chronic management of asthma. Various preparations are available either by dry powder inhaler or metered-dose inhaler. Table 2 outlines the doses and route. Side effects of growth suppression and decreases in bone mineralization are dose related as well as preparation dependent. Individuals on any of the corticosteroids need to have their growth monitored and also to have instructions on mouth rinsing after inhalation to reduce fungal colonization in the oropharynx.

Leukotriene antagonists are available in oral preparations. These offer some advantage in pediatric patients in that they do not require good inhalation technique and can be given once a day. This may improve compliance and offer benefit in asthma as well as allergic rhinitis. They are not as effective as inhaled corticosteroids but offer some benefit in mild disease or as an adjunct to inhaled corticosteroids.

Cromolyn (Intal) and nedocromil (Tilade) are available as inhaled medications. Both of these drugs are mast cell stabilizers and appear to be most effective in allergic patients. These drugs should be taken three to four times a day, which makes their compliance more difficult. There are no significant side effects to these medications, however, and they are used in children because of their safety profile. They are used primarily in the mildest of patients and as pretreatment before allergy exposure.

Long-acting β-agonists are characterized as controllers, but these medications cannot be taken as anti-inflammatory agents. They have an increased risk of mortality when taken alone. For this reason only the preparations that are in combination with inhaled corticosteroids should be used in children. The drug preparations contain varying doses of inhaled corticosteroid with one standard dose of long-acting β-agonist.

Oral corticosteroids have been used for asthma since they were developed. They were used for patients with severe or chronic asthma before inhaled steroids were available. Because oral corticosteroids have

## TABLE 2  Stepwise Approach for Managing Asthma in Children

| Classify Severity: Clinical Features Before Treatment or Adequate Control | | | Medications Required to Maintain Long-Term Control |
|---|---|---|---|
| | *Symptoms/Day* | *PEF or FEV$_1$* | |
| | *Symptoms/Night* | *PEF Variability* | *Daily Medications* |
| **Step 4** Severe persistent | Continual Frequent | <60% >30% | **Preferred treatment:** <br> • High-dose inhaled corticosteroids, *and* <br> • Long-acting inhaled β$_2$-agonists (combination preferred) *and*, if needed, <br> • Corticosteroid tablets or syrup long term (2 mg/kg/d, generally do not exceed 60 mg/d). (Make repeat attempts to reduce systemic corticosteroids and maintain control with high-dose inhaled corticosteroids.) |
| **Step 3:** Moderate persistent | Daily >1 night/wk | >60%–<80% >30% | • **Preferred treatment:** <br>  • Low- to medium-dose inhaled corticosteroids. <br> • **Alternative treatment** (listed alphabetically): <br>  • Increase inhaled corticosteroids within medium-dose range <br>  *or* <br>  • Low to medium–dose inhaled corticosteroids and either leukotriene modifier or theophylline. <br> If needed (particularly in patients with recurring severe exacerbations): <br> • **Preferred treatment:** <br>  • Increased inhaled corticosteroids within medium-dose range and add long-acting inhaled β$_2$-agonists (combination inhaler preferred). <br> • **Alternative treatment** (listed alphabetically): <br>  • Increase inhaled corticosteroids within medium-dose range, and add either leukotriene modifier or theophylline. |
| **Step 2** Mild persistent | >2/wk but <1/d >2 nights/mo | >80% 20%–30% | • **Preferred treatment:** <br>  • Low-dose inhaled corticosteroids. <br> • **Alternative treatment** (listed alphabetically): <br>  • Cromolyn (Intal). <br>  • Leukotriene modifier. <br>  • Nedocromil (Tilade) *or* sustained-release theophylline (Slo-bid Gyrocaps) to serum concentration of 5–15 µg/mL. |
| **Step 1** Mild intermittent | <2 d/wk <2 nights/mo | >80% <20% | • **No daily medication needed.** <br> • Severe exacerbations may occur, separated by long periods of normal lung function and no symptoms. A course of systemic corticosteroids is recommended. |

Note: Children <5 y cannot do adequate peak flows.

**Quick relief** All patients
- Short-acting bronchodilator: 2–4 puffs short-acting inhaled β$_2$-agonists as needed for symptoms.
- Intensity of treatment depends on severity of exacerbation; up to 3 treatments at 20-min intervals or a single nebulizer treatment as needed. Course of systemic corticosteroids may be needed.
- Use of short-acting β$_2$-agonists >2 times/wk in intermittent asthma (daily, or increasing use in persistent asthma) may indicate the need to initiate (increase) long-term-control therapy.

↓ **Step down**
Review treatment q1–6mo; a gradual stepwise reduction in treatment may be possible.

↑ **Step up**
If control is not maintained, consider step up. First, review patient medication technique, adverse effects from medications.

Notes:
The stepwise approach is meant to assist, not replace, the clinical decision-making required to meet individual patient needs.
Classify severity: Assign patient to most severe step in which any feature occurs (PEF is percentage of personal best; FEV$_1$ is percentage predicted).
Gain control as quickly as possible (consider a short course of systemic corticosteroids); then step down to the least medication necessary to maintain control.
Minimize use of short-acting inhaled β$_2$-agonists. Overreliance on short-acting inhaled β$_2$-agonists (e.g., use of approximately 1 canister/mo even if not using it every day) indicates inadequate control of asthma and the need to initiate or intensify long-term-control therapy.
Provide education on self-management and controlling environmental factors that make asthma worse (e.g., allergens and irritants).
Refer to an asthma specialist if there are difficulties controlling asthma or if step 4 care is required. Referral may be considered if care at level step 3 is required.

*Continued*

**TABLE 2** Stepwise Approach for Managing Asthma in Children—cont'd

### Usual Dosages for Long-Term-Control Medications

| Medication | Dosage Form | Child Dose |
|---|---|---|
| **Systemic Corticosteroids** | | |
| Methylprednisolone (Medrol) | 2-, 4-, 8-, 16-, 32-mg tablets | 0.25–2 mg/kg daily in single dose in AM or qod as needed for control |
| Prednisolone (Prelone) (Orapred) | 5-mg tablets 5 mg/5 mL, 15 mg/5 mL | Short-course "burst": 1–2 mg/kg/d, maximum |
| Prednisone (Orasone) | 1-, 2.5-, 5-, 10-, 20-, 50-mg tablets: 5 mg/5 mL, 5 mg/mL | 60 mg/d for 3–10 d |
| **Long-Acting β₂-agonists** | | |
| _(Do not use for symptom relief or for exacerbations.)_ | | |
| Salmeterol (Serevent) | DPI 50 μg/blister | 1 blister q12h |
| Formoterol (Foradil) | DPI 12 μg/single-use capsule | 1 capsule q12h |
| **Combine Medication** | | |
| Fluticasone/salmeterol (Advair) | DPI 100, 250, or 500 μg/50 μg | 1 inhalation bid; dose depends on severity of asthma |
| **Mast Cell Stabilizer** | | |
| Cromolyn (Intal) | MDI 800 μg/puff Nebulizer 20 mg/ampule | 1–2 puffs tid–qid 1 ampule tid–qid |
| Nedocromil (Tilade) | MDI 1.75 mg/puff | 1–2 puffs bid–qid |
| **Leukotriene Modifiers** | | |
| Montelukast (Singulair) | 4- or 5-mg chewable tablet 10-mg tablet | 4 mg qhs (2–5 y) 5 mg qhs (6–14 y) 10 mg qhs (>14 y) |
| Zafirlukast (Accolate) | 10- or 20-mg tablet | 20 mg daily (5–11 y) (10-mg tablet bid) |
| **Methylxanthines** | | |
| _(Serum monitoring is important.)_ | | |
| Theophylline (Slo-Phyllin) | Liquids, sustained-release tablets and capsules | Starting dose 10 mg/kg/d; usual maximum: <1 y: 0.2 (age in wks) + 5 = mg/kg/d >1 y: 16 mg/kg/d |

### Estimated Comparative Daily Dosages for Inhaled Corticosteroids

| Drug | Low Daily Dose | Medium Daily Dose | High Daily Dose |
|---|---|---|---|
| Beclomethasone HFA (QVAR) 40 or 80 μg/puff | 80–160 μg | 160–320 mcg | >320 μg |
| Budesonide DPI (Pulmicort) 200 μg/inhalation | 200–400 μg | 400–800 mcg | >800 μg |
| Budesonide inhalation suspension for nebulization (Pulmicort Respules) | 0.5 mg | 1.0 mg | 2.0 mg |
| Flunisolide (AeroBid) 250 μg/puff | 500–750 μg | 1000–1250 μcg | 1250 μg |
| Fluticasone (Flovent) MDI: 44, 110, or 220 μg/puff DPI: 50, 100, or 250 μg/inhalation | 88–176 μg 100–200 μg | 176–440 μg 200–400 μg | >440 μg >400 μg |
| Triamcinolone acetonide (Azmacort) 100 μg/puff | 400–800 μg | 800–1200 μg | >1200 μg |
| Mometasone fumarate (Asmanex) 220 mg | 220 μg | 440 μg | 880 μg |

_Abbreviations:_ DPI = daily permissible intake; FEV$_1$ = forced expiratory volume at 1 second; MDI = metered-dose inhaler; PEF = peak expiratory flow (rate).

significant side effects they should be used with caution. Prolonged use of systemic steroids leads to adrenal suppression, osteoporosis, and growth suppression. With prolonged use the dose should be reduced gradually. Inhaled corticosteroid effects can be similar to the systemic corticosteroids, especially if they are used at doses higher than recommended.

## OMALIZUMAB

Omalizumab (Xolair) is a monoclonal antibody that is humanized and was developed against IgE. It is expensive and requires monthly injections. It is most effective when allergies are the main trigger for asthma. It is also used in patients with severe anaphylaxis.[1] It is indicated for children with moderate to severe persistent asthma that is exacerbated by significant documented allergies. Because it is nonspecific it does not reduce specific allergies and cannot be used in patients who have no significant atopy.

## IMMUNOSUPPRESSIVE AGENTS

Various experimental studies in patients with chronic steroid-dependent asthma have used immunosuppressive agents such as methotrexate[1] (Trexall), IV gammaglobulin[1] (Gamimune N), and anti-inflammatory monoclonal antibodies against cytokines. None of these produced dramatic results and none is available or can be recommended at this time.

[1] Not FDA approved for this indication

[1] Not FDA approved for this indication

## TABLE 3 Medications for the Acute Relief of Symptoms

| Generic β-agonist | Brand Name* |
|---|---|
| Albuterol | Ventolin, Ventolin HFA, Proventil HFA, Proventil |
| Pirbuterol | Maxair, Maxair Autohaler |
| Terbutaline | Brethaire, Brethine, Bricanyl |
| Metaproterenol | Alupent |
| Levalbuterol | Xopenex |

*Many of these drugs are available in liquid, tablet, inhalation aerosol, as well as metered-dose inhalers.
Albuterol is also available in an inhaler in combination with ipratropium bromide (Combivent).

### IMMUNOTHERAPY

Specific injections of extracts of allergens to which the patient is allergic is effective for allergic rhinitis that is secondary to certain allergens. Therapy with allergy extracts is effective for pollens, and by reducing allergic rhinitis symptoms it can affect nasal breathing and therefore benefit asthma. Because of the risk of reactions to immunotherapy it should be used cautiously when the patient is having significant asthma symptoms at the time of injection. Studies in Europe suggest that in the future sublingual immunotherapy may be effective. Well-documented studies in this country have not been done and it is not approved as an FDA procedure.

## Education and Environmental Control

Education of the individual asthmatic is important. Action plans in which treatment of acute episodes is outlined is recommended. Parents and patients should be taught about the patient's triggers as well as steps they should take to increase or decrease their medications depending on symptoms. Environmental precautions such as dust mite avoidance have had some success. Pet avoidance has not worked unless the pet is totally eliminated.

### REFERENCES

Castro-Rodriguez JA, Holberg CJ, Wright AL, Martinez FD: A clinical index to define risk of asthma in young children with recurrent wheezing. Am J Respir Crit Care Med 2000;162:1403-1406.
National Institutes of Health/National Heart, Lung, and Blood Institute: NAEPP expert panel report 2: Guidelines for the diagnosis and management of asthma. Publication no. 97-4051. Bethesda, Md, The Institutes, 1997.
O'Connor GT: Allergen avoidance in asthma: What do we do now? J Allergy Clin Immunol 2005;116:26-30.
Romagnani S: Immunologic influences on allergy and the TH1/TH2 balance. J Allergy Clin Immunol 2004;113:395-400.
Spahn JD, Szefler SJ: Childhood asthma: New insights into management. J Allergy Clin Immunol 2002;109:3-13.

# Allergic Rhinitis Caused by Inhalant Factors

Method of
*Richard W. Weber, MD*

Atopy is an inherited disposition manifested by any or all of allergic rhinitis, asthma, or atopic eczema. It is closely, but not invariably, linked to the ability to generate specific allergic antibody, IgE, in greater than normal amounts. Allergic rhinitis is the most prevalent of the atopic diseases, affecting 25% to 35% of persons, depending on the population studied. The atopic disorders have become steadily more prevalent over the past century, although the exact reason for this increase is not clear.

Although allergic rhinitis is considered by nonsufferers to be a trivial disease, it delivers a significant personal impact on quality of life. It is responsible for an enormous economic burden in terms of direct medical costs for physician visits and medication and indirect costs of missed work and school and lost productivity. This cost in the United States was recently estimated at more than $2 billion annually and is now presumably even greater.

## Pathogenesis

IgE, like IgA, is a mucosal antibody, produced by plasma cells beneath the mucosal surfaces of the eyes, upper and lower airways, and the gut. IgE is a homocytotropic antibody, binding to specific high-affinity receptors on basophils in the circulation and mast cells in various tissues. Bridging by allergen of two specific IgE molecules on the cell surface is sufficient to cause activation of the basophils or mast cells. This is followed by the release of vasoactive mediators such as histamine, tryptase, leukotrienes, and prostaglandins, as well as several chemokines and cytokines. The former mediators are responsible for the immediate allergic (early-phase) reaction, manifested by sneezing, itching, rhinorrhea, and nasal congestion. Chemotactic factors result in the recruitment of inflammatory cells such as basophils, eosinophils, and polymorphonuclear leukocytes. The influx of these cells is accompanied by fresh release of vasoactive substances, culminating in the delayed (late-phase) reaction with a recrudescence of symptoms. With a single allergen exposure, the early and late phases are easily discernible, the latter occurring 4 to 6 hours after the initial reaction. With persistent exposure, such as with indoor allergens such as dust mite or animal dander, the late-phase inflammatory process is ongoing, resulting in chronic symptoms. With outdoor allergens such as pollens, the persistence of inflammation from prior exposure results in greater sensitivity to further exposures, with lesser pollen amounts resulting in greater symptoms. This is called the priming effect.

The proclivity to produce IgE is caused by a shift of helper T-cells cytokine release to a $T_H2$ profile. Two central cytokines to this allergic phenotype are IL-4 and IL-5. The former causes isotype switch in B-cells to IgE production. The latter cytokine is crucial for eosinophil activation and longevity. Once this shift to a $T_H2$ profile occurs, it tends to self-perpetuate. Atopic persons are presumably genetically predisposed to the $T_H2$ phenotype.

In the great majority of instances, allergic rhinitis sensitization is to an airborne, inhalant factor. These aeroallergens may emanate from indoor or outdoor sources and be perennial, relatively constant, or with seasonal peaks. Outdoor sources are usually of plant or fungal origin, namely, pollen grains or spores. These frequently have seasonal peaks whose timing frequently aids in diagnosing the airborne culprit. Depending on the region, tree pollens pollinate in the winter into the early spring, although certain trees shed pollen in the fall. Grasses generally pollinate from May into July, with longer seasons in the southern states, and year round in Hawaii and southern Florida. Although some weeds overlap with the grasses, most pollinate from July into the fall. Aeroallergens indoors are more likely animal in origin: dust mite or cockroach emanations or animal dander. Mold spores are possible, especially with water damage or high humidity, but less likely. The exposures are usually perennial, but there are seasonal peaks in these as well: dust mite in late summer to early fall, cat and dog dander in late winter, and cockroach in summer. A recent study showed that the allergens from dog and cat dander can be found in the dust of essentially all homes, whether pets are present or not.

## Differential Diagnosis and Co-Morbid Conditions

Irritant rhinitis was previously referred to as vasomotor rhinitis, with nasal symptoms driven by perturbations in the environment, and is as frequent as allergic rhinitis. The cause of the increased susceptibility to irritants is not fully understood, although the resultant release of mediators is similar to that seen with allergic rhinitis. A variant of irritant rhinitis is "gustatory rhinitis," where the act of eating triggers rhinorrhea. Viral infection (upper respiratory infection [URI]) is perhaps the most common cause of nasal symptoms; other infectious agents are distinctly less common. Hormonal factors such as hypothyroidism and pregnancy can lead to increased nasal congestion. Medication-induced nasal congestion was commonly seen with older hypotensive agents and is certainly seen with topical α-adrenergic agonist abuse. Intolerance to aspirin and nonsteroidal anti-inflammatory drugs (NSAIDs) may manifest as asthma, chronic sinusitis, or both. Vasculitides such as Wegener's can present with chronic sinusitis.

An expert panel convened by the World Health Organization developed a position statement, "Allergic Rhinitis and Its Impact on Asthma (ARIA)." This document emphasized several important issues. Its scope is not just industrialized countries, but developing countries as well, and it discusses resources with a global perspective. One of the major messages is the frequent concordance of allergic rhinitis and asthma. It is crucial to suspect rhinitis and inflammation of the upper airway as an aggravant in asthma, just as the lower airway should be evaluated in patients with rhinitis. The position statement also suggests that the terms *seasonal* and *perennial* be replaced by *intermittent* and *persistent* in keeping with the phraseology recommended by the National Asthma Education and Prevention Program (NAEPP) and the Global Initiative for Asthma (GINA) guidelines for management of asthma.

## Evaluation

Evaluation of rhinitis is greatly aided by a careful history: presence of itching and sneezing, severity, seasonality, and progression of symptoms, identifiable triggers, occupational exposures, alleviating factors, and medication usage. A positive family history of atopic disease is helpful. The impact of disease and medication on daily activity is likewise important. The presence of co-morbid conditions is suggested by a history of headache, loss of smell and taste, purulent discharge, cough, chest tightness or wheezing, snoring, and sleep disturbance.

Physical examination of the head may reveal characteristic findings. Dennie's lines are folds under the eyes caused by edema. Dark discoloration under the eyes, or so-called allergic shiners, is caused by venous engorgement. A transverse crease across the nose may be seen in children who chronically push their palm upward under the nose because of rhinorrhea or itching. The turbinates appearing edematous with a bluish mother-of-pearl hue is believed to be pathognomonic but may be seen in nonallergic rhinitis also. Likewise, turbinates may be engorged and erythematous. Lymphoid hyperplasia, or cobblestoning, may be seen on the posterior pharynx. Chronic mouth breathing in children caused by nasal obstruction can cause the allergic facies in the developing facial features. These include open mouth with receding chin and overbite, elongation of the face, and arching of the hard palate.

Diagnosis is frequently determined by the appropriate history and findings and supported by demonstration of specific IgE antibodies against a variety of airborne agents. Percutaneous (prick or puncture) skin testing remains the most specific and cost-effective diagnostic modality, although newer CAP-RAST (radioallergosorbent assay) testing is approaching similar sensitivity. Intradermal skin testing is more sensitive but introduces a higher false-positive rate and is not believed to add any diagnostic value to prick testing of potent pollen extracts. There may, however, be a role for intradermal testing with less potent extracts.

## Pharmacotherapy

Pharmacotherapy for allergic rhinitis is the most used mode of treatment, although perhaps not the most effective. $H_1$ antihistamines have the largest market share of rhinitis remedies, although, again, they are not the most effective. Oral first-generation $H_1$ receptor antagonists have been available for more than a half century, and many are

## CURRENT DIAGNOSIS

Appropriate history of exacerbants:
- Perennial or seasonal symptoms, with timing to identify pollens or spores
- Symptom triggering with identifiable agents such as animals

Familial history of asthma, allergic rhinitis, or atopic eczema

Medication and medical history:
- Oral aggravants such as ASA, NSAIDs, hypotensive agents
- Topical aggravants such as α-agonists
- Hypothyroidism
- Pregnancy

Physical findings:
- Rhinorrhea
- Nasal congestion
- So-called allergic facies

Corroborative findings:
- Immediate hypersensitivity skin testing
- Serum-specific IgE

Co-morbid conditions:
- Sinusitis
- Nasal polyposis
- Asthma
- Eustachian tube dysfunction and serous otitis media

*Abbreviations:* ASA = acetylsalicylic acid (aspirin); NSAIDs = nonsteroidal anti-inflammatory drugs.

obtainable as over-the counter (OTC) preparations. Typical benefits are inhibition of sneezing, itching, and rhinorrhea; oral antihistamines are notoriously ineffective for nasal congestion. Drawbacks are sedation and anticholinergic effects of overdrying. Second-generation antihistamines have the advantage of less anticholinergic effects and little to no sedation. Loratadine (Claritin) is available as an OTC formulation, whereas others such as fexofenadine (Allegra) are still prescription items. Cetirizine (Zyrtec), the active metabolite of hydroxyzine (Atarax), possesses potential for sedation. Topical azelastine (Astelin) is a twice-daily nasal spray as well as an ophthalmic preparation (Optivar). In addition to typical antihistaminic effects, it is modestly anti-inflammatory, improving nasal congestion, presumably through inhibition of ICAM-1, lipoxygenase, and leukotriene C4 synthase. It can cause sedation. Several topical ophthalmic antihistamine preparations are available for associated allergic conjunctivitis.

Leukotriene receptor antagonists were initially approved by the Food and Drug Administration (FDA) for use in asthma, but montelukast (Singulair) was more recently approved for allergic rhinitis therapy as well. However, a recent systematic review and meta-analysis showed these agents to be modestly better than placebo, as effective as antihistamines, and inferior to nasal corticosteroids in improving symptoms and quality of life in patients with seasonal allergic rhinitis. There seems little reason to use leukotriene modifier for treatment of uncomplicated allergic rhinitis. There may be some rationale for using montelukast or zafirlukast[1] (Accolate) with zileuton[1] (Zyflo) in the treatment of rhinitis complicated by sinusitis with polyposis, although evidence-based data are still missing.

Topical glucocorticoids are the most effective pharmacotherapy for allergic rhinitis. Topical corticosteroids decrease nasal $T_H2$ cytokines, IgE, and eosinophils. A meta-analysis showed superiority over antihistamines in 15 of 16 controlled trials, evaluating symptoms such as rhinorrhea, congestion, and sneezing. Another meta-analysis of nine studies again showed superiority of intranasal corticosteroids over topical antihistamines for nasal symptoms and no difference for ocular symptoms. Even if used on an as-needed basis only, nasal corticosteroids are superior for symptom relief to oral antihistamines.

In a short-term 2-week study, the combination of montelukast with cetirizine each once daily was shown to be as effective as once-daily intranasal mometasone in improvement of nasal peak flow and total nasal symptoms.

Although steroid potency based on receptor affinity is very important in the management of asthma, the dose-response curves for most topical nasal corticosteroids are such that all preparations appear to be equally effective. Choice is therefore predicated on patient preference, which is usually affected by effects of expedients. The most common side effect is epistaxis. Septal perforation is reported, presumably caused by topical vasoconstriction, but is exceedingly uncommon and appears to be adverted by proper administration technique. Concern over systemic side effects is generally not warranted. Fluticasone (Flonase) and mometasone (Nasonex) have very low levels of systemic bioavailability via the nasal route; the levels of budesonide (Rhinocort), triamcinolone (Nasacort), beclomethasone (Vancenase AQ), and flunisolide (Nasalide) are higher. Even so, reports of adverse effects are not common with nasal preparations. For severe symptoms, oral steroids such as prednisone are sometimes used for very short periods to achieve quick improvement. The well-known complications of long-term therapy are not justifiable in the management of rhinitis. In some parts of the United States, intramuscular corticosteroids are considered standard of care for severe symptoms induced by large exposures such as seen with mountain cedar fever. The wisdom of this practice is debatable.

An anticholinergic topical preparation, ipratropium bromide (Atrovent 0.06% Nasal Spray), is useful for rhinitis associated with more profuse rhinorrhea. It may be beneficial in allergic rhinitis but has a larger role in nonallergic irritant rhinitis such as cold air–induced, gustatory rhinitis, and the profuse rhinorrhea associated with viral URIs. Ipratropium has no effect on nasal congestion. Methscopolamine (Pamine) is an oral quaternary ammonium anticholinergic used as a drying agent and found primarily in combination with antihistamines such as chlorpheniramine and decongestants such as phenylephrine (Dura-vent/DA). Cromolyn (NasalCrom), a mast cell stabilizer, can be used as a topical nasal spray for allergic rhinitis but needs to be used every 4 hours for optimal efficacy.

The use of decongestants is problematic: data on oral efficacy are wanting, and benefit may be overridden by side effects. Potential for significant adverse reactions with overuse resulted in removal of phenylpropanolamine from the U.S. market. Similar problems are arising with pseudoephedrine. Phenylephrine is most often found in combination products. Overuse of topical decongestants like phenylephrine (Neo-Synephrine) and oxymetazoline (Otrivin) results in well-described rebound nasal congestion.

The use of saline nasal washes is highly recommended. A commercially available clear squeeze bottle with packets of sodium chloride and baking soda (Neilmed) is effective. This modality is especially useful in patients with complicating chronic sinusitis but is helpful for perennial allergic rhinitis as well.

## Avoidance and Environmental Controls

Although avoidance of outdoor aeroallergens can be frequently only achieved by remaining indoors, avoidance of indoor allergens is more amenable to intervention. Pets can be removed from the home, although levels of allergenic proteins may take months to subside. And many pet owners choose not to remove an allergenic animal. The value of allergen-impermeable bedding linens is either supported or disavowed by contradictory studies. Control of indoor humidity may provide the best avenue for dust mite and mold abatement. Cockroach control is very difficult to achieve, and sublethal boric acid treatment may actually increase the release of cockroach allergen.

## Allergen Immunotherapy

Allergen vaccine immunotherapy, administered via subcutaneous route, was shown by double-blind placebo-controlled studies to be effective in the treatment of allergic rhinoconjunctivitis. Extracts used include pollens such as short ragweed, timothy grass, other northern grasses, mountain cedar, and pellitory, fungi such as *Alternaria* and *Cladosporium*, house dust mites, and cat and dog dander. Immunologic changes include induction of specific IgG, blunting of specific IgE, decreased end-organ responsiveness, decreased recruitment of effector cells, shift from $T_H2$ to $T_H1$ cytokine profile, and induction of T regulatory cells. Sublingual/oral route of administration was studied extensively in Europe, requires high dose of allergen, and appears to have an excellent safety profile but is less effective than subcutaneous immunotherapy and is slower in onset of benefit.

## Biologic Modifiers

Omalizumab[1] (Xolair), the chimeric monoclonal antibody directed against IgE, is effective for allergic rhinitis, although presently approved only for use in steroid-requiring perennial allergic asthmatics. It would be an exceedingly costly way of treating hayfever, but those patients using it for asthma control could expect benefit in concomitant allergic rhinitis symptoms.

## Considerations in Pregnancy

Older antihistamines like chlorpheniramine (Chlor-Trimeton), hydroxyzine (Atarax), and tripelennamine (Pyribenzamine, PBZ) are safe in pregnancy, and data are likewise reassuring for loratadine (Claritin) and cetirizine (Zyrtec). Topical corticosteroids, especially after the first trimester, appear safe; budesonide (Rhinocort) is category B.

Cromolyn (NasalCrom) is category B also and can be used for mild disease. Pseudoephedrine (Sudafed) carries a category C, and oral decongestants are best avoided if possible. Allergen immunotherapy with stable maintenance dosing is safe.

In conclusion, pharmacotherapy is the most used therapeutic modality in allergic rhinitis because of inhalant factors. Second-generation antihistamines are preferable because of decreased sedation and

---

 **CURRENT THERAPY**

Allergen avoidance
Pharmacotherapy
- Topical corticosteroids as first-line monotherapy:
  - Mometasone (Nasonex)
  - Fluticasone (Flonase)
  - Budesonide (Rhinocort Agua)
  - Triamcinolone (Nasocort AQ)
  - Flunisolide (Nasalide)
- Oral antihistamines used as add-on therapy or alone for mild symptoms:
  - Fexofenadine (second generation) (Allegra)
  - Cetirizine (second generation) (Zyrtec)
  - Loratadine(second generation) (Claritin)
  - Hydroxyzine (Atarax)
  - Chlorpheniramine (Chlor-Trimeton)
  - Diphenhydramine (Astelin)
- Topical antihistamine (azelastine)
- Oral leukotriene modifiers (montelukast [Singulair]) as add-on only
- Oral decongestants:
  - Pseudoephedrine (Sudafed)
  - Phenylephrine (Ah-Chew D)
- Topical cromolyn (NasalCrom)
- Nasal saline irrigation (Ocean)
- Allergen immunotherapy

anticholinergic effects. Topical corticosteroids remain the best and preferred method of treatment, both for seasonal and perennial allergic rhinitis. Addition of antihistamines and antileukotrienes to topical steroids may be beneficial because of a more rapid onset of effect, and they may be withdrawn as control is achieved. Allergen avoidance is recommended but may be difficult depending on the incriminated agent. Allergen vaccine immunotherapy is effective and should be strongly considered in the face of poor response to pharmacotherapy and avoidance.

## REFERENCES

Benson M, Strannegård I-L, Strannegård Ö, Wennergren G: Topical steroid treatment of allergic rhinitis decreases nasal fluid $T_h2$ cytokines, eosinophils, eosinophil cationic protein, and IgE but has no significant effect on IFN-γ, IL-1β, TNF-α, or neutrophils. J Allergy Clin Immunol 2000;106:307-312.

Bousquet J, Van Cauwenberge P, Khaltaev N: Allergic rhinitis and its impact on asthma, J Allergy Clin Immunol 2001;108:S147-S334.

Frew AJ: Immunotherapy of allergic disease. J Allergy Clin Immunol 2003;111:S712-S719.

Incaudo GA, Takach P: The diagnosis and treatment of allergic rhinitis during pregnancy and lactation. Immunol Allergy Clin N Am 2006;26:137-154.

Kaszuba SM, Baroody FM, deTineo M, et al: Superiority of an intranasal corticosteroid compared with an oral antihistamine in the as-needed treatment of seasonal allergic rhinitis. Arch Intern Med 2001;161:2581-2587.

Pedersen S: Assessing the effect of intranasal steroids on growth. J Allergy Clin Immunol 2001;108:S40-S44.

Weber RW: Immunotherapy with allergens. JAMA 1997;278:1881-1887.

Weiner JM, Abramson MJ, Puy RM: Intranasal corticosteroids versus oral H1 receptor antagonists in allergic rhinitis: Systematic review of randomized controlled trials. BMJ 1998;317:1624-1629.

Wilson AM, O'Byrne PM, Parameswaran K: Leukotriene receptor antagonists for allergic rhinitis: A systematic review and meta-analysis. Am J Med 2004;116:338-344.

Wilson AM, Orr LO, Sims EJ, Lipworth BJ: Effects of monotherapy with intranasal corticosteroid or combined oral histamine and leukotrienes receptor antagonists in seasonal allergic rhinitis. Clin Exp Allergy 2001;31:61-68.

Yanez A, Rodrigo GJ: Intranasal corticosteroids versus topical H1 receptor antagonists for the treatment of allergic rhinitis: A systematic review with meta-analysis. Ann Allergy Asthma Immunol 2002;89:479-484.

# Allergic Reactions to Drugs

Method of
*Donald McNeil, MD*

Drug allergic reactions fall under the broader category of adverse drug reactions (ADRs), which also include toxic drug effects, drug interactions, drug intolerance, and, finally, allergic (or immunologic) drug reactions. Adverse drug reactions are common and often result in only trivial consequences. Some may be severe and life-threatening, and may result from both allergic and nonallergic causes.

The incidence of adverse drug effects is unknown but estimates of 20% of hospital admissions are not unreasonable. A skin rash is the most common manifestation; more importantly, however, severe life-threatening reactions occur, of which only a small portion have an allergic etiology. Most drug reactions are the result of unknown mechanisms. Drug intolerance, drug overdose, and side effects of drugs, as well as drug interactions, all play a significant role. These reactions should be considered both common and predictable.

Although allergic drug reactions are potentially severe, they are also the least common and least predictable. Allergic drug reactions are given particular attention because of the unpredictable, costly, and severe consequences that occasionally arise.

Several mechanisms may play a role in the underlying etiology of immunologic drug reactions. Immediate IgE-mediated reactions represent the classic allergic reaction. This is well characterized and the best understood, but other mechanisms also exist, for example, a cytotoxic reaction in which drug-induced antibodies result in hemolytic anemia. Another example is immune complex formation resulting in organ damage. This is commonly referred to as a "serum sickness" reaction and is characterized by fever, rash, and arthralgia beginning 2 to 4 weeks after initiation of drug. Finally, a delayed-type hypersensitivity reaction occurs when drug-specific T-lymphocytes react. This completes the picture of the four types of immunologic-mediated drug reactions according to the original Gell and Coombs classification. These are referred to as Type I, II, III, or IV reactions, respectively.

Cutaneous reactions comprise the most frequent type of allergic drug reaction. Approximately 94% cause a morbilliform rash and only 5% cause an urticarial reaction. Idiosyncratic reactions are still the most likely cause for a rash and occur much more frequently than a true drug-induced allergic reaction. Ampicillins in conjunction with a viral hepatitis or sulfa drugs taken in the AIDS population are common examples.

Both allergic and nonallergic reactions are known to be associated with severe reactions, including fatalities. Contrast media agents, allergic extracts, anesthetics, and antibiotics are the most commonly implicated drugs. Penicillin remains the most common cause of fatal drug reactions and accounts for up to 75% of these severe drug reactions in the United States.

An allergy to penicillin is the most frequently reported, but as many as 90% of patients labeled "penicillin allergic" are able to tolerate penicillin. This allergy is often mislabeled because of underlying illness or interaction between antibiotic and illness. Unfortunately one third to half of vancomycin (Vancocin) prescriptions in hospitals are given because of a history of "penicillin allergy." This raises the incidence of drug-resistant bacteria because of broad-spectrum antibiotic overuse. The economic impact of treating antibiotic-resistant infections is roughly $4 billion annually.

## Pathophysiology

Some drugs are capable of reacting in the body without further alteration in chemical structure, whereas others must first be metabolized to become immunogenic. Many drugs are too small to be immunogenic alone and are incapable of eliciting an immune allergic response. These drugs require binding to a high-molecular-weight protein followed by antigen processing and presentation by the macrophage in the presence of major histocompatibility complex (MHC)-specific antigen to appropriate T-cell receptors.

*Penicillin* is capable of inducing an allergic reaction in more than one manner. Benzylpenicilloyl, the major penicillin determinant, is able to produce a strong antigenic response. A commercially available product, benzylpenicilloyl-polylysine (PPL) (Pre-Pen), provides the means to reproduce the same allergic response by simple skin testing. Minor determinants are metabolic derivatives of penicillin that may also produce an immune response. The diagnostic capabilities of a penicillin allergy are strengthened by including some measure of the allergic response to the minor determinants when skin testing is conducted for penicillin (Figure 1).

Patients with a history of penicillin allergy but negative skin testing to PPL and the minor determinants rarely experience allergic reactions on re-exposure. If they should occur, these are not fatal, but rather mild and self-limited.

PPL alone will potentially miss a significant percentage of allergic reactions to penicillin. Allergy testing with fresh benzylpenicillin G, aged penicillin (reconstituted more than 24 hours) as well as skin testing with the specific penicillin in question will greatly enhance the likelihood of uncovering of penicillin allergy in a patient with a positive history.

*Cephalosporins* do not provide the same degree of certainty with respect to an allergic evaluation. Cross-reactivity with penicillin allergy patients is known to exist, and although uncommon, it is also unpredictable. To err on the side of safety, a patient with a known penicillin allergy should not be treated with a cephalosporin. A patient with a previous cephalosporin reaction with a negative penicillin skin test cannot safely receive penicillin or another cephalosporin unless

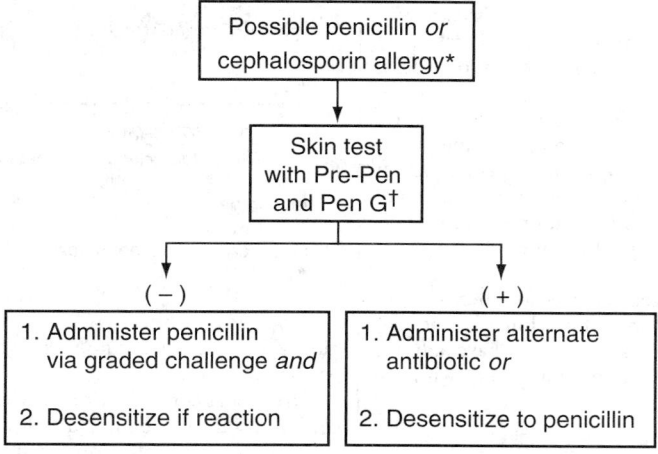

*Only 10%–20% of patients who report a penicillin allergy are actually allergic.
†Benzylpenicilloyl-polylysine (Pre-Pen) and penicillin G (Pen G) will not include all potential penicillin derivatives. The additional benefit of testing with the minor determinant mixture is impractical and usually not available.

**FIGURE 1.** Penicillin allergy evaluation.

further diagnostic measures are taken. This patient may be allergic to a side chain on the cephalosporin that has not been identified by penicillin skin testing. Others recommend a graded oral challenge using a cephalosporin with a different side chain. The latter should be done realizing that standardized procedures have not been developed for this and therefore false negative results may occur.

Successful desensitization to penicillin has permitted a similar approach with other drugs. If the drug in question is required, either intravenous or oral drug administration is possible by incremental doses given usually every 15 minutes. A 10,000-fold dilution of the initial dose is usually sufficient to begin, followed by higher doses, 2-fold or greater. The vital signs are monitored throughout the procedure with timely medical intervention if problems arise.

*Sulfonamides* typically cause cutaneous reactions, infrequently in healthy individuals but extremely common in AIDS patients. Reactions may be relatively benign in nature such as urticaria or fixed-drug eruption, but may also cause more serious reactions (Stevens-Johnson syndrome, toxic epidermal necrolysis). A variety of mechanisms may exist, alone or in combination, using IgE antibody response, T-lymphocytes, and inflammatory cytokines. Because of our inadequate understanding of these mechanisms, there are no universally acceptable means of evaluating sulfonamide hypersensitivity. Unless there has been previously severe reaction, a graded challenge with the drug in question is considered a reasonable alternative (Box 1). Although a theoretical risk exists between sulfonamides and drugs with sulfonamide derivatives (diuretics, COX-2 inhibitors), little data show this is actually true.

*Radiographic contrast media* (RCM) produce an anaphylactoid reaction by an unknown mechanism. Conventional RCM is hypertonic.

The newer nonionic RCM with lower osmolarity are associated with fewer anaphylactoid or allergic-like reactions. Complement system activation, which is capable of causing histamine release, is thought to be the method by which this reaction occurs.

In the continuum of adverse drug effects with suspected hypersensitivity, exposure to *aspirin* and other nonsteroidal anti-inflammatory drugs (NSAIDs) rarely exhibits features that are IgE mediated and allergic in nature, and are more often nonimmunologic mediated. A non–IgE-mediated event must still be approached with caution because the consequences are potentially life-threatening.

More commonly, NSAIDs are associated with the asthma triad syndrome associated with nasal polyps or rhinitis, and severe asthma. This is not an allergic drug reaction, but it represents a largely unrecognized subpopulation of asthmatics who will benefit by avoiding the use of NSAIDs.

The antibiotic *vancomycin* (Vancocin) causes a reaction referred to as *red man syndrome*. Histamine and other mast cell mediators are released, but not through vancomycin-induced IgE antibody (rare cases have been reported). Most, but not all, cases of the red man syndrome are related to the rate of the infusion, and most will subside once the medication is stopped. A graded challenge with the drug or a full course of desensitization usually permits resumption of treatment.

Angiotensin-converting enzyme (ACE) inhibitors are well known to be associated with cough and angioedema, but like NSAIDs, the mechanism is unknown. Newer ACE inhibitors have been described to cause similar reactions but at a much lower incidence. The symptoms of cough and angioedema may continue to recur for several months and up to a year after the discontinuation of the drug.

As seen from the discussion above, IgE-mediated allergic drug reactions represent only a portion of immune-mediated drug reactions. To assist in the diagnosis, a 7- to 10-day delay in the appearance of the drug reaction after initial treatment or immediate reactivation on re-exposure suggests an immunologic etiology. Oftentimes, only the history will provide this index of suspicion. Confirmation by positive skin testing with the drug in question is highly predictive of IgE-mediated hypersensitivity.

Attempts to label reactions as either IgE- or non–IgE-mediated may prove to be costly, time-consuming, and of no immediate benefit. Non-IgE reactions are capable of eliciting changes in vital signs, pulmonary function, and cutaneous effects similar to anaphylaxis and are referred to as anaphylactoid. These need to be regarded with the same degree of caution as IgE-mediated reactions. Narcotics, radiographic contrast media, and chemotherapeutic agents may directly

**BOX 1  Graded Challenge**

1. Cautious administration of medications to patient not likely allergic to drug.
2. Not to be considered equivalent to desensitization.
3. Used when insufficient evidence available to exclude drug allergy.
4. Medication administered in incremental doses beginning at 1:100 dilution of final dose.
5. Adequate medical resources exist to treat allergic reaction.

affect mast cell mediator release with the consequences listed above. Antihistamines and corticosteroids given prior to administration of these drugs are usually sufficient to prevent a reoccurrence, or at least to minimize these reactions.

Drug desensitization is indicated for those patients with positive skin tests who must receive the drug, but should not be assumed to be universally safe or protective. Some chemotherapeutic agents, such as etoposide (VePesid) and teniposide (Vumon), have a much higher incidence of anaphylactoid reactions. Readministration of these drugs in the face of a previous reaction and in spite of prophylactic measures often leads to disappointing results.

Current biologic response modifier agents, as well as others soon to arrive, are associated with adverse reactions. Monoclonal antibodies, T- and B-cell inactivators, and others may prove to have adverse immunologic effects that will only become more apparent with the experience of increased use.

## Evaluation of Drug Allergy in Practice

The importance of a reliable history in a medical evaluation is never more evident than during the initial workup of a suspected drug allergy. The timing of exposure, with the first allergic reaction occurring within days of the priming dose or immediately upon re-exposure, strongly points to an allergic etiology. Multiple exposures to the same drug on previous occasions do not preclude an allergic reaction de novo. Similarly, a previous history of an allergic drug reaction does not by itself predict a reoccurrence on re-exposure. The allergic diathesis may wane over time for drugs just as it may occur for other allergens.

Armed with this suggestive drug history and clinical findings such as a rash, fever, bronchospasm, or anaphylaxis, the evaluation becomes more straightforward. In the appropriate clinical setting, eosinophilia will also support a drug-allergic reaction.

Avoiding the implicated drug may be the simplest approach because confirmation of the diagnosis with appropriate skin testing is often unavailable. (Standardized skin testing exists only for penicillin, but even this does not provide 100% reliability.) Skin testing with the drug is questionable, but using both a positive and negative control of histamine and saline may still provide useful information. A positive skin test would certainly discourage use of this drug unless adequate precautions were taken.

If a non–life-threatening history of a reaction exists and the drug cannot be appropriately substituted, the option exists for a graded oral challenge to confirm the diagnosis. This should not be considered to be the same as desensitization because it involves higher doses and exposure over a shorter period of time than would be considered safe in a truly allergic individual. A challenge such as this should be conducted in suitable medical facilities under close medical supervision.

If the drug in question has been shown to cause an allergic reaction but still must be used, then a carefully monitored drug desensitization program should be considered. Under medical supervision, the drug should be administered orally or intravenously beginning with doses that are tenfold more dilute than the final strength. Incrementally higher doses of the drug should be administered every 15 minutes, increasing the dose twofold each time.

*Drug-induced skin reactions* are common and warrant particular attention. Early recognition is necessary to avoid an incorrect diagnosis and to institute appropriate interventional measures as soon as possible.

The following points will assist the physician in arriving at a correct diagnosis. The *timing of the onset* of the reaction in relation to the time the drug was given provides an important clue. Often signs and symptoms develop 1 to 2 weeks after time of initial drug exposure. Symptoms may develop rapidly on repeat exposure. *Pruritic urticarial lesions* strongly suggest an adverse drug reaction. A *symmetrical or truncal distribution* or a rash that occurs only in sun-exposed areas (polymorphous light eruption) also supports an ADR finding. The morphology of the reaction is helpful, although many types occur (lichenoid, morbilliform, eczematous). The histopathology of the lesion on skin

### TABLE 1 Drugs Used to Treat AIDS/HIV

| Drug | Reaction |
| --- | --- |
| Zidovudine, AZT (Retrovir) | Hyperpigmentation |
| Zalcitabine, ddC (Hivid) | Oral ulcers |
| Abacavir (Ziagen) | Severe rash/anaphylaxis |
| Nevirapine (Viramune) | Toxic epidermal necrolysis |
| Foscarnet | Urethral ulceration |
| Trimethoprim-sulfamethoxazole (TMP-SMX) (Bactrim) | Morbilliform rash or erythema multiforme |

biopsy may reveal eosinophils, which may also be detected in the peripheral blood.

Drugs that commonly cause ADRs tend to be antibiotics. The most common is the morbilliform rash when ampicillin is given in the presence of a viral infection such as infectious mononucleosis or cytomegalovirus. Rarely is this IgE mediated and it should not be regarded as a basis for a history of penicillin allergy. It should also be noted that not all ADRs are caused by prescription medications. A patient may fail to disclose over-the-counter medications that might be responsible (e.g., St. John's wort).

The *response to treatment* may aid in the recognition of an ADR. An incomplete response to topical steroids is typical of an ADR and systemic steroids may turn out to be the therapy of choice. Finally, the *response to withdrawal* of drug may range from a rapid recovery to slow clearing over many weeks, but a favorable response nonetheless.

Table 1 lists several drugs used to treat AIDS/HIV that are worthy of mention. Not all should be considered to be an allergic cause of ADR.

A careful and systematic approach to the patient with a suspected drug allergy will provide valuable information for both the immediate and the long-term management of the patient. A suspected drug allergy that is disproved will facilitate good medical care because unnecessary expense and the risk of further sensitizing the patient to a new medication will be spared if the patient is not allergic. On the other hand, a positive screen for a suspected drug allergy will result in a safe alternative. It should be emphasized, however, that neither a family history of a drug allergy nor a patient requesting a "test" for a possible drug allergy without other reason is an indication for further drug allergy evaluation because of the risk of false-negative results.

## Allergic Reactions to Insect Stings*

Method of
*David B. K. Golden, MD*

Insect bites and stings normally cause temporary localized swelling, redness, pain, and itching. Allergic swelling can also result from insect bites or stings, but stinging insects of the order Hymenoptera can cause anaphylaxis. Allergic reactions to stings from honeybees, vespids (yellow jackets, hornets, wasps), and fire ants are caused by IgE antibodies directed against the protein allergens in the venoms (but not in the bodies or saliva) of these insects. Yellow jacket and hornet venoms are almost identical and are partially cross reactive with wasp venoms, but honeybee venom and fire ant venom are each unique. Commercial venom vaccines are available for honeybee, yellow jacket, yellow hornet, white-faced hornet, and *Polistes* wasps (ALK Laboratories; Hollister-Stier Laboratories). For fire ant sting allergy, imported fire ant whole body extract is the only commercial available material.

*This work was supported by National Institutes of Health (NH) grant A108270.

Although it contains sufficient venom allergens for diagnostic use and for immunotherapy, evidence indicates that venom is superior.

Allergic reactions may be localized or systemic. Large local reactions have a late-phase inflammatory mechanism that progresses for 24 to 48 hours after the sting, causing a painful induration that is often larger than 6 inches in diameter and lasts for 5 to 10 days. A large local reaction to a sting can mimic laryngeal edema (from a sting in the mouth or throat) or cellulitis (lymphangitic drainage from the reaction on an extremity). Systemic reactions are immediate hypersensitivity reactions with manifestations distant from the site of the sting, which can include any one or more of the signs or symptoms of anaphylaxis including urticaria, angioedema, flushing, throat or chest tightness, dyspnea, dizziness, or hypotensive shock. The reported frequency of 50 to 100 fatal reactions per year in the United States is certainly an underestimate. Elevated serum tryptase and venom-specific IgE antibodies are reported in postmortem blood samples in cases of unexpected death in young individuals. Half of fatal reactions occurred in persons with no prior history of reactions to stings, and most occur in individuals older than 45 years. The population at risk is greater than generally appreciated: 3% of adults in the United States have a history of a systemic allergic reaction to insect stings, and more than 20% have IgE antibodies to venom allergens detectable in the skin or blood.

## Diagnosis

A detailed history provides the most important diagnostic information. The exact features and time course of the reaction can distinguish large local, systemic, and nonallergic reactions. Objective signs and documented clinical observations are more reliable than subjective descriptions. Venom-specific IgE antibodies can be demonstrated by skin testing or serologic methods (radioallergosorbent assay test [RAST]) but must be interpreted in the context of the clinical history. Skin testing with the five Hymenoptera venoms (or fire ant whole body extract) is recommended for patients who have had systemic allergic reactions to a sting but is not required for large local reactions. Skin tests are performed with superficial intradermal injection of 0.02 mL of each venom at concentrations starting at 0.001 µg/mL and increasing incrementally up to 1.0 µg/mL, if needed, until a positive wheal and flare reaction is elicited. Diagnostic laboratory measurement of venom-specific IgE antibodies (RAST) may be useful when skin testing is inconclusive or cannot be performed but is less sensitive than skin testing. The venom RAST is positive in 10% of affected patients with negative skin tests, and conversely, the RAST is negative in 20% of patients with positive skin tests. A positive venom skin test in an individual with no history of sting reaction is associated with a 17% frequency of systemic reaction to a subsequent sting. The level of sensitivity on skin test or RAST is not correlated consistently with the severity of the sting reaction.

Assessing the risk of a systemic reaction to a future sting is based on the detailed history of previous reactions, the presence of venom-specific IgE antibodies, and the known natural history of the condition (Table 1). In adults with positive venom skin tests and a prior history of systemic reactions, the risk of systemic reaction is 30% to 60%, with the higher risk in patients with the most severe reactions (airway

## CURRENT DIAGNOSIS

- History of systemic allergic reactions to sting
- Positive venom skin tests or radioallergosorbent assay test (RAST)
- Degree of test reaction not correlated with severity of sting reaction
- Low risk if previous large local sting reactions
- Low risk in children with mild systemic reactions
- Quality of life and frequency of exposure a consideration

obstruction, unconsciousness) and the lower frequency in patients who had cutaneous systemic signs (urticaria, angioedema) and/or mild dizziness or throat tightness. The risk declines with time, but remains at 15% to 20% even after 20 to 30 years. The risk of systemic reaction is known to be low in the general population and in some subgroups of sensitized individuals (Table 2). The majority of affected children (16 years and younger) have had systemic reactions limited to skin manifestations, including generalized hives and angioedema of the face or lips but with no tongue or throat swelling and no dyspnea or hypotension. In these children, subsequent stings cause no systemic reaction in 90%, mild cutaneous systemic reactions in 5%, and more severe systemic reaction in less than 5% of cases. Patients with large local reactions generally have strongly positive venom skin tests but have only a 5% risk of systemic reaction to future stings.

## Treatment and Avoidance of Sting Reactions

Local sting reactions can be treated symptomatically with ice and oral antihistamines. Large local reactions may require a burst of oral prednisone (e.g., 40 to 60 mg the first day, tapering over 4 to 7 days) but almost never require antibiotic treatment. Systemic reactions generally require the intramuscular administration of epinephrine (1:1000), 0.3 mg in an adult (0.01 mg/kg in children), with the availability of oxygen, intravenous fluids, or airway support if needed. Corticosteroids have no benefit in the acute stage, but despite a lack of supporting evidence are often administered in the hope of preventing late-phase manifestations. The patient should be monitored for 3 to 6 hours because more than 20% of severe cases develop biphasic or protracted anaphylaxis. Any patient judged to have a risk for anaphylaxis to future stings should have a prescription for an epinephrine injection kit and detailed instructions on when to use or not use it. Commercial kits include the EpiPen (0.3 mg epinephrine) and EpiPen Jr (0.15 mg epinephrine) (Dey Laboratories) and the Twinject (two doses of either 0.15 or 0.3 mg epinephrine) (Verus Pharmaceuticals). Such individuals should also be referred to a specialist for evaluation and discussion of risks and treatment options. Sting-allergic patients should avoid nesting areas, trash receptacles, eating or drinking outdoors, lawn mowing, or going barefoot.

**TABLE 1** Clinical Recommendations Based on History of Sting Reactions, Age, and Results of Venom Skin Test (or RAST)

| Reaction to Previous Sting | Skin Test (or RAST) | Risk of Systemic Reaction | Clinical Recommendation |
|---|---|---|---|
| No reaction | Positive | 10%–15% | Avoidance |
| Large local | Positive | 5%–10% | Avoidance |
| Cutaneous systemic | Positive: child | 5%–10% | Avoidance |
|  | Positive: adult | 15%–20% | Venom immunotherapy |
| Anaphylaxis | Positive | 30%–60% | Venom immunotherapy |
|  | Negative | 5%–10% | Repeat skin test/RAST |

*Abbreviations*: RAST = radioallergosorbent assay test.

**TABLE 2  Considerations in Stopping Venom Immunotherapy**

Severity/pattern of systemic reaction
Age (child/teen, adult, senior)
Skin tests/RAST (persistent strong)
Time/duration of venom immunotherapy
Systemic reaction during venom immunotherapy
  (to injection or sting)
Quality of life/exposure

*Abbreviation:* RAST = radioallergosorbent assay test.

**TABLE 3  Patients with Low Risk for Anaphylaxis**

| Minimal (<5%) | General adult population |
| | Patients on venom immunotherapy |
| | Children with cutaneous systemic reactions |
| Low (5%–10%) | Large local reactors |
| | Discontinued venom immunotherapy after 5 y |

# Prevention of Sting Reactions (Venom Immunotherapy)

Systemic reactions to insect stings can be prevented with up to 98% efficacy with venom immunotherapy. The indications for therapy are simply a positive history (of systemic reaction to stings) and positive venom skin tests (or RAST), although the severity of previous reactions and the patient's age at the time are also important variables (Table 3). Venom immunotherapy, and therefore skin testing, is not considered necessary for low-risk patients because more than 90% will never have a systemic reaction, such as in patients with large local reactions and in children with cutaneous systemic reactions.

Venom immunotherapy should begin with all of the venoms giving a positive skin test and follows a dose schedule described in the product package insert (ALK Laboratories; Hollister-Stier Laboratories). Injections are generally administered weekly for 8 to 26 weeks to achieve the full maintenance dose of 100 µg of each venom. More rapid treatment is not associated with more frequent adverse reactions. This dose is then repeated every 4 weeks for at least 1 year, then every 6 weeks for 1 to 2 years, and every 6 to 8 weeks thereafter. During immunotherapy, systemic reactions occur in 5% to 15% of cases, with variable degrees of urticaria, airway obstruction, or hypotension. The majority of such reactions are mild, but some require aggressive treatment for anaphylaxis. Venom injections also cause large local reactions in many patients during the first few months of therapy, but they are not predictive of systemic reactions and should not interfere with attaining the full recommended dose. All adverse reactions are much less common during maintenance treatment. The frequency of systemic reactions is similar with venom immunotherapy and immunotherapy with inhalant allergens. Periodic monitoring of venom skin test or RAST sensitivity is recommended every 2 to 5 years to determine possible early discontinuation of therapy. The level of venom-specific IgG antibodies is correlated with clinical protection and may be measured during the first 3 years of venom immunotherapy, especially to determine whether protection is adequate with single-venom therapy

and when maintenance intervals are extended. Some patients require higher doses for full protection.

The duration of venom immunotherapy remains a matter of judgment. The product package insert advises that venom immunotherapy should be continued indefinitely. Some experts advocate stopping treatment if skin tests (or RAST) become negative, but this occurs in only 25% of patients treated for 5 years and in 60% of those treated for 7 to 10 years. When venom immunotherapy is stopped after at least 5 years of maintenance treatment, the chance of reaction to a sting is 10% for each sting that occurs, even 10 to 15 years after stopping even if there are uneventful intervening stings and even if skin tests become negative. The cumulative risk of reaction is 15% to 20% more than 10 years after discontinuing treatment. The risk of a very severe reaction exists primarily in patients who had such a reaction prior to treatment, and they should therefore consider remaining on therapy indefinitely. Other high-risk patients who should consider continuing treatment beyond 5 years include those who had a systemic reaction during treatment whether to an injection or a sting. The relapse rate is also higher in honeybee allergic patients, as is the frequency of systemic reactions to venom injections and the failure rate for reaction to stings during therapy. Both the relapse rate and the level of venom-specific IgE (or skin test) are higher in patients who stop therapy after only 3 years compared to 5 years. Some investigators have suggested that lower risk patients (e.g., children with reactions of any severity and adult patients with mild reactions) might be able safely to stop after 3 years of treatment, but there are limited data published about this.

## REFERENCES

Bernstein JA, Kagan SL, Bernstein DI, Bernstein IL: Rapid venom immunotherapy is safe for routine use in the treatment of patients with Hymenoptera anaphylaxis. Ann Allergy 1994;73:423-428.
Freeman TM: Hypersensitivity to Hymenoptera stings. N Engl J Med 2004;351:1978-1984.
Freeman TM, Highlander R, Ortiz A, Martin ME: Imported fire ant immunotherapy: Effectiveness of whole body extracts. J Allergy Clin Immunol 1992;90:210-215.
Golden DBK: Insect sting allergy and venom immunotherapy: A model and a mystery. J Allergy Clin Immunol 2005;115:439-447.
Golden DBK, Kagey-Sobotka A, Norman PS, et al: Outcomes of allergy to insect stings in children with and without venom immunotherapy. N Engl J Med 2004;351:668-674.
Golden DBK, Kwiterovich KA, Kagey-Sobotka A, et al: Discontinuing venom immunotherapy: Outcome after five years. J Allergy Clin Immunol 1996;97:579-587.
Golden DBK, Marsh DG, Kagey-Sobotka A, et al: Epidemiology of insect venom sensitivity. JAMA 1989;262:240-244.
Hamilton RG: Diagnostic methods for insect sting allergy. Curr Opin Allergy Clin Immunol 2004;4:297-306.
Hoffman DR: Fatal reactions to Hymenoptera stings. Asthma Allergy Proc 2003;24:1-5.
Hunt KJ, Valentine MD, Sobotka AK, et al: A controlled trial of immunotherapy in insect hypersensitivity. N Engl J Med 1978;299:157-161.
Moffitt JE, Golden DBK, Reisman RE, et al: Stinging insect hypersensitivity: A practice parameter update. J Allergy Clin Immunol 2004;114:869-886.
Stafford CT: Hypersensitivity to fire ant venom. Ann Allergy Asthma Immunol 1996;77:87-95.

### CURRENT THERAPY

- Epinephrine Autoinjector (EpiPen or Twinject) and avoidance strategies for low-risk patients is suggested.
- Venom immunotherapy is for high-risk patients.
- Venom immunotherapy is up to 98% effective.
- Most patients can discontinue venom immunotherapy after 5 years.
- Highest risk patients may need indefinite venom immunotherapy.

# Diseases of the Skin

## Acne Vulgaris and Rosacea

Method of
*Steven R. Feldman, MD, PhD, and Alan B. Fleischer, Jr., MD*

Acne and rosacea are common conditions that share a propensity to cause red follicular papules of the face. Nonetheless, they are distinct disorders.

Acne is associated with comedones, a noninflammatory plugging of follicular orifices. Comedones may become inflamed, at least partially due to the inflammatory activity induced by the action of bacterial skin flora (*Pityrosporum* species) on lipids produced by sebaceous glands. There is a distinct tendency toward development of acne nodules with scarring.

The pathogenesis of rosacea is less well understood. Vascular dilatation and inflammation are important components of the process, with prominent flushing and blushing. Although telangiectasia can become permanent, scarring is rare. Another feature distinguishing rosacea from acne is a tendency for ocular involvement.

## Acne Vulgaris

### CLINICAL FEATURES

Acne is a common disorder of teenagers and young adults but occurs in middle age as well. The manifestations of acne are diverse. The face is characteristically involved, and the upper trunk is involved in some patients. The individual lesions can consist of comedones, inflammatory papules, pustules, and deeper inflammatory nodules mistakenly termed *cysts*. There might or might not be resulting scarring. Genetics contributes to the pattern of involvement. Environmental exposures seem less important, although some oil-based cosmetic products can induce acne comedones.

### TREATMENT

Treatments for acne address several different components of the pathogenesis of the disorder. Topical retinoids appear to have a primary effect on normalizing keratinization of the follicular ostia, reducing comedones and inflammatory papules and pustules. Topical and oral antibiotics reduce bacteria counts on the skin and can have intrinsic anti-inflammatory activity. Hormonal treatments in women reduce the production of sebaceous gland lipids. Oral retinoids (isotretinoin in particular), the most effective therapy for acne, reduces sebaceous gland activity as well.

There are no well-established evidence-based guidelines for acne treatment. There are, however, generally accepted patterns of treatment based on the type and extent of the clinical lesions. At its simplest, topical retinoids are the foundation of treatment because of their effect on comedones, the primary lesion of acne, as well as their effect on inflammatory acne papules and pustules. With increasing microbial resistance, retinoid agents work independently of direct effects on skin flora and are excellent long-term agents. Topical antibiotics, prescribed singly, in combination with antimicrobial products, or in combination with topical retinoids, are used for superficial inflammatory lesions. Oral antibiotics are used when the inflammation and potential scarring are more severe. Hormonal treatment (in the form of oral contraceptives) is used for female patients when the acne is unresponsive to both topical retinoids and topical and oral antibiotics or if there are menstrual abnormalities that suggest the acne is secondary to a primary hormonal process.

### Topical Retinoids

Topical retinoids are used for nearly all patients with acne because of their comedolytic effect and their activity on papules and pustules, as well as to spare the use of antibiotics in an age of growing antibiotic resistance. The first topical retinoid was topical tretinoin (Retin-A). It is available in cream, gel, solution, and newer slow-release particle vehicles. The main side effect of topical retinoids is the potential for drying and irritation of the skin. This is less of a problem with lower strengths of topical tretinoin (0.025% and 0.05% cream) and more of a problem with the stronger strengths (0.01% and 0.025% gel and the 0.1% cream). The drying effect may be beneficial for patients who feel their skin is too oily.

Topical tretinoin is easily oxidized and photodegraded. With the growing use of benzoyl peroxide as an anti-acne treatment, there is greater concern about the liability of topical tretinoin. Topical adapalene (Differin) gel or cream can be used as an alternative. It is equally effective as tretinoin, but it has far less potential to cause irritation. Less irritation can lead to greater compliance. It also is a robust molecule that is stable when combined with other agents, including benzoyl peroxide. Topical tazarotene (Tazorac) is another retinoid that is more effective than tretinoin and adapalene, but it is much more irritating than the other agents.

Adapalene and tazarotene may be used at any time of the day, but tretinoin should be used at night because of its photodegradation. This recommendation probably started with topical tretinoin because of the potential for photoinactivation of tretinoin.

### Topical Antimicrobial Agents

The most widely used topical antimicrobial agent is benzoyl peroxide. This biocide is available in a wide variety of inexpensive and expensive over-the-counter and prescription acne products. Benzoyl peroxide is very effective at reducing bacterial counts on the skin, and it is probably far more effective than the traditional topical antibiotics such as erythromycin (Akne-Mycin), clindamycin (Cleocin), and sulfacetamide (Klaron).

Benzoyl peroxide (in 2.5%-10% formulations) is often used in conjunction with topical retinoids or with other topical antibiotics. Combined use of benzoyl peroxide with topical erythromycin (Benzamycin) or clindamycin (BenzaClin) helps prevent development of bacterial strains resistant to the antibiotics. A combined benzoyl peroxide–erythromycin product was once widely used, but it needed to be kept refrigerated, and had a short shelf life. Newer benzoyl peroxide–clindamycin preparations (Benzaclin, Duac) are more stable, can be used once or twice daily, and have excellent efficacy.

All benzoyl peroxide products bleach clothing, bed linens, and towels. Not all vehicles are appropriate for all patients, and excellent vehicle choices can enhance compliance and clinical outcomes.

Topical azelaic acid is a useful adjunct, especially in the 15% gel formulation (Finacea). It is antimicrobial and anti-inflammatory, and it can promote pigmentary normalization. Azelaic acid can be simultaneously combined with many other agents and does not appear to be subject to microbial resistance.

A combination clindamycin–tretinoin product is now available in the United States (Ziana). Topical dapsone (Aczone) has also been approved by the FDA but is not currently marketed. Sulfacetamide is occasionally used and many forms are available (e.g., Klaron), either alone or combined with precipitated sulfur. Sulfacetamide chemically reacts with benzoyl peroxide, and these two agents should not be used simultaneously.

## Oral Antibiotics

Oral antibiotics remain widely used for acne, sometimes for short courses, other times for more prolonged periods. There are growing efforts to limit the course of these drugs in order to limit side effects and antibiotic resistance. Commonly used antibiotics include tetracycline (Sumycin), doxycycline (Doryx), minocycline (Dynacin), and erythromycin.

Of these, minocycline may be the most effective, although it has potential for uncommon and rare side effects. Common side effects include vestibular symptoms; rare ones include altered cutaenous pigmentation and lupus-like syndromes. Minocycline, in extended-release tablets (Solodyn), is the only FDA-approved antibiotic for acne treatment and has fewer vestibular side effects than other agents. This agent has an established dose-response relationship and is most effective with least toxicity at 1 mg/kg/day. It is available in 45-mg, 90-mg, and 135-mg doses.

None of the tetracycline agents should be used during pregnancy or in children younger than 12 years, because tetracycline can stain developing teeth. Erythromycin may be used in these situations; however, there are often poor gastrointestinal tolerance and marginal efficacy. Other antibiotics such as cephalexin (Kelex),[1] ampicillin,[1] or trimethoprim-sulfamethoxazole (Bactrim)[1] are alternatives that are occasionally used.

## Birth Control Pills

Oral contraceptives are somewhat effective antiacne treatments that can be used in women. Three products (Tri-Cyclen, Estrostep, and Yaz) are FDA approved for the treatment of acne. The former two are combinations of norethindrone acetate and ethinyl estradiol, although other formulations are probably also effective. Yasmin and Yaz, for instance, have an effective antiandrogenic agent, drospirone, combined with the ethinyl estradiol. Oral contraceptives should be considered as a treatment for moderate to severe acne in women (along with topical agents and oral antibiotics) before isotretinoin is used. If effective, it can spare the need to expose a woman of childbearing potential to the teratogenic isotretinoin. If this approach is not effective, the woman will already be taking an oral contraceptive when isotretinoin is started.

[1]Not FDA approved for this indication.

### Isotretinoin

Isotretinoin (Accutane, Sotret, and others) is a highly effective oral agent that can cure even very severe acne. It is given in doses of 0.5 to 2.0 mg/kg/day for 4 to 5 months. It is a potent teratogen and must be used with great caution in women of childbearing potential. Although evidence is lacking, it has been reported to cause depression in rare instances, and true informed consent is required. Other potential side effects include hair loss, decreased night vision, xerophthalmia, epistaxis, cheilitis, xerosis, arthralgias, hepatic dysfunction, and elevated cholesterol and triglycerides. Oral retinoids should not be used in conjunction with tetracycline agents because of the possible increased risk of pseudotumor cerebri.

### Behavioral Issues

Perhaps the most important environmental exposure affecting acne is behavioral: patients' tendency to pick at their acne lesions, resulting in excoriation, infection, and scarring. Psychological fixation on facial appearance is not uncommon. Patients often perceive that their follicular ostia (pores) are too large. They can manipulate their skin, resulting in excoriated lesions that mimic acne. This type of acne is not uncommon and is termed acne excoriée. The severity and extent of the lesions vary. Some patients have few lesions, others have many with considerable scarring.

Treatment of acne excoriée is difficult. Some patients respond to the suggestion that they "are spreading the infection by manipulating the skin." For other patients with more severe psychological issues, oral psychotropic medication and psychotherapy may be warranted.

Another key factor affecting outcomes of acne treatment is adherence. Patients' adherence to even short-term oral medication regimens is often poor. Adherence to topical treatment is generally worse, and adherence to chronic topical treatment is probably severely limited. Involvement of the patient in treatment planning, choosing regimens of limited complexity, and psychological interventions to promote better adherence can lead to improved treatment outcomes. Whenever possible, agents that can be administered in combination and may be used once daily are likely to promote compliance and increase efficacy.

# Rosacea

## DIAGNOSIS AND DIFFERENTIAL DIAGNOSIS

Rosacea is a common cause of a red face in adults. It must be distinguished from other conditions causing a red face, particularly seborrheic dermatitis, irritant dermatitis, and lupus. Seborrheic dermatitis, another common condition, is typically more scaly than rosacea. Seborrheic dermatitis involves the scalp (a cause of dandruff), eyebrows, nasal bridge, nasolabial and melolabial folds, and central chest. Rosacea does not typically have scale or scalp involvement of seborrhea and typically involves the cheeks and nose, sparing the fold in between. Irritant dermatitis may be confused as well, because rosacea patients report burning and stinging. Lupus is a far less common disorder and may be associated with scarring lesions of the face or a malar pattern of erythema.

## CLASSIFICATION

Rosacea is divided into four subtypes, papulopustular, erythematotelangiectatic, phymatous, and ocular. Papulopustular rosacea responds best to topical and oral therapies, ocular disease responds best to oral therapy, and erthematotelangiectatic and phymatous types respond best to physical modalities. None of these subtypes or treatment modalities is mutually exclusive. Rosacea patients with papulopustular and erythematotelangiectatic subtypes should receive counseling about gentle cleansing and use of moisturizers and sunscreens, because these improve outcomes.

# TREATMENT

## Topical Antibiotics

Most patients with papulopustular rosacea benefit from topical antibiotic therapies. There are three agents in widespread use: metronidazole, azelaic acid, and sodium sulfacetamide and sulfur preparations. Metronidazole is widely used and is available in gel, lotion (Metrolotion), and cream (Metrocream) for twice-daily use at 0.75%, and cream (Noritate) and gel (Metrogel) for once-daily use at 1%. The gel vehicle is likely the preferred for facial use, and this is a generally well-tolerated agent. The 1% product offers the advantage of single daily dosing. Some patients report mild irritation from the use of these agents. Topical azelaic acid 15% (Finacea) gel is more effective than metronidazole gel 0.75%, but appears to be equal in effectiveness to metronidazole 1% gel. Like metronidazole, it can cause mild irritation and appears slightly more irritating than metronidazole.

Sodium sulfacetamide and sulfur compounds are available as washes and topical gels and may be additional agents that can improve outcomes in treating rosacea. One product, with sodium sulfacetamide 10% and 5% sulfur with sunscreen (Rosac) was found to be at least as effective as metronidazole cream 0.75%. Small reports of the efficacy of topical clindamycin and erythromycin appear in the dermatology literature.

As with acne therapy, combinations of topical agents are more effective than monotherapy. Thus, combinations of metronidazole, azelaic acid, and sodium sulfacetamide and sulfur compounds in various combinations and permutations improve outcomes. Most patients, when counseled about appropriate use of combinations of products, with good soap-free cleansing and moisturizing products, can tolerate these agents.

## Oral Antibiotics

Oral tetracycline agents are commonly used to treat rosacea. Some employ antimicrobial doses such as tetracycline 500 mg twice daily or doxycycline 100 mg twice daily. Then the dose is tapered to the lowest dose that maintains control of the disease. A sub-antimicrobial dose doxycycline product (Oracea) has been FDA approved as a rosacea treatment. This product reduces the inflammation of rosacea and can help prevent development of organisms resistant to the antibiotic. When oral therapies are employed, efficacy of topical therapies is increased, which can decrease the need for or duration of the systemic agent.

## Isotretinoin

Isotretinoin is an effective agent in treating papulopustular rosacea, and lower doses than those employed for acne can be highly effective. With increasing difficulty in using isotretinoin due to the iPLEDGE

---

## CURRENT DIAGNOSIS

### Acne

- Determine the type of acne: Comedonal, inflammatory (papules and pustules), nodulocystic, excoriée.
- Scarring indicates need for more intensive treatment.
- In female patients, is there menstrual irregularity to suggest endocrinopathy?

### Rosacea

- Determine the type of rosacea: Papulopustular, erythematotelangiectatic, phymatous.
- Ocular involvement (itching, irritation, or redness) indicates need for oral treatment.
- Scaling of the eyebrows and nasal folds suggests seborrheic dermatitis.

---

## CURRENT THERAPY

### Acne

- Topical retinoids are used as a foundation in acne treatment to eliminate the comedones that start the disease process.
- Topical benzoyl peroxide, often in combination with topical clindamycin, is highly effective at reducing skin bacterial counts without risk of bacterial resistance.
- Oral antibiotics may best be used in short courses to control inflammatory acne.
- Oral contraceptives can be used in women with resistant disease as an acne treatment prior to starting isotretinoin.
- Controlling patients' tendency to excoriate the face is difficult, yet may be necessary to reduce the severity of the lesions.
- Adherence to topical treatments is poor, especially in the setting of chronic illness. Careful attention should be focused on maximizing patients' adherence to the treatment regimen.

### Rosacea

- Papulopustular rosacea is the form most responsive to medical treatment.
- Topical metronidazole (Flagyl), azelaic acid (Finaca), and sulfacetamide (Klaron) are the most common topical rosacea treatments.
- Oral antibiotics add further benefit and are usually needed for patients with ocular rosacea.
- Erythematotelangiectatic rosacea and rhinophyma respond best to physical modalities (laser ablation of blood vessels and surgery, respectively).

---

program, physicians might find other therapeutic alternatives more appealing.

## Physical Modalities

Although there has been a report of a series of patients with erythematotelangiectatic rosacea responding well to azelaic acid 15% gel, most patients are likely to require optical vascular destructive modalities, including vascular laser or intense pulsed light. These approaches often require multiple treatment sessions, but they do decrease erythema, flushing and blushing, and telangiectasia. Phymatous disease responds well to surgical approaches, including use of high-frequency electrosurgery with a wire loop, $CO_2$ laser, or scalpel surgery.

## REFERENCES

Gollnick H, Cunliffe W, Berson D, et al; Global Alliance to Improve Outcomes in Acne: Management of acne: A report from a Global Alliance to Improve Outcomes in Acne. J Am Acad Dermatol 2003;49(1 suppl):S1-S37.

James WD: Clinical practice. Acne. N Engl J Med 2005;352(14):1463-1472.

Leyden JJ, Shalita A, Thiboutot D, et al: Topical retinoids in inflammatory acne: A retrospective, investigator-blinded, vehicle-controlled, photographic assessment. Clin Ther 2005;27(2):216-224.

Leyden JJ, Thiboutot DM, Shalita AR, et al: Comparison of tazarotene and minocycline maintenance therapies in acne vulgaris: A multicenter, double-blind, randomized, parallel-group study. Arch Dermatol 2006;142(5):605-612.

Margolis DJ, Bowe WP, Hoffstad O, Berlin JA: Antibiotic treatment of acne may be associated with upper respiratory tract infections. Arch Dermatol 2005;141(9):1132-1136.

Ozolins M, Eady EA, Avery AJ, et al: Comparison of five antimicrobial regimens for treatment of mild to moderate inflammatory facial acne vulgaris in the community: Randomised controlled trial. Lancet 2004;364(9452):2188-2195.

Sanchez J, Somolinos AL, Almodovar PI, et al: A randomized, double-blind, placebo-controlled trial of the combined effect of doxycycline hyclate 20-mg tablets and metronidazole 0.75% topical lotion in the treatment of rosacea. J Am Acad Dermatol 2005;53(5):791-797.

Thevarajah S, Balkrishnan R, Camacho FT, et al: Trends in prescription of acne medication in the U.S.: Shift from antibiotic to non-antibiotic treatment. J Dermatolog Treat 2005;16(4):224-228.

# Diseases of the Hair

Method of
*Kimberly May Eickhorst, MD,*
*and Eyal Levit, MD*

The chief complaint of hair loss or disease is ubiquitous throughout all medical practices. Therefore it is important to have a general understanding of the normal physiologic hair growth cycle and how alterations in this cycle manifest as different hair diseases. Diagnosis and treatment of hair disease can at times be frustrating for both the physician and the patient because of a lack of unequivocal diagnostics and effective treatments. However, a thorough and appropriately directed history armed with a few key diagnostic techniques can help direct care to maximize treatment and patient satisfaction.

A hair cycles through three stages: anagen, catagen, and telogen. The duration of each cycle varies from one body area to the other. Within each body area, each follicle cycles at a different periodicity but maintains the same growth control characteristics. However, in this chapter we concentrate on the scalp. During the first stage (anagen), the bulb or hair root is located in the subcutaneous or dermal portion of the skin and actively grows for a period of approximately 2 to 5 years. As the cycle continues and the hair matures, the hair bulb begins to progress toward the scalp surface. After transiently passing through the catagen or resting phase (2 to 4 weeks), the hair enters telogen (3 to 4 months). It is in this final stage that the hair is ultimately dislodged from the follicle and shed. At any given moment, the telogen-to-anagen ratio is 85% to 15% in females and 90% to 10% in males. Hair grows at a rate of approximately 1 cm per month. An average scalp contains approximately 100,000 hairs, with no known racial or sexual differences; this translates into a completely normal hair loss of approximately 100 to 150 hairs per day, in any given individual. Alterations in this physiologic cycle often result in different types of hair loss; inherent metabolic insults or abnormalities can result in other hair disorders.

History is critical to guiding the physician toward a correct diagnosis. Table 1 lists several questions to pose to your patient when formulating a differential diagnosis. Box 1 lists some specific diagnostic techniques.

Additionally, examine all hair-bearing areas, making note of hair quality (fine, terminal, or vellus; brittle, dry, frayed, or sharp distal ends), density, distribution, and associated skin changes (erythema/inflammation/scale/scar/follicular plugging). Remember, with the exception of the palms, soles, glans, and prepuce, hair grows on all skin surfaces. A magnifying glass and side lighting can be of great assistance. Additionally, the nails, oral mucosa, and thyroid should be closely evaluated. Certain types of hair loss are associated with distinct nail findings (i.e., alopecia areata), lichen planus and lupus can have oral lesions, and thyromegaly can indicate a thyroid disorder.

If hair loss is the complaint, a hair-pull test can be extremely instrumental. This maneuver serves to estimate the number of hairs in telogen. The test is performed by gathering approximately 40 hairs between the fingers, and then while holding the hairs up away from the scalp under tension, slowly pulling along the hair shafts until the distal ends are reached. This technique should be repeated approximately seven times in different areas of the scalp and should be mildly uncomfortable to the patient if done correctly. More than six to eight hairs dislodged on any one pull indicates an increased percentage of hairs in

---

## TABLE 1  Key Questions to the Patient

**Timing**
When did you first notice changes in your hair?

**Quality**
Is the hair thinning or shedding?
Is the hair falling out from the root or breaking off?
Associated itching, pain, or burning of scalp?

**Quantity**
How much hair is lost daily? *(100–150 daily is normal)*
When did you last wash your hair? *(affects hair-pull test)*

**Associated Factors**
Have you *ever* used permanents, relaxers, hair dyes, hair picks, curlers, braiding, hot comb or curlers, hairpins, rubber bands, or worn tight hairstyles (repeat chronic use can lead to CCCA)?
Family members with similar patterns of hair loss?
Changes in medications (prescribed/OTC/herbals)?
Any recent changes in your health:
- Autoimmune disorders?
- High fever, severe illness, or surgery?
- High stress (emotional/physical)?
- Psychiatric history (depression/anxiety)?
- Pregnant (abortion, miscarriage, delivery) in the last 6 mo?
- Endocrine disorders (hirsutism, acne, irregular periods, change in voice)?
- Nutrition and significant weight loss/gain?
- Chemotherapy/radiation?

What treatments have been tried for your hair loss?

*Abbreviations:* CCCA = central centrifugal cicatricial alopecia; OTC = over the counter.

---

the telogen phase and a positive test. The classic telogen hair has a clublike root. A *caveat:* The hair-pull test is highly subjective and strongly influenced by its relation to the last shampoo/combing.

If a patient has vigorously brushed or shampooed the hair prior to the visit, a large amount of telogen hairs may have already been dislodged, thus confounding the hair-pull test with increased false-negative results. If factors exist that prohibit a valid hair-pull test, the patient can also be instructed to collect *all* hairs lost over a 1-day period and store them in a small sealable plastic bag. Over the course of 7 full days, each day's worth of lost hair should be counted by the patient, stored in an individual bag labeled with the date and hair number, and brought to the physician's office. This collection should include hair lost on the pillow, in the shower, and on combs/brushes.

The hairs harvested from the hair-pull test can also be examined under the light microscope. The proximal ends of the hairs can be

---

## BOX 1  Hair: Specific Diagnostic Techniques

- **Hair-pull test:** Gather approximately 40 hairs between the fingers, and then while holding the hairs up away from the scalp under tension, slowly pull along the hair shafts until the distal ends are reached. This technique should be repeated approximately seven times in different areas of the scalp. If more than 4–6 hairs are shed during any one of the eight pulls, the test is considered positive and indicative of an effluvium.
- **Hair parting:** Make a coronal part at the vertex. Measure the width of the part. Proceed to part other areas of the scalp and compare widths among different scalp locations. A widened coronal part with retention of the frontal hairline is seen in female androgenetic alopecia.
- **Laboratory data** and **scalp biopsy** (Table 3):
  - **Light microscope examination of hair bulb:** aids in determining stage of hair cycle during which alopecia is occurring (Figures 1A and B).

placed under a coverslip with potassium hydroxide (KOH) as background media or simply sandwiched between two glass slides and viewed under low power. The hairs can then be evaluated simultaneously for stage of cycling (anagen/telogen) and the presence of fungus. An anagen has retention of pigment at its proximal "root" as well as some remnants of root sheath, creating an irregularly shaped and glistening bulb. In contrast, a telogen hair has a more swollen, white, rounded, and cornified bulb likened to a cotton applicator tip (Figure 1). Fungus presents as hyphae or spores within or lining the hair shaft and may clinically be associated with cervical lymphadenopathy or "black dot alopecia," in which stubbles of darker hair are seen at the follicular orifices.

The scalp should also be parted in several different locations to compare the width of the parts. Parting not only helps define and compare hair density throughout the scalp but can also be a diagnostic tool. A midline widened coronal vertex part that resembles a "Christmas tree" pattern and displays central thinning while maintaining the frontal hairline is characteristic of female androgenetic alopecia.

Scalp biopsy is usually reserved as a later step in the hair disease workup when alopecia is refractory, when suspicion is high for a scarring component, or when the patient simply desires a definitive reason, specifically proof, for his or her hair disease. Scalp biopsy entails infiltrating an area of the scalp with local anesthesia and then using a 4- to 6-mm punch biopsy to obtain a full-thickness skin specimen down to the fat, where many of the hair bulbs reside. A 6-mm biopsy or two 4-mm punches are recommended over a single smaller diameter punch biopsy. It is also suggested that two biopsies from different involved scalp sites be harvested. The specimen is then sent for both vertical and horizontal sectioning. If scarring is suspected, direct immunofluorescence testing should also be considered (Table 2). Overall, a scalp biopsy is extremely useful in definitively identifying scarring versus nonscarring alopecia and the presence and type of inflammation.

Certain laboratory data (see Table 2) can also help unravel the mystery of troubling hair disease. Equipped with a thorough history and exam, one can begin to narrow the differential diagnosis of hair disease and to test and treat the suspected malady. Following is a brief discussion of some of the more commonly encountered hair disorders, as well as suggested diagnostics and treatment.

## Alopecia

Hair loss, or alopecia, is commonly divided into scarring and nonscarring alopecia (Table 3). Variants of hair loss can then be further grouped by focal or generalized involvement and acute versus chronic changes in the hair. Clinically, a scarring alopecia refers to a patch of skin where hair is not only absent but the opening of the hair follicle or orifice has also been obliterated. Oftentimes scarring alopecias present as glossy or fibrosed patches of skin. Contrastingly, nonscarring lesions maintain the integrity of the hair follicle and its opening. Although this dichotomous schema may seem quite self-explanatory, even the most adept clinician can be misled by clinical examination alone; ultimately a true scarring alopecia is defined by hair follicle fibrosis seen microscopically on scalp biopsy. Most scarring alopecias result from prior inflammation. Unfortunately, scarring alopecias hold a very poor prognosis. Once a follicle is scarred, there is no hope for renewed hair growth at the involved location. Therefore early recognition and treatment of the prescarring signs of alopecia (follicular plugging, induced traction, and follicular erythema) is critical in preventing future scarring. If any doubt exists, a scalp biopsy from the appropriate location is warranted.

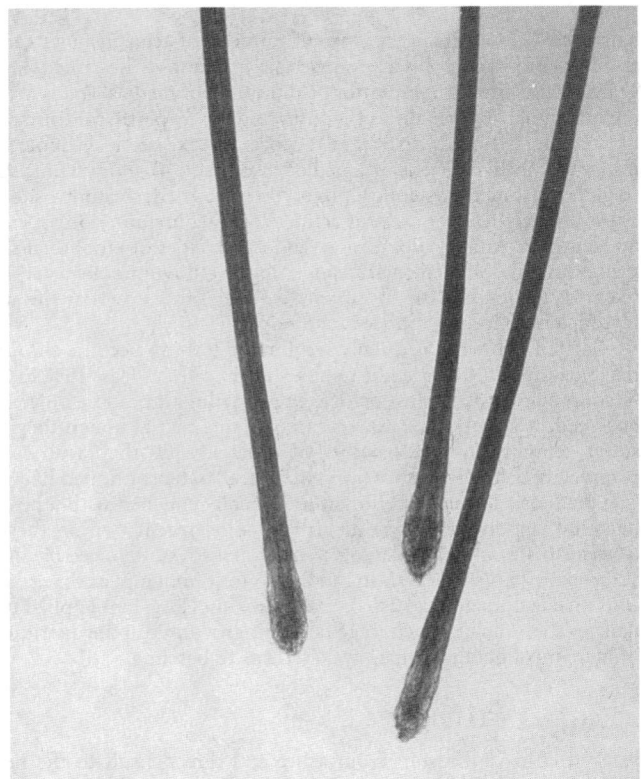

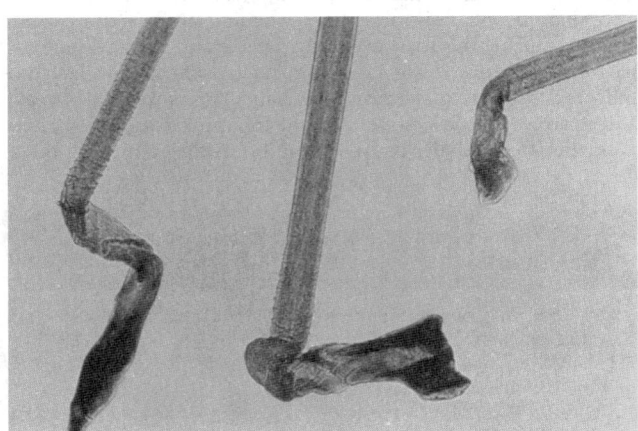

**FIGURE 1.** What to expect when examining a hair-pull test hair under the light microscope: telogen hair (**A**); anagen hair (**B**). (From Bolognia JL, Jorizzo JL, Papini RP: Dermatology, vol 1, 1st ed. Alopecias. New York, Mosby, 2003, p. 1035.)

 **CURRENT DIAGNOSIS**

- Detailed history (Table 1)
- All hair-bearing sites should be examined using specific techniques:
  - Hair quality (dry, brittle, fine, short/long, sharp or frayed distal ends)
  - Scarring versus nonscarring; diffuse versus focal involvement description
  - Hair-pull test
  - Part width measurements and comparisons
- Appropriate laboratory data collected (Table 2)
- Two 4-mm or a single 6-mm punch biopsy of the scalp helps distinguish scarring from nonscarring alopecias:
  - The specimen should be harvested from the involved edge of the scalp where some hair is still present. The specimen should then be sent for *horizontal* and *transverse* sectioning by an experienced dermatopathologist.
  - If connective tissue disease is suspected, another 3-mm biopsy should be sent for direct immunofluorescence (DIF).

**CURRENT THERAPY**

- Start aggressive treatment early. True scarring alopecias are permanent. However, if diagnosed and treated early, scarring can be prevented.
- Regarding topical Minoxidil 5% (Rogaine):
  - Once started, it must be continued indefinitely; if stopped, all the hair gained will shed, usually within the next 4–6 mo.
  - Patients should always wash their hands after scalp treatment application to prevent accidental unwanted hair growth on the face.
  - Warn patients that they may first experience a small increase in hair loss at the very beginning of treatment as the growth of new anagen hairs replaces old telogen hairs out of the hair follicle.
- Physicians should be prepared to refer patients to reputable stylists and shops that can provide alternative natural hair styling and accoutrements.

## Nonscarring Alopecias

### TELOGEN EFFLUVIUM

One of the most common causes of hair loss/shedding and thinning is telogen effluvium. This type of diffuse hair loss has both acute and chronic variants, but both are the result of a greater number of hairs (more than 10% to 20%) prematurely entering the telogen phase of the hair cycle. This shift in the overall number of telogen hairs can be clearly demonstrated by a positive hair-pull test, as described earlier. Telogen effluvium can result from a multitude of medical states including hormonal abnormalities (hypothyroidism, hyperthyroidism, pregnancy), nutritional disorders (anorexia, excessive weight loss, iron/zinc/biotin deficiencies), medications (Table 4) and systemic stress (high fever, surgery, systemic lupus erythematosus, dermatomyositis). In approximately 33% of cases of acute telogen effluvium, no trigger can be identified. Anxiety, depression, and other types of emotional stress are commonly blamed for causing telogen effluvium. However, little scientific evidence exists to support the belief that everyday life stress is sufficient to induce diffuse hair loss.

Telogen effluvium is usually self-limited but can become chronic if the triggering factors are not removed. Clinically, at least 15% to 25% of scalp hairs must be lost before telogen effluvium can be objectively observed. It is important to reassure patients that although they may suffer temporarily from decreased hair density, they will *not* go completely bald, despite what might appear to be continued hair loss. The diagnosis of telogen effluvium is usually clinched with a positive hair-pull test and a history describing some recent (within the past 6 weeks to 4 months) physiologic/emotional stress, followed by diffuse scalp hair loss/shedding. In addition to removing any persistent causative factors, topical 2% or 5% minoxidil (Rogaine) applied twice daily to the scalp can encourage new hair growth until the distribution of hairs throughout the hair cycle returns to baseline.

### ANAGEN EFFLUVIUM

Anagen effluvium results from acute and direct insult to the nearly 90% of hairs in the initial hair growth phase. Chemotherapy, followed by radiation and poisoning (e.g., arsenic), are the more common culprits. During this toxic event, the follicle and stem cells are neither harmed nor converted to a different stage in the hair cycle. However, mitosis is inhibited. The result is a hair that is proximally weakened and narrowed. As a consequence of this proximal hair shaft weakness, the affected hairs usually break off as they approach the scalp.

**TABLE 2 Suggested Laboratory Testing for Alopecia**

Rule out anemia:
- CBC
- Iron
- TIBC
- Ferritin
- MCV, RDW

Rule out autoimmune disorders:
- ANA, SSA, SSB
- Scalp biopsy for direct immunofluorescence

Rule out syphilis:
- RPR, FTA-Abs

Rule out thyroid disorder:
- TSH
- Anti-thyroglobulin Abs
- Thyroid peroxidase Abs

Rule out hormonal aberrations:
- DHEA, DHEAS (adrenal)
- LH, FSH (polycystic ovary disease)
- Free and total testosterone (ovarian/testicular)
- Antihormone binding globulin
- Morning cortisol levels
- Scalp biopsies (Bx): usually taken from involved edge; should be sent for transverse and horizontal sectioning to an experienced dermatopathologist who is familiar with transverse section reading; now considered the standard of care for proper diagnosis of alopecias
- Scalp Bx for DIF should be sent if lupus is suspected.

*Abbreviations:* ANA = antinuclear antibody (test); CBC = complete blood count; DHEA = dehydroepiandrosterone; DHEAS = dehydroepiandrosterone sulfate; FSH = follicle-stimulating hormone; FTA-Abs = fluorescence treponemal antibody absorption; LH = luteinizing hormone; MCV = mean corpuscular volume; RDW = red (blood cell) diameter width; RPR = rapid plasma reagent (test); TIBC = total iron-binding capacity; SSA = anti-Ro/single stranded DNA strand A; SSB = anti-La/single stranded DNA strand B; TSH = thyroid-stimulating hormone.

**TABLE 3 Scarring versus Nonscarring Classification of Alopecia***

| Scarring | Nonscarring |
|---|---|
| Lichen planopilaris | Androgenetic alopecia |
| Discoid lupus erythematosus | Telogen effluvium |
| Central centrifugal cicatricial alopecia (CCCA) | Alopecia areata |
| Trichotillomania/traction (chronic) | Trichotillomania/traction (acute) |
| Folliculitis decalvans | Anagen effluvium |
| | Syphilitic alopecia |

*Arranged from most to least common.

**TABLE 4 Drugs Associated with Telogen Effluvium***

Angiotensin-converting enzyme (ACE) inhibitors
Anticoagulants
β-Blockers
Interferon
Lithium
Oral contraceptives
Oral retinoids (isotretinoin, acitretin)
Valproic acid
Vitamin A excess

*Greater than 1% incidence.

Anagen hair shedding may begin approximately 1 to 2 weeks following the inciting event. But hair loss may be most evident after approximately 1 to 2 months and can be clinically profound. Patients should be assured that this condition is completely reversible and once the insult to the metabolic function of the hair follicle is removed, normal hair production and growth should resume. If chemotherapy is anticipated, a prophylactic approach to anagen effluvium involves applying a pressure cuff around the scalp during chemotherapy.

## ALOPECIA AREATA

An autoimmune, cell-mediated disorder, alopecia areata may be found in association with vitiligo, thyroid disorders, lupus, atopic dermatitis, or Down's syndrome. There may also be a strong familial predominance. However, it most commonly presents without any other disease associations. Clinically, asymptomatic or mildly pruritic ovoid patches of hair loss are seen. These patches can be small and focal (Figure 2A) or extend over large areas of skin (Figure 2B). At times there can be such diffuse focal involvement that the scalp begins to look almost "moth eaten." In this instance a rapid plasma reagent (RPR) test may be warranted to rule out syphilitic alopecia, which can take on a similar appearance.

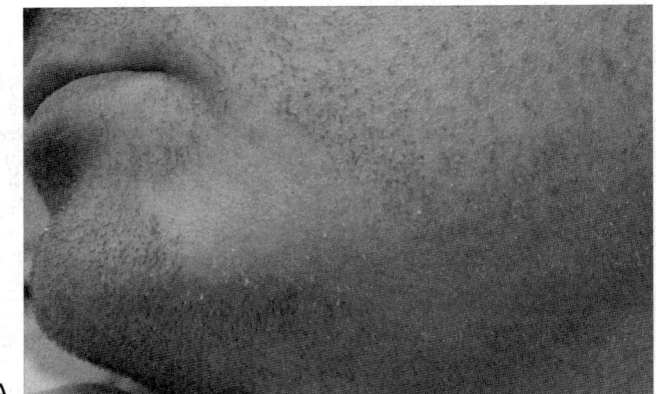

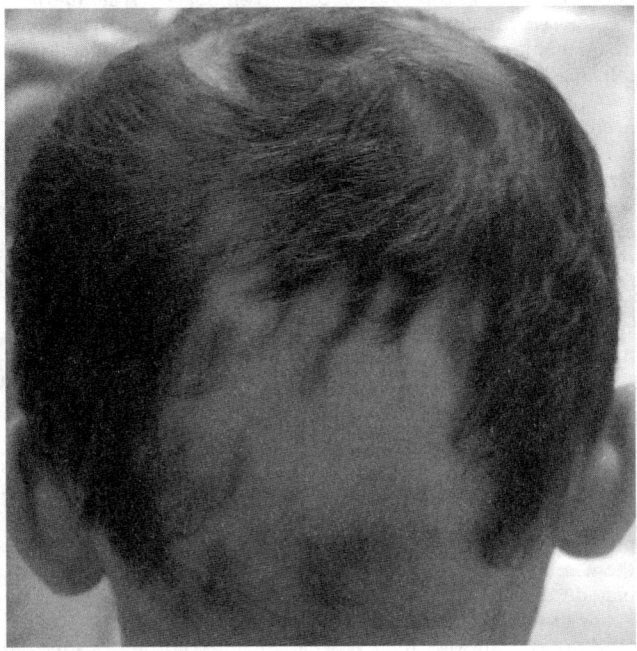

**FIGURE 2. A,** Small patches of hair loss on the chin and neck. White hairs are seen in some areas and represent signs of early hair regrowth. **B,** Large patch of alopecia areata on the occipital scalp with patches of regrowth at the edges.

When complete loss of scalp hair is seen as a result of alopecia areata, the condition is called *alopecia totalis*. When hair is absent on *all* hair-bearing areas of the body, the term *alopecia universalis* is used. *Ophiasis* describes alopecia areata in a bandlike distribution over the periphery of the temporal and occipital scalp, whereas the term *sisaipho* describes the inverse, with balding of the superior scalp. At the periphery of many of these balding patches, hair may seem loose. Forcefully dislodging these hairs can reveal a more tapered proximal end of the hair shaft. Thus, these hairs are called *exclamation hairs*. Gridlike nail pitting is another hint to the presence of alopecia areata.

Although alopecia areata may spontaneously remit, treatment is encouraged and decreases disease duration. Intralesional triamcinolone (Kenalog) is used for localized disease, but more diffuse scalp involvement usually lends itself to topical application of high potency class I topical steroids and calcineurin inhibitors like topical pimecrolimus (Elidel) or tacrolimus (Protopic). Steroid treatment demands close follow-up to avoid hypothalamic- pituitary axis (HPA) suppression or skin atrophy signs such as hypopigmentation, thinning, and telangiectasias. If these treatments fail, the use of anthralin or squaric acid dibutyl ester can be cautiously attempted with gradual increase in contact exposure time. Refractory cases may even require PUVA (oral psoralen plus UVA light treatment) or a short course of oral steroids for response. Atopic dermatitis, childhood onset, widespread involvement, ophiasis, duration longer than 5 years, and onychodystrophy tend to predict a poor prognosis.

## ANDROGENETIC ALOPECIA

Androgenetic alopecia can occur in both males and females and is by and large linked to the presence of excess androgens that subsequently cause follicular miniaturization and loss of hair. The reduction in the size of the follicle is accompanied by shortening of the anagen phase and increased telogen shedding. In males there is clinical regression of the frontal-temporal hairline, whereas in women there is retention of the frontal hairline but widening of the coronal part and decreased hair density over the vertex. In both sexes, a similar family history of patterned hair loss is often present. Interestingly, a higher risk of coronary heart disease is associated with male-patterned baldness.

Testosterone is converted to dihydrotestosterone (DHT) by the enzyme 5-α reductase (type II). In males with androgenetic alopecia, 5-α reductase (type II) activity and DHT are increased as opposed to nonbalding scalp skin. Therefore, finasteride (Propecia), a 5-α reductase (type II) inhibitor, at 1 mg orally daily, can halt or slow further hair loss in men. Pregnant women should not so much as touch this drug because pregnant women handling of finasteride (Propecia) risks feminization of the fetus. Female-patterned baldness is most commonly seen in the perimenopausal stages of life, although younger and younger patients of both sexes seem to be presenting with this complaint. Although this process may begin at any age after puberty, it usually becomes clinically apparent in men by 17 years of age and in androgenetically normal women by 25 to 30 years of age.

When younger patients, especially in the face of coexistent hirsutism, present with this classic patterned hair loss, and/or females present with a male-patterned hair loss, laboratories should be drawn to assess testosterone and dehydroepiandrosterone sulfate (DHEAS) levels. Free testosterone represents the ovarian component of hyperandrogenism, whereas DHEAS levels represent androgen contribution from the adrenals. Potential treatments for female-patterned hair loss include oral contraception with relatively higher estrogen levels or antiandrogens like spironolactone (Aldactone) at 50 to 200 mg orally daily. Although many of my female patients have had success using Finasteride (Propecia), 1 mg orally every day, a single small study by Merck failed to show statistical benefits. Topical Minoxidil 5% (Rogaine) may also be helpful, but like finasteride, it must be continued indefinitely to maintain its effect.

## TRICHOTILLOMANIA

Trichotillomania refers to the act of forcibly pulling/plucking out one's hair, resulting in patchy or full alopecia of the scalp. The scalp is the most frequent hair-pulling site, followed by the eyebrows, eyelashes, pubic area, trunk, and extremities. This type of chronic alopecia forms with more linear, well-defined borders, which include hairs of varied lengths (Figure 3). The occiput generally tends to be spared. Although patients with obsessive-compulsive disorders and neurotic personality traits are suspect for this variant of alopecia, a scalp biopsy can confirm the diagnosis with evidence of abundant catagen hairs, retained follicular pigment, and hemorrhage. Observed or reported hair-pulling behavior from family and friends may help avoid a biopsy. Such pulling can also be caused from tightly styled hair as with ponytails or braiding. Additionally, if trichotillomania is high on the differential, as a last resort, shaving a 3 × 3 cm area of the scalp may help clinch the diagnosis. Subsequent normal hair growth would support the diagnosis; these new hairs will be too short for the patient to pull out.

Treatment is difficult, and just breaking the hair-pulling habit is key. Sometimes instructing the patient to apply any salve (e.g., olive oil) to the scalp area each night under a shower cap and wearing it to bed may break the habit. Even if treatment fails, patients are often relieved to find that others pull out hair. Organizations offering educational materials and support contacts can help. Although clomipramine is the only drug that was effective in controlled trials, other selective serotonin reuptake inhibitors (SSRIs) have anecdotally led to improvement. Additionally, behavior therapy, hypnosis, insight-oriented psychotherapy, habit modification, and close, lengthy follow-up should also be treatment considerations.

## Scarring (Cicatricial) Alopecia

Scarring alopecia represents fibrosis of the hair follicle, most commonly secondary to previous inflammation. Discoid lupus erythematosus, lichen planopilaris, and central, centrifugal scarring alopecia are the most common forms of scarring hair loss. The most helpful methods to differentiate these subtypes are scalp biopsy, early in the process, and bacterial and/or fungal culture if active signs of superficial inflammation such as pustules or crusts are present. Early diagnosis is key. If the insulting inflammatory process can be halted before complete follicle fibrosis, there is still hope for improvement. However, if complete fibrosis occurs, the result is a burnt-out, noninflammatory, end-stage scarring alopecia termed pseudopelade of Brocq that has no recourse.

## Discoid Lupus Erythematosus

Discoid lupus erythematosus (DLE), a cutaneous form of lupus, manifests as sharply demarcated atrophic plaques with adherent scale and follicular plugging. Plaques are often circumscribed by a fine outline of hyperpigmentation (Figure 4). Key areas of involvement, in addition to the scalp, include the ear, perioral, and perinasal regions. Despite the often classic clinical appearance, a scalp biopsy for direct immunofluorescence (DIF) and H&E (hematoxylin & eosin) should be sent (Current Diagnosis box). Although DLE can progress to systemic lupus in approximately 5% of individuals, it is predominantly stable

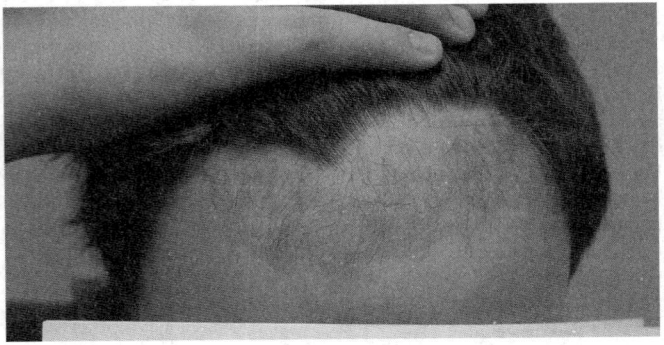

**FIGURE 3.** Traction alopecia. Hairs of varying lengths with a well-defined border.

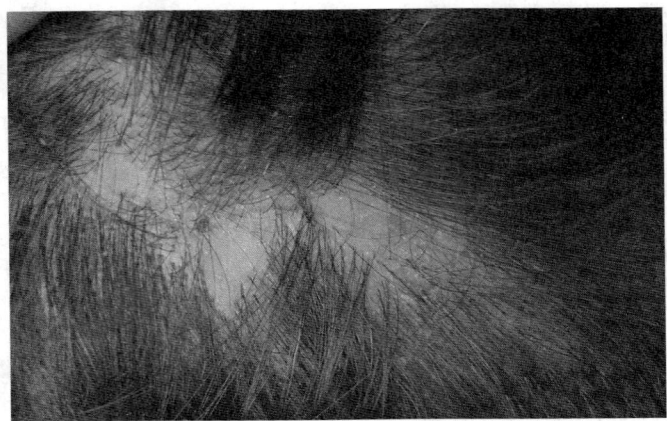

**FIGURE 4.** Discoid lupus erythematosus (DLE). Scalp showing whitish old burned-out areas and newly inflamed erythematic patches with perifollicular scale, crust, and erosions.

and can be most effectively treated with sun protection and topical and intralesional steroids. Refractory cases may also respond well to antimalarials, systemic retinoids, and dapsone.

### LICHEN PLANOPILARIS

Four more times common in women, this entity is a follicular-based variant of lichen planus. The scalp, as well as other hair-bearing areas, can be involved (Graham Little syndrome). The hair-pull test is positive for anagen hairs. Clinically this condition begins as perifollicular erythema that then leads to hyperkeratotic and spiny follicles and eventual permanent scarring. If early in the disease process, successful treatment can include potent topical and intralesional steroids as well as antimalarials.

### CENTRAL CENTRIFUGAL CICATRICIAL ALOPECIA

Largely an umbrella term for "hot comb alopecia," the "follicular degeneration syndrome," and central centrifugal scarring alopecia. Central centrifugal cicatricial alopecia (CCCA) is defined as premature desquamation of the inner root sheath eventually leading to loss of the follicular epithelium and replacement with fibrosis. Patients may be asymptomatic or complain of sensations of pruritus, pain, or pins and needles. Most commonly found in a subset of African American women, this insidious, noninflammatory primary scarring alopecia starts in the central midline scalp and spreads centrifugally over the vertex. At times polytrichia, multiple hairs exiting one hair follicle ostia, can be observed. There is little scalp bogginess or tautness, but this type of alopecia has long been associated with the hair care regimens of certain ethnic backgrounds. However, this anecdotal association remains to be scientifically validated. If treated in the early stages, the condition can be improved with both high potency topical steroids and tetracycline (500 mg orally twice a day) and cessation of any traumatic or chemical hair care practices.

### FOLLICULITIS DECALVANS

Folliculitis decalvans, a recurrent, inflammatory process, is defined by well-circumscribed patches, along which follicular papules and pustules line the advancing margins (Figures 5A and B). If progressive, these often boggy scalp areas eventually become scarred. Variants include so-called tufted folliculitis in which multiple hairs emerge from erythematous and crusted follicles resembling doll-like hair. During active disease, there is an abundance of gram-positive organisms. Hypotheses exist affirming *Staphylococcus aureus* to be the causative agent. However, the true etiology is unknown. Fungal and bacterial cultures are warranted as well as screening for potential immune deficiency. Long-term oral and topical antibiotics and/or retinoids are the mainstay of therapy.

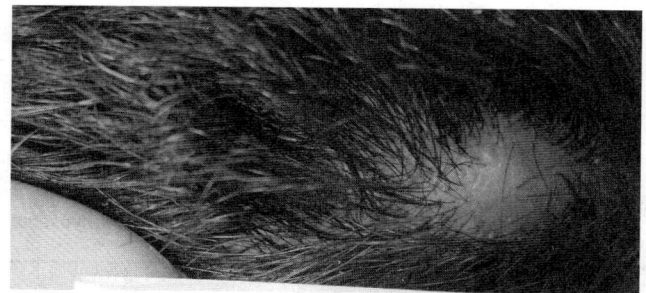

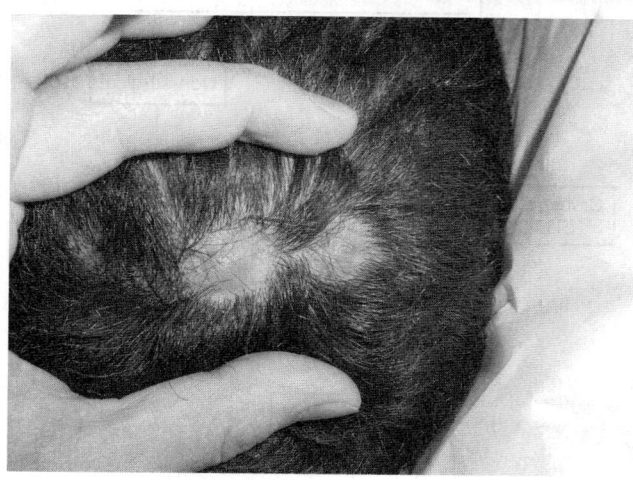

**FIGURE 5. A,** Folliculitis decalvans. Well-defined carbuncle on the scalp with overlying hair loss. **B,** Folliculitis decalvans. Well-circumscribed patches of boggy scarred scalp with few areas showing "tufted" folliculitis.

## REFERENCES

Berger RS, Fu JL, Smiles KA, et al: The effects of minoxidil, 1% pyrithione zinc and a combination of both on hair density: A randomized controlled trial. Br J Dermatol 2003;149(2):354-362.

Dawber R, Van Neste D, Dunitz M: Hair and Scalp Disorders. Common Presenting Signs, Differential Diagnosis and Treatment, 2nd ed. Philadelphia, Lippincott, 1995.

Freedberg IM, et al: Fitzpatrick's Dermatology in General Medicine, vol 1, 6th ed. Disorders of epidermal appendages and related disorders. New York, McGraw-Hill, 2003, pp 633-655.

Harrison S. Sinclair R: Telogen effluvium. Clin Exp Dermatol 2002;27(5):389-385.

Hautmann G, Hercogova J, Lotti T: Trichotillomania. J Am Acad Dermatol 2002;46(6):807-821.

Odom RB, et al: Andrews' Diseases of the Skin: Clinical Dermatology, 9th ed. Philadelphia, WB Saunders, 2000, pp 943-952.

Ross EK, Tan E, Shapiro J: Update on primary cicatricial alopecias. J Am Acad Dermatol 2005;53(1):1-37.

Sinclair R, Jolley D, Mallari R, Magee J: The reliability of horizontally sectioned scalp biopsies in the diagnosis of chronic diffuse telogen hair loss in women. J Am Acad Dermatol 2004;51(2):189-199.

Sperling LC, Solomon AR, Whiting DA: A new look at scarring alopecia. Arch Dermatol 2000;136:235-242.

# Cancers of the Skin

Method of
*Aleda A. Jacobs, MD, and Ida F. Orengo, MD*

Ultraviolet (UV) light exposure over a person's lifetime, along with other genetic factors, play critical etiologic roles in development of most skin cancers, such as squamous cell carcinoma (SCC) and basal cell carcinoma (BCC). Although argument still exists, most dermatologists today believe that these factors also contribute significantly to the dysplastic development of a nevus over time and to the development of melanoma.

A variety of host factors, including Fitzpatrick skin type, immunocompetence (or lack thereof), and genetic makeup, together with UV light exposure, determine whether acute (sunburn) and chronic cumulative UV light injuries will ultimately cause skin cancer. Other causes of skin cancer such as ionizing radiation, traumatic skin injury such as that incurred through burn insult, chemical carcinogens, and a decreased immunity (as with transplant patients) can also cause skin cancer, but these are still less often implicated in the United States as causes of skin cancer than is UV light exposure.

Many genetic disorders can also predispose patients to develop skin cancer through a variety of mechanisms. These include basal cell nevus syndrome, albinism, xeroderma pigmentosa, and epidermolysis bullosa. Patients with these syndromes typically develop multiple skin cancers at an early age and many neoplasms over a lifetime. People with these disease states lack the necessary repair mechanisms to protect their cells from UV light damage, and they often develop multiple cancers with only very minimal UV light exposure.

Viruses too, cause neoplastic conditions within the skin. Genital SCC is almost always associated with human papilloma virus (HPV), most commonly HPV-16, -18, -31, and -33. HPV can interact with sunlight to result in a potentially life-threatening SCC in a rare skin disease, epidermodysplasia verruciformis.

A great many other cancerous conditions of the skin exist, but only the most prevalent neoplastic transformations will be covered in this article.

## Clinical Features

Two of the most common skin neoplasms in which UV light is strongly implicated are BCC and SCC. Nodular BCC is the most common subtype of BCC (80%), followed by superficial BCC and then morpheaform or sclerosing BCC.

Local and regional lymph nodes should be carefully examined in patients with either type of skin cancer. Because lymph nodes are the most frequent site of SCC metastasis, questionable lymph nodes should be further investigated with fine-needle aspiration, and appropriate imaging studies should be performed to exclude metastasis in patients whose lymph node examination is abnormal.

### BASAL CELL CARCINOMA

Nodular BCC typically appears as a shiny, translucent papule or nodule, with distinct edges and visible telangiectasias. These may be either flesh colored or pigmented, and may be clinically confused with nodular melanoma. Superficial BCC (15%) usually appears as an erythematous thin, scaly macule or plaque on the trunk and often has a very subtly raised and slightly rolled border. The most challenging clinical diagnosis is that of the morpheaform or sclerotic type, which often resembles a scar.

Many dermatologists have colloquially referred to BCC as "the best type of cancer to have" if a person must have any kind of neoplasm. This is because of the long relatively latent period of slow growth of these lesions over time and their extremely low rate of metastasis. If neglected, BCC lesions, which are most often painless, can continue to grow and can destroy neighboring structures because they can be locally invasive and destructive. They can ulcerate and bleed, have a foul odor, and reach an enormous size.

## SQUAMOUS CELL CARCINOMA

SCC can be difficult to distinguish clinically from BCC. SCC lesions generally appear more solid than translucent and have a higher incidence of metastasis than BCC lesions. With SCC lesions, a keratotic scale is commonly present over the lesion, and ulceration is also common. Typically, there are no shiny borders or discrete edges as with BCC, and obvious telangiectasias are rare. SCC can appear as a small papule, but it more commonly manifests as a large and usually ulcerated nodule with a hyperkeratotic crust that ulcerates and often bleeds.

Transplant patients who receive chemotherapy to prevent organ rejection often develop many SCC lesions after years of such therapy. Renal transplant patients develop skin cancers at 10 years after transplantation, and heart and lung transplant patients develop skin cancers at 5 years after transplantation. Most likely this is due to the increased level of immunosuppression in the heart and lung transplant patients.

Patients with long-term cumulative sun exposure are at highest risk for developing these cancers (Figures 1 and 2). SCC is the most common cancer of the mucosal lip, and these lesions are even more prevalent in those who chew or smoke tobacco. Patients who also habitually drink alcohol are even more likely to develop mucosal SCC.

SCC in situ (Bowen's disease) can appear similar to superficial BCC, and simple biopsy of the lesion helps to elucidate the correct pathologic diagnosis and dictate appropriate treatment. SCC in situ on the uncircumcised penis (erythroplasia of Querat) manifests as a bright red and moist-appearing plaque with relatively discrete edges. SCC in situ can remain superficial or can invade into deeper structures and develop into invasive SCC with a strong potential to metastasize.

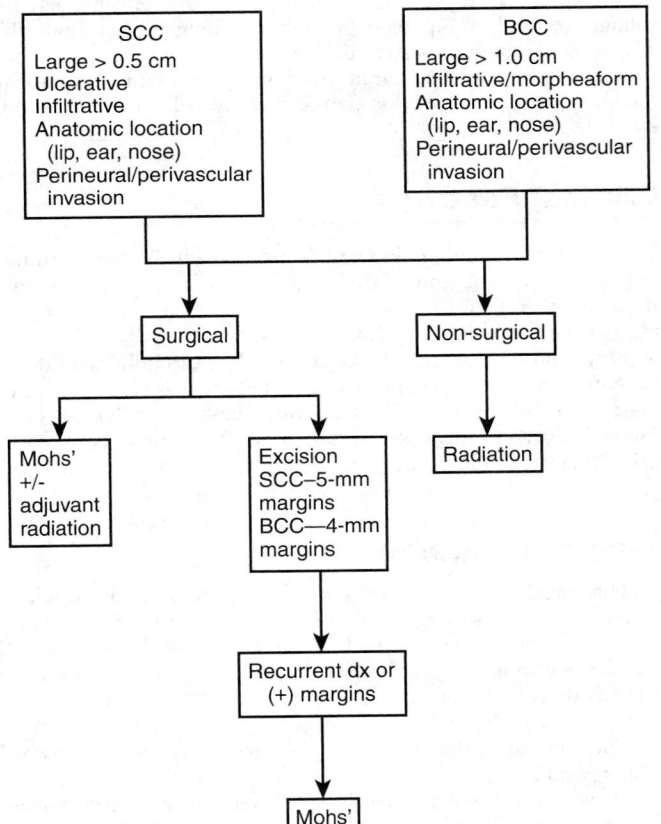

**FIGURE 1.** Diagnosis and treatment of squamous cell carcinoma (SCC) and basal cell carcinoma (BCC) in high-risk patients. *Abbreviation:* dx = diagnosis.

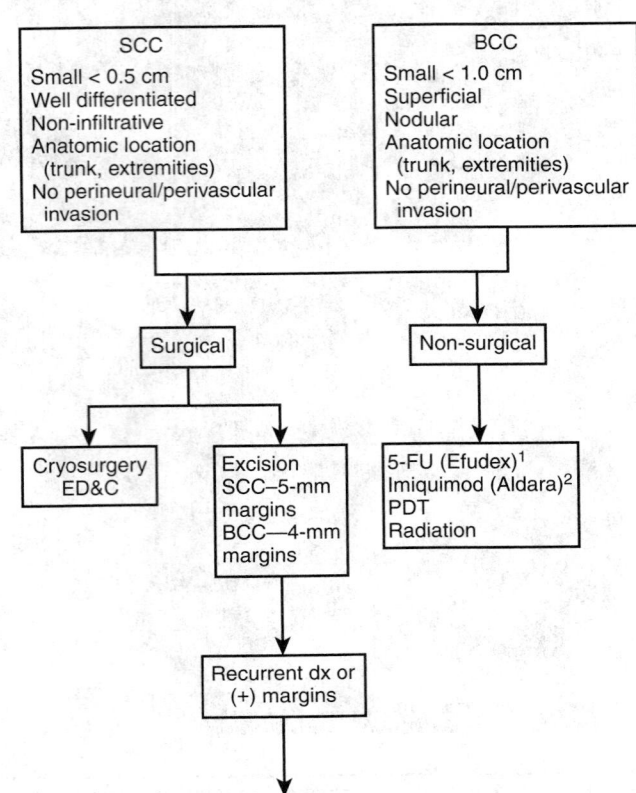

[1] FDA approved for sBCC and SCC in situ.
[2] FDA approved for sBCC.

**FIGURE 2.** Diagnosis and treatment of squamous cell carcinoma (SCC) and basal cell carcinoma (BCC) in low-risk patients. *Abbreviations:* ED&C = electrodessication and curettage; FU = fluorouracil; PDT = photodynamic therapy.

It is generally believed that some actinic keratoses (hyperkeratotic and scaly lesions termed *precancer* by many dermatologists) can develop into SCC if left untreated.

SCCs can grow slowly, but more often these tumors progress relatively quickly, and therefore treatment should be promptly initiated to reduce the size of the defect and the risk of metastasis. The keratoacanthoma, believed by most dermatologists and dermatopathologists to be a well-differentiated subtype of SCC, typically has a history of sudden rapid growth, has a central keratotic crater, and often appears cup-shaped histologically. SCC tumors larger than 2 cm in diameter often metastasize and are more likely to have perineural invasion, worsening the prognosis. This likelihood also increases if the tumor recurs.

## Treatment

### PHARMACOLOGIC THERAPY

Recently, the advent of topical immunomodulators has provided a noninvasive and very effective modality for treating superficial BCC and SCC in situ. Topical 5-FU (Efudex)[1] and topical imiquimod (Aldara) have both been employed for treatment of such cancers. They enable a person's own immune system to recognize and mount an inflammatory and immune response to cancerous cells near the application

[1] Not FDA approved for this indication.

## CURRENT DIAGNOSIS

- BCC, SCC, and melanoma can arise anywhere on the skin but are most common on areas of sun-exposed skin.
- Skin cancers can usually be diagnosed clinically based on cancer-specific features such as shiny borders and telangiectasias common to many BCCs.
- Histopathologic analysis after skin biopsy should always be considered for equivocal lesions to optimize patient management.

---

*Abbreviations:* BCC = basal cell carcinoma; SCC = squamous cell carcinoma.

of the cream. Imiquimod cream is a biological response modifier that was recently approved for treatment of nonfacial superficial BCC and is commonly also used for SCC in situ (Bowen's disease) with diameters less than 2.0 cm. It is an excellent choice for many patients unwilling or unable to undergo surgical excision.

These immunomodulators are also ideal for treating early potential cancers such as actinic keratoses. They allow treatment of an entire cancer field, thereby treating not only the lesion visible to the eye but also the usually dysplastic tissue nearby. Although these topical treatments are both very effective, patients often complain of the expected side-effect of brisk and sometimes extreme localized inflammation and erythema. These treatments are best used in patients in whom follow-up examinations of the treated areas are likely and can be expected.

## SURGICAL THERAPY

### Cryosurgery

Cryosurgery with liquid nitrogen is the workhorse of early actinic keratoses. This treatment modality relies on the destructive effect of the freeze-thaw cycle on living cells. If a lesion persists or recurs after trial with this technique, a biopsy is indicated to rule out skin cancer. Typically, the risk of scarring with hypopigmentation is the only untoward side effect with this modality. In patients with an inherent cold-sensitivity disorder, such as cryoglobulinemia, this treatment technique is contraindicated.

### Electrodesiccation and Curettage

Electrodesiccation and curettage (ED&C) remains the most frequently selected treatment modality for BCC and SCC in the United States. In fact, recent findings illustrate that curettage alone is almost as effective as ED&C, with the benefit of avoiding desiccation afterward. ED&C is highly effective for treating select tumors, although great variability exists among those who perform this technique. Cure rates of 95% for small BCCs and SCCs are reported with correct technique.

Standard technique involves curettage in three directions over a lesion until the friable tissue is completely removed. After each cycle of curettage, the remaining treated area is desiccated. Three separate cycles of each are completed.

ED&C is often the fastest treatment, is relatively inexpensive, and is ideal for areas of the body that have low recurrence rates, such as the trunk, back, and extremities. ED&C can also be effective for select lesions on the face as long as the location of the tumor is not in a hair-bearing area, because BCC and SCC tend to extend deeply into the dermis along hair follicles. Treated lesions heal by second intention and leave minimal scarring, which is later often hypopigmented.

ED&C should not be used for lesions in hair-bearing areas. For lesions that, when curetted, appear to extend deeply into the dermis or subcutaneous tissue, this method is better aborted, and the surgeon should convert to excision of the tumor.

## CURRENT THERAPY

### Noninvasive Treatment

- Relatively noninvasive modalities for destruction of malignant lesions include cryotherapy, electrodessication and curettage, and topical chemotherapy.
- These are excellent for treating small (1.0 cm diameter or less), histologically nonaggressive BCCs and SCCs that demonstrate clinically distinct margins and are not in areas with high risk of recurrence.

### Standard Surgical Excision

- Standard surgical excision is an appropriate choice for facial BCCs and SCCs that have distinct clinical margins and are in areas that have low tumor recurrence rates.
- It is also appropriate for lesions that histologically demonstrate low-risk microscopic appearance and do not invade follicular or neural structures.
- Standard excision is not appropriate for lesions on the lips, nose, or ears.

### Mohs' Micrographic Surgery

- Referral for Mohs' micrographic surgery should be considered if surgical pathology reveals perineural invasion or tumor involving the margins of a specimen after standard excision. Many such tumors extend much deeper into the dermis than is clinically apparent on the skin surface.
- Mohs' surgery has the highest statistical curative rate for BCC and SCC.
- Mohs' surgery should be the treatment of choice for primary BCC and SCC arising in high recurrence risk areas (e.g., nose, ears, eyelids, lips) and for all recurrent BCC or SCC.
- Mohs' surgery is the treatment of choice for tumors larger than 1.0 cm in diameter anywhere on the face or larger than 2.0 cm elsewhere on the body.
- Mohs' surgery is the gold standard of treatment for all tumors with aggressive histologic patterns or findings exhibiting morpheaform, micronodular, and perineural or perifollicular invasion.

### Radiation

- Radiation therapy is most commonly reserved for
  - Patients older than 50 years
  - Patients who are not good surgical candidates
  - Patients who have comorbid conditions
  - In cases when surgical treatment would result in extensive morbidity

### Sentinel Lymph Node Mapping

- Sentinel lymph node mapping for nonmelanoma skin cancers is not yet widely recommended as standard of care for treatment of such lesions.
- This is an area of current debate, and a consensus has not yet been reached for whether or not sentinel node mapping will become part of the oncologic work-up in the future.

---

*Abbreviations:* BCC = basal cell carcinoma; SCC = squamous cell carcinoma.

### Other Destructive Options

Lasers used in surgical ablation, such as the $CO_2$ and erbium:yttrium-aluminum-garnet (Er:YAG), may also be used to ablate smaller and more superficial tumors.

### Standard Surgical Excision

Basal cell carcinoma lesions with less than a 1-cm diameter and treated with excision with a 4-mm margin have a 95% cure rate. Margins for excision of SCC tumors should be 5 mm around the lesion. All excised tissue should be sent, with oriented borders, for histopathologic analysis after excision. Any positive margin should be subsequently excised. The possibility of Mohs' micrographic surgery or adjuvant radiation, or both, should be considered if appropriate.

### Mohs' Micrographic Surgery

Mohs' micrographic surgery fully integrates the interdependent roles of the dermatologic surgeon and the dermatopathologist; both roles are performed by the same person. A Mohs' surgeon is a dermatologist who is specially trained in both surgical technique and wound closure, as well as in histopathology, and can analyze tissue under the microscope.

Mohs' surgical excision has a wide range of indications and achieves the highest statistical cure rates for BCC and SCC with maximal conservation of surrounding tissue. This technique allows complete and definitive excision of the neoplastic tissue while preserving uninvolved tissue, thereby leaving the smallest possible defect in place of the cancer and facilitating closure of the resultant wound.

Indications for Mohs' surgical excision are wide ranging: Areas of high recurrence such as locations on the face (nose, lips, eyelids, and ears) or in areas where maximal tissue conservation is required are obvious choices. Additional indications include recurrent tumors, those with specifically more infiltrative and aggressive subtypes, those that demonstrate perineural invasion, those with poorly defined or equivocal margins, and those with a diameter larger than 1 cm and located on the face. Tumors located on areas other than the face, with diameters larger than 2 cm, are also arguably well suited for Mohs' surgical excision.

### OTHER MODALITIES

#### Photodynamic Therapy

Photodynamic therapy is based on the principle of activation of selectively absorbed photosensitizers by cancerous skin cells, while normal cells remain unaffected. Neoplastic cells are destroyed by the absorbed light's interaction with them, and normal tissue is undamaged. Superficial BCC and SCC in situ are both successfully treated with topically applied photosensitizers, such as amino levulonic acid, before exposure to the specialized light source. Photodynamic therapy is not yet a widely used modality for cancer treatment in the United States.

#### Radiation Therapy

In some cases, such as individual tumors extending over wide areas of the face or body surfaces, skin cancer is not amenable to curative treatment with surgical excision because adequate margins are unattainable and the remaining defect would be too large. In these situations, and in patients who are otherwise medically unfit for undergoing a surgical procedure, fractionated radiation therapy is an effective treatment, albeit costly. This modality is appropriate for treating both primary and recurrent BCC and SCC, and it has reported 90% cure rates. Fractional radiotherapy (typical total treatment dose of 4000-6000 cGy), is especially useful for treating tumors in patients with comorbid medical conditions that predispose them to a higher risk of surgical complications.

Radiation therapy as a primary treatment is not routinely considered for patients younger than 50 years old because it has a lower statistical cure rate than Mohs' surgery and the risk remains for recurrence of the tumor in the radiation portal (most commonly SCC). Therefore, radiation therapy is often used as an adjunct and very beneficial therapy for surgically treated SCC and unusually aggressive BCC that demonstrate perineural invasion, and such treatment decreases the risk of tumor recurrence.

In patients with syndromic conditions that render them unable to withstand much exposure to UV light or radiation at all (such as xeroderma pigmentosa or basal cell nevus syndrome), radiation therapy is relatively contraindicated.

## Follow-up

All patients after diagnosis of skin cancer are better managed with full-body skin examinations. These should occur biannually in the case of primary BCC and every 3 months for recurrent BCC and for primary or recurrent SCC.

All patients should be educated about safe-sun practices and advised to reduce their UV light exposure. Some patients, especially those who are immunosuppressed, may be advised to take daily oral supplemental vitamin D to compensate for decreased sun exposure; however, this issue is still not widely agreed on among dermatologists. Some patients require specialized protocols and monitoring to normalize and stabilize acceptable vitamin D levels. Close supervision with the care of a physician and timely skin examinations are still the mainstays of long-term treatment for all skin cancer patients.

Skin examinations should be repeated every 3 to 6 months for 3 years and annually thereafter. Patients with a history or diagnosis of mucosal SCC should also have a full intraoral examination biannually.

## Prevention

Although many modalities exist for treating skin cancers, prevention is still the best choice for skin cancer management, and it too often is underdiscussed. However, with cutaneous cancers such as BCC, SCC, and melanoma on the rise, new attention to this issue has pressed pharmaceutical companies and physicians to address early prevention for babies and young children as well as adults.

New formulations of sunscreen help to stabilize the protective chemicals so they are not destroyed by UV light. These new sunscreens have the added benefit that they do not need to be reapplied every two hours to have maximum preventive effect (e.g., Helioplex, Neutrogena). Educational programs such as Slip, Slap, Slop (slip on protective clothing, slap on a hat, and slop on sunscreen) have proved very effective in decreasing the overall incidence of skin cancers in Australia and are becoming increasingly accepted in the United States. As similar programs and sunless tanners gain popularity, and as tanning beds, which are well known to cause skin cancer, lose their popular following, the incidence of skin cancer in the United States will also hopefully decrease.

### REFERENCES

Autier P: Cutaneous malignant melanoma: Facts about sunbeds and sunscreen. Expert Rev Anticancer Ther 2005;5(5):821-833.

Chen TM, Rosen T, Orengo I: Treatment of a large superficial basal cell carcinoma with 5% imiquimod: A case report and review of the literature. Dermatol Surg 2002;28(4):344-346.

Fourtanier A, Moyal, D, Maccario J, et al: Measurement of sunscreen immune protection factors in humans: A consensus paper. J Invest Dermatol 2005; 125(3):403-409.

Harwood CA, Proby CM, McGregor JM, et al: Clinicopathologic features of skin cancer in organ transplant recipients: A retrospective case-control series. J Am Acad Dermatol 2006;54(2):290-300.

Hruza GJ: Mohs' micrographic surgery local recurrences. J Dermatol Surg Oncol 1994;20(9):573-577.

Lane JE, Kent DE: Surgical margins in the treatment of nonmelanoma skin cancer and Mohs' micrographic surgery. Curr Surg. 2005;62(5): 518-526.

Marmur ES, Schmults CD, Goldberg DJ: A review of laser and photodynamic therapy for the treatment of nonmelanoma skin cancer. Dermatol Surg 2004;30(2 Pt 2):264-271.

Pennington BE, Leffell DJ: Mohs' micrographic surgery: Established uses and emerging trends. Oncology (Williston Park). 2005;19(9):1165-1171.

# Cutaneous T Cell Lymphoma

Method of
*Marie-France Demierre, MD*

Cutaneous T cell lymphomas (CTCLs) are primary lymphomas of the skin belonging to the category of extranodal non-Hodgkin lymphomas. The most common type of CTCL is mycosis fungoides (MF), a malignancy of thymus-derived helper lymphocytes, usually CD4+ in phenotype, that present as patches, plaques, or tumors. Sézary syndrome (SS) is a more aggressive form of CTCL with peripheral blood involvement. Mycosis fungoides and SS account for 70% to 80% of all CTCLs diagnosed in North America. Primary cutaneous CD30+ lymphoproliferative disorders, lymphomatoid papulosis (self-healing, recurrent papules), and primary cutaneous CD30+ anaplastic large cell lymphoma (CD30+ tumors) represent 15% of CTCLs in North America. Epidemiologic data for MF only is known. Males are affected twice as often as females, and although all races appear to be affected, African Americans have a higher incidence than whites. The average age at onset is approximately 55 years. Young adults less than 20 years of age and even children can be affected.

The appropriate medical management and selection of therapeutic modalities varies with the subtype of CTCL and staging. Diagnosis, staging, and a summary of current therapies used for MF and SS patients are presented.

## Diagnosis of Mycosis Fungoides

MF often begins with subtle lesions that may be mistaken for eczema (ill-defined erythematous patches or plaques) or psoriasis (well-defined erythematous plaques). The lesions often present in sun-protected areas, the bathing trunk distribution (breast, abdomen, belt line, buttocks). Patient may have pruritus. Other presentations include hypopigmented patches, poikiloderma atrophicans vasculare with patches of telangiectasia, atrophy, pigmentation resembling radiation dermatitis, and folliculotropic mycosis fungoides with grouped follicular papules or indurated plaques devoid of hair. In large-plaque parapsoriasis, scaly, pink to dusky, sometimes slightly infiltrated patches are suggestive of MF, but full criteria for its diagnosis are lacking. Patches of MF can evolve to plaques that can be thickened, annular, serpiginous, and finally to tumors. Characteristic skin histology of MF shows numerous atypical lymphocytes with convoluted nuclei near and within the epidermis as well as clusters within the epidermis (Pautrier's microabscess).

In SS, itching is severe, and erythroderma is the hallmark. SS is accompanied by ectropion, hair loss, keratoderma, fissures, cutaneous pain, enlarged lymph nodes, and large numbers of circulating atypical lymphocytes in the peripheral blood. Molecular techniques and immunophenotyping are helpful to confirm diagnosis. In the context of clinically suspicious lesions, demonstration of dominant clonality in the skin, lymph nodes, and blood, particularly of the T cell receptor gene, represents strong evidence of malignancy, even in early-stage lesions.

### CURRENT DIAGNOSIS

- Mycosis fungoides is the most common type of cutaneous T cell lymphoma.
- Lesions can present as patches, plaques, or tumors.
- Erythroderma is the hallmark of Sézary syndrome.
- Staging is relevant to manage patients appropriately.

### CURRENT THERAPY

- Optimal treatment depends on stage of disease.
- Skin-directed therapies are for early-stage patients.
- Systemic therapy is used for more advanced disease.
- Treatment of pruritus is relevant for all patients.

## Staging of Mycosis Fungoides

Staging classification is helpful in the management of patients. The World Health Organization-European Organization for Research and Treatment of Cancer (WHO-EORTC) classification pertains to prognostic categories, indolent versus aggressive (Table 1); the TNM nomenclature permits more precise clinical staging for MF and SS (Tables 2 and 3). The extent of skin (T of TNM) and peripheral lymph node enlargement (N of TNM) involvement are significantly associated with survival in patients with CTCL. Generally, a lymph node biopsy is not obtained in patients with early patch/plaque disease because lymph nodes are rarely positive or show only dermatopathic lymphadenitis by light microscopy. In the setting of histologically proven lymph node involvement or extracutaneous lymphoma in blood (B) or viscera (M of TNM), prognosis is impacted.

Table 4 lists the tests recommended for the evaluation and staging of patients with MF or SS. Computed tomography (CT) scans are obtained in advanced disease but are not justifiable as a routine evaluation procedure in patients with early-stage disease.

## Treatment

Optimal therapy for MF and SS depends on the stage of disease, patients' co-morbidities, insurance coverage (where applicable), and accessibility (Table 5). Long remissions and possible cures are possible in patients with early disease, but current treatments are not curative in patients with more advanced disease. A National Cancer Institute (NCI) study confirmed that late-stage patients with extensive plaques, tumors, or erythroderma did more poorly when treated aggressively, usually because of increased susceptibility to superinfection.

The optimal schedules of current treatments and investigation of new therapies only occur if patients with MF and SS are entered into ongoing treatment protocols. Information regarding finding studies in progress can be obtained in the references list.

### GENERAL MEASURES

Pruritus is a common, sometimes overwhelming problem for patients with MF or SS. Moderate relief may be gained by the use of systemic antihistamines such as hydroxyzine (Atarax) at 25 mg orally every 4 hours as needed, topical emollients such as Aquaphor, or topical corticosteroids such as betamethasone, fluocinonide (Lidex), or triamcinolone (Aristocort) in ointment form applied as needed or overnight under plastic wrap occlusion. For severe itch, gabapentin (Neurontin), mirtazapine, or drugs that treat neuropathic pain are indicated.

In most cases, skin-directed therapies are used for patients with disease considered to be confined to the skin, and systemic therapy is used for more advanced disease.

### SPECIFIC MEASURES

#### Skin-Directed Therapies

##### Phototherapy

Phototherapy with ultraviolet B (UVB) treats limited patch or plaque T1 disease, resulting in up to 74% complete response rate. Psoralen ultraviolet A-range (PUVA) long-wavelength light penetrates the skin more deeply: 90% of stage IA and 76% of stage IB patients may achieve complete remission. Recently, narrowband UVB showed similar

**TABLE 1  Frequency and Disease-Specific 5-Year Survival for Primary Cutaneous Lymphomas**

| WHO-EORTC Classification | Disease-Specific 5-Year Survival (%) |
|---|---|
| **Indolent Clinical Behavior** | |
| Mycosis fungoides (MF) | 88 |
| Folliculotropic MF | 80 |
| Pagetoid reticulosis | 100 |
| Granulomatous slack skin | 100 |
| Primary cutaneous anaplastic large cell lymphoma | 95 |
| Lymphomatoid papulosis | 100 |
| Subcutaneous panniculitis-like T cell lymphoma | 82 |
| Primary cutaneous CD4+ small/medium pleomorphic T cell lymphoma[†] | 75 |
| **Aggressive Clinical Behavior** | |
| Sézary syndrome | 24 |
| Primary cutaneous NK/T cell lymphoma, nasal type | NR |
| Primary cutaneous aggressive CD8+ T cell lymphoma[†] | 18 |
| Primary cutaneous γ/δ T cell lymphoma[†] | NR |
| Primary cutaneous peripheral T cell lymphoma, unspecified[‡] | 16 |

Data are based on 1905 patients with a primary cutaneous lymphoma registered at the Dutch and Austrian Cutaneous Lymphoma Group between 1986 and 2002.
[‡]Primary cutaneous peripheral T cell lymphoma, unspecified excluding the three provisional entities indicated with a single dagger (†).
*Abbreviations:* MF = mycosis fungoides; NR = not reached; WHO-EORTC = World Health Organization-European Organization of Research and Cancer Treatment.
Data obtained from Willemze, R, Jaffe ES, Burg G, et al: WHO-EORTC classification for cutaneous lymphomas. Blood 2005;105(10):3768-3785.

response rates to PUVA without the adverse events of nausea from psoralen. However, patients with thicker plaques need frequent maintenance light treatments to maintain control along with other modalities.

### Topical Mechlorethamine

Topical application of mechlorethamine (nitrogen mustard [HN2], Mustargen) is a proven regimen for the control of early stage MF with 94% complete response rates in stage IA and 59% in stage IB.

**TABLE 2  TNM Classification for Cutaneous T Cell Lymphoma (Mycosis Fungoides and Sézary Syndrome)\***

**Skin (T)**
| | |
|---|---|
| T0 | Clinically and/or histologically suspicious lesions |
| T1 | Limited plaques, papules, or eczematous patches covering <10% of skin surface |
| T2 | Limited plaques, papules, or eczematous patches covering ≥10% of skin surface |
| T3 | Tumors (≥1) |
| T4 | Generalized erythroderma |

**Lymph Nodes (N)**
| | |
|---|---|
| N0 | No clinically abnormal peripheral lymph nodes; pathologic findings not CTCL |
| N1 | Clinically abnormal peripheral lymph nodes; pathologic findings not CTCL |
| N2 | No clinically abnormal peripheral lymph nodes; pathologic findings positive for CTCL |
| N3 | Clinically abnormal peripheral lymph nodes; pathologic findings positive for CTCL |

**Peripheral Blood (B)**
| | |
|---|---|
| B0 | Atypical circulating cells not present (<5%) |
| B1 | Atypical circulating cells present (≥5%) |

**Visceral Organ (M)**
| | |
|---|---|
| M0 | No visceral organ involvement |
| M1 | Visceral involvement (must have pathologic confirmation) |

\*Peripheral blood involvement (B) is not incorporated into the staging classification for this disorder.
*Abbreviation:* CTCL = cutaneous T cell lymphoma
Modified from Bunn PA Jr, Lamberg SI: Report of the Committee on Staging and Classification of Cutaneous T-Cell Lymphomas. Cancer Treat Rep 1979;63:725-728.

Limitations of this treatment modality include a high rate of hypersensitivity reactions (up to 20%), and the need for continuous daily application.

A liquid preparation or ointment form is used. Although there are no studies comparing the preparations, the ointment form is helpful for patients who experience significant dryness from the liquid preparation. Treatment should be carried out daily to the total body, neck down, until complete clearing, which may take several months to a year or longer. Once clear, therapy should be continued for 6 to 24 months, perhaps at a decreased frequency, and then discontinued. Many patients clear except for one or a few patches. These patients often require continuous therapy to maintain control or an alternative topical therapy. For those patients who become allergic, half can be desensitized by graded increases of diluted HN2, managed by experienced dermatologists.

### Topical Carmustine

Although less frequently used than HN2, topical carmustine (BiCNU) is an effective alternative for early-stage disease, especially in patients who became allergic to HN2. Local irritation and persistent telangiectasias usually develop. Because the drug is absorbed, patients have a risk of reversible bone marrow depression with decreased leukocytes and platelets, usually delayed for 6 weeks after use. The patient can be supplied with a stock solution by prescribing a 100-mg vial of BiCNU dissolved in 50 mL of absolute or 95% ethanol to be stored at home

**TABLE 3  Staging Classifications for Cutaneous T-Cell Lymphoma**

| Stage | Skin | Lymph Nodes | Visceral Involvement |
|---|---|---|---|
| IA | T1 | N0 | M0 |
| IB | T2 | N0 | M0 |
| IIA | T1, T2 | N1 | M0 |
| IIB | T3 | N0, N1 | M0 |
| III | T4 | N0, N1 | M0 |
| IVA | T1–T4 | N2, N3 | M0 |
| IVB | T1–T4 | N0–N3 | M1 |

Modified from Lamberg SI, Bunn PA Jr: Cutaneous T cell lymphomas: Summary of the Mycosis Fungoides Cooperative Group-National Cancer Institute Workshop. Arch Dermatol 1979;115:1103-1105.

## TABLE 4 Recommended Evaluation Procedures

| | Routine | Investigational |
|---|---|---|
| History and physical examination | X | |
| Skin biopsy | X | |
| Complete blood count and differential, renal function tests, uric acid, serum calcium, lactate dehydrogenase (LDH) | X | |
| Peripheral smear to determine the absolute lymphocyte count and percentage of Sézary cells | X | |
| Chest radiograph | X | |
| Scans and/or biopsies of organs when history or physical examination suggests abnormalities | X | |
| Lymph node biopsy* | See text | |
| Bone marrow biopsy† | | X |
| Abdominal ultrasound/computed tomography | X | |
| Positron emission tomography scans | | X |

*Lymph node biopsy would be justifiable in patients with enlarged lymph nodes (>1.5 cm in diameter) and in those with tumor stage.
†Bone marrow biopsy is indicated in those patients with peripheral blood involvement and tumor stage.

in the refrigerator. Once each day, the patient should add 5 mL of the stock to approximately 60 mL of water and paint the solution onto affected areas. Because of the potential for bone marrow suppression, treatment should only continue for 6 to 8 weeks. If the response is incomplete, this course can be followed immediately by treating individual lesions with the undiluted alcoholic stock solution up to twice daily (up to 70 mg or 35 mL/week). Alternatively, after a 6-week rest period, the patient can be retreated with twice the concentration (10 mL stock per 60 mL water) for another 6 to 8 weeks. The cycle of treatment may be repeated as necessary to suppress visible lesions.

Complete blood counts, including platelet counts, should be obtained every 2 to 4 weeks during and for 6 weeks after total body and intensive local applications.

### Topical Bexarotene Gel

Bexarotene (Targretin) gel is the topical form of the retinoid X receptor (RXR), approved by the Food and Drug Administration (FDA) for the skin manifestations of MF. Bexarotene gel is initially applied once every other day for the first week, with application frequency increased

## TABLE 5 Comparison of Treatment Options

| | Advantages | Disadvantages |
|---|---|---|
| Topical steroids | Symptomatic relief<br>Defer more definitive Rx to observe the course | Alter skin pathology<br>Questionable long-term benefit<br>No effect on infiltrated plaques |
| Phototherapy | Skin clearing in early disease<br>Side effects minimal | High relapse rate without maintenance<br>No effect on thick plaques or tumors<br>Associated with other late skin cancers (PUVA)<br>"Cure" rate low |
| Mechlorethamine (HN2, Mustargen) | Ease of use at home<br>10% long-term remission of early MF | High rate of allergic reactions<br>No effect on thick plaques or tumors |
| Carmustine (BCNU, BiCNU) | Ease of use at home<br>Response rate like that of topical HN2<br>Low rate of allergic contact dermatitis | Potential bone marrow suppression<br>Telangiectasia, pigmentation, skin tenderness |
| Bexarotene gel (Targretin) | Ease of use at home<br>Not carcinogenic | May irritate skin<br>Expensive |
| Total skin electron beam therapy | High long-term disease-free rates<br>One course of therapy | Significant cutaneous side effects<br>Expensive |
| Bexarotene (Targretin) | Benefits 30% of patients who failed prior treatments<br>Single oral dosage<br>Can be adjuvant to other treatment | Limited availability<br>Increases triglycerides and decreases TSH and $T_4$<br>Expensive |
| Interferons | May salvage late-stage disease<br>Adjuvant with other modalities | Significant side effects<br>Expensive<br>Intramuscular dosage required |
| Photopheresis | Effective in Sézary syndrome<br>Minimal side effects | Limited availability<br>Slow response to treatment<br>Expensive |
| Denileukin diftitox (Ontak) | Can treat late-stage disease (10%–35%) | Need expertise to administer<br>Possible serious side effects<br>Expensive |
| Vorinostat (Zolinza) | Can treat late stage disease (30% response rate) | Need to moniter patients closely<br>Side effects can be serious |
| Systemic chemotherapy | May maintain remissions<br>Sometimes induces remissions<br>Palliation of late stage | Significant side effects<br>Complete response unlikely<br>Increases susceptibility to infection |

Abbreviations: HN2 = nitrogen mustard; MF = mycosis fungoides; PUVA = psoralen plus ultraviolet light of A wavelength; Rx = prescription; $T_4$ = thyroxine; TSH = thyroid-stimulating hormone.

at weekly intervals to once, twice, three times, and up to four times daily, depending on individual lesion tolerance. Irritation is common. Most patients require several weeks of treatment before a response is evident. The medication is expensive; its use is reserved for resistant lesions or lesions on palms and soles.

### Radiotherapy

Mycosis fungoides is radiosensitive, and conventional orthovoltage radiation therapy has been used for decades. It can be appropriate for a single plaque or tumor. For patients with extensive skin disease or tumors, total skin electron beam (TSEB) therapy is a better consideration. The penetration of electrons can be controlled to reach depths as shallow as a few millimeters, whereas orthovoltage radiation passes deeply into tissues. A large surface dose can be given with electron beam radiotherapy without deep tissue injury or bone marrow suppression.

With TSEB therapy, most patients in early stages achieve a complete remission, and up to a third remain clear and, perhaps, cured. Therapy is usually fractionated over a period of 6 to 10 weeks to a total of approximately 3000 to 3600 cGy. All portions of the body must be treated; a higher recurrence rate was found in patients who elect scalp shielding to prevent loss of scalp hair. Acute side effects include skin edema, erythema, and fissuring. Hair, nails, and sweat gland function usually return in 3 to 6 months. Limitations of TSEB therapy include its high cost and its availability, although most large cities have medical centers capable of TSEB therapy.

### Biologic Disease Modifying Agents

#### Interferons

Interferons, especially recombinant interferon alpha-2a (Roferon-A[1]), interferon alpha-2b (Intron A[1]), and gamma-1b (Actimmune[1]), are helpful as primary treatment in early-stage CTCL and in combination with retinoids, phototherapy, or extracorporeal photopheresis in later stages. Response rates of approximately 50% are shown with 20% of patients undergoing full remission. Although low doses, 3 million U three times a week, can be offered, doses as high as 12 million U three times a week, given intramuscularly or subcutaneously, may be needed for maximal response. Toxicity depends on dose and includes fever, chills, myalgia, anorexia, and bone marrow suppression. The degree of leukopenia is the dose-limiting side effect, but recovery is rapid.

#### Retinoids

Bexarotene (Targretin) for oral use is approved by the FDA for the treatment of CTCL refractory to at least one previous course of systemic therapy. The recommended oral dose is 300 mg/m²/day, a level at which approximately a third of patients achieve at least a partial response. For a 70-kg, 6-foot person, the surface area is approximately 2m². Therefore, eight 75-mg capsules per day are required. Side effects at the recommended dosage can be significant. They often include high lipid levels that require systemic agents for control, central hypothyroidism, and signs and symptoms of retinoid therapy that may be seen with etretinate and isotretinoin, including headache, dry skin, leucopenia, pruritus, and nausea.

With antilipemic agents and thyroid replacement, side effects can be minimized. Liver function tests should be performed at baseline; after weeks 1, 2, 4; and once stable, at 8-week intervals. Thyroid function tests should be obtained at baseline and then monitored to watch for decreases in thyroid-stimulating hormone and thyroxine levels. Blood lipid levels, especially triglycerides, should be determined at baseline, weekly until the lipid response is established, and then at 8-week intervals. Alterations, especially if triglyceride levels are greater than 400 mg/dL, should be controlled with antilipemic therapy (not gemfibrozil) and dose reduction. White blood cell counts and differential should be obtained at baseline and at regular intervals.

### Extracorporeal Photopheresis

Extracorporeal photopheresis has been approved by the FDA for the treatment of CTCL since 1988. It is principally used for erythrodermic MF or SS. Complete clinical responses are 15% to 25%. In this procedure, the patient's centrifugally separated white blood cells are exposed to UVA in the presence of psoralen and then infused back into the patient. Whether because of a direct cytotoxic effect on the lymphocytes or because of an additional anti-idiotype antibody reaction induced by lymphocyte damage, a substantial reduction in the number of circulating atypical cells is seen in most patients. Skin lesions also often improve, presumably because of movement of atypical cells from the skin into the circulation, where they can be targeted. Side effects are minimal, but expertise in a hospital setting is necessary.

### Interleukin-2 Fusion Toxin

Denileukin diftitox (Ontak) is the product of the fusion of sequences of interleukin-2 (IL-2) with amino acid sequences of diphtheria toxin fragments that targets the malignant cell, the activated T-helper lymphocyte. The combination directs the cytocidal action of diphtheria toxin to cells that express the IL-2 receptor. Response rates are based on patients with at least 20% of the cells in skin lesions positive for CD25, the α-chain of the IL-2 receptor. Initial reported response rates were 30% with 10% complete response in patients who had been refractory to at least two prior therapies. Administer the drug at 9 to 18 µg/kg/day intravenously for 5 consecutive days and repeat every 3 weeks. The major side effects are a flulike syndrome, which occurs in most patients, and capillary leak syndrome, seen in 10%. Excluding patients who have a low albumin can minimize side effects.

## Oral Chemotherapy

### Histone Deacetylase Inhibitors

This new class of agents has been shown to promote an open chromatin structure and result in transcriptional activation. In 2007, vorinostat (Zolinza) was the first FDA-approved oral drug for patients with cutaneous T cell lymphoma (CTCL) who have progressive, persistent, or recurrent disease on or following two systemic therapies. Among 74 CTCL patients, the overall response rate was 30%. Principal side effects are gastrointestinal, constitutional symptoms, thrombocytopenia, and anemia.

## Systemic Chemotherapy

In resistant or progressive disease, systemic chemotherapy may be necessary. Single-agent chemotherapy, particularly low-dose methotrexate (Rheumatrex), 5 to 50 mg per week, is used for resistant plaque disease and erythrodermic MF or SS.

Chemotherapeutic agents that are effective in some cases include liposomal doxorubicin (Doxil), fludarabine (Fludara[1]), deoxycoformycin (pentostatin), gemcitabine (Gemzar[1]), CHOP (cyclophosphamide [Cytoxan], hydroxydaunomycin [Adriamycin], Oncovin [vincristine], and prednisone), and EPOCH (etoposide, prednisone, Oncovin, cyclophosphamide, and hydroxydaunomycin [doxorubicin]).

## TREATMENT BY STAGE

### Early Mycosis Fungoides Apparently Confined to the Skin

Ninety percent of patients with limited patch stage disease do not progress beyond this stage (T1 and N [any] or T2 and N0–N1 [M0]). Because most patients receive some form of therapy, it is unclear whether it is the treatment or the natural history of the disease that confers the good prognosis in patients in this group. Data from the Mycosis Fungoides Cooperative Group (MFCG) show 5-year survival

---

[1]Not FDA approved for this indication.

[1]Not FDA approved for this indication.

rates decreased to 83% in comparison to insurance data for what was expected for persons without MF of the same age and sex. Therapies are generally skin directed and include phototherapy, topical chemotherapy (nitrogen mustard, carmustine), or, more aggressively, TSEB.

### Later Stage Mycosis Fungoides Confined to the Skin

In patients with T2 and N2 or T3 (M0) (B0), although curative therapy is not likely in most instances, sustained remissions are possible. Combination of skin-directed therapies with a biologic disease modifying agent (bexarotene (Targretin), interferon,[1] extracorporeal photopheresis, denileukin diftitox [Ontak]) helps achieve remission. Maintenance therapy is necessary. Treatment of pruritus and prevention of infections are relevant. Five-year survival rates are reduced in this group of patients to 64% and for tumor stage 50% (MFCG data).

### Late Stage with Visceral Involvement, Failure of Previous Therapy, or Sézary Syndrome

Treatment in the late stage is palliative. Because aggressive systemic chemotherapy may shorten the survival of patients with late-stage disease by increasing the chance of sepsis, biologic disease modifying agents that are immunomodulators rather than immunosuppressors are better treatment options. These agents are often combined to achieve higher response rates. Examples of combination of agents include oral bexarotene with interferon[1] and extracorporeal photopheresis with interferon or with oral bexarotene. Oral bexarotene increases response rates to denileukin diftitox. Pruritus can be severe in advanced stages, and a multidisciplinary approach may be needed to treat all dimensions of the disease. Five-year survival drops to 35% in SS (stage T4) patients (MFCG data), and, if extracutaneous involvement is present (stage M1), to less than 20% (2001 Stanford data).

### REFERENCES

Foss F: Mycosis fungoides and the Sézary syndrome. Curr Opin Oncol 2004;16(5):421-428.
Girardi M, Heald PW, Wilson LD: The pathogenesis of mycosis fungoides. N Engl J Med 2004;350(19):1978-1988.
Lundin J, Osterborg A: Therapy for mycosis fungoides. Curr Treat Options Oncol 2004;5(3):203-214.
Willemze R, Jaffe ES, Burg G, et al: WHO-EORTC classification for cutaneous lymphomas. Blood 2005;105(10):3768-3785.
Information on mycosis fungoides and Sézary syndrome studies in progress can be obtained by calling the Cancer Information Service, NCI, Bethesda, MD, at 1-800-4CANCER or from the NCI Web site, http://www.cancer.gov/search/clinical_trials/

---

[1]Not FDA approved for this indication.

# Papulosquamous Disorders

Method of
*Chai Sue Lee, MD, and John Koo, MD*

## Psoriasis

Psoriasis is a genetically influenced, immune-mediated chronic disorder. It is one of the most commonly encountered conditions in dermatologic practice and is regularly seen in primary care practice. Psoriasis affects approximately 2.6% of U.S. population, or approximately 7 million people. Between 150,000 and 260,000 new cases of psoriasis are diagnosed annually. Although slightly more prevalent in women than men, psoriasis affects all ages, races, and ethnicities.

## CURRENT DIAGNOSIS

- Sharply demarcated, scaly, erythematous plaques.
- The most common sites of involvement are scalp, elbows, and knees followed by the nails, hands, feet, and trunk (including the intergluteal fold).
- Psoriatic arthritis is the major associated systemic manifestation; the most common presentation is asymmetric oligoarthritis of the small joints of the hands and feet.

Psoriasis is characterized by sharply demarcated, erythematous, scaly plaques. The most common sites of involvement are the scalp, elbows, and knees followed by the nails, hands, feet, and trunk, including the intergluteal fold.

One of the most important decisions that physicians must make is whether the patient's psoriasis can be adequately treated with topical medications alone or whether it requires phototherapy and/or systemic therapies. This critical decision should take into account the severity of psoriasis, the disease's impact on the patient's quality of life, responsiveness or lack of response to topical therapies, and the presence of or absence of psoriatic arthritis.

Psoriasis can range from mild to severe. In clinical practice, the severity of psoriasis is usually defined by the percentage of body surface area (BSA) involved. The palm of the patient's hand, including the fingers and the thumb (i.e., from the wrist to the top of the fingers), constitutes approximately 1% of the BSA. In clinical trials, severe psoriasis is defined as the presence of lesions over more than 10% of the BSA. In general, if 10% or more BSA is involved, it becomes impractical, if not unrealistic, for most patients to treat their psoriasis with topical medications. Not only does it become tedious and time consuming, it also becomes difficult to obtain sufficient quantities of topical medications. Furthermore, some of the more frequently used and effective topical treatments for psoriasis, such as superpotent topical steroids and calcipotriene (Dovonex), have limitations on the amount of medication that is allowed to be used per unit time for safety reasons. Therefore, patients with more than 10% BSA involvement should probably be managed by a dermatologist so that

## CURRENT THERAPY

Topical therapies
- Corticosteroids
- Calcipotriene (Dovonex)
- Tazarotene (Tazorac)
- Anthralin
- Tar
- Salicylic acid

Phototherapy
- Broadband UVB
- NBUVB
- PUVA

Oral therapies
- Acitretin (Soriatane)
- Methotrexate
- Cyclosporine (Neoral)

Biologic agents
- Etanercept (Enbrel)
- Efalizumab (Raptiva)
- Alefacept (Amevive)
- Infliximab (Remicade)

*Abbreviations:* NBUVB = narrowband ultraviolet light B; PUVA = psoralen plus ultraviolet light of A wavelength.

phototherapy and/or systemic therapy can be used. It is estimated that approximately 30% of psoriasis patients, or approximately 1.5 million U.S. adults, have moderate to severe psoriasis.

When determining severity the impact of psoriasis on the patient's quality of life, including both psychologic and emotional well-being, should also be taken into consideration. Psoriasis may also be deemed severe even when the BSA involved is less than 10%, and phototherapy or systemic therapy should be considered if the psoriasis proves unresponsive to optimized topical treatments. This is especially true if the psoriasis is physically debilitating or emotionally, occupationally, or socially devastating to the patient. For example, a person may only have the palms and/or soles (i.e., 2% BSA) affected by psoriasis, but the impact on quality of life may be profound if the psoriasis impairs the use of the hands or feet; aggressive therapy may be warranted.

Approximately 10% to 40% of patients with psoriasis, or approximately 1 million or more people, have psoriatic arthritis. A major clinical difference between psoriasis and psoriatic arthritis is that psoriasis does not leave behind a permanent scar as long as the patient does not excoriate or damage the skin in other ways once the psoriasis is adequately treated, whereas psoriatic arthritis, if it is severe enough, can cause irreversible bony destruction. No topical medications are known to help psoriatic arthritis, and systemic therapies such as methotrexate and etanercept (Enbrel) are FDA approved for both psoriasis and psoriatic arthritis.

There are also many different forms of psoriasis. Plaque-type psoriasis is the most common form and comprises 80% to 90% of those with psoriasis. Other less-common forms of psoriasis include pustular psoriasis, erythrodermic psoriasis, guttate psoriasis, and inverse psoriasis. When determining treatment, the form of psoriasis should also be taken into consideration because certain forms of psoriasis are more responsive to certain therapies. Trigger factors for psoriatic flares are listed in Table 1.

## TREATMENT

There are many topical and systemic medications to choose from to treat psoriasis. Our recommendation is to learn a few of these agents well, with a good understanding of appropriate patient selection, expected results, and side effects, because mastering all available agents for psoriasis is probably beyond the scope of a general practitioner.

### Topical Therapies

Topical steroids and calcipotriene (Dovonex) are two of the most useful topical agents, especially in a primary care setting, and will be discussed in some detail. Other perhaps more complicated topical agents, such as tazarotene, anthralin, and tar preparations, will be briefly described.

#### Topical Steroids

Topical steroids are best suited for a *quick fix* or rapid improvement when the patient first presents. To obtain an adequate response in psoriasis, however, the physician usually must use a stronger topical steroid than what is typically used when treating other common, chronic inflammatory conditions such as eczema or seborrheic dermatitis. Topical steroids weaker than medium potency generally are ineffective for plaque-type psoriasis, especially in nonsensitive areas such as the elbows and knees, where often a high-strength or even

**TABLE 1  Triggers for Psoriatic Flare**

- Traumatic injury to the skin
- Streptococcal infection
- Stress
- Cold weather
- Drugs: systemic corticosteroid withdrawal, β-blockers, ACE inhibitors, lithium, antimalarials, interferons
- Excessive alcohol

*Abbreviation:* ACE = angiotensin-converting enzyme.

superpotent topical steroid is necessary to control the psoriasis adequately.

The most distressing adverse effects associated with topical steroids are skin atrophy, including striae or stretch marks because of their unsightliness and irreversibility, and the risk of adrenal suppression. Steroid-sensitive areas that need special consideration include face, axillae, inframammary folds, abdominal pannus, inner thighs, and groin. If steroids must be used in high-risk areas, physicians should first try those from classes 5, 6, or 7. Topical steroids from class 4 are usually the highest potency acceptable for use in steroid-sensitive areas.

Adrenal suppression can occur with any of the medium-potent to superpotent topical steroids. The amount of superpotent topical steroid applied each week should be limited to no more than 50 to 60 g/week for an adult to avoid risk of adrenal suppression. The FDA recommends that class I, or superpotent, topical steroids such as clobetasol (Temovate) or halobetasol (Ultravate) be used for no more than 2 weeks at a time.

Topical steroid use in psoriasis is also well known to be associated with tachyphylaxis, a phenomenon in which the drugs initially work well, but efficacy gradually diminishes with continuous use. To regain efficacy, the physician needs to increase steroid potency or give the patient a *steroid holiday* lasting several months.

Whenever topical steroids are discontinued, they should be tapered off rather than abruptly stopped, because abrupt discontinuation may lead to a rebound phenomenon. In this rare phenomenon, psoriasis suddenly becomes worse than pretreatment after the medication is discontinued.

#### Calcipotriene

A topical vitamin D analogue, known as calcipotriene (Dovonex) in the United States and calcipotriol (Daivonex) in other countries, is not only the first elegant nonsteroidal alternative for the treatment of psoriasis but is also the most prescribed single agent for psoriasis worldwide. Twice daily application of calcipotriene ointment has been shown in two randomized, double-blind, multicenter studies to be more effective than a high-potency topical steroid ointment, fluocinonide (Lidex), twice daily.

One of the most important features of calcipotriene that makes it an excellent agent for primary care physicians as well as dermatologists is its safety profile. It is steroid free, and thus free from steroidal side effects such as skin thinning, striae formation, and adrenal suppression. The main side effect of calcipotriene is lesional and perilesional (around the lesion) irritation. Irritation from calcipotriene usually presents with a red ring of inflamed skin surrounding the treated lesions. Patients may report a mild stinging or burning sensation. This is usually transient and patients quickly become accustomed to it. In clinical trials of calcipotriene, only 1 in 25 research subjects had to discontinue treatment because of skin irritation. Skin irritation from calcipotriene is usually more pronounced on the face and occluded parts of the body such as the axillae and groin. This is because skin irritation appears to depend largely on the penetration of calcipotriene through the skin; the intertriginous areas are occlusive by nature and, therefore, enhance the penetration of calcipotriene through the skin. Furthermore, calcipotriene is lipophilic and more readily absorbed by skin containing oily sebaceous glands, such as the face, which also helps to explain why it tends to be more irritating on the face.

Calcipotriene irritation does not necessarily preclude its use. This can often be prevented by decreasing the penetration of calcipotriene through the skin. One way is to use the cream formulation instead of the ointment formulation. Using smaller amounts and reducing the frequency of application to once a day or every other day instead of twice a day is another method of reducing penetration and irritation. Once this regimen is tolerated, the frequency of application can be increased carefully. Another strategy used by many dermatologists at the initiation of therapy is combining calcipotriene with a topical steroid. Calcipotriene has been proven to be chemically compatible with the topical steroid halobetasol propionate (Ultravate) when mixed and applied together for up to 48 hours. Rarely, calcipotriene may cause excessive peeling and apparent expansion of erythema beyond the original border of the psoriatic lesion. If this peculiar perilesional peeling occurs, and if the patient is asymptomatic, it is best to reassure the patient that this reaction is self-limited and to encourage continued use of calcipotriene.

The systemic side effect to be aware of when prescribing calcipotriene is hypercalcemia. Hypercalcemia has been reported only in rare instances when a patient has used large amounts of this medication on the body. A good guideline to follow is to limit total weekly use of calcipotriene to no more than 100 to 120 g/week. One can instruct the patient to use no more than one large tube per week, because 120 g is the largest tube size available.

For those who wish for at least 75% or better improvement, which is what most patients would consider satisfactory response, it is good to know that the efficacy of once-daily calcipotriene is approximately half that of twice-daily use. Because many patients find time to apply topical medications only once a day, which may lead to slow onset of action and relative dissatisfaction, most dermatologists in the United States use calcipotriene not as monotherapy but rather in combination with other treatments. Combination of calcipotriene with other treatments not only increases the rate of improvement and offers greater improvement but, in the case of topical steroids, also a reduction of side effects. The topical steroid decreases the risk of skin irritation by calcipotriene, and calcipotriene prevents skin atrophy by the topical steroid.

One of the authors' favorite topical combination therapy for psoriasis is sequential therapy (Table 2).

### Other Topical Agents

Other topical agents that are either less effective, have more side effects, or involve special instructions are described in the following text.

Tazarotene (Tazorac) is the only topical retinoid approved in the United States for plaque-type psoriasis. It is available in two strengths, 0.05% and 0.1%, and two formulations, cream and gel. It is applied once daily in the evening. Tazarotene offers a somewhat longer duration of remission than other topical agents for psoriasis but tends to be significantly much more irritating. Tazarotene should be applied sparingly only to the psoriatic plaques, avoiding the surrounding normal skin. Concurrent use of a topical steroid every morning increases efficacy and reduces tazarotene irritation. Mometasone furoate (Elocon) has demonstrated a synergistic effect when used in combination with tazarotene. Tazarotene is a category X medication, which is contraindicated during pregnancy.

Anthralin has been used to treat psoriasis for more than 100 years. However, it is one of the less commonly used agents in the United States because of its tendency to stain skin, clothing, and linens; risk of irritation; and moderate efficacy. Anthralin is applied once daily to affected areas for 30 minutes to 1 hour and then washed off.

### TABLE 2 Topical Sequential Therapy

Step I (clearing phase): 2 weeks to 1 month
- Halobetasol (Ultravate)* + calcipotriene (Dovonex) bid (mixed immediately prior to application)

Step II (transitional phase): 1 month to indefinitely for some patients
- Calcipotriene (Dovonex) bid on weekdays
- Calcipotriene (Dovonex) + halobetasol (Ultravate) bid on weekends

Step III (maintenance phase): indefinitely or until clearance
- Calcipotriene (Dovonex) bid

*Generic halobetasol or clobetasol can be substituted if necessary, but chemical compatibility with calcipotriene (Dovonex) is unknown.

Coal tar is a mixture of at least 10,000 components, most of which have not been identified. Tar products are available in many different formulations and strengths. Crude coal tar in combination with phototherapy in a specialized daycare setting is still the most effective and safe treatment available for moderate to severe psoriasis since it was first described by Goeckerman in 1925. Messiness is the main drawback. Compared to other treatments, tar remains one of the safest. In response to a California lawsuit, the FDA has ruled that there is no convincing evidence of carcinogenic risk with human therapeutic use of coal tar in concentrations up to 5%.

Salicylic acid is a keratolytic agent that acts to remove excess scale and hyperkeratosis associated with psoriasis. It does not affect erythema or induration. Salicylic acid is commercially available over the counter as 6% Keralyt gel. Salicylic acid can produce local irritation and erythema. It is probably best to avoid salicylic acid in patients with diabetes, because systemic absorption of salicylic acid can inhibit gluconeogenesis and lead to hypoglycemia in diabetics.

### Systemic Therapies

For moderate to severe psoriasis, phototherapy or systemic therapy is usually required. Phototherapy options include ultraviolet B (UVB) light and psoralen plus ultraviolet light of A wavelength (PUVA). There are two types of UVB phototherapy: broadband and narrowband. Narrowband UVB (NBUVB) is more effective for psoriasis than broadband UVB therapy. Oral agents approved by the FDA for psoriasis include acitretin (Soriatane), methotrexate, and cyclosporine (Neoral) (Table 3). There are now four FDA-approved biologic agents for psoriasis: etanercept (Enbrel), efalizumab (Raptiva), infliximab

### TABLE 3 Summary of Oral Agents

| Drug | Dose | Laboratory Monitoring | Main Adverse Effects |
| --- | --- | --- | --- |
| Acitretin (Soriatane) | 10–50 mg qd | - CBC<br>- LFT<br>- Fasting lipid profile<br>- Pregnancy test | - Mucocutaneous changes<br>- Teratogenicity<br>- Hyperlipidemia<br>- Hepatotoxicity |
| Methotrexate | 15–30 mg/wk | - CBC<br>- LFT<br>- BUN and creatinine<br>- Liver biopsy<br>- Pregnancy test | - Bone marrow suppression<br>- Teratogenicity |
| Cyclosporine (Neoral) | 3–5 mg/kg/d divided bid | - CBC<br>- LFT<br>- BUN and creatinine<br>- Fasting lipid profile<br>- Urinalysis<br>- Potassium and magnesium<br>- Blood pressure | - Nephrotoxicity<br><br>- Hypertension<br>- Paresthesias<br>- Hyperlipidemia |

Abbreviations: BUN = blood urea nitrogen; CBC = complete blood count; LFT = liver function test.

## TABLE 4  Summary of Biologic Agents

| Drug | Dose | Laboratories | Adverse Events |
|------|------|--------------|----------------|
| Etanercept (Enbrel) | 50 mg biweekly for 3 months, then either 50 mg once weekly or 25 mg biweekly | | • Reactivation of TB* <br> • Multiple sclerosis* <br> • Congestive heart failure* <br> • Lupus* <br> • Bone marrow suppression* |
| Efalizumab (Raptiva) | 1 mg/kg SC weekly | CBC with platelet counts recommended but not required | • Flulike symptoms <br> • Psoriasis worsening <br> • Arthritis worsening* <br> • Thrombocytopenia* <br> • Hemolytic anemia* |
| Alefacept (Amevive) | 15 mg IM weekly for 12 weeks | CD4 counts weekly during treatment | • Decreased CD4 count if the count becomes less than 250 |
| Infliximab (Remicade) | 5 mg/kg IV at weeks 0, 2, and 6, then every 8 weeks thereafter | CBC, LFT | • Infusion reactions <br> • Infections <br> • Autoantibodies/lupus <br> • Malignancies <br> • Heart failure <br> • Hepatotoxity <br> • Hematologic events* <br> • Neurologic events* |

*Causal relationship with the drug has not been established because of the rarity of these cases.
*Abbreviations:* CBD = complete blood count; IM = intramuscularly; SC = subcutaneously; TB = tuberculosis.

(Remicade)and alefacept (Amevive) (Table 4). Specialized centers can also provide Ingram therapy (anthralin and UVB combination therapy) and Goeckerman therapy (tar and UVB combination therapy).

## Seborrheic Dermatitis

Seborrheic dermatitis is a common, chronic inflammatory scaling condition of unknown cause typically confined to the sebaceous gland-rich skin of the head and trunk. It is seen in early infancy and in adulthood and is more common in men than women. Seborrheic dermatitis affects approximately 3% to 5% of adults. Patients infected by HIV have a higher prevalence of seborrheic dermatitis.

Infantile seborrheic dermatitis typically involves the scalp, the flexural creases, and the diaper area. Thick, yellowish-white plates of scales often develop on the scalp, and this has been colloquially termed *cradle cap*. Erythematous plaques with sharply defined borders and a glazed or shiny surface are characteristic. Small erythematous papules with fine scales may be scattered around and between larger plaques. Scales may be absent in flexural areas.

Adults with seborrheic dermatitis usually have diffuse erythema and scaling of the hair-bearing portions of the scalp. Typical lesions are well-defined pink plaques with powdery scale that form in the eyebrows, glabella, nasolabial folds, and the postauricular sulci. Occasionally, the presternal, interscapular, or genital skin is affected. Pruritus may or may not be present.

Mild seborrheic dermatitis can be treated with shampoos containing tar, selenium sulfide (Selsun), or zinc pyrithione (Head & Shoulders). These may be used daily on the affected areas including scalp, face, and other involved sites until the condition is under control, then once or twice weekly for maintenance. Moderate cases often respond to shampoos or creams containing 2% ketoconazole (Nizoral), used daily until it is under control, then once or twice weekly for maintenance. Low-potency topical steroids such as 1.0% to 2.5% hydrocortisone cream (for recalcitrant cases, stronger topical steroids such as desonide [DesOwen] cream) once or twice daily may be used initially but ideally not for maintenance therapy. Topical pimecrolimus (Elidel)[1] or topical tacrolimus (Protopic)[1] can be used as steroid-sparing agents. Thick scalp scales may be loosened with overnight application of salicylic acid 6% gel under occlusion or with Derma-Smoothe/FS oil.

## Pityriasis Rosea

Pityriasis rosea is a common, acute, inflammatory dermatosis that affects mainly older children and young adults. It is characterized by a self-limited course that often starts with a primary isolated scaly patch followed by a secondary, generalized, symmetrical, papulosquamous eruption typically distributed on the trunk and proximal extremities. The disease is more prevalent in the cooler months of the year in temperate zones. The exact cause is unknown, but a viral etiology has been speculated.

Typically, most patients will initially develop a lesion referred to as the *herald patch*, which is an asymptomatic, solitary papule that enlarges rapidly in 1 to 2 days to form an oval patch 2 to 10 cm in diameter with an erythematous, salmon-colored border with fine scaling. The trunk, primarily the anterior chest, is the most common location for the herald patch. Several days later, numerous smaller patches will appear, mainly on the trunk and proximal parts of the extremities. They are typically oval, faint pink, with a collarette of delicate scales well inside the border of the lesion. On the back, longitudinal axes of the lesions run down and out relative to the orientation of the spine in a pattern that, with imagination, has been likened to a Christmas tree. The patient may have associated itching, but pruritus is often absent. The eruption usually lasts between 2 and 10 weeks and then resolves spontaneously. There are usually no complications except for occasional postinflammatory hypopigmentation or hyperpigmentation, which resolves slowly over time, often months. Recurrence of pityriasis rosea is infrequent; occurring in less than 3% of cases.

Because secondary syphilis can mimic pityriasis rosea closely, a serologic test for syphilis should be ordered in all cases of *atypical* pityriasis rosea; for example, if there is no herald patch, if the distal extremities (especially the palms and soles) are involved or if the patient is systemically ill.

Offering the patient reassurance is usually all that is necessary for this self-limited disease. Antipruritics such as calamine lotion, a mild-potency topical steroid, or oral antihistamines may be prescribed if necessary. For severe cases, UVB phototherapy has been shown to be effective in controlling the symptoms as well as in inducing a faster remission.

### REFERENCES

Feldman S, Koo J, Lebwohl M, et al: The Psoriasis and Psoriatic Arthritis Pocket Guide. Portland, OR, National Psoriasis Foundation, 2005.

[1]Not FDA approved for this indication.

Koo J, Cheung L, Lee CS: Contemporary Diagnosis and Management in Primary Care Dermatology. Newtown, PA, Handbooks in Health Care, 2002.

Koo J, Kochavi G, Kwan J: Contemporary Diagnosis and Management of Psoriasis. Newtown, PA, Handbooks in Health Care, 2004.

Koo J, Lebwohl M, Lee CS: Therapy of Mild-to-Moderate Psoriasis. New York, Taylor & Francis, 2006.

# Connective Tissue Disorders

Method of
*John Varga, MD, Susan Manzi, MD, MPH, and Gabriella Lakos, MD, PhD*

Systemic lupus erythematosus (SLE), scleroderma (or systemic sclerosis), and the inflammatory myopathies are distinct but related idiopathic autoimmune connective tissue diseases. Each of these diseases is associated with significant morbidity and mortality. Each is characterized by considerable clinical heterogeneity and a chronic and unpredictable clinical course, often with remissions and relapses. Each is more common in women than men and associated with progressive damage to multiple organs. Prominent target organs include the skin, the cardiovascular system, the lungs, and the musculoskeletal system; in SLE, the brain and the kidneys are also affected. At the tissue level, inflammation and progressive scarring are prominent. Furthermore, each of these diseases is associated with high levels of autoantibodies in the circulation. Autoimmunity, a hallmark of connective tissue diseases, reflects a fundamental breakdown in immunologic self-tolerance. Although the connective tissue diseases have no cure, many effective treatment options are currently available. Because of their clinical heterogeneity, protean multiorgan systemic manifestations, and chronic and unpredictable course, the evaluation and management of patients with connective tissue diseases present unique challenges.

## Systemic Lupus Erythematosus

Chronic inflammation and immune dysregulation characterize SLE. The precise etiology is unknown but likely results from a combination of genetic, hormonal, and environmental factors. The spectrum of manifestations in SLE is quite broad and the time course extremely variable. Some patients develop life-threatening irreversible organ damage, whereas the most incapacitating condition in others may be fatigue. Therapy should be tailored to the individual patient and designed not only to suppress disease activity but also to alleviate symptoms as well. Patients with SLE are optimally managed by a team of specialists that may include, in addition to the rheumatologist, a dermatologist, nephrologist, cardiologist, psychiatrist, psychologist, pulmonologist, gastroenterologist, orthopedic surgeon, and physical therapist.

Although a definitive cure for SLE remains elusive, recent advances, both nonpharmacologic and pharmacologic, have significantly improved survival and quality of life. According to Manzi, established treatments fall into four main categories: nonsteroidal anti-inflammatory drugs, antimalarial agents, corticosteroids, and cytotoxic and immunosuppressive agents. Choosing an appropriate treatment regimen requires careful thought in light of the complexity and marked clinical heterogeneity of the disease and the potential long-term side effects of the drugs used. Consultation with a rheumatologist or other subspecialist with expertise in lupus is recommended.

### GENERAL PRINCIPLES OF THERAPY

As patients become more information savvy, the role of health professionals in patient education becomes crucial. Physicians and their staff should assist patients in evaluating the flow of information available through modern technology such as the Internet. A patient may be alarmed by hearing or reading about worst-case scenarios. Reassurance that the manifestations and course of disease vary considerably may ease this anxiety. Providing information about support groups may also be helpful. Moreover, physicians should recognize and address the psychological impact that a diagnosis of a chronic, potentially serious disease may have on a previously healthy individual.

Although not life-threatening, fatigue is a challenge for many SLE patients. Physicians should search for contributing factors such as hypothyroidism, fibromyalgia, or depression and must emphasize the importance of adequate rest. Overexposure to ultraviolet (UV) radiation may cause systemic disease flares in addition to skin rashes. Photosensitive patients should avoid excessive exposure to sunlight and wear protective clothing and sunscreen (SPF [sun protection factor] of 35) routinely. Certain prescription drugs, including sulfa drugs and other antibiotics, can exacerbate photosensitivity as well as other lupus disease activity.

Unexplained fever should not be ignored because lupus patients are susceptible to infections. To minimize this risk, physicians should exercise caution when prescribing immunosuppressive agents and corticosteroids and consider influenza and pneumococcal immunizations. Because a disease flare during pregnancy poses risk to the fetus, pregnancies in women with lupus are considered high risk. High-dose estrogen contraceptives should generally be avoided, particularly in patients with increased risk of blood clots; low-dose estrogen, progesterone-only pills, or other effective means of contraception should be considered. Planning pregnancies during periods of disease remission and careful monitoring of both the mother and fetus can improve the chances for healthy outcomes.

Other considerations in the general management of patients with SLE include their increased risk of cardiovascular disease and osteoporosis. Patients should be screened for these conditions and be advised to adopt a cardioprotective lifestyle and take measures to ensure their bone health. These actions include smoking cessation, moderate intake of alcohol, heart-healthy diet, adequate intake of dietary calcium and vitamin D, and regular weight-bearing exercise. Although no definitive link is established between SLE and malignancy, routine gynecologic testing and breast examinations should be performed.

### NONSTEROIDAL ANTI-INFLAMMATORY DRUGS

Although nonsteroidal anti-inflammatory drugs (NSAIDs) do not have disease-modifying properties in SLE, they are used to treat fever, pleuritis, pericarditis, and musculoskeletal complaints (Figure 1). Because SLE patients may take NSAIDs for long periods of time, consideration should be given to gastroprotective agents. Furthermore, the potential adverse effects of these drugs on the kidney, liver, and central nervous system may be confused with worsening disease activity. Table 1 lists the general recommendations for monitoring NSAIDs and other commonly used agents in SLE.

### ANTIMALARIAL AGENTS

Antimalarial agents are frequently prescribed in the treatment of SLE. The most commonly used are hydroxychloroquine (Plaquenil)[1] and chloroquine (Aralen).[1] Antimalarials are regularly used in the management of cutaneous and musculoskeletal manifestations, constitutional symptoms, and in some cases serositis. Antimalarials may be used in combination when one agent by itself is ineffective because their actions can be synergistic. A particular benefit of antimalarial agents is their steroid-sparing effect. Hydroxychloroquine[1] (200 to 400 mg daily) is generally well tolerated, but it may take 6 to 8 weeks for the benefit to become apparent. Because of potential ophthalmologic toxicity, patients should have an ophthalmologic examination when they begin treatment and every 6 to 12 months thereafter. Although it is unclear whether antimalarials prevent major organ disease, they do have lipid-lowering and possible antiplatelet activities.

---

[1]Not FDA approved for this indication.

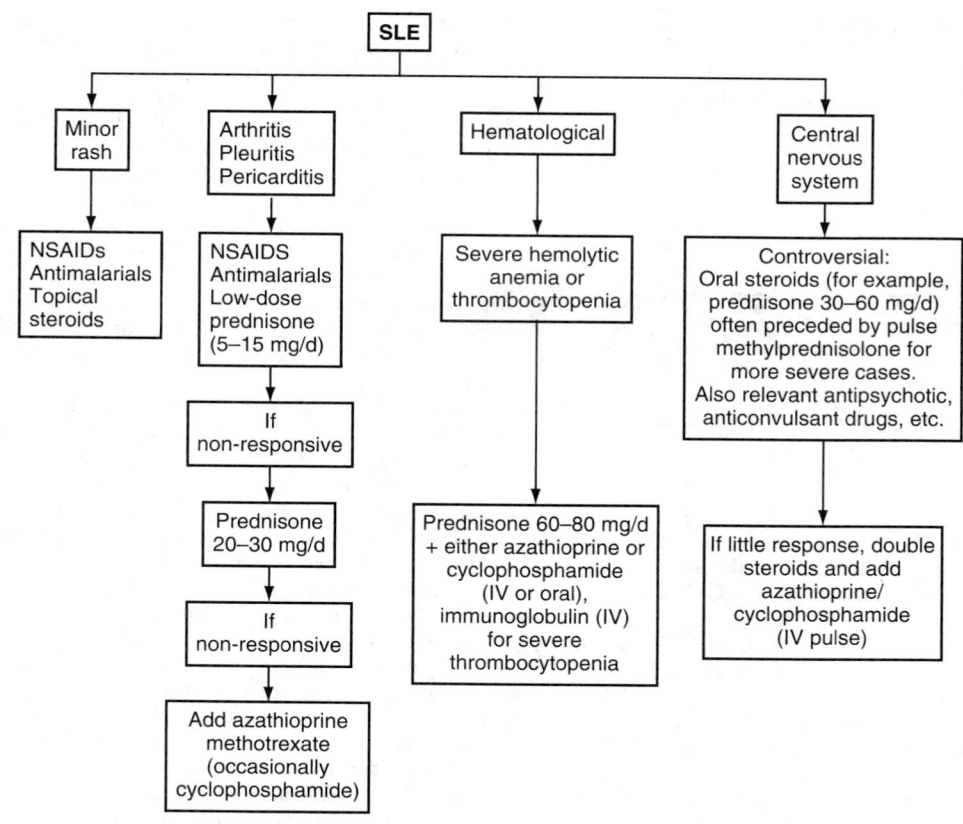

**FIGURE 1.** Management of nonrenal lupus. (Adapted from Ioannou Y, Isenberg DA: Current concepts for the management of systemic lupus erythematosus in adults: A therapeutic challenge. Postgrad Med J 2002;78:599-606.)

## CORTICOSTEROIDS

Corticosteroids are used to treat a broad spectrum of lupus manifestations. Oral administration of 5 to 30 mg of prednisone daily in single or divided doses is effective in treating constitutional symptoms, cutaneous disease, arthritis, and serositis. Once immediate relief is achieved, their dose is often tapered while slower-acting agents such as antimalarials or immunomodulatory therapy are added. For more serious organ involvement, such as nephritis, central nervous system or hematologic abnormalities, or systemic vasculitis, prednisone at higher doses (1 to 2 mg/kg) daily or parenteral corticosteroid preparations in equivalent doses are given. Pulses of methylprednisolone (1000 mg) can be given for 3 consecutive days in severe situations. According to Ionnaou and Isenberg, the infusion should be given over several hours to minimize the risk of reactions such as joint pain, flushing, headache, or tachycardia. Although high-dose corticosteroids may be required to preserve major organ function, patients who require such aggressive treatment over extended periods are subjected to highly unfavorable side effects, including emotional lability, weight gain, hypertension, hyperlipidemia, diabetes, glaucoma, risk of infection, avascular necrosis of bone, and osteoporosis. It is recommended that treating physicians attempt to taper corticosteroids to discontinuation or to a minimal dose administered daily or on alternate days once disease activity is controlled.

## CYTOTOXIC AGENTS

Aggressive therapy with cytotoxic agents is required for patients with severe disease involving major organs. In general, such therapy should be administered by specialists aware of the potential dangers involved. Cyclophosphamide (Cytoxan)[1] and azathioprine (Imuran),[1] are the agents most commonly prescribed. Methotrexate (Rheumatrex),[1]

mycophenolate mofetil (CellCept),[1] and intravenous immunoglobulin (IVIG)[1] also show promising results.

### Cyclophosphamide

According to Ortmann and Klippel, cyclophosphamide[1] is the drug of choice for treating most forms of lupus nephritis (Figure 2). Glucocorticoids in combination with intravenous bolus regimens of cyclophosphamide (0.5 to 1.0 g/m²) is more effective than glucocorticoids alone in preserving renal function. Cyclophosphamide[1] appears to be most effective in diffuse proliferative lupus nephritis, although it may also be useful in membranous nephropathy. Less severe forms of lupus nephritis are commonly treated with corticosteroids alone; however, physicians should be prepared to administer immunosuppressive agents if more severe nephritis develops or if patients develop unacceptable side effects from corticosteroids. Renal biopsy is helpful in determining the therapy of choice. Regardless of the type of immunosuppressant used, it is necessary to control blood pressure effectively to prevent irreversible organ damage. Cyclophosphamide[1] is also effective in nonrenal manifestations of SLE, such as cytopenia, central nervous system disease, pulmonary hemorrhage, and vasculitis.

Cyclophosphamide[1] has numerous undesirable side effects. Nausea, vomiting, hair loss, infertility, and bone marrow suppression are the most common. Gastrointestinal toxicity can be minimized with the administration of antiemetics, and hair loss is normally reversible when treatment is discontinued. Older age and cumulative dose appear to be the major risk factors for infertility. Adjusting the dose of cyclophosphamide[1] can often regulate leukopenia, which typically peaks 8 to 12 days after intravenous administration. Patients on cyclophosphamide[1] are also at increased risk for infections, particularly herpes zoster. Bladder carcinoma can develop even years after cyclophosphamide[1]

---

[1]Not FDA approved for this indication.

[1]Not FDA approved for this indication.

**TABLE 1  Standard Drug Therapies in Systemic Lupus Erythematosus and Recommended Monitoring Strategies**

| Drug | Toxicities Requiring Monitoring | Baseline Evaluation | Monitoring | |
|---|---|---|---|---|
| | | | System Review | Laboratory |
| Salicylates, nonsteroidal anti-inflammatory drugs | Gastrointestinal bleeding, hepatic toxicity, hypertension | CBC, creatinine, urinalysis, AST, ALT | Dark/black stool, dyspepsia, nausea/vomiting, abdominal pain, shortness of breath, edema | CBC yearly, creatinine yearly |
| Hydroxychloroquine | Macular damage | None unless patient is over 40 y of age or has previous eye disease | Visual changes | Funduscopic and visual fields q 6-12 mo |
| Glucocorticoids | Hypertension, hyperglycemia, hyperlipidemia, hypokalemia, osteoporosis, avascular necrosis, cataract, weight gain, infections, fluid retention | BP, bone densitometry, glucose, potassium, cholesterol, triglycerides (HDL, LDL) | Polyuria, polydipsia, edema, shortness of breath, BP at each visit, visual changes, bone pain | Urinary dipstick for glucose q 3-6 mo, total cholesterol yearly, bone densitometry yearly to assess osteoporosis |
| Azathioprine | Myelosuppression, hepatotoxicity, lymphoproliferative disorders | CBC, platelet count, creatinine, AST or ALT | Symptoms of myelosuppression | CBC and platelet count q 1-2 wk with changes in dose (q 1-3 mo thereafter), AST yearly, PAP test at regular intervals |
| Cyclophosphamide | Myelosuppression, myeloproliferative disorders, malignancy, immunosuppression, hemorrhagic cystitis, secondary infertility | CBC and differential and platelet count, urinalysis | Symptoms of myelosuppression, hematuria, infertility | CBC and urinalysis monthly; urine cytology and PAP test yearly for life |
| Methotrexate | Myelosuppression, hepatic fibrosis, cirrhosis, pulmonary infiltrates, fibrosis | CBC, chest radiograph within past year, hepatitis B, C serology in high-risk patients, AST, albumin, bilirubin, creatinine | Symptoms of myelosuppression, shortness of breath, nausea/vomiting, oral ulcer | CBC and platelet count, AST or ALT, and albumin q 4-8 wk, serum creatinine, urinalysis |
| Mycophenolate mofetil | Myelosuppression, gastrointestinal | CBC and differential and platelet count, creatinine, AST, ALT | Symptoms of myelosuppression, nausea, diarrhea | CBC and platelet count q1-2 wk with changes in dose (q 1-3 mo thereafter), AST, ALT, creatinine q 1-3 mo. |

*Abbreviations:* ALT = alanine transaminase; AST = aspartate transaminase; BP = blood pressure; CBC = complete blood count; HDL = high-density lipoprotein; LDL = low-density lipoprotein.
Adapted from Manzi S: Treatment of systemic lupus erythematosus. In Klippel JH, Stone J, Weyand C, Crofford LJ (eds): Primer on the Rheumatic Diseases. Atlanta, Arthritis Foundation, 2001, pp 346-352.

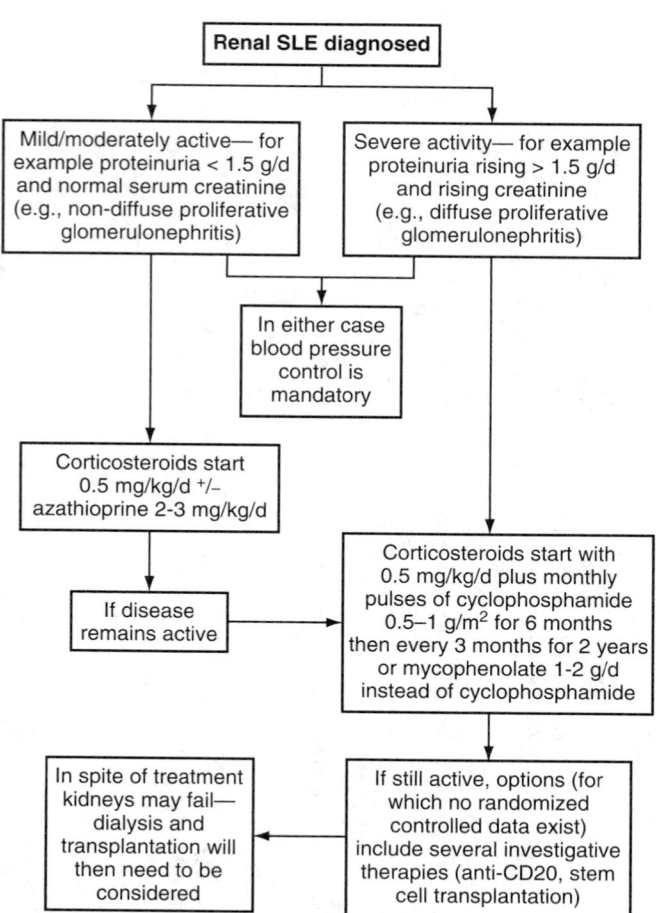

**Renal SLE diagnosed**

Mild/moderately active— for example proteinuria < 1.5 g/d and normal serum creatinine (e.g., non-diffuse proliferative glomerulonephritis)

Severe activity— for example proteinuria rising > 1.5 g/d and rising creatinine (e.g., diffuse proliferative glomerulonephritis)

In either case blood pressure control is mandatory

Corticosteroids start 0.5 mg/kg/d +/– azathioprine 2-3 mg/kg/d

If disease remains active

Corticosteroids start with 0.5 mg/kg/d plus monthly pulses of cyclophosphamide 0.5–1 g/m² for 6 months then every 3 months for 2 years or mycophenolate 1-2 g/d instead of cyclophosphamide

In spite of treatment kidneys may fail— dialysis and transplantation will then need to be considered

If still active, options (for which no randomized controlled data exist) include several investigative therapies (anti-CD20, stem cell transplantation)

**FIGURE 2.** Management of renal lupus. (Adapted from Ioannou Y, Isenberg DA: Current concepts for the management of systemic lupus erythematosus in adults: A therapeutic challenge. Postgrad Med J 2002;78:599-606.)

therapy has stopped; thus urinalysis, urine cytology, and cystoscopy are indicated in patients with hematuria.

### Azathioprine (Imuran)

Azathioprine[1] can be used for lupus nephritis, as a steroid-sparing agent in patients with nonrenal manifestations, and in patients at low risk for progressive renal failure. Azathioprine[1] is generally started at 50 mg daily and increased by 25 mg per week to a maintenance dose of 2 to 3 mg/kg daily. Azathioprine[1] is generally better tolerated than cyclophosphamide[1]; however, bone marrow, hepatic, and gastrointestinal toxicity are common.

### Methotrexate (Rheumatrex)

Much evidence supports the effectiveness of methotrexate in rheumatoid arthritis, but very few controlled studies have been conducted in SLE. Evidence suggests that methotrexate at 15 to 20 mg per week is effective in controlling cutaneous and articular manifestations. Because side effects are common at high doses, methotrexate[1] is currently used primarily as a steroid-sparing agent in milder SLE.

### Mycophenolate Mofetil (CellCept)

Mycophenolate mofetil[1] (500 to 1000 mg twice daily) appears to be effective for lupus nephritis. In one small study, it was effective in

reducing proteinuria and improving serum creatinine in severe lupus nephritis refractory to cyclophosphamide. A recent randomized, open-label, noninferiority trial supports the notion that MMF appeared to be as effective as intravenous cyclophosphamide in inducing short-term remission of lupus nephritis with a better safety profile. The role of MMF in improving long-term outcomes of lupus nephritis remains unknown. An ongoing larger, multicenter, randomized, controlled trial will examine the effectiveness of MMF compared with intravenous cyclophosphamide during induction, and MMF compared with azathioprine during the maintenance phase. MMF is a promising addition to the armamentarium for treatment for lupus nephritis, particularly in young women of childbearing potential when there are concerns of infertility.

### Intravenous Immunoglobulin

Intravenous immunoglobulin (IVIG)[1] is used most commonly for the treatment of refractory thrombocytopenia. Platelet counts rise rapidly following initiation of treatment at 400 mg/kg daily. Similar doses have produced improvements in arthritis, nephritis, fever, mucocutaneous manifestations, and immunologic parameters. Patients with SLE-associated IgA deficiency should be treated with alternative therapies. Common side effects of IVIG include fever, myalgia, arthralgia, and headache; rarely, aseptic meningitis and thromboembolism can occur.

## Immunoablation and Autologous Stem Cell Transplantation

The rationale behind immunoablation with cyclophosphamide, followed by stem cell transplantation, is to "rescue" bone marrow of the patient with autologous stem cell transplantation after receiving a high myeloablative dose of cyclophosphamide. In addition, a high-dose cyclophosphamide regimen is purported to reset the naive immune response in the bone marrow stem cells by destroying the autoreactive lymphocytes. In the retrospective analysis of 53 patients with refractory SLE who underwent immunoablation and autologous stem cell transplantation, the European group found a remission rate based on a reduction of SLE disease activity index (SLEDAI) to less than 3 in 66% of these patients. However, the one-year transplant-related mortality was high, at 12%. A recent open-label study demonstrated a reduction in disease activity by nonmyeloablative autologous hematopoietic stem cell transplantation in patients with refractory SLE. The long-term risk/benefit ratio of this treatment modality remains unclear.

## Novel Therapies

Moving away from "global" immunosuppression by traditional drug therapies for SLE, "designed" therapeutics of the future provide improved efficacy and lower toxicity by targeting specific steps in the pathogenesis of SLE while preserving immunocompetence. Many of the novel therapeutics are being developed and studied currently in clinical trials. Some of the promising novel therapies are discussed in the following overview.

### B-CELL DEPLETION

Rituximab and epratuzumab are two antibody-based agents, which target a specific cell-surface antigen on B cells and result in B-cell depletion. Rituximab is a chimeric monoclonal antibody that binds CD20 on the surface of B cells. It is the first monoclonal antibody therapy approved by the FDA for the treatment of non-Hodgkin's lymphoma and, more recently, rheumatoid arthritis. In open-label clinical studies, rituximab has been shown to be beneficial in the treatment of patients with SLE. Various dosing regiments have been used to achieve complete B-cell depletion. A multicenter randomized placebo-controlled (Phase II/III) trial has begun to study the efficacy of rituximab in patients with moderate to severe lupus flares. Another similar Phase III trial will study the efficacy of rituximab in the treatment of

---

[1]Not FDA approved for this indication.

[1]Not FDA approved for this indication.

lupus nephritis in adult patients. (Epratuzumab is a human monoclonal antibody that targets CD22 on B cells. In an open-label Phase II trial, epratuzumab showed efficacy in patients with SLE, despite causing only modest B-cell depletion.)

## INHIBITION OF B-CELL SURVIVAL

B-cell activating factor (BAFF)/B-cell stimulator (BlyS) modulates B-cell survival and maturation, and is a member of the TNF superfamily. Belimumab is a human BAFF monoclonal antibody that recognizes BlyS and reduced B-cell proliferation and differentiation in animal models. A Phase II clinical trial revealed that belimumab performed better than placebo at reducing lupus disease activity in a subset of SLE patients with elevated anti-dsDNA antibodies and low serum C3. A Phase III trial is currently under way.

## INHIBITION OF COSTIMULATORY INTERACTIONS

Abatacept is a fusion protein of CTLA4-Ig that binds to B7 molecules (CD80/CD86) on dendritic cells and blocks the binding of costimulatory molecules CD80 and CD86 with CD28 on T cells, thereby interrupting signals required for the activation of naive T cells and their downstream effects on B-cell activation. This drug has been approved by the FDA for the treatment of rheumatoid arthritis. Multicenter clinical trials are currently under way in SLE.

## CYTOKINE BLOCKADE

TNF-$\alpha$ inhibitors (etanercept, infliximab, and adalimumab) have been very successful in the treatment of rheumatoid arthritis and psoriatic arthritis. A small open-label study of infliximab in SLE showed significant improvement in patients with refractory nephritis, despite a parallel increase in levels of anti-dsDNA antibodies. However anti-TNF-$\alpha$ therapy has been associated with autoantibody production, specifically anti-dsDNA antibodies, in patients with various autoimmune conditions. Anti-TNF-$\alpha$ therapy has also been associated with several cases of demyelinating disease. Controlled clinical trials are needed to determine the long-term safety and efficacy of this therapy in SLE.

Interleukin 6 (IL-6) is another proinflammatory cytokine secreted predominantly by macrophages, and tocilizumab is a humanized monoclonal antibody against IL-6 receptor (IL-6R) that suppresses IL-6 signalling mediated by both membranous and soluble IL-6R. The results of an open-label trial of IL-6 blockade are not yet available.

Elevated serum levels of interferon-$\alpha$ are found in patients with SLE. More recent studies showed a striking interferon-$\alpha$ signature on gene expression in peripheral blood mononuclear cells of patients with SLE compared with those of controls. Interferon-$\alpha$ modulation may be another promising therapeutic target for use in the treatment of SLE.

There is an explosion of new potential drug therapies for lupus currently being testing in clinical trials. The complexity of lupus suggests that a variety of therapeutic options will be needed to successfully treat this disease.

# Scleroderma/Systemic Sclerosis

Scleroderma, or systemic sclerosis (SSc), is a chronic connective tissue disease characterized by evidence of widespread vascular injury, autoimmunity, fibroproliferative process, and variable clinical course. Localized sclerodermas (morphea and linear scleroderma) are distinct from SSc, occur more frequently in children, and are not associated with internal organ involvement. According to Mayes and colleagues, median survival in SSc is 11 years. Survival is determined by the extent of internal organ involvement. Prominent target organs include the skin, lungs, heart, kidneys, and gastrointestinal tract (Box 1). SSc has substantial clinical heterogeneity. Based on the constellation of clinical and laboratory findings present, patients are subclassified as "limited cutaneous SSc" or "diffuse cutaneous SSc" (Box 2). These two subtypes predict distinct patterns of organ involvement, clinical course, and survival. Some patients with SSc show features of overlap with other autoimmune diseases and manifest sicca syndrome, arthritis, myositis, or thyroiditis.

---

**BOX 1 Prominent Organ Involvement in Systemic Sclerosis (SSc)**

- Skin (inflammation, induration and tethering; hyper- and hypopigmentation, calcinosis)
- Lungs (alveolitis and pulmonary fibrosis; pulmonary arterial hypertension)
- Heart (restrictive cardiomyopathy, pericarditis)
- Peripheral vascular (mucocutaneous telangiectasia, Raynaud's phenomenon, digital ulcers and infarction, watermelon stomach, male erectile dysfunction)
- Gastrointestinal tract (see Box 4)
- Muscle (myositis)
- Joints (contractures, arthralgia, tendon friction rubs)

---

## GENERAL PRINCIPLES OF THERAPY

In light of the clinical heterogeneity of SSc and its variable course, treatment must be individualized according to the unique needs of each patient; some need early aggressive intervention, whereas others need a conservative symptom-based approach with close monitoring. According to Bryan and colleagues, predictors of poor outcome include older age onset (>60 years of age), anemia, evidence of significant cardiac or pulmonary involvement, tendon friction rubs, and the presence of antitopoisomerase antibodies. In general, therapies fall into two groups: those that target the underlying pathophysiologic process, and those that alleviate or reverse target organ complications. Because major internal organ involvement develops early, disease-modifying interventions should be considered before tissue damage becomes established. Because SSc is invariably a multisystem disease, a coordinated approach to evaluation and management by an integrated multidisciplinary team including a rheumatologist, pulmonologist, cardiologist, gastroenterologist, vascular or orthopedic surgeon, and physical therapist is desirable. Patients should also be given the opportunity to participate in controlled clinical trials on novel therapeutic agents.

## DISEASE-MODIFYING THERAPIES

To date, no therapy is shown conclusively to be disease modifying in SSc. Nonetheless, based on historical or anecdotal evidence or empirical considerations, many agents are used widely in an attempt to reverse or halt the progression of the immunologic, vascular, and fibrotic damage (Box 3). In light of the potential toxicities associated with these therapies and their lack of proven benefit, decisions regarding their use must be considered carefully. In patients with limited SSc and stable disease, organ-based treatments directed toward specific complications of the disease (see later) are generally more appropriate than these generalized disease-modifying treatment strategies.

---

**BOX 2 Clinical Features of Systemic Sclerosis (SSc) Subsets**

- Limited cutaneous SSc
  - Limited extent of skin induration (distal extremities and face); no truncal skin involvement; slowly progressive
  - Prominent vascular involvement (cutaneous telangiectasia, Raynaud's phenomenon, digital ulcers; pulmonary hypertension)
  - Calcinosis cutis
  - Antibodies to centromere
- Diffuse cutaneous SSc
  - Progressive and diffuse skin induration; truncal involvement frequent
  - Pulmonary fibrosis
  - Scleroderma renal crisis
  - Antibodies to topoisomerase-I

**TABLE 2  Oral Vasodilator Therapy for Raynaud's Phenomenon in Systemic Sclerosis**

| Agent | Dose |
| --- | --- |
| **Calcium Channel Blockers** | |
| Nifedipine (Procardia) | 10-30 mg three times daily |
| Diltiazem (Cardizem) | 30-120 mg three times daily |
| Amlodipine (Norvasc) | 5-20 mg daily |
| Felodipine (Plendil) | 2.5-10 mg daily |
| **Angiotensin II Receptor Antagonists** | |
| Losartan (Cozaar) | 25-100 mg daily |
| Valsartan (Diovan) | 80-320 mg daily |
| **Sympatholytic Agents** | |
| Prazosin (Minipress) | 1-5 mg daily |
| Doxazosin (Cardura) | 1-16 mg daily |
| Nitroglycerin | 2% ointment topically once daily |

Adapted from Wigley FM: Raynaud's phenomenon. N Engl J Med 2002;347(13):1001-1008.

## ORGAN-BASED TREATMENT APPROACHES

### Therapy for Skin Involvement

Skin induration can be progressive and widespread in diffuse cutaneous SSc, whereas it is generally not prominent in limited cutaneous form. Extensive skin involvement often, but not invariably, predicts severe internal organ involvement. In diffuse SSc, skin induration generally peaks in the first 2 to 4 years of SSc, after which it regresses with spontaneous softening. In early disease, inflammation of the skin dominates, with edema, erythema, and pruritus. Patients at this stage benefit form antihistamines such as hydroxyzine (Atarax),[1] 25 mg at bedtime. Low-dose glucocorticoids such as prednisone,[1] 5 mg daily, provide substantial symptomatic relief for inflammation in early SSc but should be used with caution in light of the increased risk of scleroderma renal crisis (see later); patients taking low-dose prednisone[1] should be instructed to monitor their blood pressure daily. Digital ulcers can be managed using Duoderm[1] application to promote healing and topical povidone-iodine (Betadine)[1] solution for cleansing.

### Therapy for Vascular Involvement

#### Raynaud's Phenomenon and Its Complications

Widespread damage of small and medium-sized peripheral blood vessels is virtually universal in SSc. Endothelial cell injury is associated with release of vasoconstrictors such as thromboxane and endothelin 1 (ET1), impaired production of vasodilators such as nitric oxide and prostacyclin, and platelet aggregation and thrombosis. What starts out as a reversible dysfunction of vascular smooth muscle often progresses to irreversible structural alterations characterized by intimal layer proliferation, medial hypertrophy, and adventitial fibrosis. Reduced blood flow and repeated episodes of ischemic reperfusion in the digits, kidneys, lungs, heart, and other involved organs cause tissue ischemia, progressive vascular damage, and fibrosis.

Cold-induced Raynaud's phenomenon is the most common presenting problem in SSc and may precede other manifestations of the disease by years. Repeated and increasingly severe Raynaud's episodes lead to digital ischemia, resulting in painful ulcers and nonhealing pitting scars and, in extreme cases, digital infarction and gangrene. Patients should be counseled to stop smoking and to avoid cold exposure, which triggers vasoconstriction; not only the hands but the whole body should also be kept warm. Mild Raynaud's phenomenon can be effectively treated with orally active vasodilators (Table 2) and treatment is most commonly started with calcium channel blockers. Infection complicating digital ulcers should be treated aggressively with antibiotics; such ulcers may take months to heal and may progress to osteomyelitis. The ET1 receptor blocker bosentan (Tracleer),[1] 125 mg twice daily, is effective in preventing digital ulcers. Patients with impending digital infarction may respond to intravenous epoprostenol (Flolan),[1] 0.5 to 6 µg/kg body weight per minute for 6 to 24 hours, or nonpharmacologic interventions such as sympathetic ganglion blockade and surgical digital sympathectomy. The role of statin drugs, antioxidants such as tocopherol (vitamin E)[1] (400 IU daily), and diets rich in fish oils in preventing vascular damage in Raynaud's phenomenon are not yet adequately studied.

#### Pulmonary Arterial Hypertension

Pulmonary arterial hypertension (PAH), which occurs in at least 15% of SSc patients, has a major impact on survival. PAH may complicate interstitial pulmonary fibrosis or may occur in the absence of parenchymal lung disease; the latter is indistinguishable from primary (idiopathic) and familial pulmonary hypertension. Because PAH may be asymptomatic until advanced, it was historically underdiagnosed in SSc. Moderately severe PAH is associated with exertional dyspnea, chest pain, and syncope; right-sided heart failure is seen in late-stage disease. Emphasis must be placed on early preclinical recognition of PAH. A combination of pulmonary function testing and Doppler echocardiography is appropriate for screening and should be performed yearly. Right heart catheterization is the gold standard for determining pulmonary arterial pressures and cardiac index and for excluding pulmonary embolism.

Several new classes of agents provide at least short-term symptomatic and hemodynamic improvement in PAH. Patients with New York Heart Association functional class III or IV symptoms (ordinary activity causing dyspnea, chest pain, or near syncope) should start an orally active ET1 receptor blocker such as bosentan (Tracleer). In addition, warfarin anticoagulation (to achieve an INR [international normalized ratio] of 1.5 to 2.0), low-flow oxygen therapy, diuretics, and digitalization are generally indicated. Patients who fail to respond to ET1 antagonists may benefit from parenteral prostacyclin analogues such as inhaled iloprost (Ventavis), every 2 hours up to 45 µg daily, or continuous infusions of subcutaneous treprostinil (Remodulin) 1.25 µg/kg per minute, or intravenous epoprostenol (Flolan), 2 to 10 µg/kg per minute. A major limitation of these therapies is their cost, now exceeding $30,000 per year. Furthermore, because of their short half-lives, prostacyclin analogues must be administered by continuous infusion or frequent inhalations. Epoprostenol requires long-term ambulatory central venous catheterization, which may be complicated by line sepsis and pump failure with potentially catastrophic consequences. Combinations of a prostacyclin analogue together with an ET1 antagonist or a phosphodiesterase type 5 inhibitor such as sildenafil (Viagra),[1] up to 50 mg three times daily, appear to be well tolerated and provide added benefit. Surgical options for patients unresponsive to

[1]Not FDA approved for this indication.

[1]Not FDA approved for this indication.

pharmacologic therapies include atrial septostomy and lung transplantation. In light of the complexity involved, the evaluation and management of PAH in SSc patients should be coordinated by specialized centers having appropriate expertise.

## Therapy for Interstitial Lung Disease

Some degree of interstitial lung disease is present in most patients with SSc and is a leading cause of death. The extent and progression of pulmonary fibrosis are major determinants of outcome. Combined with pulmonary function testing, high-resolution computed tomography (HRCT) scan of the chest is more sensitive for interstitial lung disease screening than chest radiography. A ground-glass appearance generally correlates with active inflammation (alveolitis). Patients with alveolitis may benefit from cyclophosphamide (Cytoxan)[1] (orally up to 50 mg daily, or intravenously as pulse therapy up to 1000 mg/m$^2$ monthly) to stabilize lung function. Low-dose prednisone[1] (up to 20 mg daily) is often used in combination with cyclophosphamide. The optimal duration of cyclophosphamide[1] treatment is uncertain, but some experts recommend at least a year. General supportive measures include pneumococcal vaccination and yearly influenza immunization, avoidance of smoking, prevention of gastroesophageal reflux, nasal oxygen supplementation, and bronchodilators. Respiratory tract infections should be treated with empirical antibiotics. For selected patients with progressive respiratory decline, lung transplantation remains an option.

## Therapy for Gastrointestinal Tract Involvement

Gastrointestinal involvement is common, can be extensive, and significantly contributes to the morbidity of SSc. Gastroesophageal reflux may be associated with dyspepsia, dysphagia, and regurgitation and can lead to chronic esophagitis and its complications (Box 4). Reflux should be managed by elevating the head of the bed, eliminating triggers such as chocolates, alcohol, and tobacco, and restricting food intake before going to sleep. Most patients require long-term treatment with proton pump inhibitors such as omeprazole (Prilosec)[1] in doses sufficient to suppress reflux symptoms (up to 160 mg daily). Prokinetic agents such as metoclopramide (Reglan)[1] (10 mg four times daily) or erythromycin[1] (250 mg three times daily) may be effective for gastroparesis. Chronic diarrhea and malabsorption caused by small bowel bacterial overgrowth can be treated with periodic courses of tetracycline[1] (500 mg four times daily) or metronidazole (Flagyl)[1] (500 mg three times daily). Some patients benefit from subcutaneous octreotide injections (Sandostatin,)[1] (50 μg one to four times daily). Nutritional assessment and support are important aspects of management. Gastric vascular ectasia (watermelon stomach) is frequent in SSc and causes recurrent occult gastrointestinal bleeding. It can be effectively treated with laser argon ablation.

## Therapy for Renal Involvement

Scleroderma renal crisis, which develops in up to 15% of patients with SSc, was uniformly fatal in the pre– angiotensin-converting enzyme

### BOX 4 Gastrointestinal Tract Complications of Systemic Sclerosis (SSc)

- Esophageal dysmotility leading to dysphagia and chronic gastroesophageal reflux; dyspepsia, esophagitis, strictures, ulcers, pulmonary aspiration; Barrett's esophagus and esophageal adenocarcinoma
- Watermelon stomach with upper gastrointestinal bleeding
- Gastroparesis and small bowel hypomotility
- Blind loop syndrome with malabsorption, weight loss, diarrhea
- Large bowel pseudo-obstruction
- Colonic perforation
- Pneumatosis cystoides intestinalis

(ACE)[1] inhibitor era. Risk factors include progressive skin induration, male sex, and glucocorticoid use. Renal crisis characteristically manifests with an abrupt rise in blood pressure, frequently associated with retinal hemorrhages, and occasionally with seizures and pulmonary hemorrhage, microangiopathic hemolysis, and rapidly progressive oliguric renal insufficiency. The key to controlling this dreaded complication of SSc is early recognition. Accordingly, high-risk patients should monitor their blood pressure daily, and if there is a rise in blood pressure, a new onset of proteinuria, or a rise in creatinine, patients should be hospitalized for close monitoring and aggressive management. Some patients (<10%) develop scleroderma renal crisis in the absence of hypertension. Treatment with increasing doses of ACE inhibitors such as captopril (Capoten)[1] (up to 200 mg daily) should be started immediately. The creatinine may continue to rise even on ACE inhibitor therapy[1] and with adequate blood pressure control. Despite aggressive treatment, progressive renal insufficiency may ensue, necessitating dialysis. Nevertheless, up to 40% of patients may ultimately recover adequate renal function to discontinue dialysis. There is insufficient evidence to support prophylactic use of ACE inhibitors[1] in SSc.

# Polymyositis/Dermatomyositis

Idiopathic inflammatory myopathies (IIM) include adult and childhood dermatomyositis (DM), polymyositis (PM), myositis associated with malignancy or other connective tissue diseases, and inclusion body myositis (IBM) (Table 3). Although the etiology of IIM is unknown, the presence of cellular infiltrates in the muscle provides strong evidence for an immune mechanism of muscle damage. In DM, the main immune effector response appears to be humoral and directed against the microvasculature, whereas in both PM and IBM, cytotoxic CD8$^+$ T cells and macrophages invade and destroy muscle fibers. Inflammatory myopathies are characterized by progressive symmetric weakness of the proximal muscles, causing difficulty walking, standing, and lifting objects. In DM, a characteristic erythematous rash on the

[1]Not FDA approved for this indication.

[1]Not FDA approved for this indication.

### TABLE 3 Clinical Characteristics of Idiopathic Inflammatory Myopathies

| Dermatomyositis | Polymyositis | Inclusion | Body Myositis |
|---|---|---|---|
| Female to male | 2:1 | 1:1 | 1:3 |
| Age (y) | 10-80 | 30-60 | 50-70 |
| Muscle atrophy | Frequent | Rare | Frequent |
| Skin rash | Yes | No | No |
| Lung disease | Frequent | Frequent | |
| Dysphagia | Frequent | Rare | Rare |
| Arthralgia | Frequent | Rare | No |
| Malignancy | 5%-17% | Rare | No |

> **BOX 5 Rationale for Using a Second-Line Immunosuppressive Agent in Idiopathic Inflammatory Myopathy (IIM)**
>
> - Increased risk of corticosteroid-related side effects (diabetes mellitus, osteoporosis)
> - Disease relapse after corticosteroid tapering attempts jeopardy
> - Corticosteroid complications (myopathy)
> - Severe or progressive myosytis
> - Serious extramuscular manifestations
> - Lack of efficiency of corticosteroid as a single agent

face, eyelids, neck, upper chest, and back is seen. Muscle biopsy is helpful in differentiating PM/DM from drug-induced myopathies and from endocrine and metabolic myopathies. Myositis-specific antibodies may be of prognostic value; patients with Jo-1 or other anti–aminoacyl-tRNA autoantibodies are at high risk for interstitial lung disease (ILD) and show poor response to therapy. The levels of serum creatine kinase (CK) are useful in assessing disease activity. Involvement of the gastrointestinal muscles can lead to dysphagia. Patients with new myositis and especially adults with dermatomyositis, should be carefully screened for malignancy.

## GENERAL PRINCIPLES OF THERAPY

Immunosuppressive therapies are the primary treatment for the IIM. Early intervention is crucial to prevent irreversible muscle damage. Because long-term administration of high doses of corticosteroids is associated with significant morbidity, a second-line agent such as methotrexate[1] or azathioprine[1] should be introduced early. Intravenous Ig therapy,[1] cyclophosphamide (Cytoxan),[1] and cyclosporine (Neoral)[1] are also used with some benefit. Rehabilitative and physical therapeutic interventions are essential to complement pharmacologic therapy. Although PM and DM can usually be controlled by immunosuppressive agents, the treatment of IBM remains unsatisfactory.

### Corticosteroids

Prednisone[1] (1 mg/kg daily) is effective as initial therapy in the majority of the cases. In patients with rapidly progressive myositis or extramuscular manifestation such as ILD, intravenous pulse methylprednisolone[1] (1 g daily for 3 days) may be used. Both muscle strength and functional status and serum levels of CK should be checked regularly. Clinical improvement usually follows a fall in CK levels. Prednisone at 10 mg daily may be needed for 6 to 12 months. Progressive weakness in the face of declining CK levels suggests steroid myopathy.

### Other Immunosuppressive Agents

In patients who fail to respond to corticosteroids, azathioprine[1] (2 mg/kg daily) or methotrexate[1] (20 mg weekly) may be used. Box 5 shows the

[1]Not FDA approved for this indication.

## CURRENT DIAGNOSIS

- Protean manifestations in multiple organs
- Marked clinical heterogeneity
- Unpredictable, often remitting-relapsing clinical course
- Diagnosis based on characteristic constellations of clinical and laboratory features (criteria)
- Accurate diagnosis, specific subset, and stage of disease must be established

## CURRENT THERAPY

- Prompt diagnosis and early intervention are desirable.
- Treatment strategies must be individualized.
- Treatment plan must consider both short-term symptom control and long-term strategies.
- Both organ-based and disease-modification approaches are used.
- Immunosuppression is often complicated by side effects.
- Management by a multispeciality team of experts is desirable.

indications for using second-line agents. Blood cell counts and liver functions should be closely monitored. Intermittent bolus IVIG (up to 2 g/kg infused every 4 to 8 weeks) may also be effective in some steroid-resistant DM patients and for severe esophageal involvement.

## Treatment of Extramuscular Manifestations

Alveolitis and ILD are frequent complications. Some experts recommend high-dose daily corticosteroids in combination with a second-line immunosuppressive agent (cyclophosphamide,[1] azathioprine,[1] or cyclosporine[1]) early in the treatment. Skin rash can be effectively treated with hydroxychloroquine (Plaquenil)[1] (200 to 400 mg daily). Patients with severe proximal dysphagia may need a feeding tube to prevent aspiration and malnutrition.

## Rehabilitative Measures

The goal of physical therapy is to preserve existing muscle function and to prevent muscle atrophy and joint contractures. Bedridden patients should receive passive exercise, stretching, and massage. As muscle strength improves, resistive exercise followed by an active aerobic conditioning regimen can be introduced. Proximal oropharyngeal dysphagia should be managed by speech therapy.

## REFERENCES

Bryan C, Knight C, Black CM, Silman AJ: Prediction of five-year survival following presentation with scleroderma: Development of a simple model using three disease factors at first visit. Arthritis Rheum 1999;42(12):2660-2665.

Dalakas MC: High-dose intravenous immunoglobulin in inflammatory myopathies: Experience based on controlled clinical trials. Neurol Sci 2003;24(Suppl 4):S256-S259.

Ionnaou Y, Isenberg DA: Current concepts for the management of systemic lupus erythematosus in adults: A therapeutic approach. Postgrad Med J 2002;78:599-606.

Isenberg DA, Allen E, Farewell V, et al: International consensus outcome measures for patients with idiopathic inflammatory myopathies. Development and initial validation of myositis activity and damage indices in patients with adult onset disease. Rheumatology (Oxford) 2004;43(1):49-54.

Manzi S: Treatment of systemic lupus erythematosus. In Klippel JH, Stone J, Weyand C, Crofford LJ (eds): Primer on the Rheumatic Diseases. Atlanta, Arthritis Foundation, 2001, pp 346-352.

Mayes MD, Lacey JV Jr, Beebe-Dimmer J, et al: Prevalence, incidence, survival, and disease characteristics of systemic sclerosis in a large US population. Arthritis Rheum 2003;48(8):2246-2255.

Oddis CV: Idiopathic inflammatory myopathies: A treatment update. Curr Rheumatol Rep 2003;5(6):431-436.

Ortmann RA, Klippel JH: Update on cyclophosphamide for systemic lupus erythematosus. Rheum Dis Clin North Am 2000;26:363-375.

Ramirez A, Varga J: Pulmonary arterial hypertension in systemic sclerosis: Clinical manifestations, pathophysiology, evaluation, and management. Treat Respir Med 2004;3(6):339-352.

Wigley FM: Raynaud's phenomenon. N Engl J Med 2002;347(13): 1001-1008.

[1]Not FDA approved for this indication.

# Cutaneous Vasculitis

Method of

*Manisha J. Patel, MD, and Joseph L. Jorizzo, MD*

Vasculitis refers to inflammation and necrosis of blood vessels. It can be local or systemic and may be primary or secondary to another disease process. In patients with systemic involvement, the kidneys, gastrointestinal (GI) tract, or peripheral nerves may be involved. The classic cutaneous manifestation of small-vessel vasculitis is palpable purpura; the clinical manifestation greatly depends on the size and type of the vessel affected.

## Clinical Presentation

The typical primary skin lesion of small-vessel cutaneous vasculitis (CV) is palpable purpura with lesions ranging in size from 1 mm to several centimeters (Figure 1). The lesions arise as a simultaneous *crop* and result from the exposure to an inciting stimulus. Usually macular in the early stages, lesions may progress to wide array of lesions including, papules, nodules, vesicles, plaques, bullae, or pustules. Secondary findings include ulceration, necrosis, and postinflammatory hyperpigmentation. Other cutaneous findings include livedo reticularis, edema,, and urticarial lesions. Lesions most commonly occur on dependent areas, such as ankles and lower legs or other areas prone to stasis.

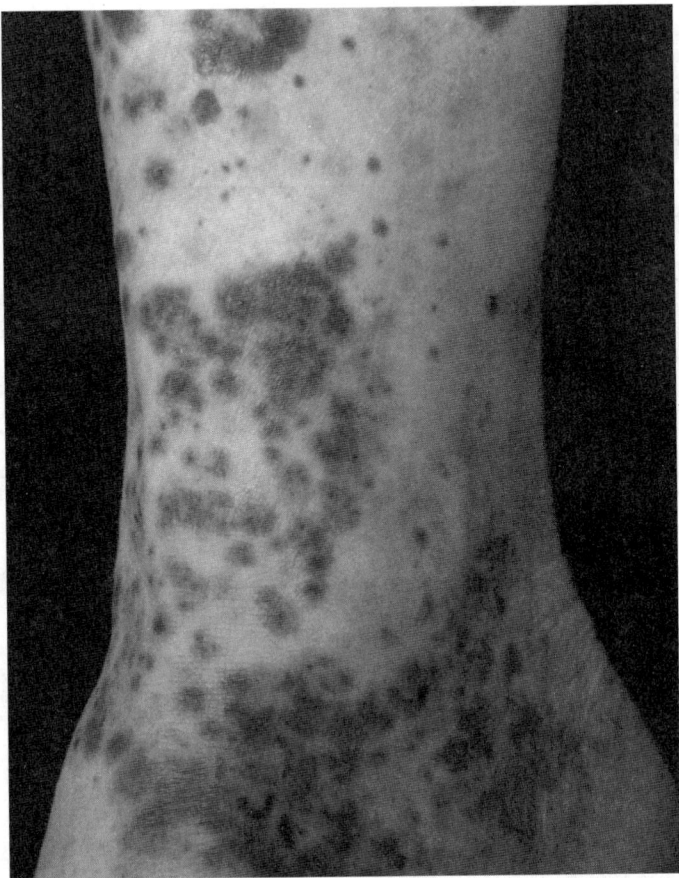

**FIGURE 1.** Small-vessel cutaneous vasculitis. Palpable purpura and early central necrosis are seen on the distal lower extremity. (Courtesy of Dr. Kelly Barham, Wake Forest University School of Medicine, Winston-Salem, NC.)

Although normally asymptomatic, local symptoms may include pruritus, pain, or burning. Systemic symptoms including fever, arthralgias, myalgias, anorexia, or GI pain should raise the suspicion that the CV may be associated with a systemic vasculitis.

Typically 50% of all patients with CV experience an acute or transient course, 30% develop chronic disease, and 20% experience relapsing disease. The percentage of patients with CV who have systemic involvement of one or more systems depends on the subspecialty of the series authors and the definition of systemic involvement. Most patients presenting to dermatologists do not have significant systemic involvement, excluding arthralgias, myalgias, fever, and serum sickness-like symptoms. It is best to consider that every patient with small-vessel CV may have systemic disease; this mandates a careful history, physical examination, and laboratory evaluation. Table 1 summarizes the key steps in evaluating suspected small-vessel CV and highlights the assessment for possible systemic involvement.

## Histopathology

The hallmark histopathologic pattern of small-vessel CV is leukocytoclastic vasculitis. The histologic specimen shows an infiltration of neutrophils within and around blood vessel walls; leukocytoclasia (degranulation and fragmentation of neutrophils leading to the production of nuclear dust); fibrinoid necrosis of the damaged vessel walls; and necrosis, swelling, and proliferation of the endothelial cells. New clinical lesions should be selected for biopsy because specimens taken too late (i.e., older than 48 hours) may show the pathology of repair more than of the initial injury. Direct immunofluorescence microscopic studies on fresh lesions frequently demonstrate perivascular deposits of IgM or activated third component of complement (C3) in the superficial dermal papillary vessels. One exception is the deposition of IgA in patients with Henoch-Schönlein purpura. Documenting leukocytoclastic vasculitis in biopsy specimens is essential to confirming the diagnosis.

## Etiology

Small-vessel CV is considered to be an aberrant immune complex response that is usually triggered by an infection, exposure to a drug, or association with an autoimmune disease; most etiologic factors identified have been incriminated by association rather than by direct demonstration. Between 50% and 60% of patients have no identifiable cause. Of the approximately 50% of patients in whom a cause is identifiable, 20% are associated with infections; and another 20% are thought to be triggered by an exposure to a drug. Bacterial infections associated with CV include streptococcus, staphylococcus, and gram-negative organisms. Several viral agents include HIV, hepatitis B and C, herpes simplex virus (HSV), and influenza. Suspected medications include antibiotics (penicillins, sulfonamides), anticonvulsants, isoniazid (Laniazid), oral contraceptives, and thiazides. Less than 5% of patients have underlying connective tissue disease. There have been patients with small-vessel CV reported rarely in patients with malignancies, especially Hodgkin's disease, mycosis fungoides, and adult T-cell lymphoma.

## Differential Diagnosis

Not all dermatoses associated with purpura are a result of vasculitis. In the differential diagnosis of vasculitis, be aware of disorders that may present with livedo or infarcted lesions secondary to vascular occlusion disorders. Some examples of vaso-occlusive disorders include cryoglobulinemia, cholesterol emboli, Sneddon's syndrome, septic emboli, and malignant atrophic papulosis (Degos' disease). The histopathology in these disorders results from either initially occlusive or mediation by antiphospholipid antibodies, and therefore, falls into the category of microvascular occlusion. The differential diagnosis also includes trauma, coagulopathies, and thrombocytopenia. Purpuras secondary to coagulopathies and thrombocytopenia are noninflammatory and often nonpalpable; they can be distinguished promptly on histologic and laboratory testing.

## CURRENT DIAGNOSIS

- Clinical spectrum of lesions ranging from purpura to palpable purpura, urticarial lesions, or ulcers: concentrated on dependent areas
- Small-vessel CV involves postcapillary venules only
- Histologic finding: leukocytoclastic vasculitis
- Pathogenesis: circulating immune complexes, neutrophils, cytokines, and adhesion molecules

*Abbreviation:* CV = cutaneous vasculitis.

Given the wide array of systemic diseases that can be associated with small-vessel CV, it is important to carefully evaluate each patient for coexistent disease; the first manifestation of large-vessel vasculitis is often small-vessel disease.

### HENOCH-SCHÖNLEIN PURPURA

Henoch-Schönlein purpura (HSP) deserves specific mention given its history and frequent occurrence. Heberden first described a single patient with HSP in 1801. Johann Schönlein and Eduard Henoch elucidated features in the mid-19th century as a tetrad of palpable purpura, arthritis, and GI renal involvement. Henoch-Schönlein purpura is defined by the Chapel Hill Consensus Conference as a vasculitis affecting small vessels, involving deposition of IgA immune complexes that characteristically involves the skin, GI system, and glomeruli with or without arthralgia or arthritis. Approximately 30% of cases follow an upper respiratory infection. The clinical outcome is excellent with fewer than 10% of patients developing chronic disease. A small percent of patients will develop persistent renal or GI disease requiring systemic immunosuppressive therapy.

### URTICARIAL VASCULITIS

Another important subtype of small-vessel CV is urticarial vasculitis. Urticarial vasculitis is a chronic disorder consisting of episodic urticarial and/or angioedematous lesions lasting longer than 24 hours that histologically manifest features of leukocytoclastic vasculitis. Urticarial vasculitis may range from patients with only urticarial skin lesions to those with urticarial vasculitis associated with hypocomplementemia with some systemic features; this meets criteria for systemic lupus erythematosus. Patients with urticarial vasculitis may also have underlying autoimmune connective tissue diseases, infections (hepatitis B and C), neoplastic processes, or medications as underlying etiologic factors. Treatment is directed at underlying etiologies and/or follows the same therapeutic ladder as for small-vessel CV (Table 2).

## Treatment

Because small-vessel CV is generally self-limited, treatment is often unnecessary except for symptomatic relief. When possible, identification and removal of a causative agent (e.g., infection, drug, chemicals, food) should be accomplished. Removal of an inciting agent is occasionally followed by rapid resolution of the lesions and no other treatment is indicated; otherwise, local and systemic therapies are recommended. Symptomatic improvement may be achieved with leg elevation, gradient support stockings, nonsteroidal anti-inflammatory drugs, and antihistamines.

**TABLE 1   Evaluation of Suspected Small Vessel Cutaneous Vasculitis**

| Confirming Histopathologic Correlation | Assessing the Extent of the Disease | Establishing Etiology |
| --- | --- | --- |
| Punch biopsy early lesion | General<br>• Myalgia<br>• Arthralgia<br>• Fever | Infection<br>• Bacterial<br>• Viral<br>• Fungal<br>• Acid-fast bacilli<br>• Other |
| Incisional biopsy for suspected larger vessel vasculitis | Renal involvement (acute and chronic renal failure)<br>• Proteinuria<br>• Hematuria<br>Nervous system<br>• Central or peripheral<br>• Diffuse or local findings | Drugs<br><br><br>Diseases associated with immune complexes<br>• Connective tissue/autoimmune diseases<br>• Malignancy (especially myelodysplastic)<br>• Inflammatory bowel disease<br>Idiopathic (50%) |
| | Musculoskeletal involvement<br>• Nonerosive polyarthritis<br>Gastrointestinal system<br>• Abdominal pain (colicky, nausea, vomiting, diarrhea)<br>• Gastrointestinal bleeding (melena or hematemesis)<br>Pulmonary involvement<br>• Pleural effusion<br>• Pleuritis<br>• Hemoptysis<br>Pericardial involvement (myocardial angiitis or pericarditis)<br>• Pericardial effusion<br>Ocular involvement (retinal vasculitis)<br>• Conjunctivitis<br>• Keratitis<br>Other | |

Modified from Barham KL et al: Rook's Textbook of Dermatology, 7th ed. Oxford, Blackwell Publishing, 2004.

**TABLE 2  Therapeutic Ladder for Small-Vessel Cutaneous Vasculitis**

| | Double-Blind Studies | Case Series | Case Reports |
|---|---|---|---|
| Skin lesions alone | Colchicine[1] | Nonsteroidal anti-inflammatory drugs<br>Dapsone[1] | Supportive therapy<br><br>• Antihistamines<br>• Pentoxifylline (Trental)[1]<br>• Hydroxychloroquine (Plaquenil)[1]<br>• Thalidomide (Thalomid)[1]<br>• Low-dose weekly methotrexate (Rheumatrex)[1] |
| Ulcerative skin lesions alone | | Prednisone[1] | |
| Systemic disease | Interferon-α and ribavirin (Rebetron) (if associated with hepatitis C) 3 million units 3/wk and 1000 mg/d, respectively | Prednisone[1]<br><br>Azathioprine (Imuran)[1]<br>  1–2.5 mg/kg/d PO as single dose or divided in half<br><br>Cyclophosphamide (Cytoxan)[1]<br>  pulsed dosing regimen, 40–50 mg/kg IV in divided doses over 2–5 d or 10–15 mg/kg IV q 7–10 d or 3–5 mg/kg IV 2/wk | Mycophenolate mofetil (CellCept)[1] 500–2000 mg PO bid<br>Cyclosporine (Neoral, Sandimmune)[1] 2.5 mg/kg/d PO divided in half qd; after 4 wk, dose may be increased 0.5 mg/kg/d at 2-wk intervals; maximum of 4 mg/kg/d<br><br>• IV gammaglobulin (Gammagard)[1]<br>• Extracorporeal immunomodulation<br>• Biologic agents: infliximab (Remicade),[1] etanercept (Enbrel)[1] (TNF-α inhibitors)<br>• Rituximab (Anti-CD20)[1] |
| | Methotrexate (Trexall)[1] 7.5–15 mg once a week* | | |

*There is no study associated with this drug.
[1]Not FDA approved for this indication.
*Abbreviations:* IV = intravenously, TNF-α = tumor necrosis factor-α.
Modified from Barham KL et al: Rook's Textbook of Dermatology, 7th ed. Oxford, Blackwell Publishing, 2004.

Small-vessel CV with persistent palpable purpura without significant internal organ complications may respond to treatment with oral colchicine[1] in doses of 0.6 mg two to three times daily. Dosing is limited by GI symptoms. This therapy is supported by anecdotal reports, but a statistically significant difference was not confirmed in a randomized controlled trial. Dapsone[1] (50 to 200 mg per day) has also been used in patients only having skin involvement.

Systemic treatment is advised for patients with small-vessel CV who have significant systemic manifestations or significant cutaneous ulceration. However, almost no double-blind, placebo-controlled prospective trials exist. Table 2 describes a therapeutic ladder for small-vessel CV. The medications discussed in Table 2 have not been FDA approved for this indication. Oral corticosteroids (Prednisone[1] 0.5 to 1 mg/kg per day) are indicated for progressive, symptomatic nodular, vesicular, or ulcerating purpura as well as systemic involvement. Once the patient's symptoms have stabilized, prednisone should be tapered gradually over 3 to 6 weeks because a rapid taper can lead to clinical disease rebound.

Small-vessel CV can manifest clinically with a spectrum of cutaneous lesions; palpable purpura is the classic presentation. The hallmark histologic appearance is a leukocytoclastic vasculitis. There is a presumed immune complex mediated pathogenesis. The therapeutic approach requires elimination of the cause (drugs, chemicals, infection) when possible. In most patients, only the skin is involved and can be treated with supportive measures. The most important step in evaluation is the full workup to find etiology and extent (systemic involvement) of the disease process. Skin manifestations alone may be managed with nonsteroidal anti-inflammatory drugs, gradient support stockings, colchicine, and dapsone. Systemic treatment is advised in small-vessel CV with significant systemic manifestations or those with significant cutaneous ulceration.

## CURRENT THERAPY

- Small-vessel CV is generally self-limited; treatment is often unnecessary except for symptomatic relief, which may be achieved with leg elevation, gradient support stockings, nonsteroidal anti-inflammatory drugs, and antihistamines.
- Skin manifestations alone may be managed with agents such as colchicine and dapsone.
- Systemic treatment is advised for patients with significant systemic manifestations or those with significant cutaneous ulceration.

*Abbreviation:* CV = cutaneous vasculitis.

## REFERENCES

Fiorentino DF: Cutaneous vasculitis. J Am Acad Dermatol 2003;48(3): 311-340.
Gonzalez-Gay MA, Garcia-Porrua C, Pujol RM: Clinical approach to cutaneous vasculitis. Curr Opin Rheumatol 2005;17(1):56-61.
Lamprecht P: TNF-alpha inhibitors in systemic vasculitides and connective tissue diseases. Autoimmun Rev 2005;4(1):28-34.
Lotti T, Ghersetich I, Comacchi C, Jorizzo JL: Cutaneous small-vessel vasculitis. J Am Acad Dermatol 1998;39(5 Pt 1):667-687.

[1]Not FDA approved for this indication.

# Diseases of the Nails

Method of
*Bianca Maria Piraccini, MD, PhD,
and Matilde Iorizzo, MD*

Nail abnormalities are frequent and their etiology extremely variable, including physiologic, inflammatory, traumatic, infective, and neoplastic causes. The diagnosis of nail diseases requires a good knowledge of nail anatomy and physiology because nail symptoms are strictly related to the portion of the nail apparatus that is affected (Table 1). The nail plate is continuously produced throughout life (at a rate of 2 to 4 mm/month for fingernails and 1 to 2 mm/month for toenails) by the matrix, which lies under the proximal nail fold. The nail plate emerges from the proximal nail fold in correspondence to the cuticle and moves distally, strictly adhering to the epithelium of the underlying nail bed. The strong nail plate nail bed adhesion is essential for the tactile, grasping, and defensive functions of the nail. The nail detaches from the nail bed at the end of the digit, in the area of the hyponychium, where the distal nail plate appears white.

The healthy nail plate is transparent and appears pink because it permits visualization of the color of the highly vascularized nail bed. The proximal part of the nail plate covers the distal matrix, which appears as a distally convex whitish crescent, the lunula.

The clinical examination of a patient with nail dystrophy includes a careful examination of all 20 nails, the skin, hair, and all the mucosae and a detailed clinical history. Optional diagnostic tools include microbiologic examinations, radiography, magnetic resonance imaging, and histopathology.

When treating nail diseases, keep in mind the following:

- Topical drugs do not reach the nail matrix, which lies beneath the nail plate and proximal nail fold.
- Because drugs do not easily penetrate the nail plate, removal of the nail plate may be indicated to treat nail bed diseases.
- Owing to the slow growth rate, complete replacement of a fingernail takes approximately 6 months and that of a toenail 1 year. For this reason improvement of nail symptoms is slow, and treatment should last longer than treatment for skin conditions. This should be clearly explained to patients to avoid unrealistic expectations and poor treatment compliance.
- Duration of systemic treatment is best chosen according to the improvement of the nail condition because nail growth rates and

treatment responses vary between patients. Follow-up of once a month or once every 2 months is the best way to achieve correct management of patients.

Table 2 lists all systemic/intralesional treatments mentioned in this article, summarizing dosages, modalities of administration, and special care measures.

## Acute Paronychia

Acute inflammation of the proximal nail fold is a common consequence of biting or chewing the periungual tissues and usually affects children. It can also be a consequence of an excessively aggressive manicure. Gram-positive bacteria, usually *Staphylococcus aureus*, invade and proliferate in the space under the fold, giving rise to the acute inflammation that may lead to abscess formation.

Differential diagnosis includes herpes simplex infection: In this case, acute paronychia occurs most commonly in adults, especially health workers; the flare is recurrent; and vesicles are often observed on the periungual skin or under the nail plate. Swabs for microbiologic study should be taken for a correct diagnosis.

## Trachyonychia

Trachyonychia, also known as 20-nail dystrophy, is a chronic disease characterized by a mild inflammation of the proximal nail matrix that results in the production of a brittle, rough, opaque nail plate. The damage is limited to the superficial layer of the nail plate because this is the portion produced by the proximal nail matrix. More common in children, it usually affects patients with severe alopecia areata, in which it is considered a nail localization of the disease. The course of trachyonychia does not parallel that of alopecia areata.

Even if several studies have shown that the pathology of patients with trachyonychia may lead to a diagnosis of psoriasis or lichen planus, the clinical features and the outcome of the disease are always the same: Nail lesions last for a long time and tend to improve slowly and spontaneously.

## Ingrowing Toenails

Ingrowing toenails are the most common nail disease of teenagers, who usually seek advice when the problem has been present for a long time and conservative treatment is no longer possible. Nail ingrowing is the final results of several factors:

## TABLE 1 Nail Symptoms Vary Depending on the Part of the Nail Apparatus Involved

| Nail Portion | Function | Symptoms When Damaged |
|---|---|---|
| Nail matrix | Nail plate production | • Nail plate abnormalities<br>• Nail plate absence |
| Nail bed/hyponychium | Nail plate attachment to underlying tissues | • Nail detachment (onycholysis)<br>• Subungual hyperkeratosis<br>• Nail uplifting |
| Proximal nail fold | Protection of the matrix through sealing the skin of the digit to the nail plate by the cuticle | • Absence of the cuticle<br>• Erythema and swelling<br>• Nail matrix damage<br>• Nail plate abnormalities |
| Nail matrix | Nail plate production | • Nail plate absence<br>• Nail detachment (onycholysis) |
| Nail bed/hyponychium | Nail plate attachment to underlying tissues | • Subungual hyperkeratosis<br>• Nail uplifting<br>• Absence of the cuticle |
| Proximal nail fold | Protection of the matrix through sealing the skin of the digit to the nail plate by the cuticle | • Erythema and swelling<br>• Nail matrix damage |

**TABLE 2** Systemic/Intralesional Treatments with Dosages, Modalities of Administration, and Special Care Measures

| Type of Treatment | Modality of Administration | Dosage | Duration | Notes |
|---|---|---|---|---|
| **Systemic Steroids** | | | | |
| Triamcinolone acetonide (Kenalog) | IM 1/mo | 0.5 mg/kg | 4–6 mo | |
| Methylprednisolone (Medrol) | PO | 32 mg/d | 2 wk | Add gastric antacids |
| **Intralesional Steroids** | | | | |
| Triamcinolone acetonide (Kenalog) | Injections into matrix or nail bed | 2–3 mL per digit of 10 mg/mL solution | 1–2 mo | • Some skills necessary<br>• Local anesthesia required |
| **Systemic Antifungals** | | | | |
| Terbinafine (Lamisil) | PO | 250 mg/d | • 2 mo fingernails<br>• 4 mo toenails | • Not effective in *Candida*<br>• Not if hepatic problems |
| Itraconazole (Sporanox) | PO | 200 mg bid × 1 wk/mo | • 2 mo fingernails<br>• 4 mo toenails | • Not if hepatic problems<br>• Possible drug interactions |
| **Systemic Retinoids** | | | | |
| Acitretin (Soriatane) | PO | 0.3–0.5 mg/kg/d | 4–6 mo | • Monitor hepatic and renal functions<br>• Contraception needed in women |
| **Systemic Steroids** | | | | |
| Triamcinolone acetonide (Kenalog) | IM | 0.5 mg/kg | 4–6 mo | |
| Methylprednisolone (Medrol) | PO | 1/mo 32 mg/d | 2 wk | Add gastric antacids |
| **Intralesional Steroids** | | | | |
| Triamcinolone acetonide (Kenalog) | Injections into matrix or nail bed | 2–3 mL per digit of 10 mg/mL solution | Once every 1–2 mo | • Some skills necessary<br>• Local anesthesia required |
| **Systemic Antifungals** | | | | |
| Terbinafine (Lamisil) | PO | 250 mg/d | • 2 mo fingernails<br>• 4 mo toenails | • Ineffective in *Candida*<br>• Not if hepatic problems |
| Itraconazole (Sporanox) | PO | 200 mg bid × 1 wk/mo | • 2 mo fingernails<br>• 4 mo toenails | • Not if hepatic problems<br>• Possible drug interactions |
| **Systemic Retinoids** | | | | |
| Acitretin (Soriatane) | PO | 0.3-0.5 mg/kg/d | 4–6 mo | • Monitor hepatic and renal functions<br>• Contraception needed in women |

*Abbreviation:* IM = intramuscularly.

- Lateral deviation of the nail plate in respect to the longitudinal axis of the digit (congenital malalignment), which predisposes to penetration of the lateral edge of the nail into the fold
- Improper cutting or manual removal of the distal edge of the nail, a frequent habit of children and teenagers, which produces a sharp nail plate edge
- Hyperhydrosis of the feet, which facilitates nail plate breaking with formation of sharp edges.

All these factors contribute to the formation of a sharp spicule on the distolateral edge of the nail plate that with walking penetrates and damages the soft tissues of the lateral fold. This produces pain and periungual inflammation (stage 1, according to Zaias' classification); with time, the injured dermis of the nail fold gives rise to a granulation tissue (pyogenic granuloma), which emerges from the lateral fold and appears as a painful bleeding nodule (stage 2). If the condition lasts longer, the granulation tissue induces the growth of a newly formed skin epithelium that partially covers the nail plate, fixing it in place (stage 3).

# Chronic Paronychia

Chronic paronychia is a common condition that typically affects predisposed persons whose hands are in frequent contact with water, humidity, detergents, and irritants, such as housewives and food handlers. Irritation and maceration of the proximal nail fold lead to inflammation and swelling of the fold with arrested production of the cuticle. Because the role of the cuticle is to protect the nail matrix from the environment by sealing the skin of the dorsal digit to the nail plate, its disappearance causes penetration of water, dirt, food particles, and microorganisms under the nail fold. This results in nail matrix damage with production of a nail plate with an irregular surface where dirt and microorganisms (*Pseudomonas aeruginosa*) easily accumulate, causing a greenish-black irregular discoloration. *Candida albicans* is frequently isolated from nails with paronychia, but the yeast is only a secondary colonizer and not the primary cause of the disease.

# Nail Fragility

Nail brittleness is a common problem for women, who complain of cosmetic and functional problems associated with the condition. Overall, it is similar to skin dryness, and results from excessive dehydration of the nail plate caused by environmental and intrinsic factors. The nail is fragile and tends to split in horizontal layers in its distal portion, causing irregularities and breakages of the free edge. Nail fragility is very difficult to cure, and predisposed individuals tend to have frequent recurrences.

## CURRENT DIAGNOSIS

**Acute Paronychia**

- Acute onset
- One digit
- Pulsating pain, swelling, and erythema of the periungual skin, usually more marked on one side

**Trachyonychia**

- Usually young patients
- One to several to all twenty nails may be affected
- Nail plate surface totally rough and scaly, as if sandpapered
- Family personal history of alopecia areata frequent

**Ingrowing Toenails**

- Great toenail(s)
- Painful periungual inflammation with/without pyogenic granulomas
- Nail plate distal margin irregular or not visible

**Chronic Paronychia**

- Fingernails
- Middle-aged women
- Swelling of the nail fold, absence of cuticle, nail plate surface abnormalities, and discoloration

**Nail Fragility**

- Fingernails
- Adult women
- Distal nail plate horizontally split and broken

**Onychomycosis**

- Toenails
- Adults and elderly people
- Onycholysis and nail bed hyperkeratosis (in distal subungual onychomycosis)
- Superficial opaque white patches (in white superficial onychomycosis)
- Tinea pedis plantaris or interdigitale often associated
- Periungual inflammation associated if a nondermatophytic mold is responsible

**Psoriasis**

- Onycholysis with erythematous border in one or more fingernails
- Salmon patches of the nail bed in one or more fingernails
- Nail plate thickening and crumbling

**Idiopathic Onycholysis**

- Fingernails
- Women
- White or greenish-black subungual space

# Onychomycosis

Onychomycosis is one of the most frequent nail disorders, usually affecting the toenails of adults. The most common form (up to 70% of the cases, according to our experience) is distal subungual onychomycosis caused by dermatophytes, where fungi invade the nail bed causing onycholysis and subungual hyperkeratosis with typical yellow-brown scales accumulated under the nail plate. White superficial onychomycosis is frequently seen in elderly people, in whom it involves several toenails and appears as white opaque patches on the superficial nail. Invasion of the nail by nondermatophytic molds is not rare in Italy, where it accounts for 15% of onychomycosis, but different figures have been reported in other countries. What characterizes mold onychomycosis (caused by *Fusarium* species, *Aspergillus* species, and *Scopulariopsis brevicaulis*)

## CURRENT THERAPY

**Acute Paronychia**

- Mechanical drainage is necessary if pus is present.
- Treatment involves topical application of creams containing antibiotics, such as mupirocin (Bactroban) for 5 to 7 days.
- When swelling and pain are severe, the association of a topical steroid, such as betamethasone cream (Diprolene), for 4 to 5 days induces a more rapid regression of symptoms.
- Systemic antibiotics (amoxicillin/clavulanate potassium tablets (Augmentin) 2 g/day for 5 days) are required in severe cases.

**Trachyonychia**

- Trachyonychia affects the nail matrix, and topical drugs are therefore ineffective. Moreover, trachyonychia is a benign condition, so medical treatment is not advisable in children and when only one or a few nails are affected. In these patients, topical application of emollients containing urea several times a day may produce cosmetic benefit, as does the use of nail lacquers.
- In adults with trachyonychia of several nails, the cosmetic discomfort may be severe, and systemic steroids may be useful in these cases (see Table 2). Trachyonychia responds well and rapidly to systemic steroids, and recurrences are rare.
- Intralesional injection of steroids (see Table 2) into the nail matrix is an option in adults when only one or two nails are involved.

**Ingrowing Toenails**

- The final goals of treatment of ingrowing toenails are to remove the spicule that penetrates and damages the lateral nail fold and to help the nail plate to grow over the distal edge of the fold. This can be easily done in stage 1, but it requires the previous removal of the pyogenic granuloma in stage 2. In our experience two modalities of treatment are effective, both needing good patient compliance and 30 to 40 days of time:
    - Uplifting the nail plate by insertion under its edge of a small cylinder of cotton gauze soaked in antiseptic, such as povidone-iodine (Betadine). The patient should then be instructed to keep the gauze in place or reinsert it if necessary until the lateral nail reaches and grows over the distolateral fold.

*Continued*

- Pushing down the lateral and distal folds with a tape sealed on the skin of the distal digit and rolled all along the digit to increase traction. The tape should be applied by the patient every night and kept on for 12 hours. This should be done until the nail has grown completely over the distal border.
- When inflammation and pyogenic granuloma are present, they can be treated by topical application of high-potency topical steroids, such as clobetasone propionate ointment (Temovate) in occlusion at bedtime followed by topical mupirocin (Bactroban) in the morning until remission.
- Severe pyogenic granuloma may also be removed by electrodesiccation or by intralesional injection of steroids (see Table 2).
- Stage 3 ingrowing toenails always require an invasive approach with chemical (phenolization) or surgical removal of the lateral portion of the matrix to obtain production of a narrower nail plate that will not ingrow any more.

### Chronic Paronychia

- Cure of chronic paronychia cannot be achieved until the patient avoids hand contact with the humid environmental condition by wearing cotton gloves under rubber gloves during manual activities.
- Topically apply medium- or high-potency steroids, such as fluocinolone (Synalar), betamethasone (Diprolene), and clobetasone propionate (Temovate) creams at bedtime followed by morning application of an antimicrobial cream, such as econazole (Spectazole).
- In severe cases, topical treatment can be preceded by a 15-day course of oral steroids (see Table 2).
- Treatment of chronic paronychia should be continued until the disease is cured, which is achieved when the cuticle has completely regrown.

### Nail Fragility

- Avoid environmental factors known to dehydrate the nail plate, including water and irritants, and nail polish and nail lacquers.
- Trim the nails short because the longer the plate, the more it tends to lose water.
- Topical moisturizers containing urea or α-hydroxy acids to be applied on the nail plate several times a day and after each hand washing.
- Oral biotin (D-Biotin) at a dose of 5 mg/day for at least 6 months.

### Onychomycosis

- Mycologic examination (KOH and cultures) is mandatory before starting therapy because treatment varies depending on type and etiology of onychomycosis.
- Onychomycoses caused by nondermatophytic molds (except for those caused by *Aspergillus* species) are difficult to treat because they usually do not respond to systemic antifungals.
- Topical treatment alone is indicated in white superficial onychomycosis caused by dermatophytes, distal subungual onychomycosis limited to the distal

one third of one digit, and onychomycosis caused by *Scopulariopsis brevicaulis* and *Fusarium* species. Suggested options include the following:

- Nail lacquers containing antifungals may be effective, such as amorolfine (Loceryl) applied once a week or ciclopirox (Penlac) applied daily.
- Another option is periodic mechanical or chemical removal of the affected portion of the nail associated with the daily application of antifungal creams. For chemical nail avulsion, we use 40% urea in petrolatum kept on the nail in occlusion for 7 days, after covering the periungual soft tissues with tape to avoid their maceration. After removal of the medication, the affected nail is soft and easy to clip away.
- Systemic treatment (see Table 2) is, in our experience, more effective when associated with topical therapy.
- Complete cure of onychomycosis (clinical and mycologic) may require a duration of systemic treatment longer than what is suggested by the manufacturer. For this reason we use a modality of treatment *à la carte*: After an initial treatment of 2 or 4 months (for fingernail and toenail onychomycosis, respectively), we perform a mycologic examination and continue therapy until its results are negative.
- Clinical cure may take more time than mycologic cure, so we continue to follow mycologically negative patients for a further 4 to 6 months.
- An annual follow-up of cured patients is advisable to check for recurrences that occur in up to 20% of patients.

### Psoriasis

- Explain to patients that psoriasis is a chronic disease with improvements and relapses that are often induced by trauma (Koebner phenomenon).
- Topical treatment is suitable only for signs of nail bed psoriasis, such as onycholysis and hyperkeratosis. After clipping away the detached nail plate, different topicals can be applied on the nail bed epithelium. Topical steroids, such as betamethasone (Diprolene) and clobetasone propionate (Temovate) creams, or the association of steroids with keratolytics (Diprosalic ointment) are effective but can be applied only for short periods of time to avoid skin atrophy. However, tazarotene cream (Tazorac) and calcipotriene cream or ointment (Dovonex) can be used for a long time. A possible treatment modality can be the alternate use of vitamin D–derived topicals from Monday to Friday with steroid creams on Saturday and Sunday.
- Intralesional steroids (see Table 2) are effective in nail matrix psoriasis and are the treatment of choice when a few fingernails are involved. Injections of steroids into the nail bed via the lateral folds can be used to treat nail bed disease.
- Severe nail matrix psoriasis and pustular psoriasis of the nails greatly improve with systemic retinoids (see Table 2). Other effective systemic treatments are methotrexate and biologicals, but they are only suitable in patients with associated severe cutaneous or arthropathic psoriasis.

## CURRENT THERAPY—cont'd

### Idiopathic Onycholysis

- The detached nail plate should be clipped away to expose the nail bed to keep it clean and dry. This is not easily accepted by patients but should be done periodically until regrowth of a totally attached plate.
- Cotton gloves inside rubber gloves should be worn when handling water and irritants.
- The nail bed should be dried carefully after each hand washing.
- Daily soaking of the affected finger in a mild antiseptic solution, such as sodium hypochlorite (Dakin's solution) for 2 to 3 minutes.
- Application of a topical steroid, such as betamethasone cream (Diprolene), at bedtime for the first 10 to 15 days, and then of a topical antiseptic in an evaporating vehicle, such as 4% thymol in chloroform.

*Abbreviation:* KOH = potassium hydroxide.

is the particular clinical feature, consisting of acute periungual inflammation associated with the findings of a severe distal subungual onychomycosis or of a proximal subungual onychomycosis. In proximal subungual onychomycosis, the nail shows a patch of subungual yellow-white discoloration that starts from under the cuticle. White superficial onychomycosis may be also caused by nondermatophytic molds: in this case, the nail plate is invaded more deeply and diffusely, and the periungual tissues are mildly erythematous.

Onychomycosis caused by *Candida* species is rare and only seen in patients with immunodeficiencies, such as HIV infection, iatrogenic immunodepression, or chronic mucocutaneous candidiasis. *Candida* invades all nail epithelia, causing a total onychomycosis characterized by paronychia, nail plate opacity and friability, and nail bed hyperkeratosis.

## Psoriasis

Nail psoriasis is not rare, even in patients without skin or scalp involvement. The nail lesions may vary considerably in different patients, and diagnosis is not always easy. Onychomycosis is the most important differential diagnosis, especially in the toenails, where psoriasis causes nondiagnostic signs such as onycholysis and subungual hyperkeratosis.

Pustular psoriasis of the nails (Hallopeau's acrodermatitis continua) is also not an infrequent occurrence: It usually involves one digit, with recurrent episodes of painful acute pustular eruptions of the nail bed and periungual tissues, leading to partial or total onycholysis.

## Idiopathic Onycholysis

Onycholysis, which is detachment of the nail plate from the nail bed, is a frequent sign of different nail diseases. The term *idiopathic onycholysis* identifies a condition common in women, possibly caused by the same environmental traumas that produce chronic paronychia. In predisposed individuals, the frequent contact with water and irritants damages the distal portion of the nail bed (the so-called onychocorneal band), where nail plate–nail bed adhesion is stronger, and causes nail plate detachment. The newly formed space under the nail plate is penetrated by water and dirt and colonized by different microorganisms that may cause discoloration.

### REFERENCES

Baran R, Kaoukhov A: Topical antifungal drugs for the treatment of onychomycosis: An overview of current strategies for monotherapy and combination therapy. J Eur Acad Dermatol Venereol 2005;19:21-29.
de Berker DA, Lawrence CM: A simplified protocol of steroid injection for psoriatic nail dystrophy. Br J Dermatol 1998;128:90-95.
Haneke E: Nail surgery. Eur J Dermatol 2000;10:227-241.
Piraccini BM, Tosti A: White superficial onychomycosis: Epidemiological, clinical, and pathological study of 79 patients. Arch Dermatol 2004;140:696-701.
Tosti A, Piraccini BM: Twenty-nail dystrophy. Curr Opin Dermatol 1997;2:82-86.
Tosti A, Piraccini BM, Ghetti E, Colombo MD: Topical steroids versus systemic antifungals in the treatment of chronic paronychia: An open, randomized double-blind and double dummy study. J Am Acad Dermatol 2002;47:72-76.
Tosti A, Piraccini BM, Lorenzi S, Iorizzo M: Treatment of nondermatophyte mold and Candida onychomycosis. Dermatol Clin 2002;2:491-497.
Uyttendaele H, Geyer A, Scher RK: Brittle nails: Pathogenesis and treatment. J Drugs Dermatol 2002;2:48-49.

# Keloids

Method of
*Tina S. Alster, MD, and Mahsa Tehrani, MA*

Patients with keloids and hypertrophic scars commonly present for dermatologic consultation due to functional and cosmetic disfigurement. Pruritus, pain, dysesthesia, ulceration, secondary infection, restricted range of motion, and psychological distress may be associated with these scars in varying degrees. The upper arms, back, chest, shoulders, cheeks, earlobes, head, and neck are regions in which these scars predominantly occur. Various ethnic backgrounds, especially in the African American and Latin American populations, have a higher incidence of keloid and hypertrophic scar development. Men and women are at equal risk for scarring, and those between the ages of 10 and 30 years are most commonly affected. Several different types of skin injury, including surgery, burns, piercing, lacerations, abrasions, tattoos, vaccinations, insect bites, and inflammatory reactions (e.g., varicella or folliculitis) can provoke a proliferative scar response.

Keloids and hypertrophic scars are often clinically distinguishable from one another. The most important distinction is that hypertrophic scars remain within the confines of the original area of dermal injury, whereas keloids transgress beyond the borders (Figures 1 and 2). Hypertrophic scars typically arise shortly after injury (within days to weeks) and regress over time. In contrast, keloids appear months to years after injury and tend to proliferate without spontaneous regression. Histopathologically, keloid collagen fibers appear larger and bulkier and occur in random orientations, whereas the fibers are more regular and aligned in parallel with the epidermis in hypertrophic scars. Additionally, in keloids, enzymes such as alanine transaminase concentrations are elevated and the ratio of type I to type III collagen is increased. In hypertrophic scars, nodular structures containing fibroblastic cells and collagen are apparent. These nodules are specific to hypertrophic scars and contain $\alpha$ smooth muscle actin-staining myofibroblasts. Hypertrophic scars tend to improve with treatment, whereas keloids are more treatment resistant and have a higher rate of recurrence.

## Pathogenesis

The exact mechanisms of keloid and hypertrophic scar pathogenesis have not been fully elucidated. There are, however, various hypotheses aimed at determining the molecular basis for the excessive fibrosis seen in these scars.

It has been demonstrated that fibroblasts in keloids function abnormally, becoming hyperstimulated and producing greater levels of collagen, elastin, fibronectin, and proteoglycans. Fibroblasts in hypertrophic

## CURRENT DIAGNOSIS

**Keloid**

CLINICAL CHARACTERISTICS

- Transgresses beyond original borders of skin injury
- Can occur months to years after injury
- Proliferates without tendency to subside

HISTOLOGIC FINDINGS

- Thick collagen fibers
- Random alignment

**Hypertrophic Scar**

CLINICAL CHARACTERISTICS

- Remains within borders of skin injury
- Occurs shortly after initial injury
- Tends to regress over time

HISTOLOGIC FINDINGS

- Less demarcated collagen bundles
- Characteristic nodular structures (contain α smooth muscle actin-staining myofibroblasts)

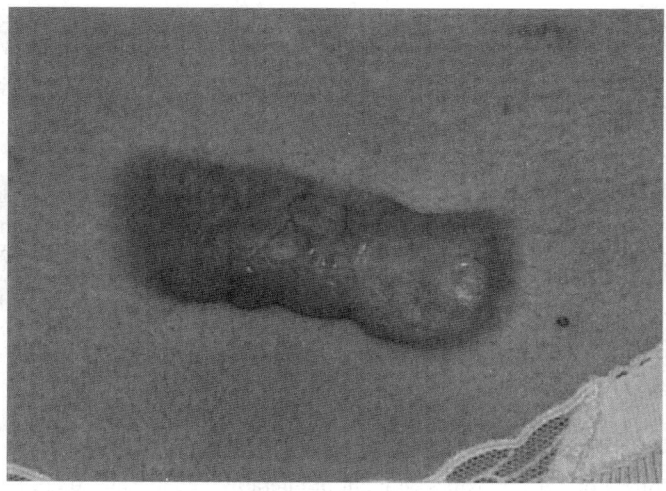

**FIGURE 2.** Keloid.

scars and normal tissue do not display this aberrant functioning. Growth factors involved in wound healing, such as transforming growth factor-β and insulin-like growth factor-1, which are associated with collagen and procollagen synthesis, respectively, have also been shown to be overexpressed in keloids.

Another etiologic hypothesis is based on studies that have demonstrated stimulation of collagen synthesis by mechanical tension. When wounds are closed under tension (particularly over bony structures or joints), collagen synthesis can be stimulated.

Most recently, based on a growing body of research confirming a significant immunologic role in keloid formation, studies are now evaluating key immunomodulators that might serve to suppress the excessive collagen production observed in keloids and hypertrophic scars.

## Treatment

Because there is no universally accepted method to treat or cure keloids and hypertrophic scars, the best strategy is prevention. If patients are predisposed to development of such proliferative scars, then elective surgical procedures should be avoided, particularly in body regions more prone to scarring.

### PHARMACOLOGIC THERAPY

#### Intralesional Corticosteroids

Intralesional corticosteroids have long been considered the gold standard for treatment of keloids and hypertrophic scars. Corticosteroids suppress collagen synthesis by decreasing gene expression within the scar. Their prophylactic use has been shown to prevent scar development in scar-prone patients. Scar recurrence rates drop below 50% when corticosteroids are used in conjunction with surgical excision. They have also been used in combination with laser treatment.

One of the most commonly administered drugs for intralesional injection is triamcinolone acetonide (Kenalog), which can be diluted

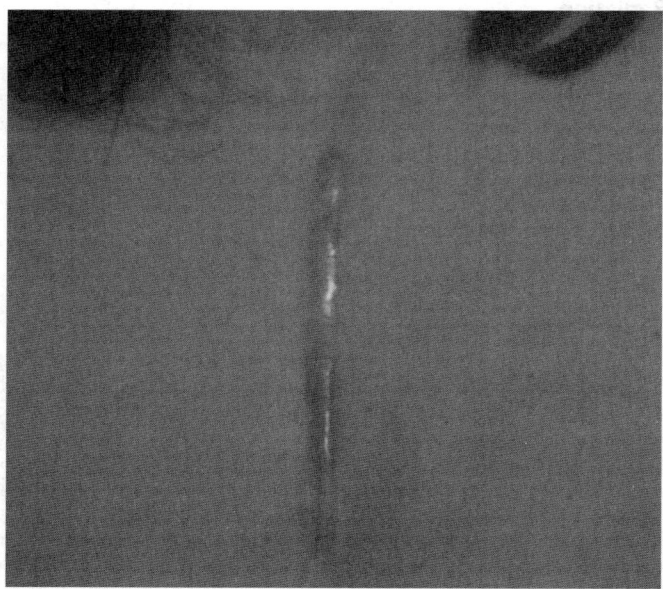

**FIGURE 1.** Hypertrophic scar.

## CURRENT THERAPY

**Medical**

- Intralesional corticosteroids (Kenalog)
- 5-Fluorouracil (Adrucil)
- Interferon

**Surgical**

- Primary excision ± grafting
- Cryosurgery
- Laser surgery

**Topical**

- Imiquimod (Aldara)
- Silicone gel
- Onion extract (Mederma)

**Other**

- Pressure therapy
- Radiation

with lidocaine to reduce the discomfort associated with dermal injection. Injections using concentrations of 10 to 40 mg/mL are typically administered at 2- to 4-week intervals. Complications of treatment include pain at the injection sites, skin atrophy, telangiectasia, and long-term hypopigmentation.

## 5-Fluorouracil

5-Fluorouracil (5-FU; Adrucil) is a pyrimidine analogue with antimetabolite activity. Intralesional 5-FU injection has been shown in limited studies to improve scars by decreasing keloid fibroblast proliferation. Injections (45-50 mg/mL) are typically administered weekly and are often combined with other treatments, including corticosteroids or laser therapy. Side effects include severe pain during injection, purpura at sites of injection, and localized superficial tissue slough.

## Interferon

Interferons are cytokines with antiproliferative and antifibrotic properties. Based on the notion that they also decrease types I and III collagen synthesis and induce apoptosis, clinical trials have studied their application in the treatment of keloids. Although up to 50% amelioration rates have been reported, recent evidence suggests that the performance of interferons as an adjuvant to surgical excision is inferior to postoperative intralesional corticosteroid injections. Additionally, adverse systemic effects, such as dose-dependent flu-like symptoms, reduce the practicality of this treatment in clinical practice.

## TOPICAL THERAPIES

### Imiquimod

Imiquimod (Aldara), an immune-response modifier, induces local cytokine production, which leads to down-regulation of collagen synthesis. A small 8-week study wherein 5% cream was applied after surgical keloid excision demonstrated no recurrence in 11 of 13 keloids at 24-week follow-up. Side effects are limited to local skin irritation and mild hyperpigmentation.

### Silicone Gel Sheeting

It has been hypothesized that the mechanism of action of silicone gel sheeting applied over scars has more to do with hydration than to the pressure or silicone in the dressing. Hydration can lead to fibroblast modification, and the dressing itself serves as a protective barrier, mimicking the stratum corneum. Clinical studies have shown that application of silicone sheeting 12 hours a day for 2 to 4 months results in scar softening and reduced pruritus. The lack of significant adverse effects of this treatment makes it a popular therapeutic option, especially in the pediatric population.

### Onion Extract

Studies of onion extract in vitro have demonstrated fibroblast-inhibiting properties. Further research has shown reduced proliferative activity and decreased production of substances in the extracellular matrix, but the exact mechanism of action whereby the onion extract exerts its effect remains unclear. In addition to its known antibacterial properties, the flavonoids (quercetin and kaempferol) in onion extract are believed to account for its fibroblast inhibition and other antiproliferative effects. The gel is prescribed for use on new scars twice daily for a period of 3 to 4 months. Scar erythema and discomfort are typically diminished, although some patients develop mild pruritus after its application.

## SURGICAL THERAPY

### Surgical Excision with or without Grafting

If used as monotherapy, lesions recur in 45% to 100% of surgically excised scars. Because the excision exposes the tissue to the same forces as the original wound, additional collagen synthesis is stimulated.

Thus, not only does the keloid recur, but it often becomes larger. Surgical closure techniques using intradermal monofilamentous sutures impose the least amount of injury to the tissue and have been shown to be somewhat helpful in reducing keloid formation.

### Cryosurgery

Cryosurgery, which involves two to three consecutive freeze-thaw cycles of 30-second durations, induces ischemia of the skin due to vascular damage and reduced microcirculation. Anoxia and eventual tissue necrosis ensue when treatments are delivered at 3- to 4-week intervals. Facial keloids and scars older than one year do not significantly improve with this modality. In addition, permanent hypopigmentation due to irreversible melanocyte destruction can result, making cryosurgery a less feasible option for patients with darker skin.

### Laser Surgery

New advances in laser technology have made vascular-specific laser therapy one of the most effective treatments for hypertrophic scars and keloids. Whereas older vaporizing lasers (such as carbon dioxide) demonstrated no advantage over scalpel excision, with high rates of scar recurrence, the newer nonablative pulsed dye lasers (PDL) have shown marked improvements in scar erythema, texture, height, and pliability without scar worsening or recurrence after two or three treatment sessions on a bimonthly basis. The clinical effectiveness of PDL irradiation on hypertrophic scars and keloids is presumably due to controlled tissue heating and hypoxia, with subsequent diminution of cellular function and inflammation. The ease of PDL treatment without significant side effects renders nonablative laser therapy a suitable choice in children and adults.

## OTHER MODALITIES

### Pressure Therapy

Although the mechanism of action of compression therapy is not completely understood, it has been hypothesized that pressure induces tissue ischemia, leading to decreased tissue metabolism and increased collagenolysis. For maximum effectiveness, 24 to 40 mm Hg of pressure should be exerted and the pressure garment worn for at least 18 hours a day for 6 months. Because many patients find pressure dressings cumbersome and uncomfortable, compliance with their regular use is patchy, limiting the ultimate benefits of treatment.

### Radiation

Radiation therapy can be used as monotherapy, but is most often delivered after surgical scar excision, effectively decreasing recurrence rates to 10% to 20%. Radiation exposure damages fibroblasts, hindering their proliferation and neoangiogenesis. Within 10 days of surgery, at least 1500 Gy are delivered in divided doses. Because of associated carcinogenicity, radiation treatment is controversial and caution must be exercised when treating children or such radiosensitive regions as the breast or thyroid gland.

## Summary

A multitude of medical and over-the-counter treatments are available for scar treatment. Although a number of outpatient scar therapies such as corticosteroid injections and laser irradiation have shown marked clinical efficacy, many common over-the-counter products purported to treat scars are based on anecdotal evidence and unsubstantiated claims. Individual differences in scar response to treatment also make it difficult to reach consensus on the single best therapeutic modality. Combination treatment regimens, including laser treatment, surgical excision, and corticosteroid injections, are proven to significantly reduce recurrence rates of keloids and hypertrophic scars. As new research is directed toward controlling aberrant collagen formation, novel and more efficacious treatments are anticipated for this difficult problem.

## REFERENCES

Al-Attar A, Mess S, Thomassen JM, et al: Keloid pathogenesis and treatment. Plast Reconstr Surg 2006 117(1):286-296.

Alster TS, Tanzi EL: Hypertrophic scars and keloids: Etiology and management. Am J Clin Dermatol 2003;4(4):235-243.

Alster TS, Zaulyanov L: Laser scar revision: A review. Dermatol Surg 2006;33(2):131-140.

Poochareon VN, Berman B: New therapies for the management of keloids. J Craniofac Surg 2003;14(5):654-657.

# Warts (Verrucae)

Method of
*Tamara Salam Housman, MD,*
*and Phillip M. Williford, MD*

Viral warts afflict approximately 10% of the population and are caused by human papillomavirus (HPV). HPV, a nonenveloped, double-stranded DNA virus, is of the papovavirus class and invades both mucous and squamous epithelium. At least 130 known types of HPV have been identified. HPV causes both clinical and subclinical infection and plays a role in certain cutaneous carcinomas, including squamous cell carcinoma (SCCa) of the anogenital area and nail unit. HPV is found in the basal layer of the epidermis but replicates only in the superficial, well-differentiated layer. The subsequent cellular proliferation gives rise to thick, hyperkeratotic lesions generally known as warts.

Cutaneous warts are mainly divided into common warts, plantar warts, flat warts, and genital warts. Common warts account for 70% of all cutaneous warts and are probably associated with HPV types 1, 2, and 4. Two thirds of untreated common warts spontaneously regress within 2 years, but these previously infected individuals have a higher rate of developing new warts than those who were never infected. Treatment of warts with salicylic acid and/or cryotherapy has demonstrated a 60% to 80% cure rate.

Transmission is via skin-to-skin contact, including sexual, and is seen with greater frequency where groups of people are in close contact, including in school-age children, with a frequency of 20% for common warts. Extent of infection is determined by the immune response, and immunocompromised hosts are at increased risk. Symptoms may include pain and bleeding, and warts may interfere with daily functioning, especially if located on the palms, soles, or digits. Warts can be professionally and socially stigmatizing, especially if located on the hands or fingers of patients who must touch others on a daily basis.

## Types of Warts

Verrucae vulgares (common warts) are flesh-colored, hyperkeratotic, verrucous, fissured, firm papules that disrupt normal skin lines on fingers and toes. They may be distinguished from calluses and corns by paring down of the stratum corneum (the uppermost horny layer of skin) to reveal thrombosed/bleeding capillaries seen as brown/black dots. A subtype is a butcher's wart, which is seen on the hands of butchers and fish and meat handlers/ packers, and appears as large, cauliflower plaques. Differential diagnoses (DDx) include seborrheic keratosis, molluscum contagiosum, keratoacanthoma, amelanotic melanoma, SCCa in situ, and invasive SCCa. Verrucae vulgares warts are associated with HPV subtypes 1, 2, 4.

Verrucae plantares (plantar warts) are flesh-colored, hyperkeratotic, endophytic papules or plaques located on the soles of the feet that also disrupt normal skin lines and may have thrombosed capillaries manifested as brown/black dots. These can be quite painful and interfere with mobility and daily functioning, especially if located on sites of pressure. A mosaic wart occurs if multiple plantar warts

coalesce into a plaque. DDx include callus, corns, exostosis, and acral melanoma. Verrucae plantares warts are associated with HPV subtypes 1, 2, 4, 27, 57.

Verrucae planae (flat warts) are tan- to flesh-colored, flat, sharply demarcated papules located on the dorsum of hands, distal lower extremities, and face; and are often in a linear arrangement after trauma. DDx include molluscum contagiosum, epidermodysplasia verruciformis, and benign syringomas on the face. Verrucae planae warts are associated with HPV subtypes 3, 10.

Epidermodysplasia verruciformis (EDV) is a rare, autosomal recessive, hereditary disorder manifesting with extensive, flesh-colored to pink to tan, round, flat papules on the trunk, hands, upper and lower extremities, and face. These do have malignant potential, especially on the face on sun-exposed areas. Patients with EDV are usually infected with multiple types of HPV. DDx include seborrheic keratosis, actinic keratosis, basal cell carcinoma, SCCa in situ, or invasive SCCa. EDV warts are classified into more than 30 associated HPV subtypes, including types 3, 5, 8, 9, 12, 14, 15, 17, 19-25, 36-38, 47, 49, 50.

Verrucous carcinoma is a slow-growing variant of SCCa arising in three sites:

1. Oral mucosa (oral florid papillomatosis)
2. Anogenital region (giant condyloma of Buschke and Löwenstein)
3. Plantar foot (epithelioma cuniculatum)

Verrucous carcinoma warts are associated with HPV subtypes 6, 11.

## Diagnosis

Diagnosis is mainly based on clinical findings. In immunocompromised or immunosuppressed patients, biopsy should be performed in large or suspicious lesions to rule out SCCa.

## Therapy

It is well accepted that the treatment of warts must be individualized and that usually more than one therapeutic modality is required to achieve complete resolution (Table 1). Conventional destructive treatments include repeated application of topical chemotherapy (i.e., salicylic acid [Compound W], cantharidin,[2] podophyllin [Podofin], 5-fluorouracil [Adrucil], etc.), cryosurgery, surgical excision, curettage and/or electrosurgery, and laser therapy. Other approaches include immunotherapy (i.e., intralesional interferon [IFN] [Alferon N], diphencyprone[2]), tape occlusion, and observation. In 20% of immunocompetent individuals, the warts will spontaneously resolve within 3 months. Cure rates for common and plantar verrucae with salicylic acid vary from 60% to 80%. Also, overall cure rates with cryosurgery range from 60% to 80%; and with carbon dioxide and pulsed-dye laser, they range from 45% to 90%. However, these methods are usually painful and expensive. Nonetheless, with most methods, recurrence is common, and repeat visits to the physician are costly.

Intralesional IFN-$\alpha$, although promising with a 36% to 62% clearance rate of anogenital warts, requires multiple injections in the physician's office, is expensive, and may cause systemic adverse effects. Imiquimod (Aldara),[1] a self-applied topical agent that induces interferon production at the site of application, is reported to have a 50% eradication rate in the treatment of genital warts. Other treatments include:

- Hyperthermia with hot water (113°F [45°C]) immersion
- Intralesional injection of *Candida*[1]/mumps[1] antigen
- Photodynamic therapy with aminolevulinic acid (Levulan Kerastick)[1] followed by red light irradiation
- Hypnosis
- Duct tape occlusion

---

[1]Not FDA approved for this indication.
[2]Not available in the United States.

**TABLE 1  Treatment of Verrucae**

| | Available Preparations | Mechanism of Action | Application | Dosage | Disadvantages/ Adverse Effects |
|---|---|---|---|---|---|
| Salicylic acid (keratolytic) (Compound W) | Solution Gel/lotion/cream Plaster Pad 10%-60% | Destruction of infected epidermis; irritation leads to stimulation of immune response. | Patient applied. Adjunct to other treatment modalities. May pare down/shave wart then apply keratolytic to increase penetration. | qhs until clear, usually weeks to months. | Irritation |
| Cryosurgery | Liquid nitrogen (−196°C [−320.8°F]): cryospray or cotton-tipped applicator | Destruction of infected epidermis; induces inflammation leading to stimulation of immune response. | Physician applied. Paring of thick lesions; liquid nitrogen freeze for 30-60 sec to include a 1-2 mm rim around wart → let thaw → repeat × 2 cycles total. | May repeat q 3-4 wk. | Pain Erythema Vesicle/bullae Crusting Possible infection Hypopigmentation Scarring (if freeze too deep) Onychodystrophy (if not careful with periungual warts) |
| Cantharidin[1,2] | Colloidal solution, 0.7% | Destruction of epidermis and leads to blister formation; extract of blister beetle. | Adjunct to other treatment modalities. Careful with periungual warts, overlying tendons, and on lower extremities. Physician applied. Paring of thick lesions. Apply using very fine applicator only to wart then patient is to wash off in 6-8 h. Painless—good for children. | May repeat q 2-4 wk. | Vesicle/bullae Crusting Avoid face or near eyes |
| Surgical excision Curettage Electrocautery | N/A | Destruction by surgical removal of wart. | Physician applied. Surgical excision of wart or surgical removal by curetting wart then cauterizing the base. | Usually only performed once but may repeat if wart recurs. | Painful (minimal if use local anesthesia but some postoperative pain) Scarring |
| Trichloroacetic acid (Tri-Chlor) Bichloroacetic acid | Solution, up to 50% concentration | Destruction of infected epidermis. | Physician applied. | Most useful for mucosal warts. | Painful reactions |
| Lasers: Carbon dioxide Pulsed-dye Erbium:YAG | N/A | Destruction of infected epidermis. | Physician applied. | May repeat q 4-6 wk. | Expensive Risk of viral spread via laser plume Not superior to conventional therapy |
| Imiquimod | Cream, 5% | Immunomodulator: indirect in vivo antitumor and antiviral effects mediated by induction of cytokines—IFN-α, TNF-α, IL-1, -6, -8, and others. | Patient applied. On nonmucosal skin, including plantar/palmar warts, apply keratolytic, followed by occlusion in PM, followed by imiquimod in AM; may also occlude imiquimod if not getting any erythema. If irritation is severe, stop regimen for few days then resume, if possible. May initiate therapy with cryosurgery followed by keratolytic-imiquimod combination therapy for 6 wks then repeat if necessary. | 3 times/wk on mucosal skin; 5-7 times/wk on keratinized skin. | Irritation Erythema Pruritus Burning Crusting Infection Scarring |

| Drug | Formulation | Mechanism | Administration | Dose | Side effects/Comments |
|---|---|---|---|---|---|
| Cimetidine (Tagamet)[1] | Tablets: 200 mg, 300 mg, 400 mg, 800 mg; liquid: 300 mg/5 mL | Immunomodulator: at high doses may enhance immune response. | Patient initiated. | 25 to 40 mg/kg daily, divided bid to qid. | True efficacy unclear |
| DPC[1] SADBE[1] DNCB[1] | Acetone solution, 0.001-2% Acetone solution, 0.01-1% | Immunomodulator: inducing a delayed hypersensitivity reaction thus leading to stimulation of immune response. | Physician applied. Sensitize patient by applying 2%-3% solution of SADBE/DPC to 1 cm area on inner arm → may need to resensitize every 10-14 d until get local reaction (erythema/vesicle). | After sensitization, apply to wart using 0.03%-2% solution once per wk until clear. | DNCB—possibly mutagenic. May be unable to sensitize some patients. Irritation. Erythema. Vesicle/bullae |
| Retinoids | Acitretin (Soriatane),[1] 10 mg or 25 mg tabs. Isotretinoin (Accutane),[1] 10 mg, 20 mg, 40 mg tabs. Topical tretinoin (Retin-A),[1] cream/microgel | Antimitotic: interferes with epidermal differentiation and proliferation. | Patient applied/initiated. Good prevention for immunosuppressed/ immunocompromised patients with multiple warts or EDV. Topical retinoids for flat warts. | Systemic: least effective qd or qod dose. Topical: apply qhs to warts only. | Topical: local irritation, erythema, and dryness. Systemic: mucocutaneous dryness, abnormal liver function tests, elevated triglycerides, |
| Bleomycin (Blenoxane)[1] | Aqueous solution, 0.1% (1 mg/mL) | Antimitotic. | Physician applied. Intralesional. | Single dose of 0.1 mL of 1 unit/mL in 0.1% solution with normal saline (unclear if repeat q 2-3 wk). | Pain (use with local anesthesia). Tissue necrosis. Scarring. Loss of nail. Raynaud's at local site. Possible significant systemic absorption |
| 5-Fluorouracil (Adrucil) | Cream, 5% | Antimitotic: inhibition of DNA and RNA synthesis leading to keratinocyte death. | Patient applied. May be combined with topical tretinoin therapy | Once per wk. | Irritation. Erythema. Edema |

[1] Not FDA approved for this indication.
[2] Not available in the United States.

*Abbreviations:* bid = twice daily; DNCB = dinitrochlorobenzene; DPC = diphenylcyclopropenone; EDV = epidermodysplasia verruciformis; q = every; qd = every day; qhs = at bedtime; qid = four times daily; qod = every other day; SADBE = squaric acid dibutylester; YAG = yttrium-aluminum-garnet.

Special attention should be paid to immunosuppressed or immuno-compromised patients in whom there is a higher rate of malignant transformation of warts and in whom warts tend to be more resistant and more numerous and thus may require systemic retinoids as a maintenance regimen.

# Condyloma Acuminatum (Genital Warts)

Method of
*Karl R. Beutner, MD, PhD,*
*and Alice N. Do, DO*

Genital warts are the most common manifestation of infection of the genital area with the human papilloma virus (HPV). Genital HPV infection is the most common viral sexually transmitted disease. Approximately 1% of the general population has genital warts at any time.

Proliferation of HIV-infected keratinocytes results in a genital wart. More than 100 genotypes of HPV exist. Low-risk HPV types 6 and 11 cause genital warts. High-risk HPV, most often types 16 and 18, are commonly associated with squamous cell carcinoma (SCC) in situ, also known as bowenoid papulosis or vulvar intraepithelial neoplasia of the external genital area, as well as abnormal Papanicoulaou (Pap) smears including in situ and invasive SCC of the cervix. In immunocompetent hosts, in situ SCC of the skin rarely, if ever, evolves into invasive SCC. Genital skin appears not to be as susceptible to the oncogenic potential of HPV as are the transformation zones of the uterine cervix and the anal canal.

Diagnosis is clinical, so identification of various presentations of genital warts involves understanding the different genital skin types that influence wart morphology. Three types of genital skin are fully keratinized hair-bearing, fully keratinized non–hair-bearing, and partially keratinized non–hair-bearing. The later appears moist and is often mistakenly referred to as mucous membranes. However, there are no mucus glands, and it appears moist because it is partially keratinized.

Treatment can be directed by skin type and wart morphology. The four morphologic types of genital warts are:

1. Cauliflower-type, or condyloma acuminatum
2. Smooth papular type, which are skin-colored, dome-shaped, 1 to 4 mm papules
3. Keratotic type, which may mimic seborrheic keratoses or common warts
4. Flat type, which are slightly raised.

Condyloma acuminatum occurs most commonly on moist, partially keratinized skin, whereas the smooth papular and keratotic types are seen most frequently on fully keratinized areas; the flat type is seen on all types of genital skin.

Genital warts may appear on the penile shaft, scrotum, perineum or perianal areas, labia, vulva, or pubic area, or in the crural folds. They can also be found in the urethra or bladder or in the oral cavity. The oral cavity should also be examined in patients being evaluated for genital warts.

Biopsy is usually unnecessary to confirm a clinical diagnosis of external genital warts. However, a biopsy should be considered when lesions are atypical, pigmented, ulcerated, indurated, or fixed to underlying tissue; fail to respond to treatment or worsen during treatment; frequently recur; exhibit individual (noncoalescent) warts larger than 1 cm in diameter; or are suspicious for malignancy. Biopsy should also be considered when diagnosis is unclear.

Acetowhitening to aid in diagnosis of external genital warts is no longer recommended because it lacks adequate specificity and sensitivity.

Differential diagnosis includes lichen planus, skin tags, seborrheic keratoses, molluscum contagiosum, condyloma latum, pearly penile papules, sebaceous glands, lichen nitidus, Crohn's disease, and SCC in situ.

## Treatment

Genital warts may spontaneously resolve or persist. Discuss expectations of therapy with patients. The goal is to eliminate symptoms, namely visible wart lesions, rather than to address HPV infection. Rather than a treatment, a course of therapy is required to achieve a wart-free state. It is unknown whether wart elimination will decrease or eliminate the patient's infectivity to current or future sexual partners. Even after proper treatment, recurrence is due to latent HPV in the surrounding normal tissue, and not necessarily due to reinfection. Once two individuals are infected with the same HPV type, they will not continue to reinfect one another. Any given treatment carries a 40% to 75% change of clearing and a 25% to 50% chance of recurrence. Recurrence is responsible for a prolonged course for the patient. Treatment failure is commonly caused by improper selection or use of a therapeutic modality. At the present time, all treatments are comparable in effectiveness.

## Choice of Treatment

Selection of treatment is influenced by wart morphology, anatomic site, total wart area, wart count, clinician's experience, and patient preference. Not all patients respond equally well to all modalities. Proper matching of patient with modality will usually shorten treatment duration. Pregnancy and immunosuppression are associated with larger and more numerous genital wart lesions. Certain treatment modalities are more appropriate in pregnancy. Immunosuppressed patients do not respond as well to therapy and have a high recurrence rate. These patients have a higher incidence of SCC. Have a plan or set protocol, particularly when a limited number of modalities are available. In general, if after three to four treatments with a given therapy a clinically significant response is not seen, or

---

 **CURRENT DIAGNOSIS**

**Diagnosis of genital warts requires their identification on physical exam. The clinician should become adept at recognizing the various morphologies of genital warts, which are influenced by the overlying genital skin type.**

| External Wart Morphology | Description | Skin Type |
|---|---|---|
| Condyloma acuminatum | Coalescent cauliflower-like plaques | Moist/partially keratinized |
| Smooth papular | Skin-colored, dome-shaped, 1 to 4 mm papules | Fully keratinized |
| Keratotic | | Fully keratinized |
| Flat type | Discrete, warty papules Slightly raised, flat-topped papules | Moist/partially keratinized or fully keratinized |

## CURRENT THERAPY

Treatment modalities can be divided into either provider-administered or patient-applied therapies. The choice of therapy will depend on skin type, wart quantity, and location.

| Treatment | Mechanism | Good Choice for | Poor Choice for | Procedure |
|---|---|---|---|---|
| **Provider administered** | | | | |
| Cryotherapy | Direct tissue destruction | • Small, flat, few warts<br>• Dry or moist warts<br>• Pregnancy OK | • Large wart areas ($> 10$ cm$^2$) | • Liquid nitrogen applied on a large, loosely wound piece of cotton on a wooden stick; or with a cryoprobe, by the spray technique<br>• Freeze the wart and 1- to 2-mm surrounding border |
| Podophyllin resin | Arrest in mitosis leading to tissue necrosis | • Moist warts | • Dry wart areas<br>• Do not exceed 10 cm$^2$ treatment area<br>• Not for pregnancy | • Use a cotton tip and apply a thin layer to wart and allow to air-dry before the patient assumes a normal anatomic position<br>• Leave on overnight and avoid washing, bathing, and sexual contact<br>• Repeat treatment 1 week later, as needed |
| TCA (Tri-Chlor)[1] | Chemical coagulation of wart proteins | • Small, moist, few warts<br>• Pregnancy OK | • Large wart areas ($> 10$ cm$^2$)<br>• Dry warts | • Apply sparingly to the lesion, being careful not to let the solution run onto normal skin<br>• Repeat weekly or every other week, as needed |
| Surgery | Direct removal of lesions | • Large or small treatment areas<br>• Rectal lesions OK<br>• Pregnancy OK | • Bleeding disorders | • Superficial tangential scissor excision, electrodesiccation, hot cautery, curettage, or CO$_2$ laser may be used |
| **Patient applied** | | | | |
| Podofilox (Condylox) | Arrest in mitosis → tissue necrosis | • Moist warts | • Do not exceed 10 cm$^2$ treatment area<br>• Not for pregnancy<br>• Poor compliance | • Apply bid for 3 days following by a 4-day treatment-free period<br>• Repeat weekly cycles four to six times, as needed |
| Imiquimod (Aldara) | Immunomodulator | • Moist warts | • Large wart areas ($> 10$ cm$^2$)<br>• Dry warts<br>• Poor compliance | • Apply every other night on moist warts or intertriginous areas, or every night on dry warts<br>• May be used for up to 16 weeks, as tolerated |

[1]Not FDA approved for this indication.
*Abbreviations:* TCA = trichloroacetic acid.

if after six treatments no clearance is achieved, the treatment modality should be changed and the diagnosis should be re-evaluated.

## TREATMENT MODALITIES

Current treatments are divided into provider-administered and patient-applied therapies. Provider-administered therapies include cryotherapy, podophyllin resin (Podocon-25), trichloroacetic acid (Tri-Chlor)[1], and surgery. Patient-applied therapies allow the patient greater control and include podofilox (Condylox) and imiquimod

(Aldara). However, these require good compliance and that the patient be able to view and reach the warts.

## PROVIDER-ADMINISTERED THERAPIES

### Cryotherapy

Cryotherapy works well for small, flat, few warts in dry or moist areas. It can be used on the penile shaft and vulva with little scarring. It can be used during pregnancy. It is not recommended for large wart areas, which can be quite painful and cause wound-care issues. A small, tightly wound cotton swab (Q-tip) that holds inadequate amounts of liquid nitrogen cannot effectively freeze a wart. Apply liquid nitrogen with a large, loosely wound piece of cotton on a wooden stick or with a cryoprobe.

[1]Not FDA approved for this indication.

A few small warts can be frozen without an anesthetic. Patients with more warts should be offered local anesthesia, with either injection of 1% lidocaine[1] or topical application of a eutectic mixture of 2.5% lidocaine and 2.5% prilocaine (EMLA cream).[1] Freeze the wart and 1- to 2-mm surrounding border. For larger warts, two freeze-thaw cycles are effective. How *hard* to freeze the warts can be learned with experience.

Cryotherapy requires proper training. Complications are rare but inexperienced clinicians often underfreeze areas, reducing efficacy. Overfreezing increases pain and the probability of scarring and other complications. Warn patients about post-treatment pain and blistering.

## Podophyllin Resin

Podophyllin resin (Podofin, Podocon-25, Podofilm) is from the plant species *Podophyllum peltatum* or *Podophyllum emodii*. This resin contains podofilox (podophyllotoxin), 4-dimethylpodophyllotoxin, α-peltatum, and β-peltatum, which cause cellular mitotic arrest and lead to tissue necrosis. It is a good choice for moist warts and up to a 10 cm[2] surface area. It is ineffective in dry areas, such as the scrotum, penile shaft, and labia majora.

Podophyllin resin lacks a standardized preparation, but it is commonly used as a 10% to 25% solution in tincture of benzoin. Use a cotton tip and apply a thin layer directly to the wart and allow to air dry before the patient assumes a normal anatomic position. Traditionally, patients were advised to wash off podophyllin 2 to 4 hours after application, but benzoin is water insoluble and cannot be removed simply with soap and water. Another ill-advised but not uncommon practice is to create a *barrier* around the wart with Vaseline or K-Y jelly, and apply podophyllin resin to the central wart. Body temperature thins the barrier, which mixes with the podophyllin resin, and spreads over the entire area, creating an impressive irritant reaction. I advise patients to leave the podophyllin resin on overnight and avoid washing, bathing, or sexual contact until the next day. Local side effects include erythema, pain, and irritation. Systemic side effects are caused by increased toxic absorption and are associated with large treatment area (>10 cm[2]) or allowing the resin to absorb for an extended time. Avoid podophyllin resin in pregnancy.

## Trichloroacetic Acid (Tri-Chlor)[1]

Trichloroacetic acid ([TCA] Tri-Chlor)[1] chemically coagulates warts and adjacent skin. Use for small, few, moist warts. TCA[1] can be used during pregnancy. Although 30% to 70% solutions are employed, the optimal concentration is undetermined. Use extreme caution with the higher concentrations, which can be highly caustic. Apply sparingly to lesions, being careful not to let the solution run onto normal skin. Treatment can be repeated weekly, or every other week, as needed. TCA[1] can be neutralized, if needed, with soap and sodium bicarbonate.

## Surgery

Surgery renders the patient wart free with a single visit. It is a good choice for limited or large treatment areas. There is no clearly superior surgical modality. Selection of a surgical approach depends on clinician experience and availability of equipment. Good results can be achieved with superficial tangential scissors, electrodesiccation, hot cautery, curettage, or $CO_2$ laser.

## PATIENT-APPLIED THERAPIES

### Podofilox

The major active lignin in podophyllin resin is podofilox, available as a 0.5% solution or gel (Condylox). Apply to warts twice daily for 3 days followed by a treatment-free period of 4 days. Repeat this cycle four to six times to achieve wart clearance. A maximum of 10 cm[2] should be treated, and podofilox should be avoided in pregnancy.

## Imiquimod

Imiquimod (Aldara) is a 5% cream, applied three times weekly at bedtime to moist wart areas. Dry and nonintertriginous areas may respond better to daily application. It can be used for up to 16 weeks. As imiquimod stimulates an inflammatory response, however, local irritation, burning, and ulceration are expected side effects and are similar to those seen with other modalities.

## 5-Fluorouracil

5-Fluorouracil creams (Carac, Effudex),[1] used previously for genital warts, are no longer recommended because of side effects, uproven efficacy, and the availability of other treatments.

# Transmission and Prevention

HPV is a sexually transmitted disease (STD). Educate patients to tell sexual partners that they have this infection. Condoms may decrease transmission but do not completely prevent infection. Asymptomatic partners can harbor a subclinical infection, and examination for genital warts is appropriate if lesions are suspected. It is unknown whether treatment of genital wart lesions eliminates infectivity. Discuss the oncogenic potential of HPV types associated with bowenoid papulosis. Women with external genital warts or whose male partners have lesions should have a Pap smear and remain in the system for monitoring for cervical cancer. Investigations for other STDs should be done if suspected.

Acquiring an STD carries a negative social stigma and emotional trauma. Patients often fear discovery and rejection and feel guilty and victimized. They view themselves as less sexually desirable, enjoy sex less, and have concerns about transmission. Teaching and educational materials are available from the American Social Health Association (1-919-361-8422).

## REFERENCES

Beutner KR, Richwald GA, Wiley DJ, et al: External genital warts: Report of the American Medical Association consensus conference. Clin Infect Dis 1998;27:796-806.

Beutner KR, Wiley DJ, Douglas JM, et al: Genital warts and their treatment. Clin Infect Dis 1999;28(Suppl 1):S37-S56.

Habif TP: Sexually transmitted viral infections. In Hodgson S, Cook L (eds): Clinial Dermatology, A Color Guide to Diagnosis and Therapy, 4th ed. Philadelphia, Mosby 2004, pp 336-342.

Odom RB, James WD, Berger TG: Viral diseases. In Fathman EM, Geisel EB, Salmo A (eds): Andrews' Diseases of the Skin, Clinical Dermatology, 9th ed. Philadelphia, WB Saunders, 2000; pp 541-519.

# Nevi

Method of
*Raymond L. Barnhill, MD, Seth I. Felder, BA, and Brandon D. Einstein, BA*

A nevus (plural, nevi), also known as a *melanocytic nevus, nevocellular nevus,* or *mole,* is a benign neoplasm composed of melanocytes. Melanocytic nevi originate from melanoblasts that migrate from the neural crest to the epidermis. Nevi are believed to be either developmental malformations (hamartomas) or benign clonal proliferations that have a growth advantage over surrounding basilar melanocytes. This article discusses the most common acquired and congenital benign melanocytic lesions.

---

[1]Not FDA approved for this indication.

---

[1]Not FDA approved for this indication.

**TABLE 1  Clinical and Histologic Features of Common Acquired Melanocytic Nevi**

| Feature | Junctional | Compound | Dermal |
|---|---|---|---|
| Size | <6 mm | <6 mm | <10 mm |
| Color | Light to dark brown | Light to dark brown | Skin colored; light to dark brown |
| Primary lesion | Macule | Papule or plaque | Papule or nodule |
| Clinical location | Head, neck, trunk, extremities | Head, neck, trunk, extremities | Face, head, neck, trunk, extremities |
| Histologic location | Dermoepidermal junction | Dermoepidermal junction and papillary dermis | Dermis |

# Epidemiology

Acquired melanocytic nevi most commonly appear in childhood and adolescence, but they can also develop later in life. In contrast, congenital melanocytic nevi are usually presumed to be present at birth, possibly resulting from a developmental error in neuroectodermal melanocyte migration. This classification of melanocytic nevi as acquired or congenital, however, has limitations. Relatively small melanocytic nevi that fulfill clinical and histopathologic criteria for congenital nevi might not be present at birth. Such lesions can develop later as *congenital nevus–like nevi* or *tardive congenital nevi.*

Few nevi are present in early childhood, and prevalence increases until the third decade of life. Over time, melanocytic nevi commonly become less pigmented and therefore less noticeable, and some nevi actually disappear.

The incidence of nevi is related to age, race, and genetic and environmental factors. Gender is not a factor in the proclivity for developing nevi. Generally, white persons have more nevi than persons from darker-skinned ethnic groups, such as persons of Asian or sub-Saharan African ancestry. Additionally, persons with fair complexions, such as Fitzpatrick types I and II—especially those with a history of sun exposure—are most likely to acquire nevi.

The notion that benign melanocytic nevi are potentially precursors to malignancy is often misinterpreted, because most melanomas arise de novo from normal skin. Regardless of origin, a greater number of melanocytic nevi, with or without atypical features, is associated with an increased risk of developing melanoma.

# Clinical Presentations

Melanocytic nevi can manifest as macules, papules, plaques, or nodules with variable contours, patterns, and pigmentations. Despite variability of nevi morphology, distinctive attributes allow classification with high specificity using clinical, dermoscopic, and histopathologic examination. Melanocytic nevi are biologically benign lesions. That is, they arise, grow to a certain size, and then cease developing. The common denominator of all melanocytic nevi is an increased number of melanocytes within the epidermis, dermis, subcutaneous fat, or any combination of these sites.

Common acquired nevi are well-circumscribed round or ovoid lesions, generally from 2 to 6 mm in diameter. They appear orderly and symmetric, with regular, well-defined borders. *Junctional nevi* are uniform light to dark brown macules with regular borders. These lesions are characterized histologically by nests of melanocytes at the dermoepidermal junction. Nests of melanocytes confined to the dermis are referred to as *dermal nevi.* These pigmented papules or nodules are light to dark brown dome-shaped lesions. *Compound nevi* are slightly raised papules or plaques, light to dark brown, and composed of nests of melanocytes at the dermoepidermal junction and papillary dermis. There is clinical and histologic overlap among the three types of nevi (Table 1). In general, benign nevi differ from melanoma by their smaller size, overall symmetry, homogenous coloration, and well-defined borders (Box 1).

Congenital nevi are benign melanocytic proliferations present at birth or soon thereafter. They are characterized by nests of melanocytes at the dermoepidermal junction and dermis, and they often extend around blood vessels, nerves, and adnexal structures. In general, classification is based on their size: small are less than 1.5 cm in greatest diameter, medium are 1.5 cm to 19.9 cm, and large or giant are larger than 19.9 cm (Table 2). Because the potential risk of becoming malignant is probably related to the size of the congenital nevus, patients with larger nevi are at the greatest risk and should be closely monitored for changes in color or surface features. Smaller congenital nevi exhibit perifollicular hyper- or hypopigmentation on a light tan background with a soft, mammilated texture, and larger congenital nevi often have a pebbly or coarse surface.

*Atypical melanocytic nevi* (AMN; dysplastic nevi, Clark's nevi) constitute a gross morphologic and histologic continuum that ranges from common nevi at one end to melanoma at the opposite end

## CURRENT DIAGNOSIS

- The diagnosis of a nevus is based on clinical appearance.
- When a nevus is suspicious for melanoma, it must be biopsied for histopathologic examination.
- Total body skin examination is recommended and should be accomplished in light of the individual patient's personal and familial histories
- Suspicious nevi are generally asymmetric, have irregular borders, show color variegation, and are often greater than 6 mm in diameter.
- Appropriate documentation should include the lesion's location, pattern, color, and size.
- Evaluation of nevi consists of unaided visual inspection along with advanced diagnostic tools such as dermoscopy and computer-aided image analysis, which are increasingly available and supplement clinical diagnostic accuracy.
- Broad-spectrum sun protection and skin self-examination using the ABCD criteria should be discussed and encouraged.
- Baseline photography is often useful in the surveillance of high-risk patients, particularly those with multiple nevi, and allows evaluation of comparative changes over time.

## BOX 1  The ABCD Method of Clinical Evaluation of Lesions

- **A**symmetric shape
- **B**order irregularity
- **C**olor variegation
- **D**iameter >6 mm

**TABLE 2 Clinical Features of Small, Medium, and Large Congenital Nevi**

| Feature | Small and Medium | Large (Giant) |
|---|---|---|
| Size | <1.5 cm (small); 1.5-19.9 cm (medium) | >19.9 cm |
| Color | Tan to brown with perifollicular hyper- or hypopigmentation | Brown to black |
| Primary lesion | Soft, mammilated | Plaque-like, pebbly, coarse |
| Clinical location | Anywhere, especially head or neck | Anywhere |
| Histologic location | Dermoepidermal junction and dermis, often extending around blood vessels, nerves, and adnexal structures | Dermoepidermal junction and dermis, often extending around blood vessels, nerves, and adnexal structures or diffuse dermal and possibly subcutaneous involvement or deeper |

of the spectrum. Clinically, AMN are usually 5 to 12 mm in diameter (with exceptions), have a macular component, often have irregular borders or ill-defined borders, or both, and irregular coloration. Histologically, *atypical (dysplastic) melanocytic nevi* are usually characterized by irregular junctional nesting of melanocytes or lentiginous melanocytic proliferation (architectural disorder) and cytologic atypia of intraepidermal melanocytes. Elongated epidermal rete ridges, bridging of the junctional nests, papillary dermal fibrosis, and superficial perivascular lymphocytic infiltrates are commonly present. Because these acquired nevi are benign but possess one or more clinical features of melanoma, they must be examined in the context of each patient's history. Despite this, AMN rarely evolve into melanoma, and the overwhelming majority of AMN are clinically stable. The presence of AMN identifies persons at high risk for developing melanoma. Dermoscopy may be useful in evaluating AMN. Although AMN can clinically simulate melanoma, many of these lesions fall into one of the benign dermoscopic melanocytic patterns, the most common patterns being reticular, globular, and homogeneous.

A *halo nevus* results from an immunologic event in which the host response, including T lymphocytes, apparently attempts to destroy nevus cells. These lesions are characterized by a central melanocytic nevus component surrounded by a well-circumscribed annulus of hypo- or depigmented skin. Some of these lesions completely regress, leaving only a depigmented area and no residual nevus. Halo nevi are more common in adolescents than adults and are most typically located on the back. Patients older than 40 years who present with halo nevi should be examined for melanoma.

*Spitz* tumors (commonly referred to as *Spitz nevi*) are composed of large epitheloid or spindle-shaped melanocytes that are usually aggregated in nests. They appear as well-circumscribed pink to tan to dark brown dome-shaped papules, plaques, or nodules. Spitz tumors are most commonly acquired, but as many as 7% may be congenital. They occur in all age groups but are exceedingly rare beyond the ages of 40 to 50 years. Although Spitz nevi can involve any part of the body, they most often occur on the head and in the neck area or extremities. Because these lesions can histologically mimic melanoma, and some fraction of Spitz tumors demonstrate a spectrum of atypicality (atypical Spitz tumors), it is imperative to biopsy and evaluate each lesion completely.

*Blue nevi* are characterized by heavily pigmented dendritic and often spindled melanocytes disposed in discrete aggregates in the superficial dermis or, less commonly, in larger multilobular configurations dispersed throughout the reticular dermis. Blue nevi appear as well-circumscribed symmetric raised lesions, blue to blue-black, and are usually located on the dorsa of the hands and feet, the sacral region, and the scalp. Blue nevi are usually acquired but are congenital in rare

instances, and they appear most commonly in childhood and adolescence. Blue nevi that are clinically stable, located in a typical anatomic site, less than 1 cm in diameter, and have characteristic features do not require removal.

*Recurrent nevi* are defined by irregular hyperpigmentation within the scar of a previously removed nevus. Asymmetric repigmentation, which generally occurs within 6 months of the procedure, should not extend beyond the white scarred area. Therefore, establishing that a previous surgical procedure has taken place, and establishing the nature of the original lesion, is critical for arriving at a definitive diagnosis. Most recurrent nevi are stable after their development and, in general, are not associated with increased melanoma risk.

## Treatment

The indications for removing melanocytic nevi are a changing lesion, atypical clinical appearance suspicious for melanoma, cosmetic reasons (by patient request), recurrence of an old lesion, presence of a new lesion, and repeated irritation (Box 2).

When performing a proper cutaneous biopsy, it is important to obtain adequate tissue for histopathologic examination and to avoid unnecessary cosmetic defects for the patient. It is imperative to perform a complete excisional biopsy when removing a suspected malignant lesion. An excisional biopsy ensures the removal of the lesion's base along with ample tissue for histopathologic interpretation. For superficial lesions, a shave biopsy encompassing the entire lesion is an acceptable alternative procedure. Sometimes it is necessary to perform a punch biopsy, especially in areas of cosmetic concern and for inconvenient sites, such as the eyelid or lip.

---

 **CURRENT THERAPY**

- Any pigmented lesion suspicious for malignancy should be excised completely with 2-mm margins for histopathologic analysis.
- A biopsy is recommended in the following instances:
  - Lesions that evolve over time in size, shape, or color
  - Lesions demonstrating bleeding or ulceration
  - Lesions that recur with unconventional repigmentation patterns
  - Newly developing lesions
  - Lesions requested for removal by patients for cosmetic or other reasons.
- Patients should be informed that scarring following biopsy depends on the location of the lesion, the size of the resulting defect, and the patient's ability to heal.
- It is not mandatory to remove atypical nevi simply to confirm or exclude the diagnosis of atypical melanocytic nevi histologically. However, it is appropriate to monitor such patients on a regular schedule, often aided by baseline photography, dermoscopy, and digital imaging.

---

**BOX 2 Indications for Biopsy or Excision**

- Atypical clinical appearance suspicious for melanoma
- Changing lesion
- Cosmetic reasons, per patient request
- New lesion
- Recurrence of an old lesion
- Repeated irritation (ulceration, pain)

## REFERENCES

Ackerman AB, Boer A, Bennin B, Gottlieb GJ: Histologic Diagnosis of Inflammatory Skin Diseases. An Algorithmic Method Based on Pattern Analysis, 3rd ed. Fredericksburg, Pa: Ardor Scribendi, 2005.

Barnhill RL: Textbook of Dermatopathology, 2nd ed. New York: McGraw-Hill, 2004.

Barnhill RL: Pathology of melanocytic nevi and malignant melanoma. Boston: Butterworth-Heinemann, 1995.

Barnhill RL, Fitzpatrick TB, Fandrey K, et al: The Pigmented Lesion Clinic: A Color Atlas and Synopsis of Benign and Pigmented Lesions. New York: McGraw-Hill, 1995.

Barnhill RL (ed): Pathology of Melanocytic Nevi and Malignant Melanoma, 2nd ed. New York: Springer-Verlag, 2004.

Barnhill RL, Lewellyn K: Benign melanocytic neoplasms. In Bolognia JL, Jorizzo J, Rapini R (eds): Dermatology. St. Louis: Mosby, 2003, pp 1757-1787.

Crowson AN, Magro CM, Mihm MC: The Melanocytic Proliferations: A Comprehensive Textbook of Pigmented Lesions. New York: Wiley-Liss 2001.

Elder D, Elenitsas R, Jaworsky C: Lever's Histopathology of the Skin. Philadelphia: Lippincott Williams & Wilkins, 1997.

Freedberg IM, Eisen AZ, Wolff K, et al: Fitzpatrick's Dermatology in General Medicine. New York: McGraw-Hill, 2003.

Weedon D: Skin Pathology. New York: Churchill Livingstone, 2002.

# Melanoma

Method of
*Frank G. Haluska, MD, PhD*

Melanoma is the most lethal of all solid cancers: prognostically, no other tumor carries the severe implication that its diagnosis does. An early-stage, solitary 3-cm lesion for lung cancer, responsible for most cancer deaths, may confer 5-year mortality of 20% to 30% on discovery. In contrast, a primary melanoma only 1 mm in depth confers a similar prognosis spread over 10 years. Melanoma offers a constant challenge to improve prevention, detection, diagnosis, and treatment.

## Epidemiology

The incidence of melanoma is rapidly increasing with approximately 62,190 new cases projected in the United States in 2006 and 7910 deaths as a consequence. Risk factors include a changing mole, dysplastic nevi either arising in the setting of family history or sporadically, or a personal history of melanoma or congenital nevi. Sensitivity to sun and a history of sunburns and freckling are also associated with risks for melanoma. Prevention and early detection depend on taking a careful history from patients in such risk categories.

### CURRENT DIAGNOSIS

- Pigmented or unusual nonpigmented skin lesions should be carefully evaluated for ABCD:
  - *Asymmetry* or unusual contours
  - *Border* irregularity
  - *Color* that is blue, black, red, or white (regressed); is variegated or changing
  - *Diameter* that is larger than 6 mm (a pencil eraser's diameter) or is enlarging
- Elevated, ulcerated or bleeding lesions require evaluation.
- Diagnosis by biopsy must be excisional or incisional.

## Clinical Features and Diagnosis

Melanomas can arise on any cutaneous surface, on any mucous membrane, in structures of the eye, or as a metastasis lacking a primary site, but they typically arise on sun-exposed skin surfaces. The most common sites of occurrence in males are the trunk and back, and in females the lower legs and back.

The clinician should have a high index of suspicion for any lesion that is new, has changed, or is out of the ordinary. The visible features requiring further investigation include irregularity of surface texture, border contour, or coloration. Growth, manifested as an increase in diameter, nodularity or elevation, is worrisome. Surface ulceration and overt hemorrhage are also hallmarks of melanoma. The clinician should have a low threshold for biopsy for lesions with any of these characteristics. Patients should be taught the features (ABCD) as well: lesion asymmetry (A), an irregular border (B), changing or variegated color (C), and a diameter (D) larger than a pencil eraser.

An expert dermatologist can augment diagnostic accuracy at the bedside using epiluminescence microscopy or by using dermoscopy with sophisticated digital photography and image analysis. The standard for diagnosis is histopathologic evaluation by excisional biopsy of the lesion with a narrow margin. An incisional biopsy may be used when lesions are large or in a difficult anatomical site. In both instances the objective should be to allow for full-thickness histopathologic assessment of the lesion. Other biopsy techniques (e.g., shave or curettage) and local ablative therapies such as liquid nitrogen are contraindicated if melanoma is considered in the differential diagnosis. Correctly performing biopsy is critical in arriving at an accurate tissue diagnosis and providing subsequent treatment.

## Treatment

### SURGICAL THERAPY OF PRIMARY MELANOMA

Melanoma, detected early, is a curable disease; but most cases cured are by surgical, not medical, means. Surgical care encompasses primary excision integrated with regional lymph node assessment and removal.

### Planning the Primary Excision

The goals of primary surgical excision of melanoma are threefold. First, the procedure must account for the potential need for assessment of regional lymph node involvement. Second, the lesion must be completely excised with curative intent. Third, the margin of excision should be planned to minimize the risk of local recurrence.

The assessment of the regional lymph nodes is controversial. No randomized clinical trial has demonstrated that elective lymph node dissection of the draining lymph node basin influences the median survival of a population of melanoma. Regional lymph node mapping, or sentinel lymph node (SLN) biopsy, has the same findings; but technical

### CURRENT THERAPY

- Proper surgery is the mainstay of treatment.
- The primary tumor should be completely excised with recommended margins.
- A sentinel lymph node biopsy is recommended for lesions 1 mm and deeper.
- Palpable regional lymph nodes should be biopsied and resected if involved.
- There is no adjuvant medical therapy for stage I and II, but interferon alpha-2B is recommended for stage III.
- Stage IV DTIC chemotherapy and interleukin-2 cytokine therapy are FDA approved, but clinical trial entry is an important option.

accessibility, reliability, proven prognostic value, relative lack of morbidity, and the potential for therapeutic value have led to its widespread use. SLN biopsy involves injection of a blue dye and radioactive tracer, which migrate to the lymph node providing drainage of the primary site; intraoperative identification of the node with a small radiation counter; and excision for histopathologic examination. Approximately 17% of patients referred for SLN biopsy ultimately have involved sentinel lymph nodes. Patients with involved (positive) sentinel nodes should then be taken to complete lymph node dissection of the involved basin. Sentinel lymph node biopsy, at the time of excision with an intermediate thickness (1 mm or greater) melanoma and in selected cases of high-risk thinner melanomas, is now the standard of surgical care for the melanoma patient.

Initial wide local excision of a primary tumor may interfere with the normal pattern of lymphatic drainage; consequently, lymphatic mapping may be impaired or precluded. Therefore, it is important to perform SLN biopsy concurrent with wide excision. Excision of the lesion is designed to remove all melanoma at the local site. Typically, the incision used is elliptical, and the tumor should be removed en bloc with the underlying tissues to the level of the muscular fascia.

Local metastases, or satellites, can spread to the skin immediately surrounding the primary tumor, and a margin of normal tissue should be excised to minimize the risk that these metastases will manifest later as local recurrences. The most recent of five randomized clinical trials assessing adequacy of margins suggests that thicker tumors require wider margins, but none show that margins affect survival. Recommendations for excisional margins vary from center to center. Table 1 lists the surgical care guidelines used in the Massachusetts General Hospital Melanoma Center.

If local lymph nodes are palpable at the time of diagnosis, therapeutic lymph node dissection is required.

## ADJUVANT MEDICAL THERAPY OF HIGH-RISK DISEASE

The most important prognostic features obtainable at the time of diagnosis, incorporated into the American Joint Committee on Cancer (AJCC) staging system, are Breslow depth, the presence of ulceration of the primary tumor, and lymph node involvement (Table 2). The 10-year survival rate for patients with stage I melanoma (localized and 2 mm or thinner) is approximately 85%; for stage II (localized but thicker than 2 mm) survival is 55%; and for stage III (metastatic to the local skin or lymph nodes), it is 35%. Biologically, at the time of diagnosis, occult metastases are present in a subset of patients who will eventually succumb to recurrence. This provides an opportunity for early therapy in an at-risk population or adjuvant therapy.

There are no adjuvant therapies at present for stage I and stage II melanoma, providing an active area for research. The United States Food and Drug Administration (FDA) has approved interferon alpha-2b (Intron A) for patients with a high risk of systemic recurrence (T4 lesions 4 mm deep or greater, or stage III melanoma). This year-long course of adjuvant therapy is expensive with a significant side-effect profile, primarily a severe flu-like syndrome, with hepato- and myelotoxicity. Yet, interferon alpha-2b is the only therapy proven in the randomized controlled setting to alter the natural history of this disease. Interferon alpha-2b prolongs relapse-free survival reproducibly; two trials suggested improvement in overall survival of

## TABLE 2  Survival by Stage and Sentinel Node Status

| Stage | 10-yr Survival | Median Survival |
|---|---|---|
| I | 85% | - |
| II | 55% | - |
| III | 35% | - |
| IV | 8% | 8 months |
| **Sentinel Node Status** | **3-yr Disease-Free Survival** | **3-yr Overall Survival** |
| Negative | 88.5% | 96.8% |
| Positive | 55.8% | 69.9% |

approximately 10% as well, though a recent meta-analysis demonstrates this is not statistically significant.

## MEDICAL THERAPY OF ADVANCED DISEASE

The median survival of stage IV melanoma patients is approximately 8 months. Melanoma can spread to any site, but metastases most commonly involve skin, lymph nodes, brain, lung, and liver. No treatment for metastatic melanoma has ever been proven to effectively prolong survival in a randomized clinical trial; thus, for many patients, entry into a clinical study is an important option for stage IV therapy.

## CYTOTOXIC THERAPY

Like many other solid tumors, such as metastatic pancreatic or renal cell cancer, melanoma is relatively refractory to the systemic administration of cytotoxic chemotherapy. Response rates to most single agents, including alkylating agents, platinum compounds, and taxanes, range from 5% to 20%. Dacarbazine (DTIC) is the only chemotherapy agent approved for use in melanoma. Temozolomide (Temodar),[2] an oral drug metabolized to the same active agent (MTIC) as DTIC, is often used in its place. In recent randomized clinical trials using modern RECIST response-evaluation criteria, response rates for DTIC were approximately 7%. Complete response rates were low: approximately 1%. A recent European randomized trial suggested fotemustine might improve response rate compared to DTIC, but no single drug has improved the survival of treated patient populations.

Combination chemotherapy has been studied extensively. Two common regimens are as follows:

1. The Dartmouth regimen: DTIC, carmustine (BCNU), cisplatin (Platinol), and tamoxifen (Nolvadex)
2. Cisplatin, DTIC, and vinblastine (CVD)

Although single-institution studies suggest improved response rates with these regimens, in randomized trials survival rates are no better with these regimens than with single agent treatment.

## IMMUNOTHERAPY

Interleukin-2 (IL-2), recombinant (Proleukin), is a second drug approved by the FDA and available for use in patients with stage IV disease. The major toxicity of IL-2 is a systemic inflammatory state, which manifests as capillary-leak syndrome and hypotension. Most patients require pressors or intensive care during treatment. Clinicians should restrict IL-2 use to a select subset of patients with excellent performance status and features predictive of response to therapy.

Initial dramatic responses were reported with systemic IL-2 therapy, but the response rate is now approximately 15%. Patients with metastases confined to the skin demonstrate a response rate of 54%, but for patients with disease other than that confined to skin and lymph nodes, the response rate is approximately 11%. At the National Cancer Institute (NCI) approximately 3% of patients experience

## TABLE 1  Surgical Treatment of Primary Melanoma

| Breslow Depth | Margin | Sentinel Node Biopsy |
|---|---|---|
| <1.00 mm | 1 cm | Only if adverse prognostic feature* |
| 1.00–2.00 mm | 2 cm | Yes |
| >2.00 mm | At least 2 cm | Yes |

*For example, ulceration.

²Not available in the United States.

durable complete responses. But overall, IL-2 therapy is of limited benefit to most patients with visceral metastatic melanoma.

## BIOCHEMOTHERAPY

The hypothesis that combining chemotherapy and immunotherapy might join therapies having different mechanisms of action and drug resistance led to the development of biochemotherapy. Most biochemotherapy regimens include combination chemotherapy, interleukin-2, and interferon, but a variety of regimens have been tested. A randomized study of biochemotherapy compared with chemotherapy conducted at the NIH was stopped early because the outcome favored chemotherapy alone; a second single-institutional randomized study suggested an improved response rate and a marginal survival improvement from biochemotherapy but with severe toxicity (90% of patients requiring pressors). Recently, several large multi-institutional randomized studies demonstrated that biochemotherapy is more toxic but no more effective than chemotherapy alone.

## Clinical Trial Directions: Targeted Therapies, Vaccines, and New Approaches

The potential for progress in treating melanoma depends on the development of new approaches tested in clinical trials. The first area of promise is the use of small molecule inhibitors of biochemical pathways important in the pathogenesis of melanoma. The most frequent somatic mutations in melanoma involve the RAS signal transduction cascades: the BRAF protein is mutated in 60% to 70% of cutaneous melanomas. Inhibitors of this protein, including the new agent sorafenib,[1] are in clinical trials alone and in combination with other small molecules and cytotoxic agents. The BCL-2 protein has also been targeted in this disease, and continued study of antisense inhibitors of BCL-2 expression is ongoing.

The second important avenue of research is active immunotherapy, using approaches designed to augment host antitumor immunity. Approaches include the use of surgically resected autologous melanoma as vaccine (in GM-CSF-gene transduced preparations, or in conjunction with autologous heat shock proteins), allogeneic vaccines (e.g., Canvaxin and Melacine), melanoma antigen-derived peptide vaccines, lymphodepletion protocols, and antibodies to immunoregulatory molecules (anti-CTLA4). Although none of these approaches has yielded positive results in randomized trials, single-institution reports often suggest potential efficacy. A focus on immunotherapy will likely remain an important component of investigational therapy for melanoma.

## REFERENCES

Atkins MB, Lee S, Flaherty LE, et al: A prospective randomized phase III trial concurrent biochemotherapy with cisplatin, vinblastine, dacarbazine (CVD), IL-2 and interferon alpha-2b versus CVD alone in patients with metastatic melanoma (E3695): An ECOG-coordinated intergroup trial. Proc ASCO 2003;22:708.

Avril MF, Aamdal S, Grob JJ, et al: Fotemustine compared with dacarbazine in patients with disseminated malignant melanoma: A phase III study. J Clin Oncol 2004;22:1118-1125.

Balch CM, Buzaid AC, Soong SJ, et al: Final version of the American Joint Committee on Cancer staging system for cutaneous melanoma. J Clin Oncol 2001;19:3635-3648.

Chapman PB, Einhorn LH, Meyers ML, et al: Phase III multicenter randomized trial of the Dartmouth regimen versus dacarbazine in patients with metastatic melanoma. J Clin Oncol 1999;17: 2745-2751.

Gershenwald JE, Thompson W, Mansfield PF, et al: Multi-institutional melanoma lymphatic mapping experience: The prognostic value of sentinel lymph node status in 612 stage I or II melanoma patients. J Clin Oncol 1999;17:976-983.

Kirkwood JM, Manola J, Ibrahim J, et al: A pooled analysis of Eastern Cooperative Oncology Group and intergroup trials of adjuvant high-dose interferon for melanoma. Clin Cancer Res 2004;10: 1670-1677.

Krown SE, Chapman PB: Defining adequate surgery for primary melanoma. N Engl J Med 2004;350:823-825.

McMasters KM, Reintgen DS, Ross MI, et al: Sentinel lymph node biopsy for melanoma: controversy despite widespread agreement. J Clin Oncol 2001;19:2851-2855.

Middleton MR, Grob JJ, Aaronson N, et al: Randomized phase III study of temozolomide versus dacarbazine in the treatment of patients with advanced metastatic malignant melanoma. J Clin Oncol 2000;18:158-166.

Phan GQ, Attia P, Steinberg SM, et al: Factors associated with response to high-dose interleukin-2 in patients with metastatic melanoma. J Clin Oncol 2001;19:3477-3482.

# Premalignant Lesions

Method of
*Donald Clemons, MD*

## Premalignant Lesions

Premalignant lesions of the skin are those that, if left untreated, can evolve into malignant invasive and potentially metastasizing tumors. With early treatment, these lesions can be managed and the threat of malignancy averted. These premalignant diseases include actinic keratosis (AK), actinic cheilitis, Bowen's disease, bowenoid papulosis, porokeratosis, and nevus sebaceus.

Nonmelanoma skin cancer's worldwide economic and health implications are enormous, because it is the most prevalent form of cancer. However, it is also one of the most preventable cancers and, in early stages, relatively easy to diagnose and treat. We must educate our patient population to not only recognize and seek treatment for these early manifestations but to also act as public health advocates regarding modification of behavioral patterns of our at-risk population.

Premalignant lesions are most commonly located on chronic sun-exposed and sun-damaged skin in lighter-skinned individuals who easily burn, have light hair color, have blue or green eyes, and freckle. Both genetic and extrinsic factors are responsible for the development and progression of these lesions. Chronically damaged skin, such as burn scars and long-standing ulcers, infections, and areas having received ionizing radiation are also more likely to develop malignant transformation. Other factors placing patients at increased risk include chronic arsenic exposure and immunosuppression as seen in the elderly, organ transplant recipients, HIV-infected individuals, and patients receiving systemic steroid therapy. This large subset of patients is more likely to rapidly develop malignant transformation and show aggressive behavior in their lesions. They should be closely monitored and considered for long-term prophylactic care.

## Actinic Keratosis

Actinic keratosis, a form of squamous cell carcinoma (SCC) in situ, is usually found on photo-damaged skin and is characterized clinically by rough adherent scale on an erythematous nonindurated occasionally friable and tender base. The background is usually telangiectatic with areas of dyspigmentation. Hyperpigmented and atrophic variations can be seen. They may be palpated easier than visualized but can progress to thickened hyperkeratotic plaques. Rapidly enlarging lesions or those that are excessively hyperkeratotic or indurated should be biopsied to rule out malignant progression to SCC. Histologically, AKs are characterized by a partial thickness disordered windblown maturation of atypical epidermal keratinocytes and a thickened compact stratum corneum. The hair acrotrichium and sweat duct acrosyringium are spared involvement and no invasion is seen. The epidermis can be thickened or atrophic.

### TREATMENT OF ACTINIC KERATOSIS

Treatment can be by physical disruptions or chemically applied methods. Among the physical methods, liquid nitrogen cryosurgery is most

## CURRENT DIAGNOSIS

Actinic keratosis
- Tender, rough adherent scale on erythematous base
- Background of photo-damaged skin
- Suspect SCC if indurated or hyperkeratotic

Actinic cheilitis
- Protuberant lower lip mucosa, fair skin, photo damage
- Often history of pipe or chewing tobacco use
- Up to 25% metastatic incidence with invasion

Bowen's disease
- Erythematous sharply demarcated plaque with variable scale
- Involves hair follicles
- Frequently recurs if inadequately treated
- May affect genital mucosal skin

Bowenoid papulosis
- Clinically indistinguishable from warts
- Genital skin
- Histologically indistinguishable from Bowen's disease
- Associated with HPV-16

Porokeratosis
- Papules or annular plaques with thin peripheral collarette of scale
- Discrete or linear
- Sun damaged skin or palms or soles
- Coronoid lamella seen histologically

Nevus sebaceus
- Perpetual elevated often inapparent plaques usually on head or neck
- Postpubertal evolve into yellow-orange papillomatous plaques devoid of hair
- Malignancies are usually low grade

*Abbreviations:* HPV-16 = human papilloma virus type 16; SCC = squamous cell carcinoma.

## CURRENT THERAPY

Actinic keratosis
- Cryotherapy, light curettage, dermabrasion, or chemical peels
- Topical or systemic tretinoin (Retin-A), fluorouracil (Efudex), diclofenac (Solaraze), imiquimod (Aldara), or PDT

Actinic cheilitis
- Cryotherapy, fluorouracil, imiquimod
- Vermilionectomy, laser, PDT

Bowen's disease
- All methods used for actinic keratosis
- Excision to include Mohs' surgery

Bowenoid papulosis
- Same as Bowen's
- Imiquimod may be treatment of choice

Porokeratosis
- Cryosurgery, salicylic plaster and fluorouracil, topical tretinoin[1]
- Imiquimod

Nevus sebaceus
- Watchful waiting with appropriate biopsies
- Excision

[1]Not FDA approved for this indication.
*Abbreviations:* PDT = photodynamic therapy

---

commonly used. Care must be taken to adequately freeze and destroy the lesion yet minimize significant pigment alteration or scarring. The length of the freeze time will vary by size, thickness, and location of the tumor, ethnic skin color, and concomitant systemic illness such as lupus erythematosus or cryoglobulinemia.

Light curettage, medium-depth chemical peels, and dermabrasion can be used for more extensive lesions. Carbon dioxide ($CO_2$) and Er:YAG (erbium:yttrium-aluminum-garnet) lasers, although more expensive and having more potential complications, are effective methods of treatment. Surgical excision is usually reserved for clinically suspicious discrete lesions or treatment recalcitrant lesions.

The topically applied chemical methods include topical tretinoin (Retin-A, Differin, Tazorac[1]), fluorouracil cream or solution (Efudex, Fluoroplex, Carac), diclofenac sodium gel (Solaraze), imiquimod cream (Aldara), or 20% aminolevulinic acid (ALA) (Levulan) with photodynamic therapy. Tretinoin[1] cream or gel is applied daily to photo-damaged skin indefinitely. Results are usually not clinically evident for 4 to 6 months of therapy. Side effects of dryness and scaling can be improved by judicious use of medication; moisturizers; and initially alternate- or every-third-day therapy, gradually increasing as tolerated. Ultraviolet A (UVA) and ultraviolet B (UVB) blocking sunscreens are critical to retard further skin damage.

Fluorouracil can be found in a 0.5%, 1%, or 5% cream or 1% solution and is applied once or twice daily for up to 8 weeks as tolerated. It is highly effective; but side effects of redness, pain, erosion, and allergic reaction may limit its usefulness. Side effects often persist for weeks after therapy has ceased. Diclofenac gel is applied twice daily for 2 to 3 months; although better tolerated clinically, it is expensive, requires

compliance, and can have side effects similar to fluorouracil as well as photosensitive and anticoagulative effects. Imiquimod cream 0.5% is a new class of immunomodulator drug that is applied once daily 2 to 5 times per week for 4 to 6 weeks.[2] It can cause erythema, scaling, and erosion but is usually relatively painless and resolves as the lesions clear. It is expensive but may offer more long-term clearing and may be effective against concomitant superficially invasive cancers.

Topical photodynamic therapy (PDT) is the most recent addition to the treatment arm. After acetone pretreatment, 20% ALA (Levulan) is applied and allowed to incubate for 1 to 3 hours. It is activated by a light source such as a blue light, an intense pulsed light, or a long pulse dye laser causing destruction of individual lesions and cosmetic improvement of photo-damaged skin. One to three treatments at 3-week intervals are needed. The therapy is expensive, requires equipment, causes 24- to 36-hour photosensitivity, and is variably uncomfortable. This therapy is also highly effective, and cosmetic downtime is lessened. Lack of scarring or dyspigmentation and less noncompliance issues combined with superior cosmetic photodamage repair make this a useful alternative treatment. Hypertropic extremity lesions can be pretreated for 5 days with fluorouracil before PDT.

Oral tretinoin (acitretin)[1] 25 mg or 0.4 mg/kg/day as tolerated can be an effective treatment for chronic AKs in immunosuppressed individuals minimizing the progression to invasive SCC. Benefits cease with disruption of therapy.

## Actinic Cheilitis

Actinic cheilitis (leukokeratosis or leukoplakia of the lip) usually occurs on the lower lip mucosa. Predisposing factors include chronic photodamage, fair skin, protuberant lower lip, and pipe or chewing tobacco use. This disease is essentially AK, and much of what was previously discussed about AK applies here. Unfortunately, the incidence of invasion is higher and the subsequent chance of metastatic

[1]Not FDA approved for this indication.
[2]Exceeds dosage recommended by the manufacturer.

spread may approach 25%. Clinically, actinic cheilitis can appear as a tender whitish plaque adherent to the mucosa. Erosion, induration, and erythema should be evaluated further because these are often signs of invasion; a biopsy of the most clinically affected area may be necessary to rule invasion out.

## TREATMENT OF ACTINIC CHELITIS

Treatment is often accompanied by pain, discomfort, erosion, and slow healing. The most commonly used method of treatment is liquid nitrogen spray. If fluorouracil or imiquimod (Aldara) are used, only 2 to 3 weekly applications may be tolerated; treatment may be necessary for 6 to 8 weeks with erosion persisting for many weeks afterward.

Surgical advancement of normal mucosa (vermilionectomy) with removal of affected tissue or $CO_2$ laser ablation can be performed, but these procedures are technically difficult and potentially scarring. Recently, another form of photodynamic therapy using 20% ALA incubated for 2 to 3 hours followed by activation with a pulse dye laser 595 nm long pulsed has been reported very effective with minimal discomfort and erosive side effects. This therapy might be an alternative treatment, if this laser is available.

## Bowen's Disease

Bowen's disease is a form of SCC in situ that differs histologically from AK by involving the full thickness of the epidermis to include involvement of the hair follicle acrotrichium. Because of hair follicle involvement, superficial treatments that are effective on actinic keratosis often fail when treating Bowen's disease. Recurrence as well as development of invasive squamous cell carcinoma may occur. Bowen's disease occurring on non–sun-exposed hair-bearing skin is suggestive of arsenic exposure; concomitant lymphoreticular or gastrointestinal malignancies may develop. Bowen's disease on mucosal surfaces of the penis or labia (erythroplasia of Queyrat) has a higher incidence of invasion and metastasis (20% to 30%) and, therefore, should be managed more aggressively and closely monitored. Clinically, these lesions appear as an erythematous sharply demarcated plaque with light to moderate scale on sun-damaged skin. It can often be mistaken for eczema or psoriasis. On mucosal surfaces, it may be more indurated and velvety. Care must be taken to ensure that there is no involvement of the urethral meatus.

## TREATMENT OF BOWEN'S DISEASE

Treatment modalities include aggressive liquid nitrogen therapy, topical fluorouracil (Efudex) two times a day for 6 to 8 weeks[2], and curettage; but there is a significant risk of recurrence on hair-bearing skin. Topical imiquimod (Aldara) 3 to 5 times weekly for 6 to 8 weeks may be more effective, especially on mucosal skin, but long-term cure rates are uncertain. Simple excision, or Mohs' surgery, probably affords the most effective and curative method available; but there is significant potential for scarring and may result in a mutilating procedure on genital skin.

## Bowenoid Papulosis

Bowenoid papulosis represents SCC in situ on genital skin associated primarily with human papilloma virus type 16 (HPV-16) that can progress to invasive SCC. Clinically, these lesions are indistinguishable from common warts, or condyloma acuminatum, and present as tan or reddish-brown papules or plaques. Histologically, viral changes are absent and show classic features of Bowen's disease.

## TREATMENT OF BOWENOID PAPULOSIS

The same treatment modalities used in Bowen's disease are effective; although imiquimod may be the treatment of choice to cure additional clinically inapparent or distal lesions on cervix or vaginal mucosa. Daily application 3 times weekly[2] for 8 weeks has shown cure.

In addition, PDT activated by a Diode laser and topical cidofovir (Vistide)[1] may also have use in recalcitrant lesions.

## Porokeratosis

Porokeratosis presents as papules or annular plaques, which may be discrete or linear and occur on photo-damaged skin or on palms or soles. Clinically, they show central flattening and a peripheral fine thin collarette of scale and may show centrifugal spread. These lesions may be congenital or acquired and are represented by five distinct variants with several types sometimes present in one patient. They may evolve into invasive SCC. Histologically, they are all characterized by having a thin angled parakeratotic column over a focus of dyskeratotic cells without a granular cell layer (coronoid lamella), which represents the advancing margin.

## TREATMENT OF POROKERATOSIS

Successful treatment of these lesions is often difficult. Hard cryosurgery is effective but may scar. Topical tretinoin[1] 0.1% gel daily for 4 months or a combination of salicylic acid plaster pads (Mediplast)[1] in the morning and fluorouracil in the afternoon or evening has been successful. Topical 5% imiquimod 3 times weekly for at least 3 weeks may be used as well as topical or systemic fluorouracil, as tolerated.

## Nevus Sebaceus

Nevus sebaceus is a congenital hamartoma of infancy comprised of immature sebaceous, follicular, and apocrine elements. Following puberty, benign pilosebaceous and apocrine tumors may develop as well as low-grade malignant neoplasms. Rarely, aggressive malignant sebaceous and apocrine carcinomas have been reported. Clinically, they are slightly elevated often inapparent linear plaques most often present on the head or neck. At puberty, they evolve into yellow-orange plaques devoid of hair with a velvety or papillomatous surface.

## TREATMENT OF NEVUS SEBACEUS

Treatment is by surgical excision or watchful waiting. Large lesions can be removed by staged excisions. Development of nodules or ulcerations should be biopsied to rule out tumor development.

## REFERENCES

Dereli T, Ozyurt S, Ozturk G: Porokeratosis of Mibelli: Successful treatment with cryosurgery. J Dermatol 2004;31(3):223-227.

Jones E, Korzenko A, Kriegel D: Oral isotretinoin in the treatment and prevention of cutaneous squamous cell carcinoma. J Drugs Dermatol 2004;3(5):498-502

Jorrizo J, Carney P, Ko W, et al: Treatment options in the management of actinic keratosis. Cutis 2004;74(6s):9-15.

Villa A, Berman B: Immunomodulators for skin cancer. J Drugs Dermatol 2004;3(5): 533-539.

[2]Exceeds dosage recommended by the manufacturer.

[1]Not FDA approved for this indication.

# Bacterial Diseases of the Skin

Method of
*Ronald Lee Nichols, MD*

The spectrum of bacterial diseases of the skin ranges from superficial, localized, easily recognized, and treated skin eruptions to deep, aggressive, gangrenous, or necrotizing infections that might appear innocuous at first but quickly become life threatening. The prompt recognition and treatment of these infections is paramount in limiting morbidity and mortality. A healthy respect for the aggressiveness of gangrenous and necrotizing infections of the skin and soft tissues is developed by first harboring a high index of suspicion to provide early recognition and appropriate treatment before overwhelming clinical infection occurs.

## COMMON INFECTIONS

### Impetigo

Impetigo is the most common bacterial infection of the skin. It is highly contagious and can occur at any age from infancy to adulthood, but it is most common in preschool-aged children. There are two classic forms of impetigo: nonbullous and bullous. Both forms have a predominantly staphylococcal etiology, but they present with different morphologic characteristics.

Nonbullous (crusted) impetigo can be recognized by the development of a serous, yellow-brown exudate, which dries into a golden crust. Lesions rarely elicit pain but can be associated with erythema and pruritus. They are most common on exposed areas such as the hands, feet, and legs and are often associated with a traumatic event such as an insect bite or laceration. Crusted impetigo is usually associated with a heavy mixed flora of both staphylococci and streptococci.

The bullous variety usually presents as a rapidly spreading papule, which may progress to a thin-walled vesicle if the lesion is infected with *Staphylococcus aureus*, an organism that produces an exfoliative toxin. These lesions occur most often in warm, moist areas of the body. Predisposing factors include warm ambient temperatures, humidity, poor hygiene, and crowded living conditions.

Treatment of impetigo begins with eradication or with the environmental factors thought to be influential in its development. Aggressive lesion débridement with mesh gauze sponges or brushes and antibacterial soap is encouraged. Special attention to hygiene and disinfection of towels and bedding is also necessary. Topical antibiotic treatment with mupirocin (Bactroban) has been effective in mild to moderate cases. In more extensive cases, oral antibiotic therapy with a penicillinase-resistant synthetic penicillin (oxacillin) is the treatment of choice (Table 1). However, it should be remembered that a high percentage of methicillin-resistant strains of *S. aureus* are now isolated in both institutional and community settings. Patients should be treated for at least 5 to 7 days. If no improvement is seen, lesions should be cultured and antibiotics adjusted appropriately.

Systemic complications from impetigo are very uncommon. Cellulitis has occurred but is usually susceptible to systemic antibiotic therapy. Septicemia and staphylococcal scaled skin syndrome are exceedingly rare complications of impetigo; when they occur systemic therapy is indicated.

### FOLLICULITIS

Folliculitis is a pyoderma that arises within a hair follicle. The process is known as a furuncle (boil) when the infection extends beyond the hair follicle. These lesions occur most frequently in the moist areas of the body and in areas subject to friction and perspiration. Host factors known to predispose one to folliculitis include obesity, blood dyscrasias, defects in neutrophil function, immune deficiency states (such as

## CURRENT DIAGNOSIS

- Most infections are superficial and local and not associated with systemic toxicity.
- Deeper infections may involve many layers of the soft tissues including fascia and muscle.
- Systemic toxicity is always present in the deeper infections.
- Rapid advancement of the local infection with areas of necrosis indicates more serious infections including necrotizing and gangrenous processes.
- Streptococci and clostridial microorganisms are the cause of most gangrenous infections.
- Mixed aerobic and anaerobic microflora cause most necrotizing infections.

diabetes, transplant-related immunosuppression, and AIDS), and treatment with corticosteroids or cytotoxic agents. The offending organism in most immunocompetent patients is *S. aureus*; however, when immunosuppression impairs host defenses, gram-negative organisms (*Klebsiella*, *Enterobacter*, and *Proteus* species) can be involved. *Pseudomonas* species such as *aeruginosa* or *cepacia* are associated with hot-tub folliculitis, which is usually self-limited, resolving in 7 to 10 days.

Successful treatment of folliculitis depends on correcting the predisposing factors that promote the development of this condition. For patients with localized disease, topical wound care including antibiotics such as mupirocin (Bactroban) is effective. Patients with furunculosis or multiple lesions should be treated with orally administered systemic antibiotics that are effective against *S. aureus*. Any fluctuant nodules or masses should be incised and drained, and recurrent disease should receive extended treatment.

### CELLULITIS

Cellulitis is an acute infection of the skin and underlying soft tissues. It commonly begins as a hot, red, edematous, sharply defined eruption and may progress to lymphangitis, lymphadenitis, or in severe cases, necrotizing fasciitis and gangrene. Cellulitis usually occurs in local skin trauma caused by insect bites, abrasions, surgical wounds, contusions, or other cutaneous lacerations. Immunosuppressed patients are particularly susceptible to the progression of cellulitis to regional or systemic infections, and these patients should be treated aggressively with systemic antibiotics, drainage, and débridement where indicated.

Initial presentation is that of a rapidly expanding, tender, erythematous, firm area of skin. An ascending lymphangitis may be present, especially in cellulitis involving an extremity often associated with regional lymphadenopathy. Systemic signs and symptoms

## CURRENT THERAPY

- Local care and oral antibiotics chosen for the suspected or culture proven pathogens are the usual treatment of most limited skin infections.
- Infections that show evidence of rapid advancement associated with bullae, blebs, crepitus, or necrosis require parenterally administered antibiotics and prompt surgical débridement.
- Morbidity and mortality rates associated with the deeper infections increase with delays in antibiotic therapy and surgical débridement.
- Antibiotic therapy should be guided by clinical presentation and changed if necessary when culture and sensitivity studies are available.

**TABLE 1 Suggested Antibiotic Therapy for Gram-Positive Bacterial Isolates**

| Isolate | Drugs of Choice | |
| --- | --- | --- |
| | **Oral** | **Parenteral** |
| GABHS | • Penicillin G or V<br>• Erythromycin<br>• First-generation cephalosporin | • Penicillin G<br>• Ampicillin/sulbactam (Unasyn)<br>• First-generation cephalosporin |
| *Staphylococcus aureus* (methicillin sensitive) | Penicillinase-resistant synthetic penicillin (Oxacillin) | • First-generation cephalosporin<br>• Clindamycin (Cleocin)<br>• Oxacillin |
| *Staphylococcus aureus* (methicillin resistant) | Linezolid (Zyvox) | • Vancomycin<br>• Daptomycin (Cubicin)<br>• Linezolid (Zyvox) |
| Clostridial species | • Penicillin G or V<br>• Clindamycin (Cleocin)<br>• Metronidazole (Flagyl) | • Penicillin G<br>• Clindamycin<br>• Metronidazole |

*Abbreviation:* GABHS = group A β-hemolytic *Streptococcus.*

can eventually evolve and when present, mandate hospitalization and treatment with systemic antibiotics. Offending organisms are most commonly group A β-hemolytic *Streptococcus* (GABHS) species and *S. aureus.*

Treatment of localized processes is with oral antibiotics (see Table 1). If fever, septicemia, or other signs of advancement to deeper tissues are present, the patient should be admitted to the hospital for blood and wound cultures, parenteral antibiotics (see Table 1), and observation. If a prompt response is not noted after parenteral antibiotic treatment, surgical exploration of the involved area may be indicated to rule out the presence of necrotic or gangrenous tissue. Immunosuppressed patients or patients with recurrent cellulitis should be extensively examined to exclude chronic sources of infection; and these patients should be treated with parenteral antibiotics until the cellulitis resolves, followed by 5 to 7 days of oral antibiotics.

## ABSCESS

Local skin signs and symptoms such as pain (dolor), redness (rubor), warmth (calor) and swelling (tumor) often denote an abscess. Loss of function associated with fluctuation may also indicate abscess formation. Localization of purulent fluid necessitates surgical drainage and local wound care. The administration of oral or parenteral antibiotic therapy should not be used routinely after incision and drainage of localized abscesses. They should be administered only when clinically indicated, and antibiotic therapy should be based on culture and sensitivity testing.

# Life-Threatening Infections

## GROUP A β-HEMOLYTIC STREPTOCOCCAL GANGRENE

Group A β-hemolytic streptococcal gangrene is an extremely rapid progressing skin and soft tissue infection commonly caused by *Streptococcus pyogenes.* These organisms secrete hemolysins and streptolysins O and S, which are cardiotoxic, leukocytic, and responsible for the characteristic hemolysis. Gangrene results when the cutaneous blood vessels thrombose, a finding that is often associated with intense local pain. The involved skin is initially erythematous and indurated and quickly evolves to hemorrhagic blebs with focal necrotic zones. The potential for extensive tissue loss and mortality exists, especially if treatment is delayed. Prompt, aggressive tissue débridement and antibiotic therapy are necessary for a favorable outcome (see Table 1).

## SYNERGISTIC NECROTIZING CELLULITIS

Synergistic necrotizing cellulitis (SNC) is an extremely aggressive, often lethal, polymicrobial infection of the skin and soft tissues, which exhibits progressive invasion superficial to fascial planes. This condition may initially begin as a benign process with scant indication of its impending severity. The initial lesion is typically an erythematous, tender pustule or abscess with a small area of necrosis. The benign appearance of this lesion belies the widespread and aggressive tissue destruction that has occurred beneath it.

Direct inspection through skin incisions reveals extensive gangrene of the superficial tissues and fat that very rarely involves the underlying fascia and muscles. These lesions characteristically exude a thin, brown, malodorous discharge, which presents mixed flora with abundant polymorphonuclear leukocytes on a Gram stain. Crepitus, which is caused by the accumulation of gas in the tissue produced by facultative and/or obligate anaerobes, can be palpated in 25% of patients and mandates immediate surgical attention.

The most common site of involvement is the perineum, which is involved in 50% of patients with SNC. Predisposing factors include perirectal abscess and ischiorectal abscess, both of which may track to the deeper structures of the pelvis, leading to abscess formation and subsequent septicemia. The thigh and leg are involved in approximately 40% of patients. This infection can occur after amputation and is usually associated with diabetes mellitus (75% of cases) and/or peripheral vascular disease (50% of cases). The relative immunosuppression and poor circulation that accompany these significant causes of morbidity are also responsible for upper extremity and neck SNC, which account for the remaining 10% of cases.

Synergistic necrotizing cellulitis is commonly caused by mixed flora originating in the gastrointestinal (GI) tract. Coliforms are the most prevalent aerobes (*Escherichia coli, Klebsiella, Proteus*), and anaerobic flora include *Bacteroides, Peptostreptococcus, Clostridium,* and *Fusobacterium.* The primary treatment modality is aggressive débridement of nonviable skin and subcutaneous tissues. This may involve several operations and dressing changes under general anesthesia, which should be performed until all necrotic tissue is removed. Rotation or free myocutaneous flaps and split-thickness skin grafting may cover areas of tissue loss when necessary. If the perineum is involved, fecal diversion by colostomy may be necessary to facilitate healing. Empiric parenteral antibiotics effective against polymicrobial gram-positive and gram-negative aerobic and anaerobic flora are also a mainstay of therapy. However, antibiotic coverage must be modified as soon as culture and susceptibility testing reveal specific offending organisms (Table 2) to reduce the emergence of resistant organisms.

## TABLE 2  Suggested Parenteral Antibiotic Therapy for Mixed Infections

| Organisms | Primary Choice |
|---|---|
| Aerobic: Must include an agent effective against anaerobic organisms | • Amikacin (Amikin) <br> • Aztreonam (Azactam) <br> • Ceftriaxone (Rocephin) <br> • Ciprofloxacin (Cipro) <br> • Gentamicin (Garamycin) <br> • Levofloxacin (Levaquin) <br> • Tobramycin (Nebcin) |
| Anaerobic: Must include an agent effective against aerobic organisms | • Chloramphenicol (Chloromycetin) <br> • Clindamycin (Cleocin) <br> • Metronidazole (Flagyl) |
| Aerobic and anaerobic coverage | • Ampicillin/sulbactam (Unasyn) <br> • Imipenem/cilastatin (Primaxin) <br> • Meropenem (Merrem) <br> • Piperacillin/tazobactam (Zosyn) <br> • Tigecycline (Tygacil) |

## CLOSTRIDIAL MYONECROSIS (GAS GANGRENE)

Clostridial myonecrosis is a destructive infectious process of muscle associated with infections of the skin and soft tissues. It is often associated with local crepitus and systemic signs of toxemia, which are caused by the anaerobic, gas-forming bacilli of the *Clostridium* species. This infection most often occurs after abdominal operations on the GI tract; penetrating trauma, such as gunshot wounds, and frostbite can also expose muscle, fascia, and subcutaneous tissues to these organisms. Common to all these conditions is an environment-containing tissue necrosis, low oxygen tension, and sufficient nutrients of amino acids and calcium to allow germination of clostridial spores and production of the lethal α toxin.

Clostridia are gram-positive, spore-forming, obligate anaerobes that are widely found in soil contaminated with animal excreta. They have also been isolated in the human GI tract and skin, most importantly in the perineum and oropharynx. *Clostridium perfringens* is the most common isolate (present in 80% of cases) and is among the fastest growing clostridial species, having a generation time, under ideal conditions, of approximately 8 minutes. This organism produces collagenases and proteases that cause widespread tissue destruction as well as α toxin, which is associated with the high mortality of clostridial myonecrosis. The α toxin causes extensive capillary destruction and hemolysis, leading to necrosis of the muscle and overlying fascia, skin, and subcutaneous tissues.

Historically, clostridial myonecrosis was a disease associated with battle injuries, but presently, 60% of cases now occur after trauma: 50% after automobile accidents and the remainder after crush injuries, industrial accidents, and gunshot wounds. Mortality can be the result of a failure to recognize that clostridial infection is under way, which leads to a delay in the débridement of devitalized tissues. Patients often complain of a sudden onset of pain at the site of trauma or surgical wound, which increases rapidly in severity and extends beyond the original borders of the wound. The skin initially exhibits tense edema, its pale appearance progresses to a magenta hue. Hemorrhagic bullae and a thin, watery, foul-smelling discharge are common. A Gram stain examination of wound discharge reveals abundant gram-positive rods with a paucity of leukocytes.

The diagnosis of gas gangrene is based on the appearance of the muscle on direct visualization by surgical exposure, because many changes are not apparent when inspected through a small traumatic wound. Initially, the muscle is pale, edematous, and unresponsive to stimulation. As the disease process continues, the muscle becomes frankly gangrenous, black, and extremely friable. This occurs as a late event and is often accompanied by septicemia and shock. Despite profound hypotension and impending organ failure, these patients may be remarkably alert and extremely sensitive to their surroundings. They feel their impending doom and often panic just before slipping into toxic delirium and eventually coma.

The clinical features should arouse suspicion early in the course, so the disease can be recognized and treated with aggressive surgical débridement. Gas in the wound is a relatively late finding, and by the time crepitation is observed, the patient may be near death. Approximately 15% of blood cultures are positive, but this too is a late finding. Serum creatinine kinase levels, although relatively nonspecific, are always elevated in cases with muscle involvement.

The mortality rate of gas gangrene is as high as 60%. It is highest in cases involving the abdominal wall and lowest in those affecting the extremities. Among the signs that prognosticate a poor outcome are leukopenia, thrombocytopenia, hemolysis, and severe renal failure. Myoglobinuria is common and can contribute significantly to worsening renal function. Frank hemorrhage may also be present and indicates disseminated intravascular coagulation.

Successful treatment of this life-threatening infection depends on early recognition and débridement of devitalized and infected tissues. Hyperbaric oxygen and systemic antibiotics are also important adjuncts. Surgical intervention should include wide débridement of all necrotic tissue and amputation if extremities are involved. Hyperbaric oxygen (100% $O_2$ at 3 atm) has been reported to reduce associated tissue loss and mortality; however, core treatment is surgical débridement and should never be delayed to arrange for hyperbaric oxygen treatments. A parenteral antibiotic is directed toward the offending organism (see Table 1). Cardiovascular collapse mandates careful monitoring of intravenous fluid resuscitation, which may require large volumes. Failure to adequately resuscitate these patients compromises therapy by limiting oxygen delivery and antibiotic distribution to the affected tissues and may promote progression to multisystem organ failure.

A less life-threatening form of this disease is known as clostridial cellulitis. In this process the bacterial tissue invasion is primarily superficial to the fascial layer without muscle involvement. Prompt recognition and treatment, as described earlier, can reduce morbidity and mortality.

## NECROTIZING FASCIITIS

Necrotizing fasciitis is an aggressive soft tissue infection involving the fascia with extensive undermining and tracking along anatomic planes. This process usually occurs in patients with significant co-morbidity such as diabetes mellitus or peripheral vascular disease but is also seen in obese or malnourished patients and intravenous drug abusers. Cellulitis is a frequent occurrence, and progressive necrosis to subcutaneous tissue results from thrombosis of the perforating vessels. Classically associated with GABHS and staphylococci, the disease is usually caused by a variety of organisms, including aerobic streptococci, staphylococci, and coliforms, as well as anaerobic *Peptostreptococcus* and *Bacteroides*. Ninety percent of these infections are polymicrobial in etiology, and it is common to culture up to 5 organisms from the fascial planes involved with this infection.

Necrotizing fasciitis most commonly evolves from a benign-appearing skin lesion (80% of cases). Minor abrasions, insect bites, injection sites, and perirectal abscesses have all been implicated. Rare cases have been reported in women with Bartholin's gland abscess, from which the infection has spread to fascial planes of the perineum and thigh. The remaining 20% of patients have no visible skin lesion. Surgical procedures, especially bowel resections and penetrating trauma, can be complicated by superficial wound infections that evolve into necrotizing fasciitis. The infection commonly involves the buttocks and perineum, which result from untreated perirectal abscesses or decubitus ulcers; intravenous drug abusers commonly participate in *skin popping*, which leads to infections of the upper extremities. The idiopathic form, commonly known as spontaneous necrotizing fasciitis, is particularly dangerous because of the frequent delay in diagnosis.

The initial presentation is a slowly advancing cellulitis that progresses to a firm, tense, woody feel of the subcutaneous tissues. This entity may be distinguished from other aggressive anaerobic soft tissue infections (i.e., SNC) by the brawny, pale, erythematous appearance of the skin overlying subcutaneous tissues that are unyielding, making fascial planes and muscle groups indistinguishable during palpation. Often a broad erythematous tract along the route of the underlying fascial plane can be discerned through the skin. If an open wound exists, probing the edges with a blunt instrument permits ready dissection of the superficial fascia well beyond the wound margins, and this is the most important diagnostic feature of necrotizing fasciitis. On direct inspection, the fascia is swollen and dully gray in appearance with stringy areas of fat necrosis. A thin, brown exudate can be expressed from the wound, and frank purulent drainage is rare. These wounds are remarkably insensate when found and mandate immediate débridement.

As with other gangrenous soft tissue infections, the most important component of the treatment plan is aggressive, total débridement of all devitalized and necrotic tissue. This may often necessitate frequent operations and dressing changes. Wide débridement and parenteral antibiotics have a profound effect on survival, and limited or staged débridement has no place in the treatment of this very aggressive, life-threatening infection. Parenteral antibiotics (see Table 2) should be directed against the polymicrobial aerobic and anaerobic microorganisms isolated from these infections. Every effort should be made to quickly identify the offending organisms, and antibiotic therapy should be changed accordingly.

There is a rarely reported monomicrobial form of this disease known as *idiopathic necrotizing fasciitis*. When erythema, induration, and warmth occur without trauma or other obvious cause of the infection, consider this entity, which often arises without any obvious portal of entry. Misdiagnosis and delay in diagnosis are common and associated with significant morbidity and mortality. Surgical exploration with débridement of infected and necrotic tissue, in addition to systemic antibiotic therapy, directed toward the aerobic *Streptococcus* can result in decreased morbidity and mortality (see Table 1).

# Special Circumstances

## FOURNIER'S GANGRENE

Fournier's gangrene is a necrotizing fasciitis that originates as a necrotic black area on the scrotum of male patients or the labia in females and most often has a cryptogenic origin. In the author's experience, Fournier's gangrene occurs more commonly without a predisposing event or after routine, uncomplicated hemorrhoidectomy. Less commonly, this condition has occurred after urologic manipulation or as a late complication of deep anorectal suppuration. Fournier's gangrene is characterized by necrosis of the skin and soft tissues of the scrotum and/or perineum associated with a fulminant, painful, and severely toxic infection. Definitive diagnosis is made by identification of a necrotic black area on the scrotum associated with local and systemic signs of infection. Left untreated, death ensues from uncontrolled, severe systemic sepsis and multiple organ failure. Prompt recognition and treatment can minimize tissue loss, specifically the skin and soft tissues of the scrotum, labia, and perineum, and may prevent complete loss of genitalia.

The infection is often polymicrobial, as with necrotizing fasciitis, with several species of aerobic and anaerobic bacteria predominating. Successful treatment is, again, based on early recognition and vigorous surgical débridement, occasionally including diversion of the fecal stream. Empirical treatment is appropriate until results of culture and susceptibility testing are available (see Table 2). The therapeutic benefit of hyperbaric oxygen treatments remains to be proved and should only be used as an adjunct to surgical débridement at this time.

## ECTHYMA GANGRENOSUM

Occasionally, hospitalized patients with overwhelming pseudomonal septicemia develop a patchy dermal and subcutaneous necrosis. Although sepsis caused by *Pseudomonas aeruginosa* is often indistinguishable from other types of gram-negative sepsis, a characteristic skin lesion may develop with erythematous macular eruptions that quickly become bullous with central ulceration and necrosis. This lesion may resemble a decubitus ulcer with the characteristic black eschar. There are usually multiple lesions occurring in different stages of development. They may concentrate on the extremities or the gluteal region. These lesions may be distinguished from the lesions of pyoderma gangrenosum (a noninfectious dermatosis) by their association with clinical signs of infection (i.e., fever and leukocytosis) in addition to the isolation of *P. aeruginosa* from culture of the lesion. Treatment is primarily by administration of antimicrobial therapy effective against the *Pseudomonas* organism and by débridement of the multiple lesions, which may lessen the bacterial burden, perhaps allowing greater antibiotic efficacy.

## SEA WATER INFECTIONS

Infections caused by *Vibrio vulnificus* and *Aeromonas hydrophilia* can be extremely aggressive, with necrosis often occurring within hours and necessitating rapid, wide débridement. Although infections caused by these organisms cannot be differentiated from those caused by mixed infections, a history of exposure to sea water and the rapidity with which the infection spreads often suggest the true etiology of the infection. The antibiotics of choice for *V. vulnificus* infection are doxycycline (Vibramycin) or tetracycline and an aminoglycoside. In cases with impaired renal function, chloramphenicol may be used.

# Conclusion

The wide range of soft tissue infections caused by bacteria may be distinguished by their wide variety of presenting signs, symptoms, and body location and by the time course of the pathologic processes unique to each. Early recognition is of paramount importance to the effective treatment plan, which most often includes aggressive surgical débridement and specific antimicrobial therapy. This approach can often minimize tissue damage and promote recovery.

## REFERENCES

Adinolfi MF, Voros DC, Moustoukas NM, et al: Severe systemic sepsis resulting from neglected perineal infections. South Med J 1983;76:746-749.

Craig ML, Hardin WD Jr, Fox LS, et al: Ecthyma gangrenosum: A deadly complication. Hosp Physician 1987;23:65-71.

Moustoukas NM, Nichols RL, Voros D: Clostridial sepsis: Usual clinical presentations. South Med J 1985;78:440-445.

Nichols RL: Postoperative infection in the age of drug-resistant gram-positive bacteria [review]. Am J Med 1998;104 (Suppl. 5A):11S-16S.

Nichols RL, Florman S: Clinical presentations of soft-tissue infections and surgical site infections. Clin Infect Dis 2001;33(Suppl. 2):84-93.

# Viral Diseases of the Skin

Method of
*Jacqueline M. Losi-Sasaki, MD,*
*and Angela Yen Moore, MD*

## Human Herpesviruses

### HERPES SIMPLEX VIRUS TYPES 1 AND 2

#### Etiology and Epidemiology

Herpes simplex virus types 1 (HSV-1/human herpesvirus [HHV-1]) and 2 (HSV-2/HHV-2) belong to the family Herpesviridae and the subfamily Alphaherpesvirinae. The two viruses cause clinically indistinguishable mucocutaneous findings. Classic clinical manifestations are grouped or clustered vesicles and erosions on an erythematous base, often with secondary crusting. Predilection for the mucocutaneous surfaces is the rule, with perioral and anogenital surfaces most commonly affected. Herpes simplex virus type 1 is the most common culprit of orofacial HSV, which typically presents at and around the oral surfaces. The etiology of most genital herpes infections is HSV-2 (70% to 90%), but recent reports demonstrate an increasing incidence associated with HSV-1 (10% to 30%).

Herpes simplex virus type 1 seropositivity is approximately 90% worldwide in adults 20 to 40 years old, with an estimated one third of the world's population able to transmit the virus during periods of viral shedding. Despite the high worldwide seropositivity, only 20% to 40% of infected individuals have a history of lesions, translating to a high number of infected individuals unaware of their ability to transmit disease. In the past two decades, there has been an alarming increase in the seroprevalence of HSV-2 in the United States, with approximately 1.6 million individuals acquiring primary genital HSV annually. An estimated 25% to 30% of women and 20% of men in the United States is infected with HSV-2. Factors associated with the transmission of genital herpes include the number of lifetime partners, the age of greatest sexual activity, black or Hispanic race, lower socioeconomic status, female gender, homosexuality, and HIV infection.

#### Pathogenesis

Herpes simplex virus types 1 and 2 are transmitted primarily through direct contact with active lesions, contaminated saliva, semen, or cervical secretions. More commonly, transmission occurs in patients without active disease, in whom subclinical or asymptomatic viral shedding occurs. Following viral replication at the mucocutaneous site of contact, viral nucleocapsids travel by retrograde axonal flow to the dorsal root ganglia and establish latency until reactivation. Latent virus has been recovered from trigeminal, sacral, and vaginal ganglia both ipsilateral and contralateral to the clinical lesion. Reactivation accounts for repeated episodes of viral shedding that result in further transmission or dissemination of disease. Many instances of reactivation are spontaneous, but others are caused by physical or emotional stress, fever, exposure to ultraviolet light, compromised skin barrier function (abrasion or other trauma), immune suppression, menses, or fatigue.

#### Clinical Features

Herpes simplex virus infections are variable in clinical expression, and most cases are, in fact, subclinical. In primary infections, a prodrome of fever, malaise, and lymphadenopathy as well as tingling, burning, or localized pain may be present. These symptoms are followed days later by the development of characteristic painful and grouped papules, vesicles, ulcers, or erosions on an erythematous base with secondary crusting and re-epithelialization. Lesions typically heal in 7 to 10 days without scarring. Recurrent outbreaks may be preceded by prodromal symptoms and are characterized by subsequent lesions that are decreased in number, severity, and duration.

Orofacial labialis, also known as herpes labialis, is the most common manifestation of HSV infection. Worldwide, 20% to 30% of children older than age 5 years are seropositive for HSV-1. In the United States 68% of children older than age of 12 years are seropositive for HSV-1, and 22% are seropositive for HSV-2. Primary infection with HSV-1 typically presents as herpetic gingivostomatitis in children and young adults. Sore throat and fever develop, as well as painful vesicles and erosions on the tongue, palate, gingiva, buccal mucosa, and lips. Edema, pain, and ulceration may cause associated dysphagia, anorexia, and drooling. Young adults may have an associated pharyngitis and mononucleosis-like syndrome. In men herpetic folliculitis of the beard area may occur and is often mistaken for a bacterial etiology because of its pustular appearance. Prodromal symptoms and recurrent episodes are historical clues to the diagnosis.

Primary genital herpes infection, usually caused by HSV-2 infection, produces an exquisitely painful erosive balanitis, vulvitis, or vaginitis. Involvement of the cervix, buttocks, and perineum with associated lymphadenopathy may be seen in women. Associated fever, dysuria, urinary retention, or aseptic meningitis may occur in decreasing order of frequency in 10% to 20% of affected females. The glans penis or shaft is typically involved in men. Recurrent disease may be subclinical or less severe in nature. Resolution occurs within 1 week in recurrences versus 2 to 3 weeks in primary infection. The severity of the primary infection correlates with the frequency of recurrences. Prodromal symptoms of tingling or burning may precede episodes of reactivation, with lesions typically occurring at the site of initial manifestation.

Eczema herpeticum, also known as Kaposi's varicelliform eruption, is a widespread dissemination of HSV that occurs in patients with atopic dermatitis, burns, or other underlying skin conditions. Painful, monomorphous, and crusted papules or vesicles develop over mucocutaneous surfaces including the face, extremities, or trunk. Secondary bacterial infection may be present and often hinders diagnosis. The presence of pain and grouped lesions are clues to the diagnosis.

Herpetic whitlow is HSV infection of a digit, most commonly observed in children and medical professionals, caused by direct contact or autoinoculation of HSV-1 or HSV-2.

Herpes gladiatorum occurs in contact-sport athletes such as wrestlers. Direct contact with active lesions or areas of asymptomatic shedding in an infected individual underlies this condition that is most commonly seen on the head, neck, or proximal trunk.

Herpes simplex virus keratitis is a major cause of blindness worldwide, most often caused by infection with HSV-1. Clinical manifestations are unilateral or bilateral keratoconjunctivitis with eyelid edema, photophobia, and preauricular lymphadenopathy. Fundic exam reveals branching dendritic lesions. Complications include corneal ulceration, scarring, globe rupture, and blindness.

Herpes simplex virus encephalitis most often affects the temporal lobe and presents with bizarre behavior changes and altered mental status. Fever and focal neurologic deficits may be present. Mortality is significant at 70% and long-term sequelae are often observed.

Herpes simplex virus in HIV patients is often severe and may be chronic. Bone marrow and solid organ transplant patients as well as chemotherapy patients are also vulnerable. Atypical clinical manifestations include large verrucous papules or plaques, pustules, ulcers, widespread distribution, and visceral organ involvement.

Neonatal HSV continues to be an important public health concern, with most instances transmitted by mothers unaware of their HSV-2 infection. The risk of transmission is highest in women with first-episode genital herpes at or near the time of delivery. Associated neonatal morbidity and mortality is high. Disseminated disease with liver, adrenal, or encephalopathic involvement is a poor prognostic indicator.

### VARICELLA-ZOSTER VIRUS

Varicella-zoster virus (VZV/HHV-3) is the cause of varicella (chickenpox), and herpes zoster (shingles). A widespread, pruritic vesicular eruption is highly characteristic of VZV. Following transmission via airborne droplets or direct contact with vesicular fluid, replication and viremia ensue. Epidermal invasion results from virus transmigration from the endothelial cells. Varicella-zoster virus eventually establishes latency in the dorsal root ganglia via mechanisms similar to HSV.

Before the introduction of live attenuated varicella vaccine, more than 90% of children in the United States contracted the primary infection before the age of 10 years. Since the advent of the vaccine, an overall decrease in incidence approaching 87% has been observed between 1995 and 2000. The greatest decline in varicella incidence has been observed in preschool children. This decline correlates with the reduction in the number of hospitalizations for varicella. Reports of outbreaks of varicella in highly immunized groups have shown a milder disease course with fewer lesions and fewer complications than the disease among previously unvaccinated children. These results provide support for ongoing efforts aimed at universal immunization in children in the United States.

Herpes zoster occurs in up to 20% of people infected with VZV and may present at any time after the primary varicella infection. Zoster is, in its classic form, recognized by a dermatomal distribution of blisters. This eruption is caused by reactivation of VZV from latently infected sensory ganglia and is most commonly observed in immunocompetent individuals older than 50 years old with a known prior history of varicella. Younger adults or children with herpes zoster typically experience a primary varicella infection relatively early, typically within the first year of life.

A prodrome of pain, pruritus, tingling, tenderness, or hyperesthesia often precedes the classic sensory dermatomal vesicular eruption. Pain that persists for more than 1 month after resolution of the herpes zoster rash is known as postherpetic neuralgia, a complication that is often chronic and refractory to treatments. The effect of the varicella vaccine on the incidence of postherpetic neuralgia appears to be unclear, with different studies showing both an increase and a decrease in the incidence of this complication. Other complications include secondary bacterial infection, ophthalmic zoster, meningoencephalitis, pneumonitis, and hepatitis.

Ophthalmic zoster is a serious complication that occurs in 5% to 10% of cases with an associated significant risk of blindness. Vesicles or crusted papules along the nasal tip, sidewall, or base is known as Hutchinson's sign and signifies involvement of the nasociliary branch of the trigeminal nerve. This clinical presentation is an indication for immediate empiric antiviral therapy and ophthalmology referral.

Severe or disseminated herpes zoster (>20 vesicles outside the primarily involved dermatome) is most frequently observed in the immunosuppressed population. Atypical clinical manifestations such as crusted, verrucous papules and plaques may also be noted.

## DIAGNOSIS

### Herpes Simplex Virus

Viral culture, serology, direct immunofluorescence, and molecular techniques are available laboratory tests for the diagnosis of HSV infection. Viral culture is a useful method of diagnosis in first-time genital outbreaks or few mucocutaneous lesions. The cell culture technique is most reliable at the onset of symptoms, before healing or crusting of the vesicular lesions. False negative results may occur, especially in lesions that are already healing.

Direct fluorescent antibody staining of vesicle base scrapings is 95% diagnostic and can be used to distinguish VZV from HSV. In one study direct immunofluorescence and culture were shown to be equally sensitive at 88% in detection of HSV, whereas direct immunofluorescence was four times more sensitive (100% versus 18%) than culture in the case of VZV.

The gold standard of serologic diagnosis is the Western blot test, which is 99% sensitive and 99% specific for HSV antibodies. To distinguish between HSV-1 and HSV-2, type-specific serologic assays based on type-specific glycoproteins from HSV-1 and HSV-2 are available and approved by the Food and Drug Administration (FDA).

The Tzanck smear offers a rapid and useful bedside test of HSV infection and relies on the identification of multinucleated giant cells

## CURRENT DIAGNOSIS

- Grouped or clustered vesicles and erosions on an erythematous base should prompt consideration of herpetic etiology.
- The presence of painful crusted, eroded, or vesicular lesions on the nose should prompt immediate ophthalmologic evaluation and empiric antiviral therapy (the so-called Hutchinson's sign, a diagnostic urgency implicating possible herpes keratitis).
- A high suspicion for herpetic etiology in an immunosuppressed patient is critical.
- Laboratory tests:
  - Viral culture is useful in first-time outbreaks, however time sensitive.
  - Serology
    - Western blot
    - Type-specific serologic assays based on glycoproteins
  - Direct immunofluorescence: rapid and specific
  - Tzanck smear:* rapid, but nonspecific
  - Polymerase chain reaction of cerebrospinal fluid

*This test does not differentiate between HSV-1, HSV-2, or VZV.
*Abbreviations:* HSV-1 = herpes simplex virus type 1; HSV-2 = herpes simplex virus type 2; VZV = varicella-zoster virus.

in vesicular scrapings. However, this test does not differentiate among HSV-1, HSV-2, or VZV.

On histopathologic examination, characteristic ballooning degeneration of keratinocytes, spongiosis or frank vesiculation, and nuclear molding may be observed. Intranuclear inclusion bodies may also be present.

Polymerase chain reaction (PCR) of the cerebrospinal fluid is the test of choice for HSV infections of the central nervous system.

### Varicella-Zoster Virus

A thorough history and physical examination are critical in diagnosis and often prompt initial antiviral therapy. The Tzanck smear (see previous mention) may aid in prompt diagnosis but will not distinguish between HSV and VZV. Similar limited information may be provided by histopathologic specimens of lesional skin.

Direct fluorescent antibody, viral culture, serology, and PCR may all distinguish between HSV and VZV. Viral culture is the most specific, albeit a less-sensitive test.

## CURRENT THERAPY

- Both topical and systemic antiviral treatments may be used to manage orolabial herpes in immunocompetent people.
- Systemic agents offer the best treatment for primary and recurrent genital herpes.
- Immunosuppressed individuals need more aggressive management with oral or IV antivirals.
- Early treatment and empirical therapy are critical for herpes zoster.
- Prompt ophthalmologic evaluation and empirical therapy is critical for nasal herpetic presentations.

*Abbreviation:* IV = intravenous.

## TABLE 1  Systemic Antiviral Therapy for Herpes Simplex Virus and Varicella Zoster Virus

### Herpes Simplex Virus Infection
**First episode of genital herpes**

| | |
|---|---|
| Acyclovir (Zovirax) | 400 mg PO tid for 7–10 d |
| Acyclovir | 200 mg PO 5 times/d for 7–10 d |
| Famciclovir (Famvir) | 250 mg PO tid for 7–10 d |
| Valacyclovir (Valtrex) | 1 g PO bid for 7–10 d |

**Recurrent episode of genital herpes**

| | |
|---|---|
| Acyclovir | 400 mg PO tid for 5 d |
| Acyclovir | 200 mg PO 5 times/d for 5 d |
| Acyclovir | 800 mg PO bid for 5 d |
| Famciclovir | 125 mg PO bid for 5 d |
| Valacyclovir | 500 mg PO bid for 3–5 d |
| Valacyclovir | 1.0 g PO bid for 5 d |
| Valacyclovir | 2.0 g PO bid for 1 d[3] |

**Chronic suppressive therapy**

| | |
|---|---|
| Acyclovir | 400 mg PO bid |
| Famciclovir | 250 mg PO bid |
| Valacyclovir | 500 mg PO qd (<10 outbreaks/y) |
| Valacyclovir | 1.0 g PO qd (≥10 outbreaks/y) |

**Recurrent orolabial or genital HSV in immunosuppressed patients**

| | |
|---|---|
| Acyclovir | 400 mg PO tid for 5–10 d |
| Acyclovir | 200 mg 5 times/d for 5–10 d |
| Acyclovir | 5 mg/kg intravenously q8h for 7–10 d |
| Famciclovir | 500 mg PO bid for 5–10 d |
| Valacyclovir | 1.0 g PO bid for 5–10 d |

**Chronic suppressive HSV therapy in immunosuppressed patients**

| | |
|---|---|
| Acyclovir | 400–800 mg PO bid to tid |
| Famciclovir | 500 mg PO bid |
| Valacyclovir | 500 mg PO bid |

### Varicella-Zoster Virus Infection
**Varicella**

| | |
|---|---|
| Acyclovir | 20 mg/kg (800 mg maximum dose) PO qid for 5 d |

**Zoster**

| | |
|---|---|
| Acyclovir | 800 mg PO 5 times/d for 7–10 d |
| Famciclovir | 500 mg PO tid for 7 d |
| Valacyclovir | 1 g PO tid for 7 d |
| Adult immunosuppressed patients: Acyclovir | 10 mg/kg IV q8h for 7–10 d |
| Pediatric immunosuppressed patients: Acyclovir | 10 mg/kg IV q8h for 7–10 d |

[3]Exceeds dosage recommended by the manufacturer.
*Abbreviations:* IV = intravenous; PO = orally.

Polymerase chain reaction is the test of choice for detection of VZV in the cerebrospinal fluid. Serologic tests have limited utility, because most of the population is seropositive.

## TREATMENT

Both topical and systemic antiviral treatments are useful in the management of orolabial herpes in immunocompetent people. Oral valacyclovir (Valtrex), 2 grams orally taken twice in one 24-hour period,[3] and topical 1% penciclovir result in decreased duration of pain, clinical lesions, and duration of viral shedding.

Systemic antiviral agents are the agents of choice for the treatment of primary and recurrent genital herpes (see Table 1). Three highly

[3]Exceeds dosage recommended by the manufacturer.

effective and well-tolerated antivirals are acyclovir (Zovirax), valacyclovir (Valtrex), and famciclovir (Famvir). All have been shown to shorten the duration, severity, pain, and period of viral shedding for initial and recurrent genital herpes infections. Because they inhibit only actively replicating viral DNA, these medications are not useful for the treatment of latent infection.

Intravenous (IV) acyclovir is reserved for neonatal HSV infection, severe HSV infections in immunocompromised hosts, and HSV patients with systemic complications. Immunosuppressed individuals require more aggressive management with oral or IV antivirals until complete mucocutaneous clearing is observed. For patients with greater than six outbreaks per year, chronic suppressive therapy is indicated and is associated with a 95% reduction of asymptomatic viral shedding (see Table 1).

Acyclovir-resistant HSV and VZV are increasing in frequency, especially in those who are immunosuppressed. Most commonly, a mutation in thymidine kinase is responsible. Antivirals that are thymidine kinase dependent are ineffective in such cases. Alternative antivirals include foscarnet (Foscavir) and cidofovir (Vistide).

Early treatment with antiviral agents is critical for herpes zoster, and empiric therapy is warranted (see Table 1). Acyclovir, valacyclovir, and famciclovir are FDA approved for herpes zoster and result in decreased VZV duration and pain. Adequate pain control with narcotics or other appropriate agents are required. Intravenous acyclovir is the treatment of choice for herpes zoster in patients with complications or immunosuppression.

Postherpetic neuralgia (PHN) correlates with active viral replication at the dorsal root ganglion and poses a difficult therapeutic challenge. Both famciclovir and valacyclovir are effective at reducing the duration and pain of PHN. Low-dose tricyclic antidepressants and gabapentin (Neurontin) are also shown to be effective in reducing pain and sleep disturbances. Narcotics, analgesics, capsaicin, biofeedback, and nerve blocks are other options.

# Human Parvovirus B19

A small, single-stranded DNA virus and member of the family Parvoviridae, human parvovirus B19 is transmitted through respiratory droplets with peak infection rates noted in patients between ages 4 and 15 years. Human parvovirus B19 is responsible for several clinical syndromes including the benign childhood exanthem known as erythema infectiosum, or fifth disease. Less commonly, purpuric eruptions or severe complications including aplastic anemia and hydrops fetalis may occur.

Classic clinical manifestations of erythema infectiosum include low-grade fever and mild upper respiratory symptoms that occur 2 to 3 days prior to the onset of the easily recognized *slapped cheeks* erythema over the bilateral malar cheeks with circumoral pallor. A pink lacy or reticular eruption over the trunk and extremities shortly follows. Duration is 7 to 14 days and occurs without scarring or long-term sequelae. Adolescents and other susceptible individuals may present with arthralgias or arthritis; severe disease is only seen in immunosuppressed patients, including pregnant women.

Papular purpuric gloves and socks syndrome is also associated with acute B19 infection and is most common in young adults in the spring. Burning and pruritus are associated. Fetal B19 infection may result in fetal hydrops, anemia, spontaneous miscarriage, or stillbirth.

Diagnostic confirmation of B19 infection may be confirmed by detection of serum anti-B19 IgM antibody. Polymerase chain reaction assays may also be used.

Symptomatic management of most B19 infections is adequate. Affected fetuses may require in utero blood transfusions. Intravenous immunoglobulin has been used in select cases of B19 infection in the immunosuppressed.

# Hand-Foot-and-Mouth Disease

Hand-foot-and-mouth disease is a common benign exanthem of childhood, characterized by a palmoplantar vesicular eruption and stomatitis. The causative agent is an enterovirus, most often coxsackievirus serotype A16. Transmission is via the oral–oral or fecal–oral route. A prodrome of malaise, low-grade fever, anorexia, abdominal pain, or upper respiratory symptoms may occur. Oval-shaped erythematous macules progress to small vesicles on the palms, soles, tongue, buccal mucosa, palate, and tonsillar pillars. Buttocks and perineal surfaces are rarely involved. The vesicles evolve into yellow-gray ulcerations with peripheral erythema in the same distribution. Self-limited resolution occurs without scarring. Treatment is symptomatic.

## Poxviruses

### MOLLUSCUM CONTAGIOSUM

Molluscum contagiosum is caused by the molluscipoxvirus genus of Poxviridae, a family of large, brick-shaped, double-stranded DNA viruses. Children, sexually active adults, and immunosuppressed individuals are the most frequent hosts, and transmission is via direct contact or fomites. In children molluscum contagiosum is a common, benign, self-limited eruption characterized by numerous, scattered dome-shaped pearly papules with central umbilication that show predilection for the face, trunk, and skin folds. The presence of Henderson-Patterson bodies (intracytoplasmic inclusion bodies) may be demonstrated by lesional scrapings and aid in the diagnosis.

Treatment is not required, but numerous modalities including topical cantharidin, curettage, electrodesiccation, cimetidine, topical tretinoin, and chemical peels are available. Similar cutaneous findings are observed in sexually active adults, but the distribution favors the perineal areas, lower abdomen, and thighs in this population. Immunosuppressed individuals exhibit atypical, larger eroded papules or plaques that are often widespread and deforming.

### ORF AND MILKER'S NODULES

Orf, or ecthyma contagiosum, is caused by a parapoxvirus endemic in sheep and goats. Direct contact with infected animals or fomites results in transmission to humans. The clinical presentation is typically on the dorsal digits or hands with single or multiple 1.5- to 5.0-cm discrete plaques or nodules. Initial lesions typically progress through several stages, including maculopapular, targetoid, nodular, regenerative, papillomatous, and regressive lesions prior to eventual healing 35 to 40 days later. Diagnosis is by history and physical examination. Treatment is symptomatic.

Milker's nodule (bovine papular stomatitis) is a similar clinical entity to orf and arises from a closely related parapoxvirus transmitted from infected cattle. Physical manifestations are indistinguishable from orf. Milker's condition is benign and self-limited. Treatment is supportive.

### REFERENCES

Armstrong GL, Schillinger J, Markowitz L: Incidence of herpes simplex virus type 2 infection in the United States. Am J Epidemiol 2001; 153:91-99.
Centers for Disease Control and Prevention: Sexually transmitted diseases treatment guidelines 2002. MMWR Morb Mortal Wkly Rep 2002;51(RR-6):1-80.
Corey L, Adams H, Brown A, Holmes KK: Genital herpes simplex virus infections: Clinical manifestations, course and complications. Ann Intern Med 1983;98:958-972.
Douglas MW, Johnson RW, Cunningham, AL: Tolerability of treatments for postherpetic neuralgia. Drug Saf 2004;27(15):1217-1233.
Johnson LS, Nahmias AJ, Magder RE, et al: A seroepidemiological survey of the prevalence of herpes simplex virus type 2 infection in the United States. N Engl J Med 1989;321:7-12.
Langtry LAA, Ostlere AS, Hawkins DA, Staughton RCD: The difficulty in diagnosis of cutaneous herpes simplex virus infection in patients with AIDS. Clin Exp Dermatol 1994;19:224-226.
Miron D, Lavi I, Kitov R, Hendler A: Vaccine effectiveness and severity of varicella among previously vaccinated children during outbreaks in day-care centers with low vaccination coverage. Pediatr Infect Dis J 2005;24(3):233-236.
Nahmias AJ, Lee FK, Bechman-Nahmia S: Sero-epidemiological and sociological patterns of herpes simplex virus infection in the world. Scand J Infect Dis 1990;69:19-36.
Stalkup JR, Yeung-Yue K, Brotjens M, Tyring SK: Human herpesviruses. In JL Bolognia (ed): Dermatology. Spain, Mosby, 2003, pp 1245-1253.
Takahashi M: Effectiveness of live varicella vaccine. Expert Opin Biol Ther 2004;4(2):199-216.
Vázquez M: Varicella zoster virus infections in children after the introduction of live attenuated varicella vaccine. Curr Opin Pediatr 2004;16:80-84.
Zirn JR, Tompkins SD, Huie C, Shea CR: Rapid detection, and distinction of cutaneous herpesvirus infections by direct immunofluorescence. J Am Acad Dermatol 1995;33:724-728.

# Parasitic Diseases of the Skin

Method of
*Andreas Katsambas, MD, PhD,*
*and Electra Nicolaidou, MD, PhD*

A parasite is an organism that obtains food and shelter from another organism and derives all benefits from this association. Parasites responsible for diseases with skin manifestations include protozoa, helminths, and arthropoda. Most parasitic diseases are more common in tropical and subtropical regions, but, mostly because of traveling and immigration, they are also encountered in temperate climates. Updated treatment guidelines for these diseases are available at the Centers for Disease Control (CDC) Web site, www.cdc.gov/travel/diseases.htm.

## Diseases Caused by Protozoa

### AMEBIASIS

Amebiasis is caused by *Entamoeba histolytica*. Infection occurs by ingestion of mature cysts in fecally contaminated food and water and through fecal exposure during sexual contact. Clinical presentation includes asymptomatic infection, invasive intestinal amebiasis, and invasive extra intestinal amebiasis. Cutaneous findings include purulent nodules, cysts, and sinuses. *Entamoeba histolytica* can be identified microscopically in the stool as well as in aspirates or biopsy samples obtained during colonoscopy or surgery. Treatment of choice for extraintestinal disease is metronidazole (Flagyl), 750 mg by mouth (PO) three times daily for 7 to 10 days or tinidazole (Tindamax), 2 g once daily for 5 days. Tinidazole was recently approved by the Food and Drug Administration (FDA) and appears to be as effective as and better tolerated than metronidazole. Treatment with either metronidazole or tinidazole should be followed by iodoquinol (Yodoxin), 650 mg PO three times daily for 20 days.

### LEISHMANIASIS

Leishmaniasis is caused by *Leishmania* species, which are transmitted by sandflies. In the cutaneous form of the disease, an initial solitary red papule develops into a well-demarcated ulcer with encrusted center that, if untreated, heals spontaneously with a scar. Diagnosis is based on a history of exposure to sandflies, symptoms and isolation of the organisms from the lesion aspirate, or biopsy by direct examination or culture. Treatment includes sodium stibogluconate (Pentostam),[2] 20 mg/kg/day intravenously (IV) or intramuscularly (IM) for 20 days.

### TRYPANOSOMIASIS

There are three different types of trypanosomiasis:

- American trypanosomiasis or Chagas' disease, caused by *Trypanosoma cruzi*
- East African sleeping sickness, caused by *Trypanosoma brucei rhodesiense*

[2]Note available in the United States

## CURRENT DIAGNOSIS

### Diseases Caused by Protozoa

#### AMEBIASIS

- Purulent nodules, cysts, and sinuses
- Microscopic identification of *Entamoeba histolytica* in stool or biopsy samples

#### LEISHMANIASIS

- Well-demarcated ulcer with encrusted center
- Isolation of *Leishmania* by direct examination or culture

#### TRYPANOSOMIASIS

#### CHAGAS' DISEASE

- Erythematous induration with a subcutaneous nodule (chagoma)
- Cardiomyopathy, megaesophagus, and megacolon
- Microscopic identification of *Trypanosoma cruzi* in fresh anticoagulated blood or blood smears
- Isolation of the parasite by culture

#### AFRICAN SLEEPING SICKNESS

- Painful chancre surrounded by a white halo
- Fever, lymphadenopathy, and generalized pruritic eruptions with erythematous annular plaques
- Headaches, somnolence, abnormal behavior, loss of consciousness, and coma
- Identification of trypanosomes by microscopic examination

### Diseases Caused by Helminths

#### CUTANEOUS LARVA MIGRANS

- Intense pruritus, papular lesions, and linear, minimally elevated, serpiginous tracts

#### DRACUNCULIASIS

- Erythematous papule or blister that ulcerates and may become secondarily infected
- Identification of the worm in the ulcer

### Filariasis

#### LYMPHATIC FILARIASIS

- Fever with lymphangitis and lymphadenitis, chronic pulmonary infection, and progressive lymphedema leading to massive tissue thickening, especially of the legs and scrotum (elephantiasis)

- Identification of microfilariae microscopically in blood

#### ONCHOCERCIASIS

- Subcutaneous nodules, dermatitis, depigmentation, skin atrophy, lymphadenopathy, lymphedema, and blindness
- Identification of microfilariae in skin snips

#### LOIASIS

- Pruritus, subcutaneous swelling containing the worm, serpiginous lesion on the sclera conjunctiva
- Microfilariae identified in the blood by microscopic examination

#### SCHISTOSOMIASIS

- Pruritic papular dermatitis
- Verrucous papules and nodules, secondary infection, ulceration, and development of squamous cell carcinoma
- Identification of eggs in urine or stool, enzyme-linked immunoabsorbent assay (ELISA) tests

### Diseases Caused by Arthropoda

#### SCABIES

- Intense pruritus, especially at night
- Burrows
- Scaly papules on the nipples and the male genitals
- Identification of the mite, its eggs, or its feces in skin samples

#### PEDICULOSIS

#### PEDICULOSIS CAPITIS

- Intense pruritus of the scalp
- Nape dermatitis
- Identification of lice and nits on the hair

#### PEDICULOSIS CORPORIS

- Intense pruritus, erythema, urticarial lesions, papules, nodules, and excoriations
- Identification of lice and nits on clothing

#### PEDICULOSIS PUBIS

- Pruritus
- Blue macules
- Identification of lice and nits on pubic hair

---

- West African sleeping sickness, caused by *Trypanosoma brucei gambiense*

Chagas' disease can be transmitted to humans by blood-sucking triatomae bugs as well as by blood transfusions, organ transplantation, and transplacentally. The acute reaction at the bite site may include an erythematous induration with a subcutaneous nodule, known as chagoma. The chronic stage of the disease is characterized by cardiomyopathy, megaesophagus, and megacolon. Microscopic identification of the parasite in fresh anticoagulated blood and in blood smears or its isolation by culture confirms the diagnosis. Drug of choice for the treatment of Chagas' disease is nifurtimox (Lampit),[2] 8 to 10 mg/kg/day PO in three to four doses for 90 to 120 days.

African sleeping sickness, East and West, is transmitted through an infected tsetse fly bite. A painful chancre surrounded by a white halo

can develop at the site of inoculation. This is followed by a hemolymphatic stage with fever, lymphadenopathy, and generalized pruritic eruptions with erythematous annular plaques. In the meningoencephalitic stage, invasion of the central nervous system (CNS) can cause headaches, somnolence, abnormal behavior, and lead to loss of consciousness and coma. Diagnosis is confirmed by identification of trypanosomes by microscopic examination in chancre fluid, lymph node aspirates, blood, bone marrow, or, in the late stages of infection, cerebrospinal fluid. East African sleeping sickness is treated with suramin (Metaret) (Germanin),[2] 100 to 200 mg (test dose) IV, then 1 g IV on days 1, 3, 7, 14, and 21. For late disease with involvement of the CNS, melarsoprol (Mel-B)[2] is used in the following dosage scheme: 2 to 3.6 mg/kg/day PO for 3 days; after 7 days, 3.6 mg/kg/day for 3 days, the latter repeated after 7 days. For West African sleeping sickness, the drug of choice is pentamidine

---

[2]Not available in the United States.

[2]Not available in the United States.

## CURRENT THERAPY

### Diseases Caused by Protozoa

#### AMEBIASIS

- Metronidazole (Flagyl), 750 mg PO tid for 7–10 d or
- Tinidazole (Tindamax), 2 g once daily for 5 d.
- Treatment with either metronidazole or tinidazole should be followed by iodoquinol (Yodoxin), 650 mg PO tid for 20 d.

#### LEISHMANIASIS

- Sodium stibogluconate (Pentostam),[2] 20 mg/kg/d IV or IM for 20 d.

#### TRYPANOSOMIASIS

##### CHAGAS' DISEASE

- Nifurtimox (Lampit),[2] 8–10 mg/kg/d PO in 3–4 doses for 90–120 d.

##### EAST AFRICAN SLEEPING SICKNESS

- Suramin (Germanin),[2] 100–200 mg (test dose) IV, then 1 g IV on days 1, 3, 7, 14, and 21.
- For late disease with involvement of the central nervous system (CNS), melarsoprol (Mel-B)[2] is used in the following dosage scheme: 2–3.6 mg/kg/d PO for 3 days; after 7 d, 3.6 mg/kg/d for 3 d; and the latter repeated after 7 d.

##### WEST AFRICAN SLEEPING SICKNESS

- Pentamidine isethionate (Pentam 300, NebuPent),[1] 4 mg/kg/d IM for 10 d.
- In cases of late disease with CNS involvement, either melarsoprol (Mel-B),[2] 2.2 mg/kg/d PO for 10 d, or eflornithine (Ornidyl), 400 mg/kg/d PO in 4 doses for 14 d.

### Diseases Caused by Helminths

#### CUTANEOUS LARVA MIGRANS

- Albendazole (Albenza), 400 mg daily PO for 3 d, or ivermectin (Stromectol),[1] 200 μg/kg/d for 1–2 d.

#### DRACUNCULIASIS

- Slow extraction of the worm, which is facilitated by metronidazole (Flagyl), 250 mg PO tid for 10 d.

#### FILARIASIS

##### LYMPHATIC FILARIASIS

- Diethylcarbamazine (Hetrazan), as follows: d 1: 50 mg, d 2: 50 mg tid, d 3: 100 mg tid, d 4–14: 6 mg/kg in 3 doses.

##### ONCHOCERCIASIS

- Ivermectin (Stromectol), 150 μg/kg PO q6–12mo until asymptomatic.

##### LOIASIS

- Diethylcarbamazine (Hetrazan), as follows: d 1: 50 mg, d 2: 50 mg tid, d 3: 100 mg tid, d 4–14: 9 mg/kg in 3 doses.

#### SCHISTOSOMIASIS

- Praziquantel (Biltricide), 40 mg/kg/d[3] in 2 doses for 1 day (S. haematobium and S. mansoni) and 60 mg/kg/d[3] in 3 doses for 1 day (S. japonicum).

### Diseases Caused by Arthropoda

#### SCABIES

- 5% permethrin (Nix, Elimite), applied for 10 h; application can be repeated after 10–14 d.

#### PEDICULOSIS

##### PEDICULOSIS CAPITIS

- Malathion (Ovide) 0.5% lotion, applied for 8–12 h before being washed off, or permethrin (Nix, Elimite) 1% cream rinse, applied to shampooed hair and washed off after 10 min; a second application 1 wk later is recommended.

##### PEDICULOSIS CORPORIS

- Disinfection of clothes.

##### PEDICULOSIS PUBIS

- Same treatment as pediculosis capitis.

---

[1]Not FDA approved for this indication.
[2]Not available in the United States.
[3]Exceeds dosage recommended by the manufacturer.

---

isethionate (Pentam 300, NebuPent),[1] 4 mg/kg/day IM for 10 days. In cases of late disease with CNS involvement, either melarsoprol (Mel-B),[2] 2.2 mg/kg/day PO for 10 days, or eflornithine (Ornidyl), 400 mg/kg/day PO in four doses for 14 days can be used.

## Diseases Caused by Helminths

### CUTANEOUS LARVA MIGRANS

Cutaneous larva migrans, or creeping eruption, is caused when various nematode larvae penetrate the skin and migrate through it. These larvae are unable to complete their life cycle or reach internal organs. Larvae of *Ancylostoma braziliense*, *Ancylostoma caninum*, *Ascaris suum*, *Bunostomum phlebotomus*, and others can cause creeping eruptions. Infection is acquired by exposure to contaminated soil. Initially, there is intense pruritus and papular lesions, but, as the larvae begin to migrate, the classic linear, minimally elevated, serpiginous tract becomes apparent. Excoriations and secondary infections are common. The diagnosis is usually clinical; sometimes the larva can be found within a tunnel. Treatment of choice is either albendazole (Albenza), 400 mg daily PO for 3 days, or ivermectin ((Stromectol),[1] 200 μg/kg/day for 1 to 2 days.

### DRACUNCULIASIS

Dracunculiasis, one of the oldest infections on record, is caused by *Dracunculus medinensis*. Infection occurs by drinking water that contains crustaceans of the *Cyclops* family infected with the larvae of *D. medinensis*. Crustaceans release the mature larvae in the intestine.

---

[1]Not FDA approved for this indication.
[2]Not available in the United States.

[1]Not FDA approved for this indication.

From the intestine they migrate to the subcutaneous tissue and, finally, the female worm moves into the skin, producing an erythematous papule or blister. The blister ulcerates and may become secondarily infected. The female worm can often be seen in the ulcer. Treatment of choice is slow extraction of the worm combined with wound care. Metronidazole (Flagyl), 250 mg PO three times daily for 10 days, decreases inflammation and facilitates removal of the worm.

## FILARIASIS

Filariasis is caused by nematodes (roundworms) that inhabit the lymphatics and subcutaneous tissues. The most common filarial infections include lymphatic filariasis, onchocerciasis, and loiasis.

### Lymphatic Filariasis

Lymphatic filariasis is caused by *Wuchereria bancrofti*, *Brugia malayi*, and *Brugia timori*. It is transmitted by mosquitoes. Adult worms block lymphatics and produce microfilariae. Many patients are asymptomatic, but some may develop fever with lymphangitis and lymphadenitis, chronic pulmonary infection, and progressive lymphedema leading to massive tissue thickening, especially of the legs and scrotum (elephantiasis). The overlying skin is thickened. Diagnosis is made by identifying the microfilariae microscopically in blood. Antigen detection using an immunoassay for circulating filarial antigens may also be used. Treatment is with diethylcarbamazine (Hetrazan), as follows: day 1: 50 mg; day 2: 50 mg three times daily; day 3: 100 mg three times daily; days 4 through 14: 6 mg/kg in three doses.

### Onchocerciasis

*Onchocerca volvulus* is the causative organism of onchocerciasis and transmitted by the blackflies *Simulium*. Onchocerciasis is manifested with subcutaneous nodules, dermatitis, depigmentation, and skin atrophy and, in later stages, with lymphadenopathy and lymphedema. The eyes are another favorite site for the microfilariae, and the infection can lead to blindness (river blindness). Diagnosis is based on identification of microfilariae in skin snips. The drug of choice for onchocerciasis is ivermectin (Stromectol), 150 μg/kg PO every 6 to 12 months until asymptomatic.

### Loiasis

Loiasis is caused after the transmission of the filarial parasite *Loa loa* by deerflies (*Chrysops*). It is usually manifested by pruritus and a subcutaneous swelling containing the worm. In some cases, there is subconjunctival migration of the adult worm producing a migrating serpiginous lesion on the sclera conjunctiva. Microfilariae can be identified in the blood by microscopic examination. Diethylcarbamazine (Hetrazan) is used for the treatment of loiasis, according to the following scheme: day 1: 50 mg; day 2: 50 mg three times daily; day 3: 100 mg three times daily; days 4 through 14: 9 mg/kg in three doses.

## SCHISTOSOMIASIS

*Schistosoma haematobium*, *Schistosoma japonicum*, and *Schistosoma mansoni* are the main trematodes that cause schistosomiasis in humans. All trematodes have a life cycle that involves the snail as an intermediate host. The infective cercariae leave the snail, swim, and penetrate the human skin, causing a pruritic papular dermatitis. *S. mansoni* primarily causes hepatosplenomegaly, colonic pseudopolyps, and pulmonary lesions, whereas *S. haematobium* mostly affects the bladder. *S. japonicum* primarily involves the liver, but its eggs are more likely to be found in ectopic sites, such as the spinal cord and brain. In the skin, the eggs elicit an inflammatory response with verrucous papules and nodules. Secondary infection, ulceration, and development of squamous cell carcinoma may follow. Diagnosis is established by identification of the eggs in the urine or stool. Enzyme-linked immunoabsorbent assay

(ELISA) tests are also available. The infection is treated with praziquantel (Biltricide), 40 mg/kg/day[3] in two doses for 1 day (*S. haematobium* and *S. mansoni*) or 60 mg/kg/day[3] in three doses for 1 day (*S. japonicum*).

Infection of the skin by cercariae of nonhuman schistosomes leads to *cercarial dermatitis* or *swimmers' itch*, manifested by intensely pruritic macules and papules that may coalesce and produce diffuse erythema and swelling. The rash usually disappears within a week because the cercariae only live for 2 to 3 days. Symptomatic treatment with topical steroids and oral antihistamines may be needed.

# Diseases Caused by Arthropoda

## SCABIES

Scabies is caused by the mite *Sarcoptes scabiei var humanus*, an obligate parasite to humans. Transmission requires close personal contact, such as sexual intercourse, contact between family members, sharing a bed, or holding hands. Live mites can be found in the environment of patients, where they survive for 2 to 3 days.

The fertilized female crawls through the stratum corneum creating tiny tunnels (burrows), where she lays her eggs. The eggs hatch in approximately 1 week.

Initial infestation is usually asymptomatic for approximately 6 weeks, after which an immune response develops to the mites or their feces. Reinfestation provokes symptoms within only 1 to 3 days.

The classic symptom of scabies is intense pruritus, especially at night. Papules, pustules, excoriations, and crusting can appear, especially at the interdigital spaces, the wrists, the axillary folds, the nipples, and the genitals. Pathognomonic signs of scabies include the burrows made by the female mite and the appearance of scaly papules on the nipples and the male genitals. In adults, the head is usually spared, whereas in infants involvement of the scalp, palms, and soles is common.

Crusted scabies (Norwegian scabies) is an aggressive infestation that usually occurs in immunodeficient, debilitated, or malnourished persons. The skin is inhabited by thousands of mites per square millimeter, and clinically there is a proliferative, hyperkeratotic response.

Diagnosis of scabies is confirmed by finding either an intact burrow or the mite, its eggs, and its feces in skin samples from the infected area.

Adults should be treated from the neck down; in infants the scalp should also be treated. Topical therapy of choice is with 5% permethrin (Nix, Elimite), applied for 10 hours. Application can be repeated after 10 to 14 days. Alternatively, crotamiton 10% topical (Eurax), applied once daily for 2 days, or ivermectin (Stromectol),[1] 200 μg/kg once (the dose can be repeated in 10 to 14 days), can be used. Ivermectin, either alone or in combination with a topical scabicide, is the drug of choice for crusted scabies in immunocompromised patients. All sexual and close personal and household contacts within the preceding 6 weeks should be treated at the same time, regardless of whether they have symptoms or not. Bedding and clothing should be decontaminated (i.e., either machine washed and dried using the hot cycle or dry cleaned) or removed from body contact for at least 3 days.

## PEDICULOSIS

Lice are blood-sucking insects and are obligate parasites of humans. There are three major types of lice: *Pediculus humanus capitis* (head louse), which lives on the scalp, *Pediculus humanus corporis* (body louse), which lives in a person's clothes, and *Phthirus pubis* (pubic louse), which lives mostly on pubic hair.

### Pediculosis Capitis

Pediculosis capitis is caused by *Pediculus humanus capitis*. The louse attaches its eggs or nits firmly to the hair shaft. Children and individuals with long hair are mostly affected. Transmission is accomplished either directly from human to human or through sharing combs and brushes. Clinically, there is intense pruritus of the scalp, which is

---

[3]Exceeds dosage recommended by the manufacturer

[1]Not FDA approved for this indication.

sometimes accompanied with nape dermatitis, secondary bacterial infection, and lymphadenopathy. Diagnosis is established by identification of lice and nits on the hair.

Treatment of choice for pediculosis capitis is either malathion (Ovide) 0.5% lotion, applied for 8 to 12 hours before being washed off, or permethrin (Nix, Elimite) 1% cream rinse, applied to shampooed hair and washed off after 10 minutes. A second application is recommended with permethrin 1 week later to kill hatching progeny. Alternatively, pyrethrins with piperidyl butoxide (RID) can be applied to the affected area and washed off after 10 minutes. Ivermectin (Stromectol)[1] can also be used at a dose of 200 µg/kg on days 1, 2, and 10. In combination with insecticide treatment, combing of wet hair with a fine-toothed comb every 3 to 4 days for 2 weeks, to remove all lice as they hatch, can be very helpful. Bedding and clothing should be decontaminated (as for scabies) or removed from body contact for at least 2 weeks.

## Pediculosis Corporis

Pediculosis corporis is associated with poor hygiene and unsanitary living conditions (vagabond's itch). *Pediculus humanus corporis*, the body louse, lives and lays its eggs on clothes, especially on seams. Transmission occurs mainly through contact with contaminated clothing or bedding. *P. humanus corporis* is capable of transferring several infectious diseases, especially epidemic typhus.

The infestation is manifested with intense pruritus, erythema, urticarial lesions, papules, and nodules. Excoriations, secondary infections, and lymphadenopathy may also be seen. The lice and nits usually can be found in the clothing.

For treatment, disinfection of clothes is enough. They should be washed and rinsed in hot water following by ironing. Items that cannot be washed should be removed from body contact for 2 weeks. Skin lesions can be managed with topical antipruritics or corticosteroids.

## Pediculosis Pubis

*Phthirus pubis* is usually transmitted during sexual intercourse, although any intimate personal contact suffices. Lice and nits are found mostly on pubic hair, but other body parts and, especially in children, eyelashes and the periphery of the scalp can be involved. Patients present with pruritus. Blue macules, or *maculae caeruleae*, are often found and result from intracutaneous hemorrhages whose hemoglobin has been altered by the saliva of the lice.

Pediculosis pubis can be treated in the same way as pediculosis capitis. Some recommend treatment with permethrin (Nix, Elimite) 5% or ivermectin (Stromectol),[1] as for scabies (see earlier). Infestation of eyelashes should be treated by applying occlusive ophthalmic ointment to the eyelid margins twice a day for 10 days. Bedding and clothing should be decontaminated (as for scabies) or removed from body contact for at least 2 weeks. Sexual partners within the last month should also be treated.

## REFERENCES

Braun-Falco O, Plewig G, Wolff HH, Burgdorf WHC: Diseases caused by worms. In: Dermatology, 2nd ed. Springer, Berlin Heidelberg, 2000, pp 383-402.

Ectoparasitic infections. In: Centers for Disease Control and Prevention: Sexually transmitted diseases treatment guidelines-2006. MMWR Morb Mortal Wkly Rep 2006;55(RR11):1-94.

Orion E, Matz H, Wolf R: Ectoparasitic sexually transmitted diseases: Scabies and pediculosis. Clin Dermatol 2004;22:513-519.

Braun-Falco O, Plewig G, Wolff HH, Burgdorf WHC: Protozoan diseases. In: Dermatology, 2nd ed. Springer, Berlin Heidelberg, 2000, pp 299-312.

Drugs for Parasitic Infections. The Medical Letter on Drugs and Therapeutics. The Medical Letter Inc, New Rochelle, NY, August, 2004;1-12.

Tsoureli-Nikita E, Campanile G, Hautmann G, Hercogova J: Pediculosis. In: Katsambas AD, Lotti TM (eds): European Handbook of Dermatologic Treatments, 2nd ed. Springer, Berlin Heidelberg, 2003, pp 377-381.

---

[1]Not FDA approved for this indication.

# Fungal Diseases of the Skin

Method of
*Rebecca Lewis Kelso, MD,*
*and Sharon S. Raimer, MD*

Dermatophytes may be distinguished by their genera and typical environmental hosts. The most common genera to cause superficial dermatophyte infection of skin include *Epidermophyton, Microsporum,* and *Trichophyton.* Dermatophytes may be anthropophilic, infecting humans as the primary host; zoophilic, with animals as the primary host; or geophilic, with soil as the primary host. When infecting humans, dermatophytes are dependent on the stratum corneum for growth and nutrition, which confines them to a superficial infection aside from very rare cases of dissemination.

## Diagnosis

Dermatophyte infection may be readily diagnosed in an office setting. Perhaps the most rapid method of diagnosis involves the scraping of scales onto a glass slide with a No. 15 blade, placing a drop of potassium hydroxide (KOH) onto the specimen, and placing a coverslip on top. In the case of tinea unguium, a small curette may be used to obtain subungual keratin debris from the proximal portion. If a dermatophyte is present, septated hyphae may be seen traversing the scales under light microscopy. In the case of tinea versicolor, both yeast and hyphae forms are seen with a "spaghetti and meatballs" appearance. Dermatophyte infections can also be diagnosed by fungal culture or, in the case of tinea unguium, periodic acid–Schiff (PAS) staining of a nail clipping. Use of a topical antifungal medicine prior to scraping can yield a false-negative result.

## Dermatophyte Infections of the Skin

### DIAGNOSIS

Dermatophyte infections of the skin may be classified by body site involved.

Tinea corporis involving the neck, trunk, or extremities typically appears clinically as slightly erythematous scaly patches with central clearing and an elevated advancing border. This pattern gives rise to the term *ringworm.*

Tinea pedis typically appears as scaling of the plantar aspect of the feet, classically involving the third toe web space. Maceration may also be present, and hyperhidrosis is believed to be a contributing factor. *Trichophyton rubrum* is the usual organism. The infection can involve the entire foot in a moccasin pattern. If *Trichophyton mentagrophytes* is the inciting agent, vesicles and bullae can predominate in a more inflammatory clinical pattern. Tinea pedis warrants examination for scaling of one hand, because patients sometimes have "two foot one hand syndrome."

Tinea cruris occurs more often in men on the medial aspects of the thighs, with sparing of the scrotum and penis. This is particularly seen in men who live in hot, humid environments or who wear tight clothing.

Tinea barbae describes involvement of the beard area and may be characterized by nodular or superficial pustular forms. Sparing of the upper lip is characteristic. Majocchi's granuloma is an erythematous plaque with perifollicular pustules often found on glabrous skin, particularly on the shins or wrists. Clinical distinction of these two forms of dermatophytes is important, because involvement of the hair follicles necessitates systemic antifungal therapy.

### TREATMENT

Treatment for uncomplicated cutaneous tinea infection is best accomplished by applying a cream from the allylamine or benzylamine

## CURRENT DIAGNOSIS

**Tinea Corporis**

- Erythematous scaly patches with elevated borders and central clearing

**Tinea Cruris**

- Erythematous scaly patches in the groin with elevated borders and central clearing
- Typically spares the scrotum

**Tinea Pedis**

- Erythematous scaly patches on the plantar aspects of the feet
- Third web space is most commonly infected
- Can have extensive moccasin pattern or bullous pattern

**Tinea Barbae**

- Pustules or nodules in the beard region
- Spares the upper lip

**Majocchi's Granuloma**

- Erythematous plaque with perifollicular pustules
- Commonly on shins or wrists

**Tinea Capitis**

- Erythematous scaly patches on scalp with or without alopecia
- Pustules may be present

**Tinea Unguium**

- Thickened, dystrophic nails
- Evaluate for concomitant tinea pedis infection

**Tinea Versicolor**

- Hypo- or hyperpigmented slightly scaly patches
- Typically involves back and chest; can extend to upper arms
- In fair-skinned patients, lesions can appear erythematous

**Cutaneous Candidiasis**

- Erythematous papules, typically in intertriginous areas
- Might have satellite lesions
- In men with groin involvement, can extend to involve the scrotum

groups, such as terbinafine (Lamisil) cream twice daily, butenafine (Mentax) cream once daily, or naftifine (Naftin) cream once daily for a minimum of 2 weeks. Other treatment options include the topical azoles, which have lesser activity against tinea infections but do have higher efficacy for candidal infections, or cicloprox (Loprox).

For tinea barbae, Majocchi's granuloma, or extensive tinea corporis, oral therapy is indicated. In these cases, terbinafine 250 mg orally once daily for 2 weeks is one recommended treatment. The other treatment of choice is griseofulvin (Grifulvin V), which is given 500 mg twice daily for the microsized formula or 250 mg twice daily for the ultramicrosized, formula, for 4 weeks.

Other options include oral itraconazole (Sporanox) or fluconazole (Diflucan).[1]

---

[1]Not FDA approved for this indication.

## Nondermatophyte Infections of the Skin

### DIAGNOSIS

Superficial infection may be caused by yeasts. In particular, *Candida albicans*, although often a commensal organism on the skin can overgrow under certain conditions such as warmth, moisture, or occlusion. Candidal infections of the skin typically manifest in beefy erythematous papules that can become confluent, typically in intertriginous areas such as skin folds. Satellite pustules may be present around the periphery. In contrast to tinea cruris, candidal infections of the groin often involve the scrotum. Pityriasis (tinea) versicolor, caused by *Malassezia furfur*, also can cause superficial skin infection. Clinically, hypopigmented or hyperpigmented slightly scaly patches are seen, typically on the back, chest, and arms. In patients with fair skin, the patches may be erythematous. As with *Candida albicans*, infections are seen more commonly in warm, humid environments.

### TREATMENT

Patients with cutaneous candidiasis should be encouraged to keep involved areas dry. Clotrimazole 1% (Lotrimin) cream applied twice a day for 2 weeks is recommended and may be combined with hydrocortisone cream 1% in equal parts for areas of intertrigo. Treatment of tinea versicolor may be accomplished by applying ketoconazole shampoo 2% (Nizoral) for 15 minutes, then washing off, repeating in 1 week and then in 1 month. Alternatively, patients may take a single oral dose of ketoconazole 400 mg. Patients who are predisposed to tinea versicolor are likely to have a recurrence, so periodic application of ketoconazole shampoo as prophylactic therapy may be of great value.

## Onychomycosis

### DIAGNOSIS

Fungal infection of the nail (tinea unguium) manifests with thickening and dystrophy of the nail. Usually, the infection is due to *T. rubrum* or *T. mentagrophytes* or, less commonly, yeasts or molds. Likelihood of infection increases with advanced age, diabetes mellitus, immunosuppressive states, poor peripheral circulation, and smoking.

### TREATMENT

Successful treatment of onychomycosis usually requires oral antifungal therapy. Treatment regimens include terbinafine 250 mg daily for 3 months for toenail infections or for 6 weeks for fingernail infections. Alternatively, itraconazole may be given in pulsed doses of 200 mg twice daily for 1 week per month for 2 months for fingernail infection and for 3 months for toenail infection. Therapeutic considerations must include the risk of hepatotoxicity and potential drug interactions with other medicines, and appropriate laboratory tests should be ordered. However, treatment may be warranted in those with recurrent tinea pedis, because onychomycosis can act as a reservoir of infection.

## Tinea Capitis

### DIAGNOSIS

Tinea capitis occurs most commonly in children. It may manifest as erythematous scaly patches, generally with patchy hair loss. Pustules and boggy, tender plaques (kerion) are seen occasionally. Infection is most commonly due to *Trichophyton tonsurans* or, less commonly, *Microsporum canis*. Identification of the fungus via culture is ideal, because it can affect the treatment choice.

### TREATMENT

Although griseofulvin is the only FDA-approved treatment for tinea capitis, for infections caused by *T. tonsurans*, a 2-week course of terbenafine[1] yields high cure rates. For infections caused by *M. canis*,

- Encourage patients to keep areas dry.
- Consider medicated powders such as miconazole 2% (Zeasorb AF) once the skin is clear.

**Complicated\* Cutaneous Tinea Infection**

SYSTEMIC

- Griseofulvin (Grifulvin V) 500 mg bid for ultramicrosized, 250 mg bid for microsized × 4 wk

or

- Itraconazole (Sporanox) 100 mg bid × 2wk

or

- Fluconazole (Diflucan)[1] 150mg/wk × 4 wk

or

- Terbinafine (Lamisil) 250 mg/d × 2 wk

**Uncomplicated Cutaneous Tinea Infection**

TOPICAL

- Butenafine (Mentax) cream qd × 2 wk

or

- Terbenafine cream qd × 2 wk

or

- Naftifine (Naftin) cream qd × 2 wk

ALTERNATIVE

- Oxiconazole (Oxistat) cream qd × 2-4 wk

or

- Ketoconazole (Nizoral) cream qd × 2-4 wk

or

- Econazole (Spectazole) cream qd × 2-4 wk

**Tinea Capitis**

SYSTEMIC

- Adult: Terbinafine 250 mg qd × 2 wk[1,3]

**Infections due to _Microsporum canis_**

- Griseofulvin microsized 1000 mg/d × 8 wk

or

- Griseofulvin ultramicrosized 500-750 mg/d

SYSTEMIC (PEDIATRIC)

- Griseofulvin microsized liquid 20-25 mg/kg/d[3] × 6-8 wk

or

- Griseofulvin ultramicrosized 15-20 mg/kg/d[3] × 6-8 wk

or

- Terbinafine[1] 62.5 mg (¼ tab) qd × 2 wk for children weighing ≤14 kg

or

- Terbinafine[1] 125 mg (½ tab) qd × 2 wk for children weighing 14-28 kg

or

- Terbinafine[1] 250 mg qd × 2 wk for children weighing >28 kg

TOPICAL

- Recommend concomitant therapy with medicated shampoo for several months: ketoconazole shampoo 2% or cicloprox (Loprox) or selenium sulfide (Selsun Blue) at least twice weekly

**Tinea Unguium**

SYSTEMIC

- Terbinafine 250 mg/d × 3 mo (toenails) or 6 weeks (fingernails)

ALTERNATIVE

- Itraconazole 200 mg bid for 1 wk per mo × 3 mo (toenails) or × 2 mo (fingernails)

**Tinea Versicolor**

TOPICAL

- Ketoconazole shampoo 2%. Apply to affected areas for 15 min, then rinse off, repeat in 1 wk, then repeat monthly

ALTERNATIVE

- Selenium sulfide (Selsun) lotion (2.5%) applied qhs and washed off in AM × 7 d

SYSTEMIC

- Ketoconazole 400 mg PO × 1 dose

**Cutaneous Candidiasis**

TOPICAL

- Clotrimazole (Lotrimin) cream bid × 2-4 wk

or

- Ketoconazole cream qd × 2-4 wk
- For intertriginous areas, consider combination with equal parts 1% hydrocortisone cream

SYSTEMIC

- Fluconazole 150 mg PO weekly × 2-4 wk

---

\*Severe, recalcitrant, extensive, or involving hair follicle.
[1]Not FDA approved for this indication.
[3]Exceeds dosage recommended by the manufacturer.

---

griseofulvin given daily for 8 weeks is the treatment of choice (see the Current Therapy box for medication dosages). As with all oral antifungal medicines, appropriate blood tests should be ordered and potential drug interactions should be considered

## Considerations in HIV/AIDS Patients

Although candidiasis and therefore intertrigo (macerated candidal infections of intertriginous areas) are common in patients with HIV/AIDS,

opportunistic dermatophyte infections do not occur any more frequently than in HIV-negative patients. However, they can manifest with more severe clinical disease, such as extensive moccasin-pattern tinea pedis, onychomycosis without interdigital tinea pedis, and Majocchi's granuloma. If highly active antiretroviral therapy (HAART) is given early on, and the CD4 count is 500/mL or more, there is no difference in frequency of tinea infections. If HAART is given later in the disease, and the CD4 count is greater than 100/mL, the tinea infection might improve or clear without any specific antifungal treatment. There is no difference in epidemiology or causative organisms. It is believed that perhaps the lack of an increase in tinea infections in HIV-positive patients in industrialized nations is due to frequent oral treatment with azoles or terbinafine for invasive candidal or fungal infection, which coincidentally provides prophylaxis against dermatophyte infection.

---

[1]Not FDA approved for this indication.

Treatment of HIV/AIDS patients can require a longer course of treatment or possibly oral therapy. For early disease, with a CD4 count of 500/mL or greater, for cutaneous tinea infections, treatment may include terbinafine 250 mg orally once a day for 7 days or for 2 weeks for advanced disease with CD4 count of less than 100/mL. Alternative treatment is itraconazole 200 mg orally once a day for 7 days for tinea corporis or tinea cruris, and twice a day for tinea pedis. Immunosuppressed patients might require topical therapy in conjunction with oral therapies, as well as prophylaxis once the infection is cleared. Prophylactic measures for all patient populations include eliminating any shoes that might have fungal residua, avoiding walking barefoot in public places, and using antifungal powder in shoes.

## REFERENCES

Adams BB: Tinea corporis gladiatorum. J Am Acad Derm 2002;47(2):286-290.

Foster KW, Gannoum MA, Elewski BE: Epidemiologic surveillance of cutaneous fungal infection in the U.S. from 1999-2002. J Am Acad Dermatol 2004;50:748-752.

Gupta AK, Chaudhry M, Elewski B: Tinea corporis, tinea cruris, tinea nigra, and piedra. Dermatol Clin 2003;21(3):395-400.

High W: Combating superficial cutaneous fungal infections. Prac Dermatol 2006;36-42.

Johnson RA: Dermatophyte infections in HIV disease. J Am Acad Dermatol 2000;43(5 suppl):S135-S142.

Milliken LE: Role of oral antifungal agents for treatment of superficial fungal infections in immunocompromised patients. Cutis 2001;68(1 suppl):6-14.

Roberts DT, Taylor WD, Boyle J: Guidelines for treatment of onychomycosis. Br J Dermatol 2003;148:402-410.

# Diseases of the Mouth

Method of
*Carl M. Allen, DDS, MSD*

A wide variety of disease processes other than dental caries and periodontal disease affect the oral region. These diseases may be classified based on the etiopathogenesis of the disease (e.g., viral, neoplastic); the clinical form of the lesions (e.g., plaque, vesicle, ulcer); or the anatomic region affected (e.g., lips, buccal mucosa). The clinical form and anatomic region are particularly useful for the clinician confronted by an unknown lesion. An accurate diagnosis is the most important aspect of patient management because treatment is predicated on diagnosis. The lesions that tend to affect certain oral mucosal sites preferentially are listed here according to their frequency; space limitations prohibit discussion of rare entities.

## Generalized Oral Involvement

Xerostomia is the subjective feeling of a dry mouth. In most instances, it is caused by any of a variety of medications (antihypertensives, antihistamines, psychoactive drugs), and withdrawal or substitution of the medication may be helpful. A smaller number of patients may have xerostomia secondary to autoimmune destruction of the salivary gland tissue (Sjögren's syndrome) or caused by radiation therapy of the head and neck region. Such patients may develop a number of problems. The mucosa is not as well lubricated and becomes susceptible to traumatic ulceration. The dry environment predisposes the individual to the erythematous or angular cheilitis forms of oral candidiasis. If the patient has natural teeth, a marked increase in dental caries is noted.

A number of over-the-counter artificial saliva substitutes, in both liquid and gel form, are available to help manage the symptoms of dryness. Oral ulcerations should be managed conservatively using a protective hydroxypropylcellulose medication (Zilactin),[1] applied as often as necessary. Oral candidiasis can be treated with any of several antifungal medications, although those with high sucrose content, such as nystatin pastilles (Mycostatin Oral Pastilles), should probably be avoided in dentulous patients because these agents could contribute to caries activity. A prescription-strength topical fluoride preparation, such as 1.1% neutral sodium fluoride gel (PreviDent), should be used daily by patients who have natural teeth to prevent dental decay. Application of the topical fluoride is best performed at night after brushing the teeth and before retiring. Several drops of the fluoride gel should be placed on the toothbrush and gently massaged onto the surfaces of the teeth next to the gum tissue.

## Lips

### COMMON CONDITIONS

#### Fordyce's Granules

Fordyce's granules, a variation of normal anatomy, are heterotopic sebaceous glands seen in more than 80% of adults. They occur as 1-mm yellow-white submucosal dots distributed on the lateral upper lip and the buccal mucosa. No treatment is indicated because of the completely benign nature of the condition.

#### Angular Cheilitis

Angular cheilitis is characterized by inflammation of the corners of the mouth, accompanied by fissuring and sometimes scaling. This condition was thought to be caused by B vitamin deficiency, but the vast majority of these lesions are now thought to be caused by a low-grade infection of *Candida albicans*, with or without *Staphylococcus aureus*.

These lesions can be easily treated with a topical antifungal agent such as nystatin-triamcinolone cream (Mycolog-II Cream). Another alternative is iodoquinol-hydrocortisone cream (Vytone Cream),[1] which is both antifungal and antibacterial but must be used externally. Either medication should be applied three to four times daily for at least 1 week. With recurrence, a careful search for an intraoral source of infection may be indicated, and the possibility of HIV infection may need to be ruled out. Angular cheilitis with associated intraoral candidiasis requires treatment. Topical agents include clotrimazole troches (Mycelex Oral Troches) and nystatin pastilles, each dissolved in the mouth four to five times daily for 7 to 10 days. Systemic therapy with fluconazole (Diflucan) may be more convenient for some patients because it is given orally, 200 mg the first day, followed by 100 mg daily for the next 6 days.

#### Herpes Labialis

Recurrent herpes labialis affects approximately 25% of the population. Reactivation of the virus is usually triggered by sun (ultraviolet light) exposure, with many patients experiencing an itching or tingling sensation in the prodromal phase. A cluster of vesicles then develops on the vermilion zone of the lip or on perioral skin, rupturing within 1 to 3 days and leaving a crusted area that resolves after a few more days.

No curative therapy exists for this condition, and treatment results may be difficult to interpret because of the strong placebo effect in some instances. High sun protection factor (SPF) sun-blocking agents significantly reduce the frequency of episodes triggered by exposure to ultraviolet light. Low-dose acyclovir (Zovirax)[1] or valacyclovir (Valtrex)[1] may prevent attacks if it is taken continuously (400 mg twice daily; 1 g per day, respectively), but attacks resume as usual once the medication is stopped. Systemic valacyclovir, 2-g doses 12 hours apart given during the prodromal phase, reduces lesion formation in a subset of individuals affected by this condition. Topical acyclovir ointment shows no benefit in double-blind, placebo-controlled trials in

---

[1]Not FDA approved for this indication.

immunocompetent patients, whereas topical penciclovir cream (Denavir) has only a modest effect on the course of the lesions.

### Melanotic Macule

Melanotic macule, a solitary lesion, usually develops on the vermilion zone of the lips, but it may be seen intraorally. The lesion occurs as a 1- to 5-mm macule that exhibits a uniform, well-demarcated brown to black color.

If the patient indicates the lesion has been present for several years and has not observed any change in size or color, no treatment is indicated unless the patient is concerned about cosmetic appearance. If changes in the lesion are recent, excisional biopsy is indicated to rule out the possibility of an early melanoma.

### Actinic Keratosis (Cheilitis)

Actinic keratosis is a premalignant process affecting the lower vermilion zone of the lip of fair-skinned adults with a history of chronic sun exposure. The lesions have a scaly texture and ill-defined margins.

Excision, by either scalpel or laser, or cryosurgery is indicated for treatment. Excision is often accomplished by vermilionectomy, in which the entire vermilion zone is removed as a strip for histopathologic examination. The labial mucosa is then advanced over the resulting defect. When topical chemotherapy with fluorouracil (Efudex) is used, dysplastic epithelial cells persist histologically. All patients with sun-damaged lips should be advised to use a sunscreen with high SPF, applied particularly to the lower lip when sun exposure is anticipated.

## UNCOMMON CONDITIONS

### Squamous Cell Carcinoma

The malignancy of squamous cell carcinoma affects the lower vermilion zone, typically arising in a preexisting actinic keratosis. Such lesions usually have a relatively slow, steady growth, with a roughened or ulcerated surface. The diagnosis should be established by biopsy. Wide surgical excision, obtaining at least a 1-cm margin of normal tissue, is usually adequate treatment because these lesions are rather indolent and do not metastasize until relatively late in their course.

### Reactive Cheilitis

Patients may present occasionally with a complaint of fissured, painful lips. Evaluation of the problem should include a history of onset, duration, and use of medications and cosmetics. Lipstick and artificially flavored cinnamon products may produce a contact cheilitis. Isotretinoin (Accutane) often causes exfoliative cheilitis. Solitary chronic lip fissures, which usually occur in the winter months, may respond to topical antibiotic preparations, with surgical excision reserved for resistant lesions. Many cases of reactive cheilitis appear to be factitial, although patients may be reluctant to admit their habit of licking and nibbling at the vermilion zone. Constant moistening of the lips also predisposes the individual to a superimposed candidal infection, which exacerbates the inflammatory symptoms, and petrolatum-based lip balms may contribute to the problem by trapping moisture and thereby promoting the growth of yeast.

### Telangiectasias

Superficial dilated blood vessels may occur on the vermilion zone of the lips as an isolated finding or, if multiple, as a component of either hereditary hemorrhagic telangiectasia or CREST (calcinosis, Raynaud's phenomenon, esophageal dysfunction, sclerodactyly, and telangiectasias) syndrome. Patients should be evaluated to distinguish between these two entities because their prognoses are different. Treatment of the telangiectatic lesions can be performed by laser excision, cryotherapy, or electrodesiccation.

# Labial Mucosa

## COMMON CONDITIONS

### Mucocele

The mucocele represents a collection of extravasated mucin within the submucosal connective tissue caused by the disruption of a minor salivary gland duct by minor trauma. Most mucoceles develop on the lower labial mucosa, appearing suddenly as a painless, soft, bluish, circumscribed swelling. A cycle of swelling, breaking, and swelling again is typical. Surgical excision of the mucous deposit and the associated gland usually is necessary for resolution of the problem.

### Varix

The varix, similar to varicose veins of the leg, is seen on the labial mucosa, lips, buccal mucosa, and tongue of patients older than 50 years. Patients usually describe the gradual onset of a painless purplish or bluish nodule.

Generally, no treatment is indicated. If the lesion is a cosmetic problem or if it occurs in areas likely to be traumatized, the varix may be treated by surgical excision or cryotherapy.

### Aphthous Ulcer (Canker Sore)

The aphthous ulcer is perhaps one of the most misdiagnosed, mismanaged, and misunderstood of all oral diseases. Most authorities believe that aphthous ulcers are immunologically induced. No convincing scientific data link the process to viral infection. Furthermore, studies suggesting the lesions are associated with certain foods or vitamin deficiencies have not been duplicated. Several mechanisms may initiate the abnormal immune response leading to focal destruction of the oral mucosa. The lesions are typically recurrent, ranging from 1 to 24 episodes per year. The most common form of aphthous ulcer is the minor aphthous ulcer, manifesting as a 1- to 10-mm ulceration with an erythematous periphery and smooth borders. From one to five ulcers may develop simultaneously. Aphthous ulcers are located on movable mucosa, not mucosa bound to periosteum, a situation directly opposite to recurrent intraoral herpes. The patient typically reports pain that seems out of proportion to the size of the lesion. With no treatment, minor aphthae heal within 5 to 10 days. Patients with frequent attacks should be questioned regarding ocular complaints or genital ulcerations to rule out Behçet's syndrome. Infrequently, aphthous-like oral ulcerations may be a manifestation of Crohn's disease as well.

Topical application of a relatively strong corticosteroid, such as fluocinonide (Lidex Gel),[1] betamethasone dipropionate (Diprolene Gel),[1] or clobetasol (Temovate Gel),[1] is most effective in controlling the lesions. For optimum response, small amounts of the medication should be applied as a thin film often (four to five times daily) and as early in the course of the lesion as possible.

## UNCOMMON CONDITIONS

### Major Aphthous Ulcers

Major aphthae are debilitating oral lesions that resemble minor aphthae, except they are much larger (ranging up to 3 cm), and they persist for periods of up to 6 weeks before healing. Topical application of fluocinonide,[1] betamethasone dipropionate,[1] or clobetasol[1] usually controls this process. If the lesions are in the posterior segments of the mouth, betamethasone syrup (Celestone Syrup),[1] used as a mouth rinse and swallowed (10 mL after meals and at bedtime for 7 to 10 days), often provides relief.

### Herpetiform Aphthous Ulcers

Herpetiform aphthous ulcers resemble primary herpetic gingivostomatitis, and they can be distinguished from that condition by their history

---

[1]Not FDA approved for this indication.

of recurrence. Herpetiform aphthae are most effectively treated with one of the topical corticosteroid preparations or rinses described earlier.

## Angioedema

Angioedema is thought to occur because of localized release of histamine from mast cells. Most cases are sporadic and harmless. The lips are most frequently affected, followed by the tongue. A tingling sensation usually precedes the sudden onset of rather dramatic, nontender swelling. The overlying skin appears normal, and the patient is otherwise asymptomatic; these features should help distinguish this condition from cellulitis associated with a dentoalveolar abscess. With no treatment, the condition resolves in 24 to 48 hours; however, oral antihistamine therapy seems to speed resolution. Attacks are commonly recurrent, and the precipitating factor is often difficult to identify. A rare hereditary form, caused by a deficiency of C1 esterase inhibitor, can be life-threatening if the laryngeal tissues are involved. With persistent swelling, biopsy may be indicated to rule out relatively rare conditions such as orofacial granulomatosis (cheilitis granulomatosa, Melkersson-Rosenthal syndrome).

# Buccal Mucosa

## COMMON CONDITIONS

### Linea Alba

The oral linea alba merely represents a mild thickening of the epithelium along the plane of occlusion in dentate patients. The extent to which it is evident varies tremendously from patient to patient. No treatment is indicated for this completely benign condition.

### Leukoedema

Leukoedema is considered a variation of normal. Clinically, it has a whitish, filmy, almost opalescent appearance, usually affecting the buccal mucosa. Stretching the mucosa causes the white appearance to diminish greatly or disappear completely. The surface epithelial cells histologically are edematous but otherwise normal, and no treatment is necessary for this benign condition.

### Cheek-Chewing

Cheek-chewing is a harmless chronic habit. Although the anterior buccal mucosa is the most common site, the labial mucosa and lateral tongue may also be affected. A white, ragged alteration of the mucosa is seen clinically. Actual ulceration is uncommon because only the outer layers of the epithelium (which have no nerve fibers) are nibbled. The patient usually admits to the habit if questioned. This habit is completely benign and requires no further management once it is identified.

### Fibroma (Irritation Fibroma, Focal Fibrous Hyperplasia)

The fibroma represents an accumulation of dense collagenous connective tissue at a site of irritation. For this reason, most of these lesions are found on the buccal mucosa. The lesion appears clinically as a sessile, dome-shaped, smooth-surfaced nodule. Patients may complain because they bite the lesion inadvertently.

Because this lesion cannot be definitively differentiated clinically from a wide array of other neoplasms, excisional biopsy is generally indicated. Recurrence is uncommon.

### Lichen Planus

Lichen planus is an immunologically mediated condition of unknown cause that affects adults. The oral lesions manifest in two patterns: reticular and erosive. The reticular pattern is more common and usually seen bilaterally on the posterior buccal mucosa, occurring as white fine interlacing lines or papules. The gingivae and the tongue may also be affected. The erosive form of the condition is symptomatic because of the presence of ulcerations. These ulcerations usually have a central yellow-white area of fibrin surrounded by an erythematous halo and radiating white striae.

Reticular lichen planus requires no treatment. In 20% of cases, candidiasis is present, which should be treated with an antifungal agent. Erosive lichen planus can usually be managed effectively with the more potent topical corticosteroids such as fluocinonide,[1] betamethasone dipropionate,[1] or clobetasol.[1] Application of a thin film of medicationto the lesional areas, four to five times daily, often resolves the ulcers within a few days. Other conditions, such as epithelial dysplasia, lichenoid amalgam reactions, contact stomatitis, lichenoid drug reactions, and systemic lupus erythematosus, may mimic lichen planus clinically; biopsy is thus warranted if classic clinical features are not present. Malignant transformation of reticular lichen planus is not thought likely, although erosive lichen planus could possibly be premalignant. Affected patients should be reevaluated periodically for evidence of significant mucosal change, with rebiopsy performed if necessary.

## UNCOMMON CONDITIONS

### Verrucous Carcinoma

Verrucous carcinoma is a relatively low-grade malignancy of surface epithelial origin. It appears as a diffuse, white, rough-surfaced, spreading plaquelike lesion affecting the buccal mucosa, palate, or alveolar process in patients over 65 years of age.

Treatment is complete surgical excision, via scalpel or laser, with evaluation of the lesional tissue histopathologically because 25% of verrucous carcinomas may contain foci of routine squamous cell carcinoma. The prognosis is generally good because this lesion does not metastasize.

### Oral Mucosal Cinnamon Reaction

The oral mucosal cinnamon reaction affects the buccal mucosa, the lateral tongue, and gingivae. The lesions appear as diffuse areas of mucosal erythema with varying degrees of superimposed white plaques and, less commonly, ulceration. Such lesions may be mistaken clinically for lichen planus, candidiasis, leukoplakia, or erythroplakia. Discontinuing the artificially flavored cinnamon product (usually chewing gum) resolves the lesions within 1 week. The diagnosis can be confirmed by challenging the oral mucosa with the offending agent, although patients are often reluctant to do so after their lesions clear.

# Hard Palate

## COMMON CONDITIONS

### Torus

Palatal tori are common developmental lesions representing a benign accumulation of dense bone in the midline posterior hard palate region. The diagnosis can be made clinically because no other condition manifests as a bony hard midline palatal mass. No treatment is necessary for this benign process, although denture construction may be hampered. Removal of the torus by an oral surgeon is recommended in that situation.

### Denture Stomatitis

Denture stomatitis is almost invariably associated with a maxillary removable denture worn 24 hours per day. The palatal mucosa directly beneath the denture appears red, although it is asymptomatic. The redness is confined to the denture-bearing mucosa.

In many cases, simply having the patient remove the denture at night may resolve the palatal erythema. If the patient has a complete

---

[1]Not FDA approved for this indication.

upper denture, it can be soaked in a mild sodium hypochlorite solution (Clorox) (1 teaspoon in 8 ounces of water) each night for a week to disinfect it. (Note: Chrome-cobalt metal denture frameworks should not be soaked in Clorox; severe corrosion will result and ruin the denture.) Because denture stomatitis is a benign and asymptomatic condition, treatment need not be a top priority.

## Inflammatory Papillary Hyperplasia

Inflammatory papillary hyperplasia (IPH) (denture papillomatosis) is seen almost exclusively in patients who wear ill-fitting complete upper dentures. The lesions appear as multiple, erythematous 1- to 2-mm papules typically confined to the palatal vault area. These papules are composed of dense fibrous connective tissue that has accumulated secondary to chronic irritation in the superficial mucosa.

Treatment of this benign process is somewhat controversial. Some prosthodontists prefer to have these lesions surgically removed prior to constructing a new denture, although this procedure may not be necessary in every case.

## UNCOMMON CONDITIONS

### Recurrent Intraoral Herpes

Recurrent intraoral herpes is much less common than aphthous ulcerations, a condition with which it is frequently confused. Recurrent intraoral herpes affects only the hard palate and the attached gingiva (the paler firm gum tissue directly adjacent to the teeth). Most patients experience mild symptoms and may give a history of recurrent episodes. Lesions appear as a cluster of 1- to 2-mm shallow ulcerations that heal within 1 week. Generally no treatment is necessary, although the patient should be cautioned that virus is being shed from the lesion.

### Salivary Gland Tumors

The posterior hard palate/anterior soft palate region is the most common site for the development of intraoral salivary gland neoplasia. This type of lesion presents as a slowly growing, rubbery firm, nontender mass that may or may not be ulcerated. The clinical appearance does not distinguish benign form malignant tumors, so a biopsy should be obtained that includes a margin of normal adjacent tissue. Approximately 50% of these tumors are pleomorphic adenomas, whereas the remainder represent mucoepidermoid carcinoma, polymorphous low-grade adenocarcinoma, adenoid cystic carcinoma, or acinic cell carcinoma. Complete excision is recommended for the pleomorphic adenoma, including overlying mucosa and underlying periosteum. The malignancies should be treated with a much more aggressive surgical approach, depending on the histologic type, the extent of bone involvement, and the size of the lesion. Adjunctive radiation therapy may be indicated for adenoid cystic carcinoma and high-grade mucoepidermoid carcinoma.

## Soft Palate/Tonsillar Pillars

### COMMON CONDITIONS

#### Papilloma

The squamous papilloma is the most common benign epithelial neoplasm that affects the oral mucosa, typically occurring as a solitary exophytic growth with numerous finger-like or frondlike projections on its surface. The soft palate/tonsillar pillar region is the most common site for the papilloma, and its color may range from pink to white.

Excisional biopsy, including the base of the lesion, should be performed. For those lesions of the posterior soft palate, periodic observation may be appropriate, particularly if the patient is experiencing no symptoms and the lesion is clinically characteristic.

## UNCOMMON CONDITIONS

### Pemphigus Vulgaris

Pemphigus vulgaris is an immunologically mediated condition characterized by the formation of vesicles and bullae secondary to attack of desmosomal complexes of the surface epithelium by autoantibodies. The condition usually is first seen intraorally, with painful, erosive lesions distributed diffusely on the oral mucosa. The soft palate is a primary site of involvement. Diagnosis should be established by light microscopy with direct and indirect immunofluorescence studies. Systemic immunosuppressive therapy is necessary to control this condition addressed in other areas of the text.

## Tongue

### COMMON CONDITIONS

#### Coated and Hairy Tongue

Coated and hairy tongue represents the accumulation of excess keratin on the filiform papillae of the dorsal tongue, resulting in the formation of elongated filamentous strands that superficially resemble hairs. Contrary to the description in numerous textbooks, this condition is not caused by an overgrowth of yeast.

No treatment is required, but if the patient is concerned about the appearance of the tongue, gentle daily débridement with a tongue scraper or the edge of a spoon assists in removing the accumulations of dead keratinized cells.

#### Fissured Tongue

Fissured tongue is essentially a variation of normal that usually develops sometime after the first decade of life. The patient may be concerned about the appearance of the tongue, but no symptoms are associated with the condition. The extent and pattern of fissuring can vary, and no treatment is indicated.

#### Benign Migratory Glossitis (Erythema Migrans, Geographic Tongue)

Benign migratory glossitis, a condition of unknown etiology, is seen in approximately 2% of the population. Most patients are asymptomatic, with lesions detected on routine examination. The dorsal tongue exhibits one or more well-demarcated zones of papillary atrophy that are surrounded, at least partially, by yellow-white slightly raised linear serpentine borders. The lesions typically resolve in one area and move to another, appearing in various stages of resolution and activity concurrently.

Because this is a benign condition, treatment is usually unnecessary. Approximately 5% of patients complain of sensitivity to hot or spicy foods when their lesions are active, but usually they do not require treatment. With severe symptoms, topical fluocinonide (Lidex Gel)[1] or one of the other stronger topical corticosteroids, applied as a thin film to the lesions several times daily, seems to reduce the discomfort.

#### Traumatic Ulcer

The traumatic ulcer occurs most frequently on the lateral tongue, buccal mucosa, and overlying bony prominences such as tori and exostoses. Most of these lesions are associated with relatively little pain. The traumatic ulcer manifests clinically as a defect covered by creamy white fibrin. Although most of these lesions heal within a week or so, some tend to persist, developing a rolled margin and peripheral induration.

Often no treatment is required because of the minimal degree of discomfort and the rapid healing time. If the patient complains of tenderness when eating salty or acidic foods, a protective medication (Zilactin) can be applied as needed. Topical corticosteroids should probably not be used because they may delay healing in this situation.

---

[1]Not FDA approved for this indication

If an ulcer is present for longer than 2 weeks, with or without previous treatment, a biopsy is mandatory to rule out malignancy. A possible exception to this rule might be those ulcers overlying tori because they are notoriously difficult to resolve.

### Burning Tongue Syndrome (Idiopathic Glossopyrosis)

The burning tongue syndrome seems to affect postmenopausal women predominantly. The patient often reports the rather sudden onset of a sensation that feels like the tongue was scalded. Symptoms are usually localized to the anterior tongue, although the labial mucosa and anterior hard palate may also be affected. Clinically, the mucosa appears normal. If mucosal erythema is identified, a variety of conditions should be ruled out, including candidiasis, anemia, local trauma, and erythema migrans. A culture for *Candida albicans* should be performed. If the workup shows no evidence of these conditions, a diagnosis of burning tongue syndrome can be made. Because there is no medically proven therapy, no specific treatment exists. The numerous suggested treatments in the literature have generally not been examined in controlled trials, and their efficacy is typically no more than that of the placebo effect. Reassuring patients this is a harmless condition, nothing more than a nuisance, and that the condition often resolves spontaneously after a period of months or years is usually sufficient.

## UNCOMMON CONDITIONS

### Squamous Cell Carcinoma

The lateral/ventral tongue is one of the most common sites for squamous cell carcinoma. In the early stages, the lesion is relatively asymptomatic, which underscores the importance of a regular and thorough oral mucosal examination. Slight thickening or nodularity within a white or red plaque frequently heralds the onset of invasion. As the lesion grows, the surface becomes ulcerated and symptoms of pain and tenderness develop. On palpation, squamous cell carcinomas are usually firm and show infiltrative borders. Biopsy is mandatory because other chronic ulcerative processes, such as chronic traumatic ulcer, deep fungal infections, mycobacterial infections, Wegener's granulomatosis, and other malignancies, may have a similar clinical presentation.

Treatment consists of wide surgical resection or radical radiation therapy, or both, depending on a number of factors. Prognosis is directly related to the tumor stage, although, in general, these patients do poorly because their lesions are not diagnosed until the later stages.

### Hairy Leukoplakia

Hairy leukoplakia is an HIV-related lesion, significant because it often heralds a rapid decline in the patient's immune status. The lesion affects the lateral borders of the tongue, usually bilaterally, appearing as white plaques with vertical streaks. Sometimes the degree of keratinization may be great enough to produce hairlike projections, hence the name. Because this is otherwise a benign condition, no treatment is necessary. Hairy leukoplakia is caused by Epstein-Barr virus, thus medications used against other herpes viruses, such as acyclovir (Zovirax),[1] valacyclovir (Valtrex),[1] and dihydroxypropoxymethyl guanine (DHPG) (ganciclovir [Cytovene]),[1] may produce transient resolution.

### Herpes in the Immunocompromised Host

With an immunocompromised host, the normal rules governing the location of the lesions of recurrent herpes are not applicable. The virus is not contained by the host, as in the normal individual, and the result is the formation of large, shallow, painful ulcerations with slightly elevated serpentine or scalloped margins. The diagnosis should be established by exfoliative cytology or viral culture, and treatment should be instituted immediately with systemic acyclovir, orally or intravenously, depending on the severity of the clinical infection.

[1]Not FDA approved for this indication.

## Macroglossia

Macroglossia is the term used to describe enlargement of the tongue. Among the more frequent causes of macroglossia are hemangiomas and lymphangiomas. Hemangiomas are usually present at birth or develop shortly thereafter, with the tongue the most common site. These lesions are typically red or purple in color. If no compromise in function of the involved tissue is seen, treatment should be delayed until the child is older than 6 years of age because many of these lesions regress spontaneously. For those lesions that do not regress, argon laser excision is the optimal therapy. Other methods of management include cryotherapy and sclerosing agents.

Lymphangiomas affecting the oral tissues often exhibit a characteristic so-called frog-egg or tapioca-pudding surface morphology because of the dilated lymphatic vessels that are close to the surface. Treatment is surgical excision, although the decision to treat may depend on the size and site of the lesion. Recurrence rates as high as 40% are reported in some series of cases.

Other causes of macroglossia are much less common and include amyloidosis as well as benign and malignant tumors. Biopsy would be indicated to establish a diagnosis prior to treatment planning.

# Floor of the Mouth

## COMMON CONDITIONS

### Leukoplakia

Leukoplakia is a clinical term that should be applied only to those white patches of the oral mucosa that cannot be wiped off and cannot be diagnosed as any other condition clinically. Leukoplakia is considered a premalignant condition and usually diagnosed in the sixth and seventh decades of life. Clinically, the condition appears as a well-defined white plaque that may show varying degrees of redness. The most worrisome sites of involvement include areas prone to cancer development, such as the lateral tongue, floor of the mouth, and the tonsillar pillar region.

Ideally, treatment is complete removal with microscopic evaluation of the excised specimen. Cryotherapy and laser excision may be used, but tissue may be rendered unsuitable for histopathologic examination. More concern should be given to leukoplakias found in nonsmokers, in high-risk areas for oral cancer, in lesions with a red component, in multifocal lesions, or those found in patients 20 to 50 years of age. If complete excision is accomplished, 30% of leukoplakias still recur, so careful follow-up with rebiopsy is indicated.

### Sialolithiasis

Sialolithiasis (salivary duct stones) may appear with symptoms or be discovered on routine examination. The classic presentation is sudden painful unilateral swelling of the involved salivary gland occurring at mealtime. Most stones involve the submandibular gland, and these can be palpated as a hard submucosal mass in the floor of the mouth. Treatment usually involves surgical removal of the stone with repositioning of the salivary duct opening proximally. Sialography should then be performed to assess the function of the gland, and if it appears abnormal, it should probably be removed to prevent subsequent episodes of chronic recurrent sialadenitis.

## UNCOMMON CONDITIONS

### Erythroplakia

The premalignant lesion of erythroplakia represents the nonkeratinized version of leukoplakia. Erythroplakia appears as a well-demarcated, velvety red plaque that is typically asymptomatic. Dysplastic changes are likely, and treatment should consist of complete removal by the most expedient means.

## Squamous Cell Carcinoma

The clinical appearance of squamous cell carcinoma at this site is similar to that of the lateral tongue, as is the treatment.

# Alveolar Process/Gingiva

## COMMON CONDITIONS

### Mandibular Tori/Exostoses

Mandibular tori/exostoses are benign developmental lesions that consist of dense, viable bone. Mandibular tori are located on the lingual surface of the mandible in the premolar region, whereas exostoses occur on the alveolar process in other sites. Radiographic evaluation of any asymmetric bony swelling is indicated, and the exostosis should appear as a well-defined radiopacity. Generally, no treatment is necessary unless the bony outgrowths interfere with denture construction, in which case surgical removal is indicated.

### Amalgam Tattoo

The amalgam tattoo is produced by the iatrogenic implantation of dental amalgam into the oral soft tissues. Amalgam tattoos are usually macular and range in color from gray to blue to black or brown. Periapical radiographs often show the fine radiopaque metallic particles.

No treatment is necessary if the diagnosis can be made definitively from the radiograph. If no radiopacity is seen, biopsy is generally indicated to rule out a relatively rare oral melanocytic process such as a nevus or melanoma.

### Dental Sinus Tract (Parulis)

The lesion of the dental sinus tract (parulis) represents a proliferation of granulation tissue at the drainage site of a sinus tract originating form the apical root portion of a nonvital tooth. Clinically, the parulis appears as an erythematous papule on the alveolar mucosa. Symptoms of pain may wax and wane. Treatment consists of either extraction or endodontic therapy for the offending tooth, and the prognosis is good.

### Acute Necrotizing Ulcerative Gingivitis (Trench Mouth, Vincent's Infection)

Acute necrotizing ulcerative gingivitis is a disease produced by bacteria that are normal inhabitants of the oral microflora. The condition, which occurs in the third or fourth decade of life, is associated with poor oral hygiene, poor diet, and stress. College students are especially vulnerable during final examinations, and the condition may be seen in HIV-positive patients as well. Patients invariably present with a complaint of painful, foul-smelling gingivae. Examination shows punched-out ulceration of the interdental papilla. Acute necrotizing ulcerative gingivitis is frequently confused with primary herpes, which also is associated with pain and ulceration, but the punched-out interdental papillae are not seen in herpes infection.

Débridement, often requiring topical or local anesthesia, or both, is very important. This should be combined with systemic antibiotic therapy, such as tetracycline,[1] 250 mg every 6 hours, or potassium penicillin V, 500 mg every 6 hours. HIV-infected patients should also use chlorhexidine (Peridex) mouth rinse twice daily to prevent recurrence of acute necrotizing ulcerative gingivitis. For non-HIV patients, the prognosis is reasonably good, assuming they improve their diet and oral hygiene status.

### Primary Herpetic Gingivostomatitis

Primary herpetic gingivostomatitis is caused by the initial exposure of the patient to herpes simplex virus, usually type I. Most of these infections occur during childhood, but occasionally an individual escapes contact with the virus until adulthood. Patients present with fever, cervical lymphadenopathy, malaise, and oropharyngeal pain. Examination of the oral mucosa reveals multiple shallow ulcerations distributed diffusely throughout the mouth, although the gingivae are often markedly affected. The gingival involvement is different from that of acute necrotizing ulcerative gingivitis, in that the interdental papillae do not show the punched-out ulcerations with the herpetic infection.

Patients should be managed symptomatically with analgesics, antipyretics, and topical anesthetics as indicated. Dehydration is sometimes a problem if oral pain prevents intake of fluids. Having the patient rinse with 5 mL of viscous lidocaine (Xylocaine Viscous) or dyclonine HCl (Dyclone) prior to meals provides temporary relief. Systemic acyclovir (Zovirax)[1] or valacyclovir (Valtrex)[1] may have a significant impact on the course of this disease if given during the first few days of the infection.

### Inflammatory Fibrous Hyperplasia (Denture Epulis, Epulis Fissuratum, Denture Fibroma)

Inflammatory fibrous hyperplasia is caused by low-grade irritation from an ill-fitting denture. Clinically, the lesions are seen as smooth-surfaced sessile masses that appear to arise from the mucosa of the alveolar process or vestibule. Sometimes a groove or fissure runs lengthwise across the lesion, corresponding to the denture flange. Ulceration of the surface may be seen.

Surgical excision of the lesion is indicated prior to construction of new dentures. If the lesion is removed and the patient continues to wear the old denture, inflammatory fibrous hyperplasia recurs, but it is a completely benign process that does not undergo malignant transformation.

## UNCOMMON CONDITIONS

### Pyogenic Granuloma, Peripheral Giant Cell Granuloma, and Peripheral Ossifying Fibroma

Pyogenic granuloma, peripheral giant cell granuloma, and peripheral ossifying fibroma are benign gingival lesions probably initiated by chronic irritation in most instances. Although they are histologically distinctive, their clinical appearance and biologic behavior are similar. All of these lesions appear as sessile, dome-shaped masses that develop mainly on the gingiva (although pyogenic granuloma may be seen on any surface). They range from pink to reddish purple in color and are often ulcerated. Excisional biopsy is recommended to rule out the less likely possibility of metastatic neoplasm, which may clinically appear very similar. A recurrence rate of 15% can be expected for each of these lesions.

### Generalized Gingival Hyperplasia

Generalized gingival hyperplasia usually develops as a side effect of medication: phenytoin (Dilantin), calcium channel blocking agents, or cyclosporine (Sandimmune). Only 30% to 50% of patients receiving one of these drugs show the diffuse gingival enlargement, which is usually related to the level of oral hygiene of the patient. If the drug cannot be discontinued or substituted, periodic periodontal surgery with reinforcement of oral hygiene instruction can usually control the problem. Rarely such enlargement may be associated with any of several genetic syndromes. These patients typically require periodic surgical reduction of the gingival tissues by a periodontist. Generalized gingival hyperplasia may also be a manifestation of myelomonocytic leukemia, although these patients usually complain of other signs and symptoms related to their leukemic state. Biopsy and appropriate hematologic evaluation are necessary to establish a diagnosis.

### Desquamative Gingivitis

*Desquamative gingivitis* is a descriptive term for a reaction pattern that affects the gingival tissues of adults. Patients complain of red, tender gingival mucosa that has a tendency to slough with minor manipulation. Vesicles may sometimes be reported. This condition must be biopsied

---

[1]Not FDA approved for this indication.

for light microscopic evaluation as well as direct immunofluorescence studies because it invariably represents one of several distinct entities: erosive lichen planus, cicatricial pemphigoid, linear IgA disease, pemphigus vulgaris, or chronic ulcerative stomatitis. Once the definitive diagnosis is established, the patient can be managed appropriately.

## REFERENCES

Neville BW, Damm DD, Allen CM, Bouquot JE: Oral and Maxillofacial Pathology, 2nd ed. Philadelphia, Elsevier Science, 2002.

Neville BW, Day TA: Oral cancer and precancerous lesions. CA Cancer J Clin 2002;52:195-215.

Regezi JA, Sciubba JJ, Jordan RCK: Oral Pathology. Clinical Pathologic Correlations, 4th ed. Philadelphia, Elsevier Science, 2003.

Sapp JP, Eversole LR, Wysocki GP: Contemporary Oral and Maxillofacial Pathology, 2nd ed. Philadelphia, Elsevier Science, 2004.

Scully C, Gorsky M, Lozada-Nur F: The diagnosis and management of recurrent aphthous stomatitis: A consensus approach. J Am Dent Assoc 2003;134:200-207.

# Venous Stasis Ulcers

Method of
*Tania J. Phillips, MD,*
*and Chukwuemeka N. Etufugh, MD*

## Epidemiology

Chronic venous ulceration is an increasingly important disease because of its impact on health care costs and effect on the quality of life. The estimated annual cost of ulcer treatment in the United States is reported to be $1 billion per year, with the average cost of one patient over a lifetime exceeding $40,000. An estimated 5% to 8% of the world population suffers from venous disease, and 1% of the world's population develops venous ulcers. In the United States alone, 5 million individuals have venous disease and approximately 500,000 individuals have chronic venous ulcers. Of the three main varieties of ulcer disease, arterial, venous, and neuropathic, venous ulcers account for 80% to 90% of all ulcers.

## Pathogenesis

The venous system of the lower extremity is made up of the deep, superficial, and communicating veins. During ambulation, the calf muscles contract and act as a pump that promotes the return of venous blood to the heart with one-way venous valves preventing retrograde flow. When the calf muscles contract, deep venous pressure decreases, thus moving blood from superficial veins through communicating veins into the deep venous system. The deep veins of the leg are emptied and the total volume of blood in the lower extremities is diminished. Individuals with venous disease because of incompetent valves, immobility, abnormality of calf muscle pump, or a combination of all three factors have a less than normal decrease in venous pressure during calf pump action. These individuals have elevated ambulatory venous pressure (so-called venous hypertension).

How this leads to ulcer formation is unclear. Hypotheses include the theory of pericapillary fibrin cuffs with leukocyte and growth factor trapping and cytokine release, which leads to capillary dysfunction and eventual ischemia, ulceration, and impaired healing of surrounding tissue.

## Clinical Features

Patients with chronic venous ulcers report having a feeling of heaviness of the affected limb and leg swelling and aching, which improves with elevation and is worse at the end of the day. These patients may also have a history of deep venous thrombosis (DVT) and are prone to allergic contact dermatitis to several topical medications.

Venous ulcers are generally found in the gaiter area, the area from the midcalf to the ankle. They are shallow with irregular borders and can vary in size and shape. Other clinical findings include periulcer hyperpigmentation caused by hemosiderin deposits, lipodermatosclerosis, which is a chronic fibrosing process of the dermis, and subcutaneous tissue because of venous insufficiency that makes the skin feel firm and indurated. Varicose veins, lower extremity edema, and eczema caused by either venous or stasis dermatitis also occur. With advanced venous disease, the patient may develop a so-called champagne bottle leg, where because of chronic venous obstruction, the proximal leg swells and the distal leg constricts as a result of loss of subcutaneous fat and fibrosis.

## Diagnosis and Treatment

A complete history and physical examination should be performed in all patients. Although most venous ulcer cases are diagnosed clinically, noninvasive techniques can aid in the diagnosis and evaluate the anatomy of the venous vasculature. Color duplex ultrasound scanning is the gold standard for evaluation of the anatomy of the venous system because of its accuracy and reproducibility. It can provide an analysis of venous anatomy and physiology and provide additional

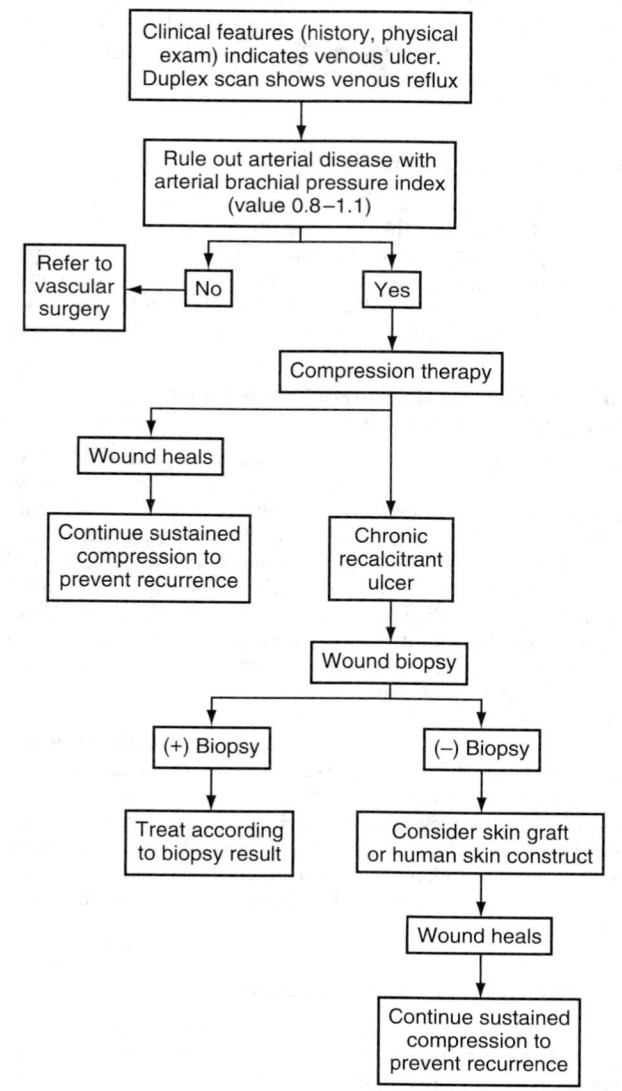

**FIGURE 1.** Scheme for treatment of venous ulcer.

**TABLE 1** Types of Compression Therapy

| Bandage | Advantage | Disadvantage |
|---|---|---|
| Elastic wraps | Inexpensive; can be reused. | Often applied incorrectly by patient. Tend to unravel. Do not maintain sustained compression. Lose elasticity after washing. |
| Self-adherent wraps | Self-adherent; maintain compression. | Expensive. Cannot be reused. |
| Unna boot | Comfortable. Protects against trauma. Full maintenance of ambulatory outpatient status. Minimal interference with regular activities. Substitute for failing pump. | Pressure changes over time. Needs to be applied by well-trained physicians and nurses. Does not accommodate highly exudative wounds. |
| Four-layered bandage | Comfortable. Can be left in place for 7 d. Protects against trauma. Maintains a constant pressure for 7 d because of the overlap and elasticity of bandages. Used for highly exudative wounds. | Needs to be applied by well-trained physicians and nurses. Expensive. |
| Graduated compression stockings | Reduces the ambulatory venous pressure. Increases the venous refilling time. Improves calf pump function. Different types of stockings accommodate different types of legs. Dressing underneath can be changed frequently. | Often cannot monitor patient compliance. Difficult to put on. |
| Orthotic device | Adjustable compression. Sustained pressure. Easily put on and removed. Comfortable. | Expensive. Bulky appearance. |
| Compression pump | Augments venous return. Improves hemodynamics and microvascular functions. Enhances fibrinolytic activity Prevents postoperative thromboembolic complications in high-risk patients. | Expensive. Requires immobility for a few hours per day. |

From Choucair M, Phillips T: Compression therapy. Dermatol Surg 1998;24:141-148.

information about other anatomic structures in the leg, which might produce signs and symptoms that mimic venous disease such as arterial aneurysms and masses. Continuous-wave Doppler, photoplethysmography, and air plethysmography also can be used. In patients with a history of DVT, screening for coagulation defects may reveal activated protein C resistance caused by a point mutation in the gene for factor V Leiden. Other mutations in the prothrombin gene, proteins C and S, and antithrombin III can also cause venous thrombosis.

## CURRENT DIAGNOSIS

All patients should be initially evaluated by a history and physical examination.

- Key features of the history should include symptoms, medications, exacerbating factors, family, travel, and social history.
- The physical examination should include shape, size, location, skin changes characteristic of ulcer base and edge, and associated physical findings such as cardiac failure.
- Clinical findings may include location in gaiter area, lipodermatosclerosis, dependent edema, varicose veins, hemosiderin pigmentation, and eczema.
- Color duplex ultrasound scanning can aid in the diagnosis by providing an analysis of venous anatomy and physiology.
- Arterial disease can coexist with venous ulcers and should be excluded by assessment of pulses and measurement of the ankle-brachial pressure index.
- Recalcitrant ulcers should be biopsied to exclude malignancy or other underlying disease.

Arterial disease, which can coexist with venous ulcers, should be excluded by the use of the ankle-brachial index (ABI) because palpation of the pedal pulses alone is not always reliable. The ABI is the ratio of systolic pressure between the ankle and the arm. An ABI in the range of 0.8 to 1.1 is considered normal, whereas a value less than 0.8 is abnormal, and the patient should be evaluated by a vascular surgeon. An ABI value of more than 1.1 suggests less compressible vasculature that is typically seen in diabetics or the elderly over 70 years of age because of vessel calcification. In these patients, the toe-brachial pressure index can be calculated by measuring the arterial pressure in the toe.

In the management of venous ulcers, compression is the mainstay of therapy. The goal of compression therapy is to counteract venous hypertension by facilitating venous return toward the heart. Several different compression devices are available, including compression pumps, elastic and nonelastic bandages, orthotic devices, and compression stockings (Table 1). Sustained graduated pressure of 30 to

## CURRENT THERAPY

- Treatment should involve optimum wound care, leg elevation, and compression therapy.
- Sustained graduated pressure of 30 to 40 mg Hg at the ankle is optimal for compression therapy.
- A variety of dressings are available that can promote wound granulation and débridement.
- Wound débridement at regular intervals can accelerate venous ulcer healing.
- Skin grafting or human skin constructs can be used to treat large slow to heal ulcers.
- Venous ulcers frequently recur.
- Compression therapy should be maintained when an ulcer is healed to prevent recurrence.

**TABLE 2**  Dressing Recommendations Based on Ulcer Type

| Type of Ulcer | Dressing Recommended |
|---|---|
| Heavy exudate | Foam, alginate, hydrofiber |
| Moderate exudate | Hydrocolloid, foam |
| Mild exudate | Hydrocolloid, hydrogel |
| Malodorous | Foam, alginate, hydrocolloid, charcoal |
| Recalcitrant | Collagen |

From Bello Y, Phillips T: Therapeutic dressings. Adv Dermatol 2000;16:253-270.

40 mm Hg at the ankle is optimal. However, it is unclear which of these compression systems is the most effective.

A variety of dressings are also used along with compression therapy in the management of venous ulcers. These dressings help promote wound granulation, promote débridement, and absorb exudate (Table 2). Some dressings that contain cadexomer iodine or silver can have antimicrobial activity without adversely affecting wound healing. Sharp débridement on a regular basis can accelerate venous ulcer healing. Drugs such as pentoxifylline, at doses of 800 mg three times a day, can accelerate healing of chronic venous ulcers.

Venous ulcers tend to heal slowly, but the majority of ulcers respond well to management with compression therapy. Large ulcer size, ABI less than 0.8, ulcer of long duration, history of venous ligation, and the presence of fibrin on more than 50% of wound surface are poor prognostic factors for healing of venous ulcers.

Large slow to heal ulcers may be treated with autologous split-thickness or pinch grafting. Another approach includes use of an allogeneic human skin construct made of keratinocytes and fibroblasts cultured in bovine type 1 collagen. Up to 40% of patients with venous ulcera have superficial venous insufficiency. In this group, ulcer recurrence can be prevented by stripping or sclerotherapy of affected veins. If the ulcer does not heal, it should be biopsied to exclude malignancy or other causes of ulceration. Once the ulcer heals, sustained compression is recommended to prevent recurrence.

## REFERENCES

Araujo T, Federman D, Kirsner R, Valencia I: Managing the patient with venous ulcers. Ann Intern Med 2003;138:326-334.

Bello Y, Phillips T: Chronic leg ulcers: Types and treatment. Hosp Pract 2000;35:101-108.

Bos J, Loots A, Mekkes J, Van der wal A: Causes, investigation and treatment of leg ulceration. Br J Dermatol 2003;148:388-401.

Callam M, Ruckley C, Harper D, Dale J: Chronic ulceration of the leg: Extent of the problem and provision of care. BMJ 1985;290: 1855-1856.

Cullum N, Fletcher A, Nelson E, Sheldon T: Compression for venous leg ulcers. Cochrane Database Syst 2004, volume (1).

Dix F, Simon D, McCollum C: Management of venous leg ulcers. BMJ 2004;328:1358-1362.

Eaglstein W, Falabella A, Kirsner R, Trent J: Venous ulcers: Pathophysiology and treatment options. Ostomy Wound Manage 2005;51:38-54.

Eaglstein W, Falabella A, Kirsner R, Valencia I: Chronic venous insufficiency and venous leg ulceration. J Am Acad Dermatol 2001;44:401-421.

Goldman M, Fronek A: The Alexander House Group: Consensus paper on venous leg ulcer. J Dermatol Surg Oncol 1992;18:592-602.

Ruckley C: Socioeconomic impact of chronic venous insufficiency and leg ulcers. Angiology 1997;46:67-69.

Vanhoutte P, Corcaud S, De Montrion C: The demographics of venous disease of the lower limbs. Angiology 1997;48:557-558.

# Pressure Ulcers

Method of
*David R. Thomas, MD*

A pressure ulcer is the visible evidence of pathologic changes in blood supply to the dermal and underlying tissues, usually because of compression of the tissue over a bony prominence.

A differential diagnosis of ulcer type is critical to treatment. Chronic ulcers of the skin include arterial ulcers, venous stasis ulcers, diabetic ulcers, and pressure ulcers. Pressure ulcers generally appear in soft tissue over a bony prominence. A classic presentation aids the diagnosis. For example, arterial ulcers occur in the distal digits or over a bony prominence, diabetic ulcers occur in regions of callus formation, and venous stasis ulcers occur on the lateral aspect of the lower leg. However, atypical presentations may occasionally obscure the etiology. The treatment of these various etiologies differs considerably. This discussion is limited to the treatment of pressure ulcers and should not be used to treat other types of ulcers.

Seven principles of management guide treatment of pressure ulcers. The chief cause of these ulcers is pressure applied to the tissues that compromises blood flow. Therefore, the first treatment principle is to relieve pressure. Pressure relief can be obtained by positioning the patient frequently at a fixed interval to relieve pressure over the compromised area. Turning and positioning may be difficult to achieve because of a patient's self-positioning or medical treatments that interfere with the ability to position the patient. Because of this difficulty, a number of medical devices are designed in an attempt to relieve pressure. These devices can be classified as static or dynamic. Static devices include air-, gel-, or water-filled containers that reduce the tissue–surface interface. Dynamic devices use a power source to fill compartments with air that support the patient's weight or alternate the pressure on different areas of the body. Choose a static device when the patient has good bed mobility. Choose a dynamic device when the patient cannot self-position in bed.

At the present time, results of reported clinical trials do not favor one device over another. The choice should be based on durability, ease of use, and patient comfort. A simple check for so-called bottoming out should be done for all devices. Your hand should be inserted palm upward under the patient's sacrum between the device and the bed surface. If there is not an air column between the patient and the bed surface, the device is ineffective and should be changed. No device is effective in reducing heel pressure, the second most common site for pressure ulcers. Bridging with pillows is effective in reducing heel pressure in immobile patients; patients with high bed mobility may require boot devices to elevate the heel off the bed surface. Patients who fail to improve or who have multiple pressure ulcers should be considered for a dynamic-type device, such as a low-air-loss bed or air-fluidized bed.

The second principle of pressure ulcer therapy is to assess pain. Pressure ulcers do not always result in pain, particularly in insensate patients. However, some pressure ulcers do result in pain and should be treated aggressively. Oral or parenteral pain medications should be used to control symptoms.

The third principle of ulcer therapy is to assess nutrition and hydration. Pressure ulcers occur in sicker individuals in whom nutrient intake may be reduced by coexisting illness. Increased intake of protein (1.2 to 1.5 g/kg/day) is associated with higher healing rates. Achievement of high protein intake may be difficult because of anorexia of aging or anorexia associated with coexisting diseases. Adequate calories, adjusted for stress (30 to 35 kcal/kg/day), should be prescribed.

## CURRENT DIAGNOSIS

- Differentiate among pressure, diabetic, venous stasis, and arterial ulcers.

Adequate dietary intake should provide adequate vitamins and minerals. No difference in healing rates is associated with supertherapeutic doses of vitamin C or zinc. If adequate dietary intake is compromised, a supplemental vitamin/mineral prescription at RDA (recommended daily allowance) doses should be considered. Adequate hydration can be maintained by 30 mL/kg/day of water. The decision to institute enteral feeding in patients with pressure ulcers who are unable to maintain adequate oral intake should not be undertaken lightly. The decision to use enteral feeding must consider the patient's wishes, overall goal of care, and the complications of enteral feeding. In several studies, the long-term result of enteral feeding was associated with poorer outcomes in patients with pressure ulcers.

The fourth principle of pressure ulcer management requires removing necrotic debris. Phagocytosis removes necrotic debris naturally. Accelerating the rate of removal may shorten healing time. Options include sharp surgical débridement, mechanical débridement with gauze dressings, application of exogenous enzymes, or autolytic débridement under occlusive dressings. Choose surgical débridement if the ulcer is infected. Surgical débridement is the fastest method but may remove some viable tissue, cause discomfort, and is the most expensive method, especially if done in an operating room. Applying moist gauze that is allowed to adhere to the ulcer bed by drying is a form of débridement. When the dry dressing is removed, nonselective tissue removal occurs. This method can be associated with discomfort, may delay healing while débridement is in progress, and is often defeated when the dressing is remoistened before removal. Enzymatic débridement can digest necrotic material. Three enzymatic preparations are available in the United States: collagenase, papain/urea, and papain/urea combined with chlorophyll. Enzyme preparations are nonselective, possibly resulting in some damage to fibroblasts, epithelial cells, or granulation tissue. Enzymatic débridement is slower, can be associated with discomfort, and should be limited in duration until a clean wound bed is obtained. Autolytic débridement is achieved by allowing autolysis under an occlusive dressing. Both enzymatic and autolytic débridement may require 2 to 6 weeks to achieve a clean wound bed. A total of five clinical trials did not show that enzymatic agents increased the rate of complete healing in chronic wounds compared to control treatment. Unless clinically infected, heel ulcers are better left undébrided because they occur in poorly vascularized tissues.

The fifth principle of pressure ulcer management is to maintain a moist wound environment. Maintaining a moist wound environment is associated with more rapid healing rates compared to dressings that are allowed to dry. Continuously moist saline gauze is the historical standard dressing for stage II through IV pressure ulcers. Care must be taken to change the gauze frequently to prevent drying because this may delay healing. Newer wound dressings provide a low moisture vapor transmission rate (MVTR), a measure of how quickly the dressing allows drying. A MVTR of less than 35 g of water vapor per square meter per hour is required to maintain a moist wound environment. Woven gauze has a MVTR of 68 $g/m^2$/hour, and impregnated gauze has a MVTR of 57 $g/m^2$/hour. By comparison, hydrocolloid dressings have a MVTR of 8 $g/m^2$/hour. Dressings with low MVTR provide a healing environment that encourages granulation tissue formation and epithelialization.

The use of occlusive-type dressings is more cost effective than gauze dressings primarily because of a decrease in nursing time for dressing changes. A meta-analysis of five clinical trials comparing a hydrocolloid dressing with a dry dressing demonstrated that treatment with a hydrocolloid dressing resulted in a statistically significant improvement in the rate of pressure ulcer healing (odds ratio: 2.6).

Occlusive dressings can be divided into broad categories of polymer films, polymer foams, hydrogels, hydrocolloids, alginates, and biomembranes. Each has advantages and disadvantages. No single agent is perfect. The choice of a particular agent depends on the clinical circumstances. Nonpermeable polymers can be macerating to normal skin. Polymer films are not absorptive and may leak, particularly when the wound is highly exudative. Most films have an adhesive backing that may remove epithelial cells when the dressing is changed. Hydrogels are hydrophilic polymers that are insoluble in water but absorb aqueous solutions and are available in amorphous gels or sheet dressings. They are poor bacterial barriers and are nonadherent to the wound. Because of their high specific heat, these dressings are cooling to the skin, aiding in pain control and reducing inflammation. Most of these dressings require a secondary dressing to secure them to the wound. Hydrocolloid dressings are complex dressings similar to ostomy barrier products. They are impermeable to moisture and bacteria and highly adherent to the skin. Hydrocolloid dressings have an accelerated healing of 40% compared to moist gauze dressings. Hydrocolloid dressings are particularly suited for areas subject to urinary and fecal incontinence. Their adhesiveness to surrounding skin is higher than some surgical tapes, but they are nonadherent to wound tissue and do not damage epithelial tissue in the wound. The adhesive barrier is frequently overcome in highly exudative wounds. Hydrocolloid dressings cannot be used over tendons or on wounds with eschar formation. Alginates are complex polysaccharide dressings that are highly absorbent in exudative wounds. This high absorbency is particularly suited to exudative wounds. Alginates are nonadherent to the wound, but if the wound is allowed to dry, damage to the epithelial tissue may occur with removal. Alginates may be used under other dressings to absorb exudate. The biomembranes are very expensive and not readily available.

Stages I and II pressure ulcers can be managed with a polymer film or hydrocolloid dressing. Stages III and IV dressings may require a wound filler, such as a calcium alginate or an amorphous hydrogel, to obliterate dead space and decrease anaerobic colonization.

Vacuum-assisted closure is used in both acute and chronic wounds. Only two randomized, controlled trials in pressure ulcers are reported. In both trials, vacuum-assisted closure was equivalent to treatment with a hydrogel or moistened gauze.

Electrotherapy is used for stages III and IV pressure ulcers unresponsive to conventional therapy. Several clinical trials suggest that electrotherapy is likely to be marginally effective. Hyperbaric oxygen, ultrasound, infrared, ultraviolet, and low-energy laser irradiation have insufficient data to recommend their use currently. No data support the use of a systemic vasodilator, hemorheologics, serotonin inhibitors, or fibrolytic agents in the treatment of pressure ulcers. Topical agents such as zinc, phenytoin,[1] aluminum hydroxide,[1] honey, sugar, yeast, aloe vera gel, or gold[1] were not effective in clinical trials.

Because the theory of augmenting ulcer healing under the newer dressings suggests that wound fluid contains favorable healing factors, it is important not to change the dressings too frequently. Unless the wound fluid seeps from under the dressing, it should not be changed more often than every 3 to 7 days.

The sixth principle of pressure ulcer treatment is to encourage granulation tissue formation and promote reepithelialization. Growth factors show promising early results, but the data do not suggest accelerated healing of pressure ulcers. It is important not to affect granulation and epithelial tissue negatively. A number of wound cleaners and antiseptics are toxic to fibroblasts and epithelial tissues, including benzalkonium chloride, povidone-iodine solution (Betadine), Dakin's solution, hydrogen peroxide, Granulex, Hibiclens, and pHisoHex. The use of these agents in a pressure ulcer should be limited to use in infected ulcers and strictly limited in duration.

The seventh principle of pressure ulcer management is to control infection. Quantitative microbiology alone is a poor predictor of clinical

---

[1]Not FDA approved for this indication.

infection in chronic wounds. All pressure ulcers are colonized with bacteria, usually from skin or fecal flora. The presence of microorganisms alone (colonization) does not indicate an infection in pressure ulcers. The diagnosis of infection in chronic wounds must be based on clinical signs: erythema, warmth, pain, edema, odor, fever, or purulent exudate. In the presence of clinical signs of infection, enteral or parenteral antibiotics should be used. In ulcers that are not progressing toward healing, an empirical trial of topical antimicrobials may be considered, although the data are inconclusive.

## REFERENCES

Thomas DR: The role of nutrition in prevention and healing of pressure ulcers. Geriatr Clin North Am 1997;13:497-512.

Thomas DR: Are all pressure ulcers avoidable? J Am Med Dir Assoc 2001;2:297-301.

Thomas DR: Improving the outcome of pressure ulcers with nutritional intervention: A review of the evidence. Nutrition 2001;17:121-125.

Thomas DR: Issues and dilemmas in managing pressure ulcers. J Gerontol Med Sci 2001;56:M238-M340.

Thomas DR: Prevention and management of pressure ulcers. Rev Clin Gerontol 2001;11:115-130.

Thomas DR: The promise of topical nerve growth factors in the healing of pressure ulcers. Ann Intern Med 2003;139:694-695.

Thomas DR: Management of pressure ulcers. J Am Med Dir Assoc 2006;7:46-59.

# Atopic Dermatitis

Method of

*Sarah L. Chamlin, MD*

Atopic dermatitis (AD) is a prevalent chronic inflammatory skin condition occurring in 7% to 17% of school-age children with most children developing the disease before they are 5 years of age. The pathophysiology of atopic dermatitis includes a complex interrelationship of genetic, environmental, skin barrier, psychological, and immunologic factors. The goals of management of AD in children include skin hydration, decreasing skin inflammation and itch, identifying and treating skin infection, and assessing the psychosocial impact of disease on the child and family.

## Diagnosis

AD is characterized by pruritus, a chronic relapsing course, an atopic history (personal or family), and a dermatitis in the typical morphology and distribution for age (facial and extensor surface in infants; flexural surfaces and lichenification in older children and adults). In addition, Table 1 lists other cutaneous features and findings present in affected patients.

### CURRENT DIAGNOSIS

Atopic dermatitis is characterized by:
- Pruritus
- Chronic relapsing course
- Atopic history both personal or family
- Dermatitis in the typical morphology and distribution for age, including facial and extensor surface in infants and flexural surfaces and lichenification in older children and adults

### CURRENT THERAPY

- Treatment of dryness should focus on hydration and lubrication to repair skin and reduce water loss. Both emollients and topical anti-inflammatory medications are recommended. Showers and baths should be no longer than 10 min using fragrance-less soap.
- Topical steroids are the first-line of therapy for treatment of the dermatitis. Ointments are often preferred to creams. Consider body location and severity of dermatitis.
- Topical therapies often relieve pruritus, but additional use of sedating antihistamines may be indicated. If nighttime sleep disruption occurs, sedating antihistamines such as diphenhydramine (Benadryl, 1 mg/kg) or hydroxyzine (Atarax, 1 mg/kg) can be given before bedtime.
- Flaring of disease caused by bacterial superinfection may improve with topical corticosteroids alone, but systemic antibiotics should be considered. A 10–14 d course is most often prescribed.

## Treatment

### DRY SKIN

Treatment of dryness is one of the most critical aspects of management. Patients with atopic dermatitis have an abnormal skin barrier that leads to increased transepidermal water loss and dryness. Treatment of dryness focuses on hydration and lubrication of the skin to repair the skin and reduce water loss. Both emollients and topical anti-inflammatory medications are most often needed for this repair. Baths or showers are recommended daily or every other day and should last no longer than 10 minutes. Recommended soaps lack fragrance and often contain a moisturizer, a humectant, and a mild synthetic surfactant (Table 2). Dryness worsens with excessive bathing or showering, exposure to detergents, and low humidity. Although ointments and creams are preferred to lotions because of increased oil content, widespread use of thick creams and ointments may not be tolerated in hot climates.

### INFLAMMATION

Topical steroids are the first line of therapy for treatment of the dermatitis and are effective and safe when used appropriately. Many parents are fearful of using of topical corticosteroids because of

### TABLE 1 Cutaneous Findings and Associated Features in Atopic Dermatitis

Xerosis
Ichthyosis vulgaris
Hyperlinear palms
Keratosis pilaris
Cutaneous infections
Hand and/or foot dermatitis
Nipple eczema
Cheilitis
Recurrent conjunctivitis
Dennie-Morgan infraorbital folds
Periorbital darkening
Midfacial pallor
Pityriasis alba
Itch when sweating
Intolerance to wool/soaps
White dermatographism
Elevated serum IgE

## TABLE 2 Bathing and Emollient Recommendations

Daily lukewarm baths or showers for 5–10 min
Sparing use of gentle shampoo for hair
Mild fragrance-free soap or soap substitute (e.g., Dove, Cetaphil)
Avoidance of harsh soaps and bubble baths
Applying emollient while still damp (e.g., petrolatum, Cetaphil Cream, Eucerin Cream)
Reapplying emollient once or twice daily
If topical corticosteroids or topical immunomodulators (TIMs) used, applying them first followed by emollient

## TABLE 4 Site-Specific Recommended Treatment

| Body Location | Topical Medication |
| --- | --- |
| Face/groin/axillae | Pimecrolimus 1% cream (Elidel)<br>Tacrolimus 0.03% or 0.1% ointment (Protopic)<br>Hydrocortisone 1% or 2.5%<br>Desonide 0.05% (DesOwen)<br>Alclometasone 0.05% (Aclovate) |
| Scalp (oil, solution, foam, or lotion) | Fluocinolone 0.01% (Synalar)<br>Hydrocortisone butyrate 0.1% (Locoid)<br>Fluocinolone 0.01% oil (Derma-Smoothe FS)<br>Betamethasone 0.12% foam (Luxiq) |
| Trunk/extremities | Triamcinolone 0.1% (Kenalog)<br>Fluocinolone 0.025% (Synalar)<br>Pimecrolimus 1% cream (Elidel)<br>Tacrolimus 0.03% or 0.1% ointment (Protopic) |
| Thickened nonfacial areas (monitored closely and used for short periods of time) | Betamethasone 0.05% (Diprosone)<br>Mometasone 0.1% (Elocon)<br>Fluocinonide 0.05% (Lidex) |

potential side effects and need reassurance that low- to mid-potency corticosteroids applied for limited periods of time are safe. Ointments are often preferred to creams because they are more moisturizing and less irritating. Consider body location and severity of dermatitis when choosing a topical corticosteroid. Low-potency corticosteroids can be safely used on the face and intertriginous areas, whereas higher potency topical corticosteroids are needed for effective treatment of dermatitis on the trunk and extremities. Liquid or foam preparations are recommended for scalp dermatitis.

Topical immunomodulators (TIMs) should be considered as second-line therapy for atopic dermatitis. Tacrolimus ointment (Protopic) 0.03% ointment is approved for use in children 2 to 15 years of age and 0.1% for use in children and adults older than 15 years. Pimecrolimus 1% cream (Elidel) is approved for patients 2 years and older. Both act via inhibition of T cell cytokine production and may have the side effects of stinging and burning with application. Short-term safety profiles remain reassuring, but long-term safety remains unknown. Sun protection is recommended while using TIMs.

Topical mid-potency corticosteroids are very effective for initial treatment of an acute flare of atopic dermatitis. When the flare is improving (5 to 7 days), treatment alternatives include low-potency topical corticosteroids or TIMs. TIMs are effective for facial dermatitis, particularly in the periocular region (Tables 3 and 4).

## PRURITUS

Controlling itch is an important step in breaking the disease-propagating itch-scratch cycle. Topical therapies often relieve pruritus, but additional use of sedating antihistamines may be indicated. If nighttime sleep disruption occurs because of pruritus, sedating antihistamines such as diphenhydramine (Benadryl, 1 mg/kg) or hydroxyzine (Atarax, 1 mg/kg) can be given prior to bedtime. The doses can be titrated to minimize daytime sleepiness. Long-standing sleep disruption because of pruritus can lead to learned behaviors and associations including nighttime awakening even when the dermatitis is in remission. To prevent these behaviors from forming, therapy with sedating antihistamines is warranted. Nonsedating antihistamines are effective for symptoms associated with allergic rhinitis and other allergic diseases, but they are less effective for relief from the itch of atopic dermatitis.

## TABLE 3 How to Apply Topical Steroids and Topical Immunomodulators (TIMs)

Apply to area affected by dermatitis (rough, red, and scaly plaques).
Coat area with thin greasy layer (it should look shiny).
Use twice daily until skin feels smooth (ignore changes in pigment).
Switch to emollients alone after treated area smooth.
If used for 2 weeks and the dermatitis not clearing:
• Medication may not be strong enough.
• Medicine is being used too sparingly.
• Skin infection may be present.

## INFECTION

The most common complication of atopic dermatitis is infection with *Staphylococcus aureus*. Bacterial infection of the skin in atopic dermatitis not only causes the clinical signs of erosion, crusting, and weeping but may also trigger a flare of the disease. The presence of infection may not be obvious or generalized and may be as subtle as a few pustules. Although flaring of disease because of bacterial superinfection may improve with topical corticosteroids alone, systemic antibiotics should be considered. Most often a 10- to 14-day course is prescribed, but a longer course may be needed for children with frequent recurrent infections. Although use of antibiotics is often required, they should be prescribed judiciously because of the increase in community-acquired methicillin-resistant *S. aureus* in the United States. Localized infection can be treated with mupirocin 2% ointment (Bactroban). A skin culture may be helpful in identifying the antibiotic sensitivity of the bacterial organism. Recommended systemic antibiotics include cephalexin (Keflex), dicloxacillin (Dynapen), and clindamycin (Cleocin).

If eczema herpeticum, herpes simplex virus superinfection, is suspected, therapy with systemic acyclovir (Zovirax) is warranted. If the patient is febrile, dehydrated, or ill appearing, hospitalization with intravenous acyclovir and fluids is indicated.

## Recalcitrant Atopic Dermatitis

A small proportion of patients with atopic dermatitis are not controlled with topical therapy. Although oral corticosteroid treatment is an effective therapy, its use is limited by its systemic toxicities and the flare of disease that often occurs after discontinuation. The use of phototherapy (UVB [ultraviolet B] and PUVA [psoralen plus ultraviolet light of A wavelength], narrow-band UVB) is often reserved for older children with recalcitrant disease. Excessive phototherapy increases risk for skin malignancies later in life, and children often miss school several times weekly for treatment, limiting its use. Systemic immunosuppressants such as cyclosporine A (Neoral[1]) may be useful in the treatment of recalcitrant atopic dermatitis. These should only be used with careful monitoring and after a thorough discussion of the short- and long-term risks and benefits.

[1]Not FDA approved for this indication.

## Psychosocial Impact

Atopic dermatitis affects the quality of life of afflicted children and their families. Childhood behavior abnormalities, parent stress and anxiety, and sleep disturbance for both the child and their parents are well documented in this population. When severity of the disease decreases, quality of life for the child improves. Physicians caring for children with atopic dermatitis should ask children and their parents about sleep quality and about the life changes that have occurred because of atopic dermatitis.

### REFERENCES

Balkrishnan R, Housman TS, Grummer S, et al: The family impact of atopic dermatitis in children: The role of the parent caregiver. Pediatr Dermatol 2003;20(1):5-10.

Chamlin SL, Frieden IJ, Williams ML, Chren MM: The effects of atopic dermatitis on young American children and their families. Pediatrics 2004;114:607-611.

Chamlin SL, Mattson CL, Frieden IJ, et al: The price of pruritus: Sleep disturbance and cosleeping in atopic dermatitis. Arch Pediatr Adolesc Med 2005;159(8):745-750.

Charman CR, Morris AD, Williams HC: Topical corticosteroid phobia in patients with atopic eczema. Br J Dermatol 2000;142:931-936.

Drake L, Prendergast M, Maher R, et al: The impact of tacrolimus ointment on health-related quality of life of adult and pediatric patients with atopic dermatitis. J Amer Acad Dermatol 2001;44: S65-S72.

Hanifin JM, Rajka G: Diagnostic features of atopic dermatitis. Acta Derm Venereol Suppl (Stockh) 1980;92:44-47.

Laughter D, Istvan JA, Tofte SJ, Hanifin JM: The prevalence of atopic dermatitis in Oregon schoolchildren. J Amer Acad Dermatol 2000;43:649-655.

Stalder JF, Fleury M, Sourusse M, et al: Local steroid therapy and bacterial skin flora in atopic dermatitis. Br J Dermatol 1994;131: 536-540.

Whalley D, Huels J, McKenna SP, Van Assche D: The benefit of pimecrolimus (Elidel, SDZ ASM 981) on parents' quality of life in the treatment of pediatric atopic dermatitis. Pediatrics 2002;110: 1133-1136.

# Erythema Multiforme, Stevens-Johnson Syndrome, and Toxic Epidermal Necrolysis

Method of
*Marcia G. Tonnesen, MD*

Historically, erythema multiforme (EM), Stevens-Johnson syndrome (SJS), and toxic epidermal necrolysis (TEN) were considered a disease spectrum, and therefore they are addressed together here. Current evidence, however, supports a clear distinction between EM, with characteristic acrally distributed target lesions and an etiologic link to herpes simplex virus (HSV) infection, and SJS/TEN, with focal to widespread skin and mucous membrane involvement, characterized by epidermal destruction, and an etiologic link to adverse drug reactions. EM is typically mild and self-limited and requires only symptomatic care. In contrast, because of the degree and extent of epidermal and mucosal involvement that occurs in SJS and TEN, careful monitoring is critical and hospitalization for supportive care often required. Thus early diagnosis is critical. Elimination of any identified or presumed precipitating factors is of prime importance. Therapy should combine symptomatic and supportive measures with observation for and treatment of associated complications, depending on the clinical characteristics and severity of the episode. Optimal therapeutic intervention is hindered because specific pathogenic mechanisms of tissue injury are not yet completely defined. In addition, few controlled studies have evaluated the effectiveness of proposed therapeutic agents. Nevertheless, recent advances elucidating unique morphologic features and novel mechanisms of epidermal necrosis enhance the likelihood of successful therapeutic intervention.

## Erythema Multiforme

EM is an acute, self-limited, but frequently recurrent, inflammatory cutaneous disorder, characterized by the sudden onset of a symmetric erythematous eruption with primarily an acral distribution. Skin lesions begin as fixed (lasting longer than 24 hours) erythematous flat macules, rapidly progress to erythematous raised papules, and then develop a pale or dusky central zone because of edema or bulla formation. This characteristic morphology is now termed *raised atypical target*. Some further evolve to form distinctive raised target lesions with at least three zones of color (dusky/bullous center, pale edematous halo, erythematous border), termed *typical target*. Individual lesions occasionally sting or itch, appear in successive crops for 24 to 72 hours, and spontaneously resolve within 1 to 4 weeks. Mucosal involvement, when present, is usually limited to the lips, buccal mucosa, and tongue.

Most recurrent EM cases are associated with herpes simplex virus (HSV) type I or II infection and typically occur 3 to 14 days after the appearance of a recurrent HSV lesion (oral, genital, or other location). Subclinical episodes of herpes can also induce EM. HSV DNA is detected in EM lesions. Herpes-associated erythema multiforme is currently believed to result from the HSV-specific host immune response.

### THERAPEUTIC APPROACH

#### Elimination of Etiologic Factor

In recurrent herpes-associated EM, a course of acyclovir (Zovirax), 200 mg orally five times daily for 5 days, should be initiated at the first symptom of HSV infection. Acyclovir therapy is not effective if initiated after the development of HSV or EM lesions.

#### Symptomatic Measures

For pruritic or painful skin lesions, systemic antihistamines or analgesics may provide symptomatic relief. Topical acyclovir and topical corticosteroids are not beneficial. Care for skin and mouth erosions is addressed in the following section.

#### Preventive Measures

Because of the common etiologic association between recurrent HSV infections and EM, measures that attempt to prevent recurrences of HSV may lessen the frequency of subsequent episodes. Avoidance of sun exposure by using sunscreens (SPF [sun protection factor] 15 or higher), sun sticks (sunscreen-containing lip balm), and UV (ultraviolet)-protective clothing and by minimizing sun exposure from 10 AM to 3 PM (the peak period for ultraviolet B [UVB]) may reduce ultraviolet light–induced HSV recurrences. Attempts should be made to minimize stress, a well-known precipitating factor of HSV. Topical antiviral preparations do not prevent or abort recurrent HSV infections.

Prophylactic administration of acyclovir abolishes recurrent HSV infections and ensuing episodes of EM. In patients with frequently recurring, debilitating, herpes-associated EM, the treatment of choice is daily oral acyclovir for a period of 6 months or longer. The recommended adult starting dose is 400 mg orally twice daily, with tapering of the dose after the disease is brought under control. Because asymptomatic subclinical HSV episodes can also trigger EM, patients with so-called idiopathic recurrent EM often benefit from prophylactic antiviral therapy. If acyclovir fails to prevent recurrences of HSV, newer antiviral agents with enhanced bioavailability, such as valacyclovir (Valtrex) or famciclovir (Famvir), should be tried. Because of the known occurrence of acyclovir resistance and the unknown long-term side effects of chronic acyclovir therapy, the drug should be stopped periodically and the need for its continuance reassessed.

## Patient Education

Patients should be reassured regarding the usual benign, self-limited course, educated regarding the frequent association of EM with recurrent HSV infections, and advised regarding preventive measures.

# Stevens-Johnson Syndrome and Toxic Epidermal Necrolysis

SJS is a severe mucocutaneous illness characterized by an extensive blistering eruption with a primarily facial and truncal distribution and extensive mucosal erosions, typically involving the mouth and conjunctivae. A prodrome with constitutional symptoms and fever usually heralds the onset of the eruption. Skin lesions begin as erythematous flat macules, frequently develop dusky central vesiculation, and may progress to bullae formation with epidermal necrosis. The current morphologic terms for these characteristic lesions are *macule with or without blister* if only one color and *flat atypical target* if two concentric zones of color are present. Epidermal detachment may involve up to 10% body surface area (BSA). Painful mucosal erosions result in characteristic hemorrhagic-crusted lips, foul-smelling mouth, and decreased oral intake. Ocular involvement with photophobia and painful conjunctival erosions may lead to residual scarring, lacrimal abnormalities, and permanent visual impairment. Disease duration is 4 to 6 weeks. Recurrences are infrequent. SJS is now recognized as strongly related to adverse drug reactions and linked to some infections, particularly *Mycoplasma pneumoniae,* but never to herpes virus infection.

TEN is characterized by widespread sheetlike necrosis and sloughing of the epidermis, involving greater than 30% of the BSA. (Epidermal detachment between 10% and 30% of the BSA is classified as SJS/TEN overlap.) Following a 1- to 3-day prodrome of fever and flulike symptoms, the cutaneous eruption characteristically begins symmetrically on the face and upper body. Initial painful erythema rapidly progresses within hours to days to widespread bulla formation. Sheetlike areas of epidermal necrosis with extensive denudation involve significant or total BSA. Alternatively, TEN may begin as erythematous or violaceous macules that then develop bullae and coalesce. Involvement of multiple mucosal surfaces is present in nearly all patients. The order of frequency is oropharynx (in severe cases extending to larynx and tracheobronchial tree), eyes, genitalia, and anus. TEN is considered a manifestation of "acute skin failure" with abnormal barrier function resulting in fluid, electrolyte, and protein loss, increased susceptibility to infection, impaired thermoregulation, altered immune status, and increased energy expenditure. Morbidity is significant, and the mortality rate is 25% to 40%. The leading cause of death is sepsis.

Adverse drug reactions are the only well-documented cause of TEN. The most common offenders (Box 1) include antibiotics, particularly sulfonamides, anticonvulsants, nonsteroidal anti-inflammatory agents (NSAIDs), and more recently antiretroviral agents, although more than 100 drugs are implicated. The greatest risk for antibiotics occurs during the initial weeks of use; for most anticonvulsants, the risk is highest during the first 2 months. Although the specific pathogenic mechanism is not fully elucidated for SJS/TEN, the characteristic epidermal necrosis is now believed to be a result of keratinocyte apoptosis. Current evidence supports important roles in the induction of keratinocyte death for Fas/Fas ligand–mediated apoptosis, cytokines such as tumor necrosis factor-α (TNF-α), and cytotoxic T lymphocytes, as well as specific genetic defects in detoxification of reactive drug metabolites. Recent novel attempts at therapeutic intervention are based on these proposed mechanisms of epidermal necrosis.

## THERAPEUTIC APPROACH

### Elimination of Etiologic Factors

Immediate withdrawal of any suspected or potential causative drug(s) is critical because cessation of the offending agent no later than the stage of early blister formation may decrease mortality. For SJS,

---

> ## BOX 1 Drugs With Highest Risk of Stevens-Johnson Syndrome/ Toxic Epidermal Necrolysis
>
> **Antibiotics**
> - Sulfonamides
> - Cephalosporins
> - Quinolones
> - Tetracycline
> - Aminopenicillins
> - Imidazole antifungals
>
> **Anticonvulsants/Antianxiety**
> - Carbamazepine
> - Chlormezanone[2]
> - Phenytoin
> - Phenobarbital
> - Valproic acid
> - Lamotrigine
> - Nonsteroidal anti-inflammatory drugs, particularly oxicams
> - Allopurinol
> - Antiretroviral agents
>
> ___
> [2]Not available in the United States.

*Mycoplasma pneumoniae* and other infections, if diagnosed, should be appropriately treated.

### Intervention with Systemic Therapy to Stop Progression

Indication for the use of systemic therapy in SJS/TEN is highly controversial because no randomized, controlled trials document efficacy of any systemic intervention. Because widespread epidermal necrosis is associated with a high mortality rate, however, early administration of systemic therapy in the progressive phase of the disease process is advocated to attempt to limit the extent of tissue damage. Use of systemic glucocorticosteroids has proved particularly controversial. There is no evidence-based documentation of their efficacy, and some retrospective studies indicate that patients treated with systemic steroids have an increased incidence of morbidity, prolonged hospitalization, and mortality. Thus other agents are currently being assessed and advocated. Case studies or uncontrolled trials involving small numbers of patients report benefit from a variety of systemic agents. Immunosuppressive therapy with oral cyclosporine (Sandimmune)[1] or high-dose intravenous cyclophosphamide (Cytoxan)[1] is claimed to help several patients. Plasmapheresis may be of some benefit. Innovative treatment is not without risk, however. For example, a double-blind, placebo-controlled trial of thalidomide, which suppresses production of TNF-α, had to be aborted because of a dramatic increase in thalidomide-related mortality.

Currently the most promising and widely advocated systemic therapy is the early administration of high-dose intravenous immunoglobulin (IVIG)[1] to inhibit epidermal apoptosis mediated by the Fas/Fas ligand death receptor. An initial landmark pilot study by Viand and colleagues of 10 TEN patients treated with IVIG demonstrates rapid cessation of disease progression and 100% survival. Subsequently, numerous case reports, retrospective analyses, and uncontrolled prospective studies support the overall safety as well as the efficacy of IVIG to decrease mortality, with only a few dissenting. Improved survival appears to depend on use of high-dose IVIG (1 g/kg/day given for 3 consecutive days, thus giving a total dose of 3 g/kg) because increased risk of mortality occurs at lower total doses (2 g/kg/day or less). A randomized placebo-controlled trial of IVIG for TEN has not yet been done and will be challenging to accomplish, given the rarity of the disease and the high mortality rate.

In the absence of documented efficacy, use of systemic therapy to limit disease progression in a specific patient remains at the discretion

___
[1]Not FDA approved for this indication.

## CURRENT DIAGNOSIS

**Erythema Multiforme**

- Symmetric erythematous acral eruption with target lesions
- Acute: Onset over 24 to 72 hours
- Unique clinical morphology: key to diagnosis
  Raised atypical target lesions
- Palpable round red with central edema/bulla
- Two concentric zones of color
  Typical target lesions
- Palpable round red with pale halo and dusky center
- Three concentric zones of color
- Mucosal involvement variable, oral only
- Self-limited: Spontaneous resolution within 1 to 4 weeks
- Recurrent EM
  Associated with HSV type I or II
  Occurs 3 to 14 days after HSV lesion

**Stevens-Johnson Syndrome**

- Severe mucocutaneous disease
  Extensive symmetrical blistering eruption
  Mucosal erosions: mouth, conjunctivae, then oropharynx, genitalia
- Characteristic erosions with hemorrhagic crust on lips
- Initial prodrome with fever and flulike symptoms
- Skin lesions: Erythematous/violaceous macules
  Often with central vesicles/bullae
  May progress to epidermal necrosis (<10% BSA)
- Unique clinical morphology: key to diagnosis
  Macules with or without blisters
- Flat nonpalpable (except central blister)

- Red or dusky
- May become confluent face/trunk
  Flat atypical target lesions
- Flat nonpalpable (except central blister)
- Round red/dusky or pale central blister
- Two concentric zones of color
- Duration 4 to 6 weeks; infrequent to no recurrences
- Severe adverse reaction to drug
  Or if infection: *Mycoplasma pneumoniae*, never HSV

**Toxic Epidermal Necrolysis**

- Severe adverse drug reaction
- Initial 1- to 3-day prodrome of fever, flulike symptoms
- Initial painful erythema of the face and upper trunk
- Rapid progression of skin involvement:
  Central, then acral
    Dusky red flat macules to flaccid blisters to large sheets of epidermal necrosis
- Unique clinical morphology: key to diagnosis
  Macules with or without blisters
- Flat nonpalpable (except central blister)
- Red or dusky
- Become confluent
  Flat atypical target lesions
- Flat nonpalpable (except central blister)
- Round red/dusky or pale central blister
- Two concentric zones of color
  Extensive areas of confluent epidermal denudation
- >30% BSA (may involve >90% BSA)
- Involvement of multiple mucosal surfaces usual
- High morbidity; mortality rate: 25% to 40%

*Abbreviations:* BSA = body surface area; EM = erythema multiforme; HSV = herpes simplex virus

---

of the physician. However, it is now clear that if systemic intervention is administered, once disease progression ceases and the wound healing process begins, or if no response is noted within 3 to 6 days, treatment should be abruptly discontinued to minimize risk of associated complications.

### Supportive Care

Because of the extensive epidermal and mucosal necrosis and detachment that can occur in SJS and TEN, careful monitoring is critical and hospitalization is often required. Early referral of severe cases to an intensive care or burn unit decreases mortality. Poor outcome can be predicted by a TEN-specific severity of illness score and correlates with the number of specific independent risk factors for mortality present within the first 24 hours after admission to an intensive care unit (Box 2).

### Skin Care

For crusted erosive discrete skin lesions, mild drying, gentle débridement, and cleansing as well as a soothing antipruritic effect is achieved with open wet to damp compresses of tepid water applied for 20 minutes three or four times per day. Lesions should be observed for signs of secondary infection, cultured when indicated, and treatment initiated with the appropriate systemic antibiotic. Topical corticosteroids are not beneficial. For pruritic or painful skin lesions, systemic antihistamines or analgesics provide symptomatic relief.

If extensive, advanced tissue necrosis occurs or is already evident (10% to 20% total BSA involvement), immediate transfer of the patient to an intensive care or burn unit under the care of an experienced dermatologist and skilled nurses is strongly advocated. Therapeutic protocols consist of the following:

- Measures to guard against iatrogenic infection, including withdrawal from systemic steroids; avoidance of indwelling lines and catheters whenever possible; limitation of antibiotic use to specific culture-proven infections; daily cultures of denuded skin, eyes, mouth, sputum, and urine; and aggressive treatment of sepsis if it occurs.
- Supportive care consisting of use of an air-fluidized bed, intravenous fluid therapy to restore fluid and electrolyte balance, tube

---

**BOX 2  SCORTEN: A Severity-of-Illness Score Predictive of Mortality in Toxic Epidermal Necrolysis**

- Age >40 y
- Presence of malignancy
- Initial epidermal detachment >10% BSA
- BUN >28 mg/dL
- Glucose >252 mg/dL
- HCO₃ slightly <20 mEq/L
- Heart rate >120 beats/min

---

*Abbreviations:* BSA = body surface area; BUN = blood urea nitrogen; HCO₃ = bicarbonate.

**CURRENT THERAPY**

## Erythema Multiforme

- Eliminate/prevent etiologic factor by initiating acyclovir (Zovirax), 200 mg orally five times daily, for 5 days at the first symptom of HSV recurrence but not after HSV or EM lesions appear.
- Reduce UV-induced HSV recurrences.
  Apply sunscreens (SPF 15 or higher).
  Use sunscreen-containing lip balm.
  Wear UV-protective clothing and minimize sun exposure from 10 AM to 3 PM.
- Consider prophylactic acyclovir if frequent severe recurrences.
  Prescribe 400 mg orally twice daily for at least 6 months.
  Taper dose after disease under control.
  Stop periodically to reassess need.

## Stevens-Johnson Syndrome/Toxic Epidermal Necrolysis

- Eliminate/prevent etiologic factor:
  Immediately stop suspected drug(s).
  Avoid exposure to causative drug and chemically related agents.
  Treat *Mycoplasma pneumoniae* if present.
- Stop progression of epidermal necrosis:
  Administer high-dose IVIG[1]
  Give total dose of 3 g/kg delivered as 1 g/kg/day for 3 consecutive days; if renal insufficiency: lower daily dose, and lengthen the duration.
  Initiate as early as possible.
  Discontinue once disease progression ceases, or if no response in 3 to 6 days, to minimize complications.

## Supportive Care

### SKIN CARE

For crusted, erosive discrete skin lesions:

- Apply open wet-to-damp compresses of sterile water for 20 minutes three to four times per day to cleanse and soothe.

- Observe for secondary infection; culture and treat with appropriate systemic antibiotic.
- Use systemic antihistamines or analgesics for discomfort.

For extensive epidermal detachment (10% to 20% BSA):

- Transfer immediately to intensive care or burn unit.
- Guard against iatrogenic infection:
  Stop all systemic steroids.
  Avoid indwelling lines and catheters.
  Limit antibiotic use to specific culture-proven infections.
  Perform daily surveillance cultures of denuded skin, eyes, mouth, sputum, and urine.
  Treat sepsis aggressively if it occurs.
- Provide supportive care:
  Try an air-fluidized bed.
  Give intravenous fluid therapy.
  Provide tube feedings.
  Provide pain relief.
  Give respiratory and physical therapy.
  Provide eye care by an ophthalmologist.
  Avoid all unnecessary medications.
  Apply wound dressings—synthetic, biologic, or silver nitrate, or use allografts/porcine xenografts.

### MOUTH CARE

- Use hygienic mouthwash of sterile normal saline every 2 hours.
- Use a pain-relief mouthwash such as viscous lidocaine or a 1:1 mixture of Kaopectate[1] and elixir of diphenhydramine (Benadryl).
- Provide a liquid/soft diet or tube feedings.

### EYE CARE

- Provide daily continuing care by an ophthalmologist:
  Use sterile irrigation and compresses.
  Perform lysis of adhesions.
  Provide instillation of topical antibiotics.

[1]Not FDA approved for this indication.
*Abbreviations:* BSA = body surface area; EM = erythema multiforme; HSV = herpes simplex virus; IVIG = intravenous immunoglobulin; SPF = sun protection factor; UV = ultraviolet.

feedings to ensure adequate caloric intake, adequate pain relief, respiratory and physical therapy as needed and tolerated, and continuing eye care by an ophthalmologist.

- Avoidance of all unnecessary medications, particularly those that are known etiologic factors of SJS/TEN, such as sulfonamides (including sulfa-containing eye preparations and topical dressings).
- Skin care with emphasis on wound dressings to protect the denuded dermis from desiccation and secondary infection and to facilitate rapid re-epithelialization. Reduced mortality and faster healing result from the use of synthetic dressings, biologic dressings, silver nitrate dressings, allografts, or porcine xenografts.

## Mouth Care

When extensive painful mouth lesions are present, good oral hygiene is critical to minimize infection and discomfort. Sterile normal saline

mouthwash every 2 hours provides cleansing and gentle débridement. Topical anesthetics, such as dyclonine, viscous lidocaine, or a 1:1 mixture of Kaopectate[1] and elixir of diphenhydramine (Benadryl), used as a mouthwash, often provides pain relief. A liquid or soft diet, usually better tolerated, contributes to the maintenance of hydration and nutrition. More aggressive nutritional support is usually required for severe oral involvement.

## Eye Care

Because of the potential for long-term sequelae resulting in loss of vision, careful monitoring of eye involvement is mandatory, and early consultation and daily continuing care by an ophthalmologist is strongly recommended. Suggested therapeutic measures might include sterile irrigation and compresses to cleanse the eye, lysis of adhesions, and instillation of topical antibiotics.

[1]Not FDA approved for this indication.

## Preventive Measures

In drug-associated SJS or TEN, future avoidance of the causative drug or chemically related agents is mandatory.

## Patient Education

For SJS and TEN, patients should be advised the course is self-limited but potentially severe and life-threatening, educated regarding the association with adverse drug reactions, and warned to avoid future use of the implicated medication(s).

## REFERENCES

Bachot N, Revuz J, Roujeau J-C: Intravenous immunoglobulin treatment for Stevens-Johnson syndrome and toxic epidermal necrolysis: A prospective noncomparative study showing no benefit on mortality or progression. Arch Dermatol 2003;139:33-36.

Bastuji-Garin S, Rzany B, Stern RS, et al: Clinical classification of cases of toxic epidermal necrolysis, Stevens-Johnson syndrome, and erythema multiforme. Arch Dermatol 1993;129:92-96.

Green JA, Spruance SL, Wenerstrom G, Piepkorn MW: Post-herpetic erythema multiforme prevented with prophylactic oral acyclovir. Ann Int Med 1985;102:632-633.

Halebian PH, Madden MR, Finklestein JL, et al: Improved burn center survival of patients with toxic epidermal necrolysis managed without corticosteroids. Ann Surg 1986;204:503-512.

Kelemen JJ, Cioffi WG, McManus WF, et al: Burn center care for patients with toxic epidermal necrolysis. J Am Coll Surg 1995; 180:273-278.

Lehrer-Bell KA, Kirsner RS, Tallman PG, Kerdel FA: Treatment of the cutaneous involvement in Stevens-Johnson syndrome and toxic epidermal necrolysis with silver nitrate–impregnated dressings. Arch Dermatol 1998;134:877-879.

Prins C, Kerdel FA, Padilla S, et al: Treatment of toxic epidermal necrolysis with high-dose intravenous immunoglobulins: Multicenter retrospective analysis of 48 consecutive cases. Arch Dermatol 2003;139:26-32.

Roujeau J-C, Kelly JP, Naldi L, et al: Medication use and the risk of Stevens-Johnson syndrome or toxic epidermal necrolysis. N Engl J Med 1995;333:1600-1607.

Tatnall FM, Schofield JK, Leigh IM. A double-blind, placebo-controlled trial of continuous acyclovir therapy in recurrent erythema multiforme. Br J Dermatol 1995;132:267-270.

Trent JT, Kirsner RS, Romanelli P, Kerdel FA: Analysis of intravenous immunoglobulin for the treatment of toxic epidermal necrolysis using SCORTEN. Arch Dermatol 2003;139:39-43.

Viard I, Wehrli P, Bullani R, et al: Inhibition of toxic epidermal necrolysis by blockade of CD95 with human intravenous immunoglobulin. Science 1998;282:490-493.

Wolkenstein P, Latarjet J, Roujeau J-C, et al: Randomized comparison of thalidomide versus placebo in toxic epidermal necrolysis. Lancet 1998;352:1586-1589.

# Bullous Diseases

Method of
*Sarah E. Dick, MD, and Victoria Werth, MD*

The autoimmune bullous diseases are a group of rare disorders with potential significant morbidity and mortality. Although our scientific knowledge of these conditions is advancing and our armamentarium of therapies is growing, evidence-based practice guidelines are still lacking. Given the rarity of these diseases and the absence of common terms and endpoints for assessing disease extent, activity, and therapeutic response, the paucity of randomized controlled studies of the bullous diseases is not surprising. Thus, the true effectiveness of the available therapies remains unclear. The following treatment recommendations are based on published data and on the authors' personal experiences with patients with bullous disease.

# Pemphigus Vulgaris

Pemphigus vulgaris (PV) is characterized by nonscarring, fragile vesicles and bullae of the mucous membranes with or without cutaneous involvement. Systemic corticosteroid use and other advances in management have dramatically decreased the mortality rate for PV from 75% in untreated cases to 5% to 10% in treated cases. At present, the primary causes of morbidity and mortality in PV are complications resulting from treatment. Thus, the goal of PV management is to induce and maintain remission with the lowest medication doses possible. Therapies can be divided into those with a rapid effect and those with a delayed effect. Treatments that act rapidly, such as systemic corticosteroids, pulse corticosteroid therapy, intravenous immunoglobulin (IVIg), and plasmapheresis, are usually used to induce remission. Therapies with a delayed effect, such as immunosuppressive medications, dapsone,[1] and antibiotics, are generally used to decrease the need for systemic steroids.

The management of PV can be divided into three therapeutic phases: control, consolidation, maintenance. During the *control phase*, the medication doses should be rapidly increased to a level at which no new lesions form and established lesions start to heal. Without this initial successful disease suppression, tapering of treatment can be difficult. In the *consolidation phase*, the current therapy should be maintained until about 80% of the established lesions are healed. During the *maintenance phase*, medications are gradually decreased to the lowest doses needed to prevent the appearance of new lesions. If multiple medications are being given, they should be tapered one at a time, with tapering of corticosteroids usually occurring first because of the significant toxicity associated with prolonged systemic corticosteroid use.

Systemic corticosteroids are the most effective and rapidly acting treatment for PV. Low to moderate doses of oral prednisone (Deltasone; 0.5 mg/kg/day) can be started for mild disease. Higher doses of prednisone (1 mg/kg/day) should be used for more severe disease. These starting doses can be increased every 1 to 2 weeks by 50% increments until disease activity is controlled. Different and/or adjuvant therapies should be considered if patients do not respond to an oral prednisone dose of 1.5 to 2 mg/kg/day. Often adjuvant immunosuppressive therapy is started concurrently with systemic corticosteroids in order to maximize disease control and minimize the steroid dose. Pulse corticosteroid therapy with intravenous methylprednisolone (Solu-Medrol) has been shown to have long-lasting benefits and should be considered in patients who are not responsive to prednisone. It is used at a dose of 1 g/day over 1 to 3 hours for 3 consecutive days. The advantage of pulse steroid therapy is that remission can be quickly achieved and long-term side effects of chronic steroid use minimized.

Once remission is achieved and maintained, prednisone doses can be tapered cautiously, with a decrease of 5 to 10 mg every 1 to 2 weeks. If a few new lesions appear during the taper, they can be treated with intralesional corticosteroids, such as triamcinolone (Kenalog), or with high-potency topical corticosteroids, such as clobetasol (Temovate), while the current dose of systemic medications is unchanged. If many new lesions appear, the dose of prednisone should be increased in increments of 25% to 50% until control is re-established.

Other rapidly acting agents for PV include IVIg (Gamimune, Gammagard) and plasmapheresis. IVIg appears to be most effective when used with immunosuppressive therapies or when used as a steroid-sparing agent. However, IVIg has also been shown to be effective as monotherapy. The usual dose is 2 g/kg over 3 to 5 days. Multiple cycles given every 4 weeks are generally needed. The effectiveness of plasmapheresis for PV is controversial. In a controlled study, plasmapheresis used in combination with prednisone was found to have no advantage over the use of prednisone alone. However, plasmapheresis in combination with immunosuppressive therapy may be a valuable treatment for severe and/or unresponsive PV. Plasmapheresis is normally performed three times per week, with approximately 2 L of plasma removed at each treatment. Concurrent use of immunosuppressive

---
[1]Not FDA approved for this indication.

medications helps prevent a rebound in the antibody concentrations that usually occurs. With both plasmapheresis and IVIg, serum antibody concentrations can be monitored to determine a response to therapy.

Immunosuppressive medications used for treatment of PV include azathioprine[1] (Imuran) at doses of 3 to 5 mg/kg/day, cyclophosphamide[1] (Cytoxan) at doses of 2 to 3 mg/kg/day or as pulse therapy of 0.5 to 1 g/m[2] monthly combined with low-dose oral cyclophosphamide,[1] mycophenolate mofetil[1] (MMF; CellCept) at doses of 2 to 3 g per day, methotrexate[1] (Rheumatrex) at doses up to 20 mg/week, chlorambucil[1] (Leukeran) at doses of 4 to 10 mg/day, and cyclosporine[1] (Neoral, Sandimmune) at doses of 3 to 6 mg/kg/day. These therapies are thought to have a lag phase of 4 to 6 weeks before they become effective. They are generally used as adjuvant therapy. In a randomized trial, cyclosporine[1] was shown to be ineffective as adjuvant therapy to corticosteroids in the treatment of PV. Nevertheless, based on case reports, some experts still believe that it may be beneficial as adjuvant therapy to corticosteroids in long-term maintenance.

Dapsone[1] (Avlosulfon) has been shown to reduce steroid dependence in PV patients. It is used at doses of 50 to 300 mg/day. It is usually started at a dose of 50 mg daily and increased by 25 mg weekly until a response is obtained.

Other treatments for PV that can be considered as alternatives to the adjuvant therapies mentioned include gold,[1] tetracycline[1] (Sumycin) with or without niacinamide,[1] and hydroxychloroquine[1] (Plaquenil).

For severe and refractory PV that has failed conventional therapies, extracorporeal photopheresis can be considered. This procedure requires collaboration with specialists.

New potential treatments for PV include rituximab (Rituxan),[1] infliximab (Remicade),[1] etanercept (Enbrel),[1] and pyridostigmine bromide (Mestinon).[1] Rituximab (Rituxan)[1] is a chimeric murine-human monoclonal antibody against CD20. It has been shown to be effective in refractory PV at a dose of 375 mg/m[2]/week for 4 weeks. Infliximab (Remicade)[1] is a chimeric murine-human monoclonal antibody against tumor necrosis factor-$\alpha$ (TNF-$\alpha$). Recent reports suggest that TNF-$\alpha$ blockade might be a short-term therapeutic option for immediate control of refractory PV. Etanercept (Enbrel)[1] is a fusion protein of TNF-$\alpha$ receptor that acts as a competitive inhibitor of TNF-$\alpha$. It may have a beneficial role in the treatment of PV. Pyridostigmine bromide[1] is an acetylcholinesterase inhibitor that is being investigated for treatment of PV.

## Pemphigus Foliaceus

Pemphigus foliaceus (PF) typically presents with nonscarring superficial, cutaneous erosions and crusts with a similar distribution as PV. In contrast to PV, there is no mucosal involvement. The principles and practice of managing PF are similar to those for PV. However, monotherapy with dapsone[1] can be effective. In addition, because PF may remain localized for several years, topical steroids such as triamcinolone (Kenalog) and clobetasol (Temovate) may suffice for many years before systemic treatment in needed.

## Paraneoplastic Pemphigus

Paraneoplastic pemphigus (PNP) is frequently associated with an underlying lymphoproliferative neoplasm (most commonly non-Hodgkin's lymphoma, chronic lymphocytic leukemia, and Castleman disease). Clinically, there are polymorphous mucocutaneous lesions. The oral lesions are typically severe and refractory to treatment. Other organs, especially the lungs, can be affected.

Management of PNP involves treatment of the underlying neoplasm as well as immunosuppression. Excision of associated benign neoplasms may result in remission, whereas excision of malignant neoplasm often does not. High-dose systemic corticosteroids, such as prednisone at doses of 1 to 2 mg/kg/day, are usually the first-line therapy. Patients rarely have a complete response to systemic corticosteroids alone. The addition of immunosuppressive therapies, such as cyclosporine, azathioprine, MMF, and cyclophosphamide, have all been used with variable success. Although there may be a concern about treatment with immunosuppression in a patient with a known malignancy, the extremely high morbidity and mortality associated with PNP warrants MMF use. Other therapies to consider for treatment of recalcitrant PNP include IVIg, plasmapheresis, immunophoresis, and photopheresis. Both rituximab and alemtuzumab (Campath)[1] are new therapies that have been shown to be beneficial in the treatment of PNP. Alemtuzumab is a humanized monoclonal antibody against CD52.

## Bullous Pemphigoid

Bullous pemphigoid (BP) usually presents as nonscarring tense blisters with a predilection for the flexural aspects of the limbs. Mucosal lesions occur in 10% to 35% of patients. Even without treatment, BP is usually a self-limited disease. Remission is likely to occur within 5 years. Despite this limited course of BP, its mortality rate appears to be between 20% and 40% with or without therapy. The aim of treatment should be to heal established lesions, halt the development of new lesions, and minimize side effects from medications.

Localized or limited disease should be treated with potent topical corticosteroids, such as clobetasol ointment twice daily. Moderate and even severe BP can also be treated with potent topical steroids. In a randomized trial, potent topical steroids used for extensive BP had a lower 1-year mortality rate compared to prednisone at a dose of 1 mg/kg/day. Nevertheless, most patients with generalized disease require systemic therapy. Systemic corticosteroids are currently the best-established treatment. They have a rapid effect (within days) and well-documented effectiveness. Prednisone alone is often sufficient as monotherapy at doses of 0.5 to 0.75 mg/kg/day. Once remission is achieved, prednisone doses can be tapered in a manner similar to that described for PV.

Immunosuppressive medications can be considered in the treatment of BP, especially for patients who cannot tolerate corticosteroids or who have severe, difficult to control disease. In randomized trials, azathioprine[1] has been shown to have a steroid-sparing effect, but it has also been associated with more side effects when used with prednisolone in comparison to prednisolone alone. It is used at doses of 2 to 3 mg/kg/day. MMF has been shown to be effective both as monotherapy and in combination with corticosteroids. It is used at doses of 2 to 3 g/day. An ongoing randomized trial is comparing azathioprine[1] and MMF.[1] Other immunosuppressive medications to consider include cyclophosphamide,[1] methotrexate,[1] chlorambucil,[1] and cyclosporine.[1]

Antibiotics have been shown to have a beneficial effect in the treatment of BP and should be considered for treatment of mild disease or as a steroid-sparing agent. In a randomized trial, the combination of tetracycline[1] and niacinamide[1] was equally as effective as prednisone alone. Tetracycline[1] is given at a dose of 500 mg four times daily with or without niacinamide[1] at a dose of 500 mg three times daily. Doxycycline[1] (Vibramycin) or minocycline[1] (Minocin) 100 mg twice daily can be given rather than tetracycline.

Dapsone[1] (50–300 mg/day) can be used as a steroid-sparing agent in the treatment of BP. It is usually started at a dose of 50 mg daily and increased by 25 mg weekly until a response is obtained.

For recalcitrant disease, IVIg and plasmapheresis can be used. Both are very costly. Randomized trials studying plasmapheresis suggest it has a steroid-sparing effect.

## Mucous Membrane Pemphigoid

Mucous membrane pemphigoid (MMP) is also known as cicatricial pemphigoid and mucosal pemphigoid. Lesions of MMP can be scarring and predominantly involve the oral cavity and conjunctiva. Limited cutaneous disease with fragile vesicles, bullae, and erosions is present in approximately one third of patients. Mucosal involvement

---

[1]Not FDA approved for this indication.

[1]Not FDA approved for this indication.

of the nasopharynx, pharynx, esophagus, larynx, trachea, genitals, and anus can occur.

Treatment of MMP is dictated by the site, extent, and severity of disease as well as by the rapidity of progression. Patients with ocular, nasopharyngeal, laryngeal, esophageal, and/or genital lesions are considered high risk because involvement of these sites can lead to blindness, airway obstruction, esophageal stricture, and urinary and sexual dysfunction. For high-risk patients with severe or rapidly progressing disease, initial treatment should consist of cyclophosphamide[1] (1-2 mg/kg/day) and prednisone (1-1.5 mg/kg/day). A small randomized controlled trial found the combination of cyclophosphamide[1] and prednisone to be more effective than prednisone alone. Azathioprine[1] or MMF[1] (at doses similar to those used for BP) given with prednisone can also be considered if cyclophosphamide[1] is ineffective or not tolerated. IVIg has been shown to have a beneficial effect and can be used for refractory MMP. Subconjunctival mitomycin can be used to help reduce mucosal fibrosis and prevent scarring. For milder disease in high-risk patients, dapsone[1] (50-300 mg daily) may be given. A small randomized controlled trial showed that cyclophosphamide[1] was superior to dapsone[1] in the treatment of severe MMP with ocular involvement. However, the study concluded that dapsone

can be beneficial for mild to moderate disease. Other treatments to consider in recalcitrant cases include methotrexate,[1] thalidomide (Thalomid),[1] etanercept,[1] and plasmapheresis. All MMP patients should be evaluated and managed in conjunction with the appropriate subspecialist (e.g., ocular involvement requires ophthalmologic monitoring) with surgical intervention as needed.

MMP patients with only oral mucosal involvement, with or without cutaneous lesions, are considered low risk. Because these patients are less likely to have mucosal scarring, a more conservative therapeutic approach can be taken. In addition to good oral hygiene, moderate- to high-potency topical corticosteroids, such as triamcinolone or clobetasol (two to four times daily), can be used for the initial treatment. An insertable prosthetic device/retainer is useful for the oral topical application of corticosteroids. Intralesional corticosteroids, such as triamcinolone, may also be beneficial for refractory oral mucosal lesions. Tetracycline[1] with or without niacinamide[1] (at doses similar to those used for BP) can be effective in managing low-risk patients. If disease control is not achieved with topical corticosteroids or oral antibiotics, other treatments to consider include dapsone[1] (50-200 mg/day) or low-dose prednisone (0.5 mg/kg/day) with or without low-dose azathioprine[1] (100-150 mg/day). For MMP with

[1]Not FDA approved for this indication.

[1]Not FDA approved for this indication.

 **CURRENT DIAGNOSIS**

**Pemphigus Vulgaris**

- Flaccid blisters: Mucocutaneous.
- Suprabasilar intraepidermal blisters.
- DIF is positive for epidermal intercellular IgG deposition.
- IIF on monkey esophagus is positive for circulating autoantibodies.
- ELISA identifies antibodies to desmoglein-3 with/ without desmoglein-1.

**Pemphigus Foliaceus**

- Flaccid blisters: Cutaneous only.
- Subcorneal intraepidermal blisters.
- DIF is positive for epidermal intercellular IgG deposition.
- IIF on guinea pig esophagus is positive for circulating autoantibodies.
- ELISA identifies antibodies to desmoglein-1 only.

**Paraneoplastic Pemphigus**

- Polymorphous lesions: Mucocutaneous.
- Intraepidermal blisters, keratinocyte necrosis, and interface dermatitis.
- DIF is positive for IgG and C3 deposition at epidermal intercellular sites and at the dermal-epidermal junction.
- IIF on rodent bladder is positive for circulating autoantibodies. Immunoblotting and immunoprecipitation identify antibodies to desmoglein and multiple plakin antigens (at a minimum, periplakin and/or envoplakin).

**Bullous Pemphigoid**

- Tense blisters: Mostly cutaneous, can be mucocutaneous.
- Subepidermal blisters with eosinophils.
- DIF is positive for IgG and C3 deposition at the dermal–epidermal junction.
- IIF on salt-split skin is positive for autoantibodies on the epidermal side (roof) of the blister. BPAg2 is the target antigen.

**Mucous Membrane Pemphigoid**

- Scarring blisters: Mucosal.
- Subepidermal blister.
- DIF is positive for IgG and C3 deposition at the dermal-epidermal junction.
- IIF on salt-split skin can be positive for autoantibodies on the epidermal side (roof) of the blister, dermal side (floor) of the blister, or both. Target antigens are BPAg2, integrin subunit $\beta_4$, and laminin-5.

**Epidermolysis Bullosa Acquisita**

- Skin fragility at sites of trauma with scarring and milia: Mostly cutaneous, can be mucosal.
- Subepidermal blister.
- DIF is positive for IgG deposition at the dermal-epidermal junction.
- IIF on salt-split skin is positive for autoantibodies on the dermal side (floor) of the blister.
- ELISA identifies antibodies to type VII collagen.

**Linear IgA Disease**

- Pruritic grouped papules: Mucocutaneous.
- Subepidermal blisters with neutrophils.
- DIF positive for linear deposition of IgA at the dermal-epidermal junction.
- IIF can be negative or detect low levels of circulating IgA autoantibodies.

**Dermatitis Herpetiformis**

- Pruritic grouped papules associated with a gluten sensitive enteropathy: Cutaneous.
- Subepidermal blisters with neutrophils.
- DIF positive for granular deposition of IgA in the dermal papillary tips.

*Abbreviations:* BPAg2 = bullous pemphigoid antigen–2; C3 = complement 3; DIF = direct immunofluorescence; ELISA = enzyme–linked immunosorbent assay; IgA = immunoglobulin A; IgG = immunoglobulin G; IIF = indirect immunofluorescence.

severe oral disease, the treatments recommended for high-risk patients may be needed.

## Epidermolysis Bullosa Acquisita

Epidermolysis bullosa acquisita (EBA) has heterogeneous clinical features. Classically, patients have skin fragility and present with bullae and/or erosions at areas of friction and trauma. However, EBA patients can also present with lesions resembling BP, linear immunoglobulin A (IgA) bullous dermatosis, or MMP. Lesions heal with scarring and milia formation. Complications similar to those with MMP, such as blindness and esophageal stricture, can occur. EBA may be associated with various systemic diseases, most commonly inflammatory bowel disease.

EBA is very difficult to treat. It appears that the classic presentation is the most resistant to therapy. Any measures that decrease friction and trauma to the skin will help. Systemic corticosteroids such as prednisone (0.5-2 mg/kg/day) can be beneficial, especially with inflammatory EBA. Dapsone[1] or colchicine[1] used as adjuvant agents or monotherapies should also be considered. Dapsone[1] (50-300 mg/day) is believed to be particularly appropriate with inflammatory EBA that has a neutrophilic predominance in histology. Colchicine[1] (0.5-2 mg/day) may not be tolerated because of gastrointestinal side effects, especially in patients with associated inflammatory bowel disease.

Cyclosporine[1], with or without systemic corticosteroids, can result in a rapid response and should be considered for the initial treatment of EBA. Doses of 3 to 9 mg/kg/day can be started and then increased or decreased as needed. Long-term toxicity of the medication limits its use.

Immunosuppressive agents, such as azathioprine[1], cyclophosphamide[1], methotrexate[1] and MMF[1], may be considered for treatment of EBA. They can be used in regimens and at doses similar to those used for PV.

IVIg can be effective when given as monotherapy or in combination with immunosuppressive agents and/or systemic corticosteroids. This treatment is expensive and is best reserved for recalcitrant cases. Extracorporeal photopheresis and plasmapheresis can also be considered for treatment of recalcitrant EBA. Plasmapheresis has been shown to be beneficial when given in combination with IVIg, systemic corticosteroids, or cyclophosphamide.[1]

As with MMP, patients with EBA should be followed by the appropriate subspecialists, such as ophthalmologists and gastroenterologists, if mucosal membranes are involved.

## Linear Immunoglobulin A Bullous Dermatosis

Linear IgA bullous dermatosis (LABD) has heterogeneous clinical features. It typically presents with annular or grouped pruritic papules, vesicles, and bullae on the elbows, knees, and buttocks. These lesions can be indistinguishable from those of dermatitis herpetiformis. However, the lesions can also resemble those of BP and EBA. Mucosal lesions resembling MMP may occur.

LABD can have an unpredictable course with occasional spontaneous remissions. Treatment with dapsone[1] usually results in a rapid dramatic response and is considered the first-line treatment of LABD. Doses as described for PV are used. Sulfapyridine[1] can also be used with similar results. The initial dose for sulfapyridine[1] is 500 mg twice daily. This can be increased by 1 g every 1 to 2 weeks until disease control, or a maximum dose of 4 g, is reached. Tetracycline[1] in combination with niacinamide[1] (at doses similar to those used for BP) has been shown to have a beneficial effect in the treatment of LABD. Prednisone can be added to these therapies when clinical responses are incomplete. Several other medications, such as MMF[1], azathioprine[1], cyclosporine[1] and methotrexate[1], have also been shown to be helpful in the management of patients with difficult to control disease. For recalcitrant cases, cyclosporine[1] (3-6 mg/kg/day) or IVIg can be used. Oral mucosal lesions may be more resistant to treatment and require therapy with topical steroids.

## CURRENT THERAPY

**Pemphigus Vulgaris**

- Rapid effect: systemic corticosteroids.
- Delayed effect: Immunosuppressive agents, dapsone,[1] and antibiotics.
- Resistant disease: Intravenous immunoglobulin, rituximab[1] (Rituxan).
- Bone prophylaxis for systemic corticosteroid use.

**Pemphigus Foliaceus**

- Similar management as pemphigus vulgaris.

**Paraneoplastic Pemphigus**

- Treat underlying neoplasm.
- High-dose systemic corticosteroids plus immunosuppressive agents.

**Bullous Pemphigoid**

- Generalized or severe disease: Systemic corticosteroids, immunosuppressive agents, dapsone.[1]
- Limited or mild disease: Topical corticosteroids, tetracycline[1] with niacinamide.[1]

**Mucous Membrane Pemphigoid**

- High-risk patients: Cyclophosphamide[1] (Cytoxan) plus prednisone.
- Low-risk patients: Topical corticosteroids, tetracycline[1] plus niacinamide,[1] dapsone.[1]

**Epidermolysis Bullosa Acquisita**

- Difficult to treat.
- Decrease friction and trauma to skin.
- Systemic corticosteroids, dapsone,[1] colchicine.[1]

**Linear IgA Disease**

- Dapsone.[1]

**Dermatitis Herpetiformis**

- Dapsone and gluten-free diet.

[1]Not FDA approved for this indication.
*Abbreviations:* IgA = immunoglobulin A.

As with MMP and EBA, patients with LABD should be followed by the appropriate subspecialists if mucosal membranes are involved.

## Dermatitis Herpetiformis

Dermatitis herpetiformis (DH) presents as intense pruritus with grouped papules and vesicles distributed on the extensor surfaces of the elbows, knees, buttocks, and back. It can be indistinguishable from LABD. DH appears to be caused by an immune response to gluten, and it is associated with a gluten-sensitive enteropathy.

Dapsone is considered the first-line therapy for DH. It usually causes a rapid and dramatic response at doses described for PV. Sulfapyridine[1] can also be used when dapsone cannot be tolerated. The initial dose of sulfapyridine is 500 mg three times daily. This can be increased by 1 g every 1 to 2 weeks until disease control, or a maximum dose of 4-6 g, is reached. Other medications have been used with variable success, including tetracycline[1] with niacinamide,[1] heparin,[1] colchicine,[1] azathioprine,[1] prednisone, and cholestyramine,[1] and can be considered for patients who are intolerant or allergic to dapsone and sulfapyridine.[1]

[1]Not FDA approved for this indication.

[1]Not FDA approved for this indication.

A gluten-free diet is important for the long-term management of DH for several reasons. First, DH symptoms improve and can allow for reduction or even discontinuation of medications. Second, associated gastrointestinal symptoms improve and can resolve. Third, the associated risk of gastrointestinal lymphoma significantly decreases and disappears after 5 to 10 years.

## REFERENCES

Ahmed AR, Dahl MV: Consensus statement on the use of intravenous immunoglobulin therapy in the treatment of autoimmune mucocutaneous blistering diseases. Arch Dermatol 2003;139:1051-1059.

Bystryn JC, Steinman NM: The adjuvant therapy of pemphigus. An update. Arch Dermatol 1996;132:203-212.

Chaffins ML, Collison D, Fivenson DP: Treatment of pemphigus and linear IgA dermatosis with nicotinamide and tetracycline: A review of 13 cases. J Am Acad Dermatol 1993;28:998-1000.

Chan LS, Ahmed AR, Anhalt GJ, et al: The first international consensus on mucous membrane pemphigoid: Definition, diagnostic criteria, pathogenic factors, medical treatment, and prognostic indicators. Arch Dermatol 2002;138:370-379.

Engineer L, Ahmed AR: Emerging treatment for epidermolysis bullosa acquisita. J Am Acad Dermatol 2001;44:818-828.

Fleischli ME, Valek RH, Pandya AG: Pulse intravenous cyclophosphamide therapy in pemphigus. Arch Dermatol 1999;135:57-61.

Garioch JJ, Lewis HM, Sargent SA, et al: 25 years' experience of a gluten-free diet in the treatment of dermatitis herpetiformis. Br J Dermatol 1994;131:541-545.

Heaphy MR, Albrecht J, Werth VP: Dapsone as a glucocorticoid-sparing agent in maintenance-phase pemphigus vulgaris. Arch Dermatol 2005;141:699-702.

Ioannides D, Chrysomallis F, Bystryn JC: Ineffectiveness of cyclosporine as an adjuvant to corticosteroids in the treatment of pemphigus. Arch Dermatol 2000;136:868-872.

Khumalo N, Kirtschig G, Middleton P, et al: Interventions for bullous pemphigoid. Cochrane Database Syst Rev 2005 (3):CD002292.

Mimouni D, Anhalt GJ, Cummins DL, et al: Treatment of pemphigus vulgaris and pemphigus foliaceus with mycophenolate mofetil. Arch Dermatol 2003;139:739-742

Werth VP: Treatment of pemphigus vulgaris with brief, high-dose intravenous glucocorticoids. Arch Dermatol 1996;132:1435-1439.

# Contact Dermatitis

Method of
*Peter C. Schalock, MD, and Kathryn A. Zug, MD*

Eczema is well described by the word's Greek roots, with "ek" meaning "out or over" and "zein" meaning "to boil." Thus, this boiling over pattern of superficial inflammatory skin diseases of the skin is one of the most common reaction pattern seen by dermatologists. Pruritus is the most characteristic skin sensation associated with eczema.

## Irritant Contact Dermatitis

Contact dermatitis (CD) is caused by exogenous substances coming into contact with the skin. Irritant contact dermatitis (ICD) is the most common form of CD, caused by frequent or chronic exposure to an irritating substance. ICD will eventually occur in any person exposed to these irritating substances in sufficient concentration. This type of reaction is the most common form of occupational skin disease and is a problem for many individuals worldwide. The most common location for ICD is the hands. Other locations commonly involved are the palms, fingers, and dorsal web spaces. As opposed to allergic contact dermatitis, the dorsal hands are most often spared from dermatitis.

# Allergic Contact Dermatitis

Two types of immune reactions are seen in allergic contact dermatitis (ACD): type I immediate-type hypersensitivity and type IV delayed-type hypersensitivity. Immediate-type reactions are most commonly caused by animal or plant proteins that are able to bind to mast cells and cause mast cell degranulation, leading to an urticarial or anaphylactic reaction. The most commonly recognized cause of this type of immediate hypersensitivity is natural rubber latex proteins. Allergy to these proteins is caused by exposure to products containing natural rubber latex, especially rubber gloves. Type IV allergy is caused by substances that are taken up by Langerhans cells in the epidermis and processed and presented to T cells in the regional lymph node, thus creating memory T cells that are capable of reacting the next time the individual is exposed to the substance. The delayed reaction is due to the time needed to mount the immune response. Frequent culprits are urushiol (poison ivy/oak), topical antibiotics, nickel, and formaldehyde/formaldehyde-releasing preservatives.

## Diagnosis

Evaluation for the etiology of CD reactions depends upon the type of allergy sought. Evaluation for type I immediate-type allergy is different than for type IV delayed-type reactions. Testing for type I allergy can be achieved by in vivo and in vitro methods. Prick testing can be performed for panels of suspected allergens. For the prick test, the skin on the flexor forearm or other area is cleaned, and a small amount of a pure dilution of the suspect protein is placed on the skin. The skin is pricked using a sterile lancet, and the patient is observed for a wheal and flare reaction. Histamine should also be used as a positive control. This type of testing can elicit an anaphylactic type of reaction and should be performed with caution. Many allergens that elicit a type I reaction can also be tested by the allergen-specific immunoglobulin E antibody test or radioallergosorbent assay test (RAST).

Type IV allergy is best evaluated by patch testing. A patch test is made with hypoallergenic tape to which Finn chambers (small metal chambers) or IQ Ultra chambers (Chemotechnique Diagnostics, Vellinge, Sweden) are placed with a purified potential allergen. The patches are placed most often on the patient's upper back and left for 48 hours. The patches are then removed, the locations of the allergens marked, and the initial reading performed. The patient is seen again in another 48 hours for the final reading. Two readings are preferable to allow assessment of some reactions that appear after the patch has been removed and of some reactions initially thought to be positive that may actually have been irritant reactions. Patch testing technique has been described in detail by Corey.

Once the patient's sensitivities are determined, the information is useful to help educate the patient regarding avoidance of the offending allergen. There is no "cure" for ACD. The Contact Allergen Replacement Database available through the American Contact Dermatitis Society is a useful tool for helping patients avoid their allergens (available at: www.contactderm.org). The patient can enter each allergen into the database, and a list of products free of the allergens is generated.

In the United States, only the 23 thin-layer rapid-use epicutaneous (TRUE) test allergens are Food and Drug Administration (FDA) approved for use. A multitude of other allergens for patch testing are available in Europe. Chemotechnique AB (Malmo, Sweden) and Hermal (Reinbek, Germany) both manufacture many standard and specialty series of allergens. Patch testing with an expanded series of allergens can be useful in identifying relevant allergens. TRUE test allergens encompass 1.4% of the more than 3700 known allergens, although 28% of patients are fully evaluated with this panel. By expanding the series to the 65 standard allergens used by the North American Contact Dermatitis Group (NACDG), 50.2% of relevant allergies are identified. Although use of the TRUE test may be a good starting point for evaluation of ACD, an expanded panel of allergens with additional testing for suspected agents to which the patient may have contact gives a much greater return on testing.

## CURRENT DIAGNOSIS

**Type I Allergy**

- Prick test
- Use test (perform with caution)
- Radioallergosorbent assay test (RAST) for specific allergens

**Type IV Allergy**

- Patch test using a broad panel of allergens and patient's personal care products most helpful
- Repeated open application test (ROAT)/use test

## Treatment

Treatment of CD hinges upon four premises: education of the patient regarding skin care and the etiology of the dermatitis, postexposure skin care, strict avoidance of the offending allergen(s), and pharmacologic therapy of active dermatitis. Patients educated on the basics of good skin care and on the cause of their ICD and ACD had less dermatitis than did those without intervention. For patient with ICD and ACD, postexposure skin care plays an important role in treatment. ICD can play a role in the development and perpetuation of ACD by allowing greater penetration of allergens. Good skin care, such as the use of appropriate barrier creams, bland emollients, and avoidance of wet work or macerating gloves, can decrease skin irritation and transepidermal water loss. Good skin care and prevention of irritation should be an integral part of preventing and treating ACD.

In cases of mild to moderate dermatitis, a medium- or high-potency topical steroid, such as triamcinolone acetonide (Aristocort A) 0.1% or desoximetasone (Topicort) 0.25%, can be used two to three times daily for monotherapy. For widespread cases, a 1-lb (454 g) jar of generic triamcinolone acetonide 0.1% is preferable. Ointments are preferable to creams because the water and preservatives present in creams may worsen the irritant reaction. Simple, greasy lubricants, such as Aquaphor or Vaseline, should be used every time the body or

---

[1]Not FDA approved for this indication.

---

## CURRENT THERAPY

- Strict avoidance of the offending allergen(s) and pharmacologic therapy for active dermatitis.
- Patient education on good skin care and prevention of irritation.
- Simple, greasy lubricants, such as Aquaphor or Vaseline, should be used every time the body or hands are washed or appear dry.
- Groin or face dermatitis: Tacrolimus (Protopic) 0.1% ointment or pimecrolimus (Elidel) 1% cream twice daily
- Mild to moderate dermatitis: Medium- or high-potency topical steroid such as triamcinolone acetonide (Aristocort A) 0.1% or desoximetasone (Topicort) 0.25% bid-tid for monotherapy.
  - Widespread dermatitis: Generic triamcinolone 0.1% cream (454-g jar) bid-tid
  - Pruritus: Hydroxyzine (Atarax) 10-50 mg PO bid–tid PRN
- Severe Dermatitis
  - Prednisone in a 4-week course with 7-day tapering steps, such as 60-40-20-10 mg
  - Open wet dressings with topical steroid application

hands are washed or appear dry. Widespread dermatitis will often improve rapidly with open wet dressings preceded and followed by a topical corticosteroid cream. For hand dermatitis, use of the steroid or of Vaseline under cotton gloves can be helpful, either for short periods or overnight. For sensitive areas such as the face and genitalia, topical calcineurin inhibitors can be useful. Either tacrolimus (Protopic) 0.1% ointment or pimecrolimus (Elidel) 1% cream twice daily can be used. For more severe cases of dermatitis, topical therapy and a corticosteroid taper can be helpful in alleviating the patient's symptoms as well as calming the dermatitis. Short prednisone tapers (i.e., "dose packs") will not always be adequate, with the patient flaring after the short taper is finished. Using prednisone in a 4-week course with 7-day tapering steps, such as 60-40- 20-10 mg, can be helpful in breaking the cycle of chronic inflammation and excoriation/pruritus. Open wet dressings with application of topical corticosteroid before and after can diminish dermatitis quickly. For patients with severe pruritus, especially at night, hydroxyzine (Atarax) 10 to 50 mg orally or doxepin[1] (Sinequan) 10 to 20 mg orally at bedtime can be helpful.

## Conclusion

Contact dermatitis is a broad diagnosis encompassing both immediate- and delayed-type hypersensitivities. Testing can be helpful in characterizing specific allergens and in guiding the patients as to which substances to avoid to prevent dermatitis. The RAST or prick test is useful for determining immediate-type hypersensitivity and patch testing for delayed-type allergy. TRUE tests will fully evaluate 28% of patients. Broadening the screen with other allergens, such as the NACDG panel, can be useful for defining ACD in patients with dermatitis. Treatment of CD consists of topical steroids, open wet dressings, moisturization, topical calcineurin inhibitors, and infrequently oral corticosteroids.

### REFERENCES

Bauer A, Kelterer D, Stadeler M, et al: The prevention of occupational hand dermatitis in bakers, confectioners and employees in the catering trades. Preliminary results of a skin prevention program. Contact Dermatitis 2001;44:85-88.

Corey G: Applying patch tests from a technician's or nurse's point of view. Am J Contact Dermat 1993;4:175-181.

Kalimo K, Kautiainen H, Niskanen T, Niemi L: "Eczema school" to improve compliance in an occupational dermatology clinic. Contact Dermatitis 1999;41:315-319.

Saripalli YV, Achen F, Belsito DV: The detection of clinically relevant contact allergens using a standard screening tray of twenty–three allergens. J Am Acad Dermatol 2003;49:65-69.

---

# Pruritus Ani and Vulvae

Method of
*Libby Edwards, MD*

Anogenital pruritus, or itching, is a symptom, not a diagnosis. The word *itching* encompasses a number of sensations, including irritation, prickling, and crawling sensations as well as a sensation of needing to scratch. Specifically excluded are burning, soreness, and other pain adjectives.

Unlike medication for pain, no nonspecific anti-itch medications are available. Thus the management of anogenital pruritus begins with an evaluation to diagnose the underlying cause, followed by specific therapy for that etiology (Box 1). The usual causes of itching are infection, dermatosis, neuropathy, or anxiety/depression. Several factors may play a role.

## BOX 1   Causes of Anogenital Itching

**Acute Itching**

*Infection*
- *Candida albicans*
- Pinworms
- Trichomoniasis
- Herpes simplex virus infection
- Mollusca contagiosa
- Genital warts, bacterial vaginosis, group B streptococcus

*Dermatoses*
- Irritant or allergic contact dermatoses
- Eczema, lichen sclerosus, psoriasis, lichen planus

**Chronic Itching (Often Multifactorial)**
- Dermatoses: Lichen simplex chronicus/eczema, lichen sclerosus, psoriasis, lichen planus
- Neuropathy
- Anxiety/depression
- Infection: Usually only a complicating factor in the face of underlying dermatosis

Acute itching is most often related to infection, especially *Candida albicans*. Herpes simplex virus infection, trichomoniasis, *Staphylococcus aureus*, and scabies are less common causes of itching. The most common dermatosis to produce sudden-onset itching is allergic or irritant contact dermatitis, in which something touching the skin (overcleaning, stool retained in skin folds, topical medications, etc.) causes itching.

Chronic itching is most often caused by skin disease, often with exacerbating factors such as secondary infection or irritation from topical medications. The most common dermatoses to cause chronic itching are eczema/lichen simplex chronicus (LSC) and lichen sclerosus (LS). Less common pruritic dermatoses that can affect anogenital skin include psoriasis and nonerosive lichen planus (LP). Although infection is almost never the primary cause of chronic anogenital itching, infection can complicate and perpetuate itching from dermatoses. Some patients exhibit chronic itching despite a normal physical examination and negative cultures. Most often these patients have subtle eczema, but itching on the basis of neuropathy or anxiety/depression can occur. These diagnoses are made by excluding infection and skin disease and by response to therapy.

# Management

The first step in management is a very careful examination of the anogenital area, including vulvar and perianal skin folds and the vaginal epithelium (Box 2). Severe symptoms sometimes are produced by subtle signs. Cultures of vaginal secretions and scrapings of scaling skin to evaluate for infection are indicated.

Acute itching on the basis of an infection can generally be cleared rapidly and definitively by treatment of the infection. All dermatoses, whether producing acute or chronic itching, can be treated with an ultrapotent topical corticosteroid ointment (e.g., clobetasol propionate [Temovate]). Ointments are less irritating than creams or gels. Although potent corticosteroids can produce atrophy, striae, and steroid dermatitis when used chronically without supervision, short-term twice-daily use produces safe and rapid control of symptoms. The frequency of application can be tapered when itching is controlled, or a lower potency medication can be substituted. Some dermatoses (LS, psoriasis) require long-term or lifetime thrice-weekly dosing of a corticosteroid to maintain control, whereas others (LSC) usually achieve remission, and medication can be discontinued, at least for prolonged times. Tacrolimus and Pimecrolimus can be beneficial for LSC, LS, and LP, but less so than Clobetasol, and current concerns for secondary squamous cell carcinoma also limit their use for LS and LP. In addition, they are slow in onset and produce burning with application. Itchy anogenital skin without evidence of an infection or a visible

## BOX 2   Treatment of Anogenital Itching

**Nonspecific Measures**
- Patient education and reassurance
- Careful evaluation for infection and dermatoses
- Elimination of irritants: Overwashing, infection, nighttime scratching, unnecessary topical medications and lubricants, infections
- Topical anesthetics: Topical lidocaine (Xylocaine) jelly 2%/ointment 5%, as needed; pramoxine (Summer's Eve Anti-itch Gel) as needed; topical benzocaine (Vagisil) and diphenhydramine (Benadryl) should be avoided
- Nighttime sedation
- Cool soaks/ice (frostbite avoided by wrapping ice in a towel)

**Specific Measures**
- Itching because of infection
  Acute itching: Treatment with standard therapy.
  Chronic itching: Evaluation for concomitant dermatosis; infection treated and suppressed long enough for skin to heal and itching to respond to therapy for concomitant process.
- Itching because of dermatoses
  Lichen sclerosus: Clobetasol propionate (Temovate) ointment two times per day until skin texture is normal, then three times per week for life (prepubertal girls occasionally experience remission at puberty; boys remit after circumcision). Or (less effective and concern regarding squamous cell carcinoma) chronic tacrolimus (Protopic) 0.1%, two times per day.
  Eczema/lichen simplex chronicus (LSC): Clobetasol propionate ointment two times per day until skin is normal and itching controlled, then frequency tapered to three times weekly, twice weekly, once weekly, then discontinued; restarted when flares occur. Or (less effective) tacrolimus (Protopic) or pimecrolimus (Elidel), two times per day.
- Itching without objective abnormalities
  Treated as for eczema/lichen simplex chronicus with clobetasol propionate for presumed subtle eczema/LSC.
  Amitriptyline (Elavil) (tapered up as high as 150 mg at bedtime), venlafaxine (Effexor) (tapered up as high as 150 mg extended release per day), gabapentin (Neurontin) (up to 3600 mg per day) for neuropathic pain
  Anxiety/depression addressed

dermatosis should be treated with a potent topical corticosteroid. If unresponsive to a steroid, the addition of medication for neuropathy (amitriptyline [Elavil], gabapentin [Neurontin], venlafaxine [Effexor]) or attention to anxiety/depression should be considered.

Whatever the cause, certain nonspecific measures can improve itching and contribute to a more rapid response to specific therapy, including the following:

- Avoidance of irritants, such as overwashing and unnecessary topical medications.
- Topical anesthetics (lidocaine [Xylocaine] jelly 2% or ointment 5%) that can temporarily improve itching and minimize ongoing

 **CURRENT DIAGNOSIS**

- Examination for skin disease
- Microscopic examinations and cultures for infection
- History of contactants and irritants

- Careful evaluation for underlying etiologies
- Specific therapies for all appropriate underlying etiologies
- Specific therapy continued long enough for the skin to heal and the itch-scratch cycle to cease
- Patient education regarding the chronic/recurrent nature of itching and the role of irritants
- Consideration of neuropathy and anxiety/depression in patients without observable disease who are resistant to topical corticosteroid therapy

irritation from scratching (but topical benzocaine [Vagisil] and diphenhydramine [Benadryl], which can be irritating and allergenic, should be avoided).

- Nighttime sedation, which can both provide well-needed respite from sleepless itchy nights and protect the skin from irritating scratching during nighttime hours. Tricyclic medications such as amitriptyline and doxepin (Sinequan) produce deeper sleep and less scratching than diphenhydramine and hydroxyzine (Atarax).

Although many clinicians use antihistamines for all itching, this class of medication has no intrinsic anti-itch properties and is generally useful only for the histamine-mediated itch of urticaria, usually a generalized rather than anogenital process.

Other, less potent measures that can be used in patients with recalcitrant symptoms include topical doxepin (Zonalon), tacrolimus (Protopic 0.1%), or pimecrolimus (Elidel). These medications are beneficial primarily in patients with mild to moderate eczema/LSC.

Patients should be advised that all causes of itching can be chronic or recurrent. Thus recurrence of itching does not necessarily reflect a failure of diagnosis or therapy but rather a need for recurrent or chronic therapy that is sufficiently prolonged for the skin to heal completely and for the itch-scratch cycle to be broken.

## REFERENCES

Bohm M, Frieling U, Luger TA, et al: Successful treatment of anogenital lichen sclerosus with topical tacrolimus. Arch Dermatol 2003; 48:444-448.

Bornstein J, Heifetz S, Kellner Y, et al: Clobetasol dipropionate 0.05% versus testosterone propionate 2% topical application for severe vulvar lichen sclerosus. Am J Obstet Gynecol 1998;178(1, Pt 1): 80-84.

Cohen AD, Masalha R, Medvedovsky E, Vardy DA: Brachioradial pruritus: A symptom of neuropathy. J Am Acad Dermatol 2003; 48(6):825-828.

Farage MA: Vulvar susceptibility to contact irritants and allergens: a review. Arch Gyneol Obstet 2005;272:167-172.

Koca R, Altin R, Konuk N, et al: Sleep distubance in patients with lichen simplex chronicus and its relationship to noctunal scratching: A case control study. South Med J. 2006;99:482-485.

Margesson LJ: Contact dermatitis of the vulva. Dermatol Ther 2004;17:20-27.

Stellon A: Neurogenic pruritus: An unrecognized problem? A retrospective case series of treatment by acupuncture. Acupunct Med 2002;20(4):186-190.

Weichert GE: An approch to the treatment of anogenital pruritus. Dermatol Ther 2004;17:129-133.

# Urticaria and Angioedema

Method of
*Eugene W. Monroe, MD*

*Urticaria* (hives) is a skin reaction pattern characterized by transient, pruritic, edematous, lightly erythematous papules or wheals, frequently with central clearing. *Angioedema* describes swellings of the deep dermis or subcutaneous tissue involving mucous membranes and loose tissues around the eyes, lips, or genitalia. Urticaria is extremely common. Approximately 15% to 20% of the general population have at least one episode of urticaria, angioedema, or both during their lives. The potential causes of urticaria are numerous, including drugs, food, infections, internal diseases, inhalants, bites/stings, contactants, immunologic processes, psychogenic factors, genetic abnormalities, and physical agents (dermographism and pressure, cholinergic, cold, solar, and heat urticaria).

## Classification

Urticaria is classified as acute or chronic, depending on the duration of the condition. Most cases of urticaria are classified as acute because they persist for only a few days to a few weeks. The incidence of acute urticaria is between 10% and 20% of the population. The etiology is usually detected, often an allergic reaction to a food or medication, or related to an acute infection. Many cases of urticaria are never seen by a physician. The initial aspect of therapy is the elimination of any suspected cause. Drug therapy should begin with the use of a so-called nonsedating $H_1$ antihistamine. In severe urticarial reactions or in cases associated with asthma or laryngeal edema, stronger medical management is required, including the use of subcutaneous injection of epinephrine or systemic corticosteroids.

When urticaria persists longer than 6 weeks, it is classified as chronic urticaria. The incidence of this form is between 0.1% and 3% of the population. The course is variable, from months to years, with 20% lasting longer than 20 years. Approximately 40% of the cases are associated with angioedema. Unfortunately, the etiology is not found in 60% to 95% of these cases, with most either idiopathic or autoimmune in nature. Treatment programs for chronic urticaria focus on measures that provide symptomatic relief.

## Diagnosis

The clinical diagnosis of urticaria is reasonably easy. Finding an underlying cause, especially for chronic urticaria, however, is usually extremely frustrating for the patient and the physician.

The most important diagnostic test in the evaluation of a patient with urticaria is a detailed history, which should include the location of lesions, morphology of lesions, pattern of attacks, precipitating factors, review of medical systems, and review of potential etiologies of urticaria. Diagnostic tests are selected on the basis of suspicions elicited by a meticulous history and physical examination. Potential minimal baseline tests might include a complete blood count with differential, a chemistry panel, and a sedimentation rate. Other possible tests based on the history might include thyroid autoantibodies, physical urticaria challenge tests, autologous serum skin testing, and so on.

## Treatment

The ideal treatment for urticaria is identification and removal of its cause. If that is not possible, the reduction of various triggering factors should be attempted, especially in cases of physical urticaria. The drug management of urticaria centers around four theoretical treatment approaches: blocking the effects of already released histamine on the receptor sites of cutaneous blood vessels; blocking the release of histamine

**TABLE 1   Comparison of Second-Generation H₁ Antihistamines**

| Drug | Recommended Dosage | Efficacy in Urticaria | Side Effects at Recommended Dosage | Side Effects at Higher than Recommended Dosage |
| --- | --- | --- | --- | --- |
| Loratadine (Claritin) | 10 mg qd | +++ | None | Mild sedation |
| Cetirizine (Zyrtec) | 10 mg qd | +++ | Mild sedation | Dose-related increases in sedation |
| Fexofenadine (Allegra) | 60 mg bid or 180 mg qd | +++ | None | None |
| Desloratadine (Clarinex) | 5 mg qd | +++ | None | Mild sedation |

*Abbreviations:* bid = twice per day; qd = every day.

and other mediators from mast cells; blocking mediators other than histamine that can cause hives; and modulating the inflammatory, cellular, and immunologic components of the urticarial process.

H₁ antihistamines remain the first line of therapy for urticaria. First-generation antihistamines such as hydroxyzine (Atarax), diphenhydramine (Benadryl), and chlorpheniramine (Chlor-Trimeton) are moderately effective in treating urticaria. The usefulness of these agents is sometimes limited by undesirable side effects, however, especially central nervous system (CNS) effects such as daytime sedation and anticholinergic effects. Because of these problems, a new class of peripherally acting second-generation antihistamines, most of which are labeled "nonsedating," are now available.

Four second-generation antihistamines are currently available on the market in the United States. In order of their FDA approval, these are loratadine (Claritin), cetirizine (Zyrtec), fexofenadine (Allegra), and desloratadine (Clarinex). Table 1 compares these agents in terms of dosing, potency, and side effects.

In clinical studies of chronic urticaria, the efficacy of the second-generation antihistamines is statistically superior to placebo and clinically comparable to the strongest of the first-generation agents such as hydroxyzine. The few clinical studies comparing the second-generation agents with each other in chronic urticaria show no statistically significant differences in efficacy.

The second-generation H₁ antihistamines are a heterogeneous group of compounds with lesser sedation than the first generation. Loratadine, desloratadine, and fexofenadine are nonsedating at the recommended dosage. Cetirizine is sedating at recommended dosage, but less than the first-generation agents. Only fexofenadine is totally nonsedating at any dosage above recommended levels.

What if monotherapy with a second-generation H₁ antihistamine does not adequately control the signs and symptoms of urticaria? Figure 1 summarizes a practical treatment algorithm for patients with chronic urticaria. The next step is to add another H₁ antihistamine to the original second-generation antihistamine, either an additional second-generation agent or a first-generation agent at night. The next option is to add an agent that blocks the H₂ receptors, either a tricyclic antidepressant such as doxepin (Sinequan) or an H₂ receptor antagonist.

The use of H₂ receptor antagonists is supported by the evidence that the cutaneous blood vessels possess H₂ receptors as well as the commonly recognized H₁ receptors, and these receptors are involved in the mediation of cutaneous vasodilatation and vascular permeability. Tricyclic antidepressants such as doxepin are potent H₁ and H₂ antihistaminic antagonists. Studies show doxepin to have comparable efficacy and side effects to hydroxyzine in the treatment of chronic urticaria. The usual initial dosage is 10 to 25 mg at night, which can be increased to two or three times daily if necessary. Several clinical studies show that the combination of an H₁ antihistamine and an H₂ antihistamine in both chronic urticaria and dermographism has added benefit compared to the use of an H₁ antihistamine alone. The dosage of the H₂ antihistamine is similar to that used for gastrointestinal disease—cimetidine (Tagamet), 300 mg four times daily, or ranitidine (Zantac), 150 mg twice daily.

Several mediators other than histamine can increase vascular permeability and thus cause hives. A few recent studies show that leukotriene receptor antagonists, such as montelukast (Singulair, 10 mg once daily) and zafirlukast (Accolate, 20 mg twice daily), may be beneficial in some cases of chronic urticaria.

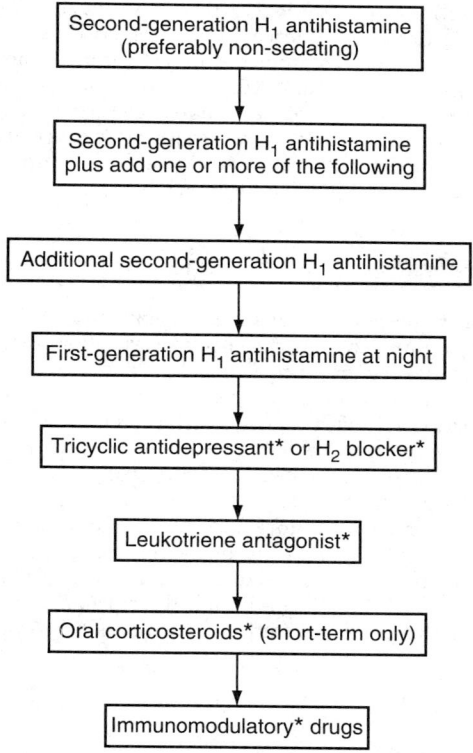

* Not FDA approved in this indication.

**FIGURE 1.** Treatment algorithm for patients with chronic urticaria.

 **CURRENT DIAGNOSIS**

The key clinical features of urticaria are the following:

- Erythematous, edematous papules or wheals, often with central clearing
- Pruritus (usually without signs of excoriation) and transient nature of individual lesions, which last 1 to 12 hours but definitely less than 24 to 48 hours.

## CURRENT THERAPY

- H₁ antihistamines remain the first choice of therapy for urticaria, both acute and chronic.
- The second-generation, so-called nonsedating antihistamines, are the treatment of choice for many patients, with urticaria because of their comparable efficacy and better safety profile compared to the first-generation antihistamines.
- Several other agents demonstrate additive value when monotherapy with H₁ antihistamines is not sufficient to control the refractory cases of chronic urticaria.

Systemic corticosteroids are sometimes indicated for the management of moderate to severe acute urticaria, pressure urticaria, or urticarial vasculitis. They have no place in extended therapy of chronic urticaria, although they may occasionally be used as a short course of therapy to break the cycle of a resistant case. A common routine is the use of prednisone beginning at 30 to 40 mg daily, tapered over 2 to 4 weeks. Systemic corticosteroids should be discontinued as soon as possible or at most maintained on an alternate-day basis.

In refractory cases of severe chronic urticaria or cases of "steroid-dependent" urticaria, other medications might be considered. Cyclosporine (Neoral, Sandimmune) in doses of 4 mg/kg per day is shown in some controlled studies to be effective in severe refractory cases of chronic urticaria or autoimmune urticaria.

In urticarial vasculitis, patients present clinically with urticaria that by skin biopsy is shown to be leukocytoclastic vasculitis. Treatment of this condition is often unsatisfactory. In addition to the use of antihistamines, other occasionally beneficial agents include nonsteroidal anti-inflammatory drugs such as indomethacin (Indocin), 25 to 50 mg three times daily; colchicine, 0.6 mg twice daily; dapsone, 50 to 300 mg daily; or hydroxychloroquine (Plaquenil), 200 to 400 mg per day. Systemic corticosteroids are also sometimes effective.

## REFERENCES

Finn AF, Kaplan AP, Fretwell R, et al: A double-blind, placebo-controlled trial of fexofenadine HCl in the treatment of chronic idiopathic urticaria. J Allergy Clin Immunol 1999;103:1071-1078.
Grattan CEH, Sabroe RA, Greaves MW: Chronic urticaria. J Am Acad Dermatol 2002;46:645-657.
Greaves M: Chronic urticaria. J Allergy Clin Immunol 2000;105: 664-672.
Kaplan AP: Chronic urticaria and angioedema. N Engl J Med 2002; 346:175-179.
Kaplan AP: Chronic urticaria: Pathogenesis and treatment. J Allergy Clin Immunol 2004;114:465-474.
Lee EE, Maibach HI: Treatment of urticaria. An evidence-based evaluation of antihistamines. Am J Clin Dermatol 2001;2:151-158.
Monroe EW: Urticaria. Curr Probl Dermatol 1993;V:113-140.
Monroe E, Finn A, Patel P, et al: Efficacy and safety of desloratadine 5 mg once daily in the treatment of chronic idiopathic urticaria: A double-blind, randomized, placebo controlled trial. J Am Acad Dermatol 2003;48:535-541.
Zuberbier T: Urticaria. Allergy 2003;58:1224-1234.

# Pigmentary Disorders

Method of
*Jacek C. Szepietowski, MD, PhD,*
*and Adam Reich, MD, PhD*

More than 1 million visits to outpatient physicians in the United States are for skin color problems. Although in most patients pigmentary disorders are not life-threatening diseases, many discolorations of the skin appear on the sun-exposed areas and thus they are visible to other people; this often evokes great embarrassment in patients suffering from dyschromias. It also implies significantly reduced quality of life in patients suffering from skin color problems.

Discoloration of the skin is sometimes a sign of an underlying serious disease (e.g., Addison's disease, incontinentia pigmenti). Therefore, patients with pigmentary disorders should be treated by the physician with great caution.

Pigmentary disorders (dyschromias) may be divided into two major groups: abnormal melanin pigmentation and deposition of pigments other than melanin in the skin.

The therapy of skin dyspigmentation often takes several months or longer. To document the progress and effectiveness of the therapy, the clinician should take photographs before and during treatment at regular intervals. A photographic record is also very helpful to show the patient the treatment's effectiveness. Pictures should be taken at the same angle and in similar lighting conditions each time.

This article concentrates on the most common pigmentary disorders, including solar lentigines, melasma, postinflammatory hyperpigmentation, drug-related dyspigmentations, and vitiligo, because they account for the vast majority of skin color problems. For discussion of less commonly observed entities, we refer all interested readers to the more specialized books.

## Solar Lentigines

### DIAGNOSIS

Solar lentigines, also called age spots, liver spots, or senile lentigines, are usually multiple, macular hyperpigmented (light to dark brown) lesions found mainly on the sun-exposed areas of skin, especially the face and forearms. They are not true lentigines but are epidermal proliferations, and they are often the first signs of photoaging of the skin. Histologically, elongated ridges with accumulation of melanin at the tips are seen; the number of melanocytes is unchanged. The incidence increases with age, affecting more than 90% of white persons older than 50 years of age. The differential diagnosis includes ephelides, lentigo simplex, melanocytic nevi, pigmented actinic keratosis, seborrheic warts, lentigo maligna, and melanoma. Whenever a question exists about the exact diagnosis, a biopsy should be performed.

### TREATMENT

#### Topical Therapy

Therapeutic approaches to the treatment of solar lentigines are divided into conservative (topical) and operative (physical) modalities. Although topical therapies take longer to achieve significant improvement than physical ones, the risk of side effects during topical treatment seems to be smaller than for ablative treatment.

A wide range of topical agents are available. The first choice is often hydroquinone or retinoic acid, either alone or in combination. Hydroquinone 2% to 4% (Ultraquin, Melanex, Glyquin) inhibits the conversion of dopa to melanin by inhibiting the activity of tyrosinase. Retinoic acid (tretinoin) (Retin A) 0.01% to 0.1% or 13-*cis*-retinoic

## CURRENT DIAGNOSIS

| Disease | Definition | Most Important Differential Diagnosis | Diagnosis |
|---|---|---|---|
| Solar lentigines | Multiple brown macules located mainly on sun-exposed skin | Ephelides, lentigo simplex, melanocytic nevi, pigmented actinic keratoses, seborrheic warts, lentigo maligna, melanoma | Based on clinical manifestation |
| Melasma | Localized facial hyper-pigmentation triggered by sunlight and hormonal changes | Phototoxic reaction to cosmetics | In cases of unclear diagnosis, perform biopsy, mainly to exclude melanoma |
| Postinflammatory hyperpigmentation | Hyperpigmentation following inflamma-tory skin diseases | Side effects of drugs that produce photo-sensitivity | Based on clinical appearance and history |
| Discoloration due to drug intake | Discoloration of skin due to drug intake | Melasma, erythema dyschromicum perstans, hyperpigmen-tation during pregnancy | Based on history and presence of lesions of underlying skin disease |
| Vitiligo | Acquired areas of hypopigmentation due to loss of functioning melanocytes from epidermis | Melasma, postinflam-matory hyperpigmen-tation, Addison's disease, Cushing's syndrome | Based on clinical appearance and history |
| | | Piebaldism, pityriasis versicolor, pityriasis alba, syphilis, scleroderma, lichen sclerosus, mycosis fungoides, postinflam-matory hypopigmenta-tion, leprosy | Based on clinical appearance and history<br>Thyroid status should be assessed to exclude hypothyroidism<br>Occasionally biopsy is necessary to exclude other diseases |

acid (isotretinoin) (Isotrex)[1] 0.05% to 0.1% causes desquamation and probably also inhibits tyrosinase transcription. Improvement in up to 80% of patients was reported in the literature.

Tazarotene 0.1% (Tazorac, Zorac), a retinoic acid derivative, and adapalene 0.1% or 0.3% (Differin),[1] a naphthoic acid derivative with potent retinoid activity, are also shown to be effective. Azelaic acid 15% to 20% (Finacea, Skinoren)[1] may be tried. Very good evidence exists also for a fixed combination of 4-hydroxyanisole 2% (mequinol) with tretinoin 0.01% (Solage cream). This preparation demonstrated a significantly better response than other topically applied treatments.

The most common adverse events from topical therapy are erythema, burning or stinging, pruritus, irritation, desquamation, and, for hydroquinone, persistent hypopigmentation when the treatment is continued over a very long period.

### Ablative Therapy

The most effective and widely used operative procedures for pigmentory disorders are cryotherapy and laser therapy.

With cryotherapy, a single freeze-thaw cycle is usually sufficient to clear the lesions. All cryotherapy techniques (liquid nitrogen, nitrous oxide, carbon dioxide) appear to be equally effective, although nitrous oxide is most commonly in use. The most frequent side effects of cryotherapy are local pain, edema, bulla formation, hypopigmentation within the lesion, and hyperpigmentation on the periphery.

Laser therapy is also widely used to treat solar lentigines. A wide range of lasers are proven effective. These include vanadate (532 nm; DioLite), argon (488-630 nm), krypton (520-530 nm; HGM K1), Nd:YAG (532 nm; neodymium-doped yttrium aluminum garnet), Q-switched ruby (694 nm), Q-switched alexandrite (755 nm), and $CO_2$ diode (10.6 μm) lasers. The treatment conditions depend on the particular type of laser.

Other ablative modalities, such as dermabrasion, intense pulse light therapy, or chemical peels, may also be tried, but they are not so well studied and should not be the treatment of first choice.

The combination of operative and topical treatments may also be of benefit. After successful therapy it is important to advise patients on regular use of sunscreens, because avoiding sun exposure can prevent development of new lesions.

## Melasma

Melasma (chloasma) is defined as localized facial hyperpigmentation triggered by sunlight and hormonal changes. About 90% of patients

---

[1]Not FDA approved for this indication.

## CURRENT THERAPY

### Solar Lentigines

- Topical therapy:
    - Mequinol 2% plus tretinoin 0.01%
    - Hydroquinone 2%
    - Tretinoin 0.01-0.1%
    - Isotretinoin[1] 0.05-0.1%
    - Tazarotene 0.1%
    - Adapalen 0.1%-0.3%
- Cryotherapy
- Laser therapy
- Sunscreens as prevention

### Melasma

- Combinational topical therapy
    - Hydroquinone 4%, retinoic acid 0.05%, topical corticosteroids
    - Chemical peels in combination with bleaching agents
- Monotherapy
    - Hydroquinone 2%-4%
    - Azelaic acid 15%-20%[2]
    - Retinoic acid 0.05%-0.1%
- Sunscreens as prevention

### Postinflammatory Hyperpigmentation

- Proper treatment of causative condition
- Topical therapy with retinoids in patients with delayed resolution
- Chemical peels or Q-switched ruby laser in refractory cases
- Sunscreens as prevention

### Medication-Related Discoloration

- Discontinuation of the treatment that provokes changes in skin color

### Vitiligo

- Narrow band ultraviolet B light (311 nm) possibly in combination with topical corticosteroids
- Alternatively, 308-nm excimer laser therapy for patients with less than 10% skin involvement

[1]Not FDA approved for this indication.

---

are women. It appears in all ethnic groups, but it is more common in people with darker skin.

The typical locations are the forehead, temples, cheeks, and upper eyelids. The color ranges from yellow-tan to brown, sometimes with a bluish hue. The lesions increase in size over time and become darker after sun exposure.

In refractory cases, cosmetic camouflage is often a good solution.

## TOPICAL THERAPY

One of the most commonly used treatments is topical hydroquinone 2% to 4%, applied alone or in combination with other topical agents (e.g., combination of hydroquinone 4%, retinoic acid 0.05%, and fluocinolone acetonide 0.01%, dexamethasone 0.1%, or triamcinolone acetonide 0.025%). The addition of retinoic acid 0.05% to 0.1% prevents the oxidation of hydroquinone, improves its epidermal penetration, and increases keratinocyte proliferation. Combination therapy with corticosteroids decreases the irritative effect of hydroquinone and inhibits melanin synthesis by decreasing the cellular metabolism. The concomitant use of sunscreens improves the response to hydroquinone.

An optimal depigmentation is achieved after 6 to 10 weeks of treatment. Prolonged use of hydroquinone often produces irritant dermatitis and hypopigmentation. Other adverse effects to hydroquinone include contact dermatitis, postinflammatory hyperpigmentation, and nail bleaching.

Other bleaching agents used to treat solar lentigines can be used to treat melasma. These include retinoic acid, isotretinoin,[1] adapalen,[1] and azelaic acid.[1] The effectiveness of 20% azelaic acid alone has been shown to be comparable with that of hydroquinone treatment. The effectiveness of azelaic acid[1] can be increased by combining it with retinoic acid 0.05% to 0.1% or with clobetasol propionate 0.05% (Temovate),[1] although very potent corticosteroids should be applied to the face with great caution, and this treatment should not last longer than 1 to 2 weeks.

Several other agents have been tried in the treatment of melasma. $N$-Acetyl-4-$S$-cysteaminylphenol is a phenol derivate with melanocytotoxic properties. In a pilot study of 12 patients, a moderate to complete improvement was noted in nearly all melasma lesions. Kojic acid 4%, which inhibits the activity of tyrosinase, combined with 5% glycolic acid showed similar effectiveness to hydroquinone 4% combined with glycolic acid 5%. However, the risk of irritation caused by therapy with kojic acid is greater than that from hydroquinone 4%.

### ABLATIVE THERAPY

Chemical peels in combination with bleaching agents seem to be the best choice for melasma. Encouraging results in melasma patients have been seen with glycolic acid 10% to 70%,[1] Jessner's solution[1] (combination of lactic acid, salicylic acid, resorcinol, and ethanol), trichloroacetic acid 10% to 25%,[1] kojic acid 10%,[1] and salicylic acid 20% to 30%.[1]

The effectiveness and the number of side effects are related to the depth of peeling. Generally, deeper peels are more effective but the risk of side effects increases significantly. Side effects include erythema, desquamation, burning, pruritus, infections, postinflammatory hyperpigmentation, and scarring.

Laser therapy may also be of benefit in the treatment of melasma, especially when combined with topical therapy.

## Postinflammatory Hyperpigmentation

Inflammatory skin lesions can remain hyperpigmented when resolving. Postinflammatory hyperpigmentation is often observed in patients with lichen planus, atopic eczema, contact eczema, acne, and photoinduced dermatoses. Ionizing and nonionizing radiation, heat, mechanical trauma, and laser therapy can also result in postinflammatory hyperpigmentation. Patients with darker skin are at greater risk for more intensive and persistent hyperpigmentation.

The first step in therapy is to prevent the development of new lesions by proper treatment of the causative disease. Patients should be advised to use adequate photoprotection to prevent the darkening of existing lesions. In many persons, postinflammatory hyperpigmentation resolves over of time, and sometimes waiting is the best option. In patients with incomplete or slow resolution, monotherapy with retinoids (retinoic acid 0.05%-0.1%, isotretinoin 0.05-0.1%,[1] tazarotene 0.1% or adapalen 0.1%[1]) seems to be the most reasonable. In case of no improvement, topical treatment options used in melasma therapy may be tried. The Q-switched ruby (694 nm) laser and chemical peels are effective in some subjects; however, these methods sometimes produce postinflammatory hyperpigmentation themselves and should be used with caution.

## Medication-Related Pigmentary Problems

Many drugs may be responsible for color problems of the skin. The list of medications that most commonly cause skin color change are listed

---

[1]Not FDA approved for this indication.

## BOX 1 Drugs and Drug Classes that Can Cause Skin Discoloration

- Hyperpigmentation (diffuse or localized) due to increase of melanin synthesis (brown to dark brown hyperpigmentation)
  - Adrenocorticotropic hormone (ACTH)
  - Antiepileptics: phenytoin (Dilantin)
  - Cytostatics: busulphan (Myleran), bleomycin (Bleoxan), cyclophosphamide (Cytoxan), 5-fluorouracil (Adrucil), doxorubicin (Adriamycin), hydroxyurea (Droxia), actinomycin D (Cosmegen), procarbazine (Matulane), mitotane (Lysodren)
  - Levodopa (Larodopa), methyldopa
  - Oral contraceptives
  - Zidovudine (Retrovir)
- Change of skin color due to deposition of drugs in the skin (the color of the skin can vary from yellow to blue to dark brown or even black)
  - Amiodarone (Cordarone) (blue-gray, brownish)
  - Antimalarias: acridine, chloroquine (Aralen), hydroxychloroquine (Plaquenil), amodiaquine[2] (brownish, brown-gray, blue-black), quinacrine[2] (yellowish)
  - Carotenoids (yellowish)
  - Chlorpromazine (Thorazine), imipramine (Tofranil) (blue-gray, brownish, grayish)
  - Clofazimine (Lamprene) ( reddish-brown)
  - Minocycline (Dynacin) (blue-gray, blue-black)
  - Mitoxantrone (Novantrone) (blue)
  - Toluidine blue (blue)
- Change of skin color due to deposition of metals
  - Arsenic (brown)
  - Bismuth (blue-gray)
  - Gold: chrysiasis (blue-gray to purplish-red)
  - Iron (brown)
  - Silver: argyria (gray, blue-gray)
- Hyperpigmentation within mucous membranes
  - Adrenocorticotropic hormone (ACTH)
  - Antimalarias: chloroquine (Aralen), amodiaquine,[2] quinacrine,[2] chinidin[2]
  - Chlorhexidine (Peridex), hexidine
  - Contraceptives
  - Cytostatics: busulfan (Myleran)
  - Metals: iron, silver, gold, bismuth, lead
  - Methyldopa
  - Minocycline (Dynacin)
  - Phenothiazines (e.g., chlorpromazine [Thorazine])
  - Zidovudine (Retrovir)
- Nail hyperpigmentation
  - Chloroquine (Aralen), hydroxychloroquine (Plaquenil)
  - Cytostatics: busulfan (Myleran), bleomycin (Blenoxane), cyclophosphamide (Cytoxan), 5-fluorouracil (Adrucil), actinomycin D (Cosmegen), melphalan (Alkeran), doxorubicin (Adriamycin), daunorubicin (Cerubidine), hydroxyurea (Hydrea)
  - Ketoconazole (Nizoral)
  - Metals: gold, silver
  - Methoxypsoralen (Oxsoralen, Uvadex)
  - Minocycline (Dynacin)
  - Phenothiazine
  - Sulfonamides
  - Zidovudine (Retrovir)
- Hypopigmentation
  - Hydroquinone (Solaquin) (topical)
  - Imatinib mesylate (Gleevec)

[2]Not available in the United States.

in Box 1. The change of skin color may be due to stimulation of melanin synthesis (e.g., methyldopa, adrenocorticotropic hormone [ACTH]) or deposition of drugs or its metabolites in the skin (e.g., tetracyclines, amiodarone). The best approach to treating the skin color changes provoked by drugs is to discontinue the drug whenever possible. Unfortunately, in many patients, skin color changes can persist for months or even years after ceasing causative treatment.

## Vitiligo

Vitiligo is the most common cause of skin hypopigmentation due to loss of functioning melanocytes, which affects about 1% of the general population. There are several types of vitiligo, including localized (focal and segmental vitiligo) and generalized forms (common, acrofacial, and universal vitiligo). Depigmentation of the skin (white patches), hair, and eyes may be observed. The etiology of vitiligo is not fully understood, but a combination of genetic predisposition, autoimmune disturbances, and neurogenic factors seems to play the major role. Although vitiligo is not a life-threatening disease, it can be a very disabling problem, especially for people with dark skin. Thus, many patients with vitiligo desire treatment from physicians because of their skin disorder, but unfortunately many doctors still handle vitiligo more as a cosmetic problem than a real disease.

Despite the many treatment options, no therapy provides truly satisfactory results. In many cases, only partial repigmentation can be achieved. So far, the best approach for vitiligo is a combination of ultraviolet (UV) irradiation and topical corticosteroids (e.g., betamethasone valerate [Diprolene],[1] clobetasole propionate [Temovate],[1] fluocinolone acetonide [Synalar][1]). However, to achieve significant improvement, the treatment should be continued for several months. Prolonged use of topical corticosteroids can cause skin atrophy, which is the most important limitation of topical therapy with corticosteroids. In case of any signs of skin atrophy, the treatment should be stopped.

An interesting alternative to topical corticosteroids are calcineurin inhibitors (tacrolimus [Protopic[1]], pimecrolimus [Elidel][1]), which, in combination with narrow-band (NB)-UVB (discussed later), showed effectiveness similar to that of corticosteroids combined with NB-UVB irradiation. However, because the long-term safety of that combination has not been studied yet, this treatment should be prescribed with caution.

Another possibility for patients who do not respond to topical corticosteroids is pseudocatalase[2] in combination with NB-UVB. Pseudocatalase, which is applied as a cream (PSCT cream), inactivates hydrogen peroxide, which was found in high levels in the skin of patients with vitiligo. Pseudocatalase has shown to be responsible for partial repigmentation of vitiligo lesions.

Regarding calcipotriol[2], (Dovonex, a vitamin D derivate) there is no sufficient evidence to support the effectiveness of this agent in vitiligo treatment, and therefore we do not recommend calcipotriol for patients with vitiligo.

NB-UVB (UVB 311 nm) irradiation appears to be a good treatment for vitiligo, especially in subjects with widely distributed lesions. PUVA (psoralens[1] with UVA irradiation) therapy showed similar effectiveness, but the risk of side effects is much greater than with NB-UVB. The UVB irradiations should be repeated 2 or 3 times per week and should last several weeks to several months (often 100 to 300 sessions in total are necessary).

A valuable alternative for NB-UVB in patients with vitiligo that encompass less than 10% of the total body surface is 308-nm excimer laser therapy, which allows selective treatment of the lesions. The treatment can be applied 1 to 3 times per week. Effectiveness is similar to that of NB-UVB and depends on the cumulative UVB dose.

Surgical procedures have been developed to treat patients who did not respond to the treatments just described. They are based on transplantation of melanocytes into hypopigmented areas from uninvolved skin. These procedures should be used only in patients with stable vitiligo, that is, patients who have not developed new lesions for at least

[2]Not available in the United States

2 years. Several treatment options already exist for transferring melanocytes. These can be divided into two main groups: implantation of an intact epidermis (epidermal blister grafts, split-thickness grafts, full-thickness grafts) and implantation of in vitro dispersed and cultured cells (monodispersed cell grafts, cultures, epidermal cell grafts). Although preliminary results are very encouraging, these methods are very time consuming and may be connected with varying side effects including scarring, infections, and hypo- and hyperpigmentation. Moreover, well-designed, controlled studies evaluating the effectiveness and safety of surgical methods are still lacking. However, these modalities seem to be very promising and they might be the treatment of choice for vitiligo in the future.

In severe and refractory cases of vitiligo, bleaching agents can be tried. These preparations are applied on normally pigmented skin around the vitiligo lesions to diminish the difference in color between involved and noninvolved skin. Cosmetic camouflage is also a good option.

## REFERENCES

Balkrishnan R, Feldman SR, McMichael AJ, et al: Racial differences in the treatment of pigmentation disorders in outpatient settings: Analysis of U.S. national practice data. J Dermatol Treat 2004;15:277-230.
Hoffer A, Hassan AS, Legat FJ, et al: Optimal weekly frequency of 308-nm excimer laser treatment in vitiligo patients. Br J Dermatol 2005;152:981-985.
Ke MS, Soriano T, Lask GP: Optimal treatment for hyperpigmentation. J Cosm Laser Ther 2006;8:7-13.
Ortonne J-P, Pandya AG, Lui H, Hexsel D: Treatment of solar lentigines. J Am Acad Dermatol 2006;54:S262-S271.
Passeron T, Ortonne J-P: What's new in hypochromy? J Dermatol Treat 2006;17:70-73.
Pianigiani E, Andreassi A, Andreassi L: Autografts and cultured epidermis in the treatment of vitiligo. Clin Dermatol 2005;23:424-429.
Rendon M, Berneburg M, Arellano I, Picardo M: Treatment of melasma. J Am Acad Dermatol 2006;54:S272-S281.
Van Geel N, Ongenae K, Haeghen YV, et al: Subjective and objective evaluation of noncultured epidermal cellular grafting for repigmenting vitiligo. Dermatology 2006;213:23-29.
Whitton ME, Ashcroft DM, Barrett CW, Gonzalez U: Interventions for vitiligo. Cochrane Database Syst Rev 2006;(1):CD003263.

# Sunburn

Method of
*Henry W. Lim, MD, and Camile Hexsel, MD*

Ultraviolet (UV) radiation is subdivided into UVC (wavelengths ranging from 270–290 nm), UVB (290–320 nm), and UVA (320–400 nm). UVA is further subdivided into UVA2 (320–340 nm) and UVA1 (340–400 nm). The stratosphere blocks most of the UVC and large amounts of the UVB rays before they reach the earth's surface; however, little or no UVA is filtered.

Sunlight at noon consists of 95% UVA and only 5% UVB. Because UVB is 1000-fold more erythemogenic compared to UVA, sunburn is predominantly a reflection of the biologic effect of UVB. UVB-induced erythema becomes visible 2 to 6 hours after irradiation, reaches a maximum in 8 to 24 hours, and fades after about 72 hours, depending on the individual's skin phototype. The erythema, which fades rapidly, is followed by delayed tanning at 72 hours.

Because UVA has long wavelengths, it penetrates deeper into the dermis compared to UVB. Approximately 10% of solar erythema is caused by UVA. UVA-induced erythema is biphasic. It becomes visible immediately after exposure, subsides by 4 hours, and reaches a second peak in 6 to 15 hours, fading within 24 to 120 hours. The predominant effect of UVA is cutaneous pigmentary alterations (pigment darkening and delayed tanning).

## CURRENT DIAGNOSIS

- Erythema, edema, and tenderness develop on sun-exposed areas 2 to 24 hours after irradiation, followed by desquamation and tanning.
- Relatively sun-protected areas, such as nasolabial folds, submental and postauricular areas, and inner aspect of arms and forearms, are spared.

Various mediators of inflammation, including histamine, eicosanoids, interleukins, tumor necrosis factor, and adhesion molecules play a role in sunburn reaction.

## Clinical Manifestations

Following excessive sun exposure, erythema, edema, warmth, and tenderness are present in the exposed areas. Pruritus may also be present. Vesicle and bullae formation with occasional erosions and ulcerations can develop within 24 to 48 hours in more severe cases. Massive UV exposure is accompanied by constitutional symptoms of headache, weakness, fever, and chills, with or without tachycardia and hypotension. The distribution of the eruption is diagnostic. It is seen exclusively in sun-exposed areas, with sharp cutoffs at areas protected by clothing. Therefore, there is accentuated involvement of the forehead, nose, chin, V area of the neck, extensor forearm, and dorsum of the hand. Areas that are naturally protected from sun exposure, such as the nasolabial folds and other skin folds, submental and postauricular areas, and the inner aspects of the arms and forearms, are spared. Resolution of the erythema is followed by desquamation and tanning, which occurs in about 1 week.

## Treatment

Because eicosanoids are a known mediator of sunburn, topical corticosteroids and nonsteroidal anti-inflammatory drugs (NSAIDs), usually used in combination, is the treatment of choice. Topical corticosteroids and NSAIDs must be started within 24 hours after the exposure and ideally within the first 4 to 6 hours. In severe cases,

## CURRENT THERAPY

- Treatment is based on symptoms and includes cool compresses, emollients, oral hydration, and rest as appropriate.
- In severe cases, topical and systemic corticosteroids and nonsteroidal anti-inflammatory drugs (NSAIDs), alone or in combination, are appropriate.
- Prevention is key to the management of sunburn (see Table 1).
- Sunscreens are regulated by the Food and Drug Administration as over-the-counter substances. They are usually a combination of more than one organic or inorganic filters that provide ultraviolet A and ultraviolet B protection.
- Cutaneous effects of excessive ultraviolet radiation are classified into acute and chronic effects. Acute effects are sunburn, vitamin D synthesis, photodermatoses, and acute photoimmunosuppression. Chronic effects are development of photoaging changes, solar lentigines, actinic keratoses, and, most importantly, skin cancers.

## TABLE 1 Preventive Measures for Sunburn

- Avoid sun exposure between 10 AM and 4 PM. If avoidance is not possible or practical, protect the skin with photoprotection measures.
- Apply broad-spectrum sunscreen with a skin-protection factor (SPF) of 15 or above.
- If possible, sunscreens should be applied at least every 2 hours and after swimming, sweating, and towel drying.
- Use of physical barriers, such as shades, wide-brimmed hats, tightly woven protective clothing, and sunglasses, is recommended.
- For individuals at risk of vitamin D insufficiency, oral vitamin D supplements are recommended.
- Photoprotection should be applied to children.
- Children younger than 6 months should be protected mainly by physical measures. Application of sunscreen to exposed areas only is probably safe.

a 7- to 10-day course of oral prednisone at a dose of 1 mg/kg, with a maximum of 80 mg, is indicated.

Oral antihistamines for treatment of sunburn have not been extensively studied, and their benefit is not completely known. A few studies reported lack of efficacy. However, they are commonly used as an antipruritic measure. Topical antihistamines should not be used because of the possibility of induction of allergic contact dermatitis.

Topical and oral antioxidants, such as polyphenols from tea, vitamin C, vitamin E, and fish oil, have been shown to decrease UV-induced inflammation in animal models and in studies involving a few human subjects. Further investigation using a larger number of subjects is needed before the benefit of antioxidants can be confirmed.

Supportive treatments, which include cool compresses, emollients, oral hydration, rest, and sun avoidance for a few days, are usually necessary. The presentation of acute sunburn is an excellent opportunity for patient education on photoprotection (see next section).

## Prevention

Preventive measures for sunburn are summarized in Table 1.

Sunscreen is an integral part of photoprotection. In the United States, UV filters are regulated as over-the-counter medications by the Food and Drug Administration (FDA). In 1999, the FDA issued a monograph listing 16 UV filters; these are the only filters that can be marketed in sunscreen products. UV filters are divided into *inorganic* (previously termed physical or nonchemical) filters and *organic* (previously termed chemical) filters. Commercially available sunscreens are often a combination of more than one agent. These agents are discussed later.

Only two inorganic filters are listed in the FDA monograph: titanium dioxide and zinc dioxide. These filters are broad-spectrum filters. The organic filters can be divided into UVA and UVB filters. The UVA filters available in the United States are the benzophenones (oxybenzone, sulisobenzone, dioxybenzone), butyl methoxydibenzoyl (avobenzone [Parsol 1789]), and meradimate (methyl anthranilate). Mexoryl and Tinosorb are UVA photostable sunscreens used in most parts of the world but are not listed in the FDA monograph. A product (Anthelios SX) containing Mexoryl SX (ecamsule) was recently approved by the FDA for marketing in the United States. UVB filters include *para*-aminobenzoic acid (PABA) derivates (PABA and padimate O or octyl dimethyl PABA), cinnamates (octinoxate and cinoxate), salicylates (octisalate or octyl salicylate, homosalate or homomenthyl salicylate, trolamine salicylate), octocrylene, and ensulizole.

## REFERENCES

Benvenuto-Andrade C, Cestari TF, Mota A, et al: Photoprotection in adolescence. Skinmed 2005;4:229-233.

Cavallo J, DeLeo VA: Sunburn. Dermatol Clin 1986;4:181-187.

Driscoll MS, Wagner RF Jr: Clinical management of the acute sunburn reaction. Cutis 2000;66:53-58.

Han A, Maibach HI: Management of acute sunburn. Am J Clin Dermatol 2004;5:39-47.

Hönigsman H: Erythema and pigmentation. Photodermatol Photoimmunol Photomed 2002;18:75-81.

Kullavanijaya P, Lim HW: Photoprotection. J Am Acad Dermatol 2005; 52: 937-958.

Lovato CY, Shoveller JA, Peters L, Rivers JK: Canadian National Survey on Sun Exposure & Protective Behaviours: Youth at leisure. Cancer Prev Control 1998;2:117-122.

Maier T, Korting HC: Sunscreens—Which and what for? Skin Pharmacol Physiol 2005;18:253-262.

Thompson L: Trying to look SUNsational? Complexity persists in using sunscreens. FDA Consum 2000;34:15-21.

# The Nervous System

## Alzheimer's Disease

Method of
*Monica Peterson Gordon, MD,*
*and L. Jaime Fitten, MD*

## Definition and Clinical Presentation

Alzheimer's disease (AD) is a progressive, neurodegenerative disorder characterized by a gradual decline of cognitive processes, such as memory, language, judgment, behavior, and global functioning. According to the *Diagnostic and Statistical Manual of Mental Disorders, Fourth Edition (DSM-IV,* 2000), dementia of the Alzheimer's type is the development of multiple cognitive deficits manifested by both memory impairment and one or more cognitive disturbances, such as aphasia, apraxia, agnosia, and disturbance in executive functioning. The deficits must cause significant impairment in social or occupational functioning and represent a decline from previous levels of functioning and cannot be due to psychiatric, systemic, substance-induced states, or delirium that cause cognitive impairment or produce the dementia syndrome. Other more detailed, research-oriented criteria also have been developed by the National Institute of Neurological and Communicative Disorders and Stroke and the Alzheimer's Disease and Related Disorders Association (NINCDS-ADRDA, 1984).

Alzheimer's disease has a gradual onset often beginning after age 60 years but most commonly after age 70 years. The rarer familial forms can have an onset as early as the fourth decade of life. Recent studies suggest that an isolated, mild but progressive forgetfulness, in the absence of functional or other cognitive impairment, signals a preclinical stage of the disease in a high percentage of cases and has been referred to as *mild cognitive impairment* of the amnestic type. Typically, AD has a 10- to 12-year progressive course. In its early stage, the disease is characterized by a declarative memory deficit that makes it difficult for patients to learn new information or recall recently experienced events. During this stage, language deficits are not always immediately apparent; however, a degree of word finding difficulty may exist. In addition, minor difficulties with visuospatial and drawing skills may be found. Mild executive dysfunction or subtle personality changes, such as reduction in spontaneity and initiative, may be present. Variations in mood may occur. As the disease progresses, memory deficits become more profound, and most of the patient's capacity for new memory formation is lost. Access to old memories becomes increasingly impaired. Language and other cognitive deficits become more pronounced, with clear

evidence of aphasia, apraxia and agnosia. The ability to manipulate concepts is lost, and thought becomes increasingly simple and concrete. During this phase, patients usually begin to exhibit behavioral and psychiatric symptoms, such as agitation, wandering, and irritability. They may experience circadian abnormalities, such as sleep cycle reversal. They may also develop psychotic symptoms such as persecutory delusions, and auditory or visual hallucinations. In the advanced stages, patients have more profound cognitive and memory deficits such that meaningful communication even at its basic level may be difficult. The loss of autonomy and the emergence of difficult to manage behavioral and psychiatric symptoms during this stage frequently lead to institutionalization. Patients invariably need full assistance for their activities of daily living and may be incontinent. Motor disturbances and difficulty walking emerge, and the patient becomes bed or chair bound in the end stages of the illness (Table 1).

Although AD accounts for more than 50% of dementias in the United States and Europe, other dementing conditions must be included in the differential diagnosis. The second and third most commonly occurring dementias are dementia with Lewy bodies and vascular dementia. Dementia with Lewy bodies can be characterized by symptoms of global cognitive impairment, including memory, and earlier neuropsychiatric disturbance than occurs in AD, with the appearance of visual hallucinations and parkinsonism. In vascular dementia, executive dysfunction is more prominent than in AD, and memory difficulties may be minimal early in the course of the illness. In contrast to AD, in which behavioral and psychiatric symptoms appear later in the progression of the illness, in vascular dementia these symptoms may appear earlier in the course. However, more than one etiologic factor may exist in patients with dementia. At autopsy, neuropathologic findings of concomitant AD and cerebrovascular disease have been reported in the brain tissue of 7% to 25% of patients who received a diagnosis of probable AD. Comorbid AD and dementia with Lewy bodies could account for as many as 20% of patients diagnosed with dementia. The frontotemporal group of dementias has a much lower incidence. These dementias occur earlier in life by a decade or two from the typical appearance of AD and often present initially with behavioral disturbances such as disinhibition, inappropriateness, apathy, and executive dysfunction. Other cognitive functions and memory become clearly impaired later in the disease process. Depression may, at times, be accompanied by cognitive impairment, producing a dementia-like clinical impression (Table 2). Elements of a diagnostic evaluation for AD are given in Table 3.

## Epidemiology

An estimated eighteen million people worldwide currently suffer from AD. This number is expected to double within the next 25 years. The current prevalence of AD in the United States has been estimated

## TABLE 1   Stages of Alzheimer's Disease

| Stage | Mild | Moderate | Severe |
|---|---|---|---|
| Folstein Mini Mental State Examination (MMSE) Score | 20–29 | 10–19 | 0–9 |
| Symptoms | Memory impairment evident<br>Early language problems (e.g., word-finding difficulty)<br>Decreased insight and scope of judgment<br>Early mood and personality changes<br>Withdrawal from more demanding activities<br>May need assistance with some instrumental ADLs | Unable to learn or recall new information<br>Worsening long-term memory and recall<br>Language, orientation, executive and other cognitive functions impaired<br>Development of behavioral and psychiatric disturbances<br>Sleep disturbance common<br>Requires help with most all instrumental ADLs | Major, broad cognitive deterioration<br>Loss of language; mutism<br>Motor disturbances and unstable gait<br>Dysphagia, frequent weight loss<br>Poor basic ADLs to complete dependence<br>Progresses to bedridden state<br>Institutionalization common |

*Abbreviation:* ADL = activity of daily living.

between 1.1 and 4.8 million cases. Although symptoms of the disease usually appear after age 60 years, the incidence of AD increases sharply and steadily after age 70 years. It has been estimated that nearly half of all people 85 years and older have some form of dementia. The National Institutes of Health estimates that, if the current trend continues, 8.5 million Americans will have AD by the year 2030.

Research has shown that the major risk factor for AD is age. Other risk factors include genetics (presenilin-1 and presenilin-2, apolipoprotein E4 status, Down syndrome), female gender, lack of education, head trauma, and myocardial infarction. The influences of presenilin on AD are based on the autosomal dominant forms of the disease, which account for 1% to 2% of all cases and result from missense mutations of genes that encode the amyloid precursor protein APP (chromosome 21) or proteolytic enzymes that cleave APP (chromosomes 1 and 14). Such mutations are associated with an increased production of β-amyloid peptide (Aβ) and result in early-onset AD. Apolipoprotein E (ApoE) status has been suggested as a risk factor for typical AD (chromosome 19). ApoE is a protein involved in cholesterol transport and has three alleles: e2, e3, and e4. Homozygous individuals who carry two ApoE e4 alleles have an increased probability of developing AD by age 85 years and do so about 10 years earlier than individuals carrying the other allelic variants. Possible mechanisms are ApoE e4 enhancement of β-amyloid deposition and amyloids reduced clearance from extracellular space.

## TABLE 2   Causes of Dementia Syndrome

| Causal Condition | Approximate Incidence* |
|---|---|
| **Common** | |
| • Alzheimer's disease | 50%–70% |
| • Dementia with Lewy bodies | 15% |
| • Vascular dementia | 10% |
| • Alzheimer's disease and vascular dementia (mixed dementia) | 10% |
| • Depression | 5%–10% |
| **Less Common** | |
| • Toxic-metabolic disorders | <5% |
| • Parkinson's disease | <5% |
| • Frontotemporal dementias | <5% |
| • Infections | <3% |
| • Space-occupying lesions | <3% |
| • Other neurodegenerations | <2% |
| • Immune inflammatory | <1% |
| • Prion diseases | <1% |

*Considerable geographic variation has been reported.

# Pathology

The brains of AD patients are atrophic with ventricular and sulcal enlargement. Histologic specimens are significant for progressive neuronal loss, β-amyloid deposition with formation of senile and neuritic plaques, and intraneuronal neurofibrillary tangles. Early changes are most abundant in the mesial temporal lobe (entorhinal cortex, hippocampus). With disease progression, parietal and frontal association areas become involved. Primary sensorimotor cortex involvement is last. The current prevailing hypothesis of AD pathogenesis contends that the initial pathogenic event is extraneuronal and intraneuronal accumulation of a misfolded protein, amyloid β-peptide, which initiates a pathogenic cascade that results in neurotoxicity, neural dysfunction, and neuronal death and culminates in the clinical syndrome of AD.

# Treatment and Management of Cognitive Symptoms

More than 30 years ago, researchers first showed decreased cholinergic markers, such as choline acetyltransferase, in the cortex of AD patients. Others subsequently demonstrated loss of basal forebrain cholinergic neurons innervating neocortex and hippocampus in AD patients. These collective findings were the basis of a cholinergic hypothesis of AD that resulted in efforts to treat AD through a variety of cholinergic interventions. Cholinesterase inhibitor (ChE-I) therapy in use today evolved from those early efforts and received FDA approval based on its good tolerability and modest efficacy. ChE-Is are believed to increase acetylcholine signaling in damaged cortical areas where neurodegeneration has occurred. Three ChE-Is are in use today: donepezil (Aricept), rivastigmine (Exelon), and galantamine (Razadyne). Tacrine (Cognex), the ChE-I first approved in 1993, is rarely used today because of its hepatotoxicity. In blinded controlled studies, donepezil treatment resulted in cognitive and global functioning benefits for up to 1 year in patients with mild to moderate AD. Patients treated with rivastigmine for 6 months also showed improvement in cognitive and global functioning. Well-controlled trials of galantamine in AD have shown comparable cognitive gains for patients treated for 5 to 6 months. More recent work has indicated that ChE-Is appear to reduce the rate of cognitive decline for periods of 6 months to 1 year or possibly longer, rather than producing a significant cognitive improvement after the start of therapy. All three agents have comparable efficacy, although their side-effect profiles and dosing schedules vary (Table 4).

Donepezil (Aricept) has an elimination half-life of about 70 hours, needing only once-daily dosing. A starting dose of 5 mg/day is given orally for 4 to 6 weeks. The dose is then increased to a maximum of

## TABLE 3 Elements of a Dementia Evaluation

### Historical Information
- Symptoms (onset, duration of cognitive, psychiatric, behavioral, and personality changes).
- Functional status (driving, cooking, finances, social contacts, other basic and instrumental activities of daily living).
- Past history (medical, neurologic, psychiatric, social functioning, family history of major medical and neuropsychiatric disorders).
- Medications.

### Mental Status Examination
- Evaluation of behavior at interaction, mood, thought content and process, psychosis, insight, and judgment, as well as cognitive evaluation that includes orientation, attention, memory, language, calculations, visuospatial abilities, executive functions.
- Folstein Mini Mental State Examination and the Clock Drawing Test are useful brief instruments.
- Neuropsychologic testing is occasionally indicated in some cases for diagnostic clarity.

### Review of Symptoms
- Falls, constipation, urinary incontinence, sensorial deficits, dentition, pain, sleep difficulties.

### Physical and Neurologic Examination
#### Laboratory evaluation
- Complete blood cell count, standard chemistry panel, vitamin $B_{12}$, folate, thyroid-stimulating hormone, neurosyphilis treponemal screen (e.g., *Treponema pallidum* hemagglutination assay), urinalysis.
- Additional tests may be indicated under specific circumstances.

#### Neuroimaging
- Magnetic resonance imaging frequently used for exclusion of other conditions and for diagnostic clarity
- Positron emission tomography may be indicated when frontotemporal dementia is in the differential diagnosis.

10 mg/day as tolerated. Donepezil is taken with or without food but preferably in the morning because vivid dreams may disturb sleep in some patients. Rivastigmine (Exelon) is given twice daily because of its shorter elimination half-life. Dosing starts at 1.5 mg twice daily and is titrated upward slowly, every 2 weeks, to a maximum of 6 to 12 mg/day. If rivastigmine is taken with food and titration occurs in 1.5-mg twice daily increments over 4-week intervals, cholinergic side effects are reduced. Dose reduction is suggested in patients with renal or hepatic impairment. Galantamine (Razadyne) also requires twice-daily dosing. Starting dose is 4 mg twice daily. After 4 weeks, the dose is slowly augmented over several weeks to a maximum of 12 mg twice daily if tolerated. Dose reduction is advised in patients with moderate renal or hepatic impairment. The total dose should not exceed 16 mg/day. Galantamine is contraindicated in patients with severe hepatic or renal impairment.

The side effects of all ChE-Is are similar. However, some agents may be better tolerated than others. The most common side effects are nausea, vomiting, diarrhea, anorexia, weight loss, vivid dreams, insomnia, and muscle cramps. Donepezil appears to have a lesser frequency of gastrointestinal side effects than do galantamine or rivastigmine. In all three agents, these side effects tend to be dose related and transient. The vagotonic effects of ChE-I therapy can cause bradycardia. Therefore, patients with a history of sick sinus syndrome, supraventricular tachycardia, congestive heart failure, and acute coronary artery disease should be monitored. The patient's ability to tolerate side effects is a major factor affecting medication adherence. However, an optimal ChE-I medication trial should consist of at least 3 to 4 months of treatment at the maximally tolerated dose prior to discontinuation of therapy for inadequate response, because that period of time is needed to establish that the patient has continued to deteriorate at the

## TABLE 4 Pharmacologic Treatment of Cognitive Impairment

| Medication | Disease Stage | Recommended Dose | Half-Life | Main Side Effects | Hepatic Cytochrome P-450 Metabolism |
|---|---|---|---|---|---|
| Donepezil (Aricept) | Mild to moderate | Start 5 mg qd for 4–6 wk then increase to 10 mg as tolerated | 70 hr | Nausea, diarrhea, insomnia, hypertension/hypotension, bradycardia, urinary obstruction | Partial inhibition by ketoconazole, quinidine Induction by carbamazepine |
| Galantamine (Razadyne, previously Reminyl) | Mild to moderate | Start 4 mg bid for 4 wk and taper slowly to a maximum of 12 mg bid | 7 hr | Nausea, vomiting, diarrhea, bradycardia, syncope Contraindicated in severe hepatic or renal disease | Partial inhibition by ketoconazole, paroxetine Clearance reduced by fluoxetine, quinidine, amitriptyline |
| Rivastigmine (Exelon) | Mild to moderate | Start 1.5 mg bid and increase slowly every 2 wk to a final dose of 6–12 mg/day | 1.5 hr | Dizziness, vomiting, headache, diarrhea, anorexia, abdominal pain; titrate slowly with hepatic or renal disease | Not affected by a wide variety of commonly used medications |
| Memantine (Namenda) | Moderate to severe | Start 5 mg qd and after 1 wk can be increased in 5-mg increments to a maximum of 20 mg daily | 60–80 hr | Hypertension, constipation, dizziness, hallucinations, headache, Stevens-Johnson syndrome | Predominantly renal metabolism and clearance |

expected nontreated rate. If the patient does not respond to one ChE-I, another can be tried.

In 2003, memantine (Namenda), a noncholinergic-related N-methyl-D-aspartate (NMDA) receptor antagonist, was approved by the FDA for treatment of moderate to severe AD based on the results of two controlled studies involving more than 600 moderately to severely demented AD patients. The first 28-week study involved memantine alone versus placebo. Results demonstrated that memantine treatment was of moderate benefit to patients in terms of both cognitive and functional measures. For 12 weeks, cognition remained stable in the memantine group then declined afterward; however, significantly less impairment was noted at endpoint in the memantine group than in the placebo group. The second study evaluated memantine in AD patients already receiving donepezil. The patients treated with donepezil plus memantine showed a modest but better therapeutic effect in cognition sustained from baseline than did the donepezil with placebo group. Treatment of mildly demented AD patients with memantine has produced less robust results, and memantine is not currently FDA approved for this use (see Table 4).

Memantine should be started at 5 mg once daily for 1 week. It can be increased in 5-mg increments per week to a maximum dose of 20 mg/day. It is then best given 10 mg twice daily. Memantine is generally well tolerated and can be taken with or without food. Because of its partial renal clearance, dosage reduction is recommended for patients with significant renal insufficiency. Potential side effects include headache, agitation, confusion, constipation, dizziness, hallucinations, and insomnia. Memantine can be used as monotherapy in patients with moderate to severe AD who do not respond to or tolerate ChE-Is. A decreased rate of cognitive decline for a period of time, as with ChE-Is, appears to be the main therapeutic effect. Best use of memantine may be in combination with a ChE-I, as benefits of the combination appear to be superior to that of either drug used alone.

# Treatment of Behavioral and Psychiatric Symptoms

Patients with AD frequently develop behavioral and psychiatric symptoms in addition to cognitive impairments. These symptoms become more prominent as the disease progresses and often lead to institutionalization. When dementia is well established, patients commonly develop some form of agitation (excessive purposeless activity), either motoric or verbal, during the day or evening hours. They may become intermittently irritable and aggressive with family members. Nearly half will develop psychosis, either as hallucinations (auditory or visual) or simple delusions of infidelity or persecution, such as believing someone is stealing from them. They may manifest apathy (loss of motivation) and disordered mood with symptoms of depression, anxiety, and irritability. Optimal management is both nonpharmacologic and pharmacologic.

## NONPHARMACOLOGIC MANAGEMENT

Often patients are confused and agitated as a consequence of temporal-spatial disorientation and need to be reassured and redirected with regularity. Environmental cues, such as the posted date and visible familiar objects and pictures of loved ones, may help. Agitated and/or aggressive behavior may be exacerbated by environmental triggers, such as insufficient (e.g., poor daytime lighting) or excessive (too much activity) sensorial stimulation. These elements can and should be adjusted. It is important to educate the patient, family, and staff (if the patient is institutionalized) regarding target behavioral symptoms and the environmental and behavioral techniques useful in their management. Implementation of a management plan can then proceed with better consistency and effectiveness wherever the patient resides. Managing AD patients is a large burden for caregivers. According to studies, caregivers have a 52% prevalence of psychiatric symptoms compared with 15% to 20% in the general population. As part of an overall management plan, caregivers will need support through reassurance, education, and referral to important community resources, such as the Alzheimer Association, caregiver support groups, day care centers, and social or legal services.

## PHARMACOLOGIC TREATMENT

Pharmacologic management of behavioral and mood symptoms depends on accurate analysis of problem moods and behaviors and should be individualized. Broadly speaking, depression and anxiety are managed with newer antidepressants (selective serotonin reuptake inhibitors [SSRIs], mirtazapine [Remeron], trazodone [Desyrel]). Dementia-related psychotic symptoms and aggression are treated with atypical antipsychotics.[1] Pure agitation without aggression can be treated with trazodone,[1] buspirone[1] (BuSpar), SSRIs,[1] or anticonvulsants.[1] Newer studies also suggest that cholinesterase inhibitors and memantine (Namenda) may be helpful in the management of this condition. Certain benzodiazepines are occasionally a useful adjunct for short-term treatment of anxiety-driven agitation or anxiety with depression (Table 5).

---

[1]Not FDA approved for this indication.

## TABLE 5 Pharmacologic Treatment of Behavioral and Mood Symptoms

| Medication | Indication | Recommended Dose | Main Side Effects | Caution |
|---|---|---|---|---|
| **Antidepressants** | | | | |
| Citalopram (Celexa) | Depression, agitation,[1] irritability,[1] anxiety[1] | 10–60 mg/day | Headache, nausea, hyponatremia, insomnia, diarrhea, somnolence | |
| Sertraline (Zoloft) | Depression, agitation,[1] irritability,[1] anxiety[1] | 50–200[3] mg/day | Headache, nausea, hyponatremia, insomnia, diarrhea, somnolence | Adjust dose in hepatic impairment |
| Mirtazapine (Remeron) | Depression, agitation,[1] irritability,[1] anxiety[1] | 15–45[3] mg/day | Somnolence, increased appetite, arrhythmia, hypercholesterolemia agranulocytosis | |
| Venlafaxine (Effexor) | Depression, agitation,[1] irritability,[1] anxiety[1] | 50–300 mg/day | Hypertension, hyponatremia, nausea, headache, nervousness, dizziness | |

[1]Not FDA approved for this indication.
[3]Exceeds dosage recommended by the manufacturer.

## TABLE 5  Pharmacologic Treatment of Behavioral and Mood Symptoms—cont'd

| Medication | Indication | Recommended Dose | Main Side Effects | Caution |
|---|---|---|---|---|
| Trazodone (Desyrel) | Agitation alone,[1] mild anxiety,[1] insomnia[1] | 25–200 mg/day | Somnolence, dizziness, headache, nausea, priapism, orthostasis | |

### Antipsychotics

| Medication | Indication | Recommended Dose | Main Side Effects | Caution |
|---|---|---|---|---|
| Haloperidol (Haldol) | Acute psychosis with agitation or aggression[1] | 0.25–3 mg/day, IM, if oral dosing not possible | Hypertension, hypotension, tachycardia, movement disorders | Parkinsonism, tardive dyskinesia, neuroleptic malignant syndrome |
| Quetiapine (Seroquel) | Subacute or chronic psychosis without or with agitation or aggression[1] | 25–200 mg/day PO | Weight gain, dizziness, headache, agitation, sedation | $QT_c$ prolongation possible, glucose intolerance, increased stroke risk? Monitor |
| Risperidone (Risperdal) | Subacute or chronic psychosis without or with agitation or aggression[1] | 0.25–2 mg/day PO | Hypotension, hyperglycemia, insomnia, agitation, headache, weight gain, extrapyramidal symptoms | $QT_c$ prolongation possible, glucose intolerance, increased stroke risk? Monitor |
| Olanzapine (Zyprexa) | Subacute chronic psychosis without or with agitation or aggression[1] | Start 2.5–5 mg/day PO, increase by 2.5 mg/wk to a maximum of 10–15 mg/day | Hyperglycemia, headache, agitation, dizziness, dyspepsia, hypotension, weight gain, somnolence | $QT_c$ prolongation possible, glucose intolerance, type 2 diabetes mellitus?, increased stroke risk? Monitor |

### Anticonvulsants

| Medication | Indication | Recommended Dose | Main Side Effects | Caution |
|---|---|---|---|---|
| Divalproex (Depakote) | Aggression with or without agitation or irritability[1] | Start 125 mg/day and may increase slowly to a maximum of 1500 mg/day | Liver toxicity, pancreatitis, thrombocytopenia, somnolence, dizziness, diarrhea, tremors, nausea, vomiting | Adjust dose for hepatic and renal impairment |

### Benzodiazepines and Other Anxiolytics

| Medication | Indication | Recommended Dose | Main Side Effects | Caution |
|---|---|---|---|---|
| Lorazepam (Ativan) | Anxiety | 1–2 mg/day | Memory impairment, sedation, dizziness, falls | For short-term use only while concomitant antidepressants are titrated to effectiveness |
| Oxazepam (Serax) | Anxiety | 15 mg/day | Hepatic dysfunction, leukopenia, dizziness | For short-term use only while concomitant antidepressants are titrated to effectiveness |
| Buspirone (BuSpar) | Anxiety, agitation only[1] | 30–60 mg/day | Dizziness, sedation | |

[1]Not FDA approved for this indication.

873

## CURRENT DIAGNOSIS

| Criteria | Description |
| --- | --- |
| Intellectual functioning | Development of multiple cognitive deficits, including memory impairment plus one or more of the following attributes:<br>■ Aphasia (language disturbance)<br>■ Agnosia (impaired recognition)<br>■ Apraxia (impaired motor activity)<br>■ Executive dysfunction (difficulties in planning and organization) |
| Functional capacity | Cognitive deficits cause significant impairment in social, occupational, or usual activities of daily living and represent a significant decline from a previous level of functioning. |
| Course of symptoms | Symptoms have a gradual or insidious onset, and patient experiences a continuous cognitive decline. |
| Absence of delirium | Cognitive deficits do not occur solely during the course of delirium. |
| Other neurologic and medical conditions excluded | Cognitive defects described are not caused by other central nervous system disorders that cause progressive deficits in memory and cognition (e.g., cerebrovascular disease, Huntington's or Parkinson's disease, subdural hematoma, normal-pressure hydrocephalus, brain tumor) or by systemic conditions known to cause the dementia syndrome (e.g., hypothyroidism, vitamin $B_{12}$ or folic acid deficiency, hypercalcemia, neurosyphilis, HIV infection) |
| Psychiatric conditions excluded | Disturbance is not caused by another major psychiatric disorder (e.g., schizophrenia, major depression, substance abuse) |

## CURRENT THERAPY

- If delirium, acute psychosis, depression, or major aggression/agitation is present initially, treat this condition first and then re-evaluate.
- If no acute psychosis, depression, or major behavioral perturbation is evident, treat cognitive symptoms with a memory enhancer such as a ChE-I or memantine (Namenda; an N-methyl-D-aspartate receptor antagonist) as appropriate for disease stage.
- Mild Alzheimer's disease: ChE-I—donepezil (Aricept), galantamine (Razadyne), or rivastigmine (Exelon).
- Moderate Alzheimer's disease: ChE-I and/or memantine (Namenda).
- Severe Alzheimer's disease: ChE-I and/or memantine.
- Consider nonpharmacologic interventions for behavioral and mood problems.
- Treat persistent psychiatric and behavioral symptoms as follows:
  - Acute psychosis with agitation/aggression: Haloperidol[1] (Haldol)
  - Subacute, chronic psychosis with or without aggression/agitation: Atypical antipsychotic
  - Depression, irritability: Second generation non-TCA antidepressant
  - Agitation alone: Trazodone[1] (Desyrel), second generation non-TCA antidepressant, nonpharmacologic intervention
  - Anxiety: Atypical antidepressant with or without short-term benzodiazepine, trazodone,[1] or buspirone[1] (BuSpar)
  - Insomnia: Trazodone,[1] short-term only benzodiazepine, or similar hypnotic

[1]Not FDA approved for this indication.
*Abbreviation:* ChE-I = cholinesterase inhibitor.

Depressive symptoms requiring treatment (e.g., withdrawal, appetite loss, worsening sleep, negativism, irritability, somatization) are more common than the classic major depressive syndrome in demented AD patients. Because of their safety profile, tolerability, and efficacy, newer antidepressants, such as the SSRIs or venlafaxine (Effexor; 50–300 mg/day) and mirtazapine (15–45 mg/day), are the mainstay of treatment. The SSRIs have comparable efficacy, but agents with low drug–drug interactions and low side-effect profiles, such as citalopram (Celexa; 10–60 mg/day) and sertraline (Zoloft; 50–200 mg/day), are preferred. Onset of action of the antidepressants may require 1 to several weeks. Patience and dose adjustments are needed. Treatment of the first episode of depression should last 1 year at the therapeutic dose before the antidepressant is tapered off. In a patient with a history of episodes of depression, therapy should be maintained indefinitely. It is useful to match the side-effect profile of the antidepressant with the patient's main symptoms. For example, for an inactive, withdrawn patient, an activating antidepressant such as venlafaxine or sertraline may be useful. On the other hand, for an anxious patient who is not sleeping or eating well, a calming agent that enhances appetite and can increase evening sedation, such as mirtazapine, may be a preferable initial choice.

The newer antidepressants are also effective in treating anxiety and irritability, both of which commonly occur in AD, although the onset of action of these agents may not be immediate. When relief of anxiety is needed more quickly, a benzodiazepine of moderately short duration of action, such as oxazepam (Serax; 15 mg/day) or lorazepam (Ativan; 1–2 mg/day), can be initiated at the same time an antidepressant at low dose is started. Over a period of 2 to 3 weeks, as the antidepressant dose is titrated upward, the benzodiazepine is tapered off to reduce exposure to possible benzodiazepine side effects, such as memory loss, falls, confusion, and behavioral disinhibition. The antidepressant should now exert a greater anxiolytic effect. For patients with mild anxiety, trazodone[1] (25–200 mg/day) or buspirone (BuSpar) can be tried.

The newer, atypical antipsychotics are helpful in treating psychosis alone and psychosis associated with aggression/agitation. These medications have demonstrated some utility in treating irritability and aggression but not agitation alone. Patients with acute psychosis who are unable to take oral medication may respond to haloperidol (Haldol) intramuscularly 0.25 to 3 mg/day, although side effects are more prominent with this conventional antipsychotic. Patients with subacute and chronic psychotic symptoms can be treated with oral risperidone[1] (Risperdal; 0.25–2 mg/day), quetiapine[1] (Seroquel; 25–200 mg/day), or olanzapine[1] (Zyprexa; 2.5–15 mg/day). Movement disorders, such as parkinsonism and tardive dyskinesia, are less frequent with atypical antipsychotics than with conventional ones. In addition to the use of atypical antipsychotics for aggression with psychosis, aggression alone or with irritability can be treated with SSRIs having low drug–drug interactions, such as citalopram[1] (Celexa; 10–60 mg/day) or sertraline[1] (Zoloft; 50–200 mg/day), with mirtazapine[1] (Remeron; 7.5–45 mg/day), or with anticonvulsants, such as divalproex[1] (Depakote; 125–1500 mg/day). Persistent male sexual aggression may benefit from treatment with medroxyprogesterone[1] (Depo-Provera) intramuscularly 150 mg biweekly or monthly. Agitation alone without psychosis or aggression may respond to environmental adjustments in combination with trazodone[1] (25–200 mg/day), buspirone[1] (30–60 mg/day), or a ChE-I. Apathy may improve in some patients with standard doses of ChE-Is.

Caution is necessary when prescribing most medications to the elderly because of their sensitivity to adverse reactions. Specifically, newer antipsychotic medications can cause $QT_c$ prolongation, weight gain, hyperlipidemia, increased glucose resistance, and type 2 diabetes mellitus. They have even been associated with a possible small increase in stroke or death risk in exposed demented populations, although additional prospective studies are needed to reach more definitive conclusions. When prescribing atypical antipsychotics to patients with a vulnerable cardiac or metabolic status, a baseline and treatment electrocardiogram, lipid panel, chemistry panel, and weight measurement should be performed, with subsequent monitoring as indicated.

In refractory patients, combination therapies may be necessary, and in such cases pharmacologic agents belonging to different classes should be combined. However, certain cautions should be observed. Only one change should be introduced at a time, and lower initial doses should be used. Avoid olanzapine (Zyprexa) and clozapine (Clozaril) in patients with diabetes. The following combinations are best avoided: clozapine (Clozaril) and carbamazepine (Tegretol); ziprasidone (Geodon) and tricyclic antidepressants; conventional antipsychotics and fluoxetine (Prozac); and conventional antipsychotics and lithium, divalproex (Depakote), or lamotrigine (Lamictal). However, divalproex and risperidone (or haloperidol) is an acceptable combination. Key therapeutic points are summarized in Current Therapy.

---

[1]Not FDA approved for this indication.

---

# Sleep Disorders

Method of
*David N. Neubauer, MD*

In recent years there has been increasing recognition of the high prevalence and significant consequences of sleep disorders and the effects of insufficient sleep. The National Sleep Foundation estimates that about 70 million Americans have problems with their sleep. Research has documented various medical and psychiatric comorbidities with sleep disorders and how sleep disturbances can increase the risk of other disorders. While the number of sleep specialists and sleep disorder centers continue to grow, primary care medicine remains the frontline in the clinical evaluation and treatment of sleep disorders. This chapter provides a broad overview of the common sleep disorders encountered in clinical practice. Sleep-disordered breathing is covered in greater detail in the article on Sleep Apnea.

The foundation of understanding sleep disorders is an appreciation of the two primary processes normally regulating the sleep-wake cycle. A *homeostatic* sleep drive determines the amount of sleep we need for alertness and vigilance during our waking hours. For most individuals, a daily sleep total of approximately 8 hours is ideal. Insufficient sleep,

whether acute or chronic, leads to increased sleepiness. The ability to achieve sufficient sleep at night and subsequent wakefulness throughout the daytime and evening is optimized by the *circadian* process, which is coordinated through the suprachiasmatic nucleus in the anterior hypothalamus with input from the photoperiod. The circadian process generates maximum arousal in the evening to offset the homeostatic sleepiness that evolves throughout the day. These two processes together promote sustained wakefulness for about 16 hours and sleep for about 8 hours in synchrony with the day-night cycle.

The homeostatic and circadian processes describe the normal pattern of alertness and sleepiness, but they also may help explain clinical problems associated with insufficient sleepiness (insomnia) and excessive sleepiness. Daytime or evening napping reduces the homeostatic sleep drive available to promote sleep onset and maintenance during a desired nighttime sleep period. This may lead a patient to complain of insomnia. Difficulty falling asleep and remaining asleep also may result from attempts to sleep outside the normal photoperiod-reinforced circadian zone of increased sleep propensity. Sleep difficulty associated with shift work is a typical example.

## Symptoms of Sleep Disorders

The evaluation of patients with sleep difficulties should begin with a thorough history of their sleep-related symptoms. How long has it been a problem? Is it intermittent, or a daily or nightly problem? What time of the day or night do the symptoms occur? Are there obvious precipitants or consequences? Is there impairment in normal functioning? What have been the typical sleep-wake hours for the individual. and what is the current pattern? Are there medical or psychiatric disorders or medications that might be influencing the sleep-related symptoms? Input from a bed partner or other informant can be invaluable. Having patients maintain sleep logs can offer a concise view of the patterns of their sleep disturbances and help demonstrate the effects of treatment strategies. Questionnaires and scales (e.g., Epworth Sleepiness Scale, Pittsburgh Sleep Quality Index) can be useful for screening patients for possible sleep disturbances.

Symptoms of sleep disorders may include an inability to sleep at desired times (insomnia), an inability to remain fully awake and attentive at desired times (excessive sleepiness), snoring and fluctuations in breathing patterns during sleep, uncomfortable sensations prior to sleep onset, abnormal movements before and during sleep, and abnormal behaviors emanating from sleep (parasomnias). Although insomnia, excessive daytime sleepiness, and parasomnias are the primary symptom clusters, individual patients may experience overlapping symptoms. For instance, sleep-disordered breathing can be associated with disrupted nighttime sleep and excessive daytime sleepiness.

## Insomnia

*Insomnia* is difficulty falling asleep or remaining asleep when people expect to be able to sleep and when there is an opportunity for them to be in bed sleeping. An insomnia disorder persists for at least 1 month and is associated with daytime impairment. Insomnia affects about 30% of the general adult population intermittently and about 10% on a chronic basis. Insomnia is a problem for more than half of patients with chronic medical conditions. Insomnia may occur idiopathically or may result from distressing circumstances; psychological conditioning; environmental factors; jet lag and shift work schedules; medication effects; and medical, psychiatric, and sleep disorders.

Treatment of insomnia may require multiple strategies that involve correction of sleep hygiene problems, bedtime routine and schedule modifications, cognitive and other psychotherapeutic techniques, strategically timed exposure to bright light, and use of medications. Additionally, optimizing the management of comorbid conditions (e.g., major depression, chronic pain, sleep-disordered breathing, and congestive heart failure) may be necessary for sleep quality improvements. General sleep hygiene recommendations are listed in Table 1. Delaying bedtime may help patients spending excessive frustrating

## TABLE 1 Sleep Hygiene Recommendations

- Try to maintain a regular sleep-wake schedule.
- Avoid afternoon or evening napping.
- Allow yourself enough time in bed for adequate sleep duration (e.g., 11 PM to 7 AM).
- Develop a relaxing evening routine for the hours approaching bedtime.
- Spend some idle time reflecting on the day's events before going to bed. Make a list of concerns and how some might be resolved.
- Reserve the bed for sleep and sex. Do not do homework, pay bills, or engage in serious domestic discussions in bed.
- Avoid evening alcohol.
- Avoid caffeine in the afternoon and evening.
- Minimize annoying noise, light, or temperature extremes.
- Consider a light snack before bedtime.
- Exercise regularly, but not late in the evening.
- Do not try harder and harder to fall asleep. If you are unable to sleep, do something else out of bed and in another room, if possible.
- Avoid smoking.

wakeful time in bed. Cognitive therapy techniques may be especially helpful for the patients who catastrophize about their sleep problems.

Significant advances in the pharmacologic treatment of insomnia have been made in recent years. Patients may experience improved sleep with sedating medications prescribed for comorbid conditions (e.g., antidepressants). The medications indicated for treatment of insomnia (Table 2) include both traditional benzodiazepines and newer nonbenzodiazepine hypnotics. All of these hypnotics function through enhancing the inhibitory responses of γ-aminobutyric acid (GABA)-A receptors. The newer medications have pharmacokinetic and pharmacodynamic characteristics that improve their safety profile. Ramelteon (Rozerem), a nonsedating, selective melatonin receptor agonist that targets activity of the circadian system, also is approved for treatment of insomnia.

The duration of action of the newer generation hypnotics ranges from the very short-acting zaleplon (Sonata) to the progressively longer-acting zolpidem (Ambien), modified-release zolpidem (Ambien CR), and eszopiclone (Lunesta). Food and Drug Administration (FDA) approval is anticipated for immediate-release indiplon,* which will join this class of relatively short-acting hypnotics.

---

*Investigational drug in the United States.

## TABLE 2 Medications Indicated for Treatment of Insomnia

| Medication | Available Doses (mg) | Duration of Action |
|---|---|---|
| **Hypnotic** | | |
| Benzodiazepines: | | |
| Estazolam (ProSom) | 1, 2 | Intermediate-long |
| Flurazepam (Dalmane) | 15, 30 | Long |
| Quazepam (Doral) | 7.5, 15 | Long |
| Temazepam (Restoril) | 7.5, 15, 22.5, 30 | Intermediate |
| Triazolam (Halcion) | 0.125, 0.25 | Short-intermediate |
| Nonbenzodiazepines: | | |
| Eszopiclone (Lunesta) | 1, 2, 3 | Intermediate |
| Zaleplon (Sonata) | 5, 10 | Very short |
| Zolpidem (Ambien) | 5, 10 | Short |
| Zolpidem (Ambien CR) extended-release | 6.25, 12.5 | Short-intermediate |
| **Melatonin Receptor Agonist** | | |
| Ramelteon (Rozerem) | 8 | Short |

The pattern of patients' sleep disturbances influences the selection of hypnotics. Exclusive sleep-onset difficulty may be treated adequately with a very short-acting medication; however, most insomnia patients have combined difficulty falling asleep and maintaining sleep. Accordingly, moderately short-acting medications that do not cause residual morning sedation generally are optimal.

Until recently, all prescription sleep-promoting medications were approved for short-term treatment of insomnia; however, beginning in 2005 the FDA began approving sleep-promoting agents simply for treatment of insomnia without the implied short-term restriction. Whereas the majority of patients taking hypnotic medications require help with their sleep only for limited periods of time, others with chronic insomnia have experienced continued improvement in nighttime sleep and daytime functioning with longer-term nightly or intermittent hypnotic use. All of the currently approved benzodiazepine receptor agonist hypnotics remain Schedule IV controlled substances. In contrast, ramelteon (Rozerem) is not classified as a controlled substance.

## Circadian Rhythm Disorders

Although the circadian system typically promotes nighttime sleep from approximately 10 to 11 PM until about 6 to 7 AM, many individuals have long-standing tendencies to experience either earlier or later sleep propensity zones. An individual's circadian phase can contribute to complaints of insomnia or excessive sleepiness, although this influence often is not recognized. Adolescents and young adults are more likely to have later sleep propensities, whereas elderly individuals tend to have an earlier onset and offset of sleepiness. People with an *advanced sleep phase* are early birds; they become sleepy earlier in the evening and then are unable to sleep later in the morning. They may complain of persistent early morning awakening as well as daytime fatigue and sleepiness. Night owls with a *delayed circadian phase* have difficulty falling asleep early and tend to sleep later in the morning. This can represent a significant clinical problem. Patients may report sleep-onset insomnia or excessive daytime sleepiness, particularly during the morning hours. Melatonin receptor agonists given prior to bedtime also may help advance and stabilize the sleep onset and morning awakening times for delayed sleep phase patients. Evening bright light exposure may help patients with a long-term predisposition for early evening sleepiness and bothersome early morning awakening. Conversely, bright light exposure upon awakening may help those with a night-owl pattern.

## Excessive Daytime Sleepiness

Excessive sleepiness during waking hours is a major public health problem most evident in associated workplace and vehicular accidents, injuries, and fatalities. Excessively sleepy patients typically complain of sleepiness for major portions of the day and report a high propensity for falling asleep during sedentary activities. In severe cases, patients may fall asleep while driving, conversing, or attending important meetings. Chronic sleepiness may lead to educational, occupational, and social difficulties. The most common cause of excessive sleepiness is insufficient sleep, whether due to work schedules or lifestyle choices. Sedating medications and other substances can lead to excessive sleepiness. Emerging evidence suggests that sleep deprivation may contribute to metabolic and immune impairment, even in healthy young individuals.

Patients complaining of difficulty remaining awake during the daytime should be evaluated at a sleep center unless there is an obvious and reversible cause. Sleep laboratory testing includes the standard nighttime polysomnography and possibly a series of daytime nap opportunities that objectively assess sleep onset latency and sleep stages. The key sleep disorders associated with excessive daytime sleepiness are narcolepsy, hypersomnolence disorders, and sleep-disordered breathing. To a limited extent, insomnia and other disorders causing frequent arousals and awakenings, or awakenings with difficulty returning to sleep, may contribute to daytime sleepiness.

The latter might include restless legs syndrome, periodic limb movement disorder, and parasomnias.

## Narcolepsy

Although *narcolepsy* is the classic disorder of excessive sleepiness, it affects only about 0.05% of the population. It is characterized by persistent sleepiness and difficulty maintaining attention. Symptoms typically begin to evolve by the late teens and continue through life. In addition to disturbed daytime wakefulness and nighttime sleep, narcolepsy patients have symptoms reflecting dysregulation of the characteristics of rapid eye movement (REM) sleep. *Cataplexy* is the loss of postural muscle tone that occurs during waking and is precipitated by heightened emotion, such as anxiety or laughter. The effects may range from a barely noticeable jaw drop to the patient lying on the ground awake but unable to move for up to several minutes. *Sleep paralysis* occurs at the transition to sleep when a person becomes aware of a complete inability to move any muscles voluntarily. It resolves spontaneously within minutes. Cataplexy and sleep paralysis both involve the intrusion of the normal paralysis that accompanies REM sleep; however, it occurs at an abnormal time. Narcolepsy patients also are more likely to experience *hypnagogic hallucinations*, which are dreamlike experiences occurring at sleep onset. Sleep laboratory testing confirms the diagnosis.

Treatment of narcolepsy begins with the establishment of therapeutic goals, typically including maximizing attention and alertness during certain hours of the day, along with the elimination of cataplexy. Narcolepsy patients should be careful to allow sufficient hours for nighttime sleep, as sleep deprivation will exacerbate their symptoms. Scheduled brief naps and periods of increased physical activity during the daytime may be very helpful. Most narcolepsy patients will require pharmacotherapy to enhance daytime alertness. Modafinil (Provigil) may be adequate for some patients; however, many will respond best to amphetamine medications. Antidepressants (e.g., venlafaxine[1] [Effexor]) may reduce cataplexy. Sodium oxybate (Xyrem), which is taken in two nighttime doses, has been shown to improve nighttime sleep, reduce cataplexy, and increase daytime alertness in narcolepsy patients.

## Hypersomnolence Disorders

In addition to narcolepsy, various central nervous system processes can cause persistent sleepiness that interferes with daytime functioning. Patients with hypersomnolence may sleep for extended periods and nap during the day, but they still never feel fully alert and refreshed. This condition may be idiopathic, or it may be related to head trauma, viral infections, encephalitis, tumors, and neurodegenerative disorders. As with narcolepsy, stimulants represent the primary treatment approach but often are less reliable in providing significant benefit for these patients.

## Sleep-Disordered Breathing

This topic is covered in greater detail in the article on Sleep Apnea. *Sleep-disordered breathing* involves fluctuations in airflow during sleep. Most commonly it is due to an obstructive process involving an abnormal collapsibility of the upper airway, which may result in recurrent episodes of hypopneas and apneas. Alternately, it may involve a decreased respiratory drive associated with central mechanisms, as can occur with congestive heart failure with a prolonged circulation time. Sleep apnea can cause frequent arousals that undermine sleep quality and lead to excessive sleepiness during the daytime.

---

[1]Not FDA approved for this indication.

## Restless Legs Syndrome and Periodic Limb Movements

Although the primary discomfort of restless legs syndrome (RLS) occurs prior to sleep, it is considered a sleep disorder because it is associated with delayed and disrupted sleep and because the irresistible urge to move the legs follows a circadian pattern with increasing symptoms as bedtime approaches. As the condition worsens over time, the sense of restlessness may begin earlier in the afternoon or morning. The discomfort is most bothersome when patients are at rest. Moving the legs offers only very brief relief. In severe cases, patients often experience such intense restlessness that they are unable to sleep for long periods and often will pace until exhaustion finally allows sleep. During sleep, about 80% of RLS patients exhibit periodic limb movements. In some patients, these involuntary jerking movements occur frequently and cause arousals that further undermine sleep quality. Occasionally patients have periodic limb movements during sleep without the pre-sleep restlessness.

Although RLS often occurs idiopathically, there also is a significant familial component. Other risk factors are iron deficiency, peripheral neuropathies, renal failure, and use of certain medications, including most antidepressants, sedating antihistamines, and centrally acting dopamine antagonists. Pregnancy may be associated with a temporary worsening of symptoms.

Iron supplementation may be beneficial for RLS patients with low ferritin levels (<50 ng/mL). Otherwise, the first-line approach consists of dopamine agonists, such as ropinirole (Requip). Selected patients may benefit from opiates (e.g., propoxyphene[1] [Darvon] and methadone[1] [Dolophine]), benzodiazepines (e.g., clonazepam[1] [Klonopin]), or gabapentin[1] (Neurontin).

## Parasomnias

Behaviors and other symptoms emanating from sleep are considered *parasomnias*. Although most parasomnias are relatively benign, occasionally injuries to patients or bed partners result from these behaviors. Evaluation of patients with parasomnias should include a consideration of sleep-disordered breathing as a possible precipitant to the abnormal behaviors. Most parasomnias can be categorized according to their association with non-REM or REM sleep.

Slow-wave sleep, classified as non-REM stages 3 and 4, generally occurs during the first few hours of sleep. Children have the most slow-wave sleep, and the amount declines with age. Compared with other sleep stages, it is most difficult to awaken from these stages. *Sleep terrors, sleepwalking, sleep-related eating disorder,* and *confusional*

---

[1]Not FDA approved for this indication.

 **CURRENT DIAGNOSIS**

- Patient should be screened routinely for problems associated with sleep and wakefulness.
- Ask patients and bed partners about difficulty falling and staying asleep, movements and behaviors during sleep, and snoring and breathing irregularities during sleep.
- The most common sleep disorders encountered in primary care settings are insomnia, sleep-disordered breathing, and restless legs syndrome. Parasomnia, narcolepsy, and other hypersomnolence disorders are relatively uncommon.
- Excessive sleepiness is a potentially dangerous condition that should be evaluated aggressively. Sleep laboratory testing is appropriate for cases not easily explained by sleep deprivation.

## CURRENT THERAPY

- Patients with persistent insomnia may benefit from improved sleep hygiene measures, cognitive-behavioral therapy, and pharmacologic agents.
- Sleep-promoting medications approved by the Food and Drug Administration include benzodiazepine and nonbenzodiazepine hypnotics, and a selective melatonin receptor agonist.
- Iron supplementation may benefit patients with restless legs syndrome and low ferritin levels. Otherwise, dopamine agonists are the first-line treatment.
- Narcolepsy can be treated with central nervous system stimulants, rapid eye movement suppressants, and sodium oxybate (Xyrem).
- Parasomnia behaviors should be treated when they frequently disrupt sleep or represent a danger to the patient or bed partners.

*arousals* all represent incomplete awakenings. Often people experiencing these parasomnias have no recollection of them the following morning. These parasomnias may be exacerbated by sleep insufficiency when there is an increase in slow-wave sleep intensity during recovery sleep. Sleep terrors may be especially dramatic. When they are frequent or involve dangerous behaviors, then treatment with a benzodiazepine receptor agonist may be appropriate.

REM sleep is associated with the most intense dreaming experiences and markedly decreased skeletal muscle tone. It occurs intermittently throughout the night but for the longest periods during the last few hours of the night. *Nightmares* are distressing awakenings from REM sleep with the awareness of frightening dream content. *REM sleep behavior disorder*, which is more common among elderly individuals, involves an incomplete muscle paralysis during REM sleep leading patients to move during REM sleep. Patients seem to be acting out intense dream experiences. The results can be dangerous because patients may thrash about in bed, fall out of bed, or even attack bed partners before awakening. Bedtime clonazepam[1] (Klonopin) has been the standard treatment; however, recent studies suggest melatonin[1] also may be beneficial.

## Summary

Sleep disorders can have a significant impact on a patient's quality of life and on comorbid conditions. Initial screening for sleep-wake cycle disturbances is as simple as asking patients how they are sleeping and whether they feel awake and alert throughout the daytime. Most sleep disorders can be identified with a thorough history in a primary care setting; however, consultation with a sleep specialist and sleep laboratory testing may be helpful in the evaluation and management of complex insomnia, hypersomnia, and parasomnia patients.

## REFERENCES

The International Classification of Sleep Disorders: Diagnostic & Coding Manual, ICSD-2, 2nd ed. Westchester, IL, American Academy of Sleep Medicine, 2005.

Chokroverty S: Sleep Disorders Medicine: Basic Science, Technical Considerations, and Clinical Aspects. Boston, Butterworth-Heinemann, 1994.

Earley CJ: Clinical practice: Restless legs syndrome. N Engl J Med 2003;348:2103-2109.

Kryger MH, Roth T, Dement WC: Principles and Practice of Sleep Medicine, 4th ed. Philadelphia, Elsevier/Saunders, 2005.

Mahowald MW, Bornemann MC, Schenck CH. Parasomnias. Semin Neurol 2004;24:283-292.

Neubauer DN: Understanding Sleeplessness: Perspectives on Insomnia. Baltimore, Johns Hopkins University Press, 2003.

Reid KJ, Zee PC: Circadian rhythm disorders. Semin Neurol 2004;24: 315-325.

Thorpy M: Current concepts in the etiology, diagnosis and treatment of narcolepsy. Sleep Med 2001;2:5-17.

# Intracerebral Hemorrhage

Method of
*J. Claude Hemphill III, MD, MAS*

Spontaneous nontraumatic intracerebral hemorrhage (ICH) accounts for 10% to 15% of acute stroke in most case series. It is consistently associated with a high mortality rate (usually around 40%) and is more likely to result in death or major disability than cerebral infarction or subarachnoid hemorrhage (SAH). Currently, without an approved treatment of proven benefit, recent clinical trials have helped to define surgical indications and suggest new interventions for ICH.

## Epidemiology and Etiology

Of the 700,000 strokes occurring annually in the United States, more than 70,000 are ICH (Box 1). ICH is more common among minority groups, including Asians and African Americans. Whether this represents a genetic predisposition or a result of less access to preventive health care is not completely clear. The average age of ICH patients is younger than for ischemic stroke, and only 20% of ICH patients are functionally independent a year after their stroke.

### HYPERTENSION

Hypertension remains the most common, and most treatable, cause of acute ICH. At least 60% of ICH is caused by the chronic effects of hypertension on the small penetrating arteries of the brain. Typical sites of hypertensive ICH are the basal ganglia (especially the putamen), the thalamus, the pons, and the cerebellum. An ICH occurring in other locations (e.g., lobar ICH) or in a young person without a prior history of hypertension should prompt a diagnostic evaluation for other causes of ICH. Aggressive treatment of hypertension prevents a substantial portion of ICH from occurring in the first place, and this is the mainstay of primary and secondary prevention for ICH.

---

**BOX 1   Etiologies of Primary Intracerebral Hemorrhage**

**Common**

Arteriovenous malformations
Cerebral amyloid angiopathy
Chronic hypertension
Coagulopathy (warfarin-related)
Drugs of abuse (cocaine, methamphetamine)

**Rare**

Cerebral vasculitis
Coagulopathy (von Willebrand's)
Moyamoya syndrome

---

[1]Not FDA approved for this indication.

## CEREBRAL AMYLOID ANGIOPATHY

Cerebral amyloid angiopathy (CAA) is an increasingly recognized cause of primary intracerebral hemorrhage, especially lobar ICH. Occurring almost exclusively in patients older than 65 years, CAA is associated with dementia and recurrent lobar ICH, especially in carriers of the apolipoprotein E ε4 gene allele. Magnetic resonance imaging (MRI) using gradient echo sequences can demonstrate prior microhemorrhages and is a useful diagnostic test in the setting of lobar hemorrhage in older patients. There is currently no treatment for CAA.

## COAGULOPATHY, VASCULAR MALFORMATIONS, AND DRUGS OF ABUSE

Warfarin (Coumadin)-related ICH is increasing in incidence and accounts for 5% to 15% of ICH. Mortality from warfarin-related ICH is substantially higher than for noncoagulopathic ICH. Additionally, hematoma expansion is even more common in the setting of an elevated international normalized ratio (INR) (<1.4) and can continue for up to a day after ICH onset unless coagulopathy is corrected back to normal.

Vascular malformations are a relatively uncommon cause of ICH, but they account for a substantial portion of young patients with ICH and for ICH in patients without hypertension. Arteriovenous malformations (AVMs), cavernous malformations, dural arteriovenous fistulas (dAVFs), and saccular aneurysms can all cause acute ICH.

Diagnostic evaluation with MRI and magnetic resonance angiography (MRA) is recommended in patients with lobar hemorrhage and in patients younger than 45 years without an obvious other cause. CT angiography (CTA) is increasingly being used instead of MRA. Diagnostic catheter angiography remains the gold standard for AVMs and dAVF, but it does not detect cavernous malformations. Because the ICH hematoma can obscure a small vascular anomaly, delayed MRI after hematoma resorption (2-3 months) may be necessary. Primary and metastatic tumors can bleed, mimicking primary ICH, and therefore a delayed MRI is useful if there is no other systemic evidence of a tumor.

Sympathomimetic drugs of abuse are an increasing cause of ICH, especially in younger patients. A urine toxicology screen for cocaine and methamphetamine should be a routine part of the ICH work-up in all patients. A positive toxicology screen is not necessarily ultimately diagnostic because these drugs can precipitate hemorrhage from an underlying vascular anomaly such as an AVM or aneurysm.

Numerous other less common etiologies of ICH exist, including cerebral vasculitis, moyamoya syndrome, and secondary hemorrhage into an arterial or venous infarct. Many times the pattern of hemorrhage on head CT scan or other associated findings on physical or laboratory examination provides clues to one of these less common etiologies.

## CURRENT DIAGNOSIS

- Obtain an emergency head CT scan immediately on hospital arrival.
- Extravasation on contrast CT might predict hematoma expansion.
- Check INR and determine if the patient is on anticoagulant therapy.
- Obtain history: Check for hypertension, dementia, prior stroke.
- MRI, MRA, CTA, or angiography for patients younger than 45 years or with lobar ICH.

*Abbreviations:* CT = computed tomography; ICH = intracerebral hemorrhage; INR = international normalized ratio; MRA = magnetic resonance angiography; MRI = magnetic resonance imaging.

## Diagnosis

Patients with ICH present with what appears to be an acute stroke, although level of consciousness is often more diminished than with ischemic stroke. An urgent head CT scan is an essential part of the diagnostic evaluation of all acute stroke patients. Noncontrast head CT scanning has traditionally been performed, but recent studies suggest that the addition of contrast may be useful, because contrast extravasation predicts mortality, likely due to hematoma enlargement. Also, CTA can be performed concurrently to evaluate for an underlying vascular anomaly.

A rapid coagulation panel (prothrombin time [PT], INR, and partial thromboplastin time [PTT]) should be obtained in all patients, as should a urine toxicology screen. Because history may be limited at the time of initial evaluation, these laboratory tests can provide unexpected clues as to etiology and identify urgent interventions needed.

The importance of early hematoma expansion is now recognized in ICH. Previously, enlargement of an ICH was believed to indicate systemic coagulopathy or underlying AVM, but it is now recognized that a significant portion of all ICH patients will suffer early hematoma expansion. Hematoma expansion tends to happen early in the clinical course, with hematomas enlarging by at least one third in 30% to 40% of patients who present within 3 hours of symptom onset. Hematoma expansion to this degree is usually associated with neurologic deterioration.

Numerous studies have identified a range of clinical and neurologic imaging factors that predict outcome. The ICH Score (Table 1) is one simple clinical grading scale that can be used to risk stratify patients for 30-day mortality based on age, Glasgow Coma Scale score, hematoma volume and location, and presence of intraventricular hemorrhage on CT scan.

## Treatment

The revised 2007 guidelines from the Stroke Council of the American Heart Association address numerous aspects of ICH management, with the recognition that there is limited evidence to guide many of these treatments (Table 2).

**TABLE 1** The ICH Score

| Component | ICH Score Points |
| --- | --- |
| **Glasgow Coma Scale Score*** | |
| 3-4 | 2 |
| 5-12 | 1 |
| 13-15 | 0 |
| **ICH Volume (mL)†** | |
| ≥30 | 1 |
| <30 | 0 |
| **Intraventricular Hemorrhage‡** | |
| Yes | 1 |
| No | 0 |
| **Infratentorial Origin of ICH** | |
| Yes | 1 |
| No | 0 |
| **Age (years)** | |
| ≥80 | 1 |
| <80 | 0 |
| **Total** | **0-6** |

*GCS score on discharge from the emergency department.
†ICH volume on the initial CT scan was calculated using the ABC/2 method, where A is the greatest diameter of the hemorrhage (by CT scan), B is the diameter 90 degrees to A, and C is the CT slice thickness (cm) times the approximate number of CT slices that include hemorrhage.
‡Presence of any intraventricular hemorrhage on initial CT.
*Abbreviations:* CT = computed tomography; GCS = Glasgow Coma Scale; ICH = intracerebral hemorrhage.

## CURRENT THERAPY

- Remember the ABCs (airway, breathing, circulation).
- Reverse warfarin (Coumadin) coagulopathy immediately with a prothrombin complex concentrate or recombinant factor VIIa (NovoSeven); also give fresh-frozen plasma and vitamin K.
- Lower blood pressure to mean arterial pressure less than 110 mm Hg or combined blood pressure less than 160/90.
- Surgery for cerebellar hemorrhage and possibly lobar hemorrhage.
- Clinical monitoring for re-bleeding or neurologic worsening for the initial 24 hours.
- Do not use corticosteroids.

## INITIAL EVALUATION AND TRIAGE

Because level of consciousness is often diminished in acute ICH patients, early attention to airway protection is essential to avoid aspiration and hypoxia. Intubation may be necessary. Most patients with acute ICH should be managed in an intensive care unit for at least 24 hours.

## BLOOD PRESSURE MANAGEMENT

Most patients with ICH are acutely hypertensive, sometimes to very extreme levels. The 2007 ICH guidelines recommend lowering the blood pressure to achieve a mean arterial pressure (MAP) less than 110 mm Hg or a combined blood pressure less than 160/90. The guidelines also recommend maintaining a cerebral perfusion pressure (CPP) of 60-80 mm Hg in patients with elevated intracranial pressure (ICP). Lowering blood pressure to limit hematoma expansion is intuitively appealing, but studies of the influence of high blood pressure on hematoma expansion have had conflicting results. Prior concerns that blood pressure lowering might create perihematoma ischemia appear largely unfounded. Clinical trials are currently under way in the United States and Australia to determine whether acute blood pressure lowering improves outcome after ICH.

## SURGICAL HEMATOMA EVACUATION

Prior studies of ICH hematoma evacuation have included no more than 100 patients. Thus, the recent completion and publication of the results of the STICH (Surgical Trial in Intracerebral Haemorrhage)

study represent a major step both in understanding the role of surgical hematoma evacuation and in demonstrating that large clinical trials in intracerebral hemorrhage can be undertaken.

The STICH study was a randomized, controlled trial designed to test the hypothesis that early surgical evacuation in supratentorial spontaneous intracerebral hemorrhage was superior to initial conservative treatment. Overall, 1033 patients from 27 different countries were randomized. About one half of patients had lobar intracerebral hemorrhage and one half had deep (thalamic or basal ganglia) hemorrhages. At 6 months, there was no difference in the fraction of patients with good functional outcome (early surgery 26%, initial conservative treatment 24%; $P = 0.4$) and no difference in mortality (early surgery 36%, initial conservative treatment 37%; $P = 0.7$). However, 26% of the patients randomized to initial conservative treatment underwent surgical hematoma evacuation later in their hospital course based on the discretion of their treating surgeon. The subgroup of STICH patients with lobar hematomas within 1 cm of the cortical surface had a strong trend toward better outcome with surgical evacuation, and the new STICH II trial is examining surgical evacuation in this group of patients.

STICH included only patients with supratentorial ICH. Cerebellar hemorrhages are considered by most to be surgically appropriate lesions, despite the lack of a randomized trial studying this group of patients. The 2007 ICH guidelines recommend surgery for deteriorating patients with cerebellar hemorrhages larger than 3 cm.

## PREVENTING HEMATOMA EXPANSION

The safety and efficacy of recombinant factor VIIa (NovoSeven)[1] were tested in a randomized, blinded, placebo-controlled phase II study of patients with acute ICH. Hematoma growth (the primary study outcome measure) was significantly less in the patients who received recombinant factor VIIa (pooled across three doses tested, $P = 0.01$). Three-month mortality (secondary outcome) was significantly less in those treated with recombinant factor VIIa (18% vs. 29%; pooled $P = 0.02$), and functional outcome was better as well. However, a recently completed phase III trial of recombinant factor VIIa in ICH did not demonstrate clinical benefit despite less hematoma growth compared with placebo.

## COAGULOPATHY-RELATED INTRACEREBRAL HEMORRHAGE

Because of the especially high risk of ongoing hematoma expansion and increased morbidity and mortality in the setting of warfarin-related ICH, immediate correction of coagulopathy (to an INR ≤1.4) is absolutely essential. Studies have demonstrated that protocols that use only fresh-frozen plasma (FFP) and vitamin K (Phytonadione) might not reverse coagulopathy sufficiently fast. International guidelines recommend prothrombin complex concentrate (PCC) in addition to FFP and vitamin K. There are also reports of the successful use of recombinant factor VIIa in this setting.

## OTHER MANAGEMENT ISSUES

The use of prophylactic anticonvulsants is controversial. Some advocate administration in all ICH patients or just in lobar hemorrhage, and others treat with anticonvulsants only after a seizure. Prior small trials of corticosteroids in ICH suggested no benefit and an increase in systemic complications. Deep venous thrombosis prophylaxis is essential. Use of sequential compression devices (SCDs) and stockings should be instituted at hospital admission; subcutaneous heparin or heparinoids are likely safe to administer 72 to 96 hours after ICH onset, unless the patient has an intracranial pressure monitor in place, in which case they may be deferred in favor of SCDs.

---

**TABLE 2  Highlights of the 2007 Intracerebral Hemorrhage Treatment Guidelines**

| Management Issue | Recommendations |
| --- | --- |
| Blood pressure | Maintain MAP < 110 mm Hg or BP < 160/90 |
| Surgical hematoma evacuation | Cerebellar ICH >3 cm<br>Consider lobar ICH in young patient if deteriorating<br>Structural lesions (e.g., AVM) |
| Intracranial pressure (ICP) monitoring | Treat elevated ICP with analgesia and sedation, osmotic diuretics, CSF drainage. Maintain CPP 60-80 mm Hg. |
| Anticonvulsants | Consider prophylaxis |
| Glucocorticoids | No |
| Temperature | Maintain normothermia |

*Abbreviations:* AVM = arteriovenous malformation; GCS = Glasgow Coma Scale; ICH = intracerebral hemorrhage; MAP = mean arterial pressure.

---

[1]Not FDA approved for this indication.

## REFERENCES

Becker KJ, Baxter AB, Bybee HM, et al: Extravasation of radiographic contrast is an independent predictor of death in primary intracerebral hemorrhage. Stroke 1999;30:2025-2032.

Broderick J, Connolly S, Feldmann E, et al: Guidelines for the management of spontaneous intracerebral hemorrhage in adults: 2007 update: A guideline from the American Heart Association/American Stroke Association Stroke Council, High Blood Pressure Research Council, and the Quality of Care and Outcomes in Research Interdisciplinary Working Group. Stroke 2007;38:2001-2023.

Brott T, Broderick J, Kothari R, et al: Early hemorrhage growth in patients with intracerebral hemorrhage. Stroke 1997;28:1-5.

Hemphill JC 3rd, Bonovich DC, Besmertis L, et al: The ICH score: A simple, reliable grading scale for intracerebral hemorrhage. Stroke 2001;32:891-897.

Kothari RU, Brott T, Broderick JP, et al: The ABCs of measuring intracerebral hemorrhage volumes. Stroke 1996;27:1304-1305.

Mayer SA, Brun NC, Begtrup K, et al: Recombinant activated factor vii for acute intracerebral hemorrhage. N Engl J Med 2005;352:777-785.

Mendelow AD, Gregson BA, Fernandes HM, et al: Early surgery versus initial conservative treatment in patients with spontaneous supratentorial intracerebral haematomas in the international surgical trial in intracerebral haemorrhage (STICH): A randomised trial. Lancet 2005;365:387-397.

Qureshi AI, Tuhrim S, Broderick JP, et al: Spontaneous intracerebral hemorrhage. N Engl J Med 2001;344:1450-1460.

# Ischemic Cerebrovascular Disease

Method of
*Elzbieta Wirkowski, MD*

A rupture of a blood vessel causes a hemorrhagic stroke. A hemorrhagic stroke can be either intracerebral or subarachnoid, and together it makes up 25% of all strokes.

An ischemic stroke is caused by an acute blood vessel occlusion and can be divided into three categories: lacunar, embolic, and atherothrombotic. A rapid distinction between hemorrhagic and ischemic strokes is crucial because each requires a different therapeutic approach.

Stroke is the third leading cause of death in the United States behind cancer and heart disease. It is the second leading cause of death worldwide, surpassed only by heart disease. An estimated 730,000 new or recurrent strokes occur every year in the United States.

Cerebral ischemia is caused by diminished blood flow. This interrupts the oxidative metabolic pathways in the brain ultimately leading to the destruction of neurons and glial cells. The extent of the tissue damage depends on the size of the occluded vessel, the patency of collaterals, and the speed of occlusion. When the cerebral blood flow falls below 10 mL/100 g/minute even for a few minutes, it results in permanent brain tissue damage. This area is called the core of the infarct. The surrounding tissue, with cerebral blood flow in the range of 10 to 20 mL/100 g/minute, is still potentially salvageable and called the ischemic penumbra. An understanding of the ischemic penumbra is extremely important in the development of new diagnostic techniques and therapeutic approaches.

Computed tomography (CT) is based on image reconstruction from a set of quantitative X-ray measurements through the brain. CT is especially useful for identifying an acute hemorrhage. An ischemic stroke may not be detectable for several hours. Early radiographic signs of stroke include a loss of gray–white matter differentiation, a loss of insular ribbon, and a dense vessel sign. After several days from the time of onset, one can find a hypodensity that ultimately obtains a well-defined dark appearance of CSF (cerebrospinal fluid).

A newer technique, CTA (CT angiography) and CTP (CT perfusion), can be very helpful in an early diagnosis of stroke. CTA can image the vascular anatomy of the neck and brain vessels. It requires intravenous (IV) contrast but is not as invasive as a formal angiogram. The CT perfusion scan when performed at stroke onset detects perfusion failure and therefore ischemia immediately.

Using a combination of noncontrast CT to exclude hemorrhage, followed by CTA to check for vascular occlusion and finally CTP to confirm ischemia, is particularly useful before the administration of tissue plasminogen activator (t-PA) in patients who have defibrillators or pacemakers.

MRI (magnetic resonance imaging) uses magnetic properties of the tissue that are displayed as maps of signal intensity. It provides a better definition of anatomic structures, especially the posterior fossa and the brainstem. MRI has several disadvantages: need for the patient's cooperation, inability to use in patients with pacemakers, defibrillators, and foreign metallic bodies. In spite of that, MRI is the modality of choice for the diagnosis of acute ischemic stroke. The ability to acquire diffusion-weighted imaging (DWI) and perfusion-weighted imaging (PWI) can identify salvageable ischemic penumbra within minutes of the stroke. In the future this may help extend the therapeutic window for acute thrombolysis.

MRA (magnetic resonance angiography) can determine the patency of the main vessels of the neck and brain without the need to administer potentially nephrotoxic contrast. Neurosonology plays yet another very important role in the diagnosis of acute stroke. MRA and duplex sonography of the carotid arteries are the most common methods used for an evaluation of carotid stenosis. The formal cerebral angiogram carries a significant number of risks for stroke (0.3% to 5.7%). In older patients with atherosclerotic disease, this number can increase two- to threefold.

Main indications for TCD (transcranial Doppler) use are sickle cell disease, right to left shunt, patent foramen ovale (PFO), intracranial stenosis, monitoring during acute thrombolysis, and detection of vasospasm.

TCD is particularly useful in the detection of PFO with sensitivity and specificity above 95% for paradoxical emboli detection. TCD can test autoregulation and vasomotor reactivity, which can help select patients for extracranial-intracranial (EC-IC) bypass surgery or endarterectomy. The main drawback of the technique is an inadequate acoustic window that limits insonation in 5% to 20% of patients.

## ATHEROTHROMBOTIC STROKE AND CAROTID DISEASE

Carotid occlusive disease is responsible for 25% of ischemic strokes. The main risk factors are hypercholesterolemia, smoking, hypertension, and diabetes. Clinical presentation may be preceded by the brief loss of vision in one eye on the side of stenosis. Carotid bruit may suggest a presence of carotid stenosis, but there is no correlation between the degree of stenosis and the presence or absence of the bruit.

Carotid endarterectomy is currently the accepted standard of treatment for carotid occlusive disease. The North American Symptomatic Carotid Endarterectomy Trial (NASCET) reported an unequivocal benefit of surgery over the best medical management in symptomatic patients with carotid stenosis of 70% or more. The surgical intervention reduced the 2-year risk of any ipsilateral stroke from 26% to 9%. The overall rate of perioperative stroke was 6.5%. The results of the European Carotid Surgery Trial (ECST) were in accordance with NASCET.

The results of carotid stenting vary. In the Stenting and Angioplasty with Protection in Patients at High Risk for Endarterectomy (SAPPHIRE) trial, perioperative stroke and death rates were 7.3% for surgery and 4.4% for stenting. SAPPHIRE data analysis showed long-lasting effectiveness of the stent. The Carotid Revascularization Endarterectomy versus Stent Trial (CREST) is ongoing. Stenting therapy may need to pass the learning curve in the same way that carotid endarterectomy did.

For the intracranial stenosis of the large vessels of the circle of Willis, aspirin appears to be adequate and safe.

## CARDIOEMBOLIC STROKE

Cardioembolic stroke accounts for 20% to 57% of all ischemic strokes. The main risk factors for cardioembolic stroke are mechanical prosthetic valve, mitral stenosis with atrial fibrillation (AF), AF (other than lone AF) left atrial thrombus, sick sinus syndrome, recent myocardial infarction (MI), left ventricular thrombus, dilated cardiomyopathy, akinetic left ventricular segment, atrial myxoma, and infective endocarditis.

Anticoagulation is recommended in AF with the exception of patients younger than 75 years old with lone AF, when aspirin can be acceptable.

## CURRENT DIAGNOSIS

- Neurologic exam consistent with stroke is reliable.
- Presence or absence of bleeding on the head CT guides therapy.
- Hyperintensity on DWI (diffusion-weighted images) MRI is diagnostic.
- Presence of flow in the major neck or brain vessels determines the therapy.

*Abbreviations:* CT = computed tomography; MRI = magnetic resonance imaging.

Warfarin (Coumadin) is otherwise recommended with an international normalized ratio (INR) between 2.0 and 3.0. In patients with MI and mural thrombus, anticoagulation with INR 2, 0 to 3.0 is recommended for 3 months to 1 year. To prevent a secondary ischemic coronary event, aspirin is frequently added. Adding aspirin to the warfarin can double the risk of bleeding complications. The Combination Hemotherapy and Mortality Prevention (CHAMP) trial compared aspirin 162 mg to warfarin (mean INR: 1.8) plus aspirin 81 mg after MI. The combination has not been better in the prevention of death, recurrent MI, or stroke. The possibility of a major hemorrhage was significantly increased in the combination therapy group. For patients with mechanical prosthetic heart valves, oral anticoagulation with INR 2.5 to 3.5 is recommended.

PFO and atrial sepal aneurysm (ASA) are common, occurring in 25% of the general population. They are associated with unexplained ischemic strokes in younger patients less than 55 years. An evaluation for the presence of sepal defects with TCD or transesophageal echocardiography (TEE) should be a part of the standard workup of stroke in the younger population. If the hypercoagulable state is not an issue, antiplatelet therapy should be the initial treatment for secondary stroke prevention in younger patients with cryptogenic stroke and isolated PFO. In patients older than 55 years, even in the presence of PFO, other risk factors play more important roles in the occurrence of the stroke.

## LACUNAR STROKES

Lacunar strokes occur because of the occlusion of small so-called end vessels in the brain (Table 1). Antiplatelet therapy is the treatment of choice for this type of ischemic stroke. The best treatment, however, is primary prevention by controlling the most prevalent risk factors: hypertension, diabetes, smoking, excessive drinking, and a sedentary lifestyle.

Secondary prevention includes aspirin, the combination of aspirin with extended-release dipyridamole (Aggrenox), and clopidogrel (Plavix) (Table 2). Positive statistically significant effects of aspirin therapy in stroke, MI, or vascular death prevention are documented in many trials.

The Warfarin Aspirin Recurrent Stroke Study (WARSS) did not show statistical benefits of warfarin compared to aspirin in noncardioembolic stroke, including antiphospholipid antibodies syndrome, PFO, or aspirin failure. Warfarin posed a slightly higher hazard in patients with hypertension, moderate stroke, and brainstem infarcts.

The European Stroke Prevention Study (ESPS2) trial compared aspirin 50 mg daily to a combination of 50 mg of aspirin and dipyridamole 400 mg (ER-DP). The aspirin/ER-DP combination showed a 23% relative risk reduction (RRR) compared to aspirin for stroke prevention. The main concern with this low dose of aspirin is the potential lack of protection against concomitant coronary artery disease. Fortunately, in this subgroup of patients, aspirin/ER-DP achieved a relative risk reduction for MI comparable to aspirin.

### TABLE 1  Clinical Syndromes of Lacunar Stroke

Silent (asymptomatic)
Pure motor hemiparesis
Ataxic hemiparesis
Sensory hemiparesis
Sensory motor
Clumsy hand dysarthria

### TABLE 2  Current ACCP Guidelines for Noncardioembolic Stroke Prevention

Every patient who has experienced a noncardioembolic stroke or transient ischemic attack (TIA)
should receive treatment with an antiplatelet agent (grade 1A)
Acceptable options for initial therapy:
- Aspirin (50–325 mg)
- Combination of aspirin and ER-dipyridamole (Aggrenox) (25/200 mg bid)
- Clopidogrel (Plavix), 75 mg/d
Recommend antiplatelet agents over oral anticoagulation (grade 1A)
Suggest the use of the combination of aspirin and ER-dipyridamole over aspirin (grade 2A) and clopidogrel over aspirin (grade 2B)

*Abbreviations:* ACCP = American College of Chest Physicians.

The Clopidogrel versus Aspirin in Patients at Risk for Ischemic Event (CAPRIE) study compared the effectiveness of aspirin versus clopidogrel in patients with stroke, MI, and PVD (peripheral vascular disorder). Clopidogrel showed an 8.7% overall risk reduction for cluster but did not reach statistical significance in stroke prevention.

The Management of Atherothrombosis with Clopidogrel in High-Risk Patients with Recent Transient Ischemic Attack (MATCH) trial showed that adding aspirin to clopidogrel did not provide any additional protective value compared with clopidogrel monotherapy. There was a significant increase in major bleeding complications in the clopidogrel plus aspirin group.

For patients with acute ischemic stroke, the use of full-dose anticoagulation is not recommended. The exceptions are: a high degree of carotid stenosis, a dissection of the cerebral arteries, and sinus vein thrombosis.

Regardless of the etiology of the ischemic stroke, thrombolysis with IV t-PA is currently the Food and Drug Administration (FDA)-approved way of the acute stroke treatment (Table 3). Only a small fraction of stroke victims receive t-PA. Treatment is demanding and requires an organized, team approach. The crucial information that needs to be obtained before the administration of t-PA is the last time the patient was seen well, a head CT to rule out a bleed, blood pressure control, and the size of the stroke. There are many misconceptions about t-PA. It is thought to be a very risky drug, yet 11 more patients out of 100 who received t-PA had a resolution of symptoms. Patients who receive t-PA have a higher risk of bleeding complications (6%); however, they still have better survival and recovery rates.

### TABLE 3  Use of t-PA in Ischemic Stroke

| Indication for t-PA | Contraindications for t-PA |
| --- | --- |
| Ischemic stroke | Time of onset >3 h |
| Onset of symptoms <3 h | Evidence of intracranial hemorrhage, mass effect, or edema on CT scan |
| | Clinical presentation that suggests subarachnoid hemorrhage |
| | Known bleeding diathesis |
| | Coumadin with INR >1.5; PTT >1.5 control |
| | Platelets <100,000 mm$^3$ |
| | Major surgery, trauma, GI and GU hemorrhage in the previous 2 wk |
| | History of previous stroke in the last 3 mo |
| | Intracranial or intraspinal surgery in the last 2 mo |
| | Glucose <50 and >400 mg/dL |

*Abbreviations:* CT = computed tomography; GI = gastrointestinal; GU = genitourinary; INR = international normalized ratio; PTT = partial thromboplastin time; t-PA = tissue plasminogen activator.

## CURRENT THERAPY

- Maintain proper perfusion using isotonic fluids.
- Involve a stroke team for best recovery results.
- Initiate t-PA if symptoms are <3 h and no hemorrhage is seen.
- Start antiplatelet agent in every nonhemorrhagic stroke unless t-PA is given or the patient has atrial fibrillation.

*Abbreviation:* t-PA = tissue plasminogen activator.

The intra-arterial (IA) use of thrombolytics has not been universally approved and is still considered experimental. The combined IA and IV use showed no difference in clinical outcomes in spite of better recanalization in the IV/IA group.

The Merci Retriever device offers acute intervention beyond 3 hours. Unfortunately the Mechanical Embolus Removal in Cerebral Ischemia (MERCI) trial showed that the rates of nonhemorrhagic complications (primarily embolization and dissection) were 5.7%. The hemorrhage rates were 9%.

## The Neurocritical Care of Stroke

Close to 70% of patients with acute stroke have an elevation of blood pressure (BP) more than 170/100 with spontaneous decline by day 4. BP control in acute brain ischemia is controversial, and some studies favor lowering the BP by 20%, whereas others favor aggressive pressor therapy. Current American Stoke Association (ASA) guidelines recommend treatment if systolic BP is more than 220 and diastolic BP is more than 120. Patients who undergo thrombolysis require better BP control with systolic BP less than 180. Normothermia as well as glucose control and admission to a dedicated stroke unit improves outcomes.

## REFERENCES

AHA 2002 Heart and Stroke Statistical Update.
Antithrombotic Trialists Collaboration: Collaborative meta-analysis of randomised trials of antiplatelet therapy for prevention of death, myocardial infarction, and stroke in high risk patients. BMJ 2002;324:71-86.
Adams HP Jr, Adams RJ, Brott T, et al: Guidelines for the early management of patients with ischemic stroke: a scientific statement from the Stroke Council of the American Stroke Association. Stroke 2003;34:1056-1083.
Diener HC, Cunha L, Forbes C, et al: European Stroke Prevention Study. 2. Dipyridamole and acetylsalicylic acid in the secondary prevention of stroke. J Neurol Sci 1996;143:1-13.
Dyken M: Stroke risk factors in presentation of stroke. In Norris JW, et al (eds): New York, Springer-Verlag, 1991, pp 83-102.
Foulkes MA, Wolf PA, Price TR, et al: The NINDS Stroke Data Bank: Design, methods, and baseline characteristics. Stroke 1988;19:547-554.
Merritt's Neurology, 11th ed. Philadelphia, Lippincott Williams and Wilkins, 2005.
Mohr JP, Thompson JL, Lazar RM, et al: A comparison of warfarin and aspirin for the prevention of ischemic stroke. N Engl J Med 2001;345:1444-1451.
Risk factors for stroke and efficacy of antithrombotic therapy in atrial fibrillation. Analysis of pooled data from 5 randomized control trials. Arch Intern Med 1994;154:1449-1457.

# Rehabilitation of the Stroke Patient

Method of
*Karl J. Sandin, MD*

Of the approximately 700,000 Americans who will have a stroke this year, an estimated half of them will need some sort of rehabilitation effort to maximize function. Whether because of thromboembolic disease, subarachnoid hemorrhage, or intracerebral hemorrhage, stroke is the third leading cause of disability in the United States. Although typically ineffective or unnecessary for either the minimally affected or tremendously impaired stroke survivor, for the large middle cohort of individuals with mild, moderate, or severe disability after stroke, rehabilitation programs provide improvements in outcome over natural recovery alone.

Rehabilitation is a coordinated program that provides reliable, conscientious, patient-centered restorative care to minimize impairment, disability, and handicap caused by a particular set of medical conditions. *Impairment* is any loss or abnormality of psychological, physical, or anatomic structure or function. *Disability* is any restriction to perform an activity in the manner within the range considered normal for a human being. *Handicap* is a social disadvantage that results from impairment or disability that limits fulfillment of a normal role. After stroke, a patient may have hemiparesis (impairment) that limits ambulation (disability), subsequently affecting ability to work (handicap). Some authors prefer to emphasize functions that remain after stroke, so they speak of ability and participation instead of disability and handicap. When rehabilitation is delivered by a well-functioning team, it provides a level of service excellence greater than the sum of its parts.

Rehabilitation settings include acute-care hospitals, acute rehabilitation hospitals and units, skilled nursing facilities, outpatient facilities and departments, the community (including the home, licensed residential care facilities, and assisted living centers), and transitional living facilities. Typically a patient with stroke is admitted through the emergency department to the hospital, preferably to a dedicated stroke unit. Use of these specialized service areas decreases morbidity and mortality after stroke and sets the stage for maximal recovery. From there patients with a substantial level of disability, yet good endurance for rehabilitation efforts and a reasonable prognosis to achieve a functional level that will allow them to live in a community setting, are referred to acute comprehensive stroke rehabilitation. Patients with less endurance or community discharge uncertainty are often referred to skilled nursing facilities for a less intensive program of rehabilitation. Some patients with less disability are referred directly from hospital care to outpatient or home health programs. Patients move from setting to setting as their medical condition and rehabilitation needs demand; services should continue in the least restrictive setting possible until the patient reaches a plateau. Younger stroke survivors, for whom community and vocational reentry is paramount, benefit greatly from transitional living center care. Gresham and colleagues in *Post-Stroke Rehabilitation* (in Chapter 5) effectively summarize decision trees to help choose a rehabilitation setting.

Apart from the patient and family, rehabilitation team clinical members include physicians (especially physiatrists—medical doctors specializing in physical medicine and rehabilitation—internists, and neurologists), nursing personnel of all levels, therapists (physical, occupational, recreational), speech/language pathologists, counselors (vocational, psychological), case/program managers, and others (dietitians, pharmacists, chaplains, etc.). The degree of involvement of each team member depends primarily on the setting and the stroke survivor's rehabilitation needs. In general, doctors are very involved in stroke rehabilitation as primary physician and team captain in acute rehabilitation settings but less so in community-based programs. Therapists are often more peripheral in intensive care unit settings but integral in home- and community-based treatment.

The antiquated term *cerebral vascular accident* (CVA) should never be used to describe a stroke. Accidents happen without warning or foreknowledge, whereas definable, manageable risk factors for stroke include homocystinemia, cardiac rhythm disturbances such as atrial fibrillation, obesity, dyslipidemia, nicotine dependence/tobacco use, stress, cocaine use, hypertension, diabetes, and autoimmune disease. Although nonmodifiable risk factors for stroke exist such as age (the older the person the higher the risk), gender (women die more of stroke than men, but men have more strokes), ethnicity (even controlled for other risk factors, people of color have more strokes than whites), and family history, primary and secondary stroke risk can be managed. Using the best medical care, family counseling, and education, stroke rehabilitation efforts should always seek to prevent future stroke. Secondary prevention of stroke through diet, exercise, cessation of smoking, and compliance with medical regimens remains a primary rehabilitation concern.

Prevention and early recognition of medical complications of stroke maximize neurologic and functional recovery. Thromboembolic disease, respiratory complications, cardiac problems, neurologic change, bowel and bladder dysfunction, skin breakdown, and pain can particularly affect stroke rehabilitation. All rehabilitation providers have the opportunity to recognize the signs and symptoms of these obstacles to improvement. Prompt recognition and diagnosis of medical problems improve patient care and outcome.

After stroke, deep venous thrombosis (DVT) and pulmonary embolism (PE) occur 40% to 50% and 9% to 15% of the time, respectively. These phenomena are the fourth most common cause of death in the first 30 days after stroke. Risk factors for their development include venous stasis, hypercoagulability, and endothelial injury. The first two are typically present in the stroke survivor because of immobility and acute-phase reaction. Primary prevention of these complications is critical. Stroke survivors not on systemic anticoagulation need either heparin or inferior vena caval filter placement. Because of lower morbidity compared with standard heparin, most stroke patients (including those with CNS [central nervous system] hemorrhage not requiring neurosurgical evacuation) receive low-molecular-weight fractionated heparin (enoxaparin sodium [Lovenox], 40 mg every day). Heparin prophylaxis continues until thromboembolic risk is minimized, typically defined as walking without physical assistance for 200 feet at a time. Pragmatically, prophylaxis is often stopped at institutional discharge but should be continued for at least 3 weeks after stroke. Intermittent pneumatic compression has little relevance in rehabilitation programs because patients are spending considerable time out of bed; elastic stockings provide no DVT/PE prevention. Recognition of failure of prevention requires clinical vigilance and forethought because 50% of DVT cases are clinically silent. A low threshold to check for DVT using Doppler ultrasound or other noninvasive testing or for PE using spiral chest computed tomography (CT) should inform the physician caring for the stroke survivor.

Pneumonia is the third major cause of death in the first 30 days after stroke. An estimated 32% of all stroke survivors develop pneumonia, especially after subarachnoid hemorrhage and in patients with coma because of stroke. Common risk factors include aspiration of oral contents, including saliva, liquids, and food, decreased chest wall compliance, poor expiratory muscle strength, decreased immune response after stroke, and general debility. Although pneumonia classically presents with shaking chills, hemoptysis, and pleuritic pain, in the stroke survivor the only symptom(s) may be low-grade fever, lethargy, loss of neurologic or functional status, or malaise. Prevention of pneumonia requires early assessment for and treatment of dysphagia, strict oral hygiene, such as sterilizing the mouth with an oral antiseptic (chlorhexidine gluconate [Peridex] on a foam-tipped mouth brush every 8 hours, preventive respiratory care including frequent incentive spirometry and inspiratory muscle training, and supervised posturally appropriate eating. Treatment of pneumonia includes rest, antibiotics, and tracheobronchial hygiene and may interrupt the stroke rehabilitation program.

At least 75% of patients with stroke have cardiac disease, which may have caused the stroke (e.g., atrial fibrillation) and may affect stroke recovery (e.g., cardiomyopathy). Cardiac disease is the second leading cause of early mortality and the leading cause of late mortality after stroke. Of stroke patients, 66% have coronary artery disease, 50% have dysrhythmias, and 20% have congestive heart failure (CHF). Effective management of CHF improves function after stroke. Cardiovascular and neurovascular disease commonly exist together, so stroke rehabilitation providers should assume all stroke survivors younger than 70 years have at least latent heart disease. Regardless of rehabilitation setting, patients should be monitored for vital signs and for signs and symptoms of well-being at the inception of the exercise components of stroke rehabilitation (and to some degree throughout).

Neurologic conditions may change or appear after stroke. Seizures complicate less than 10% of strokes; half occur in the first few days after stroke. Patients who seize after stroke typically have more brain damage and therefore a worse prognosis. Many patients with large

bland infarcts or intracerebral and subarachnoid hemorrhage are placed on antiseizure agents as a prophylaxis against seizures. This controversial practice may impair the function of surviving normal brain and is discouraged in rehabilitation settings. A short (1-week) course of seizure prophylaxis is warranted after craniotomy. Bland infarcts may hemorrhagically transform, often presenting with changes in neurologic or functional status. A low threshold for repeat neurologic imaging (especially brain CT) should uncover this phenomenon and enable transfer, as is typically required, to a higher level of medical care. Change in neurologic status because of new stroke or intolerance of medications is not unusual during rehabilitation.

Neuromuscular conditions aggravate and facilitate stroke rehabilitation. After stroke, many survivors are initially hypotonic. As a result, their joints are poorly protected, so normal assistance moving in bed can result, for example, in shoulder trauma and pain. In the first few months after stroke, flaccidity is typically replaced with spasticity, a symptom complex of resistance to passive stretch, brisk reflexes, and hypertonicity because of loss of descending inhibition of spinal interneurons. Although spasticity can have its benefits, such as causing lower extremity rigidity that provides knee and ankle stiffness and allows a stable circumducted gait, it also can cause pain, contracture, and loss of function. Physical exercises, medications (dantrolene sodium [Dantrium], up to 100 mg four times daily), chemodenervation (botulinum toxin A [Botox]), and neuro destructive techniques seek to preserve some level of tone, thereby allowing maximal motor control. Yet much of the disability after stroke is caused by underlying weakness or sensory disturbances, losses not impacted by spasticity control.

Most stroke survivors have bowel and bladder dysfunction. Bladder problems include infection, incontinence, retention, and preexisting genitourinary disease, and they are often complicated by impairments in cognition, language, and mobility in the stroke patient. Continence, a complex feat of awareness, control, mobility, and dexterity, is vulnerable at many points to the direct and indirect effects of stroke. Cortical lesions can cause symptoms of urinary urgency at low urine volumes because of an unstable detrusor, the most common finding on urodynamic testing of stroke survivors with persistent incontinence. Brainstem strokes can cause detrusor sphincter dyssynergia. Patients with large strokes that cause aphasia, alteration in consciousness, or high levels of physical disability are typically bladder incontinent during initial stroke care. Patients with postvoid urinary retention (demonstrated by ultrasound postvoid measurement of bladder volume) have higher rates of incontinence and infection. Urinary tract infection occurs in almost all stroke survivors and responds well to targeted antibiotic therapy. Incontinence rates drop in the first 3 months after stroke. Stroke survivors often require bladder retraining with timed voiding every 2 to 3 hours around the clock, elimination of medications with anticholinergic side effects that cause increased sphincter tone, and voiding trials in upright rather than recumbent positions to regain continence. Bowel dysfunction is common after stroke because of physical inactivity, inadequate fluid and/or dietary fiber, direct effect of a neurologic lesion of central defecation centers, side effects of medication, or impaction because of prolonged constipation. Conversely, some patients have diarrhea after stroke because of antibiotic side effects including *Clostridium difficile* infection, overstimulation of the colon with laxative, or obstipation. To normalize bowel function, stroke survivors require proper fluid, nutrition, fiber, and opportunity to eliminate in an upright position on their normal schedule. Often patients require a stimulant laxative (senna [Senokot], 2 to 4 tablets) followed 8 hours later by a postprandial rectal suppository (bisacodyl [Dulcolax]). Excessive use of bulk-forming agents does not help restore bowel regularity in the stroke survivor with altered mobility.

Neuropathic and nociceptive pain are common after stroke. Most worrisome is shoulder-hand syndrome (reflex sympathetic dystrophy, CPRS [Complex Regional Pain Syndrome, type 1]) that presents with pain in the eponymous parts, edema, dystrophic skin, and vasomotor instability. Triple-phase radionuclide bone scanning complemented by diagnostic and therapeutic blockade confirm the diagnosis. Additional therapies include transdermal clonidine, contrast baths, and axial loading extremity exercises. Most shoulder pain after stroke is caused by contracture, glenohumeral subluxation, rotator cuff disease, or bicipital tendonitis. Many stroke survivors have co-morbid conditions, such as osteoarthritis, which flare symptomatically with restorative efforts. True neuropathic pain because of stroke (central poststroke pain) is rare and difficult to treat.

Impairments after stroke include weakness (hemiparesis), loss of coordination (ataxia), hemisensory loss, visual deficits, agnosia, apraxia, disorders of language, and cognitive losses. After stroke, weak extremities often swell, usually because of flaccidity, loss of muscle control, or clot. If a thrombus is ruled out, extremity swelling requires elevation, such as for the upper extremity on a hemilap tray, or an external pressure gradient such as a 25 to 35 mm Hg below-knee compression stocking. Stroke survivors may have loss of light touch, pinprick, temperature, proprioception, kinesthetic, or vibratory sense, singularly or in combination. Even with normal strength, the patient with sensory loss may be very disabled. Visual deficits after stroke include field cuts, disregard, and disorders of perception. Anecdotal reports of improvement in visual functioning through behavioral optometry are not supported by well-designed studies. Agnosia (a deficit in afferent processing or inability to interpret or recognize information in one sensory modality when the end-organ is intact) particularly involves vision, touch, and hearing. Apraxia (a deficit in efferent processing or the inability to perform purposefully despite normal coordination and motor function) can involve language, dressing, or construction. Language problems include aphasia (impairment of the capacity to interpret and formulate multimodal language symbols), dysarthria (imprecise or poorly coordinated speech production with decreased articulation and intelligibility without problems in word retrieval or comprehension), and speech apraxia (a verbal or oral impairment of voluntary execution of complex speech-motor activities). Cognitive sequelae of stroke are inattention, memory loss, and loss of insight and judgment, which in combination may result in inability to initiate, plan, and complete (executive functioning) daily tasks. Various rehabilitation techniques such as transfer of training, neurodevelopmental technique (NDT) of Bobath, cutaneous stimulation of Rood, proprioceptive neuromuscular facilitation (PNF) of Voss and Knott, and motor relearning have particular disciples and adherents, although most rehabilitation therapists use a combination of various theories to improve function.

Strict attention to patient safety vis-à-vis falls and swallowing limits morbidity after stroke. Stroke survivors, regardless of location, have high fall rates. Falls can be prevented by placing the patient near the nurse's station, using bed movement alarms and mobility monitors, eliminating wet or uneven surfaces, providing one-to-one supervision, and avoiding polypharmacy, especially with cognitively impairing medications. Approximately 50% of stroke survivors have dysphagia because of deficits in oral, pharyngeal, or esophageal stages of swallowing. Of those, one third aspirate (some silently), defined as entrance of material into the airway below the level of the true vocal folds.

## CURRENT THERAPY

- Stroke rehabilitation improves outcome over natural recovery alone.
- Stroke rehabilitation is most effective when team members work together on shared functional goals.
- Reduction of future stroke risk is a primary stroke rehabilitation concern.
- Most common medical problems after stroke include DVT/PE, pneumonia, UTI, and CHF, conditions that can usually be prevented, and if they occur must be managed well to secure stroke rehabilitation success.

*Abbreviations:* CHF = congestive heart failure; DVT/PE = deep venous thrombosis/pulmonary embolism; UTI = urinary tract infection.

Although the history and physical offer some tools to identify and treat swallowing problems, most rehabilitation therapists use functional endoscopic or videofluoroscopic swallowing studies to determine swallowing ability and guide management of dysphagia. Stroke survivors with dysphagia should eat only in highly structured, distraction-free environments using techniques such as double swallow and chin tuck to mitigate risk of aspiration. At time of advancement to more difficult diet textures or consistencies, strokes survivors should receive special attention to ensure a safe transition.

In the past, stroke rehabilitation paradigms focused almost exclusively on disability limitation. Today, changes in medical and societal perspective and improved neuroscience understanding are leading to newer techniques of care that seek to first improve physical function, automatically lessening disability. Examples of such efforts in stroke rehabilitation include partial weight-bearing treadmill training, constraint-induced movement therapy, and residential aphasia training. Although there is some overlap with disability treatment, a primary goal of these interventions is to avoid or eliminate learned nonuse, demanding maximal performance of the CNS for the physical or cognitive task at hand. At a cellular level, stroke rehabilitation improves outcome in two major ways: synaptogenesis and uncovering of dormant or vestigial CNS pathways.

Enthusiasm for constraint-induced movement therapy (CIMT) appears warranted. Wolf reported on a large series of 222 individuals who had stroke of various types in the preceding 3 to 9 months with CIMT. These stroke survivors were randomized to receive routine care (a very mixed treatment group) and CIMT, with the intention of meaningfully improved upper extremity function. The individuals functioned at relatively high levels at study entrance: MMSE was ≥24, and each individual had some upper extremity movement (divided into higher functioning and lower functioning groups). The intervention was

> taught to apply an instrumented protective safety mitt and encouraged to wear it on their less-impaired upper extremity for a goal of 90% of their waking hours over a two-week period, including two weekends, for a total of 14 days. On each week day, participants received shaping (adaptive task practice) and standard task training of the paretic limb for up to six hours per day.*

They concluded, "among patients who had a stroke within the previous 3 to 9 months, CIMT produced statistically significant and clinically relevant improvements in arm motor function that persisted for at least 1 year."

Neuropharmacology augments the stroke rehabilitation process. Deficits in attention can be decreased by stimulants (methylphenidate [Ritalin], up to 10 mg twice daily). The addition of dextroamphetamine (Dextrostat) biweekly to speech/language pathologist language retraining improves aphasia and verbal apraxia compared to therapy alone. Although no controlled studies exist, many practitioners use acetylcholinesterase inhibitors designed to treat dementia (donepezil [Aricept], 5 to 10 mg every day) for cognitive disorders after stroke. Selective serotonin reuptake inhibitor (SSRI) and serotonin-norepinephrine reuptake inhibitor (SNRI) antidepressants effectively treat poststroke depression and may directly improve neural recovery after stroke.

Regardless of setting, stroke rehabilitation affects outcome beneficially. Major outcome measurement tools include the National Institutes of Health (NIH) stroke scale, a 14-item assessment scoring various impairments. Functional (disability) scales are the bedrock of analysis of stroke rehabilitation success and include, most prominently, the Barthel index and the Functional Independence Measure (FIM). Few scales assess participation, although arguably ability to return to active community living best reflects stroke rehabilitation success. Using diagnostic and demographic data and FIM scores, stroke survivors undergoing acute comprehensive rehabilitation paid by Medicare are assigned to a case-mix group (CMG) from which

*Wolf SL, Winstein CJ, Miller JP, et al: Effect of constraint-induced movement therapy on upper extremity function 3 to 9 months after stroke: The EXCITE randomized clinical trial. JAMA 2006;296:2095-2104.

prospective payment derives. Payment for stroke rehabilitation is a controversial topic because rehabilitation hospitals, skilled nursing facilities, outpatient departments, and home health agencies all believe current funding schemes under-reimburse their services.

Perhaps the biggest burden after stroke is psychosocial. Depression and anxiety are common after stroke, with an incidence of approximately 40% each at 6 months. Many standard tests for these psychological conditions require normal cognitive and language function, so they have limited usefulness in the stroke survivor. Emotionalism (emotional lability) is present up to 1 year after stroke in 21% of patients. Social problems after stroke include economic strain (46%), social isolation (53%), decreased community involvement (43%), disruption of family function (52%), poor motivation, dependency, and loss of control. Social isolation is more common in women and those with higher educational achievement. Families are often called on to provide care for stroke survivors, but they may have neither the emotional nor physical ability to do so. As a result, caregivers burn out, culminating in severe situations with neglect or abuse. The incidence of depression in spouses of stroke patients is three times that of controls. To maximize the chances of a satisfying life for stroke survivors and their families, liberal use of community services within the entire first year after stroke should be encouraged. If the challenges of resuming a meaningful life are not met, patients and their families may respond with illness and maladaptive behaviors (Current Therapy Box).

## REFERENCES

Bode RK, Heinemann AW, Semik P, Mallinson T: Patterns of therapy activities across length of stay and impairment levels: Peering inside the "black box" of inpatient stroke rehabilitation. Arch Phys Med Rehabil 2004;85(12): 1901-1908.

Bogey RA, Geis CC, Phillip R, et al: Stroke and neurodegenerative disorders: III. Stroke: Rehabilitation management. Arch Phys Med Rehabil 2004; (Suppl 1)85(3):15-20.

Da Cunha IT Jr, Lim PA, Qureshy H, et al: Gait outcomes after acute stroke rehabilitation with supported treadmill ambulation training: A randomized controlled pilot study. Arch Phys Med Rehabil 2002;83: 1258-1265.

Dettmers C, Teske U, Hamzei F, et al: Distributed form of constraint-induced movement therapy improves functional outcome and quality of life after stroke. Arch Phys Med Rehabil 2005;86(2): 204-209.

Gresham GE, Duncan PW, Stason WB, et al: Post-Stroke Rehabilitation. Clinical Practice Guideline, No. 16. Rockville, Md, U.S. Department of Health and Human Services. Public Health Service, Agency for Health Care Policy and Research. AHCPR Pub. No. 95-0662. May 1995.

McLean DE: Medical complications experienced by a cohort of stroke survivors during inpatient, tertiary-level stroke rehabilitation. Arch Phys Med Rehabil 2004;85:466-469.

Sandin KJ, Mason KD: Manual of Stroke Rehabilitation. Boston, Butterworth-Heinemann, 1996.

# Seizures and Epilepsy in Adolescents and Adults

Method of
*Erik K. St. Louis, MD,*
*and Mark A. Granner, MD*

Epilepsy is a common public health problem afflicting approximately 2.5 million Americans and 30 million persons worldwide. Epilepsy is equally prevalent between the sexes until older age, where the increased incidence of epilepsy in elderly men mirrors that of cerebrovascular disease.

Epilepsy was recognized in antiquity, described by Hippocrates as "the falling sickness." The etymology of epilepsy stems from the Greek *epilepsia,* "to be seized or taken hold of," derived from the erroneous belief and unfortunately persistent stigma that epileptic seizures result from supernatural or spiritual, rather than medical causes. Such historical misunderstandings, coupled with limited availability of effective treatments, have instilled fear of epilepsy for centuries in patients, their families and caregivers, and society. Fortunately, an evolving medical understanding of epilepsy and its many causes and imitators has enabled improved diagnostic testing and an ever-expanding palette of effective, tolerable antiepileptic drug and surgical therapies over the last three decades. All clinicians should be familiar with epilepsy not only because of its prevalence, but because its treatments are increasingly adopted for a wide variety of neurologic and psychiatric conditions including migraine, pain, and mood disorders.

## Seizures and Epilepsy Defined

An epileptic seizure is a sudden, transient alteration in behavior caused by an abnormal, excessive neuronal discharge in the cerebral cortex. Everyone has a seizure threshold and holds the potential to have a seizure. Only a small subset of the population, however, experiences spontaneous seizures or develops epilepsy. The lifetime prevalence of experiencing a single seizure is approximately 10%, but only approximately 30% of incipient seizures recur and become epilepsy.

Seizures are most often provoked by an extrinsic (systemic) or intrinsic (brain) factor. Table 1 lists the causes of provoked seizures. An individual may have recurrent provoked seizures without developing epilepsy. In most cases, a provoked seizure does not recur when the provoking factor is successfully corrected, avoided, or removed. The tendency toward recurrent provoked seizures speaks either to the root cause (e.g., recurrent episodes of alcohol withdrawal seizures) or to a heightened sensitivity to seizures in the individual (e.g., a lower than average seizure threshold).

Epilepsy is characterized by recurrent, unprovoked seizures. The prevalence of epilepsy in the general population is approximately 1%. The principal clinical symptoms and signs of epilepsy include ictal (during a seizure), postictal (immediately following seizure termination), and interictal (between seizure episodes) manifestations. Behavioral alterations accompanying epileptic seizures are diverse, ranging from subjective feelings reported by the patient, to objectively witnessed behavioral arrest, unresponsiveness, or involuntary movements. The nature of the ictal behavioral disturbance depends on the location of seizure onset in the brain and its pattern of propagation.

## Diagnosis of Seizure Type and Epilepsy Syndrome

A seizure is only a symptom of brain dysfunction, and the seizure type is not in itself an etiologic diagnosis. A diversity of underlying causative pathologies may result in identical phenotypes of clinical seizure behavior and electroencephalographic (EEG) manifestations. The patient's prognosis and treatment are directed by a diagnosis of the underlying epilepsy syndrome, which incorporates an understanding of the cause of the seizures as well as the clinical and EEG characteristics. Epilepsy syndromes are regarded as idiopathic, symptomatic, or cryptogenic.

The International League Against Epilepsy (ILAE) has created consensus terminology defining different seizure types and, in parallel, descriptions of epilepsy syndromes. Diagnosis of ILAE seizure type and epilepsy syndrome is based on electroclinical criteria, including the description of seizure behavior and EEG manifestations. Most experts now also use neuroimaging to diagnose the most likely seizure type and epilepsy syndrome. The seizure type and epilepsy syndrome diagnoses are crucial steps in the approach to the patient with epilepsy because this information determines the patient's prognosis, which type of antiepileptic drug (AED) therapy is indicated, and whether surgical therapies can potentially be offered if AEDs are ineffective.

## TABLE 1 Common Causes of Provoked Seizures

**Drugs of Abuse**
Alcohol
- Severe acute alcohol intoxication
- Alcohol withdrawal

Amphetamine and methamphetamine
Cocaine
Lysergic acid diethylamide (LSD)
Phencyclidine

**Iatrogenic (Prescription Drugs)**
Antibiotics
- High-dose intravenous penicillin
- Imipenem

Antiarrhythmic agents
- Lidocaine (Xylocaine)
- Procainamide (Pronestyl)
- Propafenone (Rythmol)

Insulin overdose
Pain medications
- Opiate analgesics, especially meperidine (Demerol)
- Tramadol (Ultram)

Psychotropic drugs
- Antidepressants
  - Clomipramine (Anafranil)
  - Bupropion (Wellbutrin)
- Antipsychotics
  - Clozapine (Clozaril)

Stimulants
- Amphetamines mixed (Adderall), methylphenidate (Ritalin)

**Infection**
Brain abscess
Cerebritis
- Lyme disease
- Neurosyphilis

Encephalitis
- Cytomegalovirus
- Herpes simplex virus type 1
- Varicella-zoster virus
- West Nile virus

Acute meningitis
- Bacterial
- Fungal
- Viral

**Metabolic Disorders**
Hypocalcemia
Hypoglycemia
Hyperglycemia
- Nonketotic hyperosmolar state
- Diabetic ketoacidosis

Hypomagnesemia
Hyponatremia
Hypernatremia
Hypophosphatemia

**Herbal Products**
Guarana
Ma Huang

The two principal varieties of epileptic seizures are partial (also known as focal or localization-related) and generalized seizures. Partial seizures begin in one brain region, whereas generalized seizures have their onset simultaneously in both cerebral hemispheres. Differentiating epileptic seizure type and syndrome is often difficult in new-onset epilepsy. Many partial seizures present clinically as a secondarily generalized tonic–clonic seizure without focal features, and patients usually present for evaluation after only one or a few seizures have occurred, so the full spectrum of their epilepsy is not yet apparent.

Partial seizures are subclassified as simplex, complex, and secondarily generalized seizures. A simple partial seizure is restricted at onset to one focal cortical region and does not impair consciousness. Simple partial seizures are synonymous with the term *aura* and involve autonomic, gustatory, cognitive, somatosensory, or involuntary motor activity depending on where they begin in the brain. When a simple partial seizure propagates beyond the initial seizure focus, it may evolve into a complex partial or secondarily generalized seizure. A complex partial seizure is defined by the feature of altered consciousness (although often not full loss of consciousness) and may involve behavioral arrest, blank staring, oral automatisms such as chewing or swallowing, limb automatisms including aimless fumbling movements of the hands, and amnesia. A complex partial seizure may or may not be preceded by an aura, and it may propagate to the whole brain to become a generalized tonic–clonic seizure. There may be considerable variability of behavioral characteristics between different patients with partial seizures or even within a given patient (although a patient's personal seizures tend to be rather monomorphic). Table 2 provides a summary of characteristic auras and behavioral manifestations of partial seizures according to the region of seizure onset. An EEG during a partial seizure usually demonstrates focal rhythmic activity overlying the region of seizure onset.

Generalized seizures involve simultaneous seizure onset in both cerebral hemispheres. By definition, consciousness is impaired from seizure onset, although myoclonic seizures may be too brief to detect an alteration in consciousness. Absence seizures, frequently confused with complex partial seizures because both were previously (and unfortunately) referred to as petit mal seizures, are brief episodes (typically less than 10 seconds) of behavioral arrest, staring with unresponsiveness, and oral or limb automatisms. Absence seizures lack an aura or postictal state. Tonic seizures involve symmetric tonic posturing of the extremities and, if prolonged, may have prominent autonomic instability. Atonic (also known as astatic) seizures involve loss of tone and may lead to falls. Generalized tonic–clonic seizures involve an initial phase of tonic posturing, generally lasting less than 20 seconds, followed by symmetric clonic movements of the limbs for 1 to 3 minutes. Ictal EEG during generalized seizures demonstrates generalized epileptiform patterns of repetitive spike-wave discharges, polyspikes, or background attenuation.

The accurate diagnosis of an epilepsy syndrome in each patient is an important tenet in epilepsy care; whereas diagnosis of the habitual seizure type describes the ictal seizure characteristics, an epilepsy syndrome diagnosis reaches further, inferring knowledge of the underlying etiology and therefore determining the prognosis and most appropriate therapy. Despite rigorous diagnostic testing, many times the epilepsy syndrome remains ambiguous in new-onset epilepsy cases.

Partial seizures and their associated epilepsy syndromes are most common in adolescents and adults, representing approximately 70% of all epilepsy in these age groups. Most partial epilepsy is related to known acquired etiologies such as head injury, cerebrovascular disease, or tumors. Conversely, idiopathic or cryptogenic partial epilepsies and idiopathic generalized epilepsies are often inherited. The basis of inherited epilepsies is a rapidly evolving field. Many of the known gene effects relate to ion channelopathies.

## The Differential Diagnosis of Paroxysmal Spells

The differential diagnosis of epilepsy is wide. Numerous paroxysmal non-neurologic and neurologic disorders may closely mimic the behavioral alterations of an epileptic seizure. Table 3 differentiates commonly confused seizure types and nonepileptic paroxysmal spells by behavioral characteristics, duration, and usual ictal EEG findings. Although most of these conditions are reviewed elsewhere in this text, psychological mimicry of epilepsy is particularly common. Psychogenic nonepileptic spells (also known as pseudoseizures) are most often an expression of a conversion disorder with subconsciously motivated spells of behavioral unresponsiveness or unusual movements that may closely resemble epileptic seizures. Psychogenic spells, however, frequently involve behavioral characteristics of eye closure, nonphysiologic patterns of movements, prominent pelvic thrusting, prolonged duration (often over 5 to 10 minutes), lack of stereotypy between

**TABLE 2  Typical Partial Seizure Characteristics According to Region of Seizure Onset**

| | Simple Partial | Complex Partial | Secondary Generalized |
|---|---|---|---|
| Frontal | Focal clonic motor or none | Amnestic<br>Automatisms<br>Hypermotor common | Frequent |
| Temporal | Mesial (none possible)<br>• Autonomic<br>• Dysmnesic<br>  • Déjà vu<br>  • Jamais vu<br>• Gustatory | Amnestic<br>Automatisms | Less frequent |
| | Lateral/posterior neocortical<br>Auditory<br>Complex visual | Amnestic<br>Automatisms | |
| Parietal | Somatosensory or none | Amnestic<br>Automatisms | Frequent |
| Occipital | Simple visual or none | Amnestic<br>Automatisms | Frequent |

**TABLE 3  Differentiating Epileptic Seizures from Nonepileptic Spells**

| | Premonitory Symptoms | Behavioral Characteristics | Duration | Postictus Symptoms | Ictal EEG Findings |
|---|---|---|---|---|---|
| Absence seizure | None | Staring, automatisms | <10 sec | None | Generalized 3-Hz spike wave |
| Partial complex seizure | Aura variable; if sensory march, brief over 10–30 sec | Staring, automatisms, posture often preserved | 30–180 sec | Common; amnesia, aphasia, sleepiness, ± incontinence | Focal rhythmic activity |
| Generalized tonic–clonic seizures | Aura variable | Sequence of tonic limb posturing for 10 sec, then clonic movements | 1–3 min | Invariable; frequently amnesia, sleep, incontinence, tongue biting | Repetitive spikes (tonic phase); spike wave (clonic phase) |
| Psychogenic nonepileptic spells (pseudoseizures) | Variable | Variable; behavioral unresponsiveness Nonstereotypy, and unusual movements common | Variable; may be prolonged (>10 min) | Variable; often none | None, other than movement artifact |
| Syncope | Common; lightheadedness | Falling, eye closure, variable convulsive movements, incontinence | Minutes | None to brief confusion; no postical amnesia | Suppression |
| Migraine | Prolonged; sensory march over minutes | "Positive" symptoms (e.g., tingling paresthesias) | 20–30 min | None | Slowing/suppression |
| Transient ischemic attack (TIA) | Sensory march rapid (<10 sec) | More often "negative" (e.g., anesthetic numbness, weakness) | Variable; <1 h | None | Slowing/suppression |
| Sleep disorders:<br>Cataplexy | Emotional provocation | Behavioral sleep | Minutes | None | REM stage sleep |
| Parasomnias | None | Sleep-onset only | Minutes | Brief confusion | Onset in REM/NREM sleep |

*Abbreviations:* EEG = electroencephalogram; NREM = nonrapid eye movement (sleep); REM = rapid eye movement (sleep).

episodes, and failure to respond to antiepileptic drugs. Because true epileptic seizures may also share all of these characteristics, the diagnosis of psychogenic nonepileptic spells is necessarily a diagnosis of exclusion and requires diagnostic ictal video-EEG monitoring for confirmation.

# Clinical Approach to the Patient with Seizures

The fundamental goals in epilepsy care are both diagnostic and therapeutic: to understand the underlying cause of epilepsy and determine the epilepsy syndrome when possible; to strive for seizure freedom without adverse side effects of treatment whenever feasible (or, at the very least, to minimize disabling, injurious seizures and limit adverse effects); and to identify and treat interictal co-morbidities in epilepsy.

## THE INTERICTAL STATE IN SEIZURES AND EPILEPSY

Recent studies have shown that quality of life in epilepsy is largely determined by the interictal state. Although reducing seizure burden is an integral determinant of patient quality of life, interictal mood disorders such as depression or bipolar affective disorder, cognitive impairments, and adverse effects of antiepileptic drugs more often affect how patients feel on a daily basis between their seizure episodes, and have great impacts on perceived quality of life. Physicians should thus proactively inquire regarding altered mood and adverse affects in patients with epilepsy. The approach to new-onset seizures and chronic care of the patient with established epilepsy is now considered.

## THE SINGLE SEIZURE AND NEW-ONSET EPILEPSY

The focus during the approach to new-onset seizures is different than in chronic epilepsy. The emphasis for new-onset seizures is prompt diagnosis of the underlying cause because it is imperative to ensure there is no symptomatic etiology requiring further diagnosis or therapy (e.g., brain mass or vascular malformation). Diagnostic tests also help determine the epilepsy syndrome diagnosis and judge the prognosis for future seizure recurrence.

After an apparent single seizure, the physician should take a detailed history from the patient and any available collateral historians about the presenting event. Although serum laboratory values are frequently obtained after a first seizure, these tests actually have little value in the diagnosis of most uncomplicated first seizures in adolescents and adults. Electrolytes and complete blood count may assure overall general health and serve as a baseline prior to contemplation of antiepileptic drug therapy. A serum or urine drug screen is often appropriate to exclude drug abuse or intoxication as a cause of provoked seizures in adolescents and adults.

The two most important diagnostic tests in the initial evaluation of new-onset seizures are a magnetic resonance image (MRI) of the brain and an EEG; the former provides a measure of structure and the latter a complementary measure of function. A computed tomography (CT) of the head is insufficient to disclose subtle epileptogenic pathology in the brain. The only reason to obtain a head CT after a new-onset seizure is for emergency exclusion of acute neurologic catastrophes requiring urgent attention, such as cerebral hemorrhage or infarction. If a patient has recovered to baseline and neurologic examination is normal, head CT can often be deferred if a definitive brain MRI and neurologic consultation may be obtained promptly (i.e., within 1 week following the seizure). If there is a question of head or neck trauma, head CT should be performed emergently, and cervical radiographs may be necessary. EEG is particularly valuable when brain MRI is normal because it may disclose functional evidence for a heightened epileptogenic potential by demonstrating interictal epileptiform discharges that help determine risk of seizure recurrence after a single seizure or diagnose the epilepsy syndrome when there have been recurrent spells.

Additional diagnostic studies such as ictal video-controlled EEG (V-EEG) monitoring, positron emission tomography (PET) of the brain, magnetoencephalography (MEG), and neuropsychological testing may be used later in the course of a patient's evaluation if empirical medical therapy is unsuccessful and if surgical candidacy is questioned, but they are of generally limited value in new-onset seizure disorders. V-EEG is appropriate when psychogenic nonepileptic spells are the suspected diagnosis to exclude epilepsy and to allow prompt triage to appropriate psychological care, thereby sparing the patient from an errant diagnosis and the potential risks of unnecessary antiepileptic drug therapy.

The risk of seizure recurrence following a single seizure is approximately 30% when both MRI and EEG are normal. Multiple seizures occurring over a single day should still be considered as a single seizure episode. The risk of recurrence following a second remote seizure is variable, ranging from roughly 50-80%. Evidence is conflicting on the precise prognostic value of an abnormal EEG following a first seizure, but most experts consider EEG abnormalities to raise the risk of seizure recurrence substantially, especially when the EEG shows generalized epileptiform discharges.

Following a second unprovoked seizure, most experts diagnose epilepsy and recommend treatment. Treatment may be considered even following a first seizure if a structural cortical lesion is found because the risk of seizure recurrence is more than 50% in such instances, or if the patient leads a lifestyle where a second seizure would be highly undesirable (such as dependency on driving or a risky occupation).

All patients with new-onset epilepsy must be counseled regarding safety and driving. All patients with consciousness-impairing seizures should be instructed to avoid work, hobbies, or sports activities exposing them to heightened risk of personal injury until seizures are controlled for at least 3 to 6 months. Driving is a critical personal and public safety concern with legal implications to both patient and physician. Because laws vary between states, clinicians must ensure intimate familiarity with the law governing epilepsy in their own jurisdiction and counsel patients appropriately, then document their discussion in the medical record. A few states require physicians to report epilepsy patients.

## CHRONIC EPILEPSY CARE AND DETERMINATION OF REFRACTORY EPILEPSY

The approach to the patient with chronic epilepsy is to determine whether the epilepsy is benign or refractory (also known as medically intractable, pharmacoresistant). Following from the tenet in new-onset epilepsy evaluation, determination of the patient's epilepsy syndrome directs the choice of AED therapy most likely to control seizures successfully and allows prognosis for future remission or commitment to long-term AED therapy. Symptomatic or cryptogenic partial or generalized epilepsies and juvenile myoclonic epilepsy rarely remit and usually require long-term AED treatment. Idiopathic partial epilepsy or unclassified epilepsy syndromes more frequently remit after 2 to 5 years of treatment, suggesting future AED withdrawal is worth considering. Drug withdrawal is a complicated decision that is best made in consultation with a neurologist.

Determination of the epilepsy syndrome is more readily achieved during longitudinal continuity of care, given information derived from observations of seizure episodes and further opportunities to obtain interictal or ictal EEG recordings. With repeated or prolonged interictal EEG recording, the yield of identifying interictal epileptiform discharges increases. However, even after repeated outpatient EEGs, or with intensive inpatient V-EEG recording, approximately 20% of those with eventually proven epilepsy lack definite interictal EEG abnormalities. It is important to realize that the diagnosis of epilepsy remains at heart a clinical determination. The absence of abnormalities on MRI or interictal laboratory EEGs does not exclude an epilepsy diagnosis. If MRI or EEG has not been performed prior to evaluation, it is helpful to begin with these investigations to determine the patient's epilepsy syndrome and to exclude symptomatic pathology. Inpatient V-EEG is the gold standard for establishing a diagnosis of epilepsy and should be considered when patients are refractory to one to two empirical AED treatment trials. Even if a patient has infrequent seizures while maintained on AED therapy, admitting patients to an epilepsy monitoring unit allows an opportunity for withdrawal of medication in a safe, carefully supervised environment with a goal of increasing seizure frequency so that one or more habitual clinical seizures may be recorded. Ambulatory EEG or outpatient V-EEG are also available at many centers but have lower yield, given limitations of the inability to withdraw AEDs safely, to conduct behavioral testing or capture video, and to accomplish a technically adequate recording.

Patients continuing to experience breakthrough seizures may have refractory epilepsy. Just more than 10% of patients who have an efficacy failure on their first AED ever become seizure free during future AED trials, suggesting the need for vigilance toward achieving the clinical goals of seizure freedom without AED side effects. If a patient fails to achieve seizure freedom following one to two AED monotherapy trials, referral to a comprehensive epilepsy center should be strongly considered to permit appropriate seizure classification and consideration of surgical options.

Approximately one-third of those with epilepsy, approximately 750,000 in the United States, have medically refractory epilepsy (i.e., epilepsy that is resistant to AEDs with continued breakthrough seizures and intolerable AED adverse effects). Those afflicted with refractory epilepsy consistently report lower quality of life for multiple reasons, including lost productivity at work or school, inability to drive, self-injury, and the fear of living with the constant uncertainty of when their next seizure may occur. Even more alarming, growing evidence indicates that patients with refractory epilepsy are at a heightened risk for mortality from sudden unexplained death in epilepsy (SUDEP). Even in patients who are well controlled on their drug treatment, approximately half of those surveyed are not satisfied with their current regimen of AEDs, in most instances because of unpleasant or disabling drug-related side effects. A determination of refractory epilepsy from breakthrough seizures or intolerable AED adverse effects should be made relatively early in the course of treatment to permit other potentially more effective care options to be considered. Because of the limitations of current AEDs, both patients and their physicians may be lulled into a dangerous complacency by the desperation of chronic refractory epilepsy, perhaps figuring that any further efforts toward improvement of the situation will prove futile. However, given the severe morbidity and potential mortality of refractory epilepsy, clinicians must aspire beyond the status quo of a so-called acceptable seizure burden and educate their patients that intensive evaluation may lead to more effective treatment for their seizures. Patients who may benefit from referral to a comprehensive epilepsy center include those with these situations:

- An uncertain diagnosis of spells (i.e., the diagnosis of epilepsy is still in question)
- Failure to achieve complete seizure control
- Adverse effects on current AED therapy
- Injury from their seizures
- Lost productivity at work or school because of seizures or adverse effects
- A complicated regimen of concurrent medications and/or other confounding medical, psychiatric, or psychosocial conditions

## Epilepsy Therapies

The goals of all epilepsy therapies are to achieve seizure freedom without adverse effects of treatment. Choosing between the numerous options available for epilepsy treatment can be daunting for physicians and patients alike. The last two decades have seen the release of a number of newer AEDs into clinical use, many of which offer improved tolerability and safety profiles. Another advent is vagus nerve stimulation (VNS), the first device using the novel approach of electrical stimulation in epilepsy approved by the Food and Drug Administration (FDA). Centers offering expert evaluation for epilepsy surgery have also become more widely available.

Guidelines for choosing among epilepsy therapies are currently lacking. Until evidence-based guidelines are developed, optimal therapeutic triage must be highly individualized by synthesizing available data, clinical wisdom, and the patient's preference.

All AEDs have the potential to cause dose-related neurotoxic adverse effects. Fortunately, these may be obviated in most patients by dose reduction or substituting for a better tolerated AED.

### ANTIEPILEPTIC DRUG THERAPY

Table 4 itemizes specific AEDs with accompanying information on clinical spectrum of uses, pharmacokinetics, typical dosing and blood levels, and cardinal adverse effects. There are currently no clear evidence-based algorithms to guide the temporal sequencing of different AED trials. Nonetheless, common treatment principles underlie the choosing, dosing, sequencing, and monitoring of AED therapy in epilepsy care. Here are several basic principles:

- Choose AED therapy appropriate for the epilepsy syndrome.
- Consider patient characteristics and co-morbidities when choosing AEDs.
- Employ AED monotherapy at the lowest effective dosage to achieve seizure freedom.
- Reserve AED polytherapy (combining two or more AEDs) for refractory patients and minimize total drug load to limit adverse effects.
- Treat according to the patient's clinical response, not the AED level.
- Monitor for long-term complications of older AED therapy and consider withdrawal of therapy when appropriate.
- Choose affordable AED therapy.

Choosing an AED appropriate for the patient's epilepsy syndrome is an important tenet of epilepsy care. AEDs have different spectrums of efficacy for various seizure types within epilepsy syndromes. Some AEDs are narrow in their spectrum of efficacy, whereas others are broader, treating a variety of different seizure types well. Broad-spectrum AEDs may be favored when the epilepsy syndrome diagnosis is ambiguous because they offer potential efficacy against most seizure types and have less potential to aggravate some epilepsy syndromes. To some degree, the spectrum of efficacy of an AED is related to its postulated mechanism of action. AEDs that chiefly antagonize sodium channel ionophores or promote γ-aminobutyric acid (GABAergic) neurotransmission are generally most effective in partial-onset seizures, whereas drugs that combine these and other mechanisms of action may have broader efficacy in primary generalized seizure types.

Evidence from prospective, blinded, randomized clinical trials is only available for certain AEDs for monotherapy use. Gabapentin (Neurontin), oxcarbazepine (Trileptal), and lamotrigine (Lamictal) possess randomized controlled trial evidence for monotherapy treatment of partial-onset seizures, and topiramate (Topamax) has evidence for monotherapy use in new-onset epilepsy. All older AEDs and other newer AEDs have either comparator trial or anecdotal monotherapy evidence. All marketed newer AEDs have randomized controlled trial evidence for use as adjunctive treatment in partial-onset seizures, whereas older AEDs have comparator trial evidence.

Patient characteristics and co-morbidities may affect the choice of an AED. For example, weight is an important consideration. Valproate (Depakene), pregabalin (Lyrica), and carbamazepine (Tegretol) may contribute to weight gain, whereas topiramate (Topamax) and zonisamide (Zonegran) may include weight loss among their adverse effect profile. The patient with both epilepsy and migraine might favor topiramate or valproate, drugs that are efficacious for both conditions.

In general, AED monotherapy is just as effective—or more effective—than polytherapy. Monotherapy limits the potential for adverse effects and drug interactions. AED dosing must be individualized to achieve optimal results. Our strategy is to titrate the AED toward a target dose that has proven effective for most individuals in clinical studies and in our experience. Dose adjustment can then be made in the event of adverse drug reactions or recurrent seizures. If the endpoint of seizure freedom is preserved, maintaining a lower but clinically therapeutic AED dosage is entirely acceptable. If a patient continues to experience breakthrough seizures, raising the AED dose to the maximal dose tolerated is sometimes necessary, although recent

## TABLE 4 Properties of the AEDs

| | Spectrum of Effect | Daily Adult Dosage/Interval | Usual Level (μg/mL) | Severe Adverse Effects | Idiosyncratic Toxicities | Interactions |
|---|---|---|---|---|---|---|
| **Older AEDs** | | | | | | |
| Carbamazepine (Tegretol) | Partial | 400–1600+ mg (bid–qid) | 4–12+ | Diplopia, dizziness, ataxia, hyponatremia | Yes | Bidirectional (AEDs, OC, AC, many) |
| Ethosuximide (Zarontin) | Absence | 500–1500+ mg (bid) | 40–100+ | Nausea, sedation | Yes | Unidirectional |
| Phenobarbital | Partial | 90–180+ mg (qd) | 15–40 | Sedation, psychomotor slowing | Yes | Bidirectional (AEDs, OC, AC, many) |
| Phenytoin (Dilantin) | Partial | 200–400+ mg (qd–bid) | 8–20+ | Sedation, dizziness, ataxia, gingival hyperplasia | Yes | Bidirectional (AEDs, OC, AC, many) |
| Primidone (Mysoline) | Partial | 500–1500+ mg (bid–tid) | 5–12 (measure phenobarbital) | Sedation, psychomotor slowing | Yes | Bidirectional (AEDs, OC, AC, many) |
| Valproate (Depakene) | Broad | 750–2500+ mg (qd–tid) | 50–100+ | Nausea, tremor, hair loss, weight gain | Yes | Bidirectional (AEDs) |
| **Newer AEDs** | | | | | | |
| Carisbamate | Partial (? Broad) | 100–200 mg | ? | ? | ? (None in clinical trials) | ? Bidirectional (AEDs, OC) |
| Felbamate (Felbatol) | Broad | 1800–4800+ mg (bid–tid) | 30–100+ | Irritability, insomnia, weight loss | Yes | Bidirectional (AEDs, OC, AC) |
| Gabapentin (Neurontin) | Partial | 900–3600+ mg (tid–qid) | 4–20++ | Sedation, dizziness, weight gain | No | None |
| Lacosamide | Partial (? Broad) | 200–600 mg | ? | Sedation, fatigue | ? (None in clinical trials) | None known |
| Lamotrigine (Lamictal) | Broad | 300–600+ mg (qd–bid) | 1–20+ | Dizziness, rash | Yes | Bidirectional (AEDs, OC) |
| Levetiracetam (Keppra) | Broad | 1000–3000++ mg (bid) | 5–40++ | Sedation, dizziness | No | None |
| Oxcarbazepine (Trileptal) | Partial | 600–3600+ mg (bid) | 10–40+ (MHD) | Sedation, dizziness | Yes | Bidirectional (AEDs, OC) |
| Pregabalin | Partial | 150–600+ mg (bid) | 2–10 | Sedation, dizziness, weight gain | No | None |
| Tiagabine (Gabitril) | Partial | 16–64 mg (bid–tid) | 100–300 μg/mL | Sedation, weight gain | No | Unidirectional |
| Topiramate (Topamax) | Broad | 100–600+ mg (qd–bid) | 10–20+ | Sedation, cognitive complaints, paresthesias, weight loss, rare nephrolithiasis | No | Bidirectional (AEDs, OC at high doses) |
| Zonisamide (Zonegran) | Broad | 100–600+ mg (qd–bid) | 10–40+ | Sedation, paresthesias, weight loss, rare nephrolithiasis | Yes | Unidirectional |

*Notes:* AED = antiepileptic drug; + = higher doses/levels often additionally effective, as tolerated; ++ = considerably higher doses/levels sometimes additionally effective in intractable patients, as tolerated; MHD = 10, 11 Monohydroxy derivative active metabolite of oxcarbazepine. Interactions: Unidirectional indicates that other AEDs or drugs may affect this AED; bidirectional indicates that other drugs may affect this AED, and this AED affects other drugs; OC = oral contraceptives, AC = anticoagulants; many = many other non-AEDs.
? = Available information incomplete and based on pre-marketing published data from clinical trials.

evidence demonstrates that only a minority of patients become seizure free when dosed above the usual therapeutic range, so a practical viewpoint of treatment futility should be realized when patients experience frequent breakthrough seizures despite adequate AED dosages. Therapeutic change should be made when seizure freedom is not maintained at AED doses effective for most patients. Overlapping AEDs in transitional polytherapy (where the baseline AED is maintained at the current dose to limit breakthrough seizures, the newly added AED is titrated to a protective dose, then the original drug is tapered and discontinued) is the preferred method when introducing a new AED monotherapy. Abruptly stopping the existing AED increases the risk of seizures (and perhaps status epilepticus), whereas introducing the new AED too rapidly may induce adverse effects that taint the patient's perception of what could be an effective therapy.

Many medically refractory epilepsy patients require chronic polytherapy. Overall, only a small minority of refractory patients can be rendered seizure free with AED polytherapy, but they may benefit substantially by reduction of seizure burden. Although no good evidence for specific AED polytherapy combinations exists, augmenting monotherapy with an AED offering a different or complementary mechanism of action may be considered. Great care must be taken to avoid excessive drug dosing and drug–drug interactions. Initiating and maintaining AED polytherapy is difficult and requires oversight by a neurologist with extensive knowledge of clinical pharmacology.

AED dosing should be adjusted to achieve the clinical goals of seizure freedom without adverse effects. This may indeed be a delicate balancing act for some patients because all AEDs have the potential to cause dose-related so-called neurotoxic adverse effects.

Fortunately, adverse effects may be obviated in most patients by dose reduction or substituting for a better tolerated AED.

Philosophies on the use of AED blood level monitoring differ, but most agree that blood levels should in most cases be considered only a guideline to treatment. AED levels should not be perceived as an absolute indication for altering AED dosing, divorced from clinical judgment of the patient's seizure control or adverse effects. Blood-level monitoring can help guide therapy, but so-called therapeutic levels are derived from treatment of populations. An individual patient may require a lower or higher intensity of AED therapy to achieve optimal results. For example, some patients develop breakthrough seizures even at supratherapeutic or toxic levels, others may experience adverse effects within the usual therapeutic range, whereas some patients become seizure-free on levels in a subtherapeutic range. The danger of overreliance on AED blood levels is twofold: levels may lead both physicians and patients to a false sense of therapeutic adequacy or may lead to errant manipulation of AEDs in patients who require no adjustments. Typical clinical scenarios where clinicians should obtain AED levels include the following:

1. After reaching steady-state administration of an AED, to establish a patient's individual personal baseline against which future comparisons can be made in event of breakthrough seizures.
2. While titrating individual AEDs in complex polypharmacy regimens, when drug interactions may influence either the new adjunctive AED or baseline antiepileptic and other medications.
3. Adjusting for alterations in AED metabolism during aging, disease states, and during each trimester of pregnancy when AED levels can fluctuate substantially based on altered drug absorption, metabolism, protein binding, and clearance. With some heavily protein-bound drugs, especially phenytoin (Dilantin), obtaining free drug levels is necessary to discern the biologically active fraction of the drug, especially in chronically or critically ill patients.
4. When trying to determine the AED responsible for adverse effects in a patient receiving polytherapy.

In summary, AED levels are most useful when testing a clinical hypothesis. We discourage the use of routine or scheduled levels, an exception being chronic phenytoin therapy in institutionalized patients (where zero-order kinetics from nonlinear hepatic metabolism may lead to drug accumulation and toxicity).

With chronic AED therapy, intermittent blood testing for monitoring of liver function tests and hematologic functions is reasonable although not of proven value. The highest risk of idiosyncratic reactions associated with AEDs such as serious rash, hepatotoxicity, and hematologic dyscrasias is during the first 6 to 12 months of therapy and extremely rare thereafter. There is, however, mounting concern that patients on chronic maintenance therapy with older AEDs are at risk for osteopenia and osteoporosis. Any enzyme-inducing AED (carbamazepine [Tegretol], phenytoin [Dilantin], phenobarbital, primidone [Mysoline], and oxcarbazepine [Trileptal]) has the potential to decrease bone density. Valproate (Depakote) may also lead to decreased bone density. Chronic phenytoin exposure is of particular concern, given its rare association with cosmetic adverse effects including gingival hyperplasia (which may be severe enough to warrant repeated gingivectomies), peripheral neuropathy, and irreversible cerebellar ataxia. Considering AED withdrawal in appropriate candidates or transition to another newer AED therapy without such untoward effects is often reasonable.

AED cost is a crucial social issue that may trump all other medical principles in selection and maintenance of AED therapy in patients who lack adequate medical insurance. Choosing expensive AEDs that a patient cannot afford may erode the patient's adherence to treatment and trust in the physician. Insurance and financial status must therefore be considered, so that available resources (i.e., indigent federal- or state-sponsored insurance or corporate pharmaceutical assistance programs) can be summoned if a prohibitively expensive newer AED is the best therapeutic choice. Some of the patents of newer AEDs will expire by publication of this book, leading to increased availability of generic drug formulations that could reduce the impact of medication cost, but the pharmacokinetic reliability of these generic formulations must also be established before their widespread use is recommended.

Withdrawal from chronic AEDs is a difficult consideration in the older adolescent or adult with epilepsy because seizure recurrence may impact driving and work abilities. In general, it is worthwhile to consider an attempt at withdrawing AED therapy when the patient has been seizure free for an arbitrary period between 2 and 5 years. Available data suggest that approximately 25% to 70% of patients experience seizure recurrence with AED withdrawal. The decision to withdraw AED therapy must be discussed in the context of the patient's lifestyle and responsibilities because driving and work considerations may be paramount and trump the medical prognosis. Neurologic consultation should be strongly considered when AED withdrawal is contemplated.

## EPILEPSY SURGERY

Evaluation for epilepsy surgery should be strongly considered in patients with refractory partial epilepsy. A syndrome particularly amenable to surgical intervention is mesial temporal-lobe epilepsy (MTLE), characterized by medically refractory complex partial seizures, often a history of complex febrile seizures in infancy, and hippocampal sclerosis on brain MRI.

Resective surgery for epilepsy has been performed for over a century, and advances in EEG and neuroimaging have increased the widespread application of epilepsy surgery. A pivotal clinical trial established the clear superiority of anterior temporal lobectomy over medical therapy for chronically refractory MTLE in carefully selected patients.

Identification of potential candidates for epilepsy surgery remains the biggest challenge for tertiary care epilepsy centers. Some have estimated that nearly 75,000 potential surgical candidates in the United States remain under care in primary care settings with ongoing seizures, yet only 3000 or fewer surgical procedures for epilepsy are performed annually.

Potential candidates for resective epilepsy surgery have refractory epilepsy with ongoing seizures that have been resistant to at least two to three appropriately administered AEDs. The precise seizure burden meriting an aggressive, invasive approach remains a subject of conjecture, but even one to two consciousness-impairing seizures annually may be highly disabling in patients who aspire to work and drive.

The basic approach in epilepsy surgery involves identification and precise localization of the epileptogenic zone, the region of the brain that is necessary and sufficient to cause clinical seizures; determining whether the patient possesses appropriate functional reserve for safe removal of that seizure focus; and subsequent operative resection of this area.

A variety of investigations must be performed at specialized comprehensive epilepsy centers to determine if epilepsy surgery would be effective and safe for an individual patient. The most useful and important initial investigations are a high-resolution volumetric brain MRI (with thin cut coronal plane acquisition perpendicular to the hippocampal long axis) and inpatient prolonged ictal V-EEG monitoring that permits intimate correlation and offline, post hoc detailed analysis of the ictal behavior and EEG to localize the patient's habitual clinical seizures. Additional techniques that help localize the epileptic focus preoperatively include functional imaging techniques such as single photon emission computed tomography (SPECT) and PET, magnetoencephalography, and neuropsychological testing. An intracarotid sodium amytal test is necessary in all patients to lateralize memory functions accurately and estimate functional reserve prior to surgery. In some cases, invasive EEG recording with surgically implanted subdural or parenchymal strips or grids of electrodes is necessary to confirm the seizure focus precisely and allow mapping of eloquent functional cerebral cortex to reduce operative morbidity.

When a structural epileptogenic mesial temporal brain lesion evident on MRI is concordant with well-localized habitual clinical seizures by ictal V-EEG, there is a 60% to 90% chance that surgery will produce seizure freedom. Resection in neocortical epilepsies offers a 30% to 80% chance of achieving a seizure-free outcome, depending largely on whether a MRI lesion concordant with the seizure focus is present. Surgical efficacy contrasts with a 5% or less chance that additional AED therapy will render the refractory patient seizure free. Favorable seizure outcome must be balanced with a 3% or less risk of major morbidity (i.e., hemorrhage, infection, stroke, memory, language, or hemianopic visual field deficit) incurred by surgery. Risk may be higher in extratemporal epilepsy surgery for postoperative motor, sensory, and visual deficits, depending on the location of the seizure focus. Memory or language deficits may occur in temporal lobe operations.

## OTHER ALTERNATIVE THERAPIES

Some patients with refractory partial epilepsy are not suitable epilepsy surgical candidates because of diffuse or unlocalizable epileptic foci, whereas others may choose not to undergo brain surgery despite suitable candidacy. In these cases, other options may still exist.

The vagus nerve stimulator (VNS) is the only electrical device currently approved as an adjunctive treatment for partial-onset seizures. A battery-operated generator and programmable computerized stimulator are placed surgically in a subcutaneous pocket on the left anterior chest. The device looks much like a cardiac pacemaker and has electrical leads connected to the left vagus nerve in the neck. Once implanted, the device is programmed by means of a radiofrequency wand in the physician's office and provides a small electrical current to the nerve at preset intervals and amounts. The patient also has the opportunity to trigger a stronger current to attempt to abort or lessen an oncoming seizure by means of a magnet that is passed externally over the device.

The efficacy of VNS for seizure reduction is roughly comparable to that of AEDs; approximately 40% of patients experience a 50% or greater reduction in their seizures, and up to 15% of patients become seizure free. Although there are no current evidence-based guidelines for the best timing of VNS placement, we reserve VNS for patients who are not resective surgery candidates or who refuse surgery and those who have failed most older and newer AEDs. In addition to reducing seizure burden, VNS may improve a patient's quality of life by improving alertness, mood, and memory. Predictors of which patients are most likely to benefit from VNS, and the optimal dosing of the device once it is implanted, are yet to be defined in prospective clinical trials. Additional neurostimulation therapies are being evaluated. The efficacy and safety of more specific neurostimulation modalities such as deep brain and cortical stimulation therapies are currently being evaluated in large randomized clinical trials. Two recent randomized controlled trials of transcranial magnetic stimulation (TMS) have yielded conflicting findings concerning efficacy; one study targetting patients with MRI-visible cortical malformations demonstrated TMS efficacy for seizure reduction.

Specialized diets may be a useful adjunctive treatment for epilepsy. The best studied of these is the ketogenic diet, a high-fat, low-protein, low-carbohydrate diet that induces systemic ketosis, which has an antiepileptogenic effect on the brain. The ketogenic diet is most often successfully used in children, but it may also be tried in adolescents and adults. Unfortunately, unless rigid compliance is assured, the ketogenic diet produces little benefit and, in general, most adolescents and adults have limited tolerance of the diet. However, highly motivated and desperately refractory epilepsy patients may benefit from the ketogenic diet. An alternative that is often more tolerable, but not yet robustly studied, is the modified Atkins diet, a high-fat, moderate-protein, low-carbohydrate diet that induces mild ketosis.

Identifying and treating seizure aggravators is an important consideration. Recent studies have suggested that obstructive sleep apnea syndrome (OSAS) is a frequent co-morbidity in refractory epilepsy, and nasal central positive airway pressure in patients with refractory epilepsy and co-morbid OSAS may lead to seizure reduction. Primary sleep disorders such as restless legs syndrome and periodic limb movements of sleep may fragment sleep and worsen seizure burden in patients with refractory epilepsy. If a primary sleep disorder is suspected, a diagnostic polysomnogram should be ordered, and aggressive treatment for the sleep disorder should be initiated.

Although most complementary and alternative therapies in epilepsy have not been rigorously studied, a variety of behavioral stress reduction techniques, meditation, yoga, or naturopathic treatments may be considered. Most of these therapies have few risks and occasionally benefit individual patients. Botanical extracts for epilepsy therapy that possess potent in vitro antiepileptogenic properties and wide therapeutic windows are currently being investigated as another avenue of therapy for refractory patients.

## STATUS EPILEPTICUS: IDENTIFICATION AND MANAGEMENT

Status epilepticus is a prolonged, unremitting epileptic seizure that constitutes a medical emergency. Until the last decade, status epilepticus was defined as a seizure lasting 30 minutes or longer (from onset through the end of the ictal period, exclusive of the postictal recovery phase that may in itself last well over 30 minutes). However, more recent data suggest that most seizures that self-terminate do so by 3 minutes after onset, indicating that longer lasting seizures are unlikely to stop without intervention.

Status epilepticus may be convulsive or nonconvulsive. Status epilepticus frequently begins with a prolonged generalized tonic–clonic or partial motor seizure, followed by a minimally convulsive or nonconvulsive phase with or without subtle motor features such as facial or eyelid twitching, or nystagmus. Status epilepticus thus evolves in a manner analogous to a lethal cardiac dysrhythmia, proceeding from clinically overt convulsive movements toward an eventual electromechanical dissociative state where the epileptic seizure continues as a subclinical electrographic discharge evident only during EEG monitoring.

Management of status epilepticus begins with securing the airway, respiration, and circulation and placement of two large-bore intravenous catheters for drug administration and fluid resuscitation. Obtaining a stat glucose is appropriate before rapid administration of thiamine, followed by intravenous dextrose (to avoid Wernicke encephalopathy in malnourished patients). If intravenous access is not readily available, rectal diazepam (Diastat) or intramuscular fosphenytoin (Cerebyx) can be used. Rectal diazepam is also useful in the out-of-hospital treatment of prolonged seizures or seizure clusters in adolescents and adults, potentially obviating escalation into status epilepticus and preventing an emergency department visit.

Initial pharmacotherapy of status epilepticus begins with intravenous lorazepam (Ativan) given at 2 mg/minute to a goal of 0.1 mg/kg (or 8 mg total) with cautious respiratory monitoring, then loading with phenytoin (Dilantin) at 20 mg/kg, given no faster than 50 mg/minute to avoid hypotension, with ECG and hemodynamic monitoring. Phenytoin should be given through a dedicated peripheral intravenous line because of potential for cardiotoxicity and to avoid precipitation by other drugs. Intravenous phenytoin, a highly insoluble alkaline solution, may lead to substantial soft-tissue toxicity (including the much feared purple-glove phenomenon). An alternative is fosphenytoin, which may be administered at up to 150 mg/min, and is not associated with tissue injury if extravasation occurs.

The success of treatment of status epilepticus can be measured clinically, but if the patient remains unresponsive after the convulsive movements stop, an urgent EEG may be needed to exclude nonconvulsive status epilepticus. Refractory status epilepticus can be treated with midazolam (Versed),[1] propofol (Diprivan),[1] pentobarbital (Nembutal), sodium pentothal (Thiopental), or phenobarbital.[1] Case series reports suggest that intravenous valproate and levetiracetam may also be tried. An advantage of short-acting agents such as midazolam and propofol is the rapidity with which pharmacologically induced coma can be reversed to examine the patient, whereas valproate and levetiracetam offer the advantage of avoiding hemodynamic or respiratory complications. An expanding armementarium for status epilepticus is expected, in that intravenous forms of the novel drug lacosamide and the older AED, carbamazepine, are currently being developed.

# Conclusion

Epilepsy is characterized by recurrent, spontaneous seizures. Epilepsy has many causes and represents a collection of syndromes that have varying natural histories and responses to therapy. Diagnosis is based on the history and may be supported by physical examination. The two

---

[1]Not FDA approved for this indication.

most important investigations in initial evaluation of the patient with new-onset seizures or epilepsy are high-resolution brain MRI and EEG. There are many mimickers of epilepsy requiring careful differential diagnosis. When confronted with spells of an uncertain type, evaluation with VEEG may secure the correct diagnosis.

The past decade has seen tremendous expansion in available AED therapies, many of which are more tolerable and safer for long-term use. Choice of AED in an individual patient depends on the epilepsy syndrome, consideration of available efficacy evidence, patient characteristics and co-morbidities, and cost. AED monitoring should reinforce, and not replace, clinical judgment. Chronic complications of certain older AEDs may include osteopenia, adverse cosmetic effects, weight gain, and neuropathy. Withdrawal of AEDs in selected seizure-free patients or transition to AEDs without chronic toxicities should be considered in such instances.

Unfortunately, despite advances in available AEDs, more than a third of patients with epilepsy are refractory. Early determination of refractory epilepsy and triage to intensive diagnostic and therapeutic resources at a comprehensive epilepsy care center is critical. Epilepsy surgery may render carefully selected patients seizure free, and VNS is a viable alternative when surgery is not possible, leading to reduced seizure burden and improved quality of life. Physicians should approach their patients with epilepsy with enthusiasm and hope for effecting an improvement in their condition.

## REFERENCES

French JA, Kanner AM, Bautista J, et al: Efficacy and tolerability of the new antiepileptic drugs: I. Treatment of new-onset epilepsy: Report of the Therapeutics and Technology Assessment Subcommittee and Quality Standards Subcommittee of the American Academy of Neurology and the American Epilepsy Society. Neurology 2004;62(8):1252-1260.

French JA, Kanner AM, Bautista J, et al: Therapeutics and Technology Assessment Subcommittee of the American Academy of Neurology; Quality Standards Subcommittee of the American Academy of Neurology; American Epilepsy Society. Efficacy and tolerability of the new antiepileptic drugs: II. Treatment of refractory epilepsy: Report of the Therapeutics and Technology Assessment Subcommittee and Quality Standards Subcommittee of the American Academy of Neurology and the American Epilepsy Society. Neurology 2004;62(8):1261-1273.

Kwan P, Brodie MJ: Early identification of refractory epilepsy. N Engl J Med 2000;342(5):314-319.

St. Louis EK, Gidal BE, Henry TR, et al: Conversions between monotherapies in epilepsy: Expert consensus. Epilepsy and Behavior 2007;11(2):222-234.

Wiebe S, Blume WT, Girvin JP, Eliasziw M: A randomized, controlled trial of surgery for temporal-lobe epilepsy. N Engl J Med 2001;345:311-318.

# Epilepsy in Infancy and Childhood

Method of
*Raj D. Sheth, MD*

## Definition

Seizures are a sudden self-limited clinical event that results from abnormal and excessive firing of cortical neurons. Paroxysmal events that are not cerebral in origin may mimic seizures, and in infants these commonly include breath-holding spells, vasovagal syncope, or cardiac arrhythmias.

## Classification

Seizures can be classified based on their onset as either *partial* (starting in a focal area of the brain), *partial with secondary generalization* (starting as a partial seizure but then secondarily spreading to other areas of the brain, usually involving both cerebral hemispheres), or *primary generalized* (involving all of the brain from the onset of the seizure) (Box 1). Partial seizures may be either simple partial, if consciousness is preserved during the seizures, or complex partial, if impairment of consciousness or confusion occurs during the seizure. Partial seizures typically present with brief motor movement, sensation, or autonomic symptoms.

Such a classification scheme, which works well in a child older than 7 years, may be difficult to apply to a younger child or infant. This feature adds considerable difficulty in determining if an event is an epileptic seizure or simply a behavioral phenomenon. For example, a young child with staring spells might simply be daydreaming or might be having an epileptic seizure such as an absence seizure or a complex partial seizure. Useful features to distinguish these events are that seizures may occur in both active and passive modes, whereas behavioral staring events are typically only seen in a passive mode (e.g., while watching television).

Generalized seizures include absence seizures, myoclonic seizures, or primary generalized tonic-clonic seizures.

## Provoking Factors

Seizures may be acutely provoked by a fever (febrile seizures) or be symptomatic of an underlying acute cerebral insult such as a severe head injury, central nervous system infection, electrolyte imbalance, or metabolic derangement. In these patients, treatment is directed at the underlying cause of the seizure. Patients with acute symptomatic seizures may require temporary seizure medication to control seizures but may not need long-term treatment with seizure medication.

## Idiopathic and Symptomatic Epilepsy

Epilepsy is the occurrence of two or more unprovoked seizures and indicates an underlying tendency toward seizures. Epilepsy that does not appear to be caused by an underlying cerebral abnormality (normal neurologic examination and cognitive function and a normal cranial magnetic resonance imaging [MRI] scan) is referred to as idiopathic epilepsy. Approximately 50% of childhood cases are idiopathic. The prognosis for idiopathic epilepsy is usually good for either spontaneous remittance of seizures or for their control. Idiopathic epilepsy is frequently related to a genetic multifactorial tendency toward the disorder. When it is a symptom of underlying remote cranial trauma, congenital cerebral malformations, tumors, or vascular anomalies, it is referred to as symptomatic epilepsy. Approximately two thirds of these patients have difficult to control seizures. When a cause cannot be identified but cognitive impairment is present, epilepsy is called cryptogenic. Patients with cryptogenic epilepsy have a similar prognosis as those with symptomatic epilepsy.

---

**BOX 1   Seizure Classification**

**Partial (or focal)**
- Simple partial
    Motor
    Sensory
    Autonomic
- Complex partial
    Focal or generalized secondarily

**Generalized**
- Absence
    Typical or atypical absence
- Myoclonic
- Tonic/clonic or tonic–clonic
    Atonic

## Epidemiology

Approximately 3% to 5% of all children experience a single seizure, with febrile seizures the most frequent. The incidence of seizures is highest in the first year of life, particularly in the neonatal period (first 4 weeks of life). Approximately 1% of these children have unprovoked seizures, and half of those have two or more seizures and are said to have epilepsy. Of those with epilepsy, approximately half have generalized seizures. Half of all children have epilepsy that is symptomatic of an underlying brain lesion, with the remainder having idiopathic epilepsy indicative of a genetic tendency.

## Diagnosis

The first priority is to determine if the event the patient experienced was a seizure or a nonepileptic paroxysmal event. Nonepileptic events in children include breath-holding spells, temper tantrums, vasovagal syncope, night terrors, hyperventilation, and panic attacks. The history is often sufficient to differentiate these events from seizures.

Evaluation of seizures requires a careful history, with particular attention given to the onset of the seizure (eye deviation, fear) and any focal weakness following the seizure to determine if the seizure was partial. The neurologic examination is very useful. When a child exhibits neurologic deficits, it strongly suggests the seizure resulted from a focal brain lesion and warrants a cranial MRI.

### ELECTROENCEPHALOGRAM

The electroencephalogram (EEG) is central to the evaluation of seizures and should be obtained in all patients who had a seizure other than those with a simple febrile seizure. The EEG can help diagnosis and guide treatment by helping classify seizures, and it also offers some indication about prognosis. Generally, two features on the EEG are helpful in the evaluation: the background EEG activity and the epileptiform discharges. Background activity may be in either the normal or slow range. Normal background activity typically suggests idiopathic epilepsy, whereas background slowing is more indicative of seizures that are symptomatic of an underlying cerebral abnormality. Epileptiform discharges can occur even when the patient is not acutely seizing and are seen in approximately two thirds of patients known to have epilepsy. They are also seen in approximately 1% of children who have never experienced a seizure. Importantly, epileptiform discharges can help differentiate between partial and generalized seizures, thereby guiding treatment. Focal epileptiform discharges are present in one part of the brain and indicate partial epilepsy. Generalized epileptiform discharges occur throughout the brain. Specific generalized seizures can be diagnosed: 3-Hz generalized spike-and-wave activity (indicative of absence seizures) or polyspike-and-wave activity (indicative of myoclonic or tonic–clonic seizures) are suggestive of generalized epilepsy. Severe forms of epilepsy, including infantile spasms, are associated with hypsarhythmia, and the Lennox-Gastaut syndrome, associated with slow spike-and-wave activity, can be diagnosed with the EEG.

### CRANIAL IMAGING

In an acute situation, a cranial computed tomography (CT) can help evaluate urgently for intracranial blood or trauma, although a comprehensive evaluation requires an MRI scan in most patients. New-onset seizures may require evaluation with gadolinium enhancement to exclude a brain tumor. Patients with temporal lobe epilepsy require specific studies, which include a temporal lobe protocol to determine if there is mesial temporal sclerosis.

### DIFFERENTIAL DIAGNOSIS

Movement in the neonatal period can be difficult to differentiate from seizures. In an intensive care unit (ICU) setting, approximately 90% of events thought to be epileptic seizures turn out to be nonepileptic. Jitteriness can be separated from seizures because seizures can be stopped by changing the position of the limb. Clonic movements are the most specific for epileptic seizures. An EEG is very helpful at this point. A consistent precipitant suggests nonepileptic events. Breath holding can be associated with brief nonepileptic convulsive activity. Importantly, seizures are stereotypic. Parental home videos of the events can be helpful in better characterization.

In children older than age 5 years and adolescents, complicated migraine, sleep disorders, and syncope may be difficult to separate from seizures. Hyperventilation and panic events should also be considered. When there is doubt about the diagnosis, an EEG may be very helpful, with approximately 70% of patients showing epileptiform discharges between seizures.

## Epilepsy Syndromes

### FEBRILE SEIZURES

Febrile seizures occur between ages 6 months and 5 years, with the majority presenting by age 3 years. Simple febrile seizures last less than 15 minutes, with a single seizure within a 24-hour period, and they are not associated with Todd's paralysis. All other seizures are complex and may require further evaluation. Antipyretic measures and therapy are often recommended, although no evidence indicates this strategy prevents recurrence. Approximately one third of patients experience a recurrence. Rectally administered diazepam (Diastat) may help reduce the length of a seizure and is typically recommended for seizures that last longer than 5 minutes. Phenobarbital and valproate (Depakene) are effective in preventing recurrence of febrile seizures, although given the adverse effect of chronic therapy they are rarely indicated. Patients with prior febrile seizures who subsequently experience a seizure without fever should be evaluated for epilepsy.

### INFANTILE SPASMS AND LENNOX-GASTAUT SYNDROME

Infantile spasms and Lennox-Gastaut syndrome, although uncommon, are severe epilepsies and should be evaluated promptly. Infantile spasms occur between ages 3 and 18 months, and Lennox-Gastaut syndrome is typically diagnosed after that. Untreated infantile spasms often transition into Lennox-Gastaut syndrome.

Spasms are typically brief, lasting 1 to 5 seconds, with symmetric contraction of the trunk, extension of the arms, and tonic extension of the legs. Spasms, which occur in clusters, are associated with irritability and often seen as the child awakens or transitions to sleep. The EEG is hypsarrhythmic, showing a markedly abnormal and chaotic background with multifocal epileptiform discharges. The triad of infantile spasms, hypsarrhythmia, and developmental regression is referred to as West's syndrome. An underlying etiology is present in 80% of infants and usually associated with a poorer outcome than those in whom an etiology is not found. Corticotropin (ACTH)[1] treatment frequently results in control of spasm, improvement in EEG background, and an improvement in development. Vigabatrin (Sabril)* is an oral agent that can control infantile spasms, particularly those associated with tuberous sclerosis.

Lennox-Gastaut syndrome develops in 50% of children with infantile spasms. The EEG shows a diffuse slow spike-and-wave pattern. Patients have a combination of tonic, myoclonic, and atypical absence seizures. Seizures are intractable to medical treatment and the outcome is poor, with mental retardation seen in up to 90% of patients.

### ABSENCE EPILEPSY

Absence seizures resemble staring spells, although they may occur in both an active or passive state. Fifty seizures a day are typical, with subtle behavioral arrest that may be associated with eyelid twitching. The EEG shows 3-Hz generalized spike and waves. Absence seizures

---

[1]Not FDA approved for this indication.
*Investigational drug in the United States.

occur in childhood absence, juvenile absence, and juvenile myoclonic epilepsy.

*Childhood absence epilepsy* develops between 4 and 10 years of age and remits in most patients by 10 years of age. Seizures are easily treated with ethosuximide (Zarontin), although valproate (Depakote) and lamotrigine (Lamictal) can also be used.

*Juvenile absence epilepsy* develops between ages 6 and 10 years and usually does not remit. Unlike the childhood form, seizures do not remit and may be associated with tonic–clonic seizures. Ethosuximide is usually not effective for the tonic–clonic seizures, and valproate or lamotrigine are usually considered.

*Juvenile myoclonic epilepsy,* the most common epilepsy syndrome seen in children of normal intellect, has a similar age of onset as juvenile absence epilepsy and does not remit. The EEG shows generalized polyspike-and-wave discharges. Valproate is an effective medication for this epilepsy, although lamotrigine can also be considered. The latter is not as effective as valproate in controlling myoclonic seizures, although it has a better side-effect profile compared to valproate.

## BENIGN PARTIAL EPILEPSY WITH CENTROTEMPORAL SPIKE

Benign partial epilepsy with centrotemporal spike (BECTS) accounts for approximately 15% of epilepsy in childhood. Seizures are partial, with face twitching, of which the child is usually aware. Generalized tonic–clonic seizures may occur at night. The EEG shows a normal background with epileptiform spikes in the centrotemporal regions. If the child is only experiencing simple partial seizures, treatment may be withheld. Seizures remit in the vast majority of children. Control of seizures is seen with low-dose medication, and carbamazepine (Tegretol) or oxcarbazepine (Trileptal) are both effective treatment options.

# Treatment

After a careful diagnosis of epileptic seizures, treatment decisions are made to reduce the risk of seizure-associated injury, prevent the risk of prolonged seizures (status epilepticus), reduce the adverse cognitive effects of frequent seizures, and deal with social factors, such as driving.

Decisions should be discussed with the child and family, weighing the benefits with the risks of treatment. Factors that help guide treatment include seizure type, etiology, frequency, duration, and impact on the patient's life, along with age and level of activity.

The goal of treatment is prevention of seizures; therefore, assessment of the recurrence risk should be made. Following a first unprovoked seizure, there is a 50% risk of a second seizure. With the second seizure, the risk of the third increases to 80%. A normal neurologic examination, MRI, and EEG are all factors that lower the risk to 25% to 33%, whereas abnormalities found in these tests and a family history of epilepsy increase the recurrence risk to 75%. An EEG that shows 3-Hz generalized spike wave discharges seen in absence of seizures, however, increases that risk to virtually 100%. Treatment is often suggested after a patient has a second unprovoked seizure.

The underlying principles guiding treatment are that the patient should be free from both seizures and the adverse effects of medications (Table 1). Choosing among the different medications requires an understanding of adverse effects and efficacy. Seizures that respond well to treatment include the benign syndromes discussed earlier. In these patients, the lowest dose of recommended medication should be tried and gradually titrated depending on response (Table 2).

Medications should be titrated slowly to minimize adverse effects. Medication serum levels can help guide treatment, but medications should be titrated to response. Serum levels can be helpful in deciding if breakthrough seizures are a result of noncompliance or lack of efficacy. Some patients require more than one medication to control seizures. Unfortunately, many patients, despite multiple medications, continue to have seizures.

## WHEN MEDICATIONS FAIL TO CONTROL SEIZURES

Approximately 33% of patients' seizures are not controlled by medication, and alternative approaches can be considered. Options include the vagus nerve stimulator, the ketogenic diet, and epilepsy surgery. The first two measures typically reduce but do not abolish seizures. These decisions are best made using a multidisciplinary approach and require referral to a comprehensive epilepsy center. Patients who do not respond to a first medication choice should be referred for consultation.

## TABLE 1  Commonly Used Antiepileptic Medications

| Agent | Pediatric Dose (mg/kg/d) | Half-life (h)* | Dosing Schedule | Side Effects |
|---|---|---|---|---|
| Carbamazepine (Tegretol) | 10-35 | 25-65 (initial) 12-17 (chronic) | bid-qid | r, hep, bd, s, n dip, hypn, ost |
| Clonazepam (Klonopin) | 0.01-0.2 | 18-50 | bid-tid | s, a, h, b |
| Ethosuximide (Zarontin) | 10-15 (initial) 15-40 (maint) | 30-40 | qd-tid | gi, n, an, s, d, b, r, bd |
| Gabapentin (Neurontin) | 30-60 | 5-7 | tid-qid | s, d, a, ny, wg |
| Lamotrigine (Lamictal) | | | | |
| Off valproate | 0.6 (initial) 5-15 (maint) | 7 | bid | r, hep, d, a, s, n |
| On valproate | 0.15 (initial) 1-5 (maint) | 45 | qd-bid | |
| Levetiracetam (Keppra)† | 20-60 | 6-8 | bid | s, d, ha, b |
| Oxcarbazepine (Trileptal) | 8-10 (initial) 20-50 (maint) | 8-10 | bid | r, hep, s, diz, n dip, a, ha, hypn |
| Topiramate (Topamax) | 1-3 (initial) 5-9 (maint) | 18-30 | bid | s, an, ks, ps, wl |
| Valproic acid (Depakote) | 15-60 | 9-20 | bid-qid | hep, bd, n, s, d, wg, hl, r, gi |
| Zonisamid (Zonegran)† | 2-4 (initial) 4-8 (maint) | 50-70 | qd-bid | r, bd, hep, s, diz, an, n, ha, wl, ks |

*Half-life is based on monotherapy and assumes normal renal function.
†Not FDA approved for this indication in children.
*Abbreviations:* a, ataxia; an, anorexia; b, behavioral difficulties; bd, blood dyscrasia; d, dizziness; dip, diplopia; gi, gastrointestinal distress; h, hyperactivity; ha, headache; hep, hepatotoxicity; hl, hair loss; hypn, hyponatremia; ks, kidney stones; maint, maintenance; n, nausea; ny, nystagmus; ost, osteomalacia; ps, psychomotor slowing; r, rash; s, sedation; wg, weight gain; wl, weight loss.

## TABLE 2 Which Medications for Which Seizure Types?

| Seizure Type | First-Line Therapy | Second-Line Therapy | Third-Line Therapy |
|---|---|---|---|
| Partial (all types) | CBZ, OXC | LTG, VPA, GBP, TPM, PHT | TGB, LEV,[A] ZNS,[A] PB |
| **Generalized** | | | |
| Tonic-clonic | VPA | LTG, TPM, PHT | PB, ZNS[A] |
| Myoclonic | VPA | LTG, CZP | PB, ZNS[A] |
| Tonic | VPA | LTG | CZP, TPM, ZNS[A] |
| Absence (before age 10) | ESM* | VPA, LTG | ZNS, TPM |
| (after age 10) | VPA | LTG | ESM, TPM, ZNS[A] |
| **Epilepsy Syndromes** | | | |
| CAE | ESM | VPA, LTG | ZNS, TPM |
| JAE | VPA | LTG | ESM, TPM, ZNS[A] |
| JME | VPA, LTG | TPM, ZNS[A] | CZP, PHT |
| Lennox-Gastaut | VPA | LTG, TPM | CZP, ZNS,[A] FBM |
| Infantile spasms | ACTH, VGB[†] | VPA, TPM, TGB, CZP | FBM, ZNS[A] |
| BECTS | CBZ, OXC | VPA, PHT, CBZ | LTG, TPM |

*Assuming no convulsive seizures.
*Abbreviations:* ACTH, adrenocorticotropic hormone; BECTS, benign epilepsy of childhood with centrotemporal spikes; CAE, childhood absence epilepsy;
  CBZ, carbamazepine (Tegretol); CZP, clonazepam (Klonopin); ESM, ethosuximide (Zarontin); FBM, felbamate (Felbatol); GBP, gabapentin (Neurontin);
  JAE, juvenile absence epilepsy; JME, juvenile myoclonic epilepsy; LEV, levetiracetam (Keppra); LTG, lamotrigine (Lamictal); OXC, oxcarbazepine (Trileptal);
  PB, phenobarbital; PHT, phenytoin (Dilantin); TGB, tiagabine (Gabitril); VGB, vigabatrin (Sabril); ZNS, zonisamide (Zonegran).
[A]Not FDA approved for this indication in children.
[†]Investigational drug in the United States.

## STOPPING MEDICATIONS

Discontinuing medications depends on the type of seizures and epilepsy. Generally, when a patient is seizure free for 2 years, discontinuing medication can be considered. With this strategy, 60% to 75% of patients remain seizure free. However, a higher relapse rate is seen in remote symptomatic epilepsy, epileptiform discharges on EEG, and structural cerebral lesions on MRI. Recurrences usually occur in the first year, but late recurrence is also seen. Discontinuing medications should be considered before adolescents start driving because once patients are driving the decision to stop medication becomes much more complicated.

# Attention Deficit Hyperactivity Disorder

Method of
*Timothy Wilens, MD, Thomas Spencer, MD, and Joseph Biederman, MD*

Attention deficit hyperactivity disorder (ADHD; the term used in this article refers to previously used definitions including hyperkinesis and ADD with or without hyperactivity) is the most common emotional, cognitive, and behavioral disorder that pediatricians, family physicians, neurologists, and psychiatrists treat in children. It is a major clinical and public health problem because of its associated morbidity and disability. Epidemiologic studies indicate that ADHD is prevalent throughout the world, with a general consensus that from 6% to 9% of youth and 4% of adults have the disorder. Follow-up studies of ADHD children into adolescence and early adulthood indicate that ADHD is associated with significant psychopathology, school and occupational failure, and peer and emotional difficulties throughout the life span. Although previously thought to remit in early adolescence, ADHD is now seen as a chronic condition continuing into adolescence in approximately three quarters of cases and into adulthood in approximately half of childhood cases. These higher persistence findings are related to more recent information indicating that whereas many of the overt hyperactive-impulsive symptoms diminish over time, the bulk of attentional problems continue and are correlated with later difficulties. For example, in one study, 90% of ADHD adults presenting for treatment endorsed functionally impairing inattentive symptomatology. Predictors of ADHD persistence include prominent hyperactivity or impulsivity, aggression, co-occurring psychiatric and learning disorders, and a family history of ADHD.

## Diagnosis

The diagnosis of ADHD is made by careful clinical history applying *Diagnostic and Statistical Manual of Mental Disorders, Fourth Edition* (*DSM IV*) criteria available in a user-friendly primary care version. Youth with ADHD are characterized by a considerable degree of inattentiveness, distractibility, impulsivity, and often hyperactivity that is inappropriate for the developmental stage of the child.

 **CURRENT DIAGNOSIS**

**Cognitive Disturbance(s)**

- Inattention (focus, vigilance, arousal)*
- Distraction (shifting, modulating, filtering)*
- Working memory (manipulation, problem solving)
- Executive function deficits (organization, time management, sequential work)

**Behavioral Difficulties**

- Impulsivity (rash decisions, interrupting, poor judgment)*
- Hyperactivity (fidgety, overactive, restlessness)*
- Talkativeness*
- Easily frustrated*
- Oppositionality/rigidity
- Immaturity
- Moodiness

*Denotes *Diagnostic and Statistical Manual of Mental Disorders, Fourth Edition* (DSM-IV) core symptom criterion.

Other common symptoms include low frustration tolerance, shifting activities frequently, difficulty organizing, and daydreaming. These symptoms are usually pervasive; however, they may not all occur in all settings. Children with predominantly inattention may have more difficulties in school and in completing homework but not manifest difficulties with peers or family. Conversely, children with excessive hyperactive or impulsive symptoms may perform acceptably academically but have difficulties at home or in situations of less guidance and structure. Adults tend to present with prominent attentional difficulties affecting work, schooling, and relationships. ADHD adults frequently also manifest residua of impulsivity (intrusiveness, impatience) and hyperactivity (fidgetiness, restlessness).

Children, adolescents, and adults who have the cognitive features of the disorder (i.e., inattention, distractibility, shifting activities, etc.) but lack hyperactive or impulsive features are considered to have ADHD. Previously anchored by overactivity and impulsivity, connected to brain dysfunction and damage, the disorder has been reconceptualized based on *impaired cognition* as a core feature. Hence, depending on what symptoms predominate, *DSM-IV* recognizes three subtypes of ADHD (percentage occurrence): a combined subtype (50% to 75% of cases), a predominantly inattentive subtype (20% to 30%), and a predominantly hyperactive-impulsive subtype (less than 15%).

Although not diagnostic, rating scales, checklists, and neuropsychiatric batteries may be helpful in providing evidence for the disorder and accompanying co-morbid conditions. Rating scales such as the Vanderbilt (downloadable from www.AAP.org) can be useful in assessing and monitoring ADHD. Although neuropsychological testing is not relied on to diagnose ADHD, testing may serve to identify particular weaknesses within ADHD or specific learning disabilities along with ADHD.

More than half of youth with ADHD are at risk for the development of co-occurring psychiatric disorders. Common co-occurring disorders include oppositional (40% to 60% of ADHD cases), conduct (10% to 20%), anxiety (30% to 40%), depression (20% to 30%), and bipolar disorder (less than 20%). For example, whereas only a minority of ADHD individuals develop mood disorders, an excess of ADHD is noted in depressed (20% to 30%) and bipolar youth (50% to 90%). ADHD and its associated co-morbid conditions also are a significant risk for higher rates and earlier ages of onset of cigarette smoking and alcohol and drug abuse. Not surprisingly, recent data suggest that these adolescents and young adults may be self-medicating mood and sleep issues with substances of abuse.

Males are more commonly affected with ADHD than females; although underidentification in girls remains a major concern. ADHD females share with their male counterparts the prototypical features of the disorder such as inattention, impulsivity and hyperactivity, high rates of school failure, and high levels of familial connection. Compared to boys, girls with ADHD have lower rates of disruptive behavior including conduct and oppositional disorders—common flags to ADHD in youth.

Although its precise neural and pathophysiologic substrate remains unknown, a large literature suggests the presence of abnormalities in (pre)frontal networks or frontal-striatal dysfunction. Studies generally show reduced corpus callosum, cerebellum, and caudate volumes and reduced prefrontal cortex and anterior cingulate activity, with recent imaging studies demonstrating reversal in baseline abnormalities in ADHD adults with stimulant administration. Both dopaminergic and noradrenergic dysfunction appear to be important in the underlying neurochemistry of ADHD. Data from family—genetic, twin, and adoption studies as well as segregation analysis—suggest a genetic origin for some forms of the disorder. Molecular genetic studies have implicated the dopamine D2, D4, and the dopamine transporter, as well as a serotonin receptor and storage protein (SNAP) as candidate genes. Studies evaluating the relationship between genetic subtypes or vulnerabilities and the expression of the ADHD and response and side effects to treatment are currently under way.

## Treatment

The management of ADHD includes consideration of two major areas: nonpharmacologic (educational remediation, individual and family psychotherapy) and pharmacotherapy. Support groups for ADHD are invaluable and an inexpensive way for families to learn about ADHD and resources available for their children or themselves. Support groups can be accessed by calling an ADHD hot line, large support group organization, or on the Internet (e.g., www.CHADD.org).

Specialized educational planning based on the child's difficulties is necessary in a majority of cases. Identification of co-morbid learning disorders, found in approximately a third of ADHD youth, should translate into the development of appropriate remediation plans. Parents should be encouraged to work closely with the child's school guidance counselor, who can provide direct contact with the child as well as a valuable liaison with teachers and school administration. The school's psychologist can be helpful in providing cognitive testing as well as assisting in the development and implementation of the individualized education plan. Educational adjustments should be considered in ADHD youth with difficulties in behavioral or academic performance. Increased structure, predictable routine, learning aids, resource room time, and checked homework are among typical educational considerations in these youth. Similar modifications in the home environment should be undertaken to optimize the child's ability to complete homework. Frequent parental communication with the school about the child's progress is essential.

Focused therapies incorporating cognitive-behavioral features are reportedly effective in children, adolescents, and adults with ADHD; however, the long-term benefit of these treatments independent of pharmacotherapy is yet to be determined. Behavioral modification with the child and parents is useful in cases of co-occurring disruptive behaviors, inflexibility, anxiety, or outbursts. More traditional insight-oriented psychotherapy should be considered in ADHD cases with evidence of self-esteem issues, adjustment problems, or depression. Social skills remediation for improving interpersonal interactions and coaching for improving organization and study skills are useful adjuncts to treatment.

## Pharmacotherapy

Medications remain a mainstay of treatment for ADHD. In fact, large multisite studies support that medication management of ADHD is the most important variable in outcome in context to multimodal treatment. Stimulants, adrenergic agents, arousal agents, antihypertensives, and antidepressants comprise the available agents for ADHD.

### STIMULANTS

The stimulants are considered among the first-line agents for ADHD based in part on their extensive efficacy and safety data. Recent work has demonstrated the efficacy and safety of stimulants in preschoolers and adolescents. Stimulants are sympathomimetic drugs that increase intrasynaptic catecholamines (dopamine and norepinephrine) by inhibiting the presynaptic reuptake mechanism and releasing presynaptic catecholamines. The most commonly used compounds in this class include *d,1*-methylphenidate (Ritalin [LA], Concerta, Metadate, methylphenidate transdermal patch [MTS, Daytrana]), *d*-methylphenidate (Focalin [XR]), amphetamine compounds (Adderall [XR]), and *d*-amphetamine (Dexedrine). A recently FDA-approved amphetamine prodrug, lisdexamfetamine, is now also available. The stimulants are available in immediate-release short-acting preparations that last 2 to 4 hours and extended-release forms that last from 8 to 12 hours. Differences among the constellation of the stimulants exist (e.g., racemic and single isomer, different release mechanisms, different "early" and "late" day concentrations with extended release).

Despite the findings on efficacy of the stimulants, studies also report consistently that typically a third of ADHD individuals do not respond or cannot tolerate this class of agents. Although methylphenidate is the best studied stimulant, the literature suggests more similarities than differences in response to the various available stimulants. However, based on marginally different mechanisms of action, some patients who lack a satisfactory response or manifest adverse effects to one stimulant may respond favorably to another.

Stimulants should be initiated at the lowest available dosing once daily and increased every 3 to 7 days until a response is noted or adverse effects emerge. Parameters for upward daily dosing of the stimulants typically are 1 mg/kg/day for the amphetamines and 2 mg/kg/day for methylphenidate (1 mg/kg/day for transdermal or *d*-methylphenidate).

Predictable short-term adverse effects include reduced appetite, insomnia, edginess, and gastrointestinal (GI) upset. A number of controversial issues are related to chronic stimulant use. Although stimulants may produce anorexia and weight loss, their effect on ultimate height is less certain. Although initial reports suggested a persistent stimulant-associated decrease in growth in height in children, other reports failed to substantiate this finding, and still others questioned the possibility that growth deficits may represent maturational delays related to ADHD itself rather than to stimulant treatment. Stimulants may precipitate or exacerbate tic symptoms in ADHD children. Recent work suggests that up to a third of children with tics may have worsening of their tics with stimulant exposure. Long-term exposure to stimulant treatment of ADHD appears to decrease the risk of subsequent substance abuse; however, diversion and misuse of immediate-release stimulants in older adolescents and young adults remains a concern.

## NORADRENERGIC AGENTS

### Antidepressants

The antidepressants are not approved by the Food and Drug Administration (FDA) for ADHD and are considered second-line agents. Bupropion (Wellbutrin, Zyban[1]) is an antidepressant with indirect dopamine and noradrenergic effects that was effective for ADHD in controlled trials of children and adults. Given its usefulness in reducing cigarette smoking, improving mood, lack of monitoring requirements, and tolerability, bupropion is often used for complex ADHD patients with substance abuse or an unstable mood disorder. Adverse events include activation, irritability, insomnia, and rarely seizures. The serotonin reuptake inhibitors (e.g., fluoxetine [Prozac][1]) are not useful for core symptoms of ADHD. The tricyclic antidepressants[1] are also effective in treating ADHD but require electrocardiogram (ECG) and blood monitoring and have substantial adverse effects (dry mouth, constipation, cardiac). Both bupropion and tricyclics may require up to 6 weeks to see a full therapeutic effect.

### Atomoxetine

Atomoxetine (Strattera) is a potent norepinephrine-specific reuptake inhibitor that was studied in more than 1800 youths with ADHD. In contrast to stimulants, atomoxetine does not increase dopamine availability in the nucleus accumbens or striatum, which may explain why it is not associated with euphoria. Although useful in uncomplicated ADHD, atomoxetine is particularly useful in ADHD co-morbid with oppositional, tic, anxiety, and substance use disorders. Dosing of atomoxetine is up to 1.8 mg/kg/day and should be reduced if patients are on concomitant medications that interfere with its metabolism (e.g., fluoxetine). Adverse effects associated with atomoxetine include GI upset, change in sleep pattern, nausea, irritability, and rare hepatitis and suicidal ideation (0.37%). Atomoxetine also had no long-term effect (less than 3 years) on growth in height and weight. Recent data show continued effectiveness and good tolerability in children and adolescents up to to 2 years.

## ANTIHYPERTENSIVES

The antihypertensives clonidine (Catapres)[1] and guanfacine (Tenex)[1] are used to treat the hyperactive-impulsive symptoms of ADHD. Clonidine is a relatively short-acting compound with usual daily dose ranges from 0.05 mg to 0.4 mg. Guanfacine is longer acting and less potent than clonidine with usual daily dose ranges from 0.5 mg to 3 mg. The antihypertensives are used for the treatment of ADHD as well as associated tics, aggression, and sleep disturbances, particularly in younger children. Two multisite studies suggest that α-agonists may be useful in ADHD plus tics, alone and in combination with stimulants. Although sedation is more commonly seen with clonidine, both agents may cause depression and rebound hypertension. Older reports have implicated the combination of clonidine plus methylphenidate in the deaths of four children; however, many mitigating and extenuating circumstances were operative, making these cases uninterpretable. A new once-daily form of guanfacine is currently under development. Cardiovascular monitoring (vital signs, ECG) remains optional.

## AROUSAL AGENTS

Modafinil (Sparlon)[1] is a nonstimulant shown effective for pediatric ADHD. Trials have shown efficacy in both the cognitive and hyperactive-impulsive symptoms in ADHD children. Despite efficacy, the precise mechanism or areas of action of modafinil in relation to the treatment of ADHD is not fully understood. Modafinil seems to exert effects on the hypothalamus and attenuates cholinergic, cathecolaminergic and monoaminergic components of the ascending reticular activating system. Activation of the frontal cortex and anterior cingulate may be directly related to the positive effect on ADHD symptoms. Modafinil may be particularly useful in addressing the various aspects of attentional dysfunction in ADHD such as impaired vigilance, arousal, motivation, and executive functioning. There may be a delayed onset to full effect, and adverse effects include reduced appetite, insomnia, and headaches. Long-term studies indicate similar tolerability to that described with stimulants. Although relatively free of drug interactions, modafinil reduces the effectiveness of some oral birth control pills.

Combined pharmacologic approaches can be used for the treatment of co-morbid ADHD, as augmentation strategies for patients with insufficient response to a single agent, pharmacokinetic synergism, and for the management of treatment-emergent adverse effects. Examples include the use of atomoxetine plus methylphenidate to enhance treatment responsivity, an antidepressant plus a stimulant for ADHD and co-morbid depression (fluoxetine [Prozac] plus methylphenidate), the use of clonidine to ameliorate stimulant-induced insomnia, and the use of a mood stabilizer or atypical antipsychotic plus an anti-ADHD agent to treat ADHD co-morbid with bipolar disorder (e.g., divalproex [Depakote] plus amphetamine compounds).

Unfortunately, a number of individuals either do not respond to or are intolerant of the adverse effects of medications used to treat their ADHD. Youth who are nonresponders to one stimulant should be considered for another stimulant trial or for a nonstimulant. If two stimulant trials are unsuccessful, a nonstimulant should be considered starting with atomoxetine (Strattera), and later considering modafinil (Sparlon)[1] or bupropion (Wellbutrin)[1] and the tricyclic antidepressants.[1] Antihypertensives may be useful for younger children or those with prominent hyperactivity, impulsivity, aggressiveness, or tics/Tourette's disorder. Cognitive activators such as donepezil may be considered for refractory youth.

In summary, there is increasing recognition that ADHD is a heterogeneous disorder that persists in a number of cases through adolescence into adult years. The scope of co-morbidity has expanded to include not only disruptive disorders but also mood, anxiety, and substance use disorders as well. Emerging findings support a genetic and neurobiologic basis for ADHD with catecholaminergic dysfunction as a central finding. An extensive literature supports the effectiveness of pharmacotherapy not only for the core behavioral symptoms of ADHD but also improvement in linked impairments including cognition, social skills, and family function. Similarities between juveniles and adults in the characteristics, biology, and pharmacologic responsivity of ADHD supports the continuity of the disorder across the life span.

---

[1]Not FDA approved for this indication.

[1]Not FDA approved for this indication.

## CURRENT THERAPY

### Medications Used in Attention Deficit Hyperactivity Disorder

| Generic Medication | Brand Name | Daily Dose (mg/kg)[3] | Common Adverse Effects |
|---|---|---|---|
| **Stimulants** | | | All age groups: |
| Methylphenidate | Ritalin (LA*) | 1.0–2.0 | ■ Insomnia, decreased appetite, weight loss, dysphoria |
| | Concerta* | 0.5–1.0 | |
| | Metadate (CD*) | 0.3–1.5 | |
| | MTS (patch)*[4] | (1 mg/kg/day) | |
| D-methylphenidate | Focalin (XR*) | (1 mg/kg/day) | ■ Possible reduction in growth velocity with chronic use |
| **Amphetamines** | | | |
| Dextroamphetamine | Dexedrine | (1 mg/kg/day) | ■ Rebound phenomena with immediate release |
| Lisdexamfetamine | Vyvanse | (1 mg/kg/day) | |
| Amphetamine compound | Adderall (XR*) | (1 mg/kg/day) | |
| **Noradrenergic Agents** | | | |
| Atomoxetine | Strattera | 0.5–1.8 | ■ GI upset |
| | | | ■ Hypersomnia and insomnia |
| | | | ■ Irritability/activation |
| **Arousal Agents** | | | |
| Modafinil[1] | Provigil | 200–400 (mg/d) | ■ Insomnia |
| | | | ■ Appetite suppression |
| | | | ■ Headache |
| **Antidepressants** | | | All age groups: |
| Bupropion[1] | Wellbutrin (SR, XL) | 3–6 (mg/kg/day) | ■ Irritability, insomnia, seizure risk |
| | | | ■ Contraindicated in bulimics |
| Tricyclics (TCA)[1] | | | ■ Dry mouth, constipation |
| Imipramine, Desipramine; | Tofranil, Norpramin, | 2.0–5.0 | ■ Weight loss |
| Nortriptyline | Pamelor | 1.0–3.0 | ■ Vital sign and ECG changes |
| | | | ■ Nausea |
| | | | ■ Sedation |
| **Antihypertensives** | | | Juveniles only: |
| Clonidine[1] | Catapres | 3–10 μg/kg | ■ Sedation, depression, confusion |
| | | | ■ Rebound hypertension |
| | | | ■ Dermatitis with patch |
| Guanfacine[1] | Tenex | 30–100 μg/kg | Similar to clonidine but less sedation |

[1]Not FDA approved for this indication.
[3]Exceeds dosage recommended by the manufacturer.
[4]Not yet approved for use in the United States.
*Denotes extended-release preparation of stimulant.

## REFERENCES

A 14-month randomized clinical trial of treatment strategies for attention-deficit/hyperactivity disorder. The MTA Cooperative Group. Multimodal Treatment Study of Children with ADHD [see comments]. Arch Gen Psychiatry 1999;56(12):1073-1086.

Barkley R: Attention-Deficit/Hyperactivity Disorder: A Handbook for Diagnosis and Treatment, 3rd ed. New York, Guilford Press, 2006.

Biederman J, Newcorn J, Sprich S: Comorbidity of attention deficit hyperactivity disorder with conduct, depressive, anxiety, and other disorders. Am J Psychiatry 1991;148:564-577.

Biederman J, Spencer T, Wilens T: Evidence based pharmacotherapy for attention deficit hyperactivity disorder. Int J Neuropsychopharmacol 2004;7(1):77-97.

Castellanos FX, Lee PP, Sharp W, et al: Developmental trajectories of brain volume abnormalities in children and adolescents with attention-deficit/hyperactivity disorder. JAMA 2002;288(14):1740-1748.

Faraone SV, Biederman J: Neurobiology of attention deficit hyperactivity disorder. In Charney DS, Nestler EJ (eds): Neurobiology of Mental Illness, 2nd ed. New York, Oxford University Press, 2004.

Greenhill L, Kollins S, Abikoff H, et al: Efficacy and safety of immediate-release methylphenidate treatment for preschoolers with ADHD. J Am Acad Child Adolesc Psychiatry. 2006;45:1284-1293.

Hinshaw SP: Preadolescent girls with attention-deficit/hyperactivity disorder: I. Background characteristics, comorbidity, cognitive, and social functioning, and parenting practices. J Consult Clin Psychol 2002;70(5):1086-1098.

Kurlan R: Treatment of ADHD in children with tics: A randomized controlled trial. Neurology 2002;58:527-536.

Michelson D, Faries D, Wernicke J, et al: Atomoxetine in the treatment of children and adolescents with attention-deficit/hyperactivity disorder: A randomized, placebo-controlled, dose-response study. Pediatrics 2001;108(5):E83.

Spencer T, Biederman J, Wilens T: Growth deficits in ADHD children. Pediatrics 1998;102(Suppl 2):501-506.

Wilens T, Faraone S, Biederman J, Gunawardene S: Does stimulant therapy of ADHD beget later substance abuse: A metanalytic review of the literature. Pediatrics 2003;11(1):179-185.

# Gilles de la Tourette Syndrome

Method of
*Cathy L. Budman, MD*

Gilles de la Tourette syndrome, or Tourette's syndrome, is an inherited neuropsychiatric disorder of childhood onset characterized by the presence of repetitive, nonrhythmic, stereotypic movements and vocalizations (tics) that wax and wane in severity and change in location.

In 1825, Jean Itard first described the ticcing and cursing symptoms of the 26-year-old Marquise de Dampierre, noting the peculiar contrasts between her peculiar disinhibited behavior and her otherwise preserved intellect and propriety. Sixty years later this association of tics with behavioral symptoms, including obsessions, compulsions, mood lability, and phobias was again described by the French neurologist Gilles de la Tourette, after whom this disorder is named. The complex interplay of neurologic, psychological, and environmental influences on tics contributes to the wide variation in their severity, form, frequency, and intensity. Once believed to be rare, it is now clear that milder cases of Tourette's syndrome are common, often unrecognized, and commonly misdiagnosed.

## Clinical Features

Historically, tic symptoms have been classified as either motor or vocal, depending on whether sounds are produced via moving air through the nose, mouth, or throat. Tics are further subclassified as either simple or complex.

*Simple motor tics* are characterized by repetitive, sudden, brief, isolated movements of a single muscle group. Examples include eye blinking, facial grimacing, and head jerking. Slower, sustained tonic movements, such as neck twisting and abdominal or buttock tensing, also occur and are called *dystonic tics*.

*Complex motor tics* consist of more coordinated, complicated movements involving several muscle groups such as twirling around, squatting, and hopping. Certain complex motor tics such as touching, tapping, smelling, copropraxia (obscene gestures), and echopraxia (mimicking others' movements) may be confused with volitional behavior or compulsions.

*Simple vocal tics* include a variety of inarticulate noises and sounds ("ooh" "tsk" "eh"), as well as throat clearing and humming. Although technically a simple motor tic, repetitive sniffing is also included in this category. Such symptoms might go unnoticed or be misattributed to seasonal allergies or nervous habits.

*Complex vocal tics* are phonic ejaculations with linguistic meaning, consisting of full or truncated words. Complex tics include echolalia (repeating the words of others), palilalia (repeating one's own words), and coprolalia (involuntary utterance of obscene words). Although coprolalia is a dramatic and distressing symptom, it occurs in only a minority of people with Tourette's syndrome and is certainly not necessary for establishing the diagnosis.

The tic itself is often experienced as an irresistible urge, a psychic itch that can usually be suppressed temporarily but at the expense of a buildup of inner tension relieved only by the tic. Because tics can be suppressed for minutes to hours at a time, the term *involuntary* is not completely accurate; tics are actually unvoluntary in nature, that is, the movement relieves the tension. *Premonitory symptoms*, characterized by patterns of uncomfortable somatic sensations such as pressure, tickle, or warmth that are localized to specific body regions, often precede the tic performance and may be more distressing and distracting than the tic itself.

Tics are increased by excitement, anxiety, fatigue, and concurrent medical illness but are often attenuated while the ticquer is performing absorbing activities. Tics typically occur in bouts: Periods of tic exacerbation can last days or weeks followed by other periods during which tics are relatively diminished or even absent. Tic symptoms also classically change in type and location over time, often progressing in a rostral-caudal fashion. Hence, episodes of repetitive eye blinking or facial grimacing can occur for several weeks, disappear for a period, then be replaced by repetitive head shaking or shoulder shrugging. This classic waxing-waning course, change in tic character, and capacity for temporary tic suppression contribute to the delay in Tourette's syndrome diagnosis.

## Natural History and Epidemiology

Although Tourette's syndrome has been identified worldwide in all ethnic groups and appears to be uniformly distributed across socioeconomic classes, it occurs 3 to 4 times more frequently in male patients than in female patients. It is currently estimated that Tourette's syndrome affects 0.5% to 1% of school-age children. Most tics manifest between ages 2 and 18 years, with an average age of tic onset at 6 to 7 years. Tics tend to peak in severity between ages 11 and 12 years, just before puberty, and in most cases they diminish by late adolescence or early adulthood. Tic severity in early childhood is not a good predictor of later tic persistence. However, the presence of severe tics in late adolescence appears associated with persistent tic symptoms into adulthood.

Some adults with Tourette's syndrome report several years, even decades, of relative tic quiescence or remission that are curiously punctuated by sudden, unexpected episodes of tic exacerbations in mid-life or later life. The explanations and risk factors for such recurrences are not clear and may be related to a combination of physiologic, psychological, and environmental factors. In the majority of Tourette's cases, however, it is not tic symptoms per se that most negatively affect quality of life but the presence and persistence of associated comorbid psychiatric conditions.

## Differential Diagnosis

At this time there is no biological marker or test that can be performed to confirm the diagnosis of Tourette's syndrome. Hence, physicians must rely on a careful, detailed history of symptoms and on clinical examination, employing the *Diagnostic and Statistical Manual of Mental Disorders*, fourth edition (text revision) (DSM-IV TR) diagnostic criteria.

Primary tic disorders generally have an onset before age 18 years and cannot be attributed to the direct physiologic effects of a substance or general medical condition (Box 1).

The primary tic disorders include chronic motor or vocal tic disorder, transient tic disorder, Tourette's disorder, and tic disorder not otherwise specified (TDNOS). Chronic motor or vocal tic disorders differ from Tourette's syndrome in that either motor or vocal tics, but not both, are present for longer than 1 year. Transient tic disorder is diagnosed when the duration of tic symptoms is less than 1 year. Tourette's disorder (used interchangeably with the term Tourette's syndrome) is characterized by motor and one or more vocal tics that have been present at some time during the illness, although not necessarily concurrently, and a course of tics that occurs nearly every day or intermittently throughout a period of more than 1 year. The category of tic disorder not otherwise specified is reserved for tic phenomena

---

**BOX 1  DSM-IV TR Classification of Tic Disorders**

- Tourette's disorder
- Chronic motor and vocal tic disorder
- Transient tic disorder
- Tic disorder not otherwise specified

*Abbreviation:* DSM-IV TR = *Diagnostic and Statistical Manual of Mental Disorders,* fourth edition (text revision).

## BOX 2   Differential Diagnosis of Tics

**Abrupt**
- Myoclonus chorea
- Paroxysmal dyskinesia
- Seizure

**Premonitory Symptoms**
- Dystonia
- Restless legs

**Suppressibility**
- All hyperkinesias

**Increased Distraction or Focus**
- Akathisia
- Chorea
- Psychogenic hyperkinesias

**Decreased Stress or Relaxation**
- Most hyperkinesias

**Present during Sleep**
- Myoclonus seizures
- Periodic movements

## BOX 3   Pharmacologic Management of Tics

**Antihypertensives**
- Clonidine (Catapres)[1]
- Guanfacine (Tenex)[1]

**Atypical Antipsychotics**
- Aripiprazole (Abilify)[1]
- Olanzapine (Zyprexa)[1]
- Quetiapine (Seroquel)[1]
- Risperidone (Risperdal)[1]
- Ziprasidone (Geodon)[1]

**Neuroleptics**
- Fluphenazine (Prolixin)[1]
- Haloperidol (Haldol)
- Pimozide (Orap)

---

[1]Not FDA approved for this indication.

that do not meet diagnostic criteria for a specific primary tic disorder, such as, for example, tics that occur with an onset after age 18 years or tics that first occur following a severe head trauma.

Primary tics must be distinguished from other stereotypic repetitive movement disorders, such as myoclonus, tardive dyskinesia, and dystonias (e.g., blepharospasm, torticollis) (Box 2). Stereotypic movements (stereotypies) associated with mental retardation, psychosis, autism, or congenital blindness or deafness may be difficult to distinguish from motor tics, and tics and sterotypies often co-occur in this population. The tendency to wax and wane in severity, change in location, and presence in context of other typical tic symptoms can be helpful in differentiating these two phenomena.

Secondary tics can result from infection, head trauma, carbon monoxide poisoning, and illegal substance abuse and can also occur in a number of neurologic disorders including Huntington's disease, Parkinson's disease, progressive supranuclear palsy, neuroacanthocytosis, Meige's syndrome, startle disorders, and developmental basal ganglia syndrome. An intriguing and highly controversial theory posits that some cases of Tourette's syndrome or obsessive-compulsive disorder (OCD) are immune-mediated secondary to group A β-hemolytic streptococci (GABHS) infection. The PANDAS (*pediatric autoimmune neuropsychiatric disorders associated with streptococcal infection*) hypothesis proposes that antibodies produced against GABHS cross-react with critical brain tissues, leading to a characteristically explosive onset or exacerbations of tic symptoms. However, there is currently conflicting basic science and clinical evidence both supporting and refuting the PANDAS hypothesis, and apart from treating culture-positive streptococcal infections with a course of antibiotics, no specific interventions are yet recommended outside research settings.

## Treatment

In the majority of Tourette's syndrome cases, tic symptoms tend to be mild and medication intervention is not necessary. Psychoeducation for patients, family members, peers, and school staff about Tourette's syndrome and its associated psychiatric disorders, appropriate modifications of the educational environment, and psychotherapy to improve adaptive functioning are the recommended initial therapeutic interventions for such cases. Pharmacotherapy should be considered once it has been determined that the tics are functionally disabling and not remediable by psychosocial interventions.

The goal in treating tics is generally to achieve a satisfactory *attenuation* (not elimination) of tic symptoms with the minimum, and tolerable, medication side effects (Box 3).

### $\alpha_2$-ADRENERGIC RECEPTOR AGONISTS

Initial medication for tic intervention typically employs an $\alpha_2$-adrenergic receptor agonist at a therapeutic dosage for a 4- to 6-week trial.

Clonidine (Catapres)[1] is started at 0.05 mg at bedtime and increased by 0.05-mg increments every few days to a maximum of 0.4 to 0.6 mg total daily, divided in a three- or four-times-daily dosing schedule. Many responders take 0.05 to 0.1 mg three or four times daily. Sedation and dry mouth are the most commonly encountered adverse effects. Transdermal clonidine[1] is an alternative dosing form, particularly for children who cannot swallow pills, but this formulation can cause skin irritation and is impractical during summer months.

Guanfacine (Tenex)[1] has the advantages of once- or twice-daily dosing and is usually less sedating. It is initiated at 0.5 to 1 mg at bedtime and increased by 0.5-mg increments every few days to a maximum daily dosage of 4 mg, which is split into a twice-a-day dosing schedule (e.g., 0.5-2.0 mg bid). When clonidine or guanfacine is to be discontinued, the drug should be tapered over 7 to 10 days to prevent withdrawal phenomena, such as tachycardia or rebound hypertension.

### ATYPICAL ANTIPSYCHOTICS

The newer atypical antipsychotics have generally supplanted the conventional antipsychotics as second-line tic suppressants due to their improved adverse-effects profile. With the atypical antipsychotics, extrapyramidal effects—drug-induced parkinsonism, akathisia, tardive dyskinesia, and acute dystonic reactions—are reduced. However, these agents can cause significant extrapyramidal side effects too, particularly at higher doses. Furthermore, there is increasing evidence that these agents can cause the metabolic syndrome as well as untoward endocrine effects in adults and children.

The atypical neuroleptics can generally be given in a single bedtime dose. Atypical antipsychotics with reported tic-suppressing actions include risperidone[1] (Risperdal) 0.25 to 4 mg/day, olanzapine[1] (Zyprexa) 2.5-15 mg/day, and ziprasidone[1] (Geodon) 20-120 mg/day. Case reports have described tic-suppressant efficacy with the atypical antipsychotics aripiprazole[1] (Abilify) and quetiapine[1] (Seroquel). Significant weight gain is a common and problematic side effect with most of these agents and that can be limited somewhat by strict diet control and increased physical activity.

---

[1]Not FDA approved for this indication.

## CONVENTIONAL ANTIPSYCHOTICS

When the atypical antipsychotics are ineffective or not tolerated, a trial of a conventional antipsychotic may be indicated. Pimozide (Orap) is an effective tic suppressant that appears to be better tolerated than haloperidol (Haldol). It is initiated at 0.5 mg daily and can be titrated up to approximately 6 mg total daily dosage. Common extrapyramidal side effects associated with dopamine-2 receptor blockade as well as a propensity toward prolongation of the QT interval on cardiac conduction (which is further worsened when combined with other medications that cause QT prolongation) can limit its use.

Haloperidol (Haldol) remains one of the most commonly employed conventional neuroleptics for treating tics, although most patients stop using it because of its unacceptable side effects. Haloperidol is initiated at 0.25 mg daily at bedtime. When the patient can continue taking it, a favorable tic response usually occurs with 3 mg/day or less.

If haloperidol is unsuccessful either due to lack of efficacy or excessive side effects, one can then switch to another conventional neuroleptic.

## OTHER TREATMENTS

Other medication strategies for suppressing tics are listed in Box 4. These agents have not been studied as extensively as the conventional and atypical antipsychotics, but in general they have a somewhat milder side-effect profile.

Although most medication interventions are nonspecific in their abilities to suppress tics, focal intramuscular injections of botulinum toxin (Botox)[1] have been used to treat patients with painful dystonic tics and might offer a unique possibility to target a specific tic.

If these preliminary attempts to attenuate tic symptoms are not successful, consultation and possibly referral to an experienced Tourette's syndrome specialist should be considered.

## Associated Psychiatric Disorders

Although tic symptoms contribute to the colorful, sometimes dramatic presentation of Tourette's syndrome, careful clinical assessment and treatment intervention for comorbid psychiatric disorders and psychosocial problems are of paramount concern. Comorbid psychiatric disorders such as obsessive-compulsive disorder (OCD), attention-deficit/hyperactivity disorder (ADHD), affective disorders (depression, bipolar spectrum disorders, non-OCD anxiety disorders), and impulse-control disorders are commonly encountered when treating Tourette's syndrome in the clinical setting. Recent studies have demonstrated that up to 50% of outpatients with Tourette's syndrome suffer from behavioral and emotional symptoms that would meet threshold criteria for a comorbid psychiatric disorder. Because distress and impairment caused by psychiatric comorbidities in Tourette's syndrome often surpass those caused by tics, active screening and specific treatment of associated emotional and behavioral symptoms are of paramount importance.

---

[1]Not FDA approved for this indication.

---

### BOX 4   Other Treatments for Tics

- Substituted benzamides: Tiapride[2], sulpiride[2]
- Nicotine: Nicotine patch (Nicoderm CQ)[1]
- Dopamine agonists: Pergolide (Permax)[1]
- Dopamine depleters: Tetrabenazine (Nitoman)[2]
- Botulinum toxin type A[1] (Botox) for dystonic tics

---

[1]Not FDA approved for this indication.
[2]Not available in the United States.

---

Such complex Tourette's syndrome cases often necessitate a referral to a specialist with expertise in the treatment of Tourette's syndrome and its psychiatric comorbidities. Cognitive behavior therapy (CBT), parent skills training, social skills training, family therapy, and anger management training are important nonpharmacologic interventions for Tourette's syndrome associated psychiatric disorders. (Zinner's article gives an excellent overview of the management of Tourette's syndrome and its psychiatric comorbidities.)

## REFERENCES

American Psychiatric Association: Diagnostic and Statistical Manual of Psychiatric Disorders, 4th ed, text revision. Washington, DC: American Psychiatric Association, 2000.

Coffey B, Park K: Behavioral and emotional aspects of Tourette syndrome. Neurol Clin 1997;15:277-289.

Jankovic J: Botulinum toxin in the treatment of tics associated with Tourette's syndrome. Neurology 1993;43(suppl 2):A310.

Jankovic J, Stone L: Dystonic tics in patients with Tourette's syndrome. Mov Disord 1991;6:248-252.

Kurlan R, Behr J, Medved L, et al:. Severity of Tourette's syndrome in one large kindred: Implication for determination of disease prevalence rate. Arch Neurol 1987;44:268-269.

Kurlan R, Lichter D, Hewitt D: Sensory tics in Tourette's syndrome. Neurology 1989;39:731-734.

McMahon WM, Leppert M, Filloux F, et al: Tourette symptoms in 161 related family members. Adv Neurol 1992;58:159-165.

Robertson M: Tourette syndrome, associated conditions and the complexities of treatment. Brain 2000;32:436-447.

Scahill LD, Leckman JF, Marek KL: Sensory phenomena in Tourette's syndrome. Adv Neurol 1995; 65:273-280.

Swedo SE, Leonard HL, Garvey M, et al: Pediatric autoimmune neuropsychiatric disorders associated with streptococcal infections: Clinical description of the first 50 cases. Am J Psychiatry 1998;155:264-271.

Tanner CM: Epidemiology. In Kurlan R (ed): Handbook of Tourette's Syndrome and Associated Tic and Behavioral Disorders. New York: Marcel Dekker, 2005, pp 399-410.

The Tourette Syndrome Classification Study Group: Definitions and classification of tic disorders. Arch Neuol 1993;50:1013-1016.

Zinner SH: Tourette syndrome: Much more than tics. Contemp Pediatr 2004;21:38-49.

# Headache

Method of
*R. Michael Gallagher, DO*

---

Headache is a disturbing and sometimes fearsome affliction that has plagued humankind throughout recorded history. It often is debilitating and particularly disturbing to the sufferer because the pain is located in the head, the very center of the body's cognitive and control functions. With its accompanying pain and debilitating symptoms, stress can mount and the headache can become all consuming.

Headache is experienced by all age groups from young children to the elderly. It is more common than asthma, diabetes, mental illness, and rheumatoid arthritis. In fact, the World Health Organization identifies severe migraine, along with psychosis and quadriplegia, as "one of the most debilitating chronic conditions." Although the majority of Americans experience tension-type headaches at some time in their lives, approximately 30 million experience migraine headache: 13% of women and 6% of men, predominantly in their most productive years between the ages of 13 and 55 years. Prepubescent boys and girls suffer equally; however, boys often outgrow their migraine attacks as they mature, and they are less subjected to hormonal influences. Smaller percentages of people, by comparison, suffer with other chronic headaches, such as cluster headache and chronic daily headache.

No sure diagnostic tests are available to differentiate headache types. The headache condition can progress over time in frequency, severity, and debilitation. Each sufferer can be different and may require a detailed evaluation and individualized treatment plan; more frequent or prolonged attacks often necessitate a more comprehensive treatment plan. Thus, the headache problem can be a challenge for both the sufferer and the clinician.

During the 20th century, dramatic advancements were made in medicine. Longevity and quality of life improved for many individuals. Unfortunately, for headache sufferers, most of these advances were for maladies that killed or maimed rather than for non–life-threatening conditions. It was not until the 1960s that even a reasonable preventive medication, propranolol (Inderal), was introduced, and by the 1980s only a handful of medications were available for wide use. Physicians had to improvise with medications and treatments that were originally designated for other medical conditions.

In the late 1980s and 1990s, epidemiologic, psychosocial, and pharmacologic research resulted in an increase in available headache information and treatment possibilities. The development of the triptans, serotonin agonists, brought a new awareness to both physicians and sufferers. Today, seven triptans and two relatively new preventive medications are available. In spite of this, a minority of migraine sufferers use these options, and more than 50% continue to self-treat without benefit of professional care.

In the past, patients wanted the physician to believe their headache problem was real. They hoped that they would be taken seriously and that the physician would make a sincere attempt to help them. The headache patient has changed. The headache sufferer who seeks treatment today is more knowledgeable and interested in rapid relief and tolerability of medication.

## Evaluation and Diagnosis

An accurate diagnosis is essential for effective management of patients with the more commonly encountered headaches. Because no biologic markers or diagnostic tests exist to determine headache type, the history is the single most important element in the evaluation of the headache patient. Various headache types sometimes have similar initial presentations, or patients may suffer with more than one type of headache (e.g., migraine and tension-type headache), which can be confusing at first, but the careful history usually differentiates the headache type. In general, little in the way of diagnostic testing is needed unless a physical cause is suspected. Some physicians prefer to perform simple laboratory tests to establish a baseline for medication toleration and monitoring as necessary (Table 1).

The headache complaint on occasion can be a sign of a more serious medical condition, such as a tumor, infection, or aneurysm. For this reason, the clinician always must be cautious and diligent in establishing an accurate and timely diagnosis. Certain so-called red flags in the history require immediate attention. These include any complex of symptoms or history that does not fit a typical headache type; report of a significant neurologic deficit; late-onset migraine (patient older than 30 years); sudden onset of a new head pain without history of similar headaches; changes in headache character; headache associated with elevated temperature; or completely unresponsive attacks in the absence of analgesic or caffeine overuse. When any of these symptoms are present or physical examination reveals significant findings, further diagnostic evaluation with imaging studies and consultation is imperative.

The appropriate headache patient evaluation includes a thorough history, physical examination with special attention to the head and the neurologic, cardiovascular, and musculoskeletal systems, and diagnostic tests when appropriate. The history should include headache onset, location, pain character (e.g., pressure, throb), frequency, duration, associated symptoms, aura or prodrome, triggers, previous treatment, and family history. Certain clues in the history may lean toward the diagnosis of migraine, such as motion sickness, absence of headache during pregnancy, and headache relationship to menses, sun glare, oversleep, fatigue, fasting, foods, or alcohol.

Various diagnostic screening questionnaires and tools have been developed over the years to assist busy clinicians in establishing the diagnosis of migraine. Most are long and cumbersome and do not easily become a part of routine patient evaluation. A simple three-question screener for migraine is helpful for generalist clinicians. A "yes" answer to all three questions indicates a strong possibility of the migraine diagnosis:

1. Do you experience headaches severe enough to see a physician?
2. Are your headaches accompanied by other symptoms?
3. Are your headaches intermittent (i.e., nondaily)?

*Note:* This screener should not be substituted for a complete history; it should be used only for screening purposes.

### TENSION-TYPE HEADACHE

Tension-type headache (TTHA) is the most common of headaches and first was believed to be caused by sustained muscle contraction of the neck, jaw, scalp, or facial muscles. However, it is now thought that the sustained muscle contraction can, in fact, be an epiphenomenon to possible central disturbances rather than a primary process. Evidence suggests that altered levels of serotonin, substance P, and neuropeptide Y in the serum or platelets of patients with TTHA are responsible.

## TABLE 1  Current Diagnosis

| Symptoms | Frequency | Duration |
|---|---|---|
| **Tension-Type Headache** | | |
| Bilateral variable pain | Variable | Hours to days |
| Squeezing or bandlike | Often related to known precipitant | |
| Tightness of head and shoulders | | |
| **Migraine Headache** | | |
| Unilateral mostly | 1–6 mo | Hours to days |
| Throbbing or constant pain | Sometimes cyclic | |
| Nausea, vomiting | | |
| Photophobia/phonophobia | | |
| Fluid disturbances | | |
| Mood changes | | |
| Can be associated with aura | | |
| **Cluster Headache** | | |
| Unilateral severe boring pain | Multiple daily | 45–90 min |
| Ipsilateral lacrimation, scleral injection, rhinorrhea | Near-daily | Cycles of attacks |
| Eyelid droop | | |
| Restlessness | | |

**CURRENT DIAGNOSIS**

- Seizures may be partial (focal or localization-related) or generalized in onset. Clinical history, EEG, and imaging data assist the clinician in determining the seizure type and epilepsy syndrome.
- The most important initial diagnostic tests for evaluating new-onset epilepsy in adolescents and adults are high-resolution brain magnetic resonance imaging and EEG.
- In refractory epilepsy or spells of an uncertain type, the patient should be referred for video-EEG monitoring to document and localize the seizure type.

TTHA is characterized by intermittent or persisting bilateral pain, usually described as a squeezing pressure or a bandlike sensation around the head. Most patients experience their symptoms in the frontal, temporal, or occipital areas of the head. Location frequently varies with the attack, and tightness of the neck and shoulders is common. Intensity varies greatly. The attacks can last from hours to days, and in some extreme cases they may last for months. Aura, nausea, photophobia and phonophobia, and incapacitation are not typically associated with TTHA.

Many TTHA sufferers easily recognize the origin of their attacks. TTHA typically results from emotional upset, periods of stress, and major life changes. Anxiousness, poor adaptation skills, and anxiety and depression often are present. Physical causes, such as degenerative joint disease, trauma to the head or neck, poor posture, or temporomandibular joint dysfunction, also can precipitate attacks. Persons older than 50 years are prone to excessive muscle contraction because of arthritis of the neck and jaw, poor posture, or stress. TTHA that is consistently precipitated by tension or pathology of the neck frequently is referred to as a *cervicogenic headache*. In contrast to migraine headache, TTHA is more likely to begin in later life.

## MIGRAINE HEADACHE

Migraine headache is a familial disease characterized by unilateral or bilateral paroxysmal headache lasting hours to days. Adult women experience attacks more than men by a ratio of 3:1. Children and the elderly experience migraine equally. Attacks occur from as infrequently as one or two per year to several times weekly. Associated symptoms usually occur and frequently include throbbing, nausea, vomiting, photophobia, phonophobia, fluid retention, and mood changes.

The two basic types of migraine headache are *migraine with aura* (previously called classic migraine) and *migraine without aura* (previously called common migraine). Migraine with aura is preceded by an aura, a transient neurologic symptom that usually is visual, such as scotoma, teichopsia, tunnel vision, or visual field deficit, lasting 10 to 30 minutes. Migraine without aura is more commonly experienced and comes on gradually or is present on awakening from sleep. In some patients, these headaches are associated with a nonspecific prolonged prodrome, such as mood changes, food cravings, or fluid retention hours before the pain.

The underlying cause of migraine headache is not clearly established, and various theories are proposed. Migraine appears to be of genetic origin and to be an inflammatory disease that causes disturbances in serotonin use and activity. Strong evidence indicates the migrainous attack originates in the central nervous system by stimulation of the locus ceruleus and dorsal raphe nuclei. Resultant changes alter cerebral and extracranial blood flow, activate the trigeminovascular system, and cause vascular dilation, neurogenic inflammation, and pain. Various precipitants are known, and many sufferers report that migraine attacks frequently are associated with menstruation or are triggered by foods containing vasoactive amines, strong odors, too much or too little sleep, sun glare, stress, altitude, weather changes, exertion, or fasting (Boxes 1 and 2, Table 2).

---

**BOX 1  Migraine Dietary Triggers**

- Dairy: Ripened cheese (cheddar, brie, camembert, half-cup of sour cream)
- Meats: Processed lunch meats, hot dogs, sausage, bologna, salami, chicken liver
- Fish: Pickled or dried herring
- Grains: Sourdough bread
- Fruits: Bananas, raisins, figs, avocado, half-cup limit of citrus
- Vegetables: Broad and fava beans, onions, snow peas
- Other: Chocolate, nuts, peanut butter, pickled foods, Chinese food with monosodium glutamate (MSG)
- Beverages: Most wines and alcohol, 200-mg daily limit of caffeine
- Additives: MSG, soy sauce, meat tenderizers, aspartame, sulfites, garlic

---

Some physicians classify migraine according to its precipitant or description (e.g., menstrual migraine, exertional migraine, coital migraine, cervicogenic migraine, cyclic migraine, acephalic migraine). Regardless, the fundamentals of evaluation and treatment are the same.

## CLUSTER HEADACHE

The cause of cluster headache is unknown, and little credible research is available. Various possibilities or theories are suggested and include, but are not limited to, disturbances in histamine production or use; hypothalamic biorhythm dysfunction; or serotonin and neurotransmitter mechanisms similar to those of migraine. Some authorities consider cluster headache one of the most severe pain conditions known to humankind.

Cluster headache predominantly affects men, with a male-to-female ratio of 6:1. It occurs in well under 0.5% of the population. Onset later in life (after age 30 years) is common, and patients sometimes report head injury or a traumatic event occurring months before onset. Attacks occur on a daily or near-daily basis for weeks or months at a time and mysteriously disappear for months to years regardless of treatment, only to recur and cycle again. Although nonspecialist physicians only occasionally encounter the patient with cluster headaches, it is important to consider cluster headaches in the differential diagnosis.

The typical patient with a cluster headache experiences relatively brief attacks (45–90 minutes) of horrible unilateral head pain associated with ipsilateral lacrimation, scleral injection, rhinorrhea, or eyelid droop. The hallmark of the syndrome is its associated symptoms and

---

**BOX 2  Migraine Triggers**

- Altitude
- Alcohol
- Caffeine withdrawal
- Fluorescent or flickering lights
- Sun glare
- Weather changes
- Stress, stress letdown
- Foods
- Skipping meals
- Smoky environment
- Noisy environment
- Strong odors
- Lack of sleep, oversleep
- Exertion
- Hormonal changes

## TABLE 2  Current Therapy

| Headache Type | PRN | Prophylaxis |
|---|---|---|
| Tension | OTC*<br>NSAIDs<br>Muscle relaxants<br>Combination<br>  analgesics | Stress/precipitant<br>  avoidance<br>Stretching<br>Warm packs<br>Relaxation<br>  techniques<br>NSAIDs<br>Muscle relaxants<br>Antidepressants |
| Migraine | NSAIDs*<br>Triptans*<br>Ergotamine*<br>Dihydroergotamine*<br>Isometheptene*<br>Combination<br>  analgesics | Biofeedback<br>β-Blockers*<br>Divalproex<br>  sodium*<br>Topiramate*<br>TCA<br>  antidepressants<br>Calcium channel<br>  blockers |
| Cluster | Oxygen<br>Triptans<br>Dihydroergotamine<br>Ergotamine | No alcohol<br>Calcium<br>  channel blockers<br>Divalproex sodium<br>NSAIDs<br>Lithium<br>Steroids |

*FDA indication.
*Abbreviations:* NSAID = nonsteroidal anti-inflammatory drug;
OTC = over-the-counter; TCA = tricyclic antidepressant.

its severe and intense pain. During attacks, most cluster patients move about, trying unsuccessfully to get more comfortable, similar to renal colic, in contrast to migraine sufferers, who prefer to lie quietly in a dark quiet room. Few triggers are identified, and alcohol almost always precipitates an attack during a cluster "on" cycle. A rare form of cluster headache does not cycle and continues on a daily or near-daily basis without cessation.

## Treatment

The doctor–patient relationship frequently is the key to successful treatment in the headache patient. Although to some this statement seems an obvious truism, its importance cannot be overemphasized. Patients who experience frequent, near-daily, or daily headaches invariably require a comprehensive treatment program that necessitates good communication. Anxious patients sometimes do not comprehend medical explanations or instructions; busy doctors sometimes do not have or take the time to ensure that the patient understands.

The two elements of headache treatment are *abortive treatment*, directed at attacks once they have begun, and *prophylactic treatment*, directed at preventing or reducing the frequency of attacks. In general, the abortive approach is used for patients who suffer infrequent attacks and for those who experience breakthrough attacks while undergoing prophylactic therapy. Prophylactic therapy should be instituted when headaches are frequent, when headaches are unresponsive to abortive medication, or when there are contraindications to abortives (Table 2).

Headache treatment can include nonpharmacologic measures, such as physical exercise, stretching, stress avoidance, relaxation exercises, biofeedback, manipulation, massage, or cold/warm packs. Pharmacologic therapies can include a vast array of medicaments from over-the-counter (OTC) drugs to prescription drugs such as triptans, other vasoconstrictors, β-blockers, antiepileptic agents, antidepressants, nonsteroidal anti-inflammatory drugs (NSAIDs), analgesics, muscle relaxants, anxiolytics, and others.

Treatment, whether prophylactic or abortive, should follow a definite plan incorporating the clinician and patient into a team focused on reducing the headache frequency, severity, and disability. As mentioned earlier, impressions and physical findings should be explained to the patient in as much detail as necessary to ensure the patient's complete understanding. The complexity of the headache condition needs to be explained, emphasizing its chronicity, rather than its curability, and that the goal of treatment is disease control.

The comprehensiveness of the treatment plan depends on the frequency of the patient's attacks. The more frequent and severe the attacks, the more detailed plan may be necessary. Patients experiencing infrequent attacks (e.g., once or twice monthly) may require only an abortive medication and little else. Patients with more frequent attacks may benefit from dietary restrictions, psychosocial intervention, biofeedback relaxation training, manipulation, and physical modality intervention, in addition to medication.

### TENSION-TYPE HEADACHE TREATMENT

TTHA often is associated with emotional stress and muscle strain or tension of the shoulders and neck. Simple self-administered measures, such as stress avoidance, stretching, warm packs, or relaxation techniques, can be helpful in reducing or relieving attacks. More comprehensive professional intervention, such as manipulation, physical therapy, local injections, or biofeedback training, are considerations for more frequent or severe cases.

Prophylactically, the use of OTC or prescription medications can be considered in addition to nonmedicinal measures for reducing the frequency and duration of attacks. NSAIDs, muscle relaxants, or antidepressants (tricyclic antidepressant [TCA], selective serotonin reuptake inhibitor [SSRI]), at the lowest effective doses, are more commonly used.

Daily use of the longer-acting NSAIDs, such as naproxen[1] (Naprosyn) or celecoxib[1] (Celebrex), in the appropriately screened patient over a 2- to 3-week period, can be an effective preventative. TCAs, such as nortriptyline[1] (Pamelor) or amitriptyline[1] (Elavil), in low doses at night over 1 to 3 months, are frequently effective, especially in patients with anxiety or mild depression. The SSRI drugs, such as fluoxetine[1] (Prozac) or sertraline[1] (Zoloft), similarly can be useful. The muscle relaxant cyclobenzaprine[1] (Flexeril), at low doses, with a similar mechanism to the TCAs, can be administered at night for limited periods. Other muscle relaxants occasionally can be effective. Potential side effects can limit the use of NSAIDs (gastrointestinal irritation) and the TCAs (fatigue and weight gain).

Abortive or symptomatic treatment of TTHA can include simple OTC medications (e.g., aspirin or acetaminophen), NSAIDs (short-acting), muscle relaxants, combination analgesics, and, in some cases, opioid or opioidlike drugs. Caution should be exercised in prescribing potentially habituating drugs. Daily or near-daily use of analgesics can lead to analgesic rebound headache, which can compound the patient's headache problem.

Botulism toxin[1] (Botox) reportedly is helpful in the treatment of tension-type and migraine headache, but controlled studies are limited. In this treatment, a diluted solution of botulism toxin is injected into various muscles of the face, scalp, neck, or shoulders. Because this treatment frequently is used in headache specialty and pain centers, simultaneous comprehensive measures and medication may contribute to positive results. Side effects from botulism toxin are low when injected properly.

### MIGRAINE TREATMENT

Migraineurs are unique individuals, and the effectiveness and tolerance of medications can vary from patient to patient. Medication changes, combinations of medications, and trial and error may be necessary in the early stages of treatment.

Nonmedicinal measures for migraine sufferers include biofeedback stress reduction, caffeine and dietary restrictions, regimentation of

---

[1]Not FDA approved for this indication.

## TABLE 3 Triptans

| Medication | Brand Name | Half-life | Form/Strength |
|------------|------------|-----------|---------------|
| Sumatriptan | Imitrex | 1.5 hr | Oral: 25, 50, 100 mg; NS: 20 mg; injection: 6 mg, 4 mg |
| Naratriptan | Amerge | 6 hr | Oral: 2.5 mg |
| Zolmitriptan | Zomig | 3 hr | Oral: 2.5, 5 mg; Melt: 2.5, 5 mg; NS: 5 mg |
| Rizatriptan | Maxalt | 2–3 hr | Oral: 5, 10 mg; Melt: 10 mg |
| Almotriptan | Axert | 3–4 hr | Oral: 6.25, 12.5 mg |
| Frovatriptan | Frova | 25 hr | Oral: 5 mg |
| Eletriptan | Relpax | 4 hr | Oral: 20, 40 mg |

[1]Not FDA approved for this indication.
*Abbreviations:* Melt = oral disintegrating; NS = nasal steroid.

meals and sleep, rest, exercise, stretching, and avoidance of work or activity overload. Limiting caffeine to less than 200 mg/day is important to prevent the caffeine headache (rebound headache). Elimination of vasoactive foods, such as chocolate, aged cheese, and processed meats, and avoidance of fasting for more than 4 hours can be helpful for patients with more frequent attacks (Table 3). Regular exercise and stretching, planned relaxation, regular sleep schedules, and following a healthy lifestyle are frequently included in a comprehensive treatment regimen. In some patients, especially children and adolescents, biofeedback stress reduction or psychotherapeutic intervention may be necessary.

The more commonly used medications for prophylaxis are β-blockers, calcium channel blockers, antiepileptics (neurostabilizers), and the antidepressants. Treatment should be continued for a 4- to 8-week trial before discontinuation for ineffectiveness. Determination of which medication to use depends on comorbidities, interactions with concomitant medications, and tolerability.

β-Blockers such as propranolol (Inderal) and timolol (Blocadren) are nonselective and are approved by the Food and Drug Administration (FDA) for migraine prevention. Other β-blockers, such as nadolol[1] (Corgard), metoprolol[1] (Lopressor), and atenolol[1] (Tenormin), also can be effective. The mechanism of action in migraine is not wholly understood, but it is thought to involve anxiolytic effects as well as vascular changes and stabilization. The usual dosage is recommended (e.g., timolol 10–30 mg/day, propranolol 120–160 mg/day), and many consider the nighttime dose the more significant.

Calcium channel antagonists are well tolerated in general and can be as effective as the β-blockers. They are believed to alter serotonin release and inhibit platelet serotonin uptake and release within the brain. Verapamil[1] (Calan) is considered the more effective and is commonly recommended to patients. Dosage can vary from 120 to 480 mg/day. Nimodipine[1] (Nimotop) is equally effective, but it is rarely used in the United States because of its high cost.

Antiepileptic medications such as phenytoin[1] (Dilantin) and carbamazepine[1] (Tegretol) have been prescribed for migraine prevention over the years, with mixed results. Their use is now limited with the advent of newer, more easily tolerated agents, such as divalproex sodium (Depakote) and topiramate (Topamax).

Divalproex sodium is effective in reducing migraine attacks and is particularly useful in patients with coexisting head injury, seizure disorders, and bipolar disorders. It is thought to improve inhibitory and excitatory amino acid imbalance in the brain. It is best to start

with a lower dose and to gradually increase as needed and tolerated. The dosage of 500 to 1000 mg/day is more frequently prescribed. A commonly experienced side effect is sedation, which can sometimes be used to the patient's advantage when anxiolytic effects are needed.

Topiramate is the most recent preventive medication approved by the FDA for migraine prophylaxis. It has multiple mechanisms of action, but its exact mechanism in migraine headache is unknown. Its effectiveness is believed to involve sodium ion channel stabilization, calcium ion channels, GABA (γ-aminobutyric acid) receptors, and neuronal membrane stabilization. The average daily dose is variable and ranges from 30 to 100 mg/day. A most unusual side effect of weight loss or appetite suppression can be used to the patient's advantage in preventing weight gain, which frequently accompanies migraine prophylactic medications.

The TCAs can be useful in patients who experience frequent attacks and in those who experience anxiety and depression. The TCAs inhibit synaptic reuptake of serotonin, thereby reducing neuron firing and release of neurotransmitters. Starting with a low dose in the evening and titrating up to efficacy and tolerability is recommended. Significant anticholinergic and sedation effects sometimes limit their use. The SSRIs[1] are reported helpful in some patients, but their use in migraine prevention is limited.

In general, prophylactic medications should be taken for 6 to 8 weeks to determine efficacy. If effective, a course of 4 to 6 months is recommended before an attempt is made to discontinue medication.

A variety of abortive treatment options are available for migraine sufferers. Although the triptans (Table 3) have generated much interest and are frequently prescribed, other medications continue to be used, including ergotamine and its derivatives, isometheptene, and NSAIDs. Many of the abortive medications carry significant prescribing limitations that must be taken into consideration. Vasoconstrictor medications are contraindicated in patients with cardiovascular or peripheral vascular disease. NSAIDs should not be used in those with gastrointestinal or bleeding disorders. As with all medications, the clinician must consider appropriate prescribing, contraindications, and side-effect information.

The vasoconstrictor ergotamine is available in oral, rectal (Ergocaff PB), and sublingual forms (Ergomar). Ergotamine has a relatively long half-life and duration of action (up to 3 days) and should be used no more frequently than every 4 to 5 days to avoid ergotamine rebound headache. The ergot derivative dihydroergotamine (DHE-45, Migranal NS) is available for intramuscular (IM), subcutaneous (SC), intravenous (IV), and intranasal use. IV dihydroergotamine (DHE-45) sometimes is used for intractable migraine (status migrainosus) in emergency departments and inpatient settings. The intranasal form (Migranal) is an effective treatment when administered correctly by the patient. Unfortunately, dihydroergotamine is not absorbed by the gastrointestinal tract, and, unlike other abortive nasal sprays, any swallowed medication will be wasted. Dihydroergotamine has a low headache recurrence rate of approximately 12%. All forms of ergotamine and dihydroergotamine are more effective when taken early in attacks.

Isometheptene is used in combination with dichloralphenazone and acetaminophen (Midrin, Duradrin). It is slow acting and more effective when taken early in attacks and when used for attacks preceded or accompanied by stress and muscle tension of the neck. Although isometheptene is considered less potent than ergotamine and triptans, it is preferred by many patients whose headaches have features of both migraine and TTHA.

At the present time, seven serotonin agonists (triptans) are approved for abortive migraine treatment in the United States (see Table 3). As a category, the triptans are approximately 65% to 70% effective in published clinical trials. Their similarities are greater than their differences, but each triptan is not necessarily effective for all patients, and familiarity with their differences can be helpful to the treating physician. Half-life, onset and duration of action, adverse events, tolerability, recurrence of headache, and routes of administration may vary and allow the physician to match the medication to the individual patient. For example, a slower onset of action and longer-lasting triptan may be appropriate for slow-onset, longer-lasting migraine attacks.

[1]Not FDA approved for this indication.

[1]Not FDA approved for this indication.

Like other treatments, oral triptan tablets are more effective in the early phases of migraines. It is thought that peripheral sensitization—allodynia—is a sign of later phase migraine, and treating the attack before this phenomenon occurs is important. When treatment is delayed or the patient awakens with severe migraine, the injection, nasal spray, or rapidly acting triptans may be more beneficial. Although triptans as a group are very effective, recurrence of headache, after initial relief, requiring retreatment is common and can be as high as 40%. The recurrence rate tends to be less with triptans having a longer half-life.

The ergots and triptans are contraindicated in patients with ischemic heart disease, uncontrolled hypertension, and cerebrovascular disease. Physicians initially were extremely cautious about recommending triptans to their patients when the triptans were first introduced in the United States. However, significant human exposure to the triptans has revealed that catastrophic myocardial infarction or serious ischemia is rare. Chest pain following triptan use affects a small percentage of patients, and because the significance of this finding is not clear, refraining from future triptan use in these patients is recommended.

Sumatriptan (Imitrex), the first triptan approved in the United States, is available in nasal spray (20 mg), SC (6 mg, 4 mg), and oral formulations (25, 50, 100 mg). Its half-life is approximately 1.5 hours, and its duration of action is less than 4 hours. The injectable form produces rapid relief in 70% to 80% of patients, and it appears to be the most effective of all the available triptan forms. Conversely, it appears to cause the most side effects, and, for this reason, it should be used only for the more severe attacks. The oral forms are more favorable with regard to adverse effects, and their effectiveness is similar to that of other triptans (approximately 65%). Because of sumatriptan's short half-life and duration of action, recurrence of headache is common, necessitating repeat dosing.

Zolmitriptan (Zomig) is available in 2.5- and 5-mg oral and oral disintegrating tablets (ZMT) and as a 5-mg nasal spray. The efficacy of oral zolmitriptan is approximately 65% and that of the nasal form is 70%. The half-life of oral zolmitriptan is 3 hours, and its duration of action is longer than the nasal form, which improves on the need to re-medicate. The nasal spray has a biphasic absorption curve, which accounts for its favorable adverse effect profile over the 5-mg oral tablet.

Naratriptan (Amerge) was the first to be approved of the gradual-onset, longer-acting triptans. It is available as oral 2.5-mg tablets and has a half-life of 6 hours. Naratriptan is well tolerated by patients and often is used by patients with slow-onset migraine. Some specialists prescribe daily naratriptan for limited periods for treatment of menstrual or intractable migraine attacks.

Rizatriptan (Maxalt) is available as oral 5- and 10-mg tablets and as an oral disintegrating form (MLT). It has a relatively rapid onset of action and a favorable one-dose 2-hour response rate. Patients who are undergoing concomitant treatment with propranolol should take the lesser 5-mg rizatriptan dose because of higher resultant rizatriptan plasma levels.

Almotriptan (Axert) is available in 6.25- and 12.5-mg tablets. It has a half-life of 3.5 hours and, because of a broad $T_{max}$ (time of maximal concentration) range of 1.4 to 3.8 hours, a relatively rapid onset of action. Almotriptan has favorable adverse effect and headache recurrence profile. Chest pain symptoms after almotriptan use are similar to placebo in clinical trials.

Frovatriptan (Frova) is a long-acting triptan available in 2.5-mg oral tablets. It has the longest half-life of 25 hours and a favorable recurrence rate. Frovatriptan is frequently used for treatment of menstrual migraine and for attacks of longer duration. Some specialists prescribe daily frovatriptan for a limited period for menstrual and prolonged migraine attacks.

Eletriptan (Relpax) is the most recently approved triptan. It is available in 20- and 40-mg oral tablets and has a half-life of nearly 5 hours. Eletriptan has a relatively rapid onset but a longer duration of action and a favorable recurrence rate. In studies, some patients who were unresponsive to other triptans responded to eletriptan.

Various attempts have been made to compare triptans. Head-to-head trials mostly have compared one triptan to sumatriptan. A meta-analysis of 53 clinical trials published in 2001 compared the efficacy, recurrence, duration of action, and tolerability of all available triptans. Almotriptan and eletriptan were rated favorably across the major parameters of onset of action, efficacy, adverse events, and recurrence. In spite of efforts to adjust for variations in protocols and placebo response, specialists reached no clear consensus as to the validity or value of the meta-analysis or the preferability of one triptan over another.

NSAIDs frequently are recommended for treatment of acute migraine and can be effective when taken early. Their effects on the physiology of pain, inflammation, and platelets are believed to be the mechanisms responsible. Various agents are used, but none of the rapid-acting NSAIDs appears to have significant efficacy superiority. OTC ibuprofen (Motrin) and aspirin, in combination with caffeine and acetaminophen (Excedrin Migraine), is approved by the FDA for treatment of migraine.

Symptomatic treatment of pain may be necessary in patients who do not respond to recommended abortive treatment. Any effective analgesic can be appropriate, provided it is used infrequently and not on a daily or near-daily basis. In general, the more effective analgesics have anti-inflammatory and sedative properties.

## CLUSTER HEADACHE TREATMENT

Cluster headache is one of the more unusual pain conditions occasionally encountered by physicians. Pain onset is rapid, and the duration of the attack is brief. For this reason, prophylactic treatment usually is the most practical. Abortive prescriptions frequently are given, but, for the most part, the cluster attack is resolving by the time medication is absorbed.

Nonmedicinal prophylactic measures are extremely limited. The reduction of cigarette smoking, the addressing of individual stress and hostility issues when appropriate, and the complete cessation of alcohol consumption during cluster periods should be part of any treatment program. Prophylactic medications include the calcium channel blockers verapamil[1] (Calan) and nimodipine[1] (Nimotop), the neurostabilizers valproate[1] (Depakote) and topiramate[1] (Topamax), various NSAIDs, ergotamine,[1] lithium[1] (Eskalith), and, in extreme cases, short intervals of steroids.[1] These medications are used in average therapeutic doses, and combinations of medications are commonly needed (Table 4). The preventatives should be used during the cluster cycle and discontinued during off-cycle periods.

Abortive treatment is less preferred for cluster headache, as noted previously. However, inhalation oxygen via facial mask at 6 L terminates cluster attacks in 75% to 80% of sufferers within 12 minutes. Other possibilities include sumatriptans (Imitrex) SC or nasal spray,[1] zolmitriptan (Zomig ZMT) nasal spray,[1] ergotamine (Ergomar) sublingual, or dihydroergotamine injection (DHE-45) or nasal spray[1] (Migranal).

---

[1]Not FDA approved for this indication.

### TABLE 4  Cluster Headache Prophylactic Medications

| Medication | Brand | Average Daily Dose |
|---|---|---|
| Verapamil[1] | Calan, Isoptin, Verelan | 240–420 mg |
| Divalproex[1] | Depakote | 500–1500 mg |
| Topiramate[1] | Topamax | 50–200 mg |
| Indomethacin[1] | Indocin | 100–150 mg |
| Naproxen[1] | Naprosyn | 1000–1500 mg |
| Lithium[1] | Lithobid | 600–1200 mg* |
| Ergotamine[1] | Bellergal[†] | 1 tablet bid[†] |
| Prednisone[1] | — | 100 mg, decrease to 0 |

[1]Not FDA approved for this indication.
*With serum level monitoring.
[†]Ergotamine 0.6 mg with phenobarbital 40 mg and 0.2 mg L-alkaloids of belladonna.

The occasional patient reports relief with the oral triptans or analgesics. When triptans, ergotamine, or analgesics are used, appropriate prescribing and frequency guidelines should be followed. In general, with the exception of oxygen, daily as-needed medications should be avoided.

Headache continues to present a challenging problem for clinicians as well as for suffering patients. In spite of recent treatment advances and more public awareness, millions continue to needlessly endure pain and debilitation. At first glance, the headache problem appears complex and difficult when, in actuality, most sufferers experience straightforward, easily diagnosed headaches. The interested generalist or specialist who takes the time to elicit a careful history can establish the headache diagnosis and direct a simple treatment plan that can make a tremendous difference in the headache sufferer's life.

## REFERENCES

Astin JA, Ernst E: The effectiveness of spinal manipulation for the treatment of headache disorders: A systematic review of randomized clinical trials. Cephalalgia 2002;22:617-623.

Diamond ML, Dalessio DJ (eds): Diamond and Dalessio's The Practicing Physician's Approach to Headache, 5th ed. Philadelphia, WB Saunders, 1999.

Ferrari MD, Roon KI, Lipton RB, et al: Oral triptans (serotonin 5HT-IB/ID-agonists) in acute migraine treatment: A meta-analysis of 53 trials. Lancet 2001;358:1668-1675.

Gallagher RM, Kunkel R: Migraine medication attributes important for patient compliance: Concerns about side effects may delay treatment. Headache: J Head Face Pain 2003;43:36-43.

Goadsby PJ, Lipton RB, Ferreri MD: Migraine current understanding and treatment. N Engl J Med 2002;346:257-270.

Silberstein SD, Lipton EB, Dalessio DJ: Wolff's Headache and Other Head Pain, 7th ed. New York, Oxford University Press, 2001.

Vernon H, McDermaid C, Hagino C: Systematic review of randomized clinical trials of complementary/alternative therapies in the treatment of tension-type and cervicogenic headache. Complement Ther Med 1999;7:142-155.

# Viral Meningitis and Encephalitis

Method of
*Mark J. Abzug, MD*

Viral meningitis is the most common cause of aseptic meningitis, an inflammatory process involving the meninges in which usual bacterial etiologies cannot be identified. Encephalitis is an inflammatory process that affects the brain parenchyma, typically producing more severe illness. Many viral infections of the central nervous system produce inflammation of both the meninges and brain tissue (meningoencephalitis). Encephalitis may result from acute viral invasion of the brain and a concomitant inflammatory response or from a postinfectious, autoimmune process characterized by demyelination following a viral illness or vaccination (acute disseminated encephalomyelitis). The majority of the approximately 8000 to 13,000 cases of aseptic meningitis and approximately 20,000 cases of encephalitis reported annually in the United States are caused by viral infections.

## Clinical Features

Regardless of etiology, most cases of viral meningitis present similarly. Infants and young children display nonspecific symptoms, such as fever, irritability, lethargy, anorexia, and emesis. More specific findings suggestive of meningeal inflammation, such as nuchal rigidity, bulging fontanelle, and photophobia, are often absent. In older children and adults, nuchal rigidity and photophobia, along with fever, headache, and emesis, are more frequent. Focal neurologic findings and seizures are uncommon presenting findings in viral meningitis, although approximately 10% of children hospitalized with viral meningitis may develop acute complications such as obtundation, seizures, increased intracranial pressure, and inappropriate antidiuretic hormone secretion. Illness can last up to 1 to 2 weeks, with protracted headache not uncommon in adults.

Encephalitis is distinguished from meningitis by a change in sensorium and/or by focal neurologic findings. In younger children, encephalitis typically presents with irritability and/or lethargy, often after a febrile illness. Older children may manifest headache, disorientation, unusual behavior, abnormal speech, bizarre movements, and disorientation in addition to fever, nausea, emesis, myalgias, and photophobia. Generalized or, less commonly, focal neurologic abnormalities, including seizures and motor deficits, may be present. Progression to extreme lethargy, stupor, or coma may ensue.

## Etiology

In recent studies, a specific etiologic agent was identified in 55% to 70% of presumed cases of viral meningitis and in only 25% to 65% of cases of encephalitis despite thorough investigation. The list of implicated viruses is extensive (Table 1). Enteroviruses (EVs) are the most common cause of both viral meningitis and encephalitis of proven etiology. Other important agents include arboviruses (transmitted by arthropod vectors such as mosquitoes or ticks), herpes simplex virus (HSV), influenza virus, Epstein-Barr virus, varicella-zoster virus, adenovirus, and rabies virus.

## Diagnosis

Important diagnostic clues may come from history (respiratory or gastrointestinal symptoms, family exposures, seasonality, prevalent diseases, travel, animal and insect exposure, and recreational activities) and physical examination (see Table 1). The presence of a rash may suggest specific agents, such as varicella-zoster virus or EVs. Whereas identification of a mucocutaneous vesicle in a neonate may be key to the diagnosis of HSV infection, cold sores in older children and adults are *not* predictive of HSV encephalitis. The combination of findings of encephalitis and myelitis in the same patient is suggestive of infection with an EV (especially EV 71), West Nile virus, or Japanese encephalitis virus. Although focal signs are present in the majority of older children and adults with HSV encephalitis, the positive predictive value of focal findings for HSV is low.

Examination of the cerebrospinal fluid (CSF) is indicated in suspected meningitis or encephalitis unless contraindicated by concern for a space-occupying lesion or increased intracranial pressure. CSF in viral meningitis typically has a low-grade pleocytosis (100–1000 white blood cells [WBCs]/mm³, range <100 to ≥2000 WBC/mm³). Polymorphonuclear leukocytes may predominate early then become mononuclear within 8 to 48 hours. In general, CSF protein is normal or slightly increased, and the glucose concentration is normal or slightly decreased, although exceptions occur. The CSF in encephalitis typically has a predominantly mononuclear pleocytosis, increased protein, and normal glucose, although CSF may be normal in 3% to 5% or more of cases, especially early in the course. Certain viruses, including influenza and parvovirus B19, typically cause encephalopathies characterized by the absence of pleocytosis.

Imaging and electroencephalography (EEG) are useful adjuncts, particularly for encephalitis. Magnetic resonance imaging generally has better sensitivity than does computed tomography, especially early in disease. Characteristic imaging findings may suggest specific pathogens (see Table 1), and imaging can exclude alternative diagnoses; for example, a parameningeal focus or tumor. EEG is the most sensitive tool for confirming encephalitis and can distinguish infection from metabolic encephalopathy.

Viral culture, polymerase chain reaction (PCR), and serology are the major techniques for specific virologic diagnosis. Sensitivity of CSF

## TABLE 1   Epidemiology and Clinical Features of Viral Meningitis and Encephalitis

### Enteroviruses
#### Epidemiology
- Most common proven cause of viral meningitis and encephalitis (up to 85%–95% of viral meningitis and 80% of viral encephalitis).
- Majority of meningitis and encephalitis occurs in children <1 year old; incidence of meningitis exceeds that of encephalitis.
- Epidemic in warm seasons in temperate climates.
- Poliovirus infection decreased with widespread immunization.
- Enterovirus 71 frequently occurs in regional outbreaks, e.g., Asia since the late 1990s. Severe disease occurs primarily in children <5 years old.

#### Clinical Features
- Meningitis and severe encephalitis more common in younger children, especially neonates. Encephalitis may be part of systemic illness in newborns.
- Encephalitis typically generalized, although focal seizures and other abnormalities may occur, especially in neonates.
- May have biphasic febrile course; meningeal and encephalitic symptoms occur during second phase.
- Rash (macular, maculopapular, petechial, vesicular), enanthem, conjunctivitis, respiratory symptoms, pleurodynia, pericarditis, myocarditis, diarrhea, myalgias may accompany.
- Chronic meningoencephalitis with waxing and waning neurologic symptoms and high fatality rate occur in hypogammaglobulinemic patients.
- Enterovirus 71 associated with hand-foot-and-mouth disease, herpangina, and neurologic disease (meningitis, brainstem encephalitis, myelitis/acute flaccid paralysis, Guillain-Barré syndrome).
  - Signs of brainstem encephalitis include myoclonic jerks, tremors, ataxia, cranial nerve palsy, limb weakness, altered consciousness, seizures, increased intracranial pressure.
  - Imaging reveals high-intensity lesions in the midbrain, brainstem, and spinal cord anterior horn cells and ventral roots.
  - Pulmonary edema/hemorrhage, cardiac failure, shock may develop rapidly.

### Herpes Simplex Virus
#### Epidemiology
- ~1%–3% of viral meningitis.
  - Predominantly associated with primary type 2 HSV genital infection and less frequently with primary type 1 HSV genital infection, nonprimary HSV genital infection (either type), or without recent genital disease.
  - Mollaret's meningitis (recurrent, benign aseptic meningitis) mostly associated with type 2 infection without signs of genital infection and occasionally with type 1 HSV or with Epstein-Barr virus.
- ~10%–20% of encephalitis in the United States.
  - Encephalitis primarily due to type 2 HSV in neonates and type 1 HSV in older age groups.
  - Encephalitis occurs in ~50% of neonatal HSV infections.
  - ~33%–50% of non-neonatal HSV encephalitis is caused by primary HSV infection and ~50%-67% is caused by HSV reactivation.
  - Most common focal viral encephalitis in nonepidemic settings; most common sporadic fatal encephalitis.

#### Clinical Features
- Neonatal encephalitis characterized by seizures (focal and generalized), lethargy, irritability, tremors, anorexia, temperature instability, bulging fontanelle.
  - Central nervous system–only disease frequently begins in temporal lobe and then becomes bitemporal.
  - Encephalitis with disseminated disease more commonly is diffuse.
- Non-neonatal encephalitis characterized by fever and focal encephalitis with necrosis and hemorrhage.
  - Tropism for temporal lobe: Aphasia, anosmia, temporal lobe seizures, other focal findings.
  - Findings include headache, emesis, altered consciousness, bizarre behavior, personality changes, disorientation, ataxia, hallucinations, hemiparesis.
  - Focal findings are not always present; bilateral disease, widespread disease, or brainstem encephalitis may occur.
  - Elevated red blood cell count may be present in CSF; CSF protein levels may be normal early and increase over time.
  - Focal abnormalities on imaging studies, especially involving one or both temporal lobes, are suggestive of HSV disease. However, focal disease may occur with other viruses, other regions of the brain may be affected by HSV, and imaging may be normal in early HSV.
  - Temporal lobe focality on electroencephalography, especially with periodic lateralizing epileptiform discharges, is characteristic of HSV but is not specific.
  - Rapid progression is common; however, atypical and mild, slowly progressive cases are increasingly being reported.

### Arboviruses
#### Epidemiology
- ~5% of viral meningitis and important cause of encephalitis.
- Prevalent during warm and/or wet seasons; incidence related to mosquito or tick exposure.
- Leading agents in the United States:
  - West Nile virus: U.S. outbreaks since late 1990s; July to December predominance. Lower incidence and severity in children. Risk factors for severe neurologic disease include older age and immune compromise.
  - La Crosse virus: Central, eastern United States. Incidence of encephalitis approximately equal to that of meningitis; affects children more than adults.

- St. Louis encephalitis virus: Central, western, southern United States. Incidence of encephalitis less than that of meningitis; lower incidence and severity of encephalitis in children.
- Japanese encephalitis virus: Most common cause of epidemic encephalitis worldwide; causes encephalitis more than meningitis. Prevalent in Asia and Australia; affects children more than adults.
- Other important viruses
  - Eastern equine encephalomyelitis virus: Causes encephalitis more than meningitis.
  - Western equine encephalomyelitis virus: Causes encephalitis more than meningitis.
  - Venezuelan equine encephalomyelitis: Causes encephalitis more than meningitis.
  - Colorado Tick Fever virus: Rocky Mountains; tickborne. Meningitis in up to 18% of cases; encephalitis uncommon.
  - Powassan, Rocio, Murray Valley, Kyasuma Forest, Jamestown Canyon, California encephalitis, tickborne encephalitis, Ilheus, Snowshoe Hare, Rift Valley viruses.

### Clinical Features
- West Nile virus
  - ~20% of infections are symptomatic; West Nile fever in majority of these infections.
  - Neurologic illness in ~1/150 infected; of these, meningitis in ~30% and encephalitis in ~65%. Neurologic manifestations also include acute asymmetrical flaccid paralysis, polyradiculitis, transverse myelitis, Guillain-Barré syndrome, optic neuritis, and chorioretinitis.
  - Encephalitis is characterized by altered consciousness, cranial nerve palsies (brainstem involvement), generalized or focal motor deficits (weakness, tremor, myoclonus), movement disorders, sensory deficits, and ataxia. Focal temporal lobe disease may mimic HSV. Case fatality rate ~10%.
  - Fever, emesis, maculopapular rash (especially in children) frequently accompany neurologic disease.
- Japanese and Eastern equine encephalitides
  - Thalamic, midbrain, basal ganglia, brainstem lesions characteristic.

## Influenza Virus
### Epidemiology
- Rare cause of meningitis.
- Cause of 8%–10% of encephalitis.
  - More commonly associated with influenza A than with influenza B.
  - Encephalitis may be acute or postinfectious.
  - Acute necrotizing encephalopathy reported primarily in 1- to 5-year-old children in Asia since the late 1990s.
- Neurologic spectrum includes Reye's syndrome (influenza B), myelitis, Guillain-Barré syndrome.

### Clinical Features
- Acute necrotizing encephalopathy
  - Fever, altered consciousness, prolonged seizures; rapid progression to coma.
  - Elevated CSF protein, usually without pleocytosis.
  - Magnetic resonance imaging: Bilateral thalamic lesions and multifocal symmetrical lesions (brainstem, putamina, medulla, periventricular white matter, cerebellum).
  - Mortality ~30%; severe sequelae among survivors.

## Varicella-Zoster Virus
### Epidemiology and Clinical Features
- Chickenpox associated with cerebellar ataxia, meningitis, encephalitis, postinfectious encephalitis/ADEM, transverse myelitis, Guillain-Barré syndrome.
- Zoster associated with encephalitis, granulomatous hemiparesis, myelitis, cranial neuritis (including Bell's palsy). Neurologic complications may occur with rash, weeks to months after rash or without rash (especially in immune-compromised patients).

## Epstein-Barr Virus
### Epidemiology and Clinical Features
- Neurologic complications occur in 1%–5% of primary infections.
- Etiology of 2%–5% of acute viral encephalitis.
- Spectrum includes meningitis, encephalitis, ADEM, cranial nerve palsy (including Bell's palsy), transverse myelitis, and Guillain-Barré syndrome. Alice in Wonderland syndrome, consisting of visual seizures with metamorphopsia, may accompany encephalitis.
- Neurologic disease more frequent in immune compromised hosts.
- Typical features of infectious mononucleosis, atypical lymphocytosis, and heterophile antibody often absent in Epstein-Barr virus neurologic syndromes.

## Cytomegalovirus
### Epidemiology and Clinical Features
- Encephalitis primarily in congenitally infected neonates and immune-compromised hosts.
- Insidious progression.

## Human Herpesvirus 6
### Epidemiology and Clinical Features
- Meningoencephalitis occasionally occurs with primary infection.
- Increased incidence of encephalitis in immune-compromised hosts.
- Confusion, headache, seizures may accompany encephalitis; disease may be focal and mimic HSV encephalitis.

*Continued*

**TABLE 1   Epidemiology and Clinical Features of Viral Meningitis and Encephalitis—cont'd**

### Adenovirus
**Epidemiology and Clinical Features**
- Neurologic spectrum includes acute encephalitis, postinfectious encephalitis, Reye's syndrome-like encephalopathy, and transient encephalopathy.
  - Acute encephalitis is characterized by seizures, CSF pleocytosis, and severe disease.
  - Transient encephalopathy is characterized by obtundation, normal CSF, and complete recovery within several days.

### Lymphocytic Choriomeningitis Virus
**Epidemiology and Clinical Features**
- Transmission by rodent secretions.
- Meningitis and encephalitis more commonly occur in developing countries.
- Spectrum includes encephalitis, hydrocephalus, transverse myelitis.

### Human Immunodeficiency Virus
**Epidemiology and Clinical Features**
- Transient meningitis and, more rarely, encephalitis may accompany primary infection (acute retroviral syndrome).
- Chronic infection may be associated with subacute encephalopathy (loss of developmental milestones in young children, dementia).
- Acute encephalitis may accompany treatment failure during chronic infection (uncommon).

### Rabies Virus
**Epidemiology and Clinical Features**
- Relatively uncommon in United States; major sources are bats, raccoons, foxes, skunks.
- Important cause of encephalitis in developing countries; important sources are dogs and cats.
- Incubation period can vary from weeks to months to years. Pain, pruritus, or paresthesias at bite wound is followed by prodromal fever and anxiety and then by encephalitis.

### Measles, Mumps, Rubella Viruses
**Epidemiology and Clinical Features**
- Meningitis occurs in ~30% of measles infections; measles also causes acute encephalitis, postinfectious encephalitis, and delayed subacute sclerosing panencephalitis.
- Mumps was the leading cause of meningitis in the prevaccine era.
- Meningitis and encephalitis due to each virus dramatically decreased with widespread immunization in developed countries.

### Other Viral Agents
- Parainfluenza virus, respiratory syncytial virus, human metapneumovirus, rhinovirus, coronavirus, parvovirus B19, rotavirus, encephalomyocarditis virus, hepatitis C virus, simian herpes B virus, human T-lymphotropic virus, JC virus, Lassa fever virus, yellow fever virus, Hendra virus, Nipah virus, Australian bat Lyssavirus.

### Acute Disseminated Encephalomyelitis
**Epidemiology**
- Implicated in 10%–15% of cases of encephalitis in the United States.
- Increased incidence in infants and children.
- Onset days to weeks after respiratory tract infection (influenza, enteroviruses, measles, mumps, rubella, *Mycoplasma pneumoniae*, and others), gastroenteritis (rotavirus), and other infections (HSV, Epstein-Barr virus, varicella-zoster virus, human herpesvirus 6, cytomegalovirus).
- History of preceding infection or vaccination elicited in up to two thirds of cases.
- Winter–spring predominance in some series.

**Clinical Features**
- Diffuse, often multifocal symptoms reflecting regions of brain affected. Spectrum includes motor deficits, cranial nerve palsies, optic neuritis, cerebellar ataxia, altered consciousness, psychosis, seizures, transverse myelitis, peripheral neuritis.
- Multifocal, asymmetrical demyelinating lesions in imaging studies, with predilection for white matter.
- CSF cytology may be normal or show pleocytosis; CSF protein elevated in 50%–70%.
- Typically monophasic; occasionally relapses occur.
- Acute hemorrhagic leukoencephalitis is a rare entity representing the fulminant end of the spectrum. It primarily affects young adults and is characterized by seizures, coma, cerebral edema, and a rapid, often fatal course.

*Abbreviations:* ADEM = acute disseminated encephalomyelitis; CSF = cerebrospinal fluid; HSV = herpes simplex virus.

## CURRENT DIAGNOSIS

Differential diagnosis of meningitis and encephalitis is broad and includes:

- Bacteria: *Streptococcus pneumoniae, Neisseria meningitidis, Haemophilus influenzae, Listeria monocytogenes, Mycobacterium tuberculosis, Borrelia burgdorferi, Mycoplasma pneumoniae, Mycoplasma hominis, Bartonella henselae,* syphilis, leptospirosis, brucellosis, rickettsial and ehrlichial infections
- Parasites: Neurocysticercosis, toxoplasmosis, amebic encephalitis
- Fungi: *Cryptococcus neoformans, Coccidioides immitis*
- Parameningeal focus: Brain abscess or subdural or epidural empyema
- Kawasaki disease
- Sarcoidosis
- Connective tissue disease: Systemic lupus erythematosus, cerebral vasculitis, Wegener's granulomatosis, Hashimoto's disease
- Medication-induced meningitis: Nonsteroidal anti-inflammatory drugs, sulfa antibiotics, immune globulin, cytosine arabinoside (Cytarabine), muromonab- CD3 (Orthoclone OKT3), carbamazepine (Tegretol)
- Metabolic derangements: Inborn errors of metabolism, leukodystrophy, uremia, hepatic encephalopathy, Reye's syndrome
- Cerebrovascular hemorrhage and/or infarct
- Malignancy
- Drug toxicity (e.g., neuroleptic malignant syndrome)
- Toxins

Historical information may suggest specific etiologic viruses:

- Respiratory symptoms: Influenza virus, adenovirus, other respiratory viruses
- Gastrointestinal symptoms: Rotavirus
- Family exposure: Influenza virus, EV

- Seasonality and prevalent diseases in the community: EV, West Nile virus, other arboviruses, influenza virus, other respiratory viruses
- Travel to areas with endemic or epidemic disease: West Nile virus, EV 71, Japanese encephalitis virus, other arboviruses
- Animal exposure: Rabies virus, lymphocytic choriomeningitis virus
- Mosquito exposure: West Nile virus, other arboviruses
- Tick exposure: Colorado tick fever virus, Powassan virus
- Recreational activities: Spelunking-associated bat exposure and rabies infection, hiking-associated mosquito and tick exposure and arbovirus infection

Useful laboratory evaluations for viral meningitis and encephalitis include CSF examination, imaging (especially magnetic resonance imaging), and electroencephalography. Imaging abnormalities may suggest certain pathogens (see Table 1). CSF PCR, serum IgM assays, and viral culture/antigen detection/PCR of mucosal specimens are especially useful specific diagnostic tests.

- CSF PCR is a more sensitive technique than viral culture for detection of viruses such as EVs; HSV; varicella-zoster virus, cytomegalovirus, human herpesvirus 6, Epstein-Barr virus, and JC virus in immune-compromised patients; measles virus; parvovirus B19; and human immunodeficiency virus. CSF PCR for other viruses, such as adenovirus, influenza virus, and arboviruses (including West Nile virus), have low or variable sensitivity. PCR of saliva has high sensitivity for rabies virus (other testing includes immunostain of a nape of neck biopsy, corneal impression, buccal mucosa, or brain tissue).
- The etiology of encephalitis is elusive in many cases. Extensive investigations ultimately are able to identify a specific etiologic agent in only 25% to 65% of cases.

*Abbreviations:* CSF = cerebrospinal fluid; EV = enterovirus; PCR = polymerase chain reaction.

---

viral culture is better for meningitis than for encephalitis. Sensitivity reaches 65% to 75% for EVs, and CSF culture may be positive in young infants lacking pleocytosis. CSF culture is positive in 25% to 40% of neonates with HSV encephalitis but in less than 2% of older children and adults. CSF PCR is generally more sensitive than culture in both meningitis and encephalitis. CSF PCR for EVs has greater than 95% sensitivity and specificity. Sensitivity and specificity of CSF PCR for HSV are between 75% and 100% in neonatal HSV encephalitis and 91% and 98% in older children and adults with HSV encephalitis. Importantly, HSV PCR may be falsely negative within the first 3 to 4 days of illness in up to 25% of cases; repeat testing 4 to 7 days later is generally positive. In many viral encephalitides, viral cultures, antigen detection tests, and PCR of non-CSF specimens have better yields than do CSF culture and PCR (e.g., throat and stool/rectum for EV 71, for which CSF culture and PCR are more often negative, and respiratory specimens for influenza, adenovirus, and other respiratory viruses). Detection of serum and CSF antibodies can be performed for many viruses (e.g., most arboviruses and lymphocytic choriomeningitis virus), frequently requiring acute and convalescent specimens. Serum and CSF IgM assays can be diagnostic for West Nile virus, Japanese encephalitis virus, Epstein-Barr virus, and EV 71. A brain biopsy should be considered in a patient with symptoms that are progressive or do not improve, with an uncertain diagnosis, and with a focal, accessible lesion.

## Treatment

The mainstay of therapy for viral meningitis and encephalitis is supportive care. In patients in whom there is difficulty distinguishing between bacterial and viral meningitis (e.g., young children, especially those younger than 1 year), hospitalization and parenteral antibiotics (vancomycin [Vancocin] plus a third-generation cephalosporin such as cefotaxime [Claforan] or ceftriaxone [Rocephin]) are administered until bacterial cultures are negative and/or an alternative diagnosis is made. Additionally, newborns or other immune-compromised patients with EV meningitis may require supportive therapy for severe disseminated disease (e.g., hepatitis, coagulopathy, or myocarditis). A presumptive diagnosis of viral meningitis can often be made in older children and adults who are not very ill based on clinical and CSF examination (low-grade pleocytosis with mononuclear predominance initially or 8–24 hours later, normal to slightly depressed glucose concentration, normal to slightly increased protein level). Lumbar puncture may alleviate symptoms such as headache, irritability, and emesis. Therefore, in older children and adults, hospitalization and/or empirical antibiotic treatment are indicated for patients who appear ill, including those requiring parenteral hydration and/or analgesics, those in whom viral and bacterial infection cannot be readily distinguished, and those who manifest findings of encephalitis. Presumptive therapy for *Mycobacterium tuberculosis* may be indicated if the

## CURRENT THERAPY

- General supportive measures for patients with severe meningitis or encephalitis include:
  - Analgesics for headache, antiemetics, intravenous fluids and medications for patients with depressed consciousness, anticonvulsants for seizures, provision of a quiet environment
  - Intensive care for severely ill patients, including tracheal intubation for airway protection, respiratory support, cardiorespiratory monitoring
  - Mild fluid restriction for cerebral edema or inappropriate antidiuretic hormone secretion
  - Head of bed elevation, hyperventilation, osmotic (mannitol) and loop diuretics, and control of temperature, pain, and seizures for increased intracranial pressure
- Specific antiviral agents available for meningoencephalitis include acyclovir (Zovirax) for HSV and varicella-zoster virus, ganciclovir (Cytovene) for cytomegalovirus and human herpesvirus 6, foscarnet (Foscavir) for cytomegalovirus and human herpesvirus 6, amantadine (Symmetrel) for influenza A, rimantadine (Flumadine) for influenza A, and oseltamivir (Tamiflu) for influenza A and B.
- Rehabilitative therapy and neurodevelopmental follow-up are frequently necessary after the acute phase of encephalitis regardless of the etiologic agent.
- Prognosis for viral meningitis is generally favorable without long-term sequelae, although fatigue, decreased concentration, and irritability may last for several weeks.
- Prognosis for viral encephalitis is variable and may be difficult to predict, especially early in the course of illness. In general, a worse prognosis is associated with extremes of age (infants <1 year and older adults), specific etiologies (HSV, enterovirus 71, West Nile virus, Japanese encephalitis virus, rabies), more severe illness (lower Glasgow Coma Scale) and extensive brain involvement, and, in the case of HSV, longer duration prior to initiation of treatment.

*Abbreviation:* HSV = herpes simplex virus.

---

exposure history, clinical presentation, CSF examination, and imaging findings are suggestive of this agent.

There are few proven specific antiviral therapies for meningitis and encephalitis. Acyclovir[1] (Zovirax) can hasten recovery from HSV meningitis, although HSV meningitis without encephalitis generally has an excellent outcome without antiviral treatment. Valacyclovir[1] (Valtrex) and famciclovir[1] (Famvir) are also available for oral therapy of HSV meningitis associated with genital HSV in immune-competent patients.

For children and adults with encephalitis, empirical therapy with acyclovir (30 mg/kg/day up to 45–60 mg/kg/day intravenously divided every 8 hours) should generally be initiated pending diagnostic studies, particularly in the presence of fever and any evidence of focal neurologic abnormality (clinical examination, imaging, or electroencephalography). Treatment for 14 to 21 days* is indicated if HSV infection is confirmed or if clinical and diagnostic findings are strongly suggestive in the absence of other proven etiologies; a 21-day

---

course is generally favored for more severe disease. Acyclovir (60 mg/kg/day intravenously divided every 8 hours) should be presumptively administered to newborns with encephalitis with focal or generalized findings. Treatment of proven or highly suspect neonatal HSV encephalitis is generally continued for 21 days and until an end-of-therapy CSF PCR is negative, although proof that extending therapy until the PCR is negative is beneficial is lacking. Whether higher doses (60 mg/kg/day) or longer courses (21 days) confer additional benefit outside the neonatal period is not established. Relapse within the first 1 to 3 months after therapy of neonatal and childhood/adult HSV encephalitis has been reported with variable incidence, in some cases correlated with lower daily dose and treatment duration. Whether relapses reflect active viral replication or an immune-mediated phenomenon is controversial, although CSF PCR positivity in some cases suggests the former.

Whether encephalitis associated with varicella-zoster virus is due more often to direct viral infection or an immune-mediated parainfectious process is not established. Thus, although acyclovir is frequently used for varicella-zoster virus encephalitis, including cerebellar ataxia, the role of antiviral therapy is unproven. Ganciclovir (Cytovene) and foscarnet (Foscavir) are used for meningoencephalitis in immune-compromised hosts caused by cytomegalovirus and human herpesvirus 6.

Pleconaril (Picovir) is an experimental agent that has been studied for treatment of EV meningitis and encephalitis, including chronic meningoencephalitis in hypogammaglobulinemic patients, with some evidence of benefit; however, the agent is not currently available. Intraventricular, intrathecal, and intravenous administration of immune globulin[1] have been used to suppress or stabilize chronic EV meningoencephalitis in immune-compromised patients. The mainstays of management of severe EV 71 neurologic disease are close monitoring, fluid restriction, osmotic diuretics, and cardiorespiratory support. Various agents, including pleconaril, interferon α,[1] intravenous immune globulin, and corticosteroids have been tried, but none has been proven to be effective.

Influenzal encephalitis is frequently treated with oral antivirals, including amantadine (Symmetrel) for influenza A, rimantadine (Flumadine) for influenza A, and oseltamivir (Tamiflu) for influenza A and B; corticosteroids and immune globulin[1] have also been tried. However, none of these agents has been proven to be effective for influenzal encephalitis. A combination of antiviral treatment, corticosteroids, and intravenous immune globulin has been suggested to reduce mortality due to influenzal acute necrotizing encephalopathy. There currently are no established therapies for West Nile virus encephalitis. Ribavirin (Rebetol),[1] interferon, high-titer immune globulin, and corticosteroids have been used, and therapeutic trials are currently ongoing. No specific therapies have been proven to be effective for encephalitis due to other arboviruses or for rabies; successful use of coma-inducing therapy plus the antivirals ribavirin and amantadine was reported in one patient. Corticosteroids, intravenous immune globulin, and plasmapheresis have been used for acute disseminated encephalomyelitis, but efficacy trials have not been performed.

## REFERENCES

Beaman MH, Wesselingh SL: Acute community-acquired meningitis and encephalitis. Med J Aust 2002;176:389-396.

Chang L, Hsia S, Wu C, et al: Outcome of enterovirus 71 infections with or without stage-based management: 1998-2002. Pediatr Infect Dis J 2004;23:327-331.

Glaser CA, Gilliam S, Schnurr D, et al: In search of encephalitis etiologies: Diagnostic challenges in the California encephalitis project, 1998-2000. Clin Infect Dis 2003;36:731-742.

Huang C, Morse D, Slater B, et al: Multiple-year experience in the diagnosis of viral central nervous system infections with a panel of polymerase chain reaction assays for detection of 11 viruses. Clin Infect Dis 2004;39:630-635.

Kennedy PGE: Viral encephalitis: causes, differential diagnosis, and management. J Neurol Neurosurg Psychiatry 2004;75(Suppl 1):i10-i15.

---

[1]Not FDA approved for this indication.
*Exceeds duration recommended by the manufacturer.

---

[1]Not FDA approved for this indication.

Kimberlin DW: Herpes simplex virus infections of the central nervous system. Semin Pediatr Infect Dis 2003;14:83-89.

Rotbart HA: Viral meningitis. Semin Neurol 2000;20:277-292.

Watson JT, Gerber SI: West Nile virus: A brief review. Pediatr Infect Dis J 2004;23:355-358.

Weitkamp J, Spring MD, Brogan T, et al: Influenza A virus-associated acute necrotizing encephalopathy in the United States. Pediatr Infect Dis J 2004;23:259-263.

Whitley RJ, Gnann JW: Viral encephalitis: Familiar infections and emerging pathogens. Lancet 2002;359:507-514.

Willoughby RE Jr, Tieves KS, Hoffman GM, et al: Survival after treatment of rabies with induction of coma. N Engl J Med 2005;352:2508-2514.

# Multiple Sclerosis

Method of
*Randall T. Schapiro, MD*

Multiple sclerosis (MS) has been called a primary demyelinating disease of the central nervous system, but that is somewhat inaccurate. Charcot's description of MS included damage to the axon, which has been especially emphasized in the past decade. Today MS is described not only as a disease of myelin, but also of the cell that makes myelin (oligodendrocyte) and also the axon. All these are primary targets in the destructive process that appears to be directed by the immune system, and thus MS is more properly called an immune-mediated disorder. The immune system can cause direct destruction and inflammation. It also can program the targets (cells, axons) to self-destruct over time (apoptosis).

The pathology of MS has been elucidated more thoroughly in the past several years thanks to international projects that began with descriptions of biopsied specimens from brain lesions of patients with the disease. Some individuals had a high involvement of the immune system; a minority had less. Four different varieties are separable. These types (I through IV) provide a way to separate the disease potentially into different categories. This combination of possibilities puts MS into both the inflammatory and degenerative categories. Much work is left to do in this area, but in the next decade treatments may be dictated by the variety of pathologic processes occurring as the disease changes over time.

While describing MS at a microscopic level, it is easy to lose sight of the fact that, at a global level, it is a disease of people with all of their complexities. The person with MS is typically diagnosed early in the third decade of life and has a family, work, and responsibilities in the community, making this potentially disabling disease one of the most important acquired, nontraumatic neurologic diseases in the world.

Relative to the past, MS today is a disease with very active treatment strategies aimed in three general directions. The ideal goal is to slow or stop the disease itself. Disease management is now routine, with six Federal Drug Administration (FDA)-approved medications available to slow MS. Symptom management remains one of the principal directions of treatment in MS. Superimposed on these two very obvious directions is the psychological support necessary to keep people with neurologic dysfunction performing at their highest level. The psychological area is often ignored in the office but is of equal importance in offering a quality of life for those with the disease.

## Etiology

The cause of multiple sclerosis remains unknown. Despite numerous advances, the discussion of MS causation has changed little in the past decade. No simple explanation is available for why MS occurs. For more than 40 years, a population gradient to MS has been understood. As one moves away from the equator north and south, the number of MS cases increases. Much of that may be because of the ethnic origin of the people in those areas. They tend to be northern European and Scandinavian, but migration studies demonstrate that the disease spreads beyond ethnic backgrounds when generations remain in the targeted geographic regions. Studies in the Faeroe and Shetland/Orkney islands off the coast of Scotland and other regions give credence to the possibility of a viral or other infectious influence. Despite decades of modern viral isolation techniques, no virus has stood the test of time in MS. Each decade has produced its own target virus. In the 1970s, it was the measles virus, in the 1980s, the herpesvirus, and in the 1990s, the retroviruses of tropical spastic paraparesis. Then, one after another, the human herpesvirus type 6 and the chlamydia bacteria were implicated. None appeared conclusive, although many continue under investigation.

What does seem clear is the involvement of the immune system in MS. The understanding of the influence of the immune system continues to evolve as newer and better techniques to explore this complex area develop. MS is now described as an immune-mediated disease to distinguish it from a classic autoimmune disease. The immune system clearly is more active toward a central nervous system antigen. Just what that antigen is remains mysterious, but several candidates have emerged, including myelin and it components, the oligodendrocyte, the axon, and other surrounding tissues and cells. For the immune system to attack the nervous system, something must trigger it. That is likely the environmental influence, and after it is programmed to attack a nervous system element, it must make its way through the blood–brain barrier to find the target. It is the very complexity of the process that may make it susceptible to intervention. Strategies are being or have been developed to interfere with the initial reaction of the antigen-presenting cell (macrophage) to the antigen, the passage through the blood-brain barrier, and the reaction once in the central nervous system.

The immune system appears to be the genetic link in MS. Although MS is said to be nonhereditary, it clearly has a genetic component. The likelihood of getting MS with no one in the family having it is approximately 0.2%. If a parent has the disease and the child is a girl, the risk jumps to 3% to 4%. If the child is a boy, the risk is 2%. If an identical twin has MS, the risk to the sibling is 30%. But if MS were wholly a hereditary disease, it would be 100%.

Thus the cause of MS is unknown, but it must be a multifactorial process. It takes a susceptible individual who has an immune system capable of being genetically stimulated by an exogenous factor, and all these factors must be at the right time in the right place.

## Course of the Disease

The disease has numerous presentations. Virtually any symptom that can result from an irritated central nervous system may be present in MS. Fatigue is the single most common symptom, but numbness, tingling, dizziness, visual distortion, weakness, clumsiness, pain, urinary, bowel, sexual, and psychological effects are often present as well. The course of MS is also very unpredictable and variable. Today MS is divided into four broad categories. Approximately 80% of MS begins with a fluctuating course with relapses of neurologic deficit followed by periods of relative quiet, termed *relapsing-remitting MS*.

Over time, half of those untreated with relapsing-remitting MS stop fluctuating and slowly get worse. This is called *secondary progressive MS*. If the course of secondary progressive MS fluctuates, it is called *secondary progressive with relapses*. The common feature of the progressive variety is that it progresses between relapses if relapses are present.

Approximately 10% of MS gets worse from the beginning, which is called *primary progressive*, and approximately 5% begins progressive and then has a relapse or two and is labeled *progressive-relapsing*.

Even though MS is divided into categories, it remains MS, which is especially true of the relapsing-remitting and secondary progressive types that are almost certainly the same process. Primary progressive and progressive-relapsing may be variants, but the two of them are also almost certainly the same process.

Approximately 20% of people with MS do fairly well, with their disease accumulating little disability over time, even untreated.

The exact number is controversial, but even autopsy studies demonstrate repeatedly that MS appears without clinical evidence much more than would be expected. Those autopsied died from other causes and did not even recognize they had MS.

Many experts believe MS is a spectrum of diseases that appear clinically similar. Little actual data support the theory, but in the past few years when researchers at the Mayo Clinic, together with many others around the world, looked at biopsied specimens of lesions that turned out to be MS, they saw great variability among them. This discovery has prompted a new classification based on the pathology that divides MS into four broad categories. At one end is a very immunologically based pathology, at the other end is a very degenerative pathology, and in between are two that blend between the extremes. Thus MS is highly diverse, both clinically and pathologically, and yet there is also much similarity.

## Diagnosis

Under normal circumstances, MS typically is not difficult to diagnose when following simple clinical dictums. There are three criteria in the clinical diagnosis of MS:

1. The person should be relatively young, between the ages of 15 and 55 years.
2. She or he should have neurologic symptoms that fluctuate.
3. The neurologic examination should demonstrate multiple abnormalities within the central nervous system, hence the name *multiple* sclerosis.

Other obvious reasons for the clinical picture should be ruled out, and then the diagnosis of MS can be made very accurately. Schumacher codified these criteria in the 1970s before the days of elaborate testing. When evoked potentials and spinal fluid tests became more accurate, Poser and his committee added the use of those modalities to allow for a diagnosis when a clinical piece is missing. Magnetic resonance imaging (MRI) advanced the cause rapidly, allowing for more precision in diagnosis, and recently the McDonald committee added its use to speed the diagnostic process. The MRI scan has to show significant specific abnormalities to be substituted for a clinical loss, and to be effective, all these criteria still depend on the initial clinical presentation.

Despite the emphasis on the clinical picture in diagnosing MS, laboratory testing continues to play a role in confirming the diagnosis. Evoked potentials are electrical potentials stimulated within the brain by a stimulus (visual, auditory, or somatosensory). They can be measured via electrodes placed on the scalp. With the aid of computerized signal averaging, normal transmission can be separated from abnormal, thus extending the neurologic examination to find more subtle abnormalities of the sensory system. The spinal fluid can be analyzed in a very sophisticated way for immune abnormalities. Detection of unique oligoclonal banding in the IgG spectrum is characteristic of MS. Increased production of IgG and the presence of myelin basic protein are also common.

Blood (and sometimes cerebrospinal fluid) should be analyzed to eliminate mimicking diseases such as lupus, Sjögren's, sarcoid, $B_{12}$ deficiency, Lyme disease, vasculitis, and other autoimmune processes.

## Management

The complexity and variability of multiple sclerosis make it a classic example of a disease best managed by a team approach. The team may require participation from physicians, nurses, rehabilitation professionals, psychologists, and social workers. The extent of participation should be determined by the complexity of the individual situation. It is not necessary or appropriate for all professionals to be involved with all patients, but an educated team makes the management of complicated patients much more effective.

With the advent of immune-modulating medication, treatment has expanded greatly. These medications have revolutionized the medical approach toward the disease, but their expense and their lack of total efficacy must be taken into consideration when determining their use.

It is abundantly clear that patients cannot get back what is lost in the destruction of the central nervous system. Thus the goal of management is to prevent loss and maintain function. In MS the immune system becomes programmed to attack the myelin, oligodendrocyte, or other nerve component. Whether that programming antigen is a virus or other stimulus does not change the fact that an antigen-presenting cell (usually a macrophage) engulfs the antigen and presents it. This causes a stimulation of T-helper cells, which separate into the highly inflammatory Th1 and the anti-inflammatory Th2 cells. In MS there is a shift of the balance, with increased Th1 allowing for increased destruction. The programmed cells then cross the blood–brain barrier looking for the part of the nervous system that resembles their programming. Stopping this from occurring has become the principal treatment strategy. The interferons appear to keep the flow of Th1 cells from crossing the blood–brain barrier, thus decreasing their likelihood of destruction. Glatiramer acetate appears to cross the barrier and stimulate increased Th2 production, changing the balance of immune regulation toward a more modulating course. Another agent awaiting approval (Natalizumab, Antegren) works to shore up the blood–brain barrier by preventing it transport across via inhibition of adhesion molecule movement.

Keeping an activated immune system from getting to the myelinated central fibers appears to slow the process of demyelination in MS. Therefore the principle of treatment in MS today revolves around immune modulation. Over the past dozen years more scientifically proven treatments for MS have evolved than in all other years combined. Today five FDA-approved medications are available.

Interferons are proteins that the body makes in response to a foreign stimulation. Thus with a viral infection the body makes interferons that modulate the immune system. The three main categories of interferon are alfa ($\alpha$), beta ($\beta$), and gamma ($\gamma$). Interferon $\gamma$ stimulates the immune system and makes MS worse, whereas interferon $\beta$ calms the system down and decreases attack rates, increases the time between attacks, and decreases the damage seen on MRI scans.

Studies done in various ways show approximately one third of the attacks in an actively affected MS population can be diminished during the first 2 years. The preponderance of information leads to the conclusion that the higher the dose of interferon, the more potent the response. Many studies show that in the appropriate person, with the appropriate dose, interferons change the course of the disease. The potent anti-inflammatory effects of interferons have a dramatic effect on the MRI, with a decrease in T2 and T1 contrast-enhancing lesions. These human gene interferons come in two formulations: interferon beta-1a (Avonex, Rebif) made in a hamster and interferon beta-1b (Betaseron) made in bacteria. The recommended doses of Rebif and Betaseron appear to be equivalent (three to four times per week); that of Avonex is significantly lower (once per week).

**CURRENT DIAGNOSIS**

- Clinical history of fluctuating neurologic symptoms (exacerbations and remissions)
- Multiple abnormalities seen on neurologic examination
- Absence of other systemic disorder (e.g., lupus, Lyme, other autoimmune processes)
- Confirmatory laboratory studies of benefit: MRI (using McDonald criteria); CSF, looking for increased immune activity including oligoclonal IgG banding, increased IgG synthesis, and index; abnormal evoked potentials indicating multiple abnormalities potentially not found on routine neurologic examination

*Abbreviations:* CSF = cerebrospinal fluid; MRI = magnetic resonance imaging.

Glatiramer acetate is a polypeptide that appears to fool the immune system. As noted earlier, it shifts the Th1-Th2 balance toward the Th2. Appearing to mimic myelin, it may also decrease the attack by blocking the cells headed toward myelin and preventing damage. It, too, appears to decrease attack rates by approximately a third in the first 2 years of use.

All of these medications are administered parentally. They all have side effects and are all costly. The β-interferons may be toxic to the blood and liver and can exaggerate depression in a susceptible individual that is generally mild but should be monitored. Glatiramer acetate has less toxicity but can cause a systemic reaction that mimics a heart attack, although it is not, and clears in 20 minutes. Although rare, this reaction can be frightening. All of the drugs can produce skin reactions except for the intermuscular interferon beta-1a (Avonex).

All of these agents were studied in the relapsing forms of MS. Although this does not preclude effectiveness in more progressive forms, there is a paucity of data for that use. Clinical experience, together with evidence-based data, gives a picture of the high-dose interferons having the most potent effect, followed by glatiramer acetate, and then low-dose interferon.

Based on the aggressiveness of the MS and the lifestyle of the patient, the physician should select the agent. The goal must include maintaining the person on the medication and preventing noncompliance. Although patients must be included in the decision making, they should not be given the choice without a recommendation from the health professional. Many neurologists tend to abdicate the decision making to patients, who are not prepared to make such a decision.

Knowing that approximately 20% of patients do well without treatment and many more do well for a significant period of time without treatment begs the question of how early to treat. As stated earlier, it is impossible to retrieve damaged neurons consistently. The issue is whether to treat 100% of patients with MS immediately at the time of diagnosis if only 80% will need to be treated eventually. If the drugs were curative, time limited, or inexpensive, all would agree on treating all patients. Given the fact they are not, who should be treated and when is an issue.

All experts agree that early treatment is necessary, but the question is how to define "early." Much controversy surrounds the question of whether it is advisable to wait and see into what group an individual falls. Studies on so-called pre-MS, what is called the "clinically isolated syndrome," do not answer the question. The clinically isolated syndrome is a first attack, usually accompanied by an abnormal MRI. Two attacks are required for diagnosis. Studies clearly show that the second attack, leading to the diagnostic label, can be delayed by treatment, but that says nothing about long-term disability. This dilemma is especially pertinent because often the disease quiets after diagnosis and can go decades or more before reactivating. Attempts to look at that issue scientifically have come up short. The CHAMPS (Controlled High Risk Avonex Multiple Sclerosis) study looked at people with a first attack who did not meet the criteria for clinically definite MS. The study showed that the immune treatment (interferon beta-1a [Avonex]) did delay the second attack, but it says nothing about whether such early treatment changes disability later in life, a very important question that remains unanswered. A European study (ETOMS [Early Treatment of MS] with interferon beta-1a [Rebif]) leaves the same question.

Prognostic indicators can help predict whether a more aggressive course is impending. A large burden of disease on initial MRI scanning and the presence of weakness, ataxia, cognitive problems, frequent attacks, and spinal cord symptoms all point to a worse prognosis and should lead to earlier treatment. Numbness, tingling, blurred vision, dizziness, pain, and fatigue do not usually evolve into the more aggressive forms of MS, and immediate treatment may not be as necessary. All experts agree with the National Multiple Sclerosis Society's practice guideline, which states that if the disease is *active*, treatment should be instituted with one of the four agents.

Thus prevention is the key, but despite best efforts, breakthrough attacks do occur. People, treated or untreated, may develop new symptomatology, which is deemed a relapse. The use of the potent anti-inflammatory cortisone agents has been used to settle attacks for many decades. There are many regimens that individual experts use

depending on the severity of the attack. If the attack is relatively minor and not encroaching on function, a hand-holding approach with no steroids is recommended. If the attack is slightly more severe, two dose packs of methylprednisolone may be given simultaneously. If the attack is even more severe with increased disability, 1000 mg of methylprednisolone may be administered each day for 3 to 5 days. If the attack is such that aggressive inpatient rehabilitation is warranted, a dose of dexamethasone beginning at 64 mg with a taper over 1 week is given. After either the outpatient high-dose or the inpatient high-dose steroid plan, a 1-month taper of oral methylprednisolone is included. All of these are based on experience rather than evidence-based data.

Once the decision is made that the person has active disease, requiring ongoing immunomodulation, a decision about which agent to use becomes paramount. If the disease is highly inflammatory with aggressive relapses and/or MRI evidence of blood–brain barrier breakdown (contrast-enhancing lesions), a high-dose β-interferon is used. If the person's lifestyle cannot tolerate that, an adjustment of medication to a less anti-inflammatory agent (glatiramer acetate or interferon beta-1a, at a lower dose) is suggested. If the disease is less aggressive but the patient is experiencing much depression, glatiramer is preferred. The use of medication is not random but represents the best fit of the drug to the situation. This is with the understanding that high-dose interferon β (Betaseron, Rebif) is the most potent, with glatiramer acetate (Copaxone) following and low-dose interferon beta-1a (Avonex) next.

If the disease cannot be controlled with the four immunomodulating medications, as seen by ongoing progression of disability with continued relapses, immunosuppression with mitoxantrone (Novantrone) is administered. The MRI scan can be of some help in the decision making but correlates poorly with the clinical picture. Thus it should not be the most important factor in decision making. Mitoxantrone is administered intravenously in a regimen of 12 mg/m$^2$. There is a total lifetime dose of 140 mg/m$^2$ before heart damage becomes a major concern. Examination of the heart at appropriate levels for ejection fraction and function is necessary. A typical course is 1 year of therapy and then continued evaluations without further mitoxantrone until (or if) progression resumes.

The use of oral immune suppressants including azathioprine (Imuron) and methotrexate (Rheumotrex) were more popular before the newer agents became available. They are still used as adjunct therapy in difficult cases of progressive disease.

Natalizumab (Tysabri, previously called Antegren) is a monoclonal antibody that prevents immune cells from moving from the blood to the central nervous system by blocking integrin, the adhesion molecule. It was originally approved by the FDA on the basis of impressive data obtained in the first year of a 2-year study. There is a dramatic lowering of relapse rate and a significant decrease in MRI activity. This treatment is a once-monthly intravenous infusion. Two large studies were conducted. One was Tysabri versus placebo and the second was Tysabri plus Avonex versus placebo plus Avonex. Unfortunately, shortly after release of the treatment by the FDA, two cases of progressive multifocal leukoencephalopathy (PML) were found in the Avonex and Tysabri group and one died and the other became much more disabled. A third case of PML was discovered in a Tysabri-treated patient with Crohn's disease. As a result, the distribution of Tysabri was halted pending further evaluation. Now it is back on the market with restrictions to be used only in patients failing all other therapies. It really has never been studied in this group. The risk of progressive multifocal leukoencephalopathy has not been fully ascertained, thus caution is advised.

Studies on intense immunosuppression with bone marrow transplantation (autologous and stem cell) continue but are not positive enough to recommend its use.

Despite the time, effort, and success given to slow the disease, the bulk of a clinician's time with multiple sclerosis is devoted to symptomatic management. The tools available include pharmacologic, rehabilitative, and psychological approaches. Fatigue is the single most common and most disabling symptom seen in MS. Five different "fatigues" are apparent in MS: normal, neuromuscular, deconditioning, fatigue of depression, and lassitude (MS-related fatigue). Normal fatigue is the same that occurs in everyone who tires after working hard.

## CURRENT THERAPY

- Education and psychological support
- Symptomatic management of appropriate symptoms
- Immune modulation with interferon beta-1a, interferon beta-1b, or glatiramer acetate early in the active disease course and ongoing
- Regular follow-up with clinical examination and magnetic resonance imaging if additional information is needed

Neuromuscular fatigue is the tiring of muscles when they are required for activities such as walking. The fatigue of deconditioning is the result of a lack of sufficient activity to maintain endurance. Depression can result in poor sleep and ongoing fatigue. The most common fatigue is a tiredness that occurs without significant activity. It comes on spontaneously and is likely the result of a neurochemical imbalance in the brain. Neurochemically active drugs including amantadine and modafinil are helpful in its management. Occupational therapy can teach energy conservation and improve activities of daily living to increase efficiency and decrease fatigue. In managing fatigue the health professional must rule out a sleep disturbance or other contributing confounding problem and then develop a plan based on the specific fatigue present.

Spasticity is managed with a multicentered approach. Noxious stimuli are minimized initially because they can increase muscle tone. An exercise program emphasizing stretching and range of motion is instituted. If more management is necessary, baclofen, tizanidine, benzodiazepines, and gabapentin may be added to appropriate doses. Failing all of the preceding, intrathecal administration of baclofen via a pump or selected muscle weakening with botulinum toxin is effective.

The bladder and bowel are often involved with MS. Bladders may become hypertonic, small, and fail to store or they may become hypotonic, large, and fail to empty. Sometimes the bladder and the sphincter become dyssynergic. Anticholinergic medication often helps the small bladder and controls the bladder spasms. Catheterization techniques may help the large bladder (self, intermittent, and indwelling). Combinations of therapy can aid the dyssynergic bladder including α-adrenergic blocking agents. A bowel program can lead to improved independence by scheduling the bowel movement rather than allowing it to be entirely spontaneous. Taking advantage of the gastrocolic reflex, attempting evacuation following a meal with the judicious use of bulking agents, stool softeners, and suppositories is the start to taking charge.

Sexual function may require attention. Erectile dysfunction in men is managed with Viagra, Levitra, or Cialis. Injection of prostaglandin (Caverject) is clearly more potent than the oral agents but requires the ability to directly inject the penis. Prostaglandin suppository (Muse) places the medication within the urethral orifice but is less potent than the injection. Women often experience decreased libido, decreased sensation, decreased lubrication, or sometimes pain. The use of various vibrators along with external water-soluble lubricants with the gentle application of cold can be helpful. Many of the commonly used antidepressant medications can decrease sexual desire and may need adjustment.

Neuropathic type pain is surprisingly common in MS (50%). The newer anticonvulsants, including gabapentin, Trileptal, Topamax, and Lamictal, are commonly dosed sufficiently to decrease the pain. Amitriptyline can be helpful, especially at night.

Cognitive problems likewise occur in approximately 50% of those with MS. Watching for depression and the contribution of other medications to the problem is essential. Keeping people in society and not allowing them to withdraw may decrease the secondary exaggeration of the symptom.

Ataxia, tremor, and balance problems often go together and are very difficult to manage. Although a number of medications can help any one person, none are consistent. Bracing across a joint can be helpful.

Compensatory training for balance sometimes helps that symptom.

A number of paroxysmal symptoms relatively unique to MS are managed with anticonvulsant medications. These include spasms of an extremity. Sensory aberrations rapidly coming and going may include the pain of trigeminal neuralgia or fluctuating pain in an extremity. Paroxysmal visual blurring or speech slurring can be seen. These fluctuations may occur many times a minute, only to settle down for hours.

Ambulation can be affected through many mechanisms including weakness and ataxia. Ambulatory support through the appropriate use of devices (canes, crutches, walkers, and ankle-foot orthoses) is recommended to enhance mobility. If ambulation becomes too difficult, other mobility devices should be used freely. One of the major answers to disability is maintaining mobility.

Progressive resistive exercises must take into account the strength of innervation of the specific muscle. Fatigue results from the overzealous use of strengthening exercises. If a muscle is not used, however, atrophy results. Thus an intelligent strengthening program can be helpful if not overdone.

The role of aerobic exercise has evolved significantly over the past 2 decades, and an appropriate training program can benefit an individual if tailored to his or her deficits. The program must emphasize the slow buildup of intensity of the exercise over as much time as it takes to prevent fatigue from becoming overwhelming with each session.

Because of the individuality of the disease for each person, generalizations are hard to make. What is clear is that simply having the diagnosis causes a ripple effect even in the patients with the mildest symptoms. The family experiences the problems of their loved ones and thus this becomes a family disease like few others. The age of the patient influences vocational planning. It also influences family roles and child rearing. Thus counseling may be a very necessary component of a well-rounded approach. The complexity of all of this has made MS centers a popular choice for many who have issues surrounding the MS. These allow for experienced therapists to communicate with the medical professionals and the patients to develop a comprehensive management strategy.

The diagnosis and management of MS has drastically evolved over the past 2 decades. It has gone from a disease characterized by the late Labe Scheinberg, MD, as "diagnose and adios" to one in which physicians are arguing about how early and how aggressively treatment strategies should be applied. We have come a long way but still have far to go to find the cause and eventual cure to this very difficult problem.

## REFERENCES

Jacobs LD, Cookfair DL, Rudick RA, et al: Intramuscular interferon beta-1a for disease progression in relapsing multiple sclerosis. Ann Neurol 1996, 39(3):285-294.

Johnson KP, Brooks BR, Cohen JA, et al: Copolymer 1 reduces relapse and improves disability in relapsing-remitting multiple sclerosis: Results of a phase III multi-center, double-blind, placebo-controlled trial. Neurology 1995;45:1268-1276.

Petajan JH, White AT: Recommendations for physical activity in multiple sclerosis. Sports Med 1999;27(3):179-191.

PRISMS Study Group and University of British Columbia MS MRI Analysis Group: PRISMS-4: Long-term efficacy of interferon-beta 1a in relapsing MS. Neurology 2001;56:1628-1636.

Rao S, Leo GT, Bernardin L, Unverzagt F: Cognitive dysfunction in multiple sclerosis: I. Frequency, pattern and predictors. Neurology 1991;41(5): 685-691.

Sadovnik AD, Remick RA, Allen J, et al: Depression and multiple sclerosis. Neurology 1996;46:628-632.

Schapiro RT: The Management of MS Symptoms. New York, Demos Medical Publishing, 2003.

The IFNB Multiple Sclerosis Group, University of British Columbia MS/MRI Analysis Group: Interferon beta-1b in the treatment of multiple sclerosis: Final outcome of the randomized controlled trial. Neurology 1995;45: 1277-1285.

# Myasthenia Gravis and Related Disorders

Method of
*Jenice Robinson, MD,*
*and Milind J. Kothari, DO*

Myasthenia gravis (MG) is a relatively uncommon disease of the postsynaptic neuromuscular junction (NMJ). Most patients with myasthenia have an acquired immunologic abnormality, but other uncommon inherited forms of myasthenia may result from structural abnormalities of the NMJ. The following discussion focuses on acquired (autoimmune) MG.

The physiologic abnormality in autoimmune MG results from the reduction in concentration of the nicotinic acetylcholine receptor (AChR) on the endplates of somatic muscles at the NMJ. Although the cause of the disorder is unknown, the pathogenesis of autoimmune MG is now well understood. Two antigens have been described: AChR and muscle-specific receptor tyrosine kinase (MuSK). Antibodies against AChR are found in 80% to 90% of patients with MG. Antibodies against MuSK are found in 40% of the remaining patients. Strong evidence supports the role of antibodies in the pathogenesis of MG. Anti-AChR antibodies cause disruption of myotubes in culture and cause myasthenic symptoms when transferred to experimental animals. Removal of anti-AChR antibodies results in clinical improvement. The thymus plays an important but incompletely understood role in MG.

## Clinical Features

The hallmark of MG is fluctuating or fatigable weakness. MG presents with ocular symptoms of ptosis or diplopia in 60% of patients. Diplopia may not fluctuate, and an ocular misalignment may appear fixed. This presentation may mimic a neuropathy of the third, fourth, or sixth cranial nerves, or an internuclear ophthalmoplegia. Abnormalities of pupillary function should not be present in MG. Patients may present initially to an optometrist or ophthalmologist for these problems. Ocular symptoms eventually develop in almost all patients with MG. Presenting symptoms are bulbar (dysarthria, dysphagia, or facial weakness) in 10%, leg weakness in 10% to 20%, and generalized weakness in 10%. Symptoms often worsen with exercise and improve with rest. Symptoms are often most prominent late in the day. Weakness in MG arises from fluctuating strength of the voluntary muscles and always causes a functional deficit, such as an inability to hold the arms above the head when washing the hair or leg weakness resulting in sudden falls. If a patient has only generalized fatigue or tiredness, MG is unlikely. Chronic pain and sensory complaints are not features of MG. Respiratory dysfunction is the initial presenting symptom in only 1% of patients but, if present, requires admission to the hospital for monitoring and treatment because respiratory failure may occur rapidly. Weakness in MG can be worsened by infection, physical stress such as surgery, emotional stress, and medications. Medications that reportedly worsen strength in MG are listed in Table 1.

The prevalence of MG is estimated to be 14 per 100,000 people. MG may present at any age, but the most common ages of onset are in the second and third decades in women and in the seventh and eighth decades in men. In the past MG was more common in women than men, but with aging of the population, MG now is more common in men. Associated autoimmune diseases, such as thyroid disease, rheumatoid arthritis, lupus, and pernicious anemia, are present in 5% to 10% of patients. Approximately 10% of MG patients have an associated thymoma, and 50% to 70% of patients have thymic hyperplasia. Familial occurrence of autoimmune MG is rare, although the incidence of autoimmune diseases in first-degree relatives of patients with MG may be increased.

---

**TABLE 1 Medications Reported to Exacerbate Myasthenia Gravis**

**Antibiotics**
Aminoglycosides, ampicillin sodium, ciprofloxacin hydrochloride (Cipro), erythromycin, imipenem (Primaxin), kanamycin sulfate (Kantrex), pyrantel (Antiminth), chloroquine (Aralen)

**Cardiovascular Agents**
β-Blocking agents (propranolol hydrochloride [Inderal], oxprenolol hydrochloride[2] [Trasicor], timolol maleate [Blocadren]), procainamide (Procanbid), verapamil hydrochloride (Calan), propafenone hydrochloride (Rythmol), quinidine
Penicillamine (Cuprimine)
Corticosteroids (transiently when initiating therapy)
Magnesium salts and lithium carbonate (Eskalith)
Phenothiazine antipsychotics
Phenytoin sodium (Dilantin)

**Neuromuscular Blocking Agents**
Vecuronium bromide (Norcuron), succinylcholine chloride (Anectine)

**Ocular Drugs**
Timolol maleate (Timoptic), proparacaine hydrochloride (Alcaine), tropicamide (Mydriacyl)

**Anticholinergic Agents**
Trihexyphenidyl hydrochloride (Artane)
Acetazolamide (Diamox)

[2]Not available in the United States

---

## Diagnosis

An accurate diagnosis prior to initiating treatment for MG is crucial. A critical assessment of the patient's symptoms is the most important initial step in evaluation. The differential diagnosis of MG is quite limited in most patients. Disorders that may mimic MG are listed in Table 2.

All patients suspected of having MG should undergo testing consisting of a complete blood count (CBC), erythrocyte sedimentation rate, thyroid-stimulating hormone and thyroxine levels, rheumatoid factor concentration, and liver and renal profiles. Autoimmune thyroid disease may mimic or accompany MG. In addition to excluding other diagnoses, these tests are important because treatments of MG may have adverse effects on the bone marrow, liver, and kidneys.

The role of specific testing for MG is to confirm the clinical diagnosis. For a patient with ptosis, the ice test is easy and convenient. A small amount of ice is placed over the ptotic lid for a few minutes. Improvement of the ptosis with cooling is suggestive of a defect of neuromuscular transmission. Further testing should then be pursued.

### EDROPHONIUM CHLORIDE (TENSILON) TEST

The edrophonium (Tensilon) test is readily available, but the result may be invalid if the test is not properly performed. A defined clinical endpoint is needed, and vague patient reports of improvement in strength are not acceptable. Cranial nerve deficits, such as ptosis, dysconjugate gaze, and limitation of extraocular movements, provide the most reliable endpoints. The test should be performed in a location where syncope, hypotension, or respiratory failure can be managed, as these complications can rarely occur in supersensitive individuals. Atropine sulfate 0.4 mg should be available in case of symptomatic bradycardia. An intravenous line is often started for the test, although some practitioners use a butterfly needle for administration. Edrophonium 10 mg (1 mL) is drawn up in a syringe. The strength or maximum excursion of the target muscles is assessed immediately prior to administration of the edrophonium. A 2-mg (0.2-mL) test dose is given to ensure that the patient is not supersensitive to the drug. If no respiratory or cardiac side effects occur, 3 mg (0.3 mL) of edrophonium is given. Re-examination of the target muscle is performed. If no definite improvement is observed at 60 seconds, the

## CURRENT DIAGNOSIS

- Hallmark of MG is fluctuating or fatigable weakness.
- Initial symptom is ptosis or diplopia in 60% of patients.
- Generalized fatigue or tiredness alone is not a symptom of MG.
- Diagnostic evaluation includes:
  - Laboratory evaluation: Thyroid-stimulating hormone level, complete blood count, erythrocyte sedimentation rate, rheumatoid factor, liver and renal function studies
  - Edrophonium chloride (Tensilon) test: >90% sensitivity, but be certain to choose a defined clinical endpoint (e.g., improvement in ptosis)
  - Antibody testing: Send AChR binding antibodies first. Binding antibodies are found in ~90% of patients with generalized MG, and 50% with ocular MG. If negative, send AChR modulating antibodies. If both are negative, send muscle-specific receptor tyrosine kinase antibody.
- All patients with suspected MG should undergo chest computed tomography with contrast for thymoma
- If antibodies are negative or if searching for evidence of generalized MG in a patient with pure ocular symptoms, obtain electromyography with repetitive nerve stimulation. This test result is abnormal in >70% of patients with generalized MG but is less sensitive in patients with pure ocular symptoms
- If diagnosis remains unclear, refer to neuromuscular specialist.

*Abbreviations:* AChR = acetylcholine receptor; MG = myasthenia gravis.

**TABLE 2 Clinical Presentations and Diagnostic Considerations in Myasthenia Gravis**

| Site of Predominant Weakness | Alternative Diagnoses |
| --- | --- |
| Ocular | Brainstem and cranial nerve disorders due to processes such as neoplasm, stroke, and multiple sclerosis |
| | Horner syndrome |
| | Oculopharyngeal muscular dystrophy |
| | Kearns-Sayre syndrome |
| | Graves' disease |
| | Congenital myasthenia |
| | Botulism (if symptom onset is acute) |
| | Miller-Fischer variant of GBS |
| Bulbar | Brainstem and multiple cranial nerve dysfunction due to processes such as neoplasm, stroke, and multiple sclerosis |
| | Bulbar-onset ALS |
| | Obstructive lesion of the oropharynx or laryngeal lesion |
| | Botulism (if symptom onset is acute) |
| Proximal extremity weakness | Inflammatory myopathies (e.g., polymyositis, dermatomyositis) |
| | LEMS |
| | GBS |
| | Periodic paralysis |
| | Acid maltase deficiency |
| Isolated respiratory weakness | ALS |
| | Polymyositis |
| | LEMS |
| | Myotonic dystrophy |
| Isolated neck weakness | ALS |
| | Inflammatory myopathies |
| | Paraspinous myopathy |

*Abbreviations:* ALS = amyotrophic lateral sclerosis; GBS = Guillain-Barré syndrome; LEMS, Lambert-Eaton myasthenic syndrome.

remaining 5 mg (0.5 mL) of edrophonium is given. If unequivocal improvement in the strength of the target muscle occurs within 60 seconds of administration of a dose of edrophonium, the test is considered positive. Edrophonium 10 mg will not weaken normal muscles, but the full dose may induce weakness in a patient with a defect in neuromuscular transmission. For this reason, the medication should be given in the manner described so that any improvement in muscle strength is not missed.

The edrophonium (Tensilon) test is positive in more than 90% of patients with MG, but a positive result is not specific for MG. Positive edrophonium tests have been reported in patients with the Lambert-Eaton myasthenic syndrome, motor neuron disease, lesions of the oculomotor nerves, and conditions affecting the extraocular muscles.

### ANTIBODY TESTING

Acetylcholine receptor antibodies (AChR-Ab) are present in 90% of patients with generalized MG and in approximately 50% to 60% of patients with ocular myasthenia. They are the most specific test for MG. False-positive results can occur but are rare. Antibody levels are not predictive of the severity of MG in an individual patient.

Three different tests for AChR-Ab are available commercially: binding, modulating, and blocking antibodies. The binding antibody is the antibody most commonly found in MG and should be tested first. If the test result is negative, a modulating antibody test should be performed because this may be positive in a small number of patients who do not have binding antibodies. The blocking antibody titer adds little additional diagnostic value and is not generally indicated.

Recently, antibodies against muscle-specific receptor tyrosine kinase (MuSK-Ab) have been described in approximately 40% of patients with "seronegative" MG. Evidence indicates that MuSK is involved in the proper distribution of AChR at the muscle endplate, and some evidence indicates that MuSK-Abs are pathogenic in these patients. The MuSK-Ab test is commercially available. Patients with MuSK-Ab are almost always seronegative for AChR-Ab. For this reason, the MuSK-Ab test should be sent only if the patient has already been tested for AChR-Ab and is seronegative. MG in patients with MuSK-Ab may have a different natural history and response to treatment, and this is an area of active investigation. Patients with MuSK-Ab are more likely to be young women and present with bulbar, neck, or respiratory symptoms. Edrophonium (Tensilon) testing is less likely to yield a positive result. Whether thymectomy should be performed in patients with MuSK-Ab is unclear.

Striational antibodies are a marker for thymoma, although false-positive and false-negative results are common. Chest computed tomography (CT) with contrast to evaluate for possible thymoma is indicated for all patients diagnosed with MG. The added value of performing striational antibodies has not been definitely demonstrated.

### ELECTROPHYSIOLOGIC TESTING

Electrophysiologic testing is indicated for evaluation of possible MG if the AChR-Ab test is negative. In antibody-positive patients, electrophysiologic testing is often not necessary unless the test is being performed to evaluate for evidence of generalized disease in those with purely ocular symptoms. Typically, routine nerve conduction studies and needle electromyography (EMG) are normal. These tests are performed to ensure that other disorders of the peripheral nerves or muscles are not present. Repetitive nerve stimulation (RNS) is then performed if the study was ordered to evaluate for an NMJ disorder. RNS has a sensitivity of approximately 50% to 60% in all patients with MG, with a higher yield in patients with generalized MG and a lower yield in patients with pure ocular MG. RNS of the spinal accessory and facial nerves may increase the yield of testing. It should be emphasized that abnormal RNS is not specific for MG, and routine nerve conduction studies and needle EMG must be performed to exclude other conditions. Single-fiber EMG (SFEMG) is a highly specialized and demanding technique with a sensitivity of approximately 90% to 95% in patients with MG. SFEMG is abnormal in many neuromuscular diseases and therefore should be performed only in the correct clinical context and after a routine EMG with RNS has been performed. Because of the demanding nature of the study, SFEMG is usually performed by a neuromuscular specialist.

## OTHER INVESTIGATIONS

Currently all patients diagnosed with MG should undergo a CT scan of the chest with contrast to evaluate for an associated thymoma. Routine chest radiography or determination of antistriational antibodies is not an adequate substitute.

# Prognosis

The natural history of MG is highly variable. Ocular symptoms are the presenting symptoms in approximately 50% to 60% of MG patients. Weakness subsequently develops in other muscles in most patients. Weakness remains restricted to the extraocular muscles for the entire course of MG in 15% to 20% of patients (pure ocular myasthenia). Patients with initial ocular involvement typically develop weakness in other muscles within the first year of having the disease. If no generalized symptoms develop after 2 years, subsequent generalization is unlikely. The maximal weakness from MG occurs within the initial 3 years of symptoms in 70% of patients. Mortality from MG is now low because of advances in critical care; however, quality of life is often affected by MG. Long-lasting remission occurs spontaneously in approximately 10% to 15% of patients if no immunosuppressive agents are used. Spontaneous remissions may be more frequent in patients with pure ocular myasthenia.

# Treatment

## CHOLINESTERASE INHIBITORS AS FIRST-LINE THERAPY

Cholinesterase inhibitors (ChEIs) are first-line therapy in all patients with MG. The commonly available ChEIs are listed in Table 3.

Acetylcholinesterase (AChE) is anchored in the synaptic cleft on the postsynaptic membrane. AChE normally cleaves acetylcholine (ACh) released from the presynaptic nerve terminal, which normally prevents repeat binding of ACh to the AChR. ChEIs reduce the hydrolysis of ACh and increase the amount of ACh available at the postsynaptic membrane. ChEIs used for treatment of MG are reversible inhibitors of AChE and cause few central nervous system side effects because they do not cross the blood–brain barrier efficiently. Absorption from the gastrointestinal tract is inefficient, and oral bioavailability is low.

Pyridostigmine bromide (Mestinon) is the most widely used ChEI. Onset of action is within 15 to 30 minutes of an oral dose, with peak action at 1 to 2 hours and gradual wearing off at 3 to 4 hours. All ChEI medications have muscarinic side effects, including cramping, diarrhea, salivation, lacrimation, and bradycardia. For this reason, the medication should always be introduced in low dose, preferably on the weekend. Pyridostigmine tablets are double scored and can be easily split. Start the patient with a half tablet (30 mg) of pyridostigmine once daily in the morning. The dose is then increased by a half tablet each day to a dose of a half tablet (30 mg) four times daily. Subsequently, the dose can be increased further to a full tablet (60 mg) four times daily. If necessary for symptom relief, pyridostigmine can be increased to a maximum dose of 120 mg every 3 to 4 hours, but 60 mg every 4 hours usually provides optimum benefit. If a patient has weakness while eating, pyridostigmine doses can be timed to be taken 1 hour before meals. If a patient has significant weakness upon awakening, the extended-release formulation of pyridostigmine (Mestinon Timespan) can be given at bedtime; however, absorption is too unpredictable for daytime use. If a patient requires parenteral dosing of medications, intravenous pyridostigmine is given at 1/30 the oral dose (usually 1–2 mg intravenously) every 3 to 4 hours.

When symptoms are not controlled with 60 to 120 mg of pyridostigmine every 4 hours, possible initiation of an immunosuppressive agent must be discussed fully with the patient. Most patients with generalized MG will require immunosuppressive treatment in order to induce a remission of symptoms. Pyridostigmine is often initially very effective, but therapeutic efficacy usually gradually diminishes. The immunosuppressive agents used in MG are corticosteroids, azathioprine[1] (Imuran), mycophenolate mofetil[1] (CellCept), cyclosporin A[1] (Neoral), and cyclophosphamide[1] (Cytoxan). Each of these agents is discussed separately in Table 4. Important considerations are the clinical severity of the MG, the patient's perception of his or her disability, any coexisting medical conditions, as well as the patient's age, gender, and overall lifestyle. For example, a physically active patient will be less tolerant of weakness than a patient with a sedentary lifestyle.

---

[1]Not FDA approved for this indication.

## TABLE 3 Commonly Available Cholinesterase Inhibitors

| Medication | Route of Administration | Unit Dose | Average Dose (Adult) | Children's Dose |
|---|---|---|---|---|
| Pyridostigmine bromide tablet (Mestinon) | Oral | 60-mg tablets, double-scored for splitting | 30–60 mg every 4–6 hours, maximum 120 mg every 3 hours | 1 mg/kg every 4–6 hours |
| Pyridostigmine bromide syrup | Oral | 12 mg/mL | 30–60 mg every 4–6 hours | 1 mg/kg every 4–6 hours |
| Pyridostigmine bromide sustained-release (Mestinon Timespan) | Oral | 180-mg tablet (not crushable) | 1 tablet at bedtime | — |
| Pyridostigmine bromide | Intravenous | 5 mg/mL ampules | 1/30 of usual oral dose, i.e., 1–2 mg every 3–4 hours | — |
| Neostigmine bromide (Prostigmin) | Oral | 15-mg tablets | 7.5–15 mg every 3–4 hours | |
| Edrophonium (Tensilon) | Intravenous | | Used for diagnosis | Used for diagnosis |

**TABLE 4  Oral Immunosuppressive Agents Used on Myasthenia Gravis**

| Medication | Starting Dose | Therapeutic Dose | Time to Clinical Effect | Laboratory Monitoring | Side Effects | Advantages |
|---|---|---|---|---|---|---|
| Prednisone[1] | 60–80 mg daily (see text) | 60–80 mg daily (or 120 mg every other day) | Days to weeks | May need to follow blood glucose level; follow bone density every 6 mo | Many serious long-term side effects (see text); always start with calcium 1500 mg/day and vitamin D 400 IU/day; may also require bisphosphonate | Short time to clinical effect; long clinical experience in MG; not teratogenic; relatively safe in pregnancy; no increase in malignancy |
| Azathioprine[1] (Imuran) | 50 mg daily | 2–3 mg/kg/day in divided doses | 4–12 mo | CBC, LFT weekly as dose increased; may then check once per month; if WBC <2500, stop azathioprine | ~10% fever, nausea, abdominal pain during first weeks of treatment; increased risk of malignancy with long-term use; teratogenic | Long clinical experience; predictable; fewer long-term side effects than prednisone |
| Mycophenolate mofetil[1] (CellCept) | 500 mg twice daily | 1000–1500 mg twice daily | 2–6 mo | CBC monthly, but significant myelosuppression is uncommon | Diarrhea; risk of malignancy with long-term use is currently unclear; should not be used in pregnancy because safety is unknown; clinical experience in MG is limited—randomized study is ongoing | Usually well tolerated; few serious side effects; faster onset of clinical effect than azathioprine |
| Cyclosporine[1] (Sandimmune, Neoral) | 3–5 mg/kg/day in divided doses | 3–5 mg/kg/day in divided doses | 2–6 mo | Renal function, trough cyclosporine levels, electrolytes monthly; follow blood pressure | Significant renal toxicity is common and is a frequent reason to stop the drug; hypertension; should not be used in pregnancy; many drug interactions; use only under guidance of neuromuscular specialist | Faster onset of clinical effect than azathioprine |
| Cyclophosphamide[1] (Cytoxan) | 25 mg/day orally; parenteral administration may be used in severe, refractory MG | 2–5 mg daily | | CBC monthly | Significant myelosuppression, hemorrhagic cystitis, risk of opportunistic infections; increased risk of malignancy; absolutely contraindicated during pregnancy; use only under guidance of neuromuscular specialist | May be effective in patients refractory to other treatments |

[1]Not FDA approved for this indication.
*Abbreviations:* CBC = complete blood count; LFT = liver function test; MG = myasthenia gravis; WBC = white blood cell count.

# CURRENT THERAPY

Be certain of the diagnosis
- Ocular symptoms only or mild weakness: Cholinesterase inhibitors
- Moderate to severe weakness:
    - Cholinesterase inhibitors, and
    - Thymectomy for patients younger than 60 years (with complete removal of the gland)
- If symptoms are uncontrolled with cholinesterase inhibitors, use immunosuppression:
    - Prednisone if urgent or severe
    - Azathioprine[1] (Imuran) or mycophenolate mofetil[1] (CellCept)
        - As a steroid-sparing agent to facilitate prednisone taper
        - Prednisone fails to elicit patient response
        - Prednisone contraindicated
        - Excessive prednisone side effects
- Plasma exchange or intravenous immune globulin[1]
    - Myasthenic crisis
    - Preoperative (i.e., before thymectomy)
- If the above measures fail:
    - Refer to neuromuscular specialist

---

[1]Not FDA approved for this indication.

## TREATMENT OF PURE OCULAR MYASTHENIA GRAVIS

From 15% to 20% of patients with MG have only visual symptoms for the entire course of their disease. Visual symptoms in patients with MG result from ptosis or ocular misalignment. Approximately 50% of patients will experience significant relief of visual symptoms with ChEIs alone and will be satisfied with their treatment. The effect on symptoms should be clear within 1 month of beginning pyridostigmine (Mestinon) therapy. In general, pyridostigmine provides significant relief of ptosis and is less helpful for ocular misalignment.

Among the 50% of patients who achieve significant control of ocular symptoms using pyridostigmine, this may be the only treatment necessary. If symptoms are not controlled, the patient's perception of his or her disability and lifestyle are very important to treatment. A patient who is unable to work because of visual misalignment will require further treatment. Nonpharmacologic options for symptom management include eyelid taping or eyelid crutches for ptosis and eye patching for ocular misalignment.

If the patient requests further treatment, prednisone[1] can be started at 10 mg/day, with an increase of 5 mg every other day until a dose of 40 to 60 mg/day is reached. This dose should be continued for approximately 1 month. The vast majority of patients will improve. At 1 month, a taper at 5 mg/wk can be started; at 20 mg the taper should be slowed to improve the chances of maintaining remission.

The role of corticosteroids in the treatment of pure ocular MG is controversial. Some data suggest that corticosteroids decrease the chance of developing generalized MG. However, corticosteroids have many undesired effects. In general, corticosteroids are used for ocular myasthenia only when the symptoms are significant to the patient and are uncontrolled by ChEIs.

## CORTICOSTEROIDS

Corticosteroids are usually the first-line immunosuppressive agent. After 6 weeks of treatment with a corticosteroid, approximately 90%

of patients have improvement in symptoms. Approximately 30% of patients treated with prednisone obtain remission, and 50% experience marked improvement. Paradoxically, 50% of patients have an initial increase in weakness during the first weeks of treatment with corticosteroids. The reasons for this effect are not well understood. Some practitioners begin treatment at the full therapeutic dose of prednisone 60 to 80 mg/day, with careful monitoring for increased weakness. If weakness worsens, the patient may require hospitalization and treatment with plasma exchange or intravenous immune globulin[1] (IVIG; Gamimune N). Others begin treatment at a lower dose with a gradual increase to the target dose over 1 month with the goal of avoiding the initial worsening of strength. An example of this method begins with a dose of prednisone 20 mg once daily. The dose is increased by 5 mg every third day until the target dose of 60 to 80 mg/day is reached. Alternate-day dosing with a target dose of 100 to 120 mg every other day can also be used. When beginning prednisone, calcium, vitamin D, and a bisphosphonate medication should be started at the same time unless a contraindication is present. This is appropriate because most patients will require long-term therapy with prednisone.

A clinical effect is typically seen within 6 weeks. If a remission is achieved, the full dose should be maintained for 6 weeks, followed by a slow taper. Initially the daily prednisone dose can be decreased by 5 mg/month. When the daily dose reaches 30 mg/day. the taper should be slowed, with further decreases in dose of 2.5 mg/month. Clinical exacerbations are frequent when the daily dose of prednisone reaches 20 to 30 mg/day, and a slower taper may prevent this problem. If an exacerbation occurs, the daily prednisone dose should be increased by 5 to 10 mg. The new dose can be maintained for 6 weeks, followed by a slower taper. Some practitioners use alternate-day dosing, with tapering from an initial dose of 100 to 120 mg every other day.

Long-term use of corticosteroids is associated with serious complications, including osteoporosis, fractures, medication-induced diabetes mellitus, obesity, glaucoma, cataracts, gastric and duodenal ulcers, anxiety or depression, myopathy, opportunistic infections, and avascular necrosis of the large joints. Most patients are not able to completely discontinue prednisone and require a minimum dose to maintain improvement of their MG. The decision to start a steroid-sparing agent is often not clear-cut. In general, if a patient has more than one relapse when tapering off steroids, therapy with a steroid-sparing agent should be considered. If a patient does not have a remission with steroids, combined therapy with a steroid-sparing agent should be considered. In the older patient population, treatment with a steroid-sparing agent should be considered early in the course. In a young patient, particularly a woman in her childbearing years, steroid-sparing drugs should be avoided when possible because of teratogenicity and the increased risk of lymphoma with long-term use of these agents.

## OTHER IMMUNOSUPPRESSIVE AGENTS

Azathioprine[1] (Imuran) has been extensively used in MG, usually as a steroid-sparing medication. Azathioprine is an inhibitor of purine synthesis and therefore affects rapidly dividing cell populations, such as lymphocytes. A large double-blind, randomized study demonstrated improvement in steroid tapering with the use of azathioprine. The major drawback of azathioprine is that a clinical effect may not be seen until 12 months. Side effects are less common than with steroids. Approximately 10% of patients have an idiosyncratic reaction in the first weeks of therapy, with fever, nausea, vomiting, and abdominal pain. Symptoms resolve with cessation of the drug but usually recur if azathioprine is restarted. Azathioprine may cause leukopenia or thrombocytopenia, vomiting, or hepatic dysfunction. Mild leukopenia occurs in 25% of patients but is usually not significant. Elevation of hepatic enzyme levels occurs in 5% of patients but is usually reversible with cessation of the drug. The risk of lymphoma increases slightly after 10 years of use. Azathioprine is potentially teratogenic and should be avoided in women of childbearing age. The initial dose is 50 mg/day

---

[1]Not FDA approved for this indication.

(or 1 mg/kg/day). The dose is increased over a few months until the therapeutic dose of 2 mg/kg/day in divided doses is reached. CBC with differential and liver function tests initially should be tested weekly and monthly after the target dose has been reached. Leukopenia may develop even after several years of treatment. If the white blood cell count drops below 2500 cells/mm³ or the absolute neutrophil count below 1000 cells/mm³, the drug should be stopped. Overall, approximately 50% of patients improve with azathioprine therapy. Relapse after discontinuation of azathioprine occurs in more than 50% of patients.

Mycophenolate mofetil[1] (CellCept) is a newer immunosuppressant that inhibits proliferation of T and B lymphocytes by blocking de novo purine synthesis. Lymphocytes are selectively affected because they are unable to use the purine salvage pathway. The major advantages of mycophenolate are its relatively fast onset of clinical effect and its favorable side-effect profile. Side effects are usually mild and include diarrhea, abdominal pain, nausea, peripheral edema, and mild leukopenia. The long-term risk of malignancy with use of mycophenolate is unclear; however, an elderly MG patient who developed primary central nervous system lymphoma in association with mycophenolate use has been recently reported. Treatment trials of patients with MG are ongoing. Some practitioners use mycophenolate to induce remission without the concomitant use of steroids. Others use mycophenolate only as a steroid-sparing agent in steroid-dependent patients. The standard starting dose is 500 mg twice daily. The therapeutic dose for treatment of MG is 1000 to 1500 mg twice daily. Significant myelosuppression is uncommon; however, a monthly check of CBC with differential is standard practice.

Cyclosporine[1] (Sandimmune, Neoral) is an inhibitor of T-helper cell function through blockade of calcineurin-mediated cytokine signaling. Cyclosporine is of limited use for treatment of MG because of renal toxicity. Cyclosporine is used for cases of severe MG when steroids and azathioprine are not tolerated or are ineffective. The standard dosage for treatment of MG is 3 to 5 mg/kg/day in divided doses. Anecdotally, a lower target dose of 2 mg/kg/day may decrease the incidence of renal insufficiency while still achieving clinical improvement. A clinical effect is usually seen within the first 6 months of treatment. Renal function and trough cyclosporine levels should be followed monthly. Creatinine levels greater than 50% of the pretreatment levels are an indication to stop the drug. A rise in creatinine level typically occurs after several years of use. Hypertension is a frequent side effect, and blood pressure must be monitored regularly. In general, this medication should be used for treatment of MG under the guidance of a neuromuscular specialist.

Cyclophosphamide[1] (Cytoxan) is an alkylating agent that acts on DNA, inhibiting cell proliferation. Cyclophosphamide has limited use in MG because of multiple serious toxicities. Cyclophosphamide is used in patients with severe MG when steroids and azathioprine are ineffective or not tolerated. It appears effective at inducing remission when used in this manner. Cyclophosphamide has been used in combination with steroids for patients with severe disease who have not responded to steroids alone. The risk of side effects from cyclophosphamide is high. Cyclophosphamide may cause severe bone marrow suppression, severe opportunistic infections, bladder toxicity, and increased risk of neoplasm. Cyclophosphamide is a chemotherapeutic agent at higher doses, and parenteral high-dose administration has occasionally been used for patients with refractory, severe MG. In general, this medication should be used for treatment of MG only under the guidance of a neuromuscular specialist.

## SHORT-TERM IMMUNOTHERAPY: PLASMA EXCHANGE AND INTRAVENOUS IMMUNE GLOBULIN

Plasma exchange (i.e., plasmapheresis) is a well-established intervention that produces short-term clinical improvement in patients with MG. Plasmapheresis is typically used in a MG patient with rapid worsening of weakness or myasthenic crisis. Plasma exchange treatments may be performed prior to an elective surgical procedure, such as thymectomy, to decrease the likelihood of a myasthenic exacerbation. Rarely a patient is refractory or intolerant of all long-term therapies and requires periodic plasma exchange on an ongoing basis. Typical treatment of a myasthenic exacerbation consists of five exchanges of 3 to 4 L each over a period of approximately 2 weeks. The effect is rapid and improvement is seen within days of starting therapy, but the effect is short lived. Typically the beneficial effects of plasma exchange last only a few weeks. Central venous access, typically with a large-bore catheter, is required. Complications of plasma exchange are usually related to the vascular access. Patients are at risk for significant iatrogenic infections, particularly because many of these patients are undergoing long-term therapy with immunosuppressive agents. Hematoma at the site of line placement, pulmonary embolism from venous thrombosis, electrolyte imbalance, pneumothorax, and hypotension during plasma exchange treatments can occur.

IVIG[1] is used for identical indications as plasma exchange. The standard dose is 400 mg/kg/day for 5 days. The only large, randomized study of IVIG in MG found IVIG equivalent to plasmapheresis for treatment of myasthenic crisis. Some practitioners anecdotally believe plasma exchange produces more rapid improvement in strength. The advantages of IVIG are that it is generally more widely available than is plasmapheresis, and it does not require central venous access. The most common side effects are headache and transient flulike symptoms. However, IVIG may cause volume overload, vascular events such as ischemic stroke, and venous thrombosis. IVIG should be used with caution in patients with risk factors for these conditions. IVIG cannot be used in patients with IgA deficiency, a relatively frequent condition. An IgA level must be determined prior to the first IVIG treatment to avoid a potentially serious allergic reaction. Anecdotally, some patients refractory to IVIG will have a good response to plasma exchange.

## THYMECTOMY

Thymectomy has been standard therapy for treatment of MG for more than 50 years, but it has never been evaluated in a large, prospective, randomized controlled trial. Thymectomy appears to be effective in improving the course of MG in patients without thymoma. If a thymoma is present, thymectomy is mandatory. The procedure is not a cure for MG, but it appears to increase the likelihood of clinical remission, particularly if performed within the first year of symptom onset. Approximately 75% of patients appear to receive some benefit from the procedure, but the effect may be apparent only after several years. Thymectomy appears to be more effective in younger patients, which may reflect the involution of the thymus with aging. Patients younger than 60 years with moderate to severe MG are candidates for thymectomy. Patients with pure ocular myasthenia do not usually undergo thymectomy unless a thymoma is suspected. Thymic tissue may be present throughout the neck and the mediastinum. The majority of surgical centers perform a combined transsternal–transcervical exposure with en bloc removal of the thymus to ensure complete removal of the gland. Incomplete resections have been followed by persistent symptoms that were later relieved by removal of residual thymus at reoperation. Referrals for thymectomy should be made to an experienced surgeon willing to perform a maximal resection. In the days preceding thymectomy, patients often undergo plasma exchange to decrease the likelihood of an exacerbation due to the surgery. The surgery involves sternotomy and a 4- to 6-week convalescence. Serious complications are uncommon when the surgery is performed at an experienced center by anesthesiologists and neurologists familiar with the perioperative management of MG.

## TREATMENT OF MYASTHENIC CRISIS

A myasthenic crisis is an exacerbation of MG producing respiratory weakness or profound muscle weakness. Myasthenic crisis is a neurologic emergency. Patients with worsening weakness should undergo tests including chest radiograph, blood and urine cultures, CBC with

---

[1]Not FDA approved for this indication.

[1]Not FDA approved for this indication.

differential, and serum chemistries to screen for concurrent infections. The patient's medication list should be scrutinized and any recent additions or changes noted. Patients occasionally increase their ChEI dose to toxic levels without consulting their physician, resulting in increased muscle weakness and a "cholinergic crisis." This event is relatively uncommon, but recent consumption of ChEI must be determined in all myasthenic patients with increasing weakness. Signs of cholinergic crisis include abdominal cramps, diarrhea, nausea and vomiting, excessive secretions, and miotic pupils; these are not characteristics of myasthenic crisis. If cholinergic crisis is a consideration, the ChEI must be stopped. A patient in myasthenic crisis should be admitted to an intensive care unit if any signs of respiratory failure are present because respiratory deterioration may occur quickly. The vital capacity and peak negative inspiratory force should be followed as measures of respiratory strength. As a rule, elective intubation should be performed when the vital capacity falls below 15 mL/kg and peak negative inspiratory force below −20 cm $H_2O$. Arterial blood gas measurements do not accurately reflect the degree of respiratory muscle weakness in MG. $PCO_2$ and $pO_2$ measurements may be normal until just prior to respiratory collapse. While a patient is ventilated, it is reasonable to discontinue pyridostigmine (Mestinon) because this medication may increase respiratory secretions. Any immunosuppressive agents should be continued. If the patient is a new-onset myasthenic, it is appropriate to begin prednisone therapy 60 to 80 mg/day while the patient is ventilated. Options for improving strength during crisis are plasma exchange treatments and IVIG (discussed earlier). Readiness for weaning from the ventilator can be assessed using the vital capacity and peak negative inspiratory force measurements. Weaning from the ventilator may otherwise be performed according to standard protocols. Once the patient is successfully extubated, treatment with ChEIs can be resumed. A treatment plan to prevent future myasthenic crises should be developed.

## Other Issues

### TRANSIENT NEONATAL MYASTHENIA

Transient neonatal myasthenia occurs in 10% of infants of mothers with autoimmune MG. Following delivery, the infant has a weak cry or suck, appears floppy, and may require mechanical ventilation. The symptoms result from maternal antibodies transferred across the placenta to the infant in utero and resolve within a few weeks. Infants with severe weakness can be treated with oral pyridostigmine 1 to 2 mg/kg every 2 hours.

### LAMBERT-EATON MYASTHENIC SYNDROME

Lambert-Eaton myasthenic syndrome (LEMS) is an uncommon autoimmune disorder of the presynaptic NMJ. LEMS is characterized by fluctuating proximal extremity weakness. Symptoms typically include difficulty walking, standing up from a chair, and climbing stairs. Patients may complain of autonomic symptoms, such as dry mouth, blurry vision, anhidrosis, or constipation. Unlike MG, in LEMS ptosis, diplopia, dysphagia, and dysarthria are usually not prominent. Respiratory failure may occur but is uncommon. Patients may report improvement in muscle strength after sustained activity. Other frequent symptoms include myalgias, muscle stiffness, paresthesias, and a metallic taste in the mouth.

On examination, patients typically have proximal muscle weakness, more prominent in the lower extremities. The objective weakness may be less than expected given the patient's symptoms. Characteristically, muscle stretch reflexes are absent. Sustained muscle grip strength often increases over the first several seconds (Lambert's sign).

LEMS is a paraneoplastic syndrome in 60% of patients, most often due to a small cell carcinoma of the lung. In patients without malignancy, LEMS is often associated with other autoimmune conditions. Male patients older than 40 years are more likely to have an associated malignancy, whereas patients without malignancy are more often young women. All patients with suspected LEMS should undergo a thorough evaluation for malignancy, however. If no malignancy is found, the evaluation should be repeated at regular intervals. Presentation of LEMS may antedate the discovery of a malignancy by up to 2 years.

LEMS is believed to result from autoantibodies against the presynaptic voltage-gated calcium channels of cholinergic nerve terminals. At the NMJ, decreased release of acetylcholine from the presynaptic nerve terminal results in muscle weakness. The cholinergic nerve terminals of the autonomic nervous system are also affected. Seventy-five percent of patients with LEMS have detectable serum IgG antibodies against voltage-gated P/Q calcium channels. The diagnosis of LEMS should always be confirmed by electrophysiologic studies. Nerve conduction studies reveal diffusely low compound motor action potential (CMAP) amplitudes with normal sensory responses. RNS shows a CMAP decrement with slow rates of stimulation but marked increment of the CMAP response after brief exercise. A similar increment is seen with fast rates of RNS.

In LEMS with an associated malignancy, treatment of the malignancy may lead to improvement of LEMS symptoms. For symptomatic treatment, some patients achieve improvement with use of ChEIs such as pyridostigmine (Mestinon). 3,4-Diaminopyridine (DAP) increases release of ACh from the presynaptic nerve terminal by decreasing potassium conductance. 3,4-DAP is not approved by the Food and Drug Administration (FDA) for use in the United States. In countries where 3,4-DAP is approved, it represents the first-line symptomatic therapy for LEMS. The typical starting dose is 10 mg every 4 to 6 hours. In patients with disabling symptoms, immunosuppressive therapies such as long-term corticosteroids, plasma exchange treatments, and IVIG[1] can be used.

## REFERENCES

Chaudry V, Cornblath DR, Griffin JW, et al: Mycophenolate mofetil: a safe and promising immunosuppressant in neuromuscular diseases. Neurology 2001;56:94-96.

Drachman DB: Myasthenia gravis. N Engl J Med 1994;330:1797-1810.

Gajdos PH, Chevret S, Clair B, et al: Clinical trial of plasma exchange and high-dose intravenous immunoglobulin in myasthenia gravis. Ann Neurol 1997;41:789-796.

Jaretzki A, Steinglass KM, Sonett JR: Thymectomy in the management of myasthenia gravis. Semin Neurol 2004;24:49-62.

Kaminski HJ (ed): Current Clinical Neurology: Myasthenia Gravis and Related Disorders. Totowa, NJ, Humana Press, 2002.

Katirji B, Kaminski HJ: Electrodiagnostic approach to the patient with suspected neuromuscular junction disorder. Neurol Clin 2002; 20:557-586.

Palace J, Newsom-Davis J, Lecky B: A randomized double-blind trial of prednisolone alone or with azathioprine in myasthenia gravis. Neurology 1998;50:1778-1783.

Pascuzzi RM, Coslett HB, Johns TR: Long-term corticosteroid treatment of myasthenia gravis: Report of 116 patients. Ann Neurol 1984;15: 291-298.

Richman DP, Agius MA: Treatment of autoimmune myasthenia gravis. Neurology 2003;61:1652-1661.

Saperstein DS, Barohn RJ: Management of myasthenia gravis. Semin Neurol 2004;24:41-48.

Seybold ME, Drachman DB: Gradually increasing doses of prednisone in MG. N Engl J Med 1974;290:81-84.

Vincent A, Leite MI: Neuromuscular junction autoimmune disease: Muscle specific kinase antibodies and treatments for myasthenia gravis. Curr Opinion Neurol 2005;18:519-525.

---

[1]Not FDA approved for this indication.

# Trigeminal Neuralgia

Method of
*Ronald F. Young, MD*

Trigeminal neuralgia (TN) is one of the most devastating pain conditions that people endure. The pain is frequently misdiagnosed as being of dental or paranasal sinus origin. Unnecessary dental procedures, such as root canals and extractions or sinus surgery, are often performed in misguided attempts to treat the pain. The condition is also referred to as *tic douloureux* because of the sudden facial grimacing that may be seen as a reaction to the pain. The illness is estimated to affect about 1 in 20,000 people and becomes more frequent with advancing age. TN may be of primary (idiopathic) origin or secondary origin due to a variety of structural conditions, such as tumors (meningiomas and vestibular schwannomas in particular), multiple sclerosis (MS), vascular malformations, and cysts of the posterior cranial fossa. The exact etiology of TN is still debated, but it is generally accepted that most cases of idiopathic TN are due to compression of the trigeminal nerve root near its entry into the brainstem at the pons by adjacent blood vessels, most commonly arteries. Such compression is thought to result in segmental demyelination due to the constant pulsatile forces directed against the nerve root. The underlying pathology is thought to be related to the aging process wherein arteries (particularly the superior cerebellar artery) that normally course superior to, but not in contact with, the nerve root gradually come into contact and then compress and distort the nerve root as a result of constant pulsatile pressure. Such pressure causes localized demyelination and loss of the normal insulating function of the myelin. Ephaptic or nonsynaptic transmission and abnormal local depolarization are then postulated to result in ectopic impulse generation. Such impulses are thought to activate nerve fibers in the trigeminal nerve root that generate the pain of TN. Ephaptic transmission is also thought to account for the "triggering" of pain by usually innocuous stimuli, such as lightly touching the face or brushing the teeth.

## Diagnosis

In spite of modern technology, TN is a diagnosis based almost exclusively on the medical history. Neither laboratory nor imaging studies establish the diagnosis conclusively, although properly formatted magnetic resonance imaging (MRI) scans recently have been thought to contribute to the correct diagnosis if they demonstrate arterial compression of the trigeminal nerve root. Three aspects of the history are critical to the diagnosis: (1) the type of pain, (2) the location of the pain, and (3) the factors that trigger or activate the pain. The pain of TN is sharp, sudden, severe, and brief in character, usually lasting only a few seconds but often occurring in repeated bursts. The pain is often described as feeling like an electric shock or ice pick jabbing into the face. Pains that are of longer duration and described as burning, aching, boring, or like pressure are not typical of TN; when such

symptoms are described, an alternative diagnosis should be considered. The pain of TN is confined within one or more of the major three peripheral divisions of the trigeminal nerve: the first division encompassing the anterior two thirds of the scalp, the forehead, the eye, and the upper portion of the nose; the second division encompassing the edges of the nares, the upper lip and cheek, the upper teeth, gums, and mucosal lining of the mouth; and the third division encompassing the skin over the mandible, including the lower lip as well as the lower teeth, gums, and anterior two thirds of the tongue. Pain that is located in the mastoid or occipital region, deep within the ear canal, extending below the edge of the mandible onto the neck or traversing the midline is not trigeminal in origin. TN is almost exclusively a unilateral condition. Bilateral pain is estimated to occur in less than 1% of cases; when bilateral, the pain on the two sides is often different with regard to the age of the patient at onset and the location of the pain. Most cases of bilateral TN occur in patients with MS wherein the pain is due to demyelination in the trigeminal nerve root secondary to an MS plaque. One of the most characteristic historical features of TN is the triggering of jabs or jolts of pain by stimuli that usually are innocuous. Such triggers include a variety of light mechanical stimuli, such as touching the face lightly, brushing the teeth, talking, attempting to eat and drink, and even a light breeze blowing against the face. Light, gentle stimuli are often more effective in eliciting the pain than are more forceful ones. Facial pain, even severe pain, probably is not TN if trigger phenomena are not described. The time course of TN is marked by unexplained, erratic exacerbations and remissions that may last days, weeks, months, or even years. The exacerbations tend to be less severe and shorter in duration at the onset of the illness and tend to become more severe and longer in duration and marked by shorter interval remissions as the illness persists over time. Patients who complain of persistent, unremitting facial pain, often with durations of weeks, months, or even years, probably do not suffer from TN. TN is often misdiagnosed as being of dental or paranasal sinus origin, but conversely other forms of facial pain are often misdiagnosed as TN. Most commonly misdiagnosed is so-called atypical facial pain. Such pain, often seen in young or middle-aged women but seen in men as well, usually is described as a strong, unremitting pressure or burning sensation that encompasses an area of the head and/or neck outside of the distribution of the trigeminal nerve, unassociated with trigger phenomena, often of prolonged durations (years), and usually unresponsive to a variety of medical interventions. Patients with atypical facial pain often express feelings of depression and hopelessness. Such pain is unresponsive to surgical intervention, and ill-advised surgical procedures often aggravate the pain and may leave the patient with new medical problems due to complications of the surgical procedures.

## Physical Examination

In classic, or idiopathic, TN due to vascular compression of the trigeminal nerve root, the physical examination is usually completely unremarkable. Specifically, at least by the usual clinical examination techniques, facial sensation including the corneal reflex is normal. When loss of facial sensation to innocuous or painful stimuli is detected, a structural cause of TN should be sought. Tumors, vascular malformations, and MS are usually accompanied by other abnormal neurologic examination findings, including double vision, unilateral hearing loss, and facial weakness. MRI scanning is recommended in all patients with a suspected diagnosis of TN because even in some cases of TN caused by structural lesions, the examination may be normal, and the diagnosis of TN may be strengthened if an MRI scan demonstrates arterial compression of the trigeminal nerve root. Occasionally, an MRI scan discloses a completely unexpected cause of TN, such as a tortuous vertebrobasilar artery complex compressing the nerve root or even a large contralateral tumor or cyst displacing the brainstem. Such findings may radically alter any surgical recommendations made for treatment of TN. Patients who are unable to undergo MRI scanning because they have a cardiac pacemaker, for instance, should undergo thin-section computed tomography scanning, which cannot detect arterial vascular compression and small tumors but can

### CURRENT DIAGNOSIS

- Sudden, sharp, severe pain on one side of the face
- Confined to the cutaneous or intraoral distribution of the trigeminal nerve
- Triggered by otherwise innocuous stimulation of the face or mouth
- Usually due to arterial compression of the trigeminal nerve root but may be due to multiple sclerosis, tumors, or vascular malformations

detect larger tumors, vascular malformations, and vertebrobasilar artery compression.

# Treatment

## MEDICAL TREATMENT

The anticonvulsant family of drugs is the mainstay of medical treatment of TN. Carbamazepine (Tegretol) and oxcarbazepine (Trileptal)[1] are the best drugs for initial medical treatment of TN. Both should be started in relatively low doses, for example, 100 to 200 mg once or twice daily and then increased gradually and slowly until either satisfactory control of the pain or intolerable side effects occur. Such side effects include drowsiness, weakness, difficulty with recent memory, and unsteadiness of gait. Older patients are particularly sensitive to such side effects, and the initial dose and maximum tolerable dose are usually lower in older patients, particularly those in their 70s and older. From 5 to 7 days should elapse between dosing increments in order to allow development of a stable blood level of medication. Additional increments of 100 to 200 mg/day are recommended. Laboratory tests of serum levels of the medications are of little or no help in the treatment of TN. In order to establish a consistent blood level of these medications and to provide the best chance for achieving lasting pain relief with minimum side effects, counseling of the patient by the physician regarding the correct dosing regimen is essential. Patients often regard these medications as analgesics and vary the dosage on an as-needed basis, some days taking little or no medication and other days taking large amounts. Because of their pharmacokinetics, these medications must be taken in a consistent dosage on a daily basis in order to maximize the chance of success. It is surprising how hard it may be for patients to understand and adhere to such a regimen, but maintaining the regimen is essential for successful pain relief. Gabapentin (Neurontin)[1] has become popular for the treatment of TN, but experience indicates it is a secondary medication only. It may be useful when pain control cannot be achieved with carbamazepine (Tegretol) or oxcarbazepine (Trileptal) or when those medications cannot be tolerated because of side effects. Other potential second-line medications include a variety of other anticonvulsants (e.g., lamotrigine [Lamictal],[1] phenytoin [Dilantin][1]) as well as baclofen (Lioresal) A variety of toxicities, including liver dysfunction, bone marrow suppression, and allergic reactions, may accompany use of these medications, so appropriate laboratory surveillance should be performed per manufacturers' recommendations.

## SURGICAL TREATMENT

In the past, surgery was reserved for patients who did not respond to medical management of TN because the medication was ineffective or the side effects or toxicities were intolerable. However, some studies suggest that the longer the illness persists, the smaller the chance for

[1]Not FDA approved for this indication.

## CURRENT THERAPY

- Usually responds to oral anticonvulsant medications, such as carbamazepine (Tegretol) or oxcarbazepine (Trileptal).[1]
- Early radiosurgical treatment offers a good chance of curing the illness with minimal side effects.
- Microvascular decompression is the most effective surgical treatment of TN, but it is associated with the greatest risk of serious complications.

[1]Not FDA approved for this indication.

lasting successful surgical relief of the pain. Many patients considered the potential side effects and complications of the surgical procedures unacceptable, and neurologists often referred patients for surgical procedures only as a last resort. With the advent of radiosurgery as a viable, successful, and safe surgical treatment of TN, consideration of surgical intervention earlier rather than later in the disease course may be better. Microvascular decompression (MVD) is the most effective, yet most dangerous, of the surgical procedures for TN. About 90% of patients will achieve immediate relief of TN after MVD, but this success rate drops to about 75% in long-term follow-up. MVD is the only surgical procedure that treats the putative cause of TN, namely, vascular compression of the trigeminal nerve root. In the MVD procedure, a small posterior fossa craniotomy is performed. The trigeminal nerve root is visualized using the operating microscope, any compressing vessels are dissected free of the nerve, and future contact is prevented by placing a shock-absorbing material, usually shredded Teflon felt, between the vessel and the nerve. Fatal complications may occur in up to 1% of patients undergoing the MVD procedures. From 15% to 20% of patients who undergo MVD experience some complication of the procedure, such as cerebellar edema, brainstem infarction, subdural and epidural hematomas, facial paralysis, unilateral hearing loss, cerebrospinal fluid leakage, meningitis, and infection. Percutaneous procedures (e.g., radiofrequency electrocoagulation, glycerol rhizolysis, balloon compression) are considerably safer than MVD, but loss of facial sensation usually accompanies such procedures. Loss of facial sensation should be avoided in order to prevent secondary complications such as anesthesia dolorosa and loss of the corneal reflex with subsequent corneal ulceration or loss of vision. The initial success rate is about 90% with the percutaneous procedures, but recurrences are frequent. Serious side effects, such as meningitis, brain abscess or hematoma, and carotid artery to cavernous sinus fistulas, occasionally occur. One of the attractive features of percutaneous procedures is that they can be repeated fairly easily if pain recurs. Radiosurgery is gaining increased acceptance as a surgical method for treating TN. Although considered a form of surgery, the procedure is accomplished without an incision, instead using either gamma rays (Gamma Knife, Elekta, Inc.) or high-energy x-rays (linear accelerator [LINAC]) that are focused on the trigeminal nerve root adjacent to the brainstem. The treatment is planned using MRI or computed tomography scanning, and the radiation is guided to the target at the trigeminal nerve root in such a way as to avoid injury to adjacent structures. The procedure provides pain relief in about 60% of patients with TN without the need for medication; another 15% to 20% of patients experience pain relief with small tolerable doses of medication. Radiosurgery is attractive to patients and referring physicians because of the ease of performing the procedure and the minimum risk of side effects. Radiosurgery is a destructive form of treatment of TN, but the degree of damage to the nerve root is usually minimal enough that normal facial sensation is maintained. Permanent losses of facial sensation may occur in as few as 5% of patients treated with radiosurgery, depending on the dose of radiation used for the treatment. Drawbacks of radiosurgery include delayed onset of pain relief after treatment (usually a few months) and recurrences. Radiosurgery can be repeated in the event of initial failure of the treatment or in case of recurrence after an initially successful treatment. The reasonable success rate, the ease of performance of the procedure, and the minimal risk of side effects make radiosurgery a treatment that can be recommended early in the treatment of TN, once the diagnosis has been well established, because it may provide permanent cure of the disease with minimal risk.

## REFERENCES

Bagheri SC, Fairhdvash F, Perciaccante VJ: Diagnosis and treatment of patients with trigeminal neuralgia. Am Dent Assoc 2004;135:1713-1717.

Kres B, Schindler M, Rasche D, et al: MRI volumetry for the preoperative diagnosis of trigeminal neuralgia. Eur Radiol 2005;15:1344-1348.

Liu JK, Apfelbaum RI: Treatment of trigeminal neuralgia. Neurosurg Clin North Am 2004;15:319-334.

Shetter AG, Aabramisk JM, Speiser BL: Microvascular decompression after gamma knife surgery for trigeminal neuralgia: intraoperative findings and treatment outcomes. J Neurosurg 2000;102(Suppl.):259-261.

Young RF: Stereotactic procedures for facial pain. In Apuzzo M (ed): Brain Surgery: Complication Avoidance and Management. New York, Churchill Livingstone, 1993, pp 2097-2114.

Young RF: Radiosurgery versus microsurgery for trigeminal neurlagia: current techniques in neurosurgery. In Salcman M (ed): Current Medicine. New York, Springer, 1998, pp 35-43.

Young RF, Vermeulen SS, Grimm P, et al: Gamma knife radiosurgery for treatment of trigeminal neuralgia: Idiopathic and tumor related. Neurology 1997;48:608-614.

Young RF, Vermeulen SS, Posewitz A: Gamma knife radiosurgery for treatment of trigeminal neuralgia. Stereotact Funct Neurosurg 1998;70:192-199.

# Bell's Palsy (Idiopathic Acute Peripheral Facial Paralysis)

Method of
*W. Cooper Scurry, Jr., MD, Jon E. Isaacson, MD, and Fred G. Fedok, MD, FACS*

## Epidemiology

Facial nerve paralysis has an extensive differential diagnosis but is most commonly idiopathic (Box 1). Although most facial paralysis is of unknown etiology, more serious causes are ruled out by careful evaluation. Each case requires cautious management to avoid secondary sequelae such as eye exposure.

Facial nerve paralysis that is rapid in onset and idiopathic in origin is referred to as *Bell's palsy*. The Scottish surgeon Charles Bell first identified and described the motor function of the facial nerve in 1821. Facial nerve paralysis that is gradually worsening in nature or has a known cause such as trauma or tumor should not be referred to as Bell's palsy.

The incidence of Bell's palsy is 20 to 30 cases per 100,000 persons per year. This condition accounts for 60% to 75% of all cases of unilateral facial paralysis. Approximately 40,000 cases occur in the United States each year, and one in 60 people will be affected during their lifetime. Bell's palsy can occur at any age; however, the median age at onset is 40 years, and the incidence is highest in people older than 70 years. Men and women are affected equally, and left and right sides are affected equally as well. Pregnant women are at significantly increased risk for developing Bell's palsy, and patients with diabetes mellitus and hypertension are at a slightly increased risk.

## Pathogenesis

The facial nerve (cranial nerve VII) leaves the brainstem and enters the temporal bone of the skull via the internal auditory canal. On exiting the internal auditory canal, and throughout the temporal bone, the facial nerve travels through the bony fallopian canal. This represents the longest intraosseous course of any of the cranial nerves. The labyrinthine segment of the nerve runs through the narrowest portion of the fallopian canal, measuring only 0.6 mm. It is at this segment where inflammation and swelling of the nerve against the bony confines of the canal lead to ischemia and subsequent neural conduction block.

Although Bell's palsy has been a synonym for idiopathic facial paralysis, a viral etiology was first suggested by McCormick in 1972. In 1996, Murakami's group identified DNA fragments of herpes simplex virus type 1 (HSV-1) in the perineural fluid of 11 of 14 patients undergoing facial nerve decompression surgery during the acute phase of an illness.

Not only have scientific experiments demonstrated evidence for a viral etiology, but recent clinical work also shows an advantage to the use of antivirals in the treatment of Bell's. In a double-blind study of 99 Bell's palsy patients treated with either acyclovir-prednisone or placebo-prednisone, Adour reported on the superior final outcome of acyclovir-prednisone compared with prednisone alone. Other studies regarding the benefit of antivirals in the management of Bell's palsy are ongoing and include a 500-patient randomized, controlled trial in Scotland that finished enrolling patients in June 2006.

## Clinical Evaluation

Patients with Bell's palsy present to a variety of caregivers. The most important aspect of the evaluation is obtaining a clear history, whether in an emergency department, primary care setting, or subspecialty setting. The provider needs to ascertain the time of onset and whether the paresis is getting better or worse. If the paralysis is complete, one should determine how long it took to evolve to completion. Bell's palsy usually manifests over only hours to days. A slowly progressive paralysis that worsens over weeks to months is not Bell's palsy and should be worked up otherwise. One should rule out a history of malignancies of the head and neck in patients with Bell's palsy. Cutaneous malignancies of the face, scalp, and auricle are especially pertinent.

Seventy percent of Bell's palsy patients will have had a preceding viral-type illness such as an upper respiratory tract infection. Other symptoms accompanying facial paralysis include otalgia, paresthesias,

---

**BOX 1   Differential Diagnosis of Acute Facial Nerve Paralysis**

- Bell's palsy
- Herpes zoster (Ramsay Hunt syndrome)
- Guillain-Barré syndrome
- Autoimmune disease
- Lyme disease
- HIV
- Kawasaki disease
- Trauma (temporal bone fracture, facial injury)
- Otitis media (acute, chronic, cholesteatoma)
- Sarcoidosis
- Melkersson-Rosenthal syndrome
- Diabetes mellitus
- Hypertension
- Sjögren's syndrome
- Eclampsia
- Amyloidosis
- Parotid tumor
- Vestibular schwannoma
- Malignancy

---

**CURRENT DIAGNOSIS**

- Acute-onset facial paresis is evaluated with a full head and neck and neurologic physical examination as soon as possible to establish the extent of facial weakness and determine a House-Brackmann score.
- History and physical examination include evaluation of the affected eye.
- All facial paresis patients need full audiometric testing.
- If a patient with facial paralysis demonstrates no improvement at 2 to 3 months, appropriate imaging is obtained.

cephalgia, dysgeusia, and phonophobia. The facial nerve also carries parasympathetic nerve fibers and thus Bell's palsy patients might have decreased saliva and tear production ipsilateral to their palsy. Other history questions should be asked to help rule out other etiologies of a facial nerve paralysis such as Lyme disease, Ramsay Hunt syndrome, and Melkersson-Rosenthal syndrome.

A thorough head and neck examination is performed in each patient presenting with facial paralysis. Palpation of the neck and parotid is performed to rule out a mass impinging the facial nerve. Such a mass might be palpated over the mastoid bone, the parotid gland, or in the soft tissues of the face on the affected side. A complete cranial nerve examination is performed in addition to a general neurologic examination. If, on examination, the patient with facial paralysis exhibits sparing of the upper face, a central etiology such as an infarct or tumor should be considered and a contralateral central process must be ruled out by imaging.

The House-Brackmann scale provides a unique scoring system for assessing facial weakness, allowing interphysician communication (Box 2). Though the scale has inherent weaknesses, it is the most universally acknowledged scale for the description of facial nerve function.

The diagnosis of Bell's palsy is strictly clinical and does not require any imaging or further testing in its initial presentation. Most patients show signs of significant recovery within 6 weeks. Patients with Bell's palsy that has not shown some return of facial function by 3 months should undergo imaging. A gadolinium-enhanced magnetic resonance imaging (MRI) study images the entire nerve, highlights inflammation of the facial nerve, and rules out other lesions. A dedicated temporal bone computed tomography (CT) demonstrates superior bone detail and often complements MRI. Because significant sensorineural hearing loss in the presence of facial nerve paralysis suggests the possibility of Ramsay Hunt syndrome or a skull base tumor, all facial paresis patients should undergo full audiometric testing.

Electrical testing is a controversial topic in the work-up of Bell's palsy. Although some authors rely heavily on electrical testing to stratify patients in treatment algorithms, few practitioners regularly order testing. Electrical testing, specifically electroneurography (ENog), is performed by stimulating the facial nerve as it exits the temporal bone at the stylomastoid foramen. ENog measures the peripheral muscle compound action potential response to an electrically evoked stimulus of the facial nerve on the paralyzed side as compared with the action potential on the normal side of the face. Patients should be sent for ENog between days 3 and 14 after developing a complete facial paralysis. Greater than 90% nerve degeneration by ENog combined with no voluntary motor unit potentials detectable on electromyography (EMG) leads some surgeons to recommend surgical decompression.

## Treatment

Treatment of Bell's palsy is controversial and has historically varied from expectant management, to multiple medical therapies, to intracranial surgical decompression of various portions of the fallopian canal. Studies describing the natural history of Bell's palsy established that 71% of untreated patients recover completely and an additional 13% achieve near-normal function. Empiric treatment of all patients who present with Bell's palsy has been widely adopted because there is no ideal test to predict which patients will recover completely.

### PHARMACOLOGIC THERAPY

Many studies support the use of steroids to counteract the facial nerve swelling documented during decompression surgery. A randomized, double-blind, placebo-controlled trial demonstrated a higher rate of recovery of facial function among 35 patients treated with prednisone as compared with 41 patients given placebo. Meta-analyses have also substantiated the use of steroids to improve outcomes for patients with Bell's palsy. Steroid therapy

---

### BOX 2 House-Brackmann Facial Nerve Grading System

**Grade I: Normal Function**
- Normal facial function in all areas

**Grade II: Mild Dysfunction**
- Gross
  - Slight weakness noticeable on close inspection
  - Might have very slight synkinesis
- At rest
  - Normal symmetry and tone
- Motion
  - Forehead: Moderate to good function
  - Eye: Complete closure with minimum effort
  - Mouth: Slight asymmetry

**Grade III: Moderate Dysfunction**
- Gross
  - Obvious but no disfiguring difference between the two sides
  - Noticeable but no severe synkinesis, contracture, and/or hemifacial spasm
- At rest
  - Normal symmetry and tone
- Motion
  - Forehead: Slight to moderate movement
  - Eye: Complete closure with effort
  - Mouth: Slightly weak with maximum effort

**Grade IV: Moderately Severe Dysfunction**
- Gross
  - Obvious weakness and/or disfiguring asymmetry
- At rest
  - Normal symmetry and tone
- Motion
  - Forehead: None
  - Eye: Incomplete closure
  - Mouth: Asymmetric with maximum effort

**Grade V: Severe Dysfunction**
- Gross
  - Only barely perceptible motion
- At rest
  - Asymmetry
- Motion
  - Forehead: None
  - Eye: Incomplete closure
  - Mouth: Slight movement

**Grade VI: Total Paralysis**
- No movement

---

consists of a starting dose of 1 mg/kg (or 60-80 mg) of oral prednisone[1] for 7 days and then tapering (Figure 1).

Since the establishment of the herpes simplex virus as the likely etiologic agent in the pathogenesis of Bell's palsy, many have sought to demonstrate the clinical efficacy of antiviral therapy. Although antiviral therapy for Bell's palsy makes clinical sense, no study has yet firmly established clear evidence for its benefit. Grogan and Gronseth and the Quality Standards Subcommittee of the American Academy of Neurology have recently summarized the roles of steroids, acyclovir[1] (Zovirax), and surgery for Bell's palsy in an evidence-based review. They conclude that early treatment with acyclovir in combination with prednisone is *possibly* effective to improve facial functional outcomes

---

[1]Not FDA approved for this indication.

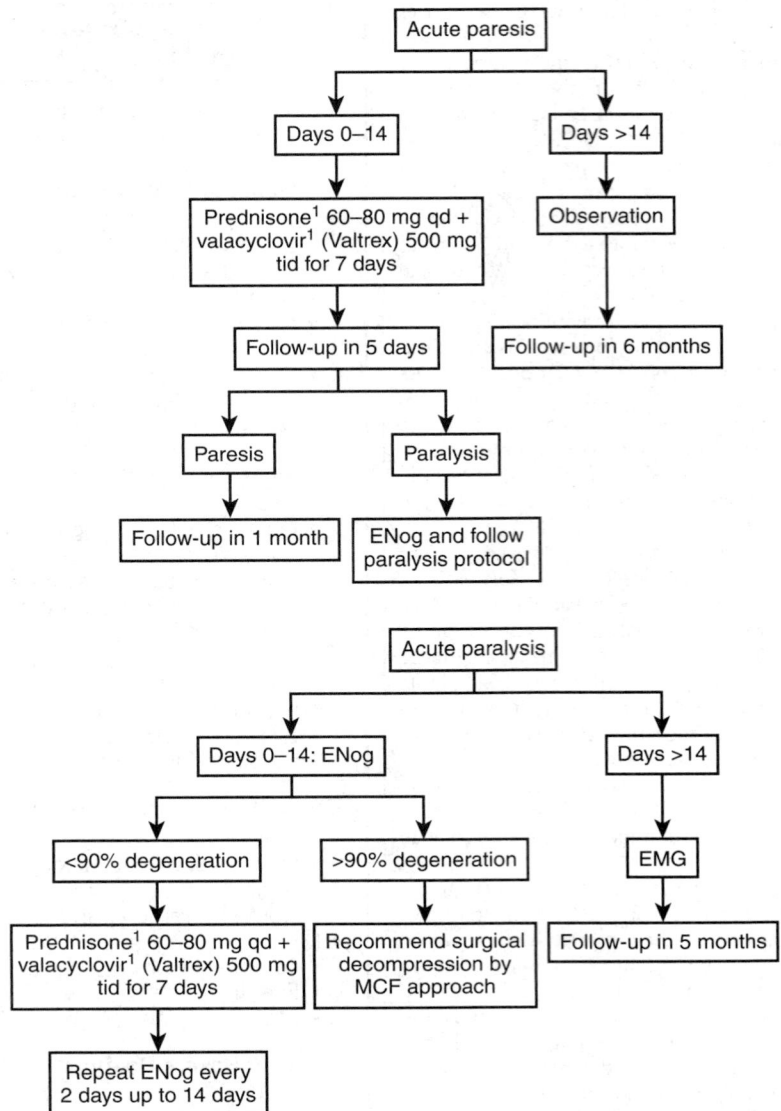

**FIGURE 1.** Algorithm for management of acute idiopathic facial palsy. *Abbreviations:* EMG = electromyography; ENog = electroneurography; MCF = middle cranial fossa.

with Level C evidence. Early treatment with oral steroids is *probably* effective with Level C evidence. A typical regimen for antiviral therapy in the treatment of Bell's palsy is to prescribe valacyclovir[1] 500 mg three times per day for 1 week.

In addition to treatments proposed to facilitate the recovery of facial motion, medical therapies must also be prescribed to prevent damage to an exposed eye. Eye care for the patient with facial paresis or paralysis consists of frequent (hourly) daytime ocular artificial tear drops (Refresh) and nighttime use of ocular ointment and a protective moisture chamber.

### SURGICAL THERAPY

Beginning in 1982, surgeons at the University of Iowa, University of Michigan, and Baylor University began prospectively enrolling patients meeting their criteria for surgical decompression. Patients with greater than 90% denervation by ENog and no voluntary motor unit potentials detectable on EMG testing were offered middle cranial fossa facial nerve decompression. In 1999, their study compared the outcomes at

## CURRENT THERAPY

- On the diagnosis of Bell's palsy, administration of prednisone[1] (start 1 mg/kg) for 1 week then tapered and valacyclovir (Valtrex)[1] (500 mg) daily for 1 week is recommended.
- Three days after the onset of acute facial paralysis, electroneurography (ENog) is performed. If before day 14 after acute facial paralysis ENog demonstrates greater than 90% nerve degeneration, referral for discussion of surgical decompression is warranted.
- Eye care for the patient with facial paresis or paralysis consists of frequent (hourly) daytime ocular artificial tear (Refresh) drops and nighttime use of ocular ointment and a protective moisture chamber.

[1]Not FDA approved for this indication.

[1]Not FDA approved for this indication.

7 months for these patients with control patients with similar electrical findings who elected steroid therapy. The results of this study demonstrated that 91% of the surgical patients achieved a good result (House-Brackmann score of I or II), whereas only 42% of patients electing medical therapy achieved a good result.

The Gantz study emphasizes the importance of the middle cranial fossa approach for decompression surgery to allow appropriate exposure of the narrowest portion of the fallopian canal. Furthermore, the study points out the importance of following ENog with EMG, which demonstrates nerve regeneration, with polyphasic potentials predicting good prognosis. No patients in the Gantz study received antiviral therapy.

One of the management difficulties in the care of Bell's palsy is that the surgical specialist rarely sees the patient within the first 2 weeks (see Figure 1). Decompression surgery for Bell's palsy is not routinely offered by all neurologic surgeons. According to the Grogan and Granseth report, there is insufficient evidence to make recommendations regarding the use of facial nerve decompression to improve facial functional outcomes.

Permanent facial nerve paralysis is a physically and emotionally debilitating condition. Fortunately, most cases of facial nerve paralysis manifest as virally induced, short-lived Bell's palsy from which greater than 80% of patients regain satisfactory facial function. Determining which patients fail to regain full facial nerve function remains the most difficult aspect in the management of these patients. All patients must be carefully managed to prevent the sequelae of exposure keratopathy. Patients who remain debilitated by facial paralysis are candidates for facial reanimation procedures.

## Acknowledgments

Thank you to Lisa McCully of the Department of Surgery at the Hershey Medical Center for preparation of our algorithm.

Thank you to Dr. Bruce Gantz of the University of Iowa for permission to modify and publish their algorithm from the Acute Facial Paralysis (Bell's Palsy) chapter in the 2006 edition of *Conn's Current Therapy*.

## REFERENCES

Adour KK, Ruboyianes JM, Von Doersten PG, et al: Bell's palsy treatment with acyclovir and prednisone compared with prednisone alone: A double-blind, randomized, controlled trial. Ann Otol Rhinol Laryngol 1996;105:371-378.

Adour KK, Wingerd J: Idiopathic facial paralysis (Bell's palsy): Factors affecting severity and outcome in 446 patients. Neurology 1974;24:1112-1116.

Austin JR, Peskind SP, Austin SG, et al: Idiopathic facial nerve paralysis: A randomized double blind controlled study of placebo versus prednisone. Laryngoscope 1993;103:1326-1333.

Gantz BJ, Rubinstein JT, Gidley P, et al: Surgical management of Bell's palsy. Laryngoscope 1999;109:1177-1188.

Gilden DH: Clinical practice: Bell's palsy. N Engl J Med 2004;351:1323-1331.

Grogan PM, Gronseth GS: Practice parameter: Steroids, acyclovir, and surgery for Bell's palsy (an evidence-based review): Report of the Quality Standards Subcommittee of the American Academy of Neurology. Neurology 2001;56:830-836.

House JW, Brackmann DE: Facial nerve grading system. Otolaryngol Head Neck Surg 1985;93:146-147.

Murakami S, Mizobuchi M, Nakashiro Y, et al: Bells palsy and herpes simplex virus: Identification of viral DNA in endoneurial fluid and muscle. Ann Intern Med 1996;124:27-30.

Peitersen E: Bell's palsy: The spontaneous course of 2,500 peripheral facial nerve palsies of different etiologies. Acta Otolaryngol Suppl (Stockh) 2002:4-30.

Schirm J, Mulkens PS: Bell's palsy and herpes simplex virus. APMIS 1997;105:815-823.

Scurry WC Jr, Isaacson JE, Fedok FG: New-onset facial paralysis and undiagnosed recurrence of cutaneous malignancy: Evaluation and management. Am J Otolaryngol 2006;27:139-142.

# Parkinsonism

Method of
*Julie Leegwater-Kim, MD, PhD,
and Cheryl Waters, MD*

The term *parkinsonism* refers to a syndrome characterized by any of a combination of six clinical features: rest tremor, bradykinesia, rigidity, postural instability, flexed posture, and freezing (motor blocks). The most common cause of parkinsonism is idiopathic Parkinson's disease (primary parkinsonism), a neurodegenerative disease first described by Dr. James Parkinson, an English physician, in 1817. The onset of Parkinson's disease is insidious, with approximately 70% of patients presenting with an asymmetrical 3- to 5-Hz resting tremor, usually of the upper extremity. Patients exhibit bradykinesia, or slowing of movement, which manifests as difficulties with fine finger movements (e.g., tying shoelaces, buttoning buttons), decreased arm swing, hypophonia, and hypomimia. Cogwheel rigidity, a ratchet-like resistance to passive movement, also develops. Over time, the disease progresses to involve the contralateral side of the body, and postural instability, flexed posture, and freezing of gait eventually develop. In addition to the motor symptoms of idiopathic Parkinson's disease (IPD), patients frequently experience autonomic symptoms, such as constipation, urinary urgency, and orthostatic hypotension. Depression occurs in approximately 50% of patients, and dementia can develop, especially in individuals with older age at onset.

The mean age at onset of IPD is 60 years. Disease prevalence and incidence increase with age, with 1% of the population older than 60 years affected. IPD affects men more than women, with a male-to-female ratio of 3:2. Onset of primary parkinsonism before age 20 years is referred to as *juvenile parkinsonism*, whereas onset between ages 20 and 40 years is known as *young-onset parkinsonism*.

## Pathogenesis

The etiology is unknown in the vast majority of cases of IPD (sporadic Parkinson's disease), but epidemiologic data and the identification of novel genes linked to heritable forms of the disease implicate a combination of environmental and genetic factors. The finding that l-methyl-4-phenyl-1,2,3,6-tetrahydropyridine (MPTP) intoxication can cause levodopa-responsive parkinsonism has suggested that similar environmental toxins play a role in the pathogenesis of IPD. Exposure to pesticides and herbicides, living in a rural environment, and drinking well water have been associated with an elevated risk of IPD. Cigarette smoking and consumption of caffeine appear to reduce the risk of developing IPD.

From 5% to 10% of cases of IPD are familial, and a number of genes have been identified in the pedigrees studied: α-synuclein (autosomal dominant), LRRK2 (autosomal dominant), parkin (autosomal recessive), DJ-1 (autosomal recessive), and PINK1 (autosomal recessive). Several of these genes encode proteins that appear to play roles in protein degradation (see following).

Pathologically, IPD is characterized by degeneration of the dopaminergic neurons in the substantia nigra. Because these neurons project to the striatum (caudate and putamen), there is a progressive loss of striatal as well as nigral dopamine. The symptoms of IPD become evident upon an approximately 60% reduction of dopamine in the substantia nigra pars compacta and an approximately 80% reduction of dopamine in the striatum. Lewy bodies (eosinophilic intracytoplasmic inclusions that contain many proteins, including α-synuclein) are seen in the surviving neurons and can be found in other structures, such as the dorsal motor nucleus of the vagus, locus ceruleus, limbic structures, and cortex.

Studies of toxic models of IPD and the genes implicated in inherited forms of IPD point to two major pathogenetic mechanisms: (1) misfolding and aggregation of proteins and (2) mitochondrial dysfunction leading to oxidative stress. Several genes identified in familial IPD (α-synuclein, parkin, and ubiquitin carboxy-terminal hydrolase L1 [UCH-L1]) encode for proteins involved in the ubiquitin-proteosome system, which is responsible for the normal degradation and clearance of proteins in eukaryotic cells. Mutations in these genes appear to be linked to mishandling and accumulation of proteins, which in turn lead to cell death. The potential role of mitochondrial dysfunction and subsequent oxidative stress in the pathogenesis of IPD was first suggested by the discovery that administration of MPTP, a mitochondrial electron transport chain inhibitor, to rodents and primates, produced a phenotype similar to that seen in IPD. Inhibition produces toxic products, including harmful reactive oxygen species that can cause cellular damage by reacting with proteins, lipids, and nucleic acids. It is important to recognize that these theories are not mutually exclusive, and they could be involved sequentially in causing cell death. For example, oxidative stress to α-synuclein can enhance its ability to misfold and aggregate, and the aggregates eventually accumulate because of proteosomal dysfunction.

## Differential Diagnosis

Because no diagnostic laboratory test for IPD is available, the diagnosis remains a clinical one. Distinguishing IPD from other causes of parkinsonism is paramount because prognosis and treatment options vary according to disease. The most helpful clinical signs supporting a diagnosis of IPD are asymmetry of presentation, presence of resting tremor, absence of atypical clinical features (i.e., cerebellar dysfunction, pyramidal signs), and clear improvement with carbidopa/levodopa (Sinemet) therapy. A number of neurologic diseases can often mimic IPD and therefore deserve mention (Table 1).

Drug-induced parkinsonism (DIP) can occur with exposure to dopamine receptor-blocking agents, such as antipsychotic medications (e.g., haloperidol [Haldol]) and antiemetic agents (e.g., metoclopramide [Reglan]). Because DIP can be reversed with discontinuation of the offending drug, it is important to carefully review the patient's current medications when investigating possible causes of parkinsonism. When DIP is suspected, the dopamine receptor-blocking agent should be stopped, if possible, or substituted with an atypical neuroleptic with a low incidence of extrapyramidal side effects (e.g., quetiapine [Seroquel]). The symptoms of DIP usually resolve within weeks to months after discontinuation of the drug.

Essential tremor (ET) is a disorder characterized by a 4- to 12-Hz tremor usually beginning in the arms. Unlike Parkinson's disease, the tremor of ET is a kinetic tremor (brought on by an action such as finger-to-nose testing). There is often a postural tremor as well, which is usually bilateral at onset. Common presenting complaints include

### TABLE 1   Classification of Parkinsonism

**Primary Parkinsonism (Idiopathic Parkinson's Disease)**
- Sporadic
- Familial

**Secondary Parkinsonism**
- Drug-induced (i.e., dopamine receptor–blocking agents)
- Vascular
- Normal pressure hydrocephalus
- Toxin-induced (i.e., manganese)
- Infectious
- Postencephalitic
- Structural lesion (i.e., tumor)

**Parkinson-Plus Syndromes/Atypical Parkinsonism**
- Progressive supranuclear palsy
- Multiple system atrophy
- Corticobasal ganglionic degeneration
- Dementia with Lewy bodies

**Heredodegenerative Disorders**
- Frontotemporal dementia
- Wilson's disease
- Huntington's disease

## CURRENT DIAGNOSIS

- *Parkinsonism* refers to a syndrome characterized by any of a combination of six clinical features: resting tremor, bradykinesia, rigidity, postural instability, flexed posture, and freezing (motor blocks).
- Idiopathic Parkinson's disease (IPD) is the most common cause of parkinsonism.
- The vast majority of cases of IPD are sporadic. The etiology of IPD is hypothesized to involve a complex interaction between environmental and genetic factors.
- The pathologic hallmarks of IPD are loss of dopaminergic neurons in the substantia nigra pars compacta and the presence of Lewy bodies (intracytoplasmic eosinophilic inclusions).
- Asymmetry of presentation, presence of resting tremor, absence of atypical signs (i.e., ataxia, pyramidal signs), and clear response to carbidopa/levodopa (Sinemet) are important features in distinguishing IPD from other forms of parkinsonism.

difficulty drinking from a cup or spoon or spilling while pouring. The handwriting of patients with ET is large and tremulous, not micrographic. In 30% to 50% of patients, tremor may spread to involve the neck (head); in rare cases there is isolated head tremor. A family history of tremor in an autosomal dominant pattern is common. Another distinguishing feature of ET is that the tremor can often be temporarily improved by alcohol. Bradykinesia, rigidity, and loss of postural reflexes are absent.

The Parkinson-plus syndromes—progressive supranuclear palsy, multiple system atrophy, corticobasal ganglionic degeneration, and dementia with Lewy body disease—are rare neurodegenerative diseases that are often confused with IPD, especially in their early stages. The presence of atypical clinical features and the lack of response to levodopa therapy are key in helping to distinguish between these diseases and IPD. Progressive supranuclear palsy typically presents with postural instability and recurrent falls. A supranuclear gaze palsy, usually affecting downgaze first, develops, and truncal rigidity with nuchal extensor rigidity predominates. Patients often have an "astonished" facial expression and deepened nasolabial folds. Multiple system atrophy is a sporadically occurring neurodegenerative disease characterized by a variable combination of parkinsonism, cerebellar dysfunction, pyramidal signs, and autonomic dysfunction. Unlike IPD, autonomic dysfunction occurs early in the clinical course and tends to be severe. Stridor can develop, and some patients exhibit the "cold hands sign": dusky violaceous fingers with delayed capillary refill after blanching. Corticobasal ganglionic degeneration typically presents asymmetrically with gradual development of stiffness, jerking, and cortical sensory loss in a limb, usually the arm. Cortical reflex myoclonus and apraxia develop in the affected limb. Over time, other limbs become involved. Dementia with Lewy body disease (DLBD) is characterized by parkinsonism and dementia. Although dementia can also be seen in IPD, the dementia of DLBD occurs early on in the disease course and is associated with prominent hallucinations and delusions and fluctuations in mental status.

Normal pressure hydrocephalus and vascular parkinsonism typically present with predominantly lower body parkinsonism. Normal pressure hydrocephalus is classically defined by a clinical triad of gait disturbance, urinary incontinence, and dementia, although many cases can present with isolated gait disturbance. The gait is usually wide based and shuffling, with features of gait apraxia and prominent retropulsion. Gait dysfunction can improve after a large-volume lumbar puncture or lumbar drain trial. Vascular parkinsonism results from multiple lacunar infarcts of the basal ganglia. Patients often have a wide-based apraxic gait with frequent freezing. Neither normal pressure hydrocephalus nor vascular parkinsonism demonstrates a significant clinical response to levodopa therapy. When these diseases are suspected, brain magnetic resonance imaging (MRI) should be obtained as part of the workup.

Other rarer causes of parkinsonism should be considered if indicated by history. Toxin exposure (i.e., carbon monoxide poisoning, manganese intoxication), head trauma, structural brain lesions, and infection can produce parkinsonism. Brain imaging is important in ruling out these etiologies.

The differential diagnosis of parkinsonism in pediatric patients and young adults should include heredodegenerative and metabolic diseases. Wilson's disease, an autosomal recessive disorder characterized by abnormal copper metabolism, should be considered in all young-onset cases of parkinsonism because the disease is treatable. Dysarthria, dystonia, and ataxia are common accompanying symptoms. Ophthalmologic examination with slit lamp to rule out Kayser-Fleischer rings (present in 100% of Wilson's disease patients with neurologic symptoms), serum ceruloplasmin, and 24-hour urine copper should be obtained to rule out this disorder. Brain MRI can reveal evidence of copper deposition within the basal ganglia. Pantothenate kinase-associated neurodegeneration (formerly called Hallervorden-Spatz disease), a genetic disorder involving a disturbance of iron metabolism, can present with parkinsonism. Dystonia is also a prominent feature. Brain MRI should be obtained to look for evidence of iron deposition in the basal ganglia. Genetic testing for PANK2, a gene implicated in pantothenate kinase-associated neurodegeneration, is now available. Juvenile Huntington's disease, unlike the adult-onset form, often presents with parkinsonism and should be considered in any patient with a family history suggestive of this disorder. Genetic testing is diagnostic.

# Treatment

Treatment of IPD includes both nonpharmacologic and pharmacologic therapies (Table 2). A regular exercise regimen is important for both medical and psychologic well-being, and physical therapy is helpful in maintaining range of motion and flexibility and in gait and balance training. Speech therapy can improve dysarthria and hypophonia. Psychologic support to patients and families is critical and support groups are important resources. Pharmacologic treatment of IPD comprises neuroprotective strategies and symptomatic treatment of both motor and nonmotor symptoms.

## NEUROPROTECTION

To date, no drug has been categorically proven to retard the progression of or reverse the course of IPD. Selegiline (Eldepryl),[1] a monoamine oxidase type B inhibitor, and vitamin E were evaluated in the Deprenyl and Tocopherol Antioxidative Therapy of Parkinsonism (DATATOP) study, a placebo-controlled trial that studied the potential neuroprotective effects of each drug separately and in combination in patients with early IPD. Vitamin E conferred no neuroprotective benefit in IPD. Selegiline delayed the onset of disability and levodopa therapy, but this finding was confounded by the fact that selegiline has mild symptomatic effects. Rasagiline (Azilect) was recently approved as monotherapy and adjunctive treatment in PD. A one-year extension of the TEMPO trial (Rasagiline Mesylate TVP-1012) as Early Monotherapy in PD Outpatients) employed a randomized delayed start design to detemine if teatment with rasagiline had a long-term impact on PD beyond its short-term symptomatic effects. The change in UPDRS from baseline to final visit for the difference between rasagiline and placebo was 2.29 UPDRS points. Additional studies will be needed to clarify the long-term effects and mechanism of action of rasagiline. Coenzyme Q10[1,*] was studied in a small, double-blind, placebo-controlled trial, which showed a trend toward slowed symptom progression in early IPD at a dose of 1200 mg/day. However, larger and longer-term studies are needed to confirm this finding.

---

[1]Not FDA approved for this indication.
*Available as a dietary supplement.

## TABLE 2  Treatment Strategies in Idiopathic Parkinson's Disease

### Nonpharmacologic
- Regular exercise
- Physical therapy
- Speech therapy
- Psychosocial support
- Occupational therapy

### Pharmacologic
#### Motor symptoms
- Carbidopa/levodopa (Sinemet)
- Dopamine agonists
- Anticholinergics
- Selegiline (Eldepryl)
- Amantadine (Symmetrel)
- Rasagiline (Azilect)

#### Motor fluctuations
- Wearing-off
  - More frequent carbidopa/levodopa (Sinemet) dosing
  - Extended-release carbidopa/levodopa (Sinemet CR)
  - Dopamine agonist
  - Catechol-O-methyltransferase inhibitor
  - Selegiline (Eldepryl), rasagiline*
  - Rasagiline
- On–off phenomena
  - Liquefied carbidopa/levodopa (Sinemet)
  - Intraduodenal infusion of levodopa[1]
  - Apomorphine (Apokyn)
- Dyskinesias
  - Reduce carbidopa/levodopa (Sinemet) dose
  - Amantadine (Symmetrel)
  - Clozapine (Clozaril)[1]

#### Nonmotor symptoms
- Orthostatic hypotension
  - Increase salt and fluid intake
  - Midodrine (ProAmatine)
  - Fludrocortisone (Florinef)[1]
- Urinary urgency/frequency
  - Oxybutynin (Ditropan)
- Constipation
  - High-fiber diet
  - Stool softeners, laxatives
- Depression
  - Selective serotonin reuptake inhibitor antidepressants
  - Tricyclic antidepressants
  - Serotonin-norepinephrine reuptake inhibitors
  - Bupropion (Wellbutrin)
- Psychosis
  - Quetiapine (Seroquel), clozapine (Clozaril)[1]
- Dementia
  - Cholinesterase inhibitors

---

[1]Not FDA approved for this indication.
*Investigational drug in the United States.

## SYMPTOMATIC TREATMENT OF MOTOR SYMPTOMS

Pharmacologic treatment of IPD should be initiated when motor symptoms are sufficiently bothersome or cause functional disability. In general, tremor, bradykinesia, and rigidity are responsive to treatments, whereas postural instability, flexed posture, and freezing of gait are more intractable to treatment. The two mainstays of therapy are carbidopa/levodopa (Sinemet) and the dopamine agonist (DA) drugs, as these medications have the greatest symptomatic benefit. Selegiline (Eldepryl) monotherapy[1] has mild symptomatic benefit. It can be started as a 5-mg dose at breakfast for one week and thereafter

---

[1]Not FDA approved for this indication.

## CURRENT THERAPY

- Treatment of idiopathic Parkinson's disease (IPD) consists of improving motor symptoms and treating nonmotor symptoms, such as autonomic dysfunction, depression, psychosis, dementia, and sleep disturbance.
- Pharmacologic therapy for early IPD should begin when motor symptoms become disabling or sufficiently bothersome.
- Treatment of motor symptoms in early IPD usually begins with either carbidopa/levodopa (Sinemet) or dopamine agonist (e.g., pramipexole [Mirapex]) monotherapy because these drugs provide the greatest symptomatic benefit. In general, dopamine agonist monotherapy is preferred in younger patients, whereas carbidopa/levodopa (Sinemet) monotherapy is preferred in elderly patients (>70 years).
- As IPD progresses, motor complications develop, including wearing-off, on–off phenomena, and dyskinesias. A variety of approaches can be used to smooth out motor fluctuations. Wearing-off can be treated with more frequent levodopa dosing, use of extended-release carbidopa/levodopa (Sinemet CR), addition of a catechol-O-methyltransferase inhibitor, or addition of a dopamine agonist. On–off phenomena can be treated with liquefied carbidopa/levodopa (Sinemet). Dyskinesias can be reduced by lowering the levodopa dose or by adding amantadine (Symmetrel) or clozapine (Clozaril).[1]
- Surgical therapy for IPD includes deep brain stimulation and ablative techniques. Appropriate selection of patients for these procedures is crucial. Clinical features that have been associated with successful outcomes include clinically definite IPD, good clinical response to levodopa, persistent, disabling medically intractable motor fluctuations, intact cognitive status, and younger age.

[1]Not FDA approved for this indication.

increased to two 5-mg doses taken in the morning and at noon. Rasagiline (Azilect) was recently approved for initial monotherapy in early IPD. Optimal therapeutic dose is 0.5 to 1.0 mg daily. Patients taking this medication should be instructed to avoid tyramine-rich foods to prevent a potentially dangerous increase in blood pressure. Amantadine (Symmetrel), an N-methyl-D-aspartate (NMDA) antagonist, provides modest symptom relief in approximately two-thirds of patients with early IPD. Amantadine (Symmetrel) can be given at a dose of 100 mg up to four times per day. Selegiline (Eldepryl) monotherapy[1] has mild symptomatic benefit. Amantadine (Symmetrel), an N-methyl-D-aspartate (NMDA) antagonist, provides modest symptom relief in approximately two thirds of patients with early IPD. Amantadine (Symmetrel) can be given at a dose of 100 mg up to four times per day. Anticholinergic drugs such as trihexyphenidyl (Artane) can be especially effective for tremor but should be used with caution in the elderly because of the tendency of anticholinergic drugs to cause confusion and cognitive disturbance. Trihexyphenidyl (Artane) can be started at 2 mg/day and increased to 2 to 5 mg three times per day.

The choice of whether to start carbidopa/levodopa (Sinemet) or a DA in patients with early IPD is controversial. Important consideration should be given to the patient's age, cognitive status, lifestyle, and degree of impairment. Because DAs are less likely to induce dyskinesia and have good symptomatic efficacy in mild disease, DA monotherapy is preferred in younger patients with early IPD, as this population is more prone to the development of levodopa-induced motor fluctuations and dyskinesias. In addition, the side effects of DAs (hallucinations, somnolence) are usually better tolerated by younger patients. Conversely, levodopa monotherapy is the preferred first-line treatment in elderly patients (older than 70 years).

DAs directly stimulate dopamine receptors and do not require conversion to active metabolites. The available DAs—pramipexole (Mirapex), ropinirole (Requip), pergolide (Permax), cabergoline (Dostinex),* bromocriptine (Parlodel),* rotigotine (Neupro), and apomorphine (Apokyn)—all activate the D2 receptors. Bromocriptine, pergolide, and cabergoline are ergot derivatives and carry the rare but serious risk of retroperitoneal, pulmonary, and cardiac valve fibrosis. A yearly transthoracic echocardiogram is advised to monitor for valvular disease. Among the nonergot DAs, pramipexole and ropinirole are used most commonly. Pramipexole (Mirapex) is started at 0.125 mg three times per day and increased slowly over 4 to 5 weeks to 3 mg/day. Pramipexole dose can be increased to a maximum of 6 mg/day and ropinirole may be titrated to a maximum dose of 24 mg/day. Ropinirole (Requip) is started at 0.25 mg three times per day and is usually titrated to 12 mg/day over a 7-week period. Cabergoline (Dostinex) has the longest half-life of the DAs; it is used in Europe but is not approved for IPD in the United States. Apomorphine (Apokyn), a potent D1/D2 agonist, is not available in oral form and must be injected. Recently, it has been developed as a "rescue" therapy in IPD patients with "off" periods. Rotigotine (Neupro), a non-ergot DA, was recently approved as the first transdermally delivered DA in PD. The once-daily patch is available in three strengths: 2 mg/24 hr, 4 mg/24 hr, and 6 mg/24 hr.

DAs have similar side-effect profiles, including nausea, sleepiness, orthostatic hypotension, leg edema, hallucinations, and obsessive-compulsive behaviors. Both pramipexole (Mirapex) and ropinirole (Requip) carry the rare risk of sleep attacks. Obsessive-compulsive behaviors include compulsive eating, spending, hypersexuality, hoarding, and gambling. Because these behaviors are not often volunteered by the patient and can be harmful to both the patient and his or her family, the physician should always ask the patient and the caregiver or spouse about these potential side effects. The side-effect spectrum of DAs varies among patients, so if one DA is not tolerated, another should be tried.

Carbidopa/levodopa (Sinemet) remains the most potent drug used for treatment of the symptoms of IPD. Levodopa, the precursor of dopamine, is administered with carbidopa, a peripheral decarboxylase inhibitor that inhibits the conversion of levodopa to dopamine. Side effects of carbidopa/levodopa (Sinemet) include nausea, vomiting, orthostasis, somnolence, and hallucinations. Long-term levodopa use has been linked to the development of motor fluctuations and dyskinesias. Carbidopa/levodopa (Sinemet) is available in standard-release (Sinemet 10/100, 25/100, 25/250) and extended-release forms (Sinemet CR 25/100, 50/200) as well as a disintegrating tablet form (Parcopa 10/100, 25/100, 25/250). The extended-release form provides a longer plasma half-life and lower peak plasma levels by slowly releasing the drug from a matrix. Standard-release carbidopa/levodopa (Sinemet) is started at half to one tablet 25/100 three times daily and increased gradually to a dose that gives optimal symptomatic benefit. Alternatively, extended-release carbidopa/levodopa (Sinemet CR) can be started at 25/100 three times daily and titrated to benefit. Despite the longer half-life, extended-release carbidopa/levodopa (Sinemet CR) has not been shown to delay the development of levodopa-induced motor complications. In elderly patients, extended-release carbidopa/levodopa (Sinemet CR) may be preferred because the lower rate of absorption and lower peak plasma level decrease the likelihood of peak-dose confusion or somnolence. Levodopa-associated nausea and vomiting can often be relieved by administration of carbidopa/levodopa (Sinemet) with meals. If this is unsuccessful, addition of carbidopa (Lodosyn) can be helpful. Carbidopa (Lodosyn) is

[1]Not FDA approved for this indication.

*Not available in this form.

available in 25-mg tablets and can be given with each carbidopa/levodopa (Sinemet) dose. At doses of 150 mg/day, carbidopa (Lodosyn) may enter the brain and block central conversion of levodopa to dopamine, so care should be taken not to exceed this value. Domperidone (Motilium),[2] a peripheral dopamine antagonist, can also be given with carbidopa/levodopa (Sinemet) to relieve nausea and vomiting. Hallucinations and delusions can be troublesome side effects of both carbidopa/levodopa (Sinemet) and the DAs, and they can be effectively treated with the atypical neuroleptics quetiapine (Seroquel)[1] and clozapine (Clozaril).[1]

The development of motor fluctuations in IPD is well known, and management of these complications can be challenging. Approximately 25% to 50% of patients taking levodopa will develop motor fluctuations after 5 years of therapy, and this risk increases substantially with younger age of onset. Early on, motor complications occur in a predictable pattern. The earliest symptom is end-of-dose "wearing-off," in which the same dose of levodopa lasts for a shorter period, and the antiparkinson effect wears off before the next dose is taken. Patients become slower, stiffer, and more tremulous. In addition, they may have nonmotor wearing-off symptoms, including cognitive changes, depression, and autonomic and sensory disturbances. Over time, patients may develop "on–off" phenomena, consisting of sudden, unpredictable shifts between mobility and immobility. Dyskinesias are involuntary movements that can occur after years of levodopa therapy. Peak-dose dyskinesia, the most common type, consists of choreiform movements of the head, trunk, and limbs. Diphasic dyskinesias occur in 15% to 20% of patients receiving chronic levodopa therapy and consist of dyskinetic movements that occur at the beginning and end of each dose.

A number of different strategies reduce motor fluctuations and "smooth out" the patient's clinical course. Wearing-off can be treated in a variety of ways. Perhaps the simplest approach is to give levodopa more frequently. Another option is to substitute extended-release carbidopa/levodopa (Sinemet CR) for regular carbidopa/levodopa (Sinemet). The major disadvantage to this approach is that absorption of the extended-release form is often unpredictable. Catechol-O-methyltransferase (COMT) inhibitors function to lengthen the half-life of levodopa by inhibiting its catabolism. The available COMT inhibitors are entacapone (Comtan) and tolcapone (Tasmar). Tolcapone (Tasmar) is the more potent inhibitor, but rare cases of acute hepatotoxicity have limited its use. Liver function tests must be monitored closely, every 2 to 4 weeks in the first year of use. Explosive diarrhea has been associated with tolcapone (Tasmar). Entacapone (Comtan) can cause a benign orange discoloration of the urine. Tolcapone (Tasmar) can be administered 100 to 200 mg three times per day. Entacapone (Comtan) is available in 200-mg tablets and can be given up to eight times per day. Recently, a combination tablet of carbidopa/levodopa/entacapone (Stalevo) was approved and is available in 12.5/50/200 (Stalevo 50), 25/100/200 mg (Stalevo 100), and 37.5/150/200 mg (Stalevo 150). DAs can also be added to smooth out motor complications. They should be used with caution in the elderly. Because DAs enhance the effects of levodopa, levodopa doses may need to be decreased gradually with titration of DA. Rasagiline has been shown to reduce levodopa-induced motor complications as well. Two recent phase III trials (Lasting Effect in Adjunct Therapy with Rasagiline Given Once Daily [LARGO] and Parkinson's Rasagiline: Efficacy and Safety in the Treatment of "Off" [PRESTO]) have found that adjunctive rasagiline therapy in patients with levodopa-induced motor fluctuations reduced the off state by at least 1 hour per day. In a recent double-blind randomized trial of Zydis selegiline,[‡] a dissolvable form of selegiline that undergoes pregastric absorption, patients taking the drug were found to have significant reduction in daily off time when compared with placebo. Currently, the adenosine $A_{2A}$ receptor antagonist istradefylline[*] (KW-6002) is being studied as a potential agent in reducing wearing-off periods.

Treatment of on–off phenomena and "yo-yoing" (a combination of fluctuations and dyskinesias) can be challenging and relies on smooth activation of dopamine receptors throughout the day. One approach involves use of liquefied carbidopa/levodopa (Sinemet). The patient makes a solution of carbidopa/levodopa (Sinemet) and takes small sips of the solution throughout the day. carbidopa/levodopa (Sinemet) is not stable at room temperature unless it is in an acidified solution. Patients can dissolve tablets in ascorbic acid solution or dietetic soda. Liquefied carbidopa/levodopa (Sinemet) should be prepared fresh daily in a 1 mg/1 mL concentration (four tablets of 25/250 carbidopa/levodopa in 1 L of liquid). A more invasive strategy for treating on–off phenomena involves infusion of levodopa through an intraduodenal pump.[1]

Sudden off periods and dose failures can be treated with liquefied carbidopa/levodopa (Sinemet) or subcutaneous apomorphine (Apokyn). Administration of apomorphine (Apokyn) requires treatment with an antiemetic for 3 days before injection. Onset of action is relatively rapid (<20 minutes) and lasts up to 40 minutes. Side effects include hypotension, chest discomfort, dyskinesias, and yawning.

Effective therapies for dyskinesias include reduction of the levodopa dose and addition of amantadine or clozapine. Amantadine (Symmetrel) has been shown to reduce dyskinesias in patients with advanced IPD by 60% when compared with placebo. Its antidyskinetic effect has been attributed to inhibition of the NMDA receptor. Clozapine (Clozaril)[1] has also been shown to suppress levodopa-induced dyskinesias. In a recent double-blind, placebo-controlled trial of 50 patients, there was a significant reduction in "on" levodopa-induced dyskinesias at a mean dosage of 39.4 mg/day. The main drawback to clozapine (Clozaril) administration is the 1% to 2% risk of agranulocytosis, which warrants frequent blood monitoring.

## SYMPTOMATIC TREATMENT OF NONMOTOR SYMPTOMS

In addition to motor symptoms, patients with IPD experience nonmotor complications, such as autonomic disturbances, sleep disorders, depression, psychosis, and dementia. Autonomic symptoms include orthostatic hypotension, urinary frequency and urgency, constipation, and sexual dysfunction. Orthostatic hypotension can occur as a result of IPD itself or as a complication of levodopa and DA therapies. Increased salt and fluid intake should be tried first. If these conservative measures are unsuccessful, medications such as fludrocortisone (Florinef)[1] 0.1 to 0.5 mg/day or midodrine (ProAmatine) 2.5 to 10 mg three times per day can be tried. Urinary symptoms are usually a result of detrusor hyperreflexia and can be helped by a peripheral anticholinergic medication such as oxybutynin (Ditropan) 5 to 10 mg/day. Low-dose amitriptyline (Elavil) 25 mg at bedtime can also be considered in a patient with concomitant depression or insomnia.[1] Both drugs should be avoided in the elderly population because anticholinergic effects can lead to cognitive disturbance. Constipation is a frequent complaint in patients with IPD. Regular exercise and adequate fluid and fiber intake should be encouraged. Stool softeners, such as docusate sodium (Colace) 100 mg two to three times per day and polyethylene glycol (MiraLax) 17 g per day, are also effective. Sexual dysfunction is not uncommon in patients with IPD, but its occurrence is frequently not volunteered by the patient. Oral medications, such as sildenafil (Viagra), can be helpful but may exacerbate hypotension.

Sleep difficulties in patients with IPD are common and can be due to rapid eye movement (REM) sleep behavior disorder, periodic leg movements of sleep, restless legs syndrome, motor symptoms (e.g., difficulty turning in bed), and daytime somnolence. A nighttime dose of clonazepam (Klonopin)[1] 0.5 mg is helpful in treating REM behavior disorder. Propoxyphene (Darvon)[1] and ropinirole (Requip) have been effective in treating restless legs syndrome. A dose of extended-release carbidopa/levodopa (Sinemet CR) 25/100 or 50/200 can help relieve nighttime motor symptoms.

---

[1]Not FDA approved for this indication.
[2]Not available in the United States.
[*]Not available in this form.

---

[1]Not FDA approved for this indication.

Daytime somnolence is a common complaint and can be a result of IPD itself or of certain medications. The activating agent modafinil (Provigil)[1] can be useful in combating daytime sleepiness. As mentioned previously, sleep attacks have been reported as a rare side effect of pramipexole (Mirapex) and ropinirole (Requip). If sleep attacks occur, driving should be curtailed, and the medication should be changed.

Depression is common in individuals with IPD, affecting nearly half of all patients. The causes are likely twofold: reactive depression and depression secondary to disease pathology. The selective serotonin reuptake inhibitors (SSRIs) serotonin-norepinephrine reuptake inhibitors (SNRIs), and bupropion (Wellbutrin) can be tried. Tricyclic antidepressants are less commonly used because their anticholinergic and antiadrenergic effects can cause confusion and hypotension, respectively. In the patient refractory to medication treatment, electro-convulsive shock therapy may be necessary.

Psychosis in IPD is usually due to antiparkinsonian medications, but intercurrent illness should always be considered as a cause. DAs, carbidopa/levodopa (Sinemet), anticholinergic drugs, and amantadine (Symmetrel) can all cause hallucinations. Management of psychosis should include discontinuing anticholinergic drugs, amantadine (Symmetrel), and DAs and using the lowest effective levodopa dose possible. If an antipsychotic medication is needed, the atypical neuroleptic medications quetiapine (Seroquel)[1] or clozapine (Clozaril)[1] should be started, as these agents have a low risk of exacerbating parkinsonism. Because clozapine (Clozaril) requires regular blood monitoring to prevent the serious risk of agranulocytosis, quetiapine (Seroquel) is the antipsychotic prescribed by most practitioners. Quetiapine (Seroquel) is started at 12.5 to 25 mg and should be given at night because of its potential to cause drowsiness. The dose can be titrated until symptomatic benefit is achieved. If quetiapine (Seroquel) is ineffective or cannot be tolerated, clozapine (Clozaril) should be tried next, starting with 12.5 mg at bedtime and titrating to effect. Baseline white blood cell (WBC) and differential counts must be obtained before clozapine (Clozaril) treatment. During treatment, WBC counts should be monitored every week for the first 6 months, every 2 weeks for the next 6 months, and monthly thereafter. Recent studies comparing the atypical neuroleptics and placebo in the treatment of elderly demented patients with behavioral disorders found a 1.6- to 1.7-fold increase in mortality in patients taking the atypical antipsychotics. Patients should be warned about this possible side effect, and both quetiapine (Seroquel) and clozapine (Clozaril) should be used at the minimum effective dose.

Dementia is encountered frequently in patients with IPD, with prevalence of approximately 40%. Risk factors include advanced age, longer duration of disease, and older age at onset of disease. Recent data suggest that cholinesterase inhibitors can improve cognitive function in IPD patients with dementia without significantly worsening IPD symptoms. The available cholinesterase inhibitors are donepezil (Aricept),[1] rivastigmine (Exelon),[1] and galantamine (Razadyne).[1] The main side effects (nausea, vomiting, and diarrhea) are related to the cholinergic action of these agents. Memantine (Namenda),[1] an NMDA receptor antagonist, has recently been approved for moderate to severe Alzheimer's dementia. A double-blind, placebo-controlled trial is currently under way to evaluate the efficacy of memantine (Namenda) in the treatment of cognitive impairment in Parkinson's disease patients with dementia.

## SURGICAL THERAPY

Advances in the understanding of both the pathophysiology of IPD and the circuitry of the basal ganglia have led to the development of surgical treatments of IPD. Recent surgical approaches have included ablative techniques and deep brain stimulation (DBS). Ablative procedures have gradually been replaced by DBS, as the latter is a reversible procedure and can be performed bilaterally. Moreover, the stimulation parameters are adjustable. In DBS, high-frequency stimulation is delivered to a precise target in the basal ganglia, effectively mimicking a lesion.

The exact mechanism by which DBS exerts its effects is unclear. Thalamic DBS, like thalamotomy, has been shown to be very effective in the relief of tremor, with no significant benefit with regard to other symptoms of IPD. The main side effect of stimulation of the ventral intermediate nucleus of the thalamus is dysarthria, which occurs in 20% of patients. DBS of the internal globus pallidus improves all of the cardinal motor symptoms of IPD and suppresses levodopa-induced dyskinesia. Complications associated with DBS of the internal globus pallidus include rare reports of mood disorder and cognitive decline. DBS of the subthalamic nucleus, like stimulation of the internal globus pallidus, is effective in alleviating all the motor symptoms of IPD. Moreover, stimulation of the subthalamic nucleus has been associated with reduced levodopa requirements after surgery. However, stimulation of the subthalamic nucleus has been associated with more reports of adverse effects on mood and cognition. Although no prospective randomized double-blind trials have compared stimulation of the internal globus pallidus with stimulation of the subthalamic nucleus, stimulation of the subthalamic nucleus has become the preferred choice because it appears to be the best target for controlling bradykinesia and allows for subsequent reduction of the levodopa dosage.

The efficacy of surgical therapy for Parkinson's disease is critically dependent on the appropriate selection of patients. Patients with a clear response to levodopa therapy and clinically definite IPD have better outcomes with surgical therapy. Patients with medically intractable motor fluctuations, drug-induced dyskinesias, and on–off phenomena may have good response to surgery. The cognitive status of all patients should be assessed by neuropsychologic testing prior to surgery, because patients with significant cognitive impairment tend to have worse outcomes. Any premorbid psychiatric disturbances (depression, anxiety) should be adequately treated before surgery. In general, younger patients tend to do better after surgery because of fewer comorbid illnesses, but there is no absolute age cutoff. Finally, because DBS requires close clinical follow-up for parameter adjustment, a history of good patient compliance and adequate family support are critical.

## REFERENCES

Fahn S: Description of Parkinson's disease as a clinical syndrome. Ann NY Acad Sci 2003;991:1-14.
Jankovic JJ, Tolosa E (eds): Parkinson's Disease and Movement Disorders, 5th ed. Philadelphia, Lippincott, Williams & Wilkins, 2006.
Pahwa R, Lyons KE, Koller WC (eds): Handbook of Parkinson's disease, 4th ed. New York, Marcel Dekker, 2006.
Walter BL, Vitek J: Surgical treatment for Parkinson's disease. Lancet Neurol 2004;3:719-728.
Waters CH: Diagnosis and Management of Parkinson's Disease. New York, Professional Communications, 2005.

# Peripheral Neuropathies

Method of
*Kerrie Schoffer, MD, FRCPC*

Disorders of the peripheral nerve system (PNS) include pathology affecting the spinal cord roots (radiculopathies), the dorsal root ganglia (neuronopathies), the brachial, lumbar, and sacral plexuses (plexopathies), and the terminal nerve (mononeuropathies) or nerves (polyneuropathies). They are among the most common and challenging problems in medical practice, with literally hundreds of conceivable causes. An organized diagnostic approach consists of first categorizing the neuropathy based on clinical and electrophysiologic assessments and then performing a tailored diagnostic evaluation. However astute the diagnostician, the cause of a neuropathy might not found in up to 20% of patients.

[1]Not FDA approved for this indication.

# Anatomy

Four types of fibers are found in the PNS: motor, large fiber sensory, small fiber sensory, and autonomic. Motor fibers extend peripherally to the neuromuscular junction of their respective muscles and have their cell bodies in motor neurons located in the spinal cord. Conversely, sensory fibers receive information from peripheral sensory receptors and transfer this to cell bodies in the dorsal root ganglia, located near, but outside, the spinal cord. Large, myelinated sensory fibers supply information regarding position and vibration. Small myelinated axons, composed of autonomic and sensory fibers, are responsible for light touch, pain, temperature, and parasympathetic and sympathetic information.

Damage can occur to the cell bodies (neuronopathy), nerve fibers (axonopathy), or to the surrounding myelin sheath (myelinopathy). Myelinopathies principally affect only the coating around the nerve, and an axonopathy results in degeneration of both the axon and myelin. The most distal segments usually degenerate first, in a process termed *Wallerian degeneration*, resulting in a dying-back neuropathy and a stocking and glove clinical pattern. Neuronopathies affect either the motor neuron or dorsal root ganglion and result in degeneration of both peripheral and central processes.

## Five-Step Approach to Neuropathies

When evaluating neuropathy, the differential diagnosis can be limited by asking five key questions:

- What is the *fiber type* involved (motor, large sensory, small sensory, autonomic, combination)?
- What is the *pattern of distribution* (distal or proximal, symmetric or asymmetric)?
- What is the *temporal course* (acute, chronic, progressive, stepwise, relapsing remitting)?
- Are there any *key features* pointing to a specific etiology?
- What is the *pathology* (axonal, demyelinating)?

### FIBER TYPE

The PNS produces symptomatology in only two ways: negative symptoms (weakness, numbness), which reflects loss of nerve signaling; or positive symptoms (tingling, burning) due to inappropriate spontaneous nerve activity. Box 1 lists symptoms and signs that suggest localization to the peripheral nerves and point specifically to motor, sensory, or autonomic involvement. When inquiring about symptoms, it is important to ask the patient to be as specific as possible. Many patients simply describe an area as numb when, in fact, they are experiencing tingling or even weakness.

A detailed motor examination should include inspection for atrophy, particularly in the distal extensor digitorum brevis and first dorsal interosseous muscles, and for fasciculations (visible twitches of muscle), which are best seen using tangential light. Strength should be tested against resistance, as well as with active maneuvers such as walking on the heels and toes to assess distal strength, and rising from a squatting position to examine proximal muscles. Facial muscles should also be tested. When assessing deep tendon reflexes, ensure the reflex is truly absent by asking the patient to concurrently perform a Jendrassic maneuver (pulling against interlocking fingers) or clench the jaw. Note that the reflex arc consists of large-diameter afferent sensory input as well as motor nerve output, so that dysfunction of either can impair reflexes. Tone is sometimes reduced in peripheral nerve diseases.

On sensory examination, sensation should be tested with a pin and a 128-Hz vibratory tuning fork, beginning at the big toe level and moving progressively more proximal. Likewise, position testing should begin distally, with fingers placed on the lateral sides of the big toe and progressively smaller movements tested. Severe loss of position sense can result in athetoid movements of the fingers when the eyes are closed (pseudoathetosis) or a positive Romber's sign.

---

**BOX 1  Signs and Symptoms of Peripheral Nervous System Disease by Fiber Type**

**Motor**
- Cramps
- Fasciculations
- Hyporeflexia
- Hypotonia
- Muscle atrophy
- Myokymia
- Pes cavus
- Weakness

**Large Fiber Sensory**
- Decreased vibration and position
- Hyporeflexia
- Pins and needles
- Tingling
- Unsteady gait, especially at night or with eyes closed

**Small Fiber Sensory**
- Burning
- Decreased pain sensation
- Decreased temperature sensation
- Jabbing

**Autonomic**
- Decreased or increased sweating
- Heat intolerance
- Impotence
- Postural hypotension
- Urinary retention

---

Temperature can be tested informally by placing a cold tuning fork on the skin. Foot injuries may be apparent with severe sensory loss.

Other important signs include high arches and hammertoe deformities, which suggest a long-standing neuropathy causing differences in muscular force. Demyelinating neuropathies, amyloidosis, and leprosy can cause nerve thickening, which is felt best in the dorsal cutaneous nerve of the foot or the great auricular nerve. Superficial nerves, such as the ulnar nerve at the elbow, can be palpated when appropriate. Postural blood pressure should be assessed for a blood pressure drop more than 20 mm Hg systolic or more than 10 mm Hg diastolic, following 5 minutes of supine rest at a minimum, to test autonomic functioning.

Several other levels of the nervous system can mimic symptoms of PNS disease. Myelopathy and motor neuron disease can manifest with weakness similar to motor neuropathies, although upper motor neuron features such as spasticity and increased reflexes are clues. Myopathies can also cause weakness, but usually more proximal than distal and without any sensory impairment. Isolated sensory involvement should be a red flag that the dorsal root ganglia may be the site of involvement rather than the peripheral nerve, particularly important because neuronopathies have a limited differential.

### PATTERN OF DISTRIBUTION

The pattern of distribution should be classified in two ways: symmetric or asymmetric and distal or proximal. Putting this together with the fiber type, six patterns of PNS disorders can be appreciated, with specific differentials (Table 1).

The symmetric distal sensorimotor neuropathy (pattern 1) manifests in a stocking-and-glove distribution and is the most common type of polyneuropathy. Once the level of the upper calves is reached, fibers of the same length in the fingertips begin to be affected. Sensorimotor polyneuropathies that affect both the distal and proximal nerves (pattern 2) should alert the physician to think of inflammatory

## TABLE 1   Causes of Neuropathy by Pattern Type

| Causes | Potentially Useful Tests |
|---|---|
| **Sensorimotor** | |
| ***Symmetric and Distal*** | |
| Metabolic disorders | OGTT, LFT, creatinine, TSH, vitamin B$_{12}$ |
| Hereditary disorders (CMT) | EMG/NCS |
| Infections (HIV, leprosy) | HIV test, review of medical |
| Toxins (drugs, alcohol, arsenic, thallium) | and social history |
| ***Symmetric and Proximal and Distal*** | |
| Inflammatory neuropathies (GBS, CIDP) | EMG/NCS, CSF |
| ***Asymmetric*** | |
| Mononeuropathy, radiculopathy, plexopathy | EMG/NCS |
| Mononeuritis multiplex Vasculitis | ANA, RF, ESR, ANCA, nerve bx |
| Diabetes | OGTT |
| HIV | HIV test |
| Multifocal CIDP | CSF |
| Rare: Porphyria, leprosy, HNPP | |
| **Pure Motor** | |
| ***Proximal*** | |
| Diabetic amyotrophy | OGTT |
| MMNCB | EMG/NCS |
| Motor variants of GBS, CIDP, MGUS | CSF, SPE, IF |
| Lymphoma | CBC |
| ***Distal*** | |
| Rare: Lead toxicity, porphyria | |
| **Pure Sensory** | |
| ***Neuropathies*** | |
| Nonsystemic vasculitis neuropathy | Nerve bx |
| Chronic gluten enteropathy | Antigliadin antibodies |
| Vitamin E deficiency | Vitamin E level |
| Distal, demyelinating, symmetric neuropathy | SPE, IF |
| Rare: Primary biliary cirrhosis, Crohn's disease | |
| ***Neuronopathies*** | |
| Paraneoplastic neuronopathy | Anti-Hu/CV2, Imaging |
| Sjögren's syndrome | Lip biopsy |
| HIV-related sensory neuronopathy | HIV test |
| Miller Fisher variant | EMG/NCS |
| Drugs (see Box 4) | Medication review |
| **Autonomic** | |
| Diabetes | OGTT |
| GBS | EMG/NCS |
| Paraneoplastic sensory neuropathy | Anti-Hu, CV2, imaging |
| HIV-related neuropathy | HIV test |
| Vincristine (Oncovin) | Medication review |
| Thiamine deficiency | Alcohol history |
| Rare: Porphyria, hereditary autonomic neuropathy, amyloidosis | |

*Abbreviations:* ANA = antinuclear antibodies; ANCA = antineutrophilic cytoplasmic antibodies; bx = biopsy; CBC = complete blood count; CIDP = chronic inflammatory demyelinating polyneuropathy; CMT = Charcot-Marie-Tooth disease; CSF = cerebrospinal fluid; EMG/NCS = electromyography/nerve conduction studies; ESR = erythrocyte sedimentation rate; GBS = Guillain-Barré syndrome; HIV = human immunodeficiency virus; HNPP = hereditary neuropathy with liability to pressure palsies; IF = immunofixation; LFT = liver function tests; MGUS = monoclonal gammopathy of unknown significance; MMNCB = multifocal motor neuropathy with conduction blocks; OGTT = oral glucose tolerance test; RF = rheumatoid factor; SPE = serum protein electrophoresis; TSH = thyroid-stimulating hormone.

---

neuropathies, such as Guillain-Barré syndrome (GBS) and chronic inflammatory demyelinating polyneuropathy (CIDP).

Asymmetric patterns (pattern 3) are often a result of trauma or compression, such as that seen in mononeuropathies, radiculopathies, and plexopathies. A pattern that affects multiple anatomically separated nerves is termed *mononeuritis multiplex* and is usually the result of a more diffuse process, such as diabetes or vasculitis.

Predominant motor neuropathies (pattern 4) are often proximal, such as diabetic amyotrophy. An exception is lead neuropathy, which affects motor fibers in a distal radial and peroneal distribution. Pure sensory neuropathies (pattern 5) are more likely to be distal, with the exception of a rare few such as Tangier disease, which manifests with a bathing-suit pattern. Neuropathies with autonomic impairment have a limited differential (pattern 6).

Additionally, involvement of the cranial nerves is only seen in a few causes of neuropathy. GBS, CIDP, Lyme disease, sarcoidosis, HIV-associated neuropathy, and Tangier disease are examples.

### TEMPORAL COURSE

Acute neuropathies are relatively rare and suggest an etiology such as GBS, acute intermittent porphyria, ischemia, toxins (thallium toxicity), drugs, or infections (diphtheric neuropathy). Subacute onset (>8 weeks) is seen in nutritional deficiencies, metabolic neuropathies, paraneoplastic syndromes, and CIDP. A chronic course is typical of hereditary neuropathies, a stepwise pattern can be seen in mononeuropathy multiplex, and a relapsing-remitting course occurs with intermittent exposure to a toxin or drug and in CIDP.

### KEY SIGNS

Sometimes, there is a key classic feature on history or examination that significantly narrows the differential immediately. Box 2 includes a checklist of items for inquiry and observation during assessment of neuropathy.

### PATHOLOGY AND THE ROLE OF NEUROPHYSIOLOGY

Nerve conduction studies (NCSs) and electromyography (EMG) are highly specialized tests that are performed principally by neurologists. NCSs electrically activate peripheral nerves at particular sites and then assess for abnormal transmission from the stimulation point to the final muscle response. EMG involves placing a small needle into the muscle to observe both the sound and appearance of the muscle at rest and with motor units firing. Because NCSs can only be performed at points where the nerve is superficial (most often distal), EMG is needed to assess for more proximal damage such as radiculopathy. EMG can also rule out other mimics of PNS disease, such as myopathy.

For the general physician, the most important thing is being able to interpret the results of these tests. Often, a report will be received back such as: "There is evidence of a symmetric distal axonal sensorimotor neuropathy." An NCS/EMG study should be able to specify the distribution and if motor or sensory fibers are involved. Autonomic and small sensory fibers are not tested well by EMG, so the diagnosis of these types of neuropathies is often clinical or requires more specialized testing. Thus, a normal NCS/EMG does not rule out neuropathy.

A further feature that electrophysiology can add is whether the pathology is demyelinating or axonal. Demyelination is characterized by slowed conduction velocity, temporal dispersion of the muscle action potential, and conduction block. Hereditary demyelinating neuropathies, such as Charcot-Marie-Tooth disease, do not show the latter two features, which are only seen in acquired neuropathies. Axonal disease is characterized by modest slowing of velocities, and more marked reduction in the amplitudes of the muscle and sensory action potentials. On EMG, there are fibrillations within 3 weeks of the neuropathic injury, indicating spontaneous firing of denervated muscle. Enlarged and prolonged motor unit potentials indicate subsequent regeneration, which occurs after several weeks to months.

Demyelination has a limited differential (Box 3), and often a better prognosis, because myelin can start to regenerate within a few days.

## BOX 2 Key Diagnostic Features

**Medical History**
- Connective tissue disease
- Diabetes
- Renal disease
- Thyroid disease

**Surgical History, Trauma**
- Compression neuropathies

**Medication History**
- Drug-induced neuropathy

**Family History, High Arches**
- Inherited neuropathy

**Nutrition, Alcohol Use**
- Alcoholic neuropathy
- Vitamin deficiency

**Occupational Exposures**
- Toxic neuropathy

**History of Weight Loss**
- Amyloidosis
- HIV
- Malignancy

**Recent Infection, Travel**
- Diptheria
- Guillain-Barré syndrome
- HIV
- Leprosy
- Lyme disease

**Dry Eyes and Mouth**
- Sarcoidosis

**Severe Pain**
- Amyloidosis
- Diabetes
- Guillain-Barré syndrome
- HIV
- Vasculitis

**Skin Lesions**
- Anaesthetic patches (leprosy)
- Bullous lesions (porphyria)
- Hyperpigmentation (osteosclerotic myeloma)
- Mee's lines (arsenic or thallium poisoning)
- Orange tonsils (Tangier disease)
- Angiokeratomas (Fabry's disease)

## BOX 3 Demyelinating Neuropathies

- Charcot-Marie-Tooth disease
- Hereditary neuropathy with liability to pressure palsies
- Inflammatory neuropathies
- Monoclonal gammopathies and paraproteinemias
- Multifocal motor neuropathy with conduction block
- Neuropathies caused by drugs such as amiodarone (Cordarone) and suramin[2]
- Neuropathies caused by infections (diptheria) or toxins (arsenic)

---

[2]Not available in the United States.

---

improve diagnostic accuracy. These metabolites can be falsely increased with hypovolemia, renal insufficiency, hypothyroidism, and increased age, but a return to normal levels 1 to 2 weeks after beginning replacement therapy indicates this is the cause. The combination of elevated gastrin and anti–parietal cell antibodies may be used to diagnose pernicious anemia. The yield of general testing for other vitamin deficiencies in polyneuropathy is relatively low.

Antinuclear antibodies (ANA) probably are usually only significant in the context of suggestive features (abrupt onset, mononeuropathy multiplex pattern, arthralgia or arthritis, fevers, rash, or renal abnormalities) because they are positive in about 3% of normal patients. However, referral to a rheumatologist should be considered with a very high titer (>1:1280).

The erythyrocyte sedimentation rate (ESR) is often elevated, especially in older patients. Rates greater than 70 mm/hour tend to be more meaningful, particularly with a mononeuritis multiplex pattern.

Serum protein electrophoresis lacks sensitivity, and immunofixation should be ordered if there is high suspicion of a paraproteinemia. If an elevated monoclonal antibody is found, a 24-hour urine test for Bence Jones proteinuria, skeletal survey, CBC, renal function tests, and serum calcium should be ordered. If the M protein is greater than 2.5 g/dL or if abnormalities are detected on these tests, referral to a hematologist for bone marrow aspiration is required. Polyclonal antibodies are not associated with neuropathy.

If there is suspicion of amyloidosis, a rectal, abdominal fat, or sensory nerve biopsy can be undertaken. Sural nerve biopsy is reserved for difficult diagnostic situations because it causes a permanent area of numbness with possible dysesthesias over the biopsied area. Suspicion of vasculitis is the most common indication, but pathology can also be seen in leprosy and with tumor infiltrate.

In approximately 20% of patients, an underlying cause of neuropathy is not found. These patients are said to have a cryptogenic sensory or sensorimotor neuropathy. A distinct clinical picture has emerged, most commonly of a patient in the sixth or seventh decade, manifesting with distal dysesthesias and possibly with mild weakness and sensory ataxia. These patients tend not to develop significant disability, and treatment is mainly for neuropathic pain.

---

Axonal regeneration proceeds at a far slower rate of 1 to 3 μm/day, and nerves with proximal lesions must go a long distance to reinnervate their muscle and might never reach their goal.

## Investigations

Once the neuropathy has been subclassified, investigations for the specific causes in that pattern class should be undertaken (see Table 1). Several recent papers suggest that 2-hour oral glucose tolerance testing (OGTT) is the best test for glucose intolerance due to the relatively low sensitivity of serum glucose levels and glycosylated hemoglobin (HbA1c). Likewise, vitamin B12 levels have a low sensitivity, and serum metabolites methylmalonic acid (MMA) and homocysteine (Hcy) should be measured in patients with a result less than 300 pg/mL to

## CURRENT DIAGNOSIS

- The five-step approach to classify neuropathies based on fiber type, pattern of distribution, temporal course, pathology, and key features allows a tailored diagnostic evaluation.
- Electrodiagnostic testing provides a useful adjunct to the clinical evaluation.
- The cause of neuropathy might not be found in 20% of patients, but there are treatments for several known etiologies, as well as specific medications to treat neuropathic pain.

# Treatment

## MONONEUROPATHIES

The most common cause of mononeuropathy is nerve compression, and surgical treatment is often a consideration for these patients. The four most common locations are median neuropathy at the wrist (carpal tunnel syndrome), ulnar neuropathy at the elbow, peroneal neuropathy at the fibular head, and facial nerve palsy (Bell's palsy).

Carpal tunnel syndrome manifests with pain and numbness principally in the first three digits, although it is often poorly localized. Classic features include pain at night and shaking out the hand to relieve pain. For milder symptoms, a nighttime splint, which prevents wrist flexion and high pressure in the carpal tunnel, is often helpful. Local corticosteroid injections can provide relief, and surgical decompression has a very high success rate.

Ulnar neuropathy manifests with numbness of the fourth and fifth digits and wasting of the interosseous muscles, often with pain localized to the elbow. Peroneal neuropathies manifest with foot drop and numbness on the dorsum of the foot. In both cases, avoidance of pressure over the nerve often leads to improvement. Surgery might improve symptoms, but less reliably so than carpal tunnel surgery.

Bell's palsy is an inflammatory rather than compressive process, presumably due to a viral etiology. Treatment is controversial, but early (within 14 days) use of prednisone[1] 60 mg daily, decreasing by 10 mg steps every 2 days, along with acyclovir (Zovirax)[1] 800 mg five times daily for 7 days has been advocated. About 15% of patients have residual facial weakness.

## GUILLAIN-BARRÉ SYNDROME

GBS often begins following gastroenteritis with *Campylobacter jejuni*, or an upper respiratory tract infection, due to a presumed autoimmune response directed against myelin. The incidence is 1 or 2 per 100,000 persons per year. Characteristic features are ascending weakness, areflexia, and sensory and autonomic symptoms progressing over a few days up to 4 weeks. Facial diplegia and pain can occur. Electrophysiology shows acute demyelination with conduction blocks, and cerebrospinal fluid (CSF) reveals an increase in protein with a cell count of less than 5 white blood cells (cytoalbuminologic dissociation) in more than 80% of patients after 2 weeks. A CSF pleocytosis of more than 10 lymphocytes/mm³ should alert the physician to another cause such as sarcoidosis, Lyme disease, or early HIV.

The Miller-Fisher variant is characterized by specific clinical features of sensory ataxia, areflexia, and ophthalmolplegia. *C. jejuni* infection has been correlated with more severe variants, such as acute motor axonal neuropathy (AMAN) and acute motor and sensory axonal neuropathy (AMSAM), which damage axons in addition to myelin. *C. jejuni*–related GBS correlates with anti-GM1 antibodies, although they are not prognostic or specific. Recovery can take months to years. Only 20% of patients are left without residual deficit. About 5% to 10% have significant persistent disability, and the mortality rate is 5%.

During early treatment, patients might require admission to intensive care, with close monitoring of pulmonary function tests for respiratory compromise. Diaphragmatic weakness correlates with neck flexion and extension and shoulder abduction. The patient should be intubated when the forced vital capacity (FVC) declines to less than 15 mL/kg or when negative inspiratory flow (NIF) is less than −20 to −30. Monitoring of the cardiac rhythm is important due to dysautonomia.

The preferred treatment is intravenous immunoglobulin (IVIg)[1] at a dose of 0.4 g/kg/day for 5 days. This is generally well tolerated, and adverse side effects such as myalgia, headache, or flu-like symptoms often resolve with a reduced infusion rate. If IVIg is contraindicated (renal failure, IgA deficiency), plasmapheresis can be initiated with four alternate-day exchanges over 7 to 10 days for a total of 200 to 250 mL/kg. Both plasmapheresis and IVIg continue to work for several weeks after the treatment period, but if patients experience a secondary worsening after successful treatment, a second dose may be initiated. Steroids were reviewed recently by a Cochrane systematic review and were not found to be of benefit in GBS.

## CHRONIC INFLAMMATORY DEMYELINATING POLYNEUROPATHY

This neuropathy is pathologically similar to GBS, but progression is longer than 8 weeks, often with a relapsing-remitting course. Symmetric distal and proximal weakness and sensory impairment, hyporeflexia, and cytoalbumingergic dissociation in the CSF is the classic presentation, although there are variants.

Treatment is either IVIg[1] or prednisone. IVIg is given initially at 0.4 g/kg/day for 5 days, then the dose and frequency are reduced over time. Prednisone is given 1 mg/kg/day until improvement, followed by a slow tapering of 5 mg every 2 to 3 weeks over a period of months. Response is usually seen within 4 weeks. Refractory patients have been treated with repeated plasmapheresis treatments or immunosuppressive therapy with cyclosporine (Sandimmune).[1]

## MULTIFOCAL MOTOR NEUROPATHY

Multifocal motor neuropathy (MMN) is not a common disorder but is important not to mistake for motor neuron disease because it has a very different prognosis and treatment. Patients present with progressive asymmetric distal weakness, often of the arm, without sensory loss and with less atrophy than would be expected for the degree of weakness. Unlike motor neuron disease, there are no upper motor neuron signs. It is different from multifocal acquired demyelinating sensory and motor neuropathy (MADSAM), an asymmetric variant of CIDP, in that loss of reflexes and weakness involves only the affected limb, there is a relatively normal CSF protein concentration, and sensory nerve conduction studies are normal. Diagnosis is supported by finding conduction blocks in sites not usually associated with compression. The GM1 antibody is elevated in 60% of cases. Repeated treatments with IVIg[1] or cyclophosphamide (Cytoxan)[1] are common choices. Rituximab (Rituxan),[1] a monoclonal antibody, has also been used. Prednisone classically worsens the condition.

## DIABETIC NEUROPATHY

Diabetes is one of the most common causes of neuropathy. Patients can present with a symmetric distal neuropathy, autonomic proximal diabetic neuropathy, mononeuritis multiplex, compressive and cranial neuropathies, and trunk polyradiculopathies.

The distal symmetric sensory polyneuropathy (DSPN) correlates with the duration of the diabetes, control of hyperglycemia, and presence of retinopathy and nephropathy. The exact etiology is unknown, but theories include a metabolic process involving aldose reductase, ischemic damage, or an immunologic disorder. Typical symptoms include lancinating pains or burning, worse at night, and possible dysautonomia. Atrophy may be noted in the foot muscles, but severe weakness is atypical. NCS may be normal because small fibers are primarily affected. Treatment includes blood sugar control to limit progression and symptom control for neuropathic pain. Gabapentin (Neurontin)[1] and tricyclic antidepressants are common choices (see later). Drugs such as QR-333, a topical compound that contains quercetin, a flavonoid with aldose reductase–inhibitor effects, are being investigated specifically for diabetic neuropathy.

Autonomic neuropathy is treated symptomatically, with fludrocortisone (Florinef)[1] 0.1 mg/day for orthostatic hypotension, metoclopramide (Reglan) 10 mg before meals for gastroparesis, and sildenafil (Viagra) 25 mg 1 hour before sexual intercourse for impotence.

Proximal diabetic neuropathy (diabetic amyotrophy) manifests typically with unilateral pain in the anterior thigh followed by stepwise progression over weeks to months of quadriceps weakness, atrophy of the proximal leg muscles, and a reduced knee reflex, with occasional

---

[1]Not FDA approved for this indication.

[1]Not FDA approved for this indication.

contralateral leg involvement. The erythrocyte sedimentation rate (ESR) may be elevated and CSF protein mildly increased (120 mg/dL on average). NCS and EMG reflect multifocal active axonal damage (fibrillations) to the lumbar plexus and roots. Small retrospective studies have reported that IVIg[1] and other forms of immunosuppressive therapy are effective in treating patients with proximal diabetic neuropathy. A short course of corticosteroids (prednisone[1] 50 mg/day for 1 week, then tapering by 10 mg/week) can be used to ease pain in severe cases, with close monitoring of the glucose level, but overall prognosis is quite good, ranging from 1 to 18 months of recovery phase (mean of 6 months) and partial or complete restoration of strength in approximately 70% of patients.

## PARAPROTEINEMIC NEUROPATHIES

Multiple myeloma, Waldenström's macroglobulinemia, cryoglobulinemia, osteosclerotic myeloma (POEMS syndrome), and monoclonal gammopathy of unknown significance (MGUS) are associated with monoclonal antibodies directed at PNS components, such as myelin-associated glycoprotein (MAG). Neuropathies associated with an immunoglobulin (Ig)M monoclonal protein (approximately 60%) are typically distal, demyelinating, and symmetric, whereas IgG (30%) and IgA (10%) gammopathies can be axonal or demyelinating. In terms of treatment, the distal demyelinating neuropathy of IgM paraproteinemias tends to be treatment refractory. IgG and IgA gammopathies can mimic the demyelination pattern seen in CIDP, and patients with any antibody and this pattern should receive immunotherapy as recommended for CIDP (see earlier). Axonal neuropathies and IgM, IgG, or IgA gammopathies have a less clear relationship and are typically not responsive to treatment.

## HEREDITARY NEUROPATHIES

Charcot-Marie-Tooth (CMT) disease is among the most common of genetic neuromuscular disorders, and more than 30 genes have been identified. Clues are a history of difficulty running in childhood, high arches, hammertoes, ankle weakness, and nerve hypertrophy developing in teenage years. Depending on the subtype, the neuropathy may be axonal or demyelinating, but the most common type (CMT-1) is caused by an autosomal dominant gene encoding peripheral myelin protein 22 and is easily diagnosed by the relatively uniform slowing on nerve conduction velocities (<25% of lower limits of normal). Patients have a mild course and remain ambulatory throughout life in most cases.

Hereditary neuropathy with liability to pressure palsies (HNPP) is another dominantly inherited neuropathy in which patients have recurrent episodes of isolated mononeuropathies, typically affecting, in order of decreasing frequency, the common peroneal, ulnar, radial, and median nerves. Most attacks are sudden onset, painless, and followed by complete recovery. There is no treatment other than preventive measures.

## TOXIC AND NUTRITIONAL NEUROPATHIES

Treatment of toxic and nutritional neuropathies involves detection and removal of the underlying cause. A thorough review of medications, occupational exposures, and nutritional risk factors is essential (Box 4). Drug toxicity is much more common than environmental toxicity. Incidence of neuropathy does not always correlate with the dosage and duration of exposure. For instance, amiodarone neuropathy has been reported with dosages as low as 200 mg/day and durations as short as 1 month. Symptoms might not improve, or might even worsen, for several weeks after the drug is stopped before improvement starts, a phenomenon known as *coasting*.

Cisplatin can cause a neuropathy that overlaps in symptomatology with paraneoplastic sensory neuronopathy, and dapsone is associated with a motor axonopathy. Gold neuropathy can have prominent myokymia and can mimic GBS.

---

### BOX 4  Causes of Toxic and Nutritional Neuropathies

**Drug Toxins**
*Axonal*
- Colchicine
- Dapsone
- Disulfiram
- Ethambutol
- Hyralazine
- Isoniazid
- Metronidazole
- Nitrofurantoin
- Nitrous oxide
- Nucleosides
- Paclitaxel
- Phenytoin
- Tacrolimus
- Vincristine

*Demyelinating*
- Amiodarone (Cordarone)
- Chloroquine (Aralen)
- Gold
- Suramin[2]

*Neuronopathy*
- Cisplatin (Platinol-AQ)
- Pyridoxine (vitamin $B_6$)
- Thalidomide (Thalomid)

**Environmental Toxins**
- Acrylamide (plastics)
- Allyl chloride (insecticides)
- Arsenic
- Carbon disulfide (cellophanes)
- Ethylene glycol (antifreeze)
- Ethylene oxide (sterilizer)
- Hexacarbons (glue)
- Lead
- Mercury
- Methyl bromide (fumigant)
- Organophosphates (insecticides)
- Thallium (pesticides)
- Trichloroethylene (drycleaning)
- Vacor (rodenticide)

**Vitamin Deficiencies**
- $B_1$ (alcoholism)
- $B_3$ (alcoholism)
- $B_6$ (isoniazid use)
- $B_{12}$ (vegans, pernicious anemia)
- E (cholestasis and abetalipoproteinemia)

---
[2]Not available in the United States.

---

Specific treatments for drug-induced neuropathies include cyanocobalamin (vitamin $B_{12}$)[1] for nitrous oxide neuropathy and pyridoxine (vitamin $B_6$)[1] for hydralazine and isoniazid neuropathies. Excessive vitamin $B_6$ can also *cause* a neuropathy. Glutamine[7] and vitamin E[1] 300 mg twice a day has shown promise for paclitaxel neuropathy, and neuroprotective agents such as nerve growth factor are being investigated for cisplatin-induced neuropathy. Tacrolimus can cause a CIDP-like neuropathy that responds to IVIg[1] or plasmapheresis.

---
[1]Not FDA approved for this indication.

---
[1]Not FDA approved for this indication.
[7]Available as a dietary supplement.

One of the most common nutritional neuropathies is caused by thiamine deficiency and is associated with alcohol consumption of at least 100 g per day. Patients present with burning feet, and early alcohol abstinence and treatment with thiamine denotes better chance of recovery. Vitamin $B_{12}$ deficiency is vital not to miss and can manifest with a subacute combined degeneration, whereby patients have a superimposed myelopathy and neuropathy (spasticity but reduced reflexes). Sudden-onset symptoms, particularly in the feet and hands simultaneously, are also suggestive.

## METABOLIC AND INFECTIOUS NEUROPATHIES

Peripheral neuropathy can complicate renal failure, hypothyroidism, biliary cirrhosis, porphyria, Tangier disease, Fabry's disease, and mitochondrial diseases.

Early in the course, HIV can manifest as a GBS-like syndrome, although with CSF pleocytosis. This typically responds to IVIg[1] and plasmapheresis. In later stages, patients might develop a distal symmetric polyneuropathy, although it is important to determine if this might be due to nucleoside reverse transcriptase inhibitors, nutritional deficiency, or infection. Cranial neuropathies, sensory neuronopathy, lumbosacral polyradiculopathies, and mononeuritis multiplex also occur.

Leprosy is the most common treatable neuropathy worldwide. Tuberculoid leprosy leads to hypopigmented patches with loss of pain and temperature sensation. Lepromatous leprosy, a more severe form seen in immunosuppressed persons, can cause ulnar, common peroneal, and facial neuropathies. Treatment involves a long-term multidrug regimen of dapsone and rifampin (Rifadin).[1]

Herpes zoster can cause a postherpetic neuralgia, defined as pain persisting for more than 6 weeks after the rash appears. Early treatment with acyclovir (Zovirax) (800 mg five times daily for 7 days) can reduce the duration of the acute phase. Chronic discomfort is treated with medications for neuropathic pain (see later).

Lyme disease, caused by *Borrelia burgdorferi*, begins with erythema migrans, followed by multifocal peripheral and cranial neuropathies, particularly facial diplegia. CSF lymphocytic pleocytosis plus serologic demonstration of *B. burgdorferi* infection on serum or CSF are the diagnostic features. Early stages are treated with a 3-week course of doxycycline[1] 100 mg twice daily, and intravenous penicillin G[1] should be given in the late stages.

---

[1]Not FDA approved for this indication.

## CARCINOMATOUS NEUROPATHY

Tumors can cause neuropathy by compression, metastatic spread, paraneoplastic antibodies, hemorrhage, and treatment with chemotherapy or radiation therapy. A distal sensorimotor neuropathy is associated with many different tumors and seldom precedes tumor diagnosis. Pathogenesis can include toxic, nutritional, and immunologic causes. A sensory neuronopathy is less common, but often precedes tumor diagnosis, thus warranting a careful work-up. Lung, breast, ovary, and gastrointestinal tract cancers are the most likely associated types. Imaging and paraneoplastic antibodies (particularly anti-Hu and anti-CV2, most commonly associated with lung cancer) may help in making the diagnosis. Treatment focuses on the underlying neoplasm.

## VASCULITIC NEUROPATHY

Vasculitis can be primary (polyarteritis nodosa, Wegener's granulomatosis, Churg-Strauss syndrome, microscopic polyangitis) or secondary (connective tissue diseases, systemic infections, drug reactions). It classically manifests with a painful mononeuritis multiplex with asymmetric patchy features, reflecting multifocal ischemic damage. If the patient's vasculitis is restricted to the PNS, serologic testing for these disorders is often negative. In this case, a sural nerve biopsy might reveal fibrinoid necrosis and perivascular inflammation.

Treatment needs to be carefully undertaken with intravenous methylprednisolone (Solu-Medrol)[1] for 3 days followed by oral prednisone. In many cases, other immunosuppressive drugs are eventually used.

# Neuropathic Pain

Often pain is the most predominant and distressing feature of neuropathy. Several classes of medications can be tried (Table 2), although it is important to counsel the patient that complete abolition of pain is unlikely. A trial period should be for at least 6 to 8 weeks before concluding that the patient does not respond. A combination of agents with different mechanisms can have an advantage over monotherapy for the nonresponsive patient.

First-line treatment is generally with tricyclic antidepressants. Serotonin and noradrenaline reuptake inhibitors such as amitriptyline[1] (Elavil), imipramine[1] (Tofranil), and clomipramine[1] (Anafranil)

---

[1]Not FDA approved for this indication.

## TABLE 2  Select Neuropathic Pain Medications

| Drug | Dosage | Side Effects |
| --- | --- | --- |
| Amitriptyline (Elavil)[1] | 10 mg/d, increasing weekly by 10 mg, up to 150 mg/d | Dry mouth, sedation, urinary retention, cardiac arrhythmias, orthostatic hypotension, constipation, weight gain<br>Contraindications: cardiac arrhythmias, CHF, recent MI, narrow angle glaucoma, urinary retention |
| Capsaicin (Zostrix) | 0.075% cream applied tid to qid | Sneezing, coughing, rash, skin irritation |
| Carbamazepine (Tegretol)[1] | 100 mg bid, increasing by 100 mg weekly<br>Max: 1200 mg/d | Somnolence, dizziness, nausea, gait changes, urticaria, hyponatremia, pancytopenia, hepatic dysfunction<br>Obtain baseline and 6-wk CBC and LFT |
| Gabapentin (Neurontin)[1] | 300 mg on d 1, 600 mg on d 2, 900 mg on day 3<br>Max: 3600 mg/d. | Sedation, fatigue, dizziness, confusion, tremor, weight gain, peripheral edema, headache<br>Reduce dose in renal insufficiency |
| Lamotrigine (Lamictal)[1] | 25 mg at night for 2 wk, increasing weekly by 25-50 mg<br>Max: 400 mg/d | Severe rash (especially if increased too quickly), dizziness, unsteadiness, drowsiness, diplopia |
| Tramadol (Ultram) | 50 mg bid<br>Titrate 50 mg every 3-7 d, using a tid or qid schedule<br>Max: 100 mg qid | Constipation, headache, nausea<br>Risk of seizures with neuroleptics and antidepressants<br>Reduce dose with hepatic or renal dysfunction |

[1]Not FDA approved for this indication.
*Abbreviations:* CBC = complete blood count; CHF = congestive heart failure; LFT = liver function test; max = maximum; MI = myocardial infarction.

may be marginally more effective than those with relatively selective noradrenergic effects such as desipramine and nortriptyline. However, nortriptyline and desipramine are less sedating. Selective serotonin reuptake inhibitors appear to be less effective. Second-line antidepressants include venlafaxine[1] (Effexor), bupropion[1] (Wellbutrin), and the recently approved duloxetine (Cymbalta), which have the advantage of better tolerability due to less muscarinic, histaminergic, and α-adrenergic affinity.

The typical next class of medications to try is the antiepileptics. Gabapentin[1] is a common choice and is generally well tolerated. Pregabalin (Lyrica) is a newer related agent that, unlike gabapentin, exhibits linear pharmacokinetics and can be initiated at a therapeutic dose without a long titration. Second-line choices include lamotrigine[1] (Lamictal), carbamazepine[1] (Tegretol), and topiramate[1] (Topamax). Valproate[1] (Depacon) and zonisamide[1] (Zonegran) have limited evidence, and phenytoin[1] (Dilantin) can cause neuropathy. Oxcarbazepine[1] (Trileptal), like carbamazepine, slows the recovery rate of voltage-activated sodium channels, but it also inhibits high-threshold N-type and P/Q-type calcium channels and reduces glutamatergic transmission. As a result, it can modulate both peripheral and central neuropathic pain pathways, and several studies into its efficacy are under way.

Topical creams, such as capsaicin (Zostrix), an extract of chili, can be tried. Capsaicin works by depleting substance P and can temporarily worsen pain by causing a burning sensation. Lidocaine[1] (Xylocaine) can be also used topically.

Other agents for severe neuropathies include opioid agents, such as tramadol (Ultram), which has low-affinity binding for μ-opioid receptors coupled with mild inhibition of norepinephrine and serotonin reuptake. Slow-release opioids, such as oxycodone (OxyContin) 30 to 60 mg/day, can help, and risk of addiction is low in this population. Glutamate antagonists, such as dextromethorphan[1] (Delsym), have shown benefit in some studies, as has mexiletine[1] (Mexitil), a class IB antiarrhythmic agent and oral analogue of lidocaine. Nonpharmacologic therapies, such as transcutaneous electrical nerve stimulation (TENS) and acupuncture, might also provide adjunctive relief.

## REFERENCES

Donofrio PD, Albers JW: AAEM minimonograph 34: Polyneuropathy: Classification by nerve conduction studies and electromyography. Muscle Nerve 1990;13:889-903.

Dworkin RH, Backonja M, Rowbotham MC, et al: Advances in neuropathic pain: Diagnosis, mechanisms, and treatment recommendations. Arch Neurol 2003;60:1524-1534.

Grant I, Benstead TJ: Differential Diagnosis of Peripheral Neuropathy. In Dyck PJ, Thomas PK (eds): Peripheral Neuropathy. Philadelphia: Saunders, 2005.

Poncelet, AN: An algorithm for the evaluation of peripheral neuropathy. Am Fam Physician 1997;57(4):755-764.

Stewart JD: Focal peripheral neuropathies. New York: Raven, 1993.

# Management of Head Injuries

Method of
*Todd W. Vitaz, MD*

Traumatic brain injury (TBI) most commonly results from motor vehicle crashes (MVC) and typically affects males in the 2nd through 4th decades of life. These sudden random acts can have long-lasting effects on the patient and family, but these events also impact society as a whole when a young, viable working-age individual becomes

---

[1]Not FDA approved for this indication.

suddenly disabled and dependent on the care of others. TBI has no regard for age or gender, however, and can be seen in infants as a result of nonaccidental trauma as well as in geriatric patients following falls. The management of these patients can become extremely complicated and often requires the close interaction of numerous different health care providers ranging from trauma, orthopedic, and neurologic surgeons to nurses, social workers, speech, occupational, and physical therapists. Unfortunately, current interventions are still limited to the avoidance or minimization of secondary injury and rehabilitative intervention. However, when these patients are managed with aggressive, comprehensive, multidisciplinary approaches, the outcomes at times can be rewarding.

TBI can be categorized based on numerous factors. Most commonly it is differentiated based on mechanism and injury type (closed versus penetrating), whether it has occurred with or without systemic injuries (isolated versus multisystem), and the severity (mild, moderate, severe). The Glasgow Coma Scale (GCS) (Table 1), which was initially developed as a prognostic indicator following closed head injury, has become the principal triage tool for evaluating these patients. Patients are scored based on their best response in each of the three categories (eye opening, verbal responses, and motor score) and then subdivided into mild (13 to 15), moderate (9 to 12), and severe (3 to 8). One caveat to this assessment tool is that it can be affected by numerous alterations: hypoxia, hypotension, hypothermia, intoxication, infection, and other metabolic derangements, which are commonly seen in the trauma population.

## Pathology

Another common classification system following TBI is based on pathophysiologic findings. Concussion commonly occurs following mild or moderate TBI as the result of transient (typically seconds to minutes) neurologic dysfunction in the setting of a normal computed tomography (CT) scan. Brief loss of consciousness, commonly with amnesia regarding the event, is not uncommon and is often associated with nausea, vomiting, headache, dizziness, and transient visual obscuration. These symptoms may persist for several hours to weeks as part of the *postconcussive syndrome* and, in rare instances, especially following repetitive injury, these alterations may become long-lasting. As a result of these persistent problems, in addition to a better understanding of the neurocognitive effects following this type of injury, there has been an enormous emphasis placed on their prevention (see text following).

Skull fractures may occur in isolation or be associated with other types of brain injuries. They are commonly classified based on whether they are open (overlying laceration) or closed, linear or comminuted, nondepressed or depressed. Skull fractures occur either as the result of a large force directed to a small area (i.e., depressed skull fracture following a blow to the head with a golf club) or when larger forces are dissipated throughout the skull resulting in fracture through the weakest area (linear fractures through frontal skull base, petrous, or squamous temporal bone). Linear fractures are commonly associated

**TABLE 1  Glasgow Coma Scale**

| Best Motor Score | Best Verbal Response | Best Eye Opening |
| --- | --- | --- |
| 6 Obeys commands | 5 Normal speech | 4 Spontaneous |
| 5 Localizes to pain | 4 Confused | 3 To voice |
| 4 Withdraws to pain | 3 Inappropriate words | 2 To pain |
| 3 Flexor posturing | 2 Incomprehensible sounds | 1 No eye opening |
| 2 Extensor posturing | 1 No verbal response | |
| 1 No motor reponse | Intubated patients receive a 1 with the suffix T added to score | |

with raccoon eyes (frontal skull base fractures), Battle's sign (posterior skull base fracture), cerebrospinal fluid leak (otorrhea or rhinorrhea) or olfactory, facial or acoustic nerve injury (amnesia, facial palsy, sensorineuronal deafness).

In addition, temporal bone fractures may also be associated with epidural hematomas (EDHs). These extra-axial blood clots are most commonly caused by laceration of the middle meningeal artery and result in accumulation of *high-pressure arterial bleeding* in the potential space between the dura and skull. EDHs are more commonly seen in younger individuals probably because of the decreased skull thickness and lack of adhesions between the skull and dura mater in this population. Commonly, these lesions appear on CT scan as lens-shaped, extra-axial hematomas most often in the temporal region and can be rapidly expansive secondary to the high-pressure arterial bleeding. The clinical course in these patients is classically described by a brief loss of consciousness from the initial concussion, followed by a "lucid interval" in which the patient may be awake and alert, which then gives way to another episode of decreased mental status that may be rapidly progressive and associated with signs of brain stem compression (flexor or extensor posturing, dilated nonreactive pupil). EDHs are usually treated surgically unless they are extremely small and constitute one of the few true neurosurgical emergencies where mere minutes may make an enormous difference in the patient's outcome.

Unlike EDHs, subdural hematomas (SDHs) are often associated with other types of brain injury and thus typically involve an altered level of consciousness (LOC) from the onset. SDHs are typically caused by bleeding from bridging veins that get torn when the brain moves within its cerebrospinal fluid (CSF) buffer while the veins remain tethered at their dural insertions; however, other causes such as venous or arterial hemorrhage from a brain laceration also exist. CT scanning reveals that these lesions commonly appear more crescent-shaped but never cross the dural boundaries (falx or tentorium). Unlike the high-pressure EDHs, SDHs typically expand at a slower rate but still cause devastating neurologic dysfunction from compression of the underlying brain. In addition mortality rates tend to be higher with worse outcome for SDH as a result of the common underlying brain injury. Once again these extra-axial clots frequently require surgical evacuation unless they are small and fail to have substantial compression on the underlying brain, where they are managed with serial imaging and close neurologic observation. In patients for whom a small SDH is not treated surgically, the physician must remain cognizant of the fact that a small proportion of these will increase in size between 1 and 4 weeks following the trauma and can be a cause of delayed deterioration or increased headache and new neurologic findings.

Intraparenchymal hematomas occur quite commonly following TBI and can be either hemorrhagic or nonhemorrhagic. These lesions range in size from 1 to 2 mm, up to several centimeters, and can cause a full range of symptoms and neurologic findings based on their location, size, and degree of compression on surrounding structures. Just like extra-axial hematomas, these lesions may increase in size and commonly coalesce or mature and *blossom* during the first 12 to 24 hours following the trauma. In addition, larger hematomas incite an inflammatory reaction in the surrounding brain resulting in increased edema around the lesion, which may result in increases in the intracranial pressure (ICP) (commonly seen on postinjury days [PIDs] 3 to 7). Management of these lesions depends on their size, location, and associated findings and ranges from serial observation and repeat imaging, surgical evacuation of the hematoma, or decompressive craniectomy with or without lobectomy.

The final category of pathologic abnormalities following TBI occurs as the result of shear injury to the axons themselves, called diffuse axonal injury (DAI). This is caused by either acceleration and deceleration or rotational forces to the axons resulting in micro- or macroscopic areas of injury and axonal transection. Most commonly this is encountered in the setting where a patient clinically has signs of a severe TBI, often with a GCS score less than 6; however, the CT scan is either unimpressive or shows only small areas of petechial hemorrhage. In addition ICP recording typically shows normal or only slightly elevated values. Magnetic resonance imaging (MRI) is commonly used in this subset of patients and can be used as a predictive indicator for determining the severity of injury, especially if CT is negative. MRI commonly shows areas of increased intensity on fluid attenuation inversion recovery (FLAIR) and T2-weighted sequences in the brainstem, diencephalon, deep white matter tracts, or corpus callosum. Recovery following this type of injury is variable and depends more on the injury location (reticular activating system of brainstem versus supratentorial white matter tracts) rather than the injury volume.

In addition to these abnormalities, patients with TBI are also at risk for damage to the spinal cord and vertebral and carotid arteries. Thus, patients with altered LOC should be assumed to have spinal instability and possible spinal cord injury (SCI); they should remain immobilized until the absence of these can be confirmed. The incidence of carotid and vertebral artery injury associated with severe TBI is unknown, but patients with facial or cervical fractures and those with soft tissue neck or chest injury (seat belt sign) have been found to be at higher risk. The appropriate screening for and treatment of these injuries have become a topic of intense debate in recent years but should be suspected in a patient with focal neurologic findings without identifiable cause on other imaging.

## INTRACRANIAL PRESSURE AND THE MONROE-KELLIE DOCTRINE

Regardless of the pathophysiologic type of injury, the end result commonly is the generation of increases in the ICP, which can then lead to secondary brain injury. ICP dynamics are easily understood if one considers the principles of the volume pressure relationships outlined by the Monroe-Kellie doctrine. The basis of this principle resides on the fact that the skull is a fixed and rigid volume; because of this any changes to the volume of its contents will directly affect the pressure within this rigid space. In simplest terms the intracranial cavity contains blood, water, and tissue. Blood may be intravascular (IV) or extravascular (EV) in the case of extra-axial blood clots; water includes not only cerebrospinal fluid, which may build up in cases of hydrocephalus, but also edema following traumatic injuries; brain parenchyma typically compromises the tissue component but in select instances tumors or cysts may also fall into this category.

As increases in any or all three of these categories occur, the pressure inside the cranial cavity increases proportionally. At first compensatory changes occur, which accommodate for these increases, resulting in only mild pressure changes; however, eventually a critical volume is reached where the compensatory mechanisms are saturated, resulting in rapid and dramatic pressure changes. The following scenario illustrates these principles. A patient is involved in a motor vehicle crash and suffers a head injury with a small epidural hematoma. Initially he is awake and alert without any focal neurologic findings. The epidural hematoma creates an increase in the EV blood

---

## CURRENT DIAGNOSIS

**Classification of Head Injuries**

- Closed versus penetrating
- Isolated versus multisystem injuries
- Severity
  - Mild (GCS 13-15)
  - Moderate (GCS 9-12)
  - Severe (GCS 3-8)

**Pathologic Findings with Closed Head Injuries**

- Skull fractures
- Epidural hematomas
- Subdural hematomas
- Parenchymal contusions
- Intraparenchymal hematomas
- Diffuse axonal injury

component of the Monroe-Kellie doctrine; however, compensatory changes in intracranial CSF volume result in decreases in ICP. However, the water component, thus preventing significant changes in ICP. However, the hematoma continues to enlarge, causing increases in ICP exhibited clinically by slow deterioration in the patient's level of consciousness. The patient is now intubated and mildly hyperventilated causing vasoconstriction, therefore decreasing the intravascular blood component and reducing ICP with an improvement in the patient's neurologic condition. Unfortunately, as the operating room (OR) is being prepared, the patient suffers a rapid decrease in his level of conscious, becoming unresponsive with flexor posturing and a nonreactive pupil. Although the hematoma has expanded at a constant rate over time, the rapid change in the patient's condition is the result of him reaching the critical point where all compensatory mechanisms have been exhausted, thus causing profound rapid changes in the patient's ICP.

## Treatment of Elevated Intracranial Pressure

Acute changes in ICP result in altered LOC, and at times other localizing neurologic findings such as *blown* (dilated, nonreactive) pupils and flexor or extensor posturing, and such findings may be the sign of impending herniation and death without immediate intervention. In a patient without a ventricular drain already in place, hyperventilation is the most rapid mechanism for acutely lowering elevated ICP. Currently, aggressive hyperventilation ($PCO_2 < 30$) is recommended only for short durations in cases of impending cerebral herniation while patients are being stabilized. As stated previously, hyperventilation causes vasoconstriction, which reduces intravascular blood within the cranial vault and almost instantaneously lowering ICP. However, several studies have now shown that the routine use of aggressive hyperventilation in the management of patients with severe closed head injury (CHI) results in decreased outcomes because of hypoxic injury and possible stroke caused by the sustained hyperventilation. Our current practice is to maintain $PCO_2$ values between 35 and 38 with controlled ventilation in all patients with severe CHI; because of this we leave all these patients intubated and mechanically ventilated until their ICPs normalize and all other therapies are withdrawn.

Adequate sedation and pain control are also important elements of ICP control. Patients who are restless and agitated will have higher ICPs than similar patients who are resting quietly in bed. Another important point is the prevention of venous congestion. This occasionally is evident in cervical collars, which are fastened too tight or with the use of trach ties that are wrapped too tightly around the neck to hold the endotracheal tube in place.

Several medications are available for the treatment of elevated ICP with the most common one being mannitol. Although this agent acts as an osmotic diuretic and helps pull excess interstitial fluid into the vascular space and thus lower ICP, there are several other hypothetical mechanisms that probably also increase its efficacy such as increasing

### CURRENT THERAPY

**Management of Elevated Intracranial Pressure**

- Prevention of venous engorgement
- $CO_2$ control (mild hyperventilation)
- Sedation and pain control
- Cerebrospinal fluid drainage
- Mannitol
- Lasix
- Hypertonic saline
- Decompressive craniectomy
- Pentobarbital coma

RBC flexibility, decreasing RBC and platelet clumping in small arterioles and capillaries, and increasing intravascular volume, thus improving cardiac function. Other diuretics such as furosemide (Lasix)[1] or urea (Ureaphil) may also be used but have less dramatic effects on ICP. Hypertonic saline (NaCl 3% to 5%)[1] has also been used more recently by some physicians and has been shown to have many of the same effects as mannitol.

CSF diversion is one of the simplest, quickest acting methods for decreasing ICP especially if a ventricular drain is already in place. The emergent surgical evacuation of mass lesions such as large epidural, subdural, or intraparenchymal hematomas is also extremely effective for controlling ICP, and in many instances it is also life-saving. However, in some instances, underlying brain injury or stroke from prolonged brain compression may be exhibited as massive intraoperative brain swelling and in these instances may necessitate that the bone flap be left off (craniectomy).

## Management of Severe Closed Head Injury

The current recommendations of the Brain Trauma Foundation Guidelines for the management of closed head injuries call for the placement of ICP monitors in all patients who fall into the severe category (GCS score < 9). At our institution we routinely place combination intraventricular monitors and drains in all patients with a postresuscitation GCS score of less than 7. Monitors are inserted into patients with a GCS score of 7 to 9 on an individual basis depending on whether there are distracting reasons, such as intoxication, to cause the altered LOC. If patients are intubated and not following commands but are purposeful in their movements, we will sometimes elect not to place a ventriculostomy and follow the patient's clinical course over several hours. Other factors include CT findings and the need to go to the operating room during the acute period for the treatment of other life-threatening injuries, age, or for heavy sedation secondary to other injuries or pulmonary problems. At times patients in this GCS range will be given 6 to 12 hours and treated medically to see whether or not they improve prior to placement of an ICP monitor.

Once an ICP monitor and drain have been placed elevations in ICP are treated in a systematic order. Target values include attempts to keep ICP less than 15 to 20 and cerebral perfusion pressure (CPP) greater than 60. Low CPP (CPP = mean arterial blood pressure [MAP] − ICP) is caused by either elevated ICP or low MAP. For patients with low MAP or uncontrolled ICP, vasopressors may be used to increase blood pressure (BP) and central venous pressure. At the University of Louisville, dopamine (Intropin) is used as a first line agent, followed by phenylephrine (Neo-Synephrine) and norepinephrine (Levophed) in refractory cases. ICP elevations are initially treated with adequate sedation and pain control, such as midazolam (Versed),[1] propofol (Diprivan), and/or morphine (Lioresal),[1] to prevent agitation and elevated airway pressures, which can further increase ICP and intermittent CSF diversion. In cases where this fails to control ICP, mannitol is then added to the treatment protocol along with more continuous CSF diversion and finally chemical paralysis. Mannitol is administered as a bolus infusion in doses ranging from 0.25 to 1.0 mg/kg body weight every 4 to 8 hours with the endpoints being either ICP control or measured serum osmolarity greater than 315 mOsmL.

Patients who continue to have sustained increases in their ICP despite these interventions are considered to have refractory ICP and at our facility are considered for one of two potential salvage treatments. Pentobarbital (Nembutal)[1] coma has been used successfully on occasion in young patients without mass lesions to decrease the metabolic demands of the brain during these periods of sustained ICP. Patients need to be chosen wisely for this therapy because it carries enormous risks in addition to the possibility of preserving the patient in a long-term, nonfunctional, persistent vegetative state. Initiation of pentobarbital (Nembutal)[1] coma causes severe hypotension, and patients almost always require the use of pressors in addition to

---

[1]Not FDA approved for this indication.

volume expansion. At our facility we also place all of these patients on a Rotorest bed in an attempt to minimize the pulmonary complications that frequently occur with the use of this technique.

The second salvage therapy is decompressive craniectomy. This procedure involves the removal of a significant area of skull, typically almost an entire hemisphere or both frontal regions with opening of the dura. This permits the injured swollen brain to herniate through the opening and is the only intervention that increases the volume of the intracranial compartment, thereby reducing pressure. In addition this technique allows for the evacuation of large hemorrhagic contusions, or in cases of extreme ICP elevations it can be coupled with either frontal or temporal lobectomy. Once again, patients must be selected carefully for this intervention. Decompressive craniectomy is used much more frequently than pentobarbital (Nembutal)[1] coma at our institution. We use this strategy for patients with elevated ICP—more than 30 to 40 for more than 30 minutes—or a significant change in neurologic condition that is nonresponsive to all other interventions. In order for either of these two salvage approaches to be effective, they must be used at the first signs of refractory ICP prior to the occurrence of complications such as ischemic infarcts or brainstem compression or hemorrhage.

Patients treated with decompressive craniectomies are at risk for significant alterations in CSF dynamics that may result in delayed deterioration. Signs of hydrocephalus either in the form of ventriculomegaly or extra-axial or interhemispheric CSF fluid collections will be evident in 50% to 80% of these patients. When necessary these patients will be treated with external ventricular or subdural drains followed by early cranioplasty (replacement of the bone plate). In many instances these changes will resolve following cranioplasty and therefore avoid the need for ventriculoperitoneal shunting, with its associated risks and complications.

All patients with abnormal head CT scans (regardless of GCS score) are treated with close neurologic observation most commonly in an intensive care unit (ICU) setting, serial CT scans (4 to 6 hours later and on PID 1), and placed on 7 days of phenytoin (Dilantin). Temkin and colleagues showed that patients with post-traumatic intracranial hemorrhage were at increased risk of suffering seizures in the acute period; treatment with antiepileptics beyond 7 days did not decrease the risk of these patients from developing epilepsy or delayed seizures but there were increased risks associated with side effects from medication administration. Patients who experience a seizure following CHI (with the exception of acute post-traumatic seizures) should be maintained on antiepileptics for at least 3 to 6 months and possible indefinitely depending on their clinical condition and EEG results. Patients with acute post-traumatic seizures (within the first several minutes following the event) are not felt to be at increased risk for developing further seizures and receive the routine 7-day treatment. At the University of Louisville we have found that changing phenytoin dosing to a weight-based schedule (15 mg/kg load, 2 mg/kg every 8 hours unless elderly [≥70 years old], then 2 mg/kg every 12 hours) increases the chance of achieving a therapeutic dose earlier in the treatment course and lowers the costs of monitoring these agents.

Finally, the treatment of these patients requires a tight-knit group of specialists and ancillary service providers with open communication channels. We have found that the use of a time-independent phased outcome clinical pathway helps maximize the level of patient care and maintain cost-effectiveness. By using such an approach all routine interactions are initiated at the time of admission and each care provider has a clear role and responsibility; one of the most important aspects of this system is the creation of a clinical coordinator whose responsibility includes ensuring that all aspects of patient care and family education are completed at the appropriate intervals. We believe another key component of this is our philosophy toward early feeding (prior to PID 3) and early tracheotomy and percutaneous endoscopic gastrostomy (PEG) feeding tube placement in a majority of these individuals (PID 4). We have shown that such an aggressive approach to these issues helps reduce infectious complications and minimizes length of ICU stay.

# Treatment of Mild and Moderate Traumatic Brain Injury

In many circumstances patients with moderate TBI are treated almost as though they had severe TBI, with the exception of invasive ICP monitoring. Many patients will be intubated at the time of admission and require sedation and adequate pain management. This can be difficult because it is of utmost importance to maintain the ability to perform serial neurologic examinations. Therefore, we commonly use a combination of propofol (Diprivan) infusions and intermittent morphine (Lioresal)[1] injections in these patients, thereby allowing hourly assessment of neurologic function. We have found that a subset of patients (older than age 45 years, multisystem trauma, presence of early pneumonia) with moderate TBI requires more aggressive treatment with early tracheostomy and PEG tube placement and at times ICP monitors.

The subset of patients with moderate TBI who are not intubated at the time of admission are also watched closely in the ICU. Once again, close monitoring of neurologic function and vigorous pulmonary toilet is of key importance because some patients may be lethargic and are at risk of pulmonary decompensation. We have found ipratropium (Atrovent)[1] and albuterol (Proventil)[1] nebulizers and early mobilization minimize pulmonary problems. Patients with progressive lethargy, worsening neurologic function, hypoxia, hypercapnia, or the inability to protect their airways are intubated and placed on mechanical ventilation. Once again, patients unable to tolerate a diet by PID 3 have a nasogastric feeding tube placed to allow for early enteral nutritional support; however, PEG tubes are not placed until later in the hospital course in the predischarge phase because many patients in this category will improve throughout their hospitalization and be able to tolerate an oral diet by the time of discharge.

Patients with mild TBI are treated over a much wider continuum, ranging from discharge from the emergency room (ER) with appropriate adult supervision to observation in the ICU to immediate surgical treatment of surgical mass lesions. The two most important factors in determining treatment algorithms for these patients are presence or absence of abnormal CT findings and neurologic function, with associated symptoms such as nausea, vomiting, dizziness, or visual problems. Headache is a common complaint in all of these patients and must be taken in context with other complaints and imaging results. Patients with severe headaches, dizziness, and vomiting (postconcussive syndrome) may commonly require a brief hospital stay to allow for delayed imaging and at least partial resolution of some of the complaints.

# Early and Delayed Neurologic Changes

Any patient suffering a significant neurologic injury requires close neurologic monitoring. Although most patients remain unchanged or show gradual improvement in the early phases, a small percentage will show signs of neurologic deterioration. At first these signs may be subtle (agitation, mild increase in lethargy, protracted vomiting); but eventually they may become more profound and can be precursors to impending neurologic demise and death. When these changes are the result of either expanding mass lesions or increases in ICP, treatment instituted in the early phases is more likely to be more successful compared to instances when interventions are performed under conditions associated with cerebral herniation syndromes. Thus any patient showing persistent signs of neurologic decline should be promptly evaluated by a physician and many may also require repeat CT scanning.

However, not all neurologic changes are the result of changes in ICP or expansion of mass lesions, and such irregularities may be caused by a long list of other metabolic or neurologic conditions. Some of the more common causes are seizures, strokes (especially from

---

[1]Not FDA approved for this indication.

[1]Not FDA approved for this indication.

carotid or vertebral dissections), electrolyte imbalances, hypoxia, hypercarbia, fever, excess sedation, or drug and/or alcohol withdrawal.

## Concussions and Sports-Related Injuries: Return to Play Guidelines

Over the past 2 decades, the knowledge regarding the detrimental effects of repetitive mild head injuries has led to intense public debate concerning whether athletes should be allowed to return to play following such injuries. Concussions are not uncommon among participants of competitive sports including football, hockey, baseball, and soccer. Concerns regarding the full negative impact of repetitive, almost innocuous injury have led many youth soccer leagues to ban or modify rules regarding *heading* of the ball. In addition, other concerns exist following more severe concussions such as development of other life-threatening neurologic injuries such as subdural or epidural hematomas, development of the double-impact syndrome (rapid uncontrolled increases in ICP following sequential minor traumas), and the long-term neuropsychological impact of these injuries. As a result of these concerns, the guidelines concerning when and if an athlete should be allowed to return to play have undergone modification since development of the earlier criteria. Because of these frequent changes, readers are encouraged to check with their local medical agencies or recent publications and Internet sources if faced with these issues. In short, if a player loses consciousness or has persistent symptoms (>15 to 20 minutes), they should not be allowed to return to play on that day or even not for 1 to 2 weeks following the complete resolution of all symptoms. It should also be stressed that an individual may have a concussion without loss of consciousness and that concussion is defined as any transient change in mental status. To this end many organizations including the National Football League have developed a sideline neuropsychological screening test that can often help illustrate these deficits even when the athlete appears normal.

## Restorative Therapies

Patients suffering any type of TBI can have long-lasting cognitive, psychological, and emotional dysfunction in addition to their functional and neurologic deficits. Although most people assume that the resolution of decreased alertness and consciousness symbolizes resolution of the overall neurologic injury, this is not the case in most patients. In our series of patients with moderate TBI, we found that almost 50% of patients at median follow-up of 27 months complained of persistent emotional or cognitive problems that interfered with their lifestyle despite the fact that they all were discharged from the hospital with a GCS score of 14 to 15. Long-term speech and cognitive therapies as well as individual, group, and family counseling will be helpful for many of these patients.

In the late hospital and early rehabilitative stages, numerous pharmacologic agents may be helpful to overcome some of the neurologic side effects following TBI. Patients with autonomic storms (intermittent episodes of diaphoresis, tachycardia, fever, agitation) may respond to adrenergic antagonists such as clonidine (Catapres)[1] or propanolol (Inderal),[1] in addition to volume resuscitation, morphine (Lioresal),[1] baclofen,[1] and bromocriptine (Parlodel).[1] Patients with hypoarousal are treated with amantadine[1] (Symmetrel), 100 mg at 8 AM and 12 PM, and bromocriptine,[1] 5 to 15 mg every day. Trazodone (Desyrel), 50 to 100 mg at bedtime, may be helpful in restoring sleep-wake cycles, whereas risperidone (Risperdal),[1] olanzapine (Zyprexa),[1] and quetiapine (Seroquel)[1] may be helpful to control agitation and combativeness during the subacute recovery phases.

---

[1]Not FDA approved for this indication.

## Future Considerations

The previously mentioned treatment strategies include what is considered common practice at the University of Louisville; however, newer, more aggressive treatments and monitoring capabilities are always being developed. Some of the newer monitoring systems under development include cerebral oximetry measurements (frequently through invasive indwelling catheters) or cerebral microdialysis systems, in which continuous assessments are performed to determine the concentrations of critical markers such as lactate in the brain or CSF. Both of these methods provide physiologic feedback for the metabolic environment of the brain, are sensitive enough to predict changes in regional oxygenation, and have been found to be correlated with outcomes in small nonrandomized studies.

### REFERENCES

Brain Trauma Foundation: Management and Prognosis of Severe Traumatic Brain Injury. New York, Brain Trauma Foundation, 2000.

Mcilvoy L, Spain DA, Raque G, et al: Successful incorporation of the Severe Head Injury Guidelines into a phased-outcome clinical pathway. J Neurosci Nurs 2001;33(2):72-78, 82.

Miller PR, Fabian TC, Bee TK, et al: Blunt cerebrovascular injuries: Diagnosis and treatment. J Trauma 2001;51(2):279-286.

Temkin NR, Dikmen SS, Wilensky AJ, et al: A randomized, double-blind study of phenytoin for the prevention of post-traumatic seizures. N Engl J Med 1990;323:497-502.

Vitaz TW, McIlvoy L, Raque GH, et al: Development and implementation of a clinical pathway for severe traumatic brain injury. J Trauma 2001;51(2):369-375.

Vitaz TW, McIlvoy L, Raque GH, et al: Development and implementation of a clinical pathway for spinal cord injuries. J Spinal Disord 2001;14(3):271-276.

Vitaz TW, Jenks J, Raque GH, Shields CB: Outcome following moderate traumatic brain injury. Surg Neurol 2003;60(4):285-291.

# Traumatic Brain Injury in Children

Method of
*Stephen R. Deputy, MD*

---

Traumatic brain injury (TBI) is one of the leading causes of death and disability among children, adolescents, and young adults. An estimated 185 per 100,000 children (ages 0 to 14 years) and 550 per 100,000 adolescents (ages 15 to 19 years) are hospitalized each year for TBI. The etiology of TBI varies depending on the age of the patient, with younger children more likely to be injured from falls and pedestrian injuries, and adolescents more often injured in motor vehicle accidents and assaults. Inflicted TBI (shaking-impact syndrome of infancy) is the leading cause of injury-related deaths in children younger than 4 years of age and accounts for 80% of deaths from head trauma in children younger than 2 years of age.

## Types and Severity of Head Injury

*Closed head injury* is the most common type of TBI seen in children. Forces from rapid deceleration are applied diffusely throughout the brain and consciousness is frequently impaired. *Open head injuries*, in which the dura is breached, are caused by focal penetrating forces, and the risk of post-traumatic epilepsy is relatively high.

*Primary brain injury* is caused by the mechanical forces of the trauma itself. Diffuse axonal injury is an example of primary brain injury. During rapid deceleration, angular forces applied to the head cause the brain to rotate about its center of gravity. Shifting regions of differing densities within the brain itself result in shearing along planes such as the gray-white junction, corpus callosum, and brainstem. The shearing of axons effectively serves to "disconnect" the cortex from the brainstem and consciousness becomes impaired. Translational (straight-line) forces applied to the head produce impact-loading contact phenomena, resulting in focal injuries to the scalp, skull, and brain, such as lacerations, skull fractures, cerebral contusions, and epidural hematomas. *Subdural hematomas* may occur because of tearing of fragile dural bridging veins during rapid decelerations.

*Secondary brain injury* follows and is the consequence of primary injury. Examples include hypoxic-ischemic injury (secondary to low cerebral perfusion pressure or anoxia), disrupted cerebral autoregulation, seizures or status epilepticus, diffuse cerebral edema, hydrocephalus, and raised intracranial pressure. The goal of treatment for TBI is to reduce or prevent secondary brain injury from occurring because the primary brain injury has already happened at the time of trauma and cannot be altered.

The severity of TBI can be broken down into mild, moderate, and severe. *Mild* TBI is defined as head trauma with an initial Glasgow Coma Scale (GCS) score of 13 to 15. *Moderate* TBI occurs with an initial GCS score of 9 to 12. *Severe* TBI occurs with an initial GCS score of 8 or less. The GCS is modified for use in infants under the age of 36 months (Table 1).

Special attention should be given to those infants with TBI who do not show evidence of external facial or head trauma and who may not be presented by their caregivers as having a history of head injury. The *shaking-impact syndrome* is usually found in infants younger than 3 years of age with a peak incidence in infants younger than 1 year of age. Presenting symptoms include irritability, lethargy, or coma, apnea or breathing irregularities, and seizures. Retinal hemorrhages may be found in from 65% to 95% of these patients and should be actively looked for with a dilated funduscopic examination in any case where head trauma is suspected. Computed tomography (CT) imaging most commonly shows evidence of acute or remote subdural hematomas with or without evidence of cerebral infarction. Workup should include a skeletal survey to look for evidence of skull, posterior rib, or long bone fractures of different healing stages. Infants may be more susceptible to shaking-impact syndrome given their relatively large head size compared to their underdeveloped neck musculature. Infants also have thinner skulls, and translational forces may cause more severe contusions. Relatively longer subdural veins that bridge the infant's enlarged subarachnoid spaces can be easily lacerated from angular forces, resulting in subdural hematomas.

# Management of Traumatic Brain Injury in Children

## MILD TRAUMATIC BRAIN INJURY

Mild TBI accounts for more than 90% of all pediatric admissions for TBI. Children in this category should have a GCS score of 15 upon arrival to the emergency room, no focal neurologic deficits, and no signs of increased intracranial pressure (ICP). These children may have had a brief loss of consciousness (less than 1 minute), amnesia for the event, an immediate impact seizure, vomiting, or lethargy (as long as the GCS score is 15 during the evaluation). Children without loss of consciousness or amnesia may be observed or sent home with competent caregivers without performing neuroimaging studies. Vigilance for any change in the child's neurologic status should be maintained for up to 72 hours after the injury. If there has been a brief loss of consciousness or amnesia for the event, the risk of intracranial hemorrhage is still relatively low, and it is up to the discretion of the treating physician whether CT imaging is warranted.

Clinical predictors of intracranial hemorrhage are less reliable for children under the age of 2 years, and nonaccidental trauma also comes into consideration in this age group. Therefore, most children under the age of 2 years with TBI should undergo CT imaging followed by careful observation.

## MODERATE TRAUMATIC BRAIN INJURY

Patients who fall within the moderate category generally need more intensive monitoring and medical management to avoid secondary brain injuries. As with all critical illness, attention should first be paid to following the ABCs (airway, breathing, circulation).

### Airway

Patients with a GCS score of 9 or greater usually do not require endotracheal intubation for airway protection, although they should be kept NPO (nothing by mouth) in case of clinical deterioration.

### Breathing

Hypoxemia and hypoventilation may increase ICP, so supplemental oxygen by nasal cannula may be helpful.

### Circulation

It is important to avoid hypotension to maintain adequate cerebral perfusion pressure (CPP). Isotonic intravenous fluids should be provided with care to avoid fluid overload, hypoglycemia, or hyperglycemia. Careful attention should be paid to fluid and sodium balance because these patients may be at risk for developing diabetes insipidus. Likewise, the head of the bed should be raised to 30 degrees and the patient's head kept midline to optimize venous return from the cranium to the right side of the heart. Sedation with short-acting sedatives (propofol [Diprivan] or midazolam [Versed]) or opioids may be necessary to avoid agitation, which can also reduce venous return to the heart.

Early post-traumatic seizures are fairly rare in children with moderate TBI. The need for empirical anticonvulsant therapy in this group remains controversial and should be reserved for those patients in whom raised intracranial pressure is of concern. Likewise, empirical use of mannitol has little clinical support for this group.

**TABLE 1  Glasgow Coma Scale for Children**

| Score | Eyes Open | Best Verbal Response | Best Verbal Response | Best Motor Response (<36 mo) | Best Motor Response (<36 mo) |
|---|---|---|---|---|---|
| 6 | — | — | — | Follows commands | Normal spontaneous movements |
| 5 | — | Oriented and converses | Coos and babbles | Localizes pain | Withdraws to touch |
| 4 | Spontaneously | Confused | Irritable to pain | Withdraws to pain | Withdraws to pain |
| 3 | To verbal commands | Inappropriate words | Cries to pain | Flexor posturing | Flexor posturing |
| 2 | To painful stimuli | Nonspecific sounds | Moans to pain | Extensor posturing | Extensor posturing |
| 1 | None | None | None | No response | No response |

## SEVERE TRAUMATIC BRAIN INJURY

Patients in the severe group are at the highest risk for secondary brain injuries. The following additional interventions are recommended.

### Airway

By definition, these patients have a GCS score of 8 or lower and require endotracheal intubation for airway protection.

### Breathing

Hyperventilation with a goal $P_{CO_2}$ of 26 to 30 mm Hg should be performed only if there is impending brainstem herniation or to bridge the gap until more definitive neurosurgical intervention can be performed to lower intracranial pressure. The benefit of hyperventilation is generally short lived (1 to 24 hours) and may worsen local ischemia following trauma or acute stroke.

### Circulation

In the setting of suspected raised intracranial pressure, the goal of fluid and blood pressure management should be to maintain the cerebral perfusion pressure greater than 50 to 70 mm Hg. Recall that CPP equals MAP (mean arterial blood pressure) minus ICP. Because children generally have a lower MAP than adults, it is not always necessary to provide vasopressor therapy to keep the CPP above 70 mm Hg unless there is evidence of raised ICP. Invasive intracranial pressure monitoring should be considered if the GCS score is lower than 8 or in the setting of elevated ICP to optimize CPP.

## Other Techniques to Lower Intracranial Pressure

### NEUROSURGICAL

Obvious mass lesions, such as hydrocephalus, subdural and epidural hematomas, and contused cortical tissue should be surgically evacuated whenever feasible. CT scanning is able to identify most of these surgical lesions. Decompressive craniectomy is now used more frequently to relieve pressure when multifocal contusions or diffuse cerebral edema is present. As mentioned earlier, ICP monitoring is usually warranted for all severe TBI patients.

### OSMOTHERAPY

Mannitol (20% solution) may be given as an initial bolus of 0.5 to 1 g/kg. Repeat doses of 0.25 to 0.5 g/kg are given every 6 to 8 hours as needed to maintain the serum osmolality and sodium levels to less than or equal to 320 mOsmL and 150 mEq, respectively. Osmotic diuretics should be used with caution in patients with renal insufficiency. The beneficial effects occur within minutes, peak at 1 hour, and last 4 to 24 hours. Potential disadvantages include worsening of focal cerebral edema in areas where the blood-brain barrier is disrupted.

## CURRENT DIAGNOSIS

- Children under the age of 2 years with traumatic brain injury (TBI) may require neuroimaging because clinical predictors of intracranial hemorrhage are less reliable in this age group.
- Children under the age of 1 year presenting with lethargy, irritability, apnea, or seizures should be evaluated with computed tomography (CT) imaging and a dilated funduscopic examination to rule out shaking-impact syndrome.

## CURRENT THERAPY

- Children with mild TBI and a GCS score of 15 at presentation can usually be observed clinically without the need for neuroimaging.
- The goal of treatment for TBI is to minimize *secondary* brain injury.
- In the setting of raised ICP, it is important to maintain CPP above 50 to 70 mm Hg.
- Early post-traumatic seizures are relatively frequent in open head injury and in severe TBI. They should be empirically treated in any patient in whom raised ICP is a concern.
- Direct intracranial pressure monitoring should be considered in any TBI patient with a GCS score of 8 or less.

*Abbreviations:* CPP = cerebral perfusion pressure; ICP = intracranial pressure; GCS = Glasgow Coma Scale; TBI = traumatic brain injury.

## BARBITURATES

Sedating agents may lower ICP by reducing pain as well as by making the brain metabolically less active. Pentobarbital is given as a loading dose of 5 to 20 mg/kg, followed by a continuous infusion of 1 to 4 mg/kg per hour. Continuous EEG monitoring to maintain a burst suppression pattern is warranted with this therapy. Potential disadvantages include systemic hypotension and a long half-life that may interfere with the declaration of brain death.

## ANTICONVULSANT THERAPY

Children with severe TBI are at a high risk for early post-traumatic seizures, which can further elevate the ICP. It is generally recommended empirically to load these children with 20 mg/kg of intravenous phenytoin (Cerebyx). Maintenance therapy can be achieved with 5 mg/kg per day divided every 8 hours with target blood levels of 10 to 20 mg/dL.

## HYPOTHERMIA

More centers are including hypothermia as an option for patients with elevated ICP not responsive to medical or surgical management. The best method of cooling (i.e., whole body versus head only) and the optimal core temperature are not established for children.

Of note, apart from neurosurgical interventions, none of the techniques just described are shown definitively to reduce morbidity or mortality in children with severe TBI.

## REFERENCES

Annegers JF, Grabow JD, Grover RV, et al: Seizures after head trauma: A population study. Neurology 1980;30:683-689.
Bruce DA, Zimmerman RA: Shaken impact syndrome. Pediatr Ann 1989;18:482-494.
Committee on Quality Improvement, American Academy of Pediatrics: The management of minor closed head injury in children. Pediatrics 1999;104(6):1407-1415.
Deputy SR: Shaking-impact syndrome of infancy. Semin Pediatr Neurol 2003;10(2):112-119.
Kraus JF, Nourjah P: The epidemiology of uncomplicated brain injury. J Trauma 1988;28:1637-1643.
Schutzman SA, Barnes P, et al: Evaluation and management of children younger than two years old with apparently minor head trauma: Proposed guidelines. Pediatrics 2001;107:983-993.

# Brain Tumors

Method of
*Ashwatha Narayana, MD, and*
*Eve S. Ferdman, BA*

Primary brain tumors accounted for an estimated 18,400 new cases diagnosed and 12,690 deaths in the year 2004 in the United States. Several histopathologically different tumors arise in the brain, reflecting the diversity of phenotypically distinct cells within the central nervous system (CNS) that have a capacity for neoplastic transformation. Gliomas, the most common tumors, are considered first in this article, followed by a description of many of the principles of brain tumor management. Then less common tumors are briefly presented, and the article closes with a discussion about managing metastatic brain tumors.

## Gliomas

### INCIDENCE

Malignant gliomas make up 35% to 45% of primary brain tumors, and of these, nearly 85% are glioblastoma multiforme. The incidence of anaplastic astrocytoma peaks in children younger than 10 years of age and then remains constant in each subsequent decade of life. In contrast, the incidence of glioblastoma multiforme increases dramatically after the age of 40 years. Low-grade astrocytomas make up 5% to 15% of primary brain tumors and 67% of low-grade gliomas. The remainder of low-grade gliomas are mixed oligoastrocytomas (19%) and oligodendrogliomas (13%). Unlike their malignant counterparts, low-grade gliomas are most common between the ages of 20 and 40 years and rarely occur after the age of 50 years.

### GENETICS AND ETIOLOGY

Genetic abnormalities are demonstrated for 50% to 75% of adult astrocytomas. It is hypothesized that p53 gene mutations are associated with the transition to grade II tumors. Malignant progression to anaplastic astrocytoma is associated with loss of heterozygosity (LOH) for chromosomes 9p, 13q, or 19q and CDK4 gene amplification. Subsequent LOH on chromosome 10 and amplification of the epidermal growth factor receptor genes characterize further progression to glioblastoma multiforme. A second, p53-independent, pathway that leads more directly to glioblastoma multiforme development is also described.

Losses of genetic information from chromosomes 1p and 19q are commonly seen in oligodendroglioma specimens, whereas losses on 17p and p53 gene mutations are notably less frequent, suggesting that early events in their oncogenesis are distinct from those associated with astrocytic tumors.

Although some environmental factors are linked with brain tumor development, they do not appear responsible for most brain tumors. Radiation-induced gliomas are reported, mainly in children with acute leukemia who received prophylactic cranial irradiation and chemotherapy. The hereditary syndromes associated with an increased risk of brain tumors include neurofibromatosis type 1 and neurofibromatosis type 2, tuberous sclerosis, Li-Fraumeni syndrome, familial polyposis, Turcot's syndrome, Gardner's syndrome, and von Hippel-Lindau disease.

### PATHOLOGY

CNS tumors are generally classified as follows (Table 1):

- Gliomas
- Neuronal/glioneuronal neoplasms
- Embryonal neoplasms
- Meningeal neoplasms
- Miscellaneous nonglial neoplasms

Reliance on a pathologic classification of brain tumors is a requisite for treatment. Indeed, histopathology is more important than anatomic staging in determining the clinical behavior and prognosis of these tumors. Neuropathologists do not all agree on a uniform classification system for astrocytic gliomas. The World Health Organization system, which divides astrocytic tumors into four grades—from grade I, corresponding to pilocytic astrocytomas, to grade IV, corresponding to the glioblastoma multiforme—is used more often.

Low-grade astrocytomas are well-differentiated tumors that display increased cellularity compared with normal brain tissue and have mild to moderate nuclear pleomorphism (Figure 1). The cytoplasmic processes that extend from the astrocytes contain a characteristic filamentous protein, glial fibrillary acidic protein (GFAP), which provides an immunohistochemical marker for these tumors. Over time, at least 50% of these tumors transform into more anaplastic lesions. The characteristic histopathologic features of anaplastic astrocytomas include moderate hypercellularity, moderate cellular and nuclear pleomorphism, variable mitotic activity, and microvascular proliferation. The presence of tumor necrosis is the hallmark that distinguishes anaplastic astrocytoma from glioblastoma multiforme (Figure 2).

Oligodendrogliomas, in contrast, are composed of small uniform cells with round central nuclei and distinct cytoplasmic borders. Formalin fixation causes a perinuclear halo that produces a "fried egg" or "honeycomb" appearance. The cells lack fibrillary cytoplasmic processes. Calcification is a frequent feature.

### CLINICAL PRESENTATION

The presenting symptoms and signs of brain tumors include those associated with a mass effect and increased intracranial pressure and those that are focal. The most common presenting symptom with gliomas is headache. Approximately two thirds of adult patients with low-grade astrocytomas and 20% of patients with malignant tumors present with seizures but are otherwise neurologically intact. Others exhibit a slowly progressive neurologic syndrome consisting of headache, vomiting, motor deficit, visual or sensory loss, language disturbance, or personality change. Symptoms may be present for months or years before the diagnosis is made.

### ROUTES OF SPREAD

The most common route of spread for gliomas is through local extension. As they enlarge, malignant gliomas extend directly into adjacent lobes and disseminate along anatomically defined nerve fiber pathways. Multicentric gliomas are found in less than 5% of patients. Dissemination by seeding through the CPF pathways occurs in approximately 10% of cases but is usually a late event. Metastases rarely arise outside the CNS.

### DIAGNOSTIC STUDIES

Computed tomography (CT) and magnetic resonance imaging (MRI) play indispensable roles in the management of brain tumors. CT is a reliable screening and diagnostic method for suspected supratentorial brain tumor lesions. MRI, now more frequently used in patients with malignant brain tumors, is the screening procedure of choice for diagnosing and localizing tumors in the brainstem, posterior fossa, and spinal cord. Ordinary astrocytomas appear as diffuse, poorly defined, low-density, nonenhancing lesions. Approximately 40% of ordinary astrocytomas enhance, and calcification is found in 10% of cases. Although the majority of malignant gliomas enhance with contrast media, as many as 30% of anaplastic astrocytomas present as nonenhancing lesions. In both low-grade and malignant gliomas, parenchymal infiltration by isolated tumor cells may be present in regions of T2-weighted abnormality that appear normal on CT (Figures 3 and 4). Positron emission tomography (PET), single-photon emission computed tomography (SPECT) with thallium-201 ($^{201}$Tl), and magnetic resonance spectroscopy (MRS) are other imaging approaches used in brain tumor management.

**TABLE 1** Histopathology of Brain Tumors

| Major Classification | Variants | WHO Grade |
|---|---|---|
| **Gliomas** | | |
| Astrocytic: circumscribed | Pilocytic astrocytoma | I |
| | Subependymal giant cell astrocytoma (SEGA) | I |
| | Pleomorphic xanthoastrocytoma (PXA) | II |
| Astrocytic: diffuse | Astrocytoma | II |
| | Anaplastic astrocytoma | III |
| | Glioblastoma multiforme | IV |
| Oligodendroglial | Oligodendroglioma | II |
| | Anaplastic oligodendroglioma | III |
| Mixed gliomas | Oligoastrocytoma | II |
| | Anaplastic oligoastrocytoma | III |
| Ependymal | Subependymoma | I |
| | Myxopapillary ependymoma | I |
| | Ependymoma | II |
| | Anaplastic ependymoma* | III |
| Choroid plexus | Choroid plexus papilloma | I |
| | Choroid plexus carcinoma* | III |
| **Cranial and Peripheral Nerve Tumors** | Schwannoma | I |
| **Neuronal and Glioneuronal Tumors** | Gangliocytoma/ganglioglioma | I–III |
| | Desmoplastic infantile ganglioma (DIG) | I |
| | Dysplastic cerebellar gangliocytoma | I |
| | Central neurocytoma | I |
| | Dysembryoplastic neuroepithelial tumor | I |
| | Paraganglioma | I |
| **Pineal Parenchymal Tumors (PPTs)** | Pineocytoma | II |
| | PPT with intermediate differentiation | III |
| | Pineoblastoma | IV |
| **Embryonal Tumors** | Medulloepithelioma* | IV |
| | Primitive neuroectodermal tumor (PNET),* including medulloblastoma and variants* | IV |
| | Atypical teratoid/rhabdoid tumor (AT/RT) | IV |
| | Cerebral neuroblastoma/ganglioneuroblastoma | IV |
| | Ependymoblastoma* | IV |
| | Olfactory neuroblastoma (esthesioneuroblastoma) | IV |
| **Meningeal Tumors** | Meningioma | I |
| | Atypical meningioma | II |
| | Anaplastic (malignant) meningioma | III |
| **Germ Cell Tumors** | Hemangiopericytoma† | II–III |
| | Germinoma | NA |
| | Mature teratoma | NA |
| | Nongerminomatous germ cell tumors | NA |
| **Tumors of the Sellar Region** | Craniopharyngioma: adamantinomatous | I |
| | Craniopharyngioma: papillary | I |
| **Hemopoietic Neoplasms** | Primary central nervous system lymphoma (PCNSL) | NA |
| | Secondary lymphoma/leukemia | NA |
| | Histiocytic tumors and histiocytoses | NA |
| **Secondary Tumors/Metastases** | Carcinomas and sarcomas | NA |

*Indicates those tumors with a tendency to disseminate throughout the central nervous system (CNS).
†The origin of hemangiopericytoma is uncertain.
*Abbreviations:* WHO = World Health Organization; NA = not applicable.

## STAGING

No accepted staging system exists for primary brain tumors. The American Joint Committee on Cancer proposed a staging scheme for primary brain tumors based on tumor size and metastases as well as tumor grade. Because this system was not generally adapted to clinical use, it was subsequently removed.

## PROGNOSTIC FACTORS

Age, histologic appearance, Karnofsky performance score (KPS), mental status, duration of symptoms, neurologic functional class, extent of surgery, and radiation dose are identified as significant partitioning covariates in clinical trials. This information is important for correctly interpreting the results of studies comparing different treatment regimens and for assessing the potential of new therapeutic methodologies.

## STANDARD THERAPEUTIC APPROACHES FOR GLIOMAS

### Surgery

The combination of surgery, radiation therapy, and chemotherapy represents the standard approach to the treatment of gliomas. The goals of surgery are to provide a histologic diagnosis, to alleviate

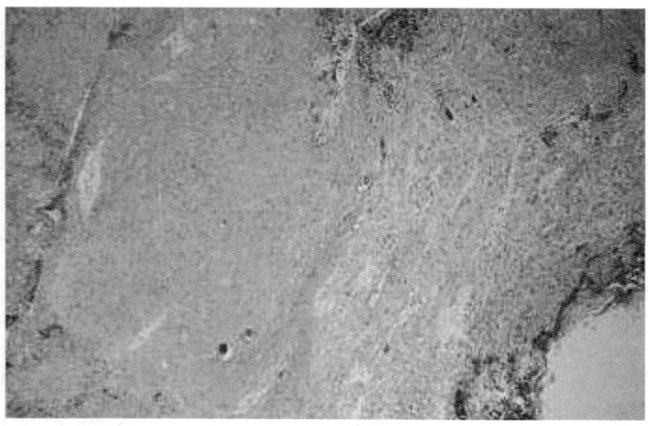

**FIGURE 1.** Low-grade astrocytoma showing mildly increased cellularity with uniform cells and nuclei.

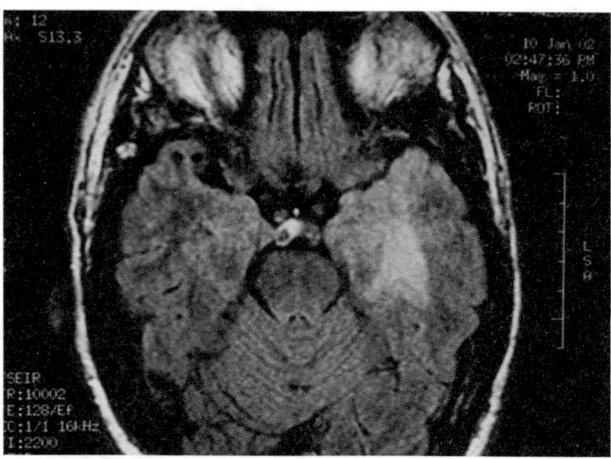

**FIGURE 3.** Axial magnetic resonance imaging scan of low-grade astrocytoma of left temporal lobe.

intracranial hypertension and focal neurologic deficits because of a mass effect, and to permit rapid corticosteroid dose tapering. Pilocytic astrocytomas are relatively well circumscribed, and 60% to 80% are amenable to total removal. Resection of the more common diffuse astrocytomas is limited by the lack of clear demarcation between the infiltrating tumor and normal brain tissue. Evidence suggests that patients with more complete resections live longer and have an improved functional status compared with those who undergo a biopsy or partial resection only. Advances in neurosurgery, including diagnostic ultrasound, lasers, ultrasonic tissue aspirators, cortical mapping, functional imaging, and computer-assisted stereotactic laser techniques, have improved the ability of neurosurgeons to radically remove intracranial tumors.

### Radiation Therapy

Limited radiation fields are used for the treatment of gliomas. Three-dimensionally designed complex treatment plans with multiple fields are used whenever appropriate to limit the high-dose volume and to minimize the risk of long-term radiation sequelae. Doses of 50.4 to 54 Gy are usually recommended for low-grade gliomas and 59.4 to 60 Gy for high-grade gliomas. Rapid fractionation schemes (such as 30 to 36 Gy) may be appropriate for some elderly or poor performance status patients with glioblastoma multiforme who have relatively short survival expectancies.

In low-grade gliomas, the role of radiation therapy is debatable. Although it improves disease-free survival, overall survival is not altered, indicating that deferring postoperative therapy is an option for selected group of patients. Evidence also indicates that lower doses of radiation therapy are probably as effective as higher doses of radiation for low-grade gliomas.

Randomized trials provide seminal evidence that external beam irradiation favorably affects the outcome of malignant gliomas. These trials demonstrate both a significant survival advantage and ability to maintain a full or partial working capacity for irradiated patients.

### Chemotherapy

Chemotherapy has little established role in adult low-grade astrocytomas, but adjuvant chemotherapy is part of the standard therapeutic regimen for malignant gliomas. The addition of chemotherapy to radiation therapy improves the 1-year survival by 10% and the 2-year survival by 8.6%. The nitrosoureas, especially BCNU (N,N'-bis(2-chloroethyl)-N-nitrosourea, carmustine), are the most active single agents. No benefit of chemotherapeutical agents such as

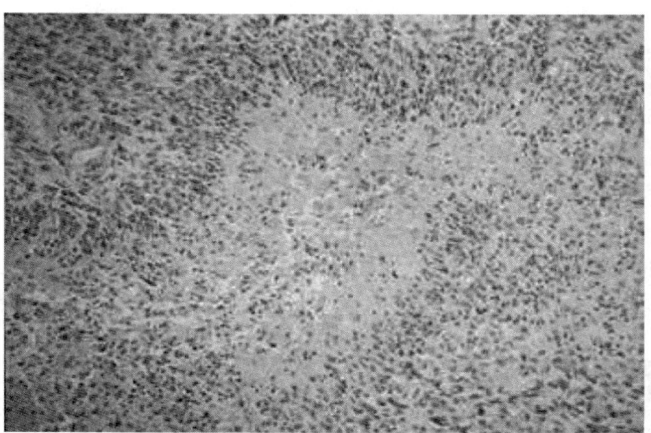

**FIGURE 2.** Glioblastoma multiforme with the hallmark features of necrosis with peripheral pseudopalisading of neoplastic nuclei.

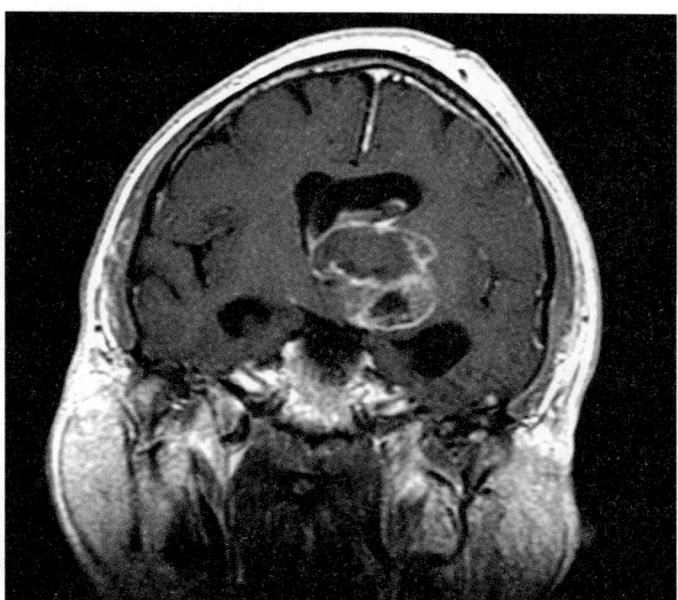

**FIGURE 4.** Coronal magnetic resonance imaging scan of high-grade astrocytoma of left internal capsule and brainstem region.

tirapazamine, topotecan (Hycamtin), paclitaxel (Taxol), B-IFN (Avonex), and thalidomide (Thalomid) is noted when used with standard radiation in clinical trials. Temozolomide (Temodar) is an alkylating agent that demonstrates an improvement in survival by an additional 2 to 3 months when given concurrently with radiation in high-grade gliomas. Anaplastic oligodendrogliomas are chemosensitive tumors. PCV (procarbazine, lomustine [CCNU], and vincristine) chemotherapy regimens produce response rates of 50% to 75% in both recurrent and newly diagnosed anaplastic oligodendrogliomas. Unfortunately, improved response to chemotherapy does not translate into improved survival for these tumors.

Some of the newer biologic agents explored today in gliomas include tyrosine kinase inhibitors, matrix metalloproteinase inhibitors, and antitenascin antibodies.

### Outcome

The 5-year recurrence-free survival rates of patients with low-grade astrocytomas or mixed oligoastrocytomas who undergo total or radical subtotal tumor resection range from 52% to 95%. The median survival times for high-grade gliomas using conventional radiation therapy alone or with chemotherapy consistently range from 9 to 14 months. The median survival for patients with glioblastoma multiforme is 10 to 12 months, whereas the 3-year survival rate is only 6% to 8%. The median survival for patients with anaplastic astrocytoma is 36 months, and the 3-year survival rate is approximately 50%.

# Uncommon Primary Brain Tumors

## PRIMARY CENTRAL NERVOUS SYSTEM LYMPHOMA

Primary CNS lymphomas (PCNSLs) represent approximately 2% to 5% of all intracranial neoplasms. During the last 2 decades, the incidence has increased in both the AIDS and immunocompetent general population. PCNSLs most frequently arise in the supratentorial paraventricular region of the brain. Multifocal tumors are present at diagnosis in 25% to 50% of immunocompetent patients and in 60% to 80% of AIDS patients. Cytologic examination of CPF reveals malignant cells in up to two thirds of immunocompetent patients and in nearly all AIDS patients. The neoplastic cells are similar to those of non-Hodgkin's lymphoma arising in extranodal sites. Single or multiple uniformly contrast-enhancing lesions in the paraventricular regions, basal ganglia, thalamus, or corpus callosum on MRI are characteristic findings.

The role of surgery is to establish a tissue diagnosis only. Primary CNS lymphomas respond dramatically to corticosteroid therapy. At least 90% of patients improve clinically, whereas 40% of lesions shrink considerably. Whole-brain irradiation with corticosteroids is the standard treatment for PCNSL. Recommended doses range from 36 to 45 Gy. Several reports document improved survival when chemotherapy is added to radiation therapy. The outcome is better with high-dose methotrexate-based regimens, often combined with intrathecal chemotherapy.

Survival times for primary CNS lymphoma with no treatment or steroids alone are approximately 1 to 4 months. The median survival for radiotherapy alone varies from 12 to 20 months. Median survival times for treatment programs that include high-dose methotrexate-based chemotherapy range from 33 to 42 months.

## EPENDYMOMA

Ependymomas represent approximately 5% of all intracranial gliomas. The incidence peaks at 5 years and again at 34 years of age. Approximately 60% to 70% of ependymomas arise in the infratentorial brain. Ependymomas are separated into low-grade and high-grade lesions. The 5-year survival for low-grade tumors ranges from 60% to 80%, whereas it varies from 10% to 47% for high-grade tumors. Supratentorial ependymomas generally have a poorer prognosis than their infratentorial counterparts.

Most ependymomas cannot be completely excised because of their location and growth characteristics. Postoperative irradiation improves local tumor control and survival and is an accepted part of the standard treatment for these tumors. Although most ependymomas are slow growing, others are more aggressive and may disseminate throughout the CSF pathways. Current therapy for high-grade ependymomas after surgical debulking is with local fields to a dose of 59.4 Gy. The value of chemotherapy in adults with ependymomas and anaplastic ependymomas is not well defined.

## BRAINSTEM GLIOMA

Brainstem gliomas account for less than 2% of brain tumors. Children constitute approximately two thirds of the reported cases. Diagnostic imaging is sufficient for the majority of the cases. The role of surgery is minimal and limited to biopsy only if there are questions about the diagnosis. Radiation therapy alone by conventional fractionation to 54 Gy in symptomatic or large brainstem lesions is recommended. Chemotherapy does not show any benefit in the management of brainstem gliomas. The median survival time is 9 to 12 months.

## MEDULLOBLASTOMA

Medulloblastoma accounts for a third of pediatric brain tumors and is the most common tumor arising in the posterior fossa in children. It arises from the roof of the fourth ventricle or from the vermis. The presenting symptoms include headache, vomiting, and imbalance. On microscopic examination, small blue undifferentiated cells are noted consistent with primitive neuroectodermal tumor. CSF involvement is noted in 25% to 40% of the patients. Five-year survival rates range from 50% to 80%, and 10-year rates vary from 40% to 55%.

Surgery involves maximal resection of the tumor. Radiation therapy to the entire craniospinal axis is essential. The dose to the craniospinal axis is 23.4 to 36 Gy. A boost of 18 to 31.4 Gy is given to the posterior fossa to bring the total to 54 Gy. The role of chemotherapy is to decrease the craniospinal radiation dose and to improve the survival in poor-risk patients. Combinations of vincristine, CCNU, and cis-platinum are used.

# Brain Metastases

## EPIDEMIOLOGY

Metastases to the brain occur in as many as 30% of patients with systemic cancer and represent the most common type of intracranial tumor. Brain metastases exert a profound effect on the quality and length of survival, and despite the best current management, they represent the direct cause of death in 25% to 30% of affected patients. Melanoma and carcinomas of the lung, breast, and colorectum have a higher propensity to metastasize to the brain. Approximately 50% of patients present with a solitary lesion. Most brain metastases, particularly those that arise from primary sites other than the lung, occur at a late stage when metastatic dissemination is present elsewhere in the body.

## STANDARD TREATMENT APPROACHES

Because the majority of patients with metastatic brain lesions have or will soon develop widely disseminated disease, treatment is dictated by the need to achieve immediate short-term palliation and the desire for durable symptom-free remission. The median survival of patients with symptomatic brain metastases is approximately 1 month without treatment and 2 months with corticosteroid administration. Survival is longer and the quality of life better if brain metastases are treated.

### Corticosteroids

Corticosteroids rapidly ameliorate many symptoms of brain metastasis and should be used at the onset for all symptomatic patients. Symptomatic but stable patients can begin with approximately 16 mg of dexamethasone daily in two to four divided doses. Patients who are receiving whole-brain irradiation should receive steroids for at least 48 hours before treatment. Steroid tapering may begin during week 2 of radiotherapy. For patients receiving 16 mg of dexamethasone, the drug should be tapered by 2 to 4 mg every fifth day.

## Surgery

Surgery establishes the diagnosis of metastatic brain disease when it is uncertain and serves as a treatment for single metastases. Surgery can provide better local control and immediate relief of neurologic signs and symptoms because of a mass effect. Surgically treated patients also live longer, have fewer recurrences of cancer in the brain, and enjoy a better quality of life compared with those treated by radiotherapy alone. Only 10% of patients are ideal candidates for surgical extirpation, however.

## Whole-Brain Radiation Therapy

Radiotherapy is the appropriate treatment for most patients with brain metastases, including those with multiple lesions and those with single metastases who are not candidates for surgery. The standard approach is to treat the whole brain to 30 Gy in 10 daily fractions over 2 weeks. Depending on the symptom, the response rate varies from 70% to 90%. Neurologic function is improved overall in 50% of patients. The median survival with radiation therapy is 4 to 6 months. Overall, 75 to 80% of remaining life is spent in an improved or stable neurologic state.

## Stereotactic Radiosurgery

Stereotactic radiosurgery (SRS) is an excellent alternative to surgical extirpation of solitary and multiple brain metastases. The procedure involves the delivery of a single large dose of radiation to a small volume of the brain region under stereotactic frame guidance. Recently, data from a large randomized trial show that addition of SRS to whole-brain radiation therapy improves both the survival and the quality of life in patients with limited brain metastases. Although surgery and SRS have never been compared directly in a clinical trial, local control, survival, and quality of life in selected patients seem comparable in retrospective trials.

## Chemotherapy

Chemotherapy can be considered in selected patients who progress locally after whole-brain irradiation. Systemic chemotherapy shows a response rate of 25% to 50%. Temozolomide shows promise both as an adjuvant to whole-brain radiation therapy and in patients who fail radiation therapy.

## REFERENCES

Andrews DW, Scott CB, Sperduto PW, et al: Whole brain radiation therapy with or without stereotactic radiosurgery boost for patients with one to three brain metastases: Phase III results of the RTOG 9508 randomised trial. Lancet 2004;363:1665-1672.

Deangelis LM, Hormigo A: Treatment of primary central nervous system lymphoma. Semin Oncol 2004;31:684-692.

Henson JW, Gaviani P, Gonzalez RG: MRI in treatment of adult gliomas. Lancet Oncol 2005;6:167-175.

Jemal A, Tiwari RC, Murray T, et al: Cancer statistics, 2004. CA Cancer J Clin 2004;54:8-29.

Kleihues P, Cavenee WK: Pathology and Genetics: Tumours of the Nervous System, 2nd ed. Lyon, France, IARC Press, 2000, pp 6-7.

Narayana A, Leibel SA: Primary and metastatic brain tumors in adults. In Leibel SA, Philips TL (eds): Textbook of Radiation Oncology, 2nd ed. Philadelphia, WB Saunders, 2004, pp 463-496.

Patchell RA, Tibbs PA, Regine WF, et al: Postoperative radiotherapy in the treatment of single metastases to the brain: A randomized trial. JAMA 1998; 280:1485-1490.

Reifenberger G, Collins VP: Pathology and molecular genetics of astrocytic gliomas. J Mol Med 2004;82:656-670.

# The Locomotor System

## Rheumatoid Arthritis

Method of
*Eric L. Matteson, MD, MPH*

Rheumatoid arthritis (RA) is a common chronic disease of the immune system characterized by polyarthritis and a variety of systemic features. It often leads to articular cartilage and bone damage, physical dysfunction, and work disability. The disease affects 1% to 2% of persons worldwide, typically developing in the fourth to sixth decades, with predominance among women of approximately 2.5:1. RA may be associated with extra-articular inflammatory features, including fatigue, subcutaneous nodules, pleuritis and pericarditis, interstitial lung disease, vasculitis, and Sjögren's syndrome. Patients with RA have excess mortality due principally to extraarticular disease and increased atherosclerotic cardiovascular disease. Other concerns in RA patients are listed in Box 1.

Steady decline in joint function caused by progressive cartilage damage, bone erosions, and tendon rupture as well as systemic features are responsible for work disability rates among patients with RA that are more than 50% within 10 years of disease onset. Joint damage begins early, and bone erosions are detectable within 2 years of disease onset in as many as 70% of patients. In some patients, RA progresses rapidly, leading to early work disability if effective therapy is not started to control the inflammatory response and joint damage.

Initial treatment of the polyarthritis is with a combination of nonsteroidal anti-inflammatory agents (NSAIDs) and when needed corticosteroids to provide sufficient time to confirm the persistence of joint inflammation and complete the diagnostic evaluation. Disease-modifying antirheumatic drugs (DMARDs) are then added, because over the long term they lessen joint damage and disability. DMARDs (Box 2) are defined by the ability to reduce the signs and symptoms as well as slow the progression of joint damage, as measured by radiographic changes in the amount of bone erosions and joint space narrowing.

Prompt DMARD treatment is critical to improve disease control and outcome. The goals of treatment include:

- Early diagnosis and intervention
- First-line therapy with DMARDs that reduces progressive joint damage followed by adding to or changing DMARDs if disease activity persists
- Management of comorbidities such as disease- and treatment-related osteoporosis

DMARDs that can be used effectively alone or in combination represent an important advance in treatment. Still, RA remains a chronic illness, usually requiring lifelong anti-inflammatory and immunomodulating treatment to limit joint damage and minimize disability (see Box 2).

## Diagnosis

In the absence of a definitive diagnostic test, the diagnosis of RA is based on clinical features and supportive laboratory tests. The American College of Rheumatology (ACR) 1987 criteria require at least four of seven features to be present for longer than 6 weeks to classify a patient as having RA for the purpose of clinical research (Table 1). The ACR criteria are highly sensitive (95%) but only modestly specific (75% to 89%) for making the clinical diagnosis of RA in patients with established disease.

Characteristic radiographic lesions are only present in up to 70% of patients within the first 2 years of disease. Recently, both musculoskeletal ultrasound (US) and magnetic resonance imaging (MRI) have been shown to detect erosive lesions early in the disease course, in

---

**BOX 1    General Medical Concerns in Rheumatoid Arthritis**

- Infection
  - Immunizations
  - Prompt treatment of infections
  - Tuberculosis and hepatitis screenings
- Lifestyle
  - Control of blood pressure (corticosteroids, NSAIDs, cyclosporine, extraarticular disease all contribute to hypertension)
  - Control of lipids
  - Smoking cessation
- Prevention of GI bleeding
  - Antacids
  - Coxibs where appropriate
  - $H_2$-blockers
  - Proton pump inhibitors
  - Avoid NSAIDs whenever possible
- Osteoporosis treatment and prevention (osteoporosis is common in rheumatoid arthritis)
  - Calcium 1200-1500 mg/day
  - Vitamin D 400 IU/day
  - Consider an antiresorptive agent such as a bisphosphonate for all patients on long-term corticosteroids, including men
- Moisturization for patients with sicca symptoms

## BOX 2   Drugs Used to Treat Rheumatoid Arthritis

### Traditional DMARDs

- Azathioprine (Imuran)
- Cyclosporine (Neoral)
- Gold (intramuscular or oral) (Myochrysine, Auranofin)
- Hydroxychloroquine (Plaquenil)
- Leflunomide (Arava)
- Methotrexate (Trexall)
- Minocycline (Dynacin)
- Sulfasalazine (Azulfidine)

### Biological Response Modifiers

- Anti B-cell therapy: Rituximab (Rituxan)
- Anti-TNF monoclonal antibodies
  - Adalimumab (Humira)
  - Infliximab (Remicade)
- Soluble TNF receptor
  - Etanercept (Enbrel)
- IL-1 receptor antagonist
  - Anakinra (Kineret)
- T-cell signaling inhibitor: Abatacept (Orencia)

*Abbreviations:* DMARD = disease-modifying antirheumatic drug; IL = interleukin; TNF = tumor necrosis factor.

many cases before they are evident on plain radiographs. Antibodies to cyclic citrullinated peptides (anti-CCP) detected in serum aid the diagnosis. They are more specific but less sensitive for the diagnosis of RA than serum rheumatoid factor (RF). The presence of RF or anti-CCP increases the diagnostic sensitivity for RA to more than 80%; the presence of both increases diagnostic sensitivity to more than 95%.

## TABLE 1   American College of Rheumatology Criteria for Rheumatoid Arthritis Diagnosis*

| Criterion | Definition |
| --- | --- |
| Morning stiffness | In and around joints, lasting at least 1 h before maximal improvement |
| Arthritis in at least three joint areas | Simultaneously involved by soft tissue swelling or fluid observed by a physician |
| Arthritis of hand joints | At least one area swollen: wrist, MCP, PIP |
| Symmetric arthritis | Simultaneous involvement of the same joint areas on both sides of the body |
| | Bilateral involvement of PIPs, MCPs, or MTPs acceptable without absolute symmetry |
| Rheumatoid nodules | Subcutaneous nodules over bony prominences, extensor surfaces, or in extraarticular regions observed by a physician |
| Serum rheumatoid factor | Abnormal amounts by any method for which the result has been positive in <5% of normal control subjects |
| Radiographic changes | Typical of RA on posteroanterior hand and wrist radiographs, which must include erosions or unequivocal bony decalcification localized or most obvious adjacent to involved joints (osteoarthritis changes alone do not qualify) |

*Abbreviations:* MCP = metacarpophalangeal; MTP = metatarsalphalangeal; PIP = proximal interphalangeal; RA = rheumatoid arthritis.
*Patient must satisfy four of the seven criteria listed. Criteria 1 through 4 must be present for at least 6 weeks.

Primary care providers play an important role in the diagnosis of RA. Recognition of inflammatory arthritis and prompt referral to rheumatologists lead to early initiation of effective joint-protective therapies. Early inflammatory polyarthritis might not always meet diagnostic criteria for RA; however, approximately 30% of these cases of undifferentiated arthritis ultimately evolve into RA (see Table 1).

The importance of early accurate diagnosis of RA has grown with evidence that early DMARD therapy can alter the natural history of the disease. Strategies using single or a combination of initial DMARD therapies are employed. Studies of initial combinations of traditional DMARDs such as methotrexate (Trexall), sulfasalazine (Azulfidine), and hydroxychloroquine (Plaquenil) have shown that early introduction of combination therapy with and without corticosteroids improves long-term radiographic outcomes. The more intensive use of DMARDs, especially methotrexate and the biological response modifiers, has lessened disability and improved survival in patients with RA. Treatment with the more aggressive use of DMARDs has resulted in a decreasing need for joint surgery in recent years.

## Treatment

### THERAPEUTIC GOALS

Successful treatment of RA is predicated on reductions in symptomatic joint pain and swelling, relief of joint stiffness, return of lost function, and prevention of joint damage (Figure 1). Clinically, response to therapy can be determined by examining joints for tenderness and swelling, obtaining laboratory measures of inflammation (erythrocyte sedimentation rate [ESR] and C-reactive protein [CRP]), and assessing patient-reported outcomes using questionnaires, such as the Health Assessment Questionnaire (HAQ), or visual analogue scales of global well-being. Long-term therapy goals include reducing joint damage (joint erosions and joint space narrowing), missed work days, delaying disability, and decreasing early mortality (see Figure 1).

Both short- and long-term goals can be reached using DMARDs, which reduce joint inflammation and retard the development of radiographic joint damage. The most commonly used DMARD, methotrexate, has a long track record of efficacy and acceptable toxicity and is often the treatment with which other agents or regimens are compared. Other DMARDs used previously for the treatment of RA, such as gold salts, penicillamine (Cuprimine), azathioprine (Imuran), and cyclophosphamide (Cytoxan),[1] are rarely used today because of either relatively poor efficacy or excessive toxicity.

Biological response modifiers (BRMs) have been a major advance in RA therapy for many patients with RA, with improved safety and efficacy profiles. The Current Therapy box summarizes the current treatment approaches to RA. Box 3 summarizes drug therapy for RA.

### METHOTREXATE

Methotrexate (MTX) is a purine antimetabolite that reduces symptoms of joint inflammation and decreases radiographic joint damage in patients with RA. MTX is the most common anchor DMARD. It is generally well tolerated. Most patients still use the drug after 5 years of treatment.

Side effects may be minor, including nausea, diarrhea, mucosal ulcerations, and alopecia. Serious complications include hepatotoxicity and bone marrow suppression. Hepatotoxicity is typically characterized by fibrosis and cirrhosis, which occur rarely with frequent monitoring for possible toxicity. Minor toxicities are an infrequent cause of MTX discontinuance and can often be managed with folic acid supplementation or by switching from oral to parenteral administration. ACR guidelines recommend monitoring hepatic transaminases and serum albumin at 4- to 8-week intervals and reserving liver biopsy for an otherwise unexplained decrease in albumin or persistent or recurrent elevation of transaminases.

MTX-induced pneumonitis is rare. It typically develops early after initiation and is characterized by cough, dyspnea, and fever. Chest

---

[1]Not FDA approved for this indication.

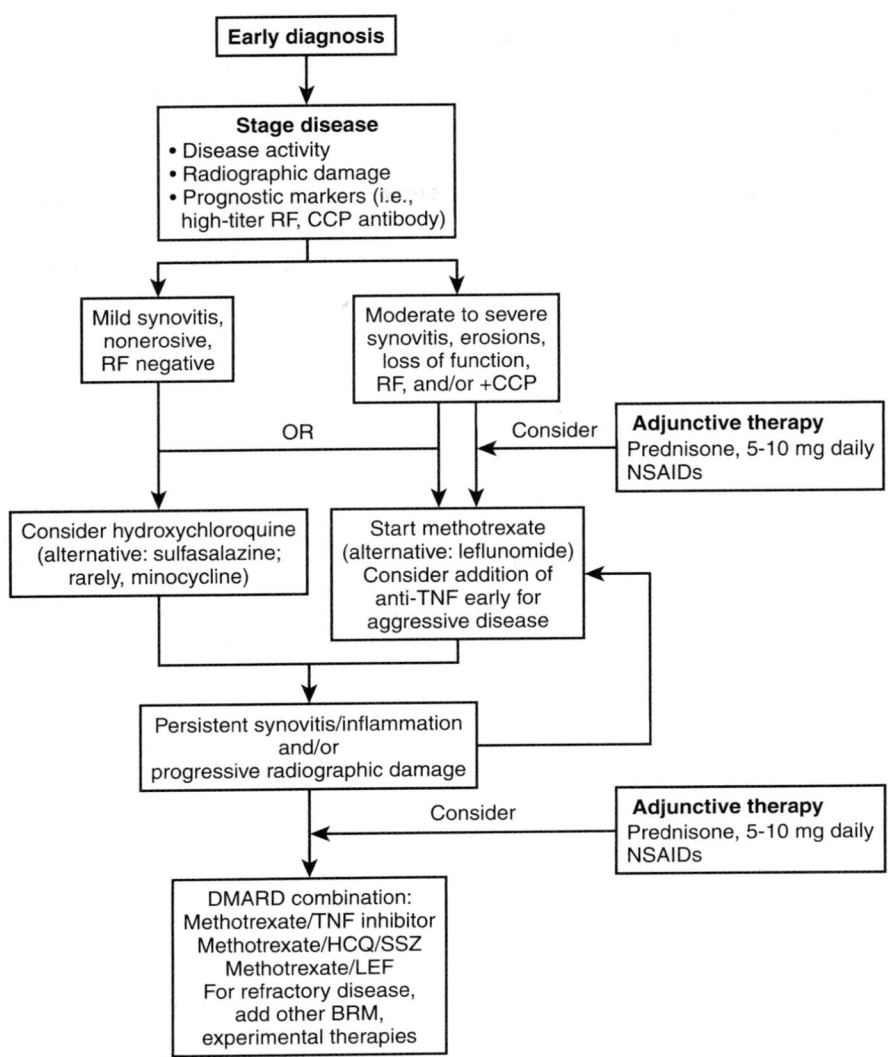

**FIGURE 1.** This flow diagram illustrates key decision points for rheumatoid arthritis therapy and has been adapted from the recommendations of the American College of Rheumatology. *Abbreviations:* BRM = biological response modifier; CCP = anticyclic citrullinated antibody; DMARD = disease-modifying, antirheumatic drug; HCQ = hydroxychloroquine; LEF = leflunomide; MTX = methotrexate; NSAID = nonsteroidal anti-inflammatory drug; RA = rheumatoid arthritis; RF = rheumatoid factor; SSZ = sulfasalazine; TNF = tumor necrosis factor. (From the American College of Rheumatology Subcommittee on Rheumatoid Arthritis Guidelines: Guidelines for the management of rheumatoid arthritis: 2002 update. Arthritis Rheum 2002;46:328-323.)

---

| BOX 3 Drug Therapy for Rheumatoid Arthritis |
|---|

**Control of Symptoms: Pain and Swelling, Loss of Function**
*NSAIDs and Other Analgesics as Needed*
- Consider patient age, sex, past medical history (GI bleeding, etc.).
- Consider cost and convenience (dosing frequency).
- These are not disease modifying.

*Corticosteroids*
- Oral.
  - It is controversial whether corticosteroids are disease modifying. In general, less is better.
  - Severe polyarticular disease: 2-15 mg/d, often in divided doses (e.g., 2 mg tid). Use split dosing because of the short half-life of the anti-inflammatory effect of oral steroids. It is desirable but often not possible to avoid continuous corticosteroid therapy.
  - Serious systemic disease (vasculitis, scleritis): 40-60 mg/d, tapering according to response.
- Intraarticular for single recalcitrant joints.

**Control of Disease with DMARDs**
  DMARDs may be used with NSAIDs. Corticosteroids may be given if needed.

*Continued*

## BOX 3 Drug Therapy for Rheumatoid Arthritis—cont'd

### Initiating DMARD Therapy

- Start DMARD therapy as soon as the diagnosis is strongly suspected or established.
  - Mild disease: MTX is preferred; hydroxychloroquine and sulfasalazine are also useful.
  - Moderate disease: MTX or leflunomide (±hydroxychloroquine, sulfasalazine, others). Use bridge therapy: Initially treat with a combination of DMARDs ±corticosteroids, tapering off steroids and DMARDs as disease is better controlled. Biological response modifiers may be considered at this point.
  - Severe or recalcitrant disease: Combination therapies of two or three DMARDs. Add biological response modifier therapy; consider experimental therapies.
- In general, the effect of DMARDs is apparent in 1 to 4 wk (BRMs) to 1 to 2 mo (MTX, leflunomide). It can take 3 to 6 mo to know whether hydroxychloroquine or sulfasalazine are effective.
- Add to or change DMARDs within 3 to 4 mo of initiating therapy if there has not been an adequate response.

### Tapering DMARD Therapy

- Rheumatoid arthritis is a chronic condition. The goal of therapy is long-term disease control and prevention of joint and organ damage. DMARDs can only infrequently be stopped without disease recrudescence.
- When symptoms are well controlled, taper corticosteroids, then taper the NSAIDs (or use NSAIDs on an as-needed basis).
- Continue with DMARD therapy indefinitely. If the patient does well and has no signs of active disease for 6 to 12 mo, the DMARD therapy can be carefully tapered.
- If the patient is doing well on combination DMARD therapy, attempt to taper one of these drugs. MTX is often viewed as anchor therapy and generally is continued long term if the patient is on baseline MTX.
- If a patient is on combination therapy, consider tapering one of the DMARDs if the patient has been in remission for at least 6 mo.
- DMARD therapy should not be completely discontinued until a patient has been in complete remission for at least 1 y on treatment. Even then, a very few patients with bona fide, seropositive rheumatoid arthritis remain in treatment-free remission.

### Extra-articular Disease

- Serositis, vasculitis, and scleritis require systemic corticosteroids and might require immunosuppressive agents such as cyclophosphamide[1] or cyclosporine.
- Consider BRMs, especially anti-B-cell therapy, for severe extraarticular disease.

---

[1]Not FDA approved for this indication.
*Abbreviations:* BRM = biological response modifier; DMARD = disease-modifying antirheumatic drug; MTX = methotrexate; NSAID = nonsteroidal anti-inflammatory drug.

---

radiographs reveal diffuse interstitial changes. Pneumonitis should be managed by immediately discontinuing the drug and considering corticosteroid treatment in severe cases. Pneumonitis often recurs with rechallenge; therefore, patients experiencing this complication should be treated with an alternative DMARD. MTX is contraindicated in patients with impaired renal function, because delayed clearance increases drug levels and, hence, the risk of side effects.

MTX is administered in once-weekly doses. It is important to maximize the beneficial effects of MTX by titrating to 20 to 25 mg[3] per week, because lower doses are often less effective. There has been little additional benefit observed in patients treated with doses greater than 25 mg per week; however, toxicities become more common at these higher doses. Folic acid (folate), generally 1 mg daily, reduces the occurrence and frequency of some toxicities (Table 2).

## INHIBITORS OF TUMOR NECROSIS FACTOR-α

TNF-α is a pleiotropic cytokine expressed by activated T lymphocytes and macrophages. It upregulates production of other proinflammatory cytokines, including interleukin 1 (IL-1) and IL-6, matrix metalloproteinases, and reactive oxygen intermediates, that provoke inflammation and injure articular cartilage and bone. In addition, TNF-α is an important promoter of immune-competent cells including receptor activation of nuclear factor-κB ligand (RANK ligand) expression that leads to differentiation and activation of osteoclasts. In RA, osteoclasts are responsible for articular bone loss characterized by erosions and osteopenia. TNF-α also has a role in the differentiation of

synoviocytes into a fibroblastic phenotype that confers invasive, tumor-like qualities on these cells. Fibroblast-like synoviocytes form the synovial pannus, a tumor-like mass unique to rheumatoid joints that invades and damages cartilage.

Clinical studies of several TNF-inhibiting agents have demonstrated the therapeutic benefits of TNF blockade on RA disease activity and joint damage. The three TNF-inhibiting drugs approved for the treatment of RA—etanercept (Enbrel), infliximab (Remicade), and adalimumab (Humira)—appear similarly efficacious for the treatment of this disease, but they have not been directly compared in clinical trials. Many clinical trials have compared treatment using TNF inhibitors and MTX to placebo-control patients on MTX alone. In these trials, 40% to 60% of patients on anti-TNF agents met ACR-20 criteria for improvement at week 20 (Box 4). Approximately 10% to 20% of patients improved even more, reaching ACR-70 criteria.

The TNF-blocking agents are generally well tolerated. However, an increased risk of reactivation of latent tuberculosis has led to the recommendation in the United States and certain other countries that a purified protein derivative (PPD) skin test should be performed before the patient begins taking a TNF inhibitor. A chest radiograph should be obtained in patients with a history of tuberculosis exposure, positive PPD, or emigration from countries where tuberculosis is endemic. Patients who have a positive PPD or history of tuberculosis should be treated with appropriate therapy before initiating anti-TNF agents.

Clinical trials of TNF inhibitors in patients with advanced congestive heart failure and multiple sclerosis suggest that these conditions may be exacerbated by these drugs. Demyelinating syndromes have been reported rarely in association with therapeutic TNF blockade. TNF inhibitors have been associated in trials with a slight increase in

---

[3]Exceeds dosage recommended by the manufacturer.

**TABLE 2  Disease-Modifying Antirheumatic Drug Monitoring**

| DMARD | Tests | Interval |
|---|---|---|
| Methotrexate (MTX, Trexall) | Hepatic transaminases, serum creatinine, CBC, albumin | Baseline and every 4-8 wk |
| | CXR, HBV and HCV serology, β-hCG | Baseline |
| Leflunomide (Arava) | Hepatic transaminases, serum creatinine, CBC, albumin, HBV and HCV serology, β-hCG | Baseline |
| | ALT | Monthly for 6 mo, then every 6-8 wk |
| | Hepatic transaminases, serum creatinine, CBC, albumin | Every 6-8 wk |
| TNF inhibitors: etanercept (Enbrel), infliximab (Remicade), adalimumab (Humira) | PPD, CXR (if positive PPD, emigration from TB-endemic country, or TB exposure history), CBC | Baseline, thereafter undetermined |
| Sulfasalazine (Azulfidine) | CBC, hepatic transaminases, creatinine | Baseline and then every 2 wk for 1-3 mo, then every 4 wk for 3 mo, then every 12 wk |
| Hydroxychloroquine (Plaquenil) | Ophthalmologic evaluation: visual acuity and retinal function tests | Baseline and then yearly |
| Cyclosporine (Neoral) | Serum creatinine, hepatic transaminases, CBC, potassium, BP | Baseline and then every 2 wk until dosage is stable, then every mo |
| Azathioprine (Imuran) | CBC, hepatic transaminases, creatinine | Baseline and then every 2 wk for 2-3 mo, then monthly for 3 mo, then every 2-3 mo |
| Anakinra (Kineret) | CBC | Baseline, then undetermined |
| Rituximab (Rituxan) | CBC, screen PPD, CXR, HBV and HCV serology | Baseline, then undetermined |
| Abatacept (Orencia) | CBC, screen PPD, CXR, HBV and HCV serology | Baseline, then undetermined |

*Abbreviations:* ALT = alanine aminotransferase; BP = blood pressure; CBC = complete blood count; CXR = chest radiograph; DMARD = disease-modifying antirheumatic drug; G6PD = glucose-6-phosphatase deficiency; HBV = hepatitis B virus; hCG = human chorionic gonadotropin; HCV = hepatitis C virus; PPD = purified protein derivative; TB = tuberculosis.

minor infections (primarily upper respiratory), although concerns about increased overall risk of infection with TNF therapy remains undefined. Postmarking surveillance suggests that infections with organisms that promote granulomatous inflammatory responses, such as histoplasmosis, coccidioidomycosis, and listeriosis might occur more often in patients treated with TNF inhibitors. There have been rare reports of lupus-like syndromes characterized by rash, serositis, and development of antinuclear and anti–double-stranded DNA autoantibodies.

Three TNF-inhibiting agents are commercially available. Etanercept is a soluble TNF-receptor type II (p75)-to-Fc fusion protein. Infliximab is a chimeric human-to-mouse monoclonal anti-TNF antibody, and adalimumab is a fully human anti-TNF monoclonal antibody. Etanercept (Enbrel) is administered by a subcutaneous injection at a dose of 25 mg twice weekly or 50 mg once weekly. Adalimumab is administered subcutaneously at a dose of 40 mg every 2 weeks. Infliximab is given as an intravenous infusion. Standard initial dosing for infliximab calls for 3 mg/kg to be given at 0, 2, and 6 weeks, followed by regular infusions at 8-week intervals. The dosage may vary among patients from 3 to 10 mg/kg, and the interval may be adjusted between 4 and 8 weeks, depending on the patient's clinical response.

Although TNF inhibitors may be used as monotherapy, more commonly, they are added to MTX or other DMARD therapy to improve disease control and possibly reduce some antibody formation, especially with infliximab. However, clinical trials in early RA suggest that combining MTX with a TNF inhibitor may be more effective than either therapy alone.

## OTHER DISEASE-MODIFYING ANTIRHEUMATIC DRUGS

Other DMARDs may be used alone or in combination to treat RA. Some traditional DMARDs such as gold and D-penicillamine are now rarely used because of poor efficacy and toxicity. In some cases of mild RA, agents such as hydroxychloroquine or minocycline (Dynacin)[1] may be useful. Hydroxychloroquine is an antimalarial drug that may be used alone in early and mild RA or as part of a combination regimen (see Box 3). It is typically prescribed at doses of 5 to 7.5 mg/kg/day (200-400 mg daily). The primary serious side effect, although rare, is retinal toxicity, so routine (at least annual) ophthalmologic evaluation is suggested. Gastrointestinal side effects and skin rashes can also occur.

Leflunomide (Arava) is a pyrimidine antimetabolite that has been shown in clinical trials to be as efficacious as MTX. The recommended starting dose is 20 mg/day. The dose may be reduced to 10 mg/day when used in combination with MTX or if the starting dose is not tolerated. Leflunomide side effects are typically observed beginning 2 to 4 weeks after starting treatment. The most important serious toxicities are hepatoxicity and cytopenias. Therefore, laboratory monitoring (see Table 2) of hepatic transaminases and a complete blood count should be performed at 4- to 8-week intervals. Some patients

---

**BOX 4  American College of Rheumatology Criteria for Improvement in Rheumatoid Arthritis**

- Requires 20% improvement in the following two:
  - Tender joint count (68 joints)
  - Swollen joint count (66 joints)
- Requires 20% improvement in each of the first three:
  - Patient assessment of pain (10 cm visual analogue scale)
  - Patient assessment of disease activity (10 cm visual analogue scale)
  - Physician global assessment of disease activity (10 cm visual analogue scale)
  - Patient assessment of physical function (HAQ score)
  - Serum CRP or erythrocyte sedimentation rate

*Abbreviations:* CRP = C-reactive protein; HAQ = Health Assessment Questionnaire; RA = rheumatoid arthritis.

---

[1]Not FDA approved for this indication.

## CURRENT THERAPY

- The goals of therapy are the control of symptoms, prevention of joint destruction and loss of function, and prevention and management of disability.

**Classes of Agents**

- Analgesics and NSAIDs, including coxibs and aspirin
- Second-line or slow-acting antirheumatic drugs (DMARDs)
  - Hydroxychloroquine, methotrexate, sulfasalazine, gold, azathioprine, leflunomide
  - Biological response modifiers (including TNF-antagonists): etanercept, infliximab, adalimumab
  - Anakinra (IL-1 receptor agonist)
  - T-cell signaling inhibitor abatacept
  - B-cell lysis: rituximab
- Others
  - Experimental and chemotherapeutic agents including cyclophosphamide, cyclosporine; minocycline
  - D-Penicillamine[1] and gold now rarely used
- Glucocorticosteroids

**Treatment Strategy: Early in the Disease**

- Proper diagnosis is essential
- Physical modalities
  - Physical therapy, occupational therapy consultation
  - Joint protection and functional enhancement
  - Splints, orthotics, adaptive and adequate footwear, adaptive devices
  - Range-of-motion exercises for affected joints
  - Appropriate stretching, strengthening, and conditioning exercises
- Disease education
  - Disease treatment and prognosis
  - Vocational and avocational counseling
  - Lifestyle and family counseling
  - Self-esteem
  - Home modifications

---

[1]Not FDA approved for this indication.
*Abbreviations:* coxib = selective cyclooxygenase-2 inhibitor; DMARD = disease-modifying antirheumatic drug; GI = gastrointestinal; IL = interleukin; NSAID = nonsteroidal anti-inflammatory drug.

---

develop hypertension and peripheral neuropathy related to the drug. Leflunomide is an alternative to MTX as a first-line DMARD in patients intolerant of MTX or with mild renal insufficiency. Leflunomide may be used in combination with TNF inhibition.

Other DMARDs include sulfasalazine and cyclosporine (Neoral). With respect to efficacy, these agents are comparable with MTX as monotherapy, and they improve control of synovitis when combined with MTX. Sulfasalazine treatment is started at 500 mg twice daily and may be titrated gradually to 3.0 gm/day,[3] divided in two or three doses. Gastrointestinal toxicity can limit the dose. Interval monitoring for hepatotoxicity and cytopenias is also required (see Table 2). Cyclosporine is used at doses of 100 to 400 mg a day depending on body weight and tolerance. It is started at 2.0 to 2.5 mg/kg/day in two divided doses. It may be titrated to 4.5 to 5 mg/kg/day,[3] but the dose may be limited by hypertension or renal toxicity. Long-term side effects such as nephrotoxicity and hirsutism make it difficult for most patients to maintain therapy with cyclosporine for long periods.

---

[3]Exceeds dosage recommended by the manufacturer.

---

Gold salts are now infrequently initiated for RA and have a generally unfavorable efficacy and safety profile. Many patients are forced to discontinue gold because of side effects that include cytopenia, nephropathy, and cutaneous hypersensitivity.

Anakinra (Kineret), a recombinant IL-1 receptor antagonist (IL-1ra), is a biological agent that blocks the proinflammatory activities of IL-1. IL-1 shares many of the proinflammatory actions of TNF-α in promoting the symptoms of arthritis and joint damage in RA. Anakinra is a naturally occurring anti-inflammatory molecule that competes with soluble IL-1β for binding to cells expressing the IL-1 receptor type 1. It reduces joint pain and swelling when administered in combination with MTX to patients with RA that is refractory to MTX monotherapy. Anakinra is given by self-administered daily subcutaneous injection (100 mg/day). Many patients develop local injection site reactions, but these are self-limited and usually subside over time. Anti-TNF agents are generally preferred over anakinra for reasons of efficacy and safety. The costs of all BRMs are substantial.

Azathioprine and cyclophosphamide are traditional cytotoxic agents that have demonstrated efficacy in RA, but their use is limited by toxicity. Cyclophosphamide in particular is usually reserved for life-threatening, extraarticular manifestations of RA such as interstitial lung disease or vasculitis.

## ABATACEPT

Abatacept (Orencia; CTLA-4Ig) is a recombinant fusion protein that blocks T-cell activation by means of signaling inhibition. T-cell activation requires two signals, the first of which is related to antigen presentation through a major histocompatibility complex peptide and the second of which acts by binding of a T-cell costimulatory receptor to the antigen presenting cell (APC). This costimulatory signal occurs by CD28-CD80/86 (B7) binding to the ligand on the APC. With T-cell activation, cytotoxic T-lymphocyte associated antigen (CTLA-4) becomes expressed, leading to deactivation of T-cells. Competitive binding of CTLA-4 to CD80 and CD86 prevents this interaction between CD28 and CD80, thereby interfering with the second costimulatory signaling required for T-cell activation.

Studies of abatacept have demonstrated significant improvement in ACR20 responses used in patients with refractory disease. The drug is administered by 30-minute infusion, with the second infusion given at 2 weeks following the first infusion, then at 4 weeks following the first infusion, and then every 4 weeks thereafter. The dose is 500 to 1000 mg per infusion, depending on body weight. Side effects include hypersensitivity and possible increased risk of infections. It is not clear whether the drug predisposes to malignancy. Drug monitoring is, as yet, undefined. The drug may be used with conventional DMARDs but should not be used with other biological response modifiers.

## RITUXIMAB

Rituximab (Rituxan) is a chimeric murine/human monoclonal antibody directed against the CD20 antigen on B-lymphocytes, leading to B-cell lysis. Like T cells, B cells play an important role in the pathophysiology of rheumatoid arthritis and are important to T-cell activation, cytokine production, and production of rheumatoid factor. Rituximab use results in prompt depletion of peripheral B-lymphocytes, which can remain depleted for months and even years following therapy. Standard treatment in rheumatoid arthritis is an initial dose of rituximab at 1000 mg given at 2-week intervals. Patients often require re-treatment after a varying amount of time, generally after 6 months. The B cells may be peripherally depleted even with recrudescence of disease, so they have not been useful parameters to follow for disease remission or recrudescence.

Rituximab is usually administered together with methotrexate. Acute infusion reactions can occur; methylprednisolone (Solu-Medrol), 100 mg IV is recommended 30 minutes before each infusion to reduce the probability and severity of infusion reactions. Rituximab can lead to severe hypersensitivity reactions and possibly infections. However, serious infections have not been demonstrated to be more common in rituximab-treated patients than in placebo-treated patients.

## COMBINATION THERAPY

Although many patients' disease appears to be well controlled using a simple DMARD, persistent synovitis or progressive radiographic joint damage is common with such an approach. The current treatment paradigm favors a rapid step-up strategy, which calls for the addition of a second or third DMARD if synovitis persists despite adequate dosing with a single DMARD (see Box 3). One approach is to add a TNF inhibitor to MTX. Another approach is triple therapy, which consists of sulfasalazine and hydroxychloroquine in addition to MTX. Biologic response modifiers should not be combined with each other. Available data suggest that combination therapy improves radiographic and functional outcomes for patients with RA inadequately controlled with a single DMARD.

## CORTICOSTEROIDS

Corticosteroids are potent anti-inflammatory agents used since 1948 for controlling signs and symptoms of synovitis in RA. The use of corticosteroids in RA is limited by the side effects associated with long-term therapy and by concerns about their effectiveness as true DMARDs. For short periods, higher doses (0.25-0.5 mg/kg/day) may be used to control severe flare-ups of arthritis (see Box 3). However, corticosteroids are most commonly used in low daily doses (5 to 10 mg/day) as bridge treatment while a concomitantly administered DMARD takes effect or as adjuvant therapy to control persistent symptoms in patients with DMARD-refractory disease.

In clinical studies, low-dose corticosteroids can reduce the number of radiographic erosions that develop early after disease onset. These doses are rarely sufficient to completely control synovitis and are, therefore, most commonly used in conjunction with traditional DMARDs or biological agents. Low-dose corticosteroids are generally well tolerated, but complications, particularly osteoporosis and diabetes, are possible and the patient should be carefully monitored for them. Intraarticular injection of corticosteroids is useful for managing individual inflamed joints or joints responding slowly to systemic therapies.

## NONSTEROIDAL ANTI-INFLAMMATORY DRUGS

NSAIDs are widely used to reduce pain, swelling, and stiffness in joints affected by RA. Although NSAIDs are useful adjunctive agents, they are not considered disease-modifying drugs. Traditional NSAIDs inhibit cyclooxygenase (COX) enzymes and thereby block the conversion of arachidonic acid into prostaglandins, molecules that can stimulate inflammation. There are two major forms of COX enzymes, COX-1 and COX-2. COX-1 is expressed constitutively in the gastric mucosa, where it functions to protect the stomach from luminal acid secretion, and in the kidney, where it serves to maintain renal perfusion. COX-2 is expressed at sites of inflammation and is also expressed constitutively in the kidney.

Traditional NSAIDs, which block the function of both COX-1 and COX-2, have anti-inflammatory effects, but they also produce gastrointestinal toxicity that can manifest as gastritis, peptic ulcers, and hemorrhage, or enteritis. NSAID toxicity may be significantly reduced by proton pump inhibitor therapy. NSAIDs that specifically antagonize COX-2 activity, termed *coxibs* (celecoxib [Celebrex]), have anti-inflammatory efficacy similar to that of the nonselective NSAIDs, but they cause less gastrointestinal toxicity. The gastrointestinal benefits of coxibs may be reduced by the concurrent use of aspirin. Coxibs have a variable propensity to increase the risk of cardiovascular and cerebrovascular events.

## Summary

The effectiveness of RA treatment has improved dramatically with recent advances in early diagnosis, the development of less toxic and more effective disease-modifying treatments, and more intensive DMARD regimens that control persistent synovitis and progressive radiographic damage. Recognition of the impact of associated disorders including osteoporosis and atherosclerotic disease, in addition to appropriate therapeutic intervention for these disorders, will likely result in improved morbidity and mortality rates among patients with RA. Most patients today are able to live productively with RA because of the timely use of effective DMARDs, including BRMs, to control the signs and symptoms of disease. The future holds an improved diagnostic and therapeutic armamentarium, which promises to afford even better disease control and less disability.

## REFERENCES

Arnett FC, Edworthy SM, Bloch DA, et al: The American Rheumatism Association in 1987 revised criteria for the classification of rheumatoid arthritis. Arthritis Rheum 1988;31:315-324.

Emery P, Fleischmann R, Filipowicz-Sosnowska A, et al: The efficacy and safety of rituximab in patients with active rheumatoid arthritis despite methotrexate treatment: Results of a phase IIB randomized, double-placebo-controlled, dose-ranging trial. Arthritis Rheum 2006;54:1390-1400.

Fries JF, Williams CA, Morfeld D, et al: Reduction in long-term disability in patients with rheumatoid arthritis by disease-modifying antirheumatic drug–based treatment strategies. Arthritis Rheum 1996;39:616-622.

Genovese NC, Becker JC, Schiff M, et al: Abatacept for rheumatoid arthritis refractory to tumor necrosis factor alpha inhibition. N Engl J Med 2005;353:1114-1123.

Kremer JM, Genovese MC, Cannon GW, et al: Concomitant leflunomide therapy in patients with active rheumatoid arthritis despite stable doses of methotrexate: A randomized, double-blind, placebo-controlled trial. Ann Intern Med 2002;137:726-733.

Landewe RB, Boers M, Verhoeven AC, et al: COBRA combination therapy in patients with early rheumatoid arthritis: Long-term structural benefits of a brief intervention. Arthritis Rheum 2002;46:347-356.

Lee D, Schur PH: Clinical utility of the anti-CCP assay in patients with rheumatic diseases. Ann Rheum Dis 2003;62:870-874.

Matteson EL: Extraarticular features of rheumatoid arthritis and systemic involvement. In Hochberg MC, Silman AJ, Smolen JS, et al (eds): Rheumatology, 3rd ed. Edinburgh: Mosby, 2003, pp 781-792.

O'Dell JR, Haire CE, Erickson N, et al: Treatment of rheumatoid arthritis with methotrexate alone, sulfasalazine and hydroxychloroquine, or a combination of all three medications. N Engl J Med 1996;334:1287-1291.

St. Clair EW, Wagner CL, Fasanmade AA, et al: The relationship of serum infliximab concentrations to clinical improvement in rheumatoid arthritis: Results from ATTRACT, a multicenter, randomized, double-blind, placebo-controlled trial. Arthritis Rheum 2002;46:1451-1459.

van Everdingen AA, Jacobs JW, Siewertsz Van Reesema DR, Bijlsma JW: Low-dose prednisone therapy for patients with early active rheumatoid arthritis: Clinical efficacy, disease-modifying properties, and side effects: A randomized, double-blind, placebo-controlled clinical trial. Ann Intern Med 2002;136:1-12.

# Juvenile Idiopathic Arthritis

Method of
*Terry L. Moore, MD*

Juvenile rheumatoid arthritis (JRA), now mainly known by the International League of Associations of Rheumatologists (ILAR) classification as juvenile idiopathic arthritis (JIA), is a protean disorder whose variable modes of onset and patterns of disease course are accompanied by a myriad of diverse signs, symptoms, and manifestations. JIA affects approximately 250,000 children in the United States. No distinct race predilection is noted at this time. It is the most common disease cause of children missing school in the United States. It is also the second leading cause of eye pathology in children. JIA presents a difficult diagnostic problem because of its lack of specific serologic abnormalities. This represents a dual problem to a clinician in that it makes it difficult to establish an early diagnosis of JIA when the clinical picture is not clear, and even after the diagnosis is established, it is difficult to know when the disease has remitted or an exacerbation is beginning. The diagnosis of JIA is usually made clinically. Serologic studies can be informative, but in the past no routine laboratory tests have been diagnostic.

## CURRENT DIAGNOSIS

- Diagnose early and treat aggressively.
- Reduce inflammation and symptoms.
- Suppress joint activity and reduce erosions to prevent disability.
- Establish a team approach with pediatric rheumatologist, ophthalmologist, physical therapist, and occupational therapist.

Diagnostic criteria for JIA include children younger than 16 years with persistent arthritis of one or more joints for at least 6 weeks. Arthritis is defined as swelling of a joint or limitation of motion with heat, pain, and tenderness.

## JIA Subtypes

These are the seven basic subgroups or categories of JIA:

1. **Polyarthritis (RF positive)**: 19S IgM rheumatoid factors (RF) are present in the peripheral blood on testing and usually anticyclic citrullinated peptide antibodies (αCCP Ab). This group is manifested by arthritis in five or more joints in the first 6 months of disease. The joints most commonly affected are peripheral joints, including the knees, ankles, wrists, and fingers, but all synovial joints can become involved. There may also be an associated tendonitis. The classical joints involved are predominantly the metacarpophalangeal (MCP) and proximal phalangeal (PIP) joints producing fusiform-shaped swelling of the fingers. The knees are usually the first joints to limit function. They may exhibit deformity and flexion contractures. Polyarthritis (RF positive) is seen in approximately 5% to 10% of the children with JIA. The incidence of this type increases with age with the highest incidence found in adolescent females. The disease course in these children is generally believed to be one of a lifelong constantly active, or recurrent, relapsing pattern. It is associated with subcutaneous nodules and a higher incidence of vasculitis than the other forms of JIA. Radiograph films may show erosions with greater frequency than other forms of arthritis in children and may be helpful in diagnosis. Antinuclear antibodies (ANA) are present in approximately 80%.

2. **Polyarthritis (RF negative)**: This group by definition also has arthritis in five or more joints involved during the first 6 months; however, RF testing is negative, but αCCP Ab may be present. The disease pattern is similar to that of the RF-positive polyarthritis group. The course of these patients may be long term; however, most improve over a period of time. This type of onset occurs in approximately 20% to 30% of children with JIA. This type also shows female predominance.

3. **a. Oligoarthritis (pauclarthritis) with iridocyclitis** (inflammation of the iris and ciliary body in the posterior uveal tract of the eye): Oligoarthritis is manifested by arthritis of one or more joints involved in the first 6 months, but less than five joints. This type of onset is seen in approximately 50% of children with JIA and again shows female predominance. The most common children presenting are younger than 4 years at onset and have ANA present on testing. The ANA positivity is found in approximately 90% of the children developing chronic iridocyclitis. This group

has a very good prognosis with little residual joint damage. There may be occasional asymmetric growth and leg length differences that develop; however, the process usually produces no long-term abnormalities. Approximately 50% of these children develop some type of iridocyclitis. Most children with iridocyclitis are easily controlled with anti-inflammatories such as naproxen, local steroid drops, or mydriatics (dilators). Therefore, any child being considered for a diagnosis of JIA requires frequent slit-lamp examinations by an ophthalmologist. **b. Extended oligoarthritis**: This type has an oligoarticular onset and then becomes more widespread, developing polyarthritis with five or more joints involved after the first 6 months of disease.

4. **Enthesitis related**: This category is predominantly seen in males who may later develop sacroiliitis and ankylosing spondylitis. This type of onset is associated with an enthesitis such as Achilles tendonitis or arthritis of the lower extremities again involving fewer than five joints in the first 6 months. The large joints, such as knees, ankles, hips, and sacroiliac joints, are usually involved. Anterior uveitis may be associated. The onset type is predominantly male, usually from 8 to 14 years of age, and may progress on to true ankylosing spondylitis. It is seen in approximately 10% to 15% of children with JIA. There is a high incidence of familial predisposition in these patients with an 80% to 95% occurrence of the HLA-B27 antigen found. Sacroiliitis is often present on radiographs before symptoms develop and precedes the development of real limitation of motion of the spine.

5. **Systemic arthritis**: Initially seen with daily temperatures rises usually late afternoon from normal to exceeding 39°C (103°F) in an intermittent, spiking pattern. This usually occurs for more than 2 weeks. The onset of this type may include a salmon-colored, transient skin rash, lymphadenopathy, splenomegaly, hepatomegaly, pleuritis, pericarditis, or abdominal pain. It is seen in approximately 20% of children with JIA. RF, αCCP Ab, and ANA are usually negative, but white blood cell counts may exceed 30 to 40,000/mm³. Erythrocyte sedimentation rate (ESR) and C-reactive protein (CRP) are elevated and anemia may rapidly develop. This group also shows a male predominance. Approximately 50% of children develop an oligoarticular pattern and remit quickly, but many of the children go on to develop a long-term symmetric polyarthritis. This type of onset causes the most consternation in the diagnosis because it may mimic severe localized infections, sepsis, or neoplasms, such as lymphomas or leukemias.

6. **Psoriatic arthritis**: Arthritis and psoriasis or dactylitis with nail pitting and onycholysis. Usually there is a first-degree relative with a psoriasis. RF is negative.

7. **Other arthritis**: Children with arthritis of unknown cause that persists for at least 6 weeks and does not fulfill criteria for any of the other categories or fulfills criteria for more than one of the other categories.

## JIA Evaluation

The workup on a JIA patient includes a complete blood count (CBC) that may show an anemia, leukocytosis, and thrombocytosis in systemic onset. ESR and CRP are quite high in systemic and polyarticular disease but may be minimally elevated or normal in oligoarticular disease. RF is only positive in the late-onset polyarticular patients and αCCP Ab also mainly appears in this group but may be seen in a small number of RF-negative polyarticular and oligoarticular patients. ANA are found in the polyarticular group and also in the oligoarticular group, associated with the presence of iridocyclitis. Other immunologic testing and liver, muscle, and kidney function tests should be in the normal range. Radiographs should be performed of involved joints looking for periarticular demineralization, joint space narrowing, and/or erosions.

## JIA Prognosis

The course and outcome of JIA is generally good, however, the disease needs to be treated early and aggressively to prevent asymmetrical skeletal development, osteopenia, chronic eye disease, or systemic manifestations. Approximately 75% of the children do well long term, with the oligoarticular group rarely having any residual damage. Approximately 25%, usually found in the polyarthritis and systemic groups, develop continuous arthritis with some long-term disability.

## JIA Therapy

The therapy of JIA begins with the use of physical and occupational therapy (PT/OT). The object of PT is to strengthen muscles, improve range of motion, and decrease the impact loading on the joints. The object of OT is to improve body mechanics, posture, and other modalities to decrease any kind of impact loading on the joints. Medical therapy begins with the judicious use of nonsteroidal anti-inflammatory drugs (NSAIDs). Oligoarthritis patients are usually placed on a NSAID, usually naproxen (Naprosyn), at a dosage of 10 to 20 mg/kg in two divided doses. Naproxen has an advantage over other NSAIDs in that it comes in both a tablet and a liquid form at 125 mg/5 mL and has a long half-life so it can be given in two doses, which is more amenable to taking before and after school for compliance. The other nonsteroidal in tablet form generally used is tolmetin sodium (Tolectin) at a dosage of 20 to 30 mg/kg in three to four divided doses. One other medication, meloxicam (Mobic), which comes in a tablet and a liquid form, was recently approved by the Food and Drug Administration (FDA). It has an advantage of a long half-life and can be given once daily at dosages of 0.125 to 0.25 mg/kg. The liquid form is 7.5 mg/5 mL. Two other medications are approved for the use of children with JIA including aspirin (dosages of 80 to 120 mg/kg in four divided doses) and ibuprofen at 30 to 40 mg in three or four divided doses. A liquid preparation comes at 100 mg/5 mL. Other NSAIDs recently used in trials in JIA but not FDA approved include nabumetone (Relafen),[1] at 30 mg/kg. This medication has an advantage in that it is only once a day and also can be used in a liquid form by crushing the tablet and dissolving in warm water. Other agents are occasionally used such as oxaprozin (Daypro), at 10 to 20 mg/kg in one to two doses; fenoprofen (Nalfon), at 40 to 50 mg/kg[3] three to four times per day; diclofenac sodium (Voltaren), 20 to 40 mg/kg[3] twice to three times per day; sulindac (Clinoril), 4 to 6 mg/kg in a twice daily dosage; or celecoxib (Celebrex), a cyclooxygenase-2 (COX-2) inhibitor, at 4 to 6 mg/kg in two doses. Laboratory studies including CBC, urinalysis, and comprehensive metabolic panel should be drawn every 4 months to monitor medication toxicity.

Children who have erosions on radiograph or show more aggressive disease at time of onset, usually those with polyarthritis, with systemic disease with polyarthritis, or with very aggressive oligoarticular disease, benefit greatly by combination therapy to reduce long-term disability. This means being aggressive with therapy in the first 2 years of disease. The first 2 years of disease are the period in which the most erosions and joint damage occurs. Combination therapy has become the standard of care of patients with JIA. The most common combination is the use of two or more of the disease-modifying antirheumatic agents (DMARDs), which include methotrexate (MTX), hydroxychloroquine (Plaquenil) [HCQ], or some of the new biologic preparations. MTX, a purine inhibitor, in dosages of 10 to 20 mg/m$^2$ once weekly along with folic acid at 400 µg to 1 mg daily is a very efficacious DMARD with little toxicity. MTX can

be given orally or by intramuscular (IM) or subcutaneous (SC) injection. Orally, the liquid preparation at 25 mg/mL can be given in 0.1 mL/2.5 mg increments from 5 mg (0.2 mL) to 20 mg (0.8 mL) or in pill form of 2.5 mg tablets from 5 mg (2 tablets) to 20 mg (8 tablets) once per week. Dosages more than 20 mg should always be administered IM or SC. These children, however, do need to be monitored monthly to every 6 weeks with CBC, urinalysis, and liver and kidney function tests to monitor the medication toxicity. The combination of MTX and HCQ is the most common with the addition of HCQ in dosages of 6 mg/kg as an excellent adjunct along with the NSAID. Eye exams every 6 months to monitor HCQ toxicity are indicated. MTX is also monitored once a year with a chest radiograph and also if any cough is present. The toxicities of these medications are relatively minimal in patients with JIA. Other DMARDs, although not approved in children, are cyclosporine (Neoral)[1] at 2.5 to 3 mg/kg, intramuscular gold[1] at a dosage of 1 mg/kg weekly for 20 weeks, and sulfasalazine (Azulfidine) (SSZ) at doses of 50 mg/kg beginning at 500 mg per day and up to 2 g twice a day.[3] These are used with efficacy in JIA patients. Also, leflunomide (Arava)[1], a pyrimidine synthetase inhibitor, is effective in children. It also has liver toxicity, so it should be monitored like MTX. Abdominal complaints such as diarrhea are the most common side effects. The drug has a long half-life and potential teratogenicity, so it should be used with caution in females of childbearing age. Recently, the use of biologics or anticytokines in JIA has brought about a great deal of improvement in some of the patients. One medication is etanercept (Enbrel) at 0.4 mg/kg SC two times per week or 0.8 mg/kg SQ once per week. It has brought about marked improvement in many patients with long-standing polyarthritis. Efficacy has been sustained for up to 9 years now. This medication has caused marked decrease in joint swelling, tenderness, decreased sedimentation rate, and marked improvement in fatigue. The mechanism of action is that of blocking tumor necrosis factor (TNF), a cytokine that increases the inflammatory response in joints. Etanercept is produced to function like the p75 receptor for TNF. It binds to TNF and keeps it from binding to its own receptor and increasing the inflammatory response. It is the only biologic approved for JIA by the FDA. It is well tolerated with the main side effect injection site reactions. TNF blockers can exacerbate an underlying tuberculosis infection, so before starting the medication a chest radiograph and purified protein derivative (PPD) skin test should be performed and then yearly while on the medication. Its counterpart, infliximab (Remicade), a chimeric monoclonal antibody to TNF, also is very efficacious in JIA. It is used as an intravenous (IV) preparation at 3 mg/kg given at baseline, 2 weeks, 6 weeks, and 8 eight weeks thereafter in an IV infusion over a 2-hour period. The dosage may be increased to 5 to 8 mg/kg and the interval shortened to every 4 to 6 weeks if needed. This agent markedly decreases the inflammatory response. It has mainly been used in older children with polyarticular disease. A fully humanized monoclonal antibody to TNF, adalimumab (Humira), is still in trials in children at 20 to 40 mg SC every 2 weeks. Also, studies are being run on the interleukin (IL)-1 receptor antagonist, Anakinra (Kineret), in children. It is given daily at 1 to 2 mg/kg SC up to 100 mg SC per day. This medication shows a more favorable response in children with systemic-onset than with polyarticular or oligoarticular disease. A high number of children experience injection site reactions. Other biologic medications are in trials, including an IL-6 receptor antagonist (tocilizumab)[2] in systemic onset JIA, anti-B cell therapy (rituximab) (Rituxan), or T-cell therapy (abatacept) (Orencia).

Prednisone still may be used in severe systemic disease to control fever, rash, and/or other systemic manifestations in dosages of 1 to 2 mg/kg. The possibility of long-term side effects such as growth retardation, avascular necrosis, osteoporosis, weight gain, and acneiform lesions from steroids make their long-term use tentative in children. If disease is controlled, steroids should be tapered. Steroid eye drops may be used at times for severe iridocyclitis or orally in those patients with severe eye disease. Intra-articular (IA) steroids may be used in all onset-types if one or more joints are severely involved at one point in time.

---

[1]Not FDA approved for this indication.

[1]Not FDA approved for this indication.
[2]Not available in the United States.
[3]Exceeds dosage recommended by the manufacturer.

## CURRENT THERAPY

- Anti-inflammatory agents (NSAIDs: naproxen [Naprosyn], ibuprofen [Advil], tolmetin [Tolectin], meloxicam [Mobic]) and intra-articular steroids for oligoarticular disease
- NSAIDs, disease-modifying agents (methotrexate [Rheumatrex], hydroxychloroquine [Plaquenil], sulfasalazine [Azulfidine], etc.) and/or biologics (etanercept) for polyarticular and systemic disease

*Abbreviation:* NSAIDs = nonsteroidal anti-inflammatory drugs.

Local injections of 10 to 40 mg of triamcinolone hexacetonide may provide symptomatic relief in one specific joint. In the long course of the disease, other immunosuppressives such as cyclophosphamide (Cytoxan), azathioprine (Imuran), and chlorambucil (Leukeran)[1] are used in certain cases of severe systemic or polyarthritis, but the use of these has waned with the new biologic medication.

The use of PT and OT is indicated at the first onset of disease. The child, after being evaluated, is sent to PT for instructions in the use of moist heat to the joints such as hot packs, the judicial use of rest, and two to three periods each day of passive or active assisted exercises performed by the patient or aided by the parent. Splints that protect joints may be prescribed to decrease the development of deformities. Splints can be made out of lightweight plastic that is molded while warm to fit the child in the desired position. The wrists and knees are the most amenable to splinting, but finger splints may hold the entire hand in slight dorsiflexion to decrease ulnar drift. If flexion contractures occur, splints can be used to hold the joint in maximum extension. The use of OT begins with the instructions for the patient in posture, body mechanics, improvement in activities of daily living, and instructions in joint protection. These instructions help the patient learn to protect and not increase the impact loading on the joints. Exercises are important in all stages of the care of the child with arthritis. During appearance of disease activity, excessive exercises exacerbate the inflammation. In these stages, passive range of motion exercise should maintain range of motion along with active assistive exercise. As joints improve and the inflammation is reduced, the exercise should be increased to a more active form. Resistive and strengthening exercises should be introduced along with isometric exercises to help provide muscle tone. Swimming or hydrotherapy or water aerobics for exercise may greatly aid in improving muscle strength. The use of regular cycling exercises may also be helpful. If the child has a lot of morning stiffness in the hands, the use of paraffin baths may be of great help, and the use of Theraputty to squeeze and improve muscle strength in the hands is indicated.

In conclusion, children with JIA should be diagnosed as soon as possible and treated aggressively. It is not a benign condition if left partially treated or untreated. Early treatment prevents further disease progression, maintains range of motion of the joints, and promotes normal growth and development. Combination therapy of NSAIDs, DMARDs, and/or biologics should be used early in those patients identified with aggressive disease. The team approach of the pediatric rheumatologist, ophthalmologist, and physical and occupational therapists will best benefit the JIA patient for a good long-term outcome.

### REFERENCES

Cassidy JT, Petty RE: Chronic arthritis. In Cassidy JT, Petty RE (eds): Textbook of Pediatric Rheumatology. Philadelphia, WB Saunders, 2005, pp 206-341.

Kietz DA, Pepmueller PH, Moore TL: Therapeutic use of etanercept in polyarticular course juvenile rheumatoid arthritis over a two-year period. Ann Rheum Dis 2002;61:171-173.

Lovell D, Giannini EH, Reiff A, et al: Etanercept in children with polyarticular juvenile rheumatoid arthritis. N Engl J Med 2000;342:763-769.

Low JM, Chauhan AK, Kietz DA, et al: Determination of anti-cyclic citrullinated peptide antibodies in sera of patients with juvenile idiopathic arthritis. J Rheumatol 2004;31:1829-1833.

Moore TL: Immunopathogenesis of juvenile rheumatoid arthritis. Curr Opin Rheumatol 1999;11:377-383.

Petty JE, Southwood TR, Manners P, et al: International League of Associations for Rheumatology classification of juvenile idiopathic arthritis; Second revision, Edmonton, 2001. J Rheumatol 2004;31:390-392.

Wallace CA, Huang B, Bandeira M, et al: Patterns of clinical remission in select categories of juvenile idiopathic arthritis. Arthritis Rheum 2005;52:3554-3562.

# Ankylosing Spondylitis

Method of
*Finbar D. O'Shea, MB, MRCPI,*
*and Robert D. Inman, MD*

Ankylosing spondylitis (AS) is a chronic inflammatory rheumatic disease characterized by inflammatory back pain due to sacroiliitis and spondylitis, restricted spinal mobility due to the formation of syndesmophytes, and often peripheral arthritis, enthesitis, and acute anterior uveitis (iritis). Symptoms commonly begin in late adolescence and early adulthood. With an estimated prevalence of 0.9% in northern European white populations, AS is a significant health burden to the community.

AS has long been a therapeutic challenge for the clinician. Exercise and nonsteroidal anti-inflammatory drugs (NSAIDs) have been the mainstays of symptom control for decades, but there has until recently been a dearth of effective disease-modifying treatments. The advent of biological treatments (specifically anti–tumor necrosis factor [TNF] agents) is currently revolutionizing the management of AS.

AS belongs to a group of related diseases termed *spondyloarthropathies* (SpA), which also comprises conditions such as arthritis/spondylitis associated with psoriasis, arthritis/spondylitis associated with inflammatory bowel disease, reactive arthritis, and undifferentiated spondyloarthritis (uSpA). They share many clinical manifestations and an association with human leukocyte antigen (HLA)-B27. The SpA group as a whole is one of the most common rheumatic diseases, with a prevalence of up to 1.9%, and this makes them at least as common as rheumatoid arthritis. The most common subgroups of SpA are AS and uSpA. It appears that all SpA subsets can progress to full-blown AS.

## Diagnosis

### DIFFICULTIES AND DELAYS IN DIAGNOSIS

Among the inflammatory rheumatic diseases there is a long delay between the onset of symptoms and the time of diagnosis for AS; in several studies an average duration of about 7 years has been reported. The mean age at onset of symptoms is in the mid-20s, thus at the normally most productive time of life. If AS is undiagnosed and untreated, or not treated effectively, continuous pain, stiffness, and fatigue are the consequences. Furthermore, a potentially progressive loss of spinal mobility and function cause a reduction in the quality of life and an increase in direct and indirect medical costs.

There are two major reasons for the long delay in the diagnosis of AS. First, the established classification criteria for AS, which date back more than 20 years, rely on the combination of clinical symptoms plus unequivocal radiographic sacroiliitis of at least grade 2 bilaterally or grade 3 unilaterally (see Box 1 for the modified New York criteria for the diagnosis of AS). The radiographs are often normal when symptoms arise, and it usually takes several years for definite radiographic

## BOX 1  Modified New York Criteria for Ankylosing Spondylitis

**Clinical Criteria**
- Low back pain and stiffness for more than 3 months that improves with exercise but is not relieved by rest
- Limitation of motion of the lumbar spine in both the lateral and frontal planes
- Limitation of chest expansion relative to normal values correlated for age and sex

**Radiographic Criterion**
- Sacroiliitis, grade ≥2 bilaterally or grade 3 to 4 unilaterally

*Note: The condition is definitely AS if the radiographic criterion is associated with at least 1 clinical criterion.*

sacroiliitis to evolve. Second, there is no unique clinical symptom or laboratory test to make the diagnosis of AS; thus it is a huge challenge to attempt to identify the estimated 5% of patients with SpA (including AS) among the great number of patients with chronic low back pain seen by the primary care physician.

Efforts have been made to try to address these issues. MRI has been used successfully to detect the presence of spinal and sacroiliac inflammation in early disease. However, until MRI detection of sacroiliitis is shown to be sensitive and specific for early AS, and until the availability of MRI greatly improves, most clinicians are left with plain radiography as the diagnostic test.

### CLINICAL FEATURES

Choosing clinical parameters for screening patients for underlying AS is attractive because their determination is not expensive. The clinical symptom of inflammatory back pain has been suggested as a cardinal symptom for AS for years, and assessment requires neither laboratory testing nor x-ray. It has been estimated that when symptoms of inflammatory back pain are present in a patient with chronic low back pain, the post-test probability for this patient of having axial SpA is 14%.

Recent refinement of these clinical features has identified a new set of criteria for inflammatory back pain. The new criteria consist of morning stiffness for longer than 30 minutes, improvement in back pain with exercise but not with rest, awakening because of back pain during the second one half of the night only, and alternating buttock pain. These features were defined by a study that sought to identify the most sensitive and specific combination of parameters for inflammatory back pain using a cohort of patients with an established diagnosis of AS. Fulfillment of at least two of these four parameters yielded a sensitivity of 70% and a specificity of 81%, with a positive likelihood ratio of 3.7. If at least three of the four parameters were fulfilled, the positive likelihood ratio increased to 12.4. However, how these discriminating features perform in a large non-specific back pain population has yet to be examined.

## Treatment

Until recently, the treatment options for AS were limited. Regular physiotherapy and treatment with NSAIDs were the only available options. Approximately one half of AS patients are adequately managed with this regimen. However, conventional disease-modifying antirheumatic drugs, which are effective in other chronic inflammatory diseases such as rheumatoid arthritis, have only a very limited effect on spinal inflammation. Local injections of corticosteroids can be used effectively if inflammation is confined to a small number of joints. Thus, although an early and accurate diagnosis has been recognized as important in these patients, this seemed less urgent for many physicians because of the lack of therapeutic options.

This treatment approach has now changed. NSAIDs should probably be taken more regularly once a diagnosis has been made. Tumor necrosis factor (TNF) blockers offer an exciting new possibility for effective treatment and possibly for arresting disease progression. It has recently been shown that the anti-TNF agents infliximab (Remicade), etanercept (Enbrel), and adalimumab (Humira) have a prompt and robust effect on almost all aspects of active disease—most notably pain and fatigue, but also function, spinal mobility, peripheral arthritis, enthesitis, bone density, and acute inflammation as reflected by acute-phase reactants and MRI. In studies using these three compounds, a 50% improvement of the disease activity could be demonstrated in about one half of the treated patients whose disease had proved refractory to NSAIDs and physiotherapy. In 72% of patients with a disease duration of less than 10 years there was at least 50% improvement of the Bath AS Disease Activity Index (BASDAI), clearly higher than patients with a longer disease duration. This finding supports the essential need for early diagnosis.

### CURRENT DIAGNOSIS

- Screen all patients younger than 40 years who have back pain longer than 3 months for features of IBP. IBP features include:
  - Early morning stiffness longer than 30 min
  - Improved back pain with exercise, not rest
  - Nocturnal pain, especially the second half of the night
  - Alternating buttock pain
- Screen for history of psoriasis, inflammatory bowel disease, iritis and any family history of these conditions
- Search for restriction in spinal mobility
  - Forward flexion (Schober's test)
  - Lateral spinal flexion
  - Chest expansion
- AP pelvic x-ray if IBP suspected for presence or absence of sacroiliitis
- If conventional radiography is not diagnostic and clinical suspicion remains, consider MRI (STIR sequence required). MRI allows direct visualization of inflammation in the spine and sacroiliac joints before conventional radiography shows any abnormality.

*Abbreviations:* AP = anteroposterior; IBP = inflammatory back pain; MRI = magnetic resonance imaging; STIR = short T1 inversion recovery.

### CURRENT THERAPY

- Physical therapy and a regular stretching program are important in all AS patients.
- NSAIDs are first-line therapy.
- Use a second NSAID even if the first has not achieved control of symptoms.
- Consider local corticosteroid injection if few joints involved.
- Ongoing disease activity is best reflected by the Bath Ankylosing Spondylitis Disease Activity Index (BASDAI). If the patient scores at least 4 out of 10 despite a full trial of two NSAIDs, an anti-TNF agent should be considered.

*Abbreviations:* NSAID = nonsteroidal anti-inflammatory drug; TNF = tumor necrosis factor.

Recent studies have shown a sustained response among AS patients with the anti-TNF agents superior even to that seen in rheumatoid arthritis. Short- to medium-term data show them to be well tolerated. On the basis of the MRI changes, it is believed that the anti-TNF agents will have a positive effect on long-term radiographic progression; however, this has yet to be proved.

Infliximab and adalimumab are monoclonal antibodies directed against the proinflammatory cytokine TNF-α. Etanercept is a fusion protein of the p75 TNF receptor linked to the Fc portion of an immunoglobulin (Ig) G1 molecule that binds and inactivates TNF-α. Inflixiamb is administered intravenously in three loading doses and then every 8 weeks at a dose of 3 to 5 mg/kg. Etanercept is administered subcutaneously once weekly (50-mg injection). Adalimumab is administered subcutaneously every other week (40-mg injection). All three agents appear to have similar efficacy and tolerability. The most serious potential side effect with any of these agents is infection, specifically tuberculosis (TB). This has been greatly minimized by screening for any evidence of latent TB infection with a chest x-ray and a TB skin (PPD) test before commencing these agents. The issue of altered rates of malignancies with these agents in AS has not been resolved and is being addressed with monitoring of biologics registries in several countries.

## Prognosis and Long-Term Outcomes

AS is a chronic condition with no predictable pattern of progression, and the disease does not follow a single defined course. Although many outcomes are possible, findings from previous prospective studies suggest that a pattern of AS emerges within the first 10 years of disease. About 74% of patients who had mild spinal restriction after 10 years did not progress to severe spinal involvement. In contrast, 81% of patients who had severe spinal restriction had been severely restricted within the first 10 years. What differentiates the rapid progression group has not been completely resolved. Hip involvement has repeatedly been shown to be an indicator of more severe disease. Other predictors of a poor outcome include a raised erythrocyte sedimentation rate (ESR), poor response to NSAIDs and peripheral oligoarthritis. Cigarette smoking is associated with worse clinical, functional, and radiologic outcomes. Early age at onset has been recently shown to be associated with a worse prognosis.

Men are afflicted with AS approximately 2 to 3 times more often than women. The disease pattern also varies by sex. The spine and pelvis are more commonly affected in men. In contrast, women have less severe involvement of the spine and more symptoms in the knees, ankles, and hips. It has been shown that women have a later age at onset. It was previously believed that women also had milder disease than men, but this view has been questioned recently.

With the advent of new effective therapies for AS, it has become important to identify predictors of response to these agents. This is important because the anti-TNF agents are expensive for the health care system and have potential side effects for the patient. It has been shown that younger patients with shorter disease duration, raised acute phase markers, and a higher disease activity at initiation do better. However, it has also been shown that patients with long-standing disease and established radiographic changes can also respond to these agents, and these patients should be also afforded a trial if conventional treatments have proved inadequate.

## REFERENCES

Davis JC, van der Jeijde DM, Braun J, et al: Sustained durability and tolerability of etanercept in ankylosing spondylitis for 96 weeks. Ann Rheum Dis 2005;64(11):1557-1562.

Maksymowych WP, Landewe R: Imaging in ankylosing spondylitis. Best Pract Res Clin Rheumatol 2006;20(3):507-519.

Rudwaleit M, van der Heijde D, Khan MA, et al: How to diagnose axial spondyloarthritis early. Ann Rheum Dis 2004;63:535-543.

Rudwaleit M, Metter A, Listing J, et al: Inflammatory back pain in ankylosing spondylitis: A reassessment of the clinical history for application as classification and diagnostic criteria. Arthritis Rheum 2006;54(2):569-578.

Sieper J, Braun J, Rudwaleit M, et al: Ankylosing spondylitis: An overview. Ann Rheum Dis 2002;61(suppl 3): iii8-iii18.

Sieper J, Rudwaleit M: Early referral recommendations for ankylosing spondylitis (including pre-radiographic and radiographic forms) in primary care. Ann Rheum Dis 2005;64:659-663.

Sieper J, Rudwaleit M, Khan MA, Braun J: Concepts and epidemiology of spondyloarthritis. Best Pract Res Clin Rheumatol 2006;20(3):401-417.

Stone M, Warren RW, Bruckel J, et al: Juvenile-onset ankylosing spondylitis is associated with worse functional outcomes than adult-onset ankylosing spondylitis. Arthritis Rheum 2005;53(3):445-451.

van der Heijde D, Dijkmans B, Geusens P, et al: Efficacy and safety of infliximab in patients with ankylosing spondylitis: Results of a randomized, placebo-controlled trial (ASSERT). Arthritis Rheum 2005;52(2):582-591.

van der Heijde D, Kivitz A, Schiff MH, et al: Efficacy and safety of adalimumab in patients with ankylosing spondylitis: Results of a multicenter, randomized, double-blind, placebo-controlled trial. Arthritis Rheum 2006;54(7):2136-2146.

van der Linden S, Valkenburg HA, Cats A: Evaluation of diagnostic criteria for ankylosing spondylitis: A proposal for modification of the New York criteria. Arthritis Rheum 1984;27(4):361-368.

Zochling J, van der Heijde D, Burgos-Vargas R, et al: ASAS/EULAR recommendations for the management of ankylosing spondylitis. Ann Rheum Dis 2006;65:442-452.

# Temporomandibular Disorders

Method of
*Charles S. Greene, DDS*

## History

The group of musculoskeletal disorders currently known as *temporomandibular disorders* (TMDs) has been through many taxonomic and conceptual changes over the past 70 years. Single-disease labels such as *temporomandibular joint syndrome* and *myofascial pain–dysfunction syndrome* have been discarded because these disorders are not simply variations on one theme. Instead, TMDs are now regarded as a collection of joint and muscle diseases or dysfunctions that are similar to other orthopedic problems. This shift in thinking has also been described as moving from a dental model to a medical model, because the early dental theories of misaligned jaws or faulty bite relationships have largely been discarded. In their place we now see TMDs being studied and treated with a medical perspective about orthopedic problems, combined with a biopsychosocial understanding of chronic pain disorders. In addition, many TMD patients have been found to be suffering from other functional disorders such as interstitial cystitis, irritable bowel syndrome (IBS), and pelvic pain, and others have reported multiple sites of pain throughout their bodies. These high levels of comorbidity with other conditions have led to hypotheses about centrally mediated dysregulatory problems producing multiple symptoms in susceptible patients.

The dental profession's interest in TMDs began as a lateral transfer of responsibility from otolaryngologists to dentists in the early 1930s. Although some articles had appeared in the dental literature before that time, it was the pronouncements of J. B. Costen that established the temporomandibular joint (TMJ) as a separate source of facial pain and about 11 other symptoms, most of which turned out later to be impossible to connect anatomically with the TMJ. It is not important to belabor the details of Costen's concepts, but their main impact was to lay the foundation for two propositions that dominated the field for many years:

- These so-called TMJ problems were the result of structural malalignments (dental, skeletal, or both) between the mandible and the skull.
- Only dentists could take care of TMJ problems because of the structural corrections that would be required.

Terms such as *overclosed vertical dimension, condylar malposition, trapped mandibles, occlusal disharmony,* and *neuromuscular imbalance* all were variants of this initial conceptual framework, and the treatments to correct all of them became part of the lexicon of dental therapies for many years. Whatever one may think of these concepts, it is clear that they were the basis for a dentally oriented etiologic viewpoint, and that the related therapies were seen as being antietiologic. Indeed, the word *definitive* often was used to describe the curative value of these TMD treatment approaches, which included such procedures as bite opening, occlusal adjustments, major restorative dentistry, orthodontics, and even surgeries.

Another structural concept of TMD etiology has been proposed by various physical therapists, chiropractors, and dentists, based on the notion that "bad" craniocervical relationships may be causing TMDs. Although this type of etiologic theory has enjoyed some popularity in the past (and is still popular in some regions of the world), several studies have demonstrated that there are no consistent postural findings that differentiate TMD patients from normal subjects. There can be some degree of comorbidity between TMDs and neck pain, but these are usually functional relationships rather than structural ones. In addition, the convergence of cervical and cranial sensory nerves in the brainstem nuclei can result in heterotopic (referred) pain in these areas.

## Etiology and Diagnosis

In more recent years, other etiologic factors besides structural ones have been recognized and discussed as a result of large studies of patient populations. For example, trauma at both the macro and micro levels has been noted in the history of certain TMD patients, with rather clear associations with onset of symptoms in many cases.

### PSYCHOPHYSIOLOGIC THEORY

The most significant changes in etiologic theorizing began in the 1950s and 1960s when the Columbia University group and the University of Illinois group proposed a psychophysiologic basis for many TMDs, especially those involving myofascial pain and dysfunction (MPD). These concepts arose from large studies of TMD patient populations in which a variety of psychometric approaches were used to assess personality characteristics and various state-trait variables. In addition, a large number of experimental stress provocation studies showed that TMD and MPD patients differed from normal subjects in many of their responses, and several psychophysical measurement studies demonstrated other significant physiologic differences between the groups.

## CURRENT DIAGNOSIS

- TMDs are musculoskeletal problems; therefore, symptoms of pain should be accompanied by symptoms and signs of dysfunction. Otherwise, the clinician should consider other craniofacial pain diagnoses.
- There are two major classes of TMDs: myogenous (extracapsular) and arthrogenous (intracapsular). The latter group includes anatomic derangements of the articular disk as well as degenerative diseases such as arthritis.
- Diagnosis depends heavily on good history taking, supplemented by appropriate physical examination of the TMJs, masticatory muscles, and adjacent tissues.
- Imaging of the TMJ should not be considered as a primary diagnostic modality; rather, it is required only when the clinical diagnosis is unclear or incomplete without further data.

*Abbreviations:* TMD = temporomandibular disorder; TMJ = temporomandibular joint.

Although Laskin's classic article about the etiology of MPD served as the basis for much of this experimental and analytical work, eventually his psychophysiologic theory proved to be incomplete as an etiologic explanation for the development of myofascial pain. Based on their research findings as well as those from other centers, the University of Illinois group published an important article in 1982 to express these reservations.

Today, the importance of psychological factors in the onset, progression, treatment, and persistence of various TMDs is well recognized as foundational knowledge in this field. However, the reasons some patients exhibit TMD symptoms and others do not remain unexplained by the psychophysiologic theory of etiology.

### BIOPSYCHOSOCIAL THEORY

Most recently, the combination of biological and psychological perspectives in etiologic theories about TMD has been given the name *biopsychosocial*. Another approach to describing the complicated nature of etiologies is to invoke the word *multifactorial*, thereby indicating an awareness that many extrinsic factors in the environment, as well as various intrinsic factors within the patient, might be involved in the development of symptomatic TMDs. Both of these labels are intellectually attractive in the sense that they suggest an appreciation of complexity, but do they imply a deeper understanding of what is actually happening to patients with TMDs?

Obviously, it is important to consider the true meaning of words such as *biopsychosocial* and *multifactorial* as expressions of etiologic thinking in the TMD field. In doing so, the reader should question their application at two levels of patient analysis: How do they help us understand *groups* of TMD patients? How do they help us understand *individual* patients?

A reasonable answer to these questions is as follows, adapted from the discussion of this issue by Okeson. The word *biopsychosocial* is actually a combination of three words, producing an excellent descriptor of the world that most patients with pain (and especially patients with chronic pain) are living in from day to day. They have a *biological* problem (i.e., activation of pain pathways, with or without a demonstrable pathologic condition) that can have *psychological* antecedents as well as behavioral consequences. This situation exists in a *social* framework that includes interpersonal relationships with friends, families, and health care providers, which almost always produces major negative experiences for the patients as well as their immediate families.

How can we assess all of these variables at the individual patient level with the crude physical and psychometric tools that are currently available? At this time it is not possible to do so with any degree of precision or certainty, and therefore this type of concept is valuable only at the group level.

## Treatment

Despite the current gaps in the profession's knowledge or ability to measure etiologic factors, most TMDs can be managed clinically based entirely on applying research-based treatment protocols to specific TMD diagnostic categories, an approach that requires little or no attention to individual etiologic factors. Although some clinicians may disagree, current scientific evidence suggests that this is what most of them really are doing when they provide treatment for most of their TMD patients, regardless of protestations to the contrary (Table 1). Even in the face of known etiologies, many TMD patients cannot be treated anti-etiologically simply because the causative factor or event cannot be undone (e.g., traumatic injuries to the mandible or spontaneous displacements of the articular disk) or because the disease process is irreversible (e.g., arthritis). Therefore, clinicians must have an intellectual framework that enables them to provide good care for their TMD patients while recognizing the limitations of the current state of knowledge.

Almost all of the current authoritative review articles and guidelines for treating the most common TMDs (masticatory muscle pain, disk derangements, and osteoarthritis) suggest a conservative, reversible approach to initial therapy. This approach includes the use of well-known

**TABLE 1**  Relationships Among Diagnosis, Etiology, and Treatment in Temporomandibular Disorders

| Standard | Diagnosis | Etiology | Treatment | Prevalence |
|---|---|---|---|---|
| **IDEAL** | Clear and correct Measurable Demonstrable | Specific Measurable Treatable | Anti-etiologic Definitive Successful | Not achievable at this time |
| **ACCEPTABLE** | Presumptive Probably correct Categoric labels | Unclear Complex Reversible | Empirically validated Matched to diagnosis Conservative | Frequently achievable Represents best current practice |
| **WRONG OR BAD** | Parochial specialty labeling Technologic diagnosis Possibly correct | Favorite theory Morphofunctional analysis Mechanical concept | Prolonged appliance wear Bite-changing procedures Jaw repositioning | Most common current practice, despite lack of scientific foundation |
| **OUTRAGEOUS** | Misdiagnosis of pain Neglect of serious pathologic conditions Neglect chronicity | Guru or cult concepts Quackery concepts Parochial specialty concepts | Whole-body procedures Quackery procedures Extreme dental procedures | All too common Represents fringe of current practice |

From Greene CS: The etiology of temporomandibular disorders: Implications for treatment. J Orofac Pain 2001;15(2):93-105

and widely accepted conservative treatment modalities, including various medications, oral appliances, physical therapies, and home care procedures, as well as a cognitive behavior information program that teaches patients about their condition and how it should be managed.

In a 1992 article on initial therapy, Greene argued that good primary care as described here should not be regarded as the first phase of a two-step program, as some of the structural theories have advocated. Instead, it is the actual treatment program that most TMD patients require, and one that will be quite successful for many of them. In that article, the dangers of various irreversible treatment approaches and improper escalation of therapy were described. Many other researchers in this field have proposed a similar viewpoint, and the long-term research on clinical outcomes from around the world supports the use of conservative and reversible treatments as the *only* appropriate way to treat the vast majority of TMD patients. It is interesting that the same concepts are echoed in a major review article dealing with the management of lower back pain.

Several prominent behavioral researchers in the TMD field have recommended a cognitive behavior approach to educating and treating TMD patients, and they have clearly demonstrated its effectiveness. This approach offers the dual benefit of teaching patients how to self-manage many of their symptoms while enhancing the feeling of empowerment (locus of control) that comes from such skills.

---

### ⓒ   CURRENT THERAPY

- Treatment of TMDs should always be preceded by a proper explanation of what is happening and also by offering a generally favorable prognosis for improvement.
- The menu of therapies should include one or more of the following:
  - Analgesic, anti-inflammatory, and/or muscle relaxant medications
  - Physical therapy, both home-based and professional
  - Oral orthotics (splints) that do not produce permanent changes in jaw position or dental occlusion
  - Cognitive behavior counseling of the patient to obtain maximum cooperation with self-care procedures
- Chronic and nonresponding TMD patients usually require more complex multidisciplinary pain management; therefore, they should be referred to orofacial pain specialists in university or hospital clinics.

---

*Abbreviation:* TMD = temporomandibular disorder.

As pointed out earlier, this is not an etiologic issue but a tactical one. Good clinicians need to be sensitive to the psychological ramifications of pain in both patients with acute TMD and those with chronic TMD, and they must expect to encounter significant psychological issues such as anxiety and depression, more often in the latter group. Only by developing this kind of awareness can clinicians avoid the mistakes of escalation to either surgery or major dental treatment instead of referring their nonresponding patients for the kind of complex chronic pain management that is much more likely to be appropriate. In the end, it is this awareness that defines the biopsychosocial approach to the diagnosis and treatment of patients with TMDs (see Table 1).

## Future Directions

The future of the TMD and orofacial pain field will be determined by the progress that is made in the larger field of pain management. Multitudes of researchers around the world are looking at both basic science and clinical paradigms that will change the way we look at pain in general. At this time, there are three main areas of focus for these investigations:

### GENETICS

Evidence is accumulating about the role that genetics can play in determining who is susceptible to developing various pain conditions, as well as how individuals respond to having pain. Some studies already have demonstrated a genetic difference in people's reactions to experimental pain, and other studies have shown that it may be possible to predict who will have painful conditions arise later or whose pain problems will become chronic. The implications of these findings for the management of pain patients are only beginning to be understood. Even in the absence of genetic manipulation, which may be a futuristic strategy, clinicians can use current modalities and strategies more wisely if they know whom they are dealing with.

### PATHOPHYSIOLOGY

It seems that every new edition of the major pain journals brings more information about the molecular chemistry and biology of various types of pain. In the case of the TMD, the discovery of inflammatory mediators and neurochemicals within the joint has led to a much better understanding of what is happening in painful conditions, and already some therapies are being tested for controlling these factors. The same is true for muscular pain, although the pathophysiology of that type of pain is less well understood at this time. As more information emerges, treatments directed at the underlying pathophysiology of painful conditions will inevitably be more successful than treatments that only suppress pain or inflammation.

## PREDICTIVE FACTORS

Some success has already been reported in identifying physical and psychological factors in orofacial pain patients that might predict their responses to therapy. Currently, a major focus is on trying to prevent acute pain conditions from developing into chronic ones, and this will require good early treatment strategies as well as better predictors of who is more likely to develop such problems. The search for more predictors should enhance the ability of clinicians to develop appropriate treatment plans that are individualized for each patient.

Chronic pain is a condition that, to paraphrase Benjamin Crue's definition, no longer has much to do with whatever caused it to begin in the first place. The implications of this fact are profound for chronic TMD pain sufferers, because it means that clinicians should try to avoid specific and aggressive treatments that will "cure" their problems. Instead, strategies directed at their centrally maintained pain conditions as well as their psychosocial well-being need to be tailored to their individual problems. This approach is already being applied in many academic centers and special pain management programs, but it also needs to be understood by frontline practitioners in both medicine and dentistry so that they also can provide appropriate care in their offices.

## Summary

The field of temporomandibular disorders has been transformed greatly by the research findings about pain in general, as well as by specific advances made within that field. As a result, they now are seen as a subset of musculoskeletal pain conditions, which requires a medical perspective for both understanding and managing TMD patients. Because of their location in the head and neck region, which is so richly innervated, differential diagnosis of TMDs can be difficult at times. Therefore, clinicians need to learn how to discriminate between vascular, neurogenic, and musculoskeletal pains in order to classify and manage orofacial pain patients appropriately. In addition, they must be prepared to deal with the psychosocial issues that so often accompany chronic pain states.

## REFERENCES

Aaron LA, Burke MM, Buchwald D: Overlapping conditions among patients with chronic fatigue syndrome, fibromyalgia, and temporomandibular disorder. Arch Intern Med 2000;160:221-227.

Alstergen P, Kopp S: Prostoglandin E$_2$ in temporomandibular joint synovial fluid and its relation to pain and inflammatory disorders. J Oral Maxillofac Surg 2000;58:180-186.

Diatchenko L, Slade GD, Nackley AG, et al: Genetic basis for individual variations in pain perception and the development of a chronic pain condition. Hum Mol Genet 2005;14:135-143.

de Leeuw R, Klasser GD, Albuquerque RJ: Are female patients with orofacial pain medically compromised? J Am Dent Assoc 2005;136(4):459-468.

Dworkin SF, Turner JA, Wilson L, et al: Brief group cognitive-behavioral intervention for temporomandibular disorders. Pain 1994;59:175-187.

Forsell H, Kalso E, Vehmanen R, et al: Occlusal treatments in temporomandibular disorders: A qualitative review of randomized controlled trials. Pain 1999;83:549-560.

Greene CS: Managing TMD patients: Initial therapy is the key. J Am Dent Assoc 1992;123:43-45.

Greene CS: Concepts of TMD etiology: Effects on diagnosis and treatment. In Laskin DM, Greene CS, Hylander WL (Eds): Temporomandibular Disorders: An Evidence-Based Approach to Diagnosis and Treatment. Chicago: Quintessence Publishing, 2006, pp 219-228.

Korszun A, Papadopolous E, Demitrack M, et al: The relationship between temporomandibular disorders and stress-associated syndromes. Oral Surg Oral Med Oral Pathol Oral Radiol Endod 1998;86:416-420.

Ohrbach R: Biobehavioral therapy. In Laskin DM, Greene CS, Hylander WL (eds): Temporomandibular Disorders: An Evidence-Based Approach to Diagnosis and Treatment. Chicago: Quintessence Publishing, 2006, pp 391-402.

Ren K, Dubner R: Focus Paper: Central nervous system plasticity and persistent pain. J Orofac Pain 1999;13:155-163.

Sessle BJ: The neural basis of temporomandibular joint and masticatory muscle pain. J Orofac Pain 1999;13:238-245.

Stohler CS, Zarb GA: On the management of temporomandibular disorders: A plea for a low-tech, high-prudence therapeutic approach. J Orofac Pain 1999;13:255-261.

# Bursitis, Tendinitis, Myofascial Pain, and Fibromyalgia

Method of
*Andrew L. Wong, MD, and Emil R. Heinze, MD*

Rheumatologic diseases include a vast number of soft tissue disorders, both regional and diffuse, affecting the muscles, tendons, bursae, nerves, and fascia. The etiologies of these syndromes include mechanical abnormalities, sports- or work-related repetitive activities, mild trauma, altered pain perception, and occasionally systemic disease. Diagnosis is made with a diligent history and a focused physical examination, with a limited role for imaging and laboratory evaluation. Most of these syndromes can be evaluated and managed by the primary care physician, with the more refractory or diagnostically challenging cases referred to the rheumatologist. The primary care physician should therefore be adept at recognizing, diagnosing, and taking a stepwise approach to managing these conditions.

## Bursitis and Tendinitis

Bursae are synovial-lined sacs containing a thin film of viscous synovial fluid adjacent to tendinous insertions and other points of friction in the body. Under normal circumstances, bursae contain very little fluid. Conditions such as overuse, mechanical stress, and occasionally inflammatory and crystalline disease lead to inflammation, pain, and fluid accumulation in the bursae. Infection can occasionally complicate bursitis. Tendons are bands of tough fibrous tissue that connect muscle to bone. Tendinitis is reactive inflammation usually due to microtrauma or inflammatory disease, resulting in pain with use.

There is a close relation between tendons and bursae, and inflammation often occurs in both at any given location. There are hundreds of bursae and tendons in the body, all of which are subject to inflammation under the right circumstances. Management of bursitis and tendinitis follows many of the same principles; therefore, these two conditions are considered together in this article. This article focuses on the diagnosis and management of the most commonly seen disorders by region, but it should not be considered all-inclusive.

### SHOULDER

#### Subacromial Bursitis and Rotator Cuff Tendinitis

The subacromial bursa is located under the acromion process. It protects the superior aspect of the rotator cuff tendons from the undersurface of the acromion process during overhead reaching activities. Repetitive overhead activities such as lifting, pushing or pulling, or throwing a baseball can lead to reactive inflammation of the bursa and significant pain. This is often associated with tendinopathy of the rotator cuff (especially the supraspinatous tendon) due to the close proximity and shared stresses of impingement.

Patients complain of pain over the lateral shoulder with abduction of the arm. Physical examination reveals pain with direct palpation at the anterior aspect of the subacromial space or bursa. Normal strength with abduction of the shoulder implies an intact rotator cuff tendon. However, a partial tear of the supraspinatus tendon can result in pain and weakness when testing for resisted shoulder abduction at 90 degrees (drop arm test).

For subacromial bursitis or supraspinatus tendinitis, management should begin with conservative measures including temporary elimination of exacerbating activities, nonsteroidal anti-inflammatory drugs (NSAIDs), ice, and physical therapy. If conservative measures fail after a 1- to 2-week trial, then prompt relief is often achieved with an injection of corticosteroids and lidocaine (Box 1).

---

[1]Not FDA approved for this indication.

## BOX 1   Techniques for Injection of Common Bursitis and Tendinitis Conditions

**Injection Principles**

- All injections are to be done with aseptic technique.
- Equivalent doses of other long-acting injectable steroids may be used in place of triamcinolone (Kenalog) 40 mg/mL.
- Ethyl chloride topical spray or a subcutaneous wheal of 1% lidocaine is recommended for surface anesthesia before injection.
- The injection should flow freely, never injecting against resistance, because this can indicate intratendinous needle insertion.
- Avoid steroid tracking back into the skin to prevent hypopigmentation and dimpling at the injection site.

**Injection Technique**

### Subacromial Bursitis

- Inject 20 mg triamcinolone (20 mg/mL) with 1-2 mL 1% lidocaine using a 1.5-in 25-gauge needle.
- Insert laterally 1-2 cm inferior to the undersurface of the midacromion process at the point of maximal tenderness and perpendicular to the skin.

### Supraspinatus Tendinitis

- Inject 20 mg triamcinolone with 1-2 mL lidocaine using a 1.5-in 25-gauge needle.
- Insert laterally 1-2 cm inferior to the undersurface of the mid-acromion process with a 10-degree upward angle deep into the subacromial space.

### Biceps Tendinitis

- Inject 10-20 mg triamcinolone with 1-2 mL lidocaine using a 1.5-in 25-gauge needle.
- Insert at the anterior shoulder toward the biceps tendon with a 45-degree upward angle.

### Lateral Epicondylitis

- Inject 10 mg triamcinolone with 0.5-1 mL lidocaine using a 0.625-in (⅝-in) 25-gauge needle.
- Insert at the point of maximal tenderness perpendicular to the skin.
- When the needle touches the lateral epicondyle, withdraw 1 mm, then inject.

### De Quervain's Tenosynovitis

- Inject 5-10 mg triamcinolone with 0.5-1 mL lidocaine using a 0.625-in (⅝-in) 25-gauge needle.
- Insert at the lateral wrist almost parallel to the skin, just distal to the radial styloid.
  Aim proximally toward the palpable inflamed extensor tendon following the tendon's course.

### Trigger Finger

- Inject 5 mg triamcinolone with 0.5-1 mL of lidocaine using a 0.5-in 27-gauge needle (PPD syringe).
- Insert just distal to proximal flexor crease of the digit toward the tender nodule using a 30-degree angle.
- Have the patient flex and extend the digit; the needle will move when engaged with the tendon.
  Withdraw 1 mm, then inject.

### Carpal Tunnel Syndrome

- Inject 10-20 mg triamcinolone with 0.5-1 mL 1% lidocaine using a 1-in 25-gauge needle.
- Insert at the intersection of the flexor crease of the wrist and the palmaris longus tendon.
- Advance 1 cm, using a 45-degree angle, aiming toward the middle finger, and inject.
  Reposition the needle if pain radiates in the distribution of the median nerve.

### Pes Anserine Bursitis

- Inject 10-20 mg triamcinolone with 1-2 mL lidocaine using a 1-in 25-gauge needle.
- Insert perpendicular to the skin, aiming toward the point of maximal tenderness.
- When the needle touches the tibia, withdraw 1 mm, then inject.

### Trochanteric Bursitis

- The patient is positioned lying on the side with the affected hip pointing up.
- Inject 20-40 mg triamcinolone with 3-5 mL lidocaine using a 1.5-in 25-gauge needle. A 22-gauge 3-in or 4-in spinal needle is often needed in heavy patients.
- Insert the needle perpendicular to the skin, dropping the needle down toward the point of maximal tenderness.
- When the needle touches the trochanter, withdraw 1 mm and inject.
  May reposition and inject several times in a half-dollar-sized distribution to ensure even coverage of corticosteroid injected.

### Plantar Fasciitis

- Inject 10-20 mg triamcinolone with 1-2 mL lidocaine using a 1.5-in 25-gauge needle.
- Insert parallel to the floor at the medial side of the foot, aiming toward the medial tubercle of the calcaneus.
- Inject into the space just above the proximal insertion of the plantar fascia.

## Biceps Tendinitis

Bicipital tendinitis occurs with heavy or forcible lifting activities. Patients complain of pain over the anterior shoulder. Examination reveals tenderness at the anterior bicipital groove exacerbated by resisted supination of the forearm (Yergason's maneuver). Management includes temporary limitation of lifting with the affected arm, NSAIDs, ice, and physical therapy. Careful corticosteroid injection of the biceps tendon sheath is considered if 1 to 2 weeks of conservative measures fail (see Box 1).

## ELBOW

### Olecranon Bursitis

The olecranon bursa is located along the posterior aspect of the olecranon process. Bursitis results from acute elbow trauma or from repetitive activities such as leaning on or applying pressure to the elbows (as occurs in carpet layers, students, etc.). Inflammation in this bursa is also commonly encountered in patients with gout, pseudogout, and rheumatoid arthritis. Patients complain of pain over the posterior aspect of the elbow, and significant swelling with fluctuance of the bursa is typically found on physical examination. Given its superficial nature, it is more likely than deeper bursae to be complicated by infection heralded by expanding erythema, intense pain, and increased swelling.

Management should include aspiration of the bursa fluid using a 20- or 22-gauge needle, entering from a posterior (horizontal) aspect to prevent a chronic draining tract. Bursa fluid analysis should include cell count and differential, crystal analysis, Gram stain, and culture. The patient should avoid aggravating activities; wear an elastic (Ace) wrap to apply slight external compression to the bursa, preventing further fluid accumulation; apply ice; and take NSAIDs. For refractory cases, the bursa can be injected with corticosteroids if infection has been ruled out. If infection is present, then appropriate intravenous antibiotic therapy should be used along with complete drainage of the bursa.

### Medial and Lateral Epicondylitis

The lateral epicondyle of the elbow is the attachment point of the extensor and supinator muscles of the forearm. Overuse is classically described in tennis players (tennis elbow), but it often occurs with other activities common to service industries and computer users. Patients complain of pain radiating from the elbow into the forearm and wrist, occasionally associated with subjective paresthesias. Physical examination is significant for pain with palpation 1 cm distal to the lateral epicondyle, and pain is exacerbated with resisted wrist extension (lift chair test) or resisted extension of the third finger. Symptoms are usually relieved with temporary elimination of exacerbating activities, a tennis elbow brace or band, ice, and NSAIDs. Corticosteroid injection can be considered for refractory cases (see Box 1). Occasionally, surgical intervention is needed to débride the damaged or inflammatory tissue.

The medial epicondyle of the elbow is the attachment point of the flexor and pronator muscles of the forearm. Overuse is classically described in golfers (golfer's elbow), but it also occurs in other persons playing other sports such as baseball (pitching) and even tennis (serving), as well as in construction workers due to tool use (screwdrivers and hammers). Patients complain of pain at the medial aspect of the elbow, often associated with paresthesias down the distal forearm. Physical examination reveals pain with palpation 1 cm distal to the medial epicondyle; this is reproduced with resisted flexion or pronation of the wrist. Occasionally, weakness or numbness is found in the distribution of the ulnar nerve due to its proximity to the medial epicondyle. Management includes elimination of exacerbating activities, counterforce bracing, physical therapy, ice, and NSAIDs. Corticosteroid injection can be considered for refractory cases, taking particular care to avoid injection of the ulnar nerve. Surgical intervention is rarely needed.

## CURRENT DIAGNOSIS

**Tendinitis and Bursitis**

- History of repetitive motion or strain to affected tendon or adjacent bursa
- Localized pain with palpation at a tendinous insertion increased with active ROM and provocative maneuvers for tendinitis
- Localized swelling and fluctuance noted at the site of a superficial bursa (especially olecranon, prepatellar, and superficial Achilles) for bursitis
- Minimal pain with passive ROM, especially with internal and external rotation of the adjacent joint (implying the joint is not inflamed)
- No focal weakness on resisted muscle testing (implying intact tendons)

**Myofascial Pain**

- Trigger point in a muscle, often with focal induration (knot)
- Palpation reproduces the regional trigger point pain

**Fibromyalgia**

- History of widespread pain longer than 3 months (above and below the waist and on both sides of the body, including axial locations)
- Pain with digital palpation in 11 of 18 defined tender points (Figure 1)
- Frequently associated with poor sleep, fatigue, headaches, IBS, anxiety, and depression
- Normal limited laboratory evaluation (CBC, chemistry panel, LFTs, TSH, CPK, and ESR)
- Avoid ordering routine ANA, RF, or Lyme titer unless these are clearly indicated from physical examination findings
- No signs of systemic autoimmune disease such as rashes, synovitis, unexplained weight loss, or fevers

*Abbreviations:* ANA = antinuclear antibody; CBC = complete blood count; CPK = creatine phosphokinase; ESR = erythrocyte sedimentation rate; IBS = inflammatory bowel syndrome; LFTs = liver function tests; RF = rheumatoid factor; ROM = range of motion; TSH = thyroid-stimulating hormone.

## HAND

### De Quervain's Tenosynovitis

De Quervain's tenosynovitis occurs due to repetitive pinching or grasping with the thumb and index finger. This condition is particularly common with activities involving gardening, knitting or needlepoint, video game playing, using hand-held e-mail devices (BlackBerry thumb), tending to an infant by new mothers, and repetitive grasping motions in factory workers. It is a result of inflammation in the tendon sheaths of the abductor pollicis longus and extensor pollicis brevis. Patients complain of pain along the dorsal surface of the proximal thumb at the radial styloid. Finkelstein's test is positive (the patient closes a fist over the thumb and the examiner deviates the wrist toward the ulna reproducing the pain). Treatment includes thumb gutter splinting, ice, NSAIDs, and physical therapy. Steroid injection is very effective in cases that fail to respond to conservative measures after several weeks (see Box 1).

### Trigger Finger

Trigger finger is caused by inflammation and stenosis of the tendon sheaths of the flexor digitorum superficialis and profundus.

Patients complain of locking or triggering of the affected digit, especially in the morning. A palpable tender nodule can be felt at or just proximal to the metacarpophalangeal (MCP) joint on the palmar surface of the affected digit. This condition is typically caused by overuse activities, but is also commonly associated with diabetes, inflammatory arthritis, and osteoarthritis. Treatment includes warm compresses, splinting the affected digit in extension at night, NSAIDs, and modification of activities. If conservative therapy fails, patients often get prompt relief of symptoms with a local corticosteroid injection into the tendon sheath (see Box 1).

### Carpal Tunnel Syndrome

Carpal tunnel syndrome is caused by compression of the median nerve in the narrow carpal tunnel of the wrist. This is a neurologic disorder but is important to mention in this article because it is a common cause of hand pain and is often associated with tenosynovitis of the digital flexor tendons in the carpal tunnel, leading to the nerve compression. There are many causes of carpal tunnel syndrome; repetitive activities, osteoarthritis with osteophyte formation, pregnancy, diabetes, and inflammatory arthritis are some of the most common.

Patients complain of burning pain, numbness, and tingling in the distribution of the median nerve including the thumb, index finger, middle finger, and radial half of the fourth finger. Pain is often noticed during repetitive activities and at night, classically waking the patient from sleep.

Examination reveals a positive Tinel's sign (symptoms are reproduced by tapping over the carpal tunnel at the wrist) and Phalen's sign (symptoms are exacerbated by flexing the wrist to 90 degrees for 1 minute). In more severe, chronic cases, wasting of the thenar muscles and weakness of grip and opposition can be observed. Nerve conduction testing of the affected extremity is helpful in confirming the diagnosis as well as grading the severity.

Treatment begins with splinting the wrist in a neutral position, avoiding exacerbating activities, and taking NSAIDs for pain. It is important for the patient to wear the splint at night, because inadvertent wrist flexion and exacerbation of the symptoms often occurs during sleep. Refractory cases require injection of corticosteroids into the carpal tunnel (see Box 1). If symptoms continue, surgical release of the transverse carpal ligament may be necessary.

## KNEE

### Prepatellar and Infrapatellar Bursitis

The prepatellar bursa is located superficially in the soft tissues overlying the patella. Bursitis occurs most commonly as a result of repetitive kneeling activities as seen with carpet layers, tile workers, and plumbers (housemaid's knee). The infrapatellar bursa is found in the superficial soft tissues above the patellar tendon. Bursitis occurs in this location secondary to frequent kneeling in an upright position (clergyman's or prayer's knee). Patients complain of pain in these locations with kneeling or direct palpation. Obvious swelling is usually appreciated on examination. Like olecranon bursitis, infection is more common in these bursae due to their superficial location, and therefore a high index of suspicion is necessary. Management includes avoiding exacerbating activities, aspirating the bursa fluid to rule out infection or crystal deposition, using an elastic wrap to apply external compression to the bursa, applying ice, and taking NSAIDs. Occasionally, corticosteroid injection is needed if conservative therapy fails.

### Quadriceps and Patellar Tendinitis

The quadriceps tendon is located directly above the patella, and the patellar tendon is located below the patella inserting into the proximal tibia. Tendinitis in these tendons is commonly due to sports requiring frequent running and jumping such as basketball, volleyball, and soccer. Microtrauma to the tendon is likely responsible for the subsequent pain and swelling. Patients complain of pain in the respective locations with flexion of the knee. Management includes rest, ice, NSAIDs, and physical therapy. Recovery can take up to 6 months; however, moderate activities can often be reinstated before

that time. Steroid injections are generally contraindicated in these locations due to the risk of tendon rupture.

### Pes Anserine Bursitis

The pes anserine bursa is located at the common tendinous insertion of the gracilis, semitendinosus, and sartorius muscles along the medial tibia approximately 4 to 5 cm below the joint line. It commonly occurs in overweight, middle-aged women and often coexists with osteoarthritis of the knee (the bursitis is often overlooked, and the pain is attributed to the osteoarthritis). Pain is noted on climbing stairs and is commonly bilateral. Examination reveals point tenderness over the bursa. Management includes ice, NSAIDs, and physical therapy referral for gait evaluation, hamstring stretching, and quadriceps strengthening. Early injection of the bursa with lidocaine and corticosteroids often provides prompt relief of symptoms (see Box 1).

### Biceps Femoris and Semimembranosus Tendinitis

The biceps femoris muscle makes up the lateral half of the hamstring with its distal tendinous insertion at the fibular head. The semimembranosus muscle comprises a large part of the medial hamstring and inserts distally into the medial femoral condyle. These muscles are responsible for bending the knee and flexing the hip as they cross two major joints, the hip and the knee. Overuse injuries such as running, and sudden accelerations and decelerations as those seen in sprinters, are responsible for tendinitis occurring at these locations.

In biceps femoris tendinitis, patients complain of pain at the lateral knee at the insertion of the tendon into the fibular head. The pain is reproduced by resisted knee flexion. In semimembranosus tendinitis, chronic irritation as the tendon slides over the medial femoral condyle results in pain in the posteromedial aspect of the knee. This pain is reproduced by resisted knee flexion or repetitive flexion and extension while weight bearing. Treatment for these two types of tendinitis includes rest, ice, NSAIDs, and physical therapy, including gradual stretching and training modification. Steroid injection is usually not necessary.

### Iliotibial Band Syndrome

The iliotibial band (ITB) is a band of fascia that extends from the lateral iliac crest to the lateral knee, inserting into the lateral tibial tubercle and patella. ITB syndrome is due to inflammation of the distal ITB as it crosses the lateral knee. It is caused by overuse and is often seen in runners and cyclists. Patients complain of pain over the lateral knee with exercise, and they sometimes experience pain along the more proximal portions of the ITB at the thigh and hip.

Examination reveals tenderness over the ITB at the lateral knee most notable 2 cm proximal to the joint line. Having the patient stand with knees partially flexed might reproduce the pain. Ober's test involves having the patient lie on his or her side, with the unaffected side down. The affected leg is flexed to 90 degrees at the knee and fully abducted, following which the hip is extended. Then the leg is released and allowed to drop toward the examining table (adducted beyond midline). If pain is reproduced or the knee does not cross the midline, this implies tension and inflammation in the ITB.

Management includes physical therapy for specific stretching exercises targeted at the ITB, NSAIDs, ice, and modification of physical activities. Corticosteroid injection can be used in conservative treatment failures. Surgery for partial release may be beneficial in refractory cases.

## HIP

### Trochanteric Bursitis

Three bursae lie around the femoral trochanter. Trochanteric bursitis most commonly occurs in the gluteus maximus bursa found at the posterior aspect of the femoral trochanter. It occurs more commonly in women and results from excessive exercise, gait abnormalities, and coexisting osteoarthritis (OA) of the hip.

Patients complain of a deep pain in the lateral aspect of the hip exacerbated by walking, stair climbing, and lying on the affected side.

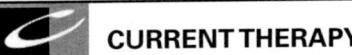 **CURRENT THERAPY**

**Bursitis and Tendinitis**

- Temporary elimination of exacerbating activities
- Splinting or bracing to provide immobilization and rest
- Ice three times a day to the affected area
- Nonsteroidal anti-inflammatory drugs (NSAIDs): Ibuprofen (Motrin) 600 mg PO tid, or naproxen (Naprosyn) 500 mg PO bid, and consider GI protection such as lansoprazole (Prevacid) 15 or 30 mg PO qd. May also try other NSAIDs.
- Physical therapy to stretch and strengthen corresponding muscle groups.
- Injection: Triamcinolone (Kenalog) 5-20 mg with 1 mL of 1% lidocaine into bursa or around tendon sheaths (if conservative therapy fails after 1-2 weeks). Should not encounter any resistance with injection (resistance implies intratendinous needle insertion). See Box 1 for technique and steroid dose for specific conditions. Steroid injection at the patellar, quadriceps, or Achilles tendon is generally contraindicated due to risk of tendon rupture.

**Myofascial Pain**

- Temporary elimination of exacerbating activities.
- Consider referral to physical therapy for local therapy.
- Injection: 1-2 mL of 1% lidocaine directly into the trigger point.

**Fibromyalgia**

- The key is to take a multidisciplinary approach to management, demonstrate compassion and understanding, and focus on the most problematic symptoms, including improving restorative (Stage 4) restful sleep.
- Education: Explain that the disease is one of increased pain sensitivity and is not progressive or deforming. Good therapy does exist and results in markedly improved quality of life.
- Graded exercise program: Essential for good outcome (best if structured by physical therapist to facilitate compliance). Start with brisk walking, stationary cycling, or swimming for 5 to 10 minutes, 3 times weekly. Increase to goal of 30 minutes every other day or 4 times weekly. Patients often experience increased pain initially but usually develop benefit in 1 to 2 months.
- Tricyclic antidepressants (TCAs): Amitriptyline (Elavil)[1] 10 mg PO 1 hour before bedtime. Begin with a very low dose and titrate every 2 to 4 weeks based on response to find lowest effective dose and minimize side effects. The usual effective dose is 25-100 mg/day. Alternatively, try doxepin (Sinequan)[1] 10 mg PO 1 hour before bedtime and titrate up similarly. If the patient cannot tolerate TCAs, try trazodone (Desyrel)[1] 25 mg 1 hour before bedtime and titrate up similarly. Used for treating insomnia, pain, and depression.
- Selective serotonin reuptake inhibitors (SSRIs): Fluoxetine (Prozac) 10 mg PO qAM (often need doses of 20-60 mg qd for benefit). Alternatively, try sertraline (Zoloft) 25 mg/day (often need doses of 50-150 mg qd). SSRIs are effective as monotherapy but can have additional benefit in combination with TCAs. Used for treating pain and depression.
- Muscle relaxants: Cyclobenzaprine (Flexeril)[1] 5 mg PO qhs. Titrate up by 5 mg every 2 weeks to find the effective dose. The usual effective dose is 10 mg qhs up to 10 mg tid. Used for treating pain and insomnia.
- Analgesics: Try gabapentin (Neurontin)[1] 300 mg PO qhs. Titrate up by 300 mg every two weeks to find the effective dose. The usual effective dose is 300 mg tid to 600 mg tid. Alternatively, try pregabalin (Lyrica)[1] 50 mg PO qhs. The usual effective dose is 300 mg to 450 mg daily. Can try tramadol (Ultram) 50 mg PO q6h as needed for pain. May also try acetaminophen (Tylenol) or low-dose NSAID therapy for mild analgesia.
- Minimize use of narcotic analgesics. There is no evidence to support the use of systemic corticosteroids.
- Consider serotonin-norepinephrine reuptake inhibitors (SNRIs) instead of TCAs: Venlafaxine (Effexor)[1] 75-150 mg PO daily, or duloxetine (Cymbalta)[1] 40-60 mg PO daily, because they often have a better side effect profile than the TCAs.
- Refer to the Arthritis Foundation, website www.arthritis.org, for patient information and local fibromyalgia self-help programs.
- Consider referral for cognitive behavior therapy.

---

[1] Not FDA approved for this indication.

---

Physical examination reveals tenderness to palpation at the lateral hip directly over the greater trochanter. Pain can often be elicited with resisted abduction of the affected leg. Examination of the true hip joint should be normal unless there is concomitant OA. Management includes limiting exacerbating activities, taking NSAIDs, and injecting with corticosteroids and lidocaine (see Box 1).

## Ischial Bursitis

The ischial bursa overlies the ischial prominence. It can become inflamed due to prolonged sitting (weaver's bottom). Pain initially occurs with sitting but progresses to pain while supine as the bursa becomes more inflamed. Sciatica can occur due to irritation of the nearby sciatic nerve. Physical examination reveals tenderness with direct palpation over the ischial prominence. Management includes sitting on a cushion with cutouts for the ischial tuberosity, NSAIDs, and hip-to-chest stretching

exercises. Corticosteroid injection is used for refractory cases, but care should be taken to avoid injection of the sciatic nerve.

## FOOT AND ANKLE

### Plantar Fasciitis

The plantar fascia is a thick band of fibrous tissue that inserts proximally into the medial tubercle of the calcaneus and distally into the proximal phalanges. It functions to support the arch of the foot. Risk factors for plantar fasciitis include running, obesity, pes planus, and prolonged standing and walking. It is sometimes seen in association with a seronegative spondyloarthropathy.

Patients complain of progressive pain over the plantar surface of the foot, most notable with the first few steps in the morning or when walking barefoot on hard surfaces. Physical examination reveals tenderness along the plantar fascia that is most notable at the insertion into the calcaneus and pain with passive dorsiflexion of the forefoot.

Treatment includes avoiding aggravating activities, physical therapy including ice, massage and passive stretching of the plantar fascia, NSAIDs, and appropriate footwear providing cushioned arch support. Refractory cases benefit from corticosteroid injection at the insertion of the plantar fascia (see Box 1).

### Retrocalcaneal Bursitis

Two bursae are located at the insertion of the Achilles tendon into the calcaneus, one deep to the tendon and the other superficial. Superficial bursitis occurs most commonly with friction over the posterior calcaneus from poor-fitting shoes, especially with high heels. Deep bursitis occurs most commonly in association with inflammatory and crystalline-induced arthritis.

Patients complain of pain over the posterior heel that is increased with dorsiflexion of the foot. Physical examination may reveal swelling of the bursa. Some involvement of the Achilles tendon is not uncommon.

Management includes proper-fitting shoes, occasionally requiring a stretch widening or cutout of the heel. Additionally, rest, ice, and NSAIDs may be beneficial. Steroid injection is generally not attempted due to risk of Achilles tendon rupture unless guided by imaging, such as ultrasound, to ensure the steroid is injected only into the bursa.

### Achilles Tendinitis

Achilles tendinitis can be caused by trauma, overuse, or running on an incline, and it can be associated with an inflammatory arthritis such as seronegative spondyloarthropathies, rheumatoid arthritis (RA), and gout. Achilles tendinitis and rupture can occur as a rare side effect of fluoroquinolone antibiotics.

Examination reveals tenderness at the insertion of the Achilles tendon that increases with dorsiflexion of the foot. Thompson's test (squeezing the posterior gastrocnemius while the patient is lying prone and observing for plantar flexion of the foot) is performed to confirm an intact (unruptured) Achilles tendon.

Management includes modification of exacerbating activities, NSAIDs, physical therapy for stretching exercises, and heel padding to decrease tension on the tendon. Steroid injection is generally contraindicated because of risk of tendon rupture.

### Posterior Tibial Tendinitis

The posterior tibial tendon courses behind the medial malleolus, inserts into the navicular, and functions to stabilize the arch and to plantarflex and invert the foot. Running or walking while overpronating the foot leads to tendinitis.

Patients complain of pain posterior to the medial malleolus radiating up the medial leg. Examination can reveal palpable swelling and tenderness posterior to the medial malleolus and pain that is reproduced with resisted inversion of the foot.

Management includes rest, ice, NSAIDs, and cushioned arch support. Careful steroid injection into the posterior tibial tendon sheath is sometimes performed in refractory cases.

## Myofascial Pain Syndrome

Myofascial pain syndrome is sometimes considered a form of localized fibromyalgia, defined by the presence of trigger points in specific muscle regions of the body that produce a characteristic pattern of referred pain on palpation. Risk factors include acute trauma, repetitive actions, poor conditioning, and sedentary lifestyle. Patients complain of deep, boring pain located in a specific muscular region of the body usually involving the neck, shoulder, lower back or hip region. Examination reveals one or more palpable tender nodules or knots in the affected muscle belly that reproduces the regional pain and might produce a twitch response when pressed. Treatment includes modifying exacerbating activities and injecting trigger points with lidocaine. Prognosis is good and complete recovery is generally anticipated.

## Fibromyalgia

Fibromyalgia is a very common cause of diffuse musculoskeletal pain characterized by diffuse pain and tender points. It affects up to 4% or 10 million Americans, approximately 75% of whom are women. Patients typically present with a long history of chronic pain over the entire body and often complain of fatigue, sleep disorders, irritable bowel symptoms, headaches, Raynaud-like symptoms, depression, anxiety, and memory disturbances.

The American College of Rheumatology (ACR) proposed criteria for diagnosis include at least 3 months of diffuse widespread pain involving bilateral upper and lower body with axial involvement and at least 11 of 18 tender points on examination (Figure 1). The underlying etiology is not well defined but appears to involve abnormalities in central nervous system pain processing, including the serotonin pathway, and an inappropriate heightened response to stress. Other triggers have also been associated including trauma, infections (parvovirus, Epstein-Barr virus, hepatitis C, HIV, Lyme disease), and chronic emotional stress. Fibromyalgia can also be the initial presenting manifestation of an underlying autoimmune disease such as RA or systemic lupus erythematosus (SLE), and therefore, if indicated, a focused history and physical examination evaluating for evidence of these disorders are appropriate.

Physical examination of patients with fibromyalgia is generally unremarkable except for the presence of multiple tender points. The examiner should apply enough pressure to each of the tender points with the force (4 kg/cm$^2$) necessary to blanch the thumbnail. A basic

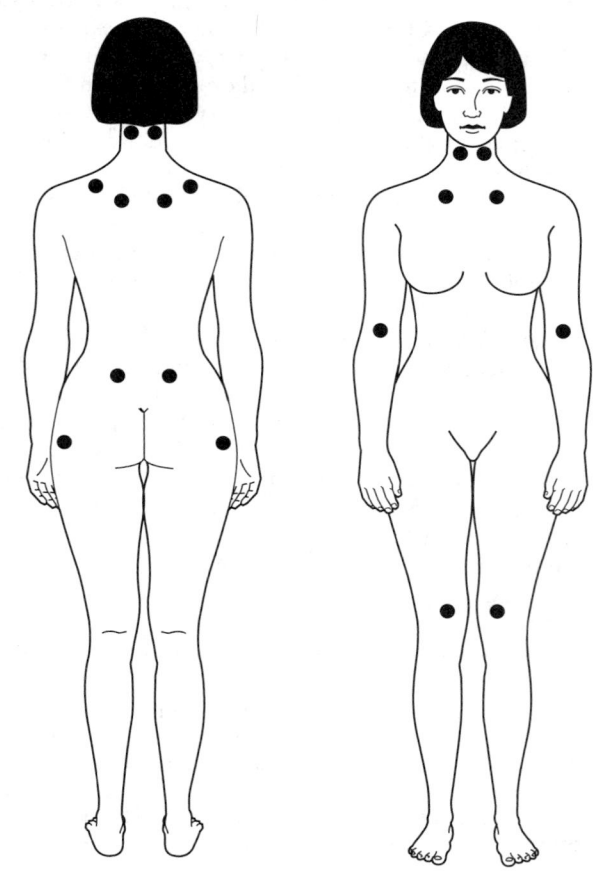

**FIGURE 1.** The location of the nine paired tender points that compose the 1990 American College of Rheumatology criteria for fibromyalgia. From the National Institute of Arthritis and Musculoskeletal and Skin Diseases: Questions and Answers about Fibromyalgia. Bethesda, MD: National Institute of Arthritis and Musculoskeletal and Skin Diseases, 2004. Available at http://www.niams.nih.gov/hi/topics/fibromyalgia/fibrofs.htm (accessed June 15, 2007).

laboratory evaluation including a complete blood count, chemistry panel, liver function tests, thyroid-stimulating hormone, creatine phosphokinase, and erythrocyte sedimentation rate is appropriate. In general, checking an antinuclear antibody, rheumatoid factor, or Lyme titer is usually not helpful, unless there is a clear suspicion from the history or physical examination of another coexisting rheumatic disease. Furthermore, nonselective rheumatologic testing can confound or delay the diagnosis and treatment of fibromyalgia by leading to further unnecessary medical evaluation, because these tests are often low positive or false positive in the normal population.

Management of fibromyalgia begins with an accurate diagnosis. Most patients are relieved to have a medical diagnosis for their symptoms and learn that it is not a dangerous or deforming arthritic disease. A multidisciplinary approach is key to achieving symptom relief and is outlined in the Current Therapy box. The physician should focus therapy on the symptoms that are most problematic for the patient and in improving restorative (Stage 4) restful sleep. Reassure the patient that most fibromyalgia patients do find some relief with therapy and can still live normal lives, despite interferences from symptom flares. Frequent physician's office visits and referrals to appropriate ancillary services often provide much needed support for the patient and lead to symptomatic improvement. Referral to a local fibromyalgia or arthritis self-help program through the Arthritis Foundation can be of much benefit.

## REFERENCES

Blundo JJ Jr: Regional rheumatic pain syndromes. In Klippel JH, Crofford LJ, Stone JH, Weyand CM (eds): Primer on the Rheumatic Diseases, 12th ed. Atlanta: Arthritis Foundation, 2001, pp 174-188.

Canoso JJ: Soft tissue and sports rheumatology. In Lahita R, Weinstein A (eds): Educational Review Manual in Rheumatology, 2nd ed. New York: Castle Connolly Graduate Medical Publishing, 2003, pp 1-85.

Clauw DJ: Fibromyalgia and diffuse pain syndromes. In: Klippel JH, Crofford LJ, Stone JH, Weyand CM eds): Primer on the Rheumatic Diseases, 12th ed. Atlanta: Arthritis Foundation, 2001, pp 188-193.

Goldenberg DL: Fibromyalgia and related syndromes. In Hochberg MC, Silman AJ, Smolen JS, et al (eds): Practical Rheumatology, 3rd ed. Philadelphia: Mosby, 2004, pp 255-266.

Goldenberg DL: Update on the treatment of fibromyalgia. Bull Rheum Dis 2004;53:1-7.

Hallegua DS, Wallace DJ: Managing fibromyalgia: A comprehensive approach. J Musculoskel Med 2005;22:382-390.

Liang KP, Matteson EL: Bursitis: Common condition, uncommon challenge. J Musculoskel Med 2006;23:513-522.

Malyak M: Fibromyalgia. In West S (ed): Rheumatology Secrets, 2nd ed. Philadelphia: Hanley & Belfus, 2002, pp 428-440.

Vogelgesang SA: Regional musculoskeletal disorders. In West S (ed): Rheumatology Secrets, 2nd ed. Philadelphia: Hanley & Belfus, 2002, pp 440-448.

Wolfe F, Smythe HA, Yunus MB, et al: The American College of Rheumatology 1990 criteria for the classification of fibromyalgia. Report of the Multicenter Criteria Committee. Arthritis Rheum 1990;33(2):160-172.

# Osteoarthritis

Method of
*George E. Ehrlich, MD*

In some respects, the term *osteoarthritis* is a misnomer because it refers only to a subset of joint changes—those accompanied by inflammation. An older, and still popular name in some parts of the world, is osteoarthrosis, which implies a condition of the joints without inflammation, and perhaps this should be revived for a majority of cases, in which pain is minimal at worst. A former synonym, degenerative joint disease, has been largely discarded, as it implies a specificity that cannot be supported. The confusion arises from the fact that no adequate definition of the term exists, and osteoarthritis occurs in almost all individuals past middle life, as well as in many individuals who are younger, but symptomatic osteoarthritis afflicts only a minority of these. Part of the reason no adequate definition exists derives from the roentgenographic criteria; a narrowing of "joint space" implies loss of cartilage (there is no real space in a joint, only the distance between the bones, composed of cartilage, which is radiolucent unless it contains crystals or metabolic derivatives), but other attributes, such as marginal osteophytes, are part of the repair process, and geodes (cysts in the subchondral bone) may even be part of the pathogenesis. The pathologist's definition includes diminished cartilage, fibrillation of cartilage, cartilaginous debris, the osteophytes and geodes, eburnation (smoothing of exposed bone denuded of its cartilage), and, in many instances, angiogenesis and increased vascularity. The clinician is confronted chiefly by symptomatic osteoarthritis, although roentgenograms taken for any purpose that include diarthrodial joints may disclose joint changes that can delude one into attributing symptoms to these; this is particularly true of spinal changes at the discs and intervertebral neural foramina.

From the standpoint of therapy, only symptomatic osteoarthritis requires treatment, and even much of that remains under dispute. Prevention would obviously be best, if it could be achieved, but in such a slowly developing process as osteoarthritis, it would require a lifetime of effort and may still not be attainable. Osteoarthritis, then, is not a disease but a final common pathway for all insults, overuse, and abuse of a joint, begun by trauma, diseases of metabolism, heritable and genetic predisposition, hormonal influences, and inflammatory diseases of the joints. The initial insult may well have occurred in childhood, but the expression as osteoarthritis takes years to develop (faster when the insult is severe, as in athletic injury, slower if because of repetitive minor trauma, and slower yet if the inception was minimal). When it becomes symptomatic, however, osteoarthritis fits the definition of disease and challenges treatment paradigms.

Osteoarthritis must be viewed as a reparative process, as confirmed by its antiquity: it is found in skeletons of prehistoric animals and early hominids and afflicted all vertebrates that lived long enough. At that, it is not a manifestation of aging, only a slowly developing process that requires time and is, therefore, more common in elderly individuals. Weather changes influence symptoms but not the process itself. There is no particular geographic predilection. Although some patterns are more common in some populations (e.g., interphalangeal osteoarthritis, which, except as a consequence of trauma, is rarely found in Africans and East Asians), that applies chiefly to interphalangeal osteoarthritis in which rows of joints are involved, and not to single large joints. Obesity has been cited as a precursor, a reasonable contention for affliction of weight-bearing joints, but equally true for interphalangeal osteoarthritis, where it should theoretically play no role. Increased bone density seems to parallel osteoarthritis, but whether causal or consequential needs to be determined (similarly, osteoporosis and osteoarthritis tend to be mutually exclusive, but again cause and effect are problematic). Some investigators have looked for causes in the bone. Subchondral microfractures and bone marrow edema have been cited, but again the relationship to expression remains controversial. Box 1 lists some of the known precursors, and Box 2 lists some of the presumed risk factors. Ultimately, osteoarthritis is thought to be a disease of chondrocyte fatigue, accelerated when the weakened chondrocytes can no longer replace proteoglycans, leading to structural alterations. Chondrocalcinosis, with deposition of hydroxy apatite or calcium pyrophosphate dihydrate, commonly accompanies symptomatic osteoarthritis, but may play more of a role in causing symptoms than contributing to pathogenesis. Although some would classify osteoarthritis as primary or secondary, it probably is always secondary, even if the inception is remote in the past and long forgotten. Remember that osteoarthritis is not an acute disease, even if punctuated by acute painful episodes in approximately 15% to 20% of those in whom roentgenographic evidence of osteoarthritis exists.

## Regional Issues

Patterns differ and give clues to pathogenesis. The knees are more frequently afflicted in women, perhaps because the broader pelvis leads to genu valgum and predisposes to knee afflictions.

## BOX 1   Precursors of Osteoarthritis

- Congenital
  Slipped femoral epiphysis
  Legg-Calvé-Perthes disease
- Bone dysplasias
  ? Kashin-Beck disease
  ? Mseleni joint disease
  ? Familial Mediterranean fever
- Metabolic
  Ochronosis
  Hemochromatosis
  Calcium pyrophosphate deposition disease
  Gout
- Traumatic
  Acute (e.g., athletic injury)
  Chronic (repetitive trauma)
- Endocrine
  Diabetes mellitus
  Acromegaly
  ? Obesity (cofactor?)
- Idiopathic
  Rheumatoid arthritis
  Septic arthritis disease
  Joint disease
- Vascular
  Avascular necrosis
- Neurologic
  Charcot joint
  Charcot-Marie-Tooth disease
- Bone disease
  Paget's disease (osteitis deformans)

## BOX 2   Risk Factors

| | |
|---|---|
| Aging | Time duration; weak muscle control (lower extremities) |
| Sex | Women: interphalangeal osteoarthritis, predilection knees in valgus |
| Obesity | May be cofactor (interphalangeal, knees in women) |
| Genetics | Symmetric Heberden's nodes, Ehlers-Danlos syndrome, genetic collagen abnormalities |
| Endocrine | Elevated growth hormone concentrations (postmenopause?) |
| Diet? | |
| Bone density | Increased bone density; osteoporosis |
| Race | Site predilections that may be racially related |
| Occupation | Jackhammers and similar tools, habitual usage (e.g., specific finger joints in knitting shop workers, elbows in foundry workers, knees in professional football running backs, shoulders in baseball pitchers) |
| Avocation | Knees and hips in joggers and runners on hard surfaces (not those who continue but those who drop out) |
| Inflammation | Calcium pyrophosphate dihydrate, hydroxy apatite, other crystal depositions |
| Trauma | Acute and severe, repetitive but mild to moderate |

However, although cartilage loss on the gliding surface of the patella generally results in symptoms, even major cartilage loss in the opposing surfaces of the femur and tibia may not, and the anatomic features fail to correlate with symptomatic expression. Although proprioceptive changes were thought to play a role in the pathogenesis of knee osteoarthritis, recent studies refute this contention.

The hips tend to be more often afflicted in men. The classic FABERE maneuver (flexion, abduction, external rotation, and extension) reveals limitations of motion and elicits pain. However, in time, knee and hip osteoarthritis are nearly gender equal.

Osteoarthritis of the distal interphalangeal (DIP) joints (Heberden's nodes) and proximal interphalangeal joints (PIP), usually symmetric, occurs in white women at about the time of menopause (earlier after total hysterectomies) and implies genetic predisposition; nonsymmetric involvement of these joints is often a consequence of specific traumas or work exposure. The symmetric variety often bares erosive changes at the joint margins, and is accompanied by the traditional signs of inflammation at presentation: redness, heat, swelling, pain, and functional deficits. The joints at the bases of the thumbs (first carpometacarpal, or trapeziometacarpal joints) tend also to be involved, and even the metacarpophalangeal joints, which rarely develop osteoarthritis in other circumstances. In these women, accompanying osteoarthritis at other joints is unrelated to the hereditary familial variety, bearing a casual, not causal, relationship.

The encroachment of osteophytes on the intervertebral foramina in the movable sections of the spine (cervical and lumbar) leads to referred pain in the areas served by the appropriate nerves. The shoulders are rarely a site of osteoarthritis, but sometimes severe destructive changes (the Milwaukee shoulder) do occur. Elbows are generally spared, but "cystic" protrusions through the joint capsules of distended fluid-filled joints lead to antecubital "cysts," the corollaries of the popliteal cysts at the knees; the latter can rupture, simulating thrombophlebitis in the calves. Wrists and ankles are almost always spared, because the mosaic distribution of the small bones diffuses forces. The first metatarsophalangeal joint is subject to osteoarthritis (the bunion) but rarely other joints of the toes (thought to be spared because shoes act as splints).

Although several studies claim that jogging and running do not predispose to osteoarthritis, these studies dealt with individuals who habitually exercised and not with those who gave up exercising, so they may well not conclusively prove the advantages of exercise for the majority of patients.

I have left out the molecular biology, the catalytic enzymes and debris, and even the synovial fluid changes, as these are of greater interest to the investigator than to the clinician responsible for counseling and treating patients. They are giving us some clues to better treatments in the future, however, and a later version of this article might well give them more prominence. Of greatest importance is not necessarily to ascribe symptoms to osteoarthritis detected on imaging; false attributions can delay correct diagnoses and appropriate treatment.

# Management

## PREVENTION

As osteoarthritis is the culmination of all life events at the joints, it cannot really be prevented. Attempts to use bovine cartilage extracts and other substances failed to retard progression and have been largely abandoned. However, as osteoarthritis is consequent to trauma or inflammation, aggressive treatment of this initial insult might delay its onset years later, but this remains unproven. Attention must be paid to the risk factors (see Box 2), minimizing them as much as possible; weight reduction obviously decreases the load on knee and hip joints in overweight individuals. Keeping joints supple through exercising and not exposing them to shear factors (particularly in sports), jogging on soft surfaces rather than on unyielding pavement, wearing supportive footwear (spike heels may not lead to osteoarthritis per se but can lead to accidents that do, and flat heels put excessive strain on the calf muscles and later the knees), and in general maintaining physical fitness are all helpful. Despite recently published studies that isometric exercises, especially of the quadriceps, probably cannot prevent osteoarthritis of the knees, these apply chiefly to radiographic changes and not to symptoms; it is still wise to recommend exercises that strengthen the muscles that move a joint, because function will be retained even if the anatomic changes continue. Osteoarthritis found on radiographs taken for another purpose, if asymptomatic, requires no treatment; the old dictum, "treat the patient, not the radiograph," applies. Architectural barriers should be avoided; ramps are particularly troublesome for knee and hip osteoarthritis, especially descending (that applies to stairs as well, as descent requires knee extension, which increases joint discomfort).

Symptomatic osteoarthritis occasions discomfort at times of weather changes, but the symptoms are often mild and tolerated. Many people treat themselves for these, before seeing a physician. It is important to know what they may be taking, as they often do not consider these as medicines, and potential drug interactions can occur.

## COMPLEMENTARY AND ALTERNATIVE TREATMENTS

Analgesics, such as acetaminophen (Tylenol and other unbranded generics) and aspirin, and several nonsteroidal anti-inflammatory drugs are readily available on supermarket shelves and pharmacies. In these days of global travel and ethnic migrations, other approaches also are common. Ayurvedic medicine is another system, popular in Southeast Asia and spreading from there; its medicines are based on plant extracts. Ayurvedic schools are found in India and the medicines themselves are carefully prepared and tested. The most popular treatment for osteoarthritis is composed of winter cherry, Indian frankincense, turmeric, and ginger (Artrex).

Herbal medicines available chiefly in health food stores have become popular throughout the United States. These are exempted by law from testing and approval by the FDA, and their safety and efficacy remain problematic. Potential interactions with prescribed drugs have not been studied. Ginger is especially popular, but among the other preparations are boron,[1] borage oil,[1] evening primrose oil,[1] and avocado soybean saponifiables,[1] all of which are claimed to be anti-inflammatory.

Yoga is currently being studied as a potential treatment for knee osteoarthritis, and acupuncture is said to provide considerable pain relief. Chiropractic adjustment is popular, especially for back pain attributed to osteoarthritis. However, the placebo effect is very striking in most osteoarthritis; even follow-up telephone calls from the doctor's office inquiring about the health of the patient lead to improvement. Do not slight the placebo effect, though—it is, after all, an effect.

## GENERAL PRINCIPLES

A recent symposium on osteoarthritis concluded that osteoarthritis is all about biomechanics, and normalization thereof yields better results than drug therapy (that means splints, braces, canes, shoe corrections, abolition of unsound architectural and style features). Joint damage is not the main determinant of pain, but psychosocial factors, compensation systems, and inaccurate labeling play a major role. Also, people who have osteoarthritis, because of the long duration of its inception, tend to be elderly and therefore more likely to tolerate drug therapy and surgery poorly, and because many have concurrent problems under treatment, are prone to untoward drug interactions.

As stated, only approximately 15% to 20% of individuals have sufficient pain to seek medical attention. This pain waxes and wanes, and considerable controversy addresses the best approaches to treatment. A much cited study compared acetaminophen 4 g per day with ibuprofen 1200 and 2400 μg a day during a span of 4 weeks, and concluded that there was no difference in results. However, the span is short, and proves only that analgesics are analgesic. Most patients prefer a

nonsteroidal anti-inflammatory drug (NSAID), especially in anti-inflammatory dosage, as confirmed in epidemiologic and observational studies. Physical and occupational therapy can help joint-sparing mobility, ergonomic principles help at the work site, and sexual counseling, for those afflicted with hip involvement in particular, should be part of the treatment program.

For inflammatory erosive osteoarthritis of the fingers, the overnight wearing of nylon and spandex stretch gloves can inhibit nodose deformities if started early enough, before these excrescences become bony and function is compromised.

## DRUG THERAPY

The severe pain of osteoarthritic joints—knees, hips, and fingers, chiefly—may be the result of secondary inflammation, caused by cartilaginous debris inciting cytokine response. A whole array of nonsteroidal anti-inflammatory drugs is available by prescription (from indomethacin [Indocin] and ibuprofen [Motrin, Advil, generics] through naproxen [Naprosyn, Aleve] and diclofenac [Voltaren], with doses usually lower than those for rheumatoid arthritis), and others, not available in the United States, may be taken by patients who purchased them abroad (e.g., tiaprofenic acid[2]). These inhibit cyclooxygenase, an enzyme necessary for prostaglandin synthesis that has been found to have at least two components, COX-1, which helps protect against gastric erosion and other consequences, and COX-2, which is evoked by inflammatory mediators and may lead to adverse gastric mucosal effects (a COX-3 has been proposed as well). To avoid the latter complication, misoprostol (Cytotec) may be prescribed or incorporated into a combination formulation with diclofenac (Arthrotec), but that is not without its own complications, namely, diarrhea and cramps. To avoid the adverse effects, a series of selective (at least in recommended dosage) COX-2 inhibitors were developed (e.g., celecoxib [Celebrex, 200 μg per day]). Lumiracoxib (Prexige),[2] 100 to 200 μg per day, was recently approved for short-term relief in osteoarthritis outside the United States. As of this writing, recommended doses may vary, so the package insert should always be consulted to determine the current appropriate dose. Gastric mucosal protection appears to be better, but there are renal consequences associated with its use and other problems are imputed. It must be stated that compounds considered safer are usually given to the patients most at risk, so the profiles do not address comparable populations. Moreover, the coxib NSAIDs are currently more expensive and not approved by all medical payment plans. Other NSAIDs, such as sulindac (Clinoril) and nabumetone (Relafen), are prodrugs, converted after absorption and hepatic biotransformation. Etodolac (Lodine) seems to work by a different mechanism; nimesulide is popular in Europe under a variety of trade names, but not available in the United States, is more COX-2 selective but less expensive, and may be brought back by travelers. Licofelone (as below) is awaiting approval in Europe. The choice of NSAIDs is relatively arbitrary; patients may respond well to one and not to another. In most instances, the most severe symptoms can be brought to a level patients will tolerate within a few days to weeks, and long-term therapy may not be necessary.

Aspirin, once the mainstay of treatment, has largely been superseded. Gastrointestinal intolerance, irreversible inhibition of platelet aggregation, and animal studies that show it to be deleterious to cartilage may be the reasons, but nonacetylated salicylates, such as salsalate (Disalcid) and choline magnesium trisalicylate (Trilisate), and simple analgesics, such as propoxyphene (Darvon)[1] and tramadol (Ultram), alone or in combination, are given alone or with NSAIDs. Narcotics are best avoided because of the potential for addiction.

Gastric mucosal erosions are found by endoscopy but usually do not translate into clinical problems. Similarly, elevation of hepatic enzymes is noncongruent with hepatotoxicity. Adverse effects on gastric mucosa are the most common; however, liver, kidney, and bone marrow complications, although uncommon, need also to be guarded against.

In most parts of the world, NSAIDs are available in creams and ointments for topical administration. The FDA is not convinced that

---

[1]Not FDA approved for this indication.

[1]Not FDA approved for this indication.
[2]Not available in the United States.

this is more than a placebo effect so these formulations are not currently available in the United States. However, topical capsaicin, the spice in pepper plants, has been approved for use in osteoarthritis and is available under a number of trade names over the counter (a prescription no longer is necessary). During the initial period of administration, localized burning is usual. Capsaicin is also available on a patch, which is especially popular in Asia.

## INTRA-ARTICULAR THERAPY

For nearly 50 years, cortisol derivatives have been injected into joints, usually after removal of the excess synovial fluid through arthrocentesis. When even symptomatic osteoarthritis was deemed not to be inflammatory, many clinicians cautioned that the resultant lack of pain indicated an insensitivity that could lead to further joint destruction, similar to the neuropathic Charcot joint. This fear has not been borne out and now arthrocentesis and corticosteroid instillation, preferably of a depot compound, in appropriately calibrated dosage, depending on the size of the joint, can effect long-lasting relief. However, patients should be admonished not to overuse the joint, at least for the first 3 days, as the lesions have not healed, even if the symptoms have abated. A general rule for counseling: do no more than when it hurt.

On the assumption that lubrication of the joint is impaired and corticosteroids are strictly palliative, preparations of hyaluronate have been approved for intra-articular instillation. While this procedure is called viscosupplementation, there is as yet little evidence that the instilled material is long retained in the joint or that it improves lubrication. Nevertheless, the results usually are as good as those with corticosteroids, and the duration of effect often long-lasting. The two preparations currently available are sodium hyaluronate (Hyalgan) and hylan G-F 20 (Synvisc), administered as a short series of three to five weekly injections; why they should work is problematic, and some controlled trials concluded that they were no more effective than placebo. This has been claimed for many preparations, however, because the placebo effect on pain is quite potent. Functional impairment remains, in most instances, especially at the hip, but often also at the knee. Hyaluronic acid is not indicated for interphalangeal injection, although small doses of corticosteroid into these tiny joints can sometimes lead to dramatic relief.

## GLUCOSAMINE AND CHONDROITIN SULFATE

Oral glucosamine[1] is said to be as analgesic as NSAIDs and acetaminophen. Multicenter controlled trials seem to agree, but there is still much skepticism about this treatment. There is no rationale to explain why it should be analgesic, but all studies show glucosamine to be superior to placebo or reference compounds, even if not statistically in all cases. It appears to be harmless, with no untoward interactions, and the hypothesis that it might aggravate diabetes mellitus has not been borne out. Most preparations are available over the counter. The likelihood exists that any patient with symptomatic osteoarthritis is taking glucosamine, and so are many rheumatologists, empirically trusting that it has a salutary effect. Chondroitin sulfate[1] has not been shown to add anything, except in some poorly designed studies. However, the combination of glucosamine and chondroitin sulfate is marketed more frequently than either compound alone, and whole shelves in markets and pharmacies are devoted to these.

## DISEASE MODIFICATION

By the time osteoarthritis becomes symptomatic and fulfills roentgenographic criteria, it is already well established. Thus, it is too late to think of "disease modification," as is now possible in rheumatoid arthritis. Nevertheless, the search for disease-modifying osteoarthritis drugs (DMOADs) goes on. All the compounds cited as possible DMOADs have been tested in animals only; no satisfactory assessment exists for studies in humans. Tetracycline derivatives, such as doxycycline,[1] seem to have merit. Drugs that work on the inner

mechanisms of cells, such as chloroquine (Aralen),[1] are also under study on theoretical grounds, but have not yet proved themselves. Antioxidant vitamins, tamoxifen (Nolvadex),[1] nitric oxide inhibitors, metalloproteases, and the aforementioned nutraceuticals have all been mentioned, but no reliable protocol exists that can measure their effect on cartilage and the joint. Specialized radiography that requires positioning is too crude for the purpose; magnetic resonance imaging and ultrasound have yet to be validated and standardized for this condition.

Studies are currently underway in Europe of diacerein (Diadar)[2] and growth factors, including insulin-like growth factor β, somatomedins, fibroblast growth factor, chondrocyte growth factor, and cartilage-derived and transforming growth factors. The problem of what to study and what outcome measures to use, and the duration of the trial, also bedevil these studies. While it is true that these are experimental treatments, not currently in use, and may never come to pass, they are mentioned here to counter the argument that the neurologist diagnoses untreatable disease and the rheumatologist treats untreatable disease. If not these, other treatments deriving from our better understanding of arthritis and its pathogenesis surely are in the offing. Included among these are mesenchymal stem cells that can produce site-specific tissue, thus restoring lost cartilage and bone, but how can that be done while mechanical impediments remain? The same is true for gene manipulation, and if new cartilage and bone are created, even with no counterpressures, how will the new attach to the older remnants and what will determine that? Cartilage transplants and chondrocyte transfer and stimulation are also being investigated. A polymer of glucosamine is also available (POLY-Nag).

## SURGERY

Surgery is the consequence of failure of medicine. Our inability to effect healing and repair leads to treatments that would be forestalled if we could anticipate who, and under what circumstances, develops symptomatic disease and offer appropriate medical treatments. Barring that, the surgical treatment of osteoarthritis has made remarkable progress during the past 40 years. By and large, the osteotomies that were formerly performed have faded into well-deserved oblivion. Arthroscopy was hailed as a less invasive way to deal with motion-impeding osteophytes and derangements and meniscal tears, especially if combined with lavage, but the results do not materially differ from those achieved with placebos. Indeed, removal of the meniscus seems to hasten the development of the ultimate osteoarthritic lesion. The major advance was the total joint replacement, first for hips, then knees and even fingers and other small joints of the hands. These have given back life content and quality of life to myriad recipients, more than 100,000 people annually in the United States alone! While surgery is clearly not a last resort, it has successfully addressed the functional deficits and pains and permitted recipients to resume their life styles. Shut-ins are liberated. Despite the trepidation of orthopedists, travel, skiing, tennis, and golf become achievable, even with bilateral surgery. Newer materials and methods of bonding have improved the longevity of these interventions.

Osteoarthritis remains an enigma, despite the major scientific advances of the past few years. Paradoxically, we have become more effective in treating advanced osteoarthritis and symptomatic disease (because of our better understanding of inflammation and the recognition that it plays a major role in evoking symptoms) than in addressing the variety of presentations. Symptomatic relief is achievable, and restoration of function; roentgenographic and pathologic changes may fulfill the definition but do not necessarily demand treatment. The removal of infectious and other killer diseases that curtailed life expectancy in the past has paradoxically resulted in the emergence of more chronic disorders. As stated in the World Health Organization's catalogue of disabilities, the killer diseases remove the consumer shortly after the consumer ceases to be a producer; the crippling diseases leave the consumer long after the consumer ceases to be a producer. The expense and increased suffering require a humane and scientifically sound understanding.

[1]Not FDA approved for this indication.

[1]Not FDA approved for this indication.

# Polymyalgia Rheumatica and Giant-Cell Arteritis

Method of
*Gideon Nesher, MD*

## Diagnosis

### GIANT-CELL ARTERITIS

Giant-cell arteritis (GCA) involves the major branches of the aorta, with a predilection for the extracranial branches of the carotid artery, such as the temporal arteries. The aorta itself can also be involved. GCA is often associated with polymyalgia rheumatica (PMR), a syndrome of bilateral aching and stiffness of the shoulder girdle and sometimes of the neck and hip girdle. More commonly, PMR manifests as an isolated disease without GCA. Both GCA and PMR occur in persons older than 50 years. Women are more commonly affected. Their clinical features and laboratory abnormalities are presented in Box 1.

Color duplex ultrasonography of the temporal arteries can aid in the diagnosis of GCA. A recent meta-analysis concluded that when the pretest probability of GCA is low, negative results of ultrasonography practically exclude GCA. It appears that ultrasonography better serves to rule out GCA, whereas a positive test needs to be confirmed by biopsy of the temporal arteries. However, because GCA affects the

### CURRENT DIAGNOSIS

#### Giant-Cell Arteritis

- Typical clinical manifestations (headache, tenderness over temporal arteries, jaw claudication, polymyalgia rheumatica, acute vision loss, low-grade fever) in an elderly patient.
- Laboratory markers of inflammation include elevated erythrocyte sedimentation rate and C-reactive protein, anemia of inflammation, and thrombocytosis.
- Color duplex ultrasonography of the temporal arteries can aid in GCA diagnosis. When the pretest probability of GCA is low, negative results of ultrasonography practically exclude GCA.
- Temporal artery biopsy showing vasculitis, often with giant cells, confirms the diagnosis. In cases with negative biopsy, rule out other conditions and rely on the clinical presentation and laboratory abnormalities together with the typical prompt response to steroid therapy.

#### Polymyalgia Rheumatica

- The chief symptom is bilateral aching of the shoulder girdle, and sometimes the neck and hip girdle, in an elderly patient. Morning stiffness is a prominent feature. Onset may be acute or gradual. PMR may be isolated or may be associated with GCA.
- Laboratory markers of inflammation include elevated sedimentation rate and C-reactive protein and sometimes anemia of inflammation.
- Prompt response to low-dose steroid therapy is typical and sometimes used to confirm the diagnosis.

*Abbreviations:* GCA = giant-cell arteritis; PMR = polymyalgia rheumatica.

---

## BOX 1   Clinical and Laboratory Features of Giant-Cell Arteritis

**Common**
- Elevated erythrocyte sedimentation rate and C-reactive protein, anemia of inflammation, thrombocytosis, elevated alkaline phosphatase
- Headache, scalp tenderness
- Jaw claudication
- Polymyalgia rheumatica
- Prominent temporal arteries
- Systemic symptoms: fever, malaise, fatigue, anorexia, and weight loss

**Uncommon**
- Aortic arch syndrome, aortic-valve insufficiency, aortic aneurysm and dissection.
- Involvement of other arteries (e.g., coronary, femoral)
- Peripheral neuropathies
- Respiratory symptoms (cough, sore throat, hoarseness)
- Scalp or tongue infarction
- Stroke, transient ischemic attacks, and other neuropsychiatric manifestations
- Vestibuloauditory manifestations (hearing loss, tinnitus)
- Vision loss, diplopia, and other ophthalmic manifestations

vessels focally, histologic examination is normal in about 15% of patients. A threshold size of 1 cm of temporal artery specimen is associated with increased diagnostic yield. It is preferable to perform the biopsy before therapy, but in most cases therapy should not be delayed pending the biopsy or its results (see later). There may be signs of arteritis even after 2 to 4 weeks of treatment.

There are no criteria to determine whether GCA is present when temporal artery biopsy is negative. The American College of Rheumatology (ACR) criteria for the classification of GCA can assist in diagnosis (Table 1). However, classification criteria work best in studying groups of patients, and they work less well when used for diagnosing individual cases. Meeting classification criteria is not equivalent to making the diagnosis in individual patients; the diagnosis should be based on all clinical and laboratory findings.

### POLYMYALGIA RHEUMATICA

There is no single diagnostic test for PMR, but sets of diagnostic criteria have been suggested by several groups of investigators. Two commonly used sets of criteria are presented in Table 1.

### GIANT-CELL ARTERITIS IN POLYMYALGIA RHEUMATICA PATIENTS

There is a wide range (4%-31%) of reported incidence of GCA in patients presenting with PMR. The two conditions can occur together, but they sometimes are separated by long intervals, and either one can manifest first. Aside from the typical features of GCA (see Box 1), severe systemic symptoms, severe degrees of anemia, thrombocytosis and ESR elevation, and poor clinical response to low-dose glucocorticoid therapy, with persistent abnormalities in laboratory parameters of inflammation all suggest GCA in patients presenting with PMR symptoms. In such cases, ultrasonography or biopsy of the temporal arteries should be performed to rule out GCA.

## Treatment

Glucocorticoids are the treatment of choice for PMR and GCA (Boxes 3 and 4). Symptoms typically begin to abate within 1 to 3 days

**TABLE 1** Suggested Criteria for Diagnosis of Polymyalgia Rheumatica and Classification of Giant-Cell Arteritis

| | Diagnosis of PMR | | Classification of GCA |
|---|---|---|---|
| Criteria | Bird et al, 1979 | Chuang et al, 1982 | ACR Criteria (Hunder et al, 1990) |
| Age (y) | >65 | >50 | >50 |
| Onset and duration | Onset <2 wk | Duration >1 mo | Not required |
| Area of pain | Shoulders | Two areas of the neck or torso, shoulders or proximal arms, hips or proximal thighs | Headache (new onset) |
| Tenderness | Upper arms | Not required | On palpation of TA or decreased pulsation of TA |
| Morning stiffness | >1 h | >30 min | Not required |
| Other features | Weight loss, depression | Not required | TA biopsy: vasculitis with mononuclear-cell infiltrates, often with giant cells |
| ESR | >40 mm/h | >40 mm/h If ESR is not elevated, look instead for other evidence to support the diagnosis | >50 mm/h |
| Requirements for diagnosis | ≥3 criteria: sensitivity 92%, specificity 80% | All criteria must be present | ≥3 criteria: sensitivity 93%, specificity 91%. |

*Abbreviations:* ACR = American College of Rheumatology; ESR = erythrocyte sedimentation rate; GCA = giant-cell arteritis; PMR = polymyalgia rheumatica; TA = temporal artery.
Based on Bird HA, Esselinckx W, Dison ASJ, et al: An evaluation of criteria for polymyalgia rheumatica. Ann Rheum Dis 1979;38:434-439; Chuang TY, Hunder GG, Ilstrup DM, Kurland LT: Polymyalgia rheumatica: A 10-year epidemiologic and clinical study. Ann Intern Med 1982;97;672-680; and Hunder GG, Bloch DA, Michel BA, et al: The American College of Rheumatology 1990 criteria for the classification of giant cell arteritis. Arthritis Rheum 1990;33:1122-1128.

of commencing therapy. This dramatic improvement is characteristic of both PMR and GCA. Prompt treatment is crucial in GCA to prevent irreversible complications of acute vision loss and stroke.

Levels of erythrocyte sedimentation rate (ESR) and C-reactive protein (CRP) do not always correlate with disease activity. Elevation of these levels while the patient is asymptomatic is not an indication to increase the dose of prednisone. In such cases, it is preferable to slow the rate of dose tapering and continue to watch closely for recurrence of symptoms. The dose should be increased if symptoms recur, even when ESR or CRP remain within the normal range.

The average duration of treatment is 2 to 3 years, but in some patients it is necessary to continue low doses of prednisone (5-10 mg/day) for longer periods. Relapses are experienced by 25% to 65% of patients, mostly during the first year of treatment or after discontinuing glucocorticoids. Most relapses are mild, but some GCA patients develop vision loss or stroke while tapering steroid dosage or after discontinuing therapy.

---

**BOX 2 Guidelines for Steroid Therapy in Giant-Cell Arteritis***

**Starting Daily Dose of Prednisone**
- Prednisone 40-60 mg for 2-4 wk
- Patients with vascular ischemic complications (stroke, vision loss) or imminent ischemic complications (transient ischemic attacks, amaurosis fugax, diplopia) are treated initially with higher prednisone doses (up to 120 mg[3]) or 500-1000 mg/d[3] of intravenous methylprednisolone (Solu-Medrol) for 3 consecutive d in an attempt to prevent additional ischemic complications

**Tapering and Maintenance**
- Reduce by 5-10 mg every 2-4 wk until dose is 20 mg, then reduce by 2.5-5 mg every 2-4 wk until the dose is 10 mg, and then reduce by 1 mg every mo
- If symptoms recur, increase the dose to the previous level or slightly above it for several weeks, then resume tapering
- In case of recurrent ischemic symptoms restart treatment with full dose

**Additional Therapies**
- Aspirin 100 mg/d to decrease the rate of vision loss and stroke
- Calcium, vitamin D, and bisphosphonates to prevent osteoporosis

---

[3]Exceeds dosage recommended by the manufacturer
*Individual cases vary greatly. The exact doses and the duration of treatment should be adjusted to the needs of the individual patient, considering both disease manifestations and steroid adverse effects. According to this schedule, treatment may be completed in 1-2 years.

---

**BOX 3 Guidelines for Steroid Therapy in Polymyalgia Rheumatica***

**Starting Daily Dose of Prednisone**
- 15-20 mg for 2-4 wk

**Tapering and Maintenance**
- Reduce by 2.5-5 mg every 2-4 wk until the dose is 10 mg, then by 1 mg every mo
- If symptoms recur, increase dose to the previous level or slightly above it for several weeks, then resume tapering.

**Additional Therapies**
- Calcium, vitamin D, and bisphosphonates to prevent osteoporosis.

---

*Individual cases vary. The exact doses and the duration of treatment should be adjusted to the needs of the individual patient, considering both disease manifestations and steroid adverse effects. According to this schedule, treatment may be completed in about 1 year.

## CURRENT THERAPY

- Glucocorticoids are the treatment of choice for both GCA and PMR. No steroid-sparing agent is proven widely effective thus far.
- Rapid improvement of clinical manifestations following treatment initiation is characteristic.
- Prompt treatment is crucial in GCA to prevent irreversible complications of acute vision loss and stroke. Addition of low-dose aspirin can further prevent these complications.
- The average duration of treatment is 2 to 3 years. Relapses are common but often mild.

*Abbreviations:* GCA = giant-cell arteritis; PMR = polymyalgia rheumatica.

Steroid-related adverse effects can become a source of great morbidity. No steroid-sparing agent is proven widely effective. Thus, the preferred approach to limit steroid side effects is to use the lowest possible dose for the shortest period, while avoiding disease relapses.

Low-dose aspirin (100 mg/day) has been shown to significantly decrease the rates of vision loss and stroke during the course of steroid therapy, probably mediated by its antiplatelet effect.

Aortic complications in the thoracic segment (aneurysms, dissection) can occur late in the course of GCA, sometimes after the completion of treatment. The thoracic aorta should be evaluated in all GCA patients during the follow-up period and after completion of treatment.

### REFERENCES

Bird HA, Esselinckx W, Dison ASJ, et al: An evaluation of criteria for polymyalgia rheumatica. Ann Rheum Dis 1979;38:434-439.

Chuang TY, Hunder GG, Ilstrup DM, Kurland LT: Polymyalgia rheumatica: A 10-year epidemiologic and clinical study. Ann Intern Med 1982;97;672-680.

Hachulla E, Boivin V, Pasturel-Michon U, et al: Prognostic factors and long-term evolution in a cohort of 133 patients with giant cell arteritis. Clin Exp Rheumatol 2001;19:171-176.

Hunder GG, Bloch DA, Michel BA, et al: The American College of Rheumatology 1990 criteria for the classification of giant cell arteritis. Arthritis Rheum 1990;33:1122-1128.

Karassa FB, Matsagas MI, Schmidt WA, Iannidis JP: Meta-analysis: Test performance of ultrasonography for giant cell arteritis. Ann Intern Med 2005;142:359-369.

Nesher G, Berkun Y, Mates M, et al: Low-dose aspirin and prevention of cranial ischemic complications in giant cell arteritis. Arthritis Rheum 2004;50:1332-1337.

Nesher G, Rubinow A, Sonnenblick M: Efficacy and adverse effects of different corticosteroid dose regimens in temporal arteritis: A retrospective study. Clin Exp Rheumatol 1997;15:303-306.

Nesher G, Sonnenblick M, Friedlander Y: Analysis of steroid related complications and mortality in temporal arteritis: A 15-year survey of 43 patients. J Rheumatol 1994;21:1283-1286.

Proven A, Gabriel SE, Orces C, et al: Glucocorticoid therapy in giant cell arteritis: Duration and adverse outcomes. Arthritis Rheum 2003;49:703-708

Weyand CM, Fulbright JW, Evans JM, et al: Corticosteroid requirements in polymyalgia rheumatica. Arch Intern Med 1999;159:577-584.

# Osteomyelitis

Method of
*Luca Lazzarini, MD*

Osteomyelitis is a complex disease often associated with high morbidity and considerable health care costs. This condition can be classified by duration (acute or chronic), pathogenesis (hematogenous or contiguous spread), site, extent, and by the type of patient (infant, child, adult, or compromised host). The Waldvogel classification system subdivides osteomyelitis as being either hematogenous or secondary to a contiguous focus of infection. Contiguous focus osteomyelitis has been further subdivided into osteomyelitis with or without vascular insufficiency. An alternative to the Waldvogel classification system has been developed by Cierny and Mader. The Cierny-Mader staging system is based on the anatomy of the bone infection and the physiology of the host (Box 1). The anatomic types of osteomyelitis are medullary (stage 1), superficial (stage 2), localized (stage 3), and diffuse (stage 4). Stage 1 infection is confined to the medullary surface of the bone. Hematogenous osteomyelitis and infected intramedullary rods are examples of this anatomic type. Stage 2 is a contiguous focus infection occurring when an exposed infected necrotic surface of bone lies at the base of a soft tissue wound. Stage 3 is usually characterized by a full-thickness, cortical sequestration that can be removed surgically without compromising bony stability. Stage 4 is a through-and-through process that usually requires an intercalary resection of the bone to arrest the disease process. Further, the patient

---

**BOX 1  The Cierny-Mader Staging System for Osteomyelitis**

**Anatomic Type**
- Stage 1: medullary osteomyelitis
- Stage 2: superficial osteomyelitis
- Stage 3: localized osteomyelitis
- Stage 4: diffuse osteomyelitis

**Physiologic Class**
- A:  normal host
- B:  compromised host
- Bs: systemically compromised
- Bl: locally compromised
- C:  treatment worse than the disease

**Factors Affecting Host Status**
- Systemic
  Malnutrition
  Renal and hepatic failure
  Diabetes mellitus
  Chronic hypoxia
  Immune disease
  Malignancy
  Extremes of age
  Immunosuppression
- Local
  Chronic lymphedema
  Venous stasis
  Major vessel compromise
  Arteritis
  Extensive scarring
  Radiation fibrosis
  Small-vessel disease
  Neuropathy
  Tobacco use

**TABLE 1 Principal Antibiotics Used in the Initial Intravenous Treatment of Osteomyelitis**

| | |
|---|---|
| Staphylococci, methicillin sensitive | Nafcillin (Unipen) 2 g q4-6h (+ rifampin[Rifadin][1] 600 mg qd PO) |
| Staphylococci, methicillin resistant | Vancomycin (Vancocin) 1 g q12h (+ rifampin [Rifadin][1] 600 mg qd PO) |
| Streptococci | Penicillin[1] 2 MU q4h |
| Anaerobes, gram-positive | Clindamycin[1] (Cleocin) 900 mg q8h |
| Anaerobes, gram-negative | Metronidazole[1] (Flagyl) 500 mg q8h |
| Enterobacteriaceae, *Pseudomonas* | Ciprofloxacin (Cipro) 400 mg q12h |

[1]Not FDA approved for this indication.
*Abbreviations:* PO = orally; q = every; qd = every day.

is classified as an A, B, or C host. An A host represents a patient with normal physiologic, metabolic, and immunologic capabilities. The B host is either systemically compromised, locally compromised, or both. When the morbidity of treatment is worse than that imposed by the disease itself, the patient is given the C host classification. This classification system aids in the understanding, diagnosis, and treatment of bone infections in children and adults (Table 1).

## Etiology

In hematogenous osteomyelitis, a single pathogenic organism is almost always recovered from the bone. In infants *Staphylococcus aureus*, *Streptococcus agalactiae*, and *Escherichia coli* are most frequently isolated from blood or bones. However, in children more than 1 year of age, *S. aureus*, *Streptococcus pyogenes*, and *Haemophilus influenzae* are most commonly isolated. The incidence of *H. influenzae* infection decreases after age 4 years. However, the overall incidence of *H. influenzae* as a cause of osteomyelitis is decreasing because of the new *H. influenzae* vaccine now given to children. In adults, *S. aureus* is the most common organism isolated. Multiple organisms are usually isolated from the infected bone in contiguous focus osteomyelitis. *S. aureus* remains the most commonly isolated pathogen. However, gram-negative bacilli and anaerobic organisms are also frequently isolated. Other microorganisms, such as mycobacteria and fungi, can be involved as well.

## Clinical Manifestations

### SIGNS AND SYMPTOMS

Hematogenous osteomyelitis in children may present with acute signs of infection including abrupt fever, irritability, lethargy, and local signs of inflammation. However, 50% of children present with vague complaints, including pain of the involved limb of 1 to 3 months in duration and minimal, if any, temperature elevation.

Adults with hematogenous osteomyelitis usually present with vague complaints consisting of nonspecific pain and few constitutional symptoms lasting 1 to 3 months. However, acute clinical presentations with fever, chills, swelling, and erythema over the involved bone(s) are occasionally seen. The source of bacteremia may be from a trivial skin infection or from a more serious infection such as acute or subacute bacterial endocarditis. Hematogenous osteomyelitis that involves either long bones or vertebrae is an important complication of injection drug abuse.

Patients with contiguous focus osteomyelitis often present with localized bone and joint pain, erythema, swelling, and drainage around

## CURRENT DIAGNOSIS

- Clinical signs
- Plain radiographs
- CT, NMR, and bone scans obtained in selected cases
- Cultures from sinus tract are unreliable
- Perform bone biopsy for culture and histology whenever possible

*Abbreviations:* CT = computed tomography; NMR = nuclear magnetic resonance.

the area of trauma, surgery, or wound infection. Signs of bacteremia such as fever, chills, and night sweats may be present in the acute phase of osteomyelitis, but not in the chronic phase.

The sedimentation rate is usually elevated, reflecting chronic inflammation, but the leukocyte count is usually normal. The chronic disease is usually either not progressive or slowly progressive. If a sinus tract becomes obstructed, the patient may present with a localized abscess and or an acute soft tissue infection. A sedimentation rate that returns to normal during the course of therapy is a favorable prognostic sign.

### MICROBIOLOGY

The diagnosis and determination of the etiology of long bone osteomyelitis rests on the isolation of the pathogen(s) from the bone lesion or blood or joint culture. Except in hematogenous osteomyelitis, where positive blood or joint fluid cultures may suffice, antibiotic treatment of osteomyelitis should be based on meticulous cultures of bone taken at débridement surgery or from deep bone biopsies. If possible, cultures should be obtained before antibiotics are initiated. Sinus tract cultures are unreliable for predicting which organisms will be isolated from infected bone; however, those growing *S. aureus* show a positive correlation with bone cultures.

### RADIOLOGY

In hematogenous osteomyelitis, radiographic changes usually correlate with the destructive process and are usually seen when at least 50% to 75% of the bone matrix is destroyed. This happens at least 2 weeks after the infection was initiated. The earliest radiologic changes are swelling of the soft tissue, periosteal thickening and/or elevation, and focal osteopenia. Radiographic improvement may lag behind clinical recovery, even when the patient is receiving appropriate antimicrobial therapy. In contiguous focus osteomyelitis, the radiographic changes are subtle, often found in association with other nonspecific radiographic findings, and require a careful clinical correlation to achieve diagnostic significance. Computed tomography (CT) may play a role in the diagnosis of osteomyelitis. Increased marrow density occurs early in the infection, and intramedullary gas has been reported in patients with hematogenous osteomyelitis. The CT scan can also help identify areas of necrotic bone and assess the involvement of the surrounding soft tissues. One disadvantage of this study is the scatter phenomenon, which occurs when metal is present in or near the area of bone infection. Magnetic resonance imaging (MRI) has been recognized as a useful modality for diagnosing the presence and scope of musculoskeletal infection. The resolution of MRI makes it useful in differentiating between bone and soft tissue infection, often a problem with radionuclide studies. Radionuclide scans may be obtained when the diagnosis of osteomyelitis is ambiguous or to help gauge the extent of bone and soft tissue inflammation.

## Treatment

Therapy of osteomyelitis is both surgical and medical and includes adequate drainage and débridement, obliteration of dead space, soft

## CURRENT THERAPY

- Stabilization (if needed) and surgical débridement
- Antibiotic treatment of 4 to 6 weeks after surgical débridement
- Select antimicrobial according to in vitro sensitivity tests; consider toxicity, allergy, costs
- Antibiotic suppressive therapy in selected cases

tissue coverage, and specific antimicrobial treatment. If the patient is a compromised host, an effort is made to correct or improve the host defect.

## ANTIBIOTIC TREATMENT

According to the results of animal studies, the optimal duration of antibiotic treatment is 4 to 6 weeks. The time needed for bone revascularization after débridement surgery is approximately 3 weeks. Shorter durations are probably successful when the infection is superficial (stage 2) and a complete débridement is performed and when ablative surgery (amputation above the infected region) is performed.

Antibiotic treatment for osteomyelitis is traditionally administered by the intravenous (IV) route. To reduce hospitalization and health care costs, outpatient IV therapy is currently used. This modality of administration reduces treatment cost and improves patient quality of life.

Antistaphylococcal penicillins (nafcillin [Unipen],[1] oxacillin [Prostaphlin][1]) are used for the treatment of methicillin-sensitive staphylococcal osteomyelitis. A first-generation cephalosporin, cefazolin (Ancef), is effective in the treatment of staphylococcal osteomyelitis. The glycopeptides vancomycin (Vancocin)[1] and the oxazolidinone antibiotic linezolid (Zyvox)[1] are used to treat methicillin-resistant staphylococcal osteomyelitis. Several third- and forth-generation cephalosporins, such as cefotaxime (Claforan)[1] or cefepime (Maxipime)[1] can be used to treat osteomyelitis because of gram-negative bacilli.

Oral antibiotics have also been successfully used to treat osteomyelitis. Several oral drugs, such as clindamycin (Cleocin),[1] rifampin (Rifadin),[1] cotrimoxazole (Bactrim),[1] and fluoroquinolones (e.g., ciprofloxacin [Cipro] and levofloxacin [Levaquin][1]) are currently used in the treatment of osteomyelitis. Clindamycin (Cleocin), a lincosamide antibiotic active against most gram-positive bacteria, possesses an excellent bioavailability and is currently used orally, after an initial IV treatment of 2 weeks. Oral therapy using quinolones for gram-negative organisms is used in adult patients with osteomyelitis. The current quinolones have variable *S. aureus* and *Staphylococcus epidermidis* coverage. Pediatric patients should not be given the quinolone class of antibiotics because of possible damage to cartilage.

The initial treatment of most cases of osteomyelitis usually starts on an empirical basis. After cultures are obtained, a parenteral antimicrobial regimen is begun, covering the clinically suspected pathogens. Once the organism is identified, different antibiotics can be selected by appropriate sensitivity methods. If possible, antibiotics should not be initiated until the results of the bone bacterial culture and sensitivities are known.

## ANTIBIOTIC TREATMENT BY CIERNY-MADER STAGE

Stage 1 osteomyelitis in children usually responds to antibiotics alone. Stage 1 osteomyelitis in adults is more refractory to therapy and is usually treated with antibiotics and surgery. The patient is treated for 4 to 6 weeks with appropriate antimicrobial therapy, dated from the initiation of therapy or after the last major débridement surgery. If after 48 hours there is no clinical improvement, surgical treatment

may be needed in conjunction with another 4-week course of antibiotics.

In stage 2 osteomyelitis shorter courses of antibiotics, such as 2 weeks, are usually given. In stages 3 and 4 osteomyelitis the patient is treated with 4 to 6 weeks of antimicrobial therapy dated from the last major débridement surgery. This long treatment is needed because even when all necrotic tissue has been adequately débrided, the remaining bed of tissue must be considered contaminated with the responsible pathogen(s).

## SUPPRESSIVE ANTIBIOTIC THERAPY

When surgical treatment of osteomyelitis is not feasible, a long-term antibiotic therapy is usually given to control the disease and to prevent flare-ups. Oral antibiotics are usually used. Suppressive therapy has been studied extensively in the setting of infected orthopedic implants. The efficacy of suppressive treatment in osteomyelitis without implants has not been determined. Suppressive therapy is usually administered for 6 months. If recurrence of the infection occurs after discontinuation, a new, culture-directed suppressive regimen is begun and administered indefinitely.

## SURGICAL TREATMENT

Surgical treatment of osteomyelitis includes adequate drainage, extensive débridement of all necrotic tissue, obliteration of dead spaces, adequate soft tissue coverage, and restoration of an effective blood supply.

Adequate débridement may leave a large bony defect termed *dead space*. The goal of dead space management is to replace dead bone and scar tissue with vascularized tissue. Local tissue flaps or free flaps may be used to fill dead space. An alternative technique is to place cancellous bone grafts beneath local or transferred tissues where structural augmentation is necessary. Antibiotic-impregnated acrylic beads may be used to sterilize and temporarily maintain dead space. The beads are usually removed within 2 to 4 weeks and replaced with a cancellous bone graft. The most commonly used antibiotics in beads are vancomycin (Vancocin),[1] tobramycin,[1] and gentamicin.[1] Because beads act as a biomaterial surface to which bacteria adhere, infection associated with the use of beads has been described.

If movement is present at the site of infection, measures must be taken to achieve permanent stability of the skeletal unit. Stability may be achieved with plates, screws, rods, and/or an external fixator. External fixation is preferred more than internal fixation because of the tendency of medullary rods to become secondarily infected and to spread the extent of the infection. The Ilizarov fixator is a type of external fixator that allows reconstruction of segmental bone defects and difficult infected nonunions. The technique is used for difficult cases of osteomyelitis when stabilization and bone lengthening is necessary.

Adequate soft tissue coverage of the bone is often necessary to arrest osteomyelitis. Small soft tissue defects may be covered with a split thickness skin graft. In the presence of a large soft tissue defect or with an inadequate soft tissue envelope, local muscle flaps and free vascularized muscle flaps may be placed in a one- or two-stage procedure. Local muscle flaps and free vascularized muscle transfers improve the local biologic environment by bringing in a blood supply important in host defense mechanisms, antibiotic delivery, and osseous and soft tissue healing.

## REFERENCES

Cierny G, Mader JT, Pennick JJ: A clinical staging system for adult osteomyelitis. Contemp Orthop 1985;10:17-37.

Lew DP, Waldvogel FA: Osteomyelitis. Lancet 2004;364:369-379.

Shuford JA, Steckelberg JM: Role of oral antimicrobial therapy in the management of osteomyelitis. Curr Opin Infect Dis 2003;16:515-519.

Simpson AH, Deakin M, Latham JM: Chronic osteomyelitis. The effect of the extent of surgical resection on infection-free survival. J Bone Joint Surg Br 2001;83:403-407.

---

[1]Not FDA approved for this indication.

---

[1]Not FDA approved for this indication.

# Common Sports Injuries

Method of
*Suraj Achar, MD, and Alexander Espinoza, MD*

Patients with sports-related injuries commonly present to primary care physicians. With more than 30 million children playing organized sports, more than one third of school-age children will sustain an sports injury severe enough to require a doctor or nurse visit. The yearly costs have been estimated to be more than $1.8 billion in direct health care costs. The incidence and cost of care for adult sports-related injuries far exceed those for our school-age children. To diagnose and treat these injuries, providers must take a focused history, carefully examine the musculoskeletal system, use radiologic and physical therapy resources, and occasionally refer to appropriate specialty services.

## Evaluation

The evaluation of all sports injuries begins with the history. Sir William Osler has been credited with giving the greatest importance to history. Even today with advanced diagnostics such as magnetic resonance imaging (MRI), computed tomography (CT), and bone scanning, the history is fundamental.

Obviously, the duration and mechanism of the injury are key factors. An acute knee effusion that develops within an hour of injury is more likely to represent an anterior cruciate ligament (ACL) tear or osteochondral fracture than a meniscal tear, where the effusion often develops over a period of 24 hours.

Age is a critical factor because a child is more susceptible to growth plate injuries than ligament injuries. In children, growth plate fractures and apophysitis are more common than severe ligamentous disruptions and tendonitis. Child abuse must also be considered in our youngest children when multiple bones are broken or the history is not compatible with the injury.

## Diagnosis

The level of sports participation is critical for diagnosis and treatment. Obviously, an X-games skateboarder is more likely to suffer higher impact forces and subsequent fractures. On occasion, for professional and elite athletes, the diagnostic evaluation needs to be completed without delay to determine if the athlete can return to play. With our minors, on the other hand, injury evaluation must be deliberate to prevent recurrent injury. Care is customized at all levels of sports medicine. Sometimes with an older athlete we wait longer to refer to orthopedics for the same meniscal tear that in an adolescent requires urgent referral for possible repair.

Today's diagnosis of sports-related injuries often includes radiologic studies. X-rays should be ordered in cases where trauma leads to large joint effusions, tenderness to palpation, inability to actively move the joint through a full range of motion, or inability to bear weight. Age plays a role. Growing adolescents need x-rays to diagnose growth plate injuries and older adults need x-rays to diagnose insufficiency fractures due to osteopenia or osteoporosis. Some special rules have been used to help physicians know when they do not need to order x-rays in the trauma situation. The Ottawa knee and ankle rules have been carefully studied and if followed properly will not lead to missed fracture diagnosis (Box 1).

Advanced diagnostic tests are needed in special cases. MRI is best used to diagnose and evaluate soft tissue tendon and ligament injuries and to grade or diagnose osteochondral injuries. When ordering an MRI, the physician should have a differential diagnosis in mind and should discuss with the patient the possibility of surgical referral if the MRI shows a lesion that will be amenable to surgery. If the patient is not at all interested in surgical referral, advanced diagnostics may be

---

**BOX 1   Ottawa Knee and Ankle Rules**

- An ankle x-ray is required for patients with any of the following:
  - Bone tenderness to palpation along the posterior edge or tip of the lateral or medial malleolus
  - Bone tenderness to palpation at the base of the fifth metatarsal or at the navicular
  - Inability to bear weight both immediately after the injury and for four steps in the emergency department or doctor's office
- A knee x-ray is required for patients with any of the following:
  - Isolated tenderness to palpation of the patella (i.e., no bone tenderness of the knee other than the patella)
  - Tenderness to palpation at the head of the fibula
  - Inability to flex to 90 degrees
  - Inability to bear weight both immediately after the injury and for four steps in the emergency department or doctor's office

From Bachmann LM, Kolb E, Koller MT, et al: Accuracy of Ottawa ankle rules to exclude fractures of the ankle and mid-foot: Systematic review. BMJ 2003;326:417; and Stiell IG, Wells GA, Hoag RH, et al: Implementation of the Ottawa knee rule for the use of radiography in acute knee injuries. JAMA 1997;278: 2075-2079.

deferred pending response to conservative management. Bone scanning and CT scanning also have particular roles. Bone scanning can help diagnose stress fractures that are not apparent on plain radiography, and CT scanning is particularly useful to evaluate fractures.

## Treatment

The most important treatment principle in sports medicine is active rest. Often, with injured bones, joints, tendons, and muscles rest is employed to help healing. However, with the epidemic of obesity and the rapid onset of stiffness in acute injuries, total rest is deleterious to the patient. Active rest, where the patient exercises noninjured parts of the body, helps healing, improves sense of control, and gives the patient an avenue for energy. While one area is injured, we crosstrain in another. A perfect example is swimming as crosstraining for an athlete with a stress injury of the tibia.

The rest of the rehabilitation protocol can be summarized in the mnemonic PRICE. P stands for protection, such as splinting an injured ligament. R stands for active rest. I represents ice. C stands for compression, and E stands for elevation.

## Pediatric Sports Injuries

### SLIPPED CAPITAL FEMORAL EPIPHYSIS

#### Epidemiology

Outside of trauma, slipped capital femoral epiphysis (SCFE) is the number one cause of adolescent limp. It occurs in approximately 1 in 10,000 children in the United States. It is more common in boys than girls by 1.5 to 1 and is three times more common in Latin American and African American children than in white children. For unknown reasons, SCFE is more common in the left hip. It is bilateral at presentation in 20% of children and can affect the unaffected hip over the next 6 to 18 months in nearly 50% of children. The peak incidence of SCFE occurs during the early adolescent growth spurt, which is earlier in girls, at approximately 12 years, than boys at approximately 13 years of age.

## Etiology

The etiology of SCFE is secondary to the basic biological susceptibility of the adolescent physis with the added forces of obesity leading to a mechanical shear effect. Genetics plays a role, with a report of four cases occurring in one family. Multiple endocrinopathies such as the metabolic syndrome, hypothyroidism, and growth hormone disorders have also been linked to an increased risk of SCFE.

## Diagnosis

The usual history of SCFE includes a dull hip pain that often radiates to the knee. Pain usually is increased during activity. In some cases, and especially with the opposite affected hip, the patient can be asymptomatic.

The physical examination often shows decreased range of motion on internal and external rotation and even occasionally obligate external rotation when the hip is passively flexed. The best diagnostic test is anteroposterior (AP) pelvis and frog leg lateral x-rays (Figures 1 and 2). On the AP pelvis, a Klein line should be drawn along the lateral femoral cortex and should intersect with at least 20% of the lateral femoral head. The frog leg lateral is even more sensitive and can show subtle lateral displacement of the femoral neck.

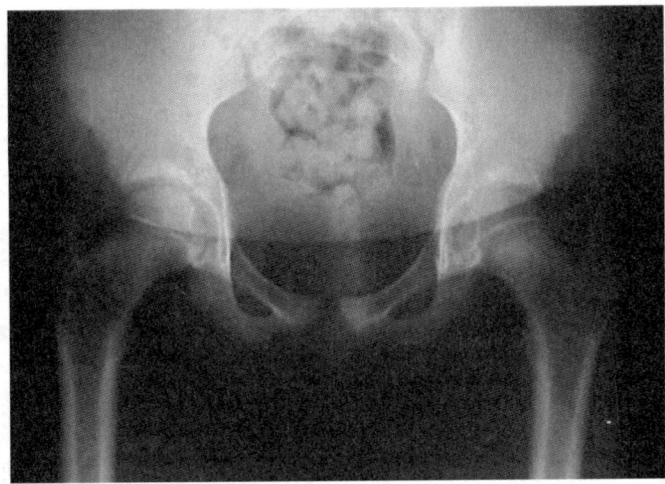

**FIGURE 1.** Anteroposterior view of the pelvis showing a slipped capital femoral epiphysis. A Klein line drawn along the lateral femoral cortex should intersect with at least 20% of the lateral femoral head.

Radiographs can also be used to grade SCFE cases. Mild slips have less than one third of the metaphyseal width involved, moderate slips involve one third to one half of the width, and severe slips involve more than one half the width. Although radiographs are the preferred initial diagnostic tools, MRI can be useful in occult preslips where widening of the physis with surrounding edema is a reliable early sign. CT and ultrasound are less useful.

## Treatment

The treatment of SCFE begins with the diagnosis. Immediately, patients should be made non–weight bearing. Ideally, a pediatric

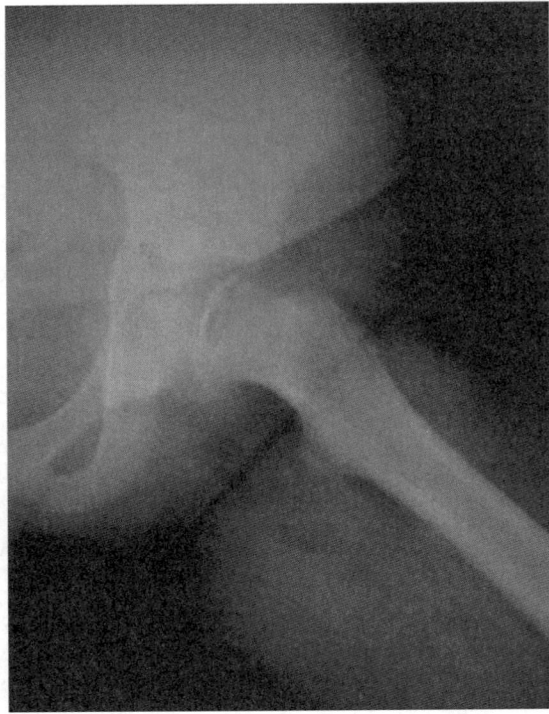

**FIGURE 2.** Frog leg lateral view of the pelvis showing a slipped capital femoral epiphysis. The frog leg lateral view is even more sensitive than the anteroposterior view and can show subtle lateral displacement of the femoral neck.

## CURRENT THERAPY

### Slipped Capital Femoral Epiphysis

- Once slipped capital femoral epiphysis is considered, immediate non–weight bearing is required until surgery can be performed to stabilize the slip.
- Order follow-up x-rays in the contralateral hip, which can have an asymptomatic slip or a slip that occurs within the next 18 months.

### Little League Elbow

- Reduced valgus strain, including throwing, is the key to recovery.
- Avulsion greater than 5 degrees often requires surgical intervention.
- Look for occult osteochondritis dissecans on the lateral elbow.

### Osteochondritis Dissecans

- Treatment is determined by level of symptoms and activity.
- Age is also a determining factor.
- More randomized studies for newer transplantation techniques are needed.

### Scaphoid Fractures

- Early immobilization in patients with suspected scaphoid fracture even with negative x-rays is the standard of care.
- Repeat x-rays in 2 weeks for those whose x-rays are initially negative.
- Liberally refer scaphoid fractures, especially those that are mid or proximal, to orthopedics because of high rates of nonunion and avascular necrosis.

### Iliotibial Band Syndrome

- Conservative treatment with rehabilitation and modified activity is standard.
- Surgery with Z-plasty is rarely indicated.

### Meniscal Tears of the Knee

- Customization of care for the treatment of meniscal tears is critical for the high-level or professional athlete to be able to return to play safely and quickly.
- Sports-specific activities such as running, jumping, twisting, and cutting should determine grade of conservative versus operative treatments.
- Conservative treatment is chosen for small stable meniscal tears and nonactive patients.

orthopedic surgeon can be consulted and surgical fixation can be arranged. Further weight bearing after diagnosis can lead to further slip and ultimately increased risk of avascular necrosis of the hip. Hospitalization should be arranged for the acute unstable cases.

Postoperative management includes a period of limited weight bearing with crutches or a walker. Follow-up should be arranged for all patients with unilateral slips because of the high incidence of eventual development of SCFE in the contralateral hip, which can occur up to 18 months after the initial hip involvement. Close follow-ups with hip examinations and possible x-rays are usually continued until the child finishes growing and the femoral growth plates close.

### Prognosis

The prognosis of SCFE depends on the severity of the acute injury. Avascular necrosis occurs in 2% of mild slips and 19% of severe slips.

## LITTLE LEAGUE ELBOW

### Epidemiology

*Little league elbow* is a term used to describe a group of medial elbow problems that result from valgus traction strain on the elbow in growing children. Initially, it was described as an avulsion fracture of the medical epicondyle growth plate. Today, it is synonymous with apophysitis of the medial elbow growth plate that occurs with throwing sports. The same valgus stress and symptoms occur in nonthrowing sports, including wrestling and gymnastics.

### Etiology

Risk factors for little league elbow include pitching fewer than 300 pitches a season or more than 600 pitches a season, pitching more than 8 months a year, and averaging over 80 pitches per game. Risk factors also include the early use of the curve ball and slider, which put more valgus strain on the medial side. More than 50% of adolescent throwers have either elbow or shoulder pain. Catchers may be at the most risk because no one keeps track of their throws, and they typically play the same position every game.

### Diagnosis

Symptoms of little league elbow include medial elbow pain, weakness, decreased throwing speed, and decreased throwing distance. On physical examination, tenderness to percussion is noted at the medial epicondyle, with pain on resisted wrist flexion and forearm pronation. Occasionally, for acute injuries, bruising and valgus instability or even an elbow contracture are noted if symptoms have been chronic.

AP and lateral x-rays must be ordered because there may be a widening, avulsion fragmentation, separation, and asymmetry of the medial epicondyle. For early or mild changes, the contralateral elbow can be used for comparison. Comparison might not be valid in athletes such as gymnasts, who might have changes in both elbows. It is important to look at the lateral elbow on x-rays because contralateral osteochondritis dissecans (OCD) can sometimes be seen secondary to microtrauma.

The main differential diagnosis of little league elbow is ulnar collateral ligament strains or tears. Initially, as children progress through their active growth spurt, the growth plate is weaker than the ligaments. However, if the x-rays show closure of the medial apophysis, then ulnar collateral ligament injury is likely. In this case, an MRI of the elbow can help define the extent of ulnar collateral ligament involvement in significantly injured athletes. MRI should also be used to define and grade any contralateral OCD lesion.

### Treatment

Treatment includes active rest. Athletes are encouraged to maintain cardiovascular conditioning drills without throwing or straining the medial elbow for 4 to 6 weeks. Ice and nonsteroidal anti-inflammatory drugs (NSAIDs) may be used for symptomatic early therapy, and physical therapy and strengthening programs may be used once pain is resolved. For small avulsions with less than 5 mm of distraction, casting may be useful; a flexion contraction that will need physical therapy is expected. For large or wide avulsions more than 5 mm of distraction, referral to pediatric orthopedics is required.

## OSTEOCHONDRITIS DISSECANS

OCD remains a rare joint disorder. As early as 1888, when Konig first described OCD as a loose-body formation associated with articular cartilage and subchondral bone formation, several advances have been developed to diagnose and treat these chronic lesions. Diagnosis can be made in the clinical setting with the aid of imaging techniques. Different grades exist. Generally, grades 1 and 2 lesions are stable and grades 3 and 4 lesions are unstable. Goals must be individualized according to symptoms and the patient's level of activity.

## Etiology and Epidemiology

OCD is defined by osteochondral fracture. It is a form of osteochondrosis of the articular epiphysis. As a result of compression, the articular epiphysis fails, most likely from trauma and ischemia. Trauma, either from impaction fractures or repetitive mictrotrauma, is most likely the primary insult, with ischemia being a secondary injury. Injury of articular cartilage allows an influx of synovial fluid into the epiphysis, which creates a subchondral cyst. The subchondral cyst and increased joint pressure prevent adequate healing. Idiopathic osteonecrosis may be another factor, most likely genetic, but not well understood.

The prevalence in the United States is unknown. No race or gender predilections have been reported. OCD tends to affect young patients, with age ranges somewhere between 4 and 50 years, the average being the second decade of life.

## Sites of Pathology

Overall, the knee is most often involved. The lateral aspect of the medial femoral condyle is the most commonly involved site (75%). Other sites include the weight-bearing surfaces of the medial (10%) and lateral femoral (10%) condyles and the anterior intercondylar groove or patella (5%).

The most common site for OCD in the elbow joint is the anterolateral aspect of the capitellum.

In the ankle, by far the most common site is the talus. Talar dome lesions are found on the posteromedial aspect (56%) and the anterolateral aspect (44%).

Others sites are rare but include the tibial plafond, tarsal navicular, hip joint (femoral capital epiphysis), shoulder (humeral head or glenoid), and wrist (scaphoid).

## Diagnosis

OCD lesions most often occur after injury such as in the ankle, with inversion injuries to the lateral ligamentous complex. Patients typically present with chronic ankle pain, intermittent swelling, and possibly weakness, stiffness, catching or locking, or instability. In general, joint line tenderness and effusions are present. Patients usually report pain at the range of motion extremes.

Start with plain radiographs. If plain films are negative, consider repeating them in 2 to 4 weeks. MRI should then be ordered to stage the lesion according to Anderson classification (Box 2.) Bone scanning is especially useful to determine if an early stage lesion has good potential to heal. Increased blood pool on delayed phases of the bone scan helps identify osteochondral lesions that are likely to heal. Sonography has been used to evaluate OCD in the humeral capitellum, with the advantage being dynamic scanning with the motion of the evaluated joint.

## Treatment

Nonoperative treatments for early stage lesions include discontinuation of the injurious activity, protected immobilization, administration of NSAIDs, and surgery. There is no evidence that non–weight-bearing casts offer improved results over weight-bearing casts.

---

> ### BOX 2  The Anderson MRI Classification
>
> - Stage I: Bone marrow edema
> - Stage IIA: Subchondral cyst formation
> - Stage IIB: Incomplete separation of the osteochondral fragment
> - Stage III: Fluid around an undetached, undisplaced osteochondral fragment
> - Stage IV: Displaced osteochondral fragment
>
> ---
>
> *Abbreviation:* MRI = magnetic resonance imaging.

---

Also, there is no evidence that patients need to be immobilized if they are kept non–weight bearing.

Surgical treatments include débridement or curettage and drilling. Newer techniques include bone grafting, autologous osteochondral grafting, and autologous chondrocyte transplantation. Special consideration is given to the younger patients who still have open growth plates, because drilling can cause growth failure. Children with open growth plates and stable OCD lesions of stage 1 and possibly stage 2 heal at a much greater rate with nonsurgical management than adults do.

# Common Adult Sports Injuries

### SCAPHOID FRACTURES

## Epidemiology

A fall on an outstretched hand (FOSH) is a common sports injury. The most common injured bone in the wrist is the distal radius, and the next most common is the scaphoid. The scaphoid accounts for approximately 70% of carpal fractures.[1] It is more common in men than women and often occurs in adolescents and young adults 15 to 30 years of age. The scaphoid bone is particularly important from a medicolegal standpoint, because 2% to 5% of injuries are missed on initial presentation, and even when they are discovered, nonunion and avascular necrosis are common.[2]

## Diagnosis

Fractures typically occur with FOSH injuries with the hand dorsiflexed. On physical examination, swelling may be absent, but tenderness to palpation is noted at the anatomic snuffbox and often at the scaphoid tubercle. Unless the bone is displaced, range of motion is often preserved, but grip strength should be decreased. A high index of suspicion and any tenderness on percussion at the snuffbox requires x-rays and treatment.

In suspected scaphoid fractures, radiographs should include posteroanterior (PA), lateral, and scaphoid views. The scaphoid view is a PA view of the scaphoid in full pronation and ulnar deviation. Lateral views are helpful to demonstrate the scapholunate angle, but the scaphoid view is the most sensitive. Negative x-rays with positive clinical suspicion necessitate either advanced diagnostic tests such as a bone scan or MRI or immobilization and follow-up films in 2 weeks. CT scanning can also be used and has been shown to be more sensitive and specific than bone scanning. High spatial resolution sonography has recently been shown to be very specific and sensitive to detect fractures.

## Treatment

Treatment of scaphoid fractures depends on the degree of injury, location of the fracture, and necessity to return to sports and activities. Initial management of those with negative x-rays and clinical suspicion of a fracture includes immobilization in a short- or long-arm splint. Splinting is preferable to casts in acute arm fractures due to edema, although casts with valves and spacers are useful. Although elbow supination and pronation allow motion at the fracture site, it is generally reasonable to use a short-arm splint with a thumb spica to treat suspected fractures that are not seen on initial x-rays. Initial immobilization in the case of suspected fractures does carry the risk of unnecessary immobilization in 75% to 90% of patients.

Fracture healing depends on blood supply. Unfortunately, the blood supply to the scaphoid runs distal to proximal, which leads to high rates of nonunion and complications in those with proximal or displaced fractures. Generally, the more distal the fracture the faster it heals and the less likely it will need prolonged immobilization or surgery. Liberal orthopedic referrals for proximal or midbody scaphoid fractures are in order for clinicians who are less experienced or comfortable managing the injury.

Immobilization times range from 4 to 6 weeks in a distal pole nondisplaced fracture to up to 20 weeks in a proximal pole fracture. Immobilization for proximal and midbody pole fractures should also include the elbow with long arm splints and casts. All fractures that are displaced or those with changes in the scapholunate angle should be immobilized and referred for orthopedic evaluation.

## ILIOTIBIAL BAND SYNDROME

Iliotibial band (ITB) syndrome remains one of the easily diagnosed but difficult to treat lateral knee pain syndromes. It is caused by inflammation or chronic tendinosis of the proximal or distal portion of the ITB. The ITB is a confluence of fascia from the hip flexors, extensors, and abductors, which ultimately inserts at Gerdy's tubercle over the lateral aspect of the proximal tibia.

The ITB has four main anatomic functions. It helps with hip abduction. It contributes to internal rotation of the hip when the hip is flexed to 30 degrees. It assists with knee extension when the knee is in less than 30 degrees of flexion, and it assists with knee flexion when the knee is at greater than 30 degrees of flexion.

### Knee Pain

#### Epidemiology

ITB lateral knee pain is caused by recurrent friction over the lateral femoral condyle during knee flexion and extension. Several observational studies have identified potential risk factors for the development of ITB syndrome (Box 3).

#### Etiology

ITB syndrome makes up 12% of all running-related injuries. Several studies of Marine Corps recruits undergoing basic training showed incidence varying from 5.3% to 22.2%. Other causes include cycling, improper athletic shoes or worn-out shoes, improper warm-up or stretching, increasing the quality and quantity of training sessions too quickly, and lower limb and foot misalignment (Box 4).

#### Diagnosis

The athlete might walk with the knee extended, because this gait pattern avoids motion in which the tendon rubs on the lateral femoral condyle. There is point tenderness on palpation over the lateral femoral epicondyle as well as with palpation of a site 2 to 4 cm above the lateral joint line and at Gerdy's tubercle.

Provocative tests include Ober's and Renne's maneuvers. With Ober's test, have the athlete lie on the unaffected side, with the hip and knee flexed at 90 degrees. Next, while stabilizing the pelvis, abduct and extend the affected leg until it is aligned with the rest of the body. The affected leg is lowered into adduction. Ober's test is positive if the affected leg remains in the abducted position or the athlete complains of lateral knee or hip pain. With Renne's test, have the athlete do a weight-bearing squat at 45 degrees of knee flexion. Pain is caused by pressure over the lateral femoral condyle.

### Snapping Hip Syndrome

#### Epidemiology

There are no U.S. data on prevalence or incidence. Coxa saltans affects female patients more often than male patients, with an age distribution

---

### BOX 3 Increasing Potential for Developing the ITB Syndrome

- Preexisting ITB tightness
- High weekly mileage
- Time spent walking or running on the track
- Interval training
- Muscle weakness of knee flexors or extensors and hip abductors

---

*Abbreviation:* ITB = iliotibial band.

---

### BOX 4 Other Causes of Lateral Knee Pain*

- Lumbosacral radiculopathy
- Patellofemoral syndrome
- Popliteal tendinopathy
- Biceps femoris tendinopathy
- Myofascial pain
- Discoid lateral meniscus
- Degenerative joint disease
- Superior tibiofibular joint sprain
- Gastrocnemius tear or strain
- Common peroneal nerve injury
- Stress fracture
- Lateral collateral sprain
- Meniscal tear

---

*Listed in order of prevalence.

---

of 15 to 40 years. It is common in ballet dancers: The sudden loading of the hip from a jump places the ITB anteriorly as the hip is flexed, then it snaps back as the dancer recovers and extends the hip.

#### Etiology

Snapping hip syndrome (coxa saltans) is the ITB syndrome at the proximal anatomic region of the hip. As with ITB syndrome at the lateral knee, snapping hip syndrome is caused by friction, this time with the ITB rubbing and snapping over the greater trochanter of the hip. It is characterized by an audible snap or click in and around the hip region, which may be painful or painless. Most patients seek medical attention when pain persists.

#### Diagnosis

The gait assessment can appear dramatic as if the patient is subluxing the hip. The patient has pain with palpation along the ITB over the proximal attachment and at the greater trochanter. Passive internal and external rotation of the hip in the side-lying position causes pain.

Plain films are not regularly needed. Other diagnostic tests may include bone scintigraphy, dynamic ultrasound, and MRI. Treatments in the acute phase include modifying activity and using ice, NSAIDs, iontophoresis, ITB strapping, and cortisone injection. Stretching and massage with a foam roller may be beneficial in the subacute setting.

Improving the hip abductors seems to play a major role in recovery. Fredericson and colleagues compared 24 runners with ITB syndrome with 30 healthy runners. Injured runners enrolled in a 6-week program to strengthen the gluteus medius. At 6 weeks, 22 of 24 were pain free with all exercises and returned to running. At 6-month follow-up, there were no reports of recurrence.

Surgery with the Z-plasty incision over the affected ITB is uncommon.

### Treatment

ITB syndrome is common in running, cycling and dancing. It remains easily diagnosed yet difficult to treat. More randomized studies are needed to look at treatment modalities. Rehabilitation remains the mainstay therapy in the improvement of ITB syndrome.

## MENISCAL TEARS OF THE KNEE

### Epidemiology and Etiology

The meniscus is a C-shaped fibrocartilage structure important in shock absorption, stability, and protection of the articular joint cartilage of the knee. A large percentage of our weight is distributed through the meniscus as we walk, run, and jump, with transmission of 50% to 70% of weight-bearing load in extension and 85% in

90-degree flexion. Meniscal tears in the athletic population most likely result from trauma, usually a twist or hyperextension event. In the anterior cruciate ligament (ACL)–deficient knee, the combination of instability and tear commonly leads to early osteoarthritis. Degenerative tears occur in older patients and often are atraumatic.

The incidence of meniscal tears is 60 to 70 per 100,000 population. Peak incidence in the acute traumatic setting is 20 to 30 years for male patients and 11 to 20 years for female patients. The male-to-female ratio is 3:1. One third of all tears are associated with ACL injury. Lateral tears are more common in acute ACL tears, and medial tears more common with chronic ACL tears. Acute trauma, degenerative processes, tibial plateau fractures, and femoral shaft fractures are the most common causes of meniscal tears.

## Diagnosis

A good history of the acute injury and progression of symptoms, joint line pain with flexion with McMurray's test, and effusion are the keys to clinical diagnosis. Several events can cause the meniscus to become damaged, from an acute twist or hyperextension to simply getting up from a squatting position. Certain meniscal tears occur gradually over a long period. In older patients, especially those older than 50 years, meniscal tears might be degenerative meniscal tears and might not be symptomatic. There are many types of meniscal tears, including vertical longitudinal (bucket handle), oblique (flap or parrot beak), complex (degenerative), transverse (radial), and horizontal.

Symptoms include pain, effusion, locking, catching, and loss of range of motion, especially blocked full extension secondary to mechanical block. Tenderness is elicited by deep palpation along medial and lateral joint lines. Check for effusion and range of motion. McMurray's test is done by flexing the knee beyond 90 degrees with one hand and applying an external and internal force to the lower leg. Apley's compression test is done by having the patient lie prone, then flexing the knee to 90 degrees and applying an axial load along with internal and external rotation of the lower leg. Perimeniscal cysts, such as Baker's cysts, can develop following meniscal tears.

Meniscal tears do not show up on plain films because the meniscus does not contain calcium, as bones do. Nevertheless, PA, lateral, and Merchant's views are ordered in the acute setting to rule out further injury. Weight-bearing views are also helpful to assess joint space narrowing. MRI remains the gold standard noninvasive test. A normal meniscus on MRI is demonstrated by a low signal structure. Intrasubstance changes are high signal structures and are common in children and with increases in age. These changes on MRI are often a common cause of over-reading.

## Treatment

Criteria for repair include complete vertical tears longer than 1 cm, a tear within 3 mm of the periphery, or a tear within 3 to 4 mm of the meniscocapsular junction. Some patients can live with a meniscal tear without significant worsening over time, but others are unable to return to preinjury form. In general, tears do not heal on their own, but stable partial-thickness vertical tears shorter than 1 cm can heal if the knee is stable. Therefore, a tear with an associated concurrent ligament instability, such as an ACL-deficient knee, is an indication for surgery.

Determining how active the patient is and whether the tear is stable or unstable are also important factors. Customization of care for the treatment of meniscal tears is critical for the high-level or professional athlete to be able to return to play safely and quickly. Sports-specific activities such as high-impact running, jumping, twisting, and cutting should determine the grade of conservative versus operative treatments.

Conservative treatment is chosen for small stable meniscal tears and nonactive patients. When repair of the meniscus is indicated, partial menisectomy is performed with the goal of retaining as much viable meniscal tissue as possible to prevent increased peak loads and development of early osteoarthritis. In the athlete with an ACL-deficient knee, ACL reconstruction allows protection of the meniscal tear, and some believe that a repairable meniscal tear is in itself an indication for ACL reconstruction. Newer techniques include meniscal transplantation where MRI is used to match donor size and recipient to within 5% of ligament size.

Postsurgery rehabilitation protocol is dictated by the presence or absence of concurrent ligament reconstruction. Full weight bearing is acceptable. A hinged knee brace is worn for 4 to 6 weeks, and the patient can usually return to play after 3 months.

## REFERENCES

Adirim TA, Cheng TL: Overview of injuries in the young athlete. Sports Med 2003;33(1):75-81.

Bachmann LM, Kolb E, Koller MT, et al: Accuracy of Ottawa ankle rules to exclude fractures of the ankle and mid-foot: Systematic review. BMJ 2003;326:417.

Berndt AL, Harty M: Transchondral fractures (osteochondritis dissecans) of the talus. J Bone Joint Surg Am 1959;41:988-1020.

Bray RC, Dandy DJ: Meniscal lesions and chronic anterior cruciate ligament deficiency: Meniscal tears occurring before and after reconstruction. Bone Joint Surg Br 1989;71(1):128-130.

Breederveld RS, Tuinebreijer WE: Investigation of computed tomographic scan concurrent criterion validity in doubtful scaphoid fracture of the wrist. J Trauma 2004;57:851-854.

Dobyns JH, Beckenbaugh RD, Bryan RS, et al: Fractures of the hand and wrist. In Flynn, JE (ed): Hand Surgery, 3rd ed. Baltimore: Williams & Wilkins, 1982, pp 111-180.

Dorsay TA, Major NM, Helms CA: Cost-effectiveness of immediate MR imaging versus traditional follow-up for revealing radiographically occult scaphoid fractures. AJR Am J Roentgenol 2001;177: 1257-1263.

Douglas G, Rang M: The role trauma in the pathogenesis of the osteochondroses. Clin Orthop Relat Res 1981;(158):28-32.

Eggli S, Wegmüller H, Kosina J, et al: Long term results of arthroscopic meniscal repair: An analysis of isolated tears. Am J Sports Med 1995;23(6): 715-720.

Fredericson M, Cookingham CL, Chaudhari AM, et al: Hip abductor weakness in distance runners with iliotibial band syndrome. Clin J Sport Med 2000;10:169-175.

Fredericson M, White JJ, Macmahon JM, Andriacchi TP: Quantitative analysis of the relative effectiveness of 3 iliotibial band stretches. Arch Phys Med Rehabil 2002;83:589-592.

Hauger O, Bonnefoy O, Moinard M, et al: Occult fractures of the waist of the scaphoid: Early diagnosis by high-spatial-resolution sonography. AJR Am J Roentgenol 2002;178:1239-1245.

Irvine GB, Glasgow MM: The natural history of the meniscus in anterior cruciate ligament insufficiency: Arthroscopic analysis. J Bone Joint Surg Br 1992;74(3):403-405.

Jingushi S, Hara T, Sugioka Y: Deficiency of a parathyroid hormone fragment containing the midportion and 1,25-dihydroxyvitamin D in serum of patients with slipped capital femoral epiphysis. J Pediatr Orthop 1997;17:216-219.

Kempers MJ, Noordam C, Rouwe CW, Otten BJ: Can GnRH-agonist treatment cause slipped capital femoral epiphysis? J Pediatr Endocrinol Metab 2001; 14:729-734.

Khan K, Cook J: The painful nonruptured tendon: Clinical aspects. Clin Sports Med 2003;22:711-725.

Lehmann CL, Arons RR, Loder RT, Vitale MG: The epidemiology of slipped capital femoral epiphysis: An update. J Pediatr Orthop 2006;26(3): 286-290.

Loder RT: The demographics of slipped capital femoral epiphysis: An international multicenter study. Clin Orthop Relat Res 1996;(322):8-27.

Loder RT, Starnes T, Dikos G: The narrow window of bone age in children with slipped capital femoral epiphysis: A reassessment one decade later. J Pediatr Orthop 2006;26(3):300-306.

Loomer R, Fisher C, Lloyd-Smith R, et al: Osteochondral lesions of the talus. Am J Sports Med 1993;21:13-19.

Lyman S, Fleisig GS, Andrews JR, Osinski ED: Effect of pitch type, pitch count, and pitching mechanics on risk of elbow and shoulder pain in youth baseball pitchers. Am J Sports Med 2002;30(4):463-468.

Messier SP, Edwards DG, Martin DF, et al: Etiology of iliotibial band friction syndrome in distance runners. Med Sci Sports Exerc 1995;27: 951-960.

Moreira JF, Neves MC, Lopes G, Gomes AR: Slipped capital femoral epiphysis: A report of 4 cases occurring in one family. Int Orthop 1998;22:193-196.

Olsen SJ 2nd, Fleisig GS, Dun S, et al: Risk factors for shoulder and elbow injuries in adolescent baseball pitchers. Am J Sports Med 2006;34:905-912.

Pillai A, Jain M: Management of clinical fractures of the scaphoid: Results of an audit and literature review. Eur J Emerg Med 2005;12(2): 47-51.

Rattey T, Piehl F, Wright JG: Acute slipped capital femoral epiphysis: Review of outcomes and rates of avascular necrosis. J Bone Joint Surg Am 1996;78:398-402.

Rosenberg LS, Sherman MF: Meniscal injury in the ACL deficient knee: A rationale for clinical decision making. Sports Med 1992;13:423-432.

Stiell IG, Wells GA, Hoag RH, et al: Implementation of the Ottawa knee rule for the use of radiography in acute knee injuries. JAMA 1997;278: 2075-2079.

Umans H, Liebling MS, Moy L, et al: Slipped capital femoral epiphysis: A physeal lesion diagnosed by MRI, with radiographic and CT correlation. Skeletal Radiol 1998;27:139-144.

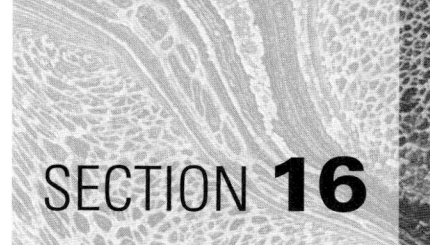

# Obstetrics and Gynecology

## Antepartum Care

Method of
*Kirk D. Ramin, MD, and Jessica P. Swartout, MD*

### Antepartum Care

Ideally, antepartum care commences 3 months before actual conception with the recommendation that women who are sexually active and not using contraception should begin taking daily multivitamin or folic acid supplements. The most convincing trials of this were performed in Europe and China when it was concluded that women of reproductive age should take multivitamin supplements containing 0.4 mg of folate daily. Women with histories of children with neural tube defects or other anomalies should increase this dose to 4 mg of folate in the periconceptional period to reduce risks of recurrence.

Preconception counseling should also include an accurate assessment of preexisting maternal medical conditions. This is the ideal time to stress changes in factors that respond to early intervention: quitting smoking, refraining from alcohol or drug abuse, treating gum disease, and avoiding teratogens. Alcohol is a known teratogen. Immunization status should be reviewed and vaccines should be administered as appropriate. Special consideration is given to patients with thyroid disease. Concern focuses on associations with low intelligence quotients (IQs) in children conceived by hypothyroid mothers. Patients with diabetes should be counseled that the increased risk of birth defects is directly related to the level of glucose control at conception.

High-risk obstetric referrals may be offered to women with potential for obstetric complications suggested by conditions listed in Box 1. Identification of the high-risk patient is critical to avoiding adverse outcomes.

In most cases, a woman's pregnancy is a normal event that is complicated by potentially dangerous disease in a minority of cases. The physician who manages pregnant patients must follow the normal changes that occur during antepartum care, so that abnormalities can be recognized and treated appropriately. Additionally, routine prenatal care offers multiple opportunities for patient education, primary intervention, and appropriate monitoring of the low-risk pregnancy in the setting of the family and community. For some women, antepartum care is part of their own continuum in a long-term primary care relationship with caregivers.

## Timeline of Routine Antepartum Care

### FIRST VISIT AND EARLY CARE

#### History

After pregnancy is confirmed, it is extraordinarily important to determine the duration of pregnancy and the estimated date of confinement (EDC). Further care is heavily predicated on this estimate. The history begins with ascertaining the first day of the last menstrual period and calculating the EDC by assuming duration of pregnancy averages 280 days (40 weeks).

The documentation of prior obstetric history includes prior complications, route of delivery, and estimated birth weights. Maternal medical disorders are often exacerbated by pregnancy; cardiovascular, renal, and endocrine disorders require evaluation and counseling concerning possible treatments required. A history of previous gynecologic surgery, including cesarean delivery, is important to consider. A family history of twinning, diabetes mellitus, familial disorders, or hereditary disease is relevant.

Current medications (prescription and nonprescription) are reviewed. Certain prescription medications are known teratogens and should be discontinued. Examples include isotretinoin (Accutane), tetracycline (Sumycin), quinolone antibiotics (ciprofloxacin [Cipro], levofloxacin [Levaquin]), and warfarin (Coumadin). Angiotensin-converting enzyme (ACE) inhibitors should not be used during the second and third trimesters, and the FDA has recently raised doubt

---

**BOX 1   Potential Indications for High-Risk Referral**

- Current disease involving renal, cardiac, or endocrine systems
- Fetal anomalies
- History of preterm delivery
- Incompetent cervix
- Isoimmunization
- Known carrier of genetic disorder
- Multiple gestation
- Placenta previa after 28 weeks
- Prior intrauterine fetal demise or stillbirth
- Systemic diseases such as hypertension, diabetes, or asthma
- Third-trimester bleeding

about their use in the first trimester. According to the approved label, ACE inhibitors are labeled pregnancy category C for the first trimester and pregnancy category D during the second and third trimesters. On June 8, 2006, the FDA issued an alert that infants whose mothers had taken an ACE inhibitor during the first trimester had an increased risk of major congenital malformations.

Honest discussion of substance abuse (alcohol, tobacco, and illicit drugs) is an integral part of the patient interview. Counseling patients about smoking cessation is vital in early pregnancy. Smoking increases the risk of fetal death or damage in utero. It is also associated with increased risk of placental abruption and placenta previa, each of which put both mother and child at risk.

## Examination

Physical examination begins with a thorough general examination to assess maternal well-being including body mass index (BMI) and blood pressure (BP). The BMI is calculated by dividing weight in kilograms by height in meters squared. The BMI of a patient is categorized as underweight (under 19.8), normal weight (19.8 to 25), overweight (25 to 30), or obese (over 30). A brief fundoscopic examination might reveal signs of hypertension-induced changes.

Breast examination may be significant for changes in pregnancy that result from hormonal responses by the mammary ducts. These changes include engorgement and vascular prominence, occasionally resulting in mastodynia. Enlargement of areolar sebaceous glands (Montgomery's tubercles) occurs between 6 and 8 weeks' gestation.

A pelvic examination is performed with attention to the adequacy of pelvis and evaluation for adnexal masses. Numerous changes in the pelvic organs occur in pregnancy. For example, congestion of the pelvic vasculature (Chadwick's sign) causes bluish discoloration of the vagina and cervix. Softening of the cervix due to increased vascularity of the cervical tissue (Goodell's sign) can occur as early as 4 weeks. The uterus is palpable at the pubic symphysis at 8 weeks.

Portable devices using Doppler effect will reliably detect fetal heart tones at a rate of 120 to 160 beats per minute as early as 8 weeks.

## Laboratory Studies

Routine laboratory studies ordered at the first visit include complete blood count (CBC) with differential, ABO and Rh typing, red cell antibody screen, rubella immunoglobulin (Ig)G, hepatitis B surface antigen (HBsAg), syphilis serology, and HIV 1 and HIV 2 antibody screens. Patients may refuse HIV testing, but all patients are counseled and offered the option for screening. A Papanicolaou (Pap) smear is performed in conjunction with cultures for chlamydia and gonorrhea.

A midstream urinalysis checks for the presence of protein or glucose. A microscopic examination of the urine is performed to rule out infection or asymptomatic bacteriuria. A baseline 24-hour urine protein collection and serum creatinine should be collected from all patients with hypertension, diabetes, or other preexisting renal disease.

## Other Studies

Special-purpose studies are also considered in early gestation. First-trimester screening with nuchal translucency should be offered to all women older than 35 years between 11 and 14 weeks. The first-trimester screen uses the nuchal translucency and maternal serum-free β–human chorionic gonadotropin (hCG) and pregnancy-associated plasma protein A (PAPP-A) and detects up to 85% of Down syndrome and trisomy 18 cases.

Chorionic villus sampling (CVS) may be offered at 10 to 13 weeks to women older than 35 years, to those with abnormal first-trimester screens, and to those with abnormal pedigrees. From this, placental tissue may be subjected to chromosomal, metabolic, or DNA study. CVS cannot be used for diagnosis of neural tube defects, because this requires measuring alpha fetoprotein (AFP) levels in maternal serum at a later date.

Patients with tuberculosis exposure may be assessed for active tuberculosis with skin testing (if not vaccinated with bacille Calmette-Guérin [BCG]) and chest x-ray. Serologic assessment for toxoplasmosis, cytomegalovirus, and varicella immunity is not routinely indicated.

Screening for genetic disorders may be undertaken if concern exists based on racial or ethnic background (hemoglobinopathies, β-thalassemia, α-thalassemia, Tay-Sachs disease) or familial background (cystic fibrosis, fragile X, Duchenne's muscular dystrophy).

## Follow-up

Follow-up visits are scheduled once monthly until 28 weeks' gestation, and then patients are followed twice monthly until 36 weeks. Visits are then scheduled at weekly intervals until delivery. At each visit, weight gain, edema, BP, fundal height, Leopold's maneuvers, and fetal heart tones are recorded. Because BP tends to decrease during the second trimester, increases of 30 mm Hg systolic or 15 mm Hg diastolic over first trimester pressures are abnormal. Interval history includes questions about diet, sleeping patterns, and fetal movement. Warning signs such as bleeding, contractions, leaking of fluid, headache, or visual disturbances are reviewed.

## 15 TO 18 WEEKS' GESTATION

### Alpha Fetoprotein Testing

Maternal serum AFP testing is offered for all pregnancies at 16 to 18 weeks as a means of screening for open neural tube defects or chromosomal trisomy. In pregnancy, AFP is produced in sequence by the fetal yolk sac, the fetal gastrointestinal tract, and the fetal liver. AFP in the maternal serum occurs via placental exchange and transamniotic diffusion.

High levels of AFP are associated with various fetal anomalies including neural tube defects, multiple gestations, and ventral wall defects. Unexplained elevation of AFP has been associated with poor fetal growth, fetal loss, and preeclampsia. In cases with unexplained elevation of AFP, maternal and fetal surveillance should be increased. Low levels of AFP are associated with increased risk of Down syndrome.

The interpretation of this test depends on the gestational age; even if timed correctly, it is known to have a moderate level of false-positive results. Expanded serum markers of AFP, unconjugated estriol, inhibin A, and β-hCG are available to more accurately screen for Down syndrome, but detection is only about 60%, and false-negative results remain at 5%.

### Amniocentesis

A more certain diagnosis is available via ultrasound-guided transabdominal amniocentesis at 16 to 18 weeks. Chromosomes from fetal cells are subjected to fluorescent in-situ hybridization (FISH) analysis, which detects trisomies 13, 18, 21, and abnormal numbers of sex chromosomes.

### Physical Findings

Interval changes in the physical examination now include the start of colostrum secretion, which can begin as early as 16 weeks' gestation.

Chloasma is darkening of the skin over the forehead, bridge of the nose, or cheekbones and is more obvious in those with dark complexions. It can begin to manifest at this time, and is intensified by exposure to sunlight. Darkening of the skin in the areolae and nipples becomes more accentuated. A darkened line appears in the lower midline of the abdomen from the umbilicus to the pubis (linea nigra). The basis of these changes is stimulation of melanophores by increased melanocyte-stimulating hormone.

At 15 to 20 weeks, abdominal enlargement can appear more rapid as the uterus rises out of the pelvis and into the abdomen.

## 18 TO 20 WEEKS' GESTATION

### Physical Findings

The mother might detect fetal movements (quickening) at around 20 weeks. The uterus is palpable at 20 weeks at the umbilicus, and ballottement reveals a fetus floating in amniotic fluid. Measurements that are 2 cm smaller than expected for week of gestation are suspicious for oligohydramnios, intrauterine growth restriction, fetal anomaly, or abnormal fetal lie. Conversely, measurements 2 cm larger than expected can indicate multiple gestation, polyhydramnios, or fetal macrosomia. These rules apply for the gestational ages of 18 to 32 weeks. Either condition can be fully evaluated with ultrasound examination.

## Laboratory Studies

Increased surveillance for preeclampsia includes testing for urine protein in patients with BP greater than 140/90 mm Hg or in those with weight gains greater than 3 pounds/week. Evaluation is also necessary for clinical signs of upper extremity edema, right upper quadrant tenderness, headaches, or vision changes. Proteinuria of more than 300 mg in 24 hours can indicate renal dysfunction or the onset of preeclampsia.

## Ultrasonography

Sonography has long established itself as the single most useful technology in monitoring pregnancy and diagnosing complications. It is for this reason that basic level ultrasound is offered at 18 to 20 weeks to evaluate growth, placentation, amniotic fluid volume, and fetal anatomy. If earlier dating of the pregnancy is uncertain, this is an opportunity to confirm or refute prior estimates. If anomalous conditions are discovered, more comprehensive ultrasonography becomes necessary.

## 28 WEEKS' GESTATION

### Physical Findings

New physical examination findings at this time include the onset of stretch marks (striae) of the breasts and abdomen. These are caused by separation of underlying collagen tissue, a response to increased adrenocorticosteroid. The ligamentous structures of the pelvis also undergo slight but definite relaxation of the joints, a progesterone effect. As the uterus enlarges, it often rotates to the right. Fundal size roughly correlates with the estimated gestational age at 26 to 34 weeks. Braxton Hicks contractions, characterized as painless uterine tightening, increase in regularity. The fetal outline can be easily palpated through the maternal abdominal wall.

### Laboratory Studies

A CBC for anemia and a 1-hour glucose tolerance test (after ingestion of 50 g of glucose) is scheduled to detect patients at risk for developing gestational diabetes. If the screening test is abnormal, a 3-hour test is performed to confirm the diagnosis. Two or more abnormal values on this test are considered diagnostic of gestational diabetes mellitus.

A repeat Rh antibody is checked at this time in Rh-negative mothers. Those who remain unsensitized in the third trimester receive a first dose of Rho(D) immune globulin (RhoGAM) to prevent maternal isoimmunization to fetal red blood cells. A 300 μg dose is sufficient for 15 mL of red cells (equivalent to 30 mL of whole blood).

### Follow-up

Return visits at 2-week intervals are now initiated, and the patient is oriented to the labor and delivery ward. Precautions are given regarding the onset of conditions listed in Box 2. The onset of any of these should prompt immediate medical attention.

## 36 WEEKS' GESTATION

### Physical Findings

Patients might complain of increased vaginal discharge at this time in their pregnancy, a physiologic consequence of hormone stimulation. The discharge consists mainly of epithelial cells and cervical mucus and is treated with reassurance. Discharge accompanied by itching, burning, or malodor should be evaluated and treated accordingly, however.

---

**BOX 2    Warning Signs and Symptoms Prompting Medical Attention**

- Burning with urination
- Chills or fever
- Prolonged vomiting or inability to keep liquids down
- Pronounced decrease in fetal movements
- Rhythmic cramping pains (>6/h)
- Rupture of membranes
- Severe abdominal, pelvic, or back pain
- Signs of preeclampsia (headache, edema, right upper quadrant pain)
- Vaginal bleeding

---

### Laboratory Studies

Vaginal and rectal cultures are collected to evaluate for the presence of group B streptococcus (GBS) at 35 to 37 weeks. GBS organisms are implicated in preterm labor, amnionitis, endometritis, and wound infection. If cultures are positive, the patient will be given antibiotic prophylaxis during active labor in efforts to protect the newborn against vertical transmission, resulting in newborn sepsis.

### Follow-up

Follow-up visits are planned on a weekly basis with emphasis on weight gain, BP, and signs of preeclampsia. Review of precautions regarding infection, pregnancy loss, and symptoms of preeclampsia completes the visit.

## POST-TERM GESTATION

About 3% to 12% of pregnancies continue beyond 43 weeks of gestation and are considered post-term. Although some of these may be due to inaccurate dating, some patients clearly progress to excessively long gestations that are a significant risk to the fetus. Increased antepartum surveillance by cervical examination, fetal heart rate testing (see the discussion of contraction stress testing), and biophysical profile should be initiated between 41 and 42 weeks. Even if fetal testing is reassuring, patients with reliable dating greater than 41 weeks are candidates for induction of labor.

# Common Concerns of the Antenatal Period

## BLEEDING

About one half of pregnant women experience some form of bleeding during the pregnancy; often this is benign. Patients also have a heightened awareness of symptoms that previously may have gone unnoticed in the nonpregnant state. Efficient and competent evaluation, followed by compassion and reassurance when prudent, allays many fears and provides clear direction. Spotting due to bleeding at the implantation site occurs from the time of implantation (about 6 days after fertilization) until 29 to 35 days after the last menstrual period in many women. Some women have unexplained cyclic bleeding throughout pregnancy. Usually, cardiac activity on ultrasound and appropriate β-hCG levels confirm a viable early pregnancy. First-trimester bleeding in lieu of these findings may be a sign of spontaneous miscarriage or ectopic pregnancy. Vaginal bleeding in late pregnancy is covered in other articles.

## NAUSEA

Nausea is a common symptom that occurs in most pregnancies. It is heightened before 14 weeks' gestation and is largely benign. The etiology is not well understood but likely is related to elevating levels of β-hCG. Its moniker "morning sickness" is misleading, because nausea of pregnancy can occur at any time during the day. Aggravating factors vary with the individual patient; success varies with interventions designed to reduce symptoms.

Uncomplicated nausea may be responsive to small nonfatty portions at mealtime. Pyridoxine (vitamin B$_6$)[1] tablets 12.5 mg twice a day or doxylamine (Unisom)[1] 12.5 mg twice a day are safe in pregnancy and may be helpful. Antiemetic drugs in the outpatient setting are a measure of last resort.

Inability to control protracted vomiting in conjunction with clinical dehydration can require hospitalization for intravenous fluids and treatment of hyperemesis gravidarium. Extreme nausea and vomiting or nausea and vomiting that persists beyond 18 to 20 weeks' gestation may be signs of multiple gestation, thyroid disease, or molar pregnancy.

## NUTRITION AND WEIGHT GAIN

The mother's nutrition is a vital factor in the development of the fetus from preconception through the postpartum period. Therefore, the pregnant woman should be advised to eat a balanced diet and should be informed of the additional 300 kcal/day needed during pregnancy. The American College of Obstetricians and Gynecologists (ACOG) recommends a target weight gain of 10 to 12 kg (22-27 lb) during pregnancy. They also advise that underweight women might need to gain more and obese women should gain less. Nutritional requirements for protein are 80 g/day, for calcium are 1500 mg/day, for iron are 30 mg/day, and for folate are 0.4 mg/day (4 mg/day in some cases). Patients with seizure disorders managed with valproic acid (Depakene) or carbamazepine (Tegretol) are also at risk and might benefit from the higher dose of folate.

## HEARTBURN

Heartburn in the form of reflux esophagitis is caused by the enlarging uterus displacing the stomach and by progesterone's relaxation of the lower esophageal sphincter. Treatment consists of taking antacids, decreasing exacerbating factors such as spicy foods, eating more frequently but in smaller quantities, limiting eating before bedtime, and taking H$_2$-receptor inhibitors.

## URINARY SYMPTOMS

Urinary frequency, nocturia, and bladder irritability are common complaints due to progesterone-mediated relaxation of smooth muscle and subsequent altered bladder function. Later in pregnancy, urinary frequency becomes even more prominent from pressure on the bladder by the enlarging uterus and the fetal presenting parts, such as when the fetal head descends into the pelvis.

Dysuria, however, is often a sign of infection that requires antibiotic treatment. Bacteriuria combined with urinary stasis from altered bladder function predisposes the patient to pyelonephritis. Although simple urinary tract infections are treated on an outpatient basis, pyelonephritis remains the most common nonobstetric cause for hospitalization during antenatal care.

Patients with a diagnosis of pyelonephritis require hospitalization, aggressive fluid replacement, and IV antibiotics until they remain afebrile for longer than 24 hours. Close monitoring of maternal respiratory status is important because these women are at risk for acute respiratory distress syndrome (ARDS). All patients should complete a 10-day course of antibiotic treatment. After treatment has been completed, suppressive therapy should be continued until delivery.

## INFECTION

Two infections of special note are HIV and bacterial vaginosis (BV). HIV transmission to the newborn can be reduced significantly with appropriate infectious disease and maternal-fetal medicine specialty management. Appropriate treatment of BV in women at high risk for preterm delivery or recurrent loss can significantly reduce either of

these untoward outcomes. Debate exists as to whether or not low-risk women should be screened.

*Chlamydia trachomatis* is an obligate intracellular bacterium and is the most common sexually transmitted bacterial infection in women of reproductive age. It may be associated with urethritis, mucopurulent cervicitis, and acute salpingitis, or it may be clinically silent. Perinatal transmission is clearly associated with neonatal conjunctivitis (leading to blindness) and pneumonia and is likely associated with preterm delivery, premature rupture of membranes, and perinatal mortality. Diagnosis is confirmed by polymerase chain reaction (PCR) during routine screening. Doxycycline should be avoided in pregnancy, and erythromycin is associated with gastrointestinal upset, so treatment with azithromycin is often appropriate.

Gonococcal infection is associated with concomitant chlamydia infection in about 40% of infected pregnant women. It is usually limited to the lower genital tract, including the cervix, urethra, and periurethral or vestibular glands. Because of an association between gonococcal cervicitis and septic spontaneous abortion, and because preterm delivery, premature rupture of membranes, and postpartum infection are more common with gonococcal infection, routine cultures are appropriate at the first antenatal visit. Because some strains have rendered some β-lactam drugs ineffective for therapy, the recommendation for uncomplicated gonococcal infection is intramuscular ceftriaxone 125 mg.

Vaginosis due to *Candida albicans* can become symptomatic with caseous white discharge and vaginal itching or burning, and it may be associated with red satellite lesions on the vulva. Marked inflammation of the vagina and introitus may be noted. Topical application of over-the-counter antifungal creams such as miconazole nitrate (Monistat) or nystatin (Mycostatin) is generally helpful in controlling the imbalance of vaginal flora.

Cytomegalovirus is a ubiquitous DNA herpes virus that is transmitted horizontally between humans by droplet infection. It is transmitted vertically from mother to fetus and is the most common cause of perinatal infection. The virus becomes latent after primary infection, with periodic reactivation and viral shedding. Infection is usually clinically silent. Many of the affected infants have died from infection, and most of the survivors have severe handicaps, including mental retardation, blindness, and deafness. Serious sequelae are more common among primary infections. The syndrome of congenital cytomegalovirus infection includes low birth weight, microcephaly, intracranial calcifications, chorioretinitis, mental and motor retardation, sensorineural deficits, hepatosplenomegaly, jaundice, hemolytic anemia, and thrombocytopenic purpura. Confirmation of primary infection is suggested by a fourfold increase of IgG titers in paired acute and convalescent sera or by detecting IgM cytomegalovirus antibodies. There is no effective therapy for maternal infection.

Human parvovirus B19 causes erythema infectiosum, or fifth disease. This is a single-stranded DNA virus that is heralded by the appearance of clinical findings of bright red macular rash and accompanying arthralgias. Acute infection is confirmed by IgM-specific antibody and can prompt adverse pregnancy outcomes, including spontaneous miscarriage and fetal death.

Rubella, also known as German measles, is directly responsible for spontaneous miscarriage and severe congenital malformations. Although large epidemics of rubella are nonexistent in the United States because of immunization, the disease can still affect the up to 25% of susceptible women. Absence of rubella antibody indicates susceptibility. Vaccination involves an attenuated live virus (MMR) and therefore is avoided in pregnancy. Vaccination of nonpregnant susceptible women (including those during the postpartum period) and hospital personnel continues to be the mainstay of therapy. Detection by IgM-specific antibody confirms recent infection. Congenital rubella syndrome (CRS) is a severe example of antenatal infection and includes one or more of the conditions listed in Box 3.

Varicella-zoster virus, the etiologic agent of childhood chickenpox, is a DNA herpes virus that remains latent in the dorsal root ganglia and may be reactivated years later to cause herpes zoster or shingles. Infection early in pregnancy can lead to severe congenital malformations including chorioretinitis, cerebral cortical atrophy, hydronephrosis, and cutaneous and bony leg defects. Varicella-zoster

---

[1]Not FDA approved for this indication.

## BOX 3  Conditions Associated with Congenital Rubella Syndrome

- Central nervous system defects (meningoencephalitis)
- Chromosomal abnormalities
- Chronic diffuse interstitial pneumonitis
- Eye lesions
  - Cataracts
  - Glaucoma
  - Microphthalmia
- Heart disease
  - Patent ductus arteriosus
  - Septal defects
  - Pulmonary artery stenosis
- Hepatic dysfunction
  - Hepatitis
  - Hepatosplenomegaly
  - Jaundice
- Osseous changes
- Retarded growth
- Sensorineural deafness
- Thrombocytopenia and anemia

immunoglobulin (VZIg) 125 U/10 kg can attenuate varicella infection if given within 96 hours.

Genital herpes simplex virus (HSV) may be confirmed by tissue culture if active lesions are present; in this event, cesarean delivery is indicated because the fetus is at risk for acquiring the virus during passage through the birth canal. Oral or topical acyclovir can improve symptoms. If no lesions and no prodromal symptoms are present, vaginal delivery is recommended.

*Trichomonas vaginalis* can be found in 20% to 30% of pregnant patients, but only a small number complain of discharge or irritation. This flagellated, oval, motile organism can be seen on normal saline wet prep and is evident clinically by presence of a foamy or greenish discharge accompanied by multiple cervical petechiae. Treatment is oral metronidazole.

Prenatally acquired infection caused by the protozoan parasite *Toxoplasma gondii* can result in the presence of abnormalities such as microcephalus or hydrocephalus at birth, development of jaundice with hepatosplenomegaly or meningoencephalitis in early childhood, or delayed appearance of ocular lesions such as chorioretinitis in later childhood. Exposure to the parasite is through eating undercooked meat, gardening in soil that is potentially contaminated by mammalian feces, or cleaning a cat's litter box.

## VARICOSE VEINS

Pressure by the enlarged uterus on venous return from the legs and progesterone-mediated vasodilation can lead to prominent varicosities and edema of the legs or vulva. Any concern for deep vein thrombosis should be ruled out by examination for erythema, edema, cords, or tenderness. Doppler ultrasound may be indicated in equivocal findings of the lower extremities. Benign varicosities almost invariably return to normal after delivery, thus limiting the need for intervention in the antepartum period. Edema of the lower extremities is common, responds to elevation, and must be differentiated from facial or hand edema accompanying preeclampsia. Hemorrhoids are manifestations of the varicosities of the rectal veins. Treatment focuses on stool softeners, sitz baths, and over-the-counter topical preparations.

## CONSTIPATION

Bowel transit time and relaxation of intestinal smooth muscle are both increased due to progesterone effects, resulting in overall slowing of bowel function. If pronounced, this can lead to constipation. Dietary management of this condition is centered around recommendations for increased fluids and high-fiber foods. Enemas and laxatives are avoided.

## UPPER EXTREMITY DISCOMFORT

Periodic numbness and tingling of the fingers is due to exacerbations of carpal tunnel compression exacerbated by tissue edema. Splinting of the affected hand at night is indicated, with anticipation of resolution during postpartum diuresis.

## BACKACHE AND PELVIC DISCOMFORT

Endocrine relaxation of ligamentous structures coupled with an offset center of gravity create exaggerated spinal curve, joint instability, and

 **CURRENT DIAGNOSIS**

- Pregnancy evaluation should begin 3 months before conception with optimization of underlying medical conditions and commencement of prenatal vitamins with 400 μg of folic acid.
- Preconception counseling with a specialist in high-risk pregnancies should be considered in all patients with underlying medical conditions, if possible.
- The first prenatal visit should include a review of the medical and obstetric histories, current medications, herbal remedies, and tobacco, alcohol, and drug use.
- Prenatal laboratory studies should be done at the first visit after a pregnancy is confirmed with a urine pregnancy test. These studies include hemoglobin, platelet count, type and screen, rubella status, and hepatitis B testing. All women should be offered screening for HIV. High-risk patients should be screened for hepatitis C, gonorrhea, and chlamydia.
- Genetic screening should be offered based on ethnic background and family history.
- Both first-trimester screening (nuchal translucency combined with maternal serum PAPP-A/free β-hCG) and second-trimester quadruple screen should be offered to all patients. These tests aid in diagnosis of chromosome abnormalities. If a patient opts for a first-trimester screen, it is important to perform an AFP screen in the second trimester to screen for neural tube defects.
- Appropriate weight gain in pregnancy depends on maternal BMI before pregnancy. In patients with a normal BMI, a 25- to 35-pound weight gain is recommended. Underweight patients are encouraged to gain 30 to 40 pounds, and overweight patients are encouraged to gain no more than 25 pounds.
- Prenatal visits should begin at 8 to 12 weeks' gestation and continue monthly until 24 weeks. Visits should then be every 2 weeks until 36 weeks and then weekly. Each visit should include assessment of maternal weight, BP, urinalysis for protein and glucose, fundal height measurement, documentation of fetal heart tones, and review of symptoms of preterm labor and preeclampsia.
- All patients should undergo a glucose challenge test at 24 to 28 weeks. This is done by administering a 50-g load of glucose and obtaining a serum sample 1 hour after administration. A level greater than 140 mg/dL is considered abnormal, and a 3-hour glucose tolerance test is indicated. If a woman demonstrates abnormalities in two of the four values, gestational diabetes is diagnosed.

*Abbreviations:* AFP = alpha fetoprotein; BMI = body mass index; BP = blood pressure; hCG = human chorionic gonadotropin; PAPP-A = pregnancy-associated plasma protein A.

## CURRENT THERAPY

- Administration of the inactivated influenza vaccine (Fluzone, Fluvirin, Fluvarix) is recommended in all pregnant patients, regardless of trimester, who will be pregnant during the flu season.
- Folic acid supplementation should begin before conception. The recommended dose is 400 µg daily. In patients with a previous pregnancy complicated by a neural tube defect, 4 mg daily is recommended to prevent recurrence of a neural tube defect.
- Pyelonephritis requires hospitalization and IV antibiotics in all pregnant patients. IV antibiotics should be continued until the patient is afebrile for longer than 24 hours. Oral antibiotics should then be commenced to complete a 10-day course. All patients should continue on suppressive antibiotic therapy until delivery.
- All patients with HIV should be treated with antiretroviral therapy regardless of gestation. Intrapartum zidovudine is recommended for all patients with HIV.

compensatory back pain. Most women experience some form of this discomfort as pregnancy progresses. Advice given for improvements in posture, local heat, acetaminophen, and massage may be helpful. Minimizing the time spent standing can have a positive effect. Round ligament pain usually occurs during the second trimester and is described as sharp bilateral or unilateral groin pain. It may be exacerbated by change in position or rapid movement and might respond to similar measures. These routine aches and pains of pregnancy must be differentiated from rhythmic cramping pains originating in the back. The latter may be a sign of preterm labor requiring appropriate evaluation.

### LEG CRAMPS

Leg cramps in the form of recurrent muscle spasms in pregnancy are believed to be due to lower levels of serum calcium or higher levels of serum phosphorus. The calves are most commonly involved and attacks are more frequent at night and in the third trimester. There are no data from controlled trials to show benefit over placebo for treatment targeted toward reduced phosphate and increased calcium or magnesium intake. Local heat, putting the affected muscle on stretch, acetaminophen, and massage can be helpful in acute events.

### INTERCOURSE

In general, intercourse is considered safe in pregnancy. The exception to this rule is found in patients who are experiencing uterine bleeding, or postcoital cramps, and spotting. It may be wise to avoid intercourse in couples who are at risk for special circumstances. Firmer recommendations can be made in instances of placenta previa or known rupture of membranes; in these instances intercourse should not occur.

### DENTAL CARE

Ideally, women should have dental care completed before conception. However, dental procedures under local anesthesia may be carried out at any time during the pregnancy. Use of nitrous oxide inhalants is to be avoided, however. Long procedures should be postponed until the second trimester. Antibiotics are given for dental abscesses and in cases of rheumatic heart disease or mitral valve prolapse.

### X-RAYS, IONIZING RADIATION, AND IMAGING

The adverse effects of ionizing radiation are dose dependent, but there is no single diagnostic procedure that results in a dose of radiation high enough to threaten the fetus or embryo. Diagnostic radiation of less than 5000 mrad is considered by ACOG to have minimal teratogenic risk, and if medically indicated, x-ray imaging may be performed safely. For example, patients may undergo chest x-rays as indicated; a dose of 0.05 mrad is typical exposure. Patients receiving dental x-rays are additionally protected by a lead apron. Still, the need for x-ray films should be evaluated for risks and potential benefits in the individual pregnant patient to conservatively protect the mother and fetus from theoretical genetic or oncogenic risk. MRI is considered safe due to its mechanism of action, which is a nonionizing form of radiation. Radioactive iodine ($^{131}$I) is contraindicated in pregnancy.

### IMMUNIZATION

Live virus vaccines must be avoided during pregnancy because of possible effects on the fetus. These include measles, mumps, rubella (MMR) and yellow fever (VF-Vax). The risks to the fetus from the administration of rabies vaccine (RabAvert, IMOVAX) are unknown. The varicella vaccine (Varivax) is not recommended in pregnancy.

Diphtheria and tetanus toxoid (Td) may be administered in pregnancy if exposure to pathogens is likely. The hepatitis B vaccine (Engerix B, Recombivax HB) series is safe and may be given in pregnancy to women at risk. The inactivated influenza vaccine (Fluzone, Fluvirin, Fluvarix) is also recommended in all women during any trimester they will be pregnant during the flu season.

## Tests of Fetal Well-Being

A primary goal in antepartum care is the competent management of patient care extended to both mother and baby in order to reduce the risk of fetal demise after 24 weeks, ensure optimal conditions for term delivery after 37 weeks, and intervene for evolving conditions threatening the well-being of either patient. Any pregnancy that may be at increased risk for antepartum fetal compromise is a candidate for tests of fetal well-being performed weekly, beginning at 28 to 32 weeks. Some conditions requiring antepartum testing are listed in Box 4.

### NONSTRESS TEST

The nonstress test consists of fetal heart rate monitoring in the absence of uterine contractions. A reactive tracing is one in which heart rate accelerations of 15 bpm above the baseline of 120 to 160 bpm are of at least 15 seconds' duration. Two of these accelerations must be observed in a 20-minute period. False-positive nonreactive tracings are more common before 28 weeks' gestation.

### CONTRACTION STRESS TEST

The requirements for a reactive tracing are combined with tocodynamometer recordings of three contractions of 40 seconds or more duration in a 10-minute period. If no contractions are present, they may be induced via nipple stimulation or intravenously administered oxytocin. Relative contraindications to this test are preterm premature rupture of membranes, classic uterine incision scar, placenta previa, and unexplained vaginal bleeding. The results of the contraction stress test are categorized in Table 1.

---

**BOX 4   Conditions that Prompt Further Testing**

- Decreased fetal movements
- Fetal growth restriction
- Hypertensive disorders
- Insulin-dependent diabetes mellitus
- Multiple gestation with discordant fetal growth
- Oligohydramnios or polyhydramnios
- Post-term pregnancy
- Prior loss or stillbirth

## TABLE 1 Possible Results of the Contraction Stress Test

| Result | Description |
| --- | --- |
| Negative | No late decelerations |
| Positive | Late decelerations follow 50% of contractions |
| Equivocal | Intermittent or variable decelerations |
| Unsatisfactory | <3 contractions in 10 minutes |

## BIOPHYSICAL PROFILE

The biophysical profile consists of a nonstress test with ultrasound observations. A total of ten points is given for the following elements (two points each):

- Reactive nonstress test
- Presence of fetal breathing movements of 30 seconds or more in 30 minutes
- Fetal movement defined as three or more discrete body or limb movements within 30 minutes
- Fetal tone defined as one or more episodes of fetal extremity extension and return to flexion
- Quantification of amniotic fluid volume, defined as a pocket of fluid that measures at least 2 cm by 2 cm

## Antepartum Hospitalization

Pregnant patients with complications requiring hospitalization are admitted to a high-risk antepartum floor in close proximity to the labor and delivery area. Specialists in maternal-fetal medicine are intimately involved in the care plans of these patients.

## REFERENCES

American College of Obstetricians and Gynecologists: Compendium of Selected Publications. Atlanta: American College of Obstetricians and Gynecologists, 2007.

Carpenter MW, Coustan DR: Criteria for screening tests for gestational diabetes. Am J Obstet Gynecol 1982;144(7):763-773.

Centers for Disease Control and Prevention: Influenza: Information for Health Professionals. Available at http://www.cdc.gov/flu/ (accessed July 13, 2007).

Cunningham FG, Leveno KL, Bloom SL, et al: Williams Obstetrics, 22nd ed. New York: McGraw-Hill, 2005.

Lopez A, Dietz VJ, Wilson M, et al: Preventing congenital toxoplasmosis. MMWR Recomm Rep 2000;49(RR-2):59-68.

Wald NJ, Rodeck C, et al: First and second trimester antenatal screening for Down's syndrome. The results of the Serum, Urine and Ultrasound Screening Study. J Med Screen 2003;10(2):56-104.

# Ectopic Pregnancy

Method of
*Gary H. Lipscomb, MD*

In the United States, the incidence of ectopic pregnancies has increased dramatically during the last several decades. Commonly cited risks include prior pelvic inflammatory disease (PID), previous tubal surgery, intrauterine device (IUD) use, previous ectopic pregnancy, ovulation induction and in vitro fertilization, progestin-containing contraceptives, smoking, previous abdominal surgery, in utero diethylstilbestrol (DES) exposure, and previous induced abortion.

A high degree of suspicion is necessary for the early diagnosis of an ectopic pregnancy. Almost all ectopic pregnancies have episodes of vaginal bleeding or lower abdominal pain prior to rupture. Such patients are appropriate candidates to evaluate for ectopic pregnancy. Figure 1 illustrates a diagnostic algorithm that is useful in efficiently coordinating and interpreting the tests used in the diagnosis of ectopic pregnancy.

## Diagnosis

Serum progesterone levels are helpful as an initial screening test for ectopic pregnancy. Levels higher than 25 ng/mL are associated with ectopic pregnancy in only 1% to 2% of cases; levels less than 5 ng/mL are associated with a nonviable pregnancy (either intrauterine or ectopic) more than 99% of the time. If progesterone levels are not readily available in a timely manner, however, human chorionic gonadotropin (hCG) levels alone may be used.

Levels of hCG rise in an essentially linear fashion until after 41 days of gestation. By this gestational age, an intrauterine pregnancy (IUP) should be seen on ultrasound. In 85% of normal pregnancies, hCG doubles approximately every 2 days, rising at least 66% in 48 hours. However, 15% of normal IUPs rise less than this in 48 hours. Conversely, 15% of ectopic pregnancies rise more than 66%. But a rise of less than 50% is associated with an abnormal pregnancy 99.9% of the time.

Because the interassay variability of hCG is 15%, a change of less than this amount is considered a plateau. Plateaued levels are the most predictive of ectopic pregnancy. The use of a urine pregnancy test to rule out the possibility of phantom hCG is strongly recommended prior to surgical or medical treatment. This phenomenon, caused by heterophilic serum antibodies, produces false-positive hCG levels usually less than 1000 IU/L.

The sonographic identification of an intrauterine gestational sac essentially excludes an ectopic pregnancy. A viable IUP should always be visualized at an hCG titer of 2000 IU/L by transvaginal scan and by 6500 IU/L with transabdominal ultrasound. An adnexal mass, in a patient with a presumed ectopic pregnancy and hCG levels less than 2000 IU/L, should not automatically be assumed to be an ectopic without the presence of a yolk sac, fetal pole, or cardiac activity. Such masses are frequently corpus luteum cysts associated with an early IUP.

Except in the rare case of heterotopic pregnancy, the identification of chorionic villi in uterine contents essentially eliminates the diagnosis of ectopic pregnancy. The use of dilation and curettage (D&C) also eliminates giving methotrexate unnecessarily to a patient with a failed IUP.

A D&C is particularly important in patients with hCG titers below the discriminatory zone of ultrasound. In these patients, the appropriate use of hCG doubling times and serum progesterone levels is necessary to avoid interrupting a viable IUP. Patients with hCG titers that plateau (less than 15% change) or an hCG rise of less than 50% in 48 hours should undergo D&C to differentiate between a failed IUP and an ectopic pregnancy. Villi is absent on final histology in up to 50% of these cases. Because only the presence of villi is diagnostic,

## CURRENT DIAGNOSIS

- Screening for symptomatic patients or those with risk factors
- Diagnostic algorithm to coordinate testing
- hCG titers every 48 hours
- Ultrasound at hCG level of 2000 mIU/mL
- D&C for inappropriate hCG rise (<50% in 48 hours) below 2000 mIU/mL

*Abbreviations:* D&C = dilation and curettage; hCG = human chorionic gonadotropin.

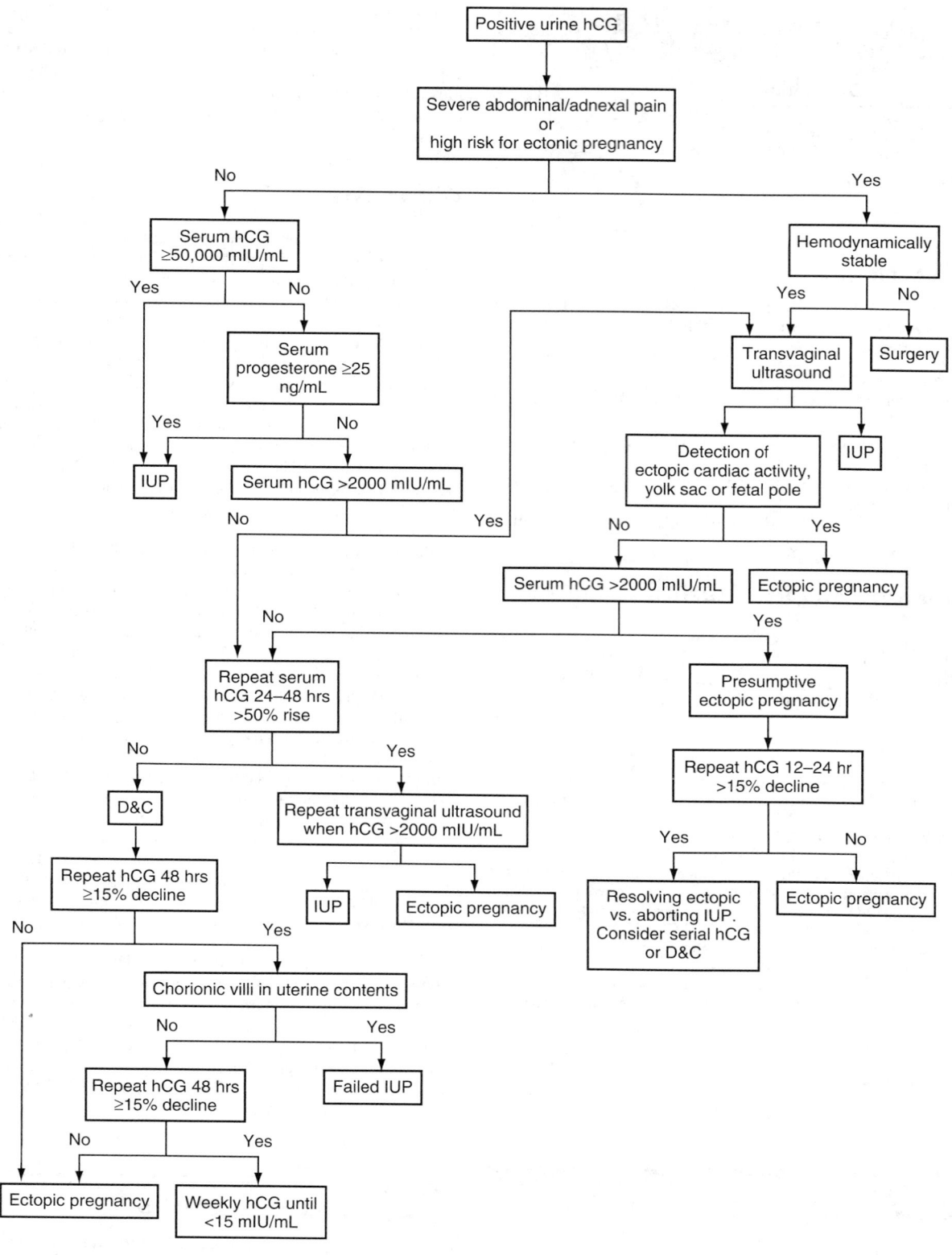

**FIGURE 1.** University of Tennessee Diagnostic Algorithm. D&C = dilation and curettage; hCG = human chorionic gonadotropin.

## CURRENT THERAPY

- Surgery: treatment of choice for unstable patients
- Methotrexate success: correlation with hCG levels
- Multidose methotrexate: 1 mg/kg body weight IM alternate days with leucovorin 0.1 mg/kg IM until hCG declines 15%
- Multidose treatment follow-up: daily hCG until decline, then weekly
- Single-dose methotrexate: 50 mg /m² based on actual body weight
- Single-dose treatment follow-up: hCG on days 1, 4, 7, then weekly if 15% decline between days 4 and 7

*Abbreviations:* hCG = human chorionic gonadotropin; IM = intramuscularly.

those without villi require serial hCG titers. While awaiting final histologic pathology, hCG titers are also followed. As noted in the ectopic algorithm, a serum hCG drawn after D&C is followed by a repeat level in 12 to 24 hours. Rising or inappropriately falling levels after D&C are considered diagnostic of an ectopic pregnancy.

Laparoscopy remains the gold standard for the diagnosis of ectopic pregnancy. It should be employed in any patient with suspected ectopic rupture, unreliable patients, or any others suspected of ectopic pregnancy for which the diagnostic algorithms are inappropriate.

## Treatment

Surgery is the classic treatment for ectopic pregnancy and remains the treatment of choice in hemodynamic unstable patients, those desiring no further pregnancies, or those who are unsuitable or unwilling to risk medical therapy.

Medical therapy with methotrexate[1] is an acceptable option to surgical therapy. Reported success rates range from 75% to 96%, with an average of approximately 90%. Whether a multidose or single-dose methotrexate protocol is most effective remains debatable, but single-dose methotrexate is the most popular because of its ease of use and low incidence of side effects.

Contraindications to medical therapy remain ill defined, but Boxes 1 and 2 note frequently used contraindications. The hCG level is the single factor most predictive of failure. With hCG levels of 5000 to 9999, success rates fall to approximately 87%, further dropping to 82% for levels 10,000 to 14,999 and 68% if more than 15,000. These levels can be used to counsel patients about the risk of failure.

### MULTIDOSE METHOTREXATE

Intramuscular methotrexate, 1 mg/kg of actual body weight, alternating with citrovorum rescue factor (Leucovorin), 0.1 mg/kg, is given daily and

---

[1]Not FDA approved for this indication.

---

### BOX 1 Generally Accepted Contraindications to Medical Therapy

White blood count <1500 cells/mL
Alanine aminotransferase (ALT) >twice upper limit normal
Creatinine >twice upper limit normal
Ectopic size >4 cm
Ectopic size >3.5 cm if cardiac activity present the upper limit of normal, hemodynamically unstable
Immunocompromised status

### BOX 2 Relative Contraindications to Medical Therapy

Ectopic cardiac activity*
Serum hCG level >15,000†

*Controversial; however, when corrected for hCG level, no longer a risk factor.
†Acceptable if patients are counseled on failure rate.
*Abbreviation:* hCG = human chorionic gonadotropin.

continued until a 15% decline in two consecutive daily hCG titers. Human chorionic gonadotropin levels are then followed weekly. A repeat course of methotrexate/citrovorum is given if levels fall to less than 15% or rise between two consecutive hCG titers.

### SINGLE-DOSE METHOTREXATE PROTOCOL

Methotrexate, 50 mg/m² based on actual body weight, is given intramuscularly. The day methotrexate is given is considered day 1. A repeat hCG is performed on days 4 and 7. If there is an appropriate decline, hCG levels are followed weekly. If the hCG level declines less than 15% between days 4 and 7, a second dose of methotrexate is given and the protocol restarted at a new day 1. Although this protocol is referred to as "single-dose methotrexate," approximately 20% of patients require more than one treatment cycle.

In conclusion, the incidence of ectopic pregnancy has reached epidemic proportions in the United States. Nevertheless, the mortality associated with this disease is steadily declining. This decline is primarily because of earlier diagnosis that allows treatment prior to rupture. This earlier diagnosis is the result of improved assays for progesterone, hCG, transvaginal ultrasound, and the use of diagnostic algorithms that do not require the use of laparoscopy. Once diagnosed, numerous treatment options are now available, including the option of medical therapy. Future developments ideally will provide for an even earlier diagnosis as well as data on the optimum candidates for each form of treatment.

### REFERENCES

Brenaschek G, Rudelstorfer R, Csaicsich P: Vaginal sonography versus serum human chorionic gonadotropin in early detection of pregnancy. Am J Obstet Gynecol 1988;158:608-612.
Kadar N, Freedman M, Zacher M: Further observation on the doubling time of human chorionic gonadotropin in early asymptomatic pregnancy. Fertil Steril 1980;54:783-787.
Lipscomb GH, McCord ML, Huff G, et al: Predictors of success of methotrexate treatment in women with tubal ectopic pregnancies. N Engl J Med 1999;341:1874-1878.
Lipscomb GH, Stovall TS, Ling FW: Nonsurgical treatment of ectopic pregnancy. N Engl J Med 2000;343:1325-1329.
Stovall TS, Ling FW, Buster JE: Nonsurgical diagnosis and treatment of tubal pregnancy. Fertil Steril 1990;54:537-538.
Stovall TG, Ling FW, Gray LA, et al: Methotrexate treatment of unruptured ectopic pregnancy: A report of 100 cases. Obstet Gynecol 1991;77:749-753.

---

# Vaginal Bleeding in Late Pregnancy

Method of
*Jami Star Zeltzer, MD*

Vaginal bleeding in late pregnancy complicates approximately 6% of pregnancies and is associated with increased maternal and fetal morbidity and mortality. Excluding labor, the most likely causes are placenta previa and placental abruption, followed by uterine rupture and vasa previa; less common etiologies include trauma, cervical lesions, and coagulopathy. The primary focus in obstetric hemorrhage, regardless of cause, is maternal hemodynamic assessment and stabilization. Given the extraordinary blood flow to the uterus at term (600 to 800 mL/min), exsanguination can occur rapidly. Additionally, redistribution of maternal blood flow may lead to fetal hypoxia.

Early maternal signs of hemodynamic compromise include tachycardia and tachypnea; later, hypotension, weakened pulses, and oliguria ensue, along with evidence of fetal compromise. Further decompensation can ultimately result in the death of both mother and fetus. Guidelines for restoration of maternal circulating volume are approximately 3 mL of intravenous crystalloid, (i.e., normal saline or Ringer's solution) per 1 mL of blood lost (often underestimated). Laboratory evaluation includes a complete blood count, blood type, and crossmatch; in the setting of thrombocytopenia (less than 100,000 platelets), coagulation studies (prothrombin time [PT], partial thromboplastin time [PTT], fibrinogen, fibrin degradation products [FDPs]) are recommended. Packed red blood cells, fresh-frozen plasma, platelets, and/or cryoprecipitate are given to maintain maternal hemoglobin near 10 g/dL and correct coagulopathy (unlikely if whole blood is observed to clot in less than 8 minutes). Additional measures include administration of oxygen, lateral displacement of the uterus and, rarely, vasopressors. Fetal evaluation and treatment, including consideration of delivery, follow stabilization of the mother.

## Placenta Previa

Placenta previa, or the implantation of the placenta adjacent to or covering the internal os, complicates approximately 0.5% of all deliveries. The degree of placenta previa may be:

- Complete (internal os covered entirely)
- Partial (portion of internal os covered)
- Marginal (placental edge at cervix or less than 2 cm away)
- Low lying (not a true previa, where the placental edge implants in the lower uterine segment but doesn't reach the cervix)

Box 1 lists the risk factors. The pathophysiology appears to involve endometrial damage, with resulting limitation of healthy uterine tissue for implantation.

The hallmark symptom is painless vaginal bleeding, presumably initiated by development of the lower uterine segment. Usually, this occurs by 29 to 30 weeks of gestation, although in approximately 33% of cases, there is no bleeding until labor. The first bleed may be self-limited, but rebleeding complicates approximately 60% of cases. The diagnosis is often made in the absence of symptoms on routine ultrasound. The incidence of placenta previa is 5% to 10% in mid-gestation; this resolves in most cases with development of the lower uterine segment (*placental migration*). When asymptomatic, expectant management is appropriate, although vaginal precautions after 28 weeks' gestation may be advised.

When a patient presents with third-trimester bleeding, speculum exams are contraindicated until placenta previa is ruled out. The most accurate method of diagnosis is transvaginal ultrasound, which is safe in experienced hands; transperineal or transabdominal ultrasound carry greater risks of false-positive and false-negative results.

Observation in the hospital is recommended following a bleed, during which time approximately 50% of patients will deliver. Steroids are indicated for enhancement of fetal lung maturation. Tocolysis can be administered if the mother and fetus are stable, but betasympathomimetics should be avoided in order to minimize cardiovascular effects. Outpatient management is acceptable if bleeding ceases, as long as the patient is compliant and has ready access to a hospital. Serial ultrasound assessment is recommended because there is an increased risk of intrauterine growth restriction. Transfusion should be offered to maintain hemoglobin greater than 10 mg/dL.

Urgent delivery by cesarean section is indicated when there is ongoing maternal hemorrhage or evidence of fetal compromise. In the stable patient, a planned cesarean section can be performed at 35 to 36 weeks, generally after an amniocentesis is performed to confirm fetal lung maturity. Vaginal delivery is preferable in the setting of fetal demise; it may be attempted if delivery is imminent, or with marginal previa, although a *double setup* for emergent cesarean section is advised.

Placenta previa predisposes to postpartum hemorrhage, either from atony of the lower uterine segment or inability to remove the placenta because of absence of the decidua basalis. The most common form of this latter condition is placenta accreta, where the trophoblast adheres to the myometrium. Less common forms include placenta increta (the trophoblast invades the myometrium) and placenta percreta (trophoblast invades uterine serosa and/or adjacent organs). The primary risk factor for placenta accreta is the number of previous cesarean sections, with an incidence approaching 40% in patients with two prior cesarean sections and a placenta previa. Other risk factors include age, parity, and history of curettage. Color Doppler ultrasound and magnetic resonance imaging (MRI) are helpful but not always definitive for diagnosis. If placenta accreta is suspected, preparations can be made for scheduled delivery with trained personnel and blood products available. At delivery, the placenta should be left in place if a cleavage plane cannot be developed easily. Cesarean–hysterectomy is often required for hemostasis, although conservative management, including preoperative and intraoperative selective embolization and/or use of methotrexate, has been reported. With placenta percreta, bladder invasion may require cystoscopy and urologic repair.

## Vasa Previa

Vasa previa is a rare condition (estimated 1 in 2500 deliveries) in which fetal blood vessels cross over the membranes in advance of the presenting part. This is most often associated with velamentous insertion of the umbilical cord (vessels reach the placenta after coursing through the membranes rather than by direct insertion); Box 2 lists the risk factors. Vasa previa carries a profound risk of fetal mortality from exsanguination, particularly at the time of membrane rupture (fetal blood volume at term is approximately 250 mL). Even in the absence of bleeding, vessel compression may result in compromise of the fetal circulation.

Signs include hemorrhage, as well as fetal heart rate abnormalities. A high index of suspicion is required, and advances in imaging techniques (color Doppler, transvaginal ultrasound) make prenatal diagnosis possible. If there is unexplained bleeding, an Apt test or Kleihauer-Betke test can identify fetal red blood cells. If the diagnosis of vasa previa is strongly suspected at term, or if hemorrhage is significant, prompt cesarean delivery is recommended, followed by neonatal resuscitation.

---

| BOX 1 | Risk Factors for Placenta Previa |
|---|---|

- Advancing maternal age
- Ethnic background (increased in Asians)
- Multiparity
- Multiple gestation
- Previous curettage
- Prior cesarean section (increases with number of sections)
- Prior placenta previa
- Smoking

---

| BOX 2 | Risk Factors for Vasa Previa |
|---|---|

- Bilobed placenta
- In vitro fertilization
- Low-lying placenta
- Multiple pregnancy
- Succenturiate lobe
- Velamentous insertion of umbilical cord

## BOX 3    Uterine Rupture

**Risk Factors**

Previous cesarean section (especially classical)
Use of oxytocin, prostaglandins, or misoprostol
Multiparity
Midforceps application
Breech version/extraction
Placental abruption
Shoulder dystocia
Placenta percreta
Müllerian duct anomalies
History of pelvic radiation

**Differential Diagnoses**

Appendicitis
Biliary colic
Pancreatitis
Peptic ulcer disease
Intestinal obstruction
Ovarian torsion
Placental abruption
Urinary tract disorders

## Uterine Rupture

Most often reported following prior cesarean section, uterine rupture can also occur in an unscarred uterus (1 in 8000 to 1 in 15,000 deliveries). This phenomenon implies complete separation of the uterine wall (as compared to uterine dehiscence), with or without expulsion of the fetus. Box 3 lists risk factors and differential diagnoses.

Common signs and symptoms include abdominal pain/tenderness and vaginal bleeding; additional complaints include epigastric or shoulder pain, abdominal distention, and constipation. The fetal tracing may show sudden variable decelerations or abrupt and prolonged bradycardia, often accompanied by recession of the presenting part. Maternal and fetal morbidity and mortality are high, particularly with delayed diagnosis. Treatment is urgent cesarean delivery, with repair of the uterus and/or hysterectomy as needed. Repeat cesarean section is advised in the future because of the risk for recurrence.

## Placental Abruption

Abruption of the placenta, or separation of the normally implanted placenta before birth, complicates 1% to 2% of pregnancies. Bleeding into the decidua basalis, with subsequent separation of varying amounts of placental tissue from the endometrium, may result in fetal compromise and/or demise. The exact pathophysiology is unclear. Box 4 lists the risk factors.

Vaginal bleeding in the second half of pregnancy is assumed to be caused by placental abruption, once placenta previa and other rare causes are ruled out. Concealed hemorrhage, present in 10% to 20% of cases, can complicate the diagnosis. Abdominal pain, back pain, uterine contractions (often described as low amplitude, high frequency), hypertonus, uterine tenderness, and/or idiopathic premature labor may be present. While ultrasound can identify placenta previa, it cannot be relied upon to definitively diagnose abruption, as clot is sonographically visible in less than 50% of cases. The differential diagnoses include uterine rupture, appendicitis, and chorioamnionitis, as well as other causes of abdominal pain.

Most commonly, bleeding is not profuse and, if the episode is self-limited, expectant management of a preterm gestation includes observation, serial fetal growth assessment, fetal well-being testing, and steroid therapy to accelerate fetal lung maturation. With ongoing significant blood loss, stabilization of the mother, fetal assessment, and laboratory evaluation are indicated. Coagulopathy is rare in the absence of fetal demise. If tocolysis is required, betasympathomimetics should be avoided, as they may mask maternal cardiovascular decompensation.

Vaginal delivery is appropriate if mother and fetus are stable. Amniotomy may decrease extravasation of blood into the myometrium by head compression. Not uncommonly, effacement will precede dilatation; oxytocin (Pitocin) is acceptable for labor dysfunction. In the event of an intrauterine demise, vaginal delivery is preferred. Acute hemorrhage requires immediate cesarean delivery, with blood and coagulation factor replacement as needed.

Potential complications of abruption include hemorrhagic shock, disseminated intravascular coagulation (unlikely unless there is greater than 2000 mL blood loss and/or fetal demise), ischemic necrosis of maternal organs (especially kidney), and Couvelaire uterus (extravasation of blood into uterine muscle). Recurrence is approximately 5% to 15%, increasing with each subsequent event. There are no known preventive measures other than correcting modifiable risk factors. Research into the association between thrombophilia and abruption is ongoing, but in absence of other risk factors, a work-up for hypercoagulability may be considered.

## BOX 4    Risk Factors for Placental Abruption

- Chorioamnionitis
- Cocaine use
- Ethnic background (highest in blacks)
- Hypertension
- Male fetal gender
- Multiple gestation
- Parity
- Polyhydramnios (rapid decompression at membrane rupture and/or therapeutic amniocentesis)
- Preterm premature rupture of membranes
- Previous cesarean section
- Smoking
- Trauma, including domestic violence
- Unexplained elevated second trimester alpha-fetoprotein
- Uterine anomalies/short umbilical cord

# Hypertensive Disorders of Pregnancy

Method of
*David G. Weismiller, MD*

Hypertension is the most common medical disorder during pregnancy. It occurs in 6% to 8% of pregnancies and contributes significantly to stillbirths and to neonatal morbidity and mortality. Hypertensive disorders during pregnancy are the second leading cause of maternal mortality in the United States after thromboembolism, accounting for almost 15% of such deaths. For this reason, strategies to diagnose, prevent, treat, and reduce the risk for hypertensive disorders of pregnancy receive considerable attention.

## Classification of the Hypertensive Disorders of Pregnancy

The most important factor to consider in classifying disease in which blood pressure rises abnormally in pregnancy is whether the hypertensive disorder antedates the pregnancy or whether it is a potentially more ominous disease peculiar to pregnancy: preeclampsia. Elevated blood pressure is the cardinal pathophysiologic feature in chronic hypertension, whereas in preeclampsia, increased blood pressure is important primarily because it signals the underlying disorder and is a potential cause of maternal morbidity.

According to the National High Blood Pressure Education Program, increased blood pressure in pregnancy is divided into four main categories:

- Preeclampsia-eclampsia
- Chronic hypertension
- Preeclampsia superimposed on chronic hypertension
- Gestational hypertension (transient or chronic)

## PREECLAMPSIA-ECLAMPSIA

Preeclampsia-eclampsia usually occurs after 20 weeks of gestation. The rate of preeclampsia ranges from 2% to 7% in healthy nulliparous women and is substantially higher in women with twin gestation (14%) and those with previous preeclampsia (18%). The disorder may occur earlier with trophoblastic diseases such as hydatidiform mole or hydrops. Preeclampsia is determined by increased blood pressure accompanied by proteinuria in a woman who is normotensive before 20 weeks (Box 1). The finding of proteinuria usually correlates with 30 mg/dL (1+ dipstick) or greater in a random urine determination with no evidence of urinary tract infection. Because of the discrepancy between random protein determinations and 24-hour urine protein in preeclampsia (which may be either higher or lower), it is recommended that the diagnosis be based on a 24-hour urine, if at all possible, or a timed collection corrected for creatinine excretion, if a 24-hour urine is not feasible.

In the absence of proteinuria, preeclampsia is highly suspect when increased blood pressure is accompanied by the symptoms of headache, blurred vision, and abdominal pain or when it is accompanied by abnormal laboratory tests, specifically low platelet counts and abnormal liver enzymes. Diastolic blood pressure is determined by the disappearance of sound (Korotkoff 5). Gestational blood pressure elevation should be defined on the basis of at least two determinations. No randomized controlled trial evidence supports the use of ambulatory blood pressure monitoring during pregnancy.

In the past, an increase of 30 mm Hg systolic or 15 mm Hg diastolic blood pressure was used as a diagnostic criterion in preeclampsia, even when absolute values were below 140/90 mm Hg. But this diagnostic criterion is not included in the classification criteria set forth by the National High Blood Pressure Education Program. The only available evidence demonstrates that women in this group are not likely to suffer increased adverse outcomes. Still, some experts believe that women who have a rise of 30 mm Hg systolic or 15 mm Hg diastolic blood pressure warrant close observation, especially if proteinuria and hyperuricemia of 6 mg/dL or more are also present. Edema is also removed as a marker in hypertension schemes because it occurs in too many normal pregnant women to be discriminant.

Eclampsia is the occurrence of seizures that cannot be attributed to other causes in a woman with preeclampsia. Up to 40% of eclamptic seizures occur before delivery. Approximately 16% occur more than 48 hours after delivery.

Preeclampsia always presents potential danger to the mother and the fetus. As the certainty of the diagnosis of preeclampsia increases, the requirements for careful assessment and consideration for delivery also increase (Table 1).

## CHRONIC HYPERTENSION

Chronic hypertension is defined as hypertension that is present and observable before week 20 of gestation, with hypertension defined as a blood pressure of 140 mm Hg systolic or 90 mm Hg diastolic or greater. Hypertension diagnosed for the first time during pregnancy that does not resolve postpartum is also classified as chronic hypertension.

## SUPERIMPOSED PREECLAMPSIA

Superimposed preeclampsia complicates almost 25% of pregnancies in women with chronic hypertension. The prognosis for mother and fetus is worse than with either condition alone. The incidence of superimposed preeclampsia is even higher in women who have underlying renal insufficiency, chronic hypertension that has been present 4 or more years, or who have had a hypertensive disorder complicate a previous pregnancy. Distinguishing superimposed preeclampsia from worsening chronic hypertension is a challenge (Table 2).

---

**TABLE 1  Findings That Increase Certainty of Diagnosis of Preeclampsia Syndrome**

| Findings | Value |
| --- | --- |
| Blood pressure | 160 mm Hg or more systolic or 110 mm Hg or more diastolic. |
| Proteinuria | 2.0 g or more in a 24-hour urine collection ($2^+$ or $3^+$ g on qualitative examination). The proteinuria should occur for the first time in pregnancy and regress after delivery. |
| Serum creatinine | Greater than 1.2 mg/dL unless known to be previously elevated. |
| Platelet count | Less than 100,000 cells/mm³ and/or evidence of microangiopathic hemolytic anemia (with increased lactic acid dehydrogenase). |
| Hepatic enzymes | Elevated ALT or AST. |
| Central nervous system | Persistent headache or other cerebral or visual disturbances. |
| Abdomen | Persistent epigastric pain. |

*Abbreviations:* ALT = alanine aminotransferase; AST = aspartate aminotransferase.

---

**TABLE 2  Findings That Increase Certainty of Diagnosis of Preeclampsia Superimposed Upon Chronic Hypertension**

| Finding | Value |
| --- | --- |
| Proteinuria | New-onset proteinuria (in women with hypertension and no proteinuria prior to 20 weeks' gestation) defined as the urinary excretion of 300 mg protein or greater in a 24-hour specimen or in women with hypertension and proteinuria before 20 weeks' gestation or sudden increase in proteinuria |
| Blood pressure | Sudden increase in blood pressure in a woman whose hypertension has been previously well controlled |
| Platelet count | Thrombocytopenia with a platelet count of less than 100,000 cells/mm³ |
| Hepatic enzymes | Increase in ALT or AST to abnormal levels |

*Abbreviations:* ALT = alanine aminotransferase; AST = aspartate aminotransferase.

---

### BOX 1  Criteria for Diagnosis of Preeclampsia

- Blood pressure of 140 mm Hg systolic or higher or 90 mm Hg diastolic or higher that occurs after 20 weeks of gestation in a woman with previously normal blood pressure.
- Proteinuria, defined as urinary excretion of 0.3 g protein or higher in a 24-hour urine specimen.

## GESTATIONAL HYPERTENSION

Gestational hypertension refers to blood pressure elevation without proteinuria that is detected for the first time after midpregnancy. The hypertension may be accompanied by other signs of the preeclampsia syndrome, which impacts management. The final determination that the woman does not have the preeclampsia syndrome is made retrospectively postpartum. Gestational hypertension is subdivided into two types. If preeclampsia has not developed and blood pressure has returned to normal by 12 weeks postpartum, the diagnosis of transient hypertension of pregnancy is assigned. If the blood pressure elevation persists, the woman is diagnosed as having chronic hypertension.

# Pathophysiology of Preeclampsia

Preeclampsia is a syndrome with well-defined maternal and fetal manifestations. The maternal disease is characterized by vasospasm, activation of the coagulation system, and derangement in many humoral and autacoid systems that are associated with volume and blood pressure control. Oxidative stress and inflammatory-like responses may also be important in the pathophysiology of this syndrome. The pathologic changes are primarily ischemic in nature and affect the placenta, brain, liver, and kidney. Several of the so-called nonhypertensive complications can be life-threatening, even in the face of otherwise mild blood pressure elevations. Risk factors for preeclampsia are related to medical conditions, such as antiphospholipid antibody syndrome and nephropathy, or they may be related to the pregnancy itself or may be specific to the mother or father of the fetus (Box 2).

The etiology of most cases of hypertension during pregnancy, particularly preeclampsia, remains unknown. Many consider the placenta the pathogenic focus for all manifestations of preeclampsia because delivery is the only definitive cure of the disease. Much research centers on the changes in the maternal blood vessels that supply blood to the placenta. Discoveries on how alterations in the immune response at the maternal interface might lead to preeclampsia address the link between placental and maternal disease. A nonclassical human leukocyte antigen (HLA), HLA G is expressed in normal placental tissue and may play a role in modulating the maternal immune response to the immunologically foreign placenta.

---

### BOX 2   Risk Factors for Preeclampsia

**Pregnancy-Associated Factors**
- Chromosomal abnormalities
- Hydatidiform mole
- Hydrops fetalis
- Multifetal pregnancy
- Oocyte denotation or donor insemination
- Structural congenital abnormalities
- Urinary tract infection

**Maternal-Specific Factors**
- Age greater than 35 years
- Age less than 20 years
- Black race
- Family history of preeclampsia
- Nulliparity
- Preeclampsia in a previous pregnancy
- Specific medical conditions: gestational diabetes mellitus, type I diabetes, obesity, chronic hypertension, renal disease, thrombophilias
- Stress

**Paternal-Specific Factors**
- First-time father
- Previously fathered a preeclamptic pregnancy in another woman

---

Additional evidence for alterations in immunity in pathogenesis includes the disease's prominence in nulliparous gestations with subsequent normal pregnancies, a decreased prevalence after heterologous blood transfusions, long cohabitation before successful conception, and observed pathologic changes in the placental vasculature in preeclampsia that resemble allograft rejection.

## BLOOD PRESSURE CHANGES

Women with preeclampsia typically do not develop frank hypertension until the second half of gestation, but vasoconstrictor influences may be present earlier. Alterations in vascular reactivity may be detected by gestational week 20, and numerous surveys suggest that women destined to develop preeclampsia have slightly higher "normal" blood pressure (e.g., diastolic levels more than 70 mm Hg) as early as the second trimester, confirmed by ambulatory blood pressure monitoring techniques. Blood pressure normalizes postpartum, usually within the first few days of the puerperium, but may take as long as 2 to 4 weeks, especially in severe cases.

## CARDIAC CHANGES

Typically the heart is not affected in preeclampsia. The decrements in cardiac performance represent a normally contracting ventricle against a markedly increased afterload.

## RENAL CHANGES

The renal lesion characteristic of preeclampsia is termed *glomerular endotheliosis*. The glomeruli become enlarged and swollen. Both glomerular filtration rate and renal blood flow decrease in preeclampsia, leading to a decrease in filtration fraction. Because renal function normally rises 35% to 50% during pregnancy, creatinine levels in women with preeclampsia may still be below the upper limits of normal for pregnancy (0.8 mg/dL). Fractional urate clearance decreases, producing hyperuricemia. Although an elevated serum uric acid level (6.0 mg/dL) represents a useful confirmatory test for the diagnosis of preeclampsia, it has very poor predictive value among patients without preexisting hypertension. But when the patient has chronic hypertension, the serum uric acid level may be of some value. One investigator has reported that a serum uric acid level of 5.5 mg/dL or greater could identify women with an increased likelihood of having superimposed preeclampsia, which is an important marker of preeclampsia. Proteinuria may appear late in the clinical course and tends to be nonselective. Preeclampsia is associated with hypocalciuria, in contrast with the increased urinary calcium excretion observed during normal pregnancy. Even when edema is marked, plasma volume is lower than that of normal gestation, and there is evidence of hemoconcentration, believed to be caused, in part, by extravasation of albumin into the interstitium. Oliguria, commonly defined as less than 500 mL in 24 hours, also may occur, secondary to the hemoconcentration and decreased renal blood flow.

## COAGULATION SYSTEM CHANGES

Thrombocytopenia is the most common hematologic abnormality in preeclampsia. Circulating fibrin degradation products occasionally may be elevated, and unless the disease is accompanied by placental abruption, plasma fibrinogen levels are unaffected. Platelet counts below 100,000 cells/mm³ signal serious disease, and if delivery is delayed, levels may continue to fall precipitously. The cause of thrombocytopenia is unclear.

## HEPATIC CHANGES

Liver damage accompanying preeclampsia may range from mild hepatocellular necrosis with serum enzyme abnormalities (aminotransferase and lactate dehydrogenase) to the ominous hemolysis, elevated liver enzymes, and low platelet count (HELLP) syndrome, with markedly elevated enzyme levels and even subcapsular bleeding or hepatic rupture. HELLP represents serious disease and is associated with significant maternal morbidity. A disproportionate elevation of lactate dehydrogenase (LDH) levels in serum may be a sign of hemolysis.

## CENTRAL NERVOUS SYSTEM CHANGES

Eclampsia is the convulsive phase of preeclampsia and remains a significant cause of maternal mortality. Other central nervous system manifestations are headache and visual disturbances, including blurred vision, scotomata, and, rarely, cortical blindness. Focal neurologic signs occasionally develop, which should prompt radiologic investigation.

# Clinical Considerations

Expectant mothers with hypertension are predisposed to the development of potentially lethal complications, notably abruptio placentae, disseminated intravascular coagulation, cerebral hemorrhage, hepatic failure, and acute renal failure. The clinical spectrum of preeclampsia ranges from mild to severe forms. In most women, progression through this spectrum is slow, and the disorder may never proceed beyond mild preeclampsia. In others, the disease progresses more rapidly, changing from mild to severe in days or weeks. In the most serious cases, progression may be rapid and fulminant, with mild disease progressing to severe preeclampsia or eclampsia.

## DIAGNOSIS

Decisions regarding hospitalization and delivery that have significant impact on maternal and fetal health are often based on whether the patient is believed to have preeclampsia or a more benign hypertensive disorder of pregnancy, such as chronic or gestational hypertension.

The period in gestation when hypertension is first documented is helpful to consider in determining the correct diagnosis. Documentation of hypertension before conception, or before gestational week 20, favors a diagnosis of chronic hypertension (either essential or secondary). High blood pressure presenting at midpregnancy (weeks 20 to 28) may be caused by early preeclampsia (rare before 24 weeks), transient hypertension, or unrecognized chronic hypertension. Blood pressure normally falls in the initial trimesters, and this physiologic decrement may even be exaggerated in patients with essential hypertension, masking the diagnosis in pregnancy. Hypertension may be noted later in pregnancy, however, as part of the normal third trimester rise in blood pressure or when superimposed preeclampsia occurs.

## LABORATORY EVALUATION

Laboratory tests recommended to diagnose or manage hypertension in pregnancy serve primarily to distinguish preeclampsia from either chronic or transient hypertension. They are also useful in assessing the severity of disease, particularly in the case of preeclampsia, which is usually associated with laboratory abnormalities that deviate significantly from those of normal pregnant women. The same measurements are usually normal in women with uncomplicated chronic or transient hypertension. Efforts to identify an ideal screening or predictive test for preeclampsia are not successful to date. At present, no single screening test is considered reliable and cost effective for predicting preeclampsia. Numerous clinical, biophysical, and biochemical tests are proposed for the prediction or early detection of preeclampsia. Most of these tests suffer from poor sensitivity and poor predictive values, although this situation may be changing. Low levels of placental growth factor (PGF) predict subsequent development of preeclampsia. Decreased urinary PGF at midgestation is strongly associated with subsequent early development of preeclampsia.

The laboratory evaluation of hypertensive disorders can be approached by classifying women into one of three categories:

1. High-risk patients presenting with normal blood pressure
2. Patients presenting with hypertension before gestation week 20
3. Patients presenting with hypertension after midpregnancy

## High-Risk Patients Presenting With Normal Blood Pressure

Pregnant women whose gestations are considered high risk for preeclampsia benefit from a database of laboratory tests performed in early gestation. Those who are at high risk for preeclampsia include women who have a history of high blood pressure before conception or in a previous gestation (especially before week 34); women with diabetes, collagen vascular disease, underlying renal vascular disease, or renal parenchymal disease; and women with a multifetal pregnancy.

Tests that by later comparison assist in establishing an early diagnosis of preeclampsia (pure or superimposed) include hematocrit and platelet count as well as serum creatinine and uric acid levels. Observation of 1+ protein by routine urine analysis, documented by a clean-catch specimen, should be followed by a 24-hour collection for measurement of protein, as well as creatinine content, to determine accuracy of collection and to permit calculation of the creatinine clearance. High-risk patients require accurate dating and assessment of fetal growth. If circumstances are not optimal for clinical dating, sonographic dates should be established as early in the pregnancy as possible. A baseline sonogram for evaluating fetal growth should be considered at 25 to 28 weeks in these circumstances.

## Patients Presenting With Hypertension Before Gestation Week 20

Most women presenting with hypertension before gestation week 20 have (or will develop) essential hypertension. Women with hypertension should be evaluated before pregnancy to define the severity of their hypertension and to plan for potential lifestyle changes that a pregnancy may require. As recommended by the Joint National Committee on Prevention, Detection, Evaluation, and Treatment of High Blood Pressure (JNC VII Report), the diagnosis should be confirmed by multiple measurements and may incorporate home or other out-of-office blood pressure readings. If hypertension is confirmed, and particularly if it is severe (stage 3, systolic pressure of 180 mm Hg or more and diastolic pressure of 110 mm Hg or more), a woman should be evaluated for potentially reversible causes.

## Patients Presenting With Hypertension After Midpregnancy

Table 3 summarizes the recommended laboratory tests in the evaluation of women with hypertension after midpregnancy and the rationale for testing them biweekly or more often, if clinical circumstances lead to hospitalization of the patient. Such tests help distinguish preeclampsia from chronic and transient hypertension and are useful in assessing disease progression and severity. Note that in women with preeclampsia, one or more laboratory abnormalities may be present, even when blood pressure elevation is minimal.

# Prevention of Preeclampsia

Preventing preeclampsia is a challenge because of the limited knowledge of its etiology. During the past two decades, numerous clinical reports and randomized trials described the use of various methods to reduce the rate and/or severity of preeclampsia. Table 4 summarizes current opinion and data on the prevention of preeclampsia. Prevention focuses on identifying women at higher risk and conducting close clinical and laboratory monitoring, to recognize the disease process in its early stages. Although these measures do not prevent preeclampsia, they may be helpful for preventing some adverse maternal and fetal sequelae.

# Management of Hypertensive Disorders of Pregnancy

Three factors underlie any management scheme in hypertension and pregnancy. First, delivery is always appropriate therapy for the mother

**TABLE 3** Laboratory Evaluation and Rationale for Women Who Develop Hypertension After Midpregnancy

| Test | Rationale |
| --- | --- |
| Hemoglobin or hematocrit | Hemoconcentration supports the diagnosis of preeclampsia, and it is an indicator of severity. Note that values may be decreased if hemolysis accompanies the syndrome. |
| Platelet count | Thrombocytopenia suggests severe preeclampsia. |
| Quantification of protein excretion | Gestational hypertension with proteinuria should be considered preeclampsia (pure or superimposed), until it is proved otherwise. |
| Serum creatinine level | Abnormal or rising serum creatinine levels, especially in association with oliguria, suggest severe preeclampsia. |
| Serum uric acid level | Increased serum uric acid levels suggest the diagnosis of preeclampsia (>6.0 mg/dL). |
| Serum transaminase levels | Rising serum transaminase values suggest severe preeclampsia with hepatic involvement. |
| Serum albumin, lactic acid dehydrogenase, blood smear, and coagulation profile | For women with severe disease, these values indicate the extent of endothelial leak (hypoalbuminemia), presence of hemolysis (lactic acid-dehydrogenase level increase, schizocytosis, spherocytosis), and possible coagulopathy, including thrombocytopenia. |

**TABLE 4** Effectiveness of Agents in Prevention of Preeclampsia

| Agent | Prevention |
| --- | --- |
| Low-dose aspirin prophylaxis | Minimal to no reduction in the incidence of preeclampsia. The prevailing opinion is that women without risk factors do not benefit from treatment. Overall, administration of low-dose aspirin to women at risk leads to a 19% reduction in the risk of developing preeclampsia. On average, for every 69 women treated, 1 case is prevented. Starting aspirin before 12 weeks and/or using higher doses cannot be recommended for clinical practice until more information is available about safety. As the reductions in risk are small to moderate, relatively large numbers of women need to be treated to prevent a single adverse outcome. |
| Calcium supplementation | No data indicate that dietary supplementation with calcium prevents preeclampsia in low-risk women in the United States. Randomized trials of calcium supplementation in women considered at high risk of gestational hypertension (teenagers, previous preeclampsia, women with increased sensitivity to angiotensin II, preexisting hypertension) and in communities with low dietary calcium intake (mean intake equals 900 mg per day) demonstrate significant reductions in incidence of preeclampsia. |
| Magnesium supplementation | Prophylactic magnesium is not beneficial in preventing preeclampsia. |
| Zinc supplementation | No benefit in preventing preeclampsia. |
| Fish oil supplementation | No reduction in the incidence of preeclampsia. |
| Antioxidant therapy (vitamin C[1] and vitamin E[1]) | Limited data show some promise in preventing preeclampsia. |
| Salt restriction | No benefit in preventing preeclampsia. |
| Diuretic therapy[1] | No benefit in preventing preeclampsia. |

[1]Not FDA approved for the indication.

but may not be for the fetus. Second, the pathophysiologic changes of severe preeclampsia indicate that poor perfusion is the major factor leading to maternal physiologic derangement and increased perinatal morbidity and mortality. Third, the pathogenic changes of preeclampsia are present long before clinical diagnostic criteria are manifest.

For maternal health, the goal of therapy is to prevent eclampsia as well as other severe complications of preeclampsia. If there is a rationale for management other than delivery, it is to palliate the maternal condition to allow fetal maturation and cervical ripening.

## ANTICONVULSIVE THERAPY

Anticonvulsive therapy is usually indicated either to prevent recurrent convulsions in women with eclampsia or to prevent convulsions in women with preeclampsia. There is universal consensus that women with eclampsia should receive anticonvulsive therapy. Several randomized studies indicate that parenteral magnesium sulfate reduces the frequency of eclampsia more effectively than phenytoin (Dilantin). Parenteral magnesium sulfate is given during labor and delivery and for variable durations postpartum. There is no clear agreement concerning the use of prophylactic magnesium for women with preeclampsia. Although parenteral magnesium sulfate should be given peripartum to women with severe preeclampsia, its benefits with mild gestational hypertension or preeclampsia remain unclear.

Women with eclampsia require prompt intervention. When an eclamptic seizure occurs, the woman should be medically stabilized. First, it is important to control convulsions and prevent their recurrence with intravenous or intramuscular magnesium sulfate. One protocol is a 4- to 6-g loading dose diluted in 100 mL fluid and administered intravenously for 15 to 20 minutes, followed by 2 g per hour as a continuous intravenous infusion.

## ANTIHYPERTENSIVE THERAPY

### Therapy in Acute Hypertension

Antihypertensive therapy is indicated when blood pressure is dangerously high or rises suddenly in women with preeclampsia, especially intrapartum. Pharmacologic treatment with antihypertensives can be withheld as long as maternal pressure is only mildly elevated. Some experts treat persistent diastolic blood pressure of 105 mm Hg or above. Others withhold treatment until the diastolic blood pressure reaches 110 mm Hg. Table 5 summarizes the medications used to treat acute elevations in blood pressure. The goal of blood pressure reduction in emergency situations should be a gradual reduction to the normal range.

**TABLE 5  Medications to Treat Acute Severe Hypertensive Crises in Pregnancy**

| | Route of Dose | Pharmacologic Agent | Administration Notes |
|---|---|---|---|
| Arterial vasodilator (hydralazine: e.g., Apresoline) | IV or IM | 5 mg over 1-2 min | After 20 min, subsequent doses are dictated by initial response; once desired response, repeat as necessary (usually 3 h) |
| β-Blockers (labetalol: e.g., Normodyne or Trandate) | IV | 20-40 mg bolus or 1 mg/kg infusion (max 220 mg) | If effect is suboptimal to initial 20 mg IV, give 40 mg 10 min later and 80 mg every 10 min for additional two doses. Avoid in women with asthma and in those with congestive heart failure (CHF). |
| Calcium antagonists (nifedipine: e.g., Adalat, Procardia) | PO | 10 mg PO and repeat in 30 min, if necessary | The JNC VII recommends rapidly acting nifedipine not be used for treating hypertension or hypertensive emergencies. |
| Sodium nitroprusside (Nipride) | IV | 0.25 µg/kg/min to a maximum of 5 µg/kg/min | After failure of hydralazine, nifedipine, and labetalol. Fetal cyanide poisoning may occur if used more than 4 h. |

*Abbreviations:* IM = intramuscularly; IV = intravenously; JNC VII = Joint National Committee on Prevention, Detection, Evaluation, and Treatment of High Blood Pressure; PO = by mouth.

## Therapy in Chronic Hypertension

The role of antihypertensive therapy for pregnant women with mild to moderate chronic hypertension (stage 1 or 2 hypertension, defined as systolic blood pressure of 140 to 179 mm Hg or diastolic blood pressure of 90 to 109) is unclear. Among women with stage 1 to 2 preexisting essential hypertension and normal renal function, most pregnancies have good maternal and neonatal outcomes. Because there is no immediate need to lower blood pressure, the rationale for treatment is that it will prevent or delay progression to more severe disease, thereby benefiting the woman and/or her infant and reducing consumption of health service resources. In addition to reducing blood pressure, these drugs are believed to reduce the risk of preterm delivery and placental abruption and improve fetal growth. A wide variety of drugs are advocated, and each group has different potential side affects and adverse effects (Table 6). More importantly, these women are candidates for nonpharmacologic therapy because to date no evidence indicates that pharmacologic treatment results in improved neonatal outcomes. Because blood pressure usually falls during the first half of pregnancy, hypertension may be easier to control with less or no medication.

The value of continued administration of antihypertensive medications to pregnant women with chronic hypertension continues to be debatable. Although it may be beneficial for the mother with hypertension to reduce her blood pressure, lower pressure may impair uteroplacental perfusion and thereby interfere with fetal development. On the basis of available data, some centers currently manage women with chronic hypertension by stopping antihypertensive medications under close observation. In patients who have had hypertension for several years, show evidence of target organ damage, or take multiple antihypertensive agents, medications may be tapered on the basis of blood pressure readings, but medications should be continued if they are needed to control blood pressure. The end point for reinstituting treatment includes exceeding threshold blood pressure levels of 150 to 160 mm Hg systolic or 100 to 110 mm Hg diastolic or the presence of target organ damage. Methyldopa (Aldomet) is preferred by most practitioners. Women who are well controlled on antihypertensive therapy before pregnancy may be kept on the same agents during pregnancy, with the exception of angiotensin-converting enzyme inhibitors and angiotensin II receptor antagonists.

For women with severe hypertension (stage 3 hypertension, usually defined as 160 to 170 mm Hg or more systolic blood pressure or 110 mm Hg or more diastolic blood pressure), there is a risk of direct arterial damage, so antihypertensive medications are indicated to lower blood pressure (see Table 6). The most effective antihypertensive drug is unclear.

# Fetal Assessment

## FETAL ASSESSMENT IN PREECLAMPSIA

Nonstress testing (NST), ultrasound assessment of fetal activity and amniotic fluid volume (biophysical profile [BPP]), and fetal movement counts constitute the most common fetal surveillance techniques. Although weekly to biweekly assessment usually suffices, daily testing is appropriate for women with severe preeclampsia who are being managed expectantly. If fetal surveillance (nonreactive NST, oligohydramnios, nonreassuring BPP) indicates possible fetal compromise, the decision to deliver must be significantly weighted by fetal age (Box 3).

## FETAL ASSESSMENT IN CHRONIC HYPERTENSION

Much of the increased perinatal morbidity and mortality associated with chronic hypertension can be attributed to superimposed preeclampsia and/or fetal growth restriction. A plan of antepartum fetal assessment is directed by these findings. Thus efforts should be directed toward the early detection of superimposed preeclampsia and fetal growth restriction. If these conditions are excluded, extensive fetal antepartum testing is less essential.

Most authorities recommend an initial sonographic assessment of fetal size and dating at week 18 to 20 of gestation. Fetal growth should be carefully assessed thereafter. If this assessment is not possible with usual clinical estimation of fundal height, sonographic assessment should be performed at 28 to 32 weeks and every 4 weeks until term. If growth restriction is evident, fetal well-being should be assessed by nonstress tests or biophysical profiles as usual for the growth-restricted fetus. Similarly, if preeclampsia cannot be excluded, fetal assessment as appropriate for the fetus of a woman with preeclampsia is mandatory. If the infant is normally grown and preeclampsia can be excluded, however, these studies are not indicated.

# Maternal Assessment

## MATERNAL ASSESSMENT IN PREECLAMPSIA

Antepartum monitoring has two goals. The first goal is to recognize preeclampsia early; the second is to observe progression of the condition, both to prevent maternal complications by delivery and to determine whether fetal well-being can be safely monitored with the usual intermittent observations. Current clinical management of preeclampsia is directed by overt clinical signs and symptoms. Although rapid weight

## TABLE 6 Antihypertensive Drug Selection

| Drug | Example | Usual Dose Range in mg/day (Daily Frequency) | Notes |
|---|---|---|---|
| Central α₂-agonists | Methyldopa (e.g., Aldomet) | 250-1000 (2) | First-line therapy on the basis of reports of stable uteroplacental blood flow and fetal hemodynamics. |
| β-Blockers | Labetalol (e.g., Normodyne, Trandate) | 200-800 (2) | There is a suggestion that β-blockers prescribed early in pregnancy, specifically atenolol (Tenormin), may be associated with growth restriction. None of these agents are associated to date with any consistent ill effect. |
| Calcium antagonists | Nifedipine long-acting (e.g., Adalat CC, Procardia XL) | 30-60 (1) | Experience is limited, with most reported uses late in pregnancy. |
| Diuretic | Hydrochlorothiazide (e.g., HydroDIURIL) | 12.5-50 mg (1) | Use is controversial; however, if their use is indicated, they are safe and efficacious agents; they can markedly potentiate the response to other antihypertensive agents, and they are not contraindicated, except in settings where uteroplacental perfusion is already reduced (preeclampsia and IUGR). |
| ACE inhibitors | Captopril (e.g., Capoten) | Contraindicated | Contraindicated because of association with fetal growth restriction, oligohydramnios, neonatal renal failure, and neonatal death. Fetal risks with ACE inhibitors depend on timing and dose. |
| Angiotensin II receptor antagonists | Losartan (e.g., Cozaar) | Contraindicated | Data are limited. Adverse effects likely to be similar to those reported with ACE inhibitors, and these agents should be avoided. |

*Abbreviations:* ACE = angiotensin-converting enzyme; IUGR = intrauterine growth retardation.

increase and facial edema may indicate the fluid and sodium retention of preeclampsia, they are neither universally present nor uniquely characteristic of preeclampsia. These signs are, at best, a reason to monitor blood pressure and urinary protein more closely. Early recognition of impending preeclampsia is based primarily on blood pressure increases in the late second and third trimesters. Once blood pressure starts to rise, a repeat examination within 1 to 3 days is recommended. The woman should be evaluated for symptoms suggestive of preeclampsia and undergo laboratory testing for platelet count, renal function, and liver enzymes. Quantification of a 12- to 24-hour urine sample for proteinuria is recommended. The frequency of subsequent observations is determined by the initial observations and the ensuing clinical progression. If the condition appears stable, weekly observations may be appropriate.

## MATERNAL ASSESSMENT IN CHRONIC HYPERTENSION

No consensus exists as to the most appropriate fetal surveillance test(s) or interval and timing of testing in women with chronic hypertension. Testing should be individualized, based on clinical judgment and on the severity of disease. There are no conclusive data to address either the benefits or the harms of various monitoring strategies for pregnant women with chronic hypertension. Box 3 lists the current proposed recommendations for antepartum monitoring. When chronic hypertension is complicated by intrauterine growth retardation (IUGR) or preeclampsia, fetal surveillance is warranted.

# Indications for Delivery

## INDICATIONS FOR DELIVERY IN PREECLAMPSIA-ECLAMPSIA

Delivery is the only definitive treatment for preeclampsia; Box 4 lists some suggested indications for delivery. All women with the diagnosis of preeclampsia should be considered for delivery at 40 weeks' gestation. Delivery may be indicated for women with mild disease and a

favorable cervix at 38 weeks' gestation and should be considered in women who have severe preeclampsia beyond 32 to 34 weeks' gestation. Prolonged antepartum management with severe preeclampsia is possible in a select group of women with fetal gestational age between 23 and 32 weeks but should be attempted only at centers equipped to provide close maternal and fetal surveillance. Vaginal delivery is preferable to cesarean delivery, thus avoiding the added stress of surgery to multiple physiologic aberrations. Labor induction should be carried out aggressively once the decision for delivery is made. In a gestation that is remote from term in which delivery is indicated and fetal and maternal conditions are

 **CURRENT DIAGNOSIS**

- The most important factor to consider in classifying disease in which blood pressure rises abnormally in pregnancy is whether the hypertensive disorder antedates the pregnancy or arises during the pregnancy.
- Preeclampsia–eclampsia usually occurs after 20 weeks of gestation. Chronic hypertension is defined as hypertension that is present and observable before the 20th week of gestation.
- Gestational blood pressure elevation is defined as a blood pressure greater than 140 mm Hg systolic or 90 mm Hg diastolic in a woman normotensive before 20 weeks.
- Proteinuria in pregnancy is defined as the urinary excretion of 300 mg protein or greater in a 24-hour specimen.
- Laboratory tests recommended to diagnose or manage hypertension in pregnancy serve primarily to distinguish preeclampsia from either chronic or transient hypertension.
- No single screening test is considered reliable and cost effective for predicting preeclampsia.

## BOX 3   Fetal Monitoring in Hypertensive Disorders

- Gestational hypertension—Hypertension only without proteinuria, with normal laboratory test results, and without symptoms.
  1. Perform estimation of fetal growth and amniotic fluid status at diagnosis. If results are normal, repeat testing only if a significant change occurs in maternal condition.
  2. Perform NST at diagnosis. If NST is nonreactive, perform BPP. If BPP value is 8 or if NST is reactive, repeat testing only if a significant change occurs in maternal condition.
- Mild preeclampsia—Mild hypertension plus proteinuria (300 mg or more per 24-hour period), normal platelet count, normal liver enzymes values, and no maternal symptoms.
  1. Perform estimation of fetal growth and amniotic fluid status at diagnosis. If results are normal, repeat testing every 3 weeks.
  2. Perform NST, BPP, or both at diagnosis. If NST is reactive or if BPP value is 8, repeat weekly. Repeat testing immediately if abrupt change in maternal condition occurs.
  3. If estimated fetal weight by ultrasound is less than 10th percentile for gestational age, or if there is oligohydramnios (amniotic fluid index equals or is less than 5 cm), perform testing at least twice weekly.
- Severe preeclampsia—Severe hypertension in association with abnormal proteinuria; hypertension in association with severe proteinuria (at least 5 g per 24-hour period); presence of multiorgan involvement such as pulmonary edema, seizures, oliguria (less than 500 mL per 24-hour period), thrombocytopenia (platelet count less than 100,000/mm³), abnormal liver enzymes in association with persistent epigastric or right upper quadrant pain; persistent severe central nervous system symptoms (altered mental status, headaches, blurred vision, or blindness).
  1. Term
     Hospitalize, prevent seizures, control hypertension, and proceed with delivery.
  2. Remote from term
     Provide care in a tertiary-care setting.
     Perform laboratory evaluation and fetal surveillance (as outlined for mild preeclampsia earlier) daily depending on the severity and progression of the disorder.[1]
- Chronic hypertension—Mild hypertension (BP more than 140/90 mm Hg) or severe hypertension (BP equal or more than 180/110 mm Hg) present before the 20th week of pregnancy or hypertension present before pregnancy.
  1. Perform baseline ultrasonography at 18 to 20 weeks and repeat at 28 to 32 weeks of gestation and monthly thereafter until delivery, to monitor fetal growth.
  2. If growth restriction is detected or suspected, monitor fetal status frequently with NST or BPP.[1]
  3. If growth restriction is not present and superimposed preeclampsia is excluded, these tests are not indicated.[1]

[1]Not FDA approved for this indication.
*Abbreviations:* BPP = biophysical profile; NST = nonstress test.

## BOX 4   Indications for Delivery in Preeclampsia

**Maternal**
- Gestational age ≥38 wk
- Platelet count <100,000 cells/mm³
- Progressive deterioration in hepatic and/or renal function
- Suspected abruption placentae
- Persistent central nervous system (CNS) manifestations: headaches or visual changes
- Persistent severe gastric pain, nausea, or vomiting

**Fetal**
- Severe fetal growth restriction
- Nonreassuring fetal testing results
- Oligohydramnios

stable enough to permit pregnancy to be prolonged 48 hours, glucocorticoids can be safely administered to accelerate fetal pulmonary maturity.

The patient with eclampsia should be delivered in a timely fashion. Once the patient is stabilized, the method of delivery should depend, in part, on gestational age, fetal presentation, and cervical examination findings.

## INDICATIONS FOR DELIVERY IN CHRONIC HYPERTENSION

Pregnant women with uncomplicated chronic hypertension of a mild degree generally can be delivered vaginally at term; most have good maternal and neonatal outcomes. Cesarean delivery should be reserved for other obstetric indications. Women with mild hypertension during pregnancy and a prior adverse pregnancy outcome (e.g., stillbirth) may be candidates for earlier delivery after documentation of fetal lung maturity (as long as fetal status is reassuring). Women with severe chronic hypertension during pregnancy most often either deliver prematurely or have to be delivered prematurely for fetal or maternal

## CURRENT THERAPY

- Prevention focuses on identifying women at higher risk and conducting close clinical and laboratory monitoring to recognize the disease process in its early stages.
- Delivery is always appropriate therapy for the mother but may not be for the fetus.
- For maternal health, the goal of therapy is to prevent eclampsia as well as severe complications of preeclampsia. Parenteral magnesium sulfate is given during labor and delivery and for variable durations postpartum to women with eclampsia and severe preeclampsia. Its benefits in mild gestational hypertension or preeclampsia remain unclear.
- Antihypertensive medications are indicated to lower blood pressure for women with severe hypertension, usually defined as 160 to 170 mm Hg or more systolic blood pressure or 110 mm Hg or more diastolic blood pressure.
- Antihypertensive therapy is indicated intrapartum when diastolic blood pressure is persistently 105 to 110 mm Hg or above.
- The goal of blood pressure reduction in emergency situations should be a gradual reduction of blood pressure to the normal range.

indications. Delivery should be considered in all women with superimposed severe preeclampsia at or beyond 28 weeks of gestation and in women with mild superimposed preeclampsia at or beyond 37 weeks of gestation. Magnesium sulfate should be used for women with superimposed preeclampsia to prevent seizures.

## Postpartum Management

Acute hypertensive changes induced by pregnancy usually dissipate rapidly, within the first several days after delivery. Resolution of hypertension is more rapid in patients with gestational hypertension and may lag in those with preeclampsia, especially those with longer duration of preeclampsia and greater extent of renal impairment. Oral antihypertensive agents may be needed after delivery (see Table 6) to help control maternal blood pressure, particularly for women who were hypertensive before pregnancy. If prepregnancy blood pressures were normal or unknown, it is reasonable to stop oral medication after 3 to 4 weeks and observe the blood pressure at 1- to 2-week intervals for 1 month, then at 3- to 6-month intervals for 1 year. If hypertension recurs, it should be treated. If the abnormalities persist, the pathology will probably be chronic.

Limited data are available on which to base our knowledge of the natural history and pathogenesis of postpartum hypertension. The women who appear to be at greatest risk for postpartum hypertension are those with antenatal preeclampsia, particularly those with higher urinary protein, serum uric acid, and blood urea nitrogen. For previously normotensive women, the risk of postpartum hypertension appears lower. Beyond the postnatal period, it is not known whether women with isolated postpartum hypertension are at increased risk of chronic hypertension.

## Risk of Recurrence

Women who have had preeclampsia are more prone to hypertensive complications in subsequent pregnancies. Risk is best established for multiparas with a history of preeclampsia; the magnitude of the recurrence rate increases the earlier the disease manifested during the index pregnancy. The recurrence rate for women with one episode of HELLP is 5%. Recurrence rates are higher for those experiencing preeclampsia as multiparas compared with nulliparous women. Risk is also increased in multiparas who conceive with a new father, even when their first pregnancy was normotensive, the incidence being intermediate between that of primiparous women and monogamous multiparous women who have not had a preeclamptic pregnancy.

### REFERENCES

Abalos E, Duley L, Steyn DW, Henderson-Smart DJ: Antihypertensive drug therapy for mild to moderate hypertension during pregnancy (Cochrane Review). In The Cochrane Library, Issue 4. Chichester, UK, John Wiley, 2004.
Agency for Healthcare Research and Quality: Management of chronic hypertension during pregnancy. Evidence Report/Technology assessment no. 14. AHRQ Publication No. 00-E011. Rockville, Md, Author, 2000.
American College of Obstetricians and Gynecologists: ACOG Practice Bulletin No. 29. Chronic hypertension pregnancy. Obstet Gynecol 2001;98:177-185.
Atallah AN, Hofmeyr GJ, Duley L: Calcium supplementation during pregnancy for preventing hypertensive disorders and related problems (Cochrane Review). In The Cochrane Library, Issue 4. Chichester, UK.: John Wiley, 2004.
Bergel E, Carroli G, Althabe F: Ambulatory versus conventional methods for monitoring blood pressure during pregnancy (Cochrane Review). In The Cochrane Library, Issue 4. Chichester, UK, John Wiley, 2004.
Cunningham FG, Gant NF, Leveno KJ, et al: Hypertensive disorders in pregnancy. In Cunningham FG (ed): Williams Obstetrics, 21st ed. New York, McGraw-Hill, 2001, pp 567-618.
Duley L, Henderson-Smart DJ: Drugs for treatment of very high blood pressure during pregnancy (Cochrane Review). In The Cochrane Library, Issue 4. Chichester, UK, John Wiley, 2004.
Joint National Committee: The Seventh Report of the Joint National Committee on Prevention, Detection, Evaluation, and Treatment of High Blood Pressure (JNC VII). JAMA 2003;289:2560-2571.
Levine RJ, Thadhani RT, Qian C, et al: Urinary placental growth factor and risk of preeclampsia. JAMA 2005;293:77-85.
Lim KH, Friedman SA, Ecker JL, et al: The clinical utility of serum uric acid measurements in hypertensive diseases of pregnancy. Am J Obstet Gynecol 1998;178:1067-1071.
Lucas JL, Leveno KJ, Cunningham FG: A comparison of magnesium sulfate with phenytoin for the prevention of eclampsia. N Engl J Med 1995; 333:201-205.
Magee L, Sadeghi S: Prevention and treatment of postpartum hypertension (Cochrane Review). In The Cochrane Library, Issue 4. Chichester, UK, John Wiley, 2004.
Report of the National High Blood Pressure Education Program: Working group report on high blood pressure in pregnancy. Am J Obstet Gynecol 2000;183:S1-S22.
Sibai BM: Prevention of preeclampsia: A big disappointment. Am J Obstet Gynecol 1998;179:1275-1278.

# Postpartum Care

Method of
*Lisa R. Nash, DO*

The postpartum period, or puerperium, is defined as the time needed for the anatomic and physiologic changes of pregnancy to revert to the normal state, lasting from immediately after delivery of the placenta to 6 to 8 weeks following birth.

## The First 4 to 6 Hours

During the first few hours after delivery, blood pressure (BP), pulse, respiratory rate, temperature, vaginal bleeding, urination, and pain should be monitored every 15 minutes until the patient is stable. Complications that can occur during this time include hypotension, hemorrhage, dyspnea, fever, hypertensive disorders of pregnancy, and urinary retention. Table 1 describes the differential diagnosis and management of these disorders. Table 2 lists oxytocics used to control uterine atony.

Early skin-to-skin contact between the mother and her healthy infant should be ensured to facilitate bonding. Early breast-feeding should be encouraged. The first breast-feeding should occur prior to transfer of the healthy newborn to the nursery in facilities where rooming-in is unavailable.

## The First 24 to 72 Hours

Hospitalization generally lasts 24 to 48 hours after an uncomplicated vaginal delivery and up to 72 hours after a typical cesarean delivery. During this time, the following should be addressed:

- Signs and symptoms of potential complications described in Table 1
- Transition of lochia to diminishing reddish-brown discharge
- Fundal height below umbilicus by 24 hours postpartum
- Perineal inflammation or edema and proper perineal hygiene
- Signs and symptoms suggesting deep venous thrombosis
- Resumption of normal ambulation
- Return of bowel/bladder function
- Lactation establishment
- Pain management
- Maternal mood, bonding, and family adjustment
- Contraceptive planning
- Any special requirements such as administration of $Rh_0(D)$ immune globulin (RhoGAM) or rubella vaccine

Symptoms of breast engorgement for mothers who will not breast-feed may be relieved by breast support, ice packs, and nonsteroidal anti-inflammatory medications.

**TABLE 1** Potential Complications of the Immediate Postpartum Period : Key Diagnostic and Treatment Considerations

| Condition | Differential Diagnosis | Management |
|---|---|---|
| Hypotension | Vagal response<br>Hypovolemia<br>Reaction to anesthesia<br>Blood loss | For All: Supportive – Trendelenburg position, 500 – 1000 mL IV crystalloid (normal) saline or lactated Ringer's solution<br>For blood loss: packed RBCs |
| Immediate hemorrhage | Uterine atony (most common) | See Table 2 for oxytocics |
| | Retained placental tissue or blood clots | Evacuation, oxytocics, surgical assistance as appropriate |
| | Laceration or hematoma | Repair |
| | Bleeding disorders | Blood products |
| Delayed hemorrhage (>24 hours after delivery) | | IV crystalloids and blood products for all etiologies, as appropriate |
| | Subinvolution of former placental site | Oxytocics, as needed |
| | Retained placental tissue or blood clots | Evacuation, oxytocics, surgical assistance as appropriate |
| Dyspnea | Amniotic fluid embolism | Respiratory and cardiovascular support, treatment of disseminated intravascular coagulation |
| | Pulmonary embolus | Antithrombolytics, anticoagulation |
| | Exacerbation of asthma | Nebulized albuterol |
| Temperature >38 degrees Centigrade (100 degrees Fahrenheit) on any 2 days beyond first 24 hours OR temparature >39 degrees Centigrade (102.2 degrees Fahrenheit) at any time | Endometritis | Clindamycin (Cleocin) 900 mg IV q8h + gentamicin (Garamycin) 100 mg (2 mg/kg) IVPB then 80 mg (1.0-1.5 mg/kg) IVPB q8h OR 2nd/3rd generation cephalosporin ± metronidazole (Flagyl) |
| | Breast engorgement (<48 hours after delivery) | Ice packs to relieve vascular congestion (note: if >48 hrs after delivery, increase breastfeeding and/or pumping) |
| | Septic pelvic thrombophlebitis | Anticoagulation with heparin |
| | Other: abdominal wound or perineal infection, UTI, DVT, pneumonia | Antibiotic as appropriate for source |
| Hypertensive disorders: postpartum preeclampsia, postpartum eclampsia | | Magnesium sulfate 4 g slowly IV over 15 – 30 min, followed by 1 to 3 g/h to keep serum magnesium levels between 4 and 7 mEq/L<br>IV hydralazine (Apresoline) titrated to maintain blood pressure about 130/80 |
| Urinary retention | Trauma of delivery<br>Anesthesia | In-and-out bladder catheterization if spontaneous voiding does not occur within 6 h of delivery |

Routine hospital discharge instructions should include direction to contact the physician for any of the following: heavy uterine bleeding; purulent lochia; worsening perineal pain; abdominal or breast pain; redness, warmth, tenderness, or swelling of the lower legs/calves; dysuria; fever (temperature >38°C [100°F]) and/or chills; presence of depression or problems with family adjustment. The patient should be instructed to maintain pelvic rest (nothing in the vagina) for 4 to 6 weeks, and encouraged to resume normal activities and diet.

# The 2-Week Newborn Check

The 2-week newborn check provides a good opportunity to reassess the maternal condition. Persistence of any depressive symptoms should be explored. Postpartum *blues* generally resolve by the 10th postpartum day. Although rare, postpartum psychosis generally manifests in this same time period and requires emergent intervention because of the risks of suicide and infanticide. Additional areas to assess include family adjustment, breast-feeding progress or problems,

**TABLE 2** Oxytocics Used for Control of Uterine Atony

| Drug | Dose | Maintenance | Contraindications |
|---|---|---|---|
| Oxytocin (Pitocin) | 10 U IM or infuse 10 to 40 U in 1 L of IV fluid | IV infusion maintained 1-4 h | None |
| Methylergonovine (Methergine) | 0.2 mg IM | Repeat q 2-4 h | Hypertension, toxemia |
| PGF$_{2\text{-alpha}}$ carboprost; (Hemabate) | 0.25 mg IM | Repeat q 15-90 min | Cardiac or pulmonary disease |
| PGE$_2$ (Prostin E$_2$) | 20 mg suppository inserted into rectum | Repeat q 2-4 h | Hypotension (use PGF$_{2\text{-alpha}}$ instead) |

*Abbreviations:* IM = intramuscular; IV = intravenous; PG = prostaglandin.

urinary incontinence, anticipated time of return to sexual intimacy, and contraceptive plans. If early postpartum complications were experienced, a repeat complete blood count or urinalysis may be indicated.

## The Traditional Postpartum Assessment

This assessment is generally scheduled at 6 weeks after delivery. Assessment should include vital signs and physical examination of the thyroid gland, breasts, heart, lungs, abdomen, perineum, pelvis (uterus and ovaries), and lower extremities. Papanicolaou smear should be obtained. Items listed previously for the 2-week assessment should be readdressed.

## Postpartum Depression

Postpartum depression is common, occurring in approximately 20% of parturients. Postpartum thyroid dysfunction may present with similar or overlapping symptoms and should be investigated when postpartum depression is suspected. Management may be supportive and could include individual or group psychotherapy or medication. Antidepressant medications acceptable for breast-feeding mothers include sertraline (Zoloft), paroxetine (Paxil), amitriptyline (Elavil), and desipramine (Norpramin).

## Family Adjustment

Many women experience transient feelings of vulnerability, inadequacy, and anxiety during the family adjustment that occurs following the addition of a new infant. Feelings of attachment may vary initially but usually increase over time. Conflicting emotions elicited by increased responsibility for meeting the demands of the expanded family are common. Significant changes in lifestyle, relationships, and careers often must be made. Assessment of emotional, tangible (financial, household, childcare, etc.), and informational support can identify families who may benefit from referral to additional resources. Men typically have concerns about infant care skills, decreased personal time, changes in the marital relationship, financial security, and the health of their partner and the newborn. Common sibling responses to arrival of the new infant include behaviors that are imitating, aggressive, solicitous, or anxious. Siblings may also withdraw or become more independent. Many authorities recommend that siblings have contact with the mother during the postpartum hospitalization. Allowing siblings to assist (as age permits) in infant care and maintaining

separate time for siblings to interact with parents (such as the newborn's nap time) may reduce adjustment problems. Reading children's books about new babies and discussing feelings with siblings are additional options.

## Return to Sexual Activity and Contraception

The return to sexual activity and contraception should be discussed. Most couples will resume sexual activity between 6 weeks and 3 months postpartum, although some will do so sooner if perineal discomfort has resolved. The most common barriers to resumption of sexual activity include perineal pain (25%), lack of interest (more common in breast-feeding than bottle-feeding mothers), and fatigue. Anticipatory guidance is helpful for negotiating this time of transition. Breast-feeding mothers should be advised they may require a vaginal lubricant because of the hormonal changes related to breast-feeding.

Postpartum anovulatory infertility persists for 5 weeks in nonlactating women and 8 weeks or more in lactating women. The anticipated time to resume sexual activity and infant feeding plans should be considered in determining the best time to initiate contraceptive measures postpartum.

Contraceptive effects of lactational amenorrhea provide approximately 98% protection in the first 6 months if there is little or no supplemental feeding. Other options for postpartum contraception include natural family planning, barrier methods, oral contraceptives, contraceptive patch (Ortho Evra) and ring (NuvaRing), the injectable contraceptive medroxyprogesterone acetate (Depo-Provera), intrauterine device, and sterilization (Table 3).

The usual amount of time off work allowed for employed mothers is 6 weeks.

## Special Circumstances

### THE SINGLE PARENT

The single parent often experiences financial and time pressures exceeding those of two-parent families. Enlisting an extended support network of family and friends in addition to a supportive and empathic physician will be helpful.

### ADOPTING PARENT(S)

Adopting parent(s) usually have experienced stressful approval and unpredictable placement processes. They may have as little as a few hours' notice to make plans for the arrival of their newborn. Loss issues related to infertility may exist at various stages of resolution. Other issues may include decisions about timing and telling the adoption story to the child(ren) as well as ethnic and cultural considerations when parents and child(ren) have different backgrounds.

### PERINATAL GRIEVING

Perinatal grieving occurs both for parents experiencing the death of an infant and parents of a child with a serious illness or congenital anomaly.

---

**CURRENT DIAGNOSIS**

- Hypo- or hypertension, tachypnea, fever, excessive vaginal bleeding, inability to void, and excessive abdominal or perineal pain are potential indicators of postpartum complications.
- Return to normal ambulation, bowel and bladder function, establishing lactation, and family adjustment and bonding are tasks for the first 24 to 72 hours postpartum.
- Persistence of depressive symptoms, family adjustment, breast-feeding progress or problems, urinary incontinence, return to sexual intimacy, and contraceptive plans should be addressed at the 2- and 6-week postpartum visits.
- Single parents, adopting parents, and parents experiencing a perinatal loss or the birth of a child with a serious illness or congenital anomaly will likely require additional/special information, services, and resources.

---

**CURRENT THERAPY**

- Specific interventions for potential complications of the immediate postpartum period are outlined in Tables 1 and 2.
- The anticipated time to resume sexual activity and infant feeding plans should be considered in the choices of contraceptive method and when to initiate contraceptive measures postpartum.

**TABLE 3  Postpartum Contraception**

| Method | Earliest Initiation | Special Considerations |
|---|---|---|
| Lactational amenorrhea | Immediately postpartum | Additional measures required for any of the following: >6 mo postpartum, supplemental infant feeding initiation or resumption of menses |
| Natural family planning | Depends on return of normal menstrual cycle | |
| Barrier methods: condom diaphragm | 3 w postpartum (coincident with earliest recommended time to resume sexual activity) 6 w postpartum | Requires full uterine involution AND refitting for patients who previously used this method |
| Medroxyprogesterone acetate (Depo-Provera) | Prior to hospital discharge | Does not diminish lactation Many physicians delay to 2 wk postpartum because of the potential risk for prolonged bleeding |
| Progesterone-only pills (Micronor) | Prior to hospital discharge | Same as medroxyprogesterone acetate (Depo-Provera) |
| Combination oral contraceptives | Non–breast-feeding women: 3 wk postpartum Breast-feeding women: 1 mo after lactation becomes well established | May diminish lactation |
| Contraceptive patch (Ortho Evra), ring (NuvaRing) | Same as combination oral contraceptives | Same as combination oral contraceptives |
| Intrauterine device (Mirena, ParaGard) | Within 20 min of delivery of placenta OR 6 wk postpartum | Full uterine involution must be achieved |
| Sterilization | After delivery/prior to hospital discharge OR 6 wk postpartum | Full uterine involution must be achieved |

Physicians can be helpful in this process by providing information and acknowledging when an answer is unknown. The medical team should recognize the infant as a person by using his or her name, encouraging the family's involvement in care of the infant as much as possible and providing opportunities for family members to express and discuss emotions. Parents experiencing a perinatal death should be encouraged to touch and hold their infant and photographs should be offered. Physicians should assist parents with plans for notifying siblings, friends, and relatives. Identifying available community and medical resources such as parent support groups can also be very helpful.

## REFERENCES

Anderson GC, Moore E, Hepworth J, Bergman N: Early skin-to-skin contact for mothers and their healthy newborn infants. Cochrane Database Syst Rev 2003(2);CD003519.

Anonymous: Postpartum care of the mother and newborn: A practical guide. Technical Working Group, World Health Organization. Birth 1999;26(4):255-258.

Baxley E: Postpartum biomedical concerns. In Ratcliffe SD, Byrd JE, Sakornbut EL (eds): Handbook of Pregnancy and Perinatal Care in Family Practice: Science and Practice, Philadelphia, Hanley & Belfus, 1996, pp 430-446.

Driscoll CE: Postpartum Care. In Rakel RE, Bope ET (eds): Conn's Current Therapy 2004, Philadelphia, WB Saunders, 2003, pp 1076-1078.

Gabbe SG, Niebyl JR, Simpson JL (eds): Obstetrics: Normal & Problem Pregnancies, 4th ed. New York, Churchill Livingstone, 2002, pp 753-779.

Hatcher RA, Nelson AL, Zieman M, et al: A pocket guide to managing contraception. Tiger, Georgia, Bridging the Gap Foundation, 2003, p 27.

Killeen I, Osborn C: Postpartum care: Psychosocial concerns. In Ratcliffe SD, Byrd JE, Sakornbut EL (eds): Handbook of Pregnancy and Perinatal Care in Family Practice: Science and Practice. Philadelphia, Hanley & Belfus, 1996, pp 447-458.

Levitt C, Shaw E, Wong S, et al: Systematic review of the literature on postpartum care: Selected contraception methods, postpartum Papanicolaou test, and rubella immunization. Birth 2004;31(3):203-212.

Montgomery, AM: Breast-feeding and postpartum maternal care. In Larimore WL (ed): Primary Care: Clinics in Office Practice. Update in Maternity Care, Vol. 27, No. 1. Philadelphia, WB Saunders, 2000, pp 237-250.

# Resuscitation of the Newborn

Method of
*Derek S. Wheeler, MD,*
*and Martin J. McCaffrey, MD*

Numerous and dramatic changes must occur more or less in sequential order around the time of birth, at which time the fetal cardiovascular and respiratory systems must undergo an instantaneous transition to life outside the liquid-filled uterine environment. Several events occurring prior to or at the time of delivery may preclude this transition and lead to problems ranging from mild respiratory distress to shock, organ dysfunction, and death. Fortunately, the vast majority of term newborns require no resuscitation beyond routine warming, drying, suctioning of the airway, and mild stimulation. However, rapid identification and resuscitation of those newborns experiencing a difficult transition to extrauterine life may dramatically improve outcome. Neonatal resuscitation is a team effort and requires the coordinated execution of several, simultaneous psychomotor and procedural skills. Adequate knowledge of the normal fetal, transitional, and neonatal physiology, as well as prior planning and preparation is essential to achieving the most favorable outcomes following neonatal resuscitation.

## Fetal, Transitional, and Neonatal Circulations

The fetal circulation is characterized by parallel circulations, the presence of intracardiac and extracardiac shunts, a high pulmonary vascular resistance, and a relatively low systemic vascular resistance (attributed to the low-resistance placental circulation). Conversely, on delivery, the right and left ventricles are in series, shunts functionally close, pulmonary vascular resistance decreases, and systemic vascular resistance increases. During intrauterine life, gas exchange occurs in the placenta; but during extrauterine life, gas exchange occurs in the lungs. An understanding and appreciation for these differences is essential to the optimal care and resuscitation of the newborn infant.

The fetal cardiac anatomy differs from that of the normal newborn infant. The fetal circulation contains the two atria, two ventricles, and two great arteries but is further complemented by a foramen ovale, ductus arteriosus, and ductus venosus. In utero there exist two large anatomic shunts. One occurs between the right and left atria (the foramen ovale). The second exists between the pulmonary artery and aorta (the ductus arteriosus). The origin of blood flowing through these shunts is crucial. A streaming pattern of fetal blood flow is observed at the level of the right atrium. Less oxygenated blood from the lower body streams along the lateral wall of the inferior vena cava (IVC), crosses the tricuspid valve, and enters the right ventricle. The right ventricle also receives poorly oxygenated blood from the superior vena cava (SVC) (from the brain and upper body) and coronary sinus (from the heart). Because of the high pulmonary vascular resistance (PVR) during intrauterine life, little of the blood pumped from the right ventricle enters the pulmonary circulation. Rather, the right ventricle ejects this poorly oxygenated blood (approximately two thirds of total cardiac output) into the main pulmonary artery and into the descending aorta via the ductus arteriosus, thereby reaching the placenta (via the paired umbilical arteries) where the blood is reoxygenated. In contrast, oxygenated blood from the umbilical-placental circulation (via the single umbilical vein) bypasses the liver via the ductus venosus and travels along the medial wall of the IVC. The majority of this relatively oxygenated stream is directed across the foramen ovale into the left atrium, crosses the mitral valve, and enters the left ventricle. Although the left ventricle also receives a small percentage of poorly oxygenated blood from the lungs, the majority is well oxygenated. In sum, blood in the fetal left ventricle is 20% more saturated than the blood in the right ventricle. The left ventricle ejects this blood (approximately one-third of total cardiac output) into the ascending aorta to supply the heart, brain, and upper fetal body with relatively well-oxygenated blood. A smaller percentage of left ventricular output crosses the aortic arch to the descending aorta. Therefore, the fetal right and left ventricles are functionally arranged in parallel, such that the right ventricle supplies the lower portion of the body, including the placenta, and the left ventricle supplies the upper portion of the body, including the brain. This arrangement assures that the brain receives blood with relatively higher oxygen content than does the placenta.

During birth, a number of complex events occur simultaneously. Clamping of the umbilical cord removes low-resistance placental capillary bed from the systemic circulation, and blood flow to the placenta ceases abruptly, resulting in an increase in systemic vascular resistance (SVR). The fluid-filled lungs rapidly expand and fill with air with the first few breaths. Initiation of respirations is followed by a marked fall in PVR, and blood flow to the lungs dramatically increases. The increase in SVR results in an increase in left-sided heart pressures. The further increase in left atrial pressure resulting from increased pulmonary venous return results in closure of the foramen ovale, because left atrial pressure exceeds the right atrial pressure. Functional closure of the ductus arteriosus occurs and shunting of blood from the pulmonary artery to the aorta ceases. The fall in PVR and functional closure of the ductus arteriosus depend on several factors, the most important of which are initiation of respirations with subsequent lung inflation and increased oxygen saturation. In the majority of cases, the transition from intrauterine to extrauterine life occurs smoothly and uneventfully. However, up to 10% of all newborn infants will require some degree of intervention (e.g., positioning, suctioning, and/or stimulation to breathe) to assist with this transition. A smaller percentage will require more intensive resuscitative efforts. Certain high-risk conditions (Box 1) may preclude a smooth transition, and further resuscitation may be required to restore and support cardiopulmonary function. For example, several recent studies suggest that approximately 1% of newborns in the delivery room will require assisted ventilation.

## Perinatal Asphyxia

Perinatal asphyxia occurs when oxygen delivery is insufficient to meet metabolic demands, resulting in hypoxia, hypercarbia, and metabolic

---

### BOX 1 Risk Factors for Neonatal Resuscitation

| Maternal Factors | Intrapartum Factors |
|---|---|
| Chronic or pregnancy-induced hypertension | Size for date discrepancy |
| Diabetes mellitus | Polyhydramnios or oligohydramnios |
| Previous fetal or neonatal death | Breech presentation |
| Maternal age >35 y or <18 y | Decreased fetal movement |
| Anemia | Prolonged labor (>24 h) |
| Rh isoimmunization | Prolonged rupture of membranes (>12 h) |
| Prematurity (<37 wk gestation) | Meconium-stained amniotic fluid |
| Postmaturity (>42 wk gestation) | Placental abruption |
| Premature rupture of the membranes | Prolapsed cord |
| Malnutrition or poor weight gain | Fetal distress (fetal heart rate abnormalities, fetal acidosis) |
| Lack of prenatal care | Emergent operative delivery |
| Substance abuse (including alcohol) | |
| Antepartum hemorrhage | |
| Multiple gestation | |
| Chronic disease (cardiovascular, rheumatologic, neurologic, etc.) | |

---

acidosis. Initial compensatory mechanisms, including tachycardia and vasoconstriction, may allow adequate oxygen delivery to the vital organs for a time. However, without resolution or treatment, these compensatory mechanisms will eventually fail, leading to a fall in heart rate and blood pressure (BP) with eventual cardiopulmonary arrest. World Health Organization (WHO) estimates from 1995 conclude that birth asphyxia is responsible for 19% of the 5 million neonatal deaths that occur annually. Intrauterine asphyxia manifests as alterations in fetal heart rate (late decelerations, bradycardia), passage of meconium (see text following), fetal gasping, and eventual apnea, termed *primary apnea*. This initial period of apnea is followed by further gasping, which gradually weakens in intensity, eventually terminating in what is termed *secondary apnea*. In the delivery room, spontaneous respirations can be elicited in newborns with primary apnea by stimulation (vigorous warming and drying) or a brief trial of positive-pressure ventilation (PPV). Newborns with secondary apnea, on the other hand, have suffered a prolonged period of inadequate oxygen delivery and require aggressive resuscitation to prevent further decompensation, cardiac arrest, and death. The longer the delay in initiating resuscitation for primary apnea, the longer the time required to establish spontaneous respirations following PPV. Because there is no definitive method of differentiating between primary and secondary apnea following delivery, the neonatal resuscitation team must promptly recognize and institute proper treatment for all newborn infants with apnea and suspected perinatal asphyxia.

## Neonatal Resuscitation

Neonatal resuscitation is directed toward assuring a smooth transition to extrauterine life by achieving the following goals:

1. Maintaining or restoring normal body temperature
2. Maintaining or establishing effective ventilation and oxygenation
3. Maintaining or restoring adequate cardiac output and tissue perfusion
4. Avoiding hypoglycemia

Neonatal resuscitation follows an orderly sequence known as the "ABCs" (airway, breathing, circulation) of resuscitation. Concurrently, the overall physiologic status of the newborn is continuously monitored via a cycle of repeated assessment and intervention ("assess-intervene-assess").

Unique to newborn infants is an increased ratio of body surface area to volume; and they are at risk for significant heat loss and temperature instability. Temperature instability and cold stress will increase oxygen consumption and may impede an effective resuscitation. Therefore, initial efforts should be directed toward minimizing heat loss. On delivery the infant should be placed on a radiant warmer. Other heat sources, such as a heating lamp may be used if a radiant warmer is not available. Heated bags of intravenous (IV) fluid should be avoided because they may cause burns. The infant is then dried vigorously with a warm, sterile towel. To minimize conductive heat losses, wet linens should be removed as soon as possible. Use of a polyethylene bag may help reduce heat loss and maintain body temperature during resuscitation of very-low-birth weight (VLBW) infants. If the newborn is otherwise stable, he or she may be placed naked against the mother's skin and covered with a clean blanket or towel.

Initial resuscitative efforts are directed toward maintaining the airway ("A = AIRWAY"). Properly positioning the infant on his or her back, with the head and neck in a neutral, midline position will assist in opening the airway. A towel roll may be placed beneath the shoulders to assist in opening the airway. Hyperextension, may lead to airway obstruction and should be avoided. The mouth and nose should be suctioned with a bulb syringe in order to remove any secretions that may contribute to airway compromise.

Drying, positioning, and suctioning will usually provide sufficient stimulation to help the newborn initiate effective breathing. If respirations are adequate and cyanosis is present, supplemental oxygen should be administered, using an appropriately sized facemask. Preclinical studies suggest that administration of 100% oxygen adversely affects the developing lung and brain, although at present there is insufficient evidence to advocate resuscitation with room-air (21% oxygen) versus 100% oxygen. Current guidelines, however, recommend administering supplemental oxygen at a sufficient concentration ($FiO_2$ 0.21-1.00) to maintain peripheral oxygen saturations at approximately 90% in neonates less than 32 weeks gestational age. The oxygen concentration should be decreased for oxygen saturations greater than 95%. Acrocyanosis (bluish discoloration of the hands and feet), on the other hand, is a normal physical finding that is often present in the first few minutes of life and does not require oxygen supplementation. Using a bag-valve-mask, positive pressure ventilation is indicated for those infants with either absent (apnea) or slow, gasping respiratory movements ("B = BREATHING"). In addition, because one of the most common causes of bradycardia is lack of sufficient oxygen, positive pressure ventilation is indicated when the heart rate is below 100 beats per minute (bpm).

Both neonatal-sized self-inflating bags and anesthesia bags (Figure 1) are acceptable for administering positive pressure ventilation in the delivery room. The main advantages to using an anesthesia bag are that these devices are capable of delivering 100% blow-by oxygen or continuous positive airway pressure (CPAP). Inspiratory pressures can be controlled and titrated with the use of an in-line manometer when using an anesthesia bag. The use of an anesthesia bag requires practice, and some centers preferentially use a self-inflating bag due to its ease of use. The main disadvantages to the self-inflating bag are that these devices require an additional oxygen reservoir attachment and inspiratory pressures cannot be closely titrated. Both devices are acceptable for use in neonatal resuscitation provided that staff is familiar with the requirements of each device.

Proper placement and sizing of the face mask are required to produce an effective seal around the mouth and nose (Figure 2). Adequate ventilation is assured using a rate of 40 to 60 breaths per minute, with a tidal volume sufficient enough to produce adequate, symmetric expansion of the chest. Initially, inspiratory pressures as high as 30 cm $H_2O$ or more may be required for adequate lung inflation. Smaller pressures (generally 20 cm $H_2O$ or less) are generally sufficient for subsequent breaths. An 8 or 10 F orogastric tube may be placed to decompress the stomach and improve ventilation. Ventilation via the bag-valve-mask is relatively simple to perform and can be lifesaving. An increase in heart rate is the primary sign of effective PPV during resuscitation. Additional signs of effective PPV include improving color, spontaneous breathing, or improving muscle tone. Endotracheal intubation should be considered if bag-valve-mask ventilation is ineffective after

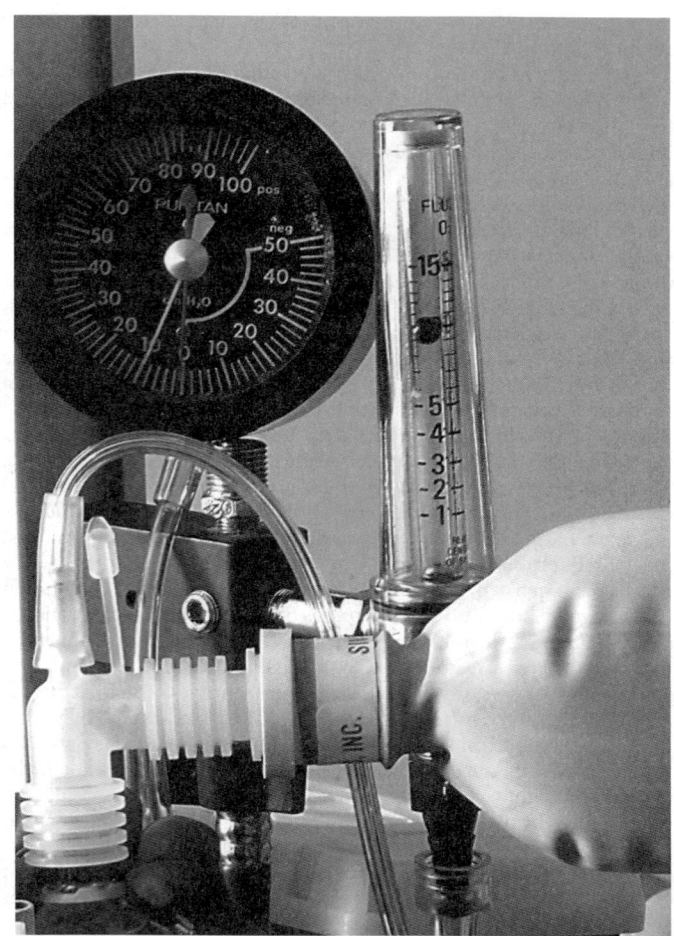

**FIGURE 1.** Anesthesia bag preparation. Setting the initial flow rate to 8 to 10 L/minute and the end-respiratory pressure to 8 to 10 cm $H_2O$ allows for effective bag filling while providing positive-pressure ventilation. Copied with permission from Golden SM. Resuscitation of the Neonate. Rakel RE, Bope ET (eds): *Conn's Current Therapy*, 2004. W.B. Saunders Co., 2003, p. 1082 (Figure 1).

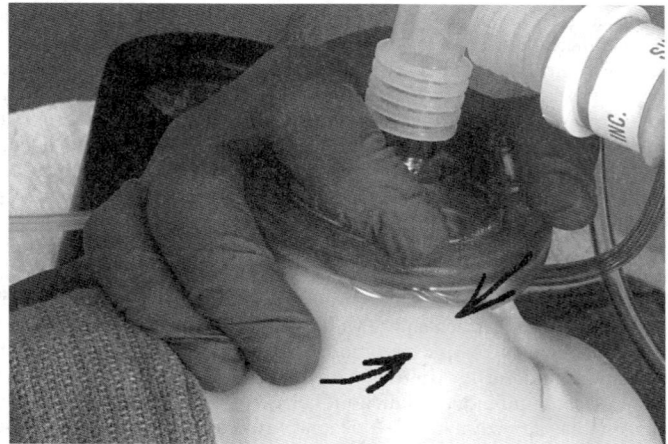

**FIGURE 2.** Proper placement and seal of face mask. The thumb and third finger (which is on the mandible or ramus of the mandible) are being squeezed toward each other in a *C hold*. Copied with permission from Golden SM. Resuscitation of the Neonate. Rakel RE, Bope ET (eds): *Conn's Current Therapy*, 2004. W.B. Saunders Co., 2004, p. 1082 (Figure 2).

attempts to optimize, if it appears that prolonged ventilation will be required, or if an intravascular route for epinephrine administration is unattainable. However, intubation should only be attempted by providers experienced with the management of the neonatal airway. Intubation of a newborn requires careful assessment to determine that the tube has been properly placed. Use of a disposable $CO_2$ indicator should be considered to confirm proper endotracheal tube placement initially and during the course of the resuscitation. The laryngeal mask airway (LMA) is an effective alternative for providing PPV when either bag-valve-mask ventilation fails or attempts at endotracheal intubation are unsuccessful.

Once adequate ventilation and oxygenation are assured, attention is directed toward the circulatory system ("C = CIRCULATION"). Heart rate is assessed by palpating the brachial pulse, palpating the pulse at the base of the umbilical cord, or by auscultation of cardiac sounds with a stethoscope. The heart rate in a newborn normally ranges from 100 to 170 beats per minute. As mentioned previously, PPV should be initiated for infants whose heart rates are less than 100 bpm. However, chest compressions should be performed immediately if the heart rate is less than 60 bpm after 30 seconds of effective PPV with supplemental oxygen (Box 2). Chest compressions are performed using either the two-thumb technique (Figure 3) or two-finger technique (Figure 4), but the two-thumb technique is thought to provide a more controlled depth of compression and better cardiac output. Team members should coordinate ventilations with chest compressions. After three

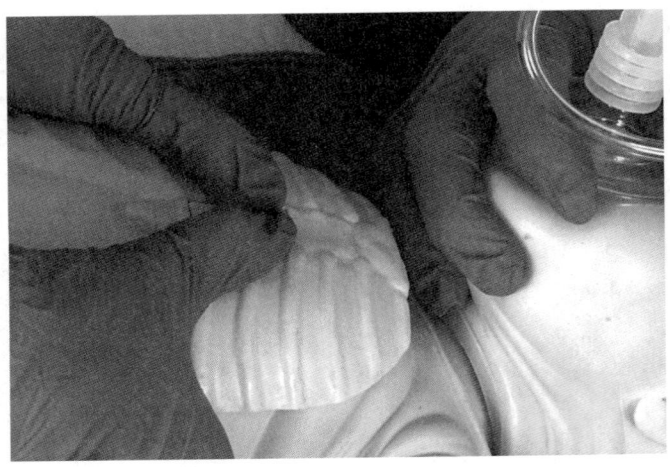

**FIGURE 3.** Two-thumb chest-encircling external cardiac massage technique. This is the preferred technique. Note that the thumbs are above the xyphoid process in the midsternum region. Copied with permission from Golden SM. Resuscitation of the Neonate. Rakel RE, Bope ET (eds): *Conn's Current Therapy*, 2004. W.B. Saunders Co., 2003, p. 1083 (Figure 4).

compressions, a positive pressure breath with supplemental oxygen should be administered (for a compression to breath ratio of 3:1). Chest compressions should be continued until the heart rate is greater than 60 bpm.

Resuscitation medications (Table 1) should be administered if the heart rate remains less than 60 bpm despite 30 seconds of chest compressions and adequate PPV. Vascular access should be established at this time, as drug (e.g., epinephrine), fluid, and dextrose administration may be necessary, but endotracheal administration of drugs may be the most accessible route. The medication is either flushed through the endotracheal tube with 0.5 to 1 mL normal saline or pushed through a 5 F feeding tube passed to the tip of the endotracheal tube. Both methods of drug administration should be followed by several positive-pressure breaths.

Vascular access may be achieved most readily via umbilical vein cannulation. The umbilical vein is easily identified and cannulated and is therefore the preferred site of vascular access in the newborn. The umbilical vein is identified as a single, thin-walled, larger vessel compared to the small, thick-walled pair of umbilical arteries (Figure 5). A 3.5 or 5.0 F catheter is inserted until the tip of the catheter

## BOX 2  Newborn Resuscitation Equipment for the Emergency Department

### Airway
- Bulb syringe
- DeLee suction catheter
- Meconium aspirator
- Laryngoscope and straight blades (sizes 0, 1)
- Endotracheal tubes, uncuffed (sizes 2.5, 3.0, 3.5, and 4.0 mm)
- Stylet
- Suction catheters (5 F, 8 F, 10 F)
- Suction source with manometer
- Nasogastric tube
- Feeding tubes (8 F, 10 F)

### Breathing
- Face masks (premature, newborn, and infant sizes)
- Self-inflating ventilation bag (450 to 750 mL), with oxygen reservoir and manometer
- Oxygen source
- Chest tubes (8 F and 10 F)

### Circulation
- Sterile umbilical vessel catheterization tray
- Umbilical catheters (3.5 F, 5.0 F)
- Three-way stopcocks
- Syringes (tuberculin, 1, 3, 10, and 20 mL)
- Medications and fluids:
  - Epinephrine 1:10,000 concentration
  - Naloxone hydrochloride
  - Sodium bicarbonate (0.5 mEq/mL or 4.2% solution)
  - Normal saline
  - Lactated Ringer's
  - 10% Dextrose
  - 5% Albumin

### Miscellaneous Equipment
- Radiant warmer or heat lamps
- Sterile towels
- Pulse oximeter
- Cardiorespiratory monitor with small electrocardiographic leads
- Sterile gowns, gloves
- Resuscitation chart

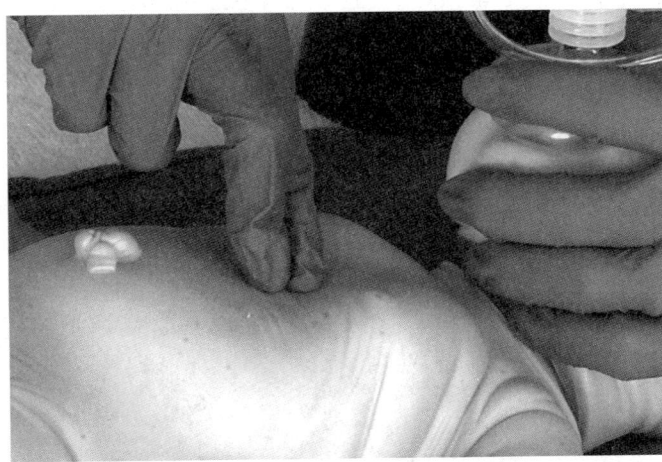

**FIGURE 4.** Two-finger external cardiac massage technique. Fingers are above xyphoid process; approximately one finger width beneath the nipple line. Copied with permission from Golden SM. Resuscitation of the Neonate. Rakel RE, Bope ET (eds): *Conn's Current Therapy*, 2004. W.B. Saunders Co., 2003, p. 1083 (Figure 5).

## TABLE 1 Drugs for Resuscitation/Stabilization

| Medication | Concentration | Dosage/Route | Indications | Comment |
|---|---|---|---|---|
| Epinephrine | 1:10,000 | 0.1-0.3 mL/kg IV<br>0.3-1 mL/kg ETT | Asystole<br>Bradycardia that is unresponsive to PPV and chest compressions | No studies for ETT route<br>Repeat dose Q 3-5 min |
| Volume expanders | Lactated Ringer's<br>0.9% normal saline<br>O-negative blood | 10 mL/kg IV | Hypovolemia<br>Shock | Cross-match to mother if possible |
| Glucose | 10% (D$_{10}$W) | 2 mL/kg IV | Hypoglycemia | May need to repeat |
| Sodium bicarbonate | 0.5 mEq/mL | 2 mL/kg IV | Documented severe metabolic acidosis or prolonged resuscitation with no response to other interventions | Administer slowly (approx. 2 mL/min) |
| Naloxone | | 0.1 mg/kg IV | Continued respiratory depression AFTER PPV has restored a normal heart rate and color AND History of maternal narcotic administration in past 4 hours | May precipitate, acute, life-threatening withdrawal in neonates born to drug-abusing mothers |

*Abbreviations:* ETT = endotracheal tube; IM, intramuscularly; IV = intravenously; PPV = positive pressure ventilation; q = every.

is below the skin or until blood can readily be aspirated. This should be done sterilely if possible. If not placed sterilely, however, after stabilization the catheter must be replaced to avoid potential complications. A peripheral intravenous (IV) line is also perfectly acceptable but may be difficult to establish by inexperienced providers.

Epinephrine is the drug used most frequently during resuscitation of the newborn. It may be administered via the IV or endotracheal routes for either asystole or heart rate less than 60 bpm despite effective ventilations and chest compressions. Generally, the dose is 0.01 to 0.03 mg/kg (0.1 to 0.3 mL/kg of the 1:10,000 solution) administered as needed every 3 to 5 minutes. If the endotracheal route is used, a higher dose (up to 0.1 mg/kg) is preferred. Volume expanders are also used frequently and are indicated for the treatment of hypovolemia. Generally, 10 mL/kg of either normal saline or lactated Ringer's are administered through an IV catheter over 5 to 10 minutes. If there is concern for significant anemia in the fetus or newborn, O-negative blood, crossmatched with the mother if possible, should be considered as a volume expander. If time does not allow, emergent-release O-negative blood should be used to initially resuscitate

the severely anemic infant. Naloxone (Narcan) is no longer recommended during the primary steps of resuscitation with the current guidelines. Narcan is indicated when continued respiratory depression is present after PPV has restored a normal heart rate and color, AND, when there is a history of maternal narcotic administration within the past 4 hours. The IV route is the preferred route of administration. Intravenous glucose (2 mL/kg D$_{10}$W) is administered for suspected or documented hypoglycemia. Sodium bicarbonate should only be given in cases of documented severe acidosis or in prolonged resuscitations with no response to other described interventions. Finally, surfactant preparations (e.g., Survanta, Infasurf) may be administered in the delivery room to preterm newborns with respiratory distress.

It should be emphasized that resuscitation proceeds according to the above protocols, and not according to the result of the Apgar score. The Apgar score is based on five objective signs (Table 2) and was designed to provide an easily reproducible measure of the status of a newborn shortly after birth. Scores are usually determined at 1 and 5 minutes of life. Resuscitation should *not* be delayed while awaiting the results of the 1-minute Apgar score.

## Meconium Staining of the Amniotic Fluid

Meconium is a viscous, greenish-black substance consisting of gastrointestinal (GI) secretions, blood, bile acids, amniotic fluid, and cellular debris present in the fetal GI tract. In the majority of cases, meconium is cleared from the GI tract with the first few bowel movements. However, in approximately 10% to 15% of all deliveries, meconium is passed prior to birth, leading to meconium staining of the amniotic fluid, which increases an infant's risk of developing the meconium aspiration syndrome (MAS), a disease with serious morbidity and mortality. Historically, routine intrapartum oropharyngeal and nasopharyngeal suctioning with a DeLee suction catheter was universally recommended. Recent evidence suggests that this is no longer necessary, and routine intrapartum suctioning is no longer recommended in the current guidelines. After the infant is delivered, if the amniotic fluid contains meconium and the infant has absent or depressed respirations, decreased muscle tone, or heart rate <100 bpm, the infant is tracheally intubated and the trachea is suctioned using a meconium aspirator attached directly to the endotracheal tube. Resuscitation is then performed in the usual sequence, if required. If the infant is vigorous, tracheal suctioning is not necessary.

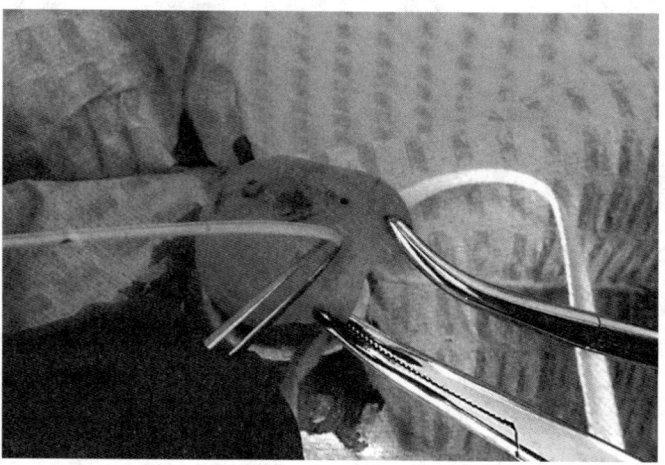

**FIGURE 5.** Umbilical vein catheterization. The umbilical vein is the preferred route for immediate venous access for drug medication and volume administration. Copied with permission from Golden SM. Resuscitation of the Neonate. Rakel RE, Bope ET (eds): *Conn's Current Therapy,* 2004. W.B. Saunders Co., 2003, p. 1084 (Figure 6).

## TABLE 2 The Apgar Score*

| Sign | 0 | 1 | 2 |
|---|---|---|---|
| Heart rate | Absent | Slow (less than 100 bpm) | Greater than 100 bpm |
| Respirations | Absent | Slow, irregular | Good, crying |
| Muscle tone | Limp | Some flexion | Active motion |
| Reflex irritability (catheter in nares) | No response | Grimace | Cough or sneeze |
| Color | Blue or pale | Acrocyanosis | Pink |

*A score of 0, 1, or 2 is assigned in each category at 1 and 5 minutes of life.
*Abbreviations:* bpm beats per minute.

# Newborn Resuscitation Outside the Delivery Room

Ideally, newborn resuscitation should take place in the delivery room setting. Unfortunately, many newborns are born outside the delivery room setting, such as in the home, en route to the hospital, or in the emergency department. Many mothers who deliver either outside the hospital setting or in the emergency department are more likely to represent high-risk groups (multiparous births, trauma-induced labor,

## CURRENT DIAGNOSIS

- Intrauterine asphyxia manifests as alterations in fetal heart rate (late decelerations, bradycardia), passage of meconium, fetal gasping, and eventual apnea, termed *primary apnea*. This initial period of apnea is followed by further gasping, which gradually weakens in intensity, eventually terminating in what is termed *secondary apnea*.
- Spontaneous respirations can be elicited in newborns with primary apnea by stimulation (vigorous warming and drying) or a brief trial of PPV. Newborns with secondary apnea, on the other hand, have suffered a prolonged period of inadequate oxygen delivery and require aggressive resuscitation to prevent further decompensation, cardiac arrest, and death.
- The longer the delay in initiating resuscitation for primary apnea, the longer the time required to establish spontaneous respirations following PPV. Because there is no definitive method of differentiating between primary and secondary apnea following delivery, the neonatal resuscitation team must promptly recognize and institute proper treatment for all newborn infants with apnea and suspected perinatal asphyxia.
- Neonatal resuscitation is directed toward assuring a smooth transition to extrauterine life by achieving the following goals:
  - Maintaining or restoring normal body temperature
  - Maintaining or establishing effective ventilation and oxygenation
  - Maintaining or restoring adequate cardiac output and tissue perfusion
  - Avoiding hypoglycemia
- Neonatal resuscitation consists of a cycle of repeated assessment and therapeutic intervention (assess-intervene-assess) until cardiorespiratory and hemodynamic stability are achieved.

*Abbreviation:* PPV = positive-pressure ventilation.

lack of prenatal care, adolescent pregnancy, placental abruption, etc.). Therefore, all emergency providers should be familiar with the resuscitation of the newborn. Resuscitation of the newborn infant presents several unique challenges to emergency care providers that are infrequently found during resuscitation of either the adult or child.

In many cases, deliveries in the emergency department will occur with little prior notice. Therefore, advanced preparation and an organized approach to resuscitation are essential. In addition to a standard obstetric tray, airway, vascular access, and other supplies and equipment unique to newborn resuscitation should be readily available (see Box 2). There is often insufficient time to obtain a complete prenatal history from the mother; however, three key pieces of information are often helpful in determining the initial priorities of resuscitation. First, if labor is premature (i.e., less than 37 weeks' gestation), a lengthy resuscitation with a possible need for prolonged PPV can be anticipated. Second, if twins are expected, two resuscitation teams and two sets of equipment should be available. Finally, if the membranes have ruptured, the presence of meconium will indicate the need for an additional, more specialized resuscitation sequence (see previous discussion).

## Ongoing Assessment

Neonatal resuscitation consists of a cycle of repeated assessment and therapeutic intervention ("assess-intervene-assess") until cardiorespiratory and hemodynamic stability are achieved. The cycle of "assess-intervene-assess" should continue once the critically ill newborn has stabilized. During stabilization, a complete blood cell count (CBC), serum electrolytes, blood urea nitrogen (BUN), creatinine, blood glucose, and an arterial blood gas to assess acid-base status should be obtained. A chest radiograph should be obtained to confirm proper placement of the endotracheal and orogastric tubes. Additional vascular access should be obtained. In the tracheally intubated patient, further deterioration should prompt rapid, close assessment for potential endotracheal tube complications. These complications can be easily recalled at the bedside by the mnemonic *DOPE*:

Dislodged: Has the endotracheal tube moved distally into the right or left main bronchus?
Obstructed: Is the endotracheal tube obstructed with inspissated secretions or blood?

## CURRENT THERAPY

- Initial efforts should be directed toward minimizing heat loss. On delivery, the infant should be placed on a radiant warmer. The infant is then dried vigorously with a warm, sterile towel.
- Properly positioning the infant on his or her back, with the head and neck in a neutral, midline position will assist in opening the airway. The mouth and nose should be suctioned with a bulb syringe to remove any secretions that may contribute to airway compromise.
- If respirations are adequate and cyanosis is present, supplemental oxygen should be administered.
- PPV, using a bag-valve-mask is indicated for those infants with either absent (apnea) or slow, gasping respiratory movements, and when the heart rate is below 100 bpm.
- Chest compressions should be performed immediately if the heart rate is less than 60 bpm after 30 seconds of effective PPV with 100% oxygen using either the two-thumb technique (preferred) or two-finger technique.
- Resuscitation medications should be administered if the heart rate remains less than 60 bpm despite 30 seconds of chest compressions and adequate PPV.

*Abbreviations:* bpm = beats per minute; PPV = positive-pressure ventilation.

*Pneumothorax:* Is there a pneumothorax?

*Esophagus:* Is the endotracheal tube in the esophagus?

In conclusion, the dramatic changes in cardiovascular and respiratory physiology that occur around the time of birth pose several potential problems that could lead to an unfavorable outcome. Proper education and training in neonatal resuscitation are imperative for all health care providers working in the deliver room and nursery setting. Health care providers in these settings, as well as those physicians working in the emergency department who may also be called on to resuscitate newborn infants should have advanced knowledge and understanding of normal fetal, transitional, and neonatal physiology so that potential problems can be recognized and treated early. Only through the early recognition, resuscitation, and stabilization of the critically ill newborn will the best possible outcome be realized.

## REFERENCES

American Heart Association and American Academy of Pediatrics: 2005 American Heart Association (AHA) guidelines for cardiopulmonary resuscitation (CPR) and emergency cardiovascular care (ECC) of pediatric and neonatal patients: Neonatal resuscitation guidelines. Pediatrics 2006; 117:e1029-e1038.

Apgar V: A proposal for a new method of evaluation of the newborn infant. Anesth Analg 1953;32:260-267.

Gelfand SL, Fanaroff JM, Walsh MC: Meconium stained fluid: Approach to the mother and the baby. Pediatr Clin North Am 2004; 51:655-667.

Palme-Kilander C: Methods of resuscitation in low-Apgar-score newborn infants: A national survey. Acta Pediatr 1992; 81:739-744.

Robertson NJ: Air or 100% oxygen for asphyxiated babies? Time to decide. Crit Care 2005; 9:128-130.

Saugstad OD: Practical aspects of resuscitating newborn infants. Eur J Pediatr 1998; 157(suppl 1):S11-S15.

Saugstad OD: Room air resuscitation: Two decades of neonatal research. Early Hum Dev 2005; 81:111-116.

Vain NE, Szyld EG, Prudent LM, et al: Oropharyngeal and nasopharyngeal suctioning of meconium-stained neonates before delivery of their shoulders: Multicentre, randomised controlled trial. Lancet 2004; 364;597-602.

Wiswell TE, Gannon CM, Jacob J, et al: Delivery room management of the apparently vigorous meconium-stained neonate: Results of the multicenter, internatinoal collaborative trial. Pediatrics 2000; 105:1-7.

# Care of the High-Risk Neonate

Method of
*Dilcia McLenan, MD*

Despite advances in prenatal care and diagnosis, the overall prematurity rate has not changed in the last two decades. The rate remains at 10% to 12% of all births in the United States. Although the overall mortality rate and the short-term morbidity rate have improved with the advances in neonatal care, premature births are still responsible for 75% to 85% of neonatal deaths. Congenital anomalies are associated with 20% to 30% of perinatal deaths. The early identification of the high-risk neonate is essential to improve outcome. The goal is to prevent the development or progression of more serious illnesses and to minimize the risk of both morbidity and mortality.

The definition of the high-risk neonate can be applied in the prenatal, perinatal or postnatal period. Approximately 75% of risk factors affecting the fetus are identified in the prenatal period. Maternal high-risk factors include age, race, socioeconomic status, nutrition and past obstetric history, current pregnancy problems, and maternal drug use. Maternal acute and chronic illness can also adversely affect the fetus. The placenta is considered fetal tissue; all conditions that affect the placenta will also affect the fetus, and vice versa. Fetal factors are limited to genetic conditions (chromosomal and nonchromosomal), and metabolic.

The prenatal diagnosis of the high-risk neonate uses many tools, such as chorionic villus sampling (CVS), amniocentesis, maternal serum screening, and cordocentesis. With the use of cytogenetics, molecular biology, and the fluorescence in situ hybridization, many genetic disorders and infectious conditions can be diagnosed. Fetal ultrasonography is another valuable tool in diagnosing high-risk conditions, including fetal growth abnormalities, which are associated with increased perinatal morbidity and mortality. The Doppler can assess blood velocity in the umbilical and fetal vessels. There is increased morbidity and mortality in fetuses with absent umbilical artery flow or with reverse end diastolic flow. The measurement of the nuchal translucency, done between 10 and 14 weeks of gestation by fetal ultrasound (US) in conjunction with the maternal serum markers, increases the detection rate of Down syndrome and other chromosomal and genetic syndromes, fetal structural malformations, and adverse pregnancy outcome.

Prenatal care facilitates the diagnosis and care of the high-risk neonate through a multidisciplinary approach. This multidisciplinary approach sets the stage for counseling, referrals, and the plan of care pre- and postnatally. When counseling the family, consider the gestational age at diagnosis, effect on maternal outcome and neonatal prognosis with or without therapy, plans for delivery, intrapartum management, and surgical intervention when applicable. General discussion with the parents during the intrapartum period regarding the preterm or high-risk neonate will include such things as anticipated birth weight and gestational age, the need for respiratory support, procedures to be expected, the need for transfusion of blood products, short- and long-term complications of each problem or condition, the need for other specialists, and morbidity and mortality. Involving the neonatologist in the counseling can aid families in making difficult decisions. One should also explain the need for transport, if delivered at a nontertiary care center, and the role the parents will have while their infant is in the neonatal intensive care unit (NICU).

The delivery management of the high-risk neonate is influenced by the factors identified in the antepartum and intrapartum period. In the intrapartum period, neonatal resuscitation facilitates the transition from the intrauterine to the extrauterine life. Approximately 5% to 10% of all newborns need help making this transition; 1% of all newborns need a more extensive intervention. The fetus is dependent on its mother and the placenta for the delivery of oxygen and nutrients as well as removal of carbon dioxide. After the umbilical cord is clamped and cut, the newborn needs to expand its lungs, establishing respirations and convert from a fetal (parallel) to an adult (in series) circulation for a successful transition, and avoid the development of asphyxia.

Resuscitation aims at facilitating the transition and reversing the process of asphyxia by clearing the airway, providing adequate oxygenation and ventilation, ensuring adequate cardiac output, and keeping oxygen consumption to the minimum. These objectives can be achieved by adhering to the initial steps and the four principles of neonatal resuscitation.

## Principles of Neonatal Resuscitation

The American Heart Association (AHA) and the American Academy of Pediatrics (AAP) Neonatal Resuscitation Program (NRP) have defined the following principles of neonatal resuscitation:

- **Anticipation.** Risk factors in the antepartum and intrapartum history help identify instances that may potentially require intervention (Box 1).
- **Preparation.** In preparing the area, equipment should be assembled and checked, and drugs should be readied.
- **Availability of qualified personnel.** At every delivery there should be at least one person skilled in neonatal resuscitation whose only responsibility is the newborn; skills include the proper use of the bag and mask. In cases of emergency or if further intervention is needed, additional competent personnel should be immediately available.
- **Organized response to the emergencies—evaluation, decision, and action.** The ABCs (airway, breathing, and circulation) of

to diagnose conditions that might have contributed to the need for further resuscitation, such as congenital abnormalities of the airway, heart, gastrointestinal (GI) tract, genitourinary (GU) system, or secondary cardiopulmonary disorders. Infants with Apgar scores below 7 at 10 minutes should be admitted to the NICU for further observation and management.

## Asphyxia

Asphyxia is the result of prolonged decrease of oxygen delivery to the tissues. During the event, there is redistribution of blood flow to the heart, brain, and adrenals. The continuation of the insult results in bradycardia, impaired gas exchange, and reduced tissue perfusion. These series of events can occur prenatally, intrapartum, or postnatally. In severe cases of asphyxia almost every organ of the body is affected:

- Central nervous system (CNS): hypoxic ischemic encephalopathy
- Cardiovascular: myocardial dysfunction
- Renal: renal dysfunction and or acute renal failure
- GI: liver dysfunction and increased risk of necrotizing enterocolitis
- Hematologic: coagulopathy
- Pulmonary: activation of the mechanisms that cause persistent pulmonary hypertension of the newborn, surfactant (Survanta) deficiency, and meconium aspiration syndrome (MAS)
- Metabolic: acidosis, hypoglycemia, and hypocalcemia

After birth the normal newborn goes through a period of transition that lasts for several hours. During this period the cardiovascular, pulmonary, and sympathetic systems regulate themselves to adjust to extrauterine life. During the transition, abnormalities in color, respirations, heart rate, sleep state, motor activity, GI function, and temperature stability can be identified and will require care in the NICU. Clinical manifestations of abnormal transition include persistent tachypnea, nasal flaring, grunting, retractions, persistent cyanosis, apnea and bradycardia, pallor, temperature instability, blood pressure (BP) instability, lethargy, and other neurologic symptoms.

## Postnatal Care

The postnatal care of the high-risk neonate is extremely important. There are interventions and supportive care that are common to the high-risk neonates to ensure the best possible outcome. These include thermoregulation, nutrition, developmental care, and parental involvement. Notwithstanding, individualized care that will address specific needs of each infant should always be kept in mind.

### THERMOREGULATION

Thermoregulation is the balance between heat production and heat loss. It is closely linked to morbidity and mortality. In the neonate, heat loss can exceed heat production because of larger surface area to body mass ratio, decreased subcutaneous (SC) tissue or fat, increased permeability to water and small radius of curvature of exchange surfaces.

The newborn generates heat by nonshivering mechanisms—brown fat, increased muscular activity, flexion, and increased metabolic rate with increased oxygen consumption. The newborn loses heat through conduction, convection, evaporation, and radiation (Table 2).

In the neonate there is always a combination of types and mechanism of heat loss. The prevention of cold stress and hypothermia is critical for intact survival of the neonate (Figure 1).

Heat production is a result of metabolic processes that generate energy by oxidative metabolism of glucose (most efficient in the premature infant), fat, and protein. In the newborn, heat or energy production is low relative to heat or energy losses. Brown adipose tissue generates more energy than any other tissue in the body. The brown adipose tissue cells begin to differentiate by 26 to 30 weeks of gestation and continue to develop until 3 to 5 weeks after birth; they constitute 10% of the adipose tissue in term infants.

resuscitation is the order in which assessment and needed intervention will be evaluated. The evaluation assesses the breathing, heart rate, and color, then the decision or diagnosis is made followed by the action or treatment.

The initial steps of resuscitation provide the support needed to make the transition from the intrauterine to the extrauterine life (Table 1).

Shortcutting these steps prolongs the resuscitation process, increases the risk for asphyxia, and increases the likelihood of morbidity and mortality. In cases where further intervention is needed beyond the initial steps of resuscitation, a thorough evaluation should be done

**TABLE 1  At Birth**

| Initial Step | Objective |
|---|---|
| Provide warmth. | Prevent heat loss, maintain oxygen consumption at a minimum, and prevent hypoglycemia. |
| Position, clear the airway (as necessary). | Establish an airway. |
| Dry stimulate and reposition. | Initiate breathing and open the airway. |

**TABLE 2   Thermoregulation: Types, Mechanisms, and Management**

| Type/Definition | Mechanism | Prevention |
| --- | --- | --- |
| Conduction, transfer of heat from the body core to surface, and object in contact with body. | Cold surfaces, cold objects in contact with the body | Use rubber mattresses, warm blankets, and warm mattresses. |
| Convection, heat transfer from the body surface to the surrounding air. | Cool rapid air flow, cold oxygen flow | Swaddle using a cap, warm oxygen, and placing infant away from draft. Servo control air or skin incubators, warm room temperature. |
| Evaporation, moisture on the body surface or respiratory tract evaporates. Major source of heat loss after delivery or during bath. Inversely related to gestational age. | Wet skin, increase of activity, tachypnea, under radiant warmer and phototherapy | Dry infant immediately after birth and bath; increase humidity; use warm soaks and solutions; use polyethylene wraps, warm and humidified oxygen. |
| Radiation, transfer of heat from the body to surrounding cooler surfaces not in contact with the infant. | Dependent on ambient temperature, air speed and other heat loss mechanisms | Double-wall incubators, radiant warmer, and heat shield. |

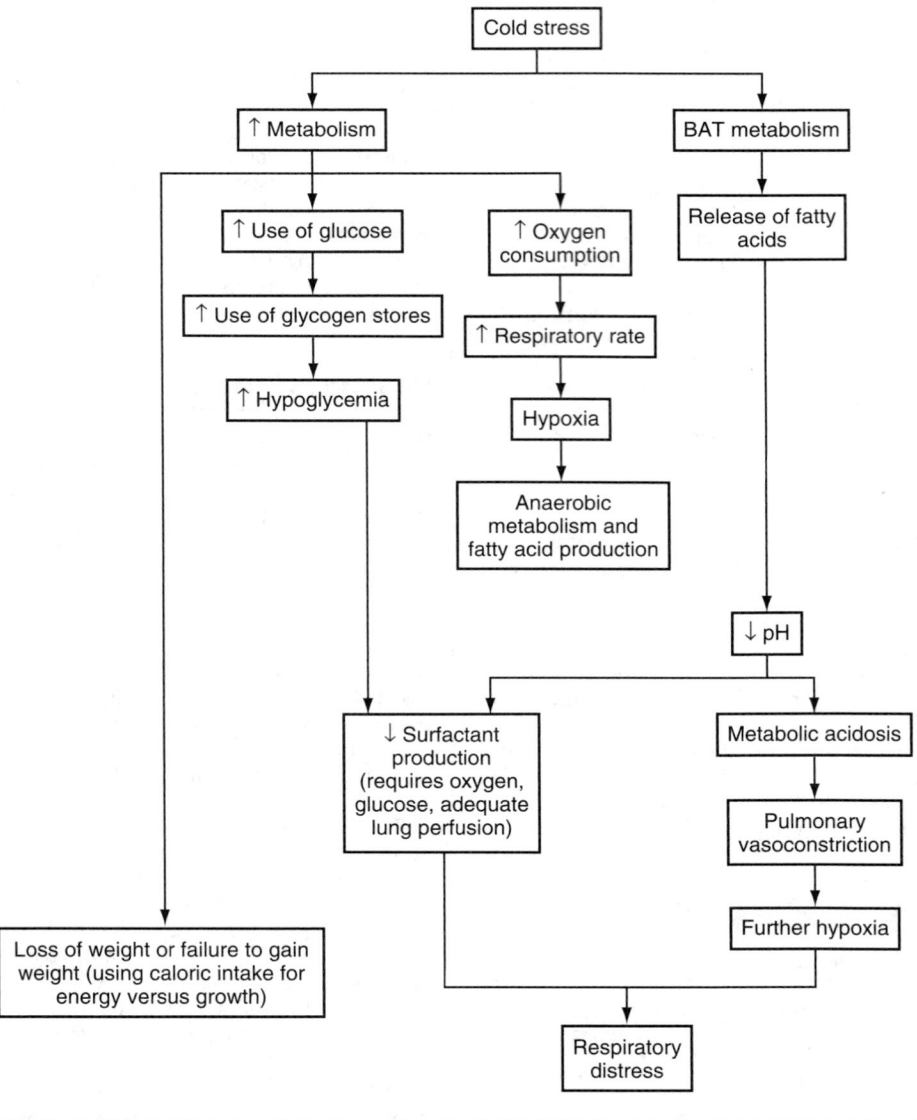

**FIGURE 1.** Physiologic consequences of cold stress. BAT = Brown adipose tissue.

Thermoregulation is achieved by providing the appropriate thermal environment to prevent heat loss, hypothermia, and cold stress. The neutral thermal environment (NTE) is an idealized range of ambient temperature at which the body temperature is normal, metabolic rate or oxygen consumption is minimal, and thermoregulation is achieved by basal nonevaporative physical processes. It promotes growth and stability and minimizes heat (energy) and water loss. Newborns have a narrow control range that make them vulnerable to alterations in the thermal environment. The NTE is achieved for the:

- Term infant at 32°C (89.6°F) to 33.5°C (92.3°F)
- Preterm infant greater than 1500 g at 34°C (93.2°F) to 35°C (95°F)
- Preterm infant less than 1500 g at 36.7°C (98.1°F) to 37.3°C (99.1°F)

The two common methods of supporting thermoregulation are the radiant warmer and the incubator (Table 3).

## NUTRITION

Proper nutrition is essential for adequate growth, development, and healing. Protein and lipid stores are decreased in the neonate, who has a higher baseline energy requirement compared to children and adults. The low-birth-weight (LBW) infant and the premature infant have even higher baseline requirements. The premature infant has minimal stores of fat and carbohydrates and rapidly develops nutritional deficiencies in calcium, phosphorus, iron trace elements, and vitamins. Nutritional requirements of calories and protein increase even further in the critically ill neonate with overwhelming infections, severe lung disease, and major surgical conditions. These conditions obviate the enteral route of delivering adequate nutrition as well as the immature digestive pathways of the GI tract. In these cases parenteral nutrition is the only option. In premature infants nutritional support is aimed at achieving an intrauterine growth pattern of 15 to 30 g per day. To achieve comparable weight at term-corrected age, compared to a term infant, the daily growth rate would have to be higher to achieve catch-up growth. When there is early positive nitrogen balance, weight loss is less, there is a better rate of growth, and healing and recovery are faster.

With parenteral nutrition the fluid requirement starts at 80 mL/kg per day and increases daily up to 150 mL/kg per day. Infants with increased fluid losses, in addition to their maintenance fluid requirement, will require replacement fluid with specific electrolytes to offset their losses. The caloric requirement varies from 80 kcal to 120 kcal/kg per day. Higher caloric needs of 20% to 30% more are required in the extremely premature infants and in the critically ill neonate. To achieve the expected postnatal growth pattern, the total nonprotein calories requirement should be at least 70 to 105 kcal/kg per day; and the protein intake should be 2.7 to 3.5 g/kg per day of protein for positive nitrogen balance, adequate nitrogen accretion, and good neurodevelopmental outcome. Protein is given in the form of an amino acid solution.

These amino acids are the building blocks required for growth, preservation of skeletal muscle protein mass, tissue repair, and appropriate inflammatory response. Protein intake starts at the recommended daily intake of 3 to 4 g/kg per day. Critically ill neonates will also require an increase in protein intake by 10% to 20%.

Calories or energy is given through carbohydrates and fat. Glucose is the carbohydrate used in parenteral nutrition and is the preferred substrate for the brain. It provides 3.4 cal/g of glucose. Fat is given as a 20% lipid emulsion solution, and it provides 2 cal/mL. The use of the lipid emulsion will prevent essential fatty acid deficiency, improve protein use and will not increase significantly $CO_2$ production or metabolic rate compared to glucose. This is an important factor in infants with chronic lung disease and retention of carbon dioxide. The infusion rate of fat begins at 0.5 g/kg per day and is advanced by 0.5 g daily up to 2 to 3 g/kg per day. Close monitoring of triglycerides is required. A level above 250 mg/dL is considered high, so the rate of infusion should then be cut back. Adequate energy intake will promote or facilitate positive nitrogen balance and nitrogen accretion. Other components of parenteral nutrition are calcium, phosphorus, vitamins, and trace minerals. Sodium and potassium are added based on the serum electrolyte results. Carnitine is added when premature infants are on prolonged parenteral nutrition with no enteral feedings.

The task of providing adequate nutrition is multidisciplinary; the neonatologist, pharmacist, and nutritionist form part of the team. Close metabolic monitoring for glucose, electrolytes, urea, lipids, and acid–base balance is an integral part of the nutritional management of the high-risk neonates. This will help assess and meet nutritional needs as well as monitor for complications such as metabolic acidosis, electrolyte imbalance, cholestatic jaundice, increased triglyceride levels, and infection. When enteral feeding is possible, human milk should be considered. Although it may not provide adequate caloric and protein intake, it has many other assets that are important in promoting healing, neurodevelopment, and protection against infection.

## DEVELOPMENTAL CARE

The NICU environment plays a major role in the growth and development of the high-risk neonate and may contribute to the morbidity of these fragile infants. The amount of abnormal sensory stimulus that these fragile beings are exposed to is the source of overwhelming stress at sensitive periods of their development, and in turn will modify their brain development. The cortex of the brain is part of the sensory system, and both deprivation and overstimulation can modify its development. The sensitive period when this occurs is between 28 and 40 weeks of gestation. Therefore the NICU environment is crucial as part of the care of the sick newborn infant. These infants are subject to numerous stress factors, unpleasant procedures, continuously disrupted sleep, frequent noxious oral stimulus, noise, and bright lights. Stress causes autonomic instability, with secretion of cortisol and catecholamines. These hormones in turn interfere with tissue healing and growth.

**TABLE 3 Measures to Promote Thermoregulation in Incubators and Radiant Warmers**

| Bed | Basis | Measures |
|---|---|---|
| Incubator | Decrease evaporative water and heat loss | Increase humidity<br>Plastic heat shield<br>Thermal blanket<br>Semiocclusive dressings or emollients |
| | Reduce radiant and convective losses | Double-walled incubator<br>Heat shield<br>Thermal blanket |
| | Promote conductive heat gain | Heated mattress |
| Radiant warmer | Decrease evaporative water and heat loss | Heat shield<br>Plastic wrap<br>Thermal blanket |
| | Reduce radiant or convective losses | Heat shield<br>Plastic wrap<br>Thermal blanket |

Modified from Sinclair, J. (1992). Management of the thermal environment. In J.C. Sinclair and M.B. Brocker (eds). Effective care of the newborn infant. Oxford: Oxford University Press.

When considering the NICU environment and the input or stimuli that could be beneficial to these high-risk neonates, one has to take into consideration the in utero environment and how the sensory stimulus would have been perceived in that environment, and the normal development of the sensory system for planned interventions. The hierarchical organization, maturation, and integration of the sensory system is as follows:

- Tactile
- Vestibular
- Gustatory
- Olfactory
- Auditory
- Visual

The visual sensory system is the least mature at term and maturation continues after birth. There is overlapping regarding when a sensory system maturation begins and ends, but there is clear evidence that disruption of one sensory system will affect the maturation of the system that has not yet developed. The same is true when a later sensory system is stimulated earlier than expected.

The interventions that support the development of the sensory system are as follows:

- Minimal handling
- Clustering of care
- Soft swaddling
- Stroking, rocking, and holding when appropriate
- Non-nutritive sucking
- Positioning prone or on the side
- Nesting
- Placing the infant in an infant seat; then swaddle and nest
- Soothing, soft, simple repetitive, and harmonic sounds with limited dynamic range
- Limit ambient light
- Shield eyes and chest from bright lights
- Limit the initial visual stimulus to the human face
- Massage therapy

These suggested interventions should take into consideration the gestational age and the clinical acuity of the high-risk patient. The goal is to improve growth and neurodevelopmental outcome of the high-risk neonate.

### PARENTAL INVOLVEMENT

When looking at specific high-risk situations, one can appreciate the scope of support needed by these high-risk neonates from various subspecialists and ancillary health care professionals. One of the things often forgotten is the major role the parents play in the healing and development of their sick infant. Parents have a sense of loss from the time their sick newborn has to be resuscitated and/or is admitted to the NICU. They have a sense of loss for delivering prematurely, for not having a healthy full-term infant, loss of self-esteem, and social status as parents. Involving the parents in the care of their infant will provide some emotional, psychosocial, and spiritual support to the parents. The literature continues to support the need for and the benefits of parental involvement in the NICU as part of the care of the high-risk neonate.

Kangaroo care, or skin-to-skin contact between the parent and the infant, provides sustained multimodal stimulation of tactile, vestibular, proprioceptive, olfactory, and auditory sensory systems. Physiologic benefits such as stable temperature; stable oxygen consumption; higher saturation levels; increased quiet sleep, which lowers cortisol levels resulting in fewer infections; and better growth have been described. It promotes non-nutritive sucking, and there is a better letdown in breast-feeding mothers. Kangaroo care acts as a behavioral organizer or facilitator, decreases motor activity, increases the quiet state in stable preterm infants, and reduces the effect of painful stimuli. These infants are also discharged sooner.

Parents can also participate in massage therapy. It has a calming effect on infants; they express fewer stress behaviors, are more alert, actively respond to face and voice, and show more organized limb movements on the Brazelton behavioral scale. Better weight gain and early discharge have been reported. At 8 months these infants continue to show better weight gain and higher scores on the Bayley Scales of Infant Development.

## Conditions Associated With Abnormal Transition

A few conditions associated with abnormal transition are described in the following text.

### HYALINE MEMBRANE DISEASE

Hyaline membrane disease (HMD) is the result of surfactant deficiency. Surfactant reduces the surface tension of the alveoli and prevents them from collapsing. This disorder is common to preterm infants. The clinical presentation of HMD is that of respiratory distress characterized by grunting, retractions, and flaring. Grunting is used to maintain the intra-alveoli pressure and prevent it from collapsing. The blood gas typically has hypoxemia and to a lesser degree respiratory acidosis. Radiographically the lungs have a ground glass appearance (this represents microatelectasis) and air bronchograms (the contrast of the air-filled bronchi against the collapse parenchyma). These infants are managed with ventilator support and/or continuous positive airway pressure (CPAP), and surfactant (Survanta) replacement therapy. The use of antenatal steroids has decreased the incidence of HMD and the need for exogenous surfactant in the premature newborn, especially in infants who are 28 weeks' gestation or more.

### TRANSIENT TACHYPNEA OF THE NEWBORN

Transient tachypnea of the newborn (TTN) is described as the retention of lung fluid or transient pulmonary edema. In some cases, there may be mild surfactant deficiency. During labor the increased level of prostaglandins causes dilation of the lymphatic vessels in the lungs promoting the absorption of the pulmonary interstitial fluid. After birth, this process is further accelerated by the expansion of the lungs with air-filled alveoli and increased pulmonary circulation. Any delay in this process will result in tachypnea and occasional grunting and flaring. This is common after elective cesarean section. The arterial blood gas shows various degrees of respiratory acidosis and some hypoxemia. The typical chest radiographic findings reveal increased interstitial marking with fluid in the fissure and on occasion pleural effusion. This condition is self-limited, resolving in 1 to 2 days. These infants are managed with oxygen support by hood and rarely require ventilator support.

### MECONIUM ASPIRATION SYNDROME

Meconium staining of the amniotic fluid occurs in 10% to 25% of all deliveries. It is seen in fetuses beyond 35 weeks of gestation. Passage of meconium in utero is often the result of a hypoxemic event. Meconium can be aspirated before, during, or after delivery. Once aspirated it can cause obstruction of the airway and pulmonary air leak, chemical pneumonitis and secondary bacterial infection, secondary surfactant deficiency, and pulmonary hypertension of the newborn (PPHN) if hypoxemia persists. After birth, a depressed neonate with poor or no respiratory effort should be intubated and suctioned immediately after being placed under the radiant warmer. This action will clear the airway and prevent aspiration or any further aspiration. The key in preventing meconium aspiration in neonates who did not have in utero aspiration is suctioning of the airway at the perineum by the obstetrician as soon as the head is delivered. The severity of the disease varies. The arterial blood gas pictures vary from mild respiratory acidosis with mild hypoxemia to severe respiratory failure with marked hypoxemia. The classic radiographic finding of the lungs is that of patchy infiltrates throughout the lung fields with areas of hyperlucency; air leak is seen in 10% to 20% of these cases. Postnatal management consists of support to minimize all factors that will perpetuate asphyxia and trigger pulmonary hypertension. Decrease energy loss and oxygen consumption by providing warmth, oxygen, and glucose. Aggressive respiratory support is needed, providing high concentration of oxygen in a hood or through the ventilator. In cases associated with severe PPHN, inhaled nitric oxide (iNO [INO$_{max}$]), and ultimately extracorporeal membrane oxygenation (ECMO) may become part of the management.

## PERSISTENT PULMONARY HYPERTENSION OF THE NEWBORN

Persistent pulmonary hypertension of the newborn is the result of severe hypoxemia because of right-to-left shunting through the foramen ovale and ductus arteriosus, without associated structural heart abnormality. The pulmonary hypertension results from increased pulmonary vasoreactivity and increased muscle mass of the pulmonary arterial vessels. The increase in pulmonary smooth arterial muscle mass seen in term infants is triggered by intrauterine stress or hypoxemia. The vasoreactive response seen after birth is caused by alteration of the balance between the circulating pulmonary vasodilator (endothelium-derived relaxing factor or endogenous nitric oxide) and pulmonary vasoconstrictors (endothelin). This vasoreactive response is seen also in preterm and term infants with primary lung disease, such as surfactant deficiency, pneumonia, or MAS. Tachypnea and cyanosis is the clinical presentation. The blood gas has severe hypoxemia and combine metabolic and respiratory acidosis. In primary PPHN, the chest radiograph is normal; in secondary PPHN, it will be characteristic of the disease in question. The diagnosis of PPHN is made with the aid of the echocardiogram, which will exclude structural heart disease, measure the pulmonary artery pressure and resistance and visualize the right-to-left shunts, and tricuspid regurgitation that is commonly present.

The management of neonates with PPHN can be challenging. The goal is to correct the hypoxemia and acidosis, both of which cause pulmonary vasoconstriction. The acidosis can be managed with hyperventilation using conventional or high-frequency ventilator (to achieve a PaCO$_2$ close to 30 mm Hg) and/or infusion of sodium bicarbonate to maintain the arterial pH around 7.40. The hypoxemia is more difficult to manage because these infants do not always respond to high concentrations of oxygen with high ventilator support. The PaO$_2$ should be maintained above 80 mm Hg. Concurrent metabolic derangement, such as hypoglycemia and hypocalcemia, and polycythemia should be corrected. The systemic arterial BP should be maintained in the high range of normal. The use of vasopressor agents (dopamine [Intropin] or dobutamine [Dobutrex]) is recommended in achieving this goal, as opposed to volume expansion. The increase in the systemic BP may decrease the right-to-left shunt through the ductus arteriosus and improve pulmonary blood flow and in turn improve the hypoxemia.

When the previously described management fails, the use of iNO at a dose of 20 ppm or less will cause selective pulmonary vasodilatation. Because many infants respond to iNO, the need for ECMO has decreased. Extracorporeal membrane oxygenation is available only in a few medical centers for those cases that fail to respond to maximum ventilator support and iNO.

# The Infant with Surgical Conditions

Infants before, during, or after surgery require special consideration regarding management and support of the cardiopulmonary system, thermoregulation, fluid and electrolyte management, nutritional support, and infection control.

## GASTROSCHISIS

The combined incidence of omphalocele and gastroschisis is 1:4000 live births. Of these two abdominal wall defects, gastroschisis is the more common. It is a cleft in the abdominal wall to the right of the umbilical cord with herniation of the bowel. The association of other congenital and chromosomal anomalies is rare compared with omphalocele. Common associated problems seen in gastroschisis are malrotation of the bowel, undescended testes, stenosis, and atresia of the bowel, all of which are the result of vascular injury. In 20% of the patients, necrotizing enterocolitis has been reported postoperatively.

Gastroschisis can be diagnosed in the prenatal period. This will allow for proper counseling of the family as well as the plans for intrapartum and postnatal management. The intrapartum and postnatal management consist of preventing further injury to the bowel, temperature stabilization, fluid and electrolyte management, antibiotic therapy, nutritional support, and surgical correction. The exposed bowel is at risk for further circulatory compromise. This may be avoided by having the infant lie on his or her side. Because there is a large surface area exposed to the environment, heat and fluid losses are increased. The bowel should be wrapped in cephalexin (Keflex) soaked in warm normal saline, and then covered with a plastic barrier. The prolonged exposure of the bowel to the amniotic fluid causes a severe inflammatory response that results in ileus. In addition to the increased fluid losses through the exposed bowel, there is intraluminal loss of fluid and electrolyte because of the severe ileus. In these patients 1.5 to 2 times their fluid maintenance is needed for fluid resuscitation. The bowel should be decompressed using a nasogastric or orogastric tube connected to intermittent low suction. Close monitoring of vital signs, intake and output, and serum electrolytes will give indications of the fluid and electrolyte status of these infants.

Nutritional support in infants with gastroschisis is crucial for healing and to decrease morbidity and mortality. Prior to parenteral nutrition, the mortality in these infants was very high, malnutrition and complications associated with infection being major causes. These infants may go for several weeks before enteral feedings can be attempted or tolerated. Early placement of central venous access will facilitate the long-term nutritional support and the overall management. Long-term parenteral nutrition is the key for full recovery of these infants.

The surgical approach considers two options: primary or secondary closure. Secondary closure creates an enclosed hernia, a silo with the bowel content. The bowel is then slowly returned to the abdominal cavity over several days. Antibiotics are continued until the abdominal wall is closed. Primary closure returns the bowel into the abdominal cavity in one step. It is not uncommon, especially with large defects, to have respiratory compromise requiring ventilator support. Be conscious of the need for pain management in these infants, more so in those with respiratory compromise. Other complications seen with primary closure are further bowel compromise with bloody drainage, acidosis, infection, and increased intra-abdominal pressure that causes decrease renal and or central venous perfusion.

## CONGENITAL DIAPHRAGMATIC HERNIA

The incidence of congenital diaphragmatic hernia (CDH) is 1:2000 to 5000 live births. This condition can be diagnosed in the prenatal period. When diagnosed in the prenatal period the plan of management begins. The infant should be delivered at a tertiary care center experienced in counseling and treatment of CDH. In these patients, further workup should be done to exclude other malformations of the heart, GI tract, GU system, and CNS and chromosomal anomalies. Associated malformations should be taken into account when counseling the family and when developing the postnatal plan of management. Plans to deliver at term, and at a center where there is a pediatric surgeon, capability for iNO (INO$_{max}$) and ECMO is desired. Once delivered, the infant should be intubated immediately, venous access obtained in case of needed circulatory support, and a nasogastric or orogastric tube placed to decompress the bowel. Bowel distention can further compromise respiration and cardiac function.

The infant should be transferred to the NICU, an arterial line should be placed and blood obtained for blood gas and crossmatch. Obtain a chest and abdominal radiograph to confirm the diagnosis and line placement. An echocardiogram should be done to assess for structural abnormalities of the heart and to estimate the degree of pulmonary hypertension. A head US should be obtained if the infant will be placed on ECMO, because of the risk of intracranial hemorrhage in patients on ECMO.

Skilled ventilator management is important because of the coexisting pulmonary hypertension. Barotrauma and volutrauma should be avoided in these patients. Permissive hypercapnia is permitted once there is adequate preductal oxygenation (preductal oxygenation is measured or obtained from the right upper extremity; the preductal blood perfuses the heart and brain). The highest rates of survival result in patients in whom barotrauma and volutrauma are avoided and permissive hypercapnia is allowed.

A patient is considered unstable or to have failed ventilator support when the pH is <7.25, a peak inspiratory pressure of >30 cm $H_2O$ is needed, and preductal saturation is <90% on 60% oxygen. The use of iNO ($INO_{max}$) may be considered in these cases, but the direct effect on pulmonary vascular resistance and right heart function need to be monitored closely. Therapy should be discontinued if no response is demonstrated. Extracorporeal membrane oxygenation is a reasonable choice for patients that have received maximum medical intervention. A venous-venous shunt is preferred unless there is significant cardiac instability.

Surgical correction is done if the infant is stable after the honeymoon period (the first 24 hours). Achievement of 90% survival is possible in a nonselect group of patients with the combination of careful ventilator management, attention to the pulmonary hypertension, delayed surgery, and aggressive early nutrition support. Survival rates are also dependent on the presence or absence of associated abnormalities and their severity. Long-term follow-up beyond the neonatal period is necessary for accurate estimation of morbidity and mortality in patients who are placed on ECMO.

# The Extremely Low Birth Weight Infant

A premature infant is a neonate who is delivered before 37 completed weeks of gestation. These infants can be further classified according to their birth weight:

- Low birth weight (LBW) if less than 2500 g
- Very low birth weight (VLBW) if less than 1500 g
- Extremely low birth weight (ELBW) if less than 1000 g

Within the ELBW infants is a subgroup called the micropremie, if birth weight is less than 750 g. The need for intrapartum and postnatal intervention and support is inversely proportional to gestational age as well as the morbidity and mortality associated with these infants. The increased risks for asphyxia, heat and water loss, intraventricular hemorrhage, and respiratory distress increase with decreasing gestational age. In the delivery room, the initial steps of resuscitation will support transition by preventing heat and water loss and asphyxia. The use of surfactant (Survanta) should be considered in ELBW infants. In infants more than 1000 g, surfactant replacement therapy should be done as soon as the neonate presents a clinical picture of surfactant deficiency (HMD). Surfactant should be given with the proper ventilator support and, it is not uncommon to require multiple doses. With delay in therapy the morbidity and mortality associated with HMD increases.

The ELBW infants are a special group within the premature infants because the advances in health care and technology seem to have had less of an impact on this group of infants. The overall morbidity and mortality continue to be comparatively high in these infants and more so in the micropremie or infants less than 27 weeks of gestation. Table 4 lists the common problems faced by the ELBW infants and their management.

## Special Therapy

Although there are continued attempts to provide care for the ELBW infant, there are infants outside the scope of *viability*—infants with complex congenital malformations, including those labeled as *incompatible with life*, and those whose condition is irreversible and ultimately will lead to death. For such infants, we see the need for comfort care or palliative care. In these situations both the health care professional and parents find themselves in an awkward position. The family remains

---

**TABLE 4 Common Problems and Management of the Extremely Low Birth Weight Infant**

| Problems | Management |
|---|---|
| **Delivery Room.** It is anticipated that a complete team will be needed for resuscitation: neonatal nurse, respiratory therapist, and neonatologist. | Prevent heat loss, provide respiratory support, prevent asphyxia, and avoid trauma. Place under radiant warmer and dry well, use warm blankets and cap. Use bag and mask properly and prompt intubation when needed. Properly position the ETT; avoid high inspiratory pressure with overdistention of the lungs. Follow the ABCs of resuscitation. |
| **NICU.** The management in the delivery room and the first hours of life sets the stage for the rest of the NICU care. | In the NICU, the infant is placed under a radiant warmer for easy access and thermoregulation. Connect to all monitors, insert umbilical venous and arterial catheters for fluid management, BP monitoring, and to facilitate blood draw. Obtain chest and abdominal radiograph to assess the severity of lung disease and position of the ETT, venous, and arterial catheters. Cover infant with plastic wrap to decrease evaporative heat and fluid loss. Frequent weighing with a bed scale will estimate hydration status. There should be minimal handling and clustered care in the first week of life. |
| **Fluid and Electrolytes.** The high insensible water loss in the ELBW infant increases the risk for dehydration, hypernatremia, and hyperkalemia | Fluid requirements range from 100 to 150 mL/kg/d, given as D5W with no added electrolytes in the first 24-48 h. Monitoring of the electrolytes and strict I&O will estimate the hydration status. Monitor blood draw and replace with PRBC from a single donor, CMV negative, when 10% of blood volume is removed. Hypernatremia is caused by increased water loss and corrected with increased intake of free water. Risk of hyperkalemia is caused by water loss and increases if there is extravascular blood collection; this is corrected using insulin infusion with glucose, correcting acidosis with sodium bicarbonate, calcium gluconate to stabilize the myocardium, and a cation exchange resin per rectum—sodium polystyrene sulfonate (Kayexalate). |

| Problems | Management |
|---|---|
| **Nutrition.** Long-term parenteral nutrition is required in these infants. Good nutritional support is necessary for growth and neurodevelopment. | Beginning early parenteral nutrition within the first 24 h in stable infants will provide a source of energy (glucose), protein to decrease the risk of negative nitrogen balance, calcium, vitamins, and trace minerals. Placement of percutaneous CVC should be done early in the course. Please refer to the section on nutrition in this article for further nutrition management. |
| **CNS.** There is an increased risk of developing IVH in unstable infants in the first few days of life. | To prevent IVH, stressful conditions like cold stress, hypoxemia, acidosis swing in BP, and increased intrathoracic pressure should be avoided. Initial US in the first 3 d if unstable and at the end of the first week if stable. Follow-up will depend on findings. Infants with no IVH should have a repeat at 36 weeks postmenstrual age. The use of sedation in the first week of life has not shown significant changes in the incidence of IVH. |
| **Respiratory.** HMD is the most common condition. Avoid complications associated with the disease (air leaks and pulmonary emphysema, pulmonary hemorrhage, ICH, and CLD). | Use of exogenous surfactant when indicated and rapid weaning of PIP and $O_2$ and close monitoring to avoid complications. Blood gas is obtained 10-15 min after each change. Use high ventilator rate and the lowest PIP to maintain saturation 93%-95%, permissive hypercapnia ($Paco_2$ 50-60), mild acidosis (pH 7.25-7.35), and $Po_2$ 50-70 are the goal. When stable, extubate to NCPAP. Apnea is common in these infants; they are treated with caffeine citrate (Cafcit). An initial bolus of 20 mg/kg is given followed by maintenance of 5 mg/kg every 24 h. |
| **Cardiovascular.** PDA occurs in >50% of ELBW infants. Appearing when the lung disease is improving, clinically there is increased need for respiratory support associated with desaturation, active precordium, bounding pulses, and wide pulse pressure. The diagnosis is confirmed by echocardiogram. The ductus arteriosus of the preterm responds less to the vasoconstrictive effect of oxygen. | Medical treatment consists of fluid restriction, maintenance of hematocrit around 40%, and the use of indomethacin (Indocin IV). Complications of indomethacin (Indocin IV) are decreased GFR causing fluid retention, and platelet dysfunction (contraindicated in renal failure, bleeding disorders, and low platelets). The dose is 0.2 mg/kg for four doses and a diuretic such as furosemide (Lasix) at 1 mg/kg/dose to try to prevent oliguria. If there is no response, additional dosing or courses can be given. The definitive treatment would be ligation of the ductus. Some centers use prophylactic indomethacin (Indocin IV). |
| **Skin.** Underdevelopment of the stratum corneum cause increase transepidermal water loss→dehydration→ electrolyte imbalance and evaporative heat loss. Traumatized skin is the port of entry for many infectious organisms. Acceleration of skin maturation occurs after birth over the next 10-14 d. | Use of plastic shields, increased humidity, and topical skin emollient will decrease heat and water loss and may be protective to the skin. |
| **Glucose.** Hyperglycemia is secondary to high glucose-infusion rates. When an infant becomes hyperglycemic on a stable glucose-infusion rate, consider infection and or IVH. Early hypoglycemia is common in this group of infants due to poor glycogen stores and immature hormonal adaptation of the endocrine system. | Glucose level should be >40 mg/dL in the first 48-72 h and >45 mg/dL after 72 h. When hypoglycemic, a bolus of D10W at 200 mg/kg (2 mL/kg) is given. Glucose level is obtained in 30 min, frequent monitoring is continued every 1-3 h, and further boluses are given as needed. Maintenance fluid provides 4-6 mg/kg/min of glucose infusion. This rate of infusion should be increased by 2 mg/kg/min with every need for D10W bolus. Refer to specific text for detailed management. |
| **Calcium.** The stores of calcium are limited and the reserves are rapidly depleted after birth. | Higher intake of calcium with adequate phosphorus intake is required for bone formation and growth. |
| **Jaundice.** These infants are at increased risk for brain toxicity from high bilirubin levels. High bilirubin level develops due to hepatic immaturity, shorter RBC life span, extravasation of blood, and increased enterohepatic circulation, coupled with lower serum albumin level. | The level that causes toxicity is lower in these infants. A crude method to determine the need for phototherapy at 50% the weight in kg: A 0.9 Kg infant is placed under phototherapy for a bilirubin level of 4.5 mg/dL. Exchange level is determined by the weight, in this case 9 mg/dL. The risk for toxicity increases in the unstable infant, the reason why lower levels should be used when managing. Fluid intake should be increased 15%-20% in infants under phototherapy. |

*Abbreviations:* ABC = airway, breathing, and circulation; BP = blood pressure; CLD = chronic lung disease; CMV = cytomegalovirus; CVC = central venous catheter; ELBW = extremely low birth weight infant; ETT = endotracheal tube; GFR = glomerular filtration rate; HMD = hyaline membrane disease; I&O = intake and output; ICH = intracranial hemorrhage; IV = intravenous; IVH = intraventricular hemorrhage; NCPAP = nasal continuous positive airway pressure; NICU = neonatal intensive care unit; PDA = patent ductus arteriosus; PIP = peak inspiratory pressure; PRBC = packed red blood cells; RBC = red blood cell; US = ultrasound.

## CURRENT DIAGNOSIS

- Review of risk factors: antenatal, perinatal, and postnatal
- Assessment of infants in the delivery room: airway, breathing and circulation—respiration, heart rate, and color
- Continued assessment in the nursery: respirations, heart rate, color, temperature, and CNS
- Common problems: pulmonary, circulatory, gastrointestinal, metabolic, surgical, and temperature instability

*Abbreviation:* CNS = central nervous system.

hopeful based on the perceived information that the health care professional gives, or the family goes through turmoil when interventions seem endless in a situation that they perceive as hopeless.

The decision for palliative care is made through collaboration between the health care team and the parents. The two factual considerations in making the decision for palliative care are pertinent medical facts (diagnosis, response to treatment given, potential response to other treatments, and prognosis) and the human value (what the parents anticipate, expect, and desire for their infant) and what motivates these values in the parents. The values of the health care team involved in the care of the infant are also considered.

Palliative care, as defined by the World Health Organization (WHO), is care for patients for whom cure is no longer a reasonable expectation or possibility. It is an active and comprehensive management of the entire patient, and not abandonment of care.

Practical considerations that need to be taken into account, and specific components of the palliative care that are appropriate for each individual high-risk neonate, are considered before a specific plan can be put in place. The application of palliative care in the NICU is not only possible, but necessary.

## CURRENT THERAPY

- Use functioning equipment and qualified personnel in the delivery room: initial steps and ABCs of neonatal resuscitation.
- Provide neutral thermal environment.
- Respiratory and cardiovascular support: oxygen, mechanical ventilation, vasopressor agent (dopamine).
- Infuse bolus of D10W and glucose at 6-8 mg/kg per minute or higher if needed.
- Use phototherapy for early jaundice and the bruised ELBW infant.
- Transfer to appropriate level of care when indicated.
- Monitor closely fluid and electrolytes and decreased IWL. Provide good nutritional support beginning in the first 24 hours and closely monitor for complications and tolerance.
- Provide family-centered care and appropriate environment to promote growth and development.
- Benefit special cases, especially those deemed futile, with a multidisciplinary approach.

*Abbreviations:* ABC = airway, breathing, and circulation; ELBW = extremely low birth weight; IWL = insensible water loss.

## REFERENCES

Aly H: Respiratory disorders in the newborn: Identification and diagnosis. Pediatr Rev 2004;25:201-208.

Avery GB, Fletcher MA, Macdonald MG (eds): Neonatology: Pathophysiology and Management of the Newborn, 5th ed. Philadelphia, Lippincott Williams & Wilkins, 1999, pp 143-173.

Blackburn ST: Maternal, Fetal, and Neonatal Physiology: A Clinical Perspective, 2nd ed. Philadelphia, WB Saunders, 2003, pp 707-730.

Carter BS: Comfort care principles for the high-risk newborn. NeoReviews 2004;e484-e490.

Chescheir NC, Harsen WF: What's new in perinatology. Pediatr Rev 1999;20: 57-63.

Downard CD, Wilson JM: Current therapy of infants with congenital diaphragmatic hernia. Semin Neonatol 2003;8:215-221.

Field TM: Stimulation of preterm infants. Pediatr Rev 2003;24:4-10.

Heird WC: Determination of nutritional requirements in preterm infants, with special reference to "catch-up" growth. Semin Neonatol 2001;6:365-375.

Klaus MH, Fanaroff MB: Care of the High-Risk Neonate, 5th ed. Philadelphia, WB Saunders, 2001, pp 195-215.

Kattwinkel J (ed): Neonatal Resuscitation Textbok, 5th ed. American Heart Association, American Academy of Pediatrics, Elk Grove Village, Ill.

Kleinman RE (ed): Pediatric Nutrition Handbook, 5th ed. American Academy of Pediatrics, Elk Grove Village, Ill, 2004, pp 23-55.

Thureen PJ, Deacon J, O'Neill P, Hernandez JA: Assessment and care of the well newborn. Philadelphia, WB Saunders, 1999, pp 83-113.

Welch KK, Malone FD: Advances in prenatal screening: Nuchal translucency ultrasonography in the first trimester. NeoReviews 2002;3:e202-e208.

Welch KK, Malone FD: Advances in prenatal screening: Maternal serum screening for Down syndrome. Neoreviews 2002;3:e209-e213.

# Normal Infant Feeding

Method of
*Meg Begany, RD, CSP, LDN, and
Maria Mascarenhas, MBBS*

Adequate and appropriate nutrition is especially critical during infancy. Infancy, defined as birth to 1 year of age, is characterized by the period of most rapid growth and development during the life cycle. In addition, recent research shows that nutrition during infancy can influence risk factors for disease at other stages of the life cycle.

## Infant Feeding

For the healthy term infant, the suck-swallow and rooting reflexes are present at birth, and thus liquid feedings can be initiated almost immediately following delivery.

### BREAST-FEEDING

The American Academy of Pediatrics (AAP) recommends human milk as the feeding of choice for nearly all infants whenever possible and mutually desirable for the mother and infant. Successful lactation and breast-feeding requires a supportive environment for the mother provided by the medical practitioner, including instruction and counseling. The World Health Organization (WHO) Expert Consultation on the Optimal Duration of Exclusive Breastfeeding, which considered the results of a systematic review of the evidence, concluded that human milk is recommended as the exclusive source of nutrition for the first 6 months and continuing human milk in combination with complementary foods until at least 12 months of age. The nutrient needs of the full-term normal birth weight infant can be met by human milk alone, with few exceptions, for the first 6 months if the mother is well nourished. The benefits of breast-feeding over formula feeding are well established and include enhanced maturity and motility of the gastrointestinal tract; maternal–infant bonding; monetary savings; facilitated fat, protein, and carbohydrate digestion and absorption; passive immunity; improved cognitive development; and decreased incidence of otitis media and respiratory and gastrointestinal disease. Further potential benefits, such as lower risk of overweight in children and adults, as well as decreased risk of cardiovascular disease in adulthood, were demonstrated in recent research.

Breast-feeding should be offered as early as possible after birth and then every 2 to 3 hours until satiety for approximately 10 to 15 minutes per breast during the first few weeks. Less frequent feedings may occur once breast-feeding is established. Intervals of more than 5 hours in between breast-feeding should be avoided during the first few weeks, including at night. Adequacy of breast-feeding is demonstrated when the infant has feedings 8 to 12 times per day, at least 6 to 8 wet diapers per day, regular stooling pattern, and is growing along established growth curves.

The composition of breast milk varies from individual to individual, as well as within the same individual, with composition changes occurring with stage of lactation, time of day, maternal diet, and time elapsed since feeding began. Milk production tends to be higher during the daytime, and fat content is increased toward the end of a feeding. On average, breast milk provides approximately 20 calories per ounce.

Contraindications to breast-feeding include maternal infections by organisms known to be transmitted to the infant via breast milk (e.g., HIV); maternal exposure to drugs, foods, or environmental agents that are excreted in human milk and harmful to the infant; and inborn errors of metabolism that are exacerbated by components present in human milk (e.g., galactosemia).

## INFANT FORMULA

When a mother chooses not to breast-feed or human milk is not an option, infant formula is an appropriate substitute. Although the composition of infant formula does not exactly duplicate that of breast milk, the composition of infant formulas continues to evolve in an effort to do so. The addition of docosahexaenoic acid (DHA) and arachidonic acid (ARA) is a recent modification to infant formula. Unlike breast milk, infant formulas prior to 2002 contained only the precursor essential fatty acids, linoleic and α-linolenic acids, from which DHA and ARA had to be synthesized. Multiple studies in both preterm and term infants have demonstrated significantly lower levels of DHA and ARA in the erythrocytes of formula-fed infants compared to their breast-fed counterparts. This suggested that infant formula containing only the precursors, α-linolenic acid and linoleic acid, could be ineffective in allowing adequate synthesis of DHA and ARA. Thus multiple studies have been published comparing visual acuity, developmental outcomes, and growth of infants fed DHA and ARA supplemented and unsupplemented formula or breast milk. Some of these studies, but not all, found short-term improvements in visual and cognitive functions in both preterm and term infants. However, no long-term benefits were demonstrated. Although the single supplementation of DHA alone resulted in ARA deficiency status and poor growth in premature infants, the balanced supplementation of both DHA and ARA consistently do not show any adverse effect on growth.

Both iron-fortified and low-iron formulas are commercially available. The AAP has stated that there is no role for the use of low-iron formulas in infant feeding and recommends that all formulas fed to infants be fortified with iron. Well-controlled studies failed to show a benefit, in terms of feeding tolerance, related to the use of low-iron formula. The amount of iron present in iron-fortified formulas meets the iron requirements through the entire first year.

Infant formula should be prepared and stored with careful attention to the manufacturer's guidelines to prevent the risk of bacterial growth.

## VITAMIN AND MINERAL SUPPLEMENTATION

The majority of vitamin and mineral requirements for infants are met in full by breast milk or infant formula. Guidelines for supplementation of vitamin K, vitamin D, iron, and fluoride are established. A single dose of vitamin K is typically given to all infants intramuscularly at birth to prevent hemorrhagic disease of the newborn.

For the breast-fed infant, the AAP recommends a supplement of 200 IU of vitamin D by 2 months of age. A multivitamin or tri-vitamin preparation can be used; solitary vitamin D supplements are not practical because of cost and dosing.

The iron requirements for formula-fed infants are met through iron-fortified formula. Although the iron content of human milk is minimal, its bioavailability is high. However, the iron body stores of the breast-fed infant diminish by 4 to 6 months of age, and thus an additional iron source is recommended at this age. Iron needs of the breast-fed infant can be met with the introduction of complementary foods when foods with good sources of iron are included (e.g., meat, fish, iron-fortified cereal, whole grains, and dark leafy green vegetables).

Fluoride supplementation is recommended at 6 months of age for both breast-fed infants and formula-fed infants who receive exclusively ready-to-feed formulas or whose water supply contains less than 0.3 ppm of fluoride.

## INTRODUCTION OF COMPLEMENTARY FOODS

At approximately 6 months of age, human milk or infant formula can no longer supply all of an infant's nutrition requirements, and complementary foods are needed to ensure adequate nutrition and growth. It is the micronutrients, rather than energy and protein, which are likely to become lacking. The ability to digest and absorb carbohydrates, proteins, and fats is mature by 6 months of age. Trypsin and chymotrypsin activities increase during the first 4 months of life. Age should not be the only factor in determining the timing of introduction of complementary feeding, but rather the timing should be determined by individual physical and psychological readiness of the infant, as well as rate of maturation of the nervous system, intestinal tract, and kidneys. Before spoon feedings are introduced, the infant should exhibit trunk stability, head control, and disappearance of the extrusion reflex. At approximately 5 to 6 months, an infant is able to indicate a desire for food by leaning forward and opening his or her mouth to indicate hunger and leaning back and turning away to show disinterest or satiety. Muraro et al. state that introduction of complementary feedings prior to 4 months of age is associated with an increased risk of atopic eczema and cow's milk protein allergy. There are presently no controlled studies showing an allergy preventative effect of restrictive diets after 6 months of age. Studies suggest that introducing complementary foods prior to 6 months does not result in increased caloric intake and has no growth advantage because the infant will displace breast milk to maintain the same level of caloric intake. Although it is possible to meet the nutrition needs of the infant solely from infant formula through the entire first year, delay of introduction of solids can lead to feeding aversions and food refusal. All infants need exposure to a variety of tastes, textures, and foods to develop appropriate feeding practices and a wider acceptance of new foods. In addition to adequate nutrition, the feeding relationship between the infant and caregiver is vital for normal growth and development.

To observe for symptoms of intolerance, only one new food should be introduced every 3 days. Because of its hypoallergenicity, infant rice cereal is often introduced as the first feeding. However, if spoon feeding is initiated at 6 months of age, gastrointestinal and renal development is mature enough to allow feedings from multiple food groups. Despite enhanced bioavailability, breast milk is relatively low in iron and zinc. Because low liver reserves of zinc at birth may predispose some infants to zinc deficiency, similar to the situation for iron, meat may be the ideal first food to provide these nutrients at the levels needed. Dr. Samuel Fomon states that unless there is a strong family history of allergy, introduction of soft-cooked red meats is desirable by 5 to 6 months of age. Furthermore, the proportion of Dietary Reference Intakes that needs to be supplied by complementary foods is highest for iron, zinc, phosphorus, and magnesium. Regardless of the food choice for the first feeding, the consistency should be thin and liquid/pureed. Thinning foods with breast milk or infant formula

## CURRENT THERAPY

**Infant Formula Composition and Indications**

| FORMULA | EXAMPLES | INDICATIONS | CHARACTERISTICS |
|---|---|---|---|
| Milk based | Enfamil LIPIL<br>Similac Advance<br>Enfamil LactoFree LIPIL<br>Similac Lactose Free<br>Enfamil AR LIPIL<br>  (prethickened)<br>Good Start Supreme | Breast milk substitute<br>  for term infants | Ready to feed, powder,<br>  or liquid concentrate<br>Variable whey: casein<br>20 kcal/oz<br>Contain DHA/ARA |
| Soy based | ProSobee<br>Isomil<br>Good Start Supreme Soy<br>Isomil DF | Breast milk substitute<br>  for infants with lactose<br>  intolerance or milk<br>  protein allergy* | Lactose free; some<br>  sucrose free<br>Ready to feed, powder,<br>  or liquid concentrate<br>20 kcal/oz<br>Contain DHA/ARA<br>May contain fiber |
| Premature (hospital grade) | Enfamil Premature LIPIL<br>Similac Special CareAdvance | Breast milk substitute<br>  for low birth weight<br>  hospitalized preterm<br>  infants | Low lactose<br>60:40 whey-to-casein<br>  ratio<br>High calcium and<br>  phosphorus<br>Contain MCT<br>20 and 24 cal/oz<br>Contain DHA/ARA<br>Ready to feed only |
| Human milk fortifiers | Similac HMF<br>Enfamil HMF | Fortification of human<br>  milk for low birth<br>  weight preterm infants | Increase calorie,<br>  protein, and<br>  vitamin/mineral content<br>  of breast milk<br>Contain MCT |
| Premature transitional | NeoSure Advance<br>EnfaCare LIPIL | Breast milk substitute<br>  for preterm infants<br>  >2.5 kg or discharge<br>  formula for preterm<br>  infants (used until<br>  6–12 mo corrected<br>  age or until catch-up<br>  growth is completed) | 22 kcal/oz<br>Ready to feed or powder<br>Contain DHA/ARA<br>Vitamin and mineral<br>  content between that of<br>  term and premature<br>  formulas |
| Hypoallergenic/protein<br>  hydrolysate | Nutramigen | Milk or soy protein<br>  allergy | Hydrolyzed protein<br>Ready to feed, powder, or<br>  liquid concentrate<br>Sucrose free<br>Lactose free<br>No MCT |
| Protein hydrolysate with<br>  MCT | Alimentum<br>Pregestimil | Malabsorption<br>Short bowel syndrome<br>Allergy | Lactose free<br>Hydrolyzed protein<br>Contain MCT<br>Ready to feed or powder |
| Amino acid based | Neocate<br>EleCare | Malabsorption<br>Short bowel syndrome<br>Allergy | Lactose free<br>Free amino acids<br>Powder only |
| Fat modified | Portagen (no longer<br>  recommended for<br>  infants)<br>Alimentum<br>Pregestimil | Defects in digestion,<br>  absorption, or<br>  transport of fat | Contain increased % of<br>  kcal as MCT |

## CURRENT THERAPY — cont'd

**Infant Formula Composition and Indications**

| FORMULA | EXAMPLES | INDICATIONS | CHARACTERISTICS |
|---|---|---|---|
| Carbohydrate modified | RCF<br>Product 3232 A | Simple sugar intolerance | Requires addition of complex carbohydrate to be complete |
| Amino acid modified | Multiple products (e.g., Cyclinex, MSUD Analog, Phenyl-Free) | Inborn errors of metabolism | Low or devoid of specific amino acids that cannot be metabolized |
| Electrolyte modified | Similac PM 60/40 | Renal or other disease state requiring low renal solute load | Decreased potassium content<br>Decreased calcium and phosphorus content |

*Children allergic to milk protein may also be allergic to soy protein.
*Abbreviations:* ARA = arachidonic acid; DHA = docosahexaenoic acid; HMF = human milk fortifier; MCT = medium chain triglycerides; MSUD = maple syrup urine disease.

---

can enhance acceptability of the food by the infant. Repeated exposure to a new food may be necessary before it is accepted.

By 9 months of age, finely chopped foods and finger foods can be added to the infant's diet. At 12 months of age, rotary chewing is well controlled, and many infants can progress to table foods. Choking hazards that are round and hard, such as grapes, nuts, popcorn, hot dogs, and hard candy, should be avoided.

For the average healthy infant, meals of complementary foods should be provided two to three times per day from 6 to 8 months of age and three to four times per day from 9 to 12 months of age, with addition of nutritious snacks once or twice per day as desired. Vegetarian diets cannot meet nutrient needs at this age unless fortified products or nutrient supplements are provided. Estimates of the energy gap that must be filled by complementary food in industrialized countries is approximately 130 kcal/day at 6 to 8 months, 310 kcal/day at 9 to 11 months and 580 kcal/day at 12 to 23 months of age.

Juice is not a necessary component of the diet and may displace the intake of nutrient-dense breast milk or formula. In addition, offering juice by bottle can contribute to dental caries. If juice is provided, it should be limited to 4 to 8 ounces per day and should not be given prior to 6 months of age.

Whole cow's milk should not be introduced before 12 months of age because of its low iron content, high renal solute load, potential for causing gastrointestinal bleeding, and increased risk of cow's milk protein allergy. Furthermore, cow's milk is a poor source of vitamin C, vitamin E, and essential fatty acids. Breast-fed infants weaned before 12 months of age should receive an iron-fortified infant formula rather than cow's milk.

## Nutritional Requirements

Because of the rapid rate of growth and development during infancy, nutrient needs per unit of body weight are very high in comparison to that of the older child or adult. Energy needs for the healthy term infant are 108 kcal/kg from birth to 6 months of age. From 6 to 12 months of age, caloric needs are 98 kcal/kg. The Recommended Daily Allowance (RDA) for protein is 2.2 g/kg from birth to 6 months of age and 1.6 g/kg from 6 to 12 months of age. Caloric distribution during infancy is recommended to be 40% to 50% fat, 7% to 11% protein, and 40% to 55% carbohydrate. The water-to-energy ratio should be 1.5 mL/kcal. Both human milk and infant formulas are models of this distribution. Hydration requirements are met by breast milk or infant formula without further addition of water to the diet, except potentially during periods of illness with fever, diarrhea, or emesis.

## Growth

Weight, length, and head circumference should be monitored serially during infancy and plotted on the gender-specific 2000 CDC (Centers for Disease Control and Prevention) Growth Charts. Breast-fed infants tend to gain less weight and usually are leaner than formula-fed infants in the second half of infancy. This difference does not seem to be the result of nutritional deficits but rather infant self-regulation of energy intake.

Obesity is increasing among children in the United States. High rates of weight gain during the first few months of life are associated with obesity in childhood and early adulthood. Optimal nutrition and growth during infancy should be promoted by encouraging healthy eating patterns in the infant to prepare for a healthy lifestyle later in life. Early identification and intervention may be a key component for establishing appropriate weight gain patterns.

Although no consensus exists on universal criteria to define failure to thrive, careful evaluation should occur when weight is less than the 5th percentile or falls more than two major percentiles from a previously established growth channel. In addition, relationship of weight to height must be considered. Prompt intervention with nutritional rehabilitation is essential to prevent illness, growth stunting, cognitive delay, and social and behavioral problems.

For the treatment of either over- or undernutrition, a multidisciplinary team approach involving the physician, dietitian, psychologist, and social worker, along with community services, can often be beneficial and necessary.

In conclusion, infant feeding during the first year of life is a complex process, and guidelines are based on developmental, nutritional, and social factors. Human milk is superior to infant formula and should be the feeding of choice for all infants. Although infant formulas do not exactly duplicate breast milk, the composition of infant formulas continues to evolve in an effort to do so. Complementary foods should be introduced at 6 months of age. Cow's milk should not be introduced until 1 year of age. Careful attention should be paid to growth and nutritional status throughout infancy, with prompt attention to any deviation from expected growth patterns.

## CURRENT DIAGNOSIS

**Expected Growth Velocity during Infancy**

| AGE | WEIGHT GAIN (g/d) | LENGTH (cm/mo) | HEAD CIRCUMFERENCE (cm/wk) |
|---|---|---|---|
| 0–3 mo | 25–35 | 2.5–3.5 | 0.3–0.6 |
| 3–6 mo | 15–21 | 1.6–2.5 | 0.2–0.5 |
| 6–12 mo | 10–13 | 1.2–1.7 | 0.1–0.4 |

## REFERENCES

American Academy of Pediatrics, Committee on Nutrition: Iron fortification of infant formulas. Pediatrics 1999;104:119-123.

American Academy of Pediatrics, Section on Breastfeeding: Breastfeeding and the use of human milk. Pediatrics 2005;115:496-506.

Dewey KG: Nutrition, growth and complementary feeding of the breastfed infant. Pediatr Clin North Am 2001;48:87-104.

Foman SJ: Feeding normal infants: Rationale for recommendations. J Am Diet Assoc 2001;101:1002-1005.

http://www.cdc.gov/growthcharts

Kleinman RE (ed): Pediatric Nutrition Handbook, 5th ed. Elk Grove Village, Ill, American Academy of Pediatrics, Committee on Nutrition, 2003.

Michaelsen KF: Cows' milk in complementary feeding. Pediatrics 2000;106: 1302-1303.

Muraro A, Dreborg S, Halken S, et al: Dietary prevention of allergic diseases in infants and small children. Part III: Critical review of published peer-reviewed observational and interventional studies and final recommendations. Pediatr Allergy Immunol 2004;15:291-307.

PAHO and WHO: Guiding Principles for Complementary Feeding of the Breastfed Child. Washington, DC, Pan American Health Organization and World Health Organization, 2003.

Samour PQ, King K (eds): Handbook of Pediatric Nutrition, 3rd ed. Sudbury, Mass, Jones and Bartlett, 2005.

Slaughter CW, Bryant AH: Hungry for love: The feeding relationship in the psychological development of young children. Permanente J 2004;8:23-29.

WHO Working Group on the Growth Reference Protocol and the WHO Task Force on Methods for the Natural Regulation of Fertility: Growth of healthy infants and the timing, type, and frequency of complementary foods. Am J Clin Nutr 2002;76:620-627.

# Diseases of the Breast

Method of
*Paniti Sukumvanich, MD,*
*and Patrick Borgen, MD*

## Benign Diseases of the Breast

Benign diseases of the breast historically are subdivided into proliferative and nonproliferative lesions (Table 1). In a study by Dupont and Page, patients with breast biopsies yielding nonproliferative lesions had no increased risk of subsequent breast cancer. In contrast, proliferative lesions were associated with a minimal to a fivefold increased risk of breast cancer. In clinical practice, of the proliferative lesions, only atypical epithelial lesions increase breast cancer risk significantly. Appropriate treatment and counseling of patients depends on the risk of breast cancer associated with these benign breast diseases.

## Nonproliferative Lesions

Nonproliferative lesions comprise mild hyperplasia without atypia, squamous or apocrine metaplasia, duct ectasia, mastitis, and cysts. In the study of 3303 patients by Dupont and Page, only 2.2% of patients with nonproliferative lesions had breast cancer following a benign breast biopsy with a mean follow-up time of 17 years (Figure 1).

### BREAST CYSTS AND FIBROCYSTIC BREAST DISEASE

Fibrocystic breast disease is a benign process in which generalized microcystic formation with stromal proliferation leads to increased breast nodularity. Cysts within the breast are most common in perimenopausal women 50 to 59 years of age as well as premenopausal women. Postmenopausal women not on hormone replacement therapy are unlikely to develop cysts in their breasts. Benign cysts are often

**TABLE 1   Benign Diseases of the Breast**

|  | Increase in Breast Cancer Risk |
|---|---|
| **Nonproliferative Lesions** | |
| Mild hyperplasia without atypia | None |
| Squamous or apocrine metaplasia | None |
| Duct ectasia | None |
| Mastitis | None |
| Cysts | None |
| **Proliferative Lesions** | |
| Fibroadenoma | None |
| Moderate or florid hyperplasia | Minimal |
| Microglandular adenosis | Minimal |
| Sclerosing adenosis | Minimal |
| Papilloma | Minimal |
| Atypical ductal hyperplasia | 4- to 5-fold |
| Atypical lobular hyperplasia | 5.8-fold |

tender and fluctuate in size with the menstrual cycle. Cysts may be detected either on physical examination as a palpable, smooth, mobile nodule or by breast ultrasound. They may appear as a solitary nodule or in a cluster. Ultrasonographic appearance of simple benign cysts is that of an anechoic, round or oval, well-circumscribed mass with posterior enhancement. If the mass has all four criteria, the accuracy of ultrasound is close to 100% for the diagnosis of a simple benign cyst. Cysts that appear complex, with internal echoes, thick septations, and irregular walls, are suspicious for breast carcinoma and should be examined surgically or with an ultrasound-guided biopsy. Confirmation of the diagnosis can be made by fine-needle aspiration (FNA) of the cystic fluid. Bloody fluid may be an indication for a biopsy. In a study of 6782 cyst aspirates, Ciatto and colleagues found that cytologic examination identified atypical cells in 1677 specimens. Of these specimens, only 0.3% of these cases had clinically and radiologically negative intracystic papillomas. Cytologic examination was positive in

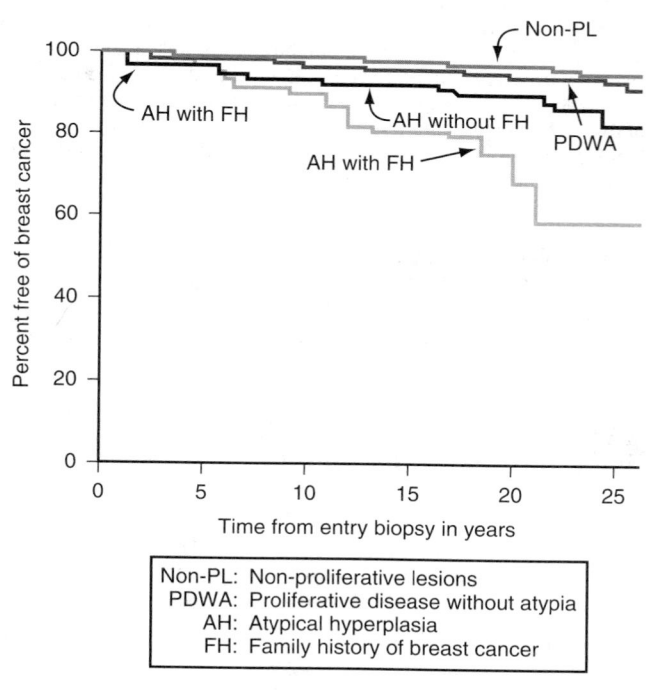

Non-PL: Non-proliferative lesions
PDWA: Proliferative disease without atypia
AH: Atypical hyperplasia
FH: Family history of breast cancer

**FIGURE 1.** Nonproliferative lesions in breast cancer.

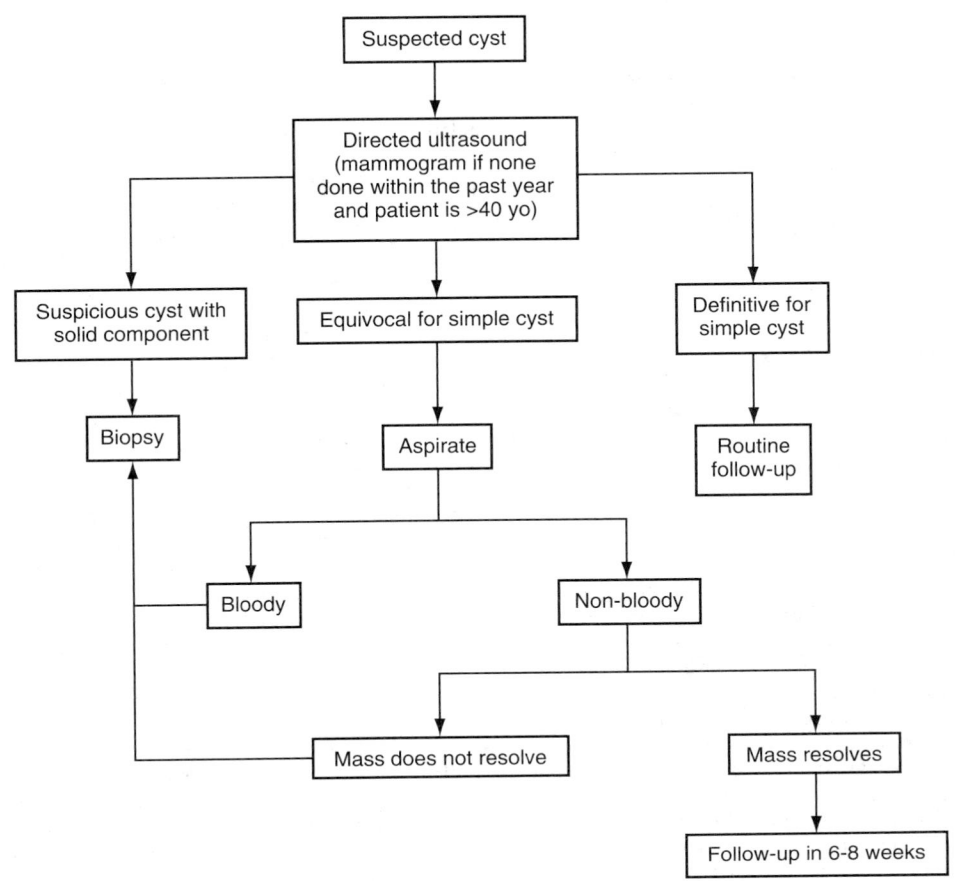

**FIGURE 2.** Algorithm for the management of suspected cysts.

only 0.1% of these cases. Thus fluid from cyst aspirations are not sent routinely for cytologic examination. Figure 2 describes the management of suspected cysts.

## MASTITIS AND DUCT ECTASIA

Mastitis is divided into lactational or nonlactational. Lactational mastitis can occur from the reflux of bacteria into the breast during breast-feeding. The causative bacteria are usually gram-positive cocci. Patients should be treated with antibiotics with the appropriate coverage and can continue to nurse or pump the breast to prevent engorgement. Nursing mothers can continue to breast-feed because the infant is not at risk for infection. Nonlactational (periductal) mastitis can be caused by duct ectasia, which occurs when the milk ducts become congested with secretions and debris, resulting in a periductal inflammation. These patients may present with greenish nipple discharge, nipple retraction, and subareolar noncyclical pain. The treatment of nonlactational mastitis includes broad-spectrum antibiotics to cover for gram-positive cocci and skin anaerobes. Total duct excision and eversion of the nipple may be necessary to treat recurrent periductal mastitis.

# Proliferative Benign Breast Diseases

Proliferative breast diseases include moderate or florid hyperplasia, microglandular and sclerosing adenosis, papilloma, fibroadenoma, and atypical ductal and lobular hyperplasia. All proliferative lesions have an increased risk of subsequent breast cancer after biopsy except for fibroadenoma. Overall, with a median follow-up of 17 years, 5.3% of patients with proliferative lesions develop breast cancer. This percentage increases to 12.9% in the presence of atypia (see Figure 1). Patients with

moderate or florid hyperplasia, sclerosing adenosis, and solitary papilloma without atypia carry a minimal increase in risk of developing breast cancer over the general population. These patients are not classified as high risk. But the risk of subsequent breast cancer is increased by four- to fivefold in the presence of atypia. Atypical lobular hyperplasia carries a higher risk than atypical ductal hyperplasia, with a relative risk as high as 5.8. This increased risk applies to the contralateral breast because subsequent breast carcinomas are evenly divided between both breasts.

## PROLIFERATIVE LESIONS WITH NO INCREASED RISK OF SUBSEQUENT CANCER: FIBROADENOMA

Fibroadenomas are benign tumors commonly found in young women (less than 30 years of age with a peak incidence at 21 to 25 years of age). They are characteristically detected on physical examination as well-circumscribed, rubbery, highly mobile, palpable masses. On mammograms, these lesions may appear as a well-circumscribed mass. Involution of fibroadenomas in the elderly can lead to hyalinization and dense popcorn-like calcification on mammograms. Fibroadenomas pose no increased risk of breast cancer and do not mandate surgical removal unless desired by the patient. Pregnancy can increase the size of these lesions; thus it may be reasonable to remove them prior to a planned pregnancy. Removal may facilitate follow-up, given the inability to follow breast masses adequately during pregnancy. Other types of fibroadenomas include juvenile and giant fibroadenomas. Juvenile fibroadenomas occur in adolescent women and can grow larger than 5 cm in diameter. These lesions are not malignant; given their large size, however, surgical excision may be needed to prevent asymmetry of the breasts. Giant fibroadenomas are large fibroadenomas found in the lactating breast or in the breasts of pregnant patients. These lesions may regress in size once hormonal stimulation subsides. Lesions that remain large can be excised surgically. Fibroadenomas and phyllodes tumors may be linked. Any rapidly enlarging fibroadenoma should be considered for surgical excision to rule out phyllodes tumor because it is difficult clinically to differentiate fibroadenoma from phyllodes tumor.

## PROLIFERATIVE LESIONS WITH MINIMAL INCREASED RISK OF SUBSEQUENT BREAST CANCER

### Multiple Peripheral Papillomas

Multiple peripheral papillomas are lesions that occur in the peripheral ducts. They most commonly present as a mass but may also present with nipple discharge. Complete excisional removal should be considered to rule out a papillary carcinoma of the breast. Approximately 10% to 33% of patients have subsequent breast cancer; thus close follow-up of these patients is warranted.

### Sclerosing and Microglandular Adenosis

Sclerosing adenosis occurs as result of the proliferation of stromal tissue along with small terminal ductules. Often these lesions are picked up incidentally, but they may also present as microcalcifications on mammogram or as a mass (termed *adenosis tumor*). Sclerosing adenosis may be confused with a tubular carcinoma. Staining with immunohistochemical (IHC) markers such as actin, smooth muscle myosin heavy chain p63, or calponin may be helpful in distinguishing between the two lesions because only sclerosing adenosis contains myoepithelial cells. Microglandular adenosis is an uncommon lesion that may be mistaken for tubular carcinoma on histologic examination, and it can increase the patient's subsequent breast cancer risk. Concomitant breast cancer has been reported, so complete surgical excision should be considered for these lesions.

## PROLIFERATIVE LESIONS WITH A FOUR- TO FIVEFOLD RISK OF SUBSEQUENT BREAST CANCER: ATYPICAL DUCTAL AND LOBULAR HYPERPLASIA

Atypical ductal and lobular hyperplasia are very similar to their in situ counterparts. These lesions are termed *atypical hyperplasia* because they lack some of the microscopic features of in situ disease. The distinction between atypical hyperplasia and carcinoma in situ is sometimes hard to make. In a study by Rosai, five expert breast cancer pathologists reviewed 17 cases of ductal or lobular lesions. In no case did all five agree on a diagnosis. Four out of the five were able to agree on a diagnosis in three cases (18%). In one third of the patients, the diagnosis ran the gamut from hyperplasia without atypia to carcinoma in situ. Despite such difficulty, the diagnosis of atypical hyperplasia is on the rise as mammographic screening becomes more popular. Atypical hyperplasia, which is detected secondary to microcalcifications or by serendipity, carries the highest risk of subsequent breast carcinoma among all proliferative lesions of the breast, with a four- to fivefold increased risk over the general population. Atypical lobular hyperplasia carries a higher risk than atypical ductal hyperplasia, with a relative risk as high as 5.8. This risk applies to the contralateral breast as well as the ipsilateral breast. Surgical excision of atypical hyperplasia on a core biopsy is recommended because 20% of patients are found to have breast cancer at time of surgical excision for atypical hyperplasia. It is not necessary to achieve negative margins for these lesions.

## OTHER BENIGN BREAST LESIONS: FAT NECROSIS, HAMARTOMA, MONDOR'S DISEASE, RADIAL SCARS, AND PSEUDOANGIOMATOUS STROMAL HYPERPLASIA

Other benign lesions of the breast include fat necrosis, hamartoma, Mondor's disease, radial scars, and pseudoangiomatous stromal hyperplasia (PASH). Trauma to the breast may lead to fat necrosis and can be mistaken for carcinomas on clinical examination. Fat necrosis lesions present clinically as painless, irregular masses with or without associated skin changes such as skin thickening. These lesions can be normal or may have rim calcifications on mammograms. No further treatment is needed when a core biopsy definitively makes the diagnosis of fat necrosis.

Hamartomas are benign lesions that are often picked up on a mammogram. The fatty composition of the mass makes these lesions clinically occult. They can be mistaken for fibroadenomas on mammograms. Hamartomas can be left alone without histologic confirmation if diagnosed definitively on a mammogram.

Mondor's disease is a thrombophlebitis of the superficial breast veins that presents as a palpable tender cord leading to the axilla. In a study of 63 cases, 8 patients (25%) had an underlying malignancy; thus a mammogram should be done to rule out the presence of breast carcinoma.

Radial scars are benign lesions whose etiology is unknown. They are often mistaken for breast carcinoma on mammograms because of their stellate appearance. Radial scars may also mimic breast carcinoma histologically. Staining for myoepithelial cells can help distinguish between invasive carcinoma and a radial scar. Radial scars carry a 1.5-fold increase in risk of subsequent breast carcinoma, so these lesions should be considered markers of future disease.

First described in 1986, PASH is a benign proliferative lesion that may present as an incidental finding or a mobile breast mass. It can occur in all ages and also in men. On a mammogram, PASH appears as a round noncalcified mass. Histologically, PASH may be mistaken for low-grade angiosarcoma. Unlike angiosarcoma, however, there should be no evidence of mitosis or cytologic atypia in PASH specimens. The role of hormones in the pathogenesis of PASH is controversial. Although these lesions tend to occur in young patients or in elderly patients on hormone therapy, most cases tend to be negative for estrogen receptors. The treatment for PASH is complete surgical excision. Approximately 7% of cases recur despite adequate treatment.

## Risk Factors for Breast Cancer

An estimated 80% of women in whom breast cancer develops have no documented risk factors or determinants. Risk factors cannot be changed, whereas risk determinants can be altered to decrease a person's risk of subsequent breast cancer. Common risk factors include a familial history of breast cancer, personal breast biopsy history, menarche before 12 years of age, menopause after 55 years of age, increasing age, geographical location, and mutations of the BRCA1 or BRCA2 genes. Women known to have the BRCA1 or BRCA2 genetic mutation have an 85% lifetime risk of breast cancer as well as an increased risk of ovarian cancer. BRCA1 carriers are at a higher risk for developing ovarian cancer than BRCA2 (60% versus 20%, respectively). The risk determinants for breast cancer include reproductive factors such as nulliparity and first pregnancy after the age of 30 years and previous radiation exposure. Previous therapy for lymphoma, especially during adolescence, elevates a woman's risk of subsequent breast cancer.

## Screening Techniques

Screening for breast cancer includes mammography, ultrasound, breast self-examination (BSE), and physical examination by a physician. Multiple studies such as the Göthenborg and Malmö trials show a reduction in breast cancer mortality from 30% to 40% in patients 40 to 49 years of age who undergo screening mammograms. A meta-analysis of six randomized trials indicates a 30% reduction in breast cancer mortality in patients 50 to 69 years of age. The sensitivity of mammograms depends on the patient's age and ranges from 53% to 81% in women 40 to 49 years of age to 73% to 81% in patients 50 years of age or older. An estimated 10% to 15% of breast cancer cases are not detectable on screening mammography, thus emphasizing the importance of physical breast examination by a physician and BSE that include both visual inspection and manual examination of the breast.

On inspection, signs of breast malignancy include skin or nipple retraction or discoloration, nipple discharge/crusting, or peau d'orange edema of the breast. On palpation, any asymmetric mass of the breast or axilla may be regarded as a potential malignancy that deserves further evaluation.

Current recommendations are for a woman to start performing BSE at 18 years of age, have a yearly physical exam, and initiate annual mammography at 40 years of age. Little data exist on what should be the upper age limit of mammogram screening. Given that breast density decreases with age and breast cancer increases with age, mammograms should be even more sensitive and specific in the older age group. For these reasons, mammograms may be continued in very elderly patients as long as the patient is not suffering from any major co-morbidities. In patients who have a very high risk of breast cancer, such as BRCA carriers, screening should start 10 years earlier than the age of onset of an affected relative or at the age of 35. Kriege screened 1909 patients (including 358 BRCA mutation carriers) who had more than a 15% lifetime risk of developing breast cancer. These patients had a biannual breast exam as well as annual mammogram and breast magnetic resonance imaging (MRI). In this population, mammograms had a sensitivity of 33% with a specificity of 95%. Breast MRI had significantly higher rates of sensitivity and specificity at 80% and 90%, respectively. Given these findings, breast MRI should be a part of the screening exam for these high-risk patients. MRI is recommended as a standard screening test in BRCA heterozygotes. Routine surveillance in high-risk patients includes a 6-month interval alternating between breast MRI and mammograms. Patients with a history of mantle radiation for lymphoma should start annual screening at 25 years of age and biannual screening 10 years after receiving radiation therapy.

## Workup of a Breast Mass

### DOMINANT PALPABLE MASS

The workup of a dominant palpable breast mass depends on the patient's menopausal status and the degree of suspicion. It is not unreasonable to follow a premenopausal patient with a nonsuspicious mass over one menstrual cycle and then reexamine her. Suspicious lesions present as a hard, nontender, irregular mass or as a mass in a high-risk patient. Palpable masses in postmenopausal patients may also warrant a workup. FNA should not be performed prior to diagnostic imaging because it may result in a hematoma that could obscure the image of the mass. Certain benign lesions on core biopsy should be excised, including lobular carcinoma in situ (LCIS), atypical ductal hyperplasia (ADH), radial scars, sclerosing papillary lesions, columnar cell hyperplasia with atypia, and PASH (Figure 3). Twenty percent of surgeries performed for atypical ductal hyperplasia have concurrent carcinoma in the specimen. Patients with a high-risk proliferative lesion should have close follow-up after surgery including physical examinations. Negative findings on a mammogram do not preclude the diagnosis of cancer because 10% of cancers are occult mammographically. This number drops to 3% when a lesion is occult both mammographically and ultrasonographically. An alternative to core biopsies in younger women is the use of the triple test: a physical exam in conjunction with breast imaging (mammogram or ultrasound) and FNA. When all three components indicate the mass is benign, the negative predictive value is 100%. In a study by Morris, a triple test score assigns points to each component of the test. One point is given for benign findings, 2 points for suspicious findings, and 3 points for

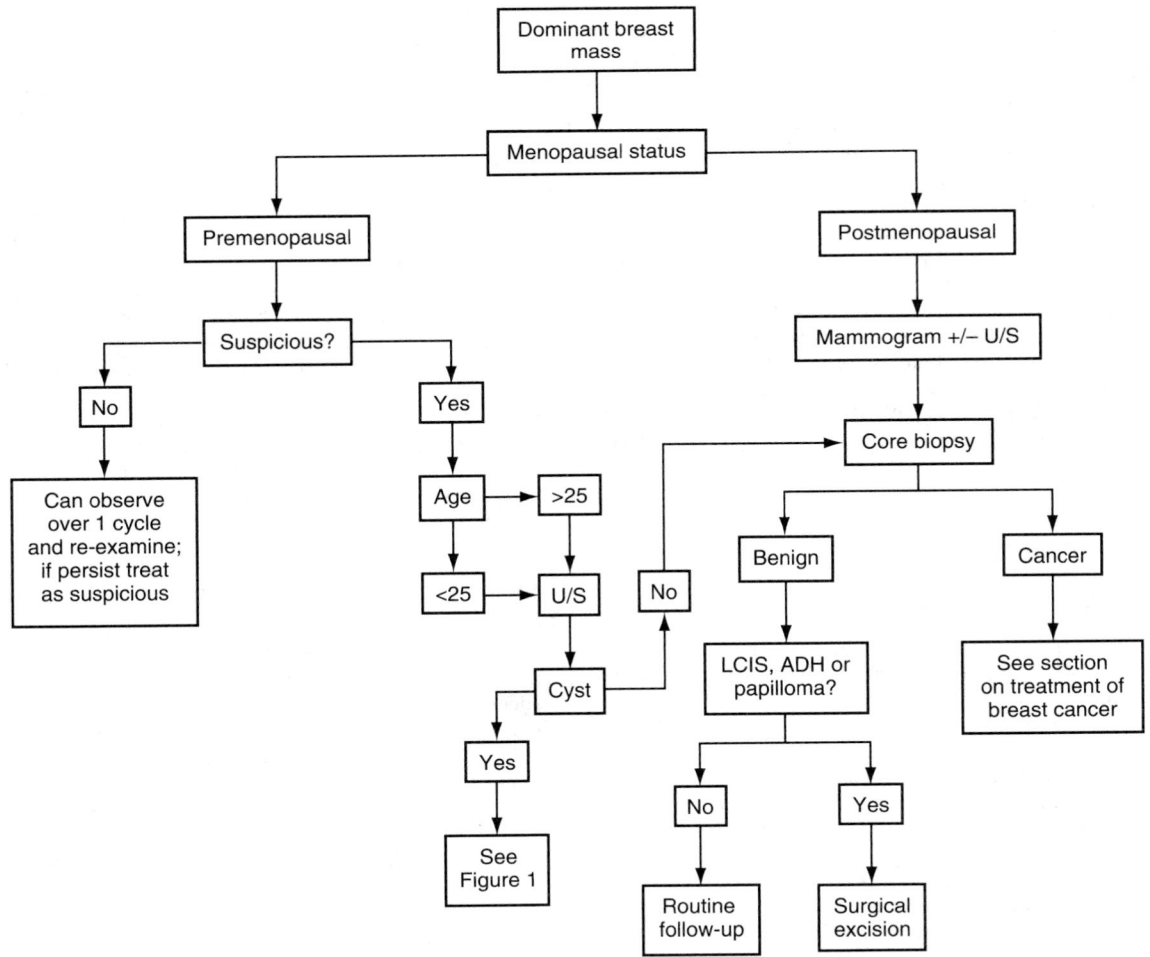

**FIGURE 3.** Algorithm for workup of a breast mass. ADH = atypical ductal hyperplasia; LCIS = lobular cancer in situ; U/S = ultrasound.

## TABLE 2 BI-RADS Mammography Classification

| BI-RADS Category | Definition | Risk of Malignancy | Recommended Follow-Up |
|---|---|---|---|
| 0 | Incomplete assessment | N/A | Further workup |
| 1 | Negative study | N/A | Repeat mammogram in 1 y |
| 2 | Benign | N/A | Repeat mammogram in 1 y |
| 3 | Probably benign | <2% | Repeat mammogram in 6 mo |
| 4 | Suspicious | 20% | Biopsy should be considered |
| 5 | Highly suggestive of malignancy | 90% | Appropriate action should be taken |
| 6 | Known biopsy-proven malignancy | N/A | Appropriate action should be taken |

*Abbreviation:* BI-RADS = Breast Imaging Reporting and Data System.

malignant findings. When added together, masses with scores of 4 or less are found to be benign. The triple test should only be used in women 40 years of age or younger because the incidence of breast cancer increases dramatically after that cutoff.

## MASSES REVEALED ON SCREENING MAMMOGRAMS

The American College of Radiology's classification lexicon, the Breast Imaging Reporting and Data System (BI-RADS), is used in breast imaging (Table 2). BI-RADS 0 means the assessment is incomplete and more workup is needed. BI-RADS 1 indicates a normal mammogram. Mammograms with BI-RADS 2 signify benign findings. Patients with BI-RADS 3 have a 1% to 2% risk of malignancy and should have short-term follow-up with another mammogram in 6 months. BI-RADS 4 indicates the presence of suspicious lesions with a 20% to 40% probability of a malignant lesion. BI-RADS 5 is highly suggestive of cancer with a greater than 95% chance of harboring an underlying malignant lesion. BI-RADS 6, recently added as a category, indicates known malignant disease. BI-RADS 4 and 5 both indicate a biopsy.

A core biopsy via ultrasound guidance may be attempted first. A stereotactic core biopsy should be considered if this is not possible. Stereotactic biopsies may be impossible in patients with lesions that are very superficial or close to the chest wall or in patients with very small breasts that compress to less than 3 cm or who are unable to lie still for the procedure. In such situations, surgical excision with needle localization is warranted. In studies comparing surgical excision to core biopsies, the concordance rate is close to 100%. The surgeon can obviate the need for multiple surgeries in the same patient by performing a core biopsy for diagnosis. High-risk proliferative lesions, such as LCIS, atypical ductal hyperplasia, radial scars, sclerosing papillary lesions, columnar cell hyperplasia with atypia, and PASH, should be considered for an excisional biopsy if the diagnosis is made by a core biopsy.

# In Situ Diseases

## LOBULAR CARCINOMA IN SITU

Lobular carcinoma in situ (LCIS) should be considered a marker for future breast cancer risk and not an early noninvasive lobular cancer. This disease is most commonly seen in premenopausal women, with a peak incidence in women 40 to 50 years of age. Only 10% of LCIS occurs in postmenopausal women. Unlike ductal carcinoma in situ, LCIS is often found incidentally because typically no clinical or radiologic abnormalities are seen at time of diagnosis. In 50% of patients, LCIS is a multifocal finding. In 30% of patients, it can be found in the contralateral breast. Patients with LCIS are at 8 to 10 times the risk of the general population for subsequent breast cancer. Their overall lifetime risk is as high as 30% to 40% for the development of invasive breast cancer. In a meta-analysis, 15% of patients developed breast cancer in the ipsilateral breast, and 9.3% of patients developed cancer in the contralateral breast. The type of breast cancer can be either ductal or lobular, although the majority is ductal.

## DUCTAL CARCINOMA IN SITU

Ductal carcinoma in situ (DCIS), or intraductal carcinoma, is a noninvasive breast cancer and designated stage 0. Historically, DCIS represented only approximately 5% of breast cancer cases, whereas today it constitutes 20% to 30% of all cases. This rise is predominantly attributed to the increasing use of screening mammography because DCIS is most often detected as mammographic microcalcifications. It tends to occur at a later age than LCIS and is not considered a multifocal or bilateral disease. Unlike LCIS, DCIS should be considered a true precursor lesion because if left untreated, approximately 60% to 100% of DCIS cases progress to invasive carcinoma.

## TREATMENT FOR IN SITU DISEASE

### Lobular Carcinoma in Situ

LCIS should be treated as a marker for increased breast cancer risk. Surgery in an attempt to achieve negative margins is not warranted for LCIS. The NSABP P-1 (the National Surgical Adjuvant Breast and Bowel Project) randomized trial examined the role of tamoxifen (Nolvadex) as a chemopreventive agent in high-risk patients, including those with LCIS. Women taking tamoxifen had a 50% reduction in the subsequent risk of breast cancer without any improvement in overall survival. The main risks of tamoxifen include increased risk of thromboembolic disease and endometrial cancer. The rate of pulmonary embolism was 3 in 1000 patients in the tamoxifen group versus 1 in 1000 in the placebo group. The rate of deep-vein thromboembolism was 5 in 1000 patients in the tamoxifen group versus 3 in 1000 in the placebo group. Endometrial cancer was seen in 9 in 1000 patients in the tamoxifen group versus 3.5 in 1000 in the placebo group. The decision to use tamoxifen as a chemopreventive agent should be made on an individual basis given these side effects. The highest reduction in breast cancer occurred in the LCIS group with a 70% reduction in risk. Despite this, no difference in survival was seen between the tamoxifen and placebo group.

### Ductal Carcinoma in Situ

Treatment of DCIS has evolved from simple mastectomy to lumpectomy with radiation therapy. A simple mastectomy is associated with a 1% local recurrence rate. Thus it is still considered a viable option in patients who do not desire or are ineligible for breast conservation therapy (BCT). No difference in survival is seen in patients treated with mastectomy versus BCT. The NSABP B-17 randomized trial examined the role of lumpectomy with and without radiotherapy for the treatment of DCIS. The addition of radiotherapy decreased the recurrence rate from 16.4% to 7% with 8 years of follow-up. More importantly, it decreased the rate of invasive carcinoma from 8% to 2%. The 5-year event-free survival with lumpectomy and radiation is 84%. Limited data support excision alone in small well-differentiated DCIS with surgical margins of at least 1 cm. Silverstein showed in retrospective studies that the recurrence rate in such patients is approximately 4%. Routine axillary lymph node dissection (ALND) is not recommended for DCIS because only 1% of patients have positive axillary nodes. Recent studies, however, show that sentinel lymph node biopsy may have a role in the management of selected patients with DCIS. This is especially true in patients receiving a mastectomy as definitive treatment or if there is a question of microinvasion on the core biopsy. Patients with DCIS and microinvasion can have anywhere from a 3% to 20% incidence of nodal involvement. Indications for a sentinel node biopsy include extensive calcifications, a palpable lesion, patients undergoing mastectomy as treatment for DCIS, and lesions for which the pathology reads "can not rule out microinvasion." Tamoxifen (Nolvadex) can also be considered in cases of DCIS that are estrogen receptor positive. The NSABP B-24 randomized trial examined the utility of tamoxifen in patients treated with lumpectomy and radiotherapy. Ipsilateral tumor recurrences decreased from 13.4% without tamoxifen to 8.2% with tamoxifen. The incidence of invasive cancer was reduced by 47%. No difference in survival was observed between the placebo and the tamoxifen group. Side effects are similar to that of the NSABP P-1 trial.

# Invasive Breast Cancer

## INCIDENCE

An estimated 1 in 9 women living in the United States if they survive to 90 years of age will develop breast cancer. The average age at diagnosis is 64 years of age and increases along with age.

The American Joint Committee on Cancer TMN (tumor, metastasis, node) system designates breast cancer as stage 0, I, II, III, or IV. This system categorizes breast cancer by its invasive or noninvasive character, tumor size, axillary lymph node status, and the presence of metastatic disease (see Table 2). Overall survival with breast cancer is related to stage (Table 3).

## HISTOLOGY

The most common type of infiltrating carcinoma is ductal carcinoma-not otherwise specified (IFDC-NOS), which represents 85% of all invasive breast cancer. Infiltrating lobular carcinoma originates from the lobular structures of the breast and accounts for 15% of all invasive breast cancer. Other less common subtypes represent less than 10% and include tubular, medullary, mucinous, and papillary carcinoma. Additional rare subtypes of breast cancer include inflammatory carcinoma, malignant phyllodes tumor, sarcoma, lymphoma, and Paget disease.

## BREAST CANCER STAGING

In 2003 the American Joint Committee on Cancer (AJCC) revised their staging system on breast cancer. This latest revision stresses the importance of nodal status as a prognostic factor by making several

### TABLE 3  Overall Survival in Breast Cancer Patients

| Stage | 10-Year Overall Survival | 15-Year Overall Survival |
|---|---|---|
| I | 74%-95% | 64% |
| II | 76% | 62% |
| IIA | 81% | 72% |
| IIB | 70% | 52% |
| III | 50% | 40% |
| IIIA | 59% | 49% |
| IIIB | 36% | 18% |
| IIIC | 36% | 18% |
| IV | 18% | 18% |

Adapted from Rosen PP, et al: J Clin Oncol 1989;355-366; Woodward WA, Strom EA, Tucker SL, et al: Changes in the 2003 American Joint Committee on Cancer staging for breast cancer, dramatically affect stage-specific survival. J Clin Oncol 2003;21:3244-3248.

changes in how it is classified within the staging system. Major changes to the staging system include the following:

- Designation is made for isolated tumor cells (ITCs), which are differentiated from micrometastasis and defined as "single tumor cells or small cell clusters not greater than 0.2 mm, usually detected only by IHC (immunohistochemistry) or molecular methods, but which may be verified on H&E (hematoxylin-eosin) stains. ITCs do not usually show evidence of malignant activity, e.g., proliferation or stromal reaction." ITCs are designated as pN0 with modifiers for positive or negative IHC (i–, i+) and molecular findings (mol–, mol+).
- Internal mammary nodes (IMNs) are reclassified based on how they are detected and whether or not there is concomitant axillary lymph node metastasis. Detection of IMNs by sentinel node biopsy alone is classified as pN1b in the absence of positive axillary nodes or pN1c in the presence of positive axillary nodes. Internal mammary nodes detected by imaging studies (excluding lymphoscintigraphy) or by clinical exam are classified as pN2b in the absence of positive axillary nodes or pN3b in the presence of positive axillary nodes.
- Supraclavicular nodal involvement is now reclassified as N3 disease; thus a patient with supraclavicular nodal involvement does not automatically have stage IV disease.
- Infraclavicular nodal involvement is added as N3 disease.
- Axillary lymph node involvement is now classified by the number of nodes involved. Involvement of 1 to 3 axillary nodes is considered pN1 disease. Involvement of 4 to 9 axillary nodes is considered pN2 disease. Involvement of greater than 10 axillary nodes is considered pN3 disease.

Staging of breast cancer can be divided into clinical staging versus pathologic staging. Factors used for clinical staging include the size of the tumor within the breast, presence or absence of pathologically confirmed lymph nodes, and presence or absence of distant metastasis. There are five stages for breast cancer. Stage 0 is defined as the presence of in situ disease only, without evidence of nodal or distant metastasis. Stage I is considered breast cancer confined to the breast, regardless of tumor size. Exception to this general characterization includes tumors with extension to the chest wall or skin or inflammatory breast cancers. These tumors are at least stage IIIB. Stage II is considered a breast cancer of any size with pathologically positive ipsilateral mobile axillary nodes. Stage IIIA is considered a breast cancer of any size with pathologically positive ipsilateral fixed axillary nodes or clinically apparent internal mammary nodes in the absence of positive axillary nodes. Also any large tumors (bigger than 5 cm) with any type of positive axillary or internal mammary nodes are considered stage IIIA. Stage IIIB tumors are breast tumors with extension to the skin or chest wall or inflammatory breast cancer. Involvement of the pectoralis major or minor muscle does not constitute chest wall involvement. Stage IIIC tumors are breast cancers of any size with either positive infraclavicular or supraclavicular nodes or positive internal mammary nodes in the presence of positive axillary nodes. Stage IV connotes any breast cancers with distant metastasis (see Figure 3).

Pathologic staging of breast cancer is more complicated and differs from clinical staging in that the number of nodes involved as well as how nodal metastasis is detected are used in stage designation of nodal status (Figures 4 and 5).

## SURGICAL TREATMENT OF THE BREAST

A significant paradigm shift in the treatment of breast cancer has occurred over the past several decades. The Halsted paradigm, popularized at the beginning of the 20th century, hypothesized that breast cancer spreads in a contiguous fashion from the breast to the axillary lymph nodes and then to distant sites elsewhere in the body. The Fisher paradigm, which views breast cancer as systemic from very early in the

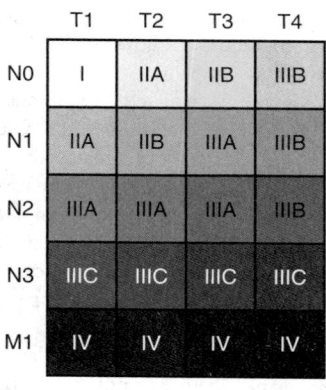

|      | T1   | T2   | T3   | T4   |
|------|------|------|------|------|
| N0   | I    | IIA  | IIB  | IIIB |
| N1   | IIA  | IIB  | IIIA | IIIB |
| N2   | IIIA | IIIA | IIIA | IIIB |
| N3   | IIIC | IIIC | IIIC | IIIC |
| M1   | IV   | IV   | IV   | IV   |

**FIGURE 4.** Pathologic staging of breast cancer.

course of the disease, modified this theory; the axillary lymph nodes act not as a barrier but as indicators of disease aggressiveness. Both paradigms are correct and incorrect. At a certain point in the evolution of a breast cancer, the disease changes from a local disease to a systemic disease. The Halsted paradigm promotes more intensive local treatment to eradicate the cancer, whereas the Fisher paradigm promotes less aggressive local treatment with the addition of systemic treatment in most women, even with relatively early disease. Because of this philosophy change and the detection of earlier disease through diligent screening techniques, surgical treatment of breast cancer is progressing toward less radical surgery and more adjuvant therapy, with equal or better outcomes. Recent mammograms of both breasts should be reviewed for any other suspicious lesions. There may be a slight increase in synchronous breast cancer in patients with invasive lobular cancer, although the rate of contralateral breast cancer is equal to that of invasive ductal carcinoma over the lifetime of the patient. The risk of distant metastasis is 25% to 50% in patients with inflammatory breast cancer.

# Breast Conservation Therapy

Most small noninvasive and invasive breast cancers are treated by BCT, which consists of wide local excision with negative surgical margins and irradiation of the breast. The NSABP B-06, Milan I and Milan II, as well as other clinical trials, show no statistically significant difference in patient survival with mastectomy or BCT.

The addition of radiation treatment to wide local excision in patients with noninvasive and invasive carcinoma is currently the standard of treatment. The NSABP B-06 randomized trial evaluated local recurrence of small invasive tumors with and without irradiation after lumpectomy. It found that patients who did not undergo radiation therapy had significantly higher rates of local recurrence. With BCT, incidence of recurrence in the treated breast is 7% at 5 years, 14% at 10 years, and 20% at 20 years. Local recurrence rate is much lower in patients treated with mastectomy, with an overall incidence of 5% to 10%. The majority of recurrences occur in the first 3 years after surgery. Contraindications to BCT include tumor of any size that can not be adequately excised with significant deformity to the breast, multicentric disease, noncompliant patient, first- or second-trimester pregnant patient, history of significant collagen vascular disease, and history of previous radiation therapy to the chest wall. If both BCT and mastectomy are viable options, the patient's preference should also play a role in the decision to proceed with BCT versus a mastectomy.

## MASTECTOMY

A patient with contraindications to breast conservation should have a mastectomy with or without immediate reconstruction. Total mastectomy surgically removes the breast parenchyma, pectoral fascia, nipple, and the areola complex. A modified radical mastectomy includes axillary dissection. A radical mastectomy, rarely done today, includes removal of the pectoralis major and minor muscles and axillary dissection.

## BREAST RECONSTRUCTION

Any patient recommended to have a mastectomy should be offered the option of immediate or delayed reconstruction and referred to a

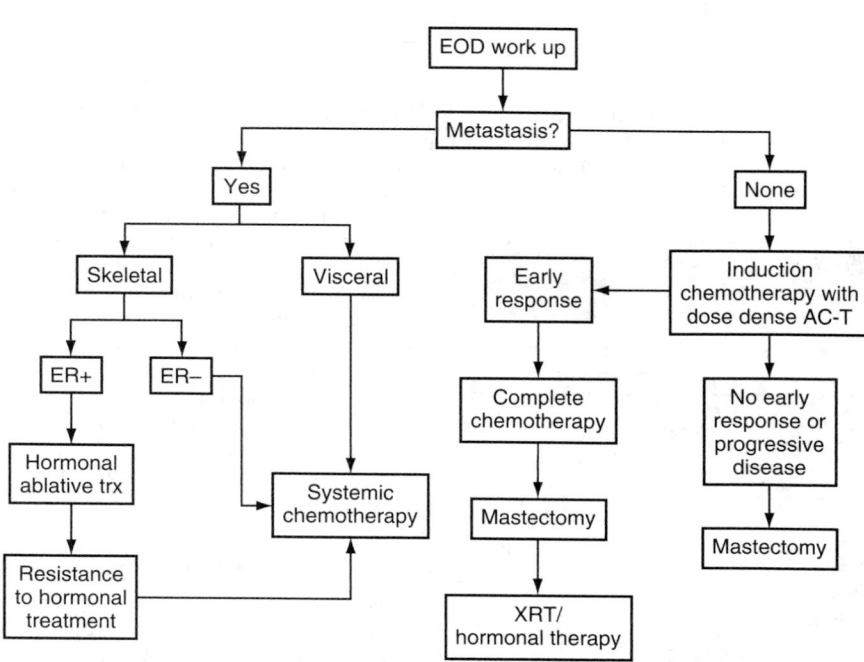

**FIGURE 5.** Algorithm for treatment of locally advanced breast cancer (LABC). AC-T = Adriamycyin and cyclophosphamide plus Taxol; EOD = extent-of-disease; trx = treatment; XRT = x-radiation therapy.

plastic and reconstructive surgeon to discuss which techniques are appropriate. One commonly used method of breast reconstruction is a tissue expander breast implant. A tissue expander is placed beneath the pectoralis muscles, and expansions are performed over a period of several weeks to months to stretch the subpectoral pocket to accommodate the permanent implant. The permanent saline or silicone implant is then inserted as a secondary procedure.

Another method of breast reconstruction is the transverse rectus abdominis myocutaneous (TRAM) flap, which involves the transfer of skin, fat, and muscle from the lower part of the abdomen to create a reconstructed breast. This procedure can be performed as a free flap with the arterial and venous supply anastomosed to vessels in the axilla or as a pedicle flap with the arterial and venous supply from the superior epigastric vessels. Other types of flap reconstructions include latissimus dorsi or gluteal flaps. Reconstruction of the nipple and areola is often performed as a later procedure.

## SURGICAL TREATMENT OF THE AXILLA

The status of the axilla should be assessed for metastases in any patient with invasive breast cancer for several reasons. The status of the axillary lymph nodes is important in determining the patient's stage of disease. The presence or absence of axillary lymph node metastasis is predictive of the prognosis and facilitates decisions by the medical oncology team regarding adjuvant therapy. Relapse-free survival is closely related to the number of lymph nodes that are positive. In a study of 2873 patients, Hilsenbeck found that the relapse-free survival at 5 years was 80% in patients with node-negative disease. This number decreased to 70%, 60%, and 40% with 1 to 3 positive nodes, 4 to 9 positive nodes, and more than 10 positive nodes, respectively. Nodal status is now incorporated into the sixth revision of the AJCC staging system. Surgical removal of metastatic nodes in the axilla significantly decreases the possibility of axillary recurrence. ALND may improve overall survival, but this issue is debated in the medical literature.

### Sentinel Lymph Node Biopsy

Axillary dissection traditionally was performed on all patients with invasive breast cancer. Today, sentinel lymphadenectomy, or sentinel lymph node (SLN) biopsy, identifies the first, or sentinel, lymph node or nodes in the axillary chain to receive drainage from the breast cancer and thus the most likely to contain metastases. The SLN biopsy is performed by injecting isosulfan blue dye and/or radioactive isotope to localize the sentinel lymph node.

The sentinel node can be identified in 95% of all cases. Multiple studies show that SLN biopsy can predict accurately the presence of axillary metastases in T1-2 breast cancer with a false-negative rate of 5% and an accuracy rate of 95%. The false-negative rate of SLN biopsy can be decreased to 1% to 3% if any palpable node is removed along with any hot or blue nodes. The SLN biopsy, a less invasive way to assess the status of the axilla, is associated with fewer complications than an axillary node dissection. Areas of controversy in SLN biopsy include T3, palpable suspicious axillary lymph nodes, and previous neoadjuvant therapy. In a study by Specht, 25% of palpable suspicious axillary lymph nodes proved benign on final pathology. Previous axillary dissection is not a strict contraindication per se because 75% of these patients can still have an identifiable sentinel node. The success rate depends on the number of nodes previously removed, with a success rate of 87% when fewer than 10 nodes are removed versus a success rate of 47% when more than 10 nodes are removed. Contraindications to SLN biopsy include T4 breast cancer and pregnancy. SLN biopsy is contraindicated in pregnancy because of the lack of data regarding fetal safety, although computer models suggest the amount of radiation exposure to the fetus is negligible.

### Axillary Dissection

Patients who have metastatic cells on SLN biopsy typically undergo complete ALND. Alternatively, if a patient is not a candidate for SLN biopsy, ALND should be considered. Axillary dissection involves the removal of 10 to 30 lymph nodes from the axilla. The potential risk of axillary dissection includes the accumulation of a seroma, ipsilateral arm lymphedema, and numbness around the area of the intercostal brachial innervation if the nerve is sacrificed at the time of surgery. Because of the lifetime increased chance of arm lymphedema and possible infection, patients should avoid any trauma or procedures such as venipuncture or blood pressure measurements on the ipsilateral arm.

## Adjuvant Therapy

Adjuvant therapy is used to treat patients with a demonstrable likelihood for the development of metastatic disease. Most medical oncologists consider this risk sufficient in node-negative patients with a tumor diameter of 1 cm or larger and in those with nodal metastases to justify adjuvant chemotherapy or hormonal therapy. Most commonly used cytotoxic regimens include CMF (cyclophosphamide [Cytoxan], methotrexate, and 5-FU [fluorouracil]) for 6 cycles or AC-T for 8 cycles (4 cycles of doxorubicin [Adriamycin] and cyclophosphamide followed by 4 cycles of paclitaxel [Taxol]). There appears to be a slight improvement of 3% in overall survival favoring the anthracycline-containing regimen over the CMF regimens. In the elderly population, the CMF regimen may be easier to tolerate than the AC-T regimens. In a recent study, a dose dense regimen of AC-T results in a slight improvement of disease-free and overall survival. Dose-dense regimen involves giving the chemotherapy in cycles every 2 weeks, with bone marrow support such as G-CSF (Neupogen), as opposed to the traditional cycles every 3 weeks. The improvement in survival is approximately 3%. In the Early Breast Cancer Trialists' Collaborative Group (EBCTCG) meta-analysis, adjuvant chemotherapy appears the most beneficial for women younger than 50 years of age. Combination chemotherapy resulted in the improvement of 10-year-overall survival from 71% in node-negative patients not receiving chemotherapy to 78% in those that did receive chemotherapy. This increase was even more dramatic in node-positive patients, with an improvement of overall survival from 42% to 53%. A much smaller effect was seen in patients older than 50 years of age. In this group of patients, survival was increased from 67% to 69% when node-negative patients not receiving chemotherapy were compared to those receiving chemotherapy. In node-positive elderly patients, improvement in overall survival was also minimal, with an increase of survival from 47% to 49% with chemotherapy.

Hormonal therapy, such as tamoxifen, is a commonly used adjuvant treatment in early breast cancer patients with estrogen receptor–positive tumors. The EBCTCG meta-analysis looking at the role of tamoxifen in the premenopausal patients found that tamoxifen results in an absolute improvement of 10-year overall survival of 5.6% in node-negative patients and 10.9% in node-positive patients. This effect is even greater in the postmenopausal population, with a 26% proportional reduction in 10-year mortality rates. The recommended length of treatment for node-negative patients is 5 years. Additionally, tamoxifen can be used as a chemopreventive agent to decrease the chance of an additional ipsilateral tumor developing in patients undergoing breast conservation or to decrease the possibility of contralateral breast cancer.

More recently, three large randomized trials of aromatase inhibitors, such as anastrozole (Arimidex), exemestane (Aromasin), and letrozole (Femara), was published. In the ATAC (Arimidex, Tamoxifen, Alone or in Combination) trial, patients on anastrozole had a statistically significant longer disease-free interval when compared with patients on tamoxifen alone (hazard ratio of 0.83). No difference in survival was seen between the two groups. In another large study, patients on tamoxifen for 2 to 3 years were randomized to continuing tamoxifen versus switching to exemestane for a total of 5 years of therapy. There appeared to be an improvement in disease-free survival in the aromatase inhibitor arm (hazard ratio of 0.68). No difference in survival was seen, and given the early stoppage and cross-over of patients, no survival data will be obtainable from this study. Yet another large double-blinded randomized trial involved patients who had finished a 5-year course of tamoxifen and were then randomized to receiving letrozole versus placebo. The trial was stopped at a mean follow-up of 2.4 years secondary to a significant improvement in disease-free survival in the letrozole arm (hazard ratio of 0.57). Again, no difference in survival was seen. Aromatase inhibitors are useful only in postmenopausal patients. Premenopausal patients may benefit from an aromatase inhibitor only after ovarian ablation.

Recommendations regarding tamoxifen, aromatase inhibitors, and chemotherapy depend on the clinical judgment of the treating medical oncologist. In general, if adjuvant chemotherapy is given, it should take place prior to the initiation of radiotherapy. Consideration should be given to the likelihood of systemic recurrence based on nodal status, tumor size, and tumor grade. Estrogen receptor positivity of the tumor is predictive of a response to hormonal therapy, and *HER2-neu* may determine the type of appropriate chemotherapy. Another factor is the patient's age and any co-morbid diseases that would decrease the patient's tolerance to a course of chemotherapy.

## Surveillance After a Diagnosis of Breast Cancer

Surveillance should continue alter diagnosis and treatment of breast cancer to detect local recurrence or a new primary breast cancer in either the ipsilateral or contralateral breast. The National Comprehensive Cancer Network guidelines recommend that patients continue diligent monthly self-examinations and that a physician perform a physical examination at 6-month intervals to assess for evidence of local recurrence and symptoms of metastatic disease. The ipsilateral arm should be evaluated to detect early signs of lymphedema and initiate appropriate management. Bilateral mammograms should be obtained every year. Bone and computed tomographic scans and other tumor markers should be performed only on patients with symptomatic systemic disease because of the lack of evidence of improved survival with early detection of distant metastases.

## Special Topics in Breast Disease

### PHYLLODES TUMOR

Phyllodes tumor (cystosarcoma phyllodes) is a fibroepithelial lesion that can be either benign or malignant. It is a rare tumor of the breast accounting for 1% of all cases. The mean age of patients is 54 years of age. These tumors often present as a breast mass on clinical and mammographic examination., and they are considered benign or malignant depending on stromal cellularity, mitotic activity, presence of necrosis, and type of borders. Treatment is complete excision without axillary node dissection. Metastases secondary to malignant phyllodes are hematogenous and primarily travel to the lungs. It is important to obtain negative margins. A mastectomy occasionally may be warranted for large lesions. Patients with malignant phyllodes have an 80% chance of 5-year survival as opposed to more than 95% for benign phyllodes.

### NIPPLE DISCHARGE

Nipple discharge can occur at any age and presents as a bloody, serous, or milky discharge. Only 6% to 12% of patients with a nipple discharge are found to have an underlying malignancy. This risk is slightly elevated if the discharge is bloody. The most common cause of serous or serosanguineous nipple discharge is a benign intraductal papilloma. Numerous drugs can also cause nipple discharge, such as phenothiazine, tricyclic antidepressants, reserpine, butyrophenones, cimetidine (Tagamet), verapamil (Calan), metoclopramide (Reglan), thiazides, and hormone replacement therapy. The most common underlying malignancy is DCIS. Ductograms may be useful in locating the papilloma. When the nipple discharge is unilaterally persistent, spontaneous, or postmenopausal, further workup may be considered. Other suspicious nipple discharges are those confined to one duct or that are bloody or serous. In general, the evaluation of nipple discharge should begin with a clinical examination and a mammogram. Cytologic examination of the discharge has a low sensitivity for detection of underlying malignancy and should be not be used in the workup. Treatment consists of a major duct excision.

## GYNECOMASTIA

Gynecomastia is the unilateral or bilateral benign enlargement of male breast tissue. The etiology is often related to various substances, including exogenous hormones, cimetidine (Tagamet), thiazides, digoxin, theophylline, phenothiazines, alcohol, and marijuana use; it may also be idiopathic. The main concern is to rule out the diagnosis of male breast cancer. Once breast cancer is excluded, no treatment is indicated. If medication and lifestyle etiologies are eliminated without remission of the gynecomastia, the excess breast tissue may be surgically removed for cosmetic considerations or for breast pain.

## MALE BREAST CANCER

Carcinoma of the male breast represents 1% of all breast cancers. Because men are not routinely screened for breast cancer, the diagnosis is often delayed. The most common manifestation of male breast cancer is a painless, firm, subareolar breast mass. The differential diagnosis includes gynecomastia. Breast imaging with mammography and/or ultrasound may be helpful in rendering a diagnosis inasmuch as the appearance of male breast cancer is a stellate, irregular solid mass. Any suspicious breast mass in a male patient should undergo diagnostic biopsy. If a malignancy is diagnosed, standard treatment is mastectomy with assessment of the axillary nodes by SLN biopsy or ALND. Most cases of male breast cancer are estrogen receptor positive, and recommendations for adjuvant chemotherapy or hormonal therapy should be based on criteria similar to those for breast cancer in female patients.

## BREAST CANCER IN PREGNANCY

Pregnancy-associated breast cancer represents less than 2% of all breast cancer diagnoses. The breast cancer frequently is diagnosed at a late stage because of the difficulty of examining the breast in pregnant women and the avoidance of mammography during pregnancy. Any suspicious lesion noted during pregnancy should be subjected to biopsy in the same fashion as in a nongravid woman. Radiation therapy should not be administered during pregnancy, so breast conservation is generally contraindicated unless the diagnosis is made within a few weeks of delivery. Surgical treatment with mastectomy and ALND is the standard treatment of breast cancer during pregnancy. Adjuvant chemotherapy can be delivered with selective agents during the second and third trimesters. The prognosis is similar to that of nongravid women in whom breast cancer is diagnosed at a comparable stage.

## INFLAMMATORY BREAST CANCER

The classic manifestation of inflammatory breast cancer is erythema, edema, peau d'orange, and color of the breast resembling an infectious process. Malignant cells within the dermal lymphatic vessels of the breast confirm the diagnosis. The usual pathology of the associated carcinoma is IFDC-NOS. Inflammatory carcinoma is a very aggressive type of breast cancer, with over 90% of patients having positive axillary lymph nodes at diagnosis. The recommended treatment is multimodality therapy, with chemotherapy preceding surgery. Surgical treatment is mastectomy followed by radiation therapy and often additional chemotherapy.

## LOCALLY ADVANCED BREAST CANCER

Patients with N2 or N3 nodal status or those with four or more positive axillary nodes, T3 or T4 tumors, or involvement of the pectoralis fascia have locally advanced breast cancer (LABC). The recommended treatment for patients is neoadjuvant chemotherapy, which is administered before surgical treatment, although it has no impact on overall survival. An extent-of-disease (EOD) workup should be done in patients with LABC and includes a computed tomography (CT) of the chest, abdomen, and pelvis along with a bone scan. Figure 5 provides an algorithm for the treatment of LABC.

# Endometriosis

Method of
*David L. Olive, MD*

Endometriosis is one of the most common diseases encountered by the practicing gynecologist, yet it is also one of the most vexing. Researchers have been searching for answers to even the most fundamental questions regarding this disease for well over a century; even today huge gaps remain in the understanding of this disorder.

## Definition

Endometriosis is defined as the presence of endometrial glands and stroma outside the endometrial cavity and uterine musculature. The requirement for both glands and stroma is an arbitrary standard, and it is unclear whether either component of endometrium alone, if placed ectopically, can result in the symptoms and signs of endometriosis.

Two related diseases are also frequently observed. Adenomyosis is the presence of endometrial glands and stroma within the myometrium. This disorder is epidemiologically and pathogenically distinct from endometriosis, but the resulting symptoms (and medical treatments) are similar. Endosalpingiosis is identical to endometriosis in location and appearance but histologically resembles tubal glands and stroma. This latter abnormality has been poorly studied, and to date, little is known regarding the distinction between endometriosis and endosalpingiosis.

## Genetics

Evidence continues to accumulate that endometriosis has a genetic basis. Evidence for this includes familial clustering, concordance in monozygotic twins, and increased prevalence among first-degree relatives. A search was recently undertaken to identify the gene or genes responsible for susceptibility to endometriosis. Although suggestive linkages were discovered, no genes have been firmly identified as instrumental in this disorder. It is hoped, however, that genetic research will eventually uncover information critical to understanding the molecular and cellular basis of this disease.

## Pathogenesis

The pathogenesis of endometriosis is a controversial subject inspiring many researchers to investigate it. Over the last 25 years considerable advancement has been made, providing solid clues to the understanding of the disease process. Today, a clear picture is beginning to emerge regarding how women develop endometriosis.

### HISTOGENESIS

Leading researchers in the field have proposed numerous theories of histogenesis. The primary theory of histogenesis is transplantation of shed uterine endometrium to ectopic locations. A number of routes of dissemination of the tissue are proposed, including lymphatic dissemination, vascular spread, iatrogenic transplantation, and retrograde menstruation.

A critical aspect of this theory is that cast-off endometrium cells remain viable and capable of implanting. Furthermore, it proposes that the tissue distribution has the capacity to sustain implantation. Considerable research has established that shed endometrial cells are viable in vitro. In vitro studies of endometrial attachment to peritoneum also support the concept of transplantation, attachment, and invasion.

Additional theories of histogenesis include coelomic metaplasia and induction of endometriosis. However, little scientific evidence indicates that either route is a viable etiology of the disease, much less a common method for development.

### ETIOLOGY AND MAINTENANCE

Retrograde menstruation is a well-established phenomenon. Data available from women undergoing peritoneal dialysis and laparoscopy at the time of menses suggest that 76% to 90% of women have retrograde flow. This mechanism is considered a critical first step in the initiation of much if not most endometriosis by a wide variety of epidemiologic and anatomic data. However, the majority of women do not have endometriosis. The question that arises is "Why not?"

Because the placement of menstrual debris into the peritoneal cavity happens with each menses, a mechanism must exist to eliminate this tissue. The prime candidate for removal of endometrial cells is cell-mediated cytotoxicity. Deficient cytotoxic response to ectopic endometrium is suggested as a mechanism for allowing implantation and growth. It is also postulated that factors positively affecting growth and maintenance may be altered to enhance the risk of endometriosis. Current evidence suggests that a variety of cytokines, including monocyte chemotactic protein-1, interleukin-8, and regulated on activation, T-cell expressed and secreted (RANTES) are overexpressed in women with endometriosis, resulting in the attraction and activation of macrophages. The source of this cytokine increase could be one or more of several tissues: Endometrium, peritoneal mesothelium, and macrophages themselves could be the primary aberrancy by which this cascade is begun.

Other abnormalities are speculated to promote endometriosis. These include abnormal expression of matrix metalloproteinases and the enzyme aromatase, which could locally produce a hyperestrogenic proimplantation environment. The mechanisms by which these abnormalities may cause disease as well as the source of such alterations are under investigation.

## Prevalence and Epidemiology

Endometriosis is a disease found almost exclusively in reproductive-age women. The mean age at diagnosis is reported to be from 25 to 29 years, although this figure depends on the diagnostic method. Because traditional diagnosis requires laparoscopy, it is likely that the disease is frequently present in even younger patients for whom many gynecologists do not readily schedule surgery.

Although rare in the premenarcheal female, adolescent endometriosis is a relatively common entity. Endometriosis is found in 47% to 65% of women younger than 20 years with chronic pelvic pain or dyspareunia.

Endometriosis is associated with increased exposure to menstruation typified by earlier menarche, more frequent menses, longer menses, fewer pregnancies, later initial pregnancy, and less breast-feeding. In addition, factors known to decrease the amount of menses or lower estrogen levels also reduce the risk: oral contraceptive use, irregular menses/oligomenorrhea, stress, exercise, and cigarette smoking (Box 1).

Postmenopausal endometriosis seldom occurs; this age group represents only 2% to 4% of all women requiring laparoscopy for

---

**BOX 1  Epidemiology of Endometriosis**

Increased risk with:
- Menses >6 d
- More menses

Decreased risk with:
- Increased parity
- Irregular menses
- Oral contraceptives
- Late menarche
- Exercise
- Smoking

endometriosis. The majority of such cases are a sequela to reactivation of disease by hormone replacement therapy; this is not true in all cases.

## Clinical Presentation

Endometriosis is associated with a wide array of presenting signs and symptoms, although many women with physical manifestations of the disease remain completely asymptomatic. Commonly, the severity of symptoms does not correlate with the stage of endometriosis; extensive disease sometimes causes only minimal symptoms, and in others, minimal disease can be associated with severe symptoms. Some symptoms may strongly suggest the presence of endometriosis, but none are pathognomonic of this disorder. Because endometriosis most commonly involves the pelvis, infertility, dysmenorrhea, pelvic pain, dyspareunia, and menstrual dysfunction are common clinical presentations. When the ovary is severely involved, an ovarian cyst or pelvic mass may be the initial sign of endometriosis.

Pelvic pain is the most frequent complaint for endometriosis patients. This generally presents as secondary dysmenorrhea, worsening primary dysmenorrhea, dyspareunia, or even noncyclic lower abdominal pain, chronic pelvic pain, and backaches. In addition, pain may be site specific when endometriosis is found in unusual locations outside of the pelvis.

Only rarely are physical findings specific for endometriosis. Localized cul-de-sac and uterosacral ligament tenderness may frequently be detected. Thickened, nodular uterosacral ligaments or rectovaginal masses may be palpable. Adnexal enlargement or tenderness may reflect ovarian involvement. Retroverted fixation of the uterus may be noted with posterior cul-de-sac obliteration by the disease.

Cutaneous manifestations may be present, with apparent lesions on the perineum or vagina, or, less commonly, in the inguinal region, the umbilical area, or at the site of surgical scars. They should be suspected whenever a scar or lesion is associated with cyclical pain, tenderness, swelling, or bleeding.

## Diagnosis

The current gold standard for the definitive diagnosis of endometriosis is laparoscopy. However, because of the heterogeneity in appearance of endometriosis lesions, the accuracy of laparoscopic diagnosis is variable and depends on the ability of the surgeon to recognize the disease. Although histologic confirmation would be ideal to ensure the presence of disease, this is infrequently accomplished because of the reticence of surgeons to excise endometriosis lesions.

Ultrasound is most useful for the detection of ovarian endometriomas, although the appearance of a cystic structure with heightened echogenicity is certainly not limited to this form of endometriosis. Structures often confused with endometriomas include corpora lutea, hemorrhagic cysts, unilocular dermoid cysts, and other benign cystic neoplasias. Ultrasound is not currently useful for identifying focal implants.

Magnetic resonance imaging (MRI) demonstrates significant potential in the diagnosis of endometriosis. MRI is clearly of value in diagnosing the ovarian endometrioma, and as technology improves, the potential for detecting peritoneal lesions will increase.

### CURRENT DIAGNOSIS

■ Symptoms associated with endometriosis are primarily those of pain and infertility, although site-specific symptoms and signs may exist when the disease is in unusual locations.

■ The standard for diagnosis is laparoscopic visualization; however, this method has a high false-positive and false-negative rate. The only method to confirm the disease absolutely is excisional biopsy.

## Treatment

### MEDICAL THERAPY

The first drug to be approved for the treatment of endometriosis in the United States was danazol (Danocrine), a derivative of testosterone. It was originally thought to produce a pseudomenopause, but subsequent studies have revealed that the drug acts primarily by diminishing the midcycle luteinizing hormone (LH) surge, creating a chronic anovulatory state. The recommended dosage of danazol for the treatment of endometriosis is 600 to 800 mg/day; however, these doses have substantial androgenic side effects such as increased hair growth, mood changes, adverse serum lipid profiles, deepening of the voice (possibly irreversible), and, rarely, liver damage (possibly irreversible and life threatening) and arterial thrombosis. Studies of lower doses as primary treatment for endometriosis-associated pain have been uncontrolled or with small numbers and thus contain information of limited value.

Progestogens are a class of compounds that produce progesterone-like effects on endometrial tissue. A large number of progestogens exist, ranging from those chemically derived from progesterone (progestins), such as medroxyprogesterone acetate (MPA), to 19-nortestosterone derivatives such as norethindrone and norgestrel. The proposed mechanism of action of these compounds causes initial shedding of endometrial tissue followed by eventual atrophy. The most extensively studied progestational agent for the treatment of endometriosis is medroxyprogesterone (dep-subQ Provera 104), which is currently approved by the Food and Drug Administration (FDA) for use in treating endometriosis in a depot subcutaneous form. A common side effect is transient breakthrough bleeding, which occurs in 38% to 47% of patients. This is generally well tolerated and, when necessary, can be adequately treated with supplemental estrogen or an increase in the progestogen dose. Other side effects include nausea (0% to 80%), breast tenderness (5%), fluid retention (50%), and depression (6%). A recent approach to treating endometriosis with progestogen is the use of a progestogen-containing intrauterine contraceptive device[1] (Mirena).

The combination of estrogen and progestogen for therapy of endometriosis, the so-called pseudopregnancy regimen, has been used for 40 years. The most commonly used pseudopregnancy regimen today is the oral contraceptive pill[1] (OCP); in fact, it is the most commonly prescribed treatment for endometriosis symptoms. Like progestational therapy, pseudopregnancy is believed to produce initial decidualization and growth of endometrial tissue, followed in several months by atrophy.

Gonadotropin-releasing hormone (GnRH) agonists are analogues of the hormone GnRH. This hypothalamic hormone is responsible for stimulating the pituitary gland to secrete follicle-stimulating hormone (FSH) and LH, two hormones necessary for normal ovarian function.

---

[1]Not FDA approved for this indication.

### CURRENT THERAPY

■ Both medical and surgical therapies are efficacious in the treatment of endometriosis-associated pain. It is unclear which offers the better approach.

■ Combined medical/surgical therapy may offer an advantage over surgery alone, if the medication is used at least 6 months postoperatively.

■ Medical therapy has no role in the treatment of endometriosis-associated infertility.

■ Surgical therapy for endometriosis-associated infertility appears to be of value for all stages of disease, but its relative value compared to assisted reproduction is not yet determined.

GnRH is secreted in a pulsatile manner; the correct pulse results in stimulation of FSH and LH release, whereas too high or too low a pulse rate results in a decrease in pituitary hormone secretion. GnRH agonists are modified forms of GnRH that bind to the pituitary receptors and remain for a lengthy period. Thus, they are identified by the pituitary as rapidly pulsatile GnRH, and after initial stimulation of FSH and LH secretion, result in a shutdown (down-regulation) of the pituitary and no stimulation of the ovary. The result is a hypoestrogenic state similar to that of menopause, producing endometrial atrophy and amenorrhea. The agonist can be given intranasally (naferelin [Synarel]), subcutaneously (goserelin [Zoladex]), or intramuscularly (IM) (leuprolide acetate [Lupro Depot]), depending on the specific product, with frequency of administration ranging from twice daily to every 3 months. The side effects are those of hypoestrogenism such as transient vaginal bleeding, hot flashes, vaginal dryness, decreased libido, breast tenderness, insomnia, depression, irritability and fatigue, headache, osteoporosis, and decreased skin elasticity; these are dose dependent.

A recent modification of GnRH agonist treatment is to add back small amounts of steroid hormone in a manner similar to that used in the treatment of postmenopausal women. The theory is that the requirement for estrogen is greater for endometriosis than is needed by the brain (to prevent hot flashes), the bone (to prevent osteoporosis), and other tissues deprived of this hormone. With this approach there is an equivalent rate of pain relief with far fewer side effects than GnRH agonist alone. Estrogen as a solitary add-back, however, is less effective and thus not indicated.

## SURGICAL THERAPY

Most surgeons performing surgery for endometriosis must choose one of two possibilities: conservative surgery, where the patient's future fertility remains an option, or definitive surgery. The latter procedure generally involves removal of the female gonads, a hysterectomy, or a combination of the two. The general perception is that definitive surgery is more effective over time than conservative treatment, but it must be reserved for patients in whom fertility or continued endocrine function is deemed less important than relief of pain symptoms.

When conservative surgery is desired, the first technical issue confronted is method of access. Traditionally, laparotomy was used for endometriosis surgery. However, recently, most surgeons performing extensive surgery for endometriosis have favored a laparoscopic approach because of improved magnification of disease with a resulting increase in surgical precision.

Surgical destruction of endometriosis lesions can be accomplished in a variety of ways: Excision, vaporization, and fulguration/desiccation have all been used. Excision is generally thought to be the most complete of these techniques, but no comparative trials have assessed the relative efficacy of each approach.

Endometriomas, or ovarian cysts formed from endometriosis, are commonly present in the patient with endometriosis. The ovaries should first be freed of all adhesions when operating on endometriomas. The endometrioma may open spontaneously during this process; if not, incision and drainage is indicated. At this point, the cyst wall may be stripped, excised, or drained.

## TREATMENT RESULTS

Medical therapy is effective against endometriosis-associated pain. Placebo-controlled randomized clinical trials (RCTs) have proven that danazol and medroxyprogesterone reduce pain significantly better than no treatment for up to 6 months following discontinuation of the drug. No good data exist for longer follow-up periods. Numerous randomized trials have compared medical therapies to one another. In 15 RCTs comparing danazol to GnRH agonists, no difference was demonstrated between the two as first-line drugs. Similarly, little difference was seen when GnRH agonists were compared to oral contraceptives, progestogens, or gestrinone.

Several trials have addressed the efficacy of combined add-back therapy and GnRH agonist treatment during 6-month treatment periods. In general, pain was relieved as effectively with the combination as

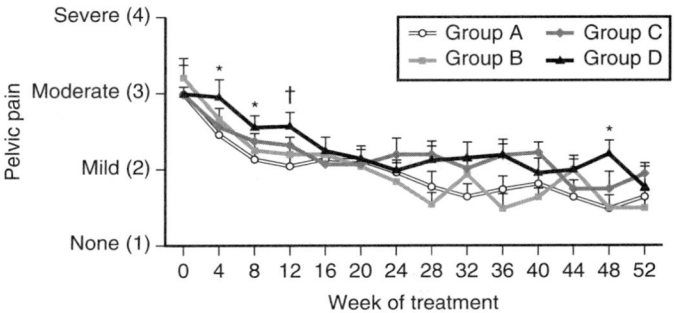

**FIGURE 1.** Pain relief from gonadotropin-releasing hormone (GnRH) agonist (Group A) and three different add-back therapies. (High dose progestin, low dose estrogen/progestin, higher dose estrogen/progestin). No difference is seen among the groups in the amount of pain relief. (From Hornstein MD, Surrey ES, Weisberg GW, Casino LA: et al: Leuprolide acetate depot and hormonal add-back in endometriosis: A 12-month study. Lupron Add-Back Study Group. Obstet Gynecol 1998;91(1):16-24).

with GnRH agonist alone, and it significantly reduced the side effects of the GnRH agonist. The results were similar in three longer trials of approximately 1-year duration (Figure 1). The amelioration of side effects with maintenance of efficacy seems to be even when the add-back therapy is begun during the first month of treatment, suggesting that an add-back-free interval at the beginning of a treatment cycle is unnecessary.

Although the studies just described randomize patients for initial therapy of endometriosis-associated pain, one study examined the value of GnRH agonist in patients failing primary therapy. Ling and colleagues treated women having failed to obtain relief with OCPs with either GnRH agonist or placebo. Those treated with active drug responded significantly better than those given placebo, with more than 80% experiencing pain relief in 3 months (Figure 2). Of interest is the fact that the therapy seemed to be beneficial whether or not endometriosis was seen at laparoscopy.

Most of the established medical therapies used to treat endometriosis have been applied to the problem of subfertility in women with this disease.

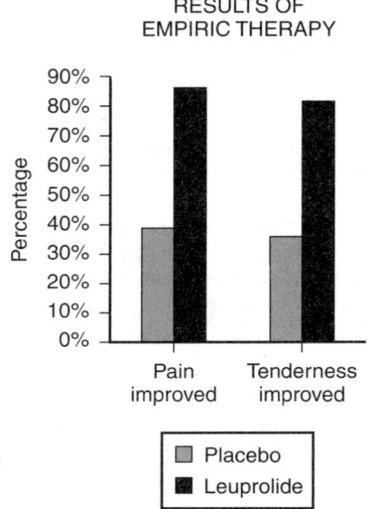

**FIGURE 2.** Patients with pain relief from empirical gonadotropin-releasing hormone (GnRH) agonist or placebo.

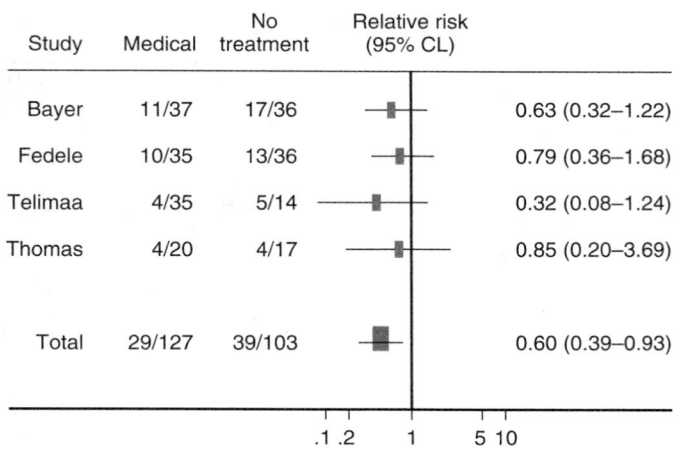

| Study | Medical | No treatment | Relative risk (95% CL) | |
|---|---|---|---|---|
| Bayer | 11/37 | 17/36 | | 0.63 (0.32–1.22) |
| Fedele | 10/35 | 13/36 | | 0.79 (0.36–1.68) |
| Telimaa | 4/35 | 5/14 | | 0.32 (0.08–1.24) |
| Thomas | 4/20 | 4/17 | | 0.85 (0.20–3.69) |
| Total | 29/127 | 39/103 | | 0.60 (0.39–0.93) |

**FIGURE 3.** Meta-analysis of all randomized trials comparing medical therapy versus no treatment or placebo for endometriosis-associated infertility. Note that the untreated group has a significantly better pregnancy rate.

These medications inhibit ovulation, and thus they are used to treat the disease for a period of time prior to allowing an attempt at conception. Five randomized trials with six treatment arms have compared one of these medical treatments for endometriosis to placebo or no treatment with fertility as the outcome measure. Another eight RCTs compared danazol to a second medication. These latter trials were summarized by a meta-analysis by Hughes et al. and modified by Olive and Pritts to include loss of fertility while on the medications (Figure 3). The data clearly show that medical therapy for endometriosis has not proven to be of value, and in fact may be counterproductive, to the subfertile patient.

Only two studies have investigated surgery for endometriosis-associated pain versus sham surgery. Sutton and colleagues assessed the efficacy of laser laparoscopic surgery in the treatment of pain associated with minimal, mild, or moderate endometriosis. They found that there was no difference in pain at 3 months follow-up, but by 6 months a clear-cut advantage was seen for surgery. Abbott and colleagues evaluated excision of endometriosis versus diagnostic laparoscopy and had nearly identical results at 6 months. Thus, both techniques were proven better than no therapy.

Conservative surgery was used extensively in an attempt to enhance fertility. Most studies, however, are uncontrolled and of poor quality. Two randomized trials were performed to examine the value of ablation of early-stage endometriosis versus sham surgery, with contradictory results. When combined into a meta-analysis, surgical treatment of early-stage endometriosis still appears to provide a significant improvement in pregnancy rates. No such trials exist for more extensive disease; expert opinion would suggest that surgery will enhance fertility but may be inferior to advanced reproductive technologies.

The use of medical therapies for endometriosis is not restricted to their use as stand-alone agents. Clinicians frequently have used drugs in combination with surgical treatment of the disease. Numerous trials have examined the issue of postoperative medical therapy as an effective adjunct for pain. Those that have treated patients for at least 6 months after surgery showed efficacy, but in those studies where only 3 months of postoperative treatment was performed, no benefit was seen. Results are similar for all medications (Table 1).

In summary, endometriosis is an enigmatic disease that has long frustrated clinicians and patients. However, great strides in the understanding of this disorder are being made. The coming years are likely to produce a plethora of new treatment approaches targeting the biologic basis of this disease. In this regard, better understanding will undoubtedly result in renewed hope for the patient suffering from the ravages of endometriosis.

### TABLE 1  Postoperative Medical Therapy

| Drug | Duration of Treatment | Studies | Findings |
|---|---|---|---|
| OCPs | 6 mo | 1 | NS at 24, 36 mo |
| Medroxy-progesterone, 100 mg/d | 6 mo | 1 | $p < 0.05$ at 6 mo |
| Danazol, 600 mg/d | 3 mo | 1 | NS at 6 mo |
| Danazol, 600 mg/d | 6 mo | 1 | $p < 0.05$ at 6 mo |
| Danazol, 100 mg/d | 6 mo | 1 | $p < 0.05$ at 24 mo |
| GnRH-a | 3 mo | 1 | NS at 6 mo |
| GnRH-a | 6 mo | 2 | $p = 0.008$ at 12 mo |

*Abbreviations:* GnRH = gonadotropin-releasing hormone; NS = no sample; OCP = oral contraceptive pill.

### REFERENCES

Abbott JA, Hawe J, Hunter D, et al: Laparoscopic excision of endometriosis: A randomized, placebo controlled trial. Fertil Steril 2004;82:878-884.

Hornstein MD, Surrey ES, Weisberg GW, Casino LA, Lupron Add-Back Study Group: Leuprolide acetate depot and hormonal add-back in endometriosis: a 12-month study. Obstet Gynecol 1998;91:16-24.

Hughes E, Ferorkow D, Collins J, Vandekerckhone P: Ovulation suppression for endometriosis (Cochrane review). The Cochrane Library (issue 1): Oxford, England: Update Software, 2000.

Jacobson TZ, Barlow DH, Koninclex PR, et al: Laparoscopic surgery for subfertility associated with endometriosis. Cochrane Database Syst Rev 2002;(4):CD001398.

Jansen RPS, Russel P: Nonpigmented endometriosis: Clinical, laparoscopic and pathologic definition. Am J Obstet Gynecol 1986;155:1154.

Ling FW: Randomized controlled trial of depot leuprolide in patients with chronic pelvic pain and clinically suspected endometriosis. Obstet Gynecol 1999;93:51-58.

Moghissi KS, Schlaff WD, Olive DL, et al: Goserelin acetate (Zoladex) with or without hormone replacement therapy for the treatment of endometriosis. Fertil Steril 1998;69:1056-1062.

Olive DL, Pritts EA: The treatment of endometriosis: a review of the evidence. Ann NY Acad Sci 2002; 955:360-372.

Olive DL, Pritts EA: Treatment of endometriosis. N Engl J Med. 2001;345:266-275.

Sampson JA: Perforating hemorrhagic (chocolate) cysts of the ovary. Arch Surg 1921;3:245.

Sutton CJG, Ewen SP, Whitelaw N, Haines P: Prospective, randomized, double-blind, controlled trial of laser laparoscopy in the treatment of pelvic pain associated with minimal, mild, or moderate endometriosis. Fertil Steril 1994;62:696.

# Dysfunctional Uterine Bleeding

Method of
*Beth W. Rackow, MD, and*
*Aydin Arici, MD*

Abnormal uterine bleeding is a common disorder among reproductive-age women. Dysfunctional uterine bleeding, defined as bleeding that occurs with no identifiable anatomic pathology, affects 33% to 50% of women with abnormal bleeding. Normal menstrual bleeding predictably occurs at the end of an ovulatory cycle because of estrogen and progesterone withdrawal, and lasts up to 7 days, with a cycle interval of 21 to 35 days. Any imbalance of either hormone, estrogen or progesterone, may lead to dysfunctional bleeding. Thus bleeding may occur from estrogen withdrawal because of bilateral oophorectomy or the midcycle fall in estrogen prior to ovulation; from estrogen breakthrough, such as with prolonged estrogen stimulation from chronic anovulation; from progesterone withdrawal after a short or long course of progestin therapy; and from progesterone breakthrough in the setting of a high ratio of progesterone to estrogen, such as with estrogen-progestin and progestin-based contraceptives. Dysfunctional uterine bleeding is a diagnosis of exclusion and requires elimination of other congenital and acquired abnormalities.

Evaluation of the woman with abnormal uterine bleeding must consider a broad differential diagnosis that includes a complication of pregnancy, cervical and uterine pathology (polyps, fibroids, adenomyosis, malignancies, chronic endometritis, congenital anomalies), infectious etiologies (sexually transmitted diseases, vaginitis), endocrinopathies (thyroid or androgen disorders, hyperprolactinemia), medications (exogenous hormonal therapy, anticoagulants, antibiotics, glucocorticoids, tamoxifen [Nolvadex], herbal supplements), bleeding diathesis, systemic illness (liver or renal disease), and genital trauma or foreign bodies. A thorough menstrual history is essential and should include details about past and present length of intermenstrual intervals, regularity of menses, volume and duration of bleeding, onset of abnormal bleeding, factors associated with change in bleeding (postcoital, contraceptive method, postpartum, new medical diagnosis, change in weight), and associated symptoms (premenstrual symptoms, dysmenorrhea, dyspareunia, pelvic pain, hirsutism, galactorrhea). A complete medical history, list of medications, and review of systems helps identify any systemic illness or medication effect contributing to the abnormal bleeding. The physical exam should include careful inspection of the external genitalia, vagina, and cervix and a bimanual exam to palpate the uterus and adnexa to assess size, contour, and tenderness.

Laboratory evaluation provides further information. A negative pregnancy test (preferably quantitative) rules out bleeding because of a pregnancy complication. A complete blood count evaluates for anemia and thrombocytopenia, and is important with prolonged or heavy bleeding. A serum progesterone timed to the luteal phase of the cycle determines if the patient is ovulatory; a level greater than 3 pg/mL is consistent with recent ovulation. Endocrine testing includes serum thyroid stimulating hormone, prolactin, testosterone levels, and further evaluation as indicated. Coagulation studies (prothrombin, partial thromboplastin, bleeding time, and von Willebrand's testing) should be performed in adolescents, women with unexplained menorrhagia, and those with a personal or family history concerning for a bleeding disorder. In the setting of a systemic disorder such as chronic liver or renal disease, appropriate testing should be performed.

An endometrial biopsy should be performed in women at high risk for hyperplasia and cancer based on age (35 years and older) and duration of unopposed estrogen exposure. Young women (less than 35 years old) with chronic anovulation, thus prolonged estrogen exposure, should also undergo endometrial biopsy because they can develop endometrial hyperplasia and cancer. If the biopsy (preferably done in the luteal phase) reveals secretory, not proliferative, endometrium, ovulation has occurred. A pap smear, cervical cultures, and wet mount should also be performed as indicated.

A history of regular menstrual cycles with an increasing amount or duration of bleeding, or intermenstrual bleeding, is suggestive of an anatomic cause of abnormal bleeding. Transvaginal ultrasound provides detailed assessment of the uterus and endometrium. Pathology such as fibroids and polyps can be identified, and size and location determined. Although an endometrial biopsy may not be necessary if the endometrium is thin (less than 5 mm), clinical suspicion of endometrial pathology takes precedence. Sonohysterography (or saline-infusion sonography) involves ultrasound assessment of the uterus and endometrium while sterile saline distends the uterine cavity. This procedure has high sensitivity and specificity for identifying uterine and endometrial pathology and is comparable to hysteroscopy.

Hysteroscopy can simultaneously diagnose and treat intrauterine pathology, but involves an invasive procedure. During assessment of uterine anatomy, it is important to recognize when anatomic abnormalities, such as fibroids, are present but not contributing to the bleeding.

# Anovulatory Dysfunctional Uterine Bleeding

A menstrual history that reveals irregular, infrequent, unpredictable bleeding, a varying amount and duration of bleeding, and no reliable symptomatology is often sufficient to diagnose anovulatory bleeding. Considered a systemic disorder, anovulatory bleeding occurs because of a variety of endocrinologic, neurochemical, and pharmacologic processes. Estrogen breakthrough is the most common scenario: persistently high estrogen levels stimulate overgrowth of an endometrium that is fragile without the stabilizing, growth-limiting effects of progesterone, and focal areas of the endometrium breakdown, bleed, and subsequently heal because of estrogen effect. This dysfunctional bleeding is common in women with polycystic ovary syndrome or obesity, in postmenarchal adolescents, and in perimenopausal women. Other conditions associated with anovulation include thyroid disorders, hyperprolactinemia, androgen disorders, psychological or physical stress, eating disorders, dramatic weight changes, and insulin resistance.

Management of anovulatory bleeding involves treating both the cause of anovulation and the abnormal bleeding. Progestins are the foundation of this medical therapy. Cyclic progestins stabilize the estrogen-stimulated endometrium and result in withdrawal bleeding after the progestin course. Medications used for a 10-day course every 4 to 6 weeks include medroxyprogesterone acetate (Provera), 5 to 10 mg, and norethindrone acetate (Aygestin), 5 mg. If bleeding does not occur after progestin withdrawal, the woman may also be hypoestrogenic, and further evaluation is indicated. Estrogen-progestin contraceptives are advantageous for women with intermittent ovulation who require contraception, and they also effectively decrease the amount of bleeding. Combined contraceptives are available in pill, patch, and vaginal ring preparations. Medroxyprogesterone acetate (Depo-Provera),[1] 150 mg intramuscularly every 3 months, can also be used to manage anovulatory bleeding, especially if women cannot take combined contraceptives. This therapy may cause irregular bleeding in the first few months, but 50% of women report amenorrhea by 12 months of use. Treatment of prolonged heavy anovulatory bleeding can be achieved with either low-dose monophasic combined contraceptives,[1] one pill twice daily for 5 to 7 days until the bleeding slows or stops, followed by routine daily use if desired, or with a higher-dose course of progestin therapy. Once the heavy bleeding is controlled, further evaluation is warranted.

Estrogen therapy is indicated for the treatment of dysfunctional bleeding with a thinned endometrium because of low estrogen levels or prolonged bleeding. This can be accomplished with conjugated estrogens (Premarin),[1] 1.25 mg, or micronized estradiol (Estrace),[1] 2 mg daily for 7 to 10 days. Similarly, estrogen (a 7- to 10-day course) can be used to treat progesterone breakthrough bleeding in the setting of low-dose combined contraceptives or long-acting progesterone therapy (medroxyprogesterone acetate [Depo-Provera]).

# Ovulatory Dysfunctional Uterine Bleeding

Heavy or prolonged bleeding may occur during ovulatory cycles, and often no specific etiology is identified. Local defects in endometrial hemostasis are implicated. A number of medical and surgical therapies are effective in this situation. Nonsteroidal anti-inflammatory drugs (NSAIDs), such as ibuprofen (Motrin),[1] naproxen (Aleve),[1] or mefenamic acid (Ponstel),[1] decrease menstrual blood loss by inhibiting

---

[1]Not FDA approved for this indication.

## CURRENT DIAGNOSIS

- Detailed medical and menstrual history
- Thorough physical and gynecologic examination
- Pregnancy test for all reproductive-age women
- Determination of ovulatory status by history, laboratory tests
- Laboratory evaluation: complete blood count, endocrine studies, coagulation profile
- Endometrial sampling if high risk for hyperplasia or cancer
- Imaging studies to evaluate anatomy

## CURRENT THERAPY

- Progestins
  - Cyclic or intermittent use
  - Prolonged therapy
  - Progestin-releasing intrauterine device (IUD) (Mirena)[1]
- Estrogens[1]
  - Intermittent use
  - High-dose course for acute heavy bleeding
- Estrogen-progestin contraceptives[1]
  - Cyclic use
  - High-dose course with taper for heavy bleeding
- Other therapies
  - Nonsteroidal anti-inflammatory drugs[1]
  - Tranexamic acid (Cyklokapron)[1]
  - Danazol (Danocrine)[1]
  - Gonadotropin-releasing hormone agonists
- Surgical options
  - Endometrial ablation
  - Myomectomy
  - Uterine artery embolization
  - Hysterectomy

[1]Not FDA approved for this indication.

prostaglandin synthesis, and thus altering the balance of factors required for endometrial hemostasis. NSAIDs may decrease blood loss by 20% to 40%, and should be initiated just prior to the onset of menses and continued for 3 to 5 days. Similarly, combined contraceptives can reduce menstrual flow by 40% to 60%. Another option is the levonorgestrel-releasing intrauterine system (Mirena)[1]; the local progestin effect on the endometrium is profound and can reduce menstrual blood loss by 75% to 90% in women with heavy bleeding. Although cyclic progestins are often ineffective in this setting, a course of progestin (norethindrone acetate, 5 mg three times daily) from days 5 to 26 of the cycle can suppress heavy ovulatory bleeding. Gonadotropin-releasing hormone agonists produce a hypoestrogenic state and thus cause amenorrhea as well as shrinkage of fibroids, if present. This therapy is best reserved for short-term management of heavy bleeding and severe anemia prior to a surgical procedure because of its cost and significant side effects such as menopausal symptoms and bone demineralization. Less commonly employed therapies include tranexamic acid (Cyklokapron),[1] an antifibrinolytic agent used in Europe to treat menorrhagia (1 g every 6 hours for the first few days of bleeding), and danazol (Danocrine),[1] a therapy that inhibits ovulation and decreases menstrual blood loss but involves androgenic side effects (200 mg daily).

Intermenstrual bleeding can also occur during ovulatory cycles. This dysfunctional bleeding may be caused by anatomic abnormalities, infection, or the preovulatory decline in estrogen. Conjugated estrogens (Premarin),[1] 1.25 mg, or micronized estradiol (Estrace), 2 mg for 2 to 3 days midcycle or 7 to 10 days for persistent breakthrough bleeding, are effective.

For patients who fail medical therapy or for those who do not desire future fertility, surgical management is appropriate. The definitive procedure is hysterectomy, but this surgery carries a significant risk of complications and involves longer recovery time. Endometrial ablation by hysteroscopic, thermal, or cryosurgical techniques is a less invasive procedure for the management of abnormal bleeding in women who do not desire future fertility. These techniques can result in significantly reduced bleeding and dysmenorrhea, and even amenorrhea, but approximately 20% of patients require additional procedures. Patients with menorrhagia attributed to uterine fibroids can be managed with myomectomy (hysteroscopic, laparoscopic, or abdominal procedures as indicated) or uterine artery embolization. Pregnancy is not recommended after the latter option because little data are available on postprocedure pregnancy outcomes.

## Uterine Hemorrhage

Acute heavy bleeding requires high-dose estrogen therapy. Women who need inpatient management should receive conjugated estrogens (Premarin), 25 mg intravenously every 4 hours for 24 hours or until the bleeding decreases. A Foley catheter balloon (30 cc) can be placed in the uterine cavity to tamponade the bleeding. Additionally, dilation

and curettage can be performed to help stop acute uterine hemorrhage. If stable for outpatient management, women can receive conjugated estrogens (Premarin),[1] 1.25 mg, or micronized estradiol (Estrace),[1] 2 mg every 4 to 6 hours for 24 hours, and when the bleeding is controlled, the dose is tapered to once daily for 7 to 10 days. Another effective regimen uses high-dose combination contraceptives[1] (3 to 4 pills daily) until the bleeding is decreased, followed by a taper to 1 pill daily for several weeks. Estrogen therapy should be followed by progestins or combined contraceptives to stabilize the estrogen-stimulated endometrium.

Because dysfunctional uterine bleeding is a diagnosis of exclusion, a thorough history and evaluation, including determination of ovulatory status, is essential. A number of medical and surgical options exist for the management of dysfunctional bleeding. However, treatment failures require further evaluation.

## REFERENCES

American College of Obstetricians and Gynecologists: Management of anovulatory bleeding. ACOG Practice Bulletin, no. 14, March 2000.

Bayer SR, DeCherney AH: Clinical manifestations and treatment of dysfunctional uterine bleeding. JAMA 1993;269:1823-1828.

Berek JS (ed): Benign diseases of the female reproductive tract. In Berek JS, ed: Novak's Gynecology. Philadelphia, Lippincott Williams & Wilkins, 2002, pp 351-373.

Farquhar CM, Lethaby A, Sowter M, et al: An evaluation of risk factors for endometrial hyperplasia in premenopausal women with abnormal menstrual bleeding. Am J Obstet Gynecol 1999;181:525-529.

Kouides PA, Conard J, Peyvandi F, et al: Hemostasis and menstruation: Appropriate investigation for underlying disorders of hemostasis in women with excessive menstrual bleeding. Fertil Steril 2005;84:1345-1351.

Munro MG: Dysfunctional uterine bleeding: Advances in diagnosis and treatment. Curr Opin Obstet Gynecol 2001;13:475-489.

Munro MG: Medical management of abnormal uterine bleeding. Obstet Gynecol Clin North Am 2000;27:287-304.

Shwayder JM: Pathophysiology of abnormal uterine bleeding. Obstet Gynecol Clin North Am 2000;27:219-234.

Speroff L, Fritz M: Dysfunctional uterine bleeding. In Clinical Gynecologic Endocrinology and Infertility. Philadelphia, Lippincott Williams & Wilkins; 2005, pp 548-571.

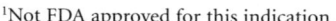

[1]Not FDA approved for this indication.

# Infertility

Method of
*Steven R. Williams, MD*

Absence of desired conception despite 12 months of unprotected intercourse generally defines infertility. Historical and physical factors allow the physician to adjust this definition to the individual patient. For example, women with longstanding amenorrhea or known distal hydrosalpinges should consider intervention before 12 months, time has elapsed. However, the couple, 22 years of age, with a negative history can be encouraged to try a bit longer than 12 months before evaluation begins. After 6 months of trying, approximately 45% of couples achieve pregnancy, and after 12 months of trying, approximately 85% will conceive. Pregnancy can occur with sex 6 days before ovulation, although one study found no pregnancies were conceived from sex the day after ovulation. Thus we recommend couples trying for a baby should plan to be active together every other day starting about 6 days before ovulation is expected (cycle day 8) until 2 to 3 days after ovulation has happened (cycle day 18). If the mood were to strike more often, that's fine with us; if the mood strikes less often, we can still be comfortable given the 6-day interval previously described. As in all of medicine, important historical points can guide the direction of the evaluation and treatment of the infertile couple.

Male-factor historical points include fathering past pregnancies or miscarriages, sexual function, urologic or hernia surgery, infections, medications, and tobacco use. Semen analysis remains the most important test for male factor evaluation. The World Health Organization (WHO) reports normal males to have more than 20 million sperm per cc with greater than 50% motility. It is probably best to advise 48 hours of abstinence before collection of the sample. A urologic exam and evaluation is indicated with abnormal counts. Modern in vitro fertilization (IVF) treatments can achieve pregnancies as long as any sperm at all can be isolated, even if that means surgical aspiration. Before pursuing assisted reproduction for severely low counts, genetic testing will be recommended because severely low counts can predict higher rates of cystic fibrosis carrier status, balanced translocation, and perhaps microdeletions of the Y chromosome.

A women's age has a strong correlation with fertility success. Figure 1 compares the live birth rate when IVF patients used their own eggs fertilized with their partner's sperm compared to the rate when young oocyte donor's eggs are fertilized with the IVF patient's partner's sperm and the resultant embryos transferred into the IVF patient's uterus. One must conclude from these data that the majority of the decline in success is related to oocyte quality, as anyone can expect the success of a woman 25 years of age who uses the oocytes from a woman 25 years of age! Follicle-stimulating hormone (FSH) measured on day 3 of the menstrual cycle correlates well with ovarian reserve and is commonly ordered for women more than 30 years of age with infertility. In our office, day-3 FSH values lower than 9 mU/mL are reassuring with respect to ovarian reserve, whereas values greater than 20 mU/mL are rarely associated with future fertility success using that patient's eggs.

Previous full-term deliveries are reassuring, whereas recurrent abortions or preterm deliveries can predict a uterine issue. Pelvic infections, intrauterine device (IUD) use, previous abdominal surgery, dysmenorrhea, or dyspareunia can predict tubal obstruction. This is explored with hysterosalpingography (HSG). After sterile preparation of the cervix, a sterile cannula is inserted, and under fluoroscopic guidance radiograph contrast is injected. The dye reveals the contour of the uterine cavity and displays uterine septa and intracavitary lesions such as fibroids or polyps. It then fills into the fallopian tubes and spills into the abdominal cavity. Most women describe the discomfort of the test as a severe menstrual cramp that lasts for several minutes. Pain is reduced by slow injection of the dye, gentle tissue handling, and pretreatment with nonsteroidal anti-inflammatory drugs (NSAIDs). Many authors suggest that the procedure itself has a fertility-enhancing effect. The American College of Obstetricians and Gynecologists (ACOG) suggests prophylaxis with doxycycline (Vibramycin)[1] 100 mg twice daily orally for 5 days after HSG if dilated tubes are demonstrated; no prophylaxis is indicated in a normal study. Abnormal uterine cavities can be further evaluated with saline infusion hysterograms or magnetic resonance imaging (MRI). Many uterine abnormalities can be treated completely with hysteroscopic surgery. Unilateral tubal disease noted on the HSG predicts subtle decreases in future fertility in these women compared with women with normal tubes. Bilateral tubal disease discovered on HSG predicts dramatic declines in fertility. Tubal patency established by HSG does not rule out peritubal adhesions that can affect fertility. Laparoscopy is an outpatient surgical procedure that can be used to further evaluate tubal abnormalities seen on HSG or to look for undetected peritubal adhesions. Laparoscopy also will detect endometriosis.

Endometriosis is noted in approximately 1 in 30 laparoscopies performed for tubal ligation (presumably for fertile women), although one third of women undergoing infertility evaluations will have endometriosis. Surgical treatment of minimal or mild endometriosis does appear to help with subsequent fertility somewhat. A prospective study of infertile women found to have mild or minimal endometriosis noted at laparoscopy showed a 31% pregnancy rate in the next 9 months for patients randomized to treatment versus a 17% pregnancy rate in the next 9 months for women randomized to no treatment.

Irregular menstruation generally indicates irregular ovulation and diminished fertility. Even with regular menstruations, serum progesterone measurements in the luteal phase (6 to 8 days after ovulation) should be greater than 10 ng/mL for the "most fertile" of ovulations. If it is not, thyroid and prolactin studies should be ordered and induction of ovulation with clomiphene citrate (Clomid) considered. Clomiphene citrate in a 50-mg dose is taken orally for 5 days starting on menstrual day 3. Serum luteal phase progesterone is drawn 7 days after ovulation and is expected to be greater than 10 ng/dL. If it is, refills for 2 more months of treatment are written. If it is not, we recommend increasing the dose of clomiphene citrate to 100 mg daily for 5 days and repeating the luteal phase progesterone assay. If still not greater than 10 ng/dL, clomiphene citrate at 150 mg daily can be tried. If the patient is still anovulatory, referral to a gynecologist or reproductive endocrinologist is considered. For resistant patients, adjunctive treatments with the clomiphene citrate can include ultrasound monitoring with HCG injections when mature follicles are noted or adding insulin-sensitizing agents or glucocorticoids. Clomiphene ovulation induction yields approximately a 70% ovulation rate and, in young couples, approximately an 8% pregnancy rate per month. One in ten clomiphene citrate pregnancies are twins, although triplets and quadruplets are very rare on this therapy.

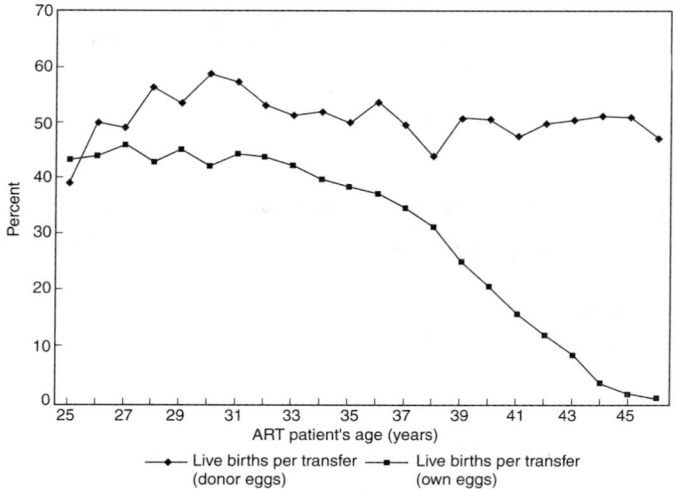

**FIGURE 1.** Live births per transfer for ART cycles using fresh embryos from own and donor eggs, by ART patient's age, 2002. ART = assisted reproductive technology.

[1]Not FDA approved for this indication.

## CURRENT DIAGNOSIS

- Medical history can guide fertility testing.
- Simple laboratory and radiograph tests can determine infertility causes.

Side effects of clomiphene citrate include hot flushes, emotional lability, mittelschmerz, headache, and sleep disturbance. Discontinue the drug if the patient experiences severe visual disturbance. Because the majority of clomiphene citrate pregnancies happen early in treatment, referral to reproductive specialists should be considered if the patients is not pregnant after 3 months of treatment.

Gonadotropin ovulation induction is available for women who failed to ovulate using clomiphene citrate or did not conceive on that therapy. This medication is the natural hormone used to initiate ovulation; therefore, response and pregnancy rates are better than with clomiphene citrate. Unfortunately, dramatic increases in multiple pregnancy are associated with these medications, and often they are quite expensive. One large study reviewed success and multiple pregnancy rates in patients treated with gonadotropin ovulation induction. The authors concluded the protocols employed with gonadotropin ovulation induction lead to an unacceptably high incidence of higher-order multiple pregnancies and raised the question whether that treatment could be replaced by IVF.

IVF involves induction of ovulation with gonadotropin in hopes of retrieving multiple oocytes. Ovarian response is monitored with pelvic ultrasounds and serum estradiol measurements. When the oocytes are mature, HCG is given to trigger the completion of oocyte development. Then transvaginal ultrasound is used to guide an aspirating needle through the posterior cul-de-sac and into the ovaries for aspiration of the oocytes. The procedure takes approximately 15 minutes under local anesthesia and is often performed in an office setting. Oocytes are then inseminated in the lab with the husband's sperm and cultured. In certain circumstances (vey low sperm count, surgically aspirated sperm, previous failed fertilization) the oocytes can be directly injected with the sperm via intracytoplasmic sperm injection (ICSI). The resultant embryos are then cultured for 2 to 5 days and then transferred into the uterus via a simple transcervical approach. IVF thus allows embryo development without tubal ovarial interaction, making it a great choice for patients with tubal disease or endometriosis. In fact, nothing we can find at laparoscopy that was not discovered by pelvic ultrasound and HSG will affect IVF success (Figure 2). We are developing protocols that reduce the numbers of embryos transferred for couples at high risk for multiple pregnancy to one. I believe that in the future IVF will replace both gonadotropin ovulation induction and the need for laparoscopy for treatment of infertility. The 2001 Centers for Disease Control (CDC) report on assisted reproductive technology (ART) success reported national average live birth rates in the high 30% per cycle start for women younger than 35 years of age. Some individual centers are reporting live birth rates in the 50% range. IVF is a very effective and increasingly safer alternative to older treatments for refractory infertility.

## CURRENT THERAPY

- Clomiphene citrate is a low risk treatment option when indicated.
- Assisted reproduction is delivering more and more babies with fewer multiples.

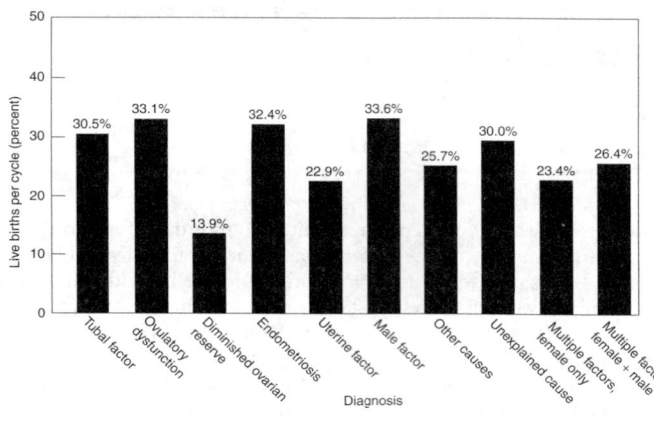

**FIGURE 2.** Live birth rates among women who had ART cycles using fresh nondonor eggs or embryos, by diagnosis, 2002. ART = assisted reproductive technology.

## REFERENCES

American College of Obstetrics and Gynecology: Antibiotic prophylaxis for gynecologic procedures. ACOG Practice Bulletin 2003;23.

Centers of Disease Control: 2002 Assisted reproductive technology success rates, National summary and fertility clinic reports. Atlanta, Center for Disease Control, 2002.

Gleicher N, Oleske DM, Tur-Kaspa I, et al: Reducing the risk of higher order multiple pregnancy after ovarian stimulation with gonadotropins. N Engl J Med 2000;343:2-7.

Jain T, Soules MR, Collins JA: Comparison of basal follicle-stimulating hormone versus the clomiphene citrate challenge test for ovarian reserve testing. Fertil Steril 2004;82:180-185.

Jordan J, Craig K, Clifton DK, et al: Luteal phase defect: The sensitivity and specificity of diagnostic methods in common clinical use. Fertil Steril 1995;63:427-428.

Marcoux S, Maheux R, Berube S: Laparoscopic surgery in infertile women with minimal or mild endometriosis. Canadian collaborative group on endometriosis. N Engl J Med 1997;337:217-222.

Mol BW, Swart P, Bossuyt BM, et al: Is hysterosalpingography an important tool in predicting fertility outcome? Fertil Steril 1997;67:663-669.

Schwabe MG. Shapiro SS, Haning RV Jr: Hysterosalpingography with oil contrast medium enhances fertility in patients with infertility of unknown etiology. Fertil Steril 1983;40:604-606.

Trimbos JB, Trimbos-Kemper GC, Peters AA, et al: Findings in 200 consecutive asymptomatic women, having a laparoscopic sterilization. Arch Gynecol Obstet 1990;247:121-124.

Wilcox AJ, Weinberg CR, Baird DD: Timing of sexual intercourse in relation to ovulation. Effects on the probability of conception, survival of the pregnancy, and sex of the baby. N Engl J Med 1995;333:1517-1521.

# Amenorrhea

Method of
*Vickie Martin, MD, and Robert L. Reid, MD*

Amenorrhea, simply put, is the absence of menses. It can be classified as either primary (when a woman of reproductive age has never had menstruation) or secondary (when amenorrhea occurs after menstruation has been established). There are normal situations in which amenorrhea is expected (physiologic amenorrhea): during pregnancy, during lactation, and at the onset of menopause. Approximately 5% of reproductive-age women experience amenorrhea at times other than these, which warrants investigation. Women with amenorrhea often present with significant apprehension and anxiety. Thus, an appropriate but timely work-up and diagnosis are required. The clinician must have a systematic approach for evaluating such women to ensure that important causes of amenorrhea are identified. As always, a detailed history, a targeted physical examination, and selective use of simple diagnostic tests are required.

## Definition

Amenorrhea may be defined as the absence of menstruation for 3 or more months in women with past menses (secondary amenorrhea) or the absence of menarche by the age of 16 years in girls who have never menstruated (primary amenorrhea). Infrequent menstruation, termed *oligomenorrhea*, may have similar causes and also warrants investigation.

## Menstrual Cycle

A clear working knowledge of the menstrual cycle and its physiology is mandatory for the clinician in these circumstances. Menstruation normally results when a cascade of hormonal signals from the hypothalamus (gonadotropin-releasing hormone [GnRH]) to cause pituitary release of luteinizing hormone (LH) and follicle-stimulating hormone (FSH). These in turn stimulate the development of an egg-containing ovarian follicle. Estrogen from this follicle results in steady growth of the endometrial lining over a 2-week period (follicular phase). When ovulation occurs, the follicle (now called the corpus luteum) develops the ability to produce a second hormone, progesterone.

The secretion of estrogen and progesterone for the next 2-week period causes the endometrial lining to become lush (decidualized) in preparation for implantation of a pregnancy. If pregnancy fails to occur, the corpus luteum undergoes a spontaneous demise, the endometrium no longer has adequate hormonal support to survive, and the tissue is sloughed synchronously over the next 5 to 7 days as menstrual flow. The final steps of this process require a means of egress for blood, implying a normal uterus with a patent cervix and vagina (the outflow tract).

## Etiology

Different classification systems have been employed. One system defines the type of amenorrhea based on the level of FSH in circulation. For example, high FSH levels indicate that the hypothalamus and pituitary are fully functioning but that the ovary is not responding (similar to menopause). The gonadotropin (FSH) levels are high and the ovary (gonad) is not functioning, which is termed *hypergonadotropic hypogonadism*. *Hypogonadotropic hypogonadism* refers to the situation where FSH levels are very low due to some central disturbance of hypothalamic or pituitary function. The problem with this classification is that normal FSH levels are often low and the distinction between hypogonadotropic and eugonadotropic causes of amenorrhea can be difficult.

A simple way to consider causes of amenorrhea is to divide the processes that regulate menstruation (the hypothalamic-pituitary-ovarian axis [HPO axis]) into compartments (Figure 1) and then consider possible contributory factors for disruption of normal processes at each of these levels. Always consider the possibility that amenorrhea may be due to unexpected pregnancy before moving on to a full investigation.

### HYPOTHALAMIC COMPARTMENT

The hypothalamus integrates a wide variety of signals from the brain and is ultimately responsible for turning on or off the hormonal cascade necessary for triggering ovulatory and menstrual function. In adolescents, the development of breasts (thelarche) between ages 8 and

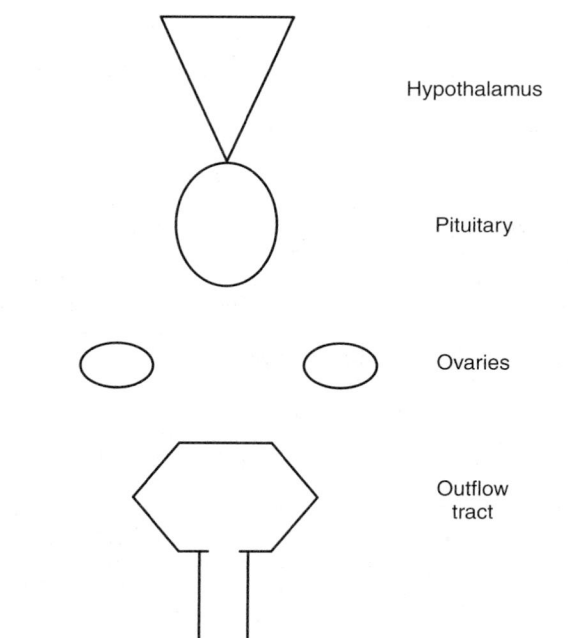

**FIGURE 1.** The four compartments to consider when evaluating amenorrhea.

10 years is usually the first sign that the HPO axis has turned on and first menstruation (menarche) typically follows within 3 to 5 years. All girls with primary amenorrhea by age 14 years, particularly if 5 or more years have passed since the first evidence of pubertal development, warrant careful investigation, because girls with primary amenorrhea on the basis of constitutional delay cannot readily be differentiated on clinical history from the two thirds of patients with primary amenorrhea who have irreversible causes of reproductive failure.

### Constitutional Delay

One third of young women presenting with primary amenorrhea have constitutional delay of puberty, meaning that they are undergoing a normal sequence of pubertal development at a rate that falls 2.5 standard deviations behind the mean. Girls with constitutional delay often present between ages 13 and 16 with primary amenorrhea and only early signs of breast development. Investigation reveals low to low-normal levels of gonadotropins and an otherwise negative work-up.

### Congenital Causes

A variety of unusual congenital conditions result in hypogonadotropic hypogonadism and primary amenorrhea. These conditions may be caused by deficiency of GnRH production or by abnormalities of the GnRH receptor. A Kallman's-like syndrome has been identified in some affected women who present with anosmia and a complete lack of pubertal development.

### Acquired Causes

Acquired diseases can lead the hypothalamus to shut down the reproductive hormonal cascade, resulting in amenorrhea, which may be primary or secondary, depending on when they develop. Nutritional deprivation (including eating disorders), excessive caloric demand due to participation in demanding sports, and extreme psychological stress are common reasons for delayed activation of reproductive processes by the hypothalamus. Less commonly, systemic illnesses, including malabsorption states, active autoimmune diseases, and rare hypoxemic states related to congenital heart malformations or severe anemias (sickle cell disease), can lead to amenorrhea.

## PITUITARY COMPARTMENT

Lesions of the pituitary stalk that interrupt normal delivery of GnRH to the pituitary include those resulting from head trauma, rare stalk tumors such as craniopharyngiomas, or from the surgery to remove these.

Pituitary causes of amenorrhea are almost always due to oversecretion of prolactin. Hyperprolactinemia resulting in amenorrhea, if associated with central retro-orbital headache and bitemporal hemianopia, can result from a prolactin-producing tumor.

Other causes of hyperprolactinemia originate outside the pituitary. For example, primary hypothyroidism, breast or chest wall lesions (or piercings) in the T4-6 dermatome, renal failure, and a variety of medications have all been linked to hyperprolactinemia. Medications that can cause hyperprolactinemia include dopamine receptor antagonists (phenothiazines, butyrophenones, thioxanthenes, risperidone, metoclopramide, sulpiride,[2] pimozide), dopamine-depleting agents (e.g., methyldopa, reserpine), $H_2$-blockers (cimetidine), opiates, and cocaine.

Rarely, other pituitary conditions result in amenorrhea. In empty sella syndrome, radiologic examination reveals an apparently empty sella due to pituitary regression from some vascular or other insult. Other conditions include Sheehan syndrome (postpartum pituitary necrosis), pituitary apoplexy (massive pituitary infarction), and radiation-induced hypopituitarism. In each of these situations, amenorrhea is usually part of a larger picture of endocrine disruption.

## OVARIAN COMPARTMENT

Depletion of eggs from the ovary before or after puberty results in primary or secondary amenorrhea, respectively. FSH levels are markedly elevated in these cases, as the hypothalamus and pituitary try to elicit follicular development from the unresponsive ovary. Destruction of oocytes by any of several environmental insults, including ionizing radiation, various chemotherapeutic (especially alkylating) agents, and certain viral infections can accelerate follicular atresia.

Primary amenorrhea in a woman with evidence of gonadal failure should elicit a search for a chromosomal abnormality. It is known that two intact X chromosomes are needed for maintenance of ovarian function. A variety of X chromosome structural abnormalities have been identified in women with premature ovarian failure, including complete absence of one X chromosome (Turner's syndrome).

Elevated FSH occurs in association with a normal karyotype. These women have normal 46,XY or 46,XX karyotypes without the phenotypic abnormalities of Turner's syndrome. Those with a Y chromosome should have their gonads removed because of the potential for malignant transformation.

Several rare inherited enzymatic defects also may be associated with premature ovarian failure. These include partial deficiencies in four enzymes in the steroidogenic pathway—17α-hydroxylase, 17, 20-desmolase, 20,22-desmolase, and aromatase—and galactosemia.

Premature ovarian failure may be associated with a number of autoimmune disorders. Most commonly associated with thyroiditis, ovarian failure also occurs in women with polyglandular failure, including hypoparathyroidism, hypoadrenalism, and mucocutaneous candidiasis.

Though it is not exclusively an ovarian disorder, it is useful to consider polycystic ovary syndrome (PCOS) in the ovarian compartment for the purpose of completeness in considering possible diagnoses. PCOS is one of the most common causes of secondary amenorrhea. Typically, women suffering from this condition are overweight (although one third have normal body weight) and have clinical features of hyperandrogenism (acne and hirsutism), hyperinsulinism (acanthosis nigricans), and hyperestrogenism (watery cervical mucus). Months of amenorrhea may be punctuated by episodes of heavy and prolonged menstrual bleeding as an estrogen-thickened endometrium sheds irregularly over several weeks.

---

[2]Not available in the United States.

## OUTFLOW TRACT COMPARTMENT

Congenital abnormalities of development of the reproductive outflow tract can cause amenorrhea. Complete absence of a uterus can be due to isolated müllerian agenesis or it can manifest in phenotypic females with a 46,XY karyotype who have complete androgen insensitivity. Developmental abnormalities can include cervical atresia, tranverse vaginal septum, and imperforate hymen. These latter abnormalities may be associated with cyclic menstrual pain in the absence of bleeding (cryptomenorrhea). Similarly, monthly cramps can occur with cervical stenosis following trachelectomy or conization. Uterine synechiae due to a vigorous curettage in the face of a postpartum or postabortion endometritis can result in obliteration of the uterine cavity and secondary amenorrhea with or without monthly menstrual-like cramps.

## OTHER CAUSES

Pregnancy must always be considered in a sexually active female patient presenting with secondary amenorrhea. Hormonal suppression of the endometrium can be accomplished with a variety of medications. The progestin component of the cyclic oral contraceptive gradually results in a thinner and thinner endometrium, which can ultimately result in pill-withdrawal amenorrhea. Other medications, including danazol, medroxyprogesterone, and long-acting GnRH agonists can result in amenorrhea.

# Diagnosis

### HISTORY

A search for clues as to the etiology should start with a personal developmental history in the amenorrheic teen and with a menstrual and reproductive history in the older amenorrheic woman. Events in the 3 to 6 months preceding the onset of amenorrhea are often critical. Rapid weight gain or loss or a marked change in energy expenditure through exercise may be important. Systems review should examine possible disruption to any of the compartments (Box 1). Inquiry about general health, risk of pregnancy, and use of medication (including illicit drugs) is important.

---

 **CURRENT DIAGNOSIS**

- Always consider the possibility of pregnancy in any woman presenting with secondary amenorrhea.
- Secondary amenorrhea is most commonly the result of some significant lifestyle change (weight gain or loss, stress, excessive exercise) or illness (with marked weight loss) in the preceding 6 months.
- Obesity and features of androgen excess are most often related to polycystic ovary syndrome (PCOS).
- Because constitutional delay of puberty is found in only one third of girls presenting with delayed menarche, an investigation should be initiated at the time of presentation rather than waiting until the girl is 16 years old (meeting the definitional criteria).
- Primary amenorrhea, particularly with the absence of other features of pubertal development (breasts and pubic and axillary hair) suggests ovarian failure.
- When amenorrhea due to ovarian failure (high FSH) occurs before age 35 years, a karyotype is indicated. If Y chromosome material is identified on karyotype, gonadectomy is required to reduce the risk of malignancy in the gonadal tissues.

---

## BOX 1  A Compartmental Approach to Systems Review

**Hypothalamic Compartment**
- Changes in temperature regulation, sleep, appetite, thirst
- Headache or visual field defects

**Pituitary Compartment**
- Central retro-orbital headache, bitemporal hemianopia
- Galactorrhea
- Features of hypothyroidism
- Medications affecting prolactin

**Ovary Compartment**
- Hot flushes
- Insomnia
- Night sweats
- Vaginal dryness

**Outflow Compartment**
- Cyclic cramps
- Possibility of pregnancy
- Recent gynecologic procedures (dilation and curettage, cervical laser or conizadon)

## PHYSICAL EXAMINATION

Height, weight, and body mass index (BMI) should be determined. Body habitus often provides an important clue to which patients are amenorrheic due to excessive physical or nutritional stress (eating disorder or malnutrition). In primary amenorrhea, examination for the stage of breast and pubic hair development (Tanner staging) can indicate whether there has been delay or disruption to the entire process of pubertal development. Restriction of later visual fields to examination by confrontation, the presence of galactorrhea, or evidence of recent scars or lesions in the region of the breast (such as zoster) can implicate hyperprolactinemia. The thyroid gland should be palpated and features of hypothyroidism sought. A lower abdominal mass may be due to pregnancy, hematocolpos or hematometra.

The gynecologic examination should be tailored to the patient. The external genitalia should be evaluated for pubic hair, acanthosis nigricans, and clitoral size. The hymen should be visualized; an imperforate hymen usually shows a bluish central bulge. Estrogenization of the tissues (presence of leukorrhea, thickened mucosa, or watery cervical mucus) can be assessed with speculum examination (choosing a speculum size appropriate to the sexual maturity of the patient). Visualization of the cervix in most circumstances is sufficient to rule out an outflow compartment problem.

## INVESTIGATIONS

### Initial Investigations

Initial investigation for any patient with amenorrhea or oligomenorrhea includes follicle-stimulating hormone (FSH), prolactin (PRL), thyroid stimulating hormone (TSH), and a sensitive pregnancy test if pregnancy is a possibility.

Ultrasonography can be helpful when an internal examination cannot be performed. When a congenital anomaly is considered, magnetic resonance imaging (MRI) can provide more definitive information.

### Follow-up Investigations

A low normal FSH in the presence of a normal outflow tract should elicit a more detailed search for hypothalamic disruptors (such as nutritional, physical, or psychological stress). In a patient who has low

FSH in conjunction with an elevated PRL and who is not taking medications known to increase PRL and whose TSH is normal, lesions of the hypothalamus or pituitary should be excluded with CT or MRI.

An elevated FSH indicates ovarian failure and should elicit a search for possible explanations such as past surgery, exposure to radiation or chemotherapy, or genetic causes. With an elevated FSH, a karyotype is usually indicated unless there is some obvious cause for loss of ovarian function. If the karyotype reveals any Y chromosome material, then, at the appropriate age, referral to a gynecologist is necessary for counseling and gonadectomy to reduce the risk of gonadoblastoma and dysgerminoma.

Evidence of outflow tract obstruction on pelvic examination or the possibility of cervical stenosis (cyclic dysmenorrhea without bleeding after a cervical surgical procedure such as a loop excision, cone biopsy, or trachelectomy) or Asherman's syndrome (obliteration of the endometrial cavity following a postpregnancy or postabortion dilation and curettage) merits referral to a gynecologist for further assessment and management.

Secondary amenorrhea related to weight gain or obesity, particularly when associated with features of acne and hirsutism, suggests the polycystic ovary syndrome. Management depends on whether the patient is seeking menstrual cycle regulation and relief from hirsutism (cyclic progestational therapy or an oral contraceptive plus an antiandrogen) or pregnancy (weight loss and fertility medication such as clomiphene citrate [Clomid]).

### REFERENCES

Rebar RW: Evaluation of amenorrhea, anovulation and abnormal bleeding (March 26, 2006). Available at http://endotext.org/female/female4/femaleframe4.htm (accessed June 15, 2007).

Reid RL: Amenorrhea. In Copeland L, Jarrell J, McGregor J (eds): Textbook of Gynecology, 2nd ed. Philadelphia: WB Saunders, 1997: 365-390.

Reindollar R, Lalwani S. Abnormalities of female pubertal development (November 21, 2002). Available at http://endotext.org/female/female2/femaleframe2.htm (accessed June 15, 2007).

# Dysmenorrhea

Method of
*Laeth S. Nasir, MBBS*

Dysmenorrhea, or pain accompanying menses, is a leading cause of morbidity among women and accounts for substantial short-term disability. Prevalence rates among women of reproductive age are reported to be higher than 90%. In some women, dysmenorrhea is significant enough to impair their quality of life to the same extent as health conditions such as angina and osteoarthritis.

Prostaglandin production during menses, resulting in tetanic uterine contractions and ischemia, plays a central role in the production of symptoms. Menstrual fluid from women who suffer from dysmenorrhea contains much higher prostaglandin levels than those who do not. Evidence also suggests that increased stress and cognitive factors such as catastrophic pain are associated with greater menstrual pain intensity.

Primary dysmenorrhea is defined as pelvic pain not associated with macroscopic pelvic pathology; whereas secondary dysmenorrhea is the presence of menstrual pain coexisting with pelvic pathology.

## Primary Dysmenorrhea

Primary dysmenorrhea typically presents with the onset of ovulatory cycles, which are present in 80% of adolescents by 4 to 5 years after menarche. The pain is often described as intermittent, cramping

## CURRENT DIAGNOSIS

- Colicky midline suprapubic pain radiates to lower back and thighs.
- Pain begins at onset of menses and lasts 12–72 h.
- May be accompanied by malaise, fatigue, diarrhea, vomiting, and other systemic symptoms.

## CURRENT THERAPY

- Nonsteroidal anti-inflammatory drugs
- Hormonal manipulation
- Complementary therapies

suprapubic pain, which may be severe and radiate to the back or inner thighs. Systemic symptoms such as fatigue, malaise, anxiety, dizziness, diarrhea, and nausea and vomiting are frequently present. Symptoms may persist for 48 to 72 hours.

## DIAGNOSIS

In patients with primary dysmenorrhea, the history, including gynecologic review of systems, is usually unremarkable. Patients who present with a typical history and unremarkable past medical history do not generally require extensive evaluation at the initial visit. In sexually naive patients, a rectoabdominal exam may provide sufficient information if the clinician feels that an evaluation of the pelvic organs is in order. Patients with an atypical history or who may be at risk for conditions such as pelvic inflammatory disease (PID) should undergo a focused clinical examination, including a pelvic exam with microscopic examination of vaginal fluid. Microbiologic testing and other tests or procedures such as ultrasound or laparoscopy may be necessary if indicated by elements of the history or physical exam.

## TREATMENT

The three major treatment approaches to the management of primary dysmenorrhea are nonsteroidal anti-inflammatory drugs (NSAIDs), hormonal treatment, and complementary therapies. Therapy can be initiated using any of these methods according to patient preferences or the clinical situation. In subsequent follow-up, incomplete response, side effects, or patient preference can lead to combining therapies or changing treatment modalities.

The majority of patients have tried self-care using NSAIDs before coming to the physician. Frequently, however, inappropriately low doses and irregular dose intervals of NSAID are used. The physician often supports patients' self-care efforts through reassurance and modifications of the patient's medication regimen. The goal of NSAID treatment of dysmenorrhea is aimed primarily at preempting the production of prostaglandins. The major principle of treatment is to start the medication prophylactically and use sufficient doses to

maximally suppress prostaglandin production. Ideally, the NSAID should be started 24 to 48 hours prior to the onset of expected menses and continued for an additional 24 to 48 hours. Clinicians sometimes recommend an initial loading dose of NSAID, followed by regular doses for the subsequent 24 to 48 hours. In patients without special needs, it is often best to choose the least expensive, most readily available NSAID to start with (Table 1). Suboptimal response to a NSAID may necessitate a trial of a different NSAID class. Traditionally, clinicians have recommended to patients that three cycles be monitored prior to evaluation of regimen efficacy.

Patients who desire contraception and have no contraindications may be candidates for hormonal therapy of dysmenorrhea. Suppression of ovulation leads to a thinning of the endometrial lining of the uterus with subsequent reduction of fluid contents of the uterus during menses. Prostaglandin levels in menstrual fluid are also reduced. Hormonal therapy usually consists of oral contraceptive pill[1] (OCP) or depot-medroxyprogesterone acetate[1] (Depo-Provera). Monophasic OCPs are believed to be more effective than triphasic formulations and hormonal patches in this regard. Women taking OCPs may elect to use the so-called long cycle method by skipping placebo pills and allowing menses to occur once every 3 months. The major disadvantage of this approach is the breakthrough bleeding that occurs in many women.

Rarely, therapies that suppress ovarian function more fully, such as the use of leuprolide acetate (Lupron[1]) or danazol (Danocrine[1]), may be considered. However, these have significant side effects and are very expensive. These should be considered once other causes of dysmenorrhea are ruled out and the cost-benefit ratio against other treatments is evaluated.

## COMPLEMENTARY THERAPIES

Complementary therapies can be subdivided into pharmacologic methods, dietary modification or supplements, and physical modalities. Pharmacologic therapies that are efficacious in reducing symptoms but are infrequently used include nitroglycerin patches[1] (Nitro-Dur) and oral nifedipine[1] (Procardia).

---

[1]Not FDA approved for this indication.

---

### TABLE 1  Nonsteroidal Anti-inflammatory Drugs (NSAIDs) for Treatment of Dysmenorrhea

| Drug | Formulation (mg) | Dosage |
|---|---|---|
| **Propionic Acids** | | |
| Ibuprofen (Motrin, Advil) | 200, 400, 600, 800 | 400 mg q4-6h; max 2400 mg/d |
| Ketoprofen (Orudis, Oruvail) | 12.5, 25, 50, 75,100 | 25–50 mg PO q6–8h; max 300 mg/d |
| Naproxen (Naprosyn) | 250, 375, 500 | 500 mg first dose, then 250 mg q6–8h prn; max 1250 mg/d |
| Naproxen sodium (Anaprox) | 275, 550 | 550 mg PO first dose, then 275 mg PO q6–8h; max 1375 mg/d |
| **Fenamates** | | |
| Mefenamic acid (Ponstel) | 250 | 500 mg first dose, then 250 mg PO q6h prn; max 3 d |
| Meclofenamate | 50, 100 | 100 mg PO tid; max 300 mg/d for 6 d |
| **Cyclooxygenase-2 (COX-2) Selective Inhibitors** | | |
| Celecoxib (Celebrex) | 100, 200, 400 | 400 mg PO first dose, then 200 mg PO bid; may take additional 200 mg on d 1 |

*Abbreviations:* max = maximum; PO = orally.

Effective dietary or supplementation interventions are reported to include a low-fat vegetarian diet and an increased intake of omega-3 fatty acids as fish oil (one trial reported significant improvement with consumption of 2 g of fish oil daily). One study reported that 100 mg of thiamine[1] daily was highly effective in reducing dysmenorrhea, but 90 days of treatment was required before an effect was apparent. Two randomized controlled trials reported that 200 international units (IU) twice daily or 500 IU of vitamin E[1] once daily taken starting 48 hours before the onset of menses and continued for a total of 5 days were both effective in reducing symptoms.

A number of physical modalities are reported to be efficacious in the treatment of dysmenorrhea. A randomized, controlled, and blinded trial showed that acupuncture was highly effective in reducing symptoms. Acupressure and high-frequency transcutaneous electrical nerve stimulation (TENS) are also reported to reduce symptoms of cramping and pain significantly. A topically applied heating patch that maintained a temperature of approximately 38.9°C (102°F) for 12 hours a day was found to be as effective as ibuprofen (Advil) in reducing pain.

Although a Cochrane Review found insufficient evidence for benefit, invasive treatments such as nerve blocks, presacral neurectomy, uterosacral nerve ablation, and hysterectomy are rarely used in cases of severe primary dysmenorrhea resistant to conservative treatment.

## Secondary Dysmenorrhea

Diagnosis of secondary dysmenorrhea may be made in patients who have significant pain with the onset of menses (when initial cycles are likely to be anovulatory), who develop increasingly severe dysmenorrhea after several years of stable menstrual symptoms, or those who fail to respond to conventional treatments such as NSAIDs or oral contraceptives. A history of atypical pelvic pain pattern such as the onset of pain several days before the onset of menses or persistence of pain after menses resolve is also suggestive of a secondary cause of dysmenorrhea. Common causes of secondary dysmenorrhea include endometriosis, pelvic inflammatory disease (PID), and anatomical abnormalities such as cervical stenosis, endometrial or endocervical polyps, or congenital obstructive müllerian anomalies.

Menstrually exacerbated nongenital causes of pelvic pain such as interstitial cystitis, irritable bowel syndrome, and psychogenic disorders seldom correspond to a history of symptoms in the menstrual cycle.

### REFERENCES

ACOG Practice Bulletin Number 11. Medical Management of Endometriosis. December 1999.

Akin MD, Weingand KW, Hengehold DA, et al: Continuous low-level topical heat in the treatment of dysmenorrhea. Obstet Gynecol 2001;97:343.

Helms JM: Acupuncture for the management of primary dysmenorrhea. Obstet Gynecol 1987;69:51.

Proctor ML, Farquhar CM, Sinclair OJ, Johnson NP: Surgical interruption of pelvic nerve pathways for primary and secondary dysmenorrhea. In The Cochrane Library, Issue 3. Oxford, Update Software, 2003. Review.

Proctor ML, Roberts H, Farquhar CM: Combined oral contraceptive pill (OCP) as treatment for primary dysmenorrhoea. Cochrane Database Syst Rev 2001;(4):CD002120. Review.

Proctor ML, Smith CA, Farquhar CM, Stones RW: Transcutaneous electrical nerve stimulation and acupuncture for primary dysmenorrhea. Cochrane Database Syst Rev 2002;(1):CD002123. Review.

Smith RP: The dynamics of nonsteroidal anti-inflammatory therapy for primary dysmenorrhea. Obstet Gynecol 1987;70:785.

Sulak PJ, Cressman BE, Waldrop E, et al: Extending the duration of active oral contraceptive pills to manage hormone withdrawal symptoms. Obstet Gynecol 1997;89:179.

Wilson ML, Murphy PA: Herbal and dietary therapies for primary and secondary dysmenorrhoea. Cochrane Database Syst Rev 2001;(3):CD002124.

Ziaei S, Faghihzadeh S, Sohrabvand F, et al: A randomised placebo-controlled trial to determine the effect of vitamin E in treatment of primary dysmenorrhea. BJOG 2001;108:1181.

[1]Not FDA approved for this indication.

# Premenstrual Syndrome

Method of
*Ellen W. Freeman, PhD*

The premenstrual syndromes (PMS) are characterized by mood, behavioral, and physical symptoms that occur from several days to 2 weeks before menses and remit with the menstrual flow. The term *PMS* as used by clinicians and the general public is generic, imprecise, and commonly applied to numerous symptoms. Included symptoms range from the mild and normal physiologic changes of the menstrual cycle to clinically significant symptoms that limit or impair normal functioning. In recent years, randomized controlled trials and other well-designed studies have defined diagnostic criteria for PMS and identified effective treatments for this disorder.

Based on scientific evidence at this time, serotonergic antidepressants are considered the primary treatment for clinically significant PMS, and particularly its severe form termed premenstrual dysphoric disorder (PMDD). This review focuses on PMS and its treatment with serotonergic antidepressants. It is not a comprehensive review of all treatments or associated literature. Other recent reviews may guide the reader to further information and other treatments for PMS and PMDD.

## Symptoms

Numerous symptoms were traditionally attributed to PMS. This plethora is related in part to the absence of a clear diagnosis that distinguishes PMS from other co-morbid conditions. Many disorders, both physical and psychiatric, are exacerbated premenstrually or occur as a co-morbid disorder with PMS. When a careful diagnosis is made to distinguish PMS from other conditions, a much smaller group of symptoms appear to be typical of the disorder (Box 1).

Mood symptoms are usually the main complaint (irritability, anxiety, tension, mood swings, feeling out of control, depression), but behavioral symptoms (e.g., decreased interest, fatigue, poor concentration, poor sleep) and physical symptoms, most commonly breast tenderness and abdominal swelling, are also present. Several recent studies suggest that irritability is the cardinal symptom of PMS. Although depressive symptoms such as low mood, fatigue, sleep difficulties, and poor concentration are frequent complaints of women with PMS, the growing evidence indicates that PMS is not a simple variant of depression but has distinct mechanisms that differ from those of depressive disorders.

---

**BOX 1  Symptoms of Premenstrual Syndrome**

Affective
- Irritability
- Anxiety
- Angry outbursts
- Confusion
- Social withdrawal
- Depression

Somatic
- Bloating
- Swelling
- Breast tenderness
- Headache

From American College of Obstetricians and Gynecologists (ACOG) Practice Bulletin 15, 2001.

## Prevalence

Surveys indicate that PMS is among the most common health problems reported by reproductive-age women. Current estimates from epidemiologic data indicate that approximately 25% of women experience severe and clinically significant premenstrual symptoms, although only 6% to 8% of menstruating women meet the stringent and predominantly dysphoric criteria for PMDD.

## Morbidity

The morbidity of PMS is related to its severity, chronicity, and resulting distress that affect work, personal relationships, or daily activities. The level of impairment is significantly above community norms and similar to that of other health problems such as major depressive disorder. Studies consistently demonstrate that the greatest impairment or distress resulting from PMS is in relationships with the partner or children and in the effectiveness of work.

## Etiology

The etiology of PMS remains undefined, although the monthly cycling of the reproductive hormones appears to have an essential role in the disorder. While circulating levels of the hormones are in normal range, the dominant theory is that some women have an underlying vulnerability to the normal fluctuations of one or more of these hormones. It is further believed that PMS involves central nervous system–mediated interactions of the reproductive steroids with neurotransmitters. The principal research evidence at this time supports the involvement of reproductive hormones, serotonergic dysregulation, and possibly dysregulation of GABAergic receptor functioning.

## Diagnosis

A diagnosis of PMS is determined primarily by the *timing* and the *severity* of the symptoms. These factors, together with an assessment of whether other physical or psychiatric disorders may account for the symptoms, are more important for the diagnosis than the particular symptoms, which are typically nonspecific and must be assessed for their relationship to the menstrual cycle.

Box 2 lists the diagnostic criteria for PMS presented by the American College of Obstetricians and Gynecologists in 2000. These criteria indicate that PMS symptoms must be experienced during the 5 days before menses and abate during the menstrual flow.

### CURRENT DIAGNOSIS

- Confirm that symptoms occur premenstrually and abate following menses.
- Confirm that symptoms are clinically significant and impair daily activities and/or cause problems for the woman.
- Obtain a medical history and conduct a physical examination to determine that other disorders are not causing the symptoms.
- Query depression, stress, substance abuse, and other diagnoses that could cause the symptoms.
- Ask the woman to maintain a daily symptom report for two or more menstrual cycles to confirm the reported symptoms and their relation to the menstrual cycle.
- Perform laboratory tests only as needed to confirm general good health or rule out other suspected conditions.

---

**BOX 2   Diagnosis of Premenstrual Syndrome**

Presenting symptoms:
- Consistent with premenstrual syndrome
- Restricted to the luteal phase
- Cause impairment or distress
- Not an exacerbation of another disorder
- Confirmed by 2 cycles of daily symptom rating

From American College of Obstetricians and Gynecologists (ACOG) Practice Bulletin 15, 2001.

---

The symptoms should cause identifiable impairment or distress, be confirmed by prospective reports recorded daily by the woman for at least two menstrual cycles, and not be accounted for by other disorders.

The diagnostic criteria for premenstrual dysphoric disorder (PMDD) are listed in the *Diagnostic and Statistical Manual of Mental Disorders, Fourth Edition* (*DSM-IV*). Importantly, the Food and Drug Administration (FDA) has approved medications only for the indication of PMDD and not for the indication of PMS at the present time. The PMDD criteria are intended to diagnose a severe, dysphoric form of PMS and require 5 of 11 listed symptoms including at least one of the mood symptoms. Physical symptoms, regardless of the number, are considered a single symptom in meeting the diagnostic criteria. The 11 PMDD symptoms are depressed mood, anxiety or tension, mood swings, anger or irritability, decreased interest, concentration difficulties, fatigue, appetite change or food cravings, sleep disturbance, feeling overwhelmed, and physical symptoms. At least five of these symptoms must each be severe premenstrually and abate with the menstrual flow. The symptoms must markedly interfere with functioning, be confirmed by daily symptom reports for at least two menstrual cycles, and not be an exacerbation of another physical or mental disorder.

To diagnose PMS, a medical history should be obtained and a complete physical with gynecologic examination performed. PMS is understood to occur in ovulatory menstrual cycles; cycles that are irregular or outside the normal range are an indication for further gynecologic investigation. Co-morbid conditions such as dysmenorrhea, endometriosis, uterine fibroids, pelvic inflammatory disease, thyroid disorders, migraine, diabetes, mood disorders, substance abuse, and numerous other possibilities should be identified. It may be difficult to determine whether the symptoms under investigation are an exacerbation of a co-morbid condition or superimposed on another condition. In either case, the usual recommendation is to treat the ongoing condition first, then reassess and possibly add treatment for the symptoms that arise premenstrually.

No laboratory test identifies PMS and none should be routinely performed for diagnosis. Laboratory tests that indicate or confirm other possible disorders are useful if suggested by the individual woman's symptom presentation or medical findings.

The key diagnostic tool for evaluating premenstrual symptoms is the daily symptom report. The diagnostic criteria for both PMS and PMDD include a daily symptom report that is kept by the woman for at least two menstrual cycles to confirm that the woman's reported symptoms are linked to the menstrual cycle in the requisite pattern. Numerous symptom reports appropriate for this diagnosis are identified in the medical literature on PMS and PMDD. It is important that the ratings indicate the severity of each symptom (and not simply check the presence or absence of symptoms).

It is informative to use two visits for the diagnostic evaluation. Although counterintuitive, seeing the patient following menses when PMS symptoms have abated is instructive. If symptoms are absent, it provides strong evidence for the diagnosis. If symptoms are present in the follicular phase, the type and severity of the symptoms are important diagnostic information for identifying other physical or mental disorders that may be the primary focus of treatment.

## CURRENT THERAPY

| SSRI | Range Studied (mg) | Mean Dose (mg/d) |
|------|------|------|
| Citalopram (Celexa[1]) | 10–30 | 20 |
| Escitalopram (Lexapro[1]) | 10–20 | 15 |
| Fluoxetine (Prozac,[1] Sarafem*) | 10–60 | 20 |
| Paroxetine (Paxil[1]) | 10–30 | 20 |
| Paroxetine-CR* (Paxil-CR) | 12.5, 25 | NA[†] |
| Sertraline (Zoloft*) | 50–150 | 75 |
| SNRI | | |
| Venlafaxine (Effexor[1]) | 37.5–200 | 112.5 |

[1]Not FDA approved for this indication
*FDA approved for the indication of premenstrual dysphoric disorder (PMDD).
[†]Not applicable because of fixed-dose study.

# Treatment

## SELECTIVE SEROTONIN REUPTAKE INHIBITORS

Serotonergic antidepressants are the primary treatment for severe PMS and PMDD at this time. Modulating serotonergic function is consistent with a leading theoretical view that the normal gonadal steroid fluctuations of the menstrual cycle are associated with an abnormal serotonergic response in vulnerable women. A meta-analysis of randomized controlled trials of selective serotonin reuptake inhibitors (SSRIs) in treatment of PMS and PMDD determined that these drugs were an effective first-line therapy, with both a statistically significant and clinically meaningful difference from placebo. The FDA has approved fluoxetine (Sarafem), sertraline (Zoloft), and paroxetine (Paxil) for the indication of PMDD. Other randomized, placebo-controlled, double-blind trials showed efficacy for citalopram (Celexa[1]), venlafaxine (Effexor[1]) (a selective serotonin-norepinephrine reuptake inhibitor [SNRI]), and clomipramine (Anafranil[1]) (a tricyclic antidepressant) for treatment of PMS and PMDD.

Effective doses of SSRIs are consistently at the low end of the dose range for depressive disorders in all reports of PMS and PMDD treatments. Significant response is often seen in the first menstrual cycle of treatment, with smaller increments with or without dose adjustments in the second and third treatment cycles. If there is not sufficient response in the first treated menstrual cycle, the dose should be increased in the next cycle unless precluded by side effects.

Side effects are common with the initiation of an SSRI but are usually transient and abate within 1 to 2 weeks of continued treatment. The most common side effects include headache, nausea, insomnia, fatigue or lethargy, diarrhea, decreased concentration, dizziness, and decreased libido or delayed orgasm. The sexual side effects of SSRIs have received considerable attention, although it is often difficult to determine the extent to which sexual effects are related to the medication or to preexisting conditions. The incidence of decreased sexual interest or delayed orgasm in the few published reports of PMS patients is approximately 9% to 16%, which is notably lower than the rates reported with the use of SSRIs by depressed patients. Another important issue is the lack of any well-controlled clinical trials of SSRI treatment for PMS and PMDD in adolescents. Whether SSRIs are safe and effective for this indication in women younger than 18 years is not demonstrated.

## Luteal Phase Dosing

The use of medication only in the symptomatic luteal phase of the menstrual cycle is particularly important in PMS because of the cyclic pattern of the symptoms, which occur only in the premenstrual phase and abate following menses. Efficacy of luteal phase administration of the SSRIs is demonstrated in multiple trials: three large multicenter, randomized, placebo-controlled trials that examined fluoxetine (Sarafem), paroxetine (Paxil), and sertraline (Zoloft); a trial that directly compared continuous and luteal phase administration of sertraline; and multiple preliminary studies.

Luteal phase administration of an SSRI is typically initiated 14 days prior to the expected onset of menstrual bleeding and concluded within several days of bleeding, using a taper for increased doses. As with continuous dosing, the SSRI doses are usually at the low end of the dose range.

One preliminary study compared symptom-onset dosing (mean of 6 days before menses) to luteal phase dosing and found no difference between the two dosing regimens in improvement overall, although there was suggestion that women with more severe symptoms may respond better to full luteal phase dosing.

Side effects may be less frequent with an intermittent dosing regimen because they may not occur when not taking the medication. However, some women experience recurring side effects when dosing is resumed, and discontinuation symptoms might also occur with the stop-start dosing pattern. At this time, no systematic data confirm discontinuation symptoms with the intermittent dosing regimen.

## Insufficient Response to Selective Serotonin Reuptake Inhibitors

Approximately 60% of PMS and PMDD patients in controlled studies respond well to an SSRI. There are no clear predictors of response. An adequate trial of an SSRI for PMS and PMDD is at least two menstrual cycles at a dose level of demonstrated efficacy, with a third cycle when there is partial response. If a woman has an insufficient response or unacceptable side effects, it is reasonable to try another SSRI. Although the SSRIs are similar in their structure and have similar response rates and side-effect profiles, an individual patient may respond better to one SSRI versus another.

Other approaches to a poor treatment response include augmenting the SSRI with another medication to address the nonresponding symptoms, but there is no systematic information on this in PMS or PMDD treatment. Switching to another class of medication, such as anxiolytics, is suggested, but no data indicate whether nonresponders to SSRIs will respond to another class of medication. Nonresponse may also be related to other co-morbid disorders. A thorough review of the diagnosis and adjustments of the premenstrual doses of medication for both the primary disorder and PMS should be considered before pursuing other treatments.

## OTHER TREATMENTS

### Hormonal

In spite of the evidence for hormonal involvement in PMS and PMDD, traditional oral contraceptives (OCs) do not show efficacy for the disorder. However, recent data indicate that shortening or omitting the placebo week in the traditional OC pill pack may effectively treat PMS and PMDD. The FDA has approved the oral contraceptive YAZ, a 24/4-day combination pill, to treat PMDD.

Gonadotropin-releasing hormone (GnRH) agonists such as depot leuprolide[1] (Lupron) and buserelin[2] (Suprefact) are effective for PMS and PMDD but are of limited usefulness because of the risks associated with low estrogen levels that result from these treatments. Although add-back therapy using low-lose estrogen and progesterone together with the GnRH agonist did not appear to reduce efficacy in a

[1]Not FDA approved for this indication.

[1]Not FDA approved for this indication.
[2]Not available in the United States.

meta-analysis, there are no definitive data on the safety and efficacy of this approach in long-term treatment. The historic use of progesterone has failed to show efficacy for the mood and behavioral symptoms of PMS in numerous controlled trials.

## Anxiolytics

Alprazolam[1] (Xanax) and buspirone[1] (Buspar) showed modest efficacy for PMS in some studies but not others. Although these medications offer an alternative to antidepressants, the response rates appear much lower, and it is not known whether a PMS patient who does not respond to antidepressants will respond to an anxiolytic. The risk of dependency with alprazolam should be considered. Dosing should be strictly limited to the luteal phase, and the patient should have no history of substance abuse.

## Nonpharmacologic

Calcium supplementation[1] (600 mg twice daily) reduced PMS symptoms significantly more than placebo. Calcium offers a dietary supplement approach that may be beneficial for some women with PMS, although there are no predictors of which women will respond well to this therapy. Other complementary and alternative therapies may be helpful for some women, but there is no convincing evidence of their efficacy for PMS.

Behavioral treatments that facilitate coping or reduce stress may reduce PMS symptoms. Cognitive-behavioral therapy is effective for PMS, and in one study it was as effective as the SSRI fluoxetine after 6 months of treatment.

## TREATMENT DURATION

All published studies of treatment efficacy for PMS and PMDD are based on acute treatment of 2 to 3 months' duration. Several small pilot investigations suggest that PMS symptoms are likely to return within several months after medication is stopped. It also appears that PMS symptoms do not resolve spontaneously but continue for many years. These observations of PMS as a chronic condition and the swift return of symptoms following the cessation of medication suggest that treatment can be expected to be long term; notably, there are no data from long-term maintenance studies at this time.

The SSRIs are currently the first-line treatment for severe PMS and PMDD. Continuous dosing and luteal phase dosing regimens are similarly effective for these disorders when the symptoms are clearly limited to the luteal phase of the menstrual cycle. Hormonal treatments have lacked consistent scientific evidence of their efficacy or safety or both for PMS treatment. Several new oral contraceptives that decrease or omit the placebo interval may provide an effective alternative to antidepressant medications. Preliminary evidence indicates that long-term maintenance of the medication may be required for PMS and PMDD, but currently, there are no studies of the effectiveness, costs, and benefits of long-term treatment.

## REFERENCES

ACOG Practice Bulletin: Premenstrual syndrome. Int J Gynecol Obstet 2001; 73(2):183-190.

Dell DL: Premenstrual syndrome, premenstrual dysphoric disorder, and premenstrual exacerbation of another disorder. Clin Obstet Gynecol 2004; 47(3):568-575.

Dimmock PW, Wyatt KM, Jones PW, O'Brien PM: Efficacy of selective serotonin-reuptake inhibitors in premenstrual syndrome: A systematic review. Lancet 2000;356(9236):1131-1136.

Freeman EW: Luteal phase administration of agents for the treatment of premenstrual dysphoric disorder. CNS Drugs 2004;18(7):453-468.

Girman A, Lee R, Kligler B: An integrative medicine approach to premenstrual syndrome. Am J Obstet Gynecol 2003;188(5 Suppl):S56-S65.

Grady-Weliky TA: Premenstrual dysphoric disorder. N Engl J Med 2003; 348(5):433-438.

---

[1]Not FDA approved for this indication.

Halbreich U: The etiology, biology, and evolving pathology of premenstrual syndromes. Psychoneuroendocrinology 2003;28(Suppl 3):55-99.

Johnson SR: Premenstrual syndrome, premenstrual dysphoric disorder, and beyond: A clinical primer for practitioners. Obstet Gynecol 2004;104(4): 845-859.

Stevinson C, Ernst E: Complementary/alternative therapies for premenstrual syndrome: A systematic review of randomized controlled trials. Am J Obstet Gynecol 2001;185(1):227-235.

# Menopause

Method of
*Irina Burd, MD, PhD, Stacey A. Scheib, MD, and Krystene I. Boyle, MD*

Menopause is the physiologic process characterized by a marked decrease in the number of oocytes, subsequent follicular depletion, decreased ovarian estrogen secretion, and finally cessation of menses. For 95% of women, menopause occurs between the ages of 45 and 55, with a mean age of 51. Time of menopause is influenced by genetic as well as environmental factors (Box 1). Menopause before age 40 years is considered premature ovarian failure.

## Diagnosis

Menopause is defined clinically as 12 months of amenorrhea following the last menstrual period in the absence of other causes. The Staging of Reproductive Aging Workshop (STRAW) has provided a beneficial staging system to help categorize patients (Box 2).

The differential diagnosis for menopause includes thyroid disease, pregnancy, hyperprolactinemia, medications, carcinoid, pheochromocytoma, or underlying malignancy, which are important in considering the diagnosis algorithm (Box 3). Follicle-stimulating hormone (FSH) and estradiol are commonly measured to diagnose menopause and are often misleading because they can fluctuate vastly in the perimenopausal period.

## Systemic Manifestations of Menopause

### VASOMOTOR SYMPTOMS

Hot flushes are the most common symptom associated with menopause. They are self-limited sensations of generalized heat that

---

**BOX 1  Factors that Influence the Timing of Menopause**

- Alcohol abuse
- Chemotherapy
- Cigarette smoking
- Contraception
- Family history of early menopause
- Galactose consumption
- Obesity
- Parity
- History of pelvic irradiation
- Physiologic and psychological stresses (e.g., living at high altitudes, depression)
- Race
- Shorter cycle length during adolescence
- Type 1 diabetes mellitus

## CURRENT DIAGNOSIS

- For women older than 45 years who have menopausal symptoms, no further work-up is necessary unless there are symptoms of hyperthyroidism.
- For women younger than 45 years, proceed with an oligomenorrhea or amenorrhea work-up: Check serum hCG, prolactin, TSH, and FSH.
- Women younger than 40 years should have a complete evaluation for premature ovarian failure.
- Common symptoms of menopause include abnormal bleeding, hot flushes, genitourinary complaints, sleep disturbances, mood disturbances, joint pain, and difficulty concentrating.
- FSH and estradiol levels can be misleading and so should not be used to make the diagnosis.

*Abbreviations:* FSH = follicle-stimulating hormone; hCG = human chorionic gonadotropin; TSH = thyroid-stimulating hormone.

---

**BOX 3  Algorithm for the Diagnosis of Menopause**

**Older than 45 years**
- No symptoms suggestive of hyperthyroidism:
  No further diagnostic evaluation
- With symptoms suggestive of hyperthyroidism:
  Check serum TSH, T3, free T4

**Younger than 45 years**
- Oligomenorrhea or amenorrhea work-up: Check serum hCG, prolactin, TSH, FSH

**Younger than 40 years**
- Complete evaluation for premature ovarian failure

*Abbreviations:* FSH = follicle-stimulating hormone; hCG = human chorionic gonadotropin; T3 = triiodothyronine; T4 = thyroxine; TSH = thyroid-stimulating hormone.

---

last 2 to 4 minutes and vary widely among people and across cultures. Without treatment, they resolve within 1 to 5 years.

## SLEEP DISTURBANCES

Sleep disturbances often occur in menopause as a result of hot flushes arousing the woman from sleep. When the hot flushes are treated, sleep usually improves. Persistent sleep disturbances can lead to more serious symptoms such as difficulty concentrating, fatigue, mood disturbances, depression, and other psychological symptoms.

## GENITOURINARY SYMPTOMS

Estrogen deficiency leads to atrophy of the urethral and vaginal epithelium. Vaginal atrophy can result in vaginal dryness, itching, irritation, and dyspareunia. The pH in the vagina also increases and, with vaginal atrophy, can lead to recurrent vaginal infections. Decreasing elasticity of the vaginal wall elasticity can result in a shorter and narrower vagina, especially without continued sexual activity. The lack of estrogen affects blood flow to the vagina and vulva, which in turn causes decreased lubrication and neuropathy. These are both reversible with estrogen replacement therapy, especially vaginal therapy.

Incontinence incidence increases with age but has not been clearly associated with menopause. The theory is that atrophy of the urethral epithelium results in diminished urethral mucosal seal, loss of compliance, and irritation. These are believed to contribute to stress and urge incontinence. These patients also report recurrent urinary tract infections; this is probably related to the increase in vaginal pH.

## ABNORMAL BLEEDING

Even though most postmenopausal bleeding is due to atrophy, during the perimenopausal period the endometrium may be exposed to unopposed estrogen that can result in anovulatory bleeding or endometrial hyperplasia. If this occurs, endometrial biopsy is needed to rule out endometrial hyperplasia or cancer. A transvaginal ultrasound can also be used as a screening tool first and then be followed by an endometrial biopsy if the endometrial thickness is greater than 4 mm.

## MOOD DISTURBANCES

In the Study of Women's Health Across the Nation (SWAN), higher risks of mood symptoms were found in perimenopausal women. The strongest risks of depression associated with menopause are a prior history of depression and premenstrual syndrome. Depression might not be entirely related to the physiology of menopause but may be a result of stressors concomitantly occurring around the time of menopause, such as children leaving home, dealing with aged parents, and midlife adjustment.

## MENSTRUAL MIGRAINES

Menstrual migraines are believed to be related to decreased estrogen levels around the time of menses. Because menopause is related to a decrease in estrogen, menstrual migraines can increase in intensity and frequency.

## BALANCE AND OSTEOPOROSIS

Estrogen deficiency can have an effect on the central nervous system by impairing balance. Along with osteoporosis, loss of balance remains one of the big causes of fractures in menopausal women. There are multiple risk factors for osteoporosis, modifiable and nonmodifiable (Box 4).

## OTHER EFFECTS

Other long-term issues that are believed to be related to menopause include cardiovascular disease and dementia.

# Treatment

## HORMONE REPLACEMENT THERAPY

Until relatively recently, long-term estrogen and combined estrogen and progestin therapy was routinely given to postmenopausal women. Hormone replacement therapy (HRT) was believed to prevent

---

**BOX 2  STRAW Staging System**

- Perimenopause
  - Stage −2 (early): Variable cycle length (>7 days from normal cycle)
  - Stage −1 (late): ≥2 skipped cycles and amenorrhea interval ≥60 days
- Menopause
  - Stage +1 (early): First 5 years after final menstrual period
  - Stage +2 (late): 5 years after final menstrual period until death

*Abbreviation:* STRAW = Stages of Reproductive Aging Workshop.

## BOX 4  Risk Factors for Osteoporosis

**Modifiable Risk Factors**
- Chronic corticosteroid use
- Cigarette smoking
- Early menopause (before age 45 years)
- High alcohol intake
- High caffeine intake
- Low body weight (<127 pounds)
- Low dietary calcium intake
- Low vitamin D intake
- Premenopausal amenorrhea (>1 y)
- Sedentary lifestyle

**Nonmodifiable risk factors**
- Dementia
- Family history of osteoporosis
- Poor general health
- White or Asian ethnicity

cardiovascular disease and osteoporosis. The Women's Health Initiative (WHI) was a set of clinical trials, whose results were first published in 2002, that resulted in a dramatic change in clinical practice. The study was designed to see if there was a decrease in cardiovascular risk with conjugated equine estrogen (CEE [Premarin]) in patients without a uterus or in combination with medroxyprogesterone acetate (MPA [Provera]). The CEE-MPA (Prempro) arm of the trial was stopped early after 5 years because of the increased risks for breast cancer, coronary heart disease (CHD) (29%), stroke (41%) and venous thromboembolism (VTE) (33%), even though there was a reduction in risk of hip and vertebral fractures and colon cancer. There was also an increased risk of stroke (39%) and VTE (33%) in the CEE-alone arm after 7-year follow-up, but there was no difference in heart disease.

The Heart and Estrogen/progestin Replacement Studies (HERS I and II trials) looked at secondary prevention in postmenopausal women with known CHD, which showed that there was not a reduction of CHD events with CEE-MPA. Both the WHI and HERS studies revealed an increase in the number of VTEs.

## CURRENT THERAPY

- CEE or 17-β estradiol plus MPA, as either continuous or cyclic short-term therapy lasting no more than 5 years is a first-line treatment for vasomotor symptoms in a patient with no contraindications.
- Locally active estrogen-containing compounds are available for treating urogenital symptoms.
- SERMs provide an alternative for treating menopausal symptoms, specifically osteoporosis. Raloxifene has less antiresorptive action than the bisphosphonates (e.g., alendronate) and should be given to patients who do not tolerate bisphosphonates.
- Alendronate increases BMD in the vertebral spine and femoral neck more than raloxifene, but patients taking both alendronate and raloxifene increased their BMD the most.
- More research is needed in the use of androgen replacement in menopause, although some evidence suggests that it might improve libido.

*Abbreviations:* BMD = bone mineral density; CEE = conjugated equine estrogen; MPA = medroxyprogesterone acetate; SERM = selective estrogen-receptor modulator.

In the WHI Memory Study (WHIMS), with CEE and CEE-MPA there was an increased risk of dementia compared with placebo, but this was in an older postmenopausal population. Epidemiologic studies indicate that estrogen may be neuroprotective if initiated earlier. Therefore, therapy should not initiated after age 65 years.

As a result of these studies and the recommendations of the North American Menopause Society, the only use for estrogen therapy, either alone or combined with progestin, is for control of menopausal symptoms, particularly hot flushes, vaginal dryness, urinary symptoms, joint pain, skin changes, and emotional lability. Studies are inconclusive whether CEE alone or CEE-MPA is beneficial for incontinence. Contraindications to estrogen therapy are a history of endometrial cancer, liver disease, breast cancer, CHD, history of VTE or stroke, or high risk of any of the above. In the Nurses' Health Study, an increased incidence of new onset of asthma that may be dose related and development of systemic lupus erythematosus might result from estrogen therapy.

The absolute risk of an adverse event is extremely low. For a 50-year-old woman on combined estrogen-progestin, estimated risk is 1:1000 at 1 year and 1:200 at 5 years. This absolute risk doubles for a 60 year-old woman. The goal of treatment is a short-term therapy, lasting no more than 5 years. Therapy should be tapered, decreasing by one pill every 1 or 2 weeks, so that there is no rebound in menopausal symptoms.

Progestin should be added to HRT for any woman with a uterus in order to prevent endometrial hyperplasia and cancer. The Postmenopausal Estrogen/Progestin Interventions (PEPI) trial showed a statistically significant reduction in the incidence of simple, complex, and atypical endometrial hyperplasia with CEE-MPA therapy compared with CEE alone. The only recommended progestin at this time is MPA 2.5 mg/day. Alternative progestin doses, less frequent administration, and alternative routes of administration have not been studied and thus might not be able to prevent endometrial hyperplasia or cancer; if these are used, closer endometrial surveillance is necessary.

Women with premature ovarian failure should be given hormonal therapy, and risks and benefits should be reassessed at age 50 years.

More research is needed the in use of androgen replacement in menopause, although some evidence suggests that it might improve libido.

Alternative therapy has been proposed for menopausal symptoms (Table 1 and Box 5).

## BISPHOSPHONATES

Bisphosphonates impair osteoclastic bone resorption and are used to treat osteoporosis (Box 6). The most common side effects are bone pain and upper gastrointestinal disorders such as dysphagia, esophagitis, and esophageal or gastric ulcer. They are contraindicated in patients with renal impairment, uncorrected hypocalcemia, or sensitivity to the drug components. There have been no randomized, controlled studies comparing one type of bisphosphonate with another.

## SELECTIVE ESTROGEN RECEPTOR MODULATORS

Selective estrogen receptor modulators (SERMs) provide an alternative for treating menopausal symptoms, specifically osteoporosis (Box 6). SERMs bind to the estrogen receptor, but they have tissue-specific properties. The two SERMs that have been studied the most are raloxifene (Evista) and tamoxifen (Nolvadex). Raloxifene's mechanism for tissue-specific activity is not fully clear. Tamoxifen probably works by variable gene expression in different cell types.

### Raloxifene

Two major double-blinded, placebo-controlled trials, one in the United States and one in Europe, have looked at raloxifene versus placebo, measuring bone mineral density (BMD), markers of bone turnover, and serum lipid levels. In all treatment arms in both studies, BMD was significantly increased and serum concentrations of both total and low-density lipoprotein (LDL) cholesterol were significantly decreased compared with placebo. In both trials there was no difference

## TABLE 1 Treatment of Vasomotor Symptoms

| Treatment | Suggested Dose | Possible Side Effects |
|---|---|---|
| **Hormones** | | |
| CEE (Premarin) or 17-β estradiol, plus MPA (Provera), either continuous or cyclic | CEE 0.3 mg/d *or* Estradiol 0.5 mg PO qd *or* Estradiol 0.05 mg patch qd *plus* MPA 2.5 mg /d or for 12-14 d/mo | See text |
| MPA | 20 mg/d[3] oral or 150 mg IM (Depo-Provera)[1] q3mo | Mood disturbances, breast tenderness, alopecia |
| Megestrol acetate (Megace)[1] | 20 mg bid | Vomiting, diarrhea, flatulence |
| **Selective Serotonin Reuptake Inhibitors** | | |
| Paroxetine (Paxil, Paxil CR)[1] | 10-20mg/d or 12.5-25 mg CR/d | Fatigue, dry mouth, nausea, decreased libido |
| Fluoxetine (Prozac)[1] | 20 mg/d | |
| Venlafaxine (Effexor, Effexor XR)[1] | 37.5-75 mg XR/d | |
| **Other Medications** | | |
| Gabapentin (Neurontin)[1] | 300-900 mg/d | Dizziness, somnolence, peripheral edema |
| Clonidine (Catapres TTS)[1] | 0.1 mg/24 h wk patch | Orthostatic hypotension, drowsiness |
| **Dietary Supplements** | | |
| Vitamin E[1] | 800 IU/d | Fatigue, weakness, diarrhea |
| Black cohosh[7] | | Gastrointestinal complaints, dizziness |
| Evening primrose oil[7] | | |
| **Other Interventions** | | |
| Acupuncture or accupressure | | |
| Exercise | | |
| Lifestyle interventions (e.g., layered clothing, fans, air conditioners) | | |

[1]Not FDA approved for this indication.
[3]Exceeds dosage recommended by the manufacturer.
[7]Available as a dietary supplement.
*Abbreviations:* CEE = conjugated equine estrogen; MPA = medroxyprogesterone acetate.

in complaints of breast pain or vaginal bleeding and no difference in endometrial thickness.

In the longer-term Multiple Outcomes of Raloxifene Evaluation (MORE) study, there was a relative risk reduction in vertebral fractures but not for nonvertebral fractures. The risk of invasive, but not noninvasive, breast cancer appeared to decrease, most likely due to the antagonistic effect of raloxifene. There was no increase in endometrial cancer. The relative risk of thromboembolic disease was 3.1 compared with placebo, but it appears that the risk is less than that with tamoxifen. There was no difference in cardiovascular events, except there was a decrease in the subset of women at greatest risk.

In a study looking at osteoporosis in postmenopausal women, patients on alendronate (Fosamax) increased their BMD in the vertebral spine and femoral neck more than patients on raloxifene, but patients taking both medications increased their BMD the most. CEE had a better effect on BMD compared with raloxifene in hysterectomized postmenopausal women. Raloxifene has less antiresorptive action than the bisphosphonates (e.g., alendronate) and should be given to patients who do not tolerate bisphosphonates.

Raloxifene significantly increased the occurrence of hot flushes compared with placebo in all the studies. Other side effects of raloxifene noted were influenza-like symptoms, peripheral edema, and leg cramps. It does not appear to affect vaginal symptoms, urinary symptoms, gallbladder disease, cognitive decline, or cataracts.

The recommended starting dose is 60mg/day.

### Tamoxifen

Tamoxifen[1] has demonstrated some benefit for osteoporosis, but estrogen and bisphosphonates have shown a greater increase in lumbar spine BMD. In the National Surgical Adjuvant Breast and Bowel

---

[1]Not FDA approved for this indication.

---

### BOX 5 Treatment of Urogenital Atrophy Symptoms

- Systemic estrogen therapy alone or combined with progestin
- Estrogen cream (Estrace Vaginal, Premarin Vaginal): 0.5-1 g biw-tiw
- Estradiol vaginal tablet (Vagifem): 1 tablet tiw
- Estrogen-containing vaginal ring (Estring): 1 ring inserted every 3 mo
- Lubricants with intercourse as needed

### BOX 6 Treatments for Osteoporosis

**Bisphosphonates**
- Alendronate (Fosamax) 70 mg/wk or 70-mg oral solution weekly or 10 mg/d
- Risedronate (Actonel) 35 mg/wk
- Ibandronate (Boniva) 150 mg/mo or 3-mg injection once every 3 mo

**Selective Estrogen-Receptor Modulators**
- Raloxifene 60 mg/d

- Perform annual gynecologic examinations.
- Monitor for signs or symptoms of endometrial hyperplasia or cancer.
- Investigate any abnormal vaginal symptoms.
- Reassess use if atypical hyperplasia develops and proceed with appropriate gynecologic management.
- Discontinue tamoxifen after 5 years because benefit has not been demonstrated beyond 5 years of use.

*Abbreviation:* ACOG = American College of Obstetricians and Gynecologists.

Project (NSABP) P-1 Trial, women on tamoxifen had fewer hip, wrist, and vertebral fractures at 7-year follow-up. In this study there was not a significant difference in the occurrence of cardiovascular events. Total and LDL cholesterol were significantly decreased on tamoxifen.

In combination with adjuvant therapy for estrogen receptor–positive breast cancer, tamoxifen can decrease the risk of recurrence and death and aid those with metastatic disease.

As with raloxifene, patients taking tamoxifen have a greater risk for VTE. This association is found particularly in patients who are concomitantly receiving chemotherapy.

The main difference between raloxifene and tamoxifen is that tamoxifen use is associated with a greater risk of endometrial cancers, especially uterine sarcoma. This risk depended on length of treatment. As a result, the American College of Obstetrics and Gynecologists (ACOG) has recommendations regarding monitoring women taking tamoxifen (Box 7), but these are not evidence based. For prevention, an intrauterine levonorgestrel could be placed. Even though there is evidence to suggest that tamoxifen is effective in preventing and treating osteoporosis, it is not approved by the FDA except for the prevention and treatment of breast cancer.

## REFERENCES

American College of Obstetricians and Gynecologists: Tamoxifen and endometrial cancer. ACOG Committee Opinion 232. Washington, DC: American College of Obstetricians and Gynecologists, 2000.

American College of Obstetricians and Gynecologists Task Force: Hormone Therapy. Obstet Gynecol 2004;104(suppl 4):S1-S129.

Barnabei VM, Cochrane BB, Aragaki AK, et al: Menopausal symptoms and treatment-related effects of estrogen and progestin in the Women's Health Initiative. Obstet Gynecol 2005;105:1063-1073.

Barrett-Connor E, Cauley JA, Kulkarni PM, et al: Risk-benefit profile for raloxifene: 4-Year data from the Multiple Outcomes of Raloxifene Eveluation (MORE) randomized trial. J Bone Miner Res 2004;19:1270-1275.

Grady D, Herrington D, Bittner V, et al: Cardiovascular disease outcomes during 6.8 years of hormone therapy: Heart and Estrogen/Progestin Replacement Study follow-up (HERS-II). JAMA 2002;288:49-57.

Hulley S, Grady D, Bush T, et al, for the Heart and Estrogen/Progestin Replacement Study (HERS) Research Group: Randomized trial of estrogen plus progestin for secondary prevention of coronary heart disease in postmenopausal women. JAMA 1998;280:605-613.

North American Menopause Society: Treatment of menopause-associated vasomotor symptoms: Position statement of The North American Menopause Society. Menopause 2004;11:11-33.

Soules MR, Sherman S, Parrott E, Rebar R: Executive summary: Stages of Reproductive Aging Workshop (STRAW). Fertil Steril 2001;76:874-878.

Women's Health Initiative Steering Committee: Effects of conjugated equine estrogen in postmenopausal women with hysterectomy. JAMA 2004; 291:1707-1712.

Writing Group for the PEPI Trial: Effects of estrogen or estrogen/progestin regimens on heart disease risk factors in postmenopausal women. The Postmenopausal Estrogen/Progestin Interventions (PEPI) Trial. JAMA 1995;273:199-208.

Writing Group for the Women's Health Initiative Investigators: Risks and benefits of estrogen plus progestin in healthy postmenopausal women: Principal results from the Women's Health Initiative randomized controlled trial. JAMA 2002;288:321-333.

# Vulvovaginitis

Method of
*David A. Baker, MD*

Vulvovaginitis brings large numbers of women to see their health care provider. Over the last several decades with the availability of numerous over-the-counter preparations, most patients medicate themselves to treat their symptoms. However, it is clear that the majority of patients make the wrong diagnosis. They use the wrong medications and delay bringing their symptoms and complaints to the attention of the clinician; as a result, many women will experience complications from their vaginal infection. Therefore, the clinician needs to take this condition (vulvovaginitis) seriously and view the patient as one with a significant medical, physiologic, and social problem that may lead not only to significant medical conditions and complications but also to significant interpersonal problems.

An accurate diagnosis is required to provide proper and correct treatment of this condition. Symptoms presented to the health care provider by phone can be very nonspecific and may lead to an improper diagnosis and treatment. The three major categories of vaginitis in the United States (Figure 1) are those caused predominantly by candidiasis, trichomoniasis, and bacterial vaginosis (BV). Of these three abnormal symptomatic manifestations, BV is the most common in the United States. Many patients mistake BV for *Candida* infections and take over-the-counter antifungal preparations, which are costly and ineffective. Patients do not appreciate the significance of this most common condition: BV may lead to important medical complications not only during pregnancy but also when the patient is not pregnant. Of the three conditions, the only one that is considered a sexually transmitted disease (STD) is trichomoniasis. BV is associated with other STDs.

The goal of therapy is to not only treat or control the organism that is abnormally colonizing or growing in the vagina but also return the vagina to normal vaginal colonization. This objective may be difficult, and one of the major problems of recurrent vaginal infection is our inability to colonize the lower genital tract with healthy bacteria. The normal vagina has an acidic pH that is produced by a combination of normal host flora and the genus *Lactobacillus*, which produces lactic acid. The importance of *Lactobacillus* strains that produce not only lactic acid but also hydrogen peroxide cannot be overemphasized; they maintain the lower genital tract flora and act as a protective barrier to the acquisition of certain STDs, including HIV. It is therefore the goal of the treating clinician to eradicate the patient's symptoms, control the abnormal vaginal colonization, and try to propagate normal lower genital tract flora. Women with normal lower genital tract flora containing lactobacilli producing lactic acid and hydrogen peroxide were less likely to contract chlamydiosis, trichomoniasis, and symptomatic candidiasis. In addition, the prevalence of gonorrhea, chlamydiosis, and trichomoniasis was significantly lower in women who had normal vaginal *Lactobacillus* flora during pregnancy.

## Bacterial Vaginosis

The term given to abnormal colonization of the lower genital tract with anaerobic bacteria is bacterial vaginosis. However, a more meaningful definition of BV may be one that includes an inflammatory component of this anaerobic bacterial overgrowth. Currently, approximately 50% of women in the United States who visit a clinician for treatment of vaginitis have BV. It is a polymicrobial infection involving an increase in anaerobic bacteria, loss of the normal *Lactobacillus* flora, and consequently, an imbalance in the vaginal ecosystem. The absence or a decreased number of lactobacilli facilitates the overgrowth of pathogenic organism, which are predominantly anaerobic bacteria.

The exact factors that trigger the overgrowth of anaerobic bacteria are still not fully understood. Douching can lead to a disturbance in the delicate balance of lower genital tract organisms. Other risk factors

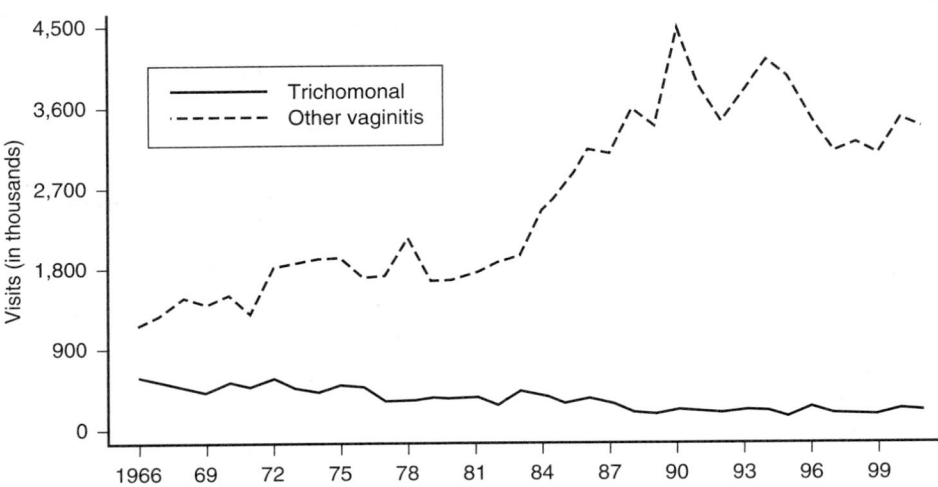

**FIGURE 1.** Major categories of vaginitis are candidiasis, trichomoniasis, and bacterial vaginosis.

for BV include trichomoniasis, other STDs, early sexual experience, multiple sexual partners, and the use of an intrauterine contraceptive device.

## DIAGNOSIS

Proper diagnosis is important for the treatment and eradication of BV. The diagnosis can be made during vaginal examination and does not require expensive and elaborate techniques. The current 2002 Centers for Disease Control and Prevention (CDC) STD treatment guidelines require three of the following symptoms or signs for diagnosis: a homogeneous, white, noninflammatory discharge that coats the vaginal walls smoothly; the presence of clue cells on microscopic examination; a pH of vaginal secretions of less than 4.5; and a fishy odor of the vaginal discharge before or after the addition of 10% KOH (the whiff test). Gram stain is an acceptable laboratory method for diagnosing BV. However, culture is not recommended as a diagnostic tool. In addition, cervical Papanicolaou (Pap) tests have limited clinical utility for the diagnosis of BV because of low sensitivity. Other commercially available tests add to the cost and rarely aid the clinician in diagnosing this vaginal infection.

## TREATMENT

The goal of therapy is to not only control this anaerobic infection but also relieve vaginal symptoms, lessen the risk of infectious complications after procedures, and reduce the risk of development of other infectious complications, HIV, and other STDs. All women who have symptomatic disease require treatment. Because of the increased risk of postoperative infectious complications associated with BV, it is suggested that before surgical procedures are performed on women, they be screened and treated for BV, in addition to undergoing other routine prophylactic measures.

BV during pregnancy has been associated with adverse pregnancy outcomes, including preterm labor, premature rupture of membranes, and postpartum infections. Therapy during pregnancy has the potential of reducing these potential risks, as well as reducing the risk of acquiring STDs and HIV during pregnancy. The CDC has given recommendations for the treatment of nonpregnant and pregnant women with BV (Table 1). Patients need to be informed that clindamycin (Cleocin) cream and ovules are oil-based preparations that may interfere with the efficiency of latex condoms and diaphragms. In addition, oral and topical metronidazole (Flagyl) regimens are equally efficacious. Studies of vaginal clindamycin cream appear to demonstrate that it is less efficacious than metronidazole regimens. Short-course therapy for BV in the form of metronidazole, 2 g orally in a single dose, has been proposed. The clinician must recognize that metronidazole, 2 g in a single dose, is an alternative regimen because of

its lower efficacy in the treatment of BV. Unfortunately, at the current time, no preparation, either intravaginal or oral, is able to induce reversion to the normal lower genital tract vaginal flora.

BV is not considered an STD, and therefore routine treatment of sex partners is not currently recommended. When using clindamycin and metronidazole, one must differentiate between side effects and allergic reactions. Metronidazole gel (MetroGel) may be appropriate for patients who have side effects with oral metronidazole, but it should not be used in a patient allergic to metronidazole.

Oral regimens are recommended (see Table 1) for pregnant women. Topical clindamycin (Cleocin vaginal cream) is contraindicated in pregnancy because of the potential overgrowth of gram-negative aerobic bacteria (*Escherichia coli*) in the vagina. Patients who have BV should be offered testing for HIV and other STDs. Patients with HIV should be screened and treated for BV with the same regimens as those who are HIV negative.

---

**TABLE 1 Bacterial Vaginosis: Treatment Regimens**

**Recommended Regimens, Nonpregnant**
Metronidazole (Flagyl), 500 mg orally twice a day for 7 d
*or*
Metronidazole (Metro-Gel), 0.75% gel, 1 full applicator (5 g) intravaginally once a day for 5 d
*or*
Clindamycin (Cleocin), 2% cream, 1 full applicator (5 g) intravaginally at bedtime for 7 d

**Alternative Regimens, Nonpregnant**
Metronidazole, 2 g orally in a single dose
*or*
Clindamycin, 300 mg orally twice a day for 7 d
*or*
Clindamycin ovules, 100 g intravaginally once at bedtime for 3 d

**Recommended Regimens, Pregnant**
Metronidazole, 250 mg orally three times a day for 7 d
*or*
Clindamycin, 300 mg orally twice a day for 7 d

---

*Note:* Patients should be advised to avoid consuming alcohol during treatment with metronidazole and for 24 hours thereafter. Clindamycin cream and ovules are oil based and might weaken latex condoms and diaphragms: Refer to condom product labeling for additional information.
From Centers for Disease Control and Prevention: Sexually transmitted diseases treatment guidelines 2002. MMWR Morb Mortal Wkly Rep 2002;51:42-48.

# Trichomoniasis

The incidence of trichomoniasis has slowly declined in the United States since the mid 1960s and has remained at a low level over the past decade. Trichomoniasis is caused by the protozoan *Trichomonas vaginalis*. Women who are infected usually have a vaginal discharge and specific symptoms, in contrast to men, who are generally asymptomatic. *T. vaginalis* is a pear-shaped flagellated protozoon that is usually identified in wet mounts by a rapid swaying motion and the presence of polymorphonuclear leukocytes. Growth is typically enhanced by anaerobic conditions and an elevated pH. The incubation period ranges from 4 to 28 days. The clinician needs to recognize that infection with this organism occurs not only in the vagina but also in the urethra, Skene's glands, and the bladder. In men, the urethra is the most common site. However, the prostate and epididymis may also be infected, and the organism may be detected in semen and urine. Trichomoniasis is an STD transmitted through sexual contact, with infection documented in 85% of female partners of infected men. Risk factors for trichomoniasis are the presence of other STDS, an increased number of sexual partners, the presence of BV, smoking, and a vaginal pH over 4.5.

## DIAGNOSIS

The patient usually has a discharge, odor, and vulvar itching with or without dysuria. The discharge is yellow-green with a frothy appearance. Further evaluation of the patient reveals that the pH of the vagina is over 4.5, the amine test may be positive, and on wet preparations, the organism and an increase in the white blood cell count (greater than 10 per high-power field) are usually found. Wet preparations and Pap smears have an approximately 50% to 60% sensitivity and greater than 90% specificity. Other techniques are in development that should better enable the clinician to diagnose this infection. Trichomoniasis in pregnant women has been associated with adverse pregnancy outcomes, specifically, preterm rupture of membranes, preterm labor, and preterm delivery. In addition, studies have shown that the presence of trichomoniasis is associated with an increased risk of acquiring HIV, so patients in whom trichomoniasis has been diagnosed should be screened for other STDs, and HIV testing should be encouraged.

## TREATMENT

Current CDC treatment guidelines are presented in Table 2. The metronidazole regimen recommended has resulted in cure rates of approximately 90% to 95%. Because trichomoniasis is an STD, treatment of sexual partners is mandatory. Metronidazole gel has an efficacy of approximately 50% for the treatment of trichomoniasis. Because the organism may be found in locations other than the vagina, such treatment is less efficacious and not recommended. Women who fail oral therapy may repeat a 7-day course of therapy with topical metronidazole. Because metronidazole is currently the only approved therapy in the United States, patients with allergic reactions to metronidazole may be managed by desensitization. Tinidazole has been recently approved for the treatment of vaginal trichomoniasis. This newer medication may be of assistance in patients with the emerging problem of metronidazole-resistant trichomoniasis.

## TABLE 2  Trichomoniasis: Treatment Regimens

**Recommended Regimen**
Metronidazole (Flagyl), 2 g orally in a single dose

**Alternative Regimen**
Metronidazole, 500 mg twice a day for 7 d

From Centers for Disease Control and Prevention: Sexually transmitted diseases treatment guidelines 2002. MMWR Morb Mortal Wkly Rep 2002;51:42-48.

## TABLE 3  Classification of Vulvovaginal Candidiasis (VVC)

| Uncomplicated | Complicated |
|---|---|
| Sporadic or infrequent VVC *or* Mild-to-moderate VVC *or* Likely to be *Candida albicans* *or* Nonimmunocompromised women | Recurrent VVC *or* Severe VVC *or* Non-*albicans* candidiasis *or* Women with uncontrolled diabetes, debilitation, or immunosuppression or those who are pregnant |

From Centers for Disease Control and Prevention: Sexually transmitted diseases treatment guidelines 2002. MMWR Morb Mortal Wkly Rep 2002;51:42-48.

# Candidiasis

Most patients think that their symptoms are associated with a yeast infection, but in reality, studies show that 75% of patients with chronic candidiasis have another etiologic agent responsible for their problems. However, candidiasis is still one of the most common vaginal infections and is usually treated initially with over-the-counter or alternative regimens. Patients who cannot control the infection or experience recurrent symptoms generally seek medical assistance. The CDC has classified vulvovaginal candidiasis (VVC) as uncomplicated VVC or complicated VVC (Table 3). This classification is based on clinical findings, microbiology, host factors, and response to therapy. Approximately 10% to 20% of women will have complicated VVC.

## DIAGNOSIS AND TREATMENT

Pruritus and an inflammatory reaction suggest the diagnosis of candidal vaginitis. A white, cheesy discharge is usually what drives the patient to buy an over-the-counter antifungal preparation. The clinician needs to use additional modalities for diagnosis, including a wet preparation with 10% KOH, Gram stain or culture, and determination of vaginal pH (less than 4.5). Because a significant number of women are colonized with *Candida*, culture in the absence of symptoms is not clinically relevant. Most patients with uncomplicated VVC have no precipitating factor; however, VVC commonly develops after antibiotic use. The CDC has recommended numerous regimens (Table 4) for the treatment of uncomplicated VVC, including 14 topical regimens and 1 single-dose oral regimen. VVC is not acquired through sexual activity, and therefore treatment of the partner is not usually recommended.

Complicated VVC is usually defined as four or more episodes of symptomatic VVC each year and should occur in only a small percentage of women. Most patients with recurrent VVC have no apparent predisposing or underlying conditions. Culture may be important in determining the appropriate treatment and management of these patients. Non-*albicans* species of *Candida* are found in only 10% to 20% of patients with recurrent VVC. Different therapeutic regimens for a longer duration may be of benefit in treating recurrent VVC. The use of antifungals for maintenance therapy or in specific daily or weekly recommended regimens can be considered for up to 6 months. However, side effects and the toxicity of oral medications need to be taken into account. Once maintenance therapy is discontinued, VVC will recur in upward of 40% of women.

Nonfluconazole azole drugs are recommended as first-line therapy for non-*albicans* VVC. In this specific clinical situation, 600 mg of boric acid* by capsule intravaginally once daily for 2 weeks may be beneficial.

*Not available in the United States. May be compounded by pharmacists.

## TABLE 4  Vulvovaginal Candidiasis: Recommended Treatment Regimens

### Intravaginal Agents

Butoconazole (Mycelex), 2% cream, 5 g intravaginally for 3 d*
or
Butoconazole 2% cream, 5 g (butoconazole—sustained release), single intravaginal application
or
Clotrimazole (Gyne-Lotrimin), 1% cream, 5 g intravaginally for 7-14 d*
or
Clotrimazole, 100-mg vaginal tablet for 7 d
or
Clotrimazole, 100-mg vaginal tablet, 2 tablets for 3 d
or
Clotrimazole, 500-mg vaginal tablet, 1 tablet in a single application
or
Miconazole (Monistat), 2% cream, 5 g intravaginally for 7 d*
or
Miconazole, 100-mg vaginal suppository, 1 suppository for 7 d*
or
Miconazole, 200-mg vaginal suppository, 1 suppository for 3 d*
or
Nystatin, 100,000-U vaginal tablet, 1 tablet for 14 d or
Tioconazole (Vagistat), 6.5% ointment, 5 g intravaginally in a single application*
or
Terconazole (Terazol), 0.4% cream, 5 g intravaginally for 7 d
or
Terconazole, 0.8% cream, 5 g intravaginally for 3 d
or
Terconazole, 80-mg vaginal suppository, 1 suppository for 3 d

### Oral Agent

Fluconazole (Diflucan), 150-mg oral tablet, 1 tablet in a single dose

---

*Note:* The creams and suppositories in these regimens are oil based and may weaken latex condoms and diaphragms. Refer to condom product labeling for further information.

*Preparations for intravaginal administration of butoconazole, clotrimazole, miconazole, and tioconazole are available over the counter (OTC). Self-medication with OTC preparations should be advised only for women in whom VVC has previously been diagnosed and who have a recurrence of the same symptoms. Any woman whose symptoms persist after using an OTC preparation or who has a recurrence of symptoms within 2 months should seek medical care. Unnecessary or inappropriate use of OTC preparations is common and can lead to a delay in treatment of other etiologies of vulvovaginitis that could result in adverse clinical outcomes.

From Centers for Disease Control and Prevention: Sexually transmitted disease treatment guidelines 2002. MMWR Morb Mortal Wkly Rep 2002;51:42-48.

Specific investigation to evaluate for pregnancy, HIV infection, and systemic immunocompromising conditions such as diabetes is important in managing vulvovaginitis.

## REFERENCES

Sobel JD, Nyirjesy P, Brown W: Tinidazole therapy for metronidazole-resistant vaginal trichomoniasis. Clin Infect Dis 33(8):1341-1346, 2001.

# Chlamydia trachomatis

Method of
*Catherine Stevens-Simon, MD*

## The Scope of the Problem

Responsible for more than 3 million infections each year in the United States, *Chlamydia trachomatis* poses a public health problem of epidemic proportions. Because of the large reservoir of undiagnosed, asymptomatic infections, the number of reported cases significantly underestimates the true prevalence of this infection. Nonetheless, *C. trachomatis* is not only the most commonly reported bacterial sexually transmitted disease (STD) in the United States but also the nation's most commonly reported bacterial infection. It is difficult to give meaningful prevalence figures because the proportion of infected individuals depends on the characteristics of the population studied and how they are studied. In addition, whereas passive surveillance systems indicate that the prevalence of this infection has risen precipitously over the last decade, studies conducted at sentinel surveillance sites demonstrate a decline, which suggests that expanded screening, increased reporting, and improved test sensitivity mask a true decrease in prevalence in some sectors of American society. The epidemiologic characteristics and clinical manifestations of chlamydial infections in the United States reflect the fact that most infections are sexually transmitted and that prevalent stereotypes have an affinity for columnar epithelium. Teenage girls are most susceptible to these infections because of the following factors:

- At their age, the columnar epithelium is prominent on the ectocervix.
- Some experience a high level of unprotected, serially monogamous sexual activity with older men whose sexual risk profiles they rarely investigate.

With these two factors combined, teenage girls are at maximal biologic and social risk. Although the national prevalence of chlamydial infections in this population is unknown, school- and clinic-based studies suggest a range of 8% to 26% (compared to 3% to 5% in sociodemographically similar young adult women), with the highest age-specific prevalence reported among adolescents ages 14 to 15 years. Although readily eradicable, the economic and human costs of these infections are staggering. Annual expenditures are estimated to exceed $1.5 billion, with 75% of the cost devoted to treating sequelae of cervical infections that were initially uncomplicated. Because the majority of severe consequences of untreated infections occur in women, and as much as 66.6% of tubal factor infertility and 33.3% of ectopic pregnancies in the United States are attributed to chlamydial infections, it is estimated that every dollar spent on screening and treating asymptomatic young women and their sex partners saves approximately $12. Although this uniquely positions primary health care providers to prevent the costly sequelae of chlamydial infections, given their prevalence among teenagers, expansion of screening and treatment programs to nontraditional settings such as schools, juvenile detention centers, and drug treatment facilities is likely to be a critical component of any national strategy to ontrol this infection.

## Clinical Presentation

Chlamydial infections are an excellent example of the dependence of the clinical manifestations of disease on the intrinsic properties of the pathogen and host. In Western industrialized countries, virtually all chlamydial infections are either sexually transmitted or vertically transmitted at birth. They are caused by nonlymphogranuloma venereum stereotypes that have an affinity for columnar epithelium and can only survive by a cytotoxic, replicative cycle that evokes a variable immune response in the host. Hence, in the United States, the endocervix, urethra, rectum, and conjunctiva are preferentially affected, and clinical manifestations range from asymptomatic to florid inflammatory conditions with severe reproductive consequences. *Chlamydia* should be suspected in these populations:

- Women and men with dysuria and pyuria
- Women with dyspareunia; abnormal vaginal discharge; postcoital, irregular menstrual, or breakthrough contraceptive bleeding; and lower abdominal or pelvic pain
- Infants with conjunctivitis or a staccato cough

These signs and symptoms are neither a sensitive nor a specific indication of infection, however. Indeed, because nearly 90% of chlamydial infections are asymptomatic and *C. trachomatis* is isolated from less than 33.3% of women with mucopurulent cervicitis and less than 50% of men with nongonococcal urethritis, such complaints are unreliable predictors of infection. In women, the most common sign is mucopurulent cervicitis, a nonspecific clinical syndrome characterized by erythema, edema, and friability of the ectocervix and purulent endocervical exudate. Mucopurulent cervicitis, however, is also caused by other STDs and noninfectious factors (i.e., cyclical fluctuations in gonadal hormones), which increase the size of the cervical ectropion or the resident population of cervical leukocytes. Other clinical manifestations of lower genital tract chlamydial infections in women include urethritis and bartholinitis. Although pelvic inflammatory disease (PID) is a polymicrobial infection, *C. trachomatis* is also often involved, and, conversely, PID is the most common complication of chlamydial cervicitis. The estimated incidence ranges from 10% to 40% in untreated women. Young age and prolonged or recurrent infection significantly increase, whereas treatment of asymptomatic infections significantly decreases both disease severity and sequelae, such as salpingo-oophoritis, perihepatitis (Fitz-Hugh-Curtis syndrome), infertility, ectopic pregnancy, and chronic pelvic pain. Adverse outcomes associated with chlamydial infections during pregnancy include preterm labor, premature rupture of the placental membranes, low-birth-weight delivery, neonatal death, postpartum or postabortal endometritis, and vertical transmission to infants. In the infected infants, 30% to 50% develop conjunctivitis, 15% to 20% develop nasopharyngitis, and 5% to 10% develop pneumonia.

In men, the most common clinical manifestation is urethritis, the symptoms of which typically commence 1 to 3 weeks after exposure and range from mild dysuria to frank penile discharge. Other clinical syndromes in men include epididymitis, prostatitis, acute proctocolitis, and Reiter syndrome (urethritis, conjunctivitis, arthritis, and mucocutaneous lesions). These suppurative complications rarely require inpatient therapy and are far less common than those encountered in women. Nonetheless, sequelae ranging from urethral strictures to infertility do occur. Nongenital clinical manifestations, such as conjunctivitis, tenosynovitis, and arthritis, are uncommon among adults in the United States.

## Diagnosis and Screening

In the United States, testing for both symptomatic and asymptomatic chlamydial infections is done with ligase chain reaction (LCR), polymerase chain reaction (PCR), and other nucleic acid amplification techniques (NAATs) because they do not require the presence of intact organisms. Urine, cervical, vaginal, or urethral fluids can be used as the analyte for these tests; specimens are stable and easy to transport; and results can be obtained within a day. This is a major advantage over the stringent collection, transport, and 3-day growth period culturing requirements associated with this fastidious organism. Although nonculture assays, non-NAATs, and rapid diagnostic tests capable of making a diagnosis within 30 minutes are available, these assays are too insensitive to be recommended for routine testing.

The signs and symptoms of chlamydial infection are nonspecific and often persist for weeks after documented eradication of the pathogen. Because of this, leukocyte, esterase-positive urine dipsticks,

## CURRENT DIAGNOSIS

- Signs and symptoms are neither a sensitive nor a specific indication of chlamydial infection and often persist for weeks after documented eradication of the pathogen.
    Most chlamydial infections are asymptomatic.
    *Chlamydia trachomatis* is isolated from less than half of women and men with the most common signs and symptoms (mucopurulent cervicitis and urethritis).
- *Chlamydia* should be suspected in:
    Women and men with dysuria and pyuria.
    Women with dyspareunia, abnormal vaginal discharge, abnormal bleeding, and lower abdominal or pelvic pain; infants with conjunctivitis or a staccato cough
- Routine periodic screening with nucleic acid amplification techniques (NAATs) is the only reliable way to diagnose this infection.

leukocyte-laden vaginal wet mounts, and endocervical Gram stains should be regarded as no more than a trigger for testing. Although concerns about the consequences of underdiagnosis and undertreatment typically overshadow concerns about the consequences of overdiagnosis and overtreatment, therapeutic decisions should not be based on these poorly standardized tests. Indeed, given their low positive predictive value for chlamydial infections, the adverse psychological effects of being diagnosed with an STD, and the serious public health problems that the indiscriminate use of antibiotics creates—even in settings where the prevalence of chlamydial infections is high and patient follow-up is uncertain and in resource-poor clinics where NAATs are unavailable—enthusiasm for the practice of diagnosing chlamydial infections empirically. This must be tempered by the knowledge that to prevent one individual from suffering the sequelae of an untreated infection, hundreds will needlessly suffer the adverse psychosocial consequences of an STD diagnosis. This is true even when the diagnosis is made based on characteristic symptom complexes, suggestive leukocyte esterase urine dipsticks, and/or vaginal wet mounts. Thus, with sensitivities and specificities fluctuating approximately 98% on male urethral and urine specimens as well as on female cervical specimens, NAATs are currently the best chlamydial tests available. However, because the sensitivity of these assays for detecting infections in women is significantly lower when urine (80% to 95%) or patient- or provider-collected vaginal fluid (70% to 85%) is the analyte, endocervical specimens should be used, except in screening situations where it is impractical to perform pelvic examinations. Thus every case diagnosed on a urine or vaginal specimen is a bonus.

Despite consensus about how to screen, uncertainty continues about whom to screen and how frequently to screen them. Pregnant women and sexually active women younger than 25 years of age are the only groups for whom there is good evidence that the benefits of screening outweigh the harms. Specifically, when prevalence rates exceed 2%, testing and treating these individuals for asymptomatic chlamydial infections is a cost-effective preventive measure that:

- Averts PID and associated medical complications.
- Reduces transmission to sex partners.
- Reduces the risk of acquiring HIV.
- Lowers the prevalence of *Chlamydia* in the community.

It is unlikely that these benefits reflect factors other than screening (i.e., increased condom use) because knowledge of sexual risk behavior adds nothing to predictive algorithms that include age and prior STD history. However, because of the highly infectious nature of this bacterium, the lack of a vaccine, and the failure of the human immune system to build up resistance to the bacteria, reinfection of effectively treated individuals tends to diminish short-term efficacy, making long-term periodic screening a prerequisite of cost efficacy.

The only other caveat is that most cost-effectiveness analyses are based on culture-proven disease and therefore may reflect a larger inoculum than infections diagnosed by NAAT assays, which can detect extremely low levels of viable and nonviable organisms. Thus further research is needed to determine if and how inoculum size affects disease presentation and to define the clinical and public health significance of NAAT-detectable infections. Specifically, studies comparing transmission rates and the clinical consequences of infections that are detected only by NAAT assay versus those that are detected by traditional assays are still needed to prove that routine, periodic, urine-based screening of asymptomatic individuals is a cost-effective way to control chlamydial infections at the population level. Moreover, because identifying infected individuals is only the first step in effective disease control, it is also important to demonstrate that once identified, the majority of these asymptomatically infected individuals and their sex partners can be contacted and treated. The randomized trial data that determine how frequently community members should be screened to lower chlamydial infections at the population level are lacking; however, observational studies consistently indicate that among sexually active teens the median time between first and repeat infections is approximately 6 months. Based on these data, biannual screening seems reasonable for women at this age (older than 25 years). Because the risk of reinfection is inversely related to age, it is unclear if this recommendation should be extended to young adults. Nevertheless, a history of prior infection predicts reinfection regardless of sexual risk behavior, and in women repeat infections are implicated in the pathogenesis of upper genital tract damage. It may be wise, therefore, to rescreen all women who were treated for chlamydial infections at 6-month intervals.

Developing selective screening criteria is a vigorously pursued public health goal. With the exception of age, however, no single demographic or behavioral risk factor or combination of risk factors consistently identifies a group of young, sexually active women who should not be screened. The utility of more selective screening is limited by the high proportion of missed infections.

Parallel evidence to support screening asymptomatic men may be lacking because before the introduction of urine screening men were not routinely tested for chlamydial infection. But because the cost of treating men is lower than the cost of treating women, a greater proportion of infected men are symptomatic than women, and the harm associated with misdiagnoses is not inconsequent, it will undoubtedly be more difficult to justify routine periodic male screening. However, false-negative test results create a reservoir of untreated disease that is likely to contribute disproportionately to the spread of *C. trachomatis*; but the psychosocial consequences of false-positive test results can range from dysphoric feelings and decreased self-esteem to the disruption of romantic relationships and domestic violence. Moreover, if treatment is initiated inappropriately, the adverse effects of drug reactions and bacterial resistance caused by antibiotic overuse must be taken into account. Thus, until more data become available, the United States Preventive Services Task Force recommends symptom-based screening for all men and for women older than 25 years of age who do not exhibit other characteristics associated with a high prevalence of chlamydial infections (i.e., unmarried status, African American race, a history of STDs, a history of new or multiple sex partners, cervical ectopy, and inconsistent condom use).

## Treatment

Recommendations for antibiotic treatment of chlamydial infections depend on the clinical syndrome. Box 1 summarizes the options for outpatient therapy of uncomplicated genital tract infections in men and women. However, because humans do not develop a natural immunity to chlamydia, treated patients remain at risk for reinfection. For this reason therapy should not be considered complete until all recent sexual contacts are treated and the patient is counseled about

---

**BOX 1** *Chlamydia trachomatis:* **Recommended Treatment Regimens by Clinical Syndrome**

**Asymptomatic, cervicitis, urethritis\***
- First-choice regimen
- Azithromycin (Zithromax), 1 g orally in a single dose

*or*
- Doxycycline (Vibramycin), 100 mg orally twice a day for 7 days

**Alternative Regimens (One of the Following)**
- Erythromycin base (E-Mycin), 500 mg orally four times a day for 7 days
- Erythromycin ethylsuccinate (EES), 800 mg orally four times a day for 7 days
- Ofloxacin (Floxin), 300 mg orally twice a day for 7 days
- Levofloxacin (Levaquin),[1] 500 mg orally for 7 days
- Epididymitis
- Ceftriaxone (Rocephin),[1] 250 mg intramuscularly (single dose)

*or*
- Doxycycline,[1] 100 mg orally twice a day for 7 days

**Outpatient Pelvic Inflammatory Disease**
- Ofloxacin, 400 mg orally twice a day for 14 days

*or*
- Levofloxacin,[1] 500 mg orally for 14 days
*with or without*
- Metronidazole (Flagyl), 500 mg orally twice a day for 14 days

**Alternative Regimens**
- Ceftriaxone, 250 mg intramuscularly (single dose)

*or*
- Cefoxitin (Mefoxin), 2 g intramuscularly (single dose)
*plus*
- Probenecid, 1 g orally
*plus*
- Doxycycline, 100 mg orally twice a day for 14 days
*with or without*
- Metronidazole, 500 mg orally twice a day for 14 days

**Inpatient Pelvic Inflammatory Disease†**
- Cefotetan (Cefotan), 2 g intravenously every 12 hours

*or*
- Cefoxitin, 2 g intravenously every 6 hours
*plus*
- Doxycycline,[1] 100 mg orally or intravenously every 12 hours

**Alternative Regimens**
- Clindamycin, 900 mg intravenously every 8 hours
*plus*
- Gentamicin,[1] 2 g/kg of body weight loading dose, then 1.5 mg/kg of body weight every 8 hours. Treatment should be continued for 24 to 48 hours after significant clinical improvement occurs and then should consist of oral therapy with doxycycline, 100 mg orally twice a day for 14 days, or clindamycin, 450 mg orally four times a day, for a total of 14 days.

---

[1]Not FDA approved for this indication.
\*Pregnancy: Doxycycline, erythromycin estolate (Ilosone), and ofloxacin are contraindicated, and repeat testing 3 weeks after completion of therapy is recommended because antibiotics may be less efficacious. HIV infection: Patients who have chlamydial infection and who also are infected with HIV should receive the same treatment regimen as those who are HIV-negative.
†Studies indicate that the efficacy of inpatient and outpatient treatment is comparable in terms of fertility and other long-term health outcomes (e.g., ectopic pregnancy and chronic pelvic pain). Therefore, inpatient therapy is no longer recommended except for individuals who do not respond to outpatient regimes or develop tubo-ovarian abscesses or other manifestations of severe upper genital tract disease.

## CURRENT THERAPY

- Antibiotic treatment is easy to summarize in tabular form but is ineffective if given in isolation of sexual network.
    - Large reservoir of asymptomatically infected partners and potential partners undermines the effectiveness of individual treatments.
    - Half of all chlamydial infections occur in previously treated persons.
- Therapy is not complete until all recent sexual contacts are treated and patient counseled about disease prevention.
- Prevalence of *Chlamydia trachomatis* in the sexual network is the best predictor of infection.
- Who an individual has sexual intercourse with puts them at higher risk for acquisition of this infection than how they do so.
- For disease prevention—condoms are plan B—plan A is choosing low-risk sexual partners.

future disease prevention. An estimated 70% of the male partners of women with chlamydial cervicitis are infected, and, conversely, approximately 30% of the female partners of *Chlamydia*-infected men are infected. Treatment is recommended for the most recent sex partner and all other individuals who had sexual contact with the infected person during the 60 days preceding the onset of symptoms or diagnosis. Also, partners should abstain from sexual intercourse for a week after they complete treatment.

Although patient-delivered partner treatment is as effective as partner notification, partners are more likely to be treated if informed by physicians rather than by the patients. This is because only 65% (approximately) of women with known chlamydial infections refer their sex partners for therapy, and even fewer (approximately 45%) infected men do so. Because the cure rate for single-dose azithromycin (Zithromax) therapy is close to 100% and the medication can easily be administered under medical supervision, a test of cure 3 weeks after treatment—NAATs remain positive for this long despite successful eradication of infection—is only recommended for pregnant women (among whom antibiotic efficacy may be reduced) and when compliance is in doubt.

Approximately 50% of all chlamydial infections occur in previously treated persons. Demographic characteristics, such as age and a past history of chlamydial infection, are better predictors of infection than behavioral risk factors, such as multiple sexual partners and the failure to use condoms consistently. Being involved with a sexual network in which *Chlamydia* is hyperendemic appears to put individuals at greater risk for infection than unsafe sexual behavior in the general population. Hence, to control the spread of *C. trachomatis*, it may be necessary to:

- Extend screening and treatment beyond recent partners to include the group of core transmitters in the infected individual's sexual network.
- Help STD patients learn to choose less risky sex partners by promoting sexual health communication within partnerships.

Although the debate about the content and duration of counseling necessary to achieve this goal is ongoing, there is a growing consensus that brief (5 minutes), personalized (provider-delivered and client-centered) counseling sessions—aimed at personal risk reduction and increasing awareness of partner risk behavior—are more effective than the conventional didactic approach to STD prevention education. They are certainly as effective as more prolonged sessions, which are difficult to conduct in busy public health clinics.

## REFERENCES

Aral SO, Hughes JP, Stoner B, et al: Sexual mixing patterns in spread of gonococcal and chlamydial infections. Am J Pub Health 1999;89:825-833.

Biro F, Workowski K, Blythe MJ, Lara-Torre E: NASPAG/JPAG roundtable discussion annual clinical meeting 2003—Philadelphia, PA: Sexually transmitted diseases (STD) treatment guidelines 2002. J Pediatr Adolesc Gynecol 2004;17:143-146.

Cates W Jr: Contraception, unintended pregnancies, and sexually transmitted diseases: Why isn't a simple solution possible? Am J Epidemiol 1996;143:311-318.

Critchlow CW, Wolner-Hanssen P, Eschenbach DA, et al: Determinants of cervical ectopia and cervicitis: Age, oral contraception, specific cervical infection, smoking, and douching. Am J Obstet Gynecol 1995;173:534-543.

Duncan B, Hart G, Scoular A, Bigrigg A: Qualitative analysis of psychosocial impact of diagnosis of *Chlamydia trachomatis*: Implications for screening. BMJ 2001;322:195-199.

Ford CA, Viadro CI, Miller WC: Testing for chlamydial and gonorrheal infections outside of clinic settings. A summary of the literature. Sex Transm Dis 2004;31:38-51.

Kamb ML, Fishbein M, Douglas JM Jr, et al: Efficacy of risk-reduction counseling to prevent human immunodeficiency virus and sexually transmitted diseases: A randomized controlled trial for the Project RESPECT Study Group. JAMA 1998;280:1161-1167.

Peipert JF: Clinical practice. Genital chlamydial infections. N Engl J Med 2003;349:2424-2430.

Rietmeijer CA, Van Bemmelen R, Judson FN, Douglas JM: Incidence and repeat infection rates of *Chlamydia trachomatis* among male and female patients in an STD clinic. Sex Transm Dis 2002;29:65-72.

U.S. Preventive Services Task Force. Screening for chlamydial infection: Recommendations and rationale. Am J Prev Med 2001;20(3S):90-94.

# Pelvic Inflammatory Disease

Method of
*Adrianne Williams Bagley, MD,*
*and Maria Trent, MD, MPH*

Pelvic inflammatory disease (PID) is a spectrum of disorders characterized by an infection of the female upper genital tract. Organs that may be affected include the uterus (endometritis, parametritis), fallopian tubes (salpingitis), and ovaries (oophoritis, tubo-ovarian abscesses [TOAs]), or the infection may involve the pelvic peritoneum.

## Epidemiology

Approximately 800,000 women per year are diagnosed with PID. Up to 20% of cases occur in teenagers. Risk factors associated with development of PID mirror the risk factors that increase the likelihood of acquiring a sexually transmitted infection. These risk factors include having multiple sex partners and inconsistent or incorrect use of condoms. Douching and use of intrauterine devices are also associated with PID. Women with a prior diagnosis of PID are at higher risk of developing future episodes.

## Pathophysiology

The infection of the female upper genital tract that characterizes PID is caused by the ascent of infectious organisms from the vagina and cervix. It is postulated that the ascent of organisms may occur more readily during menses because of reflux of blood in the fallopian tubes, and studies show a temporal relationship between menses and the subsequent diagnosis of PID.

The infectious agents most often implicated in PID are the sexually transmitted organisms *Neisseria gonorrhoeae* and *Chlamydia*

- Pelvic inflammatory disease is a clinical diagnosis.
- The minimum diagnostic criterion is one or more of the following clinical findings: uterine tenderness, adnexal tenderness, *or* cervical motion tenderness in the patient in whom no other cause can be identified.
- The use of additional supportive criteria can increase the accuracy of the diagnosis.

*trachomatis*. However, PID may be a polymicrobial infection. Other contributing infectious etiologies include anaerobic bacteria such as Bacteroides and *Peptostreptococcus* species, *Gardnerella vaginalis*, *Haemophilus influenzae*, *Streptococcus* species, *Mycoplasma hominis*, *Ureaplasma urealyticum*, enteric gram-negative bacilli, and cytomegalovirus.

## Diagnosis

The diagnosis of PID is made based on clinical assessment; therefore, a detailed history, careful examination, and the use of additional supportive diagnostic tests are warranted. Patients may present with varied nonspecific complaints including lower abdominal pain, vaginal discharge, and irregular menses or bleeding with sexual intercourse. Patients may or may not be febrile, experience vomiting or diarrhea, or have urinary symptoms. The differential diagnosis includes processes that affect not only the reproductive tract but also the gastrointestinal and urinary tracts. The differential diagnosis includes but is not limited to ovarian cyst, endometriosis, dysmenorrhea, ectopic pregnancy, septic or threatened abortion, gastroenteritis, appendicitis, diverticulitis, constipation, inflammatory bowel disease, irritable bowel syndrome, urethritis, cystitis, pyelonephritis, and nephrolithiasis.

The 2006 Centers for Disease Control and Prevention (CDC) guidelines recommend empirical treatment for PID in sexually active women with minimum diagnostic criteria of uterine tenderness, adnexal tenderness, or cervical motion tenderness, in whom no other cause can be identified. Additional supportive criteria may be used to increase the specificity of diagnosis; these criteria include oral temperature greater than 38°C (101°F), abnormal cervical or vaginal mucopurulent discharge, presence of white blood cells on saline wet mount of vaginal secretions, elevated erythrocyte sedimentation rate (ESR) or C- reactive protein (CRP), and documented cervical infection with *N. gonorrhoeae* or *C. trachomatis*. However, if cervical infection with *N. gonorrhoeae* or *C. trachomatis* is not found, these organisms can still be responsible for upper genital tract infection. Additional diagnostic tests may include complete blood cell count (CBC) with differential, urine dipstick or urinalysis, urine culture, and urine pregnancy test. Pelvic ultrasonography should be obtained if there is evidence of a pelvic mass on examination or if there is adnexal tenderness in the setting of high fever, elevated white blood cell count, or elevated CRP or ESR; this constellation of findings may suggest a TOA.

## Treatment

Treatment should be initiated promptly for the patient with suspected PID to prevent complications, which include chronic pelvic pain, ectopic pregnancy, and infertility. Antibiotic treatment is broad spectrum to ensure coverage of typical pathogens, namely *N. gonorrhoeae*, *C. trachomatis*, and anaerobes. With prompt appropriate medical treatment, the future reproductive ability of the patient may be protected.

**Inpatient Treatment for Pelvic Inflammatory Disease**

Regimen A:
- Cefotetan (Cefotan), 2 g IV q12h, *or* cefoxitin (Mefoxin), 2 g IV q6h, *plus* doxycycline (Vibramycin), 100 mg PO or IV q12h

Regimen B:
- Clindamycin (Cleocin), 900 mg IV q8h, *plus* gentamicin (Garamycin) loading dose: 2 mg/kg IV/IM, followed by maintenance dose: 1.5 mg/kg IV q8h. Single daily dosing may be substituted.

Alternative Regimen:
- Ampicillin/Sulbactam (Unasyn) 3 g IV q6h *plus* doxycycline (Vibramycin) 100 mg PO or IV q12h.

Note: Parenteral therapy for PID should be considered for 24 h following clinical improvement, and patients should be discharged home on an oral course of doxycycline (Vibramycin) 100 mg PO bid, or clindamycin (Cleocin) 450 PO qid to complete 14 d.

**Outpatient Treatment for Pelvic Inflammatory Disease**

Recommended Oral Regimens:
- Ceftriaxone (Rocephin), 250 mg IM in a single dose, *or*
- Cefoxitin (Mefoxin), 2 g IM in a single dose, with probenecid, 1 g PO in a single dose, *or*
- Other parenteral third-generation cephalosporins (ceftizoxime [Cefizox] or cefotaxime [Claforan]) *plus* doxycycline (Vibramycin), 100 mg PO bid for 14 d, *with or without* metronidazole (Flagyl), 500 mg PO bid for 14 d.

Alternative Oral Regimens:
- Levofloxacin (Levaquin) 500 mg PO once daily for 14 d or ofloxacin (Floxin) 400 mg PO bid for 14 d with or without metronidazole (Flagyl) 500 mg PO bid for 14 d, if the community prevalence and individual risk of gonorrhea are low (see CDC Sexually Transmitted Disease Treatment Guidelines, 2006). Testing for N. gonorrhoeae must be performed prior to treatment. If NAAT test is positive, parental cephalosporin is recommended. If culture is positive for *N. gonorrhoeae*, treatment should be based on antimicrobial susceptibility. If antimicrobial susceptibility cannot be obtained or culture is quinolone resistant *N. gonorrhoeae* (QRNG), parenteral cephalosporin is recommended.

Note: Recommendations from the Centers for Disease Control and Prevention 2006 Sexually Transmitted Diseases Treatment Guidelines are available at http://www.cdc.giv/std/treatment.
*Abbreviations:* IM = intramuscular; IV = intravenous; PO = orally.

The Current Therapy box outlines the 2006 CDC treatment guidelines for inpatient treatment. Hospitalization for parenteral treatment is reserved for patients for whom surgical causes of abdominal pain cannot be excluded, patients who are pregnant, patients who fail outpatient regimens (unable to follow or tolerate an outpatient regimen, no clinical response to oral antibiotics after 72 hours), patients with severe illness, nausea, vomiting, or high fever, and patients with a TOA. Patients younger than 16 years and those with extenuating social circumstances may also be candidates for inpatient treatment.

Outpatient treatment for PID is appropriate in most cases for patients who do not meet the criteria for hospitalization. Metronidazole (Flagyl) is often included as part of the treatment regimen to provide anaerobic coverage, and it is an appropriate adjunct medication in patients who also have evidence of bacterial vaginosis on saline wet mount.

## FOLLOW-UP

Patients treated with outpatient therapy should be reevaluated in 48 to 72 hours to assess response to treatment. At this visit, the medical provider can review medication adherence, readdress partner notification, review the importance of safe sexual practices, discuss related family planning issues, answer questions that the patient may have about the diagnosis, and reexamine the patient to ensure that she is improving on the current therapeutic regimen. Patients who are not improving on oral antibiotics or who have been unable to adhere with the outpatient regimen may need additional diagnostic testing for complications and hospitalization for parental treatment.

Patients being treated for PID should be advised to abstain from sexual intercourse throughout the course of treatment. All sexual partners within the past 60 days should be tested and empirically treated for both *N. gonorrhoeae* and *C. trachomatis*.

## Potential Complications

Short-term complications of PID include TOA and Fitz-Hugh-Curtis syndrome. Patients with TOA require hospitalization for parenteral treatment. Fitz-Hugh-Curtis syndrome is a perihepatitis that may result from spread of *N. gonorrhoeae* or *C. trachomatis* and is characterized by right upper quadrant pain.

Long-term complications of PID include chronic pelvic pain, tubal infertility secondary to scarring, and ectopic pregnancy. Patients with a history of PID have a 6- to 10-fold increased risk of ectopic pregnancy.

## Prevention

Primary prevention of PID can be best accomplished by prevention of sexually transmitted infections. Sexually active women should undergo routine screening for gonorrhea and *Chlamydia* and be instructed about the importance of proper condom usage. Secondary prevention can be accomplished with partner notification and empirical treatment using antibiotics with adequate coverage for infections caused by *N. gonorrhoeae* and *C. trachomatis*.

## REFERENCES

American Academy of Pediatrics: Pelvic inflammatory disease. In Pickering LK (ed): Red Book: 2003 Report of the Committee on Infectious Diseases, 26th ed. Elk Grove Village, Ill, American Academy of Pediatrics, 2003, pp 468-472.

Centers for Disease Control and Prevention: Sexually transmitted disease treatment guidelines 2006. MMWR 2006;55(No. RR-11):56-61.

Ness RB, Soper DE, Holley RL, et al: Effectiveness of inpatient and outpatient treatment strategies for women with pelvic inflammatory disease: Results from the pelvic inflammatory disease evaluation and clinical health (PEACH) randomized trial. Am J Obstet Gynecol 2002;186(5):929-937.

Rein DB, Kassler WJ, Irwin KL, et al: Direct medical costs of pelvic inflammatory disease and its sequelae: Decreasing, but still substantial. Obstet Gynecol 2000;95(3):397-402.

Shrier LA: Bacterial sexually transmitted infections: gonorrhea, chlamydia, pelvic inflammatory disease, and syphilis. In Emans SJ, Laufer MR, Goldstein DP (eds): Pediatric and Adolescent Gynecology, 5th ed. Lippincott-Raven, 2004, pp 583-598.

Trent MA, Ellen JM, Walker A: Pelvic inflammatory disease in adolescents—care delivery in pediatric ambulatory settings. Pediatr Emerg Care 2005;21(7):431-436.

Trent M, Judy SL, Ellen JM, Walker A: Use of an institutional intervention to improve quality of care for adolescents treated in pediatric ambulatory settings for pelvic inflammatory disease. J Adolesc Health 2006;39(1):50-56.

Update to CDC's sexually transmitted diseases treatment guidelines, 2006: Fluoroquinolones no longer recommended for treatment of gonococcal infections. MMWR Weekly April 13, 2007;56(14):332-336.

# Uterine Leiomyomas

Method of
*Tod C. Aeby, MD,*
*and Stella Dantas, MD*

## Epidemiology

Uterine leiomyomas are the most common pelvic tumor in women. They affect approximately 20% of women older than 35 years of age and 40% of women older than 50 years of age, although they are found any time from puberty through menopause. Survey studies involving histologic examination of the uterus suggest they are present in more than 80% of women. Nulliparity, early menarche, and African American ethnicity increase the risk of developing leiomyomas. The incidence among women of African descent is not as high in countries other than the United States, which suggests possible dietary, environmental, and genetic influences on development. Risk is also increased in women with a higher body mass index, presumably because of the increased estrogen production in adipocytes. Pregnancy reduces the risk of developing leiomyomas.

## Pathophysiology

The etiology of uterine leiomyomas is not completely understood, but development is thought to be a multistep process. They are benign monoclonal tumors of the smooth muscle of the myometrium that presumably derive from a normal myocyte. Estrogen and progesterone, in concert with local growth factors, lead to a somatic mutation of normal myometrium to a leiomyoma. Some growth factors that cause leiomyoma proliferation are epidermal growth factors, insulin-like growth factors, heparin-binding growth factors, and transforming growth factor-β. Leiomyomas develop during the reproductive years and increase in size during pregnancy. Growth usually ceases in menopause, and leiomyomas then decrease in volume. This supports the theory that estrogen and progesterone promote growth.

## Symptoms and Signs

Most uterine leiomyomas are asymptomatic. They are categorized into subgroups based on their anatomic relationship and position in the uterus, and symptoms usually depend on those relationships. They can be subserosal, intramural, submucosal, or pedunculated. The most common symptom is abnormal uterine bleeding, usually menorrhagia, occurring in 30% of women with leiomyomas. The cause of the abnormal bleeding is not totally clear but may be the result of abnormal growth and function of the endometrium near the leiomyoma and local interference with normal physiologic mechanisms for hemostasis.

Pelvic pain and increasing pelvic pressure occur in 30% of women with leiomyomas. Other symptoms include dysmenorrhea, postcoital bleeding, and dyspareunia. Pain can be caused by leiomyomas outgrowing their blood supply and becoming necrotic. This red degeneration is common in pregnancy. Patients may have an increasing abdominal girth and pressure symptoms as a result of large fibroids. Pressure on adjacent organs such as the bladder or bowel can cause urinary frequency and urgency or constipation. Rarely, an enlarged uterus causes a palpable kidney secondary to hydronephrosis from ureteral obstruction. Patients also may be lethargic from anemia secondary to menorrhagia. Leiomyomas may also be associated with infertility, although the relationship is controversial.

A rapidly enlarging uterus should raise concern for malignant transformation. But leiomyosarcomas are extremely rare, occurring in less than 0.1% of women operated on for presumed leiomyomas.

### CURRENT DIAGNOSIS

- Abnormal uterine bleeding, postcoital spotting
- Pelvic pain, pressure, dysmenorrhea and dyspareunia
- Urinary frequency and urgency, constipation
- Lethargy
- Infertility
- Physical findings: Enlarged, irregular, and firm uterus
- Ultrasound: Diagnostic imaging modality of choice
- Saline infusion sonohysterography and/or hysteroscopy: Used to evaluate the uterine cavity

## Diagnosis

Uterine leiomyomas are typically diagnosed at pelvic exam when an enlarged and irregularly shaped uterus is noted. Abdominal and transvaginal ultrasound is often helpful in making the diagnosis and in differentiating leiomyomas from adnexal masses or other pelvic pathology. Serial ultrasounds also can be used to monitor their growth. During a pelvic exam, it may not be possible to palpate ovaries next to an enlarged uterus, but an adnexal tumor can be suspected if the mass moves independently of the uterus. Submucosal leiomyomas are diagnosed using saline infusion sonohysterography and hysteroscopy. Definitive diagnosis requires histologic examination.

## Management

For the most part, asymptomatic leiomyoma should be managed expectantly. The approaches to the patient experiencing problems fall into the three general categories of medical management, conservative procedures, and hysterectomy. The choice should be individualized to the patient, based on the severity of her symptoms, her plans for future childbearing, and her personal interest in retaining her uterus. Other causes of abnormal bleeding should be considered.

Current medical therapy is limited to the use of gonadotropin-releasing hormone (GnRH) analogues and antagonists (i.e., leuprolide acetate [Lupron Depot], 3.75 mg monthly; nafarelin acetate [Synarel),[1]

---

[1]Not FDA approved for this indication.

200 μg intranasally twice a day; and goserelin acetate implant [Zoladex],[1] 3.6-mg implant monthly, cetrorelix [Cetrotide]).[1] These expensive medications are shown to decrease the uterine size by up to 65%, allowing for easier or more conservative surgical treatments. The progesterone antagonist mifepristone (Mifeprex)[1] is also effective but not currently available for this purpose in the United States. GnRH therapy has significant side effects, mostly related to the induced hypo-estrogenic state. To preserve bone density the duration of therapy must be limited. Additionally, the uterus rapidly returns to its enlarged size when the therapy is discontinued. These medications are a very effective means of inducing amenorrhea to allow for correction of an anemia prior to surgery.

Conservative procedures include myomectomy or myolysis (surgical removal or destruction of the individual fibroids while preserving the uterus), uterine artery embolization, and endometrial ablation. Each of these approaches has different risks, benefits, and complications (Table 1).

Hysterectomy remains the most common treatment for women with symptomatic leiomyoma and offers the advantage of a complete and definitive cure. The uterus can be removed through the vagina (with or without the aid of laparoscopic techniques) or through an abdominal incision. The route of removal largely depends on the size of the uterus, the patient's medical and surgical history, and the experience and preference of her surgeon.

---

[1]Not FDA approved for this indication.

### CURRENT THERAPY

- Only symptomatic leiomyomas require treatment.
- Medical therapy is for temporizing and making invasive procedures easier or more effective.
- Conservative procedures include myomectomy, myolysis, hydrothermal endometrial ablation, and uterine artery embolization.
- Hysterectomy is the only definitive therapy for leiomyomata.
- Choice of treatment should be made considering the severity of symptoms and respecting the patient's preferences.

---

**TABLE 1** Comparison of Various Procedures for the Treatment of Symptomatic Uterine Leiomyoma

| Therapy | Success Rate | Complication Rate | Possibility of Future Childbearing | Comments |
|---|---|---|---|---|
| Hysterectomy | 100% | 40% | No | Recovery time varies depending on the route of removal. |
| Myomectomy and myolysis | 75% | 39% | Yes | Can be associated with significant blood loss and can result in an unplanned hysterectomy. Recurrent leiomyomas are common. |
| Myolysis | | | Yes | Several methods for myolysis are available, including bipolar electrocautery, laser energy, and cryotherapy. |
| Uterine artery embolization | 77%-91% | 5% | Not currently recommended | Complication rates are low but can be severe, including infection, sepsis, and nontarget tissue necrosis. A few deaths have been reported. |
| Hydrothermal endometrial ablation | 91%* | 1%-2% | No | Hysteroscopic resection of submucosal leiomyomas, prior to endometrial ablation, improves success rates. Pregnancies have occurred after these procedures, so contraception is still required. |

*Best estimate based on limited studies.

## REFERENCES

Buttram VC Jr, Reiter RC: Uterine leiomyomata: Etiology, symptomatology, and management. Fertil Steril 1981;36:433-445.

Felberbaum RE, Germer U, Ludwig M, et al: Treatment of uterine fibroids with a slow-release formulation of the gonadotrophin-releasing hormone antagonist Cetrorelix. Hum Reprod 1998;13(6):1660-1668.

Goldfarb HA: Bipolar laparoscopic needles for myoma coagulation. J Am Assoc Gynecol Laparosc 1995;2(2):175-179.

Lethaby A, Vollenhoven B, Sowter M: Pre-operative GnRH analogue therapy before hysterectomy or myomectomy for uterine fibroids. The Cochrane Database of Systematic Reviews 2001, Issue 2. Article CD000547. DOI: 10.1002/14651858.CD000547.

Parker WH, Fu YS, Berek JS: Uterine sarcoma in patients operated on for presumed leiomyoma and rapidly growing leiomyoma. Obstet Gynecol 1994;83:414.

Pron G, Bennett J, Common A, et al: Ontario Uterine Fibroid Embolization Collaboration Group. The Ontario Uterine Fibroid Embolization Trial: II. Uterine fibroid reduction and symptom relief after uterine artery embolization for fibroids. Fertil Steril 2003;79(1):120-127.

The Hydro ThermAblator system for management of menorrhagia in women with submucous myomas: 12- to 20-month follow-up. J Am Assoc Gynecol Laparosc 2003;10(4):521-527.

# Cancer of the Endometrium

Method of

*D. Scott McMeekin, MD, and Tashanna K.N. Myers, MD*

## Epidemiology

Endometrial cancer is the most common gynecologic cancer facing women in the United States. The lifetime risk of endometrial cancer is currently 1 in 38. In 2007, approximately 39,000 women were found to have endometrial cancer, and 7,400 (3%) women died from the disease. Endometrial cancer is the eighth leading cause of cancer death for women in the United States. African American women appear to have a poorer prognosis: Nearly twice than many (1.8:1) African American women die from endometrial cancer than white women.

Endometrial cancer primarily occurs in postmenopausal women, and the average age at onset is 60 years. Only 25% of patients are premenopausal, and of these, only 5% are younger than 40 years.

## Etiology

Endometrial cancer is classically divided into two types (Table 1). Type I, the more common form, is associated with estrogen excess and often arises in the background of a precursor lesion, atypical hyperplasia. Type II tumors are rarer and more aggressive, and they arise in a background of atrophic endometrium or polyps.

The etiology is unclear. Despite the broad generalizations of the two categories, molecular and genetic changes differentiate these two groups as well. For example, mutations of *p53* are common in papillary serous tumors and are rare in type I tumors. *PTEN* mutations are common in type I tumors but are rare in papillary serous tumors. Global gene expression profiles also differ between type I and type II tumors.

Increased exposure to endogenous or exogenous estrogen increases the risk of developing type I cancers. Since the 1970s, unopposed estrogen use has been a known risk factor, prompting the routine addition of a progestin in combination with hormone replacement therapy regimens. Endogenous exposure to estrogens associated with obesity or chronic anovulation (polycystic ovary syndrome) are believed to be more common etiologies.

## TABLE 1 Comparison Between Type I and Type II Endometrial Cancers

| Factor | Type I | Type II |
|---|---|---|
| **Clinical Features** | | |
| Risk factors | Unopposed estrogen | Age |
| Race | White > African American | White = African American |
| Differentiation | Well differentiated | Poorly differentiated |
| Histology | Endometrioid | PS, CC, Grade 3 |
| Stage | Early | Advanced |
| Prognosis | Favorable | Poorer |
| **Molecular Features** | | |
| Ploidy | Diploid | Aneuploid |
| *k-ras* over expression | Yes | Yes |
| *her-2/neu* over expression | No | Yes |
| *p53* mutation | No | Yes |
| *PTEN* mutation | Yes | No |
| Microsatellite instability | Yes | No |

*Abbreviations:* CC = clear cell; PS = papillary serous.

Other factors associated with an increased risk of developing endometrial cancer include late menopause (older than 52 years), nulliparity, diabetes, hypertension, or a diagnosis of complex atypical hyperplasia. In contrast, normal weight, oral contraceptives, progestin use, cigarette smoking, and multiparity have been associated with a decreased incidence of endometrial cancer. Type II tumors account for a small percentage of endometrial cancers, occur in an older population, and account for nearly one half of all relapses. Papillary serous, clear cell, and perhaps, grade 3 tumors fit into the type II category. Tamoxifen (Nolvadex) used in the prophylaxis of, or treatment for, breast cancer is an established risk factor for developing either type I or type II tumors.

## Presentation and Diagnosis

Patients with endometrial cancer most commonly present with abnormal bleeding. Papanicolaou (Pap) smears detect only 30% to 50% of endometrial cancers and are not useful for diagnosing endometrial cancer. The diagnosis of endometrial cancer is most commonly made by biopsy. An endometrial biopsy can usually be performed in the office and has greater than 90% diagnostic accuracy. The histologic classification of endometrial cancers is listed in Box 1. Ultrasound has also been used to evaluate abnormal bleeding. Studies show that endometrial cancers are exceedingly uncommon if the endometrial thickness is less than 5 mm on ultrasound in postmenopausal women. Symptomatic patients with a thickened endometrium or patients with persistent bleeding despite a thin lining should have a histologic evaluation.

## BOX 1 Histologic Classification of Endometrial Cancers

- Endometrioid adenocarcinoma (includes adenosquamous carcinoma)
- Mucinous carcinoma
- Serous carcinoma
- Clear cell carcinoma
- Squamous carcinoma
- Undifferentiated carcinoma
- Mixed carcinoma

## CURRENT DIAGNOSIS

- Patients with postmenopausal bleeding warrant endometrial biopsy.
- Patients at risk include those with abnormal bleeding and obesity, chronic anovulation, and unopposed estrogen or tamoxifen (Nolvadex) exposure.
- Office biopsy should be performed when possible, and D&C should be performed if office biopsy is not available or biopsy results are equivocal.
- Malignancy is unlikely if the endometrial stripe/thickness is less than 5 mm on ultrasound.

*Abbreviation:* D&C = dilation and curettage.

Currently there is no good screening test for endometrial cancer, and thus there are no screening recommendations. A high degree of suspicion should be maintained for women who have received unopposed estrogens and for patients with vaginal bleeding who are postmenopausal, obese, or taking tamoxifen. Hereditary syndromes (Lynch's) account for 3% to 5% of endometrial cancers and are seen in patients with strong familial histories of hereditary nonpolyposis colorectal, ovarian, and pancreatic cancers.

## Staging

Endometrial cancer is surgically staged according to the 1988 criteria established by the International Federation of Gynecology and Obstetrics (FIGO) (Table 2). Staging includes collection of pelvic washings for cytology, a hysterectomy with removal of bilateral fallopian tubes and ovaries, and pelvic and para-aortic lymph node dissection. Controversies currently exist as to who should undergo lymph node dissection (all, some, or few patients), the type of nodal dissection (sampling or complete lymphadenectomy), and when to use adjuvant therapies.

The most important pathologic prognostic indicators include histologic grade, depth of invasion and lymph node status. The Gynecologic Oncology Group (GOG) performed a surgical pathologic study evaluating 621 patients with endometrial cancer and demonstrated important associations between grade, depth of myometrial invasion, and nodal involvement. For example, patients with deeply invasive (extending into the outer two thirds of the myometrium) tumors had pelvic nodal metastases between 11% and 34%, depending on tumor grade.

**TABLE 2 FIGO (1988) Surgical Staging System for Endometrial Cancer**

| Stage | Description |
| --- | --- |
| IA | Tumor is confined to the endometrium |
| IB | Tumor is confined to less than one half of the myometrium |
| IC | Tumor is confined to more than one half of the myometrium |
| IIA | Cervical involvement is limited to the endocervical glands |
| IIB | Cervical involvement includes cervical stroma |
| IIIA | Tumor involves uterine serosa or adnexa or positive peritoneal cytology |
| IIIB | Vaginal metastases |
| IIIC | Tumor involves pelvic or para-aortic lymph nodes |
| IVA | Tumor involves bladder or bowel mucosa |
| IV B | Distant metastases including intra-abdominal and inguinal lymph node involvement |

*Abbreviation:* FIGO = International Federation of Gynecology and Obstetrics.

**TABLE 3 Estimates of Distribution and Survival of Endometrial Cancer by Stage**

| Stage | Distribution of Cases (%) | 5-year Survival (%) |
| --- | --- | --- |
| Stage IA | 22 | 92 |
| Stage IB | 37 | 88 |
| Stage IC | 13 | 78 |
| Stage II | 9 | 72 |
| Stage III | 15 | 53 |
| Stage IV | 4 | 10 |

Fortunately, most women with endometrial cancer have stage I disease and have a favorable prognosis (Table 3). The 5-year survival for stage I disease approaches 90%, but the 5-year survival for women with stage IV (abdominal or distant spread) disease is only about 10%.

## Treatment

### SURGICAL MANAGEMENT

Surgical management continues to evolve. The GOG has recently completed a large prospective trial evaluating the role of laparoscopic hysterectomy and nodal dissection compared with an abdominal approach. The study, evaluating more than 2500 patients, found that laparoscopic management was feasible, and 76% of the time patients randomized to laparoscopy could have the procedure performed without conversion to laparotomy. The numbers of nodes removed and the frequency of finding positive lymph nodes were similar in the two treatment arms. Despite an increased operative time, results showed that laparoscopic surgery resulted in a shorter hospital stay.

## CURRENT THERAPY

- Surgical therapy is the mainstay of endometrial cancer treatment. Laparoscopic surgery is increasingly being used.
- Surgical staging, including pelvic and para-aortic lymph node dissection, is recommended.
- The best way to define risk is to identify patients with nodal disease.
- Staging typically requires referral to a gynecologic oncologist.
- Unstaged patients may be considered for a restaging operation.
- Most patients have stage I (uterine-confined) disease.
- Low-risk patients—stages IA and IB, grades 1 or 2—require no additional therapy.
- Intermediate-risk patients—stage IB grade 3 and stage IC grades 1 or 2—require no additional therapy or vaginal cuff brachytherapy.
- High-intermediate-risk patients are those 50 years old with two risk factors or older than 70 years with one risk factor. Risk factors are:
  - Grade 2 or 3 tumor
  - Lymphovascular space involvement
  - Outer one third myometrial invasion
  - Stage I plus papillary serous or clear cell histology
- Treatment of these patients is controversial. There is no clear consensus regarding performing no additional therapy, performing vaginal cuff brachytherapy with or without chemotherapy, or performing pelvic radiation therapy.

The benefits of routine nodal dissection include better stratification of patients into high-, intermediate-, or low risk-categories, reduced use of postoperative therapies for most node-negative patients, and improved identification of a subset of patients with nodal metastases who might benefit from adjuvant therapies. Information from a lymph node dissection is prognostic, but a lymphadenectomy is potentially therapeutic. Today, the more frequent use of nodal dissection has resulted in the less-frequent use of postoperative pelvic irradiation therapy.

Without information on nodal status, physicians and patients must decide whether or not to use postoperative therapies based on perceived risk determined from the hysterectomy findings. Because of this, many have recommended that a second surgery to complete the surgical staging be performed when only a hysterectomy was performed. Laparoscopic restaging is often a feasible approach. The risk of nodal dissection must be balanced by the information provided. Serious complications related to nodal dissection include bleeding and visceral injury, and complications have been reported to occur in less than 2% of surgeries. Lower extremity lymphedema appears to be more common but is rarely severe.

## ADJUVANT THERAPY

### Early Stage Disease

Two large trials have evaluated the role of post-operative pelvic radiation in patients with early stage (stage I to occult stage II) endometrial cancer. In the PORTEC trial, 715 patients were randomized to pelvic radiation or surveillance. Lymph node dissection was not performed. Most patients had low-grade tumors (90% grade 1-2), and about 50% had superficial myometrial invasion (< 50% invasion). Results showed that although radiation could reduce local and regional recurrences (14% vs. 4% with radiation), 5-year survival was 81% with and 85% without radiation. Similarly, the GOG performed a study with 392 patients with grades 1 to 3 tumors and any amount of myometrial invasion. All patients had a specified lymph node dissection and received either pelvic radiation or no additional therapy. Results showed that radiation reduced local recurrences but did not appreciably affect survival (4-year survival was 92% with radiation, 86% without radiation).

The lack of benefit from pelvic radiation in these studies may be due to the excellent outcomes seen in the low-risk populations enrolled in these studies. For example, in the GOG trial, only 18% of

patients had grade 3 tumors, and 31% had deep myometrial invasion. The GOG trial did suggest that a subgroup of patients at higher risk for recurrence could be defined based on age, tumor grade, depth of invasion, and the presence of lymph-vascular space invasion. These high-intermediate risk patients represented one third of the total population but accounted for two thirds of recurrences, suggesting that it might be possible to identify some patients for whom radiation might offer a benefit.

The PORTEC and GOG studies also showed that vaginal cuff recurrences were the most common site of failure without radiation, and authors for both studies suggested that vaginal cuff brachytherapy might be a reasonable alternative to for pelvic radiation. Several studies have demonstrated excellent vaginal cuff control with the use of less toxic and more tolerable vaginal cuff brachytherapy. A proposed treatment algorithm is shown in Figure 1.

Patients with papillary serous and clear cell tumors are believed by many to be at particularly increased risk for recurrence. Extrauterine disease spread is common at initial presentation, making complete surgical staging especially important in these patients. Even patients with stage I disease have a risk of failure near 30% to 50%. Chemotherapy has been increasingly advocated for this group of patients.

### Advanced and Recurrent Disease

Radiation therapy (pelvic, pelvic with an extended field to treat para-aortic nodes, and whole abdominal) has been the treatment of choice for patients with disease spread outside of the uterus. Recently, the GOG presented data showing improved progression-free and overall survival when chemotherapy (doxorubicin and cisplatin) was used compared with whole abdominal radiation in patients with stage III or IV disease. As a result, chemotherapy has been increasingly used in first-line management. Combining radiation with chemotherapy is being actively explored in clinical trials.

For patients with bulky advanced or recurrent disease, hormone therapy with progestins has been a long-standing treatment. Patients with grade 1 tumors, or those with estrogen- and progesterone-receptor positive tumors have shown the greatest likelihood of benefit. Chemotherapy has been increasingly integrated in a first-line setting for many patients due to the identification of several active agents. The most active agents include paclitaxel,[1] doxorubicin,[1] and platinum analogues.[1] Combinations of these agents have resulted in improved

---

[1]Not FDA approved for this indication.

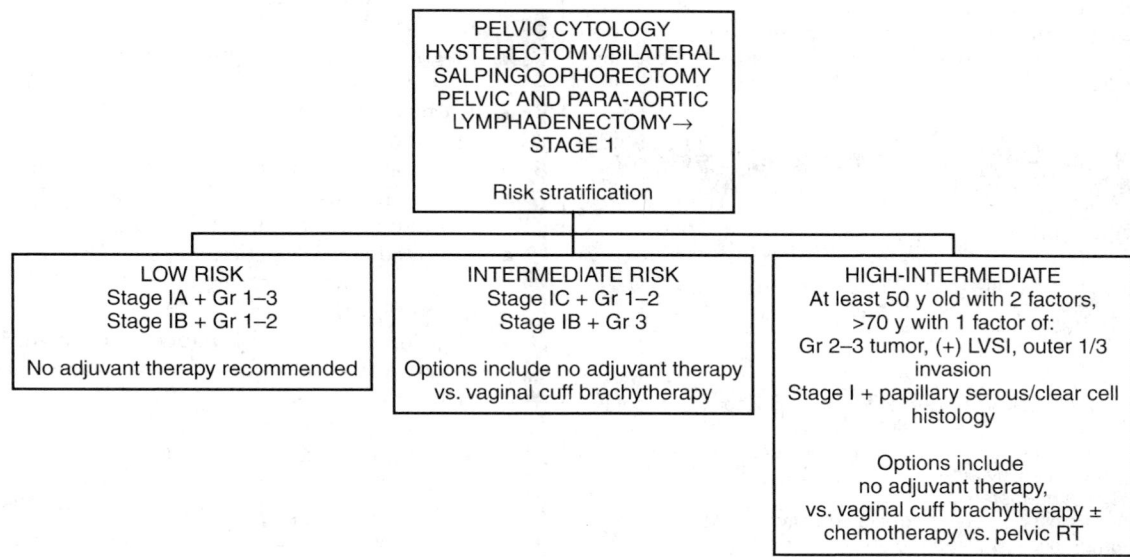

**FIGURE 1.** Postoperative treatment algorithm used at the University of Oklahoma for surgical staged endometrial carcinoma. Surgical staging allows risk stratification based on pathologic factors. *Abbreviations:* Gr = grade; LVSI = lymphovascular space involvement, RT = radiation therapy.

response rates, and the three-drug paclitaxel plus doxorubicin plus cisplatin regimen has been shown to have improved survival over the two-drug doxorubicin plus cisplatin regimen. Given the advanced age and concurrent medical comorbidities that are seen in patients with endometrial cancer, a careful balance between treatment objectives and toxicity must be made.

## Future Directions

Increasing the understanding of endometrial cancer at a genetic and molecular level is a primary goal of current research. This information might provide insights into the prognosis and predict benefits of particular therapies. Targeted biological agents are currently being explored in patients with endometrial cancer, and their use in combination with cytotoxic chemotherapy agents might result in improved outcomes, as seen in other solid tumors such as breast and colon cancers.

## REFERENCES

American College of Obstetricians and Gynecologists: ACOG practice bulletin, management guidelines for obstetrician-gynecologists, number 65, August 2005: Management of endometrial cancer. Obstet Gynecol 2005;106: 413-425.

Cragun J, Havrilesky L, Calingaert B, et al: Retrospective analysis of selective lymphadenectomy in apparent early-stage endometrial cancer. J Clin Oncol 2005;23:3668-3675.

Creasman W, Kohler M, Odicino F, et al: Prognosis of papillary serous, clear cell, and grade 3 stage I carcinoma of the endometrium. Gynecol Oncol 2004; 95:593-596.

Creasman WT, Morrow CP, Bundy BN, et al: Surgical pathologic spread patterns of endometrial cancer. Cancer 1987;60:2035-2041.

Creutzberg C, van Putten W, Koper P, et al: Surgery and post-operative radiotherapy versus surgery alone for patients with stage 1 endometrial carcinoma: Multi-center randomized trial. Lancet 2000;355:1404-411.

Fleming G, Brunetto V, Cella D, et al: Phase III trial of doxorubicin plus cisplatin with or without paclitaxel plus filgrastim in advanced endometrial cancer: A Gynecologic Oncology Group study. J Clin Oncol 2004; 22:2159-2166.

Keys H, Roberts J, Brunetto V, et al: A phase III trial of surgery with or without adjuvant external pelvic radiation therapy in intermediate risk endometrial adenocarcinoma: A Gynecologic Oncology Group study.. Gynecol Oncol 2004;92:744-751.

Kilgore LC, Partridge EE, Alvarez RD, et al: Adenocarcinoma of the endometrium: Survival comparisons of patients with and without pelvic node sampling. Gynecol Oncol 1995;56:29-33.

Randall M, Filiaci G, Muss H, et al: Whole abdominal radiotherapy versus combination doxorubicin-cisplatin chemotherapy in advanced endometrial carcinoma: A randomized phase III trial of the Gynecologic Oncology Group. J Clin Oncol 2006;24:36-44.

Straughn JM, Huh WK, Kelly FJ, et al: Conservative management of stage I endometrial carcinoma after surgical staging. Gynecol Oncol 2002; 84:191-193.

# Cancer of the Uterine Cervix

Method of
*Nader Husseinzadeh, MD*

Invasive cervical cancer accounts for 2% to 3% of all cancers in women in the United States. Incidence and mortality from cervical cancer have declined dramatically with early detection and treatment of preinvasive disease. It is estimated that approximately 9710 new cases will be diagnosed and 3700 patients died from cervical cancer in 2006 worldwide. Both incidence of and mortality from cervical cancer are second to breast cancer. Cervical cancer is a largely preventable disease with a known causative agent, the human papilloma virus (HPV), especially types 16 and 18.

---

**BOX 1  Major Risk Factors for Cervical Cancer**

- Immunosuppression (e.g., transplant, infection with HIV)
- Multiple pregnancies
- Multiple sexual partners
- Promiscuous sexual activity
- Sexually transmitted disease (herpes simplex virus, chlamydia, and human papillomavirus)
- Smoking
- Sexual activity at a young age

---

## Epidemiology

Age-specific incidences for white women are lower than those for African American women. Major risk factors for cervical cancer are listed in Box 1.

Some epidemiologic studies have shown that women using oral contraceptives tend to have more sexual contacts. Cigarette smoking has been linked to an increased risk of squamous cell carcinoma, and presence of nicotine byproduct as a carcinogen in cervical mucous or the partner's semen are possible explanations. Reduced risk of cervical cancer is noted in virgins and in women whose sexual partners were circumcised.

## Etiology and Pathogenesis

The etiology of cervical cancer is unknown. Numerous studies have indicated a close association between HPV and cervical cancer.

Although HPV appears to be the causative agent, many other changes at the molecular level have been identified that might not directly involve HPV. The molecular oncogenesis in cervical carcinoma can be explained to a degree by the regulation and function of two viral proteins, E6 and E7. The *E6* gene binds to the *p53* tumor suppressor gene and induces degradation. The *E7* gene binds another tumor suppressor, the retinoblastoma gene *(Rb)*. By binding to it, it functionally inactivates the protein, which like p53, works in cell cycle. There are more than 100 types of HPV, stratified into low-, intermediate-, and high-risk categories based on the strength of their association with invasive lesions. High-risk HPV types exhibit greater inactivation of *p53* and *Rb* genes.

The link between human leukocyte antigens (HLAs) and HPV might help to explain why the same HPV type leads to invasive cancer in one patient but not in another. It has been established that cervical dysplasia in HIV-infected women is associated with higher incidence, more rapid progression, and higher recurrence rates when compared with HIV-negative women.

## Staging

Cervical cancer is staged clinically. Surgical-pathologic staging is superior to clinical staging. It provides useful information regarding the extent of disease and status of pelvic and para-aortic lymph nodes (Box 2).

### PHYSICAL FINDINGS

The gross appearance of cervical cancer varies depending on whether the lesion is exophytic, endophytic, or ulcerative. Exophytic growths that characteristically bleed on contact are the most common type of cervical cancer. Sometimes the cancer develops entirely within the endocervical canal, manifesting as a hard, indurated, and often barrel-shaped lesion. The cancer can also appear as a small, shallow ulcer.

### HISTOPATHOLOGY

Squamous cell carcinoma is the most common type of cervical cancer. Adenocarcinoma and other carcinomas are less common (Box 3).

## PATHOPHYSIOLOGY

Cervical cancer in the early stage invades lymphatics in the parametrium and pelvic lymph nodes through tumor emboli. As the primary lesion progresses, the tumor extends to the pelvic side wall laterally, to the bladder base anteriorly, and, less frequently, to the rectum posteriorly.

## SPREAD PATTERN

Cervical cancer exhibits three spread patterns. Direct extension is to parametrial tissue and the pelvic wall (ureter), to the bladder and rectum, or to the uterine corpus and vagina. Lymphatic spread is of two kinds. The primary group involves the paracervical, obturator, hypogastric, and external iliac lymph nodes, and the secondary group involves the common iliac, inguinal, and aortic lymph nodes. Hematogenous spread is to the lung, liver, bone, and brain.

## EXAMINATION AND TESTING

The initial work-up includes history and physical examination; chest x-ray, intravenous pyelogram (IVP), or computed tomography (CT); and HIV testing (Box 4). Some centers do not routinely use IVP and CT or cystoscopy and protosigmoidoscopy for early-stage disease because of relatively low yield. In patients who are not candidates for surgery, a CT scan can be helpful in assessing nodal disease. Enlarged lymph nodes should be studied histocytologically by either surgical excision or fine-needle aspiration because of the 5% to 10% false-positive rate of a CT scan. More recently, magnetic resonance imaging (MRI) has been studied for early parametrial and nodal disease. Positron emission tomography (PET) has been reported as useful to predict para-aortic disease. Because of infrequent colon involvement, sigmoidoscopy or barium enema should be restricted to symptomatic patients or those with a positive guiac test.

# Treatment

## SURGERY AND RADIATION

In general, early-stage cervical cancer can be treated with radical hysterectomy or radiation. However, surgery is preferred for premenopausal women to preserve ovarian function and a functioning vagina following surgery. In patients with high-risk criteria—positive surgical margin, parametrial involvement, and positive pelvic nodes—cisplatin-based chemoradiation is usually recommended. Those with intermediate risk factors such as tumor size greater than 4 cm, deep cervical stromal invasion greater than 50%, or lymphovascular invasion might also benefit from chemoradiation.

Radical trachelectomy is a reasonable alternative treatment for select young patients who desire to maintain their childbearing capacity. The criteria include early-stage cervical cancer with a lesion less than 2 cm, no lymphovascular invasion, and no lymph node metastasis.

Laparoscopic-assisted radical vaginal hysterectomy (LARVH), like other surgical procedures, may be considered in select patients with early-stage cervical cancer. Reported advantages are less blood loss, better cosmetic results, shorter hospitalization, and earlier recovery.

## CHEMORADIATION THERAPY

Squamous cell carcinoma of the cervix is a chemosensitive malignancy, particularly when cisplatinum-based chemotherapy is being used. In February 1999, the National Cancer Institute published a consensus statement demonstrating superiority of platinum-based chemoradiation compared with radiation alone for locally advanced cervical cancer (stage IIB-IVA), high-risk early-stage cervical cancer (IA2-IIA2), or bulky stage IB cervical cancer (Table 1).

**TABLE 1 Concurrent Chemoradiation for Cervical Cancer**

| Reference | Study | FIGO Stages | Patients | Treatment Regimen | Overall Survival |
|---|---|---|---|---|---|
| Whitney, et al | GOG 85 | IIB-IVA | 368 | Cisplatin[1]/5-FU[1] + RT | 67% |
| | | | | Hydroxyurea[1] + RT | 57% |
| Rose, et al | GOG 120 | IIB-IVA | 526 | Weekly cisplatin + RT | 65% |
| | | | | Cisplatin/5-FU/hydroxyurea + RT | 65% |
| | | | | Hydroxyurea + RT | 47% |
| Morris, et al | RTOG 9001 | IB2-IVA* | 388 | Cisplatin/5-FU + RT | 75% |
| | | | | RT alone | 63% |
| Keys, et al | GOG 123 | IB2[†] | 369 | Weekly cisplatin + R | 83% |
| | | | | RT | 74% |
| Peters, et al | GOG 109, SWOG 8797 | IA2-IIA | 243 | Cisplatin/5-FU + RT | 81% |
| | | | | RT | 71% |

[1]Not FDA approved for this indication.
*Stages IB and IIA required positive pelvic nodes or tumor size >5 cm.
[†]Extrafascial hysterectomy followed by chemoradiation or radiation.

*References cited in the table:*
Keys HM, Bundy BN, Stehman FB, et al: Cisplatin, radiation, and adjuvant hysterectomy compared with radiation and adjuvant hysterectomy for bulky stage IB cervical carcinoma. N Engl J Med 1999;340(15):1154-1161.
Morris M, Eifel PJ, Lu J, et al: Pelvic radiation with concurrent chemotherapy compared with pelvic and para-aortic radiation for high-risk cervical cancer. N Engl J Med 1999;340(15):1137-1143.
Peters WA 3rd, Liu PY, Barrett RJ 2nd, et al: Concurrent chemotherapy and pelvic radiation therapy compared with pelvic radiation therapy alone as adjuvant therapy after radical surgery in high-risk early-stage cancer of the cervix. J Clin Oncol 2000;18(8):1606-1613.
Rose PG, Bundy BN, Watkins EB, et al: Concurrent cisplatin-based radiotherapy and chemotherapy for locally advanced cervical cancer. N Engl J Med 1999;340(15):1144-1153.
Whitney CW, Sause W, Bundy BN, et al.: Randomized comparison of fluorouracil plus cisplatin versus hydroxyurea as an adjunct to radiation therapy in stage IIB-IVA carcinoma of the cervix with negative para-aortic lymph nodes: A Gynecologic Oncology Group and Southwest Oncology Group study. J Clin Oncol 1999;17(5):1339-1348.
*Abbreviations:* FIGO = International Federation of Gynecology and Obstetrics; 5-FU = 5-fluorouracil; GOG = Gynecologic Oncology Group; RT = radiation therapy; RTOG = Radiation Therapy Oncology Group; SWOG = SouthWest Oncology Group.
Data from National Cancer Institute: Concurrent chemoradiation for cervical cancer. Clinical announcement, Washington, DC, February 22, 1999.

Since then, chemoradiation has become the standard of care, and cisplatinum has shown the best activity as a single agent in cervical cancer, with a 20% to 30% objective response. Tumor cytotoxicity is intensified when cisplatinum is combined with radiation at the same time. Clinical studies have chiefly included neoadjuvant chemotherapy or a combination of chemotherapy and radiation when given together.

Although chemoradiation is associated with higher toxicity and increased cost, there is some economic benefit from less disease recurrence and subsequent medical costs.

## THERAPY BY STAGE

### Stage IA1

Patients with no lymphovascular invasion and tumor invasion to less than 3 mm (stage IA1) have less than 1% risk of nodal metastasis. The decision to proceed with conization versus abdominal or vaginal hysterectomy is based on the patient's desire for childbearing. Women with stage IA1 cancer may be treated by conization alone, provided that all cone margins are free of disease and endocervical curettage is negative. When lymphovascular invasion is present and tumor invasion is less than 3 mm, most physicians prefer modified radical hysterectomy over radiation.

### Stage IA2

For patients with stroma invasion more than 3 mm or those with lymphovascular space involvement, the preferred treatment is modified or radical hysterectomy with pelvic lymphadenectomy. Radical trachelectomy with pelvic lymphadenectomy has been performed in women who desire further childbearing, with some women successfully becoming pregnant.

### Stage IB

Patients with stage IB1 (tumor size <4 cm) can effectively be treated by radical hysterectomy with or without pelvic or para-aortic lymphadenectomy. Radiation therapy can be used in patients with stage 1A2 or 1B, particularly in those who are not medically suitable for radical surgery.

Treatment for patients with Stage 1B2 (bulky or barrel-shaped lesions) is the same as for stage 1B1. However, many of these tumors extend anatomically beyond the curative isodose curve of the radiation field and have significant central recurrences. Therefore, preoperative radiation therapy followed by extrafascial hysterectomy has been recommended.

Because nodal metastases are present in 20% to 25% of patients with stage 1B2 cervical cancers, para-aortic lymph node dissection should be considered at the time of hysterectomy if the para-aortic nodes were not included in the preoperative radiation fields.

### Stage IIA

The optimal treatment for most patients with stage IIA cervical cancer is similar to that for stage 1B: Patients may be treated effectively by radical hysterectomy with pelvic and para-aortic lymphadenectomy and upper vaginectomy, provided that all surgical margins are free of disease. Many authors recommend postoperative whole pelvic radiation for patients with microscopic parametrial invasion, nodal metastasis, and involvement of resection margins. Morbidity from radiation therapy limited to 4500 to 5000 cGy appears acceptable; however, local recurrence is decreased, and the survival advantage, if any, is not known.

### Stages IIB to IVA

For patients with locally advanced cervical cancer, primary radiation therapy (external beam and brachytherapy) and concomitant chemotherapy is recommended. Para-aortic nodal involvement is the most important prognostic factor in patients' survival. In the absence of para-aortic nodal metastasis, transposition of both ovaries in young women should be considered.

Elective para-aortic radiation is an alternative to surgical para-aortic lymphadenectomy. The two main methods of radiation for cervical cancer are external beam radiation and brachytherapy. Brachytherapy can be performed by either the intracavity technique or

## BOX 5 Complications of Radiation Therapy in Cervical Cancer

**Intestinal**
- Abdominal cramps, diarrhea
- Malabsorption
- Nausea and vomiting
- Stricture causing bowel obstruction
- Ulceration, bleeding, and perforation causing rectovaginal fistula

**Urinary**
- Dysuria and urinary frequency
- Hematuria that can progress to perforation, causing vesicovaginal fistula or scarring, resulting in smaller bladder capacity and incontinence
- Ureteral stricture, hydroureter, and hydronephrosis

**Vaginal**
- Decreased vaginal lubrication
- Dyspareunia
- Shortening and stenosis

**Vascular**
- Fibrosis and thrombosis of pelvic vessels, causing leg edema

by the interstitial technique, using needles or after-loading catheters. Interstitial brachytherapy is used when cervical cancer cannot be optimally encompassed by intracavity applications.

Potential complications of radiation therapy can be acute occurring during treatment or they can be delayed, usually occurring 1.5 to 2 years after treatement is completed (Boxes 5 and 6).

## Recurrence

It is estimated that approximately 35% of patients with invasive cervical cancer will have recurrent or persistent disease following therapy. Recurrence can be expected in 10% to 20% of patients treated with

## BOX 6 Complications of Radical Hysterectomy in Cervical Cancer

**Intestinal**
- Ileus, bowel obstruction
- Rectal atony, rectal injury
- Rectovaginal fistula

**Urinary**
- Bladder atony, bladder injury resulting in vesicovaginal fistula
- Ureteral injury causing stricture or hydroureter and ureterovaginal fistula

**Vaginal**
- Dyspareunia
- Shortening vagina

**Vascular**
- Vascular injury, deep vein thrombosis, causing leg edema and pulmonary embolism
- Lymphocyst formation and lymphedema exist but are uncommon

radical hysterectomy and lymphadenectomy. Most recurrences are distant metastasis involving the lung, bone, abdominal cavity, and supraclavicular lymph nodes.

Prognosis for patients with recurrent disease is more favorable in those with a small (<3 cm) central recurrence, no sidewall involvement, and longer disease-free interval.

### SURGERY

Patients with central pelvic recurrences after primary treatment with radiation therapy may be salvaged with surgery. Those with small recurrences limited to the cervix or upper vagina can occasionally be treated with modified radical hysterectomy and upper vaginectomy with excellent results. Patients with larger central recurrences or those who have received previous high-dose radiation require pelvic exenteration for salvage therapy.

Recently, more attention has been directed to reconstructive procedures performed at the time of pelvic exenterations to improve quality of life. These include performing continent urinary diversion, primary colon reanastomosis, and vaginal reconstructions with myocutaneous flap.

### RADIATION THERAPY

Radiation therapy may be useful in patients with localized central pelvic recurrence after radical hysterectomy or as palliation to control symptoms such as bleeding and pelvic pain.

### CHEMOTHERAPY

Cervical cancer is a slow-growing neoplasm with poor response to chemotherapy. Cisplatinum (cisplatin)[1] remains the drug of choice for treating recurrences, although phase II trials are currently examining the efficacies of a broad range of compounds such as topotecan, paclitaxel,[1] and gemcitabine.[1] Combination therapy with agents such as paclitaxel and cisplatinum has been studied in phase II trials of recurrent or advanced squamous cell cancer of the cervix with 12% complete responses and 34% partial responses, although 61% of patients experienced severe neutropenia. Given the palliative nature of chemotherapy in recurrent disease, the quality of life and drug toxicity must be factored into the choice of agents.

The encouraging activity of topotecan plus cisplatin in phase II trials led to the comparison of this combination against single-agent cisplatin in GOG 179. The main goals of this trial were overall response rate, progression-free survival, and quality of life.

GOG 204 is a randomized phase III trial with four treatment arms designed to evaluate the efficacy and tolerability of cisplatin-based doublets in the treatment of primary stage IVB, recurrent, or persistent cervical cancer (Figure 1).

In addition to the exploration of new doublets, the incorporation of biological agents such as erlotinab[1] and bevacizumab[1] into the treatment of cervical cancer are ongoing as GOG phase II multicenter trials.

### FOLLOW-UP

Most recurrence occurs in the first 2 years following primary therapy. Therefore, physical examination with nodal assessment, abdominal examination, pelvic examination including rectovaginal examination, and Pap smear should be done at 3-month intervals for the first year, at 4-month intervals for the second year, and at 6-month intervals thereafter. After 5 years, an annual examination appears to be appropriate. Interval chest x-ray and abdominal CT scanning should be considered. Symptoms of pain, bleeding, and gastrointestinal or genitourinary dysfunction should be investigated for possible recurrence.

---

[1]Not FDA approved for this indication.

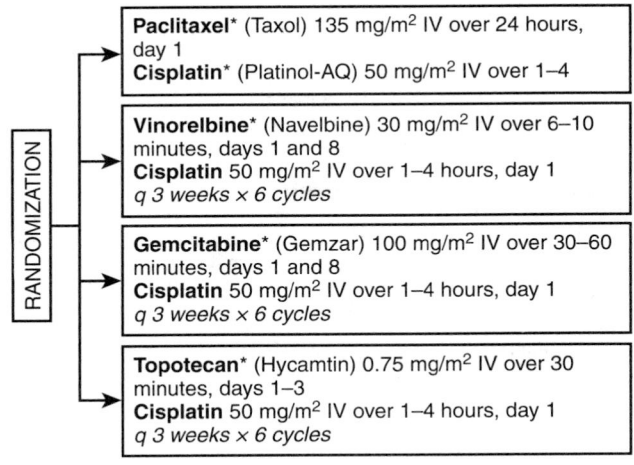

**RANDOMIZATION**

**Paclitaxel\*** (Taxol) 135 mg/m² IV over 24 hours, day 1
**Cisplatin\*** (Platinol-AQ) 50 mg/m² IV over 1–4

**Vinorelbine\*** (Navelbine) 30 mg/m² IV over 6–10 minutes, days 1 and 8
**Cisplatin** 50 mg/m² IV over 1–4 hours, day 1
*q 3 weeks × 6 cycles*

**Gemcitabine\*** (Gemzar) 100 mg/m² IV over 30–60 minutes, days 1 and 8
**Cisplatin** 50 mg/m² IV over 1–4 hours, day 1
*q 3 weeks × 6 cycles*

**Topotecan\*** (Hycamtin) 0.75 mg/m² IV over 30 minutes, days 1–3
**Cisplatin** 50 mg/m² IV over 1–4 hours, day 1
*q 3 weeks × 6 cycles*

**FIGURE 1.** Treatment schema of the Randomized Phase III Study of Paclitaxel Plus Cisplatin vs. Vinorelbine Plus Cisplatin vs. Gemcitabine Plus Cisplatin vs. Topotecan Plus Cisplatin in Stage IVB, Recurrent, or Persistent Carcinoma of the Cervix (GOG 204). *Abbreviation:* GOG = Gynecologic Oncology Group.

## Special Categories

### CARCINOMA OF THE CERVICAL STUMP

Although supracervical hysterectomy is now rarely performed, carcinoma of the cervical stump is still encountered. Stage for stage, it is treated the same as cervical carcinoma of the intact uterus; for early stages, radical cervicectomy and parametrectomy with pelvic and possible para-aortic lymphadenopathy is performed. When radiation therapy is required, the short cervix often limits the amount of intracavitary radiation, therefore requiring higher-dose external irradiation.

### INVASIVE CERVICAL CANCER AFTER HYSTERECTOMY

Occasionally, diagnosis of unsuspected invasive cervical cancer is made after a hysterectomy for a benign disease. Those with microinvasive disease do not require additional therapy. Those with invasive cancer confined to the cervix can be treated with radical parametrectomy, upper vaginectomy, and pelvic and para-aortic lymphadenopathy. The alternative is radiation therapy with or without chemotherapy.

### INVASIVE CERVICAL CANCER DURING PREGNANCY

Pregnancy does not appear to affect the prognoses of patients with cervical cancer, and the fetus is not affected by maternal cervical cancer. However, the fetus might suffer consequences from treatment.

Patients with microinvasion diagnosed with conization can continue pregnancy until term and deliver vaginally. Before fetal maturity, patients should be treated individually, and the concerns for fetal survival must be weighed against the risk of delayed therapy.

Patients with stages IA2 to IIA can be treated by radical hysterectomy and pelvic lymphadenectomy with the fetus in situ. If the patient does not want to terminate the pregnancy or if she is close to term, then the fetus can be delivered with classic cesarean section followed by radical hysterectomy and pelvic lymphadenectomy.

Patients with larger tumors or locally advanced disease can be treated with chemoradiation. Those close to term or with fetal lung maturity can be delivered by cesarean section and surgical staging followed by chemoradiation. In a patient who declines pregnancy termination, consideration may be given to neoadjuvant chemotherapy to prevent progression of disease and time for fetal lung maturity.

## ADENOCARCINOMA OF THE CERVIX

The management of adenocarcinoma of the cervix is similar to that for squamous cell carcinoma. The worse prognosis reported in some cases is attributed to a higher rate of distant metastasis.

### Adenocarcinoma In Situ

Adenocarcinoma in situ (ACIS) may be identified from investigation of an abnormal Pap smear. When diagnosed on biopsy, conization is required because ACIS can be diffuse or multifocal and may be associated with underlying adenocarcinoma. The differential diagnosis includes well-differentiated adenocarcinoma (adenoma malignum or minimal deviation adenocarcinoma) and microglandular hyperplasia, which is associated with oral contraceptives and Arias-Stella changes of pregnancy. Simple hysterectomy is the treatment of choice for women who have no desire for further childbearing. Otherwise, cone biopsy may be adequate if the margins are clear and endovervical curettage is negative.

### Microinvasive Adenocarcinoma

Patients with stage IA1 can be managed with simple hysterectomy. However, conization can be done for young women who desire to preserve fertility. Therefore, treatment should be individualized according to depth of invasion, margin of resection, and lymphovascular invasion.

### Invasive Adenocarcinoma

Invasive adenocarcinoma accounts for approximately 5% to 10% of all cervical carcinomas. Adenocarcinoma has been classified into five subtypes: endocervical, endometrioid, clear cell, adenocystic, and adenosquamous.

Cervical adenocarcinoma usually originates from the endocervical canal. Vaginal bleeding and discharge are the most common symptoms. Endocervical and endometrial curettage are essential in the evaluation of patients if the results of gross examination of the cervix, colposcopy, and cervical biopsy are negative.

The recommended treatment for stage IA2 microinvasion is modified radical hysterectomy and pelvic lymphadenectomy. For stages IB and IIA, radical hysterectomy and pelvic lymphadenopathy are recommended. Adjuvant pelvic radiation should be considered for patients with nodal metastasis, lymphovascular invasion, poorly differentiated tumor, or larger lesions. When radiation is the primary treatment, an adjuvant simple hysterectomy is recommended. Follow-up CEA (carcinoembryonic antigen) and CA-125 (cancer antigen 125) are of value in cervical adenocarcinoma.

### Adenosquamous Carcinoma

Adenosquamous carcinoma represents 20% to 30% of cervical adenocarcinomas. Overall 5-year survival and disease-free survival rates are not significantly different from those of other adenocarcinomas.

### Clear Cell Adenocarcinoma

In clear cell adenocarcinoma, the tumor occurs in two distinct groups of patients—those younger than 24 years and those older than 45 years. Cancer in the older group is unrelated to diethylstilbestrol (DES) exposure in utero. Unlike uterine clear cell adenocarcinoma, the prognosis is the same as for other adenocarcinomas.

### Glassy Cell Carcinoma

Glassy cell carcinoma is a poorly differentiated adenosquamous (or large cell undifferentiated) carcinoma with a moderate amount of cytoplasm and a typical ground glass appearance. The prognosis is poor. Reported survival for stage IB cancer treated with radical hysterectomy was 55%.

## Small Cell Carcinoma

Small cell (neuroendocrine) carcinoma is very rare, only 0.6% of cervical cancers. Small cell carcinoma histologically stains for neuroendocrine markers. These cells can synthesize amines and hence are also called amine precursor uptake and decarboxylation (APUD) cells. Small cell carcinoma has a tendency to a higher lymphovascular invasion, resulting in higher recurrence and lower survival because of their propensity for early systemic spread. Chemotherapy is usually recommended in addition to surgery and radiation.

A larger study involving 23 women compared adjuvant chemotherapy with cisplatin,[1] vinblastine,[1] and bleomycin[1] (PVB) against vincristine,[1] doxorubicin,[1] and cyclophosphamide[1] (VAC) alternating with cisplatin[1] and etoposide[1] (PE) after radical hysterectomy. The reported survival was higher in the VAC/PE group (10 of 14) compared with the PVB group (3 of 9), with median follow-up of 41 months.

# Chemoprevention and Vaccination

Due to the relatively long premalignant phase of cervical carcinogenesis (5-10 years), some investigators are studying the effect of chemoprevention or vaccination on disease progression. Investigators have focused on the retinoids as chemoprevention agents for cervical dysplasia based on their cell-differentiating properties.

Topical *trans*-retinoic acid[1] (tretinoin) in a randomized phase III clinical trial has been shown to induce regression of mild and moderate dysplasias, but not of severe dysplasias. Other suitable agents for chemoprevention include difluoromethylornithine,[5] beta-carotene,[7] and cyclooxygenase-2 inhibitors.[1]

HPV vaccines are focused on targeting the oncogenic E6/E7 proteins as therapeutic vaccines. These peptide vaccines are designed to stimulate cytotoxic T lymphocytes against specific E6/E7 epitopes. HPV16 and HPV18 together cause about 70% of cervical cancers. It is estimated that 20 million people are infected worldwide and 6.2 million people in the United States get a new infection of HPV each year. Two new vaccines, Gardasil (Merck) and Cervarix[5] (GlaxoSmithKline) reported 100% protection against HPV 16 and HPV 18 infection. To improve that effort, researchers are already working on second-generation vaccines and exploring the possibility of a therapeutic vaccine that could help prevent HPV-related cancers in those who are already being infected by the virus.

## REFERENCES

Boss EA, van Golde RI, Beerendonk CC, Massuger LE: Pregnancy after radical trachelectomy: A real option? Gynecol Oncol 2005;99(3 suppl 1): S152-S156.

Dargent D, Martin X, Sacchetoni A, Mathevet P: Laparoscopic vaginal radical trachelectomy: A treatment to preserve the fertility of cervical cancer carcinoma patients. Cancer 2000;88:1877-1882.

Delgado G, Bundy B, Zaino R, et al: Prospective surgical-pathological study of disease-free interval in patients with stage IB squamous cell carcinoma of the cervix: A Gynecologic Oncology Group study. Gynecol Oncol 1990;38:352-357.

Giacalone PL, Laffargue E: Neoadjuvant chemotherapy in the treatment of locally advanced cervical carcinoma in pregnancy: A report of two cases and review of issues specific to the management of cervical carcinoma in pregnancy including planned delay of therapy. Cancer 1999;85:1203-1204.

Hopkins MP, Lavin JP: Cervical cancer in pregnancy. Gynecol Oncol 1996; 63:293.

Jemal A, Siegel R, Ward E, et al: Cancer statistics, 2006. CA Cancer J Clin 2006; 56:106-130.

Jensen PT, Groenvold M, Klee MC, et al: Early-stage cervical carcinoma, radical hysterectomy, and sexual function: A longitudinal study. Cancer 2004; 100:97-106.

Lertsanguansinchai P, Lertbutsayanukul C, Shotelersuk K, et al: Phase III randomized trial comparing LDR and HDR brachytherapy in treatment of cervical carcinoma. Int J Radiat Oncol Biol Phys 2004;59:1424-1431.

Plante M, Renaud MC, FranÁois H, Roy M: Vaginal radical trachelectomy: An oncologically safe fertility-preserving surgery: An updated series of 72 cases and review of the literature. Gynecol Oncol 2004;94:614-623.

Roman LD, Felix JC, Muderspach LL, et al: Risk of residual invasive disease in women with microinvasive squamous cancer in a conization specimen. Obstet Gynecol 1997;90:759-764.

Sedlis A, Bundy BN, Rotman MZ, et al: A randomized trial of pelvic radiation therapy versus no further therapy in selected patients with stage IB carcinoma of the cervix after radical hysterectomy and pelvic lymphadenectomy: A Gynecologic Oncology Group Study. Gynecol Oncol 1999; 73:177-183.

Steed H, Rosen B, Murphy J, et al: A comparison of laparascopic-assisted radical vaginal hysterectomy and radical abdominal hysterectomy in the treatment of cervical cancer. Gynecol Oncol 2004;93:588-593.

# Neoplasms of the Vulva

Method of
*Susan A. Davidson, MD*

The female external genitalia includes the mons pubis, labia majora, labia minora, clitoris, perineal body, and the structures of the vaginal introitus or vestibule. Whether benign or malignant, vulvar neoplasms are uncommon, occur at all ages, and have varying characteristics. Therefore liberal use of biopsies is usually required for diagnosis and to guide treatment.

## Benign Cystic Neoplasms

Benign cystic lesions of the vulva include Bartholin's duct cyst, sebaceous and epidermal inclusion cysts, mucinous cysts, Skene duct cysts, and cysts of the canal of Nuck. Bartholin's duct cyst, located in the posterior labia near the vaginal introitus, is most common. Treatment is usually not required in asymptomatic young women (<40 years). If the cyst is symptomatic or infected, however, drainage by marsupialization or use of a Word catheter, is indicated. Bartholin's gland carcinomas are rare, especially in women younger than 40 years of age. But if the mass feels firm or nodular, it should be biopsied.

Sebaceous and epidermal inclusion cysts are also common. They are prone to infection but rarely malignant. If an infection develops, they should be incised and drained. Mucinous cysts are rare and possibly arise from the minor vestibular glands. They are located anteriorly on the vulva, typically on the inner labia minora. Skene duct cysts are located next to the urethra. Excision of these cysts is necessary only if symptomatic.

Cysts of the canal of Nuck are located in the anterior portion of the labia majora at the termination of the insertion of the round ligament. These cysts represent herniation of the peritoneum through the inguinal canal and contain peritoneal fluid. If symptomatic, excision must be accompanied by closure of the fascial defect to prevent recurrence.

## Benign Solid Neoplasms

The benign solid tumors of the vulva include fibromas, myomas, lipomas, hidradenomas, syringomas, myoblastomas, vestibular adenomas, and angiomas, among others. Benign pigmented lesions, such as nevi and seborrheic keratoses, may occasionally be found. Malignancy is rare, but most should be excised for diagnostic and therapeutic purposes.

---

[1]Not FDA approved for this indication.
[5]Investigational drug in the United States.
[7]Available as dietary supplement.

## CONDYLOMA ACUMINATUM

Vulvar condyloma acuminatum is a sexually transmitted verrucous lesion of the vulva caused by human papilloma virus (HPV), most frequently types 6 and 11. These lesions are warty growths that frequently cover large areas of the vulva. Smoking and immunosuppression are risk factors. Representative biopsies should be obtained to document disease and rule out malignancy. Wide local excision can be used for small lesions, although these growths are usually best treated by ablation.

Chemical ablative techniques include topical application of trichloroacetic acid (Tri-Chlor), podofilox (0.5%, Condylox), 5-fluorouracil[1] (1%, Fluoroplex or 5%, Efudex),[1] or imiquimod (5%, Aldara). Podophyllin can be applied twice daily for 3 days, repeated weekly for 4 weeks. Imiquimod can be applied three times per week for up to 16 weeks. Podophyllin and 5-fluorouracil should not be used in women who could become pregnant. Surgical ablative therapies include $CO_2$ laser vaporization and use of the Cavitron ultrasonic aspirator (CUSA), especially for extensive disease.

# Intraepithelial Neoplasms of the Vulva

## VULVAR INTRAEPITHELIAL NEOPLASIA

Vulvar intraepithelial neoplasia (VIN) is a dysplastic condition of the squamous epithelium whose incidence is increasing, especially in younger women. Risk factors are HPV types 16 and 18, smoking, and immunosuppression. Symptoms include pruritus (most common), pain, a noticeable lesion, and discoloration. Most patients with HPV-related disease have multifocal lesions including vaginal and cervical dysplasia. The most common location is in the area of the posterior fourchette and perineal body. Typical findings are raised white, gray, red, or mottled lesions; application of 4% acetic acid for several minutes can help identify faint lesions and outline abnormal vascular patterns. Diagnosis of VIN is made by punch biopsies through full thickness of the epithelium to rule out invasion, present in 20% of patients with VIN III (full-thickness dysplasia or carcinoma in situ). Of those patients with invasion, half (10% of VIN III) have invasion more than 1 mm.

Treatment of VIN can be categorized into excisional and ablative therapies. Patients at risk for microinvasion (unifocal disease, raised lesions, older age, and prior radiation) should have the lesion excised completely if possible. Skinning vulvectomy is rarely used because of psychological and sexual consequences related to scarring and disfigurement.

The ablative therapies can be divided into mechanical and chemical. The mechanical method most commonly used is the $CO_2$ laser, although use of the CUSA is also described. Both can ablate large or multifocal lesions successfully with an excellent cosmetic and functional outcome. The chemical method most commonly used is topical 5-fluorouracil (5%, Efudex).[1] Because of its teratogenic potential, it should not be used in women who could become pregnant. It can be applied on two consecutive nights weekly for 10 weeks. An alternative ablative therapy is use of imiquimod[1] (Aldara), as described earlier. Because of the irritation caused by these topical therapies, many patients have problems with treatment compliance. Residual disease should be excised to rule out invasion.

Patients with VIN frequently have recurrent disease, regardless of the treatment method used (Table 1). Continued smoking increases this risk, so patients should be counseled in smoking cessation. In those patients whose cancers recur and are retreated, subsequent 5-fluorouracil prophylaxis, with a single application biweekly, is used successfully to minimize further recurrences.

## PAGET'S DISEASE

Paget's disease of the vulva is an uncommon condition characterized by a patchy, eczematoid lesion that frequently covers much of the vulva. Most patients are postmenopausal and present with complaints

---

[1]Not FDA approved for this indication.

**TABLE 1 Recurrence of Vulvar Intraepithelial Neoplasia III**

| Treatment Method | % Recurrence |
| --- | --- |
| Chemical ablation | 20-40 |
| Mechanical ablation | 20-40 |
| Wide local excision | |
| Negative margin | 15-25 |
| Positive margin | 30-45 |

of pruritus. Although Paget's disease is an in situ disease process, 15% to 25% of patients have an underlying malignancy, usually an adenocarcinoma of the apocrine glands but occasionally an invasive Paget's. In addition, up to 30% of patients have a synchronous adenocarcinoma of the breast, colon, rectum, or upper genital tract. Screening for these cancers is therefore recommended. To assess for invasion, the lesion should be excised via wide local excision or simple vulvectomy with at least 5 mm of the adjacent subcutaneous tissue. Achieving negative margin status is frequently difficult. However, the risk of recurrence is approximately 30% whether margins are negative or positive. Thus expectant management, reserving treatment for symptomatic recurrences, is usually recommended.

# Invasive Vulvar Lesions

Less than 5% of gynecologic cancers arise on the vulva. Approximately 85% are squamous cell carcinomas. The etiology of this type appears mixed. Up to 50% evolve from VIN III and are usually associated with HPV-16. These women are slightly younger (age 45-52 years). Most arise in older women (mean age 60-69 years), and suggested risk factors include immunosuppression, hypertension, diabetes mellitus, obesity, and chronic vulvar inflammation. Other histologic types are melanomas (5% to 10%), basal cell carcinomas (2% to 3%), adenocarcinomas (1%), and sarcomas (1% to 2%) Most patients present with a combination of symptoms, including pruritus, discomfort, and complaints of a mass. Examination frequently reveals a suspicious lesion, which should be biopsied for diagnosis. Vulvar cancers typically spread by local extension and lymphatic dissemination. Factors that influence dissemination include tumor size (Table 2), depth of invasion (Table 3), lymphovascular space invasion, and tumor grade. Staging is surgical and classified using the tumor, nodes, and metastasis (TNM) system (Box 1) as well as the International Federation of Gynecology and Obstetrics (FIGO) system (Box 2).

## SQUAMOUS CELL CARCINOMAS AND ADENOCARCINOMAS

Surgical management of squamous cell carcinomas and adenocarcinomas depends on the size, depth of invasion, and location of the lesion. The vulvar lesion is managed with a radical excision. Management of the groins is based on depth of invasion. Lesions with invasion of <1 mm have minimal risk of lymphatic spread and do not

**TABLE 2 Incidence of Regional Node Metastases by Tumor Diameter**

| Tumor Diameter (cm) | % Positive Inguinal Nodes |
| --- | --- |
| <1 | 0-15 |
| 5-20 | |
| 25-35 | |
| 35-50 | |
| ≥50 | ≥50 |

**TABLE 3** Incidence of Regional Node Metastases by Depth of Tumor Invasion

| Depth of Invasion (mm) | % Positive Inguinal Nodes |
|---|---|
| <1 | 1-5 |
| 1-3 | 10-15 |
| 3-5 | 15-30 |
| 5-10 | 30-45 |
| >10 | >40 |

require lymphadenectomy. All others require surgical assessment of the lymph nodes. Lesions located in the midline structures require bilateral groin dissection, whereas lateral lesions are managed with ipsilateral groin dissection. This surgical approach is associated with significant morbidity including disfigurement, wound breakdown, and problems with lymphocysts and chronic lymphedema. For patients with very large lesions or lesions in sensitive areas such as the clitoris, preoperative radiation, followed by less radical excision of residual disease, may minimize problems with the vulvar wound. Current investigations are ongoing in the use of sentinel lymph node dissections as a method of minimizing the groin morbidity without sacrificing survival. Positive vulvar margins or metastases to lymph nodes are managed with postoperative radiation. Survival depends on stage at diagnosis (Table 4).

## MALIGNANT MELANOMA

Malignant melanoma is the second most common vulvar malignancy. Most patients have disease on the mucosal surfaces of the vulvar introitus, clitoris, and labia minora. The vulvar lesion is treated by radical excision, but management of the groins is controversial. The risk of spread is significant with a tumor thickness greater than 0.75 mm, but survival at 5 years is only approximately 10% with groin node metastases. Some argue against node dissection for this reason. However, given some long-term survivors with modern melanoma therapy, either lymphadenectomy or sentinel lymph node dissection, as is done for other cutaneous melanomas, appears indicated.

## VERRUCOUS CARCINOMA

Verrucous carcinoma is a large exophytic tumor that resembles giant condyloma acuminatum. It is a variant of squamous carcinomas but has an excellent prognosis because of the lack of metastases. Verrucous

---

**BOX 1  TNM Classification of Vulvar Carcinoma**

| | |
|---|---|
| T | Primary tumor |
| Tis | Carcinoma in situ |
| T1 | Confined to vulva, diameter ≤2 cm |
| T2 | Confined to vulva, diameter >2 cm |
| T3 | Adjacent spread to urethra, vagina, perineum, or anus (any size) |
| T4 | Infiltration of upper urethral mucosa, bladder, rectum, or bone |
| N | Regional lymph nodes |
| N0 | No lymph node metastases |
| N1 | Unilateral regional lymph node metastasis |
| N2 | Bilateral regional lymph node metastasis |
| M | Distant metastases |
| M0 | No clinical metastases |
| M1 | Distant metastasis (including pelvic lymph node metastasis) |

*Abbreviation:* TNM = tumor, node, metastasis.

---

**BOX 2  FIGO Classification (With Corresponding TNM Classification) for Vulvar Carcinoma**

| | |
|---|---|
| **Stage I** (T1N0M0) | Tumor confined to vulva and/or perineum, ≤2 cm in greatest dimension; nodes are negative |
| Stage IA | Stromal invasion no greater than 1 mm |
| Stage IB | Stromal invasion >1 mm |
| **Stage II** (T2N0M0) | Tumor confined to the vulva and/or perineum, >2 cm in greatest dimension; nodes are negative |
| **Stage III** | |
| T3N0M0 | Tumor of any size with adjacent spread to the lower urethra and/or the vagina or the anus |
| T3N1M0 | Unilateral regional lymph node metastasis |
| T2N1M0 | |
| **Stage IVA** | |
| T1N2M0 | |
| T2N2M0 | Tumor invades any of the following: upper urethra, bladder mucosa, rectal mucosa, pelvic bone, and/or bilateral regional node metastasis |
| T3N2M0 | |
| T4 any N M0 | |
| **Stage IVB** | |
| Any T any N M1 | Any distant metastasis including pelvic lymph nodes |

*Abbreviations:* FIGO = International Federation of Gynecology and Obstetrics; TNM = tumor, node, metastasis.

---

## CURRENT DIAGNOSIS

- Most cystic lesions are benign. Excision is reserved for symptomatic cysts and suspicious Bartholin's gland cysts, especially in women older than 40 years of age.
- All solid lesions should be biopsied for diagnostic purposes.
- Multifocal disease requires multiple biopsies to rule out invasive disease.
- Most premalignant and malignant lesions cause pruritus, discomfort, or a noticeable lesion.
- The vagina and cervix in women with dysplastic or malignant vulvar lesions should be evaluated.

---

**TABLE 4  Survival Rate by FIGO Stage for Patients With Invasive Squamous Cell Vulvar Cancer**

| FIGO Stage | % Surviving 5 years |
|---|---|
| I | 70-90 |
| II | 50-80 |
| III | 30-50 |
| IV | 10-15 |

*Abbreviation:* FIGO = International Federation of Gynecology and Obstetrics.

## CURRENT THERAPY

- Benign solid lesions should be excised.
- After ablative treatment of vulvar intraepithelial neoplasia (VIN), excise any residual lesions to rule out occult invasive disease.
- Avoid podophyllin and 5-fluorouracil in women of reproductive potential.
- Rule out synchronous neoplasms in women with Paget's disease.
- Invasion more than 1 mm requires radical excision and lymph node evaluation.

carcinomas have a high tendency to recur and should be managed with radical local excision.

## BASAL CELL CARCINOMA

Basal cell carcinomas typically occur in elderly white women, are commonly located on the labia majora, and have characteristics similar to basal cell carcinomas at other sites. Treatment is wide local excision only because metastases are rare. Basal cell carcinomas are prone to local recurrence, however. A malignant squamous component must be ruled out because it should be managed as a squamous cell carcinoma.

## SARCOMAS

Leiomyosarcoma is the most common vulvar sarcoma and usually arises in the labia majora. Malignant fibrous histiocytoma is the second most common. Management of these lesions is radical vulvar excision.

## REFERENCES

Garland SM: Imiquimod. Curr Opin Infect Dis 2003;16:85-89.
Homesley HD, Bundy BN, Sedlis A, et al: Prognostic factors for groin node metastasis in squamous cell carcinoma of the vulva (a Gynecologic Oncology Group study). Gynecol Oncol 1993;49:279-283.
Krebs HB: The use of topical 5-fluorouracil in the treatment of genital condylomas. Obstet Gynecol Clin North Am 1987;14(2):559-568.
Modesitt SC, Waters AB, Walton L, et al: Vulvar intraepithelial neoplasia III: Occult cancer and the impact of margin status on recurrence. Obstet Gynecol 1998;92(6):962-966.
Phillips GL, Bundy BN, Okagaki T, et al: Malignant melanoma of the vulva treated by radical hemivulvectomy, a prospective study of the Gynecologic Oncology Group. Cancer 1994;73:2626-2632.
Tebes S, Cardosi R, Hoffman M: Paget's disease of the vulva. Am J Obstet Gynecol 2002;187:281-284.
Trimble CL, Trimble EL, Woodruff JD: Diseases of the vulva. In Hernandez E, Atkinson BF (eds): Clinical Gynecologic Pathology. Philadelphia, WB Saunders, 1995, pp 1-90.
Wright VC, Chapman WB: Colposcopy of intraepithelial neoplasia of the vulva and adjacent sites. Obstet Gynecol Clin North Am 1993;20(1):231-255.

# Ovarian Cancer

Method of
*Amanda Nickles Fader, MD, and Jerome Belinson, MD*

Although ovarian carcinoma is only the second most common of the gynecologic malignancies, it is by far the most deadly. According to the American Cancer Society, ovarian cancer will be diagnosed annually in more than 23,000 U.S. women and an estimated 15,000 will die of their disease. Thus, ovarian cancer represents the fifth most common cause of cancer-related death in women in the United States. Although incidence rates have remained stable over the last 2 decades, the overall 5-year survival rate has only slightly improved during this time (from 37% to 44%), primarily due to the lack of effective screening strategies. As a result, more than 75% of ovarian cancers will not be diagnosed until the disease is advanced.

Most primary ovarian tumors are epithelial in origin, the most common subtype of which is papillary serous. The second most common cause of cancer in the ovaries is metastatic disease, especially from breast cancer or Krukenberg tumors (mucin-producing signet-ring cells) from the gastrointestinal tract. Most other histologic subtypes arise from the ovary and include germ cell, sex cord-stromal, and mixed-cell tumors.

The median age of patients with ovarian cancer is 60 years. The cause of epithelial ovarian cancer is still unknown, but most cases occur as a result of sporadic mutations. Risk factors include low parity, high-fat diet, obesity, family history of ovarian or breast cancer, and certain genetic mutations. Multiple pregnancies and the use of oral contraceptives can decrease a woman's risk of developing the disease by as much as 50%, perhaps because of decreased ovulation.

The lifetime risk of ovarian cancer for all U.S. women is about 1.4%, but certain women have a higher risk. Approximately 10% of epithelial ovarian cancers occur as a result of an inherited mutation, and usually arise earlier than ovarian cancers caused by sporadic mutations. Women with one or more first-degree relatives with ovarian cancer have an increased risk of 3% to 5% of developing the disease themselves. Women with known *BRCA1* and *BRCA2* gene mutations have an even greater risk of developing both ovarian and breast cancers. *BRCA1* and *BRCA2* are tumor suppressor genes found on chromosomes 17 and 13, respectively, and are inherited in an autosomal dominant fashion. The lifetime risk of a woman with a *BRCA1* mutation for developing ovarian and breast cancers is 40% and 80%, respectively, and the risk for a woman with a *BRCA2* mutation is 15% and 60%, respectively. Women of Ashkenazi Jewish ancestry have a higher incidence of germ-line mutations in *BRCA1* and *BRCA2* genes.

A second important familial disorder that increases a woman's risk of ovarian and other gynecologic and gastrointestinal cancers is the Lynch II syndrome (hereditary nonpolyposis colorectal cancer syndrome [HNPCC]). It is caused by inherited germ-line mutations in DNA-mismatch repair genes. The lifetime risk of ovarian cancer in HNPCC carriers is 5% to 10%.

Genetic counseling and testing for genetic mutations should be offered to women who have a family history of breast or ovarian cancer in either two first-degree relatives or in a first-degree and a second-degree relative, *BRCA1* or *BRCA2* gene mutations, or HNPCC. Oral contraceptives can be offered to women who desire fertility, and oophorectomy should be considered in high-risk women who have completed their childbearing, because these measures decrease the risk of developing ovarian cancer.

## Screening

Screening tests for ovarian cancer remain controversial. Although quite sensitive for diagnosing ovarian cysts and tumors, transvaginal ultrasonography is nonspecific and its use results in unnecessary surgical exploration of a large number of women with benign (and often physiologic) ovarian cysts. Another such screening test is for serum levels of CA-125 (a tumor-associated antigen). Serum levels greater than 35 U/mL are present in 80% of postmenopausal women with ovarian cancer. However, many early-stage ovarian tumors do not cause elevated levels of CA-125, whereas endometriosis, heavy menses, pelvic inflammatory disease, appendicitis, diverticulitis, benign ovarian tumors, and other benign disorders of the gastrointestinal tract may do so. Therefore, the rarity of ovarian cancer coupled with the lack of sensitivity and specificity for these two currently available tests to detect this disease make for an inability to effectively screen for ovarian cancer at this time.

Although screening is not currently recommended for women in the general public, the exception is the 5% to 10% of women who may be affected by a genetic mutation that increases their risk of ovarian cancer. Women with a potentially increased risk of a hereditary ovarian and breast cancer syndrome should be referred to a geneticist as well as a gynecologic oncologist, who can enroll appropriate candidates into an ovarian cancer screening trial and potentially offer them prophylactic surgery. For *BRCA1* or *BRCA2* mutation carriers, decision analysis indicates that prophylactic surgery or chemoprevention leads to better survival than surveillance alone.

## Diagnosis

An obstacle to diagnosing ovarian cancer is that the associated symptoms are usually nonspecific and occur relatively commonly in daily life as well as with other benign gynecologic and bowel disorders. Early-stage ovarian carcinoma is usually asymptomatic, and symptoms of late-stage disease are often vague, poorly defined, and might not be severe or specific enough to prompt a woman to seek medical attention. As a result, most cases of ovarian carcinoma are advanced at the time of diagnosis.

Advanced ovarian cancer is typically associated with abdominal distention, nausea, constipation, urinary frequency, anorexia, or early satiety due to the presence of ascites and omental or bowel metastases; dyspnea is occasionally present due to a pleural effusion. The nonspecific nature of these symptoms was illustrated by comparing survey results from women before surgery for a pelvic mass with those who visited a primary care clinic for a variety of medical issues (controls). Bloating was present in 70% of women subsequently found to have ovarian cancer, 49% of those with a benign ovarian mass, and 38% of those seeking primary care. In the control population, symptom prevalence and severity decreased with advancing age, suggesting that in young women, many of these symptoms are related to normal cyclical hormonal changes. Furthermore, ovarian cancer patients were more likely than control patients seeking primary care to have symptoms for a shorter time (onset within a few months rather than a year or more), multiple symptoms (the combination of bloating, increased abdominal girth, and urinary symptoms was present in 44%), and a greater frequency of occurrence and severity of symptoms.

If a physician suspects ovarian cancer, conducting a rectovaginal examination as part of the assessment of the pelvis is extremely important. Such an examination can lead to the discovery of the only palpable sign of ovarian disease, which would reside in the cul-de-sac. A serum CA-125 should also be drawn, and imaging studies with either transvaginal ultrasound or computed tomography of the abdomen and pelvis may be performed to help establish the diagnosis. An ovarian mass that has both solid and cystic features with Doppler flow coursing through the solid areas is concerning for ovarian cancer, especially in postmenopausal women with an elevated CA-125. Finally, if there is any suspicion that a woman may have ovarian cancer, she should be referred to a gynecologic oncologist.

## Treatment

### SURGERY

Surgery is still the cornerstone in the management of advanced epithelial ovarian cancer. With surgery, the gynecologic oncologist can confirm the diagnosis of ovarian cancer, appropriately stage the cancer, and remove as much disease as possible (primary cytoreduction). Significantly, there is substantial evidence that patients having such surgery performed by gynecologists with a special training in gynecologic oncology have a survival advantage over patients having such surgery performed by general surgeons or general gynecologists. Researchers in a recently published meta-analysis of 81 studies on the effect of maximal cytoreductive surgery on median survival in patients with advanced ovarian carcinoma concluded that referral of patients with apparent advanced ovarian cancer to gynecologic oncologists for primary surgery may be the most efficient effort currently available for improving overall survival.

### CHEMOTHERAPY

Standard treatment of ovarian cancer requires not only surgical but also medical strategies. Therapy for newly diagnosed epithelial ovarian cancer is determined primarily by the extent of disease at the time of diagnosis as described in the International Federation of Gynecology and Obstetrics (FIGO) staging system. Women with low-grade stage IA disease can generally be managed with initial surgery and observation alone. However, for most women with stage IA grade 2 disease or greater, careful staging and maximum surgical cytoreduction followed by platinum-based chemotherapy are recommended. The prognostic significance of residual disease before chemotherapy has been demonstrated in many reports, and the maxim that survival is correlated to amount of residual disease is generally accepted.

In the mid 1970s, the standard of care for advanced epithelial ovarian cancer was the combination of cyclophosphamide (Cytoxan) and doxorubicin (Adriamycin), the efficacy of which was established by studies conducted by the Gynecologic Oncology Group (GOG). Chemotherapy for this disease has evolved dramatically since that time, with the most important contribution being the discovery that platinum-containing regimens are highly active against ovarian cancer. Three randomized phase III U.S. trials (GOG 111, OV-10, and ICON 3) support the superiority of platinum therapy (either cisplatin [Platinol AQ] or carboplatin [Paraplatin]) to alternative regimens. The addition of a taxane agent to a platinum compound was further shown to improve disease-free outcomes for ovarian cancer patients, and this combination (most commonly carboplatin and paclitaxel), given intravenously, has now become standard therapy for the first-line treatment of women with advanced epithelial ovarian cancer.

---

### CURRENT DIAGNOSIS

- Most ovarian tumors are epithelial in origin, and the most common histologic subtype is papillary serous.
- Inherited mutations, such as *BRCA1* and *BRCA2*, cause 5% to 10% of ovarian cancers.
- There are no effective screening tests at this time.
- Symptoms of ovarian cancer are nonspecific.
- Physical examination should include palpation of the abdomen for masses or fluid wave, rectovaginal examination for detection of cul-de-sac lesions, and lung auscultation for pleural effusion.
- Ovarian cancer is associated with elevated serum levels of CA-125 and can appear as a complex mass (with solid and cystic features) on imaging.

---

### CURRENT THERAPY

- Women with a family history of breast or ovarian cancer should be referred to a gynecologic oncologist.
- Refer any woman with suspected ovarian cancer (by physical examination, imaging, or CA-125 criteria) to a gynecologic oncologist.
- The standard of care is adequate surgical staging, optimal cytoreductive surgery, and adjuvant chemotherapy with combination intravenous carboplatin and paclitaxel.
- Cooperative oncology group trials suggest that intraperitoneal chemotherapy is an alternative and promising primary treatment modality.
- Treatment of recurrent disease is based on sensitivity to platinum agents, toxicity, and quality-of-life considerations.

For women with stage III or IV disease, response rates approach 90%, with 75% achieving a clinical complete response.

Recent studies examining the role of intraperitoneal (IP) chemotherapy in the treatment of primary ovarian carcinoma suggest that this treatment modality might become the standard of care in the 21st century, because it may be a more effective strategy to treat a cancer that primarily remains confined to the peritoneal cavity throughout its natural course. IP therapy has several advantages for the treatment of ovarian cancer. Placing chemotherapy drugs in the peritoneal cavity takes advantage of the diffusion characteristics of some agents. This technique of dose intensification can allow a several-fold increase in drug concentration in the abdominal cavity compared with systemic IV administration. Depending on the particular drug, the chemotherapy is more slowly absorbed by capillaries, thereby prolonging time of contact with the actual tumor.

Several phase III trials of cisplatin IP[1] chemotherapy as a first-line therapeutic strategy for optimally debulked stage III cancer have been conducted in the last decade. These trials compared chemotherapy administration through IP with IV routes. The best evidence supporting IP chemotherapy is derived from three large multicenter randomized GOG trials. These trials differ in their design but have consistently shown a survival benefit with IP chemotherapy administration. Although toxicities were more commonly seen in the IP arms (catheter complications and increased short-term toxicities), there was no increase in deaths from toxicity, and quality of life measures were similar between the IV and IP arms 1 year after therapy was complete.

Unfortunately, despite the high initial response to platinum-based chemotherapy (80%-90%), most patients with advanced-stage ovarian cancer experience relapse and eventually die of progressive, chemotherapy-resistant disease. However, after recurrence, many patients can be managed in a chronic disease mode by careful selection of therapies and with close monitoring of drug toxicities. The concept of ovarian cancer as a chronic condition has led to a new paradigm in the management of patients with this disease. Prolonged survival with disease is possible in a subset of ovarian cancer patients, and goals of therapy have now become long-term control of disease while minimizing toxicity and maximizing patient quality of life.

Although platinum and paclitaxel remain the standards for primary therapy for ovarian cancer in the United States, many other compounds possess activity against the disease. Patients with a recurrence after a 1-year disease-free interval are typically referred to as *platinum sensitive* and can be re-treated with one or both of the initial drugs. Commonly used second- or third-line agents in the treatment of platinum-resistant recurrent disease include liposomal doxorubicin, gemcitabine, topotecan, and etoposide.[1]

---

[1]Not FDA approved for this indication.

The occurrence of bowel dysfunction due to intraabdominal tumor also commonly adds a management dilemma in patients with recurrent disease, but dietary management (low-residue diets and liquids) can help avert bowel obstruction in these cases.

Considerable effort has been invested in new treatment strategies for ovarian cancer. Current clinical trials continue to investigate novel cytotoxic agents as well as the role of incorporating biological agents with an emphasis on molecularly targeted therapy into the treatment of ovarian and other cancers. Promising biologicals currently under investigation include antiangiogenesis agents that target the vascular endothelial growth factor receptor and agents that target other growth factor receptors commonly overexpressed in human tumors. Moreover, intense investigation to develop new screening strategies is ongoing.

## REFERENCES

Armstrong DK, Bundy B, Wenzel L, et al; Gynecologic Oncology Group: Intraperitoneal cisplatin and paclitaxel in ovarian cancer. N Engl J Med 2006;354:34-43.

Bristow RE, Tomacruz RS, Armstrong DK, et al: Survival effect of maximal cytoreductive surgery for advanced ovarian carcinoma during the platinum era: A meta-analysis. J Clin Oncol 2002;20:1248-1259.

Colombo N, Guthrie D, Chiari S, et al: International Collaborative Ovarian Neoplasm trial: A randomized trial of adjuvant chemotherapy in women with early-stage ovarian cancer. J Natl Cancer Inst 2003;95:125-132.

Earle CC, Bodurka D, Bristow RE, et al: Effect of surgeon specialty on processes of care and outcomes for ovarian cancer patients. J Natl Cancer Inst 2006;98(3):172-180.

Goff BA, Mandel LS, Melancon CH, Muntz HG: Frequency of symptoms of ovarian cancer in women presenting to primary care clinics. JAMA 2004;291(22):2705-2712.

Hacker NF, Berek JS, Lagasse LD, et al: Primary cytoreductive surgery for epithelial ovarian cancer. Obstet Gynecol 1983;61:413-420.

International Collaborative Ovarian Neoplasm Group: Paclitaxel plus carboplatin versus standard chemotherapy with either single-agent carboplatin or cyclophosphamide, doxorubicin, and cisplatin in women with ovarian cancer: The ICON3 randomised trial. Lancet 2002;360:505-515.

Jemal A, Siegel R, Ward E, et al: Cancer statistics, 2006. CA Cancer J Clin 2006;56:106-130.

McGuire WP, Hoskins WJ, Brady MF, et al: Cyclophosphamide and cisplatin versus paclitaxel and cisplatin: A phase III randomized trial in patients with suboptimal stage III/IV ovarian cancer. N Engl J Med 1996;334:1-6.

Ozols RF, Bundy BN, Greer BE, et al; Gynecologic Oncology Group: Phase III trial of carboplatin and paclitaxel compared with cisplatin and paclitaxel in patients with optimally resected stage III ovarian cancer: A Gynecologic Oncology Group study. J Clin Oncol 2003;21:3194-3200.

Paulsen T, Kjaerheim K, Kaern J, et al: Improved short-term survival for advanced ovarian, tubal, and peritoneal cancer patients operated at teaching hospitals. Int J Gynecol Cancer 2006;16 suppl 1:11-17.

Pecorelli S, Benedet JL, Boyle P, et al: FIGO Annual Report on the Results of Treatment in Gynecological Cancer, vol 24. J Epidemiol Biostat 2001;6:1-184.

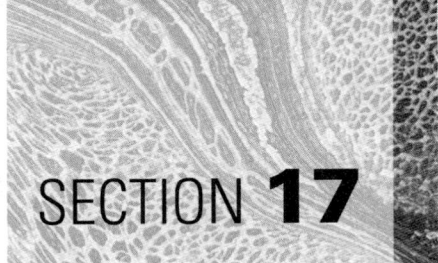

# Psychiatric Disorders

## Alcoholism

Method of
*Richard N. Rosenthal, MD*

## Epidemiology

Alcohol-use disorders are among the most prevalent mental disorders in the population, occurring at frequencies that rival those of mood and anxiety disorders. In any year, almost 8½% of the U.S. population older than 18 years meets criteria for a formal alcohol use disorder (alcohol abuse or dependence), and almost 4% meets criteria for alcohol dependence.

## Economic and Medical Sequelae

Alcohol use disorders are important to identify and treat for several reasons. The first is the direct negative impact of chronic heavy alcohol exposure on cognitive, physical, social, and vocational functioning. The second is the well-described long-term medical sequelae of alcohol dependence such as hepatic cirrhosis, pancreatitis, and dementia. Chronic heavy drinking, even in the absence of a formal diagnosis of alcohol dependence, is associated with an increased risk of diabetes mellitus, hypertension, gastrointestinal bleeding, hemorrhagic stroke, and several forms of carcinoma. The third reason for identification and treatment is the public impact of alcohol use disorders, which covers associated traumatic injuries from motor vehicle and job-related accidents, alcohol-related crime, and their associated economic costs. More than $180 billion is lost to the U.S. economy each year due to alcohol-related crime, injury, health care costs, and lost productivity in the workplace.

## Screening

### SCREENING RATIONALE

Screening for alcohol problems arrays patients on a continuum from abstinence to dependence and is a highly efficient way to identify patients who are at acute risk for the effects of alcohol abuse and dependence as well as those who do not currently meet formal alcohol-related diagnoses but who are at risk for long-term medical and social consequences of heavy alcohol exposure (Box 1). The U.S. Preventative Services Task Force (USPSTF) found that screening could accurately identify patients whose levels or patterns of alcohol consumption do not meet criteria for alcohol dependence but that place them at risk for increased morbidity and mortality. The USPSTF also found good evidence that brief interventions that consist of behavioral counseling and follow-up can reduce alcohol consumption for 6 to 12 months or longer and that the benefits outweigh any potential harms. Thus, it is recommended that alcohol screening and brief interventions be performed in primary care settings to reduce alcohol problems for adults, including pregnant women.

### BRIEF SCREENING

Every patient should be asked about alcohol use. Because drinking is normative in the United States, if drinking is denied, it is useful to determine if the patient used to drink but has stopped because of a past problem. After determining if a patient currently uses any alcohol, the simplest strategy is to ask about the number of heavy drinking days in the past year, where heavy drinking is defined as more than four drinks for men and more than three drinks for women in one day. If that threshold is reached, which corresponds to at-risk or hazardous drinking, then further evaluation of alcohol-related problems is indicated through the use of screening instruments. A standard drink is the same amount of alcohol contained in different volumes of alcoholic beverages (Box 2).

---

**BOX 1    Current Risk Terms**

**Abstinence**
- No alcohol use

**Moderate Drinking**
- Men: No more than 2 standard drinks per drinking d
- Women: No more than 1 standard drink per drinking d
- Elderly persons (>65 y): No more than 1 standard drink per drinking d

**Risky or Hazardous Drinking**
- Men
  - More than 4 standard drinks per drinking d
  - More than 14 standard drinks per wk
- Women
  - More than 3 standard drinks per drinking d
  - More than 7 standard drinks per wk
- Elderly persons (>65 y):
  - More than 3 standard drinks per drinking d
  - More than 7 standard drinks per wk

## BOX 2  Standard Drinks

Each equivalent drink contains about 14 g of pure alcohol:
- 12 oz of beer or wine cooler
- 8-9 oz of malt liquor
- 5 oz of wine
- 3 to 4 oz of fortified wine (e.g., port)
- 1½ oz of 80-proof distilled spirits (or 1 jigger of liquor before mixing)

The Alcohol Use Disorders Identification test (AUDIT) (Table 1) is a 10-item screen developed by the World Health Organization. Given its length, the AUDIT can be used as a self-report screener that patients can fill out in the waiting area before seeing the clinician. The minimum score is 0 and the maximum score is 40. A score of 8 or more for men or 4 or more for women, adolescents, and persons older than 65 years, like a positive endorsement of any heavy drinking days, indicates the need for further evaluation of alcohol use and an increased risk of an alcohol use disorder. For brevity, the AUDIT-C, a truncated version of the AUDIT consisting of the first three AUDIT questions focused on alcohol consumption, can be used as a part of a waiting-room health history form. A score of 6 or more for men or 4 or more for women on the AUDIT-C indicates a need for further evaluation.

Asking about alcohol consumption during a routine clinical interview is best bundled with other questions about lifestyle and health, such as diet, smoking, and exercise. In addition to giving the patient a pre-examination questionnaire to fill out such as the AUDIT, another screening strategy is to ask the CAGE questions (Box 3) during the clinical examination. A positive answer to any of these questions also indicates the need for further evaluation of alcohol use. Two or more CAGE questions answered affirmatively identifies a patient at high risk for alcohol dependence. Because the CAGE screens for consequences, it is not as sensitive for risky drinking.

There are other question sets that are more sensitive than the CAGE in specific demographic subsets, and these can also be easily asked during a routine history. The five-item TWEAK questionnaire (Table 2) may be a more optimal screening questionnaire for identifying women (including pregnant women) with risky drinking or alcohol-use disorders in racially mixed populations. The CRAFFT (Box 4) is a 6-item question set that has high sensitivity in screening adolescents for alcohol and other substance-abuse problems. For patients older than 65 years, the Short Michigan Alcoholism Screening Test—Geriatric (S-MAST-G) (Box 5) is useful in identifying those at risk for alcohol problems, because these patients might not need the same volumes of alcohol intake as others to develop alcohol-related problems. To complete the initial screening, one should compute the average number of drinks per week by multiplying the days per week on average that the patient drinks by the number of drinks consumed on a typical drinking day.

Laboratory testing for elevations of alanine aminotransferase (ALT), aspartate aminotransferase (AST), γ-glutamyltransferase (GGT), or carbohydrate-deficient transferrin (CDT) have no incremental sensitivity over those of validated screening instruments, and they may be better suited to monitoring patients already in treatment for alcohol-use disorders. The patient must still be asked about quantity and frequency of alcohol use. However, laboratory testing can provide indicators of covert heavy drinking (e.g., elevated GGT and CDT) when the patient does not reveal the extent of alcohol intake. CDT, which is perturbed less than other indices by nonalcoholic liver disease, may be a more specific and sensitive indicator of heavy drinking.

## TABLE 1  Alcohol Use Disorders Identification Test (AUDIT)

| Questions | Scoring | | | | |
|---|---|---|---|---|---|
| | 0 | 1 | 2 | 3 | 4 |
| **Consumption (AUDIT-C)** | | | | | |
| How often do you have a drink containing alcohol? | Never | Monthly or less | 2 to 4 times a mo | 2 to 3 times a wk | 4 or more times a wk |
| How many drinks containing alcohol do you have on a typical day when you are drinking? | 1 or 2 | 3 or 4 | 5 or 6 | 7 to 9 | 10 or more |
| How often do you have five or more drinks on one occasion? | Never | Less than monthly | Monthly | Weekly | Daily or almost daily |
| **Personal Consequences** | | | | | |
| How often during the last year have you found that you were not able to stop drinking once you had started? | Never | Less than monthly | Monthly | Weekly | Daily or almost daily |
| How often during the last year have you failed to do what was normally expected of you because of drinking? | Never | Less than monthly | Monthly | Weekly | Daily or almost daily |
| How often during the last year have you needed a first drink in the morning to get yourself going after a heavy drinking session? | Never | Less than monthly | Monthly | Weekly | Daily or almost daily |
| How often during the last year have you had a feeling of guilt or remorse after drinking? | Never | Less than monthly | Monthly | Weekly | Daily or almost daily |
| How often during the last year have you been unable to remember what happened the night before because of your drinking? | Never | Less than monthly | Monthly | Weekly | Daily or almost daily |
| **Social Consequences** | | | | | |
| Have you or someone else been injured because of your drinking? | No | | Yes, but not in the last y | | Yes, during the last y |
| Has a relative, friend, doctor, or other health care worker been concerned about your drinking or suggested you cut down? | No | | Yes, but not in the last y | | Yes, during the last y |

**Scoring and Interpretation**
Add all scores to obtain a total: >8 points for men or >4 points for women indicates a high risk of alcohol use disorder.
AUDIT-C (first three AUDIT questions): >6 points for men or >4 points for women indicates a need for further evaluation.

## Diagnosis

Screening can identify those who are at risk for the sequelae of risky or hazardous drinking and who might benefit from a brief intervention conducted in the primary care office, but only a diagnostic evaluation can confirm the clinician's suspicion that the patient's use of alcohol meets syndromal criteria and warrants specific medical and psychosocial treatment beyond the brief intervention. If, during the last 12 months, alcohol has contributed to repeated episodes of failure to fulfill obligations at home, school or work, episodes of increased risk of physical harm, arrests or other legal problems, or recurrent problems with significant others, then the patient has a diagnosis of alcohol abuse, according to *Diagnostic and Statistical Manual of Mental Disorders*, fourth edition (text revision) (DSM-IV TR) criteria (Table 3). The patient has a diagnosis of alcohol dependence if he or she has three or more of the following criteria over a 12-month period: physical tolerance, symptoms of withdrawal, repeatedly drinking more than intended, unsuccessful reduction or quit attempts, increased time drinking or recovering from drinking, reduced time in other pleasurable or important activities, and continued drinking despite physical or psychological problems.

Rates of co-occurring mood and anxiety disorders are especially high among those with alcohol-use disorders. Untreated mood and anxiety disorders tend to have a negative impact on alcoholism recovery. Among treatment-seeking patients in the National Epidemiologic Survey on Alcohol and Related Conditions (NESARC) sample with a current alcohol use disorder, 40% had at least one current independent mood disorder, and more than one third had at least one current independent anxiety disorder. Heavy alcohol intake can also induce symptoms of mood and other mental disorders. To differentiate alcohol-induced symptoms from independent disorders, it is optimal to reassess symptoms of a mental disorder several weeks after cessation or significant reduction of alcohol intake.

## Brief Intervention

### INTENTION

Although risky or hazardous drinking is not a formal diagnosis, it describes a group with a higher likelihood to develop alcohol problems with risk for accidents, injuries, and social and health problems compared with the general population (see Box 1). Thus, even without a formal diagnosis, it is beneficial to help the patient with risky drinking to change his or her drinking behavior. Several well-described short interchanges between the clinician and the patient, organized under the rubric of *brief interventions*, have been validated in randomized trials as decreasing alcohol intake in those who drink too much but do not have a diagnosis of alcohol dependence. Brief intervention has been demonstrated to reduce weekly alcohol use, frequency of binging, liver enzymes associated with heavy drinking, blood pressure, emergency department visits, hospital days, and psychosocial problems, typically for 6 to 12 months, and to reduce drinking and hospital days at up to 4 years in one study. Because most at-risk patients seen in primary care settings are subsyndromal for alcohol-use disorders, the typical clinical interaction related to alcohol will be that of screening and then a brief intervention for positive cases. The two are typically referred to together under the acronym SBI (screening and brief intervention).

The basic intention of a brief intervention is to educate the patient about the risks of heavy alcohol use in such a way as to motivate him or her to reduce weekly alcohol consumption. The standard initial brief intervention takes about 15 minutes and consists of feedback, advice, and goal setting. It can be performed wholly in the primary care setting by the physician or other members of the health delivery team. Including alcohol screening, the USPSTF suggests five As to conducting SBI: *assess* the patient's alcohol consumption with a screening tool and clinical evaluation as indicated; *advise* reduction of alcohol consumption to appropriate levels, including abstinence if indicated; *agree* on individual goals for reducing alcohol use, including abstinence if indicated; *assist* patients in obtaining the motivation, skills, or supports needed to institute changes in drinking; and *arrange* for follow-up support, including specialty treatment referral for dependent patients. The most effective interventions are multicontact ones that provide ongoing assistance and follow-up.

### PROCEDURE

#### Assess

Screen patients with the AUDIT or with the CAGE, TWEAK, CRAFFT, or S-MAST-G questionnaires as appropriate, and compute average drinks per week.

#### Advise

Give feedback in the form of expression of concern, direct conclusions, and recommendations. Present medical findings, such as elevated liver enzymes, to back up conclusive statements such as "I'm concerned that your alcohol intake exceeds safe limits." Show the patient information comparing use with population norms and the associated health risks. Educate the patient about how alcohol can lead to medical, psychosocial, and legal consequences. Where possible, link the patient's current symptoms to alcohol use. Recommend appropriate and specific changes in behavior, such as "I strongly recommend you cut down your drinking," or in the case where any drinking places the patient at high risk, "I strongly suggest you quit drinking."

#### Agree

Determine the patient's readiness to change drinking behavior, such as asking, "Do you think that cutting down on your drinking is

**TABLE 2  TWEAK Questionnaire**

| Feature | Question | Answer | Score |
|---|---|---|---|
| **T**olerance | How many drinks does it take before you begin to feel the first effects of alcohol? | ≥3 | 2 |
| **W**orry | Have your friends or relatives worried or complained about your drinking in the past year? | Yes | 2 |
| **E**ye-opener | Do you sometimes take a drink in the morning when you first get up? | Yes | 1 |
| **A**mnesia | Are there times when you drink and afterward you can't remember what you said or did? | Yes | 1 |
| **K**ut | Do you sometimes feel the need to cut down on your drinking? | Yes | 1 |

Scoring and interpretation: Two or more points indicate a possible alcohol problem.

## CURRENT DIAGNOSIS

### Risky or Hazardous Drinking (Need Further Evaluation)

- Men who drink more than four standard drinks per day or 14 standard drinks per week
- Women and those older than 65 years who drink more than three standard drinks per day or more than seven standard drinks per week
- Drinking concurrent with any medical condition where alcohol is contraindicated

### Alcohol Abuse

- Repeated failure to fulfill obligations at home, school or work
- Increased risk of physical harm
- Legal problems or interpersonal problems in any year.

### Alcohol Dependence (Three or More in Any Year)

- Cannot cut down or stop
- Decreased time spent in other usual activities
- Drinking despite physical or psychological consequences
- Drinking more than intended
- Physical tolerance
- Preoccupied with drinking
- Withdrawal episodes

---

something you are willing to talk about?" If the patient is ambivalent, avoid labeling the patient's behavior with a diagnosis at this stage, which can increase resistance to change, but encourage the patient to reflect on the positive reasons for drinking and the negative consequences of drinking. Offer concerns that continued drinking at the same level will impede the patient's achievement of goals such as decreased gastric distress or improved sleep patterns.

Empathic listening is generally more effective than a confrontational approach, and it is useful to express optimism about the patient's capacity to change. Elicit what the patient's concerns are about cutting down or quitting. Avoid arguing or challenging when the patient is unready to change, but schedule a follow-up visit to continue the dialogue and reassess drinking behavior. Restate your commitment to help when the patient is ready and that you remain open to questions.

When the patient concurs that a change in drinking would be beneficial, agree on a specific goal to cut down to particular daily and weekly limits for low-risk drinking or to stop drinking, if indicated, for a specific period of time. The agreement should be recorded and a

---

### BOX 4 CRAFFT Questionnaire

- Have you ever ridden in a **C**ar driven by someone (including yourself) who was high or had been using alcohol or drugs?
- Do you ever use alcohol or drugs to **R**elax, feel better about yourself, or fit in?
- Do you ever use alcohol or drugs while you are **A**lone?
- Do you ever **F**orget things you did while using alcohol or drugs?
- Do your **F**amily or **F**riends ever tell you that you should cut down on your drinking or drug use?
- Have you ever gotten into **T**rouble while you were using alcohol or drugs?

One yes response indicates need for further assessment. Two yes responses indicate risk of alcohol-use disorder.

---

### BOX 5 S-MAST-G Questionnaire

- When talking with others, do you ever underestimate how much you actually drink?
- After a few drinks, have you sometimes not eaten or been able to skip meals because you didn't feel hungry?
- Does having a few drinks help decrease your shakiness or tremors?
- Does alcohol sometimes make it hard for you to remember parts of the day or night?
- Do you usually take a drink to relax or calm your nerves?
- Do you drink to take your mind off your problems?
- Have you ever increased your drinking after experiencing a loss in your life?
- Has a doctor or nurse ever said that they were worried or concerned about your drinking?
- Have you ever made rules to manage your drinking?
- When you feel lonely, does having a drink help?

Two or more yes responses indicate a probable alcohol problem

---

*Abbreviation:* S-MAST-G = Short Michigan Alcoholism Screening Test—Geriatric.

---

copy given to the patient both as a reminder and motivator for behavioral change.

### Assist

Work with the patient to formulate concrete steps to implement the drinking reduction plan. These steps include how to avoid high-risk drinking situations, how to keep a record of alcohol intake, and who can support the patient in meeting his or her goals. Provide resources in the form of patient educational materials, examples of which can be downloaded from the National Institute of Alcohol Abuse and Alcoholism (NIAAA) Web site (www.niaaa.nih.gov).

### Arrange

Set up follow-up support and counseling visits or refer patients meeting dependence criteria for specialty treatment. Advise the patient to seek immediate medical treatment if withdrawal symptoms occur.

## Treatment

### DETOXIFICATION

Put simply, detoxification is medical stabilization that offers an opportunity to engage patients in alcoholism treatment, but it is not in itself treatment for alcohol dependence. Patients who drink more than 250 grams of alcohol daily are likely to experience physiologic withdrawal symptoms on cessation of drinking, but volume is not the only predictor of withdrawal severity. Although often mild, untreated alcohol withdrawal can result in seizures or delirium tremens (DTs), with increased risk of mortality.

### Assessment

The Clinical Institute Withdrawal Assessment—Alcohol Revised (CIWA-Ar) is a public domain scale that scores 10 signs and symptoms of withdrawal by severity ranging from not present to severe (Box 6). A score of less than 8 indicates mild withdrawal, characterized by increased autonomic activity with low-grade anxiety, diaphoresis, agitation, nausea, and elevated blood pressure, temperature, and heart rate. Scores of 8 to 15 indicate moderate withdrawal, and scores of

## TABLE 3 Diagnosis of Alcohol-Use Problems

| Criteria | Typical Symptoms and History |
|---|---|
| **Alcohol Abuse (≥1 in the last 12 mo)** | |
| ***Alcohol has caused or contributed to repeated:*** | |
| Failure to fulfill obligations at home, school, or work | Hangovers at work, truancy at school, missing appointments |
| Episodes of increased risk of physical harm | Drinking and driving, swimming, or operating machinery |
| Arrests or other legal problems | Public intoxication, DUI or DWI |
| Problems with significant others | Spousal strife, physical fights |
| **Alcohol Dependence (≥3 in the last 12 mo)** | |
| Development of physical tolerance | Drinks more for the same effect |
| Episodes of withdrawal syndrome (see below) | Morning shakes, nausea, anxiety |
| Drinking more than intended repeatedly | Binging episodes |
| Unsuccessful efforts to cut down or stop drinking | Failed New Year's resolution |
| Increased time planning for drinking, drinking, or recovering from drinking | Instead of being with kids, spends weekend mornings sleeping in |
| Reduced time in other pleasurable or important activities | Stopped socializing with friends, withdrew from hobby group |
| Drinking persists despite physical or psychological problems | Developed depressed mood, but kept on drinking |
| **Alcohol Withdrawal (≥2 within h to d after lowered blood alcohol levels)** | |
| Autonomic hyperactivity | Heart rate >100 bpm, diaphoresis |
| Hand tremor | Hands shake when extended |
| Insomnia | Difficulty falling asleep |
| Nausea or vomiting | Feels queasy |
| Anxiety | Spontaneous report of fear |
| Psychomotor agitation | Inability to keep still, pacing |
| Hallucinations or illusions | Reports visual disturbances |
| Seizures | Tonic-clonic movements |

15 or more indicate more severe withdrawal states. In severe withdrawal, in the context of autonomic hyperarousal, the patient can become disoriented and have a clouded sensorium, the hallmarks of delirium.

Prior history of severe withdrawal, such as DTs, is a reasonable predictor of similar future responses to alcohol withdrawal. Risk for withdrawal delirium is increased if the patient has a heart rate of greater than 120 bpm before treatment, a current infectious disease,

withdrawal symptoms in the context of a blood alcohol concentration greater than 100 mg/dL, a prior history of either delirium or seizures, or a high CIWA-Ar score, indicating severe autonomic hyperactivity. Patients who have severe withdrawal symptoms, who are at high risk for seizures, or who have a medical condition likely to be exacerbated by withdrawal, such as type 1 diabetes or coronary artery disease, should have medically supervised inpatient detoxification.

## CURRENT THERAPY

### All At-Risk Patients

- Assess: Screen patients with standard instruments and compute average standard drinks per week.
- Advise: Give feedback, express concern, present findings and conclusions, and recommend specific behavioral changes.
- Agree: Determine the patient's readiness to change, encourage reflection, listen empathically, elicit patient concerns, avoid arguing, express optimism, set a specific reduction or abstinence goal.
- Assist: Formulate concrete implementation plan, including avoiding high-risk situations, recording alcohol intake, and eliciting family and community support for patient goals.
- Arrange: Set up follow-up visits and refer patients meeting dependence criteria for specialty treatment.

### Additionally for Alcohol-Dependent Patients

- Offer or arrange for detoxification if indicated.
- Offer or arrange for specialty alcoholism treatment and/or mutual help groups.
- Offer pharmacotherapy to support maintenance of abstinence: naltrexone, acamprosate, or disulfiram.
- Offer medication management support during follow-up visits.

### Pharmacologic Therapy

Alcohol withdrawal is best treated with sedative hypnotic medications that are cross-tolerant with alcohol, such as benzodiazepines. Longer-acting benzodiazepines such as diazepam (Valium) and chlordiazepoxide (Librium) are easier to titrate against withdrawal symptoms and give a gradual offset in plasma concentration, but shorter-acting benzodiazepines such as lorazepam (Ativan)[1] are less likely to oversedate the patient. Rapid-onset benzodiazepines have a higher abuse liability and are generally best avoided. However, patients with severe hepatic impairment (elevated total bilirubin) are best treated with benzodiazepines that are not oxidized by the liver, such as oxazepam (Serax) or lorazepam.

Typical dosing is chlordiazepoxide 50 to 100 mg, diazepam 10 to 20 mg, oxazepam 20 to 40[3] mg, or lorazepam[1] 2 to 4 mg. The typical front-loading style of dosing is to administer medication at the higher end of the dose range every 1 to 2 hours so that the CIWA-Ar score is less than 8 for 24 hours.

With long-acting medications, once symptoms subside, there is often no need to taper doses. The short-acting benzodiazepines and long-acting benzodiazepines given to patients at high-risk for seizures or DTs are best given on a fixed-dose regimen of four times daily for the first 24 hours, with the patient reassessed 1 to 2 hours after each dose, and additional medication given as needed. On days 2 and 3, 50% of the dose can be given four times daily.

Long-acting barbiturates, such as phenobarbital,[1] can be also used on a fixed-dose regimen of 60 mg every 4 to 6 hours, with a loading dose of 120 mg orally or intramuscularly every hour for acute

---

[1] Not FDA approved for this indication.
[3] Exceeds dosage recommended by the manufacturer.

## BOX 6   Clinical Institute Withdrawal Assessment of Alcohol Scale, Revised (CIWA-Ar)

Patient:_____ Date: _____ Time: _____ (24 hour clock, midnight = 00:00)

Pulse or heart rate, taken for one minute:_____ Blood pressure:_____ mm Hg

**Nausea and Vomiting** — Ask "Do you feel sick to your stomach? Have you vomited?" Observation:

0  no nausea and no vomiting
1  mild nausea with no vomiting
2
3
4  intermittent nausea with dry heaves
5
6
7  constant nausea, frequent dry heaves, and vomiting

**Tremor** — Arms extended and fingers spread apart. Observation:

0  no tremor
1  not visible, but can be felt fingertip to fingertip
2
3
4  moderate, with patient's arms extended
5
6
7  severe, even with arms not extended

**Paroxysmal Sweats** — Observation:

0  no sweat visible
1  barely perceptible sweating, palms moist
2
3
4  beads of sweat obvious on forehead
5
6
7  drenching sweats

**Anxiety** — Ask "Do you feel nervous?" Observation:
0  no anxiety, at ease
1  mild anxious
2
3
4  moderately anxious, or guarded, so anxiety is inferred
5
6
7  equivalent to acute panic states as seen in severe delirium or acute schizophrenic reactions

**Tactile Disturbances** — Ask "Have you any itching, pins and needles sensations, any burning, any numbness, or do you feel bugs crawling on or under your skin?" Observation:

0  none
1  very mild itching, pins and needles, burning, or numbness
2  mild itching, pins and needles, burning, or numbness
3  moderate itching, pins and needles, burning, or numbness
4  moderately severe hallucinations
5  severe hallucinations
6  extremely severe hallucinations
7  continuous hallucinations

**Auditory Disturbances** — Ask "Are you more aware of sounds around you? Are they harsh? Do they frighten you? Are you hearing anything that is disturbing to you? Are you hearing things you know are not there?" Observation:

0  not present
1  very mild harshness or ability to frighten
2  mild harshness or ability to frighten
3  moderate harshness or ability to frighten
4  moderately severe hallucinations
5  severe hallucinations
6  extremely severe hallucinations
7  continuous hallucinations

**Visual Disturbances** — Ask "Does the light appear to be too bright? Is its color different? Does it hurt your eyes? Are you seeing anything that is disturbing to you? Are you seeing things you know are not there?" Observation:

0  not present
1  very mild sensitivity
2  mild sensitivity
3  moderate sensitivity
4  moderately severe hallucinations
5  severe hallucinations
6  extremely severe hallucinations
7  continuous hallucinations

**Headache, Fullness in Head** — Ask "Does your head feel different? Does it feel like there is a band around your head?" Do not rate for dizziness or lightheadedness. Otherwise, rate severity:

0  not present
1  very mild
2  mild
3  moderate
4  moderately severe
5  severe
6  very severe
7  extremely severe

## BOX 6  Clinical Institute Withdrawal Assessment of Alcohol Scale, Revised (CIWA-Ar)—cont'd

**Agitation** — Observation:

0  normal activity
1  somewhat more than normal activity
2
3
4  moderately fidgety and restless
5
6
7  paces back and forth during most of the interview or constantly thrashes about

**Orientation and Clouding of Sensorium** — Ask "What day is this? Where are you? Who am I?"

0  oriented and can do serial additions
1  cannot do serial additions or is uncertain about date
2  disoriented for date by no more than 2 calendar d
3  disoriented for date by more than 2 calendar d
4  disoriented for place or person

Total CIWA-Ar Score _____
Rater's Initials _____
Maximum Possible Score: 67

The CIWA-Ar *is not* copyright and may be reproduced freely. This assessment for monitoring withdrawal symptoms requires approximately 5 minutes to administer.

From Sullivan JT, Sykora K, Schneiderman J, Naranjo CA, Sellers EM: Assessment of alcohol withdrawal: The revised Clinical Institute Withdrawal Assessment for Alcohol scale (CIWA-Ar). Br J Addiction 1989;84:1353-1357.

---

withdrawal symptoms (e.g., pulse >110 bpm) or a CIWA-Ar score of 10 or more.

Anticonvulsants such as carbamazepine (Tegretol),[1] valproate (Depakote),[1] or gabapentin (Neurontin)[1] have also been used effectively in uncomplicated withdrawal, but they are unproved in preventing withdrawal-related seizures and in treating DTs.

Although phenothiazines and haloperidol are somewhat effective compared with benzodiazepines in reducing withdrawal symptoms such as agitation, they are not as protective against seizures or delirium and thus are not recommended.

Thiamine (Vitamin $B_1$) supplementation of 100 mg/day for 3 days can counteract the thiamine deficiencies that are common in alcoholic patients.

## PSYCHOSOCIAL INTERVENTIONS FOR ALCOHOL DEPENDENCE

In addition to brief interventions for risky alcohol use, the most opportune and practical psychosocial intervention that the primary care office can provide is clinical behavioral support for pharmacotherapy for alcohol dependence. Simply put, medication management support consists initially of feedback to the patient of screening and medical evaluation results and the negative health effects of continued heavy drinking, as in a brief intervention. The patient is then given the basis for the diagnosis of alcohol dependence, the rationale for abstinence, and recommendation for pharmacotherapy. The patient is given information about medication and the appropriate prescriptions and is encouraged to seek community support for sobriety in mutual help groups such as Alcoholics Anonymous or to follow a plan such as Rational Recovery. Follow-up visits consist of assessment of medication side effects, patient adherence to the medication regimen, assessment of abstinence or quantity and pattern of alcohol intake, and assessment of overall functioning. Problems with medication adherence are identified and addressed.

There are evidence-based psychosocial interventions that are typically performed in the context of specialty programs for alcohol dependence, but they can be offered by clinical personnel in the context of the physician's office. Cognitive behavior therapy, network therapy, behavioral family therapy, and motivational interviewing are effective approaches for the treatment of alcohol dependence. Motivational interviewing is especially adaptable for use in primary care settings in that it is an approach to interacting with the alcohol-dependent patient that can be learned quickly and executed by any staff with clinical contact. A motivational enhancement manual can be accessed at the NIAAA Web site (http://www.niaaa.nih.gov/)

## MEDICATION MANAGEMENT OF ALCOHOL DEPENDENCE

There are currently four FDA-approved medications for the treatment of alcohol dependence. Any of these medications can and should be given concurrently with other interventions such as psychosocial treatment or mutual help groups.

Disulfiram (Antabuse) works by inhibiting the metabolism of ethyl alcohol, causing a buildup of acetaldehyde, a noxious substance, which causes a strong stereotypic aversive response (flushing, diaphoresis, nausea, tachycardia) in the patient. Standard dosing is 250 mg/day (range, 125-500 mg). The major clinical concern with disulfiram is patient noncompliance with the medication regimen. Thus, it is most likely to be effective when there is a concrete method for supporting compliance in place, such as directly observed therapy by a spouse or in a clinic.

More recently, the opioid antagonist naltrexone (ReVia, Depade) was approved for the treatment of alcohol dependence. It is dosed at 50 mg once daily. Naltrexone reduces days of heavy drinking and can reduce alcohol craving. Naltrexone in a long-acting intramuscular formulation (Vivitrol) allows once-monthly dosing (380 mg) and reduces the risk of noncompliance. It reduces heavy drinking overall and helps maintain abstinence in those who are abstinent at initial drug administration. Both oral and IM naltrexone formulations carry FDA black-box warnings related to findings of reversible elevations of liver enzymes at three to six times the standard dosage; however, naltrexone is safe at the recommended dose.

Acamprosate (Campral) is a taurine analogue that has been demonstrated to reduce relapse to any drinking as well as reducing heavy drinking in nonabstinent patients. It is dosed as two 333-mg tablets three times a day to patients who have ceased alcohol intake. It is excreted unchanged through the kidneys and has no interactions with other medications. Side effects are benign, and the most frequent is loose stools, which are mild to moderate and self-limited.

## REFERENCES

American Psychiatric Association: Diagnostic and Statistical Manual of Mental Disorders, 4th ed, text revision. Washington, DC: American Psychiatric Association, 2000.

---

[1]Not FDA approved for this indication.

Bertholet N, Daeppen J-B, Wietlisbach V, et al: Reduction of alcohol consumption by brief alcohol intervention in primary care systematic review and meta-analysis. Arch Intern Med 2005;165:986-995.

Bradley KA, Boyd-Wickizer J, Powell SH, Burman ML: Alcohol screening questionnaires in women: A critical review. JAMA 1998;280:166-171.

Chang G, Kosten TR: Detoxification. In Lowinson JH, Ruiz P, Millman RB, Langrod JG (eds), Substance Abuse: A Comprehensive Textbook. Philadelphia: Lippincott Williams & Wilkins, 2004, pp 579-587.

Fleming MF, Mundt MP, French MT, et al: Brief physician advice for problem drinkers: Long-term efficacy and cost-benefit analysis. Alcohol Clin Exp Res 2002;26:36-43.

Grant BF, Stinson FS, Dawson DA, et al.: Prevalence and co-occurrence of substance use disorders and independent mood and anxiety disorders: Results from the National Epidemiologic Survey on Alcohol and Related Conditions. Arch Gen Psychiatry 2004;61:807-816.

Knight JR, Sherritt L, Shrier LA, et al: Validity of the CRAFFT substance abuse screening test among adolescent clinic patients. Arch Pediatr Adolesc Med 2002;156(6):607-614.

Maisto SA, Saitz R: Alcohol use disorders: Screening and diagnosis. Am J Addict 2003;12(suppl 1):S12-S25.

McCaul ME, Petry NM: The role of psychosocial treatments in pharmacotherapy for alcoholism. Am J Addict 2003;12(Suppl 1):S41-S52.

National Institute on Alcohol Abuse and Alcoholism: Helping Patients Who Drink Too Much: A Clinician's Guide. Rockville, MD: National Institute on Alcohol Abuse and Alcoholism, 2005. Available at http://pubs.niaaa.nih.gov/publications/Practitioner/CliniciansGuide2005/guide.pdf (accessed June 15, 2007).

Saitz R: Unhealthy alcohol use. N Engl J Med 2005;352:596-607.

Saunders JB, Aasland OG, Babor TF, et al. Development of the Alcohol Use Disorders Screening Test (AUDIT). WHO collaborative project on early detection of persons with harmful alcohol consumption. Addiction 1993;88:791-804.

Sullivan JT, Sykora K., Schneiderman J, et al: Assessment of alcohol withdrawal: The revised Clinical Institute Withdrawal Assessment for Alcohol scale (CIWA-Ar). Br J Addict 1989;84:1353-1357.

U.S. Preventive Services Task Force: Screening and behavioral counseling interventions in primary care to reduce alcohol misuse: Recommendation statement. Ann Intern Med 2004;140:554-556.

# Drug Abuse

Method of
*Joyce A. Tinsley, MD*

The U.S. Department of Health and Human Services reported that in 2001 nearly 7% of the population, or 16 million Americans age 12 and older, were actively using illegal drugs. The combination of drug and alcohol use costs taxpayers a staggering sum; an estimated $143 billion per year is spent on associated health care costs, extra law enforcement, motor vehicle accidents, crime, and lost productivity. The president's fiscal year 2003 budget included $4.4 billion for all substance abuse–related activities, with $127 million earmarked for treatment services. The abuse of legal drugs, such as prescription medications and nicotine, is also a serious problem. Nicotine dependence is responsible for more morbidity and mortality than any other abused substance and is so highly addictive that quitting eludes many who try to stop.

Many addicts in need of treatment do not get it. Reasons for this include a lack of treatment and recovery resources, the stigma surrounding drug use, and pessimism about recovery from addictions. Unfortunately, much of the clinical pessimism about addiction treatment is based on an inadequate or outdated knowledge base. At a minimum, clinicians should be familiar with the common drugs of abuse; signs of intoxication, withdrawal, and overdose; management of simple detoxification; and contemporary treatment options.

## Diagnosis

In the *Diagnostic and Statistical Manual of Mental Disorders, 4th ed., Text Revision (DSM-IV-TR)*, published by the American Psychiatric Association, disorders are classified as either abuse or dependence.

These criteria may be applied to any drug within the major classes of addictive substances. Inherent to the definition of dependence is the concept of impaired control. In other words, the addict cannot predictably control when or how much of a substance he or she will use. In both abuse and dependence, the individual continues to use the substance even though it causes problems in one or more important life areas. The diagnosis is based on behaviors surrounding the drug abuse rather than the amount consumed. Substance dependence, synonymous with addiction, is the more advanced disorder.

It is often challenging to diagnose drug abuse. Patients may be hesitant to reveal illegal drug abuse or the misuse of prescription drugs. Clinicians should ask questions that are perceived to be nonjudgmental. For instance, asking, "Has anyone ever been concerned about your drug use?" is less likely to be met with resistance than initial questions that ask about quantity or frequency of use. Supplemental history from significant others and objective data from urine drug screens can help clarify the diagnosis. Some addicts readily admit their addictions. For instance, heroin users have been known to overestimate their use in order to receive a more generous opiate dose for detoxification or maintenance. Heroin and cocaine addicts with advanced dependence often acknowledge their addictions because of devastating social, legal, or physical consequences. In addition, a majority of cigarette smokers express a desire to stop smoking and attempt to get help.

## Nicotine

Nicotine dependence is similar to other drug addictions in that it is best viewed as a chronic disease that requires ongoing attention. It is the addiction on which primary care clinicians may have the greatest impact. An estimated 25% of adults in the United States smoke cigarettes, and 70% of current smokers would like to quit. In view of the lethal nature of smoking, the high percentage of smokers who want to quit, and the number of individuals affected, the clinician should be prepared to encourage smoking cessation.

The nicotine withdrawal syndrome is a serious obstacle for patients who want to stop smoking. Withdrawal symptoms often begin within hours after the last cigarette, peak within 2 to 3 days, and may continue for several weeks. Nicotine cravings last much longer. Early abstinence is characterized by irritability, anxiety, restlessness, depressed mood, inattention, and insomnia. A nicotine replacement product is effective in ameliorating many of the withdrawal symptoms.

Brief counseling improves smoking cessation rates, especially when directed toward the patient's unique situation. The U.S. Public Health Service recommends easy-to-follow strategies that clinicians can use in counseling patients to quit smoking (Table 1). The "5 As" represent a strategy particularly helpful to the clinician who wants to initiate discussion about a patient's tobacco use. The "5 Rs" may be used if the patient lacks motivation to stop smoking. Finally, an action plan known by the mnemonic STAR is a guide for those ready to make a quit attempt.

There is solid evidence that several medications are effective in improving smokers' quit rates (Table 2). Unless there are contraindications to the use of these medications, a first-line agent, either a nicotine replacement product or bupropion (Zyban), should be recommended to patients who want to stop smoking. If initial agents are ineffective or contraindicated, the clinician should consider recommending a second-line agent, specifically clonidine (Catapres)[1] or nortriptyline (Pamelor).[1] The Public Health Service provides additional information to clinicians who want to learn more about how to help patients stop smoking on their Web site http://www.surgeongeneral.gov/tobacco.

---

[1]Not FDA approved for this indication.

**TABLE 1  Office-Based Interventions for Smoking Cessation**

| Initial Intervention: 5 As | Motivational Intervention: 5 Rs | Action Plan: STAR |
|---|---|---|
| Ask about tobacco use.<br>Advise the patient to quit.<br>Assess readiness to quit.<br>Assist in the quit attempt.<br>Arrange follow-up. | Relevance: Why stop?<br>Risks: Personalize them.<br>Rewards: Potential benefits.<br>Roadblocks: Identify and address barriers.<br>Repetition: Repeat message at the next visit. | Set a quit date.<br>Tell others of plan.<br>Anticipate difficulties.<br>Remove tobacco products. |

Adapted from: U.S. Public Health Service: Treating tobacco use and dependence—clinician's packet. A how-to guide for implementing the Public Health Service clinical practice guideline. March 2003. http://www.surgeongeneral.gov/tobacco/clinpack.html

## Marijuana

Marijuana, or cannabis, is the most commonly used illegal drug in the United States. Despite purported medical uses, it is not a benign substance. Individuals who become addicted often experience impairment in multiple life areas. The active ingredient in marijuana is tetrahydrocannabinol (THC). THC is classified as a hallucinogen, which it can be in large quantities or in highly sensitive individuals. More often intoxication brings relaxation, euphoria, a dreamy state, time-space distortion, and impaired attention. Perceptual disturbances may impair driving. Anxiety and paranoia are also common effects. Like other addictive substances, marijuana abuse can interfere with the assessment and treatment of psychiatric symptoms. No specific medical management is warranted for either cannabis intoxication or withdrawal.

Teenagers are among the most vulnerable users. Common signs of problematic use during adolescence include changes in sleeping and eating habits, declining school performance, changes in the adolescent's peer group, and moodiness. Physical signs include increased appetite, dry mouth, and injected conjunctiva. The University of Michigan's Monitoring the Future survey of U.S. high school students has been tracking teenage substance use for the past 25 years. In 2000, they found that by the age of 18 years, 80% of U.S. youth had used alcohol and 54% had used illicit drugs. Their drug of choice was marijuana. One in five high school seniors and nearly as many tenth graders reported marijuana use during the previous month. Treatment for marijuana abuse and dependence in adolescents or adults consists of psychotherapeutic approaches.

## Cocaine and Other Stimulants

Cocaine is a highly addictive drug that is extracted from the coca leaf. Amphetamine, which is structurally similar to cocaine, is a synthesized product used to suppress hunger, improve energy or alertness, and improve mood. The euphoria that cocaine elicits is probably caused by increased dopamine activity. Physical effects include elevated heart rate and blood pressure, mediated by stimulation of the sympathetic

**TABLE 2  Pharmacotherapy of Smoking Cessation**

| | Instructions | Dose | Advantages | Disadvantages |
|---|---|---|---|---|
| Nicotine gum/over-the-counter (Nicorette) | Chew until peppery taste, then park between cheek and gum. | 2 or 4 mg per piece. Maximum 24 pieces per day. Use for up to 6 mo. | Flexibility with scheduled and/or prn doses to relieve cravings. Delivery is more rapid than the patch. | Incomplete absorption when chewed incorrectly. Cannot eat or drink while using. Caution with dental or jaw problems. |
| Transdermal nicotine patch/over-the-counter (Nicoderm) | Apply to skin daily. Available as 16-h or 24-h patch. Do not smoke while using. | Start 21 mg × 6 wk (14 mg if weight <100 lb or smoking <1/2 ppd). Taper to 14 mg, then 7 mg × 2-4 wk. Use for 2-3 mo total. | Easy to use. Few side effects. Releases steady dose of nicotine to reduce cravings. Can use in combination with gum. | Releases nicotine more slowly. No response for sudden cravings. Can cause skin irritation. Consider lower dosing in known cardiac disease. |
| Nasal spray/prescription (Nicotrol NS) | Use every 1-2 h. Take deep breath, spray into each nostril, and exhale through mouth. | From 8 to 40 times per day. Use for 3 mo with gradual taper. | Fastest delivery of nicotine. Good at reducing sudden cravings. | Nose and sinus irritation common at first. Caution with allergies or asthma. |
| Nasal inhaler/prescription (Nicotrol Inhaler) | Inhale nicotine by bringing inhaler to mouth when desired. | From 6 to 16 cartridges per day for first 3-6 wk. Use for 3 mo with gradual taper. | Delivers nicotine as quickly as gum. Satisfies hand-to-mouth habit. Few side effects. | May cause mouth or throat irritation. Caution with asthma or chronic lung disease. |
| Bupropion HCl/prescription (Zyban) | Take 1 pill in the morning, 1 in late afternoon. Start 2 wk before quit date. | 150 mg SR bid. Continue for 7 to 12 weeks after quitting. | Easy to use, few side effects. May be more helpful when used with the patch. | Contraindicated in seizure, eating disorders, patients taking Wellbutrin or MAOIs, pregnancy, or breast-feeding. |

*Abbreviations*: bid = twice daily; MAOIs = monoamine oxidase inhibitors; ppd = packs per day; prn = as needed; SR = slow release.
Adapted from: American Cancer Society: Set yourself free; deciding how to quit, a smoker's guide. 1999.

nervous system. All stimulants possess these qualities, though in varying degrees and with variable risks. In overdose, these effects are intensified so that myocardial infarction, arrhythmia, stroke, and psychosis may occur. In those situations, therapeutic measures are supportive and aimed at reversing specific ill effects.

Physiologic withdrawal is not a major problem, and no medical management is indicated. However withdrawal from cocaine produces symptoms known as a *crash*. A crash may begin within hours of the last use and intensify over the next several days. During this time the addict feels extreme fatigue. Depression can be severe and carries a risk of suicidal ideation and behavior. Relapse is common during withdrawal because return to use provides quick and reliable relief.

The person who abuses cocaine may use it by snorting, injecting, or smoking. The rate at which the drug reaches the brain correlates with its addictive potential. Therefore, users with more advanced addictions commonly report a progression from snorting to intravenous use or the most rapid form of administration, smoking crack cocaine. Intravenous users are at risk for contracting hepatitis and HIV, as well as developing phlebitis and endocarditis. Treatment relies on psychotherapeutic approaches such as self-help, contingency management, and cognitive-behavioral therapy. Despite multiple medication trials, no drug effectively treats cocaine dependence.

## Opiates

Among the opiates, heroin may be the most widely recognized drug of abuse. In 2000, there were an estimated 1,000,000 heroin addicts. There is concern that this number will increase because heroin has become less expensive in some parts of the country. All opiates have some abuse potential depending upon a specific drug's potency and its route of administration. Not only are illicit opiates abused, but the abuse of opiate analgesics such as methadone, hydromorphone (Dilaudid), oxycodone (OxyContin), and fentanyl (Duragesic) is also common.

Signs of intoxication include sedation, mild euphoria, pinpoint pupils, bradycardia, and low blood pressure. Overdose on drugs within the opiate class produces a reduced level of consciousness that may progress to coma and respiratory depression. When overdose is suspected, naloxone (Narcan), a synthetic opioid antagonist, can be administered to reverse the opiate's effects; the initial dose of 0.4 mg intravenously (IV) (0.01 mg/kg) can be repeated every 2 to 3 minutes as clinically indicated. Naloxone may be administered intramuscularly or subcutaneously if necessary. If the patient does not respond to a dose of 5 to 10 mg, opiate overdose is doubtful.

There is a well-defined withdrawal syndrome that occurs when an opiate is discontinued in one who is physiologically dependent (Table 3). Symptoms of withdrawal from a short-acting drug such as heroin begin within a few hours; withdrawal symptoms from a long-acting opiate such as methadone begin within 3 to 4 days. Opiate withdrawal is not a medical emergency in otherwise healthy adults. However, it is uncomfortable and may be a strong trigger for continued drug use.

There are several ways to address opiate withdrawal. In the context of a prescription medication being stopped too abruptly, the simplest approach is to restart the medication and reduce it more slowly. Planned detoxification is often accomplished by substituting methadone (Dolophine), a long-acting opioid agonist, for the shorter-acting opiate. With this method, the patient is stabilized on a methadone dose that blocks significant withdrawal. A dose of 40 mg given in divided doses during the day is adequate to block significant withdrawal symptoms in most patients. The stabilizing dose is tapered over several days. Clonidine (Catapres)[1] is a nonopiate that can be used to treat opiate withdrawal. It is a centrally acting $a_2$-agonist that reduces autonomic symptoms such as vomiting, diarrhea, and sweating (Table 4).

Methadone maintenance is the mainstay treatment for dependence on illicit opiates. The Food and Drug Administration (FDA) approved methadone for opioid maintenance therapy in 1972. Federal regulations placed tight restrictions on methadone programs that include special state and federal licensing. These restrictions have had an unintended effect of limiting treatment access for some opiate-addicted patients. Methadone maintenance treatment is criticized for a number of reasons:

- There is a risk that dispensed methadone will be sold on the street.
- Daily administration is inconvenient for patients.
- Some facilities offer inadequate adjunctive psychosocial or therapy services.

Despite concerns, methadone maintenance is effective in reducing criminal activity among heroin addicts, in decreasing the risk of HIV and hepatitis acquired through needle-sharing, and in returning some addicts to functional lifestyles.

Another synthetic opiate agonist, levomethadyl (Orlaam), is approved for maintenance therapy. This agent is also federally regulated. It has an advantage of a long half-life, allowing for less frequent dosing than methadone. However, it can prolong the QT interval, and this may account for the reluctance of some approved facilities to prescribe it.

Alternatively, an opiate antagonist may be useful for treatment of opiate addiction. Naltrexone (ReVia) blocks the euphoric effects of opiates. This medication should only be prescribed once a patient is opiate-free for 7 to 10 days, in order to avoid a precipitated withdrawal syndrome. The typical dose of naltrexone is 50 mg daily, often initiated at 25 mg daily to reduce the risk of sedation and nausea. One group that has benefited from naltrexone maintenance is health care professionals who participate in a comprehensive recovery plan and are carefully monitored by state licensing boards.

Buprenorphine (Subutex) is a mixed opioid agonist-antagonist that was recently approved for the treatment of opiate addiction. A product (Suboxone) that combines buprenorphine with the opioid-antagonist naloxone reduces the risk of medication diversion for intravenous use. Office-based clinicians, including primary care physicians, may prescribe buprenorphine for treatment of opiate addiction after taking an approved training course and receiving a special waiver from the Drug Enforcement Agency. It is unclear to what extent approval of this newest agent will improve the care of opiate addicts. The potential advantages include greater convenience for patients, decreased risk of drug diversion, additional options for less severely addicted individuals, and fewer federal regulations for practitioners.

Patients at greatest risk for prescription opiate dependence include those who abuse other substances and those with a history of illicit opiate abuse. Patients with chronic pain are at risk for opiate dependence when increasing doses of medication are needed to control pain. It is advisable for clinicians who are unsure about prescribing opiates to seek the opinions of other professionals, especially when treating patients with chronic, nonmalignant pain.

## TABLE 3  Symptoms of Opiate Withdrawal

|  | Objective | Subjective |
|---|---|---|
| Early | Lacrimation | |
| | Rhinorrhea | |
| | Diaphoresis | |
| | Yawning | |
| Middle | Dilated pupils | Restlessness |
| | Piloerection | Irritability |
| | | Insomnia |
| Late | Tachycardia | Bone pain |
| | Increased blood pressure | Nausea |
| | Vomiting | Abdominal cramps |
| | Diarrhea | Depression |
| | Mood lability | |

[1]Not FDA approved for this indication.

## TABLE 4  Opioid Treatment Summary*

### Treatment of Opioid Overdose

| Drug | Administration |
| --- | --- |
| Naloxone (Narcan) | Initial dose 0.4 mg IV (0.01 mg/kg)<br>Repeat every 2-3 minutes as indicated by symptoms<br>Re-evaluate diagnosis if no response to 5-10 mg Total |

### Sample Methadone Detoxification†

| Day | Drug | Administration |
| --- | --- | --- |
| Day 1 | Methadone 40 mg (Dolophine) | Give initial dose of methadone 20 mg<br>Additional doses of 10 or 20 mg may be given if withdrawal symptoms persist after 4 hours<br>Maximum 40 mg total dose<br>Reduce dose by 25% daily |
| Day 2-3 | Methadone 25-30 mg | |
| Day 4 | Methadone 20 mg | |
| Day 5 | Methadone 10 mg | |
| Day 6 | Methadone 5 mg | |
| Day 7 | Discontinue | |

### Sample Clonidine Detoxification‡

| Day | From Short-Acting Opioid | Day With or Without Naltrexone (ReVia) Induction | From Methadone |
| --- | --- | --- | --- |
| Day 1-2 | 0.3-0.6 mg | 12.5 mg | 0.3-0.6 mg |
| Day 3 | 0.3-0.8 mg | 25 mg | 0.4-0.6 mg |
| Day 4-5 | 0.6-1.2 mg<br>Then reduce total daily dose by 50% each day, not to exceed 0.4 mg/d | 50 mg<br>Continue maintenance therapy | 0.5-0.8 mg |
| Day 6-10 | | | 0.6-1.2 mg<br>Then reduce total daily dose by 50% each day, not to exceed 0.4 mg/d |

*All treatment must be individualized to meet specific patient needs and adjusted based on response to treatment.
†May be used in combination with clonidine (Catapres) or other as-needed medications. Catapres is not FDA approved for this indication.
‡Give a test dose of clonidine 0.1 mg. Continue only if blood pressure is >85/55. Clonidine 0.1-0.2 mg every 2-4 hours, hold for systolic blood pressure <85 or diastolic blood pressure <55.

# Benzodiazepines

Benzodiazepines are used most often in the outpatient setting for the treatment of anxiety and insomnia. They have replaced barbiturates as the sedative-hypnotic of choice because of a greater safety profile in overdose. Benzodiazepines act on the brain's γ-aminobutyric acid (GABA) receptors, which results in relaxation and mild sedation. Signs of intoxication with benzodiazepines are similar to those experienced with alcohol, with higher doses producing greater sedation, slurred speech, and ataxia. However, benzodiazepines may be used as anesthetics, whereas alcohol is lethal in very high doses. In serious overdoses where benzodiazepines are suspected to play a role, the benzodiazepine antagonist flumazenil (Romazicon) may be administered at a dose of 0.2 mg IV over 30 seconds and repeated up to a 3-mg total dose. There is a risk of seizures in sedative-dependent individuals and in patients taking benzodiazepines as part of an antiepileptic regimen.

Benzodiazepines are effective in treating alcohol withdrawal. The symptoms of sedative withdrawal and alcohol withdrawal are similar—insomnia, anxiety, tachycardia, elevated blood pressure, and fever. In addition, seizures and delirium can be serious sequelae of an untreated alcohol- or sedative-withdrawal syndrome. Whereas opiate withdrawal is not a life-threatening condition unless it occurs in the context of medical frailty, untreated benzodiazepine withdrawal may result in death.

When a patient is addicted to a benzodiazepine and needs detoxification, it is common practice to substitute a long-acting benzodiazepine for a short-acting one. Table 5 gives an approximation of equivalent doses to ease the conversion from one medication to another. Once the patient is comfortable on the long-acting benzodiazepines, the dosage is gradually reduced and discontinued. However withdrawal does not always go smoothly and medication adjustments may be needed. The reduction schedule varies depending upon the severity of the addiction, the duration of benzodiazepine use, and the dosage used.

Hospitalized patients who are addicted to high doses of benzodiazepines often do well when converted to an equivalent dose of a long-acting agent such as clonazepam (Klonopin) or chlordiazepoxide

## TABLE 5  Approximate Benzodiazepine Dose Equivalency

| Generic Name (Trade Name) | Dose Equivalents (mg)* | Short- or Long-Acting |
| --- | --- | --- |
| Alprazolam (Xanax) | 1 | Short |
| Chlordiazepoxide (Librium) | 25 | Long |
| Clonazepam (Klonopin) | 0.5 | Long |
| Diazepam (Valium) | 10 | Long |
| Flurazepam (Dalmane) | 30 | Long |
| Lorazepam (Ativan) | 2 | Short |
| Oxazepam (Serax) | 30 | Short |
| Prazepam (Centrax) | 10 | Long |
| Temazepam (Restoril) | 20 | Short |
| Triazolam (Halcion) | 0.25 | Short |

*Doses are approximately equivalent to phenobarbital 30 mg.

(Librium). Then the dose may be reduced on a 10% per day schedule. In these patients it is necessary to monitor vital signs every 4 hours and have additional doses of benzodiazepine ordered for signs of withdrawal. Such signs include tremulousness, diaphoresis, blood pressure higher than 150/100, and heart rate more than 100. Outpatients may require several weeks to months for detoxification. Some treatment centers use anticonvulsants, specifically valproic acid (Depakote)[1] and carbamazepine (Tegretol),[1] to prevent or minimize withdrawal symptoms.

## Other Drugs of Abuse

Clinicians may deal with any number of abused substances. The popularity of particular drugs changes over time. However, there are several types of substances that come up frequently enough to warrant inclusion here. One example is the inhalants. The agents that make up this group are inexpensive and accessible in common household products such as glue, shoe polish, paint thinners, aerosols, and correction and cleaning fluids. Intoxication on these agents most resembles alcohol intoxication. Acute overdose is rare but can result in death from asphyxiation or cardiac arrhythmia. The brain, kidneys, and liver are susceptible to damage from repeated inhalant exposure. The result over the long term may be chronic delirium, psychosis, or renal failure. An estimated 15% of young adults have tried an inhalant. However, it is estimated that less than 1% are addicted to inhalant use.

Hallucinogens are another group of abusable drugs. Management of intoxication on these drugs is supportive in most cases. Lysergic acid diethylamide (LSD) is a well-known drug in this class. Like most hallucinogens it produces visual hallucinations and increases sensory awareness. Intoxication can also cause dilated pupils, facial flushing, tachycardia, and increased blood pressure. 3,4-Methylenedioxymethamphetamine (MDMA), or ecstasy, may be classified as either a hallucinogen or a stimulant because it has properties of both. It is generally considered a dangerous drug because of its potential for long-term brain damage. It may also be toxic to the heart and liver.

Phencyclidine (PCP) intoxication can have a frightening presentation. The patient may become agitated and unpredictable, requiring physical and chemical restraints to ensure the safety of the patient and those around him or her. Medication may not be necessary if the patient is placed in a quiet, supportive setting. If medications are used, benzodiazepines are typically chosen first. If antipsychotics are required, agents with low anticholinergic activity are preferred. Toxic doses of PCP can produce a life-threatening condition with severe autonomic instability in which hypertension, hyperthermia, convulsions, and coma may become serious medical management problems.

## Treatment

While medication management is increasingly important in the treatment of alcohol and drug dependence, nonpharmacologic approaches are the mainstay of substance abuse treatment. Alcoholics Anonymous (AA) helped many alcoholics recover before physicians had treatment techniques to offer. AA remains a proven resource, and other self-help groups are modeled after it. Narcotics Anonymous (NA) and Cocaine Anonymous (CA), similar to AA, are pivotal in the recovery of some drug abusers. The caveat is that one group may be very different from another.

There are significant problems in some self-help groups. Patients may have concerns about heavy cigarette-smoking in meetings, about attendees who actively use or sell drugs, and about criticism of prescribed psychotropic medications. Therefore, when a patient finds one group unsatisfactory for some reason, the clinician can suggest he or she try another group. Some patients object to the religious tone of traditional 12-step groups. For these individuals alternative groups such as Women for Sobriety and Rational Recovery may be more acceptable. In addition, self-help groups are free of charge, which is a factor for some patients.

Most professional addiction treatment occurs in an outpatient setting. However, higher levels of care are available in hospital, residential, or partial hospital programs if there are chaotic living situations, or pressing psychiatric or other medical needs. Social interventions are crucial for patients faced with unemployment, legal consequences, and housing dilemmas. Psychiatric disorders occur with a high frequency in drug-abusing populations, and both disorders should be treated to optimize the patient's chances for recovery. Therefore, a multidisciplinary approach to treatment often works best.

Psychiatric symptoms in patients who abuse drugs are easy to recognize. Mood lability, depression, and anxiety are common. The challenge lies in sorting out whether these symptoms are caused by the use of a mood-altering substance or represent a separate mood or anxiety disorder. Psychiatric expertise may be needed to assist in sorting out this diagnostic dilemma. Patients with schizophrenic and bipolar disorders are also at high risk for drug abuse, which can exacerbate psychoses.

The cognitive aspects of professional treatment often include educational, motivational, cognitive–behavioral, relapse prevention, and 12-step strategies. Most treatment programs try to get the patient to more fully recognize the problems associated with his or her drug use, identify reasons to change, acknowledge obstacles to sobriety, become aware of triggers to relapse, and consider ways to build a sober support network. Patients with addictive disorders do get better, and treatment of patients with drug abuse can be highly rewarding. It is important to recognize this problem as one of many chronic, relapsing conditions seen in medicine today.

[1]Not FDA approved for this indication.

## TABLE 6  Benzodiazepine Treatment Summary*

### Treatment of Overdose

| Drug | Administration |
|---|---|
| Flumazenil (Romazicon) | Initial dose 0.2 mg IV over 30 seconds. Repeat every minute up to a 3-mg total dose. Re-evaluate diagnosis if no response after 3-5 minutes. |

### Detoxification Guidelines

| Day | Action |
|---|---|
| Day 1 | Long-acting benzodiazepine until symptom control is achieved. Common upper limits are clonazepam (Klonopin), 6-8 mg per 24 hours or chlordiazepoxide (Librium), 400 mg per 24 hours. |
| Day 2–Completion | Taper by 25% every 1-2 days Monitor vital signs every 4 hours Have PRN doses available, i.e., clonazepam, 1 mg, chlordiazepoxide, 25 mg, for signs or symptoms of withdrawal (tremulousness, diaphoresis, systolic blood pressure >150, diastolic blood pressure >100, or heart rate >100). Consider adding anticonvulsants. |

*All treatment must be individualized to meet specific patient needs and adjusted based on response to treatment.

# Anxiety Disorders

Method of
*Jacqueline Carinhas McGregor, MD*

Anxiety disorders are the most common psychiatric disorders in the world among both children and adults. In the United States, 30 million people or approximately one of every four meet the criteria for an anxiety disorder in their lifetimes. It is estimated that the annual cost of anxiety disorders in 1998 dollars was more than $63 billion. More than half of these costs were due to nonpsychiatric direct medical costs, which include undiagnosed, misdiagnosed, or inadequately treated anxiety disorders. It is clear that much of the emotional and economic burden caused by these disorders could be alleviated by improving diagnosis and treatment.

Genetics, temperament, and life stressors can all be contributors to anxiety disorders. Norepinephrine and serotonin are thought to be the major neurotransmitters involved in mediating anxiety symptoms whereas the sympathetic nervous system also plays an important role. The onset of anxiety disorders can usually be traced to childhood, adolescence, or young adulthood. With the exception of obsessive-compulsive disorder, women are more likely than men to suffer from anxiety disorders. Anxiety disorders occur across racial groups without distinction.

Anxiety is characterized by subjective feelings of worry, dread, or anticipation and can include hypervigilance, excessive negativity, and a myriad of somatic symptoms. These symptoms can include diaphoresis, palpitations, shortness of breath, dizziness, chest pain, tremulousness, gastrointestinal complaints, fatigue, dry mouth, sleep problems, hot flashes, polyuria, and restlessness. Because of the wide variety of physical complaints, underlying organic causes and disorders secondary to substances use must first be ruled out (Box 1). A detailed history of present illness, past medical history, substance history, and review of symptoms is essential. If a patient initially presents with anxiety symptoms in middle or late adulthood, has no family history of anxiety disorders, has no temporally related stressors, and does not respond to psychiatric intervention, a closer investigation of organic causes of anxiety should be undertaken.

In patients describing chest pain, cardiovascular causes such as angina, mitral valve prolapse, arrhythmias, and pulmonary embolism should be ruled out. Pulmonary ailments such as asthma, chronic obstructive pulmonary disorder, and pneumonia should be considered in patients describing shortness of breath. Hyperthyroidism,

pheochromocytoma, and Cushing's syndrome are examples of endocrine disorders that can mimic anxiety disorders. Other disorders to consider include anemia, delirium, menopause, and gastroesophageal reflux. Medications such as stimulants (including herbal supplements and caffeine), decongestants, antipsychotics, theophylline, steroids, calcium channel blockers, and anticholinergics should all be considered. Alcohol and illicit drug use or withdrawal are other possible causes of anxiety symptoms.

The most common diagnoses of anxiety disorders include generalized anxiety disorder (GAD), panic disorder, social anxiety disorder, obsessive-compulsive disorder (OCD), posttraumatic stress disorder (PTSD), and specific phobias. Those suffering from anxiety disorders are likely to have another co-morbid psychiatric disorder such as a mood disorder or substance dependence. These patients also have a higher risk for suicidal behaviors. It is important to distinguish anxiety disorders from each other, as well as from other psychiatric disorders because the specific diagnosis may have significant impact on treatment decisions. Simple phobias, for example, are not responsive to medication and require cognitive behavioral intervention. OCD requires significantly higher doses of antidepressants than other disorders. Patients with GAD and panic disorder need lower starting doses of antidepressants to avoid iatrogenically exacerbating their symptoms. In the case of patient with comorbid bipolar disorder, special care should be used with antidepressants to prevent the induction of a manic episode.

Psychotherapeutic interventions are often considered the first line of intervention in anxiety disorders, particularly for patients with mild symptoms, those who prefer nonpharmacologic treatment, and for children. Cognitive behavior therapy (CBT) is a specific type of psychotherapy that combines behavioral therapy with cognitive therapy and has the best evidence-based research supporting its use in anxiety disorders. The behavioral component of CBT includes exposure and ritual prevention whereas the cognitive aspect includes identifying false, irrational thoughts and the automatic responses to them. It is important to find skilled therapists with specialized training in these modalities in order to facilitate helpful referrals.

The pharmacologic treatment of most anxiety disorders usually includes selective serotonin reuptake inhibitors (SSRIs) serotonin-norepinephrine reuptake inhibitors (SNRIs), and/or benzodiazepines. The SSRIs fluoxetine (Prozac) and paroxetine (Paxil) are both potent inhibitors of cytochrome P450 2D6, and significant interactions can occur with other drugs that a patient may be taking. Escitalopram (Lexapro) has the most favorable SSRI side effect profile with the least protein-binding and cytochrome-P450 interactions. The most common side effects of SSRIs are nervousness, insomnia, restlessness, nausea, and diarrhea. Venlafaxine (Effexor) has a lower risk of significant drug interactions compared to the SSRIs; however, patients prescribed venlafaxine (Effexor) should have their blood pressure monitored as it can cause or worsen existing hypertension. Benzodiazepines should be used carefully because of their addictive potential and should be avoided in patients with a history of substance abuse.

As with any drug, it is important to discuss the risk and benefits of medication options with patients before coming to a treatment decision. The dosage of a medication should be carefully titrated to minimize side effects while providing adequate symptom response. The Food and Drug Administration (FDA) issued a labeling change request in October 2004 for a black box warning on antidepressant medications about the *possible* association of SSRIs with suicidality in the treatment of major depressive disorder. The antidepressant side effect of agitation has been known to trigger suicidal behavior in those with or without premorbid depression. A physician should exercise special care in using SSRI medications, especially with those younger than 18 years of age. Frequent follow-up visits are recommended to monitor side effects and treatment response. Three of the most prevalent and burdensome anxiety disorders are GAD, OCD, and panic disorder. The remainder of this article will focus on the diagnosis and treatment of GAD and OCD disorders. Panic disorder is discussed in another article.

---

## BOX 1 Organic Causes of Anxiety Symptoms

| | |
|---|---|
| Cardiopulmonary | Angina, mitral valve prolapse, pulmonary embolism, COPD, asthma |
| Endocrine | Hyperthyroidism, pheochromocytoma, Cushing's syndrome, menopause |
| Gastrointestinal | Gastroesophageal reflux, irritable bowel syndrome, gastritis |
| Neurologic | Dementia, substance intoxication or withdrawal, seizure disorder, migraine |
| Medications | Stimulants, herbal supplements, decongestants, steroids, antipsychotics, theophylline, calcium channel blockers, anticholinergics |

*Abbreviation:* COPD = chronic obstructive pulmonary disease.

# Generalized Anxiety Disorder

## DIAGNOSIS

According to the *Diagnostic and Statistical Manual of Mental Disorders IV-TR*, individuals with GAD suffer from uncontrollable, excessive anxiety and worry involving several areas of functioning on most days in a 6 month period. It must be associated with three or more of the following symptoms: restlessness, fatigue concentration difficulties, irritability, muscle tension, or sleep problems. The anxiety cannot be the result of another Axis I disorder; it must cause a significant impairment in functioning, and it cannot be due to substance abuse, a medical disorder, or occur exclusively in the context of a mood disorder, psychotic disorder, or pervasive developmental disorder.

The 12-month prevalence for GAD is 3.1%, and the lifetime prevalence is close to 5%. Women are twice as likely as men to suffer from GAD. GAD usually develops sometime during late adolescence or early adulthood, its symptoms tend to have a chronic duration, and there is a high incidence of comorbid psychiatric disorders (especially depression) associated with it.

GAD can be difficult for the physician to diagnose because patients can be reluctant to discuss their anxiety or be unable to identify it as the source of their concerns. Patient complaints of fatigue, insomnia, somatic symptoms, or chronic pain should be a signal for the physician to ask more about anxiety symptoms.

## TREATMENT

Psychotherapy, pharmacotherapy, and their combination can be successfully used to treat GAD. Psychotherapy, particularly cognitive-behavior therapy and applied relaxation, are effective treatment strategies for GAD. Psychotherapy can be used concomitantly with pharmacotherapy, often with better result than if either were used alone.

There are a variety of psychopharmacologic interventions that can be used for patients with GAD (Table 1). An antidepressant or the 5-HT$_{1A}$ partial agonist, buspirone (BusPar), is considered the first line of drug treatment. Paroxetine (Paxil), escitalopram (Lexapro), and venlafaxine (Effexor) are the only antidepressants that have an FDA indication for GAD, although there is evidence that both imipramine (Tofranil)[1] and sertraline (Zoloft)[1] are effective drugs in the treatment of GAD. SSRIs are usually considered the antidepressant of choice because of their safety and relatively modest side effects. Use tricyclic antidepressants such as imipramine (Tofranil) with care because of their more troublesome side-effect profile, proarrhythmic properties, and potential lethality in overdose. The most commonly noted side effects of buspirone (BusPar) are dizziness, nausea, headache, nervousness, and insomnia. Benzodiazepines can play an important role in the treatment of GAD. It is important to keep in mind the addictive potential of these medications before using them. In the first weeks of treatment with SSRIs, it can be helpful to use benzodiazepines to address acute anxiety symptoms while allowing sufficient time for the SSRI to

[1]Not FDA approved for this indication.

achieve its effect. As symptoms begin to respond, the physician should consider tapering and discontinuing the benzodiazepine.

After an 8- to 10-week course of treatment with an antidepressant, if there has been an insufficient response at an adequate dose, the clinician should consider switching to or augmenting with another drug (e.g., another antidepressant, buspirone [BusPar] or a benzodiazepine). Patients need significant support and encouragement from their physician to be compliant with daily medication regimes and to continue their medication once they begin to experience symptom relief. There is little data on the length of treatment or whether pharmacologic intervention can prevent future relapse. It is common practice to continue treatment for at least 6 to 12 months after resolution of symptoms before stopping medications. At that time a gradual tapering of the medication dose can be considered.

| TABLE 1 Pharmacotherapy in the Treatment of Generalized Anxiety Disorder | | |
|---|---|---|
| **Drug** | **Starting Dose** | **Target Dose** |
| **SSRIs** | | |
| Paroxetine (Paxil CR)* | 10 mg qd | 10-60 mg qd |
| Escitalopram (Lexapro)* | 5-10 mg qd | 10-20 mg qd |
| Sertraline (Zoloft) | 12.5-25 mg qd | 50-200 mg qd |
| Fluoxetine (Prozac) | 10 mg qd | 20-40 mg qd |
| **SNRIs** | | |
| Venlafazine (Effexor XR)* | 37.5 mg qam | 150-300 mg qam |
| **OTHER** | | |
| Buspirone (BusPar) | 5 mg bid-tid | 10 mg bid to tid |

*FDA indication for generalized anxiety disorder (GAD)
*Abbreviations:* bid = twice daily; qam = every morning; qd = every day; tid = three times daily.
SNRIs = serotonin-norepinephrine reuptake inhibitors; SSRIs = selective serotonin reuptake inhibitors.

# Obsessive Compulsive Disorder

## DIAGNOSIS

The *Diagnostic and Statistical Manual of Mental Disorders IV-TR* outlines the criteria for OCD as having obsessions and/or compulsions. Obsessions are defined as recurrent, persistent thoughts, impulses, or images that are experienced as intrusive and inappropriate and cause significant distress. They cannot be excessive worries about realistic or reasonable concerns. The individual attempts to ignore the obsessions or counteract them with another thought or action and understands that the obsessions are a product of his or her

## CURRENT THERAPY

| | First Intervention | Second Intervention | Third Intervention |
|---|---|---|---|
| **GAD** | CBT | SSRI OR venlafaxine (Effexor) OR buspirone (BusPar) OR | Change to different antidepressant or buspirone (BusPar) OR Augment with a different antidepressant class, buspirone (BusPar), or benzodiazepine |
| **OCD** | CBT | High dose SSRI (push to maximum dose in 4 to 8 weeks) | Change to another SSRI or clomipramine (anafranil) OR Augment with atypical antipsychotic |

*Abbreviations:* CBT = cognitive behavior therapy; GAD = generalized anxiety disorder; OCD = obsessive-compulsive disorder; SSRI = selective serotonin reuptake inhibitor.

own mind. Compulsions are defined as repetitive behaviors or mental acts that the individual feels compelled to perform in response to an obsession. The compulsion is aimed at reducing distress or preventing some dreaded event, but is not clearly connected to the distress or event or is clearly excessive. Except in the case of children, at some point in the course of the disorder the individual recognizes that the obsessions or compulsions are unreasonable. This last point is important in distinguishing OCD from obsessive compulsive personality disorder. The obsessions or compulsions must cause significant impairment and, if another Axis I disorder coexists, the obsessions and/or compulsions cannot be restricted only to the content of that disorder (e.g., preoccupations with food in the case of an eating disorder, hair pulling in the case of trichotillomania). As in the case of GAD, the symptoms cannot occur because of the effects of a substance or secondary to a general medical disorder.

It is not uncommon for OCD to occur with other psychiatric disorders including major depressive disorder, other anxiety disorders, eating disorders, and tic disorders. In children, streptococcal infections are associated with the development of obsessions and compulsions. Psychotic disorders can have obsessive or compulsive behaviors, but these are typically much more bizarre, and the individual has little insight into his or her behavior. It is also important to consider illnesses that can have OCD-like symptoms such as basal ganglia disorders (e.g., Huntington's disease) or tic disorders.

OCD usually appears in late adolescence or early adulthood and has a waxing and waning course. Unlike other anxiety disorders there is an equal occurrence in males and females. The lifetime prevalence rate of OCD is 2% to 3% of the population. Neuroimaging studies of OCD suggest that there are structural and functional problems in the orbitofrontal-subcortical circuitry.

People with OCD often avoid seeking treatment for their illness. Diagnosis often requires explicit questioning regarding specific behaviors such as perfectionism, rituals, washing, counting, checking, or hoarding. The physicians should also be on the lookout for excessively red or raw hands, recurring request for reassurance about medical illnesses, frequent emergency room visits, or usual repetitive behaviors observed in the examining room such as tic-like motions or tapping.

## TREATMENT

There are a variety of treatment approaches that can be used for OCD. As with GAD, psychotherapy can be utilized effectively. There is significant research that supporting cognitive behavioral therapy that incorporates exposure-response prevention is a successful treatment for obsessions and compulsions. In more severe cases of OCD, optimal treatment uses a combination of cognitive behavioral therapy and medication.

Several studies demonstrated the efficacy of SSRIs in OCD. A reasonable trial of SSRIs in OCD can be longer and requires higher doses than what would be expected in GAD or major depressive disorder. Setraline (Zoloft), fluoxetine (Prozac), paroxetine (Paxil), and fluvoxamine (Luvox) are SSRIs with FDA indications for OCD.

For those with an inadequate response to treatment with SSRIs, the clinician should consider changing SSRIs, switching to the tricyclic antidepressant, clomipramine (Anafranil), or to the SNRI, venlafaxine (Effexor).[1] The most common side effects of clomipramine (Anafranil) include dry mouth, sedation, dizziness, and weight gain, however, more serious, less common side effects include hypertension and cardiac arrhythmias. Augmentation with a dopamine agonist such as risperidone (Risperdal)[1] or olanzapine (Zyprexa) has been shown to be an effective treatment approach as has the addition of buspirone (BusPar)[1] or benzodiazepines (Table 2).

There is some evidence to support the use of monoamine oxidase inhibitors (MAOIs) in treatment-resistant OCD, but because of the significant side effects, potential drug and food interactions, and toxicity, they are considered an option only when other medication options have proven unsuccessful. For those who fail psychotherapy and psychopharmacology and continue to have significant functional impairment, transcranial magnetic stimulation and neurosurgery are considered treatments of last resort.

Treatment of OCD can usually be accomplished on an outpatient basis; however, in severe refractory cases, inpatient treatment at a facility that specializes in OCD may be necessary. Whatever treatment strategy is employed, the physician should be mindful of the fact that the patient's family often needs to be involved in the treatment. Families often unknowingly reinforce a patient's OCD behaviors by going along with their rituals or participating in excessive reassurance.

Anxiety disorders are quite common and cause a significant burden to individuals as well as to society. The differential diagnosis of anxiety disorders is quite extensive given that anxiety symptoms are often nonspecific. Anxiety disorders often go undiagnosed or are inadequately treated and are likely to occur together with other psychiatric disorders. Primary care physicians are more likely to have the opportunity to detect anxiety disorders and, in fact treat more of these disorders than mental health care practitioners. Effective treatments for anxiety including psychotherapeutic as well as psychopharmacologic interventions are shown in Box 2.

**BOX 2 Helpful Resources for Anxiety Disorders**

| | |
|---|---|
| National Alliance for the Mentally Ill | www.nami.org |
| National Institute of Mental Health | www.nimh.org |
| Anxiety Disorders Association of America | www.adaa.org |
| Obsessive-Compulsive Foundation | www.ocfoundation.org |

## REFERENCES

American Psychiatric Association: Diagnostic and Statistical Manual of Mental Disorders, 4th ed, text rev. Washington, DC, American Psychiatric Association, 2000.

Baer L, Rauch SK, Ballantine T, et al: Cingulotomy for intractable obsessive-compulsive disorder. Arch Gen Psych 1995;52:384-392.

Borkovec T, Costello E: Efficacy of applied relaxation and cognitive-behavioral therapy in the treatment of generalized anxiety disorder. Journal of Consulting and Clinical Psychology 1993;61(4):611-619.

Food and Drug Administration: FDA labeling change request letter for antidepressant medications, 2004.

**TABLE 2 Pharmacotherapy in the Treatment of Obsessive-Compulsive Disorder**

| Drug | Starting Dose | Target Daily Dose |
|---|---|---|
| **SSRI** | | |
| Sertraline (Zoloft)* | 25-50 mg qd | 100-300 mg[3] |
| Paroxetine (Paxil CR)* | 12.5 mg qd | 25-50 mg |
| Fluoxetine (Prozac)* | 10 mg qd | 20-60 mg |
| Fluvoxamine (Luvox)* | 25-50 mg qd | 100-300 mg |
| **SNRI** | | |
| Venlafaxine (Effexor XR) | 37.5 mg qam | 150-300 mg |
| **TCA** | | |
| Clomipramine* (Anafranil) | 25 mg qhs | 100-300 mg |

*FDA indication for obsessive-compulsive disorder (OCD)
[3]Exceeds dosage recommended by the manufacturer.
*Abbreviations:* qam = every morning; qd = every day; qhs = at bed time.

[1]Not FDA approved for this indication.

Greenberg BD, George MS, Martin DJ, et al: Effect of prefrontal repetitive transcranial stimulation in obsessive-compulsive disorder: A preliminary study. Am J Psychiatry 1997;154:867-869.

Greenberg PE, Sisitsky T, Kessler RC, et al: The economic burden of anxiety disorders in the 1990s. J Clin Psychiatry 1990;60:427-435.

Jenike MA, Baer L, Minichiello WE (eds): Obsessive-compulsive disorders: practical management 3rd ed. St Louis, Mosby, 1998.

Karno M, Golding JM, Sorenson SB, et al: The epidemiology of obsessive-compulsive disorder in five US communities. Arch Gen Psychiatry 1988;45(12): 1094-1099.

Kessler RC, McGonagle KA, Zhao S: Lifetime and 12-month prevalence of DSM-III-R psychiatric disorders in the United States. Arch Gen Psychiatry 1994;51(1):8-19.

Kobak KA, Griest JH, Jefferson JW, et al: Behavioral versus pharmacologic treatment of obsessive compulsive disorder: A meta-analysis. Psychopharmacology (Berl) 1998;136:205-216.

Koran LM, Rinhold AL, Elliot MA: Olanzapine augmentation in obsessive compulsive disorder refractory to selective serotonin reuptake inhibitors: An open label case series. J Clin Psychiatry 2000;61:514-517.

Ladouceur R, Dugas MJ, Freeston MH, et al: Efficacy of a cognitive behavioral treatment for generalized anxiety disorder evaluation in controlled clinical trial. J Consult Clin Psychol 2000;68(6):957-964.

Liebowitz MR, DeMartinis NA, Weihs K, et al: Efficacy of sertraline in severe generalized social anxiety disorder: results of a double-blind, placebo-controlled study. J Clin Psychiatry 2003;64(7):785-792.

McDougle CJ, Epperson CN, Pelton GH, et al: A double blind placebo controlled study of risperidone addition in serotin reuptake inhibitor-refractory obsessive compulsive disorder. Arch Gen Psych 2000;57:794-801.

Rickels K, Downing R, Schweizer E, et al: Antidepressant for the treatment of generalized anxiety disorder: a placebo controlled comparison of imipramine, trrazodone, and diazepam. Arch Gen Psychiatry 1993;50:884-895.

Rickels K, Schweizer E: The spectrum of generalized anxiety in clinical practice: The role of short term intermittent treatment. Br J Psychiatry 1998;173(Suppl 34):49-54.

Saxena S, Bota RG, Brody AL: Brain-behavior relationships in obsessive-compulsive disorder. Semin Clin Neuropsychiatry 2001;6(2):82-101.

# Bulimia Nervosa

Method of
*David B. Herzog, MD, and Kamryn T. Eddy, PhD*

Bulimia nervosa is a prevalent eating disorder most commonly observed in late adolescent and young adult women and often associated with psychiatric co-morbidity and medical sequelae. The course of the disorder may be chronic and relapsing, and patients may demonstrate early ambivalence regarding treatment. There is often a considerable delay between onset of symptoms and presentation for treatment that may reflect shame, control issues, and fear of change (e.g., weight gain). Currently, psychosocial treatments—particularly cognitive behavioral therapy—are considered the first-line of treatment for the disorder, having demonstrated the most successful outcomes, but psychopharmacologic interventions are also promising.

## Diagnosis and Clinical Features

### DIAGNOSIS

Bulimia nervosa was first recognized formally as a clinical diagnosis in 1979 by Gerald Russell. The disorder is currently defined in the *Diagnostic and Statistical Manual of Mental Disorders, Fourth Edition* (*DSM-IV*) on the basis of recurrent binge eating and compensatory behaviors and related cognitions. Binge eating is defined as the consumption of a large amount of food (typically 2000 to 4000 calories) within a discrete period of time accompanied by loss of control overeating. Loss of control overeating involves the subjective experience of being unable to control what or how much one is eating and

may be characterized by eating more rapidly than usual and consuming calorie-dense foods that are typically avoided outside of binge episodes. Compensatory behaviors are designed to counteract the effects of binge eating and can be classified as purging (self-induced vomiting, misuse of laxatives, diuretics, and enemas) and nonpurging (excessive exercise, fasting). The *DSM-IV* specifies that the binge eating and compensatory behaviors occur on average at least twice weekly during a 3-month period. In addition to the behavioral components, the *DSM-IV* indicates a cognitive component of overevaluation of the importance of weight and shape on sense of self. Weight is not part of the bulimia nervosa criteria; although most patients with bulimia nervosa are within an average weight range, patients may be overweight, obese, or even underweight.

Patients with bulimia nervosa can be grouped into purging and nonpurging types based on the compensatory behaviors used. Notably, purging type appears to be predominant; less research exists on the nonpurging type.

According to the *DSM-IV* hierarchy rules, a diagnosis of bulimia nervosa is not made if the binge and compensatory behaviors occur exclusively during a period of anorexia nervosa. Similarly, a diagnosis of binge eating disorder (currently recognized in the *DSM-IV* as an eating disorder not otherwise specified) can be appropriate if recurrent binge eating is present in the absence of any compensatory behaviors.

Although the current diagnostic system is useful, limitations exist. For example, there appears to be heterogeneity within the diagnostic category of bulimia nervosa on the basis of psychosocial functioning, personality style, and co-morbidity, which may have treatment implications. Furthermore, a large subset of patients present for treatment in clinical settings with symptom profiles that closely resemble that of a patient with bulimia nervosa but do not meet all of the diagnostic criteria. For example, although a formal diagnosis of bulimia nervosa stipulates a twice-weekly binge/compensatory behaviors frequency criterion, patients often present to eating disorder clinics for the treatment of bingeing and/or purging that occurs less frequently. Thus, this treatment review derives from the literature on bulimia nervosa but can be considered applicable across patients with a spectrum of bulimic symptoms.

### DIFFERENTIAL DIAGNOSIS

Consideration of a range of conditions that may be characterized by features similar to bulimia nervosa is necessary in the initial assessment. Neurologic disorders impacting appetite regulation and eating behaviors (e.g., pituitary or hypothalamic brain tumors, Kleine-Levin or Klüver-Bucy syndromes), hormonal disorders relating to malnutrition and hypometabolism (e.g., adrenal disease, diabetes mellitus, pituitary dysfunction, hyperthyroidism), and gastrointestinal (GI) disorders (e.g., malabsorption, enteritis) should be considered. Psychiatric disorders including major depression and borderline personality disorder should be considered because they may be associated with binge eating even though compensatory behaviors and cognitive features of bulimia nervosa are absent.

### MEDICAL COMPLICATIONS

Patients with bulimia nervosa are generally within the normal weight range, but they may show signs of malnutrition. Medical complications secondary to bingeing and purging behaviors and malnutrition are common. Patients often present with transient facial swelling, peripheral edema, weakness and fatigue, dental problems, and abrasions on the dorsal surface of the hand (Russell's sign). Medical assessment should be based on current symptom presentation and should include complete blood count, serum electrolytes, serum blood urea nitrogen (BUN)/creatinine levels, urinalysis, and an electrocardiogram (ECG). Electrolyte and acid-based complications secondary to purging are common and may include hypochloremia, hyponatremia, and hypokalemia. Hypokalemia is related to significant cardiac problems including arrhythmias. Long-term ipecac use may lead to cardiomyopathy. Edema may be present and related to laxative and diuretic abuse. Dental complications related to chronic regurgitation of gastric contents can include enamel erosion and caries. Swelling of the parotid glands is also common. GI difficulties ranging from constipation and bloating to esophageal disorders may also be present. Many of these symptom-related complications remit when the purging is discontinued, but additional treatment and monitoring can be warranted for some patients.

## CO-MORBIDITY

Bulimia nervosa is often associated with psychiatric co-morbidity including mood, anxiety, and substance use disorders. Approximately half of patients with bulimia nervosa report a lifetime history of depression. Similarly, anxiety disorders including social phobia and obsessive-compulsive disorder are commonly reported. Although depression may precede the onset, have simultaneous onset, or follow the eating disorder onset, anxiety disorders most often precede the onset of the eating disorder. A substantial minority of patients with bulimia nervosa also reports a lifetime history of substance use disorders, with alcohol abuse being the most common.

Personality styles have received considerable attention in patients with bulimia nervosa. Research indicates that a subset of patients with bulimia can be characterized as multi-impulsive or dysregulated across multiple domains including eating, affect, interpersonal functioning, and sexuality, for example. Bulimic patients with dysregulated personality styles are more likely to present with co-morbid substance use disorders, cluster B axis II disorders, self-destructive and self-injurious behaviors, and kleptomania.

## Epidemiology

Population surveys indicate a 1% to 4% lifetime prevalence rate for bulimia nervosa. However, subthreshold binge/purge symptoms and overvaluation of weight and shape are more common. Further, rates of bulimia nervosa are generally higher within given population subsets including college females, for example. Typical age of onset is in late adolescence or early adulthood and may occur during a time of transition (e.g., high school to college) or psychosocial stress. Approximately 90% of patients presenting for treatment of bulimia nervosa are female. Current research indicates that bulimia nervosa is prevalent across ethnicity and socioeconomic status. Notably, however, eating disorders are more commonly seen in industrialized nations where a thin female appearance is valued.

## Etiology

A large body of research has considered the etiology of bulimia nervosa, implicating psychological, biological, and social factors. Psychological factors include general personality traits such as perfectionism and difficulty with emotion regulation, difficulty dealing with conflict, and pervasive low self-esteem. It is hypothesized that these variables represent vulnerability factors that are triggered by biological and environmental variables (e.g., transition, parent eating disorder, family conflict). The biological model of bulimia nervosa is supported by the higher concordance of monozygotic than dizygotic twins, which suggests genetic factors are implicated. Further, the biological model suggests that patient-induced dietary restraint leads to binge eating. The implication of social factors is supported by the increased prevalence of bulimia nervosa in industrialized nations. The images of ideal beauty portrayed by the media are inundating in Western society, and yet they are unrealistically thin for most women; women with a childhood history of overweight and obesity may be at particular risk. This leads to internalization of a thin body ideal and associated body dissatisfaction, both of which predict bulimic symptoms. It is likely that the confluence of multiple psychological, biological, and sociocultural factors predicts the development of bulimia nervosa. Early warning signs that may be observed by family members or primary care physicians are changes in eating behaviors and weight-related concerns (e.g., not eating with the family, nighttime eating, increased body concerns in normal or underweight females), physical changes (e.g., weight loss, amenorrhea), changes in social behaviors

(e.g., avoidance of activities, isolation), and mood-related changes (e.g., loss of self-esteem, depressed mood, irritability).

## Treatment Options

Treatment for bulimia nervosa often involves multiple components, the most common of which are psychosocial and pharmacologic. The primary aims of treatment for bulimia nervosa are to reduce and eliminate binge/purge behaviors, modify unhealthy attitudes toward weight and shape, and encourage healthier coping styles. Most patients with bulimia nervosa can be treated on an outpatient basis; however, hospitalization may be necessary for patients who are medically unstable (e.g., because of complications secondary to bulimia nervosa or medical morbidity such as diabetes), severely depressed, or treatment-refractory.

## ASSESSMENT

A comprehensive assessment is needed to determine an appropriate and individualized treatment course. Assessment should provide detailed information regarding:

- Eating disorder symptom severity (i.e., frequency, type, history)
- Medical issues and bulimia-related complications
- Developmental history
- Psychiatric history
- Treatment history
- Family history

For a subset of patients bulimia nervosa may be complicated by a concomitant medical condition; in these cases prioritizing the severity of various medical problems is necessary as a piece of the assessment.

Patients with bulimia nervosa tend to manifest shame and embarrassment about their binge/purge symptoms. There is often considerable ambivalence in these patients who, on the one hand, describe feeling out of control with their eating behaviors and perhaps wish for immediate relief and therefore may be interested in beginning a treatment that will help them regain stability over their eating. Yet, they may be hesitant to implement recommendations, demonstrating significant fears that discontinuing the binge/purge cycle will result in weight gain, which they believe would be unbearable. Determining motivation and readiness to change is an important phase of the assessment process.

### Psychosocial

Several psychosocial interventions have received empirical support for the treatment of bulimia nervosa, and currently psychotherapy is regarded as the first-line of treatment for the disorder.

Cognitive behavioral therapy (CBT) is one such approach that has received the strongest empirical support. CBT has been widely studied: in clinical trials it achieves 80% reductions in bingeing and purging behavior in patients and leads to full recovery in approximately 50% of patients. CBT for bulimia nervosa works on a model in which dietary restraint leads to binge eating and subsequent compensatory behaviors; both reinforce concern about eating, weight, and shape and in turn drive the bulimic cycle. CBT aims to intervene in this cycle by targeting dietary restraint to reduce and eliminate binge eating and purging and simultaneously address dysfunctional eating, weight, and shape cognitions. Core treatment components include psychoeducation around healthy eating and the implications of disordered eating behaviors, the prescription of *regular* eating, self-monitoring (in the form of daily food logs), and cognitive restructuring around eating, weight, and shape concerns. CBT is typically short-term focused treatment comprising 15 to 20 sessions held during a 4 to 5 month period. CBT can be delivered in an individual, group, or self-help manual format. Meta-analytic review indicates that individual treatment confers an advantage over group treatment. Additionally CBT-focused self-help and guided self-help approaches have also demonstrated efficacy. Although response rates with self-help are not as high as individual CBT, advantages include the wide availability and low cost.

Interpersonal psychotherapy (IPT) has also demonstrated efficacy in the treatment of bulimia nervosa, achieving rates of improvement and recovery comparable to those of CBT but somewhat less quickly. In the treatment of bulimia nervosa, IPT was first tested as a *viable control* treatment in clinical trials of CBT for bulimia nervosa. In contrast to CBT, which directly addresses the maladaptive eating disordered behaviors and cognitions, IPT focuses on interpersonal functioning. The IPT model of bulimia nervosa hypothesizes that interpersonal difficulties lead to low self-esteem and dysphoria and that bingeing and purging are used as coping mechanisms to regulate affect. The treatment focuses on addressing interpersonal difficulties in a short-term structured treatment, which leads to improvements in bulimic symptoms that often accrue even post-treatment.

In spite of the efficacy of CBT and IPT treatments, approximately 50% of patients in clinical trials do not achieve full recovery post-treatment. Presently treatment trials are aiming to deconstruct CBT and IPT approaches to identify mechanisms of change as well as understand why treatment does not work for all patients. Integrated therapies, which incorporate elements of different treatment modalities, are often used in clinical practice and attempts to study them in controlled treatment trials are underway. One such example is an enhanced version of CBT (CBT-E), which incorporates cognitive behavioral principles, interpersonal aspects, regulation strategies taken from dialectical behavior therapy, and other techniques all in an individualized approach as they apply to the patient. Preliminary findings suggest high rates of improvement and recovery for difficult-to-treat patients.

A limitation of these clinical trials for bulimia nervosa is that patient samples are most often adults; the generalizability of these findings to adolescents with the disorder is unclear. Two randomized controlled clinical trials for adolescents with bulimia nervosa have recently been completed. Both studies supported the use of family-based therapy, using the Maudsley model, in the treatment of adolescents with bulimia nervosa, and one indicated that CBT focused guided self-help was also effective and available at a lower cost.

These empirically supported treatments are described in detail in treatment manuals available for use by treating clinicians.

## Pharmacotherapy

Psychotropic medication can be helpful for patients with bulimia nervosa in reducing bingeing and purging symptoms. Controlled trials have indicated that a range of antidepressants demonstrate efficacy in reducing bulimic symptoms, with the research finding post-treatment reductions in bingeing and purging symptoms for approximately 50% of patients and post-treatment abstinence rates of 30%. Currently, the only medication that has received FDA approval in the treatment of bulimia nervosa is fluoxetine (Prozac) at a recommended dose of 60 mg every day. Studies have suggested other selective serotonin reuptake inhibitors (SSRIs) may be equally effective but controlled clinical trials and long-term follow-up data are unavailable. In particular, patients with co-morbid anxiety disorders may benefit from paroxetine (Paxil)[1] or sertraline (Zoloft).[1] Additionally, earlier studies suggested tricyclic antidepressants, particularly desipramine (Norpramin),[1] were useful in reducing bulimic symptoms, but research indicates the SSRIs may be better tolerated. Monoamine oxidase inhibitors (MAOIs) are typically avoided because they may be dangerous in patients with erratic eating patterns and nutritional instability because of bingeing and purging. Similarly, bupropion (Wellbutrin) is contraindicated in patients with bulimia nervosa because of an increased risk of seizures.

Notably, the mechanism of action in the utility of antidepressant medication in reducing bulimic behaviors is unclear. Antidepressants seem to be equally effective in patients without depressive co-morbidity, arguing against an antidepressant effect. Given the role of serotonin in appetite regulation, it has been hypothesized that certain antidepressants may act on serotonin to reduce bingeing behaviors. Additionally, several other medications have been examined in patients with bulimia nervosa demonstrating moderate efficacy, including the opiate antagonist naltrexone (ReVia),[1] and the anticonvulsant Topiramate (Topamax).[1]

There is also some indication that anxiolytic and sleep medications may also be useful for patients with bulimia nervosa.

Thus psychotropic medications, particularly antidepressants, can be helpful for patients with bulimia nervosa, but they are typically less effective than cognitive behavioral therapy. Further, there is some indication that medication in combination with psychotherapy confers an advantage, but this finding is not consistent. Similar to the psychotherapy literature, however, clinical trials including adolescent patients are limited and the applicability of these findings to younger patients is unclear.

## Adjunctive Treatments

A medical assessment is indicated in patients with bulimia nervosa, and ongoing medical management may be useful particularly to treat patients with complications or those discontinuing laxative and/or diuretic abuse. Nutritional counseling may also be helpful to provide additional structure, support, and education for patients who have difficulty meal planning and regulating their eating. Nutritional psychoeducation is often a component of psychotherapy (e.g., CBT), but additional support may be needed for some patients. Additionally, supportive group therapy can be useful for some patients, particularly in helping them feel less isolated by interacting with that others who experience similar feelings and symptoms.

## Impact of Co-Morbidity on Treatment

The role of psychiatric co-morbidity in the treatment of bulimia nervosa is unclear. Generally, improvement of bulimic symptoms is associated with an improvement in mood and anxiety, but further treatment to target co-morbidity is often warranted. Pharmacologic intervention studies indicate that antidepressants improve mood in patients with bulimia who are depressed in addition to targeting bulimic symptoms.

## Course and Outcome

The longitudinal course of bulimia nervosa is variable but can be chronic and relapsing. Long-term follow-up studies suggest that 50% to 75% of patients with bulimia nervosa will achieve full recovery from their eating disorder, but approximately 33% of them will go on to relapse. A small minority of patients seem to present with chronic bulimia nervosa. It appears that a longer duration of illness, history of unsuccessful treatment attempts, co-morbid substance abuse, and cluster B personality disorders are predictive of a worse outcome for patients with bulimia nervosa.

 **CURRENT DIAGNOSIS**

- *DSM-IV* defines bulimia nervosa on the basis of binge/compensatory behaviors and associated maladaptive cognitions.
- Binge eating is defined as the consumption of an objectively large amount of food within a discrete period of time accompanied by uncontrolled overeating.
- Compensatory behaviors include purging (self-induced vomiting, misuse of laxatives, diuretics, enemas) and nonpurging (excessive exercise, fasting).
- Binge/compensatory behaviors must occur on average twice weekly over a 3-month period.
- Cognitive component of overvaluation of weight and shape on sense of self.
- Differential diagnosis must consider medical and psychiatric conditions.

*Abbreviations: DSM-IV = Diagnostic and Statistical Manual of Mental Disorders, Fourth Edition.*

---

[1]Not FDA approved for this indication.

## CURRENT THERAPY

- Goals of treatment for bulimia nervosa are to reduce and eliminate binge/compensatory behaviors, modify maladaptive eating- and body-related cognitions, and improve coping skills.
- Psychotherapy is considered first-line treatment. Psychotherapies receiving empirical support for the treatment of bulimia nervosa include CBT and IPT. Additional promising treatments include integrative psychotherapy approaches and family psychotherapy.
- Pharmacotherapy can also be helpful in targeting bulimic symptoms. Antidepressants have received the most empirical support. Fluoxetine (Prozac) at 60 mg qd is the only medication currently approved by the FDA in the treatment.
- CBT and IPT are effective in achieving reductions in binge/compensatory behaviors for the majority of patients and recovery in approximately 50% of patients. Antidepressant therapy leads to reductions in binge/compensatory behaviors for half of patients and recovery in approximately 30% of patients.
- Additional treatment research is warranted to address bulimic symptoms in the considerable subset of patients who remain ill following treatment.

*Abbreviations:* CBT = cognitive behavioral therapy; FDA = Food and Drug Administration; IPT = interpersonal psychotherapy.

Currently, viable psychosocial and pharmacologic treatments exist for the treatment of bulimia nervosa. Psychosocial approaches, particularly cognitive behavioral therapy, lead to substantial improvement in the majority of patients. Antidepressant therapy may also be useful for a subset of patients, but alone it does not seem to be as effective as psychotherapy. Self-help and guided self-help approaches with a cognitive behavioral focus may also be helpful for patients who have difficulty accessing care. Although these psychosocial and psychopharmacologic treatments are promising and helpful for most patients, approximately 50% of patients do not achieve full recovery even following treatment. Additional treatment research with adolescent and adults patients is needed.

## REFERENCES

Agras WS, Walsh T, Fairburn CG, et al: A multicenter comparison of cognitive-behavioral therapy and interpersonal psychotherapy for bulimia nervosa. Arch Gen Psychiatry 2000;57(5):459-466.
Apple RF: Interpersonal therapy for bulimia nervosa. J Clin Psychol 1999;55:715-725.
Casper RC: How useful are pharmacological treatments in eating disorders? Psychopharmacol Bull 2002;36(2):88-104.
Fairburn CG, Cooper Z, Shafran R: Cognitive behaviour therapy for eating disorders: A "transdiagnostic" theory and treatment. Behav Res Ther 2003;41(5):509-528.
Fairburn CG, Marcus MD, Wilson GT: Cognitive-behavioral therapy for binge eating and bulimia nervosa: A comprehensive treatment manual. In Fairburn CG, Wilson GT (eds): Binge Eating: Nature, Assessment, and Treatment. New York, Guilford, 1993.
Fairburn CG, Wilson GT (eds): Binge eating: Nature, assessment and treatment. New York, Guilford Press, 1993, pp 361-404.
Kotler LA, Walsh BT: Eating disorders in children and adolescents: Pharmacological therapies. Eur Child Adolesc Psychiatry 2000; 9(Suppl 1):I108-I1016.
Le Grange D, Crosby RD, Rathouz PJ, et al: A randomized controlled comparison of family-based treatment and supportive psychotherapy for adolescent bulimia nervosa. Arch Gen Psychiatry 2007; 64(9):1049-1056.
Le Grange D, Lock, J: Treating bulimia in adolescents. Guilford Press, New York, 2007.
Mitchell JE, de Zwaan M, Roerig JL: Drug therapy for patients with eating disorders. Curr Drug Targets CNS Neurol Disord 2003;2(1):17-29.
Peterson CB, Mitchell JE: Psychosocial and pharmacological treatment of eating disorders: A review of research findings. J Clin Psychol 1999; 55:685-697.
Schmidt U, Lee S, Beecham J, et al: A randomized controlled trial of family therapy and cognitive behavior therapy guided self-care for adolescents with bulimia nervosa and related disorders. Am J Psychiatry 2007;164:591-598.
Shapiro JR, Berkman ND, Brownley KA, et al: Bulimia nervosa treatment: A systematic review of randomized controlled trials. Intl J Eat Disord 2007;40:321-336.
Steffen KJ, Roerig JL, Mitchell JE, et al: Emerging drugs for eating disorder treatment. Expert Opin Emerg Drugs 2006;11:315-336.
Thompson-Brenner H, Westen D, Glass S: A multidimensional meta-analysis of psychotherapy for bulimia nervosa. Clin Psychol Rev 2003; 10:269-287.
Wilson GT, Fairburn CC, Agras WS, et al: Cognitive-behavioral therapy for bulimia nervosa: Time course and mechanisms of change. J Consult Clin Psychol 2002;70:267-274.

# Delirium

Method of
*Soenke Boettger, MD*

Delirium is a neuropsychiatric syndrome characterized by the abrupt onset of changes in consciousness, attention, cognition, and perception, which tend to fluctuate throughout the day and have an underlying physiologic etiology. Delirium is recognized as a medical condition where psychiatrists have a prominent role in treatment given their expertise in using antipsychotic medications and their familiarity with other conditions that resemble delirium. Subtypes of delirium specified by the *Diagnostic and Statistical Manual of Mental Disorders*, fourth edition (text revision) (DSM-IV TR) include delirium resulting from a general medical condition, substance intoxication, substance withdrawal, and multifactorial etiologies (Box 1). Delirium can be further classified as hyperactive (or hyperdynamic) and hypoactive (or hypodynamic.) Other terms used for delirium are *acute confusional state*, *encephalopathy*, and *organic brain syndrome*. Although delirium is a transient state and may be self-resolving, its recognition and management are of utmost importance to minimize patient distress, reduce caregiver burden, and mitigate complications, including hospitalization.

---

### BOX 1 DSM-IV Criteria for Delirium (Modified)

- Disturbance of consciousness (i.e., reduced clarity of awareness of the environment) with reduced ability to focus, sustain, or shift attention
- Change in cognition (e.g., memory deficit, disorientation, language disturbance, or perceptual disturbance) that is not better accounted for by a preexisting, established, or evolving dementia
- The disturbance develops over a short time (usually hours to days) and tends to *fluctuate* during the course of the day
- Delirium due to general medical condition
- Delirium due to substance intoxication
- Delirium due to substance withdrawal
- Delirium due to multiple etiologies

*Abbreviation:* DSM-IV TR = *Diagnostic and Statistical Manual of Mental Disorders*, fourth edition (text revision).

## BOX 2 Predisposing Factors in Delirium

**General**
- Alcoholism
- Male sex
- Older age
- Severity of physical illness

**Cardiopulmonary**
- Anemia
- Arrhythmia
- Myocardial infarction
- Respiratory failure

**Central Nervous System**
- Cerebrovascular disease and stroke
- Head trauma
- Presence and severity of dementia and degenerative disease
- Primary brain tumor or metastatic spread to CNS

**Metabolic**
- Dehydration
- Hepatic and renal impairment
- Hypoalbuminemia
- Metabolic abnormalities
- Nutritional deficiencies

**Systemic**
- Hematologic abnormalities
- Infection
- Neoplasm

**Other**
- Functional dependence and immobility
- Hip fracture
- Visual impairment

*Abbreviation:* CNS = central nervous system.

## BOX 3 Precipitating Factors in Delirium

**General**
- High number of hospital procedures
- Intensive care unit admission
- Severe, acute illness

**Cardiopulmonary**
- Cardiac surgery
- Hypoxia
- Myocardial infarction
- Pneumonia
- Shock

**Central Nervous System**
- Bleeding
- Narcotics
- Seizures
- Stroke

**Metabolic**
- Acid-base disturbances
- Dehydration
- Endocrinopathies
- Hyponatremia, hypercalcemia, and other electrolyte imbalances

**Systemic**
- Urinary tract infection
- Other infections

**Other**
- Drugs of abuse
- Medications
- Noncardiac surgery
- Orthopedic surgery
- Pain
- Physical restraint

## Epidemiology and Etiology

Due to its diverse etiology, the incidence and prevalence of delirium vary from 1% in the community to as much as 80% in the severely ill population. Predisposing factors are those that increase a patient's risk of developing delirium; precipitating factors are those that trigger delirium.

Advanced age and premorbid brain function may be the most important predisposing factors for developing delirium (see Box 2 for predisposing factors of delirium). Particularly in the elderly population, the treatment of delirium should be pursued aggressively due to prolonged hospitalization, increased morbidity and mortality, and risk of cognitive decline. Precipitating factors for developing delirium include acute and chronic illness, medications (especially polypharmacy, which is common in the elderly or severely ill), and drugs of abuse whether the patient is in a state of intoxication or withdrawal.

Boxes 3 and 4, respectively, list medical conditions and medications known to trigger delirium. Table 1 lists select medications in managing delirium.

## Pathophysiology

The current pathophysiologic model for delirium developed by Trzepacz implies an imbalance in the neurotransmitters acetylcholine and dopamine. The acetylcholine level is reduced, as seen in the prototypic anticholinergic delirium, but dopamine levels may be elevated (seen in delirium with stimulating agents) or reduced (seen in hypoactive delirium, which can improve through the use of dopaminergic agents alone.) The deficit in anticholinergic transmission explains why the elderly are predisposed to develop delirium because these patients have reduced acetylcholine function at baseline. Through brain imaging and lesion studies, areas in the right hemisphere have been implicated in a common final pathway of delirium.

Delirium caused by alcohol withdrawal has as its pathophysiology an imbalance in γ-aminobutyric acid (GABA)-ergic and glutamatergic transmission; treatment (essential to reduce mortality associated with delirium tremens) differs accordingly (Figure 1).

## Diagnosis

The diagnosis of delirium is made by evaluating a patient in light of DSM-IV TR criteria. Delirium represents an acute change in mental status, specifically level of consciousness and cognitive ability. The patient presents with disturbances in arousal and awareness, abrupt cognitive changes such as decreased attention, concentration, and memory, as well as hallucinations and delusions, sleep-wake cycle disturbances, psychomotor changes like apathy or agitation, and mood changes resembling anxiety and depression. Hallucinations are more often visual rather than auditory. Tactile hallucinations are often associated with substance intoxication and withdrawal. Screening for abrupt, unexpected changes in mental status, cooperation, and behavior is the first step toward an accurate diagnosis of delirium.

## BOX 4 Medications that Can Cause Delirium

**Medications with High Anticholinergic Activity**

**Analgesics**
- Codeine, Dipyridamole (Persantine)
- Prednisone (Deltasone)
- Theophylline (Uniphyl)

**H₂-Receptor Antagonists**
- Cimetidine (Tagamet)
- Ranitidine (Zantac)

**Heart Disease Medications**
- Captopril (Capoten)
- Digoxin (Lanoxin)
- Furosemide (Lasix)
- Isosorbide dinitrate (Isordil)
- Nifedipine (Adalat)
- Triamterene with thiazide (Dyazide)
- Warfarin (Coumadin)

**Psychotropic Medications**
- Antipsychotics (e.g., chlorpromazine [Thorazine])
- Benztropine (Cogentin)
- Biperiden (Akineton)
- Tricyclic antidepressants
- Trihexyphenidyl (Artane)

**Other Medications Associated with Delirium**
- Antibiotics
- Antiparkinsonian agents (e.g., L-dopa)
- Benzodiazepines
- Laxatives
- Narcotics
- Nonsteroidal anti-inflammatory drugs

**Over-the-Counter Medications**
- Antidiarrheal agents (containing belladonna)
- Chlorpheniramine (e.g., Piriton)
- Diphenhydramine (e.g., Benadryl)
- Irritable bowel syndrome treatments with hyoscine (e.g., Buscopan)
- Promethazine (Phenergan)

## TABLE 1 Select Medications In Managing Delirium

| Drug | Approximate Daily Dosage Range | Route |
|---|---|---|
| **Neuroleptics** | | |
| Chlorpromazine (Thorazine)[1] | 12.5-50 mg eq4-12h | PO, IV, IM |
| Haloperidol (Haldol)[1] | 0.5-5 mg q2-12h | PO, IV, SC, IM |
| **Atypical Neuroleptics** | | |
| Aripiprazole (Abilify)[1] | 5-30 mg q24h | PO |
| Olanzapine (Zyprexa)[1] | 2.5-20 mg q12-24h | PO |
| Quetiapine (Seroquel)[1] | 12.5-200 mg q6-24h | PO |
| Risperidone (Risperdal)[1] | 0.5-3 mg q12-24h | PO |
| Ziprasidone (Geodon)[1] | 10-80 mg q12-24h | PO, IM |
| **Benzodiazepines** | | |
| Diazepam (Valium)[1] | 2-10 mg q4-6h | PO, IV, IM |
| Lorazepam (Ativan)[1] | 0.5-2.0 mg q1-4h | PO, IV, IM |
| **Barbiturates (for alcohol withdrawal *only*)** | | |
| Phenobarbital[1] | 30-60 mg q4-6h | PO |

[1]Not FDA approved for this indication.
*Maximum IM dose is 40 mg/d.

accurate diagnosis of delirium. Unfortunately, delirium continues to be underdiagnosed and undertreated.

## Treatment

The delirious patient may harm him/herself or others through agitation or combativeness. Such harm may arise through pulling out lines, falls from bed, and interruption of medical treatment. Patient safety is ensured by treatment of delirium through both pharmacologic and nonpharmacologic approaches. The most important step in treatment is to identify and eliminate, where possible, precipitating factors. Interventions include a thorough physical examination and comprehensive analysis of blood (including ammonia), urine, perhaps CSF, to rule out infection (UTI, pneumonia) and electrolyte and metabolic abnormalities. Infections must be treated and other abnormalities corrected. EEG and brain imaging may be needed if no causes are found by the preceding. In some cases, the etiology of delirium may not be clearly identified; in others, the cause may be apparent but not correctable; in still others, there may be several causes working at once. In any event, active treatment is needed to protect the patient and caregivers. Nonpharmacologic approaches include providing a safe, consistent environment with frequent reorientation by caregivers, if necessary the use of a companion. A low threshold should be maintained with regard to the use of pharmacologic approaches, which include mostly neuroleptics, occasionally benzodiazepines, and rarely cholinergics, depending on the nature of delirium. The prototypic anticholinergic delirium should be treated primarily with cholinergics such as physostigmine and acetylcholinesterase inhibitors; neuroleptics may be indicated in treatment-refractory cases or where there is a significant behavioral disturbance. Delirium due to medical conditions is generally best treated with neuroleptics with or without adjunctive benzodiazepines. Benzodiazepines alone are usually contraindicated due to their hypnotic and amnestic properties; their use may worsen delirium. Delirium associated with substance intoxication should be treated by discontinuing (often tapering) the substance and controlling symptoms with neuroleptics and benzodiazepines. It is essential to monitor

## Differential Diagnosis

The differential diagnosis of delirium includes dementia, depression, anxiety, mania, intoxication, and psychosis, given the overlap in symptoms delirium shares with these maladies. Most challenging is distinguishing delirium from dementia as both disorders present with cognitive changes. In both disorders anticholinergic transmission is reduced. Both disorders have a high degree of comorbidity. Whereas dementia develops slowly in a relatively stable (or stepwise) process, delirium is characterized by an abrupt onset, often within 24 hours, and fluctuations within its course. Delirium involves a disturbance of consciousness, something generally not seen in dementia. It is, of course, possible for delirium to be superimposed on dementia. Anxiety, depression, mania, and psychosis may resemble delirium as the latter may involve changes in affect and behavior and the presence of hallucinations and delusions. The former may be distinguished by the absence of disturbances in consciousness, the lack of impaired cognition, and the nature of symptom onset. Delirium caused by substance intoxication and withdrawal should be also differentiated as a different course of treatment is indicated. Delirium due to substance intoxication and withdrawal involves vital sign changes such as tachycardia and hypertension. Thorough history taking, good clinical observation, and the search for precipitating factors are the keys to the

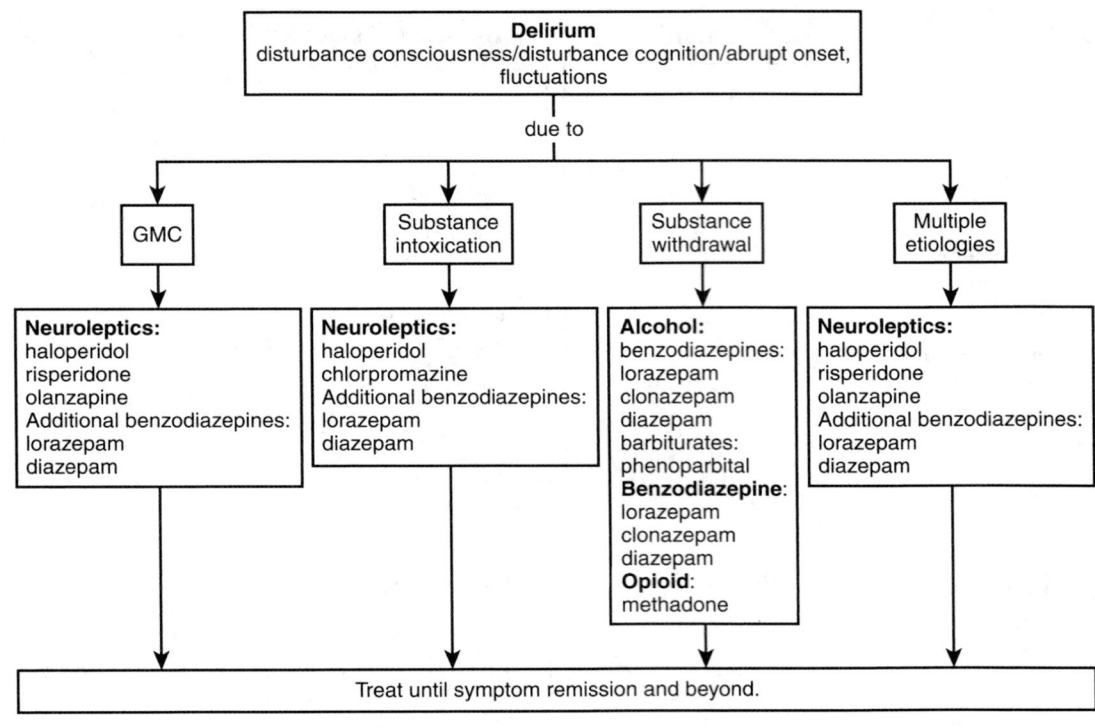

**FIGURE 1.** Treatment algorithm for delirium. *Abbreviation:* GMC = general medical condition.

for and treat withdrawal in a chemically dependent patient. Delirium due to substance withdrawal usually requires substitution of the used substance with a cross-tolerant medication. Frequent monitoring of vital signs provides information as to the state of withdrawal. Alcohol withdrawal, which has a risk of mortality if it proceeds to delirium tremens, requires generous use of GABA-ergic agents such as benzodiazepines and barbiturates. The use of neuroleptics adjunctively may be helpful, but treatment with neuroleptics alone increases mortality in cases of DT. Multifactorial delirium or delirium with unclear etiology should be treated with neuroleptics and adjunctive benzodiazepines similarly to the delirium due to general medical condition.

The "gold standard" neuroleptic for the treatment of delirium is haloperidol (Haldol),[1] even in light of the risk of acute dystonia, pseudo parkinsonism, akathisia, and tardive dyskinesia associated with all first-generation neuroleptics, regardless of dose or duration. So called "atypical" neuroleptics have been broadly used in the treatment of delirium with good results and a lower incidence of side effects. Risperidone (Risperdal) [1] and olanzapine (Zyprexa)[1] are examples of newer agents for which studies exist demonstrating efficacy. Such use is "off label" however, and there is remote controversy over a possible increased risk of cerebrovascular events, which should not prevent their use. Other agents in this class include quetiapine (Seroquel),[1] ziprasidone (Geodon),[1] and aripiprazole (Abilify).[1] Both olanzapine and quetiapine are more sedating than risperidone, ziprasidone, and aripiprazole; this favorable side effect profile may be advantageous in the agitated delirious patient. None of the atypical neuroleptics currently comes in an intravenous application, thus making the use of haloperidol[1] (or chlorpromazine[1] when haloperidol fails) necessary. All neuroleptics (and many other agents) can prolong QTc interval and a baseline and repeat EKG are recommended. Other less studied adjunctive interventions in the treatment of hypoactive delirium due to general medical condition or multifactorial delirium are the use of dopaminergic agents (such as methylphenidate (Ritalin)[1]) and cholinergic agents (acetylcholinesterase inhibitors).

## Course and Prognosis

Delirium is often a transient self-resolving state, thus symptoms may clear with monitoring only and no further intervention. The elimination of underlying etiologic factors may be sufficient to promote resolution; at times, however, this is impossible and pharmacologic treatment should be initiated. Once pharmacologic treatment has been started, symptoms often resolve in the first 48 to 72 hours; treatment should be continued for up to one week to prevent recurrence of symptoms. In the younger population, delirium is usually a transient state with no residual effects. In the older population, delirium can contribute to unnecessary suffering, increased morbidity and mortality, and yield persistent cognitive deficits, which may interfere with independent living. In alcohol withdrawal, the mortality associated with delirium tremens represents the greatest threat to the patient's life; alcohol withdrawal must be treated appropriately. Following a case of DT, there may be minor brain damage in the form of excitotoxicity. Additionally, the risk of subsequent DT is increased.

If correctly recognized, diagnosed, and treated, delirium is a manageable, reversible condition with no or few long-term effects. In many settings however, delirium remains underdiagnosed and under-treated, inflicting unnecessary suffering and complications on the individual patient. Thus, improving the recognition and treatment of delirium will contribute to better medical care for the patient, caregivers, and medical staff.

## REFERENCES

American Psychiatric Association: Diagnostic and Statistical Manual of Mental Disorders, 4th ed. Washington, DC: American Psychiatric Association, 1994, pp 124-127.

Boettger S, Breitbart W: Atypical antipsychotics in the management of delirium: A review of the empirical literature. Palliat Support Care 2005;3(3):227-237.

Boettger S, Friedlander M, Breitbart W: Delirium. In Blumenfeld M, Strain J (eds): Textbook of Psychosomatic Medicine. Philadelphia: Lippincott Williams & Wilkins 2006, pp 493-512.

Breitbart W, Marotta R, Platt MM, et al: A double-blind trial of haloperidol, chlorpromazine, and lorazepam in the treatment of delirium in hospitalized AIDS patients. Am J Psychiatry 1996;153(2):231-237.

---

[1]Not FDA approved for this indication.

Bucht G, Gustafson Y, Sandberg O: Epidemiology of delirium. Dement Geriatr Cogn Disord 1999;10(5):315-318.

Inouye SK: Delirium in hospitalized older patients: Recognition and risk factors. J Geriatr Psychiatry Neurol 1998;11(3):118-125.

Inouye SK, Bogardus ST Jr, Charpentier PA, et al: A multicomponent intervention to prevent delirium in hospitalized older patients. N Engl J Med 1999;340(9):669-676.

Inouye SK, Charpentier PA: Precipitating factors for delirium in hospitalized elderly persons: Predictive model and interrelationship with baseline vulnerability. JAMA 1996;20;275(11):852-857.

Karlsson I: Drugs that induce delirium. Dement Geriatr Cogn Disord 1999;10(5):412-415.

Lipowski ZJ: Delirium (acute confusional states). JAMA 1987;258(13): 1789-1792.

Rockwood K, Cosway S, Carver D, et al: The risk of dementia and death after delirium. Age Ageing 1999;28(6):551-556.

Trzepacz PT: Update on the neuropathogenesis of delirium. Dement Geriatr Cogn Disord 1999;10(5):330-334.

Trzepacz PT, Breitbart W, Franklin J, et al: Practice guideline for the treatment of patients with delirium. American Psychiatric Association. Am J Psychiatry 1999;156(5 Suppl):1-20.

Tune LE: Serum anticholinergic activity levels and delirium in the elderly. Semin Clin Neuropsychiatry 2000;5(2):149-153.

# Mood Disorders

Method of
*Melanie W. Conway, MD,*
*and Merry N. Miller, MD*

Mood disorders are common. Depressed mood is the fourth most common presenting complaint in a primary care setting. Approximately 1 of 10 patients seen by a primary care physician has a major depressive disorder (MDD), with a 10% to 25% lifetime prevalence for women and a 5% to 12% lifetime prevalence for men. Prevalence for bipolar disorder ranges from 1% to 5%. Mood disorders worsen the morbidity and mortality rates of other medical disorders, and in fact, 68% of so-called service overutilizers of medical care have had a major depression diagnosis. Moreover, up to 15% of people with untreated depression kill themselves. Because nonpsychiatrists prescribe 80% of antidepressants, it is essential that the primary care physician be acquainted with the diagnosis and treatment of mood disorders.

## Diagnosing Mood Disorders

As stated previously, mood disorders are very common, have high morbidity and mortality rates, and are highly treatable, but studies show that only a third to a half of those with major depressive episodes are properly recognized by practitioners, and fewer than a third of patients with bipolar disorder are in treatment. One reason might be that although mood disorders are not transitory reactions to external stressors, 70% of those who have a major depression could cite a stressor that preceded their depressive episode. A common occurrence is that both the patient and the physician focus on the stressor. This focus on the stressor generally elicits an internalized reaction from the physician, for example, "That is not bad enough to get depressed about," or conversely, "If that were happening, I would be depressed, too"; both of these reactions decrease the probability that the physician will elicit depressive symptomatology and treat a possible mood disorder.

Also, many patients do not tell the physician that they are "depressed." In fact, a lot of men use the words "stressed out." Children and adolescents may commonly present with behavioral disturbances, and the elderly (65 years and older) with somatic complaints.

So key words that might clue the physician into a mood disorder are "irritated," "short fused," "stressed," "not acting right," "not myself," "don't care," "no energy," "can't think, focus, or concentrate," or a plethora of vague physical complaints.

Table 1 summarizes the diagnostic criteria, and a decision-making algorithm can be followed as presented in Figure 1. First, the physician suspecting depression should ask about depressed mood and/or decreased interests and SIGECAPS (**S**leep, **I**nterest, **G**uilt, **E**nergy, **C**oncentration, **A**ppetite, **P**sychomotor, **S**uicide*). Primary care physicians should routinely ask about sleep and appetite and consider depression when these are altered: With depression these may change in either direction, although it is more common for depressed patients to report decreased sleep and appetite. In addition, depressed patients report decreased interests (ability to enjoy usual activities, changes in energy (usually decreased), and difficulty concentrating. The latter symptom may cause the patient to develop problems with short-term memory, and it is not unusual for depressed patients to fear they are losing their mind or becoming demented owing to difficulty concentrating and remembering. They may show psychomotor slowing or alternatively, they may become agitated. Most seriously, patients with depression may develop suicidal ideation. They also may experience feelings of guilt about real or imagined sins, and may become preoccupied with feelings of worthlessness.

The physician must first address the management of any potential suicidal risk (see later discussion of suicide). Then the physician

---

*Carey Gross, MD, originally developed this mnemonic for depression.

---

## TABLE 1 Diagnostic Criteria for Depressive and Manic Episodes

| Major Depressive Episode | Manic Episode |
|---|---|
| Five or more of the following symptoms present most of the time for 2 weeks:<br>■ Depressed or irritable mood*<br>■ Diminished interest or pleasure (anhedonia)*<br>■ Disturbance of appetite<br>■ Insomnia or hypersomia<br>■ Psychomotor agitation or retardation<br>■ Fatigue or loss of energy<br>■ Feelings of worthlessness or guilt<br>■ Diminished ability to concentrate<br>■ Recurrent thoughts of death/suicidal ideation/suicide attempt | At least 3 (or 4 if mood is only irritable) of the following symptoms for at least a 1-wk period or any duration if hospitalization required:<br>■ Elevated, expansive, or irritable mood*<br>■ Inflated self-esteem or grandiosity<br>■ Decreased need for sleep<br>■ Hyperverbal<br>■ Racing thoughts/flight of ideas<br>■ Distractibility<br>■ Increased activity or psychomotor agitation<br>■ Excessive involvement with pleasurable activities with risk for painful consequences |

*For a major depressive episode diagnosis, the symptom for either depressed mood or anhedonia must be present. For a manic episode diagnosis, the altered mood symptom must be present.

## CURRENT DIAGNOSIS

- Look for symptoms (SIGECAPS) in patients with suspected depression regardless of the presence of stressors.
- Always screen for a history of mania in patients who present for depression.
- Always ask about suicidality, including the presence of thoughts, specific plans, intent, and a history of attempts.
- Be prepared to hospitalize, including involuntarily, if patients are actively suicidal.
- Look for medical conditions and medications that may precipitate or worsen depression.
- Check T4, TSH, and CBC in all patients with mood symptoms if not recently done.
- Always ask about use of alcohol and illicit drugs in patients presenting with depression.

*Abbreviations:* CBC = complete blood count; SIGECAPS = **S**leep, **I**nterest, **G**uilt, **E**nergy, **C**oncentration, **A**ppetite, **P**sychomotor, **S**uicide; T4 = thyroxine; TSH = thyroid-stimulating hormone.

answers this question: "Does this patient have depressed mood or loss of interests or pleasure in usual activities with four other neurovegetative symptoms most of the day, nearly every day, for at least 2 weeks or not?" If the answer is yes, the patient has a major depression regardless of the presence or absence of stressors.

If instead a patient reports a recent stressor but does not meet the full criteria for a major depression, the patient has an adjustment disorder. This distinction is important because first-line treatment recommendations differ between an adjustment disorder and MDD.

If a person is determined to have a major depressive episode, it is incumbent on the physician to ask about manic symptoms as well because the prevalence of bipolar disorder is now thought to be higher than previously documented. Antidepressants alone in a depressed patient with bipolar disorder can switch them into a mania even if they were never manic before. Useful screening questions include, "Have you ever felt the opposite of what you do now, like on top of the world?" or "Have you ever had a period in which you felt you did not need sleep, or very little sleep, and still had plenty of energy?" If they answer yes, then the rest of the mania answers can be elicited with the useful mnemonic DIGFAST (**D**istractibility, **I**nsomnia, **G**randiosity, **F**light of ideas, **A**ctivities, **S**peech, **T**houghtfulness*).

However, a word of caution: mania is very difficult to diagnose accurately retrospectively. It would not be difficult to get affirmative

*William Falk, MD, originally developed this mnemonic for mania.

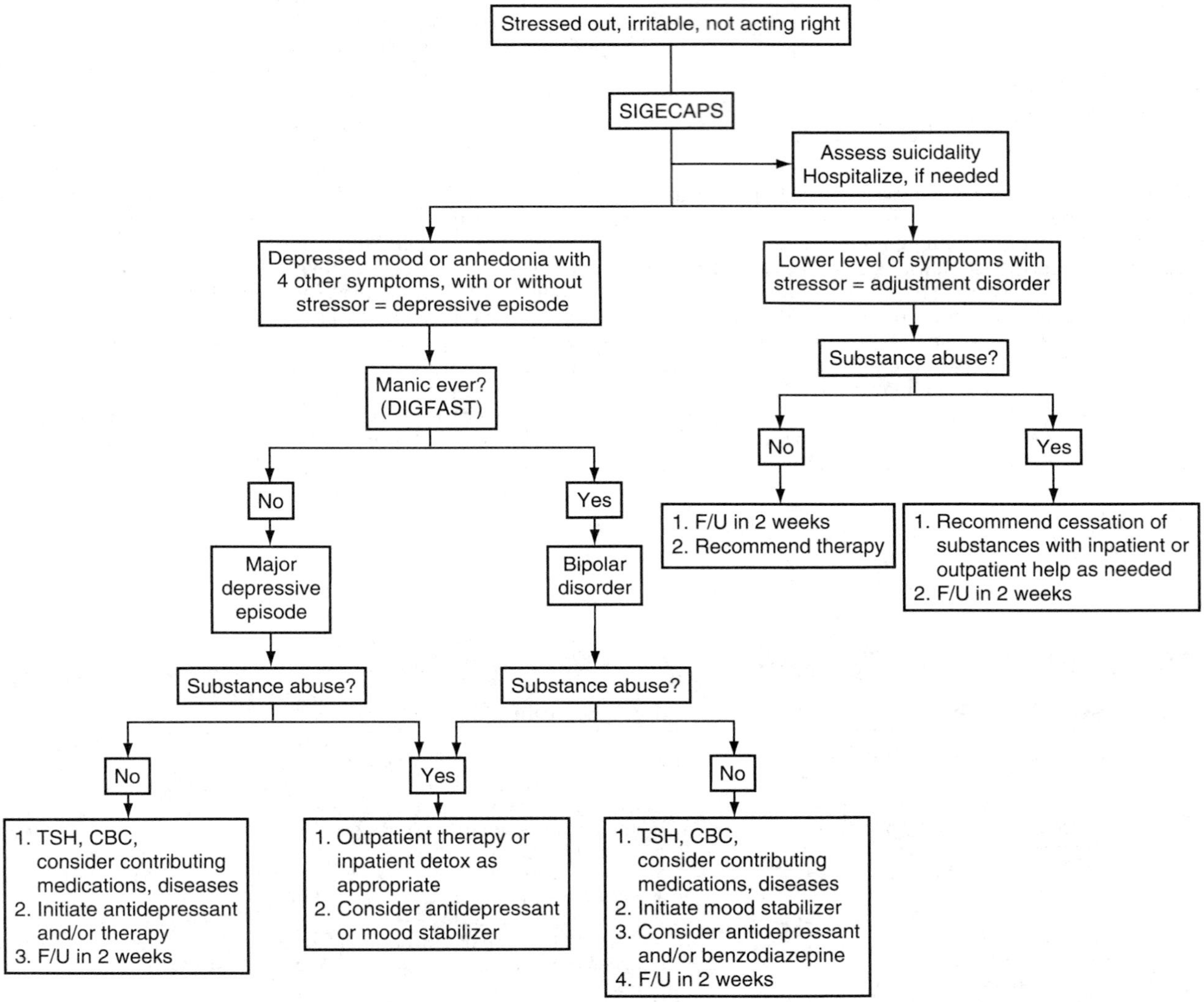

**FIGURE 1.** Basic algorithm for diagnosis and treatment of mood disorders. *Abbreviations:* CBC = complete blood count; DIGFAST = **D**istractibility, **I**nsomnia, **G**randiosity, **F**light of ideas, **A**ctivities, **S**peech, **T**houghtfulness; F/U = follow up; SIGECAPS = **S**leep, **I**nterest, **G**uilt, **E**nergy, **C**oncentration, **A**ppetite, **P**sychomotor, **S**uicide; TSH = thyroid-stimulating hormone.

answers to such questions as "Have you ever spent more money than usual?" or "Have you ever had more energy than usual?" from most people asked the questions in the mania criteria. By definition (according to the *Diagnostic and Statistical Manual of Mental Disorders, Fourth Edition [DSM-IV]*), a mania has to be a distinctly different period than normal where "the mood disturbance is sufficiently severe to cause marked impairment in occupational functioning or in usual social activities or relationships with others" that must last at least 1 week (less if hospitalized) or with a hypomanic episode last at least 4 days and be "an unequivocal change in functioning that is uncharacteristic of the person when not symptomatic." The symptoms should occur together in the same 1-week period. Sometimes a severely depressed person answers yes to mania symptomatology when describing not a mania, but rather a baseline level of functioning as compared to the depression. The distinction is important because of its implications about treatment (see treatment discussion).

Other depressive disorders that should be screened for are dysthymic disorder and premenstrual dysphoric disorder (PMDD). In dysthymic disorder, patients have a chronic low-grade level of depression (not enough to qualify for MDD) that exists for more than 2 years. Women with PMDD experience depressive symptoms that occur exclusively during the premenstrual portion of the menstrual cycle and then resolve after the onset of menses. Another variation of depression is premenstrual exacerbation of depression in which women with MDD experience worsening of the mood premenstrually that does not fully resolve with the onset of menses. These variations of depressive disorder may be treated with antidepressants, and PMDD responds to intermittent dosing (i.e., only during the premenstrual phase). A diagnostic and treatment review of other types of mood disorders is beyond the scope of this chapter.

## SUICIDE

If you are considering a diagnosis of a mood disorder, and especially if you prescribe medications for a mood disorder, you must *always* ask about suicide because two thirds of all depressed patients contemplate suicide at some point. Studies show that 50% of all people who commit suicide see their primary care physician within 1 month of the suicide and 40% within 1 week of the suicide.

Suicidal ideation, just like radiating chest pain, is a medical emergency and should be treated as such, especially when being presented to the physician the first time. Critical considerations that increase the level of risk are these: (1) Does the patient have a plan and means? How lethal is the plan? (Gunshots and hanging are the most lethal and most concerning plans.) Has the patient considered acting on the plan? (2) History of suicide attempts: Were high-risk methods used in the past, and how likely was the patient to be rescued? (3) Lack of social supports or recent losses (e.g., job, relationships); (4) Chronic medical illnesses; (5) Substances abuse, especially in the intoxicated or withdrawal state.

Consulting with a family member, with the patient's consent, is a very good way not only to elicit information but also to garner needed social support should the decision be made to treat the patient on an outpatient basis or to support an inpatient recommendation.

If the physician does not consider the patient's risk to be imminent and the decision is made to continue treatment on an outpatient basis, a psychiatric referral should be made and the physician should see the patient often; at least until the patient is seen by the psychiatrist. Contracting for safety with the patient has some psychological value, although doing so grants no legal protection to the physician.

In every area of the United States there is the equivalent of a mobile response team with a psychiatric backup that can be called in case no psychiatrist is available for consultation or if the patient or the patient's family is against an inpatient recommendation and you are very concerned about suicide risk. These telephone numbers should be readily available to the physician so during a time of crisis valuable time does not have to be spent searching for them.

Although there is some variation among the states, if the patient (and/or family) is unwilling for the patient to wait for the mobile crisis evaluation or go to the emergency department and the patient shows evidence of being dangerous to himself or others, he or she can be

## CURRENT THERAPY

- Choose an antidepressant based on how the side-effect profile fits with the symptoms of depression (e.g., a sedating medication for insomnia).
- Make sure to use an *adequate dose for an adequate duration* (at least 4–6 wk) before judging the effectiveness of an antidepressant.
- Watch for signs of antidepressant-induced switching to mania.
- If ineffective after an adequate trial, consider another antidepressant, possibly from another class.
- If still ineffective, consider augmentation of antidepressant with another class of medication; for example, lithium or thyroid hormone.
- For bipolar patients, start a mood stabilizer first. If the patient remains depressed, consider a possible antidepressant after the mood stabilizer dosage is therapeutic.
- When withdrawing antidepressants, taper the dose gradually to avoid the discontinuation syndrome.
- For patients with depression that does not respond to medication, consider electroconvulsive therapy (ECT).
- Always assess for suicidality throughout treatment for depression.

involuntarily committed. Every physician should know the commitment criteria for one's own state. If the patient's current symptoms meet these criteria, the police/security should be called to detain or apprehend the patient if necessary, and the patient should be held against his or her will until further evaluation by mobile crisis or an emergency department physician can be done. Although ideally rare, this set of events often garners extreme emotions and occasionally litigious threats. Most patients later are able to appreciate the concern that led to their hospitalization. Legal precedent tends to fall in favor of the physician who acted with due diligence rather than the physician whose patient was let go who went on to kill themselves. Regardless of the in/outpatient status of the patient, careful documentation of the symptoms, decision-making process, and plan is essential.

## MEDICAL CONDITIONS AND DRUGS ASSOCIATED WITH MOOD DISORDERS

Fifty percent of those with psychiatric illness also have substance abuse problems. Substance use alone could cause mood disorders such as depression in chronic ethanol, benzodiazepine, barbiturate, and opiate use, cocaine withdrawal, or mania in methamphetamine or cocaine intoxication. However, many times it is difficult to separate which came first, the substance abuse or the mood disorder. Useful questions are these: (1) When did the mood disorder symptoms start? When did the substance abuse start? (2) What has been your longest period of nonuse of any alcohol or illicit substances (drugs)? During that time (especially if it was more than 1 year), how was your mood?

Many prescribed substances can also evoke mood symptoms such as anesthetics, analgesics, anticholinergics, anticonvulsants, antihypertensives, antiparkinsonian medications, antiulcer medications, cardiac medications (especially β-adrenergic antagonists), isotretinoin (Accutane), oral contraceptives, muscle relaxants, anabolic steroids, corticosteroids, and sulfonamides. Heavy metals and toxins also can cause mood symptoms. This list is not exhaustive, and the patient's medication list always should be examined in search of temporal associations between newly prescribed agents and the onset or exacerbation of mood complaints.

Also, a long list of medical conditions can be associated with depression or mania, or a mood disorder can be the presenting symptom. The list is huge, but two deserve special mention. One medical condition is poststroke depression. At both 15-month and 10-year follow-ups, patients with poststroke major or minor depression are between four and eight times more likely to die than are nondepressed stroke patients. The second medical condition is cardiovascular disease. Even when one controls for smoking (depressed patients are more likely to smoke) and other factors, a large study showed that at 6 months, 17% of depressed patients had died versus 3% of the nondepressed patients. There was a 42% reduction in combined endpoint of death or recurrent myocardial infarction with antidepressant use.

## LABORATORY TESTS

Again, although the list of medical illnesses that can cause or exacerbate a depression is extensive, two of the most common illnesses etiologically related to mood disorders are thyroid disease and anemia. Either hypothyroidism or hyperthyroidism can be associated with depressive symptoms. Therefore, obtaining a thyroxine/thyroid-stimulating hormone (T4/TSH) and a complete blood count (CBC) are standard in a mood disorder workup. Other laboratory tests may be indicated based on the medication chosen (see Treatment section).

# Treatment

First, a physician must address any etiologic or contributing factors such as medical conditions or substance use. If substances are used, treatment for such must be addressed first because mood disorder symptoms may be related to their use alone, and even if mood disorder symptoms are primary (many substance abusers state they are "self-medicating"), the benefit of antidepressant or mood stabilizer pharmacotherapy will be reduced by continuing use. The standard used to be that clinicians waited to medicate until the patient had been sober many months, but recent studies show that pharmacotherapy does have a modest effect on abstinence rates.

For adjustment disorders, the recommended treatment is psychotherapy, and as with the other mood disorders, the patient is advised to return to see the physician within 2 weeks. At the later appointment, SIGECAPS should be reevaluated for progressing to a major depressive episode, and the recommendation for psychotherapy is repeated if necessary.

The majority of patients with major depressive episodes, whether of the unipolar or bipolar type, are best treated with a combination of psychotherapy and medication. Cognitive-behavioral therapy and interpersonal therapy is as effective as medication in mild to moderate depression. In addition to individual psychotherapy, group and marital and family therapy may be useful depending on the patient's circumstances. It may be best to delay the use of marital or family therapy in a depressed patient until some improvement begins to occur. Psychotherapy produces longer lasting benefits than medication. Many patients have an individual preference for either psychotherapy or medication or may have logistical difficulty in participating in therapy, so the treatment plan should be developed in conjunction with the patient with mindfulness of patient preference. If the patient should initially choose medication management alone and does not garner the full benefits he or she expected from an adequate trial of medication(s), psychotherapy should definitely be reconsidered.

## ANTIDEPRESSANTS

No particular antidepressant or class of antidepressants is more efficacious than the rest. However, effectiveness does differ because the older agents, tricyclic antidepressants (TCAs) and monoamine oxidase inhibitors (MAOIs), are less tolerable owing to side effects and lifestyle restrictions. Their use should not be ruled out because TCAs are generally inexpensive and are used to treat a variety of other medical conditions and MAOIs tend to work when other drugs have not.

Many factors need to be considered in picking an antidepressant, but there are three initial factors to consider in a treatment-naive patient. First, sleep-mood disorders do not get better if sleep does not improve, so, in treating someone who is not sleeping enough, one may consider a sedating antidepressant or a nonsedating one with a sleep agent.

In treating someone who is sleeping too much or is anergic, the physician may consider a stimulating antidepressant. Second, side effects are one of the most common reasons for treatment failure because of lack of compliance. Two of the most common side effect concerns tend to be gender linked. Women are more likely to stop a drug if they feel it is making them gain weight. Therefore, in general, it is best to avoid antidepressants with higher rates of weight gain in the weight-conscious patient. Men may be more likely to stop a drug secondary to sexual side effects. Although they initially may not care about this possible side effect secondary to their depressive state, 2 or 3 months later they tend to change their mind, putting the clinician in the precarious position of either changing the antidepressant and risking relapse of the depressed state or adding agents such as yohimbine (Yocon) or sildenafil (Viagra) to help counter the sexual side effects. The third factor is cost because a minimum recommended duration of antidepressant treatment is approximately 1 year (see Patient Education section), and patients will not take or continue to take what they cannot afford to buy. That is why the TCAs are still useful to consider in some populations because of reduced cost. It is important to know your patient's resources and your sample closet. Also, many pharmaceutical companies have programs for those in need.

In the recurrent mood disorder patient, it is essential to obtain a more detailed history of what antidepressants the patient has tried, the length of treatment, the maximum dose, and the patient's view of the helpfulness of the agent. Many times antidepressant trials are not successful because of an inadequate length of treatment (generally 1 month or less) or inadequate dose. A partial response may have occurred in which the medication was not increased to a full therapeutic dose, or over time the effectiveness of the medication may have dwindled, which is common in selective serotonin reuptake inhibitors (SSRIs), and the dose not subsequently increased. In general, if it has worked before, it will probably work again with adjustments to dose. Another useful piece of information (in the treatment-naive patient as well) is family history of response to medication. A general rule of thumb is that if one family member has responded to a particular antidepressant agent, the patient seeking treatment may also respond to that agent. All that being said, with the wide selection of antidepressants available, there is no reason to fight the uphill battle of trying to get patients to take a medication they do not want to take regardless of their reasons. Convincing them in the short term will probably only lead to noncompliance later. Tables 2 through 5 summarize the currently available antidepressants.

### Selective Serotonin Reuptake Inhibitors

The SSRIs (Table 2) are currently considered first-choice antidepressants for many patients with depression. These medications share the mechanism of blocking serotonin reuptake. As a group, they have the advantages of being relatively low in side effects, safer than the tricyclics (nonlethal in overdose), easy to administer, and efficacious. The most common side effects of the SSRIs are nausea and diarrhea during early treatment, and if these occur, they usually resolve within a week or two. Some patients experience increased energy or jitteriness soon after SSRIs begin, which can be desirable for patients with fatigue or can be uncomfortable but usually diminishes within a few weeks. Sexual dysfunction is another side effect sometimes seen with SSRIs and may include decreased libido, impotence, delayed ejaculation, or anorgasmia. Medication interactions are seen with certain SSRIs that inhibit the cytochrome P-450 liver enzyme systems, especially fluoxetine (Prozac) and paroxetine (Paxil), so caution should be used in patients taking other medications. A discontinuation syndrome is described that is most likely to occur with paroxetine and includes flulike symptoms such as nausea, vomiting, fatigue, headache, and myalgia. Slow tapering at discontinuation may prevent this syndrome.

### Other Newer Antidepressants and Novel Agents

A number of other antidepressants (Table 3) have been developed that differ in mechanism from the SSRIs. Trazodone (Desyrel) and nefazodone (Serzone) block serotonin reuptake and also block

## TABLE 2  Selective Serotonin Reuptake Inhibitors (SSRIs)

| Drug | Effective Dose | Comments |
|---|---|---|
| Fluoxetine (Prozac, Prozac weekly, Sarafem) | 20–80 mg/d; weekly capsule 90 mg | Longest half-life, good for noncompliant patients, many drug interactions |
| Sertraline (Zoloft) | 50–200 mg/d | Least potential for cytochrome-related drug interactions of SSRIs |
| Paroxetine (Paxil) | 20–50 mg/d | Benefit for anxious depression; discontinue slowly |
| (Paxil CR) | 25–62.5 mg/d | |
| Citalopram (Celexa) | 20–60 mg/d | Least highly protein bound so fewer drug interactions |
| Escitalopram (Lexapro) | 10–20 mg/d | S-enantiomer of citalopram |
| Fluvoxamine (Luvox) | 50–250 mg/d | Potentiates caffeine and theophyllines |

5-hydroxytryptamine 2 (5-HT2) receptors. Trazodone is often used for its sedative effect. The use of nefazodone has declined dramatically after being found to be the etiologic agent in some deaths secondary to hepatic failure.

Bupropion (Wellbutrin) is an effective antidepressant that acts to boost the neurotransmitters norepinephrine and dopamine. It has the potential benefits of being less likely to induce mania and less likely to cause sexual dysfunction than the SSRIs. It should be avoided in patients with a history of eating disorders because it can induce seizures in those patients.

Antidepressants with dual noradrenergic and serotonergic mechanisms include venlafaxine (Effexor) and duloxetine (Cymbalta). Venlafaxine actually has a mechanism that varies with its dose: At lower doses it blocks serotonin reuptake, whereas when the dose exceeds 150 mg/day, it blocks increasingly higher amounts of norepinephrine. Venlafaxine may increase blood pressure, especially at high doses, and should be monitored. Duloxetine is effective for major depression and also for pain that may coexist with depression.

Mirtazapine (Remeron) blocks α-2 and serotonin receptors. It has a low rate of sexual dysfunction, is sedating, and causes weight gain. It has the unusual feature of a decrease in side effects associated with increasing dose. It may be especially helpful for patients with melancholic depression who have poor sleep and appetite.

A transdermal selegiline patch (Ensam) has been approved by the FDA for depression and consists of a selective MAO-B inhibitor that is believed at high doses to inhibit both MAO-A and MAO-B in the brain, while at the same time preserving the gastrointestinal MAO-A barrier that breaks down ingested tyramine. Vagus nerve stimulation (VNS), also FDA approved, requires a surgical procedure to wrap an electrode around the vagus nerve and implant a stimulator, which on average delivers 30 seconds of current to the vagus nerve every 5 minutes. Theoretically, the stimuli, carried via afferent fibers in the vagus nerve to mood-regulating centers in the brain, alleviate some cases of previously refractory depression. Repetitive transcranial magnetic stimulation, whereby non-seizure-inducing magnetic pulses stimulate the cerebral cortex, is being investigated for the treatment of depression.

### Tricyclic Antidepressants

TCAs (Table 4) are as efficacious as the newer agents but less effective because of side effects. These side effects include antihistaminic effects (sedation and weight gain), anticholinergic effects (dry mouth, dry eyes, constipation), and antiadrenergic effects (orthostatic hypotension, which is a significant problem in the elderly (65 years and older) owing to increased fall risk). Cardiac conduction problems are of concern because the TCAs can provoke bradyarrhythmias, lengthen the QT interval, and induce symptomatic conduction delays in patients with conduction delays and bundle-branch block. The most serious problem with TCA therapy is lethality in overdose. As little as a 10-day supply can cause cardiac arrhythmias, seizures, and death. Other agents should also be considered in patients with narrow-angle glaucoma because of the TCA's anticholinergic properties. TCAs are also thought to switch depressed patients into mania at a higher rate than the other antidepressants.

All of this being said, TCAs have been used for decades for treatment of depression. Patients should receive a pretreatment electrocardiogram (ECG), and subsequent ECGs should be ordered, particularly with dosage increases. TCAs also have several other indications, including pain disorders, and sometimes simply increasing the TCA dose helps with pain and depression instead of adding a second antidepressant. This recommendation is especially important to keep in mind because TCA levels can increase two- to threefold with some SSRIs, especially fluoxetine (Prozac) and paroxetine (Paxil). Many TCAs also have the distinct advantage of the physician being able to obtain clinically relevant serum drug levels. Most TCAs show an onset of clinical effects occurring at serum levels between 150 and 200 µg/mL with little therapeutic benefit and increased side effects above these ranges. The exception is nortriptyline (Pamelor), which appears to have a therapeutic window of between 50 and 150 µg/mL.

## TABLE 3  Other Antidepressants (non-SSRIs)

| Drug | Effective Dose | Comments |
|---|---|---|
| Bupropion (Wellbutrin, Zyban) | 225–450 mg in 3 divided doses; do not give after 5 PM | Maximum single dose: 150 mg; seizure risk if dose excessive; contraindicated in bulimia and anorexia |
| Bupropion SR (Wellbutrin SR) | 200–450 mg in 2 divided doses; do not give after 5 PM | Maximum single dose: 200 mg |
| Bupropion XL (Wellbutrin XL) | 150–450 mg once daily | Less risk of sexual dysfunction than other antidepressants |
| Mirtazapine (Remeron) | 15–45 mg at bedtime | Sedating, causes weight gain; low rates of sexual dysfunction |
| Venlafaxine (Effexor, Effexor XR) | 75–225 mg/d once daily (extended release) or 2–3 doses (immediate release) | Monitor blood pressure; low protein binding so less drug interactions |
| Duloxetine (Cymbalta) | 40–60 mg/d in 1–2 doses | Benefit for co-morbid pain |

*Abbreviations:* SSRI = selective serotonin reuptake inhibitor.

## TABLE 4  Tricyclic Antidepressants

| Drug | Dosage Range (mg/d) |
| --- | --- |
| Amitriptyline | 25–300 |
| Clomipramine | 50–250 |
| Desipramine | 25–300 |
| Doxepin | 25–300 |
| Imipramine | 25–300 |
| Maprotiline | 50–225 |
| Nortriptyline | 25–150 |
| Protriptyline | 20–60 |
| Trimipramine | 75–300 |

### Monoamine Oxidase Inhibitors

Although very effective, especially in cases of refractory or atypical depression, MAOIs are used very rarely, even in the hands of a specialist, owing to their medication interactions and dietary restrictions. However, physicians should be aware of this class, and drug interaction profiles should be run on any patient who is on a MAOI before another medication is prescribed.

### Patient Education

The physician must spend a few minutes educating the patient for an antidepressant trial to be successful. As stated earlier, one of the major reasons for antidepressant trial failure is noncompliance. People stop taking antidepressants for a number of reasons including a so-called antibiotic view of medications: "Once I feel better I can stop." Anxious people, scared of initial side effects, may abruptly stop a medication. To address these, the physician needs to spend approximately 2 to 3 minutes saying something like this (tempered by the education and sophistication of the patient): "I am recommending that you take an antidepressant called _____. All antidepressants take 4 to 8 weeks to get a full effect, and you will not really know if this will work for you until you have been on it that long, although you may get a partial response sooner. Unfortunately, you may get side effects in the first few weeks before you get most of the good effects. Although there can be different side effects for different people, the most common ones for _____ are _____. I expect you to have at least one or two of these. If you have not had at least one side effect by 2 weeks, you need to call me. You can expect the side effects to be at their worst initially, then

to decrease. The therapeutic benefit may not occur until a full month or more has passed, so it is important to keep taking it. If you respond to this medication, you will need to be on it at least a year to reduce your risk of a relapse." This short statement addresses two of the biggest obstacles to compliance: anxiety over side effects and duration of treatment.

It must be added, to the suicidal patient especially, that any emergence or worsening of suicidal ideation should be reported to the physician immediately because energy and concentration generally improve before mood, which would make the still depressed patient more capable of carrying out a plan. This explanation has been the historical reasoning for the tie between suicide and antidepressant treatment, and susceptible patients should be closely monitored, especially during the first month of treatment. In fact, the Food and Drug Administration (FDA) has now issued a black box warning for children and adolescents about the potential for emerging suicidal ideation with antidepressants and is considering extending this warning to all populations. Although this should not keep the clinician from prescribing needed treatment, it might lower the bar for specialist referral.

## MOOD STABILIZERS

Lithium, lamotrigine, olanzapine, quetiapine, and fluoxetine-olanzapine combination have shown reasonable evidence they work for bipolar depression. Antidepressants are receiving mixed to negative views in the treatment of bipolar depression and, in particular, tricyclics and venlafaxine seem to cause more switching from depression into mania than other antidepressants. If used, antidepressants should only be used in combination with an antimanic agent and in contrast with unipolar depression, the antidepressant should be withdrawn when the depressive episode is over while the antimanic agent is continued.

Lithium, divalproex, carbamazapine, haloperidol, aripiprazole, olanzapine, quetiapine, ziprasidone and risperdal have shown reasonable evidence they work in acute mania. The newer anticonvulsants gabapentin (Neurontin), lamotrigine, and topiramate (Topamax) have not shown evidence they work in acute mania. Lamotrigine, as mentioned, is indicated for bipolar depression, whereas gabapentin is used as an adjunct for anxiety and pain and topiramate for help with weight gain for antimanic agents. The only FDA-approved medication for pediatrics is lithium, although there are some data to suggest that the other above agents have efficacy in children as well.

Lithium is generally started at 300 mg two to three times per day in the nonrenally impaired patient. An initial trough level can be

## TABLE 5  Mood Stabilizers

| Drug | Effective Dose | Comments |
| --- | --- | --- |
| Lithium (Lithobid, Eskalith) | Start 300 mg bid–tid; maintain 900–1200 mg/d | See text. |
| Divalproex (Depakote, Depakote ER) | Titrate up to 20 mg/kg/d, usually 500 mg bid–tid or 1000 to 1500 mg extended release | See text. |
| Carbamazepine (Tegretol, Tegretol XR) | Start 200 mg bid up to maximum of 1600 mg/d | See text. |
| Lamotrigine (Lamictal) | 25 mg qd × 2 wk, 50 mg qd × 2 wk, 50-mg increases weekly thereafter | Effective in depression. ½ dose for combination with Depakote (see text). |
| Aripiprazole (Abilify) | 5–30 mg qd | Little sedation. |
| Olanzapine (Zyprexa, IM and Zydis forms) | 5–20 mg/d (tab and Zydis) IM: 10 mg up to tid | More likely to cause weight gain, metabolic syndrome. |
| Quetiapine fumarate (Seroquel) | 100–800 mg/d | Low rate of EPS, more effective at >300 mg/d. |
| Risperidone (Risperdal, Risperdal Consta) | 2–3 mg qd initially, maximum 6 mg/d, Consta injection 25 mg IM q2wk in combination with oral for 2–3 mo | Slightly more likely to cause EPS, prolactinemia, especially at doses >6 mg/d. |
| Ziprasidone (Geodon) | 20 mg bid with food; maximum dose: 160 mg | Discontinue if QTc >500 msec, less weight gain. Take with food. |

Abbreviations: EPS = extrapyramidal side effect; IM = intramuscular.

obtained 4 to 5 days from initiation with a target blood level between 0.8 and 1.0 mEq/L. The effectiveness of lithium is decreased by its side effects, which include the following:

1. Tremor: Best evidenced when the patient's hands and fingers are outstretched; may benefit from mild dosage reduction or β-blockers.
2. Renal: Lithium is metabolized in the kidney, and interactions with the kidney can cause polyuria with secondary polydipsia in 25% of cases. Anything that affects the kidney can affect lithium metabolism. Although the list is extensive, certain nonsteroidal medications and diuretics, particularly thiazide diuretics, decrease the clearance of lithium and could cause lithium toxicity.
3. Thyroid: 5% of patients (more often women) develop hypothyroidism during chronic lithium treatment.
4. Cardiac: Lithium can cause T-wave flattening or inversion owing to displacement of intracellular potassium.
5. Weight gain.
6. Cognitive: Mental slowing, memory problems, and apathy.
7. Hematologic: Benign leukocytosis that does not require intervention.
8. Birth defects: Not recommended in pregnancy, but only in the second or third trimester by a specialist if no other option is available.
9. Gastrointestinal: Initial nausea, vomiting, and diarrhea common.
10. Toxicity: Small therapeutic window; levels above 1.5 mEq/L are toxic.

Overdose, drug interactions, and dehydration can cause toxicity. Symptoms of toxicity include nausea, vomiting, tremor, diarrhea, confusion, and ataxia; at higher levels, toxicity can lead to seizures, coma, or death. Pretreatment, it is recommended that an ECG, blood urea nitrogen (BUN), creatinine, CBC, electrolytes, pregnancy test, and thyroid studies be done as well as an evaluation of the patient's medication list. Thyroid tests, renal tests, and trough (10 to 13 hours after the evening dose and before the morning dose) levels should be obtained every 2 to 3 months during the first 6 months of maintenance therapy and then every 6 months thereafter or when clinically indicated. A common practitioner mistake is to obtain random and not trough levels. Because this is relevant to lithium, divalproex (Depakote), and carbamazepine (Tegretol), it is important to understand that all therapeutic values are based on trough levels, so obtaining a random level is virtually useless.

Divalproex (Depakote) is generally started at 500 mg twice daily, but a loading dose of approximately 20 mg/kg can be given in acutely manic patients with an initial trough level obtained after 4 to 5 days with a target blood level between 50 and 125 µg/mL. Divalproex is generally thought to be better tolerated than lithium, but common dose-related side effects include sedation, nausea, vomiting, and diarrhea, especially upon initiation. Divalproex can cause thrombocytopenia and rarely can cause fatal hepatotoxicity, hemorrhagic pancreatitis, and agranulocytosis. Also, because divalproex is highly protein bound and only the free portion reaches the central nervous system (CNS), in cases of hypoalbuminemia or in combination with other highly protein-bound drugs, it is recommended that clinicians obtain free plasma levels. Divalproex can cause neural tube defects in pregnancy. Therefore, it is recommended that liver function tests (LFTs), pregnancy tests, CBC, electrolytes, and prothrombin time be obtained pretreatment. Drug trough levels should also be done 5 days after initial therapy or after dosage change, CBC and LFTs monthly for 6 months, then CBC, LFTs, and prothrombin times quarterly for the next 6 months. Androgen and amylase need to be checked if symptoms arise.

Carbamazepine (Tegretol) is generally started at 200 mg twice daily, with an initial trough level to be obtained after 4 to 5 days with a target blood level between 4 and 12 µg/mL. Most common dose-related side effects include gastrointestinal effects (nausea, vomiting, cramps, and diarrhea) and CNS effects (confusion, drowsiness, ataxia, hyperreflexia/clonus, and tremor). Uncommon, but potentially lethal, side effects include transient leukopenia and mild thrombocytopenia, which in rare cases can progress to aplastic anemia and agranulocytosis. From 10% to 30% of people develop an elevation of liver enzymes from chemical hepatitis, elevation of bilirubin and alkaline phosphatase, and hyponatremia and hypo-osmolality from an antidiuretic hormone-like effect. Therefore, patients should be warned to call their physician if they experience any symptoms of hepatitis such as malaise, anorexia, nausea/vomiting, edema, or abdominal pain. Of great importance is carbamazepine's propensity to speed up its own metabolism and that of a number of other drugs through induction of hepatic enzymes. This induction results in lowering of the serum drug levels and can cause it and particularly oral contraceptives not to work. Because carbamazepine can also cause neural tube defects, this interaction is of particular importance. Therefore, pretreatment hepatic functioning, a pregnancy test, and a CBC should be obtained with trough level and CBC every 2 to 3 months and hepatic enzymes when clinically indicated.

Lamotrigine (Lamictal) is started at 25 mg every day and increased to 50 mg after 2 weeks with 50-mg increment increases weekly up to 500 mg.[1] If combined with Depakote, the initial dosing is 25 mg every other day with 25-mg increments to a maximum dosage of 200 mg.[1] The slow dosage titration is related to the risk of Stevens-Johnson syndrome, especially when Lamictal is titrated up too quickly and/or combined with Depakote. The atypical antipsychotics, including aripiprazole, olanzapine, quetiapine, risperdal, and ziprasidone all have indications for acute mania and in combination with lithium or divalproex showed an efficacy rate of approximately 62% for the combined treatment versus a 42% response rate for lithium or divalproex alone. The major side effects surrounding the atypicals center on the increased risk for inducing the metabolic syndrome, which increases the cardiovascular risks and mortality rates, although ziprasidone seems to have the least risk among these agents. Because of these risks, laboratory work should be done as indicated in Table 6.

---

[1]Not FDA approved for this indication.

## TABLE 6  SECOND-GENERATION ANTIPSYCHOTICS (except Clozapine) - Aripiprazole (Abilify), Olanzapine (Zyprexa), Quetiapine (Seroquel), Risperidone (Risperdal), Ziprasidone (Geodon)

| | Baseline | 4 wk | 8 wk | 12 wk | Quarterly | Yearly | If sx arise | Every 5 y |
|---|---|---|---|---|---|---|---|---|
| Pregnancy test* | X | | | | | | X | |
| Weight/BMI | X | X | X | X | X | | | |
| Waist circumference | X | | | | | X | | |
| Blood pressure (BP)** | X | | X | | | X | | |
| Fasting glucose/ Glycosylated hemoglobin (HbA1c)*** | X | | X | | | X | | |
| Fasting lipid profile*** | X | | X | | | | | X |
| Prolactin | | | | | | X | | |
| ECG**** | X | | | | | X | | |

\* In women of childbearing age
\** Orthostatic in elderly
\*** More frequent assessment in the event of marked weight gain
\**** In patients taking ziprasidone, which may cause QT prolongation (may also consider checking potassium and magnesium, as hypokalemia and hypomagnesemia can increase risk of QT prolongation)
From Biological Therapies in Psychiatry, Sept. 2006, Vol 29: 9, on Second-Generation Antipsychotics.

## Patient Education

Compliance is a major factor in treatment success. There are more suicides secondary to bipolar depressive episodes than unipolar depressive episodes. A major study found the prophylactic effects of lithium to be so great it added 7 years to the life expectancy. However, nonadherence rates range from 33% to 64% within 1 month from initiation of treatment, primarily because of denial of illness and need for treatment, especially in the substance-abusing population. With education, bipolar patients can learn to recognize the symptoms of an impending episode and avoid hospitalizations by working closely with their physician.

## ELECTROCONVULSIVE THERAPY

Electroconvulsive therapy (ECT) is the most effective available treatment for mood disorders. It surpasses treatment efficacy of all the other modalities and is used in fragile populations such as pregnant women and the elderly (65 years and older). There are no absolute contraindications to ECT, and it is the treatment of choice when a patient is refractory to all other therapies.

## REFERENCES

Bauer MS: Mood disorders: bipolar (manic-depressive) disorders. In Tasman A, Kay J, Lieberman JA (eds): Psychiatry, 2nd ed. Chichester, England, Wiley & Sons, 2003, pp 1237-1270.

Blazer G: Depression in Late Life. St. Louis, Mosby-Year Book, 1993.

Cohen BJ: Theory and Practice of Psychiatry. New York, Oxford University Press, 2003.

Dubovsky SL, Davies R, Dubovsky AN: Mood disorders. In Hales RE, Yudofsky SC (eds): Textbook of Clinical Psychiatry, 4th ed. Washington, DC, American Psychiatric Association, 2003, pp 439-542.

Gelenberg AJ: A concise guide to psychotropic medications: Laboratory testing, patient warnings, and drug interactions, Part I of II. Biological Therapies in Psychiatry newsletter, 29(9), September 2006, p. 39.

Ghaemi SN: Mood Disorders. Philadelphia, Lippincott Williams & Wilkins, 2003.

Greist JH, Jefferson JW: Depression and Its Treatment. Washington, DC, American Psychiatric Association, 1992.

Gruenberg AM, Goldstein RD: Mood disorders: Depression. In Tasman A, Kay J, Lieberman JA (eds): Psychiatry, 2nd ed. Chichester, England, Wiley & Sons, 2003, pp 1207-1236.

Mondimore FM: Depression: The Mood Disease. Baltimore, Md, Johns Hopkins University Press, 1993.

Pies RW: Handbook of Essential Psychopharmacology, 2nd ed. Washington, DC, American Psychiatric Association, 2005.

Sadock BJ, Sadock VA: Mood disorders. In Sadock BJ, Sadock VA (eds): Kaplan & Sadock's Synopsis of Psychiatry, 9th ed. Philadelphia, Lippincott Williams & Wilkins, 2003, pp 534-590.

Stahl SM: Essential Psychopharmacology: The Prescriber's Guide. Cambridge, England, Cambridge University Press, 2005.

U.S. Department of Health and Human Services: Depression in Primary Care. Vol 1: Detection and Diagnosis. Rockville, Md, Agency for Health Care Policy and Research, 1993.

# Schizophrenia

Method of
*Adriana Foster, MD, and Peter Buckley, MD*

Schizophrenia is a chronic debilitating illness, affecting 1% of the population, with an economic burden of $32.5 billion per year in the United States. Its implications include lost human potential because of inability to function personally, socially, and professionally, disability, risk of suicide, and impact on families.

The etiology of schizophrenia is still elusive. The neurodevelopmental hypothesis prevails and postulates that illness starts in utero with abnormal neuronal development. The knowledge about potential

## CURRENT DIAGNOSIS

- Impairment in reality testing: delusions and hallucinations
- Negative symptoms: anhedonia, alogia, avolition, affective flattening
- Disorganized thought and behavior
- Cognitive and executive dysfunction
- Symptoms lasting >6 mo
- Significant impairment in professional, social function, and personal relationships
- Onset in early 20s in men and early 30s in women
- Psychosis because of drugs, general medical condition, or major mood disorder ruled out.

genetic loci for schizophrenia is yet limited but it is known that dizygotic twins have a 12% chance of developing schizophrenia if one twin is affected, whereas for monozygotic twins the risk increases to 50%. Genetic predisposition is thus a major risk factor—but by no means the only risk factor—for schizophrenia. It is currently thought that individuals with genetic predisposition to schizophrenia are especially vulnerable to in utero factors like hypoxia, rubella, maternal influenza, birth during late winter and spring, and maternal malnutrition. The pathologic brain abnormalities thought to be resulting from this interaction (smaller prefrontal cortex and hippocampus, enlarged ventricles) appear to be static in nature and occur without evidence of gliosis, commonly found in neurodegenerative disorders. At the molecular level, it is thought that genetic factors converge, leading to abnormal neuronal connectivity and synaptic signaling, and they may alter the dopaminergic and the glutamatergic pathways of the brain. There is early evidence of altered gene expression profiles for a variety of neurotrophic factors involved in brain development and regulation. A causal relationship and a mechanism by which susceptibility genes can predispose to schizophrenia are still to be identified.

The neurodegenerative hypothesis of schizophrenia is based on longitudinal studies showing that morphologic brain changes progress, especially early, during the first 5 years of illness, even before the clinical manifestations of schizophrenia are apparent. A recent trend in schizophrenia research is the study of the prodromal period and family members of probands with schizophrenia, in an effort to understand the effect of brain changes thought to be induced by untreated illness. In parallel, we are trying to treat the illness as early as possible to avoid the potential for neuronal damage, which some claim may result from episodes of florid psychosis. However, this approach is contentious because it proposes treatment of a population in their early twenties with antipsychotic medications, associated with noxious side effects of abnormal movements or metabolic disturbances.

A summary of the recent knowledge about neurotransmitter changes in schizophrenia (Table 1) is necessary to understand the postulated mechanism of action for antipsychotic drugs.

Some patients may have a prodromal period, with peculiarities of thought and behavior, followed by onset of full-blown psychosis. The illness has a relapsing course. During acute episodes patients lose contact with reality and often attend and respond to internal stimuli (hallucinations). Behavior may be motivated by commands from voices or delusional beliefs. The patients' thought processes can be loose and disorganized leading to like behavior, with disregard to self-care, isolation and social withdrawal, sometimes aggression, and hostility. The course may become less acute as patients advance in age (residual type schizophrenia). However, deficits of attention and working memory, executive dysfunction with decrease in goal-directed behavior, planning, flexibility and self-monitoring, as well as poor insight and judgment, persist. Significant suicide risk is present, associated with delusions, command hallucinations, or superimposed depression. Co-morbidity with alcohol and drug abuse is significant. Noncompliance with medication is common and requires extensive psychosocial intervention. The patients have major difficulty

## TABLE 1 Neurotransmitter Abnormalities in Schizophrenia

| Neurotransmitter | Dysfunction | Localization | Normal Function | Antipsychotic Effect |
|---|---|---|---|---|
| Dopamine (DA) | Hyperactivity | Nigrostriatal tract | Extrapyramidal system, controlling movement. | Movement disorders. |
| | | Mesolimbic tract | Memory, stimulus processing, motivation (internal and external stimuli are postulated to have exaggerated motivational and emotional relevance in psychosis). | Reduce psychosis. |
| | | Mesocortical tract | Cognition, executive function. | Reduce psychosis. Can induce akathisia. |
| | | Tuberoinfundibular tract | Controls prolactin release. | Increased prolactin, galactorrhea, sexual dysfunction. |
| Serotonin (5-HT) | | Same distribution with dopaminergic neurons | Serotonergic stimulation in the striatum decreases DA release. | 5-HT$_2$ antagonism reduces psychosis and decreases DA-related movement disorders. |
| Glutamate (excitatory neurotransmitter) | Corticostriatal glutamate hypoactivity leads to DA hyperactivity (e.g., psychosis related to phencyclidine, an antagonist of the NMDA glutamate receptor) | Widespread in the brain | Synaptic plasticity, learning, memory. Under traumatic or ischemic conditions, glutamate concentrations rise to excitotoxic levels (it is postulated that obstetric complications generate a toxic glutamatergic release and thus the brain development becomes abnormal in-utero). | Not a primary mechanism of action for any current antipsychotic. |

accessing medical care, following recommendations, and complying with treatment for their psychiatric and medical conditions, as illustrated next.

## Case 1

A man with schizophrenia was admitted after being forcefully evicted from his apartment. He maintained that he owned the place and referred to his relationship with God. He complained of difficulty urinating and squatted on the unit at times. As part of his routine laboratory tests, his prostate-specific antigen (PSA) value returned in the thousands. He invoked delusional beliefs when he refused a prostate biopsy. His family, after numerous attempts to care for him, was not available to do so any longer. An emergency guardianship was obtained, and a prostate biopsy was performed in the operating room under general anesthesia. The results showed cancer of the prostate, and the urologist offered treatment with hormone injections. The patient passively accepted the treatment but never agreed that he had cancer.

## Case 2

A smoker with hypertension (HTN), chronic obstructive pulmonary disease (COPD), and paranoid schizophrenia requested to change doctors because he felt that his psychiatrist was part of a plot against him, along with people at his supported housing facility. He came in stating he felt "depressed" and demanded that his new psychiatrist be paged. He appeared somnolent and short of breath. The records showed visits to the emergency department (ED) twice in the past week, with vague complaints of fatigue; he was offered treatment for respiratory symptoms and left before any treatment was administered. At arrival in the ED, the patient's oxygen saturation was 79% and at a psychiatrist's insistence, he eventually agreed to be examined by the ED physician. He was admitted to the intensive care unit, intubated, and underwent treatment for community-acquired pneumonia.

Upon discharge from the hospital he thanked the psychiatrist for "saving my life" but continued to refuse his antipsychotic medication.

Many patients with schizophrenia, after brief hospitalizations, become clients of state-sponsored and federal outpatient mental health systems, where case management, day treatment, substance rehabilitation, vocational and incentive therapy, employment, and housing programs are accessible. The most refractory and noncompliant patients may respond to assertive community treatment, an intensive outreach approach by multidisciplinary teams available around the clock. Often the relationships with their families are under strain because of the burden on caretakers or the patient's delusional mistrust. Counseling and peer support for families of patients with schizophrenia at illness onset is key and helps them maintain involvement for the patient's lifetime. The National Alliance for Mentally Ill (NAMI) is a remarkable resource for self-help, support, and advocacy for patients and families of people with severe mental illnesses. NAMI provides education, combats stigma, promotes increased funding for research, and advocates tirelessly at the local and national level for health insurance, housing, rehabilitation, and jobs for people with mental illnesses (www.nami.org). It is a challenge to integrate the broad range of outpatient services needed to fulfill the needs of the patients with schizophrenia. An innovative approach is to include peer support specialists (trained individuals who are themselves in recovery from mental illness) to act as a support (analogous to the Alcoholics Anonymous [AA] sponsorship approach) and to help the patient focus on meaningful goals for his or her recovery. Table 2 presents the two classes of antipsychotics currently in clinical use.

Co-morbidity of schizophrenia with substance use disorders is common (estimated prevalence of 47%), nearly three times higher than in the general population, and can lead to frequent rate of relapse and hospitalization, treatment noncompliance, and poor overall response to treatment. Alcohol has a prevalence rate of 33.7% and other substance use a rate of 27.5%, with cannabis and cocaine the most common. Patients with co-morbid substance abuse have an increased risk of violence and suicide and contribute to the increased overall economic burden of schizophrenia by extensive use of the

## TABLE 2  Summary of Antipsychotics in Clinical Use

| First Generation | Mechanism of Action | Side Effects | Administration Forms |
|---|---|---|---|
| Chlorpromazine (Thorazine), thioridazine (Mellaril), perphenazine (Trilafon), trifluoperazine (Stelazine), haloperidol (Haldol), fluphenazine (Prolixin), pimozide (Orap) | Dopamine D2 receptor blockade | Extrapyramidal side effects (dystonia, parkinsonism treated with anticholinergics) Akathisia (treated with β-blocker or benzodiazepine), neuroleptic malignant syndrome (rare but life threatening), tardive dyskinesia (involuntary movements potentially irreversible) Hyperprolactinemia manifested as sexual dysfunction, menstrual irregularities, gynecomastia, galactorrhea, weight gain, and increased risk for diabetes; dyslipidemia and decreased bone mineral density; QT$_c$ prolongation with thioridazine; anticholinergic effects for thioridazine and chlorpromazine | Oral for all; injectable forms available for haloperidol (can be given IM and IV) and fluphenazine. Haloperidol and fluphenazine available in long-acting injection form. |
| **Second generation** | | | |
| Risperidone (Risperdal) | D2 antagonism and 5-HT2 antagonism | Dose dependent EPS and Hyperprolactinemia; risk of CVA in elderly with dementia treated for behavioral symptoms | Oral (including rapid dissolving tablet Risperdal Soltab) and long acting injection (Risperdal Consta) |
| Olanzapine (Zyprexa) | D2 antagonism and 5-HT2 antagonism | Weight gain, abnormal glucose and lipid metabolism | Oral (including rapid dissolving tablet Zydis) and IM |
| Quetiapine (Seroquel) | Lowest D2 antagonism | Sedation and orthostatic hypotension at therapeutic dose | Oral |
| Ziprasidone (Geodon) | D2 antagonism and 5-HT2 antagonism, 5-HT1 agonist | QT prolongation, discontinue in patients with QTc > 500 ms | Oral and IM |
| Aripiprazole (Abilify) | Partial D2 agonist and antagonist | Warnings common to all atypical | Oral (including rapid dissolving tablet Abilify Discmelt) and IM |
| Clozapine (Clozaril) | Low D2 antagonist and high 5-HT2 antagonist | Agranulocytosis, weight gain, seizures; fatalities due to myocarditis have been reported; highest risk in the first month of therapy | Oral (including rapid dissolving tablet FazaClo) |
| Paliperidone (Invega) | D2 antagonism and 5-HT2 antagonism | Risk of CVA in elderly with dementia treated for behavioral symptoms | Oral |

*Abbreviations:* IM = intramuscular; IV = intravenous.

social, institutional services, and EDs. Preliminary data exist about the possible role of second-generation antipsychotic drugs (clozapine [Clozaril], quetiapine [Seroquel], and olanzapine [Zyprexa]) in reducing the substance use in patients with schizophrenia. An estimated 58% to 90% of patients with schizophrenia smoke in comparison with the general population (28% to 30%).

## Medical Co-morbidity

Patients with schizophrenia are at high risk for cardiovascular disease because of high rates of cigarette smoking, obesity, diabetes, and hypertriglyceridemia. Thioridazine, an older drug, has now only limited use because of its QT$_c$ prolongation effect, which is associated with the development of torsades de pointes and sudden death. Dose-related QT$_c$ prolongation with ziprasidone (Geodon) is reported, but it is not clinically relevant unless other risk factors occur, like hypokalemia, hypomagnesemia, or concomitant use of quinolone antibiotics (sparfloxacin [Zagam], moxifloxacin [Avelox], and gatifloxacin [Tequin]). Myocarditis can be associated with clozapine, especially in the first month of therapy.

Diabetes and obesity are 1.5 to 2 times more common in patients with schizophrenia than in the general population. Obesity (body mass index [BMI] = 30 kg/m) is common in patients with schizophrenia, especially women. Histamine-1 and serotonin-2C receptor antagonists and increased leptin levels may underlie the antipsychotic-induced weight gain. In addition to the common risks associated with obesity, coronary heart disease, and stroke, the patients with weight gain are more likely to face stigma and increased cost of health care. Treatment should include education of the patient and family or caregiver about nutrition, exercise, symptoms of diabetes, and results of neglecting one's

## CURRENT THERAPY

- Lifelong approach
- Families involved as support system
- Complex psychosocial intervention
- Availability of crisis intervention and inpatient care
- Medication management customized for patient's co-morbid status and compliance level
- Ongoing monitoring of compliance and side effects in collaboration with primary care provider

medical care. Presently clinicians opt to switch antipsychotic if the weight gain is 5% over initial weight or if there is worsening of dyslipidemia or hyperglycemia, rather than adding antiobesity or lipid-lowering agents. Medications with additive weight gain effect should be avoided.

Patients with schizophrenia have an increased risk of abnormal glucose regulation with increased insulin resistance even without treatment with antipsychotics, which can further induce weight gain, reduce sensitivity to insulin, affect glucose transporters, and damage pancreatic islet cells.

Lipid abnormalities in schizophrenia occur as a result of antipsychotic treatment, with elevations in triglycerides and total cholesterol. Phenothiazine (chlorpromazine) and dibenzodiazepine (clozapine, olanzapine) derivatives increase serum triglycerides and total cholesterol. There is an intermediate effect from quetiapine. Risperidone (Risperdal) and ziprasidone lowered the baseline values of cholesterol and triglycerides in a landmark 18-month study comparing effectiveness of older agents with second-generation antipsychotics. The metabolic syndrome is highly prevalent in patients with schizophrenia and increases their cardiovascular risk, especially in women. The American Diabetes Association, American Psychiatric Association, and American Association of Clinical Endocrinologists developed monitoring guidelines for obesity, diabetes, and lipid abnormalities for patients on antipsychotic drugs. The patient's personal and family history should be taken before the treatment starts and annually; weight should be monitored monthly for the first 3 months and then quarterly; waist circumference, blood pressure, and fasting plasma glucose should be obtained at baseline, 3 months, then annually; and fasting lipid profile at baseline, 3 months, and then every 5 years.

Co morbidity with HIV affects 3.1% of patients with schizophrenia (eight times the prevalence in the general population). Hepatitis C affects 8.5% of psychiatric inpatients versus 1.8% of the general population. Some of the medications administered as part of the highly active antiretroviral treatment (HAART) may exacerbate psychosis. Interferon and ribavirin may induce or exacerbate depression. Cytochrome P450 2D6 and 3A4 interactions occur between antipsychotics and HAART (e.g., increased exposure to given doses of olanzapine and risperidone). Clozapine should be used with caution in patients with HIV because of possible agranulocytosis and seizures. Cognitive-behavioral therapy leads to lifestyle modifications in patients with schizophrenia; however, it has to be ongoing. Risk factors for noncompliance with treatment are poor insight, substance abuse, lack of social support, and poor therapeutic alliance. The coordination of care between medical and psychiatric staff is essential.

In using antipsychotics, psychiatrists have to bear in mind the characteristics of individual patients, appreciate the side-effect profile, and monitor carefully during the maintenance therapy. Their collaboration with primary care providers is vital in addressing the side effects when they occur. Algorithms were developed to guide the choice of antipsychotic and other somatic therapies (like electroconvulsive therapy [ECT]) at various stages of treatment.

Noncompliance is managed with long acting injectable and rapid dissolving forms of medication (Table 2) and through the psychiatrist's collaboration with the patient's family and caretakers. For refractory patients whose noncompliance exposes them at risk of hurting themselves or others, assertive community treatment and even involuntary treatment can be employed.

## REFERENCES

American Diabetes Association, American Psychiatric Association, American Association of Clinical Endocrinologists, North American Association for Studies on Obesity: Consensus development conference on antipsychotic drugs and obesity and diabetes. J Clin Psychiatry 2004;65(2):267-272.

Buckley PF, Fenley G, Mabe A, et al: Recovery and schizophrenia. Schizophrenia and Related Psychoses. 2007;11:96-100

Cournos F, McKinnon K, Sullivan G: Schizophrenia and comorbid human immunodeficiency virus or hepatitis C virus. J Clin Psychiatry 2005;66(Suppl 6):27-33.

Glassman A: Schizophrenia, antipsychotic drugs and cardiovascular disease. J Clin Psychiatry 2005;66(Suppl 6):5-10.

Green A: Schizophrenia and comorbid substance use disorder: Effects of antipsychotics. J Clin Psychiatry 2005;66(Suppl 6):21-26.

Harrison PJ, Weinberger DR: Schizophrenia genes, gene expression, and neuropathology: On the matter of their convergence. Mol Psychiatry 2005;10(1):40-68.

Lieberman JA, Stroup TS, McEvoy JP, et al: Effectiveness of antipsychotic drugs in patients with chronic schizophrenia. N Engl J Med 2005;353(12): 1209-1223.

McEvoy JP, Meyer JP, Goff DC, et al: Prevalence of the metabolic syndrome in patients with schizophrenia: Baseline results from the clinical antipsychotic trials of intervention effectiveness (CATIE). Schizophrenia Research 2005;80:19-32.

Miller A, Hall CS, Buchanan RW, et al: The Texas Medication Algorithm Project Antipsychotic Algorithm for Schizophrenia, 2003 Update. J Clin Psychiatry 2004;65(4):500-508.

Practice Guideline for the Treatment of Patients with Schizophrenia, 2nd ed. Am J Psychiatry 2004;161(2)(Suppl).

Sadock BJ, Sadock VA: Schizophrenia and other psychotic disorders. In Sadock BJ, Sadock VA (eds): Kaplan and Sadock's Comprehensive Textbook of Psychiatry, 8th ed. Philadelphia, Lippincott Williams and Wilkins, 2005.

Velakoulis D, Wood SJ, Wong MTH, et al: A magnetic resonance imaging study of chronic schizophrenia, first episode psychosis and ultra-high-risk individuals. Arch Gen Psychiatry 2006;63(2):139-149.

# Panic Disorder

Method of
*Alexander Bystritsky, MD, PhD, and Kira Williams, MD*

## Diagnosis

Panic disorder (PD) and related agoraphobia (AG) are very prevalent and disabling conditions affecting 3% to 8% of the world population. Panic disorder is characterized by sudden episodes of acute apprehension or intense fear that occur *out of the blue* without any apparent cause-panic attacks. Intense panic usually lasts no more than a few minutes, but, in rare instances, can return in *waves* for a period of up to 2 hours. During the panic itself, any of the symptoms listed in Box 1 may occur.

The attack is spontaneous, unexpected, and occurs for no apparent reason. The word *agoraphobia* means fear of open spaces; however, under many instances agoraphobia is a fear of panic attacks. Patients suffering from agoraphobia are afraid of being in situations from which escape might be difficult, or in which help might be unavailable if they suddenly had a panic attack. Many agoraphobics not only fear having panic attacks but also fear embarrassment should they be seen

---

**BOX 1  Symptoms of Panic Attack**

- Dizziness, unsteadiness, or faintness
- Fear of dying
- Fear of going crazy or losing control
- Feeling of choking
- Feeling of unreality—as if you're not all there
- Heart palpitations—pounding heart or accelerated heart rate
- Hot and cold flashes
- Nausea or abdominal distress
- Numbness, pain, or tingling in hands, feet, arms, legs, fingers, toes, lips, face
- Pain or discomfort in chest, upper back, shoulder blades
- Shortness of breath or a feeling of being smothered
- Sweating
- Trembling or shaking

## BOX 2  Some of the More Common Situations Feared by Agoraphobics

- Being at home alone
- Crowded public places such as grocery stores, department stores, restaurants
- Enclosed or confined places such as tunnels, bridges, or the hairdresser's chair
- Public transportation such as trains, buses, subways, planes

## BOX 3  Differential Diagnosis and Co-morbidity of Panic Disorder

1. Cardiac conditions
   a. Arrhythmias[a,c,d]
   b. Supraventricular tachycardia[a,c,d]
   c. Mitral valve prolapse[b,c,d]
2. Endocrine disorders
   a. Thyroid abnormality[a,b,c,d]
   b. Hyperparathyroidism[b,c,d]
   c. Pheochromocytoma[d]
   d. Hypoglycemia[a,c,d]
3. Vestibular dysfunctions[a,b,c,d]
4. Seizure disorders (temporal lobe epilepsy)[a,b,c,d]
5. Other psychiatric conditions
   a. Affective disorders
      (1) Major depression[d,e,f]
      (2) Bipolar disorder[b,d,e,f]
   b. Other anxiety disorders
      (1) Acute stress disorder[a,b,c,d,e,f]
      (2) Obsessive–compulsive disorder[a,b,c,d,e,f]
      (3) Post-traumatic stress disorder[a,b,c,d,e,f]
      (4) Social phobia[a,c,d,e,f]
      (5) Specific phobia[a,c,d,e,f]
   c. Psychotic disorders[a,d,e,f]
   d. Substance abuse and dependence
      (1) Withdrawal from central nervous system depressants[a,b,c,d,e,f]
         (a) Alcohol abuse (present in 40% of panic disorder patients)
         (b) Barbiturates
      (2) Stimulants[a,b,c,d,e,f]
         (a) Cocaine
         (b) Amphetamines
         (c) Caffeine
      (3) Cannabis[a,b,c,d,e,f]
      (4) Hallucinogens[a,b,c,d,e,f]

[a]The disorder can mimic panic disorder (PD).
[b]The disorder can cause or worsen PD through a variety of physiologic mechanisms.
[c]The disorder's symptoms could serve as triggers of panic attacks.
[d]The disorder could coexist with PD as an independent disorder.
[e]The disorder could be a co-morbid disorder with symptoms that intermingle with PD.
[f]The disorder could lead to PD or be a sequela of PD.

having a panic attack. It is common for the agoraphobic to avoid a variety of situations (Box 2). The fear usually results in travel restrictions, or a need to be accompanied by others when leaving home. They may avoid certain situations such as waiting in a line, being in crowded places (malls, theaters) and even using transportation, including driving a car. In the end, agoraphobic patients often end up completely housebound.

## Impact and Cost

Panic attacks are very common events. Some studies show that lifetime prevalence of panic or panic-like episodes is somewhere from 15% to 45%. PD characterized by frequent, disturbing panic attacks accompanied by at least 1 month of persistent fear of having another attack is less frequent. Epidemiologic studies throughout the world indicate the lifetime prevalence of PD (with or without AG) ranges between 1.5% and 3.5%. Twice as many women as men suffer from panic disorder. Studies have suggested high co-morbidity, showing that 63% to 73% of PD patients have had at least one other mental health condition, including major depressive disorder, obsessive–compulsive disorder, or another anxiety disorder during their lifetime. Panic patients also tend to seek relief from their anxiety by self-medicating with alcohol and drugs (prescription and/or illicit). The professional life of a PD patient is also likely to suffer. The majority of these patients admit that the quality of their work diminished as a result of their anxiety. Those who are financially dependent and those who receive either welfare or disability benefits constitute a considerable 27% of all PD patients. Furthermore, there seems to be a lower life expectancy among PD patients because of an increased risk of developing some cardiovascular disease or because of suicidal behavior, although the evidence for this is not consistent. The actual costs of PD are difficult to evaluate because they are indirect and hidden, but it is estimated that they are quite extensive. Because of the physical nature of panic attack symptoms, most PD patients repeatedly consult their family physicians, internists or other health professionals. Current estimates of cost of these conditions in U.S. society are more than $44 billion per year, a figure comparable to the cost of cardiovascular disorders.

## Differential Diagnoses

Box 3 summarizes the differential diagnoses for PD. The relationship between panic disorder and the other disorders listed in the table can be very complex, for example:

- Another disorder can mimic PD.
- Another disorder can cause or worsen PD through a variety of physiologic mechanisms.
- Another disorder's symptoms could serve as triggers of panic attacks.
- Another disorder could coexist with PD as an independent disorder.
- Another disorder could be a co-morbid disorder with symptoms that intermingle with PD.
- Another disorder could lead to PD or be a sequela of PD.

One such example of this interaction is cardiac arrhythmias. Although it is uncommon, an arrhythmia can coexist with panic disorder as an independent condition, and a sudden increase of heart rate could potentially provoke panic in a patient with PD. However, arrhythmia accompanied by fear could mimic a panic attack, and patients with potentially dangerous arrhythmias may receive inappropriate treatment as the result of misdiagnosis. Another possible association is mitral valve prolapse (MVP) in patients with PD, which is a frequent finding thought to be of doubtful clinical significance. However, recent research suggested that it is possible that these two disorders in some patients are linked genetically (via chromosome 13) in a syndrome characterized by β-adrenergic hyperactivity, MVP, panic, and kidney problems. Careful initial medical and psychiatric evaluation is recommended in panic patients. However, prolonged and repetitive testing should be discouraged.

## Theoretical Framework

Different theories, including cognitive-behavioral and biomedical, have been used in an attempt to describe the biologic mechanisms of panic. A brief synthesis of these theories reveals that PD is likely a combination of:

- An increase in alarm reaction
- An error in information processing (catastrophic thinking)
- Abnormal coping strategies to relieve anxiety and provide a sense of security (safety rituals and avoidance)

**TABLE 1** Theory of Panic

| Stages of Panic Disorder | Neuronal Circuits | Possible Treatments |
|---|---|---|
| Panic attacks (alarm reactions) | Periaqueductal gray amygdala, hippocampus | SSRI, SNRI, benzodiazepines, interoceptive exposure |
| Catastrophic thoughts (abnormal information processing) | Orbital frontal cortex, cingulum, hippocampus | SSRI, SNRI, cognitive restructuring, neuroleptics |
| Precaution rituals and avoidances | Prefrontal and temporal cortex | SSRI, SNRI, neuroleptics<br>Exposure and response prevention |

*Abbreviations*: SNRI = serotonin-norepinephrine reuptake inhibitor; SSRI = selective serotonin reuptake inhibitor.

The disorder represents a sequential process where the symptoms start with the physical symptoms of panic and progress through the stages of abnormal thinking, rituals, and, finally, avoidance (Table 1). These symptom clusters may be wired through different neuronal circuits and respond preferentially to different treatments. However, this theoretical frame work is incomplete, as the intricacy of the neuronal circuits and neurotransmitters is not fully understood.

## Treatment Algorithm

The treatment of PD is a stepwise process that starts with treatments of proven efficacy that are capable of ameliorating symptoms and decreasing avoidance behaviors. Figure 1 provides an algorithm of the treatment steps.

Step 1 starts with a first-line medication of a selective serotonin reuptake inhibitor (SSRI) or a therapeutic approach with cognitive

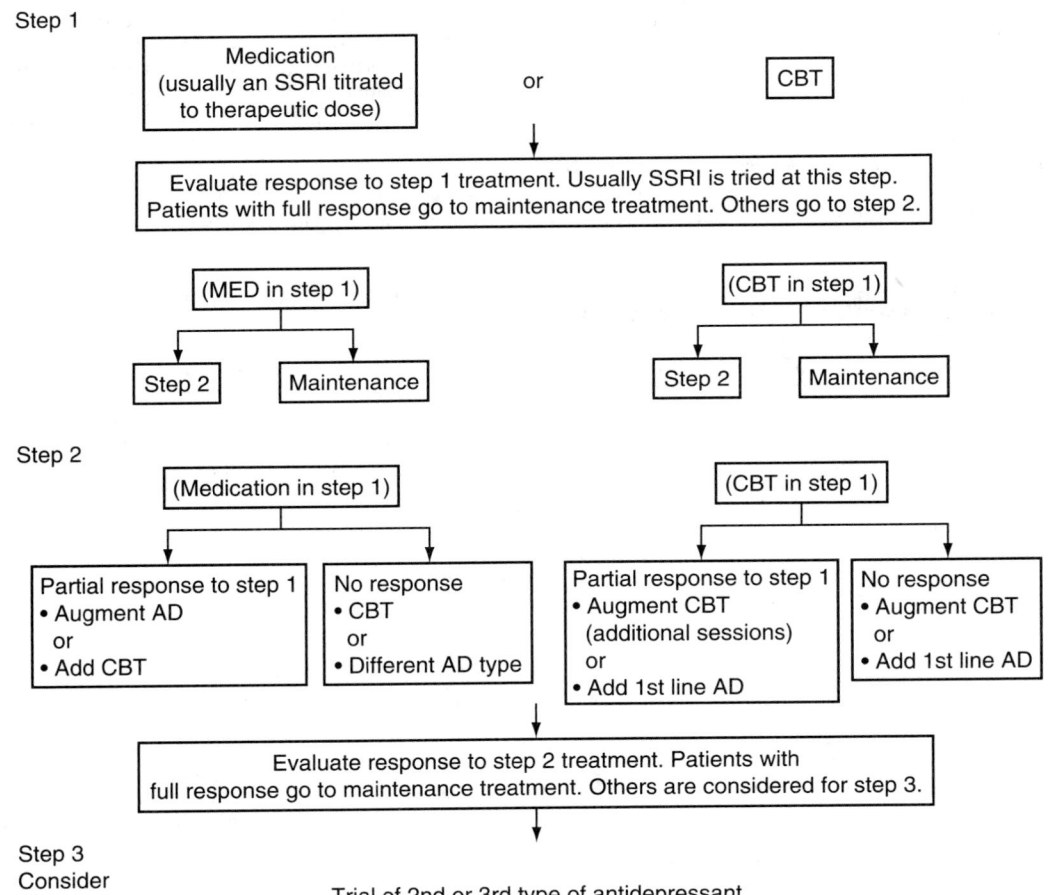

**FIGURE 1.** Treatment of panic disorder. AD = antidepressant; CBT = cognitive behavior therapy; MED = medication; PTSD = post-traumatic stress disorder; SSRI = selective serotonin reuptake inhibitor.

## BOX 4 Cognitive Behavioral Therapy

- Assessment
- Cognitive restructuring (de-catastrophizing thinking)
- Coping enhancement
- Education
- Exposure and response prevention (to phobic situations)
- Interceptive exposure (exposure to internal sensation)
- Relapse prevention
- Self-monitoring

behavior therapy (CBT). Both treatments have demonstrated efficacy between 70% and 90% in multiple studies. The treatment choice is based on the initial patient session with the physician, in which patients usually express their preference for either medication or psychotherapy. When availability and cost of the therapy is an issue, medication is the simplest way of treating PD. If, after two trials, the SSRI is deemed unsuccessful, step 2 begins.

Step 2 should start with a discussion with the patient about his/her preference for adding another medication or switching to another treatment modality (e.g., psychotherapy).

Step 3 involves treatment with more intensive CBT or with medications or combinations of treatments that have not yet been tried. Unusual and alternative treatments may be considered at that point (an expert consultation is usually recommended).

### BEHAVIORAL THERAPY

Behavior therapy can be effective in as few as four sessions and can significantly reduce a patient's distress. Box 4 gives the stages of CBT. The treatment is based on desensitizing patients to their internal sensations and external phobic situations via exposure, reduction of catastrophic thinking, and improvement in coping strategies. However, patients who have very severe anxiety accompanied by depression are frequently unable to follow the therapist's instructions and may need to be started on antidepressants early.

### MEDICATION

Selection of medication depends on whether patients have received prior pharmacotherapy for the treatment of a mood or anxiety disorder, on their previous reaction to medication, and on the severity and acuity of their panic state. An SSRI is the treatment of choice for patients who have never received pharmacotherapy and have at least moderate severity of illness. In addition to treating anxiety, SSRIs will treat a co-morbid major depressive episode (MDE) and lower the risk of future MDEs. All of the SSRIs are thought to be effective in the treatment of the four major anxiety disorders (including PD, obsessive–compulsive disorder, generalized anxiety disorder, and social anxiety disorder) and have little differences except for subtle differences in side-effect profiles and differences in their effects on the cytochrome P450 liver enzyme system (Table 2). In general, selection among antidepressants should be based on the patient's anxiety symptom profile (one should avoid medications with side effects that mimic panic symptoms) and a history the side effects of medications previously taken. Table 3 can be used as a guide. For example, in the patient with severe insomnia, one might select a sedating tricyclic, such as nortriptyline (Pamelor),[1] or perhaps mirtazapine (Remeron).[1] Paroxetine (Paxil), fluvoxamine (Luvox),[1] or citalopram (Celexa)[1] would be the SSRI of choice for patients with prominent activation. For the patient with prominent gastrointestinal (GI) side effects, one would avoid sertraline (Zoloft), and paroxetine would be the SSRI of choice. For patients with prominent palpitations and problems with weight gain, one would avoid tricyclics, paroxetine, and mirtazapine.

[1]Not FDA approved for this indication.

## TABLE 2 Antidepressants Used in Treatment of Panic

| Antidepressant | Anxiolytic Efficacy* | Advantages | Disadvantages |
|---|---|---|---|
| Fluoxetine (Prozac) | Panic[†] and PTSD | Generic form Long half-life (no withdrawal) | Most stimulating Longer half-life |
| Fluvoxamine (Luvox)[1] | Panic, GAD, and SAD | No P450 2D6 effects | Effects on P4501A2, 2C9, and 3A4 |
| Paroxetine (Paxil) | Panic,[†] GAD,[†] SAD,[†] PTSD[†] | Least stimulating No P4503A4 effects | Most anticholinergic Most sedating |
| Sertraline (Zoloft) | Panic,[†] GAD, SAD,[†] PTSD[†] | Least P450-2D6 effects Minimal P450-3A4 effects Intermediate half-life (less withdrawal) | Most diarrhea |
| Citalopram (Celexa)[1] Escitalopram (Lexapro)[1] | Panic | No P450 effects | Least studied |
| Venlafaxine ER (Effexor XR)[1] | Panic, GAD,[†] SAD,[†] PTSD | No P450 effects | Short half-life Withdrawal with missed dose or sudden discontinuation—increased BP at >225 mg |
| Nefazodone (Serzone)[1] | No controlled studies Open reports in panic, PTSD, SAD | Sedation, can take at bedtime | Prominent P450 3A4 effects Rare reports of fatal hepatotoxicity |
| Mirtazapine (Remeron)[1] | No controlled studies Rare open reports | Sedation | Oversedation Increased appetite and weight gain Rare agranulocytosis |
| Nortriptyline (Pamelor)[1] | No controlled trials, but for other TCAs (imipramine), controlled evidence in panic, GAD, PTSD | Sedation, can take at bedtime | Too many SEs |

[1]Not FDA approved for this indication.
*Data obtained from randomized clinical trials.
[†]FDA approved for this indication.
*Abbreviations:* BP = blood pressure; GAD = generalized anxiety disorder; PTSD = post-traumatic stress disorder; SAD = social anxiety disorder; SEs = side effects; TCAs = tricyclic antidepressants.

## TABLE 3 Adverse Effects of the Antidepressants*

| Adverse Effect | Fluoxetine (Prozac) | Sertaline (Zoloft) | Paroxetine (Paxil) | Fluvoxamine (Luvox) | Escitalopram (Lexapro) | Citalopram (Celexa) or Nortriptyline (Pamelor) | Venlafaxine† |
|---|---|---|---|---|---|---|---|
| Headache | ↑ | - | - | - | ↑ | ↓ | - |
| Agitation/anxiety | ↑↑ | ↑ | ↑ | - | | ↑↑ | ↑↑ |
| Tremor | ↑ | | ↑ | | | ↓ | ↑↑ |
| Insomnia | ↑↑ | ↑↑ | - | ↑↑ | | ↑↑ | ↑↑ |
| Drowsiness | ↑ | ↑ | ↑↑ | ↑↑ | | ↑↑ | ↑ |
| Fatigue | ↑ | - | ↑↑ | - | | ↑↑ | |
| Confusion | - | - | ↑ | | | ↑ | ↑ |
| Dizziness | - | - | ↑ | - | | ↑↑↑ | ↑ |
| Anticholinergic‡ | - | - | ↑ | - | | ↑↑ | ↑↑ |
| Sweating | ↑ | ↑ | ↑ | ↑ | | ↑↑ | ↑↑ |
| Weight gain | ↑ | ↑↑ | - | ↑↑ | | | ↑↑ |
| Gastrointestinal | ↑ | ↑↑ | - | ↑ | | - | ↑↑ |
| Sexual | ↑↑ | ↑↑ | ↑↑ | ↑ | ↑ | ↑ | ↑↑ |

*↑ indicates the drug increases the occurrence of the adverse effect; ↓ indicates that it decreases the occurrence.
†Can increase blood pressure; must be monitored.
‡Anticholinergic side effects include dry mouth, constipation, urinary hesitancy or retention, blurred vision.

Benzodiazepines are not the first choice because of tolerance, dependency potential, and possible interference with CBT (especially with as-needed use). They should be reserved for emergency situations (initial panic attacks), for the reduction in extreme anxiety, or infrequent phobic situations (airplanes, elevators, etc.) before the beginning of the CBT. Finally, they can be used for maintenance of chronic patients with unremitting anxiety. If the benzodiazepines are used chronically, they should be prescribed using a pharmacokinetically appropriate schedule to minimize daily withdrawal or interdose anxiety. As-needed use of benzodiazepines should be avoided and history of alcohol and drug abuse should be assessed before beginning treatment.

### TREATMENT RESISTANCE

If the patient is nonresponsive or has side effects to two prior SSRI trials, the choice is then between:

- A serotonin–norepinephrine reuptake inhibitor (SNRI)
- A newer antidepressant (e.g., venlafaxine [Effexor],[1] nefazodone [Serzone],[1] mirtazapine [Remeron][1])
- A tricyclic
- A γ-aminobutyric acid (GABA) agent (e.g., gabapentin [Neurontin][1]) (step 2)

A final consideration (step 3) involves the management of anxiety and other symptoms with a concomitant medication that would not ordinarily be a first-line treatment choice for anxiety disorders.

This involves the use of sedating atypical neuroleptics such as olanzapine (Zyprexa)[1] and quetiapine (Seroquel).[1] At this point one could consider the use of monoamine oxidase inhibitors (MAOIs), which boast very impressive data supporting their efficacy. These medications require dietary restrictions and stopping concomitant antidepressants. Combining intensive CBT (several times a week) with medication augmentation strategies may also bring a desired effect. Other strategies are under development for the treatment of this resistant population, but none of them have moved past an early experimental stage.

## Long-Term Management

While in some patients panic attacks stop in the course of a few months, PD is usually a chronic, waxing and waning condition. Some patients may completely recover, while others may be left with symptoms of other disorders initially masked by the panic attacks. If CBT is initiated, it is important to coordinate the medication treatment with the therapy. Completely blocking anxiety may impair patients' learning in therapy and discourage them from developing new coping techniques. Gradual reduction and stopping medication can be attempted after 2 or 3 months of complete resolution of symptoms. Approximately 20% of patients will not respond to any treatment and need to be maintained in the most comfortable state with medication or therapy or a combination thereof.

[1]Not FDA approved for this indication.

[1]Not FDA approved for this indication.

# Physical and Chemical Injuries

## Burn Treatment Guidelines

Method of
*Barbara A. Latenser, MD*

The initial management of the severely burned patient follows guidelines established by the American College of Surgeons (ACS). It is crucial that the patient be managed properly in the early hours after injury because the initial management of a seriously burned patient can significantly affect the long-term outcome. Optimal burn-care criteria have been established and refined by the American Burn Association (ABA) over the past 20 years.

Because of regionalization, it is common for the initial care of the seriously burned patient to occur outside the burn center. Burns are a specialized form of trauma. Therefore, the ABCs (airway, breathing, circulation) are the same as for the trauma patient: airway with cervical spine immobilization if appropriate, breathing, circulation, disability, and exposure. Also, the burn patient could be a victim of associated trauma. It is easy to be sidetracked by the obvious thermal injury. Only after the primary and secondary surveys have been performed should you evaluate the severity of the burn injury. Obtain as much information as possible regarding the incident and about the patient. An easy way to remember the information is the mnemonic AMPLE:

- Allergies
- Medications
- Past medical history
- Last meal
- Events

Universal precautions appropriate for each burn patient must be implemented by every member of the health care team.

The most commonly used guide for making an initial estimate of the second- and third-degree burns is the Rule of Nines (Figure 1). Various anatomic regions are roughly 9% of the total body surface area (TBSA) or multiples thereof. To calculate scattered burn areas, the patient's palm, including fingers, represents approximately 1% of the TBSA. A much more precise estimate of TBSA burn is provided by the Lund-Browder Classification (Figure 2). By drawing in the areas that are burned, the TBSA burn necessary for calculating resuscitation requirements can be determined. The consensus formula for the first 24 hours postburn is:

$$4 \text{ mL lactated Ringer's} \times \text{body weight in kg} \times \text{percent BSA burn}$$

Half the calculated amount is given in the first 8 hours and the rest over the remaining 16 hours. Patients with burns on more than 20% TBSA are prone to gastric dilatation and should have a nasogastric (NG) tube. To determine hourly urine output, a urinary catheter is necessary. Intravenous (IV) morphine sulfate is indicated for control of pain associated with burns. Intramuscular (IM) or subcutaneous (SC) routes of drug administration should not be used as absorption is erratic. To calculate fluid needs, weigh the patient or estimate the preinjury weight. Reliable peripheral veins should be used to establish an IV line. Use vessels underlying burned skin if necessary. If it is impossible to establish peripheral IV access, a central line may be necessary.

The burn wound should be covered with a clean, dry sheet to prevent air currents from causing pain in partial-thickness burns and to decrease fluid losses and hypothermia. Although there are many common topical antimicrobials in use, the optimal dressing prior to burn center transfer is plastic wrap such as Saran Wrap. Topical antimicrobials will just have to be washed off on arrival to the burn center, causing patient discomfort and mechanical trauma to the wound. Cold applications are appropriate only in small burns because they rapidly lead to hypothermia. Ice should never be applied because it will deepen the zone of ischemia in a thermal injury.

Escharotomies and/or fasciotomies are rarely required prior to burn center transfer, unless transfer is delayed beyond 24 hours. Patients most at risk are those with large TBSA burns, circumferential full-thickness burns, and those with electrical injury. Circumferential chest/abdominal burns may restrict ventilatory excursion. A child has a more pliable rib cage and may need an escharotomy earlier than an adult burn. If you are considering performing an escharotomy, confer with the accepting burn physician before proceeding.

So how do you know which patients should be referred to a burn center? To guide your decision making there are currently 10 burn unit referral criteria. You should have a written transfer agreement in place with a referral burn unit. The agreement should specify which patients will be referred, what stabilization is expected, who arranges transportation, and what the patient will need during transport.

## Partial-Thickness Burns on More Than 10% Total Body Surface Area

Second-degree or partial-thickness burns involve a variable portion of dermis. The skin may be red, blistered, and edematous. Because sensory nerves are damaged and/or exposed, these wounds are typically extremely painful. Healing time is proportional to the depth of dermal injury. Scarring is minimal if healing occurs in 14 days or less. With closure time beyond 3 weeks, scarring will occur, the degree being greater in darker skinned individuals.

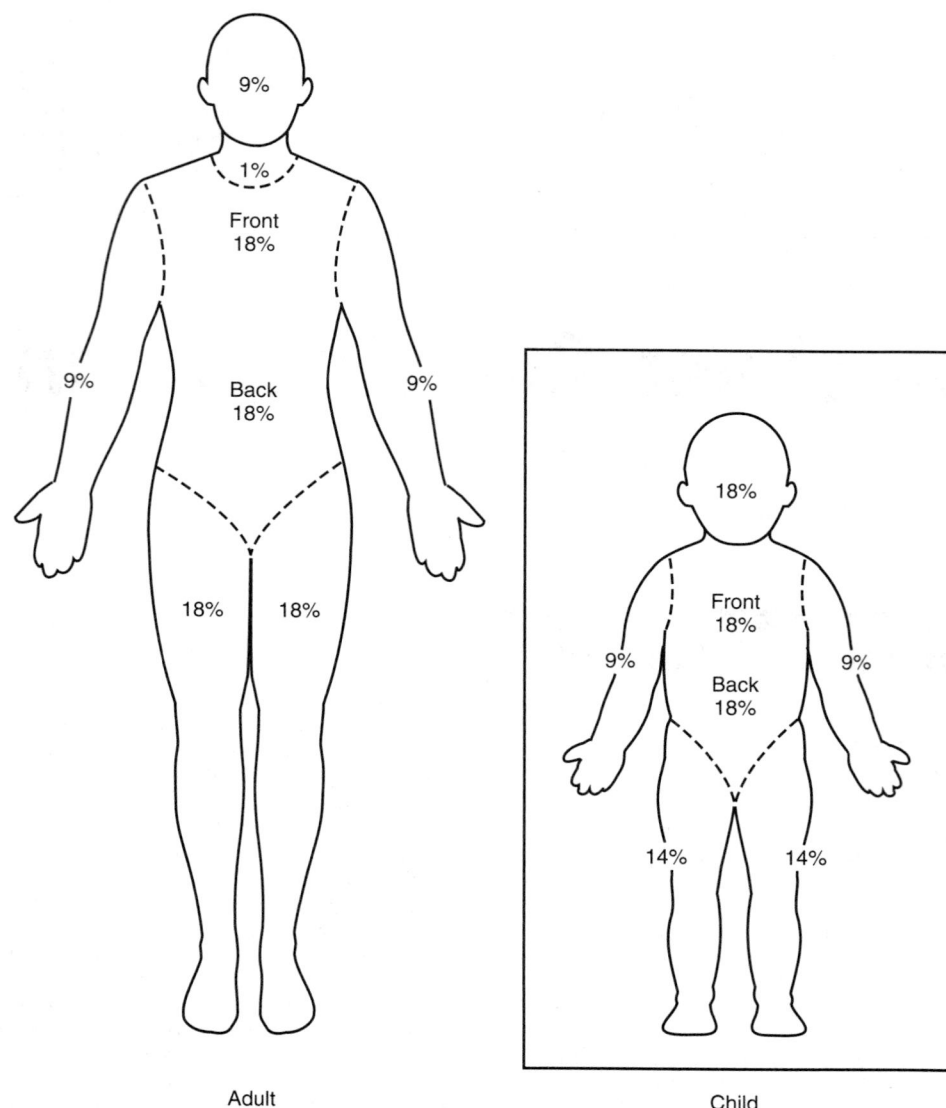

**FIGURE 1.** Rule of Nines.

Proper fluid management is critical to the survival of patients with extensive burns. Fluid resuscitation is aimed at maintaining tissue perfusion and organ function while avoiding the complications of inadequate or excessive fluid therapy. Shock and organ failure, most commonly acute renal failure, may occur as a consequence of hypovolemia in a patient with an extensive burn who is inadequately resuscitated. The increase in capillary permeability caused by the burn is greatest in the immediate postburn period and diminution in effective blood volume is most rapid at that time. A marked increase in peripheral vascular resistance accompanied by a decrease in cardiac output occurs in the first 18 to 24 hours postinjury.

In the presence of increased capillary permeability, colloid content of the resuscitation fluid exerts little influence on intravascular retention during the initial hours postburn. Crystalloid fluid is the initial resuscitation of burn patients. *Always* remember, estimates are inexact. Each patient reacts differently to burn injury and resuscitation. The actual volume of fluid infused should be varied from the calculated volume as indicated by physiologic monitoring. The patient's general condition reflects the adequacy of fluid resuscitation and should be assessed and reassessed. Mental status, anxiety, and restlessness may be signs of hypoxemia, hypovolemia, or pain.

Although urine output does not guarantee tissue perfusion, it remains the most readily available and generally reliable guide to resuscitation. Adults should produce 0.5 mL/kg per hour of urine. Children should produce 1.0 mL/kg per hour of urine, and infants 12 months or younger should produce 2.0 mL/kg per hour of urine. Oliguria is most

frequently the result of inadequate fluid administration. Diuretics are contraindicated; the rate of resuscitation should be increased. During the first 24 hours, neither the hemoglobin nor the hematocrit is a reliable guide to resuscitation, and using either leads to over-resuscitation.

Measuring blood pressure (BP) by a sphygmomanometer may be misleading in a burned limb with progressive edema formation. As the swelling increases, the signal becomes diminished. If fluid infusion is increased based on this finding, edema formation may be exaggerated. Even intra-arterial monitoring may be unreliable in patients with massive burns because of peripheral vasoconstriction secondary to marked elevation of catecholamines. Heart rate is also of limited usefulness in monitoring fluid therapy. The level of tachycardia depends on the normal heart rate in each child.

## Burns That Involve the Face, Hands, Feet, Genitalia, Perineum, or Major Joints

Facial burns are considered a serious injury. The possibility of respiratory tract damage must be considered. Because of the rich blood supply and loose areolar tissue of the face, facial burns are associated with extensive edema formation. To minimize this edema, keep the head of the bed elevated at 30°. Cool saline compresses on the face may also help. Careful examination of the eyes should be completed as soon

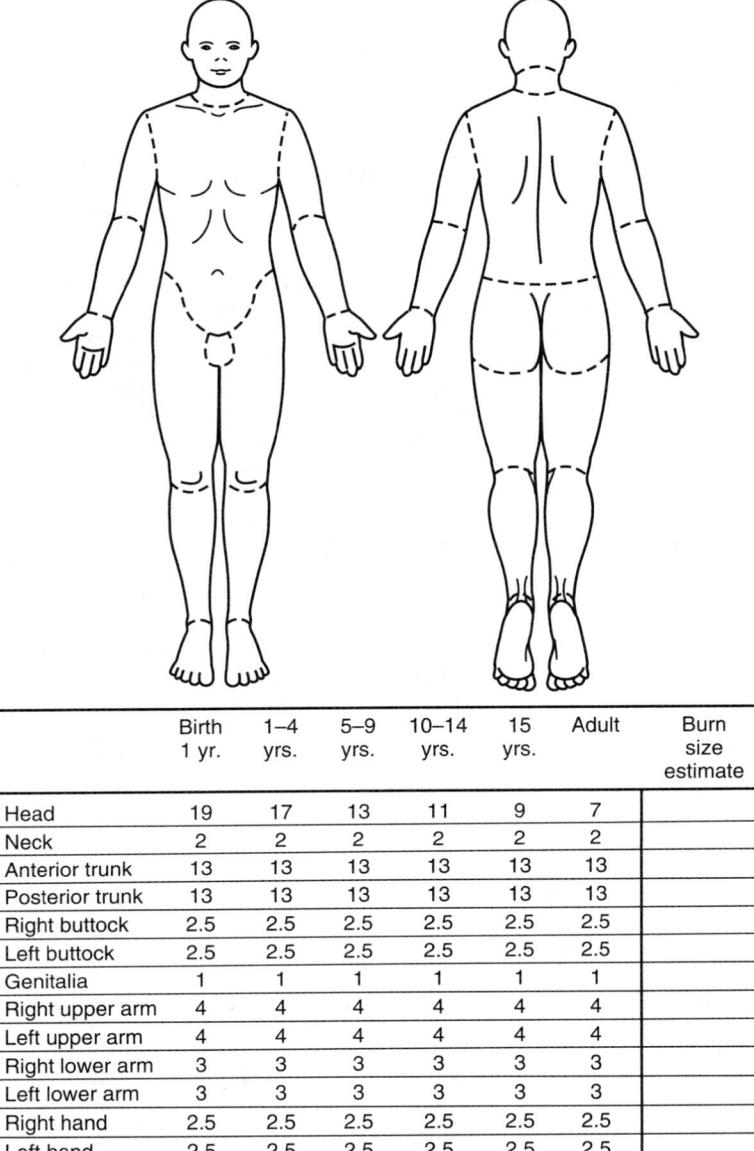

| | Birth 1 yr. | 1–4 yrs. | 5–9 yrs. | 10–14 yrs. | 15 yrs. | Adult | Burn size estimate |
|---|---|---|---|---|---|---|---|
| Head | 19 | 17 | 13 | 11 | 9 | 7 | |
| Neck | 2 | 2 | 2 | 2 | 2 | 2 | |
| Anterior trunk | 13 | 13 | 13 | 13 | 13 | 13 | |
| Posterior trunk | 13 | 13 | 13 | 13 | 13 | 13 | |
| Right buttock | 2.5 | 2.5 | 2.5 | 2.5 | 2.5 | 2.5 | |
| Left buttock | 2.5 | 2.5 | 2.5 | 2.5 | 2.5 | 2.5 | |
| Genitalia | 1 | 1 | 1 | 1 | 1 | 1 | |
| Right upper arm | 4 | 4 | 4 | 4 | 4 | 4 | |
| Left upper arm | 4 | 4 | 4 | 4 | 4 | 4 | |
| Right lower arm | 3 | 3 | 3 | 3 | 3 | 3 | |
| Left lower arm | 3 | 3 | 3 | 3 | 3 | 3 | |
| Right hand | 2.5 | 2.5 | 2.5 | 2.5 | 2.5 | 2.5 | |
| Left hand | 2.5 | 2.5 | 2.5 | 2.5 | 2.5 | 2.5 | |
| Right thigh | 5.5 | 6.5 | 8 | 8.5 | 9 | 9.5 | |
| Left thigh | 5.5 | 6.5 | 8 | 8.5 | 9 | 9.5 | |
| Right leg | 5 | 5 | 5.5 | 6 | 6.5 | 7 | |
| Left leg | 5 | 5 | 5.5 | 6 | 6.5 | 7 | |
| Right foot | 3.5 | 3.5 | 3.5 | 3.5 | 3.5 | 3.5 | |
| Left foot | 3.5 | 3.5 | 3.5 | 3.5 | 3.5 | 3.5 | |

Total BSAB _____

**FIGURE 2.** Lund-Browder Classification Burn Size and Diagram.

as possible because the rapid onset of eyelid swelling will make this difficult. Fluorescein should be used to identify corneal injury. Chemical burns to the eyes should be rinsed with copious amounts of saline. Burns of the ears require examination of the external auditory canal and ear drum before swelling occurs.

Minor burns of the hands may result in only temporary disability and inconvenience. More extensive thermal injury may cause permanent loss of function. Monitoring the digital and palmar pulses with an ultrasonic flowmeter is the most accurate means of assessing perfusion of the tissues in the hand. The burned extremity should be elevated above the heart to minimize edema formation. Digital escharotomies are not indicated prior to transfer to a burn center.

Contact the accepting burn center physician if you are concerned about the extent of the digital injury. As with burns of the upper extremity, it is important to assess the circulation and neurologic function of the feet on an hourly basis.

## Third-Degree Burns in Any Age Group

A full-thickness or third-degree burn occurs with destruction of the entire epidermis and dermis, leaving no dermal elements to repopulate. A characteristic initial appearance is a waxy white color.

Full-thickness injuries require emergent management. In most cases, treatment of the wound requires surgical skin grafting. Deep partial-thickness and full-thickness burns heal with severe scarring if not treated by surgical excision and skin grafting for optimal recovery. Disfigurement is common, and long-term functional problems can persist for years. There is also a high risk of infection, because an unexcised full-thickness burn behaves like an undrained abscess.

## Electric Burns, Including Lightning Injury

Electrical burns can be divided into flash (typical thermal injury) and high-tension injury. The latter, caused by more than 1000 volts, produces clinically characteristic entry and exit wounds. They are usually ischemic, painless, and dry; wounds of entry may appear charred and the exit explosive. Deep-muscle injury may be present even when skin appears normal. Findings that suggest electrical injury include loss of consciousness, paralysis or mummification of an extremity, loss of peripheral pulses, flexor surface burns, myoglobinuria, serum creatine kinase (CK) more than 1000, and cardiopulmonary arrest at the scene. Electrical injuries can produce vascular thrombosis, muscle tetany causing fractures, and internal organ damage. In addition to other interventions, obtain a 12-lead electrocardiogram (ECG), cardiac enzymes, and evaluate the urine for myoglobin. If there is evidence of myoglobin from muscle damage, the urine output should be maintained at 2 mL/kg per hour until the urine grossly clears to prevent acid hematin deposition in the kidney and irreversible renal damage. Compartment pressures must be monitored. If a compartment syndrome develops, contact your burn center physician because fasciotomy may be required. The most serious immediate problem associated with electrical injuries is ventricular fibrillation, asystole, or other dysrhythmias. Life-threatening arrhythmias are treated according to advanced cardiac life support (ACLS) protocols. Survival of contact with voltage greater than 70,000 volts is uncommon.

The approximate electrical potential of a lightning bolt is 20 million volts. Lightning injury can produce an enormous spectrum of clinical symptoms and signs ranging from common (cardiac asystole, respiratory arrest, arborescent markings) to the rare (disseminated intravascular coagulation [DIC], intracerebral hemorrhage). Immediate neurologic manifestations include agitation, amnesia, loss of consciousness, or motor disturbances. The eyes are particularly vulnerable to injury from electrical current, and symptoms closely correlate with the extent of the central nervous system (CNS) injury. Vitreous hemorrhage, iridocyclitis, retinal tear, macular puncture, and retinal detachment have been reported.

Lightning injuries are not usually associated with deep burns but most often with superficial injury to the skin and underlying soft tissue called *ferning*. The feathering type of burn appears as an arborescent, branching skin marking that disappears within a few hours. Pathognomonic of lightning injury, they may be of great diagnostic value in a comatose patient. Often the respiratory arrest lasts longer than the cardiac arrest. Severely injured victims often present in asystole or ventricular fibrillation. Cardiac resuscitation may occasionally be successful; but direct brain trauma as well as blunt trauma, skull fracture, and intracranial injuries, are common in these patients. The prognosis for recovery in this group is usually poor.

## Chemical Burns

Health care providers must wear protective clothing when caring for patients with potential chemical injury. The initial appearance of a chemical burn is usually deceptively benign. The severity of a chemical injury is related to the agent, concentration, volume, duration of contact, and mechanisms of action of the agent. Immediate irrigation decreases the concentration and duration of contact, reducing the severity of injury. If the agent is a powder, brush it off and irrigate with water. Irrigation should continue through emergency evaluation in the hospital and in general until evaluation in a burn center, especially for an alkali or if an unknown agent. Neutralizing agents are contraindicated because of the potential for heat generation, thereby giving the patient both a chemical and a thermal injury!

Acid burns are less severe than alkali burns. They are found in many household products including bathroom cleansers, drain cleaners, and swimming pool acidifiers. Tissue is damaged by coagulation necrosis and protein precipitation. Once a layer of eschar is formed, the burning process is self-limiting. The exception to this rule is hydrofluoric acid (HA), which is used to etch glass, make Teflon, and to remove rust. The pathogenesis of tissue damage in HA burns is distinct from other acids. HA readily crosses lipid membranes and has a potent diffusing capacity into the tissues. The molecule releases the freely dissociable fluoride ion, which produces extensive liquefactive necrosis of the soft tissues. Fluoride rapidly binds free calcium in the blood, and death from hypocalcemia may occur. Treatment is intra-arterial calcium gluconate[1] (or calcium chloride)[1] administered until the characteristic *pain out of proportion to the burn* has resolved. Even small areas of contact may result in profound hypocalcemia and death. Cardiac monitoring and frequent serum calcium determinations are indicated.

Alkalis damage tissue by liquefaction necrosis and protein denaturation. Tissue pH abnormalities may persist for 12 hours postburn, allowing deeper spread of the chemical and more severe burns. Examples would include the hydroxides, caustic sodas, and ammonium compounds found in oven cleaners, fertilizer, and cement. Wet cement damages skin in three ways: allergic dermatitis as a reaction to chromate ions, abrasions caused by the gritty nature of the cement, and as an alkali with a pH of 12.5. The ability of cement to cause such injury is not well recognized, even by professional users. With the increased media interest in do-it-yourself projects, it is likely this problem will increase.

Organic compounds such as creosote and petroleum products produce contact chemical burns as well as systemic toxicity. Gasoline and diesel fuel are petroleum products that may produce a full-thickness burn that initially appears as only partial thickness. Organic compounds cause cutaneous damage by delipidation because of their fat solvent action on cell membranes. After a motor vehicle crash involving petroleum products, always look for petroleum exposure in the lower extremities, back, and buttocks. Systemic effects include elevated liver enzymes and decreased urinary output.

## Inhalation Injury

Smoke inhalation injuries are the leading cause of fatalities from burn injuries, accounting for some 80% of all fire-related deaths. The major forms of inhalation injuries are carbon monoxide (CO) toxicity, injury to the upper airway, and pulmonary parenchymal damage. Each has different symptoms and signs, treatment, and prognosis. The compromised airway is protected by tracheal intubation, and respiratory failure is treated with assisted ventilation. Inhalation injury is manifested by the pathology and dysfunction that rapidly become evident in the airways, lungs, and respiratory system after inhaling the products of incomplete combustion. Patients receiving massive fluid resuscitation can develop upper airway edema with subsequent asphyxiation.

Immediate medical attention and diagnosis depend on a high index of suspicion, an appropriate history, careful examination of the upper airway, the presence of clinical symptoms, and suggestive arterial blood gases. An inhalation injury is suspected in any patient with full-thickness facial burns or with any burns combined with a history of being confined within an enclosed space. Other classic signs are soot or carbonaceous sputum, stridor or hoarseness, or blistering of the pharynx or vocal cords. Late signs include grunting, nasal flaring, retractions, wheezes, and rales. Use of prophylactic antibiotics and steroids is discouraged.

The effect of CO poisoning may be exhibited by respiratory symptoms and CNS findings such as altered level of consciousness, seizures, or coma. Cardiovascular effects include diminished cardiac output

---

[1]Not FDA approved for this indication.

evidenced by decreased perfusion and hypotension. There is much controversy regarding hyperbaric oxygen therapy, but there are no objective data proving the efficacy of hyperbaric oxygen in CO poisoning. At this time, hyperbaric oxygen treatment for acute CO toxicity should be restricted to randomized prospective studies. The correct treatment is administering 100% oxygen, thereby decreasing the CO half-life from 4 hours to 45 minutes.

## Burn Injury in Patients with Preexisting Medical Disorders That Could Complicate Management, Prolong Recovery, or Affect Mortality

Peripheral vascular disease can lead to a decrease in wound blood flow. Diabetes, through high glucose, will impede capillary flow. Optimum control of the blood glucose is needed to optimize blood flow. A local decrease in wound-tissue oxygen tension is recognized to be a major wound-healing impediment because all phases of healing are oxygen dependent, including local infection control. Most common causes are a decrease in systemic blood volume and oxygen delivery, decrease in hemoglobin saturation, eschar on the wound surface, or infection. Treatment modalities need to focus first on correction of systemic abnormalities: correct cardiovascular and lung function, correct large vessel obstructive disease impeding wound flow, aggressive wound debridement, and eliminate tissue exudates. Patients with preexisting cardiac disease are particularly sensitive to fluids and may tolerate the necessary fluid resuscitation poorly.

## Any Patient With Burns and Concomitant Trauma (Such as Fractures) in Which the Burn Injury Poses the Greatest Risk of Morbidity and Mortality

In such cases, if the trauma poses the greater immediate risk, the patient may be initially stabilized in a trauma center before being transferred to a burn unit. Physician judgment will be necessary in such situations and should be in concert with the regional medical control plan and triage protocols.

Most burn-trauma publications cite a 5% frequency of burn-trauma patient. Because burn trauma is rare outside of a major conflict or disaster, most centers see only a few patients annually. By definition, child abuse falls into the burn-trauma category. It may be the burn injury that prompts relatives or neighbors to bring the child to the hospital or report the family to authority. The visibility of the injury may instigate corrective action. In a 44-month review we saw 120 cases of burns and trauma. Although motor vehicle crashes (MVCs) can result in fracture, soft tissue, and thermal injury, unique to this burn-trauma population was that the MVC injury was frequently a result of assault. With the graying of America, elder abuse may become a larger societal problem.

## Burned Children in Hospitals Without Qualified Personnel or Equipment for the Care of Children

Each year more than 2500 children die and 10,000 more sustain permanent disability from thermal injury. Children are not just little adults! They respond differently than adults to severe trauma, maintaining normal vital signs longer but decompensating rapidly. Because of the smaller cross-sectional diameter of the pediatric airway, it takes much less edema to compromise a pediatric airway. If intubation is required, the most experienced pediatric airway manager should

## CURRENT DIAGNOSIS

- Maintain a high index of suspicion
- Remember the ABCs
- Rule out concomitant trauma
- Establish size and depth of burn
- Be wary of chemical and electrical burns, which may be misleading
- Establish resuscitation requirements

*Abbreviations:* ABC = airway with cervical spine immobilization if appropriate, breathing, circulation, disability, and exposure.

intubate the child because repeated attempts may create sufficient airway edema as to cause obstruction. Anatomical airway differences make intubation by the inexperienced even more difficult.

The greater surface area per unit of body mass of children necessitates the administration of relatively greater amounts of resuscitation fluid. The surface area/body mass relationship of the child also defines a lesser intravascular volume per unit surface area burned. This makes the burned child more susceptible to fluid overload and hemodilution. Hypoglycemia may occur if the limited glycogen stores of the child are rapidly exhausted by the early postburn elevation of circulating levels of steroids and catecholamines. Infants should receive maintenance fluids with 5% dextrose in addition to the resuscitation fluids outlined in the consensus formula. Children younger than 2 years of age have disproportionally thin skin so that exposures that would produce only partial-thickness burns in older patients produce full-thickness injuries. Children have a relatively small muscle mass, hampering intrinsic heat generation. Children younger than 6 months of age are unable to shiver and thus are even more prone to develop hypothermia.

Stress for the burned child not only includes the body surface area (BSA) burn and the pain that is involved but also the separation from parents and loved ones. This escalates especially if the parents were also burned in the fire. Emergency management of each pediatric burn patient requires an individual care plan. Early consultation with the burn center physician is advised.

## Burn Injury in Patients Who Will Require Special Social, Emotional, and/or Long-Term Rehabilitative Intervention

Failure to recognize the thermal manifestations of child abuse not only negates protection of the child but predicates potential lethal injury. Awareness of the patterns of abuse, the behavior patterns of the parents, and the physical manifestations will protect the child by early recognition and reporting. Physical child abuse victims frequently present with thermal injuries of varying degrees. The history of injury should correlate with the physical findings. The history also becomes important in identifying repetitious hospital visits for accidental injury. Not infrequently, the hospital visits will be made at different hospitals to avoid disclosure and identification.

The events leading to an injury are extremely important in the initial evaluation of an infant or child. *Always* consider the potential for child abuse. The incidence of child abuse is approximately 10% of all children presenting to an emergency department (ED), with a mortality rate less than 1%. Abused children present with a higher median Injury Severity Score, more severe injuries of the head and integument, longer hospital lengths of stay, and a high mortality rate.

A burn of any magnitude can be a serious injury. Health care providers must be able to assess the injuries rapidly and develop a priority-based plan of care. The plan of care is determined by the type, extent, and degree of burn as well as by available resources.

## CURRENT THERAPY

- Communicate with your burn center early and often
- Remember the ABCs
- Cover the wound with Saran Wrap
- Prevent hypothermia
- Transport to the burn center

*Abbreviations:* ABC = airway with cervical spine immobilization if appropriate, breathing, circulation, disability, and exposure.

Burn care is complex. It involves a multisystem assessment and appropriate intervention. The first 24 hours of management are perhaps the most critical for patient survival. Burn centers provide optimal care in a cost-effective, multidisciplinary manner. Every health care provider must know how and when to contact the closest burn center. If the attending physician determines that the patient should be treated at the burn center, the extent of treatment provided at the referring hospital—and the method of transport to the burn center—should be decided in consultation with the burn center physician. A complete list of verified burn centers is available at http://ameriburn.org.

## REFERENCES

Advanced Burn Life Support Course, American Burn Association, 625 N. Michigan Ave., Suite 1530, Chicago, IL. 60611. 2001.
American College of Surgeons Committee on Trauma: Resources for optimal care of the injured patient: 1999. Chicago, American College of Surgeons, 1999.
Andrews CJ, Cooper MA, Darveniza M, Mackerras D (eds): Lightning injuries: Electrical, medical, and legal aspects. Boca Raton, Fla, CRC Press, 1992, pp 62-63, 82-85, 88-98, 101-110.
Burd A: Hydrofluoric acid—revisited. Burns 2004;30(7):720-722.
Chang DC, Knight V, Ziegfeld S, et al: The tip of the iceberg for child abuse: The critical roles of the pediatric trauma service and its registry. J Trauma 2004;57(6):1189-1198.
Heimbach DM: Regionalization of burn care: A concept whose time has come. J Burn Care Rehabil 2003;24(3):173-174.
Latenser BA, Iteld L: Smoke inhalation injury. Seminars in Respiratory and Critical Care Medicine. 2001;22(1):13-22.
Luce EA (ed): Clinics in Plastic Surgery. An International Quarterly. Burn Care and Management. Philadelphia, WB Saunders, 2000; 27(1): 133-143.
Varghese TK, Kim AW, Kowal-Vern A, Latenser BA: Frequency of burn-trauma patients in an urban setting. Arch Surg. 2003;138:1292-1296.

# High-Altitude Illness

Method of
*James A. Litch, MD, DTMH*

Decreased partial pressure of oxygen at high altitude results in pronounced physiologic responses that range from beneficial to pathologic. Slow ascent normally leads to acclimatization. High-altitude illness is a collective term for a cluster of acute clinical syndromes that are a direct consequence of rapid ascent to high altitude above 2500 m. The acute syndromes affecting the brain include acute mountain sickness (AMS) and high-altitude cerebral edema (HACE). The acute syndrome affecting the lung is high-altitude pulmonary edema (HAPE). All unacclimatized sojourners to high altitude are potentially at risk. The characteristic cerebral and pulmonary abnormalities are not subtle, but when unrecognized or ignored, they may progress to death. Each year millions travel to high-altitude locations on every continent, resulting in morbidity and mortality with associated economic consequences.

## Normal Acclimatization

It is not uncommon for normal acclimatization of novice healthy visitors to high altitude to cause concern that they are experiencing a health problem. Normal acclimatization includes immediate hyperventilation, shortness of breath with moderate excursion, and a decreased work capacity. These are followed by diuresis, disturbed sleep (including periodic breathing), and peripheral/facial edema. It is important to recognize the signs of normal acclimatization so reassurance and education may be appropriately provided.

## Incidence and Risk Factors

Determinants of whether high-altitude illness will occur are individual susceptibility, rate of ascent, altitude reached, and sleep altitude. Incidence rates of AMS reported in literature are difficult to compare because of variability in methodology and rates of ascent. Reported incident figures for AMS following ascent by hiking, vehicle, or flying range from 10% to 40% at 2700 to 3000 m, and from 40% to 95% at 3800 to 4000 m. HACE and HAPE are both far less common than mild AMS, but actual incident rates are unavailable. HAPE can occur as low as 2500 m. HACE is rare below 3600 m. Most cases of HACE and HAPE are preceded by AMS.

Risk factors for altitude illness include a history of previous high-altitude illness, residence at altitude below 1000 m, physical exertion, and preexisting cardiopulmonary conditions. Traveling in a large group presents a risk because a tight itinerary often does not allow time for acclimatization, and members are reluctant to declare symptoms for fear of being left behind. Children appear to carry the same risk for altitude illness as adults, but persons over 50 years of age seem less susceptible, possibly because of a more cautious ascent profile. There appears to be little or no gender difference for AMS, but women may be less susceptible to HAPE. Heavy physical exertion at exceedingly high altitude appears to be an important risk factor for HAPE. Rapid ascent, especially by flying or driving to altitude, places sojourners at risk for altitude illnesses.

## Prevention of Altitude Illnesses

Gradual ascent to altitude over several days to allow for acclimatization reduces the likelihood of acute mountain sickness. Ascent rates of less than 300 m per day at altitudes of more than 2500 m is a common recommendation; but individuals will still experience altitude illness when abiding to this recommendation. However, the critical understanding to prevent serious life-threatening altitude illness (HAPE and HACE) is to halt further ascent until symptoms resolve.

Medications are available to help prevent the symptoms of AMS when rapid ascent (<24 hours) to altitudes more than 3000 m is anticipated, or for those with a past history of AMS with a similar ascent profile. These agents are started the evening before ascent and continued for 2 to 3 days. The most commonly used medications are acetazolamide (Diamox) (125 to 250 mg twice a day), acetaminophen[1] (325 mg four times a day), or aspirin[1] (325 mg three times a day). Acetazolamide (Diamox) is particularly useful because it actually improves oxygenation, has a positive impact on the quality of sleep at high altitude, and is effective for periodic breathing that occurs during sleep. However, these medications do not protect against the development of life threatening altitude illness: HAPE and HACE. Other medications have been suggested for use in preventing altitude illness. Randomized double blinded placebo-controlled trails of ginkgo biloba[1] and acetazolamide (Diamox) have shown no benefit from ginkgo biloba over placebo, and reduced incidence and severity of

[1]Not FDA approved for this indication.

AMS symptoms from acetazolamide (Diamox). Dexamethasone (Decadron),[1] a potent steroid, is generally best avoided as a prevention measure against AMS during ascent so it may be used, if needed, for treatment of HACE along with descent.

Nifedipine (Adalat, Procardia)[1] has been studied for use in prevention of HAPE and found to be of benefit for persons with a history of recurrent HAPE. Studies are underway to evaluate sildenafil citrate (Viagra),[1] an agent that selectively lowers pulmonary artery pressure, in the prevention of HAPE. In addition, inhaled salmeterol (Serevent)[1] has been found effective for the prevention of HAPE in a small group of climbers who had previously shown susceptibility to HAPE. However, these high-risk individuals would do far better with cautious gradual ascent, rather than relying on a medication with limited effect for a life-threatening condition.

Several nonmedication measures that can prevent or ameliorate symptoms of high-altitude illness include the following:

- Begin a high-carbohydrate diet one or two days before the climb and maintain during the ascent
- Adapt plans to realistically reflect the decreased work capacity at high altitude
- Reschedule or slow the ascent should an upper respiratory or other active infection present
- Avoid overexertion during ascent by maintaining a reasonable pace and not overloading with nonessential gear
- Maintain adequate hydration on the climb to offset increased fluid loss at altitude
- Avoid nonessential medications and remedies
- Provide good ventilation for camp stoves used in confined places
- Allow for several days of altitude exposure the week prior to ascent to high altitude

## Acute Mountain Sickness and High-Altitude Cerebral Edema

AMS is defined as a headache in the setting of recent altitude gain and typical symptoms which include anorexia, nausea, vomiting, insomnia, dizziness, or fatigue (Current Diagnosis box). Symptoms are nonspecific, and there is an absence of physical findings. The differential diagnosis is extensive and other conditions should be considered (Box 1). Pulse oximetry values may be high, normal, or low for the altitude and do not correlate to severity of symptoms. A careful and detailed history is essential to steer diagnostic decision making. Often in outdoor settings multiple conditions can be present such as AMS and dehydration. Rapid resolution of symptoms during treatment with oxygen is very specific to AMS. Early recognition of AMS is a key principle in remote areas with limited support.

AMS is not life threatening, but ignoring it can be. Progressive neurologic deterioration may occur over hours or days as dangerous collections of fluid develop in the brain leading to HACE. HACE presents with truncal ataxia, confusion, and hallucination in the setting of recent altitude gain. The period of time from initial ataxia and confusion to onset of coma may be as little as 8 to 12 hours. If descent or oxygen supplementation is not accomplished within hours, coma and death can ensue from brain herniation. A presumptive and/or rigid diagnosis of HACE in the setting of progressive neurologic deterioration has led to tragic situations when other life-threatening conditions were actually present (see Box 1). Details of the initial presentation, response to immediate descent/supplemental oxygen, and recognition of additional signs can guide clinical decision making while maintaining a high index of suspicion for other neurologic conditions. Patients with persistent symptoms after descent require prompt evacuation and thorough evaluation. In addition, HAPE may develop concurrently with HACE resulting in

---

### BOX 1 Differential Diagnosis of High-Altitude Illnesses

**Acute Mountain Sickness and High-Altitude Cerebral Edema**

- Alcohol intoxication
- Brain tumor
- CO inhalation
- CNS infection
- Cerebral vascular accident
- Dehydration
- Diabetic ketoacidosis
- Exhaustion
- Hypoglycemia and insulin shock
- Hyponatremia
- Hypothermia
- Migraine
- Narcotics
- Poisoning
- Psychosis
- Sedatives overdose
- Seizures
- Subarachnoid hemorrhage
- Transient ischemic attack

**High-Altitude Pulmonary Edema**

- Adult respiratory distress syndrome
- Asthma
- Bronchitis
- Congestive heart failure
- Myocardial infarction
- Pneumonia (infection or aspiration)
- Poisoning
- Pulmonary embolus
- Respiratory failure

*Abbreviations:* CNS = central nervous system; CO = carbon monoxide.

---

shortness of breath while at rest and a further reduction of oxygen delivery to the body.

Definitive diagnosis is available using imaging studies such as CT and MRI. However, these have limited application, because the condition should have greatly improved from oxygen/descent before the opportunity presents to obtain the study. Neuroimaging demonstrates vasogenic edema in individuals with moderate to severe AMS or HACE.

Management of AMS is directed at limiting further hypoxia by halting ascent, and providing additional oxygen should symptoms persist or progress to HACE. Acetazolamide (Diamox) is helpful for the treatment of AMS. For the management of HACE improved oxygenation is the definitive treatment. There are several methods of oxygen delivery: (1) descent, (2) supplemental oxygen via cylinder or concentrator, and/or (3) portable hyperbaric bag. These may be combined or applied in series depending on resources, location, and logistic support. Concomitant pharmacologic treatment with dexamethasone (Decadron)[1] and acetazolamide (Diamox) aid recovery. Persons with suspected HACE who do not rapidly recover during treatment or those with focal neurologic deficits should be hospitalized and undergo comprehensive neurologic evaluation including magnetic resonance imaging (MRI). The Current Therapy box summarizes management of HACE.

---

[1]Not FDA approved for this indication.

[1]Not FDA approved for this indication.

## CURRENT DIAGNOSIS

- Acute Mountain Sickness—In the setting of a recent gain in altitude, the presence of headache and at least one of the following: GI symptoms (anorexia, nausea, or vomiting), fatigue or weakness, dizziness or lightheadedness, or difficulty sleeping
- High-Altitude Cerebral Edema—In the setting of a recent gain in altitude, the presence of a change in mental status and/or ataxia in a person with AMS, or the presence of both mental status change and ataxia in a person without AMS
- High-Altitude Pulmonary Edema—In the setting of a recent gain in altitude, the presence of at least two of the following symptoms: dyspnea at rest, cough, weakness or decreased exercise performance, chest tightness, or congestion; and two of the following signs: rales or wheezing in at least one lung field, central cyanosis, tachypnea, or tachycardia

*The Lake Louise Consensus on the Definition and Quantification of Altitude Illness.
*Abbreviations:* AMS = acute mountain sickness; GI = gastrointestinal.

## High-Altitude Pulmonary Edema

HAPE is defined as noncardiogenic edema resulting from hypoxia-induced changes in the pulmonary circulation. HAPE is commonly preceded by AMS, and 20% of individuals with HAPE develop HACE. Early symptoms of HAPE include decreased exercise performance beyond that expected for the altitude, often accompanied with a dry cough (see Current Diagnosis Box). Progression is rapid with even minimal continued physical activity without descent. The hallmark of progression requiring prompt action is dyspnea at rest. Rales are present at this stage. Resting pulse oximetry reveals below-normal oxygen saturation for the altitude. Tachypnea and tachycardia beyond that expected for the altitude also are present. Pink, frothy sputum develops late in the illness. Early diagnosis is important because progression of the illness further limits oxygenation and worsens the degree of hypoxemia causing the condition.

HAPE is a life-threatening emergency; immediate improvement in oxygenation is critical to arrest the progression and is the definitive treatment. In medical facilities high-flow supplemental oxygen while at rest and sitting in an upright position should be initiated immediately during the initial assessment of the patient. Response may be assessed by pulse oximetry and resting respiratory rate. Despite prompt improvement during the first few hours of treatment, maintenance of oxygenation (oxygen saturation greater than 90%) with low-flow supplemental oxygen and rest is often required for 2 to 3 days unless descent is achieved. For vacationers to high-altitude resort areas, this oxygen requirement can be maintained outside the hospital using a cylinder or concentrator as an alternative to descent for informed individuals that wish to remain in the locale of family and friends. A continued requirement of high-flow oxygen of 4 to 5 L per minute or more to maintain oxygen saturation greater than 90%, or concurrent HACE, requires hospitalization. Antibiotics are indicated if infection is suspected. Endotracheal intubation and mechanical ventilation are rarely indicated. The differential diagnosis is extensive, and a high index of suspicion for other conditions should be maintained throughout the treatment course (see Box 1).

In remote areas oxygen may be administered by:

- Descent with minimal exertion
- Supplemental oxygen via cylinder or concentrator
- Portable hyperbaric bag placed on an incline to keep the head elevated

## CURRENT THERAPY

**Acute Mountain Sickness**
- Halt ascent, do not exceed light activity level, oral hydration.
- Administer acetazolamide (Diamox) 250 mg PO bid.
- Administer analgesics and antiemetics.
- If readily available, administer oxygen 1 to 2 L per minute as needed to resolve symptoms.
- If no improvement after 24 hours, descend to altitude where person last slept without symptoms until fully recovered.

**High-Altitude Cerebral Edema**
- Administer oxygen 2 to 4 L per minute.
- In remote mountain areas, prepare for immediate descent of at least 600 m by ground or aircraft, and if oxygen unavailable, use portable hyperbaric chamber.
- Monitor at all times, and replenish/maintain hydration as needed.
- Administer dexamethasone (Decadron) 8 mg IM, IV, or PO × 1 dose, then 4 mg q6h.
- Administer acetazolamide (Diamox) 250 mg PO bid.

**High-Altitude Pulmonary Edema**
- Administer oxygen initially 4 to 6 L per minute, then titrate to keep arterial oxygen saturation more than 90%.
- In remote mountain areas, prepare for immediate descent of at least 600 m by ground or aircraft; and if oxygen unavailable, use portable hyperbaric chamber on incline with head end elevated.
- Sit upright at 45 degree angle, strict rest, and monitor at all times.
- Administer nifedipine (Adalat, Procardia) 10 mg PO initially, then 30 mg extended release q12h *IF* oxygen unavailable *AND* IV fluid resuscitation immediately available.
- Administer salmeterol (Serevent) inhaler, 1 puff bid *OR* albuterol (Proventil) inhaler, 4 to 6 puffs q4h.
- Administer dexamethasone (Decadron) 8 mg IM, IV or PO × 1 dose, then 4 mg q6h *IF* suspect or unsure if HACE is also present.

*Abbreviations:* bid = twice daily; IM = intramuscular; IV = intravenous; PO = orally; q = every.

Because of a lack of equipment, immediate descent may be the only option available. In late stages more than one oxygen modality may need to be employed concurrently. These efforts place great strain on the limited resources of groups traveling in remote areas. It is common for the shared concern and cooperation among group members (tourists/staff/porters) to disintegrate or for groups to discover that they are woefully unequipped to handle HAPE. As a result fatal outcomes are common when HAPE presents in remote settings.

Pharmacologic treatment is directed at agents that reduce pulmonary artery pressure and thereby may improve oxygenation in HAPE. Medications including nifedipine (Adalat, Procardia),[1] nitric oxide (INO$_{max}$),[1] epoprostenol (Flolan),[1] and sildenafil (Viagra)[1] have been studied for use in treatment of HAPE. Current clinical experience warrants consideration of nifedipine (Adalat, Procardia) as an adjunct

[1]Not FDA approved for this indication.

treatment for HAPE when immediate supplemental oxygen is unavailable or descent is delayed. Vascular access and intravenous (IV) fluid should be immediately available if nifedipine (Adalat, Procardia) is administered because patients are often intravascularly depleted and risk a severe hypotensive event that could be devastating in the setting of concomitant HACE. Sildenafil citrate (Viagra)[1] can also selectively lower pulmonary artery pressure with less effect on systemic blood pressure, and is under study for the treatment of HAPE. Inhaled β-agonists, salmeterol (Serevent),[1] and albuterol (Proventil)[1] are currently under study for treatment of HAPE because β-agonists increase the clearance of fluid from the alveolar space and might lower pulmonary artery pressure. The Current Therapy Box summarizes the management of HAPE.

## Reascent After Altitude Illness

Mild AMS is common and indicative of an ascent rate that is too rapid for a given person. Further ascent should not resume until full resolution of all symptoms. Future trips with similar ascent profiles warrant consideration of prophylaxis with acetazolamide (Diamox).

After episodes of HACE and HAPE resolve fully, reascent has been successful for many patients, some reaching exceptionally high summits. Caution is warranted, however. Persons should be advised to ascend more slowly and to recognize and act appropriately for early signs of altitude illness. Persons with multiple episodes of HAPE may benefit during subsequent ascent from prophylaxis with nifedipine (Adalat, Procardia)[1] and potentially with salmeterol (Serevent)[1] while stressing the value of cautious gradual ascent over medication. Recurrent HAPE or HAPE occurring at altitudes below 3000 m should prompt evaluation to rule out cardiac or pulmonary shunts, valvular disease, or pulmonary hypertension.

## REFERENCES

Bartsch P, Merki B, Hofstetter D, et al: Treatment of acute mountain sickness by simulated descent: A randomized controlled trial. BMJ 1993;306: 1098-1101.

Chow T, Browne V, Heileson HL, et al: Ginkgo biloba and acetazolamide prophylaxis for acute mountain sickness: A randomized placebo-controlled trial. Arch Intern Med 2005;165:296-301.

Consensus Group: The Lake Louise Consensus on the Definition and Quantification of Altitude Illness. In JR Sutton, G Coates, CS Houston: Hypoxia and Mountain Medicine. Burlington, Vt, Queen City Printers, 1992, 327-330.

Litch JA: Endotracheal intubation and mechanical ventilation following respiratory arrest from high altitude pulmonary edema. West J Med 1999;170(3):174-176.

Litch JA, Basnyat B, Zimmerman M: Subarachnoid hemorrhage at high altitude. West J Med 1997;167(3):180-181.

Litch JA, Bishop RA: Re-ascent following resolution of high altitude pulmonary edema (HAPE). High Alt Med Biol 2001;2(1):53-55.

Litch JA, Bishop RA: Oxygen concentrators for the delivery of supplemental oxygen in remote high altitude areas. Wilderness Environ Med 2000; 11(3):189-191.

Larson EB, Roach RC, Schoene RB, Hornbein TF: Acute mountain sickness and acetazolamide—Clinical efficacy and effect on ventilation. JAMA 1982; 248: 328-332.

Oelz O, Maggiorini M, Ritter M, et al: Prevention and treatment of high altitude pulmonary edema by a calcium channel blocker. Int J Sports Med 1992; 13(Suppl 1):S65-S68.

Pollard AJ, Niermeyer S, Barry P, et al: Children at high altitude: An international consensus statement by an ad hoc committee of the International Society of Mountain Medicine. High Alt Med Biol 2001;2(3):389-403.

Rabold MB: Dexamethasone for prophylaxis and treatment of acute mountain sickness. West J Med 1992;3:54-60.

Sartori C, Allemann Y, Duplain H, et al: Salmeterol for the prevention of high-altitude pulmonary edema. N Engl J Med 2002;346(21):1631-1636.

---

[1]Not FDA approved for this indication.

# Disturbances Due to Cold

Method of
*Frederick K. Korley, MD, and Jerrold B. Leikin, MD*

## Accidental Hypothermia

Hypothermia is classically defined as a reduction in the body's core temperature below 95.0°F (35.0°C). Most reported cases of hypothermia are due to exposure to low ambient temperatures (accidental hypothermia). Other causes of hypothermia include sepsis, severe hypothyroidism, diabetic ketoacidosis, multisystem trauma, and prolonged cardiac arrest.

### EPIDEMIOLOGY

Risk factors for developing hypothermia include extremes of age (the elderly might not be able to remove themselves from cold environments, and young children lose heat more rapidly due to their increased total body surface area), major trauma, homelessness, psychiatric illness, and drug and alcohol abuse (Box 1). Cold-related deaths also are reported in military combatants and outdoor winter sports participants. Several drugs and chemicals can predispose to hypothermia (Box 2). Alcohol is the most common intoxicant associated with hypothermia due to its ability to cause cutaneous vasodilation, impairment of shivering, and impairment of adaptive behavior.

Between 1979 and 2002, a total of 16,555 deaths in the United States, an average of 689 per year, were attributed to exposure to low environmental temperatures. In 2002, of the 646 hypothermia-related deaths reported, 66% occurred in male patients, 52% of all decedents were aged 65 years or younger, 45% of the deaths occurred among white male patients, and 14% occurred among black male patients. The states of Alaska, New Mexico, North Dakota, and Montana had the largest overall death rates due to hypothermia in 2002. The lowest recorded core temperature in a pediatric survivor of accidental hypothermia is 57.9°F (14.4°C) and the lowest is 56.7°F (13.7°C) in an adult survivor.

### PATHOPHYSIOLOGY

The normal range of human core temperature is 97.5°F (36.4°C) to 99.5°F (37.5°C). Humans are thus warm-blooded and are normally able to maintain their body temperature by heat-generating mechanisms and heat-conserving behavior. These compensatory responses, however, can be overwhelmed under extreme environmental conditions, leading to hypothermia.

The anterior hypothalamus coordinates the nonshivering heat conservation and dissipation mechanisms, and the posterior hypothalamus coordinates shivering thermogenesis. Heat loss usually occurs by four mechanisms: About 55% to 65% of heat is lost by radiation, 25% to 30% by evaporation from the skin and respiratory tract, and 10% to 15% by conduction and convection. The amount of heat lost via conduction is markedly increased in cold-water immersion (by about 32 times). Each organ system is affected uniquely by hypothermia.

#### The Cardiovascular System

One of the initial heat-conserving mechanisms is peripheral vasoconstriction to decrease blood flow to the skin. There are also initial increases, in heart rate and blood pressure due to a catecholamine surge. At core temperatures below 82.4°F (28.0°C), bradycardia can occur. The myocardium also becomes irritable, predisposing it to arrhythmias. Atrial arrhythmias can occur with a slow ventricular response and they can precede ventricular arrhythmias and asystole at core temperatures below 77.0°F (25.0°C). The characteristic Osborn or J waves (a hump seen at the QRS-ST junction) may be seen on the electrocardiogram (ECG) at core temperatures below 89.6°F (32.0°C).

## BOX 1   Factors Predisposing to Hypothermia or Frostbite

### Physiologic
**Decreased Heat Production**

Age extremes (infants, elderly)
Dehydration or nalnutrition
Diaphoresis or hyperhidrosis
Endocrinologic insufficiency
Hypoxia
Insufficient fuel
Overexertion
Physical conditioning
Prior cold injury
Trauma (multisystem or extremity)

**Increased Heat Loss**
Burns
- Dermatologic malfunction
- Cold infusions
- Emergency resuscitation
- Poor acclimatization or conditioning
- Shock
- Vascular diseases

**Impaired Thermoregulation**
- Central nervous system trauma or disease
- Metabolic disorders
- Pharmacologic or toxicologic agents
- Sepsis
- Spinal cord injury

### Psychological
- Fatigue
- Fear or panic
- Hunger
- Intense concentration on tasks
- Intoxicants
- Mental status or attitude
- Peer pressure

### Environmental
- Altitude with or without associated conditions
- Ambient temperature or humidity
- Duration of exposure
- Heat loss (conductive, evaporative, radiative, convective)
- Quantity of exposed surface area
- Wind chill factor

### Mechanical
- Constricting or wet clothing or boots
- Inadequate insulation
- Immobility or cramped positioning

### The Renal System

Renal blood flow is increased by peripheral vasoconstriction, leading to cold-induced diuresis. Antidiuretic hormone activity is usually inhibited. This results in intravascular volume depletion, subsequent vasodilation, to increase renal blood flow, and ultimately acute renal failure.

### The Respiratory System

At core temperatures below 82.4° F (28°C), minute ventilation is reduced; bronchorrhea can occur, with a loss of cough and gag reflexes leading to an increased risk for aspiration. Apnea can then result.

### The Central Nervous System

Cerebral metabolism is depressed 6% to 7% per 1°C decrease in core temperature. Cerebrovascular autoregulation remains intact until below 77.0°F (25.0°C), which helps maintain cortical blood flow. Electroencephalographic activity is clearly not prognostic, and it silences around 66.2°F to 68.0°F (19.0°C-20.0°C).

### CLINICAL PRESENTATION

Accidental hypothermia is classified as mild at body temperatures of 90°F (32.2°C) to 95°F (35°C), moderate at body temperatures of 82.4°F (28.0°C) to 90°F (<32.2°C), or severe at body temperatures less than 28°C (82.4°F).

In general, a patient's symptoms depend on the severity of the temperature drop. Patients with mild hypothermia can develop vigorous shivering and cold diuresis. Those with moderate hypothermia can have a paradoxical decrease in shivering, slurred speech, hyporeflexia, and confusion. They may have Osborn J waves on the ECG. They are also at risk for intravascular thrombosis. Splanchnic vasoconstriction, gastric erosions, hepatic necrosis, and pancreatitis can occur.

During severe hypothermia, shivering gives way to rigor, minute ventilation decreases, and heart rate and cardiac output decrease. Cardiac instability can be seen at this stage and can manifest in the form of arrhythmias, heart blocks, and eventually asystole. Neurologically, the patient's mental status declines. He or she might attempt to undress (paradoxical undressing) and might respond only to painful stimuli, have decreased gag reflexes, and eventually become apenic. Generally, at about 68.0°F (20.0°C), patients become totally neurologically unresponsive, lose corneal and ocular reflexes, and can have a flat electroencephalograph (EEG).

### EMERGENCY DEPARTMENT EVALUATION

Typically, the source of hypothermia is revealed from the patient's history; however, it is very important to rule out secondary causes of hypothermia such as sepsis, hypothyroidism, central nervous system (CNS) lesions, and hypoglycemia among others. All patients arriving in the emergency department with hypothermia need a complete evaluation to rule out traumatic injuries and drug or toxin ingestion or overdose.

As in all resuscitation, attention should be paid to the ABCs (airway, breathing and circulation). Respiratory failure should be treated with endotracheal intubation and mechanical ventilation. Hypotension can be treated initially with warmed fluids. Placing the patient in a warm environment, removing all cold and wet clothes, and remembering to cover up the patient after he or she has been exposed should help avoid further heat loss.

The temperature should be confirmed by checking a core temperature (e.g., rectal, bladder, or esophageal), using a thermometer capable of recording very low temperatures. Patients should be placed on a cardiac monitor and an ECG should be obtained. Laboratory testing is especially useful in the postresuscitative period when complications begin. Laboratory tests should include a complete blood count (CBC), a chemistry panel, creatine phosphokinase (CPK) to evaluate for rhabdomyolysis, a coagulation profile, blood type and screen, an arterial blood gas (ABG), and a drug screen. A Foley catheter should be placed to access urinary output.

### REWARMING STRATEGIES

There are several methods of rewarming. The method of choice usually depends on the severity of hypothermia. During rewarming, the patient should be placed on a cardiac monitor with frequent measurements of blood pressure and temperature (via a rectal probe) for easy detection of complications of rewarming such as rewarming-related hypotension, arrhythmias, and core temperature after-drop.

## BOX 2 Drugs and Chemicals that Can Cause Hypothermia

**Medicinals**
Acetaminophen (Tylenol)
Amphotericin B (Fungizone)
Azithromycin (Zithromax)
Baclofen (Lioresal)
Barbituates
Benzodiazepines
β-Adrenergic blocking agents
Bethanechol (Urecholine)
Biperiden (Akineton)
Bromocriptine (Parlodel)
Carbamazepine (Tegretol)
Chloral hydrate (Noctec)
Chlorpromazine (Thorazine)
Clonidine (Catapres)
Colchicine
Diltiazem (Cardizem)
Ethchlorvynol (Placidyl)
Ethyl alcohol
Fenoprofen (Nalfon)
Fluphenazine (Prolixin)
Fosphenytoin (Cerebyx)
Gallium nitrate (Ganite)
Glutethimide (Doriden)[2]
Guanabenz (Wytensin)
Guanfacine (Tenex)
Haloperidol (Haldol)
Heroin
Ibuprofen (Advil, Motrin)
Insulin preparations
Interferon-β-1b (Betaseron)
Lithium (Eskalith, Lithobid)
Loxapine (Loxapac, Loxitane)
Magnesium sulfate
Maprotiline (Ludiomil)
Mefenamic acid (Ponstel)
Methyldopa (Aldomet)
Methyprylon (Noludar)[2]

Moricizine (Ethmozine)
Morphine sulfate
Naphazoline (Naphcon)
Omeprazole (Prilosec)
Oxymetazoline (Afrin)
Phencyclidine
Phenol
Phenytoin (Dilantin)
Pilocarpine (Salagen)
Prazosin (Minipress)
Propoxyphene (Darvon)
*Rauwolfia serpentine*
Reserpine
Salicylate
Terazosin (Hytrin)
Tetracycline (Sumycin)
Tetrahydrozoline (Visine, Opti-
   Clear)
Thioridazine (Mellaril)
Tretinoin (Topical) (Retin A)
Tricyclic antidepressants
Valproic acid and derivatives
   (Depakene)
Zinc sulfate

**Nonmedicinals**
Acrylamide
Aldicarb
Amitraz
Barium
Bromophos
Carbon disulfide
Carbon monoxide
Chloralose
Chlorfenvinphos
Chloryrifos
Coumaphos
Cyanide

Diazinon
Dichlorvos
Dicrotophos
Dioxathion
Disulfoton
Ether
Ethion
Fensulfothion
Fenthion
Hexachlorobenzene
Hydrogen sulfide
Isopropyl alcohol
Lewisite
Malathion
Methidathion
Methiocarb
Methomyl
Methylparathion
Nickel
Parathion
Profenofos
Pyrimidifen
Sodium azide
Terbufos
Tetraethly pyrophosphate

**Biologicals**
Ackee fruit poisoning
Ciguatera food poisoning
Delphinium
Lobelia
Marijuana *(Cannabis)*
Monkshood
Nutmeg
Star of Bethlehem *(Hippobroman*
   *longiflora)*
Tetrodotoxin food poisoning
White chameleon

[2]Not available in the United States.

### Passive External Warming

Passive external warming is ideal for patients with mild hypothermia who are otherwise healthy. It uses the patient's endogenous heat production for rewarming and it involves simple, logical passive maneuvers that minimize heat dissipation. When using this method, all wet clothing should be removed, the ambient core temperature should exceed 70.0°F (21.0°C), and the patient should be covered with insulating materials. Patients warmed easily using this method can be safely discharged.

### Active External Rewarming

Active external rewarming is controversial. It involves exposing the skin of the patient to exogenous heat sources. Radiant heat, thermal mattresses, electric heating blankets, and forced-air heating blankets are some of the available techniques.

This method has a number of disadvantages. First, burn injuries can occur to the vasoconstricted skin. Second, any sort of immersion can hinder monitoring and other resuscitative activities. Finally and most important, active external rewarming produces a phenomenon called *core temperature after-drop*. This refers to a drop in core temperature as a result of sudden peripheral vasodilation. This causes cold, acidic blood to return to the core. Hypotension and potentially fatal dysrhythmias can result. Focusing on rewarming the trunk only (rather than the trunk and extremities) can prevent these temperature gradients.

In general, active external rewarming is used in conjunction with active core rewarming.

### Active Core Rewarming

Active core rewarming involves techniques to deliver direct heat internally. It should be used in patients with moderate to severe hypothermia. The simplest method entails the administration of heated,

 **CURRENT DIAGNOSIS**

- Accidental hypothermia may be classified as mild, moderate, or severe.
- The measured temperature should be the core body temperature.
- The method of rewarming depends on the severity of the temperature drop.
- The complications of rewarming include arrhythmias, rewarming-related hypotension, core temperature after drop, and rhabdomyolysis.
- Patients can only be declared dead after they are warm and dead.

humidified oxygen at 107.6°F to 114.8°F (42.0°C-46.0°C) and intravenous saline solution warmed to 109.4°F (43.0°C). Saline should be administered via a central line at 150 to 200 mL/hour. Gastric, bladder, and colonic irrigations have been used but their relatively small surface areas usually limit their effect.

Another method of active core rewarming is pleural irrigation using two large-bore (36 F or greater) thoracostomy tubes. One tube is placed at the midclavicular line and is connected to saline to 107.6°F (42.0°C). The other tube is placed at the posterior axillary line and connected to a chest tube drainage kit.

A more aggressive method of active core rewarming is via peritoneal lavage and dialysis. This can be accomplished using a standard diagnostic peritoneal lavage (DPL) kit and introducing an 8-F catheter into the peritoneum using Seldinger's technique. The crystalloid diasylate should be warmed to 104.0°F to 113.0°F (40.0°C-45.0°C). This method affords the added advantage of allowing the serum potassium level to be adjusted.

The most efficient and physiologic active core rewarming method is via extracorporeal warming or heated cardiopulmonary bypass. This is the method of choice for the most severe cases, patients with severe rhabdomyolysis, and for patients who require cardiopulmonary resuscitation.

Most arrhythmias are corrected by rewarming. Atropine is typically ineffective for associated bradydysrhythmias. Ventricular tachycardia and fibrillation require electrocardioversion and the use of bretylium,[2] if it is available. The safety of amiodarone (Cordarone) in these situations is questionable. Dopamine (Intropin) may be an effective vasopressor. Empiric antibiotics may be given. However, the empiric use of levothyroxine (Synthroid)[1] and corticosteroids may be hazardous. Phenytoin (Dilantin)[1] might have cardiac-depressant qualities in the moderately hypothermic patient. Box 3 demonstrates drugs with possible decreased metabolism or clearance with increase in toxicity in hypothermia.

Indicators of grave prognosis include development of profound hyperkalemia (serum potassium >10 mEq/L), underlying medical conditions, intravascular thrombosis (fibrinogen <59 mg/dL), pH less than 6.5, and a core temperature less than 50.0°F to 53.6°F (10.0°C-12.0°C).

# Peripheral Cold Injuries

Peripheral cold injuries span a spectrum ranging from minimal to severe tissue damage. Freezing and nonfreezing syndromes can cause these injuries. Frostnip and frostbite are caused by exposure to freezing temperatures. *Frostnip* refers to the numbness and blue-white discoloration of the face and extremities that occur during exposure to freezing temperatures. It is a precursor to frostbite. It is characterized by reversible skin changes including blanching and numbness with no permanent tissue damage, unlike frostbite. Nonfreezing injuries depend on whether the ambient environment during exposure was wet (trench or immersion foot) or dry (pernio or chilblain).

## PATHOPHYSIOLOGY

During exposure to cold temperatures, the core body temperature is preserved to the detriment of the extremities. Frostbite occurs in four stages: prefreeze, freeze-thaw, vascular stasis, and late ischemic stages. The prefreeze phase occurs when the temperature of the extremities falls below 50.0°F (10.0°C) and cutaneous sensation is lost. Vasoconstriction also occurs along with leakage of intracellular fluid into the interstitium. The freeze-thaw phase begins at the freezing point of water (32.0°F or 0°C) with the formation of ice crystals extracellularly. This further enhances the exit of water from the intracellular space under osmotic forces, resulting in cell shrinkage and ultimately damage. During the vascular stasis phase, plasma leakage and formation of ice crystals continue. Arachidonic acid break down products are then released from underlying damaged tissue.

---

[1]Not FDA approved for this indication.
[2]Not available in the United States.

---

## BOX 3 Drugs Displaying Reduced Metabolism or Clearance in Hypothermia

- Atropine
- Digoxin
- D-Tubocurarine
- Fentanyl (Sublimase, Duragesic)
- Gentamicin (Garamycin)
- Lidocaine (Xylocaine)
- Phenobarbital
- Procaine
- Propranolol (Inderal)
- Sulfanilamide (AVC Cream)
- Suxamethonium (Succinylcholine, Anectine)

---

Both prostaglandin $F_{2\alpha}$ and thromboxane $A_2$ produce platelet aggregation, leukocyte immobilization, and vasoconstriction. Endothelial cells are sensitive to cold injury, and the microvasculature becomes distorted and clogged, leading to tissue ischemia. The late ischemic phase is characterized by ischemia, thrombosis, continued shunting, gangrene, autonomic dysfunction, and denaturation of tissue proteins. The tissue can eventually mummify and demarcate more than 60 to 90 days later.

## CLINICAL PRESENTATION

The face and ears are the most common sites prone to cold injury, followed by the hands and feet.

### Frostnip and Frostbite

Patients with frostnip usually have blanching and numbness of their fingertips. Frostbite has been classified as superficial, affecting the skin and subcutaneous tissue, or deep, affecting the bones, joints, and tendons. When a superficial frostbite is rewarmed, the skin can form a clear blister; however, when a deep frostbite is rewarmed, it can form a hemorrhagic blister. This classification, however, has no therapeutic or prognostic value given that frostbites can initially appear benign. Many weeks can pass before the demarcation between viable and nonviable tissues becomes apparent.

Although no prognostic factors can be entirely predictive, favorable factors include retained sensation, normal skin color, and clear rather than cloudy fluid in the blisters, if present. Poor prognostic features include nonblanching cyanosis, firm skin, and dark, fluid-filled blisters. Patients can present with pain, numbness, and a clumsy "chunk of wood" sensation in the affected extremity. The pain is initially described as a dull ache and evolves to become a throbbing sensation in about 48 to 72 hours.

### Chilblain

Chilblain results from repetitive exposure to cold dry air. It manifests as erythematous or cyanotic lesions often referred to as *cold sores*. These lesions usually develop on exposed surfaces after a delay of 12 to 14 hours and are characterized by pruritus and burning paresthesias. Young women, especially those with Raynaud's phenomenon, are at risk.

### Trench Foot and Immersion Foot

Trench foot occurs as a result of prolonged exposure to a damp, cold, nonfreezing environment. It has been classically described among soldiers in World War I, many of whom were confined to cold and damp trenches for prolonged periods. Symptoms include numbness and painful paresthesias that can progress to a throbbing and burning sensation. Initial evaluation reveals a cold, pale extremity, with or without vesicles or bullae.

Immersion foot may be considered the sailor's counterpart to trench foot. It occurs after prolonged immersion in cold water at temperatures above freezing.

## CURRENT THERAPY

**Mild Hypothermia: 32.2°C (90°F) to 35°C (95°F)**

- Passive external rewarming
  - Remove wet clothing.
  - Ambient temperature should exceed 21.0°C (70.0°F).
  - Cover patient with insulating material.

**Moderate Hypothermia: 28°C (82.4°F) to 32.2°C (90°F)**

- Active external rewarming
  - Radiant heat
  - Thermal mattresses
  - Electric heating blankets
  - Forced-air heating blankets
- Active core rewarming
  - Warmed humidified oxygen
  - Warmed intravenous saline
  - Bladder, colonic, and gastric irrigation
  - Pleural cavity lavage

**Severe Hypothermia: Less than 28°C (82.4°F)**

- Aggressive active core rewarming
  - Warmed, humidified oxygen
  - Warmed intravenous saline
  - Bladder, colonic, and gastric irrigation
  - Pleural cavity lavage
  - Peritoneal lavage or dialysis
  - Extracorporeal warming or heated cardiopulmonary bypass

**Frostnip**

- Gentle rewarming
- Usually self-resolving

**Frostbite**

- Warm-water immersion
- Débride broken vesicles
- Apply topical aloe vera or antibiotic ointment
- Use NSAIDs for pain
- Update tetanus status

**Chilblain**

- Gentle rewarming
- Nifidipine (procardia)

**Trenchfoot**

- Dry the foot
- Gentle rewarming

*Abbreviation:* NSAID = nonsteroidal anti-inflammatory drug.

## TREATMENT

Treatment of frostbite should begin with removing all wet or frozen clothing. For patients with moderate and severe hypothermia as described above, initial resuscitative efforts should be geared toward raising their core temperature. The patient should be moved to a warm environment and all wet clothing should be removed. The frozen extremity should be rewarmed by immersion in circulation water at 104.0°F to 108.0°F (40.0°C-42.0°C) for about 15 to 30 minutes. Given the risks of thermal injury, the frozen parts should not be exposed to direct or dry heat (such as hair dryers, heating pads, or heat lamps). Do not rub or massage the affected area. The process should be continued until the extremity appears warm and well perfused. Due to the pain associated with reperfusion, there may be the temptation to abruptly

abort the rewarming process. This can, however, promote further tissue damage. Parenteral analgesic medications (nonsteroidal anti-inflammatory drugs [NSAIDs] and opioids) may be administered as needed to make this process more tolerable.

Almost all authors agree that hemorrhagic blisters should not be débrided because of the risk of secondary desiccation of deep dermal layers, extending the injury. Débriding broken vesicles or bullae is also widely accepted; however, clear, intact vesicles may be broken and débrided or left intact. Topical aloe vera ointment (Dermaide Aloe) (a thromboxane inhibitor) or topical antibiotic ointments may be applied. The injured tissue should be loosely covered with sterile, dry, nonadherent dressing. Hands and feet may be splinted and elevated to reduce edema. Because the damaged tissue is tetanus prone, patients whose tetanus status has not been updated need a tetanus shot (Td).

Adjunctive agents that have been used for their antithrombotic and vasodilative properties with varying success include heparin,[1] steroids,[1] NSAIDs,[1] dimethylsulfoxide (DMSO),[1] nonionic detergents,[1] dipyridamole (Persantine),[1] calcium channel blockers,[1] pentoxifylline (Trental),[1] and phenoxybenzamine (Dibenzyline).[1]

Surgical consultation is appropriate for guiding long-term management, because some patients might need débridement of infections or skin grafts for nonhealing wounds. A sympathetic nerve block can relieve painful and refractory vasospasms.

Chilblain (pernio) may be treated with nifidipine (Procardia)[1] at an oral dose of 20 to 60 mg daily.

### SEQUELAE

Late sequelae of frostbite include cold hypersensitivity, numbness, pain, and decreased sensation. This is a result of early neuronal damage and abnormal sympathetic tone. Patients with chronic symptoms should be advised to avoid nicotine and cold exposure while using NSAIDs. Tissue demarcation can occur 60 to 90 days after initial injury. Amputation decisions should be deferred unless there is supervening sepsis or gangrene. The ultimate tissue salvage after a spontaneous slough usually far exceeds the most optimistic initial estimates.

## Therapeutic Hypothermia

Therapeutic hypothermia for reducing anoxic brain injury has been increasingly used in clinical practice in post–cardiac arrest states. The usual scenarios for such a practice are in patients with suspected postanoxic injuries following cardiopulmonary resuscitation, traumatic brain injuries associated with elevation of intracranial pressure, stroke, and various perioperative situations (such as vascular surgery). Hypothermia can reduce the metabolic oxygen utilization rate in the brain by 6% for every 1°C reduction in brain temperature (over 82.4°F or 28°C) due to reduced normal cerebral electrical activity and suppression of chemical reactions (such as free radical and glutamate production along with calcium shifts) associated with reperfusion injury. Cooling is usually initiated within 6 hours following return of spontaneous circulation, with moderate hypothermia (82.4°F to 90°F or 28°C to 32.2°C) for induction. Intravenous cooling techniques (infusion of 30 mL/kg of crystalloid solution at 4°C over 30 minutes) or extracorporeal cooling methods have been used. An intravascular heat-exchange device has also been developed. Shivering is prevented via neuromuscular blockade and sedation. Temperature can be monitored by a bladder temperature probe or through a central pulmonary catheter.

### REFERENCES

Aslam AF, Aslam AK, Vasavada BC, Khan IA: Hypothermia: Evaluation, electrocardiographic manifestations, and management. Am J Med 2006; 119(4):297-301.

Bhagat H, Bithal PK, Chouhan RS, Arora R: Is phenytoin administration safe in a hypothermic child? J Clin Neurosci 2006:13 (9):953-955.

---

[1]Not FDA approved for this indication.

Centers for Disease Control and Prevention (CDC): Hypothermia-related deaths—United States, 2003-2004. MMWR Morb Mortal Wkly Rep 2005;54(7):173-175.

Danzl DF: Hypothermia. Semin Respir Crit Care Med 2002;23(1):57-68.

Danzl DF, Pozos RS: Accidental hypothermia. N Engl J Med 1994;331(26): 1756-760.

Ervasti O, Juopperi K, Ketlumen P, et al: The occurance of frostbite and its risk factors in young men. Int J Circumpolar Health 2004;63(1):71-80.

Gilbert M, Busund R, Skagseth A, et al: Resuscitation from accidental hypothermia of 13.7 degrees C with circulatory arrest. Lancet 2000;355(9201): 375-376.

Lloyd EL: Accidental hypothermia. Resuscitation1996;32:111-124.

McCauley RD, Smith DJ, Robson MC, et al: Frostbite and other cold-induced injuries. In Auerbach PS (ed). Wilderness Medicine: Management of Wilderness and Environmental Emergencies, 3rd ed. St Louis: Mosby, 1995, pp 129-145.

McDonagh DL, Allen IN, Keifer JC, Warner DS: Induction of hypothermia after intraoperative hypoxic brain insult. Anesth Analg 2006;103(1):180-181.

Nolan JP, Morley PT, Vanden Hoek TL, Hickey RW, et al; International Liaison Committee on Resuscitation: Therapeutic hypothermia after cardiac arrest: An advisory statement by the advanced life support task force of the International Liaison Committee on Resuscitation. Circulation 2003; 108:118-121.

Ulrich AS, Rathlev NK: Hypothermia and localized cold injuries. Emerg Med Clin North Am 2004;22(2):281-298.

# Disturbances Caused by Heat

Method of
*John F. Coyle II, MD*

## Exertional Heat Stroke

Heat stroke is an illness caused by failure of thermoregulation with elevation of core temperature to 40.6°C (105°F) or more, associated with central nervous system dysfunction. Heat stroke is traditionally subdivided into *exertional* and *classic* (or nonexertional) forms.

Exertional heat stroke is a sporadic illness triggered by exercise in warm environmental conditions that add to the thermal load produced by muscular contraction. It mainly strikes manual laborers, soldiers in training, and athletic competitors; indeed, it is the third leading cause of death among high school and college athletes in the United States. Exertional heat stroke may occur at moderate temperatures, especially if humidity is high, but both exertional and classic heat strokes most likely develop in conditions of high heat. The incidence of heat stroke increases exponentially when heat stress exceeds a boundary value. Appearance of the first case should sound an alarm that conditions have become dangerous, and more cases should be anticipated. The typical heat stroke victim is highly motivated, poorly conditioned, obese, and not acclimatized. Fatigue and sleep deprivation are commonly encountered, and recent or ongoing febrile or dehydrating illness increases risk. Dehydration may play a role, especially if severe. The use of certain medicines also increases risk, most notably those that decrease cardiac output (β-blockers), promote dehydration (diuretics), affect hypothalamic control (major tranquilizers, neuroleptics, alcohol), inhibit sweating (anticholinergics, tricyclic antidepressants, antihistamines), or increase thermogenicity (amphetamines, cocaine).

*Prevention* is the ideal treatment. Because behavior is the most powerful thermoregulatory mechanism, education and empowerment have the greatest preventive potential. To avoid exertional heat stroke, organizers should schedule vigorous exercise in the coolest hours of the day (shortly after dawn or after nightfall, in difficult seasons). Exercise level should be governed by athlete fitness, acclimatization, hydration status, and freedom from intercurrent illness. Clothing should be appropriate for exercise conditions. Medication use that might interfere with effective thermoregulation should be recognized, and medical personnel must be charged with the responsibility for stopping any participant who appears to be decompensating.

*Triage* of those with exertional heat stroke is highly variable. Runners who are plunged unconscious into an ice water bath at the end of a race often respond promptly to treatment, reawaken, and are sometimes sent home without hospitalization. A less-favorable response necessitates hospital admission.

## Classic (Nonexertional) Heat Stroke

Classic (nonexertional) heat stroke usually occurs during heat waves that cause passive warming by exposure to unrelenting hot and humid conditions, afflicting urban dwellers who are elderly, infirm, solitary, and poor. Heat waves tend to be "silent and invisible killers of silent and invisible people." Their housing lacks air-conditioning or they do not use it because of expense or confusion. Alcoholism and chronic illness, especially mental illness, predispose people to heat stroke. Young children are susceptible, reflecting their high surface-to-volume ratio, relatively inefficient sweat glands, and dependent status. Classic heat stroke requires preventive measures at the community level. Those with chronic illness and substance abuse history are at highest risk, and they may be the most difficult to contact. Although ventilation fans are of little help in hot and humid conditions, a few hours spent in air-conditioned rooms each day can significantly reduce the likelihood of heat stroke. Whether this is primarily a physiologic or a sociologic effect is unclear. Patients with classic heat stroke usually respond slowly to treatment and require hospital admission.

## Pathophysiology

The pathophysiology of heat stroke is incompletely understood. Although a vast number of runners in a marathon may develop dehydration and a high core temperature, very few proceed to heat stroke. Excessive heat is a noxious agent that causes direct cell injury. The severity of heat stroke is related to the degree and duration of temperature elevation above 41.6°C (106.9°F). Exercise lowers the thermal threshold for heat stroke because of hormonal effects and

---

 **CURRENT DIAGNOSIS**

- Heat stroke often occurs in the first 2 hours of exercise and may occur in so-called moderate heat stress conditions.
- Heat stroke may occur in sedentary urban dwellers during heat waves, especially in the presence of drug or alcohol use, senility, or in young children.
- Abnormal mental status (coma, delirium, agitation, confusion, combativeness) is a constant feature of heat stroke.
- Rectal temperature should be checked immediately. Axillary and aural temperatures may be misleadingly low. A rectal temperature of 40.6°C (105°F) or more is required for diagnosis of heat stroke, but delayed measurement may produce a misleadingly low temperature.
- The trap of proceeding with complex diagnostic procedures (such as computed tomographic scans) before core temperature is assessed and lowered to less than 39°C (102.2°F) should be avoided.
- After cooling measures are instituted, blood samples should be obtained to assess coagulation status, hepatic function, renal function, likelihood of infection, acid-base status, and muscle injury.

competing demands of organ systems as blood flow is directed away from the viscera to the active muscles and the skin. Gut ischemia may result in release of bacterial polysaccharides into the blood. What happens next is a complex interplay of factors including cytokines, bacterial polysaccharides, and heat shock proteins. As endothelial abnormalities accumulate, there is precipitation of a cascade of events including activation of the coagulation system and vascular dilation, resulting in hypotension and coagulation disorders. These events in many respects mimic sepsis.

Because the brain is extremely sensitive to heat stress, the first signs of heat stroke are neurologic. Judgment is impaired, and the chance for self-diagnosis is greatly reduced. After loss of consciousness, muscular activity is markedly diminished, but temperature may remain elevated for hours. Multisystem injury may follow, with the possibility of neurologic, pulmonary, cardiac, hepatic, renal, vascular, hematologic, and immunologic damage. A high percentage of classic heat stroke patients suffer infection within 36 hours of hospital admission.

## Treatment

Treatment of heat stroke can be summarized easily:

- Lower rectal temperature immediately to 39°C (102.2°F).
- Support organ systems injured by heat, hypotension, inflammation, and coagulopathy.

There is a *golden hour* after the onset of heat stroke in which therapy can be extremely effective. When treating a patient outside of the hospital, the patient should be moved to a shaded area, clothes removed, and the person covered with water and fanned. When resources become available, the simplest treatment appears to be cold-water immersion in a shallow tub, with patient head, arms, and lower legs outside the tub. The high efficiency of this method comes from two properties of water: It has 25 times the thermal conductivity of air, and it makes perfect contact with all skin surfaces. In addition, the hydrostatic properties of water tend to reduce the risk of hypotension. Other methods of cooling include skin wetting with fanning, application of total-body ice packs (24 ice packs, with special emphasis on the neck, armpits, and groin), or use of a body-cooling unit (evaporation and convection).

*Assessment* of the patient with presumed heat stroke should be delayed pending initiation of cooling. Determination of rectal temperature, heart rate, and blood pressure can be carried out while the patient is being cooled. Oral and tympanic membrane temperatures cannot be used because they may be misleadingly low. Rectal temperature should be measured every 5 to 10 minutes, and the patient should be removed from cooling when 39°C (102.2°F) is reached, to avoid overshoot hypothermia. Hydration with normal saline or lactated Ringer's solution should be started after initiation of cooling, and most patients require 1 L in the first hour of treatment. Further rehydration needs to be guided by estimated water losses, and in difficult cases placement of a central venous monitoring catheter may be needed. Overhydration may promote cerebral edema, pulmonary edema, and hyponatremia.

Seizures, which occur commonly, should be managed with diazepam (Valium), 5 mg intravenously (IV). Shivering may also be treated with diazepam. The patient must be monitored closely with use of this medication, which occasionally promotes hypotension. Hypotension should be treated with cooling and volume expansion. If blood pressure remains depressed, pressors may be needed. For patients with prolonged exertional heat stroke, mannitol, 0.25 g/kg, or furosemide (Lasix), 0.5 to 1 mg/kg, should be given after volume expansion is carried out to minimize the adverse effects of rhabdomyolysis on renal function.

In patients with severe multiorgan damage, disseminated intravascular coagulation (DIC) is a common finding. Bleeding in DIC should be treated with transfusion of fresh-frozen plasma, cryoprecipitate, and platelet concentrates as needed. There is no role for heparin or thrombolytics in DIC in this setting. Adult respiratory distress syndrome tends to occur in conjunction with DIC, and prolonged ventilator support may be required. Hepatic failure in heat stroke is

- Injury because of heat stroke is related to both the magnitude and duration of core temperature elevation.
- After elevated rectal temperature is documented, treatment should not be delayed. In particular, it should not be delayed to start an intravenous line or to carry out advanced testing such as computed tomography or other radiograph study.
- Ideal treatment for heat stroke is cold-water immersion in a low tub, such as a child's wading pool, with the patient's arms, legs, and head hanging out of the tub.
- If low tub immersion is not available, constant flowing of cold water from a tap over the patient with drainage through a slotted Gurney cart in the presence of constant high-velocity electric fanning can be effective.
- Applying ice packs to the axillae, groins, trunk, and as many other skin surfaces as possible can be useful, but this method of cooling is not as efficient as cold-water immersion or constant cold-water flow because of reduced contact surface and limited thermal gradient.
- Rectal temperature should be checked every 5 minutes during cooling. Cooling measures are discontinued when rectal temperature reaches 39°C (102.2°F) to avoid excessive cooling. Clinicians should watch for rebound temperature elevation after cooling is discontinued.
- Clinicians should be prepared to support the patient through multisystem organ failure. Hemorrhage should be treated with transfusion of red blood cells, platelets, fresh-frozen plasma, and clotting factors. Heparin has no role in treatment of this consumptive coagulopathy. Volume expansion may be needed. Prolonged ventilator support and hemodialysis may be required.
- Medications that may be needed are diazepam (Valium), 5 mg intravenously (IV), for seizures; pressors; and mannitol, 0.25 g/kg IV, and furosemide (Lasix), 0.5 to 1.0 mg/kg IV, for renal protection from rhabdomyolysis, but only after adequate volume expansion is achieved.

usually transient. Renal failure may necessitate emergency hemodialysis. No evidence supports use of anti-inflammatory agents or antipyretic agents in heat stroke. Use of strategies that are helpful in sepsis may ultimately find a role in treatment of heat stroke, but such treatments should be considered experimental at this time.

*Prognosis* can be estimated by time to recovery of consciousness (shorter is better) and elevation of liver enzymes (lactate dehydrogenase [LDH] at 24 hours less than three times normal is a good prognostic sign).

Heat stroke should usually be regarded as an accident, like drowning. The population at highest risk is readily defined, but because of the rarity of this ailment it is difficult to maintain a high level of preparedness for its prevention and treatment. Once encountered, heat stroke must be treated with much the same urgency as cardiac arrest because prompt cooling can sometimes make the crisis little more than an inconvenience. After the process of systemic injury becomes established, heat stroke's cascade of microvascular dysfunction can take on a life of its own, eventuating in a desperate struggle against multisystem failure and a high mortality rate.

## REFERENCES

Bouchama A, Knochel JP: Heat stroke. N Engl J Med 2002;346(25):1978-1988.

Crandall CG, Vongpatanasin W, Victor RG: Mechanism of cocaine-induced hyperthermia in humans. Ann Intern Med 2002;136(11):785-791.

Dematte JE, O'Mara K, Buescher J, et al: Near-fatal heat stroke during the 1995 heat wave in Chicago. Ann Intern Med 1998;129(3):173-181.

Eichner ER: Treatment of suspected heat illness. Int J Sports Med 1998;19(Suppl 2):S150-S153.

Epstein Y, Moran DS, Shapiro Y: Exertional heatstroke in the Israeli Defence Forces. In Pandolf KB, Burr RE (eds): Medical Aspects of Harsh Environments. U.S. Defense Dept., Army, Office of the Surgeon General, 2001, pp 281-292. Available free online: http://www.bordeninstitute. army.mil/medaspofharshenvrnmnts/

Gaffin SL, Hubbard RW: Pathophysiology of heatstroke. In Pandolf KB, Burr RE (eds): Medical Aspects of Harsh Environments. U.S. Defense Dept., Army, Office of the Surgeon General, 2001, pp 161-208. Available free online: http://www.bordeninstitute. army.mil/medaspofharshenvrnmnts/

Gardner JW, Kark JA: 2001. Clinical diagnosis, management and surveillance of exertional heat illness. In Pandolf KB, Burr RE (eds): Medical Aspects of Harsh Environments. U.S. Defense Dept., Army, Office of the Surgeon General, 2001, pp 221-279. Available free online: http://www.bordeninstitute. army.mil/medaspofharshenvrnmnts/

Klinenberg E: Review of heat wave: Social autopsy of disaster in Chicago. N Engl J Med 2003;348(7):666-667.

Shephard RJ, Shek PN: Immune dysfunction as a factor in heat illness. Crit Rev Immunol 1999;19(4):285-302.

# Spider Bites and Scorpion Stings

Method of
*Rachel Haroz, MD, and James R. Roberts, MD*

## Spider Bites

Most of the approximately 34,000 species of spiders are considered to be venomous, but their short and delicate jaws generally prevent significant human envenomation. Approximately 200 species, however, do possess the ability to envenomate humans, resulting in symptoms ranging from minor to occasionally serious skin lesions to neurotoxicity, systemic illness, multiorgan dysfunction, and death. Spider identification after a bite is desirable but usually impossible. Here we discuss features, symptoms of envenomation, and treatment for bites from the *Loxosceles, Latrodectus,* and tarantula spiders.

### *LOXOSCELES* ENVENOMATION

Relatively small (approximately 1.5 cm in leg span), *Loxosceles* spiders are light brown in color with darker brown markings on their dorsal surface. The most distinctive identifying characteristic appears on the female brown recluse (*L. reclusa*), which is described as violin shaped. Eleven native species of *Loxosceles* exist in the United States in the southern, southwestern, and central states. Most confirmed necrotic arachnidism in the United States is caused by *L. reclusa. Loxosceles* spiders have six eyes, which differs from the typical eight eyes found in most other spiders. Females are usually larger than males, which are rarely considered venomous. Considered nonaggressive and nocturnal, most *Loxosceles* bites occur when the spider is inadvertently caught between clothing or bedding and the victim's skin. Perineal and genital bites can occur in outhouses. The bite may be minimally painful or go totally unnoticed.

The initial skin manifestation is a small, erythematous, flat lesion surrounded by a light-colored ring. Within hours to days this lesion becomes bluish with a deepening of the color of the ring and progressing to a blister/bleb. A necrotic eschar with an ulcerative base may develop, which rarely becomes quite extensive. The lesion is minimally painful but often takes several weeks to heal, occasionally requiring extensive débridement or skin grafting. Some ulcerated wounds (approximately 10%) produce permanent scarring. *Loxosceles* venom contains various toxic enzymes, most notably sphingomyelinase D, that contribute to cellular destruction and tissue damage.

Systemic symptoms are rare (1% to 3% of all bites) but may include hemolysis, platelet aggregation, hemoglobinuria, myoglobinuria, maculopapular rash, nausea, vomiting, renal failure, disseminated intravascular coagulation, fever, seizures, coma, and death. These symptoms are more common in children and following South American *Loxosceles* bites.

There is little the clinician can do to affect favorably the course of a *Loxosceles* bite, with the ultimate outcome dependent on the amount and potency of the venom and host factors. Local wound care includes antisepsis, immobilization, and elevation of the affected extremity, cool compresses, appropriate analgesics, antihistamines for itching, and tetanus prophylaxis. Envenomation is difficult to differentiate from infection, but antibiotics may be necessary for secondarily infected wounds. Debridement of necrotic tissue is performed as needed. Delayed excision and wound grafting may be indicated. Once recommended, early wound excision and intrawound steroid injections should be avoided. Several other treatments to ameliorate tissue necrosis are advocated, including dapsone,[1] colchicine,[1] topical nitroglycerin,[1] high-dose vitamin C,[1] electric shock therapy, cyproheptadine (Periactin),[1] and hyperbaric oxygenation, but none has proven effective. Patients exhibiting systemic symptoms should be hospitalized and receive supportive care.

Absent a witnessed attack, a spider bite is usually a clinical diagnosis made by exclusion. *Loxosceles* and other spider bites are overreported and occur far less frequently than suspected by the lay public or diagnosed by clinicians. Outside of the endemic areas, *Loxosceles* bites are highly unlikely. Importantly, if the spider was not positively identified, a differential diagnosis should be entertained. Entities confused with a spider bite include clandestine drug injection (especially cocaine and amphetamines), methicillin-resistant *Staphylococcus aureus* (MRSA) skin infections, early shingles lesions, other bug bites, self-induced trauma, and infectious embolic lesions (such as endocarditis and gonococcemia).

### NON-*LOXOSCELES* NECROTIC ARACHNIDISM

Several other species of spiders in the United States (*Cheiracanthium* species and *Tegenaria agrestis* [hobo] spiders) are associated with necrotic lesions. *Cheiracanthium* spiders are widespread and usually found indoors (e.g., in the folds of curtains or on warm windowsills). They are aggressive night foragers and produce painful, pruritic bites, usually resolving within several days. Their bites rarely result in ulceration and necrosis. Hobo spiders inhabit the Pacific Northwest to where they recently emigrated from Western Europe. They are large, aggressive, and inhabit woodpiles, subfloors, and baseboards. Their bites are usually painless but may lead to multiple ruptured blisters within 1 to 2 days and a necrotic wound. Hobo spider bites are probably responsible for necrotic arachnidism in the colder areas of the United States where the brown recluse spider is not found. Treatment of hobo spider bites is similar to that of *Loxosceles* bites.

### *LATRODECTUS* ENVENOMATION

*Latrodectus* species (widow spiders) are found worldwide. In the United States, five widow spiders are endemic. These spiders are generally dark with various ventral patterns; the most well known is the red hourglass figure found on the female black widow spider. Females are larger (16- to 20-mm leg span) and more venomous than males. *Latrodectus* spiders generally inhabit outdoor dark spaces and are nonaggressive, but they do bite if provoked. The initial bite may be mildly painful, resulting in a small raised wheal. The neurotoxicity associated with these bites results from α-latrotoxin in the venom that causes a large calcium-dependent presynaptic terminal release of neurotransmitters including norepinephrine, glutamate, acetylcholine, and dopamine. The reuptake of choline is simultaneously inhibited. Symptoms begin approximately 30 minutes to an hour after the bite,

---

[1]Not FDA approved for this indication.

## CURRENT DIAGNOSIS

- *Loxosceles* spider bites generally result in local symptoms, whereas *Latrodectus* and scorpion stings have predominantly systemic manifestations, which may be severe.
- The spider or scorpion should be identified if at all possible.
- Not all necrotic wounds are spider bites; therefore a differential diagnosis should be entertained.

and patients can appear quite ill. Muscle cramps and pain spread from the bite site and can be severe. Facial contortion and periorbital swelling, *facies latrodectismica*, may occur. Abdominal rigidity mimicking an acute abdomen, thoracic muscle spasm leading to hypoventilation and respiratory failure, diaphoresis, hypertension, nausea, vomiting, diffuse skin erythema, tremor, priapism, headache, tachycardia, paresthesias, and coma have been described. Lower extremity pain and diaphoresis, even in upper extremity bites, seem to be characteristic features. Symptoms resolve over 3 to 7 days, and death is rare.

Local wound care includes thorough cleansing, appropriate analgesics, ice application, and tetanus prophylaxis. Severe pain and muscle spasms are treated with intravenous opioids and benzodiazepines. Intravenous calcium, although recommended in the past, is ineffective. *Latrodectus* antivenom (antivenin *Lactrodectus mactans*) is horse based and may cause anaphylaxis and serum sickness in allergic persons. It should be reserved for patients with severe systemic symptoms or those with potential for complications, such as the elderly, young children, pregnant patients, and patients with severe cardiovascular disease. Patients who manifest refractory pain, autonomic instability, respiratory distress, or significant neurologic changes should be treated with antivenom. The clinical response to antivenom can be dramatic even when administered 24 hours or more after envenomation.

## TARANTULAS

Approximately 1500 species of tarantulas are found worldwide, with 40 species endemic to the southwestern United States. Tarantulas are also now popular household pets because many are considered harmless and nonvenomous. Relatively large spiders (18- to 24-cm leg span), tarantulas live in underground burrows and are night foragers. Tarantula envenomations in humans often cause mild pain with some surrounding inflammation, but necrotic wounds and systemic symptoms are rare. Bites in dogs, however, are usually rapidly fatal.

Several tarantula species possess urticating hairs, which they launch to incapacitate their enemy. These hairs may penetrate the human skin and cause intense inflammation or lodge in the cornea leading to keratitis, uveitis, and ophthalmia nodosa, a condition characterized by

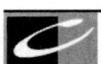

## CURRENT THERAPY

- Conservative wound care is essential in all envenomations, particularly for a *Loxosceles* spider bite.
- Particular care should be given to the very young, elderly, and patients with co-morbidity. In the setting of significant systemic symptoms, the administration of antivenom, if available, should be considered.
- Patients with ocular symptoms after exposure to a tarantula spider must be promptly referred to an ophthalmologist.
- Supportive care is often more valuable than antivenom administration, particularly considering the relatively high rate of both immediate and delayed hypersensitivity reactions.

granulomatous lesions in the cornea. Case reports generally describe patients who developed eye symptoms after cleaning tarantula cages or handling the tarantulas. Treatment involves wound care including cleansing, elevation, and immobilization of the affected extremity, tetanus prophylaxis, and appropriate analgesics. Hairs embedded in the cornea that are readily identified should be removed and the patient promptly referred to an ophthalmologist. Antihistamines and corticosteroids may be necessary for pruritus and inflammation. Patients with ophthalmia nodosa may require prolonged topical corticosteroids. Tarantula owners should be cautioned to wear gloves and eye protection when handling their pets and to wash their hands and avoid any eye rubbing after such interactions.

# Scorpion Stings

Scorpions range in size from several millimeters to 15 cm. They have a lobster-like appearance with a small head, two front claws, eight paired legs, and a segmented abdomen ending in a venom-containing tail consisting of a storage vesicle and a stinger. Scorpions are typically night stalkers and often found hidden under rocks, in shallow burrows, and in shoes, clothing, and cooking pots. Most of the severe envenomations in the United States are caused by stings by *Centruroides exilicauda (sculpturata)*, a small (4 to 7 cm long) yellowish brown scorpion.

Scorpion stings are usually very painful, quickly causing local paresthesias and edema. In adults, this usually resolves in several hours. Systemic effects are usually seen in the elderly and in infants and children. Scorpion venom blocks sodium and potassium channels and causes marked acetylcholine and catecholamine release. This leads to an initial cholinergic toxidrome characterized by the SLUDGE syndrome: salivation, lacrimation, urination, defecation, gastroenteritis, and emesis. Subsequently, catecholamine release leads to anxiety, tachycardia, hypertension, pulmonary edema, confusion, dystonic and myoclonic movements, seizures, ataxia, hyperglycemia, hyperpyrexia, and pancreatitis. Myocardial depression, myocardial infarctions without thrombosis, and ischemic strokes are rarely described.

Wound care should encompass thorough cleansing, elevation and immobilization of the affected extremity, cool compresses, tetanus prophylaxis, and appropriate analgesics. Patients should be observed for a period of 6 hours after the sting for the development of systemic symptoms.

Supportive care is the mainstay of treatment. Sympathetic symptoms should be blunted aggressively. Benzodiazepines, β-blockers, diuretics, digoxin (Lanoxin),[1] and nitroprusside (Nitropress) are successful. Dopamine (Intropin) and dobutamine (Dobutrex) may be necessary for the hypotensive patient, and mechanical ventilation may be required for respiratory failure. Angiotensin-converting enzyme inhibitors, opioids, and nifedipine may be detrimental and should be avoided.

Goat-derived antivenom use is controversial. It is not FDA approved and its availability is limited to the state of Arizona. The incidence of immediate and delayed hypersensitivity is relatively high (3% and 60%, respectively). The antivenom is species specific and must be administered within 1 hour of the exposure. Although helpful with pain, antivenom does not reverse cardiovascular and respiratory compromise because these are secondary to massive catecholamine release.

## REFERENCES

Blaikie AJ, Ellis J, Sanders R, et al: Eye disease associated with handling pet tarantulas: Three case reports. BMJ 1997;314:1524-1525.

Clark RF, Wethern-Kestner S, Vance MV, et al: Clinical presentation and treatment of black widow spider envenomations: A review of 163 cases. Ann Emerg Med 1992;21:782-787.

Diaz HJ: The global epidemiology, syndromic classification, management, and prevention of spider bites. Am J Trop Med Hyg 2004;71:239-250.

---

[1]Not FDA approved for this indication.

Hered RW, Spaulding AG, Sanitato JJ, et al: Ophthalmia nodosa caused by tarantula hairs. Ophthalmology 1988;95:166-169.

LoVecchio F, Welch S, Klemens J, et al: Incidence of immediate and delayed hypersensitivity to Centruroides antivenom. Ann Emerg Med 1999;5:615-619.

Mazzei de Davila CA, Davila DF, Donis JH: Sympathetic nervous system activation, antivenin administration and cardiovascular manifestations of scorpion envenomation. Toxicon 2002;40:1339-1346.

Merchant ML, Hinton JF, Geren CR: Effect of hyperbaric oxygen on sphingomyelinase D activity of brown recluse spider (*Loxosceles reclusa*) venom as studied by [31]P nuclear magnetic resonance spectroscopy. Am J Trop Med Hyg 1997;56:335-338.

Mold JW, Thompson DM: Management of brown recluse spider bites in primary care. J Am Board Fam Pract 2004;17:347-352.

Saucier JR: Arachnid envenomation. Emerg Med Clin North Am 2004;22:405-422.

Suntorntham S, Roberts JR, Nilsen GJ: Dramatic clinical response to the delayed administration of black widow spider antivenom. Ann Emerg Med 1994;24:1198-1199.

Swanson DL, Vetter RS: Bites of brown recluse spiders and suspected necrotic arachnidism. N Engl J Med 2005;352:700-707.

# Snakebite

Method of
*Craig S. Kitchens, MD*

The combination of fear of snakes and the unfamiliarity of most physicians with the management of snakebite often leads to an ill-founded perception of danger on the part of practitioners. It should be kept in mind that approximately 10,000 poisonous snakebites in the United States occur every year, yet fewer than 10 victims die.

In the past, treatment was often empirical and shrouded by folklore. Because survival is a near statistical certainty, various therapies including alcohol, application of ice, electric shock therapy, wide surgical débridement, or even providing no therapy have appeared efficacious. Treatment has now evolved from this disorganized state to a scientifically supported therapeutic regimen based on both the availability of antivenin and the experience garnered by large series of patients by clinical investigators. Morbidity and mortality are minimized by appropriate therapy.

Here we discuss care of patients bitten by North American poisonous snakes. In the United States, approximately 95% of poisonous snakebites are inflicted by pit vipers (family Crotalidae), which comprise multiple species of rattlesnakes as well as water moccasins and copperheads. Approximately 1% to 2% of all U.S. snakebites involve coral snakes (family Elapidae). Another 2% to 3% of snakebites are inflicted by exotic poisonous snakes that are either appropriately housed in zoos or owned by professional snake handlers or inappropriately kept as pets by amateurs. Treatment of persons bitten by exotic snakes is beyond the scope of this chapter. It is suggested that in such encounters a Poison Control Center should be consulted because antivenin to treat exotic snake bites is not commercially available in the United States; reputable handlers of such snakes usually have a supply of their own specific antivenin.

## Diagnosis

It is of prime importance to know the species of the offending snake because prognosis and treatment both heavily depend on this information. Undue risk should not be assumed by either the victim or others, yet identification of the snake is important and, if possible, the snake should be brought to the treatment facility for identification. The species of snake is actually more important than is its size in terms of prognosis. Primary care practitioners and emergency department personnel should have at least a modicum of information for

## CURRENT THERAPY

- IV access and administer crystalloid as indicated.
- Obtain CBC, PT, PTT, platelet count q6–12h for 1 d, then daily if abnormal.
- Estimate severity of envenomation.
  - Species of snake
  - Age and health status of victim
  - Rate of progression of signs/symptoms
- Administer CroFab as per Table 2.
- Determine tetanus vaccination status.
- Seek consultation from experts or a Poison Control Center, especially if one is treating envenomation for the first few times.

*Abbreviations:* CBC = complete blood count; IV = intravenous; PT = prothrombin time; PTT = partial thromboplastin time.

identification of local poisonous snakes. Bites from the pygmy rattlesnake (*Sistrurus miliarius*) have not resulted in a documented human death, and envenomations by the copperhead (*Agkistrodon contortrix*) and water moccasin (*A. piscivorus*) generally result in moderate envenomation syndromes with death rarely occurring. The Eastern diamondback (*Crotalus adamanteus*), Western diamondback (*C. atrox*), and Mojave rattlesnake (*C. scutulatus*) each have a higher degree of toxicity and indeed account for most of the fatalities in the United States.

The coral snake (*Micrurus fulvius*) accounts for only 1% to 2% of all snakebite cases in North America but has a higher than expected mortality based on its characteristic and severe neurotoxicity. Treatment of coral snake envenomation is not discussed further here. Suffice it to say that the neurotoxicity is the cause of morbidity and mortality from envenomation by the coral snake, usually through aspiration pneumonia and cessation of breathing. Accordingly, these severe manifestations can be attended by respiratory support and the natural history (i.e., without antivenin therapy), which usually is approximately a week before it reverses. Also important regarding coral snake envenomation is the absence of any signs of local pain, swelling, or discoloration, which are characteristic of pit viper envenomation. Patients cannot be assumed to have eluded envenomation by a coral snake because they lack these symptoms. That symptoms are often delayed for 8 to 24 hours must be anticipated, so 1 or 2 days of hospitalization for observation is frequently suggested.

The vast majority (approximately 80%) of envenomations by pit vipers are nonaccidental; that is, they are the result of poor judgment or senseless behavior, often in combination with intoxication with any of various substances. Most snakebite victims not only see and correctly identify the snake as poisonous but feel compelled to play with, taunt, or capture the animal and in the process may well be bitten. Fewer than 20% of snakebites are actually what most persons would call accidental.

Pit vipers are easily recognized by the so-called pit (an infrared heat-detection organ) approximately midway between the nostril and the eye. All North American pit vipers have pupils shaped like those of a cat, as opposed to round pupils characteristic of nonpoisonous snakes (with the exception of the coral snake). Pit vipers have large fangs through which a considerable volume of venom is injected, often deeply, into the victim. Because fangs are continually replaced, there may be one, two, three, or even four puncture wounds at one time that may leave a similar number of puncture wounds.

Pit viper venom is extremely complex, containing a broad range of proteolytic enzymes designed to digest protein, fat, connective tissue, nucleic acids, and other biologic material. It also contains numerous small peptides, which probably accounts for autonomic symptoms such as tachycardia, diaphoresis, diarrhea, and vomiting. There is a great variability in this complex poison with variability not only between species but also within species, and even within a single specimen if it is observed over years. Variability of the venom most likely accounts for the variability of the signs, symptoms, and prognosis in envenomation syndromes because of various species of pit vipers.

For instance, the hematologic abnormalities seen in North American pit viper envenomation occur through certain principles in pit viper venom. The Eastern diamondback rattlesnake contains a thrombin-like enzyme that partially cleaves fibrinogen, clearing it from the circulation, with the concomitant production of huge amounts of fibrin degradation products with only modest thrombocytopenia. The venom of the Western diamondback rattlesnake contains a principle that directly activates plasminogen to plasmin with resulting hyperfibrinolysis. Although through differing mechanisms, bites of each of these rattlesnakes may result in dramatic alterations of the prothrombin time (PT) and partial thromboplastin time (PTT) but little bleeding. Whereas envenomation by the Eastern or Western diamondback rattlesnake produces a minimal elevation of serum creatinine kinase (CK), myonecrosis with marked CK elevations are the hallmark of the canebrake rattlesnake (*C. horridus atricaudatus*) to include a brisk elevation of the CK-MB band yet with negative assays for either troponin I or T consistent with the lack of cardiac muscle myonecrosis. The bite of the Mojave rattlesnake produces myonecrosis similar to that of the canebrake rattlesnake as well as neurologic symptoms but minimal coagulation abnormalities. Severe thrombocytopenia usually refractory to platelet transfusion is seen in envenomation by the timber rattlesnake (*C. horridus horridus*). Thus, one can see that many envenomations have a signature, so to speak, that is slowly being unraveled (Table 1).

Approximately 20% of persons bitten by a positively identified pit viper are fortunate enough not to be envenomated by the snake and are considered to have a "dry bite." For these fortunate victims, the administration of antivenin obviously is not indicated. Dry bites are often deduced by the normality of the patient with the near complete absence of any pain, swelling, or discoloration within 1 to 2 hours of the bite.

## Treatment

It is most important to distinguish the severity of the bite to determine the need for and extent of antivenin therapy. Good supportive therapy should be instituted with the establishment of at least one large intravenous (IV) line and the infusion of saline or similar crystalloid for volume and blood pressure indications.

It is difficult to overestimate the importance of sensing the *rate of change of signs and symptoms* in determining the severity of bites. It is of more clinical significance that a patient bitten 20 minutes ago has a rapidly swelling arm than a patient bitten 3 hours ago has an even larger yet not still enlarging arm. Such a philosophy is also important in judging the efficacy of any administration of antivenin because one cannot expect prior damage to include swelling and discoloration to

## CURRENT THERAPY

- Confirm patient was bitten by a venomous snake.
- Determine snake species if possible.
- Evaluate for local signs of envenomation:
  - Pain
  - Swelling
  - Discoloration
- Evaluate for systemic signs of envenomation:
  - Alterations in vital signs
  - Nausea, vomiting, diarrhea, and diaphoresis
  - Fasciculations
  - Coagulation abnormalities
  - Altered mental status

subside promptly, but rather one determines whether such symptoms cease to progress or progress at such a slow rate that continued therapy may not be indicated. It is clear that the efficacy of the antivenin is a function of the time lapsed since the bite. It is ideal to treat bites that should be treated as soon as possible, and I prefer to initiate administration of antivenin prior to 6 or 12 hours after a bite, and essentially I never initiate treatment after 24 hours because what damage is going to be done is done and cannot be reversed.

*Dry bites* comprise approximately 20% of snakebites, and there is no evidence of any envenomation either locally or by laboratory evolutions. No treatment is indicated (Table 2).

*Minimal envenomations* are characterized by pain, swelling, and discoloration that are caused by the dissolution of underlying tissue. In general, there are no systemic signs, symptoms, or laboratory abnormalities, although anxiety is almost universal and, in the case of envenomation for rattlesnakes, notorious for their hematologic manifestations. Laboratory alterations of the coagulation system may be present, but in and of themselves they are not indications, in our experience, for the administration of antivenin.

The primary differentiation between minimal envenomations and *moderate envenomations* is not only the extent but particularly the rate of development and progression of pain, swelling, and discoloration because one may see a doubling of these symptoms within the initial hour of evaluation and care administered to the patient. Such patients should be administered antivenin to halt or lessen such progression. In general, these patients do not have severe alterations of vital signs or laboratory findings, although coagulation abnormalities may be quite dramatic with unclottable PTs and PTTs and modest thrombocytopenia on the order of 30,000 to 100,000/mm³. Most of these patients are treated with antivenin, especially if they are children, elderly, or have significant co-morbidity.

## TABLE 1 Distinguishing Clinical Characteristics of Envenomation by Selected *Crotalus* Species

| Common Name | Scientific Name | Distribution | Neurologic Symptoms | Coagulopathic Findings | Rhabdomyolysis |
|---|---|---|---|---|---|
| Eastern diamondback | *Crotalus adamanteus* | Southeastern United States | + | Prolonged PT/PTT | + |
| Canebrake | *C. horridus atricaudatus* | Eastern United States | — | — | ++++ |
| Mojave | *C. scutulatus* | Desert Southwest United States | +++ | — | ++++ |
| Timber | *C. horridus horridus* | Eastern United States | — | Prolonged PT/PTT; moderate to severe thrombocytopenia | — |

*Abbreviations:* PT = prothrombin time; PTT = partial thromboplastin time.
— = nil; + = mild; ++ = moderate; +++ = pronounced; ++++ = severe.

## TABLE 2   Grades of Severity of Envenomation by Pit Vipers

| Grade | Frequency (%) | Initial Findings | CroFab Vials in First 24 H |
|---|---|---|---|
| No envenomation | 0–15 | No local, systemic, or laboratory abnormalities 2 h after bite | 0 |
| Minimal envenomation | 20–40 | Local and slowly progressive swelling without systemic or severe laboratory abnormalities | 0–6 |
| Moderate envenomation | 20–40 | Rapidly progressive local swelling; systemic symptoms of nausea, vomiting, diarrhea, diaphoresis, fasciculations, moderate hypotension, and moderate hemostatic abnormalities but without bleeding | 6–12 |
| Severe envenomation | 5–10 | Severe systemic symptoms as above plus severe hypotension and lethargy; severe hemostatic abnormalities and possible bleeding | 12—24 or more |

Essentially all patients with *severe envenomation* are treated with antivenin. These are patients with severe alterations of vital signs, including hypotension, a peculiar unpleasant taste in the mouth, marked diaphoresis, universal diarrhea and vomiting, and frequently a stupor or inattention revealing alterations in mental status. Often the bite is in a highly vascular muscle (thenar, hypothenar, calf, or arm muscle) rather than the comparatively less vascular hand or foot. The coagulation abnormalities may again be quite remarkable. In our experience, most severe envenomations are obviously severe soon after the bite (10 to 30 minutes) with only a very small minority progressing from lesser degrees to severe.

Clinically relevant bleeding is rarely seen despite the marked alterations in coagulation tests. The explanation for this is that with North American pit viper envenomations, thrombin generation is intact so what little fibrinogen and platelets are available are used to maintain effective hemostasis. In other words, this is not disseminated intravascular coagulation (DIC) but chiefly a syndrome whose laboratory values mimic DIC. Exotic snakes may directly activate prothrombin (*Echis* species and *Bothrops* species) and/or factor X (*Vipera* species and *Dispholidus* species) leading to a true DIC with marked organ dysfunction related to thrombosis of organs with subsequent death.

Bleb formation at the site of a bite is not an important sign in and of itself, although it generates much attention.

Compartment syndromes are seen quite rarely, with surgical intervention indicated in only 1% to 5% of envenomated patients. Of interest, marked swelling itself is not often a sign of a compartment syndrome because in a true compartment syndrome, swelling is limited owing to the anatomic restriction by fibrous tissue, such as seen in the lateral anterior compartment of the lower leg or in the palm of the hand. The chief sign for a true compartment syndrome is the intense hardness of these areas and dysfunction of muscles within the compartment.

The administration of fresh-frozen plasma (FFP), platelet concentrates, or other blood products is rarely necessary in North American pit viper envenomation. We advocate a permissive posture with regard to the prolongation of the PT and PTT as long as there is no clinical bleeding. Should bleeding be present, the lack of fibrinogen is best treated with infusions of 8 to 10 bags of cryoprecipitate and monitored by serial determination of the fibrinogen level. This maneuver typically corrects the PT and PTT. Severe thrombocytopenia, implying platelet counts of less than 10,000/mm³, may well be an indication for platelet transfusion, particularly if an invasive or surgical procedure is planned. It has not been our experience that patients have significant hemorrhage. Leakage of blood into swollen tissues, dilution from crystalloid administration, and hemolysis of red blood cells from hemolysins in the venom account for most decreases in hematocrit values.

Emergency management in the field consists primarily of getting the patient to a medical facility. It is there that directed therapy should start. The use of tourniquets, cut-and-suck methodology, electric shock therapy, and the application of ice or administration of alcohol do not work and only serve to delay adequate evaluation and treatment. The victim should be kept calm and at rest during transport to the hospital. It is advised that should ice or tourniquets be in place on arrival at the hospital, it be documented in the report and removed.

The mainstay of treatment for North American pit viper envenomation is Crotalidae polyvalent immune Fab (ovine) antivenin (CroFab), which is an ovine-based preparation of immunoglobulins that is chemically treated so that only the Fab portion of the immunoglobulins is infused because the Fc fragment has been cleaved. Because the Fc fragment accounts for the majority of immunologic reactions, the Fab product appears to be much less allergenic than the prior equine-based product of intact immunoglobulins. Pretreatment skin or conjunctival testing is not required prior to administration of CroFab. Additionally, the smaller Fab molecule appears to give the advantage of facilitated penetration deep into affected tissues, but conversely, it has a rather short half-life of only several hours as opposed to several days with the previously available equine antivenin. This may be problematic in that an envenomation syndrome may appear by all accord to have been controlled with the cessation of the progression of swelling, normalization of vital signs, and the beginning of normalization of laboratory studies, only to have a relapse of these findings a few hours or days after antivenin administration. Readministration (as opposed to the initiation of antivenin administration) may very well be indicated. Because we hold that the defibrination syndrome is so benign in the first place, we do not regard the common reappearance of defibrination and secondary prolongation of the PT and PTT without evidence of clinical bleeding as an independent free-standing reason for antivenin readministration.

CroFab is administered as an IV solution starting slowly to alert for any possible adverse reaction. If such is not encountered, six vials are typically infused over 1 hour. If local and systemic findings cease or slow, the syndrome is deemed to be controlled. If not, two more vials, each over 6 hours, are suggested for a total of 12 vials in the first 24 hours. The rare severe and/or relapsing case may require up to 24 or more vials over several days.

Antibiotics are generally not employed but are indicated in wounds that were manipulated in the field, such as with a knife. Determination of which antibiotic to administer should include anaerobic bacterial coverage. Tetanus vaccination status should be determined and acted on appropriately. The extremities should be cleansed. Many find outlining the edges of the enlarging wound with a pen helpful in following the rate of change of progression of the swelling. We do not advocate determination of intercompartmental pressures routinely. The extremities should be slightly elevated above the level of the heart. The wound should not be covered or bound; it should be easily observable.

In-hospital therapy is usually given in closely monitored areas beginning with the emergency department and progressing to the intensive care unit (ICU), although ICU therapy is not necessarily a standard of care. Patients should be observed closely; particularly victims of coral snake bites or those who are deemed most likely to have dry bites. If signs, symptoms, or other evidence for envenomation do not occur within 24 to 36 hours, the patient can be discharged. We do not hold that all patients need admission to the hospital if it is very clear, within several hours, that envenomation did not occur, or if it did, it was minimal, such as with a pygmy rattlesnake bite. Because our patients typically are intoxicated, that in itself is more often than not a possible reason to keep the patient in the hospital for a day or so.

Nearly all swelling and tissue destruction is transient with North American pit viper envenomation. Edema that results from the dissolution of capillaries and particularly lymphatics may take as long as 1 to 2 months to resolve but may even be permanent in older or debilitated patients. In general, there is a total return of function to the bitten extremity, although a weakness or stiffness may be experienced by some patients for up to a year. A loss of tissue, to include fingers or limbs, is exceptionally rare and usually is accompanied by prehospital use of tourniquets and/or ice, extremely delayed therapy, over-aggressive surgical procedures, or neural damage in rare cases where a fasciotomy may have been indicated. Unfortunately, patients who are bitten by snakes tend to retain those habits that led to this envenomation and therefore may be seen again.

## REFERENCES

Bond RG, Burkhart KK: Thrombocytopenia following timber rattlesnake envenomation. Ann Emerg Med 1998;31:139-141.

Boyer LV, Seifert SA, Cain JS: Recurrence phenomena after immunoglobulin therapy for snake envenomations: Part 2. Guidelines for clinical management with Crotaline Fab antivenom. Ann Emerg Med 2001;37:196-201.

Carroll RR, Hall EL, Kitchens CS: Canebrake rattlesnake envenomation. Ann Emerg Med 1997;20:45-48.

Dart RC, Hurlbut KM, Garcia R, et al: Validation of a severity score for the assessment of crotalid snakebite in the United States. Ann Emerg Med 1996; 27:321-326.

Farstad D, Thomas T, Chow T, et al: Mojave rattlesnake envenomation in southern California: A review of suspected cases. Wilderness Environ Med 1997;8:89-93.

Kitchens CS: Hemostatic aspects of envenomation by North American snakes. Hematol/Oncol Clin North Am 1992;6:1189-1195.

Kitchens CS: From ETOH to FAB: The medicalization of therapy for pit viper envenomation. Trans Am Clin Climatol Assn 2001;112:117-135.

Kitchens CS, van Mierop LHS: Mechanisms of defibrination in humans after envenomation by the eastern diamondback rattlesnake. Am J Hematol 1983;14:345-353.

Kitchens CS, van Mierop LHS: Envenomation by the Eastern coral snake (*Micrurus fulvius fulvius*). A study of 39 victims. JAMA 1987;258:1615-1618.

# Marine Trauma, Envenomations, and Intoxications

Method of
*John E. Gough, MD, FACEP*

More than 70% of the Earth's surface is covered by water, and within these waters reside greater than 80% of the planet's living organisms. Many of these marine creatures have developed various systems for both attack and defense that can cause morbidity and mortality to humans. Although injuries and illnesses caused by marine creatures have been described since ancient times, many factors continue to contribute to frequent encounters. Some factors are the increased utilization of marine environments for both recreational and economic purposes, the popularity of seafood consumption, the growing interest in exotic animals in private and public aquariums, and the ability of air travel to make the movement of people and seafood to and from such environments more accessible.

Although there may be some overlap, for the purposes of this discussion, encounters with marine organisms are divided into the following general headings:

1. Nonvenomous trauma
2. Envenomations
3. Toxic ingestions

Nonvenomous trauma is mainly composed of bites. Treatment consists of the ABCs (airway, breathing, and circulation) of resuscitation, wound care, and prevention and treatment of infection. Envenomations may present with minor skin irritations or with life-threatening cardiovascular and respiratory compromise. Treatment is directed at resuscitation, supportive care, pain management, and administration of antidotes if available. Toxic ingestions often involve self-limited gastrointestinal conditions but, as with envenomations, may present with life-threatening symptoms. Treatment is mainly supportive.

## Nonvenomous Trauma

### SHARK ATTACKS

Sharks have existed for more than 400 million years, predating dinosaurs by more than 200 million years. Attacks on humans have been well documented in fiction and folklore. Although these attacks are often reported widely in the media, it is estimated that approximately 50 to 100 attacks occur annually worldwide. In the United States, fewer than 100 proven attacks have occurred over the past 8 years, with a dozen fatalities. The sharks most often implicated in human attacks are the great white, mako, bull, gray reef, and bull. Sharks have powerful crescent-shaped jaws with multiple (usually five or six) rows of sharp, triangular teeth that can cause significant soft tissue and bony injuries. Deaths from attacks are usually the result of exsanguinations and drowning.

Prevention of shark attacks involves avoiding shark-infested waters, not swimming at dusk or at night, and avoiding turbid waters, especially around waste outlets. Bright-colored bathing suits are believed to be attractants. Swimming with open wounds is not recommended. Although the majority of attacks occur in shallow waters, the most dangerous appear to occur in deeper waters.

The management of shark attacks is predicated on the ABCs of trauma care. Aggressive airway management, control of hemorrhage, and volume replacement are standards. Opiate medications may be necessary for pain control. Tetanus immunization including tetanus immunoglobulin (BayTet 250–500 U) as well as tetanus toxoid (Td; 0.5 cc IM) should be administered. Wound irrigation, débridement, and exploration for foreign bodies should be undertaken. Wounds are often packed and delayed primary closures performed. Organisms such as *Aeromonas, Vibrio,* and *Clostridia* are often encountered; therefore, antibiotics with activity against both aerobic and anaerobic organisms are often administered. Suitable choices of antibiotic agents are trimethoprim-sulfamethoxazole (Septra, Bactrim) 1 double-strength PO/400 mg IV; ciprofloxacin (Cipro) 500 to 750 mg PO/400 mg IV; imipenem-cilastatin (Primaxin) 500 to 750 mg IM; ceftriaxone (Rocephin) 1 to 2 g IV; and ceftazidime (Fortaz) 1 g IV or IM.

### BARRACUDA

Barracuda may reach sizes of 2.5 m in length and 50 kg in weight; however, most are less than 1.5 m long. The great barracuda (*Sphyraena barracuda*) is the only one of the 22 species of barracuda implicated in attacks against humans. Attacks occur in tropical waters in the Atlantic from Brazil to Florida and in the Indo-Pacific from the Red Sea to Hawaii. Although barracuda attacks usually are from solitary fish, attacks from schools have been reported. Attacks are very quick and may be fierce. The barracuda possesses knifelike sharp teeth resulting in V-shaped injuries that are similar to shark bites but not as severe. Treatment priorities are the same as for shark bites.

### MORAY EEL

Moray eels are bottom dwellers that typically reside in holes and crevices in rocks and corals. They inhabit tropical and temperate waters. Eels usually attack humans when they feel they are cornered or threatened. Attacks frequently occur when divers places their hand in one of the crevices and surprise the eel. Injuries have also been known to occur when the eel is accidentally entangled in fishing nets or when they are handled in an aquarium. The eel has powerful viselike jaws and sharp fangs that can cause significant soft tissue damage. The eel hangs on tenaciously, and further injury often occurs while the patient is struggling to remove the eel. Removal in some cases has required decapitation and breaking of the eel's jaws. Treatment strategies are similar to those for shark and barracuda bites.

# Envenomations

## INVERTEBRATES

### Phylum Cnidaria (Coelenterates)

The phylum coelenterates consists of approximately 10,000 species of invertebrates, of which approximately 100 are dangerous to humans. Included in this phylum are organisms that may account for some of the most dangerous envenomations known. This phylum is typically divided into three classes: (1) Hydrozoa (fire corals, hydroids, Portuguese man-of-war), (2) Scyphozoa (jellyfish), and (3) Anthozoa (sea anemones)

Members of the coelenterates envenomate through the use of nematocysts. Nematocysts are venom-filled organelles located in specialized endothelial cells known as crinocytes. The nematocysts reside in these crindocytes and are located either in tentacles or around the mouth of the organism. Inside the nematocyst are crindoblasts, which contain venom and an eversible tube. The nematocyst responds to both physical and chemical triggers, which can cause ejection of the tube into the prey, with injection of the toxin. The toxin of the coelenterates varies among the species but is usually heat labile, with direct and indirect effects on the autonomic nervous system. The venom has been shown to destabilize cell membranes through interference with the sodium–potassium pump. Other effects of the venom may include hemolysis, cardiac toxicity, muscle paralysis, and dermatonecrosis. The venom can often be degraded by proteolytic substances.

### Hydrozoa

The hydroids and stinging corals generally cause varying degrees of dermatitis and usually only require symptomatic local treatment. The most dangerous of the Hydrozoa is the Portuguese man-of-war (*Physalia physalis*) found in the Atlantic Ocean and the Gulf of Mexico. One species of Portuguese man-of-war is found in the Pacific Ocean (*Physalia utriculus*). The Pacific variety is smaller and contains only one tentacle (approximately 15 m in length). Envenomations with the Pacific variety are not as severe as with the Atlantic varieties. Envenomations typically occur during the summer months.

The pneumatophore or float is the portion of the Portuguese man-of-war that is visible above the water. The pneumatophore acts like a sail that propels the animal through the water. Dangling from the pneumatophore are the tentacles that contain the nematocysts. The tentacles are numerous and may reach up to 30 m in length. The tentacles in a single animal may contain literally thousands of nematocysts. Envenomations often occur as a swimmer or diver becomes entangled

in the tentacles; however, they can also occur from contact with a dead Portuguese man-of-war that is washed ashore.

The nematocysts respond to physical and chemical stimuli. Injection of the venom causes immediate stinging pain. Struggling to escape the tentacles frequently leads to entanglement and further envenomation. The pain is followed by the development of a local rash with papules in a linear pattern often described as "beaded." Over the next 2 hours and lasting for approximately 24 hours, the rash may then progress to erythematous welts. Systemic symptoms are nonspecific and include nausea, vomiting, myalgias, headache, respiratory distress, acute renal failure, anaphylaxis, cardiovascular collapse, and death.

Treatment is supportive. In addition to basic first aid measures, one of the initial goals is to prevent further envenomation. Undischarged nematocysts should be removed. Care should be taken while removing nematocysts to prevent accidental envenomation to the patient or rescuer. Ideally the area should be washed with heated sea water, as fresh water may stimulate nematocysts to inject further venom. Heated water is preferable to help degrade the heat-labile toxin. Commercial preparations designed for salt water aquariums can be used. Acetic acid (vinegar) is also recommended to inactivate the venom. Alternatives that have been used include aluminum sulfate 20%/surfactant (Stingose), isopropyl alcohol, Adolph's Meat Tenderizer (papain), and even Pepsi-Cola. The nematocysts can be removed by using shaving cream or a paste made of baking soda and scraping the nematocysts off with a razor. Any object with a sharp edge can be used, including credit cards and cardboard. Once the nematocysts are removed, local anesthetics may be soothing. Application of a pressure immobilization dressing can also be used. The patient's tetanus status should be ascertained and updated as needed. Pain medications and antihistamines should be administered if necessary. Prophylactic antibiotics are not recommended.

### Scyphozoa (Jellyfish)

Scyphozoa include many species of jellyfish, some of which are very dangerous to man. Jellyfish can vary in size from a few millimeters to 2 m across the main portion of the body, known as the bell. Some species have tentacles up to 40 m in length. They range from transparent to multicolored. As with the Portuguese man-of-war, the jellyfish are free-floating creatures that depend on the wind and tides for movement. Also as with the Portuguese man-of-war, envenomations can occur from both live and dead jellyfish. Scyphozoans are widely distributed through the Atlantic, Pacific, Caribbean, Indian, and even the Arctic oceans. Envenomations may be mild, limited to minimal skin irritation; moderate, which includes stinging, pruritus, and skin eruptions; and severe, which may manifest with varying degrees of systemic symptoms involving neurologic, gastrointestinal, ocular, and cardiovascular reactions. Chronic sequelae, such as keloids, hyperpigmentation, muscle spasms, contractures, and gangrene, have been reported.

The most dangerous of the jellyfish is the box jellyfish (*Chironex fleckeri*), which inhabits the South Pacific waters mainly off Australia. It is considered the most venomous of sea creatures. A much less lethal variety of the box jellyfish is found in the Chesapeake Bay off the U.S. Mid-Atlantic states. Envenomations by *Chironex fleckeri* can be fatal in as little as seconds to minutes. An adult box jellyfish contains enough venom (approximately 10 cc) to kill three adult humans. The box jellyfish is a large transparent jellyfish weighing approximately 6 kg and measuring up to 30 cm across its bell. The *Chironex* may possess as

## CURRENT DIAGNOSIS

- Intense pain at site
- Localized reactions
    - "Beaded" papules
    - Erythematous welts
- Systemic symptoms
    - Nausea, vomiting
    - Myalgias, headache
    - Respiratory distress
    - Acute renal failure
    - Anaphylaxis
    - Cardiovascular collapse
    - Death

## CURRENT THERAPY

- ABCs of resuscitation
- Pain control
- Tetanus immunization
- Wound irrigation/débridement
- Delayed primary closure
- Antibiotics

many as 60 tentacles, which can be up to 3 m in length and contain millions of nematocysts. Stings can occur at any time but most commonly in the summer months (September through May). Attacks usually occur in shallow water and often involve children.

Stings can be minor, but massive envenomations can be fatal. The venom is neurotoxic, and the action is not completely understood. Death can occur from respiratory failure, cardiotoxicity, or paralysis of the cardiac muscle. Often the victim becomes unconscious before he or she can leave the water. The venom also has dermatonecrotic actions that lead to patches of full-thickness skin necrosis and permanent scarring.

Symptoms include severe localized pain that may continue to increase even with the removal of the tentacles. Large erythematous areas occur where the skin has come in contact with the tentacles, and the size of the areas may give an indication as to the amount of envenomation. Systemic symptoms include difficulty breathing, swallowing, and speaking. In severe cases, the patient may become hypotensive, lose consciousness, and exhibit cardiac dysrhythmias or even cardiac arrest. First aid measures include removing the patient from the water, supporting the ABCs (including cardiopulmonary resuscitation if necessary), soaking the tentacles in vinegar for at least 30 seconds before removing them (in an attempt to inactivate the venom), applying a pressure immobilization dressing, administering analgesia (narcotics and muscle relaxers are recommended), and providing rapid transport. An antivenom from sheep immunoglobulin (box jellyfish antivenin) is available, and 20,000 U (one vial) should be administered as soon as possible for treatment of severe envenomations. Intravenous administration is the preferred route, but if intravenous access is not immediately available, the intramuscular route is acceptable so as not to delay administration. Indications for antivenom administration include cardiac dysrhythmias, cardiac arrest, difficulty with breathing or speaking, and severe pain. Even with apparent mild envenomations, the patient should be observed for at least 6 to 8 hours to ensure no progression of symptoms.

It is thought that many types of jellyfish may cause the Irukandji syndrome (rapid-onset pulmonary edema and respiratory failure); however, the one species known to cause this syndrome is *Carukia barnesi*. *Carukia barnesi* is a small (<2 cm in diameter across the bell) jellyfish found off North Queensland, Australia. Other similar species have been seen elsewhere in the Pacific and even off the Florida coast. Symptoms of Irukandji syndrome include muscular chest and neck pain, sweating, anxiety, nausea, vomiting, headaches, tachycardia, hypotension, pulmonary edema, and cardiopulmonary collapse. Symptoms may persist for hours to days and are similar to those resulting from massive catecholamine release. Treatment is mainly supportive. Vinegar should be used acutely to aid in removal of tentacles and to prevent further envenomation. Analgesia should be given as needed. Box jellyfish antivenom does not appear to be effective.

## Anthozoa

Sea anemones are flower-like, sessile creatures found in shallow waters and tidal pools. They range in size from a few millimeters to 0.5 m in diameter. Their multicolored appearance can attract unwary swimmers to handle them. They possess tentacles and have nematocysts similar to the Portuguese man-of-war. Envenomations are similar to the Portuguese man-of-war but generally not as severe. The "hell's fire anemone" (*Actinodendron plumosum*) produces significant local effects that have earned the animal its colorful name. Treatment is similar to that for the Portuguese man-of-war.

## Echinodermata

Fire corals (*Millepora* species) are not true coral. They are found living on rocks and other corals. Fire corals are brushlike creatures that generally range from 5 to 10 cm in length but can reach up to 2 m. Syndromes after contact include pruritus, urticaria, and severe burning pain. The pain is usually short lived (1–2 hours); however, the

urticarial wheals may become hyperpigmented and persist for several months. Treatment is similar to that of jellyfish stings. Long-term steroids can be used to treat the skin hyperpigmentation.

Sea urchins are free-living, hard-shelled creatures of the class *Echinoida*. They possess multiple, irregular, brittle spines that may or may not contain venom. Envenomation frequently occurs when the creature is handled by swimmers, fishermen, and divers. Sea urchins whose spines do not contain venom have jawed pedicellaria that may latch on so that venom can be injected. The venom causes an immediate local reaction that is marked by severe pain. The spines also contain a blue–black dye that may stain the skin but is of no medical significance. The brittle spines break off easily and contaminate the wound. Treatment consists of immersion in hot water to inactivate the venom and local débridement to clean the wound. Radiographs may be useful in detecting occult presence of spines. Care must be taken to remove the spines, which are brittle and crumble in the wound. Portions of spines remaining in the wound may lead to long-term dermatologic sequelae such as granulomas. Antibiotics and corticosteroids can be used for treatment of wounds.

## STINGING VERTEBRATES

### Stingrays

The stings and envenomations of stingrays have been recognized and recorded since ancient times. Aristotle referred to them as "devilfish." It is reported that the spear Theolonius used to kill Odysseus had the barb of a stingray on its head. Stingrays, like sharks, are cartilaginous fish and usually range from a few millimeters to 1 to 2 m in length. Some species have attained lengths of 5 to 6 m. Although stingrays are one of the fishes most implicated in envenomations to humans (approximately 2000 stings annually worldwide), they are actually docile and only attack when startled or provoked. The most common mechanism of injury is a swimmer or fisherman accidentally stepping on the stingray while it is partially covered in sand at the bottom of shallow waters. The stingray reflexively whips its tail around and strikes the unsuspecting victim, usually in the lower leg but possibly also involving the upper extremities and torso. The venom-coated barb, which is located on the tail, is serrated and can cause significant lacerations. The venom is heat labile and composed of several compounds, including serotonin, phosphodiesterases, and 5'-nucleosidase. Symptoms include immediate intense stinging pain that is out of proportion to the apparent wound. The pain usually reaches maximal intensity in about 90 minutes. Systemic symptoms are not diagnostic and may include muscle weakness, cramping, nausea, vomiting, peripheral vasoconstriction, cardiac dysrhythmias, seizures, respiratory distress, coma, and even death.

Treatment of envenomations is focused on rapid stabilization, pain control, venom neutralization, and wound care. Initially the wound should be copiously irrigated with cool normal saline. Cool temperatures are thought to cause some vasoconstriction and to delay or decrease uptake of more venom. Local anesthesia applied to the wound site and potent narcotics are recommended for patient comfort. Once the initial irrigation has been completed, the wound should be immersed in hot water (113°F [45°C]) for 30 to 90 minutes to help destabilize the heat-labile venom. Care should be taken when attempting to débride and remove all pieces of the barb from the wound. The wound should not be closed primarily. Tetanus immunization should be administered if indicated. Prophylactic antibiotics are recommended.

### Catfish

There are more than 1000 specifies of fresh and salt water catfish, many of which can envenomate humans. Catfish can introduce venom through glands on their dorsal and pectoral fins. In some cases, envenomations occur through crinotoxins present on the fish, with venom entering victims through abraded skin or puncture wounds inflicted by the catfish spines. The proteinaceous venom possesses dermonecrotic and vasoconstrictive factors. Symptoms of envenomation include pain and paresthesias that may last from minutes to

---

several days. Erythema, edema, cyanosis, and hemorrhage are also seen. Rare systemic effects include weakness, fever, hypotension, syncope, and respiratory distress. Death from envenomations has been recorded but is rare.

Treatment includes pain control and wound management. The area should be immersed in hot water (110°F [43°C]) to inactivate the venom and reverse vasospasm and muscle cramping. Pain management can be accomplished with local anesthetics and possibly analgesia. Wounds should be copiously irrigated. Radiographs should be obtained to rule out foreign bodies. Tetanus immunization should be administered as necessary. Antibiotics should be considered, especially for deep puncture wounds.

### Scorpion Fish

Scorpion fish are divided into three groups based on their venom apparatus: (1) *Pterois* (zebrafish, lionfish), (2) *Scorpaena* ("true" scorpion fish), and (3) *Synanceja* (stonefish). All have hard armor plating and are found in the shallow reef waters of the Florida Keys, Gulf of Mexico, southern California, and Hawaii. Envenomations have occurred when unsuspecting victims step on the scorpion fish. The venom glands are located on the dorsal, pectoral, and anal spines. Because of their beautiful colors, scorpion fish are now sought by many private aquariums, thus increasing the potential for envenomations. The venom has pronounced neurotoxic effects and has been likened to that of cobra venom.

Symptoms depend on the species, amount of venom injected, and underlying health of the victim. The most common initial symptom is intense pain that peaks at 90 minutes and persists for up to 12 hours. Other local symptoms include erythema, edema, and swollen lymph nodes. Paresthesias may occur and persist for weeks. Severe envenomations, particularly those seen with stonefish, may present with hypotension, cardiovascular collapse, and even death within hours. Treatment consists of immersion in hot water for 30 to 90 minutes, pain control, wound irrigation, and débridement. Tetanus immunizations should be administered when indicated. Prophylactic antibiotic use is recommended. An antivenin to stonefish venom is manufactured in Australia and is available from several sites in the United States.

### Sea Snakes

There are at least 52 species of sea snakes (*Hydrophiidae*), with at least 11 implicated in human fatalities. Most are located in the Indo-Pacific waters off Australia, but an Atlantic species (*Pelamis platurus*) inhabits the coastal waters of South America. Sea snakes have two to four fangs associated with paired venom glands. The fangs are short and easily broken. Many bites do not result in envenomations. This is fortunate because the venom of sea snakes is considered to be more potent than that of most terrestrial snakes, including the cobra and krait.

Bites are not particularly painful, and onset of symptoms may be immediate or, more commonly, delayed by minutes to hours. Often multiple (up to 20) puncture wounds from fangs are seen. Initial symptoms may include muscle cramping, muscle spasms, myosis, papillary dilation, weakness of extraocular movements, slurred speech, and paralysis. Hemoglobinuria and myoglobinuria may occur and lead to acute renal failure. Death may result from respiratory failure. Treatment is similar to that of terrestrial snakebites, and the Australian pressure immobilization technique is recommended as with terrestrial elapids. A polyvalent antivenin (Sea Snake Antivenom) is produced in Australia. Antivenin administration as soon as possible is recommended, but delays at long as 36 hours have been reported but still associated with positive outcomes. If specific sea snake antivenin is not available, tiger snake antivenin can be used.

### Blue-Ringed Octopus

The blue-ringed octopus (*Hapalochlaena* species) is found mainly off the waters of Australia. Its color is usually yellow-brown, with the striking blue rings appearing when the animal is disturbed. These animals are found in shallow tidal pools, and envenomations occur when the octopus is handled or stepped on. The venom contains tetrodotoxin and affects the neuronal sodium channels. Symptoms include weakness, paresthesias, respiratory distress, and possibly respiratory failure.

There is no specific treatment, although the pressure immobilization technique is recommended. No antivenin is available. The mainstay of treatment is supportive care. Endotracheal intubation may be necessary.

## Toxic Ingestions

### CIGUATERA

Ciguatera is the most common nonbacterial form of food poisoning. Furthermore, it is the most common poisoning associated with fish ingestion. Ciguatera has been associated with more than 500 different species of fish, many of which serve as food sources for man. Some of the more commonly implicated species are sea bass, grouper, barracuda, snapper, jack, parrot fish, and surgeon fish. The ciguatoxin is found in dinoflagellates, protozoa, and blue–green algae. This toxin is eaten by smaller fish, which in turn are eaten by larger fish, depositing the toxin in the flesh. The concentration of ciguatoxin increases as the fish moves up the food chain. The toxin does not appear to be harmful to the fish. The toxin is heat stable, is tasteless, and does not appear to be affected by refrigeration or cooking. The toxin has cholinergic and acetylcholinesterase properties. However, its main effect appears to be on calcium regulation through the sodium channels on the cell membranes.

Symptoms generally occur within 6 to 12 hours but may be delayed for more than 24 hours. Gastrointestinal symptoms are common and include nausea, vomiting, diarrhea, and abdominal cramping. The gastrointestinal symptoms tend to resolve more quickly than the neurologic complaints. Neurologic manifestations include pain, weakness, paresthesias, headaches, ataxia, and peripheral and central nerve palsies. An unusual complaint that these patients may volunteer is reversal of hot and cold sensations. These symptoms are generally self-limited, and there is no specific treatment other that symptomatic and supportive care.

### SCOMBROID

Scombroid is the second most common poisoning associated with the ingestion of fish. Scombroid is most often seen with dark-meat fish, such as tuna, bluefish, mackerel, skipjack, and bonito. Unlike ciguatera, scombroid is related to improper refrigeration of the fish prior to eating. Organisms on the surface of the fish, particularly *Klebsiella* species, *Aerobacter aerogenes*, *Escherichia coli*, and *Proteus morganii*, may elaborate histidine decarboxylase, which converts histidine to histamine. The presence of scombroid does not appear to affect the smell or taste of the fish, although a peppery taste has been described.

Symptoms usually occur within a few minutes to several hours. Because the symptoms are histamine regulated, they are often confused as allergic in origin. Nausea, vomiting, diarrhea, abdominal cramping, erythema, pruritus, and bronchospasm may occur. Treatment includes gastrointestinal decontamination, IV hydration, antihistamines, steroids, and epinephrine, and all may be used when appropriate. These symptoms are generally self-limiting; however, the severity may be affected by the underlying health of the patient.

### TOXIC SHELLFISH

Humans who consume shellfish (mussels, oysters, clams, crabs) that have ingested dinoflagellates may contract toxic shellfish poisoning. The toxins do not appear to injure the shellfish, but ingestion by humans of as few as one to three of these infected animals may cause death. Symptoms may appear to be allergic, such as pruritus and respiratory distress. Gastrointestinal manifestations may include nausea, vomiting, diarrhea, and abdominal discomfort. Furthermore, saxitoxin, a potent neurotoxin, may be present and lead to respiratory failure. No specific antidote is available, and treatment is mainly supportive.

The toxin is heat stable and water soluble, and it has curare-like properties. Symptoms may include headache, abnormal proprioception, paresthesias, and disturbance of deep tendon reflexes and may eventually progress to flaccid paralysis.

## REFERENCES

Blomkalis AL, Otten EJ: Catfish spine envenomation: A case report and literature review. Wilderness Environ Med 1999;10:242-246.

Bonnet MS: The toxicology of Octopus maculosa: The blue-ringed octopus. Br Homeopath J 1999;88:166-171.

Currie BK: Marine antivenoms. J Toxicol Clin Toxicol 2003;41:301-308.

Isbister GK: Venomous fish stings in tropical northern Australia. Am J Emerg Med 2001;19:561-565.

Nimorakiotals B, Winkel KD: Marine envenomations. Part one. Aust Fam Physician 2003;32:969-974.

Nimorakiotals B, Winkel KD: Marine envenomations. Part two. Aust Fam Physician 2003;32:975-979.

O'Reily GM, Isbister GK, Lawrie PM, et al: Prospective study of jellyfish stings from tropical Australia including the major box jellyfish Chironex fleckeri. Med J Aust 2001;175:652-655.

Seymour J, Carrette T, Cullen P, et al: The use of pressure immobilization bandages in the first aid management of cubozoan envenomings. Toxicon 2002;40:1503-1505.

Sobel J, Painter J: Illnesses caused by marine toxins. Clin Infect Dis 2005; 41:1290-1296.

# Medical Toxicology: Ingestions, Inhalations, and Dermal and Ocular Absorptions

Method of
*Howard C. Mofenson, MD, Thomas R. Caraccio, PharmD, Michael McGuigan, MD, and Joseph Greensher, MD*

## Introduction and Epidemiology

According to the national Toxic Exposure Surveillance System (TESS), over 2.4 million potentially toxic exposures were reported last year to Poison Control Centers throughout the United States. Poisonings were responsible for 1183 deaths and more than 500,000 hospitalizations. Poisoning accounts for 2% to 5% of pediatric hospital admissions, 10% of adult admissions, 5% of hospital admissions in the elderly (>65 years of age), and 5% of ambulance calls. In one urban hospital, drug-related emergencies accounted for 38% of the emergency department visits. An evaluation of a medical intensive care unit and step-down unit over a 3-month period indicated that poisonings accounted for 19.7% of admissions.

The largest number of fatalities resulting from poisoning reported to the TESS are caused by analgesics. The other principal toxicologic causes of fatalities are antidepressants, sedative hypnotics/antipsychotics, stimulants/street drugs, cardiovascular agents, and alcohols. Less than 1% of overdose cases reaching the hospitals result in fatality. However, patients presenting in deep coma to medical care facilities have a fatality rate of 13% to 35%. The largest single cause of coma of inapparent etiology is drug poisoning.

Pharmaceutical preparations are involved in 50% of poisonings. The number one pharmaceutical agent involved in exposures is acetaminophen. The severity of the manifestations of acute poisoning exposures varies greatly depending on whether the poisoning was intentional or unintentional. Unintentional exposures make up 85% to 90% of all poisoning exposures. The majority of cases are acute, occurring in children younger than 5 years of age, in the home, and resulting in no or minor toxicity. Many are actually ingestions of relatively nontoxic substances that require minimal medical care. Intentional poisonings, such as suicides, constitute 10% to 15% of exposures and may require the highest standards of medical and nursing care and the use of sophisticated equipment for recovery. Intentional ingestions are often of multiple substances and frequently include ethanol, acetaminophen, and aspirin. Suicides make up 54% of the reported fatalities. About 25% of suicides are attempted with drugs. Sixty percent of patients who take a drug overdose use their own medication and 15% use drugs prescribed for close relatives. The majority of the drug-related suicide attempts involve a central nervous system (CNS) depressant, and coma management is vital to the treatment.

## Assessment and Maintenance of the Vital Functions

The initial assessment of all patients in medical emergencies follows the principles of basic and advanced cardiac life support. The adequacy of the patient's airway, degree of ventilation, and circulatory status should be determined. The vital functions should be established and maintained. Vital signs should be measured frequently and should include body core temperature. The assessment of vital functions should include the rate numbers (e.g., respiratory rate) and indications of effectiveness (e.g., depth of respirations and degree of gas exchange). Table 1 gives important measurements and vital signs.

Level of consciousness should be assessed by immediate AVPU (Alert, responds to Verbal stimuli, responds to Painful stimuli, and Unconscious). If the patient is unconscious, one must assess the severity of the unconsciousness by the Glasgow Coma Scale (Table 2).

If the patient is comatose, management requires administering 100% oxygen, establishing vascular access, and obtaining blood for pertinent laboratory studies. The administration of glucose, thiamine, and naloxone, as well as intubation to protect the airway, should be considered. Pertinent laboratory studies include arterial blood gases (ABG), electrocardiography (ECG), determination of blood glucose level, electrolytes, renal and liver tests, and acetaminophen plasma concentration in all cases of intentional ingestions. Radiography of the chest and abdomen may be useful. The severity of a stimulant's effects can also be assessed and should be documented to follow the trend.

The examiner should completely expose the patient by removing clothes and other items that interfere with a full evaluation. One should look for clues to etiology in the clothes and include the hat and shoes.

## Prevention of Absorption and Reduction of Local Damage

### EXPOSURE

Poisoning exposure routes include ingestion (76.8%), dermal (8%), ophthalmologic (5%), inhalation (6%), insect bites and stings (4%), and parenteral injections (0.5%). The effect of the toxin may be local, systemic, or both.

Local effects (skin, eyes, mucosa of respiratory or gastrointestinal tract) occur where contact is made with the poisonous substance. Local effects are nonspecific chemical reactions that depend on the chemical properties (e.g., pH), concentration, contact time, and type of exposed surface.

Systemic effects occur when the poison is absorbed into the body and depend on the dose, the distribution, and the functional reserve of the organ systems. Shock and hypoxia are part of systemic toxicity.

### DELAYED TOXIC ACTION

Therapeutic doses of most pharmaceuticals are absorbed within 90 minutes. However, the patient with exposure to a potential toxin may be asymptomatic at this time because a sufficient amount has not

**TABLE 1** Important Measurements and Vital Signs

| Age | Body Surface Area (m²) | Weight (kg) | Height (cm) | Pulse (bpm) Resting | Blood Pressure Hypotension | Hypertension Significant | Hypertension Severe | Respiratory Rate (rpm) |
|---|---|---|---|---|---|---|---|---|
| Newborn | 0.19 | 3.5 | 50 | 70-190 | <60/40 | >96 | >106 | 30-60 |
| 1 mo-6 mo | 0.30 | 4-7 | 50-65 | 80-160 | <70/45 | >104 | >110 | 30-50 |
| 6 mo-1 y | 0.38 | 7-10 | 65-75 | 80-160 | <70/45 | >104 | >110 | 20-40 |
| 1-2 y | 0.50-0.55 | 10-12 | 75-85 | 80-140 | <74/47 | >112/74 | >118/82 | 20-40 |
| 3-5 y | 0.54-0.68 | 15-20 | 90-108 | 80-120 | <80/52 | >116/76 | >124/84 | 20-40 |
| 6-9 y | 0.68-0.85 | 20-28 | 122-133 | 75-115 | <90/60 | >122/82 | >130/86 | 16-25 |
| 10-12 y | 1.00-1.07 | 30-40 | 138-147 | 70-110 | <90/60 | >126/82 | >134/90 | 16-25 |
| 13-15 y | 1.07-1.22 | 42-50 | 152-160 | 60-100 | <90/60 | >136/86 | >144/92 | 16-20 |
| 16-18 y | 1.30-1.60 | 53-60 | 160-170 | 60-100 | <90/60 | >142/92 | >150/98 | 12-16 |
| Adult | 1.40-1.70 | 60-70 | 160-170 | 60-100 | <90/60 | >140/90 | >210/120 | 10-16 |

Data from Nadas A: Pediatric Cardiology, 3rd ed. Philadelphia, WB Saunders, 1976; Blumer JL (ed): A Practice Guide to Pediatric Intensive Care. St Louis, Mosby, 1990; AAP and ACEP: Respiratory Distress in APLS Pediatric Emergency Medicine Course, 1993; Second Task Force: Blood pressure control in children–1987, Pediatr 79:1, 1987; Linakis JG: Hypertension. In Fliesher GR, Ludwig S (eds); Textbook of Pediatric Emergency Medicine, 3rd ed. Baltimore, Williams & Wilkins, 1993.

## TABLE 2 Glasgow Coma Scale

| Scale | Adult Response | Score | Pediatric, 0-1 Years |
|---|---|---|---|
| Eye opening | Spontaneous | 4 | Spontaneous |
| | To verbal command | 3 | To shout |
| | To pain | 2 | To pain |
| | None | 1 | No response |
| Motor response | | | |
| To verbal command | Obeys | 6 | |
| To painful stimuli | Localized pain | 5 | Localized pain |
| | Flexion withdrawal | 4 | Flexion withdrawal |
| | Decorticate flexion | 3 | Decorticate flexion |
| | Decerebrate extension | 2 | Decerebrate flexion |
| | None | 1 | None |
| Verbal response: adult | Oriented and converses | 5 | Cries, smiles, coos |
| | Disoriented but converses | 4 | Cries or screams |
| | Inappropriate words | 3 | Inappropriate sounds |
| | Incomprehensible sounds | 2 | Grunts |
| | None | 1 | Gives no response |
| Verbal response: child | Oriented | 5 | |
| | Words or babbles | 4 | |
| | Vocal sounds | 3 | |
| | Cries or moans to stimuli | 2 | |
| | None | 1 | |

Data from Teasdale G, Jennett B: Assessment of coma impaired consciousness. Lancet 2:83, 1974; Simpson D, Reilly P: Pediatric coma scale. Lancet 2:450, 1982; Seidel J: Preparing for pediatric emergencies. Pediatr Rev 16:470, 1995.

yet been absorbed or metabolized to produce toxicity at the time the patient presents for care.

Absorption can be significantly delayed under the following circumstances:

1. Drugs with anticholinergic properties (e.g., antihistamines, belladonna alkaloids, diphenoxylate with atropine [Lomotil], phenothiazines, and tricyclic antidepressants).
2. Modified release preparations such as sustained-release, enteric-coated, and controlled-release formulations have delayed and prolonged absorption.
3. Concretions may form (e.g., salicylates, iron, glutethimide, and meprobamate [Equanil]) that can delay absorption and prolong the toxic effects. Large quantities of drugs tend to be absorbed more slowly than small quantities.

Some substances must be metabolized into a toxic metabolite (acetaminophen, acetonitrile, ethylene glycol, methanol, methylene chloride, parathion, and paraquat). In some cases, time is required to produce a toxic effect on organ systems (*Amanita phalloides* mushrooms, carbon tetrachloride, colchicine, digoxin [Lanoxin], heavy metals, monoamine oxidase inhibitors, and oral hypoglycemic agents).

### Initial Management

1. Stabilization of airway, breathing, and circulation and protection of same.
2. Identification of specific toxin or toxic syndrome.
3. Initial treatment: D50W; consider thiamine, naloxone (Narcan), oxygen, and antidotes if needed.
4. Physical assessment.
5. Decontamination: Gastrointestinal tract, skin, eyes.

### DECONTAMINATION

In the asymptomatic patient who has been exposed to a toxic substance, decontamination procedures should be considered if the patient has been exposed to potentially toxic substances in toxic amounts.

Ocular exposure should be immediately treated with water irrigation for 15 to 20 minutes with the eyelids fully retracted. One should not use neutralizing chemicals. All caustic and corrosive injuries should be evaluated with fluorescein dye and by an ophthalmologist.

Dermal exposure is treated immediately with copious water irrigation for 30 minutes, not a forceful flushing. Shampooing the hair, cleansing the fingernails, navel, and perineum, and irrigating the eyes are necessary in the case of an extensive exposure. The clothes should be specially bagged and may have to be discarded. Leather goods can become irreversibly contaminated and must be abandoned. Caustic (alkali) exposures can require hours of irrigation. Dermal absorption can occur with pesticides, hydrocarbons, and cyanide.

Injection exposures (e.g., snake envenomation) can be treated with venom extracts. Venom extractors can be used within minutes of envenomation, and proximal lymphatic constricting bands or elastic wraps can be used to delay lymphatic flow and immobilize the extremity. Cold packs and tourniquets should not be used and incision is generally not recommended. Substances of abuse may be injected intravenously or subcutaneously. In these cases, little decontamination can be done.

Inhalation exposure to toxic substances is managed by immediate removal of the victim from the contaminated environment by protected rescuers.

Gastrointestinal exposure is the most common route of poisoning. Gastrointestinal decontamination historically has been done by gastric emptying: induction of emesis, gastric lavage, administration of activated charcoal, and the use of cathartics or whole bowel irrigation. No procedure is routine; it should be individualized for each case. If no attempt is made to decontaminate the patient, the reason should be clearly documented on the medical record (e.g., time elapsed, past peak of action, ineffectiveness, or risk of procedure).

### Gastric Emptying Procedures

The gastric emptying procedure used is influenced by the age of the patient, the effectiveness of the procedure, the time of ingestion (gastric emptying is usually ineffective after 1 hour postingestion), the patient's clinical status (time of peak effect has passed or the patient's condition is too unstable), formulation of the substance ingested (regular release versus modified release), the amount ingested, and the rapidity of onset of CNS depression or stimulation (convulsions). Most studies show that only 30% (range, 19% to 62%) of the ingested toxin is removed by gastric emptying under optimal conditions. It has not been demonstrated that the choice of procedure improved the outcome.

A mnemonic for gathering information is STATS:

S—substance
T—type of formulation
A—amount and age
T—time of ingestion
S—signs and symptoms

The examiner should attempt to obtain AMPLE information about the patient:

A—age and allergies
M—available medications
P—past medical history including pregnancy, psychiatric illnesses, substance abuse, or intentional ingestions
L—time of last meal, which may influence absorption and the onset and peak action
E—events leading to present condition

The intent of the patient should also be determined.

The Regional Poison Center should be consulted for the exact ingredients of the ingested substance and the latest management. The treatment information on the labels of products and in the Physician's Desk Reference are notoriously inaccurate.

## Ipecac Syrup

Syrup of ipecac–induced emesis has virtually no use in the emergency department. Although at one time it was considered most useful in young children with a recent witnessed ingestion, it is no longer advised in most cases. Current guidelines from the American Association of Poison Control Centers have significantly limited the indications for inducing emesis because the risk most often exceeds the benefit derived from this procedure. The Poison Control Center should be called if inducting emesis is being considered.

Contraindications or situations in which induction of emesis is inappropriate include the following:

- Ingestion of caustic substance
- Loss of airway protective reflexes because of ingestion of substances that can produce rapid onset of CNS depression (e.g., short-acting benzodiazepines, barbiturates, nonbarbiturate sedative-hypnotics, opioids, tricyclic antidepressants) or convulsions (e.g., camphor [Ponstel], chloroquine [Aralen], codeine, isoniazid [Nydrazid], mefenamic acid, nicotine, propoxyphene [Darvon], organophosphate insecticides, strychnine, and tricyclic antidepressants)
- Ingestion of low-viscosity petroleum distillates (e.g., gasoline, lighter fluid, kerosene)
- Significant vomiting prior to presentation or hematemesis
- Age under 6 months (no established dose, safety, or efficacy data)
- Ingestion of foreign bodies (emesis is ineffective and may lead to aspiration)
- Clinical conditions including neurologic impairment, hemodynamic instability, increased intracranial pressure, and hypertension
- Delay in presentation (more than 1 hour postingestion)

The dose of syrup of ipecac in the 6- to 9-month-old infant is 5 mL; in the 9- to 12-month-old, 10 mL; and in the 1- to 12-year-old, 15 mL. In children older than 12 years and in adults, the dose is 30 mL. The dose can be repeated once if the child does not vomit in 15 to 20 minutes. The vomitus should be inspected for remnants of pills or toxic substances, and the appearance and odor should be documented. When ipecac is not available, 30 mL of mild dishwashing soap (not dishwasher detergent) can be used, although it is less effective.

Complications are very rare but include aspiration, protracted vomiting, rarely cardiac toxicity with long-term abuse, pneumothorax, gastric rupture, diaphragmatic hernia, intracranial hemorrhage, and Mallory-Weiss tears.

## Gastric Lavage

Gastric lavage should be considered only when life-threatening amounts of substances were involved, when the benefits outweigh the risks, when it can be performed within 1 hour of the ingestion, and when no contraindications exist.

The contraindications are similar to those for ipecac-induced emesis. However, gastric lavage can be accomplished after the insertion of an endotracheal tube in cases of CNS depression or controlled convulsions. The patient should be placed with the head lower than the hips in a left-lateral decubitus position. The location of the tube should be confirmed by radiography, if necessary, and suctioning equipment should be available.

Contraindications to gastric lavage include the following:

- Ingestion of caustic substances (risk of esophageal perforation)
- Uncontrolled convulsions, because of the danger of aspiration and injury during the procedure
- Ingestion of low-viscosity petroleum distillate products
- CNS depression or absent protective airway reflexes, without endotracheal protection
- Significant cardiac dysrhythmias
- Significant emesis or hematemesis prior to presentation
- Delay in presentation (more than 1 hour postingestion)

### Size of Tube

The best results with gastric lavage are obtained with the largest possible orogastric tube that can be reasonably passed (nasogastric tubes are not large enough to remove solid material). In adults, a large-bore orogastric Lavacuator hose or a No. 42 French Ewald tube should be used; in young children, orogastric tubes are generally too small to remove solid material and gastric lavage is not recommended.

The amount of fluid used varies with the patient's age and size. In general, aliquots of 50 to 100 mL per lavage are used in adults. Larger amounts of fluid may force the toxin past the pylorus. Lavage fluid is 0.9% saline.

Complications are rare and may include respiratory depression, aspiration pneumonitis, cardiac dysrhythmias as a result of increased vagal tone, esophageal-gastric tears and perforation, laryngospasm, and mediastinitis.

## Activated Charcoal

Oral activated charcoal adsorbs the toxin onto its surface before absorption. According to recent guidelines set forth by the American Academy of Clinical Toxicology, activated charcoal should not be used routinely. Its use is indicated only if a toxic amount of substance has been ingested and is optimally effective within 1 hour of the ingestion. Because of the slow absorption of large quantities of toxin, activated charcoal may be beneficial after 1 hour postingestion.

Activated charcoal does not effectively adsorb small molecules or molecules lacking carbon (Table 3). Activated charcoal adsorption may be diminished by milk, cocoa powder, and ice cream.

### TABLE 3  Substances Poorly Adsorbed by Activated Charcoal

| | |
|---|---|
| C | Caustics and corrosives |
| H | Heavy metals (arsenic, iron, lead, mercury) |
| A | Alcohols (ethanol, methanol, isopropanol) and glycols (ethylene glycols) |
| R | Rapid onset of absorption (cyanide and strychnine) |
| C | Chlorine and iodine |
| O | Others insoluble in water (substances in tablet form) |
| A | Aliphatic hydrocarbons (petroleum distillates) |
| L | Laxatives (sodium, magnesium, potassium, and lithium) |

There are a few relative contraindications to the use of activated charcoal:

1. Ingestion of caustics and corrosives, which may produce vomiting or cling to the mucosa and falsely appear as a burn on endoscopy.
2. Comatose patient, in whom the airway must be secured prior to activated charcoal administration.
3. Patient without presence of bowel sounds.

*Note*: Activated charcoal was shown not to interfere with effectiveness of *N*-acetylcysteine in cases of acetaminophen overdose, so it is no longer contraindicated as was thought in the past.

The usual initial adult dose is 60 to 100 g and the dose for children is 15 to 30 g. It is administered orally as a slurry mixed with water or by nasogastric or orogastric tube. *Caution:* Be sure the tube is in the stomach. Cathartics are not necessary.

Although repeated dosing with activated charcoal may decrease the half-life and increases the clearance of phenobarbital, dapsone, quinidine, theophylline, and carbamazepine (Tegretol), recent guidelines indicate there is insufficient evidence to support the use of multiple-dose activated charcoal unless a life-threatening amount of one of the substances mentioned is involved. At present there are no controlled studies that demonstrate that multiple-dose activated charcoal or cathartics alter the clinical course of an intoxication. The dose varies from 0.25 to 0.50 g/kg every 1 to 4 hours, and continuous nasogastric tube infusion of 0.25 to 0.5 g/kg/h has been used to decrease vomiting.

Gastrointestinal dialysis is the diffusion of the toxin from the higher concentration in the serum of the mesenteric vessels to the lower levels in the gastrointestinal tract mucosal cell and subsequently into the gastrointestinal lumen, where the concentration has been lowered by intraluminal adsorption of activated charcoal.

Complications of treatment with activated charcoal include vomiting in 50% of cases, desorption (especially with weak acids in intestine), and aspiration (at least a dozen cases of aspiration have been reported). There are many cases of unreported pulmonary aspirations and "charcoal lungs," intestinal obstruction or pseudoobstruction (three case reports with multiple dosing, none with a single dose), empyema following esophageal perforation, and hypermagnesemia and hypernatremia, which have been associated with repeated concurrent doses of activated charcoal and saline cathartics. Catharsis was used to hasten the elimination of any remaining toxin in the gastrointestinal tract. There are no studies to demonstrate the effectiveness of cathartics, and they are no longer recommended as a form of gastrointestinal decontamination.

### Whole-Bowel Irrigation

With whole bowel irrigation, solutions of polyethylene glycol (PEG) with balanced electrolytes are used to cleanse the bowel without causing shifts in fluids and electrolytes. The procedure is not approved by the U.S. Food and Drug Administration for this purpose.

#### Indications

The procedure has been studied and used successfully in cases of iron overdose when abdominal radiographs reveal incomplete emptying of excess iron. There are additional indications for other types of ingestions, such as with body-packing of illicit drugs (e.g., cocaine, heroin).

The procedure is to administer the solution (GoLYTELY or Colyte), orally or by nasogastric tube, in a dose of 0.5 L per hour in children younger than 5 years of age and 2 L per hour in adolescents and adults for 5 hours. The end point is reached when the rectal effluent is clear or radiopaque materials can no longer be seen in the gastrointestinal tract on abdominal radiographs.

#### Contraindications

These measures should not be used if there is extensive hematemesis, ileus, or signs of bowel obstruction, perforation, or peritonitis. Animal experiments in which PEG was added to activated charcoal indicated that activated charcoal-salicylates and activated charcoal-theophylline combinations resulted in decreased adsorption and desorption of salicylate and theophylline and no therapeutic benefit over activated charcoal alone. Polyethylene solutions are bound by activated charcoal in vitro, decreasing the efficacy of activated charcoal.

Dilutional treatment is indicated for the immediate management of caustic and corrosive poisonings but is otherwise not useful. The administration of diluting fluid above 30 mL in children and 250 mL in adults may produce vomiting, reexposing the vital tissues to the effects of local damage and possible aspiration.

Neutralization is not proven to be either safe or effective.

Endoscopy and surgery have been required in the case of body-packer obstruction, intestinal ischemia produced by cocaine ingestion, and iron local caustic action.

## Differential Diagnosis of Poisons on the Basis of Central Nervous System Manifestations

Neurologic parameters help to classify and assess the need for supportive treatment as well as provide diagnostic clues to the etiology. Table 4 lists the effects of CNS depressants, CNS stimulants, hallucinogens, and autonomic nervous system anticholinergics and cholinergics.

Central nervous system depressants are cholinergics, opioids, sedative-hypnotics, and sympatholytic agents. The hallmarks are lethargy, sedation, stupor, and coma. In exception to the manifestations listed in Table 4, (a) barbiturates may produce an initial tachycardia; (b) convulsions are produced by codeine, propoxyphene (Darvon), meperidine (Demerol), glutethimide, phenothiazines, methaqualone, and tricyclic and cyclic antidepressants; (c) benzodiazepines rarely produce coma that will interfere with cardiorespiratory functions; and (d) pulmonary edema is common with opioids and sedative-hypnotics.

The CNS stimulants are anticholinergic, hallucinogenic, sympathomimetic, and withdrawal agents. The hallmarks of CNS stimulants are convulsions and hyperactivity.

There is considerable overlapping of effects among the various hallucinogens, but the major hallmark manifestation is hallucinations.

## Guidelines for In-hospital Disposition

Classification of patients as high risk depends on clinical judgment. Any patient who needs cardiorespiratory support or has a persistently altered mental status for 3 hours or more should be considered for intensive care.

Guidelines for admitting patients older than 14 years of age to an intensive care unit, after 2 to 3 hours in the emergency department, include the following:

1. Need for intubation
2. Seizures
3. Unresponsiveness to verbal stimuli
4. Arterial carbon dioxide pressure greater than 45 mm Hg
5. Cardiac conduction or rhythm disturbances (any rhythm except sinus arrhythmia)
6. Close monitoring of vital signs during antidotal therapy or elimination procedures
7. The need for continuous monitoring
8. QRS interval greater than 0.10 second, in cases of tricyclic antidepressant poisoning
9. Systolic blood pressure less than 80 mm Hg
10. Hypoxia, hypercarbia, acid–base imbalance, or metabolic abnormalities
11. Extremes of temperature
12. Progressive deterioration or significant underlying medical disorders

**TABLE 4    Agents with Central Nervous System (CNS) Effects**

| Agents | General Manifestations | Agents | General Manifestations |
|---|---|---|---|
| **CNS Depressants** | | **Hallucinogens** | |
| Alcohols and glycols (S-H) | Bradycardia | Amphetamines‡ | Tachycardia and dysrhythmias |
| Anticonvulsants (S-H) | Bradypnea | Anticholinergics | Tachypnea |
| Antidysrhythmics (S-H) | Shallow respirations | Cardiac glycosides | Hypertension |
| Antihypertensives (S-H) | Hypotension | Cocaine | Hallucinations, usually visual |
| Barbiturates (S-H) | Hypothermia | Ethanol withdrawal | Disorientation |
| Benzodiazepines (S-H) | Flaccid coma | Hydrocarbon inhalation (abuse) | Panic reaction |
| Butyrophenones (Syly) | Miosis | Mescaline (peyote) | Toxic psychosis |
| β-Adrenergic blockers (Syly) | Hypoactive bowel sounds | Mushrooms (psilocybin) | Moist skin |
| Calcium channel blockers (Syly) | | Phencyclidine | Mydriasis (reactive) |
| Digitalis (Syly) | | | Hyperthermia |
| Opioids | | | Flashbacks |
| Lithium (mixed) | | | |
| Muscle relaxants | | **Anticholinergics** | Tachycardia, dysrhythmias (rare) |
| Phenothiazines (Syly) | | Antihistamines | Tachypnea |
| Nonbarbiturate/benzodiazepine | | Antispasmodic gastrointestinal | |
| glutethimide, methaqualone, | | preparations | Hypertension (mild) |
| methyprylon, sedative-hypnotics | | Antiparkinsonian preparations | Hyperthermia |
| (chloral hydrate, ethchlorvynol, bromide) | | Atropine | Hallucinations ("mad as a hatter") |
| Tricyclic antidepressants (late Syly) | | Cyclobenzaprine (Flexeril) | |
| | | Mydriatic ophthalmologic agents | Mydriasis (unreactive) |
| | | Over-the-counter sleep agents | ("blind as a bat") |
| **CNS Stimulants** | | Plants (Datura spp)/mushrooms | Flushed skin ("red as a beet") |
| Amphetamines (Sy) | Tachycardia | | Dry skin and mouth ("dry as a bone") |
| Anticholinergics* | Tachypnea and dysrhythmias | Phenothiazines (early) | Hypoactive bowel sounds |
| | | Scopolamine | Urinary retention |
| | | Tricyclic/cyclic antidepressants (early) | Lilliputian hallucinations ("little people") |
| Cocaine (Sy) | Hypertension | | |
| Camphor (mixed) | Convulsions | **Cholinergics** | |
| Ergot alkaloids (Sy) | Toxic psychosis | Bethanechol (Urecholine) | Bradycardia (muscarinic) |
| Isoniazid (mixed) | Mydriasis (reactive) | Carbamate insecticides (Carbaryl) | Tachycardia (nicotinic effect) |
| Lithium (mixed) | Agitation and restlessness | Edrophonium | Miosis (muscarinic) |
| Lysergic acid diethylamide (H) | Moist skin | Organophosphate insecticides | Diarrhea (muscarinic) |
| Hallucinogens (H) | Tremors | (Malathion, parathion) | |
| Mescaline and synthetic analogs | | Parasympathetic agents | Hypertension (variable) |
| Metals (arsenic, lead, mercury) | | (physostigmine, pyridostigmine) | |
| Methylphenidate (Ritalin) (Sy) | | Toxic mushrooms (Clitocybe spp.) | Hyperactive bowel sounds |
| Monoamine oxidase inhibitors (Sy) | | | Excess urination (muscarinic) |
| Pemoline (Cylert) (Sy) | | | Excess salivation (muscarinic) |
| Phencyclidine (H)† | | | Lacrimation (muscarinic) |
| Salicylates (mixed) | | | Bronchospasm (muscarinic) |
| Strychnine (mixed) | | | Muscle fasciculations (nicotinic) |
| Sympathomimetics (Sy) | | | Paralysis (nicotinic) |
| (phenylpropanolamine, | | | |
| theophylline, caffeine, thyroid) | | | |
| Withdrawal from ethanol, | | | |
| β-adrenergic blockers, | | | |
| clonidine, opioids, | | | |
| sedative-hypnotics (W) | | | |

*Abbreviations:* H = hallucinogen; S-H = sedative–hypnotic; Sy = sympathomimetic; Syly = Sympatholytic; W = withdrawal.
*Anticholinergics produce dry skin and mucosa and decreased bowel sounds.
†Phencyclidine may produce miosis.
‡The amphetamine hybrids are methylene dioxymethamphetamine (MDMA, ecstasy,"ADAM") and methylene dioxyamphetamine (MDA, "Eve"), which are associated with deaths.

## Use of Antidotes

Antidotes are available for only a relatively small number of poisons. An antidote is not a substitute for good supportive care. Table 5 summarizes the commonly used antidotes, their indications, and their methods of administration. The Regional Poison Control Center can give further information on these antidotes.

## Enhancement of Elimination

The acceptable methods for elimination of absorbed toxic substances are dialysis, hemoperfusion, exchange transfusion, plasmapheresis, enzyme induction, and inhibition. Methods of increasing urinary excretion of toxic chemicals and drugs have been studied extensively, but the other modalities have not been well evaluated.

In general, these methods are needed in only a minority of cases and should be reserved for life-threatening circumstances when a definite benefit is anticipated.

### DIALYSIS

Dialysis is the extrarenal means of removing certain substances from the body, and it can substitute for the kidney when renal failure occurs. Dialysis is not the first measure instituted; however, it may be lifesaving later in the course of a severe intoxication. It is needed in only a minority of intoxicated patients.

Peritoneal dialysis uses the peritoneum as the membrane for dialysis. It is only 1/20 as effective as hemodialysis. It is easier to use and less hazardous to the patient but also less effective in removing the toxin; thus it is rarely used except in small infants.

Hemodialysis is the most effective dialysis method but requires experience with sophisticated equipment. Blood is circulated past a semipermeable extracorporeal membrane. Substances are removed by diffusion down a concentration gradient. Anticoagulation with heparin is necessary. Flow rates of 300 to 500 mL/min can be achieved, and clearance rates may reach 200 or 300 mL/min.

Dialyzable substances easily diffuse across the dialysis membrane and have the following characteristics: (a) a molecular weight less than 500 daltons and preferably less than 350; (b) a volume of distribution less than 1 L/kg; (c) protein binding less than 50%; (d) high water solubility (low lipid solubility); and (e) high plasma concentration and a toxicity that correlates reasonably with the plasma concentration. Considerations for hemodialysis and hemoperfusion are cases of serious ingestions (the nephrologist should be notified immediately), and cases involving a compound that is ingested in a potentially lethal dose and the rapid removal of which may improve the prognosis. Examples of the latter are ethylene glycol 1.4 mL/kg 100% solution or equivalent and methanol 6 mL/kg 100% solution or equivalent. Common dialyzable substances include alcohol, bromides, lithium, and salicylates.

The patient-related criteria for dialysis are (a) anticipated prolonged coma and the likelihood of complications; (b) renal compromise (toxin excreted or metabolized by kidneys and dialyzable chelating agents in heavy metal poisoning); (c) laboratory confirmation of lethal blood concentration; (d) lethal dose poisoning with an agent with delayed toxicity or known to be metabolized into a more toxic metabolite (e.g., ethylene glycol, methanol); and (e) hepatic impairment when the agent is metabolized by the liver, and clinical deterioration despite optimal supportive medical management. Table 6 gives plasma concentrations above which removal by extracorporeal measures should be considered.

The contraindications to hemodialysis include the following: (a) substances are not dialyzable; (b) effective antidotes are available; (c) patient is hemodynamically unstable (e.g., shock); and (d) presence of coagulopathy because heparinization is required.

Hemodialysis also has a role in correcting disturbances that are not amenable to appropriate medical management. These are easily remembered by the "vowel" mnemonic:

A—refractory acid–base disturbances
E—refractory electrolyte disturbances
I—intoxication with dialyzable substances (e.g., ethanol, ethylene glycol, isopropyl alcohol, methanol, lithium, and salicylates)
O—overhydration
U—uremia

Complications of dialysis include hemorrhage, thrombosis, air embolism, hypotension, infections, electrolyte imbalance, thrombocytopenia, and removal of therapeutic medications.

### HEMOPERFUSION

Hemoperfusion is the parenteral form of oral activated charcoal. Heparinization is necessary. The patient's blood is routed extracorporeally through an outflow arterial catheter through a filter-adsorbing cartridge (charcoal or resin) and returned through a venous catheter. Cartridges must be changed every 4 hours. The blood glucose, electrolytes, calcium, and albumin levels; complete blood cell count; platelets; and serum and urine osmolarity must be carefully monitored. This procedure has extended extracorporeal removal to a large range of substances that were formerly either poorly dialyzable or nondialyzable. It is not limited by molecular weight, water solubility, or protein binding, but it is limited by a volume distribution greater than 400 L, plasma concentration, and rate of flow through the filter. Activated charcoal cartridges are the primary type of hemoperfusion that is currently available in the United States.

The patient-related criteria for hemoperfusion are (a) anticipated prolonged coma and the likelihood of complications; (b) laboratory confirmation of lethal blood concentrations; (c) hepatic impairment when an agent is metabolized by the liver; and (d) clinical deterioration despite optimally supportive medical management.

The contraindications are similar to those for hemodialysis.

Limited data are available as to which toxins are best treated with hemoperfusion. Hemoperfusion has proved useful in treating glutethimide intoxication, phenobarbital overdose, and carbamazepine, phenytoin, and theophylline intoxication.

Complications include hemorrhage, thrombocytopenia, hypotension, infection, leukopenia, depressed phagocytic activity of granulocytes, decreased immunoglobulin levels, hypoglycemia, hypothermia, hypocalcemia, pulmonary edema, and air and charcoal embolism.

### HEMOFILTRATION

Continuous arteriovenous or venovenous hemodiafiltration (CAVHD or CVVHD, respectively) has been suggested as an alternative to conventional hemodialysis when the need for rapid removal of the drug is less urgent. These procedures, like peritoneal dialysis, are minimally invasive, have no significant impact on hemodynamics, and can be carried out continuously for many hours. Their role in the management of acute poisoning remains uncertain, however.

### PLASMAPHERESIS

Plasmapheresis consists of removal of a volume of blood. All the extracted components are returned to the blood except the plasma, which is replaced with a colloid protein solution. There are limited clinical data on guidelines and efficacy in toxicology. Centrifugal and membrane separators of cellular elements are used. It can be as effective as hemodialysis or hemoperfusion for removing toxins that have high protein binding, and it may be useful for toxins not filtered by hemodialysis and hemoperfusion.

Plasmapheresis has been anecdotally used in treating intoxications with the following agents: paraquat (removed 10%), propranolol (removed 30%), quinine (removed 10%), L-thyroxine (removed 30%), and salicylate (removed 10%). It has been shown to remove less than 10% of digoxin, phenobarbital, prednisolone, and tobramycin. Complications include infection; allergic reactions including anaphylaxis; hemorrhagic disorders; thrombocytopenia; embolus and thrombus; hypervolemia and hypovolemia; dysrhythmias; syncope; tetany; paresthesia; pneumothorax; acute respiratory distress syndrome; and seizures.

*Text continued on page 1160.*

**TABLE 5**  Initial Doses of Antidotes for Common Poisonings

| Antidote | Use | Dose | Route | Adverse Reactions/Comments |
|---|---|---|---|---|
| **N-Acetyl Cysteine (NAC, Mucomyst):** Stock level to treat 70 kg adult for 24 h: 25 vials, 20%, 30 mL | Acetaminophen, carbon tetrachloride (experimental) | 140/mg/kg loading, followed by 70 mg/kg every 4 h for 17 doses. | PO | Nausea, vomiting. Dilute to 5% with sweet juice or flat cola. |
| | | 150 mg/kg in 200 mL of D₅W over 1 hr, then 50 mg/kg in 500 mL of D₅W over 4 hr, then 100 mg/kg in 1 liter D₅W over 16 hrs | IV | Useful for those who cannot tolerate oral route |
| **Atropine:** Stock level to treat 70 kg adult for 24 h: 1 g (1 mg/mL in 1, 10 mL) | Organophosphate and carbamate pesticides: bradydysrhythmics, β-adrenergics, calcium channel blockers/nerve agents | *Child:* 0.02-0.05 mg/kg repeated q5-10 min to max of 2 mg as necessary until cessation of secretions *Adult:* 1-2 mg q5-10 min as necessary. Dilute in 1-2 mL of 0.9% saline for ET instillation. *IV infusion dose:* Place 8 mg of atropine in 100 mL D₅W or saline. Conc. = 0.08 mg/mL; dose range = 0.02-0.08 mg/kg/h or 0.25-1 mL/kg/h. Severe poisoning may require supplemental doses of IV atropine intermittently in doses of 1-5 mg until drying of secretions occurs. | IV/ET | Tachycardia, dry mouth, blurred vision, and urinary retention. Ensure adequate ventilation before administration. |
| **Calcium Chloride (10%):** Stock level to treat 70 kg adult for 24 h: 10 vials 1 g (1.35 mEq/mL) | Hypocalcemia, fluoride, calcium channel blockers, β-blockers, oxalates, ethylene glycol, hypermagnesemia | 0.1-0.2 mL/kg (10-20 mg/kg) slow push every 10 min up to max 10 mL (1 g). Since calcium response lasts 15 minutes, some may require continuous infusion 0.2 mL/kg/h up to maximum of 10 mL/h while monitoring for dysrhythmias and hypotension. | IV | Administer slowly with BP and ECG monitoring and have magnesium available to reverse calcium effects. Tissue irritation, hypotension, dysrhythmias from rapid injection. Contraindications: digitalis glycoside intoxication. |
| **Calcium Gluconate (10%):** Stock level to treat 70 kg adult for 24 h: 20 vials 1 g (0.45 mEq/mL) | Hypocalcemia, fluoride, calcium channel blockers, hydrofluoric acid; black widow envenomation | 0.3-0.4 mL/kg (30-40 mg/kg) slow push; repeat as needed up to max dose 10-20 mL (1-2 g). | IV | Same comments as calcium chloride. |
| **Infiltration of Calcium Gluconate** | Hydrofluoric acid skin exposure | Dose: Infiltrate each square cm of affected dermis/subcutaneous tissue with about 0.5 mL of 10% calcium gluconate using a 30-gauge needle. Repeat as needed to control pain. | Infiltrate | |

| | | Route | Dose | Comments |
|---|---|---|---|---|
| **Intra-arterial Calcium Gluconate** | Hydrofluoric acid skin exposure | | Infuse 20 mL of 10% calcium gluconate (not chloride) diluted in 250 mL D₅W via the radial or brachial artery proximal to the injury over 3-4 hours. | Alternatively, dilute 10 mL of 10% calcium gluconate with 40-50 mL of D₅W. |
| **Calcium Gluconate Gel:** Stock level: 3.5 g | Hydrofluoric acid skin exposure | Dermal | 2.5 g USP powder added to 100 mL water-soluble lubricating jelly, e.g., K-Y Jelly or Lubifax (or 3.5 mg into 150 mL). Some use 6 g of calcium carbonate in 100 g of lubricant. Place injured hand in surgical glove filled with gel. Apply q4h. If pain persists, calcium gluconate injection may be needed (above). | Powder is available from Spectrum Pharmaceutical Co. in California: 800-772-8786. Commercial preparation of Ca gluconate gel is available from Pharmascience in Montreal, Quebec: 514-340-1114. |
| **Cyanide Antidote Kit:** Stock level to treat 70 kg adult for 24 h: 2 Lilly Cyanide Antidote kits | Cyanide<br>Hydrogen sulfide (nitrites are given only)<br>Do not use sodium thiosulfate for hydrogen sulfide<br>Individual portions of the kit can be used in certain circumstances (consult PCC) | Inhalation | Amyl nitrite: 1 crushable ampule for 30 secs of every min. Use new amp q3min. May omit step if venous access is established. | If methemoglobinemia occurs, do not use methylene blue to correct this because it releases cyanide. |
| | Cyanide<br>Hydrogen sulfide (nitrites are given only)<br>Do not use sodium thiosulfate for hydrogen sulfide<br>Individual portions of the kit can be used in certain circumstances (consult PCC) | IV | Sodium nitrite: *Child:* 0.33 mL/kg of 3% solution if hemoglobin level is not known, otherwise based on tables with product. *Adult:* up to 300 mg (10 mL). Dilute nitrite in 100 mL 0.9% saline, administer slowly at 5 mL/min. Slow infusion if fall in BP. | If methemoglobinemia occurs, do not use methylene blue to correct this because it releases cyanide. |
| | Do not use sodium thiosulfate for hydrogen sulfide<br>Individual portions of the Kit can be used in certain circumstances (consult PCC) | IV | Sodium thiosulfate: *Child:* 1.6 mL/kg of 25% solution, may be repeated every 30-60 min to a maximum of 12.5 g or 50 mL in adult. Administer over 20 min. | Nausea, dizziness, headache. Tachycardia, muscle rigidity, and bronchospasm (rapid administration). |
| **Dantrolene Sodium (Dantrium):** Stock level to treat 70 kg adult for 24 h: 700 mg, 35 vials (20 mg/vial) | Malignant hyperthermia | IV/PO | 2-3 mg/kg IV rapidly. Repeat loading dose every 10 minutes, if necessary up to a maximum total dose of 10 mg/kg. When temperature and heart rate decrease, slow the infusion | Hepatotoxicity occurs with cumulative dose of 10 mg/kg. Thrombophlebitis (best given in central line). Available as 20 mg lyophilized dantrolene powder for |

*Continued*

**TABLE 5** Initial Doses of Antidotes for Common Poisonings—cont'd

| Antidote | Use | Dose | Route | Adverse Reactions/Comments |
|---|---|---|---|---|
| | | 1-2 mg/kg every 6 hours for 24-28 h until all evidence of malignant hyperthermia syndrome has subsided. Follow with oral doses 1-2 mg/kg four times a day for 24 h as necessary. | | reconstruction, which contains 3 g mannitol and sodium hydroxide in 70-mL vial. Mix with 60 mL sterile distilled water without a bacteriostatic agent and protect from light. Use within 6 hours after reconstituting. |
| **Deferoxamine (Desferal):** Stock level to treat 70 kg adult for 24 h: 17 vials (500 mg/ampl). | Iron | IV infusion of 15 mg/kg/h (3 mL/kg/h: 500 mg in 100 mL D₅W) max 6 g/d Rates of >45 μg/kg/h if conc >1000 μg/dL. | Preferred IV: avoid therapy >24 h | Hypotension (minimized by avoiding rapid infusion rates) DFO challenge test 50 mg/kg is unreliable if negative. |
| **Diazepam (Valium):** Stock level to treat 70 kg adult for 24 h: 200 mg, 5 mg/mL; 2,10 mL | Any intoxication that provokes seizures when specific therapy is not available, e.g., amphetamines, PCP, barbiturate and alcohol withdrawal. Chloroquine poisoning. | Adult, 5-10 mg IV (max 20 mg) at a rate of 5 mg/min until seizure is controlled. May be repeated 2 or 3 times. Child, 0.1-0.3 mg/kg up to 10 mg IV slowly over 2 min. | IV | Confusion, somnolence, coma, hypotension. Intramuscular absorption is erratic Establish airway and administer 100% oxygen and glucose. |
| **Digoxin-Specific Fab Antibodies (Digibind):** Stock level to treat 70 kg adult for 24 h: 20 vials. | Digoxin, digitoxin, oleander tea with the following: (1) Imminent cardiac arrest or shock, (2) hyperkalemia >5.0 mEq/L. (3) serum digoxin >5 ng/mL (child) at 8-12 h post ingestion in adults, (4) digitalis delirium, (5) ingestion over 10 mg in adults or 4 mg in child, (6) bradycardia or second- or third-degree heart block unresponsive to atropine, (7) life threatening digitoxin or oleander posioning. | (1) If amount ingested is known total dose × bioavailability (0.8) = body burden. The body burden + 0.6 (0.5 mg of digoxin is bound by 1 vial of 38 mg of FAB) = # vials needed. (2) If amount is unknown but the steady state serum concentration is known in ng/mL: Digoxin: ng/mL: (5.6 L/kg Vd) × (wt kg) = μg body burden. Body burden + 100 = mg body burden/0.5 = # vials needed. Digitoxin body burden = ng/mL × (0.56 L/kg Vd) × (wt kg) Body burden + 1000 = mg body burden/0.5 = # vials needed. (3) If the amount is not known, it is administered in life-threatening situations as 10 vials (400 mg) IV in saline over 30 min in adults. If cardiac arrest is imminent, administer 20 vials (adult) as a bolus. | IV | Allergic reactions (rare), return of condition being treated with digitalis glycoside. Administer by infusion over 30 min through a 0.22-μ filter. If cardiac arrest is imminent, may administer by bolus. Consult PCC for more details. |

**Dimercaprol (BAL in Peanut Oil):**
Stock level to treat 70 kg adult for 24 h: 1200 mg (4 amps—100 mg/mL 10% in oil in 3 mL amp)

Chelating agent for arsenic, mercury, and lead.

3-5 mg/kg q4th usually for 5-10 d

Deep IM

Local infection site pain and sterile abscess, nausea, vomiting, fever, salivation, hypertension, and nephrotoxicity (alkalinize urine).

**2,3 Dimercaptosuccinic Acid (DMSA Succimer):**
100 mg/capsule: 20 capsules

Used as a chelating agent for lead, especially blood lead levels >45 µg/dL. May also be used for symptomatic mercury exposure

10 mg/kg 3 × daily for 5 days followed by 10 mg/kg 2 × daily for 14 days.

PO

Precautions: monitor AST/ALT; use with caution in G6PD-deficient patients. Avoid concurrent iron therapy. Relatively safe antidote, rarely severe, uncommon minor skin rashes may occur.

**Diphenhydramine (Benadryl):**
Antiparkinsonian action. Stock level to treat a 70 kg adult for 24 h: 5 vials (10 mg/mL, 10 mL each)

Used to treat extrapyramidal symptoms and dystonia induced by phenothiazines, phencyclidine, and related drugs.

*Children:* 1-2 mg/kg IV slowly over 5 minutes up to maximum 50 mg followed by 5 mg/kg/24 h orally divided every 6 hours up to 300 mg/24h
*Adults:* 50 mg IV followed by 50 mg orally four times daily for 5-7 days
Note: Symptoms abate within 2-5 min after IV.

IV

Fatal dose: 20-40 mg/kg. Dry mouth, drowsiness.

**Ethanol (Ethyl Alcohol):**
Stock level to treat 70 kg adult for 24 h: 3 bottles 10% (1 L each)

Methanol, ethylene glycol

10 mL/kg loading dose concurrently with 1.4 mL/kg (average) infusion of 10% ethanol (consult PCC for more details)

IV

Nausea, vomiting, sedation. Use 0.22 µm filter if preparing from bulk 100% ethanol.

**Flumazenil (Romazicon):**
Stock level to treat 70 kg adult for 24 h: 4 vials (0.1 mg/mL, 10 mL)

Benzodiazepines (may also be beneficial in the treatment of hepatic encephalopathy)

Administer 0.2 mg (2 mL) IV over 30 sec (pediatric dose not established, 0.01 mg/kg), then wait 3 min for a response, then if desired consciousness is not achieved, administer 0.3 mg (3 mL) over 30 sec, then wait 3 min for response, then if desired consciousness is not achieved, administer 0.5 mg (5 mL) over 30 sec at 60-sec intervals up to a maximum cumulative dose of 3 mg (30 mL) (1 mg in children). Because effects last only 1-5 hours, if patient responds monitor carefully over next 6 hours for resedation. If multiple repeated doses, consider a continuous infusion of 0.2-1 mg/h.

IV

Nausea, vomiting, facial flushing, agitation, headache, dizziness, seizures, and death. It is not recommended to improve ventilation. Its role in CNS depression needs to be clarified. It should not be used routinely in comatose patients. It is **contraindicated** in cyclic antidepressant intoxications, stimulant overdose, long-term benzodiazepine use (may precipitate life-threatening withdrawal), if benzodiazepines are used to control seizures, in head trauma.

*Continued*

**TABLE 5** Initial Doses of Antidotes for Common Poisonings—cont'd

| Antidote | Use | Dose | Route | Adverse Reactions/Comments |
|---|---|---|---|---|
| **Folic Acid (Folvite):** Stock level to treat 70 kg adult for 24 h: 4 100-mg vials | Methanol/ethylene glycol (investigational) | 1 mg/kg up to 50 mg q4h for 6 doses. | IV | Uncommon |
| **Fomepizole (4-MP, Antizol):** Stock level to treat 70 kg adult: 4 1.5-mL vials (1 g/mL) | Ethylene glycol Methanol | Loading dose: 15 mg/kg (0.015 mL/kg) IV followed by maintenance dose of 10 mg/kg (0.01 mL/kg) every 12h for 4 doses, then 15 mg/kg every 12h until ethylene glycol levels are <20 mg/dL. Fomipazole can be given to patients undergoing hemodialysis (dose q4h). | IV | Suggested: co-administer folate 50 mg IV (child 1 mg/kg), thiamine 100 mg/d (child 50 mg), and pyridoxine 50 mg IV/IM q6h until intoxication is resolved. Monitor for urinary oxalate crystals. Adverse reactions include headache, nausea, and dizziness. Antizole should be diluted in 100 mL 0.9% saline or D5W and mixed well. Antizole should not be given undiluted. |
| **Glucagon:** Stock level to treat 70 kg adult for 24 h: (10 vials, 10 units) | β-Blocker, calcium channel blocker | 3-10 mg in adult, then infuse 2-5 mg/h (0.05-0.1 mg/kg in child, then infuse 0.07 mg/kg/h) Large doses up to 100 mg/24h used | IV | Use D5W, not 0.9% saline, to reconstitute the glucagon (rather than diluent of Eli Lilly, which contains phenol). Vomiting precautions. |
| **Magnesium Sulfate:** Stock level to treat 70 kg adult for 24 h: approx 25 g (50 mL of 50% or 200 mL of 12.5%) | Torsades de pointes | Adult: 2 g (20 mL or 20%) over 20 min. If no response in 10 min, repeat and follow by continuous infusion 1 g/h. Children: 25-50 mg/kg initially and maintenance is (30-60 mg/kg/24h) (0.25-0.5 mEq/kg/24h) up to 1000 mg/24h. (Dose not studied in controlled fashion.) | IV | Use with caution if renal impairment is present. |
| **Methylene Blue:** Stock level to treat 70 kg adult for 24 h: 5 amps (10 mg/10 mL) | Methemoglobinemia | 0.1-0.2 mL/kg of 1% solution, slow infusion, may be repeated every 30-60 min | IV | Nausea, vomiting, headache, dizziness. |
| **Naloxone (Narcan):** Stock level to treat 70 kg adult for 24 h: 3 vials (1 mg/mL, 10 mL) | Comatose patient; decreased respirations <12; opioids | In postoperative opioid depression reversal, IV 0.1-0.5 µg/kg every 2 min as needed and may repeat up to a total dose of 1 µg/kg In **suspected overdose**, administer IV 0.1 mg/kg in a child younger than 5 years of age up to 2 mg, in older children and adults administer 2 mg every 2 min up to a total of 10-20 mg. Can also be administered into the | IV, ET | **Larger doses** of naloxone may be required for more poorly antagonized synthetic opioid drugs: buprenorphine (Buprenex), codeine, dextromethorphan, fentanyl, pentazocine (Talwin), propoxyphene (Darvon), diphenoxylate, nalbuphine (Nubain), new potent "designer" drugs, or long-acting opioids such as methadone (Dolophine). **Complications.** Although naloxone is safe and effective, there are rare reports of |

endotracheal tube. If no response by 10 mg, a pure opioid intoxication is unlikely.

**If opioid abuse** is suspected, **restraints** should be in place before administration; **initial dose** 0.1 mg to avoid withdrawal and violent behavior. The initial dose is then doubled every minute progressively to a total of 10 mg.

**A continuous infusion** has been advocated because many opioids outlast the short half-life of naloxone (30-60 min). The **naloxone infusion hourly rate** to produce a response is equal to the effective dose required (improvement in ventilation and arousal). An additional dose may be required in 15-30 min as a bolus.

complications (<1%) of pulmonary edema, seizures, hypertension, cardiac arrest, and sudden death.

The infusions are titrated to avoid respiratory depression and opioid withdrawal manifestations.

Tapering of infusions can be attempted after 12h and when the patient's condition is stable.

---

**Physostigmine (Antilirium):** Stock level to treat 70 kg adult for 24 h: 2-4 mg (2 mL each)

Anticholinergic agents (not routinely used, only indicated if life-threatening complications).

*Child:* 0.02 mg/kg slow push to max 2 mg q30-60 min; *Adult:* 1-2 mg q5 min to max 6 mg.

IV

Bradycardia, asystole, seizures, bronchospasm, vomiting, headaches. Do not use for cyclic antidepressants.

---

**Pralidoxime (2PAM, Protopan):** Stock level to treat 70 kg adult for 24 h: 12 vials (1 g per 20 mL)

Organophosphates/nerve agents

Child ≤12 y, 25-50 mg/kg max (4 mg/min); >12 y, 1-2 g/dose in 250 mL of 0.9% saline over 5-10 min. Max 200 mg/min. Repeat q6-12h for 24-48h. Max adult 6 g/d.
Alternative: Maintenance infusion 1 g in 100 mL, of 0.9% saline at 5-20 mg/kg/h (0.5-12 mL/kg/h) up to max 500 mg/h or 50 mL/h. Titrate to desired response. End point is absence of fasciculations and return of muscle strength.

IV

Nausea, dizziness, headache; tachycardia, muscle rigidity, bronchospasm (rapid administration).

---

**Pyridoxine (Vitamin B₆):** Stock level to treat 70 kg adult for 24 h: 100 mg/mL 10% solution. For a 70 kg patient, 10 g = 10 vials

Seizures from isoniazid or *Gyromitra* mushrooms; ethylene glycol

*Isoniazid: Unknown amt ingested:* 5 g (70 mg/kg) in 50 mL D₅W over 5 min + diazepam 0.3 mg/kg IV at rate of 1 mg/min in child or 10 mg dose at rate up to 5 mg/min in adults. Use different site (synergism). May repeat q5-20 min until seizure controlled.

IV

After seizure is controlled, administer remainder of pyridoxine 1 g/1 g isoniazid total 5 g as infusion over 60 min. Adverse reactions uncommon; do not administer in same bottle as sodium bicarbonate. For *Gyromitra* mushrooms, some use PO 25 mg/kg/d early when mushroom ingestion is suspected.

*Continued*

**TABLE 5** Initial Doses of Antidotes for Common Poisonings—cont'd

| Antidote | Use | Dose | Route | Adverse Reactions/Comments |
|---|---|---|---|---|
| | | Up to 375 mg/kg have been given (52 g). *Known amount:* 1 g for each gram isoniazid ingested over 5 min with diazepam (dose above) *Gyromitra mushroom:* Child 25 mg/kg or 2-5 g, adults IV over 15-30 min to max 20 g. | | |
| **Sodium Bicarbonate (NaHCO₃):** Stock level to treat 70 kg adult for 24 h: 10 ampules or syringes (500 mEq) | Tricyclic antidepressant cardiotoxicity (QRS >0.12 sec; ventricular tachycardia, severe conduction disturbances); metabolic acidosis; phenothiazine toxicity *Salicylate:* to keep blood pH 7.5-7.55 (not >7.55) and urine pH 7.5-8.0. Alkalinization recommended if salicylate conc. >40 mg/dL in acute poisoning and at lower levels if symptomatic in chronic intoxication. 2 mEq/kg will raise blood pH 0.1 unit | *Ethylene glycol:* 100 mg IV daily, 1-2 mEq/kg undiluted as a bolus. If no effect on cardiotoxicity, repeat twice a few minutes apart<br><br>*Adult* with clear physical signs and laboratory findings of acute moderate or severe salicylism: Bolus 1-2 mEq/kg followed by infusion of 100-150 mEq NaHCO₃ added to 1 L of 5% dextrose at rate of 200-300 mL/h *Child:* Bolus same as adult followed by 1-2 mEq/kg in infusion of 20 mL/kg/h 5% dextrose in 0.45% saline. Add potassium when patient voids. Rate and amount of the initial infusion, if patient is volume depleted: 1 h to achieve urine output of 2 mL/kg/h and urine pH 7-8. | IV | Monitor sodium, potassium, and blood pH because fatal alkalemia and hyponatremia have been reported.<br><br>Monitor both urine and blood pH. Do not use the urine pH alone to assess the need for alkalinization because of the paradoxical aciduria that may occur. Adjust the urine pH to 7.5-8 by NaHCO₃ infusion. After urine output established, add potassium 40 mEq/L. |

In mild cases without acidosis and urine pH >6 administer 5% dextrose in 0.9% saline with 50 mEq/L or 1 mEq/kg NaHCO₃ as maintenance to replace ongoing renal losses. If acidemia is present and pH <7.2, add 2 mEq/kg as loading dose followed by 2 mEq/kg q3 to 4h to keep pH at 7.5-7.55. If acidemia is present, recommend isotonic NaHCO₃, 3 ampules to 1 L of D₅W @ 10-15 mL/kg/h or sufficient to produce normal urine flow and a urine pH of 7.5 or higher.

*Long-acting barbiturates:* Phenobarbital and primidone (Mysoline) Note: Alkalinization is ineffective for the short- or intermediate-acting barbiturates

NaHCO₃: 2 mEq/kg during the first hour or 100 mEq in 1 L of D₅W with 40 mEq/L potassium at rate of 100 mL/h in adults. Adequate potassium is necessary to accomplish alkalinization

**Thiamine:**
100 mg/mL, 2 vials

Thiamine deficiency, ethylene glycol poisoning, alcoholism

IV/IM

100 mg IV followed with 100 mg V/IM for 5-7 days in an alcoholic and followed by 100 mg/d orally.

IV — Additional sodium bicarbonate and potassium chloride may be needed. Adjust the urine pH to 7.5-8 by NaHCO₃ infusion.

**Vitamin K₁ (Aqua Mephyton):**
10 mg/1-5 mL; 5 mg tablets

Warfarin anticoagulant or rodenticide toxicity

PO/SC, IV

Oral 0.4 mg/kg/dose child, 10-25 mg adults. If evidence of bleeding administer vitamin K₁ SC, IV 0.6 mg/kg/dose child and up to 25-50 mg adults for 6 hours depending on severity.

Give vitamin K daily until PT/INR are normal. Examine stools and urine for evidence of bleeding.

*Abbreviations:* ALT = alanine aminotransferase; amp = ampule; AST = aspartate aminotransferase; BAL = British anti-Lewisite; BP = blood pressure; Conc. = concentration; ECG = electrocardiogram; ET = endotracheal; G6PD = glucose-6-phosphate dehydrogenase; IM = intramuscular; IV = intravenous; PCC = poison control center; PO = oral; PT = prothrombin time; SC = subcutaneous.

**TABLE 6  Plasma Concentrations Above Which Removal by Extracorporeal Measures Should Be Considered**

| Drug | Plasma Concentration | Protein Binding (%) | Volume Distribution (L/kg) | Method of Choice |
|---|---|---|---|---|
| Amanitin | NA | 25 | 1.0 | HP |
| Ethanol | 500-700 mg/dL | 0 | 0.3 | HD |
| Ethchlorvynol | 150 μg/mL | 35-50 | 3-4 | HP |
| Ethylene glycol | 25-50 μg/mL | 0 | 0.6 | HD |
| Glutethimide | 100 μg/mL | 50 | 2.7 | HP |
| Isopropyl alcohol | 400 mg/dL | 0 | 0.7 | HD |
| Lithium | 4 mEq/L | 0 | 0.7 | HD |
| Meprobamate (Equanil) | 100 μg/mL | 0 | NA | HP |
| Methanol | 50 mg/dL | 0 | 0.7 | HD |
| Methaqualone | 40 μg/dL | 20-60 | 6.0 | HP |
| Other barbiturates | 50 μg/dL | 50 | 0-1 | HP |
| Paraquat | 0.1 mg/dL | poor | 2.8 | HP > HD |
| Phenobarbital | 100 μg/dL | 50 | 0.9 | HP > HD |
| Salicylates | 80-100 mg/dL | 90 | 0.2 | HD > HP |
| Theophylline | | 0 | 0.5 | |
| Chronic | 40-60 μg/mL | | | HP |
| Acute | 80-100 μg/mL | | | HP |
| Trichlorethanol | 250 μg/mL | 70 | 0.6 | HP |

*Abbreviations*: HD = hemodialysis; HP = hemoperfusion; HP > HD hemoperfusion preferred over hemodialysis.
*Note*: Cartridges for charcoal hemoperfusion are not readily available anymore in most locations, so hemodialysis may be substituted in these situations.
  In mixed or chronic drug overdoses, extracorporeal measures may be considered at lower drug concentrations.
Data from Winchester JF: Active methods for detoxification. In Haddad LM, Winchester JF (eds). Clinical Management of Poisoning and Drug Overdose, 2nd ed. Philadelphia, WB Saunders, 1990; Balsam L, Cortitsidis GN, Fienfeld DA: Role of hemodialysis and hemoperfusion in the treatment of intoxications. Contemp Manage Crit Care 1:61, 1991.

# Supportive Care, Observation, and Therapy for Complications

## ALTERED MENTAL STATUS

If airway protective reflexes are absent, endotracheal intubation is indicated for a comatose patient or a patient with altered mental status. If respirations are ineffective, ventilation should be instituted, and if hypoxemia persists, supplemental oxygen is indicated. If a cyanotic patient fails to respond to oxygen, the practitioner should consider methemoglobinemia.

## HYPOGLYCEMIA

Hypoglycemia accompanies many poisonings, including with ethanol (especially in children), clonidine (Catapres), insulin, organophosphates, salicylates, sulfonylureas, and the unripe fruit or seed of a Jamaican plant called ackee. If hypoglycemia is present or suspected, glucose should be administered immediately as an intravenous bolus. Doses are as follows: in a neonate, 10% glucose (5 mL/kg); in a child, 25% glucose 0.25 g/kg (2 mL/kg); and in an adult, 50% glucose 0.5 g/kg (1 mL/kg).

A bedside capillary test for blood glucose is performed to detect hypoglycemia, and the sample is sent to the laboratory for confirmation. If the glucose reagent strip visually reads less than 150 mg/dL, one administers glucose. Venous blood should be used rather than capillary blood for the bedside test if the patient is in shock or is hypotensive. Large amounts of glucose given rapidly to nondiabetic patients may cause a transient reactive hypoglycemia and hyperkalemia and may accentuate damage in ischemic cerebrovascular and cardiac tissue. If focal neurologic signs are present, it may be prudent to withhold glucose, because hypoglycemia causes focal signs in less than 10% of cases.

## THIAMINE DEFICIENCY ENCEPHALOPATHY

Thiamine is administered to avoid precipitating thiamine deficiency encephalopathy (Wernicke-Korsakoff syndrome) in alcohol abusers and in malnourished patients. The overall incidence of thiamine deficiency in ethanol abusers is 12%. Thiamine 100 mg intravenously should be administered around the time of the glucose administration but not necessarily before the glucose. The clinician should be prepared to manage the anaphylaxis that sometimes is caused by thiamine, although it is extremely rare.

## OPIOID REACTIONS

Naloxone (Narcan) reverses CNS and respiratory depression, miosis, bradycardia, and decreased gastrointestinal peristalsis caused by opioids acting through μ, κ, and δ receptors. It also affects endogenous opioid peptides (endorphins and enkephalins), which accounts for the variable responses reported in patients with intoxications from ethanol, benzodiazepines, clonidine (Catapres), captopril (Capoten), and valproic acid (Depakote) and in patients with spinal cord injuries. There is a high sensitivity for predicting a response if pinpoint pupils and circumstantial evidence of opioid abuse (e.g., track marks) are present.

In cases of suspected overdose, naloxone 0.1 mg/kg is administered intravenously initially in a child younger than 5 years of age. The dose can be repeated in 2 minutes, if necessary up to a total dose of 2 mg. In older children and adults, the dose is 2 mg every 2 minutes for five doses up to a total of 10 mg. Naloxone can also be administered into an endotracheal tube if intravenous access is unavailable. If there is no response after 10 mg, a pure opioid intoxication is unlikely. If opioid abuse is suspected, restraints should be in place before the administration of naloxone, and it is recommended that the initial dose be 0.1 to 0.2 mg to avoid withdrawal and violent behavior. The initial dose is then doubled every minute progressively to a total of 10 mg. Naloxone may unmask concomitant sympathomimetic intoxication as well as withdrawal.

Larger doses of naloxone may be required for more poorly antagonized synthetic opioid drugs: buprenorphine (Buprenex), codeine, dextromethorphan, fentanyl and its derivatives, pentazocine (Talwin), propoxyphene (Darvon), diphenoxylate, nalbuphine (Nubain), and long-acting opioids such as methadone (Dolophine).

Indications for a continuous infusion include a second dose for recurrent respiratory depression, exposure to poorly antagonized opioids, a large overdose, and decreased opioid metabolism, as with impaired liver function. A continuous infusion has been advocated because many opioids outlast the short half-life of naloxone (30 to 60 minutes). The hourly rate of naloxone infusion is equal to the effective dose required to produce a response (improvement in ventilation and arousal). An additional dose may be required in 15 to 30 minutes as a bolus. The infusions are titrated to avoid respiratory depression and opioid withdrawal manifestations. Tapering of infusions can be attempted after 12 hours and when the patient's condition has been stabilized.

Although naloxone is safe and effective, there are rare reports of complications (less than 1%) of pulmonary edema, seizures, hypertension, cardiac arrest, and sudden death.

## AGENTS WHOSE ROLES ARE NOT CLARIFIED

Nalmefene (Revex), a long-acting parenteral opioid antagonist that the Food and Drug Administration has approved, is undergoing investigation, but its role in the treatment of comatose patients and patients with opioid overdose is not clear. It is 16 times more potent than naloxone, and its duration of action is up to 8 hours (half-life 10.8 hours, versus naloxone 1 hour).

Flumazenil (Romazicon) is a pure competitive benzodiazepine antagonist. It has been demonstrated to be safe and effective for reversing benzodiazepine-induced sedation. It is not recommended to improve ventilation. Its role in cases of CNS depression needs to be clarified. It should not be used routinely in comatose patients and is not an essential ingredient of the coma therapeutic regimen. It is contraindicated in cases of co-ingestion of cyclic antidepressant intoxication, stimulant overdose, and long-term benzodiazepine use (may precipitate life-threatening withdrawal) if benzodiazepines are used to control seizures. There is a concern about the potential for seizures and cardiac dysrhythmias that may occur in these settings.

# Laboratory and Radiographic Studies

An electrocardiogram (ECG) should be obtained to identify dysrhythmias or conduction delays from cardiotoxic medications. If aspiration pneumonia (history of loss of consciousness, unarousable state, vomiting) or noncardiac pulmonary edema is suspected, a chest radiograph is needed. Electrolyte and glucose concentrations in the blood, the anion gap, acid–base balance, the arterial blood gas (ABG) profile (if patient has respiratory distress or altered mental status), and serum osmolality should be measured if a toxic alcohol ingestion is suspected. Table 7 lists appropriate testing on the basis of clinical toxicologic presentation. All laboratory specimens should be carefully labeled, including time and date. For potential legal cases, a "chain of custody" must be established. Assessment of the laboratory studies may provide a clue to the etiologic agent.

## ELECTROLYTE, ACID-BASE, AND OSMOLALITY DISTURBANCES

Electrolyte and acid–base disturbances should be evaluated and corrected. Metabolic acidosis (usually low or normal pH with a low or normal/high $PaCO_2$ and low $HCO_3$) with an increased anion gap is seen with many agents in cases of overdose.

The anion gap is an estimate of those anions other than chloride and $HCO_3$ necessary to counterbalance the positive charge of sodium. It serves as a clue to causes, compensations, and complications. The anion gap (AG) is calculated from the standard serum electrolytes by subtracting the total $CO_2$ (which reflects the actual measured bicarbonate) and chloride from the sodium: $(Na - [Cl + HCO_3]) = AG$. The potassium is usually not used in the calculation because it may be hemolyzed and is an intracellular cation. The lack of anion gap does not exclude a toxic etiology.

The normal gap is usually 7 to 11 mEq/L by flame photometer. However, there has been a "lowering" of the normal anion gap to $7 \pm 4$ mEq/L by the newer techniques (e.g., ion selective electrodes or

**TABLE 7 Patient Condition/Systemic Toxin and Appropriate Tests**

| Condition | Tests |
| --- | --- |
| Comatose | Toxicologic tests (acetaminophen, sedative-hypnotic, ethanol, opioids, benzodiazepine), glucose. |
| Respiratory toxicity | Spirometry, $FEV_1$, arterial blood gases, chest radiograph, monitor $O_2$ saturation |
| Cardiac toxicity | ECG 12-lead and monitoring, echocardiogram, serial cardiac enzymes (if evidence or suspicion of a myocardial infarction), hemodynamic monitoring |
| Hepatic toxicity | Enzymes (AST, ALT, GGT), ammonia, albumin, bilirubin, glucose, PT, PTT, amylase |
| Nephrotoxicity | BUN, creatinine, electrolytes (Na, F, Mg, Ca, $PO_4$), serum and urine osmolarity, 24-hour urine for heavy metals if suspected, creatine kinase, serum and urine myoglobin, urinalysis and urinary sodium |
| Bleeding | Platelets, PT, PTT, bleeding time, fibrin split products, fibrinogen, type and match |

*Abbreviations*: ALT = alanine aminotransaminase; AST = aspartate aminotransaminase; BUN = blood urea nitrogen; ECG = electrocardiogram; $FEV_1$ = forced expiratory volume at 1 second; GGT = γ-glutamyltransferase; PT = prothrombin time; PTT = partial thromboplastin time.

colorimetric titration). Some studies have found anion gaps to be relatively insensitive for determining the presence of toxins.

It is important to recognize anion gap toxins, such as salicylates, methanol, and ethylene glycol, because they have specific antidotes, and hemodialysis is effective in management of cases of overdose with these agents.

Table 8 lists the reasons for increased anion gap, decreased anion gap, or no gap. The most common cause of a decreased anion gap is laboratory error. Lactic acidosis produces the largest anion gap and can result from any poisoning that results in hypoxia, hypoglycemia, or convulsions.

Table 9 lists other blood chemistry derangements that suggest certain intoxications.

Serum osmolality is a measure of the number of molecules of solute per kilogram of solvent, or mOsm/kg water. The osmolarity is molecules of solute per liter of solution, or mOsm/L water at a specified temperature. Osmolarity is usually the calculated value and osmolality is usually a measured value. They are considered interchangeable where 1 L equals 1 kg. The normal serum osmolality is 280 to 290 mOsm/kg. The freezing point serum osmolarity measurement specimen and the serum electrolyte specimens for calculation should be drawn simultaneously.

The serum osmolal gap is defined as the difference between the measured osmolality determined by the freezing point method and the calculated osmolarity. It is determined by the following formula:

$$(Sodium \times 2) + (BUN/3) + (Glucose/20)$$

(where BUN is blood urea nitrogen).

This gap estimate is normally within 10 mOsm of the simultaneously measured serum osmolality. Ethanol, if present, may be included in the equation to eliminate its influence on the osmolal gap (the ethanol concentration divided by 4.6; Table 10).

The osmolal gap is not valid in cases of shock and postmortem state. Metabolic disorders such as hyperglycemia, uremia, and dehydration increase the osmolarity but usually do not cause gaps greater than 10 mOsm/kg. A gap greater than 10 mOsm/mL suggests that

## TABLE 8  Etiologies of Metabolic Acidosis

| Normal Anion Gap Hyperchloremic | Increased Anion Gap Normochloremic | Decreased Anion Gap |
|---|---|---|
| Acidifying agents | Methanol | Laboratory error[†] |
| Adrenal insufficiency | Uremia* | Intoxication—bromine, lithium |
| Anhydrase inhibitors | Diabetic ketoacidosis* | Protein abnormal |
| Fistula | Paraldehyde,* phenformin | Sodium low |
| Osteotomies | Isoniazid | |
| Obstructive uropathies | Iron | |
| Renal tubular acidosis | Lactic acidosis[†] | |
| Diarrhea, uncomplicated* | Ethanol,* ethylene glycol* | |
| Dilutional | Salicylates, starvation solvents | |
| Sulfamylon | | |

*Indicates hyperosmolar situation. Studies have found that the anion gap may be relatively insensitive for determining the presence of toxins.
[†]Lactic acidosis can be produced by intoxications of the following: carbon monoxide, cyanide, hydrogen sulfide, hypoxia, ibuprofen, iron, isoniazid, phenformin, salicylates, seizures, theophylline.

unidentified osmolal-acting substances are present: acetone, ethanol, ethylene glycol, glycerin, isopropyl alcohol, isoniazid, ethanol, mannitol, methanol, and trichloroethane. Alcohols and glycols should be sought when the degree of obtundation exceeds that expected from the blood ethanol concentration or when other clinical conditions exist: visual loss (methanol), metabolic acidosis (methanol and ethylene glycol), or renal failure (ethylene glycol).

A falsely elevated osmolar gap can be produced by other low molecular weight un-ionized substances (dextran, diuretics, sorbitol, ketones), hyperlipidemia, and unmeasured electrolytes (e.g., magnesium).

*Note:* A normal osmolal gap may be reported in the presence of toxic alcohol or glycol poisoning, if the parent compound is already metabolized. This situation can occur when the osmolar gap is measured after a significant time has elapsed since the ingestion. In cases of alcohol and glycol intoxication, an early osmolar gap is a result of the relatively nontoxic parent drug and delayed metabolic acidosis, and an anion gap is a result of the more toxic metabolites.

The serum concentration is calculated as mg/dL = mOsm gap × MW of substance divided by 10.

## TABLE 9  Blood Chemistry Derangements in Toxicology

| Derangement | Toxin |
|---|---|
| Acetonemia without acidosis | Acetone or isopropyl alcohol |
| Hypomagnesemia | Ethanol, digitalis |
| Hypocalcemia | Ethylene glycol, oxalate, fluoride |
| Hyperkalemia | β-Blockers, acute digitalis, renal failure |
| Hypokalemia | Diuretics, salicylism, sympathomimetics, theophylline, corticosteroids, chronic digitalis |
| Hyperglycemia | Diazoxide, glucagon, iron, isoniazid, organophosphate insecticides, phenylurea insecticides, phenytoin (Dilantin), salicylates, sympathomimetic agents, thyroid, vasopressors |
| Hypoglycemia | β-Blockers, ethanol, insulin, isoniazid, oral hypoglycemic agents, salicylates |
| Rhabdomyolysis | Amphetamines, ethanol, cocaine, or phencyclidine, elevated creatine phosphokinase |

## RADIOGRAPHIC STUDIES

Chest and neck radiographs are useful for suspected pathologic conditions such as aspiration pneumonia, pulmonary edema, and foreign bodies and to determine the location of the endotracheal tube. Abdominal radiographs can be used to detect radiopaque substances.

The mnemonic for radiopaque substances seen on abdominal radiographs is CHIPES:

C—chlorides and chloral hydrate
H—heavy metals (arsenic, barium, iron, lead, mercury, zinc)
I—iodides
P—PlayDoh, Pepto-Bismol, phenothiazine (inconsistent)
E—enteric-coated tablets
S—sodium, potassium, and other elements in tablet form (bismuth, calcium, potassium) and solvents containing chlorides (e.g., carbon tetrachloride)

## TOXICOLOGIC STUDIES

Routine blood and urine screening is of little practical value in the initial care of the poisoned patient. Specific toxicologic analyses and quantitative levels of certain drugs may be extremely helpful. One should always ask oneself the following questions: (a) How will the result of the test alter the management? and (b) Can the result of the test be returned in time to have a positive effect on therapy?

Owing to long turnaround time, lack of availability, factors contributing to unreliability, and the risk of serious morbidity without supportive clinical management, toxicology screening is estimated to affect management in less than 15% of cases of drug overdoses or poisonings. Toxicology screening may look specifically for only 40 to 50 drugs out of more than 10,000 possible drugs or toxins and more than several million chemicals. To detect many different drugs, toxic screens usually include methods with broad specificity, and sensitivity may be poor for some drugs, resulting in false-negative or false-positive findings. On the other hand, some drugs present in therapeutic amounts may be detected on the screen, even though they are causing no clinical symptoms. Because many agents are not sought or detected during a toxicologic screening, a negative result does not always rule out poisonings. The specificity of toxicologic tests is dependent on the method and the laboratory. The presence of other drugs, drug metabolites, disease states, or incorrect sampling may cause erroneous results.

For the average toxicologic laboratory, false-negative results occur at a rate of 10% to 30% and false-positives at a rate of 0% to 10%. The positive screen predictive value is approximately 90%. A negative toxicology screen does not exclude a poisoning. The negative predictive value of toxicologic screening is approximately 70%. For example, the following benzodiazepines may not be detected by some routine immunoassay benzodiazepine screening tests: alprazolam (Xanax), clonazepam (Klonopin), temazepam (Restoril), and triazolam (Halcion).

**TABLE 10** Conversion Factors for Alcohols and Glycols

| Alcohols/Glycols | 1 mg/dL in Blood Raises Osmolality mOsm/L | Molecular Weight | Conversion Factor |
|---|---|---|---|
| Ethanol | 0.228 | 40 | 4.6 |
| Methanol | 0.327 | 32 | 3.2 |
| Ethylene glycol | 0.190 | 62 | 6.2 |
| Isopropanol | 0.176 | 60 | 6.0 |
| Acetone | 0.182 | 58 | 5.8 |
| Propylene glycol | not available | 72 | 7.2 |

*Example*: Methanol osmolality. Subtract the calculated osmolality from the measured serum osmolarity (freezing point method) = osmolar gap × 3.2 (one-tenth molecular weight) = estimated serum methanol concentration.
*Note*: This equation is often not considered very reliable in predicting the actual measured blood concentration of these alcohols or glycols.

The "toxic urine screen" is generally a qualitative urine test for several common drugs, usually substances of abuse (cocaine and metabolites, opioids, amphetamines, benzodiazepines, barbiturates, and phencyclidine). Results of these tests are usually available within 2 to 6 hours. Because these tests may vary with each hospital and community, the physician should determine exactly which substances are included in the toxic urine screen of his or her laboratory. Tests for ethylene glycol, red blood cell cholinesterase, and serum cyanide are not readily available.

For cases of ingestion of certain substances, quantitative blood levels should be obtained at specific times after the ingestion to avoid spurious low values in the distribution phase, which result from incomplete absorption. The detection time for drugs is influenced by many variables, such as type of substance, formulation, amount, time since ingestion, duration of exposure, and half-life. For many drugs, the detection time is measured in days after the exposure.

## Common Poisons

### ACETAMINOPHEN (PARACETAMOL, *N*-ACETYL-PARAAMINOPHENOL)

#### Toxic Mechanism

At therapeutic doses of acetaminophen, less than 5% is metabolized by P450-2E1 to a toxic reactive oxidizing metabolite, *N*-acetyl-p-benzo-quinoneimine (NAPQI). In a case of overdose, there is insufficient glutathione available to reduce the excess NAPQI into nontoxic conjugate, so it forms covalent bonds with hepatic intracellular proteins to produce centrilobular necrosis. Renal damage is caused by a similar mechanism.

#### Toxic Dose

The therapeutic dose of acetaminophen is 10 to 15 mg/kg, with a maximum of five doses in 24 hours for a maximum total daily dose of 4 g. An acute single toxic dose is greater than 140 mg/kg, possibly greater than 200 mg/kg in a child younger than age 5 years. Factors affecting the P450 enzymes include enzyme inducers such as barbiturates and phenytoin (Dilantin), ingestion of isoniazid, and alcoholism. Factors that decrease glutathione stores (alcoholism, malnutrition, and HIV infection) contribute to the toxicity of acetaminophen. Alcoholics ingesting 3 to 4 g/d of acetaminophen for a few days can have depleted glutathione stores and require *N*-acetylcysteine therapy at 50% below hepatotoxic blood acetaminophen levels on the nomogram.

#### Kinetics

Peak plasma concentration is usually reached 2 to 4 hours after an overdose. Volume distribution is 0.9 L/kg, and protein binding is less than 50% (albumin).

Route of elimination is by hepatic metabolism to an inactive nontoxic glucuronide conjugate and inactive nontoxic sulfate metabolite by two saturable pathways; less than 5% is metabolized into reactive metabolite NAPQI. In patients younger than 6 years of age, metabolic elimination occurs to a greater degree by conjugation via the sulfate pathway.

The half-life of acetaminophen is 1 to 3 hours.

#### Manifestations

The four phases of the intoxication's clinical course may overlap, and the absence of a phase does not exclude toxicity.

- Phase I occurs within 0.5 to 24 hours after ingestion and may consist of a few hours of malaise, diaphoresis, nausea, and vomiting or produce no symptoms. CNS depression or coma is not a feature.
- Phase II occurs 24 to 48 hours after ingestion and is a period of diminished symptoms. The liver enzymes, serum aspartate aminotransferase (AST) (earliest), and serum alanine aminotransferase (ALT) may increase as early as 4 hours or as late as 36 hours after ingestion.
- Phase III occurs at 48 to 96 hours, with peak liver function abnormalities at 72 to 96 hours. The degree of elevation of the hepatic enzymes generally correlates with outcome, but not always. Recovery starts at about 4 days unless hepatic failure develops. Less than 1% of patients with a history of overdose develop fulminant hepatotoxicity.
- Phase IV occurs at 4 to 14 days, with hepatic enzyme abnormalities resolving. If extensive liver damage has occurred, sepsis and disseminated intravascular coagulation may ensue.

Transient renal failure may develop at 5 to 7 days with or without evidence of hepatic damage. Rare cases of myocarditis and pancreatitis have been reported. Death can occur at 7 to 14 days.

#### Laboratory Investigations

The therapeutic reference range is 10 to 20 µg/mL. For toxic levels, see the nomogram presented in Figure 1.

Appropriate and reliable methods for analysis are radioimmunoassay, high-pressure liquid chromatography, and gas chromatography. Spectroscopic assays often give falsely elevated values: bilirubin, salicylate, salicylamide, diflunisal (Dolobid), phenols, and methyldopa (Aldomet) increase the acetaminophen level. Each 1 mg/dL increase in creatinine increases the acetaminophen plasma level 30 µg/mL.

If a toxic acetaminophen level is reached, liver profile (including AST, ALT, bilirubin, and prothrombin time), serum amylase, and blood glucose must be monitored. A complete blood cell count (CBC); platelet count; phosphate, electrolytes, and bicarbonate level measurements; ECG; and urinalysis are indicated.

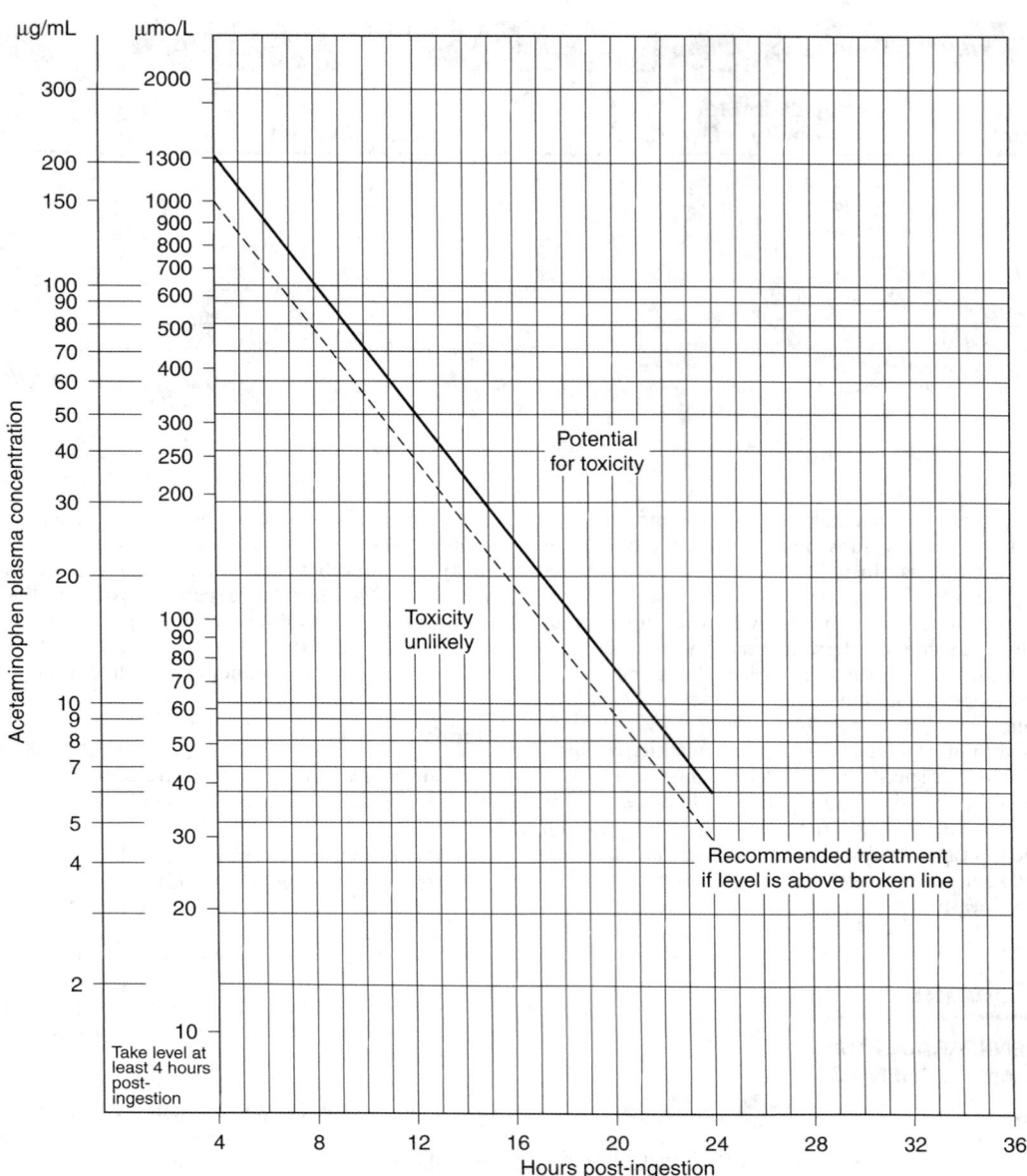

**FIGURE 1.** Nomogram for acetaminophen intoxication. *N*-acetylcysteine therapy is started if levels and time coordinates are above the lower line on the nomogram. Continue and complete therapy even if subsequent values fall below the toxic zone. The nomogram is useful only in cases of acute single ingestion. Levels in serum drawn before 4 hours may not represent peak levels. (From Rumack BH, Matthew H: Acetaminophen poisoning and toxicity. Pediatrics 55:871, 1975.)

## Management

### Gastrointestinal Decontamination

Although ipecac-induced emesis may be useful within 30 minutes of ingestion of the toxic substance, we do not advise it because it could result in vomiting of the activated charcoal. Gastric lavage is not necessary. Studies have indicated that activated charcoal is useful within 1 hour after ingestion. Activated charcoal does adsorb N-acetylcysteine (NAC) if given together, but this is not clinically important. However, if activated charcoal needs to be given along with NAC, separate the administration of activated charcoal from the administration of NAC by 1 to 2 hours to avoid vomiting.

### N-Acetylcysteine (Mucomyst)

NAC (Table 11), a derivative of the amino acid cysteine, acts as a sulfhydryl donor for glutathione synthesis, as surrogate glutathione, and may increase the nontoxic sulfation pathway resulting in conjugation of NAPQI. Oral NAC should be administered within the first 8 hours after a toxic amount of acetaminophen has been ingested. NAC can be started while one awaits the results of the blood test for acetaminophen plasma concentration, but there is no advantage to giving it before 8 hours. If the acetaminophen concentration result after 4 hours following ingestion is above the upper line on the modified Rumack-Matthew nomogram (see Figure 1), one should continue with a maintenance course. Repeat blood specimens should be obtained 4 hours after the initial level is measured if it is greater than 20 mg/mL, which is below the therapy line, because of unexpected delays in the peak by food and co-ingestants. Intravenous NAC (see Table 11) is approved in the United States.

There have been a few cases of anaphylactoid reaction and death by the intravenous route.

### Variations in Therapy

In patients with chronic alcoholism, it is recommended that NAC treatment be administered at 50% below the upper toxic line on the nomogram.

**TABLE 11** Protocol for *N*-Acetylcysteine Administration

| Route | Loading Dose | Maintenance Dose | Course | FDA Approval |
|---|---|---|---|---|
| Oral | 140 mg/kg | 70 mg/kg every 4 h | 72 h | Yes |
| Intravenous | 150 mg/kg over 15 min | 50 mg/kg over 4 h followed by 100 mg/kg over 16h | 20 h | Yes |

If emesis occurs within 1 hour after NAC administration, the dose should be repeated. To avoid emesis, the proper dilution from 20% to 5% NAC must be used, and it should be served in a palatable vehicle, in a covered container through a straw. If this administration is unsuccessful, a slow drip over 30 to 60 minutes through a nasogastric tube or a fluoroscopically placed nasoduodenal tube can be used. Antiemetics can be used if necessary: metoclopramide (Reglan) 10 mg per dose intravenously 30 minutes before administration of NAC (in children, 0.1 mg/kg; maximum, 0.5 mg/kg/d) or ondansetron (Zofran) 32 mg (0.15 mg/kg) by infusion over 15 minutes and repeated for three doses if necessary. The side effects of these antiemetics include anaphylaxis and increases in liver enzymes.

Some investigators recommend variable durations of NAC therapy, stopping the therapy if serial acetaminophen blood concentrations become nondetectable and the liver enzyme levels (ALT and AST) remain normal after 24 to 36 hours.

There is a loss of efficacy if NAC is initiated 8 or 10 hours postingestion, but the loss is not complete, and NAC may be initiated 36 hours or more after ingestion. Late treatment (after 24 hours) decreases the rates of morbidity and mortality in patients with fulminant liver failure caused by acetaminophen and other agents.

Extended relief formulations (*ER* embossed on caplet) contain 325 mg of acetaminophen for immediate release and 325 mg for delayed release. A single 4-hour postingestion serum acetaminophen concentration can underestimate the level because ER formulations can have secondary delayed peaks. In cases of overdose of the ER formulation, it is recommended that additional acetaminophen levels be obtained at 4-hour intervals after the initial level is measured. If any level is in the toxic zone, therapy should be initiated.

It is recommended that pregnant patients with toxic plasma concentrations of acetaminophen be treated with NAC to prevent hepatotoxicity in both fetus and mother. The available data suggest no teratogenicity to NAC or acetaminophen.

Indications for NAC therapy in cases of chronic intoxication are a history of ingestion of 3 to 4 g for several days with elevated liver enzyme levels (AST and ALT). The acetaminophen blood concentration is often low in these cases because of the extended time lapse since ingestion and should not be plotted on the Rumack-Matthew nomogram. Patients with a history of chronic alcoholism or those on chronic enzyme inducers may also present with elevated liver enzyme levels and should be considered for NAC therapy if they have a history of taking acetaminophen on a chronic basis, because they are considered to be at a greater risk for hepatotoxicity despite a low acetaminophen blood concentration.

Specific support care may be needed to treat liver failure, pancreatitis, transient renal failure, and myocarditis.

Liver transplantation has a definite but limited role in patients with acute acetaminophen overdose. A retrospective analysis determined that a continuing rise in the prothrombin time (4-day peak, 180 seconds), a pH of less than 7.3 2 days after the overdose, a serum creatinine level of greater than 3.3 mg/dL, severe hepatic encephalopathy, and disturbed coagulation factor VII/V ratio greater than 30 suggest a poor prognosis and may be indicators for hepatology consultation for consideration of liver transplantation.

Extracorporeal measures are not expected to be of benefit.

### Disposition

Adults who have ingested more than 140 mg/kg and children younger than 6 years of age who have ingested more than 200 mg/kg should receive therapy within 8 hours postingestion or until the results of the 4-hour postingestion acetaminophen plasma concentration are known.

## AMPHETAMINES

The amphetamines include illicit methamphetamine ("Ice"), diet pills, and formulations under various trade names. Analogues include MDMA (3,4 methylenedioxymethamphetamine, known as "ecstasy," "XTC," "Adam") and MDA (3,4-methylenedioxyamphetamine, known as "Eve"). MDA is a common hallucinogen and euphoriant "club drug" used at "raves," which are all-night dances. Use of methamphetamine and designer analogues is on the rise, especially among young people between the ages of 12 and 25 years. Other similar stimulants are phenylpropanolamine and cocaine.

### Toxic Mechanism

Amphetamines have a direct CNS stimulant effect and a sympathetic nervous system effect by releasing catecholamines from α- and β-adrenergic nerve terminals but inhibiting their reuptake.

Hallucinogenic MDMA has an additional hazard of serotonin effect (refer to serotonin syndrome in the SSRI section). MDMA also affects the dopamine system in the brain. Because of its effects on 5-hydroxytryptamine, dopamine, and norepinephrine, MDMA can lead to serotonin syndrome associated with malignant hyperthermia and rhabdomyolysis, which contributes to the potentially life-threatening hyperthermia observed in several patients who have used MDMA.

Phenylpropanolamine stimulates only the β-adrenergic receptors.

### Toxic Dose

In children, the toxic dose of dextroamphetamine is 1 mg/kg; in adults, the toxic dose is 5 mg/kg. The potentially fatal dose of dextroamphetamine is 12 mg/kg.

### Kinetics

Amphetamine is a weak base with pKa of 8 to 10. Onset of action is 30 to 60 minutes, and peak effects are 2 to 4 hours. The volume distribution is 2 to 3 L/kg.

Through hepatic metabolism, 60% of the substance is metabolized into a hydroxylated metabolite that may be responsible for psychotic effects.

The half-life of amphetamines is pH dependent—8 to 10 hours in acid urine (pH <6.0) and 16 to 31 hours in alkaline urine (pH >7.5). Excretion is by the kidney—30% to 40% at alkaline urine pH and 50% to 70% at acid urine pH.

### Manifestations

Effects are seen within 30 to 60 minutes following ingestion.

Neurologic manifestations include restlessness, irritation and agitation, tremors and hyperreflexia, and auditory and visual hallucinations. Hyperpyrexia may precede seizures, convulsions, paranoia, violence, intracranial hemorrhage, psychosis, and self-destructive behavior. Paranoid psychosis and cerebral vasculitis occur with chronic abuse.

MDMA is often adulterated with cocaine, heroin, or ketamine, or a combination of these, to create a variety of mood alterations.

This possibility must be taken into consideration when one manages patients with MDMA ingestions, as the symptom complex may reflect both CNS stimulation and CNS depression.

Other manifestations include dilated but reactive pupils, cardiac dysrhythmias (supraventricular and ventricular), tachycardia, hypertension, rhabdomyolysis, and myoglobinuria.

### Laboratory Investigations

The clinician should monitor ECG and cardiac readings, ABG and oxygen saturation, electrolytes, blood glucose, BUN, creatinine, creatine kinase, cardiac fraction if there is chest pain, and liver profile. Also, one should evaluate for rhabdomyolysis and check urine for myoglobin, cocaine and metabolites, and other substances of abuse. The peak plasma concentration of amphetamines is 10 to 50 ng/mL 1 to 2 hours after ingestion of 10 to 25 mg. The toxic plasma concentration is 200 ng/mL. When the rapid immunoassays are used, cross-reactions can occur with amphetamine derivatives (e.g., MDA, "ecstasy"), brompheniramine (Dimetane), chlorpromazine (Thorazine), ephedrine, phenylpropanolamine, phentermine (Adipex-P), phenmetrazine, ranitidine (Zantac), and Vicks Inhaler (L-desoxyephedrine). False-positive results may occur.

### Management

Management is similar to management for cocaine intoxication. Supportive care includes blood pressure and temperature control, cardiac monitoring, and seizure precautions. Diazepam (Valium) can be administered. Gastrointestinal decontamination can be undertaken with activated charcoal administered up to 1 hour after ingestion.

Anxiety, agitation, and convulsions are treated with diazepam. If diazepam fails to control seizures, neuromuscular blockers can be used and the electroencephalogram (EEG) monitored for nonmotor seizures. One should avoid neuroleptic phenothiazines and butyrophenone, which can lower the seizure threshold.

Hypertension and tachycardia are usually transient and can be managed by titration of diazepam. Nitroprusside can be used for hypertensive crisis at a maximum infusion rate of 10 μg/kg/minute for 10 minutes followed with a lower infusion rate of 0.3 to 2 mg/kg/minute. Myocardial ischemia is managed by oxygen, vascular access, benzodiazepines, and nitroglycerin. Aspirin and thrombolytics are not routinely recommended because of the danger of intracranial hemorrhage. It is important to distinguish between angina and true ischemia. Delayed hypotension can be treated with fluids and vasopressors if needed. Life-threatening tachydysrhythmias may respond to an α-blocker such as phentolamine (Regitine) 5 mg IV for adults or 0.1 mg/kg IV for children and a short-acting β-blocker such as esmolol (Brevibloc) 500 μg/kg IV over 1 minute for adults, or 300 to 500 μg/kg over 1 minute for children. Ventricular dysrhythmias may respond to lidocaine or, in a severely hemodynamically compromised patient, immediate synchronized electrical cardioversion.

Rhabdomyolysis and myoglobinuria are treated with fluids, alkaline diuresis, and diuretics. Hyperthermia is treated with external cooling and cool 100% humidified oxygen. More extensive therapy may be needed in severe cases. If focal neurologic symptoms are present, the possibility of a cerebrovascular accident should be considered and a CT scan of the head should be obtained.

Paranoid ideation and threatening behavior should be treated with rapid tranquilization using a benzodiazepine. One should observe for suicidal depression that may follow intoxication and may require suicide precautions.

Extracorporeal measures are of no benefit.

### Disposition

Symptomatic patients should be observed on a monitored unit until the symptoms resolve and then observed for a short time after resolution for relapse.

## ANTICHOLINERGIC AGENTS

Drugs with anticholinergic properties include antihistamines (H₁ blockers), neuroleptics (phenothiazines), tricyclic antidepressants, antiparkinsonism drugs (trihexyphenidyl [Artane], benztropine [Cogentin]), ophthalmic products (atropine), and a number of common plants.

The antihistamines are divided into the sedating anticholinergic types, and the nonsedating single daily dose types. The sedating types include ethanolamines (e.g., diphenhydramine [Benadryl], dimenhydrinate [Dramamine], and clemastine [Tavist]), ethylenediamines (e.g., tripelennamine [Pyribenzamine]), alkyl amines (e.g., chlorpheniramine [Chlor-Trimeton], brompheniramine [Dimetane]), piperazines (e.g., cyclizine [Marezine], hydroxyzine [Atarax], and meclizine [Antivert]), and phenothiazine (e.g., Phenergan). The nonsedating types include astemizole (Hismanal), terfenadine (Seldane), loratadine (Claritin), fexofenadine (Allegra), and cetirizine (Zyrtec).

The anticholinergic plants include jimsonweed (*Datura stramonium*), deadly nightshade (*Atropa belladonna*), henbane (*Hyoscyamus niger*), and antispasmodic agents for the bowel (atropine derivatives).

### Toxic Mechanism

By competitive inhibition, anticholinergics block the action of acetylcholine on postsynaptic cholinergic receptor sites. The toxic mechanism primarily involves the peripheral and CNS muscarinic receptors. H₁ sedating-type agents also depress or stimulate the CNS, and in large overdoses some have cardiac membrane–depressant effects (e.g., diphenhydramine [Benadryl]) and α-adrenergic receptor blockade effects (e.g., promethazine [Phenergan]). Nonsedating agents produce peripheral H₁ blockade but do not possess anticholinergic or sedating actions. The original agents terfenadine (Seldane) and astemizole (Hismanal) were recently removed from the market because of the severe cardiac dysrhythmias associated with their use, especially when used in combination with macrolide antibiotics and certain antifungal agents such as ketoconazole (Nizoral), which inhibit hepatic metabolism or excretion. The newer nonsedating agents, including loratadine (Claritin), fexofenadine (Allegra), and cetirizine (Zyrtec), have not been reported to cause the severe drug interactions associated with terfenadine and astemizole.

### Toxic Dose

The estimated toxic oral dose of atropine is 0.05 mg/kg in children and more than 2 mg in adults. The minimal estimated lethal dose of atropine is more than 10 mg in adults and more than 2 mg in children. Other synthetic anticholinergic agents are less toxic, and the fatal dose varies from 10 to 100 mg.

The estimated toxic oral dose of diphenhydramine (Benadryl) in a child is 15 mg/kg, and the potential lethal amount is 25 mg/kg. In an adult, the potential lethal amount is 2.8 g. Ingestion of five times the single dose of an antihistamine is toxic.

For the nonsedating agents, an overdose of 3360 mg of terfenadine was reported in an adult who developed ventricular tachycardia and fibrillation that responded to lidocaine and defibrillation. A 1500-mg overdose produced hypotension. Cases of delayed serious dysrhythmias (torsades de pointes) have been reported with doses of more than 200 mg of astemizole. The toxic doses of fexofenadine (Allegra), cetirizine, and loratadine (Claritin) need to be established.

### Kinetics

The onset of absorption of intravenous atropine is in 2 to 4 minutes. Peak effects on salivation after intravenous or intramuscular administration are at 30 to 60 minutes.

Onset of absorption after oral ingestion is 30 to 60 minutes, peak action is 1 to 3 hours, and duration of action is 4 to 6 hours, but symptoms are prolonged in cases of overdose or with sustained-release preparations.

The onset of absorption of diphenhydramine is in 15 minutes to 1 hour, with a peak of action in 1 to 4 hours. Volume distribution is 3.3 to 6.8 L/kg, and protein binding is 75% to 80%. Ninety-eight percent of diphenhydramine is metabolized via the liver by *N*-demethylation.

Interactions with erythromycin, ketoconazole (Nizoral), and derivatives produce excessive blood levels of the antihistamine and ventricular dysrhythmias.

The half-life of diphenhydramine is 3 to 10 hours.

The chemical structure of nonsedating agents prevents their entry into the CNS. Absorption begins in 1 hour, with peak effects in 4 in 6 hours. The duration of action is greater than 24 hours.

These agents are metabolized in the gastrointestinal tract and liver. Protein binding is greater than 90%. The plasma half-life is 3.5 hours. Only 1% is excreted unchanged; 60% of that is excreted in the feces and 40% in the urine.

## Manifestations

Anticholinergic signs are hyperpyrexia ("hot as a hare"), mydriasis ("blind as a bat"), flushing of skin ("red as a beet"), dry mucosa and skin ("dry as a bone"), "Lilliputian type" hallucinations and delirium ("mad as a hatter"), coma, dysphagia, tachycardia, moderate hypertension, and rarely convulsions and urinary retention. Other effects include jaundice (cyproheptadine [Periactin]), dystonia (diphenhydramine [Benadryl]), rhabdomyolysis (doxylamine), and, in large doses, cardiotoxic effects (diphenhydramine).

Overdose with nonsedating agents produces headache and confusion, nausea, and dysrhythmias (e.g., torsades de pointes).

## Laboratory Investigations

Monitoring of ABG (in cases of respiratory depression), electrolytes, glucose, and the ECG should be undertaken. Anticholinergic drugs and plants are not routinely included on screens for substances of abuse.

## Management

For patients in respiratory failure, intubation and assisted ventilation should be instituted. Gastrointestinal decontamination can be instituted. Caution must be taken with emesis in cases of diphenhydramine (Benadryl) overdose because of the drug's rapid onset of action and risk of seizures. If bowel sounds are present for up to 1 hour after ingestion, activated charcoal can be given. Seizures can be controlled with benzodiazepines (diazepam [Valium] or lorazepam [Ativan]).

The administration of physostigmine (Antilirium) is not routine and is reserved for life-threatening anticholinergic effects that are refractory to conventional treatments. It should be administered with adequate monitoring and resuscitative equipment available. The use of physostigmine should be avoided if a tricyclic antidepressant is present because of increased toxicity. Urinary retention should be relieved by catheterization to avoid reabsorption of the drug and additional toxicity.

Supraventricular tachycardia should be treated only if the patient is hemodynamically unstable. Ventricular dysrhythmias can be controlled with lidocaine or cardioversion. Sodium bicarbonate 1 to 2 mEq/kg IV may be useful for myocardial depression and QRS prolongation. Torsades de pointes, especially when associated with terfenadine and astemizole ingestion, has been treated with magnesium sulfate 4 g or 40 mL 10% solution intravenously over 10 to 20 minutes and countershock if the patient fails to respond.

Hyperpyrexia is controlled by external cooling. Hemodialysis and hemoperfusion are not effective.

## Disposition

### Antihistamine H₁ Antagonists

*Antihistamine H$_1$ Antagonists*

Symptomatic patients should be observed on a monitored unit until the symptoms resolve, then observed for a short time (3 to 4 hours) after resolution for relapse.

### Nonsedating Agents

*Nonsedating Agents*

All asymptomatic children who acutely ingest more than the maximum adult dose and all symptomatic children should be referred to a health care facility for a minimum of 6 hours' observation as well as cardiac monitoring. Asymptomatic adults who acutely ingest more than twice the maximum adult daily dose should be monitored for a minimum of 6 hours. All symptomatic patients should be monitored for as long as there are symptoms present.

## BARBITURATES

Barbiturates have been used as sedatives, anesthetic agents, and anticonvulsants, but their use is declining as safer, more effective drugs become available.

## Toxic Mechanism

Barbiturates are γ-aminobutyric acid (GABA) agonists (increasing the chloride flow and inhibiting depolarization). They enhance the CNS depressant effect of GABA and depress the cardiovascular system.

## Toxic Dose

The shorter-acting barbiturates (including the intermediate-acting agents) and their hypnotic doses are as follows: amobarbital (Amytal), 100 to 200 mg; aprobarbital (Alurate), 50 to 100 mg; butabarbital (Butisol), 50 to 100 mg; butalbital, 100 to 200 mg; pentobarbital (Nembutal), 100 to 200 mg; secobarbital (Seconal), 100 to 200 mg. They cause toxicity at lower doses than long-acting barbiturates and have a minimum toxic dose of 6 mg/kg; the fatal adult dose is 3 to 6 g.

The long-acting barbiturates and their doses include mephobarbital (Mebaral), 50 to 100 mg, and phenobarbital, 100 to 200 mg. Their minimum toxic dose is greater than 10 mg/kg, and the fatal adult dose is 6 to 10 g. A general rule is that an amount five times the hypnotic dose is toxic and an amount 10 times the hypnotic dose is potentially fatal. Methohexital and thiopental are ultrashort-acting parenteral preparations and are not discussed.

## Kinetics

The barbiturates are enzyme inducers. Short-acting barbiturates are highly lipid-soluble, penetrate the brain readily, and have shorter elimination times. Onset of action is in 10 to 30 minutes, with a peak at 1 to 2 hours. Duration of action is 3 to 8 hours. The volume distribution of short-acting barbiturate is 0.8 to 1.5 L/kg; pKa is about 8. Mean half-life varies from 8 to 48 hours.

Long-acting agents have longer elimination times and can be used as anticonvulsants. Onset of action is in 20 to 60 minutes, with a peak at 1 to 6 hours. In cases of overdose, the peak can be at 10 hours. Usual duration of action is 8 to 12 hours. Volume distribution is 0.8 L/kg, and half-life is 11 to 120 hours. The pKa of phenobarbital is 7.2. Alkalinization of urine promotes its excretion.

## Manifestations

Mild intoxication resembles alcohol intoxication and includes ataxia, slurred speech, and depressed cognition. Severe intoxication causes slow respirations, coma, and loss of reflexes (except pupillary light reflex).

Other manifestations include hypotension (vasodilation), hypothermia, hypoglycemia, and death by respiratory arrest.

## Laboratory Investigations

Most barbiturates are detected on routine drug screens and can be measured in most hospital laboratories. Investigation should include barbiturate level; ABG; toxicology screen, including acetaminophen; glucose, electrolyte, BUN, creatinine, and creatine kinase levels; and urine pH. The minimum toxic plasma levels are greater than 10 μg/mL for short-acting barbiturates and greater than 40 μg/dL for long-acting agents. Fatal levels are 30 μg/mL for short-acting barbiturates and 80 to 150 μg/mL for long-acting agents. Both short-acting and long-acting agents can be detected in urine 24 to 72 hours after ingestion, and long-acting agents can be detected up to 7 days.

## Management

Vital functions must be established and maintained. Intensive supportive care including intubation and assisted ventilation should dominate the management. All stuporous and comatose patients should have glucose (for hypoglycemia), thiamine (if chronically alcoholic), and naloxone (Narcan) (in case of an opioid ingestion) intravenously and should be admitted to the intensive care unit. Emesis should be avoided especially in cases of ingestion of the shorter-acting barbiturates. Activated charcoal followed by MDAC (0.5 g/kg) every 2 to 4 hours has been shown to reduce the serum half-life of phenobarbital by 50%, but its effect on clinical course is undetermined.

Fluids should be administered to correct dehydration and hypotension. Vasopressors may be necessary to correct severe hypotension, and hemodynamic monitoring may be needed. The patient must be observed carefully for fluid overload. Alkalinization (ion trapping) is used only for phenobarbital (pKa 7.2) but not for short-acting barbiturates. Sodium bicarbonate, 1 to 2 mEq/kg IV in 500 mL of 5% dextrose in adults or 10 to 15 mL/kg in children during the first hour, followed by sufficient bicarbonate to keep the urinary pH at 7.5 to 8.0, enhances excretion of phenobarbital and shortens the half-life by 50%. Diuresis is not advocated because of the danger of cerebral or pulmonary edema.

Hemodialysis shortens the half-life to 8 to 14 hours, and charcoal hemoperfusion shortens the half-life to 6 to 8 hours for long-acting barbiturates such as phenobarbital. Both procedures may be effective in patients with both long-acting and short-acting barbiturate ingestion. If the patient does not respond to supportive measures or if the phenobarbital plasma concentration is greater than 150 μg/mL, both procedures may be tried to shorten the half-life.

Bullae are treated as a local second-degree skin burn. Hypothermia should be treated.

## Disposition

All comatose patients should be admitted to the intensive care unit. Awake and oriented patients with an overdose of short-acting agents should be observed for at least 6 asymptomatic hours; overdose of long-acting agents warrants observation for at least 12 asymptomatic hours because of the potential for delayed absorption. In the case of an intentional overdose, psychiatric clearance is needed before the patient can be discharged. Chronic use can lead to tolerance, physical dependency, and withdrawal and necessitates follow-up.

## BENZODIAZEPINES

Benzodiazepines are used as anxiolytics, sedatives, and relaxants.

### Toxic Mechanism

The GABA agonists produce CNS depression and increase chloride flow, inhibiting depolarization.

Flunitrazepam (Rohypnol; street name "roofies") is a long-acting benzodiazepine agonist sold by prescription in more than 60 countries worldwide, but it is not legally available in the United States.

### Toxic Dose

The long-acting benzodiazepines (half-life >24 hours) and their maximum therapeutic doses are as follows: chlordiazepoxide (Librium), 50 mg; clorazepate (Tranxene), 30 mg; clonazepam (Klonopin), 20 mg; diazepam (Valium), 10 mg in adults or 0.2 mg/kg in children; flurazepam (Dalmane), 30 mg; and prazepam, 20 mg.

The short-acting benzodiazepines (half-life 10 to 24 hours) and their doses include the following: alprazolam (Xanax), 0.5 mg, and lorazepam (Ativan), 4 mg in adults or 0.05 mg/kg in children, which act similar to the long-acting benzodiazepines.

The ultrashort-acting benzodiazepines (half-life <10 hours) are more toxic and include temazepam (Restoril), 30 mg; triazolam (Halcion), 0.5 mg; midazolam (Versed), 0.2 mg/kg; and oxazepam (Serax), 30 mg.

In cases of overdose of short- and long-acting agents, 10 to 20 times the therapeutic dose (>1500 mg diazepam or 2000 mg chlordiazepoxide) have been ingested with resulting mild coma but without respiratory depression. Fatalities are rare, and most patients recover within 24 to 36 hours after overdose. Asymptomatic unintentional overdoses of less than five times the therapeutic dose can be seen. Ultrashort-acting agents have produced respiratory arrest and coma within 1 hour after ingestion of 5 mg of triazolam (Halcion) and death with ingestion of as little as 10 mg. Midazolam (Versed) and diazepam (Valium) by rapid intravenous injection have produced respiratory arrest.

### Kinetics

Onset of CNS depression is usually in 30 to 120 minutes; peak action usually occurs within 1 to 3 hours when ingestion is by the oral route. The volume distribution varies from 0.26 to 6 L/kg (LA, 1.1 L/kg); protein binding is 70% to 99%. For flunitrazepam, the onset of action is in 0.5 to 2 hours, oral peak is in 2 hours, and duration 8 hours or more. The half-life of flunitrazepam is 20 to 30 hours, volume distribution is 3.3 to 5.5 L/kg, and 80% is protein bound. Flunitrazepam can be identified in urine 4 to 30 days after ingestion.

### Manifestations

Neurologic manifestations include ataxia, slurred speech, and CNS depression. Deep coma leading to respiratory depression suggests the presence of short-acting benzodiazepines or other CNS depressants. In elderly persons, the therapeutic doses can produce toxicity and can have an additive effect with other CNS depressants. Chronic use can lead to tolerance, physical dependency, and withdrawal.

### Laboratory Investigations

Most benzodiazepines can be detected in urine drug screens. Quantitative blood levels are not useful. Some of the immunoassay urinary screens cannot detect all of the new benzodiazepines currently available. A consultation with the laboratory analyst is warranted if a specific case occurs in which the test result is negative but benzodiazepine use is suspected by the patient's history. Situations in which benzodiazepines may not be detected include ingestion of a low dose (e.g., <10 mg), rapid elimination, and a different or no metabolite. Some immunoassay methods can produce a false-positive finding for the benzodiazepines when nonsteroidal anti-inflammatory drugs (tolmetin [Tolectin], naproxen [Aleve], etodolac [Lodine], and fenoprofen [Nalfon]) are used. If this is a concern, the laboratory analyst should be consulted.

In cases in which "date rape" drugs such as flunitrazepam are suspected, a police crime or reference laboratory should be consulted for testing.

### Management

Emesis and gastric lavage should be avoided. Activated charcoal can be useful only if given early before the peak time of absorption occurs. Supportive treatment should be instituted but rarely requires intubation or assisted ventilation.

Flumazenil (Romazicon) is a specific benzodiazepine receptor antagonist that blocks the chloride flow and inhibitor of GABA neurotransmitters. It reverses the sedative effects of benzodiazepines, zolpidem (Ambien), and endogenous benzodiazepines associated with hepatic encephalopathy. It is not recommended to reverse benzodiazepine-induced hypoventilation. The manufacturer advises that flumazenil be used with caution in cases of overdose with possible benzodiazepine dependency (because it can precipitate life-threatening withdrawal), if cyclic antidepressant use is suspected, or if a patient has a known seizure disorder.

### Disposition

If the patient is comatose, he or she must be admitted to the intensive care unit. If the overdose was intentional, psychiatric clearance is needed before the patient can be discharged.

## TABLE 12  Pharmacologic and Toxic Properties of β-Blockers

| Blocker | Maximum Solubility | Therapeutic Plasma Level | Lipid Solubility | Intrinsic Sympathomimetic Activity (Partial Agonist) | Membrane Stabilizing Effect β-Selective β₁ | β₂ | Cardiac Selectivity α-Selective |
|---|---|---|---|---|---|---|---|
| Acebutolol (Sectral) | 800 mg | 200-2000 ng/mL | Moderate | + | + | + | + |
| Alprenolol² | 800 mg | 50-200 ng/mL | Moderate | 2+ | + | – | – |
| Atenolol (Tenormin) | 100 mg | 200-500 ng/mL | Low | – | – | 2+ | – |
| Betaxolol (Kerlone) | 20 mg | NA | Low | + | – | + | – |
| Carteolol (Cartrol) | 10 mg | NA | No | + | – | – | – |
| Esmolol (Brevibloc) (Class II antidysrhythmic, IV only) | | | Low | – | – | + | – |
| Labetalol (Trandate) | 800 mg | 50-500 ng/mL | Low | + | +/– | – | + |
| Levobunolol (AKBeta eyedrop) (Eye drops 0.25% and 0.5%) | 20 mg | NA | No | – | – | – | – |
| Metoprolol (Lopressor) | | | Moderate | – | – | 2+ | – |
| Nadolol (Corgard) | 320 mg | 20-40 ng/mL | Low | – | – | – | – |
| Oxprenolol² | 480 mg | 80-100 ng/mL | Moderate | 2+ | + | – | – |
| Pindolol (Visken) | 60 mg | 50-150 ng/mL | Moderate | 3+ | +/– | – | – |
| Propranolol (Inderal) (Class II antidysrhythmic) | 360 mg | 50-100 ng/mL | High | – | 2+ | – | – |
| Sotalol (Betapace) (Class II antidysrhythmic) | 480 mg | 500-4000 ng/mL | Low | – | – | – | – |
| Timolol (Blocadren) | 60 mg | 5-10 ng/mL | Low | – | +/– | – | – |

²Not available in the United States.

## β-ADRENERGIC BLOCKERS (β-BLOCKERS)

β-Blockers are used in the treatment of hypertension and of a number of systemic and ophthalmologic disorders. Properties of β-blockers include the factors listed in Table 12.

Lipid-soluble drugs have CNS effects, active metabolites, longer duration of action, and interactions (e.g., propranolol). Cardioselectivity is lost in overdose. Intrinsic partial agonist agents (e.g., pindolol) may initially produce tachycardia and hypertension. Cardiac membrane depressive effect (quinidine-like) occurs in cases of overdose but not at therapeutic doses (e.g., with metoprolol or sotalol). α-Blocking effect is weak (e.g., with labetalol or acebutolol).

## Toxic Mechanism

β-Blockers compete with the catecholamines for receptor sites and block receptor action in the bronchi, the vascular smooth muscle, and the myocardium.

## Toxic Dose

Ingestions of greater than twice the maximum recommended daily therapeutic dose are considered toxic (see Table 12). Ingestion of 1 mg/kg propranolol in a child may produce hypoglycemia. Fatalities have been reported in adults with 7.5 g of metoprolol. The most toxic agent is sotalol, and the least toxic is atenolol.

## Kinetics

Regular-release formulations usually cause symptoms within 2 hours. Propranolol's onset of action is 20 to 30 minutes and peak is at 1 to 4 hours, but it may be delayed by co-ingestants. The onset of action with sustained-release preparations may be delayed to 6 hours and the peak to 12 to 16 hours. Volume distribution is 1 to 5.6 L/kg. Protein binding is variable, from 5% to 93%.

## Metabolism

Atenolol (Tenormin), nadolol (Corgard), and santalol (Betapace) have enterohepatic recirculation. The duration of action for regular-acting agents is 4 to 6 hours, but in cases of overdose it may be 24 to 48 hours. The duration of action for sustained-release agents is 24 to 48 hours.

The regular preparation with the longest half-life is nadolol, at 12 to 24 hours, and the one with the shortest half-life is esmolol, at 5 to 10 minutes.

## Manifestations

See "Toxic Properties" and Table 12.

Highly lipid soluble agents produce coma and seizures. Bradycardia and hypotension are the major cardiac symptoms and may lead to cardiogenic shock. Intrinsic partial agonists initially may cause tachycardia and hypertension. ECG changes include atrioventricular conduction delay or asystole. Membrane-depressant effects produce prolonged QRS and QT interval, which may result in torsades de pointes. Sotalol produces a very prolonged QT interval. Bronchospasm may occur in patients with reactive airway disease with any β-blocker because the selectivity is lost in overdose. Other manifestations include hypoglycemia (because β-blockers block catecholamine counter-regulatory mechanisms) and hyperkalemia.

## Laboratory Investigations

Measurements of blood levels are not readily available or useful. ECG and cardiac monitoring should be maintained, and blood glucose and electrolytes, BUN, and creatinine levels should be monitored, as well as ABG if there are respiratory symptoms.

## Management

Vital functions must be established and maintained. Vascular access, baseline ECG, and continuous cardiac and blood pressure monitoring should be established. A pacemaker must be available. Gastrointestinal decontamination can be undertaken initially with activated charcoal up to 1 hour after ingestion. MDAC is no longer recommended, based on the latest guidelines. Whole-bowel irrigation can be considered in cases of large overdoses with sustained-release preparations, but there are no studies evaluating the efficacy of intervention.

If there are cardiovascular disturbances, a cardiac consultation should be obtained. Class IA antidysrhythmic agents (procainamide, quinidine) and III (bretylium) are not recommended. Hypotension is treated with fluids initially, although it usually does not respond. Frequently, glucagon and cardiac pacing are needed. Bradycardia in asymptomatic, hemodynamically stable patients requires no therapy. It is not predictive of the future course of the disease. If the patient is unstable (has hypotension or a high-degree atrioventricular block), atropine 0.02 mg/kg (up to 2 mg) in adults, glucagon, and a pacemaker can be used. In case of ventricular tachycardia, overdrive pacing can be used. A wide QRS interval may respond to sodium bicarbonate. Torsades de pointes (associated with sotalol) may respond to magnesium sulfate and overdrive pacing. Prophylactic magnesium for prolonged QT interval has been suggested, but there are no data. Epinephrine must not be used because an unopposed α effect may occur.

Hypotension and myocardial depression are managed by correction of dysrhythmias, Trendelenburg position, fluids, glucagon, or amrinone (Inocor), or a combination of these. Hemodynamic monitoring with a Swan-Ganz catheter or arterial line may be necessary to manage fluid therapy.

Glucagon is the initial drug of choice. It works through adenyl cyclase and bypasses catecholamine receptors; therefore, it is not affected by β-blockers. Glucagon increases cardiac contractility and heart rate. It is given as an intravenous bolus of 5 to 10 mg[C] over 1 minute and followed by a continuous infusion of 1 to 5 mg/h (in children, 0.15 mg/kg followed by 0.05 to 0.1 mg/kg/h). In large doses and in infusion therapy $D_5W$, sterile water, or saline should be used as a dilutant to reconstitute glucagon in place of the 0.2% phenol diluent provided with some drugs. Effects are seen within minutes. It can be used with other agents such as amrinone.

Amrinone (Inocor) inhibits phosphodiesterase enzyme, which metabolizes cyclic AMP. It is administered as a bolus of 0.15 to 2 mg/kg (0.15 to 0.4 mL/kg) intravenously, followed by infusion of 5 to 10 μg/kg/min.

Hypoglycemia should be treated with intravenous glucose. Life-threatening hyperkalemia is treated with calcium (avoid if digoxin is present), bicarbonate, and glucose or insulin. Convulsions can be controlled with diazepam or phenobarbital. If bronchospasm is present, $\beta_2$ nebulized bronchodilators are given.

Extraordinary measures such as intra-aortic balloon pump support can be instituted. Extracorporeal measures can be undertaken. Hemodialysis for cases of atenolol, acebutolol, nadolol, and sotalol (low volume distribution, low protein binding) ingestion may be helpful, particularly when there is evidence of renal failure. Hemodialysis is not effective for propranolol, metoprolol, and timolol.

Prenalterol[A] has successfully reversed both bradycardia and hypotension but is not currently available in the United States.

## Disposition

Asymptomatic patients with history of overdose require baseline ECG and continuous cardiac monitoring for at least 6 hours with regular-release preparations and for 24 hours with sustained-release preparations. Symptomatic patients should be observed with cardiac monitoring for 24 hours. If seizures or abnormal rhythm or vital signs are present, the patient should be admitted to the intensive care unit.

## CALCIUM CHANNEL BLOCKERS

Calcium channel blockers are used in the treatment of effort angina, supraventricular tachycardia, and hypertension.

### Toxic Mechanism

Calcium channel blockers reduce influx of calcium through the slow channels in membranes of the myocardium, the atrioventricular nodes, and the vascular smooth muscles and result in peripheral, systemic, and coronary vasodilation, impaired cardiac conduction, and depression of cardiac contractility. All calcium channel blockers have vasodilatory action, but only bepridil, diltiazem, and verapamil depress myocardial contractility and cause atrioventricular block.

### Toxic Dose

Any ingested amount greater than the maximum daily dose has the potential of severe toxicity. The maximum oral daily doses in adults and toxic doses in children of each are as follows: amlodipine (Norvasc), 10 mg for adults and more than 0.25 mg/kg for children; bepridil (Vascor), 400 mg for adults and more than 5.7 mg/kg for children; diltiazem (Cardizem), 360 mg for adults (toxic dose > 2 g) and more than 6 mg/kg for children; felodipine (Plendil), 40 mg for adults and more than 0.56 mg/kg for children; isradipine (DynaCirc), 40 mg for adults and more than 0.4 mg/kg for children; nicardipine (Cardene), 120 mg for adults and more than 0.85 mg/kg for children; nifedipine (Procardia), 120 mg for adults and more than 2 mg/kg for children; nimodipine (Nimotop), 360 mg for adults and more than 0.85 mg/kg for children; nitrendipine (Baypress),[A] 80 mg for adults and more than 1.14 mg/kg for children; and verapamil (Calan), 480 mg for adults and 15 mg/kg for children.

### Kinetics

Onset of action of regular-release preparations varies: for verapamil it is 60 to 120 minutes, for nifedipine 20 minutes, and for diltiazem 15 minutes after ingestion. Peak effect for verapamil is 2 to 4 hours, for nifedipine 60 to 90 minutes, and for diltiazem 30 to 60 minutes, but the peak action may be delayed for 6 to 8 hours. Duration of action is up to 36 hours. The onset of action for sustained-release preparations is usually 4 hours but may be delayed, and peak effect is at 12 to 24 hours. In cases of massive overdose, concretions and prolonged toxicity can develop.

Volume distribution varies from 3 to 7 L/kg. Hepatic elimination half-life varies from 3 to 7 hours. Patients receiving digitalis and calcium channel blockers run the risk of digitalis toxicity, because calcium channel blockers increase digitalis levels.

### Manifestations

Cardiac manifestations include hypotension, bradycardia, and conduction disturbances occurring 30 minutes to 5 hours after ingestion. A prolonged PR interval is an early finding and may occur at therapeutic doses. Torsades de pointes has been reported. All degrees of blocks may occur and may be delayed up to 16 hours. Lactic acidosis may be present. Calcium channel blockers do not affect intraventricular conduction, so the QRS interval is usually not affected.

Hypocalcemia is rarely present. Hyperglycemia may be present because of interference in calcium-dependent insulin release. Mental status changes, headaches, seizures, hemiparesis, and CNS depression may occur.

### Laboratory Investigations

Specific drug levels are not readily available and are not useful. Monitor blood sugar, electrolytes, calcium, ABG, pulse oximetry, creatinine, and BUN, and also use hemodynamic monitoring, ECG, and cardiac monitoring.

### Management

Vital functions must be established and maintained. Baseline ECG readings should be obtained and continuous cardiac and blood

---

[A]Not available in the United States.
[C]Exceeds dosage recommended by the manufacturer.

[A]Not available in the United States.

pressure monitoring maintained. A pacemaker should be available. Cardiology consultation should be sought.

Gastrointestinal decontamination with activated charcoal is recommended. If a large dose of a sustained-release preparation was ingested, whole-bowel irrigation can be considered, but its effectiveness has not been investigated.

If the patient is symptomatic, immediate cardiology consult must be obtained, because a pacemaker and hemodynamic monitoring may be needed. In the case of heart block, atropine is rarely effective and isoproterenol (Isuprel) may produce vasodilation. The use of a pacemaker should be considered early.

Hypotension and bradycardia can be treated with positioning, fluids, and calcium gluconate or chloride, glucagon, amrinone (Inocor), and ventricular pacing. Calcium salts must be avoided if digoxin is present. Calcium usually reverses depressed myocardial contractility but may not reverse nodal depression or peripheral vasodilation. Calcium chloride can be given in a 10% solution, 0.1 to 0.2 mL/kg up to 10 mL in an adult, or calcium gluconate in a 10% solution 0.3 to 0.4 mL/kg up to 20 mL in an adult. Administration is intravenous, over 5 to 10 minutes. One should monitor for dysrhythmias, hypotension, and the serum ionized calcium. The aim is to increase calcium 4 mg/dL to a maximum of 13 mg/dL. The calcium response lasts 15 minutes and may require repeated doses or a continuous calcium gluconate infusion 0.2 mL/kg/h up to maximum of 10 mL/h.

If calcium fails, glucagon can be tried for its positive inotropic and chronotropic effect, or both. Amrinone (Inocor), an inotropic agent, may reverse the effects of calcium channel blockers. An effective dose is 0.15 mg to 2 mg/kg (0.15 to 0.4 mL/kg) by intravenous bolus followed by infusion of 5 to 10 µg/kg/min.

In case of hypotension, fluids, norepinephrine (Levophed), and epinephrine may be required. Amrinone and glucagon have been tried alone and in combination. Dobutamine and dopamine are often ineffective.

Extracorporeal measures (e.g., hemodialysis and charcoal hemoperfusion) are not useful, but extraordinary measures such as intra-aortic balloon pump and cardiopulmonary bypass have been used successfully.

For cases of calcium channel blocker toxicity that fail to respond to aggressive management, recent studies demonstrate that insulin and glucose have therapeutic value. The suggested dose range for insulin is to infuse regular insulin at 0.5 IU/kg/h with a simultaneous infusion of glucose 1 g/kg/h, with glucose monitoring every 30 minutes for at least the first 4 hours of administration and subsequent glucose adjustment to maintain euglycemia (70 to 100 mg/dL). Potassium levels should be monitored regularly, as they may shift in response to the insulin.

## Disposition

Patients who have ingested regular-release preparations should be monitored for at least 6 hours and those who have ingested sustained-release preparations should be monitored for 24 hours after the ingestion. Intentional overdose necessitates psychiatric clearance. Symptomatic patients should be admitted to the intensive care unit.

## CARBON MONOXIDE

Carbon monoxide is an odorless, colorless gas produced from incomplete combustion; it is also an in vivo metabolic breakdown product of methylene chloride used in paint removers.

## Toxic Mechanism

Carbon monoxide's affinity for hemoglobin is 240 times greater than that of oxygen. It shifts the oxygen dissociation curve to the left, which impairs hemoglobin release of oxygen to tissues and inhibits the cytochrome oxidase enzymes.

## Toxic Dose and Manifestations

Table 13 describes the manifestations of carbon monoxide toxicity. Exposure to 0.5% for a few minutes is lethal. Sequelae correlate with

**TABLE 13  Carbon Monoxide Exposure and Possible Manifestations**

| CoHB Saturation (%) | Manifestations |
|---|---|
| 3.5 | None |
| 5 | Slight headache, decreased exercise tolerance |
| 10 | Slight headache, dyspnea on vigorous exertion, may impair driving skills |
| 10-20 | Moderate dyspnea on exertion, throbbing, temporal headache |
| 20-30 | Severe headache, syncope, dizziness, visual changes, weakness, nausea, vomiting, altered judgment |
| 30-40 | Vertigo, ataxia, blurred vision, confusion, loss of consciousness |
| 40-50 | Confusion, tachycardia, tachypnea, coma, convulsions |
| 50-60 | Cheyne-Stokes, coma, convulsions, shock, apnea |
| 60-70 | Coma, convulsions, respiratory and heart failure, death |

the patient's level of consciousness at presentation. ECG abnormalities may be noted. Creatine kinase is often elevated, and rhabdomyolysis and myoglobinuria may occur.

The carboxyhemoglobin (CoHB) expresses in percentage the extent to which carbon monoxide has bound with the total hemoglobin. This may be misleadingly low in the anemic patient with less hemoglobin than normal. The patient's presentation is a more reliable indicator of severity than the CoHB level. The manifestations listed in Table 13 for each level are in addition to those listed at the level above. The CoHB may not correlate reliably with the severity of the intoxication, and linking symptoms to specific levels of CoHB frequently leads to inaccurate conclusions. A level of carbon monoxide greater than 40% is usually associated with obvious intoxication.

## Kinetics

The natural metabolism of the body produces small amounts of CoHB, less than 2% for nonsmokers and 5% to 9% for smokers.

Carbon monoxide is rapidly absorbed through the lungs. The rate of absorption is directly related to alveolar ventilation. Elimination also occurs through the lungs. The half-life of CoHB in room air (21% oxygen) is 5 to 6 hours; in 100% oxygen, it is 90 minutes; in hyperbaric pressure at 3 atmospheres oxygen, it is 20 to 30 minutes.

## Laboratory Investigations

An ABG reading may show metabolic acidosis and normal oxygen tension. In cases of significant poisoning, the ABG, electrolytes, blood glucose, serum creatine kinase and cardiac enzymes, renal function tests, and liver function tests should be monitored. A urinalysis and test for myoglobinuria should be obtained. Chest radiograph can be useful in cases of smoke inhalation or if the patient is being considered for hyperbaric chamber. ECG monitoring should be maintained, especially if the patient is older than 40 years, has a history of cardiac disease, or has moderate to severe symptoms. Which toxicology studies are used is based on symptoms and circumstances. CoHB should be monitored during and at the end of therapy. The pulse oximeter has two wavelengths and overestimates oxyhemoglobin saturation in carbon monoxide poisoning. The true oxygen saturation is determined by blood gas analysis, which measures the oxygen bound to hemoglobin. The co-oximeter measures four wavelengths and separates out CoHB and the other hemoglobin binding agents from oxyhemoglobin. Fetal hemoglobin has a greater affinity for carbon monoxide than adult hemoglobin and may falsely elevate the CoHB as much as 4% in young infants.

## Management

The first step is to adequately protect the rescuer. The patient must be removed from the contaminated area, and his or her vital functions must be established.

The mainstay of treatment is 100% oxygen via a non-rebreathing mask with an oxygen reservoir or endotracheal tube. All patients receive 100% oxygen until the CoHB level is 5% or less. Assisted ventilation may be necessary. ABG and CoHB should be monitored and the present CoHB level determined. *Note:* A near-normal CoHB level does not exclude significant carbon monoxide poisoning, especially if the measurement is taken several hours after termination of exposure or if oxygen has been administered prior to obtaining the sample.

The exposed pregnant woman should be kept on 100% oxygen for several hours after the CoHB level is almost 0, because carbon monoxide concentrates in the fetus and oxygen is needed longer to ensure elimination of the carbon monoxide from fetal circulation. The fetus must be monitored, because carbon monoxide and hypoxia are potentially teratogenic.

Metabolic acidosis should be treated with sodium bicarbonate only if the pH is below 7.2 after correction of hypoxia and adequate ventilation. Acidosis shifts the oxygen dissociation curve to the right and facilitates oxygen delivery to the tissues.

The decision to use the hyperbaric oxygen chamber must be made on the basis of the ability to handle other acute emergencies that may coexist in the patient and of the severity of the poisoning. The standard of care for persons exposed to carbon monoxide has yet to be determined, but most authorities recommend using the hyperbaric oxygen chamber under any of the following conditions:

- If the patient is in a coma or has a history of loss of consciousness or seizures
- If there is cardiovascular dysfunction (clinical ischemic chest pain or ECG evidence of ischemia)
- If the patient has metabolic acidosis
- If symptoms persist despite 100% oxygen therapy
- In a child, if the initial CoHB is greater than 15%
- In symptomatic patients with preexisting ischemia
- If there are signs of maternal or fetal distress regardless of CoHB level (infants and fetus are a special problem because fetal hemoglobin has greater affinity for carbon monoxide)

Although controversial, a neurologic-cognitive examination has been used to help determine which patients with low carbon monoxide levels should receive more aggressive therapy. Testing should include the following: general orientation memory testing involving address, phone number, date of birth, and present date; and cognitive testing, involving counting by 7s, digit span, and forward and backward spelling of three-letter and four-letter words. Patients with delayed neurologic sequelae or recurrent symptoms up to 3 weeks may benefit from hyperbaric oxygen chamber treatment.

Seizures and cerebral edema must be treated.

## Disposition

Patients with no or mild symptoms who become asymptomatic after a few hours of oxygen therapy and have a carbon monoxide level less than 10%, and normal physical and neurologic-cognitive examination findings can be discharged, but they should be instructed to return if any signs of neurologic dysfunction appear. Patients with carbon monoxide poisoning requiring treatment need follow-up neuropsychiatric examinations.

## CAUSTICS AND CORROSIVES

The terms *caustic* and *corrosive* are used interchangeably and can be divided into acids and alkalis. The U.S. Consumer Product Safety Commission Labeling Recommendations on containers for acids and alkalis indicate the potential for producing serious damage, as follows:

- Caution—weak irritant
- Warning—strong irritant
- Danger—corrosive

Some common acids with corrosive potential include acetic acid, formic acid, glycolic acid, hydrochloric acid, mercuric chloride, nitric acid, oxalic acid, phosphoric acid, sulfuric acid (battery acid), zinc chloride, and zinc sulfate. Some common alkalis with corrosive potential include ammonia, calcium carbide, calcium hydroxide (dry), calcium oxide, potassium hydroxide (lye), and sodium hydroxide (lye).

### Toxic Mechanism

Acids produce mucosal coagulation necrosis and may be absorbed systemically; they do not penetrate deeply. Injury to the gastric mucosa is more likely, although specific sites of injury for acids and alkalis are not clearly defined.

Alkalis produce liquefaction necrosis and saponification and penetrate deeply. The esophageal mucosa is likely to be damaged. Oropharyngeal and esophageal damage is more frequently caused by solids than by liquids. Liquids produce superficial circumferential burns and gastric damage.

### Toxic Dose

The toxicity is determined by concentration, contact time, and pH. Significant injury is more likely with a substance that has a pH of less than 2 or greater than 12, with a prolonged contact time, and with large volumes.

### Manifestations

The absence of oral burns does not exclude the possibility of esophageal or gastric damage. General clinical findings are stridor; dysphagia; drooling; oropharyngeal, retrosternal, and epigastric pain; and ocular and oral burns. Alkali burns are yellow, soapy, frothy lesions. Acid burns are gray-white and later form an eschar. Abdominal tenderness and guarding may be present if perforation has happened.

### Laboratory Investigations

If acid ingestion has taken place, the patient's acid–base balance and electrolyte status should be determined. If pulmonary symptoms are present, a chest radiograph, ABG measurement, and pulse oximetry are called for.

### Management

It is recommended that the container be brought to the examination, as the substance must be identified and the pH of the substance, vomitus, tears, or saliva tested.

If the acid or alkali has been ingested, all gastrointestinal decontamination procedures are contraindicated except for immediate rinse, removal of substance from the mouth, and dilution with small amounts (sips) of milk or water. The examiner should check for ocular and dermal involvement. Contraindications to oral dilution are dysphagias, respiratory distress, obtundation, or shock. If there is ocular involvement one should immediately irrigate the eye with tepid water for at least 30 minutes, perform fluorescein stain of eye, and consult an ophthalmologist. If there is dermal involvement, one should immediately remove contaminated clothes and irrigate the skin with tepid water for at least 15 minutes. Consultation with a burn specialist is called for.

In cases of acid ingestion, some authorities advocate a small flexible nasogastric tube and aspiration within 30 minutes after ingestion.

Patients should receive only intravenous fluids following dilution until endoscopic consultation is obtained. Endoscopy is valuable to predict damage and risk of stricture. The indications are controversial, with some authorities recommending it in all cases of caustic ingestions regardless of symptoms, and others selectively using clinical features such as vomiting, stridor, drooling, and oral or facial lesions as criteria. We recommend endoscopy for all symptomatic patients or patients with intentional ingestions. Endoscopy may be performed immediately if the patient is symptomatic, but it is usually done 12 to 48 hours postingestion.

The use of corticosteroids is considered controversial. Some feel they may be useful for patients with second-degree circumferential burns. They recommend starting with hydrocortisone sodium succinate (Solu-Cortef) intravenously 10 to 20 mg/kg/d within 48 hours and changing to oral prednisolone 2 mg/kg/d for 3 weeks before tapering the dose. We do not usually recommend using corticosteroids because they have not been shown to be effective.

Tetanus prophylaxis should be provided if the patient requires it for wound care. Antibiotics are not useful prophylactically. Contrast studies are not useful in the first few days and may interfere with endoscopic evaluation; later, they can be used to assess the severity of damage.

Emergency medical therapy includes agents to inhibit collagen formation and intraluminal stents. Esophageal and gastric outlet dilation may be needed if there is evidence of stricture. Bougienage of the esophagus, however, has been associated with brain abscess. Interposition of the colon may be necessary if dilation fails to provide an adequate-sized passage.

Management of inhalation cases requires immediate removal from the environment, administration of humid supplemental oxygen, and observation for airway obstruction and noncardiac pulmonary edema. Radiographic and ABG evaluation should be obtained when appropriate. Intubation and respiratory support may be required.

Certain caustics produce systemic disturbances. Formaldehyde causes metabolic acidosis, hydrofluoric acid causes hypocalcemia and renal damage, oxalic acid causes hypocalcemia, phenol causes hepatic and renal damage, and picric acid causes renal injury.

### Disposition

Infants and small children should be medically evaluated and observed. All symptomatic patients should be admitted. If they have severe symptoms or danger of airway compromise, they should be admitted to the intensive care unit. After endoscopy, if no damage is detected, the patient may be discharged when he or she can tolerate oral feedings. Intentional exposures require psychiatric evaluation before the patient can be discharged.

## COCAINE (BENZOYLMETHYLECGONINE)

Cocaine is derived from the leaves of *Erythroxylum coca* and *Truxillo coca*. "Body packing" refers to the placement of many small packages of contraband cocaine for concealment in the gastrointestinal tract or other areas for illicit transport. "Body stuffing" refers to spontaneous ingestion of substances for the purpose of hiding evidence.

### Toxic Mechanism

Cocaine directly stimulates the CNS presynaptic sympathetic neurons to release catecholamines and acetylcholine, while it blocks the presynaptic reuptake of the catecholamines; it blocks the sodium channels along neuronal membranes; and it increases platelet aggregation. Long-term use depletes the CNS of dopamine.

### Toxic Dose

The maximum mucosal local anesthetic therapeutic dose of cocaine is 200 mg or 2 mL of a 10% solution. Although CNS effects can occur at relatively low local anesthetic doses (50 to 95 mg), they are more common with doses greater than 1 mg/kg; cardiac effects can occur with doses greater than 1 mg/kg. The potential fatal dose is 1200 mg intranasally, but death has occurred with 20 mg parenterally.

### Kinetics

Cocaine is well absorbed by all routes, including nasal insufflation, and oral, dermal, and inhalation routes (Table 14). Protein binding is 8.7%, and volume distribution is 1.5 L/kg.

Cocaine is metabolized by plasma and liver cholinesterase to the inactive metabolites ecgonine methyl ester and benzoylecgonine. Plasma pseudocholinesterase is congenitally deficient in 3% of the population and decreased in fetuses, young infants, the elderly, pregnant people, and people with liver disease. These enzyme-deficient individuals are at increased risk for life-threatening cocaine toxicity.

Ten percent of cocaine is excreted unchanged. Cocaine and ethanol undergo liver synthesis to form cocaethylene, a metabolite with a half-life three times longer than that of cocaine. It may account for some of cocaine's cardiotoxicity and appears to be more lethal than cocaine or ethanol alone.

### Manifestations

The CNS manifestations of cocaine ingestion are euphoria, hyperactivity, agitation, convulsions, and intracranial hemorrhage. Mydriasis and septal perforation can occur, as well as cardiac dysrhythmias, hypertension, and hypotension (with severe overdose). Chest pain is frequent, but only 5.8% of patients have true myocardial ischemia and infarction. Other manifestations include vasoconstriction, hyperthermia (because of increased metabolic rate), ischemic bowel perforation if the substance is ingested, rhabdomyolysis, myoglobinuria, and renal failure. In pregnant users, premature labor and abruptio placentae can occur.

Body cavity packing should be suspected in cases of prolonged toxicity.

Mortality can result from cerebrovascular accidents, coronary artery spasm, myocardial injury, or lethal dysrhythmias.

### Laboratory Investigations

Monitoring of the ECG and cardiac rhythms, ABG, oxygen saturation, electrolytes, blood glucose, BUN, creatinine, and creatine kinase levels should be maintained. One should monitor cardiac fraction if the patient has chest pain, as well as the liver profile, and the urine for myoglobin. Intravenous drug users should have HIV and hepatitis virus testing.

**TABLE 14  The Different Routes and Kinetics of Cocaine**

| Type | Route | Onset | Peak (min) | Half-life (min) | Duration (min) |
|------|-------|-------|-----------|-----------------|----------------|
| Cocaine leaf | Oral, chewing | 20-30 min | 45-90 | NA | 240-360 |
| Hydrochloride | Insufflation | 1-3 min | 5-10 | 78 | 60-90 |
|  | Ingestion | 20-30 min | 50-90 | 54 | Sustained |
|  | Intravenous | 30-120 sec | 5-11 | 36 | 60-90 |
| Free base/crack | Smoking | 5-10 sec | 5-11 | — | Up to 20 |
| Coca paste | Smoking | Unknown | — | — | — |

Urine should be tested for cocaine and metabolites and other substances of abuse, and abdominal radiographs or ultrasonogram should be ordered for body packers. If the urine sample was collected more than 12 hours after cocaine intake, it will contain little or no cocaine. If cocaine is present, cocaine has been used within the past 12 hours. Cocaine's metabolite benzoylecgonine may be detected within 4 hours after a single nasal insufflation and for up to 114 hours. Cross-reactions with some herbal teas, lidocaine, and droperidol (Inapsine) may give false-positive results by some immunoassay methods.

## Management

Supportive care includes blood pressure, cardiac, and thermal monitoring and seizure precautions. Diazepam (Valium) is the drug of choice for treatment of cocaine toxicity agitation, seizures, and dysrhythmias; doses are 10 to 30 mg intravenously at 2.5 mg per minute for adults and 0.2 to 0.5 mg/kg at 1 mg per minute up to 10 mg for a child.

Gastrointestinal decontamination should be instituted, if the cocaine was ingested, by administration of activated charcoal. MDAC may adsorb cocaine leakage in body stuffers or body packers. Whole-bowel irrigation with polyethylene glycol solution (PEG) has been used in body packers and stuffers if the contraband is in a firm container. If the packages are not visible on plain radiographs of the abdomen, a contrast study or CT scan can help to confirm successful passage. Cocaine in the nasal passage can be removed with an applicator dipped in a non–water-soluble product (lubricating jelly) if this is done within a few minutes after application.

In body packers and stuffers, venous access must be secured, and drugs must be readily available for treating life-threatening manifestations until the contraband is passed in the stool. Surgical removal may be indicated if the packet does not pass the pylorus, in an asymptomatic body packer, or in the case of intestinal obstruction.

Hypertension and tachycardia are usually transient and can be managed by careful titration of diazepam. Nitroprusside may be used for severe hypertension. Myocardial ischemia is managed by oxygen, vascular access, benzodiazepines, and nitroglycerin. Aspirin and thrombolysis are not routinely recommended because of the danger of intracranial hemorrhage.

Dysrhythmias are usually supraventricular (SVT) and do not require specific management. Adenosine is ineffective. Life-threatening tachydysrhythmias may respond to phentolamine (Regitine) 5 mg IV bolus in adults or 0.1 mg/kg in children at 5- to 10-minute intervals. Phentolamine also relieves coronary artery spasm and myocardial ischemia. Electrical synchronized cardioversion should be considered for patients with hemodynamically unstable dysrhythmias. Lidocaine is not recommended initially but may be used after 3 hours for ventricular tachycardia. Wide complex QRS ventricular tachycardia may be treated with sodium bicarbonate 2 mEq/kg as a bolus. β-Adrenergic blockers are not recommended.

Anxiety, agitation, and convulsions can be treated with diazepam. If diazepam fails to control seizures, neuromuscular blockers can be used. The EEG should be monitored for nonmotor seizure activity. For hyperthermia, external cooling and cool humidified 100% oxygen should be administered. Neuromuscular paralysis to control seizures will reduce temperature. Dantrolene and antipyretics are not recommended. Rhabdomyolysis and myoglobinuria are treated with fluids, alkaline diuresis, and diuretics.

If the patient is pregnant, the fetus must be monitored and the patient observed for spontaneous abortion.

Paranoid ideation and threatening behavior should be treated with rapid tranquilization. The patient should be observed for suicidal depression that may follow intoxication and may require suicide precautions. If focal neurologic manifestations are present, one should consider the possibility of a cerebrovascular accident and obtain a CT scan.

Extracorporeal clearance techniques are of no benefit.

## Disposition

Patients with mild intoxication or a brief seizure that does not require treatment who become asymptomatic may be discharged after 6 hours with appropriate psychosocial follow-up. If cardiac or cerebral ischemic manifestations are present, the patient should be monitored in the intensive care unit. Body packers and stuffers require care in the intensive care unit until passage of the contraband.

## CYANIDE

Hydrogen cyanide is a byproduct of burning plastic and wools in residential fires. Hydrocyanic acid is the liquefied form of hydrogen cyanide. Cyanide salts can be found in ore extraction. Nitriles, such as acetonitrile (artificial nail removers) are metabolized in the body to produce cyanide. Cyanogenic glycosides are present in some fruit seeds (such as amygdalin in apricots, peaches, and apples). Sodium nitroprusside, the antihypertensive vasodilator, contains five cyanide groups.

### Toxic Mechanism

Cyanide blocks the cellular electron transport mechanism and cellular respiration by inhibiting the mitochondrial ferricytochrome oxidase system and other enzymes. This results in cellular hypoxia and lactic acidosis. *Note:* Citrus fruit seeds form cyanide in the presence of intestinal β-glucosidase (the seeds are harmful only if the capsule is broken).

### Toxic Dose

The ingestion of 1 mg/kg or 50 mg of hydrogen cyanide can produce death within 15 minutes. The lethal dose of potassium cyanide is 200 mg. Five to 10 mL of 84% acetonitrile is lethal. Infusions of sodium nitroprusside in rates above 2 μg/kg per minute may cause cyanide to accumulate to toxic concentrations in critically ill patients.

### Kinetics

Cyanide is rapidly absorbed by all routes. In the stomach, it forms hydrocyanic acid. Volume distribution is 1.5 L/kg. Protein binding is 60%. Cyanide is detoxified by metabolism in the liver via the mitochondrial thiosulfate-rhodanase pathway, which catalyzes the transfer of sulfur donor to cyanide, forming the less toxic irreversible thiocyanate that is excreted in the urine. Cyanide is also detoxified by reacting with hydroxocobalamin (vitamin $B_{12a}$) to form cyanocobalamin (vitamin $B_{12}$).

The cyanide elimination half-life from the blood is 1.2 hours. The elimination route is through the lungs.

### Manifestations

Hydrogen cyanide has the distinctive odor of bitter almonds or silver polish. Manifestations of cyanide intoxication include hypertension, cardiac dysrhythmias, various ECG abnormalities, headache, hyperpnea, seizures, stupor, pulmonary edema, and flushing. Cyanosis is absent or appears late.

### Laboratory Investigations

The examiner should obtain and monitor ABGs, oxygen saturation, blood lactate, hemoglobin, blood glucose, and electrolytes. Lactic acidemia, a decrease in the arterial-venous oxygen difference, and bright red venous blood occurs. If smoke inhalation is the possible source of cyanide exposure, CoHB and methemoglobin (MetHb) concentrations should be measured.

Cyanide levels in whole blood, red blood cells, or serum are not useful in the acute management because the determinations are not readily available. Specific cyanide blood levels are as follows: smokers have less than 0.5 μg/mL; a patient with flushing and tachycardia has 0.5 to 1.0 μg/mL, one with obtundation has 1.0 to 2.5 μg/mL, and one in coma or who has died has more than 2.5 μg/mL.

### Management

If the cyanide was inhaled, the patient must be removed from the contaminated atmosphere. Attendants should not administer mouth-to-mouth resuscitation. Rescuers and attendants must be protected. Immediate administration of 100% oxygen is called for and oxygen should be continued during and after the administration of the antidote. The clinician must decide whether to use any or all components of the cyanide antidote kit.

The mechanism of action of the antidote kit is twofold: to produce methemoglobinemia and to provide a sulfur substrate for the detoxification of cyanide. The nitrites make methemoglobin, which has a greater affinity for cyanide than does the cytochrome oxidase enzymes. The combination of methemoglobin and cyanide forms cyanomethemoglobin. Sodium thiosulfate provides a sulfur substrate for the rhodanese enzyme, which converts cyanide into the relatively nontoxic sodium thiocyanate, which is excreted by the kidney.

The procedure for using the antidote kit is as follows:

Step 1: Amyl nitrite inhalant perles is only a temporizing measure (forms only 2% to 5% methemoglobin) and it can be omitted if venous access is established. Alternate 100% oxygen and the inhalant for 30 seconds each minute. Use a new perle every 3 minutes.

Step 2: Sodium nitrite ampule is indicated for cyanide exposures, except for cases of residential fires, smoke inhalation, and nitroprusside or acetonitrile poisonings. It is administered intravenously to produce methemoglobin of 20% to 30% at 35 to 70 minutes after administration. A dose of 10 mL of 3% solution of sodium nitrite for adults and 0.33 mL/kg of 3% solution for children is diluted to 100 mL 0.9% saline and administered slowly intravenously at 5 mL/min. If hypotension develops, the infusion should be slowed.

Step 3: Sodium thiosulfate is useful alone in cases of smoke inhalation, nitroprusside toxicity, and acetonitrile toxicity and should not be used at all in cases of hydrogen sulfide poisoning. The administration dose is 12.5 g of sodium thiosulfate or 50 mL of 25% solution for adults and 1.65 mL/kg of 25% solution for children intravenously over 10 to 20 minutes.

If cyanide symptoms recur, further treatment with nitrites or the perles is controversial. Some authorities suggest repeating the antidotes in 30 minutes at half of the initial dose, but others do not advise this for lack of efficacy. The child dosage regimen on the package insert must be carefully followed.

One hour after antidotes are administered, the methemoglobin level should be obtained and should not exceed 20%. Methylene blue should not be used to reverse excessive methemoglobin.

Gastrointestinal decontamination of oral ingestion by activated charcoal is recommended but is not very effective because of the rapidity of absorption. Seizures are treated with intravenous diazepam. Acidosis should be treated with sodium bicarbonate if it does not rapidly resolve with therapy. There is no role for hyperbaric oxygen or hemodialysis or hemoperfusion.

Other antidotes include hydroxocobalamin (vitamin $B_{12a}$) (Cyanokit), which has proven effective when given immediately after exposure in large doses of 4 g (50 mg/kg) or 50 times the amount of cyanide exposure with 8 g of sodium thiosulfate. Hydroxocobalamin has FDA orphan drug approval.

## Disposition

Asymptomatic patients should be observed for a minimum of 3 hours. Patients who ingest nitrile compounds must be observed for 24 hours. Patients requiring antidote administration should be admitted to the intensive care unit.

## DIGITALIS

Cardiac glycosides are found in cardiac medications, common plants, and the skin of the Bufo toad.

## Toxic Mechanism

Cardiac glycosides inhibit the enzyme sodium/potassium-adenosine triphosphatase (NA+, K+, ATPase), leading to intracellular potassium loss and increased intracellular sodium, and producing phase 4 depolarization, increased automaticity, and ectopy. There is increased intracellular calcium and potentiation of contractility. Pacemaker cells are inhibited, and the refractory period is prolonged, leading to atrioventricular blocks. There is increased vagal tone.

## Toxic Dose

Digoxin total digitalizing dose, the dose required to achieve therapeutic blood levels of 0.6 to 2.0 ng/mL, is 0.75 to 1.25 mg or 10 to 15 μg/kg for patients older than 10 years of age; 40 to 50 μg/kg for patients younger than 2 years of age; and 30 to 40 μg/kg for patients 2 to 10 years of age.

The acute single toxic dose is greater than 0.07 mg/kg or greater than 2 or 3 mg in an adult, but 2 mg in a child or 4 mg in an adult usually produces only mild toxicity. One to 3 mg or more may be found in a few leaves of oleander or foxglove. Serious and fatal overdoses are more than 4 mg in a child and more than 10 mg in an adult.

Acute digitoxin ingestion of 10 to 35 mg has produced severe toxicity and death. Digitoxin therapeutic steady state is 15 to 25 ng/mL. In cases of chronic or acute-on-chronic ingestions in patients with cardiac disease, more than 2 mg may produce toxicity; however, toxicity can develop within therapeutic range on chronic therapy.

Patients at greatest risk of overdose include those with cardiac disease, those with electrolyte abnormalities (low potassium, low magnesium, low $T_4$, high calcium), those with renal impairment, and those on amiodarone (Cordarone), quinidine, erythromycin, tetracycline, calcium channel blockers, and β-blockers.

## Kinetics

Digoxin is a metabolite of digitoxin. In cases of oral overdose, the typical onset is 30 minutes, with peak effects in 3 to 12 hours. Duration is 3 to 4 days. Intravenous onset is in 5 to 30 minutes; peak level is immediate, and peak effect is at 1.5 to 3 hours.

Volume distribution is 5 to 6 L/kg. The cardiac-to-plasma ratio is 30:1. After an acute ingestion overdose, the serum concentration is not reflective of tissue concentration for at least 6 hours or more, and steady state is 12 to 16 hours after last dose.

Sixty percent to 80% of the parent compound is excreted unchanged in the urine. The elimination half-life is 30 to 50 hours.

## Manifestations

Onset of manifestations is usually within 2 hours but may be delayed up to 12 hours.

Gastrointestinal effects of nausea and vomiting are frequently present in cases of acute ingestion but may also occur in cases of chronic ingestion. The "digitalis effect" on ECG is scooped ST segments and PR prolongation; in cases of overdose, any dysrhythmia or block is possible but none are characteristic. Bradycardia occurs in patients with acute overdose with healthy hearts; supraventricular tachycardia occurs in patients with existing heart disease or chronic overdose. Ventricular tachycardia is seen only in cases of severe poisoning.

The CNS effects include headaches, visual disturbances, and colored halo vision. Hyperkalemia occurs following acute overdose and correlates with digoxin level and outcome. Among patients with serum potassium levels of less than 5.0 mEq/L, all survive. If the level is 5 to 5.5, 50% survive, and if the level is greater than 5.5, all die. Hypokalemia is commonly seen with chronic intoxication. Patients with normal digitalis levels may have toxicity in the presence of hypokalemia.

Chronic intoxications are more likely to produce scotoma, color perception disturbances, yellow vision, halos, delirium, hallucinations or psychosis, tachycardia, and hypokalemia.

## Laboratory Investigations

Continuous monitoring of ECG, pulse, and blood pressure is called for. Blood glucose, electrolytes, calcium, magnesium, BUN, and creatinine levels should also be monitored. An initial digoxin level should be measured on patient presentation and repeated thereafter. Levels should be measured more than 6 hours postingestion because earlier values do not reflect tissue distribution. Digoxin clinical toxicity is usually associated with serum digoxin levels of greater than 3.5 ng/mL in adults.

An endogenous digoxin-like substance cross-reacts in most common immunoassays (not with high-pressure liquid chromatography) and values as high as 4.1 ng/mL have been reported in newborns, patients with chronic renal failure, patients with abnormal immunoglobulins, and women in the third trimester of pregnancy.

## Management

A cardiology consult should be obtained and a pacemaker should be readily available.

In undertaking gastrointestinal decontamination, excessive vagal stimulation should be avoided (e.g., emesis and gastric lavage). Activated charcoal should be administered, and if a nasogastric tube is required for the activated charcoal, pretreatment with atropine (0.02 mg/kg in children and 0.5 mg in adults) should be considered.

Digoxin-specific antibody fragments (Fab, Digibind) 38 mg binds 0.5 mg digoxin and then is excreted through the kidneys. The onset of action is within 30 minutes. Problems associated with Fab therapy are mainly from withdrawal of digoxin and worsening heart failure, hypokalemia, decrease in glucose (if the patient has low glycogen stores), and allergic reactions (very rare). Digitalis administered after Fab therapy is bound and may be inactivated for 5 to 7 days.

Absolute indications for Fab therapy include the following:

- Life-threatening malignant (hemodynamically unstable) dysrhythmias
- Ventricular dysrhythmias, unstable severe bradycardia, or second- or third-degree blocks unresponsive to atropine or rapid deterioration in clinical status
- Life-threatening digitoxin and oleander poisonings
- Relative indications for Fab therapy include the following:
- Ingestions greater than 4 mg in a child and 10 mg in an adult
- Serum potassium level greater than 5.0 mEq/L
- Serum digoxin level greater than 10 ng/mL in adults or greater than 5 ng/mL in children 6 hours after an acute ingestion
- Digitalis delirium and thrombocytopenia response

Digoxin-specific Fab fragments therapy can be administered as a bolus through a 22-μm filter if the case is a critical emergency. If the case is less urgent, then it can be administered over 30 minutes. An empiric dose is 10 vials in adults and 5 vials in a child for an unknown amount ingested in a symptomatic patient with history of a digoxin overdose.

To calculate the dose in the case of a known ingestion, the following equation is used:

$$\text{Amount (total mg)} \times (0.8) = \text{body burden}$$

If liquid capsules were taken or the substance was given intravenously the 80% bioavailability figure is not used. Instead, the body burden divided by 0.5 (0.5 mg digoxin is bound by 1 vial of 38 mg of Fab) equals the number of vials needed.

If the amount is unknown but the steady state serum concentration is known, the following equations are used:

For digoxin

$$\text{Digoxin ng/mL} \times (5.6 \text{ L/kg Vd}) \times (\text{wt kg}) = \text{mg body burden}$$

$$\text{Body burden} \div 1000 = \text{mg body burden}$$

$$\text{Body burden}/0.5 = \text{number of vials needed}$$

For digitoxin

$$\text{Digitoxin ng/mL} \times (0.56 \text{ L/kg Vd}) \times (\text{wt kg}) = \text{mg body burden}$$

$$\text{Body burden} \div 1000 = \text{mg body burden}$$

$$\text{Body burden}/0.5 = \text{number of vials needed}$$

Antidysrhythmic agents or a pacemaker should be used only if Fab therapy fails. For ventricular tachydysrhythmias, electrolyte disturbances should be corrected by the administration of lidocaine or phenytoin. For torsades de pointes, magnesium sulfate 20 mL 20% IV can be given slowly over 20 minutes (or 25 to 50 mg/kg in a child), titrated to control the dysrhythmia. Magnesium should be discontinued if hypotension, heart block, or decreased deep tendon reflexes are present. Magnesium is used with caution if the patient has renal impairment.

Unstable bradycardia and second-degree and third-degree atrioventricular block should be treated by Fab first. A pacemaker should be available if necessary. Isoproterenol should be avoided because it causes dysrhythmias. Cardioversion is used with caution, starting at a setting of 5 to 10 joules. The patient should be pretreated with lidocaine, if possible, because cardioversion may precipitate ventricular fibrillation or asystole.

Potassium disturbances are caused by a shift, not a change, in total body potassium. Hyperkalemia (>5.0 mEq/L) is treated with Fab only. Calcium must never be used, and insulin/glucose and sodium bicarbonate should not be used concomitantly with Fab because they may produce severe life-threatening hypokalemia. Sodium polystyrene sulfonate (Kayexalate) should not be used. Hypokalemia must be treated with caution because it may be cardioprotective. Treatment can be administered if the patient has ventricular dysrhythmias or a serum potassium level less than 3.0 mEq/L and atrioventricular block.

Extracorporeal procedures are ineffective. Hemodialysis is used for severe or refractory hyperkalemia.

One must never use antidysrhythmic types Ia (procainamide, quinidine, disopyramide [Norpace], amiodarone [Cordarone]), Ic (propafenone [Rythmol], flecainide [Tambocor]), II (β-blockers), or IV (calcium channel blockers). Class Ib drugs (lidocaine, phenytoin [Dilantin], mexiletine [Mexitil], and tocainide [Tonocard]) can be used.

## Disposition

Consultation with a poison control center and a cardiologist experienced with digoxin-specific Fab fragments is warranted. All patients with significant dysrhythmias, symptoms, elevated serum digoxin concentration, or elevated serum potassium level should be admitted to the intensive care unit.

## ETHANOL

Table 15 lists the features of alcohols and glycols.

### Toxic Mechanism

Ethanol has CNS depressant and anesthetic effects. Ethanol stimulates the γ-aminobutyric acid (GABA) system. It promotes cutaneous vasodilation (contributes to hypothermia), stimulates secretion of gastric juice (gastritis), inhibits the secretion of the antidiuretic hormone, inhibits gluconeogenesis (hypoglycemia), and influences fat metabolism (lipidemia).

### Toxic Dose

A dose of 1 mL/kg of absolute ethanol (100% ethanol, or 200 proof) gives a blood ethanol concentration of 100 mg/dL. A potentially fatal dose is 3 g/kg for children or 6 g/kg for adults. Children are more prone to developing hypoglycemia than adults.

### Kinetics

Onset of action is 30 to 60 minutes after ingestion; peak action is 90 minutes on empty stomach. Volume distribution is 0.6 L/kg. The major route of elimination (>90%) is by hepatic oxidative metabolism. The first step is by the enzyme alcohol dehydrogenase, which converts ethanol to acetaldehyde. Alcohol dehydrogenase metabolizes ethanol at a constant rate of 12 to 20 mg/dL/h (12 to 15 mg/dL/h in nondrinkers, 15 to 30 mg/dL/h in social drinkers, 30 to 50 mg/dL/h in

**TABLE 15 Summary of Alcohol and Glycol Features**

|  | Methanol | Isopropanol | Ethanol | Ethylene Glycol |
|---|---|---|---|---|
| Principal uses | Gas line antifreeze, Sterno, windshield de-icer | Solvent, jewelry cleaner, rubbing alcohol | Beverage, solvent | Radiator antifreeze, windshield de-icer |
| Specific gravity | 0.719 | 0.785 | 0.789 | 1.12 |
| Fatal dose | 1 mL/Kg 100% | 3 mL/kg 100% | 5 mL/kg 100% | 1.4 mL/kg |
| Inebriation | ± | 2+ | 2+ | 1+ |
| Metabolic change |  | Hyperglycemia | Hypoglycemia | Hypocalcemia |
| Metabolic acidosis | 4+ | 0 | 1+ | 2+ |
| Anion gap | 4+ | ± | 2+ | 4+ |
| Ketosis | Ketobutyric | Acetone | Hydroxybutyric | None |
| Gastrointestinal tract | Pancreatitis | Hemorrhagic gastritis | Gastritis |  |
| Osmolality* | 0.337 | 0.176 | 0.228 | 0.190 |

*1 mL/dL of substances raises freezing point osmolarity of serum. The validity of the correlation of osmolality with blood concentrations has been questioned.

heavy drinkers, and 25 to 30 mg/dL/h in children). At very low blood ethanol concentration (<30 mg/dL), the metabolism is by first-order kinetics. In the second step, acetaldehyde is metabolized by acetaldehyde dehydrogenase to acetic acid, which is metabolized by the Krebs cycle to carbon dioxide and water. The enzyme steps are nicotinamide adenine dinucleotide-dependent, which interferes with gluconeogenesis. Less than 10% of ethanol is excreted unchanged by the kidneys. The relationship between blood ethanol concentration (BEC) and dose (amount ingested) can be calculated as follows:

$$\text{BEC (mg/dL)} = \text{amount ingested (mL)} \times \% \text{ ethanol product} \times \text{SG (0.79)} / \text{Vd (0.6 L/kg)} \times \text{body wt (kg)}$$

$$\text{Dose (amount ingested)} = \text{BEC (mg/dL)} \times \text{Vd (0.6)} \times \text{body wt (kg)} / \% \text{ ethanol} \times \text{specific gravity (0.79)}$$

## Manifestations

Table 16 lists the clinical signs of acute ethanol intoxication.

Chronic alcoholic patients tolerate higher blood ethanol concentration, and correlation with manifestations is not valid. Rapid interview for alcoholism is the CAGE questions:

- C—Have you felt the need to Cut down?
- A—Have others Annoyed you by criticism of your drinking?
- G—Have you felt Guilty about your drinking?
- E—Have you ever had a morning Eye-opening drink to steady your nerves or get rid of a hangover?

Two affirmative answers indicate probable alcoholism.

## Laboratory Investigations

The blood ethanol concentration should be specifically requested and followed. Gas chromatography or a breathanalyzer test gives rapid reliable results if no belching or vomiting is present. Enzymatic methods do not differentiate between the alcohols. ABG, electrolytes, and glucose should be measured, the anion and osmolar gaps determined (measure by freezing point depression, not vapor pressure), and a check for ketosis made.

## Management

The examiner should inquire about trauma and disulfiram use. The patient must be protected from aspiration and hypoxia. Vital functions must be established and maintained. The patient may require intubation and assisted ventilation.

Gastrointestinal decontamination plays no role in the management of ethanol intoxication.

If the patient is comatose, glucose should be administered intravenously, 1 mL/kg 50% glucose in adults and 2 mL/kg 25% glucose in children. Thiamine, 100 mg intravenously, is administered if the patient has a history of chronic alcoholism, malnutrition, or suspected eating disorders to prevent Wernicke-Korsakoff syndrome. Naloxone (Narcan) has produced a partial inconsistent response but is not recommended for known alcoholics.

General supportive care includes administration of fluids to correct hydration and hypotension and correction of electrolyte abnormalities and acid–base imbalance. Vasopressors and plasma expanders may be necessary to correct severe hypotension. Hypomagnesemia is frequent in chronic alcoholics. In case of hypomagnesemia, a loading dose of 2 g magnesium sulfate 10% is administered by intravenous solution over 5 minutes in the intensive care unit with blood pressure and cardiac monitoring and calcium chloride 10% on hand in case of overdose. This is followed with constant infusion of 6 g of 10% solution over 3 to 4 hours. Caution must be taken with the use of magnesium if renal failure is present.

**TABLE 16 Clinical Signs in the Nontolerant Ethanol Drinker**

| Ethanol Blood Concentration (mg/dL)* | Manifestations |
|---|---|
| >25 | Euphoria |
| >47 | **Mild incoordination,** sensory and motor impairment |
| >50 | Increased risk of motor vehicle accidents |
| >100 | Ataxia (legal toxic level in many localities) |
| >150 | ***Moderate incoordination,*** slow reaction time |
| >200 | Drowsiness and confusion |
| >300 | Severe incoordination, stupor, blurred vision |
| >500 | ***Flaccid coma,*** respiratory failure, hypotension; may be fatal |

*Ethanol concentrations sometimes reported in %.
*Note*: mg% is not equivalent to mg/dL because ethanol weighs less than water (specific gravity 0.79). A 1% ethanol concentration is 790 mg/dL and 0.1% is 79 mg/dL. There is great variation in individual behavior at different blood ethanol levels. Behavior is dependent on tolerance and other factors.

Hypothermic patients should be warmed. See the section on disturbances caused by cold.

Hemodialysis can be used in severe cases when conventional therapy is ineffective (rarely needed).

Repeated or prolonged seizures should be treated with diazepam (Valium). The brief "rum fits" do not need long-term anticonvulsant therapy. Repeated seizures or focal neurologic findings may warrant skull radiographs, lumbar puncture, and CT scan of the head, depending on the clinical findings. Withdrawal is treated with hydration and large doses of chlordiazepoxide (Librium) 50 to 100 mg or diazepam (Valium) 2 to 10 mg intravenously; these doses may be repeated in 2 to 4 hours. Very large doses of benzodiazepines may be required for delirium tremens. Withdrawal can occur in presence of elevated blood ethanol concentration and can be fatal if left untreated.

Chest radiograph is warranted to determine whether aspiration pneumonia is present. Renal and liver function tests and bilirubin level measurement should be made.

## Disposition

Clinical severity (e.g., intubation, assisted ventilation, aspiration pneumonia) should determine the level of hospital care needed. Young children with significant unintentional exposure to ethanol (calculated to reach a blood ethanol concentration of 50 mg/dL) should have blood ethanol concentration obtained and blood glucose levels monitored for hypoglycemia frequently for 4 hours after ingestion. Patients with acute ethanol intoxication seldom require admission unless a complication is present. However, intoxicated patients should not be discharged until they are fully functional (can walk, talk, and think independently), have suicide potential evaluated, have proper disposition environment, and have a sober escort.

## ETHYLENE GLYCOL

Ethylene glycol is found in solvents, de-icers, radiator antifreeze (95%), and air-conditioning units. Ethylene glycol is a sweet-tasting, colorless, water-soluble liquid with a sweet aromatic fragrance.

### Toxic Mechanism

Ethylene glycol is oxidized by alcohol dehydrogenase to glycolaldehyde, which is metabolized to glycolic acid and glyoxylic acid. Glyoxylic acid is metabolized to oxalic acid via a pyridoxine-dependent pathway to glycine and by thiamine and magnesium-dependent pathways to $\alpha$-hydroxy-ketoadipic acid. The metabolites of ethylene glycol produce a profound metabolic acidosis, increased anion gap, hypocalcemia, and oxalate crystals, which deposit in tissues (particularly the kidney).

### Toxic Dose

The ingestion of 0.1 mL/kg 100% ethylene glycol can result in a toxic serum ethylene glycol concentration of 20 mg/dL. Ingestion of 3.0 mL (less than 1 teaspoonful or swallow) of a 100% solution in a 10-kg child or 30 mL of 100% ethylene glycol in an adult produces a serum ethylene glycol concentration of 50 mg/dL, a concentration that requires hemodialysis. The fatal amount is 1.4 mL/kg of 100% solution.

### Kinetics

Absorption is via dermal, inhalation, and ingestion routes. Ethylene glycol is rapidly absorbed from the gastrointestinal tract. Onset is usually in 30 minutes but may be delayed by co-ingestion of food and ethanol. The usual peak level is at 2 hours. Volume distribution is 0.65 to 0.8 L/kg.

For metabolism, see *Toxic Mechanism*.

The half-life of ethylene glycol without ethanol is 3 to 8 hours; with ethanol, it is 17 hours, and with hemodialysis it is 2.5 hours. Renal clearance is 3.2 mL/kg/minute. About 20% to 50% is excreted unchanged in the urine. The relationship between serum ethylene glycol concentration (SEGC) and dose (amount ingested) can be calculated as follows:

$$0.12 \text{ mL/kg of } 100\% = \text{SEGC } 10 \text{ mg/dL}$$

## Manifestations

### Phase I

The onset of manifestations is 30 minutes to several hours longer after ingestion with concomitant ethanol ingestion. The patient may be inebriated. Hypocalcemia, tetany, and calcium oxalate and hippuric acid crystals in urine can be seen within 4 to 8 hours but are not always present. Early, before metabolism of ethylene glycol, an osmolal gap may be present (see *Laboratory Investigations*). Later, the metabolites of ethylene glycol produce changes starting 4 to 12 hours following ingestion, including an anion gap, metabolic acidosis, coma, convulsions, cardiac disturbances, and pulmonary and cerebral edema. Because fluorescein is added to some antifreeze, the presence of fluorescence may be a clue to ethylene glycol exposure. However, it has been shown that fluorescent urine is not a reliable indicator of ethylene glycol ingestion and should not be used as a screen.

### Phase II

After 12 to 36 hours, cardiopulmonary deterioration occurs, with pulmonary edema and congestive heart failure.

### Phase III

Phase III occurs 36 to 72 hours after ingestion, with pulmonary edema and oliguric renal failure from oxalate crystal deposition and tubular necrosis predominating.

### Phase IV

Neurologic sequelae may occur rarely, especially in patients who fail to receive early antidotal therapy. The onset ranges from 6 to 10 days after ingestion. Findings include facial diplegia, hearing loss, bilateral visual disturbances, elevated cerebrospinal fluid pressure with or without elevated protein levels and pleocytosis, vomiting, hyperreflexia, dysphagia, and ataxia.

## Laboratory Investigations

Blood glucose and electrolytes should be monitored. Urinalysis should look for oxalate ("envelope") and monohydrate ("hemp seed") crystals. Urine fluorescence is not reliable as a screen. ABG, ethylene glycol, and ethanol levels, plasma osmolarity (using freezing point depression method), calcium, BUN, and creatinine should be measured. A serum ethylene glycol concentration of 20 mg/dL is toxic (ethylene glycol levels are very difficult to obtain). If possible, a glycolate level should be obtained. Cross-reactions with propylene glycol, a vehicle in many liquids and intravenous medications (phenytoin [Dilantin], diazepam [Valium]), other glycols, and triglycerides may produce spurious ethylene glycol levels. False-positive ethylene glycol values may occur with colorimetric or gas chromatography using an OV-17 column in the presence of propylene glycol.

The following equations can be used to calculate the osmolality, osmolal gap, and ethylene glycol level:

$$2(\text{Na+ mEq/L}) + (\text{Blood glucose mg/dL})/20 + (\text{BUN mg/dL})/3 = \text{Total calculated osmolality (mOsmL/L)}$$

$$\text{Osmolar Gap} = \text{measured osmolality (by freezing point depression method)} - \text{calculated osmolality}$$

A gap greater than 10 is abnormal. *Note:* if ethanol is involved, add ethanol level/4.6 to the calculated equation.

An increased osmolal gap is produced by the following common substances: acetone, dextran, dimethyl sulfoxide, diuretics, ethanol, ethyl ether, ethylene glycol, isopropanol, paraldehyde, mannitol, methanol, sorbitol, and trichloroethane. Table 10 gives the conversion factors for these substances.

Although a specific blood level of ethylene glycol in milligrams per deciliter can be estimated using the equation below, this is not considered to be a reliable method and should not take the place of obtaining a measured ethylene glycol blood concentration.

$$\text{osmolar gap} \times \text{conversion factor} = \text{serum concentration}$$

*Caution:* The accuracy of the ethylene glycol estimated decreases as the ethylene glycol levels decrease. The toxic metabolites are not osmotically active, and patients presenting late may show signs of severe toxicity without an elevated osmolar gap.

The anion gap can be calculated using the following equation:

$$Na - (Cl + HCO_3) = \text{anion gap}$$

The normal gap is 8 to 12. Potassium is not used because it is a small amount and may be hemolyzed. Table 8 lists factors that may account for an increased or a decreased anion gap.

## Management

Vital functions should be established and maintained. The airway must be protected, and assisted ventilation can be used, if necessary. Gastrointestinal decontamination has a limited role. Only gastric aspiration can be used within 60 minutes after ingestion. Activated charcoal is not effective.

Baseline measurements of serum electrolytes and calcium, glucose, ABGs, ethanol, serum ethylene glycol concentration (may be difficult to obtain readily in some institutions), and methanol concentrations should be obtained. In the first few hours, the measured serum osmolality should be determined and compared to calculated osmolality (see osmolality equation, earlier). If seizures occur, one should measure serum calcium (preferably ionized calcium) and treat with intravenous diazepam. If the patient has hypocalcemic seizures, he or she should also be treated with 10 to 20 mL 10% calcium gluconate (0.2 to 0.3 mL/kg in children) slowly intravenously, with the dose repeated as needed. Metabolic acidosis should be corrected with intravenous sodium bicarbonate.

Ethanol therapy should be initiated immediately if fomepizole (Antizol) is unavailable (see next paragraph). Alcohol dehydrogenase has a greater affinity for ethanol than ethylene glycol. Therefore, ethanol blocks the metabolism of ethylene glycol. Ethanol therapy is called for if there is a history of ingestion of 0.1 mL/kg of 100% ethylene glycol, serum ethylene glycol concentration is greater than 20 mg/dL, there is an osmolar gap not accounted for by other alcohols or factors (e.g., hyperlipidemia), metabolic acidosis is present with an increased anion gap, or there are oxalate crystals in the urine. Ethanol should be administered intravenously (the oral route is less reliable) to produce a blood ethanol concentration of 100 to 150 mg/dL. The loading dose is 10 mL/kg of 10% ethanol intravenously, administered concomitantly with a maintenance dose of 10% ethanol of 1.0 mL/kg/h. This dose may need to be increased to 2 mL/kg/h in patients who are heavy drinkers. The blood ethanol concentration should be measured hourly and the infusion rate should be adjusted to maintain a blood ethanol concentration of 100 to 150 mg/dL.

Fomepizole (Antizol, 4-methylpyrazole) inhibits alcohol dehydrogenase more reliability than ethanol and it does not require constant monitoring of ethanol levels and adjustment of infusion rates. Fomepizole is available in 1 g/mL vials of 1.5 mL. The loading dose is 15 mg/kg (0.015 mL/kg) IV; maintenance dose is 10 mg/kg (0.01 mL/kg) every 12 hours for four doses, then 15 mg/kg every 12 hours until the ethylene glycol levels are less than 20 mg/dL. The solution is prepared by being mixed with 100 mL of 0.9% saline or D₅W (5% dextrose in water). Fomepizole can be given to patients requiring hemodialysis but should be dosed as follows:

Dose at the beginning of hemodialysis:

- If <6 hours since last Antizol dose, do not administer dose
- If >6 hours since last dose, administer next scheduled dose

Dosing during hemodialysis:

- Dose every 4 hours

Dosing at the time hemodialysis is completed:

- If <1 hour between last dose and end of dialysis, do not administer dose at end of dialysis
- If 1 to 3 hours between last dose and end of dialysis, administer one half of next scheduled dose
- If >3 hours between last dose and end of dialysis, administer next scheduled dose

Maintenance dosing off hemodialysis:

- Give the next scheduled dose 12 hours from the last dose administered

Hemodialysis is indicated if the ingestion was potentially fatal; if the serum ethylene glycol concentration is greater than 50 mg/dL (some recommend at levels of >25 mg/dL); if severe acidosis or electrolyte abnormalities occur despite conventional therapy; or if congestive heart failure or renal failure is present. Hemodialysis reduces the ethylene glycol half-life from 17 hours on ethanol therapy to 3 hours. Therapy (fomepizole and hemodialysis) should be continued until the serum ethylene glycol concentration is less than 10 mg/dL, the glycolate level is nondetectable (not readily available), the acidosis has cleared, there are no mental disturbances, the creatinine level is normal, and the urinary output is adequate. This may require 2 to 5 days.

Adjunct therapy involving thiamine, 100 mg/d (in children, 50 mg), slowly over 5 minutes intravenously or intramuscularly and repeated every 6 hours and pyridoxine, 50 mg IV or IM every 6 hours, has been recommended until intoxication is resolved, but these agents have not been extensively studied. Folate, 50 mg IV (child 1 mg/kg), can be given every 4 hours for 6 doses.

## Disposition

All patients who have ingested significant amounts of ethylene glycol (calculated level above 20 mg/dL), have a history of a toxic dose, or are symptomatic should be referred to the emergency department and admitted. If the serum ethylene glycol concentration cannot be obtained, the patient should be followed for 12 hours, with monitoring of the osmolal gap, acid–base parameters, and electrolytes to exclude development of metabolic acidosis with an anion gap. Transfer should be considered for fomepizole therapy or hemodialysis.

## HYDROCARBONS

The lower the viscosity and surface tension of hydrocarbons or the greater the volatility, the greater the risk of aspiration. Volatile substance abuse has produced the "Sudden Sniffing's Death Syndrome," most likely caused by dysrhythmias.

### Toxicologic Classification and Toxic Mechanism

All systemically absorbed hydrocarbons can lower the threshold of the myocardium to dysrhythmias produced by endogenous and exogenous catecholamines.

Aliphatic hydrocarbons are branched straight chain hydrocarbons. A few aspirated drops are poorly absorbed from the gastrointestinal tract and produce no systemic toxicity by this route. However, aspiration of very small amounts can produce chemical pneumonitis. Examples of aliphatic hydrocarbons are gasoline, kerosene, charcoal lighter fluid, mineral spirits (Stoddard's solvent), and petroleum naphtha. Mineral seal oil (signal oil), found in furniture polishes, is a low-viscosity and low-volatility oil with minimum absorption that never warrants gastric decontamination. It can produce severe pneumonia if aspirated.

Aromatic hydrocarbons are six carbon ring structures that are absorbed through the gastrointestinal tract. Systemic toxicity includes CNS depression and, in cases of chronic abuse, multiple organ effects such as leukemia (benzene) and renal toxicity (toluene). Examples are benzene, toluene, styrene, and xylene. The seriously toxic ingested dose is 20 to 50 mL in adults.

Halogenated hydrocarbons are aliphatic or aromatic hydrocarbons with one or more halogen substitutions (Cl, Br, Fl, or I). They are highly volatile and are abused as inhalants. They are well absorbed from the gastrointestinal tract, produce CNS depression, and have metabolites that can damage the liver and kidneys. Examples include methylene chloride (may be converted into carbon monoxide in the body), dichloroethylene (also causes a disulfiram [Antabuse] reaction known as "degreaser's flush" when associated with consumption of ethanol), and 1,1,1-trichloroethane (Glamorene Spot Remover, Scotchgard, typewriter correction fluid). An acute lethal oral dose is 0.5 to 5 mL/kg.

Dangerous additives to the hydrocarbons can be summed up with the mnemonic CHAMP: C, camphor (demothing agent); H, halogenated hydrocarbons; A, aromatic hydrocarbons; M, metals (heavy); and P, pesticides. Ingestion of these substances may warrant gastric emptying with a small-bore nasogastric tube.

Heavy hydrocarbons have high viscosity, low volatility, and minimal gastrointestinal absorption, so gastric decontamination is not necessary. Examples are asphalt (tar), machine oil, motor oil (lubricating oil, engine oil), home heating oil, and petroleum jelly (mineral oil).

## Laboratory Investigations

The ECG, ABG, pulmonary function, serum electrolytes, and serial chest radiographs should be continuously monitored. Liver and renal function should be monitored in cases of inhalation of aromatic hydrocarbons.

## Management

Asymptomatic patients who ingested small amounts of aliphatic petroleum distillates can be followed at home by telephone for development of signs of aspiration (cough, wheezing, tachypnea, and dyspnea) for 4 to 6 hours. Inhalation of any hydrocarbon vapors in a closed space can produce intoxication. The victim must be removed from the environment, have oxygen administered, and receive respiratory support.

Gastrointestinal decontamination is not advised in cases of hydrocarbon ingestion that usually do not cause systemic toxicity (aliphatic petroleum distillates, heavy hydrocarbons). In cases of ingestion of hydrocarbons that cause systemic toxicity in small amounts (aromatic hydrocarbons, halogenated hydrocarbons), the clinician should pass a small-bore nasogastric tube and aspirate if the ingestion was within 2 hours and if spontaneous vomiting has not occurred. Some toxicologists advocate ipecac-induced emesis under medical supervision instead of small-bore nasogastric gastric lavage; we do not.

Patients with altered mental status should have their airway protected because of concern about aspiration. The use of activated charcoal has been suggested, but there are no scientific data as to effectiveness and it may produce vomiting. Activated charcoal may, however, be useful in adsorbing toxic additives such as pesticides or co-ingestants.

The symptomatic patient who is coughing, gagging, choking, or wheezing on arrival has probably aspirated. The clinician should provide supportive respiratory care and supplemental oxygen, while monitoring pulse oximetry, ABG, chest radiograph, and ECG. The patient should be admitted to the intensive care unit. A chest radiograph for aspiration may be positive as early as 30 minutes after ingestion, and almost all are positive within 6 hours. Negative chest radiographs within 4 hours do not rule out aspiration.

Bronchospasm is treated with a nebulized β-adrenergic agonist and intravenous aminophylline if necessary. Epinephrine should be avoided because of susceptibility to dysrhythmias. Cyanosis in the presence of a normal arterial PaO$_2$ may be a result of methemoglobinemia that requires therapy with methylene blue. Corticosteroids and prophylactic antimicrobial agents have not been shown to be beneficial. (Fever or leukocytosis may be produced by the chemical pneumonitis itself.)

Most infiltrations resolve spontaneously in 1 week; lipoid pneumonia may last up to 6 weeks. It is not necessary to surgically treat pneumatoceles that develop because they usually resolve. Dysrhythmias may require α- and β-adrenergic antagonists or cardioversion.

There is no role for enhanced elimination procedures.

Methylene chloride is metabolized over several hours to carbon monoxide. See treatment of carbon monoxide poisoning. Halogenated hydrocarbons are hepatorenal toxins; therefore, hepatorenal function should be monitored. *N*-acetylcysteine therapy may be useful if there is evidence of hepatic damage.

Extracorporal membrane oxygenation (ECMO) has been used successfully for a few patients with life threatening respiratory failure. Surfactant used for hydrocarbon aspiration was found to be detrimental.

## Disposition

Asymptomatic patients with small ingestions of petroleum distillates can be managed at home. Symptomatic patients with abnormal chest radiographic, oxygen saturation, or ABG findings should be admitted. Patients who become asymptomatic and have normal oxygenation and a normal repeat radiograph can be discharged.

## IRON

There are more than 100 iron over-the-counter preparations for supplementation and treatment of iron deficiency anemia.

## Toxic Mechanism

Toxicity depends on the amount of elemental iron available in various salts (gluconate 12%, sulfate 20%, fumarate 33%, lactate 19%, chloride 21% of elemental iron), not the amount of the salt. Locally, iron is corrosive and may cause fluid loss, hypovolemic shock, and perforation. Excessive free unbound iron in the blood is directly toxic to the vasculature and leads to the release of vasoactive substances, which produces vasodilation. In cases of overdose, iron deposits injure mitochondria in the liver, the kidneys, and the myocardium. The exact mechanism of cellular damage is not clear but is thought to be related to free radical formation.

## Toxic Dose

The therapeutic dose is 6 mg/kg/d of elemental iron. An elemental iron dose of 20 to 40 mg/kg may produce mild self-limited gastrointestinal symptoms, 40 to 60 mg/kg produces moderate toxicity, more than 60 mg/kg produces severe toxicity and is potentially lethal, and more than 180 mg/kg is usually fatal without treatment. Children's chewable vitamins with iron have between 12 and 18 mg of elemental iron per tablet or 0.6 mL of liquid drops. These preparations rarely produce toxicity unless very large quantities are ingested and have never caused death.

## Kinetics

Absorption occurs chiefly in the upper small intestine. Ferrous (+2) iron is absorbed into the mucosal cells, where it is oxidized to the ferric (+3) state and bound to ferritin. Iron is slowly released from ferritin into the plasma, where it binds to transferrin and is transported to specific tissues for production of hemoglobin (70%), myoglobin (5%), and cytochrome. About 25% of iron is stored in the liver and spleen. In cases of overdose, larger amounts of iron are absorbed because of direct mucosal corrosion. There is no mechanism for the elimination of iron (elimination is 1 to 2 mg/d) except through bile, sweat, and blood loss.

## Manifestations

Serious toxicity is unlikely if the patient remains asymptomatic for 6 hours and has a negative abdominal radiograph. Iron intoxication can produce five phases of toxicity. The phases may not be distinct from one another.

### Phase I

Gastrointestinal mucosal injury occurs 30 minutes to 12 hours postingestion. Vomiting starts within 30 minutes to 1 hour of ingestion and is persistent; hematemesis and bloody diarrhea may occur; abdominal cramps, fever, hyperglycemia, and leukocytosis may occur. Enteric-coated tablets may pass through the stomach without causing symptoms. Acidosis and shock can occur within 6 to 12 hours.

### Phase II

A latent period of apparent improvement occurs over 8 to 12 hours postingestion.

### Phase III

Systemic toxicity phase occurs 12 to 48 hours postingestion with cardiovascular collapse and severe metabolic acidosis.

### Phase IV

Two to 4 days postingestion, hepatic injury associated with jaundice, elevated liver enzymes, and prolonged prothrombin time occur. Kidney injury with proteinuria and hematuria occur. Pulmonary edema, disseminated intravascular coagulation, and *Yersinia enterocolitica* sepsis can occur.

### Phase V

Four to 8 weeks postingestion, pyloric outlet or intestinal stricture may cause obstruction or anemia secondary to blood loss.

## Laboratory Investigations

Iron poisoning produces anion gap metabolic acidosis. Monitoring should include complete blood cell counts, blood glucose level, serum iron, stools and vomitus for occult blood, electrolytes, acid–base balance, urinalysis and urinary output, liver function tests, and BUN and creatinine levels. Blood type and match should be obtained.

Serum iron measurements taken at the proper time correlate with the clinical findings. The lavender top Vacutainer tube contains EDTA, which falsely lowers serum iron. One must obtain the serum iron measurement before administering deferoxamine. Serum iron levels of less than 350 $\mu$g/dL at 2 to 6 hours predict an asymptomatic course; levels of 350 to 500 $\mu$g/dL are usually associated with mild gastrointestinal symptoms; those greater than 500 $\mu$g/dL have a 20% risk of shock and serious iron toxicity. A follow-up serum iron measurement after 6 hours may not be elevated even in cases of severe poisoning, but a serum iron measurement taken at 8 to 12 hours is useful to exclude delayed absorption from a bezoar or sustained-release preparation. The total iron-binding capacity is not necessary.

Adult iron tablet preparations are radiopaque before they dissolve by 4 hours postingestion. A "negative" abdominal radiograph more than 4 hours postingestion does not exclude iron poisoning.

Patients who develop high fevers and signs of sepsis following iron overdose should have blood and stool cultures checked for *Yersinia enterocolitica*.

## Management

Gastrointestinal decontamination should involve immediate induction of emesis in cases of ingestions of elemental iron of greater than 40 mg/kg if vomiting has not already occurred. Activated charcoal is ineffective. An abdominal radiograph should be obtained after emesis to determine the success of gastric emptying. Children's chewable vitamins and liquid iron preparations are not radiopaque. If radiopaque iron is still present, whole-bowel irrigation with polyethylene glycol solution should be considered. In extreme cases, removal by endoscopy or surgery may be necessary because coalesced iron tablets produce hemorrhagic infarction in the bowel and perforation peritonitis.

Deferoxamine (Desferal) in a dose of about 100 mg binds 8.5 to 9.35 mg of free iron in the serum. The deferoxamine infusion should not exceed 15 mg/kg/h or 6 g daily, but faster rates (up to 45 mg/kg) and larger daily amounts have been administered and tolerated in extreme cases of iron poisoning (>1000 mg/dL). The deferoxamine-iron complex is hemodialyzable if renal failure develops.

Indications for chelation therapy are any of the following:

- Very large, symptomatic ingestions
- Serious clinical intoxication (severe vomiting and diarrhea [often bloody], severe abdominal pain, metabolic acidosis, hypotension, or shock)
- Symptoms that persist or progress to more serious toxicity
- Serum iron level greater than 500 mg/dL

Chelation should be performed as early as possible within 12 to 18 hours to be effective. One should start the infusion slowly and gradually increase to avoid hypotension.

Adult respiratory distress syndrome has developed in patients with high doses of deferoxamine for several days; infusions longer than 24 hours should be avoided.

The endpoint of treatment is when the patient is asymptomatic and the urine clears if it was originally a positive "vin rosé" color.

For supportive therapy, intravenous bicarbonate may be needed to correct the metabolic acidosis. Hypotension and shock treatment may require volume expansion, vasopressors, and blood transfusions. The physician should attempt to keep the urinary output at greater than 2 mL/kg/h. Coagulation abnormalities and overt bleeding require blood products or vitamin K. Pregnant patients are treated in a fashion similar to any other patient with iron poisoning.

Hemodialysis and hemoperfusion are ineffective. Exchange transfusion has been used in single cases of massive poisonings in children.

## Disposition

The asymptomatic or minimally symptomatic patient should be observed for persistence and progression of symptoms or development of toxicity signs (gastrointestinal bleeding, acidosis, shock, altered mental state). Patients with mild self-limited gastrointestinal symptoms who become asymptomatic or have no signs of toxicity for 6 hours are unlikely to have a serious intoxication and can be discharged after psychiatric clearance, if needed. Patients with moderate or severe toxicity should be admitted to the intensive care unit.

## ISONIAZID

Isoniazid is a hydrazide derivative of vitamin $B_3$ (nicotinamide) and is used as an antituberculosis drug.

### Toxic Mechanism

Isoniazid produces pyridoxine deficiency by increasing the excretion of pyridoxine (vitamin $B_6$) and by inhibiting pyridoxal 5-phosphate (the active form of pyridoxine) from acting with L-glutamic acid decarboxylase to form $\gamma$-aminobutyric acid (GABA), the major CNS neurotransmitter inhibitor, resulting in seizures. Isoniazid also blocks the conversion of lactate to pyruvate, resulting in profound and prolonged lactic acidosis.

### Toxic Dose

The therapeutic dose is 5 to 10 mg/kg (maximum 300 mg) daily. A single acute dose of 15 mg/kg lowers the seizure threshold; 35 to 40 mg/kg produces spontaneous convulsions; more than 80 mg/kg produces severe toxicity. A fatal dose in adults is 4.5 to 15 g. The malnourished patients, those with a previous seizure disorder, alcoholic patients, and slow acetylators are more susceptible to isoniazid toxicity. In cases of chronic intoxication, 10 mg/kg/d produces hepatitis in 10% to 20% of patients but less than 2% at doses of 3 to 5 mg/kg/d.

### Kinetics

Absorption from intestine occurs in 30 to 60 minutes, and onset is in 30 to 120 minutes, with peak levels of 5 to 8 $\mu$g/mL within 1 to 2 hours. Volume distribution is 0.6 L/kg, with minimal protein binding.

Elimination is by liver acetylation to a hepatotoxic metabolite, acetyl-isoniazid, which is then hydrolyzed to isonicotinic acid. In slow acetylators, isoniazid has a half-life of 140 to 460 minutes (mean 5 hours), and 10% to 15% is eliminated unchanged in the urine. Most (45% to 75%) whites and 50% of African blacks are slow acetylators, and, with chronic use (without pyridoxine supplements), they may develop peripheral neuropathy. In fast acetylators, isoniazid has a half-life of 35 to 110 minutes (mean 80 minutes), and 25% to 30% is excreted unchanged in the urine. About 90% of Asians and patients with diabetes mellitus are fast acetylators and may develop hepatitis on chronic use.

In patients with overdose and hepatic disease, the serum half-life may increase. Isoniazid inhibits the metabolism of phenytoin (Dilantin), diazepam, phenobarbital, carbamazepine (Tegretol), and prednisone. These drugs also interfere with the metabolism of isoniazid. Ethanol may decrease the half-life of isoniazid but increase its toxicity.

## Manifestations

Within 30 to 60 minutes, nausea, vomiting, slurred speech, dizziness, visual disturbances, and ataxia are present. Within 30 to 120 minutes, the major clinical triad of severe overdose includes refractory convulsions (90% of overdose patients have one or more seizures), coma, and resistant severe lactic acidosis (secondary to convulsions), often with a plasma pH of 6.8.

## Laboratory Investigations

Isoniazid produces anion gap metabolic acidosis. Therapeutic levels are 5 to 8 μg/mL and acute toxic levels are greater than 20 μg/mL. These levels are not readily available to assist in making decisions in acute overdose situations. One should monitor the blood glucose (often hyperglycemia), electrolytes (often hyperkalemia), bicarbonate, ABGs, liver function tests (elevations occur with chronic exposure), BUN, and creatinine.

## Management

Seizures must be controlled. Pyridoxine and diazepam should be administered concomitantly through different IV sites. Pyridoxine (vitamin $B_6$) is given in a dose of 1 g for each gram of isoniazid ingested. If the dose ingested is unknown, at least 5 g of pyridoxine should be given intravenously. Pyridoxine is administered in 50 mL $D_5W$ or 0.9% saline over 5 minutes intravenously. It must not be administered in the same bottle as sodium bicarbonate. Intravenous pyridoxine is repeated every 5 to 20 minutes until the seizures are controlled. Total doses of pyridoxine up to 52 g have been safely administered; however, patients given 132 and 183 g of pyridoxine have developed a persistent crippling sensory neuropathy.

Diazepam is administered concomitantly with pyridoxine but at a different site. They work synergistically. Diazepam should be administered intravenously slowly, 0.3 mg/kg at a rate of 1 mg/min in children or 10 mg at a rate of 5 mg/min in adults. After the seizures are controlled, the remainder of the pyridoxine is administered (1 g/1 g isoniazid) or a total dose of 5 g.

Phenobarbital or phenytoin is ineffective and should not be used.

In asymptomatic patients or patients without seizures, pyridoxine has been advised by some toxicologists prophylactically in gram-for-gram doses in cases of large overdoses (<80 mg/kg per dose) of isoniazid, although there are no studies to support this recommendation. In comatose patients, pyridoxine administration may result in the patient's rapid regaining of consciousness. Correction of acidosis may occur spontaneously with pyridoxine administration and correction of the seizures. Sodium bicarbonate should be administered if acidosis persists.

Hemodialysis is rarely needed because of antidotal therapy and the short half-life of isoniazid, but it may be used as an adjunct for cases of uncontrollable acidosis and seizures. Hemoperfusion has not been adequately evaluated. Diuresis is ineffective.

## Disposition

Asymptomatic or mildly symptomatic patients who become asymptomatic can be observed in the emergency department for 4 to 6 hours. Larger amounts of isoniazid may warrant pyridoxine administration and longer periods of observation. Intentional ingestions necessitate psychiatric evaluation before the patient is discharged. Patients with convulsions or coma should be admitted to the intensive care unit.

## ISOPROPANOL (ISOPROPYL ALCOHOL)

Isopropanol can be found in rubbing alcohol, solvents, and lacquer thinner. Coma has occurred in children sponged for fever with isopropanol. See Table 10 for ethanol features of alcohols and glycols.

### Toxic Mechanism

Isopropanol is a gastric irritant. It is metabolized to acetone, a CNS and myocardial depressant. It inhibits gluconeogenesis. Normal propyl alcohol is related to isopropyl alcohol but is more toxic.

### Toxic Dose

A toxic dose of 0.5 to 1 mg/kg of 70% isopropanol (1 mL/kg of 70%) produces a blood isopropanol plasma concentration of 70 mg/dL. The CNS depressant potency is twice that of ethanol.

### Kinetics

Onset of action is within 30 to 60 minutes, and peak is 1 hour postingestion. Volume distribution is 0.6 kg/L. Isopropyl alcohol metabolizes to acetone. Its excretion is renal.

*Note:* The serum isopropyl concentration and amount ingested can be estimated using the same equation as is used in ethanol kinetics and substituting the specific gravity of 0.785 for isopropyl alcohol.

### Manifestations

Ethanol-like inebriation occurs, with an acetone odor to the breath, gastritis, occasionally with hematemesis, acetonuria, and acetonemia without systemic acidosis.

Depression of the CNS occurs: lethargy at blood isopropyl alcohol levels of 50 to 100 mg/dL, coma at levels of 150 to 200 mg/dL, potentially death in adults at levels greater than 240 mg/dL.

Hypoglycemia and seizures may occur.

### Laboratory Investigation

Monitoring of blood isopropyl alcohol levels (not readily available in all institutions), acetone, glucose, and ABG should be maintained. The osmolal gap increases 1 mOsm per 5.9 mg/dL of isopropyl alcohol and 1 mOsm per 5.5 mg/dL of acetone. The absence of excess acetone in the blood (normal is 0.3 to 2 mg/dL) within 30 to 60 minutes or excess acetone in the urine within 3 hours excludes the possibility of significant isopropanol exposure.

### Management

The airway must be protected with intubation, and assisted ventilation administered if necessary. If the patient is hypoglycemic, glucose should be administered. Supportive treatment is similar to that for ethanol ingestions.

Gastrointestinal decontamination has no role in the treatment of isopropanol ingestion. Hemodialysis is warranted in cases of life-threatening overdose but is rarely needed. A nephrologist should be consulted if the bloodisopropanol plasma concentration is greater than 250 mg/dL.

### Disposition

Symptomatic patients with concentrations greater than 100 mg/dL require at least 24 hours of close observation for resolution and

## TABLE 17 Occupations Associated with Lead Exposure

| | |
|---|---|
| Lead production or smelting | Demolition of ships |
| Production of illicit whiskey | and bridges |
| Brass, copper, and lead | Battery manufacturing |
| foundries | Machining/grinding lead |
| Radiator repair | alloys |
| Scrap handling | Welding of old painted |
| Sanding of old paint | metals |
| Lead soldering | Thermal paint stripping |
| Cable stripping | of old buildings |
| Worker or janitor at a firing | Ceramic glaze/pottery |
| range | mixing |

Modified from Rempel D: The lead-exposed worker. JAMA 262:533, 1989.

## TABLE 18 CDC Questionnaire: Priority Groups for Lead Screening

1. Children age 6–72 months (was 12–36 months) who live in or are frequent visitors to older, deteriorated housing built before 1960.
2. Children age 6–72 months who live in housing built prior to 1960 with recent, ongoing, or planned renovation or remodeling.
3. Children age 6–72 months who are siblings, housemates, or playmates of children with known lead poisoning.
4. Children age 6–72 months whose parents or other household members participate in a lead-related industry or hobby.
5. Children age 6–72 months who live near active lead smelters, battery recycling plants, or other industries likely to result in atmospheric lead release.

should be admitted. If the patient is hypoglycemic, hypotensive, or comatose, he or she should be admitted to the intensive care unit.

## LEAD

Acute lead intoxication is rare and usually occurs by inhalation of lead, resulting in severe intoxication and often death. Lead fumes can be produced by burning of lead batteries or use of a heat gun to remove lead paint. Acute lead intoxication also occurs from exposure to high concentrations of organic lead (e.g., tetraethyl lead).

Chronic lead poisoning occurs most often in children 6 months to 6 years of age who are exposed in their environment and in adults in certain occupations (Table 17). In the United States, the prevalence in children aged 1 to 5 years with a venous blood lead greater than 10 µg/dL decreased from 88.2% in a 1976-1980 survey to 8.9% in a 1988-1991 survey as a consequence of measures to reduce lead in the environment, particularly leaded gasoline. However, an estimated 1.7 million children between 1 and 5 years of age and more than 1 million workers in over 100 different occupations still have blood lead levels greater than 10 µg/dL.

### Toxic Dose

In cases of chronic lead poisoning, a daily intake of more than 5 µg/kg/d in children or more than 150 µg/d in adults can give a positive lead balance. In 1991, the Centers for Disease Control and Prevention (CDC) recommended routine screening for all children younger than 6 years of age. In children a venous blood level greater than 10 µg/dL was determined to be a threshold of concern. The average venous blood level in the United States is 4 µg/dL. In cases of occupational exposure (see Table 17), a venous blood level greater than \40 µg/dL is indicative of increased lead absorption in adults.

### Toxic Mechanism

Lead affects the sulfhydryl enzyme systems, the immature CNS, the enzymes of heme synthesis, vitamin D conversion, the kidneys, the bones, and growth. Lead alters the tertiary structure of cell proteins by denaturing them and causing cell death. Risk factors are mouthing behavior of infants and children and excessive oral behavior (pica), living in the inner city, a poorly maintained home, and poor nutrition (e.g., low calcium and iron). The CDC questionnaire given in Table 18 is recommended at every pediatric visit. If any answers to the CDC questionnaire are "positive," a blood screening test for lead should be administered. To be more accurate, however, identifying lead exposure studies have suggested that the questionnaire will have to be modified for each individual community because it has had poor sensitivity (40%) and specificity (60%) as it stands.

Table 19 lists sources of lead. The number one source is deteriorating lead-based paint, which forms leaded dust. Lead concentrations in indoor paint were not reduced to safer (0.06%) levels until 1978. Lead can also be produced by improper interior or exterior home renovation (scraping or demolition). It is found in pre-1960 built homes. The use of leaded gasoline (limited in 1973) resulted in residue from leaded motor vehicle emissions. Lead persists in the soil near major highways and in deteriorating homes and buildings. Vegetables grown in contaminated soil may contain lead.

Oil refineries and lead-processing smelters produce lead residue. Food cans produced in Mexico contain lead solder (95% do not in United States). Lead water pipes (until 1950) and lead solder (until 1986) deliver lead-containing drinking water (calcium deposits, however, may offer some protection). Water at a consumer's tap should contain less than 15 parts per billion (ppb) of lead (Table 20).

For occupational exposure, see Table 17. The Occupational Safety and Health Administration (OSHA) standards require employers to provide showering and clothes changing facilities for personnel working with lead; however, businesses with fewer than 25 employees are exempt from the regulation. The OSHA lead standard of 1978 set a limit of 60 µg/dL for occupational exposure to lead. At a blood lead level of 60 µg/dL, a worker should be removed from lead exposure and not allowed back until his or her lead level is below 40 µg/dL. Many authorities believe that this level should be lower. The lead residue on the clothes of the workers may represent a hazard to the family. Other occupations that are potential sources of lead exposure include plumbers, pipe fitters, lead miners, auto repairers, shipbuilders, printers, steel welders and cutters, construction workers, and rubber product manufacturers.

Leaded pots to make molds for "kusmusha" tea represent lead exposure. Imported pottery lined with ceramic glaze can leach large amounts of lead into acids (e.g., citrus fruit juices).

## TABLE 19 Sources of Lead

| Product | Lead Content (%) by Dry Weight |
|---|---|
| Paint | 0.06 |
| Solder | 0.6 |
| Plastic additives | 2.0 |
| Priming inks | 2.0 |
| Plumbing fixtures | 2.0 |
| Pesticides | 0.1 |
| Stained glass cames | 0.1 |
| Wine bottle foils | 0.1 |
| Construction material | 0.1 |
| Fertilizers | 0.1 |
| Glazes, enamels | 0.06 |
| Toys/recreational games | 0.1 |
| Curtain weights | 0.1 |
| Fishing weights | 0.1 |

## TABLE 20  Agency Regulations and Recommendations Concerning Lead Content

| Agency | Specimen | Level | Comments |
| --- | --- | --- | --- |
| CDC | Blood (child) | 10 µg/dL | Investigate community |
| OSHA | Blood (adult) | 60 µg/dL | Medical removal from work |
| OSHA | Air | 50 µg/m³ | PEL* |
| | Air | 0.75 µg/m³ | Tetraethyl or tetramethyl |
| ACGIH | Air | 150 µg/m³ | TWA† |
| EPA | Air | 1.5 µg/m³ | Three-month average |
| EPA | Water | 15 µg/L (ppb) | 5 ppb circulating |
| EPA | Food | 100 µg/d | Advisory |
| FDA | Wine | 300 ppm | Plan to reduce to 200 ppm |
| EPA | Soil/dust | 50 ppm | |
| CPSC | Paint | 600 ppm (0.06%) by dry weight | |

*Abbreviatons:* ACGIH = American Conference of Governmental Industrial Hygienists; CDC = Centers for Disease Control and Prevention; CPSC = Consumer Product Safety Commission; EPA = Environmental Protection Agency; FDA = Food and Drug Administration; OSHA = Occupational Safety and Health Administration.
*PEL = permissible exposure limit (highest level over an 8-hour workday).
†TWA = time-weighted average (air concentration for 8-hour workday and 40 hour workweek).

Hobbies associated with lead exposure are listed in Box 1. Some "traditional" folk remedies or cosmetics that contain lead include the following:

- "Azarcon por empacho" ("Maria Louisa" 90 to 95% lead trioxide): a bright orange powder used in Hispanic culture, especially Mexican, for digestive problems and diarrhea.
- "Greta" (4% to 90% lead): a yellow powder "por empacho" ("empacho" refers to a variety of gastrointestinal symptoms), used in Hispanic cultures, especially Mexican.
- "Pay-loo-ah": an orange-red powder used for rash and fever in Southeast Asian cultures, especially among Northern Laos Hmong immigrants.
- "Alkohl" (Al-kohl, kohl, suma 5% to 92% lead): a black powder used in Middle Eastern, African, and Asian cultures as a cosmetic and an umbilical stump astringent.
- "Farouk": an orange granular powder with lead used in Saudi Arabian culture.
- "Bint Al Zahab": used to treat colic in Saudi Arabian culture.
- "Surma" (23% to 26% lead): a black powder used in India as a cosmetic and to improve eyesight.
- "Bali goli": a round black bean that is dissolved in "grippe water," used by Asian and Indian cultures to aid digestion.

Cases of substance abuse involving lead poisoning have been reported, in which the patient sniffs leaded gasoline or uses improperly synthesized amphetamines.

## BOX 1  Hobbies Associated with Lead Exposure

Casting of ammunition
Collecting antique pewter
Collecting/painting lead toys (e.g., soldiers and figures)
Ceramics or glazed pottery
Refinishing furniture

Making fishing weights
Home renovation
Jewelry making, lead solder
Glass blowing, lead glass
Bronze casting

Print making and other fine arts (when lead white, flake white, chrome yellow pigments are involved)
Liquor distillation
Hunting and target shooting
Painting
Car and boat repair
Burning/engraving lead-painted wood
Making stained leaded glass
Copper enameling

## Kinetics

Absorption of lead is 10% to 15% of the ingested dose in adults; in children, up to 40% is absorbed, especially in cases of iron deficiency anemia. With inhalation of fumes, absorption is rapid and complete. Volume distribution in blood (0.9% of total body burden) is 95% in red blood cells. Lead passes through the placenta to the fetus and is present in breast milk.

Organic lead is metabolized in the liver to inorganic lead. Its half-life is 35 to 40 days in blood; in soft tissue, the half-life is 45 days and in bone (99% of the lead), the half-life is 28 years. The major elimination route is the stool, 80% to 90%, and then renal 10% (80 g/d) and hair, nails, sweat, and saliva. Nine percent of organic lead is excreted in the urine per day.

## Manifestations

Adverse health effects are given in Table 21 and include the following.

### Hematologic

Lead inhibits γ-aminolevulinic acid dehydratase (early in the synthesis of heme) and ferrochelatase (transfers iron to ferritin for incorporation of iron into protoporphyrin to produce heme). Anemia is a late finding. Decreased heme synthesis starts at >40 µg/dL. Basophilic stippling occurs in 20% of severe lead poisoning.

### Neurologic

Segmental demyelination and peripheral neuropathy, usually of the motor type (wrist and ankle drop), occurs in workers. A venous blood level of lead greater than 70 µg/dL (usually >100 µg/dL), produces encephalopathy in children (symptom mnemonic "PAINT": P, persistent forceful vomiting and papilledema; A, ataxia; I, intermittent stupor and lucidity; N, neurologic coma and refractory convulsions; T, tired and lethargic). Decreased cognitive abilities have been reported with a venous blood level of lead greater than 10 µg/dL, including behavioral problems, decreased attention span, and learning disabilities. IQ scores may begin to decrease at 15 µg/dL. Encephalopathy is rare in adults.

### Renal

Nephropathy as a result of damaged capillaries and glomerulus can occur at a venous blood level of lead greater than 80 µg/dL, but recent studies show renal damage and hypertension with low venous blood levels. A direct correlation between hypertension and venous blood level over 30 µg/dL has been reported. Lead reduces excretion of uric acid, and high-level exposure may be associated with hyperuricemia

## TABLE 21 Summary of Lead-Induced Health Effects in Adults and Children

| Blood Lead Level (µg/dL) | Age Group | Health Effect |
|---|---|---|
| >100 | Adult | Encephalopathic signs and symptoms |
| >80 | Adult | Anemia |
|  | Child | Encephalopathy |
|  |  | Chronic nephropathy (e.g., aminoaciduria) |
| >70 | Adult | Clinically evident peripheral neuropathy |
|  | Child | Colic and other gastrointestinal symptoms |
| >60 | Adult | Female reproductive effects |
|  |  | CNS disturbance symptoms (i.e., sleep disturbances, mood changes, memory and concentration problems, headaches) |
| >50 | Adult | Decreased hemoglobin production |
|  |  | Decreased performance on neurobehavioral tests |
|  | Adult | Altered testicular function |
|  |  | Gastrointestinal symptoms (i.e., abdominal pain, constipation, diarrhea, nausea, anorexia) |
|  | Child | Peripheral neuropathy* |
| >40 | Adult | Decreased peripheral nerve conduction |
|  |  | Hypertension, age 40–59 years |
|  |  | Chronic neuropathy* |
| >25 | Adult | Elevated erythrocyte protoporphyrin in males |
| 15-25 | Adult | Elevated erythrocyte protoporphyrin in females |
| >10 | Child | Decreased intelligence and growth |
|  |  | Impaired learning |
|  |  | Reduced birth weight* |
|  |  | Impaired mental ability |
|  | Fetus | Preterm delivery |

*Controversial.
From Anonymous: Implementation of the Lead Contamination Control Act of 1988. MMWR Morb Mortal Wkly Rep 41:288, 1992.

and "saturnine gout," Fanconi's syndrome (aminoaciduria and renal tubular acidosis), and tubular fibrosis.

### Reproductive

Spontaneous abortion, transient delay in the child's development (catch up at age 5 to 6 years), decreased sperm count, and abnormal sperm morphology can occur with lead exposure. Lead crosses the placenta and fetal blood levels reach 75% to 100% of maternal blood levels. Lead is teratogenic.

### Metabolic

Decreased cytochrome P450 activity alters the metabolism of medication and endogenously produced substances. Decreased activation of cortisol and decreased growth is caused by interference in vitamin conversion (25-hydroxyvitamin D to 1,25 hydroxyvitamin D) at venous blood levels of 20 to 30 µg/dL.

### Other Manifestations

Abnormalities of thyroid, cardiac, and hepatic function occur in adults. Abdominal colic is seen in children at doses greater than 50 µg/dL.

"Lead gum lines" at the dental border of the gingiva can occur in cases of chronic lead poisoning.

### Laboratory Investigations

Serial venous blood lead measurements are taken on days 3 and 5 during treatment and 7 days after chelation therapy, then every 1 to 2 weeks for 8 weeks, and then every month for 6 months. Intravenous infusion should be stopped at least 1 hour before blood lead levels are measured. Table 22 gives a classification of blood lead concentrations in children.

One should evaluate CBC, serum ferritin, erythrocyte protoporphyrin (>35 µg/dL indicates lead poisoning as well as iron deficiency and other causes), electrolytes, serum calcium and phosphorus, urinalysis, BUN, and creatinine. Abdominal and long bone radiographs may be useful in certain circumstances to identify radiopaque material in bowel and "lead lines" in proximal tibia (which occur after prolonged exposure in association with venous blood lead levels greater than 50 µg/dL).

Neuropsychological tests are difficult to perform in young children but should be considered at the end of treatment, especially to determine auditory dysfunction.

### Management

The basis of treatment is removal of the source of lead. Cases of poisoning in children should be reported to local health department and cases of occupational poisoning should be reported to OSHA. The source must be identified and abated, and dust controlled by wet mopping. Cold water should be let to run for 2 minutes before being used for drinking. Planting shrubbery (not vegetables) in contaminated soil will keep children away.

Supportive care should be instituted, including measures to deal with refractory seizures (continued antidotal therapy, diazepam, and possibly neuromuscular blockers), with the hepatic and renal failure, and intravascular hemolysis in severe cases. Seizures are treated with diazepam followed by neuromuscular blockers if needed.

## TABLE 22 Classification of Blood Lead Concentrations in Children

| Blood Lead (µg/dL) | Recommended Interventions |
|---|---|
| <9 | None |
| 10-14 | Community intervention |
|  | Repeat blood lead in 3 months |
| 15-19 | Individual case management |
|  | Environmental counseling |
|  | Nutritional counseling |
|  | Repeat blood lead in 3 months |
| 20-44 | Medical referral |
|  | Environmental inspection/abatement |
|  | Nutritional counseling |
|  | Repeat blood lead in 3 months |
| 45-69 | Environmental inspection/abatement |
|  | Nutritional counseling |
|  | Pharmacologic therapy |
|  | DMSA succimer oral or CaNa₂EDTA parenteral |
|  | Repeat every 2 weeks for 6-8 weeks, then monthly for 4-6 months |
| >70 | Hospitalization in intensive care unit |
|  | Environmental inspection/abatement |
|  | Pharmacologic therapy |
|  | Dimercaprol (BAL in oil) IM initial alone |
|  | Dimercaprol IM and CaNa₂EDTA together |
|  | Repeat every week |

*Abbreviations:* BAL = British anti-Lewisite; CaNa₂EDTA = Edetate calcium disodium; DMS = dimercaptosuccinic acid; IM = intramuscular.

Lead does not bind to activated charcoal. One must not delay chelation therapy for complete gastrointestinal decontamination in severe cases. Whole-bowel irrigation has been used prior to treatment. Some authorities recommend abdominal radiographs followed by gastrointestinal decontamination if necessary before switching to oral therapy. Chelation therapy can be used for patients in whom venous blood level of lead is greater than 45 µg/dL in children and greater than 80 µg/dL in adults or in adults with lower levels who are symptomatic or who have a "positive" lead mobilization test result (not routinely performed at most centers) (Table 23).

Succimer (dimercaptosuccinic acid, DMSA, Chemet), a derivative of British anti-Lewisite (BAL), is an oral agent for chelation in children with a venous blood level of greater than 45 µg/dL. The recommended dose is 10 mg/kg every 8 hours for 5 days, then every 12 hours for 14 days. DMSA is under investigation to determine its role in children with a venous blood level less than 45 µg/dL. Although not approved for adults, it has been used in the same dosage. Monitoring should be maintained by CBC, liver transaminases, and urinalysis for adverse effects.

D-Penicillamine (Cuprimine) is another oral chelator that is given in doses of 20 to 40 mg/kg/d not to exceed 1 g/d. However, it is not FDA approved and has a 10% adverse reaction rate. Nevertheless, D-penicillamine has been used infrequently in adults and children with elevated venous blood lead levels.

Edetate calcium disodium (ethylene diaminetetra-acetic acid or CaNa$_2$EDTA Versenate) is a water-soluble chelator given intramuscularly (with 0.5% procaine) or intravenously. The calcium in the compound is displaced by divalent and trivalent heavy metals, forming a soluble complex, which is stable at physiologic pH (but not at acid pH) and enhances lead clearance in the urine. EDTA usually is administered intravenously, especially in severe cases. It must not be administered until adequate urine flow is established. It may redistribute lead to the brain; therefore, BAL may be given first at a venous blood lead level of greater than 55 µg/dL in children and greater than 100 µg/dL in adults. Phlebitis occurs at a concentration greater than 0.5 mg/mL. Alkalinization of the urine may be helpful. CaNa$_2$EDTA should not be confused with sodium EDTA (disodium edetate), which is used to treat hypercalcemia; inadvertent use may produce severe hypocalcemia.

Dimercaprol (BAL) is a peanut oil–based dithiol (two sulfhydryl molecules) that combines with one atom of lead to form a heterocyclic stable ring complex. It is usually reserved for patients in whom venous blood lead is greater than 70 µg/dL, and it chelates red blood cell lead, enhancing its elimination through the urine and bile. It crosses the blood–brain barrier. Approximately 50% of patients have adverse reactions, including bad metallic taste in the mouth, pain at the injection site, sterile abscesses, and fever.

A venous blood lead level greater than 70 µg/dL or the presence of clinical symptoms suggesting encephalopathy in children is a potentially life-threatening emergency. Management should be accomplished in a medical center with a pediatric intensive care unit by a multidisciplinary team including a critical care specialist, a toxicologist, a neurologist, and a neurosurgeon. Careful monitoring of neurologic status, fluid status, and intracranial pressure should be undertaken if necessary. These patients need close monitoring for hemodynamic instability. Hydration should be maintained to ensure renal excretion of lead. Fluids, renal and hepatic function, and electrolyte levels should be monitored.

While waiting for adequate urine flow, therapy should be initiated with intramuscular dimercaprol (BAL) only (25 mg/kg/d divided into 6 doses). Four hours later, the second dose of BAL should be given intramuscularly, concurrently with CaNa$_2$EDTA 50 mg/kg/d as a single dose infused over several hours or as a continuous infusion. The double therapy is continued until the venous blood level is less than 40 µg/dL.

As long as the venous blood level is greater than 40 µg/dL, therapy is continued for 72 hours and followed by two alternatives: either parenteral therapy with two drugs (CaNa$_2$EDTA and BAL) for 5 days or continuation of therapy with CaNa$_2$EDTA alone if a good response is achieved and the venous blood level of lead is less than 40 µg/dL. If one cannot get the venous blood lead report back, one should continue therapy with both BAL and EDTA for 5 days. In patients with lead encephalopathy, parenteral chelation should be continued with both drugs until the patient is clinically stable before changing therapy. Mannitol and dexa-methasone can reduce the cerebral edema, but their role in lead encephalopathy is not clear. Surgical decompression is not recommended to reduce cerebral edema in these cases.

If BAL and CaNa$_2$EDTA are used together, a minimum of 2 days with no treatment should elapse before another 5-day course of therapy is considered. The 5-day course is repeated with CaNa$_2$EDTA alone if the blood lead level rebounds to greater than 40 µg/dL or in combination with BAL if the venous blood level is greater than 70 µg/dL. If a third course is required, unless there are compelling reasons, one should wait at least 5 to 7 days before administering the course.

Following chelation therapy, a period of equilibration of 10 to 14 days should be allowed and a repeat venous blood lead concentration should be obtained. If the patient is stable enough for oral intake, oral succimer 30 mg/kg/d in three divided doses for 5 days followed by 20 mg/kg/d in two divided doses for 14 days has been suggested, but there are limited data to support this recommendation. Therapy should be continued until venous blood lead level is less than 20 µg/dL in children or less than 40 µg/dL in adults.

Chelators combined with lead are hemodialyzable in the event of renal failure.

### Disposition

All patients with a venous blood lead level of greater than 70 µg/dL or who are symptomatic should be admitted. If a child is hospitalized, all lead hazards must be removed from the home environment before

## TABLE 23 Pharmacologic Chelation Therapy of Lead Poisoning

| Drug | Route | Dose | Duration | Precautions | Monitor |
|------|-------|------|----------|-------------|---------|
| Dimercaprol (BAL in oil) | IM | 3-5 mg/kg q4-6h | 3-5 days | G6PD deficiency Concurrent iron therapy | AST/ALT enzymes |
| CaNa$_2$EDTA (calcium disodium. versenate) | IM/IV | 50 mg/kg per day | 5 days | Inadequate fluid intake Renal impairment Penicillin allergy | Urinalysis, BUN Creatinine Urinalysis, BUN |
| D-Penicillamine (Cuprimine) | PO | 10 mg/kg per day increase 30 mg/kg over 2 weeks | 6-20 weeks | Concurrent iron therapy; lead exposure Renal impairment | Creatinine, CBC |
| 2,3-Dimercap-tosuccinic acid (DMSA; succimer) | PO | 10 mg/kg per dose 3 times daily 10 mg/kg per dose twice daily for 14 days | 19 days | AST/ALT Concurrent iron therapy G6PD deficiency lead exposure | AST/ALT |

*Abbreviations*: ALT = alanine aminotransferase; AST = aspartate transaminase; BAL = British anti-Lewisite; bid = twice daily; BUN = blood urea nitrogen; CBC = complete blood count; G6PD = glucose-6-phosphate dehydrogenase; IM = intramuscular; IV = intravenous; PO = oral; tid = three times daily.

allowing the child to return. The source must be eliminated by environmental and occupational investigations. The local health department should be involved in dealing with children who are lead poisoned, and OSHA should be involved with cases of occupational lead poisoning. Consultation with a poison control center or experienced toxicologist is necessary when chelating patients. Follow-up venous blood lead concentrations should be obtained within 1 to 2 weeks and followed every 2 weeks for 6 to 8 weeks, then monthly for 4 to 6 months if the patient required chelation therapy. All patients with venous blood level greater than 10 μg/dL should be followed at least every 3 months until two venous blood lead concentrations are 10 μg/dL or three are less than 15 μg/dL.

## LITHIUM (ESKALITH, LITHANE)

Lithium is an alkali metal used primarily in the treatment of bipolar psychiatric disorders. Most intoxications are cases of chronic overdose. One gram of lithium carbonate contains 189 mg (5.1 mEq) of lithium; a regular tablet contains 300 mg (8.12 mEq) and a sustained-release preparation contains 450 mg or 12.18 mEq.

### Toxic Mechanism

The brain is the primary target organ of toxicity, but the mechanism is unclear. Lithium may interfere with physiologic functions by acting as a substitute for cellular cations (sodium and potassium), depressing neural excitation and synaptic transmission.

### Toxic Dose

A dose of 1 mEq/kg (40 mg/kg) of lithium will give a peak serum lithium concentration about 1.2 mEq/L. The therapeutic serum lithium concentration in cases of acute mania is 0.6 to 1.2 mEq/L, and for maintenance it is 0.5 to 0.8 mEq/L. Serum lithium concentration levels are usually obtained 12 hours after the last dose. The toxic dose is determined by clinical manifestations and serum levels after the distribution phase.

Acute ingestion of twenty 300-mg tablets (300 mg increases the serum lithium concentration by 0.2 to 0.4 mEq/L) in adults may produce serious intoxication. Chronic intoxication can be produced by conditions listed below that can decrease the elimination of lithium or increase lithium reabsorption in the kidney.

The risk factors that predispose to chronic lithium toxicity are febrile illness, impaired renal function, hyponatremia, advanced age, lithium-induced diabetes insipidus, dehydration, vomiting and diarrhea, and concomitant use of other drugs, such as thiazide and spironolactone diuretics, nonsteroidal anti-inflammatory drugs, salicylates, angiotensin-converting enzyme inhibitors (e.g., captopril), serotonin reuptake inhibitors (e.g., fluoxetine [Prozac]), and phenothiazines.

### Kinetics

Gastrointestinal absorption of regular-release preparations is rapid; serum lithium concentration peaks in 2 to 4 hours and is complete by 6 to 8 hours. The onset of toxicity may occur at 1 to 4 hours after acute overdose but usually is delayed because lithium enters the brain slowly. Absorption of sustained-release preparations and the development of toxicity may be delayed 6 to 12 hours.

Volume distribution is 0.5 to 0.9 L/kg. Lithium is not protein bound. The half-life after a single dose is 9 to 13 hours; at steady state, it may be 30 to 58 hours. The renal handling of lithium is similar to that of sodium: glomerular filtration and reabsorption (80%) by the proximal renal tubule. Adequate sodium must be present to prevent lithium reabsorption. More than 90% of lithium is excreted by the kidney, 30% to 60% within 6 to 12 hours.

### Manifestations

The examiner must distinguish between side effects, acute intoxication, acute or chronic toxicity, and chronic intoxications. Chronic is the most common and dangerous type of intoxication.

Side effects include fine tremor, gastrointestinal upset, hypothyroidism, polyuria and frank diabetes insipidus, dermatologic manifestations, and cardiac conduction deficits. Lithium is teratogenic.

Patients with acute poisoning may be asymptomatic, with an early high serum lithium concentration of 9 mEq/L, and deteriorate as the serum lithium concentration falls by 50% and the lithium distributes to the brain and the other tissues. Nausea and vomiting may occur within 1 to 4 hours, but the systemic manifestations are usually delayed several more hours. It may take as long as 3 to 5 days for serious symptoms to develop. Acute toxicity and acute on chronic toxicity are manifested by neurologic findings, including weakness, fasciculations, altered mental state, myoclonus, hyperreflexia, rigidity, coma, and convulsions with limbs in hypertension. Cardiovascular effects are nonspecific and occur at therapeutic doses, flat T or inverted T waves, atrioventricular block, and prolonged QT interval. Lithium is not a primary cardiotoxin. Cardiogenic shock occurs secondary to CNS toxicity. Chronic intoxication is associated with manifestations at lower serum lithium concentrations. There is some correlation with manifestations, especially at higher serum lithium concentrations. Although the levels do not always correlate with the manifestations, they are more predictive in cases of severe intoxication. A serum lithium concentration greater than 3.0 mEq/L with chronic intoxication and altered mental state indicates severe toxicity. Permanent neurologic sequelae can result from lithium intoxication.

### Laboratory Investigations

Monitoring should include CBC (lithium causes significant leukocytosis), renal function, thyroid function (chronic intoxication), ECG, and electrolytes. Serum lithium concentrations should be determined every 2 to 4 hours until levels are close to therapeutic range. Cross-reactions with green-top Vacutainer specimen tubes containing heparin will spuriously elevate serum lithium concentration 6 to 8 mEq/L.

### Management

Vital function must be established and maintained. Seizure precautions should be instituted and seizures, hypotension, and dysrhythmias treated. Evaluation should include examination for rigidity and hyperreflexia signs, hydration, renal function (BUN, creatinine), and electrolytes, especially sodium. The examiner should inquire about diuretic and other drug use that increase serum lithium concentration, and the patient must discontinue the drugs. If the patient is on chronic therapy, the lithium should be discontinued. Serial serum lithium concentrations should be obtained every 4 hours until serum lithium concentration peaks and there is a downward trend toward almost therapeutic range, especially in sustained-release preparations. Vital signs should be monitored, including temperature, and ECG and serial neurologic examinations should be undertaken, including mental status and urinary output. Nephrology consultation is warranted in case of a chronic and elevated serum lithium concentration (>2.5 mEq/L), a large ingestion, or altered mental state.

An intravenous line should be established and hydration and electrolyte balance restored. Serum sodium level should be determined before 0.9% saline fluid is administered in patients with chronic overdose because hypernatremia may be present from diabetes insipidus. Although current evidence supports an initial 0.9% saline infusion (200 mL/h) to enhance excretion of lithium, once hydration, urine output, and normonatremia are established, one should administer 0.45% saline and slow the infusion (100 mL/h) for all patients.

Gastric lavage is often not recommended in cases of acute ingestion because of the large size of the tablets, and it is not necessary after chronic intoxication. Activated charcoal is ineffective. For sustained-release preparations, whole-bowel irrigation may be useful but is not proven. Sodium polystyrene sulfonate (Kayexalate), an ion exchange resin, is difficult to administer and has been used only in uncontrolled studies. Its use is not recommended.

Hemodialysis is the most efficient method for removing lithium from the vascular compartment. It is the treatment of choice for patients with severe intoxication with an altered mental state, those with seizures, and anuric patients. Long runs are used until the serum lithium concentration is less than 1 mEq/L because of extensive re-equilibration. Serum lithium concentration should be monitored every 4 hours after dialysis for rebound. Repeated and prolonged hemodialysis may be necessary. A lag in neurologic recovery can be expected.

## Disposition

An acute asymptomatic lithium overdose cannot be medically cleared on the basis of single lithium level. Patients should be admitted if they have any neurologic manifestations (altered mental status, hyper-reflexia, stiffness, or tremor). Patients should be admitted to the intensive care unit if they are dehydrated, have renal impairment, or have a high or rising lithium level.

## METHANOL (WOOD ALCOHOL, METHYL ALCOHOL)

The concentration of methanol in Sterno fuel is 4% and it contains ethanol, in windshield washer fluid it is 30% to 60%, and in gas-line antifreeze it is 100%.

## Toxic Mechanism

Methanol is metabolized by alcohol dehydrogenase to formaldehyde, which is metabolized to formate. Formate inhibits cytochrome oxidase, producing tissue hypoxia, lactic acidosis, and optic nerve edema. Formate is converted by folate-dependent enzymes to carbon dioxide.

## Toxic Dose

The minimal toxic amount is approximately 100 mg/kg. Serious toxicity in a young child can be produced by the ingestion of 2.5 to 5.0 mL of 100% methanol. Ingestion of 5-mL 100% methanol by a 10-kg child produces estimated peak blood methanol of 80 mg/dL. Ingestion of 15 mL 40% methanol was lethal for a 2-year-old child in one report. A fatal adult oral dose is 30 to 240 mL 100% (20 to 150 g). Ingestion of 6 to 10 mL 100% causes blindness in adults. The toxic blood concentration is greater than 20 mg/dL; very serious toxicity and potential fatality occur at levels greater than 50 mg/dL.

## Kinetics

Onset of action can start within 1 hour but may be delayed up to 12 to 18 hours by metabolism to toxic metabolites. It may be delayed longer if ethanol is ingested concomitantly or in infants. Peak blood methanol concentration is 1 hour. Volume distribution is 0.6 L/kg (total body water).

For metabolism, see *Toxic Mechanism*.

Elimination is through metabolism. The half-life of methanol is 8 hours, with ethanol blocking it is 30 to 35 hours, and with hemodialysis 2.5 hours.

## Manifestations

Metabolism creates a delay in onset for 12 to 18 hours or longer if ethanol is ingested concomitantly. Initial findings are as follows:

- 0 to 6 hours: Confusion, ataxia, inebriation, formaldehyde odor on breath, and abdominal pain can be present, but the patient may be asymptomatic. Note: Methanol produces an osmolal gap (early), and its metabolite formate produces the anion gap metabolic acidosis (see later). Absence of osmolar or anion gap does not always exclude methanol intoxication.
- 6 to 12 hours: Malaise, headache, abdominal pain, vomiting, visual symptoms, including hyperemia of optic disc, "snow vision," and blindness can be seen.
- More than 12 hours: Worsening acidosis, hyperglycemia, shock, and multiorgan failure develop, with death from complications of intractable acidosis and cerebral edema.

## Laboratory Investigation

Methanol can be detected on some chromatography drug screens if specified. Methanol and ethanol levels, electrolytes, glucose, BUN, creatinine, amylase, and ABG should be monitored every 4 hours. Formate levels correlate more closely than blood methanol concentration with severity of intoxication and should be obtained if possible.

## Management

One should protect the airway by intubation to prevent aspiration and administer assisted ventilation as needed. If needed, 100% oxygen can be administered. A nephrologist should be consulted early regarding the need for hemodialysis.

Gastrointestinal decontamination procedures have no role.

Metabolic acidosis should be treated vigorously with sodium bicarbonate 2 to 3 mEq/kg intravenously. Large amounts may be needed.

Antidote therapy is initiated to inhibit metabolism if the patient has a history of ingesting more than 0.4 mL/kg of 100% with the following conditions:

- Blood methanol level is greater than 20 mg/dL
- The patient has osmolar gap not accounted for by other factors
- The patient is symptomatic or acidotic with increased anion gap and/or hyperemia of the optic disc.

The ethanol or fomepizole therapy outlined below can be used.

### Ethanol Therapy

Ethanol should be initiated immediately if fomepizole is unavailable (see *Fomepizole Therapy*). Alcohol dehydrogenase has a greater affinity for ethanol than ethylene glycol. Therefore, ethanol blocks the metabolism of ethylene glycol.

Ethanol should be administered intravenously (oral administration is less reliable) to produce a blood ethanol concentration of 100 to 150 mg/dL. The loading dose is 10 mL/kg of 10% ethanol administered intravenously concomitantly with a maintenance dose of 10% ethanol at 1.0 mL/kg/h. This dose may need to be increased to 2 mL/kg/h in patients who are heavy drinkers. The blood ethanol concentration should be measured hourly and the infusion rate should be adjusted to maintain a concentration of 100 to 150 mg/dL.

### Fomepizole Therapy

Fomepizole (Antizol, 4-methylpyrazole) inhibits alcohol dehydrogenase more reliably than ethanol and it does not require constant monitoring of ethanol levels and adjustment of infusion rates. Fomepizole is available in 1 g/mL vials of 1.5 mL. The loading dose is 15 mg/kg (0.015 mL/kg) IV, maintenance dose is 10 mg/kg (0.01 mL/kg) every 12 hours for 4 doses, then 15 mg/kg every 12 hours until the ethylene glycol levels are less than 20 mg/dL. The solution is prepared by being mixed with 100 mL of 0.9% saline or D5W. Fomepizole can be given to patients requiring hemodialysis but should be dosed as follows:

Dose at the beginning of hemodialysis:

- If less than 6 hours since last Antizol dose, do not administer dose
- If more than 6 hours since last dose, administer next scheduled dose

Dosing during hemodialysis:

- Dose every 4 hours

Dosing at the time hemodialysis is completed:

- If less than 1 hour between last dose and end dialysis, do not administer dose at end of dialysis
- If 1 to 3 hours between last dose and end dialysis, administer one half of next scheduled dose

- If more than 3 hours between last dose and end dialysis, administer next scheduled dose

Maintenance dosing off hemodialysis:

- Give the next scheduled dose 12 hours from the last dose administered

Hemodialysis increases the clearance of both methanol and formate 10-fold over renal clearance. A blood methanol concentration greater than 50 mg/dL has been used as an indication for hemodialysis, but recently some toxicologists from the New York City Poison Center recommended early hemodialysis in patients with blood methanol concentration greater than 25 mg/dL because it may be able to shorten the course of intoxication if started early. One should continue to monitor methanol levels and/or formate levels every 4 hours after the procedure for rebound. Other indications for early hemodialysis are significant metabolic acidosis and electrolyte abnormalities despite conventional therapy and if visual or neurologic signs or symptoms are present.

A serum formate level greater than 20 mg/dL has also been used as a criterion for hemodialysis, although this is often not readily available through many laboratories. If hemodialysis is used, the infusion rate of 10% ethanol should be increased 2.0 to 3.5 mL/kg/h. The blood ethanol concentration and glucose level should be obtained every 2 hours.

Therapy is continued with both ethanol and hemodialysis until the blood methanol level is undetectable, there is no acidosis, and the patient has no neurologic or visual disturbances. This may require several days.

Hypoglycemia is treated with intravenous glucose. Doses of folinic acid (Leucovorin) and folic acid have been used successfully in animal investigations to enhance formate metabolism to carbon dioxide and water. Leucovorin 1 mg/kg up to 50 mg IV is administered every 4 hours for several days.

An initial ophthalmologic consultation and follow-up are warranted.

## Disposition

All patients who have ingested significant amounts of methanol should be referred to the emergency department for evaluation and blood methanol concentration measurement. Ophthalmologic follow-up of all patients with methanol intoxications should be arranged.

## MONOAMINE OXIDASE INHIBITORS

Nonselective monoamine oxidase inhibitors (MAOIs) include the hydrazines phenelzine (Nardil) and isocarboxazid (Marplan), and the nonhydrazine tranylcypromine (Parnate). Furazolidone (Furoxone) and pargyline (Eutonyl)[2] are also considered nonselective MAOIs. Moclobemide,[2] which is available in many countries but not the United States, is a selective MAO-A inhibitor. MAO-B inhibitors include selegiline (Eldepryl), an antiparksonism agent, which does not have similar toxicity to MAO-A and is not discussed. Selectivity is lost in an overdose. MAOIs are used to treat severe depression.

## Toxic Mechanism

Monoamine oxidase enzymes are responsible for the oxidative deamination of both endogenous and exogenous catecholamines such as norepinephrine. MAO-A in the intestinal wall also metabolizes tyramine in food. MAOIs permanently inhibit MAO enzymes until a new enzyme is synthesized after 14 days or longer. The toxicity results from the accumulation, potentiation, and prolongation of the catecholamine action followed by profound hypotension and cardiovascular collapse.

---

[2]Not available in the United States.

## Toxic Dose

Toxicity begins at 2 to 3 mg/kg and fatalities occur at 4 to 6 mg/kg. Death has occurred after a single dose of 170 mg of tranylcypromine in an adult.

## Kinetics

Structurally, MAOIs are related to amphetamines and catecholamines. The hydrazine peak levels are at 1 to 2 hours; metabolism is hepatic acetylation; and inactive metabolites are excreted in the urine. For the nonhydrazines, peak levels occur at 1 to 4 hours, and metabolism is via the liver to active amphetamine-like metabolites.

The onset of symptoms in a case of overdose is delayed 6 to 24 hours after ingestion, peak activity is 8 to 12 hours, and duration is 72 hours or longer. The peak of MAO inhibition is in 5 to 10 days and lasts as long as 5 weeks.

## Manifestations

Manifestations of an acute ingestion overdose of MAO-A inhibitors are as follows:

### Phase I

An adrenergic crisis occurs, with delayed onset for 6 to 24 hours, and may not reach peak until 24 hours. The crisis starts as hyperthermia, tachycardia, tachypnea, dysarthria, transient hypertension, hyperreflexia, and CNS stimulation.

### Phase II

Neuromuscular excitation and sympathetic hyperactivity occur with increased temperature greater than 40°C (104°F), agitation, hyperactivity, confusion, fasciculations, twitching, tremor, masseter spasm, muscle rigidity, acidosis, and electrolyte abnormalities. Seizures and dystonic reactions may occur. The pupils are mydriatic, sometimes nonreactive with "ping-pong gaze."

### Phase III

CNS depression and cardiovascular collapse occur in cases of severe overdose as the catecholamines are depleted. Symptoms usually resolve within 5 days but may last 2 weeks.

### Phase IV

Secondary complications occur, including rhabdomyolysis, cardiac dysrhythmias, multiorgan failure, and coagulopathies.

Biogenic interactions usually occur while the patient is on therapeutic doses of MAOI or shortly after they are discontinued (30 to 60 minutes), before the new MAO enzyme is synthesized. The following substances have been implicated: indirect acting sympathomimetics such as amphetamines, serotonergic drugs, opioids (e.g., meperidine, dextromethorphan), tricyclic antidepressants, specific serotonin reuptake inhibitors (SSRI; e.g., fluoxetine [Prozac], sertraline [Zoloft], paroxetine [Paxil]), tyramine-containing foods (e.g., wine, beer, avocados, cheese, caviar, chocolate, chicken liver), and L-tryptophan. SSRIs should not be started for at least 5 weeks after MAOIs have been discontinued.

In mild cases, usually caused by foods, headache and hypertension develop and last for several hours. In severe cases, malignant hypertension and severe hyperthermia syndromes consisting of hypertension or hyperthermia, altered mental state, skeletal muscle rigidity, shivering (often beginning in the masseter muscle), and seizures may occur.

The serotonin syndrome, which may be a result of inhibition of serotonin metabolism, has similar clinical findings to those of malignant hyperthermia and may occur with or without hyperthermia or hypertension.

Chronic toxicity clinical findings include tremors, hyperhidrosis, agitation, hallucinations, confusion, and seizures and may be confused with withdrawal syndromes.

## Laboratory Investigations

Monitoring of the ECG, cardiac monitoring, CPK, ABG, pulse oximeter, electrolytes, blood glucose, and acid–base balance should be maintained.

## Management

In the case of MAOI overdose, ipecac-induced emesis should not be used. Only activated charcoal alone should be used.

If the patient is admitted to the hospital and is well enough to eat, a nontyramine diet should be ordered.

Extreme agitation and seizures can be controlled with benzodiazepines and barbiturates. Phenytoin is ineffective. Nondepolarizing neuromuscular blockers (not depolarizing succinylcholine) may be needed in severe cases of hyperthermia and rigidity. If the patient has severe hypertension (catecholamine mediated), phentolamine (Regitine), a parenteral β-blocking agent, 3 to 5 mg intravenously, or labetalol (Normodyne), a combination of an α-blocking agent and a β-blocker, 20-mg intravenous bolus, should be given. If malignant hypertension with rigidity is present, a short-acting nitroprusside and benzodiazepine can be used. Hypertension is often followed by severe hypotension, which should be managed by fluid and vasopressors. *Caution:* Vasopressor therapy should be administered at lower doses than usual because of exaggerated pharmacologic response. Norepinephrine is preferred to dopamine, which requires release of intracellular amines.

Cardiac dysrhythmias are treated with standard therapy but are often refractory, and cardioversion and pacemakers may be needed.

For malignant hyperthermia, dantrolene (Dantrium), a nonspecific peripheral skeletal relaxing agent, is administered, which inhibits the release of calcium from the sarcoplasm. Dantrolene is reconstituted with 60 mL sterile water without bacteriostatic agents. Glass equipment must not be used, and the drug must be protected from light and used within 6 hours. Loading dose is 2 to 3 mg/kg intravenously as a bolus, and the loading dose is repeated until the signs of malignant hyperthermia (tachycardia, rigidity, increased end-tidal $CO_2$, and temperature) are controlled. Maximum total dose is 10 mg/kg to avoid hepatotoxicity.

When malignant hyperthermia has subsided, 1 mg/kg IV is given every 6 hours for 24 to 48 hours, then orally 1 mg/kg every 6 hours for 24 hours to prevent recurrence. There is a danger of thrombophlebitis following peripheral dantrolene, and it should be administered through a central line if possible. In addition one should administer external cooling and correct metabolic acidosis and electrolyte disturbances. Benzodiazepine can be used for sedation. Dantrolene does not reverse central dopamine blockade; therefore, bromocriptine mesylate (Parlodel) 2.5 to 10 mg should be given orally or through a nasogastric tube three times a day.

Rhabdomyolysis and myoglobinuria are treated with fluids. Urine alkalinization should also be treated.

Hemodialysis and hemoperfusion are of no proven value.

Biogenic amine interactions are managed symptomatically, similar to cases of overdose. For the serotonin syndrome cyproheptadine (Periactin), a serotonin blocker, 4 mg orally every hour for three doses, or methysergide (Sansert), 2 mg orally every 6 hours for three doses, should be considered. The effectiveness of these drugs has not been proven.

## Disposition

All patients who have ingested more than 2 mg/kg of an MAOI should be admitted to the hospital for 24 hours of observation and monitoring in the intensive care unit because the life-threatening manifestations may be delayed. Patients with drug or dietary interactions that are mild may not require admission if symptoms subside within 4 to 6 hours and the patients remain asymptomatic. Patients with symptoms that persist or require active intervention should be admitted to the intensive care unit.

## OPIOIDS (NARCOTIC OPIATES)

Opioids are used for analgesia, as antitussives, and as antidiarrheal agents and are illicit agents (heroin, opium) used in substance abuse. Tolerance, physical dependency, and withdrawal may develop.

## Toxic Mechanism

At least four main opioid receptors have been identified. The μ receptor is considered the most important for central analgesia and CNS depression. The κ and δ receptors predominate in spinal analgesia. The σ receptors may mediate dysphoria. Death is a consequence of dose-dependent CNS respiratory depression or secondary to pulmonary aspiration or noncardiac pulmonary edema. The mechanism of noncardiac pulmonary edema is unknown.

Dextromethorphan can interact with MAOIs, causing severe hyperthermia, and may cause the serotonin syndrome (see *Selective Serotonin Reuptake Inhibitors*). Dextromethorphan inhibits the metabolism of norepinephrine and serotonin and blocks the reuptake of serotonin. It is found as a component of a large number of nonprescription cough and cold remedies.

## Toxic Dose

The toxic dose depends on the specific drug, route of administration, and degree of tolerance. For therapeutic and toxic doses, see Table 24. In children, respiratory depression has been produced by 10 mg of morphine or methadone, 75 mg of meperidine, and 12.5 mg of diphenoxylate. Infants younger than 3 months of age are more susceptible to respiratory depression. The dose should be reduced by 50%.

## Kinetics

Oral onset of analgesic effect of morphine is 10 to 15 minutes; the action peaks in 1 hour and lasts 4 to 6 hours. With sustained-release preparations, the duration is 8 to 12 hours. Opioids are 90% metabolized in the liver by hepatic conjugation and 90% excreted in the urine as inactive compounds. Volume distribution is 1 to 4 L/kg. Protein binding is 35% to 75%. The typical plasma half-life of opiates is 2 to 5 hours, but that of methadone is 24 to 36 hours. Morphine metabolites include morphine-3-glucuronide (inactive) and morphine-6-glucuronide (active) and normorphine (active). Meperidine (Demerol) is rapidly hydrolyzed by tissue esterases into the active metabolite normeperidine, which has twice the convulsant activity of meperidine. Heroin (diacetylmorphine) is deacetylated within minutes to 6-monacetylmorphine and morphine. Propoxyphene (Darvon) has a rapid onset of action, and death has occurred within 15 to 30 minutes after a massive overdose. Propoxyphene is metabolized to norpropoxyphene, an active metabolite with convulsive, cardiac dysrhythmic, and heart block properties. Symptoms of diphenoxylate overdose appear within 1 to 4 hours. It is metabolized into the active metabolite difenoxin, which is five times more active as a regular respiratory depressant agent. Death has been reported in children after ingestion of a single tablet.

## Manifestations

Initially, mild intoxication produces miosis, dull face, drowsiness, partial ptosis, and "nodding" (head drops to chest then bobs up). Larger amounts produce the classic triad of miotic pupils (exceptions below), respiratory depression, and depressed level of consciousness (flaccid coma). The blood pressure, pulse, and bowel activity are decreased.

Dilated pupils do not exclude opioid intoxication. Some exceptions to the miosis effect include dextromethorphan (paralyzes iris), fentanyl, meperidine, and diphenoxylate (rarely). Physiologic disturbances including acidosis, hypoglycemia, hypoxia, and postictal state, or a co-ingestant may also produce mydriasis.

Usually, the muscles are flaccid, but increased muscle tone can be produced by meperidine and fentanyl (chest rigidity). Seizures are rare but can occur with ingestion of codeine, meperidine, propoxyphene, and dextromethorphan. Hallucinations and agitation have been reported.

Pruritus and urticaria are caused by histamine release by some opioids or by sulfite additives.

Noncardiac pulmonary edema may occur after an overdose, especially with intravenous heroin abuse. Cardiac effects include

**TABLE 24** Doses and Onset and Duration of Action of Common Opioids

| Drug | Adult Oral Dose | Child Oral Dose | Onset of Action | Duration of Action | Adult Fatal Dose |
|---|---|---|---|---|---|
| Camphored tincture of opium | 25 mL | 0.25-0.50 mL/kg (0.4 mg/mL) | 15-30 min | 4-5 h | NA |
| Codeine | 30-180 mg | 0.5-1 mg/kg | 15-30 min | 4-6 h | 800 mg |
| | >1 mg/kg is toxic in a child, above 200 mg in adult >5 mg/kg fatal in a child | | | | |
| Dextromethorphan | 15 mg 10 mg/kg is toxic | 0.25 mg/kg | 15-30 min | 3-6 h | NA |
| Diacetylmorphine; street heroin is less than 10% pure | 60 mg | NA | 15-30 min | 3-4 h | 100 mg |
| Diphenoxylate natiopine (Lomotil) | 5-10 mg | NA | 120-240 min | 14 h | 300 mg |
| | 7.5 mg is toxic in a child, 300 mg is toxic in adult | | | | |
| Fentanyl (Duragesic) | 0.1-0.2 mg | 0.001-0.002 mg/kg | 7-8 min | Intramuscular: 1/2-2 h | 1.0 mg |
| Hydrocodone with APAP (Lortab) | 5-30 mg | 0.15 mg/kg | 30 min | 3-4 h | 100 mg |
| Hydromorphone (Dilaudid) | 4 mg | 0.1 mg/kg | 15-30 min | 3-4 h | 100 mg |
| Meperidine (Demerol) | 100 mg | 1-1.5 mg/kg | 10-45 min | 3-4 h | 350 mg |
| Methadone (Dolophine) | 10 mg | 0.1 mg/kg | 30-60 min | 4-12 h | 120 mg |
| Morphine | 10-60 mg | 0.1-0.2 mg/kg | <20 min | 4-6 h | 200 mg |
| | Oral dose is 6 times parenteral dose, MS Contin sustained release prep | | | | |
| Oxycodone APAP (Percocet) | 5 mg | NA | 15-30 min | 4-5 h | NA |
| Pentazocine (Talwin) | 50-100 mg | NA | 15-30 min | 3-4 h | NA |
| Propoxyphene (Darvon) | 65-100 mg | NA | 30-60 min | 2-4 h | 700 mg |

vasodilation and hypotension. A heart murmur in an intravenous addict suggests endocarditis. Propoxyphene can produce delayed cardiac dysrhythmias.

Fentanyl is 100 times more potent than morphine and can cause chest wall muscle rigidity. Some of its derivatives are 2000 times more potent than morphine.

## Laboratory Investigations

For patients with overdose, one should obtain and monitor ABG, blood glucose, and electrolyte levels; chest radiographs; and ECG. For drug abusers, one should consider testing for hepatitis B, syphilis, and HIV antibody (HIV testing usually requires consent). Blood opioid concentrations are not useful. They confirm diagnosis (morphine therapeutic dose, 65 to 80 ng/mL; toxic, <200 ng/mL), but are not useful for making a therapeutic decision. Cross-reactions can occur with Vick's Formula 44, poppy seeds, and other opioids (codeine and heroin are metabolized to morphine). Naloxone 4 mg IV was not associated with a positive enzyme multiplied immunoassay technique urine screen at 60 minutes, 6 hours, or 48 hours.

## Management

Supportive care should be instituted, particularly an endotracheal tube and assisted ventilation. Temporary ventilation can be provided by a bag-valve mask with 100% oxygen. The patient should be placed on a cardiac monitor, have intravenous access established, and have specimens for ABG, glucose, electrolytes, BUN, and creatinine levels, CBC, coagulation profile, liver function, toxicology screen, and urinalysis taken.

For gastrointestinal decontamination, emesis should not be induced, but activated charcoal can be administered if bowel sounds are present.

If it is suspected that the patient is an addict, he or she should be restrained first and then 0.1 mg of naloxone (Narcan) should be administered. The dose should be doubled every 2 minutes until the patient responds or 10 to 20 mg has been given. If the patient is not suspected to be an addict, then 2 mg every 2 to 3 minutes to total of 10 to 20 mg is administered.

It is essential to determine whether there is a complete response to naloxone (mydriasis, improvement in ventilation), because it is a diagnostic therapeutic test. A continuous naloxone infusion may be appropriate, using the "response dose" every hour. Repeat doses of naloxone may be necessary because the effects of many opioids can last much longer than naloxone does (30 to 60 minutes). Methadone ingestions may require a naloxone infusion for 24 to 48 hours. Half of the response dose may need to be repeated in 15 to 20 minutes, after the infusion has been started.

Acute iatrogenic withdrawal precipitated by the administration of naloxone to a dependent patient should not be treated with morphine or other opioids. Naloxone's effects are limited to 30 to 60 minutes (shorter than most opioids) and withdrawal will subside in a short time.

Nalmefene (Revex), an FDA-approved long-acting (4 to 8 hours) pure opioid antagonist, is being investigated, but its role in cases of acute intoxication is unclear and it could produce prolonged withdrawal. It may have a role in place of naloxone infusion.

Noncardiac pulmonary edema does not respond to naloxone, and the patient needs intubation, assisted ventilation, positive end-expiratory pressure, and hemodynamic monitoring. Fluids should be given cautiously in patients with opioid overdose because opioids stimulate the antidiuretic hormone.

If the patient is comatose, 50% glucose (3% to 4% of comatose opioid overdose patients have hypoglycemia) and thiamine should be given prior to naloxone. If the patient has seizures that are unresponsive to naloxone, one administers diazepam and examines for metabolic (hypoglycemia, electrolyte disturbances) causes and structural disturbances.

Hypotension is rare and should direct a search for another etiology. If the patient is agitated, hypoxia and hypoglycemia must be excluded before opioid withdrawal is considered as a cause. Complications to consider include urinary retention, constipation, rhabdomyolysis, myoglobinuria, hypoglycemia, and withdrawal.

## Disposition

If a patient responds to intravenous naloxone, careful observation for relapse and the development of pulmonary edema is required, with cardiac and respiratory monitoring for 6 to 12 hours. Patients requiring repeated doses of naloxone or an infusion, or those who develop pulmonary edema, require intensive care unit admission and cannot be discharged from the intensive care unit until they are symptom free for 12 hours. Intravenous overdose complications are expected to be present within 20 minutes after injection, and discharge after 4 symptom-free hours has been recommended. Adults with oral overdose have delayed onset of toxicity and require 6 hours of observation. Children with oral opioid overdose should be admitted to the hospital for observation because of delayed toxicity. Some toxicologists advise restraining a patient who attempts to sign out against medical advice after treatment with naloxone, at least until the patient receives psychiatric evaluation.

## ORGANOPHOSPHATES AND CARBAMATES

Cholinergic intoxication sources are insecticides (organophosphates or carbamates), some medications, and some mushrooms. Examples of organophosphate insecticides are malathion (low toxicity, median lethal dose [$LD_{50}$] 2800 mg/kg), chlorpyrifos, which has been removed from market (moderate toxicity), and parathion (high toxicity, $LD_{50}$ 2 mg/kg). Carbamate insecticides include carbaryl (low toxicity, $LD_{50}$ 500 mg/kg), propoxur (moderate toxicity, $LD_{50}$ 95 mg/kg), and aldicarb (high toxicity, $LD_{50}$ 0.9 mg/kg). Pharmaceuticals with carbamate properties include neostigmine (Prostigmin) and physostigmine (Antilirium). Cholinergic compounds also include the "G" nerve war weapons tabun (GA), sarin (GB), soman (GB), and venom X (VX).

## Toxic Mechanism

Organophosphates phosphorylate the active site on red cell acetylcholinesterase and pseudocholinesterase in the serum, neuromuscular and parasympathetic neuroeffector junctions, and in the major synapses of the autonomic ganglia, causing irreversible inhibition. There are two types of organophosphate intoxication: (a) direct action by the parent compound (e.g., tetraethylpyrophosphate), or (b) indirect action by the toxic metabolite (e.g., parathoxon or malathoxon).

Carbamates (esters of carbonic acid) cause reversible carbamylation of the active site of the enzymes. When a critical amount, greater than 50%, of cholinesterase is inhibited, acetylcholine accumulates and causes transient stimulation at cholinergic synapses and sympathetic terminals (muscarinic effect), the somatic nerves, the autonomic ganglia (nicotinic effect), and CNS synapses. Stimulation of conduction is followed by inhibition of conduction.

The major differences between the carbamates and the organophosphates are as follows: (a) carbamate toxicity is less and the duration is shorter; (b) carbamates rarely produce overt CNS effects (poor CNS penetration); (c) carbamate inhibition of the acetylcholinesterase enzyme is reversible and activity returns to normal rapidly; (d) pralidoxime, the enzyme regenerator, may not be necessary in the management of mild carbamate intoxication (e.g., carbaryl).

## Toxic Dose

Parathion's minimum lethal dose is 2 mg in children and 10 to 20 mg in adults. The lethal dose of malathion is greater than 1375 mg/kg and that of chlorpyrifos is 25 g; the latter compound is unlikely to cause death.

## Kinetics

Absorption is by all routes. The onset of acute ingestion toxicity occurs as early as 3 hours, usually before 12 hours and always before 24 hours. Lipid-soluble agents absorbed by the dermal route (e.g., fenthion) may have a delayed onset of more than 24 hours. Inhalation toxicity occurs immediately after exposure. Massive ingestion can produce intoxication within minutes.

Metabolism is via the liver. With some pesticides (e.g., parathion, malathion), the effects are delayed because they undergo hepatic microsomal oxidative metabolism to their toxic metabolites, the -oxons (e.g., paroxon, malaoxon).

The half-life of malathion is 2.89 hours and that of parathion is 2.1 days. The metabolites are eliminated in the urine and the presence of p-nitrophenol in the urine is a clue up to 48 hours after exposure.

## Manifestations

Many organophosphates produce a garlic odor on the breath, in the gastric contents, or in the container. Diaphoresis, excessive salivation, miosis, and muscle twitching are helpful clues to diagnosis.

Early, a cholinergic (muscarinic) crisis develops that consists of parasympathetic nervous system activity. DUMBELS is the mnemonic for defecation, cramps, and increased bowel motility; urinary incontinence; miosis (mydriasis may occur in 20%); bronchospasm and bronchorrhea; excess secretion; lacrimation; and seizures. Bradycardia, pulmonary edema, and hypotension may be present.

Later, sympathetic and nicotinic effects occur, consisting of MATCH: muscle weakness and fasciculation (eyelid twitching is often present), adrenal stimulation and hyperglycemia, tachycardia, cramps in muscles, and hypertension. Finally, paralysis of the skeletal muscles ensues.

The CNS effects are headache, blurred vision, anxiety, ataxia, delirium and toxic psychosis, convulsions, coma, and respiratory depression. Cranial nerve palsies have been noted. Delayed hallucinations may occur.

Delayed respiratory paralysis and neurologic and neurobehavioral disorders have been described following certain organophosphate ingestions or dermal exposure. The "intermediate syndrome" is paralysis of proximal and respiratory muscles developing 24 to 96 hours after the successful treatment of organophosphate poisoning. A delayed distal polyneuropathy has been described with ingestion of certain organophosphates, such as triorthocresyl phosphate, bromoleptophos, and methomidophos.

Complications include aspiration, pulmonary edema, and acute respiratory distress syndrome.

## Laboratory Investigations

Monitoring should include chest radiograph, blood glucose (nonketotic hyperglycemia is frequent), ABG, pulse oximetry, ECG, blood coagulation status, liver function, hyperamylasemia (pancreatitis reported), and urinalysis for the metabolite alkyl phosphate paranitrophenol. Blood should be drawn for red blood cell cholinesterase determination before pralidoxime is given. The red blood cell cholinesterase activity roughly correlates with clinical severity. Mild poisoning is 20% to 50% of normal, moderate poisoning is 10% to 20% of normal, and severe poisoning is 10% of normal (>90% depressed). A post-exposure rise of 10% to 15% in the cholinesterase level determined at least 10 to 14 days after the exposure confirms the diagnosis.

## Management

Protection of health care personnel with clothing (masks, gloves, gowns, goggles) and respiratory equipment or hazardous material suits, as necessary, is called for. General decontamination consists of isolation, bagging, and disposal of contaminated clothing and other articles. Vital functions should be established and maintained. Cardiac and oxygen saturation monitoring are needed. Intubation and assisted ventilation may be needed. Secretions should be suctioned until atropinization drying is achieved.

Dermal decontamination involves prompt removal of clothing and cleansing of all affected areas of skin, hair, and eyes. Ocular decontamination involves irrigation with copious amounts of tepid water or 0.9% saline for at least 15 minutes. Gastrointestinal decontamination, if the ingestion was recent, involves the administration of activated charcoal.

Atropine sulfate can be given as an antidote. It is both a diagnostic and a therapeutic agent. Atropine counteracts the muscarinic effects but is only partially effective for the CNS effects (seizures and coma). Preservative-free atropine (no benzyl alcohol) should be used. If the patient is symptomatic (bradycardia or bronchorrhea), a test dose should be administered, 0.02 mg/kg in children or 1 mg in adults, intravenously. If no signs of atropinization are present (tachycardia, drying of secretions, and mydriasis), atropine should be administered immediately, 0.05 mg/kg in children or 2 mg in adults, every 5 to 10 minutes as needed to dry the secretions and clear the lungs. Beneficial effects are seen within 1 to 4 minutes and maximum effect in 8 minutes. The average dose in the first 24 hours is 40 mg, but 1000 mg or more has been required in severe cases. Glycopyrrolate (Robinul) can be used if atropine is not available. The maximum dose should be maintained for 12 to 24 hours, then tapered and the patient observed for relapse. Poisoning, especially with lipophilic agents (e.g., fenthion, chlorfenthion), may require weeks of atropine therapy. An alternative is a continuous infusion of atropine 8 mg in 100 mL 0.9% saline at rate of 0.02 to 0.08 mg/kg/h (0.25 to 1.0 mL/kg/h) with additional 1 to 5 mg boluses as needed to dry the secretions.

Pralidoxime chloride (Protopam) has both antinicotinic and antimuscarinic effects and possibly also CNS effects. Successful treatment with pralidoxime chloride may allow a reduction in the dose of atropine. Pralidoxime acts to reactivate the phosphorylated cholinesterases by binding the phosphate moiety on the esteritic site and displacing it. It should be given early before "aging" of phosphate bond produces tighter binding. However, recent reports indicate that pralidoxime chloride is beneficial even several days after the poisoning. Improvement is seen within 10 to 40 minutes. The initial dose of pralidoxime chloride is 1 to 2 g in 250 mL 0.89% saline over 5 to 10 minutes, maximum 200 mg/minute, in adults or 25 to 50 mg/kg, maximum 4 mg/kg/minute, in children younger than 12 years of age. The dose can be repeated every 6 to 12 hours for several days. An alternative is a continuous infusion of 1 g in 100 mL 0.89% saline at 5 to 20 mg/kg/h (0.5 to 12 mL/g/h) up to 500 mg/h and titrated to desired response. Maximum adult daily dose is 12 g. Cardiac and blood pressure monitoring are advised during and for several hours after the infusion. The end point is absence of fasciculations and return of muscle strength.

Contraindicated drugs include morphine, aminophylline, barbiturates, opioids, phenothiazine, reserpine-like drugs, parasympathomimetics, and succinylcholine.

Noncardiac pulmonary edema may require respiratory support. Seizures may respond to atropine and pralidoxime chloride but often require anticonvulsants. Cardiac dysrhythmias may require electrical cardioversion or antidysrhythmic therapy if the patient is hemodynamically unstable. Extracorporeal procedures are of no proven value.

## Disposition

Asymptomatic patients with normal examination findings after 6 to 8 hours of observation may be discharged. In cases of intentional poisoning, the patients require psychiatric clearance for discharge. Symptomatic patients should be admitted to the intensive care unit. Observation of milder cases of carbamate poisoning, even those requiring atropine, for 6 to 8 hours symptom-free may be sufficient to exclude significant toxicity. In cases of workplace exposure, OSHA should be notified.

## PHENCYCLIDINE (ANGEL DUST)

Phencyclidine is an arylcyclohexylamine related to ketamine and chemically related to the phenothiazines. Originally a "dissociative" anesthetic banned in United States since 1979, it is now an illicit substance, with at least 38 analogs. It is inexpensively manufactured by "kitchen chemists" and is mislabeled as other hallucinogens. Improper phencyclidine synthesis may release cyanide when heated or smoked and can cause explosions.

## Toxic Mechanism

The mechanism of phencyclidine is complex and not completely understood. It inhibits some neurotransmitters and causes a loss of pain sensation without depressing the CNS respiratory status. It stimulates $\alpha$-adrenergic receptors and may act as a "false neurotransmitter." The effects are sympathomimetic, cholinergic, and cerebellar.

## Toxic Dose

The usual dose of phencyclidine mixed with marijuana joints is 100 to 400 mg of phencyclidine. Joints or leaf mixtures contain 0.24% to 7.9% of PCP, 1 mg of PCP/150 leaves. Tablets contain 5 mg (the usual street dose). CNS effects at doses of 1 to 6 mg include hallucinations and euphoria, 6 to 10 mg produces toxic psychosis and sympathetic stimulation, 10 to 25 mg produces severe toxicity, and more than 100 mg has resulted in fatalities.

## Kinetics

Phencyclidine is a lipophilic weak base, with a pKa of 8.5 to 9.5. It is rapidly absorbed when smoked and snorted, poorly absorbed from the acid stomach, and rapidly absorbed from the alkaline middle small intestine. It has an enterogastric secretion and is reabsorbed in the small intestine. The onset of action when smoked is 2 to 5 minutes, with a peak in 15 to 30 minutes. With oral ingestion, the onset is in 30 to 60 minutes and when taken intravenously it is immediate. Most adverse reactions in cases of overdose begin within 1 to 2 hours. Its duration of action at low doses is 4 to 6 hours and normality returns in 24 hours; in large overdoses, fluctuating coma may last 6 to 10 days.

Volume distribution is 6.2 L/kg. Phencyclidine concentrates in brain and adipose tissue. Protein binding is 70%. The route of elimination is by gastric secretion, liver metabolism, and 10% urinary excretion of conjugates and free phencyclidine. Renal excretion may be increased 50% with urinary acidification. The half-life is 1 hour (in cases of overdose, it is 11 to 89 hours).

## Manifestations

The classic picture is bursts of horizontal, vertical, and rotary nystagmus, which is a clue to diagnosis (occurs in 50% of cases), miosis, hypertension, and fluctuating altered mental state. There is a wide spectrum of clinical presentations.

Mild intoxication with 1 to 6 mg produces drunken and bizarre behavior, agitation, rotary nystagmus, and blank stare. Violent behavior and sensory anesthesia make these patients insensitive to pain, self-destructive, and dangerous. Most are communicative within 1 to 2 hours, are alert and oriented in 6 to 8 hours, and recover completely in 24 to 48 hours.

Moderate intoxication with 6 to 10 mg produces excess salivation, hypertension, hyperthermia, muscle rigidity, myoclonus, and catatonia. Recovery of consciousness occurs in 24 to 48 hours and complete recovery in 1 week.

Severe intoxication with 10 to 25 mg results in opisthotonus, decerebrate rigidity, convulsions, prolonged fluctuating coma, and respiratory failure. Patients in this category have a high rate of medical complications. Recovery of consciousness occurs in 24 to 48 hours, with complete normality in a month. Medical complications include apnea, aspiration pneumonia, cardiac arrest, hypertensive encephalopathy, hyperthermia, intracerebral hemorrhage, psychosis, rhabdomyolysis and myoglobinuria, and seizures. Loss of memory and "flashbacks" last for months. Phencyclidine-induced depression and suicide have been reported.

Fatalities occur with ingestions of greater than 100 mg and with serum levels greater than 100 to 250 ng/mL.

## Laboratory Investigations

Marked elevation of creatine kinase level may occur. Values greater than 20,000 units have been reported. Urinalysis should be monitored and urine tested for myoglobin. One should monitor the blood for creatine kinase, uric acid (an early clue to rhabdomyolysis), BUN, creatinine, electrolytes (hyperkalemia), blood glucose (20% of patients have hypoglycemia), urinary output, liver function tests, ECG, and ABG if the patient has any respiratory manifestations. Measurement of phencyclidine in the gastric juice is called for because concentrations are 10 to 50 times higher than in blood or urine. Phencyclidine blood concentrations are not helpful. Phencyclidine may be detected in the urine of the average user for 10 days to 3 weeks after the last dose. In chronic users, it can be detected for over 1 month. The analogs of phencyclidine may not produce positive test results for phencyclidine in the urine. Cross-reactions with bleach and dextromethorphan may cause false-positive urine test results on immunoassay, and cross-reaction with doxylamine may produce a false-positive finding on gas chromatography.

## Management

The patient should be observed for violent, self-destructive, bizarre behavior and paranoid schizophrenia. Patients should be placed in a low sensory environment and dangerous objects should be removed from the area.

Gastrointestinal decontamination is not effective because phencyclidine is rapidly absorbed from intestines. Overtreating the mild intoxication should be avoided. There is insufficient evidence to support the use of MDAC. In cases of severe toxicity (stupor or coma), continuous gastric suction can be tried (with protection of the airway) because the drug is secreted into the gastric juice. The value of this procedure is controversial because of limited data.

The patient must be protected from harming himself or herself or others. Physical restraints may be necessary, but they should be used sparingly and for the shortest time possible because they increase risk of rhabdomyolysis. Metal restraints such as handcuffs should be avoided. For behavioral disorders and toxic psychosis, diazepam is the agent of choice. Pharmacologic intervention includes diazepam (Valium) 10 to 30 mg orally or 2 to 5 mg intravenously initially and titrated upward to 10 mg; however, up to 30 mg may be required. "Talk down" technique is usually ineffective and dangerous. Phenothiazines and butyrophenones should be avoided in the acute phase because they lower the convulsive threshold; however, they may be needed later for psychosis. Haloperidol (Haldol) administration has been reported to produce catatonia.

Seizures and muscle spasm are managed with diazepam, from 2.5 mg up to 10 mg. Hyperthermia (>38.5°C [101.3°F]) is treated with external cooling measures. Hypertension is usually transient and does not require treatment. In the case of emergent hypertensive crisis (blood pressure >200/115 mm Hg) nitroprusside can be used in a dose of 0.3 to 2 $\mu$g/kg/min. Maximum infusion rate is 10 $\mu$g/kg/min for only 10 minutes.

Acid ion trapping diuresis is not recommended because of the danger of myoglobin precipitation in the renal tubules. Rhabdomyolysis and myoglobinuria are treated by correcting volume depletion and insuring a urinary output of greater than 2 mL/kg/h. Alkalinization is controversial because of reabsorption of phencyclidine.

Hemodialysis is beneficial if renal failure occurs; otherwise, the extracorporeal procedures are not beneficial.

## Disposition

All patients with coma, delirium, catatonia, violent behavior, aspiration pneumonia, sustained hypertension greater than 200/115, and significant rhabdomyolysis should be admitted to the intensive care unit until asymptomatic for at least 24 hours. If patients with mild intoxication are mentally and neurologically stable and become asymptomatic (except for nystagmus) for 4 hours, they may be discharged in the company of a responsible adult. All patients must be assessed for suicide risk before discharge. Drug counseling and psychiatric follow-up should be arranged. Patients should be warned that episodes of disorientation and depression may continue intermittently for 4 weeks or more.

# PHENOTHIAZINES AND NONPHENOTHIAZINES (NEUROLEPTICS)

## Toxic Mechanism

Neuroleptics have complex mechanisms of toxicity, including (a) block of the postsynaptic dopamine receptors; (b) block of peripheral and central $\alpha$-adrenergic receptors; (c) block of cholinergic muscarinic receptors; (d) quinidine-like antidysrhythmic and myocardial depressant effect in cases of large overdose; (e) lowering of the convulsive threshold; (f) effect on hypothalamic temperature regulation (Table 25).

## Toxic Dose

Extrapyramidal reactions, anticholinergic effects, and orthostatic hypotension may occur at therapeutic doses. The toxic amount is not established, but the maximum daily therapeutic dose may result in significant side effects, and twice this amount may be potentially fatal. Chlorpromazine (Thorazine), the prototype, may produce serious hypotension and CNS depression at doses greater than 200 mg (17 mg/kg) in children and 3 to 5 g in an adult. Fatalities have been reported after 2.5 g of loxapine (Loxitane) and mesoridazine (Serentil) and 1.5 g of thioridazine (Mellaril).

## Kinetics

These agents are lipophilic and have unpredictable gastrointestinal absorption. Peak levels occur 2 to 6 hours postingestion and have enterohepatic recirculation.

The mean serum half-life in phase 1 is 1 to 2 hours and the biphasic half-life is 20 to 40 hours. Volume distribution is 10 to 40 L/kg; protein binding is 92% to 98%. Chlorpromazine taken orally has an onset of action in 30 to 60 minutes, peak in 2 to 4 hours, and duration of 4 to 6 hours. With sustained-release preparations, the onset is in 30 to 60 minutes and duration is 6 to 12 hours.

Elimination is by hepatic metabolism, which results in multiple metabolites (some are active). Metabolites can be detected in urine months after chronic therapy. Only 1% to 3% is excreted unchanged in the urine.

## Manifestations

In cases of phenothiazine overdose, anticholinergic symptoms may be present early but are not life-threatening. Miosis is usually present (80%) if the phenothiazine has strong $\alpha$-adrenergic blocking effect (e.g., chlorpromazine), but anticholinergic activity mydriasis may occur. Agitation and delirium rapidly progress into coma. Major problems are cardiac toxicity and hypotension. The cardiotoxic effects are seen more commonly with thioridazine and its metabolite mesoridazine. These agents have produced the largest number of fatalities in patients with phenothiazine overdose. Cardiac conduction disturbances include prolonged PR, QRS, and QTc intervals, U- and T-wave abnormalities, and ventricular dysrhythmias, including torsades de pointes. Seizures occur mainly in patients with convulsive disorders or with administration of loxapine. Sudden death in children and adults has been reported.

Idiosyncratic dystonic reactions are most common with the piperidine group. Reactions are not dose-dependent and consist of opisthotonos, torticollis, orolingual dyskinesia, or oculogyric crisis (painful upward gaze). These reactions are more frequent in children and women. Neuroleptic malignant syndrome occurs in patients on chronic therapy and is characterized by hyperthermia, muscle rigidity, autonomic dysfunction, and altered mental state. There is one case reported with acute overdose. The loxapine syndrome consists of seizures, rhabdomyolysis, and renal failure.

## Laboratory Investigations

Monitoring should include arterial blood gases, renal and hepatic function, electrolytes, blood glucose, and creatine kinase and myoglobinemia in neurol-eptic malignant syndrome. Most of these agents are

**TABLE 25** Neuroleptics and Properties

| Compound | Antipsychotic | Anticholinergic | Extrapyramidal | Hypotensive and Cardiotoxic | Sedative |
|---|---|---|---|---|---|
| **Phenothiazine** | | | | | |
| Aliphatic | 1+ | 3+ | 2+ | 2+ | 3+ |
|   Chlorpromazine (Thorazine) | | | | | |
|   Promethazine (Phenergan) | | | | | |
| Piperazine | 3+ | 1+ | 3+ | 1+ | 1+ |
|   Fluphenazine (Prolixin) | | | | | |
|   Perphenazine (Trilafon) | | | | | |
|   Prochlorperazine (Compazine) | | | | | |
|   Trifluoperazine (Stelazine) | | | | | |
| Piperidine | 1+ | 2+ | 1+ | 3+ | 3+ |
|   Mesoridazine (Serentil) | | | | | |
|   Thioridazine (Mellaril) | | | | | |
| **Nonphenothiazine** | | | | | |
| Butyrophenone | 3+ | 1+ | 3+ | 1+ | 1+ |
|   Haloperidol (Haldol) | | | | | |
| Dibenzoxazepine | 3+ | 1+ | 3+ | 1+ | 2+ |
|   Loxapine (Loxitane) | | | | | |
| Dihydroindolone | 3+ | 1+ | 3+ | 1+ | 1+ |
|   Molindone (Moban) | | | | | |
| Thioxanthenes | 3+ | 1+ | 3+ | 3+ | 1+ |
|   Thiothixene (Navane) | | | | | |
|   Chlorprothixene (Taractan) | | | | | |

1+ = very low activity; 2+ = moderate activity; 3+ = very high activity.

detected on routine screening. Quantitative serum levels are not useful in management. Cross-reactions with enzyme multiplied immunoassay technique tests occur with cyclic antidepressants. Phenothiazines give false-negative results on pregnancy urine tests using human chorionic gonadotropin as an indicator, and give false-positive results for urine porphyrins, indirect Coombs test, urobilinogen, and amylase.

## Management

Vital functions must be established and maintained. All overdose patients require venous access, 12-lead ECG (to measure intervals), cardiac and respiratory monitoring, and seizure precautions. One should monitor core temperature to detect poikilothermic effect. If the patient is comatose, intubation and assisted ventilation may be required, as well as 100% oxygen, intravenous glucose, naloxone (Narcan), and thiamine.

Emesis is not recommended. Activated charcoal can be administered if ingestion was within 1 hour. MDAC has not been proven beneficial. A radiograph of the abdomen may be useful, if the phenothiazine is radiopaque. Haloperidol (Haldol) and trifluoperazine (Stelazine) are most likely to be radiopaque. Whole-bowel irrigation may be useful when a large number of pills are visualized on radiograph or if sustained-release preparations were taken, but whole-bowel irrigation has not been evaluated in patients with phenothiazine overdose.

Convulsions are treated with diazepam or lorazepam (Ativan). Loxapine (Loxitane) overdose may result in status epilepticus. If nondepolarizing neuromuscular blockade is required, pancuronium (Pavulon) or vecuronium (Norcuron) should be used (not succinylcholine [Anectine], which may cause malignant hyperthermia), and EEG should be monitored during paralysis.

Patients with dysrhythmias should be monitored with serial ECGs. Unstable rhythms can be treated with electrical cardioversion. Class 1a antidysrhythmics (procainamide, quinidine, and disopyramide [Norpace]) must be avoided.

Hypokalemia predisposes to dysrhythmias and should be corrected aggressively. Supraventricular tachycardia with hemodynamic instability is treated with electrical cardioversion. The role of adenosine has not been defined. Calcium channel and β-blockers should be avoided.

Prolongation of the QRS interval is treated with sodium bicarbonate 1 to 2 mEq/kg by intravenous bolus over a few minutes. Torsades de pointes is treated with magnesium sulfate IV 20% solution 2 g over 2 to 3 minutes. If there is no response in 10 minutes, the dose is repeated and followed by a continuous infusion of 5 to 10 mg/min or given as an infusion of 50 mg/minute for 2 hours followed by 30 mg/minute for 90 minutes twice a day for several days, as needed. The dose in children is 25 to 50 mg/kg initially and maintenance dose is 30 to 60 mg/kg per 24 hours (0.25 to 0.50 mEq/kg per 24 hours) up to 1000 mg per 24 hours. Serum magnesium levels should be monitored.

To treat ventricular tachydysrhythmias in a stable patient, lidocaine is used. If the patient is unstable, electrical cardioversion is used. Patients with heart block with hemodynamic instability should be managed with temporary cardiac pacing.

Hypotension is treated with the Trendelenburg position and 0.9% saline. If the condition is refractory to treatment or there is a danger of fluid overload, vasopressors are administered. The vasopressor of choice is α-adrenergic agonist norepinephrine (Levophed), titrated to response. Epinephrine and dopamine should not be used because β-receptor stimulation in the presence of α-receptor blockade may provoke dysrhythmias and phenothiazines are antidopaminergic.

Hypothermia and hyperthermia are treated with external warming and cooling measures, respectively. Antipyretic drugs must not be used.

Management of the neuroleptic malignant syndrome includes the following actions:

- Immediately discontinuing the offending agent
- Hyperventilating the patient, using 100% humidified, cooled oxygen at high gas flows (at least 10 L/min) because of rapid breathing

- Administering a benzodiazepine to control convulsions and facilitate cooling measures
- Initiating appropriate mechanical cooling measures, which may include intravenous cold saline (not lactated Ringer's), ice baths, cold lavage of the stomach, bladder, and rectum, and a hypothermic blanket
- Correcting acid–base and electrolyte disturbances and treating significant hyperkalemia with hyperventilation, calcium, sodium bicarbonate, intravenous glucose, and insulin; hemodialysis may be necessary

In addition, dysrhythmias usually respond to correction of the underlying acid–base disturbances and hyperkalemia. If antidysrhythmic agents are required, calcium channel blockers must be avoided because they may precipitate hyperkalemia and cardiovascular collapse. Dantrolene sodium (Dantrium), which is a phenytoin derivative, inhibits calcium release from the sarcoplasmic reticulum and results in decreased muscle contraction. Dantrolene acts peripherally and does not reverse the rigidity or psychomotor disturbances resulting from the central dopamine blockade; it therefore is often used in combination with bromocriptine. Bromocriptine mesylate (Parlodel) acts centrally as a dopamine agonist, as does amantadine hydrochloride (Symmetrel). Bromocriptine and dantrolene have been reported to be successful in combination with cooling and good supportive measures in malignant hyperthermia.

Dosing for these agents is as follows: dantrolene sodium at 2 to 3 mg/kg IV as a bolus, then 1 mg/kg/ minute to a maximum of 10 mg/kg or until the tachycardia, rigidity, increased end-tidal $CO_2$, and temperature elevation are controlled. *Note:* Hepatotoxicity occurs with doses greater than 10 mg/kg. To prevent symptom recurrence, 1 mg/kg should be administered every 6 hours for 24 to 48 hours after the episode. After that time, oral dantrolene can be used at a dose of 1 mg/kg every 6 hours for 24 hours as necessary. The patient should be observed for thrombophlebitis following intravenous dantrolene. It is best administered via a central line. Bromocriptine mesylate at 2.5 to 10 mg orally or via a nasogastric tube, three times a day, should be used in combination with dantrolene.

Idiosyncratic dystonic reaction can be treated with diphenhydramine (Benadryl) 1 to 2 mg/kg/dose intravenously over 5 minutes up to maximum of 50 mg intravenously; a response is noted within 2 to 5 minutes. This can be followed with oral doses for 4 to 6 days to prevent recurrence.

Extracorporeal measures (hemodialysis, hemoperfusion) are not effective in removing these agents.

### Disposition

Asymptomatic patients should be observed for at least 6 hours after gastric decontamination. Symptomatic patients with cardiotoxicity, hypotension, and convulsions should be admitted to the intensive care unit and monitored for 48 hours.

## SALICYLATES (ACETYLSALICYLIC ACID, SALICYLIC ACID)

### Toxic Mechanism

The primary toxic mechanisms include (a) direct stimulation of the medullary chemoreceptor trigger zone and respiratory center; (b) uncoupling oxidative phosphorylation; (c) inhibition of the Krebs cycle enzymes; (d) inhibition of vitamin K dependent and independent clotting factors; (e) alteration of platelet function; and (f) inhibition of prostaglandin synthesis.

### Toxic Dose

Acute mild intoxication occurs at a dose of 150 to 200 mg/kg, moderate intoxication at 200 to 300 mg/kg, and severe intoxication at 300 to 500 mg/kg. Acute salicylate plasma concentration greater than 30 mg/dL (usually >40 mg/dL) may be associated with clinical toxicity. Chronic intoxication occurs at ingestions greater than 100 mg/kg/d for more than 2 days because of accumulation kinetics. Methyl salicylate (oil of wintergreen) is the most toxic form of salicylate. A dose of 1 mL of 98% contains 1.4 g of salicylate. Fatalities have occurred with ingestion of 1 teaspoonful in children and 1 ounce in adults. It is found in topical ointments and liniments (18% to 30%).

### Kinetics

Acetylsalicylic acid and salicylic acid are weak acids with a pKa of 3.5 and 3.0, respectively. Acetylsalicylic acid is absorbed from the stomach, from the small bowel, and dermally. Onset of action is within 30 minutes. Methyl salicylate and effervescent tablets are absorbed more rapidly. Salicylate plasma concentration is detectable within 15 minutes after ingestion and peaks in 30 to 120 minutes. The peak may be delayed 6 to 12 hours in cases of large overdose, overdose with enteric-coated or sustained-release preparations, and development of concretions. The therapeutic duration of action is 3 to 4 hours but is markedly prolonged in cases of overdose.

Volume distribution is 0.13 L/kg for salicylic acid but increases as the salicylate plasma concentration increases. Protein binding is greater than 90% for salicylic acid at pH 7.4 and a salicylate plasma concentration of 20 to 30 mg/dL, 75% at a salicylate plasma concentration greater than 40 mg/dL, 50% at a salicylate plasma concentration of 70 mg/dL, and 30% at a salicylate plasma concentration of 120 mg/dL.

The half-life for salicylic acid is 3 hours after a 300 mg dose, 6 hours after a 1 g overdose, and greater than 10 hours after a 10-g overdose. Elimination includes Michaelis-Menten hepatic metabolism by three saturable pathways: (a) glycine conjugation to salicyluric acid (75%); (b) glucuronyl transferase to salicyl phenol glucuronide (10%); and (c) salicyl aryl glucuronide (4%). Nonsaturable pathways are hydrolysis to gentisic acid (<1%). Ten percent is excreted unchanged.

Acidosis increases the severity of the intoxication by increasing the non-ionized salicylate that can cross membranes and enter the brain cells. In kidneys, the unionized salicylic acid undergoes glomerular filtration, and the ionized portion undergoes tubular secretion in proximal tubules and passive reabsorption in the distal tubules. Renal excretion of salicylate is enhanced by alkaline urine.

### Manifestations

The ingestion of concentrated topical salicylic acid preparations (e.g., wart remover) can cause mucosal caustic injury to the gastrointestinal tract. Occult salicylate overdose should be considered in any patient with unexplained acid–base disturbance.

The manifestations of acute overdose of salicylates are as follows:

#### Minimal Symptoms

Tinnitus, dizziness, and deafness may occur at high therapeutic salicylate plasma concentrations of 20 to 30 mg/dL. Nausea and vomiting may occur immediately because of local gastric irritation.

**Phase I.** Mild manifestations occur at 1 to 12 hours after ingestion with a 6-hour salicylate plasma concentration of 45 to 70 mg/dL. Nausea and vomiting followed by hyperventilation are usually present within 3 to 8 hours after acute overdose. Hyperventilation, an increase in both rate (tachypnea) and depth (hyperpnea), is present but it may be subtle. It results in a mild respiratory alkalosis with a serum pH greater than 7.4 and urine pH greater than 6.0. Some patients may have lethargy, vertigo, headache, and confusion. Diaphoresis may be noted.

**Phase II.** Moderate manifestations occur at 12 to 24 hours after ingestion with a 6-hour salicylate plasma concentration of 70 to 90 mg/dL. Serious metabolic disturbances, including a marked respiratory alkalosis with anion gap metabolic acidosis, dehydration, and urine pH less than 6.0, may occur. Other metabolic disturbances include hypoglycemia or hyperglycemia, hypokalemia, decreased ionized calcium, and increased BUN, creatinine, and lactate. Mental disturbances (confusion, disorientation, hallucinations) may occur. Hypotension and convulsions have been reported.

**Phase III.** Severe intoxication occurs more than 24 hours after ingestion with a 6-hour salicylate plasma concentration of 90 to 130 mg/dL.

In addition to the above clinical findings, coma and seizures develop and indicate severe intoxication. Pulmonary edema may occur. Metabolic disturbances include metabolic acidemia (pH <7.4) and aciduria (pH <6.0). In adults, alkalosis may persist until terminal respiratory failure.

In children younger than 4 years of age, a mixed metabolic acidosis and respiratory alkalosis develop earlier (within 4 to 6 hours) than in adults because children have less respiratory reserve and accumulate lactate and other organic acids. Hypoglycemia is more common in children.

Fatalities occur at 6-hour salicylate plasma concentrations greater than 130 to 150 mg/dL and result from CNS depression, cardiovascular collapse, electrolyte imbalance, and cerebral edema.

Chronic salicylism is more serious than acute intoxication and the 6-hour salicylate plasma concentration does not correlate well with the manifestations in both acute and chronic cases of intoxication. Chronic intoxication usually occurs with therapeutic errors in young children or the elderly with underlying illness, and the diagnosis is delayed because it is not recognized. Noncardiac pulmonary edema is a frequent complication in the elderly. The mortality rate is about 25%. Chronic salicylate poisoning in children may mimic Reye syndrome. It is associated with exaggerated CNS findings (hallucinations, delirium, dementia, memory loss, papilledema, bizarre behavior, agitation, encephalopathy, seizures, and coma). Hemorrhagic manifestations, renal failure, and pulmonary and cerebral edema may occur. The metabolic picture is hypoglycemia and mixed acid–base derangements. A chronic salicylate plasma concentration greater than 60 mg/dL with metabolic acidosis and an altered mental state is very serious.

## Laboratory Investigations

All patients with intentional salicylate overdoses should have acetaminophen plasma level measured after 4 hours.

One should continuously monitor ECG, urine output, urine pH, and specific gravity. Every 2 to 4 hours in cases of severe intoxication, salicylate plasma concentration, glucose (in a case of salicylism, CNS hypoglycemia may be present despite normal serum glucose), electrolytes, ionized calcium, magnesium and phosphorous, anion gap, ABGs, and pulse oximeter should be monitored. Daily monitoring of BUN, creatinine, liver function tests, and prothrombin time should take place.

The therapeutic salicylate plasma concentration is less than 10 mg/dL for analgesia and 15 to 30 mg/dL for anti-inflammatory effect. Cross-reaction with diflunisal (Dolobid) will give a falsely high salicylate plasma concentration. The Done nomogram is not considered accurate in evaluating acute or chronic salicylate intoxications.

## Management

Treatment is based on clinical and metabolic findings, not on salicylate levels. Continuous monitoring of the urine pH is essential for successful alkalinization treatment. One should always obtain an acetaminophen plasma level.

Vital functions must be established and maintained. If the patient is in an altered mental state, glucose, naloxone, and thiamine are administered in standard doses. Depending on the severity, the initial studies include an immediate and a 6-hour postingestion salicylate plasma concentration, ECG and cardiac monitoring, pulse oximeter, urine (analysis, pH, and specific gravity), chest radiograph, ABGs, blood glucose, electrolytes and anion gap calculation, calcium (ionized), magnesium, renal and liver profiles, and prothrombin time. Gastric contents and stool should be tested for occult blood. Bismuth and magnesium salicylate preparations may be radiopaque on radiographs. Consultation with a nephrologist is warranted in cases of moderate, severe, or chronic intoxication.

For gastrointestinal decontamination, activated charcoal is useful (each gram of activated charcoal binds 550 mg of salicylic acid) if a toxic dose was ingested up to 4 hours postingestion. MDAC is not recommended for salicylate poisoning.

Concretions may occur with massive (usually >300 mg/kg) ingestions. If blood levels fail to decline, prompt contrast radiography of the stomach may reveal concretions that have to be removed by repeated lavage, whole-bowel irrigation, endoscopy, or gastrostomy.

Fluids and electrolyte treatment of salicylate poisonings is given in Table 26. For shock, perfusion and vascular volume should be established with 5% dextrose in 0.9% saline, then the treatment can proceed with correction of dehydration and alkalinization.

For cases of acute moderate or severe salicylism (see Table 26), adults should receive a bolus of 1 to 2 mEq/kg of sodium bicarbonate ($NaHCO_3$) followed by an infusion of 100 to 150 mEq $NaHCO_3$ added to 500 to 1000 mL of 5% dextrose and administered over 60 minutes. Children should receive a bolus of 1 to 2 mEq/kg of $NaHCO_3$ followed by an infusion of 1 to 2 mEq/kg added to 20 mL/kg of 5% dextrose administered over 60 minutes. Potassium is added after the patient voids. The goal is to achieve a urine output of greater than 2 mL/kg/hr and a urine pH of greater than 8. The initial infusion is followed by subsequent infusions (two to three times normal maintenance) of 200 to 300 mL/h in adults or 10 mL/kg/h in children. If the patient is acidotic and has a serum pH of less than 7.15, an additional 1 to 2 mEq/kg of $NaHCO_3$ is given over 1 to 2 hours; persistent acidosis may require 1 to 2 mEq/kg of bicarbonate every 2 hours. The infusion rate, the amount of bicarbonate, and the electrolytes should be adjusted to correct serum abnormalities and to maintain the targeted urine output and urinary pH. Diuresis is not as important as the alkalinization.

---

**TABLE 26** Fluid and Electrolyte Treatment of Salicylate Poisoning

| Type of Salicylism | Metabolic Disturbance | Blood pH | Urine pH | Hydrating Solution | Amount of $NaHCO_3$ (mEq/L) | Amount of Potassium (mEq/L) |
|---|---|---|---|---|---|---|
| **Mild** | Respiratory alkalosis | >7.4 | >6.0 | 5% Dextrose, 0.45% saline | 50 (adult) 1 mEq/kg (child) | 20 |
| **Moderate** Chronic Child <4 Years | Respiratory alkalosis Metabolic acidosis | >7.4 or <7.4 | <6.0 | 5% Dextrose in water | 100 (adult) 1-2 mEq/kg (child) | 40 |
| **Severe** Chronic Child <4 years | Metabolic acidosis Respiratory alkalosis | <7.4 | <6.0 | 5% Dextrose in water | 150 (adult) 2m Eq/kg (child) | 60 |
| **CNS** Depressant Co-ingestant | Respiratory acidosis | <7.4 | <6.0 | 5% Dextrose in water | 100-150* | 60 |

*Correct hypoventilation.
Modified from Linden CH, Rumack BH: The legitimate analgesics, aspirin and acetaminophen. In Hansen W Jr (ed): Toxic Emergencies. New York, Churchill Livingstone, 1984.

Careful monitoring for fluid overload should take place for patients at risk of pulmonary and cerebral edema (e.g., the elderly) and because of inappropriate secretion of the antidiuretic hormone.

In patients with mild intoxication who are not acidotic and have a urine pH greater than 6, 5% dextrose in 0.45% saline should be administered as maintenance to replace ongoing fluid loss. Some toxicologists may consider adding sodium bicarbonate 50 mEq/L or 1 mEq/kg in some cases.

To achieve alkalinization, sodium bicarbonate is administered to produce a serum pH 7.4 to 7.5 and a urine pH greater than 8. Carbonic anhydrase inhibitors (acetazolamide [Diamox]) should not be used. If the patient is acidotic, additional bicarbonate may be required. About 2 mEq/kg raises the blood pH 0.1. In children, alkalinization may be a difficult problem because of the organic acid production and hypokalemia. Hypokalemic and fluid-depleted patients cannot be adequately alkalinized. Alkalinization is usually discontinued in asymptomatic patients with a salicylate plasma concentration less than 30 to 40 mg/dL but is continued in symptomatic patients regardless of the salicylate plasma concentration. A decreased serum bicarbonate but normal or high blood pH indicates respiratory alkalosis predominating over metabolic acidosis, and the bicarbonate should be administered cautiously. An alkalemic pH of 7.40 to 7.50 is not a contraindication to bicarbonate therapy because these patients have a significant base deficit in spite of elevated blood pH.

Potassium is added, 20 to 40 mEq/L, to the infusion after the patient voids. In cases of severe, late, and chronic salicylism, 60 mEq/L of potassium may be needed. When the serum potassium is below 4.0 mEq/L, 10 mEq/L should be added over the first hour. If the patient has hypokalemia less than 3 mEq/L and flat T waves and U waves, 0.25 to 0.5 mEq/kg up to 10 mEq/h is administered. Potassium should be administered under ECG monitoring. Serum potassium is rechecked after each rapidly administered dose. A paradoxical urine acidosis (alkaline serum pH and acid urine pH) indicates that potassium is probably needed.

Convulsions are treated with diazepam or lorazepam, but hypoglycemia, low ionized calcium, cerebral edema, and hemorrhage should first be excluded with a CT scan. If tetany develops, the NaHCO$_3$ therapy is discontinued and calcium gluconate 0.1 to 0.2 mL/kg 10% administered.

Pulmonary edema management consists of fluid restriction, high FIO$_2$, mechanical ventilation, and positive end-expiratory pressure.

Cerebral edema management consists of fluid restriction, elevation of the head, hyperventilation, osmotic diuresis, and administration of dexamethasone. Vitamin K$_1$ is administered parenterally to correct an increased prothrombin time (>20 seconds) and coagulation abnormalities. If the patient has active bleeding, fresh plasma and platelets are administered as needed. Hyperpyrexia is managed by external cooling measures, not antipyretics.

Hemodialysis is the choice for removal of salicylates because it corrects the acid–base, electrolyte, and fluid disturbances as well. The indications for hemodialysis include the following:

- Acute poisoning with salicylate plasma concentration greater than 100 mg/dL without improvement after 6 hours of appropriate therapy
- Chronic poisoning with cardiopulmonary disease and a salicylate plasma concentration as low as 40 mg/dL with refractory acidosis, severe CNS manifestations (coma and seizures), and progressive deterioration, especially in elderly patients
- Impairment of vital organs of elimination
- Clinical deterioration in spite of good supportive care and alkalinization
- Severe refractory acid–base or electrolyte disturbances despite appropriate corrective measures

### Disposition

There are limitations of salicylate plasma levels and patients are treated on the basis of clinical and laboratory findings. Patients who are asymptomatic should be monitored for a minimum of 6 hours, and

longer if enteric-coated tablets or massive overdose was taken or if there is suspicion of concretions. Those who remain asymptomatic with a salicylate plasma concentration less than 35 mg/dL may be discharged following psychiatric evaluation, if indicated. Chronic salicylate-intoxicated patients with acidosis and an altered mental state should be admitted to the intensive care unit. Patients with acute ingestion and a salicylate plasma concentration less than 60 mg/dL and mild symptoms may be able to be treated in the emergency department. Patients with moderate and severe intoxications should be admitted to the intensive care unit.

## SELECTIVE SEROTONIN REUPTAKE INHIBITORS

Selective serotonin reuptake inhibitors (SSRIs) are primarily prescribed as antidepressants. SSRIs include fluoxetine (Prozac), paroxetine (Paxil), and sertraline (Zoloft).

### Toxic Mechanism

The SSRIs interfere with the neuron reuptake of serotonin (5-hydroxytryptamine) at the presynaptic ganglia sites in the brain, increasing the activity of serotonin. SSRIs should not be used within 5 weeks of when a MAOI is given, nor should MAOI therapy be initiated or discontinued within 5 weeks of SSRI therapy.

### Toxic Dose

The therapeutic oral dose of fluoxetine is 20 to 80 mg/d. No toxicity is seen in children with up to 3.5 mg/kg/dose orally. A fatal dose for adults is 6 g. The therapeutic dose for paroxetine is 20 to 50 mg/d. In 35 adult patients, none developed serious side effects after the ingestion of 10 to 1000 mg, and a study involving 35 children failed to demonstrate serious adverse effects at doses less than 180 mg. The therapeutic dose for sertraline is 50 mg to 200 mg/d. Patients have ingested up to 2.6 g without serious side effects. Overdose involving children who ingested less than 100 mg failed to cause adverse events.

### Kinetics

Fluoxetine is well absorbed from the gastrointestinal tract, and has a peak plasma concentration at 6 to 8 hours. Volume distribution is 20 to 42 L/kg; 95% is protein bound. The half-life is 4 days (for the demethylated active metabolite norfluoxetine, the half-life is 7 to 15 days). Elimination is 80% renal. Fluoxetine and other serotonin inhibitors are inhibitors of the cytochrome P450, CYP 2D6 enzyme. Therefore interactions may occur with many other medications, such as antidysrhythmic class IC drugs (quinidine), phenytoin (Dilantin), haloperidol, lithium, tricyclic antidepressants (TCAs), β-blockers, codeine, and carbamazepine (Tegretol).

Paroxetine is almost completely absorbed from the gastrointestinal tract, with a peak in 2 to 8 hours. Protein binding is greater than 90%; volume distribution is 13 L/kg. Paroxetine undergoes extensive first-pass liver metabolism by oxidation and methylation to inactive metabolites. It inhibits the P450 system (see fluoxetine metabolism). The average half-life is 21 hours.

Sertraline peaks in 8 to 12 hours. Its volume distribution is 20 L/kg and protein binding is 98%. The average half-life of sertraline is 26 hours. It is metabolized to form a less-active metabolite, N-desmethylsertraline (half-life of 62 to 104 hours).

### Manifestations

All SSRIs may cause serotonin syndrome, a potentially life-threatening reaction, if they are administered concurrently with an MAOI. Serotonin syndrome is caused by cerebral serotonergic stimulation and can cause severe hyperthermia, myoclonus, rhabdomyolysis, confusion, tremors, and a variety of psychological disturbances. In addition, cardiovascular complications and extrapyramidal side effects, including akathisia, dyskinesia, and Parkinson-like syndromes may occur. Also, increased suicidal ideation, seizures, sexual disorders, and hematologic disorders (platelet serotonin activity blockade leading to prolonged bleeding times) may develop. Inappropriate secretion of antidiuretic hormone resulting in hyponatremia may occur when SSRIs are administered to the elderly. This effect is usually seen within the first week of therapy.

Overdose effects are similar to the serotonin syndrome.

## Laboratory Investigations

One should obtain a complete blood count (CBC), electrolytes, glucose levels, a coagulation profile, liver function tests, creatine kinase level, and an ECG.

## Management

There is no specific antidote to SSRI intoxication.

Initial management consists of stabilizing vital functions, including thermoregulation. Supportive therapy and anticipation of potential life-threatening manifestations (hypotension, hyperthermia, seizures, coma, disseminated intravascular coagulation, ventricular tachycardia, and metabolic acidosis), are essential. Vital signs, EEG, creatine kinase, and blood chemistry should be monitored.

Benzodiazepines are administered to prevent and control muscle hyperactivity (diazepam [Valium] for seizures, clonazepam [Klonopin] for myoclonus). If benzodiazepine therapy fails to control muscle activity or seizures, anesthesia or nondepolarizing neuromuscular blockade may be necessary.

Electrolyte abnormalities and acid–base balance should be corrected. Fluids are used to maintain a urine output of greater than 2 mL/kg/h if there is a risk of myoglobinuria.

There are no data to support the use of gastrointestinal decontamination, although activated charcoal may be used if an ingestion has occurred within 1 hour. Hemodialysis and charcoal hemoperfusion are unlikely to be beneficial. Haloperidol (Haldol), phenothiazines, and other highly protein-bound drugs are to be avoided.

Benzodiazepine and cooling therapy can be used for hyperthermia. Serotonin antagonists, such as cyproheptadine (Periactin), may be useful in treating serotonin syndrome, although there are no controlled data. Dantrolene (Dantrium) and bromocriptine (Parlodel) are not recommended and may actually precipitate serotonin syndrome.

## Disposition

Cases of ingestions in children up to 5 years of age of less than 180 mg of paroxetine (Paxil), less than 3.5 mg/kg of fluoxetine (Prozac), or less than 100 mg of sertraline (Zoloft) can be observed at home. Symptomatic patients should be admitted to the intensive care unit until asymptomatic for 24 hours. Asymptomatic patients should be observed for 6 hours. All patients should be assessed for risk of suicide before discharge. When taken chronically, SSRIs may increase cholesterol and triglycerides and decrease uric acid, so these test results should be followed.

## THEOPHYLLINE

Theophylline (Slo-Phyllin) is a methylxanthine alkaloid similar to caffeine and theobromine. Aminophylline is 80% theophylline. Theophylline is used in the acute treatment of asthma, pulmonary edema, chronic obstructive pulmonary disease, and neonatal apnea.

## Toxic Mechanism

The proposed mechanisms of action include phosphodiesterase inhibition, adenosine receptor antagonism, inhibition of prostaglandins, and increase in serum catecholamines. Theophylline stimulates the central nervous, respiratory, and emetic centers and reduces the seizure threshold. It has positive cardiac inotropic and chronotropic effects, acts as a diuretic, relaxes smooth muscle, and causes peripheral vasodilation but cerebral vasoconstriction. Gastric secretions, gastrointestinal motility, lipolysis, glycogenolysis, and gluconeogenesis are all increased.

## Toxic Dose

A single dose of 1 mg/kg produces a theophylline plasma concentration of approximately 2 µg/mL. The therapeutic range usually is 10 to 20 µg/mL. An acute, single dose greater than 10 mg/kg causes mild toxicity, a dose greater than 20 mg/kg causes moderate toxicity, and a dose greater than 50 mg/kg causes serious, possibly fatal toxicity. Fatalities occur at lower doses in patients with chronic toxicity, especially those with risk factors (see *Kinetics*).

## Kinetics

The pKa is 9.5. Absorption from the stomach and upper small intestine is complete and rapid, with onset in 30 to 60 minutes. Peak theophylline plasma concentration occurs within 1 to 2 hours after ingestion of liquid preparations, 2 to 4 hours after ingestion of regular tablets, and 7 to 24 hours after ingestion of slow-release formulations. Volume distribution is 0.3 to 0.7 L/kg. Protein binding is 40% to 60% in adults, mainly to albumin (low albumin increases free active theophylline).

Elimination is 90% by hepatic metabolism to an active metabolite, 2-methyl xanthine. The half-life is 3.5 hours in a child and 4 to 6 hours in an adult. The half-life is shorter in smokers and patients taking enzyme-inducing drugs. Only 8% to 10% of the drug is excreted unchanged in the urine.

Risk factors that produce a longer half-life include age younger than 6 months or older than 60 years, use of enzyme-inhibitor drugs (calcium channel blockers, oral contraceptives, cimetidine [Tagamet], ciprofloxacin [Cipro], erythromycin, macrolide anti-biotics, isoniazid), illness (persistent fever >38.9°C [>102°F]), viral illness, liver impairment, heart failure, chronic obstructive pulmonary disease, and influenza vaccination.

## Manifestations

Acute toxicity generally correlates with blood levels; chronic toxicity does not (Table 27).

In the case of an acute, single, regular-release overdose, vomiting and occasionally hematemesis occur at low theophylline plasma concentrations. CNS stimulation includes restlessness, muscle tremors, and protracted tonic–clonic seizures, but coma is rare. Convulsions are a sign of severe toxicity and usually are preceded by gastrointestinal symptoms (except with sustained-release and chronic intoxications). Cardiovascular disturbances include cardiac dysrhythmias (supraventricular tachycardia) and transient hypertension with mild overdoses, but hypotension and ventricular dysrhythmias with severe intoxications. Rhabdomyolysis and renal failure are occasionally seen. Children tolerate higher serum levels, and cardiac dysrhythmias and seizures occur at theophylline plasma concentrations greater than 100 µg/mL. Possible metabolic disturbances include hyperglycemia, pronounced hypokalemia, hypocalcemia, hypomagnesemia, hypophosphatemia, increased serum amylase, and elevation of uric acid.

Chronic intoxication, defined as multiple doses of theophylline over 24 hours, or cases in which interacting drugs or illness interfere with theophylline metabolism are more serious and difficult to treat. Cardiac dysrhythmias and convulsions may occur at theophylline plasma concentrations of 40 to 60 µg/mL and there is no correlation with TPC. The seizures occur without warning and are protracted and repetitive and may produce status epilepticus. Vomiting and typical metabolic disturbances do not occur.

Differences with slow-release preparations are that few or no gastrointestinal symptoms occur, peak concentrations and convulsions may be delayed 12 to 24 hours postingestion, and convulsions occur without warning.

## Laboratory Investigations

Monitoring includes vital signs, pulse oximeter, ABG, hemoglobin, hematocrit (for gastrointestinal hemorrhage), ECG and cardiac monitor, renal and hepatic function, electrolytes, blood glucose, acid–base

## TABLE 27   Theophylline Blood Concentrations and Acute Toxicity

| Plasma Concentration (μg/mL) | Toxicity Degree | Manifestations |
|---|---|---|
| 8-10 | None | Bronchodilation |
| 10-20 | Mild | Therapeutic range: nausea, vomiting, nervousness, respiratory alkalosis, tachycardia |
| 15-25 | | 35% have mild manifestations of toxicity |
| 20-40 | Moderate | Gastrointestinal complaints and central nervous system stimulation Transient hypertension, tachypnea, tachycardia; 80% will have some manifestations of toxicity |
| 60 | Severe | Convulsions, dysrhythmias |
| 100 | | Hypokalemia, hyperglycemia Ventricular dysrhythmias, protracted convulsions, hypotension, acid–base abnormalities |

Reprinted and modified from Linden CH, Rumack BH, In Toxic Emergencies (Honser W Jr [ed]): The legitimate analgesics, aspirin and acetaminophen, copyright 1984, with permission from Elsevier.

balance, and serum albumin. Gastric contents and stools should be tested for occult blood. Samples for theophylline plasma concentration measurement should be drawn within 1 to 2 hours after ingestion of liquid preparations, 2 to 4 hours after ingestion of regular-release formulations, and 4 hours after ingestion of slow-release formulations. One should check the serum albumin level because a decrease in albumin levels may cause manifestations of toxicity despite normal theophylline plasma concentration. A single theophylline plasma concentration reading may be misleading; therefore, theophylline plasma concentration measurement should be repeated every 2 to 4 hours to determine the trend until a declining trend is reached and then monitored every 4 to 6 hours until it is below 20 μg/mL.

### Management

Vital functions must be established and maintained. If the patient is in a coma or has convulsions or vomiting, he or she should be intubated immediately. The theophylline plasma concentration is obtained and repeated every 2 to 4 hours to determine peak absorption, and a theophylline bezoar should be considered if the theophylline plasma concentration fails to decline. Consultation with a nephrologist about charcoal hemoperfusion is recommended.

Gastrointestinal decontamination is warranted in the case of an acute overdose, but emesis must not be induced. Activated charcoal is the choice decontamination procedure in a dose of 1 g/kg to all patients, followed with MDAC 0.5 g/kg every 2 to 4 hours until the theophylline plasma concentration is less than 20 μg/mL. MDAC is effective in treating acute, chronic, and intravenous overdoses. Activated charcoal shortens the half-life of theophylline by about 50% and may be indicated up to 24 hours following ingestion.

Whole-bowel irrigation with polyethylene-electrolyte solution has been recommended for cases of massive overdose, possible

concretions, and ingestion of sustained-release preparations. If intractable vomiting occurs, the antiemetic metoclopramide (Reglan) (0.1 mg/kg adult dose), droperidol (Inapsine) (2.5 to 10 mg IV), or ondansetron (Zofran) (8 to 32 mg IV) is administered. Ondansetron, however, inhibits metabolism of theophylline after a few doses.

Convulsions are controlled with lorazepam (Ativan) or diazepam (Valium) and phenobarbital. Phenytoin (Dilantin) is ineffective. The convulsions in patients with chronic intoxication are often refractory and may require, in addition to anticonvulsants, neuromuscular paralyzing agents, sedation, assisted ventilation, and EEG monitoring.

Hypotension is treated with fluids and vasopressors, if necessary. Norepinephrine (Levophed) 0.05 μg/kg/min is preferred as the vasopressor over dopamine.

Supraventricular tachycardia with hemodynamic instability requires cardioversion. Low-dose β-blockers may be used but should not be used in patients with reactive airway disease or hypotension. Adenosine (Adenocard) is ineffective. For ventriculardys rhythmias, electrolyte disturbances should be corrected. Lidocaine is the treatment of choice but has the potential to cause seizures at toxic concentrations. Cardioversion may be needed.

Hematemesis is managed with sucralfate (Carafate) 1 g four times daily and/or Maalox TC 30 mL every 2 hours and blood replacement, if necessary. H$_2$ antihistamine blockers that are enzyme inhibitors are not used.

Fluid and metabolic disturbances should be corrected. Hyperglycemia does not require insulin therapy. Hypokalemia should be corrected cautiously, as it may be largely an intracellular shift and not total body loss. Usually adding 40 mEq potassium to a liter of fluid will suffice. The serum potassium level must be monitored closely.

Charcoal hemoperfusion is the management of choice for patients with serious intoxications. Hemoperfusion can increase the clearance twofold to threefold over hemodialysis, but hemodialysis can be used if hemoperfusion is not available. Criteria for charcoal hemoperfusion are as follows:

- Life-threatening events such as convulsions or dysrhythmias
- Intractable vomiting refractory to antiemetics
- Acute intoxications with a theophylline plasma concentration greater than 80 μg/mL or greater than 70 μg/mL 4 hours after overdose with a sustained-release formulation and greater than 40 μg/mL in the case of chronic intoxication
- Acute or chronic overdoses with a theophylline plasma concentration greater than 40 μg/mL, especially if the patient has risk factors that lengthen the half-life of the drug (see Kinetics).

### Disposition

Patients with mild symptoms and a theophylline plasma concentration less than 20 μg/mL can be treated in emergency department and discharged when asymptomatic for a few hours. Any patient with acute ingestion and a theophylline plasma concentration greater than 35 μg/mL should be admitted to a monitored bed with seizure precautions and suicide precautions, if needed. If neurologic or cardiotoxic effects or a theophylline plasma concentration greater than 50 μg/mL is present, the patient should be admitted to the intensive care unit. A patient with an overdose of a sustained-release preparation, regardless of symptoms or initial theophylline plasma concentration, requires admission, monitoring, activated charcoal, and MDAC. In patients on chronic therapy, toxicity may occur at a lower theophylline plasma concentration, and these patients should not be discharged until they are asymptomatic for several hours.

### TRICYCLIC AND CYCLIC ANTIDEPRESSANTS

Historically, tricyclic antidepressants are an important cause of pharmaceutical overdose fatalities. The mortality rate was reduced from 15% in the 1970s to less than 1% in the 1990s because of a better understanding of the pathophysiology of these agents and improvements in management (Table 28).

## TABLE 28 Cyclic Antidepressants, Daily Dose and Their Major Properties

| Generic Name | Adult Daily Dose (mg) | Therapeutic Range (ng/mL) | Half-life (hours) | Toxicity* | | |
| --- | --- | --- | --- | --- | --- | --- |
| | | | | Antichol | CNS | Cardiac |
| **Tertiary Amines** | | | | | | |
| Amitriptyline (Elavil) | 75-300 | 120-250 | 31-46 | 3+ | 3+ | 3+ |
| Imipramine (Tofranil) | 75-300 | 125-250 | 9-24 | 3+ | 3+ | 2+ |
| Doxepin (Sinequan) | 75-300 | 30-150 | 8-24 | 3+ | 3+ | 2+ |
| Trimipramine (Surmantil) | 75-200 | 10-240 | 16-18 | 3+ | 3+ | 2+ |
| **Secondary Amines** | | | | | | |
| Nortriptyline (Pamelor) | 75-150 | 50-150 | 18-93 | 2+ | 3+ | 3+ |
| Desipramine (Norpramin) | 75-200 | 75-160 | 14-62 | 1+ | 3+ | 3+ |
| Protriptyline (Vivactil) | 20-60 | 70-250 | 54-198 | 2+ | 3+ | 3+ |
| **Newer Cyclic Antidepressants** | | | | | | |
| Teracyclic | | | 30-60 | 1+ | 2+ | 3+ |
| Maprotiline (Ludiomil) | 75-300 | — | 30-60 | 1+ | 2+ | 3+ |
| Trizolopyridine, a noncyclic, produces less serious cardiac and CNS toxicity | | | | | | |
| Trazodone (Desyrel) | 50-600 | 700 | 4-7 | 1+ | 1+ | 1+ |
| **Monocyclic Aminoketones** | | | | | | |
| Bupropion (Wellbutrin) | 200-400 | — | 8-24 | 1+ | 3+ | 1+ |
| Dibenzazepine | | | | | | |
| Clomipramine (Anafranil) | 100-250 | 200-500 | 21-32 | 2+ | 2+ | 2+ |
| **Dibenoxazepine** | | | | | | |
| Amoxapine (Ascendin) | 150-300 | 200-500 | 6-10 | 1+ | 3+ | 2+ |

*Antichol = anticholinergic effect; CNS = central nervous system effect primarily seizures; Cardiac = cardiac effect.
Other drugs with similar structures are cyclobenzaprine, a muscle relaxant (similar to amitriptyline), and carbamazepine, an anticonvulsant (similar to imipramine); however, they cause less cardiac toxicity.

## Toxic Mechanism

The major mechanisms of toxicity of the tricyclic antidepressants are (a) central and peripheral anticholinergic effects; (b) peripheral α-adrenergic blockade; (c) quinidine-like cardiac membrane stabilizing action blockade of the fast inward sodium channels; and (d) inhibition of synaptic neurotransmitter reuptake in the CNS presynaptic neurons. The tetracyclics, monocyclic aminoketones, and dibenzoxazepines possess convulsive activity and less cardiac toxicity in overdose than the older tricyclic antidepressants. Triazolopyridine has less serious cardiac and CNS toxicity.

## Toxic Dose

The therapeutic dose of imipramine (Tofranil) is 1.5 to 5 mg/kg; a dose greater than 5 mg/kg may be mildly toxic; 10 to 20 mg/kg may be life threatening, although less than 20 mg/kg has produced few fatalities; greater than 30 mg/kg carries a 30% mortality rate; and at a dose greater than 70 mg/kg, patients rarely survive. In children 375 mg and in adults as little as 500 mg have been fatal. In adults, five times the maximum daily dose is toxic and 10 times is potentially fatal. Although major overdose symptoms are associated with plasma concentrations greater than 1 μg/mL (>1000 ng/mL), plasma tricyclic levels do not correlate well with toxicity; clinical signs and symptoms should guide therapy.

The relative dosage or potency equivalents are as follows: amitriptyline (Elavil) 100 mg = amoxapine (Asendin) 125 mg = desipramine (Norpramin) 75 mg = doxepin (Sinequan) 100 mg = imipramine (Tofranil) 75 mg = maprotiline (Ludiomil) 75 mg = nortriptyline (Pamelor) 50 mg = trazodone (Desyrel) 200 mg. This allows one to determine an equivalent dosage of an agent compared with another (see Table 28).

## Kinetics

The tricyclic and cyclic antidepressants are lipophilic. They are rapidly absorbed from the alkaline small intestine, but absorption may be prolonged and delayed in cases of massive overdose owing to anticholinergic action. Onset varies from less than 1 hour (30 to 40 minutes) to, rarely, 12 hours. The peak serum levels are reached in 2 to 8 hours and the peak effect is in 6 hours but may be delayed 12 hours because of erratic absorption. The clinical effects correlate poorly with plasma levels.

Cyclic antidepressants are highly protein-bound to plasma glycoproteins, 98% at a pH 7.5 and 90% at 7.0. Volume distribution is 10 to 50 L/kg. The elimination route is by hepatic metabolism. The tertiary amines are metabolized into active demethylated secondary amine metabolites. The active secondary amine metabolites undergo a 15% enterohepatic recirculation and are metabolized over a period of days into nonactive metabolites. The intestinal bacterial flora may reconstitute the metabolites, which are active.

The half-life varies from 10 hours for imipramine to 81 hours for amitriptyline and 100 hours for nortriptyline. The active metabolites have longer half-lives.

Only 3% of the ingested dose is excreted in the urine unchanged.

## Manifestations

There are reports of asymptomatic patients who, upon arrival to an emergency department, suddenly have a seizure, develop hemodynamically unstable dysrhythmias, and die shortly thereafter from ingestion of a tricyclic antidepressant. Most patients with severe toxicity develop symptoms within 1 to 2 hours, but symptoms may be delayed 6 hours after overdose.

Small overdoses produce early anticholinergic effects, agitation, and transient hypertension, which are not life-threatening. Large overdoses produce depression of the CNS and myocardium, convulsions, and hypotension. Death can occur within the first 2 to 6 hours following ingestion.

Some ECG screening tools for predicting cardiac or neurologic toxicity from ingestion of a tricyclic antidepressant have been developed: (a) A QRS greater than 0.10 second may produce seizures, and if greater than 0.16 second, 50% of patients may develop ventricular dysrhythmias (20% of these may be life-threatening) and seizures; (b) a terminal 40 msec of the QRS axis greater than 120 degrees in the right frontal plane may be associated with toxicity; or (c) a large R wave greater than 3 mm in ECG lead aVR may predispose the patient to toxicity. The quinidine cardiac membrane stabilizing effect produces depression of myocardium, conduction, and ECG changes. The peripheral α-adrenergic blockade produces hypotension.

The secondary amines are metabolized to inactive metabolites. The tetracyclics produce a high incidence of cardiovascular disturbances and seizures. Monocyclic aminoketones produce seizures in doses greater than 600 mg. Dibenzoxazepines produce a syndrome of convulsions, rhabdomyolysis, and renal failure.

## Laboratory Investigations

If the patient has altered mental status or ECG abnormalities, ABG, ECG, chest radiograph, blood glucose, serum electrolytes, calcium, magnesium, blood urea nitrogen, and creatinine levels, liver profile, creatine kinase level, urine output, and, in severe cases, hemodynamic monitoring are indicated. Levels of the tricyclic and cyclic antidepressants less than 300 ng/mL are therapeutic; levels greater than 500 ng/mL indicate toxicity, and levels greater than 1000 ng/mL indicate serious poisoning and are associated with QRS widening.

## Management

Vital functions must be established and maintained. Even if the patient is asymptomatic, intravenous access should be established, vital signs and neurologic status monitored, and baseline 12-lead ECG and continuous cardiac monitoring obtained for at least 6 hours from admission or 8 to 12 hours postingestion. QRS interval should be measured on a limb lead ECG every 15 minutes for 6 hours postingestion.

For gastrointestinal decontamination, emesis should not be induced and gastric lavage should not be used. Activated charcoal is preferable. If the patient is in an altered mental state, the airway must be protected. Activated charcoal 1 g/kg is recommended up to 1 hour postingestion. Benefit from MDAC has not been demonstrated.

Alkalinization does not control seizures; diazepam or lorazepam should be used. Status epilepticus may require high-dose barbiturates or neuromuscular blockers with intravenous diazepam. If not successful, the patient can be paralyzed with short-term nondepolarizing neuromuscular blockers such as vecuronium (Norcuron), intubation, and assisted ventilation. A bolus of sodium bicarbonate is recommended as an adjunct to correct the acidosis produced by the seizures.

Sodium bicarbonate is administered in a dose of 1 to 2 mEq/kg undiluted as a bolus and repeated twice a few minutes apart, if needed, for "sodium loading" and alkalinization, which may increase protein binding from 90% to 98%. The sodium loading overcomes the sodium channel blockage and is more important than the alkalinization. Indications include (a) a QRS complex greater than 0.12 second, (b) ventricular tachycardia, (c) severe conduction disturbances, (d) metabolic acidosis, (e) coma, and (f) seizures. A continuous infusion of sodium bicarbonate is of limited usefulness for controlling dysrhythmias. Bolus therapy should be used as needed.

Hyperventilation alone has been recommended, but the pH elevation is not as instantaneous and there is compensatory renal excretion of bicarbonate; therefore, we do not recommend it. The combination of hyperventilation and sodium bicarbonate has produced fatal alkalemia and is not recommended. One should monitor serum potassium level (the sudden increase in blood pH can aggravate or precipitate hypokalemia), serum sodium, and ionized calcium levels (hypocalcemia may occur with alkalinization) and blood pH.

Specific cardiovascular complications should be treated as follows: Hypotension is treated with norepinephrine, a predominantly α-adrenergic drug, which is preferred over dopamine. Hypertension that occurs early rarely requires treatment. Sinus tachycardia usually does not require treatment. Supraventricular tachycardia in a patient who is hemodynamically unstable requires synchronized electrical cardioversion, starting at 0.25 to 1.0 watt-second per kg, after sedation. Ventricular tachycardia that persists after alkalinization requires intravenous lidocaine or countershock if the patient is hemodynamically unstable. Ventricular fibrillation should be treated with defibrillation. Torsades de pointes is treated with magnesium sulfate IV 20% solution, 2 g over 2 to 3 minutes, followed by a continuous infusion of 1.5 mL 10% solution or 5 to 10 mg per minute. For the treatment of bradydysrhythmias, atropine is contraindicated because of the anticholinergic activity. Isoproterenol 0.1 µg/kg/minute, used with caution, may produce hypotension. If the patient is hemodynamically unstable, a pacemaker is used.

Extraordinary measures, such as aortic balloon pump and cardiopulmonary bypass, have been successful.

Investigational treatments include FAB fragments specific for tricyclic antidepressant, which have been successful in animals. Prophylactic NaHCO₃ to prevent dysrhythmias is also being investigated.

Physostigmine has produced asystole, and flumazenil has produced seizures. Both are contraindicated.

## Disposition

A patient with an antidepressant overdose who meets any of the following criteria should be admitted to the intensive care unit for 12 to 24 hours: (a) ECG abnormalities except sinus tachycardia, (b) altered mental state, (c) seizures, (d) respiratory depression, and (e) hypotension. Low-risk patients include those in whom the above symptoms are absent at 6 hours postingestion, those who present with minor transient manifestations such as sinus tachycardia who subsequently become and remain asymptomatic for a 6-hour period, and asymptomatic patients who remain asymptomatic for 6 hours. These patients may be discharged if the ECG remains normal, they have normal bowel sounds, and they undergo psychiatric disposition.

Even if the patient is asymptomatic upon presentation to the health care facility, intravenous access should be established, vital signs and neurologic status monitored, a baseline 12-lead ECG obtained, and cardiac monitoring continued for at least 6 hours. *Caution:* in 25% of fatal cases, the patients were initially alert and awake at presentation. However, in most cases of fatality initially deemed as sudden cardiac death, the patient, upon reexamination, actually had symptoms that were missed.

Children younger than 6 years of age with non-intentional (accidental) exposures to amitriptyline (Elavil), desipramine (Norpramin), doxepin (Sinequan), imipramine (Tofranil), or nortriptyline (Aventyl) in a dose less than 5 mg/kg, who are asymptomatic and have what are deemed reliable caregivers, can be observed at home, with close poison control follow-up for 6 hours. Parents or caregivers should be given instructions regarding signs and symptoms to be alert for. Children who are symptomatic, or who ingested greater than 5 mg/kg, should be referred to the emergency department for monitoring, observation, and activated charcoal treatment.

# Appendices and Index

## Reference Intervals for the Interpretation of Laboratory Tests

Method of
*Laura J. McCloskey, PhD*

Most of the tests performed in a clinical laboratory are quantitative; that is, the amount of a substance present in blood or serum is measured and reported in terms of concentration, activity (e.g., enzyme activity), or counts (e.g., blood cell counts). The laboratory must provide reference intervals to assist the clinician in the interpretation of laboratory results. These reference intervals represent the physiologic quantities of a substance (concentrations, activities, or counts) to be expected in healthy persons. Deviation above or below the reference range may be associated with a disease process, and the severity of the disease process may be associated with the magnitude of the deviation. Unfortunately, a sharp demarcation rarely exists to distinguish between physiologic and pathologic values, and the time of transition between the two is often gradual as the disease process progresses.

## Defining Normal Values

The terms "normal" and "abnormal" have been used to describe laboratory values that fall inside and outside the reference range, respectively. Use of these terms is inappropriate because no good definition of normality exists in the clinical sense, and the term "normal" may be confused with the statistical term "gaussian." Reference ranges are established from statistical studies in groups of healthy volunteers. These study subjects must be free of disease, but they may have lifestyles or habits that result in variations in certain laboratory values. Examples of these variables include diet, body mass, exercise, and geographic location. Age and gender can also affect reference values.

When the data from a large cohort of healthy subjects fit a gaussian distribution, the usual statistical approach is to define the reference limits as 2 standard deviations (SD) above and below the mean. By definition, the reference range excludes the 2.5% of the population with the lowest values and the 2.5% with the highest values. Nongaussian distributions are handled by different statistical methods, but the result is similar, in that the reference range is defined by the central 95% of the population. In other words, the probability that a healthy person has a laboratory result falling outside the reference range is 1 in 20. If 12 laboratory tests are performed, the probability that at least one of the results is outside the reference range increases to about 50%, which means that all healthy persons are likely to have a few laboratory results that are unexpected. The clinician must then integrate these data with other clinical information, such as the history and physical examination, to arrive at an appropriate clinical decision.

The reference intervals for many tests (especially enzyme and immunochemical measurements) vary with the method used. Accordingly, each laboratory must establish its own reference intervals that are appropriate for the methods used.

## International System of Units

During the 1980s, a concerted effort was made to introduce the International System of Units (Systéme International d'Unités; SI units). The rationale for conversion to SI units is sound. Laboratory data are scientifically more informative when the units are based on molar concentration rather than on mass concentration. For example, the conversion of glucose to lactate and pyruvate or the binding of a drug to albumin is more easily understood in units of molar concentration. Another example is illustrated as follows:

| Conventional Units | SI Units |
|---|---|
| 1.0 g of hemoglobin: | 4.0 mmol of hemoglobin: |
| Combines with 1.37 mL of oxygen | Combines with 4.0 mmol of oxygen |
| Contains 3.4 mg of iron | Contains 4.0 mmol of iron |
| Forms 34.9 mg of bilirubin | Forms 4.0 mmol of bilirubin |

The use of SI units would also enhance the standardization of nomenclature to facilitate global communication of medical and scientific information. The units, symbols, and prefixes used in the international system are shown in Tables 1, 2, and 3.

**TABLE 1** Base SI Units

| Property | Unit | Symbol |
|---|---|---|
| Length | Meter | m |
| Mass | Kilogram | kg |
| Amount of substance | Mole | mol |
| Time | Second | s |
| Thermodynamic temperature | Kelvin | K |
| Electrical current | Ampere | A |
| Luminous intensity | Candela | cd |
| Catalytic amount | Katal | kat |

*Abbreviation:* SI = International System of Units.

## TABLE 2 Derived SI Units and Non-SI Units Retained for Use with SI Units

| Property | Unit | Symbol |
|---|---|---|
| Area | Square meter | $m^2$ |
| Volume | Cubic meter | $m^3$ |
| | Liter | L |
| Mass | Kilograms per cubic meter | $kg/m^3$ concentration |
| | Grams per liter | g/L |
| Substance concentration | Moles per cubic meter | $mol/m^3$ |
| | | mol/L |
| Temperature | Degree Celsius | C = K−273.15 |

*Abbreviation:* SI = International System of Units.

Unfortunately, problems have arisen with the implementation of SI units in the United States. The introduction of this system in 1987 prompted many medical journals to report laboratory values in both SI and conventional units in anticipation of complete conversion to SI units in the early 1990s. The lack of a coordinated effort toward this goal forced a retrenchment on the issue. Physicians continue to think and practice with laboratory results expressed in conventional units, and few, if any, hospitals or clinical laboratories in the United States use SI units exclusively. Complete conversion to SI units is not likely to occur in the foreseeable future, but most medical journals will probably continue to publish both sets of units. For this reason, the values in the tables of reference ranges in this appendix are given in both conventional units and SI units.

## TABLE 3 Standard Prefixes

| Prefix | Multiplication Factor | Symbol |
|---|---|---|
| yocto | $10^{-24}$ | y |
| zepto | $10^{-21}$ | z |
| atto | $10^{-18}$ | a |
| femto | $10^{-15}$ | f |
| pico | $10^{-12}$ | p |
| nano | $10^{-9}$ | n |
| micro | $10^{-6}$ | μ |
| milli | $10^{-3}$ | m |
| centi | $10^{-2}$ | c |
| deci | $10^{-1}$ | d |
| deca | $10^{1}$ | da |
| hecto | $10^{2}$ | h |
| kilo | $10^{3}$ | k |
| mega | $10^{6}$ | M |
| giga | $10^{9}$ | G |
| tera | $10^{12}$ | T |

# Tables of Reference Intervals

Some of the values included in the tables that follow have been established by the Clinical Laboratories at the Thomas Jefferson University Hospital in Philadelphia and have not been published elsewhere. Other values have been compiled from the sources cited in the suggested readings. These tables are provided for information and educational purposes only. Laboratory values must always be interpreted in the context of clinical data derived from other sources, including the medical history and physical examination. One must exercise individual judgment when using the information provided in this appendix.

## REFERENCES

American Medical Association: Drug Evaluations Annual. Chicago: American Medical Association, 1994.

Bick RL (ed): Hematology: Clinical and Laboratory Practice. St Louis: Mosby–Year Book, 1993.

Borer WZ: Selection and use of laboratory tests. In Tietz NW, Conn RB, Pruden EL (eds): Applied Laboratory Medicine. Philadelphia: WB Saunders, 1992, pp 1-5.

Campion EW: A retreat from SI units. N Engl J Med 1992;327:49.

Friedman RB, Young DS: Effects of Disease on Clinical Laboratory Tests, 3rd ed. Washington, DC: American Association for Clinical Chemistry Press, 1997.

Henry JB: Clinical Diagnosis and Management by Laboratory Methods, 19th ed. Philadelphia: WB Saunders, 1996.

Hicks JM, Young DS: DORA 97-99: Directory of Rare Analyses. Washington, DC: American Association for Clinical Chemistry Press, 1997.

Jacob DS, Demott WR, Grady HJ, et al (eds): Laboratory Test Handbook, 4th ed. Baltimore: Williams & Wilkins, 1996.

Kaplan LA, Pesce AJ: Clinical Chemistry: Theory, Analysis, and Correlation, 3rd ed. St Louis: Mosby–Year Book, 1996.

Kjeldsberg CR, Knight JA: Body Fluids: Laboratory Examination of Amniotic, Cerebrospinal, Seminal, Serous and Synovial Fluids, 3rd ed. Chicago: ASCP Press, 1993.

Laposata M: SI Unit Conversion Guide. Boston: NEJM Books, 1992.

Scully RE, McNeely WF, Mark EJ, McNeely BU: Normal reference laboratory values. N Engl J Med 1992;327:718-724.

Speicher CE: The Right Test: A Physician's Guide to Laboratory Medicine, 3rd ed. Philadelphia: WB Saunders, 1998.

Tietz NW (ed): Clinical Guide to Laboratory Tests, 3rd ed. Philadelphia: WB Saunders, 1995.

Wallach J: Interpretation of Diagnostic Tests: A Synopsis of Laboratory Medicine, 6th ed. Boston: Little, Brown, 1996.

Young DS: Effects of Preanalytical Variables on Clinical Laboratory Tests, 2nd ed. Washington, DC: American Association for Clinical Chemistry Press, 1997.

Young DS: Effects of Drugs on Clinical Laboratory Tests, 4th ed. Washington, DC: American Association for Clinical Chemistry Press, 1995.

Young DS: Determination and validation of reference intervals. Arch Pathol Lab Med 1992;116:704-709.

Young DS: Implementation of SI units for clinical laboratory data. Ann Intern Med 1987:106:114-129.

## Reference Intervals* for Hematology

| Test | Conventional Units | SI Units |
|------|--------------------|----------|
| Acid hemolysis (Ham test) | No hemolysis | No hemolysis |
| Alkaline phosphatase, leukocyte | Total score, 14-100 | Total score, 14-100 |
| Cell counts | | |
|    Erythrocytes | | |
|       Males | 4.6-6.2 million/mm$^3$ | 4.6-6.2 × 10$^{12}$/L |
|       Females | 4.2-5.4 million/mm$^3$ | 4.2-5.4 × 10$^{12}$/L |
|       Children (varies with age) | 4.5-5.1 million/mm$^3$ | 4.5-5.1 × 10$^{12}$/L |
|    Leukocytes, total | 4500-11,000/mm$^3$ | 4.5-11.0 × 10$^9$/L |
| Leukocytes, differential counts* | | |
|    Myelocytes | 0% | 0/L |
|    Band neutrophils | 3-5% | 150-400 × 10$^6$/L |
|    Segmented neutrophils | 54-62% | 3000-5800 × 10$^6$/L |
|    Lymphocytes | 25-33% | 1500-3000 × 10$^6$/L |
|    Monocytes | 3-7% | 300-500 × 10$^6$/L |
|    Eosinophils | 1-3% | 50-250 × 10$^6$/L |
|    Basophils | 0-1% | 15-50 × 10$^6$/L |
|    Platelets | 150,000-400,000/mm$^3$ | 150-400 × 10$^9$/L |
|    Reticulocytes | 25,000-75,000/mm$^3$ (0.5%-1.5% of erythrocytes) | 25-75 × 10$^9$/L |
| Coagulation Tests | | |
|    Bleeding time (template) | 2.75-8.0 min | 2.75-8.0 min |
|    Coagulation time (glass tube) | 5-15 min | 5-15 min |
|    D dimer | <0.5 µg/mL | <0.5 mg/L |
|    Factor VIII and other coagulation factors | 50-150% of normal | 0.5-1.5 of normal |
|    Fibrin split products (Thrombo-Welco test) | <10 µg/mL | <10 mg/L |
|    Fibrinogen | 200-400 mg/dL | 2.0-4.0 g/L |
|    Partial thromboplastin time, activated (aPTT) | 20-25 s | 20-35 s |
|    Prothrombin time (PT) | 12.0-14.0 s | 12.0-14.0 s |
| Coombs' Test | | |
|    Direct | Negative | Negative |
|    Indirect | Negative | Negative |
| Corpuscular values of erythrocytes | | |
|    Mean corpuscular hemoglobin (MCH) | 26-34 pg/cell | 26-34 pg/cell |
|    Mean corpuscular volume (MCV) | 80-96 µm$^3$ | 80-96 fL |
|    Mean corpuscular hemoglobin concentration (MCHC) | 32-36 g/dL | 320-360 g/L |
| Haptoglobin | 20-165 mg/dL | 0.20-1.65 g/L |
| Hematocrit | | |
|    Males | 40-54 mL/dL | 0.40-0.54 g/L |
|    Females | 37-47 mL/dL | 0.37-0.47 g/L |
|    Newborns | 49-54 mL/dL | 0.49-0.54 g/L |
|    Children (varies with age) | 35-49 mL/dL | 0.35-0.49 g/L |
| Hemoglobin | | |
|    Males | 13.0-18.0 g/dL | 8.1-11.2 mmol/L |
|    Females | 12.0-16.0 g/dL | 7.4-9.9 mmol/L |
|    Newborns | 16.5-19.5 g/dL | 10.2-12.1 mmol/L |
|    Children (varies with age) | 11.2-16.5 g/dL | 7.0-10.2 mmol/L |
| Hemoglobin, fetal | <1.0 of total | <0.01 of total |
| Hemoglobin A1c | 3-5% of total | 0.03-0.05 of total |
| Hemoglobin A2 | 1.5-3.0% of total | 0.015-0.03 of total |
| Hemoglobin, plasma | 0.0%-5.0 mg/dL | 0.0-3.2 µmol/L |
| Methemoglobin | 30%-130 mg/dL | 19-80 µmol/L |
| Erythrocyte sedimentation rate (ESR) | | |
|    Westergren: | | |
|       Males | 0-15 mm/h | 0-15 mm/h |
|       Females | 0-20 mm/h | 0-20 mm/h |
|    Wintrobe: | | |
|       Males | 0-5 mm/h | 0-5 mm/h |
|       Females | 0-15 mm/h | 0-15 mm/h |

*Conventional units are percentages; SI units are absolute cell counts.
*Abbreviation:* SI = International System of Units.

## Reference Intervals* for Clinical Chemistry (Blood, Serum, and Plasma)

| Analyte | Conventional Units | SI Units |
|---|---|---|
| Acetoacetate plus acetone | | |
| Qualitative | Negative | Negative |
| Quantitative | 0.3-2.0 mg/dL | 30-200 µmol/L |
| Acid phosphatase, serum (thymolphthalein monophosphate substrate) | 0.1-0.6 U/L | 0.1-0.6 U/L |
| ACTH (see Corticotropin) | | |
| Alanine aminotransferase (ALT), serum (SGPT) | 1-45 U/L | 1-45 U/L |
| Albumin, serum | 3.3-5.2 g/dL | 33-52 g/L |
| Aldolase, serum | 0.0-7.0 U/L | 0.0-7.0 U/L |
| Aldosterone, plasma | | |
| Standing | 5-30 ng/dL | 140-830 pmol/L |
| Recumbent | 3-10 ng/dL | 80-275 pmol/L |
| Alkaline, phosphatase (ALP), serum | | |
| Adult | 35-150 U/L | 35-150 U/L |
| Adolescent | 100-500 U/L | 100-500 U/L |
| Child | 100-350 U/L | 100-350 U/L |
| Ammonia nitrogen, plasma | 10-50 µmol/L | 10-50 µmol/L |
| Amylase, serum | 25-125 U/L | 25-125 U/L |
| Anion gap, serum calculated | 8-16 mEq/L | 8-16 mmol/L |
| Ascorbic acid, blood | 0.4-1.5 mg/dL | 23-85 µmol/L |
| Aspartate aminotransferase (AST), serum (SGOT) | 1-36 U/L | 1-36 U/L |
| Base excess, arterial blood, calculated | 0±2 mEq/L | 0±2 mmol/L |
| Bicarbonate | | |
| Venous plasma | 23-29 mEq/L | 23-29 mmol/L |
| Arterial blood | 21-27 mEq/L | 21-27 mmol/L |
| Bile acids, serum | 0.3-3.0 mg/dL | 0.8-7.6 mmol/L |
| Bilirubin, serum | | |
| Conjugated | 0.1-0.4 mg/dL | 1.7-6.8 µmol/L |
| Total | 0.3-1.1 mg/dL | 5.1-19.0 µmol/L |
| Calcium, serum | 8.4-10.6 mg/dL | 2.10-2.65 mmol/L |
| Calcium, ionized, serum | 4.25-5.25 mg/dL | 1.05-1.30 mmol/L |
| Carbon dioxide, total, serum or plasma | 24-31 mEq/L | 24-31 mmol/L |
| Carbon dioxide tension ($P_{CO_2}$), blood | 35-45 mm Hg | 35-45 mm Hg |
| β-Carotene, serum | 60-260 µg/dL | 1.1-8.6 µmol/L |
| Ceruloplasmin, serum | 23-44 mg/dL | 230-440 mg/L |
| Chloride, serum or plasma | 96-106 mEq/L | 96-106 mmol/L |
| Cholesterol, serum or EDTA plasma | | |
| Desirable range | <200 mg/dL | <5.20 mmol/L |
| Low-density lipoprotein (LDL) cholesterol | 60-180 mg/dL | 1.55-4.65 mmol/L |
| High-density lipoprotein (HDL) cholesterol | 30-80 mg/dL | 0.80-2.05 mmol/L |
| Copper | 70-140 µg/dL | 11-22 µmol/L |
| Corticotropin (ACTH), plasma, 8 AM | 10-80 pg/mL | 2-18 pmol/L |
| Cortisol, plasma | | |
| 8:00 AM | 6-23 µg/dL | 170-630 µmol/L |
| 4:00 PM | 3-15 µg/dL | 80-410 µmol/L |
| 10:00 PM | <50% of 8:00 AM value | <50% of 8:00 AM value |
| Creatine, serum | | |
| Males | 0.2-0.5 mg/dL | 15-40 µmol/L |
| Females | 0.3-0.9 mg/dL | 25-70 µmol/L |
| Creatine kinase (CK), serum | | |
| Males | 55-170 U/L | 55-170 U/L |
| Females | 30-135 U/L | 30-135 U/L |
| Creatinine kinase MB isoenzyme, serum | <5% of total CK activity | <5% of total CK activity |
| | <5% of ng/mL by immunoassay | <5% of ng/mL by immunoassay |
| Creatinine, serum | 0.6-1.2 mg/dL | 50-110 µmol/L |
| Erythrocytes | 145-540 ng/mL | 330-120 nmol/L |
| Estradiol-17β, adult | | |
| Males | 10-65 pg/mL | 35-240 pmol/L |
| Females | | |
| Follicular | 30-100 pg/mL | 110-370 pmol/L |
| Ovulatory | 200-400 pg/mL | 730-1470 pmol/L |
| Luteal | 50-140 pg/mL | 180-510 pmol/L |
| Ferritin, serum | 20-200 ng/mL | 20-200 µg/L |
| Fibrinogen, plasma | 200-400 mg/dL | 2.0-4.0 g/L |
| Folate, serum | 3-18 ng/mL | 6.8-4.1 nmol/L |
| Follicle-stimulating hormone (FSH), plasma | | |
| Males | 4-25 mU/mL | 4-25 U/L |
| Females, premenopausal | 4-30 mU/mL | 4-30 U/L |
| Females, postmenopausal | 40-250 mU/mL | 40-250 U/L |
| Gastrin, fasting, serum | 0-100 pg/mL | 0-100 mg/L |
| Glucose, fasting, plasma or serum | 70-115 mg/dL | 3.9-6.4 nmol/L |
| γ-Glutamyltransferase (GGT), serum | 5-40 U/L | 5-40 U/L |
| Growth hormone (hGH), plasma, adult, fasting | 0-6 ng/mL | 0-6 µg/L |

## Reference Intervals* for Clinical Chemistry (Blood, Serum, and Plasma)—cont'd

| Analyte | Conventional Units | SI Units |
| --- | --- | --- |
| Haptoglobin, serum | 20-165 mg/dL | 0.20-1.65 g/L |
| Immunoglobulins, serum (see table, Reference Intervals for Tests of Immunologic Function) | | |
| Iron, serum | 75-175 µg/dL | 13-31 µmol/L |
| Iron-binding capacity, serum | | |
| Total | 250-410 µg/dL | 45-73 µmol/L |
| Saturation | 20-55% | 0.20-0.55 |
| Lactate | | |
| Venous whole blood | 5.0-20.0 mg/dL | 0.6-2.2 mmol/L |
| Arterial whole blood | 5.0-15.0 mg/dL | 0.6-1.7 mmol/L |
| Lactate dehydrogenase (LD), serum | 110-220 U/L | 110-220 U/L |
| Lipase, serum | 10-140 U/L | 10-140 U/L |
| Lutropin (LH), serum | | |
| Males | 1-9 U/L | -9 U/L |
| Females | | |
| Follicular phase | 2-10 U/L | 2-10 U/L |
| Midcycle peak | 15-65 U/L | 15-65 U/L |
| Luteal phase | 1-12 U/L | 1-12 U/L |
| Postmenopausal | 12-65 U/L | 12-65 U/L |
| Magnesium, serum | 1.3-2.1 mg/dL | 0.65-1.05 mmol/L |
| Osmolality | 275-295 mOsm/kg water | 275-295 mOsm/kg water |
| Oxygen, blood, arterial, room air | | |
| Partial pressure (PaO$_2$) | 80-100 mm Hg | 80-100 mm Hg |
| Saturation (SaO$_2$) | 95-98% | 95-98% |
| pH, arterial blood | 7.35-7.45 | 7.35-7.45 |
| Phosphate, inorganic, serum | | |
| Adult | 3.0-4.5 mg/dL | 1.0-1.5 mmol/L |
| Child | 4.0-7.0 mg/dL | 1.3-2.3 mmol/L |
| Potassium | | |
| Serum | 3.5-5.0 mEq/L | 3.5-5.0 mmol/L |
| Plasma | 3.5-4.5 mEq/L | 3.5-4.5 mmol/L |
| Progesterone, serum, adult | | |
| Males | 0.0-0.4 ng/mL | 0.0-1.3 mmol/L |
| Females | | |
| Follicular phase | 0.1-1.5 ng/mL | 0.3-4.8 mmol/L |
| Luteal phase | 2.5-28.0 ng/mL | 8.0-89.0 mmol/L |
| Prolactin, serum | | |
| Males | 1.0-15.0 ng/mL | 1.0-15.0 µg/L |
| Females | 1.0-20.0 ng/mL | 1.0-20.0 µg/L |
| Protein, serum, electrophoresis | | |
| Total | 6.0-8.0 g/dL | 60-80 g/L |
| Albumin | 3.5-5.5 g/dL | 35-55 g/L |
| Globulins | | |
| $\alpha_1$ | 0.2-0.4 g/dL | 2.0-4.0 g/L |
| $\alpha_2$ | 0.5-0.9 g/dL | 5.0-9.0 g/L |
| $\beta$ | 0.6-1.1 g/dL | 6.0-11.0 g/L |
| $\gamma$ | 0.7-1.7 g/dL | 7.0-17.0 g/L |
| Pyruvate, blood | 0.3-0.9 mg/dL | 0.03-0.10 mmol/L |
| Rheumatoid factor | 0.0-30.0 IU/mL | 0.0-30.0 kIU/L |
| Sodium, serum or plasma | 135-145 mEq/L | 135-145 mmol/L |
| Testosterone, plasma | | |
| Men | 300-1200 ng/dL | 10.4-41.6 nmol/L |
| Women | 20-75 ng/dL | 0.7-2.6 nmol/L |
| Pregnant | 40-200 ng/dL | 1.4-6.9 nmol/L |
| Thyroglobulin | 3-42 ng/mL | 3-42 µg/L |
| Thyrotropin (hTSH), serum | 0.4-4.8 µIU/mL | 0.4-4.8 mIU/L |
| Thyrotropin-releasing hormone (TRH) | 5-60 pg/mL | 5-60 ng/L |
| Thyroxine, free (FT$_4$), serum | 0.9-2.1 ng/dL | 12-27 pmol/L |
| Thyroxine (T$_4$), serum | 4.5-12.0 µg/mL | 58-154 nmol/L |
| Thyroxine-binding globulin (TBG) | 15.0-34.0 µg/mL | 15.0-34.0 mg/L |
| Transferrin | 250-430 mg/dL | 2.5-4.3 g/L |
| Triglycerides, serum, after 12-h fast | 40-150 mg/dL | 0.4-1.5 g/L |
| Triiodothyronine (T$_3$), serum | 70-190 ng/dL | 1.1-2.9 nmol/L |
| Triiodothyronine uptake, resin (T$_3$RU) | 25-38% | 0.25-0.38 |
| Troponin I | 0.05-0.50 ng/mL | 0.05-0.50 ng/mL |
| Urate | | |
| (FT$_4$) Males | 2.5-8.0 mg/dL | 150-480 µmol/L |
| (FT$_4$) Females | 2.2-7.0 mg/dL | 130-420 µmol/L |
| Urea, serum or plasma | 24-49 mg/dL | 4.0-8.2 nmol/L |
| Urea nitrogen, serum or plasma | 11-23 mg/dL | 8.0-16.4 nmol/L |
| Viscosity, serum | 1.4-1.8 ∞ water | 1.4-1.8 ∞ water |
| Vitamin A, serum | 20-80 µg/dL | 0.70-2.80 µmol/L |
| Vitamin B$_{12}$, serum | 180-900 pg/mL | 133-664 pmol/L |

*Reference values can vary depending on the method and sample source used.
*Abbreviations:* EDTA = ethylenediaminetetraacetic acid; SI = International System of Units.

## Reference Intervals for Therapeutic Drug Monitoring (Serum or Plasma)*

| Analyte | Therapeutic Range | Toxic Concentrations | Proprietary Analyte Name(s) |
|---|---|---|---|
| **Analgesics** | | | |
| Acetaminophen | 10-40 µg/mL | >150 µg/mL | Tylenol, Datril |
| Salicylate | 100-250 µg/mL | >300 µg/mL | Aspirin, Bufferin |
| **Antibiotics** | | | |
| Amikacin | 20-30 µg/mL | Peak >35 µg/mL<br>Trough >10 µg/mL | Amkin |
| Gentamicin | 5-10 µg/mL | Peak >10 µg/mL<br>Trough >2 µg/mL | Garamycin |
| Tobramycin | 5-10 µg/mL | Peak >10 µg/mL<br>Trough >2 µg/mL | Nebcin |
| Vancomycin | 5-35 µg/mL | Peak >40 µg/mL<br>Trough >10 µg/mL | Vancocin |
| **Anticonvulsants** | | | |
| Carbamazepine | 5-12 µg/mL | >15 µg/mL | Tegretol |
| Ethosuximide | 40-100 µg/mL | >250 µg/mL | Zarontin |
| Phenobarbital | 15-40 µg/mL | 40-100 ng/mL (varies widely) | Luminal |
| Phenytoin | 10-20 µg/mL | >20 µg/mL | Dilantin |
| Primidone | 5-12 µg/mL | >15 µg/mL | Mysoline |
| Valproic acid | 50-100 µg/mL | >100 µg/mL | Depakene |
| **Antineoplastics and Immunosuppressives** | | | |
| Cyclosporine A | 150-350 ng/mL | >400 ng/mL | Sandimmune |
| Methotrexate, high-dose, 48 h | Variable | >1 µmol/L, 48h after dose | |
| Sirolimus (within 1 h of 2-mg dose) | 4.5-14 ng/mL | Variable | Rapamune |
| Sirolimus (within 1 h of 5-mg dose) | 10-28 ng/mL | Variable | Rapamune |
| Tacrolimus (FK-506), whole blood | 3-20 µg/L | >15 µg/L | Prograf |
| **Bronchodilators and Respiratory Stimulants** | | | |
| Caffeine | 3-15 ng/mL | >30 ng/mL | Elixophyllin |
| Theophylline (aminophylline) | 10-20 µg/mL | >30 µg/mL | Quibron |
| **Cardiovascular Drugs** | | | |
| Amiodarone (obtain specimen more than 8 h after last dose) | 1.0-2.0 µg/mL | >2.0 µg/mL | Cordarone |
| Digoxin (obtain specimen more than 6 h after last dose) | 0.8-2.0 ng/mL | >2.4 ng/mL | Lanoxin |
| Disopyramide | 2-5 µg/mL | >7 µg/mL | Norpace |
| Flecainide | 0.2-1.0 µg/mL | >1 µg/mL | Tambocor |
| Lidocaine | 1.5-5.0 µg/mL | >6 µg/mL | Xylocaine |
| Mexiletine | 0.7-2.0 µg/mL | >2 µg/mL | Mexitil |
| Procainamide | 4-10 µg/mL | >12 µg/mL | Pronestyl |
| Procainamide plus NAPA (N-acetyl procainamide) | 8-30 µg/mL | >30 µg/mL | |
| Propranolol | 50-100 ng/mL | Variable | Inderal |
| Quinidine | 2-5 µg/mL | >6 µg/mL | Cardioquin, Quinaglute |
| Tocainide | 4-10 ng/mL | >10 ng/mL | Tonocard |
| **Psychopharmacologic Drugs** | | | |
| Amitriptyline | 120-150 ng/mL | >500 ng/mL | Elavil, Triavil |
| Bupropion | 25-100 ng/mL | Not applicable | Wellbutrin |
| Desipramine | 150-300 ng/mL | >500 ng/mL | Norpramin |
| Imipramine | 125-250 ng/mL | >400 ng/mL | Tofranil |
| Lithium (obtain specimen 12 h after last dose) | 0.6-1.5 mEq/L | >1.5 mEq/L | Lithobid |
| Nortriptyline | 50-150 ng/mL | >500 ng/mL | Aventyl, Pamelor |

*Values can vary depending on the method and sample collection device used. Always consult the reference values provided by the laboratory performing the analysis.

## Reference Intervals* for Clinical Chemistry (Urine)

| Analyte | Conventional Units | SI Units |
|---|---|---|
| Acetone and acetoacetate, qualitative | Negative | Negative |
| Albumin | | |
|   Qualitative | Negative | Negative |
|   Quantitative | 10-100 mg/24 h | 0.15-1.5 µmol/d |
| Aldosterone | 3-20 µg/24 h | 8.3-55 nmol/d |
| δ-Aminolevulinic acid (δ-ALA) | 1.3-7.0 mg/24 h | 10-53 µmol/d |
| Amylase | <17 U/h | <17 U/h |
| Amylase-to-creatinine clearance ratio | 0.01-0.04 | 0.01-0.04 |
| Bilirubin, qualitative | Negative | Negative |
| Calcium (regular diet) | <250 mg/24 h | <6.3 nmol/d |
| Catecholamines | | |
|   Epinephrine | <10 µg/24 h | <55 nmol/d |
|   Norepinephrine | <100 µg/24 h | <590 nmol/d |
|   Total free catecholamines | 4-126 µg/24 h | 24-745 nmol/d |
|   Total metanephrines | 0.1-1.6 mg/24 h | 0.5-8.1 µmol/d |
| Chloride (varies with intake) | 110-250 mEq/24 h | 110-250 mmol/d |
| Copper | 0-50 µg/24 h | 0.0-0.80 µmol/d |
| Cortisol, free | 10-100 µg/24 h | 27.6-276 nmol/d |
| Creatine | | |
|   Males | 0-40 mg/24 h | 0.0-0.30 mmol/d |
|   Females | 0-80 mg/24 h | 0.0-0.60 mmol/d |
| Creatinine | 15-25 mg/kg/24 h | 0.13-0.22 mmol/kg/d |
| Creatinine clearance (endogenous) | | |
|   Males | 110-150 mL/min/1.73 m$^2$ | 110-150 mL/min/1.73 m$^2$ |
|   Females | 105-132 mL/min/1.73 m$^2$ | 105-132 mL/min/1.73 m$^2$ |
| Cystine or cysteine | Negative | Negative |
| Dehydroepiandrosterone | | |
|   Males | 0.2-2.0 mg/24 h | 0.7-6.9 µmol/d |
|   Females | 0.2-1.8 mg/24 h | 0.7-6.2 µmol/d |
| Estrogens, total | | |
|   Males | 4-25 µg/24 h | 14-90 nmol/d |
|   Females | 5-100 µg/24 h | 18-360 nmol/d |
| Glucose (as reducing substance) | <250 mg/24 h | <250 mg/d |
| Hemoglobin and myoglobin, qualitative | Negative | Negative |
| Hemogentisic acid, qualitative | Negative | Negative |
| 17-Hydroxycorticosteroids | | |
|   Males | 3-9 mg/24 h | 8.3-25 µmol/d |
|   Females | 2-8 mg/24 h | 5.5-22 µmol/d |
| 5-Hydroxyindoleacetic acid | | |
|   Qualitative | Negative | Negative |
|   Quantitative | 2-6 mg/24 h | 10-31 µmol/d |
| 17-Ketogenic steroids | | |
|   Males | 5-23 mg/24 h | 17-80 µmol/d |
|   Females | 3-15 mg/24 h | 10-52 µmol/d |
| 17-Ketosteroids | | |
|   Males | 8-22 mg/24 h | 28-76 µmol/d |
|   Females | 6-15 mg/24 h | 21-52 µmol/d |
| Magnesium | 6-10 mEq/24 h | 3-5 mmol/d |
| Metanephrines | 0.05-1.2 ng/mg creatinine | 0.03-0.70 mmol/mmol creatinine |
| Osmolality | 38-1400 mOsm/kg water | 38-1400 mOsm/kg water |
| pH | 4.6-8.0 | 4.6-8.0 |
| Phenylpyruvic acid, qualitative | Negative | Negative |
| Phosphate | 0.4-1.3 g/24 h | 13-42 mmol/d |
| Porphobilinogen | | |
|   Qualitative | Negative | Negative |
|   Quantitative | <2 mg/24 h | <9 µmol/d |
| Porphyrins | | |
|   Coproporphyrin | 50-250 µg/24 h | 77-380 nmol/d |
|   Uroporphyrin | 10-30 µg/24 h | 12-36 nmol/d |
| Potassium | 25-125 mEq/24 h | 25-125 mmol/d |
| Pregnanediol | | |
|   Males | 0.0-1.9 mg/24 h | 0.0-6.0 µmol/d |
|   Females | | |
|     Proliferative phase | 0.0-2.6 mg/24 h | 0.0-8.0 µmol/d |
|     Luteal phase | 2.6-10.6 mg/24 h | 8-33 µmol/d |
|     Postmenopausal | 0.2-1.0 mg/24 h | 0.6-3.1 µmol/d |
| Pregnanetriol | 0.0-2.5 mg/24 h | 0.0-7.4 µmol/d |
| Protein, total | | |
|   Qualitative | Negative | Negative |
|   Quantitative | 10-150 mg/24 h | 10-150 mg/d |
|   Protein-to-creatinine ratio | <0.2 | <0.2 |

Continued

## Reference Intervals* for Clinical Chemistry (Urine)—cont'd

| Analyte | Conventional Units | SI Units |
| --- | --- | --- |
| Sodium (regular diet) | 60-260 mEq/24 h | 60-260 mmol/d |
| Specific gravity | | |
| Random specimen | 1.003-1.030 | 1.003-1.030 |
| 24-h collection | 1.015-1.025 | 1.015-1.025 |
| Urate (regular diet) | 250-750 mg/24 h | 1.5-4.4 mmol/d |
| Urobilinogen | 0.5-4.0 mg/24 h | 0.6-6.8 µmol/d |
| Vanillylmandelic acid (VMA) | 1.0-8.0 mg/24 h | 5-40 µmol/d |

*Values can vary depending on the method used.
*Abbreviation:* SI = International System of Units.

## Reference Intervals for Toxic Substances

| Analyte | Conventional Units | SI Units |
| --- | --- | --- |
| Arsenic, urine | <130 µg/24 h | <1.7 µmol/d |
| Bromides, serum, inorganic | <100 mg/dL | <10 mmol/L |
| Toxic symptoms | 140-1000 mg/dL | 14-100 mmol/L |
| Carboxyhemoglobin, blood | Saturation, percent | |
| Urban environment | <5% | <0.05 |
| Smokers | <12% | <0.12 |
| Symptoms | | |
| Headache | >15% | >0.15 |
| Nausea and vomiting | >25% | >0.25 |
| Potentially lethal | >50% | >0.50 |
| Ethanol, blood | <0.05 mg/dL, <0.005% | <1.0 mmol/L |
| Intoxication | >100 mg/dL, >0.1% | >22 mmol/L |
| Marked intoxication | 300-400 mg/dL, 0.3%-0.4% | 65-87 mmol/L |
| Alcoholic stupor | 400-500 mg/dL, 0.4%-0.5%, | 87-109 mmol/L |
| Coma | >500 mg/dL, >0.5% | >109 mmol/L |
| Lead, blood | | |
| Adults | <20 µg/dL | <1.0 µmol/L |
| Children | <10 µg/dL | <0.5 µmol/L |
| Lead, urine | <80 µg/24 h | <0.4 µmol/d |
| Mercury, urine | <10 µg/24 h | <150 nmol/d |

*Abbreviation:* SI = International System of Units.

## Reference Intervals for Tests Performed on Cerebrospinal Fluid

| Test | Conventional Units | SI Units |
| --- | --- | --- |
| Cells | <5 mm$^3$; all mononuclear | <5 × 10$^6$/L, all mononuclear |
| Protein electrophoresis | Albumin predominant | Albumin predominant |
| Glucose | 50-75 mg/dL (20 mg/dL less than in serum) | 2.8-4.2 mmol/L (1.1 mmol/L less than in serum) |
| IgG | | |
| Children <14 y | <8% of total protein | <0.08 of total protein |
| Adults | <14% of total protein | <0.14 of total protein |
| IgG index | 0.3-0.6 | 0.3-0.6 |
| Oligoclonal banding on electrophoresis | Absent | Absent |
| Pressure, opening | 70-180 mm H$_2$O | 70-180 mm H$_2$O |
| Protein, total | 15-45 mg/dL | 150-450 mg/L |

*Abbreviations:* Ig = immunoglobulin; SI = International System of Units.

## Reference Intervals for Tests of Gastrointestinal Function

| Test | Conventional Units |
|------|-------------------|
| Bentiromide | 6-h urinary arylamine excretion >57% excludes pancreatic insufficiency |
| β-Carotene, serum | 60-250 ng/dL |
| Fecal fat estimation | |
|   Qualitative | No fat globules seen by high-power microscope |
|   Quantitative | <6 g/24 h (>95% coefficient of fat absorption) |
| Gastric acid output | |
|   Basal | |
|     Males | 0.0-10.5 mmol/h |
|     Females | 0.0-5.6 mmol/h |
|   Maximum (after histamine or pentagastrin) | |
|     Males | 9.0-48.0 mmol/h |
|     Females | 6.0-31.0 mmol/h |
|   Ratio: basal/maximum | |
|     Males | 0.0-0.31 |
|     Females | 0.0-0.29 |
| Secretin test, pancreatic fluid | |
|   Volume | >1.8 mL/kg/h |
|   Bicarbonate | >80 mEq/L |
| D-Xylose absorption test, urine | >20% of ingested dose excreted in 5 h |

## Reference Intervals for Tests of Immunologic Function

| Test | Conventional Units | SI Units |
|------|-------------------|----------|
| **Autoantibodies, Serum, Adult** | | |
| Anti-CCP antibody | 0-19 U | |
| Anti-dsDNA antibody | 0-40 IU | 0-40 IU |
| Antinuclear antibody | <1:40 | |
| Rheumatoid factor (total IgG, IgA, IgM) | 0-30 mg/dL | |
| **Complement, Serum** | | |
| C3 | 85-175 mg/dL | 0.85-1.75 g/L |
| C4 | 15-45 mg/dL | 150-450 mg/L |
| Total hemolytic (CH$_{50}$) | 150-250 U/mL | 150-250 U/mL |
| **Immunoglobulins, Serum, Adult** | | |
| IgA | 70-310 mg/dL | 0.70-3.1 g/L |
| IgD | 0.0-6.0 mg/dL | 0.0-60 mg/L |
| IgE | 0.0-430 ng/dL | 0.0-430 mg/L |
| IgG | 640-1350 mg/dL | 6.4-13.5 g/L |
| IgM | 90-350 mg/dL | 0.90-3.5 g/L |

Helper-to-suppressor ratio: 0.8-1.8
*Abbreviations:* anti-CCP = anticyclic citrullinated peptide; dsDNA = double-stranded DNA; Ig = immunoglobulin; SI = International System of Units.

## Reference Intervals for Lymphocyte Subsets, Whole Blood, Heparinized

| Antigen(s) Expressed | Cell Type | Percentage | Absolute Cell Count |
|---------------------|-----------|-----------|--------------------|
| CD2 | E rosette T cells | 73-87% | 1040-2160 |
| CD3 | Total T cells | 56-77% | 860-1880 |
| CD3 and CD4 | Helper-inducer cells | 32-54% | 550-1190 |
| CD3 and CD8 | Suppressor-cytotoxic cells | 24-37% | 430-1060 |
| CD3 and DR | Activated T cells | 5-14% | 70-310 |
| CD16 and CD56 | Natural killer (NK) cells | 8-22% | 130-500 |
| CD19 | Total B cells | 7-17% | 140-370 |

## Reference Values for Semen Analysis

| Test | Conventional Units | SI Units |
|------|-------------------|----------|
| Volume | 2-5 mL | 2-5 mL |
| Liquefaction | Complete in 15 min | Complete in 15 min |
| pH | 7.2-8.0 | 7.2-8.0 |
| Leukocytes | Occasional or absent | Occasional or absent |
| **Spermatozoa** | | |
| Count | 60-150 × 10$^6$ mL | 60-150 × 10$^6$ mL |
| Fructose | >150 mg/dL | >8.33 mmol/L |
| Morphology | 80-90% normal forms | >0.80-0.90 normal |
| Motility | >80% motile | >0.80 motile |

*Abbreviation:* SI = International System of Units.

# Toxic Chemical Agents Reference Chart: Symptoms and Treatment

Method of
*James J. James, MD, DrPH, MHA, and*
*James M. Lyznicki, MS, MPH*

Toxic chemical agents are poisonous vapors, aerosols, gasses, liquids, or solids that have toxic effects on people, animals, or plants. Most of these agents are liquid at room temperature and are disseminated as vapors and aerosols. They may be released as bombs, sprayed from aircraft and boats, or disseminated by other means to intentionally create a hazard to people and the environment. Some of these agents are highly toxic and persistent, features that can render a site uninhabitable and require costly and potentially hazardous decontamination and remediation. Health effects range from irritation and burning of skin and mucous membranes to rapid cardiopulmonary collapse and death.

Efficient deployment of hazardous materials (HazMat) teams is critical to control a chemical agent attack. Although all major cities and emergency medical systems have plans and equipment in place to address this situation, physicians and other health professionals must be aware of principles involved in managing a patient or multiple patients exposed to these agents. Chemical weapon agents have a high potential for secondary contamination from victims to responders. This requires that medical treatment facilities have clearly defined procedures for handling contaminated casualties, many of whom will transport themselves to the facility. Precautions must be used until thorough decontamination has been performed or the specific chemical agent is identified. Health care professionals must first protect themselves (e.g., by using protective suits, respiratory protection, and chemical-resistant gloves) because secondary contamination with even small amounts of these substances (particularly nerve agents such as VX) may be lethal.

Primary detection of exposure to chemical agents will be based on the signs and symptoms of the potential victim (Table 1). Confirmation of a chemical agent, using detection equipment or laboratory analyses, will take considerable time and will not likely contribute to the early management of mass casualty victims. Several patients presenting with the same symptoms should alert physicians and hospital staff to the possibility of a chemical attack. If a chemical attack occurs, most victims will likely arrive within a short time. This situation differentiates a chemical attack from a biological attack involving infectious microganisms. Additional diagnostic clues include:

- Unusual temporal or geographic clustering of illness
- Any sudden increase in illness in previously healthy persons
- Sudden increase in non-specific syndromes (e.g., sudden unexplained weakness in previously healthy persons; dimmed or blurred vision; hypersecretion, inhalation, or burn-like syndrome)

A coordinated communication network is critical for transmitting reliable information from the incident scene to treatment facilities. Any suspicious or confirmed exposure to a chemical weapons agent should be reported to the local health department, local Federal Bureau of Investigations office, and the Centers for Disease Control and Prevention (1-770-488-7100).

## TABLE 1 Quick Reference Chart on Chemical Weapon Agents

| Chemical Agent | Diagnostic Considerations | Treatment Considerations* |
|---|---|---|
| **Cyanides**<br>Cyanogen chloride (CK)<br>Hydrogen cyanide (AC) | • Symptom onset: rapid, seconds to minutes<br>• Odor: bitter almond, musty, or chlorine-like<br>• Nonspecific hypoxic and hypoxemic symptoms<br>• Binds cellular cytochrome oxidase causing chemical asphyxia<br>• Respiratory: shortness of breath, chest tightness, hyperventilation, respiratory arrest<br>• GI: nausea, vomiting<br>• Cardiovascular: ventricular arrhythmias, hypotension, cardiac arrest, shock<br>• CNS: anxiety, headache drowsiness, weakness, apnea, convulsions, seizure, coma<br>• CNS effects may be confused with carbon monoxide and hydrogen sulfide poisoning<br>• Metabolic acidosis and increased concentration of venous oxygen (patient also may present with cyanosis)<br>• Laboratory testing: cyanide, thiocyanate, serum lactate levels; venous and arterial partial oxygen pressure | • Immediate treatment of symptomatic patients is critical<br>• Antidote: sodium nitrite and sodium thiosulfate; repeat one-half initial doses of both agents in 30 minutes if there is inadequate clinical response<br>• Amyl nitrate capsules are available for first aid until intravenous access is achieved<br>• Cyanide antidone kits are commercially available<br>• Investigational in the United States, available in Europe: hydroxycobalamin (vitamin $B_{12a}$) administered with thiosulfate<br>• Activated charcoal[A] for oral exposure<br>• Mechanical ventilation as needed<br>• Circulatory support with crystalloids and vasopressors<br>• Metabolic acidosis corrected with IV sodium bicarbonate<br>• Seizures controlled with benzodiazepines |
| **Incapacitating Agents**<br>Agent 15<br>3-quinuclidinyl benzilate (BZ) | • Symptom onset: hours<br><br>0-4 h: parasympathetic blockade and mild CNS effects<br>4-20 h: stupor with ataxia and hyperthermia<br>20-96 h: full-blown delirium<br>Resolution phase: paranoia, deep sleep, reawakening, crawling, climbing automatisms, eventual reorientation | • Antidote: physostigmine salicylate (Antilirium)[A]<br>• Support, intravenous fluids |

[A]Not FDA approved for this indication.
*Different situations may require different treatment and dosage regimens. Please consult other references as well as a regional poison control conter (1-800-222-1222), medical toxicologist, clinical pharmacologist, or other drug information specialist for definitive dosage information, especially dosages for pregnant women and children.
*Abbreviations:* CNS = central nervous system; GI = gastrointestinal.

**TABLE 1** Quick Reference Chart on Chemical Weapon Agents—cont'd

| Chemical Agent | Diagnostic Considerations | Treatment Considerations* |
|---|---|---|
| **Nerve Agents**<br>Cyclohexyl sarin (GF)<br>Sarin (GB)<br>Soman (GD)<br>Tabun (GA)<br>VX | • Odorless<br>• Competitive inhibitor of acetylcholine muscarinic receptor<br>• Mydriasis, blurred vision, dry mouth, dry skin, possible atropine-like flush, initial rise in heart rate, decreased level of consciousness, confusion, disorientation, visual hallucinations, impaired memory<br>Symptom onset: vapor (seconds), liquid (minutes or hours); symptom onset may be delayed up to 18 hours particularly for localized exposures<br>• Odor: none (GB, VX), fruity (GA), camphor-like (GD)<br>• Most toxic of known chemical agents<br>• Irreversible acetylcholinesterase inhibitors<br>• Eyes: excessive lacrimation, miosis may be present<br>• Respiratory: rhinorrhea, bronchospasm, respiratory failure<br>• GI: hypersalivation, nausea, vomiting, diarrhea<br>• Skin: localized sweating<br>• Cardiac: sinus bradycardia<br>• Skeletal muscles: fasciculations followed by weakness, flaccid paralysis<br>• CNS: loss of consciousness, convulsions, apnea, seizures<br>• May be confused with organophosphate and carbamate pesticide poisoning<br>• Laboratory testing: erythrocyte or serum cholinesterase activity to confirm exposure | • Rapid establishment of patent airway<br>• Antidote: Atropine[A] and pralidoxime[A] chloride (Protopam chloride, 2-PAM); additional doses until bronchial secretions are cleared and ventilation improved<br>• Early administration of 2-PAM is critical to minimize permanent agent inactivation of acetylcholinesterase (i.e., "aging")<br>• Benzodiazepines to control nerve agent-induced seizures<br>• Airway and ventilatory support as needed<br>• Atropine,[A] pralidoxime,[A] and diazepam[A] are available in autoinjector kits through the U.S. military |
| **Pulmonary or Choking Agents**<br>Acrolein<br>Ammonia ($NH_3$)<br>Chlorine (CL)<br>Choloropicrin (PS)<br>Diphosgene (DP)<br>Nitrogen oxides ($NO_x$)<br>Perflouroisobutylene (PFIB)<br>Phosgene (CG)<br>Sulfur dioxide ($SO_2$) | • Symptom onset: rapid or delayed; 1-24 h (rarely up to 72 h)<br>• Odor (CG): freshly mown hay or grass<br>• Easily absorbed via mucous membranes of eyes, nose, oropharynx. Degree of water solubility of the agent influences onset and severity of respiratory injury.<br>• Eye and airway irritation, dyspnea, chest tightness, rhinorrhea, hypersalivation, cough, wheezing<br>• High dose inhalation may produce laryngospasm, pneumonitis, and acute lung injury with delayed onset (≤48 h) of acute respiratory distress syndrome<br>• Chest radiograph: hyperinflation, noncardiogenic pulmonary edema<br>• May be confused with inhalation exposure to industrial chemicals (e.g., HCl, $Cl_2$, $NH_3$) | • No specific antidote<br>• Supportive measures; specific treatment depends on the agent<br>• IV fluids for hypotension; no diuretics<br>• Ventilation with or without positive airway pressure<br>• Bronchodilators for bronchospasm<br>• Methylprednisolone[A] may be effective in preventing noncardiogenic pulmonary edema |
| **Riot Control Agents**<br>Mace (CN)<br>Tear gas (CS) | • Symptom onset: immediate<br>• Odor: apple blossom (CN); pepper (CS)<br>• Metallic taste<br>• $SN_2$ alkylating agents<br>• Burning and pain on mucosal membranes and skin<br>• Eyes: irritation, pain, tearing, blepharospasm<br><br>• Airways: burning in nose and mouth, respiratory discomfort, bronchospam (may be delayed 36 h)<br>• Skin: tingling, erythema<br>• Nausea and vomiting common<br>• CN can cause corneal opacification<br>• No specific laboratory tests | • Supportive care<br>• Irrigation as necessary<br>• Persons with asthma, emphysema may need oxygen, inhaled bronchodilators, steroids, assisted ventilation<br>• Lotions, such as calamine,[A] for persistent erythema |
| **Vesicant or Blister Agents** | • Symptoms onset: immediate (L, CX); delayed 2-48 h (H, HD)<br>• Primary liquid hazard<br>• May be confused with skin exposure to caustic irritants (e.g., sodium hydroxide, ammonia)<br>• Intracellular enzyme and DNA alkylating agents | • Immediate decontamination<br>• Supportive care<br>• Thermal burn-type treatment<br>• Symptomatic management of lesions |

*Continued*

## TABLE 1  Quick Reference Chart on Chemical Weapon Agents—cont'd

| Chemical Agent | Diagnostic Considerations | Treatment Considerations* |
|---|---|---|
| Sulfur mustard (H)<br>Distilled mustard (HD) | • Clinical effects dependent on extent and route of exposure; effects may be delayed, appearing hours after exposure<br>• Odor: garlic, horseradish, or mustard<br>• Skin: erythema and blisters (may be delayed ≤8 h), pruritus<br>• Eye: irritation, conjunctivitis, corneal damage, lacrimation, pain, blepharospasm<br>• Respiratory: mild to marked acute airway damage, pneumonitis within 1-3 d, respiratory failure<br>• GI effects (nausea, vomiting diarrhea) may be present<br>• Bone marrow stem cell suppression leading to pancytopenia and increased susceptibility to infection<br>• Fever, sputum production<br>• Combination with Lewisite (called mustard-Lewisite or HL) results in rapid effects of Lewisite and delayed effects of mustard agents | • No specific antidote<br>• Skin: silver sulfadiazine[A]<br>• Eye: homatropine[A] ophthalmic ointment<br>• Pulmonary: antibiotics, bronchodilators, steroids<br>• Colony stimulating factor may be helpful for leukopenia<br>• Systemic analgesic and antipruritics<br>• Early use of positive-end expiratory pressure or continuous positive airway pressure<br>• Maintain fluid and electrolyte balance (do not excessively fluid resuscitate as in thermal burns) |
| Lewisite (L) | • Odor: fruity or geranium<br>• More volatile than mustard<br>• Damages eyes, skin, and airways by direct contact<br>• Skin: gray area of dead skin within 5 min, erythema within 30 min, blistering 2-3 h, immediate irritation or burning pain on contact, severe tissue necrosis<br>• Eye: pain, blepharospasm, conjunctival and lid edema<br>• Airway: pseudomembrane formation, nasal irritation<br>• Intravascular fluid loss, hypovolemia, shock, organ congestion, leukocytosis | • Antidote: British Anti-Lewisite (BAL or Dimercaprol) |
| Phosgene Oxime (CX) | • Odor: freshly mown hay<br>• Urticant, nonvesicant agent<br>• Vapor extremely irritating; vapor and liquid cause tissue damage upon contact<br>• Immediate burning, irritation, wheal-like skin lesions, eye and airway damage, conjunctivitis, lacrimation, lid edema, blepharospasm<br>• No distinctive laboratory findings | • No antidote<br>• Parenteral methylprednisolone[A] may be effective in preventing noncardiogenic pulmonary edema<br>• Experimental: aerosolized dexamethasone[A] and theophylline[A] for pulmonary involvement |
| **Vomiting (Arsine-Based) Agents**<br>Adamsite (DM)<br>Diphenylchlorarsine (DA)<br>Diphenylcyanoarsine (DC) | • Symptom onset: All rapidly acting within minutes<br>• Odor: none (DA), garlic (DC), burning fireworks (DM)<br>• Primary route of absorption is through respiratory system<br>• Arsine gas depletes erythrocyte glutathione and causes hemolysis<br>• Eyes: conjunctival irritation, tearing, and blepharospasm<br>• Airways: sneezing, mucosal lung irritation, edema, progressive cough, wheezing<br>• Cardiac: tachypnea, tachycardia<br>• GI: intestinal cramps, emesis, diarrhea<br>• Skin: erythema, edema at the site of dermal contact<br>• CNS: depression, syncope<br>• Chest radiograph to rule out chemical pneumonitis | • Supportive care<br>• Monitor for hemolysis<br>• Wheezing or dyspnea; may need albuterol inhalation<br>• Eye irrigation (water, normal saline, lactated Ringer's solution) in patients sustaining ocular exposure<br>• Treat repetitive emesis with IV hydration and antiemetics<br>• Blood transfusion may be required<br>• Exchange transfusion may be required<br>• Hemodialysis may be useful in decreasing arsenic level and treating renal failure |

# Biologic Agents Reference Chart—Symptoms, Tests, and Treatment

Method of

*James J. James, MD, DrPh, MHA, and*
*James M. Lyznicki, MS, MPH*

Biologic weapons are devices used intentionally to cause disease or death through dissemination of microorganisms or toxins in food and water, by insect vectors, or by aerosols. Potential targets include human beings, food crops, livestock, and other resources essential for national security, economy, and defense. Unlike nuclear, chemical, and conventional weapons, the onset of a biological attack will probably be insidious. For some infectious agents, secondary and tertiary transmission may continue for weeks or months after the initial attack.

Initial detection of an unannounced biological attack will likely occur when an astute health professional notices an unusual case or disease cluster and reports his or her concerns to local public health authorities. Physicians and other health professionals should be alert to the following:

- Unusual temporal or geographic clustering of illnesses
- Sudden increase of illness in previously healthy persons
- Sudden increase in non-specific illnesses (e.g., pneumonia, flulike illness; bleeding disorders; unexplained rashes, particularly in adults; neuromuscular illness; diarrhea)

To enhance detection and treatment capabilities, physicians and other health professionals in acute care settings should be familiar with the clinical manifestations, diagnostic techniques, isolation precautions, treatment, and prophylaxis for likely causative agents (e.g., smallpox, pneumonic plague, anthrax, viral hemorrhagic fevers). Table 1 provides a quick summary of diagnostic and treatment considerations for various infectious and toxic biological agents. For some of these agents, delay in medical response could result in a potentially devastating number of casualties. To mitigate such consequences, early identification and intervention are imperative. Front-line physicians must have an increased level of suspicion regarding the possible intentional use of biological agents as well as an increased sensitivity to reporting those suspicious to public health authorities, who, in turn, must be willing to evaluate a predictable increase in false positive reports.

Medical response efforts require coordination and planning with emergency management agencies, law enforcement, health care facilities, and social services agencies. Health care agencies should ensure that physicians know whom to call with reports of suspicious cases and clusters of infectious diseases, and should work to build a good relationship with the local medical community. Resource integration is absolutely necessary to:

- Establish adequate capacity to initiate rapid investigation of an outbreak
- Educate the public
- Begin mass distribution of antibiotics and vaccines
- Ensure mass medical care
- Control public anger and fear

In an epidemic, overwhelming numbers of critically ill patients will require acute and follow-up medical care. Both infected persons and the *worried well* will seek medical attention, with a corresponding need for medical supplies, diagnostic tests, and hospital beds. The impact — or even the threat — of an attack can elicit widespread panic and civil disorder, overwhelm hospital resources, and disrupt social services.

Any suspicious or confirmed exposure to a biological weapons agent should be reported immediately to the local health department, local Federal Bureau of Investigation office, and the Centers of Disease Control and Prevention (1-770-488-7100).

**TABLE 1** Quick Reference Chart on Biological Weapon Agents

| Disease/Agent | Diagnostic Considerations | Treatment Considerations[1] | Prophylaxis |
|---|---|---|---|
| **Bacteria** | | | |
| Anthrax<br>*Bacillus anthracis* | Incubation period: 1-5 d (perhaps ≤60 d)[2]<br>*Cutaneous:*<br>• Evolving skin lesion (face, neck, arms), progresses to vesicle, dispressed ulcer, and black necrotic lesions<br>• Lethality: 20% if untreated, otherwise rarely fatal<br>*Gastrointestinal*<br>• Nausea, vomiting, abdominal pain, bloody diarrhea, sepsis<br>• Lethality: approaches 100% if untreated but data are limited; rapid, aggressive treatment may reduce mortality<br>*Inhalational*<br>• Abrupt onset of flu-like symptoms, fever with or without chills, sweats, fatigue or malaise, non- or minimally productive cough, nausea, vomiting, dyspnea, headache, chest pain, followed in 2-5 d by | Combination therapy of ciprofloxacin (Cipro) or doxycycline (Vibramycin) plus one or two other antimicrobials should be considered with inhalational anthrax[6]<br>Penicillin[A] should be considered if strain is susceptible and does not possess inducible β-lactamases<br>If meningitis suspected, doxycycline (Vibramycin) may be less optimal because of poor CNS penetration<br>Steroids may be considered for severe edema and for meningitis. | Ciprofloxacin (Cipro) or doxycycline (Vibramycin) with or without vaccination<br>If strain is susceptible, penicillin[A] or amoxicillin[A] (Amoxil) should be considered<br>Inactivated vaccine (licensed but not readily available); six injections and annual booster |

*Continued*

**TABLE 1** Quick Reference Chart on Biological Weapon Agents—cont'd

| Disease/Agent | Diagnostic Considerations | Treatment Considerations[1] | Prophylaxis |
|---|---|---|---|
| | severe respiratory distress, mediastinitis, hemorrhagic meningitis, sepsis, shock.[3]<br>• Widened mediastinum on chest radiograph is characteristic for inhalational and occasionally GI anthrax.[4]<br>• Lethality: Once respiratory distress develops, mortality rates may approach 90%; begin treatment when inhalational anthrax is suspected, do not wait for confirmatory testing.[5]<br>Gram stain and culture of blood, pleural fluid, cerebrospinal fluid, ascitic fluid, vesicular fluid or lesion exudate; sputum rarely positive; confirmatory serological and PCR tests available through public health laboratory network | | |
| **Brucellosis**<br>*B. abortus*<br>*B. canis*<br>*B. mellitensis*<br>*B. suis* | Incubation period: 5-60 d (usually 1-2 mo)<br>• Non-specific flu-like symptoms, fever, headache, profound weakness and fatigue, GI symptoms such as anorexia, nausea, vomiting, diarrhea, or constipation<br>• Osteoarticular complications common<br>• Lethality: less than 5% even if untreated; tends to incapacitate rather than kill.<br>Blood and bone marrow culture (may require 6 wk to grow *Brucella*); confirmatory culture and serological testing available through public health laboratory network | Doxycycline (Vibramycin) plus streptomycin or rifampin[A] (Rifadin)<br>*Alternative therapies:*<br>Ofloxacin (Floxin)[A] plus rifampin[A] (Rifadin)<br>Doxycycline (Vibramycin) plus gentamicin (Garamycin)<br>TMP/SMX (Bactrim,[A] Septra) plus gentamicin (Garamycin) | Doxycycline (Vibramycin) plus streptomycin or rifampin (Rifadin)<br>No approved human vaccine |
| **Inhalational (Pneumonic) Tularemia**<br>*Francisella tularensis* | Incubation period: 3-5 d (range of 1-21 d)<br>• Sudden onset of acute febrile illness, weakness, chills, headache, generalized body aches, elevated WBCs<br>• Pulmonary symptoms such as dry cough, chest pain or tightness with or without objective signs of pneumonia<br>• Progressive weakness, malaise, anorexia, and weight loss occurs, potentially leading to sepsis and organ failure<br>• Largely clinical diagnosis<br>• Lethality: ≈30-60% fatal if untreated<br>Culture of blood, sputum, biopsies, pleural fluid, bronchial washings (culture is difficult and potentially dangerous); confirmatory testing available through public health laboratory network | Streptomycin or gentamicin (Garamycin)<br>*Alternative therapies:*<br>Ciprofloxacin (Cipro)[A]<br>Doxycycline (Vibramycin)<br>Chloramphenicol[A] (Chloromycetin) | Tetracycline<br>Doxycycline (Vibramycin)<br>Ciprofloxacin (Cipro)[A]<br>Live attenuated vaccine (USAMRIID, IND) given by scarification; currently under FDA review; limited availability |

TABLE 1 Quick Reference Chart on Biological Weapon Agents—cont'd

| Disease/Agent | Diagnostic Considerations | Treatment Considerations[1] | Prophylaxis |
|---|---|---|---|
| **Pneumonic Plague** *Yersinia pestis* | Incubation period: 1-10 d (typically 2-3 d)<br>• Acute onset of flu-like prodrome: fever, myalgia, weakness, headache; within 24 h of prodrome, chest discomfort, cough with bloody sputum, and dyspnea. By day 2 to 4 illness, symptoms progressing to cyanosis, respiratory distress, and hemodynamic instability<br>• Lethality: almost 100% if untreated; 20–60% if appropriately treated within 18-24 h of symptoms; begin treatment when diagnosis of plague is suspected; do not wait for confirmatory testing<br>Gram stain and culture of blood, CSF, sputum, lymph node aspirates, bronchial washings; confirmatory serological and bacteriological tests available through public health laboratory network | Streptomycin; gentamicin (Garamycin)<br>*Alternative therapies:*<br>Doxycycline (Vibramycin)<br>Tetracycline<br>Ciprofloxacin[A] (Cipro)<br>Chloramphenicol[A] (Chloromycetin) is first choice for meningitis except for pregnant women | Tetracycline<br>Doxycycline (Vibramycin)<br>Ciprofloxacin[A] (Cipro)<br>Inactivated whole cell vaccine licensed but not readily available; injection with boosters<br>Vaccine not effective against aerosol exposure |
| **Rickettsia**<br>**Q-Fever** *Coxiella burnetii* | Incubation period: 2-14 d (may be ≤40 days)<br>• Nonspecific febrile disease, chills, cough, weakness and fatigue, pleuritic chest pain, pneumonia possible<br>• Lethality: 1-3%. Fatalities are uncommon even if untreated but relapsing symptoms may occur<br>Isolation of organism may be difficult; confirmatory testing via serology or PCR available through public health laboratory network | Tetracycline<br>Doxycycline (Vibramycin) | Tetracycline<br>Doxycycline (Vibramycin)<br>Inactivated whole cell[B] vaccine (IND)<br>Skin test to determine prior exposure to *C. burnetii* recommended before vaccination |
| **Viruses**<br>**Smallpox** Variola major virus | Incubation period: 7-17 d<br>• Prodrome of high fever, malaise, prostration, headache, vomiting, delirium followed in 2-3 d maculopapular rash uniformly progressing to pustules and scabs, mostly on extremities and face<br>• Requires astute clinical evaluation; may be confused with chickenpox, erythema multiforme with bullae, or allergic contact dermatitis<br>• Lethality: 30% in unvaccinated persons<br>Pharyngeal swab, vesicular fluid, biopsies, scab material for electron microscopy and PCR testing through public health laboratory network<br>Notify CDC Poxvirus Section at 1-404-639-2184 | Supportive care<br>Cidofovir (Vistide) shown to be effective in vitro and in experimental animals infected with surrogate orthopox virus | Live attenuated vaccinia vaccine derived from calf lymph; given by scarification (licensed, restricted supply)<br>New vaccine being developed from tissue culture<br>Vaccination given within 3-4 d following exposure can prevent or decrease the severity of disease |

*Continued*

## TABLE 1 Quick Reference Chart on Biological Weapon Agents—cont'd

| Disease/Agent | Diagnostic Considerations | Treatment Considerations[1] | Prophylaxis |
|---|---|---|---|
| **Viral Encephalitis** Eastern (EEE) Western (WEE) Venezuelan (VEE) | Incubation period: 2-6 d (VEE); 7-14 d (EEE, WEE) • Systemic febrile illness, with encephalitis developing in some populations • Generalized malaise, spiking fevers, headache, myalgia • Incidence of seizures and/or focal neurologic deficits may be higher after biological attack • White blood cell count may show striking leukopenia and lymphopenia • Clinical and epidemiologic diagnosis • Lethality: <10% (VEE); 10% (WEE); 50-75% (EEE) Confirmatory test and viral isolation available through public health laboratory network | Supportive care Analgesics, anticonvulsants as needed | Several IND vaccines, poorly immunogenic, highly reactogenic |
| **Viral Hemorrhagic Fevers (VHFs)** Arenaviruses (Lassa, Junin, and related viruses) Bunyaviruses (Hanta, Congo-Crimean, Rift Valley) Filoviruses (Ebola, Marburg) Flaviviruses (yellow fever, dengue, various tick-borne disease viruses) | Incubation period: 4-21 d • Fever with mucous membrane bleeding, petechiae, thrombocytopenia and hypotension in patients without underlying malignancies • Malaise, myalgias, headache, vomiting, diarrhea possible • Lethality: Variable depending on viral strain; 15-25% with Lassa fever to ≤ 90% with Ebola Confirmatory testing and viral isolation available through public health laboratory network Call CDC Special Pathogens Office at 1-404-639-1115 | Supportive therapy Ribavirin (Virazole)[A] may be effective for Lassa fever, Rift Valley fever, Argentine hemorrhagic fever, and Congo-Crimean hemorrhagic fever | Ribavarin (Virazole)[A] is suggested for Congo-Crimean hemorrhagic fever and Lassa fever Yellow fever vaccine is the only licensed vaccine available Vaccines for some of the other VHFs exist but are for investigational use only |
| **Biological Toxins Botulism** *Clostridium botulinum toxin* | Symptom onset: 1-5 d (typically 12-36 h) • Blurred vision, diploplia, dry mouth, ptosis, fatigue • As disease progresses, acute bilateral descending flaccid paralysis, respiratory paralysis resulting in death • Clinical diagnosis • Lethality: 60% without ventilatory support Serum and stool should be assayed for toxin by mouse neutralization bioassay, which may require several days | Intensive and prolonged supportive care; ventilation may be necessary Trivalent equine antitoxin (serotypes A,B,E, – licensed, available from the CDC) should be administered immediately after clinical diagnosis Anaphylaxis and serum sickness are potential complications of antitoxin Aminoglycosides and clindamycin (Cleocin)[A] must not be used | Pentavalent toxoid (A-E), yearly booster (IND, CDC) Not available to the public Antitoxin may be sufficient to prevent illness following exposure but is not recommended until patient is showing symptoms |
| **Enterotoxin B** *Staphylococcus aureus* | Symptom onset: 3-12 h • Acute onset of fever, chills headache, nonproductive cough • Normal chest radiograph • Clinical diagnosis • Lethality: probably low (few data available for respiratory exposure) Serology on acute and convalescent serum can confirm diagnosis | Supportive care | No vaccine available |

**TABLE 1** Quick Reference Chart on Biological Weapon Agents—cont'd

| Disease/Agent | Diagnostic Considerations | Treatment Considerations[1] | Prophylaxis |
|---|---|---|---|
| **Ricin toxin** <br> *Ricinus communis* | Symptom onset: ≤6-24 h <br> • Weakness, nausea, chest tightness, fever, cough, pulmonary edema, respiratory failure, circulatory collapse, hypoxemia resulting in death (usually within 36-72 h) <br> • Clinical and epidemiological diagnosis <br> • Lethality: mortality data not available but is likely to be high with extensive exposure <br> Confirmatory serological testing available through public health laboratory network | Supportive care <br> Treatment for pulmonary edema <br> Gastric decontamination if toxin ingested | No vaccine available |
| **T-2 Mycotoxins** <br> *Fusarium* <br> *Myrothecium* <br> *Trichoderma* <br> *Stachybotrys* | Symptom onset: minutes to hours <br> • Abrupt onset of mucocutaneous and airway irritation and pain <br> • May include skin, eyes, and GI tract; systemic toxicity may follow | Clinical support <br> Soap and water washing within 4-6 h reduces dermal toxicity; washing within 1 h may eliminate toxicity entirely | No vaccine available |
| Other filamentous fungi | • Lethality: severe exposure can cause death in hours to days <br> Consult with local health department regarding specimen collection and diagnostic testing procedures; confirmation requires testing blood, tissue, and environmental samples | No effective medications or antidotes | |

<sup>A</sup>Not FDA approved for this indication.

<sup>B</sup>Not available in the United States.

[1]Different situations may require different dosage and treatment regimens. Please consult other references and an infectious disease specialist for definitive dosage information, especially dosages for pregnant women and children.

[2]Data from 22 patients infected with anthrax in October and November 2001 indicate a median incubation period of 4 d (range 4-7 d) for inhalational anthrax and a mean incubation of 5 d (range 1-10 d) for cutaneous anthrax.

[3]Limited data from the October/November 2001 anthrax infections indicate hemorrhagic pleural effusions to be strongly associated with inhalational anthrax; rhinorrhea was present in only 1/10 patients.

[4]Chest radiograph abnormalities include paratracheal and hilar fullness and may be subtle. Consider chest computed tomography if diagnosis is uncertain.

[5]Limited data from the 2001 terrorist-related anthrax infections indicate that early treatment significantly decreased the mortality rate.

[6]Other agents with in vitro activity suggested for use in conjunction with ciprofloxacin (Cipro) or doxycycline (Vibramycin) for treatment of inhalational anthrax include rifampin (Rifadin), vancomycin (Vancocin), imipenem (Primaxin), chloramphenicol (Chloromycetin), penicillin and ampicillin, clindamycin (Cleocin), and clarithromycin (Biaxin).

*Abbreviations:* CDC = Centers for Disease Control and Prevention; CNS = central nervous system; CSF = cerebrospinal fluid; GI = gastrointestinal; IND = investigational new drug; PCR = polymerase chain reaction; TMP-SMX = trimethoprim-sulfamethoxazole; USAMRIID, U.S. Army Medical Research Institute of Infectious Diseases; WBC = white blood cell.

Adopted for *Biological Weapons: Quick Reference Guide.* American Medical Association; 2002. Available at http://www.amaassn.org/ama1/pub/upload/mm/415/quickreference0902.pdf.

Biologic Agents Reference Chart

1219

# Popular Herbs and Nutritional Supplements

Method of
*Miriam M. Chan, RPh, PharmD*

| Herb/Nutritional Supplement | Common Uses | Reasonable Adult Oral Dosage* | Precautions and Drug Interactions |
|---|---|---|---|
| Bilberry fruit[7] | Often used orally to improve visual acuity and to treat degenerative retinal conditions<br>Also used orally to treat chronic venous insufficiency, varicose veins, and hemorrhoids<br>Approved in Germany to use orally for acute diarrhea and topically for mild inflammation of the mucous membranes of the mouth and throat | For eye conditions and circulation, 80-160 mg tid of the extract standardized to at least 25% anthocyanosides<br>For diarrhea, 20-60 g/d of the dried ripe berries or as a tea preparation (5-10 g crushed dried berries in 150 mL water, brought to a boil for 10 min, then strained)<br>For external use, 10% decoction | No known side effects reported with bilberry fruit and extract<br>However, bilberry leaf taken in large quantities or used long term has been shown to cause wasting, anemia, jaundice, acute excitation, disturbances of tonus, and death in animals<br>The anthocyanidin extracts from bilberry can increase the risk of bleeding in those taking warfarin (Coumadin) or other blood thinners |
| Black cohosh root[7] | Commonly used to relieve hot flushes and other menopausal symptoms<br>Also used to treat premenstrual discomfort and dysmenorrhea | 20 mg bid of the rhizome extract standardized to triterpene glycosides<br>The German guidelines do not recommend its use for >6 mo | Black cohosh can have an estrogen-like effect and should be avoided in women with breast cancer<br>Large doses can induce miscarriage and it is contraindicated during pregnancy<br>It can cause GI disturbances, headache, and hypotension<br>International case reports of liver dysfunction are suspected to be associated with its use |
| Chamomile flower[7] | Used orally to calm nerves and treat GI spasms and inflammatory diseases of the GI tract<br>Used topically to treat wounds, skin infections, and skin or mucous membrane inflammation | 1 cup of freshly made tea 3-4 times daily (1 tbsp or 3 g dried flower in 150 mL boiling water for 5-10 min) | Chamomile can cause an allergic reaction, especially in people with severe allergies to ragweed or other members of the daisy family (e.g., echinacea, feverfew, and milk thistle)<br>Should not be taken concurrently with other sedatives, such as alcohol or benzodiazepines |
| Chaste tree berry (Chasteberry, Vitex)[7] | For normalizing irregular menstrual periods and relieving premenstrual complaints<br>For relieving menopausal symptoms<br>For restoring fertility in women<br>For treating acne associated with menstrual cycles<br>For increasing breast milk production in lactating women | For menstrual irregularities and premenstrual complaints, 30-40 mg/d of the dried berries or an equivalent amount of aqueous-alcoholic extracts (50%-70% v/v)<br>Dried fruit extract, standardized to 0.6% agnusides, is used in doses of 175-225 mg/d<br>For other conditions, no established dosage is documented | Chaste tree berry can have uterus-stimulant properties and should be avoided in pregnancy<br>Women with hormone-dependent conditions (e.g., breast, uterine, and ovarian cancers, endometriosis, and uterine fibroids) and men with prostate cancers should avoid chaste tree berry because it contains progestins<br>Side effects include intramenstrual bleeding, dry mouth, headache, nausea, rash, alopecia, and tachycardia<br>High doses (extract ≥480 mg/d) can paradoxically decrease lactation<br>Chaste tree berry is believed to have dopaminergic effects and might interact with dopamine |

| Herb/Nutritional Supplement | Common Uses | Reasonable Adult Oral Dosage* | Precautions and Drug Interactions |
|---|---|---|---|
| | | | antagonists, such as antipsychotics and metoclopramide |
| | | | Chaste tree berry can also decrease the effects of oral contraceptives and hormone replacement therapy |
| Chondroitin[7] | Orally, often used in combination with glucosamine for osteoarthritis<br>Topically, used in combination with sodium hyaluronate, as a viscoelastic agent in cataract surgery | Oral: 200-400 mg tid | Occasional mild side effects include nausea, indigestion, and allergic reactions<br>Chondroitin derived from bovine cartilage carries a potential risk of contamination with diseased animals |
| Chromium[7] | For diabetes<br>For hypercholesterolemia<br>Commonly found in weight-loss products<br>Also promoted for body building | For diabetes, 100 µg bid for ≤4 mo or 500 µg bid for 2 mo<br>For hypercholesterolemia, 200 µg tid or 500 µg bid for 2-4 mo<br>For body building, 200-400 µg/d<br>Chromium picolinate has been used in most studies, even though the chloride form is also available | Adverse effects are rare, but they include headaches, insomnia, sleep disturbances, irritability, and mood changes. Some patients also experience cognitive, perceptual, and motor dysfunction<br>Long-term use of high doses (600-2400 µg/d) can cause anemia, thrombocytopenia, hemolysis, hepatic dysfunction, and renal failure<br>Two case reports of interstitial nephritis<br>A few studies suggest that chromium can cause DNA damage<br>Chromium competes with iron for binding to transferrin and can cause iron deficiency<br>Antacids, $H_2$-blockers, and PPIs can decrease the absorption of chromium |
| Coenzyme Q10[7] | As adjunctive treatment for congestive heart failure, angina, hypertension, and diabetes<br>Also used for reducing cardiotoxicity associated with doxorubicin | For heart failure, 100 mg/d in two or three divided doses<br>For angina, 50 mg tid<br>For hypertension, 60 mg bid<br>For diabetes, 100-200 mg/d | Mild adverse events include gastric distress, nausea, vomiting, and hypotension<br>Doses >300 mg/d can cause elevated liver enzyme levels<br>Coenzyme Q10 can reduce the anticoagulation effects of warfarin<br>Oral hypoglycemic agents and HMG-CoA reductase inhibitors can reduce serum coenzyme Q10 levels |
| Cranberry[7] | To prevent and treat UTIs or *Helicobacter pylori* infections that can lead to stomach ulcers<br>To prevent dental plaque<br>As an antioxidant to prevent cardiovascular disease and cancer | For UTIs, 150-600 mL of cranberry juice daily or 300-400 mg of standardized extract bid<br>For other conditions, no dosage determined | Drinking excessive amounts of juice could cause GI upset or diarrhea<br>Prolonged use of cranberry juice in large doses can increase the risk of kidney stone formation due to its high oxalate content<br>Cranberry can interact with warfarin and cause an increase in INR<br>The effectiveness of PPIs may be reduced by cranberry due to its acidity |
| Creatine[7] | To enhance muscle performance, especially during short-duration, high-intensity exercise | Loading dose of 20 g/d for 5-7 d followed by a maintenance dose of ≥2 g/d<br>An alternative dosing of 3 g/d for 28 d has been suggested | Creatine can cause gastroenteritis, diarrhea, heat intolerance, muscle cramps, and elevated serum creatinine levels |

*Continued*

| Herb/Nutritional Supplement | Common Uses | Reasonable Adult Oral Dosage* | Precautions and Drug Interactions |
|---|---|---|---|
| | | | Creatine is contraindicated in patients taking diuretics |
| | | | Concurrent use with cimetidine, probenecid, or NSAIDs increases the risk of adverse renal effects |
| | | | Caffeine can decrease creatine's ergogenic effects |
| Dehydroepiandrosterone (DHEA)[7] | Replace low-serum DHEA levels in adrenal insufficiency<br>Treat SLE<br>Reverse aging<br>Used in many other conditions, including Alzheimer's disease, depression, diabetes, menopause, osteoporosis, impotence, and AIDS<br>Used to promote weight loss<br>Used by bodybuilders to increase muscle mass | For replacement therapy, 25-50 mg/d<br>For SLE, 200 mg/d<br>For antiaging and osteoporosis, 50 mg/d<br>For other conditions, no established dosage documented | Most common side effects are androgenic in nature and include acne, hair loss, hirsutism, and deepening of the voice<br>Cases of hepatitis have been reported<br>When used in high doses, DHEA can cause insomnia, manic symptoms, and palpitations<br>DHEA at physiologic doses increases circulating androgens in women, but not in men; it also increases circulating estrogens in both men and women<br>Use of DHEA in persons with a history of sex hormone–dependent malignancy should be avoided<br>No information on the safety of DHEA in persons <30 y<br>DHEA inhibits the cytochrome P450 3A4 isoenzyme (CYP3A4) and could increase serum concentrations of drugs metabolized by this isoenzyme (e.g., lovastatin, ketoconazole, itraconazole, and triazolam) |
| Dong quai root[7] | Commonly used for the relief of premenstrual and menopausal symptoms<br>Also used as a blood tonic and a strengthening treatment for the heart, spleen, liver, and kidneys | For premenstrual and menopausal symptoms, 3-4 g/d in three divided doses<br>For other conditions, no established dosage is documented | Dong quai should not be used in pregnant women due to its uterine stimulant and relaxant effects<br>Women with hormone-sensitive conditions (e.g., breast, uterine, and ovarian cancers, and endometriosis and uterine fibroids) should avoid dong quai because of its estrogenic effects<br>Drinking the essential oil of dong quai is not recommended because it contains a small amount of carcinogenic constituents<br>Dong quai contains psoralens that can cause photosensitivity and photodermatitis<br>Dong quai contains natural coumarin derivatives that can increase the risk of bleeding in those who are taking anticoagulant or antiplatelet drugs |
| Echinacea[7] | As an immune stimulant, particularly for the prevention and treatment of the common cold and influenza | 300 mg tid of *Echinacea pallida* root or 2-3 mL tid of expressed juice of *Echinace purpurea* herb<br>Do not use for >8 wk because | Echinacea should not be used in transplant patients and those with autoimmune disease or liver dysfunction |

| Herb/Nutritional Supplement | Common Uses | Reasonable Adult Oral Dosage* | Precautions and Drug Interactions |
|---|---|---|---|
| | Supportive therapy for lower urinary tract infections<br>Used topically to treat skin disorders and promote wound healing | echinacea can suppress immunity if used long term | Allergic reactions have been reported<br>Adverse events are rare and include mild GI effects<br>It should be discontinued as far in advance of surgery as possible<br>Echinacea can decrease effectiveness of immunosuppressants |
| Ephedra (ma huang)[7] | For diseases of the respiratory tract with mild bronchospasm<br>Commonly found in weight-loss products<br>Also marketed as a stimulant for performance enhancement | 1 tsp or 2 g of dried herb (15-30 mg of ephedrine) in 240 mL boiling water for 10 min<br>In Canada, the maximum allowable dosage of ephedrine is 8 mg per dose or 32 mg/d | Ephedra contains ephedrine, which has sympathomimetic activities; consequently, it should not be used in patients who have cardiovascular disease, diabetes, glaucoma, hypertension, hyperthyroidism, prostate enlargement, psychiatric disorders, or seizures<br>Serious adverse effects, including seizures, arrhythmias, heart attack, stroke, and death, have been associated with the use of ephedra; as a result, the FDA has banned the sale of ephedra products in the United States<br>Because of the cardiovascular effects of ephedrine, patients taking ephedra should discontinue use at least 24 h before surgery<br>Concurrent use of ephedra and digitalis, guanethidine, MAOIs, or other stimulants, including caffeine, is not recommended |
| Evening primrose oil[7] | For PMS, especially if mastalgia is present<br>For treatment of atopic eczema<br>Also used for other medical conditions, including rheumatoid arthritis, menopausal symptoms, Raynaud's phenomenon, Sjögren's syndrome, and diabetic neuropathy | For PMS, 2-4 g/d<br>For atopic eczema, 6-8 g/d<br>For rheumatoid arthritis, 2.8 g/d<br>These doses are based on products standardized to 9% γ-linolenic acid<br>Daily dose can be given in divided doses | Evening primrose oil can increase the risk of pregnancy complications<br>Side effects include indigestion, nausea, soft stools, and headache<br>Seizures have been reported in patients with schizophrenia who were taking phenothiazines and evening primrose oil concomitantly<br>Evening primrose oil can interact with anesthesia and cause seizures<br>Concomitant use of evening primrose oil with anticoagulant and antiplatelet drugs can increase the risk of bleeding |
| Fenugreek seed[7] | For diabetes and hypercholesterolemia<br>Also for constipation, dyspepsia, gastritis, and kidney ailments<br>Approved in Germany orally for loss of appetite and topically as a poultice for local inflammation | For loss of appetite, 1-2 g of the seed tid or 1 cup of tea (500 mg seed in 150 mL cold water for 3 h) several times/d<br>Maximum 6 g/d<br>For other conditions, no established dosage documented<br>For topical use, 50 g powdered seed in 250 mL of hot water to form a paste | Fenugreek can cause uterine contractions and should be avoided in pregnancy<br>Persons who have allergies to peanuts or soybeans might also be allergic to fenugreek<br>Fenugreek can cause diarrhea and flatulence; it can also make the urine smell like maple syrup<br>Hypoglycemia can occur if fenugreek is taken in large amounts |

Continued

| Herb/Nutritional Supplement | Common Uses | Reasonable Adult Oral Dosage* | Precautions and Drug Interactions |
|---|---|---|---|
| | | | Repeated external applications can result in undesirable skin reactions |
| | | | Fenugreek contains small amounts of coumarins and can interact with anticoagulants and antiplatelet drugs |
| | | | High mucilage content of fenugreek can affect the absorption of oral drugs; therefore, fenugreek should not be taken within 2 h of other drugs |
| Feverfew[7] | For migraine headache prophylaxis For treatment of fever, menstrual problems, and arthritis | 50-125 mg qd of the encapsulated dried leaf extract standardized to at least 0.2% parthenolide | Feverfew can induce menstrual bleeding and is contraindicated in pregnancy Fresh leaves can cause oral ulcers and GI irritation Sudden discontinuation of feverfew can precipitate rebound headache Feverfew can interact with anticoagulants and potentiate the antiplatelet effect of aspirin |
| Fish oils (omega-3 fatty acids)[7] | Commonly used in the treatment of hypertriglyceridemia Used to prevent CHD and stroke Also used in many noncardiac conditions, including depression, diabetes, dysmenorrhea, rheumatoid arthritis, and IgA nephropathy Used to reduce the risk of developing age-related maculopathy, Alzheimer's disease, and cancer Promote visual and mental development in children | For hypertriglyceridemia, 3-5 g/d For cardioprotection, 1 g/d for patients with CHD; oily fish at least twice a wk, or about 0.5 g/d for people with no known heart disease For other conditions, no established dosage is documented Fish oils are composed of EPA and DHA. Fish oil capsules vary widely in amounts and ratios of EPA and DHA. The most common fish oil capsules in the United States provide 180 mg of EPA and 120 mg DHA per capsule, and three capsules provide about 1 g/d of omega-3 fatty acids | Common side effects include fishy aftertaste, GI disturbances, belching, halitosis, and heartburn High doses can cause nausea and loose stools Doses >3 g/d can inhibit platelet aggregation, suppress immune function, worsen glycemia, and raise LDL cholesterol levels Long-term use may be associated with weight gain Less well-controlled preparations can contain appreciable amounts of organochloride contaminants Fish oil can increase the risk of bleeding in patients taking warfarin, an antiplatelet agent, or herbs that have antiplatelet constituents (e.g., garlic, ginkgo, red clover) Fish oils can lower blood pressure and may have additive effects with antihypertensive agents Oral contraceptives can interfere with the triglyceride-lowering effects of fish oils |
| Flaxseed[7] | Approved in Germany for chronic constipation, colon damaged by laxative abuse, irritable colon, diverticulitis, gastritis, and enteritis For hypercholesterolemia For hot flushes and breast pain | For constipation, 1 tbsp (10 g) of whole or bruised seeds in 150 mL of liquid 2-3 times daily For bowel inflammation, soak 30-50 mL (2-3 tbsp) of milled flaxseed in 200-300 mL water and strain after 30 min For hypercholesterolemia, 35-50 g of crushed seeds daily For hot flushes, 1-2 tbsp of ground flaxseed daily | Flaxseed should be taken with plenty of water to prevent intestinal blockage Patients with ileus should not take flaxseed High mucilage content of flaxseed can delay absorption of other drugs taken at the same time |

| Herb/Nutritional Supplement | Common Uses | Reasonable Adult Oral Dosage* | Precautions and Drug Interactions |
|---|---|---|---|
| Garlic[7] | To lower blood pressure and serum cholesterol<br>To prevent atherosclerosis | Fresh clove: one 4-g clove/d<br>Tablet: 300 mg bid to tid standardized to 0.6%-1.3% allicin | Intake of large quantities can lead to stomach complaints<br>Garlic has antiplatelet effects, so patients should discontinue use of garlic at least 7 d before surgery<br>Concomitant use of garlic and anticoagulants can increase the risk of bleeding |
| Ginger root[7] | As an antiemetic<br>For prevention of motion sickness | Fresh rhizome: 2-4 g /d<br>Powdered ginger: 250 mg 3 to 4 times daily<br>Tea: 1 cup tea tid (0.5-1 g dried root in 150 mL boiling water for 5-10 min) | Ginger should not be used by patients with gallstones because of its cholagogic effect<br>Can inhibit platelet aggregation; cases of postoperative bleeding have been reported<br>Large doses of ginger can increase bleeding time in patients taking antiplatelet agents |
| Ginkgo biloba[7] leaf | To slow cognitive deterioration in dementia<br>To increase peripheral blood flow in claudication<br>To treat sexual dysfunction associated with the use of SSRIs | 60-120 mg bid of extract Egb761 standardized to 24% flavonoids and 6% terpenoids | Adverse effects are rare and include mild stomach or intestinal upset, headache, or allergic skin reaction<br>Ginkgo can inhibit platelet aggregation; reports of spontaneous bleeding have been published<br>Patients should discontinue ginkgo at least 36 h before surgery.<br>Concurrent use of ginkgo and anticoagulants, antiplatelet agents, vitamin E, or garlic can increase the risk of bleeding |
| Ginseng root[7] | As a tonic during times of stress, fatigue, disability, and convalescence<br>To improve physical performance and stamina | Root: 1-2 g/d<br>Tablet: 100 mg bid of extract standardized to 4%-7% ginsenosides<br>A 2- to 3-wk period of using ginseng followed by a 1- to 2-wk rest period is generally recommended<br>Ginseng is commonly adulterated, especially Siberian ginseng products | Ginseng has a mild stimulant effect and should be avoided in patients with cardiovascular disease<br>Tachycardia and hypertension can occur<br>Overdosages can lead to ginseng abuse syndrome, characterized by insomnia, hypotonia, and edema<br>Ginseng has estrogenic effects and can cause vaginal bleeding and breast tenderness<br>Ginseng has been shown to inhibit platelets, so patients should discontinue ginseng at least 7 d before surgery<br>Ginseng should not be used with other stimulants<br>Patients taking antidiabetic agents and ginseng should be monitored to avoid the hypoglycemic effects of ginseng<br>Ginseng can interact with warfarin and cause a decreased INR<br>Siberian ginseng can increase digoxin levels |

*Continued*

| Herb/Nutritional Supplement | Common Uses | Reasonable Adult Oral Dosage* | Precautions and Drug Interactions |
|---|---|---|---|
| | | | Reports of a drug interaction between ginseng and phenelzine (an MAOI) resulting in insomnia, headache, tremulousness, and manic-like symptoms |
| Glucosamine[7] | For osteoarthritis | 500 mg tid with meals<br>Glucosamine is available in the form of sulfate, hydrochloride, or N-acetyl salt.<br>Glucosamine sulfate is the form that has been used in most clinical studies | Side effects are generally limited to mild GI symptoms, including stomach upset, heartburn, diarrhea, nausea, and indigestion<br>Glucosamine derived from marine exoskeletons can cause reactions in people allergic to shellfish<br>Glucosamine can raise blood glucose level in patients with diabetes |
| Hawthorn leaf with flower[7] | Commonly used in Germany to increase cardiac output in patients with NYHA stages I and II heart failure | 160-900 mg water-ethanol extract (30-169 mg procyanidins or 3.5-19.8 mg flavonoids) divided into 2-3 doses | Side effects include GI upset, palpitations, hypotension, headache, dizziness, and insomnia<br>Concomitant use with CNS depressants may have additive CNS effects<br>Hawthorn can potentiate effects of digoxin (Lanoxin) and vasodilators |
| Hops[7] | For mood disturbances such as restlessness and anxiety<br>For sleep disturbances<br>Commonly found in combination products with other herbal sedatives | 0.5 g of cut or powdered strobile in a single dose; can be taken as tea (0.5 g in 150 mL water), fluid extract 1:1 (0.5 mL), tincture 1:5 (2.5 mL), or dry extract 6-8:1 (60-80 mg)<br>The preparation contains at least 0.35% (v/w) essential oil | Side effects are rare but include drowsiness and allergic reactions<br>Hops is not recommended during pregnancy and lactation<br>It can potentiate the sedative effect of CNS depressants (e.g., benzodiazapines, alcohol) and other herbal tranquilizers |
| Horse chestnut seed[7] | To relieve symptoms of chronic venous insufficiency | 250 mg bid of extract standardized to 50 mg aescin in delayed-release form<br>Unsafe to ingest the raw seed, which contains significant amounts of the most toxic constituent, esculin | Mild GI symptoms, headache, dizziness, and pruritis have been reported<br>Ingestion of high doses can cause renal, hepatic, and hematologic toxicities<br>Concomitant use with anticoagulants can increase the risk of bleeding<br>Horse chestnut can potentiate the effects of hypoglycemic drugs |
| Kava kava[7] | As an anxiolytic for nervous anxiety, stress, and restlessness<br>As a sedative to induce sleep | Herb and preparations equivalent to 60-120 mg/d of kava pyrones<br>Most clinical trials have used 100 mg tid of extract standardized to 70% kava pyrones for anxiety disorders | Kava should not be used by patients with depression<br>Kava should be avoided in pregnant or nursing women<br>Kava can affect motor reflexes and judgment, so it should not be taken while driving or operating heavy machinery<br>Accommodative disturbances have been reported; kava may exacerbate Parkinson's disease<br>Extended use can cause a temporary yellow discoloration of skin, hair, and nails |

| Herb/Nutritional Supplement | Common Uses | Reasonable Adult Oral Dosage* | Precautions and Drug Interactions |
|---|---|---|---|
| | | | Reports have linked kava use to at least 25 cases of severe liver toxicity; sale of products containing kava has been banned in Canada and several European countries |
| | | | Kava has been shown to have additive CNS depressant effects with benzodiazapines, alcohol, and herbal tranquilizers |
| | | | Kava can potentiate the sedative effects of anesthetics, so kava should be discontinued at least 24 h before surgery |
| Lutein[7] | Commonly used to prevent AMD and cataracts<br>Also used to prevent skin cancer, breast cancer, and colon cancer<br>To protect against cardiovascular disease | For AMD and cataracts, 6-20 mg/d of lutein from diet<br>For other uses, no established dosage is documented<br>Foods containing high concentrations of lutein include kale, spinach, broccoli, and romaine lettuce<br>Not known if supplemental lutein is as effective as natural lutein<br>Supplemental lutein in the form of esters might require a higher fat intake for effective absorption than purified lutein | No major adverse effects or drug interactions have been reported |
| Lycopene | Commonly used to prevent and treat prostate cancer<br>Also used to prevent cancer and arthrosclerosis and to reduce asthma symptoms | For decreasing the growth of prostate cancer, 15 mg supplement bid<br>For prostate cancer prevention, at least 6 mg/d from tomato products (or ≥10 servings/wk)<br>For other uses, no established dosage is documented<br>Heat processing converts lycopene in fresh tomatoes from the *trans* to the *cis* configuration. The *cis* isomer has better bioavailability<br>Lycopene supplements usually do not specify the type and amount of isomers in their product labeling | Lycopene, when consumed in amounts found in foods, is generally considered to be safe<br>Concomitant ingestion of β-carotene can increase lycopene absorption<br>Lycopene might reduce cholesterol levels and potentiate the effects of statins |
| Melatonin[7] | For jet lag, insomnia, shift-work disorder, and circadian rhythm disorders<br>Also for other medical conditions, including depression, multiple sclerosis, tinnitus, headache, and cancer | For jet lag, 5 mg at bedtime for 2-5 d beginning the day of return<br>For sleep disorders, 0.3-5 mg taken 2 h before bedtime<br>Avoid melatonin from animal pineal gland due to possibility of contamination | Avoid use in pregnancy because melatonin decreases serum luteinizing hormone concentrations and increases serum prolactin levels<br>The common adverse reactions include headache, transient depressive symptoms, daytime fatigue and drowsiness, dizziness, abdominal cramps, irritability, and reduced alertness<br>Concomitant use of melatonin with alcohol, benzodiazepines, or other CNS depressants can cause additive sedation<br>Melatonin can affect immune function and can interfere with immunosuppressive therapy<br>Concomitant use with other herbs that have sedative properties (e.g., chamomile, goldenseal, hops, kava, valerian) can produce additive CNS-impairing effects |

*Continued*

| Herb/Nutritional Supplement | Common Uses | Reasonable Adult Oral Dosage* | Precautions and Drug Interactions |
|---|---|---|---|
| Milk thistle fruit[7] | As a hepatoprotectant and antioxidant, particularly for treatment of hepatitis, cirrhosis, and toxic liver damage<br>Used in Europe for the treatment of hepatotoxic mushroom poisoning from *Amanita phalloides* | Average daily dose is 12-15 g of crude drug or formulations equivalent to 200-400 mg of silymarin | Adverse effects are rare but include diarrhea and allergic reactions<br>Milk thistle can potentiate the hypoglycemic effect of antidiabetic agents |
| Red clover flower[7] | Commonly used for conditions associated with menopause, such as hot flushes, cardiovascular health, and osteoporosis<br>Also used for PMS, benign prostatic hyperplasia, and cancer prevention<br>Used topically to treat psoriasis, eczema, and other rashes | For hot flushes, 40 mg/d of the isoflavones extract (Promensil)<br>For other conditions, no established dosage is documented | Red clover has estrogenic activity and should be avoided during pregnancy and lactation<br>Women with hormone-dependent conditions (e.g., breast, uterine, and ovarian cancers and endometriosis and uterine fibroids) and men with prostate cancer should also avoid taking red clover<br>Side effects include headache, myalgia, nausea, and rash<br>Red clover contains coumarin derivatives and can increase the risk of bleeding in those who are taking anticoagulants or antiplatelet drugs<br>Preliminary report suggests that red clover can antagonize the effects of tamoxifen<br>Some evidence suggests that red clover can increase the levels of drugs metabolized by the cytochrome P450 3A4 isoenzyme (e.g., lovastatin, ketoconazole, itraconazole, fexofenadine, and triazolam) |
| SAMe (S-adenosyl-L-methionine)[7] | For treatment of osteoarthritis, depression, fibromyalgia, and liver disease | For osteoarthritis, 200 mg tid<br>For depression and fibromyalgia, 800 mg bid<br>For liver disease, 600-800 mg bid | Common side effects include flatulence, nausea, vomiting, and diarrhea<br>SAMe can cause anxiety in people with depression and hypomania in people with bipolar disorder<br>Concurrent use of SAMe and other antidepressants can cause serotonin syndrome |
| Saw palmetto berry[7] | To treat symptomatic benign prostatic hyperplasia and irritable bladder | 160 mg bid of extract standardized to 85%-95% fatty acids and sterols | Adverse effects are rare but include headache, nausea, and upset stomach<br>High doses can cause diarrhea |
| Soy[7] | Commonly used for cholesterol reduction in combination with a low-fat diet<br>Also used for menopausal symptoms and for prevention of osteoporosis and cardiovascular disease in postmenopausal women | For lowering cholesterol, 25-50 g/d of soy protein<br>For hot flushes, 20-60 g/d of soy protein<br>For osteoporosis, 40 g/d of soy protein containing 90 mg isoflavones | Soy, when consumed as whole foods (e.g., tofu or soy milk), has minimal adverse effects<br>Consumption of large amounts of soy can cause gastric complaints such as constipation, bloating, and nausea<br>Long-term use of soy tablets containing isoflavones (150 mg/d for 5 y) has been shown to cause endometrial hyperplasia |
| St. John's wort[7] | Effective for treatment of mild to moderate depression | 300 mg tid of hypericum extract standardized to 0.3% hypericin | St. John's wort should not be used in pregnancy |

| Herb/Nutritional Supplement | Common Uses | Reasonable Adult Oral Dosage* | Precautions and Drug Interactions |
|---|---|---|---|
| | Might have anti-inflammatory and anti-infective activities | | Side effects include dry mouth, GI upset, dizziness, fatigue, and constipation |
| | | | St. John's wort can induce photosensitivity, especially in fair-skinned persons |
| | | | It can cause serotonin syndrome if used with other antidepressants, including SSRIs, or other serotoninergic drugs |
| | | | It has been shown to induce CYP3A4 and decrease blood levels of many drugs such as indinavir (Crixivan), nevirapine (Viramune), cyclosporine (Neoral), digoxin, theophylline, simvastatin (Zocor), oral contraceptive pills, and warfarin |
| | | | St. John's wort should be discontinued at least 5 d before surgery to avoid any potential drug interactions |
| Stinging nettle root[7] | Approved in Germany for difficulty in urination in BPH stages 1 and 2 | 4-6 g/d of cut root; can be taken as tea (1.5 g in 150 mL boiling water for 10-20 min, tid), fluid extract 1:1 (1.5 mL tid), tincture 1:5 (5-7.5 mL tid), or dry extract 5.4-6.6:1 (0.22-0.33 g tid) | Occasionally, mild GI upsets occur |
| | | | No known interactions with drugs |
| Valerian root[37] | Used as a mild sedative for insomnia and anxiety | 2-3 g of dried root or 1-3 mL of tincture, qd to several times per day | Valerian has a bad odor and can cause morning drowsiness |
| | | Two clinical trials found 400-450 mg of the root extract effective for insomnia | Long-term administration can lead to paradoxical stimulation, including restlessness and palpitations |
| | | | Because of the risk of benzodiazepine-like withdrawal, valerian should be tapered over a period of several wk before surgery |
| | | | It can potentiate the sedative effect of CNS depressants (e.g., benzodiazepines, alcohol) and other herbal tranquilizers |

[7]Available as a dietary supplement.

*Doses presented in the table are adapted from the German Commission E Monographs and/or data from clinical trials. Products from different manufacturers vary considerably. A reliable product should have a label clearly stating the botanical name of the herb and milligram amount contained in the product. Standardized extracts should be used whenever possible and are often disclosed on the labels of high-quality products.

*Abbreviations:* AMD = age-related macular degeneration; BPH = benign prostatic hyperplasia; CHD = coronary heart disease; CNS, central nervous system; DHE = docosahexaenoic acid; EPA = eicosapentaenoic acid; FDA = Food and Drug Administration; GI = gastrointestinal; HMG-CoA = 3-hydroxy-3-methylglutaryl coenzyme A; INR = international normalized ratio; LDL = low-density lipoprotein; MAOI = monoamine oxidase inhibitor; NSAID = nonsteroidal anti-inflammatory drug; NYHA = New York Heart Association; PMS = premenstrual syndrome; PPI = proton pump inhibitor; SLE = systemic lupus erythematosus; SSRIs = selective serotonin reuptake inhibitors; UTIs = urinary tract infections.

## REFERENCES

Ang-Lee MK, Moss J, Yuan C: Herbal medicines and perioperative care. JAMA 2001;286:208-216.

Blumenthal M (ed): Herbal Medicines: Expanded Commission E Monographs. Austin, TX: American Botanical Council, 2000.

Blumenthal M (ed): Complete German Commission E Monographs: Therapeutic Guide to Herbal Medicines, 1st ed. Austin, TX: American Botanical Council, 1998.

Cupp MJ: Herbal remedies: Adverse effects and drug interactions. Am Fam Physician 1999;59(5):1239-1244.

Ernst E: The risk-benefit profile of commonly used herbal therapies: Ginkgo, St John's wort, ginseng, echinacea, saw palmetto, and kava. Ann Intern Med 2002;136:42-53.

Gruenwald J (ed): PDR for Herbal Medicines, 3rd ed. Montvale, NJ: Thomson Healthcare, 2004.

Jellin JM, Gregory P, Batz F, et al (eds): Pharmacist's Letter/Prescriber's Letter Natural Medicines Comprehensive Database, 3rd ed. Stockton, CA: Therapeutic Research Faculty, 2005.

Klepser TB, Klepser ME: Unsafe and potentially safe herbal therapies. Am J Health-Syst Pharm 1999;56:125-138.

Kronenberg F, Fugh-Berman A: Complementary and alternative medicine for menopausal symptoms: A review of randomized controlled trials. Ann Intern Med 2002;137:805-813.

Mar C, Bent S: An evidence-based review of the 10 most commonly used herbs. West J Med 1999;171(3):168-171.

O'Hara MA, Kiefer D, Farrell K, Kemper K: A review of 12 commonly used medicinal herbs. Arch Fam Med 1998;7:523-536.

Rotblatt MD: Cranberry, feverfew, horse chestnut, and kava West J Med 1999; 171(3):195-198.

De Smet PA: Herbal remedies. N Engl J Med 2002;347(25):2046-2056.

# New Drugs

Method of
*Miriam Chan, RPh, PharmD*

| Generic Name | Trade Name (Manufacturer) | Strength | Dosage Form | Normal Dosage Range | Pregnancy Rating* | FDA Approval Date (m/d/y) | Indication | Classification |
|---|---|---|---|---|---|---|---|---|
| Alglucosidase alfa | Myozyme (Genzyme) | 50 mg/vial | Injection | 20 mg/kg IV infusion over 4 h q2wk | B | 04/28/06 | To improve ventilator-free survival in patients with infantile-onset glycogen-storage disease (alfa-glucosidase deficiency) | Metabolic agent, enzyme replacement |
| Anidulafungin | Eraxis (Pfizer) | 50, 100 mg/vial | Injection | Candidemia and other Candida infections: 200 mg IV infusion on d 1, then 100 mg qd; continue for at least 14 d after the last positive culture  Esophageal candidiasis: 100 mg IV infusion on d 1, then 50 mg qd for a minimum of 14 d and for at least 7 d following resolution of symptoms. | C | 02/17/06 | Treatment of candidiasis of the esophagus, candidemia, and other forms of candida. infection (intra-abdominal abscess and peritonitis) | Antifungal agent, echinocandin |
| Arformoterol | Brovana (Sepracor) | 15 µg/2 mL unit-dose vial | Inhalation solution | 15 µg bid by nebulizer | C | 10/06/06 | Long-term bid maintenance treatment of bronchoconstriction in patients with COPD | Bronchodilator, β₂-adrenergic agonist |
| Avobenzone/ ecamsule/ octocrylene | Anthelios SX (LaRoche-Posay) | SPF 15/PFA 15 | Cream | Apply liberally to face, neck, hands, and other exposed areas of the body | N/A | 7/21/06 | Prevention of sunburn and protection from UVA and UVB rays | OTC sunscreen |
| Biskalcitrate/ metronidazole/ tetracycline | Pylera (Axcan Scandipharm) | 140 mg/125 mg/ 125 mg | Capsule | 1 capsule bid given with 20 mg omeprazole | D | 9/28/06 | Treatment of patients with Helicobacter pylori infection and duodenal ulcer disease | H pylori agent, antibiotic |
| Clindamycin/ tretinoin | Ziana (Medicis) | 1.2%/0.025% in 2, 30, and 60 g tubes | Topical gel | Apply to the entire face qhs | C | 11/07/06 | For the topical treatment of acne vulgaris in patients ≥12 y | Antiacne agent, antibiotic and retinoid combination |
| Ciclesonide | Omnaris (Altana Pharma) | 120 metered sprays in 12.5-g bottle | Nasal spray | 2 sprays (50 µg/spray) in each nostril once daily (200 µg/d) | C | 10/20/06 | Treatment of nasal symptoms associated with seasonal and perennial allergic rhinitis in patients ≥12 y | Intranasal steroid, nonhalogenated glucocorticoid |

*Continued*

## New Drugs Approved in 2006—cont'd

| Generic Name | Trade Name (Manufacturer) | Strength | Dosage Form | Normal Dosage Range | Pregnancy Rating* | FDA Approval Date (m/d/y) | Indication | Classification |
|---|---|---|---|---|---|---|---|---|
| Darunavir | Prezista (Ortho Biotech) | 300 mg | Tablet | 600 mg bid taken with ritonavir (Norvir) 100 mg bid and with food | B | 06/23/06 | Treatment of HIV infection in antiretroviral treatment-experienced adult patients, such as those with HIV-1 strains resistant to more than one protease inhibitor | Antiretroviral, protease inhibitor |
| Dasatinib | Sprycel (Bristol-Myers Squibb) | 20, 50, 70 mg | Tablet | 70 mg bid | D | 06/28/06 | Treatment of adults with chronic, accelerated, or myeloid or lymphoid blast phase chronic myeloid leukemia with resistance or intolerance to prior therapy, including imatinib Treatment of adults with Philadelphia chromosome–positive acute lymphoblastic leukemia with resistance or intolerance to prior therapy | Antineoplastic, tyrosine kinase inhibitor |
| Decitabine | Dacogen (MGI Pharma) | 50 mg/vial | Injection | 15 mg/m² IV infusion over 3 h q8h × 3 d; repeat cycle q6 wk for a minimum of 4 cycles | D | 5/2/06 | Treatment of patients with MDS, including previously treated and untreated, de novo and secondary MDS of all FAB subtypes and intermediate-1, intermediate-2, and high-risk IPSS groups | Antineoplastic, DNA demethylation agent |
| Etonogestrel | Implanon (Organon) | 68 mg, single-rod | Subdermal implant | Insert 1 rod subdermally in the inner side of the upper nondominant arm about 6-8 cm (2.5-3 in) above the elbow crease overlying the groove between the biceps and the triceps May replace with a new rod after 3 y if continued contraception is desired | Not indicated for use | 07/17/06 | Prevention of pregnancy | Contraceptive, progestin |

| Generic Name | Brand (Manufacturer) | Strength | Form | Dosing | Pregnancy Category | Approval Date | Indication | Classification |
|---|---|---|---|---|---|---|---|---|
| Human papillomavirus (types 6, 11, 16, and 18) recombinant vaccine | Gardasil (Merck) | 0.5-mL single-dose vial | Injection | 3-dose series given IM at 0, 2, and 6 mo after the first dose | B | 06/08/06 | Prevention of cervical cancer, genital warts, and precancerous or dysplastic lesions caused by HPV types 6, 11, 16, and 18 | Vaccine, virus antigens |
| Idursulfase | Elaprase (Shire) | 2 mg/mL, 3 mL in 5-mL vial | Injection | 0.5 mg/kg IV infusion over 1-3 h once weekly | C | 07/24/06 | Treatment of patients with Hunter's syndrome (mucopolysaccharidosis II) | Enzyme replacement |
| Insulin human (rDNA origin) inhalation powder | Exubera (Pfizer) | 1, 3-mg blister | Oral inhalation | Start premeal dose at 0.05 mg/kg × body weight (kg), round down the dose to the nearest whole mg; titrate dose per blood glucose measurements | C | 01/27/06 | Treatment of adults with diabetes mellitus for the control of hyperglycemia | Antidiabetic, insulin |
| Kunecatechins | Veregen (MediGene) | 15%, 15-g tube | Topical ointment | Apply an 0.5 cm strand of ointment tid to each external genital and perianal wart; treat until complete clearance of warts, but ≤16 wk | C | 10/31/06 | Topical treatment of external genital and perianal warts (Condylomata acuminate) in immunocompetent patients ≥18 y | Keratolytic, green tea extracts |
| Lubiprostone | Amitiza (Sucampo/Takeda) | 24 µg | Capsule | 24 µg bid with food | C | 01/31/06 | Treatment of chronic idiopathic constipation in the adult population | Laxative, chloride channel activator |
| Methylphenidate | Daytrana (Shire) | 10, 15, 20, 30 mg/9 h | Transdermal patch | Apply patch to the hip area 2 h before needed effect and remove 9 h after application; wk 1, 10 mg; wk 2, 15 mg; wk 3, 20 mg; wk 4, 30 mg; titrate dose to effect | C | 04/26/06 | Treatment of attention deficit/hyperactivity disorder in children >6 y | CNS stimulant, amphetamine related |
| Paliperidone | Invega (Janssen) | 3, 6, 9 mg | Extended-release tablet | 6 mg once daily in AM; may increase dose to a max of 12 mg/d | C | 12/19/06 | Treatment of schizophrenia | Psychotropic agent, benzisoxazole derivative |
| Panitumumab | Vectibix (Amgen) | 20 mg/mL in 5-, 10-, 20-mL vial | Injection | 6 mg/kg IV infusion over 60 min q14d; infuse doses >1000 mg over 90 min | C | 09/27/06 | Treatment of EGFR-expressing metastatic colorectal carcinoma with disease progression on or following fluoropyrimidine-, oxaliplatin-, and irinotecan-containing chemotherapy regimens | Antineoplastic, monoclonal antibody |

Continued

## New Drugs Approved in 2006—cont'd

| Generic Name | Trade Name (Manufacturer) | Strength | Dosage Form | Normal Dosage Range | Pregnancy Rating* | FDA Approval Date (m/d/y) | Indication | Classification |
|---|---|---|---|---|---|---|---|---|
| Posaconazole | Noxafil (Schering) | 40 mg/mL, 105 mL in 4-oz bottle | Oral suspension | Prophylaxis of invasive fungal infections: 200 mg tid Oropharyngeal candidiasis: 100 mg bid × 1 d, then 100 mg qd × 13 d Oropharyngeal candidiasis refractory to itraconazole and/or fluconazole: 400 mg bid | C | 09/15/06 | Prophylaxis of invasive Aspergillus and Candida infections in patients ≥13 y who are at high risk for developing these infections due to being severely immunocompromised Treatment of oropharyngeal candidiasis, including oropharyngeal candidiasis refractory to itraconazole and/or fluconazole | Antifungal, triazole |
| Ranibizumab | Lucentis (Genentech) | 10 mg/mL, 0.05 mL in a single-use vial | Injection | 0.5 mg (0.05 mL) by intravitreal injection once a mo; may reduce to once q3 mo after the first 4 injections if monthly injections are not feasible | C | 06/30/06 | Treatment of patients with neovascular (wet) age-related macular degeneration (AMD) | Ophthalmic, monoclonal antibody |
| Ranolazine | Ranexa (CV Therapeutics) | 500 mg | Extended-release tablet | Start at 500 mg bid and increase to 1000 mg bid as needed | C | 01/27/06 | Treatment of chronic angina in patients who have not achieved an adequate response with other antianginal drugs | Antianginal, piperazine acetamide |
| Rasagiline mesylate | Azilect (Teva) | 0.5, 1 mg | Tablet | Monotherapy: 1 mg once daily Adjunctive therapy: 0.5 mg once daily, may increase to 1 mg once daily | C | 05/16/06 | Treatment of signs and symptoms of idiopathic Parkinson's disease as initial monotherapy and as adjunctive therapy to levodopa | Antiparkinsonian agent, irreversible MAO type B inhibitor |
| Rotavirus vaccine, live, oral, pentavalent | RotaTeq (Merck) | 2 mL in single-dose tube | Oral suspension | 3-dose series given at 2, 4, and 6 mo of age; may give dose #1 as early as age 6 wk and dose #3 no later than age 32 wk Do not start the series later than age 12 wk; dose #2 and dose #3 may be given 4 wk after previous dose | N/A | 02/03/06 | Prevention of rotavirus gastroenteritis in infants and children caused by the serotypes G1, G2, G3, and G4 when administered as a 3-dose series to infants between the ages of 6 and 32 wk | Vaccine, live virus antigen |

Continued

| Generic name | Brand (manufacturer) | Strengths | Dosage form | Dosing | Preg. cat. | Approval date | Indication | Classification |
|---|---|---|---|---|---|---|---|---|
| Selegiline transdermal system | Emsam (Bristol-Myers Squibb) | 6, 9, 12 mg/24 h | Transdermal patch | Apply 6 mg/24 h patch once q 24 h. May increase dose at intervals of 2 wk in dose increments of 3 mg/24 h up to a max dose of 12 mg/24 h | C | 02/27/06 | Treatment of major depressive disorder | Antidepressant, monoamine oxidase type B inhibitor |
| Sitagliptin phosphate | Januvia (Merck) | 25, 50, 100 mg | Tablet | 100 mg once daily as monotherapy or in combination with metformin or PPARγ agonist (e.g., thiazolidinediones) | B | 10/16/06 | As an adjunct to diet and exercise to improve glycemic control in patients with type 2 diabetes mellitus | Antidiabetic agent, dipeptidyl peptidase IV inhibitor |
| Sunitinib malate | Sutent (Pfizer) | 12.5, 25, 50 mg | Capsule | 50 mg once daily with a cycle of 4 wk on followed by 2 wk off | D | 01/26/06 | Treatment of gastrointestinal stromal tumor after disease progression on or intolerance to imatinib; Treatment of advanced renal cell carcinoma | Antineoplastic agent, tyrosine kinase inhibitor |
| Telbivudine | Tyzeka (Novartis) | 600 mg | Tablet | ≥16 y of age: 600 mg once daily | B | 10/25/06 | Treatment of chronic hepatitis B in adults with evidence of viral replication and either evidence of persistent elevations in serum aminotransferases (ALT or AST) or histologically active disease | Antiviral, thymidine nucleoside analogue |
| Varenicline tartrate | Chantix (Pfizer) | 0.5, 1 mg | Tablet | 0.5 mg qd × 3 d, 0.5 mg bid × 4 d, then 1 mg bid; Treat for 12 wk, may repeat an additional course of 12 wk | C | 05/10/06 | As an aid to smoking cessation treatment | Smoking deterrent, nicotine receptor agonist |
| Voriconazole | Vfend (Pfizer) | 200 mg IV vial; 50, 200 mg tablet; 40 mg/mL oral suspension | Injection, tablet, powder for oral suspension | Aspergillosis, scedosporiosis, and fusariosis: 6 mg/kg IV q12h × 24 h, then 4 mg/kg IV q12h; may switch to oral dose of 200 mg q12h; Candidemia and other deep tissue Candida infections: 6 mg/kg IV q12h × 24 h, then 3-4 mg/kg IV q12h; may switch to oral dose of 200 mg | D | 3/10/06 | Treatment of invasive aspergillosis; Treatment of candidemia in non-neutropenic patients and the following Candida infections: disseminated infections of the skin and infections in the abdomen, kidneys, bladder wall, and wounds; Treatment of esophageal candidiasis | Antifungal, triazole |

## New Drugs Approved in 2006—cont'd

| Generic Name | Trade Name (Manufacturer) | Strength | Dosage Form | Normal Dosage Range | Pregnancy Rating* | FDA Approval Date (m/d/y) | Indication | Classification |
|---|---|---|---|---|---|---|---|---|
| | | | | q12h Esophageal candidiasis: 200 mg po q12h | | | Treatment of serious fungal infections caused by *Scedosporium apiospermum* and *Fusarium* spp. including *Fusarium solani* | |
| Vorinostat | Zolinza (Merck) | 100 mg | Capsule | 400 mg once daily with food If patient does not tolerant drug, decrease dose to 300 mg qd; may further reduce dose to 300 mg qd × 5 d each wk if needed | D | 10/09/06 | Treatment of cutaneous manifestations in patients with cutaneous T-cell lymphoma (CTCL) who have progressive, persistent, or recurrent disease on or following two systemic therapies | Antineoplastic, histone deacetylase inhibitor |
| Zoster vaccine, live | Zostavax (Merck) | Single-dose vial | Injection | 1 dose SC, preferably in the upper arm | C | 05/25/06 | Prevention of herpes zoster (shingles) in persons ≥60 y | Vaccine, live virus antigen |

*FDA pregnancy categories:*

A: Adequate studies in pregnant women have not demonstrated a risk to the fetus in the first trimester of pregnancy and there is no evidence of risk in later trimesters.

B: Animal studies have shown an adverse effect, but adequate studies in pregnant women have not demonstrated a risk to the fetus during the first trimester of pregnancy and there is no evidence of risk in later trimesters.

C: Animal studies have shown an adverse effect on the fetus, but there are no adequate studies in humans; the benefits from the use of the drug in pregnant women may be acceptable despite its potential risks.

D: There is evidence of human fetal risk, but the potential benefits from the use of the drug in pregnant women may be acceptable despite its potential risks.

X: Adverse reaction reports indicate evidence of fetal risk; the risk of use in a pregnant woman clearly outweighs any possible benefit.

No drug should be administered during pregnancy unless it is clearly needed and the potential benefit outweighs the potential hazard to the fetus, regardless of the pregnancy category.

*Abbreviations:* COPD = chronic obstructive pulmonary disease; FAB = French-American-British classification system; HPV = human papillomavirus; IPSS = International Prognostic Scoring System; max = maximum; MDS = myelodysplastic syndrome; OTC = over-the-counter.

## Agents Pending FDA Approval

| Generic Name | Trade Name (Manufacturer) | Indication |
| --- | --- | --- |
| Abetimus | Riquent (La Jolla Pharmaceutical) | Treatment of lupus kidney disease |
| Aliskiren | Rasilez (Novartis/Speedel) | Use as both monotherapy and combination treatment of hypertension |
| 17 α-hydroxy-progesterone caproate | Gestiva (Adeza) | Prevention of preterm delivery (before 35 wk) in women with a history of preterm delivery |
| Alvimopan | Entereg (Adolor Corp/GlaxoSmithKline) | Treatment of postoperative ileus in patients recovering from bowel surgery |
| Armodafinil | Nuvigil (Cephalon) | To improve wakefulness in patients suffering from excessive sleepiness associated with narcolepsy, shift-work sleep disorder, and obstructive sleep apnea-hypopnea syndrome |
| Certolizumab pegol | Cimzia (Celltech/UCB) | Treatment of Crohn's disease |
| Cilomilast | Ariflo (GlaxoSmithKline) | Treatment of patients with COPD who are poorly responsive to albuterol |
| Clodronate | Bonefos (Berlex Laboratories) | Adjuvant oral treatment for reducing the occurrence of bone metastases in stages II/III breast cancer patients |
| Continuous erythropoiesis receptor activator (CERA) | Mircera (Roche) | Treatment of anemia in patients with chronic kidney disease, either on dialysis or not on dialysis |
| Dalbavancin | No brand name (Vicuron Pharmaceuticals) | Treatment of complicated skin and soft tissue infections caused by gram-positive bacteria, including MRSA |
| Desvenlafaxine succinate | No brand name (Wyeth) | Treatment of major depressive disorder |
| Dextromethorphan/quinidine | Zenvia (Avanir) | Treatment of involuntary emotional expression disorder |
| Eculizumab | Soliris (Alexion Pharmaceuticals) | Treatment of paroxysmal nocturnal hemoglobinuria |
| Efaproxiral | No brand name (Allos Therapeutics) | An adjunct agent to whole-brain radiation therapy for the treatment of brain metastases in patients with breast cancer |
| Eprodisate | Kiacta (Neurochem) | Treatment of amyloid A amyloidosis |
| Everolimus | Certican (Novartis) | Prevention of rejection after heart and kidney transplantations |
| Febuxostat | No brand name (TAP) | For management of hyperuricemia in patients with chronic gout |
| Fesoterodine | No brand name (Schwarz/Pfizer) | Treatment of overactive bladder |
| Garenoxacin mesylate | Geninax (Schering) | Treatment of acute bacterial exacerbation of chronic bronchitis, acute bacterial sinusitis, community-acquired pneumonia, complicated and uncomplicated skin and skin structure infections, and complicated intra-abdominal infections |
| Lisdexamfetamine dimesylate | No brand name (New River Pharmaceuticals) | Treatment of pediatric attention-deficit/hyperactivity disorder |
| Nebivolol | No brand name (Mylan) | Treatment of hypertension |
| Oxypurinol | Oxyprim (Cardiome) | Treatment of allopurinol-intolerant hyperuricemia |
| Retapamulin | No brand name (GlaxoSmithKline) | Topical treatment for uncomplicated skin and skin structure infections due to susceptible strains of *Staphylococcus aureus* and *Streptococcus pyogenes* |
| Rotigotine transdermal system | Neupro (Schwarz Pharma) | Treatment of Parkinson's disease and restless leg syndrome |
| Roxatidine acetate | Roxin (Hoechst-Roussel) | Treatment of peptic ulcer disease |
| Ruboxistaurin | Arxxant (Eli Lilly) | To reduce risk of moderate vision loss associated with diabetic retinopathy and diabetic macular edema |
| Rufinamide | No brand name (Eisai) | Adjunctive therapy for Lennox-Gastaut syndrome in children ≥4 y and as adjunctive therapy for partial-onset seizures with and without secondary generalization in adults and adolescents ≥12 y |
| Sipuleucel-T | Provenge (Dendreon) | Treatment for prostate cancer |
| Sitaxsentan sodium | Thelin (Encysive Pharmaceuticals) | Treatment of pulmonary arterial hypertension |
| SnET2 (tin ethyl etiopurpurin) | No brand name (Miravent Medical Technologies) | Slow the progression of wet age-related macular degeneration |
| Vapreotide | Sanvar IR (H3 Pharma) | Treatment of acute esophageal variceal bleeding secondary to portal hypertension |
| Vildagliptin | Galvus (Novartis) | Treatment of type 2 diabetes |

*Abbreviations:* FDA = United States Food and Drug Administration; MRSA = methicillin-resistant *Staphylococcus aureus.*

# Index

Index

1280